LIBRARY & INFORMATION SERVICE
TEES, ESK & WEAR VALLEYS
NHS FOUNDATION TRUST
COUNTY HOSPITAL

Rutter's Child and Adolescent Psychiatry

Rutter's Child and Adolescent Psychiatry Companion CD-ROM
The CD accompanying this book contains: • The complete text • A full text search function This CD is suitable for both PC and Mac

Rutter's Child and Adolescent Psychiatry

Edited by

Michael Rutter CBE, MD, FRCP, FRCPsych, FRS, FMedSci, FBA
Professor of Developmental Psychopathology
MRC, Social Genetic and Developmental Psychiatry Centre
Institute of Psychiatry, King's College London
London, UK

Dorothy V. M. Bishop MA, DPhil, FBA, FMedSci
Professor of Developmental Neuropsychology
Department of Experimental Psychology
University of Oxford, Oxford, UK

Daniel S. Pine MD
National Institute of Mental Health (NIMH)
Intramural Research Program
National Institutes of Health
Bethesda, MD, USA

Stephen Scott FRCP FRCPsych
Professor of Child Health and Behaviour
& Consultant Child and Adolescent Psychiatrist
Department of Child and Adolescent Psychiatry
Institute of Psychiatry, King's College London
London, UK

Jim Stevenson BA, MSc, PhD, CPsychol, FBPsS
Professor of Psychology
School of Psychology
University of Southampton
Southampton, UK

Eric Taylor MA, MB, FRCP, FRCPsych, FMedSci
Professor of Child and Adolescent Psychiatry
Department of Child and Adolescent Psychiatry
Institute of Psychiatry, King's College London
London, UK

Anita Thapar MBBCH, FRCPsych, PhD
Professor of Child and Adolescent Psychiatry
Department of Psychological Medicine
Cardiff University
Cardiff, UK

FIFTH EDITION

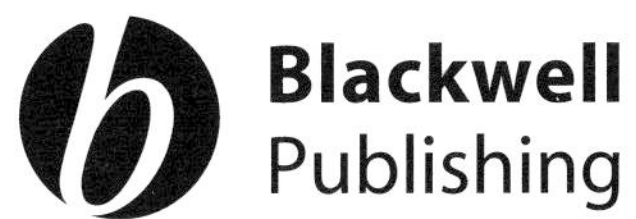

Blackwell Publishing, Inc., 350 Main Street, Malden, Massachusetts 02148-5020, USA
Blackwell Publishing Ltd, 9600 Garsington Road, Oxford OX4 2DQ, UK
Blackwell Publishing Asia Pty Ltd, 550 Swanston Street, Carlton, Victoria 3053, Australia

First published 1976
Second edition 1985
Third edition 1994
Fourth edition 2002
Fifth edition 2008
1 2008

Library of Congress Cataloging-in-Publication Data

Rutter's child and adolescent psychiatry / [edited by] Michael Rutter . . . [et al.]. – 5th ed.
p. ; cm.
Rev. ed. of: Child and adolescent psychiatry / edited by Michael Rutter, Eric Taylor. 4th ed. 2002.
Includes bibliographical references and index.
ISBN 978-1-4051-4549-7
1. Child psychiatry. 2. Adolescent psychiatry. I. Rutter, Michael, 1933– II. Child and adolescent psychiatry.
III. Title: Child and adolescent psychiatry.
[DNLM: 1. Mental Disorders. 2. Adolescent Behavior. 3. Adolescent. 4. Child. 5. Developmental Disabilities.
WS 350 R982s 2008]
RJ499.C486 2008
618.92′89–dc22

2007021160

ISBN: 978-1-4051-4549-7

A catalogue record for this title is available from the British Library

Set in 9/12pt Sabon by Graphicraft Limited, Hong Kong
Printed and bound in Singapore by Markono Print Media Pte Ltd

Commissioning Editor: Martin Sugden
Editorial Assistant: Deirdre Barry
Development Editor: Rob Blundell
Production Controller: Debbie Wyer
CD produced by Meg Barton and Nathan Harris

For further information on Blackwell Publishing, visit our website:
http://www.blackwellpublishing.com

The publisher's policy is to use permanent paper from mills that operate a sustainable forestry policy, and which has been manufactured from pulp processed using acid-free and elementary chlorine-free practices. Furthermore, the publisher ensures that the text paper and cover board used have met acceptable environmental accreditation standards.

Contents

A CD with the full text in searchable format is included at the end of the book

Contributors

Annah N. Abrams MD
Instructor in Psychiatry, Harvard Medical School; MGH Child Psychiatry Consultation Liaison Service, Massachusetts General Hospital, Boston, MA, USA

Susan Bailey MB, ChB, FRCPsych
Professor of Child & Adolescent Forensic Mental Health, University of Central Lancashire, Preston, UK

Gillian Baird MB, Bchir, FRCPCH
Consultant Paediatrician and Honorary Professor in Paediatric Neurodisability, Guy's & St Thomas' NHS Foundation Trust, London, UK

Torsten Baldeweg MD
Reader in Developmental Cognitive Neuroscience, UCL Institute of Child Health, University College London, London, UK

Sarah Kate Bearman PhD
Postdoctoral Fellow, Judge Baker Children's Center, Harvard Medical School, Boston, MA, USA

Dorothy V. M. Bishop MA, DPhil, FBA, FMedSci
Professor of Developmental Neuropsychology, Department of Experimental Psychology, University of Oxford, Oxford, UK

R. James Blair PhD
Chief, Unit on Affective Cognitive Neuroscience, Mood and Anxiety Disorders Program, National Institute of Mental Health, Bethesda, MD, USA

Michael H. Bloch MD
Child Study Center, Yale University School of Medicine, New Haven, CT, USA

Stewart Boyd MD
Department of Clinical Neurophysiology, Great Ormond Street Hospital for Children NHS Trust, London, UK

David Brent MD, MS Hyg
Academic Chief, Child and Adolescent Psychiatry Professor of Psychiatry, Pediatrics and Epidemiology, University of Pittsburgh School of Medicine, Pittsburgh, PA, USA

Maggie Bruck PhD
Professor of Psychiatry and Behavioral Sciences, John Hopkins Medical Institutions, Baltimore, MD, USA

Jan K. Buitelaar MD, PhD
Professor of Psychiatry, and Child and Adolescent Psychiatry; Head, Department of Psychiatry, UMC St Radboud, and Karakter Child and Adolescent Psychiatry University Centre, Nijmegen, The Netherlands

Richard J. Butler BSc, MSc, PhD, C.Psychol
Consultant Clinical Psychologist & Senior Associate Lecturer, Department of Clinical Psychology (Child & Adolescent Mental Health Service), Leeds Primary Care NHS Trust, Leeds, UK

Gwen Carr
Deputy Director, Medical Research Council Hearing & Communication Group, University of Manchester; Formerly Deputy CEO, Director UK Services, National Deaf Children's Society, UK

Avshalom Caspi PhD, F.Med.Sci, FBA
Professor of Personality Development, MRC, Social Genetic and Developmental Psychiatry Centre, Institute of Psychiatry, King's College London, London, UK and Duke University, Department of Psychology and Neuroscience, Durham, NC, USA

Stephen J. Ceci PhD
The Helen L. Carr Professor of Developmental Psychology, Department of Human Development, Cornell University, NY, USA

Tony Charman MA, MSc, PhD
Professor of Neurodevelopmental Disorders, Behavioural & Brain Sciences Unit, Institute of Child Health, University College London, London, UK

Sonia Chehil MD, FRCPC
Assistant Professor of Psychiatry, Division of Child and Adolescent Psychiatry, Department of Psychiatry, Dalhousie University, Halifax, Nova Scotia, Canada

Nancy J. Cohen PhD, CPsych
Director of Research, Hincks-Dellcrest Center Institute; Professor, Department of Psychiatry and Adjunct Professor, Department of Human Development and Applied Psychology, Ontario Institute for Studies in Education, University of Toronto; Adjunct Professor, Department of Psychology, York University, Toronto, Canada

E. Jane Costello PhD
Professor of Medical Psychology, Center for Developmental Epidemiology, Department of Psychiatry and Behavioral Sciences, Duke University Medical Center, Durham, NC, USA

Ronald E. Dahl MD
Staunton Professor of Psychiatry and Pediatrics, University of Pittsburgh, Pittsburgh, PA, USA

Daniel P. Dickstein MD
Section on Bipolar Spectrum Disorders, National Institute of Mental Health (NIMH), Bethesda, MD, USA

Stewart L. Einfeld MD, DCH, FRANZCP, MRACMA
Professor, Brain and Mind Research Institute, and Faculty of Health Sciences, University of Sydney, Sydney, Australia

Ivan Eisler MA, PhD, Cpsychol
Reader in Family Psychology and Family Therapy; Head of Section of Family Therapy, Institute of Psychiatry, King's College London, London, UK

Eric Emerson BSc MSc PhD
Professor of Disability & Health Research, Institute for Health Research, Lancaster University, Lancaster, UK and Visiting Professor, Faculty of Health Sciences, University of Sydney, Sydney, Australia

Christopher G. Fairburn DM, FRCPsych, FMedSci
Wellcome Principal Research Fellow and Professor of Psychiatry, Oxford University Department of Psychiatry, Warneford Hospital, Oxford, UK

Peter Fonagy PhD, FBA
Freud Memorial Professor of Psychoanalysis, University College London; Chief Executive, The Anna Freud Centre, London, UK

Jane Fortin LLB
Professor of Law, Sussex Law School, University of Sussex, Brighton, UK

Sarah Fortune PhD
Lecturer in Clinical Psychology, Academic Unit of Psychiatry and Behavioural Sciences, School of Medicine, University of Leeds, Leeds, UK

Christopher Frith PhD, FRS
Wellcome Trust Centre for Neuroimaging at University College London, London, UK

Uta Frith FmedSci, FBA, FRS
Emeritus Professor of Cognitive Development, UCL Institute of Cognitive Neuroscience, Queen Square, London, UK

Frances Gardner MPhil, DPhil
Professor of Child and Family Psychology, Centre for Evidence-Based Intervention, Department of Social Policy & Social Work, University of Oxford, Oxford, UK

Elena Garralda MD, MPhil, FRCPsych, FRCPCH DPM
Professor of Child and Adolescent Psychiatry, Academic Unit of Child and Adolescent Psychiatry, Imperial College London, London, UK

Danya Glaser MB, DCH, FRCPsych, Hon FRCPCH
Consultant Child and Adolescent Psychiatrist, Department of Child and Adolescent Mental Health, Great Ormond Street Hospital for Children, London, UK

Simon G. Gowers BSc MBBS FRCPsych MPhil
Professor of Adolescent Psychiatry, University of Liverpool; Hon Consultant Psychiatrist, Cheshire & Merseyside Eating Disorders Service for Adolescents Academic Unit, Chester, UK

Jonathan Green MA, MBBS, FRCPsych, DCH
Professor of Child and Adolescent Psychiatry, University of Manchester; Hon. Consultant in Child and Adolescent Psychiatry, Manchester Children's Hospital Trust, Manchester, UK

Paul Gringras MBChB MSc Developmental Paediatrics MRCPCH
Consultant in Paediatric Neurodisability and Honorary Senior Lecturer, Institute of Psychiatry, Guy's & St Thomas' NHS Foundation Trust, London, UK

Christina J. Groark PhD
Associate Professor of Education and Co-Director of the University of Pittsburgh Office of Child Development, Pittsburgh, PA, USA

Brenda Hale DBE, PC, MA (Cantab), LL.D (Hon), DUniv (Hon), FBA
The Rt Hon Baroness Hale of Richmond, House of Lords, London, UK

James Harris MD
Professor of Psychiatry and Pediatrics, Department of Psychiatry and Behavioral Sciences, The Johns Hopkins Hospital, Baltimore, MD, USA

Allison G. Harvey PhD
Associate Professor of Clinical Science, Department of Psychology, University of California, Berkeley, USA

Jennifer F. Havens MD
Associate Professor of Child and Adolescent Psychiatry at the New York University of Medicine, College of Physicians and Surgeons, New York, NY, USA

Keith Hawton DSc, DM, FRCPsych
Professor of Psychiatry and Director, Centre for Suicide Research, University of Oxford, Department of Psychiatry, Warneford Hospital, Oxford, UK

Andrew C. Heath MD
Spencer T. Olin Professor of Psychiatry; Director, Missouri Alcoholism Research Center, Department of Psychiatry and Siteman Cancer Center, Washington University School of Medicine, MO, USA

Jonathan Hill BA, MBBChir, MRCP, FRCPsych
Professor of Child and Adolescent Psychiatry, University of Manchester; Honorary Consultant in Child and Adolescent

Psychiatry, Central Manchester and Manchester Children's University Hospitals, Manchester, UK

Matthew Hodes BSc, MSc, PhD, FRCPsych
Senior Lecturer in Child and Adolescent Psychiatry, Academic Unit of Child and Adolescent Psychiatry, Faculty of Medicine, Imperial College London, London, UK

Chris Hollis PhD MRCPsych
Professor of Child and Adolescent Psychiatry, Developmental Psychiatry Section, Division of Psychiatry, University of Nottingham, Nottingham, UK

Jane Hood BSc, MSc, PGCE, C. Psychol
Consultant Paediatric Neuropsychologist and Educational Psychologist at Guy's and St Thomas' Hospital, London, UK

Patricia Howlin BA, MSc, PhD, FBPS
Professor of Clinical Child Psychology, Department of Psychology, Institute of Psychiatry, King's College London, London, UK

Charles Hulme MA, DPhil, FBPsS
Professor of Psychology, Department of Psychology, University of York, York, UK

Jennifer Jenkins PhD
Professor, Human Development and Applied Psychology, University of Toronto, Toronto, Canada

Shafali Jeste MD
Harvard Medical School, The Developmental Medicine Center, Laboratory of Cognitive Neuroscience, Boston Children's Hospital, Boston, MA, USA

David P. H. Jones FRCPsych, FRCPCH, DCH
Consultant Child Psychiatrist and Honorary Senior Lecturer, University of Oxford, Oxford, UK

Rachel G. Klein PhD
Fascitelli Family Professor of Child and Adolescent Psychiatry, New York University Child Study Center, New York, NY, USA

J. Zoe Klemfuss BA
Department of Human Development, Cornell University, Ithaca, NY, USA

Martin Knapp PhD
Professor of Social Policy and Director of the Personal Social Services Research Unit at the London School of Economics and Political Science; and Professor of Health Economics and Director of the Centre for the Economics of Mental Health at Institute of Psychiatry, King's College London, London, UK

Tami Kramer MBBCh, MRCPsych
Senior Clinical Research Fellow and Consultant Child & Adolescent Psychiatrist, Academic Unit of Child and Adolescent Psychiatry, Imperial College London, London, UK

Sarah Kulkofsky PhD
Department of Human Development, Cornell University, Ithaca, NY, USA

Stanley Kutcher MD, FRCPC
Professor of Psychiatry and Sun Life Financial Chair in Adolescent Mental Health; Director, WHO/PAHO Collaborating Center in Mental Health Training and Policy Development, Department of Psychiatry, Dalhousie University, Halifax, Canada

Judith Lask BA, MSc, ADFT, CQSW
Section of Family Therapy, Institute of Psychiatry, King's College London, London, UK

Ann Le Couteur BSc Psychology, MBBS, FRC Psych, FRCPCH
Professor of Child & Adolescent Psychiatry, Newcastle University, Sir James Spence Institute, Newcastle upon Tyne, UK

James F. Leckman MD
Neison Harris Professor of Child Psychiatry, Pediatrics, and Psychology, Child Study Center, Yale University School of Medicine, CT, USA

Ellen Leibenluft MD
Chief of the Section on Biopolar Spectrum Disorders, Mood and Anxiety Disorders Program, National Institute of Mental Health (NIMH), Bethesda, MD, USA

John E. Lochman PhD
Professor and Saxon Chairholder of Clinical Psychology, Department of Psychology, The University of Alabama, AL, USA

Michael T. Lynskey MD, PhD
Assistant Professor of Psychiatry Department of Psychiatry, Washington University School of Medicine, MO, USA

Barbara Maughan PhD
Professor of Developmental Epidemiology, MRC, Social Genetic and Developmental Psychiatry Centre, Institute of Psychiatry, King's College London, London, UK

Robert B. McCall PhD
Professor of Psychology and Co-Director of the University of Pittsburgh Office of Child Development, Pittsburgh, PA, USA

Helen McConachie MA, MPhil, PhD
Professor of Child Clinical Psychology, Institute of Health and Society, Newcastle University, Newcastle upon Tyne, UK

Claude Ann Mellins PhD
Associate Professor of Clinical Psychology in Psychiatry and Sociomedical Sciences, Columbia University, NY and Research Scientist, HIV Center for Clinical and Behavioral Studies, New York State Psychiatric Institute and Columbia University, NY, USA

Helen Minnis MD, PhD, MRC Psych
Senior Lecturer in Child and Adolescent Psychiatry, Section of Psychological Medicine, University of Glasgow, Glasgow, UK

Terrie E. Moffitt PhD, F.Med.Sci, FBA
Professor of Social Behaviour and Development, MRC Social Genetic and Developmental Psychiatry Centre, Institute of Psychiatry, King's College London, London, UK and Duke University, Department of Psychology and Neuroscience, Durham, NC, USA

Lynne Murray PhD
Research Professor in Developmental Psychopathology, School of Psychology, University of Reading, Reading, UK

Charles A. Nelson III PhD
Professor of Pediatrics, Harvard Medical School; Richard David Scott Chair in Pediatric Developmental Medicine Research, Children's Hospital Boston, MA, USA

Anula Nikapota FRCPsych
Senior Tutor, Institute of Psychiatry, King's College London, London, UK and Emeritus Consultant in Child and Adolescent Psychiatry, South London and Maudsley NHS Trust, London, UK

Courtenay Frazier Norbury DPhil
RCUK Fellow in Cognitive Science, Department of Psychology, Royal Holloway, University of London, London, UK

Dustin A. Pardini PhD
Department of Psychiatry, University of Pittsburgh Medical Center, Pittsburgh, PA, USA

Andrew Pickles PhD
Professor of Epidemiological and Social Statistics, Biostatistics Group, Epidemiology and Health Science, University of Manchester, Manchester, UK

Daniel S. Pine MD
National Institute of Mental Health (NIMH), Intramural Research Program, National Institutes of Health, Bethesda, MD, USA

Paul Ramchandani BM DPhil MRCPsych
Senior Research Fellow and Honorary Consultant Child and Adolescent Psychiatrist, Department of Psychiatry, University of Oxford, Oxford, UK

Judith L. Rapoport MD
Chief, Child Psychiatry Branch, National Institute of Mental Health (NIMH), Bethesda, MD, USA

Paula K. Rauch MD
Director, Child Psychiatry Consultation Service; Director, MGH Cancer Center Parenting Program, Massachusetts General Hospital; Assistant Professor of Psychiatry, Harvard Medical School, Boston, MA, USA

Alan Rushton BA, CQSW, PhD
Reader in Adoption Studies; Programme Leader, MSc in Mental Health Social Work, Section of Social Work and Social Care, Health Services Research Department, Institute of Psychiatry, London, UK

Michael Rutter CBE, MD, FRCP, FRCPsych, FRS, FMedSci, FBA
Professor of Developmental Psychopathology, Social Genetic and Developmental Psychiatry Centre, Institute of Psychiatry, King's College London, London, UK

Seija Sandberg MD, FRCPsych
Consultant and Hon. Senior Lecturer in Child and Adolescent Psychiatry, Department of Mental Health Sciences, University College London, London, UK

Stephen Scott FRCP FRCPsych
Professor of Child Health and Behaviour, & Consultant Child and Adolescent Psychiatrist, Department of Child and Adolescent Psychiatry, Institute of Psychiatry, King's College London, London, UK

Anna Seigal BA Hons
Research Assistant, Behavioural and Brain Sciences Unit, Institute of Child Health, London, UK

Michael C. Seto PhD
Law and Mental Health Program, Centre for Addiction and Mental Health, Toronto; Associate Professor, Department of Psychiatry and Centre of Criminology, University of Toronto, Toronto, Canada

Philip Shaw MD, PhD
Staff Psychiatrist, Child Psychiatry Branch, National Institute of Mental Health (NIMH), Bethesda, MD, USA

Daniel S. Shaw PhD
Professor of Psychology, University of Pittsburgh, Pittsburgh, PA, USA

Rebecca Shiner PhD
Associate Professor of Psychology, Department of Psychology, Colgate University, Hamilton, NY, USA

Emily Simonoff MD, FRCPsych
Professor of Child and Adolescent Psychiatry, Department of Child and Adolescent Psychiatry, Institute of Psychiatry, King's College London, London, UK

David H. Skuse MD, FRCP, FRCPsych, FRCPCH
Professor of Behavioural and Brain Sciences, Behavioural and Brain Sciences Unit, Institute of Child Health, London, UK

Patrick Smith PhD
Institute of Psychiatry, King's College London, London, UK

Anna T. Smyke PhD
Associate Professor of Psychiatry, Tulane University School of Medicine, Institute of Infant and Early Childhood Mental Health, Tulane University Health Sciences Center, New Orleans, LA, USA

Margaret J. Snowling PhD, DipClinPsych, FBPsS
Professor of Psychology, Department of Psychology, University of York, York, UK

Edmund J. S. Sonuga-Barke PhD
Professor of Developmental Psychopathology, Developmental Brain and Behaviour Unit, School of Psychology, University of Southampton, Southampton, UK and Child Study Center, New York University, New York, USA

Alan Stein MB, BCh, MA, FRCPsych
Professor of Child and Adolescent Psychiatry, Department of Psychiatry, University of Oxford, Oxford, UK

Jim Stevenson BA, MSc, PhD, CPsychol, FBPsS
Professor of Psychology, School of Psychology, University of Southampton, Southampton, UK

James M. Swanson PhD
Professor of Pediatrics, University of California, Irvine, CA, USA

Charlotte D. Sweeney MA
Department of Human Development, Cornell University, Ithaca, NY, USA

Mary Target MSc, PhD
Reader in Psychoanalysis, Research Department of Clinical, Educational and Health Psychology, University College London; Professional Director, The Anna Freud Centre, London, UK

Eric Taylor MA, MB, FRCP, FRCPsych, FMedSci
Professor of Child and Adolescent Psychiatry, Department of Child and Adolescent Psychiatry, Institute of Psychiatry, King's College London, London, UK

Anita Thapar MBBCH, FRCPsych, PhD
Professor of Child and Adolescent Psychiatry, Department of Psychological Medicine, Cardiff University, Cardiff, UK

Richard E. Tremblay PhD, FRS Canada
Departments of Pediatrics, Psychiatry and Psychology, University of Montreal, Montreal (Quebec), Canada

Jan van der Ende MsC
Research Psychologist, Department of Child and Adolescent Psychiatry, Erasmus MC – Sophia Children's Hospital Rotterdam, The Netherlands

Herman van Engeland MD, PhD
Professor and Director of Child and Adolescent Psychiatry, Department of Child and Adolescent Psychiatry, Rudolf Magnus Institute of Neurosciences, University Medical Center Utrecht, The Netherlands

Frank C. Verhulst MD, PhD
Professor and Director of Child and Adolescent Psychiatry, Erasmus MC-Sophia Children's Hospital, Rotterdam, The Netherlands

Essi Viding PhD
Department of Psychology and Institute of Cognitive Neuroscience, University College London, & Institute of Psychiatry, King's College London, London, UK

Frank Vitaro PhD
Professor of Developmental Psychopathology, Department of Psycho-Education, University of Montreal, Montreal (Quebec), Canada

Nora Volkow MD
Director, National Institute on Drug Abuse, National Institutes of Health, Bethesda, MD, USA

Mary Waldron MD, PhD
Research Instructor in Psychiatry, Department of Psychiatry, Washington University School of Medicine, MO, USA

V. Robin Weersing PhD
Assistant Professor, Joint Doctoral Program in Clinical Psychology, San Diego State University/University of California at San Diego, San Diego, CA, USA

John R. Weisz PhD, ABPP
President and CEO, Judge Baker Children's Center; Professor of Psychology, Harvard Medical School, Boston, MA, USA

Miranda Wolpert MA, PsychD
Director, CAMHS Evidence Based Practice Unit, University College London and Anna Freud Centre, London, UK

Anne Worrall-Davies MB, ChB (Hons), MMedSc, MRCPsych, MD
Senior Lecturer and Hon. Consultant in Child & Adolescent Psychiatry, Academic Unit of Psychiatry & Behavioural Sciences, Institute of Health Sciences, University of Leeds, Leeds, UK

William Yule MA, DipPsychol, PhD, FBPsS, C. Psychol
Emeritus Professor of Applied Child Psychology, Institute of Psychiatry, King's College London, London, UK

Charles H. Zeanah MD
Sellars Polchow Professor of Psychiatry, Tulane University School of Medicine, Institute of Infant and Early Childhood Mental Health, Tulane University Health Sciences Center, New Orleans, LA, USA

Kenneth J. Zucker PhD
Psychologist-in-Chief, Centre for Addiction and Mental Health; Head, Gender Identity Service, Child, Youth, and Family Program, Toronto, Canada

Preface to the Fifth Edition

In most respects, this Fifth Edition follows the tradition laid down by previous editions. However, it is different in several key respects. Most obviously, there has been a major increase in the number of editors. We wished to make the editorial team both international and interdisciplinary because the authorship has been both for quite some time. Most especially, we wanted to expand the range of expertise covered by the editors in order that we could have rigorous detailed peer review of all chapters. In this edition, each and every chapter (including those by editors) has had detailed critique from at least three (usually four or five) editors. As a result, all chapters have been revised to deal with editorial criticisms and suggestions. This means that chapters in this volume were peer reviewed with the same detailed rigor as would be the case for any high-standard scientific journal.

Throughout the various editions of the book, there has been a committed attempt to integrate scientific and clinical perspectives. In this edition, however, we have made a number of substantial changes in order to do this in a much more thorough fashion. The first section of the book, comprising 18 chapters, deals with conceptual approaches. The purpose of these chapters was not to provide an encyclopedic summary of what is known on different areas of science or different methods of interventions but rather to convey a lively picture of the concepts, principles and approaches in each case and to indicate why each was important and relevant for clinical practice. Some of the topics were covered in previous editions but several are new to this edition. Thus, there are chapters on how epidemiological/longitudinal methods may be used both to study causal hypotheses and to plan services. There is a chapter on what clinicians need to know about statistical methods and issues, another chapter deals with the field of health economics and another on what can be learned from structural and functional imaging. Other chapters include development and psychopathology, temperament and personality, basic psychopharmacology, psychological treatments, clinical neurophysiology and brain development. The opening chapter in this conceptual section deals with developments in child and adolescent psychiatry over the last 50 years. Previous editions have included chapters on history but this time we thought it appropriate to try to bring things up-to-date. Inevitably, in dealing with very recent history, we are having to discuss developments that are too new to have stood the test of time but we have sought to highlight what seemed to us some of the important landmarks. As before, there are chapters on classification and diagnosis, children's testimony and legal issues in the care and treatment of children with mental health problems and on culture, ethnicity and psychopathology. With respect to classification, there is a new chapter dealing with the concept of neurodevelopmental disorders that has come into increased prominence in recent times.

There is a short section with four chapters on clinical assessment in which the new approach has been focusing on the particular way in which structured techniques (with respect to interviews, questionnaires and psychometrics) can be applied in the clinical context. As before, there is a chapter on physical examination and medical investigations.

The next section of 11 chapters concerns influences on psychopathology. Most of these have parallels in previous editions but, this time, more attention has been paid to providing an understanding of the ways in which the possible influences might work and on testing for mediating effects. The section also includes a new chapter on psychopathology in refugee and asylum seeking children, as this is a group that has come to increasing attention in recent years.

The aim of all the chapters up to now has been an understanding of mechanisms rather than a detailing of effects in individual disorders, because we thought these were better covered in the separate chapters on clinical syndromes. However, in order to ensure that the chapters on specific disorders did, indeed, provide an up-to-date account of relevant findings, all authors were asked to pay particular attention to evidence on genetic influences, on imaging findings, on developmental features and on treatment methods – because for all of these there have been major advances since the last edition. The coverage of different clinical syndromes is fairly similar to that in previous editions, although it will be obvious that the information provided has moved on in important ways, but there is a new chapter on psychopathy (because its application to childhood seems to be of increasing interest) and on behavioral problems in infancy and in preschool children.

The final section of the book deals with a range of different approaches to treatment. In some respects, there were parallel, comparable chapters in previous editions but there are several innovations. Thus, community-wide and targeted interventions now have separate chapters and more attention is paid to some of the principles in these types of prevention. The chapter on physical and pharmacological treatments is complementary to that on basic psychopharmacology in that it looks at the ways in which clinicians need to think about the use of medication. There is also a new chapter on the organization of mental health services – again, focusing on the principles rather than on the details which vary so greatly across countries.

As with previous volumes, we have made quite a few changes in authorship both to bring in new blood and to include experts who have something special to offer. Well over half the chapters have a new main author and, if co-authors are also considered, the number of new authors is even greater. We are grateful to the good work provided by authors of previous editions but we also welcome the great strengths provided by the new team of authors. We feel ourselves fortunate in having succeeded in obtaining world leaders as the authors for most chapters.

Finally, Michael Rutter would like to express deep thanks to his fellow editors. The editorial team has been a pleasure to work with, has hugely helped with providing a distribution of workload but, even more importantly, has contributed ideas, fresh ways of thinking about things and a much greater breadth and depth of expertise.

The Editors

Acknowledgments

We are most appreciative of all the authors' high level of expertise and effort and of their constructive responsiveness in dealing with the many editorial suggestions on new material that needed adding, topics that required strengthening, extension of the international coverage that was desirable, clarifications that would help readability and integration across chapters. We have indeed been most fortunate in having such a strong team of leaders of the field. We would also like to take this opportunity of expressing our immense gratitude to Professor Lionel Hersov who first had the idea for this textbook, and who was a tower of strength in preparing the first three editions before he decided to stand down from the fourth. We hope that he will be pleased to see what the book has grown into.

The production of this book has been very much a team effort and the book would not have been possible without the excellent team that we have had. Most of all, special thanks are due to Sandra Woodhouse who exercised overall administrative responsibility for the complex process of working with coordinating editors, in checking chapters prior to submission to the publishers, and in dealing with the copyediting and proofreading. She was adept at spotting when problems were arising and in sorting them out. The editorial team owes much to Jenny Wickham who had the main responsibility of dealing with Michael Rutter's joint chapters and those for which he was coordinating editor. In this way, she played a key role in the overall cohesive and effective editorial team. We are also most indebted to Rob Blundell of Wiley-Blackwell who oversaw the book from start to finish and who stepped in to undertake detailed checking and rechecking of proofs when that process ran into temporary difficulties. Thanks are also due to John Forder who was an exceptionally astute and thorough proof reader and to Jonathan Burd for his professionalism in preparing the index.

Preface to the First Edition

These are exciting times for anyone working in the field of child psychiatry. A wider understanding of child development now throws a clearer light on deviations from the normal pattern; knowledge of the nature and causes of psychiatric disorders in childhood is steadily increasing; new and effective methods of treatment are evolving; and clinical and education services for children with mental disorders are growing in scope and sophistication. The first academic departments of child psychiatry in the UK are now established to meet the needs for teaching and research and to add to the existing body of knowledge. A serious concern to raise training standards in the specialty has led to recommendations on the range of content of training and a national exercise to visit and appraise all training schemes is under way.

For these reasons the time seemed ripe for a new and different textbook of child psychiatry. Our aim has been to provide an accurate and comprehensive account of the current state of knowledge through the integration of research approaches and findings with the understanding that comes from clinical experience and practice. Each chapter scrutinizes existing information and emphasizes areas of growth and fresh ideas on a particular topic in a rigorous and critical fashion, but also in practical vein to help clinicians meet the needs of individual children and their families.

In planning the book we had to decide how to choose authors of individual chapters. Obviously we wanted colleagues who had made important contributions in their fields of interest and who could write with authority and knowledge. We were fortunate in our choice and we are deeply indebted to all of them. We also decided that it would be appropriate to invite contributions from those who had worked at The Bethlem Royal and The Maudsley Hospital or its closely associated postgraduate medical school, The Institute of Psychiatry. Over the years "The Maudsley" has played a major role in training psychiatrists from all parts of the world and members of its staff have been among the leaders in both research and clinical practice. The fact that we have all worked at the same institution has produced some similarities: a firm acceptance of the value of interdisciplinary collaboration; an intense interest in new ideas and creative thinking; a commitment to the integration of academic and clinical approaches; a concern for empirical findings; and a belief in the benefits that follow from open discussion between people who hold differing views. As all of us work with children we have a common concern with developmental theories and with the process of development. However, as will also be apparent, we do not share any single theoretical viewpoint. A variety of theoretical approaches are represented in the chapters which also reflect a differing emphasis on biological, sociocultural, behavioural and psychodynamic aetiologies and formulations.

It is also fitting that this book should be based on The Joint Hospital as it has played such an important part in the development of child psychiatry. Children with psychiatric disorders were first seen at The Bethlehem Royal Hospital as long ago as 1800 and Henry Maudsley was unusual among the psychiatrists of his day in appreciating the importance of psychiatric disorders arising in childhood. In his *Physiology and Pathology of Mind*, published in 1867, he included a 34-page chapter on "Insanity of early life." The Maudsley Hospital first opened its doors just over half a century ago, children have always been included among its patients and the Children's Department became firmly established during those early years. Since then, and especially with the first British academic appointment in child psychiatry at the Institute of Psychiatry in the 1950s, it has trained many child psychiatrists who now practise in all parts of the globe.

The book is organized into five sections. The first eight chapters review different influences on psychological development in childhood and are followed by three that discuss the foremost developmental theories. A third section describes some of the crucial issues in clinical assessment and the fourth deals systematically with the various clinical syndromes and their treatment. The final section comprises six chapters that bring together knowledge on some of the main therapeutic approaches. We have sought to include most of the topics and issues that are central to modern child psychiatry, but there has been no attempt to cover all known syndromes and symptoms. Instead, the focus has been on concepts and methods with special emphasis on those areas where development of new ideas or knowledge has been greatest.

We hope that the book's contents will be of interest and use to all those professionally concerned with the care, study and treatment of children with psychiatric disorders. We will be satisfied if, in the words of Sir Aubrey Lewis, it also helps the psychiatrist in training to acquire "reasoning and understanding" and fits him "to combine the scientific and humane temper in his studies as the psychiatrist needs to."

M. Rutter
L. Hersov

Conceptual Approaches

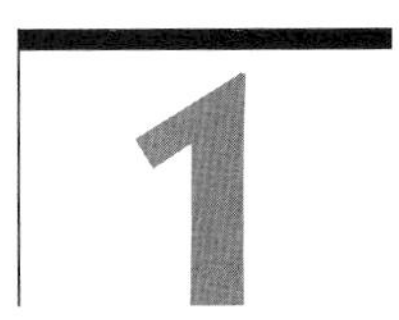

Developments in Child and Adolescent Psychiatry Over the Last 50 Years

Michael Rutter and Jim Stevenson

State of Child and Adolescent Psychiatry 50 Years Ago

The development of child and adolescent psychiatry in the first half of the 20th century was well described by Achenbach (1974), Cameron (1956), Kanner (1959), Parry-Jones (1989) and Warren (1974) with respect to both its strengths and limitations. The establishment of community child guidance clinics, much influenced by the Mental Hygiene movement, had the value of viewing psychopathology in the context of young people's real-life circumstances. The cost, however, was that there was both geographical and professional isolation from general psychiatry, pediatrics and academic research. Most treatment tended to be very open-ended and prolonged, usually without a well-defined focus (Rutter, 1982a). There tended, also, to be a rigid separation in the functioning of the unholy trinity of the psychiatrist, the psychologist and the psychiatric social worker. In addition, there was a tendency to blame parents for the disorders of their children – as indexed by concepts of the schizophrenogenic mother (Jackson, 1960) and "refrigerator" parents (Bettelheim, 1967), in relation to schizophrenia and autism, respectively. The dominant theories were the several varieties of psychoanalysis (Eisenberg, 2001), clinical practice was mostly not evidence-based, and there was a paucity of specific treatments (Chess, 1988). Furthermore, very little attention was paid to diagnosis. The prevailing terminology concerned "maladjustment" and official classifications referred only to "behavior disorders of childhood."

However, very important changes were afoot (Rutter, 1998). Although systematic diagnosis was not yet in fashion, Kanner (who wrote the first definitive English-language textbook in 1935) had already done much to foster critical thinking about different patterns of psychopathology and to encourage a questioning approach (as exemplified by his 1969 paper on differential diagnosis). Also, his first description of autism (Kanner, 1943) not only provided a model of top-level clinical observation, but established the reality of a disorder that was distinctively different from others. Similarly, approaching diagnosis psychometrically rather than clinically, Hewitt and Jenkins (1946) wrote a pioneering monograph identifying different patterns of psychopathology. The tide was beginning to turn with respect to both diagnosis and classification in both child and adult psychopathology (Meehl, 1954).

Although biological causes had only a very limited role in clinical thinking at that time, Pasamanick and Knobloch (1966), in relation to their concept of a continuum of reproductive casualty, postulated the importance of prenatal and perinatal risk factors. Studies of children with epilepsy as, for example, by Pond (1961) and by Ounsted (1955) were also influential in pointing to the interplay between biological and psychosocial risk factors. The concept of so-called "minimal brain dysfunction" was beginning to be established. It did not stand the test of empirical investigation (Rutter, 1982b) but, nevertheless, it did force people to pay attention to biological risk factors. In the realm of treatment, the value of stimulants in the treatment of children with hyperkinetic disorders was beginning to be appreciated and, in adult psychiatry, neuroleptics were starting to be developed for the treatment of schizophrenia. At about the same time, there was the birth of behavioral therapies (Wolpe, 1958). At first, these were largely considered in relation to adults, rather than children, but the application to children soon followed (Rachman, 1962; Yule & Berger, 1972).

Academic child and adolescent psychiatry scarcely existed in the 1950s although there were some chairs in the subject in North America and mainland Europe and there were the beginnings of systematic clinical research (Hersov, 1986; Remschmidt & van Engeland, 1999; Schowalter, 2000).

However, the report that probably did most to change the field in a radical fashion was Bowlby's (1951) review of "maternal deprivation" for the World Health Organization. Spitz and Goldfarb had previously drawn attention to the damaging effects of institutional care but Bowlby drew on a much wider range of evidence and did most to pull together the ideas. For quite a while, his views were treated with extreme hostility by both academic psychologists and by psychoanalysts. The former pointed to the weakness of much of the research and the latter to the heresy that the causal factors lay in real-life experiences rather than internal conflict. Despite the controversies, Bowlby's observations on young children's responses to separation from their parents led to enduring changes in hospital practice. Professionals, almost for the first time, were forced to become aware of young

Rutter's Child and Adolescent Psychiatry, 5th edition. Edited by M. Rutter, D. Bishop, D. Pine, S. Scott, J. Stevenson, E. Taylor and A. Thapar. © 2008 Blackwell Publishing, ISBN: 978-1-4051-4549-7.

children's sensitivities and of the importance of personal social relationships. The pioneering films by Robertson and Robertson (1971) were particularly influential in persuading people of the reality of many of the features that Bowlby was emphasizing.

Developments in Empirical Research Over the Last 50 Years

The fruits of empirical research over the last 50 years are considered in more detail in chapters throughout this book. Here, however, we seek to highlight some of the key developments in research strategies and research concepts, as well as giving credit to some of the pioneers who played a crucial part in taking the field forward (see also Clarke & Clarke, 1986; Hersov, 1986).

Longitudinal Studies

The value of long-term follow-up studies was most clearly established in Robins' now classic study of deviant children grown up (1966). Her findings demonstrated the important links between conduct disorders in childhood and antisocial personality disorders in adult life; they also showed for the first time how psychopathology in childhood was associated with a much increased risk of adverse environments in adulthood. The several Californian longitudinal studies were important in showing the value of prospective longitudinal studies (Elder, 1974, 1998) and the first British national birth cohort study, established by James Douglas in 1946, blazed the trail for long-term longitudinal epidemiological studies (Douglas, 1964). In more recent times, the Dunedin (Moffitt, Caspi, Rutter *et al.*, 2001) and Christchurch (Ferguson & Horwood, 2001) longitudinal studies have been particularly influential in showing the value of an hypothesis-testing approach and in demonstrating the importance of having multiple sources of measurement. Cohen's "Children in the community" longitudinal study, too, was very informative on psychopathological progressions over time (Cohen & Brook, 1987; Cohen & Cohen, 1996). Accordingly, as a consequence, there is now a substantial body of knowledge on the continuities and discontinuities between psychopathology in childhood and adult life (Rutter, Kim-Cohen & Maughan, 2006; see chapter 13, this volume). The follow-up study of the Glueck's sample of delinquent boys, undertaken by Laub and Sampson (2003) requires specific mention both because of the quite extraordinary duration of the follow-up (to age 70) and also because of its creative and rigorous combination of quantitative and qualitative approaches in order to gain an understanding, not only of risk and protective factors in relation to antisocial behavior, but also of the mechanisms through which they might operate. One key development was the recognition of the value of archival longitudinal data because of what could be gained from secondary analyses by researchers bringing new perspectives to the topic. Elder (1974, 1998) was a pioneer in that connection.

Epidemiology

With respect to epidemiology, the Isle of Wight studies (Rutter, 1989b; Rutter, Graham & Yule, 1970; Rutter, Tizard & Whitmore, 1970) showed how this could be useful for both the testing of causal hypotheses and for the planning of services. It was innovative in using systematic standardized interview techniques of tested reliability, in showing the value of using children as informants with respect to their own psychopathology, in demonstrating the frequency of mixed patterns of symptomatology (now more usually considered under the concept of comorbidity), in indicating the relatively strong associations between psychopathology and reading difficulties, in noting the differences between psychopathology beginning in childhood and that beginning in adolescence, and in observing the relatively low level of agreement among reports from different informants even when each had been shown to be reliable.

The Waltham Forest longitudinal epidemiological study was similarly important in noting that, contrary to the given wisdom of the day (and some opinions even now), psychopathological problems in the preschool period were often precursors of later psychiatric disorder (Richman, Stevenson & Graham, 1982). The clinical follow-up study undertaken later by Campbell (1994) gave the same message. More recently, a large-scale study of the prevalence of mental health problems in the UK has provided national benchmark estimates of the level of service needs in the population (Meltzer, Gatward, Goodman *et al.*, 2000). All of the epidemiological studies noted the high proportion of individuals with manifest disorders who were not receiving treatment.

Measurement

Several developments warrant mention in the domain of measurement. To begin with, there was widespread appreciation that it was essential in interviewing to use systematic standardized approaches (see chapter 19). Two rather different ways of providing standardization have been employed. In North America, this was achieved through the use of a uniform set of structured questions giving rise to "yes" or "no" answers with respect to particular well-defined elements of psychopathology. The Diagnostic Interview Schedule for Children (DISC) and Diagnostic Interview for Children and Adolescents (DICA) represent methods of this kind (Reich, 2000; Shaffer, Fisher & Lucas, 1999; Shaffer, Fisher, Lucas *et al.*, 2000). In the UK there tended to be a preference for investigator-based methods in which standardization is achieved by explicit specification of the psychopathological concepts and of the rules for their coding. This approach also differs in that the objective is the attaining of detailed descriptions of actual real-life behavior, rather than affirmative or negative answers to closed questions. Child and Adolescent Psychiatric Assessment (CAPA) provides the prototype for this approach in the field of general psychopathology (Angold, Prendergast, Cox *et al.*, 1995) and the Autism Diagnostic Interview-Revised (ADI-R) does so in the field of symptomatology associated with autism (Rutter, Le Couteur & Lord, 2003). The 1950s had seen the demonstration of the limitations of retrospective recall (Radke-Yarrow, Campbell & Burton, 1970) and this led to a preference for longitudinal data when they were possible. On the other hand, there was a recognition that, even with longitudinal data, there had to be a degree of retrospective recall. More recent reviews have shown both the value and the limitations of retrospective and prospective data (Hardt & Rutter, 2004). From a methodological point of view, Caspi, Moffitt, Thornton *et al.*'s (1996b) development of the life history calendar approach constituted an important step forward.

Somewhat similar developments took place in the design of questionnaires. On the whole, the UK preference has been for shorter scales and the US preference for longer ones. However, it has been shown that the agreement between the two tends to be quite high (Goodman & Scott, 1999) and with all scales there has been an appreciation of the importance of having measures that have parallel versions for parents, teachers and the children themselves. Key players in these developments include Achenbach and Edelbrock (1981) in the USA, and Rutter (1967) and Goodman, Ford, Simmons *et al.*, (2003) in the UK. Another development, however, was the appreciation of the need for questionnaires that focused on specific features, as well as those that focused on general psychopathology. These are considered in more detail in chapter 20.

In parallel with the interviews to assess psychopathology, there was development of interviews to assess aspects of family functioning. Brown and Rutter (1966) and Rutter and Brown (1966) showed that reliable ratings were possible on quite subtle features such as warmth and hostility and that attention needed to be paid to tone of voice as well as the words used. This led to the development of measures of marital quality (Quinton, Rutter & Rowlands, 1976) and of negative expressed emotion (Brown & Rutter, 1966; Rutter & Brown, 1966). At first, the latter was based on lengthy interviews but briefer versions of reasonable reliability and validity were later developed (Magaña, Goldstein, Karno *et al.*, 1986; Sandberg, Rutter, Giles *et al.*, 1993).

In the field of observational studies, probably the most important development was the recognition of the value of using standardized situations as a way of providing a "press" for eliciting a particular behavior. Mary Ainsworth's development of the "Strange Situation" measurement of attachment security/insecurity (Ainsworth, Blehar, Waters *et al.*, 1978) and the Autism Diagnostic Observation Schedule (Lord, Rutter, DiLavore *et al.*, 2001) for assessing autistic features constitute particularly good examples of this approach.

Binet had pioneered the measurement of intellectual level early in the 20th century. However, the field was taken forward in a major way by the scales developed by Wechsler for the measurement of intelligence in adults and in children (Wechsler, 1986, 1992). New standards were set and, through the establishment of separate verbal and visuospatial factors, the means were provided for the quantification of more specific cognitive skills and for the study of particular patterns of cognitive strengths and limitations (see chapter 21). Similarly, Neale (1958) pioneered measures of reading that differentiated between accuracy and comprehension, and Reynell (1969) did much the same with respect to her differentiation of language expression and comprehension. Basic research on memory functions was undertaken by Baddeley (1990) and by Tulving (1983) and there was the burgeoning development of a range of specialized tests of various neuropsychological functions – many at first to be used with adults and later extended to children (CANTAB, 1987; Connors, 1992; Reitan & Wolfson, 1993; Robbins, James, Owen *et al.*, 1998).

Diagnosis and Classification

In the 1950s, knowledge on diagnosis and classification in the whole of psychiatry was extremely limited. Robins and the Washington University group (Feighner, Robins, Guze *et al.*, 1972; Robins & Guze, 1970) pioneered the revolution in thinking on the topic – arguing forcefully for the importance of diagnostic distinctions, providing standardized measures of psychopathology and demonstrating how the validity of diagnostic distinctions could be put to the test. The original work concerned adult disorders but the application to mental disorders in childhood soon followed (Cantwell, 1988; Rutter, 1965). The end product was the highly systematized classifications of DSM-IV (American Psychiatric Association, 2000) and ICD-10 (World Health Organization, 1996). There can be no doubt that these constituted hugely important advances, but they carried with them the disadvantage of implying that the diagnostic differentiations were much more valid than the evidence justified. A better balance has now been achieved between an appreciation of the value of rules and operationalization of concepts on the one hand, and, on the other, a recognition that the existing schemes are no more than a best guess that will have to be modified as new research findings become available. The issues are more fully discussed in chapters 2 and 4.

Clinical Delineation of Hitherto Unrecognized Disorders

It is important to appreciate too that clinical observations have had a crucial role in the identification of diagnostic patterns. The best example of this is provided by Kanner's (1943) delineation of the syndrome of autism, with a scrupulously careful and astute detailed account of the clinical features shown by 11 children – almost all of which have been validated by subsequent systematic research. However, there are many other examples (see chapter 4). The key point is that clinical discoveries are still being made and that each of these original observations necessarily led to a two-way interplay between research and clinical practice (Rutter, 1998).

Psychosocial Influences

Several different types of advances have been important in providing an understanding of how family influences may affect psychopathology. Brown, working with adults, introduced the crucial methodological and conceptual checks needed to test for the causal impact of negative life events (Brown & Harris, 1989). Hetherington's (1989, 2005) longitudinal studies of the effects of divorce and remarriage showed the value of multimodal methods of measurement and highlighted some of the key mediating mechanisms and sources of individual differences. Harlow and Harlow's (1965) experiments with rhesus monkeys, although somewhat controversial by contemporary ethical standards (Blum, 2003), were crucially important in showing that the influences involved intimate relationships ("love" in Harlow & Harlow's language) and not just "stimulation" or feeding. Hinde's studies with the same species were equally important in a different way, through the elegance of his experimental control and his demonstration of the effects of mother–infant separation in much more ordinary naturalistic circumstances (Hinde & McGinnis, 1977). Patterson (1981) was equally pioneering in his combination of quantitative observational studies and studies of intervention with humans. The result of these various developments has been an appreciation of the reality of family influences, together with an acceptance that the magnitude of effects has been exaggerated in the past (Rutter, 2005a).

In parallel with studies of the family, a range of studies has also demonstrated the importance of school influences (Rutter, Maughan, Mortimore *et al.*, 1979; Rutter & Maughan, 2002), of peer group influences (Dodge, Dishion & Lansford, 2006) and of community effects (Sampson, Raudenbush & Earls, 1997). The old style exclusive focus on parenting has given way to a realization of the much broader operation of psychosocial influences outside, as well as inside, the family. Bronfenbrenner (1979) was especially influential in pointing to the interplay between these various social systems. More recently, there has been demonstration of the impact of prenatal, as well as postnatal stress effects (McEwan & Lasley, 2002), of prenatal effects of physical toxins (Rutter, 2005b) and of the effects in adolescence of heavy cannabis use (Arseneault, Cannon, Witton *et al.*, 2004). The sometimes long-term sequelae of physical and sexual child abuse have become better recognized (see chapters 28 and 29) and it has come to be appreciated that multiple indirect causal pathways may be involved (Rutter, 1989a), as well as more direct effects on brain functioning (Rutter, 2006b).

Testing Causal Hypotheses

Over the course of the 20th century, there accumulated a substantial literature on environmental risk and protective factors for mental disorders and, at first, it was assumed that the statistical association represented environmental risk mediation. Two key papers provided a major challenge to those associations. First, Bell (1968) noted that the associations could reflect children's influences on family interactions and functioning, as well as socialization effects deriving from children's upbringing in the family. This seminal paper had been preceded by Thomas, Chess, Birch *et al.*'s (1963) demonstration of the importance of children's temperamental features (at that time termed "primary reaction patterns"). Second, Plomin brought together an impressive body of evidence showing that some of the effects of environmental risk factors were actually genetically mediated (Plomin & Bergeman, 1991). At first, many psychosocial researchers were reluctant to accept the validity of both challenges but eventually the message was accepted and greater reliance came to be placed on the range of epidemiological and/or longitudinal designs that could deal with the possibilities of child effects and of genetic mediation (Campbell & Stanley, 1963; Rutter, 1981; Rutter, Pickles, Murray *et al.*, 2001; Rutter, 2007; Shadish, Cook & Campbell, 2002; see chapter 5). The result was a convincing demonstration of the reality of environmental risk and protective effects, combined with a realization that many of the effects were quantitatively quite small (a recognition that paralleled the comparable conclusion on the effects of individual genes – see below).

Animal Experiments

Up until very recently, child psychologists and psychiatrists have paid rather little attention to animal studies. Bowlby (1969) deserves high credit for his integration of human and animal studies in his consideration of the development of selective social attachments. Mention has already been made of the parenting studies of Harlow and Hinde. Suomi (2005) has carried the monkey studies forward in important ways through his investigation of the operation of gene–environment interactions, and Meaney (2001), through rodent studies, has revolutionized thinking on the ways in which early nurturing experiences may change gene expression – and hence alter genetic effects (Rutter, 2006a). Gross and Hen's (2004) mouse studies of the serotonergic system were important in showing how early postnatal developmental processes have a key role in later anxiety-like behavior. Amaral and Corbett's (2003) ablation studies of the amygdala in monkeys has cast new light on the role of this part of the brain in social stress reactions, and Insel and Young's (2001) studies of voles have provided vital clues on possible genetic influences on social relationships. As indicated by the important studies of Rett syndrome, animal models have also been shown to be crucially important in testing hypotheses on gene actions (Guy, Hendrich, Holmes *et al.*, 2001; Zoghbi, 2003). In addition, animal experiments have demonstrated the effects of experiences on brain structure and function (Greenough, Black & Wallace, 1987; Rosenzweig, Krech, Bennett *et al.*, 1962).

Factors Within the Child

Temperament

The last 50 years have also seen the emergence of a strong interest in temperamental features as influences on psychological development and psychopathology. Three main approaches may be identified. First, Thomas, Chess, Birch *et al.* (1963) and Thomas, Chess & Birch (1968) used an inductive approach to parent reports to develop nine individual categories concerned with adaptation to the environment, and also composite constructs of "easy" and "difficult" child features. Second, Buss and Plomin (1984) used a more psychometric approach to pick out temperamental features that were both manifest early in life and also subject to strong genetic influences. Kagan and Snidman (2004) pioneered the combination of observational and physiological measures and argued that although temperamental features could be dimensionally measured, they might operate more as categories at the extremes of the distribution. Caspi, Moffitt, Newman *et al.*, (1996a) have also been especially influential through their demonstration of the long-term continuities from as early as age 3 years. Stevenson and Graham (1982) have queried whether the differentiation between temperament and psychopathology is valid, and Rutter (1987a) has highlighted the need to study the interconnections between temperament, broader concepts of personality and constructs of personality disorder.

Cognitive Features

In the 1960s, the ingenious and creative experimental studies of Hermelin and O'Connor (1970) were pioneering in showing that experimental methods could be applied even to young, handicapped, non-verbal children with autism, and in pointing to the likelihood that cognitive deficits would underlie the social impairments that were characteristic of autism. Their research paved the way to the more recent studies of "theory of mind" deficits, lack of central coherence and impairments in executive planning (Baron-Cohen, 1997; Frith, U., 2003; Happé, 1994). Somewhat similar attempts were made to identify specific cognitive deficits thought to underlie attention deficit/hyperactivity disorders (ADHD) (see chapter 34) and schizophrenia (see chapter 45). The results of research have proved somewhat more difficult to interpret in these two fields, but there is no doubt that the study of cognitive deficits is proving to be a most fruitful line of research (Pennington, 2002). The early studies did not address the neural basis of the deficits but that has changed with the availability of functional brain imaging and the recognition that cognitive neuroscience needs to integrate brain and mind (see below).

In parallel but separate from the study of cognitive deficits, there has been investigation of the possible role of cognitive biases in the origins of antisocial behavior (Dodge, Bates & Pettit, 1990; Dodge, Pettit, Bates *et al.*, 1995), of depression (Beck, Rush, Shaw *et al.*, 1979; Teasdale & Barnard, 1993) and in the development of internal working models of attachment relationships (Bretherton, 2005; Main, Hesse & Kaplan, 2005). There is now ample evidence of the existence of biased processing, and there is recognition of the likely psychopathological importance of such biases (Rutter, 1987b), but there continues to be a remarkable paucity of studies that have put causal hypotheses regarding the possible etiological role of cognitive biases to the test. That constitutes a major unmet research challenge for the future.

Brain Imaging

Major technological advances have made it possible to undertake quantified structural and functional brain imaging studies – particularly using magnetic resonance imaging (MRI) methods (see chapter 11). Claims have sometimes been made that the functional studies show the brain in action, but this conveys a somewhat misleading impression in that they do not identify the specific neural mechanisms. What they do do, however, is show the parts of the brain involved in particular mental tasks, or influenced by particular chemical substances. Provided that the studies are undertaken with the necessary experimental controls and the necessary between-task and between-group contrasts, they are invaluable in showing differences between psychopathological groups in the ways in which tasks are dealt with (see chapter 11). Thus, the functional imaging studies of individuals with autism have been informative in showing not just weak activation of the brain areas ordinarily involved in "mind reading" (which is poor in autism), but normal functioning in areas dealing with earlier aspects of sensory processing (Frith, C., 2003). The implication is that the deficit in autism probably lies in an impairment in neural connectivity rather than a deficit in any one localized brain area. Studies comparing the activation of brain systems associated with pharmacological and psychological interventions (Goldapple, Segal, Garson *et al.*, 2004) have been informative in noting both similarities and differences in the mediation of therapeutic effects. The combination of molecular genetic and functional imaging strategies has been particularly informative in understanding inter-individual differences in human memory performance and memory-related brain activations (de Quervain & Papassotiropoulos, 2006) and in demonstrating that the moderation of responses to stress and adversity brought about by a genetic variant of the serotonin transporter promoter operates in normal individuals and not just those with clinical depression (Hariri, Drabant, Munoz *et al.*, 2005). Also, developmental studies using imaging methods are beginning to cast valuable light on the development of the brain (Gogtay, Giedd, Lusk *et al.*, 2004; Shaw, Greenstein, Lerch *et al.*, 2006) and of the changes in the brain following the onset of an overt schizophrenic psychosis (Rapoport, Addington, Frangou *et al.*, 2005).

EEG Methods

During the 1970s and 1980s, optimistic claims were made regarding the potential of neurometrics – meaning the quantified application of electroencephalographic (EEG) methods (Prichep, 1983). The optimism has not been borne out by subsequent research, but functional imaging using magnetoencephalography (MEG) is providing the means to study the temporal processing of tasks, which complements the spatial processing studies by MRI. Its use is too recent to assess its potential but it appears more promising than neurometrics. In addition, evoked potentials and a range of other EEG techniques have proved their usefulness (see chapter 17).

Neurochemistry

Neurochemistry, too, suffered from premature claims – as exemplified, for example, by the so-called "pink spot" supposed to be characteristic of schizophrenia. The problem was that most of the research constituted little more than a gigantic fishing expedition based on the most rudimentary understanding of neurochemistry. During the last 50 years, however, there has been a dramatic growth in the understanding of neurotransmitters and their functions (Andreasen, 2001) and there is now the potential for a much more focused hypothesis-testing approach which is likely to pay rich dividends (see chapter 16).

Genetics

Finally, there has been the tremendous growth in the recognition of the importance of genetic influences on psychopathology, and in the understanding of how they operate (see chapter 23). At first, there was considerable resistance to suggestions that genetic factors might be important but, over the years, the weight of evidence from twin and adoptee studies of high quality made it impossible not to recognize that there were important genetic influences on all forms of human (and animal) behavior (Plomin, DeFries, McClearn *et al.*, 2001; Rutter, 2006a). Perhaps inevitably, this was accompanied by an unfortunate genetic evangelism seeking to dismiss the role of environmental influences, and to imply a much more deterministic role of genetics than is in fact the case. Nevertheless, the reality is that there is the imprint of genetic influences on almost all aspects of psychological functioning. The difference from the evangelism concerns the appreciation that many genetic influences are indirect, operating through gene–environment correlations and interactions. Hence, rather than separating disorders into those due to nature and those due to nurture, most disorders reflect a complex multifaceted co-action between the two (Rutter, 2006a; Rutter, Moffitt & Caspi, 2006). The potential of genetics has increased enormously through the possibility of identifying individual susceptibility genes (numerous pioneers were crucial in that connection; Rutter, 2006a), and through the appreciation of the value of studying gene–environment correlation and interactions (Eaves, Last, Martin *et al.*, 1977; Plomin, DeFries & Loehlin, 1977; Rutter & Silberg, 2002). Empirical advances have come especially from the human epidemiological studies of Caspi, McClay, Moffitt *et al.* (2002), Caspi, Sugden, Moffitt *et al.* (2003) and Caspi, Moffitt, Cannon *et al.* (2005), the imaging studies of Weinberger and colleagues (Hariri & Weinberger, 2003; Hariri, Drabant & Weinberger, 2006) and the animal studies of Suomi (2005).

Randomized Controlled Trials

Preceding the work on "natural experiments" to test causal hypotheses was the recognition that, if the effects of planned interventions were to be tested in rigorous fashion, randomized controlled trials were essential, and the means to conduct them in a systematic fashion had to be developed. The key point underlying this recognition was the appreciation that it was likely that the individuals volunteering to receive some new treatment were likely to differ systematically from those who declined the treatment. The solution had to lie in random assignment to the new treatment and to the old treatment with which it was to be compared (Everitt & Pickles, 1999). In medicine as a whole, in the UK Hill (1965) was a pioneer in showing what was needed, and Cochrane (see Starr & Chalmers, 2003), also in the UK, was instrumental in pointing out the dangers of reliance only on published studies, because of the bias against publishing negative findings. Cochrane-style reviews of evaluations have come to be accepted as the standard. The USA has led the field in its recognition of the need for multicenter collaboration in order to test the effects of treatment and in its willingness to provide the funds to do this, such as the MTA trial on ADHD (see chapter 34) and the trial of antidepressants (see chapter 37). Harrington and others in the UK have also played a crucial part in undertaking randomized controlled trials and in emphasizing their importance (Harrington, Whittaker, Shoebridge *et al.*, 1998a; Harrington, Kerfoot, Dyer *et al.*, 1998b; Harrington, Whittaker & Shoebridge, 1998c). In the USA, Rapoport deserves particular credit, not just for the methodological rigor of her studies, but, more particularly, for her recognition of the need to test whether beneficial effects of medication were diagnosis-specific (Rapoport, 1980; Rapoport, Buchsbaum, Zahn *et al.*, 1978). Earlier on, Eisenberg warrants special mention for a study that showed the negative effects of withdrawal or refusal of treatment, as distinct from treatment not being available as part of a randomized controlled trial (Molling, Lockner, Sauls *et al.*, 1962). Almost all the early drugs used in psychiatry were discovered serendipitously, with little input from biological studies (Ayd & Blackwell, 1970). The field is now quite different as a result of the burgeoning of knowledge on neurotransmitters (see chapter 16).

More recently, Weisz highlighted the major differences between treatments delivered by experts in a research setting and what are supposed to be the same treatments administered on a community-wide basis by generalists rather than specialists – the results of the latter being much weaker in almost all cases (Weisz, Weersing & Henggeler, 2005). Weisz also has been influential in pointing out that only a tiny proportion of studies have included any kind of measurement of the factors mediating benefits (Weersing & Weisz, 2002a,b).

Treatment Advances

Both psychological and drug treatments have changed out of all recognition over the last 50 years. In the mid 20th century neither had much to offer, whereas now there is a substantial range of interventions bringing proven benefits. Initially, psychological methods were mainly based on a psychoanalytic approach focused almost exclusively on mental conflict and mental mechanisms rather than on real-life experiences; with a focus on the past rather than the present; and with an avoidance of any consideration of problem-solving strategies. Alternatively, they involved a rather general "supportive" function without specific focus or goals. Behavioral methods then came on the scene with their rather mechanistic application of learning principles to bring about specific changes in symptomatic behavior. They provided a huge challenge as a result of the limited evidence that they could be effective in the short term, and the much shorter duration and greater focus of the methods. In addition, they brought the claim of being based on a scientific foundation and the potential for identifying the mechanisms underlying treatment efficacy.

For some while, the psychodynamic and behaviorist camps

seemed to be in open conflict with one another. Six developments played a key part in changing that situation. First, systematic studies – such as that undertaken by Reid and Shyne (1969) – showed that, on the whole, time-limited focused psychotherapeutic methods were more effective than open-ended unfocused ones. Second, Malan (1979) argued for the value of, and pioneered the use of, briefer psychotherapeutic techniques (with adults, but the point also applies to childhood). Third, both family therapy (see chapter 65) and attachment-based concepts (Holmes, 2001) forced greater attention to the here and now of social interactions and of problematic behavior. Fourth, psychologists began to develop interventions based on problem-solving approaches of various kinds. Fifth, psychologists and psychiatrists came to recognize the important role of cognitive processes and to develop cognitive methods of behavioral treatment (see chapter 63). Sixth, behaviorists similarly came to recognize the need to take into account both thought processes, and past, as well as present, experiences. Important differences remain among psychological treatments but, to a far greater extent than previously, they have become more evidence-based and wider ranging in their methods. Amongst other things, this has meant that many interventions now include work in schools and in the community as well as work in the clinic, whether individual or family oriented.

Pharmacological treatments have undergone equally great changes. Fifty years ago dextroamphetamine was the only drug used with children (to treat hyperkinesis) and, with adults, chlorpromazine and reserpine were just about the only neuroleptics available. Neither antidepressants nor anxiolytics had come on the scene. Strikingly, then and to a considerable extent even recently, nearly all of the major classes of useful therapeutic drugs were discovered by chance rather than through basic biological research (Ayd & Blackwell, 1970). Of course, basic research into neurotransmitters has revolutionized our understanding of how drugs might work (see chapter 16) and clearly there is the potential for a much more rational development of new classes of drugs, but for the most part that has yet to happen. Later chapters review the evidence on what can be achieved by pharmacological treatments; here we simply draw attention to a few major themes.

In many respects, the most important change in therapeutic practice lies less in the details of individual methods than in the acceptance that practice needs to be evidence-based. This has led to the development of specific treatment guidelines such as those produced by the National Institute for Health and Clinical Excellence (NICE) in the UK (e.g., 2005), and in the USA by the Food and Drug Administration (FDA) (e.g., 2004), the American Academy of Pediatrics (e.g., 2001) and the American Academy of Child and Adolescent Psychiatry (e.g., Dulcan, 1997). Meta-analyses have been informative, not only in the assessment of efficacy, but also in the identification of risks, as with suicidality and antidepressant drugs (Hammad, Laughren & Racoosin, 2006).

Apart from the vast body of research on the use of stimulants to treat ADHD, most of the research with children has involved extrapolations from studies of adults. That has meant that, until very recently, drug companies have not bothered to test their products with children and very little is known on the extent to which benefits and side-effects are the same for children as for adults. The findings with antidepressants, although far from conclusive, suggest there may be important differences – as do the findings with regard to stimulants and cannabis. The effects of age differences, and the mechanisms they reflect, constitute a still largely neglected (but crucially important) research area. As a consequence of this neglect, most drugs used to treat children have not been specifically approved for use in this age group. Fortunately, the situation is being remedied in many countries and there is now at last an official pediatric formulary in the UK (*British National Formulary for Children*, Costello, 2005). The USA passed legislation in the late 1990s requiring manufacturers to assess the efficacy and safety of drugs likely to be used with children, and this led to increased drug company research on psychotropic drugs applicable to children (Wolraich, 2003).

As in adults, most psychiatric disorders in children are recurrent or chronic. Yet we know relatively little about the effects of drug treatments on long-term outcome. Also, there are sizeable groups of child disorders for which there is no very satisfactory drug treatment. That applies, for example, to autism spectrum disorders, conduct disorders, most anxiety disorders and substance abuse. Of course, there are drugs that bring about limited symptom relief in these disorders but their effects on the basic condition are unimpressive. It is notable that there are considerable international variations in the extent to which drugs are used to treat childhood psychopathology. Thus, their use in the USA is much greater than in the UK (Bramble, 2003; Wolraich, 2003).

As a result of these considerations, although we are very positive about the future of pharmacotherapy, our optimism is guarded and is accompanied by the view that if real progress is to be achieved, there will need to be much more fundamental research into drug actions in children, as well as into the neural underpinning of disorders, and also more experimental studies examining the complex (and sometimes seemingly contradictory) connections between the nature and timing of the neurochemical effects and the behavioral responses (Bundgaard, Larsen, Jorgensen *et al.*, 2006).

Perhaps an even greater need, with respect to both psychological and pharmacological treatments, concerns the development of an understanding of the mechanisms underlying the large individual differences in treatment response. Pharmacogenomics should help but its achievements so far have been quite modest.

Theories

In many respects, one of the biggest changes during the last 50 years has been the demise of the "big" theories purporting to explain the whole of life and seeking to provide support through the provision of a religious certainty. That was the style of psychoanalysis when one of us (M.R.) first entered psychiatry and it was followed by the somewhat similar style of other "universalist" theories such as family systems theories, Eriksonian lifespan theory, behaviorism and, most recently, attachment theory. Each of these has been important in bringing important insights and in highlighting important issues and findings. Current thinking has been the better for what they have contributed. Nevertheless, their faults have been profound and have rightly led to their being classified as history and not contemporary science or even a contemporary guide to clinical practice. That is because they tended to be "sold" as the explanation of all psychopathology (that which explains all probably explains nothing); because they conveyed an impression of certainty, whereas both science and clinical practice have to take on board the extent of uncertainty; because implicitly, and sometimes explicitly, they (like world religions) denied the validity of other views; and because they both lacked a sound empirical basis and failed to recognize the need for empirical data to resolve troubling questions and dilemmas.

The rejection of the "big" theories has definitely not meant a denial of the importance of theory and, even less, should it imply a reversion to "dustbowl empiricism." On the contrary, there has been an increasing strength of theory and of hypothesis testing, as exemplified throughout the chapters of this book. The difference is that these are mini-theories designed to test competing alternative hypotheses about what a particular set of empirical findings might mean – in short, a postulate about what might constitute the basic mediating mechanisms or processes. As the Nobel prize winning biologist Medawar (1982) argued, science involves in equal degrees the telling of "stories" about what might be happening and the conducting of experiments to determine which aspects of the "story" are supported and which are not. The findings in turn should lead to a further story and further testing in iterative fashion.

Some people might argue that we have "big" theories today – quoting, perhaps, genetics or neurotransmitters or developmental psychopathology as examples. In our view, none of these has the same qualities as the rejected "big" theories. Thus, genetics provides an understanding of a range of mediating and moderating mechanisms that have a major role in psychopathological development, but new mechanisms that did not derive out of genetic theory continue to be discussed, and it makes no claim to account for everything. Similarly, neurotransmitters are centrally implicated in most neural processes but the understanding of their functioning does not amount to a single theory. The situation with respect to developmental psychopathology is similar. It provides an invaluable research and conceptual perspective but it incorporates a range of mechanisms, and not just one integrative model. Moreover, its strength lies in the questions it poses and the strategies it provides for tackling research questions, and not in any one overarching model.

Developmental Psychopathology

Nevertheless, developmental psychopathology has provided an invaluable research and conceptual perspective that has proved to be as relevant for adult as for child psychiatry (Rutter, in press). There has been an explicit focusing on continuities and discontinuities in risk processes and psychopathology across the lifespan and between normality and disorder. Amongst other things, this has led to a recognition of the importance of early neurodevelopmental impairment in schizophrenia and of early life experiences in the genesis of depression, as well as the high frequency with which adult mental disorders have their first onset in childhood (see chapter 13).

The Growth of Academic Child and Adolescent Psychology and Psychiatry

As several reviews have documented, academic child and adolescent psychiatry was already being established in both Europe and North America during the first half of the 20th century (Remschmidt, 1996; Schowalter, 2000), but it really took off after World War II when it came to be recognized as a speciality in most major countries, professional appointments began to be established (so that they now exist in most, but not all, medical schools), official training standards were established during the 1960s–1980s, and there was a tremendous increase in the number of scientific publications and in the availability of research training fellowships (Hersov, 1986). In that connection, reference must be made to the role of the *Journal of Child Psychiatry and Psychology* (JCPP) and the *Journal of the American Academy of Child and Adolescent Psychiatry*. The JCPP, although developed by a pioneering psychoanalyst, Miller, was crucial in its explicit rejection of adherence to any particular theory and in its interdisciplinary coverage. It has gone from strength to strength since its launch in 1956. The American Academy journal took much longer to achieve the same breadth of approach but now it too aspires to the same aims. Both journals have been important in seeking to emphasize research–clinical links.

It is clear that a child and adolescent psychopathology has gained greatly in academic strength over the last 50 years. Several features have probably played a part. Most especially, child psychiatry has gained enormously from the central involvement of leading psychologists in most of the key research developments. Sometimes this involved interdisciplinary collaboration but, especially in the USA, the psychopathological advances took place independently of psychiatry and outside medical schools. The research contributions of psychologists have most especially concerned autism, ADHD, antisocial behavior, depression, psychological treatments, genetics and brain imaging – to give just a few examples. Some of the pioneers have been recognized already in this chapter and the role of others pervades all chapters of this book. Also, many clinicians have received formal research training – sometimes through training fellowships and sometimes through working in research units and centers. In addition, researchers have been quick to see the need and value of basic science and of methodologies derived from basic science – such as quantitative and molecular genetics, structural and functional brain imaging, and experimental strategies, as well as hypothesis-testing approaches in epidemiological and longitudinal research.

Academic impetus has come from the centers, formal and informal, established by research pioneers who fostered the careers of numerous younger researchers (usually spanning a range of disciplines). The child psychiatry research societies (providing both mutual support and leadership) set up during the 1980s in both the UK and Germany served a similar role. What is striking in viewing the field as a whole is the extent to which concepts and findings in child psychiatry have made an impact on general psychiatry, and vice versa. A degree of autonomy in child and adolescent psychiatry has clearly been beneficial but its close research integration with the rest of psychiatry, with psychology and, to a lesser extent, with pediatrics has been equally crucial.

Children's Understanding and Role in Decision-Making

Fifty years ago, scarcely anyone considered it either necessary or worthwhile to solicit children's views on their placement when their parents' marriage broke up, or on their medical treatment or on their participation in research. Today, it is widely accepted that it is essential and useful to determine children's views in relation to treatment (British Medical Association, 2000) and to research (Royal College of Psychiatrists' Working Party, 2001). The same applies to placements following family break-up. This massive change in view has derived in part from the growing body of evidence that even very young children can, and do, conceptualize and understand. Of course, compared with adults they are more limited in their ability to look back, look forward and anticipate long-term consequences, but their cognitive capacities clearly mean that their voices must be heard and taken into account as part of shared decision-making on all major issues, while at the same time recognizing that too much responsibility should not be placed on their shoulders.

All of this represents real progress, but both dilemmas and inequities remain. A key dilemma concerns the age of criminal responsibility, which varies incredibly widely across the world. The point is that whereas even preschool children have quite a well-developed sense of what is right and wrong, nevertheless, their overall ability to be fully responsible is less than that of most adults. Even more crucially, their actions will be influenced by their immaturity and their response to criminal court proceedings means that their needs should play a part in deciding how they should be dealt with (Commission of Families & the Well-Being of Children, 2005).

The chief inequity is that in many countries (including the UK and USA) it is illegal, as well as unacceptable, for adults to assault another adult but it is not illegal for parents to beat their children if "reasonable chastisement" can be claimed. In short, children have fewer human rights in that connection than do adults. The tide is turning in many European countries (as it did earlier with respect to corporal punishment in schools), but societies continue to be reluctant to abandon the notion that children are their parents' property, with their parents having very wide permission to treat them in any way that they think fit. Much remains to be done.

Ethics

Across the whole of medicine there has come an appreciation of the need to pay serious attention to ethical issues in both treatment and research, and to accept that ethical review needs to be undertaken by interdisciplinary committees that are independent from the research and the researchers. This is not something specific to child psychiatry, although there is the particular need to be aware of the possible problems in adults taking decisions on behalf of children (Royal College of Psychiatrists' Working Party, 2001). There is an awareness of the realities of research fraud and plagiarism (Giles, 2005), of experts in their court reports making unsupportable claims, of researchers destroying data to avoid them being examined when an accusation of fraud has been made (White, 2005), of acceptance of grants from grant-giving bodies having unacceptable aims (such as racism), or having a long-standing record of suppressing unwanted research findings (as with tobacco funding; Glantz, Barnes, Bero *et al.*, 1995), or concealing the source of their research funding. Strong concerns have also been expressed with regard to the role of pharmaceutical companies concealing findings, exerting influence on academic institutions and ghost-writing papers under the name of academics who have not had access to the data (Healy, 2004; but see Diller, 2006 for a balanced discussion of the issues). We accept that there have been abuses but, equally, we think that some of the concerns have been somewhat unbalanced. Moreover, the involvement of drug companies in product development is essential and many companies have responded appropriately by taking steps to ensure fair practice. Unquestionably, standards have risen in a most important way. There is an emphasis on a required transparency with respect to both the conduct of research and its funding. Also, there is a general acceptance that there must be efficient research governance to ensure that ethical standards are maintained.

Equally, however, there is now a growing appreciation that it is in everyone's interest that high-quality research be undertaken if our preventive and therapeutic services are to be improved in the future. Accordingly, there is some danger that mindless bureaucratic rules will prevent, or at the very least make very difficult, some of the types of research that are most needed (Academy of Medical Sciences, 2006). In many countries, including both the USA and the UK, consumer groups have had a very positive influence in urging that top-quality research is needed and that the challenge is to ensure that it is undertaken to the highest ethical standards. In that connection, a problem-solving approach is required. Consumer groups have also had a powerful advocacy role in pointing out the shortcomings in service provision and in making initiatives to improve services. Thus, in the UK this has been evident with respect to Young Minds (dealing with child and adolescent psychopathology generally) and both the National Autistic Society (NAS) and the Association For All Speech-Impaired Children (AFASIC) – to give but two examples of groups with more focused interests. The availability of the Internet has also meant that patients and their families are now much better able to come to clinics with both knowledge and incisive questions.

Organization of Services

The last 50 years has seen major changes in the organization and content of clinical services. It is not possible to provide a statement of universal trends because there are such great differences between countries (Remschmidt & van Engeland, 1999). Thus, for example, as Chess (1988) and Eisenberg (1986) described so vividly, in the 1950s and 1960s, American psychiatry (child and adult) was totally dominated by psychoanalysis, associated with an assumption that almost all causation was environmental, and that parents were largely to blame for the problems of their children. This was followed by a massive swing to biological models, leading Eisenberg (1986) to express concern that a "brainless" psychiatry was being replaced by a "mindless" psychiatry. Today, the use of drugs occupies a prominent place in therapeutic interventions in the USA to a degree that would have been inconceivable in the 1950s and 1960s. By contrast, despite a broadening of approaches and the development of community services, and psychodynamically oriented treatments, psychoanalysis continues to occupy a predominant position in French child psychiatry (Jeammet, 1999).

Nevertheless, despite these (and numerous other) divergencies, some important trends can be discerned that apply widely, albeit not universally. It has come to be generally accepted that there is an interplay among multiple causal influences – genetic, environmental and developmental – and that all adequate clinical services must provide a range of therapeutic interventions. Nevertheless, in most parts of the world, there is a continuing shortage of clinicians (of any discipline) who have been trained to an appropriate level in the growing list of treatments of demonstrated efficacy. Although the days are numbered for the single-therapy clinician who believes that one method serves all needs, such practitioners are still numerous.

There has also been a substantial growth in research-led specialist clinics devoted to the care of individuals with particular kinds of psychopathology and to the development of improved methods of treatment for such conditions; clinics for autism spectrum disorder, for ADHD, for conduct disturbances, for eating disorders, for obsessive-compulsive disorders and for depression all constitute examples of this kind. There can be little doubt that this constitutes a most beneficial advance, but it is important to ensure that a specific focus does not lead to neglect of a broad approach to the problems presented by individual patients. It is necessary also to consider what should be the future of the generalist clinician. We suggest that, as with the rest of medicine, it is likely that most clinicians will (and should) develop special areas of interest and expertise. We hope, however, that this will not lead to exclusionary approaches because there will always be a need to recognize that reasons for referral do not boil down to a list of predecided diagnoses.

The growth of these specialist clinics has led to an awareness that, for many conditions, it may not be desirable for an arbitrary division on age grounds between child/adolescent and adult psychiatry. Thus, a young person with a serious eating disorder needs to be assessed and treated by an eating disorder specialist who spans age groups, without regard for whether they are above or below the age of 16 (or whatever bureaucratic cut-off is in operation). There are special skills involved in dealing with children, and certainly it will usually be desirable to have in-patient units that cater specifically for different levels of maturity. Nevertheless, there is a need for an integration between child and adult psychiatry because of the research evidence that the majority of major mental disorders in adult life had their onset in childhood or early adolescence (Rutter, Kim-Cohen & Maughan, 2006).

Despite this desirable blurring of age boundaries, there has also been the growth of at least one relatively new age specialization – infant psychiatry. The positive aspect of this development has been the appreciation that very young children can and do suffer from mental disorders which require skilled assessment and treatment. The less desirable feature has been the often heavy, exclusive reliance on psychoanalysis and attachment theory, and the weak links with developmental pediatrics. It is also striking that there has *not* been the development of good services for young adults who suffer from the continuation of a neurodevelopmental disorder (see chapters 13 and 3). That is something that will have to be remedied in the years ahead.

There has been an appreciation that it is desirable that many mental health problems should be dealt with at the primary care level, without referral to specialized clinics. The use of community psychiatric nurses, school counselors and primary care consultative services are all examples. There has been a paucity of adequate evaluations of their efficacy and this is much needed, but the general notion of intervening early as part of universal services seems sound. The key challenge is to ensure that those providing these early interventions are appropriately trained and supervised, with adequate access to consultative advice when needed. It is also relevant that there have been major developments in special educational services (see chapter 74).

In some countries (such as the UK), a model of a multitier service has developed, with different levels of expertise at each tier (Hill, 1999). In principle, that sounds desirable but it is less clear how well it works in practice. It was preceded by a breaking down of the divisions that had grown up between community child guidance clinics and hospital-based psychiatric out-patient clinics. Increasingly, staff work in both settings. Once again, however, the aspiration of good integration between the two has not always resulted in the desired practice.

Two negative influences on service development need to be mentioned. First, economic goals have come to have an increasing dominance. In many places this has meant that clinicians are discouraged from participating in research because it is not a part of their clinical contract. Equally, however, clinical researchers are expected to provide clinical services that bring in funds, rather than those that make sense in relation to research and development goals. Second, in some countries (perhaps especially the UK), professional advancement for social workers and nurses has depended on their taking administrative responsibility rather than on their clinical skills as applied to the development of better methods of treatment.

Finally, we note that not all aspects of child and adolescent mental health services have developed equally strongly. In many places, forensic psychiatry, services for individuals with substance use disorders and services for those with an intellectual disability remain rather Cinderella-like subspecialties. It appears that, to a large extent, this is a consequence of a weaker integration between research and practice. There are positive developments in each of these areas but much remains to be done.

Conclusions

The last 50 years has seen an amazing revolution in child psychiatry, a revolution that parallels that in the rest of psychiatry. As a consequence, the body of knowledge, and the range of therapeutic interventions, have increased in a way that would have seemed scarcely conceivable 50 years ago. We welcome these many gains but we draw attention to four key issues. First, it is crucial to appreciate the giant strides made by the iconoclastic pioneers of half a century ago. Today, the need for researchers who will question the given wisdom of the day is just as great as it ever was. Second, the advances in basic science have opened up vital avenues of development for clinical practice, and it is essential that these are pursued in a vigorous fashion. Equally, however, we need to recognize that the pathways work in both directions. Namely, some of the creative ideas stem from clinical science as well as from basic science, and clinical science involves far more than the translation of findings from the laboratory to interventions at the bedside. Third, the supposed division between basic science and clinical science is somewhat artificial. Some of the most important science represents an amalgam of the two (Rutter, 2005c). Finally, we need to appreciate the crucial role of clinical observations. Their value has been dramatically evident in the identification of new syndromes but it is equally important in thinking about causal processes and about clinical interventions. The interplay between clinical practice and empirical research is two-way, not unidirectional.

Further Reading

Rutter, M. (in press). Scientific foundations of clinical practice. In: R. Williams, K. W. M. Fulford, & M. Shooter (Eds.), *Psychiatry in the 21st century: Principles, possibilities and challenges*. London: Gaskell.

Rutter, M. (in press). Developing concepts in developmental psychopathology. In: J. Hudziak (Ed.), *Genetic and environmental influences on developmental psychopathology*. Arlington, VA: American Psychiatric Publishing.

References

Academy of Medical Sciences. (2006). *Personal data for public good: Using health information in medical research*. London: Academy of Medical Sciences.

Achenbach, T. (1974). *Developmental psychopathology*. New York: Ronald Press.

Achenbach, T., & Edelbrock, C. (1981). Behavioral problems and competencies reported by parents of normal and disturbed children aged 4 through 16. *Monographs of the Society for Research in Child Development*, *46*, 1–82.

Ainsworth, M., Blehar, M., Waters, E., & Wall, S. (1978). *Patterns of attachment: A psychological study of the strange situation*. Hillsdale, NJ: Erlbaum Associates.

Amaral, D. G., & Corbett, B. A. (2003). The amygdala, autism and anxiety. In: Novartis Foundation Symposium 251, *Autism: Neural basis and treatment possibilities* (pp. 177–197). Chichester, UK: John Wiley & Sons Ltd.

American Academy of Pediatrics, Subcommittee on Attention-Deficit/Hyperactivity Disorder and Committee on Quality Improvement. (2001). Clinical practice guideline: Treatment of the school-aged child with attention-deficit/hyperactivity disorder. *Pediatrics*, *108*, 1033–1044.

American Psychiatric Association. (2000). *Diagnostic and statistical manual of mental disorders (DSM-IV)*, 4th edn. Text Revision. Washington, DC: American Psychiatric Association.

Andreasen, N. C. (2001). *Brave new brain*. Oxford: Oxford University Press.

Angold, A., Prendergast, M., Cox, A., Harrington, R., Simonoff, E., & Rutter, M. (1995). The child and adolescent psychiatric assessment (CAPA). *Psychological Medicine*, *25*, 739–753.

Arseneault, L., Cannon, M., Witton, J., & Murray, R. M. (2004). Causal association between cannabis and psychosis: examination of the evidence. *British Journal of Psychiatry*, *184*, 110–117.

Ayd, F. J., & Blackwell, B. (Eds.). (1970). *Discoveries in biological psychiatry*. Philadelphia, PA: Lippincott.

Baddeley, A. (1990). *Human memory*. London: Lawrence Erlbaum Associates.

Baron-Cohen, S. (1997). *Mindblindness: An essay on autism and theory of mind*. Massachusetts: The MIT Press.

Beck, A. T., Rush, A. J., Shaw, B. F., & Emery, G. (1979). *Cognitive therapy of depression*. New York: Guilford Press.

Bell, R. Q. (1968). A reinterpretation of the direction of effects in studies of socialization. *Psychological Review*, *75*, 81–95.

Bettelheim, B. (1967). *The empty fortress: Infantile autism and the birth of the self*. London: Collier-Macmillan.

Blum, D. (2003). *Love at Goon Park*. Chichester, UK: Wiley.

Bowlby, J. (1951). *Maternal care and mental health*. Geneva: World Health Organization.

Bowlby, J. (1969). *Attachment and Loss* (Vol. 1), *Attachment*. London: Hogarth Press.

Bramble, D. (2003). Annotation: The use of psychotropic medications in children: a British view. *Journal of Child Psychology and Psychiatry*, *44*, 169–179.

Bretherton, I. (2005). In pursuit of the internal working model construct and its relevance to attachment relationships. In: K. E.

Grossmann, K. Grossmann, & E. Waters (Eds.), *Attachment from infancy to adulthood* (pp. 13–47). London: Guilford Press.
British Medical Association. (2000). *Consent, rights and choices in health care for children and young people*. London: BMJ Books.
Bronfenbrenner, U. (1979). *The ecology of human development: experiments by nature and design*. Cambridge, MA: Harvard University Press.
Brown, G., & Harris, T. O. (1989). *Life events and illness*. New York: Guilford Press.
Brown, G. W., & Rutter, M. (1966). The measurement of family activities and relationships: A methodological study. *Human Relations*, *19*, 241–263.
Bundgaard, C., Larsen, F., Jorgensen, M., & Gabrielsson, J. (2006). Mechanistic model of acute autoinhibitory feedback action after administration of SSRIs in rats: Application to escitalopram-induced effects on brain serotonin levels. *European Journal of Pharmaceutical Sciences*, *29*(5), 394–404.
Buss, A. H., & Plomin, R. (1984). *Temperament: early developing personality traits*. Hillsdate NJ: Lawrence Erlbaum.
Cameron, K. (1956). Past and present trends in child psychiatry. *Journal of Mental Science*, *102*, 599–603.
Campbell, S. B. (1994). Hard-to-manage preschool boys: externalizing behavior, social competence, and family context at two-year follow-up. *Journal of Abnormal Child Psychology*, *22*, 147–166.
Campbell, D. T., & Stanley, J. C. (1963). *Experimental and quasi-experimental designs for research*. Boston, MA: Houghton Mifflin Company.
CANTAB. (1987). *The Cambridge neuropsychological test automated battery*. Cambridge: Cambridge Cognition Ltd.
Cantwell, D. P. (1988). DSM-III studies. In: M. Rutter, A. H. Tuma, & I. S. Lann (Eds.), *Assessment and diagnoses in child psychopathology* (pp. 3–36). New York: Guilford Press.
Caspi, A., McClay, J., Moffitt, T. E., Mill, J., Martin, J., Craig, I. W., *et al.* (2002). Role of genotype in the cycle of violence in maltreated children. *Science*, *297*, 851–854.
Caspi, A., Moffitt, T. E., Cannon, M., McClay, J., Murray, R., Harrington, H., *et al.* (2005). Moderation of the effect of adolescent-onset cannabis use on adult psychosis by a functional polymorphism in the COMT gene: Longitudinal evidence of a gene X environment interaction. *Biological Psychiatry*, *57*, 1117–1127.
Caspi, A., Moffitt, T. E., Newman, D. L., & Silva, P. A. (1996a). Behavioral observations at age 3 years predict adult psychiatric disorders: longitudinal evidence from a birth cohort. *Archives of General Psychiatry*, *53*, 1033–1039.
Caspi, A., Moffitt, T. E., Thornton, A., Freedman, D., Amell, J. W., Harrington, H. L., *et al.* (1996b). The Life History Calendar: A research and clinical assessment method for collecting retrospective event-history data. *International Journal of Methods in Psychiatric Research*, 6, 101–114.
Caspi, A., Sugden, K., Moffitt, T. E., Taylor, A., Craig, I. W., Harrington, H. L., *et al.* (2003). Influence of life stress on depression: Moderation by a polymorphism in the 5-HTT gene. *Science*, *301*, 386–389.
Chess, S. (1988). Child and adolescent psychiatry come of age: a fifty year perspective. *Journal of American Academy of Child and Adolescent Psychiatry*, *27*, 1–7.
Clarke, A. M., & Clarke, A. D. (1986). Thirty years of child psychology: a selective review. *Journal of Child Psychology and Psychiatry*, *27*, 719–759.
Cohen, P., & Brook, J. S. (1987). Family factors related to the persistence of psychopathology in childhood and adolescence. *Psychiatry*, 50, 332–345.
Cohen, P., & Cohen, J. (1996). *Life values and adolescent mental health*. Mahwah, NJ: Lawrence Erlbaum Associates.
Commission of Families & the Well-Being of Children. (2005). *Families and the state. Two-way support and responsibilities*. Bristol: Policy Press.
Connors, C. K. (1992). *Manual for the Connor's continuous performance task*. Toronto: Multi Health Systems.
Costello, I. (Ed.). (2005). *British National Formulary for Children*. London: BMJ Publications.
de Quervain, D. J-F., & Papassotiropoulos, A. (2006). Identification of a genetic cluster influencing memory performance and hippocampal activity in humans. *Proceedings of the National Academy of Sciences*, *103*, 4270–4274.
Diller, L. H. (2006). *The last normal child: Essays on the intersection of kids, culture and psychiatric drugs*. Westport, CT: Praeger.
Dodge, K. A., Bates, J. E., & Pettit, G. S. (1990). Mechanisms in the cycle of violence. *Science*, *250*, 1678–1683.
Dodge, K. A., Pettit, G. S., Bates, J. E., & Valente, E. (1995). Social information-processing patterns partially mediate the effects of early physical abuse on later conduct problems. *Journal of Abnormal Psychology*, *104*, 632–643.
Dodge, K. A., Dishion, T. J., & Lansford, J. E. (Eds.). (2006). *Deviant peer influences in programs for youth: Problems and solutions*. New York: Guilford Press.
Douglas, J. W. B. (1964). *The home and the school*. London: MacGibbon & Kee.
Dulcan, M. (1997). Practice parameters for the assessment and treatment of children, adolescents and adults with attention-deficit/hyperactivity disorder. *Journal of the American Academy of Child and Adolescent Psychiatry*, *36*(Suppl), 85S–121S.
Eaves, L. J., Last, K. S., Martin, H. G., & Jinks, J. L. (1977). A progressive approach to non-additivity and genotype-environmental covariance in the analysis of human differences. *British Journal of Mathematical and Statistical Psychology*, *30*, 1–42.
Eisenberg, L. (1986). Mindlessness and brainlessness in psychiatry. *British Journal of Psychiatry*, *148*, 497–508.
Eisenberg, L. (2001). The past 50 years of child and adolescent psychiatry: A personal memoir. *Journal of American Academy of Child and Adolescent Psychiatry*, *40*, 743–748.
Elder, G. H. (1974). *Children of the Great Depression*. Chicago: University of Chicago Press.
Elder, G. H. (1998). The life course as developmental theory. *Child Development*, *69*, 1–12.
Everitt, B. F., & Pickles, A. (1999). *Statistical aspects of design and analysis of clinical trials*. London: Imperial College Press.
Feighner, J. P., Robins, E., Guze, S. B., Woodruff, R. A., Winokur, G., & Muno, R. (1972). Diagnostic criteria for use in psychiatric research. *Archives of General Psychiatry*, *26*, 57–63.
Ferguson, D. M., & Horwood, L. J. (2001). The Christchurch Health and Development Study: Review of Findings on Child and Adolescent Mental Health. *Australian and New Zealand Journal of Psychiatry*, *35*, 287–296.
Food and Drug Administration. (2004). *Public Health Advisory: suicidality in children and adolescents being treated with antidepressant medications*. Retrieved from http://www.fda.gov/cder/dru/antidepressants/SSRIHA200410.htm Feb. 16, 2007.
Frith, C. (2003). What do imaging studies tell us about the neural basis of autism? In: Novartis Foundation Symposium 251. *Autism: Neural basis and treatment possibilities* (pp. 149–176). Chichester, UK: John Wiley & Sons Ltd.
Frith, U. (2003). *Autism: explaining the enigma* (2nd ed.). Oxford, UK: Blackwell Publishing.
Giles, J. (2005). Taking on the cheats. *Nature*, *435*, 258–259.
Glantz, S. A., Barnes, D. E., Bero, L., Hanauer, P., & Slade, J. (1995). Looking through a keyhole at the tobacco industry. The Brown and Williamson documents. *Journal of the American Medical Association*, *274*, 219–224.
Gogtay, N., Giedd, J. N., Lusk, L., Hayashi, K. M., Greenstein, D., Vaituzis, A. C., *et al.* (2004). Dynamic mapping of human cortical development during childhood through early adulthood. *Proceedings of the National Academy of Sciences USA*, *101*, 8174–8179.

Goldapple, K., Segal, Z., Garson, C., Lau, M., Bieling, P., Kennedy, S., *et al.* (2004). Modulation of cortical–limbic pathways in major depression: Treatment-specific effects of cognitive behavior therapy. *Archives of General Psychiatry*, *61*, 34–41.

Goodman, R., & Scott, S. (1999). Comparing the strengths and difficulties questionnaire and the child behavior checklist: is small beautiful? *Journal of Abnormal Child Psychology*, *27*, 17–24.

Goodman, R., Ford, T., Simmons, H., Gatward, R., & Meltzer, H. (2003). Using the Strengths and Difficulties Questionnaire (SDQ) to screen for child psychiatric disorders in a community sample. *International Review of Psychiatry*, *15*, 166–172.

Greenough, W. T., Black, J. E., & Wallace, C. S. (1987). Experience and brain-development. *Child Development*, *58*, 539–559.

Gross, C., & Hen, R. (2004). The developmental origins of anxiety. *Nature Reviews Neuroscience*, *5*, 545–552.

Guy, J., Hendrich, B., Holmes, M., Martin, J. E., & Bird, A. (2001). A mouse MECP2–null mutation causes neurological symptoms that mimic Rett syndrome. *Nature Genetics*, *27*, 322–326.

Hammad, H. A., Laughren, T., & Racoosin, J. (2006). Suicidality in pediatric patients treated with antidepressant drugs. *Archive of General Psychiatry*, *63*, 332–339.

Happé, F. (1994). *Autism: an introduction to psychological theory*. London: UCK Press.

Hardt, J., & Rutter, M. (2004). Validity of adult retrospective reports of adverse childhood experiences: Review of the evidence. *Journal of Child Psychology and Psychiatry*, *45*, 260–273.

Hariri, A. R., & Weinberger, D. R. (2003). Imaging genomics. *British Medical Bulletin*, *65*, 259–270.

Hariri, A., Drabant, E., Munoz, K., Kolachana, B., Venkata, S., Egan, M., *et al.* (2005). A susceptibility gene for affective disorders and the response of the human amygdale. *Archives of General Psychiatry*, *62*, 146–152.

Hariri, A. R., Drabant, E. M., & Weinberger, D. R. (2006). Imaging genetics: Perspectives from studies of genetically driven variation in serotonin function and corticolimbic affective processing. *Biological Psychiatry*, *59*, 888–897.

Harlow, H. F., & Harlow, M. K. (1965). The effect of rearing conditions on behavior. *International Journal of Psychiatry*, *13*, 43–51.

Harrington, R., Whittaker, J., Shoebridge, P., & Campbell, F. (1998a). Systematic review of efficacy of cognitive behaviour therapies in child and adolescent depressive disorder. *British Medical Journal*, *316*, 1559–1563.

Harrington, R., Kerfoot M., Dyer, E., McNiven, F., Gill, J., Harrington, V., *et al.* (1998b). Randomized trial of a home based family intervention for children who have deliberately poisoned themselves. *Journal of the American Academy of Child and Adolescent Psychiatry*, *37*, 512–518.

Harrington, R., Whittaker, J., & Shoebridge, P. (1998c). Psychological treatment of depression in children and adolescents: A review of treatment research. *British Journal of Psychiatry*, *173*, 291–298.

Healy, D. (2004). *Let them eat Prozac: The unhealthy relationship between the pharmaceutical industry and depression*. New York: New York University Press.

Hermelin, B., & O'Connor, N. (1970). *Psychological experiments with autistic children*. Oxford: Pergamon.

Hersov, L. (1986). Child psychiatry in Britain: The last 30 years. [Review.] *Journal of Child Psychology and Psychiatry*, *27*, 781–801.

Hetherington, E. M. (1989). Coping with family transitions: winners, losers and survivors. *Child Development*, *60*, 1–14.

Hetherington, E. M. (2005). Divorce and the adjustment of children. *Pediatric Review*, *26*, 163–169.

Hewitt, L. E., & Jenkins, R. L. (1946). *Fundamental patterns of maladjustment*. Springfield, IL: State of Illinois.

Hill, A. B. (1965). The environment and disease: Association or causation? *Proceedings of the Royal Society of Medicine*, *58*, 295–300.

Hill, P. (1999). Child and adolescent psychiatry in the United Kingdom. In: H. Remschmidt, & H. van Engeland (Eds.), *Child and adolescent psychiatry in Europe*. Steinkopff: Darmstadt; Springer: New York.

Hinde, A., & McGinnis, L. (1977). Some factors influencing the effect of temporary mother–infant separation: Some experiments with rhesus monkeys. *Psychological Medicine*, *7*, 197–212.

Holmes, J. (2001). *The search for the secure base: Attachment theory and psychotherapy*. London: Brunner-Routledge.

Insel, T. R., & Young, L. J. (2001). The neurobiology of attachment. *Nature Reviews: Neuroscience*, *2*, 129–136.

Jackson, D. D. (1960). A critique of the literature on the genetics of schizophrenia. In: D. D. Jackson (Ed.), *The Etiology of Schizophrenia* (pp. 37–87). New York: Basic Books.

Jeammet, P. (1999). Child and adolescent psychiatry in France. In: H. Remschmidt & H. van Engeland (Eds.), *Child and adolescent psychiatry in Europe*. Steinkopff: Darmstadt; Springer: New York.

Kagan, J., & Snidman, N. (2004). *The long shadow of temperament*. Cambridge, MA: Belknap Press of Harvard University Press.

Kanner, L. (1943). Autistic disturbances of affective contact. *The Nervous Child*, *2*, 217–250.

Kanner, L. (1959). The Thirty-Third Maudsley Lecture: Trends in child-psychiatry. *Journal of Mental Science*, *105*, 581–593.

Kanner, L. (1969). Children haven't read those books, reflections on differential diagnosis. *Acta Paedopsychiatrica*, *36*, 2–11.

Laub, J. H., & Sampson, R. J. (2003). *Shared beginnings, divergent lives: Delinquent boys to age 70*. Cambridge, MA: Harvard University Press.

Lord, C., Rutter, M., DiLavore, P. C., & Risi, S. (2001). *Autism Diagnostic Observation Schedule*. Los Angeles, CA: Western Psychological Services.

Magaña, A. B., Goldstein, M. J., Karno, M., & Miklowitz, D. J. (1986). A brief method for assessing expressed emotion in relatives of psychiatric patients. *Psychiatric Research*, *17*, 203–212.

Main, M., Hesse, E., & Kaplan, N. (2005). Predictability of attachment behavior and representational processes at 1, 6 and 19 years. In: K. E. Grossmann, K. Grossmann, & E. Waters (Eds.), *Attachment from infancy to adulthood* (pp. 245–304). London: Guilford Press.

Malan, D. (1979). *Individual psychotherapy and the science of psychodynamics*. London: Butterworths.

McEwan, B., & Lasley, E. N. (2002). *The end of stress*. Washington, DC: Joseph Henry Press.

Meaney, M. J. (2001). Maternal care, gene expression, and the transmission of individual differences in stress reactivity across generations. *Annual Review of Neuroscience*, *24*, 1161–1192.

Medewar, P. (Ed.). (1982). *Pluto's Republic*. Oxford: Oxford University Press.

Meehl, P. E. (1954). *Clinical versus statistical prediction: A theoretical analysis and a review of the evidence*. Minneapolis: University of Minnesota Press.

Meltzer, H., Gatward, R., Goodman, R., & Ford, T. (2000). *Mental health of children and adolescents in Great Britain*. London: Stationery Office.

Moffitt, T. E., Caspi, A., Rutter, M., & Silva, P. A. (2001). *Sex differences in antisocial behavior: Conduct disorder, delinquency, and violence in the Dunedin Longitudinal Study*. Cambridge, UK: Cambridge University Press.

Molling, P., Lockner, A., Sauls, R. J., & Eisenberg, L. (1962). Committed delinquent boys: The impact of perphenazine and of placebo. *Archives of General Psychiatry*, *7*, 70–76.

Neale, M. D. (1958). *Neale analysis of reading ability*. London: Macmillan.

National Institute for Health and Clinical Excellence. (2005). *Depression in children and young people: identification and management in primary, community and secondary care*. Retrieved from www.nice.org.uk or http://www.nice.org.uk/page.aspx?o=cg028) Feb. 16, 2007.

Ounsted, C. (1955). The hyperkinetic syndrome in epileptic children. *Lancet*, *ii*, 303–311.

Parry-Jones, W. L. (1989). The history of child and adolescent psychiatry: its present day relevance. *Journal of Child Psychology and Psychiatry*, *30*, 3–11.

Pasamanick, B., & Knobloch, H. (1966). Retrospective studies on the epidemiology of reproductive casualty: old and new. *Merrill-Palmer Quarterly of Behavioural Development*, *12*, 7–26.

Patterson, G. R. (1981). *Coercive family process*. Eugene, OR: Castalia Publishing.

Pennington, B. (2002). *The development of psychopathology: Nature and nurture*. New York: Guilford Press.

Plomin, R., & Bergeman, C. S. (1991). The nature of nurture: Genetic influence on "environmental" measures. *The Behavioural and Brain Sciences*, *14*, 373–427.

Plomin, R., DeFries, J. C., & Loehlin, J. C. (1977). Genotype–environment interaction and correlation in the analysis of human behavior. *Psychological Bulletin*, *84*, 309–322.

Plomin, R., DeFries, J., McClearn, G. E., & McGuffin, P. (Eds). (2001). *Behavioral genetics* (4th ed.). New York: Worth Publishers.

Pond, D. A. (1961). Psychiatric aspects of epileptic and brain-damaged children. *British Medical Journal*, *2*, 1378–1382.

Prichep, L. (1983). Neurometrics: Quantitative evaluation of brain dysfunction in children. In: M. Rutter (Ed.), *Developmental Neuropsychiatry* (pp. 213–238). Edinburgh: Churchill Livingstone.

Quinton, D., Rutter, M., & Rowlands, O. (1976). An evaluation of an interview assessment of marriage. *Psychological Medicine*, *6*, 577–586.

Rachman, S. (1962). Learning theory and child psychology: therapeutic possibilities. *Journal of Child Psychology & Psychiatry*, *3*, 149–168.

Radke-Yarrow, M. J. D., Campbell, J. D., & Burton, R. V. (1970). Recollections of childhood: A study of the retrospective method. *Monographs of the Society for Research in Child Development*, *35*, 1–83.

Rapoport, J. (1980). Diagnostic significance of drug response in child psychiatry. In: L. Eisenberg (Ed.), *Psychopathology of children and youth* (pp. 154–170). New York: Josiah Macy Jnr Foundation.

Rapoport, J., Addington, A., Frangou, S., & MRC Psych. (2005). The neurodevelopmental model of schizophrenia: Update 2005. *Molecular Psychiatry*, *10*, 434–449.

Rapoport, J., Buchsbaum, M. S., Zahn, T. P., Weingartner, H., Ludlow, C., & Mikkelsen, E. J. (1978). Dextroamphetamine: cognitive and behavioural effects in normal prepubertal boys. *Science*, *199*, 560–563.

Reich, W. (2000). Diagnostic interview for children and adolescents (DICA). *Journal of the American Academy of Child and Adolescent Psychiatry*, *39*, 59–66.

Reid, W. J., & Shyne, A. W. (1969). *Brief and extended casework*. New York: Columbia University Press.

Reitan, R. M., & Wolfson, D. (1993). *The Halstead-Reitan Neuropsychology Test Battery: Theory and clinical interpretation*. Tuscon, AZ: Neuropsychology Press.

Remschmidt, H. (1996). Changing views: New perspectives in child psychiatric research. *European Child & Adolescent Psychiatry*, *5*, 2–10.

Remschmidt, H., & van Engeland, H. (Eds.). (1999). *Child and adolescent psychiatry in Europe*. Darmstadt: Steinkopff; New York: Springer.

Reynell, J. (1969). *Reynell developmental language scales*. Windsor, UK: NFER Publishing Company.

Richman, N., Stevenson, J., & Graham, P. (1982). *Preschool to school: a behavioral study*. London: Academic Press.

Robertson, J., & Robertson, J. (1971). Young children in brief separation: A fresh look. *Psychoanalytic Study of the Child*, *26*, 264–315.

Robins, E., & Guze, S. B. (1970). Establishment of diagnostic validity in psychiatric illness: its application to schizophrenia. *American Journal of Psychiatry*, *126*, 983–987.

Robins, L. (1966). *Deviant children grown up: A sociological and psychiatric study of sociopathic personality*. Baltimore: Williams & Wilkins.

Robbins, T. W., James, M., Owen, A. M., Sahakian, B. J., Lawrence, A. D., McInnes, L., *et al.* (1998). A study of performance on tests from the CANTAB battery sensitive to frontal lobe dysfunction in a large sample of normal volunteers: implications for theories of executive functioning and cognitive aging. Cambridge Neuropsychological Test Automated Battery. *Journal of the International Neuropsychological Society*, *4*, 474–490.

Rosenzweig, M. R., Krech, D., Bennett, E. L., & Diamond, M. C. (1962). Effects of environmental complexity and training on brain chemistry and anatomy: a replication and extension. *Journal of Comparative Physiology & Psychology*, *55*, 429–437.

Royal College of Psychiatrists' Working Party. (2001). *Guidelines for researchers and for research ethics committees on psychiatric research involving human participants*. (Council Report No. CR82). London: Royal College of Psychiatrists.

Rutter, M. (1965). Classification and categorization in child psychiatry. *Journal of Child Psychology and Psychiatry*, *6*, 71–83.

Rutter, M. (1967). A children's behaviour questionnaire for completion by teachers: Preliminary findings. *Journal of Child Psychology & Psychiatry*, *8*, 1–11.

Rutter, M. (1970). Autistic children: Infancy to adulthood. *Seminars in Psychiatry*, *2*, 435–450.

Rutter, M. (1981). Epidemiological/longitudinal strategies and research in child psychiatry. *Journal of the American Academy of Child Psychiatry*, *20*, 513–544.

Rutter, M. (1982a). Psychological therapies in child psychiatry: Issues and prospects. *Psychological Medicine*, *12*, 723–740.

Rutter, M. (1982b). Syndromes attributed to "Minimal Brain Dysfunction" in childhood. *American Journal of Psychiatry*, *139*, 21–33.

Rutter, M. (1987a). Temperament, personality and personality disorder. *British Journal of Psychiatry*, *150*, 443–458.

Rutter, M. (1987b). The role of cognition in child development and disorder. *British Journal of Medical Psychology*, *60*, 1–16.

Rutter, M. (1989a). Pathways from childhood to adult life. *Journal of Child Psychology and Psychiatry*, *30*, 23–51.

Rutter, M. (1989b). Isle of Wight revisited: twenty-five years of child psychiatric epidemiology. *Journal of American Academy Child Adolescent Psychiatry*, *28*, 633–653.

Rutter, M. (1998). Practitioner review: Routes from research to clinical practice in child psychiatry: Retrospect and prospect. *Journal of Child Psychology and Psychiatry*, *39*, 805–816.

Rutter, M. (2005a). Environmentally mediated risks for psychopathology: Research strategies and findings. *Journal of American Academy of Child and Adolescent Psychiatry*, *44*, 3–18.

Rutter, M. (2005b). Adverse preadoption experiences and psychological outcomes. In: D. M. Brodzinsky, & J. Palacios (Eds.), *Psychological issues in adoption: Theory, research and application* (pp. 67–92). Westport, CT: Greenwood Publishing.

Rutter, M. (2005c). Autism research: Lessons from the past and prospects for the future. *Journal of Autism and Developmental Disorders*, *35*, 241–257.

Rutter, M. (2006a). *Genes and behavior: Nature–nurture interplay explained*. Oxford: Blackwell Publishing.

Rutter, M. (2006b). The psychological effects of early institutional rearing. In: P. J. Marshall, & N. A. Fox (Eds.), *The Development of Social Engagement* (pp. 355–392). New York: Oxford University Press.

Rutter, M. (in press). Developing concepts in developmental psychopathology. In: J. J. Hudziak (Ed.), *Genetic and environmental influences on developmental psychopathology*. Arlington, VA: American Psychiatric Publishing.

Rutter, M. (2007). Proceeding from observed correlation to causal inference: The use of natural experiments. *Perspectives on Psychological Science*, *2*, 377–395.

Rutter, M., & Brown, G. W. (1966). The reliability and validity of measures of family life and relationships in families containing a psychiatric patient. *Social Psychiatry*, *1*, 38–53.

Rutter, M., Graham, P., & Yule, W. (1970). A neuropsychiatric study in childhood. *Clinics in Developmental Medicine 35/36*. London: Heinemann/SIMP.

Rutter, M., Kim-Cohen, J., & Maughan, B. (2006). Continuities and discontinuities in psychopathology between childhood and adult life. *Journal of Child Psychology and Psychiatry*, *47*(3/4), 276–295.

Rutter, M., Le Couteur, A., & Lord, C. (2003). *ADI-R: Autism Diagnostic Interview – Revised*. Los Angeles, CA: Western Psychological Services.

Rutter, M., & Maughan, B. (2002). School effectiveness findings 1979–2002. *Journal of School Psychology*, *40*, 451–475.

Rutter, M., Maughan, B., Mortimore, P., Ouston, J., & Smith, A. (1979). *Fifteen thousand hours: Secondary schools and their effects on children*. London: Open Books; Cambridge, MA: Harvard University Press. Reprinted, 1994, London: Paul Chapman Publishers.

Rutter, M., Moffitt, T. E., & Caspi, A. (2006). Gene–environment interplay and psychopathology: multiple varieties but real effects. *Journal of Child Psychology and Psychiatry*, *47*(3/4), 226–261.

Rutter, M., Pickles, A., Murray, R., & Eaves, L. (2001). Testing hypotheses on specific environmental causal effects on behavior. *Psychological Bulletin*, *127*, 291–324.

Rutter, M., & Silberg, J. (2002). Gene–environment interplay in relation to emotional and behavioral disturbance. *Annual Review of Psychology*, *53*, 463–490.

Rutter, M., Tizard, J., & Whitmore, K. (1970). *Education, Health and Behaviour*. London: Longmans; [Reprinted 1981, Melbourne, FA: Krieger.]

Sampson, R. J., Raudenbush, S. W., & Earls, F. W. (1997). Neighborhoods and violent crime: A multilevel study of collective efficacy. *Science*, *277*, 918–924.

Sandberg, S., Rutter, M., Giles, S., Owen, A., Champion, L., Nicholls, J., *et al.* (1993). Assessment of psychosocial experiences in childhood: methodological issues and some illustrative findings. *Journal of Child Psychology and Psychiatry*, *34*, 879–897.

Schowalter, J. (2000). Child & adolescent psychiatry comes of age, 1944–1994. In: R. W. Menninger & J. C. Nemiah (Eds.), *American psychiatry after World War II* (pp. 461–480). Washington, DC: American Psychiatric Press.

Shadish, W. R., Cook, T. D., & Campbell, D. T. (2002). *Experimental and quasi-experimental designs for generalized causal inference*. Boston & New York: Houghton Mifflin Company.

Shaffer, D., Fisher, P. W., & Lucas, C. P. (1999). Respondent-based interviews. In: D. Shaffer, C. P. Lucas, & J. E. Richters (Eds.), *Diagnostic Assessment in Child and Adolescent Psychopathology* (pp. 3–33). New York: Guilford Press.

Shaffer, D., Fisher, P., Lucas, C. P., Dulcan, M. K., & Schwab-Stone, M. E. (2000). NIMH Diagnostic Interview Schedule for Children version IV (NIMH DISC-IV): description, differences from previous versions, and reliability of some common diagnoses. *Journal of the American Academy of Child and Adolescent Psychiatry*, *39*, 28–38.

Shaw, P., Greenstein, D., Lerch, J., Clasen, L., Lenroot, R., Gogtay, N., *et al.* (2006). Intellectual ability and cortical development in children and adolescents. *Nature*, *30*, 676–679.

Starr, M., & Chalmers, I. (2003). *The evolution of the Cochrane Library, 1988–2003*. UPDATE software: Oxford. Retrieved from www.update-softare.com/history/clibhist.htm Feb. 16, 2007.

Stevenson, J. P., & Graham, P. (1982). Temperament: a consideration of concepts and methods. *Ciba Foundation Symposium*, *89*, 36–50.

Suomi, S. J. (2005). Aggression and social behaviour in rhesus monkeys. *Novartis Foundation Symposium*, *268*, 216–222; discussion 222–226, 242–253.

Teasdale, J. D., & Barnard, P. J. (1993). *Affect cognition and change: Re-modelling depressive thought*. Hove, UK: Lawrence Erlbaum Associates.

Thomas, A., Chess, S., Birch, H. G., Hertzig, M. E., & Korn, S. (1963). *Behavioral individuality in early childhood*. New York: New York University Press.

Thomas, A., Chess, S., & Birch, H. G. (1968). *Temperament and behavior disorders in children*. New York: New York University Press.

Tulving, E. (1983). *Elements of episodic memory*. New York: Oxford University Press.

Volkmar, F. R., & Nelson, D. S. (1990). Seizure disorders in autism. *Journal of the American Academy of Child & Adolescent Psychiatry*, *1*, 127–129.

Warren, W. (1974). *Child Psychiatry and the Maudsley Hospital: An historical survey*. Unpublished Third Kenneth Cameron Memorial Lecture, Institute of Psychiatry Library.

Wechsler, D. (1986). *Wechsler Adult Intelligence Scales – Revised*. New York: Psychological Corporation.

Wechsler, D. (1992). *Wechsler Intelligence Scales For Children – Revised*. NewYork: Psychological Corporation.

Weersing, V. R., & Weisz, J. R. (2002a). Mechanisms of action in youth psychotherapy. *Journal of Child Psychology and Psychiatry*, *43*, 3–29.

Weersing, V. R., & Weisz, J. R. (2002b). Community clinic treatment of depressed youth: benchmarking usual care against CBT clinical trials. *Journal of Consultant Clinical Psychology*, *70*, 299–310.

Weisz, J. R., Weersing, V. R., & Henggeler, S. W. (2005). Jousting with straw men: Comment on Westen, Novotny, and Thompson-Brenner (2004). *Psychological Bulletin*, *131*, 418–426.

White, C. (2005). Christopher Gillberg, the psychiatrist at the centre. *British Medical Journal*, *331*, 180.

Wolpe, J. (1958). *Psychotherapy of reciprocal inhibition*. Stanford, CA: University Press.

Wolraich, M. L. (2003). Annotation: The use of psychotropic medications in children: an American view. *Journal of Child Psychology and Psychiatry*, *44*, 159–168.

Woodhouse, W., Bailey, A., Rutter, M., Bolton, P., Baird, G., & Le Couteur, A. (1996). Head circumference in autism and other pervasive developmental disorders. *Journal of Child Psychology & Psychiatry*, *37*, 785–801.

World Health Organization. (1996). Multiaxial classification of child and adolescent psychiatric disorders: *The ICD-10 classification of mental and behavioural disorders in children and adolescents*. Cambridge, UK: Cambridge University Press.

Yule, W., & Berger, M. (1972). Behaviour modification principles and speech delay. In: M. Rutter & J. A. M. Martin (Eds.), *The child with delayed speech* (pp. 204–219). *Clinics in Developental Medicine No 43*. London: Heinemann/Spastics International Medical Publications.

Zoghbi, H. Y. (2003). Postnatal neurodevelopmental disorders: Meeting at the synapse? *Science*, *302*, 826–830.

2 Classification

Eric Taylor and Michael Rutter

Purposes

Classifications are tools for thought and communication. They have to serve many purposes: communication among clinicians and researchers, application of research to clinical problems, guidance on practice, explanations to patients, and clinical reimbursement. For all these purposes, a good scientific classification should have the virtues of clarity, comprehensiveness, acceptability to users and fidelity to nature; also a scheme should change as understanding alters. Different purposes, however, call for different types of ordering.

Research into the psychopathology of young people requires groups of children who are reasonably homogenous with respect to what is being investigated, and replicability is crucial. It often does not matter very much if many cases are left unclassified, so long as those that are classified are classified accurately (but note the problems inherent in a focus on uncommon "pure" cases; see chapter 3). In mature sciences, a classification can itself be a scientific tool, as in cladistics, where the relations of bodily structure among animals are a means for studying evolutionary descent. This is occasionally the case in psychopathology – similarities between obsessions and stereotypies led to trials of a treatment for obsessive-compulsive disorder (OCD) in autism (Hollander, Phillips, Chaplin *et al.*, 2005), and similarities between the symptoms of mania and attention deficit/hyperactivity disorder (ADHD) led to cross-disorder studies (Tillman, Geller, Craney *et al.*, 2003). Researchers may not themselves need some of the practical implications of classification, but they do want their conclusions to guide practice, and therefore they wish to choose classes that practitioners will also recognize and use.

Clinical practitioners need to know how to apply research findings to an individual case, so a widely accepted classification scheme is indispensable. For them, a scheme leaving many cases unclassified has serious drawbacks because it cuts the bridge between their practice and the research that should inform it. Indeed, if research definitions have drifted too far from clinical ones, it may be quite misleading to generalize lessons from strictly defined research groups to broader and vaguer clinical ones. Clinical treatment has to define who does not need intervention as well as who does, so impairment is sometimes a necessary part of definition. Other clinical needs for classification – for example, in communication among clinicians, statistical record keeping and audit – mean that homogeneity of groups in severity and responsiveness to intervention may be more important than homogeneity with respect to cause.

Epidemiology and public health raise another set of requirements. Simplicity and robustness become more important than in clinical and research settings (where detailed and expert assessments are feasible). Impairment is not necessarily to be included. In defining populations at risk, or requiring early intervention, it may be important to include cases of disorder who are not yet impaired (cf. the use of statins to prevent coronary artery disease, or immunization against infections).

Communication with users and carers often has to interpret between classifications. Lay concepts of disorder are often different from those of professionals. A striking example was shown by Klasen and Goodman (2000), who elicited ideas about ADHD from parents that were based on the concept of a neurological disorder, contrasting markedly with those of primary care physicians, who used concepts of continuous variation and psychosocial influence. The public may try to make diagnoses explain the condition, whereas professionals are seeking only to describe.

Administration and management also need to classify. Those who purchase clinical care require ways of understanding costs, prices and outcomes for different kinds of clinical problem. Diagnoses are not a very good way of doing this, but other means of prediction such as "case complexity" have fared poorly and the combination of type and severity of condition remains the most widely used.

The variety of purposes has led the World Health Organization to a "family of classifications" adapted to different settings (Sartorius & Janca, 1996). They must not, however, be allowed to diverge too much. They all need to communicate with each other and to address essentially the same ideas. They all need a comparable approach to what is and what is not considered to be a disorder. They are all based upon cases and not people. There is very much more to be said about people than their casehood, and the extra requirements for a clinical formulation are dealt with in chapter 4.

Rutter's Child and Adolescent Psychiatry, 5th edition. Edited by M. Rutter, D. Bishop, D. Pine, S. Scott, J. Stevenson, E. Taylor and A. Thapar. © 2008 Blackwell Publishing, ISBN: 978-1-4051-4549-7.

DSM and ICD

ICD-10 (World Health Organization, 1996) and DSM-IV-TR (American Psychiatric Association, 2000) constitute the two major psychiatric classifications used throughout the world. Their predecessors (ICD-9 and DSM-III) were very different from one another and strenuous efforts were made to bring ICD-10 and DSM-IV much closer together. Those efforts were successful in achieving better international understanding and communication. Nevertheless, some differences remain in principle as well as in detail. DSM-IV, for example, has one scheme that is designed for both research and routine clinical usage, whereas ICD-10 has separate (but interlinked) schemes for these two rather different purposes, the research version being closer to DSM-IV. Comorbidity is dealt with in DSM-IV by making multiple diagnoses; in ICD-10 by making more use of combination categories and exclusion criteria to arrive at a single diagnosis where possible.

There is something to be said in support of deliberate differences when evidence is lacking to decide which of two alternatives is to be preferred. Further research comparing the two systems should provide for an empirically based choice in the future. For example, the two schemes differ in the rules to be followed in the diagnosis of attention deficit/hyperactivity disorder (ADHD – the term in DSM-IV) and hyperkinetic disorder (the ICD-10 term). The symptom lists are almost identical, but the two systems have different requirements for pervasiveness across situations, whether all problems or only some need to be present, and on the use of exclusion criteria in relation to comorbidity. The consequence is that ICD-10's hyperkinetic disorder is a subcategory of DSM-IV's ADHD; the grounds for translating one into the other are reasonably clear, and research findings to compare the two can be informative (Santosh, Taylor, Swanson *et al.*, 2005).

The two schemes also differ in how they deal with emotional disorders with an onset in childhood. ICD-10 makes a distinction between separation anxiety that represents an exaggeration or prolongation of a normal stage of emotional development (operationally defined as requiring an onset before age 6 years and absence of a generalized anxiety disorder), whereas DSM-IV makes the diagnosis solely on the basis of symptom pattern without regard to either age of onset or generalized anxiety. The validity of the different diagnostic approaches could be compared, although so far little research has addressed this rather fundamental question.

Unfortunately, in addition to these deliberate differences, there are other minor differences that, although trivial in themselves and seemingly inadvertent in their origins, have been found to have major implications – as shown, for example, by the findings with respect to post-traumatic stress disorder (PTSD). A difference between the two schemes in relation to just one item (numbing of general responsiveness) had a dramatic effect on concordance between the two schemes (Andrews & Slade, 1998).

In the future development of both classification schemes, we hope that international comparability can be achieved, with agreement between ICD-11 and DSM-V where that is possible; and where it is not, clear rules for translation. This chapter indicates several areas of uncertainty where research could lead to sounder judgment about how to arrange the taxons. Issues include how to conceptualize problems; how to deal with associated problems and overlapping conditions; changes related to age; and how far notice needs to be taken of advancing neurobiological knowledge.

Types

Classifications themselves can helpfully be classified into the following.

Types of Classification

Categories and Dimensions

The choice of a categorical or a dimensional system of ordering has generated much debate (Sonuga-Barke, 1998). A thoroughgoing categorical arrangement is often described, although only by its detractors, as a medical model. This is a highly misleading view of medicine, which incorporates dimensional as well as categorical approaches. One example would be that of blood pressure, which is a dimension distributed continuously in the population; elevated blood pressure (hypertension) is a diagnostic category, but it is based on the quantitative idea of the degree of elevation that entails significant risk and at which treatment is justified. Another example is that of anemia – not only are levels of hemoglobin continuously distributed, but the level that is judged to be a problem to treat will depend upon other factors, such as the cause and the society in which it is encountered.

Nevertheless, it is plain that there are many constraints on clinicians' thinking that favor a set of categories. The output from many clinical encounters is a set of categorical decisions: a child either is, or is not, prescribed a drug – or admitted into a treatment program – or taken into care. It is therefore convenient (although obviously not essential) for diagnostic thinking to fall into the same mode. The convenience may be more apparent than real. It invites an immediate abuse – in which the treatment is determined directly and exclusively by the diagnosis. This possibility becomes all too real in some types of practice. The need of busy clinicians for simple rules of thumb, and the wish of some purchasers of health care to restrict treatment to mechanically defined groups and protocols, can lead to a lack of careful planning of care for the individual case.

It is sometimes said that categorical thinking is inherent in the human mind. It arises in the first months of life (Blewitt, 1994), and characterizes the lay theories through which non-experts perceive psychological abnormality (Schoeneman, Segerstrom, Griffin *et al.*, 1993). Even if this is the natural tendency of the mind, especially when coping with complex information under pressure to make decisions, it is not necessarily the best approach. Artificial intelligence can increasingly be used to assist in handling complex information sets, and need not be constrained by human infirmity.

Categories have other practical advantages (Klein & Riso, 1996); a single term, if carefully chosen, carries a great deal of meaning very conveniently and will be much more tractable in communication with parents and teachers than a large set of dimensional scores. These advantages have ensured that diagnostic schemes are mostly categorical; and dimensional ordering is for the most part either secondary or rather tentative and speculative (e.g., Appendix B of DSM-IV).

By contrast, when dealing with genetic and environmental risk factors, researchers usually find dimensional relations between risks and manifest disorders. Individual alleles are either present or absent, but their consequences are graded. Indeed, the distinctions between categories and dimensions should not be exaggerated. Generally, each can be translated into the other. A category can be expressed as a set of dimensional scores; and a profile of dimensional scores is a category. The degree to which an individual case fits a category can itself be a dimensional construct. Sometimes it is preferable to use both ways of thinking about a single domain. IQ is better conceived as a dimension when the purpose is to predict educational achievement, but low IQ (e.g., below 50) is better thought of categorically when the purpose is to consider whether structural disorder of the brain is likely to be present (see below). Hypertension is conveniently regarded as a diagnostic category when the purpose is to select cases for treatment; as a dimension when analyzing the physiological reasons for changes in blood pressure; and as a category again when considering the different factors determining variations in the most severely affected cases at the top of the range.

In spite of the difficulties involved, the testing of assumptions about the nature of the underlying problems is useful. One classic research strategy has been to examine distributions of cases along a continuum of severity to see if there is a discontinuity between normality and pathology (such as would be implied by a bimodal distribution). This often suggests continuity – but the power of tests for mixed distributions is low (Meehl, 1995) and even very large numbers of cases can fail to give unequivocal answers.

Some investigators have compared the effect size of a continuous measure with a categorical one in predicting an external association such as outcome. For example, Fergusson, Horwood & Lynskey (1993) argued on this basis that a dimensional measure of disruptive behavior in childhood gave a better prediction of adolescent outcome than a discrete category of childhood disorder. This may say more about the power of alternative statistical methods than about taxonomy, and it ignores the possibility that a strongly predictive category of antisocial behavior may be present, but one that is based upon the type of problems rather than the severity of disruptiveness. This was the conclusion of Bergman and Magnusson (1997) in another longitudinal study, predicting antisocial outcome, which included a wider range of possible predictors, physiological as well as behavioral. Moffitt (1993) also concluded, from analysis of the longitudinal course of a population cohort of boys, that an antisocial outcome in adult life was characteristic, not so much of the boys who had been the most disruptive adolescents, but those who had had the combination of early onset and neurodevelopmental impairments.

Another research strategy has been to examine the distribution of cases against a measure of presumed etiology and to seek a point of discontinuity; for example, in comparing successive levels of definition of hyperactivity against measures of neurodevelopmental delay and reporting that the putative risk factor was more common only in the most severe subgroup of "hyperkinetic disorder" (Taylor, Sandberg, Thorley *et al.*, 1991). This strategy has not given unequivocal results. Latent class analyses, for example, have suggested not only the presence of subtypes of ADHD but also that they tended to breed true within families (e.g., Rasmussen, Neuman, Heath *et al.*, 2004). The argument was for etiologically distinct classes. On the other hand, Gjone, Stevenson and Sundett (1996) addressed a similar question by comparing group heritability with individual heritability of ADHD symptoms in a twin study using multiple regression techniques: the extent to which cotwins showed a regression to the mean in their scores did not function differently at the extremes of the distribution. This was in keeping either with a more dimensional view (with heritability similar across the whole continuum) or with a single, very common category. The issues are not resolved, even for this rather well-studied condition.

In the current state of knowledge, clinicians are likely to use a mixture of dimensional and categorical ideas. They will seek to fit a child's problems into an economical description of a pattern of disorder or several coexistent patterns. They will also grade some of their problems – the severity of the behavioral deviance, the level of impairment and the extent of risk factors. The level of IQ will be taken into account when judging whether neurodevelopmental impairments (such as those of language, attention or social communication) can be considered as deviant. The analysis of a case of schizophrenia will include differentiation of the severity of positive and negative symptoms. They should aim to elicit and record the full range of problems presented by an individual child and their context, and should not seek only to classify on a single axis.

There are many other examples in medicine of dimensional approaches being used as a supplement to a categorical classification. Oncologists regularly grade the degree of malignancy of tumors, and cardiologists measure the degree of occlusion of coronary arteries and the degree of exercise tolerance. The multiaxial system in child psychiatry (World Health Organization, 1996) provides a similar facility with respect to degree of social impairment and intellectual level, and DSM-IV provides a means of coding the severity of disorders, as well as the extent to which a disorder is in remission.

When a category is defined as a dimensional score above a cut-off, the exact cut-off chosen can seldom be defined absolutely. It may have been validated against clinicians' judgment, or by finding the level that best differentiates referred children from the ordinary population. It may vary with cultural expectations, so it is hard to give absolute or universal criteria. Accordingly, the presence of functional impairment usually needs to be added to a definition. A disorder is often defined as a "harmful dysfunction" – there needs to be both a perturbation of ordinary function, at behavioral or cognitive level, and evidence that it is indeed causing impairment to the mental and social development of the child. The idea of impairment and its assessment are taken further in chapter 4.

Multiple Taxons

Single vs. Multiple Entities

Categorical classifications can be based on allotting cases to the single category they best fit, or on multiple categorization – a case may be simultaneously classified in several ways. It can be a good discipline to try to fit multiple problems into a single pattern, but it is also important to detect a secondary condition even when it is masked by a more obvious one.

One kind of multiplicity is obviously necessary: different domains of problems need different classifications. It makes no sense to ask whether a child has asthma or intellectual disability. They constitute problems of different types, and are best considered on separate axes. Field trials of early versions of the ICD (Rutter, Lebovici, Eisenberg *et al.*, 1969; Tarjan, Tizard, Rutter *et al.*, 1972) indicated that many disagreements between clinicians were of this type, and correspondingly that reliability among diagnostic raters could be increased if they were not asked to choose between (say) autism and severe intellectual disability, but were allowed to choose both, one on an axis of psychiatric symptoms and the other on one of intellectual ability. This not only increases agreement, but provides a richer conceptualization and an opportunity to code and examine the extent to which (in this example) intellectual ability modifies the course and treatment response of autism. A multiaxial system embodies this conceptual refinement; it differs from a multicategory system in that every axis needs a coding (even if the coding is of "no abnormality"). Axes of psychiatric symptoms, somatic diseases, psychosocial stressors and severity of impairment have been incorporated in the multiaxial version of ICD-10 (WHO, 1996). Specific learning disabilities and intellectual impairments are dealt with in rather different ways by DSM-IV and ICD-10 (in which they are independent axes); the important feature is that both, in different ways, allow the clinician to record, systematically and separately, the extent to which both general and specific learning impairments are present.

Multiaxial systems of classification have become the norm in child/adolescent psychiatry for five main reasons. First, they avoid false dichotomies resulting from having to decide between two diagnoses that do not, in any meaningful sense, constitute alternatives. The example given of autism or intellectual disability illustrates the point. The first gives information on the clinical syndrome whereas the second describes the level of intellectual impairment. Second, because there has to be a coding on each and every axis, the classification provides information that is both more complete and less ambiguous. Thus, in a multicategory system the absence of a coding of intellectual disability could mean that the child had normal intelligence, or that the child was cognitively impaired but the clinician did not consider that it was relevant to the referral problem, or that the diagnosis was omitted by error. That ambiguity could not arise with a multiaxial system. Third, it avoids artifactual unreliability resulting from differing theoretical assumptions. Thus, psychosocial adversity would be coded and present by both the clinician who viewed it as the main cause and by the clinician who saw it as only a minor contributor. The same would apply to somatic conditions such as cerebral palsy or diabetes. Fourth, it provides a means by which to note systematically, not only the presenting clinical picture, but also possible causal factors (or factors likely to influence prognosis or response to treatment) and degree of overall psychosocial impairment. Fifth, because of these features it represents a style of thinking that is much closer to most clinicians' preferred style of conceptualization than is the case with a system that forces everything into the Procrustean bed of a diagnosis based only on symptom pattern.

Hierarchical Classification Systems

Most classification schemes make some use of hierarchies, based on a view that some conditions are fundamental and that, if others are present, they are likely to derive from the fundamental condition. The implication is that the former includes and accounts for the latter. Foulds (1976), for example, presented rating scale data from adult psychiatric in-patients to argue that the symptoms of people with schizophrenia usually included depression and anxiety; that those of people with depression did not usually include those of schizophrenia but did include anxiety; whereas people with anxiety did not usually show either depression or schizophrenia and were therefore at the bottom of a hierarchy of schizophrenia–depression–anxiety. There are evident dangers of circular reasoning, but with care the predictions can be tested. Clearly, this type of prediction would be unlikely to give a complete account of child psychopathology as a whole, but could be practical within groups of children sharing risk factors (such as diffuse brain damage) or with problems in a particular domain such as hyperactivity.

In this way, DSM-IV excludes the diagnosis of generalized anxiety disorder if it occurs exclusively during a mood disorder, or a psychotic disorder (such as schizophrenia) or a pervasive developmental disorder (such as autism), and ICD-10 does so if the criteria for a panic disorder or an obsessive-compulsive disorder are met. Both DSM-IV and ICD-10 exclude the diagnosis of autism if Rett disorder is present, and exclude the diagnosis of reactive attachment disorder if a pervasive developmental disorder is present. The general assumption that severe and pervasive mental disorders often give rise to secondary symptom patterns is well based; the problem is that the evidence to justify hierarchies is generally rather thin, and neither DSM-IV nor ICD-10 is consistent in its approach.

Polythetic/Monothetic Classes

Almost all medical classifications are polythetic. That is, cases are defined on the basis of having many, but not all, of a list of specified attributes in common. That is because variability in manifestation is a general biological feature, even with diseases solely due to one major gene. In the neuropsychiatric arena, such variability is evident in marked degree with conditions such as tuberous sclerosis or the Fragile X anomaly. There is similarly great variability in the manifestations of autism, even between monozygotic twins with the same genetic liability: the phenotype extends from severe handicap to quite subtle disturbances of social function. It would not therefore be reasonable to require that the disorder in any particular individual had to have *all* the diagnostic features. The trouble is that, in the absence of a diagnostic test of some kind, there are real difficulties in deciding both how varied the manifestations could be and where and how the boundaries should be drawn. Latent class analyses may help but what are really required are external validators (see below).

Prototype vs. Algorithm

In allotting cases to classes, most clinicians use a combination of two strategies. The first is a kind of pattern matching: the profile of problems presented in the case is compared with a "schema" or "prototype" in the clinician's mind. The clinical guidelines of the ICD-10 provide a set of descriptions of problems, which act as prototypes in this sense. This does not exclude a dimensional approach: a case can fit more or less well to a prototype, can be more or less typical, and can be of greater or lesser severity. Furthermore, a case may fit one or more separate prototypes (see Multiaxial Classification Systems, below). The mental processes involved are what distinguish it from the second form of case identification: the algorithmic. The research diagnostic criteria of ICD-10 and the whole of the DSM-IV system are founded upon an algorithmic approach, in which a number of possible features are recognized as present or absent. The features are then combined (often by simple addition) to determine whether a cut-off point for the disorder has been reached. This has the advantages of transparency and fidelity to the rules that are applied in research. It also provides a ready means of resolving boundary problems about whether a case does or does not reach the requisite severity for a diagnosis. The disadvantages are that it tends to lead to a large number of diagnoses being made in a single case, which may not be truly independent; and that it is hard to apply in practice because it is simply not feasible to go through the process for every diagnosis that might apply to the individual case. The replicability of the algorithmic process makes it much the preferred method for research purposes. The needs of practice tend to lead clinicians to adopt a prototypic approach. Algorithms are often applied in the specialist assessment of complex cases and in cases presenting diagnostic difficulty. Legal processes sometimes apply algorithms in an overmechanical fashion.

Lumping vs. Splitting

Grouping disorders into superordinate categories can be helpful in drawing attention to features they may have in common. This applies, for instance, to the neurodevelopmental disorders (see chapter 3). Oppositional and conduct disorders are regarded by ICD-10 as being closely linked rather than as separate disorders, with oppositional disorders representing an earlier version of the condition. The kinds of research to test this approach are *developmental*, with most conduct-disordered children having been oppositional at an earlier stage; *hierarchical*, with most conduct-disordered children showing or having shown the features of oppositional disorder; and *associational*, with both conditions having strong links with environmental adversity in family and neighborhood (see chapter 35).

The coexistence of conduct disorder with hyperkinesis is dealt with by a mixed category of hyperkinetic conduct disorder that is a subcategory of hyperkinetic disorder. This decision is based on evidence such as the developmental course, with hyperactivity predicting antisocial behavior but not vice versa; and genetic and neurobiological evidence suggesting similarity between hyperkinesis simple and hyperkinesis in the presence of conduct problems (see chapter 34). However, the appearance of conduct disorder has massive implications for substance abuse and personality problems, so the distinction is important to retain in classification.

A subdivision may need to be made for a single symptom – blood phobia has such striking differences from other phobias, in associations with fainting and slowed heart rate on exposure, that it needs a separate place. It must be admitted that many fine subdivisions – for instance, among the disorders of anxiety – are unvalidated, but only if they are made can their implications be explored.

General vs. Child-Specific

Children present in very different ways at different developmental stages. However, there are practical and conceptual difficulties entailed in changing diagnosis simply because one ages. The difficulties have increasingly led to child psychiatrists using similar categories of emotional disorder to those of adult psychiatry. Sometimes this can be misleading. Differences between depressive disorders in children and those in adults are quite marked: in heritability, in presentation and in response to medication (see chapter 37). Tricyclic medicines are known to be ineffective in childhood, yet they are often prescribed. This poor practice may be maintained by the lack of clear distinction between childhood and adult forms.

The decision about whether or not to split can increasingly be based on evidence from prospective longitudinal studies, in which people are examined both in childhood and as adults. There is, for example, a change in pattern of ADHD towards an adult presentation more of disorganization than of overactivity (see chapter 34). At the same time, the adult and childhood forms show similar cognitive changes and responses to medication. The concept resulting is of a continuity in disorder with age-related differences in presentation.

Transcultural Issues

In general, the idea of using a single classification for all countries has worked well, and many types of problem have proved to be essentially invariant across cultures (see chapter 15). Exceptions to the rule, however, need to be noted lest investigators and clinicians in non-Western cultures apply taxons and metrics uncritically.

Other differences may reflect variations in the blend of risk and protective factors. Strongly religious societies, for example, may create both supports for those with disabilities and occasions for spiritual anxieties. A high rate of obsessional symptoms focused on religion in some Muslim countries (Fontenelle, Mendlowicz, Marques *et al.*, 2004) could reflect either the opportunity for religious scrupulosity to develop or the functional value of obsessionality in promoting religious observance.

Other differences again result from differences between societies in the significance attached to particular problems. Examples come from lower concern about anxiety and more about oppositional behavior in Thailand by comparison with the USA (Weisz, Suwanlert, Chaiyasit *et al.*, 1993); and in the contrast between the low rates of ADHD in Hong Kong when identified objectively and the high rates when identified by parent and teacher concern and ratings (Luk, Leung & Ho, 2002).

Validation of Categories

The classification of child psychopathology started with the taxonomy of how behaviors correlate with each other, notably Hewitt and Jenkins' (1946) factor analysis of symptoms. Sophisticated multivariate analyses then led to the derivation of a larger number of syndromes based on symptom profiles (Verhulst & Achenbach, 1995). It was increasingly recognized that groupings based on patterns of symptomatology needed to be tested by their ability to predict criteria that are *external* to the symptomatology and that have clinical meaning and utility (Feighner, Robins, Guze *et al.*, 1972; Cantwell, 1975; Rutter, 1978).

Clinicians sometimes assume that an ideal classification should be based on etiology; however, that is not so. Most successful medical diagnoses that work well are based, instead, on the underlying pathophysiology that gives rise to the clinical syndrome. For instance, diabetes is defined in terms of the metabolic abnormality and not on which pattern of susceptibility genes is present. Most disorders are multifactorial, and elucidation of causal factors is important chiefly because it is likely to lead to an understanding of the basic pathophysiology. There is not, and cannot be, a classification according to a particular cause because there is no single cause. However, in internal medicine, there usually is a final common pathophysiological pathway that leads to the clinical disorder. The goal should be the identification of the underlying pathophysiology of mental disorders, rather than finding the single main cause. We are a long way from reaching that goal at the moment. For the same reason, there cannot be any one validating test against some hypothetical gold standard. Instead, there has to be recourse to multiple validating approaches with the hope, and expectation, that when most point in the same direction, it is likely that the diagnosis has some meaningful discriminative validity. Accordingly, we summarize such evidence briefly before seeking to draw conclusions on the current state of play on diagnostic validity.

Biological Findings

In many respects, the clearest biological distinction is between severe intellectual disability (IQ below 50), mild intellectual disability (IQ 50–69) and the range of normal intelligence (Simonoff, Bolton & Rutter, 1996; see chapter 49). Individuals who are severely cognitively impaired have a much reduced fecundity and life expectancy, most show gross neuropathological abnormalities of the brain, and most have either clinical brain disorders (such as cerebral palsy or epilepsy) or marked congenital abnormalities. Their social class background, on the other hand, is generally similar to that of the general population. By contrast with severe cognitive impairment, most people with mild impairment show a normal fertility pattern and a normal life expectancy, but to a marked extent they are disproportionately likely to come from a socially disadvantaged background. The genetic influences are more likely than in the case of severe intellectual disability to reflect many genes operating as part of a multifactorial liability, and thus constitute the end of a continuum on the dimension reflecting normal variations in intelligence. (Some individuals will nevertheless have the same major genetic mutations as those found with severe intellectual disability.)

Autism is differentiated from the broad run of other psychiatric disorders by its reduced life expectancy (mainly due to deaths associated with epilepsy; Isager, Mouridsen & Rich, 1999) and by the high rate of epilepsy (about 25%). It does not differ from intellectual disability in either respect but it does differ with respect to the age of onset of epilepsy (Rutter, 1970; Volkmar & Nelson, 1990). Neuropathological studies are few, but the findings do not reflect the gross pathology that is typical of intellectual disability (see chapter 46). Furthermore, a larger than normal head size is associated with autism, by contrast with the small head size that is more usually characteristic of intellectual disability (Fombonne, Wostear, Cooper *et al.*, 2001; Woodhouse, Bailey, Rutter *et al.*, 1996).

Biological findings are beginning to find some differentiation among other disorders. Abnormalities on both structural and functional imaging are found in many cases of hyperkinetic disorder and OCD and the findings provide a substantial case for a neural basis for the disorders (at least as a contributory factor in etiology; see chapters 34 and 43). Neurodevelopmental impairment is also more likely than in ordinary children. However, there are limitations in how far these findings can be used for validation. There are a few pointers to possible diagnostic specificity: the structural and functional changes in frontal and striate regions in hyperkinetic disorders probably differ from the limbic changes in obsessional and post-traumatic disorders, and those with bipolar disorder have more extensive abnormalities (including amygdala) than either. It is too early in investigation to be clear how robust and how generalizable such findings will turn out to be.

To some extent, similar problems apply to the associations between neurodevelopmental impairment (as indexed by motor delay and language impairment) and schizophrenia (Tosato & Dazzan, 2005): association is present, but far from universal, and found in similar forms in other disorders too. Life-course-persistent antisocial behavior differs from that which is adolescence-limited in its association with neurodevelopmental impairment and this helps to make a developmentally important distinction.

More recently, evidence has suggested that the misuse of psychoactive substances may have a coherent pathophysiology. A low striatal density of D_2 receptors predicts a much bigger subjective reaction when people are given either intravenous methylphenidate (a D_2 dopamine transporter inhibitor) or other euphoriant drugs (Volkow, Wang, Fowler *et al.*, 2002). Furthermore, a variety of different drugs, including heroin, alcohol and nicotine, all engage mesolimbic dopamine projections to the nucleus accumbens (Hyman, Malenka & Nestler, 2006). Genetic analyses are compatible with this view (see below). Therefore, it may be that substance misuse itself may come to be regarded as a mental disorder, rather than a lifestyle choice that only merits a diagnosis if it causes harm or physical dependence.

Drug Response

It might be expected that drug responses would help greatly in diagnostic validation. In general, at a scientific level they do not. As a first consideration, most drugs target multiple neurotransmitters and have several distinct therapeutic actions. For example, tricyclics have independent effects on disorders as diverse as depression, ADHD and nocturnal enuresis. Second, in many cases, the therapeutic effects are neither specific nor dramatic. There are substantial benefits at the group level but these are not sufficiently consistent at the individual level to help much in diagnosis: if someone who is depressed does not return to a normal mood following administration of antidepressants, this by no means rules out the diagnosis of depression. Marked individual variations in drug response are common throughout medicine. Third, many drugs appear to affect behaviors rather than diagnosis-specific pathophysiologies. Thus, the effects of stimulants on inattention and overactivity are qualitatively much the same (albeit quantitatively less marked) in individuals who do not have ADHD as in those who do. On the other hand, there are drugs that appear to have effects on disorders that differ from those on the healthy. Thus, lithium does not make euthymic individuals less "manic," even though it does reduce the likelihood of manic episodes in those with bipolar disorder. There are sometimes strong predictors of drug action (e.g., the val/val form of the *COMT* gene is associated with a stronger enhancement of cognitive performance by stimulants than are other forms of the gene), but these are in the realm of genotypic rather than phenotypic prediction (Mattay, Goldberg, Fera *et al.*, 2003).

In practice, the treatability of a disorder can be a strong reason for diagnosing it. The acceptable indications for drugs are usually phrased in terms of the presence of disorder rather than the presence of a target behavior. It is often said, for instance, that stimulants should not be given unless a child meets diagnostic criteria for ADHD. The great variations between countries in the rate of diagnosis of ADHD seem likely to be influenced by the extent to which clinicians desire to use the medication. Treatment needs to be decided on the basis of assessment of risks and benefits and not on whether a particular set of diagnostic criteria is met.

Genetic/Family Study Findings

Findings from twin, adoptee and family studies have been crucial in establishing some very important differences among diagnostic groups (Kendler & Prescott, 2006). Schizophrenia tends to breed relatively true, with associations that extend to schizotypal and paranoid disorders but not much wider than that. However, there is some overlap in genetic influences with bipolar disorder: it seems probable that there are both specific influences on each and common influences on both (see chapter 45). Autism and its broader phenotype breed true, and there is no evidence of any genetic association between schizophrenia and autism (see chapter 46). Affective disorders do indeed show a substantial familial loading for depression, but also for generalized anxiety disorders, with twin data suggesting a substantial shared genetic liability. Twin and family data also suggest a distinction between prepubertal depression and major depression starting in adolescence or adult life. Attention deficit disorders with hyperactivity clearly stand out as having a substantively higher heritability than that for other disorders involving disruptive behavior. They also largely share the same genetic liability – possibly because one is a risk factor for the other, but also emphasizing that the distinction is not absolute (see chapter 34). The twin findings also raise queries about the validity of a qualitatively distinct diagnosis of ADHD, in as much as the heritability of hyperactivity seems much the same throughout its range. Subtypes are being examined with a latent class type of analysis, but a clear structure is not yet evident. From a genetic perspective, there is no justification for differentiating between oppositional defiant disorder and conduct disorder (see chapter 35).

The genetic findings on Tourette syndrome are mainly of interest in relation to validity because they suggest some overlap with both multiple chronic tics and OCD. Genetic findings on other disorders all indicate a significant genetic component but they are less informative on discriminative diagnostic validity, apart from the findings in adults suggesting that the specific phobias may be relatively distinct from generalized anxiety and from panic disorder (Kendler & Prescott, 2006).

Molecular genetics is increasingly being applied to the question of validating diagnostic categories. The clearest finding has been the validation of Rett syndrome by an association with a specific genetic mutation (see chapters 24 & 46). ADHD has been robustly associated with allelic variants in the genes coding for the dopamine (D_4 and D_5) receptors and the dopamine transporter; and more provisionally with a range of other DNA variants affecting synaptic transmission. Specificity to the diagnosis of ADHD is much less clear, however, and the same variants have been associated with a range of personality changes and with anxiety states. The loci found in genome scans of people with ADHD show a strong overlap with loci provisionally detected in studies of people with autism, suggesting either that some common genetic influences exist or that phenotypic differentiation still leaves much to be desired.

Molecular and behavioral genetics have both contributed to the idea that misuse of various psychoactive substances may have a common origin. Kendler, Jacobson, Prescott *et al.* (2003), using a large adult population-based sample of male twins, found that both the genetic and the shared environmental effects on the use and misuse of six classes of illicit substances were largely or entirely non-specific in their effect – the influences were not on the tendency to use one drug rather than another, but on the misuse of all the drugs considered. One DNA variant implicated (*DRD2* gene minor Taq 1A (A_1) allele) is more common in people misusing substances than in the general population (Young, Lawford, Nutting *et al.*, 2004).

Unquestionably, genetic findings are informative on the differentiations among mental disorders but they should not determine classificatory distinctions. Thus, the genetic liability to blood phobia does not differ from that of other specific phobias, but it needs to be differentiated clinically because, unlike all the other phobias, it is associated with a fall (rather than rise) in blood pressure – leading to fainting. Generalized anxiety disorder and major depression share the same genetic liability but the implications for choice of medication are somewhat different.

Psychosocial Risk Factors

On the whole, there is relatively little diagnostic specificity with respect to the psychopathological risks associated with psychosocial stress and adversity. However, there are two important exceptions. First, severe institutional deprivation in the early years of life has a relatively specific association with syndromes involving disinhibited attachment (Rutter, Colvert, Kreppner *et al.*, 2007; see also chapter 55). Second, severe and acute stress experiences of an exceptional kind are particularly likely to lead to PTSD phenomena (see chapter 42). There is also some tendency for psychological loss stresses to lead to depression, and danger-type stresses to lead to anxiety (see chapter 26). Family conflict, discord and hostility are also more likely to lead to antisocial behavior than to emotional disturbance; the same applies to social disadvantage. Within antisocial disorders, life-course-persistent varieties show a stronger association in serious family adversities than that found with adolescence-limited varieties (see chapter 35).

Cognitive Correlates

Autism stands out as different from other psychiatric disorders both because of its particularly strong association with general cognitive impairment and its relatively specific association with theory of mind and central coherence deficits (see chapter 46). ADHD, too, is relatively distinctive through its association not only with mild cognitive impairment (which would apply to many conditions), but also with impulsive responding, altered time perception and sensitivity to delay of reward (see chapter 34). Schizophrenia is associated with a slightly below average IQ before the onset of the psychosis; there is sometimes a marked drop in IQ around the time of onset; and established cases have a higher rate of particular problems such as those in working memory (Bowie & Harvey, 2005).

Epidemiology

Age of onset and sex ratio tend to go together. Thus, disorders involving neurodevelopmental impairment (such as developmental disorders of language, autism, and ADHD, and life-course-persistent antisocial behavior) characteristically begin early in life and are much more common in males (see chapter 3). Emotional disorders beginning in adolescence (such as depression and eating disorders), by contrast, tend to be much more common in females; even antisocial behavior beginning in adolescence differs from earlier onset varieties in having a much weaker male preponderance. Rett syndrome is unique in being confined (or almost confined) to females – because the mutation is lethal in males.

Course of Disorder

The long-term course of disorders also helps to sort out diagnostic distinctions (see chapter 13). The plateau of developmental progress and loss of purposive motor skills associated with Rett syndrome make it quite distinct. Adult outcome findings are relevant in showing the major continuities between depression in adolescence and recurrent depression in adult life. Similarly, strong continuities are to be found between antisocial behavior (including conduct and oppositional/defiant disorders) and personality disorders in adult life; there is a strong persistence of autism and a relatively strong persistence of schizophrenia, of obsessive-compulsive disorders and of tics/Tourette syndrome. There are fewer data on anxiety disorders but, although there is some overlap with depression, specific phobias seem somewhat distinct.

Summary of Validity Inferences

Putting together the evidence discussed above, it is possible to arrive at a three-fold division of disorders into those that are reasonably well-validated, those with pointers suggesting probable validity and those where the evidence indicates that the categorical subdivisions are probably invalid.

The first group clearly contains autism and autism spectrum disorders (considered together), schizophrenia and schizophrenic spectrum disorders (again as a grouping), depressive disorders, hyperkinetic behavior as a feature that differentiates it from other disorders of disruptive behavior, oppositional and conduct disorders (considered together) and Rett syndrome. A range of contrasting approaches all provide good evidence of discriminative validity. The same applies to the distinction between intellectual disability (usually severe) that is associated with gross neuropathology and that (usually mild) that is not.

The second cluster of probably valid syndromes includes OCD, eating disorders (pooling anorexia and bulimia nervosa), tics and Tourette syndrome, specific phobias, PTSD, disinhibited attachment disorder, bipolar affective disorders, and the distinction between life-course-persistent and adolescent-linked antisocial behavior. As briefly noted above, in each instance there is substantial evidence of discriminative validity but it is either less consistent or it spans fewer research approaches. From a practical point of view, these provide sufficient grounds for retaining the diagnostic category, even though there are important questions to be tackled.

The third cluster of probably invalid categories is less easy to deal with, if only because of the usual problem of knowing how much weight to attach to a lack of evidence of a meaningful difference, when new research could change that situation completely. Nevertheless, it is important to be aware that our usage of prevailing classifications means that we are making distinctions that, at least currently, lack substance. For example, that applies to most of the detailed subclassifications, such as those among anxiety disorders or those among pervasive developmental disorders (PDD), Rett syndrome apart. That definitely does not mean that we should necessarily switch to some broader category. Thus, although there is no good evidence that the distinction between, say, autism and Asperger syndrome or atypical autism means much, the evidence on discriminative validity applies to the narrower category of autism and not to the broader category of PDD. Also, up to now, it has proved quite difficult to provide either a clear conceptualization or precise operationalization of the criteria for the broader category. The issue is the one that pervades psychiatry: namely, uncertainty on the boundaries of a syndrome when the defining pathophysiology is unknown. It should be added that this uncertainly applies in some (often major) degree to most of the conditions for which there is no evidence of validity.

A second group of probably invalid categories includes syndromes that are clinically striking but for which the external correlates provide little support for basic differences from other diagnostic categories. Selective mutism and conversion reactions fall into that group. In both cases the distinctiveness of the clinical picture and the particular therapeutic challenges it presents probably warrant the retention of the category. However, the same might have been said of school refusal (Hersov, 1977) and that no longer has a place in most classification schemes (Elliott, 1999). Then there are categories that derive from theoretical concepts but that lack satisfactory diagnostic criteria that would allow the testing of validity. Inhibited attachment disorder (see chapter 55) clearly is a diagnosis of that type and many would argue that borderline personality disorder is too (see chapter 50). Certainly, subdivisions among personality disorders remain rather unsatisfactory. It should be added that it is necessary to note that epidemiological findings indicate that there are quite a few children with psychosocial impairment but whose mental health problem does not fulfill any particular diagnostic category. Moreover, they have a mental health outcome, at least in the short term, that is as poor as those with a diagnosis (Angold, Costello, Farmer *et al.*, 1999a). Evidently, there is a need for some sort of residual psychopathological category.

In practice, clinicians find it useful to recognize and name some types of presentation that they do not suppose to be coherent diagnoses. Deliberate self-harm, for instance, is a behavior that can characterize several diagnoses and can be seen in people with no other diagnosis at all. However, the pragmatic implications are strong – including the need for treatment guidelines to manage the emergency presentations and the assessments of risk that are required whatever the underlying cause (see chapter 40).

Finally, it is necessary to return to the uncertainties in deciding between categorical and dimensional approaches. ADHD well illustrates this dilemma. Most of the biological validity evidence (such as the neuroimaging findings and associations with motor and language problems) applies to a relatively narrow diagnostic category, but many of the genetic findings suggest (but do not prove) a dimensional liability (Banaschewski, Hollis, Oosterlaan *et al.*, 2005). Furthermore, the risk over time for social impairment applies to the broader and milder form of ADHD as well as to a narrowly defined hyperkinetic disorder (Lahey, Pelham, Chronis *et al.*, 2006). Of course, it may well be that there is both a qualitatively distinct disorder and a risk dimension, which look similar but which differ in their pathophysiology.

Agreement

Agreement on Clinical Psychiatric Diagnoses

Diagnostic ratings by experienced clinicians show at least a modest concordance. Limited agreement within panels of independent clinicians has been found over the years – for DSM-III (Mattison, Cantwell, Russell *et al.*, 1979; Mezzich, Mezzich & Coffman, 1985; Prendergast, Taylor, Rapoport *et al.*, 1988), and for ICD-9 (Gould, Shaffer, Rutter *et al.*, 1988; Prendergast *et al.*, 1988; Remschmidt, 1988). Field trials for DSM-IV reported better agreement, but on the basis of self-selected pairs of psychiatrists who made diagnoses on selected patients. The shortcomings of this strategy were pointed out by Rutter and Shaffer (1980), who noted that one would expect clinicians working together to have similar diagnostic practices. Further work needs to be carried out before the language of child psychiatry becomes sufficiently explicit to sustain scientific progress.

On the other hand, good diagnostic agreement can be achieved by independent research teams that have agreed supplementary criteria in advance (Prendergast *et al.*, 1988). This satisfactory agreement is comparable with that obtained by studies in which two clinicians from the same center rated cases with fuller information (Stroeber, Green & Carlson, 1981; Werry, Methren, Fitzpatrick *et al.*, 1983). The conclusion seems to be that training can improve diagnostic reliability to a satisfactory level; so the goal of an adequate system is not impossibly distant. The increased clarity of diagnostic rules in ICD-10 has been reported to increase inter-rater reliability, although the overall accuracy still leaves much to be desired (Steinhausen & Erdin, 1991). Other procedures that have been reported to enhance reliability are the use of a standard coding form after interview (Beitchman, Kruidenier, Clegg *et al.*, 1989), and the use of a multiaxial system (Skovgaard, Isager & Jorgensen, 1988).

A good deal of the unreliability in routine practice can be seen therefore to stem, not from the ambiguities in classification as such, but from their application under the constraints of everyday work. In other branches of medicine, the pitfalls in diagnosis have been studied, and it seems likely that these will apply to psychiatric diagnosis also. Chief among them is the tendency of the human mind to seek confirmation of a working hypothesis rather than to seek disproof of it. The initial perception of clinical problems often proceeds by matching to a prototype that is held in the mind, and there is a tendency to overestimate the similarity of the case to the phenotype. It is therefore easy to arrive at a premature categorization; and once it has been arrived at then the mind tends to overlook aspects that do not fit. This is often called "anchoring" of the first impression; and it will also be influenced by the prior conceptions of the probability of different classes that the diagnostician carries. These prior conceptions can also be prone to illusions – for instance, a clinician tends to overestimate associations between phenomena based on the frequency with which they see it, rather than the base rates of each problem in the population. The most practical way to avoid these kinds of errors is to be aware of them. The use of checklists in diagnostic practice is helpful, even to the experienced clinician, in making sure that comprehensiveness of assessment is achieved and that one does not ignore features of the case that are not a part of the key prototype being used. In training, and in reflecting on one's clinical experience, it is important to instill a sense of the diversity of presentations as well as the most typical ones. Above all, one should be critical of one's working ideas and be prepared to change formulations as assessment and treatment proceed.

The limited agreement between raters has had some impact on the way that diagnostic schemes have been formulated. The emphasis has been on clarity and simplicity of definitions rather than on subtleties of phenomenology. Descriptions such as overtalkativeness and overactivity are common to bipolar disorder and ADHD; they therefore cause confusion to clinicians as to how they should be placed; but remedies such as defining the qualitative differences between the goal-directed energies of mania and the desultory and disorganized qualities of ADHD have been hard to achieve in reliable fashion. Poor agreement between raters can also be due to systematic variability in the child's response to different situations (such as home and school). Correspondingly, the criteria for ADHD and for hyperkinetic disorder require that the defining behaviors should be present and impairing across situations.

Co-occurrence of Different Symptom Patterns

Over the last few decades, a substantial literature on the topic of "comorbidity" has accumulated. The concept refers to the situation in which two or more separate and independent disorders are present in the same person. It is crucial to appreciate that this is by no means synonymous with the co-occurrence of different symptom patterns. It is not the same because the co-occurrence may have several other meanings. To begin with, statistical considerations deriving from referral patterns mean that clinic samples will always be likely to be misleading (Berkson, 1946). Nevertheless, even epidemiological samples show very high rates of co-occurrence of different symptom patterns (Angold, Costello & Erkanli, 1999b), so other explanations must be considered (Caron & Rutter, 1991; Rutter, 1997). First, as already noted in the section on hierarchical classifications, there is a general recognition that it is very common for many disorders to include a diverse mixture of symptoms. Even outside accepted exclusionary hierarchy rules, it must be expected that many co-occurrences are likely to reflect this diversity. Thus, it is very frequent for affective disorders to involve a mixture of anxiety and depression. Similarly, it is quite common for obsessive-compulsive features to arise only in the course of a depressive disorder, and remit with it.

Second, there are many symptoms of mental disorders that are both non-specific indications of psychopathology (the mental equivalent of fever in internal medicine) and also defining symptoms for specific disorders. Clearly, anxiety is a feature of this kind but so are depression, overactivity and inattention.

Third, the overlap may reflect imperfections in diagnostic criteria – such as the inclusion of the same symptom in two or more categories, as with overactivity in relation to both ADHD and mania. This is particularly likely to lead to artifactual overlap when using either questionnaires or structural interviews relying on respondents' "yes" or "no" answers.

Fourth, the overlap may stem from misleading assumptions in diagnostic criteria. Thus, the high frequency of co-occurrence among anxiety disorders, or among personality disorders, probably arises for this reason. Similarly, co-occurrence may arise because one disorder represents an early manifestation of another. In these circumstances, at the point of transition from one pattern to the other, artifactual co-occurrence will occur. This probably accounts for much of the co-occurrence between oppositional/defiant and conduct symptoms (see chapter 35).

Fifth, the overlap may reflect the fact that many risk factors provide risks for several disorders and from the sharing of multiple risk factors across disorders. As we have noted, few risk factors are diagnosis-specific. This non-specificity is by no means special to psychopathology; it applies to many multifactorial disorders in internal medicine (Rutter, 1997).

Sixth, the presence of one disorder may create a risk for another. Thus, someone with an autism spectrum disorder (Hutton, Goode, Murphy *et al.*, in press) or an obsessive-compulsive disorder may become depressed as a response to their predicament. Alternatively, they may behave in ways that predispose to life situations that provide risks for another. The association between antisocial disorders and the shaping of stressful environments (Champion, Goodall & Rutter, 1995; Robins, 1966) that provide an increased risk for depression would be an example of this kind.

It is apparent from these contrasting possibilities that their investigation could throw an important light on causal processes. For example, multivariate analyses of adult twin data (Kendler & Prescott, 2006) have shown that although both social anxiety and depression show similar patterns of behavioral co-occurrence with alcohol abuse, the mechanisms are different. Social anxiety constitutes a statistical mediator for alcohol abuse (implying that the presence of social anxiety leads people to seek relief through alcohol consumption), the association between depression and alcohol abuse does not reflect mediation. Rather, it largely reflects a shared genetic liability. Findings, of course, may point to multiple mechanisms. Thus, for example, as we have noted, twin findings indicated that most of the genetic influence on drug taking applies to all drugs. The implication is that the genetically influenced propensity to take drugs concerns some aspect of risk-taking rather than response to particular chemical substances. On the other hand, twin data also suggest that using marijuana creates a "gateway" influence to using other drugs with more serious dependency properties and ill-effects on health (see chapters 13 & 36). Clearly, the scientific need is for more hypothesis-testing studies of the mechanisms underlying co-occurrence of different symptom patterns, rather than further documentation that it exists, with the unwarranted assumption that it means that there is comorbidity.

In the meanwhile, classification systems have to have rules on how to deal with the co-occurrence of different symptom patterns. Both ICD-10 and DSM-IV accept the need to be able to make multiple diagnoses if it is clear that the individual truly does have two or more separate conditions. After all, in most circumstances, it cannot be supposed that the presence of one disorder protects against others (although that can happen). Accordingly, someone with, say, autism or schizophrenia, can develop another mental disorder if they experience the risk factors for it. A strict single-category system would be unworkable and neither of the main systems have such a requirement.

Nevertheless, there is a dilemma on how to classify when there is uncertainty on whether or not the two conditions are truly separate and independent. ICD-10 and DSM-IV differ somewhat in their approach. Both provide for a hierarchical approach in a few instances (see above) and both provide a few mixed categories when there is good evidence that they both represent a single disorder (e.g., mixed episode of mania and depression). However, ICD-10 has rather more mixed categories (e.g., mixed anxiety and depressive disorder and depressive conduct disorder). The rationale is that the weight of evidence suggests either that there is something distinctive about the admixture (as compared with the situation when either condition occurs on its own) or that the same disorder commonly gives rise to this admixture of symptoms. It provides an economic way of communicating and it is a practice that is common in medicine. However, it has two possible disadvantages. First, the overall placement of the combination category in the classification system carries messages that may be misleading. Thus, in ICD-10, mixed anxiety and depression is classified as a variety of anxiety disorder, although the evidence suggests that it is more likely to represent a mood disorder (see chapter 37). Depressive conduct disorder is classified as a variety of conduct disorder and that does seem to be better justified in that research findings suggest that conduct disorder has much the same set of correlates and much the same outcome irrespective of the co-occurrence of depression – although there are some differences (Simic & Fombonne, 2001). On the other hand, it seems doubtful whether the presence of conduct disorder alters the meaning of the depression (Fombonne *et al.*, 2001). Accordingly, the validity of the mixed category is called in question. Also, the mixed category limits finer distinctions (such as between the subvarieties of anxiety disorder that may be associated with either conduct disorder or major depression).

The availability of mixed categories in ICD-10 is quite limited, however, and the bigger difference from DSM-IV lies in the approach to mixed symptom patterns that are not covered by a combination category. ICD-10 is not entirely explicit in how they should be dealt with, but the implicit expectation is a profile recognition or prototypic approach. Thus, if the main picture is one of severe depression, but there are marked obsessional features that ebb and flow with fluctuations in the depression, the mood disorder only would be the expected diagnosis. By contrast, DSM-IV would code obsessional disorder in addition (if the criteria were met) unless the *content* was mood-specific (e.g., as with a guilty rumination). The ICD-10 prototypic approach probably closely approximates much ordinary clinical practice. The main problem is that it has proved difficult to make prototypes sufficiently explicit that they will always be used in the same way.

With DSM-IV the mixture of two or more symptom patterns leads to the coding of as many diagnoses as there are patterns. This has the advantage of not requiring hierarchical judgments about which pattern is primary when in reality it may be very hard to tell, and it also succeeds in retaining a good deal of information when many patterns are present and no single category would convey them all. On the other hand, there are practical drawbacks to such a scheme. It encourages an unchallenged assumption that they are indeed independent patterns and that each can be dealt with in the same way as if there were no other problems. Alternatively, after multiple diagnoses are made, the clinician may then after all resort to a superordinate single-category way of thinking in which every possible profile has its own place. The coexistence of many diagnoses can be confusing and work against the key purpose of clarity and understanding how the research literature may apply to a particular child. It does not allow for the possibility of artifactual associations (see above). Furthermore, it is cumbersome, and perhaps impossible, for a clinician to review the presence or absence of every possible category, and clinicians usually vary a good deal in their willingness to record symptom patterns that are not the main presentation (Rutter, Shaffer & Shepherd, 1975).

Future Developments

Classification will develop as knowledge grows, and especially as we achieve more knowledge on the pathogenetic processes that lead to disorder. They have been considered under "validity" and will be taken up in more detail in following chapters. We may discover specific links between cause and presentation that will yield new "diseases" to join Lesch–Nyhan and Rett syndromes. At present, however, it seems clear that, with multifactorial disorders, it will be usual for there to be multiple causes of small effect, often involving an interplay between genetic susceptibility and environmental risk and protection (Rutter, Moffitt & Caspi, 2006). Given that most forms of psychopathology are multifactorial in origin, it would make little sense to classify on the assumption of a single basic cause, because there will not be one (Rutter, 2006). Rather, the future is likely to lie in the elucidation of the underlying neurophysiology (or neurochemistry or neuropsychology or neural interconnectivity). Social scientists sometimes object on the grounds that this would ignore the importance of environmental risk mechanisms. Their objections involve a reversion to an unwarranted dualism between psyche and soma. The recognition of the importance of infectious agents in causing somatic disease led to research, and then better understanding, of the effects of such agents on the organism and on its functioning. Something closely comparable should happen with psychosocial risk factors. It may be that new knowledge will lead those working on classification systems to introduce yet more complexity, more categories and more axes. We hope that does *not* happen. The history of science is that an increased understanding of causal processes often leads to simplification, rather than an ever-expanding complexity. The same should occur with psychopathology.

Public Impact

The use of explicit diagnostic schemes has demystified some of mental health, and created a better public understanding of the processes involved. Nevertheless, substantial concerns remain. The enterprise of psychiatric diagnosis is often attacked.

Some attacks are essentially on the functions for which diagnoses are used. Educators may object to the concepts of specific learning disorder because they object to assumptions that the causes lie in the children rather than their social situations. Many European clinicians resist the use of the concept of ADHD because they reject the idea that it is a neurological disorder. These attitudes ask too much of a diagnosis; it does not usually explain a child's condition, but only describes it. We may regard the diagnosis of ADHD as valid, in part because it predicts at a group level a range of neurobiological changes. However, there should be no expectation that the diagnosis means that the individual child arrived at the condition through those changes.

Other attacks on diagnosis are upon its consequences. The stigma of mental disorder is real, and can be unwelcome to children and their parents, who fear that normal means of education and socializing will be barred to those known to have a diagnosis. Evidence for this happening, however, is hard to find. Labeling a disorder can also have helpful consequences, in obtaining appropriate resources or in relieving confusion and guilt. The behaviors that evoke a diagnostic label may also evoke much crueller vernacular labels such as "stupidity," "laziness" or "immorality." The issue should be not so much that of whether to convey a diagnostic label as how to do so in a constructive fashion that encourages problem-solving and understanding.

Other attacks on diagnosis are on its abuses. Several of these have been referred to in this chapter. Clinicians should not allow their prototype of a disorder to become a stereotype and neglect other factors in the child, and they should not ignore factors beyond the individual; these are reasons for going beyond diagnosis to formulation. One should not start to regard diagnoses as things. Such "reification" is present in arguments such as "He does not *really* have a mental disorder; the cause lies in his family and society." These are alternative and complementary descriptions, not contradictory explanations.

Classification schemes are an essential language for making sense of mental health. They allow the user to relate individual cases to others, to communicate, and therefore to learn. When a case is assigned to a powerful class, many predictions follow. The classifications of child and adolescent mental health are becoming increasingly powerful.

References

American Psychiatric Association. (2000). *Diagnostic and Statistical Manual of Mental Disorders* (4th ed.), Text Revision. Washington, DC: American Psychiatric Association.

Andrews, G., & Slade, T. (1998). Depression, dysthymia and substance use disorders: sources of dissonance between ICD-10 and DSM-IV. *International Journal of Methods in Psychiatric Research*, *7*, 116–120.

Angold, A., Costello, E. J., Farmer, E. M., Burns, B. J., & Erkanli, A. (1999a). Impaired but undiagnosed. *Journal of the American Academy of Child and Adolescent Psychiatry*, *38*, 129–137.

Angold, A., Costello, E. J., & Erkanli, A. (1999b). Comorbidity. *Journal of Child Psychology and Psychiatry*, *40*, 55–87.

Banaschewski, T., Hollis, C., Oosterlaan, J., Roeyers, H., Rubia, K., Willcutt, E., *et al.* (2005). Towards an understanding of unique and shared pathways in the psychopathophysiology of ADHD. *Developmental Science*, *8*, 132–140.

Beitchman, J. H., Kruidenier, B., Clegg, M., Hood, J., & Corradini, A. (1989). Diagnostic interviewing with children: the use and reliability of the diagnostic coding form. *Canadian Journal of Psychiatry*, *34*, 283–290.

Bergman, L. R., & Magnusson, D. (1997). A person-oriented approach in research on developmental psychopathology. *Development and Psychopathology*, *9*, 291–319.

Berkson, J. (1946). Limitations of the application of fourfold table analysis to hospital data. *Biometrics*, *2*, 47–49.

Blewitt, P. (1994). Understanding categorical hierarchies: The earliest levels of skill. *Child Development*, *65*, 1279–1298.

Bowie, C. R., & Harvey, P. D. (2005). Cognition in schizophrenia: impairments, determinants, and functional importance. *Psychiatriatric Clinics of North America*, *28*, 613–633.

Cantwell, D. (1975). A model for the investigation of psychiatric disorders of childhood: Its application in genetic studies of the hyperkinetic syndrome. In: E. J. Anthony (Ed.), *Explorations in Child Psychiatry* (pp. 57–59). New York, NY: Plenum Press.

Caron, C., & Rutter, M. (1991). Comorbidity in child psychopathology: concepts, issues and research strategies. *Journal of Child Psychology and Psychiatry*, *32*, 1063–1080.

Champion, L. A., Goodall, G. M., & Rutter, M. (1995). Behavioural problems in childhood and stressors in early adult life: A 20-year follow-up of London school children. *Psychological Medicine*, *25*, 231–246.

Elliott, J. G. (1999). School refusal: Issues of conceptualisation, assessment, and treatment. *Journal of Child Psychology and Psychiatry*, *40*, 1001–1012.

Feighner, J. P., Robins, E., Guze, S. B., Woodruff, R. A., Winokur, G., & Munoz, R. (1972). Diagnostic criteria for use in psychiatric research. *Archives of General Psychiatry*, *26*, 57–63.

Fergusson, D. M., Horwood, L. J., & Lynskey, M. T. (1993). The effects of conduct disorder and attention deficit in middle childhood on offending and scholastic ability at age 13. *Journal of Child Psychology and Psychiatry*, *34*, 899–916.

Fombonne, E., Wostear, G., Cooper, V., Harrington, R., & Rutter, M. (2001). The Maudsley long-term follow-up of child and adolescent depression. 1. Psychiatric outcomes in adulthood. *British Journal of Psychiatry*, *179*, 210–217.

Fontenelle, L. F., Mendlowicz, M. V., Marques, C., & Versiani, M. (2004). Trans-cultural aspects of obsessive-compulsive disorder: A description of a Brazilian sample and a systematic review of international clinical studies. *Journal of Psychiatric Research*, *38*, 403–411.

Foulds, G. A. (1976). *Hierarchical nature of personal illness.* London: Academic Press.

Gjone, H., Stevenson, J., & Sundett, J. M. (1996). Genetic influences on parent reported attention-related problems in a Norwegian general population twin sample. *Journal of the American Academy of Child and Adolescent Psychiatry*, *35*, 588–596.

Gould, M. S., Shaffer, D., Rutter, M., & Sturge, C. (1988). UK/WHO Study of ICD-9. In: M. Rutter, A. H. Tuma, & I. S. Lann (Eds.), *Assessment and diagnosis in child psychopathology* (pp. 37–65). New York & London: Guilford Press.

Hersov, L. (1977). School refusal. In: M. Rutter & L. Hersov (Eds.), *Child and adolescent psychiatry: Modern approaches* (pp. 455–486). Oxford: Blackwell Scientific Publications.

Hewitt, L. E., & Jenkins, R. J. (1946). *Fundamental patterns of maladjustment: The dynamics of their origin.* Illinois: Michigan Child Guidance Institute.

Hollander, E., Phillips, A., Chaplin, W., Zagursky, K., Novotny, S., Wasserman, S., *et al.* (2005). A placebo controlled crossover trial of liquid fluoxetine on repetitive behaviors in childhood and adolescent autism. *Neuropsychopharmacology*, *30*, 582–589.

Hutton, J., Goode, S., Murphy, M., Le Couteur, A., & Rutter, M. (In press). New-onset psychiatric disorders in individuals with autism. *Journal of Autism.*

Hyman, S. E., Malenka, R. C., & Nestler, E. J. (2006). Neural mechanisms of addiction: The role of reward-related learning and memory. *Annual Review of Neuroscience*, *29*, 565–598.

Isager, T., Mouridsen, S. E., & Rich, B. (1999). Mortality and causes of death in pervasive developmental disorders. *Autism*, *3*, 7–16.

Kendler, K. S., & Prescott, C. A. (2006). *Genes, environment, and psychopathology: Understanding the causes of psychiatric and substance use disorders.* New York: Guilford Press.

Kendler, K. S., Jacobson, K. C., Prescott, C. A., & Neale, M. C. (2003). Specificity of genetic and environmental risk factors for use and abuse/dependence of cannabis, cocaine, hallucinogens, sedatives, stimulants, and opiates in male twins. *American Journal of Psychiatry*, *160*, 687–695.

Klasen, H., & Goodman, R. (2000). Parents and GPs at cross-purposes over hyperactivity: A qualitative study of possible barriers to treatment. *British Journal of General Practice*, *50*, 199–202.

Klein, D. N., & Riso, L. P. (1996). Psychiatric disorders: Problems of boundaries and comorbidity. In: C. G. Costello (Ed.), *Basic Issues in Psychopathology*. New York: Guilford Press.

Lahey, B. B., Pelham, W. E., Chronis, A., Massetti, G., Kipp, H., Ehrhardt, A., *et al.* (2006). Predictive validity of ICD-10 hyperkinetic disorder relative to DSM-IV attention-deficit/hyperactivity disorder among younger children. *Journal of Child Psychology and Psychiatry*, *47*, 472–479.

Luk, E. S. L., Leung, P. W. L., & Ho, T.-P. (2002). Cross-cultural/ethnic aspects of childhood hyperactivity. In: S. Sandberg (Ed.), *Hyperactivity and Attention Disorders of Childhood* (2nd ed.), (pp. 64–98). Cambridge, UK: Cambridge University Press.

Mattay, V. S., Goldberg, T. E., Fera, F., Hariri, A. R., Tessitore, A., Egan, M. F., *et al.* (2003). Catechol O-methyltransferase val158-met genotype and individual variation in the brain response to amphetamine. *Proceedings of the National Academy of Sciences USA*, *100*, 6186–6191.

Mattison, R., Cantwell, D. P., Russell, A. T., & Will, L. (1979). A comparison of DSM-III in the diagnosis of childhood psychiatric disorders. II. Inter-rater agreement. *Archives of General Psychiatry*, *36*, 1217–1222.

Meehl, P. E. (1995). Bootstrap taxometrics: Solving the classification problem in psychopathology. *American Psychologist*, *50*, 266–275.

Mezzich, A. C., Mezzich, J. E., & Coffman, G. (1985). Reliability of DSM-III vs. DSM-II in child psychopathology. *Journal of the American Academy of Child Psychiatry*, *24*, 272–280.

Moffitt, T. E. (1993). 'Life-course-persistent' and 'adolescence-limited' antisocial behavior: A developmental taxonomy. *Psychological Review*, *100*, 674–701.

Prendergast, M., Taylor, E., Rapoport, J. L., Bartko, J., Donnelly, M., Zametkin, A., *et al.* (1988). The diagnosis of childhood hyperactivity: A US–UK cross-national study of DSM-III and ICD-9. *Journal of Child Psychology and Psychiatry*, *29*, 289–300.

Rasmussen, E. R., Neuman, R. J., Heath, A. C., Levy, F., Hay, D. A., & Todd, R. D. (2004). Familial clustering of latent class and DSM-IV defined attention-deficit/hyperactivity disorder (ADHD) subtypes. *Journal of Child Psychology and Psychiatry*, *45*, 589–598.

Remschmidt, H. (1988). German study of ICD-9. In: M. Rutter, A. H. Tuma & I. S. Lann (Eds.), *Assessment and diagnosis in child psychopathology*, (pp. 66–83). New York & London: Guilford Press.

Robins, L. (1966). *Deviant children grown up: A sociological and psychiatric study of sociopathic personality.* Baltimore: Williams and Wilkins.

Rutter, M. (1970). Autistic children: Infancy to adulthood. *Seminars in Psychiatry*, *2*, 435–450.

Rutter, M. (1978). Diagnostic validity in child psychiatry. *Advances in Biological Psychiatry*, 2, 2–22.

Rutter, M. (1997). Comorbidity: Concepts, claims and choices. *Criminal Behaviour and Mental Health*, *7*, 265–285.

Rutter, M. (2006). *Genes and behavior: Nature–nurture interplay explained.* Oxford: Blackwell.

Rutter, M., Colvert, E., Kreppner, J., Beckett, C., Castle, J., Groothues, C., *et al.* (2007). Early adolescent outcomes for institutionally deprived and non-deprived adoptees: I. Disinhibited attachment. *Journal of Child Psychology and Psychiatry*, *48*, 17–30.

Rutter, M., Lebovici, S., Eisenberg, L., Sneznevskij, A. V., Sadoun, R., Brooke, E., *et al.* (1969). A triaxial classification of mental disorders in children. *Journal of Child Psychology and Psychiatry*, *10*, 41–61.

Rutter, M., Moffitt, T. E., & Caspi, A. (2006). Gene–environment interplay and psychopathology: Multiple varieties but real effects. *Journal of Child Psychology and Psychiatry*, *47*, 226–261.

Rutter, M., & Shaffer, D. (1980). DSM-III: A step forward or back in terms of classification of child psychiatric disorder? *Journal of the American Academy of Child Psychiatry*, *114*, 563–579.

Rutter, M., Shaffer, D., & Shepherd, M. (1975). *A multi-axial classification of child psychiatric disorders.* Geneva: WHO.

Santosh, P. J., Taylor, E., Swanson, J., Wigal, T., Chuang, S., Davies, M., *et al.* (2005). Refining the diagnoses of inattention and overactivity syndromes: A reanalysis of the Multimodal Treatment study of attention deficit hyperactivity disorder (ADHD) based on ICD-10 criteria for hyperkinetic disorder. *Clinical Neuroscience Research*, *5*, 307–314.

Sartorius, N., & Janca, A. (1996). Psychiatric assessment instruments developed by the World Health Organization. *Social Psychiatry and Psychiatric Epidemiology*, *31*, 55–69.

Schoeneman, T. J., Segerstrom, S., Griffin, P., & Gresham, D. (1993). The psychiatric nosology of everyday life: Categories in implicit abnormal psychology. *Journal of Social and Clinical Psychology*, *12*, 429–453.

Simic, M., & Fombonne, E. (2001). Depressive conduct disorder: Symptom patterns and correlates in referred children and adolescents. *Journal of Affective Disorders*, *62*, 175–185.

Simonoff, E., Bolton, P., & Rutter, M. (1996). Mental retardation: Genetic findings, clinical implications and research agenda. *Journal of Child Psychology and Psychiatry*, *37*, 259–280.

Skovgaard, A. M., Isager, T., & Jorgensen, O. S. (1988). The reliability of child psychiatric diagnosis: A comparison among Danish child psychiatrists of traditional diagnoses and a multiaxial diagnostic system. *Acta Psychiatrica Scandinavica*, *77*, 469–476.

Sonuga-Barke, E. J. (1998). Categorical models of childhood disorder: A conceptual and empirical analysis. *Journal of Child Psychology and Psychiatry*, *39*, 115–133.

Steinhausen, H. C., & Erdin, A. (1991). The inter-rater reliability of child and adolescent psychiatric disorders in the ICD-10. *Journal of Child Psychology and Psychiatry*, *32*, 921–928.

Stroeber, M., Green, J., & Carlson, G. (1981). Reliability of psychiatric diagnosis in hospitalized adolescents: Inter-rater agreement using DSM-III. *Archives of General Psychiatry*, *38*, 141–145.

Tarjan, M. D., Tizard, J., Rutter, M., Becab, M., Brooke, E. M., De La Cruz F. *et al.* (1972). Classification and mental retardation: Issues arising in the Fifth WHO Seminar on Psychiatric Diagnosis, Classification and Statistics. *American Journal of Psychiatry*, *128* (Supplement), 34–45.

Taylor, E., Sandberg, S., Thorley, G., & Giles, S. (1991). *The epidemiology of childhood hyperactivity.* Maudsley Monograph No. 33. Oxford: Oxford University Press.

Tillman, R., Geller, B., Craney, J. L., Bolhofner, K., Williams, M., Zimerman, B., *et al.* (2003). Temperament and character factors in a prepubertal and early adolescent bipolar disorder phenotype compared to attention deficit hyperactive and normal controls. *Journal of Child and Adolescent Psychopharmacology*, *13*, 531–543.

Tosato, S., & Dazzan, P. (2005). The psychopathology of schizophrenia and the presence of neurological soft signs: A review. *Current Opinion in Psychiatry*, *18*, 285–288.

Verhulst, F. C., & Achenbach, T. M. (1995). Empirically based assessment and taxonomy of psychopathology: Cross-cultural applications. A review. *European Child & Adolescent Psychiatry*, *4*, 61–76.

Volkmar, F. R., & Nelson, D. S. (1990). Seizure disorders in autism. *Journal of the American Academy of Child & Adolescent Psychiatry*, *1*, 127–129.

Volkow, N. D., Wang, G. J., Fowler, J. S., Thomas, P., Logan, J., Gtley, S. J., *et al.* (2002). Brain DA D_2 receptors predict reinforcing effects of stimulants in humans: Replication study. *Synapse*, *46*, 79–82.

Weisz, J. R., Suwanlert, S., Chaiyasit, W., Weiss, B., Achenbach, T. M., & Eastman, K. L. (1993). Behavioral and emotional problems among Thai and American adolescents: Parent reports for ages 12–16. *Journal of Abnormal Psychology*, *102*, 395–403.

Werry, J., Methren, R. J., Fitzpatrick, J., & Dixon, H. (1983). The inter-rater reliability of DSM-III in children. *Journal of Abnormal Psychology*, *11*, 341–354.

Woodhouse, W., Bailey, A., Rutter, M., Bolton, P., Baird, G., & Le Couteur, A. (1996). Head circumference in autism and other pervasive developmental disorders. *Journal of Child Psychology & Psychiatry*, *37*, 785–801.

World Health Organization. (1996). *Multiaxial classification of child and adolescent psychiatric disorders: The ICD-10 Classification of mental and behavioural disorders in children and adolescents.* Cambridge, UK: Cambridge University Press.

Young, R. McD., Lawford, B. R., Nutting, A., & Noble, E. P. (2004). Advances in molecular genetics and the prevention and treatment of substance misuse: Implications of association studies of the A_1 allele of the D_2 dopamine receptor gene. *Addictive Behaviors*, *29*, 1275–1294.

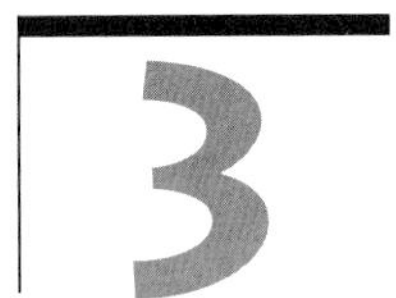

Neurodevelopmental Disorders: Conceptual Issues

Dorothy Bishop and Michael Rutter

From the beginnings of psychiatric classifications, there have been attempts to establish broad overarching groups (see chapter 2). Thus, for many years, mental disorders tended to be put into the two broad categories of "organic" and "functional" disorders. The rationale was that, with respect to causation, the disorders within each group had more in common with other disorders in the same group than with those in the alternative group. The implication was that it might be useful for research into causal processes to determine commonalities within these broad groups, rather than to assume that each diagnostic category would have a unique cause not shared by all other conditions.

One such broad grouping was the notion of "minimal brain dysfunction" (MBD), which was popular in the 1960s and 1970s (Wender, 1971). The concept has been discredited (Rutter, 1982) and is no longer in general use. The crucial flaws were that particular behaviors could not be used to infer brain pathology, and that organic brain dysfunction did not lead to a homogenous psychopathological pattern. In addition, it seemed to presuppose that all types of brain dysfunction would have similar consequences. It is clear that that is not so. The problem with this broad grouping is that it arose from a theoretical notion for which there was no good empirical support. The question that we consider in this chapter is whether the concept of neurodevelopmental disorders fares any better as a guide to the future. Our focus here is on conceptual issues in the characterization and classification of disorders, rather than on aspects of clinical management, which are dealt with in the chapters on individual disorders.

What Do We Mean by Neurodevelopmental Disorders?

Over the last two decades or so, there has been increasing use of this concept. However, there are at least four rather different ways in which the term has been used. The narrowest concept is provided by the second axis of the ICD-10 classification (World Health Organization, 1996), dealing with Specific Disorders of Psychological Development. They were placed on a separate axis because they differed from the general run of psychopathological conditions in three key respects:

1 An onset that is invariably during infancy or childhood;

2 An impairment or delay in the development of functions that are strongly related to biological maturation of the central nervous system; and

3 A steady course that does not involve the remissions and relapses that tend to be characteristic of many mental disorders.

The overall description of this group of disorders noted that there is impairment in some aspect of mental development, but the impairment tends to lessen as the children grow older; despite this, deficits tend to continue into adult life; most of the conditions are more common in males than females; and a family history of similar or related disorders is common, suggesting that genetic factors have an important role in the etiology. The subclassification within this axis comprised disorders involving language development, scholastic skills or motor function. DSM-IV (American Psychiatric Association, 2000) has a broadly comparable subclassification but the disorders are not placed on a separate axis and the overall conceptualization for grouping is not expressed so explicitly.

An alternative usage extends the term "neurodevelopmental disorders" much more broadly to include single-gene disorders such as Williams syndrome or Prader–Willi syndrome (Tager-Flusberg, 1999) or disorders deriving from prenatal insults or toxins, such as fetal alcohol syndrome (Harris, 1995). These conditions develop on the basis of neural impairment, involve cognitive deficits of various kinds, and, as with the specific disorders of psychological development, are characterized by a steady course without remissions or relapses. However, whereas the Axis 2 ICD-10 disorders are defined in terms of a profile of specific impairment of linguistic, scholastic or motor skills, these disorders are defined in terms of etiology. Although it can sometimes be fruitful to compare the deficits associated with a particular known etiology and those in a specific developmental disorder, it is potentially confusing to classify these different types of disorder together, and in this chapter we restrict consideration to those disorders with a putative multifactorial etiology. For similar reasons, we would argue against adopting a definition that includes intellectual disability, cerebral palsy, traumatic brain injury and epilepsy under the rubric of neurodevelopmental psychiatric disorders.

Rutter's Child and Adolescent Psychiatry, 5th edition. Edited by M. Rutter, D. Bishop, D. Pine, S. Scott, J. Stevenson, E. Taylor and A. Thapar. © 2008 Blackwell Publishing, ISBN: 978-1-4051-4549-7.

There are two more modest ways in which the concept of neurodevelopmental disorder can be broadened beyond specific disorders of psychological development. First, many people include both autism spectrum disorders (ASD) and attention deficit/hyperactivity disorders (ADHD) in the overall grouping of neurodevelopmental disorders. At first sight, it might be objected that there are several ways in which both of these are rather different. Thus, neither reflects a straightforward impairment in a development-based skill that is closely related to biological maturation. Also, both involve deviant functioning (i.e., that which is not normal at any age) as much as impaired functioning (i.e., that which is normal in form but impaired in level). Nevertheless, the reason why they have come to be grouped with neurodevelopmental disorders is that they share with the other disorders the facts that they are multifactorial in origin; are present from early life; tend to improve with increasing age but are also associated with disordered functioning that extends right into adult life; they involve a strong genetic influence; and both show a marked male preponderance. Furthermore, they are characterized by neuropsychological impairments, in aspects of executive function in ADHD (see chapter 34), and in social cognition, central coherence and executive function in ASD (see chapter 46). Strikingly, epidemiological and clinical studies have shown that these two disorders often co-occur with the ICD-10 Axis 2 disorders of psychological development, and genetic findings have similarly begun to point to a possible shared genetic liability (as well as a liability that is more syndrome specific). In addition, although autism may be associated with other forms of psychopathology that do show remission and relapses (Hutton, Goode, Murphy *et al.*, in press) the basic disorder is persistent rather than recurrent. Much the same applies to ADHD (see chapter 34).

A further possible broadening of the concept of neurodevelopmental disorders brings in life-course-persistent antisocial behavior (Moffitt, 1993) and schizophrenia (Rapoport, Addington, & Frangou, 2005). At one time, both of these would have been regarded as acquired disorders but there is now an abundance of evidence that schizophrenia is often associated with impairments in the development of both language and motor function and with cognitive impairments that precede the development of overt schizophrenia (see chapter 45). Similarly, unlike adolescence-limited antisocial behavior, the life-course-persistent variety of antisocial behavior begins in the preschool years and is associated with hyperactivity and impairments in information processing and social cognition (see chapter 35). For the purposes of this chapter we have not included either of these disorders under the rubric of neurodevelopmental disorders for two main reasons. First, both antisocial behavior and schizophrenia do show fluctuations in their manifestations that are more akin to the remissions and relapses associated with the broad run of mental disorders than with the relatively steady state of the specific disorders of psychological functions. Second, there is not the same evidence of a shared genetic liability. For these reasons, we prefer to conceptualize these as disorders that have their origins in a neurodevelopmental abnormality rather than as a neurodevelopmental disorder as such, and confine the term neurodevelopmental to those disorders traditionally regarded as specific developmental disorders, plus ASD and ADHD.

Are the Neurodevelopmental Disorders Distinct Conditions?

Both traditional medical, and traditional psychological, approaches have tended to operate with discrete diagnostic categories. Thus, reading disability continues to be conceptualized as "developmental dyslexia," with the implication that it is a discrete neurological condition (Démonet, Taylor, & Chaix, 2004). For many years, specific language impairment was termed developmental dysphasia (Zangwill, 1978) with the same kind of implication. This terminology has now gone out of fashion because of the recognition that impairments in language development differ in important ways from acquired disorders of language. In psychiatric classifications, both ASD and ADHD are treated as if they are conditions that are entirely separate from other disorders of psychological development. In line with this conceptualization, cognitive psychologists have looked for a single specific underlying deficit that is responsible for each disorder, the nature of the deficit differing for each one (Morton & Frith, 1995).

There are two main reasons for challenging this view of neurodevelopmental disorders as a set of independent conditions. First, there is substantial co-occurrence among them. Second, both etiological and psychological studies indicate that multiple deficit models are more consistent with the multifactorial and probabilistic etiology of such disorders (Pennington, 2006), and that significant developmental impairment may arise only when there is more than one risk factor present (Bishop, 2006). As in internal medicine, the same pathological endpoint can arise through multiple, rather different, causal pathways (cf. Rutter, 1997). In the following sections, we present evidence to support the case that rather than looking for *the* cause of each type of neurodevelopmental disorder, we need to take account of the commonalities among them, and develop more complex models that can explain the patterns of association and dissociation among deficits.

Commonalities Among Developmental Disorders

Research findings across the whole of psychopathology, both in childhood and adult life, have been consistent in showing the high frequency with which individuals have multiple, supposedly separate, disorders (Angold, Costello, & Erkanli, 1999; Caron & Rutter, 1991). This is strikingly apparent for the neurodevelopmental disorders – indeed, it has been argued that a pure disorder is the exception rather than the rule (Gilger & Kaplan, 2001; Kaplan, Dewey, Crawford *et al.*, 2001) – and is reflected in the ICD-10 category of mixed developmental disorders. Thus, there is considerable overlap between specific reading disability (SRD) and specific language impairment (SLI) (Bishop & Snowling, 2004; Eisenmajer, Ross, & Pratt, 2005), between SRD and ADHD (Dykman & Ackerman, 1991; Willcutt & Pennington, 2000) and between SLI and ADHD (Beitchman, Brownlie, Inglis *et al.*, 1996). Less work has been carried out on developmental coordination disorders (DCD), but there is evidence for an overlap between motor impairment and both SLI (Hill, 2001) and ADHD (Kadesjö & Gillberg, 1998). As far as autistic disorder is concerned, the defining criteria disallow a diagnosis of SLI in a child meeting criteria for autistic disorder, but it is clear that at the symptomatic level there is considerable overlap, with many affected children showing the kinds of structural language deficits that characterize SLI (Tager-Flusberg & Joseph, 2003). Furthermore, many children with SLI or ADHD show in milder form the kinds of social/pragmatic impairments that are characteristic of autistic disorder (Bishop & Norbury, 2002; Clark, Feehan, Tinline *et al.*, 1999; Farmer, 2000; Geurts, Verté, Oosterlaan *et al.*, 2004). SRD co-occurs with mathematical difficulties at a higher level than predicted from the prevalence of either disorder on its own (Lewis, Hitch, & Walker, 1994).

It has become accepted to refer to these patterns of co-occurrence as "comorbidity," but this is misleading because it ignores the possibility that much of the supposed comorbidity is simply a function of the invalid, and artificial, diagnostic subdivisions in classification systems (see chapter 2). Thus, for example, it seems likely that much of the co-occurrence of supposedly different anxiety disorders is simply a consequence of these disorders being slightly different manifestations of the same underlying condition (see chapter 39). Might the same apply to neurodevelopmental disorders? Clearly it could.

Thus, SLI and reading disability both comprise disorders of language – the former with respect to spoken language and the latter with respect to written language. It would be rather surprising if there was no co-occurrence between the two. That is not to argue that all cases of reading disability derive from oral language impairment, because manifestly they do not (Bishop & Snowling, 2004); but it is to suggest that co-occurrence to some degree is to be expected.

However, the co-occurrence of neurodevelopmental disorders does not apply only to language-related disorders; as noted above, there are also overlaps between language and motor impairments, attention deficit and social deficits, and these cannot readily be explained as different manifestations of a common cognitive disability. To some extent, overlaps could reflect referral bias in clinical samples: for instance, a child whose reading or language disability is accompanied by social impairment or attentional deficit would be more likely to be referred to a psychiatrist than one who had an isolated impairment. However, this cannot be the whole explanation, because overlaps are seen in epidemiological samples (e.g., Beitchman *et al.*, 1996), and second, the rates of co-occurrence are higher than would be predicted from knowledge of the frequency of individual disorders.

A "Syndrome" of Neurodevelopmental Disorder?

One might start to wonder if, rather than differentiating between neurodevelopmental disorders, it would make more sense to group them all together into an overarching category, treating them as variant forms of a common underlying disorder. However, there are sufficient differences among the neurodevelopmental disorders to preclude such a conceptualization. First, molecular genetic studies have been successful in identifying chromosomal regions associated with risk for reading disability, SLI, ADHD and ASD, but there has been little or no overlap between the linkages reported for these different disorders. For instance, Fisher (2006) noted that whereas linkages to dyslexia have been found on chromosomes 1, 2, 3, 6, 15 and 18, those to SLI have been found on chromosomes 13, 16 and 19. Fisher pointed out that we need to be careful in interpreting such findings: it would be dangerous to assume that there are highly specific pathways from genotype to phenotype, especially because few studies have used multivariate methods to look at more than one disorder at a time. Undoubtedly there are some genes whose effects are common to more than one neurodevelopmental disorder (e.g., Willcutt, Pennington, Smith *et al.*, 2002), but behavior genetic studies also usually find evidence for specific as well as common genetic influences on co-occurring disorders (e.g., Martin, Piek, & Hay, 2006). Second, there are differences among disorders in drug response. It is striking, for example, that whereas ADHD shows a marked beneficial response to stimulant medication (see chapter 34), no drugs have other than a slight inconsistent effect on the basic problems associated with ASD (see chapter 46). Similarly, although medication may provide some symptomatic improvement with the other neurodevelopmental disorders, there are not the marked benefits that are seen with ADHD. Third, although it is difficult to compare across imaging studies because of variations in the ways in which they have been conducted (Peterson, 2003), patterns in the various neurodevelopmental disorders do not seem at all closely similar: for instance, fronto-striatal systems are implicated in ADHD (see chapter 34), whereas in dyslexia there is reduced activation in left temporo-parietal cortex (see chapter 48). Fourth, at a behavioral level, there are differences among neurodevelopmental disorders in short and long-term course (Rutter, Kim-Cohen, & Maughan, 2006a). Finally, although most neurodevelopmental disorders are characterized by a preponderance of males, sex ratios vary across disorders, with the male excess being far more striking for ASD than for other neurodevelopmental disorders (Rutter, Caspi, & Moffitt, 2003). Arithmetical difficulties stand out from the rest, with boys and girls equally likely to be affected (Lewis *et al.*, 1994; Rourke, 1989; Shalev, Auerbach, Manor *et al.*, 2000).

Clearly, it is not feasible to treat the whole gamut of neurodevelopmental disorders as a single condition, but can we nevertheless identify distinct syndromes within this category, in which a pattern of deficits arises from a common neurobiological cause? Rourke's (1989) account of "non-verbal learning disability" (NLD) is such a model: a distinctive pattern of strengths and weaknesses in sensorimotor skill, scholastic achievement, and socioemotional development are seen as all originating from destruction or dysfunction of white matter in the right cerebral hemisphere. The deficits seen as characterizing NLD encompass specific arithmetical disorder, DCD and Asperger syndrome. The construct of NLD explains the co-occurrence of these deficits in terms of a specific neurobiological basis. However, the validity of the category is questionable. The different deficits certainly can and do co-occur, and the association of the symptomatology of Asperger syndrome with the neuropsychological manifestations of NLD has been empirically demonstrated (Klin, Volkmar, Sparrow *et al.*, 1995). However, the association appears too weak to justify treating it as a syndrome: this is demonstrated in studies showing that a high proportion of children with a clinical picture of NLD do not show specific deficits thought to characterize this disorder (Drummond, Ahmad, & Rourke, 2005; Pelletier, Ahmad, & Rourke, 2001). If we embrace the construct of NLD, we end up by excluding numerous cases because they do not show the anticipated combination of deficits, meaning that either we have to dilute the "syndrome" to be too general to be useful, or we have to devise additional categories to encompass the cases that do not fit. Similar problems arise if we try to fit language, literacy and speech disorders into a broader syndrome; we can find many children who show this constellation of impairments, but there are also many who do not (Bishop & Snowling, 2004; Pennington, 2006).

Neurodevelopmental disorders thus pose a considerable challenge for a classification system. On the one hand, we need to explain why there is common co-occurrence of different deficits, while at the same time allowing for dissociations between different types of deficit, and variable patterns of associated features. The causal model shown in Fig. 3.1 provides a framework for conceptualizing these questions. In this model, first put forward in the context of SLI and dyslexia, a neurodevelopmental disorder is identified on the basis of a constellation of behaviors; these result from specific cognitive deficits, which have particular neurobiological bases, which are in turn affected by genetic or environmental factors. When extending the model to cover the whole gamut of neurodevelopmental disorder, the "cognitive" level is taken to include a wide range of underlying mental operations that cannot be directly observed, but are inferred from behavior, including perceptual-motor skills, language, memory, social cognition, reasoning and executive functions. Relationships among the different levels of functioning are not one-to-one, but involve complex multifactorial influences going from etiology to neurobiology, from neurobiology to cognition, and from cognition to behavior. Viewed from this perspective, it is clear that overlaps between observed behavioral impairments may arise from shared cognitive deficits, shared neurobiological origins and/or shared etiology. We now turn to consider evidence for these different causal mechanisms.

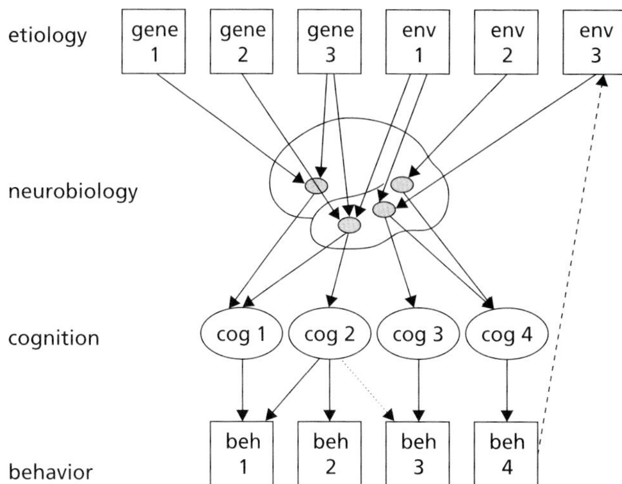

Fig. 3.1 Levels of causation for developmental disorders. The dashed line emphasizes that children's behavior (beh) can affect the environment (env) they experience. [From Bishop, D. V. M., & Snowling, M. J. (2004). Developmental dyslexia and specific language impairment: Same or different? *Psychological Bulletin*, *130*, 858–886 with permission.]

Causal Models of Neurodevelopmental Disorders

Cognitive Deficits

One goal of developmental neuropsychology is to uncover the underlying nature of deficits seen in neurodevelopmental disorders. As shown in Fig. 3.1, the same behavioral deficit may arise for different reasons, and one would hope that as our conceptual understanding advances, we might be able to categorize disorders not in terms of surface behavior, but in terms of underlying cognitive deficits. For instance, most children with reading disability have difficulties with phonological analysis which are evident even when they are tested using methods that do not require any reading or writing (see chapter 48). Other poor readers have visual difficulties, problems learning specific spellings of irregular words or poor comprehension of written texts. A focus on underlying cognitive deficits thus could help identify new subgroups. It also suggests that some of the existing distinctions among disorders may be unrealistic; for instance, increasingly speech, language and literacy problems are regarded as different manifestations of a common phonological impairment, whose behavioral correlates would vary depending on the age at which the child was observed and the severity of the impairment (Bishop & Snowling, 2004). Nevertheless, if we try to categorize disorders in terms of underlying deficit rather than observed behavior, this does not necessarily simplify our nosology, because multiple deficits are the rule rather than the exception, at the cognitive as well as the behavioral level. Thus, although one can identify children who fit the picture of "phonological dyslexia" or "surface dyslexia," most poor readers present a mixed picture (Snowling & Nation, 1997).

Even if one looks at impairments in very different domains, associated disorders are common.

Pennington (2006) conducted a series of studies comparing children with pure dyslexia, pure ADHD, and comorbid dyslexia and ADHD. He was interested in the possibility that comorbidity among these disorders might reflect the influence of one behavior on another (e.g., attentional difficulties might arise because the child who could not read well became bored and distractible; or conversely, the child's difficulty in attending could lead to scholastic deficits). If the first account were true, then the comorbid children should resemble the pure dyslexic cases in terms of underlying impairment. If the second account applied, then the comorbid children should resemble the pure ADHD cases. In fact, the pure dyslexia group had phonological deficits, the ADHD group had inhibition deficits, but the comorbid group had evidence of both phonological *and* inhibition deficits. These results are consistent with conventional wisdom that links dyslexia to poor phonology and ADHD to weak inhibition, but it leaves unexplained the co-occurrence of these two impairments.

We can summarize by saying that it was hoped that, by studying underlying impairments, we would obtain clearer distinctions between disorders and find that apparent comorbidity was a consequence of poor specification of disorders. In fact, studies such as this show that comorbidity is just as apparent at the level of cognitive impairment as it was at the level of observed behavior. This suggests that we need to seek an explanation for the associations among neurodevelopmental disorders at a different causal level.

Neurobiological Bases

Neuropsychological studies of adults highlight how fairly specific impairments in functions such as language, reading, arithmetic or motor programming can arise as a consequence of a focal brain lesion (McCarthy & Warrington, 1990). When one sees analogous impairments in children, it is tempting to assume a similar etiology via underlying brain damage, with the precise pattern of observed impairment depending on the extent, location and severity of the damage. This kind of model was put forward in the 1950s by Pasamanick and colleagues, who proposed a "continuum of reproductive casualty," suggesting that whereas major neurological insult resulting from birth trauma, intracranial hemorrhage or anoxia can lead to clear signs of neurological damage such as cerebral palsy or epilepsy, milder damage may lead to more subtle learning difficulties. However, this conceptualization of the etiology of neurodevelopmental disorders has not received much empirical support. There is good evidence that such damage often gives rise to behavioral and cognitive sequelae (Pasamanick & Knobloch, 1966), but the suggestion that neurodevelopmental disorders often arise from damage during the obstetric process has not proved to be the case. Nichols and Chen (1980) found only weak associations among neurological soft signs, hyperactivity and learning disorders, and even weaker associations between these variables and perinatal complications.

Furthermore, the notion that "birth injury" was the main risk factor fell into disrepute in view of the evidence that many of the risks supposedly associated with obstetric complications actually derived from prenatal problems. A genetically abnormal fetus is more likely to have a low birth weight and to be born following premature gestation. That probably accounts for the somewhat inconsistent association between obstetric complications and ASD (Bolton, Murphy, Macdonald *et al.*, 1997). Undoubtedly, extremely low birth weight does lead to an increased rate of motor, language, scholastic and attentional difficulties (Marlow, 2004; Marlow, Wolke, Bracewell *et al.*, 2005). However, the association is not strong when assessed in the opposite direction (i.e., by starting with children with neurodevelopmental disorders and studying their perinatal history). With the possible exception of developmental co-ordination disorder (for review see Cermak, Gubbay, & Larkin, 2002), obstetric complications do not have a particularly important association with any of the neurodevelopmental disorders. It is family history that provides the key differentiator.

The Concept of Maturational Lag

Given that neurodevelopmental disorders are, on the one hand, familial, and on the other hand, not caused by acquired brain lesions, we need to seek another causal mechanism at the neurobiological level. There is often an implicit assumption that genetic or other prenatal influences have led to some failure of neurodevelopment that leads to abnormality that is functionally equivalent to a focal brain lesion – hence the analogous syndromes seen in neurodevelopmental disorders and adult acquired disorders (Temple, 1997). According to this view, the brain of a child with a neurodevelopmental disorder has an underlying abnormality that persists through childhood. An alternative possibility is that these disorders are no more than an extreme of the normal variation in the timing of development. We know that there are huge differences in the timing of puberty in both males and females, and marked differences, too, in the timing of the eruption of teeth. In similar fashion, there is marked individual variation in the timing of speech acquisition. When such a delay is followed by later normal functioning it may be regarded as a maturational lag of some kind. The implication is that the problem involves a normal variation in the development of certain brain systems responsible for cognitive functioning, rather than in some abnormal *difference* in brain systems, and that there can be a highly selective delay in the maturation of just one brain system. Associations between neurodevelopmental disorders would then arise in cases where the maturational lag extended to encompass several brain regions, or where there is pluripotentiality (i.e., a given brain structure is involved in a range of cognitive functions; Noppeney, Friston, & Price, 2004).

A key prediction from the "lag" hypothesis is that not only should the pattern of functioning resemble that of a normal younger child but also, as children with a neurodevelopmental disorder get older, the main difference from normal functioning should be found for later-maturing functions and not for early-maturing functions (Bishop & Edmundson,

1987; Bishop & McArthur, 2004, 2005). The limited available evidence is in keeping with that expectation and runs against the outmoded static lesion notion. However, for most neurodevelopmental disorders, although there is a general tendency for gains in function with increasing age, delayed early development is *not* followed by later normal functioning (Rutter, Kim-Cohen, & Maughan, 2006a). Can a maturational lag account have any explanatory value in such cases?

Two main possible explanations, both speculative, have been proposed for why children with a neurodevelopmental disorder do not ultimately catch up. First, the persistence could derive from what Stanovich (1986) termed a "Matthew effect," whereby the poor (poor readers) get poorer (make slow progress), while the rich (good readers) get richer (make good progress) as a result of literacy experience boosting further language and literacy development. Furthermore, a poor reader may lack the necessary experiences later (i.e., reading is not usually taught in secondary schools, and such books as are available are likely to be too advanced to be intelligible). There could also be more indirect effects whereby early impairments create a negative spiral affecting other skills (e.g., the effects on intimate social relationships of communication difficulties in early childhood). Because of the importance of experiences in the development of psychological functions, there is little doubt that something of this kind could have a contributory role. What is much less certain is whether it could account for the severe problems in intimate social relationships in adult life found for many individuals with a severe receptive SLI in adult life reported by Clegg, Hollis, Mawhood *et al.* (2005) – because the relationship deficits were not a function of the severity of the earlier language deficits (at least in terms of those measured), and because the nature of the deficits appeared so different from those usually associated with social rejection. It is also noteworthy that persistence of disorder is often seen in young people with SLI who have been enrolled in special education throughout the secondary as well as primary school years (Conti-Ramsden, Botting, Simkin *et al.*, 2001; Haynes & Naidoo, 1991). Perhaps the key empirical finding is provided by Francis, Shaywitz, Stuebing *et al.*'s (1996) individual growth curves comparison of 69 children with a reading disability and 334 children with no reading problem. Nine yearly longitudinal assessments showed that *both* groups tended to plateau at about 13 years of age, with no narrowing or expansion of the gap between the groups. They differed in level but not in trajectory. The finding rather runs counter to the Stanovich (1986) proposition.

A second kind of explanation for persistence of disorder was proposed in the context of language and literacy deficits by Wright and Zecker (2004). They invoked a decline in neuroplasticity as a limiting factor, and suggested that neurobiological events at age 10 years associated with the onset of puberty halted auditory development at whatever level it has reached, so that the adolescent was left with a lasting residue of deficit. This viewpoint is consistent with evidence that there are sensitive periods for aspects of language acquisition, so that it is difficult to become fully competent in the phonology and syntax of a second language acquired after puberty (Mayberry & Lock, 2003; Oyama, 1976). However, critical periods for auditory development have not been demonstrated, and there is electrophysiological evidence that development of the auditory system (Albrecht, von Suchodoletz, & Uwer, 2000) as well as of some other cortical systems continues right up into adulthood (see chapter 12). Longitudinal studies using magnetic resonance imaging (MRI) have confirmed that brain development continues well after the onset of puberty, with higher-order association areas maturing only after lower-order somatosensory and visual areas (Gogtay, Giedd, Lusk *et al.*, 2004; see also chapter 12), and that such changes – especially in the frontal cortex – are associated with intellectual functions (Shaw, Greenstein, Lerch *et al.*, 2006a). There is considerable variation from one cortical region to another, with some showing radical changes at puberty and others unaffected (Nelson, Bloom, Cameron *et al.*, 2002). Clearly, further research is required in order to provide an understanding of both brain development (and its functional consequences) in typically developing individuals and in those with neurodevelopmental disorders. As the evidence currently stands, the postulate that the relevant brain systems lose plasticity around the time of puberty remains highly speculative, and to test it we would need studies that compare the impact of training on brain and behavior in pre- and postpubertal individuals. The trajectory findings of Francis *et al.* (1996) are compatible with the suggestion of a change in brain plasticity in adolescence but they provide no direct support.

We may sum up by concluding that there is little hard evidence in support of a maturational lag account. We need more longitudinal and neurobiological studies to evaluate this idea. In its favor, this kind of explanation has the potential to highlight parallels between causal mechanisms in normal and impaired development, and to account for changing profiles seen in neurodevelopmental disorders. It provides the impetus for studies that track neurodevelopment over time: for instance, Shaw, Lerch, Greenstein *et al.* (2006b) documented changes in cortical thickness over time in children with ADHD, with evidence of normalization in children who had a good outcome. However, a maturational account seems more plausible as an explanation for transient delays early in development than for severe and persistent neurodevelopmental disorders.

A final point to note is that it is important not to confuse the hypothesis of a developmental delay with the entirely different hypothesis that the causation of disorders of psychological development, together with ASD and ADHD (as well as numerous forms of other psychopathology), are based on dimensional genetic and environmental risk factors (Rutter, Moffitt, & Caspi, 2006b). With multifactorial disorders, dimensional liability is the rule rather than the exception. The question of whether or not the dimensional risks are the same ones that apply within the normal distribution is a separate issue and it is one that has been very little investigated up to now, although there has been some relevant research in relation to ADHD (see chapters 23 and 34).

The Neuroconstructivist Approach

The "maturational lag" account is not the only alternative to a "static lesion" model of neurodevelopmental disorders. We have become increasingly aware that the brain changes in the course of development, restructuring itself to form new neural systems, both in response to interactions between functional neuronal networks and in response to environmental input (see chapter 12). Karmiloff-Smith (1998) argued that one needs to take such evidence into account when devising explanations for neurodevelopmental disorders, and that an apparently specific deficit in a child may be the endpoint of a process that started with a relatively non-specific disruption to brain development. This "neuroconstructivist" approach emphasizes interactions between different neural systems, and to that extent would predict the existence of disorders affecting more than one domain of functioning. However, this theoretical perspective is still very young; its main contribution to date has been to question the simple parallels that are sometimes drawn between developmental and acquired disorders, and to emphasize the need to put development center stage. In order to make more specific predictions about neurodevelopmental disorders and their co-occurrence, we need to develop specific computational models of normal development, which then allow us to identify which perturbations could result in a particular profile of deficit (Thomas & Karmiloff-Smith, 2003).

Etiological Influences

For those conditions where genetically informative designs have been applied (SRD, SLI, ADHD, ASD), there is evidence of substantial genetic influences on the liability to disorder (see chapter 23). With respect to neurodevelopmental disorders (together with other multifactorial disorders), these probably usually reflect the actions of normal variants of multiple genes of small effect operating together with multiple environmental influences (Gilger & Kaplan, 2001; Rutter, Moffitt, & Caspi *et al.*, 2006b) rather than the determinative effect of major mutant genes. This view of etiology is reflected in the causal model in Fig. 3.1, in that there is no one-to-one relationship between genes and neurobiology. Rather, a specific neurological system is likely to be influenced by a range of etiological influences and the given etiology will impact on a range of brain regions. Such a model allows for both co-occurrence of deficits and the existence of pure disorder. Particular patterns of variation may reflect the influence of either specific combinations of genetic or environmental factors, or the operation of chance influences (Wolf, 1997).

This raises the question of whether patterns of co-occurrence between disorders indicate a shared liability. Klein and Riso (1993) noted that evidence for overlapping etiology of disorders can be found by looking at the familiality of disorders in pure and comorbid cases. In essence, they note that if shared etiology is implicated in causing disorders A and B, then we should see an increased risk for disorder B (with or without A) in relatives of a person with disorder A, and vice versa. Furthermore, relatives of comorbid cases should show increased risk for the single disorders A and B, as well as for the A + B combination. Note that these predictions are not made by other models of comorbidity: for instance, if the A + B combination represented a separate subtype of disorder with distinct causes, then it should "breed true," and there should be no increase in rates of disorder A in relatives of those with disorder B (or vice versa). Furthermore, the predictions hold up for any disorder that shows familiality, regardless of whether genes or shared environmental factors are more important.

If the disorders are significantly heritable, it is possible to go further using either quantitative genetic methodologies (such as twin studies) or molecular genetic studies (focusing on individual identified genes) to determine how far there is a shared genetic influence between the two disorders. Few researchers to date have adopted this approach; an exception is Pennington (2006), who studied comorbidity of SRD and ADHD in a twin sample and concluded that there was evidence for shared genetic influence on the two disorders. In a similar vein, Bishop (2002) found evidence for overlapping genetic influences on language impairment and motor immaturity in a sample selected for SLI. Molecular genetic findings also suggest that susceptibility extends beyond traditional diagnostic boundaries (Rutter, Moffitt, & Caspi, 2006b).

Research Implications of the Neurodevelopmental Disorder Concept

Probably the single most crucial research implication is that investigators need to consider the possibility that the causal influences on key features may extend across the range of neurodevelopmental disorders, rather than being specific to just one. Thus, it is striking that, with the exception of arithmetical difficulties, all the neurodevelopmental disorders show a marked male preponderance (Rutter, Caspi, Fergusson *et al.*, 2004). That stands in marked contrast to the finding that disorders with a marked female preponderance all concern syndromes typically beginning in adolescence and that involve emotional disturbance, rather than neurodevelopmental impairment, as the key feature. Baron-Cohen and Hammer (1997) have hypothesized that ASDs represent an "extreme male brain." There is a lack of good supporting evidence but, in addition, it is necessary to ask whether that same explanation should be held to apply to ADHD or SRD or SLI. It does not seem particularly likely that the causes of the male preponderance are entirely different in the case of each of the syndromes, although there may be syndrome-specific factors as part of the explanation.

A further question for research is whether studies should continue to be focused on "pure" disorders given that they do not appear to be at all typical. The answer will depend on the question that is being asked. Pure groups can be useful in identifying correlates of a specific kind of deficit without additional confounds. For instance, suppose one wants to test the hypothesis that reading disability is caused by a low-level auditory perceptual deficit. The goal is to compare a group of children with SRD and a control group on a task in which they have to listen for small differences between sounds, and make a manual response to indicate what they have heard. If the sample includes children who have substantial difficulties with language comprehension, motor dexterity or attentional control, then it may be hard to disentangle the influence of these impairments on task performance. Careful sample selection to exclude such cases may give cleaner results. Having said that, it is worth noting that those who claim to study pure cases may be including large numbers of children with additional deficits which are missed because they are not assessed. For instance, many studies of SRD fail to assess children's language or attentional skills. If a sufficiently detailed assessment battery is used, covering the whole range of neurodevelopmental disorders, the numbers of pure cases available for study may become vanishingly small. If so, it may be better to assess associated deficits, so that one can establish how far they are associated with the dependent variable of interest, rather than try to control for their effects by exclusion of comorbid cases (cf. Breier, Gray, Fletcher *et al.*, 2001).

In many research contexts, focus on pure groups is not just hard to achieve, it can be seriously misguided. In etiological studies, restricting the phenotype to those with a pure disorder may be misleading, if risk factors in fact operate across a range of neurodevelopmental disorders. As noted above, inclusion of comorbid cases can provide a rich source of evidence about the reasons for co-occurrence of disorders, both when studying underlying impairments and when the focus is on etiology. Another instance where it may be unhelpful to restrict attention to pure cases is when conducting research on intervention. For instance, a remedial package that is effective for children with a pure reading disability may not work well if there is co-occurring ADHD. Given the common overlap between disorders, we need more research that considers how the presence of a comorbid disorder affects treatment outcome, rather than simply ignoring or excluding such cases.

Implications for Clinical Practice

Perhaps the most important point to stress is the need for clinicians to be aware of the complexity of neurodevelopmental disorders. Multidisciplinary assessment is key for identifying each child's pattern of strengths and weaknesses. We are aware of cases where a child has received a diagnosis of SLI from a speech and language therapist, dyslexia from an educational psychologist, ADHD from a pediatrician, ASD from a child psychiatrist and developmental dyspraxia from an occupational therapist! In part this may be because of the different perspectives and expertise brought to the assessment by different professionals, and in part by genuine changes in the clinical presentation over time. For instance, a child whose main problem in the preschool years is unintelligible speech may become intelligible but subsequently be diagnosed as having developmental dyslexia (Bishop & Snowling, 2004). Another child who initially seems to be a case of specific receptive language disorder may subsequently merit a diagnosis of ASD (Conti-Ramsden, Simkin, & Botting, 2006). Most parents will be thoroughly confused by such multiple diagnoses, and conclude that somebody has "got it wrong." It is essential that professionals work together to ensure that the child receives a diagnosis that provides access to the most appropriate services, while at the same time assessing the whole range of areas of function that may be impaired. Intervention will need to be individually tailored to take into account the child's specific strengths and weaknesses.

It is also important that both clinicians and parents recognize that diagnostic labels are shorthand descriptors that do two things: they summarize the child's major area of deficit; and they indicate that the problem is neither part of another syndrome nor attributable to a known organic etiology. All too often, those interpreting the labels assume they imply more than this, and treat terms such as "developmental dyslexia" and "developmental dyspraxia" as if they referred to syndromes with distinctive features and clear boundaries that are distinct from normality and have a known biological basis. In practice, these diagnoses are made on the basis of quantitative difference from normality. A statement such as "My child can't read because he's dyslexic" is not an explanation, rather it is a circular redescription of the problem. Furthermore, the use of a single diagnostic label can oversimplify the complex and multifaceted nature of many neurodevelopmental disorders.

References

Albrecht, R., von Suchodoletz, W., & Uwer, R. (2000). The development of auditory evoked dipole source activity from childhood to adulthood. *Clinical Neurophysiology*, *111*, 2268–2276.

American Psychiatric Association. (2000). *Diagnostic and statistical manual of mental disorders*, (4th ed.) Text revision. Washington, DC: American Psychiatric Association.

Angold, A., Costello, E. J., & Erkanli, A. (1999). Comorbidity. *Journal of Child Psychology and Psychiatry*, *40*, 57–87.

Baron-Cohen, S., & Hammer, J. (1997). Is autism an extreme form of the "male brain"? *Advances in Infancy Research*, *11*, 193–217.

Beitchman, J. H., Brownlie, E. B., Inglis, A., Wild, J., Ferguson, B., Schachter, D., *et al.* (1996). Seven-year follow-up of speech/language impaired and control children: psychiatric outcome. *Journal of Child Psychology and Psychiatry*, *37*, 961–970.

Bishop, D. V. M. (2002). Motor immaturity and specific speech and language impairment: Evidence for a common genetic basis. *American Journal of Medical Genetics: Neuropsychiatric Genetics*, *114*, 56–63.

Bishop, D. V. M. (2006). Developmental cognitive genetics: How psychology can inform genetics and vice versa. *Quarterly Journal of Experimental Psychology*, *59*, 1153–1168.

Bishop, D. V. M. & Edmundson, A. (1987). Specific language impairment as a maturational lag: evidence from longitudinal data on language and motor development. *Developmental Medicine and Child Neurology*, *29*, 442–459.

Bishop, D. V. M., & McArthur, G. M. (2004). Immature cortical responses to auditory stimuli in specific language impairment: evidence from ERPs to rapid tone sequences. *Developmental Science*, *7*, F11–F18.

Bishop, D. V. M., & McArthur, G. M. (2005). Individual differences in auditory processing in specific language impairment: A follow-up study using event-related potentials and behavioural thresholds. *Cortex*, *41*, 327–341.

Bishop, D. V. M., & Norbury, C. F. (2002). Exploring the borderlands of autistic disorder and specific language impairment: A study using standardised diagnostic instruments. *Journal of Child Psychology and Psychiatry*, *43*, 917–929.

Bishop, D. V. M., & Snowling, M. J. (2004). Developmental dyslexia and specific language impairment: Same or different? *Psychological Bulletin*, *130*, 858–886.

Bolton, P., Murphy, M., Macdonald, H., Whitlock, B., Pickles, A., & Rutter, M. (1997). Obstetric complications in autism: Consequences or causes of the condition? *Journal of the American Academy of Child and Adolescent Psychiatry*, *36*, 272–281.

Breier, J. I., Gray, L., Fletcher, J. M., Diehl, R. L., Klaas, P., Foorman, B. R., *et al.* (2001). Perception of voice and tone onset time continua in children with dyslexia with and without attention deficit/hyperactivity disorder. *Journal of Experimental Child Psychology*, *80*, 245–270.

Caron, C., & Rutter, M. (1991). Comorbidity in child psychopathology: concepts, issues and research strategies. *Journal of Child Psychology and Psychiatry*, *32*, 1063–1080.

Cermak, S. A., Gubbay, S. S., & Larkin, D. (2002). What is developmental coordination disorder? In S. A. Cermak & D. Larkin (Eds.), *Developmental coordination disorder* (pp. 2–22). Albany, NY: Delmar.

Clark, T., Feehan, C., Tinline, C., & Vostanis, P. (1999). Autistic symptoms in children with attention deficit-hyperactivity disorder. *European Child and Adolescent Psychiatry*, *8*, 50–55.

Clegg, J., Hollis, C., Mawhood, L., & Rutter, M. (2005). Developmental language disorder: A follow-up in later adult life. Cognitive, language, and psychosocial outcomes. *Journal of Child Psychology and Psychiatry*, *46*, 128–149.

Conti-Ramsden, G., Botting, N., Simkin, Z., & Knox E. (2001). Follow-up of children attending infant language units: outcomes at 11 years of age. *International Journal of Language Communication Disorders*, *36*, 207–219.

Conti-Ramsden, G., Simkin, Z., & Botting, N. (2006). The prevalence of autistic spectrum disorders in adolescents with a history of specific language impairment (SLI). *Journal of Child Psychology and Psychiatry*, *47*, 621–628.

Démonet, J., Taylor, M. J., & Chaix, Y. (2004). Developmental dyslexia. *Lancet*, *363*, 1451–1460.

Drummond, C. R., Ahmad, S. A., & Rourke, B. P. (2005). Rules for the classification of younger children with nonverbal learning disabilities and basic phonological processing disabilities. *Archives of Clinical Neuropsychology*, *20*, 171–182.

Dykman, R. A., & Ackerman, P. T. (1991). Attention deficit disorder and specific reading disability: Separate but often overlapping disorders. *Journal of Learning Disabilities*, *24*, 96–103.

Eisenmajer, R., Ross, N., & Pratt, C. (2005). Specificity and characteristics of learning disabilities. *Journal of Child Psychology and Psychiatry*, *46*, 1108–1115.

Farmer, M. (2000). Language and social cognition in children with specific language impairment. *Journal of Child Psychology and Psychiatry*, *41*, 627–636.

Fisher, S. E. (2006). Tangled webs: tracing the connections between genes and cognition. *Cognition*, *10*, 270–297.

Francis, D. J., Shaywitz, S. E., Stuebing, K. K., Shaywitz, B. A., & Fletcher, J. M. (1996). Developmental lag versus deficit models of reading disability: A longitudinal, individual growth curves analysis. *Journal of Educational Psychology*, *88*, 3–17.

Geurts, H. M., Verté, S., Oosterlaan, J., Roeyers, H., Hartman, C. A., Mulder, E. J., *et al.* (2004). Can the Children's Communication Checklist differentiate between children with autism, children with ADHD, and normal controls? *Journal of Child Psychology and Psychiatry*, *45*, 1437–1453.

Gilger, J. W., & Kaplan, B. J. (2001). A typical brain development: a conceptual framework for understanding developmental learning disabilities. *Developmental Neuropsychology*, *20*, 465–481.

Gogtay, N., Giedd, J. N., Lusk, L., Hayashi, K. M., Greenstein, D., Vaituzis, A. C., *et al.* (2004). Dynamic mapping of human cortical development during childhood through early adulthood. *Proceedings of the National Academy of Sciences*, *101*, 8174–8179.

Harris, J. C. (1995). *Developmental neuropsychiatry*. New York and Oxford: Oxford University Press.

Haynes, C., & Naidoo, S. (1991). *Children with specific speech and language impairment* (Clinics in Developmental Medicine: Vol. 119). London: MacKeith Press.

Hill, E. L. (2001). Non-specific nature of specific language impairment: a review of the literature with regard to concomitant motor impairments. *International Journal of Language and Communication Disorders*, *36*, 149–171.

Hutton, J., Goode, S., Murphy, M., Le Couteur, A., & Rutter, M. New onset psychiatric disorders in individuals with autism. *Autism* (in press).

Kadesjö, B., & Gillberg, C. (1998). Attention deficits and clumsiness in Swedish 7-year-old children. *Developmental Medicine and Child Neurology*, *40*, 796–811.

Kaplan, B. J., Dewey, D. M., Crawford, S. G., & Wilson, B. N. (2001). The term comorbidity is of questionable value in reference to developmental disorders: data and theory. *Journal of Learning Disabilities*, *34*, 555–565.

Karmiloff-Smith, A. (1998). Development itself is the key to understanding developmental disorders. *Trends in Cognitive Sciences*, *2*, 389–398.

Klein, D. N., & Riso, L. P. (1993). Psychiatric disorders: problems of boundaries and comorbidity. In C. G. Costello (Ed.), *Basic issues in psychopathology* (pp. 19–66). New York: Guilford Press.

Klin, A., Volkmar, F. R., Sparrow, S. S., Cicchetti, D. V., & Rourke, B. P. (1995). Validity and neuropsychological characterization of Asperger syndrome: Convergence with nonverbal learning disabilities syndrome. *Journal of Child Psychology and Psychiatry*, *36*, 1127–1140.

Lewis, C., Hitch, G. J., & Walker, P. (1994). The prevalence of specific arithmetic difficulties and specific reading difficulties in 9- to 10-year-old boys and girls. *Journal of Child Psychology and Psychiatry*, *35*, 283–292.

Marlow, N. (2004). Neurocognitive outcome after very preterm birth. *Archives of Disease in Childhood*, *89*, F224–F228.

Marlow, N., Wolke, D., Bracewell, M. A. & Samara, M., for the EPICure Study Group. (2005). Neurologic and developmental disability at six years of age after extremely preterm birth. *New England Journal of Medicine*, *352*, 9–19.

Martin, N., Piek, J. P., & Hay, D. (2006). DCD and ADHD: A genetic study of their shared aetiology. *Human Movement Science*, *25*, 110–124.

Mayberry, R. I., & Lock, E. (2003). Age constraints on first versus second language acquisition: Evidence for linguistic plasticity and epigenesis. *Brain and Language*, *87*, 369–384.

McCarthy, R., & Warrington, E. (1990). *Cognitive neuropsychology*. San Diego: Academic Press.

Moffitt, T. E. (1993). Adolescence-limited and life-course-persistent antisocial behavior: A developmental taxonomy. *Psychological Review*, *100*, 674–701.

Morton, J., & Frith, U. (1995). Causal modeling: A structural approach to developmental psychopathology. In D. Cicchetti & D. J. Cohen (Eds.), *Developmental Psychopathology* (Vol. 2, pp. 357–390). New York: Wiley.

Nelson, C. A., Bloom, F. E., Cameron, J. L., Amaral, D., Dahl, R. E., & Pine, D. (2002). An integrative, multidisciplinary approach to the study of brain–behavior relations in the context of typical and atypical development. *Development and Psychopathology*, *14*, 499–520.

Nichols P. L., & Chen T. C. (1980). *Minimal brain dysfunction: A prospective study*. Hillsdale, NJ: Lawrence Erlbaum Associates.

Noppeney, U., Friston, K. J., & Price, C. J. (2004). Degenerate neuronal systems sustaining cognitive functions. *Journal of Anatomy*, *205*, 433–442.

Oyama, S. (1976). A sensitive period for the acquisition of a nonnative phonological system. *Journal of Psycholinguistic Research*, *5*, 261–283.

Pasamanick, B., & Knobloch, H. (1966). Retrospective studies on the epidemiology of reproductive casualty: old and new. *Merrill Palmer Quarterly*, *12*, 7–26.

Pelletier, P. M., Ahmad, S. A., & Rourke, B. P. (2001). Classification rules for basic phonological processing disabilities and nonverbal learning disabilities: Formulation and external validity. *Child Neuropsychology (Neuropsychology, Development and Cognition: Section C)*, *7*, 84–98.

Pennington, B. (2006). From single to multiple deficit models of developmental disorders. *Cognition*, *101*, 385–413.

Peterson, B. S. (2003). Conceptual, methodological and statistical challenges in brain imaging studies of developmentally based psychopathologies. *Development and Psychopathology*, *15*, 811–832.

Rapoport, J. L., Addington, A. M., & Frangou, S. (2005). The neurodevelopmental model of schizophrenia: update. *Molecular Psychiatry*, *10*, 434–449.

Rourke, B. P. (1989). *Nonverbal learning disabilities: The syndrome and the model*. Guilford Press: New York.

Rutter, M. (1982). Syndromes attributed to "minimal brain dysfunction" in childhood. *American Journal of Psychiatry*, *139*, 21–33.

Rutter, M. (1997). Comorbidity: concepts, claims and choices. *Criminal Behaviour and Mental Health*, *7*, 265–286.

Rutter, M., Caspi, A., Fergusson, D., Horwood, L. J., Goodman, R., Maughan, B., *et al.* (2004). Sex differences in developmental reading disability: new findings from 4 epidemiological studies. *Journal of the American Medical Association*, *291*, 2007–2012.

Rutter, M., Caspi, A., & Moffitt, T. E. (2003). Using sex differences in psychopathology to study causal mechanisms: unifying issues and research strategies. *Journal of Child Psychology and Psychiatry*, *44*, 1092–1115.

Rutter, M., Kim-Cohen, J., & Maughan, B. (2006a). Continuities and discontinuities in psychopathology between childhood and adult life. *Journal of Child Psychology and Psychiatry*, *47*(3/4), 276–295.

Rutter, M., Moffitt, T. E., & Caspi, A. (2006b). Gene–environment interplay and psychopathology: multiple varieties but real effects. *Journal of Child Psychology and Psychiatry*, *47*, 226–261.

Shalev, R. S., Auerbach, J., Manor, O., & Gross-Tsur, V. (2000). Developmental dyscalculia: prevalence and prognosis. *European Child and Adolescent Psychiatry*, *9*(Supplement 2), 58–64.

Shaw, P., Greenstein, D., Lerch, J., Clasen, L., Lenroot, R., Gogtay, N., *et al.* (2006a). Intellectual ability and cortical development in children and adolescents. *Nature*, *440*(7084), 676–679.

Shaw, P., Lerch, J., Greenstein, D., Sharp, W., Clasen, L., Evans, A., *et al.* (2006b). Longitudinal mapping of cortical thickness and clinical outcome in children and adolescents with attention-deficit/hyperactivity disorder. *Archives of General Psychiatry*, *63*, 540–549.

Snowling, M., & Nation, K. (1997). Language, phonology and learning to read. In C. Hulme & M. Snowling (Eds.), *Dyslexia: biology, cognition and intervention* (pp. 153–166). London: Whurr Publishers.

Stanovich, K. E. (1986). Matthew effect in reading: some consequences of individual differences in the acquisition of literacy. *Reading Research Quarterly*, *21*, 360–407.

Tager-Flusberg, H. (1999). *Neurodevelopmental disorders*. Cambridge, MA: MIT Press.

Tager-Flusberg, H., & Joseph, R. M. (2003). Identifying neurocognitive phenotypes in autism. *Philosophical Transactions of the Royal Society of London, Series B*, *358*, 303–314.

Temple, C. (1997). Developmental cognitive neuropsychology. *Journal of Child Psychology and Psychiatry*, *38*, 27–52.

Thomas, M., & Karmiloff-Smith, A. (2003). Modeling language acquisition in atypical phenotypes. *Psychological Review*, *110*, 647–682.

Wender, P. (1971). *Minimal brain dysfunction in children*. New York, John Wiley & Sons.

Willcutt, E. G., & Pennington, B. F. (2000). Psychiatric comorbidity in children and adolescents with reading disability. *Journal of Child Psychology and Psychiatry*, *41*, 1039–1048.

Willcutt, E. G., Pennington, B. F., Smith, S. D., Cardon, L. R., Gayan, J., Knopik, V. S., *et al.* (2002). Quantitative trait locus for reading disability on chromosome 6p is pleiotropic for attention-deficit/hyperactivity disorder. *American Journal of Medical Genetics: Neuropsychiatric Genetics*, *114*, 260–268.

Wolf, U. (1997). Identical mutations and phenotypical variation. *Human Genetics*, *100*, 305–321.

World Health Organization. (1996). *Multi-axial classification of child and adolescent psychiatric disorders: The ICD-10 classification of mental and behavioral disorders in children and adolescents.* Cambridge: Cambridge University Press.

Wright, B. A., & Zecker, S. G. (2004). Learning problems, delayed development, and puberty. *Proceedings of the National Academy of Sciences*, *101*, 9942–9946.

Zangwill, O. L. (1978). The concept of developmental dysphasia. In M. A. Wyke (Ed.), *Developmental dysphasia*. London: Academic Press.

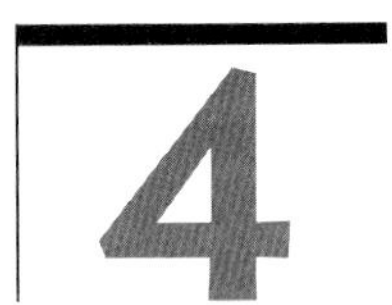

Clinical Assessment and Diagnostic Formulation

Michael Rutter and Eric Taylor

Initial Questions Regarding Referral

Clinical appointments are initiated by someone making a referral, usually with some form of focused question, although the extent to which this is made explicit varies. In the case of children, it would be rather unusual for the young people themselves to have initiated referral, but that may sometimes be the case. Although the clinician is likely to wish to organize the initial assessment around the question as to whether the child has a clinically significant disorder and, if there is such a disorder, what its nature is, that may or may not be the question that is uppermost in the mind of the person making the referral. Rather, the main issue may be what the family or school should do about a particular behavior that is causing concern in that setting. Alternatively, there may be questions over particular administrative decisions such as whether the school the child is attending is most appropriate, whether there is a need for exclusion from school, or whether the child should be removed from the family. In other cases, the referral may be to request an opinion that is relevant to some court case involving either child care or the child's responsibility for some criminal act or possible need to respond to such an act with some form of therapeutic intervention. In yet other cases, there may be an implicit query as to the meaning of the child's behavior – perhaps as to whether or not it represents an early manifestation of some serious mental disorder (such as schizophrenia or autism) that is thought to run in the family. Another possibility is that the main problem concerns disturbed family function that happens to have involved the children in some way (Shepherd, Oppenheim, & Mitchell, 1971). If so, there is the need to understand why this child has been referred at this time in this way. It is quite common, too, for different people to have quite discrepant views as to what is the problem and what needs to be done about it. Thus, the father and mother may be at loggerheads over this, their view may be different from that of the child, and all of these may differ from the perspectives of the school, the social services or the family doctor.

Because of all of these uncertainties, and the wide range of possibilities, it is crucial for any assessment to begin with some procedures designed to clarify questions about the referral (Kanner, 1957; Rutter, 1975). Who initiated the referral? Why was the referral made? Why was the referral made now? Whose problem is it? What are the key concerns or questions to which people want a response? Are there administrative decisions that hang on the assessment and, if there are, what are they?

To some extent, these questions can be clarified through obtaining relevant reports in advance of the interview for diagnostic assessment. Clearly, this needs to be carried out through discussion with the family and with their approval. Ordinarily, however, at the time of the first interview it is desirable to have available relevant reports from the school, from any social agencies that have been involved, from previous medical assessments, and from psychological and educational evaluations. Chapter 20 considers the circumstances under which it may be desirable to have structured questionnaires completed in advance of the first interview, as well as the use of more open-ended questionnaires regarding what the family wants from the referral.

As well as clarifying the reasons for referral, the initial assessment needs to be planned in such a way as to provide information on how family members interact with one another and how they deal with each other's concerns. The aim is to identify possible strengths and limitations in the family and to understand their ways of functioning in order that this may be taken into account in planning therapeutic interventions. The establishment of a relevant form of therapeutic alliance needs to be a key consideration right from the beginning of the diagnostic assessment (Green, 2006; Kazdin, Whitley, & Marciano, 2006).

Observations of the Family

Observations need to begin with the ways in which the communications (either by letter or telephone call) were dealt with prior to the first interview (Cox & Rutter, 1985). Who took the lead? What was the style used? What implications might there be for either the parents' attitudes towards their children or towards professionals? Similar questions need to be considered in relation to observations in the waiting room. If the availability of chairs provided open choice, how did the family choose to sit? What was the style of interactions among family members while waiting to be seen and how did

Rutter's Child and Adolescent Psychiatry, 5th edition. Edited by M. Rutter, D. Bishop, D. Pine, S. Scott, J. Stevenson, E. Taylor and A. Thapar. © 2008 Blackwell Publishing, ISBN: 978-1-4051-4549-7.

they respond to meeting the clinicians? How did they spend their time in waiting and what were they doing when the clinician went to collect them for interview?

Regardless of how later stages of the assessment are to be undertaken, it is usually informative to have a brief meeting with the family all together in order to clarify these sort of issues and also to explain how the assessment will be organized and who will be seeing whom for what purpose. Similar queries to those posed in relation to the waiting room arise with respect to the seating in the interview room. If the aim is to assess family interaction, it is crucial that the interview questions be addressed to the family as a whole, rather than singling out individual family members for their views. Often it may be better to put the query in the form of a questioning statement of a general kind, rather than a specific enquiry. Thus, the clinician may say something like: "I wonder how much you talked together about coming to see me today?" or there could be a general question such as "Have you had a family discussion about the reasons for coming here today?" Many parents are likely to have the cultural expectation that they (rather than the child) should answer the clinician's questions and, in interpreting how they respond, it is important to take that into account. Nevertheless, direct questions to the child in this initial family session may make him or her feel put on the spot and, thereby, uncomfortable. Again, a more general style of bringing the whole family into the interview may be preferable (for a fuller discussion of family interviewing see chapter 65). For example, if someone has responded with a firm answer on expectations or the reasons for coming, the interviewer might say something like: "I wonder whether everyone in the family sees things in this way?" It is helpful to note how much the parents provide the child with "space" to express his or her own views. How do the parents react if the child puts things in oppositional or confrontational ways? How do members of the family react when someone is expressing feelings of distress, anger or resentment? What are the patterns of eye-to-eye gaze among family members? What are their facial expressions and body gestures? Although it is usually a mistake to move quickly into interpretations, it may be helpful to make observations or express reactions as a means of getting the family to talk about the situation. Thus, the clinician may say things such as "That appears to be a very difficult situation" or "It feels as if that was awkward for you to talk about" or "It sounds as if that came as a bit of a surprise to you."

Depending on how the interview progresses, it may be appropriate to move on to direct questions about some aspect of the referral. For example, if the school or social services initiated the referral, the family may be asked how they felt about whatever it was that precipitated the referral. Was that something that they, too, were concerned about or did they see it rather differently? Similarly, if the parents have initiated referral because they were worried about some aspect of the child's behavior or emotional state, it may be important to ask the child directly whether this was something he or she was concerned about.

Younger children should not be expected to sit still during the interview and the interviewer needs to decide in advance what toys or play materials will be made available for the children. The interview provides the opportunity for seeing what the children decide to do and also whom they talk to or whom they turn to during the interview. How do the parents respond if the child seems distressed or is behaving in a disruptive way? Again, it is necessary to recognize that there may be culturally influenced expectations as to how the parents should behave. If the clinician wants the parents to be able to respond to the children it may be appropriate to say that directly by indicating "It's okay if you want to respond to (*child's name*) while we're talking" or "By all means go to (*child's name*) if you'd feel more comfortable doing that."

Elements in the Diagnostic Clinical Assessment

Interview with the Child

Interviews with older children and adolescents can follow rather similar approaches to those used with adults, but various adaptations are needed with young children. Nevertheless, in all cases, it is essential to have an individual assessment of the child. Several points warrant emphasis (see chapter 19). First, it is usually helpful to be able to assess children's behavior, styles of social interaction and ways of talking in several contrasting situations. Thus, it is usually desirable to have an opportunity of seeing the child with the rest of the family. Psychological testing will provide the quite different stimulus of a series of structured tasks requiring the child's engagement and attention. Psychological testing should always include a careful description of the child's behavior and social interactions, as well as test performance (see chapter 21). The interview with the child will be different yet again in providing a dyadic interaction opportunity but of a much less structured kind. Particularly at the beginning of the interview, the style needs to be such as to encourage children to express their own concerns (after setting the child at ease through talking about neutral topics that interest the child) and this needs to proceed to a more systematic approach to specific behaviors and feelings. Chapter 7 notes some of the considerations that apply particularly to the interviewing of young children. On the whole, free descriptions in answer to open questions provide accounts of behavior that are most accurate and least prone to distortion. On the other hand, these tend to be very lacking in detail and, almost always, it will be necessary to follow with more specific questions. It is important that this be carried out in a way that does not provide a lead to specific answers. People of all ages are open to the influence of suggestion but this is particularly the case with younger children (see chapter 7).

Variations in the style of child interview and observation are needed both when the children may be handicapped in their communication and social skills, and when the clinical issues require a focus on particular forms of behavior that may not be tapped adequately in an ordinary interview (see chapter 19). The Autism Diagnostic Observation Schedule (ADOS) provides relevant social presses (Lord, Risi, Lambrecht *et al.*, 2000). It was initially developed primarily for research purposes but specialized clinics are now increasingly using it for clinical assessments. Even if the standardized half-hour assessment is not used clinically, the principles are certainly relevant to any form of clinical diagnostic interview with children or adults for whom the diagnosis of some form of pervasive developmental disorder (autism spectrum disorder) has been raised (see chapter 46). There is a similar need to adapt interview approaches for children with seriously impaired hearing or vision, or with limited language (see chapter 59).

The need to consider how assessments should be adapted for particular purposes is exemplified by the approaches needed for the assessment of possible attachment disorders (see chapter 55). The concept of these disorders is that they are characterized by pervasive problems in selective attachment. The disinhibited variety of attachment disorder might be thought to comprise a relative lack of selective attachments and the inhibited variety both a lack of security provided by established selective attachments and by various abnormal features. So far as the disinhibited variety is concerned, there are two features that particularly require attention. The first concerns the children's response to a stranger and the degree to which this lacks the normal wariness plus the extent to which there is an inadequate appreciation of social boundaries and an unusual degree of physical closeness or contact before a relationship has been established. In addition, there may be a lack of selectivity in going to the principal caregivers for security or comfort and it is important that the children's response to family members be observed, as well as the response to a stranger. What is needed clinically is a form of assessment that provides the opportunity to assess the child's reaction to strangers (the clinicians fill that role); responses to separations from and reunions with the parents (taking the child to be seen on his or her own and returning later serves that purpose); and the child's use of the parents as a secure basis (a joint family interview is useful in that connection).

Whatever the age of the child, and whatever the clinical issue, it is important that the interview combine an appropriate degree of structure and standardization (which are essential for comparability across children) and sensitivity to the unexpected and to the individual issue. The latter have been most studied in relation to the interviewing of parents in a clinical setting (Cox, Rutter, & Holbrook, 1981; Rutter, Cox, Egert *et al.*, 1981) in which one of the most striking findings was the very high frequency of clinically significant information of an unusual kind which would be most unlikely to have been picked up by confining questioning only to predetermined topics. The same consideration certainly applies to interviews with children. It is very important for clinicians to be sensitive to the cues provided by children and these will need to be followed through in whatever way seems most appropriate to the individual situation. This need applies even more to what children say about their psychosocial circumstances than it does to what they say about psychopathology (see below).

Parental Interview

The parental interview will be particularly concerned with the assessment of psychopathology but, in planning therapeutic interventions, several other features need to be considered. To begin with, it is essential to determine what it is about the child's behavior, feelings or social interactions that is of the greatest concern to the parents. That may not necessarily be the feature that the clinician considers of the greatest psychopathological importance but, ordinarily, it is sensible that early therapeutic interventions be recognized by the parents as addressing their concerns. In addition, it will be important to find out how the parents (and other people) have tried to deal with the concern. How have they tried to respond and what success or otherwise have their approaches achieved? If adequate use is to be made of this in therapeutic planning, it will be essential to move beyond a general answer (such as admonish the child, comfort him or her, or try to be understanding) and, instead, obtain a more detailed sequential account of *how* this has been done. What did they do and what was the child's response? If certain approaches did not work, did they persist (and if so, for how long and under what circumstances) or did they keep changing? A closely related issue is the impact that the child's disturbance has had on them and on the rest of the family.

In dealing with the development of the disorder, attention will need to be paid to possible predisposing factors in life circumstances or physical state. Before proceeding with specific questioning, it is usually better to elicit the parents' views on what might have been important. There is then the somewhat different matter of the functional analysis of the behavior that is causing concern (see chapter 62). In other words, what are the features that seem to make the behaviors of concern more or less likely to occur? What circumstances seem to improve the situation? Questions regarding the degree to which behaviors are situation-specific or pervasive are important, not only for their implications with respect to severity, but also in terms of features in the environment that may act as a risk or protective factor.

There are important advantages in making sure that children are seen with their parents for part of the diagnostic assessment. However, people do not behave, or talk, in the same way when seen on their own and when seen as part of a family group. Moreover, it may be unhelpfully embarrassing for children to have to hear their problems discussed with a professional. Accordingly, it is usually desirable for part of the assessment time to be spent in seeing the child on their own and for the parents similarly to be seen separately. Not only may this provide information that would not be obtained quite so readily in a family setting, but it also makes explicit a concern to pay attention to family members as individuals as well as with them as part of a group. Some clinicians prefer to conduct the whole of the diagnostic assessment interview in a conjoint family setting but, in our view, this has disadvantages with respect to information gathering. A somewhat similar decision needs to be made as to whether both parents should be seen together or whether there should be some time with each separately. Our usual practice is to follow parental preferences in the first instance but to be alert to cues that suggest that it may be necessary to see parents on their own for a brief period in addition. In that connection, however, it should be noted that one study (Cox, Hemsley, & Dare, 1995) showed that families did not respond well to a change of style from family to individual or vice versa, when making the transition from diagnostic assessment to therapeutic intervention.

School Reports

It is always desirable to obtain a school report, preferably in advance of the first interview with the family (but after obtaining their agreement that the school may be contacted). Children may well behave differently at school from the way they do at home and it is important to obtain an account of scholastic functioning (educational difficulties are frequently associated with psychopathology). There are some advantages in using a standard questionnaire as part of the reporting from school (see chapter 20). However, a questionnaire is never adequate on its own because it is crucial for teachers to be able to express their own concerns (and that may involve features that are outside the coverage of the questionnaire), because it is important to consider changes over time and not just present behavior, and because it is important to find out how school has dealt with difficulties and how the child has responded to whatever actions were taken. Sometimes, there may be specific queries that arise out of the diagnostic assessment and, when that is the case, it may be useful for a member of the clinical team to contact the school directly in order to discuss the points that have arisen. Particularly when there seems to be a major discrepancy between the accounts of the child's behavior at home and at school, visits to both settings to observe what is happening may be informative.

Psychological Testing

Chapter 21 considers the approach that needs to be taken to psychological testing and its role in the overall diagnostic assessment. A key part of the psychological evaluation concerns the psychologist's observation of the child's behavior in relation to the tasks that have been given and in relation to the social encounter with the psychologist. This is important because of the information that it provides about the child's psychological functioning generally, and not just because of its importance in relation to the interpretation of the psychological test findings.

So far as the latter are concerned, it is essential in all cases to consider whether the scores are consistent with the account of the child's performance given by the parents and by the school, and in keeping with the clinician's observations of the child. Of course, it is to be expected that there will not be perfect agreement across all assessments but, if there are major discrepancies, that always has to be a matter for further study. If the child's performance during standardized testing was markedly better or markedly worse than that expected on the basis of other people's reports, what is the explanation? Does it reflect differences in the cognitive demands in the several situations, or does it reflect social features of the situation? What are the implications for the situational factors that seem to facilitate better performance?

A crucial part of any psychological assessment concerns the evaluation of the likely validity of the findings. Attention needs to be paid to the extent to which it was possible to engage the child in the relevant tasks, noting whether disturbed behavior may have interfered with task performance. Particularly in the case of young children for whom there is a query regarding possible severe intellectual disability, it is important to note how the child dealt with the situation as a whole, and with the task presented. A clear enquiring curiosity about the environment, a systematic problem-solving approach, and initiative combined with imagination in dealing with test materials would all cause questioning of the validity of a very low test score. Obviously, too, it will be necessary to consider whether overall task performance has been constrained because of specific difficulties in functions such as language, motor coordination or vision. In terms of the predictive validity of scores, consideration will also need to be given to the possibility that current cognitive functioning has been impaired as a result of severely disadvantageous rearing experiences that no longer apply. In short, test scores provide invaluable information but they need to be interpreted in relation to the assessment as a whole.

Medical Examination and Testing

Physical illnesses are common in the population and can cause mental disturbance, so a child mental health assessment needs to be competent to detect illness (see chapter 22). The most fundamental requirement is that a thoughtful and systematic history-taking should be used as a guide to the possibility that somatic problems might be relevant with respect to the psychopathology that has been the focus of the referral. General medical problems, as well as neurological ones, should be borne in mind – such as deafness in attention problems and endocrine dysfunction in eating problems. When there is nothing in the history to suggest the presence of a possibly relevant somatic condition, it will probably be sufficient to ensure that previous health screening has been competent, to measure the child's height and weight, and to undertake a screening neurodevelopmental examination that does not require the child to undress fully. Questions should have been asked to determine pubertal status but, unless it appears likely to be specifically relevant, there is no need to undertake a physical examination for this purpose.

When the child has a possible global or specific developmental delay, or a disorder such as autism (see chapter 46) or hyperkinetic disorder (see chapter 34), a rather fuller assessment is necessary (see chapters 22 & 49). Appropriate medical assessments will be essential when there are symptoms affecting somatic functions, because this could result from somatic disease. Early studies of so-called hysterical conversion reactions in both children (Caplan, 1970) and adults (Slater, 1965) showed the relatively high frequency with which these were wrongly diagnosed as psychogenic in origin, as indicated by the clear emergence of underlying physical disease of a directly pertinent kind during the course of follow-up. With proper clinical assessment, such misdiagnoses nowadays should be much less common, but clinicians need to be aware of the possibility (see chapter 57).

Standardization of Clinical Assessment

A key question concerns the merits and demerits of standardizing how clinical assessments are undertaken. In the past, some clinicians used methods that assumed that a particular form of treatment would invariably be required. At one time, this often concerned psychoanalytically oriented psychotherapy and somewhat later it often concerned conjoint family therapy of one kind or another. Exactly the same issues, however, apply to the assumption that the treatment will always involve use of diagnosis-specific medication (whether this be for depression or attention deficit/hyperactivity disorder [ADHD]). This approach to clinical assessment should no longer be acceptable. To begin with, single-therapy clinical practice is bad practice and any form of adequate clinical assessment must take on board the possibility of a range of appropriate therapeutic interventions. Systematic studies of interviewing (Cox & Rutter, 1985) have made it clear that systematic focused questioning is essential to obtain the relevant data for clinical diagnosis. In that connection, there is much to be said for the use of standardized interviews and standardized observations (see chapter 19). On the other hand, there are also dangers in the restriction of assessment to such diagnostic instruments.

The dangers arise from several different considerations. First, systematic studies of interviewing have shown the very high frequency with which idiosyncratic items of clinically significant importance are present (Cox & Rutter, 1985). These will be missed if assessments are constrained by predetermined areas of interest. Second, it cannot be assumed that current diagnostic concepts cover the full range of psychopathology. As Kanner aptly put it in the title of one of his papers on differential diagnosis, "The children haven't read those books" (Kanner, 1969). The point that he was making is that there is a most imperfect match between the neat diagnostic description given in textbooks and the clinical presentations seen in referred patients. The usual explanation will be that the person has a somewhat atypical variety of a well-recognized, well-validated disorder. Nevertheless, the last half-century has seen the recognition for the first time of several disorders of considerable importance that had not been noticed before. Kanner's (1943) identification of autism is the most striking example but it is closely followed by the identification of Rett syndrome (Hagberg, Aicardi, Dias *et al.*, 1983; Rett, 1966). Both Asperger syndrome (Asperger, 1944) and Wolff's concept of schizoid disorder in childhood (Wolff, 1995) constitute other variants within the realm of what might be regarded as autism spectrum disorders. "New" conditions are, however, by no means restricted to this group. Russell's (1979) identification of bulimia nervosa constitutes another example, as does that of attachment disorders (see chapter 55). More recent, and therefore less well validated, examples are also provided by the quasi-autistic pattern seen in some children who have experienced profound institutional deprivation (Rutter, Andersen-Wood, Beckett *et al.*, 1999); the social abnormalities that have been found to be associated with severe developmental disorders in receptive language (Clegg, Hollis, Mawhood *et al.*, 2005); and the autistic-like patterns seen with some cases of congenital blindness (Brown, Hobson, & Lee, 1997). Sometimes, too, the clinical recognition of a new pattern concerns a risk factor (as with the fetal alcohol syndrome; Jones & Smith, 1973) or a feature that had not been appreciated before (as with pragmatic language disorders; see chapter 47). Not all of these patterns of psychopathology constitute well-validated syndromes but the general point remains; clinicians must always be on the alert for unusual patterns that do not fit existing diagnostic conventions.

Third, the initial diagnostic assessment cannot be confined to the topic of diagnosis. It must also concern reasons for referral, factors that might be important in either the causation or course of the disorder or which influence the planning of treatment; and the assessment of factors that may be relevant for prognosis. In the remainder of this chapter, we consider the range of issues that should be covered in any adequate clinical assessment. Standardized approaches constitute an important part of such assessment but they are only one part. In other words, there is much to be said for well-articulated clinical standards but there are dangers in translating these into a rigid and restricted predetermined diagnostic protocol.

Finally, the initial diagnostic assessment must go on to provide a formulation that provides a basis for therapeutic planning. That must include not only what the pattern of symptomatology has in common with those seen in other individuals, but also the aspects that are particular to this individual child and this individual family. Formulations need to include a hypothesis of what seem to be the most important factors that are going to influence response to treatment; an articulation of what evidence will be needed to determine whether that hypothesis was, or was not, correct; and the development of a therapeutic plan as to how best the therapeutic goals may be achieved.

Presence/Absence of Clinically Significant Psychopathology

Because most psychiatric disorders do not include pathognomonic qualitatively abnormal features that cannot be found in normal children or adolescents, a key basic question has to be whether the severity or nature of psychopathology is such as to be clinically significant. Necessarily, that query comprises two somewhat different issues. First, there is the question of whether the problems being considered are causing significant suffering for the individual or significant distress for others. Second, there is the question of whether the psychopathology falls outside the normal range of behavior, or which carries with it a significant likelihood of recurrent or chronic malfunction. Clinical intervention will sometimes be indicated when the answer to one of the questions is in the affirmative but in the negative to the other. Thus, a serious grief reaction following the death of a loved one is quite common in normal individuals but it may warrant offering appropriate counseling (see chapter 26), even though it may not be a psychiatric disorder in the normal sense of the word. Similarly, many parents present at health clinics with their children's difficulties in eating or sleeping – these are essentially normal, yet are causing major family disruption. Appropriate guidance and help may well be needed in such circumstances (see chapters 53 & 54).

The issue is an important one in relation to emotional disorders because anxiety, depression and fears are a normal part of the human condition that most people experience at some time. The considerations to be taken into account include: whether there has been a substantial change from the person's usual mental state, whether the intensity of the emotions goes beyond the range of normal variation, whether the person is able to control the unpleasant emotions by means of distraction or engagement in pleasurable activities, whether the emotions intrude into and interfere with normal life functioning, and whether the emotions are pervasive across situations. Somewhat similar criteria apply to overactivity/inattention but with the difference that, because these are usually first manifest in the preschool years, there will not usually be a recognizable change from any previous normal pattern. The assessment of disruptive behavior is rather less straightforward because the child may not perceive that there is a need to control such behavior.

Assessment of Impairment

From the time of the Isle of Wight studies onwards (Rutter, Tizard, & Whitmore, 1970), the degree to which psychopathology gives rise to impairment of psychosocial functioning has been a key consideration in the assessment of clinical significance. There was a further impetus to use such a criterion from the epidemiological evidence that some forms of symptomatology, particularly specific phobias, were present in what seemed to be an absurdly high proportion of the population if impairment was not taken into account (Bird, 1999; Bird, Yager, Staghezza *et al.*, 1990). That has seemed a reasonable approach because, if psychopathology is not impairing function, there would not seem to be much need for intervention. Epidemiological findings have been consistent in showing that there are substantial differences among different forms of psychopathology in the extent to which there is associated impairment. To begin with, quite a few children show psychosocial impairment associated with psychopathology but without the required number of symptoms to fulfill the criteria for a specific diagnosis (Angold, Costello, Farmer *et al.*, 1999). When this is the case, intervention may well be justified. The presence of marked symptoms in the absence of impairment is most frequently seen in relation to specific phobias (Simonoff, Pickles, Meyer *et al.*, 1997). Conversely, it is rather unusual for there to be multiple symptoms of depression without there being any impairment (Pickles, Rowe, Simonoff *et al.*, 2001). However, the diagnosis here is made, not just on the severity of negative mood, but on associated phenomena such as self-depreciation, feelings of guilt, feelings of hopelessness about the future and suicidal thoughts or actions. The need to consider associated symptomatology constitutes a key element in diagnosis.

Clinically significant developmental disorders of language (see chapter 47) need to be differentiated from normal variations in language development on the basis of the breadth of affected language functions (e.g., including understanding as well as use of spoken language), impaired use of language-related skills in make-believe play, difficulties in the control of motor movements associated with spoken language (as with drooling) and associated socioemotional or behavioral problems (Rutter, 1987). Although impairment is certainly a useful criterion to employ, there are both logical and practical problems associated with giving it too high a priority. First, from a medical perspective, it would seem foolish to say that a person did not have a disorder because they were not impaired if there were signs or symptoms (or test findings) indicating an obviously pathological condition. Thus, someone with diabetes, whose condition has been shown by the appropriate laboratory tests, would still be diagnosed as having diabetes even if functioning was unimpaired because symptoms were well controlled by diet or the use of insulin. The same would clearly apply in the case of schizophrenia that was well controlled by appropriate medication. In these instances, however, the abnormality is evident in terms of qualitatively abnormal findings, as evidenced either by history or present status, or both. The second concern is that a person may cope successfully with their disorder to the extent that symptoms are not manifest because the situations that elicit them have been avoided. There will not be psychosocial impairment if the person's life is so organized that the issues do not arise. This most obviously applies in the case of certain phobias. Third, the degree to which there is psychosocial impairment will inevitably be influenced by social circumstances. Many decades ago Wootton (1959) pointed to the absurdity, for example, of rates of disorders going up and down according to fluctuations in the employment rate. She noted too the major difficulties in basing a diagnosis of psychiatric disorder on the extent to which it caused problems for other people. This has been a problematic issue in deciding whether conduct disorders should be regarded as psychiatric conditions (Hill & Maughan, 2001). In this case, what is a persuasive argument in favor of regarding it as a disorder is the extensive evidence of impaired personal functioning in both childhood and adult life, including an increased risk of suicide and of other forms of psychopathology.

Although qualitative abnormalities are not a feature of the majority of psychiatric disorders in childhood or adolescence, they are present in some. For example, the pattern of socioemotional deficits shown by individuals with autism is one that would be abnormal at any age (see chapter 46). The same applies to the thought disorder, negative symptoms and delusions/hallucinations found in schizophrenia (see chapter 45). The situation is not quite so clear cut with obsessive-compulsive phenomena but, although ruminations and minor checking behavior may be regarded as falling within the normal range of variation, that is not the case with overt compulsive rituals of a marked kind (see chapter 43). Somewhat similar considerations apply to Tourette syndrome and chronic multiple tics (see chapter 44). Particular care needs to be taken in eliciting detailed descriptions of such qualitatively abnormal features because, if people have not experienced these phenomena, they may interpret the questions as referring to the more normal features that were within their experience.

The existence of firm diagnostic criteria for different psychiatric disorders in the official classification systems is sometimes thought to imply that there cannot be a disorder if it does not fit into one of the specified diagnoses. Manifestly, that is not the case, as both clinical and epidemiological studies show (Angold *et al.*, 1999; Pickles *et al.*, 2001). Of course, the presence of social impairment does not in itself mean that there is a psychiatric disorder. It does suggest that something is wrong but one key diagnostic question is whether or not this is attributable to some form of physical disease. Nevertheless, even when such disease appears to be ruled out, the diagnosis of psychiatric disorder needs to be based on clear evidence of psychopathological dysfunction, even if the number and pattern of symptoms do not fit the rules of any single specified disorder.

Duration and Timing of Disorder

Classification systems have often used duration of disorder as a key criterion by which to determine whether or not psychopathology is clinically significant. For example, DSM-IV (American Psychiatric Association, 2000) has specified a minimum duration of 2 weeks for a major depressive disorder, 6 months for a conduct disorder or a generalized anxiety disorder, 2 years for a dysthymic disorder in adults and 1 year in childhood, no duration for anorexia nervosa but 3 months for bulimia nervosa. It is immediately obvious that the choice of these time periods is essentially arbitrary. Thus, most clinicians would regard 2 weeks as a rather short period of time for a major depressive disorder, and it is noteworthy that the research diagnostic criteria specify 4 weeks, rather than 2 (Mazure & Gershon, 1979). Also, a year seems a long time to require a dysthymic disorder to last in order to regard it as meeting criterion. A further problem is that, even with high-quality research interviewing that involves a specific focus on personalized timing, the reliability of the timing of onset of disorder has proved rather poor (Angold, Erkanlis, Costello *et al.*, 1996). In all probability, this is not because people find it difficult to remember some clearly identifiable time when a disorder began, but rather because many disorders do not have a clear-cut onset. Frequently, symptomatology builds up over time, with several points at which new symptoms become apparent and/or when psychosocial impairment first becomes evident (Rutter & Sandberg, 1992; Sandberg, Rutter, Pickles *et al.*, 2001). Clearly, it is important for clinicians to obtain as good an account as possible of how psychopathology developed over time and to seek to identify times that might be conceptualized as either an onset of disorder or a clear worsening of disorder. From a clinical perspective, however, it is less appropriate to follow DSM-IV rules about duration in a slavish fashion than it is to decide that the symptoms constitute something that manifestly falls outside the range of normal variation for that person and which either involves qualitative abnormalities or has interfered with psychosocial functioning to a substantial extent.

Nature of the Mental Disorder

In chapter 2 we consider some of the conceptual and practical issues concerned with varying concepts of comorbidity. Here, we need to emphasize that, regardless of which classificatory principle is followed, it is essential in clinical assessment to obtain an adequate assessment of the mix of symptomatology. That is because, irrespective of whether or not the mixture is conceptualized as comorbidity or mixed symptomatology in a single disorder, it is likely to have implications for treatment strategies. The day may come when there are drugs that are specific to particular diagnoses but that day is a long way off at the moment. Both psychological and pharmacological treatments need to focus on particular patterns of symptomatology rather than the diagnosis as such.

If the assessment has indicated that there is a significant psychopathological disorder, the next questions are what form it takes, and what diagnosis or diagnoses may be applied to it. ICD-10 (World Health Organization, 1996) and DSM-IV (American Psychiatric Association, 2000) adopt different approaches to this issue (see chapter 2). There are pros and cons with respect to how co-occurrence is handled in both these classification systems. However, the clinical need is to assess the overall mixture of psychopathology because this is likely to influence treatment decisions and prognosis, and because it may help in sorting out the meaning of the symptom patterns and the causal mechanisms that might be involved.

Also, a basic hypothesis-testing approach to diagnostic assessment is fundamental to the diagnostic enterprise. For example, although not well reflected in either of the two main classification systems, it is important to differentiate among the various causes of fecal soiling (Rutter, 1975). This may arise, for example, because the child has failed to gain bowel control. Alternatively, control may well have been achieved and maintained, with the disorder lying in the deposition of feces in inappropriate places rather than in any lack of or loss of control. A third possibility is that there has been fecal retention leading to gross distension of the bowel and partial blockage. In these circumstances, fecal soiling may arise because there has been an overflow of feces stemming from the prior distension. In order to differentiate between these possibilities, careful assessment is needed of whether or not the feces are normal in form and consistency, whether there is a history of previous normal bowel control, whether the soiling has been preceded by patterns of retention or other abnormalities in bowel functioning, and whether the deposition of feces is essentially random (according to where the child happens to be at the time that the bowels are opened) rather than selectively placed in situations having psychological meaning. Clearly, the therapeutic interventions need to be chosen on the basis of the type of disorder represented by the soiling (see chapter 56).

A decision-tree approach may also be very useful in the assessment of developmental disorders of language. When the diagnostic issue concerns some pattern of psychopathology associated with the language delay, it is helpful to tackle the decision-making in stepwise fashion (Rutter, 1985). Thus, it is usually best to begin by determining the child's overall level of cognitive functioning, going on to consider whether language skills are significantly below those of other aspects of cognitive functioning. The question then is whether the psychopathology shown is outside the range of normal behavior expected in relation to the child's overall mental age and level of language functioning. If it is outside that range, rather than move straight away to consider the complete list of possible psychiatric diagnoses, it is generally helpful to ask the question of whether the behaviors are of a kind that might be found in any child (that is, the usual run of emotional problems and disorders of disruptive behavior) or whether the pattern is qualitatively different in a way that is associated with pervasive developmental disorders. Having made that decision, it is then somewhat easier to move on to a consideration of which particular diagnostic concept best fits the picture in whichever direction the prior decision has taken.

In some cases, the clinical question may concern social usage of a skill. Thus, selective mutism (see chapter 47) is characterized by a high degree of selectivity in circumstances of talking. As in experimental studies more generally, the need is to design a situation in which children can and do succeed but do so in ways that are informative on the mechanisms involved. With selective mutism, the need is to be able to demonstrate that the children can use spoken language in particular circumstances, just as much as showing that they do not use spoken language in other situations.

Psychosocial Assessment

Psychosocial risks are important in the development of psychopathology (see chapters 25 & 26). It is important therefore that the diagnostic assessment provides an efficient, reliable and valid means of assessing the presence of psychosocial risk factors. However, the need should not be seen as exclusively related to questions of causation. In planning psychological interventions (when they are indicated), it is important to identify possible protective mechanisms as well as risk features. Moreover, it is necessary to assess risk and protective factors, not only in terms of what is happening within the family, but also what is happening within the peer group, school and community (Rutter, Giller, & Hagell, 1998; Shonkoff & Phillips, 2000). Furthermore, the psychosocial assessment needs to include both past experiences and current circumstances. On the whole, most early experiences do not have enduring effects that are independent of later psychosocial circumstances (Clarke & Clarke, 2000). Nevertheless, profoundly depriving experiences can have major sequelae that persist long after children have ceased to suffer deprivation and have had good rearing experiences in a well-functioning family (Rutter, Kreppner, O'Connor *et al.*, 2001). Similarly, there may be enduring effects of seriously abusive experiences (see chapters 28 & 29) or unusual severely traumatic experiences (see chapter 42).

A key consideration with respect to all these experiences, risk and protective, is the need to appreciate that the experiences cannot be thought of as impinging on a passive organism. Children, and adults, think and feel about what they experience and the cognitive/affective sets that they develop (or internal working models) may be very important in determining the consequences of such experiences. What this means is that the assessment needs to determine both how children have coped with their experiences (see chapter 65) and what they have thought about what has happened to them and how they view their current experiences.

Research over recent decades has made it abundantly clear that genetic factors have an important role in the origins and persistence of all forms of behavior, including all forms of psychopathology (see chapter 23). The findings are of major clinical importance for several rather different reasons. First, they show the importance of recognizing the influence of genetic susceptibilities with respect to individual differences in the liability to psychopathology. That means, amongst other things, that any adequate diagnostic assessment will need to include systematic questioning with respect to a family history of psychopathology.

Particular attention needs to be paid to disorders in parents and in siblings, not just because they are the closest relatives with respect to genetic inheritance, but also because mental disorders in the immediate family will involve environmentally mediated, as well as genetically mediated, psychosocial risks (Rutter, 1989). Thus, parental mental disorder is associated with a substantially increased risk of family discord and family breakdown, and also focused hostility on individual children (Rutter, Maughan, Meyer *et al.*, 1997). This means that it is important to assess the ways in which parental mental disorder impinges on the family and not just to be content with recognizing its presence. The risks may also involve physical risk factors in relation to substances that cross the placental barrier during pregnancy. Thus, high levels of alcohol ingestion in the early months of pregnancy may lead to the neurodevelopmental abnormalities associated with fetal alcohol syndrome (Spohr & Steinhausen, 1996; Stratton, Howe, & Battaglia, 1996). There may also be effects from taking recreational drugs or prescribed medications (Delaney-Black, Covington, Templin *et al.*, 2000; Singer, Arendt, Farkes *et al.*, 1997). The extent to which there is enquiry about mental disorders occurring in second- and third-degree relatives needs to be guided by the particular clinical problem. However, it should be routine to ask about the occurrence of major mental disorders or developmental problems on both sides of the family. Genetic testing (using cytogenetic and molecular genetic methods) is not part of routine assessment but it is important in some circumstances (see chapter 24) and could become more generally applicable in the future.

Research methods that provide systematic standardized assessments of psychosocial features are too time-consuming for use in most clinics. Nevertheless, they do provide helpful guides on how such routine clinical assessments should be undertaken. As with the assessment of psychopathology, the agreement between the reports of parents and children tends to be modest to moderate at best (Achenbach, McConaughy, & Howell, 1987; Borge, Samuelsen, & Rutter, 2001; Rutter, Tizard, & Whitmore, 1970; Simonoff *et al.*, 1997). That is partly because parents will not know about the full range of children's experiences outside the home, partly because their perspectives may not be the same and partly because some disorders may be relatively situation-specific (Cox & Rutter, 1985). The implication is that some assessment of psychosocial risk and protective experiences needs to be obtained from both parents and children. The classification of psychosocial experiences developed by the World Health Organization (van Goor Lambo, Orley, Poustka *et al.*, 1990) provides some guidance on the range of experiences that need to be considered and there are standardized interviews that cover most of the relevant experiences (Sandberg, Rutter, Giles *et al.*, 1993). However, the research findings from studies that have used designs that can separate environmental from genetic mediation (Rutter *et al.*, 2001; Rutter, 2007) suggest that the experiences carrying the greatest psychopathological risk mainly concern marked negativity in close personal relationships, a lack of continuity in personalized caregiving, a lack of appropriate learning experiences and participation in social groups with a deviant ethos, attitudes or styles of behavior (Rutter, 2000a). Although not much investigated in genetically sensitive designs, it is likely that parental monitoring and supervision of children's behavior are also important in relation to antisocial problems (Rutter, Giller, & Hagell, 1998; but see Stattin & Kerr, 2000, with respect to the role of children's disclosures). In relation to all these experiences, it is necessary to determine the ways in which such experiences impinge on individual children, and are responded to, and not just the experiences as they affect the family as a whole. Although excessive claims have been made about the preponderant importance of child-specific experiences (Reiss, Neiderhiser, Hetherington *et al.*, 2000; Rutter, 1999), it is the risks as they affect the individual child that are important, even if they impinge similarly on other children in the same family.

In that connection, the research evidence suggests that it is often useful to make direct comparisons among children in the family with respect to features such as whether one is more likely to be criticized than others, more frequently favored, or more likely to be involved in relevant risk or protective experiences in the family (Carbonneau, Eaves, Silberg *et al.*, 2002a, Carbonneau, Rutter, Simonoff *et al.*, 2002b). In addition, research has shown how much can be inferred from the ways in which a parent talks about the children. This was first demonstrated in the Camberwell Family Interview (Brown & Rutter, 1966; Rutter & Brown, 1966) but has been developed as a much briefer assessment in relation to the 5-minute speech sample (Magaña, Goldstein, Karno *et al.*, 1986). The implication is that it is important to have a time during the assessment when parents are asked neutral questions about their children, not just questions focusing on problems. Thus, it is helpful to get parents to talk about what their children are like as individuals, how easy they are to be friendly and affectionate with, what is their most striking individual characteristic, etc. The same, of course, applies to the ways in which children talk about their parents and about their siblings.

Diagnostic Formulation

Diagnoses serve the important role of providing a succinct summary of the key clinical features that are held in common with disorders experienced by others (see chapter 2). This is a most important purpose and one that is central to communication among clinicians, just as much as among researchers. Multiaxial systems of classification (World Health Organization, 1996) can go somewhat further because they can serve to classify relevant psychosocial situations that may have played a part in causation or that may be pertinent with respect to therapeutic planning, as well as intellectual level and level of adaptive functioning. By considering the information included across a complete range of axes, a lot of clinically relevant information can be summarized succinctly.

Nevertheless, that is not quite the same thing as developing hypotheses about causal processes and hypotheses about therapeutic interventions. For example, suppose it has been found that the child has cerebral palsy. As outlined in chapter 30, there is good epidemiological evidence that this is associated with a substantial increase in psychopathological risk in groups of children with this condition. However, the risk could come about through several different routes, each of which has different implications for intervention. Thus, in some instances, the main risk may derive from the electrophysiological disturbance associated with frequent, poorly controlled epileptic attacks. In other cases, the risk may stem from impaired cognitive skills and from the educational difficulties to which they may give rise. In some cases there may be relatively direct neural effects of brain dysfunction, as exemplified in so-called frontal lobe syndromes exhibiting social disinhibition that sometimes occur after severe head injuries (Rutter,

Chadwick, & Shaffer, 1983). In yet other cases, the psychopathological risk may derive from the child's negative self-image as a result of his or her physical limitations, or perhaps from parental overprotection that came about as a way of dealing with a physically handicapped child. In yet other cases, the cerebral palsy may be a relatively incidental finding that has no particular relevance with respect to the mental disorder. Of course, when dealing with a single case, it is difficult to have hard evidence that enables a choice between these alternatives, but it is important for the clinician to have a view on the likely importance of different mechanisms.

Closely comparable issues arise with respect to psychosocial risk factors. If the mother is alcoholic, did the psychopathological risk derive from the child's *in utero* exposure to high levels of alcohol, from the genetic susceptibility, or from the family disruption and poor parenting to which the alcoholism may have given rise? In considering causal processes, too, crucial distinctions need to be drawn between distal and proximal risk processes (Rutter, Giller, & Hagell, 1998) and also between influences on the initiation of the child psychopathology and the processes that are currently maintaining it. Thus, poverty and social disadvantage are associated with an increased risk of mental disorders in childhood, but most of the risks seem to be indirectly mediated. That is, the overall disadvantageous social circumstances do not, in themselves, cause psychopathology but they do make good parenting more difficult and the main risks stem from the parenting problems (see e.g. Conger, Conger, Elder *et al.*, 1992, 1993). In the same sort of way, parental loss and parent–child separations are associated with an increased risk of antisocial behavior but, again, this seems to be largely because of the associated family discord and conflict (Fergusson, Horwood, & Lynskey, 1992; Rutter, 1971). Furthermore, although family conflict is associated with an increased risk of psychopathology, it seems that this largely comes about when the conflict leads to negativity that is focused on that particular child (Reiss, Hetherington, Plomin *et al.*, 1995). Also, it is important to appreciate that the child's disorder may predispose to problems in parenting or to family conflict. In these examples, the global family situation needs to be thought of as a risk indicator, rather than an immediate risk mechanism. It is implicated in the causal processes but largely because it predisposes to other psychosocial features that constitute a more direct psychopathological risk. It is by no means easy to make these distinctions in individual cases (or even at a group level) but it is important when trying to decide how best to intervene.

The distinction between initiatory or provoking risk factors and factors concerned with the maintenance of a disorder is somewhat different. For example, an extremely traumatic experience may precipitate a post-traumatic stress disorder (see chapter 42) but some individuals recover quite quickly whereas others are affected for several years afterwards. In most cases, the difference between recovery and persistence is likely to lie less in the severity of the initial experience than in how the person thinks about that experience and how they have dealt with it. The original traumatic experience cannot be taken away but the person may be helped to deal better with both the thought patterns and emotional reactions to which the experience gave rise. In other cases, it may be helpful to differentiate between the factors that had a major role in the timing of the onset of the disorder and those that were responsible for the increased liability that led to the disorder occurring at all (see chapter 26). Thus, severely threatening life events (such as psychological loss or humiliation) may precipitate the onset of a depressive reaction or the initiation of a particular behavior such as a suicidal act (see chapter 40). On the other hand, the overall susceptibility to disorder may have more to do with the associated chronic psychosocial adversity than with the time-limited acute event itself. One of the important findings in life-events research is the high frequency with which seriously negative events derive out of chronic psychosocial adversity. Both are important but they may serve a somewhat different risk role.

Treatment Planning

In recent years, systematic literature review and consensus development conferences have led to official and unofficial guidelines for treatment planning. They are usually organized around a diagnosis, so the diagnosis given will in itself suggest treatment possibilities. Indeed, purchasers or managers of health care may insist on clinicians following the guidelines for a particular condition.

The clarification of the evidence base is very welcome, but we see dangers in the mechanical following of protocols. The current state of knowledge seldom allows the diagnosis by itself, or even several simultaneous diagnoses, to dictate intervention. Major benefits of treatment protocols include the indication to services of what methods of assessment and treatment should be made available. However, it is the individual formulation rather than the diagnostic category that should guide the treatment plan.

Clearly, the proximal risk mechanisms involved with the maintenance of the disorder must play a major part in determining the therapeutic hypotheses that constitute the basis for planning treatment. However, several other matters have to be taken into account. To begin with, it is necessary to consider possible protective mechanisms, as well as risk processes (Rutter, 1990). As in the broader consideration of features associated with resilience (Rutter 1999, 2000b, 2006), such possible protective processes may reflect a quite diverse range of features. Thus, the strengths may lie in the child's temperamental qualities and/or coping skills (Sandler, Tein, Mehta *et al.*, 2000), in the presence of a particularly good close relationship in or outside the family, of compensating good experiences at school or in the peer group, or in a possible change of pattern in family functioning. Thus, if one parent is particularly under stress, the other parent may be encouraged to take a greater role in parenting. The point is that the clinician needs to think broadly about the child's psychosocial situation in order to identify possible strengths and protective possibilities.

In planning any intervention, it is as necessary to decide which features are modifiable as it is to determine which are the risk and causal mechanisms. Thus, it is necessary to decide whether the intervention should focus primarily on working with the child, with the parents, with the family as a whole, with the school or trying to change other aspects of the broader environment. Of course, the treatment strategy may involve more than one of these avenues. One aspect of deciding about openness to modifiability concerns different perceptions of the child and of what needs to be done. Part of the same issue concerns a decision on what are realistic goals. The aim must be to provide relief for the child's suffering in the first instance, but restoration of full normality may not be a realistic goal (e.g., only rarely would it be so in the case of autism; see chapter 46). Similarly, the intervention may not necessarily focus on the hypothesized basic causal process. Again, to use the example of autism, there would be general acceptance that this is a neurodevelopmental disorder but, equally, the evidence suggests that behavioral and/or educational interventions working with parents and teachers currently provide the best opportunities for reducing handicaps, even though autism has clearly not been caused by the lack of such experiences.

Yet another decision concerns whether or not to use medication and, if medication is used, how it should be employed and when it should be introduced. There are no drugs that are curative for child psychiatric disorders but there are several conditions for which medication has been shown to produce worthwhile benefits. These include depressive disorders (see chapter 37), obsessive-compulsive disorders (see chapter 43), tics and Tourette syndrome (see chapter 44), schizophrenia (see chapter 45) and hyperkinetic disorders (see chapter 34). They may also provide symptomatic benefits in other disorders. Decisions on drug usage will be influenced, among other things, by the severity of overall impairment and the particular pattern of symptomatology. Thus, the advantage of stimulants over behavioral approaches is much less marked, or even absent, when ADHD symptomatology is mild (see chapter 34), and antidepressants are probably more likely to be effective when the depression is accompanied by vegetative symptoms such as sleep and appetite disturbance, and psychomotor retardation (see chapter 37). In most cases, medication will need to be combined with some form of psychological or educational intervention. That is because, in most cases, although medication brings marked benefits, it does not restore normality and steps may be needed to help the child and/or family cope more effectively and deal with any life situations or circumstances that provide psychopathological risk. Such steps may involve guidance or counseling of some kind but, in other cases, more intensive psychological intervention may be indicated. Decisions will need to be guided by what seem to be risk features either in the psychosocial situation or the child's style of thinking, or perhaps of behavior. It should be added, however, that the use of medication will carry psychological messages and that, unless carefully handled, these can undermine the psychological intervention (for an example in relation to dieting see Craighead, Stunkard, & O'Brien, 1981). The implication is not that different forms of intervention should not be combined but rather that the clinician needs to be concerned to present the combination in an appropriate way.

However, it should not be thought that drugs will influence only somatic features and not cognitions. The use of antidepressants in adult depression makes it clear that that is not the case (see chapter 37). Equally, it should not be supposed that psychological treatments cannot influence somatic functioning. The effects of psychological treatments in obsessive-compulsive disorder, in terms of their effects on functional imaging findings, negate that expectation (Baxter, Schwartz, Bergman *et al.*, 1992). However, recent research indicates that the effects of treatments on the brain may vary according to whether or not the treatment has been psychological or pharmacological, or whether a placebo has been used (Goldapple, Segal, Garson *et al.*, 2004). At present, it is not clear quite how these findings should be used in thinking about the diagnostic formulation, but what they do indicate is the fallacy of assuming that psychological interventions operate only on the mind and pharmacological ones only on the brain. In fact, both do both, albeit in slightly different ways. Nevertheless, in relation to hypotheses about maintaining factors, the clinician will wish to take decisions on the appropriate choice, and mixture, of therapeutic interventions. It is important that this is done in a way that carries with it predictions as to how it will be clear whether the therapeutic hypothesis is correct or needs modification as a result of the response to intervention.

A good treatment plan will include an indication of how one can tell whether it is meeting its goals. This may be an expectation of what symptoms on a rating scale will change, or a less tangible prediction for a change in family or peer relationships. Whatever the intended outcome, it should be clear enough that one can check whether it is being achieved. The spirit of hypothesis-testing, which we have emphasized throughout this chapter, implies that formulations must be able to shift in the light of review. One example would be that of a child who presented with marked inattentiveness at school, who was sleepy in the daytime and markedly sleepless at night. The initial formulation was unified: the lack of sleep was thought to cause both drowsiness and poor attention. Successful treatment of the insomnia, however, did nothing to help the tendency to fall asleep in the daytime and it became clear that the two sleep problems were in fact independent and needed different interventions.

As Hoch (1964) pointed out many decades ago, one of the key challenges in the whole of treatment, not only in psychiatry but right across medicine, is why treatments work for some individuals yet not for others. Similarly, side-effects can be really problematic in some people yet of minor importance in others. The field of pharmacogenetics (see chapter 23) carries with it the promise that genetic findings may help in this connection because of the evidence that genetic factors influence people's susceptibility to drugs and probably also their susceptibility to psychological interventions. At the moment, pharmacogenetics is a field with promise but one with, as yet, few direct clinical implications for the care of individual patients.

Research findings are not as helpful as one might wish in the choice of which particular kind of psychological treatment to use, when that is the approach that is being adopted. Although the evidence is reasonably consistent that focused goal-oriented interventions work better than open-ended, more general ones (Rutter, 1982), that would seem to suggest that the specifics of the treatment are important and that general support is not enough. On the other hand, although the range of comparisons remains more limited than one would like, the evidence does not indicate that, for any disorder, one particular style of psychological treatment is clearly generally better than others. Moreover, even when treatment is given by experienced clinicians, with an investment in more intensive treatments, studies with both young people (Le Grange, Eisler, Dare *et al.*, 1992) and adults (Wallerstein, 1986) have often shown that skilled counseling may be as effective as more intensive psychological interventions that are designed to get more into the heart of the psychological problem. Although it should certainly not be supposed that simple treatments are always to be preferred, the findings do indicate that the more complicated and intensive ones are not necessarily better. Decisions on the particular form of psychological intervention probably need to be guided by the nature of the psychological difficulties, the personal characteristics and preferences of the individual child and family, and the preferences of the clinician in terms of skills, experience and preferred mode of working. Nevertheless, cost–benefit considerations are important and the choice of a more prolonged treatment over a shorter one will always need to be justified.

Standards for Practice

Clinical practice must be performed under a variety of administrative and financial constraints. We have outlined what is needed in psychiatric assessment; health services may often wish to make some assessments of mental function that fall short of psychiatric assessment. This is often justified, and problems such as uncomplicated bedwetting, or parental discomfort at coping with young children's oppositional behavior, may well need no more than a simple screen as to whether problems are present that indicate a psychiatric assessment.

However, when problems are big enough and persistent enough to require referral, then information is needed about all the above domains – the nature of the disorder based on several sources of information, coexistent problems, impairment, course of disorder and psychosocial experiences, together with a professional judgment to synthesize them.

Assessment for Court Reports and Other Comparable Situations

Clinical assessment and diagnostic formulations tend ordinarily to be thought of in terms of what should be done with respect to a young person who is referred to a clinic because somebody feels that there is a problem and that something needs to be done to help. However, in addition, there are a variety of situations in which the clinician (whether psychiatrist, psychologist, pediatrician or social worker) is expected to serve as an expert witness in relation to some dispute that has come before the courts or some other decision-making body (see chapter 8). The assessment, rules and principles are, in essence, closely comparable to those that apply in the clinic situation (although the reporting and responsibilities are different) but there are several particular considerations that require emphasis.

To begin with, it is absolutely essential to be explicit about the expertise that one does, and does not, have. For example, the case might be one where there is litigation over whether or not a child has developed autism (or some other condition) as a result of immunization, head injury or an infection. The clinical expert can usually express well-informed views on the nature of the child's disorder, on whether its onset and course are atypical in any way that casts light on the nature of the disorder, and on what is known about the causes of the condition in question. On the other hand, psychiatrists and psychologists are not likely to be expert on particular detailed laboratory findings and the report needs to be careful to avoid straying on to conclusions based on types of evidence on which the person is not expert.

Similarly, dispute may focus on the statistical likelihood of a particular association between some postulated causal factor and the specified outcome, or on the likelihood that, when two or more children in the same family have died or suffered from a particular injury, this implies malevolent action on the part of the parent. Particular care needs to be taken on interpreting the meaning of any particular statistical likelihood, as well as the strength of the particular likelihood. As always in clinical diagnosis and assessment, it is crucial to consider competing possibilities. For example, if the occurrence of two cases of autism arising in the same family is being alleged to be a result of parental mishandling, the report would need to draw attention to the likelihood that genetic factors may have played a part. Alternatively, if the outcome is tuberculosis, it would be important to bear in mind the likelihood that multiple cases in the same family may stem from the spread of infection. Those are obvious circumstances and the dispute usually arises when causation is nowhere near so obvious. Nevertheless, the same need arises to consider the possibility that genetic factors or shared environmental factors (other than those involving parental abuse) may be responsible. Where relevant, attention needs to be drawn to what possible investigations might be undertaken that could help in resolving the issue. A further consideration is that the clinician needs to consider what is the appropriate comparison to be made. The issue will very rarely be one of simply whether multiple cases of the condition could have arisen by chance, but rather what is the relative likelihood of its having arisen through some genetic or shared environmental factor rather than parental abuse. Clinicians would need to ask themselves whether there is research evidence that has shown the likelihood of particular answers when the starting point is uncertainty of a comparable kind to the case in question. In short, the court may be asking the expert whether some particular outcome is a result of some alleged cause, but, just as in the situation where a child is referred with the question as to whether the behavior is caused by, say, schizophrenia, the duty of the clinician is to look much more broadly at the issues and not confine attention to the one alleged possibility.

A further need is to ensure that attention is drawn to findings (whether clinical or laboratory) that raise doubts about the particular opinion the expert is putting forward. In other words, it is the obligation of the clinician to make explicit the evidence for and against, and not simply come up with some *ex cathedra* assertion. When expert opinions have proved potentially misleading it is usually because either expertise has been claimed when the person does not have the relevant expertise, or attention has not been paid to possible competing explanations, or the statistical comparisons have been made against a too limiting set of alternatives, or possibly relevant evidence has been omitted from the report despite the fact that the expert knew about the evidence.

A further need is to pay careful attention to the relevant research evidence, as well as the findings in the particular case, and to make explicit the logic and reasoning that constitute the basis of the opinion being expressed. Particularly in criminal courts, the lawyers on either side are likely to press the expert for a definitive statement as to whether something did or did not occur. If such a definitive opinion is possible, that is fine, and it should be stated, but in most instances the valid conclusion is likely to be probabilistic rather than categorically determinative and that should be made explicit, regardless of pressures to come down on one side or the other.

Perhaps most frequently of all, clinicians are likely to be called upon to give evidence when there is disagreement as to whether, following the break-up of a marriage or break-up of a family, a particular child should be placed with one parent or the other, or should have this amount or that amount of time with each parent, or indeed whether it is safe for the child to have unsupervised contact with a particular parent when the evidence suggests that abuse may have taken place. In almost all circumstances that come to court, there is no ideal solution. In these circumstances, the obligation of the expert is to consider carefully the pluses and the minuses of the various alternatives and to put forward a carefully considered opinion as to what is the most desirable (or least undesirable) course to take. It is also quite common for it to be necessary to express opinions on the basis of some contingency as to how things are managed or how something is dealt with. It is the sort of thinking that ought to constitute the basis of any clinical assessment but it is a very healthy challenge for clinicians to have to be as explicit as they need to be in making overt the reasoning for their opinions and the balance of evidence on which they are having to rely.

In recent high-profile cases, senior figures in the profession have expressed grave worries about the dangers that professionals face in giving evidence in cases that involve disputes over child protection. In our view, these concerns are misplaced. It is true that there have been ill-judged and unreasonable campaigns against the opinions of some expert in particular cases. It is also, of course, not unknown for even the most careful, skilled and thoughtful assessments to be sometimes in error. We all make mistakes. What is required is that we take the greatest care in coming to decisions, to be fully honest in the way we express opinions (including doubts and uncertainties where these are present) and to be willing to change our opinion if it is made evident that either there is evidence that we did not know about or, alternatively, that there are facts or findings either in the literature or in a particular case that indicate that we have been in error.

In the British judicial system, it is explicit that the expert's duty is to the court, and not to whoever has called them to give evidence (or who has paid their fees). That is not so in all countries but, in our view, there is much to be said for having it explicit that where the expertise is being sought in relation to the needs of a particular child, the expert's loyalties are to do the best for that child and that is most easily accomplished if the expert is called by the court, rather than by one or other of the parties in dispute. At the moment, that is the exception rather than the rule and it is to be hoped that this may change in the future.

In other circumstances, the expert may be asked to give an opinion in relation to some specific skill or capacity. For example, this often arises with respect to decisions on whether or not a child can be held responsible for their actions in relation to some alleged criminal activity. In these circumstances, the clinician will need to think carefully on how to assess such responsibility and to recognize that it cannot be carried out purely on the basis of age or IQ. There are marked individual differences in children's ability to understand, even when the children are all of the same age or IQ. Moreover, understanding is likely to be influenced by children's particular experiences in relation to relevant circumstances, and the ability to understand may also be influenced by the nature and gravity of the alleged offence (Royal College of Psychiatrists, 2006).

Precisely similar issues arise with respect to decisions on whether children are, or are not, competent to give permission, or refuse permission, for particular forms of treatment (or on whether or not to participate in research – Royal College of Psychiatrists Working Party, 2001). These are not easy decisions to make and there are no entirely satisfactory tests that may be employed. On the other hand, there are some reasonable guidelines that have been put forward (British Medical Association, 2000). A rather more specific example of a related issue has concerned cases in the past where it has been alleged that children have made statements about being abused or about their wishes for some particular family arrangement and have done so through what has been called "facilitated communication." This is a circumstance in which the child is supposed to convey what they want to say through some technical device that involves the cooperation of another person. The whole topic of "facilitated communication" has proved to be a controversial one but, from an expert witness point of view, the key issue is to find a means of determining whether the statements derive from the child or from the adult who was assisting. The usual solution to this dilemma has been to set up a procedure in which the answer is influenced by what is known to the facilitator but not to the child (Rutter & Yule, 2002).

Conclusions

In this chapter we have sought to bring together some of the main considerations that need to guide the approach to diagnostic assessment and the planning of treatment. Research findings have been informative in providing guidance on some of the methods of assessment that work better than others and have undoubtedly indicated the value of a systematic approach to the degree of standardization. However, it is always necessary to be responsive to the individual needs and circumstances of each patient, to pick up cues and to adapt assessment procedures accordingly. With respect to both diagnosis and the planning of treatment, it is also important to adopt a problem-solving, hypothesis-generating, and hypothesis-testing, style. The gathering of factual data on psychopathological signs and symptoms and on risk and protective circumstances constitutes the essential basis. On that basis, it is important to seek to tell a "story" about causal processes and to use that "story" to plan a treatment strategy and to do so in a way in which the response to treatment may indicate whether or not the therapeutic hypothesis was correct.

References

Achenbach, T. M., McConaughy, S. H., & Howell, C. T. (1987). Child–adolescent behavioral and emotional problems: Implications of cross-informant correlations for situation specificity. *Psychological Bulletin*, *101*, 213–232.

American Psychiatric Association. (2000). *Diagnostic and statistical manual of mental disorders* (4th ed.) (DSM-IV-TR). Washington DC: American Psychiatric Association.

Angold, A., Erkanlis, A., Costello, E. J., & Rutter, M. (1996). Precision, reliability and accuracy in the dating of symptom onsets in child and adolescent psychopathology. *Journal of Child Psychology and Psychiatry*, *37*, 657–664.

Angold, A., Costello, E., Farmer, E. M. Z., Burns, B. J., & Erkanli, A. (1999). Impaired but undiagnosed. *Journal of the American Academy of Child and Adolescent Psychiatry*, *38*, 129–137.

Asperger, H. (1944). Die "Autistischen Psychopathen" im Kindesalter. *Archiv für Psychiatrie und Nervkrankheiten*, *117*, 76–136. Translated in U. Frith (Ed.), *Autism & Asperger syndrome* (pp. 37–92). Cambridge, UK: Cambridge University Press.

Baxter, L. R., Schwartz, J. M., Bergman, K. S., Szuba, M. P., Guze, B. H., Mazziotta, J. C., *et al.* (1992). Caudate glucose metabolic rate changes with both drug and behavior therapy for obsessive-compulsive disorder. *Archives of General Psychiatry*, *49*, 681–689.

Bird, H. (1999). The assessment of functional impairment. In D. Shaffer, C. P. Lucas, & J. E. Richters (Eds.), *Diagnostic assessment in child and adolescent psychopathology* (pp. 209–229). New York, London: Guilford Press.

Bird, H. R., Yager, T., Staghezza, B., Gould, M., Canino, G., & Rubio-Stipec, M. (1990). Impairment in the epidemiological measurement of childhood psychopathology in the community. *Journal of the American Academy of Child and Adolescent Psychiatry*, *29*, 796–803.

Borge, A., Samuelsen, S., & Rutter, M. (2001). Observer variance within families: Confluence among maternal, paternal and child ratings. *International Journal of Methods in Psychiatric Research*, *10*, 11–21.

British Medical Association. (2000). *Consent, rights and choices in health care for children and young people.* London: BMJ Books.

Brown, R., Hobson, R. P., & Lee, A. (1997). Are there autistic-like features in congenitally blind children? *Journal of Child Psychology and Psychiatry*, *38*, 693–704.

Brown, G., & Rutter, M. (1966). The measurement of family activities and relationships: A methodological study. *Human Relations*, *19*, 241–263.

Caplan, H. (1970). *Hysterical "conversion" symptoms in childhood* (M. Phil dissertation, University of London).

Carbonneau, R., Eaves, L. J., Silberg, J. L., Simonoff, E., & Rutter, M. (2002a). Assessment of the within-family environment in twins: Absolute versus differential ratings, and relationship with conduct problems. *Psychological Medicine*, *32*, 729–741.

Carbonneau, R., Rutter, M., Simonoff, E., Silberg, J. L., Maes, H. H., & Eaves, L. J. (2002b). The Twin Inventory of Relationships and Experiences (TIRE): Psychometric properties of a measure of the nonshared and shared environmental experiences of twins and singletons. *International Journal of Methods in Psychiatric Research*, *10*, 72–85.

Clarke, A. M., & Clarke, A. D. B. (2000). *Early experience and the life path.* London: Jessica Kingsley.

Clegg, J., Hollis, C., Mawhood, L., & Rutter, M. (2005). Developmental language disorder: A follow-up in later adult life. Cognitive, language, and psychosocial outcomes. *Journal of Child Psychology and Psychiatry*, *46*, 128–149.

Conger, R. D., Conger, K. J., Elder, G. H., Lorenz, F. O., Simons, R. L., & Whitbeck, L. B. (1992). A family process model of economic hardship and adjustment of early adolescent boys. *Child Development*, *63*, 526–541.

Conger, R. D., Conger, K. J., Elder, G. H., & Lorenz, F. O. (1993). Family economic stress and adjustment of early adolescent girls. *Developmental Psychology*, *29*, 206–219.

Cox, A., Hemsley, R., & Dare, J. (1995). A comparison of individual and family approaches to initial assessment. *European Child and Adolescent Psychiatry*, *4*, 94–101.

Cox, A., & Rutter, M. (1985). Diagnostic appraisal and interviewing. In M. Rutter & L. Hersov (Eds.), *Child and adolescent psychiatry: Modern approaches* (2nd ed.) (pp. 233–248). Oxford: Blackwell Scientific Publications.

Cox, A., Rutter, M., & Holbrook, D. (1981). Psychiatric interviewing techniques: V. Experimental study: Eliciting factual information. *British Journal of Preventive and Social Medicine*, *31*, 29–37.

Craighead, L. W., Stunkard, A. J. & O'Brien, R. M. (1981). Behaviour therapy and pharmacotherapy for obesity. *Archives of General Psychiatry*, *38*, 763–768.

Delaney-Black, V., Covington, C., Templin, T., Ager, J., Nordstrom-Klee, B., Martier, S., *et al.* (2000). Teacher-assessed behavior of children prenatally exposed to cocaine. *Pediatrics*, *106*, 782–791.

Fergusson, D. M., Horwood, L. J., & Lynskey, M. T. (1992). Family change, parental discord and early offending. *Journal of Child Psychology and Psychiatry*, *33*, 1059–1073.

Goldapple, K., Segal, Z., Garson, C., Lau, M., Bieling, P., Kennedy, S., *et al.* (2004). Treatment-specific effects of Cognitive Behavior Therapy. *Archives of General Psychiatry*, *61*, 34–41.

Green, J. (2006). Annotation: The therapeutic alliance – a significant but neglected variable in child mental health treatment studies. *Journal of Child Psychology and Psychiatry*, *47*, 425–435.

Hagberg, B., Aicardi, J., Dias, K., & Ramos, O. (1983). A progressive syndrome of autism, dementia, ataxia and loss of purposeful hand use in girls: Rett syndrome: report of 35 cases. *Annals of Neurology*, *14*, 471–479.

Hill, J., & Maughan, B. (Eds.). (2001). *Conduct disorders in childhood and adolescence*. Cambridge: Cambridge University Press.

Hoch, P. H. (1964). In P. H. Hoch & J. Zubin (Eds.), *The evaluation of psychiatric treatment* (pp. 55–56). New York: Grune & Stratton.

Jones, K. L., & Smith, D. W. (1973). Recognition of the fetal alcohol syndrome in early infancy. *Lancet*, *2*, 999–1000.

Kanner, L. (1943). Autistic disturbances of affective contact. *Nervous Child*, *2*, 217–250.

Kanner, L. (1957). *Child Psychiatry* (3rd ed.). Springfield, IL: Chas. C. Thomas.

Kanner, L. (1969). The children haven't read those books: Reflections on differential diagnosis. *Acta Paedopsychiatrica*, *36*, 2–11.

Kazdin, A. E., Whitley, M., & Marciano, P. L. (2006). Child–therapist and parent–therapist alliance and therapeutic change in the treatment of children referred for oppositional, aggressive and antisocial behavior. *Journal of Child Psychology and Psychiatry*, *47*, 436–445.

Le Grange, D., Eisler, I., Dare, C., & Russell, G. F. M. (1992). Evaluation of family treatments in adolescent anorexia nervosa: A pilot study. *International Journal of Eating Disorders*, *12*, 347–357.

Lord, C., Risi, S., Lambrecht, L., Cook, E. H. Jr., Leventhal, B. L., DiLavore, P. C., *et al.* (2000). The Autism Diagnostic Observation Schedule-Generic: A standard measure of social and communication deficits associated with the spectrum of autism. *Journal of Autism and Developmental Disorders*, *30*, 205–223.

Magaña, A. B., Goldstein, M. J., Karno, M., & Miklowitz, D. J. (1986). A brief method for assessing expressed emotion in relatives of psychiatric patients. *Psychiatric Research*, *17*, 203–212.

Mazure, C., & Gershon, E. S. (1979). Blindness and reliability in lifetime psychiatric diagnosis. *Archives of General Psychiatry*, *36*, 521–525.

Pickles, A., Rowe, R., Simonoff, E., Foley, D., Rutter, M., & Silberg, J. (2001). Child psychiatric symptoms and psychosocial impairment: Relationships and prognostic significance. *British Journal of Psychiatry*, *179*, 230–235.

Reiss, D., Hetherington, M., Plomin, R., Howe, G. W., Simmens, S. J., Henderson, S. H., *et al.* (1995). Genetic questions for environmental studies: Differential parenting and psychopathology in adolescence. *Archives of General Psychiatry*, *52*, 925–936.

Reiss, D., Neiderhiser, J. M., Hetherington, E. M., & Plomin, R. (2000). *The relationship code: Deciphering genetic and social influences on adolescent development*. Cambridge, MA: Harvard University Press.

Rett, A. (1966). Uber ein eigenartiges himatrophisches Syndrom bei Hyperammonamie in Kindesalter. *Weiner Medizinische Wochenschrift*, *116*, 723–726.

Royal College of Psychiatrists' Working Party. (2001). *Guidelines for researchers and for research ethics committees on psychiatric research involving human participants*. Council Report no. CR82. London: Royal College of Psychiatrists.

Royal College of Psychiatrists. (2006). *Child defendants*. (OP56). London: Royal College of Psychiatrists.

Russell, G. F. M. (1979). Bulimia nervosa: An ominous variant of anorexia nervosa. *Psychological Medicine*, *9*, 429–448.

Rutter, M. (1971). Parent–child separation: Psychological effects on the children. *Journal of Child Psychology and Psychiatry*, *12*, 233–260.

Rutter, M. (1975). *Helping troubled children*. Harmondsworth, Middlesex: Penguin Books.

Rutter, M. (1982). Psychological therapies: Issues and prospects. *Psychological Medicine*, *12*, 723–740.

Rutter, M. (1985). Infantile autism. In D. Shaffer, A. Erhardt, & L. Greenhill (Eds.), *The Clinical Guide to Child Psychiatry* (pp. 48–78). New York: Free Press.

Rutter, M. (1987). Assessment of language disorders. In W. Yule & M. Rutter (Eds.), *Language development and disorders* (pp. 295–311). Oxford: Blackwell Scientific Publications.

Rutter, M. (1989). Psychiatric disorder in parents as a risk factor in children. In D. Shaffer, I. Philips, N. Enver, M. Silverman & V. Anthony (Eds.), *Prevention of psychiatric disorders in child and adolescent: The project of the American Academy of Child and Adolescent Psychiatry*. OSAP Prevention Monograph 2 (pp. 157–189). Rockville, MD: Office of Substance Abuse Prevention, US Department of Health and Human Services.

Rutter, M. (1990). Psychosocial resilience and protective mechanisms. In J. Rolf, A. S. Masten, D. Cicchetti, K. N. Neuchterlein & S. Weintraub (Eds.), *Risk and protective factors in the development of psychopathology* (pp. 181–214). Cambridge & New York: Cambridge University Press.

Rutter, M. (1999). Resilience concepts and findings: Implications for family therapy. *Journal of Family Therapy*, *21*, 119–144.

Rutter, M. (2000a). Psychosocial influences: Critiques, findings, and research needs. *Development and Psychopathology*, *12*, 375–405.

Rutter, M. (2000b). Resilience reconsidered: Conceptual considerations, empirical findings and policy implications. In J. P. Shonkoff & S. J. Meisels (Eds.), *Handbook of early childhood intervention* (pp. 651–682). New York & Cambridge: Cambridge University Press.

Rutter, M. (2006). Implications of resilience concepts for scientific understanding. *Annals of the New York Academy of Science*, *1094*, 1–12.

Rutter, M. (2007). Proceeding from observed correlation to causal inference: The use of natural experiments. *Perspective on Psychological Science*, *2*, 377–395.

Rutter, M., Andersen-Wood, L., Beckett, C., Bredenkamp, D., Castle, J., Groothues, C., *et al.* (1999). Quasi-autistic patterns following severe early global privation. *Journal of Child Psychology and Psychiatry*, *40*, 537–549.

Rutter, M., & Brown, G. (1966). The reliability and validity of measure of family life and relationships in families containing a psychiatric patient. *Social Psychiatry*, *1*, 38–53.

Rutter, M., Chadwick, O., & Shaffer, D. (1983). Head injury. In M. Rutter (Ed.), *Developmental Neuropsychiatry* (pp. 83–111). New York: Guilford Press.

Rutter, M., Cox, A., Egert, S., Holbrook, D., & Everitt, B. (1981). Psychiatric interviewing techniques. IV. Experimental study: Four contrasting styles. *British Journal of Psychiatry*, *138*, 456–465.

Rutter, M., Kreppner, J., O'Connor, T., & the E. R. A. Research team. (2001). Specificity and heterogeneity in children's responses to profound privation. *British Journal of Psychiatry*, *179*, 97–103.

Rutter, M., Giller, H., & Hagell, A. (1998). *Antisocial behavior by young people*. New York & London: Cambridge University Press.

Rutter, M., Maughan, B., Meyer, J., Pickles, A., Silberg, J., Simonoff, E., *et al.* (1997). Heterogeneity of antisocial behavior: Causes, continuities, and consequences. In R. Dienstbier (Series Editor), & D. W. Osgood (Volume Editor), *Nebraska Symposium on Motivation* (Vol. 44), *Motivation and delinquency* (pp. 45–118). Lincoln, NE: University of Nebraska Press.

Rutter, M., Pickles, A., Murray, R., & Eaves, L. (2001). Testing hypotheses on environmental risk mechanisms. *Psychological Bulletin*, *127*, 291–324.

Rutter, M., & Sandberg, S. (1992). Psychosocial stressors: Concepts, causes and effects. *European Journal of Child and Adolescent Psychiatry*, *1*, 3–13.

Rutter, M., Tizard, J., & Whitmore, K. (1970). *Education, health and behaviour*. Longmans, London. Reprinted 1981. Melbourne: F.A. Krieger.

Rutter, M., & Yule, W. (2002). Applied scientific thinking in clinical assessment. In M. Rutter & E. Taylor (Eds.), *Child and Adolescent Psychiatry* (4th ed.) (pp. 103–116). Oxford: Blackwell Science.

Sandberg, S., Rutter, M., Giles, S., Owen, A., Champion, L., Nicholls, J., *et al.* (1993). Assessment of psychosocial experiences in childhood: Methodological issues and some illustrative findings. *Journal of Child Psychology and Psychiatry*, *34*, 879–897.

Sandberg, S., Rutter, M., Pickles, A., McGuinness, D., & Angold, A. (2001). Do high threat life events really provoke the onset of psychiatric disorder in children? *Journal of Child Psychology and Psychiatry*, *42*, 523–532.

Sandler, I., Tein, J-Y., Mehta, P., Wolchik, S., & Ayers, T. (2000). Coping efficacy and psychological problems of children of divorce. *Child Development*, *71*, 1099–1118.

Shepherd, M., Oppenheim, B., & Mitchell, S. (1971). *Childhood behaviour and mental health*. London: University of London Press.

Shonkoff, J. P., & Phillips, D. A. (2000). *From neurons to neighborhoods: The science of early childhood development*. Washington, DC: National Academy Press.

Simonoff, E., Pickles, A., Meyer, J., Silberg, J. L., Maes, H. H., Loeber, R., *et al.* (1997). The Virginia Twin Study of Adolescent Behavioral Development: Influences of age, sex and impairment in rates of disorder. *Archives of General Psychiatry*, *54*, 801–808.

Singer, L., Arendt, R., Farkas, K., Minnes, S., Huang, J., & Yamashita, T. (1997). Relationship of prenatal cocaine exposure and maternal postpartum psychological distress to child developmental outcome. *Development and Psychopathology*, *9*, 473–489.

Slater, E. (1965). The diagnosis of 'hysteria'. *British Medical Journal*, *1*, 1395–1399.

Spohr, L., & Steinhausen, C. (Eds.). (1996). *Alcohol, pregnancy and the developing child*. Cambridge, UK: Cambridge University Press.

Stattin, H., & Kerr, M. (2000). Parental monitoring: A reinterpretation. *Child Development*, *71*, 1072–1085.

Stratton, K., Howe, C., & Battaglia, F. (1996). *Fetal alcohol syndrome: Diagnosis, epidemiology, prevention, and treatment*. Washington, DC: National Academy Press.

van Goor-Lambo, G., Orley, J., Poustka, F., & Rutter, M. (1990). Classification of abnormal psychosocial situations: Preliminary report of a revision of a WHO scheme. *Journal of Child Psychology and Psychiatry*, *31*, 229–241.

Wallerstein, R. S. (1986). *Forty-two lives in treatment: A study of psychoanalysis and psychotherapy*. New York & London: Guilford Press.

Wolff, S. (1995). *Childhood and human nature: The development of personality*. London & New York: Routledge.

Wootton, B. (1959). *Social science and social pathology*. London: George Allen & Unwin.

World Health Organization. (1996). Multiaxial classification of child and adolescent psychiatric disorders. *The ICD-10 Classification of Mental and Behavioral Disorders in Children and Adolescents*. Cambridge, UK: Cambridge University Press.

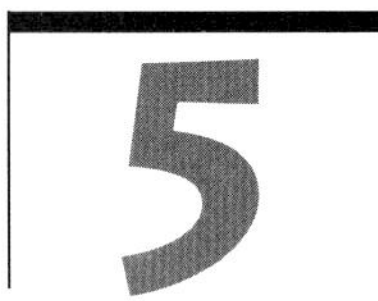

Using Epidemiological and Longitudinal Approaches to Study Causal Hypotheses

E. Jane Costello

Felix qui potuit rerum cognoscere causas.

Happy the one who has been able to learn the causes of things.

Virgil, *Georgics II*, 490

This chapter reviews what epidemiological and longitudinal research can tell us about the causes of child and adolescent mental illness. The job of epidemiology is to understand patterns of distribution of disease in time and space, so that those patterns can provide a guide to preventing disease (Kleinbaum, Kupper, & Morganstern, 1982). Not all epidemiological studies are longitudinal, and cross-sectional studies can also provide useful clues to the causes of illness. However, many epidemiological studies have studied longitudinal patterns of disease distribution over time as a test of causality; for example, to see whether smokers die younger than non-smokers (Doll & Hill, 1966). In this chapter, the main focus is on studies that are both epidemiological and longitudinal; that is, they make use of patterns in both space and time to develop and test ideas about what might be causing disorders.

Using Epidemiological Studies to Answer Causal Questions

Observation, categorization, pattern recognition, hypothesis testing, causal thinking – these are the stages through which a science tends to progress as it advances in knowledge and rigor (Feist, 2006). People tend to think of epidemiology as primarily a descriptive discipline, stuck at a fairly primitive level in its development as a science, somewhere between categorization and pattern recognition (Maldonado & Greenland, 2002). However, pattern recognition in the study of disease (how the distribution of disease deviates from random) can serve more than one purpose. Of course, descriptions of the prevalence and burden of disease in various places and at various times are critical for planning services and warning of epidemics, but studying these patterns can also generate hypotheses about what might be causing a disease or encouraging its spread. Observing the spread of a disease from one person to another across a city, a country or a continent may provide clues about its mode of transmission (by touch? sneezing? sexual contact?) and thus about what causes it, while the length of time between cases can give hints about the necessary incubation period, and thence the type of mechanism driving the disease process. In the case of psychiatric disorders, we can also use observations of the distribution of disorders across both space (why is the prevalence of schizophrenia so high in immigrants from the Caribbean to England? Eagles, 1991) and time (why is there an increase in depression in girls at puberty? Angold, Costello, & Worthman, 1999) to explore possible causes. Thus, epidemiology can be descriptive and analytic at the same time, concerned with both observation and causation.

Causation and Counterfactuals

Scientists, including epidemiologists, are taught never to equate correlation with causation without better evidence than a statistically significant association. But how do we get beyond association? How can we know that something was the effect of a certain cause? We think we know clearly enough in everyday life, but people have argued for centuries about the true definitions of cause and effect. Attempts to define them can easily become circular.

An approach that has gained popularity since the 1960s is based on an idea of the 18th century philosopher David Hume: "We may define a cause to be an object followed by another, . . . where, if the first object had not been, the second never had existed" (Hume, 2000). A 20th century reformulation of the proposition states: "Where c and e are two distinct possible events, e causally depends on c if and only

Rutter's Child and Adolescent Psychiatry, 5th edition. Edited by M. Rutter, D. Bishop, D. Pine, S. Scott, J. Stevenson, E. Taylor and A. Thapar. © 2008 Blackwell Publishing, ISBN: 978-1-4051-4549-7.

if c occurs → e occurs and c does not occur → e does not occur" (Lewis, 1973).

For the empirical researcher, the question is how to demonstrate this in a given situation. However strongly I believe that poverty is the cause of behavioral problems in the children I observe in my epidemiological study, how can I test the hypothesis that the relationship is causal; that is, that if the families had not been poor then the behavioral problems would not have occurred ("social causation"), against the alternative hypothesis that the association between poverty and behavioral problems exists because more antisocial children are born into poor families ("social selection")? (Costello, Compton, Keeler *et al.*, 2003).

The prototypical experiment involves the idea of a counterfactual. If we expose a child to a fearful stimulus, and at the same time do not expose the same child to the same stimulus, we can argue that the difference in the same child's response to the two situations was caused by the fearful stimulus. As demonstrated by Robins and others (Maldonado & Greenland, 2002; Robins, 1997), the counterfactual approach to causal inference applies equally to observational and experimental designs, and is structurally equivalent to other systems of reasoning about cause and effect. Of course, this is an impossible research model because we cannot both expose and not expose the same child at the same time. "A counterfactual is something that is contrary to fact" (Shadish, Cook, & Campbell, 2002). However, the counterfactual metaphor is a useful one, because it sets a standard against which to judge the experimental and quasi-experimental designs that we discuss in this chapter.

In the real world, we generally follow John Stuart Mill's more practical approach, which states that a causal relationship becomes more likely if:

1 The cause preceded the effect;

2 We can assume some sort of relationship between cause and effect; and

3 Our identified cause is the only logical explanation we can find for the effect (Mill, 1856).

As researchers we try to create (or observe) a situation where these three principles hold. As our knowledge of an area increases, it may be possible to strengthen the causal argument by elaborating some parts of the relationship. For example, the famous Henle–Koch principles (Koch, 1882) elaborated by Hill (1965), Susser (1991) and for psychiatry by Robins and Guze (1970), impose additional requirements that broaden their applicability beyond infectious diseases. Hill's nine conditions comprise strength of association between "cause" and disease; consistency of the association over several studies; specificity of the association; temporal precedence of cause over outcome; biological gradient (e.g., a dose–response curve); biological plausibility; coherence (i.e., the explanation does not conflict with current knowledge about the natural history of the disease); experimental evidence; and analogy with similar "causes." It is important to note that Hill did not refer to these conditions as necessary "criteria," but rather as "viewpoints from all of which we should study association before we cry causation" (Hill, 1965).

Two Kinds of Causality

There are two kinds of causal inference that epidemiological studies of causality seek to establish: specific causal inference, the ability to infer that the observed relationship is a causal one, not merely *post hoc ergo propter hoc* ("after this, therefore because of this"); and generalized causal inference, the ability to infer that whatever causal relationship was observed or tested in a given study applies more generally, outside the confines of the specific samples used. A useful study of causality will permit both kinds of inference to be made: the predicted causal factor did indeed cause the observed outcome, and the relationship between the two applies beyond this study.

Specific Causal Inference

Random assignment to treatment conditions is an excellent tool in the effort to infer that an observed relationship really is a causal one. Randomization is the nearest we can come to unbiased assignment to intervention and non-intervention groups. It simplifies controlling extraneous variables that might confuse the picture, and measuring the dose of the factor expected to be causal. However, in epidemiological studies, random allocation to "treatment" and "no treatment" groups is rarely possible (we discuss later some ways in which researchers have tried to create unbiased assignment in other ways). Other threats to internal validity (i.e., the validity of a specific causal inference) are problems for clinical as well as epidemiological research, and are discussed in the next section. For example, selection criteria for the study must not create the risk of regression artifacts (e.g., selecting participants because they score at the top of the range on a behavior problem scale, so that they are likely to score lower next time, irrespective of the treatment), and attrition must not occur at different rates or for different reasons from different groups in the study.

Generalized Causal Inference

Establishing that a causal inference is generalizable beyond a specific experiment is also a problem for both clinical and epidemiological studies. Establishing generalizability involves two tasks: matching the "surface characteristics of an operation to those that are prototypical of a construct" (Shadish, Cook, & Campbell, 2002), known more informally as establishing "construct validity"; and establishing "the extent to which causal relationships generalize over variations in persons, settings, treatments, and outcomes (external validity)" (Shadish, Cook, & Campbell, 2002). However clearly a causal relationship may be established in a laboratory experiment, this is of little practical value until it is clear that:

1 The relationship shown in the experiment applies to the construct that the experiment was designed to model; and

2 The relationship holds outside the specific subjects, laboratory and methods used in the experiment.

To quote Shadish, Cook, & Campbell (2002) again, it is necessary to specify "(a) which parts of the treatment (b) affect which parts of the outcome (c) through which causal mediating processes in order to accurately describe the components that need to be transferred to other situations to reproduce the effect." Where internal validity refers to the validity of inferences about whether an observed covariation between (a) and (b) reflects a causal relationship, construct validity refers to the validity of inferences about the higher order constructs that the procedures of the study instantiate.

Causal Inference in Epidemiology

General causal validity is one area in which quasi-experimental epidemiological studies may have the edge over laboratory experiments. The reason for this is an extension of external validity that has been labeled "ecological validity" (Bronfenbrenner, 1977). Each experiment takes place in a specific setting, at a specific time. There may be characteristics of that setting or time that interfere with the simple logic of the experiment. For example, it is notoriously difficult to study blood pressure in laboratory settings because of the "white coat" phenomenon that plays havoc with people's "resting" blood pressure in the presence of nurses and doctors. Even when a causal hypothesis is supported in laboratory studies, its effect size needs to be estimated in the real world.

Does Correlation Mean Causation or Doesn't it?

Many research papers infer causation from a simple correlational observation. Later we discuss some better research strategies; here we point out some questions that have to be answered before a causal inference can safely be drawn. More details and further examples can be found in Rutter (2007) and Shadish, Cook, & Campbell (2002).

Which Variable Came First?

Does a good education lead to a higher income, or does a higher income enable a family to buy a better education? A variant on this theme occurs when what looks like the outcome turns out to be the cause. For example, 40 years ago Richard Bell argued that "Current literature on socialization, based largely on correlations between parent and child behavior, can be reinterpreted plausibly as indicating effects of children on parents" (Bell & Harper, 1977).

Is There an Alternative Explanation for the Correlation?

Does a lack of exercise cause weight gain, or is weight gain caused by a high fat diet, which is more common in people who do not exercise? A variant on this occurs when the putative causal variable is associated with the true cause. For example, in unpublished analyses of a longitudinal community study of children and adolescents we compared the effects of growing up with a range of family structures (e.g., single, adopted or step-parent) with the effects of a disrupted family structure, via death or divorce or a new parental figure, controlling for family structure. We found that it was disruption, not family structure itself, that "caused" children's behavioral problems. However, some family structures, such as having a single parent, were much more likely to be disrupted than others, such as having two biological parents, so the "true" cause was correlated with the putative cause.

Conclusions

We have argued that proving a causal relationship is difficult whatever research design is used. Balancing specific causality against general causality can require trade-offs in research design. In the next section we consider how longitudinal designs can help.

Using Longitudinal Data to Test Causal Hypotheses

Epidemiologists will often carry out repeated surveys to estimate whether some phenomenon (e.g., smoking) has increased or decreased. The essence of using repeated measures of the same subjects for testing causal hypotheses is that the subjects serve as their own controls. This eliminates some of the uncertainty about whether differences between measurements taken before and after an event are the result of using different subjects.

The passage of time can be interpreted in different ways that have different implications for causality. For example, age at first exposure to a risk, length of time since first exposure, and duration of exposure to risk are all interrelated aspects of timing of risk that may have different implications for causality and thus for prevention.

Duration of Exposure

Sometimes, the length of exposure to a risk factor may be a key to its harmful effects. For example, Duncan, Yeung, Brooks-Gunn *et al.* (1998) and Duncan, Brooks-Gunn, & Klebanov (1994) have made use of several longitudinal data sets containing information on family income to compare the relative importance of age at exposure to poverty and duration of exposure. They found a major effect of the persistence of poverty on emotional symptoms such as "dependence, anxiety, and unhappiness" (Brooks-Gunn & Duncan, 1997), whereas current but not persistent poverty was associated with higher levels of hyperactivity and peer conflict. However, effects of duration of poverty on conduct problems were seen in two other longitudinal studies (Moffitt, 1990; Offord, Boyle, Racine *et al.*, 1992), so the picture is far from clear.

A series of papers from the English and Romanian Adoption Study Team addresses the impact of duration of risk exposure on cognition and affect some years after the risk was removed. Romanian children who had been in institutional care and were adopted before age 4 by families in the UK were compared with children born and adopted within the UK (Croft, O'Connor, Keaveney *et al.*, 2001). The key exposure was neglect by caregivers, the outcome variable was parent–child relationship, and the hypothesis tested was that developmental and/or cognitive delay, a known consequence of severe early deprivation, would mediate the relationship between early deprivation and parent–child relations. Duration of exposure to adversity was associated with more negative and less positive parent–child relations at age 4. By age 6, however, an effect was only seen in those who entered the UK after the age of 2, and who presumably suffered the most protracted exposure.

Age at Onset of Exposure

The importance of age at first exposure has been studied most intensively of all the aspects of risk over time in child psychopathology, because of the theoretical importance attached to early experiences in psychodynamic models of development. For example, researchers investigating the role of attachment in children's development have concentrated on the very early months and years of life as the crucial period during which the inability to form one or more such relationships may have damaging effects that last into childhood and perhaps even into adulthood (Sroufe, 1988). In this case the critical date of onset of risk appears to occur after 6 months, but the duration of the risk period is not yet clear.

Timing of Exposure

Sometimes, longitudinal studies can clarify the difference between age at exposure and the developmental stage that a child is going through. For example, Rutter has pointed out that once children have achieved urinary continence at around age 2, there is a period of risk for relapse into incontinence that appears to coincide with starting school (Rutter, 1985). Once this period of risk is over, the chance of developing enuresis is very slight. In this case, developmental stage at exposure is clearly the critical developmental risk factor, because no parallel increase in functional enuresis occurs at later times of stress, such as moving to middle or high school, and there is no delay between the stress and the symptoms.

The difference between timing of exposure and length of exposure can also yield clues about causation. For example, a study of insulation workers exposed to asbestos found a cumulative risk of dying of mesothelioma over a 20-year period (controlling for other causes of death) that was the same irrespective of age at first exposure (Peto, Seidman, & Selikoff, 1982). Here, *length of exposure* was the critical aspect of risk. In contrast, the risk of breast cancer following irradiation appears to be highest in girls exposed at ages 0–9, falling with age until there is little excess risk for breast cancer associated with exposure to radiation after age 40 (Howe, 1982). Cases of breast cancer attributable to irradiation begin to occur some 10 years after exposure, and continue thereafter at a roughly constant level, suggesting that the absolute excess risk increases with time since exposure. In this case, *timing* rather than *duration* is the critical aspect of the risk exposure.

Using Longitudinal Data to Create Comparison Groups

An important recent development in causal research is the use of longitudinal data to create groups that are comparable on a wide range of potential "confounders" of the causal hypothesis. In one example, Haviland and Nagin (2005) combined two recent statistical developments – trajectory modeling and propensity score modeling – to come closer to creating valid comparison groups to test the effect of an intervention. They were interested in whether joining a gang increases violence. Because youths who join gangs are known to be more violent than others before they join (Ireland, Thornberry, & Loeber, 2003; Lacourse, Nagin, Tremblay *et al.*, 2003), some way had to be found to account for this in order to be able to examine the effect of joining a gang. Haviland and Nagin first divided the sample of boys into three trajectory groups based on their self-reports of violent delinquency at ages 11, 12 and 13 (the few boys who had already joined gangs by this age were excluded from the analyses). They then used the data from age 14 to divide each trajectory group into those who did, and did not, join a gang, and compared them on a range of measures (e.g., peer and teacher ratings of aggression at age 11, percent falling behind in school at age 10) that can be expected to be correlated both with the trajectory group and with gang membership. Although there were, as expected, large differences among the three trajectory groups, there were very few differences *within* each group between those who later became gang members and those who did not. This suggested that the trajectory grouping had created a balance on prior violent delinquency. The authors were then able to look at the effect of joining a gang at age 14 on violent delinquency within each trajectory group. First-time gang membership at 14 was associated with a significant increase in violence in each trajectory group, especially in the trajectory group that was persistently violent before joining a gang. These analyses help to direct the causal arrow from joining a gang to increased violence, rather than in the opposite direction.

Research Designs for Studying Causal Relationships in Epidemiological Research

In this section we describe three types of research design whose goal is to test for causality: the randomized experiment, in which subjects are assigned at random to experimental groups; the natural experiment, in which subjects are randomly assigned to groups, but not by the experimenter; and the quasi-experiment, in which the groups are not randomly assigned.

Before exploring in more detail the use of longitudinal studies to test causal hypotheses, it is important to recognize that there are important structural limitations to what can be done to test causality using longitudinal data.

Age, Period and Cohort Effects

As time goes by, people grow older, the world changes and new generations grow up. The passage of time in relation to a disorder can be examined in terms of age (e.g., subject's age at onset of the disorder), period (the year or period of history when the disorder was assessed) and cohort (the year of birth of the sample or samples being assessed). Because of the linear dependency among these three time-related variables, if any two are fixed then the third is also fixed.

In practice, most longitudinal epidemiological studies recruit only a single cohort, so they cannot compare, for example, the effect on rates of depression of being aged 10 in 1980 and 10 in 2000 (a cohort effect). This is unfortunate, because changes from one cohort to another can give valuable suggestions about what might be driving behavior (e.g., Collishaw, Maughan, Goodman *et al.*, 2004). Period effects also appear rarely in epidemiological studies of child psychopathology, although we will present some examples. This means that most longitudinal studies of causation deal with age effects (either on exposure to risk or on the development of a disorder given risk exposure), and they rarely acknowledge the potential effects of period or cohort.

The Randomized Controlled Experiment: Why is it the Gold Standard for Causal Research Even in Epidemiology?

The randomized controlled experiment is widely accepted as the highest standard of comparison for research that aims to establish causality (Shadish, Cook, & Campbell *et al.*, 2002). Underlying the value placed on randomization is a concern that risk is not randomly distributed among comparison groups. If we want to know whether, for example, poverty predicts depression, we have to deal with the problem that poverty tends to go along with many other factors, such as medical illness, that might also predict depression. In a randomized experiment, the subject's assignment to one research condition or another (e.g., treatment or no treatment) is based on chance. This procedure makes it easier to ascribe causality to an intervention because (given a reasonable number of study subjects) it:

1 Distributes threats to validity randomly across treatment conditions;

2 Permits the assumption that at pretest the expected value of all variables (measured or not) will be the same across treatment conditions; and

3 Allows the researcher to compute a valid estimate of error variance.

Thus, the great strength of the randomized design is that it provides an unbiased estimate of the average of the experimental variable or treatment effect (Shadish, Cook, & Campbell 2002).

Two distinct characteristics of the relationship between risk and outcome can influence the probability of disease: confounding and effect modification (Miettinen, 1974).

Confounding

Confounding distorts the impact of a risk factor on the risk of disease, because of the presence of some extraneous variable. A factor may act as a confounder in one study but not in another. Consider, for example, two groups at high and low levels of genetic risk for a disease that is also affected by poverty. If everyone in one group was at high genetic risk, a "real" relationship between poverty and disease might be obscured in that community; almost everyone who was poor would also be at genetic risk, so it would not be possible to say which factor was causing the disorder. In the second community, where not all the poor were at high genetic risk and not all those at high genetic risk were poor, it would be possible to look separately at the rates of disorder in four groups (poor non-affected, rich non-affected, poor affected, rich affected), and figure the risk associated with poverty.

Effect Modification

Effect modification or synergy refers to the different impacts of a risk factor at different levels of another variable (Rothman, 1976). This relationship is not specific to any particular study or community; it is a "real" relationship among two or more risk factors. For example, if both the gene for phenylketonuria (PKU) and a diet high in phenylalanine are necessary for PKU to occur, rates of the disorder will vary in different communities, depending on how many people inherit the gene and how many eat a high phenylalanine diet. The relationship between gene and disease remains constant across sites, but diet will act as an effect modifier, controlling the phenotypic consequences of the gene. Another example is the relationship among peak height velocity (PHV: the "growth spurt" of early adolescence), change of school and depressive symptoms. The period of PHV may be a time when youngsters are particularly vulnerable to symptoms of depression (Simmons & Blyth, 1987), particularly when they have to deal with stressful events. For example, it happens that in the American school system most children move from middle school to high school between eighth and ninth grades (ages 13–14). This coincides with the time when many girls, but few boys, are at PHV. School change could thus be acting as an effect modifier, increasing the risk of depression in girls but not in boys. Both confounding and effect modification can be dealt with by randomization.

Randomized Experiments in Epidemiology

Although it is rarely possible to use random assignment at the individual level in the "real world" settings of epidemiological research, it is sometimes possible to allocate classrooms, schools, towns or other communities to treatment and control conditions using the toss of a coin or a random number table, making the assumption that the estimate of the average treatment effect will be relatively unbiased by site differences. For example, recently there has been a flurry of research on methods to improve outcomes for the children of very poor families by supplementing family income on condition that parents ensure that their children get vaccinations and attend school. Incentive-based welfare programs like this, for example, the PROGRESA (Programa de Educación, Salud y Alimentación) intervention which has been running in Mexico since 1997 (recently renamed "Opportunidades"), are "site randomized experiments," where whole communities, in this case 506 villages, are randomized to receive the intervention or not. The researchers plausibly argue that it makes sense to assign a community-wide intervention at the level of the community, rather than that of the individual.

Opportunidades has been shown to increase rates of vaccination and school attendance, but so far has not been evaluated for its impact on child psychopathology.

Problems With Random Assignment in the Real World

There are many situations in which randomization is either impossible or unethical. Little of astronomy, geology, climatology or evolutionary science is amenable to randomized controlled experiments (but we have learned a lot about causation in spite of that). Frequently in medical research the barrier to assignment without bias is an institution – a school board, an ethics committee, a panel of judges – whose members believe that it would be "unethical" to assign a treatment randomly, when some patients or clients "need" it more than others. In effect, these situations pit the cold logic of science against the hot logic of human compassion, and hot logic usually wins, even when (because this is an experiment) the intervention may not work, or may even be harmful (Dishion, McCord, & Poulin, 1999). The research community has done a poor job of educating the world of educators, social workers, judges, even doctors, and others at the battlefront of human services that a rigorous experiment may in the long run be more humane than a less rigorous one that cannot yield clear findings. Furthermore, if a non-randomized experiment shows an effect, the next step is a properly randomized experiment to be quite sure, so two sets of participants will be subjected to the research protocol instead of one.

However, there are situations in which a causal question simply cannot be answered using unbiased assignment. We cannot ethically assign children to have a parent with or without HIV/AIDS (Rotheram-Borus, Lee, Lin *et al.*, 2004), or to witness a horrendous fire in order to study the effect on their use of mental health care (Dorn, Yzermans, Kerssens *et al.*, 2006), or to have a major disaster such as 9/11 occur in the middle of their adolescence (Costello, Erkanli, Keeler *et al.*, 2004) in order to test whether predisaster psychiatric disorder makes children more vulnerable to a traumatic event. If we want to ask causal questions in such situations, then we have to use other methods. Here we describe two alternatives: quasi-experiments and natural experiments.

Quasi-experiments

What distinguishes quasi-experiments from randomized experiments is that in the former case we cannot be sure that group assignment is free of bias. In other respects – the selection of the intervention, the measures administered, the timing of measurement – the two designs may be close to identical. But the difference – inability to use random assignment – can threaten the validity of causal conclusions based on the results, for reasons discussed earlier.

There are many variants on true randomization that have taken advantage of a situation where randomization was not possible but some approximation was. We describe three such strategies that epidemiologists have used to test causal hypotheses about risk factors or risk moderators. In the diagrams O = observation, X = event, T = time.

Sample Compared Post-event to a Population Norm

If data have already been collected before the event or intervention, it may be possible to set up a pre–post, exposed–not exposed design that comes close to random assignment.

	T1	T2	T3
Sample	X	O	
Population norm	O		

This is the most common form of quasi-experiment following an unexpected catastrophe, because usually there has been no opportunity to collect "before" measures on those to whom the event will occur. Researchers try to use measures with known population norms, and compare the affected group with these. For example, Hoven, Dnarte, Lucas *et al.* (2005) compared children living in New York during the 9/11 attack on the Twin Towers with a representative population sample from nearby Stamford, CT, who had been assessed with the same instruments just before 9/11, as well as with other community samples. The New York children assessed 6 months after 9/11 had higher rates of most diagnoses.

This design is critically dependent on the comparability of the post-event sample and the sample on which the measures were normed, because otherwise the differences found might be the result of pre-existing differences rather than the event. So this tends to be the weakest of the various quasi-experiments, but it is often the only one available.

Dose–Response Measures of Exposure to an Event

	T1	T2
Sample a	X	O
Sample b	X	O

Sometimes it is possible to use a dose–response strategy to test hypotheses about whether an exposure causes an outcome. The same researchers (Hoven *et al.*, 2005) divided New York city into three areas at different geographical distances from the site of the World Trade Center and sampled children attending schools in each area, to test the hypothesis that, if physical distance from the event reduced the risk of psychiatric disorder, then the event was causally related to the disorder. They found high rates of mental disorder throughout the study area, but significantly lower rates in children who went to school in the area closest to the site of the attack. This took the researchers by surprise; their post hoc explanation was that the extent of social support and mental health care poured out after 9/11 prevented the harm that the event might have caused.

Second, they measured personal and family exposure to the attack, and compared children who had family members involved in the attack with those who were geographically close but had no personal involvement. They found, as predicted, that both personal and family involvement increased the risk of a mental disorder, but involvement of a family member was the stronger risk factor, even when the children were physically distant from the site.

These aspects of the design of this study carry more weight than the one described earlier, because they incorporate stronger and more theory-based design characteristics. However, they still lack a pretest, and cannot rule out the possibility that these groups were different before the event.

In a study that combined a dose–response measure with a comparison to national norms, Glynn, Wadhwa, Dunkel-Schetter *et al.* (2001) used a group of women who were at different stages of pregnancy, or up to 6 weeks postpartum, on the day of the Northridge, CA, earthquake in 1994 to test two ideas:

1 Women become increasingly stress-resistant across the course of pregnancy; and

2 Prenatal stress affects gestational age.

Across the three trimesters, women became progressively less responsive to the stressor, but were back to normal (same as first trimester) at 6 weeks postpartum (by which time the hypothalamic-pituitary-adrenal (HPA) axis response system is back to normal). Babies had 1.2, 0.6 and 0.6 weeks' shorter gestation than predicted from national norms (adjusted for age, race and socioeconomic status, and obstetric risk), as a function of the trimester of pregnancy in which the earthquake occurred. As there was absolutely no reason for babies at different gestational stages at the time of the earthquake to be different in any systematic way connected to the event, this was a good example of a randomly assigned intervention. However, the study lacked pre-earthquake measures of maternal stress.

Different Groups Exposed and Not Exposed, Both Tested Before and After Exposure

	T1	T2	T3
Sample a	O		O
Sample b	O	X	O

This design has the potential to come closest to a randomized design, because the same subjects are studied both before and after the event that happened to one but not to the other. However, if sample a and sample b were not randomly assigned from the same subject pool, the researcher must convince the reader that there were no differences between the two before the event on potential confounders of the causal relationship.

For example, in a longitudinal study of development across the transition to adulthood, we had been interviewing a representative sample of young people every 1–2 years since 1993. Subjects were interviewed each year on a date as close as possible to their birthday. Thus, in 2001, when the participants were aged 19–21, about two-thirds of them had been interviewed when, on 9/11, the Twin Towers and the Pentagon were struck. We continued to interview the remaining subjects until the end of the year (Costello *et al.*, 2004), but the world facing these young people was a very different one from that in which we had interviewed the first group of participants; for example, there was talk of a national draft, which would directly affect this age group.

The strength of this design is critically dependent on the comparability of the groups interviewed before and after the event. In this case we had 8 years of interviews with the participants before 2001. We compared the before and after 9/11 groups on a wide range of factors, and could demonstrate that each was a random subsample of the main sample. Thus, we had a quasi-experiment that was equivalent to randomly assigning subjects to experience vs. not to experience 9/11. We predicted that even though the participants were living 500 miles away from where the events occurred, this "distant trauma" (Terr, Bloch, Michel *et al.*, 1999) would increase levels of anxiety and, possibly, in this age group, of alcohol and drug abuse. We also thought that the potential for military conscription, which would mainly affect the boys, might further increase the young men's anxiety levels. We were wrong on both counts. There was no increase in levels of anxiety. Women interviewed after 9/11 reported higher levels of drug use in general, and cannabis in particular, with rates of reported use approaching twice the pre-9/11 level. However, men interviewed after 9/11 were *less* likely to report substance abuse, and use of all drugs was lower. There was an effect of time, such that in women the rate of drug use and abuse increased with each month following 9/11, while in men it fell each month.

We interpreted these finding in the light of evidence that when nations are at war rates of suicide and psychiatric hospitalization in the civilian population may go down (Lyons, 1979), suggesting that some people see the state of war as a challenge rather than a stressor. Perhaps the possibility of military service (or even of being subjected to drug tests) inspired the young men to get their act together, whereas it had the opposite effect on young women.

Conclusions About Quasi-experimental Designs to Test Causal Hypotheses in Epidemiology

A wide range of poor to excellent designs can be encompassed under the label "quasi-experimental," from ones that lack either pretest or control group, to designs using interrupted time series or regression discontinuity approaches (neither of which is to be found yet in child psychiatric epidemiology) that combine ecological validity with logical rigor. The examples of quasi-experimental studies described here suggest that such designs can be quite effective at discounting previously held beliefs, but are open to the risk of post hoc interpretations (as in the Costello and Hovens examples). Also, as Shadish, Cook, & Campbell (2002) point out, "they can undermine the likelihood of doing even better studies."

Natural Experiments in Epidemiology

Natural experiments are gifts to the researcher; situations that could not have been planned or proposed, but which do what a randomized experiment does: assign participants to one exposure or another without bias, and hold all other variables constant while manipulating the risk factor of interest. Sometimes, the unbiased assignment is created by events, as when one group of families in our longitudinal study received an income supplement while others did not, where race (Native American vs. Anglo) was the sole criterion (Costello *et al.*, 2003). In this case we had 4 years of assessments of children's psychiatric status before and after the introduction of the income supplement, and so could compare the children's behavior before and after the intervention in both groups. The years of measurement before the event enabled us to rule out the potential confounding of ethnicity with the children's emotional and behavioral symptoms.

A tremendously important possibility for natural experimentation occurs when genes and environment can be separated (see chapter 21). Such naturally occurring situations provided the foundation for the rise of genetic epidemiology, which "focuses on the familial, and in particular genetic, determinants of disease and the joint effects of genes and non-genetic determinants" (Burton, Tobin, & Hopper, 2005). Genetic epidemiology also has the power to contribute in important ways to our understanding of environmental causes of disease:

> "One serious problem facing mainstream epidemiology is that residual confounding by unobserved covariates could be strong enough to swamp the small aetiological effects now being sought. The distribution of alleles at any given locus tends not to be correlated either with environmental exposures or with the distribution of alleles at other loci (except those few in tight linkage disequilibrium). Therefore, the biology underpinning genetic epidemiology offers a potentially useful way to study environmental determinants in disease without residual confounding. This approach [is] often called mendelian randomization" (Burton, Tobin, & Hopper, 2005).

Mendelian Randomization

The argument is based on Mendel's second law, which states that the inheritance of any one trait is independent of the inheritance of any other trait. If it is possible to find a genetic polymorphism that influences exposure to a putative risk factor, then by Mendel's second law those who carry the polymorphism and those who do not are randomly distributed with respect to other genes influencing the disease of interest. To use an example provided by Katan, suppose that a researcher wants to know whether low serum cholesterol increases the risk of cancer by favoring tumor growth. It is known that a gradient in the apolipoprotein E (APOE) genotype is associated with a gradient in serum cholesterol levels in the population. There have been suggestions that low cholesterol increases cancer risk (Katan, 2004). If serum cholesterol level does affect cancer, we would logically expect an association between APOE and cancer. In the absence of an APOE–cancer association, the cholesterol–cancer association may well be the result of other factors, or reverse association (i.e., cancer reduces cholesterol). In effect, this is a variant of the classic mediational model, using the argument that because the gene is known to affect the "mediator" (here cholesterol), if the gene does not influence disease frequency then the "mediator" cannot be causally related to the disease. Davey Smith and Ebrahim (2005) extended this work to show that the size of the effect of an intermediate phenotype on a disease can be estimated from the ratio of the coefficients for the regression of the disease on the gene and of the intermediate phenotype on the gene. As Burton, Tobin & Hopper (2005) point out, the same logic can be applied to genetic and environmental determinants of disease.

As the number of identified associations between genotype and disease increases, this approach will be increasingly useful. However, there are still problems (Chen, Akula, Detra-Wadleigh *et al.*, 2004; Davey Smith & Ebrahim, 2005; Nitsch, Molokhia, Smeeth *et al.*, 2006). First, as Tobin, Minelli, Burton *et al.* (2004) note, "Almost all current genetic studies are statistically underpowered to detect the relatively small effects of the frequent gene variants that underlie common, complex diseases." Second, there is sometimes a risk of population stratification (i.e., confounding of genotype–disease associations by factors related to subpopulation group membership within the overall population in a study). Third, a genetic variant expressed during fetal development may influence development in such a way as to buffer against the effect of the variant, a form of developmental compensation introduced as "canalization" by Waddington (1957). Fourth, publication bias is a problem for meta-analyses of findings, because non-confirmatory studies tend not to get published. And, of course, most disorders that are fairly common in the population have complex etiologies involving multiple genes of small effect as well as multiple environmental exposures. If this were not the case, natural selection would have long since eliminated those with the disadvantageous polymorphism, unless, as appears to be the case of the hemoglobin beta (HBB) gene, which gives rise to thalassemia, some mutations may confer resistance to other disease (in this case, malaria).

Using Natural Experiments to Examine Genetic and Environmental Causes

As several papers have recently pointed out (Burton, Tobin, & Hopper *et al.*, 2005; Davey Smith & Ebrahim, 2005), genetic epidemiology and standard observational epidemiology are rapidly merging. As Burton, Tobin, & Hopper *et al.* (2005) put it, "Once it is known which of two versions of a potentially causative gene an individual possesses, looking for an association between variants in that gene and the disease of interest is fundamentally no different from an exploration of a disease–exposure association in traditional epidemiology."

Genetic research in psychiatry began with the hypothesis that genes "cause" mental illness. More recently, genetic approaches are being used to map out the role of environmental factors in the etiology of mental illness in people with different genetic profiles. The first approach privileged genes as the causal factors; in one sense rightly so, because psychiatric disorders involve behavior, and behavior comes about as a result of activity at the level of the genes. So for several decades causal research in genetic epidemiology took as its focus measuring the extent to which specific disorders were under genetic control by using genetically informative samples to partition the variance among genetic and environmental causes, primarily in order to estimate the extent of genetic involvement. But, in the words of the epidemiologists Kenneth Rothman and Sander Greenland: "Since 'environment' can be thought of as an all-embracing category that represents non-genetic causes, it is clear on a priori grounds that 100% of any disease is environmentally caused . . . Similarly, one can show that 100% of any disease is inherited." (Rothman & Greenland, 1998). Although geneticists have historically focused on establishing or measuring the genetic contribution to a given disorder, genetic designs can also be used to examine the causal role of environmental factors, controlling for genetic liability (Rutter, Pickles, Murray *et al.*, 2001).

Examples of Designs for Causal Research in Genetic Epidemiology

One thing that kept the two disciplines apart for a long time was the selection of samples. Genetic epidemiologists have used a range of research designs to get around the fact that the most direct experiment, which would modify a gene in some individuals and then compare their outcome to that of controls, is unethical in humans. Animal models of this kind have been very helpful in some areas of psychopathology, but are outside the scope of this chapter. Until recently, genetic epidemiology tended to make use of natural experiments affecting family structure – twins, children of twins, twins reared apart, adopted children, and so on – or else place of residence, as in migrant samples, to "pull apart" the aspects of the family that contribute genes and environment. Recently, direct study of individual gene variants in relation to disease outcomes has become easier and cheaper, so that singleton epidemiological samples can be used. Here we briefly review some traditional study designs for genetic epidemiology, and then look to the future.

Adoption Studies

Adoption studies separate genes from environment by separating a child from its biological parents, to be brought up by unrelated parents who provide the environment but not the genes. This avoids the passive gene–environment correlation (rGE) that is inherent in studies of children brought up by their biological parents, who pass on not only genes but also the environment in which the child grows up (Plomin, 1995). In one of the earliest of such studies, Cunningham, Cadoret, Loftus *et al.* (1975) compared two groups of adoptees, one group whose biological parents were "psychiatrically disturbed" and one whose biological parents were not. More than twice as many of the former group had psychiatric conditions requiring professional care. Because there were no differences between the adopting parent groups in levels of psychiatric disorder, this was taken as prima facie evidence that there was a genetic cause for the difference. Variants on this design include comparisons between adoptees and children raised by their biological parents (Plomin, DeFries, & Fulker, 1988), including studies of twin pairs of which one was adopted and one was not (Bergeman, Chipuer, Plomin *et al.*, 1993), and mixed families of twins, singletons and adoptees (Neiderhiser, Reiss, & Hetherington, 1996).

Adoption studies have provided evidence for a genetic component in antisocial behavior, hyperactivity, drug abuse and schizophrenia (Cadoret, 1992; Cadoret & Stewart, 1991; Cadoret, Troughton, Bagford *et al.*, 1990; Tienari, Lahti, Sorri *et al.*, 1990), but perhaps not for childhood depression (Eley, Deater-Deckard, Fombonne *et al.*, 1998). They have also been used to illuminate the causal role of environmental factors. For example, Duyme, Dumaret, & Tomkiewicz (1999) compared the IQ scores before adoption at age 4–6 and in adolescence, in groups of children adopted by families of low, medium and high socio-economic status (SES). The IQ scores of the three groups, which were similar before adoption, improved by significantly different amounts, from 7.7 points in the group adopted into low SES families to 19.5 points in those adopted into high SES families. These differences in improvement between groups with similar IQ scores a decade earlier argue for an environmental effect on an area of functioning that previous studies have shown to be under strong genetic influence (Plomin & Spinath, 2004).

Adoption studies have made tremendously important contributions to our understanding of the role of genes and environments in the development of psychopathology. However, they face serious problems (Maughan & Pickles, 1990). The meaning of adoption has changed dramatically over time, and has very different meaning in different cultures. Adoptive parents are in most societies carefully scrutinized, and as a group are low in high-risk behaviors. The amount known about birth mothers is often limited, and about birth fathers frequently nothing. In today's open adoptions the birth parent may become a part of the rearing environment, which undermines the "pulling apart" of genes and rearing environment.

Migration Studies

If people move from one country to another, bringing their genes with them, it is potentially possible to compare their history of illness with:

1 Those from the same gene pool whom they left behind; and
2 Those with whom they share a new environment.

The latter strategy was used, for example, by Dohrenwend, Levav, Shrout *et al.* (1992) to test whether the high rates of mental illness seen in impoverished Israeli immigrants was more likely to be caused by the environment or by their genetic heritage of mental illness. Dohrenwend, Levav, Shrout *et al.* used the terms "social causation" for discrimination and hardship as causes of mental illness, and "social selection" to refer to the fact that those who came from mentally ill families were more likely to move down the SES gradient. Comparing more recent immigrants from North Africa, who were struggling with discrimination as well as poverty, and European immigrants of low SES who had lived much longer in Israel, they found that schizophrenia was more common in the latter, while the North African immigrant men had more antisocial personality and substance use disorders, and the North African immigrant women had more depression. The authors argue for gender-specific modes of responding to environmental stress, while the "sorting and sifting" process had "left behind a residue of severely ill persons of advantaged European background" (Dohrenwend, Levav, Shrout *et al.*, 1992) (i.e., people with a genetic liability to schizophrenia).

Janssen, Verhulst, Bengi-Arslan *et al.* (2004) compared self-reported psychiatric symptoms of Turkish youth whose families had migrated to the Netherlands with those of two comparison groups: Native-born Dutch youth and Turkish youth living in Turkey. A genetic causal argument would predict that areas in which the two Turkish samples were the same, but different from the Dutch youth, would be areas more affected by genetics than environment. This was true of scores on anxious/depressed, withdrawn, and thought problem scales. Areas in which the two Turkish samples differed could be affected by the stress of immigration. The immigrant Turkish youth reported more delinquency, aggression and attention problems than the Turkish youth living in Turkey.

Although migrants may be more representative of the general population than adoptees, there are still problems with generalizing from such samples (Hobcraft, 2006). Different groups migrate for different reasons; sometimes they are healthier than the population they left behind, sometimes they emigrate under extreme stress. It is quite rare to have "before" measures, especially of mental health, and migration itself may impose significant stress.

Twin Studies

Since the 1920s, geneticists have used the idea of comparing the correlation between monozygotic (MZ) and dizygotic (DZ) twins as a way to estimate the heritability of disease (Bukowski, Sippola, & Brender, 1993). MZ twins, with their identical genes, provide a wonderful opportunity for research into environmental causes of disease, because differences between them must be brought about by factors other than inherited genes, whereas DZ twins brought up together share a rearing environment but only half their genes.

Before genetic risk could easily be measured directly at the molecular level, comparing the correlations of MZ and DZ twins was an important technique for measuring the extent to which a given disease or trait was heritable (Plomin, DeFries, & McClearn, 1990). Several decades of work using this approach have made it clear that there is a substantial genetic component to many psychiatric disorders as well as to most personality traits. This was a major shift in thinking about the causes of disease. By extension, it was possible to use twins to construct a scale of genetic risk by examining the disease status of the cotwin, and to use this to test for gene–environment interactions. "A child's genetic risk is highest if his or her co-twin has a diagnosis of disorder and the pair are MZ and a child's genetic risk is lowest if his or her co-twin does not have a diagnosis of disorder and the pair are MZ. DZ twins' genetic risk falls intermediate to these two groups" (Jaffee, Caspi, Moffitt *et al.*, 2005). That is, risk was highest if an MZ cotwin had a diagnosis of conduct disorder, somewhat high if a DZ cotwin had a diagnosis, lower if a DZ cotwin had no diagnosis, and lowest if an MZ cotwin had no diagnosis. In a study of the impact of parental maltreatment on later conduct problems, the researchers had to establish, first, that there was no difference between MZ and DZ twins in their concordance for maltreatment; second, that the severity of maltreatment among children who were physically maltreated was similar across high and low genetic risk; and third, that MZ and DZ twins were equally likely to have conduct problems. They then compared the level of conduct problems in the four groups of twins. There was a clear increase in conduct problems from the lowest to the highest genetic risk group, and a significant interaction with maltreatment, such that the number of conduct problems was similar in maltreated and non-maltreated low-risk groups, but rose faster with increasing genetic risk in the maltreated group. This study could not identify which genes were involved in the increased vulnerability to maltreatment in some children, but it provides an excellent example of the use of twin samples to move beyond simple heritability studies toward identifying gene–environment interaction.

Children of twins provide another interesting variant on the twin design. Children of twins are as genetically related as siblings (if the twin parents are MZ) or cousins (if the twin parents are DZ), but are reared by different mothers. D'Onofrio, Turkheimer, Emery *et al.* (2006) compared the children of twin mothers who had divorced with the children of the non-divorced cotwins. The results were consistent with a causal role of divorce in earlier sexual intercourse and emotional difficulties, and increased risk of educational problems, depressed mood and suicidal ideation. No such effect of divorce was found for early drug use. The main drawback to this ingenious design is the large sample size needed.

Twins are likely to be much more similar to the general population than are adoptees or migrants. However, there are several potential problems with the use of twin samples for causal research (Rutter, Simonoff, & Silberg, 1993). First is the problem of representative sampling. It is difficult to recruit a truly representative sample of twin families, and those studied tend to be disproportionately white and middle class. It is even more difficult to keep twin families in a longitudinal study, given the considerable reporting burden on parents, and the need to keep both children engaged. Then there is the question of how far twin families really resemble singleton families; even families with two children of different ages. A major problem for teasing apart genetic and environmental influences on behavior, for twin as well as singleton studies, is the likelihood that genes and environment are correlated (rGE). Twins, like other individuals, are likely to select environments that suit their genetic temperament (active rGE), to elicit reactions from their environment that reflect in part their own temperament (reactive rGE), and to be exposed to environmental influences provided by another individual to whom they are genetically related; for example, an intelligent parent may also provide a more than usually stimulating environment (passive rGE). These types of rGE have the effect of making what is in fact an effect of environmental factors look like a genetic effect in analyses to partition the variance, unless they are specified and measured.

Conclusions

There has been a great deal of argument in epidemiological journals recently about whether observational epidemiology can ever establish causality (e.g., Kaufman & Cooper, 1999; Krieger & Smith, 2000; Maldonado & Greenland, 2002; Parascandola & Weed, 2001; Susser, 1991). The argument could more properly be framed within a wider question: can research ever establish causality? As the earlier discussion of randomized experiments pointed out, even the gold standard of clinical research, the randomized controlled trial, is only an approximation to the un-doable "counterfactual" experiment. The various designs described in this chapter are examples of ways in which researchers have used their ingenuity to get closer to their goal, either by clever design, for example by including overlapping cohorts of subjects, or by capitalizing on chance, as in natural experiments, or by incorporating a whole new body of knowledge, as in molecular genetic epidemiology. The genomics revolution in particular has the potential to revitalize psychiatric epidemiology, adding tremendously to the value of the longitudinal studies that have been building up over time, directing the search for causality, and providing important new links with clinical psychiatry.

For the reader of academic and professional journals the challenge of sorting valid causal research from invalid claims may seem overwhelming. It is often helpful to go back to the progress of scientific maturity listed at the beginning of the chapter: observation, categorization, pattern recognition, hypothesis testing and causal explanation, and ask of a given paper where it should be placed along the pathway to causality. Much epidemiological literature is somewhere between categorization and pattern recognition. The hard task is to observe a correlational pattern, develop a hypothesis about why it should exist and develop a valid way of testing the hypothesis. This chapter describes and presents examples of several such methods, from longitudinal studies to taking advantage of natural experiments such as twins.

For policy-makers it can be very difficult to know when the scientific evidence is strong enough to warrant a new intervention. The inference to be drawn from the work reviewed here is that it is probably dangerous to initiate new programs simply on the basis of correlational data. However, policy decisions have to be based not only on scientific evidence about causality, but also on the costs and benefits of both intervening and not intervening. This is too big a topic to deal with here, but methods are available (Kraemer, 1992).

For researchers trying to "learn the causes of things," epidemiological and laboratory studies can support one another, with laboratory experiments, whether on humans or on animals, generally stronger on "specific causation" and population-based epidemiological studies stronger on "general causation." Longitudinal studies are particularly useful (subject to the cautions discussed earlier) as we struggle to find the causes of complex chronic diseases, a class that includes most psychiatric disorders. Here the key risk exposures, and their interplay with genes, are likely to vary across development (Vineis & Kriebel, 2006).

Further reading

Shadish, W., Cook, T., & Campbell, D. (2002). *Experimental and quasi-experimental designs for generalized causal inference.* Boston: Houghton Mifflin.

References

Angold, A., Costello, E. J., & Worthman, C. M. (1999). Pubertal changes in hormone levels and depression in girls. *Psychological Medicine*, *29*, 1043–1053.

Bell, R. Q., & Harper, L. V. (1977). *Child effects on adults.* Hillsdale, NJ: Lawrence Erlbaum Associates.

Bergeman, C. S., Chipuer, H. M., Plomin, R., Pedersen, N. L., McClearn, G. E., Nesselroade, J. R., *et al.* (1993). Genetic and environmental effects on openness to experience, agreeableness, and conscientiousness: An adoption/twin study. *Journal of Personality*, *61*, 159–179.

Bronfenbrenner, U. (1977). Toward an experimental ecology of human development. *American Psychologist*, *32*, 513–531.

Brooks-Gunn, J., & Duncan, G. J. (1997). The effects of poverty on children. *Future of Children*, *7*, 55–71.

Bukowski, W. M., Sippola, L., & Brender, W. (1993). *Where does sexuality come from? Normative sexuality from a developmental perspective.* In Barbaree, H., Marshall, W., Hudson, S. (Eds), *The juvenile sex offender.* New York: Guilford Press, pp. 84–103.

Burton, P. R., Tobin, M. D., & Hopper, J. L. (2005). Key concepts in genetic epidemiology. *Lancet*, *366*, 941.

Cadoret, R. J. (1992). Genetic and environmental factors initiation of drug use and the transition to abuse. In M. Glantz, & R. Pickens (Eds.), *Vulnerability to Drug Abuse* (pp. 99–113). Washington, DC: American Psychological Association.

Cadoret, R. J., & Stewart, M. J. (1991). An adoption study of attention deficit, hyperactivity, aggression and their relationship to antisocial personality. *Comparative Psychiatry*, *32*, 73–82.

Cadoret, R. J., Troughton, E., Bagford, J., & Woodworth, G. (1990). Genetic and environmental factors in adoptee antisocial personality. *European Archives of Psychiatry and Neurological Sciences*, *239*, 231–240.

Chen, Y. S., Akula, N., Detera-Wadleigh, S. D., Schulze, T. G., Thomas, J., Potash, J. B., *et al.* (2004). Findings in an independent sample support an association between bipolar affective disorder and the G72/G30 locus on chromosome 13q33. *Molecular Psychiatry*, *9*, 87–92.

Collishaw, S., Maughan, B., Goodman, R., & Pickles, A. (2004). Time trends in adolescent mental health. *Journal of Child Psychology and Psychiatry*, *45*, 1350–1362.

Costello, E. J., Compton, S. N., Keeler, G., & Angold, A. (2003). Relationships between poverty and psychopathology: A natural experiment. *JAMA*, *290*, 2023–2029.

Costello, E. J., Erkanli, A., Keeler, G., & Angold, A. (2004). Distant trauma: A prospective study of the effects of 9/11 on rural youth. *Applied Developmental Science*, *8*, 211–220.

Croft, C., O'Connor, T. G., Keaveney, L., Groothues, C., Rutter, M., Team EaRAS. (2001). Longitudinal change in parenting associated with developmental delay and catch-up. *Journal of Child Psychology and Psychiatry*, *42*, 649–659.

Cunningham, L., Cadoret, R. J., Loftus, R., & Edwards, J. (1975). Studies of adoptees from psychiatrically disturbed biological parents: Psychiatric conditions in childhood and adolescence. *British Journal of Psychiatry*, *126*, 534–549.

D'Onofrio, B. M., Turkheimer, E., Emery, R. E., Slutske, W. S., Heath, A. C., Madden, P. A., *et al.* (2006). A genetically informed study of the processes underlying the association between parental marital instability and offspring adjustment. *Developmental Psychology*, *42*, 486–499.

Davey Smith, G., & Ebrahim, S. (2005). What can mendelian randomisation tell us about modifiable behavioural and environmental exposures? *British Medical Journal*, *330*, 1076–1079.

Dishion, T. J., McCord, J., & Poulin, F. (1999). When interventions harm: Peer groups and problem behavior. *American Psychologist*, *54*, 755–764.

Dohrenwend, B. P., Levav, I., Shrout, P. E., Schwartz, S., Naveh, G., Link, B. G., *et al.* (1992). Socioeconomic status and psychiatric disorders: The causation–selection issue. *Science*, *255*, 946–952.

Doll, R., & Hill, A. B. (1966). Mortality of British doctors in relation to smoking: Observations on coronary thrombosis. *National Cancer Institute Monographs*, *19*, 205–268.

Dorn, T. M., Yzermans, C. J., Kerssens, J. J., Spreeuwenberg, P., & van der Zee, J. (2006). Disaster and subsequent healthcare utilization: A longitudinal study among victims, their family members, and control subjects. *Medical Care*, *44*, 581–589.

Duncan, G., Yeung, W. J., Brooks-Gunn, J., & Smith, J. (1998). How much does childhood poverty affect the life chances of children? *American Sociological Review*, *63*, 406–423.

Duncan, G. J., Brooks-Gunn, J., & Klebanov, P. K. (1994). Economic deprivation and early childhood development. *Child Development*, *65*, 296–318.

Duyme, M., Dumaret, A. C., & Tomkiewicz, S. (1999). How can we boost IQs of "dull children"? A late adoption study. *Proceedings of the National Academy of Sciences of the USA*, 96, 8790–8794.

Eagles, J. M. (1991). The relationship between schizophrenia and immigration: Are there alternatives to psychosocial hypotheses? *British Journal of Psychiatry*, *159*, 783–789.

Eley, T. C., Deater-Deckard, K., Fombonne, E., Fulker, D. W., & Plomin, R. (1998). An adoption study of depressive symptoms in middle childhood. *Journal of Child Psychology and Psychiatry*, *39*, 337–345.

Feist, G. J. (2006). *The psychology of science and the origins of the scientific mind*. New Hanover, CT: Yale University Press.

Glynn, L. M., Wadhwa, P. D., Dunkel-Schetter, C., Chicz-DeMet, A., & Sandman, C. A. (2001). When stress happens matters: Effects of earthquake timing on stress responsivity in pregnancy. *American Journal of Obstetrics and Gynecology*, *184*, 637–642.

Haviland, A. M., & Nagin, D. S. (2005). Causal inferences with group based trajectory models. *Psychometrika*, *70*, 557–578.

Hill, A. B. (1965). Environment and disease: Association or causation? *Proceedings of the Royal Society of Medicine*, *58*, 295–300.

Hobcraft, J. (2006). The ABC of demographic behaviour: how the interplays of alleles, brains, and contexts over the life course should shape research aimed at understanding population processes. *Population Studies*, *60*, 153–187.

Hoven, C. W., Duarte, C. S., Lucas, C. P., Wu, P., Mandell, D. J., Goodwin, R. D., *et al.* (2005). Psychopathology among New York city public school children 6 months after September 11. *Archives of General Psychiatry*, *62*, 545–552.

Howe, G. R. (1982). Epidemiology of radiogenic breast cancer. In J. J. D. Boice, & J. J. R. Fraumeni (Eds.), *Radiation carcinogenesis: Epidemiology and biological significance* (pp. 119–129). New York: Raven Press.

Hume, D. (2000). An enquiry concerning human understanding: a critical edition. In T. L. Beauchamp (Ed.), *The Clarendon edition of the works of David Hume*. New York: Oxford University Press.

Ireland, T., Thornberry, T. P., & Loeber, R. (2003). Violence among adolescents living in public housing: A two-site analysis. *Criminology and Public Policy*, *3*, 3–38.

Jaffee, S. R., Caspi, A., Moffitt, T. E., Dodge, K. A., Rutter, M., Taylor, A., *et al.* (2005). Nature X nurture: genetic vulnerabilities interact with physical maltreatment to promote conduct problems. *Development and Psychopathology*, *17*, 67–84.

Janssen, M. M., Verhulst, F., Bengi-Arslan, L., Erol, N., Salter, C., & Crijnen, A. M. (2004). Comparison of self-reported emotional and behavioral problems in Turkish immigrant, Dutch and Turkish adolescents. *Social Psychiatry and Psychiatric Epidemiology*, *39*, 133–140.

Katan, M. B. (2004). Apolipoprotein E isoforms, serum cholesterol, and cancer, 1986 [see comment]. *International Journal of Epidemiology*, *33*, 9.

Kaufman, J. S., & Cooper, R. S. (1999). Seeking causal explanations in social epidemiology. *American Journal of Epidemiology*, *150*, 113–120.

Kleinbaum, D. G., Kupper, L. L., & Morgenstern, H. (1982). *Epidemiologic research: Principles and quantitative methods*. New York, NY: Van Nostrand Reinhold.

Koch, R. (1882). Dei aetiologie der Tuberkulose. In: *Gesammelte Werke von Koch*, Schwalbe, J. (Ed.). Georh Thieme.

Koch, R. (1932). *The aetiology* of *tuberculosis*. New York City: National Tuberculosis Association.

Kraemer, H. C. (1992). *Evaluating medical tests: Objective and quantitative guidelines*. Newbury Park: Sage Publications.

Krieger, N., & Smith, G. D. (2000). Re: "Seeking causal explanations in social epidemiology". *American Journal of Epidemiology*, *151*, 831–832.

Lacourse, E., Nagin, D., Tremblay, R., Vitaro, F., & Claes, S. (2003). Developmental trajectories of boys delinquent group membership and facilitation of violent behaviors during adolescence. *Development and Psychopathology*, *15*, 183–197.

Lewis, D. L. (1973). Causation. *Journal of Philosophy*, *70*, 556–567.

Lyons, H. (1979). Civil violence: The psychological aspects. *Journal of Psychosomatic Research*, *23*, 373–393.

Maldonado, G., & Greenland, S. (2002). Estimating causal effects. *International Journal of Epidemiology*, *31*, 422–429.

Maughan, B., & Pickles, A. (1990). Adopted and illegitimate children growing up. In L. N. Robins, & M. Rutter (Eds.), *Straight and devious pathways from childhood to adulthood* (pp. 36–61). Cambridge: Cambridge University Press.

Miettinen, O. S. (1974). Confounding and effect modification. *American Journal of Epidemiology*, *100*, 350–353.

Mill, J. S. (1856). *A system of logic: Ratiocinative and inductive*. London: Routledge, 1892.

Moffitt, T. E. (1990). Juvenile delinquency and attention deficit disorder: Boys' developmental trajectories from age 3 to age 15. *Child Development*, *61*, 893–910.

Neiderhiser, J. M., Reiss, D., & Hetherington, E. M. (1996). Genetically informative designs for distinguishing developmental pathways during adolescence: Responsible and antisocial behavior. *Development and Psychopathology*, *8*, 779–791.

Nitsch, D., Molokhia, M., Smeeth, L., DeStavola, B. L., Whittaker, J. C., & Leon, D. A. (2006). Limits to causal inference based on Mendelian randomization: a comparison with randomized controlled trials. *American Journal of Epidemiology*, *163*, 397–403.

Offord, D. R., Boyle, M. H., Racine, Y. A., Fleming, J. E., Cadman, D. T., Blum, H. M., *et al.* (1992). Outcome, prognosis, and risk in a longitudinal follow-up study. *Journal of the American Academy of Child and Adolescent Psychiatry*, *31*, 916–923.

Parascandola, M., & Weed, D. L. (2001). Causation in epidemiology. *Journal of Epidemiology and Community Health*, *55*, 905–912.

Peto, J., Seidman, H., & Selikoff, I. J. (1982). Mesothelioma mortality in asbestos workers: Implications for models of carcinogenesis and risk assessment. *British Journal of Cancer*, *45*, 124–135.

Plomin, R. (1995). Genetics and children's experiences in the family. *Journal of Child Psychology and Psychiatry and Allied Disciplines*, *36*, 33–68.

Plomin, R., DeFries, J. C., & Fulker, D. W. (1988). *Nature and nurture in infancy and early childhood*. London: Cambridge University Press.

Plomin, R., DeFries, J. C., & McClearn, G. E. (1990). *Behavioral genetics: A primer* (2nd ed.). New York: W. Freeman and Company.

Plomin, R., & Spinath, F. M. (2004). Intelligence: genetics, genes, and genomics. *Journal of Personality and Social Psychology*, *86*, 112–129.

Robins, E., & Guze, S. B. (1970). Establishment of diagnostic validity in psychiatric illness: Its application to schizophrenia. *American Journal of Psychiatry*, *126*, 107–111.

Robins, J. (1997). Causal inference from complex longitudinal data. In M. Berkane (Ed.), *Latent variable modeling and applications to causality. Lecture notes in statistics* (pp. 69–117). New York: Springer Verlag.

Rotheram-Borus, M. J., Lee, M., Lin, Y-Y., & Lester, P. (2004). Six-year intervention outcomes for adolescent children of parents with the human immunodeficiency virus 10.1001/archpedi.158.8.742. *Archives of Pediatric Adolescent Medicine*, *158*, 742–748.

Rothman, K. J. (1976). Reviews and commentary: Causes. *American Journal of Epidemiology*, *104*, 587–592.

Rothman, K. J., & Greenland, S. (Eds.). (1998). *Modern epidemiology* (2nd ed.). Philadelphia: Lippincott-Raven.

Rutter, M. (1985). Resilience in the face of adversity: Protective factors and resistance to psychiatric disorder. *British Journal of Psychiatry*, *147*, 598–611.

Rutter, M. (2007). Proceeding from observed correlation to causal inference: The use of natural experiments. *Perspectives on Psychological Science*, *2*, 377–395.

Rutter, M., Pickles, A., Murray, R., & Eaves, L. (2001). Testing hypotheses on specific environmental causal effects on behavior. *Psychological Bulletin*, *127*, 291–324.

Rutter, M. L., Simonoff, E., & Silberg, J. L. (1993). How informative are twin studies of child psychopathology? In T. J. Bouchard, & P. Propping (Eds.), *Twins as a tool of behavior genetics*. (pp. 179–194). Chichester: John Wiley & Sons.

Shadish, W., Cook, T., & Campbell, D. (2002). *Experimental and quasi-experimental designs for generalized causal inference*. Boston: Houghton Mifflin.

Simmons, R. G., & Blyth, D. A. (1987). *Moving into adolescence: The impact of pubertal change and school context*. Hawthorne, NY: Aldine de Gruyter.

Sroufe, L. A. (1988). The role of infant–caregiver attachment in development. In J. Belsky, & T. Nezworski (Eds.), *Clinical implications of attachment*. Hillsdale, NJ: Lawrence Erlbaum Associates.

Susser, M. (1991). What is a cause and how do we know one? A grammar for pragmatic epidemiology. *American Journal of Epidemiology*, *33*, 635–648.

Terr, L. Bloch, D., Michel, B., Shi, H., Reinhardt, J., Metayer, S. (1999). Children's symptoms in the wake of Challenger: A field study of distant-traumatic effects and an outline of related conditions. *American Journal of Psychiatry*, *156*, 1536–1544.

Tienari, P., Lahti, I., Sorri, A., Naarala, M., Moring, J., Kaleva, M., *et al.* (1990). Adopted-away offspring of schizophrenics and controls: The Finnish adoptive family study of schizophrenia. In L. N. Robins, & M. Rutter (Eds.), *Straight and devious pathways from childhood to adulthood* (pp. 365–380). Cambridge: Cambridge University Press.

Tobin, M. D., Minelli, C., Burton, P. R., & Thompson, J. R. (2004). Commentary: Development of Mendelian randomization: from hypothesis test to "Mendelian deconfounding". *International Journal of Epidemiology*, *33*, 26.

Vineis, P., & Kriebel, D. (2006). Causal models in epidemiology: Past inheritance and genetic future. *Environmental Health: A Global Access Science Source*, *5*, 1–10.

Waddington, C. H. (1957). *The strategy of genes*. London: Allen and Unwin.

Using Epidemiology to Plan Services: A Conceptual Approach

Michael Rutter and Jim Stevenson

As Earls (1979) noted in relation to child psychiatry, epidemiology is a basic science with two rather distinct functions: first, it documents the patterns of disorder in the community as a means of planning services (Rutter, Tizard, & Whitmore, 1970); and, second, it studies the causes of disorder (Costello, Foley, & Angold, 2006; Rutter (2007); see also chapter 5). Epidemiology differs from clinical medicine primarily with respect to studying disorders in the context of a community, rather than the individual (Costello, Egger, & Angold, 2005). Analyses are based on counts of individuals but the inferences concern population risks and outcomes, rather than the development of a disorder at an individual level.

In this chapter, we focus on using epidemiology to provide data that are needed for the planning of services; chapter 5 considers its use in inferring possible causal influences. As we note, the delineation of such influences and of their patterns of variation across groups constitutes an essential element in planning services. Both uses require rigorous attention to many details of design, measurement and data analysis – which are well described in several key sources (Detels, McEwen, Beaglehole *et al.*, 2002; Fombonne, 2002; Rothman & Greenland, 1998; Susser, Schwartz, Morabia *et al.*, 2006; Verhulst & Koot, 1995).

Information Needed for Planning Services

The efficient and cost-effective planning of services involves consideration of a wide range of features. The starting point is often seen as the determination of the number of individuals in a particular population with disorders causing either current impairment or carrying risks for later hazards. That necessarily requires information on the extent to which disorders of any given type involve impairment or future risk (Costello, Egger, & Angold, 2005; Ezpeleta, Keeler, Erkanli *et al.*, 2001). Questionnaire surveys on their own generally provide an inadequate means of obtaining this information, although they may constitute a most useful step in the overall planning. However, service planners need to know several other crucial bits of information. Thus, it is necessary to know whether there are effective treatments for these disorders and, if they exist, are they ordinarily available as part of existing services?

A somewhat related issue concerns the extent to which disorders tend to be recurrent or chronic. This information may strongly influence priority setting in resource allocation for services. The long-term cost of an untreated disorder is another key piece of information of relevance to service planning (Costello, Copeland, Cowell *et al.*, 2007). For example, the significance of conduct disorder as a priority for services was given added weight when the considerable costs to a range of services (mental health, education and the justice system) were shown (Scott, Knapp, Henderson *et al.*, 2001).

A further consideration is the extent to which the professionals in existing services recognize disorders when they present. Planning services on the basis of the true prevalence of disorders as ascertained by experts is not of much use if the professionals operating existing services are unable to recognize the disorders needing intervention. Similarly, it is important to know the extent to which families appreciate the needs. Do they share the professionals' view that particular features mean that there is a disorder that could be responsive to intervention and are they willing to accept the services on offer?

Over recent decades, psychiatrists have become concerned with diagnostic distinctions. In parallel, service providers have often wanted to restrict services to individuals with a particular diagnosis. It might seem to follow, therefore, that the need is to know the frequency of the particular diagnoses that constitute passports or entry tickets to particular forms of service provision. However, that would be a cardinal error because of the extensive evidence that it is common, perhaps even usual, for individuals to show multiple features of psychopathology representing supposedly different disorders (see chapter 2). Moreover, although there are important associations between types of disorders and the types of treatment that are most effective for them, the associations are relatively modest and there are few truly specific effective treatments, either pharmacological or psychological.

Knowledge of the number of individuals for whom services ought ideally to be made available is not sufficient in itself because services need to take account of where such individuals are to be found. Are they evenly distributed throughout the community or are there particular high-risk groups or particular high-risk geographical areas? Epidemiology

Rutter's Child and Adolescent Psychiatry, 5th edition. Edited by M. Rutter, D. Bishop, D. Pine, S. Scott, J. Stevenson, E. Taylor and A. Thapar. © 2008 Blackwell Publishing, ISBN: 978-1-4051-4549-7.

has also been very useful in tracking changes over time in communities – for example, the rising rates of psychoactive medication, the altering patterns of substance use, variations over time in rates of suicide and attempted suicide, and changing rates of children being taken into care or of homelessness. It may also document changing patterns in in-patient provision or of the other residential facilities. The basic point is that epidemiology can provide an essential backcloth of factors (other than the number of children with disorders) relevant to the planning of services.

Epidemiology Comprises the Scientific Study of the Distribution of Particular Features in Populations

There is sometimes a tendency to think only in terms of the distribution of disorders and also to assume that populations must represent the entire general population. Neither assumption is warranted. To begin with, as discussed in chapter 5, the focus may be on risk factors rather than disorders. A classic paper in the field of internal medicine was titled "The epidemiology of uniforms" (Morris, Heady, & Raffle, 1956). This particular study was not concerned with the general population; rather, it was a study of the records of uniform size in bus conductors and bus drivers in order to determine the risks for heart disease associated with being overweight and with lack of exercise. Service planning ought to be influenced by knowledge of the distribution of risk factors and their association with the development of disorders requiring intervention.

In the same way, service planning needs information on the extent to which there is a disproportionately high or low rate of disorders in particular segments of the population – such as those with physical ill-health, with scholastic difficulties, or in so-called "looked after" children in residential care or family foster care. A relevant historical example is provided by the Isle of Wight study (Rutter, Graham, & Yule, 1970; Rutter, Tizard, & Whitmore, 1970). The initial prompt for the study concerned a query from the British Department of Education to Tizard (and then Tizard & Rutter) whether the strong association found in the early part of the 20th century of scholastic problems being much more frequent in children with chronic physical disabilities still applied in the latter part of the 20th century. As the epidemiological research went ahead, further queries were posed as to whether the rate of disorders was the same in inner city areas such as London as on the Isle of Wight (Rutter, 1981) and whether the rates of disorder found in the pre-adolescent years were the same as those during the teenage years (Rutter, 1979).

Sometimes there has been an assumption that service planning needs to be concerned only with chronic disorders on the grounds that if the disorder is acute, one can assume that recovery will take place without the need for intervention. However, this is a mistaken assumption for several different reasons. To begin with, disorders may be acute because they are fatal. Thus, there has been a legitimate concern over the high level of suicide in young people (see chapter 40). Concern is not because one can do anything after the person has killed themselves, but rather because the fatal act raises questions as to whether it might have been preventable if appropriate services had been provided. Even when not fatal, acute disorders may have much longer-term clinical, and therefore service, implications. Thus, episodes of mania are often relatively short lived (see chapter 38) but bipolar disorders are associated with a high rate of recurrence and a high rate of impairment. Accordingly, even a short-lived episode of mania has implications for treatment provision.

For many purposes, prevalence constitutes the most appropriate index of rates of disorder. However, in some instances it is necessary to know about incidence – the rate of new cases arising over a particular period of time. This would apply to the effects of some acute major hazard in causing disorder (such as floods, earthquakes, being taken hostage or receiving a serious head injury). Similarly, in planning services it will be important to know the age period when a first psychotic episode occurs.

Because so many questions with respect to service planning involve the need to know about longitudinal course, there has been an increasing tendency for epidemiological studies to be longitudinal (see chapter 13). Longitudinal studies have been crucial in showing that cross-sectional epidemiological studies greatly underestimate the true rate of disorders in the community because so many disorders are recurrent. The cumulative prevalence is much higher than the cross-sectional prevalence at any single point in time (Kim-Cohen, Caspi, Moffitt *et al.*, 2003).

Prevalence of Mental Disorder

Aware of the very different living conditions in developing countries, compared with the circumstances in western industrialized nations in which most epidemiological studies have been undertaken, researchers have sought to determine whether the differences have led to variations in the rates of mental disorders (Verhulst, 1995; Weisz & Eastman, 1995). As Fleitlich-Bilyk & Goodman have emphasized, the question requires an adequate sample size, a representative sampling frame, the use of standardized interview measures, and assessment of distress and impairment as well as symptoms (Fleitlich-Bilyk & Goodman, 2004). Their study in a predominantly urban municipality in Brazil found a prevalence rate for mental disorders of 13% in 7–14-year-old school children using the same instrument (Development and Well-being Assessment; DAWBA) as that employed in the British national survey (Ford, Goodman, & Meltzer, 2003; Meltzer, Gatward, Goodman *et al.*, 2000), which showed a rate of 10%. The pattern of diagnoses was broadly similar in Brazil and Britain. A comparable study of the same age group in a Russian city (Goodman, Slobodskaya, & Knyazev, 2005) produced a rate of 15.3%. Again, the general pattern of diagnoses was broadly similar to that in Britain. The family risk factors for disorder were also similar in the two countries, except that parents' socioeconomic status was largely unassociated with risk in Russia. A third comparable study, of 5–10-year-olds in Bangladesh, also gave rise to a prevalence figure of 15% (Mullick & Goodman, 2005). The pattern of diagnoses was generally similar to that in the British survey (apart from a query about a possibly higher rate of obsessive-compulsive disorder). Possibly the most important finding for service planning was that the prevalence of disorder varied by area – being highest in the slum area (19.5%), lowest in the urban area (10.0%) and intermediate in the rural area (15.4%). These differences closely paralleled the variations in psychosocial circumstances. It might be thought that the variation in prevalence in these studies between 9% and 20% has implications for service provision. In an ideal world that might be the case but what is most apparent across all the surveys is that the prevalence of disorder far exceeded the availability of services. This has been a universal finding in both developing and industrialized countries (see e.g. Costello, Mustillo, Erkanli *et al.*, 2003; Flisher, Kramer, Grosser *et al.*, 1997; Meltzer, Gatwood, Goodman *et al.*, 2000). Rather than attempt any precise estimate of service needs in relation to any given prevalence figure, the key message is that the available services everywhere fall well short of even a conservative estimate of requirements. The broad similarity of diagnostic patterns and risk factors also suggests that, for many purposes, it is likely to be legitimate to extrapolate across countries.

Family Perception of Service Need

One of the important innovations in the Isle of Wight survey was the systematic assessment of the parents' views on service need. About 7% of 10–11-year-old children were judged to have a clinically significant mental disorder (Rutter, Tizard, & Whitmore, 1970), but only 1 in 10 of these was receiving psychiatric treatment. The research assessment was that about one-third of the 7% of children with disorder needed diagnosis and advice only, one-third possibly required treatment and one-third definitely required treatment. Half the parents of children with a mental disorder stated definitely that they thought their child had a disorder that was beyond that experienced by most other children of the same age. Only 10% stated that their child had no difficulties, but 41% were indefinite or uncertain whether the child had any emotional or behavioral disorder. The proportion definitely wanting help for their children was only 18%, although spontaneous comments later in the interview indicated that some other parents would welcome help if it was offered. Whether the parents wanted help seemed to have little to do with either the severity of the disorder or its nature. Many parents seemed to be unaware of what services were available or what kinds of help could be offered. When people believe that they cannot change a situation, there is a marked tendency for them to believe that they are satisfied with it (Festinger, 1957). Also, in the small group of children receiving services, some parents were critical of the help being provided. Of course, in the 40 years or so since the surveys were undertaken, much more effective treatments have become available and people have become more aware of children's difficulties and needs. Nevertheless, the point remains that the planning of services has to take into account what people want, and will accept, as well as expert assessments of need.

Epidemiology has an important role in examining population variations in people's recognition of mental health service need. Thus, the comparisons between Thailand and the USA, and between Jamaica and the USA, undertaken by Weisz & Eastman (1995), showed that Thai adults tended to rate children's problems as less serious, less unusual and more likely to improve without intervention than were US adults. Problems involving disruptive behavior were much more likely to result in clinic referral in the USA than in Thailand, whereas emotional problems were more likely to lead to referral in Thailand. In relation to attention deficit/hyperactivity disorder (ADHD), Ho, Leung, Luk *et al.* (1996) compared the epidemiological characteristics of ADHD in the UK and Hong Kong populations. They found that in Hong Kong parents and teachers reported higher levels of hyperactivity than in the UK, although on objective measures the rates in the two populations were comparable. It is suggested that cultural expectations about children being controlled and well regulated in their behavior accounted for this effect (Luk, Leung, & Ho, 2002). However, in general at the present, the database is too limited, and the number of systematic cross-cultural comparisons too few, for any general explanation of the meaning of these variations. What is clear, however, is that they should inform the planning of services. It is a major limitation of epidemiological studies of psychopathology that very few have assessed either family views on children's problems or people's willingness to access services offered. There is as yet no standard method of assessing these attitudinal factors and such information may in any case be best obtained with methods tailor-made for specific populations (for a useful exploration of these issues see Sayal, Goodman, & Ford, 2006).

Age Variations

A key issue with respect to the planning of services concerns possible age variations, because the type of services available tends to be different for each age group. For many years, the accepted view was that the problems of preschoolers were of little clinical significance. The Waltham Forest epidemiological study in London set out to test this notion by undertaking systematic assessments of 3-year-olds who were then followed up to age 8 years (Richman, Stevenson, & Graham, 1982). The findings at age 3 showed that some 7% had a moderate or severe mental disorder and a further 15% had mild problems. From a service perspective, it was important that the rates of disorder were much higher in children who showed language delay. It might still be argued that the disorders at age 3 were likely to be evanescent and would readily remit without treatment. The findings at age 8, however, negated this view. Of those with disorder at 3, 62% showed disorder at 8, compared with 22% of those without disorder at 3. Adverse family factors were associated with the development of disorder at 3, but were only marginally associated with its persistence. Rather, the form of the disorder at 3 years was strongly predictive; outcome was more likely to be poor in the case of disorders involving restlessness and overactivity.

Since this pioneering study, better measures of psychopathology have become available (Egger, Erkanli, Keeler *et al.*, 2006). Studies using these methods have similarly shown that the rate of psychopathology in the preschool age period is broadly comparable with that in middle childhood (Egger & Angold, 2006). The limited available follow-up data on preschoolers have confirmed the early finding of substantial persistence of disorder (Campbell, 1994). It is clear that mental disorders in the preschool years *are* of clinical importance and services for this age group need to include the diagnosis and treatment of psychopathology.

A parallel question arose with respect to adolescence. It was directly tackled by means of a follow-up of the 10–11-year-olds in the Isle of Wight study (Rutter, 1979). The findings showed an increase in psychopathology, but this was largely a function of the adolescent's own reporting, rather than that of their parents. Other evidence has shown that the rising rate of mental disorder in adolescence reflects the incidence of schizophrenia, depressive disorders, substance abuse and eating disorders (Rutter, in press). It is noteworthy, too, however, that the early-onset neurodevelopmental disorders also tend to persist through adolescence into adult life (see chapter 13).

Epidemiology of Services

In considering the planning of services, evidence is needed on the current provision of services and the extent to which such current provision actually deals with psychopathology in young people. This is where, for example, surveys of mental disorders in young people as they arise in either primary care services (see chapter 72), pediatric services (see chapter 70) or special education (see chapter 74) are relevant. To attempt to best use limited resources to meet the treatment needs of the population, a system of tiered service has been developed in the UK, although systematic evaluation of its effectiveness is as yet underdeveloped (Worrall-Davies, Cottrell, & Benson *et al.*, 2004; see also chapter 71).

It remains to be seen whether this particular tier structure is the most appropriate one. In both developing and industrialized countries, the overall levels of disorder mean that a key service question concerns which types of problems can be appropriately dealt with in primary care (by family doctors, community nurses or volunteers) and which require highly trained specialists. It may also be relevant to consider when traditional healers may have an appropriate role. What are needed in these connections are systematic comparative studies (see, for example, Olds, Robinson Pettit *et al.*, 2004b), rather than assumptions that lack an adequate empirical basis.

As discussed in chapter 10, mental health problems in young people are at least as likely (if not more so) to be dealt with outside mental health services as within them. Accordingly, service planning needs to consider the extent to which this is appropriate and, in so far as it is, what use can be made of interventions in these other services – whether they be social services, schools, community nursing or pediatrics. Epidemiological evidence will not itself indicate the value of interventions in these settings (unless the researchers deliberately plan to do that), but it does emphasize that service planners need to think broadly rather than narrowly.

In that connection, epidemiological studies can be informative in demonstrating the ways in which needs, rather than bureaucratic rules, must guide planning. Throughout the world, the holders of purse strings are inclined to control costs through decisions on groups that should not be eligible for services. Thus, for example, in some parts of the UK, it has been ruled that children with an intellectual disability are ineligible to receive NHS mental health services. Epidemiological data from the Isle of Wight survey (Rutter, Tizard, & Whitmore, 1970) onwards, have been consistent in showing that such children have an increased rate of psychopathology and that, often, the disorders are complex and require skilled specialist services (see chapter 49).

In considering existing patterns of service provision, and possibilities of their strengthening or expansion, attention needs to be paid to the role of charities, consumer groups and others outside regular state provision. Particularly during recent years, there has been major growth in the influence and the role of such non-governmental organizations. This is partly in terms of their providing important "ginger" group functions in terms of pointing to needs, partly in terms of their role of providing information and partly also their direct provision of services. For example, parent-led associations have certainly been important in the development of services for young people with autism spectrum disorders, specific language impairment and with cognitive impairment.

Patterns of Disorder

One of the most important findings to emerge from the Isle of Wight epidemiological studies was the extent of overlap among disorders. This was evident at several different levels. Thus, at a psychiatric diagnostic level it was clear that, although there were important distinctions between emotional disorders and conduct disorders, many children showed features of both (Rutter, Tizard, & Whitmore, 1970). In addition, there was substantial overlap between scholastic problems of various kinds, physical ill-health and psychopathology. Moreover, it was also apparent that service needs were greatest in the case of young people with problems in several different arenas, rather than just one. This led to a recommendation that service planning needed to be based on individual needs (taking into account the overlap among problems), rather than individual diagnoses, important though they were for some purposes.

The much more recent Great Smoky Mountains study (Costello, Angold, Burns *et al.*, 1996) also showed that service planning needs to be based on individual needs. It underlined the point that there were children who showed substantial impairment in their functioning as a result of mental disorders (approximately 10%), but yet where the disorders did not meet any currently accepted criteria for any one particular diagnosis (Angold, Costello, Farmer *et al.*, 1999). The implication, again, was that planning needed to be based on impairment rather more than on whether particular diagnostic criteria were met.

Epidemiological and/or longitudinal studies have brought out the importance of considering continuities and discontinuities over time (see chapter 13). Thus, it has been found that in the majority of mental disorders in early adult life that are of a sufficient severity to involve active treatment, over half were first manifest before the age of 15. It might have been expected that there was substantial continuity in the form of the disorder, as shown at the different age periods, but there were important differences. It was particularly striking that conduct disorder in childhood constituted the form of psychopathology that was most likely to be associated with mental disorders in adult life, this tendency being evident across a broad range of diagnoses (Kim-Cohen *et al.*, 2003). Similarly, other epidemiological studies have shown the frequency and importance of psychopathological progressions – as for example between substance abuse and depression (Brook, Cohen, & Brook, 1998; Rao, Daley, & Hammen, 2000).

Epidemiological and/or longitudinal studies have also been crucial in noting that schizophrenic psychoses in adult life are frequently preceded by neurodevelopmental impairment in early childhood and by psychotic-like manifestations in late childhood/early adolescence (see chapter 13). This has raised the issue as to whether it might be possible to prevent overt schizophrenic psychoses by appropriate interventions in earlier life. The difficulty, however, is not just the limited evidence on whether interventions could be successful at this early age, but also the problems of false positive indications for treatment. Most individuals with these precursors of schizophrenia do not go on to develop schizophrenia. Hence, early preventive interventions would involve treating a large number of individuals unnecessarily. That might not matter if the interventions were without risk but this is very unlikely to be the case.

Responsivity to Treatment

As discussed in numerous chapters throughout this volume, good evidence is available on the short-term effectiveness of both pharmacological and psychological treatment for psychopathology in young people. Moreover, there is growing evidence on which treatments are most effective for which problems (see chapters 60–73). That is very encouraging but, unfortunately, it does not lead very directly to recommendations on service planning because the evidence on efficacy largely stems from interventions by experts and the results of ordinary services are much less impressive. This was particularly striking, for example, in the multicenter American study for treatment of ADHD. Most treatments in the community involved the use of stimulant medication, which proved effective in expert hands. Results, by contrast, were much worse for ordinary treatment as delivered in the community and this was especially so with disorders that involved several patterns of psychopathology (Jensen, Garcia, Glied *et al.*, 2005). Also, the particular forms of psychological treatment that had been shown to be most effective involved skills that are not widely available in ordinary services as provided in the UK or indeed in any other industrialized western country. It needs to be added that the evidence of efficacy of interventions is much better with respect to short-term benefits than it is for long-term ones.

Much the same applies in the field of universal preventive interventions. Thus, there are good studies showing the benefits of community-wide interventions focused on improving family functioning (Olds, 2002; Olds, Henderson, Cole *et al.*, 1998; Olds, Kitzman, Cole *et al.*, 2004a; Olds *et al.*, 2004b). The very large-scale British prevention program based on similar principles – "Sure Start" – does not seem to have had anything like the same success (Rutter, 2006). These are early days and it may be that the benefits are greater than suggested by early findings. Nevertheless, what is quite clear from the epidemiological evidence is that generally well-intentioned programs based on established principles may not work if adequate attention is not paid to the details of implementation (see chapter 60).

Patterns of Referral and Use of Services

An early British epidemiological study, the Buckinghamshire study, drew attention to the finding that young people's referral to mental health services was driven at least as much by problems in the family as by the children's own pattern of disorder (Shepherd, Oppenheim, & Mitchell, 1971). They concluded that the findings meant that rates of clinic referral provided a most unsatisfactory guide to the level of psychopathology in young people. Another lesson might be that the services needed to be geared to the family problems often (but not always) associated with child psychopathology as much as with the children's disorders themselves. It should be noted that this association does not necessarily mean that the family problems caused the child's disorder, but rather that it is when the two occurred together that help was most likely to be sought. With respect to uptake of services, in countries without free medical care, it has been striking that unmet needs for mental health services tend to be greatest in young people from economically disadvantaged families and from families with parental psychopathology (Flisher *et al.*, 1997).

A further point evident in almost all epidemiological studies has been the relatively weak agreement between the reports of parents and the young people themselves (Achenbach,

McConaughy, & Howell, 1987; Borge, Samuelson, & Rutter, 2001; Eaves, Silberg, Meyer *et al.*, 1997; Hewitt, Eaves, Silberg *et al.*, 1997; Rutter, 1979; Rutter *et al.*, 1970). To some extent this probably reflects differences in the perspectives of children and parents, but to a considerable extent it stems from the parents being unaware of the children's impairment. Service implication stemming from the epidemiological evidence is that, particularly in the case of adolescents, services need to have the possibility of direct access by the young people themselves without necessarily having to rely on their being brought by their parents.

Historically, child and adolescent services have tended to be rather separate, with little connection between the two. The epidemiological evidence has raised serious queries on the problems of the degree of separation according to services for different age groups. Two rather different sets of findings are relevant. First, there are the numerous, high-risk epidemiological studies showing the extent to which parental mental disorder constitutes a risk factor for psychopathology in the children (Rutter, 1989). Much of the high-risk research was predicated on the basis of the genetic risks involved but it is clear that the mediation of risks is partially environmental as well as genetic. Early epidemiological and clinical studies (see e.g., Rutter, 1966) indicated how few psychiatrists dealing with adults even asked about the children, let alone paid attention to their needs. Fortunately, that has changed to a considerable extent (although it cannot be said to be really satisfactory now) and it is clear that when one member of the family has a mental disorder, attention needs to be paid to the possibility that other family members also have mental health problems. The finding that many disorders span age periods in crucial ways is also relevant. This is obvious, for example, with respect to prodromal schizophrenia, substance abuse problems and eating disorders. Most adult psychiatrists are ill-equipped to deal with the sequelae in adult life of serious problems that develop during childhood and many child psychiatrists do not have the experience of dealing with the disorders as they are manifest in adult life. Some of the issues this raises are outlined in relation to ADHD by Asherson, Chen, Craddock *et al.* (2007). Not only is a more "joined-up" approach to services needed, but thought needs to be given to whether or not some services need to be problem focused, rather than age defined (see chapter 13).

Variations Across Groups in Rates or Patterns of Disorder

Funding agencies and policy-makers press for statistics that represent the true national rates of disorder. This is based on the totally mistaken assumption that this is what is needed for planning, but it is not. It is more important to understand the nature and origins of variation in rates within a population than to obtain ever more accurate estimates of general prevalence across an entire nation. It would make no sense, for example, to plan services on the expectation that the level and pattern of need would be the same in, say, inner London and rural Wales, or in US cities and in rural farm areas in the USA. Rather, what is needed is evidence on the extent to which rates and patterns vary across areas together with the reasons for such variation, if those can be identified (see e.g., Bird, Canino, Davies *et al.*, 2001). Numerous epidemiological studies have shown that geographical variations are indeed quite large. What has been less forthcoming has been the evidence on the causes of such variation. A complication with any proposal simply to plan services to be located in geographical locations with the highest rate of those in need is the "ecological fallacy" (Pinatadosi, Byar, & Green, 1988). This arises because there will be in sum more individuals in need outside areas of greatest concentration of needs. For this reason there will continue to be a place for screening for needs at an individual or family level and not just to plan service delivery by geographic concentration.

Of course, valuable clues have emerged from the epidemiological research but too few studies have been designed in a way that could test competing explanations about the mediating causal influences. Nevertheless, what the research has shown are some of the most important high-risk groups (see chapters 5 & 25). For example, children in residential and family foster care have consistently been found to have unusually high rates of both scholastic difficulties and psychopathology (Meltzer, Gatward, Goodman *et al.*, 2003; see chapter 32). Mental disorders are also high in homeless children (see chapter 25), asylum seekers (see chapter 31) and in those in prison or other forms of custodial care (see chapter 68).

Generalizability of Epidemiological Findings

As noted in chapter 15, epidemiological studies around the world have, on the whole, showed that the main risk and protective factors of mental disorders are broadly similar. Moreover, similarities outweigh dissimilarities even in the overall patterning and rate of disorders. Nevertheless, this does not mean that studies in industrialized western nations can be extended without question to developing countries. All too often, new surveys seem to have been planned as if the main question was whether the rates of disorder are higher or lower in some country as compared with, say, the USA or UK. Only very rarely is that the most important question. Rather, studies are needed to determine whether the patterning of risk factors has important service implications. Thus, for example, in parts of the world where serious malnutrition, HIV or malaria is common, how does that interface with risks for mental disorder? If the associations are very strong, that might mean that there should be a greater focus on pediatric care in the first instance, rather than mental health services provision. It is also relevant to know whether the community attitudes towards and perception of psychopathology vary in ways that have implications for either patterns of referral or for service provision (see chapter 15).

Highly Focused Epidemiological Studies

For many aspects of service planning, broad-based epidemiological studies using instruments that tap all the main types of psychopathology are highly appropriate. The British Office of National Statistics studies provide a good example of how this may be done and how it may be useful (Meltzer *et al.*, 2003). However, there are certain needs that are not most satisfactorily met in this way. For example, many children with intellectual disability are dealt with in child and adolescent mental health services and it is clear that the rate of associated psychopathology is quite high (see chapter 49). However, broad-based mental disorder surveys are not likely to be very suitable for determining either the rate of mild intellectual disability or the patterns of association with psychopathology, and their meaning. This requires studies that are more specifically focused on the epidemiology of cognitive impairment and its correlates (Simonoff, Pickles, Chadwick *et al.*, 2006). Much the same applies to the epidemiology of specific language impairment and of reading disability, both of which have quite strong associations with psychopathology (see chapters 47 & 48). Similar considerations apply in the case of autism spectrum disorders (see chapter 46). One of the problems here is that the epidemiological evidence is clear-cut that the manifestations extend much more broadly than the traditional diagnostic concepts. Detailed studies specifically focused on autism spectrum disorders are required – not only to determine the prevalence of this group of conditions, but also the variations in its manifestations and their correlates (see e.g., Baird, Simonoff, Pickles *et al.*, 2006). It is clear that, as diagnosed, autism spectrum disorders have become much more common over time (Rutter, 2005). This rise is, without doubt, caused in part by better ascertainment and a broadening of the diagnostic concept but it remains uncertain whether or not, in addition to these methodological considerations, there has also been a true rise brought about by some environmental hazard.

General Population Screening

The evidence that the majority of young people with a mental disorder do not receive services might seem to point to the desirability of the widespread routine application of screening methods to determine which children have disorders and hence which ones should be targeted for intervention. The possibility raises several different issues. To begin with, as discussed in chapter 20, screening questionnaires have a place as the first stage in clinical assessment. In much the same way, they may be valuable in planning systematic interventions, such as in schools. By alerting families to the presence of possible problems, they may become interested in taking up the services on offer. What would not be helpful, however, is to imply that all high scorers will receive interventions if the services are not available to provide that. Raising false expectations is not desirable.

There is, then, the rather different issue of using screening instruments at a population level to pick out children who should receive a preventive intervention because they have an increased risk of developing some serious disorder later. Thus, politicians have seized on the evidence that antisocial behavior that begins at an early age is that which is most likely to persist into adult life. Their influence is that this means that parents should be compelled to receive interventions to improve their parenting and hence to reduce the risks for the children. A key problem, however, is that epidemiological evidence indicates that although the risks associated with an early onset are real, most children showing early conduct problems do *not* go on to show a life-course-persistent pattern (Odgers, Caspi, Broadbent *et al.*, 2007). The intervention risks for false positives may not be trivial. In addition, there is uncertainty as to whether the interventions shown to be effective in treating early antisocial behavior are effective in the subgroup who are likely to continue into adult life. Somewhat similar issues arise with the prodromata of schizophrenia (see chapter 13). It will be appreciated that the concerns here arise from the problem of false positives rather than from the limitations in screening as such.

There is also the issue of using screening instruments in a total population sample as a guide to the possible overall level of disorder. There are many examples of this usage. The fact that the screening measure has only a moderate correlation with a fuller clinical assessment is not a concern with respect to population estimates, although the screen instrument cannot provide a valid diagnosis at an individual level. Nevertheless, there are three considerable problems with this use of screening. First, the presence of disorder is only one of many features on which information is needed for service planning. Moreover, most screens are not very satisfactory for the identification of unusual, highly specific disorders. Second, most emotional and/or behavioral items (whether in a questionnaire or a structured interview) involve judgments on the degree to which a child shows misery, anxiety, overactivity or some other feature. The Thailand and Hong Kong examples indicate that it cannot be assumed that raters in all cultures will make identical assumptions in making such judgments. Third, within all cultures, there is only a weak agreement among informants (such as parent, child and teacher) in their ratings. In part, this derives from differences in their opportunity to observe the relevant features but similar inter-rater disagreements arise even when they all observe the same features in the same situation. In this case, the disagreements may derive from the different raters using different comparisons (Borge, Samuelson, & Rutter *et al.*, 2001). Thus, the rating of misery or anxiety may be made by parents on the basis of a comparison with other children in the same family, by teachers on the basis of a comparison with other children in the same school class and by the child/adolescent in relation to how they felt a year ago. Surprisingly, and regrettably, epidemiologists have failed to examine these possibilities systematically. The usual solution has been to use the "or" rule – that is, a behavior is treated as present if anyone reports it. Clearly, this "works" at a rough and ready level but it causes the risk of overestimating prevalence. Alternatively, some kind of latent construct may be used in order to focus on shared variance (see e.g., Simonoff, Pickles, Meyer *et al.*, 1998). The problem with this solution is the opposite (i.e., the estimate will account for a small proportion of the total variance and hence greatly underestimate the prevalence).

We have discussed this issue at some length because the issues are poorly understood, with a resulting wrong expectation that there is some "gold standard" available if only someone would say what it is. There have been huge advances in the measurement of psychopathology, but major challenges remain.

Policy Decision-Making on Services

One further critical issue concerns patterns of policy decision-making in relation to services. The prevailing tendency in many countries today involves a view that efficacy requires competition amongst service providers. Epidemiology may well not be the best tool to identify such competition, but it can be informative in identifying the effects of market-driven inequalities in service provision.

Conclusions

In this chapter we have chosen not to focus on the many crucial technical considerations in undertaking epidemiological studies designed to be informative in the planning of services. That is certainly not because we regard methodological details as unimportant; on the contrary, they are crucial. However, our objective has been to provide an understanding for general readers of how epidemiology may be informative in service planning. Readers wishing to undertake such epidemiological studies need to turn to the various sources that provide a good account of the technicalities. We have assumed that there is a general wish for evidence-based policy-making. It has to be said that in most countries, although that may be the rhetoric, that is not actually the way decisions are made. Of course, politicians and other policy-makers need to decide on the values that they wish to use in the planning of services, but they will be foolish if they ignore the role of epidemiology in providing evidence that will enable them to consider whether the particular policies they favor are ones that will actually meet the objectives they have set. Epidemiological findings as such do not, and cannot, answer policy questions on service provision but what they can do, and can do rather well, is provide information that is essential in the overall process of planning effective services. As we have emphasized, the conceptual understanding of what is required has greatly improved in recent years. The challenges for the future are many, but the way to put all the information together for service planning is one of the most important.

References

Achenbach, T. M., McConaughy, S. H., & Howell, C. T. (1987). Child–adolescent behavioural and emotional problems: Implications of cross-informant correlations for situation specificity. *Psychological Bulletin*, *101*, 213–232.

Angold, A., Costello, E. J., Farmer, E. M. Z., Burns, B. J., & Erkanli, A. (1999). Impaired but undiagnosed. *Journal of the American Academy of Child and Adolescent Psychiatry, Special Section*, *38*, 129–137.

Asherson, P., Chen, W., Craddock, B., & Taylor, E. (2007). Adult attention-deficit hyperactivity disorder: recognition and treatment in general adult psychiatry. *British Journal of Psychiatry*, *190*, 4–5.

Baird, G., Simonoff, E., Pickles, A., Chandler, S., Loucas, T., Meldrum, D., *et al.* (2006). Prevalence of disorders of the autism spectrum in a population cohort of children in South Thames: the Special Needs and Autism Project (SNAP). *Lancet*, *15*, 210–215.

Bird, H. R., Canino, G. J., Davies, M., Zhang, H., Ramirez, R., & Lahey, B. B. (2001). Prevalence and correlates of antisocial behaviors among three ethnic groups. *Journal of Abnormal Child Psychology*, *29*, 465–478.

Borge, A. I. H., Samuelson, S. O., & Rutter, M. (2001). Observer variance within families: confluence among maternal, paternal and child ratings. *International Journal of Methods in Psychiatric Research*, *10*, 11–21.

Brook, J. S., Cohen, P., & Brook, D. W. (1998). Longitudinal study of co-occurring psychiatric disorders and substance abuse. *Journal of the American Academy of Child and Adolescent Psychiatry*, *37*, 322–330.

Campbell, S. B. (1994). Hard-to-manage preschool boys: externalizing behavior, social competence, and family context at two-year follow-up. *Journal of Abnormal Child Psychology*, *22*, 147–166.

Costello, E. J., Angold, A., Burns, B. J., Stangl, D. K., Tweed, D. L., Erkanli, A., *et al.* (1996). Great Smoky Mountains study of youth: Goals, design, methods and the prevalence of DSM-III-R disorders. *Archives of General Psychiatry*, *53*, 1129–1136.

Costello, E. J., Copeland, W., Cowell, A., & Keeler, G. (2007). Service costs of caring for adolescents with mental illness in a rural community, 1993–2000. *American Journal of Psychiatry*, *164*, 36–42.

Costello, E. J., Egger, H. L., & Angold, A. (2005). 10-year research update review: The epidemiology of child and adolescent psychiatric disorders. 1. Methods and public health burden. *Journal of the American Academy of Child and Adolescent Psychiatry*, *44*, 972–986.

Costello, E. J., Foley, D. L., & Angold, A. (2006). 10-year research update review: The epidemiology of child and adolescent psychiatric disorders. 2. Developmental epidemiology. *Journal of the American Academy of Child and Adolescent Psychiatry*, *45*, 8–25.

Costello, E. J., Mustillo, S., Erkanli, A., Keeler, G., & Angold, A. (2003). Prevalence and development of psychiatric disorders in childhood and adolescence. *Archives of General Psychiatry*, *60*, 837–844.

Detels, R., McEwen, J., Beaglehole, R., & Tanaka, H. (Eds.). (2002). *Oxford textbook of public health* (4th ed). Oxford & New York: Oxford University Press.

Earls, F. (1979). Epidemiology and child psychiatry: historical and conceptual development. *Comprehensive Psychiatry*, *20*, 256–269.

Eaves, L. J., Silberg, J. L., Meyer, J. M., Maes, H. H., Simonoff, E., Neale, M. C., *et al.* (1997). Genetics and developmental psychopathology. 2. The main effects of genes and environment on behavioral problems in the Virginia Twin Study of Adolescent Behavioral Development. *Journal of Child and Adolescent Psychiatry*, *38*, 965–980.

Egger, H. L., & Angold, A. (2006). Common emotional and behavioral disorders in preschool children: Presentation, nosology, and epidemiology. *Journal of Child Psychology and Psychiatry*, *47*, 313–337.

Egger, H. L., Erkanli, A., Keeler, G., Potts, E., Walter, B. K., & Angold, A. (2006). Test–retest reliability of the Preschool Age Psychiatric Assessment (PAPA). *Journal of the American Academy of Child and Adolescent Psychiatry*, *45*, 538–549.

Ezpeleta, L., Keeler, G., Erkanli, A., Costello, E. J., & Angold, A. (2001). Epidemiology of psychiatric disability in childhood and adolescence. *Journal of Child Psychology and Psychiatry*, *42*, 901–914.

Festinger, L. (1957). *A theory of cognitive dissonance*. Evanston, IL: Row, Peterson. (Reissued 1962. London: Tavistock.)

Fleitlich-Bilyk, B., & Goodman, R. (2004). Prevalence of child and adolescent psychiatric disorders in southeast Brazil. *Journal of the American Academy of Child and Adolescent Psychiatry*, *43*, 727–734.

Flisher, A. J., Kramer, R. A., Grosser, R. C., Alegria, M., Bird, H. R., Bourdon, K. H., *et al.* (1997). Correlates of unmet need for mental health services by children and adolescents. *Psychological Medicine*, *27*, 1145–1154.

Fombonne, E. (2002). Case identification in an epidemiological context. In M. Rutter, & E. Taylor (Eds.), *Child and adolescent psychiatry* (4th ed). Oxford: Blackwell Publishing.

Ford, T., Goodman, R., & Meltzer, H. (2003). The British child and adolescent mental health survey 1999: the prevalence of DSM-IV disorders. *Journal of American Academy Child Adolescent Psychiatry*, *42*, 1203–1211.

Goodman, R., Slobodskaya, H., & Knyazev, G. (2005). Russian child mental health: A cross-sectional study of prevalence and risk factors. *European Child and Adolescent Psychiatry*, *14*, 28–33.

Hewitt, J. K., Eaves, L. J., Silberg, J. L., Rutter, M., Simonoff, E., Meyer, J. M., *et al.* (1997). Genetics and developmental psychopathology. 1. Phenotypic assessment in the Virginia Twin Study of Adolescent Behavioral Development. *Journal of Child Psychology and Psychiatry*, *38*, 943–963.

Ho, T. P., Leung, P. W. L., Luk, E. S. L., Taylor, E., BaconShone, J., & Mak, F. L. (1996). Establishing the constructs of childhood behavioral disturbances in a Chinese population: A questionnaire study. *Journal of Abnormal Child Psychology*, *24*, 417–431.

Jensen, P. S., Garcia, J. A., Glied, S., Crowe, M., Foster, M., Schlander, M., *et al.* (2005). Cost-effectiveness of ADHD treatments: findings from the multimodal treatment study of children with ADHD. *American Journal of Psychiatry*, *162*, 1628–1636.

Kim-Cohen, J., Caspi, A., Moffitt, T. E., Harrington, H. L., Milne, B. S., & Poulton, R. (2003). Prior juvenile diagnoses in adults with mental disorder: Developmental follow-back of a prospective-longitudinal cohort. *Archives of General Psychiatry*, *60*, 709–717.

Luk, E. S. L., Leung, P. W. L., & Ho, T-P. (2002). Cross-cultural/ethnic aspects of childhood hyperactivity. In S. Sandburg (Ed.) *Hyperactivity and attention disorders of childhood* (2nd ed.), (pp. 64–98). Cambridge: Cambridge University Press.

Meltzer, H., Gatward, R., Corbin, T., Goodman, R., & Ford, T. (2003). *The mental health of young people looked after by local authorities in England*. London: HMSO.

Meltzer, H., Gatward, R., Goodman, R., & Ford, T. (2000). *The mental health of children and adolescents in Great Britain*. London: The Stationery Office.

Morris, J. N., Heady, J. A., & Raffle, P. A. B. (1956). Physique of London busmen: Epidemiology of uniforms. *Lancet*, *2*, 569–570.

Mullick, M. S. I., & Goodman, R. (2005). The prevalence of psychiatric disorders among 5–10 year olds in rural, urban and slum areas in Bangladesh. *Social Psychiatry and Psychiatric Epidemiology*, *40*, 663–671.

Odgers, C. L., Caspi, A., Broadbent, J. M., Dickson, N., Hancox, M. D., Harrington, H., *et al.* (2007). Conduct problem subtypes in males predict differential adult health burden. *Archives of General Psychiatry*, *64*, 476–484.

Olds, D. L. (2002). Prenatal and infancy home visiting by nurses: From randomized trials to community replication. *Prevention Science*, *3*, 153–172.

Olds, D. L., Henderson, C. R. Jr., Cole, R., Eckenrode, J., Kitzman, H., Luckey, D., *et al.* (1998). Long-term effects of nurse home visitation on children's criminal and antisocial behavior. *Journal of the American Medical Association*, *280*, 1238–1244.

Olds, D. L., Kitzman, H., Cole, R., Robinson, J., Sidora, K., Luckey, D. W., *et al.* (2004a). Effects of nurse home visiting on maternal life course and child development: Age 6 follow-up results of a randomized trial. *Pediatrics*, *114*, 1550–1559.

Olds, D. L., Robinson, J., Pettit, L., Luckey, D. W., Holmberg, J., Ng, R. K., *et al.* (2004b). Effects of home visits by paraprofessionals and by nurses: Age 4 follow-up results of a randomized trial. *Pediatrics*, *114*, 1560–1568.

Pinatadosi, S., Byar, D. P., & Green, S. B. (1988). The ecological fallacy. *American Journal of Epidemiology*, *127*, 893–904.

Rao, U., Daley, S. E., & Hammen, C. (2000). Relationship between depression and substance use disorders in adolescent women during the transition to adulthood. *Journal of the American Academy of Child and Adolescent Psychiatry*, *39*, 215–222.

Richman, N., Stevenson, J., & Graham, P. (1982). *Preschool to school: a behavioural study*. London: Academic Press.

Rothman, K. J., & Greenland S. (Eds.). (1998). *Modern Epidemiology* (2nd ed.). Philadelphia: Lippincott Williams & Wilkins.

Rutter, M. (1966). *Children of sick parents: An environmental and psychiatric study*. Institute of Psychiatry Maudsley Monographs No. 16. London: Oxford University Press.

Rutter, M. (1979). *Changing youth in a changing society: Patterns of adolescent development and disorder*. London: Nuffield Provincial Hospitals Trust. (1980. Cambridge, MA: Harvard University Press.)

Rutter, M. (1981). Isle of Wight and inner London studies. In S. A. Mednick, & A. E. Baert (Eds.), *Prospective longitudinal research: An empirical basis for primary prevention of psychosocial disorders*. Oxford: Oxford University Press, pp. 122–131.

Rutter, M. (1989). Psychiatric disorder in parents as a risk factor in children. In D. Shaffer, I. Philips, N. Enver, M. Silverman, & V. Q. Anthony (Eds.), *Prevention of psychiatric disorders in child adolescence: The project of the American Academy of Child and Adolescent Psychiatry*. OSAP Prevention Monograph 2 (pp. 157–189). Rockville, MD: Office for Substance Abuse Prevention, US Department of Health and Human Services.

Rutter, M. (2005). Incidence of autism spectrum disorders: Changes over time and their meaning. *Acta Paediatrica*, *94*, 2–15.

Rutter, M. (2006). Is Sure Start an effective prevention intervention? *Child and Adolescent Mental Health*, *11*, 135–141.

Rutter, M. (2007). Proceeding from observed correlation to causal inference: The use of natural experiments. *Perspectives on Psychological Science*, *2*, 377–395.

Rutter, M. (in press). Psychopathological development across adolescence. *Journal of Youth Adolescence*,

Rutter, M., Graham, P., & Yule, W. (1970). *A neuropsychiatric study in childhood*. Clinics in Developmental Medicine 35/36. London: Heinemann/SIMP.

Rutter, M., Tizard, J., & Whitmore, K. (1970). *Education, health and behaviour*. London: Longmans. (Reprinted 1981. Melbourne, FA: Krieger.)

Sayal, K., Goodman, R., & Ford, T. (2006). Barriers to the identification of children with attention deficit/hyperactivity disorder. *Journal of Child Psychology and Psychiatry*, *47*, 744–750.

Scott, S., Knapp, M., Henderson, J., & Maughan, B. (2001). Financial cost of social exclusion: follow-up study of antisocial children into adulthood. *British Medical Journal*, *323*, 191–194.

Shepherd, M., Oppenheim, A. N., & Mitchell, S. (1971). *Childhood behaviour and mental health*. London: University of London Press.

Simonoff, E., Pickles, A., Chadwick, O., Gringras, P., Wood, N., Higgins, S., *et al.* (2006). The Croydon assessment of learning study: prevalence and educational identification of mild mental retardation. *Journal of Child Psychology and Psychiatry*, *47*, 828–839.

Simonoff, E., Pickles, A., Meyer, J., Silberg, J., & Maes, H. (1998). Genetic and environmental influences on subtypes of conduct disorder behavior in boys. *Journal of Abnormal Child Psychology*, *26*, 495–509.

Susser, E., Schwartz, S., Morabia, A., & Bromet, E. J. (2006). *Psychiatric epidemiology: searching for the causes of mental disorders*. Oxford & New York: Oxford University Press.

Verhulst, F. C. (1995). The epidemiology of child and adolescent psychopathology: strengths and limitations. In F. C. Verhulst, & H. M. Koot (Eds.), *The epidemiology of child and adolescent psychopathology*. Oxford & New York: Oxford University Press.

Verhulst, F. C., & Koot, H. M. (Eds.). (1995). *The epidemiology of child and adolescent psychopathology*. Oxford & New York: Oxford University Press.

Weisz, J. R., & Eastman, K. L. (1995). Cross-national research on child and adolescent psychopathology. In F. C. Verhulst, & H. M. Koot (Eds.), *The epidemiology of child and adolescent psychopathology*. Oxford & New York: Oxford University Press.

Worrall-Davies, A., Cottrell, D., & Benson, E. (2004). Evaluation of an early intervention Tier 2 child and adolescent mental health service. *Health and Social Care in the Community*, *12*, 119–125.

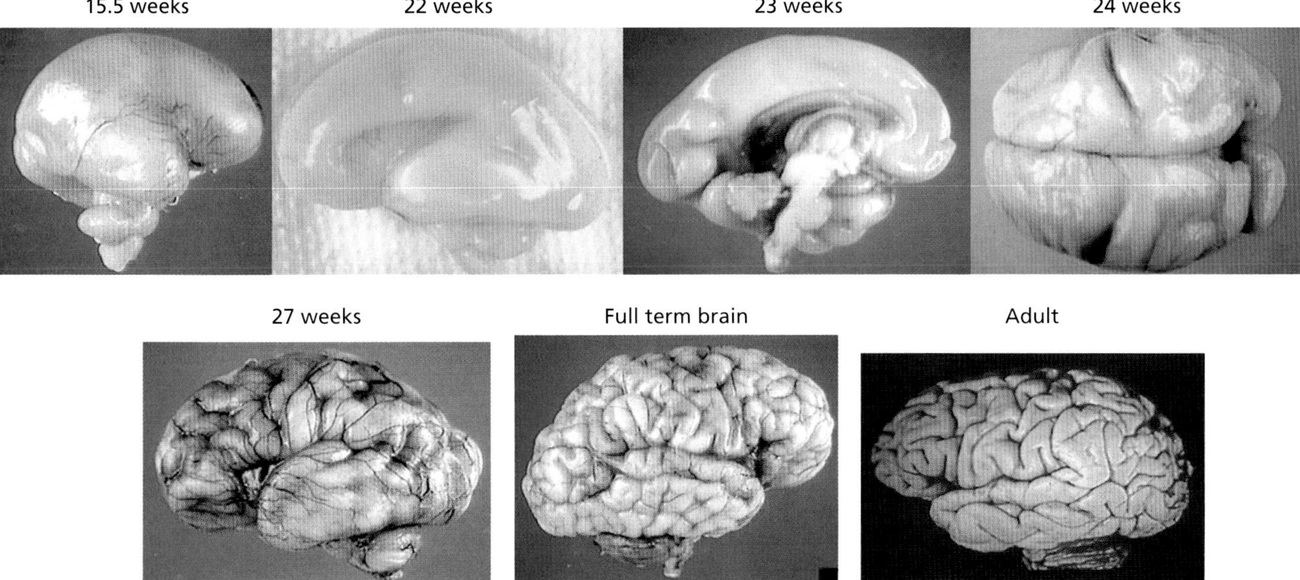

Plate 12.1 Overview of human brain development, beginning the 15th prenatal week and continuing to term and then the adult. [From Millhouse, O. E., & Stensaas, S. (n.d.). Central Nervous System. Retrieved June 6, 2005.]

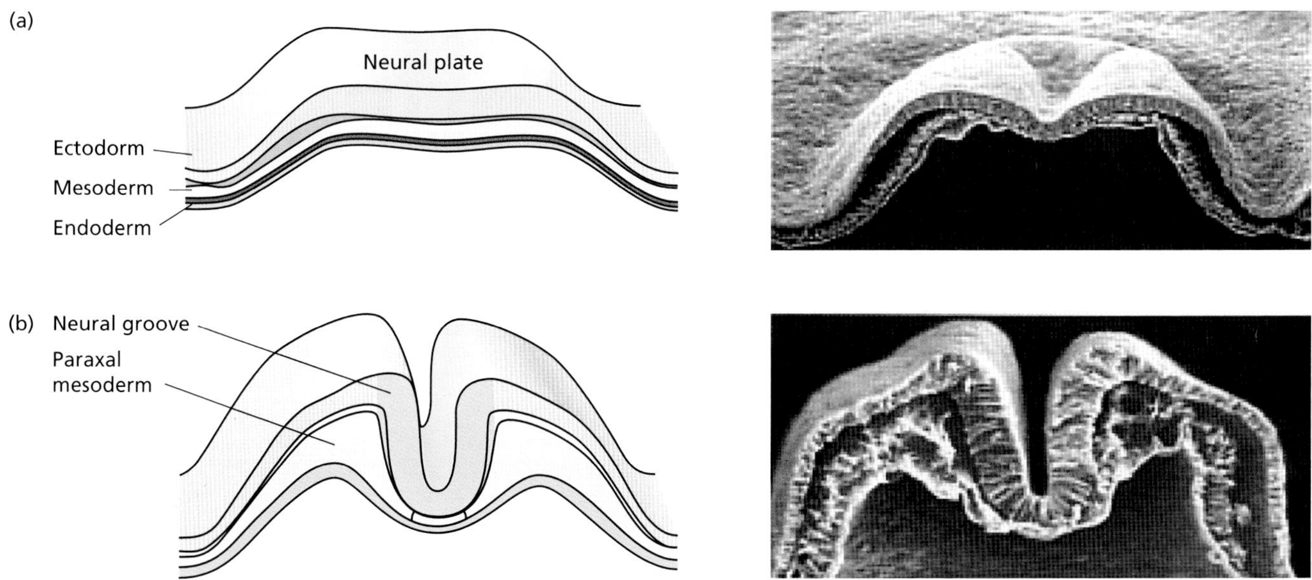

Plate 12.2 The formation of the neural tube. The left side of the figure illustrates this in cartoon form, whereas the right side displays an electron micrograph of the same process. Moving from top to bottom shows the initial formation of (a) the neural plate and (b) the neural groove.

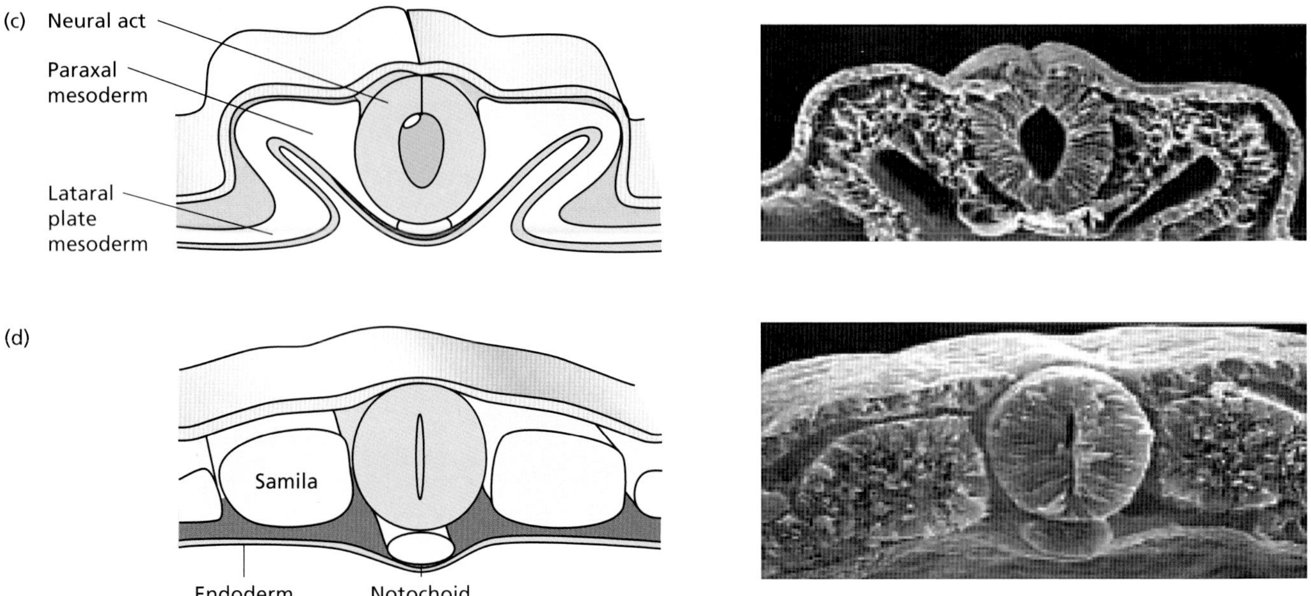

Plate 12.2 (c) & (d) Closure of the neural groove to form the neural tube. [From Jessell, T. M., & Sanes, J. R. (2000). The induction and patterning of the nervous system. In E. R. Kandel, J. H. Schwartz, & T. M. Jessell (Eds.), *Principles of neuroscience* (4th ed.) (p. 1020). USA: McGraw-Hill.]

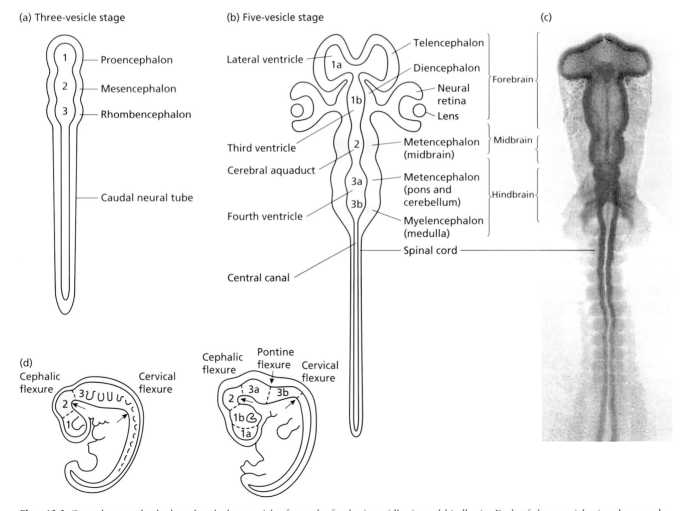

Plate 12.3 Once the neural tube has closed, three vesicles form: the forebrain, midbrain and hindbrain. Each of these vesicles is subsequently elaborated, as illustrated in panels B and C. [From Jessell, T. M., & Sanes, J. R. (2000). The induction and patterning of the nervous system. In E. R. Kandel, J. H. Schwartz, & T. M. Jessell (Eds.), *Principles of neuroscience* (4th ed.) (p. 1021). USA: McGraw-Hill.]

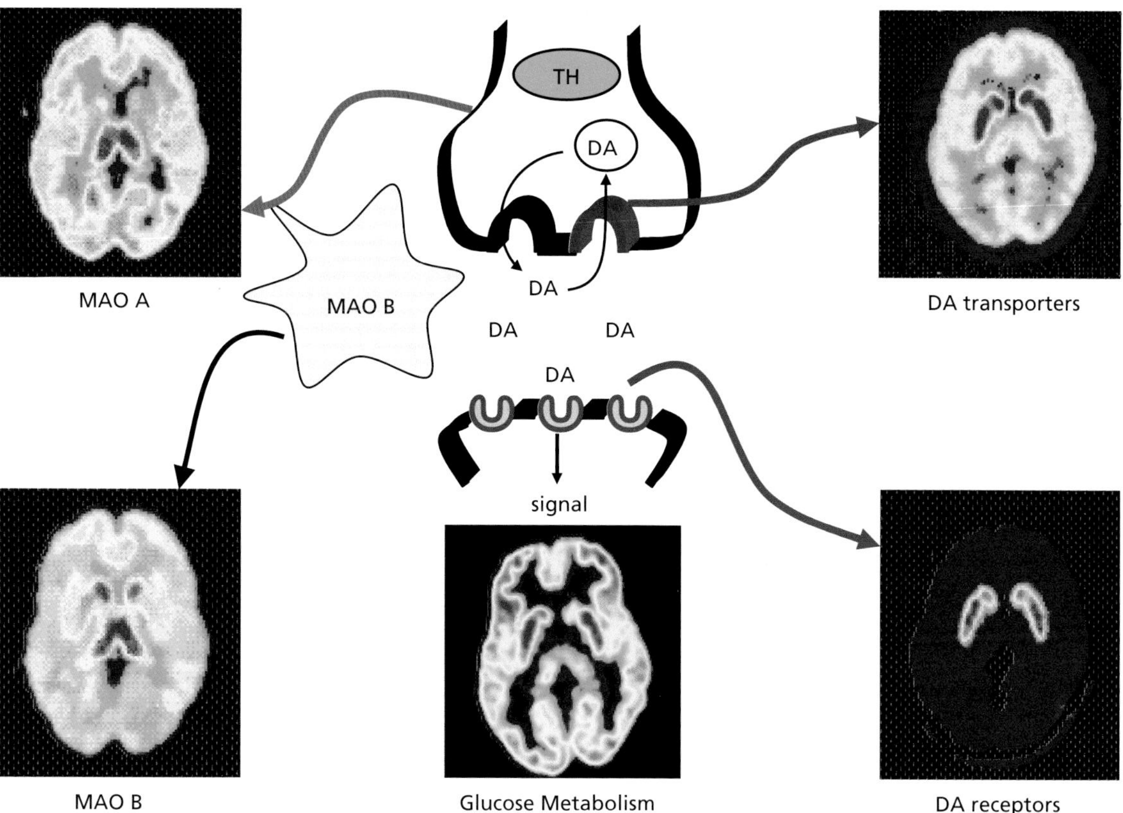

Plate 16.1 (a) A simplified diagram of the molecular targets that participate in synaptic neurotransmission and that are relevant for the effects of medications, illustrated for dopamine (DA), to show their concentration in the human brain as assessed with positron emission tomography. Courtesy of Fowler and colleagues at Brookhaven National Laboratory.

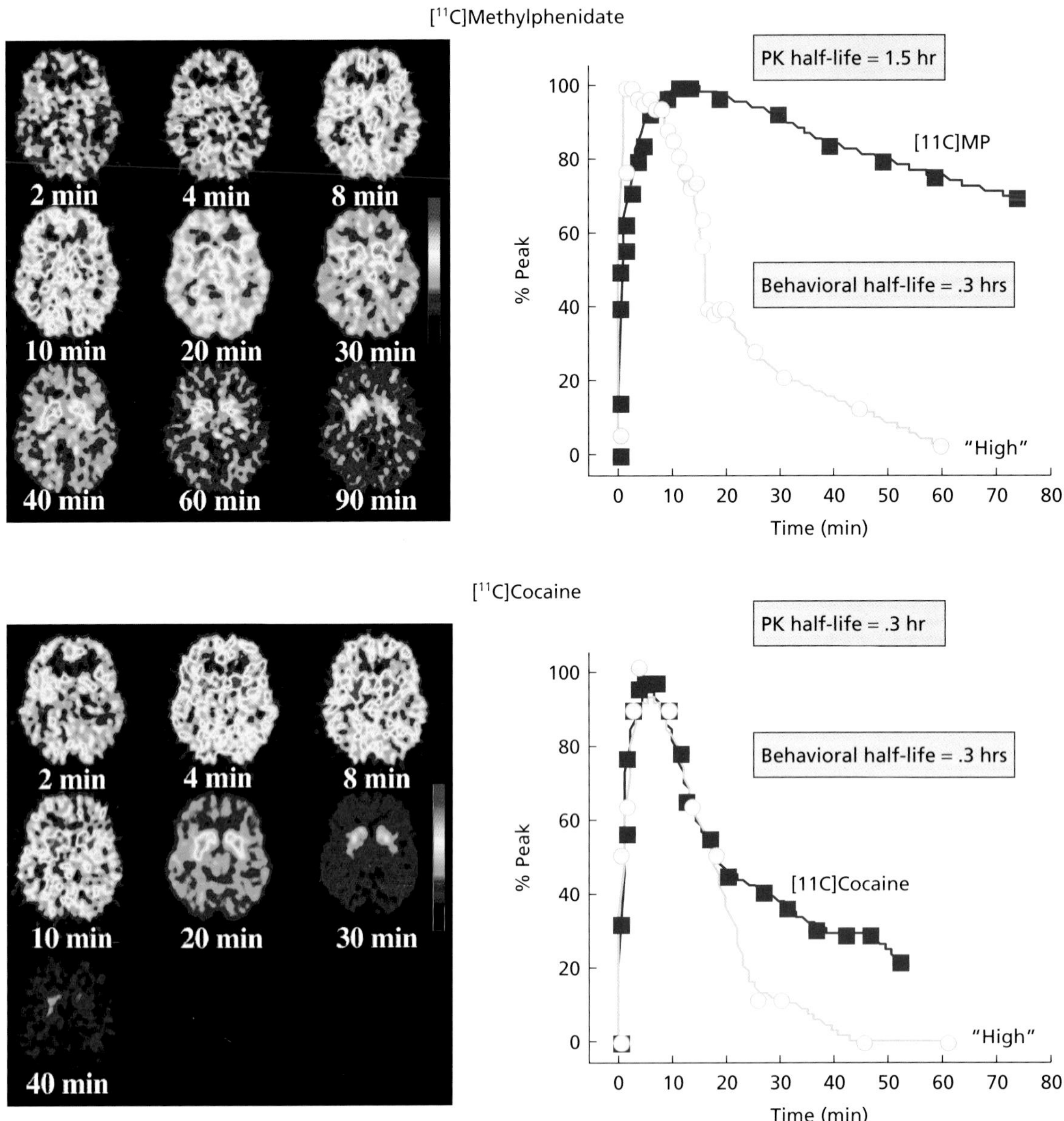

Plate 16.1 (b) Top left panel shows brain images for the distribution of [11C] methylphenidate (MPH) in the brain and right panel shows the time activity curves for [11C] MPH in striatum alongside the temporal course for the self-reports of "high" after 0.6 mg/kg i.v. MPH. Bottom left panel shows brain images for the distribution of [11C] cocaine in the brain and right panel shows the time activity curves for [11C] cocaine in striatum alongside the temporal course for the self-reports of "high" after 0.5 mg/kg i.v. cocaine. Note that, while it is the fast uptake of the drugs in brain that correlates with the "high" their rate of clearance does not. This is particularly apparent for MPH where the "high" is of short duration despite the slow clearance of the drug from the brain. After Volkow *et al.*

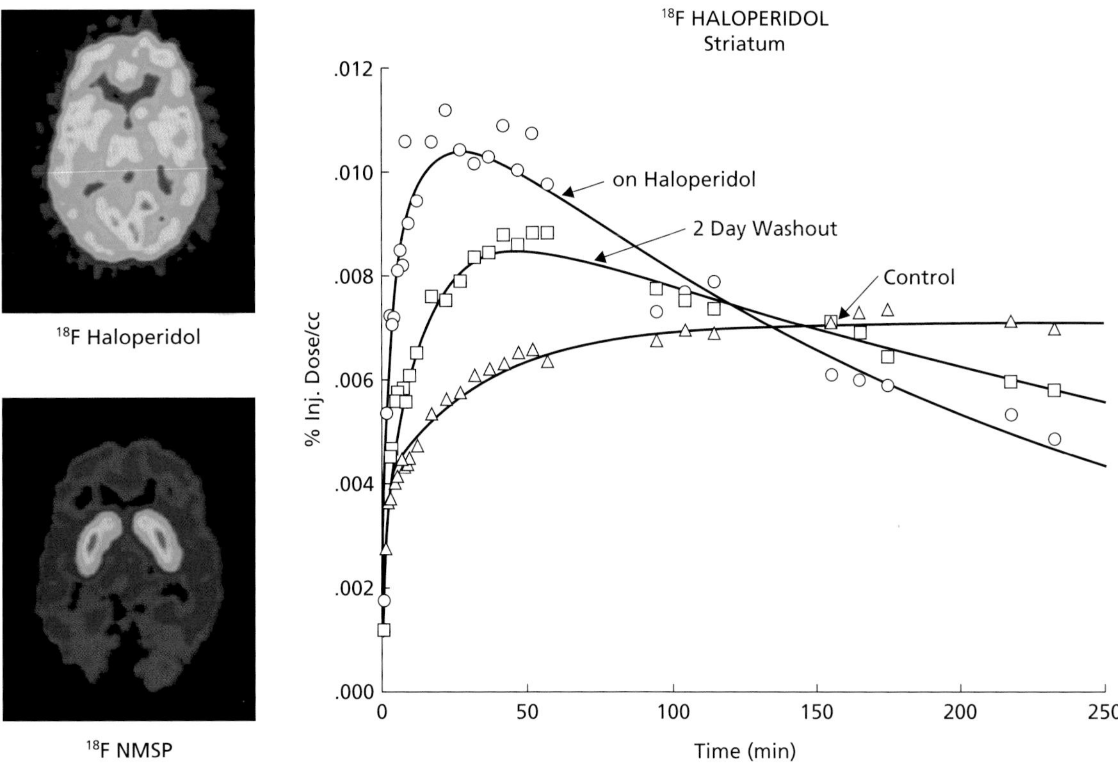

Plate 16.1 (c) Left panels show the images of the distribution of [^{18}F] haloperidol and that of the dopamine (DA) D_2 receptor radioligand [^{18}F] *N*-methyl spiroperidol (NMSP). Note the widespread binding of [^{18}F] haloperidol in brain and the restricted binding of NMSP to the basal ganglia, which is where the DA D_2 receptors are located. Right panel shows the time–activity curves of [^{18}F] haloperidol in the brain of a control subject who is not being treated with haloperidol alongside the time–activity curves of a subject who is being treated with haloperidol, tested while on the medication and 2 days after its discontinuation. Note the much faster clearance of [^{18}F] haloperidol from brain in the medicated patient from the non-treated control and also note the slowing of its clearance even after 2 days of discontinuation. NMSP images are courtesy of Brookhaven National Laboratory and [^{18}F] haloperidol data is from Schlyer *et al.* (1992).

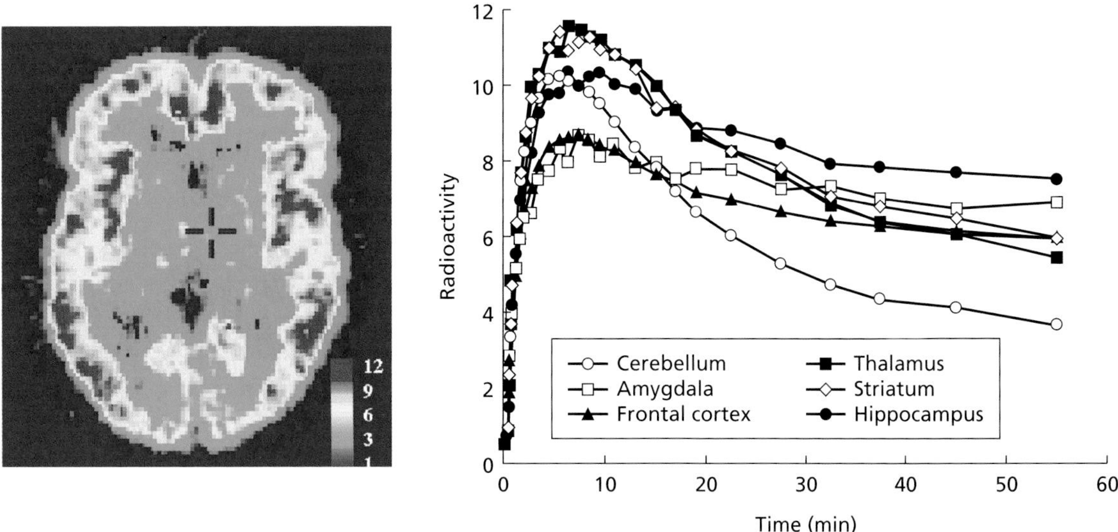

Plate 16.1 (d) Left panel shows brain images of the distribution of the antidepressant drug [^{11}C] *N*-methyl-mirtazapine and right panel shows the time–activity curves for its concentration in the various brain regions, from Marthi *et al.* (2004). With permission of Springer Science and Business Media.

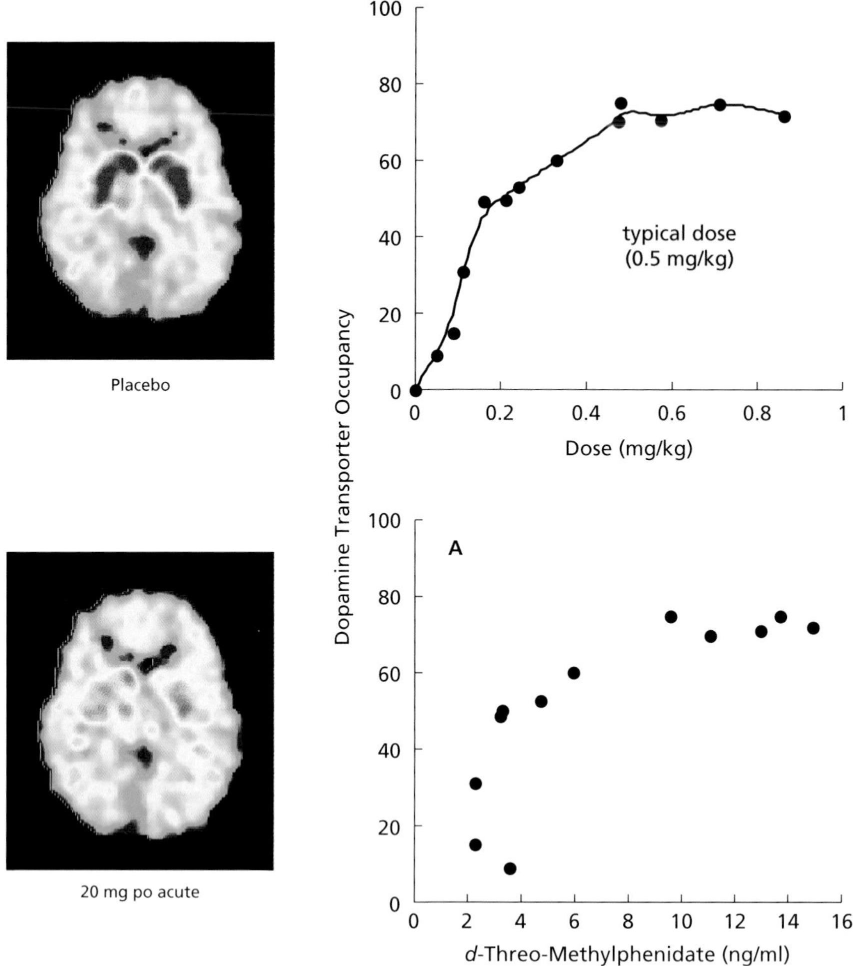

Plate 16.2 (a) Left panel shows images obtained with [^{11}C] cocaine used as a dopamine transporter ligand obtained 120 minutes after placebo and after 20 mg oral methylphenidate (MPH). Right panel shows the levels of dopamine transporter (DAT) blockade as a function of doses of oral MPH adjusted to the weight of the subjects (top) and the concentration in plasma of *d*-threo MPH (active enantiomer of MPH). Note the significant decrease in the binding of [^{11}C] cocaine in striatum even after a 20-mg oral dose of MPH. Notice also that typical doses of oral MPH blocked DAT. After Volkow *et al.* (1998).

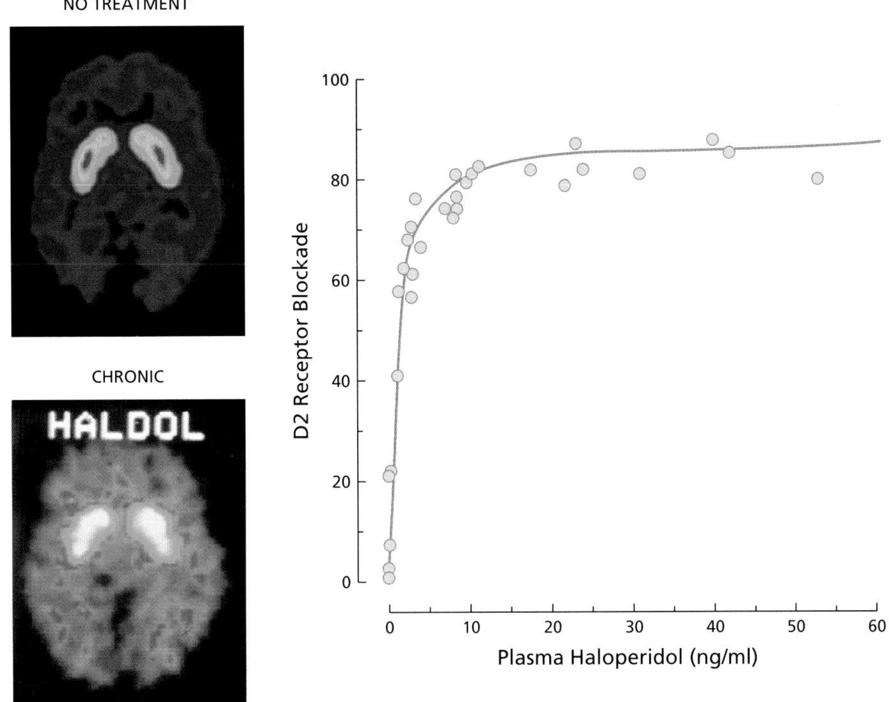

Plate 16.2 (b) Left panel shows [^{18}F] *N*-methyl spiroperidol (NMSP) images of a control and of a subject being treated chronically with haloperidol. Right panel shows the relationship between plasma haloperidol concentrations and dopamine (DA) D_2 receptor blockade.

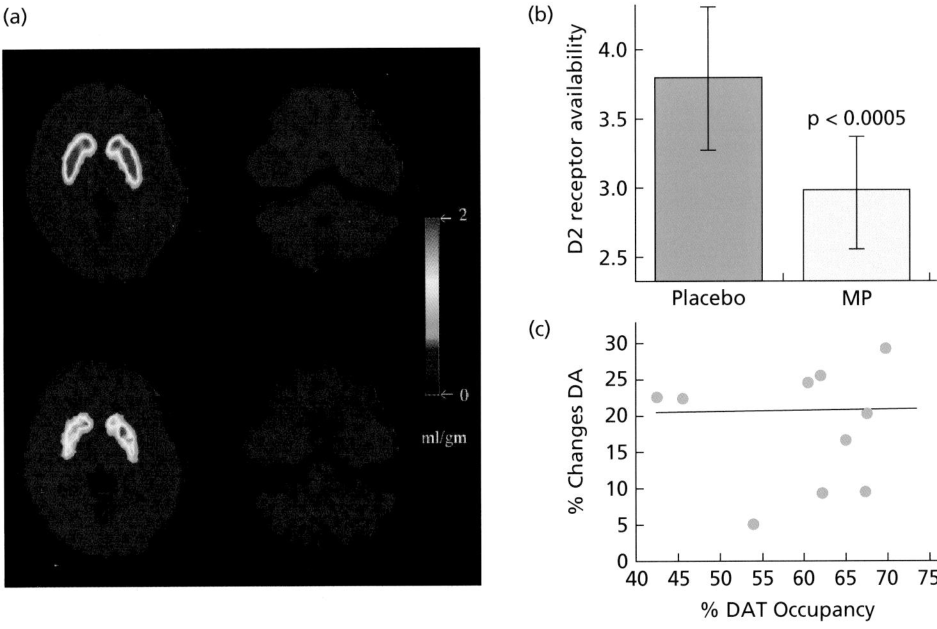

Plate 16.2 (c) Left panel shows images obtained with [^{11}C] raclopride after placebo and 120 minutes after oral MPH (60 mg). Note the decrease in the binding in striatum after MPH secondary to DA increases. Right panel shows measures of DA D_2 receptor availability in striatum after placebo and after MPH. The difference in the measures of B_{max}/Kd is used as a measure of relative changes in DA. Regression plots between the level of DAT blockade and the changes in DA induced by 60 mg oral MPH. Note that the variability in the changes in DA cannot be accounted for by the differences in DAT blockade. From Volkow *et al.*

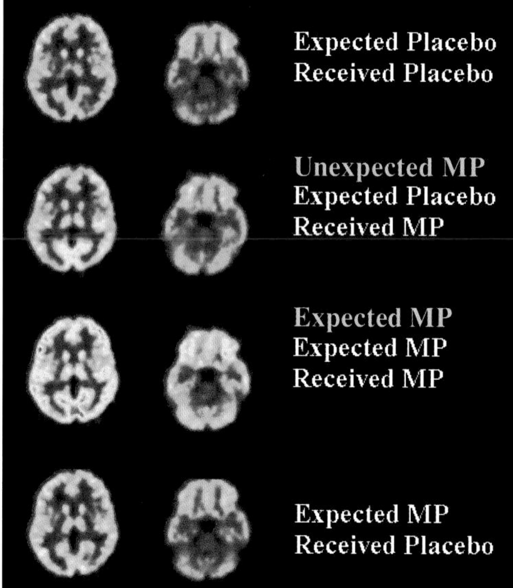

Plate 16.2 (d) Metabolic response to MPH and placebo under double-blind conditions with expectation varied. Note that MPH had a larger effect on brain metabolism when it was expected than unexpected. The overall effects were in areas devoid of dopamine transporters (cerebellar vermis, thalamus and occipital cortex) and the brain response to MPH was enhanced in the left lateral orbital–frontal cortex when the drug was unexpected, suggesting involvement of a cortical–striatal–thalamic brain circuit.

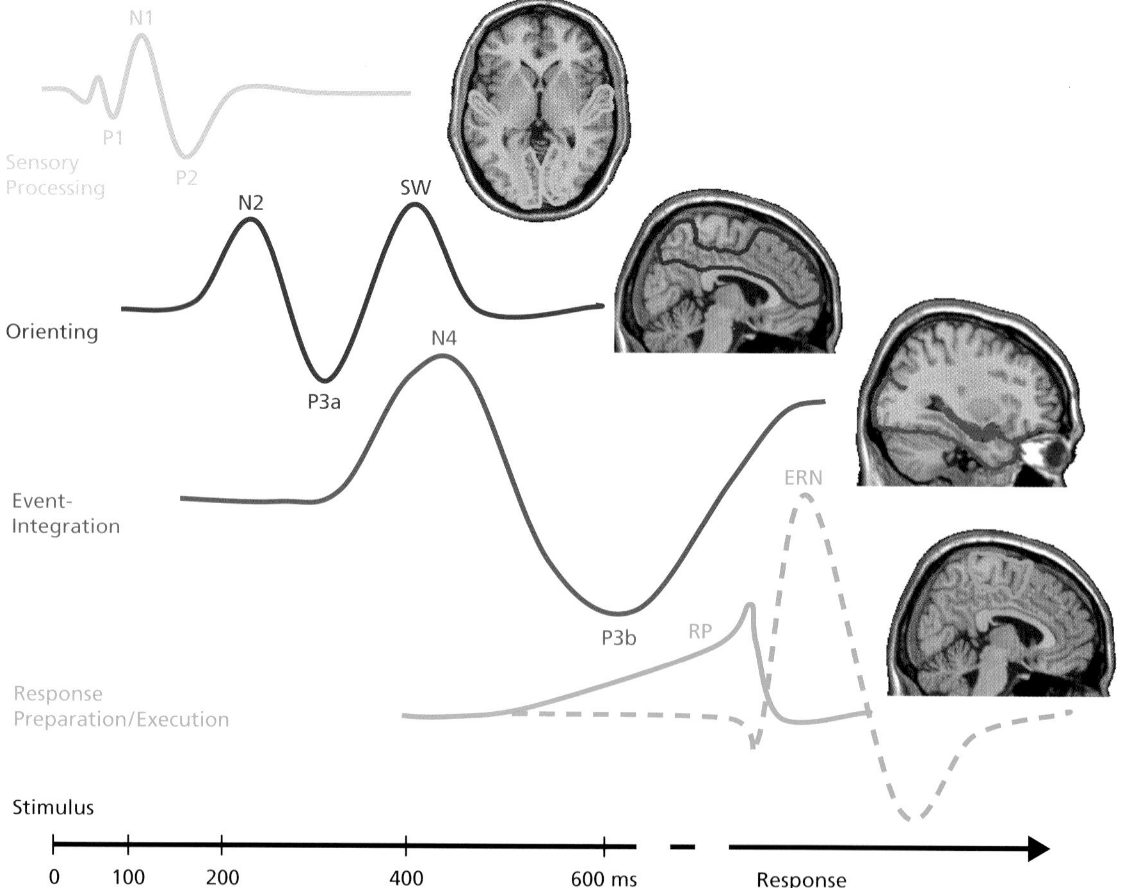

Plate 17.1 Hierarchical processing stages are characterized by distinct ERP patterns which are generated in distinct neuroanatomic regions (after Halgren & Marinkovic, 1995). The brain regions implicated in generation of specific event-related potential (ERP) components are outlined schematically in the corresponding color.

1 *Sensory ERP* components (P1, N1, P2) are generated in primary (outlined in light blue) and secondary sensory cortices.

2 An *orienting* complex, consisting of N2 (or MMN), P3a and slow wave (SW) is generated in medial (cingulate gyrus) and lateral frontal and posterior parietal cortices (outlined in dark blue).

3 Endogenous N4 and P3b components, associated with *event integration*, are generated in the hippocampus, amygdala (shaded in red) and associated inferotemporal and lateral orbitofrontal cortices (outlined in red).

4 The response-locked readiness potential (RP) during *response preparation* can be recorded in central cingulate gyrus and associated supplementary and premotor cortices (outlined in green).

5 ERP components correlated with *performance monitoring, such as* the *error-related negativity* (ERN), are generated in the anterior cingulate cortex (outlined by a broken green line).

Other ERP components mentioned in the text, such as slow cortical potential shifts (SCP) and language-related ERP are not shown here for clarity. The timescale is approximate and ERP are shown with negativity upward.

7 Children's Testimony

Maggie Bruck, Stephen Ceci, Sarah Kulkofsky, J. Zoe Klemfuss and Charlotte Sweeney

Research on children's testimony has been one of the fastest growing areas in developmental psychology. It encompasses such issues as the reliability of children's statements, children's understanding of legal concepts, courtroom preparation of child witnesses, competency tests, suggestibility, jurors' perceptions of children's credibility and detection of children's deception. In this chapter, we restrict our coverage to the subtopic of children's suggestibility, the most active topic within the research in this area, and one that cuts across many of the issues above.

Defining Suggestibility

One's recall of past experiences is rarely error free. Errors can occur for a variety of reasons such as forgetting, lapses of attention in experiencing the event or in recalling its details, blocking of the memory by other experiences, or blending of two or more different memories (Schacter, 2001). Recall of one's past can also be distorted by one's beliefs of what should have happened. Finally, recall can be distorted by suggestions – interactions with others that result in incorporation of their beliefs into one's own report.

Suggestions become incorporated into reports for a variety of social and cognitive reasons. Cognitive theories suggest that the original memory trace can be damaged, replaced or overshadowed by suggestions (Brainerd & Reyna, 2005), whereas social theories posit that although reports are consistent with the suggestions, the original accurate memory may nevertheless be maintained (McCloskey & Zaragoza, 1985). Both social and cognitive mechanisms may account for suggestibility effects: a child may initially acquiesce due to social factors (to please their interviewer) and with time this acceptance may affect memory, so that the child comes to believe falsely that the suggested incident actually occurred.

Experimental Measures of Suggestibility

In order to examine the direct influence of various types of suggestions on the accuracy of reports, a number of different paradigms have been used. These can be divided into two basic categories. In the first category, children are exposed to an event or activity about which the researcher has full knowledge of all the details. Children are asked to recall these experiences through the use of techniques that falsely suggest details that were not present during the event, or through neutral interviewing techniques that do not involve suggestion. A comparison of the errors made in the suggestive and neutral conditions allows a determination of the degree to which suggestions taint the child's reports. Because the researchers have full knowledge of the original event, they can easily determine the accuracy of the child's reports. In the second major paradigm, children are given suggestions about whole events that (according to parent reports) they have never experienced. The degree to which children provide details about non-experienced events is a measure of their suggestibility.

In this chapter, we first place the topic of children's suggestibility in a broader societal context, citing annual estimates of the number of children brought to the attention of law enforcement, attorneys and mental health specialists. We then describe a recent UK case that serves as a basis for applying the research. Finally, we show how recent research in the field of suggestibility can provide a basis for scientific examination of the nature of the children's reports and adults' acceptance of these reports.

Social Context of Child Suggestibility Research

Scope of the Problem

According to the latest statistics, in 2003 there were 2.9 million reports of child maltreatment in the USA alone, of which 906,000 were classified as founded. Of these founded cases, 537,026 resulted in court action (US Department of Health and Human Services, 2005). In addition to children who enter the legal arena for issues related to abuse and maltreatment, there are many others who come into contact each year with the juvenile and family court systems for other reasons (witnesses to domestic violence, Persons in Need of Supervision [PINS] hearings, neglect/permanency hearings and custodial disputes). In the USA alone, there is an estimated 1 million children involved in divorce proceedings annually (Emery, Otto, & O'Donohue, 2005), many of whom are interviewed as part of the custody determination (see chapter 8 for comparable UK perspectives).

Thus, the numbers of young children involved in the various branches of the justice system becomes frighteningly large. In all of these situations, children may be asked to provide

Rutter's Child and Adolescent Psychiatry, 5th edition. Edited by M. Rutter, D. Bishop, D. Pine, S. Scott, J. Stevenson, E. Taylor and A. Thapar. © 2008 Blackwell Publishing, ISBN: 978-1-4051-4549-7.

sworn or unsworn statements, they may be deposed, and sometimes they may be required to testify in court proceedings. In short, young children represent a large and growing legal constituency, one that possesses a special set of characteristics involving the development of basic cognitive, social and emotional competencies that may constrain their effective participation in the legal system.

Focus on Preschool-aged Children

In considering factors related to children's ability to provide accurate testimony about experienced events, much of the research in the past two decades has focused on preschool-aged children, and has been framed to address issues concerned with sexual abuse. There appear to be several reasons for this focus on young children. First, in the USA, where national archives are kept for each type of maltreatment, nearly 38% of reported cases of sexual abuse involve children aged 7 and younger (US Department of Health and Human Services, 2005).

Second, beginning in the 1980s, there were a number of highly visible cases in Europe, the USA, Australia, New Zealand and Canada in which young children claimed that their caretakers had abused them. The claims often included a co-mingling of plausible allegations with fantastic reports of ritualistic abuse, pornography, human and animal sacrifice, multiple perpetrators and multiple victims (e.g., California v. Raymond Buckey *et al.*, 1990; Commonwealth of Massachusetts v. Cheryl Amirault LeFave, 1999; Lillie and Reed v. Newcastle City Council & Ors, 2002; New Jersey v. Michaels, 1994; North Carolina v. Robert Fulton Kelly Jr., 1995; State v. Fijnje, 1995). When these types of cases first came to trial in the 1980s, the major issue before the jury was whether to believe the children. Prosecutors argued that children do not lie about sexual abuse, that the child witnesses' reports were authentic and that their bizarre and chilling accounts of events, which were well beyond the realm of most preschoolers' knowledge and experience, substantiated the fact that the children had actually participated in them. Furthermore, they argued that patterns of delayed disclosures, denials and recantations were typical if not diagnostic of sexual abuse in children (Summit, 1983; Summit, Miller, & Veltkamp, 1998). The defense in these cases argued that the children's reports were the product of repeated suggestive interviews by parents, law enforcement officials, social workers and therapists. Although the defense attempted to point out the potentially "suggestive" interview techniques that were used in eliciting the children's allegations, at the time there was not any direct scientific evidence to support the view that such techniques could actually lead children to make incorrect disclosures of a sexual nature. As will be shown, there is now sufficient evidence to support these views.

A Case Example: Lillie and Reed v. Newcastle City Council & Ors

To illustrate the issues that will be raised in this chapter, we provide the following case example. We chose this case because one of us (M.B.) served as an expert witness for the complainants, thus allowing us access to much of the official documentation. It was also chosen because the facts and the interviewing styles resembled those of a myriad of cases throughout the English-speaking world; these cases have given rise to much of the science on children's testimony, which in turn has been used to address issues arising in such cases.

Chris Lillie and Dawn Reed were two British daycare workers who were accused of sexually abusing 27 children at a daycare facility in Newcastle, England. The initial allegation was reported to the police by Mrs. Roberts in April 1993. She claimed that her 2-year-old son, Tim (the index child),[1] had indicated that Chris Lillie had touched him in the genital area. However, when interviewed by the police and social services a few days later, Tim denied that Chris Lillie had hurt him; physical examination also failed to show any positive evidence of abuse. Nonetheless, the investigation continued and Lillie was suspended from his duties at the daycare facility. Mrs. Roberts continued to supply the police with additional details: Tim was abused in a house with black doors and Lillie's coworker Dawn Reed was involved.

Several weeks after Mrs. Roberts' report, social services met with the parents of the daycare children and announced that one of the workers had been suspended because of an allegation of sexual abuse. Dawn Reed was officially suspended from the school soon after that meeting. Social services contacted families to determine whether the children had made any allegations or whether parents were concerned, as well as to provide parents with advice on how to question their otherwise silent children.

Approximately 29 children were interviewed at least once by the police and social services. A number of the children were interviewed two and even three times in order to elicit allegations of abuse. In June 1993 Lillie and Reed were arrested, after 4-year-old Mandy Brown claimed that she had been vaginally penetrated with a crayon at least 9 months previously. They were successfully granted bail, but just as they were leaving their cells, they were rearrested on the basis of a 5-year-old girl's allegation that she also had been abused. This child, who had not attended the daycare facility for over 1 year, made this statement after three investigative interviews. All interviews in this case were videotaped.

On the basis of a disciplinary hearing held by social services in February 1994, Lillie and Reed were dismissed from their positions at the daycare facility and, in July 1994, their criminal trial commenced. There were 11 counts involving 11 children (the index child Tim was not a witness). It was a very short trial because the judge dismissed the entire case on the grounds that the evidence was too weak to present to a jury. Lillie and Reed were legally free. However, because of the outrage of the parents and based on the city council's belief that the pair were guilty, an independent review team was

[1] The names of the children and their families have been changed to protect their identities.

set up to determine what, if anything, had gone wrong in the investigation. The review team's mandate was to examine how the allegations of abuse arose, and to investigate specific complaints made by parents. They were not asked to judge the guilt or innocence of Lillie and Reed.

In 1998, after 4 years' investigation, the review team issued its report, *Abuse in the Early Years*, and concluded: "From the evidence we have seen it is clear that Chris Lillie and Dawn Reed had conspired as a pair to abuse children and it is also clear that other people outside the nursery were involved." Lillie and Reed became the objects of public hatred, in part incited by the headlines in the local newspaper. They went into hiding. Eventually, because of the efforts of two journalists, they brought a suit against the city council, the local evening newspaper (the newspaper made an out-of-court settlement) and the review team itself. After a 6-month trial, the judge ruled in favor of the complainants, awarding them the maximum penalty of £200,000 each. The review team was found guilty of libel; the city council was not found guilty on the grounds of "qualified privilege."

We selected this case because it contains a variety of examples that have been examined in research on children and the law. In addition, it shares the following set of characteristics with other cases involving allegations of sexual abuse by young children that spurred the initial research interest in this area. First, the first child to make an allegation (the index child) did not originally make spontaneous statements but was questioned by an adult who was suspicious that something had happened to the child. When first questioned, the index child denied harm or wrongdoing; however, with repeated questioning, allegations began to emerge. Second, on the basis of the index child's uncorroborated allegations, parents of children in the daycare facility were informed that a child had been abused or that abuse was suspected. Parents were instructed to look for symptoms of abuse (bedwetting, crying, nightmares) and to question their children about specific events. Third, as was the case with the index child, children at first told their interviewers that nothing had happened; however, after repeated questioning by parents, police, social workers and/or therapists, some of these children also reported abuse. Sometimes, it took months of questioning for them to provide an acceptable report. Fourth, there were a number of contaminating factors that could account for the common allegations of the children: the same small group of professionals interviewed all of the children, provided therapy for them and evaluated them for sexual abuse. In addition, parents and children interacted with each other and spoke about the newest claims or rumors. Fifth, although there was no reliable medical evidence of sexual abuse for the most part, most parents reported changes in their children's behavior around the time of the alleged abuse, such as nightmares, bedwetting, baby-talk, resistance to going to the bathroom alone, refusal to attend daycare and much more. Finally, the children's reports became more elaborated with time; for example, after naming a specific perpetrator, children included other workers at the daycare center or other people in the town in their accusations. Over a period of time, the children's allegations became quite disturbing and bizarre; they alleged that they were penetrated with a sword, that needles were stuck into their bottoms, that there were monsters in elevators or that they were locked up in cupboards with no windows or handles. The following discussion and examples of this case are based on an analysis of the index child and six children that the prosecution had expected to testify at trial.

Scientific Analysis of the Case

There are two major competing hypotheses to account for the evolution of these children's allegations (no disclosure, denial of abuse, disclosure and sometimes recantation) and their acceptance by the parents and professional interviewers. The first hypothesis (put forward by the review team) is that the children accurately reported acts of abuse. According to this hypothesis, sexually abused children deny and recant either because they are afraid (because of threats), ashamed, believe themselves to be culpable or are confused by the events themselves. The fact that the parents were able to recall that, prior to their disclosures, the children experienced a number of behavioral symptoms that were deemed characteristic of abuse was viewed as corroborative evidence of the children's reports. The second hypothesis (put forward by the complainants) is that the children's reports were a product of a vast array of suggestive interviewing techniques that were used to elicit reports of abuse. The parents' recall of behavioral problems was not accurately dated but reflected memory errors resulting from their beliefs that their children had been abused. Each of these two major hypotheses will be evaluated in light of the scientific evidence.

Hypothesis 1: The Children were Abused

It is of primary importance to examine the evolution of the children's reports of sexual abuse. The pattern that occurred in the present case has raised the most concerns among researchers: the children were initially silent; with one ambiguous exception, none of the children made any unsolicited or spontaneous statements about abusive acts. Rather, the allegations emerged only after an adult suspected that something has occurred and started to question the children. In *Lillie & Reed*, all the children initially denied that the event happened, but with repeated questioning (in this case mainly by the parents and the investigators) the children eventually made a disclosure. Some of the children recanted these disclosures only to later restate the original allegation after further questioning. The most popular embodiment of this sequence of behaviors is Summit's (1983) description of the child sexual abuse accommodation syndrome (CSAAS). Summit intended to explain to clinicians why sexually abused children show this pattern of disclosure. The explanation rested on the assumption that these children are often frightened, confused and feel guilty. This explanation was fully accepted by the interviewers in the present case.

Because the CSAAS model was based on clinical intuitions rather than scientific findings, we recently reviewed the literature to determine its empirical support (London, Bruck, Ceci *et al.*, 2005). We identified 10 studies in which adults with histories of childhood abuse were asked to recall their disclosures in childhood. Across studies, an average of only 33% of the adults remembered disclosing the abuse in a timely fashion. In some studies, approximately 30% of adults reported that they had never told anyone before the current interview about their childhood abuse (Finkelhor, Hotaling, Lewis *et al.*, 1990; Smith, Letourneau, Saunders *et al.*, 2000). These data support the claim of the CSAAS model that sexually abused children are silent about their victimization and delay disclosure for long periods of time.

Although informative on the issue of delay of reporting, these data are silent with regard to the phenomena of denial and recantation, because the participants were never asked, "As a child, did anyone ever ask you or question you about abuse?" We have no way of knowing whether these individuals denied having been abused and then perhaps subsequently recanted their reluctant disclosures. Another set of studies provides some data relevant to this point. We identified 17 studies that examined rates of denial and recantation by sexually abused children who were asked directly about abuse when they were assessed or treated at clinics. The rates of denial at assessment interviews were highly variable (4–76%), as were the rates of recantation (4–27%). We found that the methodological adequacy of each study (e.g., the representativeness of the sampling procedures and the degree to which sexual abuse was validated) was directly related to the rates of denial and recantation: the weakest studies produced the highest rates of denial and recantation. For the six methodologically superior studies, the average rate of denial was only 14% and the average rate of recantation was 7%. Thus, although the retrospective studies of adults show that children often do not disclose their abuse, the studies of sexually abused children's responses in a formal interview indicate that if they are directly asked, they do not deny, but rather disclose that they were abused.

Over the course of the investigation, parents recalled that their children experienced a number of behavioral problems, including not wanting to go to school, sleep problems, nightmares, tantrums, inappropriate touching and being afraid of men. These symptoms were interpreted by both professionals and parents as signs that the children had been abused. However, the central assumption that there is a common constellation of symptoms that are diagnostic of sexual abuse is not supported by the scientific evidence. There are no behavioral symptoms that are diagnostic of sexual abuse. Many of the problems cited by the parents (anxiety, enuresis, fears, night terrors and even sexual behaviors) either are common in children of this age or can be associated with other types of childhood behavioral disorders (Hagen, 2003; Kendall-Tackett, Williams, & Finkelhor, 1993). For example, Maddocks, Griffiths, and Anto (1999) compared the medical histories of 107 boys with histories of sexual abuse with 107 non-abused age-matched boys. There were no between-group differences in the number or type of somatic and physical complaints (17% of sexually abused boys presented with such symptoms compared to 23% of the control boys); however, symptoms were more likely to persist for 1 year or longer among the target group (7%) than among the non-abused group (<1%). Thus, using behavioral symptoms as indicators of abuse is not scientifically supported.

Hypothesis 2: The Children's Reports Reflected Suggestive Interviewing Techniques and the Biases of their Interviewers

There is now a vast literature on the various situations and interviewing techniques that are known to produce false reports by children in experimental situations. In the present case, the children were subjected to just about every scientifically studied suggestive technique. The central driving force for the use of these techniques was the concept of interviewer bias, which we address next.

Interviewer Bias: The Central Characteristic of Suggestive Interviews

Interviewer bias refers to interviewers who hold a priori beliefs about the occurrence of certain events and, as a result of these beliefs, mold the interview to elicit statements from the interviewee that are consistent with these ideas. One of the hallmarks of "interviewer bias" is the single-minded attempt to gather only confirmatory evidence and to avoid all questions that may yield negative or inconsistent evidence. The biased interviewer does not ask questions about the allegations that might provide alternate explanations that are inconsistent with their beliefs or hypotheses. When confronted with a statement that runs counter to their beliefs, biased interviewers either ignore it or else interpret it within the framework of their initial hypothesis.

Biased interviewers' beliefs are transmitted to the child through a range of suggestive interviewing techniques that are associated with the elicitation of false reports. Consequently, the child may come to inaccurately report the belief of the interviewer rather than the child's own experience. A biased interviewer may be a police officer, a therapist or even a parent.

Below we provide two examples of scientific studies of the influence of interviewer bias on children's report accuracy.

Chester the Janitor

Thompson, Clarke-Stewart, and Lepore (1997) conducted a study in which children viewed a staged event that could be construed as either a misdeed or an innocent act. Some children interacted with a confederate named "Chester" as he cleaned some dolls and other toys in a playroom. Other children interacted with Chester as he handled the dolls roughly and in a mildly abusive manner. The children were then questioned about this event. The interviewer was:

1 "Accusatory" – suggesting that the janitor had been inappropriately playing with the toys instead of working;
2 "Exculpatory" – suggesting that the janitor was just cleaning the toys and not playing; or
3 "Neutral" and non-suggestive.

In the first two types of interviews, the questions changed from mildly to strongly suggestive as the interview progressed. Following the first interview, all children were asked to tell in their own words what they had witnessed and then they were asked questions about the event. Immediately after the interview and 2 weeks later, parents asked their children to recount what the janitor had done.

When questioned by a neutral interviewer, or by an interviewer whose interpretation was consistent with the activity viewed by the child, children's accounts were both factually correct and consistent with the janitor's script. However, when the interviewer was biased in a direction that contradicted the activity viewed by the child, those children's stories quickly conformed to the suggestions or beliefs of the interviewer. In addition, children's answers to interpretive questions (e.g., "Was he doing his job or just being bad?") were in agreement with the interviewer's point of view, as opposed to what actually happened. When asked neutral questions by their parents, the children's answers remained consistent with the interviewer's biases.

Surprise Party

Bruck, Ceci, Melnyk *et al.* (1999) showed how interviewer bias can quickly develop in natural interviewing situations, and how it not only taints the responses of child interviewees but also the reports of the adult interviewers. In this study, a special event was staged for 90 preschool children in their school. In groups of three children, and with the guidance of research assistant A, the children surprised research assistant B with a birthday party, played games, ate food and watched magic tricks. Another 30 children did not attend the birthday party but in groups of two, they simply colored a picture with research assistants A and B. These children were told that it was assistant A's birthday.

Interviewers (who were recruited from graduate degree programs in social work or counseling and who had training and experience in interviewing children) were asked to question four children about what had happened when special visitors came to the school. The interviewers were not told about the events but were simply told to find out from each child what had happened. The first three children that each interviewer questioned attended the birthday party and the fourth child attended the coloring event.

Bruck *et al.* found that the fourth child (who attended the coloring event and was interviewed last) produced twice as many errors as the children who attended the birthday party. For example, 60% of the children who only colored made false claims that involved a birthday party. This result suggests that the interviewers had built up a bias that all the children had attended a birthday party as a result of interviewing three consecutive children who actually had done so. By the time they interviewed the fourth child, they structured their interviews to elicit claims consistent with this hypothesis. Thus, if interviewers have the belief that all the children they are interviewing have experienced a certain event, then it is probable that many of the children will come to make such claims even though they were non-participants (or non-victims). Another important finding from this study was that even when the fourth child denied attending a birthday party, 84% of their interviewers later reported that all four of the children they interviewed had reported to them that they attended a birthday party. These data suggest that, regardless of what children actually say, biased interviewers inaccurately report the child's claims, making them consistent with their own hypotheses. It is also important to note that this bias likely can influence the interview in the absence of conscious manipulation on the part of the interviewer.

The Chester and Birthday Party studies and others like them (Bruck, Ceci, & Principe, 2006) provide evidence that interviewers' beliefs about an event can influence their judgments as well as their style of questioning. This, in turn, can affect the accuracy of children's testimony. Finally, interviewers' beliefs can affect their own ability to recollect accurately what the child actually told them during the interview. The findings from such studies highlight the dangers of having only one hypothesis about the event in question – especially when this hypothesis is incorrect. In applying the research on interviewer bias to a particular case, it is important to note that interviewer bias has a variety of manifestations and can occur at various levels of investigation of the case. For example, interviewer bias can be observed in a specific interview, in how an interviewer assesses the content or the impact of specific interviews or, at a higher level, interviewer (or investigator) bias is revealed by the types of evidence that are pursued or ignored at the investigational level.

Examples of Interviewer Bias in the Present Case

The investigators did not consider other explanations for reports of touching When the investigators tried to get the children to tell or to show on their bodies how they had been touched by Chris and Dawn, many of the children talked about touching in the toilet (often with their clothes on) and having a hurt bottom. It is possible that these comments reflected actual toileting practices which the children reported when they were asked about things that happened to their bottoms or genitals. Given the age of these children, the workers did perform these duties. The interviewers did not appear to consider this hypothesis in the interviews.

Investigators ignored that children did not demonstrate sexual touching accurately When children were asked to explain or to show where on their bodies they had been molested, a number of children pointed to many parts of their bodies that did not include their genitals. For example, one child stated that Chris had inserted a crayon into her vagina but it turns out, as seen below, that she may not have understood the nature of her claim:

> Interviewer: Which bits of your body was Dawn tickling?
> Child: That.
> Interviewer: What bit's that?
> Child: It was my back.

Interviewer: Your back. And was it any of the bits that Chris had tickled?
Child: Yes.

Another child showed similar confusions:

Interviewer: Which bits was he smacking?
Child: He smacked us there and he smacked us there, and he smacked us there, and he smacked us there, and he smacked us there, and he smacked us there, and he smacked us there and he smacked us there. *(Child does not point to buttocks.)*
Interviewer: And was there any bits down the back way?
Child: No.

The same child showed a similar confusion in her second formal interview. When asked, "Did he use some part of his body to hurt you?" the child pointed to her stomach. When she was asked to point to her genitals, she pointed to her back. Thus, these children's allegations about sexual touching were initially about being touched on various parts of their bodies, none of which included their buttocks and genitals. The investigators did not seem to notice the children's ignorance of such matters and their repeated questioning may have resulted in these children becoming very knowledgeable about sexual touching. Their bias that the children had been molested by Chris and Dawn may have blinded them to this possibility.

Investigators ignored children's exculpatory statements about Dawn There were a number of instances in which the children made exculpatory statements about Dawn. For example:

Interviewer: Is anybody else? Is Dawn in here or not?
Child: No.
. . .
Interviewer: And who was on the bus with you?
Interviewer: Anybody else?
Child: Not Dawn.
. . .
Interviewer: You know you mentioned somebody called Dawn. Who's that?
Child: [coughs] The girl inside Chris's [inaudible]
Interviewer: Did she do anything to you?
Child: No.

In her second of three interviews, this child made the following exculpatory statements about Dawn:

But don't say nothing to Dawn cos she wasn't silly.
She just went into jail for nothing.
Say Dawn can come out today. Say that.
Cos Dawn done nothing.

Despite these and other denials that Dawn had not done anything, the investigators concluded that Dawn had abused these children.

When the children denied abuse, the investigators would not take "no" as an answer because of their primary hypothesis that abuse had occurred and that the children were too frightened to talk about it. Consequently, children were interviewed until they simply gave in to the interviewers' requests to admit abuse. For example, one child ended the interview by moaning in her mother's lap, another child whimpered at the end of one interview; in the third and final interview the star witness for the prosecution begged her mother to stop and when she did not, the child simply left the room. The interviewers nevertheless interpreted these behaviors as further signs of resistance as reflected in their continuing to question the children. For example, one social worker interpreted Child 2's behavior during a suggestive interview as follows:

Investigator: Towards the end of the interview Child 2 appeared to become restless. I had visited Child 2 at home and not seen her display this sort of behaviour before. Although the interview had been fairly long I do not think she was tired, but rather pretending to be tired in order to avoid answering our questions. I recall that when we went out of the room Child 2 was running around and playful.

This interviewer did not consider the hypothesis that the interview was aversive to the child because she was being pressured to provide false information or information that she could not remember.

Parents' and investigators' biases in reporting and interpreting behavioral problems The primary source of evidence concerning the children's behaviors and allegations was provided to the police, social services and the review team by the children's parents. Thus, much of the primary evidence is only as reliable as the memories of these adults. Because parents recalled behaviors and conversations that had occurred months and sometimes years in the past, one might predict that there would be errors due to natural forgetting and due to other factors that allow one to reconstruct previous memories. In fact, there are many examples throughout the record that show changes in parents' memories and discrepancies between parents' and other observers' reports of the children.

One type of pattern that is observed entails parents' changing their reports over time such that the children's behaviors in the past were recalled as worse as the case proceeded. For example, Chris and Dawn cared for Ricky when he was 3 years old. Ricky's mother was interviewed by social services 15 months after he had left their care and 4 months after the investigation of abuse had begun. At that time she noted that Ricky had been disruptive and aggressive before he met Chris and Dawn and after he left their class. At present, however, she thought his behavior was much improved. She stated that she was pleased with the daycare facility, that she had a good relationship with Chris and was glad that her son had a male teacher. Two years later, she reported (to the review team) that she began to get very concerned because Ricky had become afraid of a male friend who, upon retrospect, was physically similar to Chris (Note, this had actually happened before Ricky met Chris). She reported that he began soiling at night and having more tantrums. She reported that Ricky had spent about 1 year in the red room (Note, he spent 3 months). She rarely spoke to Chris and had had a poor experience with him. She used to dread picking Ricky up from the red room and was made to always feel ashamed about her son's bad behavior. After Ricky had reported abuse, he spent a year in treatment because he was so traumatized.

The concept of *hindsight bias* could account for many of the changes in memories and reports throughout this case. Hindsight bias refers to the extent to which one changes one's memory of prior events based upon what is known in the present. This is sometimes referred to as "I knew it all along effect" or "The Monday Morning Quarterback Effect" (Hawkins & Hastie, 1990; Schacter, 2001). In a classic hindsight study, participants were asked to predict the outcome of a major political event (Fischhoff & Beyth, 1975). Two weeks after the event participants were asked to recall what they had predicted prior to the event. Although they were told to explicitly recall what they thought would happen before the event occurred, participants exhibited a significant bias, rating events that actually occurred as being more probable than they initially had. In another study, doctors were asked to make an independent diagnosis (a second opinion) for a case that had previously been worked up and diagnosed. Some of the doctors were given no information about the prior diagnosis. Other doctors were given the prior diagnostic label but were told to ignore it when arriving at their independent opinion. This latter group of doctors was more likely to make a diagnosis consistent with the first label, compared with doctors who were not given this information (Arkes, Watmann, Saville *et al.*, 1981).

In addition to interpreting past behaviors as signs of abuse, there was also the matter of the children's behaviors after they disclosed abuse. It seemed as though the children's behaviors actually became worse in some instances as the investigation proceeded. The problem was that these behaviors were interpreted as corroborative signs that abuse had occurred; they were seen as a consequence of the abuse. However, there were a number of other highly plausible explanations that were never considered. For example, the children's behaviors became worse because they were treated as victims and came to believe they were victims. The following interaction suggests how children may have become frightened or disoriented because of the interviewing practices that were used to help them reveal their abuse. It is possible that these suggestions caused the children to believe that something awful had happened to them.

Interviewer: You know, there's nothing for you to be frightened of, you know. You're not frightened are you?
Child: No.
Interviewer: You don't have to be frightened to tell us anything cos you're safe here and there's nothing to be worried about.
Child: No, there's no monsters here.
Interviewer: Of course there isn't. Has somebody been talking that there'd be monsters here?
Child: No.
Interviewer: Why do you say that?
Child: I do.
Interviewer: Are you frightened of monsters?
Child: No.
Interviewer: Who's told you about the monsters? Has somebody told you that there's monsters?
Child: No.
Interviewer: Cos mummy and daddy look after you, you know . . . You know mummy and daddy look after you and I'm just here to help you. There's nothing to be worried about. These monsters that you talk about, where do they go?
Child: [inaudible]
Interviewer: Where do they come from?
Child: Nowhere.
Interviewer: Has somebody told you a story about monsters?
Child: No.
Interviewer: You don't have to be frightened, you know. You can tell me anything. You can. Mummy says it's all right. We just want to help you. If somebody's told you about monsters, I'd like you to tell me. Cos you know, nobody can hurt you. Nobody's going to hurt you. There's nobody going to come and take you away or anything. Mummy and daddy love you and they look after you. And I'm just talking to you to try and help you, cos I care about you. And there's no monster going to come. You're safe. I just thought maybe somebody told you about them.

In another example, all of Janie's troubling behaviors were seen as consequences of abuse, although there were other factors that could have had an important role. Specifically, when Janie was with Chris and Dawn she loved school. Problems began after she left the care of Chris and Dawn, in March 1992; sleep problems increased in September 1992, and in January 1993 she did not want to go to school. Her mother initially thought these problems were related to her meeting her current partner because Janie kept asking about her dad. However, her behavioral problems began to increase after she was interviewed by the police and social services. She had terrible nightmares, she became antagonistic towards her mother's partner, and she initiated inappropriate touching with children. Although these symptoms could be trauma-related, the question that could be raised is "what trauma?" The investigators believed it was the trauma of the abuse, but it could just as well have been the trauma of pressurized interviews, a new man in the house and the false belief that she was abused. These alternative hypotheses were never considered.

In summary, as parents learned more about the case and became more concerned or convinced that their children were victims, their perceptions of the severity of the child's behaviors, prior to April 7, 1993 (the time of the initial disclosure) increased. As seen from the example above, the timing of the behavioral problems also changed so that these occurred when the children were cared for by Chris and Dawn. Thus, hindsight bias provided the parents with stronger beliefs that their children had been abused. In addition, the fact that all of the children's poor behaviors were also viewed as signs of abuse fueled the investigators' and parents' confirmatory bias that the children had been abused. It was this confirmatory bias that was central to the entire case. The ways that this was made apparent to the children are reviewed in the following section.

Suggestive Interviewing Techniques

Interviewer bias influences the entire architecture of interviews and is revealed by the methods or strategies used by interviewers to elicit the children's allegations of abuse. The following techniques were used in the interviews with the children in the current case:

- The children were given little opportunity to say in their own words what, if anything, had happened.
- Interviewers quickly resorted to the use of specific yes/no or forced-choice questions that required monosyllabic responses (e.g., "Was it this or that?").
- Interviewers' statements and questions contained sexual content and details about the case that may not have been part of children's initial knowledge.
- Questions were repeated within and across interviews.
- Interviews continued or were repeated until the child provided information consistent with sexual abuse.
- Interviewers used bribes or threats of punishment ("I will give you a treat if you tell me" or "We can't go home until you tell what happened").
- Interviewers used selective reinforcement in response to children's statements. They rewarded children for abuse consistent statements but ignored or made negative comments in response to denials of abuse or related activities.
- Interviewers made "atmospheric" statements that conveyed the theme that something bad happened (e.g., telling the child not to be afraid, that he or she should not be afraid, that he or she is being brave, that he or she is going to be protected).
- Interviewers invoked statements of other people ("Your mom told me that . . ." or, "All your friends have talked about this, now it's your turn").
- Children spoke among themselves about the allegations.
- Interviewers induced negative stereotypes of the suspected perpetrator (e.g., telling the child that the suspect does bad things, that he or she is in jail).
- Props, such as dolls, toys and drawings, were used to elicit statements about touching.

The results of the scientific literature indicate that the use of these suggestive techniques, especially by biased interviewers, can bring children to make claims about events that they have never experienced. This is especially so when these techniques are used repeatedly and in combination (as was the case in *Lillie & Reed*) because the concentration of suggestive interviewing provides the child with a clear view of the biases of the interviewer and thus promotes the risk of their complying with the perceived beliefs of their interrogators.

In the next section we provide a brief overview of the scientific literature on some of the suggestive interviewing techniques that were used in *Lillie & Reed* (for a more detailed description see Bruck, Ceci, & Principe, 2006).

Repeating Interviews and Repeating Questions

In formal investigations, children are often interviewed on many different occasions. There are numerous concerns about the influence of these repeated interviews on children's reports, especially when these are conducted by biased interviewers. In these situations, children are repeatedly exposed to (mis)leading questions and to other suggestive techniques. The results of several studies indicate that when this occurs, children's reports become highly tainted, sometimes after just one or two interviews.

For example, preschool children were interviewed on five different occasions about two true events and two false events (Bruck, Ceci, & Hembrooke, 2002). The two true events involved the child helping a visitor in the school who had tripped and hurt her ankle and a recent incident where the child was punished by the teacher or the parent. The two false events involved helping a lady find her monkey and witnessing a man steal food from the daycare facility. In the first interview, children were simply asked if each event had ever happened to them. If they said yes, they were asked to describe the event. During the next three interviews, the children were suggestively interviewed (e.g., they were asked repeated leading questions, they were praised for responses, they were asked to try to think about what might have happened, they were told that their friends had already told and now it was their turn). In the fifth interview, a new interviewer questioned each child about each event in a non-suggestive manner. Across the five interviews, all children consistently and accurately assented to the true event about helping a lady who fell in the daycare facility. However, children were at first reluctant to talk about the punishment event; many of the children denied that the punishment had occurred. With repeated suggestive interviews, the children agreed that the punishment had occurred. Similar patterns of disclosure occurred for the false events; that is, children initially denied the false events but with repeated suggestive interviews, they began to assent to these events. By the third interview, most children had assented to all true and false events. This pattern continued to the end of the study. Thus, although suggestive interviewing techniques promote the disclosure of true embarrassing events, they are equally effective in promoting false allegations.

One of the rationales for reinterviewing children is that it provides them additional opportunities to report important information that was forgotten or simply not reported in earlier interviews. Thus, it is assumed that, when children provide new details in subsequent interviews, these new reports are accurate memories that were not remembered in previous interviews. Another rationale is to allow children to rehearse, so that their memories will not fade over a period of time. However, the results of recent studies dispute this claim. One set of studies consistently shows that reports that emerge in a child's first interview with a neutral interviewer are the most accurate. When children are later interviewed about the same event and report new details not mentioned in a previous interview, these have a high probability of being inaccurate whether children are interviewed by a neutral interviewer (Peterson, Moores, & White, 2001; Pipe, Gee, Wilson *et al.*, 1999; Salmon & Pipe, 2000) or by a very suggestive interviewer (Bruck, Ceci, & Hembrooke, 2002). Thus, insertion of new but inaccurate details can be a natural memory phenomenon; it can be due to prior suggestions that become incorporated into later reports; but it can also be due to the demand characteristics of the interview. When interviewers urge children to tell them anything (that is consistent with the bias of the interviewer), these requests for additional information will sometimes result in false reports that are supplied by the children to comply with their perception of the interviewer's wishes.

Although these studies show the detrimental effects of repeated interviews, there is an important qualification to this conclusion. There are a number of studies in which children who are provided with misinformation across multiple interviews are no more likely to incorporate this information into a later report than children who receive only one suggestive interview. The major factor appears to be the timing of the suggestive interviews. If the first suggestive interview occurs soon after an event and the second interview occurs close to the final interview, then misinformation effects are maximized (Melnyk & Bruck, 2004). There are several interrelated qualifications to bear in mind. As shown in some of the studies in this chapter, one suggestive interview can destroy the reliability of a child's report, but it may also take several suggestive interviews to move the child from making simple assents to providing some elaboration to the false allegations (see Bruck, Ceci, & Hembrooke, 2002, in which repeated suggestive interviews were associated with more elaborated narratives of false events).

Just as there are risks associated with repeated interviews, there are also risks associated with repeating questions within the same interview. Biased interviewers sometimes repeatedly ask the same question until the child provides a response that is consistent with their hypothesis. Poole and White (1991) found that asking the same question within an interview, especially a yes/no question, often results in young children changing their original answer (see Cassel, Roebers, & Bjorkland, 1996, for similar effects when children are asked repeated leading questions). Furthermore, when children are asked the same question on numerous occasions, they sound increasingly confident about their statements even if these are false.

When questions are repeated within or between interviews, they need not be verbatim to produce deleterious effects. It is the repetition of questions about a specific theme (the suspected perpetrator does bad things) that compromises the reliability of children's reports. Garven, Wood, Malpass *et al.* (1998) found that preschoolers provided increasingly inaccurate responses to misleading statements and questions as a suggestive interview proceeded. In this study, children were suggestively interviewed for 5–10 minutes about a stranger who came to read their class a story. As a result of the suggestive devices used by the interviewers, children falsely claimed that the visitor said a bad word, threw a crayon, broke a toy, stole a pen, tore a book and bumped the teacher. Of particular importance, the children came to make more false claims as the interview progressed; that is, within a short, 5–10 minute interview, children made more false claims in the second half than in the first half of the interview.

In summary, if children's allegations are elicited by specific leading questions that have been repeated within the same interview or across interviews, there is a high risk that the children's statements will be unreliable. Conversely, children's answers to open-ended questions asked prior to any suggestive interviewing have a high probability of being accurate.

The following example shows how a child's denials of abuse become allegations of abuse after repeated specific questions:

Q: What about Dawn, because you had some things to tell me about Dawn as well, didn't you, eh?
Child: No.
Q: You said there were some silly things about Dawn, eh?
Child: No, that was ages ago when I come here.
Q: But you said that you got touched by Dawn and can you – I just need to know where she touched you. It's all right.
Child: On my fairy (Note, this is the term children used to refer to their vagina).

In *Lillie & Reed*, all children had repeated interviews before they made allegations of abuse. Although this analysis focuses mainly on the children's statements in the videotaped interviews, it is important to note that the children were questioned before these official interviews were recorded. The record shows that children had several to many sessions with parents, friends of parents, relatives and professionals. For example, one mother first suspected that her child had been abused in May 1993. Her child was interviewed at the police station in June 1993 but made no allegations consistent with sexual abuse. Then she was questioned many times over the next 6 months. On December 1, 1993, when she was interviewed for the second time at the police station, she made a few allegations consistent with abuse. Given the denial of wrongdoing in June, followed by an enormous amount of repeated interviewing during the next few months, the few allegations that emerged in December were not "fresh" utterances but may have been contaminated by multiple retellings and questionings.

Atmospherics or Emotional Tone of the Interview

Interviewers can use verbal and non-verbal cues to communicate their bias. These cues can set the emotional tone of the interview. Children are quick to notice the emotional tones in an interview and to act accordingly. For example, in some studies when an accusatory tone is set by the examiner (e.g. "It isn't good to let people kiss you in the bathtub," or "Don't be afraid to tell"), children are likely to fabricate reports of past events even in cases when they have no memory of any event occurring. In some cases, these fabrications are sexual in nature.

In one such study, children played with an unfamiliar research assistant for 5 minutes while seated across a table from him. Four years later, researchers asked these same children to recall the original experience (Goodman, Batterman-Faunce, Schaaf *et al.*, 2002). The researchers created "an atmosphere of accusation," telling the children that they were to be questioned about an important event and saying things like, "Are you afraid to tell? You'll feel better once you've told." Although few children had any memory of the original event from 4 years earlier, five out of the fifteen children incorrectly agreed with the interviewer's suggestive question that they had been hugged or kissed by the confederate, two of the fifteen agreed that they had had their picture taken in the bathroom, and one child agreed that she or he had been given a bath. In other words, children may give inaccurate responses to misleading questions about events for which they have no memory when the interviewer creates an emotional tone of accusation.

In *Lillie & Reed*, the children were repeatedly told not to be frightened, not to be afraid and that they were brave. In the June 22 interview with Julie, the word "frighten" was used nine times. The following excerpt shows the potentially damaging effect of this strategy, which was repeated by the police investigator (POL), the mother (MOM) and the mother's friend (FR).

POL: I was wondering if maybe Julie was frightened.
POL: Do you think she's frightened to tell me?
FR: I think so and I think I know what she's frightened of.
POL: Julie, have we got this bit right?
FR: Julie. Are you listening?
MOM: Listen, Julie, are you frightened?
POL: What of?
JULIE: Chris.
FR: What for? You're safe.

POL: We're all there to look after you and there's nothing for you to be frightened of.
FR: So that nobody can harm her, can they not, Julie?

FR: What did he do when he was naughty, Julie?
POL: I think Julie's still a little bit frightened but she doesn't have to be.
MOM: What did Chris tell you to be frightened of, Julie? Why were you frightened?
JULIE: Monsters.

Rewards and Punishment

Rewards and punishment shape the emotional tone of an interview and provide another means for the interviewer to express bias. The use of rewards and punishments in interviews with children can have beneficial as well as negative consequences. The use of these may motivate children to come to tell the truth. On the other hand, children may learn that if they produce stories that are consistent with the interviewers' beliefs, they will be rewarded by their interviewers.

The following study conducted by Garven, Wood, and Malpass (2000) illustrates how the use of rewards and punishments in an interview can quickly shape the child's behavior and have long-lasting consequences. Children between the ages of 5 and 7 years attended a special story time led by a visitor called Paco. During this 20-minute visit, Paco read the children a story, handed out treats and placed a sticker on the child's back. One week after the visit, the children were asked mundane questions ("Did Paco break a toy?") and fantastic questions ("Did Paco take you somewhere in an airplane?"). Children in the neutral–no reinforcement condition were simply asked a list of 16 questions and provided with no feedback after each question. Other children, in the reinforcement condition, were asked the same 16 questions, but in addition, they were provided with feedback after each question, as illustrated by the following example:

Interviewer: Did Paco take you somewhere on a helicopter?
Child: No (Note, this is an accurate denial).
Interviewer: You're not doing good. Did Paco take you to a farm?
Child: Yes (Note, this is an incorrect assent).
Interviewer: Great. You're doing excellent now. (*The next question is asked.*)

The reinforcement had large negative effects on the accuracy of children's responses. Children in the reinforcement condition inaccurately assented to 35% of misleading mundane questions and to 52% of the misleading fantastic questions. The comparable rates for the non-reinforcement group were 13% and 15%. In a second interview, a week later, all children were asked the same questions, without any reinforcement. The same high error rates continued for the reinforcement group. When children were challenged and asked in the second interview, "Did you see that or just hear about that?" children in the reinforcement group stated that they had personally observed 25% of the misleading mundane events and 30% of the misleading fantastic events. Children in the non-reinforcement group only made these claims 4% of the time.

These findings show how quickly reinforcing statements can shape children to provide inaccurate responses no matter how bizarre the question. Furthermore, the inaccurate responses persist upon a second questioning, with a number of children claiming that they actually observed the suggested but false event.

Rewards and punishments can take a more explicit form such as promising children a treat if they tell the right answer or threatening the children if they provide an undesirable answer. There is a long history of psychological research that shows the effects of such techniques (Ettinger, Crooks, & Stein, 1994; Zigler & Kanzer, 1962).

There were a number of examples of rewards and punishments being used in the present case. For example:

Interviewer: Well, you tell me now, what did he do? Was he naughty?
Child: I don't know.
Interviewer: Yes, you do.

Interviewer: What did you have on?
Child: This dress.
Interviewer: No, you didn't.
Child: I did.
Interviewer: You didn't have it then. Did you have your clothes on all the time?

MOM: Listen. Come here. Listen, will you talk to me before the interviewer comes back? Sh, sh, sh, sh (*trying to quiet child who is moaning*). Listen. You're being very silly aren't you? You're being very silly. Come on. Listen. You know what? Eeh, aren't you just acting like a baby? You're a big girl. You'll not get any juice, mind. Vanessa (the interviewer) will not give you if you start acting like a baby. Listen, I want to talk to you.

Peer Contamination

The effect of telling children that their friends have "already told" is a much less investigated area in the field of forensic developmental psychology. Certainly, the common wisdom is that a child will go along with a peer group. But will a child provide an inaccurate response just so he or she can be one of the crowd? Can simply discussing information between children affect their answers? The most recent and most relevant studies in the literature suggest that the answer is "yes" (Principe & Ceci, 2002; Principe, Kanaya, Ceci *et al.*, 2006).

Preschoolers in groups ranging in size from 6 to 8 took part in a contrived "dig" with a fictitious archeologist named Dr. Diggs (Principe & Ceci, 2002). Dr. Diggs led the children through an event in which they used plastic hammers to dig pretend artifacts (e.g., dinosaur bones, gold coins). Dr. Diggs also showed the children two special artifacts: a map to a buried treasure and a rock with a secret message. The children were warned not to touch these because they could be ruined. All children in the study participated in or viewed these core events. However, one-third of the children also saw Dr. Diggs ruin the two special artifacts (hereafter referred to as the target activities) and show upset about their loss. A second third of the children were the classmates of those in the first group but did not witness the extra target activities. The remaining children were not the classmates of those who witnessed the target activities, nor did they witness the target activities themselves; they thus served to provide a baseline against which to assess the effects of peer contact. Following the dig, the children were interviewed in either a neutral or a suggestive manner on three occasions. The suggestive interviews for children who did not view Dr. Diggs ruining the special artifacts provided children with this information. Children in the neutral interview were not given information about the two target events. In a later interview, children were asked questions about the dig. Children who had not reported the two absent special activities were prompted to disclose more by the interviewer's telling them that their friends had already told.

Children who were classmates of those who saw Dr. Diggs ruining the two artifacts were more likely to claim that they had viewed the target activities (i.e., they incorporated the misinformation from the previous interview) than children who did not view the special activities and were in another classroom. These data suggest that there was contamination from classroom interactions; children who had not experienced the target events learned of them from their classmates and thus were more likely to assent to false events. Finally, telling children that their friends had told increased their false assent rate.

Principe *et al.* (2006) conducted another study in which they found that children who overheard a child talking were as likely to falsely claim to have seen the event in question (a rabbit that escaped from a magician) as were peers who actually saw it escape. Moreover, in this study, the effect of suggestive questioning did not notably increase their false reports; children were as likely to report falsely if they overheard peers talking about the rabbit, regardless of whether interviewers employed suggestive questions.

In *Lillie & Reed*, children often had the opportunity to talk with each other throughout the investigation. Further, they were told that their friends had come and talked about "silly things":

Interviewer: You know your friends that you played with at nursery school? I've been talking to them. They were telling me about some silly things that happened at the nursery. Do you know about them things? . . .
Child: Don't know that.
Interviewer: Shall I help you a bit? They were telling me about their teachers, when they were in your class?

After the accusations of abuse, teachers in the daycare facility kept "disclosure logs" to record children's statements about abuse. Some of the examples show how children talked among themselves about abusive subjects in what seemed to be a very playful atmosphere.

Child 1: They had real snakes, they went SSS, they were toys in the cage outside.
Child 2: I saw the snakes and cage, but I ran up the steps, the snakes are called _____ the same as me. (Note, this is the first time Child 2 mentions snakes).
Child 2: And do you know what? Chris and Dawn kicked me.
Child 3: Why did they kick you?
Child 2: Cos they thought I was a pirate lady.
Child 1: And they slapped me cos they thought I was a doggy.
(*Both Child 1 and Child 2 laugh and begin to jump on a piece of equipment.*)

It appears that the first allegations of Child 2 and Child 3 may have emerged from these sessions.

Summary

We have provided examples of only some of the suggestive techniques used in *Lillie & Reed* (for more details see http://

www.richardwebster.net/cleared.html; http://www.hmcourts-service.gov.uk/judgmentsfiles/j1302/lillie_reed_part_1.htm). Although one can never know whether or not the children were actually abused, the materials clearly show that all children were subjected to an array of suggestive interviewing techniques. As documented in the scientific literature, these techniques can destroy the accuracy of children's reports, and they can bring children to believe the suggestions themselves.

Going Beyond Suggestive Interviewing in *Lillie & Reed*

We presented the *Lillie & Reed* case to demonstrate how the scientific literature on the reliability of children's statements addresses a variety of important issues that this and other cases raise. In this section, we address some misconceptions that have arisen and that need correcting.

Misconception 1: Suggestibility studies show that children can only be led to make false reports about unemotional, unimportant events This is incorrect. Suggestive techniques result in a wide range of false allegations. Although for ethical reasons there has never been a study in which researchers explicitly attempted to suggest to children that they were abused, nevertheless, there have been a number of studies in which children have been led to make false allegations about bodily events which, were they to occur in the real world, would cause a great deal of concern and further investigation. In research studies, children have made false claims about "silly events" that involved body contact (e.g., "Did the nurse lick your knee?" "Did she blow in your ear?"), and these false claims persisted in repeated interviewing over a 3-month period (Ornstein, Gordon, & Larus, 1992). Children falsely reported that a man put something "yuckie" in their mouth (Poole & Lindsay, 2001). Preschoolers falsely alleged that their pediatrician had inserted a finger or a stick into their genitals (Bruck, Ceci, Francoeur *et al.*, 1995), or that some man touched their friends, kissed their friends on the lips and removed some of the children's clothes (Lepore & Sesco, 1994). A significant number of children falsely reported that someone touched their private parts, kissed them and hugged them (Goodman, Rudy, Bottoms *et al.*, 1990; Goodman, Bottoms, Schwartz-Kenney *et al.*, 1991; Bruck, Melnyk, & Ceci, 2000). Children assented to suggestions that a doctor had cut out a bone in the center of a child's nose to stop the child from bleeding (Quas, Goodman, Bidrose *et al.*, 1999). Children have also elaborated their false narratives with emotional terms (e.g., "It hurt"; "I cried"; "I was happy"; Bruck *et al.*, 1995; Bruck, Ceci, Hembrooke, 2002). Thus, the suggestibility literature is a valid basis for evaluating the possibility that suggestive interviewing can result in false allegations about emotionally evocative events which may include bodily harm.

Misconception 2: The problem with suggestive interviews concerns young children; older children are immune to these techniques This is not the case. Suggestive techniques used in the studies with young children also produce tainted reports or false memories in older children, adolescents and adults (Loftus, 2003). The same principles hold across a wide variety of ages. For example, Porter, Yuille, & Lehman (1999) asked parents of college students about six categories of negative emotional events (serious medical procedures, serious animal attacks, getting seriously hurt with another child, serious indoor or outdoor accidents, and getting lost) that may have happened to their children between the ages of 4 and 10 years. Next, the college students were interviewed about one of the events that the parents said had occurred when they were children and one event that had not occurred. Over three interviews, the interviewers tried to implant a memory of the false event, instructing the subjects to engage in daily recall to try to imagine themselves in the event. Overall, 26% of participants created complete memories for the false emotional events. Another 30% provided some details of the false events, but did not produce a full narrative. Thus, a total of 56% of the college students felt that they had experienced an event that, according to their parents, had never happened.

By inference, one might assume that children in middle childhood must also be quite suggestible, given that both younger and older groups are. Recent evidence supports this view; susceptibility to suggestion is highly common in middle childhood, and under some conditions there are small to no developmental differences in suggestibility. For example, Finnila, Mahlberga, Santtilaa *et al.* (2003) staged an event (a version of the Paco visit we described earlier) for 4- to 5-year-olds and 7- to 8-year-olds. One week later, half the children were given a low-pressure interview that contained some misleading questions with abuse themes (e.g., "He took your clothes off, didn't he?"). The other children received a high-pressure interview; they were told that their friends had answered the leading questions affirmatively, they were praised for assenting to the misleading questions, and when they did not assent, the question was repeated. In both conditions, there were no significant age differences in the percentage of misleading questions answered affirmatively, although a significant number (68%) were assented to in the high-pressure condition (see also Bruck, London, Landa *et al.*, 2007). Older children are quick to notice the emotional tones in an interview (which convey bias), and to act accordingly. For example, the Goodman *et al.* (2002) study described above found that children 7–10 years of age falsely assented to misleading questions that involved inappropriate touching activities.

Conclusions

When the first high-profile child sexual abuse cases emerged more than two decades ago, the scientific community had little to say about children's susceptibility to suggestive interviewing techniques. Since then, we have discovered compelling empirical evidence that children can come to falsely report events that did not happen, and may even come to report events that are sexually themed. To compound the problem, once a child has been subjected to suggestive techniques, his or her erroneous reports are often indistinguishable from accurate reports. False reports that emerge in response to suggestive interviewing are often stylistically indistinguishable from true narratives. For example, they cannot be distinguished on the basis of linguistic markers, temporal terms or narrative coherence. Even trained experts in the field cannot, on the basis of their reports, identify which children have been suggestively interviewed (Bruck, Ceci, & Principe, 2006). In summary, there are no scientifically acceptable markers for judging the accuracy of a child's statement after exposure to suggestive interviews.

There has been a substantial research effort to develop standardized interview protocols that, if used appropriately, help interviewers avoid suggestive techniques. One such protocol was developed by Lamb, Sternberg, and Esplin (1998; see also Memorandum of Good Practice, 1992). The protocol requires trained interviewers to encourage suspected child abuse victims to provide detailed life event narratives through the guidance of open-ended questions (e.g., "Tell me what happened"; "You said there was a man; tell me about the man"). The use of specific questions is allowed only after exhaustive free recall. Suggestive questions are highly discouraged. These types of practices prevent interviewers not only from using suggestive techniques but, most importantly, from adopting a specific bias of wrongdoing.

Throughout this chapter we have focused on issues that primarily arise during investigations involving child witnesses. However, the issues we have covered apply to all adults who interact with children and who rely on children's reports as a primary source of information in making decisions or recommendations. This includes child and adolescent psychiatrists, who are not immune to the potential problems of interview bias (e.g., having a high suspicion that the child has an anxiety disorder and failing to rule out other explanations for the child's behavior) or of using suggestive interviewing techniques (e.g., repeating questions, asking leading questions, rewarding specific statements). In summary, individuals who are charged with the task of interviewing or evaluating children should be especially fastidious in their use of leading questioning and other suggestive techniques. Interviewers should do their utmost to be aware of and minimize their own biases and should be willing to consider alternative theories when questioning children.

Further Reading

Ceci, S. J., & Bruck, M. (1995). *Jeopardy in the courtroom: A scientific analysis of children's testimony*. Washington, DC: American Psychological Association.

Poole, D. A., & Lamb, M. E. (1998). *Investigative interviews of children: A guide for helping professionals*. Washington, DC: American Psychological Association.

References

Arkes, H. R., Wortmann, R. L., Saville, P. D., & Harkness, A. R. (1981). Hindsight bias among physicians weighting the likelihood of diagnoses. *Journal of Applied Psychology*, *66*, 252–254.

Brainerd, C. J., & Reyna, V. R. (2005). *The science of false memory*. New York: Oxford University Press.

Bruck, M., Ceci, S. J., Francoeur, E., & Renick, A. (1995). Anatomically detailed dolls do not facilitate preschoolers' reports of a pediatric examination involving genital touch. *Journal of Experimental Psychology: Applied*, *1*, 95–109.

Bruck, M., Ceci, S. J., & Hembrooke, H. (2002). Nature of true and false narratives. *Developmental Review*, *22*, 520–554.

Bruck, M., Ceci, S. J., & Principe, G. (2006). Forensic developmental psychology in the courtroom. In I. Sigel & K. A. Renninger (Eds.), *Handbook of Child Psychology: Psychology in Practice*. New York: Wiley.

Bruck, M., Ceci, S. J., Melnyk, L., & Finkelberg, D. (1999). The effect of interviewer bias on the accuracy of children's reports and interviewer's reports. Paper presented at the Biennial Meeting of the Society for Child Development, April 1999, Albuquerque, NM.

Bruck, M., London, K., Landa, R., & Goodman, J. (2007). Autobiographical memory and suggestibility in children with Autism Spectrum Disorders. *Development and Psychopathology*, *19*, 73–95.

Bruck, M., Melnyk, L., & Ceci, S. J. (2000). Draw it again Sam: The effect of drawing on children's suggestibility and source monitoring ability. *Journal of Experimental Child Psychology*, *77*, 169–196.

California v. Raymond Buckey et al. (1990). Los Angeles County Sup Ct # A750900.

Cassel, W. S., Roebers, C. E., & Bjorklund, D. F. (1996). Developmental patterns of eyewitness responses to repeated and increasingly suggestive questions. *Journal of Experimental Child Psychology*, *61*, 116–133.

Commonwealth of Massachusetts v. Cheryl Amirault LeFave. (1999). 430 Mass 169.

Emery, R., Otto, R., & O'Donohue, W. (2005). A flawed system with limited science. *Psychological Science in the Public Interest*, *7*, 1–29.

Ettinger, R. H., Crooks, R. L., & Stein, J. (1994). *Psychology: Science, behavior, and life* (3rd ed.). Orlando, FL: Harcourt Publishers.

Finkelhor, D., Hotaling, G., Lewis, J. A., & Smith, C. (1990). Sexual abuse in a national survey of adult men and women: Prevalence, characteristics, and risk factors. *Child Abuse and Neglect*, *14*, 19–28.

Finnila, K., Mahlberga, N., Santtilaa, P., Sandnabbaa, K., & Niemib, P. (2003). Validity of a test of children's suggestibility for predicting responses to two interview situations differing in their degree of suggestiveness. *Journal of Experimental Child Psychology*, *85*, 32–49.

Fischhoff, B., & Beyth, R. (1975). "I knew it would happen" – remembered probabilities of once-future things. *Organizational Behavior and Human Performance*, *13*, 1–16.

Garven, S., Wood, J. M., & Malpass, R. S. (2000). Allegations of wrongdoing: The effects of reinforcement on children's mundane and fantastic claims. *Journal of Applied Psychology*, *1*, 38–49.

Garven, S., Wood, J. M., Malpass, R., & Shaw, J. S. (1998). More than suggestion: Consequences of the interviewing techniques from the McMartin preschool case. *Journal of Applied Psychology*, *83*, 347–359.

Goodman, G. S., Batterman-Faunce, J. M., Schaaf, J. M., & Kenney, R. (2002). Nearly 4 years after an event: Children's eyewitness memory and adults' perceptions of children's accuracy. *Child Abuse and Neglect*, *26*, 849–884.

Goodman, G. S., Bottoms, B. L., Schwartz-Kenney, B., & Rudy, L. (1991). Children's testimony about a stressful event: Improving children's reports. *Journal of Narrative and Life History*, *1*, 69–99.

Goodman, G. S., Rudy, L., Bottoms, B., & Aman, C. (1990). Children's concerns and memory: Issues of ecological validity in the study of children's eyewitness testimony. In R. Fivush, & J. Hudson (Eds.), *Knowing and remembering in young children* (pp. 249–284). NY: Cambridge University Press.

Hagen, M. (2003). Faith in the model and resistance to research. *Clinical Psychology: Science and Practice*, *10*, 344–348.

Hawkins, S. A., & Hastie, R. (1990). Hindsight: Biased judgments of past events after the outcomes are known. *Psychological Bulletin*, *107*, 311–327.

Kendall-Tackett, K. A., Williams, L. M., & Finkelhor, D. (1993). Impact of sexual abuse on children: A review and synthesis of recent empirical studies. *Psychological Bulletin*, *113*, 164–180.

Lamb, M. E., Sternberg, K. J., & Esplin, P. W. (1998). Conducting investigative interviews of alleged sexual abuse victims. *Child Abuse and Neglect*, *22*, 813–823.

Lepore, S. J., & Sesco, B. (1994). Distorting children's reports and interpretations of events through suggestion. *Applied Psychology*, *79*(1), 108–120.

Lillie & Reed v. Newcastle City Council & Ors. (2002). EWHC 1600 (QB).

London, K., Bruck, M., Ceci, S. J., & Shuman, D. (2005). Disclosure of child sexual abuse: What does the research tell us about the ways that children tell? *Psychology, Public Policy & Law*, *11*, 194–226.

Loftus, E. F. (2003). Make believe memories. *American Psychologist*, *58*(11), 867–873.

Maddocks, A., Griffiths, L., & Anto, V. (1999). Detecting child sexual abuse in a general practice: A retrospective case–control study from Wales. *Scandinavian Journal of Primary Health Care*, *17*, 210–214.

McCloskey, M., & Zaragoza, M. (1985). Misleading postevent information and memory for events: Arguments and evidence against the memory impairment hypothesis. *Journal of experimental Psychology: General*, *114*, 1–16.

Melnyk, L., & Bruck, M. (2004). Timing moderates the effects of repeated suggestive interviewing on children's eyewitness memory. *Applied Cognitive Psychology*, *18*, 613–631.

Memorandum of Good Practice. (1992). London: Her Majesty's Stationery Office.

New Jersey v. Michaels. (1994). A.2d 579 aff'd 642 A.2d.

North Carolina v. Robert Fulton Kelly Jr. (1995). 456 S.E. 2d 861.

Ornstein, P. A., Gordon, B. N., & Larus, D. M. (1992). Children's memory for a personally experienced event: Implications for testimony. *Applied Cognitive Psychology*, *6*, 49–60.

Peterson, C., Moores, L., & White, G. (2001). Recounting the same event again and again: Children's consistency across multiple interviews. *Applied Cognitive Psychology*, *15*, 353–371.

Pipe, M. E., Gee, S., Wilson, S. J., & Egerton, J. M. (1999). Children's recall 1 or 2 years after an event. *Developmental Psychology*, *35*, 781–789.

Poole, D. A., & Lindsay, D. S. (2001). Children's eyewitness reports after exposure to misinformation from parents. *Journal of Experimental Psychology: Applied*, *7*, 27–50.

Poole, D. A., & White, L. T. (1991). Effects of question repetition on the eyewitness testimony of children and adults. *Developmental Psychology*, *27*, 975–986.

Porter, S., Yuille, J., & Lehman, D. (1999). The nature of real, implanted, and fabricated memories for emotional childhood events: Implications for the recovered memory debate. *Law & Human Behavior*, *23*, 517–537.

Principe, G. F., & Ceci, S. J. (2002). "I saw it with my own ears": The influence of peer conversations and suggestive questions on preschoolers' event memory. *Journal of Experimental Child Psychology*, *83*, 1–25.

Principe, G. F., Kanaya, T., Ceci, S. J., & Singh, M. (2006). Believing is seeing: How rumors can engender false memories in preschoolers. *Psychological Science*, *17*, 243–248.

Quas, J. A., Goodman, G. S., Bidrose, S., Pipe, M. E., Craw, S., & Ablin, D. (1999). Emotion and memory: Children's long-term remembering, forgetting and suggestibility. *Journal of Experimental Child Psychology*, *72*, 235–270.

Salmon, K., & Pipe, M. E. (2000). Recalling an event one year later: The impact of props, drawing, and a prior interview. *Applied Cognitive Psychology*, *14*, 99–120.

Schacter, D. (2001). *The seven sins of memory.* Boston, MA: Houghton Mifflin.

Smith, D. W., Letourneau, E. J., Saunders, B. J., Kilpatrick, D. J., Resnick, H. S., & Best, C. L. (2000). Delay in disclosure of childhood rape: Results from a national survey. *Child Abuse and Neglect*, *24*, 273–287.

State v. Fijnje. (1995). 11th Judicial Circuit Court, Dade Country, Florida #84-19728.

Summit, R. C. (1983). The child sexual abuse accommodation syndrome. *Child Abuse & Neglect*, *7*, 177–193.

Summit, R. C., Miller, T. W., & Veltkamp, L. J. (1998). The child sexual abuse accommodation syndrome: Clinical issues and forensic implications. In T. W. Miller (Ed.), *Children of trauma: Stressful life events and their effects on children and adolescents* (pp. 43–60). Madison, CT: International Universities Press.

Thompson, W. C., Clarke-Stewart, A., & Lepore, S. (1997). What did the janitor do? Suggestive interviewing and the accuracy of children's accounts. *Law & Human Behavior*, *21*, 405–426.

US Department of Health and Human Services, Administration on Children, Youth, and Families. (2005). *Child Maltreatment 2003.* Washington, DC: US Government Printing Office.

Zigler, E., & Kanzer, P. (1962). The effectiveness of two classes of verbal reinforcers on the performance of middle and lower-class children. *Journal of Personality*, *30*, 157–163.

8 Legal Issues in the Care and Treatment of Children with Mental Health Problems

Brenda Hale and Jane Fortin

Any child with mental health problems is likely to encounter a variety of professionals and agencies. Each of these has their own role, responsibilities and perspective. At their best, this can lead to fruitful cooperation in the best interests of the child. At their worst, this can lead to failures in communication, failure to take responsibility, failure to "own" the problem; in short to failure of the child. Every professional involved with the child has first to ask themselves what sort of a problem it is and which service or services will be best equipped to help solve it. If legal measures may also be required, a further question is whether these should be directed primarily towards the child or the child's family. We first sketch the legal position of the various agencies and professionals, and consider the role of expert witnesses, then look at the legal position of the child's family, and finally at the legal position of the children themselves. We use examples from the UK but attempt to draw out principles that hold across other judicial systems.

Different Services – Different Perspectives

Education

Education is the one universal service, free to every child of compulsory school age, irrespective of learning disability, mental illness or emotional and behavioral disorders.[1] Indeed, education is the one right specific to childhood that is spelled out in the European Convention on Human Rights: "No-one shall be denied the right to education."[2] Europe assumes that each member state offers an education service but does not lay down any particular standard. Children are entitled to be provided with the education offered by the educational system in their own country. If for whatever reason that educational system is inadequate to meet their special needs, they may have little recourse under the European Convention.[3] The United Nations Convention on the Rights of the Child (UNCRC) is more specific[4] but creates no rights enforceable in UK law because it has never been made part of domestic law.

Rutter's Child and Adolescent Psychiatry, 5th edition. Edited by M. Rutter, D. Bishop, D. Pine, S. Scott, J. Stevenson, E. Taylor and A. Thapar. © 2008 Blackwell Publishing, ISBN: 978-1-4051-4549-7.

The aspiration now is that as many children as possible will be educated in mainstream schools with special help if necessary.[5] If a school encounters problems with a child with mental health difficulties, a great deal will depend upon whether teachers define the problem as a pedagogical or a disciplinary issue (see chapter 74). If it is defined as a pedagogical problem, the solution may eventually lie in the complex process of assessing and providing the child with a statement of his or her special educational needs, which the authorities will then be under a duty to meet.[6] The legal duties attaching to educational provision are unlike those relating to health and social care because the parents of children with special educational needs have defined rights to be involved in the decision-making process and to challenge the authorities' decisions in the special educational needs and disability tribunal (SENDIST). Unlike other tribunals in the field of health and social care, SENDIST has the power to order the authorities to provide the education that it decides the child needs.

However, if the school instead classifies the child as having a disciplinary problem, the solution may be very different. It will lie in an escalating scale of formal disciplinary measures including temporary or permanent exclusion.[7] These may solve the school's immediate problems, but will do nothing to meet the long-term educational and mental health needs of the child. The children's services authority has the duty to provide an education for excluded children, but this will

[1] Education Act 1996, s 14.
[2] Protocol 1, article 2.
[3] The European jurisprudence is discussed in *Ali v. Lord Grey School* [2006] UKHL 14; [2006] 2 WLR 690; a boy who had been kept out of school when he should have been allowed back, thus losing months of his education, had no remedy because his parents had failed to take up alternatives. Nevertheless, a pupil will have a remedy if he is denied access to a minimum level of education: per Lord Hoffmann, at para 59.
[4] See article 28; the minimum is free compulsory primary education for all.
[5] Education Act 1996, s 316. These provisions date back to Warnock (1978).
[6] Education Act 1996, Part IV. See also DfES (2001).
[7] Education Act 2002, s 52 and regulations, SI 2002/3178 and SI 2002/3139.

rarely meet the standards of mainstream schools, and will carry its own stigma and disadvantage.[8] The child and his or her parents may challenge the exclusion, but here the focus is more like that in a criminal trial: was the child guilty of the conduct complained of and did the punishment fit the crime? Only indirectly will the disciplinary process be concerned with whether the school was meeting the child's needs.

The other side of the coin is that parents have an obligation to ensure that their children receive an education suitable to their age, ability, aptitude and any special educational needs they may have.[9] If a child is not going to school, the children's services authority may either prosecute the parents or take action in respect of the child. Recent well-publicized prosecutions suggest that they are increasingly insisting that parents take their responsibilities seriously.[10] However, if the child rather than the family is seen as the origin of the problem (as discussed in chapter 35), the children's services authority have few effective remedies for truancy or school refusal. In England and Wales, what used to be called the "status offences" of childhood have been abolished: being beyond parental control or in moral danger, falling into bad associations, or persistently failing to go to school are no longer virtually automatic grounds for placing a child in institutional care.[11] Today, the education officers within the children's services authority may find it difficult to persuade the children's social care section that the child's development is at such significant risk that they should take over parental responsibility for the child (see p. 101). The aim of the reform was to ensure that the education authorities took responsibility for what were fundamentally educational problems (see also DHSS, 1985, chapter 15), but with the increasing autonomy of individual schools, individual children may fall through the net.

The Criminal Justice System

The one net that children are less and less likely to avoid is the criminal justice system. Civil law recognizes that children are not yet sufficiently mature to play a full part in civil society. The criminal justice system in England and Wales, on the other hand, sees children of 10 years or over as sufficiently mature to be held fully responsible for their criminal behavior. This age is controversially low (Commission on Families and the Wellbeing of Children, 2005; Royal College of Psychiatrists, 2006). In Scotland, the age of criminal responsibility is set even lower, at 8 years, but children who plead or are found guilty are dealt with in the more child-friendly children's hearings rather than in court (McDiarmid, 2005; Scottish Law Commission, 2001). The criminal justice system aims to deter, punish and reform. The rules of the criminal law are the same for adults and children.[12] The differences lie in the court procedures and the sentences available. In the 1970s and into the 1980s, the emphasis of the juvenile justice system was on prevention and reform (Home Office, 1965, 1968).[13] Much of the responsibility for tackling juvenile offenders was passed to the social services authorities (now children's services authorities), who followed a welfare rather than a punishment model (Parsloe, 1978). The longer children could be kept out of the penal system the better. That way the system could do them no harm and they would eventually grow out of their offending behavior. By the 1990s, children were being cautioned time and time again and hardly ever brought to court. This gave the impression that they could break the law with complete impunity unless they did something really serious or became involved with an older gang. The legislative pendulum soon swung sharply back towards punishment and deterrence (Home Office, 1998). Greater efforts are also being made to get parents to take responsibility for their children's misbehavior.[14]

The principal aim of the youth justice system is still "to prevent offending by children and young persons."[15] It still aims to divert offenders away from prosecution and punishment if at all possible, but a limit has now been placed on the number of warnings that a child may be given before being taken to court.[16] Another move that has catapulted more children towards the criminal justice system is the invention of antisocial behavior orders (ASBOs).[17] These aim to deter particular types of antisocial behavior by prohibiting not only the behavior itself, but also the conditions that may lead to it, such as gathering in town centers late at night. The proceedings themselves are civil proceedings, but breach of an ASBO is a criminal offence.[18]

[8] Education Act 1996, s 19.

[9] Education Act 1996, ss 7, backed up by the offences in ss 443–444B.

[10] The penalties for a parent who knows that a child is not going to school and fails without reasonable cause to make him or her attend were increased in 2002 to include imprisonment: see Education Act 1976, s 444. Fixed penalty notices against any parent whose child fails to attend school regularly were introduced in 2004: see Education Act, 1996, s 444A.

[11] Children Act 1989, s 31, replacing Children and Young Persons Act 1969, s 1. For a discussion of the history of these provisions, see Dingwall, Eekelaar & Murray (1983).

[12] The common law presumption that a child of 10–13 years inclusive was *doli incapax* until the prosecution proved that he knew what he was doing was seriously wrong was abolished by the Crime and Disorder Act 1998, s 34.

[13] The 1968 report (*Children in Trouble*) led to Part I of the Children and Young Persons Act, 1969.

[14] Binding parents over to take proper care and exercise proper control over their children (now under the Powers of Criminal Courts [Sentencing] Act 2000, s 150) and ordering them to pay their children's fines have a long history; but parenting orders, requiring them to attend counseling or guidance programs, were introduced by the Crime and Disorder Act 1998, ss 8–10, and parenting contracts by the Anti-Social Behaviour Act 2003, s 25.

[15] Crime and Disorder Act 1998, s 37.

[16] A reprimand is given for a first offence, a final warning for the second. The third must be charged and prosecuted, irrespective of its triviality.

[17] Crime and Disorder Act 1998, s 1.

[18] In 2005, 1058 ASBOS were issued to persons aged 10–17 years, compared with 185 in 2001.

Once taken to court, the range of sentences available for juveniles is still different from those available for adults, but an offender is likely to climb the ladder from the less to the more serious disposals more quickly than he or she did before. This is one reason for the sharp rise in the numbers of children detained in secure institutions run by the penal rather than the children's services authorities.[19] Indeed, the UK locks up more young people under 18 than most other European countries (NACRO, 2003), not a record of which the UK can be proud. The UN Committee on the Rights of the Child has expressed its deep concern over "the increasing number of children who are being detained in custody at earlier ages for lesser offences and for longer sentences" (UN Committee on the Rights of the Child, 2002). These large numbers of young and juvenile detainees were also criticized more recently by the Council of Europe's Commissioner for Human Rights (Gil-Robles, 2005). Child offenders are even more likely than adults to have mental health problems, but there are far fewer resources available to meet those needs in penal establishments (young offender institutions) than there are in the local authority secure children's homes, to which a minority are sent. Although specialist mental health services in the local authority institutions are far from ideal (Kroll, Rothwell, Bradley *et al.*, 2002), those in young offender institutions are often very poor (Harrington & Bailey, 2005).

Whichever way the pendulum swings, it is universally recognized that child offenders merit a different approach from adults. The UNCRC requires member states to promote measures for dealing with children outside court and to provide a variety of dispositions "to ensure that children are dealt with in a manner appropriate to their well being and proportionate both to their circumstances and the offence."[20] While the system no longer thinks that the whole problem, and therefore the whole solution, lies with the family rather than the child, there may be other steps that could be taken to bring home some of the responsibility to the parents. Some would like to see the link with the child care system restored at least so as to enable the criminal court to require the children's services authority to investigate and decide whether social rather than penal action would be more appropriate (Butler-Sloss, 2003).

Children's Services

In England and Wales, the children's social care section of the local children's services authority has both the duty and the power to take steps to protect a child from significant harm. Unlike some other countries, other services and professionals have no mandatory duty to report cases of suspected child abuse and neglect to them. In practice, however, failure to report may be less of a problem than failure to recognize abuse when it occurs.[21] An even greater challenge may be to persuade children's social care services to take action when others think they should.

Child protection is only one of a range of social care services provided for "children in need."[22] In keeping with the family-centered philosophies of both the European Convention on Human Rights and UNCRC (see p. 99), it is the duty of the children's services authorities to "promote the upbringing of such children by their families."[23] These are target duties owed to the particular client group, rather than enforceable duties owed towards particular children or their families.[24] There is no statutory procedure, like the process of "statementing" a child with special educational needs, for identifying a child's social needs and ensuring that these are met. Those who are lucky enough to be advised by a knowledgeable lawyer may apply for a judicial review of a refusal to provide support services. This is concerned with the legality of a particular administrative decision but not its merits. It is not for the courts to take the tough decisions about the allocation of scarce resources which Parliament has entrusted to the providers of both health and social services. The courts can only ensure that service providers act within the law. This includes acting rationally and fairly. Authorities are allowed to take resources into account, but they may have to explain why they are offering a service to one person but not to another.

Nevertheless, children's services authorities do owe some duties to the individual child. Reports of suspected abuse or neglect must be investigated and action taken where necessary to protect the child (see chapters 28 & 29). Before the Human Rights Act 1998, it was held that children's social services could not be held liable either for negligently failing to protect a child or for negligently taking action to remove or keep a child away from home.[25] The European Convention, however, brings positive as well as negative obligations. There is the negative obligation to refrain from unjustified interference with the right to respect for family life, but also the positive obligation to protect a child from death or serious ill-treatment. In the light of these, courts have now held that the authorities do owe duties of care towards the child.[26]

Social care workers should therefore conduct a comprehensive assessment of the child and his or her family. Their focus will inevitably be upon the interaction between children and their families, because any compulsory intervention that they promote will operate to interfere in the legal relationship between child and family (see p. 101). They are bound, therefore, to assess the extent to which the child's problems are the product of his or her home environment. Of course, they

[19] Youth Justice Board figures indicate that in March 2006, the total under-18 population in custody was 2785 (cf. 2684 March 2005) of whom 196 were girls.

[20] UNCRC art 40.3 and 40.4.

[21] No service is immune from this, as shown in Laming (2003).

[22] Part III of the Children Act 1989.

[23] Children Act 1989, s 17(1).

[24] *R (on the application of G) v. Barnet London Borough Council* [2003] UKHL 57; [2004] 2 AC 208.

[25] *X and Others v. Bedfordshire County Council* [1995] 2 AC 633.

[26] See *JD v. East Berkshire Community NHS Trust and Others* [2005] UKHL 23; [2005] 2 AC 373.

will have to rely upon the specialist mental health services if specialist assessment is necessary at the outset and for any future treatment of the child.

Mental Health Services

The only role of the child, adolescent and family mental health services is to provide a specialist service for the child and his or her family. Unlike both the education and social care sections of children's services authorities, they have virtually no coercive powers to back up the service they wish to offer, and can rarely be obliged to offer a service that they do not wish to offer. There are a few cases where compulsory intervention under the Mental Health Act 1983, may be necessary and appropriate (see p. 107). There are also a few cases where a hospital wishes to take a particular course of action which is opposed by either the child or the family. In England and Wales, an NHS Trust could invoke the inherent jurisdiction of the High Court[27] or apply for a "specific issue" about the child's upbringing to be decided.[28] The most obvious examples involve the treatment of anorexic teenagers or giving blood transfusions to the children of Jehovah's witnesses.[29] In most cases where the relationship between the professionals and the family of a child with mental health problems breaks down, such one-off determinations are unlikely to provide a long-term solution. If the professionals think that legal proceedings should be taken against either the child or the family, they will have to refer the case for the children's services authority to take action. Children's services will then be "in the driving seat," although assessment and treatment should be a multidisciplinary endeavor.

Nor can health professionals be obliged to offer a service that they do not wish to offer. Like all professionals, they owe a duty of care to their own patients. If they negligently fail to diagnose or to treat, and the patient suffers harm as a result, they may be held liable in damages. The most obvious examples are a child psychologist who fails to diagnose dyslexia or a child psychiatrist who negligently diagnoses child abuse.[30] The courts have interpreted the scope of their legal duty, so that it is owed only to their child patient and not to the child's parents. The courts in the UK and elsewhere have been well aware that if professionals also owed a duty to the parents, they might hesitate to diagnose abuse and the child would go unprotected.[31]

That aside, parents have sometimes tried to use wardship or judicial review to oblige health authorities, hospitals or individual doctors to provide treatment that they do not wish to provide. Thus far, while the courts have been prepared to reassure the authorities in advance that a course of action that they do wish to pursue will be lawful,[32] they have not been prepared to order the medical authorities to provide treatment for an individual patient that they consider will be futile or counterproductive.[33] The Human Rights Act has not altered these fundamental principles.[34]

The main role of a mental health professional in legal proceedings is therefore not as claimant or defendant, applicant or respondent, but as an expert witness in cases brought by others. Before examining the principles of law applying to those cases, it may be helpful to examine the role of the expert witness.

Role of the Expert Witness

Expert medical witnesses fall into two broad categories. Psychiatrists and other professionals who are already working with the child and his or her family may be asked to report on the history, diagnosis and treatment to date, together with their assessment and recommendations for the future. As expert witnesses, they are entitled to offer their professional opinions as well as their factual accounts. No doubt they will bring the independence expected of any professional to that task. This should include a willingness to acknowledge that medical records are not always perfectly accurate or complete and may from time to time repeat or rely upon unverified hearsay.[35] But they are essentially witnesses of fact and the child is their patient.

They have a different role in the proceedings from that of an independent expert who has been commissioned to make a report and recommendations to the court.[36] An independent expert may be commissioned by any of the parties to the case, but the court is firmly in charge of whether and how many experts may be instructed and in which disciplines.[37] In

[27] Better known as the wardship or *parens patriae* jurisdiction derived from the Crown's guardianship over all minor children, but it can be invoked for a single issue without making the child a ward of court.
[28] Children Act 1989, s 8(1).
[29] A standard form of order has now been developed. This requires that every effort is made to avoid giving a blood transfusion, but that if there is no alternative, it may be done. Parents are generally advised not to consent, but not actively to oppose such orders.
[30] See *Phelps v. Hillingdon London Borough Council* [2001] 2 AC 619; X *and Others v. Bedfordshire County Council* [1995] 2 AC 633.
[31] See the majority view in *JD v. East Berkshire Community Health NHS Trust and Others* [2005] UKHL 23; *B and Others v. Attorney General of New Zealand* [2003] UKPC 61; [2003] 4 All ER 803.
[32] Extending the effect of the wardship jurisdiction over children to mentally disabled adults, principally to authorize the non-therapeutic sterilization of mentally disabled women and girls or the withdrawal of artificial nutrition and hydration from patients in a persistent vegetative state: see *B (A Minor) (Wardship: Sterilization)* [1988] AC 199; *Re F (Mental Patient: Sterilization)* [1990] 2 AC 1; *Airedale NHS Trust v. Bland* [1993] AC 789; *R (on the application of Burke) v. General Medical Council* [205] EWCA Civ 1003.
[33] *Re J (A Minor) (Wardship: Medical Treatment)* [1991] Fam 33.
[34] Summed up in *R (on the application of Burke) v. General Medical Council* [2006] QB 273, para 50.
[35] This concern has led some to argue that the standard of proof of the continuing conditions for detention in mental health review tribunals should be higher than the usual balance of probabilities.
[36] *Re B (Sexual Abuse: Expert's Report)* [2000] 1 FLR 871.
[37] This is provided for both in the Family Proceedings Rules 1991, rule 4.18 and the ordinary Civil Procedure Rules 1998, rule 35.4.

child protection proceedings, following the Cleveland Inquiry Report (Butler-Sloss, 1988), the object is now to prevent the child being subjected to multiple examinations and assessments. The court's expectations of an expert in child protection proceedings are laid down in the *Code of Guidance for Expert Witnesses in Family Proceedings*.[38] The expert's overriding duty is to the court and takes precedence over any duty to the party who has instructed them (see chapter 4). The court always hopes that the experts will be able to clarify, narrow and if possible agree upon the issues in the case. The common practice is for a single expert to be jointly instructed by all parties, usually led by the children's guardian who is appointed by the court to act for the child in the proceedings.[39] An assessment carried out by a jointly instructed expert is not without problems. The family may be very happy to agree with the proposed assessment before they know the result, but if they are unhappy with the result, they may want a second, third or fourth opinion. The courts try hard to resist this "expert shopping." Parents or children who have serious concerns about the accuracy or rigor of a report will face formidable difficulties if they try to challenge it without expert evidence of their own. It is no simple task to reconcile the need of the child to be spared endless and intrusive investigations with the right of both child and family to a fair trial of the issues.[40] The lack of contradiction or opposition places a heightened duty of independent professionalism upon the expert witness and of vigilance upon the court. Issues upon which there is properly room for professional disagreement should be identified at the outset, so that two experts can be appointed without adding to the delays. Expert witnesses enjoy the same immunity from suit in respect of their evidence as any other witness, but this does not include immunity from professional discipline.[41]

Another problem is that child protection law in England and Wales draws a clear distinction between an assessment of the child, which is within the court's power to direct, and what, in truth, amounts to treatment of the parents, which is not.[42] This distinction does not always reflect the realities of psychiatric practice, particularly in some of the most complex and difficult cases. It is not possible to separate the assessment of the child from the assessment of the parents. What requires assessment is the relationship between them and the capacities of the parents to meet the needs of the child. Moreover, what begins as assessment may move into assessment with therapy and move again into therapy with continuing assessment. As Dr. Kennedy of the Cassel Hospital has forcefully argued (Kennedy, 2001), doctors are assessing their patients all the time. Nice legal distinctions mean nothing to them.

None of this would matter were it not for the problems in funding the very specialist resources that some of these deeply damaged families require. The court can only require the parties – whether the local children's services authority or the legal services commission that is funding both the child's and the parents' representation – to pay for an assessment which is necessary to enable the court to perform its own function. The court's function is only to decide what order, if any, to make about the child's future. The court has no power to order either the local children's services authority or the health services to provide any particular form of treatment for the child or their family (see p. 101).

Families and Their Children

The Family and the State

The legal status of children as minors, let alone their physical and financial dependency, means that they are different from adults in two respects. First, they have claims upon other people that adults do not have: claims to be nurtured, cared for and brought up to play their full part in adult society. Second, the people with the responsibility of meeting those claims have both the right and the responsibility to make decisions on behalf of their children. As we shall see in the next section, these do not stay static throughout childhood: the claims change and the child's own autonomy grows. In some respects, a child remains a child until he or she reaches adulthood, in England and Wales at the age of 18.[43]

It is a cardinal feature of western democratic legal systems that parents and families, rather than the state, have the primary right and the primary responsibility to bring up their children: to meet their claims for nurture, care and upbringing and to decide for themselves how this will be done. "It is important in a free society to maintain the rich diversity of lifestyles which is secured by permitting families a large measure of autonomy in the way in which they bring up their children." (DHSS, 1985, para 2.13) It is the hallmark of a dictatorship to gain control of the children and distance them from the varied and subversive influences of their families (Hale, 2005a). This is why the European Convention on Human Rights, drafted in 1950 in the twin shadows of the Nazi totalitarianism of the recent past and the Stalinist totalitarianism of the then present, guarantees to everyone – parents and children alike – the right to respect for their private and family life, their home and their correspondence.[44] The UNCRC also requires states to recognizes that, "Parents or, as the case may be, legal guardians, have the primary responsibility for the upbringing and development of the child. The best interests of the child will be *their* basic concern."[45]

Historically, English common law placed this legal responsibility upon the fathers of children born to married parents and (eventually) upon the mothers of children born to unmarried

[38] Annex C to the Protocol on Judicial Case Management in Public Law Children Act Cases, June 2003 [2003] 2 FLR 719.

[39] This will usually be a Children and Family Court Advisory and Support Service (hereafter CAFCASS) officer.

[40] Protected by article 6 of ECHR as well as common law.

[41] *Meadow v. General Medical Council* [2007] 2 WLR 286.

[42] Children Act 1989, s 38(6) and *Re G (A Child) (Interim Care Order: Residential Assessment)* [2005] UKHL 68; [2006] IAC 576.

[43] Reduced from 21 by the Family Law Reform Act 1969.

[44] Article 8.

[45] Article 18.1, emphasis supplied.

parents. The position now is that if the parents are or have been married to one another at any time since the child's conception they are both legally responsible for his or her upbringing – they alone are deemed to have "parental responsibility" for the child.[46] If they are not married, the default position is that the mother alone has parental responsibility; but the father may acquire it, either by agreement with the mother, or by court order or, since December 1, 2003, simply by being registered as the father on the child's birth certificate.[47]

The state's role is to supplement and enable the parents' role. UNCRC requires state parties to render all parents "appropriate assistance . . . in the performance of their child-rearing responsibilities and shall ensure the development of institutions, facilities and services for the care of children."[48] State parties also recognize "the right of the child to the enjoyment of the highest attainable standard of health and to facilities for the treatment of illness and rehabilitation of health"[49] and "that a mentally or physically disabled child should enjoy a full and decent life, in conditions which ensure dignity, promote self-reliance and facilitate the child's active participation in the community."[50] All but two of the members of the UN have ratified this Convention.[51] Some who have ratified the Convention are relatively poor developing countries for whom these rights can only be aspirational. In the UK, they are not, or should not be, mere pious aspirations.

Intervening in Family Life

What are the professionals to do if they disagree with the child's parents about what the child needs? Everyone hopes that it will never come to this. Every effort will be made to persuade the parents to agree. If they do not, most legal systems present two possible ways of overcoming their objections.

The earliest was the threat of prosecution for child neglect or abuse. In English law, it is an offence for a person over the age of 16 who is responsible[52] for a person below that age, wilfully to assault, ill-treat, neglect, abandon or expose that child in a manner likely to cause unnecessary suffering or injury to health.[53] This entails positive obligations on the part of a parent (or other person legally liable to maintain the child): he or she is presumed to have neglected the child in such a manner if he or she fails to provide the child with adequate food, clothing, shelter or medical aid.[54] In English law, the fact that a parent has religious or conscientious objections to medical treatment is not a defense,[55] but failure to appreciate the risks could be.[56]

Some legal systems may be reluctant to go beyond the threat of prosecution to secure parental compliance, but this will not help the child unless the threat is effective. It is least likely to be effective against inadequate parents who simply do not appreciate the risks. What are the professionals to do if the parents refuse their advice? It should not be forgotten that we are talking here of the child's rights, on the one hand to appropriate health care and on the other hand the child's right to decide what should happen to his or her own body (see p. 103). In English law at least, we are not talking about the parents' own right to sue for harm done to them by the unauthorized treatment of their child. They have no right to sue for damages on their own account.[57] They could only sue on behalf of their child for the harm done *to him or her* by the unauthorized invasion of the child's own bodily integrity.

The person actually looking after the child (including a health care facility) is sometimes entitled to act without taking the matter to court. A somewhat neglected provision of the Children Act 1989,[58] states the obvious: "A person who (a) does not have parental responsibility for a particular child; but (b) has care of the child, may (subject to the provisions of this Act) do what is reasonable in all the circumstances of the case for the purpose of safeguarding and promoting the child's welfare." This is clearly enough to authorize a non-parent to provide the child with day-to-day care and also treatment in an emergency or which it is unreasonable to delay until the parents can be consulted. In some cases, discussed in detail below, the child may be competent to consent to his or her own treatment even if the parents object. For one-off treatments, the hospital or doctors might apply for a specific issue order authorizing the treatment in the child's best interests.

Children with mental health problems or learning difficulties are likely to present more long-term and complex problems. The family environment and dynamics may be an important part of the child's problems. The legal system provides machinery to enable the professionals to step in and provide the care and treatment which they believe that the child needs even if the parents resist this. Because of the principles of parental responsibility and respect for family life, there are two basic requirements, one procedural and one substantive.

[46] Children Act 1989, s 2(1).

[47] Children Act 1989, ss 2(2) and 4, as amended by the Adoption and Children Act 2002, s 111. 83.2% of births outside marriage were jointly registered by both parents in 2004. The father is liable to support the child even if he does not have parental responsibility.

[48] Article 18.2.

[49] Article 24.1.

[50] Article 23.1.

[51] The exceptions are Somalia, which has said that it will do so when it has a functioning government; and the USA, which objects to some of the Convention's principles.

[52] This includes having formal parental responsibility or actual care: Children and Young Persons Act 1933, s 17.

[53] Children and Young Persons Act 1933, s 1(1).

[54] Children and Young Persons Act 1933, s 1(2)(a).

[55] *R v. Senior* [1899] 1 QB 283.

[56] *R v. Sheppard* [1981] AC 394.

[57] The parent's right to claim against third parties who injured his child was abolished by the Law Reform (Miscellaneous Provisions) Act 1970.

[58] s 3(5). Indeed, in the light of ss 1(1) and 17 of the Children and Young Persons Act 1933, it could be argued that this should have imposed a positive duty to act where the child would otherwise be caused unnecessary suffering or injury to health.

The procedural requirement is that action can only be taken with the authority of a court order obtained by due process of law. In England and Wales, responsibility for undertaking proceedings to intervene compulsorily in family life lies, not with the health authorities, but with the children's social care departments of local children's services authorities. These are the public bodies charged with the overall responsibility of protecting children from harm. This is because the eventual outcome of most care proceedings is that the authority will have to take parental responsibility for the child. Care by a local authority may not be ideal, but at least the child should thereby have, or have access to, the full range of facilities needed to discharge those responsibilities, including the health and education services. Neither the health nor the education services are equipped to cater for everything that parents should provide for their children, nor can they find alternative families for children who need them.

The substantive requirement is that, although the welfare of the child is the paramount consideration, it must first be shown that the child is suffering or likely to suffer significant harm.[59] Harm is so widely defined[60] that it is very likely that a child with mental health problems whose health or educational needs are not being met will be suffering or likely to suffer significant harm. That is not the end of the matter. It must also be shown that this is attributable to a lack of reasonable parental care, whether because the parent cannot or will not provide it, rather than to the failure of the services themselves to deliver what the child needs.[61] Only once the harm threshold has been crossed can the court decide what will be best for the child. This includes deciding whether making an order will be better for the child than not doing so.[62]

This puts the court in a quandary. Only by looking into the future can it decide what will be best for the child. It must therefore be shown a plausible care plan for the child and have some confidence that it will be carried out. Unless there is some other individual able to take responsibility for the child, the court can only choose between a care order, a supervision order or no order at all. While a care order places the child in the care of the designated local authority, with parental responsibility being vested in that authority,[63] a supervision order merely places the child under the local authority's supervision, with the parents' own legal role being unaffected. Despite the apparent strength of a care order, the court has no power to impose conditions on it or to insist that the local authority discharge their parental responsibilities in a particular way. This can be another source of frustration for health-care professionals whose recommendations for treatment are not always adopted by the local authority looking after the child.[64] Some look back nostalgically to the days of the old wardship system, when, theoretically at least, the court could direct how the child was to be cared for and review the case at regular intervals.[65] However, the reality was often very different. Courts have neither the resources nor the expertise to act as substitute parents for children.

In most cases, the court has no choice, because the risk of leaving the child at home is now too great. The real choice is between planning to reunite children with their families and planning to place them with permanent alternative families. This raises an even greater dilemma. If the authorities intervene early, before a child suffers permanent harm, the more likely it is that he or she can be successfully placed for adoption with a new family. The later things are left, the more harm is done, and the more difficult it will be to repair the damage successfully. The dilemma is particularly acute with emotional neglect and abuse, which may take many years to result in significant harm to the child (see chapter 28). Can such early intervention be justified in human rights terms?

Influence of Human Rights Law on Child Care Law

The European Convention prohibits any interference by a public authority with the right to respect for family life unless three conditions are fulfilled.[66] First, the intervention must be in accordance with the law; it must comply with a national law that is sufficiently clear and certain for people to be able to conduct themselves accordingly. Second, it must be for a legitimate aim; in this case, for the protection of the rights and freedoms of the child. Third, and most important, it must be "necessary in a democratic society"; the means used must be proportionate to the legitimate aim pursued and the reasons given must be relevant and sufficient. The jurisprudence of the European Court of Human Rights in Strasbourg is consistent.[67] The aim of any public authority removing a child from home must generally be to reunite the family; permanent removal requires exceptional justification in the interests of the child. The reasons for cutting off children from their families of birth will be scrutinized with much more care than the reasons for initially removing them from home.

UK courts are conscious that their task is to ensure that compulsory intervention in family life is no more than is necessary to achieve its aim of protecting the child from

[59] Children Act 1989, ss 1(1) and 31(2)(a).

[60] It means ill-treatment or the impairment of health or development. Health means physical or mental health. Development means physical, intellectual, emotional, social or behavioral development. Ill-treatment includes sexual abuse and forms of ill-treatment that are not physical. Children Act 1989, s 31(9).

[61] Children Act 1989, s 31(2)(b).

[62] Children Act 1989, s 1(5).

[63] Armed with a care order, the local authority can limit the extent to which the child's parents can exercise their own parental role in relation to their child. Children Act 1989, s 33(3).

[64] The issues involved in care planning within the family justice system were discussed at the President's interdisciplinary conference in September 1997 (Thorpe & Clarke, 1998).

[65] The attempts of the Court of Appeal to devise some method of policing the care plan were firmly rejected by the House of Lords in *Re S (Children) (Care Order: Implementation of Care Plan)* [2002] UKHL 10; [2002] 2 AC 291.

[66] Article 8.2.

[67] See, for example, *KA v. Finland* (2001) 2 FLR 696, repeating what had been said in numerous earlier cases.

significant harm in the particular circumstances of the case. What is the court to do if it decides that the local authority should take steps to make possible the reunification of mother and child but the local authority fails to do this? And what is the court to do if it decides that the child needs a permanent family elsewhere but the local authority fails to take timely steps to find one?[68] The Children Act 1989, denies the court any continuing role in supervising the local authority's discharge of its parental responsibilities. Yet this may lead to breaches of either the parents' or the child's human rights. In the former situation, a parent might complain that the authority was acting in breach of either his or her own or the child's Convention rights; in the latter, the child might do so. It can certainly be argued that if the state destroys the family life of a child in his or her birth family, it has a positive obligation to use its best endeavors to supply the child with a new family.[69] In many cases there may be no-one to take action on behalf of the child.[70] The Court of Appeal tried to solve this problem by giving the court a way of ensuring that the case came back to court if major steps in the care plan were not implemented. However, in *Re S (Children) (Care Order: Implementation of Care Plan)*[71] the House of Lords decided that the Human Rights Act did not allow the courts to alter a "cardinal feature" of the Children Act by putting things into the Act which were not there.

Compulsory adoption is clearly the most drastic possible interference in the family life of a child, the parents and their wider family (see chapter 33). The UK is unusual amongst European states in allowing children to be adopted into a new family without their parents' consent.[72] So far, the issues have not been thoroughly explored in Strasbourg. There has been no direct challenge to this aspect of UK law. The European Court has scrutinized with special care the proceedings for the removal of a baby shortly after birth from a mother thought to have a factitious illness, followed very swiftly by an order freeing the baby for adoption.[73] The move towards more open adoption, already well under way in England and Wales[74] before the Human Rights Act, 1998, was motivated by the child's rather than the parents' needs. The ability of birth parents to retain some contact with their child may also help to make compulsory adoption more Convention compliant. The dilemma still remains that adoption is the preferred solution precisely when the harm (or most of it) has yet to be done. This makes the professional task of accurately assessing the future risks all the more important.

The recent House of Lords decision in *Re G (A Child) (Interim Care Order: Residential Assessment)*,[75] although concerned with the mental health of the mother rather than the child, illustrates many of these issues. The mother's second child had died in infancy having suffered multiple injuries. The court could not decide whether the mother or the father was responsible, but the risk was such that the mother's first child by an earlier relationship was removed.[76] She then formed a new and more promising relationship. Could they be allowed to parent the new baby? Initially the local authority's care plan was adoption. The court directed an assessment of their suitability for the intensive program offered by the Cassel hospital. This was successful, but who would pay for the next phase? The local NHS authorities could not fund the treatment of everyone from all over the country who might benefit from this very intensive and specialist work. The local children's services authority responsible for this child's care and safety were unwilling to devote a large proportion of their budget to funding in-patient treatment which was principally aimed at keeping the family together in a safe place while addressing the mother's problems. The legal services commission could assist in funding the evidence-gathering necessary for the legal proceedings but not the treatment necessary to enable the mother to parent the child safely. The House of Lords decided that neither the local authority nor the legal services commission could be obliged to fund the mother's treatment. Fortunately, by then the family had completed the program at the Cassel so successfully that they had been allowed home together without a court order. This was indeed "planned and purposeful delay" but not at all what the legislation intends. Without the earlier pressure from the court, the child would have been placed for adoption. In the light of the horrific injuries suffered by the older child, this might well have survived scrutiny in Strasbourg. But who can doubt that it was right to try to enable this mother to parent this child?

The Individual Child – the Ethical Dilemmas of Adolescence

Most common law legal systems contain case law emphasizing the principle that for adults, medical treatment without

[68] The very issues which the Court of Appeal had been trying to resolve in *Re S (Children) (Care Order: Implementation of Care Plan)* [2002] UKHL 10; [2002] 2 AC 291.

[69] This aspect of the Court of Appeal's judgment in the *Re S* case was not challenged in the House of Lords. See *Re W and B* [2001] EWCA Civ 757; [2001] 2 FLR 582.

[70] Hence there is now a procedure for the local authority to refer cases where the care plan has not been achieved to the Child and Family Court Advisory and Support Service (CAFCASS) so that they can consider whether to take action for the child.

[71] [2002] UKHL 10; [2002] 2 AC 291.

[72] Adoption and Children Act 2002, ss 47 and 52. Evidence given in the recent House of Lords case of *Down Lisburn Health and Social Services Trust v. H* [2006] UKHL 36 suggested that only the UK, Portugal and perhaps one other country allows this. However, adoption may take different forms in different countries, so that exact comparisons are not always possible.

[73] *P, C and S v. United Kingdom* [2002] 2 FLR 631.

[74] Apparently still uncommon in Northern Ireland, where freeing for adoption is still the common practice in contested cases.

[75] [2005] UKHL 68; [2006] 1 AC 576.

[76] See her unsuccessful appeals, first against the finding of non-accidental injury, then against the removal of the child: [2001] 1 FCR 97; [2001] 1 FLR 872.

consent involves an intolerable invasion of bodily and personal privacy.[77] But children in developed societies grow up fast. Why should they be treated differently, particularly when they reach adolescence? In most developed countries, there has been a growing realization that adolescents have a strong personal interest in taking responsibility for decisions affecting their future, perhaps including their own medical treatment. Although most countries have legislation setting a relatively high age for achieving legal maturity,[78] many legal systems have a hotchpotch of laws which also allow teenagers legal capacity to undertake various activities before they reach legal adulthood.[79] Below such fixed ages, the traditional legal approach has been to assume that parents are the appropriate people to determine what happens to their children's bodies when receiving medical treatment. Now such an approach appears outmoded.

> "Important physical, cognitive and psychological developments take place during adolescence. Adolescence begins with the onset of puberty; from puberty to adulthood, the 'capacity to acquire and utilise knowledge reaches its peak efficiency'; and the capacity for formal operational thought is the forerunner to developing the capacity to make autonomous moral judgments. Obviously, these developments happen at different times and at different rates for different people. But it is not at all surprising to find adolescents making different moral judgments from those of their parents. It is part of growing up."[80]

In the UK, a ground-breaking decision of the House of Lords[81] in the early 1980s reflected the clear view that to ignore the decision-making capacities of adolescents under the age of 16 might be counterproductive, especially given the increase in sexual activity amongst young teenagers.[82]

Paradoxically, while most doctors sympathize with the need to adopt more liberal attitudes towards adolescents' own powers of consent, they are also aware that some adolescents are particularly ill-equipped to reach decisions that affect their long-term well-being. Rather than producing greater maturity, adolescence sometimes marks the onset of psychological ill health which hampers the ability of young patients to consider treatment options with any detachment. Doctors may turn to the courts for assistance if they consider that their young patient's refusal to undergo essential medical treatment is not only ill-considered but dangerous.

Adolescents' Right to Say Yes to Medical Treatment

Consent and Adolescents Under 16

Some legal systems give specific legal authority to adolescents to take responsibility for their own medical treatment long before they attain the legal age of majority.[83] The meaning of such provisions is clear enough; on attaining the required age, teenagers gain the legal right to consent on their own behalf to the treatment specified. However, what does the law say about the legal competence of teenagers below the specified age? The House of Lords in *Gillick v. West Norfolk and Wisbech Area Health Authority*[84] emphasized that English legislation does not preclude minors below the age of 16 from consenting to any medical advice or treatment. Lord Scarman made it clear that parents lose the right to veto any decision their children may make at the point at which: "The child achieves a sufficient understanding and intelligence to enable him or her to understand fully what is proposed. It will be a question of fact whether a child seeking advice has sufficient understanding of what is involved to give a consent valid in law."[85]

This approach to assessing capacity to consent to treatment apparently gives adolescents considerable freedom regarding their own medical treatment. Indeed, Lord Scarman's *Gillick* competence formula, to all intents and purposes, provides an excellent method whereby English doctors can identify those teenage patients who are sufficiently mature to reach responsible decisions for themselves. It allows a doctor to adopt a far more intelligent approach to the concept of capacity than one merely relying on age or even on the research evidence on children's cognitive growth. The test is a functional one – whether the minor has capacity to comprehend and therefore consent to the procedure depends on the gravity of what is proposed. Even so, the difficulty implicit in the test for assessing *Gillick* competence is its deceptive simplicity (Fortin, 2003). It fails to provide doctors with any clear guidelines over the circumstances in which they should accept that an

[77] See, inter alia: *Re F (mental patient: sterilization)* [1990] 2 AC 1, per Lord Goff at p. 72. There "is the fundamental principle, long established, that every person's body is inviolate"; *Sidaway v. Board of Governors of the Bethlem Royal Hospital and the Maudsley Hospital* [1985] AC 871, per Lord Scarman, at p. 882; *Re B (adult: refusal of medical treatment)* [2002] EWHC 429 (Fam) [2002] 2 All ER 449, per Dame Elizabeth Butler-Sloss, paras 94, 104.

[78] In common with most other European countries, the legal age of majority throughout the UK is 18.

[79] For example, English law allows teenagers to consent to medical treatment, to marry (with parental consent), smoke and leave full-time education at the age of 16. At 17 they may drive a car.

[80] *R (on the application of Begum) v. Head Teacher and Governors of Denbigh High School* [2006] UKHL 15, [2007] AC 100, per Baroness Hale, para 93.

[81] *Gillick v. West Norfolk and Wisbech Area Health Authority* [1986] AC 112. See discussion below.

[82] Statistics issued in 2005 indicated that the UK has the highest teenage birth rate in western Europe, twice as high as Germany, three times as high as France and six times as high as the Netherlands.

[83] For example, the English Family Law Reform Act 1969, section 8(1) provides "The consent of a minor who has attained the age of 16 years to any surgical, medical or dental treatment which, in the absence of consent, would constitute a trespass to his person, shall be as effective as it would be if he were of full age; and where a minor has by virtue of this section given an effective consent to any treatment it shall not be necessary to obtain any consent for it from his parent or guardian." See also the Age of Legal Capacity (Scotland) Act 1991, s 2(4).

[84] [1986] AC 112.

[85] [1986] AC 112, p. 189.

adolescent may consent to a particular procedure without involving his or her parents (Brazier & Bridge, 1996). Indeed, their Lordships only offered greater clarity over the provision of contraceptive advice and treatment – detail that was rapidly adopted by health service providers.[86] In other contexts, the *Gillick* competence formula indicates merely that if doctors are satisfied that the procedure is in an adolescent's best medical interests and that he or she can adequately understand all the issues involved, the doctor can proceed with treatment. Nevertheless, doctors also risk angering some parents if they go ahead with treatment without prior consultation.

Professional guidance provided by the British Medical Association (BMA) elaborates upon the *Gillick* formula and provides doctors with more practical advice on assessing children's competence in a medical context (BMA, 2001). It uses the test of competence first established by the courts for testing the legal competence of adult patients.[87] When tackling the difficult problem of assessing the competence of a young person in the context of his or her family, it warns doctors that young people can be strongly influenced by their parents over treatment options, and suggests that older children should be given opportunities to discuss their treatment without their parents being present (BMA, 2001). Such advice is useful; without it the uncertainty of the *Gillick* test might deter doctors from proceeding with any treatment for adolescents that is not trivial, unless they can involve their parents.

Influence of Human Rights Law on Adolescents' Right to Say Yes to Medical Treatment

International human rights law recognizes that an important aspect of an adult's right to self-determination includes the right to decide what should happen to his or her own body.[88] This growing emphasis on the value to adults of autonomy is bound to impact on our ideas about children's developing maturity. Perhaps for this reason, far greater attention is currently being given to the requirements of international instruments such as the UNCRC. Its provisions encourage adults to treat children as people in their own right, rather than adjuncts of their parents and families. In particular, article 12(1) requires states to give all children who are capable of forming their own views, the right to express them freely in all matters affecting them and the right to have their view given "due weight in accordance with the age and maturity of the child."

In the UK, because it has not been incorporated into domestic law, the UNCRC is of persuasive importance only. Nevertheless, a commitment to human rights has been made explicit by the entrenchment of a charter of human rights into domestic law.[89] The Human Rights Act 1998, superimposes on the principles of common law a further layer of legal requirements. Consequently, the principles of law established before the implementation of that legislation can be challenged if they fail to match up to the demands of the European Convention on Human Rights. In recent case law, the English courts have emphasized that the notions of teenage autonomy developed by the House of Lords in *Gillick* have been reinforced by the values underlying many Convention rights. Thus, the *Gillick* competent child has this added form of legal protection, both in the context of medical treatment and in other areas of life.[90]

Meanwhile, human rights legislation also carries a potential risk for the maturing adolescent. It offers an extra source of power to parents wishing to retain control over their offspring, by reference to their own rights under such instruments. An English mother recently claimed, albeit unsuccessfully, that the *Gillick* decision had now to be reinterpreted in the light of the Human Rights Act, 1998. She argued that article 8 of the European Convention on Human Rights gave her the right to be notified by any medical professional consulted by

[86] The so-called "Fraser guidelines," promulgated by Lord Fraser in *Gillick v. West Norfolk and Wisbech Area Health Authority* [1986] AC 112, at p. 174. He stated that a doctor could proceed to provide contraceptive advice and treatment provided he was satisfied on five matters: (1) that the girl (although under 16 years of age) will understand his advice; (2) that he cannot persuade her to inform her parents or allow him to inform the parents that she is seeking contraceptive advice; (3) that she is very likely to begin or to continue having sexual intercourse with or without contraceptive treatment; (4) that unless she receives contraceptive advice or treatment her physical or mental health or both are likely to suffer; (5) that her best interests require him to give her contraceptive advice, treatment or both without the parental consent. These guidelines have been adopted in a series of official guidance documents, the latest being Department of Health (2004).

[87] The capacity test established for adult patients by Thorpe J (as he then was) in *Re C (refusal of treatment)* [1994] 1 FLR 31, at p. 33. Adopted by Wall J in *Re C (detention: medical treatment)* [1997] 2 FLR 180, at p. 195, when considering whether to overrule the refusal of an anorexic teenager to accept treatment. The test itself was later refined by Butler-Sloss LJ, in *Re MB (medical treatment)* [1997] 2 FLR 426, at p. 437. It requires the patient to show an ability to comprehend and retain treatment information relevant to the decision, especially as to the likely consequences of having or not having the treatment in question, to use it, and to weigh it in the balance when arriving at a decision. See now the similar, but more expanded test of *in* capacity adopted by the Mental Capacity Act, 2005, s 3(1). The 2005 Act authorizes decision-making on behalf of incapable adults (and minors over the age of 16 with disabilities causing incapacity lasting into adulthood) in a variety of general contexts.

[88] Inter alia: *YF v. Turkey* (2004) 39 EHRR 34: the European Court of Human Rights stressed at para [33] that article 8 of the European Convention on Human Rights, which covers the physical and psychological integrity of a person, protects against compulsory medical intervention, even if that intervention is of minor importance. "A person's body concerns the most intimate aspect of one's private life"; *Storck v. Germany* (2006) 43 EHRR 6: the European Court of Human Rights held that an adult's rights to liberty under article 5 of the European Convention on Human Rights was infringed by her being detained in a psychiatric clinic against her will on her father's authorization alone, without a court order.

[89] The Human Rights Act 1998 was implemented in the UK on October 2, 2000. A charter of human rights was entrenched into Canadian law by the Canadian Charter of Rights and Freedoms, 1982.

[90] For example, *Re Roddy (a child) (identification: restriction on publication)* [2003] EWHC 2927 (Fam), [2004] 2 FLR 949.

her daughters under the age of 16.[91] The court rejected her arguments, emphasizing that the principles established by the House of Lords in *Gillick* had survived unscathed the implementation of the Human Rights Act. The mother's right to bring up her daughters free from state interference, as guaranteed by article 8, was not so extensive that it overrode her daughters' own need for medical privacy. This was an important affirmation of adolescent autonomy. Nonetheless, the challenge demonstrates the fact that there remains an uneasy boundary between parents' rights and children's rights, making further parental challenges a distinct possibility.

Right of the Adolescent to Say Yes to Medical Confidentiality

As Brazier points out, "Doctors, like priests and lawyers, must be able to keep secrets . . . Most people do not broadcast their medical problems from the rooftop" (Brazier, 2003). Doctors' legal obligation to maintain their adult patients' medical secrets can never be absolute;[92] nevertheless, its overriding importance has been reinforced by human rights law which maintains that patients' right to personal privacy[93] embraces the right to medical confidentiality.[94]

Are doctors legally obliged to respect the confidences of young patients in the same way? Doctors should not disclose the medical details of children too young to consent to their own treatment to anyone other than those with parental responsibility over them.[95] As in the case of adult patients, such confidentiality cannot be absolute. The doctor must be prepared to pass on medical information to assist a child protection investigation into alleged abusive practices. Official guidance clearly sets out the circumstances justifying their sharing such information with other agencies, in the public interest. It suggests that in some circumstances, "Sharing confidential information without consent will *normally* be justified in the public interest. These are: *when there is evidence* that the child is suffering or is at risk of suffering significant harm; or *where there is reasonable cause to believe* that a child may be suffering or at risk of significant harm; or *to prevent significant harm* arising to children and young people or *serious harm to adults*, including through the prevention, detection and prosecution of serious crime" (HM Government, 2006, para 3.12, emphasis as written).

In many ways, medical confidentiality is far more important to the teenager than to the younger child. Teenagers are not only becoming sexually active at increasingly young ages (Parliamentary Office of Science and Technology, 2004), but a growing body of research indicates that they are deterred from seeking medical advice and treatment over sexual matters, such as contraception and abortion, by fears about lack of confidentiality and privacy (French, Joyce, Fenton *et al.*, 2005; Save the Children, 2002; Social Exclusion Unit, 1999). A teenager legally competent to consent to medical treatment certainly has a right to medical confidentiality.[96] As with younger children, child protection concerns may override a doctor's obligations to respect teenage patients' confidences and, depending on the circumstances, he or she should consider passing on such information to the relevant child protection agencies, even if they disagree with his or her doing so (HM Government, 2006, para 3.12). However, such a situation is rare.

Teenagers' overriding fear is that their doctors will inform their parents of their medical consultations (Social Exclusion Unit, 1999, para 7.7). Health agencies are well aware that unless doctors can allay such fears, the rate of teenage pregnancy will continue to rise, with girls continuing their sexual activity unprotected by contraceptive measures (Department of Health, 2004). Nevertheless, some, like Mrs. Axon (see footnote 96), urge that caring parents should be informed of their teenagers' medical consultations. As noted above, the High Court recently confirmed the commonly held view that a teenager who is sufficiently competent to consent to a medical procedure (the *Gillick* competent teenager) is also legally entitled to medical confidentiality, whether it is contraceptive advice and treatment that are being sought, or abortion advice and treatment.[97]

There seems little legal basis for the official assumption that the *Gillick incompetent* teenager is also entitled to medical confidentiality.[98] The strict legal position is a controversial one; it assumes that because such young patients cannot legally consent to any treatment, they cannot claim the legal right to confidentiality either, and that if their doctors cannot persuade them to discuss matters with their parents, the doctors can themselves disclose any medical information to the parents (see discussion in Fortin, 2003). Nevertheless, because the younger, more immature teenager is unlikely to be deterred from sexual activity by her parents learning of her request for medical advice and treatment, it is undoubtedly sensible for the official guidance to encourage doctors to respect the confidentiality of all patients under the age of 16.

[91] *R (Axon) v. Secretary of State for Health and the Family Planning Association* [2006] EWHC 37 (Admin), [2006] 2 FLR 206.

[92] There are rare circumstances where disclosure may be justified "in the public interest," for example, where failure to disclose appropriate information would expose the patient or someone else to risk of death or serious harm. The principle of disclosure "in the public interest" has its roots in the decision of Scott J, in *W v. Egdell* [1990] Ch. 359.

[93] Under article 8 of the European Convention on Human Rights.

[94] See *Z v. Finland* (1997) 25 EHRR 371, para 95 and *Campbell v. MGN Ltd* [2004] UKHL 22, [2004] 2 AC 457, especially Baroness Hale, paras 144, 145.

[95] For example, *Re C (A Minor) (Wardship: Medical Treatment) (No 2)* [1990] Fam 39.

[96] *R (Axon) v. Secretary of State for Health and the Family Planning Association* [2006] EWHC 37 (Admin), [2006] 2 FLR 206, at [91].

[97] Ibid, at para 91.

[98] In England, successive documents issued by the Department of Health have stressed that doctors who are unable to persuade teenagers under 16 to involve their parents in any treatment decisions involving contraception, sexually transmitted infections or abortion, must always maintain strict medical confidentiality (Department of Health, 2004).

Adolescents' Right to Say No to Medical Treatment

The fact that adolescents commonly experience mood swings ranging from intense exhilaration to extreme depression is probably at least in part attributable to the fact that their brains are still undergoing profound physical changes, combined with hormonal development (Cyronowski, Frank, Young *et al.*, 2000; Juvenile Justice Center, 2004; Maughan & Kim-Cohen, 2005). These developmental considerations are reviewed in chapter 13. During the teenage years, the frequency of many psychosocial disorders increases (Green, McGinnity, Meltzer *et al.*, 2005). Indeed, there seems to be a consensus that the overall prevalence rate for child and adolescent mental health problems has been rising in nearly all developed countries (Collishaw, Maughan, Goodman *et al.*, 2004). Although children of all ages clearly have a right to the "highest attainable standard of health,"[99] severe eating disorders, suicide attempts and deliberate self-harm,[100] aggression and violence obviously need urgent treatment and may even endanger others if left untreated.

What then should a medical team do if, for example, a teenager rejects life-saving treatment? The principles established by the House of Lords in *Gillick v. West Norfolk and Wisbech Area Health Authority*[101] suggest that an intelligent teenager has the legal right to determine his or her own destiny. Nevertheless, in England and Wales, doctors have obtained judicial authority to side-step such refusal. The judiciary have found it difficult to stand aside and allow teenage patients to risk death by refusing essential treatment. The Court of Appeal considered two applications, both involving adolescents with serious psychological problems.[102] It held that under its inherent jurisdiction (see p. 98), a court can override a young patient's wishes and authorize life-saving treatment[103] in his or her best interests.[104] Such a judicial response is not surprising, given that a court may find it impossible to reach the conclusion that it is in the child's best interests to be allowed to die.[105] Although this approach is not unique (Ferguson, 2004), it makes a substantial inroad into the principle of adolescent responsibility (Douglas, 1992), albeit after a legal proceeding in which the child's voice will be heard.[106] Even more controversially, the view was also expressed that *anyone* with parental responsibility for a teenage patient,[107] even if *Gillick* competent, could provide doctors with the legal authority to carry out much needed treatment, despite the teenager's own clear opposition.[108]

Such an approach is problematic. In the first place, it is doubtful that the House of Lords in *Gillick* intended to produce such an outcome. Lord Scarman's words certainly suggest that when a child attains *Gillick* competence, the parents' right to determine questions about their child's medical treatment terminates and that thereafter they cannot veto *or* override his or her wishes on such matters.[109] Nevertheless, this approach may make good sense to a doctor attempting to treat a severely ill, but uncooperative teenager. After all, because doctors only recommend treatment that is in a patient's best interests, the teenager is far more likely to risk death (or serious harm) by refusing treatment than by accepting it. To the child, however, it has produced a situation that appears illogical and which is certainly confusing. It allows a *Gillick* competent teenager to consent to medical treatment, while withholding from the teenager's parents the right to veto their son's or daughter's decision; but it also allows the parents to override that same teenager's refusal to accept such treatment. In some cases, of course, doctors will obtain no assistance from parents whose strong religious views dictate their own opposition to the treatment their child is refusing. Then doctors have no option but to seek judicial authority to go ahead with treatment against the young patient's wishes. In the past, the English courts have responded to such applications by introducing stringent requirements into assessments of young patients' legal competence. Thus, young Jehovah's Witness patients have been defined as lacking sufficient competence to reach decisions over their treatment because they do not understand the manner of their impending death, together with the pain and distress accompanying it.[110] Using this approach, a court can provide the doctors with legal authority for the treatment planned, despite there being far less stringent requirements adopted when assessing an adult

[99] UNCRC, article 24 (1).

[100] The research summarized in Mind (2005) and BMA (2006) suggests that these conditions are increasing.

[101] [1986] AC 112.

[102] *Re R (a minor) (wardship: consent to treatment)* [1992] Fam 11: the Court of Appeal authorized the compulsory use of antipsychotic drugs to treat a 15-year-old suffering from increasingly paranoid and disturbed behaviour; *Re W (a minor) (medical treatment: court's jurisdiction)* [1993] Fam 64: the Court of Appeal authorized the compulsory treatment of a 16-year-old in a dangerously anorexic state.

[103] *Re R (a minor) (wardship: consent to treatment)* [1992] Fam 11, per Lord Donaldson of Lymington MR, at p. 24.

[104] The "best interests" formula is used when the courts exercise their inherent jurisdiction in relation to children.

[105] See *Re E (a minor) (wardship: medical treatment)* [1993] 1 FLR 386, at p. 394. Per Ward J: A court "should be very slow to allow an infant to martyr himself."

[106] In complex medical cases, the child is normally represented by CAFCASS Legal.

[107] Each parent, if married and, if unmarried, the mother, plus the unmarried father, provided he has parental responsibility (see p. 100).

[108] *Re R (a minor) (wardship: consent to treatment)* [1992] Fam 11 and *Re W (a minor) (medical treatment: court's jurisdiction)* [1993] Fam 64.

[109] "As a matter of law the parental right to determine whether or not their minor child below the age of 16 will have medical treatment terminates if and when the child achieves a sufficient understanding and intelligence to enable him or her to understand fully what is proposed." Per Lord Scarman in *Gillick v. West Norfolk and Wisbech Area Health Authority* [1986] AC 112, at pp. 188–189.

[110] For example, *Re E (a minor)(wardship: medical treatment)* [1993] 1 FLR 386; *Re L (Medical treatment: Gillick competency)* [1998] 2 FLR 810; *Re S (a minor)(consent to medical treatment)* [1994] 2 FLR 1065 (McCafferty, 1999).

patient's competence to refuse treatment.[111] As critics point out, although few adults can comprehend the process of dying, the pain they would suffer, the fear they would undergo and relatives' distress in watching them die, neither doctors nor the courts are entitled to overrule their refusal to undergo treatment for similar reasons (Huxtable, 2000).

The present law is also controversial in other respects. In particular, the courts have sometimes found themselves on a slope too slippery to resist when appealed to by doctors keen to provide much-needed treatment. Thus, while it may be morally justifiable to override the wishes of a teenager to prevent his or her "death or severe permanent injury,"[112] cases where failure to treat will not produce such dire consequences are more problematic.[113] Critics also object to the way in which the minor status of the uncooperative patient is allowed to dictate the outcome of a dispute over treatment, with the patient's legal competence being treated as irrelevant.[114] They see this as an arbitrary and status-driven form of decision-making (Ferguson, 2004; Huxtable, 2000). There is the additional objection that court orders cannot obviate the use of physical force – this may be unavoidable in cases involving the treatment of an uncooperative but fully grown teenager.[115] Doctors may themselves object to overpowering physically mature patients, whatever their age. Thus, there are some who, even before the Human Rights Act 1998 dictated a greater concern with individual autonomy, were suggesting that enforced survival to adulthood might not be in every child's best interests (Bridge, 1999; Lewis, 2001).

Use of the Mental Health Legislation to Force Treatment on Adolescents Who Wish to Say No to Medical Treatment

It appears that in England attitudes to the use of the mental health legislation are beginning to change and that, particularly when treating eating disorders in older children, doctors are much more prepared to envisage its use.[116] Nevertheless, in general, those caring for mentally ill or behaviorally disturbed young people have often been reluctant to use the mental health legislation to enforce their detention and treatment (BMA, 2001). The most common objection, often accepted by the English judiciary,[117] is the perceived stigma attached to the use of compulsory powers. An individual may find it disadvantageous when older for it to become known that he or she has been treated under the mental health legislation during adolescence. Furthermore, those wishing to ensure that adolescents obtain the treatment they need have been able to turn to other methods. In the absence of parental consent, doctors have been able to turn to the courts to obtain judicial authorization for compulsory admission and treatment. This might appear preferable, because a court order may be of some comfort to doctors faced with a complex case and the child normally obtains some form of independent representation.[118] Nevertheless, a seriously ill adolescent facing compulsory admission and treatment might prefer being admitted to hospital under the mental health legislation, rather than under the parental responsibility of his or her parents or the courts. This legislation applies to all patients requiring compulsory treatment for mental disorders, irrespective of their age. It recognizes that removing an individual's liberty in order to treat them on a compulsory basis is a drastic step and it contains a set of strict legislative safeguards that apply to all mental health patients. Patients are legally protected from arbitrary restrictions on their liberty and unsupervised treatment regimes (Jones, 2005). These legal safeguards are designed to compensate for the fact that a patient's competence to consent to or refuse treatment cannot prevent treatment taking place.

Planned reform of the mental health legislation in England[119] has provoked a reassessment of the way in which teenagers with mental health problems should be dealt with under current law and practice. Perhaps prompted by a greater judicial

[111] For example, *Re C (refusal of medical treatment)* [1994] 1 FLR 31: the court respected the right of an adult paranoid schizophrenic to refuse an amputation of his leg to cure potentially fatal gangrene. There was no indication that he fully realized the implications which lay before him as to the process of dying.

[112] This was the justification provided by Balcombe LJ, in *Re W (a minor) (medical treatment: courts' jurisdiction)* [1993] Fam 64, at p. 88.

[113] For example, *Re K, W and H (minors) (medical treatment)* [1993] 1 FLR 854: a psychiatric treatment unit obtained legal authority for the use of "emergency medication" when treating three mentally disturbed teenagers; *South Glamorgan County Council v. W and B* [1993] 1 FLR 574: a local authority obtained judicial authority for the forcible removal of a disturbed 15-year-old from home and her transfer to a specialized psychiatric unit for assessment and treatment.

[114] For example, *Re M (medical treatment: consent)* [1999] 2 FLR 1097. See also *Re C (detention: medical treatment)* [1997] 2 FLR 180: Wall J indicated that he would override the anorexic girl's refusal to accept treatment irrespective of her capacity to consent on her own behalf to medical treatment.

[115] In *Re S (a minor)(consent to medical treatment)* [1994] 2 FLR 1065, at p. 1074 Johnson J acknowledged that the possible use of force was "extremely distasteful."

[116] It has now become far more commonplace for psychiatrists to use the mental health legislation as a means of treating anorexia nervosa and other eating disorders. See BMA 2001: 144. The law supports this approach. See *Riverside Mental Health NHS Trust v. Fox* [1994] 1 FLR 614, where the Court of Appeal was satisfied that anorexia nervosa was a mental disorder under the Mental Health Act, 1983, s 63 and that force-feeding an adult sufferer was a form of medical treatment for such a disorder; per Sir Stephen Brown P, at p. 619.

[117] For example, *Re W (a minor) (medical treatment: court's jurisdiction)* [1993] Fam 64, per Lord Donaldson, at p. 83. See also *Re K, W and H (minors) (medical treatment)* [1993] 1 FLR 854, per Thorpe J, at p. 857.

[118] When the inherent jurisdiction is invoked, the child is normally represented by the Children and Family Court Advisory Support Service (CAFCASS) Legal.

[119] The patient safeguards contained in the current mental health legislation are to be strengthened by amendments to the 1983 Mental Health Act. See draft Mental Health Bill 2006 and *Mental Health Bill Draft Illustrative Code of Practice* (2006) Department of Health. Please note that the text represents the law at the point of printing which was prior to the passage of the Mental Health Act 2007.

willingness to respect teenage autonomy in other contexts,[120] the government considers that medical practitioners should respect the right of competent teenagers to determine their own affairs. Detailed guidance will advise doctors to respect the wishes of *Gillick* competent teenagers, whatever their age. Doctors confronted by *competent* teenagers resisting treatment will be warned against relying on parental consent as a means of obtaining legal authority for such treatment.[121] They will be advised that unless a *Gillick* competent teenager freely consents to the treatment, detaining a child in order to administer treatment may amount to a deprivation of his or her liberty[122] and compulsion should only be attempted by using the mental health legislation, as in the case of adult patients.[123]

Official thought is less coherent regarding the way ahead for the doctor contemplating the compulsory treatment of a teenager under the age of 16 who is not *Gillick* competent. The government argues that the doctor can still rely on the case law suggesting that a teenager's resistance to treatment can be side-stepped by obtaining legal authority from his or her parents,[124] and can therefore treat the teenager as an informal patient.[125] Admittedly, doctors are to be warned about the possible limitations on parents' powers to consent on behalf of their teenage offspring.[126] Nevertheless, this regime will leave the parents of non-*Gillick* competent teenagers under the age of 16 with considerable power over decisions regarding unwanted treatment. It seems arbitrary to conclude that it is only when a non-*Gillick* competent teenager attains the age of 16 that his or her compulsory treatment acquires the need for outside scrutiny.[127] Given the new demands of the Human Rights Act 1998, the case law on which such advice rests is by no means certain to survive scrutiny in a higher court. Furthermore, if introduced as planned, the new regime will be extremely complex and produce considerable uncertainty.[128]

Whatever form the new mental health legislation eventually takes in England, doctors should reflect on the wisdom of turning to parents for legal authority to treat against the wishes of their teenage son or daughter, given how difficult parents will find it to be objective over the need for compulsory treatment. At present, a doctor's reluctance to use the mental health regime automatically results in children losing all the important safeguards deemed so essential for adult patients. On the other hand, if the new laws lead doctors to use the mental health regime for the treatment of all those over 16 and for many under that age, they risk greater numbers of young people being compulsorily detained than ever before, perhaps for relatively trivial conduct disorders. This would depend upon the breadth of the new grounds for compulsory admission, which has proved one of the most controversial areas in the government's proposals.

Influence of Human Rights Law on Adolescents' Right to Say No to Medical Treatment

When teenagers refuse much-needed or live-saving medical treatment, it is difficult for their doctors to stand aside and allow them to take the consequences. Nevertheless, a court order overriding a teenager's rejection of treatment has obvious implications for his or her physical dignity and self-respect. Court orders cannot obviate the need for physical force in some cases. However, as Gostin says, "Nothing degrades a human being more than to have intrusive treatment thrust upon him despite his full understanding of its nature and purpose and his clear will to say 'no' "(Gostin, 1992). The human rights dimension of such a dilemma is obvious. Child patients, like adults, have a right to freedom from arbitrary deprivation of liberty[129] and to protection from all forms of physical violence.[130] Meanwhile, there are many who would deplore allowing teenagers to reach decisions that might undermine their long-term health and happiness, preferring to adopt a paternalistic stance, at least during their minority (Fortin, 2006).

To date there is no English case law indicating that teenagers resisting medical treatment will succeed if they appeal to the courts arguing that the European Convention on Human Rights protects them from such an invasion of their rights. There appears to be no Strasbourg case law that would directly support such arguments[131] and challenges of this kind have been met with varying success in Canada (Ferguson, 2004). Today, an English teenager objecting to having his or her wishes

[120] For example, *R (Axon) v. Secretary of State for Health and the Family Planning Association* [2006] EWHC 37 (Admin), [2006] 2 FLR 206.

[121] Mental Health Bill Information Sheet, Children and Young People (2006) and Mental Health Bill Draft Illustrative Code of Practice (2006), Department of Health, paras 31.9 and 31.16–31.18.

[122] Under Article 5 of the European Convention on Human Rights, see below.

[123] FN121, para 31.18.

[124] See above, e.g., *Re W (a minor) (medical treatment: court's jurisdiction)* [1993] Fam 64.

[125] Thereby obviating the need to comply with the requirements of the mental health legislation when treating patients against their wishes.

[126] The draft Code of Guidance warns practitioners that parents can only authorize treatment against a teenager's wishes, if it is within the "zone of [their] parental responsibility" to do so and gives examples of the scope of this 'zone'. FN121, para 31.21 and 31.28–31.31.

[127] His treatment must then comply with the mental health legislation. FN121, para 31.26.

[128] The draft Code of Practice provides 12 pp. of guidance plus two flow charts explaining the decision-making regime governing teenagers under 18. FN121, pp. 152–164.

[129] UNCRC, article 37(b); European Convention on Human Rights, article 5.

[130] UNCRC 19(a); European Convention on Human Rights, articles 3 and 8, respectively, protect individuals of any age against inhuman and degrading treatment and against infringements of physical integrity.

[131] The decision in *Nielsen v. Denmark* (1988) 11 EHRR 175 undermines such arguments. The European Court of Human Rights controversially decided that because it was within the mother's own rights as a parent, under Article 8 of the European Convention on Human Rights, to decide her 12-year-old son's medical treatment, his rights under Article 5 of the Convention had not been infringed by his being kept against his will in a closed psychiatric ward for 5.5 months.

ignored might claim the protection of articles 3, 5, 8 and 14[132] of the European Convention on Human Rights. A more detailed assessment of the Strasbourg case law relating to adult claims[133] which might be relevant to adolescent patients should be sought elsewhere (Fortin, 2006), while Hale provides an assessment of the potential impact of the Human Rights Act 1998 on mental health law generally (Hale, 2005b). Generally speaking, the European Court takes the view that treatment that is a "medical necessity" is neither inhuman nor degrading under article 3 nor an unjustified interference with physical and mental integrity under article 8. However, an informal admission to hospital may amount to a deprivation of liberty for the purpose of article 5, in which safeguards against its arbitrary use would be required.

Conclusions

Most mental health practitioners will never need to refer to the principles reviewed above. They would certainly be wise to clarify their legal position over a proposed course of action; nevertheless, specialized treatment is often provided in circumstances that produce few concerns about the legality of the course taken. Even when disputes or challenges do arise, the legal principles governing them may provide little real assistance. The law is often too blunt an instrument to take full account of practitioners' real concerns (Kennedy, 2001; King & King, 2006). Furthermore, recourse to the law may polarize positions, making it difficult for either "side" to work purposefully together in the future, even for the sake of a young patient who requires treatment. Despite these shortcomings, the legal principles governing this area of medical practice do at least encourage practitioners to keep a young patient's interests center stage, without losing them under a welter of adult perspectives.

Further Reading

Bainham, A. (2005). *Children, the modern law*. Bristol. Family Law.

Brazier, M. (2003). *Medicine, patients and the law* (chapter 14). London: Penguin Books.

Fortin, J. (2003). *Children's rights and the developing law* (chapter 5). London: Lexis Nexis Butterworths.

General Medical Council (2007). *0–18 years: guidance for all doctors*, London: General Medical Council.

Standley, K. (2006). *Family law* (chapter 15). Basingstoke: Palgrave Macmillan.

References

BMA. (2001). *Consent, rights and choices in health care for children and young people*. London: BMJ Books.

BMA. (2006). *Child and adolescent mental health: A guide for healthcare professionals*. London: BMA Board of Science, British Medical Association.

Brazier, M. (2003). *Medicine, patients and the law*. London: Penguin Books.

Brazier, M., & Bridge, C. (1996). Coercion or caring: analysing adolescent autonomy. *Legal Studies*, *16*, 84–109.

Bridge, C. (1999). Religious beliefs and teenage refusal of medical treatment. *Modern Law Review*, *62*, 585–594.

Butler-Sloss, L. J. (Chairman). (1988). *Report of the Inquiry into Child Abuse in Cleveland 1987*, Cm 412. London: HMSO.

Butler-Sloss, E. (President of the Family Division). (2003). *Are we failing the family? Human rights, children and the meaning of family in the twenty-first century. Paul Sieghart Memorial Lecture* (unpublished).

Collishaw, S., Maughan, B., Goodman, R., & Pickles, A. (2004). Time trends in adolescent mental health. *Journal of Child Psychology and Psychiatry*, *45*, 1350–1362.

Commission on Families and the Wellbeing of Children (Chairman, Sir Michael Rutter). (2005). *Families and the state: Two-way support and responsibilities*. Bristol: Policy Press.

Cyronowski, J. M., Frank, E., Young, E., & Shear, M. K. (2000). Adolescent onset of the gender difference in lifetime rates of major depression. *Archives of General Psychiatry*, *57*, 21–27.

Department for Education and Skills. (2001). *Special educational needs code of practice*. DfES/581/2001. London: DfES.

Department of Health. (2004). *Best practice guidance for doctors and other health professionals on the provision of advice and treatment to young people under sixteen on contraception, sexual and reproductive health*, 2004/0290. London: Department of Health.

Dingwall, R., Eekelaar, J., & Murray, T. (1983). *The protection of children: State intervention and family life*. Oxford: Blackwell.

DHSS. (1985). *Review of child care law: Report to ministers of an interdepartmental Working Party*. London: HMSO.

Douglas, G. (1992). The retreat from Gillick. *Modern Law Review*, *55*, 569–576.

Ferguson, L. (2004). *The end of an age: Beyond age restrictions for minors' medical treatment decisions*. Ottawa: Law Commission of Canada.

Fortin, J. (2003). *Children's rights and the developing law*. London: Lexis Nexis Butterworths.

Fortin, J. (2006). Accommodating children's rights in a post Human Rights Act era. *Modern Law Review*, *69*, 299–326.

French, R. S., Joyce, L., Fenton, K., Kingori, P., Griffiths, C., Stone, V., *et al.* (2005). *Exploring the attitudes and behaviour of Bangladeshi, Indian and Jamaican young people in relation to reproductive and sexual health*. A Report for the Teenage Pregnancy Unit. London: UCL/BMRB.

Gil-Robles, A. (2005). *Report by Mr Alvaro Gil-Robles, Commissioner for Human Rights, on his visit to the United Kingdom 4th–12th November 2004*, Comm DH (2005) 6, Strasbourg, Council of Europe.

Gostin, L. (1992). Consent to treatment: The incapable person. In C. Dyer (Ed.), *Doctors, patients and the law*. Oxford: Blackwell Scientific Publications.

Green, H., McGinnity, A., Meltzer, H., Ford, T., & Goodman, R. (2005). *Mental health of children and young people in Great Britain, 2004*. Basingstoke: Palgrave Macmillan.

Hale, B. (2005a). Understanding children's rights: theory and practice. *Childright*, *216*, 3–8.

Hale, B. (2005b). 'What can the Human Rights Act 1998 do for my mental health?' *Child and Family Law Quarterly*, *17*, 295.

Harrington, R., & Bailey, S. with Chitsabesan, P., Kroll, L., Macdonald, W., Sneider, S., Kenning, C., Taylor, G., *et al.* (2005). *Mental health needs and effectiveness of provision for young offenders in custody and in the community*. Retrieved September 18, 2006, from htpp://www.youth-justice-board.gov.uk.

[132] Article 3 – freedom from torture or inhuman or degrading treatment or punishment; Article 5 – the right to liberty and security of person; Article 8 – the right to respect for private and family life; Article 14 – freedom from discrimination.

[133] For example, *Storck v. Germany* (2006) 43 EHRR 6 (see footnote 88).

HM Government. (2006). *Information sharing: Practitioner's guide, Integrated working to improve outcomes for children and young people.* London: DfES.

Home Office. (1965). *The child, the family and the young offender*, Cm 2742. London: HMSO.

Home Office. (1968). *Children in trouble*, Cm 3601. London: HMSO.

Home Office. (1998). *No more excuses: A new approach to tackling youth crime in England and Wales*, Cm 3809. London: HMSO.

Huxtable, R. (2000). *Re M (medical treatment: consent):* Time to remove the flack jacket? *Child and Family Law Quarterly, 12*, 83–88.

Jones, R. (2005). *Mental health act manual.* London: Sweet and Blackwell.

Juvenile Justice Center. (2004). *Adolescence, brain development and legal culpability.* American Bar Association. Retrieved September 17, 2006, from htpp://www.abanet.org/crimjust/juvjus.

Juvenile Justice Center. (2004). *Adolescence, Brain Development and Legal Culpability.* Washington: American Bar Association.

Kennedy, R. (2001). Assessment and treatment in family law: A valid distinction? *Family Law, 31*, 676–681.

King, M., & King, D. (2006). How the law defines the special educational needs of autistic children. *Child and Family Law Quarterly, 18*, 23–42.

Kroll, L., Rothwell, J., Bradley, D., Shah, P., Bailey, S., & Harrington, R. C. (2002). Mental health needs of boys in secure care for serious or persistent offending: a prospective, longitudinal study. *The Lancet, 359*, 1975–1979.

Laming, H. (2003). *The Victoria Climbié Inquiry: Report on an Inquiry by Lord Laming*, Cm 5730. London: HMSO.

Lewis, P. (2001). The Medical Treatment of Children. In J. Fionda (Ed.), *Legal concepts of childhood.* Oxford: Hart Publishing.

Maughan, B., & Kim-Cohen, J. (2005). Continuities between childhood and adult life. *British Journal of Psychiatry, 187*, 301–303.

McCafferty, C. (1999). Won't consent? Can't consent! Refusal of medical treatment. *Family Law, 29*, 335–336.

McDiarmid, C. (2005). Welfare, offending and the Scottish Children's Hearing System. *Journal of Social Welfare and Family Law, 27*, 31–42.

Mind. (2005). *Children and young people and mental health.* Retrieved September 17, 2006, from htpp://www.mind.org.uk.

NACRO. (2003). *A failure of justice: Reducing child imprisonment.* London: Nacro.

Parliamentary Office of Science and Technology. (2004). Teenage sexual health. *Postnote, 217*, 1–4. Retrieved September 17, 2006, from htpp://www.parliament.uk/post/home/htm.

Parsloe, P. (1978). *Juvenile justice in Britain and the United States: The balance of needs and rights.* London: Routledge and Kegan Paul.

Royal College of Psychiatrists. (2006). *Child defendants.* Occasional Paper OP56. London: Royal College of Psychiatrists.

Save the Children. (2002). *Get real: Providing dedicated sexual health services for young people.* London: Save the Children UK.

Scottish Law Commission. (2001). *Discussion paper on age of criminal responsibility.* Discussion Paper 115. Edinburgh: Stationery Office.

Social Exclusion Unit. (1999). *Teenage pregnancy*, Cm 4342. Retrieved September 17, 2006, from http://www.socialexclusionunit.gov.uk/page.asp?id=227.

Thorpe, M., & Clarke, E. (Eds.). (1998). *Divided duties: Care planing for children within the family justice system.* Bristol: Family Law.

UN Committee on the Rights of the Child. (2002). *Concluding observations of the Committee on the Rights of the Child: United Kingdom of Great Britain and Northern Ireland*, CRC/C/15/Add 188 2002. Geneva: Centre for Human Rights.

Warnock, H. M. (Chairman). (1978). *Special educational needs, report of the Committee of Enquiry into the Education of Handicapped Children and Young People*, Cmnd 7212. London: HMSO.

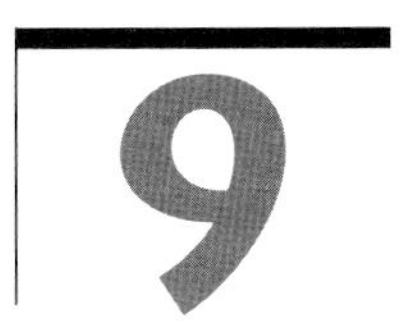

What Clinicians Need to Know about Statistical Issues and Methods

Andrew Pickles

Although as an academic discipline statistics is often associated with mathematics, from its beginnings it has also had strong links to science. Most appreciate the link as an area of application of statistics. Less well appreciated is that science has motivated methodological development in statistics. Indeed, one could argue that the whole rationale for the use of statistics is as an objective and efficient operationalization of the scientific method in a context of complex data, and in practice almost any study yields complex data. Statistical methods should achieve this in several ways. First, by requiring precise operational definitions of theories and critical differences or contrasts. Second, by providing methodology for estimating scientifically meaningful quantities as precisely as possible and freed from as many sources of bias as possible. Third, by providing a framework for determining whether data are consistent or inconsistent with a particular theory.

Some introductory statistics classes and books give the impression that statistics is much concerned with making assumptions; assumptions that appear abstract, derived from probability theory, with little meaning and anyway probably rarely met in practice. This is unfortunate, because in the great majority of cases the assumptions correspond to critical scientific simplifications of a kind that most scientists and clinicians could easily comprehend and would have considerable intuitive insight into whether they are likely to be met or not. Moreover, it is crucial for the quality of the science that it be understood that such assumptions are being made.

As an example, consider the very commonly made assumption of independence among observations. In scientific terms, this requires that no observation influence another, that sets of observations are not subject to the effects of some shared factor not explicitly accounted for in the analysis and that the sampling of one subject has not influenced the probability that another subject be sampled. Thus, this assumption would not be an appropriate one where sibships of children had been selected, instead of individual children, or where some children were picked and then their friends. In such circumstances, progress might be possible where such clusters of observations were independent. As a second example, consider the homoscedasticity or homogeneity of variance assumption required for the simple difference of means *t*-test. In scientific terms this requires that within each of the groups that are the focus of study, there is no greater variability in one group than another. Great care is often spent in collecting a carefully selected and fully characterized "case" group, whereas the "control" group is often just a group who are "not cases," drawn from the general population or a "convenience sample" – sometimes just a collection of individuals from other studies or even individuals rejected from other studies. It is therefore unsurprising that control groups are often more variable than case groups. In other circumstances, cases may be defined as the most severe in a distribution of severity, with controls drawn from the mean. Here, particularly with a distribution long-tailed at the abnormal end, the cases may be more variable than the controls (Roach, Edwards, & Hogben, 2004). Any homogeneity of variance assumption would be inappropriate.

Rutter's Child and Adolescent Psychiatry, 5th edition. Edited by M. Rutter, D. Bishop, D. Pine, S. Scott, J. Stevenson, E. Taylor and A. Thapar. © 2008 Blackwell Publishing, ISBN: 978-1-4051-4549-7.

What are we Trying to Do: Hypothesis Testing or Estimating Effects?

Child psychiatry has been strongly influenced by the practice of psychology of placing great emphasis on hypothesis testing. This approach focuses on assessing the evidence in a data set against some null hypothesis; for example, the hypothesis that "This treatment or putative risk factor has no effect." Commonly, the evidence is presented in the form of a *P* value for some measure of effect, the probability that we might have obtained an effect as large or larger than that obtained from our observed data as the result of the chance sampling of participants and events. Non-psychiatric epidemiology and the main body of medical statistics has moved away from this focus to emphasize instead the careful estimation of effects and their presentation together with a confidence interval. The confidence interval characterizes the uncertainty we have in the estimate obtained from our data, which may be high or low as the result of chance sampling of participants and events. This approach has a range of advantages, some of which we elaborate in the following sections. For now, note two advantages. First, it avoids the distinction between descriptive and theory testing studies being drawn on the basis of the statistics used. Some studies are more descriptive than others, but that relates more to the prominence and use of theory in the choice of data to present and its manipulation. Second, the hypothesis test rejects a hypothesis based on the evidence of the study being reported in isolation. Such a perspective no longer fits the industrial scale of modern research where few individual studies are thought to be individually potentially decisive. Instead, studies are seen as contributing, and hopefully through some future systematic review/overview/meta-analysis, to a pool of effect estimates that will be used as the basis for some more robust and confidently held conclusion. As a consequence, while having a large study is desirable, more important is that the study is undertaken to a sufficiently high standard that it will pass the quality criteria for eligibility for inclusion in an overview.

Common Misunderstandings, Study Design and the Natural History of "Findings"

Nonetheless, it remains a weakness of readers and editors that they are drawn to reports of significant associations and effects rather than reports of non-significant effects. As a consequence, the P value remains the statistic upon which the success or failure of a study is often seen to rest. That this is the case is a major flaw. The size of the group difference or other parameter that is estimated that measures the contrast or effect of interest is the key statistic, together with some measure of the precision with which this has been estimated, preferably a confidence interval. The confidence interval gives the reader the opportunity to reflect upon the range of possible values that might be considered as potentially consistent with the data and assess whether effects of this magnitude would be, say, of clinical importance. This last emphasizes the importance of measuring the effect of interest in units that are as meaningful as possible – indeed, more than one form may be useful. For example, treatment effects are often reported in terms of both reductions in risk and the number needed to treat in order to cure or avoid one case/death (equal to 1 over the absolute risk reduction). In other circumstances, reporting in a form to allow comparison can be important. For outcomes on a continuous scale, a commonly used effect scale for group comparisons is Cohen's d, defined as the difference between two means divided by the pooled standard deviation for those means. Cohen (1992) suggests a value of d of 0.2 is indicative of a small effect, 0.5 a medium and 0.8 a large effect.

Study size also needs to be considered in relation to assessing whether significant effects are likely to be important. Those who undertake small studies often think that if they find something significant then it must be a substantial effect because it was significant even in a small study. The more skeptical point of view starts from expecting most of the targets of interest, notably treatments, to have no effect. At the traditional $P = 0.05$ level of significance, both small and large studies have a 1 in 20 chance of finding something as appearing to have a significant effect that in fact has no effect. However, in the small study the magnitude of the estimated effect will necessarily have to be large for it to appear as significant. What happens when we consider the case of assessing a number of possible factors, only one of which in fact has a true effect? Then, although both large and small studies have the same chance of falsely identifying one of the no-effect factors as significant, the larger study has greater power to detect the effects of the one factor with a true effect – it has more chance of finding the true-effect factor as significant. Thus, of the effects found to be significant, a higher proportion of those from a small study will be false and of an exaggerated size compared to the proportion from a large study. Funnel plots (Light & Pillemer, 1984) can display this graphically. Figure 9.1 shows data from a set of acupuncture studies. It illustrates the diminution of effect size reported as the sample size increases, to the point where the largest study shows no effect. If the true effect was zero, then we would expect a collection of smaller studies to give estimates scattered symmetrically either side of zero. Fig. 9.1 has a near complete absence of study points on the left-hand side, a pattern that suggests the effects of considerable publication bias – the selective submission and acceptance of reports indicating a positive effect.

Indeed, there is a common natural history for many "findings" from small studies (Ioannidis, 2005). First, a small study finds a significant association and persuades an editor of its interest value. Much note is taken and it receives many citations. Then many small studies fail to replicate the finding, but because everyone knows that small studies have low power this comes as no surprise and, as we have seen, most do not see the light of day. By chance alone, some studies do find a positive effect and are published as apparently replicating the interesting finding. Eventually, perhaps a decade later although the timescale is shortening, the finding is tested out in a large and often more rigorous study, fails to replicate and, because the size of the study demands it be published

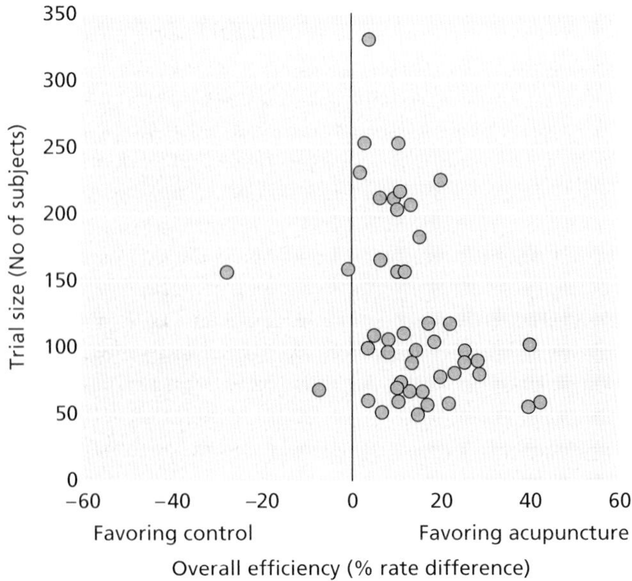

Fig. 9.1 From Tang, Zhan, and Ernst (1999).

whatever its conclusion or because this failure is now seen as overturning a received wisdom, the results are published in a prominent journal. Patients then need to be persuaded that something formerly considered effective is now considered ineffective.

In fact, sample size and publication bias are not the only reasons for this "natural history." Although there are critical exceptions, because large projects cost more and are commonly staffed by more experienced researchers, they tend to be superior on a whole range of methodological measures of quality, such as being prospective rather than retrospective, randomized rather than observational, having blind assessments, and being better analyzed and reported. Each of these factors tends to exclude possible biases that can contribute to artifact, and indeed reported effect size does seem to decline as the methodological rigor of the study increases (Schulz, Chalmers, Hayes *et al.*, 1995). More recently, some apparently robust findings from epidemiology have been tested out in randomized trials, considered by most as the ultimate test of causal effect. Results from several high-profile treatments have been not just disappointing but, in the case of hormone replacement therapy (HRT), really most worrying. The major epidemiological studies (Stampfer & Colditz, 1991) suggested beneficial effects of HRT (for cancer and coronary heart disease) but the trial findings suggested it was dangerous (Hulley, Grady, Bush *et al.*, 1998). One explanation relates to the longer treatment examined by the epidemiological studies, and would emphasize the complementary contributions of epidemiological and trials methodology. However, many worry that the discrepancy lies in the failure of the epidemiological studies to control for confounders (see below), biases arising from systematic differences in those who did and did not receive HRT treatment (e.g., inadequate control of socioeconomic position; Lawlor, Davey Smith, & Ebrahim, 2004). We are yet to see whether this general concern should apply to psychiatric epidemiology. There are some reasons to suggest it may not because many psychiatric disorders are relatively common and effect estimates for risk factors comparatively large. Moreover, some of the flaws in the rigor and objectivity of observational research may be soluble. Nonetheless, this experience does suggest the need for more critical evaluation and skepticism.

Confounding, Selection and Randomization

Rarely is an outcome of psychiatric interest related to just a single causal factor. In practice, many different processes are and have been at work to give rise to the current mental state of a child. Moreover, it is the nature of many of the factors of interest in child psychiatry that they co-occur. Poor families tend to live in poor neighborhoods, with poor educational opportunities and experience psychosocial risks and stresses that give rise to discord. Thus, a group of children identified by any one of these factors will also have an unusually high frequency of the other factors. There are at least two distinct aspects of this problem that are important. The first is that these other factors may have effects which we could attempt to account for. The second is that in our sample the variation among subjects in the factor of interest is correlated with variation in these other factors. This latter is commonly referred to as a selection effect that those who are selected to be exposed to one risk factor have commonly experienced and are experiencing other risks as well. The effect of our factor of interest will be confounded with the effects of these other risks.

Broadly speaking, we can attempt to solve our problem if we can deal with either of the two aspects of the problem. The obvious approach to dealing with the independent effects of possible confounders, that of adjustment, is addressed in the next section. The second aspect of the problem, that of selective exposure, can be dealt with if we can identify circumstances under which the exposure is assigned at random and thus in a way that is not correlated with any other factor. Random assignment is possible in experiments and trials and without dispute provides the most convincing route to estimating effects unconfounded with those of other possible exposures. In practice, it is becoming increasingly common that even trials cannot make this attribution of effect unambiguous. In psychiatry, the target disorder may itself interfere with the ability of the patient to comply with the assigned treatment and to complete the measurement protocol of the trial, and patients are less deferential and exercise their rights to switch treatment more often. As a consequence of such selective treatment exposure mechanisms, treatment received soon becomes correlated with all sorts of possible confounders. Nonetheless, as we shall see, we can continue to exploit the initial randomization to assess the causal impact of treatment.

Simple Adjustment for Measured Confounders

One way of dealing with confounding is through standardization. Intelligence scores are standardized to remove the effects of age, usually by means of a calibration sample. The standardized score measuring the extent of deviation from the norm is a particular raw score at a particular age. Standardization can also take the form of weighting age-specific sample data to correspond to a population with a standard age distribution. Point prevalence is a rate per person (or 100 or 10,000 persons) of some disorder and so for prevalence standardization means adjusting the data to correspond to that from a population with a specified number of individuals in each age category. With episodic disorders, such as depression, we commonly consider period prevalence, which includes as affected additional individuals those who, although without the disorder now, report disorder in the previous weeks or months (e.g., 3 months). Standardization of period prevalence data invariably proceeds as for point prevalence data, but will give higher rates than point prevalence. However, for incidence, which is the rate of occurrence per person per unit time, both the numbers of individuals in each age category and the time each has spent in that age category at risk of the disorder occurring are important. We therefore standardize not to a specific age distribution but to a specific distribution of

	Risk-exposed group			Risk-unexposed group		
Age category	Cases	Person-years	Rate	Cases	Person-years	Rate
5–<10	3	150	0.020	4 400	0.010	
10–<15	10	300	0.033	5 300	0.017	
15–<20	20	400	0.050	4 150	0.027	
Overall	33	850	0.039	13	850	0.015

Table 9.1 Incidence of disorder by exposure group and age (From Pickles, 1995).

person time (the product of persons and their time at risk) within each age category. Table 9.1 gives some illustrative data on the incidence of a disorder within three age categories for a risk-exposed and a risk-unexposed sample. The person-years have been calculated by summing the number of years each individual has spent at risk within that age category. The overall incidence is the number of incident cases divided by the person-years and the overall incidence rate ratio for risk-exposed to risk-unexposed is 0.039/0.015 = 2.6. However, the exposed group has more older children, for whom the incidence rate is higher; and the unexposed group more younger children, for whom the rate is lower. We can calculate standardized rates for hypothetical samples that had equal person-years of data in each age group (e.g., [0.20 + 0.033 + 0.05]/3 = 0.034 and [0.010 + 0.017 + 0.027]/3 = 0.018). This gives an incidence ratio accounting for age of 1.9. Further simple manual calculation would give a 95% confidence interval (CI) of 1.0–3.8 (see Clayton & Hills, 1993, chapter 14). This kind of adjustment for confounders is intuitive, can be presented in transparent steps and thus is easy to communicate. However, a more flexible tool is often required and for that we usually turn to some statistical model.

Regression and the Generalized Linear Model

For continuous outcome measures the familiar regression model is used to combine the effects of several factors. In this model, the expected or model predicted value of the outcome is assumed to be some linear combination of the predictor variables

$$E(Y) = \alpha + \beta_1 X_1 + \beta_2 X_2$$

and the variance of the outcome around its expected value is assumed to be constant (homoscedasticity). The X variables can be continuous or discrete (binary dummy categorical variables). This model subsumes analysis of variance (ANOVA) and analysis of covariance (ANCOVA).

Of course, there are many outcomes for which this model is not appropriate, and we then often turn to some form of the generalized linear model (McCullagh & Nelder, 1989). This allows two extensions to the ordinary regression model. First, a choice of link function that transforms the expected value of the response. For example, for a count response, such as that in Table 9.1, a log-link would be chosen such that

$$\mathrm{Log}[E(Y)] = \alpha + \beta_1 X_1 + \beta_2 X_2$$

This would ensure that all predicted counts were positive. Second, a different distribution for the variability of the observed response can be chosen. The key feature of this choice is how the variability in the observed responses might be expected to increase with its expected value. For example, in ordinary regression no increase is expected while with a Poisson distribution the variance increases with the expected value. For the data of Table 9.1, a Poisson distribution is often thought plausible for counts arising from independent events. The combination of log-link and Poisson error gives a Poisson regression model. Applied to the data of Table 9.1, a model in which both risk group and age group are included as main effects is appropriate. However, because we are wanting to examine an incidence rate, observed as a count divided by a person-years denominator, this latter must also be included in the model. As we are using a log-link function, dividing by the denominator is equivalent to subtracting the log of the denominator from the linear predictor, a procedure that in generalized linear model (GLM) terminology is known as specifying the log(person-years) as an offset. Applying this model gives an estimate for the effect of risk group of 0.67 (standard error [SE] 0.35), but this is the effect on the log scale. On the risk ratio scale, the effect is exp(0.67) = 1.9 with a 95% CI given by exp(0.67 ± 1.96 × 0.35) or (1.0–3.8), answers very close to those obtained by the standardization of the previous section.

The other commonly used GLM, particularly in child psychiatry where incidence is harder to determine than point or period prevalence, is the logistic regression model suitable for analyzing binary outcomes. This model estimates odds ratios (OR), a measure of effect that has both desirable and undesirable properties. A desirable quality is that it is the only measure of association between risk factor and binary outcome that is unaffected by oversampling risk exposed or by oversampling outcome cases (but not both of them at the same time). Thus, the OR estimate from a cohort study and a case–control study should be the same. An undesirable quality is that most readers and many authors interpret the OR as a risk ratio, something it approximates only rarely in psychiatry. An OR of 2 does not imply a doubling of the rate unless that outcome is very rare. If the rate in the unexposed group is 2% then the rate in the risk group does indeed almost double to 2 × 0.02/(1 + 0.02) = 4%, but with an unexposed group rate of 20% an OR = 2 implies a rate in the risk group of 2 × 0.2/(1

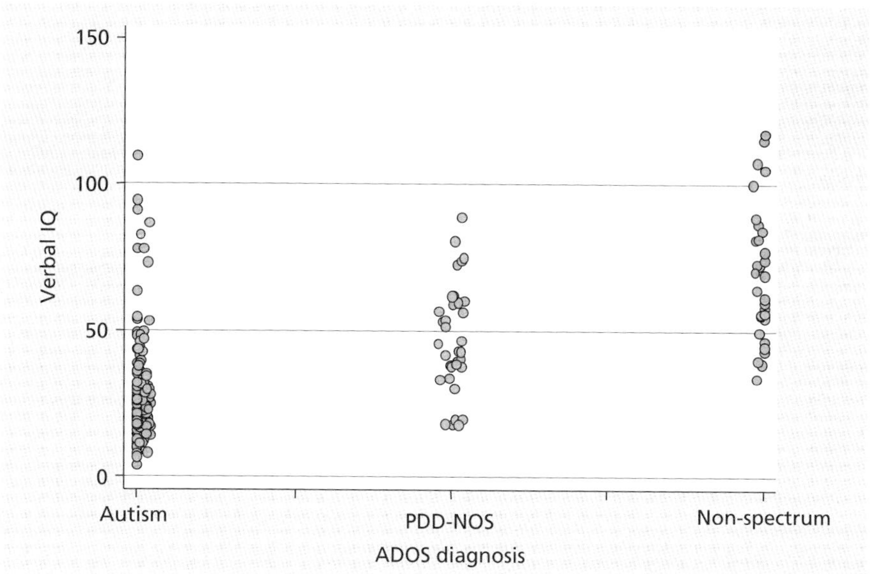

Fig. 9.2 Distribution of baseline verbal IQ and diagnostic group. PDD-NOS, autistic spectrum but not autism.

+ 0.2) = 33%, and with an unexposed group rate of 80%, then an OR = 2 implies a modest rate increase to 2 × 0.8/(1 + 0.8) = 89% in the risk group.

Regression and the more general GLM make covariate adjustment straightforward. It is therefore widely applied. However, it should not be considered as a cure-all and should always be accompanied by a process of carefully thinking through what is being assumed. A typical example is shown in Fig. 9.2 for 167 children from a prospective study of autism (Lord, Risi, DiLavore *et al.*, 2006). Figure 9.2 shows how initial verbal IQ is associated with initial diagnostic status of autism, autistic spectrum but not autism (PDD-NOS) and non-autistic spectrum (NS) as determined using an observation assessment, the ADOS (Lord, Risi, Lambrecht *et al.*, 2000). We might wish to examine how diagnosis made at age 2 is associated with outcome at age 9, measured on the ADOS social and communication score, taking into account initial verbal IQ. We could do this by covariate adjustment for verbal IQ in an ANOVA where age 2 diagnosis was a between-subjects factor, or equivalently by including both diagnosis and verbal IQ as main effects in a regression. We would obtain the answer that compared to those initially diagnosed with autism, those with PDD-NOS score –2.52 (95% CI, –4.69, –0.35) lower and those initially NS score –4.59 (95% CI, –7.20, –1.97) lower on the ADOS at age 9, and that each additional verbal IQ point is associated with a 0.102 (95% CI, 0.144–0.062) lower score. But what have we assumed in this adjustment process? We focus here on the assumption of linearity, both within and between groups, which has allowed us to make an adjustment across the whole range of IQ in the sample. A cursory examination of Fig. 9.2 shows that most of the children (in fact 71%!) with an initial diagnosis of autism have a verbal IQ below that of the child with the lowest verbal IQ in the non-spectrum group. Were we to control for verbal IQ by matching, a non-parametric approach that does not assume linearity, these children with autism and low verbal IQ would find no match in the non-spectrum group and would be dropped from the analysis. We could restrict our covariance adjustment approach to the verbal IQ range shared by all three diagnostic groups. The resulting analysis of 78 (previously 167) children gives estimates of outcome differences of –0.92 (95% CI, –4.09, 2.26) and –3.94 (95% CI, –7.37, –0.50), smaller and much less precise than the previous estimates. The covariance adjustment using the whole sample may be more powerful, but that power was gained at the expense of a more speculative assumption that the verbal IQ adjustment is correct even though in some areas of the scale that relationship is determined solely by children from one diagnosis. A compromise approach might be to allow more flexible non-linear adjustment. The results obtained using a fractional polynomial adjustment (Royston & Altman, 1994) for verbal IQ gave estimates of –1.98 (95% CI, –4.20, 0.024) and –4.28 (95% CI, –6.91, –1.64), estimates that fall between those calculated by the previous two methods.

The analyses above have assumed that the way that verbal IQ has an effect on the outcome is the same within each diagnostic group. Figure 9.3 shows the estimated relationship for each group, obtained from fitting a model that allowed an interaction term between diagnostic group and verbal IQ. Although this term was non-significant ($F[2,161] = 1.65$; $P = 0.2$), Fig. 9.3 clearly shows non-parallel lines. These imply that the difference among diagnostic groups in ADOS outcome score would depend upon the child's initial verbal IQ, that the estimates for the main effects of group difference will typically represent the difference when the covariate (verbal IQ) is zero, an uninteresting point on the scale unless verbal IQ is rescaled such that zero represents a more meaningful point, and that the answer obtained from "adjustment" for verbal IQ may represent some sort of average difference that could hide important variation. Unless designed in advance (e.g., by

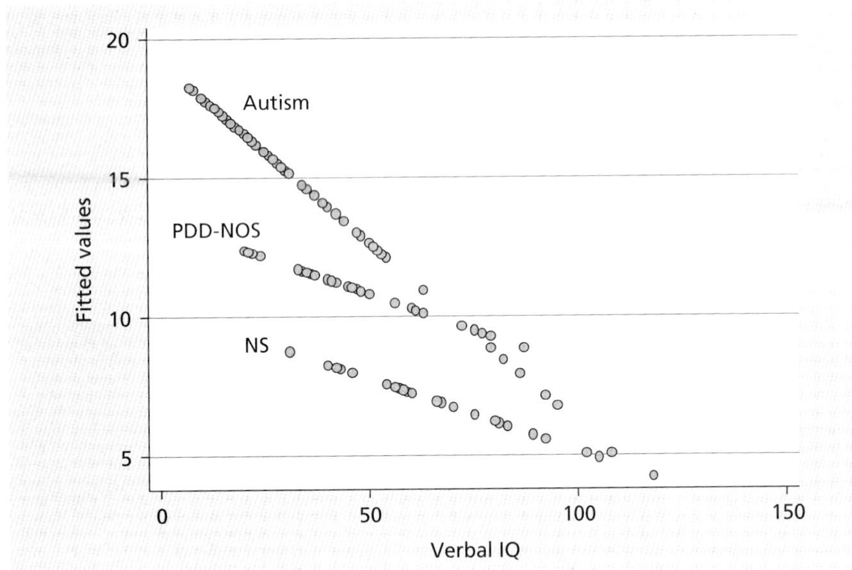

Fig. 9.3 Relationship between baseline verbal IQ and follow-up ADOS score by initial diagnosis. NS, non-autistic spectrum; PDD-NOS, autistic spectrum but not autism.

selecting only subjects who can be matched on verbal IQ), most studies do not have the power to test effectively for such variation. Unfortunately, designing a study to be powerful in this regard would make it clumsier to analyze for all but the designed contrasts. Moreover, the design would have increased power only with respect to the matched variables, and would exclude important subgroups of children, in this case the majority of autistic children who have low verbal IQs.

There remains the more general question as to what are relevant and suitable control variables. This is not a simple question to answer. We commonly find autism strongly associated with low verbal IQ. This may be partly the result of contamination, that low verbal IQ may result in an increased chance of false positive identification as being autistic using our current instruments. It may be that autism increases the risk of low verbal IQ, an association that might be expected to increase with development. Alternatively, low verbal IQ may increase the risk of autism. What is being achieved by controlling for verbal IQ, whether it is useful and how results should be interpreted, will differ according to which of these scenarios applies. Some argue that covarying for variables should only be undertaken to improve efficiency and that covarying in order to control for group differences in the covariate is entirely mistaken (Miller & Chapman, 2001). For practical research this would seem to be a counsel of despair. While rightly emphasizing the need for caution covariate adjustment, or some newer equivalents such as marginal structural modeling (see p. 120), undertaken in the context of supporting theory and evidence, is an essential and valid tool.

Mechanisms, Statistical Interactions and Effects Scales

The term interaction has distinct substantive and statistical definitions. As we shall see, because these usually relate to quite different concepts and each may be poorly defined in any particular instance, there is scope for much debate, mostly fruitless. The notion of synergy is often associated with interaction, where risk factors or characteristics have worse effects when they occur together than when each occurs by itself. The concept may be of special importance within psychiatry, where many of the features that are studied as being risk factors may in fact be risky only in certain contexts. For example, whereas high blood pressure or cholesterol levels seem to be almost universally bad for coronary heart disease, we cannot say that child antisocial behavior is universally increased as a result of:

1 Divorce, because it may be beneficial if the absenting father is themselves antisocial (Jaffee, Moffitt, Caspi *et al.*, 2003); or

2 High levels of testosterone, because while its association with leadership may confer risk in neighborhoods where deviant peers are common, elsewhere its role may be socialized (Rowe, Maughan, Worthman *et al.*, 2004).

Indeed, it is not unreasonable to expect that many behavioral responses may be adaptive or maladaptive depending upon the context. Effect modification also corresponds to synergy. In a clinical context, the effect of therapy may vary with the level of a moderator variable, such as family type. This makes resolving this confusion over interaction all the more pressing.

Where the response variable is continuous relatively little confusion arises. Thus, as in Fig. 9.3, slopes that characterized the relationship of one risk measure to an outcome score may be different in one group compared with another, and this slope variation can be tested for by a test of the interaction term. A group that has a particularly steep slope would be indicative of a form of synergy, although how it was described might also depend upon where the mean levels for the groups lay (Fig. 9.3). More problematic is the circumstance where the outcome is a binary diagnosis or an incident event where we are examining factors that might contribute to the rate of occurrence. (Rothman, 1976; Rothman & Greenland,

1986), in enlarging upon the notion of component causes, describes how for causal factors that are not too common and where no synergism occurs, the combined effect of exposure to two risk factors should be additive in the rates of outcome occurrence to either exposure alone. Where synergism occurs (e.g., where one factor increases the risk of an individual being in a state of vulnerability), from which exposure to the second risk factor increases the risk of occurrence of the final outcome of interest (a two-stage model; cf. Pickles, 1993), then the risk factors will appear to act multiplicatively. However, for analyzing binary outcomes, the common models are the log-rate models of survival analysis and the logit model for period prevalence data. Additive main effects on these log-rate and logit scales (for low rates) imply multiplicative effects on the simple rate scale. For these models the absence of an interaction can be consistent with synergy, and a significant (negative) interaction consistent with no synergy. Simply put, there is no correspondence between the need for a statistical interaction and synergy, because the former depends upon the scale in which the main effects have been combined (Blot & Day, 1979).

Our task should be to fit a parsimonious but adequately fitting model (with or without interaction terms) with easily understood and well-behaved parameters, which the logit model is, but then to support the interpretation, particularly the public health interpretation, by examining group-wise predicted outcome rates. Examining other effect measures may be helpful, such as group-wise attributable fractions (see p. 121).

Measurement Error

Psychiatry is one of the few areas of medicine that takes measurement error seriously. Nonetheless intuitive understanding of its impact on analysis is severely limited. Many researchers are familiar with the idea that if a risk factor is measured with error, then in any regression-type model where such a measure is used to predict an outcome, the estimated regression coefficient will be "attenuated" – the magnitude of the association will be lower and less significant than that obtained had the risk factor been perfectly measured. This conclusion, which is true in the simple bivariate case, is then interpreted to mean that the worst that can happen is that measurement error may reduce power and that our analyses might "miss" a few associations.

In fact, in more practical settings, where there are several possibly correlated exposures, with one or more measured with error, then such error can have far more pernicious effects. We illustrate these in the next example.

Measurement Errors in Children's Ability Scores

Ability scores were collected in children aged 6, 7, 9 and 11 years to measure continuity in general ability (Osbourne & Suddick, 1972). Summary statistics for these data are shown in Table 9.2.

Table 9.2 Summary statistics for the repeated measures of childhood ability measured by Osbourne and Suddick (1972).

	Age at measurement (years)			
	6	7	9	11
Mean	18.03	25.82	35.26	46.59
Standard deviation	6.37	7.32	7.80	10.39
Correlation matrix				
Age (years) 7	0.809			
9	0.806	0.850		
11	0.765	0.831	0.867	

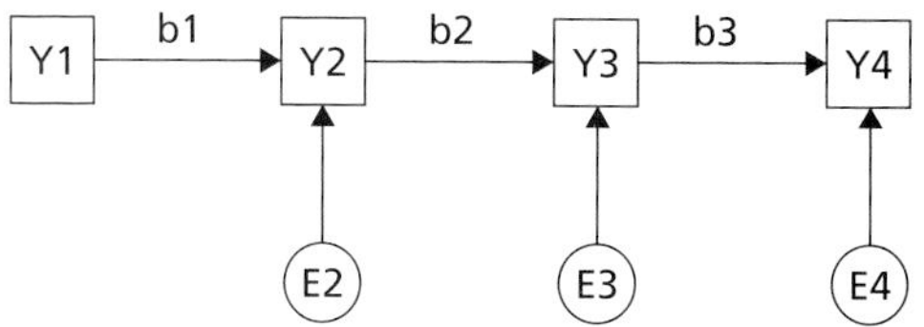

Fig. 9.4 An autoregressive model for continuity.

A plausible starting model is the first-order autoregressive model shown in Fig. 9.4, where ability at one age, having taken into account ability at the previous measurements, is not associated with any earlier measure.

A feature of such a model is that an early measure may influence a later measure but only through an intermediate measure. This is an example of "effect mediation" – the intermediate measure mediates the effect of the earlier measure. The model consists of three regressions (Y2 on Y1, Y3 on Y2 and Y4 on Y3), each with error terms that are assumed uncorrelated (E2, E3 and E4). In addition to estimating the standardized regression coefficients (0.809, 0.850 and 0.867, respectively), as one would do in standard regression modeling, we can assess the model's goodness-of-fit by comparing observed and expected covariance matrix, from which we would conclude that the autoregressive model had a very poor fit (χ^2 statistic of 61.82 with 3 degrees of freedom[1]). Something is wrong, but what? For many researchers the instinct is to conclude that additional relationships must exist (e.g., from Y1 to Y3 and Y2 to Y4). These additional relationships correspond to "sleeper effects" which have no effect on the immediately next measure but yet can influence a subsequent one. There are circumstances where such effects are plausible (e.g., where the tests vary in content and two non-adjacent tests have more similar content, say, being more mathematical), but skepticism should be retained.

We should first take the issue of measurement error seriously. In the classic measurement error model, the observed

[1] The degrees of freedom are found from the difference between the 10 observed summary statistics and the seven estimated parameters that are the variances for Y1, E2, E3 and E4 and the three regression coefficients b1, b2 and b3.

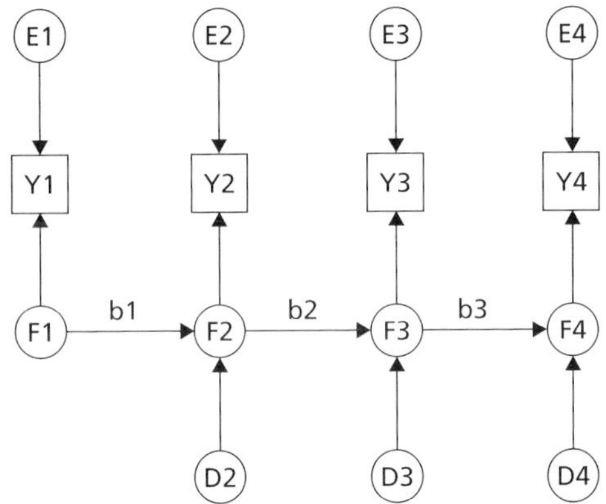

Fig. 9.5 A latent variable continuity model.

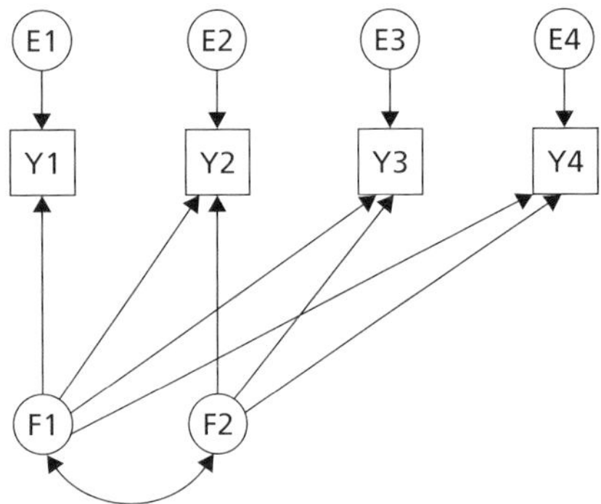

Fig. 9.6 Growth curve model with intercept and slope factors or random effects.

measurement is additively related to a "true variable" F and a measurement error E of constant variance,

$$Y = F + E$$

The "true variable" F is an example of a latent variable or factor, and in this simple case one that involves no regression coefficient or factor loading (and is also therefore a simple random effect). Usually, replicate measurements are necessary in order to identify and estimate the measurement error separately from the true variable. However, a structural equation model (SEM) of the four measurements can be fitted with constraints, enabling the variance for F and E to be identified with only single measurements per occasion (Fig. 9.5). Imposing constraints such that the measurement error variance remains the same over the four occasions achieves identification of the model and involves only one more parameter than the previous model (three regression coefficients between the factors and variances for F1, D2, D3, D4 and the single common measurement error variance for the E's). Allowing for measurement error results in a huge improvement in model fit with it now fitting well ($\chi^2 = 1.43$ with 2df). Clearly, this model has no need of any additional sleeper effect, because it already fits so well. How has this come about?

In the model corresponding to Fig. 9.4, measurement error in the Y's attenuates the coefficients estimated in each regression of one Y on the previous one, and the estimated coefficients are thus smaller than they would have been in the absence of measurement error. This underestimation results in the predicted association among the most temporally distant variables, Y1 and Y4 and which is given by the product of the standardized regression coefficients b1, b2 and b3, being even more underestimated (a 10% underestimation in each coefficient resulting in a $1 - 0.9 \times 0.9 \times 0.9 = 27\%$ underestimation of the b1 × b2 × b3 product). Allowing for measurement error corrects each regression coefficient and in so doing removes the gross underestimation of the model predicted long-term association.

There are numerous implications from this very modest example. The first is that in general, although measurement error in a covariate X1 may result in systematic underestimation of its relationship with some response, it can also give rise to overestimation of the effects of some other covariate, X2, with which X1 is correlated. Consider the often-repeated finding that current health is not only associated with contemporaneous risk factors, but also independently with the same risk factors measured earlier in childhood. Is this because the risk has its effect through an accumulation of risk exposure, or is it an artifact of measurement error in the risk measurements? This latter possibility is rarely properly explored. When examining mediation it is important that the mediator, in particular, should be either well measured or modeled as a latent variable in an SEM.

These data can be used to illustrate a further important point, namely that achieving a good model fit is not evidence for the correctness of the model, merely that it is one contender. A natural alternative model for data of this kind is a growth curve model (Rogosa & Willett, 1985) in which each child is considered as having a trajectory defined by an initial ability, represented by a latent intercept factor – or random effect – F1, and a latent rate of improvement, represented by a slope factor – or random coefficient – F2 (Fig. 9.6). The intercept factor "loads" (i.e., regresses) on all four measurements with a common regression coefficient. The growth or slope factor loads on all but the first measurement with either distinct factor loadings on each path or with constraints such that the loadings vary in proportion with the time since the initial measurement (equivalent to allowing for the linear effects of time to be random). In almost all growth situations, values at the initial starting point are correlated with subsequent growth, requiring the two latent factors or random effects to be correlated. Again, we can impose restrictions such that the measurement error variances (E1–E4) are constant. This model has one fewer parameter than the model of Fig. 9.5 and yet fits these data better, indeed extraordinarily well (χ^2 goodness-of-fit of just 0.92 with 3df).

Which of the two well-fitting models of Figs 9.5 and 9.6 should we choose? In this case, the choice is likely to rest upon theoretical considerations because we lack the data to discriminate effectively. The last model has the fewer parameters and in addition has the advantage of cleanly partitioning initial cross-sectional variation into one intercept factor from subsequent change in the second slope factor. This has appeal, especially were the model to be extended to allow for the effects of exposures to be associated with each of the intercept and slope factors. Where continuous growth or continuous decline are not expected, but instead change may be reversible, then random coefficients can be extended to a quadratic in time (or still higher order terms).

SEM with continuous and discrete variables and interactions: trajectory models

Much theory relates to groups or a categorical typology of individuals. A classic example is the three groups proposed by Moffitt (1993) in relation to antisocial behavior; these are defined in terms of their longitudinal trajectory into the life-course-persistent group, the adolescent limited group and the never-antisocial group. Practical definition of these groups may be somewhat arbitrary so a method that would identify these groups directly from the data with only general guidance from the researcher has been seen as desirable. These ideas may be operationalized within a trajectory model, a form of growth curve model in which the variations in the possible values of the intercept and growth factors are restricted to belong, in this case, to just three sets of values. Such a model can be considered as a form of latent class model or a model-based cluster analysis (Curran & Hussong, 2003). We can compare the relative fit of a model with two or four, rather than three classes to assess how gross an approximation the restriction to just three classes might be. It should not, however, be considered as a tool that can identify how many classes actually exist. Two things argue against this. First, the number of classes found as providing the best fit according to some standard information criterion (e.g., BIC or Akaike), has been found to vary with the extent of the data available to the analysis. Second, although one can continue to add more classes, both some theory (Laird, 1978) and practice have shown that there quite quickly comes a point where no further improvement in fit occurs, and that the additional new class either looks just like an already existing class or is assigned a probability of zero, implying that nobody belongs to it. This set of classes is referred to as the non-parametric maximum likelihood (NPML) estimator of the latent growth distribution. Although the NPML estimator is formed of classes, it can be shown that it fully characterizes the latent growth distribution even if that distribution is not one of classes but one of continuous variability, as in a traditional growth curve model. As a consequence, showing that a latent trajectory class model fits quite well is merely to say that we can approximate the latent growth distribution, whatever its true discrete or continuous form, by these classes and not that the classes exist. Nonetheless, this can remain a valuable achievement, allowing for an effective summary of the data and for helpful theory building and testing opportunities.

As with latent variable models, we can examine how various risk factors and confounders may be related to the latent quantity, estimating OR for the effect of these factors on latent trajectory class membership probabilities. In addition, we can calculate so-called posterior probabilities, which are estimates for each subject of the probability that they belong to each of the three classes. Such models can be estimated in programs such as the SAS procedure TRAJ, the SEM program Mplus (Muthen & Muthen, 2001) or the very general Stata procedure **gllamm** (Rabe-Hesketh, Pickles, & Taylor, 2000).

One of the major limitations of SEM path models is their inability to represent interactions. In fact, this is not a strict limitation, because multiple group methods, models that allow random coefficients for example, **gllamm** (Rabe-Hesketh, Pickles, & Skrondal, 2003) and a number of other approaches enable these to be considered. Nonetheless, few substantive applications have pursued them. Skrondal and Rabe-Hesketh (2004) describe an enormous range of models that fall within the multilevel and SEM framework.

Causal Analysis

Structural equation modeling is often referred to as causal modeling, but although it can provide a framework within which analysis specifically concerned with attempting to isolate evidence for causation can be undertaken, in practice this is rarely done. More often its use is more akin to the methods that we have already described in an earlier section for dealing with confounders, namely of covariance adjustment assuming linearity, although perhaps with the additional sophistication of allowing for measurement error.

There is, however, a quite distinct collection of methods that specifically address causal interpretation (Greenland & Brumback, 2002). We will consider two of these, propensity score weighting and its "double robust" property when used in combination with covariance adjustment, and instrumental variables, which have the capacity to control for unmeasured as well as measured confounders.

Propensity Score Approach

Consider the case where, in the population, the effect of X on the outcome Y may be confounded only by measured confounders denoted by Z (where Z is a set of variables). The setting described above is far more general than this approach can tackle. Rosenbaum and Rubin (1983) proposed the propensity score approach for estimating the causal effect of X in this circumstance. For a binary exposure of interest X, the propensity score for a subject is the conditional probability of exposure given the vector of observed confounders Z. Such a propensity score is usually estimated by logistic regression with X treated as the binary response variable and the confounders Z as the predictors. It can be shown that the point estimate of the effect of X from an analysis that also includes the propensity score, or better still matches and stratifies on the propensity score (Rosenbaum, 2002), gives unbiased estimates of the exposure effect under a wider range of conditions than an analysis that covaries for all the variables in Z. For example, if these have greater variability, or different patterns of correlation in one exposure group than another, as in Fig. 9.3, then direct covariate adjustment would increase the bias or even overcorrect.

An alternative way of using the propensity score idea, proposed by Robins and Rotnitsky (1995), is to weight individuals by the inverse of the probability of experiencing the exposure that they did (i.e., 1/propensity score for those that were exposed and 1/(1 – propensity score) for those that were not). In this weighted sample the exposure of interest is no longer correlated with the possible confounders Z and near standard analysis of such a weighted sample, a so-called marginal structural model (MSM), gives estimates of the effect of X unconfounded with the effects of Z.

The analysis thus consists of fitting the usual models for the effects of X on Y (e.g., linear or logistic regression), but with subjects weighted by weights $\{w_i\}$. This must be performed within a procedure that recognizes these weights as probability weights and requires that the procedure calculates the standard error, and thus *P* values and confidence intervals, using the sandwich or robust estimator (Binder, 1983; Huber, 1967) or some other technique (such as bootstrap) that recognizes that, although a subject may be assigned a weight of two, they nonetheless can be expected to possess the variability of a single subject.

Both the propensity score and MSM models require that the propensity score model be right. This means that we tend to err on the side of more rather than fewer variables in the set Z for estimation of the propensity scores. However, we may also include possible confounders as covariates in the model for the outcome. This then provides what Robins refers to as "double robustness," meaning that our estimate for the causal effect of X should be unbiased by confounders if either our covariate adjustment or the propensity score equation is correct – we do not need both to be correct.

In a longitudinal study we will commonly be concerned with a time-dependent exposure, $X_0, X_1 \ldots X_K$, where we might wish to estimate the effect of a cumulative exposure. With exposures confounded with $Z_0, Z_1 \ldots Z_K$ then we can again use weights for the probability of exposure, but now the weight's denominator is the conditional probability that a subject experienced their particular exposure history.

In the single period case, the practical advantage of the MSM approach over more routine covariate adjustment is not obvious. However, in the multiperiod time-dependent case, the advantage of the MSM approach is clearer. Both approaches attempt adjustment for Z_k, where Z_k is a confounder for later exposure. However, adopting the simpler covariate adjustment approach erroneously controls for the effect that earlier values of the exposure have on Z_k (i.e., the value of the confounder during period *k*). Thus, it would also wrongly partial out causal effects that should be attributed to the exposure. An example is the study of the effect of antiretroviral therapy (the exposure) and CD4 counts (the confounder) on the risk of acquired immunodeficiency syndrome (Cole, Hernan, Robins *et al.*, 2003). We have yet to see such methods used in child psychiatry.

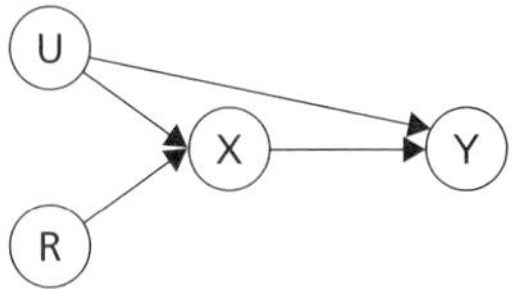

Fig. 9.7 Confounding of the causal relationship of X to Y by U and the instrumental variable R.

Instrumental Variables

The approaches described above require full information on all the confounders of the causal effect of the exposure of interest because these are needed to define the propensity score or the inverse probability weights. Almost always there are numerous possible confounders that we simply have not measured. How then do we proceed?

A way to deal with unmeasured confounding involves having data on a variable R that precedes and is related to exposure but is not directly related to the outcome or the unmeasured confounders (Fig. 9.7). A variable with these properties, if it exists, is said to be an "instrument" for the unbiased estimate of the causal effect of the exposure. If all relations are linear, then the instrumental variable estimate of the causal effect is the ratio of the coefficient in the regression of Y on R to the coefficient in the regression of X on R. With adjustment for measured confounders and multiple instruments the estimation is more complex, although programs are commonly available.

The main problem with this method is that it is rare to identify good instruments. Most examples exploit the occurrence of "natural experiments." Examples include using the Vietnam draft lottery number to examine the effects of traumatic event exposure (Hearst, Newman, & Hulley, 1986) and geographical variation in treatment provision to assess treatment impact on autism (Lord *et al.*, 2006).

More recent novel applications include an example of Mendelian randomization. In this approach (presumed) functional genes are used as instruments for phenotypes thought to cause certain diseases (Davey Smith & Ebrahim, 2005). Genotypic variation in the enzyme alcohol dehydrogenase makes some people drink much less alcohol (it becomes an unpleasant experience) while having no apparent direct effect on other behaviors, such as sociability, aggression or smoking. It thus provides a source of variation in alcohol consumption that is uncorrelated with many potential confounding variables. It has therefore been suggested as an instrument for studying the causal effects of alcohol on depression, antisocial behavior and even blood pressure.

Of course, the most obvious source of an instrument is from deliberate randomization within an actual experiment. In this context, the approach is becoming increasingly popular. The standard intention-to-treat estimator estimates the average effect of the treatment for everyone who was assigned for treatment, ignoring whether anyone actually took any of the treatment to which they were assigned or not. This declines in interest as the proportion of non-compliers with treatment increases, and we may want to know what the treatment effect would be on those who would take it if offered. Provided that the effect of being randomized to treatment was to increase exposure to the treatment of interest (and that certain other assumptions are met; cf. Dunn, Maracy, & Tormenson, 2005), then a causal effect is estimable using instrumental variable methods. However, the more complex assumptions and interpretation required for such an effect estimator means that it should supplement rather than replace the standard intention-to-treat estimate.

Reporting Results

Although statistical modeling may be increasingly used as the principal analysis tool, authors should nonetheless be expected to present tables and figures that display the essential features of the data in as raw a form as possible. For the reporting of results from trials sensible guidelines exist (e.g., CONSORT), while for epidemiological studies such guidelines are only now being drafted (e.g., STROBE). Estimates of effects should be reported in both standard form and in other ways that help interpretation. Mention has already been made of number-needed-to-treat for describing treatment effects. In observation studies, where causal interpretation is felt justified, quantities such as population attributable fraction (the fraction of cases that could be avoided if the risk exposure could be eliminated) can be helpful. More generally, comparing and describing results based on continuous-variable analysis and discrete/group based analysis is to be encouraged, because these two approaches offer quite different insights and strengths and weaknesses (Pickles & Angold, 2003).

As far as possible, results should present both the evidence for and against the principal conclusions. In this respect, we have mentioned how estimates and confidence intervals are preferred to significance levels alone.

Conclusions

This chapter has highlighted just some of the careful considerations required in undertaking, interpreting and reporting analysis. The chapter does not provide an exhaustive overview of statistical methods and there are many useful and important tools that we have omitted; for example, measures of diagnostic validity and reliability (see e.g., Dunn, 2000). The principal message is that statistical science is not a set of recipes, nor a set of hurdles that must be jumped to get to publication, but a set of concepts and principles whose application delivers better science.

Further Reading

McCartney, K., Burchinal, M., & Bub, K. L. (Eds.). (2006). Best practices in quantitative methods for developmentalists. *Monographs of the Society for Research in Child Development*, Vol. 71, serial no. 285. Boston: Blackwell Publishing.

References

Blot, W. J., & Day, N. E. (1979). Synergism and interaction: are they equivalent? *American Journal of Epidemiology*, *110*, 99–100.

Binder, D. A. (1983). On the variance of asymptotically normal estimators from complex surveys. *International Statistical Review*, *51*, 279–292.

Clayton, D. G., & Hills, M. (1993). *Statistical models in epidemiology*. Oxford: Oxford University Press.

Cohen, J. (1992). A power primer. *Psychological Bulletin*, *112*(1), 155–159.

Cole, S. R., Hernan, M. A., Robins, J. M., Anastos, K., Chmiel, J., Detels, R., *et al.* (2003). Effect of highly active antiretroviral therapy on time to acquired immunodeficiency syndrome or death using marginal structural models. *American Journal of Epidemiology*, *158*, 687–694.

Curran, P., & Hussong, A. M. (2003). The use of latent trajectory models in psychopathology research. *Journal of Abnormal Psychology*, *112*, 526–544.

Davey Smith, G., & Ebrahim, S. (2005). What can Mendelian randomisation tell us about modifiable behavioural and environmental exposures? *British Medical Journal*, *330*, 1076–1079.

Dunn, G. (2000). *Statistics in psychiatry*. London: Arnold.

Dunn, G., Maracy, M., & Tormenson, B. (2005). Estimating treatment effects from randomised clinical trials with non-compliance and loss to follow-up: the role of instrumental variables. *Statistical Methods in Medical Research*, *14*, 369–395.

Greenland, S., & Brumback, B. (2002). An overview of relations among causal modelling methods. *International Journal of Epidemiology*, *31*, 1030–1037.

Hearst, N., Newman, T. B., & Hulley, S. B. (1986). Delayed effects of military draft on mortality: A randomised natural experiment. *New England Journal of Medicine*, *314*, 620–624.

Huber, P. (1967). The behaviour of maximum likelihood estimates under non-standard conditions. *Proceedings of the Fifth Berkely Symposium on Mathematical Statistics and Probability*, Vol. 1 (pp. 221–233). Berkeley: University of California Press.

Hulley, S., Grady, D., Bush, T., Furberg, C., Herrington, D., Riggs, B., *et al.* (1998). Randomized trial of estrogen plus progestin for secondary prevention of coronoary heart disease in post-menapausal women. Heart and Estrogen/progestin Replacement Study (HERS) Research Group. *Journal of the American Medical Association*, *280*, 605–613.

Ioannidis, J. P. A. (2005). Contradicted and initially stronger effects in highly cited clinical research. *Journal of the American Medical Association*, *294*, 218–228.

Jaffee, S. R., Moffitt, T. E., Caspi, A., & Taylor, A. (2003). Life with (or without) father: the benefits of living with two biological parents depend on the father's antisocial behavior. *Child Development*, *74*, 109–126.

Laird, N. M. (1978). Nonparametric maximum likelihood estimation of a mixing distribution. *Journal of the American Statistical Association*, *73*, 805–811.

Lawlor, D. A., Davey Smith, G., & Ebrahim. S. (2004). Socioeconomic position and hormone replacement therapy: explaining the discrepancy in evidence from observational and randomized controlled trials. *American Journal of Public Health*, *94*, 2149–2154.

Light R. J., & Pillemer D. B. (1984). *Summing up. The science of reviewing research*. Cambridge, MA: Harvard University Press.

Lord, C., Risi, S., Lambrecht, L., Cook, E. H., Leventhal, B. L., DiLavore, P. C., *et al.* (2000). The Autism Diagnostic Observation Schedule–Generic: A standard measure of social and communication deficits associated with the spectrum of autism. *Journal of Autism and Developmental Disorders*, *30*, 205–223.

Lord, C., Risi, S., DiLavore, P. S., Shulman, C., Thurm, A., & Pickles, A. (2006). Autism from two to nine. *Archives of General Psychiatry*, *63*, 694–701.

McCullagh, P., & Nelder, J. A. (1989). *Generalized linear models* (2nd ed.). London: Chapman and Hall.

Miller, G. M., & Chapman, J. P. (2001). Misunderstanding analysis of covariance. *Journal of Abnormal Psychology*, *110*, 40–48.

Moffitt, T. E. (1993). Adolescence-limited and life-course persistent antisocial behavior: A developmental taxonomy. *Psychological Review*, *100*, 674–701.

Muthen, L. K., & Muthen, B. O. (2001). *Mplus users guide*. Los Angeles, CA: Muthen & Muthen.

Osbourne R. T., & Suddick, D. E. (1972). A longitudinal investigation of the intellectual differentiation hypothesis. *Journal of Genetic Psychology*, *110*, 83–89.

Pickles, A. (1993). Stages, precursors and causes in development. In D. F. Hay & A. Angold (Eds.), *Precursors and causes in development and psychopathology* (pp. 23–49). Chichester: Wiley.

Pickles, A. (1995). Statistical analysis in epidemiology. In F. C. Verhulst & H. M. Koot (Eds.), *The epidemiology of child and adolescent psychopathology* (pp. 104–121). Oxford: Oxford University Press.

Pickles, A., & Angold, A. (2003). Natural categories or fundamental dimensions: On carving nature at the joints and the re-articulation of psychopathology. *Development and Psychopathology 15*, 529–551.

Rabe-Hesketh, S., Pickles, A., & Taylor, C. (2000). GLLAMM: Generalized linear latent and mixed models. *Stata Technical Bulletin*, *53*, 47–57.

Rabe-Hesketh, S., Pickles, A., & Skrondal, A. (2003). Correcting for measurement error in logistic regression using non-parametric maximum likelihood estimation. *Statistical Modelling*, *3*, 215–232.

Roach, N. W., Edwards, V. T., & Hogben, J. H. (2004). The tale is in the tail: an alternative hypothesis for psychophysical performance variability in dyslexia. *Perception*, *33*, 817–830.

Robins, J. M., & Rotnitsky, A. (1995). Semiparametric efficiency in multivariate regression models with missing data. *Journal of the American Statistical Association*, *90*, 122–129.

Rogosa, D., & Willett, J. B. (1985). Understanding correlates of change by modelling individual differences in growth. *Psychometrika*, *50*, 203–228.

Rosenbaum, P. R. (2002). *Observational studies* (2nd ed.). New York: Springer Verlag.

Rosenbaum, P. R., & Rubin, D. B. (1983). The central role of the propensity score in observational studies for causal effects. *Biometrika*, *70*, 41–55.

Rothman, K. J. (1976). Causes. *American Journal of Epidemiology*, *104*, 587–592.

Rothman, K. J., & Greenland, S. (1986). *Modern epidemiology*. Philadelphia, PA: Lippincott-Raven.

Rowe, R., Maughan, B., Worthman, C. M., Costello, E. J., & Angold, A. (2004). Testosterone, antisocial behavior, and social dominance in boys: pubertal development and biosocial interaction. *Biological Psychiatry*, *5*, 546–552.

Royston, P., & Altman, D. (1994). Regression using fractional polynomials of continuous covariates: parsimonious parametric modelling (with discussion). *Applied Statistics*, *43*, 429–467.

Schulz, K. F., Chalmers, I., Hayes, R. J., & Altman, D. (1995). Empirical evidence of bias: Dimensions of methodological quality associated with estimates of treatment effects in controlled trials. *Journal of the American Medical Association*, *273*, 408–412.

Skrondal, A., & Rabe-Hesketh, S. (2004). *Generalised latent variable modelling*. London: Chapman and Hall.

Stampfer, M. J., & Colditz, G. A. (1991). Estrogen replacement therapy and coronary heart disease: a quantitative assessment of the epidemiologic evidence. *Preventive Medicine*, *20*, 47–63.

Tang, J-L., Zhan, S-Y., & Ernst, E. (1999). Review of randomized controlled trials of traditional Chinese medicine. *British Medical Journal*, *319*, 160–161.

10 Health Economics

Martin Knapp

For better or for worse, money is always just below the surface in policy and practice discussions. Although the professional delivering one-to-one therapy, prescribing a course of medication or arranging a group activity might not have to be concerned about the associated costs, further along the management chain someone will be watching expenditure levels and trying to balance the books. While the budget holder may be focused on avoiding a financial deficit at the end of the year, someone higher up in the health, education or social services system will need to consider wider strategic options and will be looking to achieve best value for money in the use of available resources. If a new treatment (such as a new drug or new mode of family therapy) is introduced – and known to be effective – budget holders will want to know whether it is affordable and worth what it costs to provide. If needs and their consequences are enduring, governments will want to know the associated long-term expenditure implications and how to contain them.

The underlying challenge common to all of these wants is scarcity: there are never enough resources to meet all of society's needs. This is the most fundamental, pervasive, durable and indeed important justification for a better understanding of the economics of child and adolescent mental health. Scarcity is an endemic, indeed permanent feature of all health and related systems and is the reason why choices have to be made between alternative uses of a particular resource or service. As we shall see, those choices between alternative uses give meaning to costs. Economics – and, in particular, economic evaluation – aim to provide evidence to inform both professional practice and strategic decisions about how to allocate available resources so as to get more out of them (in terms of – for example – better outcomes for children and families, or a fairer distribution of access or use of services), and about the incentives needed to help achieve those allocations.

Although the primary aim of any mental health system is to alleviate symptoms so as to improve personal functioning and promote quality of life, it is increasingly recognized that pursuit of such a laudable fundamental objective cannot proceed without regard for the economic consequences of the therapies, support arrangements or broad policy strategies put into place. Awareness of this need to improve not only the effectiveness, but also the cost-effectiveness of health care (and other sector) interventions and actions has produced various demands for economic evidence. There are requests for measures of the overall resource or cost impact of a particular health problem (often called *cost-of-illness* studies). There are demands for *cost-effectiveness* and similar analyses of particular treatments or policies, carried out either alongside trials or independently: these are evaluations that compare not only the outcomes of different interventions, but also the costs of achieving them. There are searches for new service and system reconfigurations that can improve the efficiency of use of available resources. And there are searches for improved incentive structures that could positively alter the ways that resources are deployed.

By way of illustration, Fig. 10.1 offers a highly simplified framework within which to locate some of these demands. Figure 10.1(a) is a selection of some of the many available interventions, some of the outcomes that could result from them and some of the long-term cost implications. The links between the first and second columns are the concerns of any treating professional: they want to know what are the effects of different therapeutic arrangements on the well-being of children and families. The links between the second and third columns are of particular interest to budget holders and governments: will better health and functioning reduce needs for services, and with what cost savings? Figure 10.1(b) shows the associated economic questions and how these are connected to the basic "clinical" concerns in Fig. 10.1(a). Figure 10.1 is therefore a hypothesis map: it points to the questions that tend to dominate the economics agenda in the child and adolescent mental health area – cost, cost-offset (comparing amounts expended with amounts saved) and cost-effectiveness – and each has associated with it a number of questions about incentives and disincentives. These concepts are introduced, defined and illustrated in this chapter.

Costs in Childhood

Mental health problems – if they are recognized and responded to – have cost implications. The most obvious effect will be on health service utilization, but there may be contacts with special education, social work, public housing, criminal justice

Rutter's Child and Adolescent Psychiatry, 5th edition. Edited by M. Rutter, D. Bishop, D. Pine, S. Scott, J. Stevenson, E. Taylor and A. Thapar. © 2008 Blackwell Publishing, ISBN: 978-1-4051-4549-7.

(a)

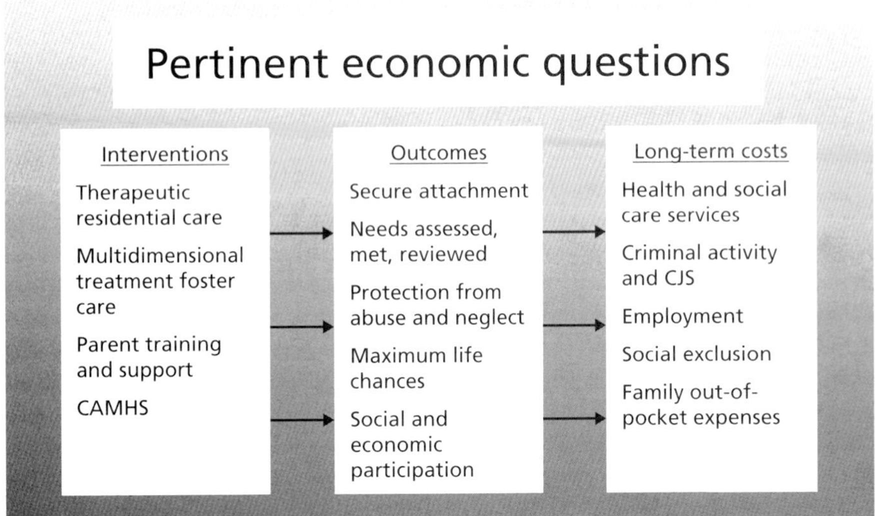

(b)

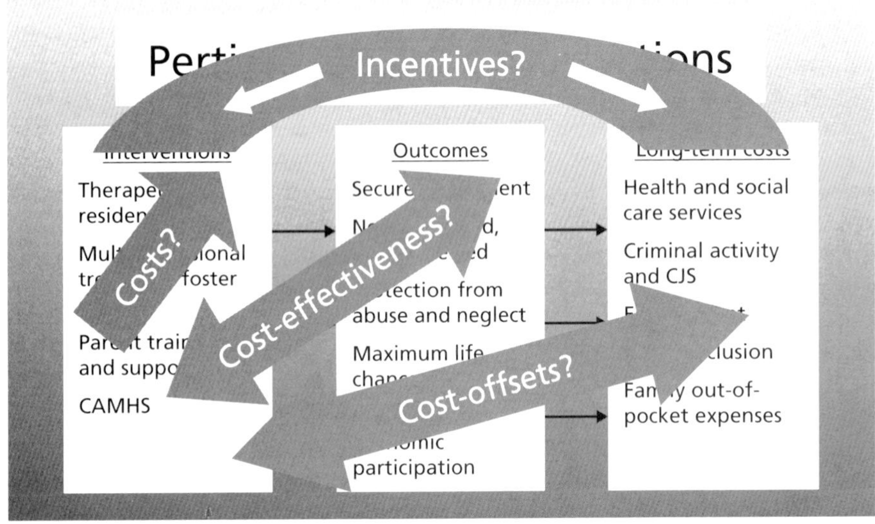

Fig. 10.1 (a) A hypothesis map. (b) Associated economic questions relating to Child and Adolescent Mental Health and other services.

and other service-delivering agencies. Indeed, the multiplicity of contacts and services is a marked characteristic of well-developed child and adolescent mental health systems (Glied & Evans Cuellar, 2003). If needs or problems are not appropriately treated, then there could be adverse effects on functioning, with implications for educational engagement and attainment, employment and income (in later years), as well as effects on families. A number of studies have described these costs during childhood and adolescence. For example, a small pilot study in London estimated the broad cost implications for services, families and the wider economy of childhood conduct disorder (Knapp, Scott, & Davies *et al.*, 1998). Over a 1-year period these costs averaged £15,282 per family (range £5411–40,896, up-rated to 2004–2005 prices). The financial impacts fell quite broadly across different sectors. In fact, although the children in this pilot study were all diagnosed as having a health problem and all were, at the time, being treated by specialist child mental health services, only 16% of the total cost fell to the National Health Service (NHS).

Romeo, Knapp, & Scott *et al.* (2006) offer a more recent estimate of costs for a similar group of children, again from south London. Eighty children aged 3–8 years referred for severe antisocial behavior to child and adolescent mental health services were found to use several services as a result of their severe antisocial behavior, provided by the NHS, education and other public sector services. There were also considerable non-service costs within the family. Mean annual cost of care was £5960 (ranging from as low as £48 for one child, to a high of £19,940 for another). Almost half of this total was borne by the family (Fig. 10.2). What this and the earlier study both show very clearly is the breadth of economic impact across a variety of service sectors and on families, although they can only measure what is provided (in terms of service-related costs) or what impacts are recognized (in terms of indirect costs).

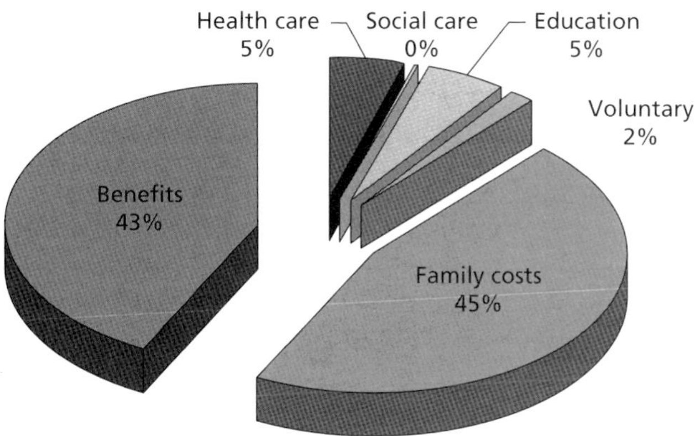

Fig. 10.2 Costs of children with persistent antisocial behavior. Total cost excluding benefits averaged £5960 per child per year, at 2000–2001 prices (benefits = £4307). From Romeo, Knapp, & Scott (2006).

We shall see in the next section that if behavioral problems in childhood or adolescence are inadequately addressed, then there are also likely to be substantial long-term costs stretching into adulthood.

A third example points to the high and enduring costs of autistic spectrum disorder. Patching together data from a number of UK studies, combined with estimates of prevalence, Järbrink and Knapp (2001) suggested that the lifetime cost of someone with autism and intellectual disability would be more than £4 million at today's cost levels. Three-quarters of this amount is for living support (particularly special accommodation) and another one-eighth of the total is for day activities. Family inputs were not properly measured in this study, but there are a range of formal services included, such as special education, hospital services and voluntary support.

The extent to which the resource (cost) consequences of childhood or adolescent mental health problems fall outside the health sector will obviously depend on how that and neighboring sectors are organized and configured: different boundaries between health, social services, education, housing and other service sectors will mean redrawing the cost map. However, it will not change the fact that many young people with mental health problems have needs in multiple life domains, each of them with economic ramifications. Foster, Jones *et al.* (2005), for example, describe the economic implications of conduct disorder among adolescents in four US communities over a 7-year period. The cost difference between youths with and without conduct disorder was nearly $70,000. The distribution of costs between budgets was different from in the UK, partly because of differences in system structures.

These multiple impacts are obviously hard to measure, and much harder still to factor into decision-making. Not only does the decision-maker in, for example, the health sector need to find out the implications of their actions for other sectors, whether positive or negative, but they also have to think through the mechanisms needed to do something about them. A major problem in many systems is "silo budgeting": resources located in specific agencies or budgets cannot easily be shifted, indeed, might be rigorously protected (Glied & Evans Cuellar, 2003). Professional rivalry, myopic budget protection, performance assessment regimes or simply slowly churning bureaucratic processes could leave one agency unwilling or unable to devote more of its own resources in order for another agency or service to achieve savings or for the broader system of treatment and support to achieve greater effectiveness or cost-effectiveness. These inter-budget considerations can be important. For example, Foster and Connor (2005) found that delivering child and adolescent mental health services as part of a system-of-care approach, while more expensive than standard services, reduced expenditure in other sectors (juvenile justice, child welfare, special education, in-patient services).

Costs Continuing into Adulthood

It is well known that mental health problems experienced in childhood or adolescence can have many and often serious adverse effects on psychosocial outcomes such as crime, relationships, substance misuse and on quality of life. Many studies have traced these connections between behavioral and emotional problems in childhood and adverse experiences of various kinds in adulthood (see chapter 13).

Many of these adulthood problems and experiences will have measurable cost consequences, and while any computed monetary indicators cannot hope to represent or cover the full set of experiences of individual children and adults, they have the virtue of expressing some of these experiences in magnitudes that are readily understood by those key policy-makers who hold the purse strings.

A few studies have explicitly explored the connections between childhood disorders and adulthood economic consequences. These latter include unusually high rates of utilization of health and other services (obviously with personal and societal costs), and impacts related to employment (such as not being economically active, being active but unemployed, being employed but frequently absent or unproductive, or working in a lower status occupation than would otherwise be expected). The latter will inevitably have impacts on earnings and could lead to individual and household poverty. Three examples can be offered.

Evidence from the Inner London Longitudinal Study

The Inner London Longitudinal Study collected data on 2281 10-year-olds in 1970 and selected 228 of them for intensive study: a random 1 in 12 sample of the population and a 1 in 2 sample of children with emotional or behavioral problems (Maughan, 1989). This group was interviewed again at age 28. Neither interview set out to collect "economic" data as such, but it was possible to construct service-related costs from the information gathered (Scott, Knapp, Henderson *et al.*, 2001). Nevertheless, the computed cost averages are undoubtedly underestimates of the full costs because the data collection did not cover all possible impacts and did not follow people continuously over time. Among the costs not measured were those associated with social work, voluntary sector service use, primary health care contacts, lost employment, divorce, undetected crime, the effects of crime on victims, the emotional impacts on other people and other transmitted effects to other family members or children. Many of these omissions are known to be substantial (see the other studies below). Notwithstanding these missing elements, conduct disorder in childhood (which was found for the most antisocial 3% of the population studied) and conduct problems (which were found for the next 9%) led to greatly elevated costs in adulthood for a number of agencies, and especially for the criminal justice system.

The links between conduct problems and conduct disorder in childhood and service-related costs in early adulthood were further explored through multiple regression analysis, adjusting for gender, parental social class, reading age and number of primary schools attended. A number of other factors were examined, but found not to be significant. Adjusting for those covariates, the estimated coefficient on the conduct disorder variable – the additional cost between the ages of 10 and 28 (aggregating across all 18 years) of having conduct disorder at age 10 compared to not having any antisocial behavior problems – was £40,784 (at 2004–2005 prices). The additional cost of having conduct problems (those who were less severely affected by antisocial behavior – the next 9% of the group) compared to having no such problems was £17,017. Given the underdeveloped and under-resourced nature of child and adolescent mental health services in the early 1970s, these cost differences might be interpreted as indicative of the economic consequences of not addressing (or inadequately addressing) antisocial behavior among 10-year-olds.

Evidence from the Maudsley Depression Study

The Maudsley long-term follow-up study of child and adolescent depression illustrates the persistent costs of comorbidity. It gathered data from people who attended child psychiatric services in south London for depression. They were followed up as adults – on average 21 years after they had been treated as children. All 149 people in the sample had received treatment for childhood depression; 53 of them had also been diagnosed with conduct disorder (Fombonne, Wostear, Cooper *et al.*, 2001). The childhood and adulthood collections of data were made at a variety of ages. For those 140 people for whom all relevant data were available, costs of health, social care and criminal justice service use in adulthood were calculated. Mean annual cost in adulthood was £1219 (2004–2005 prices; Knapp, McCrone, Fombonne *et al.*, 2002). The range was wide – from zero to £10,318. General hospital and psychiatric hospital costs accounted for just over half of the total.

Adjusting for an individual's circumstances and morbidity at the time of their treatment as a child or adolescent showed that a number of factors were significant predictors of higher adulthood costs (McCrone, Knapp, & Fombonne, 2005):

- *Age at first contact with psychiatric services* Younger age was associated with lower adulthood cost.
- *Anxiety in childhood* A higher level of anxiety was associated with higher adulthood costs.
- *Peer–sibling relationship* Children with more difficulty with such relationships had lower adulthood costs, although it is not absolutely clear how to interpret this finding (one possibility is that it might be masking greater isolation in adulthood, resulting in lower rates of service use).
- *Comorbid conduct disorder* Individuals with both depression and conduct disorder had much higher adulthood costs than those with depression alone (the difference being more than £900 per annum).

These findings demonstrate how antisocial behavior among a juvenile group with affective disorders carries an elevated risk of subsequently high service use, even after adjusting for other factors. Moreover, the comorbid group had much higher utilization rates for out-patient care, in-patient care and prison stays; in contrast, the group with depression (alone) did not make higher use of any services than would be expected for the general population.

Evidence from the Cambridge Study of Delinquent Development

The final example, again from a London sample, points to a wider set of undesirable economic consequences, in this case stemming from poor labor market attainments in early adulthood. The Cambridge Study in Delinquent Development (CSDD) sampled 411 boys born 1952–1954 (predominantly born into a working class environment) and has reinterviewed most of them eight times since, most recently at age 48 (Farrington, 2001). Healey, Knapp, & Farrington (2004) looked at the links between "troublesome behavior" in childhood and poor employment experiences (unemployment, low status employment, low earnings) at ages 18–19 and 32.

In childhood, sample members were described as "troublesome" (or not) based on peer and teacher ratings of behavior at school at age 8–10. A "troublesome" boy was one in the lowest quartile of the behavioral ratings distribution. In adolescence, a boy was defined as "delinquent" if he had a criminal conviction between the ages of 10 and 16, with data taken from the Criminal Records Office. Thereby, four mutually exclusive groups could be defined: troublesome and delinquent; non-troublesome and delinquent; troublesome and non-delinquent; non-troublesome and non-delinquent.

Among the findings from this study, childhood antisocial conduct at age 8–10 (being a troublesome boy) was associated with an increased risk of teenage unemployment and employment instability, although less strongly linked to poor employment outcomes identified at age 32. Antisocial tendencies that persisted from childhood and through adolescence (troublesome and delinquent) were strongly associated with a lower probability of employment participation at age 32, with long-term periods of unemployment in their late 20s and early 30s, and a persistent absence of success in the labor market (lack of employment participation and/or low pay job status at ages 18 and 32).

Antisocial tendencies (troublesome and delinquent) were not associated with lower weekly earnings at age 32, which may be partly a result of a wage ceiling effect for this particular cohort, given that they came from a fairly narrow socioeconomic background. Nevertheless, the link between antisocial development and *expected* earnings from employment was marked: weekly earnings (calculated at 1985 wage levels but inflated to 2004 levels) adjusted for the probability of unemployment were £205 for those described as troublesome delinquents, but £301 for the rest of the cohort.

These associations are adjusted for covariates. For example, both poor school-leaving outcomes and subsequent adult convictions appeared to be important mediating factors behind these less favorable employment outcomes. Around 89% of the "troublesome delinquent" group did not study for or pass any school examinations, compared to 47% of the remainder of the cohort. Over 85% of this same group went on to receive a criminal conviction between ages 17 and 32 compared to only 26% of the remaining boys, receiving on average around five criminal convictions during their adult years up to age 32.

Cost-Offset Considerations

A question that governments and other macro-level decision makers often want answering is whether investment in preventive measures or better treatments during, say, the early years will pay off in terms of reduced economic impacts in adolescence and in later years. This is what economists would call the *cost-offset* question: it asks about the balance between amounts expended and amounts saved.

An example comes from the well-known Fort Bragg Demonstration (Bickman, Guthrie, Foster *et al.*, 1995). The initial evaluation of the Demonstration, which introduced a continuum of care for children and adolescents with mental health problems, looked only at direct program costs narrowly defined. Subsequently, Foster and Bickman (2000) calculated a broader measure of costs, including mental health services used outside the catchment sites, other medical services used by children and services used by family members. The higher program costs of the Demonstration were found to be partially offset by reduced expenditures in these other sectors.

An earlier Swedish study by Gustafsson and Svedin (1988) looked at family therapy for children with psychosomatic or somatic disorders and its cost-offsetting properties. The calculated total cost of introducing the treatment was balanced by savings in in-patient stays for the children concerned. This and the Fort Bragg example, together with a few other studies, focus on the immediate potential for investment in a child or adolescent mental health service to "pay for itself" by reducing the need for other services.

There have also been studies that have looked at the long-term cost-offsetting properties of such investments. Cohen (1998), for example, looked at "high-risk youth" in the USA and the *potential* economic advantages from "saving" each individual by estimating costs over the lifetime associated with crime, drug misuse and dropout from school. The estimated monetary value of "saving each high-risk youth" was estimated to be between \$1.7 million and \$2.3 million. Cohen's study was based on hypothetical valuations, whereas a second example – the High/Scope Perry Preschool Study – was based on direct observations. Although not focused on children with mental health problems, this well-known and uniquely effective intervention is interesting and has been quite influential because of its finding of substantial savings in relation to crime, education and welfare payments, as well as higher taxes paid by those people who went through the preschool program (see, e.g., the summary by Schweinhart, 2004). However, these findings relate to a very small sample of individuals, and generalization from this study is far from straightforward.

In the UK, a recent report by Dretzke, Frew, Davenport *et al.* (2005) summarizes much of the evidence on the effectiveness of parent training programs for conduct disorders, and provides estimates of the cost of such programs (2005 prices):

- *Group community-based settings* Cost £633–944 per child, depending on group size.
- *Group clinic-based settings* Cost £444–660 per child, depending on group size.
- *Individual home-based settings* Cost as much as £4030 per child.

These estimates are higher than those suggested by previous authors in the USA and UK, but still look quite modest when compared with some of the estimates offered earlier in the chapter for the adulthood economic consequences of conduct disorder, measured in terms of health and social care service use, criminal justice system contacts, unemployment and earnings. In other words, there is again the strong suggestion that expenditure in childhood or adolescence in response to identified mental health needs will be more than matched by later savings because of reduced rates of use of a range of services.

Exploring Cost-Effectiveness

Knowing the costs in childhood associated with mental health problems helps decision-makers to gauge the overall societal impact of these conditions. Knowing what economic consequences these problems lead to in adulthood helps those same decision-makers focus their minds on the need for better preventive or treatment interventions in early years or subsequently. But neither of these bodies of evidence can tell a decision-maker how to make better use of available resources. For this purpose it is necessary to examine both the costs and the outcomes of different uses of those resources. This is what economists would recognize as the examination of *cost-effectiveness*.

Consider what happens following the development or introduction of a new treatment (say, a new medication intended for treating childhood depression). Decision-makers face two central questions when considering whether to use or recommend this new drug as part of the treatment range. The first is the clinical question: is the medication effective in alleviating depressive symptoms and generally improving child health? Or, when considering two or more different drugs, which of them has the better outcomes? If the answer to the clinical question is that the new medication is worse than existing treatment options, then there is usually no need to consider its use any further. However, if the new medication looks equally or more clinically effective, the decision-maker will then want an answer to a second question: is it cost-effective? That is, does the treatment achieve the improved or equivalent child outcomes at a cost that is worth paying?

These two questions (Is the treatment effective? Is it worth it?) sit at the heart of cost-effectiveness analysis. It is important to emphasize that cost-effectiveness analysis does what it says: it looks at *both* costs and effectiveness (outcomes). Comparing the costs of one intervention with the costs of another, without any evidence on outcomes, might be interesting but does not constitute an economic evaluation because it does not provide enough information to assist service professionals, managers or others to make choices between alternative uses of their scarce resources. Similarly, calculating the costs and outcomes of a single intervention could be revealing, but again is not especially helpful (and not an economic evaluation) unless comparison is made with equivalent data for another service, for otherwise the decision-maker will have no benchmark against which to judge whether the observed costs and outcomes are attractive.

Note that the second question in a cost-effectiveness analysis asks whether improved outcomes are "worth" the extra cost. Deciding what is or is not "worth" the cost is far from straightforward and not without controversy, as discussed below.

There are different variants of cost-effectiveness that can be applied to decision-making in health and related contexts. They share a common approach to the conceptualization, definition and measurement of costs, but they adopt different approaches when considering and measuring the outcome side of the evaluation, primarily because they seek to answer slightly different questions. There is, however, some potential for terminological confusion. The term "cost-effectiveness" is used to describe a specific variant of economic evaluation as well as to refer generically to the group of all such evaluations. In this chapter I am using the term in its generic sense, unless specifically stated to the contrary.

Question and Perspective

The choice of evaluative approach therefore depends on the question to be addressed. If the question is essentially clinical – what is the most appropriate treatment for a child with particular needs in particular circumstances, and whether to opt for one therapeutic package or another – then information is needed on the comparative costs of the different therapies and the comparative outcomes measured in terms of symptom alleviation, improved functioning and so on. In these circumstances, a cost-effectiveness analysis (in the narrow sense of the term) would be appropriate and sufficient (see p. 129).

If, to take a broader stance, the question is whether to invest available health system resources to treat either childhood depression or asthma, then decision-makers again need to know the relative costs of the two alternatives, but they now need a measure of effectiveness that uses a common metric across the fields of depression and asthma. The most commonly such employed measure is "utility," generated from health-related quality of life scales (see p. 130). In these circumstances a cost–utility analysis is needed (see p. 130).

To widen the perspective even further, if the question is whether to invest more money in the health system or more money in improving transport, launching a new environmental policy or bolstering a country's defense forces, then the research question becomes one of asking what are the comparative costs and merits of the different investment options, where "merit" will now need to be measured in a common unit across all of these broad areas of public policy. The usual choice of broad measure is monetary, leading to cost–benefit analysis (see p. 130).

The choice of question clearly influences the type of evaluation needed, but the choices are not mutually exclusive: a single study could support more than one type of analysis. A body of evidence that is well located within the clinical domain will be exactly what the treating professional needs but may not be appropriate for a higher level decision-making body, such as a health ministry. The broader the research question, the more demanding are the data needs: brutally summarized, cost–benefit analyses are harder to do than cost–utility analyses, which in turn are more difficult than cost-effectiveness analyses.

Linked to the specification of the question to be addressed is the *perspective* to be adopted. Is the evaluative information needed to help resource allocation within a particular agency (such as a child and adolescent mental health service) or within a particular system (such as the health care system or education system) or within the whole society? The breadth of perspective will determine the breadth of both the measurement of costs and the effectiveness or outcomes.

Cost Measurement

There are a number ways to categorize the costs associated with mental health problems. There are direct costs associated with the treatment services and associated supports, some of them delivered by non-health agencies. There are also indirect costs, which may fall to families, or may be measured in terms of lost productivity because of future disruptions to employment patterns. There may also be some unmeasured costs, perhaps reflecting the burden carried by family members, or societal concerns about antisocial behavior. In evaluations, the usual approach is to try to measure these elements as long-run marginal opportunity costs (Knapp, 1993). This helps to ensure that a long-term perspective on resource implications is employed, that only those effects on resources attributable to the program or service user are counted, and that costs are reckoned as opportunities forgone, not just money expended. How broadly the costs are measured will depend upon the perspective taken for the evaluation, which in turn depends upon the purpose of the study.

In carrying out evaluations in practice, the economist would be looking for data on service use patterns from one or more source. The data might come from organizational "billing" systems, recording the amounts that are transferred between a payer and a provider for services used by individual children or families. This is a common approach in US research, for example. In care systems without such payment mechanisms, there might nevertheless be routine information systems that record service contacts and referrals, which might provide the necessary data for an evaluation. However, in many countries there are no billing data, and organizational information systems are too rudimentary or inaccurate to provide the basis for cost calculation. In these circumstances, the usual approach is to collect information on patterns of service use through interviews with family members or service professionals (for which there are a number of tools, including the Client Service Receipt Inventory; Beecham & Knapp, 2001).

To the service use levels generated by information systems or from interviews the researcher would then attach unit cost estimates for each service (Beecham, 2000). It is not always necessary to calculate these unit costs anew. In England, for example, there is an excellent annual compendium of such unit costs which is very widely used in applied research (Curtis & Netten, 2006). This method of service use data capture (using a version of the Client Service Receipt Inventory and then attaching unit costs mostly drawn from the published annual compendium) was the approach employed in the two London cost-of-illness studies for antisocial behavior described on p. 124, whereas Foster and Bickman (2000), in their Fort Bragg study, were able to use records of financial transactions from local agencies.

Non-service costs are harder to measure than service costs, partly because of the difficulty of identifying the impacts (e.g., on parental employment patterns, or on a child's own future earning capacity) and partly because of the difficulty of then attaching a monetary value. (For further discussion of these issues see Brouwer, Rutten, & Koopmanschap, 2001; Johnston, Buxton, Jones *et al.*, 1999.)

Effectiveness Measurement

Probably the most intuitive mode of economic evaluation is cost-effectiveness analysis (CEA), now using the term in its narrower sense. It measures costs as set out above, and measures outcomes using instruments and scales familiar from clinical studies, because its focus is symptoms, behavior functioning, peer-group integration and so on. A CEA is employed to help decision-makers choose between alternative interventions available to or aimed at specific patient groups. An analysis would look at a single outcome dimension – such as change in a behavioral measure, or symptom-free days or self-esteem – and would then compute and compare the ratio of the difference in costs between two treatments to the difference in (primary) outcome (the so-called incremental cost-effectiveness ratio). For example, an evaluation of a home-based social work intervention for children and adolescents who have deliberately poisoned themselves by Byford, Harrington, Torgerson *et al.* (1999) measured suicidal ideation, hopelessness and family functioning as the main outcomes, and health, education, social care and voluntary sector services as the basis for cost measurement. Their randomized controlled trial, involving 162 children aged 16 years or under, found no significant difference in the main outcomes for costs, although parental satisfaction with treatment was significantly greater in the group that received a new social work intervention compared to those who received routine care.

A second example of a cost-effectiveness analysis is provided by Cunningham, Bremner, & Boyle (1995) who compared a large community-based parenting program for families of preschool children at risk of disruptive behavior with a clinic-based individual program. Among their outcome measures they chose adherence, behavior problems at home and child behavior more generally; their cost measures included the direct costs of the program plus costs associated with using other education and health care services. The community groups were found to report better outcomes, but they cost marginally more than the individual program.

An obvious weakness with the strict cost-effectiveness methodology is the focus on a single outcome dimension (in order to compute ratios) when people with mental health problems often have multiple needs for support and when most clinicians would expect to achieve improvements in more than one area. For this reason, cost-effectiveness ratios are sometimes computed for each of a number of outcome measures. This is sometimes called cost-consequences analysis. It has the advantage of breadth but poses a challenge if two or more ratios point to different interventions as the more cost-effective: in these circumstances, the decision-maker must weigh up the strength of evidence.

Making Trade-offs

Many evaluations of new interventions find them to be both more effective (the outcome profiles are better than for old or current interventions) but simultaneously more expensive. For example, the Cunningham, Bremner, & Boyle (1995) study found that a group-training program had better outcomes but slightly higher costs than an individual program. How is the trade-off to be made between the better outcomes and the higher expenditure necessary to achieve them?

The net benefit approach seeks to explicate the nature of the trade-off. It is most commonly seen today in the construction of *cost-effectiveness acceptability curves* (CEACs). These constructs show the probability that a new intervention will be cost-effective for each of a number of prespecified or implicit valuations of an outcome improvement by the decision-maker. To date, there is no published application of the use of the CEAC approach in child and adolescent mental health studies, but the technique has been highly instructive in other areas. An example that illustrates the approach would be the study by McCrone, Weeramanthri, Knapp *et al.* (2005) of computer-delivered cognitive–behavioral therapy (CBT) for anxiety and depression (among adults). These authors found the computer-delivered CBT to be more expensive in health service terms than standard primary care services, but also more effective in reducing depressive symptoms and anxiety. The fitted CEACs showed that, even if the value placed by society on a unit reduction in the Beck Depression Inventory was as little as £40, there was an 81% probability that the computer-delivered CBT would be viewed as cost-effective. Similarly, assigning a societal value of just £5 to each additional depression-free day would result in an 80% probability that CBT would be cost-effective. The advantage of the CEAC approach is that it makes transparent the trade-offs faced by decision-makers.

Utility Measurement

An increasingly commonly used evaluative mode that seeks to reduce outcomes to a single dimension is cost–utility analysis (CUA), which measures and then values the impact of an intervention in terms of improvements in preference-weighted, health-related quality of life. The value of the quality of life improvement is gauged in units of "utility," usually expressed by a combined index of the mortality and quality of life effects of an intervention. The best known and most robust such index is the Quality Adjusted Life Year (QALY).

CUAs have a number of distinct advantages, including using a unidimensional measure of impact, a generic measure which allows comparisons to be made across diagnostic or clinical groups (e.g., comparing psychiatry with oncology or cardiology), and a fully explicit methodology for weighting preferences and valuing health states. But these same features have sometimes been seen as disadvantages: the utility measure may be seen as too reductionist; the generic quality of life indicator may be insufficiently sensitive to the kinds of change expected in schizophrenia treatment; and a transparent approach to scale construction paradoxically opens the approach to criticism from those who question the values thereby obtained (see early reservations expressed by Chisholm, Healey, & Knapp, 1997). In particular, there are worries that the generic utility-generating instruments, such the EQ-5D (EuroQol Group, 1990) and the SF-6D (Brazier, Roberts, & Deverill, 2002), which are recommended by the National Institute for Health and Clinical Excellence (NICE), are insufficiently sensitive to the kinds of symptom and functioning change observed for people with mental health problems, and particularly for children and adolescents.

On the other hand, CUAs avoid the potential ambiguities with multidimensional outcomes in cost-effectiveness studies. The transparency of approach should obviously also be welcomed. Such an approach to economic evaluation produces an estimate of the cost per QALY-gain from one therapy or intervention and another. Estimates of this kind can then inform health care resource allocation decisions or priority setting, such as in the work of NICE, which has responsibility in England and Wales for providing national guidance on promoting good health and preventing and treating ill health.

There appears to be only one published example of a CUA in the child and adolescent mental health field, and it is unfortunately not a very strong example. Gilmore and Milne (2001) created an economic model that compared the costs and effects of methylphenidate and placebo for treating hyperactivity. Costs were calculated based on the assumption that all follow-ups would be hospital-based. Non-responders and those terminating treatment would be treated on average for 6 weeks. There would be an average of five out-patient attendances in the first year of treatment, followed by 3-monthly routine appointments. The authors acknowledged the methodological limitations of the framework used in the study, but concluded that the short-term treatment of hyperkinetic children with methylphenidate may be cost-effective. Gilmore and Milne used a cost–utility framework to structure their hypothetical model. They calculated a cost per QALY of between £7446 and £9177, depending on the severity of disorder. However, the unproven validity of currently generated QALY estimates in the child and adolescent mental health field leaves this finding as, at best, tentative.

The quandary that faces researchers and decision-makers in the UK today, and in some other countries that have chosen a strategic evidence-based approach to resource allocation in the health system, is that a generic outcome measure such as the QALY, when combined with cost estimates, can point to ways of achieving improved value for money, but if that QALY measure does not reflect the underlying effectiveness changes in the field, then it must surely be of very limited usefulness.

Benefit Measurement

Cost–benefit analysis asks whether the benefits of a treatment or policy exceed the costs. This would allow decision-makers to consider the merits not only of allocating resources within health care, but also of considering whether it would be more appropriate to invest in other sectors such as housing, education or defense. In this form of evaluation, all costs and outcomes (benefits) are valued in the same (monetary) units. If benefits exceed costs, the evaluation would provide support for the treatment, and vice versa. With two or more alternatives, the treatment with the greatest net benefit would be deemed the most efficient. Cost–benefit analyses are thus intrinsically attractive, but conducting them is especially problematic because of the difficulties associated with valuing outcomes in monetary terms.

Comparing costs incurred (e.g., on treatments) with costs saved (e.g., on future health services no longer needed) is not a cost–benefit analysis but a cost–offset comparison. This confusion is unfortunately still quite common. A cost–benefit analysis must measure outcomes (in terms of improved health or improved quality of life) and then convert them to monetary values. Consequently, studies such as that by Jacobson, Mulick, & Green (1999) of an early intensive behavioral program for children with pervasive development disorder or autism, which compared the costs of the intervention with cost savings into adulthood, are certainly interesting but not as helpful as studies that compare the costs *and* the outcomes of interventions.

The problem is that attaching values to the outcomes of child and adolescent mental health interventions is inherently complicated. Recent methodological advances in health economics may offer a way of obtaining direct valuations of health outcomes by patients, relatives or the general public. These techniques ask individuals to state the amount they would be prepared to pay (hypothetically) to achieve a given health state or health gain, or they observe actual behavior and deduce the implicit values (Olsen & Smith, 2001). They are likely to be quite difficult to apply in mental health contexts.

Another approach, which is beginning to be used more and more often to value health interventions, is "conjoint analysis": individuals are asked to rank different real world scenarios, which may consist of several dimensions (including, for instance, health outcomes, quality of life, time inputs, discomfort and stigma) and by including cost as one of these dimensions a monetary value can be elicited. While quite complex, the conjoint analysis approach has the advantage of not specifically asking individuals to put a monetary value on health states or health gain, which can make the technique easier to administer than traditional willingness-to-pay studies (Ryan, 1999).

Body of Evidence

There remain very few completed economic evaluations in the child and adolescent mental health field, and a number of those that have been undertaken have some methodological or other limitations. (Among the common problems are small sample sizes, methodological weaknesses and other design issues.) Romeo, Byford, and Knapp (2005) found only 14 published studies that could be described as economic evaluations. One or two others have been published subsequently, and there are certainly quite a number now under way, but this accumulated volume of evidence about such a fundamental issue as the efficient way to use scarce resources is clearly very disappointing. Without such evidence, decision-makers may well take decisions that are utterly inefficient, wasting resources as a result.

How are we to judge the quality of these evaluations? Two immediate checks can be made, one in relation to costs and one in relation to outcomes:

• Have all the relevant costs been taken into account? As we have seen, there are many and various inputs to a broadly defined mental health system – from health, social care, education, housing, social security and other agencies – plus economic consequences in terms of lost productivity, premature mortality and family impact. It might be necessary to measure all of these, depending on the policy or practice question that needs to be addressed and the perspective necessary for the evaluation.

• Are all the dimensions of effectiveness taken into account? Good mental health care is obviously not just about tackling clinical symptoms, but about improving an individual's ability to function in ways that are valued by them (such as performing well at school and integrating with peers) and of course about promoting quality of life.

Guidelines and quality checklists for health economist researchers and readers of their outputs are available (Drummond, Jefferson *et al.*, 1996), addressing a wider set of issues than the two suggested above.

As well as a limited number of completed evaluations, there must also be concern that most of the completed economic studies have been undertaken in North America, parts of western Europe and Australia. Unfortunately, the results of economic evaluations often do not transfer well from one health or care system to another, and therefore not between countries. This is primarily because of differences in the structure of health systems, financing arrangements, incentive structures and relative price levels. There might also be differences in the appropriate choice of comparator: a new therapeutic approach might look attractive compared to current arrangements in one country but not in comparison to what is generally the norm elsewhere. It is unfeasible and certainly unnecessary to carry out an evaluation every time a policy decision needs to be taken, but evidence-based decisions are generally thought to be better than evidence-free decisions. This could mean using the results from a study carried out in another country, updating a previous study or carrying out a modest adaptation to adjust for context.

Looking across the mental health field more generally, the accumulation of new cost-effectiveness evidence has accelerated in recent years. There have tended to be more cost-effectiveness studies in diagnostic areas when new classes of medication are launched because the pharmaceutical industry looks to economic evaluative evidence to support its marketing, and health care funding and delivery bodies also want their own independent evidence. Consequently, in other parts of the mental health territory, many economic studies of depression followed the licensing of the early selective serotonin reuptake inhibitors (SSRIs) and later antidepressants with other mechanisms of action. Similarly, the arrival of the atypical antipsychotics and the cholinesterase inhibitors stimulated much economics research on, respectively, the treatment of schizophrenia and Alzheimer disease.

Conclusions

The starting point for an interest in the economics of child and adolescent mental health is clearly scarcity: it is the recognition that there are not, and indeed there never will be, enough resources available to meet all of the needs of children and families. There is still a notion abroad in some parts of some health systems that incremental growth in budgets will gradually remove all need, but this is surely wildly overoptimistic. We cannot and must not avoid facing up to the choices that have to be made in the face of scarcity. In making those choices we would want our decision-makers to be explicit and transparent about the criteria that they are employing. Are they looking to maximize effectiveness in terms of symptom alleviation or aggregate quality of life, to redistribute resources to poorer communities within society or to ensure that access to skilled resources is equally available to every family?

Within this set of criteria, cost-effectiveness obviously has a role. The cost-effectiveness criterion should probably be seen as secondary. If, for example, a therapeutic intervention has been shown to be effective in improving the well-being of children and families, and appears to be more effective than currently available therapies, then it would be natural to ask about the relative costs of the two options and to compare those costs with the outcome gains. Balancing outcome improvements with higher costs is, however, quite a challenge. A great many economic evaluations across the health spectrum today find that new therapies (whether pharmacological, psychological or organizational) offer better outcome profiles than currently prevalent interventions, but they do so at higher cost. The decision-maker, whether this is the individual care professional working with children and families, or their line manager and budget holder, or someone near the top of the health ministry, then faces a difficult trade-off: are the better outcomes from the new intervention worth the higher cost of introducing that intervention?

There have been a number of types of request for economic insights in the child and adolescent mental health field. In this chapter I have illustrated some of those, including requests to measure the overall cost impact of a particular disorder or diagnosis (so-called cost-of-illness studies). Second, there are cost–offset studies that compare the amounts expended on interventions with the longer term savings from introducing those interventions. Third, and much the most powerful and useful, are cost-effectiveness studies (using the term generically also to include cost–benefit and cost–utility studies). These weigh up costs *and* outcomes, and therefore give a more complete and rounded view as to the consequences of introducing different interventions.

The available economics evidence base in the child and adolescent mental health field is disappointingly underdeveloped at present, but more is now being invested in the area, including a number of new studies that will – in time – offer valuable new insights into the resource consequences and cost-effectiveness properties of different interventions aimed at meeting the needs of children and families.

References

Beecham, J. K. (2000). *Unit costs: Not exactly child's play*. London: Department of Health.

Beecham, J. K., & Knapp, M. R. J. (2001). Costing psychiatric interventions. In G. Thornicroft (Ed.), *Measuring mental health needs* (2nd ed.). London: Gaskell.

Bickman, L., Guthrie, P. R., Foster, E. M., Lambert, E. W., Summerfelt, W. T., Breda, C., *et al.* (1995). *Managed care in mental health: The Fort Bragg experiment*. New York: Plenum.

Brazier, J., Roberts, J., & Deverill, M. (2002). The estimation of a preference-based single index measure for health from the SF-36. *Journal of Health Economics*, *21*, 271–292.

Brouwer, W., Rutten, F., & Koopmanschap, M. (2001). Costing in economic evaluations. In M. Drummond & A. McGuire (Eds.), *Economic evaluation in health care: Merging theory with practice*. New York: Oxford University Press.

Byford, S., Harrington, R., Torgerson, D., Kerfoot, M., Dyer, E., Harrington, V., *et al.* (1999). Cost-effectiveness analysis of a home-based social work intervention for children and adolescents who have deliberately poisoned themselves: the results of a randomised controlled trial. *British Journal of Psychiatry*, *174*, 56–62.

Chisholm, D., Healey, A., & Knapp, M. (1997). QALYs and mental health care. *Social Psychiatry and Psychiatric Epidemiology*, *32*, 68–75.

Cohen, M. A. (1998). The monetary value of saving a high-risk youth. *Journal of Quantitative Criminology*, *14*, 5–33.

Cunningham, C. E., Bremner, R., & Boyle, M. (1995). Large group community-based parenting programs for families of preschoolers at risk for disruptive behaviour disorders: utilisation, cost effectiveness, and outcome. *Journal of Child Psychology and Psychiatry*, *36*, 1141–1159.

Curtis, L., & Netten, A. (2006). *Unit costs of health and social care, 2006*. University of Kent: PSSRU.

Dretzke, J., Frew, E., Davenport, C., Barlow, J., Stewart-Brown, S., Sandercock, J., *et al.* (2005). The effectiveness and cost-effectiveness of parent training/education programmes for the treatment of conduct disorder, including oppositional defiance disorder, in children. *Health Technology Assessment*, *9*, 50.

Drummond, M. F., Jefferson, T. O. for BMJ Working Party. (1996). Guidelines for authors and peer-reviewers of economic submissions to the *British Medical Journal*. *British Medical Journal*, *313*, 275–283.

EuroQol Group. (1990). EuroQol: A new facility for the measurement of health-related quality of life. *Health Policy*, *16*, 199–208.

Farrington, D. P. (2001). Key results from the first forty years of the Cambridge Study in Delinquent Development. In T. P. Thornberry, & M. D. Krohn (Eds.), *Taking stock of delinquency*. New York: Kluwer.

Fombonne, E., Wostear, G., Cooper, V., Harrington, R., & Rutter, M. (2001). The Maudsley long-term follow-up of child and adolescent depression. *British Journal of Psychiatry*, *179*, 210–217.

Foster, E. M., & Bickman, L. (2000). Refining the cost analyses of the Fort Bragg evaluation: the impact of cost-offset and cost shifting. *Mental Health Services Research*, *2*, 13–25.

Foster, E. M., & Connor, T. (2005). Public costs of better mental health services for children and adolescents. *Psychiatric Services*, *57*, 50–55.

Foster, E. M., & Jones, D. E., Conduct Problems Prevention Research Group. (2005). The high costs of aggression: public expenditures resulting from conduct disorder. *American Journal of Public Health*, *95*, 1767–1772.

Glied, S., & Evans Cuellar, A. (2003). Trends and issues in child and adolescent mental health. *Health Affairs*, *22*, 39–50.

Gilmore, A., & Milne, R. (2001). Methylphenidate in children with hyperactivity: review and cost–utility analysis. *Pharmacoepidemiology and Drug Safety*, *10*, 85–94.

Gustafsson, P. A., & Svedin, C.-G. (1988). Cost effectiveness: family therapy in a pediatric setting. *Family Systems Medicine*, 2, 162–175.

Healey, A., Knapp, M., & Farrington, D. (2004). Adult labour market implications of antisocial behaviour in childhood and adolescence: findings from a UK longitudinal study. *Applied Economics*, *36*, 93–105.

Jacobson, J. W., Mulick, J. A., & Green, G. (1999). Cost-benefit estimates for early intensive behavioural intervention for young children with autism: General model and single state case. *Behavioural Interventions*, *13*, 201–226.

Järbrink, K., & Knapp, M. R. J. (2001). The economic impact of autism in Britain. *Autism*, *5*(1), 7–22.

Johnston, K., Buxton, M. J., Jones, D. R., & Fitzpatrick, R. (1999). Assessing the costs of healthcare technologies in clinical trials. *Health Technology Assessment*, *3*, 1–76.

Knapp, M. R. J. (1993). Principles of applied cost research. In A. Netten, & J. Beecham (Eds.), *Costing community care: Theory and practice*. Aldershot: Ashgate.

Knapp, M. R. J., Scott, S., & Davies, J. (1998). The cost of antisocial behaviour in younger children. *Clinical Child Psychology and Psychiatry*, *4*, 457–473.

Knapp, M., McCrone, P., Fombonne, E., Beecham, J., & Wostear, G. (2002). The Maudsley long-term follow-up study of child and adolescent depression: impact of comorbid conduct disorder on service use and costs in adulthood. *British Journal of Psychiatry*, *180*(1), 19–23.

Maughan, B. (1989). Growing up in the inner city: findings from the inner London longitudinal study. *Paediatric and Perinatal Epidemiology*, *3*, 195–215.

McCrone, P., Knapp, M., & Fombonne, E. (2005). The Maudsley long-term follow-up of childhood and adolescent depression: predicting costs in adulthood. *European Child and Adolescent Psychiatry*, *14*, 407–413.

McCrone, P., Weeramanthri, T., Knapp, M. R. J., Rushton, A., Trowell, J., Miles, G., *et al.* (2005). Cost effectiveness of individual vs. group psychotherapy for sexually abused girls. *Child and Adolescent Mental Health*, *10*, 26–31.

Olsen, J. A., & Smith, R. D. (2001). Theory versus practice: a review of 'willingness to pay' in health and health care. *Health Economics*, *10*, 39–52.

Romeo, R., Byford, S., & Knapp, M. (2005). Economic evaluations of child and adolescent mental health interventions: a systematic review. *Journal of Child Psychology and Psychiatry*, *46*, 919–930.

Romeo, R., Knapp, M., & Scott, S. (2006). Economic cost of severe antisocial behaviour in children – and who pays it. *British Journal of Psychiatry*, *188*, 547–553.

Ryan, M. (1999). Using conjoint analysis to go beyond health outcomes: an application to in vitro fertilisation. *Social Sciences and Medicine*, *8*, 535–546.

Schweinhart, L. J. (2004). The High/Scope Perry Preschool Study through age 40: summary, conclusions and frequently asked questions. Ypsilanti, MI: The High/Scope Educational Foundation.

Scott, S., Knapp, M., Henderson, J., & Maughan, B. (2001). Financial cost of social exclusion: follow-up study of antisocial children into adulthood. *British Medical Journal*, *323*, 191–194.

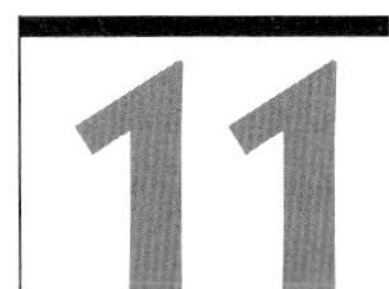

What Can We Learn from Structural and Functional Brain Imaging?

Christopher Frith and Uta Frith

Issues in the Study of Brain Imaging in Children

The study of the structure and function of the human brain was dramatically enhanced by the development of positron emission tomography (PET) and magnetic resonance imaging (MRI) in the last quarter of the last century. These methods are exciting tools for studying the development of brain structure and function throughout the lifespan. They can throw new light on developmental disorders and psychiatric conditions with their origin in childhood. As a result, an increasing number of neuroimaging studies are being published in this field. However, how have the techniques been applied and how do they influence what is being studied? We consider examples of neuroimaging studies in typical and atypical development to illustrate both the promise and the problems of these remarkable new tools.

At the outset we should point out some important limitations of brain imaging techniques often ignored in the over-enthusiastic interpretation of the compelling colored images of brains in action. Any study of abnormality in which brain structure or function in patients is compared with healthy controls is essentially correlational. If we find a significant brain difference we cannot conclude that this difference is the cause of the problem. The brain difference may result from some other factor, which has not been controlled for, or may even be a secondary consequence of the problem.

In studies of brain function, as opposed to brain structure, we can conduct genuine experiments where we can be confident that the condition we have applied is the cause of the change in brain activity. For example, we can be sure that the sight of a face is the cause of brain activity seen in inferior temporal cortex. However, we cannot invert the logic and conclude that activity in inferior temporal cortex can cause the experience of a face. To justify such conclusions we need to manipulate brain activity directly with techniques such as transcranial magnetic stimulation (TMS) or direct electrical stimulation. These issues are discussed later in this chapter.

Rutter's Child and Adolescent Psychiatry, 5th edition. Edited by M. Rutter, D. Bishop, D. Pine, S. Scott, J. Stevenson, E. Taylor and A. Thapar. © 2008 Blackwell Publishing, ISBN: 978-1-4051-4549-7.

Brain Imaging Techniques

Structural MRI

MRI is the method of choice for visualizing the structure of the human brain. This method has largely replaced computed tomography (CT) scanning because it has better resolution and does not involve exposure to harmful radiation. By placing the brain in a strong magnetic field and passing harmless, low-frequency radio waves through it, the density of hydrogen (i.e., water) at any point in the brain can be measured. Because the density of water varies systematically between the different components of the brain (white matter, gray matter, cerebral spinal fluid), this measurement builds up an image of the brain with a resolution of approximately 1 mm, which approaches the quality of a photograph of a postmortem brain slice. Such images can be obtained in approximately 15 minutes and can be used to detect changes in volume or shape in specific brain structures as well as to measure the volume of gray and white matter.

The more recently developed technique of diffusion tensor imaging (DTI) visualizes the diffusion of water molecules along white matter tracts. This method permits the tracing of long-range connections between cortical areas and can thus be used to measure anatomical connectivity (Croxson, Johansen-Berg, Behrens *et al.*, 2005). However, the technique only reveals approximate connectivity of bundles of white matter rather than single neurons. Currently, questions about the direction of flow of signals can only be answered from animal studies.

EEG and MEG (see chapter 17)

There are many methods for measuring human brain function, each with particular advantages and disadvantages. It has long been known that the basic units of brain function – the neurons – generate and propagate electrical impulses. The electroencephalograph (EEG) measures this electrical activity directly via electrodes attached to the scalp. This technique can track neural events at very short time intervals, but cannot tell very precisely where in the brain these events take place. Magneto-encephalography (MEG) measures the changing magnetic fields associated with the electrical activity of neurons using detectors placed close to the head. This technique also has very good temporal resolution and somewhat better spatial resolution than EEG, particularly for sources close to the detectors. However, the interpretation of data gathered through both techniques suffers from a fundamental problem. For any pattern of electrical or magnetic activity measured at the scalp there are many different possible sources of this activity within the brain. This is known as the inverse problem. Methods for solving this problem are currently under development (Mattout, Phillips, Penny *et al.*, 2006). The problem of localizing the source of brain activity does not arise with functional MRI (fMRI).

PET, fMRI and NIRS

These techniques use indirect methods for detecting changes in neural activity. They capitalize on the fact that, when neurons become active, they consume oxygen carried by hemoglobin in red blood cells from local capillaries. The oxygen uptake in the blood vessels can be made visible in the scanner, and this uptake reflects neural activity. The more oxygen is detected in a particular region, the greater the neural activity.

The local response to this oxygen utilization is a local increase in blood flow to regions of increased neural activity, occurring after a delay of approximately 1–5 seconds. The precise mechanism by which neural activity causes an increase in blood flow (the hemodynamic response) is unknown. Recent work suggests that most brain energy is used to power postsynaptic currents and action potentials rather than presynaptic activity. Furthermore, the hemodynamic response seems to be driven by neurotransmitter-related signaling and not directly by the local energy needs (i.e., oxygen consumption) of the brain (Attwell & Iadecola, 2002). PET measures changes in blood flow directly via injection of a radioactive tracer. Because of the risk associated with radiation, this method is rarely used with children. In contrast, fMRI is considered safe as it measures changes in blood flow without the need for any tracer. This is possible because the blood flow increase is associated with a change in the ratio of oxyhemoglobin to deoxyhemoglobin with the blood becoming more oxygenated. These two forms of hemoglobin have different magnetic properties so changes in their ratio can be detected by MRI (blood oxygenation level dependent contrast; BOLD). Studies of animals have shown that there is a good correspondence between changes in neural activity and changes in the BOLD signal (Logothetis, Pauls, Augath *et al.*, 2001).

The two forms of hemoglobin also differ in color: red as in arteries and blue as in veins. This color change can be measured by near-infrared spectroscopy (NIRS) using light transmitters and detectors close to the scalp. The value of this methodology for brain imaging is currently being established (Huppert, Hoge, Diamond *et al.*, 2006). NIRS has the advantage of being much cheaper and less cumbersome than fMRI and may prove to be particularly useful in the study of newborn infants because their thin skulls cause less attenuation of the light signal (Bartocci, Bergqvist, Lagercrantz *et al.*, 2006).

EEG/MEG and fMRI are complementary measures in that EEG/MEG tells us precisely when neural events are happening, but not precisely where they are happening, while fMRI tells us where things are happening, but with a crude time scale of seconds rather than milliseconds. Although technically demanding, it is now possible to acquire data simultaneously in these two imaging modalities. This approach is particularly relevant in the field of epilepsy (Salek-Haddadi, Diehl, Hamandi *et al.*, 2006), because EEG can detect the abnormal epileptic activity and fMRI can localize its source in the brain. However, more frequently, the two techniques are used consecutively in the same participants performing the same task. In general, fMRI can be used to locate the source of the signals, such as spikes, evoked potentials or oscillations detected by EEG/MEG. Temporal resolution is particularly important if we want to understand neural mechanisms and address questions of control when it is vital to know whether activity in one region occurs before or after activity in another region (Bar, Kassam, Ghuman *et al.*, 2006).

Connectivity

Until recently, the majority of brain imaging studies have been concerned with localization of function (functional specialization or brain mapping). However, in the long run, understanding how the brain works will depend on revealing the mechanism by which different brain regions interact with one another (functional integration). By measuring correlations across time between neural activity in different brain regions it is possible to show that certain regions are functionally connected. This pattern of connectivity will change depending upon the task being performed by the subject (Sakai & Passingham, 2003). More sophisticated analysis techniques are currently being developed that not only show that regions are functionally connected, but also assess the direction of causality associated with this interaction (Penny, Stephan, Mechelli *et al.*, 2004).

Chemical Imaging

The transmission of signals between neurons depends upon chemical messengers (neurotransmitters) rather than electrical signals. Through the use of appropriate radioactive tracers, PET can be used to measure neurotransmitter release and receptor occupancy. This technique has been of great value in the study of disorders, such as Parkinson disease, in which there is a specific loss of the neurotransmitter dopamine (Au, Adams, Troiano *et al.*, 2005). However, the use of radioactive tracers is too risky a technique to apply to children. MRI spectroscopy (MRS) cannot replace PET for the study of neurotransmitters, but it can be used to study other chemical markers of brain abnormality (Frangou & Williams, 1996). For example, the concentration of *N*-acetylaspartate (NAA) can be measured in brain tissue. This substance is thought to be a marker that decreases in processes where neurons die. MRS has been used to detect metabolic changes associated with abnormal aging (Pettegrew, Panchalingam, Moossy *et al.*, 1988) and also to monitor effects of drug treatment (Satlin, Bodick, Offen *et al.*, 1997). The spatial and temporal resolution of MRS is lower than those of fMRI, and the technique has still to prove itself (Gujar, Maheshwari, Bjorkman-Burtscher *et al.*, 2005). Nevertheless, interesting results concerning developmental disorders are al-ready beginning to emerge (Sun, Jin, Zang *et al.*, 2005). In the future, this technique will undoubtedly provide important new data for the understanding of abnormal brain development.

Genomic Imaging

There is increasing interest in studying genetic factors in brain function by looking at correlates of allelic variation (see chapter 23). For example, different forms of the serotonin (*5-HT*) transporter gene, (*5-HTT*), have been found to relate to individual differences in traits related to negative affect, leading to the suggestion that genotype might be associated with variation in amygdala activation. Canli, Omura, Haas *et al.* (2005) showed that *5-HTT* genotype was indeed associated with functional activation of the amygdala, and also with structural variation in frontal cortical regions, anterior cingulate and cerebellum. A particularly exciting possibility for the future is the imaging of local changes in gene expression. This would be an enormously powerful adjunct to the study of brain development, but it is not yet available for studying the human brain (Dijkhuizen, 2006).

To finish with a note of caution, despite claims to the contrary, all the techniques discussed above are still primarily of interest to researchers rather than clinicians, except in individual cases of gross structural abnormalities (see chapter 22). Although there is the potential for major breakthroughs in diagnosis and treatment, these are yet to be realized. Perhaps the area where these techniques have the most immediate practical value is in monitoring the effects of treatment on the brain. For example, studies of patients with obsessive-compulsive disorder (OCD) have shown that brain changes occur with psychological therapies as well as drug therapies (Brody, Saxena, Schwartz *et al.*, 1998). Imaging also has the potential to distinguish between brain changes brought about by treatment and changes relating to the natural course of the disorder (Casey & Durston, 2006).

Analysis of Imaging Data

Some fundamental problems of analysis of brain images apply to both structure and function. First, there is the problem of aligning brains from different individuals. One solution is to choose regions of interest (ROIs). For example, the amygdala can be identified and measured in each brain, and then these measurements, whether volumes or activity, are put together for analysis. The disadvantages of this approach follow, first, from the need to define the regions of interest and, second, from throwing away all the data outside the regions of interest.

At the opposite extreme are techniques such as statistical parametric mapping (SPM) in which brains are first normalized to a template and then comparisons are made on a voxel by voxel basis. A voxel is the basic element of spatial resolution, typically a cube with sides of approximately 2 mm. Such a voxel typically contains approximately 500 K neurons and several million synapses. In the case of structural images this technique is known as voxel-based morphometry (VBM). This technique is suitable for looking at fairly small-scale changes in structure, but is not applicable for large-scale changes (Ashburner & Friston, 2000). This is because each brain is first normalized to a standard template, thus eliminating large-scale differences between individuals. Techniques for identifying large-scale changes in brain structure, which are essentially differences in shape, are currently being developed but have yet to be routinely applied (Ashburner, Hutton, Frackowiak *et al.*, 1998).

Second, there is the problem of multiple comparisons. Analysis of a whole brain involves thousand of comparisons. Unless there are well-justified a priori hypotheses, strict levels of significance corrected for multiple comparisons must be applied.

The colorful brain images associated with fMRI studies must always be interpreted with caution. They are not direct reflections of brain activity, but typically show differences in brain activity between one state and another rather than absolute activity. They are usually maps of statistical differences rather than absolute measures. Thus, the brighter the blob, the greater the difference between the conditions or the people that are being compared.

Difficulties in Using Brain Scanning Techniques with Children

Before the scan begins the researcher or clinician must explain the procedure to the participants and make sure that they are free of all metallic objects. Prior practice in a "mock-up" scanner can be particularly helpful.

Even though it is non-invasive, there is no denying that having an MRI scan is not a pleasant experience. Not only does the head have to be put into a small and confined space, but the scanner produces a very loud noise. This noise is audible even through the routinely used and constantly improved earphones. Even some adults who volunteer for scanning may discover that they are claustrophobic when lying in the scanner.

Perhaps the greatest limitation as regards children is the requirement to lie completely still in the scanner. Unfortunately, keeping completely still for at least several minutes at a time is a requirement for MRI. While a structural scan can be completed in about 10–15 minutes, a functional scan could last for anything between 20 and 60 minutes or more. With young children sedation has been used in some studies. This means that the psychological tasks that are used when investigating brain activity and demand fully waking attention cannot be performed. Interestingly, very small babies can be swaddled so that they are calm and lie very still in the scanner (Dehaene-Lambertz, Dehaene, & Hertz-Pannier, 2002). Unfortunately, because of concerns with as yet unknown risks that might conceivably be associated with exposure to magnetic resonance, studies with newborns or infants have been carried out only rarely. While structural studies are increasingly applied to children from age 4 onwards (Giedd, Blumenthal, Jeffries *et al.*, 1999; Gogtay, Gield, Lusk *et al.*, 2004), functional studies have only rarely been conducted with children under the age of 8 years. This is frustrating because it is in the earlier years that the most interesting and important developmental changes in cognitive processes take place.

Brain Function and Cognitive Architecture

It is often stated that it is only by recording the activity in single neurons that we can come to an understanding of the mechanisms of brain function. Such recording is not really feasible in the human brain. The only exception occurs in cases of severe epilepsy where electrodes are sometimes implanted, typically in medial temporal cortex (Kreiman, Koch, & Fried, 2000) to allow precise location of seizure activity prior to surgery. Brain imaging as currently used means we see activity averaged across thousands, if not millions of neurons. Thus, relative to single cell recording, brain imaging techniques must appear extremely crude. However, given that the brain contains 100 billion neurons, there is clearly a place for studies at a much coarser grain in which activity across the whole brain can be observed. MRI studies can provide important guidance as to where to place electrodes for subsequent single neuron recording (Tsao, Freiwald, Tootell *et al.*, 2006). The coarse grain of brain imaging studies is also more appropriate for current levels of theorizing about cognitive processes. The language of cognition is critical for making the link between, on the one hand, physiological processes in the brain and, on the other hand, mental activity and behavior. The wealth of information available even from a coarse brain imaging study can be too much to be explained by extant cognitive theories. Studies of the mechanisms by which brain regions interact typically involve not more than three or four different brain regions (Meyer-Lindenberg, Hairi, Munoz *et al.*, 2005).

Whether activity is measured in the firing of a single neuron or indirectly from millions of neurons throughout the brain using EEG or fMRI, such studies are essentially correlational. Because we can reliably observe activity in, for example, the fusiform gyrus when subjects observe faces, this does not prove that this region is necessary for perceiving faces. Studies of the effects of brain lesions are an important complement for brain imaging studies, because lesion studies can show whether a brain region is necessary for a particular function. It is now possible to produce short-lived "lesions" in healthy volunteers with the use of TMS, in particular the repetitive version (rTMS). This procedure can reduce cortical excitability for some minutes after application. The precise mechanism of this effect is not clear, but it may result from changes in synaptic efficacy. While the exact location of the "lesion" induced by this technique is difficult to establish, the technique does provide an important experimental alternative to the study of patients with lesions (Cowey & Walsh, 2001). However, TMS is not suitable for the study of children. Although it is considered a safe method for the study of healthy adult volunteers, there is a risk of eliciting seizures, and it is not known what effects rTMS might have on the developing brain.

Brain Changes in Typical Development

The need for normal developmental information on typical brain and cognitive development is obvious, not only for its own sake, but also because we need a baseline for knowing what constitutes an abnormality (i.e., what lies beyond normal variation). All developmental scientists would agree that cross-sectional data are less informative than longitudinal data (Kraemer, Yesavage, Taylor *et al.*, 2000). The collection of data on the same child at key points in time is highly desirable, but it makes heavy demands on research time and effort. Fortunately, some examples of such studies exist already, although the timespan covered is still relatively narrow. For the reasons discussed above, it is impractical to subject healthy children to lengthy scanning procedures before middle to late childhood. Ideally, one would like to start studying the development of the brain, in terms of structure and function, straight from birth at frequent intervals. This study is still very new, but reviews of human brain maturation based on structural neuroimaging techniques, which require only brief scanning sessions, are beginning to appear (Toga, Thompson, & Sowell, 2006).

Structural Studies

Lenroot and Giedd (2006) provide a comprehensive review of studies of structural brain changes during normal development from approximately 5 years onwards. However, the most systematic studies concern brain development during adolescence (Blakemore & Choudhury, 2006; Paus, Collins, Evans *et al.*, 2001). MRI studies demonstrate that in prefrontal cortex (PFC) there is an increase in the density of gray matter (the layer of cortex that contains neurons) up to the onset of puberty followed by a subsequent rapid decrease in gray matter density from just after puberty and throughout adolescence, continuing into early adulthood. At the same time, there is an increase in the density of cortical white matter (the layer of cortex that contains the connections between neurons) from puberty throughout adolescence and into adulthood. The dorsolateral prefrontal cortex is notably late in reaching adult levels of cortical thickness. Complex patterns of change related to gender are observed in specific structures such as the amygdala and hippocampus. Such findings are difficult to interpret without a theory of what the observed changes mean.

One interesting area of speculation concerns ideas about brain reorganization at different ages. Results of earlier post-mortem investigations of human brain development suggest that the cortical changes seen in MRI mainly reflect two cellular processes occurring during infancy and adolescence: first, synaptogenesis followed by synaptic pruning, and, second, axonal myelination (Benes, 1989; Huttenlocher, 1979; Huttenlocher, de Courten, Garey *et al.*, 1982; Yakovlev & Lecours, 1967). Myelination speeds up nerve conduction and the associated cognitive processes. It has been hypothesized that synaptogenesis and pruning fine-tune neural circuitry in the PFC and other cortical regions, and thus increase efficiency of the cognitive systems they subserve. It is important to distinguish two types of neuron: feedforward or driving neurons, which carry information about the outside world, and feedback or modulatory neurons, whose function is to modulate the driving neurons. Feedforward connections run from primary sensory areas carrying sensory signals to higher level association cortex. Feedback connections run in the opposite direction and modulate the effects of the sensory signals at earlier stages of processing. Recent studies in animals have shown that the process of refining connections through synaptogenesis and pruning applies to lateral and feedback connections, but not to feedforward connections, which are established much earlier (Price, Kennedy, Dehay *et al.*, 2006).

As Paus (2005) comments, developmental studies of structural changes during adolescence are as yet at a preliminary stage and the meaning of gray matter increases or decreases is still a matter for speculation. However, through a combination of structural and functional studies it may be possible to obtain indices of critical variables such as synaptic density (Marcar, Strassle, Loenneker *et al.*, 2004).

Functional Studies

Interpretation of changes in brain activity associated with development is an order of magnitude more difficult than the interpretation of structural changes. In part, this problem springs from the lack of a framework for the understanding of the development of brain function. One of the burning questions in developmental psychology is to what extent there is regional specialization of brain functions from birth. It is generally assumed that programmed brain maturation interacts with modification by experience. Perhaps development proceeds along a path of differentiation of brain function with initially more global and more diffuse cognitive abilities being replaced by more specific and spatially localized functions. These ideas could be explored by scanning young children at those critical stages when behavioral and cognitive changes are most conspicuous.

A result that highlights very early specialization for cognitive functions, in this case speech processing, comes from a pioneering fMRI study by Dehaene-Lambertz, Dehaene, & Hertz-Pannier (2002). These researchers exposed swaddled 3-month-old infants to speech and non-speech noises. Remarkably, the left-lateralized brain structures known from adult studies to be activated preferentially by speech were also active in the babies' brains when they heard speech.

Schlaggar, Brown, Lugar *et al.* (2002) studied single word processing in 7- to 10-year-old children and adults and found differences in circumscribed frontal and extra-striate regions. Some of these differences were dependent on age rather than performance, suggesting maturational effects.

There is also evidence for changes in brain structure and function solely in response to environmental input in studies with adults. For example, Draganski, Gaser, Busch *et al.* (2004) observed a transient increase in gray matter in regions concerned with the analysis of motion in people who practiced juggling for 3 months. Paulesu, McCrory, Fazio *et al.* (2000) observed subtle differences in brain activity associated with reading, between English and Italian participants, presumably as a consequence of exposure to English or Italian orthography, respectively.

Thus, in adults at least, the learning of novel tasks is associated with a shift from activity in many areas concerned with general problem-solving (including frontal cortex) to activity in a few specialized areas (Jenkins, Brooks, Nixon *et al.*, 1994). Similar changes can be observed during development. In a simple arithmetic task, Rivera, Reiss, Eckert *et al.* (2005) found that younger subjects showed greater activity in prefrontal cortex, while adults showed greater activity in inferior parietal cortex, suggesting increased functional specialization in this area for mental arithmetic. Durston, Davidson, Tottenham *et al.* (2006) observed similar shifts with age towards increased focal activation in a cognitive control task. Passarotti, Paul, Russiere *et al.* (2003) studied face and location processing in 10- to 12-year-old children. Here again the children showed a more distributed pattern of brain activity than adults.

What Can Brain Imaging Reveal About Abnormal Development?

At first glance it seems a simple step from finding a brain abnormality to finding the cause of a neurodevelopmental disorder. But can we be sure that the abnormality we find is a cause of the disorder rather than merely a correlate or marker? Is the abnormality we find actually the way the plastic brain compensates for a developmental derailment at an earlier stage, now invisible?

Spelke (2002) points out the usefulness of functional neuroimaging methods in discovering the neural signatures of cognitive processes and by implication their change or persistence over development. The term neural signature is neutral as to whether the brain activations seen while the volunteer engages in a particular mental process are a correlate, cause or consequence of this process. Imaging techniques also provide the possibility of finding differences in this signature in children whose development is atypical. However, there are many pitfalls in explaining the cause of a disorder of development.

For instance, Morton (2004) reviewed a range of developmental disorders and showed in detailed examples that performance on psychological tests does not map in one-to-one fashion to underlying cognitive processes and by implication to underlying brain processes. Thus, when interpreting activations obtained from scanning studies, analyses have to be carried out at different levels simultaneously of behavior, cognition and brain. This is essential for understanding abnormalities of brain function when individuals are compared who may show the same performance on behavioral tests but different patterns of brain activation. We would infer that they perform the task in a different way. For the same reason, findings from brain imaging studies cannot be mapped directly to the behavioral manifestations of a disorder, but should be mapped to abnormalities in the specific neurocognitive processes that are thought to give rise to the behavior.

Success in distinguishing different developmental disorders requires a degree of specificity, but at what level should this specificity apply? For example, abnormalities of the developing brain are always likely to involve abnormal connectivity because it is connectivity that is modified by maturation and experience. In this case the specificity lies in precisely where the abnormal connections occur. Understanding of brain function at this level of detail will require considerable development in techniques for measuring connectivity and in mechanistic theories of cognition.

Compensation

It has long been thought that extensive damage that in adulthood would result in marked neuropsychological deficits, is associated with only mild deficits in children. This has been taken to mean that the developing brain is more plastic and better able to cope with brain injury than the mature brain, possibly by adapting brain systems unaffected by the injury. In the case of focal brain damage from birth or early infancy, brain regions tend to take over functions that are not normally carried out by this region (Krageloh-Mann, 2004; Stiles, Reilly, Paul *et al.*, 2005). Examples are changes in the organization of visuospatial and language processes (Lidzba, Staudt, Wilke *et al.*, 2006). Furthermore, these compensatory processes are enhanced through teaching. Thus, remedial teaching of reading strategies can change the pattern of brain activity in dyslexic children when reading (Shaywitz, Shaywitz, Blachman *et al.*, 2004) and similar results have been found for adult dyslexics (Eden, Jones, Cappell *et al.*, 2004).

Abnormality or Compensatory Adaptation?

Compensatory adaptations make the study of the abnormal brain extremely complicated. First, the same overt behavior may be achieved by different cognitive processes and associated brain systems. Brain imaging has an important role in revealing these hidden differences. An interesting example of what it means when a brain "abnormality" reflects adaptation rather than being the prime cause of the developmental abnormality comes from a study of Tourette syndrome (see chapter 44). The tics that characterize this disorder are probably caused by pathology in the basal ganglia (Peterson, Thomas, Kane *et al.*, 2003). However, abnormalities in the volume of dorsolateral prefrontal cortex (DLPFC) have also been observed. Plessen, Grüner, Lundervold *et al.* (2006) have speculated that these changes in DLPFC reflect an adaptation enabling children to suppress their tics in social situations. Thus, abnormally high activity in PFC found in this group, far from being a sign of primary abnormality, is instead a sign of high demands for inhibition. This is also a striking example of compensation during brain development.

Cause or Consequence?

Abnormal brain changes could also be a consequence rather than the cause of an abnormality. For example, a number of studies suggest that people with autism show a lack of specific activity in response to faces in the fusiform gyrus. However, this may not be a primary abnormality. Schultz (2005) has proposed that this is a consequence of a more basic lack of interest in social stimuli, which in turn may be a result of faulty amygdala functioning. A lack of social interest might plausibly cause a failure to develop expertise in face processing, and therefore might result in the absence of a specialized face processing area in the fusiform gyrus.

Clearly, in these examples, group differences in brain activations found in fMRI studies may not be a guide to the cause of the disorder, but merely reveal changes that are secondary consequences of the disorder and of compensatory changes that occurred, or the remedial actions that have been taken. These examples also remind us of the artificiality of separating structure and function in brain imaging studies. This is most obviously the case when an abnormality of structure, such as a lesion, leads to a compensatory change in function. There is a general consensus that whenever an abnormality of brain function is observed there must be an associated abnormality of structure. Of course, this abnormality need not be as obvious as a space-occupying lesion, but could be a subtle alteration in connectivity or could be manifest in neurochemical changes that might only be seen at the microscopic level of the synapse. Studies of developmental abnormalities benefit greatly from investigating both structural and functional changes. One of the advantages of MRI is that structural scans are routinely obtained in the course of functional studies. We present an example combining these techniques in the next section.

Can Neuroimaging Studies of Adults With Developmental Disorders Give Useful Information About Underlying Abnormalities?

We have mentioned a number of practical and ethical limitations that make neuroimaging studies of children rather difficult. However, we do not have to wait around for the improvement in techniques, nor do we have to rely on EEG-based approaches only, to study the neural causes and correlates of these disorders. Developmental disorders do not cease when children become adults or when behavioral problems are no longer manifest. Many useful studies of developmental disorders have been conducted with adults. An example is developmental dyslexia.

Dyslexia (see chapter 48)

Many adults with developmental dyslexia have learned to read and write to a high level of accuracy and sometimes cannot be detected by conventional reading tests. However, their problems remain manifest in slow reading and poor spelling. Dyslexia also exists in other languages. In Italian there is a highly transparent writing system that allows largely unambiguous mapping of sounds and letters. As a result, children with dyslexia who would have severe problems in learning to read English may not manifest obvious problems in learning to read Italian. Still, as adults, Italian individuals with dyslexia read significantly more slowly than their peers, just as in the case of English.

In a PET study by Paulesu, Demonet, Fazio *et al.* (2001), university students in three countries (England, France and Italy), those with developmental dyslexia and those without dyslexia, were exposed to print, which they either read aloud or perceived only as a background to another task. The difference between the groups in each of the three countries was significant in one brain region, the left posterior fusiform gyrus, sometimes referred to as the visual word-form area (Cohen & Dehaene, 2004). This region is active when people read words. For participants with dyslexia, this region was less active. A subsequent voxel-based investigation of the whole brain showed that anatomical differences between the groups, again in each of the three countries, were present in precisely this region of the cortex (Silani, Frith, Demonet *et al.*, 2005).

There were two kinds of differences, increases and decreases in gray matter density relative to control subjects. However, it was the increases in density that were significant. This was shown by their correlation with reading performance in the dyslexic groups, again observed for each country. The more gray matter in the critical region, the worse the reading impairment. Given that the decreases in gray matter density were seen in a region immediately next to the increases, the authors offer the speculative hypothesis of a failure in neural migration: some neurons ended up where they should not be, and these unwanted neurons disrupt the functioning of the word-form area. The more such neurons are present, the more the functioning is impaired. While this hypothesis is extremely speculative, it has some support from traditional neuropathological studies. The idea of migration failure in developmental dyslexia was first proposed by Galaburda, Sherman, Rosen *et al.* (1985), who found ectopic cells in the perisylvian region of the left temporal lobe when studying postmortem tissue of dyslexic brains under the microscope. Chang, Ly, Appignani *et al.* (2005) found an association with impairment in reading skills in a sample of 10 patients with epilepsy who showed neuronal migration disorder of periventricular nodular heterotopia.

However, only extremely high-field scanners would be able to detect ectopias, and the theory remains to be tested in the future, if such instruments become available for the study of human brains. In addition, for a full understanding of the behavioral and brain abnormalities in dyslexia, genetic studies would be essential. In the next section we discuss an example where such convergent evidence already exists.

Brain Imaging Studies Require Converging Evidence from Other Disciplines

We have emphasized throughout this chapter that the application of brain imaging to developmental disorders will not be informative unless interpretation of the results can be supported by convergent evidence from several other sources: evidence about causes from genetic and neuropathology and evidence about consequences from behavioral testing and cognitive theory.

Williams Syndrome

Williams syndrome (WS), also known as Williams–Beuren syndrome, is important as an example of a developmental disorder caused by a specific genetic anomaly (a microdeletion of approximately 21 genes on chromosome 7q11.23; see chapter 24). Its incidence has been estimated as 1 in 7500. In a recent comprehensive review, Meyer-Lindenberg, Mervis, and Berman (2006) summarized findings from several disciplines and pointed out the convergence of behavioral and neuroimaging studies. The genetically complex deletions on chromosome 7q11, 23 that characterize the syndrome are associated with quite specific consequences in brain structure and function. In this field, volunteers in scanning experiments are frequently adolescents or adults, as it is clear that the disorder does not go away with age.

The most obvious advantage of knowing the genetic cause of the disorder is that the study group can be defined by a genetic test. Furthermore, variations in the form and severity of the disorder can be linked to the size or location of the deletions.

Starting with anatomical abnormalities of the brain of individuals with WS, van Essen, Dierker, Snyder *et al.* (2006) reported cortical folding abnormalities, while Thompson, Lee, Dutton *et al.* (2005) also found cortical abnormalities when looking at cortical complexity and thickness. However, these rather pervasive structural abnormalities are not sufficient to explain the cognitive abnormalities that are present in WS. The behavioral abnormalities associated with WS have been studied intensively and the pattern of cognitive impairments has been well charted (Farran & Jarrold, 2003). While being associated with mild to moderate intellectual disability, WS is characterized by a distinctive cognitive profile with severe impairment in visuospatial construction tasks alongside relative strength in verbal short-term memory and language.

fMRI studies of high-functioning adult cases of WS performing visuospatial construction tasks have revealed reduced activity in the parietal lobe just in front of the intraparietal sulcus. This observation is consistent with the proposal that the visuospatial impairments in WS result from abnormalities in the dorsal visual processing stream (Atkinson, Braddick, Anker *et al.*, 2003). Structural investigations of the same WS cases, using VBM, revealed symmetrical reductions of gray matter volume in the intraparietal sulcus (Meyer-Lindenberg, Kohn, Mervis *et al.*, 2004). This observation has been confirmed in younger and more typical WS cases (Boddaert, Mochel, Meresse *et al.*, 2006). The structural abnormality revealed by these studies is immediately adjacent to the parietal region showing reduced activity during the performance of visuospatial tasks. Thus, the structural abnormality might serve as a "roadblock" preventing information flowing from visual cortex to parietal regions concerned with the representation of space. Consistent with this idea, Meyer-Lindenberg *et al.* (2004) demonstrated reduced connectivity between visual areas and parietal cortex in WS cases.

The intraparietal sulcus is not the only region of structural abnormality identified in WS. An abnormality has also been found in orbitofrontal cortex. This abnormality may be linked to the social disinhibition typical of WS (Meyer-Lindenberg *et al.*, 2005).

These studies of Williams syndrome illustrate the importance of combining brain imaging studies of structure, function and connectivity with detailed behavioral testing and cognitive analysis.

Disorders of Connectivity

Locating lesions will never be sufficient to understand abnormal brain function and the resulting cognitive and behavioral abnormalities. We need to know about how different brain regions interact with one another. A lesion will alter the way the remaining regions interact with one another (Price, Warburton, Moore *et al.*, 2001). In many developmental disorders there may not be a lesion, but rather an abnormality in the way in which brain regions interact. The development of methods for detecting abnormalities of structural and functional connectivity is at an early stage, but influential speculations have been presented about certain disorders, such as dyslexia (Pugh, Mencl, Shaywitz *et al.*, 2000) and schizophrenia (Stephan, Baldeweg, & Friston, 2006), as fundamentally disorders of neural connectivity.

Another example concerns psychopathy (see chapter 51). It has been proposed that this disorder is characterized by a lack of connectivity between the amygdala and orbitofrontal cortex leading to impaired stimulus-reinforcement learning (Mitchell, Fine, Richell *et al.*, 2006). This proposal relies on combining evidence from non-human primate studies (Baxter & Murray, 2002), human lesion studies (Mitchell *et al.*, 2006) and brain imaging studies (Gottfried, O'Doherty, & Dolan, 2003).

Autism

Autism (see chapter 46) is a prime example of the recent increase in interest in disconnection as opposed to regional abnormalities. As yet there are few structural studies of connectivity, although abnormalities of white matter have been observed (Hendry, De Vito, Gelman *et al.*, 2006). However, the convergence of data from different functional imaging studies suggesting atypical connectivity as an underlying brain abnormality in autism is impressive. Just, Cherkassky, Keller, *et al.* (2004) found indications of underconnectivity between two language areas during performance of a sentence comprehension task, and underconnectivity between frontal and parietal areas during performance of a typical executive function task (Just, Cherkassky, Keller *et al.*, 2007). Villalobos, Mizuno, Dahl *et al.* (2005) observed reduced connectivity between V1 and inferior frontal cortex. Courchesne and Pierce (2005) suggest that connectivity within the frontal lobe is excessive, while connectivity between frontal cortex and other brain systems is poor. Castelli, Frith, Happe *et al.* (2002) used PET to study individuals with high functioning autism and Asperger syndrome while they watched the movements of animated triangles, which normally compel observers to attribute mental states. The people with autism showed reduced activation in the previously established mentalizing system, comprising medial prefrontal cortex (MPFC), superior temporal cortex (STS), basal temporal regions and temporal poles. At the same time, they showed enhanced activation in extra-striate visual regions. This may be because the STS region, which is specialized for the analysis of intentionally moving agents, is failing to get the information from the regions earlier in the visual processing stream, which are specialized for analyzing more general characteristics of movement. In line with this suggestion, weak connectivity was observed between the active visual regions V3 and STS in the autism group.

While all these studies show evidence of reduced connectivity in autism, it is striking that the location of the abnormal connectivity differs from one study to another and probably is determined by the task used to elicit brain activity. It seems unlikely that there is a different abnormality for every task. Furthermore, it is not at all clear what precise form the lack of connectivity might take in physiological terms.

Schultz (2005) has proposed that in autism relevant visual information may not properly reach the dedicated face processing area (FPA) because of weak feedback connections between the amygdala and fusiform gyrus. He proposes that from early on in life the amygdala fails to send emotionally enhanced signals and that this may be the primary cause of disconnection. This line of reasoning was also considered by Castelli *et al.* (2002). They proposed the hypothesis of a top-down failure of feedback signals reaching STS from the anterior components of the mentalizing system. Top-down feedback is believed to alter connectivity. For example, when subjects attend to a particular visual feature, such as motion, connectivity between V1 and the visual motion area V5 is enhanced. This enhanced connectivity is under the control of top-down signals from parietal cortex (Friston & Buchel, 2000). Frith (2003) suggested that the reduced connectivity in autism might be caused by a lack of this top-down modulation. Anterior brain regions, such as amygdala and prefrontal cortex, normally enhance attention towards the signals being processed (e.g., by increasing connectivity between STS and earlier regions in the visual processing stream) and are thus able to signal their social significance. This top-down modulation might be faulty in autism.

This hypothesis was tested by Bird, Catmur, Silani *et al.* (2006) with a paradigm where houses and faces were presented simultaneously, but attention was directed at a single spatial location. This paradigm, introduced by Vuilleumier, Armony, Driver *et al.* (2001), had established that attentional amplification of FFA could be induced when faces appeared in the attended location, while amplification of activity in the parahippocampal place area (PPA) occurred when houses appeared in the attended location. As predicted by their hypothesis, Bird *et al.* found that in autism the amplification of activation in FFA by attention was significantly weaker than in controls. At the same time, the amplification in PPA, although reduced, was not different from normal. Faces are normally salient social stimuli, but seem to be less salient to individuals with autism. The study offers an explanation through the proposal of a failure in top-down processes.

Thus, there would be a transmission failure between basic perceptual information and higher level interpretation of the social significance of the perceptual input.

While these various studies offer different proposals for the reasons of underconnectivity, the top-down modulation hypothesis has the advantage of parsimony as it suggests a common pathology.

Failures of connectivity have also been postulated in other disorders. It remains to be seen whether the precise location and type of the disconnection can distinguish between different disorders. Clearly, if neural signatures can be identified in terms of lack of connectivity and can be related to specific disorders, then this could be helpful in the clinical diagnosis. However, we are just as far from knowing the necessary detail of the critical differences in neural connectivity as we are in knowing the critical differences in cognitive processes. This highlights the continuing importance of cognitive models in the interpretation of imaging data.

Conclusions: The Age of Pioneering rather than Definitive Studies

The examples given demonstrate that brain imaging can teach us much about the development of brain and mind as well as its disorders, even though its full potential has yet to be realized. We have mentioned a number of reasons why developmental neuroscientists have not yet been able to use neuroimaging techniques to the full. In fact, the neuroimaging studies available must still be considered pioneering rather than definitive. Nevertheless, we believe that just as in the investigation of basic neurocognitive processes in healthy adults and neuropsychological patients, huge progress can be made in our knowledge of the developing brain and its disorders. The studies we have reviewed confirm that there is exciting potential even though this potential has not yet been fully realized.

New methods are still evolving, in particular statistical methods for the analysis of the masses of data that can be obtained from activations in cortical areas and in the connections between them. There are continuous improvements in engineering, which means that pictures of increasingly higher resolution can be obtained. At the same time, efforts are being made to improve the administration of the techniques, with noise being reduced and space opened up and the ability to compensate for spontaneously occurring head movement. These technical improvements will benefit studies of children in particular.

When reviewing neuroimaging studies in disorders such as autism, attention deficit/hyperactivity disorder (ADHD), Williams syndrome and dyslexia, one is struck by the number of inconsistent findings. These can to some extent be put down to the typical use of small numbers of participants and poor matching procedures. There are warning examples when divergent results have been obtained when clinical and typical developmental groups were matched for diagnosis but not for IQ. Often, as in behavioral studies, group difference can be accounted for by IQ differences. However, poor designs are also to blame for apparent inconsistencies, because the importance of appropriate control tasks is not always realized.

Sometimes, inconsistencies arise from differing statistical thresholds used for analysis. If thresholds are set too low, then unreliable findings will swamp the literature. On the other hand, it is important to be cautious about setting thresholds too high. Findings from studies using stringent thresholds cannot be taken to mean that they have identified the only abnormality in a clinical group. While the strict statistical procedures used allow confidence in the presence of such an abnormality, they do not rule out that other differences, currently below the threshold, are not also of importance.

Finally, it is not necessarily the methods that are to blame for inconsistent findings. The heterogeneity of developmental disorders makes it very hard to avoid noise in empirical data, be they behavioral or physiological.

Given the ethical and practical considerations, it is particularly important that neuroimaging studies in children should get the most out of the limited opportunity to see the living brain in action. Here, a combination of methods from different disciplines can optimize designs and these need to be guided by hypotheses from cognition and from genetics. Fishing expeditions, where the only question is "what does the active brain look like?" cannot be justified. Studies in children, even more than adult studies, need to be constrained by theory.

Further Reading

Frackowiak, R. S. J., Friston, K. J., Frith, C. D., Dolan, R. J., Price, C. J., Zeki, S., *et al.* (Eds). (2004). *Human brain function* (2nd ed.). San Diego: Elsevier Science.

References

Ashburner, J., & Friston, K. J. (2000). Voxel-based morphometry: the methods. *Neuroimage*, *11*, 805–821.

Ashburner, J., Hutton, C., Frackowiak, R., Johnsrude, I., Price, C., & Friston, K. (1998). Identifying global anatomical differences: deformation-based morphometry. *Human Brain Mapping*, *6*(5–6), 348–357.

Atkinson, J., Braddick, O., Anker, S., Curran, W., Andrew, R., Wattam-Bell, J., *et al.* (2003). Neurobiological models of visuospatial cognition in children with Williams syndrome: measures of dorsal-stream and frontal function. *Developmental Neuropsychology*, *23*, 139–172.

Attwell, D., & Iadecola, C. (2002). The neural basis of functional brain imaging signals. *Trends in Neuroscience*, *25*, 621–625.

Au, W. L., Adams, J. R., Troiano, A. R., & Stoessl, A. J. (2005). Parkinson's disease: *in vivo* assessment of disease progression using positron emission tomography. *Brain Research: Molecular Brain Research*, *134*, 24–33.

Bar, M., Kassam, K. S., Ghuman, A. S., Boshyan, J., Schmid, A. M., Dale, A. M., *et al.* (2006). Top-down facilitation of visual recognition. *Proceedings of the National Academy of Sciences USA*, *103*, 449–454.

Bartocci, M., Bergqvist, L. L., Lagercrantz, H., & Anand, K. J. (2006). Pain activates cortical areas in the preterm newborn brain. *Pain*, *122*, 109–117.

Baxter, M. G., & Murray, E. A. (2002). The amygdala and reward. *Nature Reviews: Neuroscience*, *3*, 563–573.

Benes, F. M. (1989). Myelination of cortical–hippocampal relays during late adolescence. *Schizophrenia Bulletin*, *15*, 585–593.

Bird, G., Catmur, C., Silani, G., Frith, C., & Frith, U. (2006). Attention does not modulate neural responses to social stimuli in autism spectrum disorders. *Neuroimage*, *31*, 1614–1624.

Blakemore, S. J., & Choudhury, S. (2006). Development of the adolescent brain: implications for executive function and social cognition. *Journal of Child Psychology and Psychiatry*, *47*, 296–312.

Boddaert, N., Mochel, F., Meresse, I., Seidenwurm, D., Cachia, A., Brunelle, F., *et al.* (2006). Parieto-occipital grey matter abnormalities in children with Williams syndrome. *Neuroimage*, *30*, 721–725.

Brody, A. L., Saxena, S., Schwartz, J. M., Stoessel, P. W., Maidment, K., Phelps, M. E., *et al.* (1998). FDG-PET predictors of response to behavioral therapy and pharmacotherapy in obsessive compulsive disorder. *Psychiatry Research*, *84*, 1–6.

Canli, T., Omura, K., Haas, B. W., Fallgatter, A., Constable, R. T., & Lesch, K. P. (2005). Beyond affect: a role for genetic variation of the serotonin transporter in neural activation during a cognitive attention task. *Proceedings of the National Academy of Sciences USA*, *102*, 12224–12229.

Casey, B. J., & Durston, S. (2006). From behavior to cognition to the brain and back: what have we learned from functional imaging studies of attention deficit hyperactivity disorder? *American Journal of Psychiatry*, *163*, 957–960.

Castelli, F., Frith, C., Happe, F., & Frith, U. (2002). Autism, Asperger syndrome and brain mechanisms for the attribution of mental states to animated shapes. *Brain*, *125*, 1839–1849.

Chang, B. S., Ly, J., Appignani, B., Bodell, A., Apse, K. A., Ravenscroft, R. S., *et al.* (2005). Reading impairment in the neuronal migration disorder of periventricular nodular heterotopia. *Neurology*, *64*, 799–803.

Cohen, L., & Dehaene, S. (2004). Specialization within the ventral stream: the case for the visual word form area. *Neuroimage*, *22*, 466–476.

Courchesne, E., & Pierce, K. (2005). Why the frontal cortex in autism might be talking only to itself: local over-connectivity but long-distance disconnection. *Current Opinion in Neurobiology*, *15*, 225–230.

Cowey, A., & Walsh, V. (2001). Tickling the brain: studying visual sensation, perception and cognition by transcranial magnetic stimulation. *Progress in Brain Research*, *134*, 411–425.

Croxson, P. L., Johansen-Berg, H., Behrens, T. E., Robson, M. D., Pinsk, M. A., Gross, C. G., *et al.* (2005). Quantitative investigation of connections of the prefrontal cortex in the human and macaque using probabilistic diffusion tractography. *Journal of Neuroscience*, *25*, 8854–8866.

Dehaene-Lambertz, G., Dehaene, S., & Hertz-Pannier, L. (2002). Functional neuroimaging of speech perception in infants. *Science*, *298*, 2013–2015.

Dijkhuizen, R. M. (2006). Application of magnetic resonance imaging to study pathophysiology in brain disease models. *Methods in Molecular Medicine*, *124*, 251–278.

Draganski, B., Gaser, C., Busch, V., Schuierer, G., Bogdahn, U., & May, A. (2004). Neuroplasticity: Changes in grey matter induced by training. Newly honed juggling skills show up as a transient feature on a brain-imaging scan. *Nature*, *427*, 311–312.

Durston, S., Davidson, M. C., Tottenham, N., Galvan, A., Spicer, J., Fossella, J. A., *et al.* (2006). A shift from diffuse to focal cortical activity with development. *Developmental Science*, *9*, 1–8.

Eden, G. F., Jones, K. M., Cappell, K., Gareau, L., Wood, F. B., Zeffiro, T. A., *et al.* (2004). Neural changes following remediation in adult developmental dyslexia. *Neuron*, *44*, 411–422.

Farran, E. K., & Jarrold, C. (2003). Visuospatial cognition in Williams syndrome: reviewing and accounting for the strengths and weaknesses in performance. *Developmental Neuropsychology*, *23*, 173–200.

Frangou, S., & Williams, S. C. (1996). Magnetic resonance spectroscopy in psychiatry: basic principles and applications. *British Medical Bulletin*, *52*, 474–485.

Frith, C. D. (2003). What do imaging studies tell us about the neural basis of autism? *Novartis Found Symp*, *251*, 149–166.

Friston, K. J., & Buchel, C. (2000). Attentional modulation of effective connectivity from V2 to V5/MT in humans. *Proceedings of the National Academy of Sciences USA*, *97*, 7591–7596.

Galaburda, A. M., Sherman, G. F., Rosen, G. D., Aboitiz, F., & Geschwind, N. (1985). Developmental dyslexia: four consecutive patients with cortical anomalies. *Annals of Neurology*, *18*, 222–233.

Giedd, J. N., Blumenthal, J., Jeffries, N. O., Castellanos, F. X., Liu, H., Zijdenbos, A., *et al.* (1999). Brain development during childhood and adolescence: a longitudinal MRI study. *Nature Neuroscience*, *2*, 861–863.

Gogtay, N., Giedd, J. N., Lusk, L., Hayashi, K. M., Greenstein, D., Vaituzis, A. C., *et al.* (2004). Dynamic mapping of human cortical development during childhood through early adulthood. *Proceedings of the National Academy of Sciences USA*, *101*, 8174–8179.

Gottfried, J. A., O'Doherty, J., & Dolan, R. J. (2003). Encoding predictive reward value in human amygdala and orbitofrontal cortex. *Science*, *301*, 1104–1107.

Gujar, S. K., Maheshwari, S., Bjorkman-Burtscher, I., & Sundgren, P. C. (2005). Magnetic resonance spectroscopy. *Journal of Neuro-ophthalmology*, *25*, 217–226.

Hendry, J., DeVito, T., Gelman, N., Densmore, M., Rajakumar, N., Pavlosky, W., *et al.* (2006). White matter abnormalities in autism detected through transverse relaxation time imaging. *Neuroimage*, *29*, 1049–1057.

Huppert, T. J., Hoge, R. D., Diamond, S. G., Franceschini, M. A., & Boas, D. A. (2006). A temporal comparison of BOLD, ASL, and NIRS hemodynamic responses to motor stimuli in adult humans. *Neuroimage*, *29*, 368–382.

Huttenlocher, P. R. (1979). Synaptic density in human frontal cortex: developmental changes and effects of aging. *Brain Research*, *163*, 195–205.

Huttenlocher, P. R., de Courten, C., Garey, L. J., & Van der Loos, H. (1982). Synaptogenesis in human visual cortex: evidence for synapse elimination during normal development. *Neuroscience Letters*, *33*, 247–252.

Jenkins, I. H., Brooks, D. J., Nixon, P. D., Frackowiak, R. S., & Passingham, R. E. (1994). Motor sequence learning: a study with positron emission tomography. *Journal of Neuroscience*, *14*, 3775–3790.

Just, M. A., Cherkassky, V. L., Keller, T. A., Kana, R. K., & Minshew, N. J. (2007). Functional and anatomical cortical underconnectivity in autism: Evidence from an fMRI study of an executive function task and corpus callosum morphometry. *Cerebral Cortex*, 17, 951–961.

Just, M. A., Cherkassky, V. L., Keller, T. A., & Minshew, N. J. (2004). Cortical activation and synchronization during sentence comprehension in high-functioning autism: evidence of underconnectivity. *Brain*, *127*, 1811–1821.

Kraemer, H. C., Yesavage, J. A., Taylor, J. L., & Kupfer, D. (2000). How can we learn about developmental processes from cross-sectional studies, or can we? *American Journal of Psychiatry*, *157*, 163–171.

Krageloh-Mann, I. (2004). Imaging of early brain injury and cortical plasticity. *Experimental Neurology*, *190*(Supplement 1), S84–90.

Kreiman, G., Koch, C., & Fried, I. (2000). Category-specific visual responses of single neurons in the human medial temporal lobe. *Nature Neuroscience*, *3*, 946–953.

Lenroot, R. K., & Giedd, J. N. (2006). Brain development in children and adolescents: insights from anatomical magnetic resonance imaging. *Neuroscience and Biobehavioral Reviews*, *30*, 718–729.

Lidzba, K., Staudt, M., Wilke, M., & Krageloh-Mann, I. (2006). Visuospatial deficits in patients with early left-hemispheric lesions and functional reorganization of language: consequence of lesion or reorganization? *Neuropsychologia*, *44*, 1088–1094.

Logothetis, N. K., Pauls, J., Augath, M., Trinath, T., & Oeltermann, A. (2001). Neurophysiological investigation of the basis of the fMRI signal. *Nature*, *412*, 150–157.

Marcar, V. L., Strassle, A. E., Loenneker, T., Schwarz, U., & Martin, E. (2004). The influence of cortical maturation on the BOLD response: An fMRI study of visual cortex in children. *Pediatric Research*, *56*, 967–974.

Mattout, J., Phillips, C., Penny, W. D., Rugg, M. D., & Friston, K. J. (2006). MEG source localization under multiple constraints: an extended Bayesian framework. *Neuroimage*, *30*, 753–767.

Meyer-Lindenberg, A., Hariri, A. R., Munoz, K. E., Mervis, C. B., Mattay, V. S., Morris, C. A., *et al.* (2005). Neural correlates of genetically abnormal social cognition in Williams syndrome. *Nature Neuroscience*, *8*, 991–993.

Meyer-Lindenberg, A., Kohn, P., Mervis, C. B., Kippenhan, J. S., Olsen, R. K., Morris, C. A., *et al.* (2004). Neural basis of genetically determined visuospatial construction deficit in Williams syndrome. *Neuron*, *43*, 623–631.

Meyer-Lindenberg, A., Mervis, C. B., & Berman, K. F. (2006). Neural mechanisms in Williams syndrome: a unique window to genetic influences on cognition and behaviour. *Nature Reviews: Neuroscience*, *7*, 380–393.

Mitchell, D. G., Fine, C., Richell, R. A., Newman, C., Lumsden, J., Blair, K. S., *et al.* (2006). Instrumental learning and relearning in individuals with psychopathy and in patients with lesions involving the amygdala or orbitofrontal cortex. *Neuropsychology*, *20*, 280–289.

Morton, J. (2004). *Understanding developmental disorders: A causal modelling approach*. Oxford: Blackwell Publishing.

Passarotti, A. M., Paul, B. M., Russiere, J. R., Buxton, R. B., Wong, E. C., & Stiles, J. (2003). The development of face and location processing: an fMRI study. *Developmental Science*, *6*, 100–117.

Paulesu, E., Demonet, J. F., Fazio, F., McCrory, E., Chanoine, V., Brunswick, N., *et al.* (2001). Dyslexia: cultural diversity and biological unity. *Science*, *291*, 2165–2167.

Paulesu, E., McCrory, E., Fazio, F., Menoncello, L., Brunswick, N., Cappa, S. F., *et al.* (2000). A cultural effect on brain function. *Nature Neuroscience*, *3*, 91–96.

Paus, T. (2005). Mapping brain maturation and cognitive development during adolescence. *Trends in Cognitive Sciences*, *9*, 60–68.

Paus, T., Collins, D. L., Evans, A. C., Leonard, G., Pike, B., & Zijdenbos, A. (2001). Maturation of white matter in the human brain: A review of magnetic resonance studies. *Brain Research Bulletin*, *54*, 255–266.

Penny, W. D., Stephan, K. E., Mechelli, A., & Friston, K. J. (2004). Modelling functional integration: a comparison of structural equation and dynamic causal models. *Neuroimage*, *23*(Supplement 1), S264–274.

Peterson, B. S., Thomas, P., Kane, M. J., Scahill, L., Zhang, H., Bronen, R., *et al.* (2003). Basal ganglia volumes in patients with Gilles de la Tourette syndrome. *Archives of General Psychiatry*, *60*, 415–424.

Pettegrew, J. W., Panchalingam, K., Moossy, J., Martinez, J., Rao, G., & Boller, F. (1988). Correlation of phosphorus-31 magnetic resonance spectroscopy and morphologic findings in Alzheimer's disease. *Archives of Neurology*, *45*, 1093–1096.

Plessen, K. J., Grüner, R., Lundervold, A., Hirsch, J. G., Xu, D., Bansal, R., *et al.* (2006). Reduced white matter connectivity in the corpus callosum of children with Tourette syndrome. *Journal of Child Psychology and Psychiatry*, *47*, 1013–1022.

Price, C. J., Warburton, E. A., Moore, C. J., Frackowiak, R. S., & Friston, K. J. (2001). Dynamic diaschisis: anatomically remote and context-sensitive human brain lesions. *Journal of Cognitive Neuroscience*, *13*, 419–429.

Price, D. J., Kennedy, H., Dehay, C., Zhou, L., Mercier, M., Jossin, Y., *et al.* (2006). The development of cortical connections. *European Journal of Neuroscience*, *23*, 910–920.

Pugh, K. R., Mencl, W. E., Shaywitz, B. A., Shaywitz, S. E., Fulbright, R. K., Constable, R. T., *et al.* (2000). The angular gyrus in developmental dyslexia: task-specific differences in functional connectivity within posterior cortex. *Psychological Science*, *11*, 51–56.

Rivera, S. M., Reiss, A. L., Eckert, M. A., & Menon, V. (2005). Developmental changes in mental arithmetic: evidence for increased functional specialization in the left inferior parietal cortex. *Cerebral Cortex*, *15*, 1779–1790.

Sakai, K., & Passingham, R. E. (2003). Prefrontal interactions reflect future task operations. *Nature Neuroscience*, *6*, 75–81.

Salek-Haddadi, A., Diehl, B., Hamandi, K., Merschhemke, M., Liston, A., Friston, K., *et al.* (2006). Hemodynamic correlates of epileptiform discharges: an EEG-fMRI study of 63 patients with focal epilepsy. *Brain Research*, *1088*, 148–166.

Satlin, A., Bodick, N., Offen, W. W., & Renshaw, P. F. (1997). Brain proton magnetic resonance spectroscopy (1H-MRS) in Alzheimer's disease: changes after treatment with xanomeline, an M1 selective cholinergic agonist. *American Journal of Psychiatry*, *154*, 1459–1461.

Schlaggar, B. L., Brown, T. T., Lugar, H. M., Visscher, K. M., Miezin, F. M., & Petersen, S. E. (2002). Functional neuroanatomical differences between adults and school-age children in the processing of single words. *Science*, *296*, 1476–1479.

Schultz, R. T. (2005). Developmental deficits in social perception in autism: the role of the amygdala and fusiform face area. *International Journal of Developmental Neuroscience*, *23*, 125–141.

Shaywitz, B. A., Shaywitz, S. E., Blachman, B. A., Pugh, K. R., Fulbright, R. K., Skudlarski, P., *et al.* (2004). Development of left occipitotemporal systems for skilled reading in children after a phonologically based intervention. *Biological Psychiatry*, *55*, 926–933.

Silani, G., Frith, U., Demonet, J. F., Fazio, F., Perani, D., Price, C., *et al.* (2005). Brain abnormalities underlying altered activation in dyslexia: a voxel based morphometry study. *Brain*, *128*, 2453–2461.

Spelke, E. S. (2002). Developmental neuroimaging: a developmental psychologist looks ahead. *Developmental Science*, *5*, 392–396.

Stephan, K. E., Baldeweg, T., & Friston, K. J. (2006). Synaptic plasticity and dysconnection in schizophrenia. *Biological Psychiatry*, *59*, 929–939.

Stiles, J., Reilly, J., Paul, B., & Moses, P. (2005). Cognitive development following early brain injury: Evidence for neural adaptation. *Trends in Cognitive Sciences*, *9*, 136–143.

Sun, L., Jin, Z., Zang, Y. F., Zeng, Y. W., Liu, G., Li, Y., *et al.* (2005). Differences between attention-deficit disorder with and without hyperactivity: A 1H-magnetic resonance spectroscopy study. *Brain and Development*, *27*, 340–344.

Thompson, P. M., Lee, A. D., Dutton, R. A., Geaga, J. A., Hayashi, K. M., Eckert, M. A., *et al.* (2005). Abnormal cortical complexity and thickness profiles mapped in Williams syndrome. *Journal of Neuroscience*, *25*, 4146–4158.

Toga, A. W., Thompson, P. M., & Sowell, E. R. (2006). Mapping brain maturation. *Trends in Neuroscience*, *29*, 148–159.

Tsao, D. Y., Freiwald, W. A., Tootell, R. B., & Livingstone, M. S. (2006). A cortical region consisting entirely of face-selective cells. *Science*, *311*, 670–674.

Van Essen, D. C., Dierker, D., Snyder, A. Z., Raichle, M. E., Reiss, A. L., & Korenberg, J. (2006). Symmetry of cortical folding abnormalities in Williams syndrome revealed by surface-based analyses. *Journal of Neuroscience*, *26*, 5470–5483.

Villalobos, M. E., Mizuno, A., Dahl, B. C., Kemmotsu, N., & Muller, R. A. (2005). Reduced functional connectivity between V1 and inferior frontal cortex associated with visuomotor performance in autism. *Neuroimage*, *25*, 916–925.

Vuilleumier, P., Armony, J. L., Driver, J., & Dolan, R. J. (2001). Effects of attention and emotion on face processing in the human brain: an event-related fMRI study. *Neuron*, *30*, 829–841.

Yakovlev, P. I., & Lecours, A. R. (1967). The myelogenetic cycles of regional maturation of the brain. In A. Minkowski (Ed.), *Regional development of the brain in early life* (pp. 3–70). Oxford: Blackwell Scientific Publications.

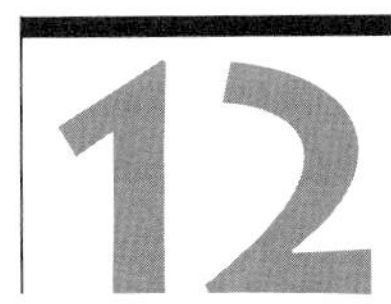

Neurobiological Perspectives on Developmental Psychopathology

Charles Nelson and Shafali Jeste

The field of developmental psychopathology is a relatively new discipline, launched slightly more than two decades ago by the publication of two papers, one by Sroufe and Rutter (1984) and another by Cicchetti (1984). As these authors eloquently pointed out, the disciplines of developmental psychology and abnormal psychology have historically traveled along parallel rather than convergent paths. However, our understanding of child mental health would improve dramatically if we adopted a true developmental framework. It was with this goal in mind that this new field of developmental psychopathology was created, and it has clearly taken root, with whole conferences and journals devoted to it. Yet imbuing the study of developmental psychopathology with biology (be it neurobiology or molecular biology) has only recently begun to gain traction (Cicchetti & Posner, 2005; Dahl & Spear, 2004; Nelson, Leibenluft, McClure *et al.*, 2005; Rutter, 2006; see also Nelson, Bloom, Cameron *et al.*, 2002). The failure to consider the linkages between developmental psychopathology and biology is unfortunate for several reasons, not the least of which is the observation that many mental health disorders have a strong genetic basis (Rutter, 2006), and the fact that mental disorders are inherently brain disorders.

This leads us to ask, why have those studying typical or atypical child development been so hesitant to consider the biological bases of development? Several possible explanations come to mind. First, the training involved in becoming a psychologist, psychiatrist or neuroscientist is long and arduous, and to master the methods and models of multiple disciplines is difficult. Second, through at least the first two-thirds of the 20th century, Freudian theory and, later, some strains of attachment theory (Sroufe, 1986; Sroufe, Carlson, Levy *et al.*, 1999; Warren, Huston, Egeland *et al.*, 1997) had a dominant influence on many aspects of developmental psychopathology. These theories focused more on the importance of environment and upbringing in development, and therefore underplayed the impact of biological factors. Additionally, investigators in that period believed that genetics seemed overly deterministic, and argued that to attribute the cause of mental disorders to atypical neural processes deflected attention away from the assumed root cause – bad parenting, adverse early experiences, and so forth.

As has been the case for child development and neuroscience (Nelson & Bloom, 1997), most contemporary views of child psychopathology are more inclusive, and few investigators would now argue that biology (be it genes or brain) is unimportant. In this chapter we sound the contemporary theme that mental processes (normal or abnormal) have their basis in neural activity. To illustrate this perspective, we begin our chapter with a tutorial on brain development. Here we include summaries of neurulation, cellular proliferation, migration and differentiation, followed by discussions of synaptogenesis and myelination. Next, because some forms of psychopathology have their origin in abnormal early experiences (e.g., abuse, neglect), and because much is known about the role of experience in brain development and brain function, we turn our attention to a discussion of neural plasticity. Finally, having laid the ground-work for how errors in brain development might contribute to psychopathology, we turn our attention to the neurobiological origins of developmental psychopathology. We begin with a general review of the link between early pre- and perinatal insults and subsequent psychopathology. We then focus this discussion on a specific developmental disorder – autism. We argue that children with classic autism and some children with histories of institutionalization share features in common, a phenotypic overlap, if you will. We consider the mechanism by which such a final common pathway can emerge despite very different etiologies and early beginnings. This brings us back to the original struggle between the influence of biology versus environment in developmental psychopathology.

Brain Development

Brain development is a protracted process. It begins after conception, and is essentially complete by the time an individual reaches his or her mid-20s. We illustrate these remarkable changes in Plate 12.1, in which the surface development of the brain is shown from just a few weeks after conception through adulthood.

How does this miracle occur? We can approach an answer to this question at multiple levels: the action of genes (the molecular level), the action of synapses (the physiological level), the functions subserved by specific structures (the anatomical

Rutter's Child and Adolescent Psychiatry, 5th edition. Edited by M. Rutter, D. Bishop, D. Pine, S. Scott, J. Stevenson, E. Taylor and A. Thapar. © 2008 Blackwell Publishing, ISBN: 978-1-4051-4549-7.

level) and the combination of all of these, in which diffuse networks of millions of neurons work synchronously in the service of behavior (the systems level).

Basic Embryology

Beginning shortly after conception, the primitive zygote undergoes multiple cell divisions that eventually lead to the formation of the blastocyst (a mass of cells), which contains an inner and an outer layer. The former will give rise to the embryo proper, whereas the latter will give rise to support structures (placenta, umbilical cord, amniotic sac). After several more cell cycles have been completed, some time between the first and second prenatal week, the inner layer subdivides out into three layers. Here the inner layer (endoderm) will give rise to most of the internal organs of the body, the middle layer (mesoderm) will give rise to support structures (e.g., bone) and the outer layer (ectoderm) will give rise to the nervous system.

Although brain development is a continuous process that begins with the formation of the neural tube and ends when the basic architecture of the brain becomes adult-like (approximately two decades later), we organize our review of brain development into those events that occur prenatally and those that begin prenatally and continue postnatally.

Prenatal Development

Neurulation

The formation of the neural tube, which is derived from the ectoderm, is considered by most to be the first stage of brain development (Plate 12.2). As cells that line the ectoderm multiply, the ectodermal layer thickens to form a pear-shaped neural plate. This plate gradually begins to fold over onto itself, forming a tube. This tube, in turn, gradually closes at the bottom and then the top, a process that is complete by roughly the end of the third week of gestation. Cells trapped inside the tube will lead to the formation of the central nervous system (CNS), whereas those trapped between the outer layer and the ectodermal wall will give rise to the autonomic nervous system (ANS).

As illustrated in Plate 12.3, the neural tube rapidly becomes a three-vesicle structure, and then a five-vesicle structure. The rear-most (caudal) portion of the tube will give rise to the hindbrain (rhombencephalon), which will consist of the medulla oblongata (which regulates basic bodily functions; importantly it is the medulla that connects the rest of the brain to the spinal cord), pons (which relays sensory information between the cerebrum and cerebellum) and cerebellum (which will subserve a variety of motor functions). The middle vesicle gives rise to the midbrain (mesencephalon), which caudally connects to the pons and rostrally connects to the diencephalon (a forebrain structure that consists of the thalamus and hypothalamus). Finally, the most rostral (top) portion of the tube will give rise to the forebrain (prosencephalon), which in turn will subdivide into the telencephalon (cerebral hemispheres), the diencephalon and the basal ganglia.

Proliferation

Once the neural tube has formed, cells that line the innermost portion of the tube (the *ventricular* zone) proliferate at a logarithmic rate. As cells in the ventricular zone multiply, a second zone is formed, the *marginal* zone, which contains axons and dendrites. This proliferative stage continues for some time, ultimately leading to the newborn brain having many more neurons than the adult brain. The overproduction of neurons is eventually compensated for by a second normative process referred to as *apoptosis*, or programmed cell death. Apoptosis is responsible for the pruning back of these neurons to adult numbers.

Cell Migration

The cortex proper – the several millimeters thick covering of the brain – is formed through a process of cell migration. Postmitotic cells that originate in the ventricular zone will migrate through the intermediate zone (essentially a zone that lies between the ventricular zone and the cortical plate), eventually reaching their final destination. These postmitotic cells move in an inside–out direction, with the earliest migrating cells occupying the deepest cortical layer, with subsequent migrations passing through the previously formed layer(s). Six months after conception, all six layers of the cortex have been formed.

Cell migration takes place using radial and tangential migratory patterns. The former refers to the propagation of cells from the deepest to the most superficial layers of the cortex. Approximately 70–80% of migrating neurons (primarily pyramidal neurons) and most glia (including oligodendrocytes and astrocytes) use this radial pathway. In contrast, cortical interneurons and nuclei of the brainstem adopt a tangential migratory pattern.

Most cell migration is complete by approximately the 25th prenatal week. Once a cell has completed its migratory journey, it can differentiate, the process we discuss next.

Differentiation

Once a neuron has migrated to its target destination, it generally proceeds along one of two roads: the cell can differentiate and develop *processes* (axons and dendrites) or it can be retracted through apoptosis. Current estimates place the number of neurons that are subsequently retracted at 40–60% (Oppenheim & Johnson, 2003). The development of axons is facilitated by *growth cones*, small structures that sit on top of an axon. The growth cone directs an axon towards some targets and away from others. This is accomplished by using a combination of molecular guidance cues (e.g., cell adhesion molecules) as well as anatomical structures that sit atop the tip of the axon (e.g., *lamellipodia* and *filopodia*).

Recent work has indicated that the gene calcium-regulated transcriptional activator (CREST) has an important role in the development of dendrites (Aizawa, Hu, Bobb *et al.*, 2004). Early dendrites appear as thick processes with few spines (small protuberances that occupy the length of the dendrite) which extend from the cell body. As dendrites mature, the number and density of the spines increase; this, in turn, increases the chance that a dendrite will make contact with a neighboring axon. The first dendrites appear approximately 15 weeks after conception, which is about the same time the first axons reach the cortical plate. At 25–27 weeks' gestation dendritic spines greatly increase in number, on both pyramidal and non-pyramidal cells.

Pre- and Postnatal Development

Synaptogenesis

A synapse is the point of contact between two neurons, frequently between an axon and a dendrite. Depending on the neuron in question, the action of a synapse can be excitatory (promoting the likelihood of an action potential) or inhibitory (reducing the likelihood of an action potential).

The first synapses are generally observed by about 23 weeks gestation (Molliver, Kostovic, & Van der Loos, 1973), although the peak of production does not occur until some time in the first year of life. As is the case with neurons, there is a massive overproduction of synapses which is followed by a gradual reduction. In the visual cortex, a synaptic peak is reached between approximately 4 and 8 postnatal months (Huttenlocher & de Courten, 1987), whereas in the middle frontal gyrus (a region of the prefrontal cortex) the peak synaptic density is not obtained until after 15 postnatal months (Huttenlocher & Dabholkar, 1997).

The process of reducing the number of synapses (pruning) is dependent in part on the communication between neurons. Following the Hebbian principle of use and disuse, the more active synapses tend to be strengthened and less active synapses tend to be weakened or even eliminated (Chechik, Meilijson, & Ruppin, 1999). An elegant example of this can be found in a paper by Le Bé and Markram (2006) who, using 12- to 14-day-old rat neocortical slices, demonstrated that pyramidal neurons spontaneously connect and disconnect from each other, and that adding an excitatory neurotransmitter (glutamate) increases the number of connections that are formed. Importantly, the adjustments that are made in the pruning of synapses can either be quantitative, with a reduction in the overall number of synapses, or qualitative, with a refinement of connections such that silent or abnormal connections are eliminated.

The process of synaptic pruning varies by brain area. For example, in the human occipital cortex the peak number of synapses occurs at 4–8 months of age, and is reduced to adult numbers by 4–6 years. Synapses in the middle frontal gyrus of the human prefrontal cortex reach their peak closer to 1–1.5 years of age, and adult numbers are not obtained until mid to late adolescence (Huttenlocher, 1979, 1994; Huttenlocher & Dabholkar, 1997; Huttenlocher & de Courten, 1987).

Myelination

Myelin is a lipid–protein substance, which, when wrapped around an axon, tends to increase the conduction velocity, or speed at which neuronal impulses travel. *Oligodendroglia* produces myelin in the CNS, whereas *Schwann cells* produce myelin in the ANS. Myelination in the peripheral nervous system, motor roots, sensory roots, somesthetic cortex, and the primary visual and auditory cortices begins prenatally. During the first postnatal year, regions of the brainstem, cerebellum and the splenium of corpus callosum myelinate. By 1 year of age myelination of all regions of the corpus callosum is under way.

In contrast to most other aspects of brain development, myelination can be studied non-invasively using magnetic resonance imaging (MRI). The attractiveness of this tool is that one can repeatedly study the same individual across time, yielding impressive developmental data. Previously, of course, all such data were obtained pathologically, through cross-sections of brains of autopsy specimens.

Although the application of MRI in the study of typical development is still quite novel, this tool has been used to examine brain anatomy, gray and white matter development, myelination and the development of white matter tracts across a range of ages. While ultrasound is most useful for the diagnosis of gross abnormalities (e.g., intraventricular or intraparenchymal hemorrhage, or major structural malformation) and can be used to view some additional details of cortical development, MRI is the gold standard for visualization of the posterior fossa, and for viewing sulcation and myelination. Prenatally, a rather accurate estimate of gestational age can be made by the pattern of sulcation seen on MRI. For instance, at 16 weeks only the parieto-occipital and calcarine sulci have been formed but, by 30 weeks, the occipito-temporal, superior and inferior frontal, and superior-temporal sulci have also appeared (Van der Knaap, van Wezel-Meijler, Barth *et al.*, 1996).

Degree and location of myelination can be accurately measured by level of signal intensity on T1 and T2 weighted MRI studies. As shown by MRI, myelination begins in the fifth fetal month with the cranial nerves, and then continues through the first two decades of life. In general, the process occurs in a caudal to cephalad and dorsal to ventral pattern. Furthermore, in any specific portion of the brain, the posterior region myelinates first. Myelination progresses most quickly in areas of the brain that are used in early life. For instance, in the brainstem, the regions needed for tactile sensation and proprioception sensation are myelinated at birth, whereas regions necessary for motor input into the cerebellum do not myelinate until later in infancy. These patterns have been consistently documented using MRI and, postnatally, the level of brain maturation is estimated based on degree and location of myelination (Barkovich, 2005a).

Gilmore and colleagues have conducted an elegant series of studies of typically developing newborns and young infants using a relatively high-field magnet (3 Tesla). They have reported that males in general have larger intracranial volumes than females, and (in an unpublished study) that in contrast to the adult, there are no sex differences in white matter in newborns (Gilmore, Zhai, Wilber *et al.*, 2004, Gilmore, Lin,

Knickmeyer, 2006). This same group has also been studying 1- to 2-year-old typically developing infants. From this work they report that there is a large increase in intracranial volume in the first year, and that by age 1 year intracranial volume is about 75% of adult volume, and at 2 years it is 80% (Gilmore *et al.*, 2006).

Moving beyond infancy, there are now a number of longitudinal studies that have examined the course of myelination from early childhood through early adulthood (for a recent review see Toga, Thompson, & Sowell, 2006). A summary of these findings suggests that there is a linear increase in white matter until 20 years of age, and non-linear changes in gray matter during this same time period. Regarding gray matter, Giedd, Blumenthal, Jeffries *et al.* (1999) have shown that there is an increase in gray matter up until about the age of 12 years in the frontal and parietal lobes, thereafter followed by a decrease. In the temporal lobes, the increase occurs until age 16, and then again is followed by a decrease.

Collectively, changes in gray and white matter continue across the first two decades of life, with gray matter reaching its peak around the age of 12, and myelination reaching its peak around the age of 20 years. Unfortunately, relatively little work has been carried out on relating these changes to behavior. One exception is recent work by Sowell *et al.* (2004). Drawing on longitudinal data collected between 5 and 11 years of age, Sowell *et al.* (2004) have shown that among these typically developing children, the cortex thins by 0.15–0.30 mm per year, particularly in the frontal and parietal regions; such thinning also occurs in the temporal and frontal regions (specifically those that are related to language functions). Intriguingly, cortical thinning in the left dorsal frontal and parietal lobes correlated with improvements in performance on a general IQ test. The authors speculated that such thinning represents a plastic process, likely driven by experience (for another example see Shaw, Greenstein, Lerch *et al.*, 2006).

Postnatal Neurogenesis

The process of neurogenesis begins shortly after the neural tube has been formed, and continues through much of gestation. For most of the 20th century it was commonly believed that our full complement of neurons is complete at or around the time of birth, and that we do not make new neurons after that, not even in response to injury. One exception to this rule was the olfactory bulb, where there were reports of postnatal neurogenesis occurring through much of life. However, the assumption of "no new neurons" began to be questioned in earnest by a number of investigators during the 1990s. Initially it was demonstrated that a region of the hippocampus – the dentate gyrus – continues to make new neurons through at least middle age (for a review see Barinaga, 2003). Such data have been replicated multiple times, so there is little reason to question their veracity.

However, far more controversial is whether other regions of the brain, the cortex in particular, also continue to make new neurons postnatally. For example, Gould and Gross (2002) have reported postnatal neurogenesis in the cingulate gyrus and segments of the parietal cortex, and Bernier, Bédard, Vinet *et al.* (2002) have reported postnatal neurogenesis in the amygdala, piriform cortex and inferior temporal cortex. However, other authors have failed to replicate these findings (for discussion see Rakic, 2002). In a seminal paper published by Bhardwaj, Curtis, Spalding *et al.* (2006) employing ^{14}C and BRDU (DNA methods that permit one to examine the birth of a cell), it now appears that the cortex does not enjoy the same privilege as the dentate gyrus: that is, all the cortical neurons we will ever have are typically present by birth, and no new neurons are made after that. Accordingly, it now appears that postnatal neurogenesis may be limited to the dentate region of the hippocampus (Kozorovitskiy & Gould, in press).

An intriguing observation about postnatal neurogenesis is that these new neurons have a relatively short half-life, and typically die within a few weeks of birth. Equally intriguing is the fact that, despite their short lifespan, these neurons differentiate (develop axons and dendrites), express neurotransmitters and possess all the functional properties of a "typical" neuron, and they are influenced by experience (Gould, Beylin, Tanapat *et al.*, 1999; Mirescu, Peters, & Gould, 2004). For example, when mice or rats are placed in contexts in which demands are placed on learning and memory, or in which exercise is encouraged, there is an increase in the number of cells produced in the dentate gyrus; importantly, this effect can be obtained among aged mice, not just young mice. For example, van Praag, Shubert, Zhao *et al.* (2005) demonstrated that when young and aged mice were housed with a running wheel, both groups showed an increase in neurogenesis in the hippocampus and a corresponding improvement in spatial memory.

In contrast to complex (or so-called "enriched") environments, stress in adulthood appears to reduce the number of postnatally derived neurons in the rat dentate gyrus. Moreover, in unpublished work by Gould (2003), when rodents are housed together, dominance hierarchies develop. Within these hierarchies, the dominant animals tend to produce more new neurons than the non-dominant animals. Interestingly, if these same animals are then housed in complex environments, there is an increase in the number of neurons born in the dentate, although the dominant animals continue to fare better than the non-dominant animals. Perhaps most intriguingly, although environmental enrichment up-regulates postnatal neurogenesis, these cells are *not* involved in spatial learning (Meshi, Drew, Saxe *et al.*, 2006; but see van Praag *et al.*, 2005). Collectively, experience appears to have an influence on postnatal neurogenesis, although it is unknown what role these new cells have in brain function.

Because the area that benefits from the process of postnatal neurogenesis lies in the hippocampus, and because the hippocampus is deeply involved in memory, some have speculated that postnatal neurogenesis will functionally benefit memory processes. This has led Aimone, Wiles, and Gage (2006) to speculate that newly born cells and prenatally born (mature) cells serve different purposes; the new cells are capable of encoding new information, but because these cells die off, this information is not retained for the long term. However, the next generation of new cells also encodes information, as does the one after that, and the one after that. As a result, postnatally derived cells serve the function of tagging information that exists over a temporal time frame. This information then communicates with more established circuits, made up of mature cells, and subsequently the temporal associations come to exist in long-term memory.

In conclusion, work on postnatal neurogenesis continues to proliferate at a rapid pace, although it remains unclear how postnatally derived cells work their way into existing circuits and influence brain function. Undoubtedly, these questions will receive considerable attention in the coming years, given that answers to these questions have the potential to revolutionize how we manage and treat a range of CNS disorders such as spinal cord injury or stroke.

Summary

It is relatively easy to determine the starting point for brain development, but ascertaining the endpoint – the transition from childhood to adulthood – is much more difficult. The basic architecture of the brain is established fairly early in life, with the surface structure closely resembling the adult brain within the first few years of life (for a recent review see White & Hilgetad, in press). However, changes in synaptogenesis and myelination continue well through adolescence, and in some regions (e.g., prefrontal cortex) into early adulthood. Throughout this time period, the engine that drives development is the interaction of genes and environment, with postnatal experience playing a prominent part, although always within the constraints imposed by genetics. Changes during adolescence are nearly as dramatic as those during infancy, particularly in the functional domain. These functional changes are undoubtedly influenced by the surge of pubertal hormones, although explicating the exact mechanism by which such hormones affect brain structure and function remains elusive (although headway has been made in animal models; for a recent overview on adolescent brain development see Dahl & Spear, 2004). This is unfortunate, as it is during puberty that many forms of psychopathology really take root (e.g., in the case of depression) or manifest themselves for the first time in obvious ways (e.g., schizophrenia). Moreover, it is also during puberty that sex differences in psychopathology first emerge (again, the case of depression comes to mind). Clearly, more research is needed to explicate changes in brain development during the adolescent period, and to relate such changes to psychopathology.

Neural Plasticity

The topic of neural plasticity has received considerable attention over the past decade, and in the context of development, Nelson and colleagues have discussed this topic extensively (Black, Jones, Nelson *et al.*, 1998; Cline, 2003; de Haan & Johnson, 2003; Nelson, 1999, 2000; Nelson & Bloom, 1997; Nelson, de Haan, & Thomas, 2006).

In its simplest terms, plasticity refers to the brain's ability to be molded by experience. Of course, because experiences can be good or bad, this means that plasticity "cuts both ways" (Greenough, personal communication). Thus, good experiences can lead to "good" brains and bad experiences can lead to "bad" brains. Moreover, experience is not merely something to which the organism is passively exposed; rather, the effects of experience on development represent a complex interplay among:

- The developmental status of the brain at the time of exposure;
- The nature of the experience;
- The degree of experience (e.g., a great deal of early stress vs. limited exposure to early stress);
- The organism's involvement with the experience, and, very likely;
- The individual's genetic background.

Some of these factors can be illustrated by the following example.

Francis, Szegda, Campbell *et al.* (2003) cross-fostered two strains of mice with one another. One was cross-fostered prenatally (here, embryos from one strain that were just a few hours old were implanted in the mothers of another strain) and the other postnatally (newborn pups from one strain were raised by mothers of the other strain). Control animals consisted of the two original (non-cross fostered) strains. All animals were tested at 3 months of age. The authors reported that the control animals differed reliably from one another on four dimensions:

1. Differences in exploration of an open field;
2. Relative time on the open arms of a plus maze;
3. Latency to find a hidden platform in the Morris water maze; and
4. Acoustic startle pre-pulse inhibition.

Cross-fostering animals prenatally *or* postnatally did not exert any effects on the expected phenotype. However, mice that had been prenatally *and* postnatally cross-fostered exhibited the same behavioral phenotype as the adopted strain, despite differing genetically from the adopted strain. The fact that mice that had been cross-fostered prenatally did not show this effect supported the contention that the effects of the combined cross-fostering must be a result of non-genetic factors, namely the powerful role of experience on gene expression. This study illustrated the dynamic interaction between genes, brain and behavior.

Sensory and Perceptual Development

In the context of developmental psychopathology, it is important to stress that the impact of experience on the brain is not constant throughout life. As the brain develops and matures, its sensitivity to experience changes. As we discuss below, there is now a plethora of examples of adult plasticity but, suffice to say, the functional properties of the developing brain are such that they are more experience-dependent than the adult brain. Below we provide examples of both developmental and adult plasticity (for a more extensive treatise on this topic in the context of development see Nelson, de Haan, & Thomas, 2006).

Developmental Plasticity

The classic examples of developmental plasticity are generally drawn from early sensory and/or perceptual development. For example, we know that between 6 and 12 months of age, the ability to discriminate phonemes from languages to which an infant is not exposed declines dramatically (for a review see Saffran, Werker, & Werner, 2006; Werker & Vouloumanos, 2001). With that said, it appears that the door does not shut completely on retaining the ability to discriminate non-native contrasts. For example, if before 12 months of age infants are given additional experience with speech sounds in a non-native language, this ability is retained (Kuhl, Tsao, & Liu, 2003). A similar phenomenon occurs in the visual domain; specifically, in the domain of face processing. Pascalis, de Haan and Nelson (2002) have reported that 6-month-olds, 9-month-olds and adults are all equally good at discriminating two human faces, but only 6-month-olds can also discriminate two monkey faces. However, it is also the case that if 6-month-olds are given 3 months' experience viewing monkey faces, they retain this ability (Pascalis, Scott, Kelly *et al.*, 2005). Thus, as is the case with speech, face processing also appears to go through a developmentally sensitive period, although one that can be extended with specific experience.

A similar phenomenon exists for visual acuity. Maurer, Lewis, Brent *et al.* (1999) have reported that among infants born with cataracts that are removed and new lenses placed within months of birth, even just a few minutes of visual experience can lead to a big improvement in visual acuity. However, the longer the cataracts are left untreated, the less favorable the outcome.

In the broad domain of visual function, we know that among Braille-reading individuals who lost their sight *after* age 16, activation of area 17 of the visual cortex is absent, whereas such activation is present among those who lost their sight *before* age 16 (Sadato, Pascual-Leone, Grafman *et al.*, 1998). Such findings are also consistent with a sensitive period for visual function.

Effects of Early Focal Lesions on Language Development

The extent to which language represents a special modular function that is hard-wired into the nervous system or represents a domain-general function that becomes domain-specific with experience continues to be debated. One element of the language literature that is particularly relevant to this debate concerns the effect of early brain injury on the development and neural organization of language. In what way is this literature relevant? If there are such things as language modules, then there should be relatively little plasticity in language systems, as other systems should be unable to absorb the functions subserved by language-dedicated areas. On the other hand, if language (speaking broadly) reflects an experience-expectant system that is heavily activity dependent, then there should be considerable plasticity in the system – although such plasticity is likely to be bounded by a sensitive period. As a result, children experiencing early damage to language-related areas should develop reasonably normal language, assuming they are reared in a language-typical environment. As we shall see below, that is exactly what happens.

Building on earlier work by Lenneberg and others (e.g., Lenneberg, 1969), the late Elizabeth Bates led a longitudinal study concerned with language development in children experiencing focal brain damage. In their project (for a review see Bates & Roe, 2001), children who experienced a stroke immediately prior to birth or in the immediate postpartum period were studied. In some cases the stroke was unilateral and in others bilateral. As the infants developed, they were studied using a battery of tasks designed to evaluate a range of language functions.

The most consistent finding reported by these researchers was that relative to typically developing controls, by school age, children with unilateral brain damage fell within the normal range on measures of productive language, and that no differences in productive language were observed between children experiencing left vs. right hemisphere damage. When compared with adults with damage to the left hemisphere, children who experienced focal brain injury were superior in all measures of language production. A virtually identical pattern of findings was obtained on measures of language comprehension.

Bates and colleagues interpreted these findings to suggest that the left hemisphere is initially committed to language development. If development proceeds normally, this hemisphere will become specialized for language; however, when brain damage occurs (as with a pre- or perinatal stroke), the right hemisphere will subsume the functions of the left hemisphere. This pattern is very different from that observed in adults, in whom damage to language-related areas typically leads to significant and persistent deficits (i.e., there is much less plasticity in recovery from brain damage). These findings also suggest that the neural substrate for language is not fixed but, rather, is simply biased in a particular direction. Should the typical trajectory be perturbed because of early brain damage, the brain's plasticity makes it possible for other neural systems to subsume the functions of the original architecture.

Social and Emotional Development and Developmental Psychopathology

Moving away from the sensory, perceptual and linguistic domains, a rather dramatic example of the effects of early experience on development can be found in an ambitious project concerned with the effects of early institutionalization on brain and behavioral development. The *Bucharest Early Intervention Project* (BEIP) is a longitudinal study contrasting three groups of children. The *institutionalized group* comprised children who had lived virtually their entire lives in institutional settings in Bucharest, Romania. The *foster care group* included children who were institutionalized at birth, and then following an extensive baseline assessment, placed in foster care (the mean age of placement was 22 months). Finally, the *never-institutionalized group* included children living with their biological families in the greater Bucharest community (for details see Zeanah, Nelson, Fox *et al.*, 2003). The neuroscientific premise underlying this project is that the deficits and developmental delays that result from institutional rearing have their origins in compromised brain development. For the brain to wire correctly requires input; a lack of input leads to the under-specification of circuits and miswiring of circuits. Children living in institutions lack input (stimulation) on a grand scale, and thus, we expect such children to experience a range of problems as a result of "errors" in brain development. Finally, we know that some domains of function are more experience-dependent than others, and in the experience-dependent functions, *the critical timing* of the experience needed to ensure healthy development will vary. Thus, the efficacy of foster care should vary by domain (e.g., language, psychopathology) and duration of deprivation.

Our findings have been reported and reviewed in a variety of outlets (for a recent overview see Nelson, Zeanah, & Fox, 2007). For the purposes of this chapter, we briefly touch on our psychopathology data.[1]

First, it is important to note at the outset that the *institutionalized group* and *foster care group* were identical in all respects at baseline (i.e., before half the sample was placed in foster care). Second, we found that at 54 months of age, approximately 56% of the *institutionalized group* met criteria for an axis I disorder, whereas this figure dropped to 36% for the *foster care group*. If we break this down further, we see that 50% of the *institutionalized group* but only 22% of the *foster care group* met the criteria for any emotional disorder; however, in the domain of behavioral disorders, there were no statistically significant differences between the *institutionalized group* and *foster care group* (where the rates are 32% and 25%, respectively).

Naturally, we were curious about specific disorders, so we broke our data down further. Here several observations are worth noting. For depression, the incidence among the *institutionalized group* and the *foster care group* was 8.5% and 3%, respectively; for anxiety, these same figures were 44% and 20%. Thus, for emotional disorders generally, there was a very high incidence of anxiety overall, and foster care appears to be effective in reducing the burden of suffering for both anxiety and depression. The picture is quite different for disruptive symptoms. Here we found that the incidence of attention deficit/hyperactivity disorder (ADHD) was 25% in the *institutionalized group* and 19% in the *foster care group* (not a statistically significant difference). For oppositional defiant disorder/conduct disorder (ODD/CD), these figures were 15% and 14%, respectively. Thus, in contrast to emotional disorders, foster care has shown no beneficial effect (as yet) on reducing the symptoms of ADHD and ODD/CD.

Collectively, this project demonstrates that early psychosocial deprivation appears to be causally related to subsequent psychopathology, and that foster care is more effective in reducing symptoms of emotional disorders than disruptive disorders. This latter observation permits us to speculate that the neural circuits that subserve attention and emotion regulation (largely prefrontal) may be established in the first 2 years of life, prior to when the children were removed from the institution and placed in foster care. However, whether this represents a true sensitive period or not is impossible to say until we see the children at a later age (as we are currently doing).

Collectively, these and other examples (for elaboration see Nelson, de Haan, & Thomas, 2006) demonstrate the role of early experience in development, and the concept of sensitive periods.

Adult Plasticity

It was once assumed that with the exception of a few isolated domains (e.g., recovery from stroke), the adult brain possessed little plasticity. However, studies by Rosenzweig and Diamond (e.g., Diamond, Lindner, Johnson *et al.*, 1975) and later by Greenough, clearly proved this view incorrect. For example, over the past 30 years Greenough and colleagues have elegantly demonstrated that rats raised in complex laboratory environments perform many cognitive tasks better than rats reared in isolation. Some of the changes observed in the brain include the following:

1 Regions within the dorsal neocortex are heavier and thicker and have more synapses.

2 The number and length of dendritic spines and branching patterns increase.

3 There is increased capillary branching, thereby increasing blood and oxygen volume (for some specific examples and overviews see Black, Jones, Nelson *et al.*, 1998; Greenough & Black, 1992; Kolb, Gibb, & Robinson, 2003).

Other examples of adult plasticity can be found in the motor and sensory domains. For example, Elbert, Pantev, Wienbruch *et al.* (1995) have reported that the somatosensory cortex representing the fingers of the left hand in highly proficient stringed instrument players is larger than: (i) the analogous area in the opposite hemisphere representing the right hand (used to bow vs. the left hand, which is used in more fine motor activity), and; (ii) than non-musicians. In addition, Draganski, Gaser, Busch *et al.* (2004) have reported that individuals who had been given 3 months to learn to juggle showed increased bilateral neural activation in certain brain regions (mid-temporal area and left posterior intraparietal sulcus). Importantly, 3 months after this group stopped juggling, there was a decrease in activation. Non-jugglers over the 6-month period showed no changes in brain activation.

Moving into more cognitive systems, Erickson, Jagadeesh, and Desimone (2000) presented adult monkeys with multicolored

[1] Note: because the critical question being addressed in this project is the efficacy of foster care in ameliorating the negative sequelae of early institutionalization, we do not report the data from the Never Institutionalized Group (NIG). However, suffice to say, the incidence of psychopathology in this group is virtually identical to that of a US comparison sample.

complex stimuli (some familiar, some novel) while brain activity was recorded from the perirhinal cortex (an area known to be involved in episodic memory). The authors reported that after only 1 day's experience viewing the stimuli, the performance of neighboring neurons became highly correlated during viewing of familiar stimuli; this was in contrast to novel stimuli, which revealed little correlated neuronal activity. The authors interpreted these findings to suggest that visual experience leads to functional changes in an area of the brain known to be involved in memory.

An even more dramatic example of how experience leads to changes in neural architecture is the now well-known study of London cab drivers. Maguire, Gadian, Johnsrude *et al.* (2000) obtained structural MRI scans from individuals with great expertise in navigating the streets of London (i.e., London cab drivers). The authors reported that, relative to non-cab drivers, the posterior hippocampus was larger; moreover, there was also a positive correlation between hippocampal volume and the amount of experience the drivers had. Alas, there is rather a chicken-and-egg problem with this work: specifically, it might be the case that individuals who choose to be cab drivers already have a larger hippocampus or possess more plasticity than non-cab drivers, thus making them more likely to show anatomical changes in response to experience. Clearly, this is an area ripe for future study.

Collectively, we now know that the adult brain is quite capable of being molded by experience. Over and above the examples provided, learning and memory represent the quintessential examples of adult plasticity. However, the behavioral domains that benefit from such experience are more limited than those that benefit from experiences earlier in development. This leads us to ask what the difference is between adult versus developmental plasticity.

What distinguishes adult plasticity from developmental plasticity?

There are a number of fundamental differences in the way plastic processes might work in the developing brain compared to the developed brain. First, at the physiological, anatomical and metabolic levels, the plastic processes that operate early in the lifespan differ from those that occur later in the lifespan. The newborn brain has more neurons and synapses than an adult brain, and many of these are not yet committed to particular circuits or functions. Thus, an axon that is growing towards its target has very different terrain to negotiate in the newborn brain than in the adult brain. Similarly, modifying synapses already committed to a particular circuit is quite different from committing synapses to a particular circuit for the first time. In other words, rewiring the brain is different from wiring the brain.

Another way to demonstrate the difference between developmental and adult plasticity is at a systems or behavioral level. For example, a goal of infant development is to establish neural circuits in the service of some behavior. However, these circuits are already in place in the adult brain, and must be retasked or reconfigured in order to serve another function; a case in point might be the difference in acquiring a first language versus learning a second or third language.

In summary, both the developing and developed brain are capable of being molded by experience, although there are many more constraints on changing the adult brain and the mechanisms that underlie plasticity likely differ between children and adults.

Biological Insults

Across developmental time the brain can be altered by experience. However, many organic insults can, and do, also alter brain development, and can sometimes lead to long-lasting damage. In this section we describe such pre- and perinatal insults, with emphasis on the fact that many different types of injury can result in similar developmental outcomes.

The central nervous system develops over a protracted course, beginning shortly after conception and continuing after birth, with refining processes (e.g., myelination and synaptogenesis) occurring throughout childhood and adolescence. As one would expect, the brain is susceptible to injury at each stage of development. Following the principles of neural plasticity outlined earlier in this chapter, we know that timing, duration, location, mechanism and extent of injury and initial clinical course all contribute to neurological outcome and extent of neurodevelopmental pathology. As we will show, the level of clinical impairment depends upon the interplay of the factors listed above (e.g., timing, extent and location of injury), with no one factor having a singularly dominant role in defining outcome.

Prenatal, or intrauterine, defects can result from malformation or destruction of brain tissue. Brain malformations can occur at every stage of prenatal development (Aicardi, 1998; Barkovich, 2005a; Swaiman, Ashwal, & Ferriero, 2006). Aberrant neural tube formation can lead to *anencephaly* (failed closure of the rostral end of neural tube, leading to incomplete formation of brain and skull), *encephalocele* (herniation of the brain outside of skull) or *myelomeningocele* (failure of closure of the caudal end of neural tube, leading to an open sac of spinal cord tissue). Later in development, abnormal segmentation and cleavage can result in *holoprosencephaly* (failure of the brain to divide into lobes), *agenesis of the corpus callosum*, or *septo-optic dysplasia* (underdevelopment of the optic nerve, hypopituitarism and absence of a midline structure called the septum pellucidum). Later still in development, disordered neuronal proliferation can cause *microcephaly* (small brain), *macrocephaly* (large brain) or can lead to abnormal *neoplastic* or *benign* cortical tumors. Disordered migration can result in *lissencephaly* (smooth brain) or *cortical heterotopias* (groups of neurons not fully migrated), while abnormal neuronal organization can result in *schizencephaly* (abnormal cortical clefts). Finally, defects in myelination result in disorders of the white matter such as *white matter hypoplasia*.

In addition, far beyond the scope of this chapter, there exist countless inherited metabolic, neurodegenerative and genetic disorders that result in brain malformations and associated developmental psychopathology. Common examples include trisomy 21, fragile X and tuberous sclerosis (see chapter 24). Extensive research in the past two decades on the genetics of brain malformations has resulted in the isolation of genes for many of the above disorders, such as the *DCX*, *LIS1* and *RELN* gene mutations found in the lissencephaly syndromes (Barkovich, 2005b).

The clinical outcome of brain malformations varies, and depends on both timing and extent of the area of brain involved. For instance, children with holoprosencephaly typically have intractable seizures, profound developmental delay and spastic quadriparesis, while those with small cortical heterotopias may only have focal seizures with no developmental disabilities. The level of impairment in children with lissencephaly depends on the extent of cortex affected, but typically children have profound neurological impairment in all realms of development.

Destructive processes, including infection, vascular injury and toxic exposures, also can occur *in utero*. With regard to infectious agents, the most common pathogens affecting the CNS include viruses such as cytomegalovirus (CMV), herpes simplex virus (HSV), varicella zoster virus (VZV), Epstein–Barr virus (EBV), human immunodeficiency virus (HIV) and rubella, parasitic infections such as toxoplasmosis, and, more rarely, bacterial infections. *In utero* infection with any of the above agents can result in significant neurological sequelae such as profound developmental delay, seizures, behavioral disturbances, autistic features, visual impairment, sensorineural hearing loss and spastic quadriparesis (Swaiman, Ashawl, & Ferriero, 2006; Volpe, 2001). Again, as with brain malformations, the extent of intraparenchymal involvement and timing of infection influence the severity of outcome. In some cases the earlier the exposure to the infectious agent, the more significant the neurological devastation. For example, a recent study compared children exposed to CMV infection in the first-trimester with those exposed later in gestation. Of the first-trimester group, 24% had sensorineural hearing loss, compared to 2.5% of the later-infection group. Of the first-trimester group, 32% exhibited at least one CNS sequela (intellectual disability, cerebral palsy, seizures) compared to 15% in the later group, and none of this later group had more than one sequela (Pass, 2006).

Moving on from infection, prenatal vascular injury usually occurs in the setting of hypoxia or ischemia, resulting from maternal disease, placental insufficiency or pathology intrinsic to the fetus. Pathologically, necrotic and cavitary lesions are most commonly seen with prenatal injury, especially lesions of the white matter such as periventricular leukomalacia (PVL). Diagnosis of these insults is often postnatal, and sometimes can be delayed for months in milder lesions. Outcome depends on extent and site of injury. For example, global hypoxia can cause profound intellectual disability and quadriparesis, while focal ischemia may result in only a mild motor impairment or seizures, depending on location of the stroke. Mild to moderate degrees of hypoxic injury, however, can sometimes exert their effects relatively selectively, leading, for example, to damage to the hippocampus, which in turn may lead to selective deficits in memory (de Haan, Wyatt, Roth *et al.*, 2006).

Finally, toxic exposures to the fetus can lead to neurodevelopmental pathology, even in the setting of normal-appearing brain parenchyma. Toxins include therapeutic drugs such as antiepileptics, or recreational drugs such as alcohol, nicotine, marijuana or cocaine. As discussed in detail in chapter 30, fetal alcohol exposure is the most common preventable chemical cause of intellectual disability in the USA (Aicardi, 1998). Long-term follow-up studies of children with fetal alcohol syndrome (FAS) show significant deficits in visuospatial functioning, verbal and non-verbal learning, attention and executive functioning. They also have behavioral problems that further affect their daily functioning (Riley & McGee, 2005).

Perinatal injury, defined as insults during or just after birth, can also cause significant neurological sequelae. The most common examples include intracerebral hemorrhage, hypoxic ischemic injury, PVL and perinatal toxic or metabolic disturbances. With these insults, timing may be less critical, and more important become location, extent of injury and level of neurological dysfunction at the time of injury. Most perinatal insults occur within the first 10 days of life.

Intracerebral hemorrhage includes subdural, intraventricular, intraparenchymal and subarachnoid bleeding. Birth trauma is the major cause of subdural and subarachnoid hemorrhage, and often can fully resolve without neurological sequelae. Sometimes children will have seizures in the acute setting, and based on the location of the hemorrhage may have some motor deficits. Intraventricular hemorrhage occurs most commonly in the preterm infant, especially before age 32 weeks, when the germinal matrix still exists. Classically, hemorrhage is graded by the extent of ventricular blood and dilatation. Grade I is the mildest, with less than 50% of the ventricle filled with blood, with grade IV, or periventricular hemorrhagic infarction, resulting in both intraventricular and intraparenchymal blood. Factors that predispose the preterm infant to intraventricular hemorrhage include labile blood pressures, sepsis, certain medications and mechanical ventilation. The neurological outcome of intraventricular hemorrhage depends on the extent of hemorrhage and the neonate's clinical status at presentation. Grade I hemorrhage often results in a normal outcome, whereas 75% of neonates with grade III–IV hemorrhage, if they survive, have profound spastic quadriparesis, intellectual disability and behavioral disturbances (Volpe, 2001).

Hypoxic ischemic encephalopathy (HIE) can occur as a result of prenatal vascular insufficiency, perinatal asphyxia, or postnatal hypoxia from respiratory failure, hypotension or other systemic illness. HIE occurs in up to 6 per 1000 live births, and results from two mechanisms: hypoxia (reduced oxygen supply to the blood), or ischemia (reduced perfusion of the brain). Both are caused by asphyxia, or hypoxia associated with hypercarbia (a build-up of carbon dioxide in the blood). The end result is a depletion of adenosine triphosphate (ATP) and a rise in lactate production in the brain, which ultimately causes brain edema and cell death. The pathology associated with HIE depends on the duration and extent of the asphyxia. Acute total asphyxia leads to bilateral lesions in the brainstem and thalamic lesions, while partial prolonged asphyxia causes more diffuse lesions with edema, mainly affecting the cortex and basal ganglia. In addition, HIE is often associated with PVL (bilateral necrosis of the white matter adjacent to the lateral ventricles). Sometimes these lesions can become hemorrhagic or cystic (Aicardi, 1998; Volpe, 2001).

Clinical impairments of HIE range from mild to severe based on the extent of pathology. Preterm infants tend to have poorer outcomes than term infants. In the milder cases, irritability and jitteriness prevail, whereas in more severe cases, obtundation and intractable seizures occur. Babies with diffuse involvement of the cortex can present in coma. When the brainstem is affected, babies may lose their ability to breathe, suck or swallow independently. The long-term prognosis depends on the severity of the clinical picture during the first days of life. Neurodevelopmental deficits are not seen if there are no initial clinical sequelae of HIE (Aicardi, 1998). In mild HIE, only some motor deficits may occur. In severe HIE, most children will have significant developmental delay along with cerebral palsy and seizure disorder.

Metabolic disturbances such as *hyperbilirubinemia* leading to *kernicterus*, or electrolyte abnormalities such as *hypoglycemia* or *hypocalcemia* can also lead to significant neurological sequelae after birth, initially with encephalopathy and seizures and ultimately with developmental delays, depending on extent and duration of exposure. Also, many inborn errors of metabolism present early in the neonatal period and lead to varying degrees of developmental delay and behavioral disturbances.

Perhaps the most common risk factor for subsequent morbidity concerns infants born prematurely and/or of low birth weight. About 55,000 children per year are born in the USA with birth weights less than 1500 g, defined as very low birth weight (VLBW) (Taylor, Minich, Klein *et al.*, 2004). In these children, the incidence of major developmental disabilities (e.g., intellectual disability, cerebral palsy, epilepsy, blindness, sensorineural hearing loss) is in the range of 15–20%. In addition, more subtle disabilities such as learning disabilities, mild cognitive impairment, ADHD and behavioral problems occur in an estimated 50–70% of such children (Hack, Klein, & Taylor, 1995).

In the CNS, hypoxic ischemic injury, intraventricular hemorrhage, PVL and infection represent the primary pathology in children of VLBW. Both white and gray matter are vulnerable to injury, and hypoxic ischemic injury leads to multifocal cortical ischemia and necrosis, especially in the sensorimotor, parieto-occipital, temporal regions adjacent to the ventricles, hippocampus and other subcortical structures (Volpe, 2001).

Neuropsychological studies of VLBW adolescents have shown deficits in multiple cognitive domains, such as visual–motor skills and memory, independent of IQ. In a recent study by Taylor, Minich, Klein *et al.* (2004), long-term follow-up of children of VLBW was performed, with neuropsychological testing performed until age 16. Analysis revealed poorest outcomes in those with lower birth weight, lower weight for gestational age and longer period of oxygen requirement. The major impairments were in visual–motor skills, spatial memory and executive function. In studies of younger children, impairments in working memory and spatial planning are consistently found, and are thought to be predicted by the presence of intraventricular hemorrhage or PVL (Frisk & Whyte, 1994).

Overall, there seems to be a correlation between birth weight and level of impairment, with the lowest birth weight children having the most impairment. Associated factors that likely determine clinical outcome include medical and neurological complications in the neonatal period. Furthermore, there is evidence that environmental factors may also have a role, with sociodemographic status and family environment likely moderating the biological effects of being VLBW (Taylor *et al.*, 2004). Therefore, like many of the other prenatal insults described in the above section, rather than one variable defining clinical outcome, it is likely the interplay of several critical factors that predicts the degree of impairment in children of VLBW. While degree of prematurity (with weight as a marker of gestational age) does have an important role, it is not clear that specific CNS pathology correlates consistently with specific neuropsychological deficits.

Summary

This brief review was designed to illustrate that many different mechanisms of biological injury can result in psychopathology, ranging from profound intellectual disability to mild developmental delay, behavioral problems or disorders on the autistic spectrum. We now discuss one specific neurodevelopmental disorder, autism, and consider how this clinical syndrome can result from many distinct biological entities (for a fuller discussion of autism see chapter 46). In this section, we use autism as a model for a discussion about biological and environmental mechanisms of developmental psychopathology. While many children with autism do not have a known underlying neuropathology, many children with the pre- and postnatal insults described earlier meet the criteria for autism; these include children with prenatal CMV infection, intracerebral hemorrhage and genetic syndromes such as tuberous sclerosis. In our discussion we illustrate that while much of the pathogenesis of this disorder remains unknown, there is adequate evidence to support underlying pathology at multiple stages of brain development.

Autism

Decades ago, it was believed that this disorder of behavior and cognition resulted from emotional deprivation in infancy. However, subsequent studies found a much higher incidence of abnormal electroencephalograms (EEGs), epilepsy and intellectual disability in children with autism, thereby arguing for a biological basis for the syndrome (Small, 1975). Because of the variability in age of diagnosis, the timing of the insult or injury was not well characterized.

As discussed in chapter 46, in the past decade, studies in neuropathology, neuroimaging, morphometrics and early behavior of children with autism suggest that abnormalities in the nervous system occur at multiple stages of brain development, from the first prenatal months through early childhood. Changes in the brain occur long before atypical behaviors become apparent, and these changes continue over the course of a lifetime. These changes are likely not static, but progressive, and may evolve over the course of brain development. For example, it may be the case that an error in brain development that occurs prenatally will not be expressed until the area affected begins to mature and subserve function (Miller, Goldman, & Rosvold, 1973); a case in point may be the prevailing view that schizophrenia, which does not typically present until late in the second decade of life, likely has it origin in errors in cell migration, an event that occurred perhaps as much as two decades earlier (see chapter 45).

Given the mounting evidence that at least some signs of autism appear well before a formal diagnosis is made, the question then arises, when and how does this insult occur? Is there one critical time of development that results in the autistic phenotype, or are there many paths to one final common phenotype? Much speculation exists regarding the role of prenatal insults in the pathogenesis of autism. Retrospective studies have shown a higher incidence of many different perinatal and prenatal factors in children with autism, such as uterine bleeding, hyperbilirubinemia, early gestational age, early fetal distress and low Apgar scores, but none have been evaluated prospectively (Glasson, Bower, Petterson *et al.*, 2004; Juul-Dam, Townsend, & Courchesne, 2001). Some argue that obstetric complications may, in fact, be an epiphenomenon or even a consequence, and not a cause, of neurodevelopmental disabilities such as autism. In other words, both autism and perinatal complications may be derived from shared risk factors, such as genetic or environmental susceptibility (Bolton, Murphy, Macdonald *et al.*, 1997). More studies are needed to resolve these issues.

Pre- and Postnatal Insults and Autism

Associations exist between autism and certain prenatal insults, including fetal exposure to alcohol, valproic acid and thalidomide, as well as congenital infections including CMV and rubella (Arndt, Stodgell, & Rodier, 2005; Miller, Strömland, Ventura *et al.*, 2005). It is also known that certain genetic syndromes, such as tuberous sclerosis, fragile X, Smith–Lemli–Opitz, and Cornelia de Lange, as well as some neurodevelopmental disorders, such as Möbius sequence and CHARGE association (colobomas, heart defects, choanal atresia, retarded growth/development, genital anomalies and ear anomalies/hearing loss) have a higher incidence of autism than the general population (Miller *et al.*, 2005).

From a neurodevelopmental perspective, what is interesting is the fact that each of the above syndromes influences the brain at different stages of fetal development, with some insults clearly occurring early in gestation. For instance, in Möbius sequence and CHARGE association, children exhibit abnormalities in cranial nerves and facial structures (such as ear development) both of which develop in the first month of gestation. The teratogenic effects of valproic acid are thought to occur early in gestation as well, as the anomalies seen in exposed children indicate defects of neural tube closure, such as craniofacial abnormalities and defects in heart, genitalia, and limb structure (Arndt, Stodgell, & Rodier, 2005). In genetic syndromes such as tuberous sclerosis, where the incidence of autism is as high as 40%, benign tumors appear in multiple organ systems, including the heart, kidney and brain, throughout fetal development. Finally, in the case of congenital CMV or rubella, timing of infection is not as well correlated with outcome, as some children with evidence of infection as late as the second and third trimesters can ultimately show clinical signs of autism.

Furthermore, as reviewed in chapter 46, there are data from pathology and neuroimaging (functional imaging, morphometrics) that abnormalities exist that can be attributed to both pre- and postnatal development. It is clear that at least some of the dysregulation of neuronal growth must occur in the early prenatal period, but then likely continues through childhood and adolescence.

Work by Courchesne and colleagues has shown evidence of dysregulation of brain growth throughout development in children with autism. In their studies, the average head circumference in children with autism was slightly smaller than normal, but during the first year of life there was an abnormally accelerated rate of brain growth, so that by age 2 the brain of a child with autism was 10% larger than average (Courchesne, Carper, & Akshoomoff, 2003; Courchesne, Redcay, & Kennedy, 2004). MRI data have shown that the enlargement represents both gray and white matter, but most prominently cortical and cerebellar white matter (Courchesne, 2002; Herbert, Ziegler, Deutsch *et al.*, 2005). Moreover, the overgrowth is consistently regional, with frontal lobes being most abnormally enlarged, while posterior regions of the brain such as the occipital lobes are normal in size. Furthermore, while the volume of brainstem and cerebellum was shown to increase with age, the overall sizes of regions of the brainstem as well as the cerebellar vermis were smaller than in the general population (Hashimoto, Tayama, Murakawa *et al.*, 1995). The phase of cortical overgrowth was followed later in childhood by a phase of abnormally slow (or arrested) growth. By adolescence, the autistic child's brain was only 1–2% larger than average. As with the localization of brain overgrowth, the growth retardation affects both white and gray matter, but most prominently cortical and cerebellar white matter (Courchesne, Redcay, Morgan *et al.*, 2005).

While the principle of brain growth dysregulation in children with autism has been well accepted, the details of the data (such as cerebellar size and the fact that the brain returns to average size by adulthood) have not been confirmed by other studies. Nevertheless, these data do support the notion that changes in the brain may occur at different and continuing time points in children with autism.

Through this discussion, one might conclude that autism is a biologically based disorder of brain development, and not a result of environmental deprivation. However, as we have emphasized throughout this chapter, brain development is affected by many factors, and there is likely an interplay of environment and biology. We now illustrate the fact that environment may also have a critical role in the development of the autistic phenotype, at least in some children. The monozygotic twin concordance rate in autism has been reported to be in the range 60–95% (Bailey, Luthert, Dean *et al.*, 1998). The fact that the concordance is not 100% has been used as evidence for the important contribution of environment in the development of the final autistic phenotype (although of course variable expression of genes can also be due to stochastic effects).

What Environmental Factors are Associated with Autism?

The relationship between environmental deprivation and the autistic phenotype has been described retrospectively. Fraiberg (1977) found that children born blind developed behavioral abnormalities similar to autism, and defined them as manifesting an "autistiform syndrome." More recently, several retrospective studies of Romanian children adopted into families after early institutionalization have been found to exhibit a similar autistic phenotype (Hoksbergen, ter Laak, Rijk *et al.*, 2005; Rutter, Anderson-Wood, Beckett *et al.*, 1999).

Rutter *et al.* (1999) evaluated a subgroup of Romanian children who were adopted from orphanages into homes in England. These children, most of whom were adopted by age 2, were reported to be severely deprived and malnourished. Their experience in the orphanages was described as ranging from "poor to appalling," left in cots all day without much interactive play, verbal communication or physical interaction with others. The children underwent screening for autism at age 4 and then age 6 using the Autism Screening Questionnaire (ASQ). The Autism Diagnostic Interview (ADI-R) was also used to interview the adoptive parents about their children's behaviors.

In their assessment, Rutter *et al.* (1999) found that 6% of these children at age 4 showed "a pattern of behavior that closely resembled childhood autism," a pattern that Rutter defined as "quasi-autistic." They had "poor reciprocity, a deviant style, poor appreciation of social cues, and a lack of normal social boundaries" as well as "indiscriminate friendliness." They also demonstrated stereotyped preoccupations with certain types of play. However, unlike children with classic autism, they maintained a high degree of social interest and they did not manifest any repetitive movements such as rocking or spinning in circles. Furthermore, these children *improved* in all realms of behavior from age 4 to 6, quite unlike the typical child with autism. While there were no clear predictors of autism in this group, two correlates that emerged were degree of cognitive impairment and duration of institutionalization.

These findings were supported by Hoksbergen *et al.* (2005), who studied 80 children from Romania adopted in the Netherlands. Using parental interview only, they described a "Post-Institutional Autistic Syndrome" in 13 of the 80 children and also described some developmental improvement after adoption. Overall, according to these studies, children facing early environmental deprivation had a higher incidence of autism. The features of autism, however, were rather atypical. They also tended to improve with amelioration of their environment.

Conclusions

Earlier in this section we reported that a variety of disorders (e.g., fragile X, tuberous sclerosis) can present as classic autism, and that a number of pre- or perinatal insults increase the probability that a child will present with autism. We concluded this section of our chapter by also reporting that a subset of children experiencing early severe privation appear quasi-autistic although, intriguingly, the symptoms of this disorder are lessened or even disappear following placement into families. Therefore, using autism as an example of a neurodevelopmental disorder, we have shown that a similar phenotype can result from a purely biological and a purely environmental insult.

How do we reconcile the fact that frank biological insult (e.g., tubers that replace normal brain tissue, as in the case of tuberous sclerosis), toxic exposures (e.g., alcohol), and exposure to early psychosocial adversity can all lead to the same disorder? To address this question, we must return to the definition of the "disorder" itself. Autism, as defined by DSM-IV (American Psychiatric Association, 2000), is a summation of specific cognitive and behavioral traits, which together create a specific phenotype. Like many behavioral and developmental disorders, the definition is based purely on clinical criteria created by clinicians and researchers. The definition assumes no specific pathogenesis or etiology, but only describes the ultimate clinical outcome. Thus, the fact that multiple causes can produce the same phenotype does not undermine or confound the definition itself. However, it does support the contention that autism encompasses a number of different – although likely related – disorders, and that as we learn more about their neuropathology, these separate syndromes will emerge from the blanket diagnosis of "autism" as independent identities. Stated rather differently, the heterogeneity of autism may, in fact, reflect biologically distinct disorders.

One could argue that most clinically defined disorders, such as ADHD, bipolar disorder and schizophrenia, face a similar underlying heterogeneity. For example, some "strains" of ADHD or depression may have a much higher genetic loading than others, some may be largely attributed to a birth injury (e.g., an intraventricular hemorrhage that occurs as a by-product of being born very prematurely) and still others may be triggered predominantly by environmental factors (such as the association between early maltreatment and depression). What we need to consider is that autism and all other forms of psychopathology are inherently brain disorders, with alterations in neurochemistry, neural circuitry or neural anatomy causing the clinical phenotype.

The cause of these alterations is likely multifactorial. For example, alterations in specific genes or gene products at particular points in development can lead to changes in brain anatomy, circuitry or chemistry. Similarly, in some cases these genes may express themselves independently of experience, whereas in others it may well take an environmental trigger to alter gene expression. In still other cases, as among children who experience profound early privation, genes may play no part in the disorder. Instead, the pathogenesis can be attributed to the brain's ability to be molded by experience – albeit molded abnormally. Ultimately, we could argue that brain development can be perturbed by both genetic and non-genetic factors, and that such perturbations can present in exactly the same way, despite different underlying causes.

Our only hope of unraveling the biological mechanisms that actually cause a disorder are to consider:

1 Both genetic and non-genetic factors simultaneously;

2 The *exact timing* of these factors; and

3 The *degree* to which these factors cause pathology (e.g., how many repeats of a given gene; the extent of early adverse experience).

We conclude our chapter with an additional recommendation for future research. If neuroscience is to shed light on psychopathology, it is imperative that we improve our phenotyping instruments. As behavioral neuroscientists have known for many years, the success in elucidating the neural underpinnings of a given behavior depends to a great degree on how carefully and specifically the behavior is described. For example, to say someone is anxious says little about the myriad of behaviors that collectively express themselves as anxiety. To improve the precision of diagnoses (by improved phenotyping), we need to improve our armamentarium of tools that permit us to look inside the developing brain. At present, the best functional tool we have to study the infant's brain is EEG, as functional imaging (fMRI, PET) requires that a child be old enough to comply with the study. Ideally, we must develop a system of co-registering these measures in order to take advantage of the strengths of each tool. For completeness, we should use multiple measures *combined with sensitive behavioral assays.*

Ultimately, as we improve our ability to characterize accurately the neuropathology underlying behavioral disorders, the way we view and perhaps even treat these disorders will change. They will evolve from being definitions created by clinical observation to precise diagnoses validated by scientific data. This evolution will not only facilitate effective therapy, but also provide insight into the biology of behavior and, essentially, the mind.

If we accept at face value that all disorders of the mind are inherently disorders of the brain, and that genes and gene products have an integral role in brain development and brain function, it is incumbent upon us to train the next generation of developmental psychopathologists accordingly.

Further Reading

Nelson, C. A., de Haan, M., & Thomas, K. M. (2006). *Neuroscience and cognitive development: The role of experience and the developing brain.* New York: Wiley.

Rutter, M. (2006). *Genes and behaviour: Nature–nurture interplay explained.* London, UK: Blackwell Publishing.

References

Aicardi, J. (1998). *Diseases of the nervous system of childhood* (2nd ed.). Cambridge, UK: Cambridge University Press.

Aimone, J. B., Wiles, J., & Gage, F. H. (2006). Potential role for adult neurogenesis in the encoding of time in new memories. *Nature Neuroscience, 9,* 723–727.

Aizawa, H., Hu, S-C., Bobb, K., Balakrishnan, K., Ince, G., Gurevich, I., *et al.* (2004). Dendrite development regulated by CREST, a Calcium-Regulated Transcriptional Activator. *Science, 303,* 197–202.

American Psychiatric Association. (2000). *Diagnostic and statistical manual of mental disorders* (4th ed.), Text Revision (DSM-IV-TR). Washington DC: American Psychiatric Association.

Arndt, T., Stodgell, C. J., & Rodier, P. M. (2005). The teratology of autism. *International Journal of Developmental Neuroscience, 23,* 189–199.

Bailey, A., Luthert, P., Dean, A., Harding, B., Janota, I., Montgomery, M., *et al.* (1998). A clinicopathological study of autism. *Brain, 121,* 889–905.

Barinaga, M. (2003). Newborn neurons search for meaning. *Science, 299,* 32–34.

Barkovich, A. J. (2005a). Magnetic resonance techniques in the assessment of myelin and myelination. *Journal of Inherited Metabolic Disease, 28,* 311–343.

Barkovich, A. J. (2005b). *Pediatric neuroimaging.* Philadelphia: Lippincott Williams and Wilkins.

Bates, E., & Roe, K. (2001). Language development in children with unilateral brain injury. In C. A. Nelson & M. Luciana (Eds.), *Handbook of developmental cognitive neuroscience* (pp. 281–307). Cambridge, MA: MIT Press.

Bernier, P. J., Bédard, A., Vinet, J., Lévesque, M., & Parent, A. (2002). Newly generated neurons in the amygdala and adjoining cortex of adult primates. *Proceedings of the National Academy of Sciences, 99,* 11464–11469.

Bhardwaj, R. D., Curtis, M. A., Spalding, K. L., Buchholz, B. A., Fink, D., Björk-Eriksson, T., *et al.* (2006). Neocortical neurogenesis in humans is restricted to development. *Proceedings of the National Academy of Sciences, 103,* 12564–12568.

Black, J. E., Jones, T. A., Nelson, C. A., & Greenough, W. T. (1998). Neuronal plasticity and the developing brain. In N. E. Alessi, J. T. Coyle, S. I. Harrison, & S. Eth (Eds.), *Handbook of child and adolescent psychiatry.* Vol. 6. *Basic Psychiatric Science and Treatment* (pp. 31–53). New York: John Wiley & Sons.

Bolton, P., Murphy, M., Macdonald, H., Whitlock, B., Pickles, A., & Rutter, M. (1997). Obstetric complications in autism: consequences or causes of the condition? *Journal of the American Academy of Child and Adolescent Psychiatry,* 36, 272–281.

Chechik, G., Meilijson, I., & Ruppin, E. (1999). Neuronal regulation: A mechanism for synaptic pruning during brain maturation. *Neural Computation, 11,* 2061–2080.

Cicchetti, D. (1984). The emergence of developmental psychopathology. *Child Development, 55,* 1–7.

Cicchetti, D., & Posner, M. I. (2005). Cognitive and affective neuroscience and developmental psychopathology. *Developmental Psychopathology, 17,* 569–575.

Cline, H. (2003). Sperry and Hebb: Oil and vinegar? *Trends in Neuroscience, 26,* 655–661.

Courchesne, E. (2002). Abnormal early brain development in autism. *Molecular Psychiatry,* 7, S21–S23.

Courchesne, E., Carper, R., & Akshoomoff, N. (2003). Evidence of brain overgrowth in the first year of life in autism. *Journal of the American Medical Association*, *290*, 337–344.

Courchesne, E., Redcay, E., & Kennedy, D. P. (2004). The autistic brain: birth through adulthood. *Current Opinion in Neurology*, *17*, 489–496.

Courchesne, E., Redcay, E., Morgan, J. T., & Kennedy, D. P. (2005). Autism at the beginning: Microstructural and growth abnormalities underlying the cognitive and behavioral phenotype of autism. *Development and Psychopathology*, *17*, 577–597.

Dahl, R. E., & Spear, P. (2004). *Adolescent brain development: Vulnerabilities and opportunities*. New York, NY: New York Academy of Sciences.

de Haan, M., & Johnson, M. H. (2003). *The cognitive neuroscience of development*. London, UK: Psychology Press.

de Haan, M., Wyatt, J. S., Roth, S., Vargha-Khadem, F., Gadian, D., & Mishkin, M. (2006). Brain and cognitive–behavioural development after asphyxia at term birth. *Developmental Science*, *9*, 350–358.

Diamond, M. C., Lindner, B., Johnson, R., Bennett, E. L., & Rosenzweig, M. R. (1975). Differences in occipital cortical synapses from environmentally enriched, impoverished and standard colony rats. *Neuroscience Research*, *1*, 109–119.

Draganski, B., Gaser, C., Busch, V., Schuierer, G., Bogdahn, U., & May, A. (2004). Changes in grey matter induced by training. *Nature*, *427*, 311–312.

Elbert, T., Pantev, C., Wienbruch, C., Rockstroh, B., & Taub, E. (1995). Increased cortical representation of the fingers of the left hand in string players. *Science*, *270*, 305–307.

Erickson, C. A., Jagadeesh, B., & Desimone, R. (2000). Clustering of perirhinal neurons with similar properties following visual experience in adult monkeys. *Nature Neuroscience*, 11, 1143–1148.

Fraiberg, S. (1977). *Insights from the blind: Comparative studies of blind and sighted infants*. New York: Basic Books.

Francis, D. D., Szegda, K., Campbell, G., Martin, W. D., & Insel, T. R. (2003). Epigenetic sources of behavioral differences in mice. *Nature Neuroscience*, *6*, 445–448.

Frisk, V., & Whyte, H. (1994). The long-term consequences of periventricular brain damage on language and verbal memory. *Developmental Neuropsychology*, *10*, 313–333.

Giedd, J. N., Blumenthal, J., Jeffries, N. O., Castellanos, F. X., Liu, H., Zijdenbos, A., *et al.* (1999). Brain development during childhood and adolescence: A longitudinal MRI study. *Nature Neuroscience*, *2*, 861–863.

Gilmore, J. H., Lin, W., Knickmeyer, R., Hamer, R. M., Smith, J. K., & Gerig, G. (2006). *Imaging early childhood brain development in humans*. Society for Neuroscience.

Gilmore, J. H., Zhai, G., Wilber, K., Smith, J. K., Lin, W., & Gerig, G. (2004). 3 Tesla magnetic resonance imaging of the brain in newborns. *Psychiatry Research*, *132*, 81–85.

Glasson, E., Bower, C., Petterson, B., de Klerk, N., Chaney, G., & Hallmayer, J. F. (2004). Perinatal factors and the development of autism: A population study. *Archives of General Psychiatry*, *61*, 618–627.

Gould, E. (2003, July). *Neurogenesis in the adult brain*. Presented at the Merck Summer Institute on Developmental Disabilities, Princeton University, Princeton, NJ.

Gould, E., Beylin, A., Tanapat, P., Reeves, A., & Shors, T. J. (1999). Learning enhances adult neurogenesis in the hippocampal formation. *Nature Neuroscience*, *2*, 260–265.

Gould, E., & Gross, C. G. (2002). Neurogenesis in adult mammals: some progress and problems. *Journal of Neuroscience*, *22*, 619–623.

Greenough, W. T., & Black, J. E. (1992). Induction of brain structure by experience: Substrates for cognitive development. In M. R. Gunnar, & C. A. Nelson (Eds.), *Minnesota symposia on child psychology*. Vol. 24. *Developmental behavioral neuroscience* (pp. 155–200). New Jersey: Lawrence Erlbaum.

Hack, M., Klein, N. K., & Taylor, H. G. (1995). Long term developmental outcomes of low birth weight infants. *Future Child*, *5*, 176–196.

Hashimoto, T., Tayama, M., Murakawa, K., Yoshimoto, T., Miyazaki, M., Harada, M., *et al.* (1995). Development of the brainstem and cerebellum in autistic patients. *Journal of Autism and Developmental Disorders*, *25*, 1–18.

Herbert, M. R., Ziegler, D. A., Deutsch, C. K., O'Brien, L. M., Kennedy, D. N., Filipek, P. A., *et al.* (2005). Brain asymmetries in autism and developmental language disorder: a nested whole-brain analysis. *Brain*, *128*, 213–226.

Hoksbergen, R., ter Laak, J., Rijk, K., van Dijkum, C., & Stoutjesdijk, F. (2005). Post-institutionalized autistic syndrome in Romanian adoptees. *Journal of Autism and Developmental Disorders*, 35, 615–623.

Huttenlocher, P. (1979). Synaptic and dendritic development and mental defect. In N. Buchwald, & M. Brazier (Eds.), *Brain mechanisms in mental retardation* (pp. 123–140). New York: Academic Press.

Huttenlocher, P. R. (1994). Synaptogenesis, synapse elimination, and neural plasticity in human cerebral cortex. In C. A. Nelson (Ed.), *Minnesota symposia on child psychology*. Vol. 27. *Cognition, perception, and language* (pp. 35–54). Hilsdale, NJ: Lawrence Erlbaum Associates.

Huttenlocher, P. R., & Dabholkar, A. S. (1997). Regional differences in synaptogenesis in human cerebral cortex. *Journal of Comparative Neurology*, *387*, 167–178.

Huttenlocher, P. R., & de Courten, C. (1987). The development of synapses in striate cortex of man. *Human Neurobiology*, *6*, 1–9.

Juul-Dam, N., Townsend, J., & Courchesne, E. (2001). Prenatal, perinatal, and neonatal factors in autism, pervasive developmental disorder-not otherwise specified, and the general population. *Pediatrics*, *107*, e63.

Kolb, B., Gibb, R., & Robinson, T. E. (2003). Brain plasticity and behavior. *Current Directions in Psychological Science*, *12*, 1–5.

Kozorovitskiy, Y. & Gould, E. (in press). Adult neurogenesis in the hippocampus. In C. A. Nelson, & M. Luciana (Eds.), *Handbook of developmental cognitive neuroscience* (2nd ed.). MIT Press: Cambridge, MA.

Kuhl, P. K., Tsao, F. M., & Liu, H. M. (2003). Foreign-language experience in infancy: effects of short-term exposure and social interaction on phonetic learning. *Proceedings of the National Academy of Sciences*, *100*, 9096–9101.

Le Bé, J-V., & Markram, H. (2006). Spontaneous and evoked synaptic rewiring in the neonatal neocortex. *Proceedings of the National Academy of Sciences*, *103*, 13214–13219.

Lenneberg, E. H. (1969). On explaining language. *Science*, *164*, 635–643.

Maguire, E., Gadian, D. G., Johnsrude, I. S., Good, C. D., Ashburner, J., Frackowiak, R. S., *et al.* (2000). Navigation-related structural change in the hippocampi of taxi drivers. *Proceedings of the National Academy of Sciences*, 97, 4398–4403.

Maurer, D., Lewis, T. L., Brent, H. P., & Levin, A. V. (1999). Rapid improvement in the acuity of infants after visual input. *Science*, *286*, 108–110.

Meshi, D., Drew, M. R., Saxe, M., Ansorge, M. S., David, D., Santarelli, L., *et al.* (2006). Hippocampal neurogenesis is not required for behavioral effects of environmental enrichment. *Nature Neuroscience*, 9, 729–734.

Miller, E. A., Goldman, P. S., & Rosvold, H. E. (1973). Delayed recovery of function following orbital prefrontal lesions in infant monkeys. *Science*, *182*, 304–306.

Miller, M. T., Strömland, K., Ventura, L., Johansson, M., Bandim, J. M., & Gillberg, C. (2005). Autism associated with conditions characterized by developmental errors in early embryogenesis: A mini-review. *International Journal of Developmental Neuroscience*, *23*, 201–219.

Mirescu, C., Peters, J. D., & Gould, E. (2004). Early life experience alters response of adult neurogenesis to stress. *Nature Neuroscience*, *7*, 841–846.

Molliver, M., Kostovic, I., & Van der Loos, H. (1973). The development of synapses in the human fetus. *Brain Research*, *50*, 403–407.

Nelson, C. A. (1999). Neural plasticity and human development. *Current Directions in Psychological Science*, *8*, 42–45.

Nelson, C. A. (2000). Neural plasticity and human development: The role of early experience in sculpting memory systems. *Developmental Science*, *3*, 115–130.

Nelson, C. A., & Bloom, F. E. (1997). Child development and neuroscience. *Child Development*, *68*, 970–987.

Nelson, C. A., Bloom, F. E., Cameron, J., Amaral, D., Dahl, R., & Pine, D. (2002). An integrative, multidisciplinary approach to the study of brain–behavior relations in the context of typical and atypical development. *Development and Psychopathology*, *14*, 499–520.

Nelson, C. A., de Haan, M., & Thomas, K. M. (2006). Neural bases of cognitive development. In W. Damon, R. Lerner, D. Kuhn, & R. Siegler (Volume Editors), *Handbook of child psychology* (6th ed., Vol. 2.). *Cognitive, perception and language* (pp. 3–57). New Jersey: John Wiley & Sons, Inc.

Nelson, C. A., Zeanah, C., & Fox, N. A. (2007). The effects of early deprivation on brain–behavioral development: The Bucharest Early Intervention Project. In D. Romer, & E. Walker (Eds.), *Adolescent psychopathology and the developing brain: Integrating brain and prevention science* (pp. 197–215). New York: Oxford University Press.

Nelson, E. E., Leibenluft, E., McClure, E. B., & Pine, D. S. (2005). The social re-orientation of adolescence: a neuroscience perspective on the process and its relation to psychopathology. *Psychological Medicine*, *35*, 163–174.

Oppenheim, R. W., & Johnson, J. E. (2003). Programmed cell death and neurotrophic factors. In L. R. Squire, F. E. Bloom, S. K. McConnell, J. L. Roberts, N. C. Spitzer, & M. J. Zigmond (Eds.), *Fundamental neuroscience* (2nd ed., pp. 499–532). New York: Academic Press.

Pascalis, O., de Haan, M., & Nelson, C. A. (2002). Is face processing species specific during the first year of life? *Science*, *296*, 1321–1323.

Pascalis, O., Scott, L. S., Kelly, D. J., Dufour, R. W., Shannon, R. W., Nicholson, E., *et al.* (2005). Plasticity of face processing in infancy. *Proceedings of the National Academy of Sciences*, *102*, 5297–5300.

Pass, R. (2006). Congenital cytomegalovirus infection following first trimester maternal infection: Symptoms at birth and outcome. *Journal of Clinical Virology*, *35*, 216–220.

Riley, E. P., & McGee, C. L. (2005). Fetal alcohol spectrum disorders: an overview with emphasis on changes in brain and behavior. *Experimental Biology and Medicine*, *230*, 357–365.

Rakic, P. (2002). Neurogenesis in adult primate neocortex: An evaluation of the evidence. *Nature Reviews Neuroscience*, *3*, 65–71.

Rutter, M. (2006). *Genes and behaviour: Nature–nurture interplay explained*. London, UK: Blackwell Publishing.

Rutter, M., Andersen-Wood, L., Beckett, C., Bredenkamp, D., Castle, J., Groothues, C., *et al.*, and the English and Romanian Adoptees (ERA) Study Team. (1999). Quasi-autistic patterns following severe early global privation. *Journal of Child Psychology and Psychiatry*, *40*, 537–549.

Sadato, N., Pascual-Leone, A., Grafman, J., Deiber, M. P., Ibanez, V., & Hallett, M. (1998). Neural networks for Braille reading by the blind. *Brain*, *121*, 1213–1229.

Saffran, J. R., Werker, J. F., & Werner, L. A. (2006). The infant's auditory world: hearing, speech and the beginnings of language. In W. Damon, R. Lerner, D. Kuhn, & R. Siegler (Volume Editors), *Handbook of child psychology* (6th ed., Vol. 2.). *Cognition, perception and language* (pp. 58–108). New Jersey: John Wiley & Sons, Inc.

Shaw, P., Greenstein, D., Lerch, J., Classen, L., Lenroot, R., Gogtay, N., *et al.* (2006). Intellectual ability and cortical development in children and adolescents. *Nature*, *440*, 676–679.

Small, J. G. (1975). EEG and neurophysiological studies of early infantile autism. *Biological Psychiatry*, *10*, 385–397.

Sowell, E. R., Thompson, P. M., Holmes, C. J., Batth, R., Jernigan, T. L., & Toga, A. W. (1999). Localizing age-related changes in brain structure between childhood and adolescence using statistical parametric mapping. *Neuroimage*, *9*, 587–597.

Sroufe, L. A. (1986). Bowlby's contribution to psychoanalytic theory and developmental psychology: attachment, separation, loss. *Journal of Child Psychology and Psychiatry*, *27*, 841–849.

Sroufe, L. A., Carlson, E. Z., Levy, A. K., & Egeland, B. (1999). Implications of attachment theory for developmental psychopathology. *Developmental Psychopathology*, *11*, 1–13.

Sroufe, L. A., & Rutter, M. (1984). The domain of developmental psychopathology. *Child Development*, *55*, 17–29.

Swaiman, F., Ashawl, S., & Ferriero, D. M. (2006). *Pediatric neurology* (4th ed.). *Principles and practice*. New York: Mosby.

Taylor, H. G., Minich, N. M., Klein, N., & Hack, M. (2004). Longitudinal outcomes of very low birth weight: neuropsychological findings. *Journal of the International Neuropsychological Society*, *10*, 149–163.

Toga, A. W., Thompson, P. M., & Sowell, E. R. (2006). Mapping brain maturation. *Trends in Neuroscience*, *29*, 148–159.

Van der Knaap, M. S., van Wezel-Meijler, G., Barth, P. G., Barkhof, F., Adèr, H. J., & Valk, J. (1996). Normal gyration and sulcation in preterm and term neonates: appearance on MR images. *Radiology*, *200*, 389–396.

van Praag, H., Shubert, T., Zhao, C., & Gage, F. H. (2005). Exercise enhances learning and hippocampal neurogenesis in aged mice. *Journal of Neuroscience*, *25*, 8680–8685.

Volpe, J. J. (2001). *Neurology of the newborn* (4th ed.). Philadelphia: W. B. Saunders.

Warren, S. L., Huston, L., Egeland, B., & Sroufe, L. A. (1997). Child and adolescent anxiety disorders and early attachment. *Journal of the American Academy of Child and Adolescent Psychiatry*, *36*, 637–644.

Werker, J. F., & Vouloumanos, A. (2001). Speech and language processing in infancy: A neurocognitive approach. In C. A. Nelson, & M. Luciana (Eds.), *Handbook of developmental cognitive neuroscience* (pp. 269–280). Cambridge, MA: MIT Press.

White, T., & Hilgetag, C. C. (in press). Gyrification and development of the human brain. In C. A. Nelson, & M. Luciana (Eds.), *Handbook of developmental cognitive neuroscience* (2nd ed.). Cambridge, MA: MIT Press.

Zeanah, C. H., Nelson, C. A., Fox, N. A., Smyke, A. T., Marshall, P., Parker, S. W., *et al.* (2003). Designing research to study the effects of institutionalization on brain and behavioral development: The Bucharest Early Intervention Project. *Development and Psychopathology*, *15*, 885–907.

13 Development and Psychopathology: A Life Course Perspective

Barbara Maughan and Michael Rutter

Across the social and biological sciences, investigators are increasingly taking a life course perspective on the development of human health, behavior and disease (Elder & Shanahan, 2006). Psychiatry is no exception to this trend; as findings from long-term longitudinal studies proliferate, so it becomes increasingly clear that many adult disorders have origins very early in development, and that many childhood disorders have sequelae that persist to adult life. Knowledge of these long-term developmental linkages has cast new light on the etiology and course of many disorders, highlighted unexpected connections across the life course and raised key questions about the mechanisms – biological, psychological and social – that underlie both continuities and discontinuities in vulnerability over time.

Although there were earlier pointers (Rutter & Garmezy, 1983), the first clear evidence of the childhood origins of adult disorder came from large-scale surveys of adult mental health. Questioned about their first episode of disorder, many adults with histories of depression, anxiety and substance use dated the start of their difficulties before age 20 (Christie, Burke, Regier *et al.*, 1988); analyses of peak hazard rates for a broader range of disorders set them too in childhood and adolescence (Burke, Burke, Regier *et al.*, 1990). Since that time, epidemiological studies in childhood have clarified typical age at onset patterns for most disorders, and highlighted two broad age at onset groups. One, with onsets very early in childhood, includes what are now regarded as neurodevelopmental disorders (see chapter 3): autism spectrum disorders, specific language impairment, dyslexia and attention deficit/hyperactivity disorder (ADHD). All of these disorders have a strong male preponderance. The second group, with onsets in adolescence, includes disorders more common in women and girls: depression, eating disorders, social phobia and panic (Costello, Foley, & Angold, 2006). Separation anxiety, specific phobias and oppositional disorders also onset in childhood; substance problems typically emerge in the teens; and conduct disorders show two onset periods, one in childhood and the second in adolescence. Charting these onset patterns has provided an essential point of departure for the study of longer-term developmental trajectories.

Rutter's Child and Adolescent Psychiatry, 5th edition. Edited by M. Rutter, D. Bishop, D. Pine, S. Scott, J. Stevenson, E. Taylor and A. Thapar. © 2008 Blackwell Publishing, ISBN: 978-1-4051-4549-7.

Childhood studies have also highlighted other themes relevant to a life course view. First, although the point prevalence of childhood and adolescent disorders centers at around 10–12%, repeated assessments produce much higher estimates. In one community study, for example, annual assessments showed that over one-third of young people had met diagnostic criteria for disorder at some stage between the ages of 9 and 16 years (Costello, Mustillo, Erkanli *et al.*, 2003). From this perspective, the childhood and adolescent "base" for later psychiatric morbidity is high. Second, persistence of disorder in childhood is also high. A 3-year follow-up of cases identified in the 1999 British Child Mental Health Survey (Meltzer, Gatward, Corbin *et al.*, 2003), for example, found that more than 40% of young people who met criteria for disorder at first assessment also did so at follow-up. In many instances this reflected *homotypic continuity* – persistence or recurrence of the same disorder over time. Not infrequently, however, earlier and later disorders were of a different kind, highlighting the importance of *sequential comorbidity* or *heterotypic continuity* in the mental health domain. As these findings suggest, developmental models need to account for both continuity and discontinuity across the life course, and to identify factors that make for both stability and change.

Evidence for longer-term continuities in disorder comes from many sources. Some of the most persuasive are prospective studies of unselected birth cohorts, set up by far-sighted investigators many years ago (Coleman & Jones, 2004). As cohorts of this kind mature, their findings offer two complementary perspectives on connections between disorder in childhood and in adult life. First, looking forwards from childhood, longitudinal data provide estimates of the extent to which children and adolescents with mental health problems are at risk for disorder later in their lives. Second, looking backwards from adulthood, they highlight early roots of adult vulnerability. Some of the most compelling evidence for long-term continuities has come from this second approach. Recent reports from the Dunedin longitudinal cohort (Kim-Cohen, Caspi, Moffitt *et al.*, 2003), for example, show that most young adults with a psychiatric disorder had diagnosable problems much earlier in life. Of those with treated mental health problems at age 26, half had first met criteria for disorder by age 15; by the late teens, that figure approached 75%.

What accounts for these long-term vulnerabilities? Although we are still far from definitive answers to this question, important pointers are beginning to emerge. This chapter draws together recent findings in this area, using examples from contrasting disorders and early risks to highlight key themes emerging from developmental research. Because long-term developmental studies pose particular challenges, we begin with an overview of the methodological issues that arise in long-term longitudinal research, and the strengths and limitations of the differing strategies that investigators have used to examine continuities and discontinuities in psychopathology. Next, we explore patterns of child–adult links in a series of specific disorders, and in relation to early risks, to illustrate the varying mechanisms now thought to contribute to continuities and discontinuities over time. Finally, we consider the implications of these long-term developmental findings for clinical practice.

Methodological Considerations

There are many ways in which evidence on continuities and discontinuities between psychopathology and experiences in childhood and adult life may be informative. From a methodological perspective, however, three main topics may be differentiated. First, there is the need to determine the outcome of childhood disorders and, most especially, the factors associated with variations in outcome and course. If comparisons can be made among outcomes of different disorders, findings may also contribute to the validation of diagnostic distinctions. Second, the interest may lie in the possibility that one form of psychopathology creates a risk for another. This arises, for example, with respect to the suggestion that antisocial behavior predisposes to substance abuse, or that anxiety in childhood predisposes to depression after puberty. Here, the research requirements differ from the study of prognosis mainly in terms of the crucial need to study the *timing* of transitions in psychopathology over its developmental course. Third, investigators have examined the effects of risk factors in childhood (whether individual characteristics or risk experiences) and psychopathology in adult life. Here, the starting point has to be in terms of postulated *risks* (rather than the presence of a diagnosed disorder); outcomes must be examined in terms of those who do not, as well as those who do, suffer from the sequelae of risk; and there must be the possibility of examining the effect of later experiences in ameliorating or mitigating the effects of early stress or adversity. Especially for this last topic, but also for the first two, longitudinal data and longitudinal analyses will usually be needed to provide definitive answers to developmental questions. Almost always, however, it will be desirable to precede longitudinal studies with other research strategies to develop relevant hypotheses. As one of the father figures of developmental studies, Baldwin put it: "A longitudinal study is the last, not the first step, in a research program. It is an absolutely essential research method if we are to get firm knowledge of psychological change, but paradoxically it is to be avoided whenever possible" (Baldwin, 1960). Because longitudinal studies are extremely costly and time-consuming, they need to be saved for use at the point when appropriate ground clearing research has been undertaken to articulate the questions to be examined. Moreover, as we will outline, longitudinal data in themselves do not provide a sufficient answer to developmental questions: in addition, they must be used in the context of appropriate designs and with appropriate methods of data analysis (Rutter, 2007; see chapter 9).

Historically, quite a diverse range of research strategies has been used to examine continuities and discontinuities over the lifespan (Rutter & Garmezy, 1983). Early researchers were innovative in building on existing records to "fast-track" their coverage of developmental time, and much early research focused on clinic-referred rather than general population groups. More recently, prospective studies of representative samples – now regarded as the gold standard in the field – have become increasingly available.

Case–Control Designs and Related Strategies

In many ways, the strategy that involves the least resource consists of bringing together existing record data on the same individuals in childhood and in adult life. That approach was usefully employed by Zeitlin (1986), investigating individuals who had been patients as both children and adults in the same postgraduate teaching hospital. His aim was to compare continuities across different diagnostic groups. The findings were informative, but they were inevitably heavily reliant on the representativeness of the individuals who were both child and adult patients. Many findings proved similar to those of prospective epidemiological studies, but those on the childhood features associated with depression in adult life have turned out to be somewhat misleading.

A different approach was provided by taking an adult patient group as the starting point and looking back to childhood using contemporaneous records. Watt (1974) used this strategy to great effect by using school records to examine childhood precursors of schizophrenia. Because the records were inevitably lacking in precision by current research standards, there is limited specificity in what was found. Nevertheless, the overall pattern of the findings has proved substantially similar to that gained from prospective longitudinal research. The main limitation was that the focus on a single disorder could show how schizophrenia differed from normality, but could not distinguish differences among different adult diagnostic groups.

The least satisfactory strategy has been to rely on retrospective recall for the assessments of childhood. Several studies used this approach to examine relationships between autism in childhood and adult schizophrenia, using the latter as a starting point (Howells & Guirguis, 1984; Petty, Ornitz, Michelman *et al.*, 1984). Continuities were claimed, but prospective studies of children with autism have shown that the conclusions were mistaken. Schizophrenia is indeed preceded by language and social abnormalities in childhood, but prospective studies of individuals with autism have been quite consistent in showing that there is not a raised rate of schizophrenia in adult life (Howlin, Goode, Hutton *et al.*, 2004; Volkmar &

Cohen, 1991). This research strategy is not to be recommended because of the major lack of precision in retrospective recall, as well as the possibility of bias.

Despite their utility, all of these designs also face one other inevitable and major constraint: adult outcomes are restricted to recognized diagnostic categories, and there is no scope for tracking unanticipated outcomes, not well encapsulated by prevailing diagnostic conventions. As we shall see, unexpected findings of this kind have been some of the most illuminating to emerge from other approaches to developmental research.

Follow-up Studies of Clinical Groups

The standard for follow-up studies of clinical groups was first set by Robins' research-based adult follow-up of children who had been seen at a child guidance clinic in middle America in the 1930s (Robins, 1966). Robins traced and interviewed these young people in adulthood, gaining a broad picture of strengths as well as difficulties in their later lives. She used a general population comparison group from the same geographic area to assess how far outcomes were specific to those with childhood disorder, and paid careful attention to differences among psychopathological groups. The findings proved hugely influential: diagnostic criteria for antisocial personality disorder were largely shaped by her findings, and the study generated numerous other developmental hypotheses that have stood the test of time.

Other researchers have used variations on this strategy to study outcomes of specific disorders. This applied, for example, to Rutter, Greenfeld, & Lockyer's (1967a,b) follow-up of children with autism, and to Harrington, Fudge, Rutter *et al.* (1990) follow-up of childhood depression. Both used clinical samples, but both were innovative in using as comparisons not general population controls, but rather children with other forms of psychopathology. The findings of both studies were striking in showing a surprising degree of diagnostic specificity in outcomes, findings that have also stood the test of time. In both cases, there were, however, inevitable limitations arising from the reliance on clinic samples and – in these particular instances – samples that lacked early research-based measures.

Prospective Studies of Clinically Defined Groups

Prospective studies of clinically defined groups differ from record-based follow-ups in three key respects. First, they have the major advantage of research-based assessments for their starting point. As a result, differentiation of the qualities of childhood psychopathology that may affect later outcomes is likely to be much more satisfactory. Second, because prospective studies can involve multiple waves of assessment, they allow better tests of the timing and patterning of symptoms as they unfold over time. Third, for the same reason, there are also better opportunities to test focused hypotheses on possible causal mechanisms.

Numerous studies have now used this strategy; many have highlighted previously quite unexpected effects. Laub and Sampson's (2003) follow-up of a juvenile delinquency sample to age 70 constitutes much the longest follow-up of this kind. It has been especially informative on the role of adult experiences, showing how developmental trajectories continue to be influenced by both negative and positive turning points well into in adult life. Clegg, Hollis, Mawhood *et al.* (2005) follow-up of children with specific language impairment involving severe comprehension difficulties constitutes a rather different example, in which one of the major findings was the very high frequency of social impairments in adulthood – impairments that did not follow traditional psychiatric diagnostic categories.

Prospective Studies of General Population Epidemiological Samples

Prospective studies of general population samples have all the advantages of prospective studies of clinically defined groups, but some key additional strengths: they provide a stronger basis for generalizability, they can examine effects of environmental risk factors, and they can also study outcomes of traits or behaviors in childhood that fall short of full diagnostic criteria. The extensive insights that have emerged from the Dunedin (http://dunedinstudy.otago.ac.nz/) and Christchurch (http://www.chmeds.ac.nz/research/chds/index.htm) longitudinal studies in New Zealand and the US Children in the Community study (http://nyspi.org/childcom) well illustrate the powerful strengths of this design. Its one important limitation, however, is that – unless based on extremely large samples – general population studies are typically in a weak position to examine effects of extreme patterns, and may only include small numbers of individuals who meet full diagnostic criteria for disorder. As a result, there is much to be said for combining general population epidemiological and/or longitudinal studies with prospective studies of more extreme groups. The former have the advantage of avoiding possible biases associated with clinical referral, while the latter have the advantage of being able to examine the effects of more extreme patterns.

Prospective Studies of High-Risk Groups

None of the above designs are particularly good for the study of more subtle abnormalities that may constitute important precursors of later psychopathology. Here, studies of groups likely to be at high risk because of genetic factors involved in familial loading come into their own. Weissman, Wickramaratne, Nomura *et al.* (2005) research into depression constitutes one good example here, illustrating the value of multiple measures over time and the utility of studying age at onset. Lyytinen, Ahonen, Eklund *et al.* (2004) prospective study of babies born into families with a familial loading for dyslexia constitutes another good example. Detailed cognitive and neurophysiological measures were obtained from early in the children's development, making it possible to explore how far at-risk children show hypothesized precursor deficits very early in development, well before they are exposed to the demands of learning to read. Owen and Johnstone's (2006) study of a high-risk schizophrenia sample, again beginning before the onset of disorder, has been similarly informative about the specifics involved in the prodromata of schizophrenia. The major limitation of this design, however, lies in uncertainties over the extent to which findings are specific to individuals with a high familial loading. In that connection, it is important to be able to combine the high-risk strategy with data from general population samples that can tap at least some of the features thought to constitute precursors of adult psychopathology.

High-risk designs can also be used to assess outcomes of hypothesized environmental risks. The longitudinal study of children experiencing profound institutional deprivation in Romania and who were subsequently adopted into UK families constitutes an example of this kind (Croft, Beckett, Rutter *et al.*, 2007; Kreppner, Rutter, Beckett *et al.*, 2007; Rutter, Colvert, Kreppner *et al.*, 2007). In this case, the main interest is not so much in testing hypotheses about environmental risk mediation (although designs of this kind do allow that), but rather in examining factors contributing to variations in outcome within a high-risk group. As with all studies of developmental pathways, it is crucial to check the representativeness of the samples being studied. In that connection, when the frequency of the postulated risk factor is sufficiently high, there is much to be said for embedding a high-risk sample within an epidemiological design. The study of children born to teenage mothers, as part of the Moffitt & the E-Risk Study Team (2002) environmental risk study, constitutes an example of this kind.

Retrospective and Prospective Measures

Whenever possible, contemporaneous measures of childhood behaviors or experiences are almost always to be preferred over measures based on retrospective recall, especially when the aim is to examine the relative timing of events or onsets. People are much better at remembering *whether* something happened than *when* it occurred, and memories of the temporal ordering of events or behaviors – often required to test causal hypotheses – are especially open to bias associated with later outcomes. Because temporal sequence is particularly important for the study of environmental risk mediation, prospective measures are ordinarily much to be preferred. Nevertheless, for memorable, easily defined and well-conceptualized happenings (e.g., parental divorce), retrospective recall may be useable for the assessment of *whether* particular experiences have occurred, but not for timing of *when* they took place (Hardt & Rutter, 2004). To date, evidence suggests that deliberate falsifications of adverse experiences are uncommon. Rather, findings suggest that the main source of bias lies in the tendency of people who are functioning well in adulthood to forget or under-report early risk experiences, rather than those with psychopathology exaggerating negative experiences in the past. Two further points need to be made about retrospective recall. First, some events – such as exposure to sexual or physical abuse within the family – cannot readily be assessed prospectively in non-referred samples because parents are unlikely to agree to their children being asked about such happenings, and ethical committees often constrain questioning. Second, even "prospective" studies will usually involve some degree of retrospective reporting, covering the periods between study contacts. Accordingly, although – other things being equal – prospective data are to be preferred, it is important not to exaggerate problems of retrospective recall. The problems are serious with respect to time sequences and also for value judgments such as severity of punishment or quality of relationships. On the other hand, retrospective reports may be more satisfactory for experiences that are prolonged, memorable for their impact and likely to have been discussed subsequently. For any experiences that are less striking than that, under-reporting will be common and retrospective reports will not provide an accurate estimate of frequency or prevalence.

Testing Causal Hypotheses

When studying causal hypotheses, longitudinal analyses focusing on within-individual change are almost always to be preferred over between-group comparisons. Nevertheless, it is essential to appreciate that longitudinal analyses alone are not adequate for testing causal hypotheses. However, they are extremely useful in sorting out the likely direction of the causal arrow – an important consideration, for example, in differentiating between child effects on the environment and environmental influences on the child (Bell, 1968). Even so, caution is needed before assuming that earlier behaviors necessarily *cause* later ones. Many studies have shown, for example, that anxiety in childhood constitutes an important precursor to depression later in life, leading to the proposal that anxiety is part of the causal process. However, an alternative possibility is that at some stages in the life course this temporal sequence is simply a function of maturational processes whereby anxiety manifests itself earlier than depression. It is relevant, therefore, that in adult life depression both precedes and follows anxiety (Rutter, Maughan, & Kim-Cohen, 2006a).

Four main alternatives to causal influences have to be considered when drawing inferences from statistical associations between postulated risk factors or precursor conditions and psychopathological outcomes (Rutter, 2007). First, both may reflect the same underlying liability. Thus, crawling precedes the onset of walking and babbling precedes the onset of spoken language, but it is most unlikely that crawling *causes* walking or babbling *causes* language. Rather, both are likely to constitute part of the same process. In the same way, the association between early conduct problems and later substance misuse is at least partially likely to reflect the same underlying liability.

The second possibility is that associations with environmental risks may reflect social selection rather than social causation. Environments are not randomly distributed, and variations in risk exposure may be a consequence, at least in part, of individuals' own behavior, rather than reflecting an independent environmental influence. Processes of this kind are likely to be widespread in psychopathology, and call for particular attempts to examine the origins, as well as the effects, of postulated environmental risks.

Third, statistical associations between later outcomes and prior risks or disorders may reflect effects of confounding. Environmental risks rarely occur in isolation, and comorbidity among disorders is high; as a result, associations with any individual early risk or prior disorder may in practice be attributable to the effects of other correlated risks. Reports from the Christchurch Health and Development study have paid particular attention to the problem of confounding. Examining early adult sequelae of adolescent depression, for example, Fergusson and Woodward (2002) reported initial associations with a wide range of adverse outcomes including depression and anxiety, suicidal behaviors, problems in employment and early parenthood. Adolescent depression was also associated with numerous other childhood and adolescent adversities. Controls for these correlated difficulties markedly refined conclusions on later outcomes: while associations with later depression and anxiety remained strong, links with all other problems in adult functioning were spurious, and reflected the effects of confounding.

The final possibility is that, although the risk effect is real, it is, at least in part, genetically rather than environmentally mediated. Thus, the association between, say, harsh discipline and child psychopathology may partially reflect genetic factors involved in the liability to use severe disciplinary strategies as well as effects of harsh discipline on the child. Twin and adoption studies provide well-accepted designs that "pull apart" influences of this kind; in addition, a much larger variety of "natural experiments" can serve much the same purpose (Rutter, 2007; Rutter, Pickles, Murray *et al.*, 2001). With ingenuity, some purchase can be gained on most causal questions.

As is implicit in the whole of this methodological discussion, the research focus has changed over time from attention to the *extent* of continuities to attempts to understand the causal mechanisms involved. In the remainder of the chapter, we consider some examples.

Developmental Findings

We begin by examining developmental findings in relation to a number of individual disorders or disorder groups. Detailed discussions of each these disorders are presented in later chapters. Our aim here is a rather different one; to use emerging findings to illustrate the more general developmental issues, principles and questions that emerge in relation to differing patterns of childhood–adult continuity.

Neurodevelopmental disorders

We begin with the group of what has come to be known as neurodevelopmental disorders (see chapter 3): autism spectrum disorders, specific language impairment (SLI), dyslexia and ADHD. Although differentiated in important ways, these disorders also share key features in common: they are diagnosed early in development, involve delay or deviance in maturationally influenced psychological features, along with some degree of cognitive impairment (specific or general), and all show relatively strong genetic liabilities. They are all also much more common in boys than in girls.

At this stage, knowledge of the long-term prognosis for individuals with these disorders is highly variable: prospective follow-ups of ADHD samples have been reported for many years, but data on adult outcomes in the other disorders remain much more limited. In each case, however, current findings suggest a clear persistence of impairments into adulthood (although often with some diminution of effects with age), but also considerable variability in adult functioning. In some instances, follow-up findings have highlighted quite unexpected features. Specific language impairment has traditionally been regarded as reflecting a relatively pure deficit in language, and follow-ups have, as expected, documented long-term sequelae in relation to both language functioning and literacy skills. In addition, however, quite unanticipated findings have emerged in relation to the later social functioning of individuals with unusually severe SLI. In one study (Clegg *et al.*, 2005), the majority of males with SLI involving an impairment in receptive language had not achieved independent living by their 30s, many had faced problems in employment, few had established cohabitations and half had impairments in non-romantic friendships; performance on theory of mind tasks also suggested deficits in social cognition. Although outcomes were better among individuals with the least severe initial language impairments, associations with language skills were quite weak. Overall, the pattern of the findings raises important questions about the conceptualization of SLI. Because it is unlikely that such extensive social impairments emerge solely in response to early language problems, it may be that, rather than being viewed as a pure deficit in language skills, SLI should more appropriately be regarded as involving much broader social and/or cognitive deficits from the outset.

Variability in long-term outcomes has been noted across the neurodevelopmental disorders: some individuals continue to show marked impairments in adulthood, while others function relatively successfully. At this stage, the basis for these variations is poorly understood. In autism, for example, IQ is clearly of importance: outcomes are universally poor in individuals with IQs below 50, and more positive adult functioning is very largely concentrated in groups within the normal IQ range. Among individuals with IQs of 70 or higher, however, specific IQ levels are of little or no prognostic value (Howlin, Goode, Hutton *et al.*, 2004), and it remains unclear whether variations in functioning within this group are predominantly attributable to the severity of the basic biological handicap, or reflect effects of the adequacy of services received either in childhood or in adult life (Mawhood & Howlin, 1999). Social factors clearly impact on outcomes in dyslexia: although underlying literacy problems are highly persistent, effects on educational and occupational outcomes are considerably mitigated for young people from more socioeconomically advantaged homes, and appropriate "niche-picking" – the selection of adult environments where literacy demands are limited, or can be met in other ways – is a clear feature of the histories of individuals with more successful later outcomes (Maughan, 1995). Finally, heritable factors are also likely to influence outcome and course. In the case of SLI, for example, heritability seems substantially greater for children with persistent language impairment than for those with more transient language delays (Bishop, Price, Dale *et al.*, 2003), and in ADHD polymorphisms in the *DRD4* and *DAT1* genes have been shown to be associated with variations in both IQ and later adult functioning (Mill, Caspi, Williams *et al.*, 2006).

On both clinical and theoretical grounds, a life course approach to the neurodevelopmental disorders requires knowledge not only of adult outcomes but also of early precursors. Although all of these disorders are typically diagnosed early in childhood, it is of considerable importance to know how early they can be detected, and whether reliable indicators of presumed underlying deficits are evident before major impairment appears. In the case of autism, marked difficulties do not typically emerge until around 18 months of age, and reliable diagnoses are often only possible at or after age 2; analyses of home movies, however, suggest that some children show evidence of abnormalities as early as the first year of life (Rutter, Le Couteur, & Lord, 2003). In ADHD, diagnostic criteria require that symptoms are present before age 7 but clinical evidence clearly shows that ADHD-related behaviors often result in major impairments well before children reach school age. Diagnosing ADHD in preschoolers has long been recognized as challenging, but systematic studies of preschoolers are beginning to show that both rates and psychosocial correlates of preschool ADHD are closely comparable to those found in school-age samples (Egger & Angold, 2006). In addition, preschool children with ADHD have been found to show deficits in executive functioning and delay aversion, now regarded as core features of the disorder (Sonuga-Barke, Dalen, & Remington, 2003), providing further pointers that the liability to ADHD is present early in development.

Probably the most extensive data on early precursors are available in the dyslexia field. Although, by definition, developmental reading problems can only become manifest once children are exposed to reading instruction, current models assume that core linguistic and cognitive deficits are present well before children begin to read. Preschoolers who go on to develop reading difficulties are now known to show delays in oral language, a lack of interest in books and reading materials, and problems in pre-reading and related cognitive skills. Studies of high-risk groups (Lyytinen *et al.*, 2004) show some differences from controls in brain responses to speech sounds even in infancy. Measures of expressive and receptive language became increasingly differentiated across early childhood, with stronger associations with later reading in the family high-risk group than among controls. Overall, the findings suggest that the cognitive and language deficits found in dyslexia are indeed evident earlier in development, but are not sufficiently distinctive to be useful at an individual diagnostic level.

Finally, mention must be made of the high rates of comorbidity with conduct and oppositional disorders found in both ADHD and dyslexia in childhood, and their implications for outcomes later in life. ADHD and dyslexia themselves show strong overlaps, largely genetically influenced. As a result, we might anticipate that associations with antisocial behavior would also show much in common. Perhaps surprisingly, current evidence is somewhat against that view. ADHD is strongly comorbid with oppositional disorders in childhood, and conduct disorders often develop from this base. Follow-up studies suggest that these risks persist: ADHD is associated with increased rates of antisocial personality disorder and substance abuse in adult life, even in the absence of marked conduct/oppositional symptomatology earlier in development, although the increase in adult psychopathology is much greater when there were conduct problems in childhood (Manuzza, Klein, & Moulton, 2003; Manuzza, Klein, Abikoff *et al.*, 2004). A variety of factors might contribute to these links. Genetic influences are strongly implicated in comorbidity in childhood, and almost certainly contribute to risks of persistence; family and peer influences seem salient, perhaps in interaction with genetic risk; and evidence also points to the importance of severe and pervasive ADHD symptomatology, especially when combined with low cognitive abilities, as a key element in the clinical picture associated with persistence. Reviewing this evidence, Thapar, van der Bree, Fowler *et al.* (2006) drew attention to the complexities involved in any more precise specification of risk pathways at this stage: despite a plethora of evidence on putative risks, current findings leave it uncertain which factors predict, which mediate and which moderate the links between ADHD and antisocial outcomes. Given the clinical and public health significance of these progressions, more detailed studies testing competing hypotheses about the key developmental pathways are clearly a major priority.

Findings in relation to dyslexia differ in several ways. First, although developmental reading problems have long been known to be associated with conduct disorder in childhood (Rutter, Tizard, & Whitmore, 1970), the mechanisms involved have remained obscure. Findings on the mediating role of inattentiveness are mixed (Maughan & Carroll, 2006), but recent twin data suggest that, in contrast to ADHD, comorbidity between dyslexia and childhood conduct problems is best explained by reciprocal phenotypic causation: conduct problems impede reading acquisition, while reading failure exacerbates disruptive tendencies (Trzesniewski, Moffitt, Caspi *et al.*, 2006). Long-term follow-ups of representative samples of poor readers remain limited. Available evidence suggests, however, that – again unlike findings in ADHD – poor readers show few increased risks of criminality or other indices of antisocial behavior in early adult life (Maughan, Pickles, Rutter *et al.*, 1996); rather than the persisting vulnerability associated with ADHD, comorbid conduct problems in dyslexia may thus reflect more time-limited responses to school failure. Although comparisons of long-term trajectories across disorders are only now beginning to be possible, examples of this kind suggest that they should prove increasingly informative for our understanding of intervening mechanisms.

Childhood Origins of Schizophrenia

Arguably, developmental findings have made the most major change to conceptualizations of disorder in relation to schizophrenia (Keshavan, Kennedy, & Murray, 2004; Murray & Lewis, 1987; Weinberger, 1987). Traditionally seen as a psychosis beginning in late adolescence or early adulthood, schizophrenia is now increasingly regarded as a developmental disorder, with roots traceable to very early vulnerabilities (Walker, Kestler, Bollini *et al.*, 2004a). This change of view has largely been prompted by follow-back findings from longitudinal studies that show mild deficits in social, motor and cognitive functioning in children and adolescents, and even infants, who go on to display psychotic symptoms. Susceptibility to schizophrenia has also been associated with a range of prenatal and perinatal risks that have the potential to affect neurodevelopmental processes. Early insults of this kind, perhaps in interaction with genetic predispositions, are now thought to lay the groundwork for vulnerable neuronal circuits whose effects can compromise brain structure and function. Not all individuals with these vulnerabilities go on to show disorder; indeed, although neuropsychological and neurodevelopmental measures differentiate high-risk individuals from healthy controls, it is schizotypal symptoms and cognitions that offer the best differentiation within high-risk groups. Final illness expression is thus likely to depend on later developmental processes (such as those associated with adolescent neuromaturation), or enhanced sensitivity to the effects of later stress.

These findings raise a series of key developmental questions. First, what is the meaning of the associations with childhood and adolescent characteristics? Although some features (in particular, delays in early motor development, and impairments in receptive language and cognitive functioning) show some diagnostic specificity with later schizophreniform disorder, childhood socioemotional disturbances clearly do not. Distinctions are often drawn between precursors to a disorder (thought to constitute risk factors) and prodromal features, seen as early manifestations of the disorder itself. Although the distinction is probably a useful one, in the case of schizophrenia over half of individuals with prodromal features do not go on to develop the disorder (Drake & Lewis, 2005), raising uncertainties over the meaning of a prodromal phase (Cannon, Kendell, Susser *et al.*, 2003). As we shall see, this pattern of clear and consistent, but far from necessary or specific, associations across development arises in a range of disorders.

That being so, a second key question concerns the factors or processes that lead to the translation of precursors and/or prodromata into overt disorder. In the case of schizophrenia, three main possibilities have been considered to date. First, developmental changes in brain structure and function in late adolescence may be crucial (Keshavan, Kennedy, & Murray, 2004), although once again it is unclear how such general developmental processes contribute to disorder onset in just a small minority of individuals. Second, certain types of social adversity (such as migration and social isolation) may also contribute (Broome, Woolley, Tabraham *et al.*, 2005). Third, consistent evidence now implicates heavy early adolescent use of cannabis with a substantial increase in risk (Arsenault, Cannon, Witton *et al.*, 2004; Henquet, Krabbendam, Spauwen *et al.*, 2005; Moore, Zammit, Lingford-Hughes *et al.*, 2007). Here, some degree of specificity does seem apparent: the risk applies mainly to individuals who have shown either precursors or prodromata of schizophrenia spectrum disorders, and is confined to those with early and heavy cannabis use. Molecular genetic findings (Caspi, Moffitt, Cannon *et al.*, 2005) suggest that it is a function of the valine allelic variation in the catechol-O-methyltransferase (*COMT*) gene. Even so, this gene–environment interaction can only account for part of the population variance in the transition to schizophrenia: most individuals with the specific allelic variation, and who use cannabis heavily, do not develop schizophrenia, while many of those who do develop disorder have not shown heavy cannabis use. Although we are beginning to identify factors important in the transition to disorder, we are far from having achieved a complete account.

Finally, it remains possible that, in addition to early neurodevelopmental abnormalities, further changes in both cognitive function and brain structure and function take place during the course of the disorder, either as a result of the disease process, or of the drugs used in its treatment (Keshavan, Kennedy, & Murray, 2004). The evidence so far is not decisive, but does suggest that further changes may take place after the development of the psychosis that may be relevant to its later course.

Depression

As in research on schizophrenia, so developmental studies have markedly changed concepts of depression in recent decades. Prior to the 1970s, depression was viewed as a predominantly adult disorder: pre-adolescent children were thought incapable of experiencing adult-like depressions, and low mood in adolescence was thought to reflect little more than "normal" adolescent mood swings. Research since the 1980s has radically changed that view. Both clinical and epidemiological studies have confirmed the reality of childhood and adolescent depressive disorders; indeed, recent evidence suggests that (with age-appropriate modifications to diagnostic criteria) depression is also seen in some preschoolers, although the high rate of comorbidity with other disorders leaves it unclear whether depressive symptom clusters at these very early ages are phenotypically similar to depression at later ages (Egger & Angold, 2006). Age and sex trends – other key features of the developmental picture – have also been clarified. Depressive disorders are rare in childhood, but rates rise markedly from the early teens (Glowinski, Madden, Bucholz *et al.*, 2003), probably associated with the hormonal changes of puberty (Angold, Costello, & Erkanl *et al.*, 1999b), related changes in brain physiology and social information processing (Nelson, Leibenluft, McClure *et al.*, 2005) and possibly an increase in gene–environment correlations (Rice, Harold, & Thapar, 2003). The female predominance typical of adult depression also emerges at this stage, to be maintained throughout the childbearing years. Much adolescent onset depression is preceded by childhood anxiety; later in development, depression can form part of more complex progressions, both preceding and following adult anxiety, and is a not uncommon outcome of both anti-social disorders and substance use.

Developmental studies of depression have explored a variety of issues, beginning with the question of whether – despite similarities in symptomatology – childhood, adolescent and adult onset depressions do indeed reflect the same underlying disorder. Medicine provides many examples – diabetes being perhaps the best known – where, despite similar clinical features, disorders with differing ages at onset show quite distinct patterns of neurobiological correlates. A variety of evidence now points to rather similar possibilities in depression. Jaffee, Moffitt, Caspi *et al.* (2002), for example, found that while "juvenile onset" depression (with onset prior to age 15) was associated with high rates of family psychopathology and disruption, neurocognitive impairments, and with a broad spectrum of emotional and behavioral problems in childhood, adult onset cases (aged 18 years and older at first reported episode) were not; indeed, the only "adverse" childhood factor clearly evident among adult onset cases was exposure to sexual abuse. Studies have also shown that neurobiological correlates of depression differ in adult and earlier onset disorders, and there are well-documented variations in response to tricyclic medication (for a review see Kaufman, Martin, King *et al.*, 2001). It remains unclear at this stage whether these differences reflect developmental variations in the maturation of relevant neurobiological systems, stage of illness factors or heterogeneity in the underlying nature of the disorder.

Second, longitudinal data have shown that, at least between adolescence and adulthood, continuities in depression are strong. Risks are elevated at least twofold (and often considerably more so) by contrast with rates in non-depressed controls; are increased in sub-threshold groups, as well as in young people meeting full diagnostic criteria for depression (Pine, Cohen, Cohen *et al.*, 1999); and remain increased when other comorbid disorders and associated childhood risks are taken into account (Fergusson & Woodward, 2002). By contrast, childhood onset samples (Harrington *et al.*, 1990; Weissman, Wolk, Wickramaratne *et al.*, 1999) show little or no increased risk for adult depression by comparison with non-depressed controls, and are at lower risk of recurrence than their adolescent onset peers. If further replicated, evidence of this kind provides additional pointers to the possibility that childhood depression differs in important ways from its later onset counterparts.

Third, investigators have highlighted a range of mechanisms that may be implicated in risk for the recurrence of depressive episodes across developmental periods. Among these, genetic factors seem almost certain to be involved. Genetic influences on depressive phenotypes are low in childhood, but rise in adolescence to levels broadly similar to those found in adult samples (Rice, Harold, & Thapar, 2002). To date, longitudinal data from genetically sensitive designs have only been reported across relatively short follow-up periods, and often in samples spanning quite wide age ranges. Bearing these limitations in mind, findings suggest that genetic factors do contribute to stability in depression scores across adolescence and early adulthood, but that new genetic and non-shared environmental influences also arise across this age period (Lau & Eley, 2006). Interplay between genetic predispositions and environmental exposures is also likely to be involved. Studies have confirmed, for example, that specific gene variants affect susceptibility to adverse life events in both adolescence (Eley, Sugden, Corsico *et al.*, 2004) and early adulthood (Caspi, Sugden, Moffitt *et al.*, 2003), and that both depressed children (Rudolph, Hammen, Burge *et al.*, 2000) and adults (Hammen, 2003) behave in ways that increase their likelihood of exposure to interpersonal stress.

Early adversities – spanning both severe exposures such as abuse and maltreatment and more chronic difficulties such as lack of adequate maternal care – have long been recognized as risk factors for adult depression. Over time, a variety of pathways have been proposed to mediate these links. As more immediate precipitants, depressive episodes are often provoked by acute or chronic stressors; one route for the effects of early adversity may thus be to increase exposure or vulnerability to these more proximal risks (Harris, Brown, & Bifulco, 1990). Childhood adversity is also associated with later difficulties in close personal relationships, and they too are implicated in risk for depression. In a retrospective study, Hill, Pickles, Burnside *et al.* (2001) found intriguing suggestions of specificity in mechanisms here: while good adult love relationships did nothing to reduce risks of depression following child sexual abuse, they made a substantial difference to risk following neglect or poor maternal care. The authors speculated that these findings may in turn reflect differential responses to differing types of adversity: while the chronic nature of neglect may affect self-views, the fright and trauma associated with abuse may have wider effects, impacting both affect regulation and neurobiological pathways (Grossman, Churchhill, McKinney *et al.*, 2003).

Finally, as suggested in a number of models, cognitive factors may also have a role in long-term vulnerability to depression, and the experience of an initial episode may itself bring about changes that affect recurrence risk. Depressogenic cognitive biases have now been identified in children as young as 5 years of age (Murray, Woolgar, Cooper *et al.*, 2001), and appear to function both as outcomes and as risks for depression in childhood (Nolen-Hoeksema, Girgus, & Seligman, 1992). Such biases are moderately stable, and contribute to the risk for recurrence of depression (Abramson, Alloy, Hankin *et al.*, 2002); at this stage, however, we still await direct longitudinal evidence of their persistence across extended developmental periods. In terms of recurrence risk, the role of precipitating stressors changes across episodes in adulthood (Kendler, Thornton, & Gardner, 2000), with vulnerability becoming increasingly autonomous from overt and severe precipitants as the number of episodes increases. Although effects of this kind have typically been interpreted as reflecting processes akin to "kindling" (Post, 1992), recent commentaries have highlighted ambiguities in that view: although illness-related factors may increase sensitivity to ever more minor stressors, the empirical evidence is also consistent with a model of *reduced* sensitivity to stress (Monroe & Harkness, 2005). Further studies are needed to clarify these competing interpretations, and to determine whether similar effects are seen in depressions beginning in adolescence.

Eating Disorders

In many respects, eating disorders represent the form of psychopathology that would most seem to require a developmental psychopathology perspective. Overt eating disorders arise for the first time in the teens, and show a highly variable long-term course; to date, however, very little is known about key childhood precursors of disordered eating, or predictors of better or poorer later outcome. In addition, core questions remain about associations among different types of eating disorder, and continuities with more common eating-related problems. Dieting and dissatisfaction with body shape and size are extremely common in adolescent girls and, on the face of it, seem to constitute a lesser variant of the much rarer overt eating disorders. However, the huge disparity in prevalence raises the possibility of an essentially qualitative discontinuity between the two. Comparable questions arise over continuities and discontinuities within the domain of overt eating disorders. Both clinic and community samples show that by far the rarest syndrome is anorexia nervosa (AN), with a rate well below 1% even within adolescent girls; the next rarest is bulimia nervosa (BN), with a prevalence in young adults of 1–2%; but much the most common is eating disorders not otherwise specified (EDNOS; Fairburn & Bohn, 2005; Fairburn, Cooper, Doll *et al.*, 2005; see also chapter 41). Over time, there is some movement across these groups, suggesting that all three may constitute variants in the manifestation of the same basic disorder. On the other hand, BN has a substantially later average age of onset than AN (early adult life, by contrast with mid-adolescence), and twin studies suggest that genetic factors are more influential in AN than BN (see chapter 41). Finally, AN typically begins in the immediate postpubertal years, but the meaning of this association remains unclear. Is onset causally associated with the hormonal changes of puberty; or is it provoked (in societies that value thinness) by adverse effects on body image and satisfaction associated with the increase in adiposity that accompanies puberty; or is the adolescent timing rather a function of the effect of depression, which rises markedly in frequency in girls at about the same time? Many of these issues were first raised in a heavily cited paper by Attie and Brooks-Gunn (1989) nearly two decades ago. Their small-scale 2-year longitudinal study of adolescent girls suggested that negative attitudes to body size and/or shape constituted the most important predictor of eating problems, with puberty an initial stimulus but not an enduring influence. As they recognized, however, the rarity of eating disorders meant that a much larger sample would be required to provide proper answers.

In principle, occupations with a particular pressure for thinness provide an additional window on the development of eating disorders. Szmukler, Eisler, Gillies *et al.* (1985), following Garner & Garfinkel (1980), drew attention to the high frequency of severe dieting in ballet dancers and the probable increase in overt AN. However, they also noted the generally good outcome among dancers, and the relative infrequency of more obviously psychopathological features such as induced vomiting or laxative abuse. They emphasized the difficulties in diagnosing eating disorders when there is a strong occupational pressure to be thin, and the dangers of drawing false psychopathological inferences. Surprisingly, there have been few attempts to examine these issues further. Neumärker, Bettle, Neumärker *et al.* (2000) found that an excessive concern with dieting, a drive for thinness and a preoccupation with weight were all more frequent in female (but not male) dancers, but found no instances of either binge eating or self-induced vomiting. Somewhat similarly, Santonastaso, Mondini, & Favaro (2002) found that although fashion models weighed significantly less than controls, few used unhealthy methods to control their weight. The database is decidedly thin, but the tentative conclusion would seem to be that although occupational pressures may provide a risk for eating problems, the risk for overt disorder is very low.

In order to examine possible continuities in the general population, it is necessary to turn to the very few large samples with longitudinal data spanning adolescence to early adult life. Kotler, Cohen, Davies *et al.* (2001), in a childhood–early adult follow-up, found high stability in bulimic symptoms between early adolescence and adult life, but the number with AN was too small for analysis. Despite this, the authors noted that it seemed that, although eating conflicts in childhood predicted AN symptoms, they did not predict BN. Leon, Fulkerson, Perry *et al.* (1999), in a 3–4-year longitudinal study of adolescents, found that negative affect and attitudes were the only robust predictors of eating disorders (mostly EDNOS); Johnson, Cohen, Brook *et al.* (2002) found that the main predictor of eating disorders was depression; and Measelle, Stice, & Hoganson (2006) reported a unidirectional relationship from depressive symptoms to eating pathology across the teens. In sum, although existing evidence is not entirely consistent, the tentative conclusion may be drawn that emotional disturbance in early adolescence constitutes the main risk factor for later eating disorder. The evidence on the putative risks stemming from eating conflicts in childhood is unconvincing.

With respect to possible continuities within the domain of overt eating disorders, the best data are provided by Fairburn and Bohn (2005). Out of a potential community sample of some 10,000, they focused on some 3000 currently dieting. Within the latter, there were 45% with a possible eating disorder, of whom 104 were found on the basis of more detailed study to have disorder (10 AN, 19 BN and 75 EDNOS). There was no follow-up of individuals who were not dieting, but the figures indicate a likely increased risk for the development of eating disorder. The most important finding concerned the risk factors for eating disorders among the dieters. In addition to low body mass index, seven stood out: frequent binge eating, eating in secret, a preoccupation with food and eating, a desire to have an empty stomach, frequent purging, a fear of losing control and a preoccupation with shape or weight. Taken together with other evidence, the tentative inference is that, whereas there is very little continuity between "ordinary" dieting and body weight and/or size dissatisfaction in adolescence and overt eating disorder, there is continuity (involving an extension outside overt disorder) when body dissatisfaction is associated with these more unusual features.

It cannot be claimed that the key developmental questions regarding eating disorders have been answered but, despite the sample size challenges, it is clear that they warrant more detailed study than they have received up to now.

Antisocial Behavior

Key aspects of the developmental profile of antisocial behavior have been known for many years. Four decades ago, Robins (1966) highlighted the pattern that has since been confirmed in numerous follow-up and follow-back studies: most severely antisocial adults have been antisocial children, but, at most, half of antisocial children go on to show marked antisocial behavior in their adult lives. Alongside this life-course picture, criminologists have also noted a highly consistent pattern of age-related change in "participation" in offending: official crime rates are low in late childhood, rise sharply in the teens, then fall back again across the adult years. Taken together, these two sets of observations suggest that any developmental account of antisocial behavior needs to "explain" at least three key phenomena: first, strong childhood–adulthood persistence among some individuals; second, the marked rise in antisocial involvement in the teens; and third, a general pattern of *desistance* in at least more overt markers of antisocial behaviors from late adolescence or early adulthood.

These developmental variations strongly suggest heterogeneity within the antisocial population. Among the many models advanced to account for this, Moffitt's (1993) developmental taxonomy has been perhaps the most influential. This taxonomy (see chapter 35) highlights age at onset as the key distinguishing marker, and proposes that early onset conduct problems are distinct from adolescent onset delinquency in both etiology and course. In brief, early onset conduct problems – male-dominated, and associated with both individual and environmental risks – are especially likely to show poor long-term outcomes. Adolescent onset problems – largely prompted by social influences, and with a less marked sex ratio – are assumed to be relatively transient, and to remit once individuals assume the responsibilities and experience the benefits of moving into adult roles. As Moffitt (see chapter 35) outlines, extensive evidence has now accumulated to support key elements of this model, although persistence of adolescent onset antisocial behavior has proved to be greater than originally anticipated.

In addition, developmental findings point to other potentially salient markers of heterogeneity. As we have seen, comorbid ADHD carries a strong risk for persistent antisocial behavior (Thapar *et al.*, 2006) and psychopathy and related callous/unemotional traits (Viding, 2004) may also be markers of poor long-term outcome; it is unclear at this stage how far these reflect differing facets of a single high-risk subgroup or separable associated risks. In addition, a number of studies have now identified subgroups with early onset conduct problems where adult outcomes are also poor, but where the pattern of later difficulties is of a markedly different kind. For these young people – estimated in some studies as approaching half of the childhood onset population – the sequelae of early conduct problems are marked not by persistence in antisocial difficulties, but by poor social functioning, social isolation, avoidance of close relationships and increased risks for emotional difficulties later in life (Moffitt, 2006). Very little is known at this stage about the early risks or later maintaining factors that differentiate young people who follow this avoidant "childhood-limited" pathway from those whose difficulties follow a more persistent "externalizing" course.

Outcome studies have also consistently highlighted a further striking feature of the sequelae of childhood conduct problems: the wide spectrum of adverse outcomes faced by young people with disruptive behavior disorders later in their lives. Fergusson, Horwood, & Ridder (2004) found that conduct problems at ages 7–9 years conveyed risk for poor educational and occupational achievements; for problems in sexual and partner relationships (including exposure to domestic violence); for early parenthood; and for elevated rates of substance use, mood and anxiety disorders and suicidal acts, as well as for crime and antisocial personality disorder. Educational and occupational difficulties seemed largely attributable to correlated early risks. For all other outcomes, the severity of childhood conduct problems continued to be associated with an increased risk after the effects of a broad spectrum of potential confounders had been taken into account. Kim-Cohen *et al.* (2003), exploring psychiatric sequelae of a range of childhood disorders, found a similar picture: alone among childhood disorders, conduct problems were associated with increased risks of *all* the adult disorders surveyed, including anxiety, depression, schizophreniform disorders and mania as well as substance abuse.

These findings raise key questions about the early risks and intervening mechanisms that contribute to this broad spectrum of adult difficulties. We focus here on possible pathways in persistence in and desistance from antisocial behavior, and effects on poor social functioning in adulthood; heterotypic continuities to other disorders are considered in a later section. First, genetic liabilities are almost certain to be implicated. Pervasive early onset antisocial behaviors – likely to carry high risks of persistence – are also known to be strongly heritable (Arseneault, Moffitt, Caspi *et al.*, 2003). As in depression, genetic effects may be as important in contributing to exposure or vulnerability to environmental adversities as in any direct "main effects" way (Rutter, Moffitt, & Caspi, 2006b). Genetic factors have been found to moderate vulnerability to childhood family adversity and maltreatment, with effects evident on measures of both childhood–adolescent conduct problems and on personality features and violent offending in adult life (Caspi, McClay, Moffitt *et al.*, 2002). In addition, genetically influenced traits may influence exposure to adverse environments. Childhood disruptive behaviors have long been known to evoke negative maintaining responses from parents (Anderson, Lytton, & Romney, 1986; Patterson, Reid, & Dishion, 1992). Recent evidence suggests that processes of this kind may be set in train very early in development (Boivin, Perusse, Dionne *et al.*, 2005). Later, genetically influenced traits are also likely to play a part in selecting antisocial young people into deviant peer groups (Fergusson, Swain-Campbell, & Horwood, 2002) and intimate partnerships (Woodward, Fergusson, & Horwood, 2002) that reinforce early difficulties, stabilizing maladaptive behaviors and interactional styles, and restricting opportunities for involvement in more positive functioning.

Cumulating consequences of this kind – also referred to as chains or cascades of risk – seem likely to be key mechanisms in the persistence of early onset conduct problems (Maughan & Rutter, 2001). Where adolescent onset antisocial behavior is followed by poor adult outcomes, similar processes also seem likely to be implicated, although this remains to be directly tested at this stage. Questions also remain over the extent to which the poor long-term prognosis for childhood onset conduct problems is at least in part attributable to more extended exposure to the cumulating consequences of early behaviors – that is, to age at onset per se – or whether effects are primarily driven by associated early risks or variations in mediating mechanisms. In addition, antisocial young people may vary in the extent to which they have access to, or perhaps can benefit from, positive later experiences associated with desistance from delinquency and crime. Stouthamer-Loeber, Wei, Loeber *et al.* (2004) found that desistance from serious delinquency was most common among young adult males with good job skills, positive earlier relationships with peers, awareness of the risks of offending and who were actively engaged in either education or employment. In a similar way, Laub and Sampson (2001, 2003; Rutter, 1996) have highlighted the role of adult "turning point" experiences in desistance, underlining the importance of adult social attachments – arising both from work involvement and supportive marital relationships – in promoting desistance from crime. While almost all offenders eventually desist, these findings – along with models suggesting the cumulative nature of many intervening risk mechanisms – provide important pointers for intervention, suggesting that chains of risk can be broken and that later opportunities can, to some extent at least, offset the effects of earlier risks.

Substance Use

Although a great many young people are involved in experimental and recreational drug use, far fewer progress to abuse or dependence (Fergusson & Horwood, 2000; Kandel, Yamaguchi, & Chen, 1992). Adolescent substance use is implicated in a nexus of other disorders across development, strongly predicted by externalizing disorders in childhood and comorbid with, and predicting to, both antisocial outcomes and affective disorders later in life. Many early psychosocial risks for drug and alcohol use overlap with family-based adversities implicated in risk for other disorders; as a result, there are major difficulties in determining how far later adverse outcomes are specific to drug-related problems or operate primarily via effects on other disorders. However, twin studies provide a most useful means of testing alternative mechanisms (Kendler & Prescott, 2006; see also chapter 2).

We take up issues associated with heterotypic continuities with other disorders below; here, we focus on the role of age at onset as a potential predictor of later adverse outcomes. Throughout the history of epidemiological studies of substance use, early initiation of drug and alcohol use – in general, before the mid-teens – has been identified as a strong marker both for progression to later stages in substance abuse pathways and for more global difficulties in adult functioning. As in the case of antisocial behavior, these findings raise the key question of whether early initiation per se contributes to these effects, or whether it functions primarily as a marker for more severe, and possibly more generalized, liability to subsequent difficulties. As will be apparent, answers to this question carry major implications for policy and practice, as well as for theoretical understanding (Rutter, 2005b). Although current evidence is not entirely unequivocal, there are increasing pointers that early onset of a range of "problem behaviors" tends to co-occur. McGue and Iacono (2005) found strong evidence for a generalized risk for early onset problems, encompassing delinquency and early sexual behaviors as well as alcohol and drug use, before age 15. Young people with this multiple problem cluster of early behaviors were at exceptionally high risk of both externalizing disorders and depression at follow-up at age 20. This in turn suggests that shared risks (genetic and environmental) underlying a general tendency to early onset difficulties may have a key role in later outcomes. Twin findings confirm the importance of shared genetic influences in this multiple problem cluster (Kendler & Prescott, 2006). Although early initiation may, in itself, carry a minor additional facilitating effect, most of the increased risk for poor functioning later in development appears to lie in shared early risks of this kind. This has been shown most clearly through discordant twin designs (Kendler & Prescott, 2006). Twins as a group show the same association between early alcohol use and later alcoholism found in singletons. However, when twins differ in their age of starting drinking they do not differ in their alcoholism outcome. The apparent early onset effect is largely an artifact of shared genetic liability.

Heterotypic Continuity and Psychopathological Progressions

As we have seen, developmental data leave no doubt that many child psychiatric disorders represent early manifestations of persisting or recurring vulnerability to mental health problems later in life. Thus far, our discussions have focused mainly on homotypic continuities – the persistence of the same disorder over time. In addition, the empirical evidence also makes clear that more complex developmental sequences are far from uncommon. Follow-back analyses of young adult disorders in the Dunedin longitudinal study (Kim-Cohen *et al.*, 2003) showed that adult anxiety disorders were predicted not only by earlier emotional difficulties, but also by ADHD and conduct disorder/oppositional defiant disorder (CD/ODD); that schizophreniform disorders were preceded by elevated rates of both emotional and behavioral disorders earlier in development; and that childhood CD/ODD was part of the developmental history of *all* of the adult disorders studied.

In studies of concurrent comorbidity, commentators have noted that because multiple disorders often co-occur, some two-way associations may be "epiphenomenal" – the product (at least statistically) of associations among other disorders. Ford, Goodman, & Meltzer (2003) found that associations between CD and anxiety were largely of this kind: each disorder showed strong links with depression, but once these were taken into account, overlaps between CD and anxiety no longer exceeded chance levels. Costello *et al.* (2003) examined year-on-year progressions in disorder across the 9–16 year age range controlling for the presence of other diagnoses in this way. Once prior comorbid conditions had been taken into account, they found that heterotypic continuities centered on transitions among a relatively limited number of disorders: from anxiety to depression and depression to anxiety; from anxiety to substance abuse/dependence; and from ADHD to ODD. In this late childhood/early adolescent period, both concurrent comorbidity and heterotypic continuity were significantly more common in girls than in boys.

To date, childhood–adult studies have not yet reported analyses involving comprehensive controls for co-occurring prior disorders in this way, although individual studies have done so in relation to particular later outcomes. As a result, some of the disorder progressions reported to date may prove to be epiphenomenal. However, many have unequivocal empirical support: progressions from ADHD to later antisocial disorders and substance use; from substance use to depression (Rutter, 2002); from CD/ODD to a spectrum of later disorders; and between anxiety and depression have all been confirmed in numerous studies. In addition, associations between schizophrenia and earlier emotional/behavioral difficulties need to be considered in this context, along with the emergence of widespread problems in social functioning identified in the adult outcomes of children with SLI.

To date, two rather different processes have been proposed as underlying these varying developmental sequences. First, some connections may reflect age-varying manifestations of the same underlying liability: in general, the term *heterotypic continuity* has been used to refer to processes of this kind. Second, some links may more properly reflect *psychopathological progressions* – instances where one disorder or its associated impairments function as risk factors for a second, distinct condition. Some of the examples documented to date fall relatively straightforwardly under one or other of these headings, while others raise more queries.

Heterotypic Continuity

Several of the patterns of continuity outlined above seem well captured by the notion that there is meaningful continuity in the course of individual disorders, but that their manifestations change with age. This is likely to be the case, for example, in relation to the associations between neurodevelopmental impairments early in childhood, psychotic-like features later in childhood and the eventual development of schizophrenia; and in the progression from prepubertal anxiety to postpubertal depression. In some instances the impairments involved are clearly closely related, so that associations across development can be expected to be high. In others, mechanisms contributing to continuities are less clear. In relation to schizophrenia, for example, although there is relative specificity in some of the developmental linkages observed, childhood precursor deficits are much more common than eventual psychotic outcomes, raising key questions over the mechanisms involved in the translation of early vulnerabilities into subsequent disorder.

Developmental progressions in anxiety and depression have attracted particular attention. Associations between these two disorders are high at all stages of development, and clearly reflect shared genetic risks (Kendler, Prescott, Myers *et al.*, 2003). The order of emergence of these phenomena does, however, appear to vary systematically across development. Between childhood and early adolescence – around the time of puberty – anxiety typically precedes depression, and the degree of diagnostic overlap between the two disorders increases strongly over the following years (Wittchen, Kessler, Pfister *et al.*, 2000). From later adolescence onwards, the temporal sequence runs in both directions: anxiety predicts to depression, but depressive disorders also predict to later anxiety (Pine, Cohen, Gurley *et al.*, 1998). To an extent, of course, the apparent specificity of the childhood–adolescent transition may simply reflect typical ages at onset of the two disorders: anxiety is common in childhood, but there is a sharp increase in depression in the early teens (Glowinski *et al.*, 2003; Hankin, Abramson, Moffitt *et al.*, 1998), whether preceded by anxiety or not. In addition, there seems little doubt that childhood anxiety does constitute a risk factor for depression (Wittchen, Beesdo, Bittner *et al.*, 2003), and possibly an age-dependent expression of the same underlying disorder (Weissman *et al.*, 2005). Twin study data lend support to this position, suggesting a common genetic etiology, and developmental findings point to a variety of possible mediating factors, including the role of pubertal hormones (Walker, Sabuwalla, & Huot *et al.*, 2004b), increased exposure to stressful life events (Silberg, Pickles, Rutter *et al.*, 1999) and negative cognitions (Nolen-Hoeksema, Girgus, & Seligman, 1992), and adolescent changes in brain functioning (Nelson *et al.*, 2005). While the presence of any childhood anxiety disorder is associated with increased depression risk (and the presence of multiple anxiety diagnoses seems especially salient), generalized anxiety disorder (GAD) appears to show the highest individual risk (Wittchen *et al.*, 2003).

As noted earlier, progressions from ADHD to later antisocial disorders also seem likely to reflect shared underlying liabilities, as do progressions from CD to substance use. Here, however, associations are not simply unidirectional: although CD is a strong predictor of adolescent substance use, both alcohol and cannabis use, early in adolescence, predict later delinquency, and alcohol dependence later in the teens seems to "ensnare" some young men into persisting in antisocial behavior (Malone, Taylor, Marmorstein *et al.*, 2004). Mediating mechanisms also vary at different stages of substance use involvement. Twin data suggest that early in the teens, when symptoms of alcohol problems are rare, associations with conduct problems are almost entirely mediated by shared environmental influences (Rose, Dick, Viken *et al.*, 2004). By late adolescence, however, shared genetic liability is by far the strongest influence on the covariation of alcohol dependence and antisocial behavior in males (Malone *et al.*, 2004), likely reflecting shared risks in personality features such as impulsivity, risk-taking and lack of behavioral restraint (Krueger, Hicks, Patrick *et al.*, 2002). Once established, substance use problems may affect persistence in antisocial behavior through somewhat different routes, including the disinhibiting effects of alcohol, psychosocial factors associated with peer influences and adverse effects on family relationships, and the need for money to support drink and drug habits.

Alongside evidence of such heterotypic continuities, we should also note instances where clinical assumptions about progressions in disorder do *not* appear to be borne out by empirical findings. One such example concerns the long-held view that separation anxiety in childhood constitutes a precursor to panic disorder later in life. Three separate large-scale prospective studies have now failed to find evidence for associations of this kind (Costello, Foley, & Angold, 2006). Although much remains to be learned about developmental variations in the manifestations of anxiety, this widely anticipated progression seems not – on current evidence at least – to be supported by empirical findings. In a rather similar way, the strong associations between depressed mood and use of a range of substances in both adolescence and adulthood have long been assumed to reflect efforts at self-medication. At least in adolescence, longitudinal evidence has cast doubt on that view: studies of teenage cannabis use find no direct effects of depressive symptomatology (Rey, Martin, & Krabman, 2004), and follow-ups of depressed samples show little elevated risk for later drug or alcohol use (Fombonne, Wostear, Cooper *et al.*, 2001). As ever more complex progressions are identified in the sequencing of many disorders, *dis*confirmations of this kind are of particular importance in refining our models of potential mediating mechanisms.

Psychopathological Progressions

While some developmental associations in disorder seem likely to reflect varying expressions of the same underlying liability, others are probably best conceptualized as psychopathological progressions, where the experience of one disorder contributes, directly or indirectly, to risk for another. The broad spectrum of psychiatric sequelae of childhood conduct problems probably includes examples of both kinds. In relation to depression, for example, origins of the increased risk in conduct-disordered samples may arise in part from shared roots in temperamental features. Zoccolillo (1992) has argued that conduct disorder should be seen as a disorder of multiple dysfunction, involving emotional as well as behavioral dysregulation. In childhood, findings from a number of studies are beginning to highlight ODD as a central focus for much comorbidity (Angold, Costello, & Erkanli, 1999a), and for progressions to affective as well as antisocial outcomes (Burke, Loeber, Lahey *et al.*, 2005). To date, most longer-term follow-ups have not differentiated outcomes of CD and ODD, leaving it uncertain how far early temperamental difficulties indexed by oppositional diagnoses may contribute to continuities currently attributed to more directly antisocial traits. In addition, psychosocial mediating mechanisms seem likely to be involved in transitions to depression. As we have seen, childhood conduct problems frequently select individuals into adverse environments (both physical and relational) later in the life course, which in their turn are likely to increase exposure to stress (Champion, Goodall, & Rutter, 1995). In addition, school failure and relationship difficulties may contribute to the development of negative cognitions and self-views (Capaldi, 1992); and for some previously conduct disordered individuals, the pharmacological effects of substance use may constitute further independent risks for depression. As our knowledge of developmental pathways becomes clearer, so equally complex linkages may emerge in relation to a range of disorders.

Long-term Effects of Early Experience

In addition to tracing continuities in disorder, the expanding longitudinal database has also underscored the long-term effects of early experience on later psychological functioning. Numerous studies have now confirmed associations between a spectrum of early adversities – prenatal as well as postnatal, and both chronic and acute – and increased risk for disorder later in the life course. The specifics of these findings are considered in detail in chapters 25–31; we focus here on the more general issues that need to be borne in mind in interpreting associations of this kind, and on current evidence on the mechanisms that may underlie such long-term links.

Several rather different trends are evident in recent research in this area. First, studies have continued to demonstrate statistical associations between adverse experiences in childhood and later psychopathological outcomes, using a range of increasingly sophisticated designs. Where much early work rested on retrospective reports of childhood circumstances, many associations have now also been demonstrated in prospective studies; where retrospective reports continue to be needed (as, for example, in studies of sexual or physical abuse, where ethical constraints preclude prospective questioning in non-referred samples), important efforts have been made to establish the reliability of retrospective reports (Hardt & Rutter, 2004). Collectively, this work has demonstrated the broad spectrum of psychopathological sequelae that follow from the more severe forms of childhood adversity, and the substantial contribution that exposures such as childhood sexual abuse have on the overall burden of mental disorder in both childhood and adult life (Andrews, Corry, Slade *et al.*, 2004). In addition, there has been a growing interest in the role of prenatal as well as postnatal exposures. Maternal smoking in pregnancy, for example, has attracted extensive attention as a risk for antisocial behavior in offspring across the life course (Wakschlag *et al.*, 2002), and evidence is also accumulating for associations of later emotional/behavioral difficulties with maternal stress in pregnancy (O'Connor, Ben-Shlomo, Heron *et al.*, 2005), and for links between prematurity/low birthweight and risk for subsequent depression (Patton, Coffey, Carlin *et al.*, 2004).

Alongside these increasingly well-replicated statistical associations, commentators have also drawn attention to the need for appropriate caution in interpreting the meaning of such links. Several different issues are of concern here. First, because early risks frequently cluster, tracking the effects of any specific early exposure inevitably presents major challenges. Prenatal smoking provides an especially telling example here. Numerous studies have now confirmed links between maternal smoking in pregnancy and antisocial outcomes in offspring (Wakschlag *et al.*, 2002), and preclinical studies provide clear and biologically plausible models for effects of nicotine exposure on development of the fetal brain. Despite these persuasive findings, uncertainties over the causal role of pregnancy smoking still remain, in part at least because prenatal smoking co-occurs so strongly with factors such as young maternal age, low maternal education, antisocial traits in parents and depression in mothers, all of which are also well-established risks for childhood conduct problems (Wakschlag *et al.*, 2002). Against that background, passive observational studies alone are unlikely to be able to identify the key pathogenic factors; instead, planned or natural experiments capable of teasing out specific smoking-related effects are needed to take the causal argument forward.

Confounding of this kind typically presents fewer difficulties in relation to postnatal exposures, but problems of interpretation may nonetheless arise. In some instances, these relate to accurate identification of the key elements of risk; in others, to their mode of operation. In relation to the first point, studies have shown that associations with relatively "distal" risk factors such as family poverty in childhood are largely mediated through more proximal indicators of family functioning or the quality of parent–child relationships (Conger, Ge, Elder *et al.*, 1994). Although poverty is indeed implicated in the risk process, its effects on child outcomes are largely indirect. In relation to the second point, genetically informative studies have been important in offering correctives to unquestioning assumptions that associations with apparently "environmental" risk factors do indeed point to environmentally mediated effects (Rutter, 2005a). Harsh parenting – well known to be associated with a plethora of adverse outcomes for children – provides a simple case in point. Although adverse parenting may indeed carry environmentally mediated risk, extensive evidence also points to two alternative possibilities: that genetically influenced child characteristics evoke negative responses from parents, and that styles of parenting are correlated with parental characteristics that also convey genetically mediated risks. Once again, passive longitudinal studies of individuals – the designs most commonly used thus far in tracking long-term developmental sequelae of early adversity – are rarely capable of disentangling these differing effects. However, more appropriate designs are now becoming available. D'Onofrio, Turkheimer, Emery *et al.* (2005) have recently used the additional leverage offered by studying the children of twins to demonstrate that environmental influences associated with parental divorce do indeed account for the higher rates of drug and alcohol use, and behavioral and emotional problems, shown by young adult children in divorcing families. Although empirical examples of the use of such designs are still limited, over time they promise important advances in our understanding of the key influences underlying exposure to early risks.

Several other general issues are also worthy of note. First, although especially severe early adversities are associated with poor outcomes in many exposed individuals (and effects of multiple adversities are typically most deleterious), most evidence also highlights individual differences in response, with some individuals apparently protected against, or resilient to, later adverse outcomes. In relation to sexual abuse, for example, current findings suggest that although the majority of affected young people show some psychiatric sequelae in adulthood, up to one-third do not (Fergusson & Mullen, 1999). In addition to variations in severity of risk exposure, positive adaptation following abuse appears to reflect interactions among heritable factors, individual characteristics (ranging from biological factors such as stress-reactivity to cognitive and personality features) and later life course experiences (including the availability of emotionally responsive parenting and positive and supportive peer relationships and intimate partnerships). However, discordant twin designs show that the strong effect of sexual abuse in childhood on later depression and later alcoholism is *not* explicable on the basis of shared genetic liability that spans both the experience and the outcome (Kendler & Prescott, 2006). The twin experiencing serious sexual abuse is the one more likely to have the psychopathological outcomes. Second, although some early theoretical discussions assumed specificity in the psychopathological sequelae of particular types of early adversity, empirical findings if anything suggest diversity in adverse outcomes; although the evidence base is too slim for firm conclusions at this stage, there are some pointers that mediating mechanisms, rather than phenotypic outcomes, will prove to show more specificity. Third, although some recent discussions have appeared to support early claims that the major effects of adverse experiences arise in the earliest years of life, when brain development is at its most rapid, the evidence is clearly against that view. Although very early adversities do indeed show long-term impacts, and some apparently sensitive period effects have been reported in relation, for example, to the effects of severely depriving early institutional care (Rutter & O'Connor, 2004), it is also clear that experiences across childhood and adolescence, and indeed in adult life, can function as risk factors for psychopathology.

Mediating Mechanisms

From both theoretical and clinical perspectives, delineating the mechanisms that contribute to the long-term sequelae of early adversity clearly constitutes a major priority. To date, direct evidence on mediating mechanisms remains limited, but a number of possible processes have been proposed (Rutter, 2005a). In some instances these reflect the development of biological or psychological vulnerabilities in childhood that are activated by exposure to further risk later in development; in others, effects may run through more immediate precipitation of disorder in childhood or adolescence, which then heightens risk for recurrence; and in others again, effects may run through selection into later risk-prone environments. Psychological mediators include the development of negative cognitive sets and dysfunctional mental representations of self, others and relationships. Exposure to maltreatment, for example, is known to be associated with problems in social information processing, and the development of hostile attributions and biases that may mediate effects on intimate relationships in adulthood (Berlin & Dodge, 2004). Findings on the sequelae of sexual abuse are of particular interest here in suggesting delayed effects in some individuals, not apparent (at least in terms of overt psychopathology) until later in the life course (Jaffee *et al.*, 2002). It has been proposed that exposure to traumatic early experience may evoke active coping strategies to regulate affect. The overgeneralized autobiographical memories reported in some depressed samples, for example, have been argued to reflect attempts to deal with painful memories associated with childhood trauma (Williams, 1996); although adaptive in childhood, such strategies may prove less functional in the context of intimate adult relationships (Hill *et al.*, 2001).

Cognitive development (Richards & Wadsworth, 2004) and coping styles may also be affected, and styles of interpersonal interaction seem especially vulnerable. Many childhood adversities are associated with later difficulties in close relationships (Paz, Jones, & Byrne, 2005); these in turn may function both to deprive individuals of the benefits of positive adult relationships and to increase the likelihood of exposure to later stress. Despite their importance, the roots of these difficulties remain poorly understood. In addition to other aspects of parenting, it is clearly essential to consider the role of attachment here. From the outset, Bowlby (1969) argued that an infant's early attachments may constitute the basis of all later social relationships, and would be crucial to later psychological development. Prospective studies of attachment from infancy to adulthood (Grossman, Grossman, & Waters, 2005) suggest that the pathways involved are likely to be complex. Alongside evidence that the sensitive supportiveness, acceptance of the child and challenging cooperation of both parents contribute to favorable models of close relationships later in life, it is also clear that taken alone, attachment security in infancy is only a weak predictor of global functioning in early adulthood; when combined with other social measures, prediction to later outcomes is strong (Sroufe, Egeland, Carlson *et al.*, 2005). This suggests that early attachment experiences work with and through other experiences – including peer relationships, later family experiences, and eventually mature intimate relationships – to contribute to later functioning. Although early relationships with mothers are most influential, they are not determinative: the quality of attachments to fathers and to other caregivers may also have domain-specific effects, and no one attachment style will work best under all contextual circumstances. It remains to be clarified quite how dyadic relationships early in development become more generalized, individual features later in the life course, and whether parental sensitivity or ongoing commitment forms the key component.

In addition to these psychosocial pathways, there is also increasing evidence for physical effects of maltreatment, with adverse outcomes on physical health suggesting that chronic early stress has effects on the cardiovascular system, the immune system and on neurobiological functioning (Paz, Jones, & Byrne, 2005). Preclinical studies now provide elegant models for the ways in which a range of early social experiences influence the brain (Champagne & Curley, 2005). Prenatally, gestational stress has been shown to affect the behavior and neuroendocrine functioning of offspring, and deprivation of maternal care in infancy has emerged as central to the development of stress responsivity associated with disruption of hypothalamic–pituitary axis functioning. Importantly, such effects are not confined to extremes of maternal care; in rats, for example, high levels of maternal licking and grooming in the postpartum period are associated with less fearful behavior in offspring, with attenuated corticosterone response to stress, and with increased levels of hippocampal glucocorticoid receptor expression. Recent evidence suggests that these effects may result from epigenetic changes in DNA methylation, providing a stable mechanism whereby the effects of early social experience persist across development. Equally important, preclinical studies also provide evidence of plasticity. Enrichment of the post-weaning environment, for example, is related to decreased corticosterone response to stress and reduced behavioral indications of anxiety among rats exposed to postnatal maternal separation, with these later social experiences apparently affecting brain development through differing, but equally stable, mechanisms (Champagne & Curley, 2005).

It is unknown at this stage how far these mechanisms are directly relevant to other species, or whether effects of early environment on human behavior involve parallel epigenetic modifications. Existing evidence does suggest, however, that susceptibility to early adversity varies depending on the individual's genotype. In the Dunedin longitudinal study, a gene–environment interaction was found whereby associations between an index of early maltreatment/adversity and risk of both childhood and adult antisocial outcomes were dependent on variations in the monoamine oxidase A gene (Caspi *et al.*, 2002); males with a lowactivity form of the gene were at high risk of antisocial outcomes when exposed to maltreatment, while those with the high-activity form appeared protected. In a similar way, gene–environment interactions have been reported in relation to risk for depression in the face of stress (Rutter *et al.*, 2006b), suggesting that genetic risk largely operates through its effects on susceptibility to risk environments. As studies of this kind are extended they promise important advances in our understanding of individual differences in the effects of early risks.

General Developmental Themes

Taken together, the findings reviewed here underscore the major advances in our understanding of the development of psychopathology achieved through the application of life course concepts and perspectives to the rapidly expanding long-term longitudinal database in psychiatric research. As they make clear, development involves both continuity and change, and an ongoing interplay between individuals and their environments; although early experience strongly shapes later developmental outcomes, opportunities for change also arise across the life course, and individual differences in response are evident throughout.

Alongside the major advances in knowledge reflected here, many issues also remain to be clarified. Although relatively robust evidence now exists on the *pattern* of continuities in many disorders, for example, and on the long-term sequelae of early adversity, understanding of the mechanisms underlying these links remains much more rudimentary. Gene–environment interplay seems likely to be central to many of these effects, but as we have seen, effects are also likely to be carried forward through psychological mechanisms, through influences on developing brain and neurobiological systems and through connections among social experiences. Much of the later impact of early disorder and adversity seems likely to run through the lasting chains of effects that they set in train in these differing developmental domains. To date, studies have primarily been concerned to highlight the range of mechanisms that may potentially be involved; a key need in the future is to pit alternative hypotheses against one another, to provide more specific pointers to particular mechanisms of risk.

Other challenges also abound. Beginning early in development, we need to know more about how early in life behavior is predictive of later psychopathology, and why, in a number of domains, early onset of disorder appears to carry such deleterious long-term effects: is early age itself a contributory factor (so that, for example, delayed involvement could ameliorate later outcomes), or are age-related variations in onset largely markers for heterogeneity in underlying risk (Rutter, 2005b)? Moving forward in development, the biological changes of puberty and the socially defined changes of adolescence are clearly associated with major changes in risk for many differing types of psychopathology, but the basis for those effects is only now beginning to be understood. Finally, one further key challenge highlighted by existing findings concerns heterotypic continuities – changes in the expression of vulnerability to disorder across age – which seem as striking in many arenas as consistency in emotional and behavioral progressions. From a scientific perspective, the tools now exist to address many of these issues, and major advances can be expected in the coming years in many of these domains. Equally importantly, developmental findings require integration into clinical practice; we conclude by highlighting some of the key implications of existing findings for practice in both the childhood and the adult fields.

Clinical Implications

The evidence on lifespan continuities and discontinuities in psychopathology clearly underlines the value of the developmental psychopathology perspective for mental disorders in all age periods, and highlights a range of issues that are relevant for services. We focus here on implications for the timing of interventions; the need to take account of risks of recurrence, as well as current symptomatology; the implications of developmental variations in response to medication; the value of support for successful coping with stress; and, perhaps most importantly, the need for co-ordination and co-operation between services for children and those for adults.

Multiphase or multistage pathways operate over time with many disorders. Different causal factors are implicated at different points on these pathways, offering different targets for intervention. For example, substance abuse disorders start with experimental, recreational use of substances; in some individuals this leads on to much heavier, regular use; and this, in turn, may lead on to pharmacological or psychological dependency and adverse physical consequences. On the whole, environmental influences are much stronger at earlier points on this pathway than in the later points involved with dependency and overt disorder. Physiological responses to the substance also have a role. Thus, individuals who are able to tolerate high dosages of alcohol without marked ill effects are more likely to go on to become dependent than those who become intoxicated more readily. The models provided by peers, parents and others are also important in the early phases of substance use. The issue of whether one substance provides a "gateway" to the use of other substances has proved a controversial one. Nevertheless, most regular heavy drug users and abusers take many different substances, and both longitudinal and genetic data suggest that regular cannabis use predisposes to the use of other substances (Rutter, 2007). It is not entirely clear why that is so. It could simply be that it brings the individual into contact with people who use other drugs, or it could mean the acquisition of an attitude of mind in which drug-taking is an accepted part of both a means of pleasure and a means of dealing with stress. Either way, the implication is that preventive measures would do well to focus on the early phases of substance use and abuse, without waiting for overt disorder to become manifest. It is also apparent that the effects of drugs may vary with age. Thus, for example, the schizophrenogenic effects of heavy cannabis use seem to apply largely or entirely to such use in adolescence, rather than adult life. An early study of stimulant drug effects (Rapoport, 1980) suggested that these tended to have a dysphoric effect in childhood in contrast to the usual euphoriant effect in adult life. This suggested that the likelihood of recreational use may be greater in adulthood than in childhood.

Somewhat different considerations derive from developmental evidence on schizophrenia. As we have seen, schizophrenia in adult life is frequently preceded by neurodevelopmental impairments in childhood. The pattern is not diagnostically specific, however, and as yet, there is no justification for intervention at this early stage – at least with respect to the use of medication that is beneficial for overt schizophrenia. The psychotic-like features that may be evident in later childhood or early adolescence are obviously much closer to the overt disorder. Even so, the base rate of these features is far higher than the rate of schizophrenia itself, and only a minority of individuals with such experiences will go on to develop overt schizophrenia. At present, it is not known which factors are involved in that transition, other than that the heavy early use of cannabis does seem to be an important predisposing factor in some cases. This means that individuals with such psychotic-like experiences are particularly vulnerable to the risks associated with early cannabis use. The clinical features described in terms of the prodromata of schizophrenia, arising in late adolescence or early adult life, are even closer to overt schizophrenia. Because there is fairly consistent suggestive evidence that the prognosis is worse when there has been a marked delay in initiating treatment, some clinicians have argued that treatment ought to be initiated at this prodromal stage. The dilemma once again is that prodromata are more common than overt schizophrenia, and not everyone with prodromata goes on to develop the disorder. The possibility of preventing progression has to be balanced against the risks associated with the possibly adverse effects of long-term psychotropic medication. At present, the weight of evidence suggests that preventive intervention should probably be restricted to individuals with a strong family history of schizophrenia and prodromata that are associated with current social malfunction. Nevertheless, the issues are far from resolved (Phillips, McGorry, Yung *et al.*, 2005) and one obvious need is for the development of services that are particularly designed for young people (older adolescents and young adults) who appear to have these prodromal problems. Further research on this group is needed in order to decide how best to intervene.

The findings on the outcome of neurodevelopmental disorders such as autism, ADHD, dyslexia, and the more severe varieties of SLI indicate the high frequency with which these early onset child disorders lead on to substantial social impairment in adult life. Services for these individuals are particularly poor because most adult psychiatrists lack expertise in dealing with the later sequelae of such disorders, and few child psychiatrists provide ongoing care once the individuals cease to be children. The development of better services for young adults who have had neurodevelopmental disorders in childhood constitutes a priority.

The findings of the sometimes long-term effects of early adverse experiences such as physical and sexual abuse raise a somewhat different set of issues. The evidence is clear that there are important long-term effects in some individuals. It is not immediately obvious, however, how that should influence treatment strategies. In a previous era, most psychological interventions were exclusively focused on the past and it definitely would not be justified to return to that approach. Current real life experiences are of major importance. Nevertheless, it would be unrealistic to suppose that the early experiences can simply be ignored as features of the past that are best forgotten and ignored. Psychological interventions need to focus on the present but, equally, they need to pay attention to predisposing experiences when the individuals were younger.

The findings on depressive disorders bring out other considerations. Traditionally, in psychiatry and psychology, therapeutic attention has focused on the relief of current suffering and the alleviation of current symptoms. That is appropriate, but most psychopathological disorders tend to be quite strongly recurrent. It is crucial to have therapeutic interventions that bring a particular episode to a close, but it is equally important to consider what sort of interventions are likely to reduce the risk of recurrence in the years ahead (Scott, 2006). Part of the attraction of cognitive–behavior therapy has lain in its claimed potential to help individuals cope better with life stressors or challenges and, thereby, to reduce risks of recurrence. It is not clear as yet how far it does in fact do that, but the aim is an appropriate one.

Awareness of recurrence risk has also led to a change in approach to the use of antidepressant medication in adults, with the practice now being continuing medication for at least 6 months, and possibly longer, after relief of symptoms. With respect to children and adolescents, recent attention has focused on apparent age differences in responses to medication, and on the risk of side-effects. It has been a puzzle that although there are strong continuities between depression in childhood/adolescence and in adult life, tricyclic medication seems much less efficacious in young people than it is in adults. The evidence on selective serotonin reuptake inhibitors (SSRIs) is less conclusive. Controlled trials have indicated worthwhile benefits, but doubts have been expressed on the extent to which these are comparable to those found in adulthood, and there has been much concern over the possible increased risks of suicidal responses. Opinions differ on the interpretation of the evidence and the jury is still out on the overall question. Nevertheless, what is clear is that there are likely to be important age-related differences in response to medication; gaining an understanding of these constitutes an important priority for research.

Across the age span, it is obvious that there are individual differences in response to stress and adversity. Gene–environment interaction constitutes an important part of the explanation for these differences (see chapter 23). Nevertheless, the findings on resilience (see chapters 25 & 26) indicate that other factors are also involved (Rutter, 2006). Thus, successful coping with stress or adversity may increase resistance to later stressors. In the past, preventive efforts have been mainly concerned with the avoidance of negative experiences; research findings now suggest that, although that is an important objective, equal attention should be paid to the strengths that may come from successful coping. It is also likely to be important how people interpret their adverse experiences and how they deal with them. Both considerations need to have a role in the planning of therapeutic interventions.

Perhaps most of all, the evidence on continuities and discontinuities in psychopathology over time emphasizes the need for better co-ordination and co-operation across services for children, adolescents and young adults than is usually available today. Clearly, special skills and experience are relevant for the provision of services for young people, and specialization is therefore needed. Also, there are good reasons for wanting in-patient services to be particularly adapted to the needs of different age groups. Ordinarily, it is not good practice to treat children on wards that are predominantly concerned with adults. Nevertheless, questions do need to be asked about the merits and demerits of focusing some services on particular psychopathological features, rather than on age groups. Thus, for example, should services for individuals with eating disorders subdivide into those for children and adolescents and those for adults, or would there be advantages to having services that span different age groups? Much the same considerations apply with respect to substance use and abuse. While endeavoring to maintain the real and important strengths of age-related specializations, we need to avoid the rigidities that can sometimes come with them and ask ourselves when they should predominate in planning services and when they should not.

Further Reading

Rutter, M., Maughan, B., & Kim-Cohen, J. (2006a). Continuities and discontinuities in psychopathology between childhood and adult life. *Journal of Child Psychology and Psychiatry*, *47*, 276–295.

References

Abramson, L. Y., Alloy, L. B., Hankin, B. L., Haeffel, G. J., MacCoon, D. G., & Gill, B. E. (2002). Cognitive-vulnerability-stress models of depression in a self-regulatory and psychological context. In I. H. Gotlib, & C. L. Hammen (Eds.), *Handbook of depression* (pp. 268–294). New York: Guilford.

Anderson, K. E., Lytton, H., & Romney, D. M. (1986). Mothers' interactions with normal and conduct-disordered boys: who affects whom? *Developmental Psychology*, 22, 604–609.

Andrews, G., Corry, J., Slade, T., Issakidis, C., Swanston, H. (2004). Child sexual abuse. In M. Ezzati, A. D. Lopez, A. Rodgers, & C. Murray (Eds.), *Comparative quantification of health risks: global and regional burden of disease attributable to selected major risk factors* (pp. 1851–1940). Geneva: World Health Organization.

Angold, A., Costello, E. J., & Erkanli, A. (1999a). Comorbidity. *Journal of Child Psychology and Psychiatry*, *40*, 55–87.

Angold, A., Costello, E. J., Erkanli, A., & Worthman, C. M. (1999b). Pubertal changes in hormone levels and depression in girls. *Psychological Medicine*, *29*, 1043–1053.

Arseneault, L., Cannon, M., Witton, J., & Murray, R. M. (2004). Causal association between cannabis and psychosis: Examination of the evidence. *British Journal of Psychiatry*, *184*, 110–117.

Arseneault, L., Moffitt, T. E., Caspi, A., Taylor, A., Rijsdijk, F., Jaffee, S., *et al.* (2003). Strong genetic effects on cross-situational antisocial behaviour among 5-year-old children, according to mothers, teachers, examiner-observers, and twins' self-reports. *Journal of Child Psychology and Psychiatry*, *44*, 832–848.

Attie, I., & Brooks-Gunn, J. (1989). Development of eating problems in adolescent girls: A longitudinal study. *Developmental Psychology*, *25*, 70–79.

Baldwin, A. L. (1960). The study of child behavior and development. In P. H. Mussen (Ed.), *Handbook of research methods in child development* (pp. 3–35). New York: Wiley.

Bell, R. Q. (1968). A reinterpretation of the direction of effects in studies of socialization. *Psychological Review*, *75*, 81–95.

Berlin, L. J., & Dodge, K. A. (2004). Relations among relationships. *Child Abuse and Neglect*, *28*, 1127–1132.

Bishop, D., Price, T., Dale, P., & Plomin, R. (2003). Outcomes of early language delay. II. Etiology of transient and persistent language difficulties. *Journal of Speech, Language, and Hearing Research*, *46*, 561–575.

Boivin, M., Perusse, D., Dionne, G., Saysset, V., Zoccolillo, M., Tarabulsy, G. M., *et al.* (2005). The genetic–environmental etiology of parents' perceptions and self-assessed behaviours towards their 5-month-old infants in a large twin and singleton sample. *Journal of Child Psychology and Psychiatry*, *45*, 612–630.

Bowlby J. (1969). *Attachment and loss*, Vol. 1. *Attachment* (2nd ed. 1982). London: Hogarth Press.

Broome, M. R., Woolley, J. B., Tabraham, P., Johns, L. C., Bramon, E., Murray, G. K., *et al.* (2005). What causes the onset of psychosis? *Schizophrenia Research*, *79*, 23–34.

Burke, J. D., Loeber, R., Lahey, B. B., & Rathouz, P. J. (2005). Developmental transitions among affective and behavioral disorders in adolescent boys. *Journal of Child Psychology and Psychiatry*, *46*, 1200–1210.

Burke, K. C., Burke, J. D., Regier, D. A., & Rae, D. S. (1990). Age at onset of selected mental-disorders in 5 community populations. *Archives of General Psychiatry*, *47*, 511–518.

Cannon, M., Kendell, R., Susser, E., & Jones, P. (2003). Prenatal and perinatal risk factors for schizophrenia. In R. Murray, P. Jones, E. Susser, J. van Os, & M. Cannon (Eds.), *The epidemiology of schizophrenia* (pp. 74–99). Cambridge: Cambridge University Press.

Capaldi, D. M. (1992). Cooccurrence of conduct problems and depressive symptoms in early adolescent boys. 2. A 2-year follow-up at grade 8. *Development and Psychopathology*, *4*, 125–144.

Caspi, A., McClay, J., Moffitt, T. E., Mill, J., Martin, J., Craig, I. W., *et al.* (2002). Role of genotype in the cycle of violence in maltreated children. *Science*, *297*, 851–854.

Caspi, A., Moffitt, T. E., Cannon, M., McClay, J., Murray, R., Harrington, H., *et al.* (2005). Moderation of the effect of adolescent-onset cannabis use on adult psychosis by a functional polymorphism in the COMT gene: Longitudinal evidence of a gene–environment interaction. *Biological Psychiatry*, *57*, 1117–1127.

Caspi, A., Sugden, K., Moffitt, T. E., Taylor, A., Craig, I. W., Harrington, H., *et al.* (2003). Influence of life stress on depression: Moderation by a polymorphism in the 5-HTT gene. *Science*, *301*, 386–389.

Champagne, F. A., & Curley, J. P. (2005). How social experiences influence the brain. *Current Opinion in Neurobiology*, *15*, 704–709.

Champion, L. A., Goodall, G. M., & Rutter, M. (1995). Behavioural problems in childhood and stressors in early adult life: A 20-year follow-up of London school children. *Psychological Medicine*, *25*, 231–246.

Christie, K. A., Burke, J. D., Regier, D. A., Rae, D. S., Boyd, J. H., & Locke, B. Z. (1988). Epidemiologic evidence for early onset of mental disorders and higher risk of drug use in young adults. *American Journal of Psychiatry*, *145*, 971–975.

Clegg, J., Hollis, C., Mawhood, L., & Rutter, M. (2005). Developmental language disorders – a follow-up in later adult life: Cognitive, language and psychosocial outcomes. *Journal of Child Psychology and Psychiatry*, *46*, 128–149.

Coleman, I., & Jones, P. (2004). Birth cohort studies in psychiatry: beginning at the beginning. *Psychological Medicine*, *34*, 1375–1383.

Conger, R. D., Ge, X. J., Elder, G. H., Lorenz, F. O., & Simons R. L. (1994). Economic-stress, coercive family process, and developmental problems of adolescents. *Child Development*, *65*, 541–561.

Costello, E. J., Foley, D. L., & Angold, A. (2006). 10-year research update review: The epidemiology of child and adolescent psychiatric disorders. II. Developmental epidemiology. *Journal of the American Academy of Child and Adolescent Psychiatry*, *45*, 8–25.

Costello, E. J., Mustillo, S., Erkanli, A., Keeler, G., & Angold, A. (2003). Prevalence and development of psychiatric disorders in childhood and adolescence. *Archives of General Psychiatry*, *60*, 837–844.

Croft, C., Beckett, C., Rutter, M., Castle, C., Colvert, E., Groothues, C., *et al.* (2007). Early adolescent outcomes of institutionally deprived and non-deprived adoptees at age 11 years. II. Language as a protective factor and a vulnerable outcome. *Journal of Child Psychology and Psychiatry*, *48*, 31–44.

D'Onofrio, B. M., Turkheimer, E., Emery, R. E., Slutske, W. S., Heath, A. C., Madden, P. A., *et al.* (2005). A genetically informed study of marital instability and its association with offspring psychopathology. *Journal of Abnormal Psychology*, *114*, 570–586.

Drake, R. J., & Lewis, S. W. (2005). Early detection of schizophrenia. *Current Opinion in Psychiatry*, *18*, 147–150.

Egger, H. L., & Angold, A. (2006). Common emotional and behavioral disorders in preschool children: presentation, nosology, and epidemiology. *Journal of Child Psychology and Psychiatry*, *47*, 313–337.

Elder, G. H. Jr., & Shanahan, M. J. (2006). The life course and human development. In R. M. Lerner (Ed.), *Handbook of child psychology*, Vol. 1 (6th ed. pp. 665–715). New York: Wiley and Sons.

Eley, T. C., Sugden, K., Corsico, A., Gregory, A. M., Sham, P., McGuffin, P., *et al.* (2004). Gene–environment interaction analysis of serotonin system markers with adolescent depression. *Molecular Psychiatry*, *9*, 908–915.

Fairburn, C. G., & Bohn, K. (2005). Eating disorder NOS (EDNOS) An example of the trouble-some "not otherwise specified" (NOS) category in DSM-IV. *Behavior Research and Therapy*, *43*, 691–701.

Fairburn, C. G., Cooper, Z., Doll, H. A., & Davies, B. A. (2005). Identifying dieters who will develop an eating disorder: A prospective, population-based study. *American Journal of Psychiatry*, *162*, 2249–2255.

Fergusson, D. M., & Horwood, L. J. (2000). Does cannabis use encourage other forms of illicit drug use? *Addiction*, *95*, 505–520.

Fergusson, D. M., Horwood, L. J., & Ridder, E. M. (2004). Show me the child at seven: The consequences of conduct problems in childhood for psychosocial functioning in adulthood. *Journal of Child Psychology and Psychiatry*, *45*, 1–13.

Fergusson, D. M., & Mullen, P. E. (1999). *Childhood sexual abuse: An evidence based perspective*. Thousand Oaks, CA: Sage Publications.

Fergusson, D. M., Swain-Campbell, N. R., & Horwood, L. J. (2002). Deviant peer affiliations, crime and substance use: A fixed effects regression analysis. *Journal of Abnormal Child Psychology*, *30*, 419–430.

Fergusson, D. M., & Woodward, L. J. (2002). Mental health, educational, and social role outcomes of adolescents with depression. *Archives of General Psychiatry*, *59*, 225–231.

Fombonne, E., Wostear, G., Cooper, V., Harrington, R., & Rutter, M. (2001). The Maudsley long-term follow-up of child and adolescent depression. *British Journal of Psychiatry*, *179*, 210–217.

Ford, T., Goodman, R., & Meltzer, H. (2003). The British child and adolescent mental health survey 1999: The prevalence of DSM-IV disorders. *Journal of the American Academy of Child and Adolescent Psychiatry*, *42*, 1203–1211.

Garner, D. M., & Garfinkel, P. E. (1980). Socio-cultural factors in the development of anorexia nervosa. *Psychological Medicine*, *10*, 647–656.

Glowinski, A. L., Madden, P. A., Bucholz, K. K., Lynskey, M. T., & Heath, A. C. (2003). Genetic epidemiology of self-reported lifetime DSM-IV major depressive disorder in a population-based twin sample of female adolescents. *Journal of Child Psychology and Psychiatry*, *44*, 988–996.

Grossman, A. W., Churchill, J. D., McKinney, B. C., Kodish, I., Otte, S. L., & Greenough, W. T. (2003). Experience effects on brain development: Possible contributions to psychopathology. *Journal of Child Psychology and Psychiatry*, *44*, 33–63.

Grossman, K. E., Grossman, K. & Waters, E. (2005). *Attachment from Infancy to Adulthood*. New York: Guilford Press.

Hammen, C. (2003). Interpersonal stress and depression in women. *Journal of Affective Disorders*, *74*, 49–57.

Hankin, B. L., Abramson, L. Y., Moffitt, T. E., Silva, P. A., McGee, R. & Angell, K. E. (1998). Development of depression from preadolescence to young adulthood: Emerging gender differences in a 10-year longitudinal study. *Journal of Abnormal Psychology*, *107*, 128–140.

Hardt, J., & Rutter, M. (2004). Validity of adult retrospective reports of adverse childhood experiences: review of the evidence. *Journal of Child Psychology and Psychiatry*, *45*, 260–273.

Harrington, R., Fudge, H., Rutter, M., Pickles, A., & Hill, J. (1990). Adult outcomes of childhood and adolescent depression. I. Psychiatric status. *Archives of General Psychiatry*, *47*, 465–473.

Harris, T., Brown, G. W., & Bifulco, A. (1990). Loss of parent in childhood and adult psychiatric disorder: a tentative overall model. *Development and Psychopathology*, *2*, 311–328.

Henquet, C., Krabbendam, L., Spauwen, J., Kaplan, C., Lieb, R., Wittchen, H. U., *et al.* (2005). Prospective cohort study of cannabis use, predisposition for psychosis, and psychotic symptoms in younger people. *British Medical Journal*, *330*, 11–15.

Hill, J., Pickles, A., Burnside, E., Byatt, M., Rollinson, L., Davis, R., *et al.* (2001). Child sexual abuse, poor parental care and adult depression: evidence for different mechanisms. *British Journal of Psychiatry*, *179*, 104–109.

Howells, J. G., & Guirguis, W. R. (1984). Childhood schizophrenia 20 years later. *Archives of General Psychiatry*, *41*, 123–128.

Howlin, P., Goode, S., Hutton, J., & Rutter, M. (2004). Adult outcome for children with autism. *Journal of Child Psychology and Psychiatry*, *45*, 212–229.

Jaffee, S. R., Moffitt, T. E., Caspi, A., Fombonne, E., Poulton, R., & Martin, J. (2002). Differences in early childhood risk factors for juvenile-onset and adult onset depression. *Archives of General Psychiatry*, *58*, 215–222.

Johnson, J. G., Cohen, P., Brook, J. S., Kotler, L., & Kasen, S. (2002). Psychiatric disorders associated with risk for the development of eating disorders during adolescence and early adulthood. *Journal of Consulting and Clinical Psychology*, *70*, 1119–1128.

Kandel, D. B., Yamaguchi, K., & Chen, K. (1992). Stages of progression in drug involvement from adolescence to adulthood: Further evidence for the gateway theory. *Journal of Studies on Alcohol*, *53*, 447–457.

Kaufman, J., Martin, A., King, R. A., & Charney, D. (2001). Are child-, adolescent-, and adult-onset depression one and the same disorder? *Biological Psychiatry*, *49*, 980–1001.

Kendler, K. S. & Prescott, C. A. (2006). *Genes, environment, and psychopathology: Understanding the causes of psychiatric and substance use disorders*. New York: Guilford Press.

Kendler, K. S., Prescott, C. A., Myers, J., & Neale, M. C. (2003). The structure of genetic and environmental risk factors for common psychiatric and substance use disorders in men and women. *Archives of General Psychiatry*, *60*, 929–937.

Kendler, K. S., Thornton, L. M., & Gardner, C. O. (2000). Stressful life events and previous episodes in the etiology of major depression in women: An evaluation of the 'kindling' hypothesis. *American Journal of Psychiatry*, *157*, 1243–1251.

Keshavan, M. S., Kennedy, J. L., & Murray, R. M. (Eds.). (2004). *Neurodevelopment and schizophrenia*. London: Cambridge University.

Kim-Cohen, J., Caspi, A., Moffitt, T. E., Harrington, H. L., Milne, B. S., & Poulton, R. (2003). Prior juvenile diagnoses in adults with mental disorder: Developmental follow-back of a prospective-longitudinal cohort. *Archives of General Psychiatry*, *60*, 709–717.

Kotler, L. A., Cohen, P., Davies, M., Pine, D. S., & Walsh, B. T. (2001). Longitudinal relationships between childhood, adolescent and adult eating disorders. *Journal of American Academy of Child & Adolescent Psychiatry*, *40*, 1434–1440.

Kreppner, J. M., Rutter, M., Beckett, C., Castle, J., Colvert, E., Groothues, C., *et al.* (2007). Normality and impairment following profound early institutional deprivation. A longitudinal follow-up into early adolescence. *Developmental Psychology*, *43*, 931–946.

Krueger, R. F., Hicks, B. M., Patrick, C. J., Carlson, S. R., Iacono, W. G., & McGue, M. (2002). Etiologic connections among substance dependence, antisocial behavior, and personality: Modeling the externalizing spectrum. *Journal of Abnormal Psychology*, *111*, 411–421.

Lau, J. Y. F., & Eley, T. C. (2006). Changes in genetic and environmental influences on depressive symptoms across adolescence and young adulthood. *British Journal of Psychiatry*, *189*, 422–427.

Laub, J. H., & Sampson, R. J. (2001). Understanding desistance from crime. *Crime and Justice: A Review of Research*, *28*, 1–69.

Laub, J. H., & Sampson, R. J. (2003). *Shared beginnings, divergent lives: Delinquent boys to age 70*. Cambridge, MA: Harvard University.

Leon, G. R., Fulkerson, J. A., Perry, C. L., Keel, P. K., & Klump, K. L. (1999). Three to four year prospective evaluation of personality and behavioral risk factors for later disordered eating in adolescent girls and boys. *Journal of Youth and Adolescence*, *28*, 181–196.

Lyytinen, H., Ahonen, T., Eklund, K., Guttorm, T., Kulju, P., Laakso, M. L., *et al.* (2004). Early development of children at familial risk for dyslexia: Follow-up from birth to school age. *Dyslexia*, *10*, 146–178.

Malone, S. M., Taylor, J., Marmorstein, N. R., McGue, M., & Iacono, W. G. (2004). Genetic and environmental influences on antisocial behavior and alcohol dependence from adolescence to early adulthood. *Development and Psychopathology*, *16*, 943–966.

Mannuzza, S., Klein, R., Abikoff, H., & Moulton, J. (2004). Significance of childhood conduct problems to alter development of conduct disorder among children with ADHD: A prospective follow-up study. *Journal of Abnormal Child Psychology*, *32*, 565–573.

Mannuzza, S., Klein, R., & Moulton, J. (2003). Persistence of attention deficit hyperactivity disorder into adulthood: What have we learned from the prospective follow-up studies? *Journal of Attentional Disorders*, *7*, 93–100.

Maughan, B. (1995). Annotation. Long-term outcomes of developmental reading problems. *Journal of Child Psychology and Psychiatry and Allied Disciplines*, *36*, 357–371.

Maughan, B., & Carroll, J. (2006). Literacy and mental disorders. *Current Opinion in Psychiatry*, *19*, 350–354.

Maughan, B., Pickles, A., Rutter, M., Hagell, A., & Yule, W. (1996). Reading problems and antisocial behaviour: Developmental trends in comorbidity. *Journal of Child Psychology and Psychiatry*, *37*, 405–418.

Maughan, B., & Rutter, M. (2001). Antisocial children grown up. In J. Hill, & B. Maughan (Eds.), *Conduct disorders in childhood and adolescence* (pp. 507–552). Cambridge: Cambridge University Press.

Mawhood, L., & Howlin, P. (1999). The outcome of a supported employment scheme for high functioning adults with autism or Asperger syndrome. *Autism: International Journal of Research and Practice*, *3*, 229–253.

McGue, M., & Iacono, W. G. (2005). The association of early adolescent problem behavior with adult psychopathology. *American Journal of Psychiatry*, *162*, 1118–1124.

Measelle, J. R., Stice, E., & Hogansen, J. M. (2006). Developmental trajectories of co-occurring depressive, eating, antisocial, and substance abuse problems in female adolescents. *Journal of Abnormal Psychology*, *115*, 524–538.

Meltzer, H., Gatward, R., Corbin, T., Goodman, R., & Ford, T. (2003). *Persistence, onset, risk factors and outcomes of childhood mental disorders*. London: The Stationery Office.

Mill, J., Caspi, A., Williams, B. S., Craig, I. W., Taylor, A., Polo-Tomas, M., *et al.* (2006). Genetic polymorphisms predict variation in intelligence and adult prognosis among children with attention-deficit hyperactivity disorder. *Archives of General Psychiatry*, *63*, 462–469.

Moffitt, T. E. (1993). Adolescence-limited and life-course persistent antisocial behavior: A developmental taxonomy. *Psychological Review*, *100*, 674–701.

Moffitt, T. E. (2006). Life course persistent versus adolescence-limited antisocial behavior. In D. Cicchetti, & D. Cohen (Eds.), *Developmental psychopathology* (2nd edn, Vol. 3, pp. 570–578). New York: Wiley.

Moffit, T. E., & the E-Risk Study Team. (2002). Teen-aged mothers in contemporary Britain. *Journal of Child Psychology and Psychiatry*, *43*, 727–742.

Monroe, S. M., & Harkness, K. L. (2005). Life stress, the 'kindling' hypothesis, and the recurrence of depression: Considerations from a life stress perspective. *Psychological Review*, *112*, 417–445.

Moore, T. M., Zammit, S., Lingford-Hughes, A., Jones, P. B., Burke, M., Lewis, G. (2007). Cannibis use and risk of psychotic or affective mental health outcomes: A systematic review. *Lancet*, 370 (9584), 319–328.

Murray, L., Woolgar, M., Cooper, P., & Hipwell, A. (2001). Cognitive vulnerability to depression in 5-year-old children of depressed mothers. *Journal of Child Psychology and Psychiatry*, *42*, 891–899.

Murray R. M., & Lewis S. W. (1987). Is schizophrenia a neurodevelopmental disorder? *British Medical Journal*, *295*, 681–682.

Nelson, E. E., Leibenluft, E., McClure, E. B., & Pine, D. S. (2005). The social re-orientation of adolescence: a neuroscience perspective on the process and its relation to psychopathology. *Psychological Medicine*, *35*, 163–174.

Neumärker, K-J., Bettle, N., Neumärker, U., & Bettle, O. (2000). Age-and gender-related psychological characteristics of adolescent ballet dancers. *Psychopathology*, *33*, 137–142.

Nolen-Hoeksema, S., Girgus, J. S., & Seligman, M. E. P. (1992). Predictors and consequences of childhood depressive symptoms: A

5-year longitudinal study. *Journal of Abnormal Psychology*, *101*, 405–422.

O'Connor, T. G., Ben-Shlomo, Y., Heron, J., Golding, J., Adams, D., & Glover, V. (2005). Prenatal anxiety predicts individual differences in cortisol in pre-adolescent children. *Biological Psychiatry*, *58*, 211–217.

Owens, D. G. C., & Johnstone, E. C. (2006). Precursors and prodromata of schizophrenia: findings from the Edinburgh High Risk Study and their literature context. *Psychological Medicine*, *36*, 1501–1514.

Patterson, G. R., Reid, J. B., & Dishion, T. J. (1992). *Antisocial boys*. Eugene, OR: Castalia.

Patton, G. C., Coffey, C., Carlin, J. B., Olsson, C. A., & Morley, R. (2004). Prematurity at birth and adolescent depressive disorder. *British Journal of Psychiatry*, *184*, 446–447.

Paz, I., Jones, D., & Byrne, G. (2005). Child maltreatment, child protection and mental health. *Current Opinion in Psychiatry*, *18*, 411–421.

Petty, L., Ornitz, E. M., Michelman, J. D., & Zimmerman, E. G. (1984). Autistic children who become schizophrenic. *Archives of General Psychiatry*, *41*, 129–135.

Phillips, L. J, McGorry, P. D., Yung, A. R., McGlashan, T. H., Cornblatt, B., & Klosterkotter, J. (2005). Prepsychotic phase of schizophrenia and related disorders: recent progress and future opportunities. *British Journal of Psychiatry*, *187*(Supplement 48), S33–S44.

Pine, D. S., Cohen, E., Cohen, P., & Brook, J. (1999). Adolescent depressive symptoms as predictors of adult depression: Moodiness or mood disorder? *American Journal of Psychiatry*, *156*, 133–135.

Pine, D. S., Cohen, P., Gurley, D., Brook, J., & Ma, Y. (1998). The risk for early-adulthood anxiety and depressive disorders in adolescents with anxiety and depressive disorders. *Archives of General Psychiatry*, *55*, 56–64.

Post, R. M. (1992). Transduction of psychosocial stress into the neurobiology of recurrent affective disorder. *American Journal of Psychiatry*, *149*, 999–1010.

Rapoport, J. (1980). Diagnostic significance of drug response in child psychiatry. In E. F. Purcell (Ed.), *Psychopathology of children and youth*. New York: Josiah Macy Jnr Foundation.

Rey, J. M., Martin, A., & Krabman, R. (2004). Is the party over? Cannabis and juvenile psychiatric disorder: the past 10 years. *Journal of the American Academy of Child and Adolescent Psychiatry*, *43*, 1194–1205.

Rice, F., Harold, G. T., & Thapar, A. (2002). Assessing the effects of age, sex and shared environment on the genetic aetiology of depression in childhood and adolescence. *Journal of Child Psychology and Psychiatry*, *43*, 1039–1051.

Rice, F., Harold, G. T., & Thapar, A. (2003). Negative life events as an account of age-related differences in the genetic aetiology of depression in childhood and adolescence. *Journal of Child Psychology and Psychiatry*, *44*, 977–987.

Richards, M., & Wadsworth, M. E. J. (2004). Long term effects of early adversity on cognitive function. *Archives of Disease in Childhood*, *89*, 922–927.

Robins, L. N. (1966). *Deviant children grown up*. Baltimore: Williams & Wilkins.

Rose, R. J., Dick, D. M., Viken, R. J., Pulkinnen, L., & Kaprio, J. (2004). Genetic and environmental effects on conduct disorder and alcohol dependence symptoms and their covariation at age 14. *Alcohol: Clinical and Experimental Research*, *28*, 1541–1548.

Rudolph, K. D., Hammen, C., Burge, D., Lindberg, N., Herzberg, D., & Daley, S. E. (2000). Toward an interpersonal life-stress model of depression: The developmental context of stress generation. *Development and Psychopathology*, *12*, 215–234.

Rutter, M. (1996). Transitions and turning points in developmental psychopathology as applied to the age span between childhood and mid-adulthood. *International Journal of Behavioral Development*, *19*, 603–626.

Rutter, M. (2002). Substance use and abuse: causal pathways considerations. In M. Rutter, & E. Taylor (Eds.), *Child and adolescent psychiatry* (4th edn. pp. 455–462). Oxford: Blackwell Science.

Rutter, M. (2005a). Environmentally mediated risks for psychopathology: research strategies and findings. *Journal of the American Academy of Child and Adolescent Psychiatry*, *44*, 3–18.

Rutter, M. (2005b). Multiple meanings of a developmental perspective on psychopathology. *European Journal of Developmental Psychology*, *2*, 221–252.

Rutter, M. (2006). Implications of resilience concepts for scientific understanding. *Annals of the New York Academy of Sciences*, *1094*, 1–12.

Rutter, M. (2007). Proceeding from observed correlation to causal inference: The use of natural experiments. *Perspectives on Psychological Science*, *2*, 377–395.

Rutter, M., Colvert, E., Kreppner, J., Beckett, C., Castle, J., Groothues, C., *et al.* (2007). Early adolescent outcomes for institutionally-deprived and non-deprived adoptees years: I. Disinhibited attachment. *Journal of Child Psychology and Psychiatry*, *48*, 17–30.

Rutter, M., & Garmezy, N. (1983). Developmental psychopathology. In P. H. Mussen (Series Editor), & E. M. Hetherington (Volume Editor), *Handbook of child psychology*. Vol. 4. *Socialization, personality, and social development* (4th edn, pp. 775–911). New York: Wiley.

Rutter, M., Greenfeld, D., & Lockyer, L. (1967a). A five to fifteen year follow-up study of infantile psychosis. I. Description of sample. *British Journal of Psychiatry*, *113*, 1169–1182.

Rutter, M., Greenfeld, D., & Lockyer, L. (1967b). A five to fifteen year follow-up of infantile psychosis. II. Social and behavioural outcome. *British Journal of Psychiatry*, *113*, 1183–1199.

Rutter, M., Le Couteur, A., & Lord, C. (2003). *ADI-R Autism Diagnostic Interview – Revised Manual*. Los Angeles: WPS Edition.

Rutter, M., Maughan, B., & Kim-Cohen, J. (2006a). Continuities and discontinuities in psychopathology between childhood and adult life. *Journal of Child Psychology and Psychiatry*, *47*, 276–295.

Rutter, M., Moffitt, T., & Caspi, A. (2006b). Gene–environment interplay and psychopathology: Multiple varieties but real effects. *Journal of Child Psychology and Psychiatry*, *47*, 226–261.

Rutter, M. & O'Connor, T. (2004). Are there biological programming effects for psychological development? Findings from a study of Romanian adoptees. *Developmental Psychology*, *40*, 81–94.

Rutter, M., Pickles, A., Murray, R., & Eaves, L. (2001). Testing hypotheses on specific environmental causal effects on behavior. *Psychological Bulletin*, *127*, 291–324.

Rutter, M., Tizard, J., & Whitmore, K. (1970). *Education, health and behaviour*. London: Longmans. (Reprinted 1981 Melbourne, FA: Krieger.)

Santonastaso, P., Mondini, S., & Favaro, A. (2002). Are fashion models a group at risk for eating disorders and substance abuse? *Psychotherapy and Psychosomatics*, *71*, 168–172.

Scott, J. (2006). Depression should be managed like a chronic disease: Clinicians need to move beyond ad hoc approaches to isolated acute episodes. *British Medical Journal*, *332*, 985–986.

Silberg, J., Pickles, A., Rutter, M., Hewitt, J., Simonoff, E., Maes, H., *et al.* (1999). The influence of genetic factors and life stress on depression among adolescent girls. *Archives of General Psychiatry*, *56*, 225–232.

Sonuga-Barke, E., Dalen, L., & Remington, B. (2003). Do executive deficits and delay aversion make independent contributions to preschool attention deficit/hyperactivity disorder symptoms? *Journal of the American Academy of Child and Adolescent Psychiatry*, *42*, 1335–1342.

Sroufe, L. A., Egeland, B., Carlson, E., & Collins, W. A. (2005). *The development of the person: The Minnesota study of risk and adaptation from birth to adulthood*. New York: Guildford Press.

Stouthamer-Loeber, M., Wei, E., Loeber, R., & Masten, A. S. (2004). Desistance from persistent serious delinquency in the transition to adulthood. *Development and Psychopathology*, *16*, 897–918.

Szmukler, G. I., Eisler, I., Gillies, C., & Hayward, M. E. (1985). The implications of anorexia nervosa in a ballet school. *Journal of Psychiatry*, *19*, 177–181.

Thapar, A., van den Bree, M., Fowler, T., Langley, K., & Whittinger, N. (2006). Predictors of antisocial behaviour in children with attention deficit hyperactivity disorder. *European Child & Adolescent Psychiatry*, *15*, 118–125.

Trzesniewski, K. H., Moffitt, T. E., Caspi, A., Taylor, A., & Maughan, B. (2006). Revisiting the association between reading achievement and antisocial behavior: New evidence of an environmental explanation from a twin study. *Child Development*, *77*, 72–88.

Viding, E. (2004). Annotation: Understanding the development of psychopathy. *Journal of Child Psychology and Psychiatry*, *45*, 1329–1337.

Volkmar, F. R., & Cohen, D. J. (1991). Comorbid association of autism and schizophrenia. *American Journal of Psychiatry*, *148*, 1705–1707.

Wakschlag, L. S., Pickett, K. E., Cook, E., Benowitz, N. L., & Leventhal, B. L. (2002). Maternal smoking during pregnancy and severe antisocial behavior in offspring: A review. *American Journal of Public Health*, *92*, 966–974.

Walker, E., Kestler, L., Bollini, A., & Hochman, K. M. (2004a). Schizophrenia: etiology and course. *Annual Review of Psychology*, *55*, 401–430.

Walker, E. F., Sabuwalla, Z., & Huot, R. (2004b). Pubertal neuromaturation, stress sensitivity, and psychopathology. *Development and Psychopathology*, *16*, 807–824.

Watt, N. F. (1974). Childhood roots of schizophrenia. In D. F. Ricks, A. Thomas, & M. Roff (Eds.), *Life history research in psychopathology* (Vol. 3, pp. 194–211). Minneapolis: University of Minnesota Press.

Weinberger, D. R. (1987). Implications of normal brain development for the pathogenesis of schizophrenia. *Archives of General Psychiatry*, *44*, 660–669.

Weissman, M. M., Wickramaratne, P., Nomura, Y., Warner, V., Verdeli, H., Pilowky, D. J., *et al.* (2005). Families at high and low risk for depression: A 3-generation study. *Archives of General Psychiatry*, *62*, 29–36.

Weissman, M. M., Wolk, S., Wickramaratne, P., Goldstein, R. B., Adams, P., Greenwald, S., *et al.* (1999). Children with prepubertal-onset major depressive disorder and anxiety grown up. *Archives of General Psychiatry*, *56*, 794–801.

Williams, J. M. G. (1996). Depression and the specificity of autobiographical memory. In D. C. Rubin (Ed.), *Remembering our past* (pp. 244–267). Cambridge: Cambridge University Press.

Wittchen, H.-U., Beesdo, K., Bittner, A., & Goodwin, R. D. (2003). Depressive episodes: Evidence for a causal role of primary anxiety disorders? *European Psychiatry*, *18*, 384–393.

Wittchen, H.-U., Kessler, R. C., Pfister, H., & Lieb, R. M. (2000). Why do people with anxiety disorders become depressed? A prospective-longitudinal community study. *Acta Psychiatrica Scandinavica*, *102*, 14–23.

Woodward, L. J., Fergusson, D. M., & Horwood, L. J. (2002). Romantic relationships of young people with childhood and adolescent onset behavior problems. *Journal of Abnormal Child Psychology*, *30*, 231–243.

Zeitlin, H. (1986). *The Natural history of psychiatric disorder in children*. Institute of Psychiatry Maudsley Monograph, 29. Oxford: Oxford University Press.

Zoccolillo, M. (1992). Co-occurrence of conduct disorder and its adult outcomes with depressive and anxiety disorders: A review. *Journal of the American Academy of Child Adolescent Psychiatry*, *31*, 547–556.

14 Temperament and Personality

Avshalom Caspi and Rebecca Shiner

Personality traits refer to individual differences in the tendency to behave, think and feel in certain consistent ways. The goal of this chapter is to describe these differences and to document how they shape children's lives. This chapter is divided into five sections. The first section describes a taxonomy of measurable individual differences in temperament and personality. We present evidence about how to organize and describe the most fundamental personality differences between children and adolescents. It is important to bear in mind that a personality taxonomy is an *evolving* classification system whose purpose is to integrate and guide research. This also means that any such system must be open to empirical refutation and modification. In this sense, there are historical parallels between the use of structural models in personality psychology and the use of a standardized model for describing and diagnosing mental illness in psychiatry. For example, prior to the advent of the *Diagnostic and Statistical Manual of Mental Disorders III* (DSM-III; American Psychiatric Association, 1980), clinicians and researchers did not have available explicit criteria to define the boundaries of diagnostic categories (see chapter 2). Clinical diagnoses were difficult to compare and cross-sample replications were hard to conduct. The development of DSM-III was a big improvement because it provided a common language with which clinicians and researchers could communicate about the disorders they were treating or investigating. DSM-III had its share of problems, and subsequent modifications testify to the need for a flexible and evolving system that can accommodate new empirical information, as do recommended modifications in anticipation of DSM-V (Kupfer, First, & Regier, 2002). We can similarly hope that the use of a generally accepted trait taxonomy will help to impose structure on research findings and advance the study of personality development across the life course.

Using this taxonomy, we move on to discuss the development of personality. The second section discusses the developmental processes by which early emerging temperamental differences are elaborated into personality traits that influence how individuals organize their behavior to meet environmental demands and new developmental challenges. The third section reviews evidence about personality continuity and change across the life course. Next we review evidence about the effects of personality traits on behavioral outcomes in different developmental contexts. We go on to discuss the links between personality traits and psychopathology, with special emphasis on contrasting models of the relations between "normal" personality variants and psychiatric disorders. Finally, we discuss the assessment and treatment relevance of personality traits.

Rutter's Child and Adolescent Psychiatry, 5th edition. Edited by M. Rutter, D. Bishop, D. Pine, S. Scott, J. Stevenson, E. Taylor and A. Thapar. © 2008 Blackwell Publishing, ISBN: 978-1-4051-4549-7.

Temperament and Personality Traits in Childhood and Adolescence

Definitional Issues

Before describing current research on children's individual differences, it is important to address the issue of what is meant by the terms *temperament* and *personality*, because these terms are used in such varied ways by different people. According to most contemporary perspectives, temperament includes individual differences in affect, activity, attention and self-regulation; although such early emerging traits have a biological basis and are in part shaped by heredity; experience and maturation also play an important part in their development (Rothbart & Bates, 2006). Although this relatively broad definition is widely accepted, it is important to note that some researchers argue for a more narrow definition of temperament. For example, Kagan and Snidman (2004) have suggested that temperament should be considered as individual differences in the reactivity of basic neural systems; this more narrow definition leaves out the self-regulatory dimensions included in other temperament models and puts the emphasis squarely on the biological basis of individual variation.

Personality is typically seen as including a wider range of individual differences than is temperament. Personality differences include personality traits such as extraversion and neuroticism, but they also encompass goals, coping styles, defensive styles, motives, attachment styles, life stories, identities and various other processes (McAdams & Pals, 2006). Although it can be useful to make distinctions between temperament and personality, particularly when considering aspects of personality beyond traits, research has demonstrated that traits from the two domains have much in common. Personality traits are like temperament traits in that they involve variations in emotion and regulation, and personality is likewise shaped by the interplay of heredity and experience (Caspi & Shiner, 2006; Nigg, 2006). Sometimes, child psychologists and psychiatrists shy away from using the term "personality" to describe individual differences in children, because of understandable but incorrect assumptions about the nature of personality traits. Although personality is often assumed to be extremely stable across time and situations and essentially unchangeable, more recent work suggests that personality differences, in transaction with environmental circumstances, organize behavior in dynamic ways over time (Caspi & Shiner, 2006). Because of the significant commonalities between temperament and personality traits, we discuss them together throughout this chapter.

Structure of Temperament and Personality Traits in Childhood and Adolescence

As all observers of the human condition know well, children and adults vary strikingly in their day-to-day patterns of thinking, feeling and behaving. An important starting point for temperament and personality research has been describing how these patterns are structured: what are the reliable patterns of covariation of behaviors or traits across individuals? Arriving at some consensus about the basic structure of temperament and personality traits is a crucial task. Although debate continues about the best ways to parse the various traits in childhood and adulthood, considerable consensus has been achieved for both temperament and personality traits.

During infancy and early childhood, children display a more limited range of traits. Temperamental differences in infants and toddlers include three higher-order traits identified by Rothbart and Bates (2006). First, *surgency/extraversion* taps young children's tendencies toward high activity, a rapid approach style, expressions of positive emotions, and pleasure and excitement in social interactions. Second, *negative emotionality* taps children's tendencies toward sadness, fear, irritability and frustration, and difficulty with being quieted after high arousal. Third, *orienting/regulation* in infancy includes soothability, cuddliness, ability to sustain attention and pleasure in low intensity situations. In the toddler years, this factor also includes more sophisticated self-regulatory abilities, such as the ability to sustain attention over time and persist at tasks.

As children's motor, cognitive, emotional and language abilities develop, the range of traits they can express similarly expands; thus, by later in childhood, children display a wider range of individual differences. Research over the last two decades has demonstrated that the basic five-factor structure of personality traits is fairly similar from childhood through adulthood. These comprise the *big five* traits of *extraversion*, *neuroticism*, *conscientiousness*, *agreeableness* and *openness to experience*, with weaker support for openness in youths than for the other four traits (Caspi & Shiner, 2006). Rothbart and Bates' (2006) work on the structure of temperament in preschoolers and school-age children has yielded evidence for three higher-order traits of surgency, negative affectivity and effortful control, as well as a trait of affiliativeness in adolescence (although these traits are not identical to the big five traits, they are conceptually similar to extraversion, neuroticism, conscientiousness and agreeableness, respectively). Thus, youths and adults manifest a remarkably similar range of individual differences, albeit with some significant changes as development proceeds. It is important to note that the big five traits tend to be correlated with each other in particular patterns that replicate across samples of children and adults (DeYoung, Peterson, Séguin *et al.*, 2006). Specifically, at a higher level of analysis, conscientiousness, agreeableness and neuroticism (reversed) cohere to form an overarching trait, as do extraversion and openness. De Young *et al.* (2006) have argued that the former "meta-trait" taps the tendency to maintain stability, whereas the latter taps the tendency toward exploration.

Some readers may be more familiar with other temperament models, specifically those of Thomas and Chess and of Cloninger. Because of widespread interest in these models, it is useful to note their links and discrepancies with the models described here. Thomas, Chess, Birch *et al.* (1963) identified nine traits in infancy and childhood in their New York longitudinal study. As discussed later in this chapter, some of these traits have proven to be very important for children's development, particularly tendencies toward irritability and frustration and toward fearful withdrawal from new situations. However, the nine-trait structure Thomas *et al.* articulated does not accurately describe the structure of traits measured by questionnaires based on their model (Shiner & Caspi, 2003); rather, these questionnaires measure a smaller set of traits that are included in the models described in this chapter – irritability, fear and inhibition, activity level, and attention.

The model developed by Cloninger, Przybeck, Svrakic *et al.* (1994) in the temperament and character inventory (TCI) has also been a popular model, particularly in research on the biological basis of personality. According to this model, personality consists of four temperament dimensions, which are seen as moderately heritable and generally stable, and three character dimensions, which are viewed as more greatly shaped by experience and more malleable. Research reviewed later in this chapter has demonstrated that, contrary to the TCI model, all traits are moderately heritable, including those often considered to be influenced primarily by experience (e.g., traits associated with self-control, diligence, empathy, aggression and prosocial tendencies). Current neuroscience research also suggests that the TCI traits do not map onto the posited underlying biological dimensions (Paris, 2005). The big five structure also appears to be more robust than that of the TCI dimensions (Markon, Krueger, & Watson, 2005). The TCI dimensions can be understood in terms of their primary links with the big five traits (Markon, Krueger, & Watson, 2005): extraversion (high reward dependence); neuroticism (high harm avoidance and low self-determination); conscientiousness (low novelty seeking and high persistence); agreeableness (high cooperativeness); and openness (high self-transcendence). Despite some of the limitations of this model, it does converge in important ways with several dimensions of the big five model and with other personality models that include an approach domain manifested in positive emotions, an avoidance domain manifested in negative emotions and a constraint domain manifested as tendencies to inhibit or express emotion or impulse.

Traits in Childhood and Adolescence: Descriptions and Underlying Processes

One of the great benefits of a consensually agreed-upon taxonomy of traits is that it allows researchers to turn their attention to the ways temperament and personality traits express themselves in daily life and to the fundamental processes underlying variations in these traits. In this section, we first describe the traits and then review some of the most interesting current work on the psychological and evolutionary underpinnings of each trait. A more detailed description of the components of these traits is found in Caspi and Shiner (2006). Because relatively less is known about the processes underlying openness in children, we do not review this trait here.

Extraversion

Children vary in their tendencies to be vigorously, actively and surgently engaged with the world around them. Extraverted children and adolescents are described in big five studies as sociable, expressive, high-spirited, lively, socially potent, physically active and energetic (Caspi & Shiner, 2006). In contrast, introverted youths are quiet, inhibited and lethargic. Extraversion is often conceptualized as the predisposition to experience positive emotions (Watson & Clark, 1997). In adults, extraversion is robustly associated with positive emotions in emotionally neutral conditions and sometimes associated with stronger positive emotional responses to pleasant events (Lucas & Baird, 2004). Similarly, preschoolers' tendencies toward "smiling, positive verbalizations, and joyful bodily movements" are one part of an overarching positive emotionality trait (Durbin, Klein, Hayden *et al.*, 2005). In a related model, extraversion is conceptualized as representing individual differences in a behavioral activation, approach or appetitive system (Caspi & Shiner, 2006; Rothbart & Bates, 2006). The biological system posited to underlie variations in extraversion is argued to have enhanced tendencies toward exploration and mating opportunities and thus may have conferred evolutionary benefits in some circumstances but created greater risks to survival in others (Nettle, 2006).

Neuroticism

Just as children vary in their predisposition toward positive emotions, they vary in their susceptibility to negative emotions and general distress. In the big five studies, children and adolescents who are high on neuroticism are described as anxious, vulnerable, tense, easily frightened, "falling apart" under stress, guilt-prone, moody, low in frustration tolerance and insecure in relationships with others (Caspi & Shiner, 2006). Fewer descriptors define the lower end of this dimension; these include traits such as stability, being "laid back," adaptability in novel situations and the ability to "bounce back" after a bad experience. As these descriptions of childhood neuroticism illustrate, the trait appears to include both the child's experience of negative emotions and the child's effectiveness at self-regulating such negative emotions. Although children and adults do appear to have a general tendency toward experiencing a wide range of negative emotions, it is often important to distinguish among a number of different likely subcomponents, because each is likely to index traits with different underpinnings and outcomes; such components are likely to include distinguishable tendencies toward fearfulness, anxiety, sadness and anger or irritation (which is also related to low agreeableness; Caspi & Shiner, 2006).

Recent research has demonstrated that higher neuroticism is associated with specific detrimental ways of appraising and coping with difficult situations. Children who are higher on negative emotionality are more likely to appraise negative life events as threatening and to use avoidant coping as a way of dealing with these life events, which in turn leads to poorer adjustment (Lengua & Long, 2002). Neuroticism in adults is likewise associated with more self-reported daily problems, stronger negative emotional reactions to everyday problems and to chronic problems, and greater negative "mood spillover" from one part of the day to the next (Suls & Martin, 2005). These findings regarding neuroticism are consistent with the claim that individual differences in neuroticism are associated with individual variation in a withdrawal, inhibition or avoidance system (Caspi & Shiner, 2006; Rothbart & Bates, 2006). The biological system underlying variations in withdrawal and avoidance is likely to have served the evolutionary purpose of protecting individuals from threats; although it is likely to be detrimental at high levels in contemporary society, it may also serve to protect individuals from risks and may confer benefits in some circumstances (Nettle, 2006). Although aspects of neuroticism have been studied in children (e.g., inhibition, anxiety), this trait as a whole warrants much more intensive developmental study, given its links with psychopathology, as discussed later in this chapter.

A temperament trait related to neuroticism that has received widespread attention is that of *behavioral inhibition* (sometimes termed "inhibition to the unfamiliar"; Fox, Henderson, Marshall *et al.*, 2005). This trait indexes variations in the tendency to withdraw and express fear in the face of stressful novel situations. Inhibition has generally been measured by children's observed behavior, including fearful responses to novel situations (e.g., a toy robot, an adult dressed as a clown) and reticent withdrawn behavior with unfamiliar adults or children. This trait has been studied extensively in terms of its biological substrates and has been hypothesized to be associated with increased amygdala function, but evidence on links with various indices of amygdala function has been mixed (Fox, Henderson, Marshall *et al.*, 2005). Recent research suggests that behavioral observations of inhibition in young children may confound temperamental differences in low approach and high negative emotions (Putnam & Stifter, 2005); in other words, there is evidence that behavioral inhibition in high intensity situations may be evoked either by low approach tendencies (related to low extraversion) or high negative emotional tendencies such as fear (related to high neuroticism). Thus, future work on inhibition is likely to benefit from considering the dimensions of approach and fear separately.

Conscientiousness

An overarching conscientiousness trait taps children's individual differences in self-control. In big five studies, highly conscientious children and adolescents are described as responsible, attentive, persistent, orderly and neat, planful, possessing high standards and thinking before acting (Caspi & Shiner, 2006). Children low on this trait are depicted as irresponsible, unreliable, careless, distractible and quitting easily. Rothbart and Bates (2006) have identified in children a similar temperament trait termed effortful control, which includes children's capacities to plan behavior, inhibit inappropriate responses, focus and shift attention, take pleasure in low intensity situations and perceive subtle external stimuli. In a series of studies, Kochanska and Knaack (2003) have developed a battery of tasks to measure children's emerging effortful control; all of the tasks require a child to exert self-control by suppressing a dominant response in favor of carrying out a subdominant response. Temperament models of effortful control thus tend to emphasize early emerging differences in attention and impulse control, whereas personality models also include aspects of control that are not evident in children until they are older, such as orderliness, dependability and motivation to meet goals and complete work.

As described later in this chapter, conscientiousness in children and adults is associated with effective self-regulation in task-focused contexts (school and work), and with social competence with peers. Researchers studying the biological basis of self-regulation have pointed to the importance of the prefrontal cortex for a variety of self-regulatory skills, including working memory, emotional processing, planning, novelty detection, resolving conflicting information, initiating action and inhibiting inappropriate responses (Banfield, Wyland, Macrae *et al.*, 2004). Rothbart and Bates (2006) consider many of these capacities to reflect individual differences in an overarching executive attention capacity.

Agreeableness

Agreeableness includes a variety of traits seen as very important by developmental psychologists; yet, historically, these traits have been left out of temperament models. The high end of agreeableness includes descriptors such as warm, considerate, empathic, generous, gentle, protective of others and kind (Caspi & Shiner, 2006). The low end of agreeableness includes tendencies toward being aggressive, rude, spiteful, stubborn, bossy, cynical and manipulative. In studies with both children and adults, agreeableness also includes being willing to accommodate others' wishes rather than forcing one's own desires and intentions on others; among children, this aspect of the trait also involves how manageable the child is for parents and teachers. Within the agreeableness trait, it is important to distinguish between prosocial tendencies and antagonistic aggressive tendencies. Although these tendencies are negatively correlated, they are not simply polar opposites and, in fact, appear to have distinct developmental origins (Krueger, Hicks, & McGue, 2001).

A number of researchers have argued that agreeableness reflects individual differences in the motivation to maintain harmonious relationships with others; from this point of view, agreeableness taps differences in the willingness to forgo individual interests out of concern for others (Graziano & Eisenberg, 1997). Agreeableness is positively associated in children and adolescents with stronger endorsement of constructive conflict tactics, such as negotiation and compromise (Jensen-Campbell, Gleason, Adams *et al.*, 2003), and high-agreeable children negotiate conflict better. When children are observed in conflict situations in the laboratory, low agreeableness is associated with higher levels of conflict and tension, as well as more destructive conflict tactics (Jensen-Campbell *et al.*, 2003). Interestingly, greater agreeableness does not predict more observed submissive behavior in children (Jensen-Campbell *et al.*, 2003); apparently, agreeable people do not simply solve their interpersonal problems by giving in to other people. In short, more agreeable youths appear to generate fewer conflicts for themselves and have a greater capacity for handling the interpersonal conflicts that do arise. Differences in empathy, warmth and nurturance may arise from a biological system designed to promote parental investment in offspring and close family bonds. Some researchers (e.g., MacDonald, 1995) have argued that evolution yielded a human biological system that typically ensures that intimate relationships and the care of close others are inherently rewarding and pleasurable and that the loss of such relationships is painful and distressing. Such a system would clearly confer adaptive benefits, because it would promote successful care of offspring through the establishment of strong attachment relationships between infants and their caregivers. Further, there is some preliminary evidence in humans that affectional bonds may activate brain areas that support positive emotions and deactivate brain areas that are linked with aggression, fear and sadness (Diamond, 2004); this finding is consistent with the emotional profile associated with agreeableness.

Personality Trait Development

Genetic Influences on Personality

Personality traits are substantially influenced by genetic factors. Bouchard and Loehlin (2001) provide a comprehensive review of this research, pointing to heritability estimates (see chapter 23) across the big five factors in the range of 0.50 ± 0.10. There are some study-to-study fluctuations, but, in general: (i) all personality superfactors appear to be influenced by genetic factors to the same extent; and (ii) genetic factors influence males' and females' personalities to the same extent.

In contrast, the search for which specific genetic variants influence which specific personality traits is much less conclusive. A meta-analysis of studies reporting data on associations between candidate genes and personality traits concluded there were few replicable associations (Munafo, Clark, Moore *et al.*, 2003), although it should be noted that differences in the personality measures used in different studies contribute to between-study heterogeneity (Sen, Burmeister, & Ghosh, 2004). Much of the initial excitement about research on molecular genetics and personality has given way to a more sober appreciation of the pitfalls involved in this kind of research (Benjamin, Ebstein, & Belmaker, 2002), as it has in the parallel field of psychiatric genetics.

Where will future research be headed? First, research on molecular genetics and the human personality will, of course, continue to be influenced by methodological advances outside of personality psychology. For example, genome-wide association studies are likely to be featured more prominently in personality research. The success of this enterprise will depend on the ability to mine the resulting data effectively and reliably, especially to the extent that non-additive or epistatic interactions are present (i.e., to the extent that the effect of a particular genotype on personality measures depends on other genotypes). Second, new research directions will be dictated by measurement and design considerations internal to the field of personality psychology (Ebstein, 2006). For example, fewer studies will continue to rely solely on self-report questionnaires. Instead, the use of "consensus trait measures", which incorporate multiple sources of information (e.g., self, peer and observational data), may be needed to reduce inter-study heterogeneity caused by the use of different measures. Third, newer studies may turn to experimental paradigms for assessing individual differences in characteristic styles of thinking, feeling and behaving. In the vanguard of such research is imaging genomics, which compares the responses of genotype groups using functional neuroimaging measures (Meyer-Lindenberg & Weinberger, 2006; see also chapter 11). There is untapped potential in other experimental personality paradigms, and we can look forward toward a new wave of investigations asking whether genotype influences humans' responsiveness to emotion-eliciting stimuli, laboratory stress paradigms and decision-making paradigms, which offer ways of indexing individual differences in personality (Caspi & Moffitt, 2006). For now, it is fair to state that there are reliable genetic influences on personality traits, but little is known about which genes are involved.

Developmental Elaboration of Personality Traits

Personality traits develop through a process of elaboration. The process of developmental elaboration refers to the processes by which those temperament attributes that are part of each individual's genetic heritage accumulate response strength through their repeated reinforcement and become elaborated into cognitive and affective representations that are quickly and frequently activated; that is, into personality traits. Here we describe five processes through which an initial disposition is elaborated so that it increasingly organizes emotion, thought and action.

The first process refers to learning. Specifically, temperament differences influence several learning mechanisms, including positive and negative reinforcement, punishment, discrimination learning and extinction. For example, extraversion may involve an approach system that is sensitive to potential rewards, and neuroticism may involve an avoidance system that is sensitive to potential threats (Caspi & Shiner, 2006). The implication is that different individuals should learn different things from common experiences.

The second process is *environmental elicitation*. Temperament differences elicit different reactions from the environment and influence how other people react to children, beginning already in the first few months of life (Bell & Chapman, 1986). Research on evocative effects of children's temperament on parents is especially well developed in relation to infants and young children with "difficult" temperaments (i.e., children who are irritable, hostile, prone to cry and hard to soothe; Crockenberg & Leerkes, 2003); more emotionally negative children evoke more negative parental responses than less emotionally negative children, even within the same family (Jenkins, Rasbash, & O'Connor, 2003). The evocative effects of children's temperaments extend beyond the family environment to other caregivers, teachers and peers. For example, as described later in this chapter, children's temperaments shape the quality of their relationships with peers. In turn, the responses that children evoke from others are likely to be internalized as part of children's emerging self-concepts. Research has begun to uncover some of the microprocesses through which children's temperament elicits responses from others. Specifically, individual differences in temperament and personality traits are reliably expressed in specific verbal and non-verbal behaviors, including vocal properties and facial expressions (Keltner, Moffitt, & Stouthamer-Loeber, 1995; Lin, Bugental, Turek *et al.*, 2002). In turn, other persons in the immediate environment react to these behaviors and use this information to make inferences and attributions about the developing person (Borkenau & Liebler, 1995; Gifford, 1994).

The third process is *environmental construal*. With the emergence of belief systems and expectations, temperament differences also begin to influence how environmental experiences are construed, thus shaping each person's "effective experience" of the environment (Hartup & van Lieshout, 1995). Research about the construal process stems from the cognitive tradition in personality psychology that emphasizes each person's subjective experience and unique perception of the world. This research focuses on what people "do" mentally (Cervone & Mischel, 2002), demonstrating that social information processing – including attention, encoding, retrieval and interpretation – is a selective process shaped by individual differences in temperament and personality (Derryberry & Reed, 2003). For example, individual differences in children's positive and negative emotionality affect the cues they notice in the environment, the goals that are salient to them and the types of potential responses they generate

(Lemerise & Arsenio, 2000). Moreover, individual differences in children's self-regulation shape the responses they select and their ability to enact those responses.

The fourth process is *environmental selection*. As children's self-regulatory competencies increase with age, they begin to make choices and display preferences that may reinforce and sustain their characteristics. Processes of environmental selection become increasingly important across the years from childhood to adulthood (Scarr & McCartney, 1983). Even among very young children, temperament is likely to shape the spheres children occupy within the environments chosen for them by adults (e.g., inhibited toddlers may avoid interactions with other children in child care, or children high on intellect may choose more stimulating activities at home). As children move into middle childhood and adolescence, they are given greater freedom to choose the environments in which they spend their time. Youths' personalities shape the activities in which they participate and the ways they choose to spend their free time (Shanahan & Flaherty, 2001) and predict the peer groups children join (Lacourse, Nagin, Vitaro *et al.*, 2006), their experiences of peer rejection and acceptance (Hay, Payne, & Chadwick, 2004) and the quality of their friendships (Pike & Atzaba-Poria, 2003). Across adulthood, individual differences in personality increasingly predict experienced life events. For example, negative emotionality puts individuals at greater risk of being exposed to stressful life events, such as divorce and unemployment (Jockin, McGue, & Lykken, 1996; Kokko, Bergman, & Pulkinnen, 2003).

The fifth process is *environmental manipulation*. Once the self-concept is firmly established, and with the development of more sophisticated self-regulatory capacities, individuals begin to alter, modify and manipulate the environments in which they find themselves in ways that are consistent with their own personalities (Buss, 1987). These processes may become particularly important as children become more skilled in regulating their own behavior and more insightful into the causes of others' behaviors.

Goodness-of-Fit: Personality-by-Context Interactions

Many researchers, clinicians and parents intuitively believe that various temperaments can yield a range of later outcomes, depending on the fit between the child and his or her context. In their early theoretical work on temperament, Thomas and Chess put forth the idea of "goodness-of-fit" (i.e., that the environment moderates the outcomes of children's early individual differences; Thomas *et al.*, 1963). Such a perspective would suggest that even young children with challenging temperaments have the potential to flourish if the context can adapt to their needs. Although the idea of personality-by-context interactions is compelling, it proved difficult to substantiate with data for many years, and in some cases a more direct link between temperament and outcomes seems to occur (Rothbart & Bates, 2006). More recent work, however, has demonstrated several replicable patterns of interactions between childhood temperament and contextual factors; in these instances, different combinations of temperament and context appear to predict whether temperament will remain stable or change and whether other outcomes (e.g., psychopathology) will be negative or positive.

Most of the research on temperament-by-context interactions has focused on parenting behavior as the context. Parenting behavior or socialization patterns can be described along at least three dimensions (Bugental & Grusec, 2006): *parental support* (which includes warmth, nurturance and affection), *psychological control* (which includes intrusive attempts to shape a child's thoughts and feelings rather than accepting and validating the child's point-of-view) and *behavioral control* (which includes making and enforcing rules and monitoring). Other aspects of the family environment have also been studied, such as family stress. Contextual factors outside the family are also likely to be important: children's school experiences, peer relationships and neighborhoods could all affect the outcomes of children's temperaments. Following are some of the patterns of temperament–parenting interactions, organized by the temperament traits studied. In all of these instances, certain temperamental tendencies appear to amplify the effects of parenting, or parenting appears to amplify the effects of temperament.

Children's tendencies toward poor self-control have been examined, with such dysregulation measured in a number of ways (e.g., low effortful control, unmanageability, impulsivity). The traits identified have generally been aspects of low conscientiousness and low agreeableness. Across a number of studies, it has been found that children with poorer self-control are more vulnerable to the negative effects of adverse parenting (including low parental support, low behavioral control and high family stress), whereas children with better self-control are less affected by parenting (Rothbart & Bates, 2006). The negative outcomes studied thus far have ranged widely but have often focused on externalizing behaviors. Similarly, highly impulsive youths who live in better-off neighborhoods or who stay in school show lesser criminal behavior than impulsive youths who live in poor neighborhoods or who drop out of school prematurely (Henry, Caspi, Moffitt *et al.*, 1999; Lynam, Caspi, Moffitt *et al.*, 2000). Thus, youths with poor self-control appear to be particularly vulnerable to the dysregulating effects of negative parenting, poverty and dropping out of school.

Other research has examined traits associated with psychopathy in childhood. Psychopathy includes a number of behavioral and personality tendencies: grandiosity, manipulativeness, low fear, and lack of empathy and remorse (Lynam & Gudonis, 2005). The associated traits generally appear to combine low agreeableness with low fear. Across a number of studies, children who are low on psychopathy are more likely to develop conduct problems when facing poor parenting than those receiving more positive parenting (Blair, Peschardt, Budhani *et al.*, 2006). In contrast, youths high on psychopathic traits appear to be less influenced by the rearing environment, which likely makes them very difficult to socialize.

Traits associated with tendencies toward negative emotionality have also received attention. First, children with high levels of negative emotions (including irritability, fearfulness and various combinations of negative emotions) appear to be vulnerable to developing behavioral and emotional problems in the face of unsupportive or intrusive parenting (Rothbart & Bates, 2006). Much of the research on negative emotionality has looked at general negative emotional tendencies, which makes the results difficult to interpret. Specific types of negative emotions are likely to have different patterns of effects; for example, in one study, high negative emotionality and high negative maternal control predicted increased externalizing behaviors when combined with low fear but predicted increased internalizing behaviors when combined with high fear (Gilliom & Shaw, 2004). Second, behaviorally inhibited children receiving intrusive, derisive or overprotective parenting remain more consistently inhibited across time than inhibited children receiving other parenting (Fox *et al.*, 2005). Non-parental care may contribute to decreasing inhibition over time (Fox *et al.*, 2005). In essence, behaviorally inhibited children appear to benefit from contextual experiences that provide opportunities to overcome their fears, whereas protection from novel situations results in more stable inhibition. Third, the combination of children's fearfulness and parenting has been examined in relation to moral development. This line of research was inspired by Kochanska's work on conscience development in children varying in fearfulness (summarized in Kochanska, 1997). Specifically, Kochanska found that fearful children show more positive conscience development when mothers use gentle discipline rather than power-assertive discipline; in contrast, relatively fearless children tend to develop stronger internalization when they are securely attached to their mothers and when their mothers are more responsive to them. These findings have not been replicated in all samples (Rothbart & Bates, 2006) and will require greater follow-up. Across numerous studies, the research on interactions of negative emotionality and context yields a complex set of patterns, depending on the particular combinations of negative emotional traits, contextual factors and outcomes examined.

All of the previously described patterns indicate that temperament can amplify the positive or negative effects of context, or that context can amplify the effects of temperament. A new line of work documents a different type of interaction, one in which children's features may affect how sensitive they are to context. Specifically, Boyce and Ellis (2005) have argued, and provided some evidence for the possibility, that high stress reactivity may promote particularly positive functioning in especially protective conditions and particularly negative functioning in adverse conditions, whereas low stress reactivity may yield less responsiveness to contextual features. Stress reactivity is conceptualized and measured at the biological level as "heightened reactivity in one or more of the neurobiological stress response systems" (Boyce & Ellis, 2005, p. 284); the links between stress reactivity and temperamental traits are not yet clear. This new work on stress reactivity requires further replication but points to the intriguing possibility that the same temperamental differences may confer benefits or disadvantages, depending on the context (see chapter 25).

Taken together, there is now robust evidence for the developmental importance of "goodness-of-fit" between children's temperaments and their contexts, at least for a subset of temperamental traits and contextual factors. Future work in this area will benefit from addressing three issues. First, it will be important to use standard, consensual ways of conceptualizing both temperament and context, in order to make results more interpretable across studies. Second, an important next step will be to focus on the processes through which such interactions exert their effects on development. Third, it is important to recognize that, for many years, goodness-of-fit effects were difficult to identify empirically. In some cases, the link between temperament and children's outcomes is more direct and is not clearly moderated by the context (Rothbart & Bates, 2006). Thus, it will be important for future research to clarify the traits and outcomes where context has a moderating role and the cases where temperamental traits have a more direct effect on children's outcomes.

Personality Continuity and Change

Differential Continuity and Change

Continuity and change are most often indexed by correlations between personality scores across two points in time (i.e., test–retest correlations). These differential, or rank-order stability correlations reflect the degree to which the relative ordering of individuals on a given trait is maintained over time. A meta-analysis of the rank-order stability of personality (organized according to the five-factor model) revealed three conclusions (Roberts & DelVecchio, 2000). First, stability correlations over time are moderate in magnitude, even from childhood to early adulthood. Second, there is a notable trend toward increasing stability of individual differences in personality with age (Fraley & Roberts, 2005); test–retest correlations increase with age, from 0.4 in childhood to 0.55 at age 30, and then reach a plateau around 0.7 between ages 50 and 70. Third, test–retest correlations do not vary markedly across the big five traits or by gender.

Two implications can be drawn from this meta-analysis. First, personality stability in childhood and adolescence is higher than proposed by many developmental theorists (Lewis, 2001), especially after age 3. Moreover, the level of stability increases in a relatively linear fashion through adolescence and young adulthood. Young adulthood has been described as demographically dense, in that it involves more life-changing roles and identity decisions than any other period in the life course (Arnett, 2000). Yet, despite these dramatic contextual changes, personality differences remain remarkably consistent during this time period. Second, personality stability in adulthood peaks later than expected. According to one prominent perspective, personality traits are essentially fixed and unchanging after age 30 (McCrae & Costa, 1994). However, the meta-analytic findings show that rank-order stability peaks some time after age 50, but at a level well below unity. Thus, individual differences in personality traits continue to change throughout adulthood, but only modestly after age 50.

Mean-Level Continuity and Change

Mean-level change refers to changes in the average trait level of a population. This type of change is thought to result from maturational processes shared by a population, and is typically assessed by mean-level differences in specific traits over time which indicate whether the sample as a whole is increasing or decreasing on a trait. A meta-analysis of mean-level changes in personality (organized according to the five-factor model) revealed four conclusions (Roberts, Walton, & Viechtbauer, 2006). First, traits belonging to the domain of neuroticism decreased most prominently in young adulthood. Second, traits belonging to the domains of agreeableness and conscientiousness increased in young adulthood and middle age. Third, the pattern of change in extraversion was complex, until this superfactor was divided into constituent elements of social dominance (assertiveness, dominance) and social vitality (talkativeness, sociability). Traits associated with social dominance increased from adolescence through early middle age, whereas traits associated with social vitality increased in adolescence and then showed decreases in young adulthood and old age. Fourth, traits from the openness-to-experience domain showed increases in adolescence and young adulthood and a tendency to decrease in old age.

Three aspects of the results are of special interest. First, the majority of mean-level personality change occurs in young adulthood, not in adolescence as one might suspect given traditional theories of psychological development. This pattern of change is not simply a recent historical phenomenon, as it was observed in different birth cohorts across the 20th century. This finding suggests that the causes of normative personality change are likely to be identified by narrowing research attention to the study of young adulthood. Second, for selected trait categories, change occurs well past young adulthood, demonstrating the continued plasticity of personality well beyond typical age markers of maturity. Third, there are no discernible sex differences in patterns of mean-level continuity and change across the big five. Apparently, men and women change in the same ways over the life course, although mean-level differences between the sexes are maintained over time. This suggests that the causes of personality continuity and change across the life course are likely to be the same for the sexes.

Personality Influences on Life Outcomes

In this section we review evidence about personality effects on relationships, status attainment and health. We provide an overview of research conducted throughout the lifespan, and emphasize both prediction models and process analyses.

How Personality Shapes Friendships and Intimate Relationships

One of the most important tasks faced by children and adolescents is the establishment of friendships and acceptance among peers (Hartup & Stevens, 1999). Among children, all of the higher-order big five traits except openness are important predictors of social competence. Agreeable and extraverted children show better social competence and experience growth in perceived social support from early to late adolescence (Asendorpf & van Aken, 2003; Branje, van Lieshout, & van Aken, 2004; Graziano, Hair, & Finch, 1997; Shiner, 2000; Shiner, Masten, & Roberts, 2003). Children high on negative emotionality or low on aspects of conscientiousness (e.g., attention and self-control) have a variety of social difficulties (Eisenberg, Fabes, Guthrie *et al.*, 2000). Perhaps so many aspects of personality predict social competence because social functioning requires a wide array of skills, including emotional expression, emotional understanding, and emotional and behavioral regulation (Rubin, Bukowski, & Parker, 2006).

Personality continues to be an important predictor of relationships in adulthood. Extraversion predicts positive relationships (Shiner, Masten, & Tellegen, 2002), whereas neuroticism and disagreeableness are the strongest and most consistent personality predictors of negative relationship outcomes – including relationship dissatisfaction, conflict, abuse and, ultimately, dissolution (Karney & Bradbury, 1995). These effects of neuroticism and low agreeableness have been uncovered in long-term studies following samples of children into adulthood, as well as in shorter term longitudinal studies of adults that collect data from dyads (Donnellan, Conger, & Bryant, 2004). One study that followed a large sample of adolescents across their multiple relationships in early adulthood discovered that the influence of neuroticism and low agreeableness on relationship quality showed cross-relationship generalization; that is, it predicted the same abusive relationship experiences across relationships with different partners (Robins, Caspi, & Moffitt, 2002).

An important goal for future research will be to uncover the proximal relationship-specific processes that mediate personality effects on relationship outcomes (Reiss, Capobianco, & Tsai, 2002). Three processes merit attention. First, personality traits influence people's exposure to relationship events (see chapters 25 & 26). For example, people high in neuroticism may be more likely to be exposed to daily conflicts in their relationships (Bolger & Zuckerman, 1995). Second, personality traits shape people's reactions to the behavior of their partners. For example, high disagreeable individuals may escalate negative affect during conflict (e.g., Gottman, Coan, Carrere *et al.*, 1998). Similarly, high agreeable people may be better able to regulate emotions during interpersonal conflicts (Jensen-Campbell & Graziano, 2001). Cognitive processes also come on line in creating trait-correlated experiences (Snyder, & Stukas, 1999). For example, highly neurotic individuals may overreact to minor criticism from their partner, believe they are no longer loved when their partner does not call or assume infidelity on the basis of mere flirtation. Third, personality traits evoke behaviors from partners that contribute to relationship quality. For example, people high in neuroticism and low in agreeableness may be more likely to express behaviors identified as detrimental to relationships: criticism, contempt, defensiveness and stonewalling (Gottman, 1994).

Given the substantial research literature about personality effects on intimate relationships, it is curious that relatively little research has examined personality effects on parenting behaviors (Belsky & Barends, 2002). Although researchers interested in psychiatric disorders have documented that maternal psychopathology can compromise effective parenting (Goodman & Gotlib, 2002; see also chapter 27), developmental researchers have been slower to recognize that parental personality forms a critical part of children's developmental context (Goldsmith, Losaya, Bradshaw *et al.*, 1994). The handful of studies that have examined personality–parenting associations – using self-reports as well as observations of parenting – suggest that extraversion and agreeableness are related to sensitive and responsive parenting, whereas aspects of neuroticism, such as anxiety and irritability, are related to less competent parenting (e.g., Clark, Kochanska, & Ready, 2000; Prinzie, Onghena, Hellinckx *et al.*, 2004). Research on personality effects on parenting is still in its early stages, and there are several important questions that have yet to be addressed. First, most of the research to date has focused on parents of very young children to the virtual exclusion of adolescents. Second, most of the research has focused on the main effects of personality and has not addressed the conditions under which particular personality attributes are more or less important in explaining parenting behavior (e.g., are personality main effects moderated by qualities of the marital relationship or by the child's temperament?). For example, there is some evidence that difficult children are particularly likely to be rejected by highly conscientious mothers during problem-solving tasks (Neitzel & Stright, 2004). Third, to our knowledge, no study has examined personality effects on parenting behavior in relation to multiple children in the same family, a design that has the power to test the cross-situational generalizability of personality effects (across offspring) and to estimate the influence of parental personality on family life independently of other family-wide environmental effects.

How Personality Shapes Performance in School and Work Settings

Personality traits from the domain of conscientiousness are the most important non-cognitive predictors of educational achievement and occupational attainment (Judge, Higgins, Thoresen *et al.*, 1999), and they predict job performance across a wide variety of measures and across nearly all types of jobs (Barrick, Mount, & Judge, 2001). Conscientiousness encompasses many traits that are necessary for completing work effectively: the capacities to sustain attention, to strive toward high standards and to inhibit impulsive behavior. In contrast, neuroticism predicts lower academic attainment (Shiner, Masten, & Tellegen *et al.*, 2002), lower adult occupational attainment (Judge *et al.*, 1999) and has small, negative effects on job performance (Barrick, Mount, & Judge *et al.*, 2001; Hurtz & Donovan, 2000). The predictive associations between temperament and personality traits and achievement are already apparent early in life, at the time that children first enroll in school (Miech, Essex, & Goldsmith, 2001). The finding that personality effects on achievement emerge early in life is important, because school adjustment and academic performance have cumulative effects over time (Entwistle & Alexander, 1993). Links between the other big five traits and academic and work achievement are less consistent and robust but are still found. Openness-to-experience/intellect predicts academic achievement in samples of school-age children, adolescents and college students (Graziano, Jensen-Campbell, & Finch, 1997; John, Caspi, Robins *et al.*, 1994), and child and adult agreeableness sometimes do as well (Shiner, 2000; Shiner, Masten, & Tellegren, 2002). Meta-analyses reveal that extraversion, agreeableness and openness predict some more limited aspects of work performance in a subset of occupations (Barrick, Mount, & Judge *et al.*, 2001).

Why are personality traits related to achievement in educational and occupational domains? The personality processes involved may vary across different stages of development, and at least four candidate processes deserve research scrutiny (cf. Schneider, Smith, Taylor *et al.*, 1998). First, the personality–achievement associations may reflect "attraction" effects, or "active niche-picking," whereby people actively choose educational and work experiences whose qualities are concordant with their own personalities. For example, people who are more conscientious prefer conventional jobs, such as accounting and farming (Gottfredson, Jones, & Holland, 1993). People who are more extraverted prefer jobs that are described as social or enterprising, such as teaching or business management (Ackerman & Heggestad, 1997). Moreover, extraverted individuals are more likely to assume leadership roles in multiple settings (Anderson, John, Keltner *et al.*, 2001). In fact, all of the big five have substantial relations with better performance when the personality predictor is appropriately aligned with work criteria. This indicates that if people find jobs that fit with their dispositions they will experience greater levels of job performance, which should lead to greater success, tenure and satisfaction across the life course (Judge, Higgins, Thoresen *et al.*, 1999).

Second, personality–achievement associations reflect "recruitment" effects, whereby people are selected into achievement situations and are given preferential treatment on the basis of their personality characteristics. These "recruitment" effects begin to appear early in development. For example, children's personalities influence their emerging relationships with teachers already at a young age (Birch & Ladd, 1998). In adulthood, job applicants who are more extraverted, conscientious and less neurotic are liked better by interviewers and are more often recommended for the job (Cook, Vance, & Spector, 2000).

Third, some personality–achievement associations emerge as consequences of "attrition" or "deselection pressures," whereby people leave achievement settings (e.g., schools or jobs) that do not fit with their personality or are released from these settings because of their trait-correlated behaviors (Cairns & Cairns, 1994). For example, longitudinal evidence from different countries shows that children who exhibit a combination of high irritability/antagonism and poor self-control are at heightened risk of unemployment (e.g., Kokko & Pulkkinen, 2000).

Fourth, personality–achievement associations emerge as a result of direct proximal effects of personality on performance. Personality traits may promote certain kinds of task effectiveness; there is some evidence that this occurs in part via the processing of information. For example, higher positive emotions facilitate the efficient processing of complex information and are associated with creative problem-solving (Ashby, Isen, & Turken, 1999; Fredrickson, 2003). In addition to these effects on task effectiveness, personality may directly affect other aspects of work performance, such as interpersonal interactions (Hurtz & Donovan, 2000). Personality traits may also directly influence performance motivation; for example, conscientiousness consistently predicts stronger goal setting and self-efficacy, whereas neuroticism predicts these positive motivations negatively (Erez & Judge, 2001; Judge & Ilies, 2002).

How Personality Shapes Health Trajectories

Personality traits contribute to the maintenance of physical integrity and health. Especially impressive are lifespan studies documenting associations between personality traits related to conscientiousness with longevity (Friedman, Tucker, Tomlinson-Keasey *et al.*, 1993). Individuals high in traits related to disagreeableness (e.g., anger and hostility) appear to be at greatest risk of disease (e.g., cardiovascular illness; Miller, Smith, Turner *et al.*, 1996). The evidence for the involvement of neuroticism in ill health is more mixed, with some research pointing to links with increased risk of actual disease and other studies documenting links with illness behavior only (Smith & Spiro, 2002).

Personality traits can affect health through at least three distinct processes (Contrada, Cather, & O'Leary, 1999; Rozanski, Blumenthal, & Kaplan, 1999). First, personality differences may be related to pathogenesis, mechanisms that promote disease. This has been evaluated most directly in studies relating various facets of disagreeableness/hostility to greater reactivity in response to stressful experiences (Smith & Gallo, 2001) and in studies relating low extraversion to neuroendocrine and immune functioning (Miller *et al.*, 1996) and greater susceptibility to colds (Cohen, Doyle, Turner *et al.*, 2003a,b). However, part of the complexity of testing hypotheses about the role of personality in the physiological processes of a disease involves the need for greater clarity about the relevant disease processes and about which processes may be affected by personality. Second, personality differences may be related to physical health outcomes because they are associated with health-promoting or health-damaging behaviors. For example, individuals high in extraversion may foster social relationships, social support and social integration, which are positively associated with health outcomes (Berkman, Glass, Brissette *et al.*, 2000). In contrast, individuals low in conscientiousness engage in a variety of health-risk behaviors such as smoking, unhealthy eating habits, lack of exercise, unprotected sexual intercourse and dangerous driving habits (Bogg & Roberts, 2004). Third, personality differences may be related to reactions to illness. This includes a wide class of behaviors, including the possibility that personality differences affect the selection and execution of coping behaviors, modulate distress reduction and shape treatment adherence (see chapter 57).

The aforementioned processes linking personality traits to physical health are not mutually exclusive. Moreover, different personality traits may affect physical health via different processes. For example, facets of disagreeableness may be most directly linked to disease processes, facets of low conscientiousness may be implicated in health-damaging behaviors and facets of neuroticism may contribute to ill health by shaping reactions to illness. In addition, it is likely that the impact of personality differences on health varies across the life course. For example, the association between conscientiousness-related traits and health-risk behaviors is especially robust and appears to be stronger among adolescents than adults (Bogg & Roberts, 2004). It is apparent from the extant research that personality traits influence outcomes at all stages of the health process, but much more work remains to be done to identify the processes that account for these effects.

Temperament, Personality and the Development of Psychopathology

Much of the early interest in temperament traits was generated by Thomas and Chess's suggestion that children's early individual differences could help set off a chain of transactions between the child and the environment that could lead eventually to the development of clinical disorders (Thomas, Chess, & Birch, 1968). Recent years have seen a tremendous increase in research about the links between temperament and personality and the development of psychopathology, in both childhood and adulthood. In this section, we address two aspects of this burgeoning literature. First, we present an overview of how to conceptualize the associations between personality and psychopathology. Second, we summarize what is known about the correlations between temperament–personality differences and the emergence of psychopathology in childhood and adolescence.

A Conceptual Model for Personality–Psychopathology Associations

Personality and psychopathology may come to be linked through a range of processes (Widiger, Verheul, & van den Brink, 1999). In a *vulnerability association*, personality is a risk factor that causes individuals to be vulnerable to the development of particular forms of psychopathology, particularly in certain environmental conditions. In this case, the psychological disorder is distinct from the risk-inducing trait or traits. The traits may set in motion processes that cause the development of disorders over time (for a more thorough discussion of these processes see Caspi & Shiner, 2006). In contrast, in a *spectrum association*, psychopathology represents the extreme end of a continuously distributed personality trait or cluster of traits. In this case, the psychological disorder is not a categorically distinct condition, but rather it is an extreme expression of a dimensional trait. Although the vulnerability and spectrum associations are presented here as if they are distinct, the line between the two is blurred. Most of the associations that have been found between personality and psychopathology could be explained equally well by either the vulnerability or the spectrum model. Some disorders may be better described as discrete entities, whereas others may be better described as dimensional conditions. Further, some aspects of the same disorder may be discrete, whereas other aspects may be dimensional.

Although vulnerability and spectrum associations have received the most attention, other links between personality and psychopathology may occur as well. In a *maintenance association*, personality may influence the manifestation, course and prognosis of a disorder once it has started. In a *resilience association*, personality may protect against the development of psychopathology in the face of stress and adversity. This is not simply the opposite of a vulnerability association. Indeed, to the extent that protective and risk factors operate dimensionally – at opposite ends of a continuum – there is little to be gained from focusing on the beneficial effects of, for example, low neuroticism than on the harmful effects of high neuroticism. But there is a great deal of value in testing two hypotheses:

1 Some personality factors provide protection in the presence of risk, even though they have no effect in the absence of such risk; and

2 Higher levels of a trait are necessary for protection under adverse conditions than are necessary for competent functioning in low-risk conditions.

A final personality–psychopathology link is that of a *scarring association*, in which the experience of significant psychopathology alters children's personalities in lasting ways. For example, the early experience of depressive symptoms may influence children's typical cognitive style, such that children who experience more depressive symptoms may begin to develop a more negative attributional style over time (Garber & Carter, 2006).

Associations Between Temperament and Personality Traits and Psychological Disorders in Childhood and Adolescence

Numerous studies have examined associations between temperament and personality differences and psychopathology, both concurrently and longitudinally. A number of recent reviews have described these associations, organized generally by findings for specific temperament or personality traits (Caspi & Shiner, 2006; Muris & Ollendick, 2005; Rothbart & Bates, 2006). In the following summary, we present an alternative view of these associations, organized instead by classes of disorders (Nigg, 2006; Tackett, 2006).

Emotional Disorders

Watson, Clark, Weber *et al.* (1995) developed a tripartite model to account for co-occurring emotional disorders in adults. According to this model, depression and anxiety tend to co-occur because both share high levels of negative affect or neuroticism, including distress and fearfulness. In addition, depression is specifically characterized by low positive affect (or extraversion) and anxiety is specifically characterized by physiological arousal. There is general support for these hypothesized associations in cross-sectional studies using a range of child populations, as well as some evidence that high negative affect predicts increases in anxiety, and low positive affect predicts increases in depression in youths (Lonigan, Vasey, Phillips *et al.*, 2004). Further, a study of preschoolers' positive emotionality (assessed through laboratory tasks and behavior observations) has provided intriguing evidence that low positive emotionality is specifically associated with maternal depression (Durbin *et al.*, 2005); comparable links were not found for the preschoolers' negative emotionality. Behavioral inhibition also poses risks for the development of anxiety disorders, particularly social anxiety, although most behaviorally inhibited children do not develop anxiety disorders (Tackett, 2006). As noted previously, because current measures of behavioral inhibition are likely to confound low approach and high fear, it is not clear which of these components (or both) is most predictive of anxiety disorders.

Although much of the research on emotional disorders has focused on positive affect (extraversion) and negative affect (neuroticism), aspects of conscientiousness and agreeableness may also be relevant. Lonigan, Vasey, Phillips *et al.* (2004) have argued for and provided some preliminary evidence that effortful control moderates the effect of high negative affect on the experience of anxiety symptoms. In other words, high negative affect predicts anxiety symptoms only when youths lack adequate levels of effortful control to be able to regulate their negative emotions and cognitive biases toward threatening information. Muris and Ollendick (2005) have presented some preliminary evidence, however, that it is the attention aspect of effortful control that is most relevant to internalizing disorders, perhaps because poor attentional control results in greater cognitive distortions. The role of attention in causing emotional difficulties is also supported by research demonstrating that greater attentional control is associated with more effective regulation of negative emotionality, beginning in infancy and continuing into later childhood (Eisenberg, Smith, Sadovsky *et al.*, 2004). Finally, aspects of excessively high agreeableness, such as excessive empathy and compliance, may be related to the development of depression, particularly in girls (Keenan & Hipwell, 2005); the current evidence for this possibility is thin but worthy of further examination.

In summary, emotional disorders in childhood and adolescence are clearly associated with high negative affect (neuroticism); the fear and distress aspects of neuroticism are likely to be most relevant. A recent meta-analysis of research with adult samples suggests that general distress may be a stronger predictor of disorders such as depression and generalized anxiety, whereas fear may be a stronger predictor of disorders such as panic disorder and the phobias. Poor attentional control may also be a significant risk factor for the development of emotional disorders when it co-occurs with high negative affect. Depression is likely to be specifically predicted by low positive affect (extraversion). The research on temperament by context interactions described previously in this chapter suggests that children's tendencies toward negative affect are more likely to worsen into emotional problems in the context of intrusive, derisive or overprotective parenting that interferes with children's ability to learn to manage their negative emotions effectively. Stressful life events may further exacerbate temperamental tendencies toward high negative emotions (Jacobs, Kenis, Peeters *et al.*, 2006).

Disruptive Disorders

A number of disruptive disorders tend to co-occur. The most likely temperamental contributor toward this disruptive spectrum is a general tendency toward disinhibition versus constraint, which includes both low conscientiousness and low agreeableness (Clark, 2005). In childhood, tendencies toward disinhibition are associated with disruptive behaviors as well. Low effortful control and similar traits are robustly associated with a variety of conduct problems (Rothbart & Bates, 2006). Although the attentional component of effortful control is likely to be most important for emotional disorders, effortful control more generally is likely to be important for disruptive disorders; in other words, children who are low in planning, cautiousness, deliberateness and self-control are at a higher risk of developing oppositional behavior, aggression and conduct problems (Caspi & Shiner, 2006; Muris & Ollendick, 2005).

Although disinhibition and poor effortful control are general risk factors for disruptive behaviors, there are likely to be subtypes of youths with conduct problems that are characterized by additional personality patterns (Frick & Morris, 2004; Nigg, 2006). First, there are disruptive youths characterized by high levels of anger, irritability and reactive aggression (Frick & Morris, 2004). Children who are easily angered but who have poor self-control may be particularly vulnerable to developing conduct problems and oppositionality; in these cases, the problem is largely one of poor emotional regulation (Frick & Morris, 2004). This personality profile appears to characterize youths with co-occurring attention deficit/hyperactivity disorder (ADHD) and conduct disorder (Cukrowicz, Taylor, Schatschneider *et al.*, 2006), as well as those who go on to develop substance abuse problems (Wills & Dishion, 2004) and problem gambling (Slutske, Caspi, Moffitt *et al.*, 2005). The previously described research on temperament by context interactions suggests that the problems of children with this constellation of traits are likely to be exacerbated by a range of contextual influences, such as unsupportive or intrusive parenting, a lack of monitoring and structure, family stress or poverty. Second, there appears to be a subset of previously described youths with psychopathic tendencies, meaning that they display aspects of low agreeableness (manipulativeness, low empathy and remorse) and low fear (Frick & Morris, 2004; Nigg, 2006). As described in the section on temperament-by-context interactions, these youths are less susceptible to socialization, and their disruptive behaviors may be less related to their context. However, Kochanska's (1997) work on conscience development suggests the possibility that an early secure attachment may help fearless children develop a stronger conscience. Third, there is a group of youths who do not evidence significant conduct problems as children but only develop such problems as adolescents (Moffitt, Caspi, Dickson *et al.*, 1996); although this group of youths with "adolescent-onset" conduct problems is difficult to identify in childhood, they appear to have adolescent personalities characterized by a lack of traditional values and a strong motivation to attract attention and wield influence over others.

Finally, Nigg (2006) has provided evidence that temperament may also be relevant to the development of ADHD. First, the inattentive-disorganized symptoms of ADHD may represent an extreme variant of low effortful control (thus, having a spectrum association with this trait), accompanied by a range of executive functioning deficits. Second, the hyperactive-impulsive symptoms of ADHD may involve extreme approach tendencies that are not restrained by good self-control or adequate fearfulness.

In summary, disruptive behavior problems are robustly associated with problems with self-control and a general tendency toward disinhibition. There are likely to be several subtypes of youths with disruptive problems: those with strong irritability and aggression and general problems with emotion regulation, likely exacerbated by negative environmental influences; those with low empathy, guilt and fear, with less consistent environmental contributors; and those with non-traditional values and high social potency, who do not develop significant behavioral problems until adolescence. Aspects of ADHD are likely to be related to low self-control as well, with attention problems associated with very low effortful control and impulsive hyperactivity associated with poorly restrained and modulated approach tendencies.

Temperament and Personality Assessment and Treatment Relevance

Assessment

Four types of measures are available to assess childhood temperament and personality, each with different strengths and weaknesses. First, questionnaires are the most commonly used measures. Although questionnaires are most often administered to parents, they can also be used to obtain reports from peers, teachers and other informants. Self-report questionnaires are available for older children. Questionnaires have a number of strengths: they aggregate information about children's behavior across a number of situations and over a period of time; they are inexpensive to administer; they efficiently gather a lot of information; and they can solicit information about relatively rare but important behaviors (see chapter 20). Questionnaires may be limited by reporter biases, including those that may be more emotionally motivated and those arising from an inability to report accurately (Funder, 2004). Parent-report temperament questionnaires have sometimes been criticized on this basis. However, research suggests that parent report still has a useful role in assessing temperament (Rothbart & Bates, 2006).

Second, peer and self-reports can be obtained through other means, specifically peer nomination measures and a puppet interview. In peer nomination measures, peers nominate other students who are "best" or "least well" described by particular items. With the Berkeley Puppet Interview, children aged 4–8 report on their traits and experiences by stating which of two puppets they are most like (Measelle, John, Ablow *et al.*, 2004). This measure can be used to assess the big five traits, as well as a range other individual differences. These two types of measures generally possess the same strengths and weaknesses as questionnaires.

Third, naturalistic observation can be used to code children's behavioral tendencies. For example, home observation systems have been developed to assess temperament or personality in preschoolers (Buckley, Klein, Durbin *et al.*, 2002). Fourth, laboratory tasks create specific situations in which children's behaviors can be observed. Tasks have been developed to assess specific individual differences, and a more comprehensive battery of laboratory tasks assessing temperament in children is available (Goldsmith, Reilly, Lemery *et al.*, 1995). Naturalistic observations and laboratory assessments have the advantages of potentially possessing ecological validity and of providing an "outsider" view of the child's behavior. Laboratory tasks also allow for fine-grained analysis of specific behaviors and for linking behaviors with brain functioning. These methods share the weaknesses of being time and labor intensive, being vulnerable to situational effects on behavior and limiting the possibility of observing rare behaviors. Further, any behavior may tap more than one underlying trait, which sometimes makes it difficult to interpret the meaning of any particular task.

Several recommendations are offered for choosing a measure for research. First, ideally more than one method should be used, to take advantage of the strengths of different methods and to counteract the weaknesses inherent in each. At the very least, it is important to include more than one informant when possible, as is true for assessing children's functioning in general. Second, more than one trait should be measured, to provide evidence of divergent validity for the trait or traits of interest. Third, it is important to evaluate which method is best for measuring a particular trait, depending on the trait or research question being pursued. For further information on finding specific measures to use, readers are referred to citations in several recent reviews (Caspi & Shiner, 2006; Rothbart & Bates, 2006; Shiner & Caspi, 2003). Detailed information about measures for assessing normal range and pathological personality traits in adolescents can be found in Shiner (2008).

Treatment

New knowledge about children's individual differences in temperament and personality has immense potential for informing treatment and prevention programs, but has yet to be fully integrated into most programs because temperament and personality traits are often wrongly assumed to be highly stable and immutable. However, there are a number of ways that greater understanding of temperament and personality can inform treatment.

Some treatment and prevention programs have the goal of modifying children's personality tendencies, whereas at other times the focus may be on helping children learn to cope better with their personality tendencies. Muris and Ollendick (2005) have argued that many cognitive–behavioral treatment programs have as their goal the improvement of children's effortful control: "Cognitive–behavioral therapy teaches techniques that help children to inhibit their maladaptive behaviors and to regulate their attention, thereby improving their effortful control" (Muris & Ollendick, 2005, p. 285). These treatment programs go about changing children's self-regulation in a variety of ways, depending on what symptoms are most problematic. Prevention work may often have a similar focus on strengthening children's basic skills in emotion regulation and self-control. In contrast, other treatments may successfully help children to learn to cope with challenging traits without directly changing those traits. For example, a recent prevention program provided education to parents of withdrawn or inhibited preschool-age children (Rapee, Kennedy, Ingram *et al.*, 2005); parents were taught how to avoid overprotection, encourage the children's exposure to feared situations and use cognitive restructuring for their own and their child's worrying. Interestingly, the program successfully diminished the likelihood of the children developing an anxiety disorder but did not appear to affect the children's level of inhibition or withdrawal. Thus, treatment and prevention may operate in two different and complementary ways: by modifying basic tendencies or by helping youths cope better with those tendencies.

Treatment procedures may need to be adapted to the personalities of particular youths to maximize treatment effectiveness. The use of punishments and rewards may need to be tailored to children's temperaments, because children will vary in what consequences they find to be positive versus aversive (Manassis & Young, 2001). For example, children with the psychopathic traits described elsewhere in this chapter may be unresponsive to typical discipline and punishment but may still respond well to positive incentives for compliance (Hawes & Dadds, 2005). The entire approach to treatment may in some cases need to be altered depending on youths' personalities, because some approaches may be unsuitable for some children. For example, some oppositional children may not benefit from typical parent training programs because they are especially low in frustration tolerance and high in inflexibility (Greene, Ablon, & Goring, 2003). Such youths may need an alternative approach to helping them learn to comply. The adaptation of treatment to children's individual personalities has great potential for improving the effectiveness of treatment.

Youths' personality strengths should be considered in treatment. Even the most troubled youths are likely to have areas of relative health in their personalities. These personality strengths are resources that can be drawn upon in treatment, and a better appreciation of youths' individual strengths can sustain a sense of optimism for the youths themselves, their caregivers and their treatment providers. There is also evidence that some traits may promote resilient functioning in youths in the face of stress and adversity, and clinicians can work with children's contexts to further promote these positive traits (Luthar, 2006).

Research on temperament and personality has demonstrated clearly the fundamental importance of these individual differences for youths' development. An important next task for the fields of psychiatry and psychology will be to integrate more fully what is known about these individual differences into best practices in treatment and prevention.

Further Reading

Caspi, A., & Shiner, R. L. (2006). Personality development. In N. Eisenberg (Ed.), *Handbook of child psychology*. Vol. 3. *Social, emotional, and personality development* (6th ed., pp. 300–365). New York: Wiley.

Nigg, J. T. (2006). Temperament and developmental psychopathology. *Journal of Child Psychology and Psychiatry*, *47*, 395–422. Review.

Rothbart, M. K., & Bates, J. E. (2006). Temperament. In N. Eisenberg (Ed.), *Handbook of child psychology*. Vol. 3. *Social, emotional, and personality development* (6th ed., pp. 99–166). New York: Wiley.

References

Ackerman, P. L., & Heggestad, E. D. (1997). Intelligence, personality, and interests. *Psychological Bulletin*, *121*, 219–245.

American Psychiatric Association. (1980). *Diagnostic and statistical manual of mental disorders*, (3rd ed.). Washington, DC: American Psychiatric Association.

Anderson, C., John, O. P., Keltner, D., & Kring, A. M. (2001). Who attains social status? Effects of personality and physical attractiveness in social groups. *Journal of Personality and Social Psychology*, *80*, 132.

Arnett, J. J. (2000). Emerging adulthood: A theory of development from the late teens through the twenties. *American Psychologist*, *55*, 469–480.

Asendorpf, J. B., & van Aken, M. A. G. (2003). Personality–relationship transaction in adolescence: Core versus surface personality characteristics. *Journal of Personality*, *71*, 629–666.

Ashby, F. G., Isen, A. M., & Turken, U. (1999). A neuropsychological theory on positive affect and its influence on cognition. *Psychological Review*, *106*, 529–550.

Banfield, J. F., Wyland, C. L., Macrae, C. N., Munte, T. F., & Heatherton, T. F. (2004). The cognitive resolution of self-regulation. In R. F. Baumeister, & K. D. Vohs (Eds.), *Handbook of self regulation: Research, theory, and applications* (pp. 62–83). New York: Guilford.

Barrick, M. R., Mount, M. K., & Judge, T. A. (2001). Personality and performance at the beginning of the new millennium: What do we know and where do we go next? *International Journal of Selection and Assessment*, *9*, 9–30.

Bell, R. Q., & Chapman, M. (1986). Child effects in studies using experimental or brief longitudinal approaches to socialization. *Developmental Psychology*, *22*, 595–603.

Belsky, J., & Barends, N. (2002). Personality and parenting. In M. H. Bornstein (Ed.), *Handbook of parenting*. Vol. 3. *Being and becoming a parent* (2nd ed., pp. 415–438). Mahwah, NJ: Lawrence Erlbaum Associates.

Benjamin, J., Ebstein, R. P., & Belmaker, R. H. (2002). *Molecular genetics and the human personality*. Washington, DC: American Psychiatric Press.

Berkman, L. F., Glass, T., Brissette, I., & Seeman, T. E. (2000). From social integration to health. *Social Science and Medicine*, *51*, 843–857.

Birch, S. H., & Ladd, G. W. (1998). Children's interpersonal behaviors and the teacher–child relationship. *Developmental Psychology*, *34*, 934–946.

Blair, R. J. R., Peschardt, K. S., Budhani, S., Mitchell, D. G. V., & Pine, D. S. (2006). The development of psychopathy. *Journal of Child Psychology and Psychiatry*, *47*, 262–274.

Bogg, T., & Roberts, B. W. (2004). Conscientiousness and health behaviors: A meta-analysis of the leading behavioral contributors to mortality. *Psychological Bulletin*, *130*, 887–919.

Bolger, N., & Zuckerman, A. (1995). A framework for studying personality in the stress process. *Journal of Personality and Social Psychology*, *69*, 890–902.

Borkenau, P., & Liebler, A. (1995). Thin slices of behavior as cues of personality and intelligence. *Journal of Personality and Social Psychology*, *86*, 599–614.

Bouchard, T. J., & Loehlin, J. C. (2001). Genes, evolution, and personality. *Behavior Genetics*, *31*, 243–274.

Boyce, W. T., & Ellis, B. J. (2005). Biological sensitivity to context: I. An evolutionary-developmental theory of the origins and functions of stress reactivity. *Development and Psychopathology*, *17*, 271–301.

Branje, S. J. T., van Lieshout, C. F. M., & van Aken, M. A. G. (2004). Relations between Big Five personality characteristics and perceived support in adolescent families. *Journal of Personality and Social Psychology*, *86*, 615–628.

Buckley, M. E., Klein, D. N., Durbin, E., Hayden, E. P., & Moerk, K. C. (2002). Development and validation of a Q-sort procedure to assess temperament and behavior in preschool-age children. *Journal of Clinical Child and Adolescent Psychology*, *31*, 525–539.

Bugental, D. B., & Grusec, J. (2006). Socialization processes. In W. Damon, & R. Lerner (Editors in Chief) & N. Eisenberg (Volume Ed.), *Handbook of child psychology*. Vol. 3. *Social, emotional and personality development* (6th ed., pp. 366–428). New York: Wiley.

Buss, D. M. (1987). Selection, evocation, and manipulation. *Journal of Personality and Social Psychology*, *53*, 1214–1221.

Cairns, R. B., & Cairns, B. D. (1994). *Lifelines and risks: Pathways of youth in our time*. New York: Cambridge University Press.

Caspi, A., & Moffitt, T. E. (2006). Gene–environment interactions in psychiatry: Joining forces with neuroscience. *Nature Reviews Neuroscience*, *7*, 583–590.

Caspi, A., & Shiner, R. L. (2006). Personality development. In W. Damon, & R. Lerner (Editors in Chief) & N. Eisenberg (Volume Ed.), *Handbook of child psychology*. Vol. 3. *Social, emotional, and personality development* (6th ed., pp. 300–365). New York: Wiley.

Cervone, D., & Mischel, W. (2002). Personality science. In D. Cervone, & W. Mischel (Eds.), *Advances in personality science* (pp. 1–26). New York: Guilford.

Clark, L. A. (2005). Temperament as a unifying basis for personality and psychopathology. *Journal of Abnormal Psychology*, *114*, 505–521.

Clark, L. A., Kochanska, G., & Ready, R. (2000). Mother's personality and its interaction with child temperament as predictors of parenting behaviour. *Journal of Personality and Social Psychology*, *79*, 274–285.

Cloninger, C. R., Przybeck, T. R., Svrakic, D. M., & Wetzel, R. D. (1994). *The Temperament and Character Inventory (TCI): A guide to its development and use*. St. Louis, MO: Center for Psychobiology of Personality, Washington University.

Cohen, S., Doyle, W. J., Turner, R. B., Alper, C. M., & Skoner, D. P. (2003a). Emotional style and susceptibility to the common cold. *Psychosomatic Medicine*, *65*, 652–657.

Cohen, S., Doyle, W. J., Turner, C. W., Alper, C. M., & Skoner, D. P. (2003b). Sociability and susceptibility to the common cold. *Psychological Science*, *14*, 389–395.

Contrada, R. J., Cather, C., & O'Leary, A. (1999). Personality and health: Dispositions and processes in disease susceptibility and adaptation to illness. In L. A. Pervin, & O. P. John (Eds.), *Handbook of personality* (2nd ed., pp. 576–604). New York: Guilford.

Cook, K. W., Vance, C. A., & Spector, P. E. (2000). The relation of candidate personality with selection-interview outcomes. *Journal of Applied Social Psychology*, *30*, 867–885.

Crockenberg, S., & Leerkes, E. (2003). Infant negative emotionality, caregiving, and family. In A. C. Crouter, & A. Booth (Eds.), *Children's influence on family dynamics: The neglected side of family relationships* (pp. 57–78). Mahwah, NJ: Erlbaum.

Cukrowicz, K. C., Taylor, J., Schatschneider, C., & Ianoco, W. G. (2006). Personality differences in children and adolescents with attention deficit/hyperactivity disorder, conduct disorder, and controls. *Journal of Child Psychology and Psychiatry*, *47*, 151–159.

Derryberry, D., & Reed, M. A. (2003). Information processing approaches to individual differences in emotional reactivity. In R. J. Davidson, K. R. Scherer, & H. H. Goldsmith (Eds.), *Handbook of affective sciences* (pp. 681–697). New York: Oxford.

DeYoung, C. G., Peterson, J. B., Séguin, J. R., Mejia, J. M., Pihl, R. O., Beitchman, J. H., *et al.* (2006). The dopamine D4 receptor gene and moderation of the association between externalizing behavior and IQ. *Archives of General Psychiatry*, *63*, 1410–1416.

Diamond, L. M. (2004). Emerging perspectives on distinctions between romantic love and sexual desire. *Current Directions in Psychological Science*, *13*, 11.

Donnellan, M. B., Conger, R. D., & Bryant, C. M. (2004). The Big Five and enduring marriages. *Journal of Research in Personality*, *38*, 481–504.

Durbin, C. E., Klein, D. N., Hayden, E. P., Buckley, M. E., & Moerk, K. C. (2005). Temperamental emotionality in preschoolers and parental mood disorders. *Journal of Abnormal Psychology*, *114*, 28–37.

Ebstein, R. P. (2006). The molecular genetic architecture of human personality: Beyond self-report questionnaires. *Molecular Psychiatry*, *11*, 427–445.

Eisenberg, N., Fabes, R. A., Guthrie, I. K., & Reiser, M. (2000). Dispositional emotionality and regulation: Their role in predicting quality of social functioning. *Journal of Personality and Social Psychology*, *78*, 136–157.

Eisenberg, N., Smith, C. L., Sadovsky, A., & Spinrad, T. L. (2004). Effortful control: Relations with emotional regulation, adjustment and socialization in childhood. In R. F. Baumeister, & K. D. Vohs (Eds.), *Handbook of self-regulation: Research, theory, and applications* (pp. 259–282). New York: Guilford.

Entwistle, D. R., & Alexander, K. L. (1993). Entry into school. *Annual Review of Sociology*, *19*, 401–423.

Erez, A., & Judge, T. A. (2001). Relationship of core self-evaluation to goal setting motivation, and performance. *Journal of Applied Psychology*, *86*, 1270–1279.

Fox, N. A., Henderson, H. A., Marshall, P. J., Nichols, K. E., & Ghera, M. M. (2005). Behavioral inhibition: Linking biology and behavior within a developmental framework. *Annual Review of Psychology*, *56*, 235–262.

Fraley, R. C., & Roberts, B. W. (2005). Patterns of continuity: A dynamic model for conceptualizing the stability of individual difference in psychological constructs across the life course. *Psychological Review*, *112*, 60–74.

Fredrickson, B. L. (2003). The value of positive emotions. *American Scientist*, *91*, 330–335.

Frick, P. J., & Morris, A. S. (2004). Temperament and developmental pathways to conduct problems. *Journal of Clinical Child and Adolescent Psychology*, *33*, 64–68.

Friedman, H. S., Tucker, J. S., Tomlinson-Keasey, C., Schwartz, J. E., Wingard, D. L., & Criqui, M. H. (1993). Does childhood personality predict longevity? *Journal of Personality and Social Psychology*, *65*, 176–185.

Funder, D. C. (2004). *The personality puzzle* (3rd ed.). New York: Norton.

Garber, J., & Carter, J. S. (2006). Major depression. In R. T. Ammerman (Ed.), *Comprehensive handbook of personality and psychopathology*. Vol. 3. *Child psychopathology* (pp. 165–216). Hoboken, NJ: Wiley.

Gifford, R. (1994). A lens-mapping framework for understanding the encoding and decoding of interpersonal dispositions in nonverbal behavior. *Journal of Personality and Social Psychology*, *66*, 398–412.

Gilliom, M., & Shaw, D. S. (2004). Codevelopment of externalizing and internalizing problems in early childhood. *Development and Psychopathology*, *16*, 313–333.

Goldsmith, H. H., Losoya, S. H., Bradshaw, D. L., & Campos, J. J. (1994). Genetics of personality: A twin study of the five-factor model and parent-offspring analyses. In C. F. J. Halverson, C. S. Kohnstamm, R. P. Marin, & R. P. Martin (Eds.), *The developing structure of temperament and personality from infancy to childhood* (pp. 241–266). Hillsdale, NJ: Erlbaum.

Goldsmith, H. H., Reilly, J., Lemery, K. S., Longley, S., & Prescott, A. (1995). Laboratory Temperament Assessment Battery: Preschool Version. Unpublished Manual, University of Wisconsin-Madison.

Goodman, S. H., & Gotlib, I. H. (2002). *Children of depressed parents*. Washington, DC: American Psychological Association.

Gottfredson, G. D., Jones, E. M., & Holland, J. L. (1993). Personality and vocational interests: The relation of Holland's six interest dimensions to five robust dimensions of personality. *Journal of Counseling Psychology*, *40*, 518–524.

Gottman, J. M. (1994). *What predicts divorce? The relationship between marital processes and marital outcomes*. Hillsdale, NJ: Lawrence Erlbaum Associates, Inc.

Gottman, J. M., Coan, J., Carrere, S., & Swanson, C. (1998). Predicting marital happiness and stability from newlywed interactions. *Journal of Marriage and Family*, *60*, 5–22.

Graziano, W. G., & Eisenberg, N. (1997). Agreeableness: A dimension of personality. In R. Hogan, J. Johnson, & S. Briggs (Eds.), *Handbook of personality psychology* (pp. 795–824). San Diego, CA: Academic Press.

Graziano, W. G., Hair, E. C., & Finch, J. F. (1997). Competitiveness mediates the link between personality and group performance. *Journal of Personality and Social Psychology*, *73*, 1394–1408.

Graziano, W. G., Jensen-Campbell, L. A., & Finch, J. F. (1997). The self as mediator between personality and adjustment. *Journal of Personality and Social Psychology*, *73*, 392–404.

Greene, R. W., Ablon, J. S., & Goring, J. C. (2003). A transactional model of oppositional behavior: Underpinnings of the Collaborative Program Solving approach. *Journal of Psychosomatic Research*, *55*, 67–75.

Hartup, W. W., & Stevens, N. (1999). Friendships and adaptation across the life span. *Current Directions in Psychological Science*, *8*, 76–79.

Hartup, W. W., & van Lieshout, C. F. M. (1995). Personality development in social context. *Annual Review of Psychology*, *46*, 655–687.

Hawes, D. J., & Dadds, M. R. (2005). The treatment of conduct problems in children with callous-unemotional traits. *Journal of Consulting and Clinical Psychology*, *73*, 737–741.

Hay, D. F., Payne, A., & Chadwick, A. (2004). Peer relations in childhood. *Journal of Child Psychology and Psychiatry*, *45*, 84–108.

Henry, B., Caspi, A., Moffitt, T. E., Harrington, H., & Silva, P. A. (1999). Staying in school protects boys with poor self-regulation in childhood from later crime: A longitudinal study. *International Journal of Behavioral Development*, *23*, 1049–1073.

Hurtz, G. M., & Donovan, J. J. (2000). Personality and job performance: The Big Five revisited. *Journal of Applied Psychology*, *85*, 869–879.

Jacobs, N., Kenis, G., Peeters, F., Derom, C., Vlietinck, R., & Van Os, J. (2006). Stress-related negative affectivity and genetically altered serotonin transporter function: Evidence of synergism in shaping risk of depression. *Archives of General Psychiatry*, *63*, 989–996.

Jenkins, J. M., Rasbash, J., & O'Connor, T. G. (2003). The role of the shared family context in differential parenting. *Developmental Psychology*, *39*, 99–113.

Jensen-Campbell, L. A., Gleason, K. A., Adams, R., & Malcolm, K. T. (2003). Interpersonal conflict, Agreeableness, and personality development. *Journal of Personality*, *71*, 1059–1085.

Jensen-Campbell, L. A., & Graziano, W. G. (2001). Agreeableness as a moderator of interpersonal conflict. *Journal of Personality*, *69*, 323–362.

Jockin, V., McGue, M., & Lykken, D. T. (1996). Personality and divorce: A genetic analysis. *Journal of Personality and Social Psychology*, *71*, 288–299.

John, O. P., Caspi, A., Robins, R. W., Moffitt, T. E., & Stouthamer-Loeber, M. (1994). The "Little Five": Exploring the five-factor model of personality in adolescent boys. *Child Development*, *65*, 160–178.

Judge, T. A., Higgins, C. A., Thoresen, C. J., & Barrick, M. R. (1999). The Big Five personality traits, general mental ability, and career success across the life-span. *Personnel Psychology*, *52*, 621–652.

Judge, T. A., & Ilies, R. (2002). Relationship of personality to performance motivation: A meta-analytic review. *Journal of Applied Psychology*, *87*, 797–807.

Kagan, J., & Snidman, N. (2004). *The long shadow of temperament*. Cambridge, MA: Belknap Press.

Karney, B. R., & Bradbury, T. N. (1995). The longitudinal course of marital quality and stability: A review of theory, method and research. *Psychological Bulletin*, *118*, 3–34.

Keenen, K., & Hipwell, A. E. (2005). Preadolescent clues to understanding depression in girls. *Clinical Child and Family Psychology Review*, *8*, 89–105.

Keltner, D., Moffitt, T. E., & Stouthamer-Loeber, M. (1995). Facial expressions of emotion and psychopathology in adolescent males. *Journal of Abnormal Psychology*, *104*, 644–652.

Kochanska, G. (1997). Multiple pathways to conscience for children with different temperaments: From toddlerhood to age 5. *Developmental Psychology*, *33*, 228–240.

Kochanska, G., & Knaack, A. (2003). Effortful control as a personality characteristic of young children: Antecedents, correlates, and consequences. *Journal of Personality*, *71*, 1087–1112.

Kokko, K., & Pulkinnen, L. (2000). Aggression in childhood and long-term unemployment in adulthood: A cycle of maladaptation and some protective factors. *Developmental Psychology*, *36*, 463–472.

Kokko, K., Bergman, L. R., & Pulkinnen, L. (2003). Child personality characteristics and selection into long-term unemployment in Finnish and Swedish longitudinal studies. *International Journal of Behavioral Development*, *27*, 134–144.

Krueger, R. F., Hicks, B. M., & McGue, M. (2001). Altruism and antisocial behavior: Independent tendencies, unique personality correlates, distinct etiologies. *Psychological Science*, *12*, 397–402.

Kupfer, D. J., First, M. B., & Regier, D. A. (2002). *A research agenda for DSM-V*. Arlington, VA: American Psychiatric Publishing.

Lacourse, E., Nagin, D. S., Vitaro, F., Cote, S., Arsenault, L., & Tremblay, R. E. (2006). Prediction of early-onset deviant peer group affiliation: A 12-year longitudinal study. *Archives of General Psychiatry*, *63*, 562–568.

Lemerise, E. A., & Arsenio, W. F. (2000). An integrated model of emotion processes and cognition in social information processing. *Child Development*, *71*, 107–118.

Lengua, L. J., & Long, A. C. (2002). The role of emotionality and self-regulation in the appraisal-coping process: Tests of direct and moderating effects. *Journal of Applied Developmental Psychology*, *23*, 471–493.

Lewis, M. (2001). Issues in the study of personality development. *Psychological Inquiry*, *12*, 67–83.

Lin, E. K., Bugenthal, D. B., Turek, V., Martorell, G. A., & Olster, D. H. (2002). Children's vocal properties as mobilizers of stress-related physiological responses in adults. *Personality and Social Psychology Bulletin*, *28*, 346–357.

Lonigan, C. J., Vasey, M. W., Phillips, B. M., & Hazel, R. A. (2004). Temperament, anxiety, and the processing of threat-relevant stimuli. *Journal of Clinical Child and Adolescent Psychology*, *33*, 8–20.

Lucas, R. E., & Baird, B. M. (2004). Extraversion and emotional reactivity. *Journal of Personality and Social Psychology*, *86*, 473–485.

Luthar, S. S. (2006). Resilience in development: A synthesis of research across five decades. In D. Cicchetti, & D. J. Cohen (Eds.), *Developmental psychopathology*. Vol. 3. *Risk, disorder, and adaptation* (2nd ed., pp. 739–795). Hoboken, NJ: Wiley.

Lynam, D. R., Caspi, A., Moffitt, T. E., Wikstrom, P. H., Loeber, R., & Novak, S. (2000). The interaction between impulsivity and neighborhood context on offending: The effects of impulsivity are stronger in poorer neighborhoods. *Journal of Abnormal Psychology*, *109*, 563–574.

Lynam, D. R., & Gudonis, L. (2005). The development of psychopathy. *Annual Review of Clinical Psychology*, *1*, 381–407.

MacDonald, K. (1995). Evolution, the five-factor model, and levels of personality. *Journal of Personality*, *63*, 525–567.

Manassis, K., & Young, A. (2001). Adapting positive reinforcement systems to suit child temperament. *Journal of the American Academy of Child and Adolescent Psychiatry*, *88*, 139–157.

Markon, K. E., Krueger, R. F., & Watson, D. (2005). Delineating the structure of normal and abnormal personality: An integrative hierarchical approach. *Journal of Personality and Social Psychology*, *88*, 139–157.

McAdams, D. P., & Pals, J. L. (2006). A new Big Five: Fundamental principles for an integrative science of personality. *American Psychologist*, *61*, 204–217.

McCrae, R. R., & Costa, P. T. J. (1994). The stability of personality: Observation and evaluations. *Current Directions in Psychological Science*, *3*, 173–175.

Measelle, J., John, O. P., Ablow, J., Cowan, P. A., & Cowan, C. P. (2004). Can children provide coherent, stable, and valid self-reports on the Big Five dimensions? A longitudinal study from ages 5–7. *Journal of Personality and Social Psychology*, *89*, 90–106.

Meyer-Lindenberg, A., & Weinberger, D. R. (2006). Intermediate phenotypes and genetic mechanisms of psychiatric disorders. *Nature Reviews Neuroscience*, *7*, 818–827.

Miech, R., Essex, M. J., & Goldsmith, H. H. (2001). Self-regulation as a mediator of the status-attainment process: Evidence from early childhood. *Social Education*, *74*, 102–120.

Miller, T. Q., Smith, T. W., Turner, C. W., Guijarro, M. L., & Hallet, A. J. (1996). A meta-analytic review of research on hostility and physical health. *Psychological Bulletin*, *119*, 322–348.

Moffitt, T. E., Caspi, A., Dickson, N., Silva, P. A., & Stanton, W. (1996). Childhood-onset versus adolescent-onset antisocial conduct in males: Natural history from age 3 to 18. *Development and Psychopathology*, *8*, 399–424.

Munafo, M. R., Clark, T. G., Moore, L. R., Payne, E., Walton, R., & Flint, J. (2003). Genetic polymorphisms and personality in healthy adults: A systematic review and meta-analysis. *Molecular Psychiatry*, *8*, 471–484.

Muris, P., & Ollendick, T. H. (2005). The role of temperament in the etiology of child psychopathology. *Clinical Child and Family Psychology Review*, *8*, 271–289.

Neitzel, C., & Stright, A. D. (2004). Parenting behaviors during child problem solving: The roles of child temperament, mother education and personality, and the problem-solving context. *International Journal of Behavioral Development*, *28*, 166–179.

Nettle, D. (2006). The evolution of personality variation in humans and other animals. *American Psychologist*, *61*, 622–631.

Nigg, J. T. (2000). Inhibition/disinhibition in developmental psychopathology: Views from cognitive and personality psychology and a working inhibition taxonomy. *Psychological Bulletin*, *126*, 220–246.

Nigg, J. T. (2006). Temperament and developmental psychopathology. *Journal of Child Psychology and Psychiatry*, *47*, 395–422.

Paris, J. (2005). Neurobiological dimensional models of personality: A review of the models of Cloninger, Depue, & Siever. *Journal of Personality Disorders*, *19*, 156–170.

Pike, A., & Atzaba-Poria, N. (2003). Do sibling and friend relationships share the same temperamental origins? *Journal of Child Psychology and Psychiatry*, *44*, 598–611.

Prinzie, P., Onghena, P., Hellinckx, W., Grietens, H., Ghesquiere, P., & Colpin, H. (2004). Parent and child personality characteristics as predictors of negative discipline and externalizing problem behaviour in children. *European Journal of Personality*, *18*, 73–102.

Putnam, S. P., & Stifter, C. A. (2005). Behavioral approach-inhibition in toddlers: Prediction from infancy, positive and negative affective components, and relations with behavior problems. *Child Development*, *76*, 212–226.

Rapee, R. M., Kennedy, S., Ingram, M., Edwards, S., & Sweeney, L. (2005). Prevention and early intervention of anxiety disorders in inhibited preschool children. *Journal of Consulting and Clinical Psychology*, *73*, 488–497.

Reiss, H. T., Capobianco, A., & Tsai, F. T. (2002). Finding the person in relationships. *Journal of Personality*, *70*, 813–850.

Roberts, B. W., & DelVecchio, W. F. (2000). The rank-order consistency of personality traits from childhood to old age: A quantitative review of longitudinal studies. *Psychological Bulletin*, *126*, 25–30.

Roberts, B. W., Walton, K., & Viechtbauer, W. (2006). Patterns in mean-level change in personality traits across the life-course: A meta-analysis of longitudinal studies. *Psychological Bulletin*, *132*, 1–25.

Robins, R. W., Caspi, A., & Moffitt, T. E. (2002). It's not just who you're with, it's who you are: Personality and relationship experiences across multiple relationships. *Journal of Personality*, *70*, 925–964.

Rothbart, M. K., & Bates, J. E. (2006). Temperament. In W. Damon, & R. Lerner (Editors in Chief) & N. Eisenberg (Volume Ed.), *Handbook of child psychology*. Vol. 3. *Social, emotional, and personality development* (6th ed., pp. 99–166). New York: Wiley.

Rozanski, A., Blumenthal, J. A., & Kaplan, J. (1999). Impact of psychological factors on the pathogenesis of cardiovascular disease and implications for therapy. *Circulation*, *99*, 2217.

Rubin, K. H., Bukowski, W. M., & Parker, J. G. (2006). Peer interactions, relationships, and groups. In W. Damon, & R. Lerner (Editors in Chief) & N. Eisenberg (Volume Ed.), *Handbook of child psychopathology*. Vol. 3. *Social, emotional, and personality development* (6th ed., pp. 571–645). New York: Wiley.

Scarr, S., & McCartney, K. (1983). How people make their own environments: A theory of genotype to environment effects. *Child Development*, *54*, 424–435.

Schneider, B., Smith, D. B., Taylor, S., & Fleenor, J. (1998). Personality and organizations: A test of the homogeneity of personality hypothesis. *Journal of Applied Psychology*, *83*, 4.

Sen, S., Burmeister, D., & Ghosh, D. (2004). Meta-analysis of the association between a serotonin transporter promotor polymorphism (5-HTTLPR) and anxiety related traits. *American Journal of Medical Genetics, Part B: Neuropsychiatric Genetics*, *127B*, 85–89.

Shanahan, M. J., & Flaherty, B. P. (2001). Dynamic patterns of time use in adolescence. *Child Development*, *72*, 385–401.

Shiner, R. L. (2000). Linking childhood personality with adaptation: Evidence for continuity and change across time into late adolescence. *Journal of Personality and Social Psychology*, *78*, 310–325.

Shiner, R. L. (2008). Personality disorders in adolescence. In E. J. Mash, & R. A. Barkley (Eds.), *Assessment of childhood disorders* (4th ed., pp. 781–816). New York: Guilford Press.

Shiner, R. L., & Caspi, A. (2003). Personality differences in childhood and adolescence: Measurement, development, and consequences. *Journal of Child Psychology and Psychiatry*, *44*, 2–32.

Shiner, R. L., Masten, A. S., & Roberts, J. M. (2003). Childhood personality foreshadows adult personality and life outcomes two decades later. *Journal of Personality*, *71*, 1145–1170.

Shiner, R. L., Masten, A. S., & Tellegen, A. (2002). A developmental perspective on personality in emerging adulthood: Childhood antecedents and concurrent adaptation. *Journal of Personality and Social Psychology*, *83*, 1165–1177.

Slutske, W. S., Caspi, A., Moffitt, T. E., & Poulton, R. (2005). Personality and problem gambling. *Archives of General Psychiatry*, *62*, 1–8.

Smith, T. W., & Gallo, L. (2001). Personality traits as risk factors for physical illness. In A. Baum, T. Revenson, & J. Singer (Eds.), *Handbook of Health Psychology* (pp. 139–174). Hillsdale, NJ: Laurence Erlbaum.

Smith, T. W., & Spiro, A. (2002). Personality, health, and aging: Prolegomenon for the next generation. *Journal of Research in Personality*, *36*, 363–394.

Snyder, M., & Stukas, A. (1999). Interpersonal processes: The interplay of cognitive, motivational, and behavioral activities in social interaction. *Annual Review of Psychology*, *73*, 273–303.

Suls, J., & Martin, R. (2005). The daily life of the garden-variety neurotic: reactivity, stressor exposure, mood spillover, and maladaptive coping. *Journal of Personality*, *73*, 1485–1510.

Tackett, J. L. (2006). Evaluating models of the personality–psychopathology relationship in children and adolescents. *Clinical Psychology Review*, *26*, 584–599.

Thomas, A., Chess, S., & Birch, H. (1968). *Temperament and behavior disorders in children*. New York: New York University Press.

Thomas, A., Chess, S., Birch, H., Hertzig, M., & Korn, S. (1963). *Behavioral individuality in early childhood*. New York: New York University Press.

Watson, D., & Clark, L. A. (1997). Extraversion and its positive emotional core. In J. Hogan, J. Johnson, & S. Briggs (Eds.), *Handbook of Personality Psychology* (pp. 767–793). San Diego, CA: Academic Press.

Watson, D., Clark, L. A., Weber, K., Assenheimer, J. S., Strauss, M. E., & McCormick, R. A. (1995). Testing a tripartite model: II. Exploring the symptom structure of anxiety and depression in student, adult, and patient samples. *Journal of Abnormal Psychology*, *104*, 15–25.

Widiger, T. A., Verheul, R., & van den Brink, W. (1999). Personality and psychopathology. In L. A. Pervin, & O. P. John (Eds.), *Handbook of personality: Theory and research* (pp. 347–366). New York: Guilford.

Wills, T. A., & Dishion, T. J. (2004). Temperament and adolescent substance abuse: A transactional analysis of emerging self-control. *Journal of Clinical Child and Adolescent Psychology*, *33*, 69–81.

15 Sociocultural/Ethnic Groups and Psychopathology

Anula Nikapota and Michael Rutter

Most modern industrialized nations have populations that are markedly heterogeneous with respect to ethnicity, first language, religion, socioeconomic status and cultural traditions. In this chapter, we seek to consider the implications of these concepts and these groupings for an understanding of psychopathological mechanisms and for the provision of services.

It will be appreciated that the terms themselves imply a rather diverse range of mediating processes. Thus, socioeconomic status and poverty both tend to put the emphasis on the constraints or opportunities provided by the broader external social and physical environment. In support, there is extensive evidence that social disadvantage and poverty are associated with increased risks for a multiplicity of health and psychological functioning outcomes (Bradley & Corwyn, 2002; Evans, 2004; Rutter & Madge, 1976). In the past, there was often an assumption that it was an absolute lack of resources that provided the risks, but there is now increasing evidence that inequalities, rather than absolute level, may provide the risk (Wilkinson, 2005; Wilkinson & Marmot, 2006).

A somewhat related set of issues applies to the observation that there are marked geographical variations in indices of physical health/illness, psychopathology and crime – differences that remain surprisingly persistent over time despite substantial turnovers in population (Rutter, 1981; Rutter, Giller, & Hagell, 1998; Rutter & Quinton, 1977; Townsend, Whitehead, & Davidson, 1992).

Finally, there is the rather different concept of culture – a term that is applied to social groups that are characterized by shared values, practices and traditions (Greenfield, Keller, Fuligni *et al.*, 2003; Shweder, Goodnow, Hatano *et al.*, 1997). Such groups may be defined on the basis of ethnicity, religion, nationality, geography or indeed any other feature that leads to group identification that provides a commonality among members of the group. The implication is not one of advantage or disadvantage, but rather one of meaningful *differences* in styles of life or styles of thinking. In this chapter, we seek to consider the varied meanings and implications associated with these concepts. The starting point needs to be evidence on social groups.

Social Groups

Humans are social beings with a strong tendency to form social groups whenever they come together for some perceived social purpose. Such groups typically involve strong loyalties and negative feelings about other groups. The classic "Robbers' Cave" experiment undertaken many years ago (Sherif, Harvey, White *et al.*, 1961) showed how quickly such social groupings arose when young people were brought together in a summer camp and divided into two competing teams. Intense feelings and identifications developed rapidly. This occurred despite the fact that those in one group had no more in common with each other than they had with those in the other group. The brevity of their acquaintance did not prevent strong group identification and strong rivalries from developing. The process was shown in this case through a quasi-experimental approach, but it is evident naturalistically in numerous other contexts. Thus, we see the same phenomenon in the fighting between supporters of competing soccer teams, and in the national rivalries in the Olympic Games, despite the fact that it is supposed to be about the success of individuals rather than the success of nations.

The supposition is that people are much influenced in their attitudes and behavior by the mores, or ethos, of the social groups within which they function. A further classic study that illustrates this effect is that undertaken by Christensen (1960), who showed that the effects of a premarital pregnancy on the timing of subsequent marriage varied markedly according to the sexual mores of the community. An early example of an experimental approach to people's susceptibility to social group influences is provided by Asch's (1952, 1956) studies involving simple decisions about the length of lines. Research accomplices were instructed to give a unanimous judgment that was patently wrong from time to time. In just over one-third of cases individuals succumbed to the implicit group pressure to make a wrong judgment. On the other hand, when even one other accomplice agreed with the subject, the compliance dropped to just 5%. More recent research has taken much further the analysis of influences on the extent to which inter-group interactions differ from inter-individual interactions

Rutter's Child and Adolescent Psychiatry, 5th edition. Edited by M. Rutter, D. Bishop, D. Pine, S. Scott, J. Stevenson, E. Taylor and A. Thapar. © 2008 Blackwell Publishing, ISBN: 978-1-4051-4549-7.

(Wildschut, Pinter, Vevea *et al.*, 2003) but the basic point that there are group effects has been well documented.

The possible relevance for psychopathology and for psychological functioning more generally is evident in the effects of school ethos on pupils' scholastic progress and behavior, and the effects of peer group influences on the same. In both cases, the basic research challenge has been to determine the extent to which the social group truly has an environmentally mediated effect on individuals, compared with the extent to which the apparent effect is just a consequence of the characteristics of the individuals who happen to make up such groups. Longitudinal studies have been required to test these competing alternatives. Thus, Rutter, Maughan, Mortimore *et al.* (1979) examined the effects of school ethos by taking account of variations in the intake to schools. Substantial effects were found for both school ethos (as determined by school policy and practice) and school balance (meaning the extent to which the pupil body was made up of predominantly advantaged or disadvantaged children).

Peer group effects have somewhat similarly been examined by determining changes in people's behavior over the time period extending from before to after joining a peer group (Kandel, 1978; Rowe, Wouldbroun, & Gulley, 1994). The findings show strong enduring effects of prior individual differences but also moderate effects of social group membership. A related strategy has been to check whether young people who join delinquent gangs commit more crimes when part of a gang than they do when outside such groups (Thornberry, 1998). The findings have shown that they do – indicating that the ethos and activities of the social group have effects on the behavior of individuals in them (Lacourse, Nagin, Tremblay *et al.*, 2003). The body of research extends far beyond the few illustrative examples provided here, and it is fair to conclude that the reality of social group effects has been shown, even if debate continues on their relative importance in varying circumstances (Rutter, 1999).

Culture

Against that background, we need to turn to the concept of culture. It has, in common with social groups, the feature of shared experiences and meanings that result in values, beliefs and practices that are distinctively different from those found in other cultures (Greenfield *et al.*, 2003). It differs with respect to the fact that cultures tend to be thought of in terms of groupings that we are born into, rather than ones that we choose to join. Thus, culture is often viewed as a function of ethnicity, race or nationality. This leads to an implicit expectation that each of us is part of just one culture that shapes our personal identity as well as our attitudes and behavior. Research findings indicate the highly misleading nature of these assumptions (Rutter & Tienda, 2005). Not only are each of the defining features complex and multifaceted, but also it is common for individuals to feel part of, and identify with, several different cultures. Moreover, it is also common for people to identify with some aspects of a culture but not others.

Thus, drawing on the large-scale British National Survey of ethnic minorities in Britain in the mid-1990s, Modood (2005) noted that many second-generation immigrants identified both with being British and with some aspect of their ethnic origin. However, the latter was not necessarily focused on the geographical origin from which their parents came. For many Caribbeans, one of their identifications was with being Black, and with many of the South Asians religion was the identifying feature. Also, over time, there was a reduced participation in distinctive cultural practices. For example, younger South Asians, when compared with their elders, were less likely to speak to family members in the South Asian language, to attend a place of worship regularly or to have an arranged marriage. Nevertheless, this did not necessarily mean any reduced identification with their cultural background. Modood drew a distinction between cultural practices and associational identity, in which the latter took the form of pride in one's origins, identification with certain group labels and sometimes political assertiveness.

Rumbaut (2005), in his major Child of Immigrants longitudinal study in Southern California and South Florida, made somewhat similar points but also noted that ethnic self-identities differed substantially according to where the immigrant parents came from. A further complicating feature, to a greater extent in the UK than in the USA, is the high frequency of intermarriage across some ethnic groups. For example, among the British-born with a partner, half of the Caribbean men and one-third of the Caribbean women had a White partner. That was very much less common among Pakistani and Bangladeshi men, and very few South Asian women had a White partner. Furthermore, it was evident that Asians in Scotland, like other Scots, tended to consider themselves in terms of their Scottishness rather than their Britishness. It is very clear that to assume that anyone is a member of just one cultural group is a highly misleading oversimplification.

It is also clear that cultural identities and social group allegiances often change over time. For example, an early study by Lieberman (1956) showed that taking on a new role could change attitudes; thus, workers who initially held much the same attitudes towards management came to hold different ones when becoming foremen or shop stewards. Siegel and Siegel (1957) showed much the same phenomenon and Newcombe (1943, 1963) described both the persistence and change in the attitudes of girls from "conservative" families who attended a "liberal" college community. In the same way, it must be expected that as second-generation immigrants experience education and careers that differ from those of their parents, they may adopt different values and attitudes. Cultural identifications are influenced both by personal experiences of a positive kind and by discriminatory responses from host communities. In addition, it is obvious that the all too common experience of war and civil conflict may both increase identifications and disrupt cultures. To an even greater extent, the pandemic of AIDS in Africa has hugely altered cultural context, family styles and caretaking patterns for many children in Africa.

Clearly, that does not imply that there are no meaningful cultural differences. Thus, it is obvious that cultures vary in the extent to which they use arranged marriages, emphasize the importance of the extended family or regard women as having a lower status and lesser rights than men, in the extent to which children are allowed autonomy, in dietary practices, in the use of fostering and other forms of child care, and in concepts of illness and agency – to mention but a few of a long list of features. Similarly, although systematic studies have found negligible correlations between perceived national stereotypes and measured personality characteristics (Terraciano, Abdel-Khalek, Ádám *et al.*, 2005), there are national differences in styles of behavior – as is obvious in terms of times of eating, having a siesta, as well as in collectivistic versus individualistic orientations.

The use of the term "culture" implies that effects on individuals derive from the values, beliefs and practices of the cultural groups. As we have noted, such effects are real. Nevertheless, it is necessary to consider the alternative mediating mechanisms. Thus, apparent effects may stem from the broader societal context rather than from features within the cultural group. Some years ago the concept of a "culture of poverty" was put forward (Lewis, 1968) – the suggestion being that the poor behaved in ways that created a self-defeating culture that perpetuated their problems. The concept fell from favor both because of a lack of supporting evidence and a growing awareness of the societal constraints provided by discriminatory housing and benefits policies. Thus, Wilson (1987) argued that many of the supposed adverse consequences of being African-American in a predominantly White society stemmed from low socioeconomic status rather than from their ethnicity as such. He pointed out the substantial expansion over time of an African-American middle class, as well as the continuing disadvantage of the underprivileged living in ghettoes (which applied to a far higher proportion of African-Americans than White people).

With respect to discrimination it is important to appreciate, too, the indirect as well as the direct effects. The latter were well demonstrated through experimental studies examining discrimination in housing and employment (Brown & Gay, 1986; Daniel, 1968). The former are more subtle but may have even greater effects because they impinge so unmistakably on individuals. For example, it could be argued that it was justifiable and rational for the police to stop and search young Black males in inner city areas rather than elderly White females in rural areas – because the crime rate in the former far exceeds the latter. Nevertheless, the consequence will be discriminatory because law-abiding individuals in the former group will suffer much more frequent police harassment than law-abiding individuals in the latter group. Equally, elderly White female criminals will escape detection more often than young Black male criminals. In brief, whenever group characteristics, rather than individual behavior, are used to justify official interventions, the effect will be unavoidably discriminatory.

Cultures and Community

Culture is sometimes extended to the related, but different, concept of community. In many countries, there is a quite marked tendency for new immigrants to choose to live in communities where there are already many people who come from the same country of origin. On the positive side, this has often provided a sense of both practical and social support that helps the newcomers to settle in their new country, and also helps them retain a sense of cultural identity (Bhugra & Becker, 2005). There has also been a negative side in so far as the areas in which such communities live have often been socially disadvantaged and have involved poor quality, overcrowded living conditions. The social support may have come at a price. A further consideration is that the key identifying characteristic of a community may be in terms of what it lacks rather than what it possesses. Thus, the study of neighborhoods in Chicago showed that the key risk factor for crime lay in the social disorganization and lack of community cohesion (Sampson, Raudenbush, & Earls, 1997). Other research has pointed to similar conclusions (Brooks-Gunn, Duncan, & Aber, 1997), and has also raised the possibility of the role of environmental hazards (Gee & Payne-Sturges, 2004). It is not appropriate to conceptualize these lacks as representing any kind of culture.

Religion

In some communities a person's religion is of little or no consequence, whereas in others it is the crucial defining characteristic. Thus, within academia in the UK only quite a small minority of people actively practice any religion and most of the time people are not even aware of what religious background others come from. That does not mean that their background is unimportant to them. For example, for many Jews, Quakers, Catholics or Muslims, although they have rejected the formal and structural aspects of religious beliefs and practices of their youth, nevertheless the values remain important and so does their cultural heritage. By contrast, there are other communities where religion is perceived as the defining characteristic. The perception may have been fueled by political and economic issues but nevertheless leads to bitter tensions – such as the rift between Catholics and Protestants in Northern Ireland, the riots and divisions that have occurred from time to time between Hindus and Muslims in Asia and between Jews and Muslims in the Middle East. However, these bitter rivalry groupings are by no means restricted to formal religions as ordinarily recognized. Thus, they have been devastating in their effects with respect to the clashes between Sunni and Shiite groups in Iraq and between tribes and sects of all kinds all over the world. Again, however, we need to emphasize the huge heterogeneity within each of these groupings. There is a tendency sometimes to identify particular religions with their fundamentalist extremes, despite the fact that the great majority of people of that religion do not support those extremes and may, indeed, be quite strongly opposed to their views and actions. Nevertheless, clashes between religions have been responsible for some of the worst atrocities in history (although other ideologies, such as exemplified by the Nazi Holocaust or the Stalinist and Maoist slaughters have been at least as destructive). The damage comes from the groups, whether religious or irreligious, regarding themselves as superior to all others and thus having the right to impose their will on everyone else. Inevitably, these clashes constitute an unavoidable background to clinical practice in countries that are multicultural and include diversity of religions (that is, most countries in the world today).

Despite these negative aspects of major religions, it is still clear that religion can provide a powerful sense of support to individuals, as well as having positive effects on their values (Josephson & Dell, 2004; Josephson & Petitt, 2004). It has been argued, not very convincingly in view of the conflicting evidence, that in the USA, religious belief fosters prosocial behavior and may therefore protect against some forms of psychopathology (Mabe & Josephson, 2004). Sometimes this will be the case but clearly there are important exceptions.

Ethnicity

The standard definition of ethnicity is that it refers to population groups "sharing a distinctive cultural and historical tradition, often associated with race, nationality, or religion, by which the group identifies itself and others recognize it" (*Shorter Oxford English Dictionary*, 2002). As is obvious from the definition, this leaves rather open which aspect should be given precedence in deciding ethnicity. It has become standard practice in both national statistics and research surveys in the UK or USA to assign ethnicity solely on the basis of the ethnic description that individuals attribute to themselves (Rutter & Tienda, 2005). The self-identification approach involves five main problems. First, at least as operated officially, people are forced to select from a predetermined set of categories that involve consequences. For example, in many countries, people of a mixed ethnic background are automatically treated as "non-White." Logically, of course, they might just as well be classified as "non-Black," or whatever terminology is being used for non-Caucasian groups. This may, or may not, coincide with the person's own concepts.

Second, the categories used to deal with ethnicity differ strikingly across countries. Thus, "Hispanics" constitute a very large, highly diverse and rapidly growing segment of the US population but it is one so small in the UK that its existence is not even recognized. Conversely, there is a very large Asian community in the UK that is subdivided along religious lines or lines of national origin, there being no direct parallel within the USA. Within England, religious affiliation as Catholic or Protestant is seldom consequential, whereas in Northern Ireland it is the defining aspect of group membership for many people. Within those of Asian background in the UK, country of origin (e.g., India, Pakistan or Sri Lanka), community (e.g., Gujerati or Punjabi) or religion (e.g., Hindu, Muslim, Sikh, Buddhist) may be crucially important.

Language is sometimes a very important differentiator; thus in Canada it matters greatly whether someone is Francophone or Anglophone, and in Belgium it matters whether someone is Flemish or French-speaking. By contrast, within England for most people it matters little what a person's first language is. In large cosmopolitan cities such as London, New York and Los Angeles the diversity of languages spoken at home is simply enormous. Census categories are often rejected by subnational populations. Within the UK, many Scottish and Welsh people clearly see themselves as meaningfully distinct ethnic groups on the grounds of both language and a different cultural heritage, but Welsh and Scottish is seldom included in different ethnic categories. In countries where there is not a large immigrant grouping, only national identity may be included in statistics but the reality is often that regional identities may be more important in terms of identity. For example, in India one is Punjabi, Gujerati or Tamil, and these identities include differences in language and culture but not always religion, although within these groupings religion may be the most important other influence for some.

Third, the use of a single category presupposes that ethnicity can be reduced to a single concept and also that designation should be categorical rather than dimensional.

Fourth, the categorical approach presupposes that each person has only a single ethnic identity, whereas research findings make it clear that many people have more than one, and indeed may have several, the relative importance of which varies by context. There is nothing contradictory in a person considering themselves simultaneously as "Black" (if that is the color of their skin), Glaswegian (if that is the part of the country in which they have grown up) and Hindu (if that is their religion).

The last problem is that a self-descriptive approach presupposes that it is each person's self-concept that matters most, whereas, at least for some psychosocial features, it may be the response of others that is most decisive.

The social construction of ethnicity may differ quite markedly from self-identifications. For example, in the UK, society's designation of "Black" includes dark-skinned Asians as well as Africans, despite the fact that neither see themselves as similar, and their historical and cultural backgrounds are as different as their genetic make-up (Rutter & Tienda, 2005). In parallel fashion, the insulting term "Paki" is applied to persons who originated from Bangladesh and India just as much as those who came from Pakistan, thus ignoring a host of differences among these groups, not the least of which is religion. Sometimes ethnicity is equated with social disadvantage or poverty. Of course, it is the case that some ethnic groups are disadvantaged in relation to the society in which they live, but that is by no means always the case. Thus, on the whole, people of Asian origin have been generally successful in the countries to which they migrated. Moreover, although research has tended to equate ethnicity with minority status, ethnically privileged groups are no less affected by ethnicity issues, as is just beginning to be acknowledged (Quintana, Aboud, Chao *et al.*, 2006).

Race

The equation of ethnicity with race has been viewed as controversial by many people. The reasons are not difficult to find, because racial concepts have so often been seen as fixed categories and to convey implications of inferiority or superiority. Nevertheless, the major racial/ethnic groups as identified in census statistics do differ, on average, in genetic make-up. Interestingly, and importantly, the genetic differences do not necessarily coincide with the cultural constructs of ethnicity (Rutter & Tienda, 2005). For example, some Asian groups cluster genetically with Europeans rather than with East Asians. Also, some ethnic groups, most especially Hispanics, are genetically admixed to a major degree. Most crucially, a high proportion of most populations have a heritage that includes a mixture of genetically different racial groups.

The positive side of a genetic focus on race differences is that there are some reasonably well-documented examples of race-related genetic differences that have psychopathological implications. For example, it is well known that some individuals of Asiatic origin have a genetic variant that means that they get a very unpleasant flushing reaction to the ingestion of alcohol – a reaction that has been found to be protective in relation to alcoholism (see chapter 36). The APOE-4 allele is known to carry a substantially increased risk of Alzheimer disease and not only does the frequency of this allele vary across race (being substantially lower among Japanese than African-Americans) but the strength of its association with Alzheimer disease varies hugely, from a factor of 33 in Japanese to 50 in Whites but only 6 in African-Americans (see chapter 23). The reasons for this variation remain unknown at present, but they are likely to have clinical implications.

There is some evidence of racial variations in the distribution of the allelic variations of the serotonin transporter gene that has been found to involve gene–environment interplay with respect to the risk of depression. Widom & Brzustowicz (2006) found that the moderating effect of the MAOA genotype on the effects of child abuse/neglect on violence/antisocial behavior in later life applied to Whites but not to non-Whites. It remains uncertain whether this reflects ethnic differences in the effects of polymorphism on MAOA expression, or other background genetic influences or the meaning of the childhood experiences. There is also limited evidence that there are racial differences in response to therapeutic medication (with regard to both efficacy and side-effects). This has led to a call for developing drugs specifically for certain racial groups. Although clearly there are important advantages in tailoring medication to individual variations in drug response, there are substantial problems in doing this solely on the basis of perceived ethnicity. That is because most individuals have a mixture of racial backgrounds and because the relevant variations in drug response are better assessed in terms of measured genes rather than perceived ethnicity.

With these broad themes as a background, six key issues need to be considered:

1 Variations in rates of disorder across sociocultural/ethnic groups;
2 The possible existence of culture-specific mental disorders;
3 Varied manifestations of disorder across different groups;
4 Similarities or differences in risk factors across groups;
5 The universal meaning of measures; and
6 The unacceptability of culturally accepted behaviors that cause serious risks.

Variations in Rates of Disorder Across Sociocultural/Ethnic Groups

Epidemiological studies, mainly based on questionnaires or structured interviews (Weisz, McCarty, Eastman *et al.*, 1997), have generally shown that rates and patterns of disorder are broadly similar across groups, although there are differences in detail. Weisz *et al.*'s (1997) comparison of psychopathology in Thailand and the USA indicated that differences in perception and expectation had quite marked effects on rates of reported disturbance, which had service implications, but the overall prevalence of psychopathology differed little. The study by Luk, Leung, & Ho (2002) brought out a similar point in relation to hyperkinetic disorder, for which there were contradictory reports on whether the rate was higher or lower in Chinese children. The research team spanned Hong Kong and the UK and examined the question by using observational and psychometric measures as well as questionnaire and interview data. The findings were illuminating in showing that although teachers in Hong Kong tended to rate slightly more children as hyperactive than was the case in the UK, observational data suggested that, if anything, the true difference ran in the opposite direction.

Nevertheless, there are forms of psychopathology or psychological functioning that show substantial differences among ethnic groups. First, findings in both the USA (Morenoff, 2005) and the UK (Smith, 2005) noted that antisocial behavior is substantially higher in African-Caribbeans and African-Americans. Conversely, offending rates tend to be low among Pakistanis and Bangladeshis in the UK and among Hispanics in the USA. It is clear that social disadvantage as such cannot be the explanation for the high crime rate, and racial discrimination does not seem to be the main explanation either, because in the UK racial discrimination is high against both African-Caribbeans and Subcontinental Asians, and yet the crime rate of the former is high whereas that of the latter is low. There are substantial problems in measurement and it is likely that some of the differences are caused by the way that crimes are processed and dealt with, but that does not appear to be sufficient explanation. The challenge is to ensure that appropriate measurement is used to compare rates of antisocial behavior but, equally, there is the challenge of determining what factors might be responsible.

Second, Taylor Gibbs (2005) has drawn attention to the curious paradox that, despite their greater exposure to psychosocial adversities, both Black and Hispanic youth in the USA have rates of suicide that are lower than that of their more advantaged White counterparts. Interestingly, however, the patterns in Black people and Hispanics differ. The findings for Black people indicate that their rate of depressive disorder and of suicidal ideation, as well as their rate of suicide, is low in comparison with White people. The main issue, therefore, is why all of those rates are relatively low. The situation with Hispanics is different in that their rates of depression and of suicidal ideation are *not* low, despite their low rate of suicide. Accordingly, for them the query is why their relatively high rate of suicidal ideation does not result in a correspondingly high rate of suicide. No good answers are as yet available and recent data suggest that the pattern may be changing, but the questions could be tackled by appropriate research.

Third, there are ethnic differences in educational attainments in both the UK (Maughan, 2005) and the USA (Hirschman & Lee, 2005). In the UK, scholastic attainments tend to be highest for African-Asians and Indians, intermediate for Pakistanis and White people, somewhat lower for Black Caribbeans and lowest of all for Bangladeshis. All ethnic groups have shown educational gains in relation to their immigrant parents, but these have been greatest for African-Asians and least for Bangladeshis. Black Caribbeans have experienced the highest rate of exclusion from school and also the highest rate of teacher–child conflict. Some have sought to explain the ethnic differences in scholastic attainment (as also in antisocial behavior) in terms of the high rate of single parent households in children of Caribbean immigrants, but the data in the UK do not support that conclusion.

Stevenson, Lee, Chen *et al.* (1990) undertook a comparative study of elementary school children in the USA, Taiwan and Japan. As found by others, attainments tended to be higher in the Chinese and Japanese groups but the groups also differed in terms of family involvement and expectations with respect to academic achievement and their explanations for success or failure. The Chinese and Japanese mothers tended to stress the importance of hard work whereas US mothers gave greater emphasis to innate ability. The study suggested the likely importance of family influences but other explanations are possible, and the study is mainly of value in indicating the utility of comparisons across groups.

Fourth, it has been found that the rate of schizophrenia is substantially higher among African-Caribbeans living in the UK than in either African-Caribbeans living in the Caribbean or White people living in the UK (Jones & Fung, 2005). The ethnic difference has been shown not to be an artifact of diagnostic practice or referral pattern and the difference is one that has been also found in the Netherlands. The elevated rate is not just confined to schizophrenia because, to a lesser degree, it also applies to mania, but there is no differential in minor psychiatric morbidity. Findings so far suggest that the higher rates of psychoses are not a result of differential migration or early brain injury and it appears that the causal influences are likely to lie in some aspect of psychosocial experiences associated with living in the UK for African-Caribbeans, but quite what these factors are has yet to be determined.

The strong message that derives from these findings is that the differences provide a means of testing competing hypotheses about possible mediating causal mechanisms. All too often, discussions about ethnicity are seen as politically unacceptable because they are so prone to degenerate into expressions of prejudice and stereotype. While that is clearly the case, it is important to recognize that such differences need to be investigated in a sensitive and discriminating way in order to understand how the differences, if confirmed, come about. The findings are likely to have implications that extend well beyond the particular ethnic groups that have been studied so far. What applies in such ethnic minorities is very likely to apply to Caucasian groups as well.

Culture-Specific Syndromes

An interest in the possibility of culture-specific syndromes first arose from the reporting of psychopathological patterns in adults in Asian and African communities that did not seem to fit the criteria for psychiatric disorders as conceptualized in standard classification systems largely developed from studies in industrialized western societies. The key question was whether these represented different manifestations of common disorders or, rather, unusual syndromes deriving from causal factors rarely encountered in western societies. A study by Guarnaccia, Martinez, Ramirez *et al.* (2005) illustrates well how the issue can be tackled. They focused on the syndrome of "ataque de nervios" – a pattern first recognized in Hispanic adults that involved screaming, crying and trembling, associated with aggressive behavior and a strong feeling of being out of control. The pattern often seemed to have been precipitated by some acute stressful experience. Guarnaccia *et al.* (2005) investigated the occurrence of these features in two samples of 4- to 17-year-old children in Puerto Rico – a general population sample and a clinical sample. The measures used included questions on the specific features of "ataque de nervios," as well as the psychopathological features associated with western diagnostic concepts. In brief, 9% of children in the community sample and 26% in the clinical sample reported the specific features, these were associated with a family history of the same, and they were also associated with depressive, anxiety and disruptive behaviors, and with psychosocial impairment, as found in western populations. It was concluded that "ataque de nervios" represented a culturally influenced expression of emotional distress, associated with affective and anxiety disorders, especially panic. The findings suggested that it was unlikely that the syndrome was fundamentally different from disorders that are highly prevalent in western societies, but they also highlighted that, in contrast to the usual concept of panic disorder, the symptoms often seemed to have a specific precipitant (Guarnaccia, Canino, Rubio-Stipec *et al.*, 1993).

Early studies had suggested that anorexia nervosa and bulimia nervosa might constitute culture-bound syndromes because of their rarity in non-western societies (Cummins, Simmons, & Zane, 2005; Keel & Klump, 2003; Lester, 2004). Systematic evidence suggests that these eating disorders are actually more prevalent in non-western societies than the early claims suggested. Nevertheless, cultural influences do appear to be operative. For example, there is one study of the effect of the introduction of television in Fiji on binge-eating and purging at a normal weight (Becker, Burwell, Gilman *et al.*, 2002). It has been pointed out that self-starvation can occur in any context, but binge-eating requires large stores of readily edible food and these would often not be available in developing countries where famine is all too common. The various studies indicate that there may also be differences in the particular patterning of eating disorders in different cultures, and it is important to pay attention to these when considering what should be regarded as the essential core of such eating disorders. Nevertheless, eating disorders do not appear to constitute culture-specific syndromes.

Dissociative identity disorder (previously termed multiple personality) seems a peculiarly North American phenomenon, although isolated cases have been reported elsewhere. Questionnaire studies have shown that features purported to index dissociative identity do occur in European samples, even though the diagnosis is made much less frequently (Gast, Rodewald, Nickel *et al.*, 2001; Lipsanen, Korkeila, Peltola *et al.*, 2004). To what extent the questionnaire responses truly reflect the postulated diagnostic category remains uncertain and, in any case, the validity of the diagnostic concept remains controversial (Merskey, 2000). Also, rates of so-called hysterical (conversion) disorders have varied greatly over time in keeping with cultural mores (Merskey, 2000). Very few data are available for any firm conclusions to be drawn, but the implication seems to be that these manifestations of psychopathology probably are influenced by culture, but whether or not they constitute culture-specific disorders of a meaningfully distinctive kind is much more questionable.

Cultural findings, like genetic findings (see chapter 23), serve to alert us to the fact that the current classification systems provide only a rough guide to the best conceptualization and grouping of disorders (see chapter 2). It would be a mistake to force all disorders into the currently prevailing rules of diagnosis, but, equally, there is no good evidence for culture-specific syndromes. Rather, we need to use the findings to ask questions about what should be the key criteria for particular disorders.

Cultural/Religious Beliefs and Psychopathology

A key clinical issue concerns the interpretation of phenomena that might be caused by mental disorder or might be normal in the individual's own culture or religion. For example, religious rituals can readily become the focus of compulsions in obsessive-compulsive disorders (Greenberg & Wiesner, 2004). The Pentecostal "speaking in tongues" may appear as thought disorder. Thinking that you are possessed by evil spirits may appear delusional. There is both the danger of assuming psychopathology in ignorance of the relevant cultural beliefs and the danger of assuming normality when in reality the phenomena reflect mental disorder. In these circumstances, it may be helpful to seek the views of an experienced person in the relevant culture or religion. Often it will be found that there is a recognition that the phenomena in the referred patient are unusual and peculiar even within the culture or religion. There is also the clinical dilemma with respect to the situation in which someone has become increasingly religious to the extent that it is interfering with daily life or leading to clashes within the family. Is this "normal," albeit unusually strong, religious devotion, or is it an indicator of psychopathology? There are no easy guidelines for making these differentiations and the main need is to be aware of the possibilities, to be sensitive to the specifics of the features in question and to consult with community or religious leaders when in doubt.

A further clinical dilemma, especially with the ultra-orthodox in any religion, concerns the religious reservations about the propriety of discussing certain matters and a worry lest this could lead to a clinical questioning of religious dogma (Greenberg & Wiesner, 2004). The needs in this situation are similar to those regarding differential diagnosis.

Varied Manifestations of Disorder Across Different Groups

Some 30 years ago, Kleinman (1977) drew attention to the finding that, in some societies, emotional disturbance is often reported in terms of somatic symptoms rather than reports of altered mood. He went on to argue (Kleinman, 1987) that it could not be assumed that psychiatric categories and diagnoses have the same meaning when carried over to a new cultural context. The point is an important one but there is a danger of assuming an outmoded dichotomy between psyche and soma, with the expectation that the psychiatric category should truly be defined in mood terms. That ignores two key features. First, mood changes are accompanied by somatic changes (both in terms of complaints and physiological alterations). It is not that one causes the other, but rather that both are part of the same phenomenon. Second, the notion that children do not express mood in somatic terms in western cultures is obviously wrong. It is a commonplace for emotional disturbances to be reported by children in terms of headache, stomach ache and the like. It is clinically most important to recognize the range of ways in which emotional disturbances may be experienced, reported and given particular attributions. The prevailing psychiatric classifications accord a priority to the mood features, and that makes good sense, but we need to appreciate the various ways in which these may be expressed.

Similarities or Differences in Risk Factors Across Groups

In so far as evidence is available, it appears that almost all the risk and protective factors that operate in one group operate somewhat similarly in other groups. It appears that child abuse and neglect are serious risk factors in all populations. Similarly, committed personal relationships that are continuous over time, matter in all cultures. Social groups pressures are universally operative as are the benefits of interactive play and conversation. Equally, separation from a close caring relationship is stressful for all children. On the other hand, there are some differences that alert one to the dangers of drawing wrong conclusions about the nature of the mediating mechanisms. For example, it might be assumed that the high rate of single parent families in African-Caribbean communities in the UK or in African-American families in the USA would be a major risk factor for adverse psychopathological outcomes. However, the evidence suggests that actually this is not the case (Maughan, 2005; Morenoff, 2005). This probably does not mean that family influences are radically different across cultures, but rather that the structure of the family is not the major mediating variable; rather it is the quality of relationships and care that has implications for psychopathology. The complicating feature is that the associations between quality and structure may well vary across cultures. It may also mean that the social selection factors that lead to single parenthood are not the same in all groups.

The commonality in major risk factors across groups does not necessarily mean that there are no variations in the way the mechanisms operate. For example, Pachter, Auinger, Palmer *et al.* (2006) compared White, Black and Latino families with children aged 6–9 years in the US National Longitudinal Study of Youth. Much the same risk factors operated in all three groups, but whereas the risk effects of maternal depression were partially mediated through parenting in the White and Latino samples, they were direct and unmediated through parenting practices in the Black sample. Similarly, neighborhood effects were present in the White and Black samples but not significant in the Latino sample. The meaning of these differences remains uncertain at the moment because of parallel uncertainties as to whether variables have precisely the same meaning in the different groups. Nevertheless, it may well be that the social context influences the ways in which more proximal risk processes operate (Rutter, 1999).

Rubin, Hemphill, Chen *et al.* (2006), using a standard paradigm developed by Kagan and colleagues, found that there were cross-cultural differences in behavioral inhibition. It is possible that these reflect biological differences, as Kagan and Snidman (2004) have suggested. However, it could also be that they reflect either cultural differences in the experience of separations or expectations with respect to emotional expression (Camras & Fatani, 2006; Wang, 2006). Greenfield *et al.* (2003) have also pointed out that parental goals may vary across cultures with respect, for example, to individuality and to social or familial interdependence.

The studies by Deater-Deckard, Dodge, & Sorbring (2005) and Lansford, Deater-Deckard, Dodge *et al.* (2004) brought public attention through its finding that whereas corporal punishment tended to be associated with more disruptive behavior in White Americans, it tended to have the reverse effect in African-Americans. However, in all groups physical abuse was a substantial risk factor. Research findings based on a twin sample have been important in showing that the risks of physical maltreatment for later psychopathology do indeed reflect an environmentally mediated process (Jaffee, Caspi, Moffitt *et al.*, 2004, 2005). The same study, however, suggested that much of the risk effect apparently associated with corporal punishment reflected genetically influenced mediation rather than an environmental effect. The evidence on the reality of the risks associated with corporal punishment remains uncertain if viewed in the context of efficacy or inefficacy (Larzelere, Kuhn, & Johnson, 2004; Larzelere & Kuhn, 2005). The public concerns over the risks associated with the regular use of corporal punishment derive from both the evidence of the risk that regular use of corporal punishment tends to predispose to a slide into physical abuse (Jaffee *et al.*, 2004), and the human rights consideration that it is not acceptable for it to be legal to beat your child whereas it is not legal to beat your spouse or neighbor (Commission on Families and the Wellbeing of Children, 2005). At the moment, there are no data on whether this risk that the regular use of physical punishment predisposes to a slide into physical abuse applies within African-American or African groups within the UK, both of whom tend to make more use of physical punishment and find it more acceptable.

A further issue is that there seem to be cultural variations in the prime goals of childrearing. Thus, Halgunseth, Ispa, & Rudy (2006) argued that in Latino families in the USA, the fostering of strong family ties and of respect for elders may be viewed as more important than the fostering of independence. As with other cultural groups, parents use control, guidance and modeling and these will impact on children's psychological development. The psychopathological effects may differ because the goals are not the same.

Universal Meaning of Measures

A somewhat related issue concerns the question of whether measures can, and do, have the same meaning in all contexts. The topic is most readily illustrated by considering context specificity for cognitive functioning (Ceci & Roazzi, 1994). Many psychologists have made the assumption that it is possible to have culture-fair tests – meaning ones that are not dependent on specific experiences or schooling. However, it is not as straightforward as that, in that problem-solving is very dependent upon the way in which questions are put. For example, Schliemann and Carraher (1994) found that proportional reasoning problems were solved better by Brazilian street vendors who had little or no schooling than by schooled individuals when the problems involved selling–purchasing operations. By contrast, the reverse was true when the same problems were couched in the language of the mathematics text used in Brazilian schools. Schliemann and Nunes (1990) found a similar sort of answer with respect to tasks in which fishermen were asked to calculate prices and quantities having to do with catching, processing and selling fish. In this case, even schooled fishermen tended to work things out in ways that did not use the proportion algorithms that they had been taught as part of their formal education.

It is important to emphasize that this situation specificity in terms of reasoning extends way beyond culture. For example, Johnson-Laird and Wason (1972; Johnson-Laird, 1983) showed that university students were very poor at a number–letter decision task when it was put in an abstract form but much better when put in a familiar practical form. This is not to argue that cognitive skills show cultural specificity, but that it makes quite a sizeable difference to cognitive performance how questions are posed and how this relates to their everyday experience. Exactly the same is likely to apply to almost any psychological feature when comparing across social groups, societies or cultures, so steps have to be taken to ensure that the meaning of measures is similar across the groups and that this has been tested for and not assumed. For obvious reasons, it would make little sense to use one social group as the standard against which all others have to be compared – although that was an assumption that was built into many early studies.

Unacceptability of Culturally Accepted Behaviors that Carry Serious Risks

There are two parallel dangers in relation to this issue. First, it is important to be aware that we are all at risk for assuming that the mores in our own culture are necessarily the right ones and, therefore, differing mores in other cultures are unacceptable. The other danger is the assumption that because something is acceptable in some cultures, it necessarily means that it is not harmful. Clearly, that is a logical non sequitur. Until relatively recently, lynching of Black people in the USA was seen as culturally acceptable in some parts of the South (that was so in 1961–1962 when one of us [M.R.] was working in New York) and, even today, beating of children is seen as culturally acceptable to many people in the UK. That definitely does not mean that either are desirable or acceptable practices. The same applies to the practice of female circumcision, or what are misleadingly termed "honor killings," and the subordination of women in some cultures around the world.

Several considerations arise from these findings and concepts. First, whether or not something is helpful or damaging needs to be based on robust empirical evidence rather than on the prevailing values in any particular society, our own or others. Second, there needs to be a recognition that the reasons why individuals engage in practices that are manifestly harmful may derive from cultural values rather than from individual psychopathology. That does not mean that they are any more acceptable, but it does mean that they need to be dealt with in a rather different way. Third, it is necessary to appreciate that with virtually all examples, there is substantial variation within cultures. There is also substantial variation across generations. This means that there needs to be a sensitivity to, for example, the way in which women are dealt with in different societies but, equally, there needs to be an appreciation that what applies to some people in particular cultures does not necessarily apply to all. The planning of therapeutic interventions needs to be done with a sensitivity to cultural mores but it should be done in a way that responds to the specifics of individual children and individual families, rather than on the basis of any assumption that everyone from any particular cultural or ethnic group is the same. Equally, sensitivity to cultural mores cannot alter situations where the risk nature of the experience has been well established.

How Can Services be Culturally Sensitive and Appropriate?

It is important not to confuse what may be appropriate with respect to service development in developing countries (Hackett & Hackett, 1999; Nikapota, 2002) with how services should become culturally appropriate within industrialized nations with reasonably good resources. So far as the former is concerned, it is necessary to make use of existing personnel rather than assume that a multidisciplinary western style of practice is needed. However, it is important to encourage the development of methods of intervention for which there is good evidence of efficacy. Of course, it cannot be assumed that what worked best in one social context will work equally well in all others; by the same token it cannot be assumed that there will necessarily be differences. The matter needs to be put to the test in a systematic fashion.

Cultural sensitivity and appropriateness are important for all service contexts. With respect to these issues within western industrialized societies, it is clear from what has already been discussed that the need is not for clinicians to learn about supposedly specific patterns and needs for each cultural or ethnic group. Also, it should not necessarily be assumed that services are always best provided by someone from the same background. What is necessary is to recognize that the use of services, and the response to service provision, are likely to be influenced by people's concepts of causation and of psychopathology. That does require service providers to be aware of such variations and the acceptability of services may well be aided by ensuring that the responsible professionals include people of varied ethnic and cultural background. There is also a research need to learn more about variations in people's expectations of services and what sort of help they wish to receive. The ways in which families are dealt with by services also need to be responsive to cultural variations in how families are expected to function.

This may be illustrated by reference to religious variations. For example, ultra-Orthodox Jews may be unwilling to sit alone in a room with a person of the opposite sex or may insist that a rabbi or other figure of authority be present throughout to ensure that the patient is protected from exposure to non-religious values (Greenberg & Wiesner, 2004). Somewhat similarly, some Muslim girls and women consider it essential to wear a full veil that conceals the whole of the face other than the eyes. Many clinicians consider that this creates a barrier that makes them feel uncomfortable. Obviously, it prevents the use of cues in facial expression. Nevertheless, there are blind clinicians who cannot see faces but who, despite this limitation, may be quite adept at picking up social cues. In both these examples, cultural sensitivity implies that the limitations should be accepted initially because confrontation with deeply held values would erect an even greater barrier between clinician and patient.

However, this sensitivity does not mean that psychopathological or therapeutic implications are ignored. We referred above to the recognition of religious obsessive-compulsive disorder (OCD) in which there is a need to help patients recognize that they are not just punctiliously religious or virtuous but rather that they have a problem. Similarly, while respecting the male dominant hierarchical structure in Muslim families and the expectation that children should obey their parents without question, it may be necessary to help parents understand that in western societies, this may present dilemmas for young people (Al-Mateen & Afzal, 2004). It may also be necessary to help parents appreciate that although physical abuse may be tolerated in some Muslim families (Al-Mateen & Afzal, 2004) it carries risks for the children. As Josephson emphasized (Josephson & Dell, 2004; Josephson & Petitt, 2004), there must be respect for the values and beliefs of each family but, equally, this must not mean an avoidance of significant risk or protective influences on psychopathology.

Some have argued that more use needs to be made of traditional cultural therapies (e.g., Cuento therapy for Puerto Rican children; Constantino, Malgady & Roglet, 1996) and it is possible that this may be useful but there need to be systematic comparisons with forms of treatment that are known to be effective in other groups. Such evidence is lacking at the moment.

Future Directions

The most important issue with respect to clinical practice concerns the need to appreciate the rich diversity (e.g., with respect to culture, ethnicity, religion, language) in most societies. Clinicians need to be sensitive to this diversity in the ways in which they approach diagnostic issues and plan therapeutic interventions. Human distress and disruptive behavior are universal but the ways in which they are expressed are immensely varied. Because the diversity within all groups is as great as that between groups, the solution does not lie in learning a set of "rules" as to how each and every group expresses their feelings. Rather, clinicians need to be alert to possible differences in emotional expression and to variations in the kinds of explanation that people have for the causes of mental disorder. Equally, clinicians need to be aware that children may not always view things in the same way as their parents, although some do. This may be a particular issue for children of first-generation immigrants.

The top research priority is the use of variations among groups in rates or types of psychopathology to tackle questions on causal mechanisms. Why is the rate of schizophrenia higher in people from the Caribbean now living in the UK or the Netherlands than it is in Whites living in the same region or in people of the same ethnic origin living in the West Indies? Similar questions can, and should, be posed with respect to group differences in antisocial behavior, scholastic attainment and suicide. If causal mechanisms are to be identified, it will be necessary to examine risk and protective processes both within and between groups, and the testing of causal inferences will be greatly facilitated by using migration as a kind of "natural experiment" that brings about change (Rutter & Tienda, 2005).

In the same vein, there needs to be a focus on the few instances in which risk factors seem to operate in different ways in different groups. It is not that it is likely that there are major differences among sociocultural or ethnic groups in the nature of risk and protective processes. Rather, it is that the differences raise questions about the meaning of associations in all groups, and similarly they raise questions about how the impact of proximal risk and protective factors may be influenced by the broader social context. The aim needs to be to use variations as a way of providing a broader understanding of the development of psychopathology in all populations. The implication is that we need to bring cultural studies into the mainstream of research, but to do so in a way that downplays their special features and emphasizes their broader value.

Although for some the question of so-called culture-specific syndromes has not been fully answered, it does not seem to provide a fruitful area of study. The "dhat" loss of semen syndrome seems likely to have about as much validity as the western concept of "masturbatory insanity" had a century or so ago. Of course, cultural beliefs can constitute sources of distress as well as providing sources of foci for people's explanatory concepts regarding the disorders they experience. Thus, this would seem to apply to anorexic and bulimic eating disorders. However, in our view, the way ahead needs to lie in the study of the possibly etiological role of attitudes to body shape and size rather than the study of group differences as an end in itself. In other words, cultural variations can be very informative but they are most likely to be so when they are part of a broader scientific enterprise.

The issue of the extent to which there are variations in symptom expression raises questions about the comparability of patterns across groups, and is another area worth further study. In essence, it needs tackling in much the same way that apparent sex or age differences in patterns of psychopathology have been investigated (Moffit, Caspi, Rutter *et al.*, 2001). The need is to compare causes, correlates, course and consequences in order to determine whether there are important valid differences that need to be recognized (Rutter, 2007). Up to now, there have been rather few studies that have done this in a systematic fashion. Assumptions about age and sex differences in psychopathology need testing just as much as do cultural variations.

Some 30 years ago, Liederman, Tulkin, & Rosenfeld (1977) noted that the comparative study of societies provided a fertile ground for hypothesis testing. They emphasized the need to understand the cultures and societies being investigated and to use measures that were sensitive to key features. They added that it was also important to appreciate that the comparisons across societies can be strengthened significantly through the study of individual differences within groups. It is necessary to discover whether or not the relationship of processes within each of the groups is relevant to any of the differences found between groups. It is evident from more recent conceptual and methodological critiques (Swanson, Spencer, Harpalani *et al.*, 2003) that all too few studies have really taken on board how those cultural and ethnic variations need to be dealt with in research.

Some might argue that there is a need to define what is meant by culture. Along with others (Canino & Guarnaccia, 1997), we disagree. That is because the concepts and differences that we have discussed in this chapter are so multifaceted and so various. There is a need to understand better how cultures develop and how they change over time and in response to altered circumstances. Surprisingly, although opinions abound, there is little systematic knowledge on these matters. It may not have great importance for psychopathology, but it is an important topic in its own right.

Further Reading

Rutter, M., & Tienda, M. (Eds). (2005). *Ethnicity and causal mechanisms*. New York: Cambridge University Press.

References

Al-Mateen, C. S., & Afzal, A. (2004). The Muslim child, adolescent and family. In A. M. Josephson, & M. L. Dell (Eds.), *Child and adolescent psychiatric clinics of North America* (pp. 183–200). Philadelphia: Saunders.

Asch, S. E. (1952). *Social psychology*. Englewood Cliffs, NJ: Prentice-Hall.

Asch, S. E. (1956). Studies of independence and conformity. 1. A minority of one against a unanimous majority. *Psychological Monographs*, 70, No. 9.

Becker, A. E., Burwell, R. A., Gilman, S. E., Herzog, D. B., & Hamburg, P. (2002). Eating behaviours and attitudes following prolonged exposure to television among ethnic Fijian adolescent girls. *British Journal of Psychiatry*, *180*, 509–514.

Bhugra, D., & Becker, M. A. (2005). Migration, cultural bereavement and cultural identity. *World Psychiatry*, *4*, 18–24.

Bradley, R. H., & Corwyn, R. F. (2002). Socioeconomic status and child development. *Annual Review of Psychology*, *53*, 371–399.

Brooks-Gunn, J., Duncan, G. J., & Aber, J. L. (1997). *Neighborhood Poverty*. Vol. 1. *Context and consequences for children*. New York: Russell Sage Foundation.

Brown, C., & Gay, P. (1986). *Racial discrimination 17 years after the Act*. London: Policy Studies Institute.

Camras, L. A., & Fatani, S. S. (2006). The development of emotional expressivity and the influence of culture. *International Society for the Study of Behavioural Development Newsletter*, *49*, 12–15.

Canino, G., & Guarnaccia, P. (1997). Methodological challenges in the assessment of Hispanic children and adolescents. *Applied Developmental Science*, *1*, 124–134.

Ceci, S. J., & Roazzi, A. (1994). The effects of context on cognition: Postcards from Brazil. In R. J. Sternberg, & R. K. Wagner (Eds.), *Mind in Context: Interactionist perspectives on human intelligence* (pp. 74–101). New York: Cambridge University Press.

Christensen, H. T. (1960). Cultural relativism and premarital sex norms. *American Sociological Review*, *25*, 31–39.

Commission on Families and the Wellbeing of Children. (2005). *Families and the State: Two-way support and responsibilities*. Bristol: Policy Press.

Constantino, G., Malgady, R. G., & Roglet, L. H. (1996). Cuento therapy: A culturally sensitive modality for Puerto Rican children. *Journal of Consulting and Clinical Psychology*, *54*, 639–645.

Cummins, L. H., Simmons, A. M., & Zane, N. W. S. (2005). Eating disorders in Asian populations: A critique of current approaches to the study of culture, ethnicity and eating disorders. *American Journal of Orthopsychiatry*, *75*, 553–574.

Daniel, W. W. (1968). *Racial discrimination in England*. Harmondsworth: Penguin.

Deater-Deckard, K., Dodge, K. A., & Sorbring, E. (2005). Cultural differences in the effects of physical punishment. In M. Rutter, & M. Tienda (Eds.), *Ethnicity and causal mechanisms* (pp. 204–226). New York: Cambridge University Press.

Evans, G. W. (2004). The environment of childhood poverty. *American Psychologist*, *59*, 77–92.

Gast, U., Rodewald, F., Nickel, V., & Emrich, H. (2001). Prevalence of dissociative disorders among psychiatric inpatients in a German university clinic. *Journal of Nervous and Mental Disease*, *189*, 249–257.

Gee, G. C., & Payne-Sturges, D. C. (2004). Environmental health disparities: A framework integrating psychosocial and environmental concepts. *Environmental Health Perspectives*, *112*, 1645–1653.

Greenberg, D., & Wiesner, I. S. (2004). Jews. In A. M. Josephson, & J. R. Peteet (Eds.), *Handbook of spirituality and worldwide clinical practice* (pp. 91–110). Washington, DC: American Psychiatric Publishing.

Greenfield, P. M., Keller, H., Fuligni, A., & Maynard, A. (2003). Cultural pathways through universal development. *Annual Review of Psychology*, *54*, 461–490.

Guarnaccia, P. J., Canino, G., Rubio-Stipec, M., & Bravo, M. (1993). The prevalence of ataques de nervios in the Puerto Rico disaster study: The role of culture in psychiatric epidemiology. *Journal of Nervous and Mental Disease*, *181*, 157–165.

Guarnaccia, P. J., Martinez, I., Ramirez, R., & Canino, G. (2005). Are *ataques de nervios* in Puerto Rican children associated with psychiatric disorder? *Journal of the American Academy of Child and Adolescent Psychiatry*, *44*, 1184–1192.

Hackett, R., & Hackett, L. (1999). Child psychiatry across cultures. *International Review of Psychiatry*, *11*, 225–235.

Halgunseth, L. C., Ispa, J. M., & Rudy, D. (2006). Parental control in Latino families: An integrated review of the literature. *Child Development*, *77*, 1281–1297.

Hirschman, C., & Lee, J. (2005). Race and ethnic inequality in educational attainment in the United States. In M. Rutter, & M. Tienda (Eds.), *Ethnicity and causal mechanisms* (pp. 107–138). New York: Cambridge University Press.

Jaffee, S. R., Caspi, A., Moffitt, T. E., Dodge, K. A., Rutter, M., Taylor, A., *et al.* (2005). Nature × nurture: Genetic vulnerabilities interact with physical maltreatment to promote conduct problems. *Development and Psychopathology*, *17*, 67–84.

Jaffee, S. R., Caspi, A., Moffitt, T. E., Polo-Tomas, M., Price, T. S., & Taylor, A. (2004). The limits of child effects: Evidence for genetically mediated child effects on corporal punishment but not on physical maltreatment. *Developmental Psychology*, *40*, 1047–1058.

Johnson-Laird, P. N. (1983). *Mental models*. Cambridge, MA: Harvard University Press.

Johnson-Laird, P. N., & Wason, P. C. (1972). A theoretical analysis of insight into a reasoning task. In P. N. Johnson-Laird, & P. C. Wason (Eds.), *Thinking: Readings in Cognitive Science*. Cambridge: Cambridge University Press.

Jones, P. B., & Fung, W. L. A. (2005). Ethnicity and mental health: The example of schizophrenia in the African-Caribbean population in Europe. In M. Rutter, & M. Tienda (Eds.), *Ethnicity and causal mechanisms* (pp. 227–261). New York: Cambridge University Press.

Josephson, A. M., & Dell, M. L. (2004). Religion and spirituality in child and adolescent psychiatry: A new frontier. *Child and Adolescent Psychiatric Clinics of North America*, *13*, 1–15.

Josephson, A. M., & Petitt, J. R. (2004). *Handbook of spirituality and worldview in clinical practice*. Washington, DC: American Psychiatric Publishing.

Kagan, J., & Snidman, N. (2004). *The long shadow of temperament*. Cambridge, MA: Belknap Press.

Kandel, D. B. (1978). Homophily, selection and socialization in adolescent friendships. *American Journal of Sociology*, *84*, 427–436.

Keel, P. K., & Klump, K. L. (2003). Are eating disorders culture-bound syndromes? Implications for conceptualizing their etiology. *Psychological Bulletin*, *129*, 747–769.

Kleinman, A. M. (1977). Depression, somatization and the "new cross-cultural psychiatry". *Social Science and Medicine*, *11*, 3–10.

Kleinman, A. M. (1987). Anthropology and psychiatry: The role of culture in cross-cultural research on illness. *British Journal of Psychiatry*, *151*, 447–454.

Lacourse, E., Nagin, D., Tremblay, R. E., Vitaro, F., & Claes, M. (2003). Developmental trajectories of boys' delinquent group membership and facilitation of violent behaviors during adolescence. *Development & Psychopathology*, *15*, 183–197.

Lansford, J. E., Deater-Deckard, K., Dodge, K. A., Bates, J. E., & Pettit, G. S. (2004). Ethnic differences in the link between physical discipline and later adolescent externalizing behaviors. *Journal of Child Psychology and Psychiatry*, *45*, 801–812.

Larzelere, R. E., & Kuhn, B. R. (2005). Comparing child outcomes of physical punishment and altlernative disciplinary tactics: A meta-analysis. *Clinical Child and Family Psychology Review*, *8*, 1–37.

Larzelere, R. E., Kuhn, B. R., & Johnson, B. (2004). The intervention selection bias: An under-recognized confound in intervention research. *Psychological Bulletin*, *130*, 289–303.

Lester, R. (2004). Commentary: Eating disorders and the problem of "culture" in acculturation. *Culture, Medicine and Psychiatry*, *28*, 607–615.

Lewis, O. (1968). The culture of poverty. In D. P. Moynihan (Ed.), *On understanding poverty*. New York: Basic Books.

Lieberman, S. (1956). The effect of changes in role on the attitudes of role occupants. *Human Relations*, *9*, 385–402.

Liederman, P. H., Tulkin, S. R., & Rosenfeld, A. (Eds.). (1977). *Culture and infancy: Variations in the human experience*. New York: Academic Press.

Lipsanen, T., Korkeila, J., Peltola, P., Jarvinen, J., Langen, K., & Lauerma, H. (2004). Dissociative disorders among psychiatric patients. *European Psychiatry*, *19*, 53–55.

Luk, E. S. L., Leung, P. W. L., & Ho, T-P. (2002). Cross-cultural/ethnic aspects of childhood hyperactivity. In S. Sandberg (Ed.), *Hyperactivity and attention disorders of childhood* (pp. 64–98). Cambridge: Cambridge University Press.

Mabe, P. A., & Josephson, A. M. (2004). Child and adolescent psychopathology: Spiritual and religious perspectives. *Child and Adolescent Psychiatric Clinics of North America*, *13*, 111–125.

Maughan, B. (2005). Educastional attainments: Ethnic differences in the United Kingdom. In M. Rutter, & M. Tienda (Eds.), *Ethnicity and causal mechanisms* (pp. 80–106). New York: Cambridge University Press.

Merskey, H. (2000). Conversion and disassociation. In M. G. Gelder, J. J. López-Ibor, & N. Andreasen (Eds.), *New Oxford Textbook of Psychiatry*, Vol. 2 (pp. 1088–1098). Oxford: Oxford University Press.

Modood, T. (2005). Ethnicity and intergenerational identities and adaptations in Britain: The socio-political context. In: M. Rutter, & M. Tienda (Eds.), *Ethnicity and causal mechanisms* (pp. 281–300). New York: Cambridge University Press.

Moffitt, T. E., Caspi, A., Rutter, M., & Silva, P. A. (2001). *Sex differences in antisocial behaviour: Conduct disorder, delinquency, and violence in the Dunedin Longitudinal Study*. Cambridge: Cambridge University Press.

Morenoff, J. D. (2005). Racial and ethnic disparities in crime and delinquency in the United States. In M. Rutter, & M. Tienda (Eds.), *Ethnicity and causal mechanisms* (pp. 139–173). New York: Cambridge University Press.

Newcombe, T. M. (1943). *Personality and social change: Attitude formation in a student community*. New York: Dryden.

Newcombe, T. M. (1963). *The acquaintance process*. New York: Holt, Rinehart & Winston.

Nikapota, A. D. (2002). Cultural and ethnic issues in service provision. In M. Rutter, & E. Taylor (Eds.), *Child and Adolescent Psychiatry* (4th ed., pp. 1148–1157). Oxford: Blackwell.

Pachter, L. M., Auinger, P., Palmer, R., & Weitzman, M. (2006). Do parenting and the home environment, maternal depression, neighborhood, and chronic poverty affect child behavioral problems differently in different racial-ethnic groups? *Pediatrics*, *117*, 1329–1338.

Quintana, S. M., Aboud, F. E., Chao, R., Contreras-Grau, J., Cross, W. E., Hudley, C., *et al.* (2006). Race, ethinicity and culture in child development: Contemporary research and future directions. *Child Development*, *77*, 1129–1141.

Rowe, D. C., Wouldbroun, E. J., & Gulley, B. L. (1994). Peers and friends as non-shared environmental influences. In E. M. Hetherington, D. Reiss, & R. Plomin (Eds.), *Separate social worlds of siblings* (pp. 159–173). Hillsdale, NJ: Erlbaum.

Rubin, K. H., Hemphill, S. A., Chen, X., Hastings, P., Sanson, A., Lo Coco, A., *et al.* (2006). A cross-cultural study of behavioral inhibition in toddlers: East-West-North-South. *International Journal of Behavioral Development*, *30*, 219–226.

Rumbaut, R. G. (2005). Assimilation, dissimilation and ethnic identities: The experience of children of immigrants in the United States. In M. Rutter, & M. Tienda (Eds.), *Ethnicity and causal mechanisms* (pp. 301–334). New York: Cambridge University Press.

Rutter, M. (1981). The city and the child. *American Journal of Orthopsychiatry*, *51*, 610–625.

Rutter, M. (1999). Social context: meanings, measures and mechanisms. *European Review*, *7*, 139–149.

Rutter, M. (2007). Proceeding from observed correlation to causal inference: The use of natural experiments. *Perspectives on Psychological Science*, *2*, 377–395.

Rutter, M., Giller, H., & Hagell, A. (1998). *Antisocial behaviour by young people*. New York and Cambridge: Cambridge University Press.

Rutter, M., & Madge, N. (1976). *Cycles of disadvantage: A review of research*. London: Heinemann Educational.

Rutter, M., Maughan, B., Mortimore, P., Ouston, J., & Smith, A. (1979). *Fifteen thousand hours: Secondary schools and their effects on children*. Cambridge, MA: Harvard University Press.

Rutter, M., & Quinton, D. (1977). Psychiatric disorder: Ecological factors and concepts of causation. In H. McGurk (Ed.), *Ecological factors in human development* (pp. 173–187). Amsterdam: North-Holland.

Rutter, M., & Tienda, M. (Eds.). (2005). *Ethnicity and causal mechanisms*. New York and Cambridge: Cambridge University Press.

Sampson, R. J., Raudenbush, S. W., & Earls, F. (1997). Neighborhoods and violent crime: A multilevel study of collective efficacy. *Science*, *277*, 918–924.

Schliemann, A. D., & Carraher, D. W. (1994). Proportional reasoning in and out of school. In P. Light, & G. Butterworth (Eds.), *Context and cognition: Ways of learning and knowing* (pp. 47–73). Hillsdale, NJ: Lawrence Erlbaum Associates.

Schliemann, A. D., & Nunes, T. (1990). A situated schema of proportionality. *British Journal of Developmental Psychology*, *8*, 259–268.

Sherif, M., Harvey, O. J., White, B. J., Hood, W. R., & Sherif, C. W. (1961). *Intergroup conflict and cooperation: The Robbers' Cave experiment*. Norman, Oklahoma: University of Oklahoma Press.

Shorter Oxford English Dictionary. (2002). Oxford: Oxford University Press.

Shweder, R. A., Goodnow, J., Hatano, G., LeVine, R. A., Markus, H., & Miller, P. (1997). The cultural psychology of development: One mind, many mentalities. In W. Damon, & R. M. Lerner (Eds.), *Handbook of child psychology*. Vol. 1. *Theoretical models of human development* (pp. 865–937). New York: Wiley.

Siegel, A. E., & Siegel, S. (1957). Reference groups, membership groups and attitude change. *Journal of Abnormal Social Psychology*, *55*, 360–364.

Smith, D. J. (2005). Explaining ethnic variations in crime and antisocial behaviour in the United Kingdom. In M. Rutter, & M. Tienda (Eds.), *Ethnicity and causal mechanisms* (pp. 174–203). New York: Cambridge University Press.

Stevenson, H. W., Lee, S-Y., Chen, C., Stigler, J. W., Hsu, C-C., & Kitamural, S. (1990). Contexts of achievement. *Monographs of the Society for Research in Child Development*, *221*, 55, nos 1–2.

Swanson, D. P., Spencer, M. B., Harpalani, V., Dupree, D., Noll, E., Ginzburg, S., *et al.* (2003). Psychosocial development in racially and ethnically diverse youth: Conceptual and methodological challenges in the 21st century. *Development and Psychopathology*, *15*, 743–771.

Taylor Gibbs, J. (2005). Ethnic variations in youth suicide. In M. Rutter, & M. Tienda (Eds.), *Ethnicity and causal mechanisms* (pp. 262–280). New York: Cambridge University Press.

Terraciano, A., Abdel-Khalek, A. M., Ádám, N., Adamovová, L., Ahn, C.-K., Ahn, H.-N., *et al.* (2005). National character does not reflect mean personality trait levels in 49 cultures. *Science*, *310*, 96–100.

Thornberry, T. P. (1998). Membership in youth gangs and involvement in serious and violent offending. In R. L. Loeber, & D. P. Farrington (Eds.), *Serious and violent juvenile offenders: Risk factors and successful interventions* (pp. 147–166). Thousand Oaks, CA: Sage.

Townsend, P., Whitehead, M., & Davidson, N. (Eds.). (1992). *Inequalities in health: The Black Report and the health divide* (2nd ed.). London: Penguin.

Wang, Q. (2006). Developing emotion knowledge in cultural contexts. *International Society for the Study of Behavioural Development Newsletter*, *49*, 8–12.

Weisz, J. R., McCarty, C. A., Eastman, K. L., Chaiyasit, W., & Suwanlert, S. (1997). Developmental psychopathology and culture: ten lessons from Thailand. In S. S. Luthar, J. A. Burack, D. Cicchetti, & J. R. Weisz (Eds.), *Developmental Psychopathology: Perspectives on adjustment, risk, and disorder* (pp. 568–592). Cambridge: Cambridge University Press.

Widom, C. S., & Brzustowicz, L. M. (2006). MAOA and the "cycle of violence": childhood abuse and neglect, MAOA genotype, and risk for violent and antisocial behavior. *Biological Psychiatry*, *60*, 684–689.

Wildschut, T., Pinter, B., Vevea, J. L., Insko, C. A., & Schopler, J. (2003). Beyond the group mind: a quantitative review of the interindividual-intergroup discontinuity effect. *Psychological Bulletin*, *129*, 698–722.

Wilkinson, R. (2005). *The impact of inequality: How to make sick societies healthier*. New York & London: The New Press.

Wilkinson, R. & Marmot, M. (Eds.). (2006). *Social inequalities of health*. Oxford: Oxford University Press.

Wilson, W. J. (1987). *The truly disadvantaged: The inner city, the underclass, and public policy*. Chicago, IL: University of Chicago Press.

16 Basic Neuropsychopharmacology

Nora Volkow and James Swanson

The use of psychotropic medications in children has increased dramatically over the past decade (Zito & Safer, 2005). An increase in clinical research followed, partly resulting from governmental regulations and legislation that encouraged studies on the safety and efficacy of drugs that are approved for use in adults but not for children, yet are widely used off-label to treat children (DeVeaugh-Geiss, March, Shapiro *et al.*, 2006). Most studies have been conducted to evaluate established clinical practices, and some have generated significant controversy – if they did not support these practices (Vitiello, 2006) or questioned their safety (US Food and Drug Administration, 2003b, 2004a, 2005).

This pattern, of research following practice, has led to a rather slow development of new pharmacological treatments with improved efficacy and safety. Basic principles and findings from the neurosciences could be better integrated into innovative, theory-driven treatment development (Vitiello, 2006). In this chapter, we summarize some basic properties of psychoactive medications used in the treatment of psychiatric disorders of childhood. The areas of neurochemistry and psychopharmacology provide extensive information that can be used to specify rational dosing regimens and to identify mechanisms of action of the commonly prescribed drugs. We describe methods from clinical pharmacology that have been successfully applied to evaluate amount (dose) and timing (dosing rate) of drug administration, and we describe methods from brain imaging that have elucidated cellular targets of some commonly prescribed medications and their effects on brain function. We focus on basic principles in neurochemistry and psychopharmacology that could help us understand how currently available psychotropic medications exert their clinical effects on the core symptoms of some childhood disorders for which cellular targets have been proposed (e.g., attention deficit/hyperactivity disorder [ADHD], major depressive disorder [MDD], anxiety disorder [ANX] and schizophrenia [SCZ]). Better basic understanding should guide us in the development of new and improved pharmacological treatments for these disorders and for others, such as autistic spectrum disorder (ASD), for which currently there is neither a proposed cellular target nor a pharmacological treatment that is effective for the reduction of the core symptoms of the disorder. We have organized the chapter into three sections.

First, we review some basic pharmacokinetic (PK) methods that describe how psychotropic drugs are delivered to the brain after administration of clinical doses, some basic pharmacodynamic (PD) analyses that model responses at sites of action in the brain, and some basic PK/PD analyses that describe the relationships between drug concentration and effect (Fig. 16.1).

Second, we discuss neurotransmitters that are the primary targets of medications used to treat ADHD, MDD (and ANX) and SCZ (and ASD), namely dopamine (DA), norepinephrine (NE) and serotonin (5-HT), and their synaptic components that participate in neurotransmission and are targets for psychotropic drugs (transporters, enzymes and receptors).

Third, we describe how positron emission tomography (PET) imaging has been used to measure directly in the human brain the concentrations of psychotropic medications, their effects on cellular targets and their functional effects on brain circuits which are involved in multiple processes associated with cognition and emotion.

To link psychopharmacology with neurochemistry, we discuss how PET imaging methods can be used to investigate the cellular mechanisms involved in response to psychotropic medications. In Plate 16.1(a), we show a schematic DA synapse, and surrounding it we present images from different PET methods that have been used to characterize the components related to the neurotransmitter DA: *transporters*, which recycle the neurotransmitter back into the neuron after its release; *enzymes*, which are involved in neurotransmitter

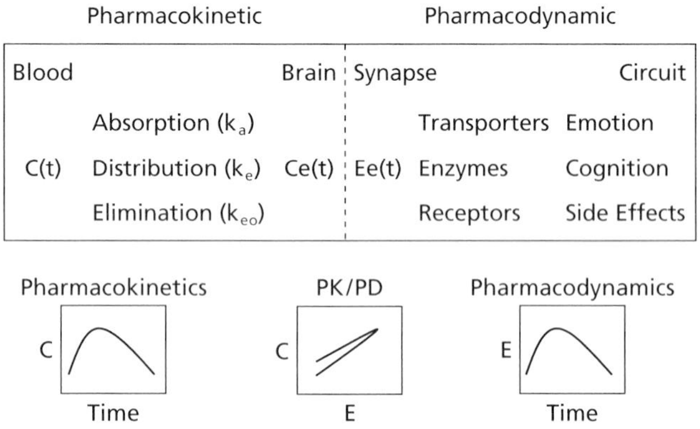

Pharmacokinetic			Pharmacodynamic		
Blood		Brain	Synapse		Circuit
	Absorption (k_a)			Transporters	Emotion
C(t)	Distribution (k_e)	Ce(t)	Ee(t)	Enzymes	Cognition
	Elimination (k_{eo})			Receptors	Side Effects

Pharmacokinetics: C / Time — PK/PD: C / E — Pharmacodynamics: E / Time

Fig. 16.1 Pharmacokinetic/pharmacodynamic (PK/PD) model of the drug in the body and at the effect sites in the brain. C, concentration; E, effect.

Rutter's Child and Adolescent Psychiatry, 5th edition. Edited by M. Rutter, D. Bishop, D. Pine, S. Scott, J. Stevenson, E. Taylor and A. Thapar. © 2008 Blackwell Publishing, ISBN: 978-1-4051-4549-7.

synthesis and metabolism; and *receptors* at postsynaptic sites, which transmit the signal when activated as well as at presynaptic sites, which regulate neurotransmitter synthesis and release. Also, we present an example of a functional PET image of *glucose metabolism*, which represents an integrated consequence of these factors operating in combination.

Figure 16.1 presents a framework for the three sections of this chapter that present information about the fate of a drug after it is administered by a given route (e.g., oral, transdermal, intranasal, intravenous). To start the processes outlined in Fig. 16.1, a clinician must make a series of choices. After the initial choice of the particular medication (which is typically related to diagnosis), further decisions are necessary about the dose (which varies between individuals and is based on titration) and the frequency of dosing (which may be controlled by the formulation). After entering the body, processes occur that define the PK and PD properties of the drug. Based on a common description from clinical pharmacology (Gupta, Hwang, Benet *et al.*, 1993), the PK processes on the left side of Fig. 16.1 reflect "what the body does to the drug," and the PD processes on the right side reflect "what the drug does to the body." Here we present some simple methods from clinical pharmacology to describe the PK processes on the left (absorption, distribution and elimination of the drug) which describe the maximum plasma concentration (C_{max}), when it occurs after dosing (T_{max}) and the plasma half-life ($t_{1/2}$). We also present some PET imaging methods that have been used to describe the PD processes shown on the right (e.g., drug effects of transporter blockade and receptor occupancy). We illustrate these methods for stimulant, selective serotonin reuptake inhibitor (SSRI) and neuroleptic medications. These examples are intended to demonstrate how the basic principles of clinical pharmacology and neurochemistry can be used to provide a fundamental understanding of how these drugs exert their clinical effects.

Psychiatric Disorders and Psychotropic Medications

A relatively small number of drugs are approved by regulatory agencies for the treatment of psychiatric disorders of childhood and adolescence, but many others not approved are used off-label (Emslie, Hughes, Crismon *et al.*, 2004; Pliszka, 2005; Wilens, 2004). Table 16.1 was adapted from the Children's Medication Chart prepared by the National Institute of Mental Health (2002), which lists the commonly prescribed medications and the approved age for their use for the treatment of classes of disorder (i.e., "Medications for ADHD," "Anti-depressant and Antianxiety Medications," "Antipsychotic Medications" and "Mood Stabilizing Medications").

We use our framework of clinical pharmacology and PET imaging to discuss some important current issues in child psychopharmacology:

1 The use of controlled delivery formulation of the stimulant medications;

2 The difficulties of demonstrating efficacy of antidepressant medications; and

3 The side-effects of antipsychotic medications.

Chapter 67 describes the use of psychotropic drugs in clinical practice.

Stimulant Medications for ADHD

The place of drug treatment in ADHD is discussed in chapter 34. Animal studies have suggested that the stimulants amphetamine (AMP) and methylphenidate (MPH) have their primary effects on two neurotransmitters: DA and NE (Solanto, 1998). The enhancement of catecholaminergic activity in the basal ganglia and prefrontal cortex increases the readiness to respond to external stimuli and the saliency of external stimuli, and these in turn increase the clinical targets of attention and executive function. In addition, adverse effects in limbic areas (including hypothalamus) decrease appetite and sleep.

The immediate-release (IR) formulations of AMP and MPH were used before the modern Food and Drug Administration (FDA) approval process was even established, and since then thousands of studies have been published about their efficacy and safety (Pliszka, 2005; Swanson, McBurnett, Wigal *et al.*, 1993). The PK properties of IR formulations of these stimulants document rapid absorption, with a t_{max} of about 1–2 hours and rapid metabolism with a $t_{1/2}$ of around 3–4 hours, with slightly greater values for AMP than MPH. The PD properties parallel the PK profiles. So, for effective treatment across the day, multiple doses of IR formulations are required, and these treatment regimes (i.e., IR MPH t.i.d. and IR AMP b.i.d.) emerged from almost a half century of clinical use (Swanson, McBurnett, Wigal *et al.*, 1993). The basic findings for school-aged children are the following: the two stimulants have large short-term effects that reduce the core symptoms of ADHD (reduction of inattention, hyperactivity and impulsivity) and some associated features if they are present (aggression and defiance); efficacy is about the same for these two stimulants (effect size about 1.0; about 80% response rate); across individuals the range of clinical doses for optimal response is large (five- to sixfold) so a titration process is used to select the best dose for each individual (see chapter 34).

Despite decades of concentrated research, there are still many critical unanswered questions about the effects of the stimulant medications, including questions about effects in age groups typically not treated with stimulants, long-term effects on efficacy and side-effects, and emergence of side-effects over time.

The use of stimulants is primarily with school-aged children (Centers for Disease Control and Prevention, 2005; Jick, Kaye, & Black, 2004), but their use to treat ADHD in adults (Spencer, Biederman, Wilens *et al.*, 1996) and preschool children (Greenhill, Beyer, Finkleson *et al.*, 2002) has been increasing over the past decade (Zito, Tobi, de Jong-van den Berg *et al.*, 2006). These reports suggest that treatment of adults and preschool children results in similar effects as in school-aged children, but with somewhat reduced effectiveness and/or greater side-effects, which may be partially due to more diagnostic uncertainty in these extreme age groups than in the

Table 16.1 Psychotropic medications, disorders and neurochemical targets.

Class of drug	Medication	Disorder	Target
Antidepressant			
Tricyclics	Desipramine	Depression	NE
	Imipramine		
SSRI	Fluoxetine	Depression	Serotonin
	Fluvoxamine	OCD	
	Paroxetine		
	Sertraline		
Neuroleptics			
Typical	Haloperidol	Schizophrenia	DA antagonist
	Thioridazime	Tourette syndrome	
	Thorazine	Aggression	
Atypical	Clozapine	Schizophrenia	
	Olanzapine		
	Risperidone		
Stimulants	Methylphenidate	ADHD	DA agonists
	Amphetamines	ADHD	
Anxiolytics	Alprazolam	Anxiety disorder	GABA agonists
	Chlorodiazepoxide		
	Clonazepam		
	Diazepam		
	Lorazepam		
Antiepileptics	Carbamazepine	Bipolar	
	Valproate	Conduct disorder	
Non-classified	Modafinil	Narcolepsy	DA
		ADHD	Hypocretin
	Atomoxetine	ADHD	NE
	Buspirone	Depression	DA
		ADHD	
		Nicotine dependence	
	Clonidine	ADHD	NE
		Tourette syndrome	
	Guanfacine	ADHD	NE
		Tourette syndrome	
	Lithium	Bipolar disorder	
		Conduct disorder	

ADHD, attention deficit/hyperactivity disorder; DA, dopamine; GABA, γ-amino butyric acid; NE, norepinephrine; OCD, obsessive-compulsive disorder.

school-aged group for which the diagnostic criteria were developed. For example, the Preschool ADHD Treatment Study (PATS) ($n = 145$) documented safety and efficacy of IR MPH in children with ADHD below the age of 6 years (Greehill, Biederman, Boellner *et al.*, 2006; Wigal, Greenhill, Chuang *et al.*, 2006), but lower rates of response, smaller benefits and greater side-effects were seen in this age group than typically observed in school-aged children with ADHD.

Long-term trials have suggested improvement over time, but whether this is related to past or continued treatment is not clear. For example, a single site study ($n = 62$) of AMP (Gillberg, Melander, von Knorring *et al.*, 1997) suggested that improvement in the first year was maintained after withdrawal of treatment, but a dual site study ($n = 103$) of MPH (Abikoff, McGough, Vitiello *et al.*, 2005) suggested that continued treatment is necessary to maintain improvement into the second year of treatment. The Multimodal Treatment Study of ADHD (MTA), a large multisite study ($n = 579$), added to the literature by documenting long-term efficacy of MPH. The benefits of IR MPH t.i.d. treatment compared with non-pharmacological (behavioral) treatment over the first year were clear and large (MTA Cooperative Group, 1999a,b). A secondary analysis of the MTA revealed that some of the beneficial effects of medication were larger for the subset of cases with pervasiveness of symptoms across home and school settings that qualified them for ICD-10 diagnoses of hyperkinetic disorder (Santosh, Taylor, Swanson *et al.*, 2005).

The evaluation of the MTA groups in a naturalistic follow-up has provided information on the persistence of effects over longer periods of time than 1 year. The relative superiority of medication was reduced by 50% at the 24-month follow-up (MTA Cooperative Group, 2004a,b) and dissipated completely at the 36-month follow-up (Jensen, Arnold, Swanson *et al.*, 2007), when no effect of prior assigned treatment or current actual treatment with stimulant medication could be documented for reduction of ADHD symptoms (Swanson, Hinshaw, Arnold *et al.*, 2007b) or emergent problems of delinquency or substance use (Molina, Flory, Hinshaw *et al.*, 2007). A statistical procedure (growth mixture modeling) was used which identified three subgroups with different trajectories of outcome (symptom severity) over time, which appeared to be independent of history of assigned or actual treatment with stimulant medication. This naturalistic follow-up of the MTA randomized clinical trial offers new and potentially important information about prognosis of the ADHD condition. First, there appears to be a general trend of improvement regardless of treatment modality (medication or behavioral). Second, there are clear short-term but not long-term relative benefits of medication of ADHD symptoms, suggesting that the beneficial effects of stimulants on symptom reduction may dissipate over a period of 2–3 years of treatment or as the treated patients become older (which were confounded in the MTA protocol).

Side-effects of the stimulant medications are typically mild and manageable, with suppression of appetite and sleep, which dissipates over time, or can be managed by adjustment of doses, timing of doses or type of stimulant (Greenhill, Pliszka, Dulcan *et al.*, 2001). Recently, the MTA follow-up (MTA Cooperative Group, 2004a; Swanson, Elliot, Greenhill *et al.*, 2007a) revived concern about stimulant-related growth suppression, which had previously been thoroughly discounted (Spencer *et al.*, 1996) and thus had not been considered worthy of an a priori hypothesis in the MTA design and analysis plan. A *post hoc* analysis of the randomized clinical trial phase of the MTA (MTA Cooperative Group, 2004b) revealed stimulant-related reduction in growth rate (by about 1 cm per year in height and 2.0 kg per year in weight) over the initial 14-month phase of supervised and randomly assigned to treatment with medication compared to behavior modification without MPH. This reduction in growth rate appeared to persist in the naturalistic follow-up (MTA Cooperative Group, 2004b), with a cumulative stimulant-related growth suppression effect of about 2.0 cm in height and 2.7 kg in weight after 3 years of continuous treatment (Swanson, Elliot, Greenhill *et al.*, 2007a). The evaluation of growth in another controlled trial, the Preschool ADHD Treatment Study (PATS), also revealed a significant stimulant-related growth suppression of height and weight in preschool children with ADHD during the initial year of a continuous and monitored treatment with IR MPH (Swanson, Greenhill, Wigal *et al.* (2006c), which was slightly larger than in the school-aged children of the MTA (Wigal, Greenhill, Chuang *et al.*, 2006). These reports from controlled trials (i.e., MTA and PATS) stand in contrast to the reports of some recent chart review studies of modern clinical practices that do not show stimulant-related growth suppression (Pliszka, Matthews, Braslow *et al.*, 2006; Spencer, Faraone, Biederman *et al.*, 2006b).

In addition, side-effects related to rare cardiac effects of the stimulant medications have been evaluated by regulatory agencies in Canada (Health Canada, 2005), the USA (US Food and Drug Administration, 2005) and in the European Union (NICE, 2005). These reviews have generated considerable controversy about whether these serious adverse events are greater than expected in the population (Anders & Sharfstein, 2006; Nissen, 2006; Rappley, Moore, & Dokken, 2006; Shader & Oesterheld, 2006).

In the mid-1990s, pharmaceutical companies initiated research programs to evaluate and improve the formulations of stimulant medications. One new development that produced a dramatic shift in clinical practice is reviewed here: the development and use of controlled-release (CR) formulations of both MPH (Concerta©, Metadate CD©, Ritalin LA©, and Focalin LA©) and AMP (Adderall XR©). The CR formulations were developed to replace specific dosing regimens of the IR formulations, including IR MPH t.i.d. for Concerta© (Swanson *et al.*, 2003), IR MPH b.i.d. for Metadate CD (Wigal, Sanchez, DeCory *et al.*, 2003) and Ritalin LA (Biederman, Quinn, Weiss *et al.*, 2003) and IR AMP b.i.d. for Adderall XR (Greenhill, Swanson, Steinhoff *et al.*, 2003). The development programs, funded by pharmaceutical companies, all used PK and PD methods to select the drug delivery profile to be established by controlled delivery systems. These PK and PD methods are described and addressed in a subsequent section of this chapter.

Two basic systems have been used that deliver an initial bolus of IR drug (mg), followed by delayed release from a reservoir of drug at a specified dosing rate (mg/hour). The first application was an osmotic release oral system (OROS) for the delivery of MPH (Concerta®). This system uses an "overcoat" of IR MPH as an initial bolus, with controlled release from a three-part reservoir consisting of a semipermeable membrane to control the entry of water, a polymer that expands to create an osmotic pump, and methylphenidate layered to be delivered over an 8-hour period of time as the system traverses the gastrointestinal tract (Swanson *et al.*, 2003). The subsequent applications for CR formulations were based on dual-beaded systems, which provide an IR bolus by uncoated beads of the drug followed by delayed release from beads with polymer coats that dissolve in the gastrointestinal tract to allow the drug to escape. This dual-beaded technology was used for MPH (Metadate CD©, Ritalin LA© and Focalin LA©) and AMP (Adderall XR©).

After the introduction of Concerta©, within a year most prescriptions in the USA for MPH were for the CR formulation instead of the multiple daily doses of IR MPH that had been accepted and used in clinical practice for decades. After the introduction of Adderall XR©, within a year most prescriptions in the USA for AMP were for the CR formulation instead of multiple daily doses of the IR formulation. This rapid acceptance of second-generation CR formulations of the stimulants stands in stark contrast to the lack of clinical acceptance of the first-generation of CR formulations (Ritalin SR© and Dexedrine Spansules©), which were considered to have reduced efficacy compared to multiple daily doses of IR formulations. The achievement of sustained efficacy by the second-generation CR formulations has been attributed to the rational dosing regimens that were chosen based on PK/PD studies and analyses, which are described in a subsequent section.

Non-stimulant Medications for ADHD

In 2000, pharmaceutical companies initiated drug development programs for non-stimulant alternatives. This was prompted in part by concerns about the stimulants, such as abuse potential, lack of efficacy in a percentage of children with ADHD and side-effect profile. The first development program was for atomoxetine (ATX), which Lilly Pharmaceuticals successfully developed as a treatment for ADHD (Allen & Michelson, 2002) and received FDA approval for this indication in late 2002. Buitelaar, Danckaerts, Gillberg *et al.* (2004) described the use in non-North American clinical populations of children. Animal studies suggested that ATX did not affect the neurotransmitter DA in the basal ganglia and its effects were primarily on the neurotransmitter NE and perhaps on DA in the frontal cortex (Bymaster, Katner, Nelson *et al.*, 2002; Swanson, Perry, Koch-Krueger *et al.*, 2006a).

The PK properties of ATX and the stimulants are similar in children (see below), but the dosing regimen is different than for IR stimulants. Some clinical trials of ATX (Buitelaar *et al.*, 2004; Michelson, Faries, Wernicke *et al.*, 2001; Michelson, Adler, Spencer *et al.*, 2003) used twice daily dosing (0.5–1.8 mg/kg/day up to 120 mg) administered in the early morning and late afternoon, but others used once daily dosing in the morning (Kelsey, Sumner, Casat *et al.*, 2004; Michelson *et al.*, 2003). These trials documented effectiveness compared with placebo based on ratings of ADHD symptoms by parents, but they did not report information from teacher ratings. Clinical impressions suggested that the magnitude of effect in typical cases with ADHD was less than for stimulants (Steinhoff, 2004). Recently, the effectiveness of ATX has been demonstrated for the treatment of children with ADHD and comorbid conditions, including anxiety (Kratochvil, Newcorn, Arnold *et al.*, 2005), tics (Allen, Kurlan, Gilbert *et al.*, 2005) and pervasive developmental disorder (PDD) (Troost, Steenhuis, Tuynman-Qua *et al.*, 2006). A review of the side-effect profile suggested that insomnia was similar to the stimulants, anorexia less than the stimulants and vomiting more common (Gibson, Bettinger, Patel *et al.*, 2006). Because ATX was classified as an antidepressant, it received the same black box warning about possible suicidality as did the antidepressant drugs (US Food & Drug Administration, 2005). The UK Committee on Safety of Medicines recommends warning families of suicide risk so that they can be vigilant.

The PK properties of ATX have been well described in children (Witcher, Long, Smith *et al.*, 2003) and adults (Sauer, Ring, & Witcher, 2005). A standard dose of 1 mg/kg produces a maximum plasma concentration of about 300 μg/L about 2 hours after dosing with a $t_{1/2}$ of about 3 hours. Polymorphism in a gene for a cytochrome enzyme (CYP-2D6) affects metabolism of the drug. One variant produces fast metabolism and a short $t_{1/2}$ (3–4 hours), and the other produces slow metabolism and a long $t_{1/2}$ (24 hours) (Witcher, Long, Smith *et al.*, 2003). Surprisingly, this PK difference did not translate into differences in titrated daily dose, efficacy or side-effect profiles (Allen & Michelson, 2002; Michelson *et al.*, 2001) so prescription based on genotype was not considered necessary. In spite of the short $t_{1/2}$, Sauer, Ring, & Witcher (2005) suggested a rationale for once daily dosing: studies on rats showed that some PD effects (inhibition of the NE transporter) may persist much longer than the short PK $t_{1/2}$ of 2 hours.

However, some recent PD studies suggest waxing and waning of effect across the day. For example, a recent PD study of children with ADHD revealed a correlation of PK and PD effects, with rapid onset and offset on surrogate measures of efficacy in a laboratory school setting (Wigal *et al.*, 2005). This study investigated the PD effects of a single daily dose of ATX (titrated up to a maximum of 1.2 mg/kg) in children with ADHD. This study showed clear acute effects of ATX that lagged but paralleled the PK profile of rising and falling blood levels, with a significant and near-maximum effect 2 hours after dosing which dissipated by 7 hours after dosing. Furthermore, slow metabolizers develop plasma concentrations about five times higher than fast metabolizers and manifest both greater efficacy and greater side-effects (increases in heart rate, blood pressure, tremor and decrease in appetite). These clinical differences can be attributed to differences in plasma ATX exposure (see Michelson, Read, Ruff *et al.*, 2007).

In 2000, another pharmaceutical company (Cephalon) initiated a program to develop modafinil (MFL) for the treatment of ADHD. MFL is a novel medication which was developed for the treatment of narcolepsy (which was once treated with stimulant medications). A maximum plasma concentration is achieved about 3 hours after dosing and the $t_{1/2}$ is about 4 hours, with a PD profile that suggests rapid onset and offset. However, in a study of once daily (300 mg) versus twice daily (100/200 or 200/100 mg) dosing to evaluate acute tolerance, administration of the full dose in the morning produced a larger overall effect than either divided dose (Biederman, Swanson, Wigal *et al.*, 2006). This offered no evidence of acute tolerance as with the stimulants, and also suggested once daily dosing.

These early studies suggested a higher dose of MFL would be required for the treatment of ADHD in children (200–400 mg) than for the treatment of narcolepsy in adults (100–200 mg), and that once daily dosing was superior to dividing the dose. Based on this, MFL was reformulated in a concentrated form (Sparlon©) to make smaller tablets for the higher doses estimated to be required for clinical treatment of children. Three clinical trials provided evidence of efficacy (Biederman,

Swanson, Wigal *et al.*, 2005; Greenhill, Biederman, Boellner *et al.*, 2006; Swanson, Greenhill, Lopez *et al.*, 2006b). The FDA review process accepted efficacy, but expressed concern about possible rare, serious dermatological side-effects, including suspected cases of Stevens–Johnson syndrome and a variety of skin rashes. The FDA requested further studies of this possibility, but the company elected instead to withdraw the application and to cancel the development of MFL for the treatment of ADHD (Cephalon, 2006).

Antidepressant and Antianxiety Medications

The use of antidepressants to treat children with psychiatric disorders is increasing (see chapter 37 for their clinical use in depression). Zito and Safer (2005) estimated that the recent treatment rate was three times higher in the USA (1.63%) than in Europe (less than 0.55%), and documented significant cross-national differences in the clinical practices, which resulted in different preferences for one class of antidepressant over the other (e.g., SSRIs are favored in the USA while tricyclics are favored in Germany).

The increase in use of SSRIs preceded studies of the efficacy of these drugs in children. Lack of efficacy of tricyclic antidepressants (Hazell, O'Connell, Heathcote *et al.*, 1995) and concern about rare but serious cardiac side-effects (Riddle, Geller, & Ryan, 1993) led to widespread clinical use of SSRIs (e.g., fluoxetine, paroxetine, sertraline) in the treatment of depression in children.

The use of SSRIs to treat depression in children was based on documented efficacy in adults, and became a common clinical practice even though these drugs were not fully evaluated and approved for use in children (Hughes, Emslie, Crismon *et al.*, 1999). Research followed clinical practice, and some trials did not find effectiveness. Reviews of the published studies of SSRIs for the treatment of childhood depression are provided by Cheung, Emslie, & Mayes (2006) and Wagner (2005), and reviews of unpublished ($n = 10$) as well as published ($n = 6$) studies are provided by the US Food and Drug Administration (2003a) and the UK Medicines and Healthcare Products Regulatory Agency (2003). Only one drug, fluoxetine (Prozac©), was shown to be superior to placebo in more than one randomized clinical trial (RCT) (Cheung, Emslie, & Mayes, 2006). Emslie, Rush, Weinberg *et al.* (1997) conducted a single-site RCT that showed a significant difference in response in the drug than the placebo condition (56% vs. 33%), and this response rate was replicated (52% vs. 37%) in a multisite study (Emslie, Heiligenstein, Wagner *et al.*, 2002). The US FDA considered these two trials and approved this SSRI (fluoxetine) for the treatment of childhood depression in 2003 (US Food and Drug Administration, 2003a). A multimodal RCT against placebo (March, Silva, Petrycki *et al.*, 2004) found a similar response rate (61% vs. 35%). Clinical recommendations are provided in chapter 37.

The review of other SSRIs is complicated by high rates of response to placebo (30–60% in various trials), different outcome measures across trials, small number of trials and a variety of other factors, including choice of dose and dosing regimen (Findling, Nucci, Piergies *et al.*, 2006). No other SSRI has reached the criterion of two positive RCTs that the FDA requires for approval, although one combined analysis of two studies provided evidence of efficacy for sertraline (Wagner, Ambrosini, Rynn *et al.*, 2003) as did one study of citalopram (Wagner, Robb, Findling *et al.*, 2004). RCTs of the other SSRIs were negative (Wagner, 2005). RCTs in adults, however, suggest that the SSRIs are equally efficacious. Cheung, Emslie, & Mayes (2006) suggested that it is unlikely that the various SSRIs differ in efficacy in children; rather, methodological differences across the studies may be responsible for the lack of significant effects in some studies.

Concern about side-effects of SSRIs related to suicidal ideation has generated considerable controversy, with multiple committees and reports from the US Food and Drug Administration (2004a,b) and the UK Medicines and Health Products Regulatory Agency (2003). Analyses of combined cases from multiple studies suggested that the relative risk is significantly greater than 1.0 in RCTs; this rare adverse event was more commonly reported in the drug (4%) than the placebo (2%) condition. Analysis of suicide rates during times of increasing use of the SSRI (Gibbons, Hur, Blaumik *et al.*, 2005), the absence of SSRI in the serum of many suicide victims (Leon, Marzuk, Tardiff *et al.*, 2004) and the absence of any suicides in the RCTs (Klein, 2006) have led some to discount the significance of this finding. However, a "black box" warning has been recommended for the package labeling of all SSRIs in the USA, and the UK Committee on Safety of Medicines recommends that SSRIs other than fluoxetine are not routinely indicated (Medicines and Health Products Regulatory Agency, 2003).

The SSRIs are the first-line pharmacological treatments for anxiety disorders in adults (Baldwin, Anderson, Nutt *et al.*, 2005), but there are few studies in children and approval by regulatory agencies has not been obtained. Nevertheless, evidence of efficacy of the SSRIs for treatment of anxiety disorders in children has been addressed by the National Institute of Mental Health (NIMH) supported Research Unit for Pediatric Psychopharmacology (RUPP) network. The first RUPP study (Walkup, Labellarte, Riddle *et al.*, 2002) of 128 children with diagnoses of anxiety documented efficacy of 8 weeks' treatment with the SSRI fluvoxamine, with 76% of the group randomly assigned to medication ($n = 63$) showing benefit versus 29% of the group randomly assigned to placebo ($n = 65$). Another RUPP study addressed the treatment of anxiety when it occurs in com-bination with ADHD: it found that adding fluvoxamine for the treatment of anxiety symptoms, after stabilization of treatment of ADHD with MPH, was no different than adding placebo (Abikoff *et al.*, 2005). A trial of another SSRI, sertraline, is now being conducted by the Child and Adolescent Anxiety Multimodal Study of the RUPP network.

Antipsychotic Medications

Antipsychotic medications are used to treat childhood onset schizophrenia, a rare but severe condition (Spencer &

Campbell, 1994; see chapter 45). The effect size (ES), the difference in standard deviation units, from drug–placebo comparisons indicates that the effects of typical or first-generation antipsychotic medications (e.g., haloperidol) are large (ES > 1.0), the difference in standard deviation units. The effects are on both positive and negative symptoms, because of potent blockade of DA D_2 receptors (Seeman & Tallerico, 1999). However, side-effects are present (weight gain and tardive dyskinesia) that limit their long-term use and may be of particular concern in children and adolescents during periods of rapid physical growth (see chapter 45).

The development of second-generation or atypical antipsychotic medications (e.g., clozapine) with different relative effects on classes of dopamine receptors (e.g., D_4 vs. D_2) improved efficacy and reduced the incidence and severity of some side-effects (e.g., tardive dyskinesia). In adults, the primary atypical antipsychotic medication, clozapine, is considered to have greater efficacy and reduced risk for tardive dyskinesia than the primary typical antipsychotic medication, haloperidol. Atypicals, however, show metabolic side-effects related to obesity and diabetes, and rare hematological hazards are present. These adverse effects are particularly strong for clozapine, so treatment guidelines (Lewis, Davies, Jones *et al.*, 2006) suggest clozapine is used only after other atypical antipsychotic medications have been tried and failed. In children, there are few data for any of the atypicals (Findling *et al.*, 2006; Glick, Murray, Vasudevan *et al.*, 2001).

Recently, a small RCT of clozapine and olanzapine was conducted on children with schizophrenia who had failed trials on typical antipsychotic medication (Shaw, Sporn, Gogtay *et al.*, 2006). Over a 7-year period, 25 subjects were identified and entered into a rigorous protocol designed to compare the differential efficacy and side-effects of these two atypical antipsychotic medications when titrated to a clinically effective dose (maximum = 900 mg for clozapine and 20 mg for olanzapine). This study demonstrated greater efficacy (ES difference approximately 0.5) for clozapine (average dose = 327 mg) than olanzapine (average dose = 18.1 mg), not only on negative symptoms (as expected) but also on positive symptoms of the disorder. Some adverse events were greater on clozapine than olanzapine in these doses (enuresis, tachycardia and hypertension), but the increase in prolactin was less.

Antipsychotic medications are also used for adolescents to treat prodromal symptoms of schizophrenia, and trials suggest that they may delay the conversion to frank schizophrenia (see chapter 45).

Antipsychotics are also used for other purposes. A summary of the recent studies on the use of antipsychotics in children and adolescents with bipolar, mood and behavioral disorders is provided by Scahill, Koenig, Carroll *et al.* (2007).

The use of antipsychotic medications to treat aggressive behavior in childhood is common but evidence of efficacy and safety in children is sparse (Schur, Sikich, Findling *et al.*, 2003). However, treatment guidelines have been developed (Pappadopulos, Macintyre, Crismon *et al.*, 2003) to guide use based on clinical experience as well as evidence from controlled trials.

The antipsychotic medication risperidone (RIS) has been used to treat autism. The first RCT was from the RUPP network (McDougle, Scahill, McCracken *et al.*, 2000), which evaluated 101 children, with 52 assigned to placebo and 49 assigned to RIS using ratings on the Aberrant Behavior Checklist. Treatment with RIS improved scores on some subscales (irritability, hyperactivity and stereotypy) but not on others related to the core features of autism (social withdrawal and inappropriate speech). A subsequent publication (McDougle, Scahill, Aman *et al.*, 2005) used a secondary measure designed to evaluate symptoms of autism (social relatedness and language); it revealed no difference between treatment with RIS and placebo on these subscales, despite differences on other scales (sensory motor, affectual reaction and sensory response). A separate industry-sponsored study by Shea, Turgay, Carroll *et al.* (2004) evaluated 79 children, with 39 assigned to placebo and 40 to RIS: it showed a similar degree of improvement on ratings of irritability and hyperactivity. Recently, an open study of ATX for the treatment of children with PDD and autistic features (Troost, Steenhuis, Tuynman-Qua *et al.*, 2006) was conducted with a small group of patients ($n = 12$). This suggested a pattern of effectiveness of a standard dose of ATX (about 1 mg/kg) as with antipsychotic medications (i.e., a reduction of ADHD-like symptoms but not core components of autism). These studies suggest that autism does not yet have a simple biochemical target to define the rationale for pharmacological intervention as for other childhood disorders.

In the studies of atypical antipsychotic medications (i.e., RIS) for the treatment of autism, the most worrisome side-effect was weight gain. In the RUPP study, the weight gain over 8 weeks was 2.7 kg in the RIS condition and 0.8 kg in the placebo condition. In the study by Shaw *et al.* (2006), over 8 weeks of treatment the weight gain in the RIS condition was 2.7 kg and 1.0 kg in the placebo condition. Correll, Penzner, Parikh *et al.* (2006) provided a summary of the adverse effects of various atypical antipsychotics, and concluded that (because of little information from head-to-head trials) no differences across medications had been established. Also, in the study of ATX for the treatment of PDD with autistic features, adverse effects were present in a high proportion (42%) of this small group (e.g., gastrointestinal symptoms, irritability, sleep problems and fatigue) which limited treatment.

Basic Principles of Clinical Pharmacology

Blood levels are not typically measured in clinical practice to determine if the dose of medication places an individual within a "therapeutic range" defined by plasma levels. Titration to effect is used to establish the dose of a drug, and usually the concentration of the drug is merely proportional to the dose and therefore does not add much to the titration process. Therefore, the use of blood levels in clinical practice is not recommended or needed to select the optimal doses for individual patients. However, the population estimates of PK and PD properties of common medications could be used for rational recommendations about dosing level and dosing frequency, and to guide the development of new formulations, as demonstrated by Swanson, Gupta, Guinta *et al.* (1999a) and Swanson *et al.* (2003) for the stimulants. Such evidence-based dosing strategies are apparently not used often, even in otherwise sophisticated randomized, placebo-controlled efficacy trials (for examples for childhood depression see Findling *et al.*, 2006).

Here we emphasize how PK analysis is important in drug development (Fleishaker & Ferry, 1995). PK parameters differ across some subgroups based on age, gender and other factors (Davis, Chen, & Glick, 2003). This provides the rationale for the requirements and guidelines from some regulatory agencies (e.g., US Food and Drug Administration) to obtain PK information in the age group for intended treatment. However, in the reactive research related to current incentives to perform studies in children, PK information has been obtained late in the stages of drug development and has not been used in the design of the clinical trials (DeVeaugh-Geiss *et al.*, 2006). Also, PK analysis has been valuable in characterizing genetic differences in the P450 enzymes that have an important role in the metabolism of many drugs and in characterizing drug interactions (Greenblatt, von Moltke, Harmatz *et al.*, 1998).

Some influential clinical pharmacologists have recommended a concentration-controlled paradigm (Peck, 1993) for clinical trials, in which dose is titrated so that all individuals have the same plasma concentration and the variation in effect is evaluated. Others have recommended the effect-controlled paradigm (Levy, Ebling, & Forrest, 1994), in which dose is titrated so that all individuals have the same effect and variation in plasma concentration is evaluated. Levy (1994) points out that individual differences in effect (the PD properties of a drug, shown on the right of Fig. 16.1) are greater than individual differences in concentrations of the drug in plasma (the PK properties of the drug, shown on the left of Fig. 16.1). In the effect-controlled trial, doses of medication are gradually increased to achieve predetermined intensities of effects, which is similar to the way clinicians titrate dose in clinical practice. For effect-controlled studies, blood samples are obtained from individuals taking different doses of medication, either using sparse sampling of a single blood sample across many individuals to characterize the PK properties in the population (Shader, Harmatz, Oesterheld *et al.*, 1999), or using dense sampling to characterize the PK properties at the effective dose (Swanson *et al.*, 2003; Wigal *et al.*, 2006).

Basic Pharmacokinetics

In clinical practice, empirical dosing regimens have been established by experience. When taken orally (the usual route of administration) in an IR formulation, the recommendation for clinical treatment for most of the drugs listed in Table 16.1 is for administration of the total daily dose in divided portions given two or three times daily (Wilens, 2004). However, long-standing clinical practices may be non-optimal (Findling *et al.*, 2006; Swanson, Agler, Fineberg *et al.*, 1999b). For example, in the development of the MTA protocol, an empirical dosing regimen was established in which IR MPH was administered at 7:30 AM, 11:30 AM and 3:30 PM, but the third dose in the three times daily regimen was reduced relative to the first dose, was established (Greenhill, Abikoff, Arnold *et al.*, 1996; Greenhill *et al.*, 2001). This was based on the assumption that once established for an individual, the optimal dose (or plasma concentration) would remain constant, and with multiple doses (i.e., three times daily, with a 4-hour interdose interval), the carry over from early doses would require lower doses to maintain the constant optimal level of the drug across the day.

Later, when acute tolerance to MPH was discovered, the opposite appeared to be true – the later doses should be the same or larger than the initial dose of the day to achieve an ascending drug (D) and plasma concentration (C). This pattern was incorporated into the controlled-release formulations of MPH (Concerta®; Swanson *et al.*, 2003) and AMP (Adderall XR©; Greenhill *et al.*, 2003). Similar evaluations with basic PK/PD methods have not been applied to optimize the delivery of antidepressant medications. Even in controlled clinical trials based on IR formulations, empirical rather than rational dosing regimens have been used, and these may not be optimal (Findling *et al.*, 2006).

The basic PK and PD principles outlined in Fig. 16.1 can be used to understand and evaluate the twice daily (b.i.d.) or three times daily (t.i.d.) dosing regimes. The starting place for PK analyses is the concentration–time graph (Fig. 16.1), which shows four important PK parameters: C_{max}, T_{max}, $t_{1/2}$ and area under the curve (AUC). The maximum concentration achieved by an oral dose (C_{max}, in ng/mL) and the time when it occurs (T_{max}, in hours) depend on absorption from the gastrointestinal tract into the blood stream. The time required for the drug concentration to fall by 50% is the elimination $t_{1/2}$ of the drug and can be estimated by taking the difference between T_{max} and the time when the concentration is 50% of C_{max}.

The calculation of the AUC is somewhat more complicated, but can be based on a simple principle, the trapezoid rule. Trapezoids are formed based on the points available, the area under each trapezoid is calculated and the AUC is the sum of these areas. AUC is expressed in units derived from the product of concentration (ng/L) and time (hours) or ((ng × hours)/L).

Volume (V) of distribution and clearance (CL) are two of the most important PK concepts for establishing the frequency of dosing (the dosing rate). V can be estimated (Hardman, Limbird, Molinoff *et al.*, 1996) by estimating the zero intercept of the concentration–time curve (C_0), and dividing it into the dose of medication (D/C_0), which yields units of volume [mg/(ng/mL) = liters]. CL is derived using the formula CL = D/AUC, so it is stated in units of volume and time (e.g., L/hour).

Dosing rate (DR) is another PK parameter with considerable potential for understanding drug delivery systems that are used in the new formulations to maintain a target concentration. For a given target concentration (C_x), the dosing rate is merely CL times the target concentration, $DR = CL \times C_x$. Because the units for CL are volume and time (ng/min or L/hour) and for C_x are amount and volume (ng/mL or mg/L), the DR is stated in units of amount and time (mg/hour). DR is crucial for optimizing drug delivery in CR formulations of medications, as well as for determining the size and frequency of doses in regimens with multiple administrations per day. For example, when the volume of distribution of the drug in the body varies across subgroups (e.g., children, adolescents and adults), but the C_{max} for titrated clinical effect is assumed to be the same, then DR should vary across age directly in proportion to CL. This concept may help the practitioner understand some actions and statements of regulatory agencies.

The age-related values of volume of distribution and clearance of MPH provide an instructive example. In the review of the application to approve Concerta® for use in adolescents, there was evidence for higher clearance in adolescents (384 L/hour) than in school-aged children (243 L/hour), but less than expected for adults (497 L/hour), which may be related to differences in body weight and volume in these groups. This led to a change in the prescribing information (see www.Concerta.net), which now contains a note that these PK factors suggest why older (and larger) adolescents may have lower exposure to MPH than younger (and smaller) school-aged children taking the same doses of the drug.

At the other end of the age spectrum, Wigal, Greenhill, Chuang *et al.* (2006) showed that CL was lower in preschool children (99 L/hour) than in school-aged children (232 L/hour), suggesting that less frequent dosing may be appropriate in preschool children than in school-aged children. Taken together, these studies suggest that on the average CL is directly proportional to age, ranging from about 500 L/hour in adults to about 100 L/hour in preschool children. Consideration of these population values of this basic PK property may help clinicians make rational choices about dosing frequency of MPH as a function of age, as suggested by the FDA review and by Wigal, McGough, McCracken *et al.* (2005).

Using these basic terms and formulas from clinical pharmacology, population PK information for a medication may be used to suggest a rational dosing regimen *without* the need to obtain blood samples or drug levels for each individual. Consider IR MPH. In clinical practice, the optimum regimen is established empirically by titration. Because PK and PD effects are closely linked, the first dose in the morning will be expected to produce its maximum effect soon after T_{max}, or about when C_{max} is achieved, so the concentration of the dose that produces the best effect about 2 hours after the initial dose would be considered optimal (C_{opt}), with some practical range (i.e., an upper and a lower limit). The effect would be expected to dissipate as the concentration of the drug falls and thus be proportional to $t_{1/2}$. For short-acting medications that do not reach steady-state levels, basic PK principles suggest that a rational choice for multiple doses would be to administer the first dose to achieve the upper limit of C_{opt}, and that the next dose be administered at a time after the first dose such that the declining concentration does not fall below the lower limit of C_{opt}. If neural adaptations occur, then the values for C_{opt} and its upper and lower limits may change over time (e.g., the limits may increase across the day in the face of acute tolerance; Swanson *et al.*, 2003).

The basic PK principles suggest that, when the optimal initial dose has been established by titration, the subsequent DR should be set to maintain plasma concentration within the upper and lower limits of C_{opt}, and that this would depend on CL. DR, given by the formula $DR = CL \times C_{opt}$, specifies the amount of medication per unit of time (e.g., mg/hour). For example, ADHD children who are responders to stimulants vary in terms of the titrated dose of MPH for optimal response, and the literature suggests that C_{max} values would vary too. For a typical 10-year-old child, the expected values for the initial morning dose would be about 10 ng/mL for a low (e.g., 10-mg) dose, 15 ng/mL for a medium (e.g., 15-mg) dose and 20 ng/mL for a high (e.g., 20-mg) dose. Because CL varies with age, different DRs as a function of age would be required to maintain this level over the day (i.e., from DR ~100 L/hour × 10 ng/mL ~1 mg/hour for preschool children up to DR ~500 L/hour × 10 ng/mL ~5 mg/hour for adults).

An understanding of these basic PK principles may help the practitioner conceptualize and explain how a flat (zero-order) or ascending (first-order) concentration profile over time is achieved, as described by Swanson *et al.* (2003). It is instructive to note that blood sampling and measurement of plasma concentrations in each patient are not necessary to apply these basic principles. For example, Swanson, Gupta, Guinta *et al.* (1999) did not obtain blood samples or use plasma concentrations in the study that proposed acute tolerance to clinical doses of methylphenidate, but instead used published PK values for use along with PD measures from a laboratory classroom setting.

From the concentration–time graph, C_{opt} and AUC can be estimated. AUC can be used to define CL for the dose administered (D/AUC). The product of C_{opt} and CL specifies DR. The desired length of duration (e.g., 10 hours) times DR gives the total daily dose (DD). Under the constraints of DR, duration and DD, a rational choice of frequency and size of multiple doses can be made on the basis of convenience and efficacy: larger doses can be given less often or smaller doses given more often for a given value of DD. The choice of size and frequency will set the upper and lower peaks and valleys in plasma concentrations between doses in the regimen.

However, it should be noted that plasma concentrations of a drug have a logical limitation, because it is the concentration at the site of action (i.e., in the brain) not in the blood that is the target of a rational dosing regimen. Basic PK principles also include methods for estimating brain levels of a drug by mathematical modeling. Compartmental PK models are used to estimate the effect site concentration (C_e). The methods for this are provided in standard books on clinical pharmacology (Gabrielsson & Weiner, 1997), and have been applied to characterize medications used in child psychiatry (Modi, Wang, Hu *et al.*, 2000; Swanson, Gupta, Guinta *et al.*, 1999a).

The example provided by Swanson *et al.* (1999a) shows how PK modeling can be used to estimate the succession of processes of the body that operate after a drug is taken – in other words, what "the body does to the drug." Based on published PK properties of MPH (Chan, Swanson, Soldin *et al.*, 1983), factors related to the drug's absorption from the gastrointestinal tract into the blood stream, distribution from the blood to the brain, and elimination were incorporated into a complex equation (in which D = dose, V = volume of distribution, t_i = time since i^{th} dose and t = time since first dose) to estimate a value at a point in time:

$$C_{e(t)} = \sum_{i=1}^{n}\left(\frac{D_i k_a k_{eo} e^{-ka \cdot t_i}}{V\, k_a(k_e - k_a)\,(k_{eo} - k_a)} + \frac{D_i k_a k_{eo} e^{-ke \cdot t_i}}{V\, k_e(k_a - k_e)\,(k_{eo} - k_e)} + \frac{D_i k_a k_{eo} e^{-keo \cdot t_i}}{V\, k_{eo}(k_a - k_{eo})\,(k_e - k_{eo})}\right)$$

Of course, these calculations would not be made in clinical practice, but they were important for the development of new CR formulations of MPH.

For MPH (as with most drugs), a time delay exists between the plasma concentration and the effect site concentration. When a lag occurs between the concentration in the blood and in the brain, and perhaps also between the concentration in the brain and the effect (as show in Figure 16.1), then the time courses of the concentration–time curve and the effect–time curve are offset. This complicates the definitionof the relationship between effect (as shown in Figure 16.1), and concentration. For example, if the effect continues to increase after the peak concentration is achieved, then a model to account for this lag between PK (plasma) and PD (brain) concentrations is necessary.

The estimated effect site concentration may not be sufficient for optimizing drug delivery, because neural adaptations are likely to occur which also must be considered. In PK/PD analyses, a "link" model provided estimates of the concentrations at the site of action (rather than in the plasma or blood) to relate to effect (E). This is described in detail by Swanson *et al.* (2003) for the example of MPH, in which additional modeling was required to adjust for acute tolerance.

Basic Pharmacodynamics

The data from measurement of the effect (E) over time can be used to graph the relationship (see right panel of Figure 16.1). This effect–time curve may be similar to the concentration–time curve (see left panel of Figure 16.1). After oral administration of a drug, there is a delay between the plasma concentration and the effect. When effect is plotted versus concentration, the effect–concentration relationship may be distorted by a counterclockwise hysteresis loop. The use of C_e, with an adjustment for the time lag, may be necessary to reveal the true effect versus concentration relationship.

The basic assumption of PD analysis is that the concentration of a drug at the site of action (C_e) produces a biochemical effect that starts a cascade of effects (E_e) (see top of Figure 16.1) that eventually result in the clinical response (i.e., symptom reduction).

The information from the concentration–time and effect–time (see left and right sides at the bottom of Figure 16.1) relationships can be used to describe the concentration–effect relationship. Logically, if the two curves were identical, the concentration–effect curve would be represented by a 45° line on a graph. However, even though they may be similar in shape, a lag in the effect–time (see middle of the bottom of Figure 16.1) curve is often present because of the time taken for the psychotropic drug in the blood to reach the site of action in the brain. In addition to the expected time lag, neural adaptations (sensitization or tolerance) may occur. When these processes are present, characteristic patterns in the concentration–effect curves are manifested as deviations from the 45° line, or hysteresis loops. The hysteresis loops are clockwise if sensitization is present and counterclockwise if tolerance is present. When time lag and neural adaptation effects are present, interpretation is difficult, and consideration of both is likely to be required to understand the relationship between C_e and E. This was necessary for PK/PD analyses of MPH (Swanson *et al.*, 2003). An example of counterclock-wise hysteresis in the concentration–effect curve that is caused by the lag between C and C_e is shown in the middle panel at the bottom of Figure 16.1. Expected distortions of the concentration–effect relationships because of a time lag or neural adaptations can be removed by modeling the relationship between C_e and E_e.

Instead of using the complicated mathematical modeling methods to estimate the drug concentrations at the effect size (C_e), it is also possible to measures C_e directly (Plate 16.1b–d), using radiolabeled drug (e.g., [^{11}C] MPH) and serial PET scans (Volkow, Wang, Fowler *et al.*, 1998). Examples from PET studies of brain PK are shown in three sections of Plate 16.1 for methylphenidate (b), haloperidol (c) and mirtazapine (d). PET methods can also be used to obtain direct measures of PD effects on intermediate response in the brain. Examples from PET studies of brain PD are shown in the four sections of Plate 16.2 for transporters (a), receptors (b), neurotransmitters (c) and circuits (d). In subsequent sections of this chapter, we focus on the modern direct measurements from PET imaging methods that inform us about how some intermediate responses occur in the brain.

PK/PD models are used to describe the relationship between the drug concentration (C_e) and effect (E_e). A simple linear function, $E = E_0 + b(C)$, where E_0 is the starting measure of effect when the concentration is zero and b is the increase in E usually does not describe the relationship. The more complex and realistic models for describing concentration–effect relationships are non-linear, because increases in dose (D) or concentration (C) rarely produce proportional increases in effect (E) across the entire range. Based on the Law of Mass Action, PD analyses are based on the assumption that at the site of action, a drug will occupy its targets proportional to C_e and the effects will be proportional to the percentage of targets occupied.

In evaluations of medications in children (or in adults), it is impractical or unethical to make observations across a wide range of concentrations, because the maximum effects of a drug are often associated with side-effects that should or must be avoided. Over a typical acceptable range of concentrations, the concentration–effect relationship may appear linear, with only minor departures from a straight line at the higher doses. Fortunately, methods to estimate the true underlying non-linear relationship are available, such as the E_{max} model, which uses the equation

$$E_i = E_0 + (E_{max} \times C)/(EC_{50} + C)$$

to describe the parabolic relationship between effect and concentration. The first part of the parabola, from 0 up toward the maximum, is often approximately linear and describes the relationship over the clinical range of doses and concentrations of a drug and effect. The E_{max} model has been applied to address important questions such as whether sensitivity to a new drug is greater than to an established standard and how sensitivity changes with increases in dose (for an example for benzodiazepines see Schoemaker, van Gerven, & Cohen, 1998).

Homeostatic mechanisms operate at the cellular (e.g., internalization of transporters and receptors) and neurocircuitry levels (modulation of neuronal firing by more than one process or neurotransmitter). These adaptive mechanisms may operate in the short term during the exposure to a single dose of short-acting medication, as well as in the long term to repeated or chronic exposure to medication. Some of these adaptations may occur rapidly, and the theory of acute tolerance offered by Swanson, Gupta, Guinta *et al.* (1999a) is an example. This neural adaptation was proposed as the underlying reason why increasingly higher concentration of stimulant medications would be required to achieve similar effects throughout the day. In other instances, adaptations occur over time. This is the mechanism thought to underlie the therapeutic effects of antipsychotics and antidepressants and does not occur until after 2–3 weeks of administration. Recently, by using serial PET imaging methods, a direct alternative for estimating brain concentrations of drugs has been applied for stimulants (Volkow, Ding, Fowler *et al.*, 1995), neuroleptics (Schlyer, Volkow, Fowler *et al.*, 1992) and antidepressants (Marthi, Jakobsen, Bender *et al.*, 2004). In the next section, these methods and these examples are discussed.

Imaging Studies on the Distribution of Drugs in the Human Brain

PET is used to measure the regional concentrations of positron-labeled radiotracers with short half-lives in the human brain. For example, using a positron emitter for carbon or fluorine, chemists can label psychoactive medications (^{11}C-methylphenidate or ^{18}F-haloperidol) without affecting their pharmacological properties. Measurement of the regional concentration of the positron-labeled drug (i.e., brain PK properties) can then be obtained non-invasively in the human brain (Plate 16.1b–d). This permits evaluation of the drug's absolute uptake and rate of entry into the brain. Relationships based on these direct measures can be compared with relationships based on values estimated by complex mathematical equations. These estimated values represent the concentration at the site of action in the brain (C_e; see Plate 16.1b–d) and the effect at the brain site of action (E_e; see Plate 16.2a–d).

The strategy of labeling psychotropic drugs and using PET for brain PK to measure the equivalent of C_e has been applied for some therapeutic drugs as well as for some drugs of abuse (e.g., cocaine, methamphetamine). Here we exemplify this PET method for brain PK analysis (Plate 16.1b–d) for each of the main classes of psychoactive medications used for the treatment of childhood psychiatric disorders (e.g., stimulants, neuroleptics and antidepressants).

Stimulant Medications

The value of the brain PK approach is illustrated for MPH (see Plate 16.1b). The pharmacokinetics and bioavailability of MPH in the human brain were investigated using PET and ^{11}C-labeled methylphenidate ([^{11}C] MPH) by Volkow, Ding, Fowler *et al.* (1995). When administered intravenously, the uptake of [^{11}C] MPH in the human brain is high (7.5% ± 1.5% of the injected dose) and fast; peak concentration in the brain (C_e) is reached within 10 minutes of its administration. The PK properties of orally administered MPH in brain are significantly slower than after intravenous administration, and peak concentration in brain is not reached until 60–90 minutes after its administration. The elimination of MPH, estimated after oral intravenous administration, showed a time to half-peak concentration that ranged from 50 to 90 minutes. The elimination of orally administered MPH could not be measured because of the short $t_{1/2}$ of ^{11}C (20 minutes).

The striatum is the brain area with the highest accumulation of MPH, where it binds to dopamine transporters (DAT). Plate 16.1b (top panel) shows the distribution of [^{11}C] MPH in the brain at different times of its administration along with the concentration–time (C_e–time) curves for its absorption, distribution and elimination. These studies were particularly useful for comparing MPH with cocaine, which has a similar potency in blocking DAT. Cocaine is believed to exert its reinforcing effects through DAT blockade (Volkow, Wang, Fowler *et al.*, 1998), and because MPH shares this effect at the site of action in the brain, there were important questions: why MPH was not as reinforcing as cocaine and why it was so infrequently associated with abuse and addiction. Specifically, these PET studies revealed that while their potencies in blocking DAT (C_{max}) and their rates of uptake into the brain (T_{max}) were similar, their rates of elimination ($t_{1/2}$) were not. By comparing the temporal course of the reinforcing effects of intravenous cocaine and of intravenous MPH with their rate of uptake and elimination from brain, this PET method revealed that it was the fast uptake of the stimulant drugs in the striatum that was associated with their reinforcing effects rather than the absolute concentration (C_e).

The much slower brain elimination of MPH than of cocaine is therefore likely to interfere with its frequent and repeated administration because it would rapidly lead to DAT saturation (Plate 16.1b, bottom panel). In contrast, the fast elimination of cocaine from brain allows repeated administration without saturation of DAT and this property is likely to contribute to its higher rate of abuse than MPH. MPH when used therapeutically is given orally, which leads to very slow uptake in brain, so this too dampens its reinforcing effects. The contrast between MPH when used for use versus abuse, including a discussion of acute tolerance that occurs in both use and abuse, has been addressed elsewhere in detail (Spencer, Biederman, Ciccone *et al.*, 2006a; Volkow & Swanson, 2003).

Neuroleptics

The value of the brain PK approach is illustrated for haloperidol (Plate 16.1c). The PK and bioavailability of this "typical" neuroleptic medication in the human brain were investigated using PET and ^{18}F-labeled haloperidol (Schlyer *et al.*, 1992). Because the haloperidol molecule contains a fluorine atom, one can use the positron emitter ^{18}F to label it. The advantage of such an approach in this case is that ^{18}F has a longer $t_{1/2}$ than ^{11}C (120 versus 20 minutes), which is particularly useful for drugs that clear from the brain slowly ($t_{1/2} > 90$ minutes). The study showed a high brain uptake of [^{18}F] haloperidol (6.6% of the injected dose), which peaked at 2 hours with minimal elimination at 10 hours, which was the time at which the last PET measurement was made.

The distribution and site of action concentration (C_e) of the drug in brain were much more extensive than would be expected by the distribution of DA D_2 receptors as revealed for example by the D_2 receptor radioligand [^{18}F] *N*-methylspiroperidol (Plate 16.1c). The cerebellum, striatum and thalamus showed a greater concentration than the cortex. This is likely to reflect not only the fact that haloperidol distributes into specific as well as non-specific binding sites, but also that it binds not only to DA D_2 receptors but also to other receptor types (e.g., acetylcholine receptors, sigma receptors, 5-HT2 receptors). The diversity among neuroleptics in affecting receptors other than the DA D_2 (i.e., D_4, 5-HT, D_1, D_3) is likely to underlie why some patients respond to some neuroleptics better than to others and why atypical but not typical neuroleptics appear to be beneficial for the treatment of negative symptoms (Reynolds, 2004).

Antidepressants

The value of the brain PK approach is illustrated for mirtazapine (Plate 16.1d), a noradrenergic and specific serotonergic antidepressant that does not block monoamine transporter and instead is believed to act at the receptor level by inhibiting α_2-adrenergic auto- and heteroceptors.

The regional brain concentrations (C_e) were assessed with PET and [^{11}C] *N*-methylmirtazapine (Marthi *et al.*, 2004). Peak levels of activity in the brain were observed at 10 minutes post-injection and half-peak elimination varied among the brain regions with a range of 30 to 50 minutes. The distribution was highest in hippocampus and amygdala followed by thalamus and with lower levels in cerebellum (Plate 16.1d).

The brain PK of this antidepressant exemplifies the dissociation that exists between the short PK of some medications and their longer lasting clinical effects. These adaptations can be further analyzed with effect–concentration analyses designed to quantify hysteresis (Gupta *et al.*, 1993; Sheiner, Stanski, Vozeh *et al.*, 1979).

Imaging Studies of the Effects of Drugs at their Cellular Targets

As outlined in Fig. 16.1, the concentration of the drug at the site of action in the brain (C) is assumed to be proportional to its effect at that site of action (E). One effect of the drug on the brain can be measured by the neurotransmitter level. The mechanics of how drugs affect neurotransmitter levels are complex. As a starting place, we present in Plate 16.1(a) a simplified view of three distinct steps:

1 Cell firing releases the neurotransmitter that has specific receptor(s) as targets;

2 A transporter recycles some of the released neurotransmitter, which regulates its temporal and spatial distribution in the extracellular space; and

3 Enzymes operate to either metabolize or synthesize the neurotransmitter, which inactivates or increases its concentration, respectively.

PET (and single photon emission computed tomography; SPECT) have been used to evaluate the potency of psychoactive drugs at their molecular target. This strategy utilizes radioligands that bind to the cellular targets of the medications (i.e., DAT for stimulant medications, D_2 receptors for neuroleptics and SERT for SSRI). When a ligand is available, PET studies can be used to measure the effects at these brain sites (Plate 16.1a).

Table 16.2 summarizes the ranges of occupancies at the relevant molecular targets. One class of target is the transporter,

Table 16.2 Ranges of target occupancies for therapeutic doses of stimulant medications, neuroleptics and antidepressants that have been measured with positron emission tomography (PET) in the human brain.

Drug	Target	Brain region	Occupancy range (%)	Dosage range (mg)	Reference
Stimulants					
Methylphenidate	DAT	Striatum	55.8	5–60	Volkow *et al.* (1998)
			12–71.5		
Neuroleptics					
Typical	DA	Striatum	75	10–150	Fitzgerald *et al.* (2000)
Haloperidol	$D_{2/3}R$	Thalamus	38–90	4–150	
		Temp. cortex	65.5	4–150	
		SN/VTA	34–80	10–150	
		Amygdala	60	10–150	
			24–85		
			59.3		
		Striatum	50.1–68.5		
Atypical	DA D_1R		75.6		Kapur *et al.* (1999);
Clozapine			67.5–83.7	4–511	Tauscher *et al.* (2004)
		Striatum			Bressan *et al.* (2003)
	DA $D_{2/3}R$	Thalamus			
Amisulpride		Temp. cortex	33.8		
		SN/VTA	2–70	3–1200	
		Amygdala			
		Hippocampus	56	10–1200	
		Anterior	3–89		
		cingulate	77.1	4–1200	
		cortex	50.7–91		
			79.6	10–20	
		Striatum	43–93.5	4–20	
Clozapine	5-$HT2_A$	Frontal	40.2	4–6	Kapur *et al.* (1999)
		cortex	27.8–52.4	4–6	
			73		
			64.2–79.5		
			81.5	4–900	
			79.5–82.5		
			78.6	37.5–300	
			69.7–88		
			73.6		
			18–100		
			80.7		
			62–98		
Antidepressants	SERT	Striatum	79	20–100	
Fluoxetine		Thalamus	67–85	20–250	Meyer *et al.* (2004)
		Anterior	83	20–100	
		cingulate	69–100	20–100	
		cortex	82	20–100	
		Prefrontal	53–100	20–100	
		cortex	85.5	20–40	
		Midbrain	80–91	20–40	
		Cuneus	92		
		Hippocampus	80–100		
		Amygdala	79.3		
Bupropion	DAT		67–92		Meyer *et al.* (2002)
		Striatum	92		
			72–100	40–300	
			94		
			82–100		
			21.3		
			12–28		

Table 16.3 Main circuits that have been directly linked to the psychopathology of the disorder.

	Executive function	Reward motivation	Attention	Emotion/ mood	Vigilance/ alertness	Memory learning
Schizophrenia		DA	DA	DA	DA	DA
Depression		DA		5-HT	NE	
ADHD		DA	DA NE			
OCD	5-HT	5-HT				
Anxiety disorder				×	GABA	
Addiction	DA	DA				DA
Autism		×	×			

DA, dopamine; GABA, γ-amine butyric acid; 5-HT, 5-hydroxytryptamine; NE, norepinephrine.

which is the target for stimulant medications and SSRIs. Another class of target is the receptor, which is the target for neuroleptic medications. In Table 16.2, we summarize the effects at the brain sites of action, shown as the percentage of occupancy measured with PET in the human brain for transporter and receptors.

Two different strategies have been used to determine the effect of the drug at its molecular target. One strategy involves pre-administration of various doses of the drug at pre-fixed times (usually at times when peak plasma concentrations are reached) prior to injection of the radioligand to determine the degree to which the various doses block the radioligand binding. The rate of radioligand blockade by the drug can be calculated after appropriate modeling (to account for metabolism of the radiotracer in blood, its delivery into the brain, its transfer into the tissue and its non-specific binding). The rate of blockage will be a function of the receptor or transporter occupancy by the drug. In the other strategy, the drug is administered after the radioligand has reached equilibrium in brain and the rate of its displacement is a function of the potency of the drug for its target. This method can provide information on the rate at which the drug binds to its target, which is obtained by measuring the time from injection of the drug to that of radioligand displacement.

Blockade of Transporters

Stimulant Medications

The value of this approach for PD analysis is illustrated for MPH (see Plate 16.2a). Occupancy of DAT (represented as E in Fig. 16.1) by therapeutic doses of MPH was measured by PET and the DAT radioligand [^{11}C] cocaine, which has a high affinity for DAT. Subjects were pretreated with various doses of MPH given 120 minutes prior to the radioligand and compared with the administration of a placebo. The study revealed that at the site of action in the brain, therapeutic doses of oral MPH induced an effect (represented as E in Fig. 16.1) characterized as a dose-dependent blockade of DAT (Volkow, Wang, Fowler *et al.*, 1998). Efficient DAT blockade was observed with 20 mg MPH (50 ± 5%), and was nearly complete with 40 and 60 mg doses (72 ± 3% and 74 ± 2%, respectively). Thus, the ED_{50} of oral MPH was estimated to be 0.25 mg/kg, and the standard dose of 0.5 mg/kg was shown to block more than 60% of DAT (Volkow, Wang, Fowler *et al.*, 1998). The framework provided by Fig. 16.1 can be used to describe these effects of MPH at the site of action. DAT occupancies (C in Fig. 16.1) were significantly correlated with the plasma concentration of *d*-threo-MPH (C in Fig. 16.1) at 120 minutes after dosing when DAT measurements were made.

PET imaging was used to estimate the plasma concentration of *d*-threo-MPH (C in Fig. 16.1) required to block 50% of the DAT (E in Fig. 16.1). The estimate, about 6 ng/mL (Plate 2a), was surprisingly low and was achieved in these adult subjects at doses in the range used clinically to treat ADHD (0.3–0.6 mg/kg). Until this study, MPH had been traditionally considered a weak psychostimulant, and the lower abuse potential (compared to cocaine) was assumed to be related to rapid metabolism of the drug to ritalinic acid, which has a weak affinity for the DAT, and therefore would have minimal pharmacological effects. The surprising results from this study indicated that after therapeutic oral doses of MPH, the drug itself does reach the brain and has about the same affinity for DAT as cocaine (Volkow, Wang, Fowler *et al.*, 1998). The difference in abuse liability has been attributed to differences in the time course of occupancy of DAT, not the level of occupancy.

A recent PET study that used a different DAT radioligand ([^{11}C] altropane) corroborated that therapeutic doses of MPH block more than 60% of the DAT (Spencer *et al.*, 2006a). In addition, this study compared the brain PK (represented by C in Fig. 16.1) and the reinforcing effects of orally administered IR MPH with the effects of CR MPH (OROS). Spencer *et al.* (2006a) accomplished this by measuring the levels of DAT blockade for a given dose of IR MPH and of OROS MPH across multiple time points after administration. They show that doses of IR MPH (40 mg) and of OROS MPH (90 mg) lead to equivalent maximum effects in the brain (which could be represented by E in Fig. 16.1), reflected by the peak levels of DAT blockade (72% for IR MPH and 68% for OROS MPH) but at different time points. The peak DAT blockade was achieved significantly faster for the 40 mg IR MPH (at 1.7 hours) than for 90 mg OROS MPH (at

5 hours). Also, the levels of DAT blockade during the first 2 hours were significantly higher and therefore were achieved faster for IR MPH than for OROS MPH. The peak level of DAT blockade achieved by 40 mg of IR MPH was associated with mild reinforcing effects (assessed with self-reports of drug liking), but the same peak effect for 90 mg OROS MP was not.

These findings corroborate that the reinforcing effects of stimulant drugs are driven by the rate at which DA increases (change in DA concentration per time unit) rather than DA level per se (for a discussion of adaptation and tolerance see Volkow & Swanson, 2003). Based on this, Spencer *et al.* (2006) speculate that delivery systems that lead to very slow rates of DAT blockade and slow rates of DA increase are likely to have less abuse liability than delivery systems that lead to faster DA changes. This study also compared differences in the duration of DAT blockade between IR and OROS and showed that it was longer for the OROS MPH than for IR MPH, so that at a constant time after dosing (e.g., 7 hours) the level of DAT blockade for OROS MPH (65%) was considerably higher than for IR MPH (40%).

Because the rate of DA change (rate of DAT blockade) is positively associated with the reinforcing effects of MPH, the slower elimination from brain and the longer occupancy of DAT when MPH is delivered by the OROS formulation than by the IR formulation are likely to limit further the rate at which MPH will be self-administered. Also, the rate at which rodents self-administer stimulant drugs has been shown to be associated with the downward slope of DA after its peak in the nucleus accumbens (Ranaldi, Pocock, Zereik *et al.*, 1999). This predicts that stimulant drugs delivered by a system (formulation) that maintains steady state or increasing plasma levels (C) and brain levels (C_e) for longer time periods are less likely to be abused than when delivered by a formulation that leads to more abrupt changes. In fact, the slow onset of CR MPH can even block the effects of other DA agonist drugs, as has recently been shown by Tiihonen, Kuoppasalmi, Foer *et al.* (2007), who documented that 54 mg CR MPH was an effective treatment for the prevention of relapse of intravenous AMP abuse.

Neuroleptics

The value of this brain PD approach is illustrated by haloperidol (Plate 16.2b). The study used fluorine-18-*N*-methylspiroperidol (FNMSP), a dopamine D_2 receptor ligand, to assess the effects of pretreatment with different doses of haloperidol. This study showed that, as expected, haloperidol blocked binding of the D_2 receptor ligand. The percent inhibition of binding (represented by E in Fig. 16.1) correlated with the plasma concentration (represented by C in Fig. 16.1) of the neuroleptic.

This study demonstrated that relatively low plasma concentrations of the neuroleptic were able to produce more than 80% inhibition of DA D_2 receptors, and that much larger plasma concentrations were required to further increase inhibition. It also showed that the quantification of plasma neuroleptic dose correlated with percent inhibition of D_2 receptors by the drug, and that the length of interaction of the neuroleptic with DA D_2 receptors (i.e., E, the effect at the site of action in Fig. 16.1) was shorter than previously described – significant recovery of D_2 receptors was seen as soon as 24 hours after discontinuation of the neuroleptic and returned to almost normal levels 7 days later. This apparent discrepancy between the faster rate for the recovery to baseline levels of D_2 receptor availability upon drug discontinuation than the time required for psychotic symptoms to return, suggests that while D_2 receptors are the targets for haloperidol, adaptations or downstream effects triggered by the receptor blockade underlie its clinical effectiveness. This would explain both why discontinuation of neuroleptic treatment does not result in an immediate relapse, and why clinical effectiveness does not occur until several days after neuroleptic administration even though effective D_2 receptor blockade is achieved within days of neuroleptic initiation.

The levels of D_2 receptor blockade (represented as E in Fig. 16.1) have been measured with PET for a wide variety of neuroleptics (Table 16.2). Based on this literature the consensus is that in the striatum typical neuroleptics require approximately 80% receptor blockade for clinical effectiveness whereas atypical neuroleptics require approximately 40–60% blockade (Bressan, Erlandsson, Jones *et al.*, 2003). In cortical regions the level of DA D_2 receptor blockade achieved with therapeutically effective doses of atypical neuroleptics is significantly higher than in striatum (Bressan *et al.*, 2003; Grunder, Landvogt, Vernaleken *et al.*, 2006).

Antidepressants

Because radioligands for the norepinephrine transporter (NERT) have only recently been developed, there are no published PET studies yet on the potencies of tricyclic antidepressants at the NERT. However, radioligands have been available for the serotonin transporter (SERT), and thus there is a literature on the effects of SSRIs on SERT (i.e., at the site of action, represented by E in Fig. 16.1). For example, the relative potencies of various SSRIs (citalopram, fluoxetine, sertraline, paroxetine or extended-release venlafaxine) at the SERT were evaluated using PET and the SERT radioligand [^{11}C] DASB (Meyer, Wilson, Sagrati *et al.*, 2004). This study showed a non-linear dose–SERT occupancy relationship that peaked at high doses, which would define the effect–concentration relationship (represented by E versus C in Fig. 16.1). It also showed that all of the SSRIs tested at therapeutic doses occupied greater than 80% of the SERT. The relevance of this study lies in the demonstration that: (i) greater than 80% SERT occupancy is required for therapeutic efficacy of SSRIs; and (ii) that differences in the clinical efficacy between the SSRIs cannot be explained on the basis of their differences in the levels of SERT blockade but are likely to reflect differences in PK and bio-availability as well as their effects on targets other than SERT.

Neurotransmitter Concentration

Receptor radioligands have relatively low affinity, so they compete for binding to the receptor with the endogenous neurotransmitter. Thus, they can be used to measure changes in neurotransmitters induced by drugs. The most widely utilized radioligand for this purpose has been [^{11}C] raclopride, which has been used to assess the effects of stimulant drugs (MPH and AMPH) on extracellular concentrations of DA (represented by E in Fig. 16.1). Because [^{11}C] raclopride competes for binding to the D_2 receptor with endogenous DA, the comparison of its binding after placebo from that after the drug can be used to estimate the relative changes in DA it induces (Volkow, Fowler, Wang *et al.*, 1993; Plate 16.2c). This strategy was used to compare the potency of AMPH with that of MPH in increasing DA in the non-human primate brain (Schiffer, Volkow, Fowler *et al.*, 2006). It revealed potency for these two drugs that parallel their relative therapeutic potencies; that is, double the dose of MPH was required to achieve the DA increases induced by AMPH.

A study in healthy adult controls to assess the relationship between the levels of DAT blockade achieved after 60 mg oral MPH and the concomitant increases in striatal DA induced by this dose (Volkow, Wang, Fowler *et al.*, 2002). The study showed that in some subjects the same level of DAT blockade induced much greater increases in DA than in others (see Plate 16.2c). This highlights that differences in the response to a drug between subjects are not necessarily explained by differences in plasma concentration (represented by C in Fig. 16.1), or even delivery into the brain and its relevant molecular targets, but to the differences in the reactivity of the neurotransmitter system (in this case activity of the DA cells). That is, for a given level of DAT blockade, subjects with low DA neuronal firing will show smaller DA increases than subjects with high neuronal firing. The variability in effects of DAT blockade also provides an explanation of why some ADHD subjects do not respond to MPH despite having adequate plasma concentrations. This may account for the large (fivefold) individual difference in dose of medication required to produce a titrated clinical response when used to treat the psychiatric disorders of childhood considered here.

DA cell firing in a given subject fluctuates in part as a function of context: DA cells fire when exposed to stress and to reinforcing, novel or unexpected stimuli. This would suggest that the effects of stimulant medications should be sensitive to the context in which they are administered. Indeed, an imaging study compared the increases in DA induced by MPH as a function of the context of its administration (Volkow, Wang, Fowler *et al.*, 2004). It showed that the DA increases were greater when MPH was given concomitant to a reinforcer (money) than when no reinforcer was available. This provides a mechanism to understand the context dependency for stimulant effects, which was first noted by Conners (1966) 40 years ago.

Effects of Drugs on Brain Function and Neural Networks

The effects of medications on neural networks reflect their downstream effects: the initial molecular targets transmit these signals predominantly through glutamatergic (stimulatory) and GABAergic (inhibitory) pathways. Most of the neurotransmitters that are the main targets for the effects of medication used in child psychiatry have been linked to neural networks (Table 16.3). For example, Alexander, Crutcher, & DeLong (1990) described neural networks as parallel segregated circuits linking cortical, striatal and thalamic brain regions. Le Moal and Simon (1991) used these circuits to propose how a specific neurotransmitter (DA) affected behavior by modulation of activity in these parallel segregated circuits and affected behavior related to psychiatric disorders such as schizophrenia, which is associated with disrupted executive function.

Functional brain imaging techniques have been used to identify the downstream effects of the pharmacological effects of drugs. In the current literature, measures of function are often derived from functional magnetic resonance imaging (fMRI) techniques and the blood oxygen level dependent (BOLD) measure. It is generally believed that the activation signal, which is generated from fMRI, is due to differences in magnetic properties of oxygenated versus deoxygenated hemoglobin (BOLD contrast). During activation of a brain region there is an excess of arterial blood delivered into the area with concomitant changes in the ratio of deoxyhemoglobin to oxyhemoglobin, which generates the signal detected by fMRI. However, functional measures can also be obtained from some PET imaging techniques. For example, as shown in Plate 16.1(a), regional changes in brain glucose utilization can be used to document the consequences of drug effects on neural circuits that are distant from the pharmacological or neurochemical site of action.

Glucose metabolism is measured using PET and the radioligand fluoro-deoxyglucose labeled with ^{18}F (FDG) (shown in Plate 16.1a) and CBF is measured with oxygen-15 labeled water (not shown). Measures of brain glucose metabolism and of CBF serve as surrogate markers of brain activity because glucose is a source of energy for the brain and its transport into the tissue is dependent on CBF. By comparing PET images obtained after placebo and the drug, the selective effects on function can be estimated.

Although initial studies targeted measures of the effects of drugs on specific brain regions, increasingly, studies are targeting the effects of drugs on regional circuits. Inasmuch as drugs target specific neurotransmitter systems, these investigations are providing knowledge on the role of neurotransmitters in the function of brain circuits. Moreover, these imaging studies are also enabling us to understand how regions interact with one another to form circuits responsible for behavior and how their disruption may occur in psychiatric diseases. For example, Seminowicz, Mayberg, McIntosh *et al.* (2004) used PET imaging studies to develop a model for major depression based on a limbic–cortical circuit with three "compartments" (sensory–cognitive, emotional–cognitive and autonomic).

While initial studies evaluated the effects of the drug under no intervention conditions (resting state), there is an increasing number of studies that have evaluated the effects of the drug on brain activation patterns as the individuals are involved in emotional or cognitive tasks. This approach sheds light on the role of neurotransmitters in the function of a given circuit and on its consequent output. We have manipulated expectation in studies of metabolic response to MPH i.v. (Plate 16.2d) in subjects with a history of stimulant (cocaine) abuse (Volkow & Swanson, 2003) and in normal control subjects (Volkow, Wang, Ma *et al.*, 2006). As shown in Plate 16.2(d), in subjects with a history of stimulant abuse (and therefore experienced in the euphoric effects of i.v. stimulants), the effects of MPH on brain metabolism were not in the basal ganglia (the site of biochemical effects presented and discussed earlier), but were primarily in the cerebellum (vermis), thalamus and occipital cortex. In addition, when MPH was unexpected, the metabolic response in the left lateral orbital–frontal cortex was enhanced. In control subjects without prior experience with i.v. stimulants, the effects of expectation on MPH response were largest in the anterior cingulate gyrus and the nucleus accumbens, which are areas related to emotional reactivity and reward. These metabolic responses were interpreted as consequences of biochemical effects concentrated in the caudate nucleus, and apparently reflect the MPH-induced activation of a cortical–striatal–thalamic circuit described by Alexander, Crutcher, & DeLong (1990) and Posner and Raichle (1994).

As more knowledge is gained from these imaging studies on how the brain functions, and in particular how various neurotransmitters overlap in their regulation of brain regions and circuits, it is becoming evident that in most instances the abnormality in a disorder does not reside solely in the one neurotransmitter modified by the medication, but in the brain regions that it regulates or the regions or other neurotransmitters that modulate its function.

Conclusions

The application of basic principles from neuropsychopharmacology has contributed considerably to our understanding of the dose–response and time–response characteristics of medications used to treat childhood psychiatric disorders. PK and PD analyses of medications listed in Table 16.1 are rare but do exist for some drugs. For example, the PK analysis of the stimulant medications, described above, altered clinical practice in terms of frequency of dosing (which moved from once daily to twice or three times daily regimens, in order to cover a longer duration with these short-acting drugs) and conditions of dosing (which moved from before meals to with or after meals, which allowed flexibility in managing the common side-effect of appetite suppression). Also, PK studies of antidepressant drugs in children have been performed (Wilens, Biederman, Baldessarini *et al.*, 1992), but the information obtained has not typically been used to set the dosing regimens used in most clinical trials. Findling *et al.* (2006) suggested that even though the clinical trials of antidepressant drugs have sometimes been unsuccessful in documenting efficacy under double-blind conditions, the efficacy of the drugs themselves should not be dismissed without consideration of their PK properties. Clinical trials should be developed that use rational or optimal drug regimens to evaluate efficacy and safety.

PD analyses have been used to evaluate dosing regimens for stimulants and for non-stimulants that are used for the treatment of ADHD, and this has influenced recent changes in clinical practice. For example, PK/PD inspired CR formulations of MPH (Swanson *et al.*, 2003) and AMP (Greenhill *et al.*, 2003; McCracken, Biederman, Greenhill *et al.*, 2003) are now the most prescribed stimulant formulations for the treatment of ADHD in the USA. PK/PD analyses have also been applied (see Wigal, McGough, McCracken *et al.*, 2005) to evaluate possible age-related differences in dose or dosing rate in the treatment of adolescents and preschool children.

Other examples of how PK/PD analyses have affected clinical practice are provided by the drug development programs for the FDA-approved use of ATX and the unapproved experimental use of MFL. In these examples, PK/PD analysis was used to evaluate the titration schedules (i.e., how rapidly increases in dose are made) and the daily dosing schedule (i.e., once daily and twice daily dosing regimens). For ATX, PK/PD analysis of ATX (Michelson *et al.*, 2007) was used to justify the recommendation for once daily dosing. For MFL, PK/PD analysis were used to evaluate the difference between slow (weekly) and fast (daily) increases in dose for titration, and resulted in the recommendation of the fast schedule that produces the same results as the slow schedule (Greenhill *et al.*, 2006; Swanson, Greenhill, Lopez *et al.*, 2006b).

In this chapter we focus on the effects of drugs on their direct targets and on downstream circuits, but we do not address parallel molecular biology studies that are shedding light on how the effects of drugs affect the transduction signals that regulate cell function, and we do not discuss the intracellular events that follow the interaction of the drug with its target (Popoli, Brunello, Perez *et al.*, 2000). Instead, we describe modern direct measurements from PET imaging methods that inform us about how some intermediate responses occur in the brain, including biochemical effects on neurotransmitter systems (transporters, enzymes, receptors, neurotransmitter release) and on functional effects on brain circuits (glucose utilization and blood flow).

We consider the use of PET for brain PK and PD analysis to be a major methodological advance in this area. Until recently, most of the knowledge on the pharmacological properties of psychoactive drugs relied on the use of preclinical models, *in vitro* measurements and on behavioral studies linking drug plasma concentrations and behavioral effects. The advent of imaging technologies has revolutionized the way we characterize medications, for these methods have enabled us not only to assess the PK properties and bioavailability of drugs directly in the human brain, but also to asses the potency of drugs at their relevant targets and their effects on neuronal circuits implicated in the neurobiology of the psychiatric disorders.

References

Abikoff, H., McGough, J., Vitiello, B., McCracken, J., Davies, M., Walkup, J., *et al.* for the RUPP Study Group. (2005). Sequential pharmacotherapy for children with comorbid attention-deficit/ hyperactivity and anxiety disorders. *Journal of the American Academy of Child and Adolescent Psychiatry*, *44*, 418–427.

Alexander, G. E., Crutcher, M. D., & DeLong, M. R. (1990). Basal ganglia-thalamocortical circuits: parallel substrates for motor, oculomotor, "prefrontal" and "limbic" functions. *Progress in Brain Research*, *85*, 119–146.

Allen, A. J., & Michelson, D. (2002). Drug development process for a product with a primary pediatric indication. *Journal of Clinical Psychiatry*, *63*, 44–49.

Allen, A. J., Kurlan, R. M., Gilbert, D. L., Coffey, B. J., Linder, S. L., Lewis, D. W., *et al.* (2005). Atomoxetine treatment in children and adolescents with ADHD and comorbid tic disorders. *Neurology*, *65*, 1941–1949.

Anders, T., & Sharfstein, S. (2006). ADHD drugs and cardiovascular risk. *New England Journal of Medicine*, *354*, 2296–2298; author reply 2296–2298.

Baldwin, D. S., Anderson, I. M., Nutt, D. J., Bandelow, B., Bond, A., Davidson, J. R., *et al.* (2005). Evidence-based guidelines for the pharmacological treatment of anxiety disorders: recommendations from the British Association for Psychopharmacology. *Journal of Psychopharmacology*, *19*, 567–596.

Biederman, J., Quinn, D., Weiss, M., Markabi, S., Weidenman, M., Edson, K., *et al.* (2003). Efficacy and safety of Ritalin LA, a new, once daily, extended-release dosage form of methylphenidate, in children with attention deficit hyperactivity disorder. *Paediatric Drugs*, *5*, 833–841.

Biederman, J., Swanson, J. M., Wigal, S. B., Kratochvil, C. J., Boellner, S. W., Earl, C. Q., *et al.* (2005). Efficacy and safety of modafinil film-coated tablets in children and adolescents with attention-deficit/hyperactivity disorder: results of a randomized, double-blind, placebo-controlled, flexible-dose study. *Pediatrics*, *116*, e777–784.

Biederman, J., Swanson, J. M., Wigal, S. B., Boellner, S. W., Earl, C. Q., & Lopez, F. A. Modafinil ADHD Study Group. (2006). A comparison of once-daily and divided doses of modafinil in children with attention-deficit/hyperactivity disorder: a randomized, double-blind, and placebo-controlled study. *Journal of Clinical Psychiatry*, *67*(5), 727–735.

Bressan, R. A., Erlandsson, K., Jones, H. M., Mulligan, R., Flanagan, R. J., Ell, P. J., *et al.* (2003). Is regionally selective D2/D3 dopamine occupancy sufficient for atypical antipsychotic effect? An *in vivo* quantitative [123I] epidepride SPET study of amisulpride-treated patients. *American Journal of Psychiatry*, *160*, 1413–1420.

Buitelaar, J. K., Danckaerts, M., Gillberg, C., *et al.* for the Atomoxetine International Study Group. (2004). A prospective, multicenter, open-label assessment of atomoxetine in non-North American children and adolescents with ADHD. *European Child and Adolescent Psychiatry*, *13*, 249–257.

Bymaster, F. P., Katner, J. S., Nelson, D. L., Hemrick-Luecke, S. K., Threlkeld, P. G., Heiligenstein, J. H., *et al.* (2002). Atomoxetine increases extracellular levels of norepinephrine and dopamine in prefrontal cortex of rat: a potential mechanism for efficacy in attention deficit/hyperactivity disorder. *Neuropsychopharmacology*, *27*, 699–711.

Centers for Disease Control and Prevention. (2005). Mental health in the United States. Prevalence of diagnosis and medication treatment for attention-deficit/hyperactivity disorder – United States, 2003. *MMWR Morbidity and Mortality Weekly Report*, *54*, 842–847.

Cephalon website. http://www.cephalon.com/

Chan, Y. P., Swanson, J. M., Soldin, S. S., Thiessen, J. J., Macleod, S. M., Logan, W. (1983). Methylphenidate hydrochloride given with or before breakfast: II. Effects on plasma concentration of methylphenidate and ritalinic acid. *Pediatrics*, *72*, 56–59.

Cheung, A. H., Emslie, G. J., & Mayes, T. L. (2006). The use of antidepressants to treat depression in children and adolescents. *Canadian Medical Association Journal*, *174*, 193–200.

Concerta website. http://www.concerta.net/ Accessed March 2007.

Conners, C. K. (1966). The effect of dexedrine on rapid discrimination and motor control of hyperkinetic children under mild stress. *Journal of Nervous and Mental Disease*, *142*, 429–433.

Correll, C. U., Penzner, J. B., Parikh, U. H., Mughal, T., Javet, T., Carbon, M., *et al.* (2006). Recognizing and monitoring adverse events of second-generation antipsychotics in children and adolescents. *Child Adolescent Psychiatry Clinics North America*, *15*, 177–206.

Davis, J. M., Chen, N., & Glick, I. D. (2003). A meta-analysis of the efficacy of second-generation antipsychotics. *Archives of General Psychiatry*, *60*, 553–564.

DeVeaugh-Geiss, J., March, J., Shapiro, M., Andreason, P. J., Emslie, G., Ford, L. M., *et al.* (2006). Child and adolescent psychopharmacology in the new millennium: a workshop for academia, industry, and government. *Journal of the American Academy of Child and Adolescent Psychiatry*, *45*, 261–270.

Emslie, G. J., Heiligenstein, J. H., Wagner, K. D., Hoog, S. L., Ernest, D. E., Brown, E., *et al.* (2002). Fluoxetine for acute treatment of depression in children and adolescents: a placebo-controlled, randomized clinical trial. *Journal of the American Academy of Child and Adolescent Psychiatry*, *41*, 1205–1215.

Emslie, G. J., Hughes, C. W., Crismon M. L., Lopez, M., Pliszka, S., Toprac, M. G., *et al.* (2004). A feasibility study of the childhood depression medication algorithm: the Texas Children's Medication Algorithm Project (CMAP). *Journal of the American Academy of Child and Adolescent Psychiatry*, *43*, 519–527.

Emslie, G. J., Rush, A. J., Weinberg, W. A., Kowatch, R. A., Hughes, C. W., Carmody, T., *et al.* (1997). A double-blind, randomized, placebo-controlled trial of fluoxetine in children and adolescents with depression. *Archives of General Psychiatry*, *54*, 1031–1037.

Findling, R. L., Nucci, G., Piergies, A. A., Gomeni, R., Bartolic, E. I., Fong, R., *et al.* (2006). Multiple dose pharmacokinetics of paroxetine in children and adolescents with major depressive disorder or obsessive-compulsive disorder. *Neuropsychopharmacology*, *31*, 1274–1285.

Fitzgerald, P. B., Kapur, S., Remington, G., Roy, P., & Zipursky, R. B. (2000). Predicting haloperidol occupancy of central dopamine D_2 receptors from plasma levels. *Psychopharmacology (Berlin)*, *149*, 1–5.

Fleishaker, J., & Ferry, J. (1995). Pharmacokinetic-pharmacodynamic modeling in drug development: Comments and applications. In H. Derendorf, & F. Hochhaus (Eds.), *Handbook of pharmacokinetic/pharmacodynamic correlation* (pp. 57–78). Boca Raton: CRC Press.

Gabrielsson, J., & Weiner, D. (1997). *Pharmacokinetic and pharmacodynamic data analysis, concepts and applications* (2nd edn.). Stockholm: Swedish Pharmaceutical Press.

Gibbons, R. D., Hur, K., Bhaumik, D. K., & Mann, J. J. (2005). The relationship between antidepressant medication use and rate of suicide. *Archives of General Psychiatry*, *62*, 165–172.

Gibson, A. P., Bettinger, T. L., Patel, N. C., & Crismon, M. L. (2006). Atomoxetine versus stimulants for treatment of attention deficit/hyperactivity disorder. *Annals of Pharmacotherapy*, *40*, 1134–1142.

Gillberg, C., Melander, H., von Knorring, A. L., Janols, L. O., Thernlund, G., Hagglof, B., *et al.* (1997). Long-term stimulant treatment of children with attention-deficit hyperactivity disorder symptoms. A randomized, double-blind, placebo-controlled trial. *Archives of General Psychiatry*, *54*, 857–864.

Glick, I. D., Murray, S. R., Vasudevan, P., Marder, S. R., & Hu, R. J. (2001). Treatment with atypical antipsychotics: new indications and new populations. *Journal of Psychiatric Research*, *35*, 187–191.

Greenblatt, D. J., von Moltke, L. L., Harmatz, J. S., & Shader, R. I. (1998). Drug interactions with newer antidepressants: Role of human cytochromes P450. *Journal of Clinical Psychiatry*, *59* (Supplement 15), 19–27.

Greenhill, L., Beyer, D. H., Finkleson, J., Shaffer, D., Biederman, J., Conners, C. K., *et al.* (2002). Guidelines and algorithms for the use of methylphenidate in children with attention-deficit/hyperactivity disorder. *Journal of Attention Disorders*, 6(Supplement 1), S89–100.

Greenhill, L. L., Biederman, J., Boellner, S. W., Rugino, T. A., Sangal, R. B., Earl, C. Q., *et al.* (2006). A randomized, double-blind, placebo-controlled study of modafinil film-coated tablets in children and adolescents with attention-deficit/hyperactivity disorder. *Journal of the American Academy of Child and Adolescent Psychiatry*, *45*, 503–511.

Greenhill, L. L., Pliszka, S., Dulcan, M. K., Bernet, W., Arnold, V., Beitchman, J., *et al.* (2001). Summary of the practice parameter for the use of stimulant medications in the treatment of children, adolescents, and adults. *Journal of the American Academy of Child and Adolescent Psychiatry*, *40*, 1352–1355.

Greenhill, L. L., Swanson, J. M., Steinhoff, K., Fried, J., Posner, K., Lerner, M., *et al.* (2003). A pharmacokinetic/pharmacodynamic study comparing a single morning dose of Adderall to twice-daily dosing in children with ADHD. *Journal of the American Academy of Child and Adolescent Psychiatry*, *42*, 1234–1241.

Greenhill, L. L., Abikoff, H. B., Arnold, L. E., Cantwell, D. P., Connors, C. K., Elliott, G., *et al.* (1996). Medication treatment strategies in the MTA study: Relevance to clinicians and researchers. *Journal of the American Academy of Child and Adolescent Psychiatry*, *35*, 1304–1313.

Greenhill, L. L., Kollins, S., Abikoff, H., McCracker, J., Riddle, M., Swanton, J., *et al.* (2006). Efficacy and Safety of Immediate-Release Methylphemidate Treatment for Preschoolers with ADHD. *Journal of the American Academy of Child and Adolescent Psychiatry*.

Grunder, G., Landvogt, C., Vernaleken, I., Buchholz, H. G., Ondracek, J., Siessmeier, T., *et al.* (2006). The striatal and extrastriatal D_2/D_3 receptor-binding profile of clozapine in patients with schizophrenia. *Neuropsychopharmacology*, *31*, 1027–1035.

Gupta, S. K., Hwang, S. S., Benet, L. Z., & Gumbleton, M. (1993). Interpretation and utilization of effect and concentration data collected in an *in vivo* pharmacokinetic and *in vitro* pharmacodynamic study. *Pharmaceutical Research*, *10*, 889–894.

Hardman, J. G., Limbird, P. B., Molinoff, P. B., Rutton, R. W., & Gilman, A. G. (Eds) Goodman & Gilman's The Pharmacological Basics of Therapeutics, Ninth Edition. New York: McGraw-Hill.

Hazell, P., O'Connell, D., Heathcote, D., Robertson, J., & Henry, D. (1995). Efficacy of tricyclic drugs in treating child and adolescent depression: a meta-analysis. *British Medical Journal*, *310*, 897–901.

Health Canada. (2005). *Health Canada suspends the market authorization of ADDERALL XR®, a drug prescribed for Attention Deficit Hyperactivity Disorder (ADHD) in children.* Ottawa: Health Canada.

Hughes, C. W., Emslie, G. J., Crismon, M. L., Wagner, K. D., Birmaher, B., Geller, B., *et al.* (1999). The Texas Children's Medication Algorithm Project: report of the Texas Consensus Conference Panel on Medication Treatment of Childhood Major Depressive Disorder. *Journal of the American Academy of Child and Adolescent Psychiatry*, *38*, 1442–1454.

Jensen, P. S., Arnold, L. E., Swanson, J., Vitiello, B., Abikoff, H. B., Greenhill, L. L., *et al.* (2007). Follow-up of the NIMH MTA study at 36 months after randomization. *Journal of the American Academy of Child and Adolescent Psychiatry*, *46*, 988–1001.

Jick, H., Kaye, J. A., & Black, C. (2004). Incidence and prevalence of drug-treated attention deficit disorder among boys in the UK. *British Journal of General Practice*, *54*, 345–347.

Kapur, S., Zipursky, R. B., & Remington, G. (1999). Clinical and theoretical implications of 5-HT2 and D2 receptor occupancy of clozapine, risperidone, and olanzapine in schizophrenia. *American Journal of Psychiatry*, *156*, 286–293.

Kelsey, D. K., Sumner, C. R., Casat, C. D., Coury, D. L., Quintana, H., Saylor, K. E., *et al.* (2004). Once-daily atomoxetine treatment for children with attention-deficit/hyperactivity disorder, including an assessment of evening and morning behavior: A double-blind, placebo-contolled trial. *Pediatrics*, *114*, 1–8.

Klein, D. F. (2006). The flawed basis for FDA post-marketing safety decisions: the example of anti-depressants and children. *Neuropsychopharmacology*, *31*, 689–699.

Kratochvil, C. J., Newcorn, J. H., Arnold, L. E., Duesenberg, D., Emslie, G. J., Quintana, H., *et al.* (2005). Atomoxetine alone or combined with fluoxetine for treating ADHD with comorbid depressive or anxiety symptoms. *Journal of the American Academy of Child and Adolescent Psychiatry*, *44*, 915–924.

Le Moal, M., & Simon, H. (1991). Mesocorticolimbic dopaminergic network: functional and regulatory roles. *Physiological Reviews*, *71*, 155–234.

Leon, A. C., Marzuk, P. M., Tardiff, K., & Teres, J. J. (2004). Paroxetine, other antidepressants, and youth suicide in New York City: 1993 through 1998. *Journal of Clinical Psychiatry*, *65*, 915–918.

Levy, G. (1994). Mechanism-based pharmacodynamic modeling. *Clinical Pharmacology and Therapeutics*, *56*, 356–358.

Levy, G., Ebling, W., & Forrest, A. (1994). Concentration- or effect-controlled clinical trails with sparse data. *Clinical Pharmacology and Therapeutics*, *56*, 1–8.

Lewis, S. W., Davies, L., Jones, P. B., Barnes, T. R. E., Murray, R. M., Kerwin, R., *et al.* (2006). Randomised controlled trials of conventional antipsychotic versus new atypical drugs, and new atypical drugs versus clozapine, in people with schizophrenia responding poorly to, or intolerant of, current drug treatment. *Health Technology Assessment*, *10*, 1–165.

March, J., Silva, S., Petrycki, S., Curry, J., Wells, K., Fairbank, J., *et al.* (2004). Fluoxetine, cognitive-behavioral therapy, and their combination for adolescents with depression: Treatment for Adolescents With Depression Study (TADS) randomized controlled trial. *Journal of the American Medical Association*, *292*, 807–820.

Marthi, K., Jakobsen, S., Bender, D., Hansen, S. B., Smith, S. B., Hermansen, F., *et al.* (2004). [*N*-methyl-11C] Mirtazapine for positron emission tomography neuroimaging of antidepressant actions in humans. *Psychopharmacology (Berlin)*, *174*, 260–265.

McCracken, J. T., Biederman, J., Greenhill, L. L., Swanson, J. M., McGough, J. J., Spencer, T. J., *et al.* (2003). Analog classroom assessment of a once-daily mixed amphetamine formulation, SLI381 (Adderall XR), in children with ADHD. *Journal of the American Academy of Child and Adolescent Psychiatry*, *42*, 673–683.

McDougle, C. J., Scahill, L., Aman, M. G., McCracken, J. T., Tierney, E., Davies, M., *et al.* (2005). Risperidone for the core symptom domains of autism: results from the study by the autism network of the research units on pediatric psychopharmacology. *American Journal of Psychiatry*, *162*, 1142–1148.

McDougle, C. J., Scahill, L., McCracken, J. T., Aman, M. G., Tierney, E., Arnold, L. E., *et al.* (2000). Research Units on Pediatric Psychopharmacology (RUPP) Autism Network. Background and rationale for an initial controlled study of risperidone. *Child and Adolescent Psychiatric Clinics of North America*, 9, 201–224.

Medicines and Health Products Regulatory Agency. (2003). Selective Serotonin Reuptake Inhibitors (SSRIs): Overview of regulatory status and CSM advice relating to major depressive disorder (MDD) in children and adolescents including a summary of available safety and efficacy data. http://www.mhra.gov.uk/home/idcplg?IdcService=SS

Meyer, J. H., Goulding, V. S., Wilson, A. A., Hussey, D., Christensen, B., Houle, S. (2002). Bupropion occupancy of the dopamine transporter is low during clinical treatment. *Psychopharmacology (Berlin)*, 163, 102–105.

Meyer, J. H., Wilson, A. A., Sagrati, S., Hussey, D., Carella, A., Potter, W. Z., *et al.* (2004). Serotonin transporter occupancy of five selective serotonin reuptake inhibitors at different doses: An [11C] DASB positron emission tomography study. *American Journal of Psychiatry*, *161*, 826–835.

Michelson, D., Faries, D., Wernicke, J., Kelsey, D., Kendrick, K., Sallee, F. R., *et al.* (2001). Atomoxetine in the treatment of children and adolescents with attention-deficit/hyperactivity disorder: a randomized, placebo-controlled, dose-response study. *Pediatrics*, *108*, E83.

Michelson, D., Adler, L., Spencer, T., Reimherr, F. W., West, S. W., Allen, A. J., *et al.* (2003). Atomoxetine in adults with ADHD: Two randomized, placebo-controlled studies. *Biological Psychiatry*, *53*, 112–120.

Michelson, D., Read, H. A., Ruff, D. D., Witcher, J., Zhang, S., & McCracken, J. (2007). CYP2D6 and clinical response to atomoxetine in children and adolescents with ADHD. *Journal of the American Academy of Child and Adolescent Psychiatry*, *46*(2), 242–251.

Modi, N. B., Wang, B., Hu, W. T., & Gupta, S. K. (2000). Effect of food on the pharmacokinetics of osmotic controlled-release methylphenidate HCl in healthy subjects. *Biopharmaceuticals and Drug Disposition*, *21*, 23–31.

Molina, B. S. G., Flory, K., Hinshaw, S. P., Greiner, A. R., Arnold, L. E., Swanson, J. *et al.* (2007). Deliquent behavior and emerging substance use in the MTA at 36 months: Prevalence, course, and treatment effects. *Journal of the American Academy of Child and Adolescent Psychiatry*, *46*, 1027–1039.

MTA Cooperative Group. (1999a). A 14-month randomized clinical trial of treatment strategies for attention-deficit/hyperactivity disorder. The MTA Cooperative Group. Multimodal Treatment Study of Children with ADHD. *Archives of General Psychiatry*, 56, 1073–1086.

MTA Cooperative Group. (1999b). Moderators and mediators of treatment response for children with attention-deficit/hyperactivity disorder: the Multimodal Treatment Study of children with Attention-deficit/hyperactivity disorder. *Archives of General Psychiatry*, *56*, 1088–1096.

MTA Cooperative Group. (2004a). National Insititute of Mental Health Multimodal Treatment Study of ADHD follow-up: 24-month outcomes of treatment strategies for attention-deficit/hyperactivity disorder (ADHD). *Pediatrics*, *113*, 754–761.

MTA Cooperative Group. (2004b). National Institute of Mental Health Multimodal Treatment Study of ADHD follow-up: changes in effectiveness and growth after the end of treatment. *Pediatrics*, *113*, 762–769.

National Institute of Mental Health. (2002). Medications. Bethesda: National Institutes of Health; p. 36. http://www.nimh.nih.gov/

Neligan (undated) (http://www.4um.com/tutorial/science/pharmak.htm)

National Institute for Health and Clinical Excellence (NICE). (2005). Methylphenidate, atomoxetine and dexamfetamine for the treatment of attention deficit hyperactivity disorder in children and adolescents. http://www.nice.org.uk/page.aspx?o=TA013

Nissen, S. E. (2006). ADHD drugs and cardiovascular risk. *New England Journal of Medicine*, *354*, 1445–1448.

Pappadopulos, E., Macintyre, I. J. C., Crismon, M. L., Findling, R. L., Malone, R. P., Derivan, A., *et al.* (2003). Treatment recommendations for the use of antipsychotics for aggressive youth (TRAAY). Part II. *Journal of the American Academy of Child and Adolescent Psychiatry*, *42*, 145–161.

Peck, C. C. (1993). Concentration-controlled versus concentration-defined clinical trials (reply) [Letter]. *Clinical Pharmacology and Therapeutics*, *53*, 385–387.

Pliszka, S. R. (2005). The neuropsychopharmacology of attention-deficit/hyperactivity disorder. *Biological Psychiatry*, *57*, 1385–1390.

Pliszka, S. R., Matthews, T. L., Braslow, K. J., & Watson, M. A. (2006). Comparative effects of methylphenidate and mixed salts amphetamine on height and weight in children with attention-deficit/hyperactivity disorder. *Journal of the American Academy of Child and Adolescent Psychiatry*, *45*, 520–526.

Popoli, M., Brunello, N., Perez, J., & Racagni, G. (2000). Second messenger-regulated protein kinases in the brain: their functional role and the action of antidepressant drugs. *Journal of Neurochemistry*, *74*, 21–33.

Posner, M., & Raichle, M. (1994). *Images of mind*. New York: Scientific American Library.

Ranaldi, R., Pocock, D., Zereik, R., & Wise, R. A. (1999). Dopamine fluctuations in the nucleus accumbens during maintenance, extinction, and reinstatement of intravenous D-amphetamine self-administration. *Journal of Neuroscience*, *19*, 4102–4109.

Rappley, M. D., Moore, J. W., & Dokken, D. (2006). ADHD drugs and cardiovascular risk. *New England Journal of Medicine*, *354*, 2296–2298; author reply 2296–2298.

Reynolds, G. P. (2004). Receptor mechanisms in the treatment of schizophrenia. *Journal of Psychopharmacology*, *18*, 340–345.

Riddle, M. A., Geller, B., & Ryan, N. (1993). Another sudden death in a child treated with desipramine. *Journal of the American Academy of Child and Adolescent Psychiatry*, *32*, 792–797.

Santosh, P., Taylor, E., Swanson, J., Wigal, S., Chuang, S., Davies, M., *et al.* (2005). Refining the diagnoses of inattention and overactivity syndromes: a reanalysis of the Multimodal Treatment study of attention deficit hyperactivity disorder (ADHD) based on ICD-10 criteria for hyperkinetic disorder. *Clinical Neuroscience Research*, *5*, 304–314.

Sauer, J., Ring, B. J., & Witcher, J. W. (2005). Clinical pharmacokinetics of atomoxetine. *Clinical Pharmakokinetics*, *44*, 571–590.

Scahill, L., Koenig, K., Carroll, D. H., Patchler, M. (2007). Risperidone approved for the treatment of serious behavioral problems in children with autism. *Journal of Child and Adolescent Psychiatry Nursing*, *20*, 188–190.

Schiffer, W. K., Volkow, N. D., Fowler, J. S., Alexoff, D. L., Logan, J., & Dewey, S. L. (2006). Therapeutic doses of amphetamine or methylphenidate differentially increase synaptic and extracellular dopamine. *Synapse*, *59*, 243–251.

Schlyer, D. J., Volkow, N. D., Fowler, J. S., Wolf, A. P., Shiue, C. Y., Dewey, S. L., *et al.* (1992). Regional distribution and kinetics of haloperidol binding in human brain: a PET study with [18F] haloperidol. *Synapse*, *11*, 10–19.

Schoemaker, R. C., van Gerven, J. M., & Cohen, A. F. (1998). Estimating potency for the Emax-model without attaining maximal effects. *Journal of Pharmacokinetics and Biopharmaceutics*, *26*, 581–593.

Schur, S. B., Sikich, L., Findling, R. L., Malone, R. P., Crismon, M. L., Derivan, A., *et al.* (2003). Treatment recommendations for the use of antipsychotics for aggressive youth (TRAAY). Part I: a review. *Journal of the American Academy of Child and Adolescent Psychiatry*, *42*, 132–144.

Seeman, P., & Tallerico, T. (1999). Rapid release of antipsychotic drugs from dopamine D_2 receptors: an explanation for low receptor occupancy and early clinical relapse upon withdrawal of clozapine or quetiapine. *American Journal of Psychiatry*, *156*, 876–884.

Seminowicz, D. A., Mayberg, H. S., McIntosh, A. R., Goldapple, K., Kennedy, S., Segal, Z., *et al.* (2004). Limbic–frontal circuitry in major depression: a path modeling meta-analysis. *Neuroimage*, *22*, 409–418.

Shader, R. I., Harmatz, J. S., Oesterheld, J. R., Parmelee, D. X., Sallee, F. R., & Greenblatt, D. J. (1999). Population pharmacokinetics of methylphenidate in children with attention-deficit hyperactivity disorder. *Journal of Clinical Pharmacology*, *39*, 775–785.

Shader, R. I., & Oesterheld, J. R. (2006). Facts and public policy: Should I keep my child on ADHD drugs? *Journal of Clinical Pharmacology*, *26*, 223–224.

Shaw, P., Sporn, A., Gogtay, N., Overman, G. P., Greenstein, D., Gochman, P., *et al.* (2006). Childhood-onset schizophrenia: A double-blind, randomized clozapine-olanzapine comparison. *Archives of General Psychiatry*, *63*, 721–730.

Shea, S., Turgay, A., Carroll, A., Schulz, M., Orlik, H., Smith, I., *et al.* (2004). Risperidone in the treatment of disruptive behavioral symptoms in children with autistic and other pervasive developmental disorders. *Pediatrics*, *114*, e634–641.

Sheiner, L. B., Stanski, D. R., Vozeh, S., Miller, R. D., & Ham, J. (1979). Simultaneous modeling of pharmacokinetics and pharmacodynamics: application to d-tubocurarine. *Clinical Pharmacology and Therapeutics*, *25*, 358–371.

Solanto, M. V. (1998). Neuropsychopharmacological mechanisms of stimulant drug action in attention-deficit hyperactivity disorder: a review and integration. *Behavioural Brain Research*, *94*(1), 127–152.

Spencer, E. K., & Campbell, M. (1994). Children with schizophrenia: diagnosis, phenomenology, and pharmacotherapy. *Schizophrenia Bulletin*, *20*, 713–725.

Spencer, T., Biederman, J., Wilens, T., Harding, M., O'Donnell, D., & Griffin, S. (1996). Pharmacotherapy of attention-deficit hyperactivity disorder across the life cycle. *Journal of the American Academy of Child and Adolescent Psychiatry*, *35*, 409–432.

Spencer, T. J., Biederman, J., Ciccone, P. E., Madras, B. K., Dougherty, D. D., Bonab, A. A., *et al.* (2006a). PET study examining pharmacokinetics, detection and likeability, and dopamine transporter receptor occupancy of short- and long-acting oral methylphenidate. *American Journal of Psychiatry*, *163*, 387–395.

Spencer, T. J., Faraone, S. V., Biederman, J., Lerner, M., Cooper, K. M., & Zimmerman, B. (2006b). Does prolonged therapy with a long-acting stimulant suppress growth in children with ADHD? *Journal of the American Academy of Child and Adolescent Psychiatry*, *45*, 527–537.

Steinhoff, K. W. (2004). Attention-deficit/hyperactivity disorder: Medication treatment-dosing and duration of action. *American Journal of Managed Care*, *10*, S99–S109.

Swanson, J., Greenhill, L., Wigal, T., Kollins, S., Stehli, A., Davies, M., *et al.* (2006c). Stimulant-related reductions of growth rates in the PATS. *Journal of the American Academy of Child and Adolescent Psychiatry*. [epub].

Swanson, C. J., Perry, K. W., Koch-Krueger, S., Katner, J., Svensson, K. A., & Bymaster, F. P. (2006a). Effect of the attention deficit/hyperactivity disorder drug atomoxetine on extracellular concentrations of norepinephrine and dopamine in several brain regions of the rat. *Neuropharmacology*, *50*, 755–760.

Swanson, J., Agler, D., Fineberg, E., Wigal, S., Flynn, D., Fineberg, K., *et al.* (1999b). University of California, Irvine, Laboratory School Protocol for Pharmacokinetic and Pharmacodynamic Studies. In L. Greenhill, & B. Osman (Eds.), *Ritalin: Theory and practice* (2nd edn.) (pp. 405–430). Mary Ann Liebert, Inc.

Swanson, J., Gupta, S., Guinta, D., Flynn, D., Agler, D., Lerner, M., *et al.* (1999a). Acute tolerance to methylphenidate in the treatment of attention deficit hyperactivity disorder in children. *Clinical Pharmacology and Therapeutics*, 66, 295–305.

Swanson, J., Gupta, S., Lam, A., Shoulson, I., Lerner, M., Modi, N., *et al.* (2003). Development of a new once-a-day formulation of methylphenidate for the treatment of attention-deficit/hyperactivity disorder: proof-of-concept and proof-of-product studies. *Archives of General Psychiatry*, 60, 204–211.

Swanson, J., McBurnett, K., Wigal, T., Pfiffner, L., Lerner, M., Williams, L., *et al.* (1993). Effect of stimulant medication on children with attention deficit disorder: A "Review of Reviews". *Exceptional Children*, *60*, 154–162.

Swanson, J. M., Elliot, G. R., Greenhill, L. L., Wigal, T., *et al.* (2007a). Effects of stimulant medication on growth rates across 3 years in the MTA follow-up. *Journal of the American Academy of Child and Adolescent Psychiatry*, *46*, 1304–1313.

Swanson, J. M., Greenhill, L. L., Lopez, F. A., Sedillo, A., Earl, C. Q., Jiang, J. G., *et al.* (2006b). Modafinil film-coated tablets in children and adolescents with attention-deficit/hyperactivity disorder: results of a randomized, double-blind, placebo-controlled, fixed-dose study followed by abrupt discontinuation. *Journal of Clinical Psychiatry*, *67*, 137–147.

Swanson, J. M., Hinshaw, S. P., Arnold, L. E., Gibbons, R., *et al.* (2007b). Secondary evaluations of MTA 36-month outcomes: Propensity score and growth mixture model analyses. *Journal of the American Academy of Child and Adolescent Psychiatry*, *46*, 1002–1013.

Tauscher, J., Hussain, T., Agid, O., Verhoeff, N. P. L. G., Wilson, A. A., Houle, S., *et al.* (2004). Equivalent occupancy of dopamine D1 and D2 receptors with clozapine: Differentiation from other atypical antipsychotics. *American Journal of Psychiatry*, *161*, 1620–1625.

Tiihonen, J., Kuoppasalmi, K., Foer, J., Tuomola, P., Kuikanmaki, O., Vorma, H., *et al.* (2007). A comparison of aripiprazole, methyphenidate, and placebo for amphetamine dependence. *American Journal of Psychiatry*, *164*, 160–162.

Troost, P. W., Steenhuis, M., Tuynman-Qua, H. G., Kalverdijk, L. J., Buitelaar, J. K., Minderaa, R. B., *et al.* (2006). Atomoxetine for attention-deficit/hyperactivity disorder symptoms in children with pervasive developmental disorders: A pilot study. *Journal of Child and Adolescent Psychopharmacology*, *16*, 611–619.

US Food and Drug Administration. (2000). Center for Drug Evaluation and Research Approval Letter. In Alza Corporation, *Final approval for Concerta Extended Release Tabs* (pp. 21–121).

US Food and Drug Administration. (2003a). *FDA approves Prozac for pediatric use to treat depression and OCD: FDA Talk Paper.* Rockville: US Food and Drug Administration.

US Food and Drug Administration. (2003b). *Reports of suicidality in pediatric patients being treated with antidepressant medications for major depressive disorder (MDD).* Public Health Advisory: US Food and Drug Administration.

US Food and Drug Administration. (2004a). *Background information on the Suicidality Classification Project.* US Food and Drug Administration.

US Food and Drug Administration. (2004b). Review of AERS data for marketed safety experience during stimulant therapy: death, sudden death, cardiovascular SAEs (including stroke). In M. D. Russell Katz (Ed.), *Letter requesting assistance with analysis of AERS data for marketed safety experience with amphetamine and/or dextroamphetamine salts.*

US Food and Drug Administration. (2005). In *Alert for Healthcare Professionals: Adderall and Adderall XR (amphetamine).* US Food and Drug Administration.

Vitiello, B. (2006). An update on publicly funded multisite trials in pediatric psychopharmacology. *Child and Adolescent Psychiatric Clinics of North America*, *15*, 1–12.

Volkow, N. D., Ding, Y. S., Fowler, J. S., Wang, G. J., Logan, J., Gatley, J. S., *et al.* (1995). Is methylphenidate like cocaine? Studies on their pharmacokinetics and distribution in the human brain. *Archives of General Psychiatry*, *52*, 456–463.

Volkow, N. D., Fowler, J. S., Wang, G. J., Dewey, S. L., Schlyer, D., MacGregor, R., *et al.* (1993). Reproducibility of repeated measures of carbon-11-raclopride binding in the human brain. *Journal of Nuclear Medicine*, *34*, 609–613.

Volkow, N. D., & Swanson, J. M. (2003). Variables that affect the clinical use and abuse of methylphenidate in the treatment of ADHD. *American Journal of Psychiatry*, *160*, 1909–1918.

Volkow, N. D., Wang, G. J., Fowler, J. S., Gatley, S. J., Logan, J., Ding, Y. S., *et al.* (1998). Dopamine transporter occupancies in the human brain induced by therapeutic doses of oral methylphenidate. *American Journal of Psychiatry*, *155*, 1325–1331.

Volkow, N. D., Wang, G. J., Fowler, J. S., Logan, J., Franceschi, D., Maynard, L., *et al.* (2002). Relationship between blockade of dopamine transporters by oral methylphenidate and the increases in extracellular dopamine: therapeutic implications. *Synapse*, *43*, 181–187.

Volkow, N. D., Wang, G. J., Fowler, J. S., Telang, F., Maynard, L., Logan, J., *et al.* (2004). Evidence that methylphenidate enhances the saliency of a mathematical task by increasing dopamine in the human brain. *American Journal of Psychiatry*, *161*, 1173–1180.

Volkow, N. D., Wang, G. J., Ma, Y., Fowler, J. S., Wong, C., Jayne, M., *et al.* (2006). Effects of expectation on the brain metabolic responses to methylphenidate and to its placebo in non-drug abusing subjects. *Neuroimage*, *32*(4), 1782–1992.

Wagner, K. D. (2005). Pharmacotherapy for major depression in children and adolescents. *Progress in Neuropsychopharmacology and Biological Psychiatry*, *29*, 819–826.

Wagner, K. D., Ambrosini, P., Rynn, M., Wohlberg, C., Yang, R., Greenbaum, M. S., *et al.* (2003). Efficacy of sertraline in the treatment of children and adolescents with major depressive disorder: two randomized controlled trials. *Journal of the American Medical Association*, *290*, 1033–1041.

Wagner, K. D., Robb, A. S., Findling, R. L., Jin, J., Gutierrez, M. M., & Heydorn, W. E. (2004). A randomized, placebo-controlled trial of citalopram for the treatment of major depression in children and adolescents. *American Journal of Psychiatry*, *161*, 1079–1083.

Walkup, J., Labellarte, M., Riddle, M. A., Pine, D. S., Greenhill, L., Fairbanks, J., *et al.* for the RUPP Anxiety Study Group. (2002). Treatment of pediatric anxiety disorders: an open-label extension of the research units on pediatric psychopharmacology anxiety study. *Journal of Child and Adolescent Psychopharmacology*, *12*, 175–188.

Wigal, S., McGough, J. J., McCracken, J. T., Biederman, J., Spencer, T. J., Posner, K. L., *et al.* (2005). A laboratory school comparison of mixed amphetamine salts extended release (Adderall XR) and atomoxetine (Strattera) in school-aged children with attention deficit/hyperactivity disorder. *Journal of Attention Disorders*, *9*, 275–289.

Wigal, S., Sanchez, D., DeCory, H., D'Imperio, J., & Swanson, J. (2003). Selection of the optimal dose ratio for a controlled-delivery formulation of methylphenidate. *Journal of Applied Research*, *42*, 1234–1241.

Wigal, T., Greenhill, L., Chuang, S., McGough, J., Vitiello, B., Skribala, A., *et al.* (2006). Safety and tolerability of methylphenidate in preschool children with ADHD. *Journal of the American Academy of Child and Adolescent Psychiatry*, *45*, 1314–1322.

Wilens, T. (2004). *Straight talk about psychiatric medications for kids* (Revised edn.). New York: Guilford Press.

Wilens, T. E., Biederman, J., Baldessarini, R. J., Puopolo, P. R., & Flood, J. G. (1992). Developmental changes in serum concentrations of desipramine and 2-hydroxydesipramine during treatment with desipramine. *Journal of the American Academy of Child and Adolescent Psychiatry*, *31*, 691–698.

Witcher, J. W., Long, A., Smith, B., Sauer, J. M., Heilgenstein, J., Wilens, T., *et al.* (2003). Atomoxetine pharmacokinetics in children and adolescents with attention deficit hyperactivity disorder. *Journal of Child and Adolescent Psychopharmacology*, *13*, 53–63.

Zito, J. M., & Safer, D. J. (2005). Recent child pharmacoepidemiological findings. *Journal of Child and Adolescent Psychopharmacology*, *15*, 5–9.

Zito, J. M., Tobi, H., de Jong-van den Berg, L. T., Fegert, J. M., Safer, D. J., Janhsen, K., *et al.* (2006). Antidepressant prevalence for youths: a multi-national comparison. *Pharmacoepidemiology and Drug Safety*, *15*, 793–798.

17 Clinical Neurophysiology

Torsten Baldeweg and Stewart Boyd

General Principles of Electroencephalography

The *electroencephalogram* (EEG) is a technique that measures the electrical activity of the brain non-invasively, from electrodes placed on the scalp. It is widely used in clinical practice and is also an important tool in basic and clinical neuroscience research. There are dramatic neurophysiological changes with age, so EEG and related methods, such as *event-related potentials* (ERP), are paramount for our understanding of the relation between brain maturation and normal as well as abnormal cognitive and behavioral development. This chapter reviews some principles of their application in clinical pediatric practice as well as in research in the developmental neurosciences.

Introduction and Historical Note

We identify three major phases in the history of neurophysiology and EEG, in particular as applied to the search for neural correlates of mental processes and their application to psychiatry:

1 The pioneering discovery of the EEG by Berger;

2 Its application to neurology, including the invention of evoked potential techniques; and

3 The present day cognitive neuroscience approach attempting to capture and understand the dynamic properties of cognitive processes and neural computations by means of EEG-based methods.

We have structured this chapter along this meandering road of discovery.

The EEG was discovered by Berger (1873–1941), a psychiatrist working in Jena, Germany, who early in his career attempted to study human mental function through physiological measurement. He began by observing changes in cerebral blood flow in patients with pulsating skull defects and by measuring temperature in neurosurgical patients during mental tasks. He was forced to give up because these techniques were too crude for the task he set out to achieve (Gloor, 1994). He then turned to electrophysiology following the pioneering work in animals by Caton (1842–1926) and in 1924 Berger succeeded in measuring the electrical activity of the human brain. Using what he called the *Electroenkephalogram*, Berger described the different brain rhythms, such as alpha waves, today also known as Berger's rhythm. By 1939 he had described all the major features of the normal and abnormal EEG, including EEG alterations in sleep and states of diminished consciousness (Berger, 1969). Although he did not fulfill his ultimate ambition to capture neural signatures of mental processes, EEG proved the most lasting of his psychophysiological methods, finding a permanent place in clinical investigations of neurological patients, particularly those with epilepsy. In the 1930s, EEG entered routine clinical diagnostics and EEG patterns associated with different seizure disorders were described by Gibbs, Davis, and Lennox in 1935.

The desire to investigate perceptual and cognitive processes resulted in the invention of the evoked potential technique by Davis, Davis, Loomis *et al.* (1939) and Dawson (1947, 1954). The discovery of this method of recording small electrical potential changes on the scalp to simple sensory stimuli had a long-term impact – again, mainly for neurological diagnosis.

The era of cognitive neurophysiological research was initiated by Walter and colleagues in 1964, who recorded slow frontal EEG potential shifts ("contingent negative variation") during stimulus–response tasks. The discovery of these "cognitive" evoked potentials, today known as ERP, has brought Berger's original idea to fruition, by identifying physiological changes associated with specific cognitive operations. Today, we witness the merging of the concepts of EEG (as a measure of brain dynamics) and ERP (as markers of cognitive processing stages) by incorporating both measures into a more unified theoretical treatment of brain function (see p. 242). We expect that this novel approach will ultimately shed more light on the subtle neurophysiological processes underlying synaptic plasticity and connectivity in the developing and mature brain and their disruption in psychopathology.

Neurophysiological Origins of EEG

The electrical activity that can be recorded using surface electrodes is a summation of the synchronous activity of thousands or millions of neurons, which communicate with each other using two major forms of electrical signals: *action potentials* propagated along *axons* to generate *postsynaptic potentials* in the *dendrite* of the receiving neuron. Action potentials are too short in duration (a few milliseconds) to produce sufficient summation of electrical potentials to be detected by surface electrodes. In contrast, the slower postsynaptic potentials (typically tens of milliseconds to over 100 ms in duration)

Rutter's Child and Adolescent Psychiatry, 5th edition. Edited by M. Rutter, D. Bishop, D. Pine, S. Scott, J. Stevenson, E. Taylor and A. Thapar. © 2008 Blackwell Publishing, ISBN: 978-1-4051-4549-7.

can produce externally detectable potentials, especially when generated in *pyramidal cells*. The elongated shape of these neurons leads to a separation of the electrically active part (mostly causing extracellular negativity) and passive parts (positivity) of the pyramidal cell. This is called an *electrical dipole* and the external electrical field is most likely to be detected at a distance if these dipoles are arranged in parallel with each other. In contrast, in cells with a spherical shape of the dendritic tree (e.g., *interneurons*) the external electrical field will cancel out because of random orientation of dipoles.

Therefore, the slow postsynaptic electrical activity of pyramidal cells in the cortex is the largest contributor to surface EEG. This activity is *volume conducted* through the overlying tissues (cerebrospinal fluid, skull and skin) with different and non-homogenous conductance, thus contributing to a substantial spread and distortion of intracerebrally generated electrical fields at the scalp. This property and the limits imposed by the physics of electromagnetism prevent an accurate reconstruction of the cortical generators of EEG and ERP. Nevertheless, techniques of topographical (spatial) EEG analysis as well as magneto-encephalography (MEG) can be used to find approximate generator estimations (see p. 243).

Classification of EEG Rhythms

EEG rhythms span a broad frequency range, from *slow oscillations* (0.5–1 Hz) and *delta waves* (1–4 Hz) dominating during sleep to the faster rhythms of wakefulness: *theta* (4–8 Hz), *alpha* (8–12 Hz), *beta* (12–30 Hz) and *gamma* frequencies (from >30 Hz to over 100 Hz). These rhythms show a characteristic scalp distribution (e.g., the alpha rhythm has a posterior maximum), while a characteristic *mu rhythm* (8–10 Hz) is found over the sensorimotor regions. There are marked developmental changes in their scalp distribution too (see p. 242).

Brain arousal states are characterized by changes in the EEG spectrum. The waking EEG is dominated by fast rhythms (alpha, beta and gamma). Eye closure augments alpha activity while eye opening suppresses this prominent posterior wave pattern (alpha-block). The onset of sleep is characterized by *sleep spindles* (7–14 Hz), while EEG in deep sleep is dominated by delta and theta waves (hence called slow wave sleep), in contrast to paradoxical or rapid eye movement (REM) sleep, where these slow oscillations are suppressed (misleadingly termed EEG "desynchronization") and replaced by fast waves (waking EEG pattern).

Maturation of EEG Activities

After birth, the normal EEG continues to mature until adolescence, although the most striking changes are seen in the first few years of life. Rhythmic precursors of prominent normal features such as mu and alpha rhythms appear in the first few months of life, and reach alpha frequencies by 1 and 3 years, respectively. The alpha rhythm continues to mature until adolescence with a gradual increase in frequencies.

Prominent features of sleep mature over the first 18 months (*K-complexes*) to 2 years (*sleep spindles*). Rhythms of drowsiness remain prominent until near puberty, while posterior temporal slowing only appears with adolescence, as does midfrontal theta activity. Still other features, such as the slow occipital transients seen in relation to eye movements, remain throughout childhood, although they peak at around 2 years. All these normal features continue to be misinterpreted as abnormalities on occasion. This point is considered further below (see p. 240).

Maturation of normal activities continues from the first appearance of EEG activities around 23–24 weeks post-conceptional age, with the most marked changes occurring throughout infancy. The activities are initially discontinuous (*trace discontinu*) but become continuous in all states except for a transient phase of quiet sleep (*trace alternant*). The adult sleep onset pattern where non-REM stages are seen before the first period of REM appears from around 44–47 weeks, associated with a maturational change in the responsiveness of *pedunculopontine neurons*.

Neurophysiological Origin of EEG Rhythms

The mechanisms underlying the generation of rhythmic background EEG activity during waking and sleep are now well understood (for reviews see McCormick, 2002; Steriade, 2006; Steriade, McCormick, & Sejnowski, 1993). The cerebral cortex and thalamus can both generate cyclical oscillations of neuronal activity, which are determined by the physiological properties of neurons and the highly interconnected nature of the brain. The major components of the oscillatory network are as follow:

1 *Cortical neurons*, receiving input from and transmitting information to

2 *Thalamocortical relay cells*, which in turn also send collaterals to

3 *Thalamic reticular cells*.

Activation of the latter inhibitory cells determines the periodicity of firing of *thalamocortical cells* and hence shapes oscillation frequency and pattern of the whole thalamocortical network. Several forms of epileptic activity appear as aberrations of the normal activity within cortical and thalamocortical circuits.

The cellular and network mechanisms of rhythm generation are known in much detail for *spindle oscillations* (7–14 Hz), which characterize light sleep as well as for the *slow oscillations* (0.5–1 Hz) in deep sleep. Both types of rhythm are characterized by inhibitory processes in thalamic and cortical neurons, thus gating sensory information and preventing the processing of such external information in the cortex. Similarly, the mechanisms behind *fast rhythms* (beta and gamma: 20–60 Hz) are increasingly understood, suggesting an essential role for inhibitory interneurons in shaping frequency and type of network behavior (Whittington & Traub, 2003).

Mechanisms of *theta wave* generation (4–7 Hz) are still not well understood. Theta waves represent an "on-line" state of the hippocampus, generated by rhythmic inputs from other limbic structures (Steriade & Llinas, 1988). Human frontal theta activity does not arise from the hippocampus directly, but is probably generated in limbic projection regions in the *cingulate cortex* and other frontal regions.

Similarly, the precise neural mechanism of *alpha wave* (8–12 Hz) generation is not known. However, it is suggested that alpha waves, which share the frequency range of sleep spindles, also emerge from the interplay of thalamocortical connections, especially of the visual cortex and *visual thalamus* (Lopes da Silva, 1991). Several sources of focal alpha activity have been detected in the parieto-occipital and *calcarine cortex* using MEG (Hari, Salmelin, Makela *et al.*, 1997). During alpha activity there is widespread cortical deactivation in frontal, parietal and occipital regions and increased thalamic activation as measured in combined EEG and functional imaging studies (Goldman, Stern, Engel *et al.*, 2002).

The *mu rhythm* is a sensorimotor rhythm in the alpha range (8–10 Hz) seen over the central regions in a relaxed awake subject. This activity is blocked by making or receiving an instruction to make a movement. MEG studies suggest that this rhythm arises mainly from the somatosensory area with contributions from the motor cortex (Hari *et al.*, 1997).

In more general terms, the period of oscillation is constrained by the size of the neuronal pool engaged in a given cycle. Higher frequency oscillations are confined (due to axon conduction and synaptic delays) to a small neuronal space, whereas very large networks are recruited during slow oscillations (Buzsaki & Draguhn, 2004).

Neuromodulatory influences on thalamocortical rhythms arising from ascending *monoaminergic and cholinergic midbrain projections* are especially important in regulating sleep stages and associated EEG rhythms (Hobson & Pace-Schott, 2002; Steriade, 2006). Cholinergic activity arising from the *tegmentum* inhibits the cells of the *reticular nucleus of thalamus*, thus releasing thalamocortical relay cells from their inhibitory influence, which results in EEG activation ("desynchronization") and arousal (sleep–waking transition).

Functional Roles of Cortical EEG Rhythms

There is continuing debate about the functional significance of spontaneous EEG oscillations, with some regarding them as epiphenomena, while recent evidence suggests that such brain rhythms during different behavioral states have distinct functional roles (for review see Buzsaki & Draguhn, 2004). These roles can be grouped as follows:

- *Input selection and plasticity* Oscillatory activity facilitates responsiveness and plastic changes in the strength of connections among neurons, supporting the process of information representation and memory storage (Steriade, 2006). The evidence for cognitive roles is best established for the hippocampal theta and cortical fast gamma and beta rhythms (Kahana, 2006).
- *Binding cell assemblies* Information in the brain has been hypothesized to be processed and stored in flexible cell assemblies, defined as distributed neuron networks that are transiently synchronized by dynamic connections. This hypothesis has been specifically formulated for gamma oscillations enabling phase-locked discharges of distributed neurons to "bind" different stimulus features into a coherent perceptual concept (Gray, Konig, Engel *et al.*, 1989). This "gamma binding hypothesis" is challenged by the observation of identical waves during slow wave sleep. A number of hypotheses about the role of gamma oscillations in psychopathology are reviewed by Herrmann and Demiralp (2005).
- *Consolidation and combination of learned information* Synaptic modifications in neural networks, which were brought about by experience and learning during wakefulness, are being "frozen" into the oscillatory dynamics during sleep to be turned into long-term memory.
- *Representation by phase information* Evidence for such function largely comes from recordings of *hippocampal place cell* firing during theta oscillations (O'Keefe, 1979). At a network level this means that neurons with stronger dendritic inputs will discharge earlier in the oscillatory cycle than neurons with weaker inputs.

Transition of Normal Rhythms into Electrical Seizures

Aberrations in the thalamo-cortical interplay that underlies EEG rhythms can lead to the emergence of seizure activity (Steriade, 2006). The occurrence of spike-and-wave seizures (absence or petit mal) is especially facilitated during transitional states from waking to slow wave sleep or during drowsiness. Abnormally strong activation of the inhibitory thalamic reticular neurons can result in the transformation of a normal sleep rhythm (spindles) into one that resembles those underlying absence seizures (3-Hz rhythms).

Seizures characterized by *3-Hz spike–wave complexes* are strongly associated with generalized, notably childhood absence, epilepsies. Originally ascribed to a "centrencephalic" system 3-Hz spike–wave complexes have recently been shown to be initiated by a cortical focus, rapidly transmitted to other (contralateral) cortical regions (within 20 to 100 ms) and the thalamus (within a few seconds). This corticofugal input has two effects on thalamic neurons:

1 Interneurons in the reticular nucleus are excited and then actively participate during seizure activity; and

2 Thalamocortical relay cells are inhibited, resulting in loss of external sensory input to the cortex, and hence explaining the loss of consciousness during absence seizures (Steriade, 2006).

The neurophysiological mechanisms behind spike and wave generation involve both excitation and inhibition in close succession: the surface negative spike is the result of excitatory *postsynaptic potential* (EPSP) generation primarily in apical dendrites of pyramidal neurons; while the longer lasting surface negative wave is generated by inhibitory postsynaptic potentials (IPSPs) predominantly on or near the soma of *pyramidal cells*. The subsequent slow component has predominantly inhibitory effects on cerebral function and is responsible for alterations in cognitive function (Shewmon & Erwin, 1988).

Spike–wave discharges can also arise in the cerebral cortex alone from disruption of a synchronized slow oscillation (<1 Hz) that occurs in sleep. These slow oscillations are the result of a cyclical interaction between recurrent cortical excitation (depolarization) and its control by inhibitory mechanisms (hyperpolarization). Again, loss of cortical inhibitory control allows this normal activity to become epileptiform. Together, the cerebral cortex and thalamus can form loops of activity that contribute to some forms of epileptic seizures (McCormick, 2002).

EEG Recording Techniques

Standard EEG Recording

This continues to form the backbone of clinical neurophysiological investigation in children with possible central nervous system (CNS) problems. Although there are many limitations in sampling the EEG activity randomly and for a limited period, this has served well for over 50 years. In younger children, a recording lasting 30–40 minutes may well include a period of spontaneous sleep, and this can be encouraged by manipulating aspects of the environment, such as lighting and laying the child on a bed wrapped in a blanket. In older children and adolescents sleep may be induced by the use of some form of sedation or by sleep deprivation (see p. 239).

In pediatrics, digital EEG recordings should be time-locked to video recording (subject to consent; see p. 239) particularly if the nature of episodic behavior changes or possible seizures (here defined as "events") is part of the question. Simultaneous recording of other physiological variables (polygraphy) such as surface electromyography (EMG), electrocardiography (ECG) and oxygen saturation may be particularly helpful. Although such recordings document attacks in children relatively often compared with adults, most recordings will be interictal, and this must be borne in mind when interpreting the result. Caution is also needed in interpreting localization on the basis of a single recording, as the apparent site of spike activity may vary between records (Kaufman, Harris, & Shaffer, 1980).

Video-EEG Telemetry

Extended EEG recordings over periods of days to around a fortnight are indicated when shorter recordings have not answered an important clinical question about the nature or frequency of events. Such video-EEG recordings, which require a ward setting, are usually carried out in specialized telemetry units. Events must be sufficiently frequent to be likely to be captured during the time available (usually 2–3 times per week to be confident of documenting an event in 4–5 days of recording). Shorter periods of telemetry can be used to ensure that a whole night-time's sleep is obtained; this may be important when clinical events are confined to particular times of day.

Ambulatory EEG Recording

Ambulatory EEG recording is carried out when the events are both frequent and markedly related to environmental factors. Recording periods are usually extended for 2–3 days at a time, indicating that events should be occurring 3–4 times per week to have a realistic hope of capturing one. The lack of simultaneous time-locked video in these circumstances means that interpretation of changes in behavior or perception, signaled by pressing the "event-button," rely upon the event diary being kept accurately.

Electrocorticography

EEG recordings performed directly from the cortical surface after surgical implantation of electrodes are an increasingly common procedure in patients with refractory focal epilepsy. Following surgical placement of the subdural arrays and/or depth electrodes, EEG telemetry is carried out for periods of days until sufficient seizures have been documented to allow detailed mapping of the sites involved in the onset and spread of the habitual seizures. Determination of the extent of functionally eloquent cortex and its relation to the seizure focus is also possible using the same electrode placements by selectively stimulating electrode pairs to elicit clinical signs. In addition to mapping the motor cortex, speech and memory functions can be tested using appropriate protocols (Lüders, 2000) similar to those used nowadays in preoperative functional imaging studies.

Magneto-encephalography

MEG is a new technique based on the physical capability of electrical currents to produce a magnetic field. This field is perpendicular to the orientation of the generating electrical current (dipole). MEG systems employ *superconducting quantum interference devices* (SQUIDs) to detect the ultra-weak magnetic fields generated by the brain's electrical activity. Apart from the cost of a superconducting medium (liquid helium) for the sensors to operate, MEG also requires a recording environment shielded from external magnetic fields. Because of the fixed size of the sensor helmet, the recording of children can be problematic (for review see Phillips, 2005). Its main advantages over EEG are:

1 Magnetic fields can be detected at a distance from the scalp (i.e., there is no need to fit electrodes to the scalp, noncontact measurement);

2 The spatial resolution of MEG is superior to that of EEG because magnetic fields are not distorted by biological tissues (scalp, skull, cerebrospinal fluid) which spread and distort the electrical potential on the scalp.

The latter property has led to MEG being used to localize the cortical generators of electrical and magnetic fields in the human brain. Its main disadvantage is the insensitivity of MEG to radial currents in the brain (generated in cortical gyri), in contrast to tangential currents, which are generated mostly in the depth of sulci. This means that a proportion of electrical brain activity will not be detected by MEG. The combined recording of EEG and MEG, however, can improve the localizing ability of neurophysiological methods, reflected in a growing number of clinical research applications in a few specialist centers, mostly for localization of interictal spikes and of eloquent (language, memory) functions.

Evoked Potentials

Evoked potentials (EPs) constitute part of the ongoing EEG that is specifically elicited by sensory stimuli (auditory, visual or somatosensory). Sensory EPs, with peaks within 50 ms post-stimulus, can be contrasted with stimulus-induced EEG changes of longer latency in response to specific psychological task instructions. These latter are ERP (see p. 243). EPs are very often much smaller in amplitude than the on-going EEG activity, and this adverse signal : noise ratio can be improved by repeating the stimulus and averaging the EEG response across many repetitions.

Despite some caveats, replicable series of averaged waveforms can be obtained in a wide range of clinical settings, and clinical EP studies have been widely used to elucidate function in particular sensory pathways. Normal values for standard clinical EPs have been established taking account of maturational changes in waveforms and latencies. EP techniques have established roles in intraoperative monitoring, particularly of the spinal cord during neurosurgical and orthopedic operations, and in specialist audiological and ophthalmological applications.

EP peaks are labeled by their polarity at the scalp (P for positive, N for negative) and the typical peak latency (i.e., time [in ms] poststimulus, at which they are elicited in the adult: N20 or P25) or by the number in a sequence of peaks (i.e., P1/N1/P2). EPs are quantified using peak latency and amplitude.

Short-latency EPs often used in clinical studies include the following.

Brainstem Auditory Evoked Potentials (BAEPs) These are a series of vertex-positive waves in the nanovolt range revealed by averaging a repeated set of simple auditory stimuli such as clicks or pure tones. These waveforms originate in auditory pathways through the brainstem and when recorded and interpreted carefully can give information about the conduction through the brainstem which is not accessible using standard EEG recordings. Apart from their obvious audiological applications, they can be useful in the intensive care unit (ICU) and in determining brainstem involvement in neurological conditions affecting white matter.

Visual Evoked Potentials (VEPs) These can be recorded from two types of visual stimuli: pattern and flash. Although both may evoke a negative–positive–negative waveform, with the positivity around 100 ms, they are essentially testing different aspects of the visual system. Pattern EPs to a reversing checkerboard are sensitive to changes in white matter and are often used in suspected demyelinating conditions in adults. However, they require the patient's active cooperation in fixating on a central target and are particularly vulnerable to fatigue. For these reasons, they are more reliable when used in older children. Flash VEPs may, by contrast, be used in children of all ages, and require no active cooperation, but the waveforms are degraded by a wide range of cortical and subcortical disorders. The flash VEP waveform does not show the consistent increase in latency of the main components with demyelination seen in the pattern VEP and interpretation is more subjective.

Somatosensory Evoked Potentials (SSEPs or SEPs) These are recorded maximally from the centro-parietal area over the primary somatosensory cortex. They also show a complex waveform but most attention is usually given to the short-latency components (N20, P25 and N30) following stimulation of the median nerve. The N20 persists after the EEG is completely suppressed by sedatives, and measurement of this component is often used to monitor patient progress in the ICU.

Activation Procedures

Overbreathing

Overbreathing is carried out for 3 minutes primarily as a method of activating epileptiform features associated with both generalized (absence) and focal (e.g., temporal lobe) epilepsy. The amplitude and to some extent frequency of the normal EEG response to overbreathing are functions mainly of age, being more marked in younger children, but neither feature of itself is a marker of abnormality. They become much less marked in adolescents, and should not be asymmetrical or focal. An initial slowing followed by recrudescence of marked slow activity (generalized, lateralized or focal) after the end of overbreathing can be evidence of vascular disease, notably *moyamoya syndrome*. If the latter is suspected, then overbreathing should be avoided because of the risk of precipitating long-term neurological deficits.

Photic Stimulation

Photic stimulation is a long-established method of provoking epileptiform changes, but the results must be interpreted with caution. Spikes confined to the occipital region have a very low risk of associated clinical seizures. Only widespread spiking (usually mixed with slow waves) carries a substantial risk of seizures, particularly if the spikes persist after the train of photic stimuli is ended (self-sustaining). However, this is a common finding around puberty and may be confined to the test situation. Furthermore, around 2–3% of the population show this risk of clinical seizures in the presence of flickering light, mostly between the rates of 16 and 25 Hz.

Sleep Recording

Sleep recording is indicated when the "events" are confined to sleep and/or when the waking EEG has been uninformative or inconclusive; this will usually be in the context of a suspected epileptic process or syndrome or other sleep disorder. Different states within sleep associated with different patterns of activity or with distinctive waveforms have been recognized for many years, the criteria of Rechtschaffen and Kales (1968) being the most widely used to score these stages. It is often difficult to differentiate drowsiness and stage 1 sleep, particularly in children. The presence of distinctive runs of spindles around the central regions associated with larger generalized biphasic slow waves (*K-complexes*) indicates that the child is finally definitely asleep (stage 2 or spindle sleep). Both focal and generalized epileptic disorders may demonstrate most epileptiform activity at this stage. This is followed by the appearance of increasing amounts of slow activity, with reduction in spindles as the child enters the deeper stages of non-REM sleep (rarely reached in routine EEG recordings), followed by an abrupt transition to a period of awake-like irregular activities associated with rapid eye movements and virtual absence of muscle activity (REM sleep). The particular focus of interest may be on drowsiness and light sleep, stage 2 sleep (*benign epilepsy with centrotemporal spikes*) or following arousal (*juvenile myoclonic epilepsy*).

Currently, several methods are used to obtain sleep, depending to some extent on the age of the child and, increasingly, on parental preferences. Induction of sleep by *melatonin* avoids the problems of conventional sedatives (EEG changes and prolonged sedation effects after the test) and is now widely used. Sleep deprivation remains an alternative when melatonin is unacceptable or has previously failed.

One particular variant of sleep recording, the *multiple sleep latency test* (MSLT), is carried out when the clinical question is that of *narcolepsy*. The child is instructed to fall asleep then awakened after 20 minutes on five or six occasions over the course of a day. The number of periods of REM sleep and the latency to sleep onset are measured. The MLST interpretation is limited if the previous night's sleep pattern has not been monitored.

Consent and Ethical Issues

Other aspects of the recording require consent from carers, particularly video recording, activation procedures (overbreathing, photic stimulation) and sleep deprivation or sedation for sleep. Sleep is often achieved by giving an age-dependent dose of melatonin at the beginning of the procedure. The carers consent to this either before or on arrival, with full information about melatonin-induced sleep given when the appointment is made. Sleep deprivation is potentially more difficult, because the patient is already sleep-deprived on arrival for the test. This often requires the clinician requesting the test to explain the procedure.

Normal and Abnormal EEG

Normal EEG Features

The continuous mixture of *"ongoing" activities* (loosely referred to as "background activity"), normally contains rhythmic elements (e.g., alpha rhythm) against which identifiable components such as normal lambda waves or abnormal epileptiform spikes are seen.

The development and functional correlates of alpha rhythm (associated with visual function) and the sensorimotor mu rhythm have been described above, and the presence of these rhythms is checked during recording by appropriate maneuvers. If the child falls asleep, the sequence of changes during drowsiness and onset of sleep are recorded. Rhythms associated with drowsiness are often difficult to assess because this involves a subjective evaluation of the amount and type of rhythmic slow activity (see p. 240). This physiological slow activity can appear in generalized bursts, and may in some cases contain sharp components. Such sharp appearances and semirhythmic groups of 2–3 occurrences are also a feature of normal K-complexes in younger children, reflecting the state of a network which may at this point be readily suborned by epileptic activity.

EEG Variants in Children and Adolescents

A group of unusual but relatively stereotyped EEG appearances remain officially designated as "variants": alpha variants, midline rhythms, rhythmic temporal theta bursts of drowsiness, breach rhythms and others. For practical purposes these may be regarded as part of the normal EEG, or at the least as not having specific pathological connotations.

Pathological EEG Features

Clear-cut and characteristic EEG abnormalities are seen consistently in a very few conditions, but in the majority of clinical situations abnormalities are non-specific and variable. Furthermore, the point is often made that "normal" is itself a statistical concept and an interpretative term when applied to EEGs. In spite of this, the EEG can be seen as a measure of global cerebral dynamics, and a general indicator of pathophysiological processes.

Discrete lesions in a single area are most likely to produce localized or focal disturbances of function. If the lesion is small and located in an area of cortex that is not eloquent, there may be no clear EEG change. However, if located in an area that transmits to a wide area of cortex, this may result in marked and widespread alterations in function, reflected in the EEG changes, much of which will appear remote from the site of the lesion itself. This is also the case with a lesion sited subcortically. Diffuse cerebral pathology and lesions affecting deep structures such as the brainstem will produce "generalized" EEG abnormalities. These EEG abnormalities will appear as either loss of activity, EEG slowing or as epileptiform activity.

Loss of Activity

Loss of activity is the most severe manifestation of cerebral pathology and, apart from deep anesthesia, is associated with severe neurological or metabolic changes when generalized, and with corresponding neurological deficits when localized.

EEG Slowing

The most common manifestation of altered cerebral function is EEG slowing, which once again may be localized or generalized. The extent to which this is seen will depend on the rate of change in the lesion as well as in the pathology itself. Therefore, a long-standing lesion may show little or no disturbance, while a rapidly expanding lesion in the same area will show marked disturbances, usually with much slowing of activities, and possibly epileptiform spiking if it involves cortex. Abnormal slow waves in the delta range are a marker of acute disturbances, and often the assessment of the degree of abnormality of the EEG will depend on the presence and amount of this type of activity as well as its response to changes in state (e.g., sudden alerting).

Differentiating different types of posterior slow activity remains one of the most difficult areas of pediatric EEG. Occipital transients following eye blinks or eye movements are normal and common between 2 and 4 years, diminishing rapidly thereafter, before disappearing in the teens. Posterior temporal slow activity is a normal finding in the young, particularly after puberty, disappearing in the early twenties. Differentiating posterior temporal slow waves that exceed the norm for the child's age remains difficult, and extreme caution is advised, unless the suspect activity is completely unilateral, mixed with unequivocal spikes or it persists through sleep and wakefulness. It most often appears as a non-specific abnormality. Rhythmic 3-second activity, sometimes associated with small spikes, may appear following eye closure in some children with absence seizures. Of itself, it does not imply a focal origin for the seizures or an adverse prognosis.

Epileptiform Activity

Epileptiform abnormalities are often the most enigmatic changes found in the EEG, especially when they occur interictally. The term "epileptiform" simply refers to waveforms that might be associated with an epileptic seizure. Epileptiform *spikes* are defined as abrupt changes in activity that stand out from the ongoing activities and last less than 70 ms, while *sharp waves* last up to 300 ms but otherwise have the same characteristics. Such distinctions are often not useful, because both may reflect a propensity for seizures to develop and the less specific term "*epileptiform activity*" is preferred here. It should be remembered, however, that some normal physiological features appear as sharp waves in particular states, such as vertex waves in early sleep. A more clear-cut epileptiform abnormality is a spike/sharp wave followed by a slower negative wave forming a *spike–wave complex* (see p. 236).

The boundaries between interictal and ictal events are sometimes difficult to define, because even brief runs of spike–waves may be associated with alterations in cognitive function (*transitory cognitive impairment*; TCI). The type of impairment is related to the site of the discharges, but lasts only a few seconds (Binnie, 2003). There is evidence that when epileptiform activities are seen interictally, they represent a successful containment of the abnormal activity. A perennial difficulty in ascribing significance to these interictal changes is that they may be seen in around 2–3% of children who never develop clinical seizures. The ictal EEG changes associated with different clinical seizure types range from sudden decrements in activity associated with infantile spasms and tonic seizures to runs of well-formed 3-s spike–wave complexes associated with typical absence seizures (see chapter 22).

Periodic phenomena are waveforms that appear at more or less regular intervals of more than 1 second and may appear focal or generalized, associated with different pathologies.

Periodic lateralized epileptiform discharges (PLEDs) are a distinctive variant seen as a focal or localized change. PLEDs can be a sign of cerebral infarcts or vasculitis, but perhaps most often reflect the incomplete resolution of a seizure. They are seen in the classic form of *herpes simplex encephalitis*, occurring as focal periodic changes over the affected temporal lobe.

Generalized periodic complexes are seen in subacute sclerosing panencephalitis as complexes of varied (bi- or polyphasic) morphology lasting 0.5–2 seconds, recurring between 4 and 15 seconds (although occasionally longer). In adults with *Creutzfeldt–Jakob disease* (CJD) they appear as sharp waves with a period of around 1 second, but are *not* found in cases of new-variant CJD.

Interpretation and Reporting

EEG reporting is still most often carried out by visual inspection of waveforms in time series, describing features in terms of their frequency, amplitude, behavioral associations and topography. Artifacts (non-cerebral scalp potentials) are more readily recognized using these techniques. The use of digital recording allows display of the relative differences in potentials between different electrodes on the head in any combination (or *montage*) and has contributed to improvements in EEG interpretation (Levy, Berg, Testa *et al.*, 1998). The EEG is usually read twice, first to describe the activities, and then to review the findings in order to attempt to relate them to the history and the clinical question.

It is important to point out that the process of visual analysis and setting into a clinical context contains a number of potentially serious flaws. The clinical setting and clinical questions arising from it may be ill-posed or not given. Many request forms still do not contain appropriate well-posed questions. Furthermore, the recording conditions may not be appropriate to directly address the question (e.g., when the events in question occur only during sleep and this is not achieved during the recording). Ultimately, the interpreter's own level of experience may bias the report. They may, for instance, be broadly aware that benign epilepsy with centrotemporal spikes is common in childhood, but may not be clear about the details of the typical clinical setting. An inappropriate report suggesting a condition that the child clearly cannot have mars the outcome of the EEG investigation. Overbreathing is often carried out and the intermittent generalized bursts of often very high amplitude, slow activity continue to be misinterpreted by those unaccustomed to working with children.

This visual approach to analysis has survived in the clinical context despite the presence of many difficulties and inherent frustrations and uncertainties, because it has allowed clearer recognition of artifacts and of patterns of abnormalities with definite clinical associations, particularly in childhood epilepsy. It also facilitates the concurrent use of postacquisition digital signal processing. There is still considerable active debate about the place of particular signal processing algorithms in aiding the reporting of EEG investigations (see p. 242) and this is particularly the case in psychiatric disorders. By combining these approaches to the interpretation of clinical records, it is hoped to reduce the large element of individual interpretation and, perhaps, lessen the need for highly specialized training and experience.

Selecting Neurophysiological Investigations in a Clinical Setting

Determining which neurophysiological investigation is the most appropriate to request depends on a number of factors, of which by far the most important is deciding the clinical question that is being posed. The most common is as an aid to the diagnosis of epilepsy. Clinicians will be aware that a "normal" EEG at a time when a child is not having seizures does not exclude epilepsy (see chapter 22 for the place of EEG in the investigation of clinical problems). Although an ictal recording documenting the events at the time of an episodic change in behavior may seem (and be) the only possible answer to the question of their underlying nature, much useful information may still be obtained from the interictal recording. Before requesting video-EEG telemetry as a first investigation, on the basis that only the capture of "events" will be significant, clinicians should consider the frequency of the events, whether or not the presence of interictal findings will suffice to permit making a rational clinical management plan (as is the case in many epilepsy syndromes), as well as the relative waiting times for the two types of investigation.

Alternatively, the question may be "Is there evidence of an organic process, such as an acute/subacute encephalopathic process?" This might be answered by finding generalized slow activities suggesting an acute or subacute process, although the finding is itself not specific for any particular diagnosis.

The interplay of EEG abnormalities representing changes related to both pathology and maturation is seen in a number of conditions often encountered in psychiatric practice. These include cerebral dysplasias, the underlying cause of learning difficulties and behavior disorders in many childhood syndromes. When these are extensive, as in the various forms of lissencephaly and pachygyria, EEG abnormalities may appear as distinctive high-amplitude rhythmic generalized activities at a mixture of frequencies in the first year of life, but may later appear as non-specific irregular slowing with or without spikes. However, clinicians will be aware that in many important psychiatric disorders, such as autism, standard clinical neurophysiological investigations are very unlikely to be informative with respect to diagnosis. There are continuing suggestions that children with pervasive developmental disorders and very frequent epileptiform spikes may have clinically detectable differences from those without such spikes (Ballaban-Gil & Tuchman, 2000), but these studies await replication.

Pediatric EEG recording may be regarded as a means of obtaining additional clinical signs, which, like any other sign, must be evaluated in the light of the clinical history and other findings, and which will have false positive and false negative results. If the answers given in the report are unexpected or unclear, there may be several reasons for this. The initial question might not have been well-posed, or posed clearly enough with sufficient clinical information given. It might not be possible to answer the question in the circumstances in which the recording was obtained.

What if the Result is Unexpected?

Some structured approach is called for to avoid missing an important point. The problem might be approached in the following way.

What is the strength and nature of the evidence obtained from the EEG?

If the child did have one of their habitual episodes and this was associated with EEG changes, then the clinical view of their underlying disorder may be confirmed. However, if the EEG is entirely unchanged during a typical event which had been strongly suspected of being epileptic in nature, then two possibilities may have to be considered. The event might indeed have an epileptic basis, but this is not seen in the EEG, either because it arises from a deep structure (as in ictal laughter associated with some hypothalamic *hamartomas*) or from cortex remote from the electrodes (frontal lobe seizures may often do this). However, the question must then be asked as to whether or not the other clinical features are quite consistent with such an explanation.

Alternatively, it may be that the event does not have an epileptic basis. Once again, the event has to be reviewed for clinical consistency and for what it may reveal about the child's behavior and attitudes, bearing in mind that children may have both epileptic and non-epileptic events, and that the child may wish to help by displaying what they believe to happen in the events. These clinical decisions may be aided by careful review of video-EEG of the event, particularly with a clinical neurophysiologist.

The discrepancy between the clinical assessment and the EEG report is often less clear-cut, with "abnormalities" being reported in a child in whom a "normal" finding was expected. Once again, it may be useful to consider the context in which the abnormalities were found, with a mild non-specific excess of slow activity in a possibly slightly drowsy child being less compelling evidence than the finding of markedly high-amplitude rhythmic slow activity abnormal for any age and state, particularly if associated with spikes. The EEG report may in these circumstances be seen as giving pointers to areas of the history that might be worth revisiting, or to other investigations that might clarify the diagnosis.

Summing up, the nature of clinical neurophysiological testing is now changing because of developments in other techniques, particularly neuroimaging. Therefore, the emphasis is now rightly more on the physiological and pathophysiological significance of any identified abnormalities (e.g., structural brain lesions). In addition to EEG recording, it can be useful to extend the clinical neurophysiological assessment of the child using EP or ERP techniques (see p. 237).

Finally, the following general points should be kept in mind. Clinical EEG recording will only tell us about the neurological underpinnings of abnormal behavior and cognition, not necessarily about the details of the underlying substrate. Conventional clinical EEG is unlikely to reveal underlying processes when these do not have a grossly organic basis such as epilepsy. In terms of exploring mechanisms of underlying brain function, standard EEG may be useful in defining sleep stages or other "states" but cannot directly illuminate the more intricate mechanisms of human cognition and their aberration in psychiatric disorders. The extent to which it is possible to look at perception, attention, memory and language using time-resolved EEG methods will be discussed in the final part of this chapter.

Application of EEG and ERP in Clinical Research

EEG – A Quantitative Measure of Cortical Dynamics

Neurophysiological techniques are currently undergoing a phase of significant innovation after a previous period of major advances that came with the introduction of digital processing capabilities of personal computers. Computerized methods of analysis have become indispensable tools for capturing the complexity of EEG rhythms and dynamics. There is also closer interaction with other neuroscience disciplines, which by now have recognized the intrinsic advantages of EEG and ERP measures as direct correlates of neuronal activity emerging in real time. This interaction builds on advances in functional and structural neuroimaging and computational neuroscience as well as experimental neurophysiology. A better knowledge of the cortical generator sites of EEG and ERP is now based on systematic studies in neurosurgical patients with indwelling electrodes. We examine examples of this interaction and their application in clinical neuroscience research further below. EEG findings in specific developmental disorders are reviewed in the chapters dealing with individual disorders.

Computerized Analysis of EEG (Quantitative EEG)

The traditional visual analysis of EEG recorded on paper has been supplemented in recent EEG systems with two innovations based on computer technology. First, digital paperless EEG is now a standard technique used in most EEG settings. Second, a number of computerized quantitative methods of EEG analysis have been introduced, aiding the process of EEG interpretation (see p. 240). One of the first computerized methods to be introduced was *spectral analysis* of brain rhythms using fast Fourier transforms. This method decomposes the time domain EEG signal into a frequency domain signal (sum of sines and cosines), which enables quantification of the spectral content of EEG into distinct frequency bands. Furthermore, the analysis of the spatial distribution of EEG across the scalp can be enhanced using methods of *topographical analysis*, such as scalp potential maps, current source density maps (i.e., the spatial derivative of electrical potential) and electrical source (dipole) modeling. In addition, the coupling of rhythms in different brain regions can be assessed using correlation or *coherence analysis*. This technique enables a quantitative assessment of neural connectivity changes in the brain to be made.

While these quantitative EEG techniques have a major role in research settings, they are used in clinical practice only in adjunct to traditional EEG interpretation by highly skilled EEG physicians (Nuwer, 1997). Certain quantitative EEG techniques are considered established only for specific clinical questions:

1 *In epilepsy* for screening for epileptic spikes or seizures in long-term EEG monitoring or ambulatory recording to facilitate subsequent expert visual EEG interpretation;
2 *In intensive care or operating theatre monitoring* for continuous EEG monitoring by frequency-trending to detect early acute intracranial complications, and for screening for possible epileptic seizures in high-risk patients.

Quantitative EEG analysis is an established technique in psychopharmacology, where affinity of drugs for certain neuromodulatory receptors (e.g., dopamine and serotonin receptor subtypes) is associated with characteristic changes in resting EEG rhythms. This method is therefore being used to characterize drug kinetics and profiles in human studies. Computerized EEG analysis has also become an integral part of sleep research and sleep medicine by providing objective criteria for the assessment of sleep architecture.

Quantitative EEG Maturation from Infancy to Adulthood

There are dramatic EEG changes with age that reflect cortical development. EEG can be used to assess cognitive functions and improve our understanding of the relation between brain maturation and behavioral development (for review see Taylor & Baldeweg, 2002). The different EEG rhythms have distinct developmental patterns. In the neonatal period, the waking EEG is dominated by slow frequencies (delta and theta) with the higher frequencies (alpha and beta) emerging with age (Gasser, Verleger, Bacher *et al.*, 1988; Harmony, Marosi, Diaz de Leon *et al.*, 1990b). The decreases in the lower frequency bands occur in the first years of life, whereas the increases in alpha typically continue until early adolescence, while beta continues to mature until adulthood. EEG coherence in childhood shows two types of change: continuous growth processes, and discrete growth spurts in specific anatomical locations and at specific postnatal periods. Using this measure, it emerged that the left and right hemispheres develop at different rates and with different postnatal onset times (Thatcher, 1992; Thatcher, Walker, & Giudice, 1987).

EEG maturation in posterior brain regions is almost twice as fast as that seen at central sites (Benninger, Matthis, & Scheffner, 1984) and is slowest over frontal regions (Gasser *et al.*, 1988), where the process continues until late adolescence. These EEG changes are in keeping with the patterns of cortical maturation derived from quantitative magnetic resonance imaging (MRI) (decreases in cortical thickness or gray matter density (Toga, Thompson, & Sowell, 2006). The latter changes may contribute to the decrease across childhood in the overall amplitude of the EEG signal, in addition to changes in skull thickness.

Quantitative EEG Findings in Developmental Disorders

The resting EEG spectral measures have been used in comparisons of children with normal cognitive development with children with learning disabilities (Harmony, Marosi, Becker *et al.*, 1995), dyslexia (Klimesch, Doppelmayr, Wimmer *et al.*,

2001) and attention deficit disorders (Barry, Clarke, Johnstone *et al.*, 2005). Generally, decreased power in the higher-frequency bands is seen in the clinical groups (Fein, Galin, Yingling *et al.*, 1986), suggesting *maturational lag*. EEG spectral measures also demonstrated maturational spurts in children with reading and writing problems, showing a good behavioral prognosis in those children who showed accelerated EEG maturation at follow-up (Harmony *et al.*, 1995). Maturational EEG group differences diminish with age, but there are still persisting differences later in adolescence and adulthood, suggesting that the maturational lag hypothesis may not be sufficient to account for developmental learning disabilities and attention deficit/hyperactivity disorder (ADHD) (Bresnahan, Anderson, & Barry, 1999; Bresnahan & Barry, 2002; see also chapter 3).

EEG coherence measures show fewer age-related changes in cognitive developmental disorders (Marosi, Harmony, Sanchez *et al.*, 1992; Marosi, Harmony, Reyes *et al.*, 1997). Children at risk for such disorders can also show abnormalities on conventional EEG (Harmony, Hinojosa, Marosi *et al.*, 1990a). This is particularly true of autism and pervasive developmental disorders, where EEG abnormalities in sleep have been found in up to 61% of autism spectrum disorders (ASD) children referred for EEG (Chez, Chang, Krasne *et al.*, 2006). Evaluations using quantitative EEG (John, Karmel, Corning *et al.*, 1977) may identify distinct EEG profiles in a large proportion of children with developmental disorders (Chabot, di Michele, Princhep *et al.*, 2001). It will be important to determine how these measures relate to modern diagnostic criteria and other neuroimaging investigations and if they predict response to treatment (Bresnahan, Barry, Clarke *et al.*, 2006). Furthermore, it is not yet known if maturational differences are specific to certain brain systems (e.g., auditory and speech processing; Bishop & McArthur, 2004), or reflect more large-scale brain maturational differences as changes in global EEG measures (spectral and intra- and interhemispheric coherence) would suggest.

Event-related Potentials – Markers of Cognitive Processing

Introduction and Basic Principles

ERPs are now an established technique in studying neural correlates of specific cognitive operations. We review some general principles of this method and give brief examples of their application in clinical research settings. The reader will find more comprehensive reviews on ERP methodology by Luck (2005) and Handy (2007). ERPs constitute the stimulus-locked part of the EEG elicited by a specific cognitive or motor event or stimulus (cf. EP; see p. 237). Therefore, ERPs are modulated by task instructions (e.g., detection of a specific target event) more than by physical properties of the eliciting stimulus.

Task-specific modulations of the ERP wave shape (i.e., increases or decreases in amplitude) are called *ERP components*, which are best identified in difference waves. ERPs are direct neural measures of functional integration in the brain which can be elicited at distinct hierarchical processing stages: from sensory perception, attention to specific stimulus features, contextual event integration (e.g., recognition memory, emotional evaluation) to the planning and execution of a motor response (see p. 244).

ERP at the Interface of Neurophysiology and Cognitive Neuroscience

Up to the 1980s ERPs had been used as a physiological addition to behavioral measures such as reaction time which allowed a further dissection of processing stages and their modulation by task instructions. Today, armed with a whole array of new methods, ERPs can be used to answer very specific questions, utilizing the unique properties of this method in comparison with functional imaging. The advantages of ERPs are chiefly their temporal resolution (in milliseconds), their direct neural origin (as opposed to the hemodynamic nature of the fMRI signal) and the relative inexpensiveness of the method. Their low spatial resolution necessitates *independent converging evidence* from other methods, if inference about activity in specific cortical regions is of interest. It is important to bear this limitation in mind when interpreting ERP studies. ERPs also allow the examination of covert (unattended) processing in the absence of a behavioral response, which is useful in studies of infants and children with behavioral problems.

Methods of ERP Registration and Analysis

ERPs are recorded using similar apparatus as conventional EEGs and EPs, except that different filter settings are used to capture some of the slower event-related changes in ERP signals, called *slow cortical potentials*. General guidelines and recommendations are available for the recording and analysis of ERPs (Picton, Bentin, Berg *et al.*, 2000).

In addition to ERP activity that is tightly time- and phase-locked to the stimulus, there are also systematic stimulus-related EEG changes that are not tightly phase-locked to the stimulus. These "stimulus-induced oscillations" (*event-related synchronization* [ERS] or *desynchronization* [ERD]) can be observed in a variety of experimental conditions and across the entire EEG spectrum, ranging from induced theta changes during memory processes to high-frequency gamma oscillations during perceptual tasks.

Estimation of ERP Generators

Using techniques such as MEG or multielectrode EEG, it is possible to estimate the likely location of cortical electrical generators from the scalp distribution of magnetic fields and electrical potentials, respectively. However, this method of inverse source modeling yields no unique solution and its application is therefore limited to research settings where converging evidence can be obtained from a priori anatomical knowledge, or increasingly obtained from functional neuroimaging.

Intracranial ERP Recordings

A more accurate estimation of cortical ERP generators is possible when electrodes are inserted directly into the brains of neurosurgical patients for whom such invasive procedure is performed for localization of epileptic seizure activity (see p. 237). *Intracranial ERPs* (iERPs) are extracted from the electrocorticogram (ECoG) in much the same way as from scalp EEGs, except that their voltage is much larger (up to 150 μV) as the attenuating influence of skull and skin is removed. Intracranial ERPs have a high spatial resolution, in contrast to scalp ERPs, with components usually visible only in very few adjacent electrode contacts, spanning a few square centimeters, with steep amplitude gradients, suggesting close proximity to the cortical generators.

In addition to providing insights into the functional anatomy of ERPs, this method is also used clinically in neurosurgical patients to provide information about the proximity of functional cortex to the site of surgical resection. For example, iERPs recorded from medial temporal regions are used as diagnostic markers of the functional integrity of the hippocampal formation before temporal lobe surgery. They reveal the laterality of verbal memory processes (Grunwald, Elger, Lehnertz *et al.*, 1995) and predict the impact of temporal lobe resection on postoperative verbal memory (Grunwald, Lehnertz, Helmstaedter *et al.*, 1998). Intracranial ERPs recorded from the cortical surface help identifying sensory cortices (Liasis, Towell, & Boyd, 1999), as well as eloquent motor and language-related regions.

Cognitive Processing Stages and Functional Anatomy of Associated ERP Components

Our knowledge of the functional neuroanatomy of ERPs has been advanced largely by systematic sampling by intracranial ERPs of a large number of brain sites in neurosurgical patients (Halgren, Baudena, Clarke *et al.*, 1995; Halgren, Marinkovic, & Chauvel, 1998). Two types of task have been used, which are also frequently used in ERP studies from the intact scalp. The first type is a simple target detection task where a sequence of frequent non-target stimuli is presented, and among them occasional (oddball) targets have to be detected. This oddball task gives rise to a well-known sequence of ERP peaks (N1, P2 to non-targets, and additional N2, P3a and P3b and slow wave to targets). Stimulus classification tasks have been used to examine the modulation of long-latency intracranial ERP components (N4, P3b) by emotional and semantic context.

The following *basic processing stages* can be delineated, characterized by distinct ERP patterns, which follow a hierarchical pattern arising from sensory cortices extending to multimodal, association and premotor cortices (Halgren & Marinkovic, 1995) (Plate 17.1). Examples of their respective applications in clinical research studies are given further below (see p. 245).

1 *Perceptual processing* in primary and secondary sensory cortices is reflected in a sequence of positive and negative polarity *sensory components* (P1, N1, P2) from approximately 50 to 200 ms poststimulus.

2 *Orienting and attention* to surprising or biologically important stimuli is reflected in a triphasic *N2–P3a–slow wave complex*. This orienting complex is generated concurrently in the cingulate gyrus and connected lateral prefrontal and posterior parietal cortices, known to subserve attentional control. Similar potentials are also elicited in the absence of attention to the stimuli (see p. 245).

3 *Event encoding* of attended semantic stimulus information and integration within the cognitive and emotional context are reflected in long-latency "endogenous" ERP components *N4* and *P3b* in the *hippocampus*, *amygdala* and associated inferotemporal and lateral orbitofrontal cortices.

4 These stimulus-locked ERP components are followed by potentials reflecting *response preparation and execution*, *readiness potentials* in the central cingulate gyrus and associated supplementary and premotor cortices. Potentials correlated with response execution are the *lateralized motor potentials* in sensorimotor regions.

5 ERP components arising immediately after response execution are correlated with *performance monitoring* of successful or erroneous actions. *Error-related negative potentials* (ERNs) are generated in medial frontal (cingulate cortex) regions involved in performance monitoring (see p. 246).

6 Sustained *slow cortical potential shifts* (SCPs), recorded mainly over prefrontal regions, reflect the *maintenance of a sustained cognitive context* during task execution.

7 Among ERPs associated with *language processing* is a late negativity recorded over central scalp electrodes (*N4*) elicited by semantic expectations in left anterior medial temporal cortex. Syntactic violations elicit a short latency (300–500 ms) *left anterior negativity (ELAN)* and a late posterior positivity (*P600*).

Developmental ERP Changes from Infancy to Adulthood

ERPs provide valuable insight into the neural maturation of sensory and cognitive processing in humans (for review see Taylor & Baldeweg, 2002). Because subject cooperation is not required to test basic sensory processing and discrimination, such studies can be performed even in neonates, infants and during sleep. Similarly, early linguistic processes (e.g., semantic concepts) can be probed using ERPs even in pre-verbal children. We will examine examples of such developmental studies below, while developmental ERP studies of other cognitive functions can be found elsewhere: attention (Sanders, Stevens, Coch *et al.*, 2006), memory (Cycowicz, 2000) and reading (Licht, Bakker, Kok *et al.*, 1992; Taylor & Keenan, 1999) and language (Friederici, 2005).

The following characteristic ERP changes are found during infant and child development:

1 Changes in *ERP morphology* (e.g., the emergence of new ERP components can signal the development of new cortical modules);

2 The *shortening of component latencies* reflecting increased processing efficiency and speed; and

3 *ERP amplitude changes* reflect the number of synaptic elements synchronously activated.

These amplitude changes can be non-linear across age, showing distinct peaks during infant development, which may index developmental periods of synapse formation and elimination.

Maturation of Auditory Cortices are Reflected in Auditory ERPs

The maturational changes of auditory ERPs have been well documented in infancy and childhood (Wunderlich & Cone-Wesson, 2006), showing a protracted time course which extends into the second decade of life. The protracted developmental course of auditory ERPs is paralleled by an extended neuroanatomical maturation of human auditory cortex. Maturity of the auditory cortical architecture is not reached until after 12 years of age, which might explain the prolonged development of certain auditory processing skills, such as frequency discrimination and speech recognition (Moore, 2002).

In children and adults, the most prominent auditory ERP component is the N1 wave, which is composed of at least three distinct subcomponents. These N1 components show different developmental changes, and hemispheric differences were found, with one of these components over the left hemisphere maturing earlier than over the right side. This precocious development of the left auditory cortex is even more pronounced for speech stimuli than for pure tones.

ERP Investigation of Developmental Disorders

In the following sections we review examples of ERP studies of auditory perceptual functions (reflected in mismatch negativity [MMN]), attention and event encoding (P3) and response execution (ERN). The objective is to demonstrate the limitations and the nature of insights that can be obtained from ERP studies. The ERP findings are not clearly shown to be specific to the disorders reviewed here, nor do they characterize all people with such developmental conditions.

Aberrant Auditory Cortical Maturation in Developmental Disorders

Some studies using ERPs to simple sound stimuli have suggested altered maturation of auditory cortices in a number of developmental disorders. Dyslexic children showed a lack of hemispheric lateralization in early auditory magnetic fields in a study by Heim, Eulitz, and Elbert (2003), perhaps related to a lack of *planum temporale* asymmetry. In children with *specific language impairment* (SLI), ERP evidence points to impaired auditory maturation (Bishop & McArthur, 2004). Furthermore, Bruneau, Roux, Adrien *et al.* (1999) reported that N1b and N1c are abnormally small in autistic children with poor verbal communication and lack the normal modulation by sound intensity, suggesting dysfunction in auditory association cortex in the lateral part of the superior temporal gyrus, especially in the left hemisphere.

Maturation of Sound Discrimination Reflected in Mismatch Negativity Potentials

When ERPs to frequently presented sounds (standards) are subtracted from those to occasional sounds deviating in any physical feature such as frequency, location or duration (deviants), the difference potentials show an early negative deflection at around 100–200 ms, called *mismatch negativity* (MMN). MMN indexes an automatic auditory change detection (discrimination) process as it is elicited in the absence of overt attention to the sounds (Naatanen, 1992). Its magnitude and latency correlate well with behavioral sound discrimination performance. MMN potentials emerge early during postnatal development, being robust by about 6 months (Jing & Benasich, 2006). There is further developmental change in MMN latency, magnitude and topography, which can index the acquisition of sound representation for the native language during infancy (Cheour, Ceponiene, Lehtokoski *et al.*, 1998). MMN has proved an important tool in the investigation of children at risk of impaired speech and sound discrimination, such as dyslexia (Maurer, Bucher, Brem *et al.*, 2003; Pihko, Leppanen, Eklund *et al.*, 1999), SLI (Shafer, Morr, Datta *et al.*, 2005; Uwer, Albrecht, & von Suchodoletz, 2002), autism (Gomot, Giard, Adrien *et al.*, 2002; Kuhl, Coffey-Corina, Padden *et al.*, 2005) and non-specific learning difficulties (Kraus, McGee, Carrell *et al.*, 1996).

Despite significant differences being found between clinical and control groups, the application of MMN to developmental disorders on an individual patient basis is still limited by low intrasubject reproducibility. Nevertheless, encouraging clinical utility of MMN has been shown in cochlear implant users (Ponton, Eggermont, Don *et al.*, 2000; Singh, Liasis, Rajput *et al.*, 2004), indicating that MMN can be used to assess the functional status and plastic potential of the auditory system in children with cochlear implants and that it may provide an objective predictor for long-term behavioral outcome.

MMN Potentials as Markers of Aberrant Cortical Plasticity

MMN is also a robust biological marker of schizophrenia (for review see Umbricht & Krljes, 2005), and shows some specificity for this disorder, in as much as MMN generation is normal in patients with bipolar (manic-depressive) illness. MMN is also reduced in relatives of patients with schizophrenia, both in childhood and adulthood, suggesting that it is a trait marker for this disorder. This is also supported by premorbid MMN deficits in children and adolescents at high risk for schizophrenia (Baker, Baldeweg, Sivagnanasundaram *et al.*, 2005; Schreiber, Stolz-Born, Kornhuber *et al.*, 1992). The considerable interest in its application to schizophrenia arose from the observation that MMN is abolished after blockade of *N*-methyl-D-aspartate (NMDA) receptor dependent synaptic transmission, a receptor system implicated in cognitive symptoms of this disorder. Furthermore, NMDA receptors are also critical for many forms of cortical plasticity. It was therefore not surprising to find that MMN deficits in schizophrenic patients correlate strongly with measures of illness severity and cognitive performance. Indeed, there is a remarkable convergence between the neurophysiological mechanism of MMN generation in supragranular layers (II/III) of the auditory cortex (Javitt, Steinschneider, Schroeder *et al.*, 1996), on the one hand, and the site of most consistent neuropathological abnormality in glutamatergic synapses located in these cortical layers in schizophrenia (Harrison, 1999). MMN is simpler than other ERPs, and can therefore be studied not only in humans but also in experimental animals (Umbricht, Vyssotki, Latanov *et al.*, 2005), offering the opportunity to study in more detail the cellular and molecular mechanisms of this important aspect of synaptic pathology of schizophrenia.

Development of Face Processing in Healthy and Autistic Children

Faces are the most important visual stimuli for social interactions and specialized neural modules for processing of human faces have been identified with intracranial ERP in inferior temporal cortex (fusiform gyrus) (Allison, Puce, Spencer *et al.*, 1999). Scalp recorded ERPs show a face-sensitive N170 component at posterior temporal leads. This N170 is sensitive to various types of facial stimuli and the emergence of such expertise has been studied in infants and children, demonstrating a prolonged maturational course of its neural substrate (i.e., shortening of N170 peak latency). Differing developmental curves for upright and inverted faces argue that the development in face processing is brought about primarily by improvement in configural processing. Of interest are reports of aberrant face ERPs in children with autism: the N170 is slower by about 20 ms and ERPs fail to differentiate between familiar and unfamiliar faces, although recognition for objects is intact. Furthermore, in 3- to 4-year-old children with ASD, ERPs failed to show a recognition effect to facial emotions (fear) which is normally present from 7 months of age (Dawson, Webb, Carver *et al.*, 2004). In summary, face ERPs can offer unique insight into maturation of specific pre-verbal cognitive skills in children and their early developmental aberration.

Deficits in Attention and Event Encoding are Reflected in P3 Potentials

P3 potentials are a family of ubiquitous long-latency positive potentials in response to biologically important or attended stimuli. Surprising and novel stimuli elicit a fronto-central positivity (P3a or *novelty P3*) at 300 ms poststimulus, while expected target events elicit a posterior parietal P3b (or *target P3*) component at 300–500 ms. The novelty P3a may be altered in children with autism, especially in response to speech sounds (Lepisto, Kujala, Vanhala *et al.*, 2006). Furthermore, there is considerable evidence that P3b generation is abnormal in schizophrenia (as well as possibly in autism and ADHD; e.g., Mathalon, Ford, & Pfefferbaum, 2000), perhaps reflecting dysfunction in an extended cortico-limbic system, centered on the hippocampus, with top-down feedback from higher level regions. In summary, endogenous ERPs, including P3 potentials, hold promise in identifying abnormally developing brain systems early during child development.

Maturation of Cognitive Control Indexed by Error Negativity Potentials

A number of ERP components are associated with cognitive control functions, such as inhibiting a prepotent response, and monitoring the outcome of actions. The stimulus-locked frontal N2 and P3a ERP components are associated with the former operations (i.e., the initiating of inhibitory control or "braking mechanism"). Performance errors are associated with a distinct error-related negativity (ERN) potential time-locked to the incorrect response. ERN is elicited in medial prefrontal cortex (dorsal anterior cingulate gyrus) within 100–200 ms of the executed motor response, indexing a very rapid comparison process between intended and executed actions (Falkenstein, Hohnsbein, Hoorman *et al.*, 1991; Gehring & Knight, 2000). ERN potentials show a protracted developmental course from childhood to adulthood (Hogan, Varga-Khadem, Kirkham *et al.*, 2005), reflecting the late maturation of executive control functions. Children with ADHD show marked deficits in eliciting ERP responses (N2 and P3a) associated with response inhibition and error detection (ERN) (Liotti, Pliszka, Perez *et al.*, 2005). The ERP data implicate an interconnected network of regions in the frontal lobe and its subcortical projections in dysfunctions of cognitive control in ADHD.

ERP as a Marker of Liability to Disorder

It has been suggested that ERPs might be useful as *endophenotypes* for the study of genetic factors affecting the risk of psychopathology. Such endophenotypes are thought to reflect the action of risk genes more reliably and directly than symptoms (Gottesman & Gould, 2003). However, it cannot be asserted that ERPs are an endophenotype (see chapter 23), not least because their heritability is not established. One study has found that a functional polymorphism in one of the candidate genes in the deleted region of chromosome 22 (the *COMT* gene involved in dopamine metabolism) affected both MMN generation and cognitive function (Baker *et al.*, 2005). This polymorphism has also been associated with increased risk of developing psychosis in this population (Gothelf, Eliez, Thompson *et al.*, 2005). Reduced MMN amplitude has been reported in some studies of relatives of schizophrenia patients during both adulthood (Michie, Innes-Brown, Todd *et al.*, 2002) and childhood (Schreiber, Stolz-Born, Kornhuber *et al.*, 1992).

The long-latency P3 component is also changed in schizophrenia (Ford, 1999), as well as in relatives of patients and could also index vulnerability to this disorder (Winterer, Egan, Raedler *et al.*, 2003), perhaps along with genes involved in dopamine transmission (Berman, Noble, Antolin *et al.*, 2006; Gallinat, Bajbouj, Sander *et al.*, 2003). Nevertheless, it is unlikely that even ERPs will directly reflect the action of single genes, given the complexity of brain systems involved in their generation. At best, they offer the potential to study the action of risk genes and their interaction with other factors at the neurophysiological level.

Considerations for the Interpretation of ERP Findings

Because of the limitations of the ERP method (e.g., in localizing activity in specific brain regions), it is necessary to ask: what can be inferred from ERP studies? The following considerations may help in providing some guidance in this complex issue.

The separation of ERPs into distinct processing stages (see p. 244) might imply that neural computations reflected in ERPs are strictly serial in nature, with activity in higher processing stages beginning after the computations in an earlier lower level stage have been completed. However, endogenous long-latency ERPs with a widespread scalp distribution, such as P3a, P3b and N4, have multiple, concurrently active intracerebral generators. This could reflect parallel and independent processes, or alternatively, interdependent processing. The experimental evidence on P3 potentials supports the notion of parallel but *interdependent processing* (Halgren, Marinkovic, & Chauvel, 1998). ERP studies in patients with discrete lesions of the medial temporal cortex, dorsolateral prefrontal cortex or posterior parietal cortex showed impaired P3a generation, correlated with deficits in orienting attention to novel events (Daffner, Scinto, Weitzman *et al.*, 2003; Knight, 1996). These findings cannot be explained if the intact cortical P3a generators operate independently of generators in regions affected by lesions; the findings therefore support the notion of at least partial interdependence of the components of the attention network involved in P3a generation. It is therefore more helpful to think of ERPs as providing insight into the neural interaction of brain systems, rather than in localizing dysfunction in specific neuroanatomical systems. We return to this notion further below.

However, ERPs are generated in more widespread areas than are necessary for the performance of a specific task (Halgren, Marinkovic, & Chauvel, 1998). For example, lesions of the hippocampus, where the largest P3b potentials are generated, do not interfere with performance in the simple oddball discrimination task used to elicit such P3b potentials (Polich & Squire, 1993). This hints at *redundancy in brain activation* to engage many potentially useful regions, even though they might not be required to perform the task. In such cases, it is only possible to infer from an ERP deficit in a particular patient group that the neural substrate involved in its generation is compromised. The nature of the compromise cannot be directly inferred, and requires independent evidence.

Indeed, it is necessary to ensure that ERPs are recorded during tasks that can be performed by all patients. Otherwise, interpretation of ERP correlates of a specific cognitive operation of interest is complicated by the possibility of dysfunction in an antecedent process. For example, if the neural substrate for event integration is of interest, as measured with P3b potentials, it is necessary to ensure that the sensory discrimination necessary to identify target stimuli from background non-target stimuli can be performed with high accuracy.

Future Directions

Integration with Other Neuroscience Methods

Neurophysiological techniques are continually developing and current trends indicate that they are increasingly being applied in combination with other neuroimaging modalities. The application of MEG is likely to increase in specialist research facilities for specific clinical applications. For example, MEG can aid in localization of cortical generators of sensory evoked potentials and epileptic spikes. Furthermore, there is tight coupling between intracortical electrical field potential generation and fMRI signal changes (Logothetis, Pauls, Augath *et al.*, 2001), which facilitates the combination of both methods (e.g., in estimating the sources of ERPs using fMRI constrained source modeling). The technology of combined EEG and fMRI meas-urement is rapidly improving and the first clinical studies were able to identify brain areas activated concurrently with interictal epileptic spikes (Krakow, Woermann, Symms *et al.*, 1999). The combination of EEG and ERP recordings with transcranial magnetic stimulation (TMS) has potential for investigations of pathological spread of activation and in evaluating if cognitive operations can be interrupted or facilitated with focal cortical stimulation. Furthermore, as our understanding of the neurophysiological mechanisms and cognitive correlates of different brain rhythms increases, there will be a need to extend the frequency range of EEG recordings beyond what is currently being used in clinical practice, from very slow (<1 Hz) to very high frequencies (>100 Hz). The latter high-frequency oscillations are of particular relevance to seizure initiation and spread (Traub, Contreras, & Whittington, 2005). In addition, further elucidation of the functional role of rhythmic activity in synaptic plasticity and shaping of neural connections will allow us to make inferences from EEG/ERP time-frequency dynamics about their role in the psychopathology of the developing and mature brain. This endeavor will be critically informed by another recent innovation, the application of methods of computational neuroscience to neurophysiology, which is summarized briefly below.

Computational Models and Synaptic Plasticity

We predict that neurophysiological methods will be instrumental in our understanding of the nature of the computations performed by the human brain. Because of the enormous complexity of brain architecture such insights are likely to be informed by theoretical perspectives afforded by computational sciences. Such an approach might enable us to understand disorders of the brain and mind that have so far eluded conventional methods of analysis. A critical step in this direction would be a deeper understanding of the principles of cortico-cortical interactions, thought to be at the core of disorders such as schizophrenia and autism. ERPs are markers of neural mass action in the brain generated concurrently in multiple brain regions and might therefore reveal the nature of cortico-cortical interaction between those distinct generators and their presumed disruption in psychopathology. Indeed, a formalized mathematic model of cortical computation has been proposed which makes direct predictions about the behavior of EEG and ERP components (Friston, 2003, 2005). This biologically constrained computational model is based on knowledge of cortico-cortical connectivity, such as feedforward, backward and lateral connections, well characterized by anatomical studies (Felleman & Van Essen, 1991) and the role of neuromodulators in dynamically shaping synaptic plasticity.

Furthermore, recent developments in statistical evaluation of EEG/ERP responses allow inferences to be made about the nature and strengths of cortical connectivity between hierarchical interconnected cortical regions. The method of dynamic causal modeling (DCM; David, Kiebel, Harrison *et al.*, 2006; Friston, Harrison, & Penny, 2003) is based on neural mass models representing hierarchically connected cortical areas and makes realistic assumptions about the neuroanatomical nature of cortico-cortical connectivity. A further critical step in understanding aberrant cortical plasticity that might underlie developmental psychopathology is the study of neuromodulation of ERP dynamics. Given the highly heritable nature of interindividual variants of the normal EEG pattern (Vogel & Propping, 1982) and the considerable proportion of neurophysiological variability (EEG frequency spectrum and P3 potentials) that is influenced by genomic variation (van Beijsterveldt & van Baal, 2002), it can be expected that a combination of genetic and ERP markers of disrupted brain physiology could guide and predict individual patient's response to treatments (Stephan, Baldeweg, & Friston, 2006). Hence, an increasing convergence of neuroscience methodologies, including neurophysiology, will aid the development of an informed view on the pathophysiology of developmental psychological disorders.

References

Allison, T., Puce, A., Spencer, D. D., & McCarthy, G. (1999). Electrophysiological studies of human face perception. I: Potentials generated in occipitotemporal cortex by face and non-face stimuli. *Cerebral Cortex*, 9, 415–430.

Baker, K., Baldeweg, T., Sivagnanasundaram, S., Scambler, P., & Skuse, D. (2005). COMT Val108/158 Met modifies mismatch negativity and cognitive function in 22q11 deletion syndrome. *Biological Psychiatry*, *58*, 23–31.

Ballaban-Gil, K., & Tuchman, R. (2000). Epilepsy and epileptiform EEG: association with autism and language disorders. *Mental Retardation and Developmental Disabilities Research Reviews*, 6, 300–308.

Barry, R. J., Clarke, A. R., Johnstone, S. J., & Oades, R. D. (2005). Electrophysiology in attention-deficit/hyperactivity disorder. *International Journal of Psychophysiology*, *58*, 1–3.

Benninger, C., Matthis, P., & Scheffner, D. (1984). EEG development of healthy boys and girls: Results of a longitudinal study. *Electroencephalography and Clinical Neurophysiology*, *57*, 1–12.

Berger, H. (1969). On the electroencephalogram of man. *Electroencephalography and Clinical Neurophysiology. Supplement*, *28*, 37.

Berman, S. M., Noble, E. P., Antolin, T., Sheen, C., Conner, B. T., & Ritchie, T. (2006). P300 development during adolescence: Effects of DRD2 genotype. *Clinical Neurophysiology*, *117*, 649–659.

Binnie, C. D. (2003). Cognitive impairment during epileptiform discharges: Is it ever justifiable to treat the EEG? *Lancet Neurology*, 2, 725–730.

Bishop, D. V., & McArthur, G. M. (2004). Immature cortical responses to auditory stimuli in specific language impairment: Evidence from ERPs to rapid tone sequences. *Developmental Science*, 7, F11–F18.

Bresnahan, S. M., Anderson, J. W., & Barry, R. J. (1999). Age-related changes in quantitative EEG in attention-deficit/hyperactivity disorder. *Biological Psychiatry*, *46*, 1690–1697.

Bresnahan, S. M., & Barry, R. J. (2002). Specificity of quantitative EEG analysis in adults with attention deficit hyperactivity disorder. *Psychiatry Research*, 112, 133–144.

Bresnahan, S. M., Barry, R. J., Clarke, A. R., & Johnstone, S. J. (2006). Quantitative EEG analysis in dexamphetamine-responsive adults with attention-deficit/hyperactivity disorder. *Psychiatry Research*, *141*, 151–159.

Bruneau, N., Roux, S., Adrien, J. L., & Barthelemy, C. (1999). Auditory associative cortex dysfunction in children with autism: Evidence from late auditory evoked potentials (N1 wave–T complex). *Clinical Neurophysiology*, *110*, 1927–1934.

Buzsaki, G., & Draguhn, A. (2004). Neuronal oscillations in cortical networks. *Science*, *304*, 1926–1929.

Chabot, R. J., di Michele, F., Prichep, L., & John, E. R. (2001). The clinical role of computerized EEG in the evaluation and treatment of learning and attention disorders in children and adolescents. *Journal of Neuropsychiatry and Clinical Neuroscience*, *13*, 171–186.

Cheour, M., Ceponiene, R., Lehtokoski, A., Luuk, A., Allik, J., Alho, K., *et al.* (1998). Development of language-specific phoneme representations in the infant brain. *Nature Neuroscience*, *1*, 351–353.

Chez, M. G., Chang, M., Krasne, V., Coughlan, C., Kominsky, M., & Schwartz, A. (2006). Frequency of epileptiform EEG abnormalities in a sequential screening of autistic patients with no known clinical epilepsy from 1996 to 2005. *Epilepsy & Behavior*, *8*, 267–271.

Cycowicz, Y. M. (2000). Memory development and event-related brain potentials in children. *Biological Psychology*, 54, 145–174.

Daffner, K. R., Scinto, L. F., Weitzman, A. M., Faust, R., Rentz, D. M., Budson, A. E., *et al.* (2003). Frontal and parietal components of a cerebral network mediating voluntary attention to novel events. *Journal of Cognitive Neuroscience*, *15*, 294–313.

David, O., Kiebel, S. J., Harrison, L. M., Mattout, J., Kilner, J. M., & Friston, K. J. (2006). Dynamic causal modeling of evoked responses in EEG and MEG. *Neuroimage*, *30*, 1255–1272.

Davis, H., Davis, P. A., Loomis, A. L., Harvey, E. N., & Hobart, G. (1939). Electrical reaction of the human brain to auditory stimulation during sleep. *Journal Neurophysiology*, *2*, 500–514.

Dawson, G. D. (1947). Central responses to electrical stimulation of peripheral nerve in man. *Journal of Neurology, Neurosurgery, and Psychiatry*, *10*, 137–140.

Dawson, G. D. (1954). A summation technique for the detection of small evoked potentials. *Electroencephalography Clinical Neurophysiology*, *6*, 65–84.

Dawson, G., Webb, S. J., Carver, L., Panagiotides, H., & McPartland, J. (2004). Young children with autism show atypical brain responses to fearful versus neutral facial expressions of emotion. *Developmental Science*, 7, 340–359.

Falkenstein, M., Hohnsbein, J., Hoormann, J., & Blanke, L. (1991). Effects of crossmodal divided attention on late ERP components. II. Error processing in choice reaction tasks. *Electroencephalography and Clinical Neurophysiology*, *78*, 447–455.

Fein, G., Galin, D., Yingling, C. D., Johnstone, J., Davenport, L., & Herron, J. (1986). EEG spectra in dyslexic and control boys during resting conditions. *Electroencephalography and Clinical Neurophysiology*, *63*, 87–97.

Felleman, D. J., & Van Essen, D. C. (1991). Distributed hierarchical processing in the primate cerebral cortex. *Cerebral Cortex*, *1*, 1–47.

Ford, J. M. (1999). Schizophrenia: the broken P300 and beyond. *Psychophysiology*, *36*, 667–682.

Friederici, A. D. (2005). Neurophysiologic markers of early language acquisition: from syllables to sentences. *Trends in Cognitive Science*, *9*, 481–488.

Friston, K. (2003). Learning and inference in the brain. *Neural Networks*, *16*, 1325–1352.

Friston, K. (2005). A theory of cortical responses. *Philosophical Transactions of the Royal Society of London. Series B, Biological Sciences*, *360*, 815–836.

Friston, K. J., Harrison, L., & Penny, W. (2003). Dynamic causal modelling. *Neuroimage*, *19*, 1273–1302.

Gallinat, J., Bajbouj, M., Sander, T., Schlattmann, P., Xu, K., Ferro, E. F., *et al.* (2003). Association of the G1947A COMT

(Val(108/158)Met) gene polymorphism with prefrontal P300 during information processing. *Biological Psychiatry*, *54*, 40–48.

Gasser, T., Verleger, R., Bacher, P., & Sroka, L. (1988). Development of the EEG of school-age children and adolescents. I. Analysis of band power. *Electroencephalography and Clinical Neurophysiology*, *69*, 91–99.

Gehring, W. J., & Knight, R. T. (2000). Prefrontal–cingulate interactions in action monitoring. *Nature Neuroscience*, *3*, 516–520.

Gibbs, F. A., Davis, H., & Lennox, W. G. (1935). The electroencephalogram in epilepsy and in conditions of impaired consciousness. *Archive of Neurology and Psychiatry*, *34*, 1133–1148.

Gloor, P. (1994). Berger lecture. Is Berger's dream coming true? *Electroencephalography and Clinical Neurophysiology*, *90*, 253–266.

Goldman, R. I., Stern, J. M., Engel, J. Jr., & Cohen, M. S. (2002). Simultaneous EEG and fMRI of the alpha rhythm. *Neuroreport*, *13*, 2487–2492.

Gomot, M., Giard, M. H., Adrien, J. L., Barthelemy, C., & Bruneau, N. (2002). Hypersensitivity to acoustic change in children with autism: Electrophysiological evidence of left frontal cortex dysfunctioning. *Psychophysiology*, *39*, 577–584.

Gothelf, D., Eliez, S., Thompson, T., Hinard, C., Penniman, L., Feinstein, C., *et al.* (2005). *COMT* genotype predicts longitudinal cognitive decline and psychosis in 22q11.2 deletion syndrome. *Nature Neuroscience*, *8*, 1500–1502.

Gottesman, I. I., & Gould, T. D. (2003). The endophenotype concept in psychiatry: etymology and strategic intentions. *American Journal of Psychiatry*, *160*, 636–645.

Gray, C. M., Konig, P., Engel, A. K., & Singer, W. (1989). Oscillatory responses in cat visual cortex exhibit inter-columnar synchronization which reflects global stimulus properties. *Nature*, *338*, 334–337.

Grunwald, T., Elger, C. E., Lehnertz, K., Van Roost, D., & Heinze, H. J. (1995). Alterations of intrahippocampal cognitive potentials in temporal lobe epilepsy. *Electroencephalography and Clinical Neurophysiology*, *95*, 53–62.

Grunwald, T., Lehnertz, K., Helmstaedter, C., Kutas, M., Pezer, N., Kurthen, M., *et al.* (1998). Limbic ERPs predict verbal memory after left-sided hippocampectomy. *Neuroreport*, *9*, 3375–3378.

Halgren, E., Baudena, P., Clarke, J. M., Heit, G., Marinkovic, K., Devaux, B., *et al.* (1995). Intracerebral potentials to rare target and distractor auditory and visual stimuli. II. Medial, lateral and posterior temporal lobe. *Electroencephalography and Clinical Neurophysiology*, *94*, 229–250.

Halgren, E., & Marinkovic, K. (1995). Neurophysiologic networks integrating human emotions. In M. Gazzaniga (Ed.), *The Cognitive Neurosciences* (pp. 1137–1151). Cambridge, MA: MIT Press.

Halgren, E., Marinkovic, K., & Chauvel, P. (1998). Generators of the late cognitive potentials in auditory and visual oddball tasks. *Electroencephalography and Clinical Neurophysiology*, *106*, 156–164.

Handy, T. C. (2007). *Event related potentials: A methods handbook.* Boston, MA: MIT Press.

Hari, R., Salmelin, R., Makela, J. P., Salenius, S., & Helle, M. (1997). Magnetoencephalographic cortical rhythms. *International Journal of Psychophysiology*, *26*, 51–62.

Harmony, T., Hinojosa, G., Marosi, E., Becker, J., Rodriguez, M., Reyes, A., *et al.* (1990a). Correlation between EEG spectral parameters and an educational evaluation. *International Journal of Neuroscience*, *54*, 147–155.

Harmony, T., Marosi, E., Becker, J., Rodriguez, M., Reyes, A., Fernandez, T., *et al.* (1995). Longitudinal quantitative EEG study of children with different performances on a reading–writing test. *Electroencephalography and Clinical Neurophysiology*, 95, 426–433.

Harmony, T., Marosi, E., Diaz de Leon, A. E., Becker, J., & Fernandez, T. (1990b). Effect of sex, psychosocial disadvantages and biological risk factors on EEG maturation. *Electroencephalography and Clinical Neurophysiology*, *75*, 482–491.

Harrison, P. J. (1999). The neuropathology of schizophrenia: A critical review of the data and their interpretation. *Brain*, *122*, 593–624.

Heim, S., Eulitz, C., & Elbert, T. (2003). Altered hemispheric asymmetry of auditory P100m in dyslexia. *European Journal of Neuroscience*, *17*, 1715–1722.

Herrmann, C. S., & Demiralp, T. (2005). Human EEG gamma oscillations in neuropsychiatric disorders. *Clinical Neurophysiology*, *116*, 2719–2733.

Hobson, J. A., & Pace-Schott, E. F. (2002). The cognitive neuroscience of sleep: Neuronal systems, consciousness and learning. *Nature Reviews. Neuroscience*, *3*, 679–693.

Hogan, A. M., Vargha-Khadem, F., Kirkham, F. J., & Baldeweg, T. (2005). Maturation of action monitoring from adolescence to adulthood: An ERP study. *Developmental Science*, *8*, 525–534.

Javitt, D. C., Steinschneider, M., Schroeder, C. E., & Arezzo, J. C. (1996). Role of cortical N-methyl-D-aspartate receptors in auditory sensory memory and mismatch negativity generation: Implications for schizophrenia. *Proceedings of the National Academy of Sciences of the USA*, *93*, 11962–11967.

Jing, H., & Benasich, A. A. (2006). Brain responses to tonal changes in the first two years of life. *Brain Development*, *28*, 247–256.

John, E. R., Karmel, B. Z., Corning, W. C., Easton, P., Brown, D., Ahn, H., *et al.* (1977). Neurometrics. *Science*, *196*, 1393–1410.

Kahana, M. J. (2006). The cognitive correlates of human brain oscillations. *Journal of Neuroscience*, *26*, 1669–1672.

Kaufman, K. R., Harris, R., & Shaffer, D. (1980). Problems in the categorization of child and adolescent EEGs. *Journal of Child Psychology and Psychiatry*, *21*, 333–342.

Klimesch, W., Doppelmayr, M., Wimmer, H., Schwaiger, J., Rohm, D., Gruber, W., *et al.* (2001). Theta band power changes in normal and dyslexic children. *Clinical Neurophysiology*, *112*, 1174–1185.

Knight, R. (1996). Contribution of human hippocampal region to novelty detection. *Nature*, *383*, 256–259.

Krakow, K., Woermann, F. G., Symms, M. R., Allen, P. J., Lemieux, L., Barker, G. J., *et al.* (1999). EEG-triggered functional MRI of interictal epileptiform activity in patients with partial seizures. *Brain*, *122*, 1679–1688.

Kraus, N., McGee, T. J., Carrell, T. D., Zecker, S. G., Nicol, T. G., & Koch, D. B. (1996). Auditory neurophysiologic responses and discrimination deficits in children with learning problems. *Science*, *273*, 971–973.

Kuhl, P. K., Coffey-Corina, S., Padden, D., & Dawson, G. (2005). Links between social and linguistic processing of speech in preschool children with autism: Behavioral and electrophysiological measures. *Developmental Science*, *8*, F1–F12.

Lepisto, T., Kujala, T., Vanhala, R., Alku, P., Huotilainen, M., & Naatanen, R. (2006). The discrimination of and orienting to speech and non-speech sounds in children with autism. *Brain Research*, *1066*, 147–157.

Levy, S. R., Berg, A. T., Testa, F. M., Novotny, E. J. Jr., & Chiappa, K. H. (1998). Comparison of digital and conventional EEG interpretation. *Journal of Clinical Neurophysiology*, *15*, 476–480.

Liasis, A., Towell, A., & Boyd, S. (1999). Intracranial auditory detection and discrimination potentials as substrates of echoic memory in children. *Brain Research. Cognitive Brain Research*, *7*, 503–506.

Licht, R., Bakker, D. J., Kok, A., & Bouma, A. (1992). Grade-related changes in event-related potentials (ERPs) in primary school children: Differences between two reading tasks. *Journal of Clinical and Experimental Neuropsychology*, *14*, 193–210.

Liotti, M., Pliszka, S. R., Perez, R., Kothmann, D., & Woldorff, M. G. (2005). Abnormal brain activity related to performance monitoring and error detection in children with ADHD. *Cortex*, *41*, 377–388.

Logothetis, N. K., Pauls, J., Augath, M., Trinath, T., & Oeltermann, A. (2001). Neurophysiologic investigation of the basis of the fMRI signal. *Nature*, *412*, 150–157.

Lopes da Silva, F. (1991). Neural mechanisms underlying brain waves: from neural membranes to networks. *Electroencephalography and Clinical Neurophysiology*, *79*, 81–93.

Luck, S. J. (2005). *An introduction to the event-related potential technique*. Boston, MA: MIT Press.

Lüders, H. O. (2000). Symptomatogenic areas and electrical cortical stimulation. In H. O. N. S. Lüders (Ed.), *Epileptic seizures: pathophysiology and clinical semiology* (pp. 131–140). New York: Churchill Livingstone.

Marosi, E., Harmony, T., Reyes, A., Bernal, J., Fernandez, T., Guerrero, V., *et al.* (1997). A follow-up study of EEG coherences in children with different pedagogical evaluations. *International Journal of Psychophysiology*, *25*, 227–235.

Marosi, E., Harmony, T., Sanchez, L., Becker, J., Bernal, J., Reyes, A., *et al.* (1992). Maturation of the coherence of EEG activity in normal and learning-disabled children. *Electroencephalography and Clinical Neurophysiology*, *83*, 350–357.

Mathalon, D. H., Ford, J. M., & Pfefferbaum, A. (2000). Trait and state aspects of P300 amplitude reduction in schizophrenia: a retrospective longitudinal study. *Biological Psychiatry*, *47*, 434–449.

Maurer, U., Bucher, K., Brem, S., & Brandeis, D. (2003). Altered responses to tone and phoneme mismatch in kindergartners at familial dyslexia risk. *Neuroreport*, *14*, 2245–2250.

McCormick, D. A. (2002). Cortical and subcortical generators of normal and abnormal rhythmicity. *International Review of Neurobiology*, *49*, 99–114.

Michie, P. T., Innes-Brown, H., Todd, J., & Jablensky, A. V. (2002). Duration mismatch negativity in biological relatives of patients with schizophrenia spectrum disorders. *Biological Psychiatry*, *52*, 749–758.

Moore, J. K. (2002). Maturation of human auditory cortex: implications for speech perception. *Annals of Otology, Rhinology, and Laryngology Supplement, 189*, 7–10.

Naatanen, R. (1992). *Attention and brain function*. Hillsdale, NJ: Erlbaum.

Nuwer, M. (1997). Assessment of digital EEG, quantitative EEG, and EEG brain mapping: report of the American Academy of Neurology and the American Clinical Neurophysiology Society. *Neurology*, *49*, 277–292.

O'Keefe, J. (1979). A review of the hippocampal place cells. *Progress in Neurobiology*, *13*, 419–439.

Phillips, C. (2005). Electrophysiology in the study of developmental language impairments: Prospects and challenges for a top-down approach. *Applied Psycholinguistics*, *26*, 79–96.

Picton, T. W., Bentin, S., Berg, P., Donchin, E., Hillyard, S. A., Johnson, R. Jr., *et al.* (2000). Guidelines for using human event-related potentials to study cognition: recording standards and publication criteria. *Psychophysiology*, *37*, 127–152.

Pihko, E., Leppanen, P. H., Eklund, K. M., Cheour, M., Guttorm, T. K., & Lyytinen, H. (1999). Cortical responses of infants with and without a genetic risk for dyslexia: I. Age effects. *Neuroreport*, *10*, 901–905.

Polich, J., & Squire, L. R. (1993). P300 from amnesic patients with bilateral hippocampal lesions. *Electroencephalography and Clinical Neurophysiology*, *86*, 408–417.

Ponton, C. W., Eggermont, J. J., Don, M., Waring, M. D., Kwong, B., Cunningham, J., *et al.* (2000). Maturation of the mismatch negativity: effects of profound deafness and cochlear implant use. *Audiology and Neurootology*, *5*, 167–185.

Rechtschaffen, A., & Kales, A. A. (1968). *Manual of standardized terminology, techniques and scoring system for sleep stages of human subjects*. Washington, DC: National Institutes of Health, Publication No 204.

Sanders, L. D., Stevens, C., Coch, D., & Neville, H. J. (2006). Selective auditory attention in 3- to 5-year-old children: an event-related potential study. *Neuropsychologia*, *44*, 2126–2138.

Schreiber, H., Stolz-Born, G., Kornhuber, H. H., & Born, J. (1992). Event-related potential correlates of impaired selective attention in children at high risk for schizophrenia. *Biological Psychiatry*, *32*, 634–651.

Shafer, V. L., Morr, M. L., Datta, H., Kurtzberg, D., & Schwartz, R. G. (2005). Neurophysiologic indexes of speech processing deficits in children with specific language impairment. *Journal of Cognitive Neuroscience*, *17*, 1168–1180.

Shewmon, D. A., & Erwin, R. J. (1988). Focal spike-induced cerebral dysfunction is related to the after-coming slow wave. *Annals of Neurology*, *23*, 131–137.

Singh, S., Liasis, A., Rajput, K., Towell, A., & Luxon, L. (2004). Event-related potentials in pediatric cochlear implant patients. *Ear and Hearing*, *25*, 598–610.

Stephan, K. E., Baldeweg, T., & Friston, K. J. (2006). Synaptic plasticity and dysconnection in schizophrenia. *Biological Psychiatry*, *59*, 929–939.

Steriade, M. (2006). Grouping of brain rhythms in corticothalamic systems. *Neuroscience*, *137*, 1087–1106.

Steriade, M., & Llinas, R. R. (1988). The functional states of the thalamus and the associated neuronal interplay. *Physiological Reviews*, *68*, 649–742.

Steriade, M., McCormick, D. A., & Sejnowski, T. J. (1993). Thalamocortical oscillations in the sleeping and aroused brain. *Science*, *262*, 679–685.

Taylor, M. J., & Baldeweg, T. (2002). Application of EEG, ERP and intracranial recordings to the investigation of cognitive functions in children. *Developmental Science*, *5*, 318–334.

Taylor, M. J., & Keenan, N. K. (1999). ERPs to orthographic, phonological, and semantic tasks in dyslexic children with auditory processing impairment. *Developmental Neuropsychology*, *15*, 307–326.

Thatcher, R. W. (1992). Cyclic cortical reorganization during early childhood. *Brain and Cognition*, *20*, 24–50.

Thatcher, R. W., Walker, R. A., & Giudice, S. (1987). Human cerebral hemispheres develop at different rates and ages. *Science*, *236*, 1110–1113.

Toga, A. W., Thompson, P. M., & Sowell, E. R. (2006). Mapping brain maturation. *Trends in Neurosciences*, *29*, 148–159.

Traub, R. D., Contreras, D., & Whittington, M. A. (2005). Combined experimental/simulation studies of cellular and network mechanisms of epileptogenesis *in vitro* and *in vivo*. *Journal of Clinical Neurophysiology*, *22*, 330–342.

Umbricht, D., & Krljes, S. (2005). Mismatch negativity in schizophrenia: a meta-analysis. *Schizophrenia Research*, *76*, 1–23.

Umbricht, D., Vyssotki, D., Latanov, A., Nitsch, R., & Lipp, H. P. (2005). Deviance-related electrophysiological activity in mice: Is there mismatch negativity in mice? *Clinical Neurophysiology*, *116*, 353–363.

Uwer, R., Albrecht, R., & von Suchodoletz, W. (2002). Automatic processing of tones and speech stimuli in children with specific language impairment. *Developmental Medicine and Child Neurology*, *44*, 527–532.

van Beijsterveldt, C. E., & van Baal, G. C. (2002). Twin and family studies of the human electroencephalogram: a review and a meta-analysis. *Biological Psychology*, *61*, 111–138.

Vogel, F., & Propping, P. (1982). Genetic variation in brain physiology (EEG) and behavior. *Progress in Clinical and Biological Research*, *103*, 433–441.

Whittington, M. A., & Traub, R. D. (2003). Interneuron diversity series: Inhibitory interneurons and network oscillations *in vitro*. *Trends in Neurosciences*, *26*, 676–682.

Winterer, G., Egan, M. F., Raedler, T., Sanchez, C., Jones, D. W., Coppola, R., *et al.* (2003). P300 and genetic risk for schizophrenia. *Archives of General Psychiatry*, *60*, 1158–1167.

Wunderlich, J. L., & Cone-Wesson, B. K. (2006). Maturation of CAEP in infants and children: A review. *Hearing Research*, *212*, 212–223.

18 Psychological Treatments: Overview and Critical Issues for the Field

John Weisz and Sarah Kate Bearman

In this chapter we provide a selective overview of the field of child and adolescent psychotherapy. We begin with a historical perspective, discuss how treatment of children[1] differs from treatment of adults, note how researchers assess the effects of treatment and then summarize some of the findings of that research. Finally, we note some strengths and limitations of the evidence base, and highlight some critical debates for the field.

Child and Adolescent Psychotherapy in Historical Context

It is not clear when psychotherapy began, but its roots can be found as early as the classical Greek era, when human discourse was used as a means of exploring and examining the life of the mind. As one example, Socrates' (469–399 BCE) philosophical dialectic, later labeled the "Socratic method," involved questioning others in order to stimulate introspection into their beliefs. Socrates believed that the philosopher's role was to "deliver" truth that resided within others, much like a midwife delivers a baby from within its mother. By asking questions of others – rather than telling them what to think – Socrates sought to plumb their capacity for feeling, desire and reasoning. This ancient "midwife thesis" still informs many modern therapists' approach to helping others. In addition, Socrates' belief that the inner life of the mind and outward behavior are inextricably connected foreshadowed a tenet of many modern therapies. Although the term *psychotherapy* is relatively new historically, the general idea harkens back to the ancient tradition of questioning, discussing and listening as means of nurturing understanding and change.

Centuries of subsequent work in philosophy, religion, medicine and other contemplative and healing traditions have given rise to a myriad of practices encompassing meditation, expert instruction, subtle suggestion, hypnosis and persuasion (Shapiro & Shapiro, 1982). Today, a vast array of non-medical interventions are considered psychotherapies, with the common objective of easing subjective distress, decreasing maladaptive behavior or increasing adaptive behavior.

The notion of psychotherapy as a profession can be traced back about a century (Freedheim, Freudenberger, & Kessler, 1992). A case can be made that contemporary psychotherapy grew out of the work of Sigmund Freud (1856–1939). Important themes in this work were the notions that early experience can be critical, and that even children may be appropriate candidates for intervention. Indeed, child psychotherapy can be credited in part to Freud's consultation with the father of "Little Hans" and the psychoanalysis of his own daughter, Anna (1895–1982), who became a prominent child analyst in her own right. Anna Freud – and others, such as Berta Bornstein (e.g., 1949) – applied psychoanalytic precepts and methods to children and adolescents well into the mid-1990s.

The rapid growth of child psychotherapy was also fueled by very different models and methods, including a radically divergent behavioral approach. Jones (1924a,b), for example, used behavioral modeling and "direct conditioning" to help a 2-year-old boy overcome fear of a white rabbit, and this helped launch a more structured, environmentally focused approach to child psychotherapy. Such behavioral therapies for young people developed alongside psychoanalysis and humanistic treatments. Later, Beck (1964, 1970, 1971) construed cognition as an antecedent to affect, constructing *cognitive therapy*, and Meichenbaum and Goodman (1971) helped launch *cognitive–behavioral therapy* for children. By the late 20th century, child psychotherapy had expanded remarkably in the variety of its forms and the extent of its reach. Recently, Kazdin (2002) identified 551 different named therapies used with children and adolescents. Even this large number greatly underestimates the diversity of approaches employed in practice, given the extent to which hundreds of thousands of practitioners eclectically blend different orientations to form distinctive combinations.

How Child and Adolescent Psychotherapy Differs from Adult Psychotherapy

Adult and child psychotherapy share a common ancestry, and therefore have many similarities. Nonetheless, some substantial differences warrant attention. First, unlike adults,

[1] In this chapter, the terms "children" and "youths" are both intended to encompass children and adolescents. Similarly, we use the terms "child psychotherapy" and "youth psychotherapy" broadly, to encompass psychotherapy for children and adolescents.

Rutter's Child and Adolescent Psychiatry, 5th edition. Edited by M. Rutter, D. Bishop, D. Pine, S. Scott, J. Stevenson, E. Taylor and A. Thapar. © 2008 Blackwell Publishing, ISBN: 978-1-4051-4549-7.

children rarely perceive themselves as "disturbed" or as needing therapy. Thus, most treatment referrals for children and adolescents are made by parents, teachers or other adults. Typically, adults contract for therapy, pay the bill and identify some or all of the goals the therapist pursues. Although children may participate to some degree, they often exert less ultimate influence than the adults involved. In short, the child in many therapies is "the patient," but the parent or another adult is often "the client." With the therapy initiated and commissioned by adults, it is not surprising that children often begin the process with less motivation for treatment and for personal change, or at least with different objectives, than those of the adults involved. Indeed, in one study in which clinically referred children and their parents were asked separately to identify the problems for which the child needed help, 63% of parent–child pairs failed to agree on even a single problem (Yeh & Weisz, 2001).

A related difference between child and adult therapy resides in the sources of information the therapist uses to plan and monitor treatment. Because the self-awareness, psychological mindedness and expressive ability of children are limited developmentally, child therapists must rely on adults for information about the youngsters they treat, and this can present several unique challenges. The accuracy of parent and teacher reports may be compromised by incomplete opportunities to observe children in multiple settings, by distorted comparison samples of child behavior, by the influence of undetected adult agendas (e.g., help-seeking, leading to high levels of reported problems, or fear of reports to child protective services, leading to underreporting of problems) or by the effects of parents' own life stresses or mental health problems (Kazdin & Weisz, 1998). Moreover, rates of agreement among different adult informants reporting on the same child tend to be low (Achenbach, McConaughy, & Howell, 1987), further muddling the picture of what most needs attention in treatment. Additionally, adults' reports of child behavior and identification of reasons for referral are apt to reflect the values, standards, practices and social ideals of their cultural reference group (Weisz, McCarty, Eastman *et al.*, 1997). Because child therapy involves multiple stakeholders (e.g., child, parents, school personnel), each of whom may have different motivations, perceptions and goals, establishing the target of intervention – and the outcomes that will be used to index treatment success – may be a complicated process, in comparison with the process for therapy with individual adult clients.

A third remarkable difference between adult and child treatment relates to environmental impact. To a much greater extent than with adults, children are captives of their externally engineered environments. The family, school and neighborhood contexts in which children live are typically determined by others. By extension, the "pathology" or "dysfunction" being treated may arise as much from a less-than-optimal environment – which the child can neither escape nor alter significantly – as from processes within the child. The powerful impact of such factors as socioeconomic status, family configuration, family conflict and life stressors on child functioning at home, school and with peers may constrain the impact of interventions that focus on the child as solo or primary participant, highlighting a need to involve key members of the child's social context in intervention (Henggeler, Schoenwald, Borduin *et al.*, 1998).

Assessing the Effects of Psychotherapy

The child therapist habitually faces a number of obstacles that are much less likely to be confronted by those who treat only adults. It would therefore be naïve to assume that an effective adult therapy will automatically succeed with children. Instead, a separate treatment literature with a separate body of treatment outcome research is required. More than 500 named therapies are practiced with youths (Kazdin, 2002), and countless other variations are created by eclectic therapists; however, only a small proportion of therapies in use have been subjected to empirical test, at least in the venerable form of randomized clinical trials (RCTs). In marked contrast to the rapid growth of psychotherapy practice over the past century, research examining the effects of psychotherapy took shape slowly. In 1952, Eysenck published his important review of studies of adult psychotherapy, raising serious doubts about whether therapy was effective. A few years later, Levitt (1957, 1963) reviewed studies that included children and concluded that rates of improvement in the youth were about the same with or without treatment. These early reviews were influential – and distressing – but the methodology of the studies they relied on was not rigorous by today's standards. Since those landmark reviews, research has grown more stringent and abundant (Durlak, Wells, Cotton *et al.*, 1995; Kazdin & Weisz, 2003). Furthermore, the focus of treatment research with children and adolescents has been honed, shifting from early studies of unspecified "treatment" for often vaguely defined youth problems to trials of well-operationalized therapies targeting specific patterns of dysfunction. Thus, we are now in a position to benefit from a large and increasingly rigorous body of evidence on youth psychotherapies and their effects.

Forms of Evidence

Evidence on the effects of child treatment comes in several forms. The most widely recognized of these is the RCT, an outcome study wherein children with a particular target problem (e.g., antisocial behavior or an anxiety disorder) are randomly assigned to groups that either receive a candidate intervention, a control condition (e.g., waitlist or an attention-only group) or sometimes an alternative intervention. After the intervention phase, outcome measures assessing the target problem are compared across the different groups. It is these RCTs that are most frequently pooled in reviews and meta-analyses (see p. 253) and constitute most of the evidence discussed in this chapter. However, other approaches to outcome assessment should be noted. In circumstances where all the children with a particular condition must receive an active treatment, multiple baseline designs, ABAB (sometimes called "reversal") designs, and related designs are useful. In multiple baseline designs, treatment onset is delayed for different periods of time for different youths (or different target problems within the same youth); if the timing of improvements corresponds to the timing of treatment, treatment benefit may be inferred. In ABAB designs, treatments are alternately introduced and withdrawn for the same youth, or the same group; if improvement corresponds to times when the treatment is in place, and improvements disappear when the treatment is withdrawn, then beneficial treatment effects may be inferred. Multiple baseline and ABAB designs – and variations on these approaches – are often used in treatment research with attention deficit/hyperactivity disorder (ADHD) youth (Pelham, Carlson, Sams *et al.*, 1993), in studies where an entire classroom needs to receive an intervention (Wurtele & Drabman, 1984) and in cases (sometimes involving rare conditions) where only one or two children are treated (McGrath, Dorsett, Calhoun *et al.*, 1988; Tarnowski, Rosen, McGrath *et al.*, 1987). These alternative outcome assessment designs have generated a rich body of outcome data that, unfortunately, still await an enterprising reviewer. For now, we focus on the clinical trials research, which has been the focus of considerable review.

Narrative and Quantitative (Meta-analytic) Approaches to Evidence Review

The ever-expanding body of RCT research has been examined periodically through both narrative and quantitative reviews of outcome findings. Narrative reviews (Kazdin, 2000; Shirk & Russell, 1996) can bring the perspectives of thoughtful experts to bear on what the outcome findings show, and the strengths and limitations of those findings. As an example, Kazdin's (2000) scrutiny of the research on youth treatment led to a detailed appraisal of what has and has not been learned, and Shirk and Russell (1996) focused their narrative review in part on what treatment research has told us about pathogenic processes and mechanisms of change in treatment. Both reviews led to useful recommendations for individualizing and improving treatment for children and adolescents.

Another approach to reviewing outcome research is quantitative review, most often in the form of *meta-analysis*. Meta-analyses provide a synthesis of the evidence, with the effects of multiple studies pooled to generate an overall picture of average treatment impact. The hard currency of meta-analysis is the effect size (ES; for group comparison studies: ES = [M treatment group – M control group]/SD outcome measure), an index of the strength and direction of treatment effects. Many in the field follow Cohen's (1988) guidelines for interpretation of effect size, wherein an ES of 0.20 may be considered a "small" effect, 0.50 a "medium" effect and 0.80 a "large" effect. Averaging across the various outcome measures used, meta-analysts can compute a mean ES for each study, or each treatment–control comparison, and in turn an overall mean ES for an entire collection of studies (Mann, 1990). Mean ES may also be compared across groups of studies that differ in potentially important ways (e.g., the types of therapy employed, or the ages of the youngsters treated).

Findings of Meta-analyses

To date, there have been four particularly broad-based youth psychotherapy meta-analyses – that is, meta-analyses in which few restrictions were imposed on the disorders of interest or types of intervention included. Casey and Berman (1985) surveyed treatment trials published between 1952 and 1983, involving children aged 12 and younger. Among the studies that included treatment–control comparisons, the mean ES was 0.71, indicating that the average treated child was doing better after treatment than 76% of the control group children. In a second meta-analysis, Weisz, Weiss, Alicke *et al.* (1987) included outcome studies published between 1952 and 1983, with youth aged 4–18 years. This synthesis yielded a mean ES of 0.79; following treatment, the average treated child was better off than 79% of control group peers. In a third meta-analysis, Kazdin, Bass, Ayers *et al.* (1990) included studies published between 1970 and 1988, with ages 4–18. For studies comparing treatment groups to no-treatment control groups, mean ES was 0.88, with the average treated child better after treatment than 81% of the no-treatment comparison group. For the subset of studies comparing treatment groups to active control groups, mean ES was 0.77, with the average treated child functioning better after treatment than 78% of the control group. In the fourth meta-analysis, Weisz, Weiss, Han *et al.* (1995) included studies published between 1967 and 1993, with ages 2–18; mean ES was 0.71; after treatment, the average treated child was functioning better than 76% of the control group.

These four meta-analyses indicate uniformly beneficial treatment effects. ES values ranged from 0.71 to 0.84 (estimated overall mean for Kazdin *et al.*, 1990), with an average just below Cohen's (1988) threshold for a "large" effect, and within the range of what has been found in two widely cited meta-analyses of mostly adult outcome studies (Shapiro & Shapiro, 1982; Smith & Glass, 1977). It should be noted, however, that: (a) analyses in Weisz *et al.* (1995) suggest that, with weighting to correct for sample size and heterogeneity of variance, ES means may be closer to "medium" rather than "large" effects; and (b) findings by McLeod and Weisz (2004) supported the notion that publication bias favoring studies that show beneficial effects may have inflated our picture of the mean impact of treatment. However, even when we focused on dissertation studies, which did not go through journal peer review, the results showed beneficial treatment effects (McLeod & Weisz, 2004).

Two other meta-analytic findings warrant attention here. First, we have found (Weisz *et al.*, 1987, 1995) that effects measured immediately after treatment are quite similar to effects measured at follow-up assessments, which average 5–6 months after post-treatment assessment points. This suggests that the benefits of treatment for youth are reasonably durable. However, a recent meta-analysis that focused specifically on treatment of depression in children and adolescents (Weisz, McCarty, & Valeri, 2006b) found beneficial effects fading out by 1 year post-treatment among the small number of studies that extended follow-up assessment that far. This may suggest a need for booster sessions to refresh coping skills, but it may also reflect the fact that major depressive disorder is episodic, such that control groups may improve over time, converging with treatment groups after many months have passed. A second point worth noting concerns the "specificity" of treatment effects. Frank (1973) and others have proposed that psychotherapy has general "non-specific" effects on diverse problems (e.g., by making people feel understood and supported). An alternative view is that therapies help in specific ways, doing the most good with the problems they are designed to address. We have found evidence for the latter view; our analyses (Weisz *et al.*, 1995) showed effect sizes about twice as large for the specific problem domains targeted by a treatment than for other, more incidental domains (e.g., anxiety treatments produced bigger effects on anxiety than on depression). Filling out the picture, Shirk and Karver's (2003) metaanalysis of 23 studies suggested that such non-specific factors as therapeutic relationship may be moderately related to treatment outcomes, particularly for such internalizing problems as anxiety. It is possible that relatively specific treatment effects may coexist with certain non-specific treatment effects; it may also be true that the relative importance of specific versus non-specific factors depends on the nature of the problem being addressed.

While narrative reviews and meta-analyses are useful in many ways, they are generally designed to characterize a body of evidence, rather than to identify specific treatments that are supported by the evidence. For that kind of identification to take place, a different type of review is needed, entailing a search for specific psychotherapies that have been supported in clinical trials. Complementing the broad-based analyses just described, some meta-analysts have addressed rather specific questions by focusing on select subsets of treatment outcome studies.

Treatments Showing Replicated Success with Commonly Treated Problems and Disorders

In this section of the chapter we complement the overall picture of treatment benefit provided through broad-based meta-analyses by identifying some specific forms of intervention that have shown replicated success in RCTs. To do this within space constraints, we focus on a manageable range of the conditions for which treatment is provided; however, we emphasize that psychotherapy for children is used to address a highly diverse array of problems and disorders – many of which we cannot discuss here. The concerns addressed in therapy encompass, for example, enuresis, Tourette disorder, bulimia, autistic disorder, learning disabilities, fire-setting, trichotillomania and even headaches. Rather than attempting to include every treated condition within our review, we focus here on four broad clusters that account for a particularly large proportion of youth referrals for clinical care in most western countries (Jensen & Weisz, 2002; Weisz, 2004) and for which a particularly extensive clinical trials literature exists:

1 Anxiety-related problems and disorders (e.g., social phobia, generalized anxiety disorder);
2 Depression-related problems and disorders (e.g., dysthymic disorder, major depressive disorder);
3 Attentional problems, impulsivity and ADHD; and
4 Conduct-related problems and disorders (e.g., oppositional defiant disorder, conduct disorder).

With a focus on these four clusters, we have searched the treatment outcome database in an effort to identify those psychotherapies for which success has been demonstrated in multiple RCTs.

To provide the most reliable evidence, we sought treatment outcome studies meeting rather uniform standards that were important for our particular purposes; this made our study collection somewhat different from those used in previous reviews. We included studies with children aged 3–18, published between 1965 and 2002. We required that the studies:

1 Include a comparison of psychotherapy to a control group (waitlist, no treatment, placebo or other process intended to be inert) or an alternative treatment;
2 Involve a prospective design and random assignment of subjects to treatment and comparison conditions;
3 Use participants selected for having psychological problems or maladaptive behavior (within the problem clusters noted above); and
4 Include a post-treatment assessment of the psychological problem(s) or maladaptive behavior for which participants were selected and treated.

To ensure a focus on psychotherapy, we selected only those studies in which participants in the groups were not assigned psychotropic medications. A total of 298 studies met our criteria for inclusion. Details of the search procedure and the studies can be found in Weisz, Hawley, and Jensen Doss (2004) and Weisz, Jensen Doss, and Hawley (2005).

Treatments for Internalizing Conditions

Anxiety, Phobias and Fears

Treatment of child anxiety has a long and rich history, and encompasses a large number of RCTs for children. Three forms of treatment have emerged over this history and have shown especially positive outcomes and particularly well-replicated success.

Modeling

One of these is *modeling*, an approach designed to disrupt the self-sustaining sequence of *feared object* → *anxious thoughts* → *aversive arousal* → *avoidance* → *relief*. The distress caused by the feared object or situation can be so powerful, and the sense of relief resulting from avoiding the object or situation can be so rewarding, that alternate forms of behavior simply are not tried – often despite the best efforts of parents and peers. One venerable approach that can help relies on observational learning – exposing the fearful youth to a model who violates the assumptions underlying the fear. The model tries the feared behavior (e.g., approaching a dog and patting it on the head), thus demonstrating that it *can* be done without the negative consequences the treated youth had feared. When this approach works, the observer emulates the behavior of the model and thus learns that no adverse effects occur. Studies have shown beneficial effects of modeling interventions, in various forms.

In *live modeling*, the anxious youngster observes a peer, the therapist or some other model engaging in the feared behavior in real time. Across the exposures, the model experiences no adverse consequences and often appears to enjoy the experience. A variation of this approach is *symbolic modeling*, in which video (or some other media product) is used to present a model to anxious youngsters. This approach allows the medium to be reused repeatedly with no worry that the model's behavior may change in some unwanted way. Finally, in *participant modeling*, the fearful youth performs the feared activities in concert with the model. The approach appears to be particularly potent. In Ollendick and King's (1998) careful review of anxiety treatments, this was the only modeling method identified as "well-established." The potency of this approach may reflect the fact that it combines observational learning with the added security of a confident partner plus active encouragement to try the exposure. Across the different variations of modeling, a frequent practice is to start at low intensity (e.g., sitting at some distance from the feared object) and add increments (e.g., moving closer, touching the object, picking it up) gradually.

Reinforced Exposure

Another approach to anxiety is *reinforced exposure*. This entails graduated steps of exposure to the feared object or situation, with the youngster rewarded for accomplishing each step. It is commonly believed that reinforced exposure is simply one form of contingency management, in which behavior is altered by changing its consequences (Ollendick & King, 1998). A challenge for the therapist is creating graduated steps of exposure that will be appropriately challenging but not so overwhelming that the youth refuses outright. For some fears of situations (e.g., darkness) the graduating procedure may involve increments in time (e.g., the amount of time the child remains in a darkened room) or degree (e.g., degree of darkness tolerated). For other fears, the gradations may involve a series of increasingly lifelike and direct exposures. As one example, Muris, Merckelbach, Holdrinet *et al.* (1998) treated spider fears in 8- to 17-year-olds by exposing them to a variety of spiders and progressing from looking at the spiders from a distance to letting the spiders walk on the youngsters' arms. In the various procedures, rewards follow successful exposures, ranging from praise to concrete incentives.

Youth-Focused Cognitive–Behavioral Therapy

Cognitive–behavioral therapy (CBT) has been used extensively to address youth anxiety; indeed, it is the most frequently tested treatment for child anxiety in the RCT literature. As the name implies, CBT entails efforts to identify and alter cognitions that contribute to the anxiety, and also to identify and alter maladaptive behavior (such as avoidance of feared situations) that may serve to sustain the condition. Some forms of CBT have been used in treatment focused on individual youths, others with youths and their family members in various combinations. Applications of CBT at the individual youth level have ranged from procedurally simple approaches using self-talk, typically addressing specific fears, to much more complex multisession programs typically used to address multisymptom anxiety disorders.

Multicomponent CBT For anxiety disorders that are more complex than simple phobias, more complex packages of CBT procedures may be needed. There are several examples of such programs, including the Coping Cat program (Kendall, Kane, Howard *et al.*, 1990) and the Transfer of Control Approach (Silverman & Kurtines, 1996) designed for children diagnosed with generalized anxiety disorder, separation anxiety disorder or social phobia. Although different programs vary in some important ways, they often follow a similar treatment course, which begins with psychoeducation regarding the nature and course of anxiety, and how to recognize the somatic, cognitive and behavioral manifestations of anxiety. During this phase, the child learns various coping strategies to manage anxious feelings, such as identifying and modifying anxious cognitions, or relaxation exercises which may include progressive muscle relaxation or deep breathing. Often, an easy-to-recall acronym is used to help children remember the sequence of identifying physical symptoms of anxiety and anxious cognitions, devising a behavioral plan to cope with these feelings, and judging the success of their plan. For example, FEAR in the Coping Cat program, (Feeling frightened? Expecting bad things to happen? Actions and attitudes that help, Rate and reward). Similarly, the acronym STOP is used in another program (Silverman & Kurtines, 1996), and serves to remind children to recognize when they are Scared, identify their anxious Thoughts, refute them with Other, more realistic thoughts, and Praise themselves.

In many CBT programs for anxiety (Albano, Marten, Holt *et al.*, 1995; Kendall *et al.*, 1990) children work with their therapist to identify and rank the feared or phobic situations, and this hierarchy serves as a measure of treatment progress and provides targets for the behavioral exposure phase of treatment. Using graduated exposure, the child and therapist collaboratively work their way through the fears on the hierarchy with the goal of decreasing the maladaptive somatic, cognitive and behavioral responses to the imagined threat.

Variations on the kind of core CBT program just described have been used in a number of creative ways to extend the application of cognitive and behavioral training. Barrett, Dadds, and Rapee (1996) created a CBT-oriented Family Anxiety Management Program to address specific youth anxiety disorders through sessions with parents and child together, and separate sessions for parents as a couple. A unique form of individual CBT has been developed to address post-traumatic stress disorder and other behavioral and emotional problems in sexually abused children (Deblinger & Heflin, 1996); the non-offending mothers of sexually abused children have been trained to play the part therapists had played in the individual child version of the treatment (Deblinger & Heflin, 1996). The general strategies of modifying anxious cognitions and confronting phobic assumptions via exposure have also been applied successfully to obsessive-compulsive disorder in children, with the added component of *response prevention* – encouraging the child not to engage in the ritual compulsions that reduce the obsession-triggered distress (Barrett, Healy, Piacentini *et al.*, 2004; March, Frances, Carpenter *et al.*, 1997).

Depressive Symptoms and Disorders

We turn now to treatment of depression, a form of dysfunction that tends to be highly correlated with anxiety. Given the close association between these two clusters, perhaps it is not surprising to find that some of the procedures used to good effect with anxiety reappear in the list for depression. Readers interested in the effects of psychotherapies for child depression are referred to a recent meta-analysis on the topic by Weisz, McCarty, & Valeri (2006b).

Cognitive–Behavioral Therapy

The most extensively tested and supported approach to youth depression treatment is youth-focused CBT. Of the CBT manuals used, the one with the most ample empirical support, to date, is the *Coping with Depression Course for Adolescents* (CWD-A; Lewinsohn, Clarke, & Hops, 1990). In keeping with its cognitive–behavioral pedigree, the CWD-A program treats depression by addressing cognitive, behavioral and affective skill deficits. To address these deficits, CWD-A therapists teach youngsters how their emotions are related to their thoughts and actions, and encourage them to monitor their moods and track mood–thought–action connections. Participants also learn to:

1 Identify activities they find mood-elevating and increase their frequency;
2 Develop and carry out a personal plan for change;
3 Identify unrealistic negative thoughts and practice replacing those thoughts with realistic, positive counter-thoughts;
4 Deal with stress by using relaxation techniques; and
5 Interrupt negative thoughts, to prevent themselves from getting stuck in unproductive rumination.

In some of their work, the CWD-A collaborators have combined treatment of adolescents with a parallel program for their parents.

Interpersonal Therapy

Relatively recent evidence points to beneficial effects of interpersonal therapy for adolescents (IPT-A). The IPT approach (Mufson, Dorta, Wickramaratne *et al.*, 2004; Mufson, Weissman, Moreau *et al.*, 1999) is based on the premise that depression occurs in an interpersonal context, and that an improved understanding and renegotiation of this context can be vital to recovery. Therapy focuses on one or two problem areas, which include grief and loss, interpersonal role disputes, role transitions and interpersonal deficits. Initially, the therapist provides education about the symptoms of depression and how depression is connected to interpersonal processes. Then therapist and youth conduct an interpersonal inventory to understand better the nature of the adolescent's interactions with significant others, in regard to both satisfying and unsatisfying aspects. A treatment contract is established, and the main problem areas are identified and discussed with the adolescent. In the middle phase, therapist and adolescent work directly on the identified problem areas, and the adolescent is encouraged to monitor depressive symptoms, link affect with interpersonal events, clarify conflicts and styles of communication, and use various strategies (e.g., role play) to try out various forms of behavior change. In the termination phase, the therapist and adolescent work to establish a sense of competence to manage future stressors.

Relaxation Training

Two studies have found that relaxation training alone produces significant relief from depression, perhaps by reducing tension and stress, or perhaps through some as yet unassessed biological change. In a common procedure, youngsters learn to alternately tense and relax muscle groups, progressing from one body region to another until most of the major muscle groups are relaxed. For tense situations that arise without warning, or situations in which the child only has a few moments to cope, children may learn techniques for quick calming; one example is "the quick Benson," which is taught as part of the CWD-A (Lewinsohn, Clarke, & Hops 1990). This method, shown in the box below, requires only that the students have a personal "relaxation word" (such as "calm" or "cool") and that they have a ready-to-use image of a favorite calming place or situation.

The Quick Benson: To calm down quickly when you are caught off guard by a tense situation

1 Check the tension level in the area where you hold tension (e.g., your neck or back). Try to relax those muscles
2 Take a deep breath and let it out slowly, while repeating your relaxation word to yourself
3 Picture yourself relaxing in your favorite calming place

Treatments for Disruptive Conditions

ADHD and Related Problems

Focusing now on the attention and hyperactivity domain, we should note at the outset that a non-psychological intervention is known to show quite positive acute effects. Stimulant medication (e.g., methylphenidate) has been shown to work well in scores of RCTs, and forms of stimulant medication that extend effects throughout a full school day (e.g., Concerta) have increased the popularity of this approach to treatment. However, most studies show that: (i) stimulant medication is not effective (or even safe) for all children; and (ii) stimulants do not eliminate all the symptoms associated with ADHD. Moreover, some parents and children are simply not going to choose medication as a treatment option. For all these reasons, the search for beneficial psychotherapies has continued, and with some success; mean effects, however, have tended to be more modest than mean effects for the other three problem clusters addressed in this chapter. Most of the psychotherapies showing significant benefit in RCTs have been behavioral and cognitive–behavioral. Some have focused treatment on children directly, but others have employed parent training, teacher training (e.g., classroom management programs) or multiple foci including child, parent and/or teacher. We provide here some examples of treatments that have shown respectable effects.

Cognitive–Behavioral Therapy

Among the treatments administered directly to youths, we found that CBT is the approach whose beneficial effects are the most widely replicated in RCTs (cf. Pelham, Wheeler, & Chronis, 1998, who reached a different conclusion, based on a different approach to evidence review). Although there were several useful precursors to CBT, many experts credit Meichenbaum and Goodman (1971) with launching this approach to youth treatment. These authors used what they then called self-instructional training to help impulsive second-graders reduce their impulsivity and improve their performance on tasks requiring concentration, including even an IQ test. Across multiple activities, the procedures were designed to teach children to identify the requirements of a task, rehearse the task mentally, guide their own performance through self-talk, and give appropriate encouragement and praise to themselves when they did well.

The Meichenbaum and Goodman (1971) article was followed by an explosion of intervention trials using elements of their procedure and contributing to the genre that has come to be called CBT. As an example, Bender (1976) found that training impulsive first-graders to guide themselves using self-talk led to slower (i.e., less impulsive) responses and fewer errors on a letter- and picture-matching task. Kendall and Wilcox (1980) used their own adaptation of self-instructional training with 8- to 12-year-olds referred by teachers for "problematic lack of self-control that interfered with both personal and classroom performance and general classroom deportment" (Kendall & Wilcox, 1980, p. 81). Children were trained across six 30–40 minute sessions to guide their own behavior on various tasks by:

1 Identifying the requirements of the task;
2 Planning a strategy;
3 Focusing attention on the task;
4 Use of coping statements when mistakes were made; and
5 Self-reinforcement for success at the task.

Afterward, blind teacher ratings indicated that this intervention improved self-control and reduced hyperactivity.

Relaxation Training, Biofeedback, Metronome Training

We were rather surprised to find that another class of child-focused interventions that showed beneficial effects on ADHD were those focused on calming or relaxation. For example, Redfering and Bowman (1981) reduced non-attending behavior in "behaviorally disturbed" 8- to 11-year-olds by simply playing tapes with relaxation-meditation instructions for the children, across five half-hour sessions. Porter and Omizo (1984) reported that group relaxation training, together with large muscle exercise followed by rest and deep breathing, significantly reduced impulsivity and improved attentiveness in hyperactive first- and second-graders. In two related studies, Omizo and Michael (1982) and Rivera and Omizo (1980) combined relaxation training with biofeedback in their work with hyperactive children. While listening to parts of a relaxation-induction audiotape, youngsters received visual and auditory feedback (e.g., clicks) from an electromyometer that measured muscle activity in the frontalis area. Children were told that their job was to keep their bodies relaxed enough that the feedback would show a sustained pattern of low activity. Just 3–4 sessions, less than half an hour each, were associated with significantly reduced impulsivity and gains in attention on a post-intervention performance task.

Behavioral Parent and Teacher Training

A widely practiced approach to the treatment of problems related to ADHD, such as disruptive and disobedient behavior, involves teaching parents to create and maintain environments in which desirable child behavior (e.g., obeying adults, thinking before acting) is rewarded and undesirable behavior (e.g., disobedience, impulsive acts) is not. This basic concept of contingency management is the centerpiece of a number of different *behavioral parent training* programs. Because so many ADHD-related problems appear in the school setting, an important complement to parent-training programs is teacher involvement, sometimes in the context of classroom-focused training programs designed to establish and maintain contingencies at school that will reinforce self-control, attention to school work and appropriate social behavior with teachers and peers. Because these programs are used for children with ADHD when it co-occurs with other disruptive behavior disorders, such as oppositional defiant disorder (ODD) or conduct disorder, we will discuss parent-training programs in greater detail in the next section.

Conduct-Related Problems and Disorders

Conduct-related problems and disorders are matters of genuine concern in most societies, as well they should be. Considerable evidence indicates that such problems and disorders can presage social dysfunction, including antisocial and criminal behavior which often lasts into late adolescence and adulthood (Moffitt, 1993). The good news is that treatment of conduct-related problems and disorders has received a great deal of attention in the research literature, and that a number of treatments have shown substantial positive effects which have been replicated in multiple RCTs. Here we focus on a few examples.

Youth-Focused Operant Treatment

Treatments placed within the operant category are those emphasizing reinforcement contingencies, including response cost and time out. For example, Autry and Langenbach (1985) succeeded in reducing disruptive fourth, fifth and sixth grade boys' levels of disruptive behavior in class by rewarding the boys with tokens for such reductions; the tokens were redeemable for items from the school store and for special class privileges, such as free time. In a very different cultural context, Moracco and Kazandkian (1977) were able to reduce disruptive behavior among teacher-referred 7- to 11-year-olds in a Beirut, Lebanon, elementary school by using operant procedures. In a series of behavioral counseling sessions, children were reinforced with praise and attention when they behaved appropriately, and were systematically ignored for inappropriate behavior, with the counselor turning her head away and looking uninterested. Another example of behavior change with operant procedures is found in Jessness's (1975) report on their use with adjudicated boys in the California Youth Authority. This program involved eight living units for 15- to 17-year-olds. Each unit employed a microeconomy in which appropriate behavior earned institutional "dollars" and points. The dollars could be used to purchase objects, services and recreational activities. Points could accumulate to earn a recommendation for parole and release. Charts showing points earned by each boy were placed in conspicuous locations as an additional form of reinforcement. The program had significant effects on both behavior ratings in the institution and recidivism after discharge.

Cognitive–Behavioral Therapy (e.g., Problem-Solving Skills)

CBT for youth conduct problems has taken a variety of forms. We illustrate the CBT approach by focusing on a particularly successful example: Problem-Solving Skills Training (Kazdin, 2003). In essence, this approach is designed to teach aggressive youngsters to use their heads before using their fists. The children, aged 7–13, go through about 20 45-minute individual sessions with a therapist to learn basic steps of problem-solving, practiced initially via familiar games. Youngsters then learn to apply these steps to interpersonal situations, including the kinds of situation that often lead to aggression. The core skills of the program are embodied in five problem-solving steps, presented as five thoughts the youth is expected to review when confronting a problem. Through these steps, children learn to identify the problem, brainstorm more than one possible solution, evaluate the proposed solutions in terms of their likely consequences, make a choice, and then evaluate how successful they were in solving the problem. Children first learn to use these steps in simple games like Checkers and Connect Four; over time the skills are applied to more and more lifelike problems, including social conflicts of the type that have caused problems in the past.

Behavioral Parent Training

Parent-focused intervention is the most extensively tested and supported form of treatment for youth conduct problems and disorders, and nearly all of the studies involved have tested *behavioral parent training*. Although each program has unique characteristics, we discuss common features of some of the programs that have demonstrated beneficial effects, including the intervention procedures developed by Patterson, Chamberlain, & Reid (1982) and Barkley's (1997) *Defiant Children: A Clinician's Manual for Assessment and Parent Training*. In these and related programs, parents learn basic behavioral principles relevant to child rearing, such as the role of attention in the recurrence of both positive and negative behaviors. Parents learn how to define, track and record rates of the antisocial and prosocial behaviors they want to target, and are coached in the design, implementation and refinement of behavior modification programs.

A core idea of these interventions is that children generally act the way they do because they have learned to act that way; much of that learning involves identifying what behaviors are rewarded in their environment, and then doing more of those behaviors. As an example, most children show some kind and generous behavior, but if that behavior is not noticed, praised or rewarded, it will decline in frequency. Most children show some aggressive, oppositional or antisocial behavior at some times; if that behavior is rewarded, even if only by increased attention from the parent, it may increase in frequency.

In behavioral parent training, parents use praise and increased attention to positive child behavior to strengthen their relationship with their child, and increase the rewarding consequences that follow appropriate behaviors by means of token or point systems that lead to tangible reinforcers. To reduce the frequency of unwanted behaviors, parents learn ways of making those behaviors less rewarding; one example is *time out*, in which the child is withdrawn from opportunities for reward.

Parent-training interventions also stress the need to reduce what are called *coercive exchanges* between parents and children. For example, some parents speak to their child in ways that lead to hurt feelings, resentment and escalation in conflict. Instead of saying, "Heather, turn off that stupid music, and get your d— homework done!" the parent could calmly ask, "Honey, it's time to turn off the music now and do your homework." Speaking of homework, because many youth problems extend to school and other out-of-home settings, these programs often include methods of extending intervention to such settings. In school, if the teacher is willing, a *school card* can be used to provide a simple daily report to parents on issues of importance in the school setting (e.g., staying on-task in class, obeying the teacher, turning in homework). Feedback from the school card can be incorporated into the contract and point system used at home.

Webster-Stratton's Video-Guided Parent Group Approach A particularly well-tested intervention is the video-guided program through which Webster-Stratton (e.g., 1984) and her colleagues convey behavioral skills to parents of young children. In the Incredible Years BASIC parent-training program, groups of 10–14 parents meet with a therapist for up to 14 weekly sessions lasting about 2 hours. Parents view a series of 1–2 minute video vignettes showing parents dealing with their children in a variety of situations, sometimes successfully, sometimes not. These videos are used to stimulate discussion of basic behavioral principles. Parents practice the principles in homework assignments. Over the series of sessions, four themes are covered: constructive use of play, using praise and reward effectively, setting and enforcing limits, and handling misbehavior. The 1–2 minute video vignettes used in the group sessions show a mixture of successful and unsuccessful parent–child interactions, each designed to prompt a lively discussion by parents. Similar to the behavior parent-training programs described above, the Incredible Years also includes assignments in which the parents try procedures discussed in groups at home and track the results (chapter 64 provides further information on applications of the Webster-Stratton approach and other parenting programs).

Parent–Child Interaction Treatments To round out the picture of the forms that behavioral treatment in a family context can take, we close with a description of parent–child interaction treatments (i.e., interventions that place parents and young children in the same room and have them interact, guided by coaching from a therapist). The general approach grows out of the unpublished work of Hanf and Kling (1974) at the University of Oregon Medical School. Two prominent current examples of the approach are *Parent–child interaction therapy* (Eyberg & Boggs, 1998) and *Helping the noncompliant child* (McMahon & Forehand, 2003). Parent–child interaction treatments are used primarily for disruptive and oppositional children in the preschool through early elementary age range. Parent and child interact in a playroom, observed by a therapist from behind a one-way glass or via a videocamera, and the therapist coaches the parent using a bug-in-the-ear device. (In a low-tech version, the therapist coaches in a soft voice from a corner of the playroom.) The nature of the interactions shifts from time to time, with some child-directed interactions in which the child selects the activities and the parent practices attending closely, reinforcing desirable child behavior through labeled praise, hugs, etc., and selectively ignoring undesirable behavior. Other interactions are set up to be explicitly parent-directed, with the parent selecting activities and setting rules for the child to follow; parents are coached to make it easy for children to obey by keeping instructions specific and direct, focusing on one behavior at a time, and waiting 5 seconds or so after instructions to give the child time to comply. When instructions follow these guidelines, most children obey most of the time. When they do not, parents are taught procedures for addressing non-compliance – they practice the best way to give the child a "time-out," for example.

Multiple Target/Multisystem Treatments Other approaches are broader in their outreach to multiple targets. For example, Chamberlain and Reid's (1998) *Multidimensional Treatment Foster Care*, for difficult youth who are being cared for through foster care placements, combines interventions targeting youths, foster parents, family and teacher. *Multisystemic Therapy* (Henggeler *et al.*, 1998) treats delinquent youths by reaching out to multiple layers of their social environment, often including siblings, parents, extended family, neighbors and neighborhood groups, peer group, school, church and juvenile justice personnel. Both the Treatment Foster Care program and Multisystemic Therapy are described in chapter 68.

Overview and Highlights of the Findings

The treatments represented in this selective review – illustrating a much larger array of interventions – have evolved over more than four decades. Although we focused only on problems and disorders in four broad clusters – anxiety, depression, ADHD and conduct – we found 298 acceptable RCTs, encompassing 326 different treatment programs that showed at lease some significant benefit relative to a control group or alternative treatment group. Neither studies, treatment programs nor treatment impact were evenly distributed across the four problem clusters. In the depression domain, we identified only 23 studies and 26 beneficial treatments; the scarcity of such studies and treatments is partly because of a late start; no youth depression trial was published until 1986. This may be partly attributable to the fact that for many years depression in children was considered an impossibility (Hammen & Rudolph, 1996).

By contrast, anxiety (94 articles, 111 beneficial treatments) and conduct problems (135 articles, 136 treatments) have been long-standing foci for treatment researchers, with considerable pay-off in terms of trials and treatments. The treatments identified (including those not detailed in this chapter) were not only numerous but diverse, crossing continental, national, cultural and ethnic boundaries. The treatments also spanned a range of targets, including youths seen individually and in groups; parents seen individually, in couples and in groups; teachers alone and with parents; whole families and parent–child combinations; and multiple systems encompassing up to a half-dozen intervention targets. Amid all this diversity, certain targets and modalities were clear favorites in certain domains. Among anxiety and depression treatments, for example, youth-focused treatments predominated, particularly those following CBT principles. Somewhat surprisingly, we also found this to be true of ADHD treatment. This prominence of CBT in randomized trials of ADHD treatment complements findings of an important previous review (Pelham, Wheeler, & Chronis, 1998) which included numerous within-group study designs and identified behavioral parent training and behavioral procedures in the classroom as the dominant forms of evidence-based intervention. Finally, we found that behavioral parent training was the most common form of empirically supported treatment for disruptive behavior problems, with the Patterson Parent Management Training – Oregon Model (PMTO) approach and Webster-Stratton's video-guided approach particularly influential.

There was also some diversity in the treatment models employed. Although youth psychotherapy may have begun with psychoanalysis, as suggested at the outset of this paper, we found that behavioral treatments, including CBT, now dominate the list of supported treatments. However, the list covered a rather broad range, encompassing interpersonal therapy for depression in adolescents and relaxation training and biofeedback for ADHD in children. This suggests that there may be considerable room for innovation in the development of beneficial treatments.

Strengths of the Evidence Base

Magnitude, Durability and Specificity of Treatment Effects

While there is much to appreciate in the evidence base on youth treatments, there are also some gaps. On the plus side, meta-analytic reviews point to mean effects of tested treatments that:

- Fall within the "medium" to "large" range (as per Cohen, 1988);
- Are relatively specific to the problems and disorders targeted in treatment, not just general improvements in overall adjustment; and
- Show substantial holding power, at least over the 5–6 month periods characteristic of most follow-up assessments.

Task force reviews by child specialist teams (Brestan & Eyberg, 1998; Kaslow & Thompson, 1998; Ollendick & King, 1998; Pelham, Wheeler, & Chronis, 1998) have identified 27 specific treatments as either "well-established" or "probably efficacious." Because some problems and disorders have not yet been addressed by task force review, and because new evidence has accumulated since these reviews, it seems likely that additional treatments now exist that would meet task force criteria.

Diverse Models of Treatment Delivery

Another strength is the increasingly rich array of treatment delivery models employed. The traditional weekly office visit model still predominates in the research base, but investigators have pushed the boundaries, with tests of more intensive approaches geared to school breaks and summer camp programs (Pelham, Greiner, Gnagy *et al.*, 1996), treatments in which core skills training is embedded in videotaped vignettes (Webster-Stratton & Reid, 2003), interventions providing behavioral training and support for foster parents (Chamberlain & Smith, 2003), treatment supplements in the form of post-therapy booster sessions (Clarke, Rohde, Lewinsohn *et al.*, 1999) and a peripatetic therapist in the youth's environment model (Henggeler *et al.*, 1998).

Breadth and Practical Relevance of Outcomes Assessed

Measurement of outcomes across the evidence base shows a relatively healthy range of approaches and content. We have found (Weisz, Jensen Doss, & Hawley, 2005) that, while 60% of the randomized trials we examined used youths themselves as informants on outcome measures, 33% also used parent reports, 29% used teacher reports and 78% used various other sources of outcome information, including trained observers. As for measurement content, in addition to a primary focus on measures of the target disorder or problem addressed in treatment, 78% of the studies we examined included at least one measure of non-target disorders or problems (thus permitting assessment of generalization of treatment effects), 28% included some measure of real-world functioning (e.g., school grades, disciplinary incidents, arrests), 8% assessed consumer satisfaction and 5% included an assessment of environmental impact of treatment (e.g., parenting stress).

Limitations of the Evidence Base Suggest Directions for Future Research

In addition to significant strengths, the evidence base on child treatment shows several limitations, highlighting directions for emphasis in future research (Table 18.1).

Strengthen the Control/Comparison Conditions against which Treatments are Tested

Our reviews of the evidence base suggest that the most common form of treatment–control group comparison in the research is arguably the weakest experimentally: active treatment versus inactive waitlist or no treatment. Passive control groups control only for the passage of time, not for attention, discussion of problems and solutions, a therapeutic relationship or various other non-specific factors that may enter into an episode of therapy. Fewer than 40% of the randomized trials we have reviewed used an active intervention control condition. Moreover, fewer than 8% used standard case management or some form of treatment-as-usual as the comparison condition. This presents a significant inferential problem which we discuss later in this chapter.

Address Gaps in Coverage of Important Forms of Dysfunction

The evidence base also reveals significant gaps in coverage of youth problems. As one example, the annual mortality rate in 15- to 24-year-old females diagnosed with anorexia is

Table 18.1 Research on child and adolescent psychotherapy: Directions for the future.

1 Strengthen the control and/or comparison conditions against which treatments are tested
2 Address gaps in coverage of important forms of dysfunction
3 Identify necessary and sufficient conditions for treatment benefit
4 Clarify the effective range of treatments (moderation)
5 Identify mechanisms of change (mediation) underlying treatment benefit
6 Make treatment research conditions more like real-world practice conditions
- Shift to a deployment-focused model of treatment development and testing
- Build the evidence base on comparisons to usual clinical care

more than 12 times the rate for this age × gender group from all other causes (Sullivan, 1995). Yet, there have been only a handful of controlled treatment trials for anorexia nervosa (for reviews see Fairburn, 2005; Le Grange & Lock, 2005) and none for the treatment of bulimia nervosa (Wilson & Sysko, 2006) in adolescent populations. Although Stice, Shaw, Burton *et al.* (2006) have shown preventive effects of psychosocial interventions on eating pathology in adolescent girls, tests of treatment protocols with clinically relevant populations are lacking, despite increasing rates of eating disordered attitudes among adolescents (Bearman, Presnell, Martinez *et al.*, 2006). In addition, with few exceptions (e.g., Azrin, Donohue, Besalel *et al.*, 1994), potent treatments for substance abusing youth are rare, particularly for users of harder drugs such as cocaine. Also with few exceptions (e.g., Borduin, Henggeler, Blaske *et al.*, 1990), the literature lacks successes in the treatment of youthful sex offenders. And despite attempts by several research teams, we still lack interventions for suicidal youth that clearly reduce the risk of further attempts (Weisz & Hawley, 2002). Finally, most of the psychosocial treatment success with ADHD has been with pre-adolescents, and some of the behavioral treatments that work within that age range may not travel so well up the developmental ramp into adolescence. Indeed, the author of a widely used behavioral parent program argues that adolescents should *not* be considered candidates for the program, as their poor responses may exacerbate family conflict (Barkley, 1997). Limited success of psychosocial treatments with ADHD in teens could make stimulant medication the evidence-based treatment (EBT) of choice for this age group, by default (Weisz & Jensen, 1999). To put the coverage issue more starkly, there are at least 150 disorders in the current DSM-IV (American Psychiatric Association, 2000) that can be applied to children and adolescents, and many more problems of living for which youngsters need help; our list of EBTs to date encompasses only a modest percentage of these.

Identify Necessary and Sufficient Conditions for Treatment Benefit

Many of our treatments are *omnibus* in style – packing a variety of procedures and training a variety of skills, but without a clear picture of which ones really matter. Despite a long tradition of "dismantling" research, we have only begun the process of identifying the specific components of our multisession, multiconcept, multiskill treatments that are necessary for good outcomes. The *full monty* nature of so many manualized treatments often renders them a poor fit to the current emphasis in real-world clinical care on session limits and maximum efficiency. There is almost certainly some excess baggage in some treatments (i.e., elements that do not actually contribute much to the outcomes achieved). Making treatment programs leaner and more efficient could enhance their attractiveness to practitioners, render the procedures more teachable, increase treatment viability in the marketplace of clinical care and thus perhaps reach more of the children who need their benefits.

Clarify the Effective Range of Treatments (Moderation)

For each treatment in the armamentarium, we need to understand the range of youth clinical and demographic characteristics within which the treatments produce benefit and outside of which benefit diminishes. Even the best-supported EBTs are good for some individuals but not others, with most clinical trials reporting substantial percentages showing poor response. It is relatively common in trials to see that 30% or more of treated children are not helped much by the treatment. One possible reason is that treatment benefit is constrained by such potential moderators as age, gender, socio-economic status (SES), comorbidity, family income, ethnicity, family configuration or other clinical and demographic factors. With relatively few exceptions (e.g., Brent, Kolko, Birmaher *et al.*, 1998; Curry, Rohde, Simons *et al.*, 2006; Kazdin & Crowley, 1997), research to date has left us rather poorly informed about such constraints. Racial, ethnic and cultural factors, for example, are embedded but unexamined in most of our treatment outcome research (Weisz, Jensen Doss, & Hawley, 2005), and this makes it difficult to know how robust most treatment effects are across various population groups. At this early stage in youth treatment development research, it is understandable that most tested treatments have not been designed to take into account the broad variations associated with different cultural traditions. However, many would agree that the interplay between such factors and treatment characteristics may influence the outcome of the treatment process, and that an understanding of these processes would enrich efforts to produce treatments that can be applied across a broad spectrum of individuals and groups (Weisz, Huey & Weersing, 1998). While there is great interest in the impact of cultural variations and other potential moderators, our reviews suggest quite variable findings across studies, without much evidence of robust moderators that are consistent in their impact across studies.

Identify Mechanisms of Change (Mediation) Underlying Treatment Benefit

We also need sustained inquiry into the change processes in treatment that account for observed outcomes. At present, we know much more about what outcomes our treatments produce than about what actually causes those outcomes (Kazdin, 2000; Shirk & Russell, 1996). If we fail to identify core causal processes, we risk a proliferation of treatments administered rather superstitiously because studies show they work, but without an understanding of the change processes therapists actually need to set in motion to produce results. To understand *how* the treatments work, we need a generation of research testing hypothesized mediators of outcome. Mediation testing procedures have been well described (Baron & Kenney, 1986; Holmbeck, 1997; Judd & Kenny, 1981), and the use of randomized clinical trials to test moderators and mediators of therapeutic change has been thoughtfully addressed by Kraemer, Stice, Kazdin *et al.* (2001) and Kraemer, Wilson, Fairburn *et al.* (2002). Some treatment researchers have already applied mediation testing procedures to good effect. Huey, Henggeler,

Brondino *et al.* (2000), for example, found that decreased affiliation with delinquent peers mediated reductions in delinquent behavior in youths treated with multisystemic therapy. Eddy and Chamberlain (2000) found that improved family management skills and reduced deviant peer associations mediated the effects of their behaviorally oriented treatment foster care program on adolescent antisocial behavior. Other investigators have probed change processes associated with other treatments (Weersing & Weisz, 2002), although not always with complete mediation test methods. We need more studies in which proposed mediators are identified a priori, measured well and tested with care (Kazdin, 2000; Kazdin & Weisz, 2003). Failure to test rigorously for mediation leaves an information vacuum that may be filled by faulty assumptions about the nature and causes of treatment benefit. Increased understanding of the actual processes underlying therapeutic improvement will improve prospects for:

- Understanding and addressing impediments, stalls, and failures in treatment;
- Training therapists by teaching them what *change processes* they need to effect rather than simply what techniques to use; and
- Identifying cross-cutting principles that can be used in designing, refining and perhaps combining interventions.

Make Treatment Research Conditions More Like Real-World Practice Conditions

For a variety of reasons, the conditions under which most EBTs have been developed and tested tend to differ markedly from the conditions under which treatments are provided to clinically referred children in everyday mental health care settings (Southam-Gerow, Weisz, & Kendall, 2003). The gap between research and clinical conditions includes:

1 Psychological and social characteristics of the treated individuals (e.g., with clinic-referred youths more severely disturbed, more likely to meet criteria for a diagnosis, more likely to have comorbidities and more likely to drop out of treatment than youths recruited for RCTs);

2 Reasons for seeking treatment (e.g., referred youths not recruited from schools or through advertisements, but referred by caregivers because of unusually serious problems or family crisis, or even court-ordered);

3 The settings in which treatment is carried out (e.g., more financial forms to complete, more bureaucracy and sometimes a less welcoming approach in the clinic);

4 The therapists who provide the treatment (e.g., not graduate students or research assistants hired by and loyal to the adviser and committed to her or his EBT program, but professionals with years of experience and their own treatment preferences);

5 The incentive system (e.g., therapists not paid by the treatment developer to deliver her or his treatment with close adherence to the manual, but paid by the clinic to see many cases and with no particular method required); and

6 The conditions under which therapists deliver the treatment (not graduate students' flexible time, but strict productivity requirements or payment per therapy hour, paperwork to complete and little time to learn a manual or prepare for each session in advance).

The gap between RCT conditions and practice conditions has contributed to the concern of many practitioners and some clinical scientists that the treatments emerging from RCTs may not be well-suited to the rigors of real-world practice (Addis & Krasnow, 2000; Westen, Novotny, & Thompson-Brenner, 2004; Weisz, 2004). Two possible responses to this concern warrant attention in this chapter.

Shift to a Deployment-Focused Model of Treatment Development and Testing

It is possible that these many differences between therapy in most RCTs and therapy in actual clinical practice are too pronounced to be bridged as simply the final step at the end of a long series of traditional RCTs. Perhaps the number of dimensions along which treatment would need to be changed to bridge the research–practice gap makes the task of moving so complex that the task needs to be made an integral part of the treatment development process. Indeed, the very real-world factors that experimentalists might view as a nuisance (e.g., child comorbidity, parent pathology, life stresses that produce no-shows and dropouts, therapists with heavy caseloads) and thus attempt to avoid (e.g., by recruiting and screening cases, applying exclusion criteria, hiring their own therapists), may in fact be precisely the factors that need to be included in research designs if researchers are to develop psychosocial treatment protocols that fit well into everyday practice. Treatments that cannot cope with these real-world factors may not fare so well in practice, no matter how beneficial they are in efficacy trials.

To address this challenge, one proposal has been that traditional RCTs exercising tight control over diverse real-world treatment factors give way to a model of treatment development and testing that brings treatments into the crucible of clinical practice early in their development and treats testing in the practice setting as a sequential process, not as a single final phase. This approach has been called the deployment-focused model (DFM) of treatment development and testing. The model (detailed in Weisz, 2004) outlines a series of steps by which the creation and testing of treatments can encompass representative practice conditions and contexts. Central to this model is the notion that to create interventions that work well in the crucible of everyday professional use, treatment developers and researchers will need to focus their work on precisely the kinds of individuals, treatment providers and clinical care contexts for which the treatments are ultimately intended.

Build the Evidence Base on Comparisons with Usual Clinical Care Another possible response to the gap between traditional research conditions and everyday clinical practice conditions focuses on the question of which comparison groups to include in research. Largely absent from the treatment research literature are comparisons that address what is arguably the most critical question for those concerned about the research–practice gap (i.e., how helpful are EBTs in comparison with the treatment that children would otherwise have received in usual clinical care?). In some respects, this is the touchstone question. Indeed, if EBTs cannot outperform the treatments children would otherwise receive in clinical care, one could question the point of all the time, effort and funding used to create those EBTs. Our evidence review (Weisz, Jensen Doss, & Hawley, 2005) found that fewer than 8% of all child RCTs used standard case management or some other form of usual care as the comparison condition, and some of these comparisons lacked the precise control (e.g., for treatment dose, or for whether usual care was in fact a "treatment") that would be needed for ideal inferential power. In a recent analysis, Weisz, Jensen Doss, and Hawley (2006a) focused on the 32 RCTs identified that compared an EBT for children to some form of usual care (e.g., everyday psychotherapy with no protocol, case management, structured community program that had not been previously tested). On average, EBTs outperformed usual care interventions, but not to an overwhelming degree. The mean effect size across all the EBT versus usual care comparisons was 0.30, falling within the small to medium range. Notably, the range of effects was quite wide across individual studies, with some showing impressive superiority of EBTs but others showing EBTs to be less effective than treatment as usual. This suggests a need for caution on the part of potential consumers of EBTs. The fact that an intervention has been tested and shown to work in clinical trials – say, in comparison to a waitlist condition – may not necessarily mean that the intervention is superior to current forms of clinical care that are untested. To address this question requires a genre of research that is quite rare to date; direct comparisons of EBTs with the most common forms of usual clinical care to which the EBTs are potential alternatives. In our view, the next era of research in the field should include a large component of EBT versus usual care testing, encompassing the creation of a taxonomy of usual care interventions and a growing body of evidence on the relative advantage (or disadvantage) of various EBTs in comparison with various forms of usual care, in the context of various child problems, disorders, and combinations thereof.

Critical Tensions and Unanswered Questions

Beyond its strengths and limitations, research on child psychotherapy can also be characterized by tension around some critical questions about which there is no consensus answer. Here we focus on a few of the questions that seem particularly central to the field (Table 18.2).

Table 18.2 Critical tensions and unanswered questions in the field.

1 Efficacy versus effectiveness of child and adolescent treatments
2 Precision versus breadth in individual treatment focus
3 Linear treatment manuals versus modular approaches
4 Common factors (e.g., therapeutic relationship) versus specific techniques
5 How to train, and how to measure skill in treatment: fidelity and beyond
6 Relation between science and practice

Efficacy versus Effectiveness of Child and Adolescent Treatments

Although we have advocated increased emphasis on treatment research that encompasses real-world characteristics, and we have proposed a deployment-focused model to guide that process, we must acknowledge that not all researchers agree on this issue. In the treatment literature, both psychotherapeutic and medical, a distinction is drawn between two very different forms of outcome research. In *efficacy designs*, experimental control is used to test treatment impact under carefully arranged idealized conditions, described above. In *effectiveness designs*, intervention effects are assessed under ordinary clinical conditions, with treatment delivered to "average" or representative patients or clients, by "average" or representative practitioners, working under conditions that reflect typical practice realities. In a recent review of youth clinical trials, Weisz, Jensen Doss, & Hawley (2005) found that about 13% of study samples consisted of clinically referred youths (many were recruited, e.g., through advertisements, or identified through screening procedures in schools); about 19% of the studies used at least one practicing clinician to deliver treatment; and only about 4% of the studies provided treatment within a clinical practice setting. In fact, only 1% of the studies involved all three elements (i.e., clinically referred youths, treated by practicing clinicians, in clinical practice settings). So, elements of effectiveness research are not very common in the treatment outcome literature. Should we be concerned about this? Some researchers believe that, at this stage in treatment development research, energy is best devoted to research that uses well-controlled conditions to generate the strongest possible treatments for specific forms of dysfunction – and thus that efficacy research needs special emphasis. Others believe that what is most needed are treatments that can address the complexity and severity of mental health problems as they appear in everyday practice, and that doing this will require increased emphasis on effectiveness research. The debate has important implications for the funding of research and, in turn, for what will be learned about treatments and the conditions under which treatments have their effects.

Precision versus Breadth in Individual Treatment Focus

Another important debate in the field concerns the degree to which treatments should be narrowly focused on single problems or disorders, versus designed to address problems in clusters, or even the "whole child." Most manual-guided treatments designed for children and teens have been focused on single problems or disorders, or at least relatively homogenous clusters. In fact, in much of the research on these treatments (but certainly not all), youths who have comorbidities that might undermine treatment success have been excluded from study samples. Even when comorbidities have been included in study samples, the treatments being tested have most often had a relatively narrow problem or diagnostic focus. On the plus side, this procedure may provide a useful context for testing treatments without interference from unwanted conditions.

However, the longer treatment development and research focus on single conditions, the longer the field is delayed in addressing a widely recognized fact about child psychopathology. Extensive evidence (e.g., Angold, Costello, & Erkanli, 1999) shows that co-occurrence of disorders and problems is quite characteristic of the youngsters seen in everyday clinical care. For example, ADHD is frequently found in concert with ODD, and often also with depressive or anxiety disorders. Rates of comorbidity, striking even in community samples, are markedly higher in clinical samples (Angold, Costello, & Erkanli, 1999). A case can be made that we need to understand: (i) the extent to which comorbidities of various kinds moderate the effects of treatments that are focused on single conditions; and (ii) the potential benefits of treating multiple conditions concurrently. More than a decade ago, Kendall and Clarkin (1992) referred to comorbidity as the "premier challenge facing mental health professionals in the 1990s" (Kendall & Clarkin, 1992, p. 833). The 1990s have now come and gone, and the challenge remains largely unaddressed by youth treatment researchers.

Linear Treatment Manuals versus Modular Approaches

A closely related debate centers on the merits of using full treatment manuals – which typically describe a linear sequence of steps, with one lesson or skill to be covered in session 1, another in session 2, etc. Some see an inherent logic in such sequences, with the information or skills covered in earlier sessions needed for movement to subsequent sessions, and with the full package required for full treatment benefit. Indeed, most treatment manuals for which there is support in RCTs have taken exactly this linear form. However, many professionals outside the world of research object to the idea of standardized intervention protocols with a series of sessions in a predetermined sequence (Addis & Krasnow, 2000; Addis, Wade, & Hatgis, 1999; Havik & VandenBos, 1996). We should note that manuals come in a variety of forms and formats, and that the manuals for some of the best-tested treatments (e.g., multisystemic therapy; Henggeler, Schoenwald, Borduin *et al.*, 1998) emphasize treatment principles and guidelines, not a lock-step sequence of session topics, and clinicians have considerable flexibility to use their own creativity and judgment to achieve desired clinical outcomes.

However, for some professionals, full treatment protocols of any kind may not be appealing. A more appealing application of evidence-based interventions may involve incorporating new practice elements into their work selectively, using their own experience and skills to decide which elements are worth trying, rather than replacing their traditional approaches wholesale. This conflicts with the extant evidence base, in which empirically supported interventions have almost always come in the form of full manualized programs, and in which some evidence from both prevention and treatment research (Durlak & Wells, 1998; Huey *et al.*, 2000) indicates that fidelity to the manual enhances outcomes.

Thus, a case can be made that, at this time and for a number of interventions, the most "evidence-based" practice involves the application of full programs in the specific forms tested in research trials. In principle, though, it seems possible that certain elements of these programs, combined in ways that fit distinctive characteristics of individuals targeted for intervention, might produce genuine benefit. The problem is that the research to date provides little guidance on how to extract specific best practices from full protocols, and lacks information as to which of these – alone or in combination – might lead to good outcomes. To compile such knowledge in the most systematic way will require that we find reliable ways of identifying separable elements of treatment protocols, logically and theoretically sound ways of turning these elements into separate modules, and clinically sensitive ways of selecting modules and combinations to fit various individuals and groups targeted for intervention. At least one approach to these steps has been documented, and a resulting "modular protocol" created, to encompass intervention for youth anxiety, depression and/or conduct problems (Chorpita, Daleiden, & Weisz, 2005a,b). Tests of the resulting modular protocol are under way. It seems likely that many years of refinement and testing lie ahead before researchers can begin to assess whether separating "best practices" and organizing them in modular fashion will match or improve on standard manuals as we now know them. The questions of interest include not only what kinds of outcomes the modular treatments produce, but also what their prospects are for dissemination to and effective implementation by practitioners in real-world clinical practice, where standard manuals face significant challenges.

Common Factors (e.g., Therapeutic Relationship) versus Specific Techniques

The current array of EBTs is strong in describing (through manuals) principles and specific procedures to apply in treatment. This is a strength to the extent that the manuals document the steps therapists need to follow to replicate treatment procedures that have been successful in randomized trials. However, it is a limitation to the extent that aspects of treatment other than the specific procedures may have played a part in treatment success. As an example of what may be missing, many who study therapy process believe that "non-specific" "common factors," such as the quality of the therapeutic relationship, account for a large proportion (even most) of the variance in outcomes (Luborsky, Rosenthal, Diguer *et al.*, 2002). Indeed, many child therapists rate the therapeutic relationship as more important than the specific techniques used in treatment (Kazdin *et al.*, 1990; Motta & Lynch, 1990; Shirk & Saiz, 1992), and some treated children may agree, even those treated by EBTs. Kendall and Southam-Gerow (1996) found that children treated for anxiety disorders using the Coping Cat program rated their relationship with the therapist as the most important aspect of treatment. Given these sources of support for the importance of the relationship and alliance, it is notable that most manuals associated with EBTs provide little guidance to therapists in building a warm empathic relationship and a strong working alliance with children and families. What we lack thus far is a strong body of evidence:

- Clearly defining what a positive therapeutic relationship consists of;
- Establishing how best to measure it;
- Identifying therapist characteristics and behaviors that foster it; and
- Testing the extent to which it actually predicts outcome when EBTs are used.

A broader question concerns the extent to which therapeutic relationship-building is a teachable skill and, if it is, how much of that skill can be captured and taught via a written treatment protocol. Many would perhaps agree that the best therapy involves tested and proven methods and procedures combined with a strong positive therapeutic relationship and working alliance between therapist and child (and parents). How to create this combination remains a matter of considerable debate in the field.

How to Train, and How to Measure Skill in Treatment: Fidelity and Beyond

Suppose we develop a new treatment, Therapy X, for Disorder X, and we do the research needed to show that Therapy X shows a large effect size across a succession of RCTs. Suppose, further, that some of those RCTs show that Therapy X outperforms some of the most common forms of usual care for Disorder X. At this point, we are ready to disseminate Therapy X to an array of clinical practitioners, most of whom are quite busy and who thus want to have only enough training to become truly effective at Therapy X. We are ready to begin training, but are we ready to determine which therapists have achieved what it takes to be effective with Therapy X? Probably not. In the current state of the art for most EBTs, the closest we can come to this holy grail is assessment of "fidelity" or "adherence" to the protocol. Operationally, this typically means coding whether therapists cover the material that is listed in the treatment manual, and sometimes whether they use the techniques that are recommended in the manual (e.g., role plays, *in vivo* exercises, quizzes). Fidelity to the treatment model is important, of course, and it may be necessary for success in many treatments. But is it sufficient? Again, probably not.

Our experience in assessing fidelity over the years has convinced us that it is possible to achieve relatively high fidelity but in ways that seem unlikely to be very effective in producing good treatment outcomes. Something more is needed, and for most treatments that "something" is not very well-defined and not easy for experts to code from treatment videotapes. Examples include ability to engage the child's interest and motivation, to bring the treatment concepts and skills to life in ways that are meaningful, and to use real-life concerns or crises presented by the child as opportunities to illustrate and practice key skills of the treatment program. In our view, identifying such "keys to effective use" of EBTs should be central to the agenda for research in the years ahead.

Relation between Science and Practice

A debate of sorts has emerged between some in the research community who favor dissemination of EBTs into clinical practice and some in the clinical practice community who favor studying everyday clinical practice to identify the most effective practices. In a sense, the debate overlooks an important fact about EBTs (i.e., that many of them emerged from successes in everyday clinical practice). As we noted earlier, the Hanf and Kling's parent training program in Oregon, which grew out of Hanf's everyday practice and supervision, led to the development of three EBTs: separate parent training programs authored by Barkley (1997), Eyberg and Boggs (1998) and McMahon and Forehand (2003). Indeed, the interplay between everyday practice and science has been quite rich at times, and quite often ordered in such a way that practice leads science. We believe there is a great deal of room for continued interaction. Science can be good for practice, helping us identify which forms of care are in fact helpful to children, and – in the best circumstances – what causal mechanisms have a role. Practice can likewise be good for science, helping us identify areas in which new knowledge and improved treatment are most needed, and grounding science in the realities of everyday clinical care.

Acknowledgments

Some of the evidence review reported in this chapter was supported through the Research Network on Youth Mental Health (Bruce F. Chorpita, Robert Gibbons, Charles Glisson, Evelyn Polk Green, Kimberly Hoagwood, Peter S. Jensen, Kelly Kelleher, John Landsverk, Stephen Mayberg, Jeanne Miranda, Lawrence A. Palinkas, Sonja Schoenwald and John Weisz), funded by the John D. and Catherine T. MacArthur Foundation. The authors were supported by the National Institute of Mental Health (R01 MH 547347). We are grateful to Andrew Colitz, Sara Fuentes, Julie Edmunds, Kaitlin Gallo and Abby Wolf for their help in various aspects of this project.

References

Achenbach, T. M., McConaughy, S. H., & Howell, C. T. (1987). Child/adolescent behavioral and emotional problems: Implications of cross-informant correlations for situational specificity. *Psychological Bulletin*, *101*, 213–232.

Addis, M. E., & Krasnow, A. D. (2000). A national survey of practicing psychologists' attitudes toward psychotherapy treatment manuals. *Journal of Consulting and Clinical Psychology*, *68*, 331–339.

Addis, M. E., Wade, W. A., & Hatgis, C. (1999). Barriers to dissemination of evidence-based practices: addressing practitioners' concerns about manual-based psychotherapies. *Clinical Psychology: Science and Practice*, *6*, 430–441.

Albano, A. M., Marten, P. A., Holt, C. S., Heimberg, R. G., & Barlow, D. H. (1995). Cognitive–behavioral group treatment for social phobia in adolescents: A preliminary study. *Journal of Nervous and Mental Disease*, *183*, 649–656.

American Psychiatric Association. (2000). *Diagnostic and Statistical Manual of Mental Disorders* (4th ed.). Text revision. Washington, DC: American Psychiatric Association.

Angold, A., Costello, E. J., & Erkanli, A. (1999). Comorbidity. *Journal of Child Psychology and Psychiatry*, *40*, 57–87.

Autry, L. B., & Langenbach, M. (1985). Locus of control and self-responsibility for behavior. *Journal of Educational Research*, *79*, 76–84.

Azrin, N. H., Donohue, B., Besalel, V. A., Kogan, E. S., & Acierno, R. (1994). Youth drug abuse treatment: A controlled outcome study. *Journal of Child and Adolescent Substance Abuse*, *3*, 1–16.

Barkley, R. A. (1997). *Defiant children: A clinician's manual for assessment and parent training*. New York: Guilford.

Baron, R. M., & Kenny, D. A. (1986). The moderator-mediator variable distinction in social psychological research: Conceptual, strategic, and statistical considerations. *Journal of Personality and Social Psychology*, *51*, 1173–1182.

Barrett, P., Healy, L., Piacentini, J., & March, J. (2004). Treatment of OCD in children and adolescents. In P. Barrett, & T. Ollendick (Eds.), *Handbook of interventions that work with children and adolescents* (pp. 187–216). Chichester, UK: Wiley.

Barrett, P. M., Dadds, M. R., & Rapee, R. M. (1996). Family treatment of childhood anxiety: A controlled trial. *Journal of Consulting and Clinical Psychology*, *64*, 333–342.

Bearman, S. K., Presnell, K, Martinez, E., & Stice E. (2006). The skinny on body dissatisfaction: A longitudinal study of adolescent boys and girls. *Journal of Youth and Adolescence*, *35*, 217–229.

Beck, A. T. (1964). Thinking and depression: Theory and therapy. *Archives of General Psychiatry*, *10*, 561–571.

Beck, A. T. (1970). Cognitive therapy: Nature and relation to behavior therapy. *Behavior Therapy*, *1*, 184–200.

Beck, A. T. (1971). Cognition, affect, and psychopathology. *Archives of General Psychiatry*, *24*, 495–500.

Bender, N. N. (1976). Self-verbalization versus tutor verbalization in modifying impulsivity. *Journal of Educational Psychology*, *68*, 347–354.

Borduin, C. M., Henggeler, S. W., Blaske, D. M., & Stein, R. (1990). Multisystemic treatment of adolescent sexual offenders. *International Journal of Offender Therapy and Comparative Criminology*, *35*, 105–114.

Bornstein, B. (1949). The analysis of a phobic child; some problems of theory and technique in child analysis. In A. Freud, H. Hartmann, & E. Kris (Eds.), *The psychoanalytic study of the child* (pp. 181–226). Oxford, UK: International Universities Press.

Brent, D. A., Kolko, D. J., Birmaher, B., Baugher, M., Bridge, J., Roth, C., *et al.* (1998). Predictors of treatment efficacy in a clinical trial of three psychosocial treatments for adolescent depression. *Journal of the American Academy of Child & Adolescent Psychiatry*, *37*, 906–914.

Brestan, E. V., & Eyberg, S. M. (1998). Effective psychosocial treatments of conduct-disordered children and adolescents: 29 years, 82 studies, 5,272 kids. *Journal of Clinical Child Psychology*, *27*, 180–189.

Casey, R. J., & Berman, J. S. (1985). The outcome of psychotherapy with children. *Psychological Bulletin*, *98*, 388–400.

Chamberlain, P., & Reid, J. B. (1998). Comparison of two community alternatives to incarceration for chronic juvenile offenders. *Journal of Consulting and Clinical Psychology*, *66*, 624–633.

Chamberlain, P., & Smith, D. K. (2003). Antisocial behavior in children and adolescents: The Oregon Multidimensional Treatment Foster Care Model. In A. E. Kazdin, & J. R. Weisz (Eds.), *Evidence-based psychotherapies for children and adolescents* (pp. 282–300). New York: Guilford.

Chorpita, B. F., Daleiden, E. L., & Weisz, J. R. (2005a). Identifying and selecting the common elements of evidence based interventions: A distillation and matching model. *Mental Health Services Research*, *7*, 5–20.

Chorpita, B. F., Daleiden, E, & Weisz, J. R. (2005b). Modularity in the design and application of therapeutic interventions. *Applied and Preventive Psychology*, *11*, 141–156.

Clarke, G. N., Rohde, P., Lewinsohn, P. M., Hops, H., & Seeley, J. R. (1999). Cognitive–behavioral group treatment of adolescent depression: Efficacy of acute treatment and booster sessions. *Journal of the American Academy of Child & Adolescent Psychiatry*, *38*, 272–279.

Cohen, J. (1988). *Statistical power analysis for the behavioral sciences* (2nd ed.). Hillsdale, NJ: Erlbaum.

Curry, J., Rohde, P., Simons, A., Silva, S. G., Vitiello, B., Kratochvil, C. J., *et al.* (2006). Predictors and moderators of acute outcome in the treatment for adolescents with depression study (TADS). *Journal of the American Academy of Child and Adolescent Psychiatry*, *45*, 1427–1439.

Deblinger, E., & Heflin, A. H. (1996). *Treating sexually abused children and their nonoffending parents: A cognitive–behavioral approach*. Thousand Oaks, CA: Sage.

Durlak, J. A., & Wells, A. M. (1998). Evaluation of indicated preventive intervention (secondary prevention) mental health programs for children and adolescents. *American Journal of Community Psychology*, *26*, 775–802.

Durlak, J. A., Wells, A. M., Cotton, J. K., & Johnson, S. (1995). Analysis of selected methodological issues in child psychotherapy research. *Journal of Clinical Child Psychology*, *24*, 141–148.

Eddy, J. M., & Chamberlain, P. (2000). Family management and deviant peer association as mediators of the impact of treatment condition on youth antisocial behavior. *Journal of Consulting and Clinical Psychology*, *68*, 857–863.

Eyberg, S. M., & Boggs, S. R. (1998). Parent–child interaction therapy: A psychosocial intervention for the treatment of young conduct-disordered children. In J. M. Briesmeister, & C. E. Schaefer (Eds.), *Handbook of parent training: Parents as co-therapists for children's behavior problems* (2nd ed., pp. 61–97). Hoboken, NJ: John Wiley & Sons, Inc.

Eysenck H. J. (1952). The effects of psychotherapy: An evaluation. *Journal of Consulting Psychology*, *16*, 319–324.

Fairburn, C. G. (2005). Evidence-based treatment of anorexia nervosa. *International Journal of Eating Disorders*, *37*, 526–530.

Frank, J. D. (1973). *Persuasion and healing: A comparative study of psychotherapy*. Baltimore: Johns Hopkins University Press.

Freedheim, D. K., Freudenberger, H. J., & Kessler, J. W. (1992). *History of psychotherapy: A century of change*. Washington, DC: American Psychological Association.

Hammen, C., & Rudolph, K. D. (1996). Childhood depression. In E. J. Mash, & R. A. Barkley (Eds.), *Child psychopathology* (pp. 153–195). New York, NY: Guilford Press.

Havik, O. E., & VandenBos, G. R. (1996). Limitations of manualized psychotherapy for everyday clinical practice. *Clinical Psychology: Science and Practice*, *3*, 264–267.

Henggeler, S. W., Schoenwald, S. K., Borduin, C. M., Rowland, M. D., & Cunningham, P. B. (1998). *Multisystemic treatment of antisocial behavior in children and adolescents*. New York, NY: Guilford Press.

Holmbeck, G. N. (1997). Toward terminological, conceptual, and statistical clarity in the study of mediators and moderators: Examples from the child-clinical and pediatric psychology literatures. *Journal of Consulting and Clinical Psychology*, *65*, 599–610.

Huey, S. J. Jr., Henggeler, S. W., Brondino, M. J., & Pickrel, S. G. (2000). Mechanisms of change in multisystemic therapy: Reducing delinquent behavior through therapist adherence and improved family and peer functioning. *Journal of Consulting and Clinical Psychology*, *68*, 451–467.

Jessness, C. F. (1975). Comparative effectiveness of behavior modification and transactional analysis programs for delinquents. *Journal of Consulting and Clinical Psychology*, *43*, 758–779.

Jensen, A. L., & Weisz, J. R. (2002). Assessing match and mismatch between practitioner-generated and standardized interview-generated diagnoses for clinic-referred children and adolescents. *Journal of Consulting and Clinical Psychology*, *70*, 158–168.

Jessness, C. F. (1975). Comparative effectiveness of behaviour modification and transactional analysis programs for delinquents. *Journal of Consulting and Clinical Psychology*, *43*, 758–779.

Jones, M. C. (1924a). A laboratory study of fear: The case of Peter. *Pedagogical Seminary*, *31*, 308–315.

Jones, M. C. (1924b). The elimination of children's fears. *Journal of Experimental Psychology*, *7*, 382–390.

Judd, C. M., & Kenney, D. A. (1981). Process analysis: Estimating mediation in treatment evaluations. *Evaluation Review*, *5*, 602–619.

Kaslow, N. J., & Thompson, M. P. (1998). Applying the criteria for empirically supported treatments to studies of psychosocial interventions for child and adolescent depression. *Journal of Clinical Child Psychology*, *27*, 146–155.

Kazdin, A. E. (2000). *Psychotherapy for children and adolescents: Directions for research and practice*. New York: Oxford University Press.

Kazdin, A. E. (2002). The state of child and adolescent psychotherapy research. *Child and Adolescent Mental Health*, *7*, 53–59.

Kazdin, A. E. (2003). Problem-solving skills training and parent management training for conduct disorder. In A. E. Kazdin, & J. R. Weisz (Eds.), *Evidence-based psychotherapies for children and adolescents* (pp. 241–262). New York: Guilford.

Kazdin, A. E., Bass, D., Ayers, W. A., & Rodgers, A. (1990). Empirical and clinical focus of child and adolescent psychotherapy research. *Journal of Consulting and Clinical Psychology*, *58*, 729–740.

Kazdin, A. E., & Crowley, M. J. (1997). Moderators of treatment outcome in cognitively based treatment of antisocial children. *Cognitive Therapy and Research*, *21*, 185–207.

Kazdin, A. E., & Weisz, J. R. (1998). Identifying and developing empirically supported child and adolescent treatments. *Journal of Consulting and Clinical Psychology*, *66*, 19–36.

Kazdin, A. E., & Weisz, J. R. (2003). *Evidence-based psychotherapies for children and adolescents*. New York, NY: Guilford Press.

Kendall, P. C., & Clarkin, J. F. (1992). Introduction to special section: Comorbidity and treatment implications. *Journal of Consulting and Clinical Psychology*, *60*, 833–834.

Kendall, P. C., Kane, M., Howard, B., & Siqueland, L. (1990). *Cognitive–behavioral therapy for anxious children: Treatment manual*. Philadelphia, PA: Temple University.

Kendall, P. C., & Southam-Gerow, M. A. (1996). Long-term follow-up of a cognitive–behavioral therapy for anxiety-disordered youth. *Journal of Consulting and Clinical Psychology*, *64*, 724–730.

Kendall, P. C., & Wilcox, L. E. (1980). Cognitive–behavioral treatment for impulsivity: Concrete versus conceptual training in non-self-controlled problem children. *Journal of Consulting and Clinical Psychology*, *48*, 80–91.

Kraemer, H. C., Stice, E., Kazdin, A., Offord, D., & Kupfer, D. (2001). How do risk factors work? Mediators, moderators, and independent, overlapping, and proxy risk factors. *American Journal of Psychiatry*, *158*, 848–856.

Kraemer, H. C., Wilson, G. T., Fairburn, C. G., & Agras, W. S. (2002). Mediators and moderators of treatment effects in randomized clinical trials. *Archives of General Psychiatry*, *59*, 877–884.

Le Grange, D., & Lock, J. (2005). The dearth of psychological treatment studies for anorexia nervosa. *International Journal of Eating Disorders*, *37*, 79–91.

Levitt, E. E. (1957). The results of psychotherapy with children: An evaluation. *Journal of Consulting and Clinical Psychology*, *21*, 189–196.

Levitt, E. E. (1963). Psychotherapy with children: A further evaluation. *Behaviour Research and Therapy*, *60*, 326–329.

Lewinsohn, P. M., Clarke, G. N., & Hops, H. (1990). Cognitive–behavioral treatment for depressed adolescents. *Behavior Therapy*, *21*, 385–401.

Luborsky, L., Rosenthal, R., Diguer, L., Andrusyna, T. P., Berman, J. S., Levitt, J. T., *et al.* (2002). The dodo bird verdict is alive and well – mostly. *Clinical Psychology: Science and Practice*, *9*, 2–12.

Mann, C. (1990). Meta-analysis in the breech. *Science*, *249*, 476–480.

March, J., Frances, A., Carpenter, D., & Kahn, D. (1997). Expert consensus guidelines: Treatment of obsessive-compulsive disorder. *Journal of Clinical Psychology*, *58*, 1–72.

McGrath, M. L., Dorsett, P. G., Calhoun, M. E., & Drabman, R. S. (1988). "Beat-the-buzzer": A method for decreasing parent–child morning conflicts. *Child and Family Behavior Therapy*, *9*, 35–48.

McLeod, B. D., & Weisz, J. R. (2004). Using dissertations to examine potential bias in child and adolescent clinical trials. *Journal of Consulting and Clinical Psychology*, *72*, 235–251.

McMahon, R. J., & Forehand, R. L. (2003). *Helping the noncompliant child: Family-based treatment for oppositional behavior* (2nd ed.). New York, NY: Guilford Press.

Meichenbaum, D., & Goodman, S. (1971). Training impulsive children to talk to themselves: A means of developing self-control. *Journal of Abnormal Psychology*, *77*, 115–126.

Moffitt, T. E. (1993). Life-course persistent and adolescent-limited antisocial behavior: A developmental taxonomy. *Psychological Review*, *100*, 674–701.

Moracco, J., & Kazandkian, A. (1977). Effectiveness of behavior counseling and consulting with non-Western elementary school children. *Elementary School Guidance & Counseling*, *11*, 244–251.

Motta, R. W., & Lynch, C. (1990). Therapeutic techniques vs. therapeutic relationships in child behavior therapy. *Psychological Reports*, *67*, 315–322.

Mufson, L., Dorta, K. P., Wickramaratne, P., Nomura, Y., Olfson, M., & Weissman, M. M. (2004). A randomized effectiveness trial of interpersonal psychotherapy for depressed adolescents. *Archives of General Psychiatry*, *61*, 577–584.

Mufson, L., Weissman, M. M., Moreau, D., & Garfinkel, R. (1999). Efficacy of interpersonal psychotherapy for depressed adolescents. *Archives of General Psychiatry*, *56*, 573–579.

Muris, P., Merckelbach, H., Holdrinet, I., & Sijsenaar, M. (1998). Treating phobic children: Effects of EMDR versus exposure. *Journal of Consulting and Clinical Psychology*, *66*, 193–198.

Ollendick, T. H., & King, N. J. (1998). Empirically supported treatments for children with phobic and anxiety disorders. *Journal of Clinical Child Psychology*, *27*, 156–167.

Omizo, M. M., & Michael, W. B. (1982). Biofeedback-induced relaxation training and impulsivity, attention to task, and locus of control among hyperactive boys. *Journal of Learning Disabilities*, *15*, 414–416.

Patterson, G. R., Chamberlain, P., & Reid, J. B. (1982). A comparative evaluation of a parent-training program. *Behavior Therapy*, *13*, 638–650.

Pelham, W. E., Carlson, C., Sams, S., Vallano, G., Dixon, J., & Hoza, B. (1993). Separate and combined effects of methylphenidate and behavior modification on boys with attention-deficit-hyperactivity disorder in the classroom. *Journal of Consulting and Clinical Psychology*, *55*, 76–85.

Pelham, W. E., Greiner, A. R., Gnagy, E. M., Hoza, B., Martin, L. E., Sams, S. E., *et al.* (1996). Intensive treatment for ADHD: a model summer treatment program. In M. Roberts (Ed.), *Model programs in child and family mental health* (pp. 193–213). Mahwah, NJ: Erlbaum.

Pelham, W. E., Wheeler, T., & Chronis, A. (1998). Empirically supported psychosocial treatments for attention deficit hyperactivity disorder. *Journal of Clinical Child Psychology*, *27*, 190–205.

Porter, S. S., & Omizo, M. M. (1984). The effects of group relaxation training/large muscle exercise, and parental involvement on attention to task, impulsivity, and locus of control among hyperactive boys. *Exceptional Child*, *31*, 54–64.

Redfering, D. L., & Bowman, M. J. (1981). Effects of a meditative-relaxation exercise on non-attending behaviors of behaviorally disturbed children. *Journal of Clinical Child Psychology*, *10*, 126–127.

Rivera, E., & Omizo, M. M. (1980). The effects of relaxation and biofeedback on attention to task and impulsivity among male hyperactive children. *Exceptional Child*, *27*, 41–51.

Shapiro, D. A., & Shapiro, D. (1982). Meta-analysis of comparative therapy outcome studies: A replication and refinement. *Psychological Bulletin*, *92*, 581–604.

Shirk, S. R., & Karver, M. (2003). Prediction of treatment outcome from relationship variables in child and adolescent therapy: A meta-analytic review. *Journal of Consulting and Clinical Psychology*, *71*, 452–464.

Shirk, S. R., & Russell, R. L. (1996). *Change processes in child psychotherapy: Revitalizing treatment and research*. New York: Guilford.

Shirk, S. R., & Saiz, C. C. (1992). Clinical, empirical, and developmental perspectives on the therapeutic relationship in child psychotherapy. Special Issue: Developmental approaches to prevention and intervention. *Development & Psychopathology*, *4*, 713–728.

Silverman, W. K., & Kurtines, W. M. (1996). Transfer of control: A psychosocial intervention model for internalizing disorders in youth. In E. D. Hibbs, & P. S. Jensen (Eds.), *Psychosocial treatments for child and adolescent disorders: Empirically based strategies for clinical practice* (pp. 63–81). Washington, DC: American Psychological Association.

Smith, M. L., & Glass, G. V. (1977). Meta-analysis of psychotherapy outcome studies. *American Psychologist*, *32*, 752–760.

Southam-Gerow, M. A., Weisz, J. R., & Kendall, P. C. (2003). Youth with anxiety disorders in research and service clinics: Examining client differences and similarities. *Journal of Clinical Child and Adolescent Psychology*, *32*, 375–385.

Stice, E. M., Shaw, H., Burton, E., & Wade, E. (2006). Dissonance and healthy weight eating disorder prevention programs: A randomized efficacy trial. *Journal of Consulting and Clinical Psychology*, *74*, 263–275.

Sullivan, P. F. (1995). Mortality in anorexia nervosa. *American Journal of Psychiatry*, *152*, 1073–1074.

Tarnowski, K. J., Rosen, L. A., McGrath, M. L., & Drabman, R. S. (1987). A modified habit reversal procedure in a recalcitrant case of trichotillomania. *Journal of Behavior Therapy and Experimental Psychiatry*, *18*, 157–163.

Webster-Stratton, C. (1984). Randomized trial of two parent-training programs for families with conduct-disordered children. *Journal of Consulting and Clinical Psychology*, *52*, 666–678.

Webster-Stratton, C., & Reid, M. J. (2003). The Incredible Years Parents, Teachers, and Children Training Series: A multifaceted treatment approach for young children with conduct problems. In A. E. Kazdin, & J. R. Weisz (Eds.), *Evidence-based psychotherapies for children and adolescents* (pp. 224–240). New York: Guilford.

Weersing, V. R., & Weisz, J. R. (2002). Mechanisms of action in youth psychotherapy. *Journal of Child Psychology and Psychiatry*, *43*, 3–29.

Weisz, J. R. (2004). *Psychotherapy for children and adolescents: Evidence-based treatments and case examples*. New York, NY: Cambridge University Press.

Weisz, J. R., & Hawley, K. M. (2002). Developmental factors in the treatment of adolescents. *Journal of Consulting and Clinical Psychology*, *70*, 21–43.

Weisz, J. R., Hawley, K. M., & Jensen Doss, A. (2004). Empirically tested psychotherapies for youth internalizing and externalizing problems and disorders. *Child and Adolescent Psychiatric Clinics of North America*, *13*, 729–815.

Weisz, J. R., Huey, S. M., & Weersing, V. R. (1998). Psychotherapy outcome research with children and adolescents: The state of the art. In T. H. Ollendick & R. J. Prinz (Eds.), *Advances in clinical child psychology*, Vol. 20, pp. 49–92). New York: Plenum.

Weisz, J. R., & Jensen, P. S. (1999). Efficacy and effectiveness of child and adolescent psychotherapy and pharmacotherapy. *Mental Health Services Research*, *1*, 125–157.

Weisz, J. R., Jensen Doss, A., & Hawley, K. M. (2005). Youth psychotherapy outcome research: A review and critique of the evidence base. *Annual Review of Psychology*, *56*, 337–363.

Weisz, J. R., Jensen Doss, A. J., Hawley, K. M. (2006a). Evidence-based youth psychotherapies versus usual clinical care: A meta-analysis of direct comparisons. *American Psychologist*, *61*, 671–689.

Weisz, J. R., McCarty, C. A., Eastman, K. L., Chaiyasit, W., & Suwanlert, S. (1997). Developmental psychopathology and culture: Ten lessons from Thailand. In S. S. Luthar, J. A. Burack, D. Cicchetti, & J. R. Weisz (Eds.), *Developmental psychopathology: Perspectives on adjustment, risk, and disorder* (pp. 568–592). New York, NY: Cambridge University Press.

Weisz, J. R., McCarty, C. A., & Valeri, S. M. (2006b). Effects of psychotherapy for depression in children and adolescents: A meta-analysis. *Psychological Bulletin*, *132*, 132–149.

Weisz, J. R., Weiss, B., Alicke, M. D., & Klotz, M. L. (1987). Effectiveness of psychotherapy with children and adolescents: A meta-analysis for clinicians. *Journal of Consulting and Clinical Psychology*, *55*, 542–549.

Weisz, J. R., Weiss, B., Han, S. S., Granger, D. A., & Morton, T. (1995). Effects of psychotherapy with children and adolescents revisited: A meta-analysis of treatment outcome studies. *Psychological Bulletin*, *117*, 450–468.

Westen, D., Novotny, C. M., & Thompson-Brenner, H. (2004). The empirical status of empirically supported psychotherapies: Assumptions, findings, and reporting in controlled clinical trials. *Psychological Bulletin*, *130*, 631–663.

Wilson, G. T., & Sysko, R. (2006). Cognitive–behavioural therapy for adolescents with bulimia nervosa. *European Eating Disorders Review*, *14*, 8–16.

Wurtele, S. K., & Drabman, R. S. (1984). "Beat-the-buzzer" for classroom dawdling: A one-year trial. *Behavior Therapy*, *15*, 403–409.

Yeh, M., & Weisz, J. R. (2001). Why are we here at the clinic? Parent–child (dis)agreement on referral problems at outpatient treatment entry. *Journal of Consulting and Clinical Psychology*, *69*, 1018–1025.

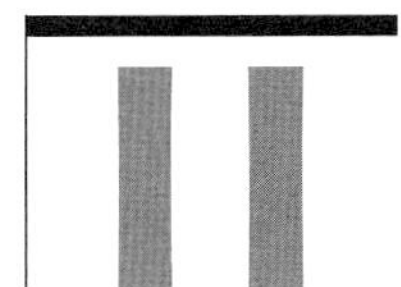

Clinical Assessment

19 Use of Structured Interviews and Observational Methods in Clinical Settings

Ann Le Couteur and Frances Gardner

There are many challenges for families, clinicians and researchers in the evaluation of clinically significant mental health problems in children and adolescents. These include distinguishing normal, temperamental and biological variations from signs of pathology, and assessing mental health in the context of transitions and developmental change, particularly in the early years. It is also important to be able to assess relevant environmental influences, including parenting and the wider family and social contexts as experienced by the child or adolescent. This chapter reviews the current use of some research-based structured interviews (SIs) and observational methods including their advantages and limitations in clinical settings. These are not fixed properties of the instruments, but depend closely on the purpose of the assessment. SIs and observational methods provide specific standardized information but do not replace clinical judgment. This is important to bear in mind when considering any assessment method.

Service Context

Best clinical practice in child and adolescent mental health (CAMH) services takes an evidence-based, multidisciplinary (MD) multiagency (MA) approach to both direct and indirect work. Clinical practices change over time in response to a variety of pressures including the prevailing theoretical knowledge base, revisions of diagnostic classification systems, local resources, referral practices and available treatment modalities. Multiple sources of information are needed to gain a realistic picture of the child's development over time (Grills & Ollendick, 2002; Silverman & Kurtines, 1996). Similarly, quality of parenting is usually assessed using a combination of systematic interviews with parents and children coupled with observations of family interactions (Mrazek, Mrazek, & Klinnert, 1995).

Children and adolescents rarely present with single disorders but rather a range of problems. Once a referral has been made, direct interviewing of parents, children and relevant adults together with specific assessments such as direct observations in different settings are necessary. However, informants do not necessarily all agree on the nature, extent and severity of the difficulties (Grills & Ollendick, 2002; Simonoff, Pickles, Meyer *et al.*, 1997). Previously, parents were thought to be the best informants regarding a child's behavior, with information from the child considered secondary (Edelbrock, Costello, Dulcan *et al.*, 1985). This view has changed significantly in the last several decades (for recent review see Grills & Ollendick, 2002). Direct observations provide a very different window on functioning, where information is not filtered through the perceptions of the involved parent, teacher or child. We show how observational methods can complement other aspects of assessment and provide specific information for treatment planning.

Standardized procedures (irrespective of whether or not research-based instruments have been used) are needed to combine all available information into a clinical formulation and intervention plan. Unfortunately, this will not always resolve the problem of discrepancies between sources of information (Goodman, Yude, Richards *et al.*, 1996; see also chapter 21).

Purposes of Clinical Assessment

A common set of information is necessary as part of an initial assessment, for subsequent follow-up reviews and for reassessment. A detailed description of the child's current functioning, abilities and behavior (including frequent and infrequent behaviors and skills) is required to establish a current baseline of capacity and need. Parents and/or principal caregivers and the child (depending on the context) are likely to welcome an opportunity to express early on their concerns, describe how they understand the "problem(s)" and share any other information they believe is relevant. The form of the assessment and choice of assessment methods need clinical judgment to consider the context of the referral, the specific questions or concerns raised, the needs of the family, the chronological and developmental age of the child, any history or evidence of existing special needs, and any circumstances that might mean the child is at particular risk or considered a "child in need" (Department of Health, 2004). Judgments will also need to be made about the frequency of particular types of referral to a clinical service and the relevance and

Rutter's Child and Adolescent Psychiatry, 5th edition. Edited by M. Rutter, D. Bishop, D. Pine, S. Scott, J. Stevenson, E. Taylor and A. Thapar. © 2008 Blackwell Publishing, ISBN: 978-1-4051-4549-7.

performance of particular assessment processes with children from different cultural and social backgrounds (e.g., whether there is an approved local translation).

Structured Interviews in Clinical Settings

"Interviewing has long been the standard method of assessing children's emotional, behavioral, and social functioning . . . Yet, it is one of the least trustworthy assessment procedures, subject to broad variations in content, style, detail and coverage" (Edelbrock & Costello, 1990).

Interviews with structure have developed for two main purposes (Del Carmen-Wiggins & Carter, 2004): contributing to the diagnostic assessment and obtaining descriptive data on children's emotional, behavioral and social problems.

Historically, structured clinical interviews with an adult informant have been considered the "gold standard" in terms of comprehensiveness and psychometric properties (Cox, Rutter, & Holbrook, 1981; McClellan & Werry, 2000). Cox, Rutter, & Holbrook (1981), investigating different interviewing styles in a clinical setting using individual interviews with the mother of the referred child, found that a high frequency of clinically important information was unique to individual families and that all techniques *if mastered well* were equally effective in eliciting emotions. However, when the interviewing styles were compared for their efficiency in eliciting good quality factual information, a process of systematic questioning was shown to be superior.

For research and clinical groups to share findings and experience, it is essential that all use the same terminology to minimize information variance. This was not possible prior to the publication of agreed international diagnostic classification systems, criteria and thus standardized measures (American Psychiatric Association, 2000; Spitzer, Endicott, & Robins, 1978; World Health Organization, 1996). The SI schedules developed over the last 20 years are mostly based on internationally agreed classification systems (DSM-IV and ICD-10), and use categorical diagnoses rather than a quantitative dimensional approach to levels of psychopathology (see chapter 20). Studies investigating the relationship between these two approaches have found only moderate convergence (Bird, Gould, & Staghezza, 1993; Boyle, Offord, Racine *et al.*, 1993).

The form and content of published interview schedules vary, but overall there is a trend for more specialization of focus such as specification of coverage, modification for different informants or for age range (for detailed reviews see Del Carmen-Wiggins & Carter, 2004; Grills & Ollendick, 2002; Shaffer, Lucas, & Richters, 1999). Such modifications are driven in part by the emphasis on evidence-based practice and disorder-specific funding for treatment services in some healthcare systems. This emphasis on specific diagnoses may not be appropriate for day-to-day clinical practice where a broad-based assessment to investigate the comorbidity of presenting problems for the child and family is the priority (Angold, Costello, & Erkanli, 1999). Moreover, individual and family vulnerabilities and strengths also show little apparent specificity between diagnostic groups (see chapters 23–33).

Current diagnostic boundaries will be revised as our understanding of the causal mechanisms for mental health disorders increases (see chapter 4). The differentiation of Rett syndrome from autism within the currently defined group of Pervasive Developmental Disorders is a recent case in point (Kerr, 2002). Furthermore, research and clinical findings have identified a broader spectrum of behaviors that extend beyond currently accepted diagnostic boundaries. These may represent milder and subclinical traits within the general population (Brugha, 2002; Melzer, Tom, Brugha *et al.*, 2002). This awareness of a broader spectrum of difficulties and the limitations of current diagnostic criteria emphasizes the need for systematic recording of clinical information irrespective of the use of existing standardized instruments.

The decision about whether to use a standardized procedure(s) in clinical practice must take into account the specific concerns and needs of the referred child and family as well as the clinical context. It is this individualized approach to clinical practice that is so important for a comprehensive assessment and for intervention planning.

Structure may be defined in a variety of ways. Traditionally, the treatment plan and therapeutic outcomes determined the interview structure. More recently, the interview style and format (respondent or investigator based), the method for recording and coding of information (paper schedule or computer), whether a live recording is made (audio or DVD), as well as the diagnostic classification system (American Psychiatric Association, 2000; World Health Organization, 1996), and the final procedures for interpreting the information and making appropriate clinical judgments about the data all determine the structure of the assessment. Some SIs use a prespecified diagnostic algorithm (e.g., Autism Diagnostic Interview [ADI-R]; Le Couteur, Lord, & Rutter, 2003) or a final rating scale (such as the Children's Yale-Brown Obsessive Compulsive Scale [CY-BOCS]; Storch, Murphy, Adkins *et al.*, 2006; see chapters 20 & 43) or the Child Global Impression (CGI) scale. Most research studies do not rely on SI generated data in isolation but as a contribution, alongside information from other standardized assessments (such as cognitive and other testing) with observation across settings to produce a "best estimate" clinical judgment. This procedure is often defined as the gold standard in research and clinical guidelines (Dunn, G., 2000; Le Couteur, 2003).

Respondent-based Interviews

Respondent-based interviews are highly structured in both the format of the interview and how the interview is delivered. The interviewer is trained to use the questions as specified in the interview and the informant is required to respond whether the symptom/behavior is present, absent or meets the criterion for a prespecified severity. There is no opportunity for clarifying the concepts used by the informant when answering the questions. It works well (in terms of inter-rater reliability of administration and codings) as long as both interviewer and informant/respondent have the same conceptual understanding of the definitions of the symptoms/behaviors considered and the distinctions needed for accurate coding. Such interviews are relatively quick to administer and interviewers require little training. Administration by trained lay people without clinical expertise can be used to collect precise data; a definite benefit for large research studies (Meltzer *et al.*, 2002; Shaffer, Fisher, Dulcan *et al.*, 1996).

However, because this type of interview requires minimal clinical judgment, one of the risks when compared with investigator-based SIs is the tendency to overdiagnose disorders (Boyle *et al.*, 1993; Shaffer, Fisher, Lucas *et al.*, Reich, 2000). There is no opportunity to adapt the interviewing style, for example to expand on a response to a question to take into account specific concerns for that family. Examples of respondent-based interviews administered to parents include the Diagnostic Interview Schedule for Children (DISC-IV, current version; Shaffer, Schwab-Stone, Fisher *et al.*, 1993; Shaffer, Fisher, Lucas *et al.*, 2000); and the Diagnostic Interview for Children and Adolescents (DICA; Reich, 2000). Both have been extensively revised over the last 20 years, with new teacher versions, translations and the development of computerized instruments (Lucas, 2003). The Children's Interview for Psychiatric Syndromes (ChIPS) (Weller, Weller, Fristad *et al.*, 2000) is a highly structured interview designed to be used by trained lay interviewers with children of normal intellectual ability aged 6–18 years to "diagnose" 20 common psychiatric disorders. As with all SIs, it relies on a cooperative informant. A parent version is also available. Administration time is described as relatively brief and Weller *et al.* (2000) report encouraging psychometric conclusions.

Investigator-based Interviews

Investigator-based interviews provide a semistructured "guided conversation" with the informant. These are more like the clinical situation but with some loss of reliability when compared with respondent-based interviews (Rijnders, van den Berg, Hodiamont *et al.*, 2000). The structure lies in the precision of the definitions of the behaviors and the codings described in the schedule or glossary. The interviewer is required to use compulsory opening questions and supplementary open-ended questions in a flexible but systematic manner, to gather sufficient detailed information to make each coding judgment (Richardson, Dohrenwend, & Klein, 1965). These detailed descriptions of actual behavior contribute to the interview diagnoses and also provide accounts of individual functioning in specific situations that can contribute to the clinician/team's formulation and intervention planning. However, SIs are usually designed for a particular purpose and thus are unlikely to cover all the aspects considered important when dealing with a clinical referral.

Some examples of investigator-based interviews (with a broad focus and others with a narrower focus of study) will be reviewed. Other broad-based interviews such as the Parent Account of Child Symptoms (PACS; Taylor, Schachar, & Hepstinall, 1993) and with a narrower focus such as the Adolescent to Adult Personality Functioning Assessment (ADAPFA; Naughton, Oppenheim, & Hill, 1996) will be considered elsewhere (see chapters 34 & 50). Investigator-based interviews have also been used to assess aspects of parenting behaviors; for example, the Stress and Coping Interview (Mrazek, Mrazek, & Klinnert, 1995) in combination with the Parenting Risk Scale (PRS; Mrazek, Mrazek, & Klinnert, 1995); and the Adult Attachment Interview (AAI; George, Kaplan, & Main, 1985). This latter instrument has been used primarily as a research instrument for measuring parental representations of their early childhood attachment relationships in their family of origin.

Advantages of Structured Interviews in Clinical Settings

SIs provide a standardized framework for obtaining information from different informants according to defined criteria and the psychometric properties of most SIs are published, so standards can be set for reliability of these measures. Most implement current diagnostic criteria, thus minimizing the risk of information variance (such as the potential for individual practitioners to ascribe differing degrees of clinical significance to particular symptoms). Overall results from reliability studies demonstrate that diagnostic consistency is enhanced with the use of SIs (McClellan & Werry, 2000; Silverman, 1991, 1994). The standardized information can also be used for treatment planning. However, there is no evidence in favor of recommending a particular interview for specific applications (Angold, 2002). If no instrument seems suitable, it might be tempting to create one. However, this process is fraught with difficulties and is not for the amateur.

Drawbacks and Limitations

SIs only provide a structure for gathering the information predefined for that instrument. Used in isolation, SIs are unlikely to provide sufficient information for a comprehensive assessment and for planning interventions.

Training staff to administer structured assessments means the investment of significant time and resources with the inevitable impact on other aspects of the service (such as length of waiting lists). However, for some SIs, accessing appropriate training can be problematic (see p. 275) and once training has been completed, achieving the required levels of accuracy and reliability may not be achievable for all trainees. Resources are also necessary for provision of protocols and other equipment (e.g., for recording), for dedicated funding for continuing post-training supervision and longer term for the maintenance of reliability to prevent interviewing and rating "drift." This level of investment is only worthwhile if the use meets a service need of the local population. For example, in the UK there are no recommendations that SIs should be included in the protocols for all care pathways as part of a comprehensive CAMH service (National Service Framework, 2004). However, training in the use of SIs (such as Kiddie-Schedule for Affective Disorders and Schizophrenia [K-SADS] and Child and Adolescent Psychiatric Assessment [CAPA] or ADI-R; see p. 276) can enhance interviewing skills, knowledge and accuracy of CAMH professionals identifying particular problems, although the instruments may require modification for regular use in busy routine CAMH settings (Le Couteur, 2003; NICE, 2005). Further, if a service provides specialist clinics for particular client groups, or for some other reason requires standardized information to be recorded, SIs provide standardized assessment procedures.

Research studies are required to report the procedures employed to achieve reliability in the use of instrument administration, how the results of administration are reviewed and what arrangements are made to maintain reliabilities between interviewers and across research sites. Similar resource-intensive precautions are also needed in clinical practice. Most published SIs have been developed in English. Several have been translated into other languages, but the reliability and validity of the instrument needs to be established for the different client groups, and for particular ethnic and cultural settings.

Finally, most SIs have specified time frame definitions (e.g., "current episode" might be defined as the last week, 4 weeks or 3 months; or the "worst episode" is over last year or a lifetime/ever rating). This may not be appropriate for an individual patient, family or clinical setting. Further, the methods used to "assist" retrospective recall of behaviors are likely to influence the recorded timing of onsets and lifetime diagnoses.

Considerations When Deciding to Use an SI and Examples of Interview Assessments

There are no specific SIs recommended as "gold standard" tools for clinical practice. The decision to use an existing SI will depend on both the clinical question and whether there is an SI "fit for purpose." This section reviews some of the most well-known and widely used SIs, but is not a comprehensive review of available interviews. The examples chosen will be used to illustrate different types and highlight the psychometric considerations and constraints (Del Carmen-Wiggins & Carter, 2004). The use of disorder-specific headings is to assist the reader and does not imply that problems for a child and family should necessarily fit a particular diagnosis. Where possible, links will be made with equivalent observational assessments.

Structured Interviews Used in General Child and Adolescent Psychiatric Practice

Diagnostic Interview Schedule for Children (DISC-I to DISC-IV)

This is an example of a highly structured respondent-based diagnostic instrument in two forms: parent and/or teacher, covering 4–17 years; and a child form for 9–17 years. It was originally developed by Costello, Edelbrock, & Costello (1985) following the development of the US National Institute for Mental Health Diagnostic Interview Schedule for adults (Robins, Helzer, Croughan *et al.*, 1981). Revised and translated over the years (Shaffer *et al.*, 1996, 2000), it takes 70–120 minutes to administer. The interview has a branching tree format with 358 "stem questions." The expectation is that the informant will answer "yes" or "no" to the questions.

DISC-IV covers more than 30 different non-hierarchical mental health disorders (in line with ICD-10 and DSM-IV), together with an assessment of impairment based on responses to six sets of questions about the effects of symptoms on the child's relationships with his or her caretakers and family, peers and school. The timescale covered has changed across the different versions. DISC-IV covers the last 4 weeks, the past year and can generate lifetime diagnoses in some formats.

Psychometric properties of DISC-IV and previous versions have been published (Shaffer *et al.*, 2000) including the performance of the instrument for children of different developmental ages, use in different study populations, and discrepancies between parent and child interviews (Bravo, Ribera, Rubio-Stipec *et al.*, 2001; Jensen, Roper, Fisher *et al.*, 1995).

The interviews are usually audio-taped. Once completed, the scores are entered electronically and DSM-IV and ICD-10 research diagnoses generated for the parent and child versions. The DISC has been used in both clinical and community-based studies, some of which have involved high-risk youth such as those in juvenile justice settings (Teplin, Abram, McClelland *et al.*, 2002).

Voice Diagnostic Interview Schedule for Children (Voice DISC)

A self-administered computerized version of the DISC-IV has been developed. It is recommended by some authors because the error rate for scoring and algorithm calculations is said to be less and the preliminary data show that the reliability of the Voice DISC is comparable to other versions of the DISC (Lucas, 2003). It generates provisional diagnoses of disorders present in the past month. As a self-administered comprehensive psychiatric assessment it may have advantages for certain client groups (Wasserman, McReynolds, Lucas *et al.*, 2002; West, Sweeting, Der *et al.*, 2003).

Kiddie-Schedule for Affective Disorders and Schizophrenia (K-SADS) (Ambrosini, 2000; Kaufman, Birmaher, Brent *et al.*, 1997)

This is a widely used, semistructured investigator-based SI for use with children aged 6–18. There are adult and child versions. It was originally published by Puig-Antich and Chambers (1978) as a modification of the Schedule for Affective Disorders and Schizophrenia (SADS; Endicott & Spitzer, 1978). The interview was primarily developed to identify children with major depressive disorders, but has been shown to be useful in assessing a broader range of psychopathologies. Several revisions have been undertaken (Ambrosini & Dixon, 1996). However, some diagnoses, such as specific and pervasive developmental disorders, are not covered. The interview is published in English (Kaufman *et al.*, 1997) and other languages (Ghanizadeh, Mohammadi, & Yazdanshenas, 2006; Kim, Cheon, Kim *et al.*, 2004; Kolaitis, Korpa, Kolvin *et al.*, 2003).

There are three DSM-IV compatible versions (K-SADS-P IVR; K-SADS-E and K-SADS-Present/Lifetime [P/L]; Ambrosini, 2000; Kaufman, Birmaher, Brent *et al.*, 1997). All provide a current diagnostic assessment. K-SADS-P IVR covers the worst episode in the last year; K-SADS-E and K-SADS-P/L provide a lifetime diagnosis. Each version has separate sets of score sheets (for details see Ambrosini, 2000). The K-SADS-P IVR score sheet has specific diagnostic domain scores that might be useful for evaluation outcome studies.

For the K-SADS-P/L, the authors recommend that parent(s) and child are interviewed separately: parent first, then child. Each interview takes approximately 1.25 hours. After the child interview, the Summary Lifetime Diagnoses Checklist and Children's Global Assessment Scale (CGAS) ratings are completed by the interviewer/clinician after synthesizing all the data and resolving any discrepancies in the informants' reports (undertaking further interviews if necessary).

The interview begins with an unstructured introductory session with opportunities to develop rapport and obtain an account of the problem. The diagnostic screening review covers 20 diagnostic areas and 82 symptom areas (for current and past episodes) using a modular interviewing technique with screening questions and a "skip structure" for symptom areas that are of insufficient intensity. It is the interviewer's responsibility to ascertain range of symptoms, types of treatments and interventions received, if any, and severity of impairment.

The final diagnoses made are based on the clinician/interviewer's overview of the interview, not an algorithm. Both K-SADS and CAPA (see below) provide detailed (DSM-IV and/or ICD-10 compatible) definitional glossaries (Angold & Fisher, 1999). However, most studies use the K-SADS diagnoses as part of a best estimate procedure.

The interviews can be downloaded from the University of Pittsburgh website for clinical and research purposes. To use the K-SADS reliably requires specific training in the use of the interview(s) and in the DSM diagnostic classification system. Recent studies have reported the use of the K-SADS with a variety of interviewers including research clinicians and lay interviewers (who attended a 4-month training program and received at least weekly supervision throughout the study; Axelson, Birmaher, Strober *et al.*, 2006). Interrater and test–retest reliability data are available for the English language versions of the K-SADS (for details of the reliability data and discussion of the validity studies see Ambrosini, 2000). Recent papers have reported preliminary data on psychometric properties for different translations and use in different populations (Ghanizadeh, Mohammadi, & Yazdanshenas, 2006; Kim *et al.*, 2004; Kolaitis *et al.*, 2003; Shanee, Apter, & Weizman, 1997).

Child and Adolescent Psychiatric Assessment (CAPA)

(Angold & Costello, 2000; Angold, Prendergast, Cox *et al.*, 1995; Angold, Costello, Erkanli, 1999)

This is a more recently published, investigator-based, semi-structured diagnostic interview (originally developed at the Institute of Psychiatry, London, UK) which has been used in international research studies and some clinical settings. The current CAPA 4.2 (2001) has versions for use with children aged 9–18 years.

The interviews take approximately 2 hours to complete. The child version does not contain an attention-deficit/hyperactivity disorder (ADHD) section. The overall structure has a number of features in common with other currently available SIs such as the K-SADS (Ambrosini, 2000). The interview is divided into three sections: introduction, overview of presenting problems and current functioning; detailed symptom review; and incapacity ratings. There are 1401 emphasized compulsory probes and 2571 discretionary probes. Interviewers are required to take notes and encouraged to make an audio-taped recording. Each section has an initial screening part and "skip" rules apply if no symptoms are reported for that section. The interview covers 30 different categorical disorders (according to ICD-10 and DSM criteria, including certain uncommon symptoms – e.g., suicidal attempts – but omits neurodevelopmental disorders such as the pervasive developmental disorders), together with sections focusing on family, peer and academic functioning, life events and service utilization (Child and Adolescent Services Assessment [CASA]; see below).

There is a current ("primary 3 month period") and a lifetime version for major episodes of certain disorders. Further developments include new Lifetime Child and Parent versions used in specific research studies (Rutter, Silberg, Colvert *et al.*, 2004; Silberg, Simonoff, & Rutter, 2003).

The authors report test–retest reliability for diagnoses. Their website refers to a 1-month course, provides a contact for enquiries about training and emphasizes the need for regular supervision and fidelity checks. No information is available about translations.

The CASA assesses the use of mental health services by children (Ascher, Farmer, Burns *et al.*, 1996; Farmer, Angold, Burns *et al.*, 1994). It has four parts and takes up to 20 minutes to administer using a mixture of respondent- and investigator-based approaches.

Preschool Age Psychiatric Assessment (PAPA)

(http://devepi.mc.duke.edu)

This is a newly developed, investigator-based, semistructured parent interview for diagnosing psychiatric disorders and symptoms in preschool children aged 2–5 years (Egger & Angold, 2004; Egger, Ascher, & Angold, 1999). It is derived from the CAPA (with mandatory and supplementary probes together with a definitions glossary) but revised for young preschool children. There is no child version of this interview. The interview covers DSM-IV disorders relevant to younger children and symptoms that do not feature in current diagnostic systems. PAPA also assesses disability, family environment and relationships, family psychosocial problems and life events. The time focus is the 3 months immediately before the interview and a lifetime framework for some symptoms. The interview is said to take 1.5–2 hours to administer.

The interview begins with a brief developmental assessment to orient the interviewer to the developmental level of the child. The sections cover topics such as family structure and function, play, peer and sibling relationships; day care/school experiences and behaviors; food-related behaviors; sleep behaviors; elimination problems; somatization; accidents; reactive attachment; life events; parental psychopathology; marital satisfaction; socioeconomic status and diagnostic modules including conduct problems, ADHD, separation anxiety; anxious affect; tics; stereotopies; depression; mania, etc. At the end of each section/domain an evaluation of resultant disability is made. Once the interview is completed it is coded and entered into a computerized database. Computerized algorithms generate various symptoms, impairments, life events and family functioning scores and diagnoses for DSM-IV disorders (Chrisman, Egger, Compton *et al.*, 2006).

The authors report test–retest reliabilities for PAPA diagnoses and scale scores and no significant differences by age, sex or race (Egger, Erkanli, Keeler *et al.*, 2006). To date, the PAPA has been used as a research diagnostic tool. If it is acceptable to families and clinicians, this modularized general diagnostic interview for preschool children may have clinical utility for practitioners working with preschool children and their families.

Structured Interviews for Specific Disorders

Described in this section are four exemplars of the types of SIs in current use in some clinical settings. They contribute to the assessment of two different specific types of disorder: pervasive developmental disorders and anxiety disorders.

Pervasive Developmental Disorders

A detailed developmental history is an essential component of a multidisciplinary and/or multiagency assessment for the differential diagnosis of pervasive developmental disorders (PDD)/autism spectrum disorders (ASD). A professional with recognized ASD training usually undertakes this. The three instruments described below all provide a standardized interview format for the systematic collection and recording of this information while providing different approaches to the topic. Although there is no evidence to date for a particular framework for history-taking within a CAMH service, the history-taking format should use ICD-10 and/or DSM-IV criteria (Le Couteur, 2003).

Diagnostic Interview for Social and Communication Disorders (DISCO, version 9) (Leekam, Libby, Wing *et al.*, 2002; Wing, Leekam, Libby *et al.*, 2002)

This is a semistructured, investigator-based schedule for use with parents and carers. It was designed to collect information on development and behavior for individuals of all ages and levels of ability, to assist clinicians in the diagnosis, differential diagnosis and management of autism spectrum and other developmental disorders affecting social interaction and communication. Unlike most published SIs it was not designed to provide a particular diagnostic category related to current international classification systems (ICD-10 and DSM-IV), but rather to cover a wide range of developmental skills and behavioral features including diagnoses beyond ASD. The interview is used in some clinical settings to help in the assessment of need and guide recommendations for interventions. The authors have reported initial inter-rater reliability data and provisional algorithms to facilitate the research use of the interview (Leekam, Libby, Wing *et al.*, 2002). The information collected can be used to make a clinical diagnosis within the autistic spectrum, a developmental disorder on the borderlines of the spectrum and a psychiatric disorder. It takes approximately 3 hours to complete. Training is required and is available in the UK through the Center for Social and Communication Disorders, National Autistic Society.

Autism Diagnostic Interview-Revised (ADI-R) (Le Couteur *et al.*, 2003; Rutter, Le Couteur, & Lord, 2003)

This investigator-based interview was designed to provide a developmental history framework for a lifetime differential diagnosis of PDD and information about current functioning (over the previous 3 months), for individuals (with a mental age of 2 years or above) from early childhood to adult life (American Psychiatric Association, 2000; WHO, 1996). It was originally developed to form part of a multidisciplinary research-based diagnostic assessment in combination with a parallel observation measure: the Autism Diagnostic Observation Schedule (ADOS; Corsello, Spence, & Lord, 2003; Lord, Risi, Lambrecht *et al.*, 2000; Lord, Rutter, DiLavore, 2001).

The interview has been used extensively for research and for some clinical purposes. Clinicians might consider using it when more information is required for a complex case including a diagnostic query regarding possible ASD or related disorders, or to assess syndrome boundaries. However, currently there are no published standard algorithm cut-off scores for "non-autism" ASDs. The ADI-R does not cover the more subtle or milder symptoms that might be considered clinically as part of the extended ASD broader phenotype but further measures are under development (Bailey, Palferman, Heavey *et al.*, 1998).

The ADI-R contains over 100 items in five main sections: early development; communication; social development and play; repetitive and restricted behaviors; and related problems. There is a standard format with behavioral definitions for each item both on the schedule and within the published manual (Rutter, Le Couteur, & Lord, 2003). Each item or section has an initial compulsory question but the interviewer needs to record detailed descriptions of behavior and activity directly onto the schedule to justify each coding decision.

The ADI-R takes 1.5–3 hours to administer and score (Rutter, Le Couteur, & Lord, 2003). The ADI-R diagnosis is not a clinical diagnosis but the result of combining coded information from the interview.

Training is essential for the reliable administration of the interview. Video training tapes and training manuals are available in English for clinical training purposes. Additional reliability training is required for the research use of the interview. The ADI-R has now been translated into several languages. At present these translations have been primarily for research purposes.

Psychometric data on the ADI-R are available (for summary see Rutter, Le Couteur, & Lord, 2003). The authors have reported good inter-rater and test–retest reliability and shown that the interview is effective in differentiating autism from intellectual disability and language impairment in people with a range of chronological ages and developmental levels. Further studies by other groups have reported both good psychometric properties (de Bildt, Sytema, Kraijer *et al.*, 2004; Lecavalier, Aman, Scahill *et al.*, 2006) and the usefulness of the ADI-R in research studies (Berument, Rutter, Lord *et al.*, 1999; Constantino & Todd, 2003; IMGSAC, 2001; South, Ozonoff, & McMahon, 2005). Recent studies have confirmed high sensitivity (83–91%) but lower specificity (56–72%) for autism (Risi, Lord, Corsello *et al.*, 2006). Recent studies have investigated the relationship between the ADI-R and the observational assessment of the ADOS (de Bildt *et al.*, 2004; Le Couteur, Haden, Hammal *et al.*, 2007; Risi, Lord, Corsello *et al.*, 2006). With increasing awareness of the broader autism spectrum, the original authors and a number of other ASD research groups are currently reanalyzing the diagnostic algorithm(s) for the ADI-R (Buitelaar, Van der Gaag, Klin *et al.*, 1999; IMGSAC, 2001; Tadevosyan-Leyfer, Dowd, Mankoski *et al.*, 2003).

Developmental, Dimensional and Diagnostic Interview (3di)

This is a recently published, computerized procedure devised for administration by trained interviewers with a parent informant using a laptop computer that generates symptom and diagnostic profiles for autism and non-autism conditions (Skuse, Warrington, Bishop *et al.*, 2004). It is an investigator-based SI with opportunities to expand the questions used depending on the parental account. It focuses mainly on current functioning. Parents can be sent a pre-interview package of questionnaires to complete. This information is entered onto the computer and allows an abbreviated interview lasting 45 minutes, compared to 90 minutes for a full interview. The 3di was primarily devised to assess autistic traits and comorbidity in normal ability range children, but may be used with those with moderate or severe intellectual disability. It has 183 items on background child and family information, 266 autism-specific items and 291 questions about current mental state. Algorithms automatically weight and sum responses within domains, and adjust scoring for age and for non-verbal subjects. A structured computer-generated report is available at the end of the interview. The authors, using comparisons with the ADI-R and DISCO to assess content and criterion validity, have published initial reliability and validity data. Training is required. The authors recommend both that the 3di is used in combination with independent observational assessments (such as the ADOS; see p. 281) and the facility to download automatically the 1300 variables to investigate dimensions of ability and impairment within clinical and non-clinical groups. This automated instrument claims to provide new opportunities for the assessment of individuals, particularly those with a range of symptoms including social impairment. The facility to generate automatic reports is likely to appeal to busy clinicians.

Anxiety Disorder

The final example of an SI is the Anxiety Disorders Interview Schedule IV (ADIS-IV), used for the investigation of anxiety disorders. These disorders are common in childhood and, given the high rates of comorbidity, a careful thorough diagnostic evaluation is necessary to establish an accurate diagnostic profile and baseline for planning intervention (see chapter 39). Such considerations are relevant for most child and adolescent assessments and many diagnostic interviews (e.g., K-SADS and DISC-IV) cover the specific symptoms of these disorders (Langley, Bergman, & Piacentini, 2002). These recent DSM-IV-based interviews, including the ADIS-IV, demonstrate acceptable to good psychometrics for these diagnoses (Langley, Bergman, & Piacentini, 2002; Silverman, Saavedra, & Pina, 2001; see chapter 39).

Anxiety Disorders Interview Schedule (ADIS-IV) (with both Child and Parent versions) (Silverman & Albano, 1996a,b; Silverman & Nelles, 1988)

This was first published in 1988 and revised in line with DSM-IV in 1996. There is a lifetime version (ADIS-IV-L) to establish past diagnoses. It also contains a timeline to assist charting onset, remission and temporal sequences of disorders. This investigator-based interview is designed specifically for the diagnosis and functional analysis of anxiety and related disorders including ADHD, phobic disorders and obsessive-compulsive disorders (OCD) in children and adolescents aged 6–18 years. The interview takes 1–1.5 hours, with initial sections for most diagnoses that can be used to screen for disorder. It is able to assess comorbidity and screen for other disorders including psychosis, selective mutism and substance misuse. There is some evidence that the interview is useful in other cultural settings (Rapee, Barrett, Dadds *et al.*, 1994). The parent version contains probes for disruptive disorders and requests greater detail. The child version provides a simpler format and wording. A visual prompt in the form of a 9-point scale "feeling thermometer" is used to assist parents and children judge the degree of impairment (Silverman & Albano, 1996a). Composite diagnoses are made by clinicians based on level of severity and agreement between the two interviews (Grills & Ollendick, 2002; Stallings & March, 1995).

Structured Observational Methods in Clinical Settings

Observational methods involve watching and systematically recording the behavior of others directly as it occurs rather than retrospectively. This contrasts with interview techniques, which typically involve recalling or making judgments about one's own behavior and that of others over a longer time period. Observational methods can be used to assess child behavior and social interactions in a range of contexts. One of their great strengths is that they provide a window on these processes in their natural setting. They can also be used in settings that are intended to mimic aspects of a natural setting, such as in a laboratory or clinic.

Observational methods have a wide range of research and clinical uses (e.g., assessing the nature and extent of a clinical problem, formulating hypotheses about social influences on behavior, evaluating treatment outcome and investigating basic research questions). Observations can be informal and unplanned, such as when observing parent–child interaction in a clinic waiting room, or they can be highly structured, such as those used in clinical research studies.

This chapter focuses on observational methods that entail imposition of some degree of structure in terms of the setting and the way in which behavior is recorded and coded. In order to understand what constitutes good-quality measurement for a given purpose, the principles behind formal structured observation will be covered. However, it is important to note that that there is a continuum from highly structured to more informal methods. Although methods that are closer to the informal end of the spectrum may be more useful in clinic settings, formal principles may be helpful in applying these techniques with greater rigor and validity to everyday clinical questions. For more detailed coverage, readers are referred to general reviews (Bakeman & Gottman, 1997; Gardner, 2000; Hartmann, Barrios, & Wood, 2004; Hops, Davis, & Langoria, 1995; Patterson, 1982; see chapter 4). Margolin, Oliver, Gordis *et al.*'s (1998) paper is particularly useful on practical considerations in using observational methods.

First, what is meant by "*structure*"? In this context it refers to two things: the nature and specification of the setting in which behavior is observed; and the formal method of measuring behavior. A highly structured setting would be one that involves a series of precise instructions to those being observed (Gardner, 2000). Sometimes these are referred to as "analog" settings (Heyman & Slep, 2004; Roberts, 2001). For example, parent and child are asked to interact in a particular ways during the "strange situation," or during a parent–child task. However, other methods specify that the setting will be as natural as possible (Gardner, Ward, Wilson *et al.*, 2003; Patterson, 1982). A highly structured measurement method would be a formal reliable coding system, used to describe and quantify behaviors or interactions of clinical interest. For example, many parenting intervention studies have used Eyberg, Bessmer, Newcomb *et al.*'s (1994) "Dyadic Parent–Child Interaction System" to quantify behavior in the home or clinic. High degrees of structure in task and measurement may go hand-in-hand (e.g., in the "Strange Situation," where both are highly specified). In contrast, many parent–child interaction observation schemes have flexible tasks but highly systematic measurement.

This distinction between types of structure has a clear parallel in interview methods: earlier, a distinction was made between the structure of the stimulus (questions) presented to the interviewee, and the structure of the coding definitions for the reported behaviors to quantify the clinical phenomena of interest. We focus primarily on formal structured observational methods that might be used in clinical research or practice, but we attempt to consider how elements of these methods might be applied realistically and more informally in practice. As with interview methods, the usefulness and feasibility of a particular method of assessment will depend to a very great extent on the purpose of the assessment and the type of question being asked.

Advantages of Observational Methods

Observational methods have a number of advantages. The first two of these are to some extent shared with interview techniques, the other two are more distinctive. First, they have a wide range of uses (e.g., to assess child problem behavior and social skills, or parenting skill, in a natural or contrived setting). They can be used to measure environmental conditions (e.g., the social interactions surrounding problem behavior, or the physical surroundings of the home, classroom or neighborhood).

Second, observational measures appear to be sensitive to treatment change (Dishion & Granic, 2004), and thus are suited to assessing outcomes of interventions for individuals, or as part of group treatment designs. They complement other measures that draw largely on participants' perceptions, and these in combination provide a "gold standard" of measurement of treatment mechanisms and outcomes in randomized controlled trials for some clinical problems, particularly where observable behavior is central (e.g., for measuring conduct problems or social skills; Gardner, Burton, & Klimes, 2006; Webster-Stratton, 1988).

Third, observational methods have high face validity; some have suggested that "what you see is what you get" (it is not this simple). Behaviors are normally observer-defined, and hence can be applied consistently across individuals, relatively uninfluenced by respondent biases, which may result from low mood, expectancy and definitional idiosyncrasies (Richters, 1992). Instead, observer bias can be a problem (Patterson, 1982), but steps can be taken to minimize this (e.g., the expectancy that behavior will change following treatment).

Fourth, observations in structured situations may be arranged so as to "press" for (elicit) clinically important behaviors or emotions (e.g., response to separation or to parental demands). This is particularly important for assessing young or socially impaired children, who cannot report on their own behavior.

Finally, observations are the only way of assessing in detail the nature of fast-moving social interactions. These are hard for participants to access themselves, yet they may be central to understanding social influences on a clinical problem. Observations provide an account of these interactions, independent of the perceptions of those taking part. This has been particularly important in understanding family processes, exemplified by Patterson's (1982) work on conduct problems and Gottman's (1995) on marital problems. Observational measurement of processes such as dyadic reinforcement, peer contagion and responsiveness has helped to build major causal theories of clinical problems, to develop interventions and to test mediating mechanisms (Gardner, Shaw, Dishion *et al.*, 2007; Rutter, 2005). This approach to observation can also be very helpful in clinical assessment, to aid formulation of parent influences on child behavior and affect.

Drawbacks and Limitations

The first drawback is shared with SIs. The time and expertise needed to learn a coding system, and collect and analyze data means that complex observation systems may be impractical for clinic use (Margolin *et al.*, 1998). However, validity depends on purpose. Brief, informal use of a parent–child observation system is helpful for generating hypotheses about family influence, providing feedback to parents on interaction style, or generating discussion and goals for intervention (Dishion & Kavanagh, 2003; Hartmann, Barrios, & Wood, 2004). Non-systematic observations may be less useful for making accurate comparisons of behavior before and after treatment, or between families. Observations can only sample small segments of behavior, measured in minutes or hours. They cannot easily measure infrequent events or summarize across multiple settings and over time. This is an important caution, given that many behaviors vary a great deal by context. Representativeness of these segments becomes a critical issue. A consequence of brevity of observations is that sampling error can also be a problem. Observer bias and reactivity can present considerable potential threats to validity (what you see is maybe not what you normally get), although these problems also affect other assessment methods. However, these problems are not insurmountable, and much thoughtful work in the field has focused on assessing the extent of error and bias, and on attempting to overcome them (Gardner, 2000; Haynes, 2001; Patterson, 1982; Stoolmiller, Eddy, & Reid, 2000). Finally, these methods can only tap observable aspects of clinical phenomena, such as behavior, emotional expression, social interaction or the physical environment. They cannot assess feelings or perceptions of a problem.

Reactivity to Being Observed

Reactivity refers to the phenomenon whereby the process of being observed affects participants' behavior, which in turn may affect generalizability from observation data to other situations. The extent to which there is an observer effect is likely to depend on several factors, including: conspicuousness of the observer; opportunity to habituate to their presence; participants' understanding of the purpose of observation; and demands and setting of the task. These factors are least likely to affect observations of young children. However, even adults may be less affected by being observed than common sense would suggest. Thus, Johnson and Lobitz (1974) found that parents in clinical samples were unable to alter their own behavior during observation (Patterson, 1982). It is encouraging that evidence from other approaches to measuring reactivity has led to a similar conclusion (for reviews see Gardner, 1997, 2000; Patterson, 1982). Nevertheless, it is worth taking steps to minimize reactivity, by allowing time for familiarization with procedures, by having the same observer for repeat observations, by limiting the number of observers present, and minimizing obtrusiveness of their behavior and equipment.

Considerations in Selecting an Instrument or Method

General Considerations

When designing a coding system, Hartmann, Barrios, & Wood (2004) suggest three golden rules: begin with a clear question; conduct pilot observations; keep coding simple. This advice equally applies to choosing from among existing systems. Every aspect of selecting a method is closely driven by the question or purpose of assessment, as well as practicality and resources. Is it for diagnosis, baseline and outcome comparison, case formulation, treatment planning or several of these? What phenomena are of interest? It is important that the purpose is thought through carefully, and that feasibility of observations is tested through piloting. Two very common problems can be revealed through piloting. First, many coding systems are too complex to be of practical use, except in large research projects. Second, many clinically interesting phenomena have a low base-rate of occurrence. Piloting helps clarify which behaviors are possible to observe and code in the context and time available.

Idiographic or "Off the Shelf"?

For research purposes, where comparability among participants is vital, it makes sense not to reinvent the wheel but to use a well-validated instrument with a manual, if there is one that fits the purpose. However, for many clinical purposes, such as to develop hypotheses about factors influencing problem behavior, or to evaluate individualized outcomes, it may be useful to design observations specially for a given clinical situation, which may be entirely idiographic ones, to suit the clinical goals for that individual. There is a lively literature within the field of behavioral assessment on the reliability and validity of individually designed observational methods (Haynes, 2001; Heyman & Slep, 2004; Mash & Foster, 2001), suggesting that rigor need not necessarily be sacrificed in order to answer individualized clinical questions.

What Behaviors to Observe?

In addition to the practical considerations above, selection of behavior to observe will depend on which clinical phenomena are of interest. It may also be linked to the theoretical underpinning of interventions. Thus, within an attachment framework one would focus on different aspects of parenting compared to a cognitive–behavioral framework. Dowdney, Mrazek, Quinton *et al.* (1984) provide a rare thorough discussion of how behaviors were selected, and for what purposes, in developing a parent–child interaction coding system. Many of the systems reviewed below can be adapted to carry out simple counts of a few common behaviors for clinical purposes (e.g., non-compliance, parent negative commands, praise and affection).

Given a particular content area of interest, the stream of social interaction may be described and split up along a number of different dimensions (e.g., a system for measuring harsh parenting might code content, affect or timing of behavior, or all of these). Two considerations are of particular importance: the level of complexity of the codes and the unit of analysis employed.

Complexity of Behavior Codes

Observed behavior can be described and coded in terms of relatively simple, discrete behaviors (e.g., hit, command, smile), or in terms of more complex, higher-order constructs (sensitive parenting, avoidant attachment, play, ritualistic behavior). More complex constructs generally need more inference to code, and as a result may be harder to learn and to code reliably. However, simpler codes may have the drawback of not adequately representing phenomena of clinical interest. Interobserver reliability, validity and resources are key considerations in deciding whether to use complex codes. It should be noted that even apparently simple behaviors require a good deal of inference to code, as social behaviors are rarely captured by definitions based on motor behavior alone.

Unit of Analysis: Splitting the Stream of Behavior

The behaviors selected will guide the process of identifying the most appropriate unit of analysis. For example, event-sampling methods, which count the frequency of behaviors of interest, are suitable for measuring occurrence of discrete events. Behaviors that tend to occur continuously over time (e.g., crying, arguing, task concentration, elaborate rituals) are more suited to timing duration, although this is hard to do for several behaviors at once. Many observational systems record neither real frequency nor duration, instead they make coding simpler by using some kind of time-sampling. This involves recording occurrence or absence of a given behavior in a set time interval. Piloting and consulting the literature are crucial, to check that the time interval is appropriate for the behaviors and the context. Many systems use 30-second intervals (e.g., Dyadic Parent–Child Interaction Coding Scheme [DPICS]); however, this may be too short for rare behaviors and too long for very frequent ones. Much work has gone into assessing the utility of these sampling methods for different purposes (Bakeman & Gottman, 1997; Hartmann, Barrios, & Wood, 2004). Many systems do not count or time behaviors, but make systematic global judgments about qualities of behavior (e.g., Deater-Deckard, Pylas, & Petrill's 1997 Parent Child Interaction System (PARCHISY); Dishion's Coder Impressions Inventory – Jabson, Dishion, Gardner *et al.* (2004)).

Selecting Task and Setting

Observational methods necessarily involve sampling only a small fraction of the tasks, settings and occasions in which interaction normally take place. They may also require families to be observed during unusual tasks or settings (e.g., playing with new toys in a laboratory, or being asked to plan a party together). Yet observational data are normally intended to be representative of the underlying base-rate or style of the given behavior. Thus, it is important to consider and choose carefully the task, setting and duration of observations, as all these have implications for how generalizable, or ecologically valid, the data may be. Caution is needed, given that there are few studies to inform us about whether observations collected in the laboratory and clinic, or during tasks imposed by the observer, are representative of interactions that typically take place in the home (for reviews see Gardner, 1997, 2000; Mori & Armendariz, 2001). This is all the more important because social behavior is strongly influenced by context. It is also vital to choose behaviors that are common enough to be observed during a brief session; otherwise the session will need lengthening. Researchers should avoid designing a system that appears clinically relevant, but where behaviors (e.g., mother "follows through" on threats; uses time-out) are unlikely to occur in a 30-minute home session.

Many different observation tasks have been used to study parent–child interaction in the home and clinic, including common mildly stressful events such as mealtime (Patterson, 1982), problem-solving tasks, tidy-up tasks (Gardner, Sonuga-Barke, & Sayal, 1999; Roberts & Powers, 1988) and tasks where the mother is busy and the child has nothing to do (Gardner *et al.*, 2006, 2007). Others include structured and free play (Forehand & McMahon, 1981). Many minimize imposition of tasks by carrying out naturalistic unstructured observation at home (Gardner *et al.*, 2003; Patterson, 1982). The selection of tasks has important implications for which behaviors will be generated. Employing brief structured tasks is more economical, and has the benefits of increasing the consistency of sampling across individuals or time, and increasing the likelihood of certain key behaviors arising. However, artificiality of tasks that "press" for particular behaviors can mean that behavior is not representative of that seen elsewhere. Although we need to be cautious about their validity, for certain purposes observations carried out in highly artificial situations may still generate sufficient information to demonstrate underlying behaviors or processes of interest (Margolin *et al.*, 1998).

Examples of Observational Assessments

Examples of observation approaches and instruments will be classified by the purpose of assessment, rather than by the diagnostic problem. This is because differences of purpose lead to markedly different kinds of assessment. It is not possible to provide an exhaustive list of instruments; instead, commonly used exemplars will be described briefly, with references to other instruments.

General Classes of Clinical or Research Purpose

To Assess Discrete, Clinically Important Parent or Child Behaviors in their Relevant Setting

For example, in order to measure their frequency before and after intervention; to compare families.

Parenting and Child Problem Behavior

The Dyadic Parent–Child Interaction Coding Scheme (DPICS; Eyberg *et al.*, 1994) is commonly used for assessing parenting and child oppositional behavior in clinical trials and practice, and has a full manual (www.hp.ufl.edu/~seyberg/measures.htm). The system captures common clinically relevant behaviors that can easily be observed and counted in the home or clinic, including child non-compliance, yelling, aggression, and parent behaviors such as praise, clear/vague/negative commands, threats, yelling, hitting. Although there are 28 categories, these can be collapsed into summary codes, or relevant behaviors selected, to reduce complexity and training time. It can be used during unstructured interactions and tasks such as clear-up or parent-directed play. The system has been validated extensively in clinical trials by Eyberg and by Webster-Stratton (see Brestan & Eyberg, 1998) and is sensitive to treatment change. It captures most basic information about positive and negative parenting and child behavior needed to evaluate interventions aimed at these targets.

Others have developed similar systems, described in an accessible way; for example, Forehand and McMahon's (1981) Behavioral Coding System (BCS), which has been used more recently in the FastTrack trial of conduct disorder prevention (Conduct Problems Prevention Research Group, 1999). Somewhat more complex systems, from which behaviors could be selected for clinical purposes, include systems by Dishion, Nelson, Winter *et al.* (2004; see Oregon Social Learning Centre www.oslc.org) and by Gardner *et al.* (1999, 2003, 2006, 2007).

Social Communication and Stereotyped and Repetitive Behaviors

Repetitive and stereotyped behaviors occur intermittently and so may not occur during the defined observation period. In the field of autism/ASD research and increasingly in clinical practice, methods of standardizing direct observations including ratings of repetitive behaviors have been used to complement information from other sources. There are several checklists and observation schedules that can be used for observing individuals. The Childhood Autism Rating Scale (CARS) provides a framework for characterizing behaviors associated with autism (DiLalla & Rogers, 1994; Schopler, Reichler, & Rochen Renner, 1986). It is widely used but was developed as an initial screening assessment and not a diagnostic tool. The ADOS was first developed together with the Autism Diagnostic Interview (ADI) as a "package" of instruments for research diagnosis. It has been revised and published in four modules (Corsello, Spence, & Lord, 2003; Lord, Rutter, DiLavore *et al.*, 2001). It provides through the specification of "social presses," standard contexts for observation of behavior in individuals (across the ability range) suspected of having a possible autism spectrum disorder, ranging from toddlers to adults. This is one of the strengths of this standardized measure. The ratings cover aspects of social behavior, communication, play and restricted and repetitive behaviors. Until recently these latter items had not been included in the diagnostic algorithms (Gotham, Risi, Pickles *et al.*, 2007). The ADOS is widely used in research and clinical settings, is translated into several languages and takes about 30–45 minutes to administer. Training and regular reliability checks are necessary (for psychometric data see de Bildt *et al.*, 2004; Lord *et al.*, 2001). Inter-rater reliability of items across modules is good (kappa ≥ 0.6). The exception is coding of some items such as some repetitive behaviors and sensory abnormalities. These occur less frequently and are therefore more difficult to code reliably. The diagnostic validity of the ADOS algorithm across modules for autism versus non-spectrum disorders, controlling for expressive language, is excellent (specificity score range 0.93–1.00). However, as expected, the distribution of item and algorithm scores between autism and the broader grouping of ASD shows considerable overlap. Differentiation of autism from Pervasive Developmental Disorders Not Otherwise Specified (PDD-NOS) is moderate (specificities 0.68–0.79; see chapter 46).

Fearful and Anxious Behavior

Various observational systems have been devised for assessing children's approach/avoidance and signs of anxiety in response to phobic or fear-provoking situations. Melamed and Siegel's (1975) Observer Rating Scale of Anxiety rates 29 possible behaviors in response to feared situations (e.g., crying, hair pulling, trembling, and behaviors assumed to indicate lower fear, including smiling, chatting). Behaviors are sampled as present or absent in each 3-minute time-sample. The system has been validated in a range of medical and dental settings, but could also be applied to other phobic situations. Another commonly used observational measure is the behavioral avoidance test. This is not a specific test, rather a set of principles for measuring approach or avoidance to a phobic situation, individualized for the child. It has also been used in a standardized manner, where all patients have the same circumscribed phobia (e.g., in a spider phobia trial; King, Muris, & Ollendick, 2005).

Social Skills

Social skills are frequently assessed in analog tasks (Spence & Marzillier, 1981; Van Hasselt, Hersen, & Bellack, 1981), for example, by asking children to role play the situations they find difficult, and coding their behaviors in a standardized manner.

To Assess Factors in the Social Environment that Influence Child Behavior

Most systems for counting parent–child behaviors can also be used to examine relationships between behaviors. This is particularly useful for formulating hypotheses about immediate functional relations between parent behavior and child symptoms. Thus, DPICS can be used to assess whether parental praise or other attention follows contingently from appropriate child behavior, or whether they tend to be elicited by child problem behavior. Gardner, Sonuga-Barke, & Sayal (1999) used observations of a parent–child clear-up task to assess timing of parental control strategies (e.g., incentives or reasons), that is, whether they "pre-empted" child non-compliance, or simply reacted to its occurrence. The pre-emptive sequence was found to be predictive of fewer conduct problems 2 years later. Such observations can be used to generate hypotheses or agree targets for intervention, as well as to monitor treatment process or outcome, examining whether these contingencies change following intervention.

There is a considerable literature on the use of idiographic observational methods tailored to suit the particular presenting problems and contextual factors relevant to that child, in relation to emotional and behavioral problems (Haynes, 2001; Heyman & Slep, 2004) and challenging behavior in learning disability (Oliver, 1995). These techniques can be used to analyze behavior in their presenting context (e.g., bedtime, mealtime, school refusal). Some clinicians make use of home videos to assess and analyze influences on these symptoms, which can be filmed by staff or parents and brought into the clinic for discussion if home visits are not feasible (Juffer, Hoksbergen, Riksen-Walraven *et al.*, 1997; Shaw, Dishion, Supplee *et al.*, 2006).

To Assess the Physical Environment Around the Child

The HOME Inventory (Caldwell & Bradley, 1984) measures the physical and social environment in home through a combination of observer ratings of resources (e.g., books, toys, general chaos) and of parent–child interaction, and an interview with the parent.

To Make Global Judgments about Qualities of Behavior or Relationship

These may be used for various purposes, including clinical description of a parent–child relationship; and comparing families in clinical research; and setting goals for intervention or evaluating change.

Global coding schemes are ones that do not count individual behaviors, but instead make global judgments about complex behaviors, in a pre-set time interval, or across an entire observation session. PARCHISY (Deater-Deckard, Pylas, & Petrill, 1997) is a global coding scheme with 13 parent and child categories rated on Likert scales. It can be used in home or clinic during brief "free play" sessions, or in structured play tasks. In a study of 62 twin-pairs, behaviors measured by the scheme were associated with children's social-emotional adjustment based on parent-report (Deater-Deckard, Pike, Petrill *et al.*, 2001). However, PARCHISY's validity has not been formally evaluated, and it uses generalizability theory approaches to assessing interobserver reliability (alpha range, 0.78–1.0). There is no published manual for PARCHISY; however, its format suggests it would be an accessible scheme to use, as it is designed to be self-explanatory. Although global ratings generate rich information, they carry the drawback of being more open to bias compared to frequency counting methods (Patterson, 1982), making it particularly important for research – or for objective monitoring of treatment progress – that observers are blind to other information.

The "strange situation" (Ainsworth, Blehar, Waters *et al.*, 1978) is a well-known example of a highly structured observation task used primarily as a research instrument for assessing attachment security. It involves observing the child's response to a series of separations and reunions with mother and with a stranger in the clinic setting. The high degree of structure has raised questions about its validity in relation to attachment behavior in more natural settings (see chapter 55).

To Give Feedback on Presenting Problems

A number of interventions involve using direct observational assessments of family interaction and child behavior in order to give feedback to families on the presenting problems. Examples where the intervention has been tested in randomized controlled trials (RCTs) include Dishion's Family Check-Up (Dishion & Kavanagh, 2003; Shaw *et al.*, 2006) and Juffer *et al.* (1997) Video Home-Training. Another example not tested in RCTs is Puckering *et al.* (1994) Mellow Parenting. Dishion's Family Check-Up uses feedback from video home observations, as well as other parent-report assessments, to motivate parents for change. This is carried out by comparing the child's behavior with norms, and with the parents' own stated goals, using motivational interviewing strategies. Video feedback is also used to decide intervention goals and stimulate collaborative discussion of effective parenting strategies. It has been used with young children and adolescents, in both preventive and treatment settings.

To Assess the Therapy Process

Systematic observations have been used to examine therapy processes (e.g., as an aid to clinical supervision and training, and more formally in order to assess treatment fidelity). Examples of coding schemes include Forgatch's Fidelity of Implementation (FIMP), which involves rating content and therapeutic skills during parent management training. Construct validity of the system is assessed by examining predictions from FIMP score to treatment outcome. Forgatch, Bullock, & Patterson (2004) found that higher adherence to the treatment model predicted better treatment outcome.

Reliability and Validity of Interview and Observational Measures

As with any measuring instrument, there are several facets of reliability and validity assessment to consider. Interobserver (or inter-rater) reliability is most commonly assessed for standardized interviews and observations (Dorsey, Nelson, & Hayes, 1986; McClellan & Werry, 2000; Rijnders *et al.*, 2000). The nature of the instrument, its clarity and complexity influence how reliable raters can become (Dunn G., 2000; Jensen & Edelbrock, 1999; Weinrott & Jones, 1984). For SIs there is also the need to consider multiple informant reliability (for review of parent–child discordance see Grills & Ollendick, 2002). Human error and bias, as well as contextual variation in behavior, limit reliability and validity (Gardner, 2000). With suitable training, bias is unlikely significantly to alter observational findings (Patterson, 1982). Nevertheless, it is good practice to keep raters blind to participant status, although this is not easy in clinical settings. Global observation ratings are particularly susceptible to influence of expectations (Lord *et al.*, 2000; Patterson, 1982). In contrast, for SIs higher reliabilities are usually obtained for ratings of global psychiatric status than for ratings of specific symptoms (Charter & Feldt, 2001; Edelbrock & Costello, 1990; Rutter, Le Couteur, & Lord, 2003). Awareness of these issues can inform the use of standardized methods, and interpretation and critical appraisal of research and clinical findings.

There are several indices of agreement, including kappa, intraclass correlation and percent agreement, which can yield different results. Thus, their choice depends on the nature of the data produced and the questions posed (Dunn G., 2000; Repp, Deitz, Boles *et al.*, 1976). Likewise, acceptable agreement level depends on the purpose of measurement and the data properties. However, in practice, many reviewers would regard a kappa or correlation of 0.7 or above as acceptable (Hodges & Cools, 1990). The intraclass correlation coefficient calculates agreement between observers on overall frequency of each behavior observed, and requires continuous data sets, such as frequency counts. For categorical data, Cohen's (1960) kappa considers point-by-point agreement, taking into account the probability of chance agreement, especially important if there is only a small number of categories. In research studies where comparability between participants is crucial, reliability should be checked periodically to prevent rater "drift" away from the original coding definitions (Patterson, 1982). Regular checks will also be important for enhancing diagnostic reliability (McClellan & Werry, 2000) and ensuring comparability across services.

Also important, although seen less frequently, are measures of test–retest reliability. These refer to the relationship between data collected on the same individual on different occasions. If a system produces consistent results across consecutive interviews or observations for the same individual it is considered to show short-term stability, or test–retest reliability. Few observational systems are subjected to evaluations of stability across sessions (Patterson, 1982), although there is evidence that increasing the number of sessions may increase the power to detect change, important in intervention studies (Gardner, 2000; Stoolmiller, Eddy, & Reid, 2000). With SIs there is the complication of attenuation of symptom reports. This is the tendency for participants to report fewer symptoms on retesting and has been seen in most forms of repeated psychiatric inquiry (Lucas, Schaffer, & Richters, 1999).

While reliability assesses if an instrument is consistent in its measurement, validity considers if is actually measuring what it purports to measure and, with observations, is affected by issues of task and setting discussed above. Most SIs use operationally defined criteria for presence of a disorder based on existing classification systems. The investigation of content and construct validity of an SI is therefore directly linked with the validation of childhood psychiatric disorders, itself an extensive and continuous process (see chapters 2 & 4). Predictive and concurrent validity of observational and interview systems is also very important to assess. Concurrent validity assesses the relationship between different measures of the same behavior, while predictive validity reflects the extent to which measures produce information that predicts a future criterion (e.g., arrest, response to treatment, risk for recurrence of disorder).

Integrating Structured Interviews and Observational Measures in Clinical Practice

SIs and observational methods have many complementary strengths and weaknesses. Using both in combination is seen as the gold standard in clinical research assessments, for example, in randomized trials of conduct problem treatment (Gardner, Burton, & Klimes, 2006; Scott, Spender, Doolan *et al.*, 2001). However, in everyday practice, clinicians use information from different sources such as parent interview, observations of child behavior and reports from school, when assessing new referrals. How the information is then brought together to understand the presenting problem and plan intervention requires clinical skill and judgment.

The level of detailed information obtained through standardized instruments may not be appropriate for everyday practice where what is required is a broad-based assessment including the individual's and family's view(s) of a problem(s), information about personal circumstances and their views about interventions and solutions. However, for CAMH services to be comprehensive and for services to be guided by best available evidence, some professionals will need higher level skills in assessment, intervention and evaluation. Training in the use of standardized measures is one way of increasing the knowledge base and clinical competencies of staff. CAMH professionals with this additional expertise can undertake more intensive assessments of complex cases and apply the broad principles of reliable and valid measurement to everyday practice through the support and supervision of other members of staff. Even for staff who rarely use standardized instruments, critical clinical skills can be gained from specific training, which are generalizable to everyday clinical assessment. Thus, training may develop their style of systematic detailed questioning; rigorous approach to observation; critical consideration of the validity of their findings. These ways of thinking critically about assessment are likely to be important for enhancing the quality of clinical assessment and intervention.

Finally, the development of robust mechanisms for the integration of different sources of information is a crucial next step for both research and clinical practice. Two recent very different approaches to this dilemma are the Development and Well-Being Assessment (DAWBA; Goodman, Ford, Richards *et al.*, 2000) and the Child and Adolescent Functional Assessment Scale (CAFCAS; Hodges, 2000). Further work in this area will allow us to advance personalized clinical care within an evidence-based approach to CAMH practice.

Conclusions

Consistent clinical assessments and the evaluations of interventions in child and adolescent mental health settings require the collection of standardized information. SIs and standardized observations provide reliable data and, importantly, may help clinicians to improve their generic assessment skills. However, they are unlikely to meet the broader-based needs of individuals seen in everyday practice. Future developments in CAMH will include an increasing emphasis on standardizing measures and the evaluation of staff skills using direct ratings of observed practice and testing of clinical competencies for professional revalidation. In this context, training in the use of specific SIs and standardized observational measures lends itself to this type of professional skills recognition. Future developments in computerized administration and coding of interviews or observations are also likely to make standardized assessment more efficient.

Acknowledgments

The authors would like to thank Nicola Burton and Jennifer Burton for their assistance.

References

Ainsworth, M. D. S., Blehar, M. C., Waters, E., & Wall, S. (1978). *Patterns of attachment: A psychological study of the Strange Situation*. Hillside, NJ: Erlbaum.

Ambrosini, P. J. (2000). Historical development and present status of the Schedule for Affective Disorders and Schizophrenia for School-age Children (K-SADS). *Journal of the American Academy of Child and Adolescent Psychiatry*, *39*, 59–66.

Ambrosini, P. J., & Dixon, M. (1996). *Schedule for Affective Disorders and Schizophrenia for School-Age Children (K-SADS)*. Philadelphia: Allegheny University of Health Sciences.

American Psychiatric Association. (2000). *Diagnostic and Statistical Manual of Mental Disorders* (4th edn.). Text Revision. Washington DC: American Psychiatric Press.

Angold, A. (2002). Diagnostic interviews with parents and children. In M. Rutter, & E. Taylor (Eds.), *Child and adolescent psychiatry* (4th edn., pp. 32–70). UK: Blackwell Science.

Angold, A., & Costello, E. J. (2000). The Child and Adolescent Psychiatric Assessment (CAPA). *Journal of the American Academy of Child and Adolescent Psychiatry*, *39*, 39–48.

Angold, A., Costello, E. J., & Erkanli, A. (1999). Comorbidity. *Journal of Child Psychology and Psychiatry*, *40*, 57–87.

Angold, A., & Fisher, P. W. (1999). Interviewer-based interviews. In D. Schaffer, C. P. Lucas, & J. E. Richters (Eds.), *Diagnostic assessment in child and adolescent psychopathology* (pp. 34–64). New York: Guildford.

Angold, A., Prendergast, M., Cox, A., Harrington, R., Siminoff, E., & Rutter, M. (1995). The Child and Adolescent Psychiatric Assessment (CAPA). *Psychological Medicine*, *25*(4), 739–753.

Ascher, B. H., Farmer, E. M. Z., Burns, B. J., & Angold, A. (1996). The Child and Adolescent Services Assessment (CASA): Description and psychometrics. *Journal of Emotional and Behavioral Disorders*, *4*(1), 12–20.

Axelson, D., Birmaher, B., Strober, M., Gill, M. K., Valeri, S., Chiappetta, L., *et al.* (2006). Phenomenology of children and adolescents with bipolar spectrum disorders. *Archives of General Psychiatry*, *63*, 1139–1148.

Bailey, A., Palferman, S., Heavey, L., & Le Couteur, A. (1998). Autism: the phenotype in relatives. *Journal of Autism and Developmental Disorders*, *28*, 369–392.

Bakeman, R., & Gottman, J. M. (1997). *Observing interaction: An introduction to sequential analysis* (2nd edn.). New York: Cambridge University Press.

Berument, S. K., Rutter, M., Lord, C., Pickles, A., & Bailey, A. (1999). Autism screening questionnaire: diagnostic validity. *British Journal of Psychiatry*, *175*, 444–451.

Bird, H. R., Gould, M. S., & Staghezza, B. M. (1993). Patterns of diagnostic comorbidity in a community sample of children aged 9 through 16 years. *Journal of the American Academy of Child and Adolescent Psychiatry*, *32*, 361–368.

Boyle, M. H., Offord, D. R., Racine, Y. A., Sanford, M., Szatmari, P., Fleming, J. E., *et al.* (1993). Evaluation of the diagnostic interview for children and adolescents for use in general population samples. *Journal of Abnormal Psychology*, *21*, 663–681.

Bravo, M., Ribera, J., Rubio-Stipec, M., Canino, G., Shrout, P., Ramirez, R., *et al.* (2001). Test–retest reliability of the Spanish version of the Diagnostic Interview Schedule for Children (DISC-IV). *Journal of Abnormal Child Psychology*, *29*, 433–444.

Brestan, E. V., & Eyberg, S. M. (1998). Effective psychosocial treatments of conduct disordered children and adolescents: 29 years, 82 studies, and 5,272 kids. *Journal of Clinical Child Psychology*, *27*, 180–189.

Brugha, T. S. (2002). The end of the beginning: A requiem for the categorization of mental disorder? *Psychological Medicine*, *32*, 1149–1154.

Buitelaar, J. K., Van der Gaag, R., Klin, A., & Volkmar, F. (1999). Exploring the boundaries of Pervasive Developmental Disorders Not Otherwise Specified: Analysis of data from the DSM-IV autistic disorder field trial. *Journal of Autism and Developmental Disorders*, *29*, 33–43.

Caldwell, B. M., & Bradley, R. H. (1984). *Home observation for measurement of the environment*. Little Rock, AR: University of Arkansas at Little Rock.

Charter, R. A., & Feldt, L. S. (2001). Meaning of reliability in terms of correct and incorrect clinical decisions: The art of decision making is still alive. *Journal of Clinical and Experimental Neuropsychology*, *23*, 530–537.

Chrisman, A., Egger, H., Compton, S. N., Curry, J., & Goldston, D. B. (2006). Assessment of childhood depression. *Child and Adolescent Mental Health*, 11, 111–116.

Cohen, J. (1960). A coefficient of agreement for nominal scales. *Educational and Psychological Measurement*, *20*, 37–46.

Conduct Problems Prevention Research Group (1999). Initial impact of the Fast Track prevention trial for conduct problems: I. The high-risk sample. *Journal of Consulting and Clinical Psychology*, *67*, 631–647.

Constantino, J. N., & Todd, R. D. (2003). Autistic traits in the general population. *Archives of General Psychiatry*, *60*, 524–530.

Corsello, C., Spence, S., & Lord, C. (2003). *Autism diagnostic observation schedule*. WPS Edition. Los Angeles, CA: Western Psychological Services.

Costello, E. J., Edelbrock, C. S., & Costello, A. J. (1985). Validity of the NIMH Diagnostic Interview Schedule for Children: A comparison between psychiatric and pediatric referrals. *Journal of Abnormal Child Psychology*, *13*, 579–595.

Cox, A., Rutter, M., & Holbrook, D. (1981). Psychiatric interviewing techniques: V. Experimental study: Eliciting factual information. *British Journal of Psychiatry*, *139*, 29–37.

Deater-Deckard, K., Pike, A., Petrill, S. A., Cutting, A. L., & O'Connor, T. G. (2001). Fast-track report: Nonshared environmental processes in social-emotional development: an observational study of identical twin differences in the preschool period. *Developmental Science*, *4*, 1–4.

Deater-Deckard, K., Pylas, M., & Petrill, S. A. (1997). *Parent–child interaction coding system*. London: Institute of Psychiatry.

de Bildt, A., Sytema, S., Kraijer, D., Ketelaars, C., Volkmar, F., & Minderaa, R. (2004). Measuring pervasive developmental disorders in children and adolescents with mental retardation. *Journal of Autism and Developmental Disorders*, *33*, 595–605.

Del Carmen-Wiggins, R., & Carter, A. (2004). *A handbook of infant, toddler and preschool mental assessment*. New York: Oxford University Press.

Department of Health. (2004). *National Service Framework: The mental health and psychological wellbeing of children and young people*. Available at www.dh.gov.uk Accessed 22nd February 2007.

DiLalla, D. L., & Rogers, S. J. (1994). Domains of the Childhood Autism Rating Scale: Relevance for diagnosis and treatment. *Journal of Autism and Developmental Disorders*, *24*, 115–128.

Dishion, T. J., & Granic, I. (2004). Naturalistic observation of relationship process. In M. Hersen, S. N. Haynes, & E. M. Heiby (Eds.), *The comprehensive handbook of psychological assessment* (Vol. 3). *Behavioral assessment* (pp. 394–446). New York: Jossey-Bass.

Dishion, T. J., & Kavanagh, K. (2003). *Intervening in adolescent problem behavior: A family centered approach*. New York: Guildford.

Dishion, T. J., Nelson, S. E., Winter, C. E., & Bullock, B. M. (2004). Adolescent friendship as a dynamic system: Entropy and deviance in the etiology and course of male antisocial behavior. *Journal of Abnormal Child Psychology*, *32*, 651–663.

Dorsey, B. L., Nelson, R., & Hayes, S. C. (1986). The effects of code complexity and of behavioral frequency on observer accuracy and interobserver agreement. *Behavioral Assessment*, *13*, 349–363.

Dowdney, L., Mrazek, D., Quinton, D., & Rutter, M. (1984). Observation of parent–child interaction with two- to three-year-olds. *Journal of Child Psychology and Psychiatry*, 25, 379–407.

Dunn, G. (2000). *Statistics in psychiatry*. London: Arnold.

Dunn, J. (2000). Mind-reading, emotion understanding, and relationships. *International Journal of Behavioral Development*, *24*, 142–144.

Edelbrock, C., & Costello, A. J. (1990). Structured psychiatric interviews for children and adolescents. In G. G. M. Hersen (Ed.), *Handbook of psychological assessment* (pp. 276–290). New York: Pergamon Press.

Edelbrock, C., Costello, A. J., Dulcan, M. K., Kalas, R., & Conover, N. C. (1985). Age differences in the reliability of the psychiatric interview of the child. *Child Development*, *56*, 265–275.

Egger, H. L., & Angold, A. (2004). The Preschool Age Psychiatric Assessment (PAPA): A structured parent interview for diagnosing psychiatric disorders in preschool children. In R. Del Carmen-Wiggins, & A. Carter (Eds.), *A handbook of infant, toddler and preschool mental assessment* (pp. 223–243). New York: Oxford University Press.

Egger, H. L., Ascher, B. H., & Angold, A. (1999). *The Preschool Age Psychiatric Assessment*: Version 1.1. (Unpublished Interview Schedule). Center for Developmental Epidemiology, Department of Psychiatry and Behavioral Sciences, Duke University Medical Center.

Egger, H. L., Erkanli, A., Keeler, G., Potts, E., Walter, B. K., & Angold, A. (2006). Test–retest reliability of the Preschool Age Psychiatric Assessment (PAPA). *Journal of the American Academy of Child and Adolescent Psychiatry*, *45*, 538–550.

Endicott, J., & Spitzer, R. L. (1978). A diagnostic interview: The Schedule for Affective Disorders and Schizophrenia. *Archives of General Psychiatry*, *35*, 837–844.

Eyberg, S., Bessmer, J., Newcomb, K., Edwards, D., & Robinson, R. (1994). *Dyadic Parent–Child Interaction Coding System – II: A manual*. Gainsville, FL: University of Florida, Department of Clinical and Health Psychology, Child Study Lab.

Farmer, E. M. Z., Angold, A., Burns, B. J., & Costello, E. J. (1994). Reliability of self-reported service use: Test–retest consistency of children's responses to the Child and Adolescent Services Assessment (CASA). *Journal of Child and Family Studies*, *3*, 307–325.

Forehand, R. L., & McMahon, R. J. (1981). *Helping the noncompliant child: A clinician's guide to parent training*. New York: Guilford Press.

Forgatch, M. S., Bullock, B. M., & Patterson, G. R. (2004). From theory to practice: Increasing effective parenting through role-play. The *Oregon* model of parent management training. In H. Steiner (Ed.), *Handbook of mental health interventions in children and adolescents* (pp. 782–814). San Francisco, CA: Jossey-Bass.

Gardner, F. (1997). Observational methods for assessing interaction: How generalisable are the findings? *Child Psychology and Psychiatry Review*, *2*, 70–75.

Gardner, F. (2000). Methodological issues in the direct observation of parent–child interaction: Do observational findings reflect the natural behavior of participants? *Clinical Child and Family Psychology Review*, *3*, 185–198.

Gardner, F., Burton, J., & Klimes, I. (2006). Randomized controlled trial of a parenting intervention in the voluntary sector for reducing child conduct problems: outcomes and mechanisms of change. *Journal of Child Psychology and Psychiatry*, *47*, 1123–1132.

Gardner, F., Shaw, D., Dishion, T., Burton, J., & Supplee, L. (2007). Randomized trial of a family-centered approach to preventing conduct problems: Linking changes in proactive parenting to boys' disruptive behavior in early childhood. *Journal of Family Psychology*, *21*, 398–406.

Gardner, F., Sonuga-Barke, E. J. S., & Sayal, K. (1999). Parents anticipating misbehavior: An observational study of strategies parents use to prevent conflict with behavior problem children. *Journal of Child Psychology and Psychiatry*, *40*, 1185–1196.

Gardner, F., Ward, S., Wilson, C., & Burton, J. (2003). Joint play and the early development of conduct problems in children: a longitudinal observational study of preschoolers. *Social Development*, *12* (Special issue: Innovative approaches to examining social processes in the development of antisocial behavior), 361–379.

George, M., Kaplan, N., & Main, M. (1985). Attachment interview for adults (Unpublished document). Berkeley, CA: University of California.

Ghanizadeh, A., Mohammadi, M. R., & Yazdanshenas, A. (2006). Psychometric properties of the Farsi translation of the Kiddie

Schedule for Affective Disorders and Schizophrenia-present and lifetime version. *BMC Psychiatry*, *6*, 1–5.

Goodman, R., Ford, T., Richards, H., Gatward, R., & Meltzer, H. (2000). The Development and Well-Being Assessment: Description and initial validation of an integrated assessment of child and adolescent psychopathology. *Journal of Child Psychology and Psychiatry and Allied Disciplines*, *41*, 645–656.

Goodman, R., Yude, C., Richards, H., & Taylor, E. (1996). Rating child psychiatric caseness from detailed case histories. *Journal of Child Psychology and Psychiatry*, *37*, 369–379.

Gotham, K., Risi, S., Pickles, A., & Lord, C. (2007). The Autism Diagnostic Observation Schedule: Revised algorithms for improved diagnostic validity. *Journal of Autism and Developmental Disorders*, *37*, 613–627.

Gottman, J. M. (1995). *What predicts divorce? The measures.* Hillsdale, NJ: Lawrence Erlbaum.

Grills, A. E., & Ollendick, T. H. (2002). Issues in parent–child agreement: The case of structured diagnostic interviews. *Clinical Child and Family Psychology Review*, *5*, 57–83.

Hartmann, D. P., Barrios, B. A., & Wood, D. D. (2004). Principles of behavioral observation. In S. N. Haynes, E. M. Heiby, & M. Hersen (Eds.), *Comprehensive handbook of psychological assessment* (Vol. 3) *Behavioral assessment* (pp. 108–128). UK: Wiley.

Haynes, S. N. (2001). Clinical applications of analogue behavioral observation: dimensions of psychometric evaluation. *Psychological Assessment*, *13*, 73–85.

Heyman, R. E., & Slep, A. M. S. (2004). Analogue behavioral observation. In M. Hersen (Ed.) & E. M. Heiby, & S. N. Haynes (Volume Eds.), *Comprehensive handbook of psychological assessment* (Vol. 3) *Behavioral assessment* (pp. 162–180). New York: Wiley.

Hodges, K. (2000). *Child and adolescent functional assessment scale*, 2nd revision. Ypsilanti: Eastern Michigan University. www.ffta.org.

Hodges, K., & Cools, J. N. (1990). Structured diagnostic interviews. In A. M. La Greca (Ed.), *Through the eyes of the child: Obtaining self-reports from children and adolescents* (pp. 109–149). Boston, MA: Allyn and Bacon.

Hops, H., Davis, B., & Longoria, N. (1995). Methodological issues in direct observation: Illustrations with the Living in Familial Environments (LIFE) coding system. *Journal of Clinical Child Psychology*, *24*, 193–203.

IMGSAC. (2001). A genomewide screen for autism: Strong evidence for linkage to chromosomes 2q, 7q and 16p. *American Journal of Human Genetics*, *69*, 570–581.

Jabson, J. M., Dishion, T. J., Gardner, F., & Burton, J. (2004). *Relationship Process Code v-2.0. training manual: A system for coding relationship interactions.* Unpublished coding manual. (Available from the Child & Family Center, 195 West 12th Avenue, Eugene, OR 97401-3408 http://cfc.uoregon.edu.

Jensen, P. S., & Edelbrock, C. (1999). Subject and interview characteristics affecting reliability of the Diagnostic Interview Schedule for Children. *Journal of Abnormal Child Psychology*, *27*, 413–415.

Jensen, P., Roper, M., Fisher, P., Piacentini, J., Canino, G., Richters, J., *et al.* (1995). Test–retest reliability of the Diagnostic Interview Schedule for Children (DISC 2.1). *Archives of General Psychiatry*, *52*, 61–71.

Johnson, S. M., & Lobitz, G. K. (1974). The personal and marital adjustment of parents as related to observed child deviance and parenting behaviors. *Journal of Abnormal Child Psychology*, *2*, 193–207.

Juffer, F., Hoksbergen, R. A. C., Riksen-Walraven, J. M., & Kohnstamm, G. A. (1997). Early intervention in adoptive families: Supporting maternal sensitive responsiveness, infant–mother attachment, and infant competence. *Journal of Child Psychology and Psychiatry*, *38*, 1039–1050.

Kaufman, J., Birmaher, B., Brent, D., Rao, U., Flynn, C., Moreci, P., *et al.* (1997). Schedule for Affective Disorders and Schizophrenia for School-Age Children – Present and Lifetime Version (K-SADS-PL): Initial reliability and validity data. *Journal of the American Academy of Child and Adolescent Psychiatry*, *36*, 980–988.

Kerr, A. (2002). Annotation: Rett syndrome: recent progress and implications and clinical practice. *Journal of Child Psychology and Psychiatry*, *43*, 277–287.

Kim, Y. S., Cheon, K. A., Kim, B. N., Chang, S. A., Yoo, H. J., Kim, J. W., *et al.* (2004). The reliability and validity of Kiddie-Schedule for Affective Disorders and Schizophrenia-Present and Lifetime Version-Korean version (K-SADS-PL-K). *Yonsei Medical Journal*, *45*, 81–89.

King, N. J., Muris, P., & Ollendick, T. H. (2005). Childhood fears and phobias: Assessment and treatment. *Child and Adolescent Mental Health*, *10*, 50–56.

Kolaitis, G., Korpa, T., Kolvin, I., & Tsiantis, J. (2003). Schedule for affective disorders and schizophrenia for school-age children-present episode (K-SADS-P): A pilot inter-rater reliability study for Greek children and adolescents. *European Psychiatry*, *18*, 374–375.

Langley, A., Bergman, R. L., & Piacentini, J. (2002). Assessment of childhood anxiety. *International Review of Psychiatry*, *14*, 102–113.

Lecavalier, L., Aman, M. G., Scahill, L., McDougle, C. J., McCracken, J. T., & Vitiello, B. (2006). The validity of the Autism Diagnostic Interview-Revised. *American Journal on Mental Retardation*, *111*, 199–215.

Le Couteur, A. (2003). *National Autism Plan for Children (NAPC).* London: National Autistic Society.

Le Couteur, A., Haden, G., Hammal, D., & McConachie, H. (2007). Diagnosing Autism Spectrum Disorders in pre-school children using two standardised assessment instruments: The ADI-R and the ADOS. *Journal of Autism and Developmental Disorders* (available online at www.springerlink.com).

Le Couteur, A., Lord, C., & Rutter, M. (2003). *Autism Diagnostic Interview-Revised (ADI-R).* Los Angeles, CA: Western Psychological Services.

Leekam, S. R., Libby, S. J., Wing, L., Gould, J., & Taylor, C. (2002). The Diagnostic Interview for Social and Communication Disorders: algorithms for ICD-10 childhood autism and Wing and Gould autistic spectrum disorder. *Journal of Child Psychology and Psychiatry*, *43*, 327–342.

Lord, C., Risi, S., Lambrecht, L., Cook, E. H., Leventhal, B. L., DiLavore, P. C., *et al.* (2000). The Autism Diagnostic Observation Schedule-Generic: A standard measure of social and communication deficits associated with the spectrum of autism. *Journal of Autism and Developmental Disorders*, *30*, 205–223.

Lord, C., Rutter, M., DiLavore, P. C., & Risi, S. (2001). *Autism Diagnostic Observation Schedule (Manual) – WPS (WPS Edition).* Los Angeles, CA: Western Psychological Services.

Lucas, C. P. (2003). The use of structured diagnostic interviews in clinical child psychiatric practice. In M. B. First (Ed.), *Standardized evaluation in clinical practice* (pp. 75–102). Washington, DC: American Psychiatric Publishing.

Lucas, C. P., Schaffer, D., & Richters, J. E. (1999). *Diagnostic assessment in child and adolescent psychopathology.* New York: Guilford Press.

Margolin, G., Oliver, P. H., Gordis, E. B., O'Hearn, H. G., Medina, A. M., Ghosh, C. M., *et al.* (1998). The nuts and bolts of behavioral observation of marital and family interaction. *Clinical Child and Family Psychology Review*, *1*, 195–213.

Mash, E. J., & Foster, S. L. (2001). Exporting analogue behavioral observation from research to clinical practice: Useful or cost-defective? *Psychological Assessment*, *13*, 86–98.

McClellan, J. M., & Werry, J. S. (2000). Introduction–research psychiatric diagnostic interviews for children and adolescents. *Journal of the American Academy of Child and Adolescent Psychiatry*, *39*, 19–27.

Melamed, B. G., & Siegel, L. J. (1975). Reduction of anxiety in children facing hospitalization and surgery by use of filmed modeling. *Journal of Consulting and Clinical Psychology*, *43*, 511–521.

Melzer, D., Tom, B. D. M., Brugha, T. S., Fryers, T., & Meltzer, H. (2002). Common mental health disorder symptom counts in populations: are there distinct case groups above epidemiological cut-offs? *Psychological Medicine*, *32*, 1195–1201.

Mori, L. T., & Armendariz, G. M. (2001). Analogue assessment of child behavior problems. *Psychological Assessment*, *13*, 36–45.

Mrazek, D. A., Mrazek, P., & Klinnert, M. (1995). The clinical assessment of parenting. *Journal of the American Academy of Child and Adolescent Psychiatry*, *34*, 272–282.

National Institute for Health and Clinical Excellence (NICE). (2005). *Depression in children and young people: Identification and management in primary, community and secondary care*. London. www.nice.org.uk Accessed 22nd February 2007.

National Service Framework for Children, Young People and Maternity Services. (2004). *The mental health and psychological well-being of children and young people*. Department of Health: London.

Naughton, M., Oppenheim, A., & Hill, J. (1996). Assessment of personality functioning in the transition from adolescent to adult life: Preliminary findings. *British Journal of Psychiatry*, *168*, 33–37.

Oliver, C. (1995). Self-injurious behavior in children with learning disabilities: Recent advances in assessment and intervention. *Journal of Child Psychology and Psychiatry*, *36*, 909–927.

Patterson, G. R. (1982). *Coercive family process*. Eugene, OR: Castalia.

Puckering, C., Rogers, J., Mills, M., & Cox, A. D. (1994). Process and evaluation of a group intervention for mothers with parenting difficulties. *Child Abuse Review*, *3*, 299–310.

Puig-Antich, J., & Chambers, W. (1978). *The Schedule for Affective Disorders and Schizophrenia for School-Age Children (Kiddie-SADS)*. New York: New York State Psychiatric Institute.

Rapee, R. M., Barrett, P. M., Dadds, M. R., & Evans, L. (1994). Reliability of the DSM-III-R childhood anxiety disorders using structured interview: Interrater and parent–child agreement. *Journal of the American Academy of Child and Adolescent Psychiatry*, *33*, 984–992.

Reich, W. (2000). Diagnostic Interview for Children and Adolescents (DICA). *American Academy of Child and Adolescent Psychiatry*, *39*, 59–66.

Repp, A. C., Dietz, D. E., Boles, S. M., Dietz, S. M., & Repp, C. F. (1976). Differences among common methods for calculating interobserver agreement. *Journal of Applied Behaviour Analysis*, *9*, 109–113.

Richardson, S. A., Dohrenwend, B. S., & Klein, D. (1965). *Interviewing: Its forms and functions*. New York: Basic Books.

Richters, J. E. (1992). Depressed mothers as informants about their children: A critical review of the evidence for distortion. *Psychological Bulletin*, *112*, 485–499.

Rijnders, C. A., van den Berg, J. F. M., Hodiamont, P. P. G., Nienhuis, F. J., Furer, J. W., Mulder, J., *et al.* (2000). Psychometric properties of the Schedules for Clinical Assessment in Neuropsychiatry (SCAN-2.1). *Social Psychiatry and Psychiatric Epidemiology*, *35*, 348–352.

Risi, S., Lord, C., Corsello, C., Chrysler, C., Szatmari, P., Cook, E., *et al.* (2006). Combining information from multiple sources in the diagnosis of autism spectrum disorders. *Journal of the American Academy of Child and Adolescent Psychiatry*, 45, 1094–1103.

Roberts, M. (2001). Clinical observations of structured parent–child interaction designed to evaluate externalizing disorders. *Psychological Assessment*, *13*, 46–58.

Roberts, M. W., & Powers, S. W. (1988). The compliance test. *Behavioral Assessment*, *10*, 375–398.

Robins, L. N., Helzer, J. E., Croughan, J., & Ratcliff, K. F. (1981). National Institute of Mental Health Diagnostic Interview Schedule: Its history, characteristics, and validity. *Archives of General Psychiatry*, *38*, 381–389.

Rutter, M. (2005). Environmentally mediated risks for psychopathology: Research strategies and findings. *Journal of the American Academy of Child and Adolescent Psychiatry*, *44*, 3–19.

Rutter, M., Le Couteur, A., & Lord, C. (2003). *ADI-R: The Autism Diagnostic Interview-Revised*. WPS Edition, Manual. Los Angeles, CA: Western Psychological Services.

Rutter, M., Silberg, J. L., Colvert, E., & Kreppner, J. M. (2004). *CAPA-C Lifetime Version developed for use in the English and Romanian Adoptees Study*. London: SGDP Centre, Institute of Psychiatry.

Schopler, E., Reichler, R. J., & Rochen Renner, B. R. (1986). *The Childhood Autism Rating Scale for diagnostic screening and classification of autism*. New York: Irvington.

Scott, S., Spender, Q., Doolan, M., Jacobs, B., & Aspland, H. (2001). Multicentre controlled trial of parenting groups for childhood antisocial behaviour in clinical practice. *British Medical Journal*, *323*, 194–203.

Shaffer, D., Fisher, P., Dulcan, M. K., Davies, M., Piacentini, J., Schwab-Stone, M. E., *et al.* (1996). The NIMH Diagnostic Interview Schedule for Children Version 2.3 (DISC-2.3): Description, acceptability, prevalence rates, and performance in the MECA study. *Journal of the American Academy of Child and Adolescent Psychiatry*, *35*, 865–878.

Shaffer, D., Fisher, P., Lucas, C., Dulcan, M., & Schwab-Stone, M. (2000). NIMH Diagnostic Interview Schedule for Children Version IV (NIMH DISC-IV): Description, differences from previous versions, and reliability of some common diagnoses. *Journal of the American Academy of Child and Adolescent Psychiatry*, *39*, 28–39.

Shaffer, D., Lucas, C. P., & Richters, J. E. (Eds) (1999). *Diagnostic assessment in child and adolescent psychopathology*. New York: Guilford.

Shaffer, D., Schwab-Stone, M., Fisher, P., Cohen, P., Piacentini, J., Davies, M., *et al.* (1993). The Diagnostic Interview Schedule for Children-Revised Version (DISC-R): I. Preparation, field-testing, interrater reliability, and acceptability. *Journal of the American Academy of Child and Adolescent Psychiatry*, *32*, 643–650.

Shanee, N., Apter, A., & Weizman, A. (1997). Psychometric properties of the K-SADS-PL in an Israeli adolescent clinical population. *Israel Journal of Psychiatry and Related Sciences*, *34*, 798–804.

Shaw, D. S., Dishion, T. J., Supplee, L., Gardner, F., & Arnds, K. (2006). Randomized trial of a family-centred approach to the prevention of early conduct problems: Two-year effects of the family check-up in early childhood. *Journal of Consulting and Clinical Psychology*, *74*, 1–9.

Silberg, J. L., Simonoff, E., & Rutter, M. (2003). *CAPA-C lifetime version developed for use in the children of twins study*. Richmond, VA: Department of Human Genetics, Medical College of Virginia, Virginia Commonwealth University.

Silverman, W. K. (1991). Diagnostic reliability of anxiety disorders in children using structured interviews. *Journal of Anxiety Disorders*, *5*, 105–124.

Silverman, W. K. (1994). Structured diagnostic interviews. In T. H. Ollendick, N. J. King, & W. Yule (Eds.), *International handbook of phobic and anxiety disorders in children and adolescents* (pp. 293–315). New York: Plenum.

Silverman, W. K., & Albano, A. M. (1996a). *The Anxiety Disorders Interview Schedule for DSM-IV: Child Interview Schedule*. San Antonio, TX: Graywind Publications.

Silverman, W. K., & Albano, A. M. (1996b). *The Anxiety Disorders Interview Schedule for DSM-IV: Parent Interview Schedule*. San Antonio, TX: Graywind Publications.

Silverman, W. K., & Kurtines, W. M. (1996). *Anxiety and phobic disorders: A pragmatic approach*. New York: Plenum Press.

Silverman, W. K., & Nelles, W. B. (1988). The Anxiety Disorders Interview Schedule for Children. *Journal of the American Academy of Child and Adolescent Psychiatry*, *27*, 772–778.

Silverman, W. K., Saavedra, L, & Pina, A. (2001). Test–retest of reliability of anxiety symptoms and diagnoses with the Anxiety Disorders Interview Schedule for DSM-IV: Child and parent versions. *Journal of the American Academy of Child and Adolescent Psychiatry*, *40*, 937–945.

Simonoff, E., Pickles, A., Meyer, J. M., Silberg, J. L., Maes, H. H., Loeber, R., *et al.* (1997). The Virginia twin study of adolescent behavioral development. Influences of age, sex, and impairment on rates of disorder. *Archives of General Psychiatry*, *54*, 801–808.

Skuse, D., Warrington, R., Bishop, D., Chowdhury, U., Lau, J., Mandy, W., *et al.* (2004). The Ddevelopmental, dimensional and diagnostic Interview (3di): A novel computerized assessment for autism spectrum disorders. *Journal of the American Academy of Child and Adolescent Psychiatry*, *43*, 548–558.

South, M., Ozonoff, S., & McMahon, W. M. (2005). Repetitive behavior profiles in Asperger syndrome and high-functioning autism. *Journal of Autism and Developmental Disorders*, *35*, 145–158.

Spence, S. H., & Marzillier, J. S. (1981). Social skills training with adolescent male offenders: II. Short-term, long-term and generalized effects. *Behavior Research and Therapy*, *19*, 349–368.

Spitzer, R. L., Endicott, J., & Robins, E. (1978). Research diagnostic criteria: Rationale and reliability. *Archives of General Psychiatry*, *35*, 773–782.

Stallings, P., & March, J. S. (1995). Assessment. In J. S. March (Ed.), *Anxiety disorders in children and adolescents* (pp. 125–147). New York: Guilford Press.

Stoolmiller, M., Eddy, M. J., & Reid, J. B. (2000). Detecting and describing preventive intervention effects in a universal school-based randomized trial targeting delinquent and violent behavior. *Journal of Consulting and Clinical Psychology*, *68*, 296–306.

Storch, E. A., Murphy, T. K., Adkins, J. W., Lewin, A. B., Geffken, G. R., Johns, N. B., Jann, K. E., & Goodman, W. K. (2006). The children's Yale-Brown obsessive-compulsive scale: Psychometric properties of child- and parent-report formats. *Journal of Anxiety Disorders*, *20*, 1055–1070.

Tadevosyan-Leyfer, O., Dowd, M., Mankoski, R., Winklosky, B., Putnam, S., McGrath, L., *et al.* (2003). A principal components analysis of the Autism Diagnostic Interview – Revised. *Journal of the American Academy of Child and Adolescent Psychiatry*, *42*, 864–872.

Taylor, E., Schachar, R., & Hepstinall, E. (1993). *Manual for parental account of childhood symptoms interview.* London: Maudsley Hospital.

Teplin, L. A., Abram, K. M., McClelland, G. M., Dulcan, M. K., & Mericle, A. A. (2002). Psychiatric disorders in youth in juvenile detention. *Archives of General Psychiatry*, *59*, 1133–1143.

Van Hasselt, V. B., Hersen, M., & Bellack, A. (1981). The validity of role play tests for assessing social skills in children. *Behavior Therapy*, *12*, 202–216.

Wasserman, G. A., McReynolds, L. S., Lucas, C., Fisher, P., & Santos, L. (2002). The voice DISC-IV with incarcerated male youths: Prevalence of disorder. *Journal of the American Academy of Child and Adolescent Psychiatry*, *41*, 314–321.

Webster-Stratton, C. (1988). Mothers' and fathers' perceptions of child deviance: Roles of parent and child behaviors and parent adjustment. *Journal of Consulting and Clinical Psychology*, *56*, 909–915.

Weinrott, M. R., & Jones, R. R. (1984). Overt versus covert assessment of observer reliability. *Child Development*, *55*, 1125–1137.

Weller, E. B., Weller, R. A., Fristad, M. A., Rooney, M. T., & Schecter, J. (2000). Children's Interview for Psychiatric Syndromes (ChIPS). *Journal of the American Academy of Child and Adolescent Psychiatry*, *39*, 76–84.

West, P., Sweeting, H., Der, G., Barton, J., & Lucas, C. (2003). Voice-DISC identified DSM-IV disorders among 15-year-olds in the West of Scotland. *Journal of the American Academy of Child and Adolescent Psychiatry*, *42*, 941–950.

Wing, L., Leekam, S. R., Libby, S. J., Gould, J., & Larcombe, M. (2002). The Diagnostic Interview for Social and Communicative Disorders: background, inter-rater reliability and clinical use. *Journal of Child Psychology and Psychiatry*, *43*(3), 307–325.

World Health Organization. (1996). Multiaxial classification of child and adolescent psychiatric disorders: *The ICD-10 classification of mental and behavioural disorders in children and adolescents.* Cambridge, UK: Cambridge University Press.

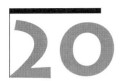

Using Rating Scales in a Clinical Context

Frank C. Verhulst and Jan Van der Ende

There has been an increase in the use of rating scales to assess child and adolescent psychopathology in routine clinical practice. (For brevity henceforward in this chapter the term child will include the adolescent age range.) This is not surprising because rating scales can assist by obtaining and organizing information on children's problems and strengths in a cost-effective way. Rating scales can aid in various decisions once a patient has been referred to a clinic, including whether assessment at this particular clinic is the most appropriate way of proceeding; if it is, what sort of diagnostic assessment should be undertaken, what type of treatment should be provided for how long, what type and degree of improvement should be expected with intervention, and what should be done after treatment? Thus, the role of rating scales to assess child psychopathology in clinical decision-making pertains to screening, treatment planning, monitoring of treatment progress and to outcomes assessment.

We consider issues specific to the use of rating scales for child psychopathology, discuss some psychometric issues and outline other criteria by which to judge which instrument best suits a particular purpose, discuss issues related to the multicultural use of rating scales in clinical practice, and consider the purposes for which rating scales may be used in routine clinical practice.

The main focus will be on scales to measure a broad spectrum of psychopathology; those for a narrower spectrum of disorders/behaviors and for psychosocial features are considered in the relevant chapter elsewhere in the book. We focus on the criteria to be employed in the evaluation of rating scales rather than discussing the pros and cons of the many scales that exist. For a detailed summary of descriptions of the most widely used rating scales to assess child/adolescent psychopathology, we refer to Verhulst and Van der Ende (2006), where over 100 rating scales are summarized.

Issues Specific to Rating Scales for Child Psychopathology

Multisource Data

Diagnostic assessment should be based on information from different sources. Diagnostic evaluations will comprise clinical observations as well as interview information. Clinicians can obtain information on the child's behavior, emotions, rapport and fantasies, as well as estimate the severity and acuteness of problems and the child's motivation for treatment. However, clinicians are capable of sampling only a small subset of behaviors that children readily show in office settings. For example, behaviors such as fire-setting, stealing or bedwetting, and even behaviors such as tics or hyperactivity will not always be observable by clinicians. Therefore, informants such as parents and teachers, who see children in different situations (home, classroom and playground), are needed to obtain a comprehensive picture of the child's functioning. Parents are usually familiar with their child's functioning in many situations and across time. Teachers have the opportunity to compare a child's functioning with that of large groups of peers. Teacher reports may reveal difficulties in a child's academic and social skills that may not be evident to parents. Also, adolescents may sometimes take the teacher into confidence and reveal significant problems to the teacher that the parents are unaware of. In addition to adults as informants, adolescents' self-reports are indispensable, especially on their own affective and other emotional problems.

However, each informant will have a different relationship with the child in different conditions; consequently they often vary in their response to the child's behavior. In a meta-analysis of 119 published samples, the average correlation between pairs of adult informants who had different roles with respect to the child was 0.28 (Achenbach, McConaughy, Howell *et al.*, 1987). The mean correlation between self-reports and reports by parents, teachers and mental health workers was even lower (0.22). In contrast, the mean correlation between pairs of similar informants (e.g., father and mother; teacher and teacher aide) was 0.60. Correlations were significantly higher for 6- to 11-year-olds than for adolescents, and for disruptive versus emotional problems, although these differences were not large. No significant differences in correlations were found for boys versus girls.

The informants' differing standards for judging the child's functioning, as well as their specific impacts on the child and the situational specificity of the child's behavior, are all reflected in cross-informant variation. Children's behavior is often much more variable than that of adults, and children are more susceptible to environmental influences.

Instead of viewing the generally low agreement between different informants as a nuisance, or discarding certain sources

Rutter's Child and Adolescent Psychiatry, 5th edition. Edited by M. Rutter, D. Bishop, D. Pine, S. Scott, J. Stevenson, E. Taylor and A. Thapar. © 2008 Blackwell Publishing, ISBN: 978-1-4051-4549-7.

of information, it is important to regard each informant as a potentially valid source of information (De Los Reyes & Kazdin, 2005). For example, in a twin study using mothers' and fathers' ratings to determine the genetic and environmental contribution to children's problem behaviors, it was concluded that mothers and fathers validly assess different aspects of the child's behavior (Van der Valk, Van den Oord, Verhulst *et al.*, 2001). Unique interactions between parent and child, or differences in duration and contexts in which one parent but not the other interacts with the child, might allow each parent to provide additional information about a child's behavior, apart from the information on which they both agree. Another twin study by Arsenault, Moffitt, Caspi *et al.* (2003) extended this finding by showing that mothers, teachers, examiner-observers and children themselves each reported unique and meaningful information beyond the information that was agreed upon.

Disagreement among informants can be valuable (Jensen, Rubio-Stipec, Canino *et al.*, 1999). For example, children who are reported to be hyperactive by both parents *and* teachers have poorer prognoses than children who are reported to be hyperactive only by parents or only by teachers (Schachar, Rutter, & Smith, 1981). Often, agreement between informants signifies poorer prognosis. However, evidence suggests that discrepancies between information from different informants may also indicate poor prognoses. For example, Ferdinand, van der Ende, & Verhulst (2004b) studied a general population sample of 15- to 18-year-olds prospectively across a 4-year period with parents' and children's self-report rating scale scores as information sources. In general, outcomes were worse if parents and children agreed about the presence of significant problems. However, for some types of problems, discrepancies between parent and child were a strong indicator of poor outcomes. For example, the larger the discrepancy in delinquency scores by parents versus child, the greater the likelihood for police/judicial contacts in young adulthood. Likewise, attention problems discrepancy scores were an important predictor of future use of mental health services, and aggressive behavior reported by parents but not by children themselves was a strong predictor of later substance abuse. Also, children who indicated problems with anxiety or depression of which their parents were not aware, had a poor prognosis. Evidence thus suggests that for most problems information from multiple sources seems to be needed.

As yet there are no fixed rules, such as the use of computer algorithms (Bird, Gould, & Staghezza, 1992), to resolve discrepancies between informants. Instead, clinicians need to evaluate whether differences in information reflect important variations in the child's functioning or differences between informants' views of the child who in fact behaves similarly in each context. Most rating scales for the assessment of child psychopathology have parallel versions for parents and teachers. Some rating scales have versions for adolescents' self-reports, although for some rating scales the self-report version is not parallel to the parent and teacher versions and may tap other domains such as personality. The advantage of rating scales with parallel parent, teacher and self-report versions is that the scores across the different informants can be compared. By comparing the level of agreement between different informants' reports on an individual child's problems with the level of agreement between similar informants typically found for large reference samples, it is possible to decide whether the reports by a particular pair of informants agree better, worse, or about the same as typically found between these informants.

An important question is how the clinician should proceed once it is known if discrepancies between informants on a particular child's problems deviate from the typical level of disagreement between similar informants in reference samples. For the clinician to decide how to proceed, it is important to acknowledge that discrepancies between reports may shed light on the children, on the informants themselves and on the interactions between the children and informants (Achenbach, 2006). Because there are no fixed rules for deciding which informant is best in each individual's case, it is the clinician's task to interpret discrepancies between reports and to decide how to proceed. For example, where certain problems are reported by only one informant and not by others, the clinician might want to ask each informant in an interview to describe the problems in greater detail. Some informants may exaggerate certain behaviors, or they may interact with the child in ways that trigger or enlarge certain problems. Consequently, the clinician may decide to make a particular informant's views of the child, or the interaction between this informant and the child a focus for intervention, for example in order to reach a problem definition that is shared by parents and child.

Developmental Considerations

Longitudinal studies have provided evidence for developmental changes both in level and in type of problems. Assessment has to take account of developmental changes in the level of problems. For example, problems such as temper tantrums or separation anxiety are common and therefore normal at a young age, but much less frequent and more likely to indicate psychopathology at older ages.

Because rating scales are inexpensive they can economically be applied to large normative samples of children from different ages. For young people within the normal range for cognitive and physical development, comparisons with normative samples of children of the same age (and sex) provide guidelines for evaluating behaviors. If the ages of children to be studied differ substantially from those in the standardization sample for the scale, valid comparisons are not possible. Although age effects on overall indices of problems usually are rather weak, they can be larger for specific syndrome scales or for individual problem items, and they are usually larger for clinical samples than for general population samples. Some rating scales employ the same version for different age groups. This has the advantage that scores obtained for children at one age can be compared with scores obtained for the same children at a later age. Provided that there are age-standardized norms, comparisons can also be made on the relative levels of problems at different ages.

Assessment also has to take account of developmental changes in the patterning of child psychopathology. For example, anxiety problems in childhood are often followed by depressive problems (Roza, Hofstra, Van der Ende *et al.*, 2003) and oppositional problems are often followed by conduct problems (McMahon & Frick, 2005). Instead of regarding these developmental changes as indicating categorical changes from one disorder into another, it may also be that etiological factors are responsible for continuities underlying such phenotypic changes. If this is the case then assessment procedures should be capable of tapping continuities. Most rating scales for assessing general psychopathology can be scored on continuous scales. Because these scales are often derived through statistical techniques, such as factor analysis, which determine the ways in which problems tend to statistically co-occur, they are independent of the relatively inflexible criteria for diagnostic categories such as employed by the DSM. Instead of either present or absent diagnostic categories, rating scales are capable of assessing problems in ways that take account of etiological continuities despite phenotypic changes.

For example, the Achenbach System of Empirically Based Assessment (ASEBA; Achenbach & Rescorla, 2001) – including the Child Behavior Checklist (CBCL) – and the Strengths and Difficulties Questionnaire (SDQ; Goodman, 1997) have scales designated as Anxious/Depressed (ASEBA) and Emotional Problems (SDQ), respectively, which consist of a combination of problems of anxiety and depression. The suggestion that vulnerabilities to a chronic disposition of anxiety and depression are closely related is supported by findings of genetic studies showing that anxiety and depression are influenced by the same genetic factors (Kendler, 1996). Using rating scales with overlapping anxiety and depression problems has the advantage that developmental changes in anxiety and depression can be assessed without losing important information, and without assuming that changes in problems are interpreted as indicating categorical changes in disorders.

It is also possible to use separate narrow-spectrum rating scales to assess developmentally related problems such as anxiety and depression. For example, the Mood and Feelings Questionnaire (MFQ; Angold, Costello, Messer *et al.*, 1995) and the Multidimensional Anxiety Scale for Children (MASC; Marsh, 1997) can be used to assess depression and anxiety separately. Likewise, the Eyberg Child Behavior Inventory (ECBI; Eyberg & Pincus, 1999) and the ADHD Rating Scale IV (DuPaul, Power, Anastopoulos *et al.*, 1998) can be used to assess disruptive behavior and attention deficit/hyperactivity disorder (ADHD) problems, respectively. This has the advantage that more detailed information of a specific problem area can be obtained. A problem with the use of separate narrow-spectrum rating scales is that although these scales are intended to assess separate problem areas, they often have overlapping items. For example, rating scales that assess depression may contain items on sleeping problems or somatic complaints that are also present in anxiety rating scales, so that viewing separate rating scale scores as information on separate disorders or problem areas may therefore be partially artifactual.

Abnormality and the Use of Norms

Clinicians spend a great deal of their time distinguishing the normal from the abnormal and between different grades of abnormality. They are confronted with many questions, such as: "Is unhappiness in this adolescent a sign of depression or is it an affective state that is normal for his or her age?" "Is this body weight a sign of anorexia nervosa or is it part of normal dieting?" Patients who are referred for specialized mental health services have been selected for special attention. As a consequence, clinicians' concepts of normality and abnormality are usually derived from experiences with small subsets of patients who do not provide representative data for quantifying abnormality. Nevertheless, a great deal of a clinician's work ends in decisions for situations such as: "Can treatment be started or does this child need further evaluation?" "Does this child need treatment or can we reassure the parents?" "What kind of treatment is best for this particular child?"

The prevailing DSM nosological approach lacks normative reference points and uses similar diagnostic criteria and cut-points for both genders and diverse ages, regardless of the source and type of information. Rating scales that have published norms can be of great help in distinguishing the normal from the abnormal, and between grades of abnormality. These norms should be specific for each gender within certain age periods, as assessed by different informants (parent, teacher and self-report). Using norms in this way makes it possible to determine whether and in what ways a child's functioning deviates from that of his or her peers.

Deviation from what is normal does not automatically signify impaired functioning. For example, a child who walks much earlier than the average child will evidently not be regarded as impaired. However, most rating scales to assess child psychopathology consist of problem items reflecting behaviors that may be a reason to seek help, and higher scores on these items usually reflect greater impairment.

Categorical and Quantitative Approaches

Many clinical phenomena such as heart rate, blood pressure, height, weight or serum chemistries are best measured on continuous scales. Likewise, most (problem) behaviors in children can best be regarded as quantitative variations rather than present/absent categories. This approach allows for inter-individual differences that are normal. Abnormality can be regarded as the quantitative extreme of the normal distribution. This quantitative approach makes it possible to assess the degree to which an individual child's problems deviate from those that are typical of the individual's age and sex. In other words, instead of asking whether a particular child has ADHD, the quantitative normative approach enables us to determine the degree to which the child's scores deviate from those of other children of the same sex and age.

In most behavioral genetic research, child psychiatric disorders are regarded as quantitative variations. Behavioral geneticists view most common psychiatric disorders as complex traits that are affected by multiple gene systems. Because multiple genes are responsible for variation throughout distributions of traits, they are apt to yield quantitative continua rather than dichotomous disorders (Plomin, DeFries, Craig *et al.*, 2003).

Despite the fact that many psychopathological phenomena in children can best be regarded as quantitative variations, the dilemma of the clinical reality is that dichotomous decisions need to be made. The use of quantitative rating scale scores does not preclude the use of categories, which can be defined by cutpoints for distinguishing between cases and non-cases. Although dividing lines for caseness may be rather arbitrary, there are methods for selecting cutpoints that serve certain purposes best. However, there is as yet little basis for perfect categorical distinctions between abnormality and normality. How can we determine which children are most likely to need help? For most rating scales this is done by comparing the distribution of scores for non-cases with the distribution of scores for cases. In the absence of an ultimate criterion for caseness, a frequently used morbidity criterion for general rating scales is whether a child has been referred for specialist mental health services. Other morbidity criteria include expert clinical judgment of caseness, diagnoses based on structured interviews, impairment (Angold, Costello, Farmer *et al.*, 1999) or highly specific criteria for certain problem areas such as movement monitor information to assess hyperactivity (Ho, Luk, Leung *et al.*, 1996).

Empirical Versus A Priori Approaches

Guided by psychometric principles, rating scales use multiple items which are aggregated into scales or syndromes. There are two main approaches, the *empirical* or bottom-up, and the *a priori* or top-down approach, to select and group items. The empirical approach employs multivariate statistical techniques, such as factor analysis and principal components analysis, which are used to identify sets of problems that tend to occur together. These co-occurring items constitute *syndromes*. Each syndrome can be quantified by summing the scores of the items that comprise the syndrome such as "hyperactivity," "anxiety" or "conduct problems." This approach starts with empirical data derived from informants who describe the behavior of children, without any assumptions about whether these syndromes reflect predetermined diagnostic categories. The empirical quantitative approach forms the basis of the empirical syndromes of most general rating scales. Before applying specific syndromes to samples that are much different from the ones from which the factor structure was derived (e.g., in other cultures or in different populations such as twins), it is important to test the factor structure in the different populations (Ivanova, Dobrean, Dopfner *et al.*, 2007).

The second, a priori, approach is to take the diagnostic categories of one of the two international nosological systems: DSM-IV (American Psychiatric Association, 2000) or ICD (World Health Organization, 1996) as the basis for scoring rating scales. This approach starts with assumptions about which disorders exist and about which symptoms define them.

Instead of disregarding one approach for the other, we hold the view that both approaches are needed, and that combining both approaches by adding information from one approach that is not captured by the other, may aid in increasing our knowledge of psychopathology (Ferdinand, Heijmens Visser, Hoogerheide *et al.*, 2004a; Jensen, Salzberg, Richters *et al.*, 1993; Kasius, Ferdinand, Van den Berg *et al.*, 1997). For example, problems in social interactions reflected by high scores on the CBCL scale designated as Social Problems are strong predictors of later psychopathology, even across 14 years, whereas the Social Problems scale does not have a clear DSM counterpart (Hofstra, Van den Berg, & Verhulst, 2000). As a consequence, if we know that an individual has significant problems in areas of functioning that are captured by empirically based assessment procedures, and that are not captured by nosological systems such as the DSM, this information may be an important addition to clinical diagnoses.

Rating Scales or Interviews

One of the great advantages of rating scales over clinical interviews is that they can be applied in a flexible, easy-to-administer and economical way. Administration time is usually modest. Most rating scales will take 10–20 minutes to be completed. They can be administered in various locations such as home, school or (mental) health settings. Rating scales are also characterized by great flexibility in the way they can be administered: in person, by telephone or by mail. Some rating scales have a computer-assisted client entry program which can facilitate administration.

Rating scales need not be administered by expensive, clinically trained professionals. These characteristics make it possible to obtain uniform data across different populations and different settings in a relatively easy and economical way. For example, rating scales can be routinely administered in (mental) health settings prior to or at intake, or can be used in large-scale epidemiological surveys. Thanks to their practicality, many rating scales have good data on reliability and validity (Verhulst & Van der Ende, 2006). This gives us detailed information on the variation that can typically be expected.

Rating scales have disadvantages too, some of which are shared by other measurement procedures. Rating scales are limited to the informant's perspective. Characteristics of the informant and the tendency toward response biases are sources of variation in ratings (Fergusson, 1997; Sawyer, Streiner, & Baghurst, 1998). Rating scales are limited to the structured scores for standardized items. Information that may be relevant but that is not covered by the items of the scale may be missed. It is not possible to explore the informant's responses and subjective experiences, nor is it possible to observe behavior directly. Misunderstandings and ambiguous answers that may be clarified in a clinical interview are missed when using rating scales. Also, slight changes in the wording of instructions, or the wording of the items themselves, may have large effects that limit comparability (Woodward, Thomas, Boyle *et al.*, 1989).

Of course, the main aim of any diagnostic assessment tool is that it measures what it is designed to measure. This is an issue of the validity of an assessment approach. If the aim of a rating scale is to determine the presence or the absence of psychiatric disorders then it is necessary to have a definitive criterion. However, given the present state of the art in the field of child psychopathology there is no infallible criterion that can serve as the "gold standard" for definitively establishing the presence or absence of most disorders, and the boundaries between them.

One way to test the validity of a rating scale is to test the relationship between rating scale scores and DSM diagnoses derived from structured or semistructured interviews (Jensen *et al.*, 1993; Kasius, Ferdinand, Van den Berg *et al.*, 1997). However, there is little empirical ground for assuming that one approach is intrinsically superior to the other. The view that we cannot a priori assume that greater diagnostic accuracy or objectivity can be obtained by using (semi)structured interviews is supported by a meta-analysis of 30 studies with information on the agreement between structured interviews and typical clinical diagnostic evaluations (Rettew, Doyle, Achenbach *et al.*, 2006 unpublished data). This metaanalysis showed that overall diagnostic agreement between (semi)structured interviews and clinical evaluations was poor, with a mean kappa of 0.21. This study could not determine which method was more problematic. Both methods have strengths and weaknesses.

Another study supporting the view that fully structured, as opposed to semistructured, psychiatric interviews cannot be regarded as superior over other assessment approaches is by Boyle, Offord, Racine *et al.* (1997), who compared the associations of a rating scale (the Ontario Child Health Study scales) versus a psychiatric interview (the revised version of the Diagnostic Interview for Children and Adolescents; DICA) to external validators. They concluded that differences between the two assessment procedures in validity were small, and where present they showed somewhat better performance for the rating scales than for the interview.

Ferdinand, Hoogerheide, Van der Ende *et al.* (2003) studied the 3-year predictive value of parents', teachers' and clinicians' judgment of problems in a clinical sample of 6- to 12-year-olds. Parent and teacher information was superior to clinical judgment regarding the prediction of prolonged out-patient treatment, school problems and police/judicial contacts. However, clinicians' observations of attentional problems in children during a semistandardized interview were needed to obtain an optimal estimation of the prognosis. Clinical observations were especially strong predictors of later use of in-patient services. Clinicians who performed the diagnostic interviews were not involved in later treatment decisions. Each of the three informants provided unique information to the prediction of outcomes. It could be concluded that none of the informants was superior to the others in all instances and all three information sources were needed to optimize the prediction of outcomes.

Multicultural Issues

Multicultural populations containing minorities, immigrants and refugees characterize many contemporary societies. When evaluating children of different cultures within one country, mental health professionals must determine whether problems merely reflect cultural differences or whether they reflect needs for professional help (Bengi-Arslan, Verhulst, van der Ende *et al.*, 1997). To help children from various cultural backgrounds we need:

1 Assessment instruments that are available in various languages;

2 Assessment procedures that generate results that are comparable across cultures; and

3 Norms based on representative samples of children living in the original home countries.

If this is the case, rating scales for identifying variations in behavioral and emotional problems can be applied by professionals under diverse conditions.

Because many cultures lack well-standardized indigenous instruments for assessing children, instruments developed in one culture are often translated and adapted for use in other cultures. To apply such instruments to other cultures, they should be tested in various ways to maximize the equivalence of data obtained in the different cultures (Bird, 1996; Canino & Bravo, 1999). Norms derived from epidemiological samples can be used for evaluating a child's problems in relation to those of peers in the child's specific culture. Children whose problems significantly exceed the norms may need more detailed assessments. Norms thus provide clinicians with information with which to evaluate each child's problems.

An important question is whether the clinician who evaluates children of different cultures should compare a child's problem scores to norms derived for representative samples of children living in the original home countries, or to norms derived for majority groups of children living in the host country (see chapter 15). Comparisons of parents' reports of problems for children in 31 cultures, of teachers' reports in 21 cultures and of youths' self-reports in 24 cultures (Rescorla, Achenbach, Ivanova *et al.*, in press; Rescorla *et al.*, 2007a; Rescorla, Achenbach, Ginzburg *et al.*, 2007b) have indicated that, when the same standardized assessment procedures are used to assess children from different cultures, cultural differences per se do not lead to big differences in reported problems. Although it was found that individual differences within each cultural group are larger than differences between cultures, differences between some cultures may be too big to disregard. For clinicians this means that decisions on whether a child needs help and, if so, what kind of help, need to be based on appropriate norms.

Obtaining information from multiple informants is especially important when there are cultural differences between mental health professionals and those who are being assessed. For example, it was found that parent-reported and self-reported problem scores for Moroccan youths were similar or even lower than scores obtained for Turkish youths and for Dutch youths in the Netherlands (Stevens, Pels, Bengi-Arslan *et al.*, 2003). However, Dutch teachers reported substantially higher levels of externalizing problems for Moroccan youths than for Turkish and Dutch youths. If parents from a particular culture systematically underreport their children's problems, clinicians may need to obtain fuller evaluations from other informants and to explore issues that may be responsible for this under-reporting, such as the parents' lack of awareness of their child's problem behavior outside the home.

Use of Rating Scales in Clinical Practice

After referral to mental health services, the clinician and patient go through a sequence of steps. Although this clinical process will vary, the typical sequence has six steps: referral, diagnostic assessment, diagnostic formulation, treatment, treatment effect monitoring and outcomes evaluation. Rating scales can be useful for obtaining and organizing the information needed for making decisions during the clinical process. When we base decisions on explicit rules that follow assessment data on individual cases, we may improve our ways of helping children and adolescents. The process from first contact of a parent with the clinic to the termination of treatment consists of a chain of decisions. Assessment data need to be tailored to the specific needs for each step that precedes a decision.

Referral and the Use of Rating Scales as Screening Tools

When parents contact a clinic about their child's behavior, the first decision is whether assessment at this particular clinic is the best way of proceeding, or whether the child and the parents should seek help elsewhere. Baseline information about the behavioral and emotional functioning of the child can be obtained in a cost-effective way by having parents and other informants complete rating scales as screening tools, for instance by mailing them. Broad-spectrum rating scales can quickly identify children in need of mental health services. Narrower spectrum rating scales may then be used for more detailed assessment of specific disorders or behaviors.

Distributions of problem scores for cases typically overlap with distributions for non-cases. As a consequence, every possible cutpoint results in some degree of misclassification (Fombonne, 2002). The effectiveness of a cutpoint can be described in terms of the rate of true positives (*sensitivity*) and the rate of true negatives (*specificity*) (Rothman & Greenland, 1998). Any cutpoint that is chosen is a trade-off between sensitivity and specificity. The accuracy of a measure can also be expressed as the extent to which being categorized as a case or as a non-case predicts the presence of the disorder. The *predictive value of a positive test* (PV+) reflects the proportion of those with a positive test who have the disorder. By contrast, the *predictive value of a negative test* (PV–) reflects the proportion of those with a negative test who do not have the disorder. These measures estimate the probability that a particular score means that an individual has a certain disorder. The predictive value of a test is strongly influenced by the prevalence of the disorder. In a sample with relatively few disordered individuals, the PV+ of even a very specific test will be low, because a "positive" result on the test will yield many false positives. If the same test is used in a sample with a much higher prevalence, the PV+ will be much higher. Although the problem of low base rates for predicting rare conditions, even with highly valid tests, was observed long ago (Meehl & Rosen, 1955), Clark and Harrington (1998) showed that few child mental health professionals who regularly use rating scales in clinical practice were aware of this problem.

However, the generally modest PV+, even for valid rating scales, shows that a single measure should not be the only source of information when important decisions must be made for individual patients. Clinicians should make decisions for individual patients after evaluating all available information, including psychiatric parent and child interviews, psychological and physical test data, and information on social competence.

The utility of a rating scale does not depend only upon its classification efficiency (Maruish, 2004). It is equally important that:

1 Rating scales are easily integrated into an agency's daily regimen of service delivery;
2 Clinicians know how to use the information obtained from the rating scales; and
3 The agency's staff are committed to the screening process.

Diagnostic Assessment

After obtaining referral data and rating scale scores on the child's emotional and behavioral problems, the next step in the sequence of clinical case management is the interview with the child, with the parents and with other relevant informants.

Interviews with parents are essential for most mental health evaluations of children. Such interviews are needed not only to obtain information for making diagnoses, but also to accomplish other important tasks that cannot be fulfilled by rating scales, such as: forming a therapeutic relationship to promote collaborative problem-solving; establishing effective communication between clinicians and parents; and formulating ideas about what the parents have done or can do to help their child. Interviews with parents also lay the groundwork for the next steps, including decisions about further evaluation and implementation of interventions. Interviews with the children themselves are also essential, while interviews with teachers and other informants may be helpful as well.

The findings to date suggest that neither interviews nor rating scales are intrinsically better for all assessment purposes. In one of the few studies on the effects of combining interview and rating scale data, Ferdinand *et al.* (2004a) tested the ability of DISC/DSM-III-R diagnoses and CBCL scores to predict poor outcome variables longitudinally. The combination of both assessment procedures provided better predictions of outcomes than either procedure separately.

Diagnostic Formulation

The next steps in the clinical process are to form an integrative conception of the case, including etiological and prognostic hypotheses, and to come up with a comprehensive diagnostic formulation (see chapter 4). The clinician not only formulates a picture of the important phenotypic features, the school situation and the environment of the child, but also formulates hypotheses about risk and prognostic factors affecting the child's functioning, and how these factors can be modified by treatment. The clinician will usually decide whether criteria are met for particular DSM or ICD diagnoses. The integrative conception of a case also involves weighting the child's competencies that may affect the outcome. The diagnostic formulation should thus ideally contain information that will facilitate the planning of specific therapeutic interventions.

Treatment Planning

After formulating a diagnosis, the clinician needs to identify targets for intervention and to determine which treatment works best for a particular type of problem. In children with multiple problems, it should be decided which aspects of the child's functioning should be treated first. Treatment planning consists of the development of a set of goals for a child and his or her family and the specific means by which the therapist will work toward those goals. In clinical practice, interviews will play an important part for targeting major goals for treatment. Rating scales for the assessment of psychopathology can aid in the treatment planning process by providing information on secondary but significant problems that might otherwise be overlooked. Because a categorical diagnosis only indicates the presence of a specific condition, it does not give us information on the *severity* of the problems. An estimate of the severity of problems will be made by the clinician using different sources of information, including information obtained through the clinical interview.

Impairment Measures

Another important aspect of a child's functioning that can help the clinician in a number of decisions, including the appropriate level of care, the appropriate therapeutic approach and the need for medication, is the extent to which the child's problems affect functioning in the family, in school, with peers, and activities such as sports or hobbies. Some broad band rating scales such as the CBCL and the SDQ contain items reflecting social competencies or prosocial behaviors which can be used as an index of general impairment. A number of scales are specifically designed to assess functional impairment (Verhulst & Van der Ende, 2006). The most commonly used scale is the Children's Global Assessment Scale (CGAS; Shaffer, Gould, Brasic *et al.*, 1983). The CGAS correlates well with other clinician-rated measures of impairment and is found to be sensitive to response to treatment in a variety of studies. Another impairment scale, the Child and Adolescent Functional Assessment Scale (CAFAS; Hodges, 2004), discriminated well between children and adolescents receiving different levels of care. Higher scores on the CAFAS were associated with more restrictive care, higher cost, more bed days and more days of service.

Treatment Effect Monitoring

After selecting a treatment, it is important to determine whether an intervention produces the desired improvements. Treatment goals can be set prior to treatment and can be defined as a certain decrease in problem scores on a rating scale from pre- to post-treatment, or as the absence of DSM diagnoses that were present prior to treatment (Hayward, Varady, Albano *et al.*, 2000). A problem with using DSM diagnoses as improvement criteria is that significant improvements within the clinical range will remain undetected. When using pre- to post-treatment rating scale scores, decisions should be made about the magnitude of change that will be regarded as sufficient improvement. A reliable change index tests whether pre- to post-treatment score differences surpass the boundaries of the standard error of measurement, usually defined as the 95% confidence interval based on test–retest reliability data. Most manuals of commonly used scales give readily available guidelines for evaluating individual children's change in scale scores.

Of course, the least costly intervention should be chosen if several interventions are equally effective (see chapter 10). If improvement is insufficient, other interventions should be tried. Actuarial tests of relations between diagnostic data and outcomes for large samples of cases may provide useful evidence.

The utility of a rating scale for treatment monitoring will depend on its sensitivity to possible changes in response to treatment. Specific information on sensitivity to change has been published for only a few broad-spectrum scales. However, in the literature numerous examples of the utility of rating scales to assess therapeutic effects are reported. The Conners' Rating Scales–Revised (CRS; Conners, 1997) have been shown to be sensitive to the effects of drug treatment of hyperactive children (Kollins, Epstein, & Conners, 2004). Both the SDQ and the CBCL have been found to be sensitive to change and to be useful for evaluating the clinical significance of therapeutic interventions (Kendall, Marrs-Garcia, Nath *et al.*, 1999). Recently, brief measures have become available which require only minutes to complete and provide information on multiple domains of functioning for evaluating treatment (Lambert, Whipple, Hawkins *et al.*, 2003). These measures can be used for ongoing assessment and monitoring of patients from the beginning to the end of treatment and using the information to chart progress and make decisions about treatment (Kazdin, 2005).

A well-known but poorly understood phenomenon that complicates the evaluation of the effects of therapeutic intervention is the repeated finding that problem scores decline from the first to the second administration of rating scales and interviews (Edelbrock, Costello, Dulcan *et al.*, 1985; Helzer, Robins, McEvoy *et al.*, 1985). This is called *test–retest attenuation*. For example, it was found that for some CBCL scales readministration resulted in a decrease in problem scores across a 1-week interval (Achenbach & Rescorla, 2001). However, the magnitude of the decline in scores was small and only present for a minority of the specific scales. It has also been found that the longer the interval between administrations, the weaker the effect of test–retest attenuation is likely to be (Verhulst & Althaus, 1988; Verhulst, Koot, & Bergen, 1990). Test–retest attenuation is a general tendency for reports of problems to decline from a first to a second assessment regardless of whether many or few problems are reported. Thus, test–retest attenuation differs from *regression toward the mean*, which reflects the tendency of extremely high or extremely low scores to subsequently become closer to the mean of the entire sample at a second assessment than at an initial assessment. Both test–retest attenuation and regression toward the mean may contribute to declines in problem scores for children who initially obtain high problem scores. Of course, this complicates the assessment of intervention effects. Consequently, children should be reassessed on more than one occasion, and evaluations of interventions should employ designs that include random assignment to an intervention and control group which is assessed repeatedly in the same ways as the intervention group before and after the intervention conditions.

Outcome Evaluations

To evaluate outcomes of child mental health services, baseline rating scale measures obtained at the time of referral can be compared with measures obtained after services have been provided. The intervals for monitoring treatment effects should be geared to the type of problem, the type of intervention and the effects that are found. By contrast, outcome evaluations are most useful when they are carried out at uniform intervals across all cases seen in a particular clinical setting. This makes it easier to draw generalizable conclusions about whether the interventions were effective. Outcomes can be determined by repeating the intake assessment measures at regular intervals, for instance after 4, 6, 12 and 18 months. Outcomes need not only pertain to problem behaviors, but may include all kinds of areas important for the child's functioning, including physical health, social functioning, school functioning and family functioning.

Research on treatment outcomes makes use of statistical analyses that differ from analyses that help clinicians decide whether sufficient treatment progress has been made. For many rating scales, information is provided that clinicians can use to judge whether changes in scale scores exceed the error of measurement. For example, if the standard error of measurement (SEM) is provided separately for samples of children by age and gender, it is possible to evaluate whether a change in scale scores exceeds the change expected by chance (Sheldrick, Kendall, & Heimberg, 2001).

Criteria for Selecting a Rating Scale

The suitability of a rating scale for certain purposes can be judged by a number of characteristics: applicability, acceptability, practicality, reliability, validity and sensitivity to change. There are many similarities between the different rating scales. Some scales cover roughly similar contents, most have evidence of adequate reliability and validity, most are user-friendly and most can be scored in a comprehensive way. However, there are some differences that may be relevant for some purposes. Answers to the following questions may aid in making a choice of which scale to use.

1 Do I need a broad- or narrow-spectrum rating scale, or both? For example, in a specialist clinic for children with eating disorders, one might need a narrow-spectrum rating scale with detailed questions on eating behaviors such as food preoccupation, dieting, vomiting and preoccupation with body weight. However, because patients with eating disorders often have other problems, it might be equally important to use a broad-spectrum scale to assess behavioral and emotional problems in addition to the narrow-spectrum scale.

2 Do I need multiple informants? If so, a scale that has separate versions should be chosen.

3 Do I need a rating scale for early assessment or screening of every individual who comes into a service, or do I need one for more extensive clinical evaluation, and will the instrument be completed for one individual or for many individuals by the same informant (e.g., all children in one classroom by one teacher)? Most scales take 10–20 minutes to complete, but there are shorter scales available.

4 Do I need a brief rating scale for monitoring treatment progress?

5 Do I need to assess problems only, or do I need a scale that has competence or adaptive functioning items as well?

6 Do I want to obtain ratings that can be scored on DSM-oriented scales, on empirically derived scales, or on both?

7 Are translations of the instrument available in the languages that I need?

8 Are there local norms available for the assessment scale to allow comparison?

Conclusions

Over the last decades, advances have been made in the development and evaluation of rating scales to assess child psychopathology. Knowledge of developmental psychopathology has benefitted from the application of measures to assess child psychopathology in systematic research. More recently, rating scales are being increasingly applied in clinical contexts. They are not a short-cut to clinical diagnosis, but an aid in obtaining and organizing information on children's problems and strengths in a cost-effective way throughout the process of case formulation, treatment planning, treatment monitoring and outcome evaluations.

Child psychiatric practice is moving away from the use of unfocused lengthy diagnostic procedures of unknown reliability and validity towards brief, problem-oriented, reliable and well-validated diagnostic procedures (see chapters 18 & 71). At the same time, the field is moving from the use of therapeutic strategies with unknown effectiveness towards evidence-based treatments with proven effectiveness. Rating scales can greatly assist in more cost-effective diagnostic assessments and treatment planning by aiding clinicians addressing referral complaints, relevant diagnostic issues and characteristics of children, parents and families. Also, rating scales can be economically used for treatment monitoring and outcome assessment.

The use of instruments that require minimal clinician time is not only cost saving, it also enables clinicians to focus on diagnostic and treatment aspects that cannot be replaced by standardized procedures. An upcoming trend is the use of computer- and Internet-based assessments. Rating scales can be completed by parents, teachers or children themselves by Internet and scored prior to the first appointment in a clinic.

Influenced by cost and time considerations, the change in the field towards more evidenced-based practice, as well as developments towards more pluralistic societies, there are a number of future challenges. There will probably be an increase in the need for brief, disorder-specific, symptom- or problem-focused narrow-band rating scales to be used for treatment monitoring and outcome assessments. Second, the increasing availability of computer-assisted techniques will result in time saving. A major challenge for the near future will be to integrate Internet-based assessments into daily clinical practice. Third, rating scales can have a role in providing closer linkage between assessments at the different stages of the clinical process, including diagnostic assessment, treatment planning, treatment monitoring and outcome evaluations. Fourth, for children from multiple cultures who live together in one society, the availability of norms based on representative samples of children living in the original home countries can greatly aid in the assessment of such children who are in need of professional help.

References

Achenbach, T. M. (2006). As others see us: Clinical and research implications of cross-informant correlations for psychopathology. *Current Directions in Psychological Science*, *15*, 94–98.

Achenbach, T. M., McConaughy, S. H., & Howell, C. T. (1987). Child/adolescent behavioral and emotional problems: Implications of cross-informant correlations for situational specificity. *Psychological Bulletin*, *101*, 213–232.

Achenbach, T. M., & Rescorla, L. A. (2001). *Manual for the ASEBA school age forms and profiles*. Burlington, VT: University of Vermont, Research Center for Children, Youth and Families.

American Psychiatric Association. (2000). Diagnostic and statistical manual of mental disorders (4th edn.), Text revision. Washington, DC: American Psychiatric Association.

Angold, A., Costello, E. J., Messer, S. C., Pickles, A., Winder, F., & Silver, D. (1995). Development of a short questionnaire for use in epidemiological studies of depression in children and adolescents. *International Journal of Methods in Psychiatric Research*, *5*, 237–249.

Angold, A., Costello, E. J., Farmer, E. M., Burns, B. J., & Erkanli, A. (1999). Impaired but undiagnosed. *Journal of the American Academy of Child and Adolescent Psychiatry*, *38*, 129–137.

Arsenault, L., Moffitt, T. E., Caspi, A., Taylor, A., Rijsdijk, F. V., Jaffee, S. R., *et al.* (2003). Strong genetic effects on cross-situational antisocial behavior among 5-year-old children according to mothers, teachers, examiner-observers, and twins' self-reports. *Journal of Child Psychology and Psychiatry*, *44*, 832–849.

Bengi-Arslan, L., Verhulst, F. C., van der Ende, J., & Erol, N. (1997). Understanding childhood (problem) behaviors from a cultural perspective: comparison of problem behaviors and competencies in Turkish immigrant, Turkish and Dutch children. *Social Psychiatry and Psychiatric Epidemiology*, *32*, 477–484.

Bird, H. R. (1996). Epidemiology of childhood disorders in a cross-cultural context. *Journal of Child Psychology and Psychiatry*, *37*, 35–49.

Bird, H. R., Gould, M. S., & Staghezza, B. (1992). Aggregating data from multiple informants in child psychiatry epidemiological research. *Journal of the American Academy of Child and Adolescent Psychiatry*, *31*, 78–85.

Boyle, M. H., Offord, D. R., Racine, Y. A., Szatmari, P., Sanford, M., & Fleming, J. E. (1997). Interview versus checklists: adequacy for classifying childhood psychiatric disorder based on parent reports. *Archives of General Psychiatry*, *54*, 793–799.

Canino, G., & Bravo, M. (1999). The translation and adaptation of diagnostic instruments for cross-cultural use. In D. Shaffer, C. P. Lucas, & J. E. Richters (Eds.), *Diagnostic assessment in child and adolescent psychopathology* (pp. 285–298). New York: Guilford Press.

Clark, A., & Harrington, R. (1998). On diagnosing rare disorders rarely: appropriate use of screening instruments. *Journal of Child Psychology and Psychiatry*, *40*, 287–290.

Conners, C. K. (1997). *Conners' rating scales: Revised technical manual*. North Tonawanda, New York: Multi Health Systems.

De Los Reyes A., & Kazdin A. E. (2005). Informant discrepancies in the assessment of child psychopathology: a critical review, theoretical framework, and recommendations for further study. *Psychological Bulletin*, *131*, 483–509.

DuPaul, G. J., Power, T. J., & Anastopoulos, A. D., & Reid, R. (1998). *ADHD rating scale-IV: Checklists, norms and clinical interpretation*. New York, Guilford Press.

Edelbrock, C. S., Costello, A. J., Dulcan, M. K., Kalas, R., & Conover, N. C. (1985). Age differences in the reliability of the psychiatric interview of the child. *Child Development*, *56*, 265–275.

Eyberg, S., & Pincus, D. (1999). *ECBI & SESBI-R Eyberg Child Behavior Inventory and Sutter–Eyberg Student Behavior Inventory – Revised: Professional manual*. Lutz, FL: Psychological Assessment Resources.

Ferdinand, R. F., Hoogerheide, K. N., Van der Ende, J., Heijmens Visser, J., Koot, H. M., Kasius, M., *et al.* (2003). The role of the clinician: three-year predictive value of parents', teachers', and clinicians' judgment of childhood psychopathology. *Journal of Child Psychology and Psychiatry*, *44*, 867–876.

Ferdinand, R. F., Heijmens Visser, J., Hoogerheide, K. N., Van der Ende, J., Kasius, M., Koot, H. M., *et al.* (2004a). Improving estimation of the prognosis of childhood psychopathology; combination of DSM-III-R/DISC diagnoses and CBCL scores. *Journal of Child Psychology and Psychiatry*, *45*, 599–608.

Ferdinand, R. F., van der Ende, J., & Verhulst, F. C. (2004b). Parent–adolescent disagreement regarding psychopathology in adolescents from the general population as a risk factor for adverse outcome. *Journal of Abnormal Psychology*, *113*, 198–206.

Fergusson, D. M. (1997). A brief introduction to structural equation models. In F. C. Verhulst, & H. M. Koot (Eds.), *The epidemiology of child and adolescent psychopathology* (pp. 122–145). Oxford: Oxford Medical Publications.

Fombonne, E. (2002). Case identification in an epidemiological context. In M. Rutter, & E. Taylor (Eds.), *Child and adolescent psychiatry* (4th edn., pp. 52–69). Oxford, UK: Blackwell Publishing.

Goodman, R. (1997). The Strengths and Difficulties Questionnaire: a research note. *Journal of Child Psychology and Psychiatry*, *38*, 581–586.

Hayward, C., Varady, S., Albano, A. M., Thienemann, M., Henderson, L., & Schatzberg, A. F. (2000). Cognitive–behavioral group therapy for social phobia in female adolescents: results of a pilot study. *Journal of the American Academy of Child and Adolescent Psychiatry*, *39*, 721–726.

Helzer, J. E., Robins, L. N., McEvoy, L. I., Spitznagel, E. L., Stolzman, R. K., Farmer, A., *et al.* (1985). A comparison of clinical and Diagnostic Interview Schedule diagnoses: physician reexamination of lay-interviewed cases in the general population. *Archives of General Psychiatry*, *42*, 657–666.

Ho, T. P., Luk, E. S., Leung, P. W., Taylor, E., Lieh-Mak, F., & Bacon-Shone, J. (1996). Situational versus pervasive hyperactivity in a community sample. *Psychological Medicine*, *26*, 309–321.

Hodges, K. (2004). Child and Adolescent Functional Assessment Scale (CAFAS). In M. E. Maruish (Ed.), *The use of psychological testing for treatment planning and outcomes assessment* (3rd edn., Vol. 1, pp. 405–441). Mahwah, NJ: Lawrence Erlbaum.

Hofstra, M. B., Van der Ende, J., & Verhulst, F. C. (2000). Continuity and change of psychopathology from childhood into adulthood: A 14-year follow-up study. *Journal of the American Academy of Child and Adolescent Psychiatry*, *39*, 850–858.

Ivanova, M. Y., Dobrean, A., Dopfner, M., *et al.* (2007). Testing the 8-syndrome structure of the child behavior checklist in 30 societies. *Journal of Clinical Child and Adolescent Psychology*, *36*, 405–417.

Jensen, P. S., Salzberg, A. D., Richters, J. E., & Watanabe, H. K. (1993). Scales, diagnoses and child psychopathology. I. CBCL and DISC relationships. *Journal of the American Academy of Child and Adolescent Psychiatry*, *32*, 397–406.

Jensen, P. S., Rubio-Stipec, M., Canino, G., Bird, H. R., Dulcan, M., Schwab-Stone, M. E., *et al.* (1999). Parent and child contributions to diagnosis of mental disorder: Are both informants always necessary? *Journal of the American Academy of Child and Adolescent Psychiatry*, *38*, 1569–1579.

Kasius, M. C., Ferdinand, R. F., Van den Berg, H., & Verhulst, F. C. (1997). Associations between different diagnostic approaches for child and adolescent psychopathology. *Journal of Child Psychology and Psychiatry*, *38*, 625–632.

Kazdin, A. E. (2005). Evidence-based assessment for children and adolescents: Issues in measurement development and clinical application. *Journal of Clinical Child and Adolescent Psychology*, *34*, 548–558.

Kendall, P. C., Marrs-Garcia, A., Nath, S. R., & Sheldrick, R. C. (1999). Normative comparisons for the evaluation of clinical significance. *Journal of Consulting and Clinical Psychology*, *67*, 285–299.

Kendler, K. S. (1996). Major depression and generalised anxiety disorder. Same genes, (partly) different environments – revisited. *British Journal of Psychiatry Supplement*, *30*, 68–75.

Kollins, S. H., Epstein, J. N., & Conners, C. K. (2004). Conners' Rating Scales – Revised. In M. E. Maruish (Ed.), *The use of psychological testing for treatment planning and outcomes assessment* (3rd edn., Vol. 2, pp. 215–233). Mahwah, NJ: Lawrence Erlbaum Associates.

Lambert, M. J., Whipple, J. L., Hawkins, E. J., Vermeersch, D. A., Nielsen, S. L., & Smart, D. W. (2003). Is it time for clinicians to routinely track patient outcome? A meta-analysis. *Clinical Psychology: Science and Practice*, *10*, 288–301.

Marsh, J. S. (1997). *MASC Multidimensional Anxiety Scale for Children*. North Tonawanda, NY: Multi Health Systems.

Maruish, M. E. (2004). Introduction. In M. E. Maruish (Ed.), *The use of psychological testing for treatment planning and outcomes assessment* (3rd edn., Vol. 1, p. 29). Mahwah, NJ: Lawrence Erlbaum Associates.

McMahon, R. J., & Frick, P. J. (2005). Evidence-based assessment of conduct problems in children and adolescents. *Journal of Clinical Child and Adolescent Psychology*, *34*, 477–505.

Meehl, P. E., & Rosen, A. (1955). Antecedent probability and the efficiency of psychometric signs, patterns, or cutting scores. *Psychological Bulletin*, *52*, 194–216.

Plomin, R., DeFries, J. C., Craig, I. W., & McGuffin, P. (2003). Behavioral genetics. In R. Plomin, J. C. DeFries, I. W. Craig, & P. McGuffin (Eds.), *Behavioral genetics in the postgenomic era*. Washington, USA: American Psychological Association.

Rescorla, L., Achenbach, T. M., Ivanova, M. Y., *et al.* (in press). Problems reported by parents of children ages 6 to 16 in 31 societies. *Journal of Emotional and Behavioral Disorders*, in press.

Rescorla, L., Achenbach, T. M., Ivanova, M. Y., *et al.* (2007a). Epidemiological comparisons of problems and positive qualities reported by adolescents in 24 countries. *Journal of Consulting and Clinical Psychology*, *75*, 351–358.

Rescorla, L., Achenbach, T. M., Ginzburg, S., *et al.* (2007b). Consistency of teacher reported problems for students in 21 countries. *School Psychology Review*, *36*, 91–110.

Rettew, D. C., Doyle, A., Achenbach, T. M., Dumenci, L., Ivanova, M. (2006). *Meta-analyses of agreement between clinical evaluations and standardized interviews*. Poster presented at the 53rd Annual Meeting of the American Academy of Child and Adolescent Psychiatry in San Diego, October 2006.

Rothman, K. J., & Greenland, S. (1998). *Modern epidemiology* (2nd edn). Philadelphia, PA: Lippincott-Raven.

Roza, S. J., Hofstra, M. B., Van der Ende, J., & Verhulst, F. C. (2003). Stable prediction of mood and anxiety disorders based on behavioral and emotional problems in childhood: a 14-year follow-up during childhood, adolescence, and young adulthood. *American Journal of Psychiatry*, *160*, 2116–2121.

Saywer, M. G., Streiner, D. L., & Baghurst, P. (1998). The influence of distress on mothers' and fathers' reports of childhood behavioral and emotional problems. *Journal of Abnormal Child Psychology*, *26*, 407–414.

Schachar, R., Rutter, M., & Smith, A. (1981). The characteristics of situationally and pervasively hyperactive children: Implications for syndrome definition. *Journal of Child Psychology and Psychiatry*, *22*, 375–392.

Shaffer, D., Gould, M. S., Brasic, J., Ambrosini, P., Fisher, P., Bird, H., *et al.* (1983). A Children's Global Assessment Scale (CGAS). *Archives of General Psychiatry*, *40*, 1228–1231.

Sheldrick, R. C., Kendall, P. C., & Heimberg, R. G. (2001). The clinical significance of treatments: A comparison of three treatments for conduct disordered children. *Clinical Psychology: Science and Practice*, *8*, 418–430.

Stevens, G. W. J. M., Pels, T., Bengi-Arslan, L., Verhulst, F. C., Vollebergh, W. A. M., & Crijnen, A. A. M. (2003). Parent, teacher and self-reported problem behavior in the Netherlands: Comparing Moroccan immigrant with Dutch and with Turkish immigrant children and adolescents. *Social Psychiatry and Psychiatric Epidemiology*, *38*, 576–585.

Van der Valk J. C., Van den Oord E. J. C. G., Verhulst F. C., & Boomsma D. I. (2001). Using parental ratings to study the etiology of 3-year-old twins' problem behaviors: Different views or rater bias? *Journal of Child Psychology and Psychiatry*, *42*, 921–931.

Verhulst, F. C., & Van der Ende, J. (2006). *Assessment scales in child and adolescent psychiatry*. Oxon, UK: Informa Healthcare.

Verhulst, F. C., & Althaus, M. (1988). Persistence and change in behavioral/emotional problems reported by parents of children aged 4–14: An epidemiological study. *Acta Psychiatrica Scandinavica Supplement*, *339*, 1–28.

Verhulst, F. C., Koot, H. M., & Berden, G. F. M. G. (1990). Four-year follow-up of an epidemiological sample. *Journal of the American Academy of Child and Adolescent Psychiatry*, *29*, 440–448.

Woodward, C. A., Thomas, H. B., Boyle, M. H., Links, P. S., & Offord, D. R. (1989). Methodologic note for child epidemiological surveys: The effects of instructions on estimates of behavior prevalence. *Journal of Child Psychology and Psychiatry*, *30*, 919–924.

World Health Organization. (1996). *Multiaxial classification of child and adolescent psychiatric disorders: The ICD-10 classification of mental and behavioural disorders in children and adolescents*. Cambridge, UK: Cambridge University Press.

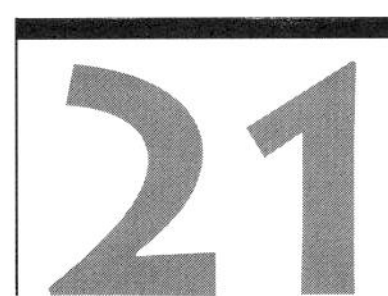

Psychological Assessment in the Clinical Context

Tony Charman, Jane Hood and Patricia Howlin

The notion that psychological assessment involves just the administration of psychometric tests is no more accurate than the definition of intelligence as being simply "what IQ tests measure." Whereas the accurate use and valid interpretation of psychometric tests serve an important function in establishing children's levels and profiles of ability, it is unusual for children to be referred solely for the purpose of establishing their IQ. Rather, psychological assessment is usually requested because of wider concerns about a child – for example, why is his or her behavior giving rise to so many problems within the classroom? Why is he or she falling behind the rest of the class, or is unable to relate to peers? The present chapter explores not only the importance of skilled psychometric assessment, but also the much wider role that psychological assessment can have in the identification and resolution of the many different types of problem that present to clinicians.

Psychological Assessment within the Broader Context

Rutter and Yule (2002) pointed out that clinical psychology training requires expertise in experimental psychology, developmental psychology, psychopathology, neurophysiology, neuroscience and biology. Psychological assessment is not merely the administration of a clinical test, but involves the identification of key clinical issues pertaining to each *individual* case; the formulation of clinical issues into testable hypotheses; the implementation of hypothesis-driven intervention strategies; the evaluation of the outcome of these strategies; and the reformulation of both the original hypotheses and intervention procedures if the predicted improvements are not achieved. They stress the role of all clinicians, including psychologists, as being that of "scientist-practitioners" (Drabick & Goldfried, 2000; Kennedy & Llewelyn, 2001). This does not imply that all clinicians should be involved in large-scale treatment or research trials. Even though these are *sometimes* possible within clinical settings (see chapter 64), service demands usually preclude research of this kind. However, on an individual client basis, the skilled practitioner will constantly be learning from past experience and applying scientific thinking to his or her practice. As Rutter and Yule (2002, p. 114) noted, this can range from "something that is little more than thoughtful questioning clinical enquiry, to a scientific investigation that approximates to a piece of research that can be applied to individual cases." In relation to clinical diagnosis, the same authors suggested that this may involve a combination of "pattern recognition" or "the ability to put together very complex sets of data, weighting different elements appropriately and considering possible interactions among risk and protective factors" (p. 105). Very similar processes also form the basis of psychological assessment and intervention.

Rutter's Child and Adolescent Psychiatry, 5th edition. Edited by M. Rutter, D. Bishop, D. Pine, S. Scott, J. Stevenson, E. Taylor and A. Thapar. © 2008 Blackwell Publishing, ISBN: 978-1-4051-4549-7.

Pre-assessment Assessments

Psychological assessment should begin long before the child sits down to complete a cognitive test. The referral letter and reports from parents, school or other professionals, are all important in describing the presenting nature of the child's problems and identifying factors that may need special consideration. For example, are there inconsistencies in the various reports of the child's behavior? It is not unusual, especially in the case of children with developmental disorders, to find very different accounts of behavior in different settings. Thus, a young child may be reported as highly disruptive at school, but not at home. Alternatively, a child who is described by parents as very difficult to manage may show few problems at school. In addition to these anecdotal accounts, brief standardized questionnaires (e.g., Conners' 1997 scales; Development and Well Being Assessment [DAWBA], Goodman, Ford, Richards *et al.*, 2000; Strengths and Difficulties Questionnaire [SDQ], Goodman, 1997), which can be completed independently by teachers and parents, can help to pinpoint areas of discrepancy. If previous assessments are unavailable, brief postal questionnaires relating to possible developmental delays or abnormalities as well as general family circumstances can provide valuable information which helps to focus the initial assessment. If a specific disorder, such as autism, is suspected parents might also be asked to complete an appropriate screening instrument (e.g., Social Communication Questionnaire [SCQ]; Rutter, Bailey, & Lord, 2003).

Clinic-based Assessment

Informal observations of the child in the waiting room can also prove an important part of the psychological assessment. Who has accompanied the child – one parent or two? If a single parent, has he or she come with another relative, such as a grandmother? Have other children also come along? How does the child relate to the accompanying family members – and how do they respond in turn? Is the child obviously disruptive, distressed, sullen, talkative, clingy, aloof? How does the child react when first approached by the clinician? The interpretation of such observations must, of course, always take into account the developmental level of the child. Screaming, clinging to the mother and refusing to accompany an unknown professional are entirely appropriate in a 3-year-old child. Taking the clinician's hand and leaving the parent without a backward glance is certainly not! Sitting well away from parents and adopting a sullen uncommunicating look is unusual in a 7-year-old, but typical of many adolescents.

Careful observation of the child should continue throughout any more structured cognitive assessment, and should be documented during formal testing. Degree of cooperation with the examiner, general behavior, activity and concentration levels, social and communication skills, specific areas of difficulty or competence all need to be monitored, summarized and reported. Do these tally with the referral reports – thereby helping to clarify the nature of the presenting problems – or does the child's behavior in the assessment setting seem very different to that described? It is not unusual, for example, to find that more able children with autism or Asperger syndrome, far from being socially withdrawn, may appear relaxed, confident and highly cooperative in a formal testing session. This does not suggest that reports of difficult behavior at home or school are inaccurate, but indicates that, in a highly structured, predictable and relatively impersonal setting, the child is able to perform at his or her best. In turn, such observations can be extremely important in planning appropriate interventions.

Informal, but informed, psychological assessment will also have an impact on the way in which testing is conducted. As is stressed later in this chapter, choice of well-standardized tests and adherence to testing protocols are important elements of the assessment procedure. However, when assessing children for whom the tests were not specifically normed (i.e. *most* children with moderate–severe intellectual disability, or children with specific developmental, physical or sensory impairments), some deviation from the prescribed format may produce findings that are of greater practical value. After all, it is rare that the ultimate aim of testing such children is to confirm their IQ score per se; rather, the general aim is to obtain an overall estimate of their potential level of functioning. Many years ago, Clark and Rutter (1979) reported that alterations to the ordering of test items, or allowing "non-standard" forms of response, resulted in improved cooperation amongst children with autism. Moreover, longer-term follow-up of children with autism assessed under somewhat modified testing conditions indicates that results can be highly predictive of performance 20 or more years later (Howlin, Goode, Hutton *et al.*, 2004).

The need for modifications to conventional protocols may also have implications for intervention. One 8-year-old boy with autism was referred because his school felt that his intellectual ability was too low for him to be appropriately placed there. At the assessment he refused all tests with a verbal component but finally showed an interest in the Ravens Progressive Matrices. However, instead of simply identifying the correct item he listed only the numbers of items that were *not* correct! This greatly extended the time taken for testing but did produce a much higher IQ score than expected on the basis of teacher reports. However, it was apparent that his functioning was significantly affected by his very stereotyped and rigid behavior and an individual intervention program was designed largely on the basis of the information gleaned during this unstandardized testing session. This consisted of making school staff aware of his potential ability, helping teachers to reduce his very fixed behavior patterns, reducing the verbal content of tasks as far as possible, using computerized teaching methods, providing him with novel tasks (on which he had had no opportunity to develop stereotyped responses) and allowing him to finish off certain tasks in his own idiosyncratic fashion once most of his work was complete.

It should also be recognized that when assessing "unusual" children, the use of a less well-standardized test may be appropriate. The Merrill–Palmer scale (Stutsman, 1948), for example, has outdated (USA-based) norms, and would be unsuitable for most typically developing children. However, long experience with lower ability children with autism indicates that there is something about the materials that can generate interest and cooperation where other tests have failed. The long-term reliability of scores from early testing on the Merrill–Palmer (as long as the child is able to complete more than one or two isolated test items) has also been shown to be good (Howlin *et al.*, 2004). One 3-year-old nonverbal child with autism was thought by his parents to be very bright because of his ability with constructional toys; in contrast, at nursery, where he showed no interest in any of the equipment available, it was felt that he should be moved to a unit for children with severe intellectual impairments. In the assessment session he showed no inclination to do anything other than spin objects on the floor; he threw the contents of the Wechsler tests across the room and although he showed some interest in the book form of the Ravens Matrices he clearly disliked the feel of the Velcro™ pads required to place the pieces. An old Merrill–Palmer test was also rejected. However, his mother pointed out that he hated any equipment that was obviously used or dirty; indeed, she believed this was the reason he ignored the nursery equipment. The family was asked to return at a later date, after a new Merrill–Palmer had been ordered. The child completed the whole test, well above the 6-year level ceiling, within minutes. On the basis of the assessment (which also illustrated the importance of parental information) the boy was moved to a specialist autism unit, where he continued to make good progress, initially in visuospatial skills and later in computing and mathematics.

Prior knowledge about specific clinical conditions may also be a crucial part of the assessment process. For example, one young girl with Williams syndrome was referred by her mainstream school because of disruptive behavior in class and highly inappropriate social interactions with male teachers. In addition to concerns about her academic progress, staff suspected that she might have been sexually abused. Her parents were outraged by this suggestion. According to them their daughter was a delightful, friendly child who, apart from mild intellectual difficulties, had no problems at all. During the initial assessment three things became clear. First, the girl's IQ was much lower (around 45) than originally thought. Second, she showed the very typical pattern of indiscriminate overfriendliness that is characteristic of children with Williams syndrome. Her superficial chattiness, especially her constant questioning, did much to disguise her lack of social understanding and her profound language problems. Third, when questioned about her special interests, it became apparent, as is not uncommon among young people with Williams syndrome, that she had an intense preoccupation with a particular pop-singer – in this case Bob Geldof. Further questioning of her parents confirmed that any man of a certain age with long hair or an Irish accent would be approached, asked if he was Geldof, have his hair stroked or requests made to sit on his knee. While the parents viewed this behavior as rather "cute," the school (where there were a number of male teachers with longish hair) interpreted the behavior very differently. The working "hypotheses" – that her "sexualized" behavior was probably related to her particular preoccupation and that her disruptive behavior in class was mainly due to her constant questioning and inability to cope intellectually – were supported by observations at school where it became clear that educationally the placement was quite unsuitable. Her move to a unit for children with mild to moderate intellectual impairments led to a significant improvement in her classroom behaviors, and as staff members were warned beforehand of her particular preoccupation, any inappropriate responses to male members of staff were prevented from the outset.

Non-clinic-based Assessment

Successful intervention necessitates a clear understanding of the factors that may be causing or maintaining problem behaviors or interfering with learning. Although the above examples illustrate how informal observations conducted around the time of the formal assessment helped to inform both understanding and intervention, in many cases psychological assessment will require more detailed and systematic data collection in the home and/or school, or other settings.

Observational data can be collected in a number of ways, including time-sampling, latency recording, duration recording, event recording and ABC (Antecedent–Behavior–Consequence) analysis. There are also several formal systems available for observing children that enable the observer to monitor change over time and evaluate the effect of interventions on behavior (e.g., Behavioral Observation of Students in Schools [BOSS]; Shapiro, 1996; and the Classroom Interaction System [CIS]; Smith & Hardman, 2003; see chapter 19).

The need for non-clinic-based assessment is especially important when there is a discrepancy between the various accounts of behavior (e.g., disagreements between parents and teachers concerning the nature or severity of the presenting difficulties, or when the behavior observed in the clinic does not tally with other reports). For example, a child referred for learning or behavioral difficulties at school may, on testing, show no obvious intellectual impairment. If more detailed assessment also fails to identify any specific cognitive/learning impairments (i.e., in language, reading, memory, executive functioning or other skills), then further investigation will be needed to explore possible home or school-based factors (family disruption, parent–child relationship problems, bullying, or emotional or mental health problems) that are affecting progress.

Children with intellectual impairments, and especially those with autism, may behave very differently in different situations or with different people. One 11-year-old boy with autism and moderate intellectual impairment was described by his teachers as the "easiest pupil in the class"; his parents requested a referral because his behavior at home was impossible to manage. School and home visits indicated that the reports from both teachers and parents were essentially accurate and that his behavior differed markedly in the two settings. However, it was also noticed that at school the child often seemed very tense and he would become upset, sometimes destroying his work, if everything was not completed perfectly. It was apparent too, that at playtime he was very reluctant to go outside, disliked team games of any kind, avoided other children as much as possible, showed many stereotyped behaviors and was clearly a source of some amusement to other pupils. Two possible causes for the problems at home were proposed:

1 Pressure to perform well in school was leading to stress which was only apparent when he was in the familiar home setting;
2 Some form of covert bullying/teasing was occurring.

Personal accounts by individuals with autism (Sainsbury, 2000) indicate that playtimes, far from being pleasurable, can be more akin to "torture" – sometimes because of bullying but also because of the child's total failure to understand the multitude of unwritten rules governing playground behavior. In this case, allowing the child to use the computer room during playtimes and team games significantly reduced his anxiety level at school (teachers completed a brief rating sheet at the end of each lesson to monitor this). Parental ratings of disruptive behavior, however, decreased only slightly. A very simple diary record indicated that the most difficult days for them occurred when he had English or design and technology for the final afternoon session. If the day finished with maths or computing he returned home much calmer. A reorganization of his timetable, so that he spent the last hour of each day working alone on maths or computing problems resulted in his arriving home much more relaxed. Although the situation at home remained difficult, his parents felt that they now had better understanding of, and hence better control over, his behavior.

Psychological assessments conducted outside the clinic may also produce unpredicted findings. For example, in group settings (home, classroom or a residential unit) reports of difficulties often focus on one particular individual. However, systematic observations may indicate that the problem is not restricted to the referral case. For example, a teacher in a school for children with moderate intellectual impairment had asked for help with a particular student who was described as being constantly off-task and disrupting other pupils. Classroom assessments included counts of on-task behaviors using very simple time sampling techniques (child not sitting at desk at 15-minute intervals). These indicated that the child concerned was off-task no more than other pupils. However, when out of his desk he had a habit of dribbling and smearing saliva and it was this specific undesirable behavior that needed to be the focus of intervention.

In families too, although one child may be the center of parental concerns, there may also be difficulties with regard to other siblings. A broad psychological assessment can be crucial in identifying these and in refocusing intervention on the wider family dynamics.

Observations made as part of the assessment process may suggest minor modifications that can help considerably. Thus, the disruption caused by one child who constantly arrived late for lessons was minimized by simply recommending that he be supplied with a desk by the door and that this desk had a drawer with basic equipment, such as paper and writing materials that he could use if he had lost (as was typical) his school bag.

Of course, psychological assessment may also reveal much more fundamental learning or behavioral problems and there may be inadequacies or inconsistencies in the ways these are dealt with at home or at school. In such cases, the initial assessment can be essential in establishing the basis for more systematic cognitive, behavioral or pharmacological interventions.

Assessing Behavioral Functions

The term "applied behavior analysis" has, in recent years, often been used synonymously with the intensive home-based programs for preschool children with autism promoted by Lovaas (1993, 1996; see chapters 46, 62 & 74). However, as reviews such as that by Baer, Wolf, and Risley (1968) indicated, the value of applied behavioral analysis in reducing behavioral problems or improving behavioral functioning has been recognized for decades. Early studies stressed the importance of the ABC model (i.e., identifying the *antecedent* events that appeared to trigger the *behavior* and the modification of the *consequences* resulting from the behavior). However, in real-life settings, establishing the true antecedents to a specific behavior may be very difficult. For example, a child may arrive at school in a disturbed state because of something that happened on the bus en route, an event the night before or even something that occurred days or weeks earlier. Thus, recent applications of behavioral analysis have tended to focus on the observable consequences of behavior. The functional analysis of behavior – identifying the functions of "challenging behaviors" especially for non-verbal, severely intellectually impaired individuals – has also had a major role in changing the way in which problem behaviors are interpreted and treated. Assessments of this kind, which are often conducted in experimental analog situations (see chapter 62), frequently reveal that so-called "maladaptive behaviors" may be extremely *adaptive* if an individual is unable to express his or her needs or feelings in any other way. Functional communication training (i.e., teaching alternative forms of communication by means of pictures/symbols/electronic devices, etc.) can then enable individuals to express their need for assistance, to obtain attention or desired objects, or to escape unwanted situations more effectively. Such strategies, as well as increasing communicative competence, frequently result in a decrease in disruptive, aggressive, stereotyped and self-injurious behaviors (for reviews see Durand & Merges, 2001; Hanley, Iwata, & McCord, 2003).

Although the majority of studies involving functional analysis have been conducted within experimental settings, it is possible to adapt this methodology to more naturalistic environments. Over the years, a variety of behavior checklists or brief observation scales have been developed to assist in the assessment of problem behaviors in children with developmental disorders (e.g., Communication Forms and Functions Scale [CFFS], Schuler, Peck, Willard *et al.*, 1989; Motivation Assessment Scale [MAS], Durand & Crimmens, 1988; Shogren & Rojahn, 2004; Functional Analysis Checklist [FAC], Sturmey, 2001; Questions about Behavioral Function [QABF], Nicholson, Konstantinidi & Furniss, 2006; Paclawskyj, Matson, Rush *et al.*, 2001). While none of these are without problems, they can provide a useful framework for behavioral assessment, forming the basis of hypotheses about causation that can then be systematically tested. Part of the FAC, for example, focuses on an hourly breakdown of the individual's typical daily schedule. Using this very simple observational format with a severely intellectually impaired child, referred for his very disruptive behaviors in a respite setting, clearly demonstrated that, for most of the day, he was left alone with very little adult interaction. It was when adults actively intervened (often inconsistently and unpredictably) that outbursts occurred. Introducing regular, brief, low-intensity interactions focused on activities that he seemed to enjoy, significantly reduced the severity and frequency of disruptive behaviors.

Assessing Intervention Effectiveness

Strategies used in psychological assessment may also be important in evaluating the effectiveness of other interventions to which the child is exposed. Certain therapies (e.g., special diets, vitamin supplements, sensory integration or facilitated communication) have attracted the attention of parents of children with developmental problems (particularly autism) because of wide publicity. Glowing testimonials on treatment websites, or DVD demonstrations of apparent "miracles" are highly seductive and it is easy to understand why parents seek out these "alternative" treatments. One such example is Facilitated Communication, in which a facilitator physically supports the client's use of a key- or letter-board to indicate his or her needs or thoughts. This technique was claimed to lead to "Communication Unbound" (Biklen, 1993). Despite evidence from over 50 studies indicating such claims are false (Simpson & Myles, 1995) and statements by the American Psychological Association (1994) and the American Academy of Pediatrics Committee on Children with Disabilities (1998) describing this as an ineffective and potentially dangerous form of treatment, its use by private therapists, and even in some schools, continues. Clinicians' dismissal of such therapies as "useless" is unlikely to be readily accepted by desperate parents. However, by adopting a psychological approach to monitoring and assessment, parents may be helped to assess the effects on their own child more objectively. For example, the parents of a young boy with Down syndrome were convinced that his weekly sensory integration sessions (which claimed to restore defective neurological processing; for review see Smith, Mruzek, & Mozingo, 2005) were of great benefit. In contrast, his school believed that the sessions resulted in his behavior deteriorating on the days following therapy and conflicts had arisen when they had asked the family to discontinue therapy. Having agreed on a specific set of behaviors that should be monitored over time, the psychologist involved (who was unaware of the days therapy was conducted) called the parents and school every morning over a period of 4 weeks to rate these. An adaptation of the Personal Questionnaire Rapid Screening Test (PQRST; Chalkely & Mulhall, 1991) is useful in such circumstances as it is very difficult for raters to remember all their baseline ratings. Over the course of the month little evidence emerged to support the school's view that the therapy resulted in a worsening of behavior; however, parental records showed no consistent improvement. The outcome was that the school ceased their complaints about treatment, leading to better relationships with the family; the family did not discontinue therapy but they became somewhat more skeptical about its effectiveness and reduced the number of sessions, thus allowing the child to take part in some extracurricular school activities such as horse riding.

In another case, the parents of a teenage boy with autism were battling with local social services about the quality of care he was receiving at home. The school was using Facilitated Communication and in these sessions he apparently demonstrated impressive scientific knowledge; his level of written English was also remarkable. The therapist claimed that his progress was being held back by his parents and that he should be removed to a residential placement. Formal psychological assessment of his cognitive, language and literacy skills indicated that his overall functioning was, at best, equivalent to a 4–5-year level. Observations at home and school did nothing to alter this judgment. Moreover, nothing to which he was exposed at home or school (books, video, TV programs or parents' educational background) could explain his highly specialized areas of knowledge. With the cooperation of the parents and therapist, the psychologist constructed a mixture of different assessment protocols, some in which the therapist and student were exposed to the same materials and asked the same questions; some in which the materials/questions given to therapist and student differed. Materials also differed in complexity. In over 90% of trials when the therapist did not have access to the same materials, the student's responses were incorrect. Only for very simple items (naming common animals) was there any evidence of independent communication. The assessment demonstrated that the therapist's conclusions about the student's level of functioning were completely misguided and the school subsequently suspended its use of Facilitated Communication. Unfortunately, the damage caused by the school's past criticisms of his parents took much longer to repair.

Psychological Assessment of Children with Rare Disorders

Psychological assessment can be particularly complicated when dealing with children with unusual or complex genetic disorders. Because of the rarity of such cases the psychologist may have far less information on which to base testable hypotheses about the causes of or treatments for behavioral disturbance. However, as well as updating knowledge of the condition as far as possible (the website of the Society for the Study of Behavioural Phenotypes, ssbp.co.uk, is helpful here), skills in "pattern recognition" (Rutter & Yule, 2002) are also important. For example, in recent years, structured and informal observations of children with Cornelia de Lange syndrome suggested that severe discomfort caused by gastroesophageal reflux (GER) might be the cause of syndrome-specific behaviors such as self-injury, nocturnal agitation and hyperactivity. Consequently, medical or surgical intervention for GER is now standard therapy, frequently leading to a significant decrease in behavioral problems (Luzzani, Macchini, Valadè *et al.*, 2003). Although in many cases of severe self-injurious behavior (SIB) the cause may be much more difficult to determine, theory-driven psychological assessment has had an important role in both identifying possible causes and developing interventions based on these.

Much of the early work on SIB in individuals with severe intellectual impairments made use of functional analysis and controlled manipulation of experimental contingencies (Iwata, Dorsey, Slifer *et al.*, 1982; Repp, Singh, Karsh *et al.*, 1991). However, such methods are expensive in time and resources. Moreover, although analog situations can be adapted to the home situation (Oliver, Demetriades, & Hall, 2002), they do not necessarily reflect real-life settings. A clinically more relevant approach to assessment is described by Moss, Oliver, Arron *et al.* (2005). Based on their wide clinical experience of Cornelia de Lange syndrome, they conducted unstructured observations in the classroom of the specific types of SIB associated with this condition (skin picking, poking, hitting and finger biting) and the settings in which these occurred. Among the eight children observed, seven showed a clear relationship between SIB and setting, although the combination of factors involved varied from child to child (for the eighth child subsequent treatment for GER reduced SIB to near zero). Identifying the settings that contribute to an increase or decrease in SIB is clearly crucial for successful intervention. In the case of children with Lesch–Nyhan syndrome (in which SIB occurs in nearly all children and is thought to be biologically based) direct observations, driven by psychological theory, indicated that environmental influences (notably levels of demand or attention) were also highly influential. In particular, the finding that SIB tended to increase during periods of low attention has significant implications for intervention.

A further important finding, again related to detailed psychological assessment of children with severe intellectual impairment and SIB, relates to the spontaneous use of self-restraint. Clinical observation, and a number of single case studies, described children using their own form of restraint (e.g., by restricting the movement of arms or hand to prevent self-harm). Subsequent research with larger samples suggested that self-restraint was greater in children who were *not* provided with protective devices (Oliver, Murphy, Hall *et al.*, 2003). Based on these observations, shaping procedures have been successfully used to reduce dependence on protective devices and also gradually to decrease the degree of self-restraint (e.g., progressing from having the arm tucked tightly into the shirt sleeve to wearing a simple wrist-band; Oliver *et al.*, 2003). For children with debilitating and sometimes life-threatening behaviors, the potential value of systematic psychological assessments such as these, conducted over time and with different disorders, is immense. The research program of Oliver and his team (Hall, Oliver, & Murphy, 2001; Moss *et al.*, 2005; Oliver, Demetriades, & Hall, 2002) illustrates how single case reports, based on observations made in the context of psychological assessment, can lead to larger case series studies and subsequently to systematic comparative investigations of self-injury in different conditions.

Value of Single Case Research

Within the hierarchy of research-based evidence, single case studies are generally viewed as the weakest form of data. Nevertheless, within the behavioral field, single case studies have, over the years, led to an increasing number of randomized controlled trials. Psychologists were amongst the first to develop statistical techniques to assess the significance of individual change (Payne & Jones, 1957) and single case methodology continues to play an important part in psychological assessment (Crawford & Garthwaite, 2004). In turn, single case publications themselves derive from psychological assessment of particular patterns of behavior, or individual responses to treatment. In our own research for example, early clinical observations and single case reports of the effectiveness of picture-based forms of communication for non-speaking children with autism (Howlin & Rutter, 1987) led to an interest in the use of a specific picture-based program (Picture Exchange Communication System [PECS]; Bondy & Frost, 1994), investigation of its implementation in special schools (Magiati & Howlin, 2003) and ultimately to a large randomized controlled trial (Howlin, Gordon, Pasco *et al.*, 2007). Similar stages – moving from successful outcomes with single clinical cases, through case series reports to efficacy and effectiveness studies – can also be traced within the fields of behavioral intervention (see chapter 62), cognitive therapy (see chapter 63) and parent training (see chapter 64).

Psychometric Assessment

Intelligence and IQ Tests – Historical Background

Since the emergence of "intelligence testing" in the late 19th century (Cattell, 1890; Galton, 1883) there has been much debate about what "intelligence" is and how to measure it. Some of this discussion has been compromised by inconsistent use of the terms "intelligence" and "intelligence quotient (IQ)," but there are also substantive arguments about psychological theory and empirical methodology (Horn & Blankson, 2005). One approach has been to side-step the sometimes acrimonious debate and simply define intelligence as "what intelligence tests measure" (Boring, 1929; Sparrow & Davis, 2000). However, there is strong empirical evidence that IQ tests do measure something meaningful about development, cognitive abilities and adaptive behavior. Thus, IQ scores show moderate (0.6) to high (0.8) stability over time (Bayley, 1949; Moffitt, Caspi, Harkness *et al.*, 1993) although stability from infancy is lower, at least in clinical samples (Bowen, Gibson, Leslie *et al.*, 1996; Charman, Taylor, Drew *et al.*, 2005). IQ scores also correlate highly with real-life outcomes, such as academic achievements, employment and income (Gottfredson & Deary, 2004).

Following on from Galton and Cattell but deviating from their emphasis on sensory and motor assessments (which are now considered more relevant for the assessment of infants; Hadders-Algra, 2005), Binet used the term intelligence to refer to "the sum total of higher mental processes" (Binet & Simon, 1905/1916). Many of the features that characterize current IQ tests were developed in the first Binet–Simon Scale (1905/1916), including items ranked by difficulty, detailed administration protocols, and the concepts of age-graded norms and mental age. Around the same time, Spearman (1904) proposed his concept of a "g" or general factor, empirically derived from factor analysis. While the subsequent century-long debate about the existence and nature of "g" has failed to reach a consensus, most contemporary theories of intelligence admit the presence of a general factor, with recent indications that this may have an identifiable brain basis (Duncan, Seitz, Kolodny *et al.*, 2000). This general factor has been characterized as "fluid reasoning ability" (Carroll, 1989; Cronbach, 1984), working memory capacity or mental complexity (Kyllonen, 1996).

Another important landmark in the history of intelligence testing was the focus on individual profile analysis, particularly with regard to verbal-performance differences or scatter (Rapaport, Gil, & Schafer, 1945/6; Wechsler, 1939). Following the development of factor analysis methodology (Cohen, 1959), Kaufman suggested a three-factor system for the Wechsler Intelligence Scale for Children–Revised (WISC-R; Wechsler, 1974): Verbal Comprehension, Perceptual Organization and Freedom from Distractibility. Although profile analysis – interpretation of patterns of peaks and troughs across individual subtests – has its advocates, others have expressed caution about the poor reliability of differences scores (Anastasi & Urbina, 1997; McDermott, Fantuzzo, Glutting *et al.*, 1992). Nevertheless, the current version of the Wechsler scales (WISC-IV; Wechsler, 2003) has developed this approach even further by replacing the Performance (PIQ) and Verbal (VIQ) summary scores with four factor-based index scores: Verbal Comprehension, Perceptual Reasoning, Working Memory and Processing Speed.

Standardized Assessments

Understanding of psychometric theory and the statistical methods used to derive standardized scores is essential for interpretation and analysis of scores derived from intelligence tests (for a cautionary note see Micceri, 1989). It is also necessary if psychologists are to be able to assess the implications of their use with particular clinical populations or individuals. Statistical methods, primarily factor analysis, have been used to derive global metrics of psychological constructs from individual test items. Many standardized tests have scaled scores with means of 100 and standard deviations of 15. Standard scores are then used to define average, below average or superior ability depending on how many standard deviations above or below the general population mean a child's performance lies (for comprehensive reviews see Anastasi & Urbina, 1997; Sattler, 2001).

Findings from standardized tests then have to be related to the taxonomy for classification within educational and clinical systems that operate in any country. These may differ from ICD-10 and DSM-IV classification systems – sometimes creating a tension between medical-led clinical teams and education-led school services. Thus, within the UK education system, an IQ between 70 and 50/55 is described as "moderate learning difficulty," whereas ICD-10/DSM-IV criteria define an IQ in this range as "mild mental retardation." The terminology used to describe children with low IQ is also inconsistent. The North American term "mental retardation" is considered pejorative in Europe where the term "intellectual disability" is preferred, even though this does not appear in the ICD-10/DSM-IV classification system (see chapter 49). Furthermore, terms such as "learning difficulty," "learning disability" and "intellectual disability" tend to be used interchangeably, and confusingly.

What Makes a "Good Test"?

In determining the applicability of any test, consideration should be given to the size, composition and diversity of the standardization sample in relation to the individual, group or setting for which it is to be used. Characteristics such as age, sex distribution, educational, social, economic and geographic backgrounds of the normative sample are all important. For example, individuals with low IQ are often omitted from school-based standardization samples (Simonoff, Pickles, Chadwick *et al.*, 2006), leading to problems in their use with children with intellectual disabilities. *When* the test was normed is also crucial because there is likely to be an increase in scores in successive cohorts of children from any one country (the so-called "cohort effect"), generally due to a combination of improvements in diet and education (Flynn, 1987; Hertzog, 1994). Sometimes, as noted above, there can be justification for using an out-of-date test but the possible effect of this on the results must be taken into account. Clinical reports should state the nature of the normative sample when this differs from the testing situation (e.g., test was normed in a different country).

Other critical test parameters are *reliability* and *validity*. The different types of reliability that are most relevant are split-half and test–retest reliability – the latter is particularly important for indicating the minimum test–retest time period that is vulnerable to practice and other learning effects. Some tests provide parallel forms to enable such difficulties to be minimized. Construct validity is usually documented by comparing test scores from the normative sample to scores on another established IQ test or to a previous version of the same test. Data on cross-validation should be provided in the test manual.

The final "test of a good test" is the *accessibility* and *relevance* of the test items to the population on whom the test is to be used. Particular considerations (e.g., on timed items) apply for children with sensory or physical limitations such as those with cerebral palsy or sight or hearing impairments. Some tests of general intelligence, such as the Wechsler tests, rely heavily on understanding verbal instructions; others specifically eliminate the need for verbal comprehension (e.g., Leiter International Performance Scale–Revised, Roid & Miller, 1997; Snijders-Oomen Non-verbal Intelligence Scale, Snijders & Snijders-Oomen, 1976; see p. 307). These considerations make some UK practitioners favor the K-ABC and Leiter for testing individuals with autistic spectrum disorders (Tsatsanis, Dartnall, Cicchetti *et al.*, 2003). However, it should be recognized that these are currently standardized only in the USA. Another consideration is how attractive and engaging the materials are, and more recent editions of many of the most widely used intelligence tests now use colorful and modern test stimuli.

Psychometric Properties of the Most Widely Used Tests of Intelligence

Most well-established tests have been standardized on large representative samples (mostly from the USA) ranging from 2200 6- to 16-year-olds for WISC-IV (Wechsler, 2003) to over 8000 children and adults (3–85 years plus) for the Stanford–Binet Test, 5th Edition (SB-5; Roid, 2003). Some measures, most notably the SB-5, have included substantial (>1200) subsamples of children with learning and behavior problems. Internal consistency, test–retest and spilt-half reliabilities for overall measures of "IQ" and for the main index or subscale scores on these tests are high (>0.80 to >0.90). Individual subtest reliabilities are lower. Many test manuals also report concurrent validity scores based on standardization subsamples completing two contemporaneous measures (see also Flanagan & Harrison, 2005). Cross-measure correlations of the most general indexes of "IQ" or "intelligence" tend to be above 0.80. This indicates – at least at the level of relatively large standardization groups – that many of these measures are tapping similar constructs (perhaps even "g"!).

Tests of General Intelligence

Among the best established tests are the SB-5 (Roid, 2003) and the suite of Wechsler tests (Wechsler Preschool and Primary Scale of Intelligence, 3rd Edition (WPPSI-III; Wechsler, 2002); WISC-IV (Wechsler, 2003); Wechsler Adult Intelligence Scale, 3rd Edition (WAIS-III; Wechsler, 1997)). The SB-5 covers the whole age range from 2 years to older adulthood, while the three Wechsler tests provide overlapping scales for preschoolers, school-age children and adults (for comprehensive reviews see Roid & Pomplun, 2005; Zhu & Weiss, 2005). The Wechsler suite of tests probably remains the most widely used in professional practice internationally and has been translated into many languages.

Both the Wechsler and Stanford–Binet tests have been criticized as being based on an outmoded historical perspective of intelligence. However, recent revisions go some way to addressing this criticism. For example, the new four-factor structure of the ability indices derived in WISC-IV (Verbal Comprehension, Perceptual Reasoning, Working Memory and Processing Speed) relates well to constructs in more contemporary theories of intelligence such as fluid reasoning and working memory (Georgas, Van de Vijver, Weiss *et al.*, 2003). The most radical change to the Wechsler tests is the de-emphasis on the PIQ and VIQ scales with the recommendation that clinical reports emphasize the global intelligence Full Scale IQ and the four processing/ability index scores. These index scores are more closely tied to empirically based theories of intelligence and are of greater remedial value in identifying individual profiles of cognitive strength and weakness.

The most recent revision of the SB-5 (Roid, 2003) has also undergone significant change. Its five-factor structure (based on the five-factor hierarchical mode of Carroll, 1993) allows for each factor (Fluid Reasoning, Knowledge, Quantitative Reasoning, Visual–Spatial Processing and Working Memory) to be measured using separate verbal and non-verbal subtests. There are also attempts (Roid & Pomplun, 2005) to identify which factor scores discriminate best between clinical groups, including children with attention deficit/hyperactivity disorder (ADHD), average IQ autism and low IQ. However, while statistical procedures, such as discriminant function analysis, can indicate how well within a particular sample scores can "classify" cases, this does not translate into a clinically utilizable metric for any individual child. Indeed, the notion that a child who scores at a particular level on one factor or subscale, or one who has a particular size of discrepancy between a score on one factor or subscale versus another, is likely to have a particular neurodevelopmental condition is misleading and inappropriate.

Many other tests of general intelligence are also available: Cognitive Assessment System (CAS; Naglieri & Das, 1997); the US standardized Differential Ability Scales II (DAS-II; Elliott, 2006) and its UK equivalent the British Ability Scales II (BAS-II; Elliott, 1997); the Kaufman Assessment Battery for Children II (KABC-II; Kaufman & Kaufman, 2004); and the Woodcock–Johnson III Tests of Cognitive Abilities (WJ-III-COG; Woodcock, McGrew, & Mather, 2001). For comprehensive summaries see Flanagan and Harrison (2005), Kaufman and Kaufman (2001) and Sattler (2001). Each has different advantages and below we highlight some of the issues relevant to the practitioner when deciding which test to use.

The DAS/BAS tests are conceptually tied to particular abilities in the Cattell–Horn–Carroll (CHC) model of intelligence, although the summary scores most commonly used include a General Conceptual Ability (GCA) index – akin to Wechsler Full Scale IQ (FSIQ) – and cluster scores of Verbal and Nonverbal Ability. Three overlapping sets of subtests are available for children aged 2:6–17:11 years and within each subset there is a Special Non-verbal Composite of subtests that can be administered without verbal instructions. The WJ-III-COG provides a battery of 31 subtests that are also tied to the hierarchical CHC model. Scores can be reported for "narrow cognitive abilities" (lexical knowledge, phonetic coding, visual memory), "broad cognitive abilities" (comprehension knowledge [Gc], fluid reasoning [Gf]), "cognitive category clusters" (verbal ability, cognitive efficiency) and "general intellectual ability."

Other tests are modeled on somewhat different theories of intelligence and are also more explicitly linked to strategies for remediation. The KABC-II (Kaufman & Kaufman, 2004) retains the theoretical emphasis of the original (KABC; Kaufman & Kaufman, 1983). The KABC-II is derived from Luria's (1966) neuropsychological model of information processing (simultaneous versus sequential) as opposed to information content (verbal versus visuospatial); Luria-based constructs of learning ability and planning ability are also included. Aside from the extended age range (3:0–18:11 years) the most significant change to the KABC-II is the incorporation of new subtests that explicitly measure aspects of the CHC model: short-term memory (Gsm), fluid reasoning (Gf) and crystallized abilities (Gc). Two different composites can be calculated: the Mental Processing Index (MPI), related to Luria's theory, and the Fluid-Crystallized Index (FCI) based on the CHC model. Kaufman, Kaufman, Kaufman-Singer *et al.* (2005) recommend that the CHC model be used as a starting point for assessment unless the child is bilingual, or has language comprehension problems or autism. Another valuable component of the Kaufman tests is the reduced reliance on verbal understanding/responding, so that non-verbal subtests can be both administered and responded to without speech.

The KABC-II is conceptually similar to the CAS (Naglieri & Das, 1997). This has been developed to model the Planning, Attention, Simultaneous and Successive (PASS) theory of intelligence – also heavily influenced by Luria's work (Naglieri, 2005; Naglieri & Das, 2005). The CAS standardization sample included over 800 children with special needs (intellectual disability/mental retardation, learning disorders, ADHD) to allow for examination of subtest profiles across clinical populations. The CAS also emphasizes strategies for remediation according to a child's profile of strengths and weakness (Naglieri & Johnson, 2000).

There are a number of brief IQ assessments available, such as the Wechsler Abbreviated Scale of Intelligence (WASI; Wechsler, 1999) and the Kaufman Brief Intelligence Test, 2nd Edition (K-BIT-2; Kaufman & Kaufman, 2006), some of which do not need to be administered by fully qualified psychologists, and others that can be administered across whole school populations, such as the Cognitive Abilities Test, 3rd Edition (CAT3; Lohman, Thorndike, Hagen *et al.*, 2001). Such measures can provide a useful indication of a child's general functioning for research purposes and can be useful clinically when a child has previously undergone extensive testing and updated assessments are required to monitor progress. However, results can be misleading if wrongly applied in clinical settings. For example, achieving a normal IQ on a brief assessment does not rule out the presence of significant specific learning difficulties; a low score does not provide detailed information about the nature of the child's difficulties.

Test Selection and Administration for Special Populations

While most well-established IQ scales have large standardization samples and good psychometric properties, caution is needed when using tests of more specific aspects of cognitive ability. These typically have smaller standardization samples, less robust validity/reliability data, and, as they are more recent, have not undergone the decades-long iterative revision processes that characterize the more widely used tests. Nevertheless, they are often very valuable for testing children with special needs.

Testing Children with Language Impairments

Among tests that have been specifically developed for children with hearing or language difficulties are the Leiter International Performance Scale–Revised (Leiter-R; Roid & Miller, 1997), the Snijders-Oomen Non-verbal Intelligence Scale (Snijders & Snijders-Ooman, 1976; Snijders, Tellegren, & Laros, 1989) and the Universal Non-verbal Intelligence Test (UNIT; Bracken & McCallum, 1997). All can be administered without spoken instructions, using demonstrations of correct responses. The UNIT comprises two subscales measuring memory and reasoning; the Leiter-R includes the two domains of ability tested by its predecessor – Reasoning and Visualization (Leiter-IPS; Leiter, 1952) – plus new domains of Ability, Attention and Memory. These tests are also useful for children from different language or cultural backgrounds. However, a full clinical assessment should include measures of language understanding and expression (in the child's own language, if possible; if not, in the language in which he or she is being educated), because communicative function (note this is not the same as spoken language) is key to adaptive learning, behavior and development (see chapter 47).

Testing Children with Low IQ

Parents whose children have learning difficulties and the teachers who work with them will often report clearly observed strengths and weaknesses in their children's skills, even if all these skills are relatively delayed for their age. Both parents and teachers are naturally keen to use children's strengths to maximize their learning. However, when children have low IQs, it is not meaningful to use standardized psychometric tests to determine whether they have any specific difficulties (i.e., to use subtest profiles and index scores to identify individual strengths and weaknesses). This is because if a child has an IQ, for example, at the 2nd centile or lower, it is not possible to have a score on any other test that is reliably significantly lower.

Many clinicians use mental age equivalents to estimate children's levels of functioning when they are below the basal level on standardized tests or subtests. While this can be useful for estimating the degree of a learning difficulty, discrepancies between age-equivalents should not be used as evidence of significant strengths and weaknesses. Skills in different areas do not always develop in a linear and comparable fashion, nor do they necessarily continue to develop throughout childhood. Ideally, comparisons between tests should only be made using evaluated statistical procedures.

Assessment of Preschool Children

Until the 1990s the use of intelligence tests with preschool children and toddlers was controversial, both because of unease about the appropriateness of such testing and concerns regarding the stability (and hence predictability) of performance at this age (Bagnato & Neisworth, 1994; Flanagan & Alfonso, 1995). However, in the past decade there has been considerable development of preschool tests. Several of the instruments reviewed above have extended the age range downwards to 2–3 years (e.g., SB-5; DAS/BAS; WJ-III-COG; WPPSI-III) and other tests specifically designed for preschoolers have been developed, such as the Bayley Scales of Infant Development (0–42 months; Bayley, 1993) and Mullen Scale of Early Learning (0–68 months; Mullen, 1995; for comprehensive reviews of preschool assessments see Lipkin & Allen, 2005; Isquith, Crawford, Espy *et al.*, 2005). There is also good evidence that early test scores are generally reliable predictors of longer term functioning (Brooks-Gunn, McCarton, Casey *et al.*, 1994; Lonigan, Burgess, & Anthony, 2000).

Tests of Other Abilities

Frequently, there is a need for more extensive testing (e.g., to examine language, visuospatial skills, executive functions, memory, attention and motor development). Eliciting relevant information from parents and school about the child's development and general adaptive functioning can indicate when assessment in specific developmental domains is required (see chapter 22).

The administration of a comprehensive neuropsychological battery can provide an indication of underlying neurological conditions, when conducted within the context of a broader neuroscientific assessment service (e.g., when results are considered in conjunction with electroencephalogram [EEG] and/or magnetic resonance imaging [MRI] data). In the absence of such provision a broad picture of the child's strengths and difficulties can be obtained by means of assessments across multiple inter-related domains. For example, if a child with behavioral difficulties is assessed as having average IQ, the assumption may be made that his or her behavior is a consequence of emotional disturbance, poor home circumstances, lack of discipline, etc. However, Mattison, Hooper, and Carlson (2006) used the NEPSY (Korkman, Kirk, & Kemp, 1997) to examine the neuropsychological profiles of primary school children with significant emotional and behavioral difficulties. They found that over half of the pupils scored at least two standard deviations below the mean on at least one domain, usually language or attention/executive functions. Scores were significantly related to academic achievement and teacher ratings of behavior and attention, and children's aggressive and disruptive behavior could often be attributed to misunderstanding of language and poor impulse control. Similarly, Ripley and Yuill (2005) found that pupils who had been excluded from school had poorer expressive language and, in the case of the youngest children, poorer auditory working memory than controls. Expressive problems were also linked to high levels of emotional symptoms. Within clinical practice it is well-established that language and attention/executive impairments are highly associated with problem behavior and several studies have found that 30–50% of children referred to child and adolescent mental health services (CAMHS) have language, reading or other learning difficulties (Cohen, Davine, Horodezky *et al.*, 1993; Humphrey, 2006; Javorsky, 1995; see chapters 47 & 48).

Assessment of Executive Functioning and Attention

Executive functioning difficulties are implicated in many different learning and neurodevelopmental disorders (e.g., autism and ADHD, Happé, Booth, Charlton *et al.*, 2006, see chapters 34 & 46; dyslexia, Helland & Asbjørnsen, 2000, see chapter 48; Tourette syndrome and obsessive compulsive disorder (OCD), Watkins, Sahakian, Robertson *et al.*, 2005, see chapters 43 & 44) and may be at the root of many children's behavioral and emotional difficulties. The term "executive functions" refers to the set of skills required for higher order thinking (e.g., problem-solving, planning and the ability to react appropriately to complex multicomponent situations using previous learning). Attention and memory skills are also involved.

The importance of evaluating executive functions is particularly relevant when there is a significant discrepancy between a child's intellectual ability and his or her adaptive functioning (Morgan, Singer-Harris, Bernstein *et al.*, 2000) or when there are difficulties with self-help and self-organization. Instruments such as the Behavioral Assessment of Dysexecutive Syndrome for Children (BADS-C; Emslie, Wilson, Burden *et al.*, 2003) can be helpful when used in conjunction with a structured parents and teacher rating scale (e.g., Adaptive Behavior Assessment System Second Edition [ABAS-II]; Harrison & Oakland, 2003) or the Vineland Adaptive Behavior Scale-II (Sparrow, Cicchetti, & Balla, 2006) for determining whether executive functioning difficulties are affecting daily functioning (Bolte & Poustka, 2002; Stein, Szumowski, Blondis *et al.*, 1995). If this proves to be the case, independence training should be implemented; a more structured home environment is also likely to be beneficial.

Testing children's executive functions and attention skills can pose significant problems because structured assessments do not necessarily reflect the child's functioning in unstructured real-life situations. Moreover, formal assessments tend to test only subcomponents of executive skills: attention switching (e.g., Trails tasks); monitoring and responding to feedback (e.g., Wisconsin Card Sorting Test); planning multistep rule-based strategies (e.g., Tower of Hanoi). Although these tests have proved useful for adults they have proved less so for children whose executive skills are still developing and in whom the differentiation between executive domains is less clear-cut (Hughes, 2002; Wright, Waterman, Prescott *et al.*, 2003).

Recent tests of executive function have been increasingly influenced by neurodevelopmental models (Karmiloff-Smith, 1998), and recognition of the need for more ecologically valid assessments. The BADS-C, for example (Emslie, Wilson, Burden *et al.*, 2003), although adapted from an adult test, more closely reflects real-life problems and may provide a better indication of the child's difficulties in everyday situations. It also provides norms for various groups of children according to age and IQ.

There is now a range of executive tests specifically for young children (3–12 years; NEPSY; Korkman, Kirk, & Kemp, 1997); others range from 8 to 80 years (Delis–Kaplan Executive Function System [D-KEFS]; Delis, Kaplan, & Kramer, 2001). Many assess a wide range of executive abilities such as working memory, planning, flexibility and inhibition (the ability to withhold an impulsive or learned response). The computerized Cambridge Neuropsychological Testing Automated Battery (CANTAB; Luciana, 2003) provides a number of measures of executive function, including planning, set-shifting and flexibility. The advantage of computerized measures is that they provide accurate and objective measures of children's skills in specific areas. The disadvantage is that they cannot provide clinical evaluations of *how* children fail tests – information that is often essential for designing interventions.

There are also scales for assessing memory (e.g., Children's Memory Scale [CMS]; Cohen, 1997); Wide Range Assessment of Learning and Memory, Second Edition (WRAML2; Sheslow & Adams, 1990); Working Memory Test Battery for Children (WMTB-C; Pickering & Gathercole, 2001). These tap skills such as immediate and delayed memory (verbal and visual), phonological loop, visuospatial sketchpad and executive memory. However, these measures tend to be based on relatively small standardization samples.

Assessments of attention include the Test of Everyday Attention in Children (TEA-Ch; Manly, Robertson, Anderson *et al.*, 1998), which measures areas such as sustained attention, switching attention and inhibition. Computerized tests, such as the Conners' Continuous Performance Test (CPT-II;

Conners, 2000), measure elements of attention including sustained attention, response speed and impulsivity.

Tests of specific skills such as memory, attention and executive function are most reliable when a child's intellectual ability is within the average range. However, referrers to neuropsychological assessment services often request more extensive testing for children with low IQs because they can observe specific strengths and weaknesses in their skills. For example, if the teacher of a child with a Full Scale IQ of 70 was reporting that the child appeared to have particular memory problems (e.g., could not remember what had been said to them or taught to them the day before), it might be tempting to assess the child's verbal memory. However, when IQ is around 70 (2nd centile) or below, interpretation of test score discrepancies is very difficult. If the child in question achieved a verbal memory score of 55 (0.1st centile), this would represent a statistically significant discrepancy between their achieved score and that predicted from their IQ. Nevertheless, in clinical terms, it would be unsafe to describe such children as having a *specific* verbal memory impairment, because they would be expected to score poorly on most tests because of their global intellectual impairment. However, within any group of pupils with mild intellectual disabilities, there will be those who stand out as being more hyperactive, less attentive or with poorer working memory and, while such observations are valid and important for informing intervention and management, conducting extensive neuropsychological assessments is not a reliable way of eliciting such information.

Achievement Tests

Both general and specific learning difficulties will affect academic progress and it is often a failure to progress academically that first brings intellectual difficulties to the attention of parents and teachers. In educational practice, school-based achievement test results are useful for identifying children who are falling behind but within the clinical setting they are no substitute for dedicated psychological assessment. Furthermore, in most countries, they focus only on circumscribed aspects of learning. Within education, a range of measures, such as the Neale reading tests (Neale, 1997), is used to monitor reading skills. However, to determine whether a child has *specific* literacy difficulties, it is necessary to use tests that provide standard scores and have been normed in conjunction with IQ measures. Such tests include the Wechsler Individual Achievement Test, 2nd Edition (WIAT-II; Wechsler, 2001), Woodcock–Johnson III Achievement Tests (WJ-III; Woodcock, McGrew, & Mather, 2001) and the Wide Range Achievement Test (WRAT-III; Wilkinson & Roberston, 2006).

Practical Issues

One question for the practicing psychologist in a CAMHS setting is which children to recommend for psychological assessment if there is not capacity to see all the children. A combination of factors such as a family history of learning difficulties, or observations from school staff detailing when children show most problem behavior (e.g., when the verbal demands are high; when there is least structure), can act as indicators for further neuropsychological assessment (Humphrey, 2006).

Another issue is how far to extend any clinical assessment, given that further assessment with one child limits the resources available to others (Yates & Taub, 2003). A pragmatic rule-of-thumb is to continue assessment until a reasonable answer to identifying likely contributing causes to an individual child's learning or behavioral problems has been reached. The current working hypothesis can then be put "on hold" until the planned intervention has had time to take effect. If intervention is successful there may be no grounds for additional assessment; if intervention fails then the hypothesis formulation-testing iterative process should continue.

Unstandardized Assessments

The importance of non-clinic assessments for both understanding and remediating children's problems was discussed in detail earlier in this chapter. Observation of the child's skills in a variety of unstructured settings can also be crucial in identifying the specific nature of a child's learning difficulties and for implementing appropriate remedial strategies. This may involve examining how the child approaches normal, everyday activities and school learning tasks in order to determine how he or she learns and responds to mediation. Here the focus is on identifying what *works* for that child, rather than simply assessing what is going wrong. Although such observations may lack scientific rigor, they should, nevertheless, be informed by a scientific approach and be as objective and systematic as possible. The advantage lies in the high validity of such observations and their direct relevance to any individual child.

Dynamic assessment, based largely on Vygotsky's theory (1978) and Feuerstein, Rand, Hoffman *et al.* (1980) Instrumental Enrichment Program of Cognitive Modifiability, represents an alternative approach to traditional cognitive assessments and is based on the concept that intelligence is constantly influenced by ongoing activity. In dynamic assessment, the psychologist attempts to assess the child's learning potential or the modifiability of his or her learning style. This involves a process of testing, intervening and retesting, and includes analysis of qualitative changes in the child's responses, a record of the mediated learning experiences, measures of test score gains and ratings of modifiability and learning strategies. A similar approach, designed to provide a link between the assessment and intervention processes, is the Response to Instruction model (Fuchs & Fuchs, 1998). Its specific aim is to provide early intervention and avoid discrimination against minority students (Fuchs, Mock, Morgan *et al.*, 2003; Vaughn & Fuchs, 2003). Advocates argue that "learning tests" provide a fairer and more valid assessment than static intelligence tests (Fabio, 2005; Guthke & Stein, 1996) and that they provide effective interventions (Tzuriel, 2000). However, this approach has remained rather marginalized (Kozulin, 2005), perhaps because it mainly relies on individual practitioners developing specific interventions for individual children, with the consequent problems of interpreting results.

Intervention

There have been few controlled studies examining the efficacy of interventions for either global or specific learning difficulties (D'Amato, Crepeau-Hobson, Leesa *et al.*, 2005) and recommendations for classroom interventions are normally made on an ad hoc basis according to the experience and ingenuity of individual psychologists and teachers. The support any individual child receives is also likely to depend more on available resources than on any evidence base (Rothlisberg, D'Amato, & Palencia, 2003; Sattler & D'Amato, 2002).

In the UK, educational psychologists increasingly use a "consultation model" in their direct work with schools (Caplan, 1970; Wagner, 2000). The consultation model aims to improve the quality of children's education and care by supporting organizational change to assist all children (Alkon, Ramler, & MacLennan, 2003) rather than trying to address the specific problems or needs of individual pupils (Collins, Mascia, Kendall *et al.*, 2003).

The use of the consultation model is intended to maximize the impact of psychologists' interventions by gaining the cooperation and commitment of everyone involved with the child and by moving away from looking for within-child factors to find solutions to problems. If feedback from the psychologist is provided simply via a written report or presented as a fait accompli, staff at all levels, from classroom assistant to headteacher, may disagree with the recommendations or feel powerless to carry them out, and may well resent the interference and imposition of the "expert," whom they may not even have met face-to-face. Psychologists need to gain the cooperation of school staff because they rarely carry out the interventions themselves but rather make recommendations to those managing the children on a daily basis. The consultation model seeks to ensure that staff and parents working with the child have a personal commitment to making interventions work and are able to develop problem-solving skills that will prepare them for future difficulties (Caplan, 1995; Sandoval, 2003). While consultation as a model of service delivery has been embraced by educational psychology services in the UK, and is also being introduced in the USA, there do not appear to be any published studies providing evidence of its efficacy in terms of its benefits for children or schools.

Intervention Case Studies

The following hypothetical brief case studies illustrate the benefits of combining observational data with assessment information. In each example the same observed behavior is discussed so that the importance of interpreting test data to identify the cause of behavioral and learning difficulties can be highlighted.

Case description

Lucy is an 8-year-old girl. Observed behavior in class: Lucy was distractible; daydreamed; misunderstood the teacher's instructions; lost her possessions; was always in the wrong place; maths and literacy skills were very weak. Her teacher believed she had poor attention and that her behavior was attention-seeking as, when an adult worked with her, she was able to perform much better. Initial observations, using time-sampling, indicated that Lucy was off-task 70% of the time. An age-matched peer was only off-task 22% of the time in the same lesson.

The following tests were included in the test battery:

- Wechsler Intelligence Scale for Children UK, 4th Edition (WISC-IV-UK)
- Children's Memory Scale (CMS)
- Working Memory Test Battery for Children (WMTB-C)
- Delis–Kaplan Executive Function System (D-KEFS)
- Behavioral Assessment of the Dysexecutive Syndrome for Children (BADS-C)

Scores are given as standard (mean: 100, average range 85–115) or scaled scores (mean: 10, average range 7–13).

Assessment results: Example 1

Lucy obtained a full-scale IQ of 95 (WISC-IV UK), but a Working Memory Index of 62. Further assessment indicated significant verbal working memory impairment (WMTB, Phonological Loop, Standard Score: 75, Central Executive: 62). Teacher reports supported clinic observations that she found it hard to retain and manipulate verbal or auditory information in her head. She confused instructions; could not sequence and hold on to ideas that she had generated herself; could not use number sequences for mental arithmetic; could not remember her ideas for writing or how to spell the words and found it hard to filter out classroom noise when the teacher was speaking.

Interventions were needed to provide external support for her weak working memory. The main aim was to reduce the amount of verbal information she had to retain by providing her with visual reminders. For example, she should use number lines and tables during maths; she should be provided with lists of instructions that she can tick off as she works; and she should plan out her stories, perhaps graphically, before attempting to write. She should sit at the front of the class to reduce distractions.

Assessment results: Example 2

Assessments show that Sophie had average intellectual ability (Full Scale IQ: 90) but very poor executive skills (e.g., D-KEFS Colour-Word Interference, scaled score: 3. Tower, scaled score: 3. BADS-C, standard score: 55). She found it hard to plan her work although she could follow individually given instructions well; she did nothing when given open-ended tasks; could not organize herself unless following a repetitive and learned routine; could not hold instructions in her head or generate an understanding of what the instructions meant in practical terms and did not know when to apply rules.

Interventions needed to focus on providing a model or framework within which Sophie could operate. At the beginning of every task she should be shown each step that she will need to take; she should be shown the endpoint of what she is trying to achieve and she should be taken through the steps needed to achieve this goal. By following this process and achieving success on several occasions, she should be able to learn how to apply the same series of steps to similar situations (i.e., she will develop a template to use in the future). When faced with changes to the task, she will need support to adapt her learned system. She should be provided with a visual timetable of the day's events and the things she needs for each session so that she can begin to learn to organize herself and see the sequence of events ahead of her.

Assessment results: Example 3

Assessment showed that Alice had a mild intellectual disability (Full Scale IQ: 63). She found it hard to learn from being told about things; she could not concentrate on the teacher's narrative, and processed language too slowly to keep up with the class. Her learning capacity was limited. She seemed to learn new information at the expense of previously learned material. She struggled with literacy and numeracy.

Interventions were needed to target Alice's learning style and slow pace of learning. She would need to learn through practical experience rather than verbal description. She would find it easiest to learn concepts that could be practically demonstrated rather than abstract concepts. Aiding her understanding should improve her concentration. She might benefit from a precision teaching approach to literacy (e.g., only teaching her a few words at a time initially rather than attempting to teach her "how to read"). Precision teaching and direct instruction would allow teachers to evaluate her rate of learning and prevent new learning "knocking out" previously learned information (Solity, Deavers, Kerfoot *et al.*, 1999). Numeracy should be taught through the use of concrete materials; standard notation of maths should be introduced gradually when basic skills are consolidated.

These examples are used to illustrate the potential dangers of an inadequately implemented hypothesis-testing model. For example, if Lucy were observed in class to have a poor attention span, the hypothesis might be that she had a primary attention deficit. If, upon administration of an attention test, she achieved low scores, the psychologist might conclude that Lucy had a specific attention difficulty. However, that conclusion could only be reached if Lucy were found to have a significant discrepancy between her IQ and attention scores and if other contributing factors such as language difficulties, hearing impairments and trauma had been excluded.

Practical Considerations

Psychometric assessment relies on the child's performance on a series of tasks conducted in the testing environment. Thus, it is essential to create an environment that allows the child to perform as well as he or she is able. An appropriate environment should be relatively free of distractions (conducting psychometric assessments in a clinic room with a sink or large open box of toys is rarely a good idea) but suitably child friendly and age appropriate. In order for the psychologist to engage optimally with the child, some "warm-up" activities (e.g., conversation, drawing, toy play) are also important. Moreover, such activities allow the clinician to determine the child's social interaction and communication style and to identify favored activities – these can be useful as "rewards" for remaining on task. However, warm-up or reward activities should not be extensive else they risk that the transition from "play" to a more structured, possibly more difficult, activity might be unsuccessful. The clinician will have to make decisions on the approach to any individual child on the basis of parental or teacher report and clinical judgment. All of these considerations can be important in maximizing the child's motivation and engagement and also to help interpret why the child might be failing on items that would seem to be well within his or her competence. Ideally, children should be tested in the absence of their parents but younger children may refuse to be separated. In such circumstances several cautions are necessary. While the parents' presence can put the child at ease it can also lead to "clingy" behavior in children who are particularly shy or nervous, or avoidant behavior when children are finding the test difficult. Parents should be positioned so that they can see what the child is being asked to do and how they are responding but not so close that they are tempted to interfere or so that the child becomes overly aware of parents' monitoring of his or her performance.

As stressed earlier in this chapter, school- or home-based assessments are often necessary to supplement the information obtained at the clinic. School visits should include observations during structured classroom activities and at break or meal times. Observation of the child working in the classroom and his or her response to adult direction can also provide information relevant to hypothesis generation and testing. Psychological assessment in the home is relevant to assessing children's behavior or relationships as these may differ considerably in different settings. However, formal assessment of cognitive abilities in the home is not usually recommended, not least because of all the distractions present in most family homes.

What to Report and How

As a consequence of their psychometric assessment, most psychologists will produce a report for fellow professionals, parents and schools. The purpose of this is to inform all those involved with the child on a regular basis about how his or her learning problems may be affecting behavior at home and/or school, the extent to which these difficulties are remediable, and the external support or additional teaching needed to maximize progress and minimize the longer term impact of these difficulties.

Although it is important that reports are written in such a way as to be accessible to all readers, whether professionals or parents, the use of vague terms, such as "below average" or "low ability," without reference to the statistical data upon which such judgments are based, should be avoided. Ideally, when reporting test results, the circumstances of testing and any limitations of the test should be made explicit.

Interpretation of scores is dependent on:

1 The clinical information available that affects the ecological validity of scores;

2 The statistical normative data that will affect content and the construct validity and reliability of scores.

Therefore, when interpreting standardized scores it is important to look at different aspects of the normative data of the particular psychometric test being used. For example, even when two reliable index scores on the same psychometric measure are statistically significantly different from each other, it is very important to check the frequency of such differences within the normative data set. For example, if a child attains a Verbal Comprehension Index on the WISC-IV within the average range and a Working Memory Index within the low range, this discrepancy might be statistically significant at the 0.05 level but examination of the frequency data shows that such a discrepancy would be expected in 25% of the population and this information will affect the interpretation of the relevance of this score.

Following the assessment (after time spent scoring and rechecking scores; e.g., by checking mental addition both backwards and forwards) the practitioner should give verbal feedback to the parent(s). This should include a general description of what the test is measuring, how the child performed and what his or her behavior was like during the session. Clinicians should check with parents (particularly when they have been present) whether the child performed as expected. Discrepancy in performance in different situations is useful not only for developing hypotheses about the child's abilities and behavior, but also for assessing parental expectations and understanding of their child's abilities. At the end of the feedback parents should always be given a chance to ask questions. Psychologists need to be aware that concepts such as IQ, and the limitations of IQ testing, are often misunderstood. Discussion between clinician and parent(s) is helpful to establish mutual understanding about the assessment findings and to help them assimilate this information.

For children of an appropriate age and maturity, it is good practice to provide them with feedback. This is useful for eliciting their views concerning any difficulties at school and gauging their own awareness of "difference" from their class peers in terms of learning or behavior. It is important to be clear to parents and teachers that problems with learning and behavior and emotional difficulties can often co-occur and the outcomes and conclusions of a "whole child" assessment should address each of these features – even when the referral is for a "cognitive assessment" only.

In their reports, psychologists should make their hypotheses about the child's difficulties explicit. This will enable other agencies working with the child, such as speech and language therapists, psychiatrists and pediatricians, to understand the formulation and add to the psychologist's gathering of evidence, as well as aiding interagency collaboration. Reports should be sufficiently detailed to enable school staff to construct a precise measurable Individual Education Plan (IEP) that not only sets targets but includes specific teaching strategies to achieve those targets. Reports should also give teachers some idea of the rate of progress that should be anticipated so that methods can be usefully evaluated.

Conclusions

In this chapter we have stressed the important role of the psychologist as "science practitioner." Cognitive assessment can be a vital part of the assessment process, and requires a rigorous and methodological approach to testing together with detailed understanding of psychological and statistical theory. Consequently, practitioners need continually to update their knowledge base as new developments arise, such as the advent of computerized testing (Berger, 2006) or new findings from emergent fields such as developmental cognitive neuroscience (Munakata, Casey, & Diamond, 2004). However, psychometric assessment is neither the psychologist's only, nor indeed primary, role. Thus, we have attempted to illustrate the crucial importance that far broader, wide ranging and theory-driven assessment plays in formulating hypotheses about a child's difficulties, systematically testing these hypotheses and, most importantly, in designing effective interventions.

Further reading

Anastasi, A., & Urbina, S. (1997). *Psychological testing*. New Jersey: Prentice Hall.

Flanagan, D. P., & Harrison, P. L. (Eds.). (2005). *Contemporary intellectual assessment: Theories, tests and issues* (2nd edn.). New York: Guilford.

Kaufman, A. S., & Kaufman, N. J. (2001). *Specific learning disabilities and difficulties in children and adolescents*. Cambridge: Cambridge University Press.

References

Alkon, A., Ramler, M., & MacLennan, K. (2003). Evaluation of mental health consultation in child care centers. *Early Childhood Education Journal*, *31*, 91–99.

American Academy of Pediatrics Committee on Children with Disabilities. (1998). Auditory integration training and facilitated communication for autism. *Pediatrics*, *102*, 431–433.

American Psychological Association. (1994). *Resolution on facilitated communication, August 1994*. Washington, DC: American Psychological Association.

Anastasi, A., & Urbina, S. (1997). *Psychological testing*. New Jersey: Prentice Hall.

Baer, D. M., Wolf, M. M., & Risley, T. R. (1968). Some current dimensions of applied behavior analysis. *Journal of Applied Behavior Analysis*, *1*, 91–97.

Bagnato, S. J., & Neisworth, J. T. (1994). A national study of the social and "treatment" invalidity of intelligence testing for early intervention. *School Psychology Quarterly*, *9*, 81–108.

Bayley, N. (1949). Consistency and variability in the growth of intelligence from birth to 18 years. *Journal of Genetic Psychology*, *75*, 165–196.

Bayley, N. (1993). *Bayley scales of infant development, 2nd Edition*. London: Psychological Corporation.

Berger, M. (2006). Computer assisted clinical assessment. *Child and Adolescent Mental Health*, *11*, 64–75.

Biklen, D. (1993). *Communication unbound: How facilitated communication is challenging traditional views of autism and ability/disability*. New York: Teachers College Press.

Binet, A., & Simon, T. (1905/1916). *The development of intelligence in children* (E. S. Kit, trans.). Baltimore: Williams & Wilkins.

Bolte, S., & Poustka, F. (2002). The relation between general cognitive level and adaptive behaviour domains in individuals with autism with and without co-morbid mental retardation. *Child Psychiatry and Human Development*, *33*, 165–172.

Bondy, A. S., & Frost, L. A. (1994). *PECS: The Picture Exchange Communication System Training Manual*. Cherry Hill, NJ: Pyramid Educational Consultants.

Boring, E. N. (1929). *A history of experimental psychology*. New York: Appleton.

Bowen, J. R., Gibson, F. L., Leslie, G. I., Arnold, J. D., Ma, P. J., & Starte, D. R. (1996). Predictive value of the Griffiths assessment in extremely low birthweight infants. *Journal of Paediatrics and Child Health*, *32*, 25–30.

Bracken, B. A., & McCallum, R. S. (1997). *Universal Nonverbal Intelligence Test (UNIT)*. Itasca, IL: Riverside.

Brooks-Gunn, J., McCarton, C. M., Casey, P. H., McCormick, M. C., Bauer, C. R., Bernbaum, J. C., *et al.* (1994). Early intervention in low-birth-weight premature infants. Results through age 5 years from the Infant Health and Development Program. *Journal of the American Medical Academy*, *272*, 1257–1262.

Caplan, G. (1970). *The theory and practice of mental health consultation*. London: Tavistock Publications.

Caplan, G. (1995). Types of mental-health consultation. *Journal of Educational and Psychological Consultation*, *6*, 7–21.

Carroll, J. B. (1989). Factor analysis since Spearman: Where do we stand? What do we know? In R. Kanter, P. L. Ackerman, & R. Gudeck, (Eds.), *Abilities, motivation and methodology: The Minnesota symposium on learning and individual differences* (pp. 43–67). Hillsdale, NJ: LEA.

Carroll, J. B. (1993). *Human cognitive abilities: A survey of factor-analytic studies*. New York: CUP.

Cattell, J. M. (1890). Mental tests and measurements. *Mind*, *15*, 373–380.

Chalkley, A. J., & Mulhall, D. J. (1991). The PQRSTUV: The Personal Questionnaire Rapid Scaling Technique – ultimate version. *British Journal of Clinical Psychology*, *30*, 181–183.

Charman, T., Taylor, E., Drew, A., Cockerill, H., Brown, J., & Baird, G. (2005). Outcome at 7 years of children diagnosed with autism at age 2: Predictive validity of assessments conducted at 2 and 3 years of age and pattern of symptom change over time. *Journal of Child Psychology and Psychiatry*, *46*, 500–513.

Clark, P., & Rutter, M. (1979). Task difficulty and task performance in autistic children. *Journal of Child Psychology and Psychiatry*, *20*, 271–285.

Cohen, J. (1959). The factor structure of the WISC at ages 7–6, 10–6 and 13–6. *Journal of Consulting Psychology*, *23*, 285–299.

Cohen, M. (1997). *Children's memory scale*. San Antonio, TX: Harcourt.

Cohen, N. J., Davine, M., Horodezky, M. A., Lipsett, L., & Isaacson, L. (1993). Unsuspected language impairment in psychiatrically disturbed children. *Journal of the American Academy of Child and Adolescent Psychiatry*, *32*, 595–603.

Collins, R., Mascia, J., Kendall, R., Golden, O., Schock, L., & Parlakian, R. (2003). Promoting mental health in child care settings: Caring for the whole child. *Zero to Three*, *23*, 39–45.

Conners, C. K. (1997). *Conners' rating scales: Revised technical manual*. North Tonawanda, New York: Multi Health Systems.

Conners C. K. (2000). *Conners' Continuous Performance Test-II (CPT-II)*. Toronto: Multi-Health Systems.

Crawford, J. R., & Garthwaite, P. H. (2004). Statistical methods for single case studies in neuropsychology: comparing the slope of a patient's regression line with those of a control sample. *Cortex*, *40*, 533–548.

Cronbach, L. (1984). *Essentials of psychological testing* (6th edn.). New York: Harper & Row.

D'Amato, R. C., Crepeau-Hobson, F., Leesa, V. H., & Geil, M. (2005). Ecological neuropsychology: An alternative to the deficit model for conceptualising and serving students with learning disabilities. *Neuropsychology Review*, *15*, 97–103.

Delis, D. C., Kaplan, E., & Kramer, J. H. (2001). *Delis–Kaplan Executive Function System (D-KEFS)*. San Antonio, TX: Harcourt.

Drabick, D. A., & Goldfried, M. R. (2000). Training the scientist-practitioner for the 21st century: putting the bloom back on the rose. *Journal of Clinical Psychology*, *56*, 327–340.

Duncan, J., Seitz, R. J., Kolodny, J., Bor, D., Herzog, H., Ahmed, A., *et al.* (2000). A neural basis for general intelligence. *Science*, *289*, 457–460.

Durand V. M., & Crimmins, D. B. (1988). Identifying the variables maintaining self injurious behavior. *Journal of Autism and Developmental Disorders*, *18*, 99–117.

Durand V. M., & Merges, E. (2001). Functional communication training: A contemporary behavior analytic intervention for problem behavior. *Focus on Autism and Other Developmental Disorders*, *16*, 110–119.

Elliott, C. D. (1997). *British Abilities Scale II (BAS-II)*. Windsor, UK: NFER Nelson.

Elliott, C. D. (2006). *Differential Abilities Scale, 2nd Edition (DAS-II)*. San Antonio, TX: Psychological Corporation.

Emslie, H., Wilson, C., Burden, V., Nimmo-Smith, I., & Wilson, B. A. (2003). *Behavioral assessment of the dysexecutive syndrome for children (BADS-C)*. Lutz, FL: Psychological Assessment Resources.

Fabio, R. A. (2005). Dynamic assessment of intelligence is a better reply to adaptive behavior and cognitive plasticity. *Journal of General Psychology*, *132*, 41–64.

Feuerstein, R., Rand, Y., Hoffman, M. B., & Miller, R. (1980). *Instrumental enrichment: An intervention programme for cognitive modifiability*. Baltimore: University Park Press.

Flanagan, D. P., & Alfonso, V. C. (1995). A critical review of the technical characteristics of new and recently revised intelligence tests for preschool children. *Journal of Psychoeducational Assessment*, *13*, 66–90.

Flanagan, D. P., & Harrison, P. L. (Eds.). (2005). *Contemporary intellectual assessment: Theories, tests and issues* (2nd edn.). New York: Guilford.

Flynn, J. R. (1987). Massive gains in 14 nations. What IQ tests really measure. *Psychological Bulletin*, *101*, 171–191.

Fuchs, L. S., & Fuchs, D. (1998). Treatment validity: A unifying concept for reconceptualizing the identification of learning disabilities. *Learning Disabilities Research and Practice*, *13*, 204–219.

Fuchs, D., Mock, D., Morgan, P. L., & Young, C. L. (2003). Responsiveness-to-intervention: Definitions, evidence, and implications for the learning disabilities construct. *Learning Disabilities Research and Practice, 18*, 157–171.

Galton, F. (1883). *Inquiries into human faculty and its development*. New York: AMS Press.

Georgas, J., Van de Vijver, F., Weiss, L., & Saklofske, D. (2003). A cross-cultural analysis of the WISC-III. In J. Georgas, L. Weiss, F. Van de Vijver, & D. Salklofske (Eds.), *Cross-cultural analysis of the WISC-III: Cultural considerations in assessing intelligence* (pp. 277–313). San Diego, CA: Academic Press.

Goodman, R. (1997). The Strengths and Difficulties Questionnaire: a research note. *Journal of Child Psychology and Psychiatry*, *38*, 581–586.

Goodman, R., Ford, T., Richards, H., Gatward, R., & Meltzer, H. (2000). The Development and Well-Being Assessment: Description and initial validation of an integrated assessment of child and adolescent psychopathology. *Journal of Child Psychology and Psychiatry*, *41*, 645–655.

Gottfredson, L. S., & Deary, I. J. (2004). Intelligence predicts health and longevity, but why? *Current Directions in Psychological Science*, *13*, 1–4.

Guthke, J., & Stein, H. (1996). Are learning tests the better version of intelligence tests? *European Journal of Psychological Assessment*, *12*, 1–13.

Hadders-Algra, M. (2005). The neuromotor examination of the preschool child and its prognostic significance. *Mental Retardation and Developmental Disabilities Research Reviews*, *11*, 180–188.

Hall, S., Oliver, C., & Murphy, G. (2001). Self injurious behavior in young children with Cornelia de Lange syndrome. *Developmental Medicine and Child Neurology*, *43*, 745–749.

Hanley, G. P., Iwata, B. A., & McCord, B. (2003). Functional analysis of problem behavior: a review. *Journal of Applied Behavior Analysis*, *36*, 147–185.

Happé, F., Booth, R., Charlton, R., & Hughes, C. (2006). Executive function deficits in autism spectrum disorders and attention-deficit/hyperactivity disorder: examining profiles across domains and ages. *Brain and Cognition*, *61*, 25–39.

Harrison, P., & Oakland, T. (2003). *Adaptive Behavior Assessment System, 2nd Edition. (ABAS-II)*. San Antonio, TX: Harcourt.

Helland, T., & Asbjørnsen, A. (2000). Executive functions in dyslexia. *Child Neuropsychology*, *6*, 37–48.

Hertzog, C. (1994). Cohort effects. In R. J. Sternberg (Ed.), *Encyclopedia of human intelligence* (Vol. 1, pp. 273–275). New York: MacMillan.

Horn, J. L., & Blankson, N. (2005). Foundations for better understanding of cognitive abilities. In D. P. Flanagan, & P. L. Harrison (Eds.) *Contemporary intellectual assessment: Theories, tests and issues* (2nd edn., pp. 41–68). New York: Guilford.

Howlin, P., Goode, S., Hutton, J., & Rutter, M. (2004). Adult outcomes for children with autism. *Journal of Child Psychology and Psychiatry*, *45*, 212–229.

Howlin, P., Gordon, K., Pasco, G., Wade, A. & Charman, T. (2007). A group randomised, controlled trial of the Picture Exchange Communication System for children with autism. *Journal of Child Psychology and Psychiatry*, *48*, 473–481.

Howlin, P., & Rutter, M. (1987). *Treatment of autistic children*. Chichester: Wiley.

Hughes, C. (2002). Executive functions and development: Emerging themes. *Infant and Child Development*, *11*, 201–209.

Humphrey, A. (2006). Children behaving badly. A case of misunderstanding? *The Psychologist*, *19*, 494–495.

Isquith, P. K., Crawford, J. S., Espy, K. A., & Gioia, G. A. (2005). Assessment of executive function in preschool-aged children. *Mental Retardation and Developmental Disabilities Research Reviews*, *11*, 209–215.

Iwata, B. A., Dorsey, M. F., Slifer, K. J., Bauman, K. E., & Richman, G. S. (1982). Towards a functional analysis of self injury. *Analysis and Intervention in Developmental Disorders*, *2*, 3–20.

Javorsky, J. (1995). An examination of language learning difficulties in youth with psychiatric disorders. *Annals of Dyslexia*, *45*, 215–231.

Karmiloff-Smith, A. (1998). Development itself is the key to understanding developmental disorders. *Trends in Cognitive Neuroscience*, *2*, 389–398.

Kaufman, A. S., & Kaufman, N. J. (1983). *Kaufman Assessment Battery for Children (K-ABC)*. Circle Pines, MN: American Guidance Services.

Kaufman, A. S., & Kaufman, N. J. (2001). *Specific learning disabilities and difficulties in children and adolescents*. Cambridge: Cambridge University Press.

Kaufman, A. S., & Kaufman, N. J. (2004). *Kaufman Assessment Battery for Children (K-ABC-II)* (2nd edn.). Circle Pines, MN: American Guidance Services.

Kaufman, A. S., & Kaufman, N. J. (2006). *Kaufman Brief Intelligence Test, 2nd Edition (K-BIT–2)*. Bloomington, MN: Pearson Assessment.

Kaufman, J. C., Kaufman, A. S., Kaufman-Singer, J., & Kaufman, N. L. (2005). The Kaufman Assessment Battery for Children, 2nd Edition and the Kaufman Adolescent and Adult Intelligence Test. In D. P. Flanagan, & P. L. Harrison (Eds.), *Contemporary intellectual assessment: Theories, tests and issues* (2nd edn., pp. 344–370). New York: Guilford.

Kennedy, P., & Llewelyn, S. (2001). Does the future belong to the scientist practitioner? *The Psychologist*, *14*, 74–78.

Korkman, M., Kirk, U., & Kemp, S. (1997). *NEPSY*. San Antonio, TX: Harcourt.

Kozulin, A. (2005). Learning potential assessment: Where is the paradigm shift? In D. B. Pillemer, & S. H. White-Sheldon (Eds.), *Developmental psychology and social change: Research, history and policy* (pp. 352–367). New York: Cambridge University Press.

Kyllonen, P. C. (1996). Is working memory capacity Spearman's *g*? In I. Dennis, & P. Tapsfield (Eds.), *Human abilities: Their nature and measurement* (pp. 49–76). Mahwah, NJ: Erlbaum.

Leiter, R. G. (1952). *Leiter International Performance Scale*. Wood Dale, Il: Stoetling.

Lipkin, P. H., & Allen, M. C. (2005). Introduction: Developmental assessment of the young child. *Mental Retardation and Developmental Disabilities Research Reviews*, *11*, 171–172.

Lohman, D. F., Thorndike, R. L., Hagen, E. P., Smith, P., Fernandes, C., & Strand, S. (2001). *Cognitive Abilities Test, 3rd Edition (CAT-3)*. London: NFER Nelson.

Lonigan, C. J., Burgess, S. R., & Anthony, J. L. (2000). Development of emergent literacy and early reading skills in preschool children: evidence from a latent-variable longitudinal study. *Developmental Psychology*, *36*, 596–613.

Lovaas, O. I. (1993). The development of a treatment-research project for developmentally disabled and autistic children. *Journal of Applied Behavior Analysis*, *26*, 617–630.

Lovaas, O. I. (1996). The UCLA young autism model of service delivery. In C. Maurice (Ed.), *Behavioral intervention for young children with autism* (pp. 241–250). Austin, TX: Pro-Ed.

Luciana, M. (2003). Practitioner Review: Computerized assessment of neuropsychological function in children: clinical and research applications of the Cambridge Neuropsychological Testing Automated Battery (CANTAB). *Journal of Child Psychology and Psychiatry*, *44*, 649–663.

Luria, A. R. (1966). *Higher cortical functions in man*. Andover, Hants: Tavistock Publications.

Luzzani, S., Macchini, F., Valadè, A., Milani, D., & Selicorni, A. (2003). Gastroesophageal reflux and Cornelia de Lange syndrome: typical and atypical symptoms. *American Journal of Medical Genetics*, *119A*, 283–287.

Magiati, I., & Howlin, P. (2003). A pilot study of the effectiveness of the Picture Exchange Communication System (PECS) for children with autism. *Autism: International Journal of Research and Practice*, *7*, 297–320.

Manly, T., Robertson, I. H., Anderson, V., & Nimmo-Smith, I. (1998). *Test of Everyday Attention for Children (TEA-Ch)*. London: Harcourt.

Mattison, R. E., Hooper, S. R., & Carlson, G. A. (2006). Neuropsychological characteristics of special education students with serious emotional/behavioural disorders. *Behavioural Disorders*, *31*, 176–188.

McDermott, P. A., Fantuzzo, J. W., Glutting, J. J., Watkins, M. W., & Baggaley, A. R. (1992). Illusions of meaning in the ipsative assessment of children's ability. *Journal of Special Education*, *25*, 504–526.

Micceri, T. (1989). The unicorn, the normal curve, and other improbable creatures. *Psychological Bulletin*, *105*, 156–166.

Moffitt, T. E., Caspi, A., Harkness, A. R., & Silva, P. A. (1993). The natural history of change in intellectual performance: Who

changes? How much? Is it meaningful? *Journal of Child Psychology and Psychiatry*, *34*, 455–506.
Morgan, A. E., Singer-Harris, N., Bernstein, J. H., & Waber, D. P. (2000). Characteristics of children referred for evaluation of school difficulties who have adequate academic achievement scores. *Journal of Learning Disabilities*, *33*, 489–500.
Moss, J., Oliver, C., Arron, K., Sloneem, J., & Petty, J. (2005). The association between environmental events and self injurious behaviour in Cornelia de Lange syndrome. *Journal of Intellectual Disability Research*, *49*, 269–277.
Mullen, E. M. (1995). *Mullen scales of early learning*. Circle Pines, MN: American Guidance Services.
Munakata, Y., Casey, B. J., & Diamond, A. (2004). Developmental cognitive neuroscience: progress and potential. *Trends in Cognitive Science*, *8*, 122–128.
Naglieri, J. A. (2005). The cognitive assessment system. In D. P. Flanagan, & P. L. Harrison (Eds.), *Contemporary intellectual assessment: Theories, tests and issues* (2nd edn., pp. 441–460). New York: Guilford.
Naglieri, J. A., & Das, J. P. (1997). *Cognitive Assessment System (CAS)*. Itasca, IL: Riverside.
Naglieri, J. A., & Das, J. P. (2005). Planning, Attention, Simultaneous, Successive (PASS) Theory. In D. P. Flanagan, & P. L. Harrison (Eds.), *Contemporary intellectual assessment: Theories, tests and issues* (2nd edn., pp. 120–137). New York: Guilford.
Naglieri, J. A., & Johnson, D. (2000). Effectiveness of a cognitive strategy intervention in improving arithmetic computation based on the PASS theory. *Journal of Learning Disabilities*, *33*, 591–597.
Neale, M. D. (1997). *Neale analysis of reading ability* (2nd edn.). Windsor: NFER Nelson.
Nicholson, J., Konstantinidi, E., & Furniss, F. (2006). On some psychometric properties of the Questions About Behavioral Function (QABF) scale. *Journal of Developmental Disability*, *27*, 337–352.
Oliver, C., Murphy, G., Hall, S., Arron, K., & Leggett, J. (2003). Phenomenology of self restraint. *American Journal on Mental Retardation*, *108*, 71–81.
Oliver, C., Demetriades, L., & Hall, S. (2002). Effects of environmental events on smiling and laughing behaviour in Angelman syndrome. *American Journal on Mental Retardation*, *107*, 194–200.
Packlawskyj, T. R., Matson, J. L., Rush, K. S., Smalls, Y., & Vollmer, T. R. (2001). Assessment of the convergent validity of the Questions about Behavioral Function scale with analogue functional analysis and the Motivation Assessment Scale. *Journal of Intellectual Disability Research*, *45*, 484–494.
Payne, R. W., & Jones, G. (1957). Statistics for the investigation of individual cases. *Journal of Clinical Psychology*, *13*, 113–121.
Pickering, S., & Gathercole, S. (2001). *Working Memory Test Battery for Children (WMTB-C)*. London: Harcourt.
Rapaport, D., Gil, M., & Schafer, R. (1945/6). *Diagnostic psychological testing*. Chicago, IL: Year Book Medical.
Repp, A. C., Singh, N. N., Karsh, K. G., & Deitz, E. D. (1991). Ecobehavioral analysis of stereotypic and adaptive behaviors: activities as setting events. *Journal of Mental Deficiency Research*, *35*, 413–429.
Ripley, K., & Yuill, N. (2005). Patterns of language impairment and behaviour in boys excluded from school. *British Journal of Educational Psychology*, *75*, 37–50.
Roid, G. H., & Miller, L. J. (1997). *Leiter International Performance Scale–Revised (Leiter-R)*. Wood Dale, IL: Stoelting.
Roid, G. H. (2003). *Stanford–Binet Test, 5th Edition (SB-5)*. Itasca, IL: Riverside.
Roid, G. H., & Pomplun, M. (2005). Interpreting the Stanford–Binet Intelligence Scales, 5th Edition. In D. P. Flanagan, & P. L. Harrison (Eds.), *Contemporary intellectual assessment: Theories, tests and issues* (2nd edn., pp. 325–343). New York: Guilford.
Rothlisberg, B. A., D'Amato, R. C., & Palencia, B. N. (2003). Assessment of children for intervention planning following traumatic brain injury. In C. R. Reynolds, & R. W. Kamphaus (Eds.), *Handbook of psychological and educational assessment of children: Personality, behavior and content* (2nd edn.). New York: Guilford.
Rutter, M., Bailey, A., & Lord, C. (2003). *Social Communication Questionnaire (SCQ)*. Los Angeles, CA: Western Psychological Services.
Rutter, M., & Yule, W. (2002). Applied scientific thinking in clinical assessment. In M. Rutter, & E. Taylor (Eds.), *Child and adolescent psychiatry: Modern approaches* (4th edn., pp. 103–116). Oxford: Blackwell Publishing.
Sainsbury, C. (2000). *Martian in the playground: Understanding the school child with Asperger's syndrome*. Bristol: Lucky Duck Publishing.
Sandoval, J. (2003). Constructing conceptual change in consultee-centered consultation. *Journal of Educational and Psychological Consultation*, *14*, 251–261.
Sattler, J. M. (2001). *Assessment of children: Cognitive applications* (4th edn.). La Mesa, CA: J. M. Sattler Publisher.
Sattler, J. M., & D'Amato, R. C. (2002). Brain injuries: Theory and rehabilitation programs. In J. M. Sattler (Ed.), *Assessment of children: Behavioral and clinical applications* (4th edn., pp. 440–469). San Diego, CA: J. M. Sattler Publisher.
Schuler, A. L., Peck, C. A., Willard, C. & Theimer, K. (1989). Assessment of communicative means and functions through interview: Assessing the communicative capabilities of individuals with limited language. *Seminars in Speech and Language*, *10*, 51–61.
Shapiro, E. S. (1996). *Academic skills problems workbook*. Oxford: Routledge.
Sheslow, D., & Adams, W. (1990). *Wide Range Assessment of Memory and Learning (WRAML)*. Wilmington, DE: Jastak Associates.
Shogren, K. A., & Rojahn, J. (2004). Convergent reliability and validity of the Questions About Behavioral Function and the Motivation Assessment Scale: A replication study. *Journal of Developmental and Physical Disabilities*, *15*, 367–375.
Simpson, R. L., & Myles, B. S. (1995). Facilitated communication and children with disabilities: An enigma in search of a perspective. *Focus on Exceptional Children*, 27, 1–16.
Simonoff, E., Pickles, A., Chadwick, O., Gringras, P., Wood, N., Higgins, S., *et al.* (2006). The Croydon assessment of learning study: prevalence and educational identification of mild mental retardation. *Journal of Child Psychology and Psychiatry*, *47*, 828–839.
Smith, F., & Hardman, F. (2003). Using computerised observation as a tool for capturing classroom interaction. *Educational Studies*, *29*, 39–47.
Smith, T., Mruzek, D. W., & Mozingo, D. (2005). Sensory integrative therapy. In J. W. Jacobson, R. M. Foxx, & J. A. Mulick (Eds.), *Controversial therapies for developmental disabilities: Fad, fashion and science in professional practice* (pp. 331–350). Mahwah, NJ: Lawrence Erlbaum Associates.
Snijders, J. T., & Snijders-Oomen, N. (1976). *Snijders-Oomen Non-verbal Intelligence Scale (SON 2.5–7)*. Groningen: Wolters-Noordhoff.
Snijders, J. T., Tellegen, P. J., & Laros, J. A. (1989). *Snijders-Oomen Non-verbal Intelligence Test (SON-R 5.5–17)*. Groningen: Wolters-Noordhoff.
Solity, J., Deavers, R., Kerfoot, S., Crane, G., & Cannon, K. (1999). Raising literacy attainments in the early years: the impact of instructional psychology. *Educational Psychology*, *19*, 373–397.
Sparrow, S. S., & Davis, S. M. (2000). Recent advances in the assessment of intelligence and cognition. *Journal of Child Psychology and Psychiatry*, *41*, 117–131.
Sparrow, S. S., Cicchetti, D. V., & Balla, D. A. (2006). *Vineland Adaptive Behavior Scales, Survey Edition* (2nd edn.). Circle Pines, MN: American Guidance Service.

Spearman, C. (1904). "General intelligence" objectively determined and measured. *American Journal of Psychology*, *15*, 201–293.

Stein, M. A., Szumowski, E., Blondis, T. A., & Roizen, N. J. (1995). Adaptive skills dysfunction in ADD and ADHD children. *Journal of Child Psychology and Psychiatry*, *36*, 663–670.

Sturmey, P. (2001). The Functional Analysis Checklist: Inter-rater and test–retest reliability. *Journal of Applied Research in Intellectual Disabilities*, *14*, 141–142.

Stutsman, R. (1948). *Merrill–Palmer Scale of Mental Tests*. Los Angeles, CA: Western Psychological Services.

Tsatsanis, K. D., Dartnall, N., Cicchetti, D., Sparrow, S. S., Klin, A., & Volkmar, F. R. (2003). Concurrent validity and classification accuracy of the Leiter and Leiter-R in low-functioning children with autism. *Journal of Autism and Developmental Disorders*, *33*, 23–30.

Tzuriel, D. (2000). Dynamic assessment of young children: Educational and intervention perspectives. *Educational Psychology Review*, *12*, 385–435.

Vaughn, S., & Fuchs, L. S. (2003). Redefining learning disabilities as inadequate response to instruction: The promise and potential problems. *Learning Disabilities Research and Practice*, *18*, 137–146.

Vygotsky, L. (1978). *Mind in society: The development of higher psychological processes*. Cambridge, MA: Harvard University Press.

Wagner, P. (2000). Consultation: developing a comprehensive approach to service delivery. *Educational Psychology in Practice*, *16*, 9–18.

Watkins, L. H., Sahakian, B. J., Robertson, M. M., Veale, D. M., Rogers, R. D., Pickard, K.M., *et al.* (2005). Executive function in Tourette's syndrome and obsessive-compulsive disorder. *Psychological Medicine*, *35*, 571–582.

Wechsler, D. (1939). *The Measurement of Adult Intelligence*. Baltimore: Williams & Wilkins.

Wechsler, D. (1974). *Wechsler Intelligence Scale for Children – Revised (WISC-R)*. San Antonio, TX: Psychological Corporation.

Wechsler, D. (1997). *Wechsler Adult Intelligence Scale, 3rd Edition (WAIS-III)*. San Antonio, TX: Psychological Corporation.

Wechsler, D. (1999). *Wechsler Abbreviated Scale of Intelligence (WASI)*. San Antonio, TX: Psychological Corporation.

Wechsler, D. (2001). *Wechsler Individual Achievement Test, 2nd Edition (WIAT-II)*. San Antonio, TX: Harcourt.

Wechsler, D. (2002). *Wechsler Preschool and Primary Scale of Intelligence, 3rd Edition (WPPSI-III)*. San Antonio, TX: Psychological Corporation.

Wechsler, D. (2003). *Wechsler Intelligence Scale for Children, 4th Edition (WISC-IV)*. San Antonio, TX: Psychological Corporation.

Wilkinson, G. S., & Robertson, G. J. (2006). *Wide Range Achievement Test 4 (WRAT4)*. San Antonio, TX: Psychological Corporation.

Woodcock, R. W., McGrew, K. S., & Mather, N. (2001). *Woodcock–Johnson III Tests of Cognitive Abilities (WJ-III-COG)*. Itasca, IL: Riverside.

Wright, I., Waterman, M., Prescott, H., & Murdoch-Eaton, D. (2003). A new Stroop-like measure of inhibitory function development: typical developmental trends. *Journal of Child Psychology and Psychiatry*, *44*, 561–575.

Yates, B. T., & Taub, J. (2003). Assessing the costs, benefits, cost-effectiveness, and cost-benefit of psychological assessment: We should, we can, and here's how. *Psychological Assessment*, *15*, 478–495.

Zhu, J., & Weiss, L. (2005). The Wechsler Scales. In D. P. Flanagan, & P. L. Harrison (Eds.), *Contemporary intellectual assessment: Theories, tests and issues* (2nd edn., pp. 297–324). New York: Guilford.

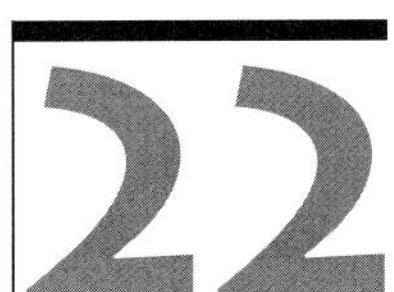

Physical Examination and Medical Investigation

Gillian Baird and Paul Gringras

This chapter describes the contribution of physical examination and subsequent investigations to the detection and assessment of any organic physical disorder in children presenting with mental health symptoms to the child and adolescent mental health services (CAMHS). Chapters 12, 24 and 30 outline brain disorders and the etiological risks that they pose for psychiatric disorders. Chapters 57 and 70 describe the impact of physical illness on psychosocial function.

The purpose of any medical assessment, including physical examination and laboratory or other tests, is to identify causative, associated or exacerbating medical problems.

Causation may be difficult to establish; but, for example, in a child with intellectual disability, identifying the etiology informs prognosis and recurrence risk counseling, and may guide subsequent therapeutic and educational intervention. For many families the need to "leave no stone unturned" can block coping mechanisms until finding the cause is addressed.

Associated medical conditions include hypothyroidism in children with Down syndrome, and conductive deafness in children with chromosome 22q11 deletions, and can strongly influence the presentation and management of developmental and psychiatric disorders.

Exacerbating medical disorders include, for example, unrecognized sensorineural deafness in an adolescent with autism, and severe iron deficiency in children with hyperactivity and learning difficulties. They are seldom causal, but if unrecognized and untreated they serve to worsen cognitive and behavioral problems in vulnerable groups of children.

The guiding principle for history-taking, physical examination and subsequent investigations is that treatable conditions need to be identified and a high priority given to any condition with genetic implications for the child or other family members. The impact of false negative and false positive tests, the discomfort associated with some examinations and investigations, and economic constraints, mean that clinicians need to know when to accept that a given child has been adequately examined and investigated. In this chapter we outline a systematic approach for using the relevant evidence to decide what makes particular aspects of history, examination and investigation worthwhile for a particular child.

Rutter's Child and Adolescent Psychiatry, 5th edition. Edited by M. Rutter, D. Bishop, D. Pine, S. Scott, J. Stevenson, E. Taylor and A. Thapar. © 2008 Blackwell Publishing, ISBN: 978-1-4051-4549-7.

Even though this chapter primarily focuses on what is reasonable to expect of the mental health professional, there are huge differences in training, seniority and experience that will affect an individual's threshold to refer to another specialist colleague, or examine and investigate personally. These factors, as well as national and international variations in the availability of specialist services and investigations, mean that the interpretation and application of didactic protocols can be difficult, despite their superficial attractiveness (Palfrey & Frazer, 2000).

Screening Programs

Most screening tests in pediatrics were designed to identify children at increased risk for certain disorders. It is expected that the natural history of the disorder is known, and that an intervention is available that can change its course.

The screening programs adopted vary internationally. Neonatal screening is rapidly growing, particularly with technologies such as tandem mass spectrometry, which allows the detection of a wide range of inborn errors of metabolism near birth. Phenylketonuria and thyroid function are particular examples of well-established neonatal screens in many western countries (National Screening Committee, 2006a,b). In the UK there has been a trend in recent years to decrease preschool screening programs and place an increasing reliance on parental concerns being brought to the appropriate professional group. In the preschool years this is usually a health visitor, and at school age either school nursing or teaching staff. Barlow, Stewart-Brown, & Fletcher (1998) conducted a critical appraisal of school-entry examination literature; disappointingly, no study provided either follow-up of children after referral to estimate the positive predictive value or yield of the screening, or follow-up of the whole cohort to identify false negative cases. The conclusion was that "Data on the effectiveness and efficiency of both the routine and selective school medical examination in accurately identifying children with new or ongoing health problems are not available at the present time" and challenged the ethics of such a program.

Unfortunately, and even in situations where routine screening has taken place, the assumption cannot be that a specific problem has been excluded. The advent of universal neonatal hearing screening does not rule out the need for subsequent hearing tests, particularly if there is parental or school concern. Late-onset sensorineural losses and middle-ear conductive problems can be acquired subsequent to birth. Any undiagnosed hearing loss can have devastating effects on a child's daytime performance, sociability and behavior. Even newborn testing for congenital hypothyroidism can miss hypopituitary hypothyroidism and primary hypothyroidism.

Faced with this variable and changing picture we suggest in the first instance that the clinician in the mental health clinic enquire about and document which routine screening tests have and have not been carried out. A negative screen may reduce the likelihood of a disorder, but this must always be outweighed by any clinical, parental or school concerns, which should trigger appropriate referral and investigations.

What is Worthwhile in History and Examination?

The approach to deciding if an activity is worthwhile applies as much to history-taking as to performing an examination or medical investigations. In all three situations the clinician needs a degree of specific local background knowledge, applicable to the population of children referred to the clinic. The concepts of availability, affordability and precision apply equally to physical examination as to medical investigations. In a busy clinic room, time is the main commodity, and aspects of history and physical investigation need to be worthwhile.

Hampton, Harrison, Mitchell *et al.* (1975) compared medical diagnosis after reading the referral letter, after taking a history and after physical examination. With history and the referral letter, the diagnosis was reached in 66 out of 80 cases. Clinical examination contributed and resulted in another seven diagnoses and laboratory investigations to another seven. Of more relevance to the specific population of children with psychiatric disorders and their comorbidities is the work of Dooley, Gordon, Wood *et al.* (2003), who prospectively assessed the impact of each component of the pediatric neurological consultation in 500 consecutive referrals to a tertiary care pediatric neurology clinic. Specifically, they found that examination and investigations were never influential for children with headaches, Tourette syndrome, developmental delay or attention deficit/hyperactivity disorder (ADHD). In children with developmental delay, examination did not alter their subsequent decision about investigation. For the majority of children, even in a specialized clinic with relatively high pre-test probabilities of neurological disorder, history influenced management in over 90% of cases, and examination in less than 6%.

Sackett, Haynes, Tugwell *et al.* (1991) have clarified the process of deciding what is worthwhile. The concept of pre-test probability requires the clinician to know or estimate the likelihood of the particular disorder being considered. Here populations differ and a child presenting to their GP with a headache for the first time has a lower "pre-test probability" of an underlying brain tumor than a child presenting to a regional pediatric neurology clinic with the same symptoms. Clinical history also affects pre-test probability of a certain diagnosis. For example, 0.4–3% of children with autism are found to also have tuberous sclerosis (Smalley, Smith, & Tanguay, 1991). When epilepsy and intellectual disability are additionally present the likelihood of also having tuberous sclerosis rises to 8–14% (Riikonen & Simell, 1990). In a cohort of children with autism the baseline chance of any child having fragile X syndrome is around 1.6%. However, a thorough physical examination that identifies key physical markers increases the likelihood of fragile X to 45% (Brown, Jenkins, Neri *et al.*, 1991). For the interested reader, Sackett *et al.* (1991) propose a convenient nomogram using Bayes' theorem that generates post-test probabilities if one knows the likelihood ratio of a given examination or test finding (Dooley, Gordon, Wood *et al.*, 2003). Results of using such a system have been published for the investigation of children with learning difficulties and potential fragile X syndrome (Hartley, Salt, Dorling *et al.*, 2002), and for children with motor delay and potential Duchenne muscular dystrophy (Dorling & Salt, 2001). In both examples it is clear which clinical findings would generate post-test probabilities that might take the clinician over a diagnosis or treatment threshold (Table 22.1).

Clinical experience, alongside the available evidence above, thus supports the need for any health professional to remain focused on the critical process of taking a good clinical history for organic disorders, before becoming distracted by lengthy examination protocols and a wide choice of modern investigations. The risks of missing a particular diagnosis are also likely to weigh heavily with clinicians in their decision-making.

The sections that follow on history and examination are by no means comprehensive, but focus on what is worthwhile.

History-Taking

Family History

We assume that a full family history for psychiatric, neurological, medical or learning difficulties and details of consanguinity is accepted as standard. We argue that a full "organic" history is worthwhile for any child presenting to CAMHS. Even when the history has been taken by a previous health care professional, it is not unusual for the family to have subsequently identified a further affected member, or remembered a significant prior illness. Furthermore, if time is short, the history is likely to be the most worthwhile area to spend time on, with examination and investigations taking much less time.

Pregnancy

An enquiry about pregnancy is expected by parents and is also worthwhile. The full range of teratogens, including tobacco, alcohol and most anticonvulsants, needs systematic enquiry, as does any history of rashes and fever during pregnancy, which may indicate exposure to a congenital viral infection.

Previous neonatal deaths or even acute life-threatening episodes in a sibling can be the most important pointer towards

Table 22.1 Examples of how factors modify pre-test probabilities for associated medical disorders in autism, influencing investigation decisions.

	Fragile X	Tuberous sclerosis	Treatable epileptic disorder in autism regression
Pre-test probability of disorder	Low (1.6%)	Low (1–4%)	Low
Factors increasing pre-test probability	IQ <70, family history, phenotypic features	Epilepsy, severe intellectual disability (increases rate to 8–14%)	Clinical epilepsy
Test	Molecular genetic testing	MRI	Sleep EEG
Likelihood of abnormal result	Low	Low	High for epileptiform abnormalities
Test sensitivity and specificity	High	Intermediate	Low
Post-test probability of disorder	High	Intermediate	Low
Chances of influencing action or treatment	High	Intermediate	Low in the absence of clinical epilepsy

EEG, electroencephalogram; MRI, magnetic resonance imaging.

an inborn error of metabolism. These rare conditions can present as unexplained learning and behavioral difficulties and are autosomal recessive with a recurrence risk of 25%.

Asking about previous spontaneous abortions may sometimes be uncomfortable for the clinician to ask, or parents to answer, but needs including in all histories. The important group is those couples who have had two or more spontaneous abortions; as many as 1 in 20 of these parents will carry a chromosome translocation or inversion. This may be associated with further viable children with unbalanced chromosomal disorders (Gardner & Sutherland, 1996).

Birth and Neonatal History

Parents are frequently concerned that any difficulty at birth is the cause of subsequent behavior or developmental problems, and therefore it is important to establish the gestational age at birth, the birth weight and whether the baby was "small for dates" (i.e., less than 10th centile at birth). Birth details need to include the type of delivery, state of the baby at birth and subsequent neonatal course. Although a history of traumatic birth may be of significance, it can also be a marker of pre-existing fetal difficulties, or be explained by recall bias. Persistent Apgar scores below 5, any symptoms of neonatal encephalopathy (e.g., fits), early imaging evidence, general metabolic disturbance, requirement for breathing support and the period for which that was needed would all be relevant in considering a difficult birth as a risk factor for subsequent developmental problems (see chapter 12).

Early Developmental History (Up to 5 Years)

We encourage the routine taking of a developmental history, alongside a behavioral history. Once again we are not in favor of the universal use of didactic developmental questionnaires. We prefer a flexible and responsive style of history-taking which uses broad probes that can quickly be refined to pursue any specific hypothesis that emerges. In this way the developmental history can be as quick as 10 minutes, to 1 hour in complex cases.

Dates of milestones are often hard for parents to recall. The advent of near universal parent-held records in the UK has proved invaluable and, where applicable, parents should be encouraged to bring these to the first assessment.

With the possible exception of remembering when a child first walked, dates of milestones need linking to key points in the family's life such as births, deaths, house moves, etc. Parents who have significant depression in the child's early life frequently find accurate recall much more difficult. Relative ages of acquisition of milestones can be easier for parents to remember, but while comparison with peers or siblings may be useful, it can also be misleading. The clinician needs to remember gender differences when comparing milestones in young children, and the huge normal range for most milestones.

Even when everything seems normal, "milestone moments" are a useful basis for discussing concerns. As a minimum we would propose the mental health professional gains an overview of the child's development and behavior during the first year of life, the expected changes in communication competence in the second year, and development and behavior during preschool placements, primary and secondary school and the transitions between them. Table 22.2 gives a simplified description of the skills expected at varying ages up to 5 years.

The age of onset of symptoms is crucial for a number of conditions, but establishing whether the pattern of development followed a normal trajectory is more difficult. Careful questioning is required to assess whether there is a loss of skills, or onset of new and different behaviors. It can be difficult to distinguish persistent continuing loss of skills from the plateauing that happens so often in children with a severe intellectual disability. The gains and plateaus of normal development

Table 22.2a Developmental examination (newborn – 13 months). Reproduced with permission from Dr. Ajay Sharma.

	Newborn	3 months	4 months	6 months	8 months	9 months	12 months	13 months
Posture/gross motor								
Supine	Head to side	Head in midline, finger play		Lifts head spontaneously				
Pull to sit	No head control		Good head control	Lifts head in anticipation				
Sitting	Flopping forward	Head held up, back curved	Straight back	Sits with hands for support	Sits with no support			
Ventral suspension		Good head control			Forward parachute			
Prone		Shoulders up on forearms		Chest off on hands				
Supported standing				Weight bears, downward parachute		Stands holding on	Walks hands held	Walks alone
Visual behavior								
Visual fixation and following	Looks towards bright light	Follows face beyond midline	Follows objects 180 degrees		Fixes on 1 mm sweets			
Hearing behavior								
Response to sound	Startle	Searches for sound		Turns head towards sound				
Personal–social								
	Smiles responsively – 6 weeks			Stranger awareness 6–7/12	Waves bye-bye	Points to ask	Points to show and share interest	
Play								
				Bangs and mouths	Looks for fallen toy, pulls string to get toy	Plays pat a cake, explores with finger	Holds phone to ear	Brushes own/mother's hair
Hand function/fine motor								
			Reaches with 1 hand 5–6/12, mouths 6/12, Transfers from hand to hand 7/12		Index finger approach	Pincer grasp 9–10/12, releases brick in a container	Mature grasp of 1 in brick	Builds tower of 2 cubes
Language and communication								
		Cooing		Babbling	Responds to own name		First word with meaning	Understands familiar names

Table 22.2b Developmental examination (15 months – 5 years).

	15 months	18 months	2 years	2.5 years	3 years	3.5 years	4 years	5 years
Play								
		Brushes doll's hair	Plays with small toys, relates 2	Symbolic use of toy (tea set, doll)	Develops short sequences with small toys	Uses "pretend" items in play	Acts out roles in play	
Hand function/fine motor								
Cubes	2 cubes 14/12	3 cubes	6 cubes	Puts 3 cubes in a row for a train	Makes a train with a chimney 39/12	3 brick bridge from a model	Steps of 6 cubes from a model	Steps of 10 cubes from a model
Pencil grasp			In prone at distal end	Middle of pencil	Mature grasp (tripod grasp)			
Drawing	Makes a mark on paper	Straight scribble	Circular scribble	Line in imitation	Copies: ○	Copies: +	Copies: □ 4–4.5 years	Copies: △
Shape sorting		Simple shapes ○ & □	○, □ & △		Completes simple jigsaw puzzles		Completes complex jigsaw puzzles	
Language								
Understanding	Simple requests in context: give me . . .	Knows 2–3 body parts	2 idea requests	Prepositions: in, on	Action words (running, eating)	Size, color, simple negatives	Follows 2 or more instructions in joined-up sentences	
Expressive	3 words		Puts 2 words together		Sentences of 3+ words, speech mainly clear; uses pronouns by 3.5 years		Uses conjunctions (and, but)	Gives complex explanations

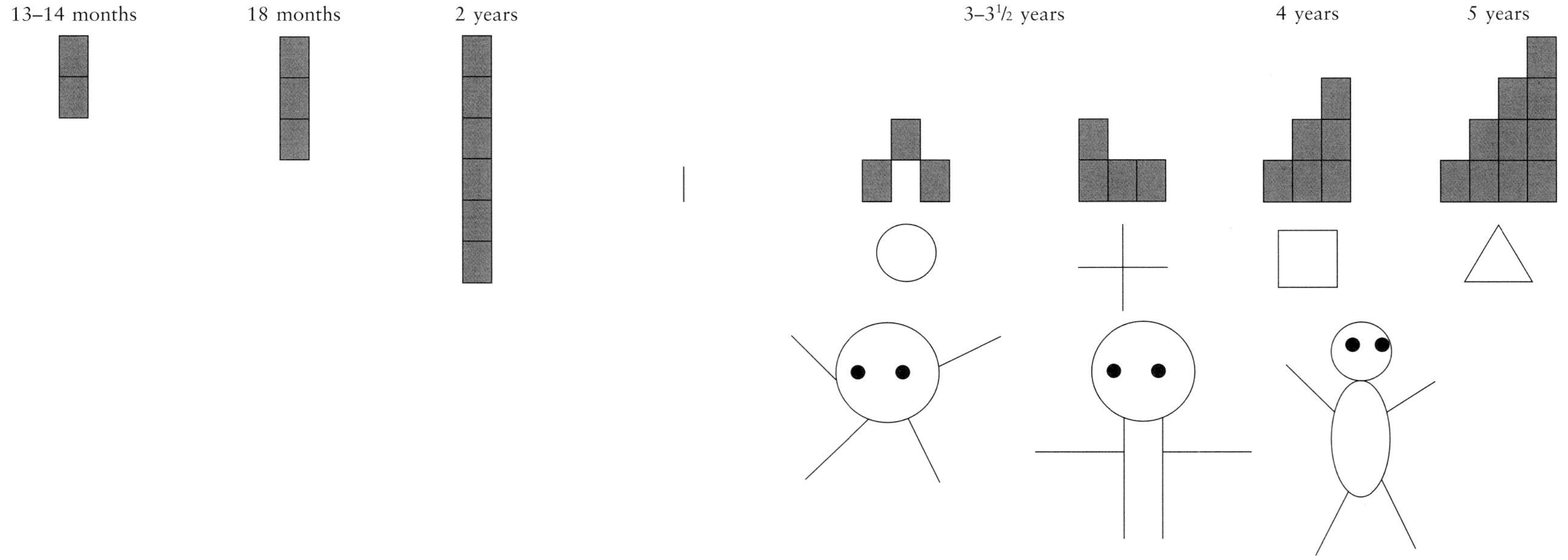

13–14 months | 18 months | 2 years | 3–3½ years | 4 years | 5 years

are often much more exaggerated in these developmentally delayed children.

Timing and trajectory are crucial for a number of conditions. It would appear that, for a number of prenatally acquired disorders, the brain is still capable of sustaining a certain amount of developmental progress before higher order functions fail. Thus, deaf children may babble normally in the first 6 months of life but then, lacking the usual language input, fail to develop further oral language skills. Some children with autism can progress well early in the first year but then show more apparent difficulties when demands on their social interaction and understanding increase. In children with Rett syndrome, early developmental skills can often appear in normal order (although usually delayed) before the process slows and there is emergence of extrapyramidal features and loss of useful hand function. In many neurological, genetic or metabolic disorders the advent of early seizures marks the beginning of developmental plateauing or decline. Seizure onset in the first 2 years is a marker of risk for developmental delay and autistic features.

Systematic Enquiry

The clinician will be aware that the separation of history and examination is necessary for the written page, but does not occur in reality. Observations of a child's general appearance, height and weight, signs of ill health and behavior are taking place before and during any period of history-taking, and may reasonably direct specific avenues of questioning.

We suggest starting with a probe into recent and past medical health with attention to hospitalizations, chronic diseases, hospital admissions and time off school with illness. General questions about physical and mental energy and enthusiasm for in-school and out-of-school activities are important, as is a discussion about whether these have recently changed.

Enquiries about appetite, weight gain or loss are important and naturally accompany the measurement and plotting of a child's height and weight centiles. Systematic enquiry is then made into concerns about motor competences, gait, hand and general co-ordination skills, sleep problems, gastrointestinal symptoms, headache, seizures, aches and pains generally, unspecified illnesses and weaknesses and any known medical problem. Fits, faints, headaches and other neurological symptoms are dealt with in specific sections that follow below.

Common disorders of childhood (e.g., asthma) should lead to an enquiry into medications that the child takes, both prescribed and over-the-counter.

Some symptoms are seen more commonly in particular disorders than in the general population, including thirst and excessive drinking in children with autism (who do not have diabetes), and constipation in many children with learning difficulties. Enquire about achievement of bowel and bladder control day and night, any day or night loss of control and history of stool withholding or opening in the nappy only (common in the autism spectrum disorders; see chapter 56). For gastrointestinal symptoms, a description of appetite, abdominal pain, vomiting, constipation and diarrhea is important, as is a discussion of the severity, frequency, timing, and exacerbating and relieving factors.

Primary sleep disorders are common in the general pediatric population and can exacerbate any emotional or behavioral symptoms (see chapter 54). Sleep disorders secondary to mood disorders are also common, and therefore this remains an important area of enquiry. Sleep difficulties can be broadly divided into problems with falling asleep, staying asleep or excessive daytime sleepiness. Insomnia, obstructive sleep apnea, restless leg syndrome and narcolepsy all impact on daytime behaviors, cognition and quality of life (Kotagal & Pianosi, 2006).

Perhaps the most difficult yet important part of history-taking is the presentation of child abuse, including factitious illness. Child abuse has protean manifestations, and without an awareness that it is common, and is often hidden for years, the diagnosis may be missed. Well-described presentations include withdrawal and depression, seizures, allergies and psychiatric symptoms. Often in the case of factitious illness the presentation of the illness or disease course does not make sense, and treatment is invariably ineffective or associated with the development of more symptoms.

We emphasize that for both these areas meticulous documentation of the history, which caregiver was being interviewed, and explanations and timings for all events is essential. It is often small but repeated inconsistencies in these cases that trigger suspicions that can prompt fuller multiagency investigations (see chapter 28).

Behavioral Phenotypes

The recognition that many genetic disorders present with both dysmorphic signs and well-characterized behavioral patterns can often guide the choice of investigations and speed diagnosis. Suspicion of a particular behavioral phenotype may begin during history-taking and then be strengthened by observations of the child (Table 22.3). The level of intellectual function of the child or young person (an essential component of the diagnostic framework), combined with specific neuropsychiatric diagnosis, will direct the clinician towards particular investigations. As in so many areas of medicine, knowledge of what phenotypes exist is the essential precondition for their recognition. Only if the Smith–Magenis syndrome phenotype is part of a clinician's diagnostic vocabulary will the self-injuring and sleepless autism spectrum child be quickly and appropriately investigated. Similarly, the disinhibited talkative child with a heart murmur presenting to an ADHD clinic may be recognized as having Williams syndrome, even if the facial dysmorphic features are subtle and would have been missed.

Examination

Although we include details of the neurological examination, we do not propose that all children presenting to mental health services need a full physical and neurological examination.

Table 22.3 Selected syndromes associated with self-injurious/challenging behavior and intellectual disability. (All are rare apart from 22q deletion (1 in 2000) and prevalence data, which are uncertain in most cases, have been omitted – this list comprises the "more common" top 10). Physical, behavioral and genetic information has been kept to a minimum to act as an *aide-memoire* without replacing any of the larger pre-existing texts and electronic databases. From Gringas (2003) with permission.

Syndrome	M : F Ratio	Physical "handles"	Behavioral "handles"	Genetics
Prader–Willi	M = F	Flat face/almond-shaped eyes/hypogenitalism	Skin-picking/voracious eating/sleep disorders	Paternal 15q11–13 (SNRP gene)
Lesch–Nyhan disease	Almost exclusively males	Motor delay and hypotonia/hyperreflexia and clonus/seizures	Pattern of self-biting of lips, tongue and fingers/aggression towards others	Xq26–27
Smith–Magenis	M = F	Brachycephaly/broad face/short broad hands	Nail-pulling/sleep disturbance/hyperactivity and autism	17q11
Rett syndrome	Usually females; rare cases of males	Hypotonia and deceleration of head growth/jerky truncal and gait dyspraxia/focal seizures	Midline hand stereotypies/hyperventilation and breath-holding	X-linked MECP2
Fragile X syndrome	X-linked but female carriers may have learning difficulties	Large ears/long face/testicular enlargement	Hyperactivity and impulsivity/gaze aversion/hand-biting and hand-flapping	FMR1
Aicardi syndrome	X-linked dominant, only seen in females	Retinal colobomas, spinal and rib abnormalities/agenesis of corpus callosum (on cerebral scan), eye lesions, infantile spasms	No communication/self-injury and aggression/frequent night waking	?Xp22
22q11-deletion syndrome	M = F		50% IQ <70. Attention deficits, non-verbal learning disability, autistic type features	22q11-deletion
Cri-du-chat	F : M 4 : 3	Hypertelorism/broad flat nose/microcephaly	High-pitched cry/hyperactivity/hand-waving/hand-sucking	5p-
Rubinstein–Taybi syndrome	M = F	Short stature and microcephaly/broad thumbs and big toes/beaked nose	Resistance to environmental change/rapid mood swings	?16p
Lowe syndrome	Males only – X-linked recessive	Congenital cataracts/renal tubular dysfunction/deep-set eyes/frontal bossing	Hand waving between eyes and light source/scratching/chewing hands/head-banging	Xq24–26
Cornelia de Lange	M = F	Miniature limbs/shortened fingers and toes/small upturned nose/anteverted nostrils	Minimal language/odd vocal sounds/face-hitting/lip-biting	?3q

This would not be supported by the available evidence, particularly in children with no intellectual impairment presenting with common emotional and behavioral problems. Much of the time a detailed examination will have been carried out previously and, unlike the history, we do not feel this always needs repeating. There are obviously certain aspects of the history, behavior or psychiatric diagnosis that may trigger specific examinations or investigations, and these are addressed separately.

General

The main purpose of physical examination in the absence of any specific organic symptoms is to look for evidence of physical abuse and neglect or a specific medical diagnosis. The general inspection is usually closely followed by a skin inspection looking for bruises and birthmarks. In older children the examination needs also to identify any signs of drug use including needle tracks, abscesses or hyperpigmentation on the arms. In those children with any degree of intellectual disability or intellectual disability, a systematic look for more dysmorphic features, including an inspection of the genitalia, may be required.

The height and weight should be plotted on appropriate centile charts. It is usually the trajectory that matters more than any one absolute measurement. Here again the parent-held record, where available, may contain earlier measurements for comparison. Changing trends and markedly discrepant weights for heights may be relevant for disorders such as Marfan syndrome, anorexia, the obesity of Prader–Willi and the adverse effects of some medications. Obesity in childhood is increasingly common and itself has major health implications. It could be a contraindication to some medications (e.g., risperidone). For some conditions, specialized growth charts are available (e.g., for children with Down syndrome) and are more informative.

There are no studies considering the impact of routine cardiovascular examination for children with mental health problems. Significant cardiac problems usually present early in life. In the absence of cardiac symptoms there is little justification for a full examination of pulses, heart sounds and blood pressure. Innocent murmurs are common in children, particularly in potentially stressful environments. In general, innocent murmurs will be asymptomatic, soft, early systolic and change with position. Pathological murmurs are more likely to be loud, symptomatic and continuous. If in any doubt a referral to a cardiologist is appropriate.

Certain medications should be monitored with regular recording of blood pressure and pulse rate from the baseline measurement. In such situations, blood pressure testing is important but the examiner needs to remember to use a cuff that covers two-thirds distance elbow to shoulder, and then interpret blood pressure with reference to age-appropriate normative values. An electrocardiogram (ECG) is indicated before starting some medications (e.g., tricyclics) but not as a routine.

Symptoms of abdominal pain or constipation should prompt abdominal examination. A distended abdomen with palpable stools suggests a degree of constipation that is capable of causing significant pain and changes in mood and can be treated.

The routine examination of vision and hearing in the child mental health setting is unlikely to be worthwhile, and has considerable potential to yield harmful false positive and false negative results (Hall & Elliman, 2006). We would be guided by parental concerns for visual problems and remember that a family history of eye disorders is often the best indicator that ophthalmological examination is required. Although there continues to be some debate, the early identification of a squint remains important (Table 22.6).

The additive impairment for any child with mental health problems of an unrecognized conductive or sensorineural hearing loss has already been discussed. The difficulty is that without the right expertise, equipment and environment there is little value in attempting hearing screening and we therefore encourage a very low threshold for referral to pediatric audiology services.

In the group of children who have problems communicating their symptoms, and where reasons for particular behaviors or changes in behavior are being sought (often those with intellectual disability and autism), a thorough physical examination becomes very important. Physical problems as straightforward as a tooth abscess, constipation or ear infections can all present with complex changes in behavior (often increased self-injury) in children with intellectual disability. Examination may have to be undertaken under sedation in a hospital in order to be certain that a physical pain does not underlie behaviors or to ensure that behaviors such as self-injury have not resulted in damage. Examples from the authors' personal experience include gastroesophageal reflux and chronic constipation as causes of challenging behavior and retinal detachment resulting from self-injury: all requiring sedated investigation in older teenagers with severe intellectual disability, autism and challenging behavior.

Dysmorphology

Much has been written about the recognition of facial dysmorphology. The advent of sophisticated electronic dysmorphology databases, while helpful, in no way replaces the opinion of experienced clinical geneticists. For many non-geneticists, the clinical history, examination and behavioral phenotype should precede and strongly influence the likelihood of attributing significance to facial features.

As in all aspects of examination, height, weight and head circumference are an important place to start. In genetic terms, these may act as pointers to many underlying conditions such as Sotos syndrome (large head, tall and often outbursts of challenging behaviors), XXX, XXY and XYY syndromes (tall, accompanying behavior and language problems) and Turner syndrome (XO) (girls with small stature and sometimes autism spectrum; see chapter 24).

The study of what is worthwhile remains the focus of our discussion, and congenital minor malformations (e.g., a pre-auricular skin tag, short fifth finger, sacral dimple, webbing of skin between toes) are a good example. Single minor

Table 22.4 Common dysmorphology and neurocutaneous syndromes that may present in the child and adolescent mental health services (CAMHS) clinic.

Neurofibromatosis type 1
Incidence 1 in 2500–4000; dominant with near-complete penetrance but 30% new mutation rate
Signs Short stature, café au lait marks after age 1 year >1.5 cm diameter, freckling in armpits after 3 years. Specific learning difficulty 40–60%, epilepsy 7%, macrocephaly common. Visual check needed for risk of optic glioma
Behavior Hyperactivity and other neuropsychiatric problems, OCD, autism, anxiety

Fragile X (X-linked)
Signs Macrocephaly, testicular enlargement, prognathic after puberty, large ears
Behavior Variable learning difficulties, mild–severe. Hyperactive, autistic features

Prader–Willi syndrome (chromosome 15)
Signs Obesity, strabismus, small stature, small hands and feet, cryptorchidism
Behavior Moderate to severe learning difficulty, rages, compulsive eating

Tuberous sclerosis
Signs Ash-leaf depigmented macules, shagreen patches, adenoma sebaceum on malar regions after 5 years, periungual fibromas, optic phakoma
Behavior Seizures including infantile spasms, autism, hyperactivity, severe learning difficulties common

Angelman syndrome (chromosome 15)
Signs Maxillary hypoplasia, deep-set eyes, large mouth and tongue, characteristic arm posture
Behavior Seizures, challenging behavior, need little sleep, severe learning difficulties with little or no speech

Sturge–Weber syndrome
Signs Port wine stain usually in trigeminal region
Behavior Seizures, learning difficulty

OCD, obsessive-compulsive disorder.

malformations are not a marker for occult major malformations. However, one-quarter of infants with three or more minor malformations will have a major malformation (Leppig, Werler, Cann *et al.*, 1987). Of these, around 15% will involve the CNS. Finding one major malformation (e.g., history of repaired cleft palate) in an adolescent presenting with psychosis should lead to the search for another major malformation such as congenital heart disease and a request for testing for abnormality in chromosome 22q11.

The surface skin features of tuberous sclerosis and neurofibromatosis are important, but again clues in the history will indicate the need for assessment. A child with developmental delay, autism and seizures should have a thorough examination including use of a Wood's light to highlight the "ash-leaf" depigmented areas. Parents (and child) will usually remember whether this has been performed and, unless it was a long time ago, it should not need repeating within a mental health clinic. If there has been no such prior examination, the decision of individual child mental health professionals whether to examine themselves or refer will depend on their confidence and experience and facilities available. The possibility of falsely reassuring or falsely worrying a family exists with physical signs, just as with investigations.

Genital physical examination in the mental health setting can be important for conditions such as Prader–Willi syndrome and fragile X, both of which can present with behaviors that may present for the first time to child mental health services (see chapter 24). However, there is no evidence to support doing this routinely without good suspicion, and in fragile X syndrome this is of little help in the prepubertal child.

Table 22.4 summarizes some features of syndromes in children presenting to mental health services. We would suggest all such examinations should take place at the end of a general process of observation and gradual physical examination, and end with the vest and pants off. During this time, in addition to parents' or carers' verbal consent, we would wish to have the child's assent and to respect their autonomy and privacy at all times.

Neurological examination

Despite the ordered precision suggested by proforma, the value of opportunistic observation cannot be overemphasized. The examination starts when the child walks towards the consulting room, climbs the stairs, manipulates the toys, gets up and down from the floor and sits in and out of chairs and talks – listen for speech abnormalities that may indicate neurological problems such as dysarthria. For a very young child, the physical examination is usually a confirmation of what has already been observed. Many movement disorders are diagnosed by the time the child has risen from a chair, walked across the room, turned round and walked back. Standing on tip-toes, hopping and walking heel–toe and on the outer edge of the feet (Fog test) only add to the precision of the diagnosis. It is important to remember that any examination of a child's gait includes an observation of how naturally the arms swing. A subtle hemiplegic cerebral palsy may well only be apparent on hopping, or observation of less spontaneous movements, or of flexed posturing of the arm on the affected side. Although some children do toe-walk normally (and often as a familial trait), it is more often seen in autism and can also be a sign of increased tone, or associated with contractures. A wide-based gait can again be simple immaturity, but raises suspicions about hypotonia or cerebellar problems. Children with neuromuscular problems such as Duchenne muscular dystrophy may present with learning or language difficulties before their motor signs become obvious. They should be observed rising from a chair and getting up from lying on the floor for signs of proximal muscle weakness. Look at the spine if there is any concern about asymmetry of movement or posture, a tuft of hair and pes cavus suggesting a hidden spinal lesion. Look for wasting in muscle groups (e.g., the calf in peroneal muscular atrophy).

Obvious dysmorphic features of the face have been discussed above. Mobility and strength may not be obviously affected in congenital hemiplegia but are in bilateral cerebral palsy. Limited movement plus dribbling, oromotor impairment and no speech may signal upper motor signs (e.g., perisylvian syndromes such as Worster–Drought syndrome; Clark, Carr, Reilly *et al.*, 2000).

Measurement of head circumference, which has already been discussed in the context of genetic disorders, is also an important part of the neurological examination. It needs to be accurately measured (best of three if possible) and then accurately plotted on an appropriate centile chart. It often reduces anxiety for the child if the parents' head circumferences are measured first, and this is anyway a necessary step. The most common cause of large and small heads is simply familial, and thus a comparison of midparental head centiles should precede interpretation of any single measurement. It is important to remember that even acceleration in head growth with centile crossing in the early years can still be familial and not imply serious underlying pathology. Abnormal head size is associated with a large number of rare disorders: Table 22.5 lists some important ones. It is important to remember that the initial increased head size, seen in some children with autism, may decrease with age and is very non-specific. The identification of an unusually large or small head centile measurement lacks sensitivity or specificity for any particular disorder, but can be useful for directing appropriate examinations and investigations. Marked microcephaly has specific genetic implications.

Table 22.5 Conditions associated with microcephaly and macrocephaly.

Conditions associated with microcephaly
Rett syndrome
Fetal alcohol syndrome
Acquired or secondary microcephaly after cerebral insult
Conditions associated with macrocephaly
Sotos syndrome
Mucopolysaccharidoses (e.g., San Filippo)
Signs Progressive macrocephaly, coarse features
Behavior Severe behavior disturbance, sleep problems

Neurological soft signs have been described as minor abnormalities in the neurological examination in the absence of other features of fixed or transient neurological disorder (i.e., hard neurological signs; Shaffer, O'Connor, & Shafer, 1983). The mere fact that the same group of signs has been associated with so many disorders (behavior problems, co-ordination difficulties, learning difficulties, bipolar disorder, prematurity, malnutrition, meningitis and schizophrenia) suggests a lack of specificity. In a study assessing mainstream schoolchildren, where half had previous meningococcal disease and half were controls, results were unhelpful (Fellick, Thomson, Sills *et al.*, 2001). Although higher scores on the soft sign battery used (graphesthesia, dysdiadokokinesis, mirror movements, motor speed and involuntary movements) were related to significantly worse performance on measures of cognition, co-ordination and behavior, the specificities and sensitivities were so poor that tossing a coin would have been of as much use.

In contrast, "hard" neurological signs contribute very precisely to diagnosis, where often the main objective is localization. In conceptual terms, the neurological history is expected to elicit what the "lesion" is, and then the examination to elicit where the "lesion" is. The detailed observation of a young child's gait or the ability to examine muscle tone and elicit deep tendon reflexes takes time to learn, but is likely to be more worthwhile than the routine use of a lengthy battery of imprecise soft neurological tests. Any neurological examination proforma, like a mental state examination, is hugely operator dependent. An experienced pediatric neurologist may elicit a brisk jaw-jerk reflex that others would miss. There are many excellent pediatric neurology textbooks towards which the interested reader is directed (e.g., Aicardi, 1992).

Table 22.6 Eye abnormalities.

Eye examination is helpful in a number of syndromes associated with learning problems and regression
The cornea is cloudy in mucopolysaccharidosis
Lens dislocation occurs in Marfan syndrome and homocystinuria
Coloboma is found in CHARGE association
Abnormal rings of color are found in Wilson disease
Abnormal eye movements are found in nystagmus, nerve palsy or apraxia
Fundal examination is indicated for atrophy, phakoma in tuberous sclerosis and pigmentary changes in Batten disease
Visual fields are abnormal in some hemiplegias and optic chiasm tumors

CHARGE, Coloboma, Heart defects, Atresia Choanae, Restricted growth and development, Genital hypoplasia, Ear abnormalities.

Neurological Motor Examination – A Rough Guide

Assessing Stance and Gait

Ask the child to stand still with eyes open then shut.

• Unsteadiness with eyes closed may indicate a sensory loss–posterior column (positive Romberg sign), peripheral neuropathy or vestibular problem (falls to one side consistently).

Watch the child walk away from you, turn and walk towards you.

• An ataxic gait is broad-based, unsteadiness is worse on "heel–toe" tightrope walk.

• Hemiparetic gait is with shoulder adducted, elbow flexed, forearm pronated and fingers flexed or fisted, foot plantar flexed, leg internally rotated and knee extended. If subtle, you may need to "stress" the system by asking the child to hop on each leg in turn.

• In a diplegic gait the legs scissor and may be crouched.

• A high-stepping slapping gait is typical of peripheral neuropathy.

Ask the child to walk on their *heels* (difficult if foot extensor or calf muscles are short or spastic), on *toes* and on the *outside* of incurled feet (Fog test).

• These walking tests assess associated movements (e.g., arm flexion, curling of both hands and fingers) which are normal up to 9 years. This is principally a test of neurological maturity, but marked asymmetry is abnormal.

Ask child to get up from floor as an easy test of proximal muscle power.

• Gower's test for weakness is positive if child has to climb up his or her own legs. This is abnormal and seen in muscle disease (e.g., Duchenne muscular dystrophy).

Tests for Cerebellar Function

Ask the child to reach with either hand to touch your finger and then return to touch their nose. Move your target finger to "stress" the system and ensure the need for the child to stretch a little.

• Past pointing and poor co-ordination may indicate cerebellar abnormality.

General observations

• Fasciculations (quivering under the skin) can signal neuromuscular disease.

• Tics are involuntary contractions in single or groups of muscles, repetitive and stereotyped.

• Myoclonus is a brief jerk in a muscle.

• Dystonia is a contraction, longer than myoclonus, resulting in spasm.

• Athetosis is spasms of writhing character, chorea is sinuous movements affecting multiple, usually distal joints.

• Hemiballismus – violent flinging movements of half the body.

• Static or intention tremors – these can signal cerebellar origin but also can be familial or due to medication.

Tone, Power and Reflexes

At the end of the above you may wish more formally to test tone, power and peripheral reflexes. If in doubt, refer.

Child Abuse Including Factitious Illness

Childhood abuse and childhood sexual abuse can present with a wide range of symptoms and signs, most of which are not, on their own, pathognomonic of abuse (see chapters 28 & 29). Psychiatric presentations can be subtle and varied including child regression, dementia-like symptoms and conversion behaviors. It is the combination, context and corroboration of information from multiprofessional opinion that usually result in successful identification and prevention of further abuse (Larcher, 2004). Specialist training is usually required as even the more obvious physical signs, including bruise types, bites and burns, can be missed unless some specific training has taken place (increasingly commonly mandatory for health care professionals). A search for more subtle signs, genital examinations and invasive procedures should take place on as few occasions as possible, preferably by an experienced team which will often include forensic expertise, police and social service support (Kellogg *et al.*, 2005).

Münchausen syndrome by proxy (or factitious illness) forms an important and increasingly commonly recognized part of the spectrum of child abuse. Many children who are victims of factitious illness have long-term morbidity resulting from the attacks themselves or complications from the medical procedures that ensue. Virtually all have serious psychological sequelae from this form of abuse. It is said that parents who act as perpetrators in these cases often seem particularly close with the medical staff, eliciting their sympathies, and seem very eager to pursue invasive and in-patient testing for their child. Given that so much of the morbidity resulting from this condition occurs in hospitals and at the hands of the treating pediatrician or mental heath professional, it is essential to consider the possibility of factitious illness in the differential diagnosis as early as possible.

Standard toxicology studies are often inadequate for detecting poisons that perpetrators give; examples include tricyclic antidepressant abuse in cases of CNS depression, and warfarin in apparent coagulopathies (Galvin, Newton, & Vandeven, 2005). It is worth measuring blood levels if a child is on medications (e.g., antiepileptics or antidepressants) as toxic levels may be causing the presenting symptoms.

Given that these children are very likely to have received care from multiple hospitals and doctors, records from all professionals need to be meticulously kept and shared if required. As in all subgroups of child abuse, the use of a multidisciplinary team (including pediatricians, social workers, the child protection team and often the police) is essential for these cases (Working Party of the RCPCH, 2002).

Investigations

Unfortunately, the attraction of newer technologies often overtakes the need for a robust evaluation of a test in a representative and controlled large-scale study. Few investigations have undergone any analysis of sensitivity or specificity in truly representative clinical populations and control groups. As

Table 22.7 Framework for considering reasons for diagnostic tests in developmentally delayed children. From Gringras (1998) with permission.

Positive	Negative
Treatment possibility Such as thyroid replacement in hypothyroidism	Physical/psychological harm from testing Such as need for general anesthetic/lumbar puncture
Genetic causation Such as fragile X with implications for extended family	False positive or false negative diagnosis Implications for child and whole family
Explanation for parents and family "Need to leave no stone unturned" for some families	Financial implications of expensive tests
Prognostic information Help carers to reach realistic future expectations	Delays appropriate "non-medical" management May slow down process of choosing right education placement or behavioral intervention
Research	

If ethical, consent/assent given and conducted on representative epidemiological sample or likely to contribute to etiology and treatment.

with history and examination, the same standard of requiring a test to be available, affordable, accurate and precise exists. Knowledge of pre-test probabilities and likelihood ratios will help determine the potential for any particular investigation to affect management.

The potential to discover a treatable condition or one that will inform future family reproductive decisions remains the most important reason to pursue testing. Other potential benefits and drawbacks of testing are summarized in Table 22.7.

Harm From Testing

Anyone who has been faced with children with developmental delay will acknowledge that for some parents the need to know is great, and therefore any investigation that may "tell us something" has to be a good thing; but if it tells us the wrong thing then it is clearly not a good thing. False positives and false negatives occur all the time, and the more investigations carried out per child, the more chance of unearthing a "borderline" result that simply worries parents and causes the child to be subject to more unnecessary tests. False positive genetic tests for fragile X when cytogenetic techniques were used affected extended families, who may have been subjected to needless screening (Gringras & Barnicoat, 1998). Furthermore, the process of blood tests, electroencephalogram (EEG) and scans can be aversive for some children (and parents).

Numbers Needed to Test

In evidence-based medicine we have found the concept of "number needed to test" in order to find one positive result that will affect management, helpful in this regard. The calculation is not too difficult but crucially depends on the prevalence of the condition in the population being tested. In some countries, if HIV testing were advocated for every child presenting with unexplained neuropsychiatric symptoms, the number needed to test would be high; in others low enough to make routine testing worthwhile. Examples exist even on a national level where in certain locations screening for lead is important and should be part of every guideline, while in other areas it would be an expensive investigation that would yield too few positive results.

Economics

It is clear that no health system will be able to sustain an approach of carrying out every test available on every child with intellectual disability or neuropsychiatric problems, regardless of cost or impact on the child. It is increasingly clear that economic considerations will affect thresholds for investigations, between countries, regions and even individual units.

Current Testing Schema

When evidence-based methods are employed, the results tend to support fewer rather than more investigations. To improve yield, investigations need to be tailored to individual populations. It is likely that a stepwise approach is effective but this needs further evaluation. If it is certain that cerebral imaging (computed tomography [CT] or magnetic resonance imaging [MRI]) will need to take place, then we would suggest performing them first as they may give enough diagnostic clarity to avoid the need for subsequent tests.

Cerebral Imaging

The decision of what cerebral imaging and when is far from easy. While, for example, MRI scans give a higher yield than CT scans, the debate is still open on whether they are worthwhile. In one study, 224 MRI scans were carried out in children with developmental delay and other problems (Bouhadiba, Dacher, Monroc *et al.*, 2000). A retrospective analysis of clinical findings and diagnostic yield found abnormalities in 109 cases, but none that resulted in any patient care modification. In some cases it was even unclear whether they represented normal variants or true abnormalities.

Cerebral or cerebellar dysgenesis is usually the most common diagnostic category in these children, and while we do not know what causes this, it implies a prenatal event which should then usefully limit further laboratory investigations for acquired or metabolic causes (Shevell, Majnemer, Rosenbaum *et al.*, 2001). In rarer cases, MRI studies can show a characteristic signature for metabolic, neurocutaneous and degenerative disorders and can even give enough information to direct subsequent genetic testing.

Attractive new technologies are constantly evolving, with functional and diffusion tensor imaging techniques currently exciting the research world. Despite their promise, they still lack any of the robust validation work in representative populations that we would suggest is prerequisite to considering their routine clinical use (see chapter 11).

Genetic Investigations

Genetic investigations continue at an astonishing pace. Many useful reviews have been written to summarize the role of genetic investigations for children with developmental delays (Poplawski, 2003). High-resolution chromosome banding still remains important for many children with intellectual disability. Specific molecular genetic tests – fMRI studies for fragile X syndrome, *MECP2* for Rett syndrome and fluoresent in-situ hybridisation (FISH) 22q11.2 studies for velocardiofacial syndrome – can confirm specific diagnoses with known natural histories and heritabilities.

Although limited by cost and time, subtelomere fluorescent *in situ* hybridisation (FISH) is receiving increasing support as a routine investigation in children with intellectual disability. Some studies report such chromosome subtelomere rearrangements occurring with a frequency of 7–10% in children with mild to moderate intellectual disability, and approximately 50% of cases are familial (Dawson, Putnam, Schultz *et al.*, 2002). Positive results from this investigation are eight times more likely than fragile X in some intellectually disabled populations.

Uniparental disomy – in which both copies of a chromosome pair or region are inherited from only one parent – is well known in the context of chromosome 15 in Angelman and Prader–Willi syndromes, and is now recognized to affect many more chromosomes with resultant physical and neurological problems. Newer and cheaper methods for genetic investigations include multiplex ligation-dependent probe amplification (MLPA). They suggest that genetic investigations will increasingly contribute towards the investigation and understanding of these children (see chapter 24).

Metabolic Investigations

The range of metabolic conditions that can be relatively easily detected, even at birth, has dramatically increased. However, there is still debate about the yield of such testing.

The most important principle in later detection of metabolic disorders is that there are clues in the history that greatly alter the pre-test probability of detecting a metabolic disorder. Key pointers in the clinical history include consanguinity, failure to thrive and episodic decompensations (often during minor illnesses). Examination findings may include coarse facial features or hepatosplenomegaly. Although the yield of metabolic testing across population studies is lower than that of MRI scans and genetic testing, the debate is not quite that simple. Metabolic screening if positive is more likely to offer a treatment possibility or recurrence information than most other investigations, and may therefore be more worthwhile (Papavasiliou, Bazigou, Paraskevoulakos *et al.*, 2000).

The authors recommend watching this area with interest, but would not recommend metabolic testing for children presenting to CAMHS unless strongly indicated by any of the above clinical clues.

Electroencephalography

The EEG examination is most commonly used as an adjunct to the diagnosis and management of epilepsy. An EEG should be carried out to support a diagnosis of epilepsy and is usually recommended after the second epileptic seizure and in certain circumstances after the first (see chapter 17). An EEG is unhelpful and not indicated if the clinical presentation suggests a non-epileptic event, and an EEG should never be used in isolation to make a diagnosis of epilepsy. Where a standard EEG has not contributed to the diagnosis or classification of the epilepsy, a sleep EEG (under sleep-deprived conditions, which enhance EEG abnormality, or sleep induced with melatonin) or video or ambulatory EEG may be used. Epileptiform activity (spike, spike–wave complexes and ictal discharges) on the EEG with coincident clinical symptomatology is the hallmark of epilepsy. Identical epileptiform activity known as interictal epileptiform discharges (IEDs), which are not associated with obvious clinical phenomena, also occur. In some studies they have been associated with altered performance on a variety of cognitive and memory tasks carried out during awake EEGs. However, their significance remains uncertain. A review of IEDs suggested that "although they can have an additional and independent effect, this is mild" (Aldenkamp & Arends, 2004).

The finding of abnormality in the EEG in otherwise normal people who have never had an epileptic seizure is common. In one study of 60 healthy student volunteers screened for neurological disorder, only 6.7% did not show any transient "abnormality" in a whole night's sleep recording of the EEG. Abnormalities were mainly sharp but also spike-like activity (Beun, van Emde Boas, & Dekker, 1998).

Many previous uses of EEG, such as the diagnosis of brain tumors, have been superseded by both CT and MRI neuroimaging. However, there are rarer examples of an EEG study helping in non-seizure-related diagnoses. These include children presenting with the characteristic physical and behavioral phenotype of Angelman syndrome, who often have characteristic EEG changes that may precede seizures and support the diagnosis. The investigation of developmental regression can be supported by identifying the distinctive patterns of periodic discharges in subacute sclerosing panencephalitis and Creutzfeldt–Jakob disease. The EEG can aid diagnosis in both infective (herpes simplex) and non-infective (Hashimoto) causes of encephalitis, and a diffuse slowing pattern is a hallmark of some metabolic encephalopathies and can be used to track progress. Finally, the EEG is often employed in presentations with coma, but interpretation is complex with marked variations dependent on cause.

Specific Clinical Scenarios

The Child with Developmental Delay

In the relatively uncommon scenario in which a detailed history and thorough examination have yielded no clues, there is a debated "minimum" raft of investigations for a child with moderate to severe delay. The outcome of this debate is the fact that even similarly trained UK pediatricians, when confronted with exactly the same hypothetical case scenario of a child with developmental delay, varied widely in the type (26 different investigations) and the number of investigations in combination they would perform (0–15) (Gringras, 1998).

Developmental Delay without Motor Signs

One larger study separated children with developmental delay into subtypes with global delay, motor delay, developmental language delay and autistic spectrum disorders (Majnemer & Shevell, 1995). The etiological yield varied across these delay subtypes: 55% for global developmental delay, 59.1% for motor delay, 4.2% for developmental language disorders and 2% for autistic spectrum disorders. Thus, the subtype of delay is important, and the yield is lowest in those children with "pure" language disorders or autism.

On most lists therefore, the investigations would appear as in Table 22.8, but even these are open to debate, as is the order we have suggested performing them.

Developmental Delay with Motor Signs

The reader is referred to the neurological examination section (see p. 327). The likelihood of an underlying cause in this group of children is much higher, and thus examination is more worthwhile. In most cases, an early referral will be appropriate if the child is not already known to pediatric neurology services. There are both treatment and important genetic implications for diagnoses such as Duchenne muscular dystrophy. Simple tics need differentiating from choreoathetoid movements but it is worth emphasizing that Wilson disease and Friedreich ataxia are extremely rare, even in pediatric neurology clinics. Huntington chorea is also rare, but the child can often present with behavioral issues, long before motor problems are identified.

Table 22.8 Investigations in developmental delay.

Creatine kinase in boys less than 3 years
Thyroid function tests irrespective of neonatal screening
Chromosomes for karyotype and molecular analysis for fragile X
MRI scan or CT scan in more severe delay

CT, computed tomography; MRI, magnetic resonance imaging.

The Child with Delayed/Impaired Speech and Language

Delayed speech and language development is common and usually part of normal developmental variation, or associated with intellectual disability, in which case investigation follows the developmental delay protocol above but with a low threshold for requesting chromosome analysis to look for sex chromosome abnormalities. Hearing assessment is obviously crucial to exclude deafness, but thereafter cases are often divided into those with severe receptive language impairment and those with speech and articulation impairments. The former may benefit from a sleep EEG to exclude Landau–Kleffner syndrome if the clinician is confident of any regression beyond the first 10-word stage and there is marked fluctuation of language skills. However, in the case where a child has not reached a 10-word stage and presents with an autistic phenotype an EEG is not informative.

For the group with speech and articulation impairment, the presence of symptoms and signs of oromotor involvement such as dribbling, chewing problems or palatal insufficiency is important. Abnormalities on neurological examination may suggest Worster–Drought syndrome and prompt an MRI brain scan looking for perisylvian abnormalities (Clark *et al.*, 2000). Palatal abnormalities should lead to consideration of genetic causes such as 22q deletion. Medical investigations are unlikely to be helpful in the absence of the above signs or symptoms.

The Child with a Possible Seizure

The prevalence of epilepsy in the UK is 0.5% in children, with 1 in 2000 children developing epilepsy each year. The National Child Development Study (Ross, Peckham, West *et al.*, 1980) found that 0.7% of all children had at least one episode of altered consciousness in their lifetime, and nearly 40% of those children had other paroxysmal episodes. The differential diagnosis of a first seizure is wide. The important factor to remember about epilepsy is that in studies of either adults or children, 10–40% are wrongly diagnosed with epilepsy. Recently, the National Centre for Clinical Excellence (NICE) in the UK produced recommendations for practice (NICE, 2004). The main recommendation is that confirmation of a diagnosis of epilepsy should be made in children by a pediatrician with specialist training and expertise in epilepsy who can undertake further investigations. In addition to the importance of an extremely good description, by somebody who has seen an episode, the increased availability of home videos has been very helpful. Together these will often allow accurate diagnostic classification and diagnosis of the type of epilepsy syndrome. For most psychiatrists the appropriate course of action would be to refer to the pediatrician rather than undertaking further investigation themselves.

The mental health professional may, however, find themselves in the position of management of young people with epilepsy taking antiepileptic drugs (AEDs) who may or may not have additional learning and neuropsychiatric problems. The clinician should bear in mind the need for someone to review the requirement for and dose of AEDs (which may exacerbate or reduce behaviors), a protocol for emergency treatment in the community for those prone to prolonged or repeated seizures, the possible interaction with oral contraceptives in girls and the risks of particular medications in pregnancy (see chapter 30).

Neuroimaging with MRI is recommended to identify structural abnormalities causing epilepsy, especially in those under 2 years, where there is any suggestion of focal epilepsy, or in those where epilepsy persists despite medication treatment.

Differently sited sustained focal epileptic activity of continuous spike–waves during sleep (CSWS) may be related to varying neuropsychological deficits in a spectrum of childhood encephalopathies with or without overt seizures (e.g., language regression syndromes such as Landau–Kleffner syndrome), cognitive regression with occipital discharges and benign Rolandic epilepsy (a common benign epilepsy with centrotemporal spikes). Support for a causative role of the epileptic discharges in causing the language regression is suggested by the start of language recovery when the sleep abnormalities disappear (Robinson, Baird, Robinson *et al.*, 2001; Wilson, Djukic, Shinnar *et al.*, 2003). Knowledge of the possibility of such epileptic phenomena will alert the clinician to a story of fluctuating cognitive and behavioral manifestations and prompt referral to the pediatric neurologist or pediatric epilepsy specialist.

The Child with Regression

Parents will occasionally report a loss of skills and this always needs taking very seriously. The difficulty often arises in deciding what may be developmental plateauing in a child whose peers have started to accelerate in one or another domain. Altered function is a feature of many other ordinary life experiences including change of school and family domestic upheaval. History and examination, including type of developmental neuropsychiatric diagnosis and whether the regression is progressive or has plateaued, help guide further investigation. There should be a low threshold for onward referral, particularly if the regression is accompanied by epilepsy or abnormal neurological findings.

Causes of regression are often grouped either by age of presentation or pattern of clinical features. Children with white matter disease are more likely to present with focal neurological deficits, spasticity and blindness, whereas those with gray matter disease initially present with seizures, personality change and dementia. If the peripheral nervous system is also involved, mitochondrial and lysosymal disorders are more likely. The presence of other organ involvement again suggests mitochondrial and lysosomal, and also peroxisomal disorders.

Detailed description of the causes and investigations for regression are the remit of pediatric neurology textbooks. We have chosen just a few salient examples to illustrate the range of causes and subtle differences in presentation.

In many countries human immunodeficiency virus (HIV) infections are becoming an important cause of regression, with neurological and neuropsychiatric manifestations usually presenting in the first 3 years of life (see chapter 58). These include loss of developmental milestones, loss of cognitive abilities and progressive, often symmetrical, motor deficits with ataxia and eventual spasticity. This presentation can be subtle or delayed, particularly if children are on retroviral medications.

Parents of a proportion (15–30% in varying series) of children with autism report language regression in the second year of life (loss of use of words after 5+ words are established for 3 months; Tuchman & Rapin, 1997). This feature of autism remains a puzzle and has been the subject of investigation without finding any positive results that have effectively influenced treatment. Landau–Kleffner syndrome has been discussed, but it is very rare and most children presenting with language regression under the age of 36 months will have autism (McVicar, Ballaban-Gil, Rapin *et al.*, 2005). In issuing its guidelines, the report of the quality standards committee of the American Neurology Association states that "the relationship between regression early or late in autism and epileptiform discharges or electrical status in slow wave sleep (ESES) remains unclear" (Filipek, Accardo, Ashwal *et al.*, 2000). Our view on the present evidence is that an EEG should be carried out as part of the investigation of *clinically* suspected epilepsy, not routinely in regression in autism (Baird, Robinson, Boyd *et al.*, 2006). Regression in autism after the age of 36 months is less common, and if there is a 2-year period of normal development it is termed childhood disintegrative disorder (CDD). As the regression frequently involves not only social and communicative and language regression, but also bowel and bladder and cognitive function, investigations are frequently undertaken; but if the diagnosis of CDD is correct and the phenotype that of autism, the yield of investigation is frustratingly low.

A study group focusing on the very rare progressive intellectual and neurological degenerative (PIND) diseases was established to collate data in the UK from May 1997 to October 2005. During the surveillance, over 90 different neurodegenerative conditions were determined. Subacute symptom onset is common and psychiatric presentations – including dysphoria, withdrawal anxiety, insomnia and loss of interest – are not unusual, particularly for degenerative neurological diseases such as the rarer variant Creutzfeldt–Jakob degenerative neurological disease. Children with those conditions will invariably develop signs of neurological dysfunction evident on thorough clinical examination. For example, there may be signs of spastic paraparesis in adrenoleukodystrophy, visual loss in neuronal ceroid lipofucinosis or extrapyramidal features in Wilson disease. Some diagnostic features, although specific, may be subtle. San Filippo is an example of a condition in which regression can occur with or without autistic symptoms but where signs may be missed. The 10 most commonly reported PIND diagnoses are listed with some basic clinical features in Table 22.9.

The Child with ADHD

Routine investigations are not recommended as part of the diagnosis. There have been inconsistent findings in the tests of thyroid function, lead levels, EEG and imaging, and

Table 22.9 Most commonly reported progressive intellectual and neurological degenerative (PIND) diagnoses and basic clinical features.

PIND diagnosis	Sample of clinical features
Mucopolysaccharidosis type III San Filippo	Facial coarsening not prominent but most have hepatomegaly. Main feature is delayed motor development towards the end of the second year. Hyperactivity and sleep disorders are seen in early childhood before progressive dementia
Neuronal ceroid lipofucinosis	Decreasing visual acuity then declining school performance and behavioral disturbance. In late juvenile type delusions and hallucinations are common
Adrenoleukodystrophy	Cerebral form usually manifests between 5 and 10 years. Often presents with an alteration in behavior and poor school performance, followed by gait and co-ordination involvement
Mitochondrial cytopathy (unspecified)	
Rett syndrome	Mainly but not exclusively girls. Characteristic deceleration of head growth, loss of purposeful hand movements before the age of 3 years replaced by midline hand wringing
Metachromatic leukodystrophy	Onset of juvenile form usually between 5 and 10 years. Cognitive regression, ataxia and speech disturbances
GM_2 gangliosidosis (Tay–Sachs)	Affected children appear normal until 3 years. Then language delay and gait disturbances followed by progressive dementia
Niemann–Pick disease type C	Normal early development in delayed onset form. Ataxia or dystonia around 3 years with vertical gaze apraxia (can move eyes upwards reflexly but not voluntarily)
Krabbe leukodystrophy	In late onset type neurological deterioration any time from infancy to adolescence. Regression accompanied by cortical blindness and spasticity
Leukodystrophy unclassified	

consequently none are routinely recommended (see chapter 34). A recent review of the value of chromosome tests in ADHD confirms that without other clinical concerns, such as intellectual disability, these should not be routinely performed (Stephen & Kindley, 2006). It is most important to enquire about sleep problems, as interference with sleep can cause symptoms indistinguishable from those of ADHD. Baseline physical examination should focus on height, weight, pulse and blood pressure.

The Child with Autism

The importance of history, checking that hearing and vision have been tested at some stage recently, and more detailed examination has already been discussed. The overall yield in medical investigations is very low when applied routinely (Battaglia & Carey, 2006). We would suggest only fMRI (for fragile X syndrome) and karyotype, and even this is likely to have a low yield unless there are other clinical indications, including intellectual disability. The yield of testing for *MECP2*, the Rett gene, when assessing children with abnormalities suggestive of the broader phenotype, including learning difficulties and regression, remains to be determined. There is no justification for EEG routinely in autism but the clinician needs to be alert to fluctuant symptoms and regression with suspicion of epilepsy, and should use the EEG only as a clinical tool that contributes to the evaluation of epilepsy. Neuroimaging is worthwhile only when there are specific neurological signs, a focus found on EEG (sometimes) or the triad of severe intellectual disability, autism and epilepsy. There is no evidence to justify routine hair analysis, celiac testing, fungal or immunological tests, lumbar puncture, micronutrients or vitamin measurements, or urinary peptide determination (Battaglia & Carey, 2006).

The Child with Tourette Syndrome

The challenge in most children with tic disorders is to be sure of the diagnosis (see chapter 44). Once again a good clinical history is fundamental to reaching a confident diagnosis. True tics are often accompanied by an urge to carry them out, can be resisted by the child for a while, but then burst out, usually with a feeling of relief. The phenomenon of tic suppression often means that a short clinic visit can pass with no tics seen in all but the most severe of cases. The era of video cameras and even video phones has helped diagnosis greatly. With careful history and observation, there is usually no confusion between tics and other movement disorders such as chorea or dystonia.

The diagnosis of uncomplicated Tourette syndrome should not trigger any further investigations in most situations. Only if there are very atypical symptoms, which go beyond the common fluctuating picture often seen in Tourette syndrome, such as a progressively worsening picture or localizing neurological signs, would we consider referring for a neurological opinion and an appropriate battery of neurological investigations.

The discovery of a streptococcal autoimmune association in certain cases of tic disorder, Tourette syndrome and obsessive-compulsive disorder promised a whole new battery of useful investigations and treatment options for these disorders. However, rates of streptococcal infections in the general population are high, as are the presence of antibodies to the streptococcus. Some detailed antibody studies have challenged the hypothesis that this population differs from controls in any immunological manner (Singer, Hong, Yoon *et al.*, 2005). This means that we are cautious in recommending the investigation of a child with tics, Tourette or obsessive-compulsive disorder with a view to treating "the PANDAS," as neither antibiotics, steroids or plasmapheresis have good evidence to support their use, and the latter two carry potential for side-effects (King, 2006).

The Child with Anorexia Nervosa

There are no epidemiological studies that justify investigating these children differently from those with other mental health disorders. However, there are case reports of occasional hypothalamic germ-cell tumors presenting with classic symptoms of anorexia, but these are very uncommon, and we suspect that neurological examination would usually have been revealing (Chipkevitch, 1994). However, this may influence an individual's threshold for neuroimaging, particularly when faced with a severe, early and atypical presentation.

The value of neuroimaging to monitor the degree of cerebral atrophy is debatable and usually forms part of non-evidence-based protocols. Otherwise, medical work-up depends on the degree of starvation and length of illness, covering the whole spectrum of tests: metabolic, hormonal and bone density.

The Child with Psychosis

Neurobiological studies during the early course of psychoses have shown brain structural alterations that are present early in the illness and may predate symptom onset. Some changes, notably those in frontal and temporal lobes, can progress during the early phases of the illness (Keshavan, Berger, Zipursky *et al.*, 2005). The importance of these findings, however, is less clear. They do not yet alter treatment or prevention options, or inform prognosis accurately.

We are aware that neuroimaging is often "routine" but like many investigations discussed in this chapter, the evidence is lacking and we would question how worthwhile this investigation is. More common basic investigations include urine toxicology screen, thyroid function tests, liver function tests, full blood count and erythrocyte sedimentation rate. Endocrine abnormalities may present with a range of neuropsychiatric symptoms in adolescence. Tests for thyroid and parathyroid function are recommended.

The Child with Fatigue, Chronic Fatigue Syndrome

The Royal College of Paediatrics and Child Health (RCPCH, 2004) has produced evidence-based guidelines for the management of Chronic Fatigue Syndrome/myalgic encephalopathy (CFS/ME). This emphasizes there is no distinct marker for CFS/ME. There are diagnostic criteria, and there is a differential diagnosis of profound fatigue (see chapter 70). A family history specifically for CFS/ME should be taken; and tests to exclude known physical causes are listed in Table 22.10.

Table 22.10 Routine tests recommended in the diagnosis of CFS/ME to exclude other causes of symptoms.

General and neurological examination
Examination for spleen, lymph node and tonsillar enlargement (for viral infection)
Palpation over sinuses
Lying and standing blood pressure (for postural hypotension)
Pain on muscle palpation (for fibromyalgia)
Routine tests: full blood count and film (to exclude anemia, iron deficiency and leukemia)
Erythrocyte sedimentation rate (ESR) and C-reactive protein (CRP) (high in systemic lupus and chronic infection)
Blood glucose for diabetes
Biochemistry, sodium and creatinine for Addison's and renal impairment
Creatinine kinase for muscle disease
Thyroid function tests

The Child with Abdominal Pain

Recurrent abdominal pain occurs in up to 10–15% of schoolchildren with wide impact on school attendance. Anxiety, mild depression and low self-esteem are common associations. Questioning needs to exclude those with bleeding and use of drugs such as anti-inflammatories. In those with bowel symptoms the type of symptom dictates the investigation; for example, frequent diarrhea may lead to stool examination (e.g., for *Giardia*). In the absence of constipation or diarrhea, recurrent abdominal pain for at least 12 not necessarily consecutive weeks in 12 months, presenting in the mental health clinic with psychiatric symptoms, should prompt consideration of a search for *Helicobacter pylori* (Nakayama, Horuichi, Kumagai *et al.*, 2006).

The Child with Headaches

Children with headaches present commonly to both pediatric and child mental health services. Chronic headaches are often comorbid with anxiety and depressive disorders and associated with somatization and school problems. Tension-type headache and migraine are the two most common types of headache in children and adolescents. However, classification systems have difficulty in separating tension-type headaches from migraine without aura in children. Although the smaller genetic effect on tension-type headache than on migraine suggests that the two disorders are distinct, many believe that tension-type headache and migraine represent the same pathophysiological spectrum. Novel clinical approaches to identifying the different types of headache have included the use of drawing by the children. These headache drawings were shown to be a simple inexpensive aid in the diagnosis of headache type, with a very high sensitivity, specificity and predictive value for migraine (drawings that contained an artistic feature consistent with migraine, e.g., pounding pain, nausea/vomiting, desire to lie down, periorbital pain, photophobia, visual scotoma) versus non-migraine headaches (Stafstrom, Rostasy, & Minster, 2002).

Headaches are diagnosed clinically rather than by any specific testing (Lewis, Ashwal, Dahl *et al.*, 2002). Parents are often concerned about the possibility of underlying brain pathology, but most can be reassured on the basis of history and examination. On history-taking the high-risk group are those headaches that have been present less than 6 months and have one other predictor from a list that includes sleep disturbing headaches, vomiting, abnormal neurological examination, seizures and a total absence of any family history of headaches or migraines. In those children where a treatable intracranial lesion was found to be responsible for the headache, the neurological examination was abnormal either because of papilledema, eye movement abnormalities or motor or gait dysfunction (Lewis & Dorbad, 2000).

The routine use of any diagnostic studies for headaches, including neuroimaging, is therefore not indicated when the clinical history is without associated risk factors and the child's examination is normal.

In a review of the presenting features of 200 cases of brain tumors in children, the most common symptom was headache. However, new onset visual, educational and behavioral symptoms (notably lethargy) were also prominent; additional symptoms were present at some stage; and 88% had neurological signs on examination (Wilne, Ferris, Nathwani *et al.*, 2006).

Conclusions

Organic physical disorders may cause, exacerbate or be associated with mental health symptoms in any child presenting to CAMHS. Many of these conditions may be treatable, and many may give important prognostic and recurrence risk information. Children with an intellectual disability and seizures need particular consideration, as the phenomenon of "overshadowing" can lead to both overlooked psychiatric diagnoses and missed physical and genetic diagnoses. The harm from false positive and false negative diagnoses, as well as economic and ethical testing considerations, should guide our choice of investigations at all times. We know that the evidence appraised in this chapter will rapidly become out of date but hope that we have provided a framework for the busy clinician to appraise any newer evidence and apply it to their own practice. The general principles of knowing when to stop investigating and reassure, and when to refer, will remain valid.

References

Aicardi, J. (1992). *Diseases of the nervous system in childhood.* London: MacKeith Press.

Aldenkamp, A., & Arends, J. (2004). Effects of epileptiform EEG discharges on cognitive function: Is the concept of transient cognitive impairment still valid? *Epilepsy and Behavior*, *5*, S25–S34.

Baird, G., Robinson, R., Boyd, S., & Charman, T. (2006). Sleep electroencephalograms in young children with autism with and without regression. *Developmental Medicine and Child Neurology*, *48*, 604–608.

Barlow, J., Stewart-Brown, S., & Fletcher, J. (1998). Systematic review of the school entry medical examination. *Archives of Disease in Childhood*, *78*, 301–311.

Battaglia, A., & Carey, J. C. (2006). Etiologic yield of autistic spectrum disorders: A prospective study. *American Journal of Medical Genetics Part C, Seminars in Medical Genetics*, *142*, 3–7.

Beun, A. M., van Emde Boas, W., & Dekker, E. (1998). Sharp transients in the sleep EEG of healthy adults: A possible pitfall in the diagnostic assessment of seizure disorders. *Electroencephalography and Clinical Neurophysiology*, *106*, 44–51.

Bouhadiba, Z., Dacher, J., Monroc, M., Vanhulle, C., Menard, J. F., & Kalifa, G. (2000). MRI of the brain in the evaluation of children with developmental delay. *Journal de Radiologie*, *81*, 870–873.

Brown, W. T., Jenkins, E., Neri, G., Lubs, H., Shapiro, L. R., Davies, K. E., *et al.* (1991). Conference report: Fourth International Workshop on the fragile X and X-linked mental retardation. *American Journal of Medical Genetics*, *38*, 158–172.

Chipkevitch, E. (1994). Brain tumors and anorexia nervosa syndrome. *Brain and Development*, *16*, 175–179.

Clark, M., Carr, L., Reilly, S., & Neville, B. G. (2000). Worster–Drought syndrome, a mild tetraplegic perisylvian cerebral palsy. *Brain*, *123*, 2160–2170.

Dawson, A. J., Putnam, S., Schultz, J., Riordan, D., Prasad, C., Greenberg, C. R., *et al.* (2002). Cryptic chromosome rearrangements detected by subtelomere assay in patients with mental retardation and dysmorphic features. *Clinical Genetics*, *62*, 488–494.

Dooley, J. M., Gordon, K. E., Wood, E. P., Camfield, C. S., & Camfield, P. R. (2003). The utility of the physical examination and investigations in the pediatric neurology consultation. *Pediatric Neurology*, *28*, 96–99.

Dorling, J., & Salt, A. (2001). Evidence based case report: Assessing developmental delay. *British Medical Journal*, *323*, 148–149.

Fellick, J. M., Thomson, A. P. J., Sills, J., & Hart, C. A. (2001). Neurological soft signs in mainstream pupils. *Archives of Disease in Childhood*, *85*, 371–374.

Filipek, P. A., Accardo, P. L., Ashwal, S., Baranek, G. T., Cook, E. H., Dawson, G., *et al.* (2000). Practice parameter: Screening and diagnosis of autism. *Neurology*, *55*, 468–479.

Galvin, H. K., Newton, A. W., & Vandeven, A. M. (2005). Update on Münchausen syndrome by proxy. *Current Opinion in Pediatrics*, *17*, 252–257.

Gardner, R. J. M., & Sutherland, G. R. (1996). Pregnancy loss and infertility. In *Chromosome abnormalities and genetic counseling. Oxford Monographs on Medical Genetics, No 29* (2nd edn., pp. 311–321). New York: Oxford University Press.

Gringras, P. (1998). Choice of medical investigations for developmental delay: A questionnaire survey. *Child: Care, Health and Development*, *24*, 267–276.

Gringas, P. (2003). Self-injurious behavior. In K. P. Nunn, & C. Dey (Eds.), *The clinician's guide to psychotropic prescribing in children and adolescents, child and adolescent mental health statewide network* (pp. 270–279). Australia: Glade Graphics.

Gringras, P., & Barnicoat, A. (1998). Retesting for fragile X syndrome in cytogenetically normal males. *Developmental Medicine and Child Neurology*, *40*, 62–64.

Hall, D. M. B., & Elliman, D. (Eds.). (2006). *Health for all children* (4th edn., revised). Oxford: Oxford University Press.

Hampton, J. R., Harrison, M. J., Mitchell, J. R., Prichard, J. S., & Seymour, C. (1975). Relative contributions of history-taking, physical examination, and laboratory investigation to diagnosis and management of medical outpatients. *British Medical Journal*, *2*, 486–489.

Hartley, L., Salt, A., Dorling, J., & Gringras, P. (2002). Investigation of children with "developmental delay". *Western Journal of Medicine*, *176*, 29–33.

Kellogg, N., & The Committee on Child Abuse and Neglect. (2005). The evaluation of sexual abuse in children. *Pediatrics*, *116*, 506–512.

Keshavan, M. S., Berger, G., Zipursky, R. B., Wood, S. J., & Pantelis, C. (2005). Neurobiology of early psychosis. *British Journal of Psychiatry*, *48*, S8–S18.

King, R. A. (2006). PANDAS: To treat or not to treat? *Advances in Neurology*, *99*, 179–183.

Kotagal, S., & Pianosi, P. (2006). Sleep disorders in children and adolescents. *British Medical Journal*, *332*, 828–832.

Larcher, V. (2004). Non-accidental injury. *Hospital Medicine (London)*, *65*, 365–368.

Leppig, K. A., Werler, M. M., Cann, C. I., Cook, C. A., & Holmes, L. B. (1987). Predictive value of minor abnormalities. 1. Association with major malformations. *Journal of Pediatrics*, *110*, 531–537.

Lewis, D. W., & Dorbad, D. (2000). The utility of neuroimaging in the evaluation of children with migraine or chronic daily headache who have normal neurological examinations. *Headache*, *40*, 629–632.

Lewis, D. W., Ashwal, S., Dahl, G., Dorbad, D., Hirtz, D., Prensky, A., *et al.* Quality Standards Subcommittee of the American Academy of Neurology, Practice Committee of the Child Neurology Society. (2002). Practice parameter: evaluation of children and adolescents with headaches. *Neurology*, *59*, 490–498.

Majnemer, A., & Shevell, M. I. (1995). Diagnostic yield of the neurologic assessment of the developmentally delayed child. *Journal of Pediatrics*, *127*, 193–199.

McVicar, K., Ballaban-Gil, K., Rapin, I., Moshé, S., & Shinnar, S. (2005). Epileptiform EEG abnormalities in children with language regression. *Neurology*, *65*, 129–131.

Nakayama, Y., Horuichi, A., Kumagai, T., Kubota, S., Taki, Y., Oishi, S., *et al.* (2006). Psychiatric somatic and gastrointestinal disorders and *Helicobacter pylori* infection in children with recurrent abdominal pain. *Archives of Disease in Childhood*, *91*, 671–674.

National Institute for Clinical Excellence (NICE). (2004). *The diagnosis and management of the epilepsies in adults and children in primary and secondary care*: *Clinical Guideline 20*. London: National Institute for Clinical Excellence.

National Screening Committee, UK. (2006a). *National Screening Committee policy – phenylketonuria (PKU) screening.* Retrieved May 3, 2007, from www.library.nhs.uk/screening/ViewResource.aspx?resID=57174

National Screening Committee, UK. (2006b). *National Screening Committee policy – congenital hypothyroidism screening.* Retrieved May 3, 2007, from www.library.nhs.uk/screening/ViewResource.aspx?resID=56895

Palfrey, J. S., & Frazer, C. H. (2000). Determining the etiology of developmental delay in very young children: What if we had a common internationally accepted protocol? *Journal of Pediatrics*, *136*, 569–570.

Papavasiliou, A. S., Bazigou, H., Paraskevoulakos, E., & Kotsalis, C. (2000). Neurometabolic testing in developmental delay. *Journal of Child Neurology*, *15*, 620–622.

Poplawski, N. K. (2003). Investigating intellectual disability: A genetic perspective. *Journal of Paediatrics and Child Health*, *39*, 492–506.

Riikonen, R., & Simell, O. (1990). Tuberous sclerosis and infantile spasms. *Developmental Medicine and Child Neurology*, *32*, 203–209.

Robinson, R. O., Baird, G., Robinson, G., & Simonoff, E. (2001). Landau–Kleffner syndrome: Course and correlates with outcome. *Developmental Medicine and Child Neurology*, *43*, 243–247.

Ross, E. M., Peckham, C. S., West, P. B., & Butler, N. R. (1980). Epilepsy in childhood: findings from the National Child Development Study. *British Medical Journal*, *280*, 207–210.

Royal College of Paediatrics and Child Health (RCPCH). (2004). *Evidence based guideline for the management of CFS/ME (chronic fatigue/myalgic encephalopathy) in children and young people.* London: Royal College of Paediatrics and Child Health.

Sackett, D. L., Haynes, R. B., Tugwell, P., & Guyatt, G. H. (1991). *Clinical epidemiology: A basic science for clinical medicine* (2nd edn.). Boston: Little, Brown and Company.

Shaffer, D., O'Connor, P. A., & Shafer, S. Q. (1983). Neurological soft signs: Their origins and significance for behavior. In M. Rutter (Ed.), *Developmental neuropsychiatry* (pp. 145–163). New York: Guilford Press.

Shevell, M. I., Majnemer, A., Rosenbaum, P., & Abrahamowicz, M. (2001). Etiologic determination of childhood developmental delay. *Brain and Development*, *23*, 228–235.

Singer, H. S., Hong, J. J., Yoon, D. Y., & Williams, P. N. (2005). Serum autoantibodies do not differentiate PANDAS and Tourette syndrome from controls. *Neurology*, *65*, 1701–1707.

Smalley, S., Smith, M., & Tanguay, P. (1991). Autism and psychiatric disorders in tuberous sclerosis. *Annals of the New York Academy of Sciences*, *615*, 382–383.

Stafstrom, C. E., Rostasy, K., & Minster, A. (2002). The usefulness of children's drawings in the diagnosis of headache. *Pediatrics*, *109*, 460–472.

Stephen, E., & Kindley, A. D. (2006). Should children with ADHD and normal intelligence be routinely screened for underlying cytogenetic abnormalities? *Archives of Disease in Childhood*, *91*, 860–862.

Tuchman, R. F., & Rapin, I. (1997). Regression in pervasive developmental disorders: Seizures and epileptiform electroencephalogram correlates. *Paediatrics*, *99*, 560–566.

Wilne, S. H., Ferris, R. C., Nathwani, A., & Kennedy, C. R. (2006). The presenting features of brain tumors: A review of 200 cases. *Archives of Disease in Childhood*, *91*, 502–506.

Wilson, S., Djukic, A., Shinnar, S., Dharmani, C., & Rapin, I. (2003). Clinical characteristics of language regression in children. *Developmental Medicine and Child Neurology*, *45*, 508–514.

Working Party of the Royal College of Paediatrics and Child Health. (2002). *Fabricated or induced illness by carers.* London: Royal College of Paediatrics and Child Health.

Influences on Psychopathology

23 Genetics

Anita Thapar and Michael Rutter

Genetic research and knowledge across medicine and science are advancing very rapidly. This process is being facilitated both by enormous advances in technology and a progressive integration of genetics with other areas of research. Despite its seeming complexity, the goal of psychiatric genetics research is essentially that of delineating the causal processes that lead to disease or disorder. The two main approaches and types of study design used in psychiatric genetics generate different kinds of results. First, there are studies that essentially focus on the degree of resemblance among relatives for a given disorder or characteristic. The study of individuals who differ in their degree of genetic relatedness (using family, twin and adoption designs) allows influences regarding the strength of genetic contributions to the liability for disorder to be inferred. Such research is now moving well beyond assessments of heritability in order to tackle important questions on causal mechanisms.

The second type of genetic design focuses at the molecular level on specific genes identified through laboratory methods. The most dramatic successes to date have been with single gene disorders (autosomal dominant, autosomal recessive or sex-linked disorders; see chapter 24) such as Huntington disease and cystic fibrosis, in which there is a direct connection between one gene or gene anomaly and a disorder. These conditions are important but rare. This success has been a major driving force for the next challenge of identifying genetic risk factors for complex disorders such as cardiovascular disease and psychiatric disorders, which represent the major global burdens of disease. In these conditions, multiple genes and environmental risk factors co-act and interact in a probabilistic rather than deterministic fashion. In recent years there have been some notable successes in identifying risk genes for these types of common, complex disorders notably Alzheimer disease, asthma, macular degeneration, schizophrenia and attention deficit/hyperactivity disorder (ADHD). However, identifying susceptibility genes is only the start. What is especially exciting about this field for clinicians working in child psychiatry services is the increasing focus on potential causal chain mechanisms that lead from genetic risk to disorder, with emerging evidence for a dynamic interplay between genes and environment (Kendler & Prescott, 2006; Rutter, 2006).

Enthusiasm about the importance and potential impact of genetics is sometimes tempered by caution or suspicion because of the previous history of the appalling misuse of genetics for political ends. There are also, quite rightly, a number of ethical issues that need careful consideration (Nuffield Council on Bioethics, 1998). However, much of the concerns over potential misuse have stemmed from misconceptions about how nature and nurture operate. In this chapter, we set out to address the key issues in genetics that are of relevance to psychopathology. We also include brief descriptions of the methods used and what is known about the science of genetics. We hope to impart to clinicians an appreciation of what genetics research can and cannot tell us and to enable them to interpret new findings in this field. Specific genetic findings are covered in the relevant chapters for each disorder.

What is a Gene and How Does it Work?

The Gene at a Molecular Level

A gene is a unit of inheritance that is made up of a stretch of DNA, more specifically a sequence of molecules called nucleotides. There are four of these nucleotides: guanine (G), cytosine (C), adenine (A) and thymine (T). The inheritance "code" encrypted in genes essentially lies in the sequence of these nucleotides. The human genome, as well as containing genes, mainly consists of non-coding sequences of nucleotides. The physical locations of these are referred to as loci. This sequence in genes and non-coding regions varies across individuals in the population but not as much as one would think. In fact, around 99% of the DNA sequence is common to all humans. However, for clinical research purposes, it is the variation that we are interested in (see p. 344). This individual variation provides genetic markers (variants or polymorphisms) across the genome, which are used to identify disease susceptibility loci. Although most of the sequence in the human genome appears to be non-coding, there is increasing interest in these non-coding regions. Recent evidence suggests that these regions are not simply redundant "junk" DNA as previously thought, but significantly contribute to human variation in different ways (e.g., by regulating and modifying the pathway from gene to protein). In other words, genes that do not code for proteins may influence the effects of those

Rutter's Child and Adolescent Psychiatry, 5th edition. Edited by M. Rutter, D. Bishop, D. Pine, S. Scott, J. Stevenson, E. Taylor and A. Thapar. © 2008 Blackwell Publishing, ISBN: 978-1-4051-4549-7.

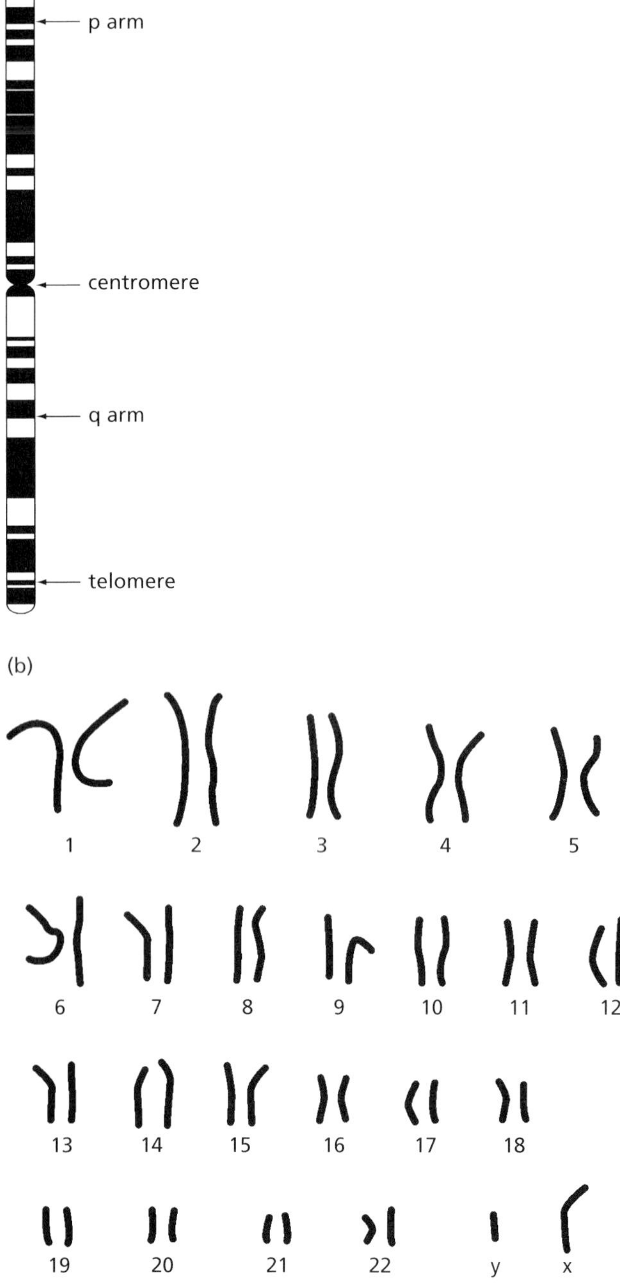

Fig. 23.1 (a) Schematic diagram of a chromosome. (b) The 23 pairs of human chromosomes.

that do through their influence on gene transcription and gene expression (Castillo-Davis, 2005). The traditional notion that there is one gene for each protein effect is misleading in so far as multiple inherited DNA elements are involved in the processes leading to gene expression.

Genes and non-coding sequences of DNA lie on chromosomes, which have a short arm (known as p), a long arm (q) and a centromere (c) in the middle (Fig. 23.1). Each chromosome is one of a pair and humans possess 46 chromosomes, of which 22 pairs are known as autosomes and 1 pair consist of the sex chromosomes (XX for females, XY for males; see chapter 24). The autosomes are numbered 1–22. To describe the physical location of a locus on a chromosome, the number of the chromosome is followed by the arm on which the gene is situated and then a number to indicate where on the arm the gene/marker is located. For example, the gene coding for the enzyme catecholamine-O-methyltransferase (COMT), involved in the breakdown of the neurotransmitters dopamine, noradrenaline and adrenaline, is located on chromosome 22q11.

Alternative forms of a gene (or non-coding) variant are known as alleles. As each chromosome is one of a pair (excepting sex chromosomes in males, who have one X and one Y chromosome), an individual possesses two alleles for a given gene (Fig. 23.1). The description of these two alleles is known as a genotype. Thus, at locus A, if there are two alleles called 1 and 2, an individual with two copies of allele 1 is said to have a genotype of 1,1.

Genes code for proteins; thus, the term gene "for" a particular disorder is misleading. The processes and pathways leading from gene to protein to brain function and structure and then to phenotype are complex. Within each gene, there are also coding and non-coding sequences known as exons and introns, respectively. The coding encrypted in the gene DNA sequence is first "read" and copied into messenger RNA (transcription). Then, sections of sequence are taken out (spliced) and the mRNA code is "read" and this message brings together the sequence of amino acids specified by the code (translation). These amino acids, of which there are a variety, are the building blocks of proteins. The genetic code is encrypted in such a way that a sequence of three nucleotides (e.g., CAG) codes for a specific type of amino acid (e.g., valine; Fig. 23.2). This provides a basic description of how a gene codes for a protein. It is now being realized that the process is far more complex than this (see p. 342). We provide some illustrations of this complexity and new research will undoubtedly continue to change current thinking.

How is knowledge about gene expression currently being applied in psychiatry and child psychiatry? Examining mRNA expression *in vitro* or in animal brains is used to test whether specific gene variants of interest (e.g., those that have been found to be associated with schizophrenia) are functional; that is, whether or not the variation results in changes to proteins. This provides one initial clue that the variant might be a causal risk factor. For example, a variant in the gene encoding the serotonin transporter (an enzyme involved in the reuptake of serotonin in the synaptic cleft) was found to have an effect on expression of this protein, thereby potentially affecting serotonin levels in the brain. A particular form of this variant has been suggested to be associated with an increased risk of depression when the individual is also exposed to life events (Caspi, McClay, Moffitt *et al.*, 2002).

There is also increasing research focusing on investigating gene expression patterns in different regions in the brain (in human postmortem brains where the individual has a specific psychiatric disorder, in animal models of psychiatric disorder

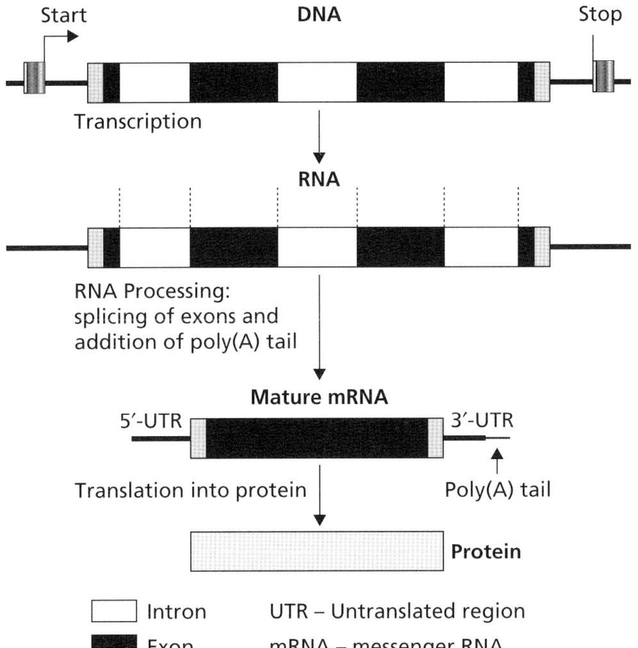

Fig. 23.2 From DNA to protein: transcription and translation.

or in animals where the focus is on examining normal traits). Here the aims are to examine how already identified gene variants might exert risk effects on disorders and identify some of the biological processes involved in the disorder to provide clues about which genes to examine in humans affected by psychiatric disorder and provide some insight into whether an associated gene is actually involved in the pathogenesis of the disorder.

Gene activity/expression is a complex process (Fig. 23.3), regulated by inherited genetic factors and mechanisms, non-inherited genetic mechanisms (epigenetics), endogenous biological factors such as hormones (e.g., stress hormones and sex hormones) and environmental factors operating externally to the individual organism (e.g., toxins, psychosocial stress).

Inherited Genetic Factors Affecting Gene Expression

Gene activity and thus protein manufacture is known to be regulated by non-coding regions of the genome. Some of these regulatory regions have been found near the gene in question; these are known as *cis* modulators (e.g., promoter regions that are sequences found at the beginning of a gene; Fig. 23.2); and also, more surprisingly, in regions that are not near the gene being regulated, known as *trans* modulators. The switching on and off and regulation of genes are not only crucial in development, but occur throughout the lifespan and provide an important means by which organisms adapt to changing environmental circumstances and so evolve. One well-known example is the gene coding for the enzyme involved in the breakdown of lactose. In many ethnic groups this gene (and thus the enzyme activity it regulates) is commonly switched off after childhood (when milk is no longer the main source of nutrition), resulting in poor tolerance to milk in adulthood. There is increasing interest in the possibility that such regulatory regions have an important role in psychiatric disorders. This is because many susceptibility gene variants do not appear to encode protein changes, whereas regulatory regions do affect protein function.

Parent-of-Origin Effects

An interesting example of non-inherited genetic influences on gene activity is the process of imprinting (see chapter 24). Here, gene expression depends on which parent the gene is inherited from, whereby one of two inherited alleles (maternal or paternal) is silenced. It is thought that imprinted genes are important in the "battle of the sexes" whereby, in evolutionary terms, paternal genes "compete" with those inherited from mother. This "battle" refers to the evolutionary advantage for a male to increase prenatal nutritional resources for his own offspring, whereas for the mother there are advantages in sharing out resources amongst all her offspring, regardless of their paternal origins. For example, imprinted genes appear to contribute to fetal and postnatal growth, with genes of paternal origin tending to increase nutritional resources being taken from the mother and genes of maternal origin reducing the demand for maternal resources. These parent-of-origin effects have been found to contribute to disorders such as Prader–Willi syndrome. However, there is increasing evidence that such influences may also be relevant in psychiatric and other complex disorders and contribute to gender differences in behavior (for examples see chapter 24).

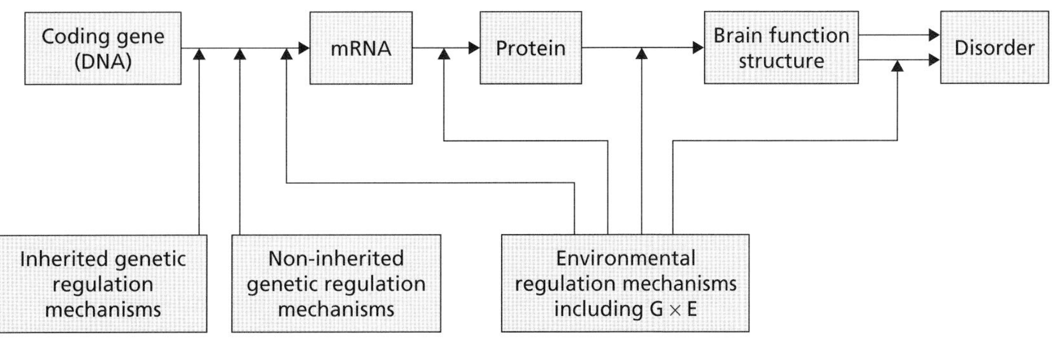

Fig. 23.3 Simplified overview of how genes and environment work together.

Environmental Influences on Gene Expression

Environmental influences interplay with genetic risk factors (Fig. 23.3) at an observable phenotypic level (see p. 343) and also have an important effect on gene activity at a cellular level. Animal studies demonstrate that exposure to early specific environmental conditions influences health and characteristics in animals through non-inherited effects on gene activity. For example, maternal caregiving behavior early in life, notably high levels of licking and grooming of rat pups, has an effect on brain glucocorticoid (a stress hormone) receptor expression and sensitivity to stress in the offspring (Meaney & Szyf, 2005). This effect is observable even when non-genetically related pups are fostered to low-licking mothers and appears to be a type of early "programming effect" that is mediated by structural modifications of DNA. Surprisingly, these non-inherited effects may persist over two generations. Biological mechanisms explaining this process (e.g., DNA methylation and histone acetylation which contribute to this "epigenetic marking" early in life) are now being discovered and in animals appear to be potentially reversible (Weaver, Champagne, Brown *et al.*, 2005).

This exciting and developing area of research highlights how the processes by which inherited and non-inherited genetic and environmental factors exert risk effects on health, behavior and psychopathology are complex and intimately intertwined.

Phenotypic Pathway from Gene to Child Psychiatric Disorder

Biological pathways and mechanisms are essential areas of research in terms of understanding the pathogenesis of disorders. For clinicians there is additional interest in the complex phenotypic pathways that lead from genes/cellular processes to psychiatric disorder. Endophenotypes have been described as measurable characteristics thought to lie along the pathway from gene to psychiatric disorder but that are closer to the gene and that are thought to have a simpler relationship with a given gene (Cannon, 2005; Gottesman & Gould, 2003). For a trait to meet the criteria as a potential endophenotype for a given disorder, it must be genetically influenced itself and associated with the disorder. It should also be familially and genetically related to the disorder in question with the endophenotype linked to the gene of interest. Finally, the endophenotype should not result from the disorder itself.

More recently, there has been a stronger interest in intermediate phenotypes (Meyer-Lindenberg & Weinberger, 2006). These differ crucially from endophenotypes with respect to the lack of any assumption that they are necessarily closely connected to gene action. Rather, they are similar with respect to the assumption that they have a key role in the causal biological processes leading to disorder. Thus, in the study of the progression from HIV to AIDS there are laboratory findings that index the stage reached in the process. This is an example of an intermediate phenotype that is not an endophenotype. Such intermediate phenotypes are most useful in investigating the effects of drug action without the need to wait for the final endpoint. There are equivalent intervening changes in carcinogenic and in allergic diseases. It may be presumed that the same is likely to apply in the field of psychopathology. The snag is the lack of any adequate understanding of the underlying neural processes in most instances. So far, the key intermediate phenotypes and putative endophenotypes of interest in psychiatry have been neuroimaging features, cognitive and emotional processing and psychophysiological measures.

For example, there is now a very large area of research that has shown that a variant in the gene coding for the enzyme COMT, which is responsible for breakdown of dopamine in the prefrontal cortex (PFC), is linked to an individual's performance on tasks assessing prefrontal cognition (Tunbridge, Harrison, & Weinberger, 2006). This gene variant is functional. That is, it affects the activity of the COMT enzyme whereby one form of the variant (the *val* allele) results in higher activity of the enzyme and thus greater clearance of dopamine in the PFC. The other form (the *met* allele) is associated with lower enzyme activity. It is the higher activity *val* allele that has been found to be linked to lower levels of dopamine in the prefrontal cortex and associated with cognitive function. The findings to date suggest that the COMT *val/met* variant influences PFC function but there is no compelling evidence yet that this represents a risk pathway for psychiatric disorders such as schizophrenia.

Another example is provided by a study that suggested that a functional variant in the serotonin transporter gene variant may be linked to amygdala reactivity to environmental stimuli (Hariri, Drabant, Munoz *et al.*, 2005; Hariri, Drabant, & Weinberger, 2006). The importance of this finding concerns the identification of a possible biological pathway and the evidence that this operates in individuals without psychopathology.

There are different schools of thought with regard to the importance of endophenotypes. Some suggest that identifying susceptibility genes for them may be easier than for psychiatric disorders themselves but, thus far, the evidence is lacking as assessed by the standard of replicated findings. An alternative view is that the focus on endophenotypes becomes more important after specific genes that influence psychiatric disorder are identified. The next question is how does that gene variant exert its risk effects? Does the gene influence psychiatric disorder through effects on brain structure or specific alterations in function such as those mediated through effects on neurotransmitters, specific cognitive mechanisms or temperamental attributes? The key point is that the value of genetic findings is crucially dependent on determination of the biological pathways involved (Meyer-Lindenberg & Weinberger, 2006). The issue of whether or not any index of that pathway is closer to the gene action is an interesting specific question but it fails to recognize that the delineation of biological pathways is as relevant to environmental risk mechanisms as genetic ones. Accordingly, our preference is for the broader concept of intermediate phenotypes rather than the narrower genetic concept of endophenotypes.

Gene–Environment Interplay at the Clinical/Phenotypical Level

There is increasing evidence that genes do not just exert risk effects by influencing specific traits, but can work indirectly by increasing an individual's vulnerability to environmental adversity (gene–environment interaction) and also have indirect risk effects by being involved in bringing about environmental adversity (gene–environment correlation).

Gene–Environment Interaction

Environmental factors not only influence gene activity at a cellular level but have also been found to modify the effects of inherited genetic liability for psychiatric and medical disorders at an observable phenotypic level (Fig. 23.3). It is well recognized by researchers and clinicians that individuals vary in their response when exposed to an environmental risk factor. The term gene–environment interaction ($G \times E$) is now widely used to describe the phenomenon whereby even where there is genetic susceptibility, an individual does not necessarily show disorder until exposed to an environmental risk factor (Rutter, Moffitt, & Caspi, 2006). This is important for researchers to appreciate, as some genes will not appear to be risk genes unless the individual is also exposed to a risk environment. Thus, $G \times E$ may account for non-replication of findings in different genetic studies. It is also a clinically relevant issue that is of potential importance to prevention and treatment approaches, because it suggests that changes in environmental factors can prevent the manifestation of genetic dispositional factors.

Investigation of $G \times E$ has been undertaken using twin and adoption strategies, and more recently in molecular genetic studies. The first group of studies allows for testing whether the association of a specific environmental risk factor with psychopathology varies depending on genetic risk for a disorder which is inferred by virtue of having a biologically affected relative with that disorder. Molecular genetic studies provide the opportunity of testing for $G \times E$ in a different way; specifically by testing whether the risk effect of a specific environmental factor varies depending on possession of an allelic variant of one specific gene. For example, in a study based on the Dunedin cohort, a variant in a gene coding for the enzyme monoamine oxidase A (MAOA), involved in the breakdown of dopamine, noradrenaline, adrenaline and serotonin (see chapter 16), was significantly associated with adult antisocial behavior but only when there had been exposure to childhood maltreatment (Caspi *et al.*, 2002). This finding of interaction between the *MAOA* gene and family adversity has been replicated in other samples (Kim-Cohen, Caspi, Taylor *et al.*, 2006), is supported by animal study findings, and imaging work supports plausible biological mechanisms linking this *MAOA* gene variant to aggression (Meyer-Lindenberg, Buckholtz, Kolachana *et al.*, 2006). In the same Dunedin sample, a serotonin transporter gene variant was found to be associated with depression but only where there had been exposure to life events (Caspi *et al.*, 2002). This finding has again been replicated by several groups although there are also non-replications (Kendler, Kuhn, Vittum *et al.*, 2005; Zammit & Owen, 2006). The findings are supported by animal and imaging studies. Clearly, given the potential pitfalls of multiple statistical testing that can increase the rate of false positives (and there are hundreds of thousands of gene variants that could be tested with many different environmental factors), testing for $G \times E$ needs to be empirically driven and findings have to be replicated. That is, the specific hypotheses need to be scientifically plausible, the environmental risk factor should ideally be causal or at least a proximal risk factor (see chapter 25), the gene variant should be functional (have an effect on proteins) and there should ideally be some information about potential biological plausibility (Moffitt, Caspi, & Rutter, 2005; Rutter, Moffitt, & Caspi, 2006). A clinically important example of $G \times E$ is individual genetic variation in the clinical response to medication. This variation between individuals can arise because of genetic differences in pharmacokinetics (Sadee & Dai, 2005; see also chapter 16); for example, variation in genes affecting the activity of metabolizing enzymes in the liver. It can also arise because of genetic variation in drug targets in the brain (pharmacodynamics); for example, neurotransmitter receptor binding. One example is the suggestion that a variant in the dopamine D3 receptor may be associated with susceptibility to medication-related tardive dyskinesia in schizophrenia (Malhotra, Murphy, & Kennedy, 2004). This area of pharma-cogenetics research is becoming of increasing interest across medicine because it holds the potential for individually tailoring treatments and better predicting response and side-effects (see chapter 16). However, at present findings remain preliminary and treatment response is likely to be influenced by many different genes as well as environmental risk factors.

Gene–Environment Correlation

This phenomenon is characterized by the co-occurrence of genetic and environmental risk factors that arises because the presence and degree of severity of an environmental risk factor is related to the individual's genetic make-up. This concept of genes and environmental risk factors going hand in hand will be familiar to clinicians and epidemiologists; given that other risk factors tend to cluster, adversities are often multiple. There are three potential sources of gene–environment correlation (Plomin, 1994).

First, children not only inherit genes from their parents, but are also exposed to environments created by these parents. When the parental genes that provide risk also shape parental behavior that influences the rearing environment, there is a passive gene–environment correlation. An example of this would be the association between parental mental disorder and family discord (Rutter, 1989). The parental genes are thereby contributing to the likelihood that the child will be exposed to risky environments. Second, children at increased genetic risk may seek out risky environments as a result of their own genetically influenced behavior. A possible example of such an active gene–environment correlation would be the case of a child with ADHD whose impulsive risk-taking behavior involves him or her in maladaptive peer groups. Finally, individuals' own genetically influenced behavior will evoke responses from other people; for example, when a child with genetic susceptibility for antisocial behavior evokes hostile responses from others. This is known as evocative gene–environment correlation. The influence of individuals on their environments has long been recognized in developmental psychology (Bell, 1968). The study of gene–environment correlations takes this concept a step further in highlighting the role of genes in this causal process.

Again, this issue is of relevance to both clinicians and researchers. First, there needs to be an appreciation that genetic and environmental risks are not mutually exclusive. Even where there is a strong family history of disorder, there may be additional risk effects from environmental factors that go hand in hand with genetic risk factors in these families and that can be modified. Second, for researchers, there needs to be an awareness that the associations between specific environmental risk factors (e.g., family conflict and antisocial behavior) can arise because of genes influencing both the risk factor and outcome ("genetic mediation"). Ideally, one needs to test whether there are risk effects of the environmental factor that are independent of genetic risk ("environmental mediation"; see p. 351) (Rutter, 2007).

There is evidence to suggest that gene–environment correlation is especially important in child psychiatry for antisocial behavior (Ge, 1996; O'Connor, 1998) and depression (Rice, Harold, & Thapar, 2003; Silberg, Pickles, Rutter *et al.*, 1999). For example, two adoption studies have shown that biologically unrelated adoptive parents of children at high genetic risk of antisocial behavior show greater negative parenting practices than adoptive parents of children at low genetic risk as indexed by disorder in the biological parents (Ge, 1996; O'Connor, 1998). The adverse parenting appeared to be provoked by the children's behavior but nevertheless still carried risk effects on the behavior, independent of the direct genetic influences.

How Genes are Inherited and Transmitted from one Generation to the Next

In this section, we consider how genes are passed onto the next generation. Mendel, an Augustinian monk, first deduced the existence of a unit of inheritance and the rules governing transmission of this unit (now known as a gene) from generation to generation. He inferred all this from a famous set of experiments on peas. This deduction was reached long before DNA and genes were discovered. Mendel's Laws are now well-established (McGuffin, Owen, & Gottesman, 2002). One law is that during gamete formation, maternal and paternal allele pairs separate and one of each is transmitted to the offspring. Another important law is that where two characteristics are influenced by two different genes (when there is simple single-gene inheritance), the two genes will be transmitted independently in the next generation. For example, if one "parent" has red flowers and smooth peas, the offspring's flower color and smoothness of its peas will be independent of each other. This is because during fertilization and meiosis, the genetic sequence from both the mother and father is shuffled (in the way that a sequence of playing cards will be changed by shuffling) by the process of recombination, whereby a chromosome crosses over with its partner chromosome at many different recombination points. It is sufficient to know that the process of recombination means that there is, on average, a 50 : 50 chance of genetic sequences being inherited together, unless they are physically located close to each other on a chromosome when there will be a departure from this Mendelian rule. The departure from this rule whereby two genetic loci tend to be co-inherited is known as "linkage disequilibrium" and is used in mapping human disease and traits.

Single-gene disorders, such as tuberous sclerosis, which can be associated with autism (see chapters 24 & 46), are sometimes known as Mendelian disorders because the transmission from generation to generation can be clearly seen to follow Mendel's Laws. Genes that increase susceptibility for complex disorders such as psychiatric disorders also follow Mendel's Laws. However, here multiple gene risk effects operate, not only in an additive fashion, but also through gene–gene interaction (epistasis) and gene–environment interplay (see p. 343). Detecting gene–gene interaction is becoming an area of research interest. Like G × E, it can explain why some risk gene variants may not behave as risk factors for disorder unless they are accompanied by other specific risk gene variants. The genetic background is thus important and may account for why risk effect sizes of susceptibility genes that influence complex diseases have been found to be relatively small and why findings vary in different studies, although there are other explanations for non-replication.

In summary, the inheritance patterns of most common disorders and traits, including psychiatric disorders, are not straightforward, which explains why many affected individuals (e.g., with autism or diabetes) may, but do not necessarily, have a known affected relative. These disorders are known as complex, polygenic (influenced by many genes) or multifactorial (influenced by different risk factors) disorders.

Molecular Genetic Research Methods

In this section we provide sufficient information for non-specialist researchers and clinicians to interpret genetic study findings and to be aware of the strengths and weaknesses of different designs.

The process of identifying genes that influence disorder or traits involves testing for links between variation in individuals' DNA and the trait or disorder in question (phenotype). The first generation of useful markers were restriction fragment length polymorphisms (RFLPs) where DNA variation consisted of different length markers after digestion of the DNA by an enzyme. The second generation consisted of microsatellite markers that were made up of repeated DNA sequences (e.g., $(CA)_n$), which are still used. The most recent group of markers are single nucleotide polymorphisms (SNPs). These are variations in single nucleotides that occur commonly. These are extremely useful markers as they are relatively cheap and more accurate to genotype, provide denser coverage of the genome and are associated with greater statistical power when testing for risk gene variants across the genome. There is now the technology for high throughput genotyping, and more recently genotyping using DNA "chips" that allow for rapid genotyping of large numbers of SNPs for large samples of people. Increasingly, this type of work is being undertaken commercially at lower and lower prices as the process is being increasingly automated. The selection of markers whereby most common genetic variation is selected is an important task, so that all possible markers do not have to be genotyped. A public database of more than 1 million SNPs (HapMap; Altshuler & Clark, 2005) and information about the patterns of linkage disequilibrium between these markers that can guide selection of "tagging SNPs" for genetic studies is now available. Most recently, another type of common variation in the genome has been recognized. This is structural variation in the genome that includes copy number variants (CNVs). These CNVs have been found to capture variation in gene expression and are likely to be important in contributing to complex diseases (Stranger, Forrest, Dunning *et al.*, 2007) such as autism (Autism Consortium Group, 2007).

Some research groups also use a type of laboratory screening approach that is easy and cheap to undertake. DNA pooling involves evaluating the "pooled" frequencies of multiple genetic marker alleles in two groups, cases and controls, rather than individually genotyping each marker. Markers that appear more commonly in cases can then be examined in a second stage by more costly individual genotyping. Such methods have been used in molecular genetic studies of IQ for example. The two main types of methods used to identify susceptibility genes are linkage and association approaches. Linkage studies involve testing whether specific genetic markers or sets of markers are co-inherited with disorder in affected families. Association studies are traditional epidemiological type designs based on testing whether the frequency of a specific marker, or sets of markers, is higher in those affected compared with a control group. In the past there have been concerns about the possibility of false positive findings (population stratification) from association studies, essentially because of inadequate matching of controls so that they differ genetically from cases for reasons other than the disorder (e.g., ethnicity differences). To circumvent this potential problem, many researchers have adopted the approach whereby parental DNA is collected, and the alleles that are not transmitted to the affected offspring are used as the controls in statistical analysis. These methods are known as family-based rather than case–control association methods and include the Transmission Disequilibrium Test (TDT) and Haplotype Relative Risk method (HRR). For later onset diseases, where collecting parental DNA is not feasible, another approach is to test for population stratification in the laboratory by examining whether random gene variants not thought to be involved in disease, differ in cases and controls.

Throughout this chapter, the risk gene variant has been considered in terms of one particular allelic risk factor. Linkage and association studies have also focused on sets of markers and for some conditions (e.g., Crohn disease) the risk variant appears to be a specific grouping of alleles across a set of different markers within the gene. This set of alleles is known as a haplotype. In psychiatry, there has been some suggestion that a haplotype derived from several markers in the *COMT* gene is functional (Bray, Buckland, Williams *et al.*, 2003) and is associated with schizophrenia (Schiffman, Bronstein, Sternfeld *et al.*, 2002).

One of the major difficulties in psychiatry is that the biological mechanisms involved in the development of psychiatric disorders are unclear and there is currently a lack of understanding of their pathophysiology. This situation contrasts with some other complex disorders such as diabetes, where it is known that a lack of insulin results in raised blood glucose levels that in turn lead to adverse consequences. It is for this reason that hypothesis-free molecular genetic strategies, which involve no assumptions about the underlying biology of psychiatric disorders and where the whole genome is systematically searched for risk variants, are attractive in psychiatry.

Linkage Studies

In whole-genome linkage studies, the goal is to identify susceptibility gene variants through positional strategies; that is, by locating specific regions in the genome that harbor disease susceptibility genes. These studies are based on samples of families consisting of multiply affected relatives. Linkage studies that involve knowing the pattern of inheritance of the disorder and that are statistically parametric in nature have been successful in identifying susceptibility genes for single-gene disorders such as Huntington chorea and tuberous sclerosis. For complex disorders, including psychiatric disorders where inheritance is not straightforward, non-parametric linkage methods are used. The most commonly used approach is to select affected sibling pairs (ASPs), where at least two siblings in a family have the disorder in question. On average, for any given marker (remembering that each individual has a pair of chromosomes), 1 in 4 full biological siblings will inherit the same pair of alleles from their parents (one from mother, one from father, identical by descent), 1 in 4 will share zero alleles and half will share two alleles. If the marker lies close to the disease susceptibility locus (when there is significant linkage), ASPs will share more of the linked marker alleles than expected. This departure from expectation occurs because the marker is in linkage disequilibrium with the disease susceptibility locus (i.e., recombination between the two loci on the chromosome is lower than expected). In whole-genome linkage studies, markers across the genome are selected, genotyped and each one is tested for linkage with the disorder. As this involves multiple testing, the currently accepted genome-wide significance level is stringent (Lander & Kruglyak, 1995). For example, in an ASP linkage study of ADHD, one region on chromosome 16p13 achieved genome-wide significance and a number of other regions reached the threshold for suggestive linkage (Smalley, Kustanovich, Minassian *et al.*, 2002). However, specific susceptibility genes within any of these regions have yet to be identified (see chapter 34).

This ASP linkage approach has until recently been the strategy of choice for molecular genetic studies of complex disorders, including schizophrenia, bipolar disorder and autism, as well as medical conditions such as diabetes, asthma, rheumatoid arthritis and Crohn disease. Another linkage strategy that has been less commonly used in psychiatry because the samples are more difficult to collect, is based on collections of smaller numbers of multiplex families in which there are usually several generations of multiply affected family members. This strategy is also more challenging where the manifestation of disorder is developmentally influenced; for example, ADHD or reading disability may be difficult to diagnose retrospectively in the grandparent generation.

Linkage studies provide an initial "broad-brush" approach to identifying susceptibility genes in that they can identify regions of the genome that may harbor these genes (significant regions of linkage may include very many genes). They are better at picking up genes of larger effect but are not able to pick up genes of small effect. There has been some impatience with linkage studies and criticisms made about the usefulness of this approach as results were not as quickly forthcoming as initially thought. With the benefit of hindsight, it is clear that early forecasts of how quickly susceptibility genes for complex disorders would be identified were unrealistically optimistic. Now, with larger samples, linkage studies are beginning to yield results. For example, linkage studies have led to replicated findings of susceptibility gene variants for schizophrenia (see chapter 45), Crohn disease and asthma.

Whole-Genome Association Studies

Until now, the most cost-effective and pragmatic approach has been to first undertake linkage studies to identify chromosomal regions of interest and then to carry out more detailed mapping with multiple markers in these regions to identify the susceptibility gene. A useful analogy here is to think of linkage studies as the equivalent of screening in epidemiology, where sensitivity in picking up the true cases may be a problem, and subsequent association studies as the detailed interviews on the selected group. For epidemiological studies, if detailed interviews could be undertaken easily and cost-effectively in large numbers, one would want to interview the whole sample. For molecular genetic studies, it is now becoming cost-effective to test thousands and thousands of markers across the genome (search for susceptibility loci in detail across the genome with high levels of sensitivity) and such studies are now yielding replicated findings. These studies, which are also hypothesis-free, are known as whole-genome association studies (WGA).

There is some excitement about this approach as it now provides a feasible systematic method of searching the whole genome for susceptibility genes of small effect size (Carlson, Eberle, Kruglyak *et al.*, 2004) and because several WGA studies of complex disorders, including bipolar disorder, published in 2007, have resulted in the identification of susceptibility loci (Wellcome Trust Case Control Consortium, 2007). Given the issues of multiple testing and the risks of false positives, very large samples sizes are likely to be needed to avoid the statistical problem of a large number of false positive findings whereby apparent susceptibility loci are found to be associated simply by chance. It is not certain exactly how large samples need to be. Theoretically, several thousand cases are desirable. However, one whole-genome association study of only 96 cases of macular degeneration and 50 controls (Klein, Zeiss, Chew *et al.*, 2005) resulted in identification of a susceptibility gene and this finding has been replicated. Large-scale sample collections are a challenge in psychiatry where establishing the phenotype is expensive and labor-intensive. At the time of this chapter going to press however, WGA studies seem to be one important way forward.

Molecular Genetic Strategies that Involve Testing Specific Hypotheses

These studies involve selecting specific genes that are thought a priori to be involved in the disease process and then examining variants within these selected "candidate" genes. These candidate genes can be either functional and/or positional. Positional candidate gene studies involve selecting genes according to evidence on position (i.e., in genomic regions of significant linkage or association, see p. 345). This type of positional candidate gene fine mapping association study following replicated linkage findings has resulted in identifying a susceptibility locus KIAA0319 for reading disability (Cope, Harold, Hill *et al.*, 2005).

Another positional strategy involves following up clues about the potential position of a susceptibility gene provided by individual families who present with a disorder and have a specific region of a chromosome disrupted. For example, a study of a family with a translocation involving a region on chromosome 1 and schizophrenia and bipolar disorder led to the identification of a susceptibility gene *DISC* for schizophrenia (Millar, Pickard, Mackie *et al.*, 2005; Owen, Craddock, & O'Donovan, 2005). Another well-known example is the description of a Dutch family where multiple members showed seriously aggressive behavior and learning disability accompanied by a mutation in the *MAOA* gene (Brunner, Nelen, van Zandvoort *et al.*, 1993). A variant in the *MAOA* gene, in the presence of environmental adversity has since been linked to antisocial behavior (Caspi *et al.*, 2002).

Functional, rather than positional, candidate gene studies are considered by many as problematic. This is because here genes are selected on the basis of an assumption that they are involved in the pathophysiology of disease and one of the aims of genetic studies is to elucidate novel biological pathways. This type of method has been partially successful in diabetes where variants in the insulin gene have been found to be associated with the disorder. However, the situation is different for psychiatric disorders where the pathophysiology is unknown. Nevertheless, despite these criticisms, functional candidate gene association studies have been successful for some disorders, notably ADHD (see chapter 34).

Clues for selecting functional candidate genes can come from a variety of research studies. These include studies of animals that show behaviors of relevance to psychiatry (e.g., hyperactivity), postmortem human and animal gene expression studies (these can shed light on which biological systems are involved in a disorder; see p. 340), psychopharmacology and imaging research. Animal studies that have guided candidate gene work have included instances in which specific genes are artificially disrupted (e.g., knockout mice or irradiated mutants) and where the animal then shows a phenotype of interest. An example relevant to child psychiatry is the dopamine transporter knockout mouse that shows marked hyperactivity and where there is some evidence from meta-analysis that a variant in the dopamine transporter gene is associated with ADHD (Faraone, Perlis, Doyle *et al.*, 2005). Another example whereby genetics research was guided by animal studies is the finding of association between variants in the *SNAP25* (synaptosomal associated protein) gene, which is involved in vesicular uptake of neurotransmitters and ADHD. This clue came from findings that the coloboma mutant mouse, which has a deletion on a segment of chromosome including the *SNAP25* gene, shows marked motor hyperactivity (Thapar, O'Donovan, & Owen, 2005b).

Other clues about which genes may be involved may come from studying behavioral phenotypes in humans who have a single gene disorder (see chapter 24). However, many would argue that the difficulty here is that the pathway to disorder in these individuals may be different, and also many of these single-gene disorders are accompanied by learning disability (lower IQ). Thus, it is not always straightforward to establish whether the apparent increased rates of a specific psychopathology (e.g., autism) arise specifically from disruption to the gene rather than from being related to lower IQ.

Once a gene variant has been found to be robustly associated with a disorder, given the potential for false positive findings, the next step required is that the finding should be independently replicated in other samples. This has been difficult in many instances and has led to criticism of psychiatric genetics. However, it must be remembered that large samples are needed to replicate findings (Goring, Terwilliger, & Blangero, 2001) and that false negative results can also be a problem. Moreover, for complex disorders, risk gene variants will interact with other gene variants and environmental factors, and it is likely that there will be phenotypic heterogeneity (e.g., because of differences in sample ascertainment). If these background factors vary in different samples, replication becomes problematic. Despite these challenges and the issues of phenotype definition, genetic findings in child and adult psychiatry are now being replicated and indeed significant evidence of association is now beginning to be yielded by meta-analyses, which some consider an overly stringent requirement. Once association has been robustly demonstrated, as in all epidemiology, the next stage involves testing whether the risk factor is causal by investigating the mechanisms by which it exerts its risk effects. In genetics, this process needs to be undertaken at a biological and phenotypic level.

Once a genetic marker/haplotype has been found to be robustly associated with a disorder, it is crucial to identify whether or not it is functional. The areas of research on gene expression profiling (transcriptomics) and proteomics that involve examining gene products are becoming increasingly important (see p. 340). However, in child psychiatry, a problem is that brain tissue to undertake such studies is usually not readily available. The next stage involves investigating the physiological mechanisms that lead to disorder, in which it is crucial for genetics research to be fully integrated with other areas of neuroscience, such as imaging. It is also becoming increasingly apparent that once it is established that a gene variant is associated with a disorder, these next stages of biological and phenotypic research are also challenging and not straightforward tasks. Animal studies provide a means of examining gene function and investigating the link between genes, biological pathways and behaviors and cognition that could increasingly inform human genetics research.

Defining the Phenotype for Genetic Studies

Diagnosis

Success in identifying susceptibility genes for complex disorders is dependent on how well the phenotype is defined. That is not always straightforward in psychiatry (an exception is Alzheimer disease), where phenotypes are defined on the basis of reported symptoms rather than on the basis of measurable pathology or physiological measures (e.g., diagnostic intestinal biopsy for Crohn disease, high blood glucose levels for diabetes). However, the use of research diagnostic interviews (see chapter 19) has meant that diagnoses can be made at least with high levels of reliability. Also, there is increasing evidence of biological and clinical validity for some disorders (see chapter 2). However, there is considerable variation in the clinical presentation of psychiatric disorders, as there is across the whole of medicine. This has led to some interest as to whether this observable variation indexes underlying etiological heterogeneity and whether inclusion of such clinical/phenotypic information can help refine the search for susceptibility genes. The evidence to date suggests that such phenotypic considerations may be useful and important. For example, linkage evidence for asthma was found to be stronger when the clinical covariate of bronchial hyper-responsiveness was included (van Eerdewegh, Little, Dupuis *et al.*, 2002). Linkage to a chromosomal region for schizophrenia was refined by including depression as a covariate (Hamshere, Williams, Norton *et al.*, 2005). One study of autism found that by including a factor representing the clinical phenotype of "insistence of sameness" genetic linkage findings were strengthened and refined (Shao, Cuccaro, Hauser *et al.*, 2003). It remains to be seen whether that can be replicated. There is also increasing evidence to suggest that consideration of the overlap of psychiatric disorders is important. For example, variants in two genes, *NRG1* and *DISC1*, appear to influence a phenotype that is a mixture of schizophrenia and bipolar affective disorder (Craddock, O'Donovan, & Owen, 2006).

Modifying Factors

Gene variants may also influence the different phenotypic manifestation of disorder (e.g., antisocial behavior in ADHD, depression in schizophrenia) as those that contribute to its origins. In some instances, the same gene variants may influence phenotypic presentation, severity and course of a disorder. In other instances, different modifying genes may be important for these clinical aspects. For example, there is consistent evidence now that the COMT *val/val* genotype influences antisocial behavior in ADHD but not ADHD itself (Caspi, Langley, Milne *et al.*, 2008; Thapar, Langley, Fowler *et al.*, 2005a; see chapter 34).

Trait Measures and Quantitative Trait Loci Studies

Traditionally, genetic studies have focused on clinical disorder, defined categorically. However, there is a strong opinion among some that it may be preferable to focus on identifying susceptibility genes for quantitative traits related to disorder (e.g., ADHD symptom scores rather than ADHD, or schizotypy rather than schizophrenia). Genes of small effect influencing continuously distributed trait measures are known as quantitative trait loci (QTL). QTL linkage and association studies have long been used successfully in plant and animal genetics, including investigating behavioral traits such as anxiety (Abiola, Angel, Avner *et al.*, 2003). Furthermore, mapping QTLs that influence gene expression in animals and linking these to specific behaviors and characteristics is well advanced such that databases of this information are now available (Web QTL; www.genenetwork.org).

The mapping of QTLs for continuously distributed measures has also been utilized in general medicine. Examples include blood pressure and cholesterol levels, which are continuously distributed trait measures that behave as risk dimensions in that they are associated with increased risk of ischemic heart disease in a continuous fashion. Another example is body mass index (BMI) because of its importance in terms of obesity. QTL studies of these risk dimensions, some of which are intermediate phenotypes, has been an important adjunct to focusing on molecular genetic studies of categorically defined clinical disorder (Abiola, Angel, Avner *et al.*, 2003; Carlson, Eberle, Kruglyak *et al.*, 2004).

Many child psychiatric disorders can also be easily conceptualized in dimensional terms or risk dimensions identified (e.g., depression or ADHD symptom scores or personality traits such as neuroticism). It has been argued that searching for QTLs for these types of continuously distributed trait measures is a more powerful strategy, both statistically and conceptually. In reality, that depends on a number of different issues. First, there needs to be consideration of the ease of phenotyping. For QTL linkage studies, extremely large sample sizes are needed although statistical power can then be increased by selection strategies; for example, by selecting high and low scorers (this approach has been used for IQ and ADHD studies) or highly concordant and discordant sibling pairs (this approach has been used for mapping studies of neuroticism; Fullerton, Cubin, Tiwari *et al.*, 2003). Where phenotyping is expensive (e.g., interviews are needed) this becomes a problem. Second, the issue of whether or not it is better to use categorical or dimensional conceptualizations of child psychopathology has received much attention and outside the realm of genetics is a topic of much discussion (Pickles & Angold, 2003; Rutter 2003; see chapters 2 & 4). However, the likelihood is that neither approach is right or wrong. What is of key importance is the nature of the relationship between the risk factor (here the gene variant) and phenotype. For example, a risk factor may influence an underlying risk dimension (e.g., a personality attribute for disorder) but not the disorder (e.g., depression). It may influence both. It may influence the disorder only and not the risk dimension given that there are numerous different risk pathways into psychiatric disorder. This will clearly not be known before the risk factor or gene variant is identified. Ideally, both approaches should be considered as they each have their strengths (Thapar, Langley, O'Donovan *et al.*, 2006). However, to date, the replicated molecular genetic evidence in child and adult psychiatry has been most consistent for traditional clinical diagnoses (e.g., ADHD, schizophrenia, depression) and the evidence has been much weaker for QTL studies of trait measures. Of course, this may be because there has been less QTL research. For example, there have been a few QTL studies of hyperactivity symptom scores in the general population but, so far, association findings with susceptibility gene variants that have been associated with and replicated for clinical ADHD have been weaker (Mill, Xu, Ronald *et al.*, 2005). On the other hand, the replicated imaging findings in relation to genetic variants do point to dimensional effects that extend across the general population. Overall, it is important to evaluate evidence as it emerges and remain open to different approaches.

Quasi-experimental Studies of Genetic Effects

In themselves, findings on susceptibility genes provide only a starting point for investigating causal processes. The potential of genetics lies in the leads it provides for other biological studies, but that potential will be realized only if such studies are integrated with genetics. In that connection, laboratory studies of gene functions will be crucial and, often, these will need to involve animal models of one kind or another. In addition, more clinically oriented quasi-experimental studies (e.g., where subjects undergo imaging after exposure to an experimental stressor) can be highly informative. Thus, structural and functional brain-imaging studies have been used to examine the differences in neural function in relation to psychological challenges associated with different genetic allelic variations (Hariri *et al.*, 2005; Heinz, Braus, Smolka *et al.*, 2005; Pezawas, Meyer-Lindenberg, Drabant *et al.*, 2005). The key findings have been that the allelic variations shown to involve G × E are indeed associated with measurable differences in neural structure and function, and that these effects apply within the general population to individuals who show no evidence of psychopathology. The crucial implication is that genes mainly influence responses to the environment rather than disorder as such.

Animal studies, as exemplified by the Suomi group findings with rhesus monkeys, are comparably informative in their demonstration of the neuroendocrine effects of allelic variations that apply only in the context of environmental adversity (Newman, Syagailo, Barr *et al.*, 2005).

Quantitative Genetic Strategies to Study Causal Processes

Family, twin and adoption studies start by examining the relative contribution of genes and environmental influences to psychiatric disorder. The same designs are now being used to address questions on causal mechanisms.

Family Studies

Family studies involve examining the rate of disorder in first- (and sometimes second-) degree relatives of those who are affected and comparing these rates to those in a control group. In psychiatry, the control group has sometimes consisted of unaffected individuals and sometimes those with a different psychiatric disorder. The latter provides a more robust test of whether or not a specific disorder runs in families. Family studies may also involve the offspring of parents with a disorder (e.g., depression or schizophrenia). These are known as "top-down" family studies. Others begin with affected child probands and examine the relatives of these children. Clearly, in such studies, adjustment needs to be made for whether or not individuals have passed through the age period of risk. Familial risk is usually expressed as a relative risk or odds ratio and the derived estimate will also depend on the estimated rate of the disorder in the general population. For example, calculations of familial risk for autism have dropped since the first set of family studies was published (see chapter 46) because estimates of the incidence of the disorder have risen.

Another note of caution is that ascertainment biases can influence findings. For example, if families who are recruited to a study on a voluntary or selected basis have more affected relatives, the estimate of familial loading will be higher than if a sample was recruited systematically. Family studies have shown that all child psychiatric disorders are familial although the degree of familial clustering varies for different disorders. For example, the familial risk in terms of odds ratios is around 2–4 for childhood depression, around 5 for ADHD and over 50 for autism. Familial clustering of a condition can arise because of relatives sharing genes. For example, first-degree relatives (such as mother–child or full biological siblings) share on average 50% of their segregating genes and environmental factors can impact on all family members in a way that increases their similarity for a given trait or disorder. This type of environment is known as shared environment. It is important to recognize that the term "shared environment" says nothing about the type of environmental risk factor involved (these have to be measured), rather it is a statistically inferred measure of non-genetic factors that make family members more similar for a disorder. Thus, social class or an infectious agent may affect all family members but is not necessarily a shared environment if it impacts differently on individuals in terms of developing a specific disorder. To disentangle genetic and shared environmental influences, twin and adoption studies are needed.

Adoption Studies

Adoption studies examine similarity for a given disorder between individuals and their biologically related relatives compared with their adoptive relatives (Rutter, Silberg, O'Connor *et al.*, 1999a,b). Where a condition is genetically influenced, we would expect greater similarity with biological relatives, whereas an important shared environment contribution would lead to resemblance to biologically unrelated adoptive relatives. Adoption studies are also a useful method for examining gene–environment interaction and gene–environment correlation.

There are three main types of adoption design. First there are studies examining the adopted-away offspring of parents with a disorder. Such early studies found that adopted-away offspring of parents with schizophrenia also showed increased rates of schizophrenia. Second, there are studies that focus on examining the biological and adoptive relatives of affected adoptees. Such studies have found that genetic influences have an important role in antisocial behavior. Finally, a particularly interesting variety of adoption study is the cross-fostering design where the rate of a disorder in children at high genetic risk who are adopted in low environmental risk families is compared with that among children who are at low genetic risk/high environmental risk and children at high genetic risk/high environmental risk. Such studies have also shown that high genetic risk and psychosocial adversity interact in substantially increasing the risk of antisocial behavior (see chapter 35) and in influencing IQ in children.

Twin Studies

Twinning occurs on average in 1 in 80 births. Twin studies provide a natural experiment to disentangle genes and shared environmental effects. The premise of the twin study design is that monozygotic (MZ) twins are genetically identical (for some caveats see p. 350) and share 100% of their genes. Dizygotic (DZ) twins, like other full biological siblings, share on average 50% of their segregating genes. For genetically influenced traits or disorders, we thus would expect to see significantly greater MZ twin similarity (expressed as a correlation coefficient, rMZ) or concordance than DZ twin similarity (rDZ) or concordance. There are a number of assumptions made in twin studies and these will be discussed in further detail.

Twin methods involve statistically inferring genetic and environmental contributions from the patterns of twin resemblance for a given trait or disorder in the population being studied. The phenotypic variance in the population is decomposed into variance explained by additive genetic factors and environmental influences of the shared and non-shared type. The proportion of additive genetic variance is known as heritability. Heritability estimates are thus simply a measure of variation. If there is no genetic variation (if there is a trait that is influenced by a single gene that everyone carries) that trait would show zero heritability. Like all measures of variance, heritability estimates are specific to the population being studied and do not provide an index of whether or not that trait is susceptible to change by intervention. A well-known example is height, which has a heritability of about 90%. Most of the individual differences in height are attributable to genetic factors. Nevertheless, it is well acknowledged that in wealthier countries the average adult height has steadily risen and that is partly attributable to better nutrition and not to a sudden change in the gene pool (Roche, 1979). MZ and DZ twin similarity can be expressed in proportions of variance as follows, where r refers to the observed twin correlation and estimates of h^2 = heritability, c^2 = shared or common environmental variance and e^2 = non-shared environmental variance can be calculated: $rMZ = h^2 + c^2$; $rDZ = 0.5\ h^2 + c^2$; $1 - rMZ = e^2$.

It can be seen that non-shared environmental variance (e^2) refers to non-inherited influences that make MZ twins dissimilar. This includes environmental influences which impact differentially on MZ twins in terms of a given phenotype, measurement error and random effects, which will appear as non-inherited differences.

Virtually all published twin studies estimate h^2, c^2 and e^2 as well as other parameters if additional data are available (e.g., parent data or specific measures of environment) using structural equation modeling techniques (see chapter 9). A hypothesized model of etiology is drawn up and this is represented by a path diagram. For computer programs such as Mx, observed data are provided and starting values for estimated parameters (e.g., h^2) are suggested by the researcher. The program iterates with different parameter estimates until the optimum statistical fit between the estimated model and the observed data is reached (e.g., maximizing a likelihood function). An estimate of how well the hypothesized model fits is derived as well as estimates of the parameters of interest. The most basic twin model will allow for estimation of h^2, c^2 and e^2, although now the focus in twin research is on answering specific questions (e.g., on comorbidity or gene–environment interplay and addressing developmental issues; see p. 352), rather than simply providing heritability estimates.

Although twin studies provide much useful research evidence on child psychopathology, there are a number of assumptions and drawbacks that need to be borne in mind when interpreting findings.

Equal Environment Assumption

The twin study design is based on the assumption that MZ and DZ twin pairs share environment (including prenatal environment; e.g., fetal nutrition) to the same extent in so far as the environment influences the trait being studied. The issue is *not* whether, in general, MZ twin pairs share environments to a greater extent than DZ twin pairs. It is obvious that they will because of active gene–environment correlations. However, the assumption is violated only if the genetically influenced environment influences phenotypic differences. Thus, it is well known that MZ twins are more likely than DZ twins to be dressed alike, but no-one supposes that this is likely to influence susceptibility for any psychiatric disorder.

Violations of the equal environment assumptions (EESs) have been tested in several different ways. First, it has been examined by using a questionnaire measure of environmental sharing (e.g., assessing whether twins share friends) and by measuring the amount of twin contact. The findings have shown that MZ pairs do share more similar environments than DZ pairs but this is unrelated to twin similarity for psychopathology or behavior. Others have addressed the issue by investigating twins who are mistaken about their zygosity. These studies have generally found that it is true zygosity rather than the perception of zygosity that seems to be important (Goodman & Stevenson, 1991). The most robust method of testing the EEA is to determine whether environmental differences within MZ pairs are systematically associated with phenotypic differences within those pairs (Rutter, 2006). The findings show that they are with respect to antisocial behavior and depression but, so far as is known, there is no violation of the EEA with respect to twin studies of schizophrenia, autism, IQ and personality traits. This indicates that it makes no sense to consider the EEA as something that applies generally; rather, it has to be considered in relation to particular phenotypes. The increased environmental sharing in MZ pairs arises because of greater MZ twin similarity in genetically influenced behavior or traits. This does not negate the meaning of twin studies. Rather, it means that there needs to be an awareness that gene–environment correlations may contribute to the heritability estimate for some disorders. It should be added that, with respect to intrauterine influences, there is some tendency for MZ twins to differ more than DZ twins (because of the transfusion syndrome in some of the former), but it is doubtful whether this has much effect on heritabilities, other than perhaps on IQ.

Placental Heterogeneity Within MZ Pairs

Although MZ twins come from the same fertilized egg, the process by which twinning occurs is complex. Non-inherited genetic changes may have an important role and there may be other changes (e.g., imprinting effects; see p. 341) such that MZ twins are not truly genetically identical. Moreover, some MZ twin pairs share the same placental chorion (monochorionic) whereas others do not (dichorionic). There is some evidence to suggest that this may be important in that monochorionic MZ twins may be more similar in IQ than dichorionic MZ twins (Jacobs, Van Gestel, Derom *et al.*, 2001). This highlights that prenatal environmental influences that are unequally shared may sometimes be important.

Comparability of Twins to Singletons

Another potential concern is whether twins are representative of the general population. Twin births are higher risk prenatally and perinatally, they are of lower birth weight, some MZ twins show fetal–fetal transfusion syndrome (where one twin receives most of the blood supply) and being one of a twinship is an unusual experience. There is also evidence to suggest that mothers of twins show increased rates of depression in the early years. However, apart from somewhat increased rates of speech and language delay that appear to be environmental in origin (Thorpe, Rutter, & Greenwood, 2003), there is no consistent evidence that rates of psychopathology are different in twins.

Another potential source of difference among twins is that increasingly multiple births are arising as a result of fertility treatment. There is some recent concern that some *in vitro* fertilization (IVF) procedures may result in an increased rate of certain medical and developmental conditions (Gosden, Trasler, Lucifero *et al.*, 2003). Families of IVF children may also differ from other families although as yet there is no evidence to suggest that twins conceived by IVF differ in rates of psychopathology (Tully, Moffitt, & Caspi, 2003) or in twin similarity compared with other twins (Goody, Rice, Boivin *et al.*, 2005).

Blended Families Design

A recent innovation has been the use of a blended families design (Reiss, Hetherington, & Plomin, 2000) in which, in addition to twins, use is made of step-siblings, half-siblings and full biological siblings who vary in their genetic relationship but share some of their rearing environment. At first sight this seems an attractive design given the frequency of divorce and remarriage, but it suffers from an inherent confound between genetic and rearing influences (Rutter *et al.*, 1999a). Thus, not only are there genetic and environmental differences associated with divorce and remarriage, but also step-siblings and half-siblings will differ from biological siblings in the timing of duration of their rearing in the same family. In addition, relationships that children have with step-parents are not the same as those with biological parents (Dunn, Deater-Deckard, Pickering *et al.*, 1998).

As Bergeman, Plomin, Pedersen *et al.* (1991) pointed out, the presence of gene–environment correlations inevitably means that the observed correlations between measured risk environments and psychopathology (or behavioral traits) could reflect genetic rather than environmental mediation. The empirical findings that they reviewed showed that, to some extent, this was indeed the case.

Twin Designs to Examine Environmental Risk Mediation

There are three main ways in which twin studies may be used to test hypotheses regarding environmental risk mediation. First, there is the children of twins (COT) design. The method is based on the fact that the offspring of MZ twins are social cousins but genetic half-siblings. This is because one of their parents from whom they receive 50% of their genetic material is genetically identical to their MZ twin aunt/uncle. The offspring of DZ twins are like ordinary cousins and share on average 1 in 8 of their segregating genes. The design is particularly appealing because it potentially allows the contrasting of environmental and genetic transmission across generations (D'Onofrio, Turkheimer, Eaves *et al.*, 2003; Silberg & Eaves, 2004). In brief, the effects of the rearing environment provided by the biological mother can be compared with the comparable environment provided by the MZ twin mother who did not rear her nephew/niece. Three features of the design require conceptual and analytic attention. First, the possibility of assortative mating needs to be considered and taken into account. This is because, although the offspring have the same genetic relationship with their aunt who is an MZ cotwin of their mother, they differ with respect to their other parent/uncle. Second, it is unlikely that the children of the twins will be comparable in age, and may differ in gender; both will need to be taken into account. Finally, there is the assumption that the phenotype in parent and offspring has the same meaning. This can be problematic for disorders in which the phenotypic manifestations change with development (e.g., ADHD) and the heritability varies with age (as with depression and antisocial behavior). To a substantial extent, these issues can be dealt with through appropriate analyses but the rich potential of the COT design has still to be put to the test in a range of studies.

Second, provided that the putative environmental risk factor can be measured in a child-specific fashion (Purcell & Koenen, 2005), it is possible to use multivariate analyses to compare genetic and environmental mediation by treating the environment as a phenotype and employing across-twins and across-trait analyses in MZ and DZ pairs.

In this way, Pike & Plomin (1996) showed that family negativity had a true environmentally mediated effect on child psychopathology, even though some of the effect was genetically mediated. Other studies have shown the same for life events (Kendler, Kessler, Walters *et al.*, 1995; Rice, Harold, & Thapar, 2003), and physical maltreatment (Jaffee, Caspi, Moffitt *et al.*, 2004).

Third, environmental mediation can be studied by examining effects within MZ twin pairs (Pike, Reiss, Hetherington *et al.*, 1996). Thus, Caspi, Moffitt, Morgan *et al.* (2004) examined the effects of maternal negative expressed emotion on antisocial behavior. The study involved two key design features that were crucial in testing causal effects in a rigorous fashion, beyond just excluding genetic mediation. To begin with, within-individual change over a 2-year time span was assessed, and this was combined with the use of different informants for the maternal expressed emotion and the child psychopathology. Both these design features are equally necessary in all the genetic designs to test environmental risk mediation, but they have only sometimes been employed. One query with respect to this design is what it was that led the mother to respond so differently to the two MZ twins. This does not affect the conclusiveness on environmental mediation but it could possibly affect the generalization of the finding to other samples.

There is also a fourth design that has sometimes been employed – the extended twin family design (Kendler, Neale, Prescott *et al.*, 1996; Meyer, Rutter, Silberg *et al.*, 2000). This uses the measures of the phenotype in parents and children, and the association of the former with the putative environmental risk factor to test for environmental risk mediation. Its use has shown the environmental impact of early parental loss on alcoholism and of family maladaption on antisocial behavior. However, it is a problematic design with respect to the assumptions involved and the difficulty in putting these to the test. As a result it has not been much used.

Twin and Adoptee Designs to Test for Gene–Environment Interaction

It is usually claimed that adoptee studies are superior to twin studies for the study of G × E because they provide a better separation of G × E. Indeed, the rationale is based on the separateness of genetic risk and environmental risk. Undoubtedly, this means that there is a "cleaner" testing of G × E, but the downside is that, by design, it will be unusual for genetic risk and environmental risk to apply to the same individuals. That is, under natural circumstances, genetic and environmental risk would not be separated in this "experimental manner," individuals would be exposed to both sets of risk. This means that the G × E effect on population variance will always be underestimated in adoption studies. Nevertheless, the findings have pointed to significant G × E with respect to antisocial behavior (Rutter, 2006; Rutter, Moffitt, & Caspi, 2006; van Os, Pedersen, & Mortensen, 2004); specifically, increased rates of antisocial behavior in the offspring of antisocial biological relatives who are also exposed to social adversity in the adoptive family compared to offspring who are at low genetic risk of antisocial behavior and those at high genetic risk but who are exposed to a positive adoptive environment.

Twin studies have been used in two different ways to study G × E. First, as shown by Kendler *et al.* (1995), genetic risk can be inferred from the concordance (degree of similarity) findings for a given disorder among MZ and DZ twins. High genetic risk was inferred when MZ twins were already concordant for a past episode of psychopathology (e.g., depression) and low genetic risk when they were discordant (one twin had an episode of depression, the other remained unaffected), DZ pairs being intermediate. They showed that the risk of a new episode of major affective disorder was highest in the presence of high inferred genetic risk and when exposed to life events – pointing to G × E. Jaffee, Caspi, Moffitt *et al.* (2004, 2005) showed the same with respect to maltreatment and antisocial behavior.

The second approach, exemplified by Silberg, Rutter, Neale *et al.* (2001), is to determine whether heritability is greater in the presence of environmental risk. This implies G × E because the G × E term is incorporated in the measure of heritability. Their findings suggested G × E with respect to life events and depression/anxiety.

It will be appreciated that the main limitation of twin and adoptee studies to test for G × E is that the effect has to be inferred and deals only with the generality of a genetic effect, rather than one that applies to specific identified gene variants. As such, twin and adoptee studies provide an invaluable filter for the situations in which true G × E is likely to apply, but the proper testing has to be undertaken through molecular genetic studies.

Variations in Heritability by Social Context

Psychiatric geneticists have always emphasized that heritability is a population and not an individual characteristic and that it is bound to vary according to environmental circumstances. Studies by Rowe, Jacobson, & Van den Oord (1999) and by Turkheimer, Haley, Waldron *et al.* (2003) aroused considerable interest in terms of their finding that heritability for IQ was much lower in the presence of environmental adversity. Unfortunately, the findings of other studies have been contradictory (Rutter, Moffitt, & Caspi, 2006; Rutter, 2006) and, although it would be extremely valuable to determine why heritability varies by social circumstance, there are several competing explanations with contrasting predictions and the findings so far are inconclusive.

Comorbidity

Psychiatric disorders commonly co-occur and symptoms covary. It remains unknown why this is the case, although there are a number of plausible mechanisms (Caron & Rutter, 1991; see also chapter 2). Twin studies provide one means of examining this issue, specifically by investigating whether a shared set of risk factors (genetic and environmental) contribute to the overlap of two or more phenotypes (e.g., both genetic and individual environmental factors contributing to the overlap of novelty seeking personality traits and cannabis use; Kendler & Prescott, 2006).

Alternatively, twin analyses can be undertaken to test whether a "risk index" mediates risk for another clinical outcome (e.g., social anxiety in females leading to alcoholism; Kendler & Prescott, 2006). Multivariate genetic analysis can be used to test this. Such studies have found that childhood anxiety and depression (Thapar & Rice, 2006) and that ADHD and conduct disorder symptoms (Silberg, Rutter, Meyer *et al.*, 1996) share a common genetic etiology. This means that the comorbidity does not reflect the causal effect of one disorder on another, but rather the fact that shared risk factors (in this case genetic) apply to both. It might be thought that genetic studies will always lead to this conclusion but that is not so. Thus, in adults, analyses have shown that anxiety disorder may have a causal effect on substance abuse (through a form of self-medication) whereas the similar association in the case of depression does not – the supposed comorbidity arising only through shared genetic risk factors (Kendler & Prescott, 2006).

Developmental Questions

More recently, longitudinal twin studies have been used to examine questions about the contribution of etiological factors to the developmental continuity, change and phenotypic progression of child psychopathology. Such studies have been consistent in showing that genetic influences appear to become more important for depression symptoms in adolescence than in childhood. There is also evidence that this increased heritability over time may be partly explained by increased active and evocative gene–environment correlation through an increase in dependent life events in adolescence (Rice, Harold, & Thapar, 2003).

Most studies have also found that genetic factors have a major contribution to continuity in disorder and symptoms over time, but that non-shared environmental factors are most important in accounting for change. This appears to be the case for ADHD. For some disorders, notably adolescent depression and ADHD, additional genetic influences can be detected at later time points, suggesting that new age-specific genetic influences (that will include gene–environment correlation and G × E effects) may contribute to developmental change in the level of symptoms. Finally, change in phenotype over time has also been examined. For example, clinical and epidemiological studies have shown that childhood anxiety often precedes adolescent depression. Twin study findings additionally suggest that childhood anxiety is a precursor to depression and show that this is mainly because of shared genetic factors contributing to anxiety earlier in time and to depression at a later time (Rice, van den Bree, & Thapar, 2004). The relationship between earlier anxiety and later depression in adolescence also appears to arise through gene–environment interaction and gene–environment correlation with life events (Eaves, Silberg, & Erkanli, 2003).

Gender Effects

Many psychiatric disorders in childhood show gender differences in prevalence (Rutter, Caspi, & Moffitt, 2003). Neurodevelopmental disorders such as autism, ADHD and childhood onset schizophrenia show a male excess (see chapter 3). Depression affects more females but this gender difference only appears in early adolescence. The explanations for these observed sex differences remain elusive (Rutter, Caspi, & Moffitt, 2003) although biological, genetic and social factors are all likely to have a role. Twin studies allow for testing whether the contribution of genetic and environmental influences to a specific form of psychopathology differs across genders. Such designs have been used to test whether the magnitude of genetic and environmental contribution varies for males and females and to investigate whether there is significant evidence of gender-specific genetic influences. Although male–female differences in the rates of many disorders are well established, such studies have in general failed to show significant gender differences in genetic etiology although this may be because of low statistical power. However, there has been increasing interest in searching for molecular genetic mechanisms such as imprinting effects and for X-linked susceptibility genes (see chapter 24) that might account for gender differences in the rates of psychopathology.

Phenotype Definition

One of the key problems in psychiatry concerns the definition of diagnostic categories and delineation of their boundaries. Although obviously this cannot, and should not, be determined only by genetic findings, such findings can be helpful. For example, both the twin and family findings on autism clearly indicate that the genetic liability extends well beyond the traditional diagnostic category of a severely handicapping disorder (Le Couteur, Bailey, Goode *et al.*, 1996; Rutter, 2005). Similarly, the findings on schizophrenia indicate that the diagnostic concept needs to be extended to include schizotypal personality disorder but, equally, it does not include many other forms of psychopathology that are sometimes associated with schizophrenia (Kendler, Masterson, Ungaro *et al.*, 1984).

Twin studies have been used to examine the extent to which genetic influences extend to variations in the general population, and the extent to which the magnitude of these influences is the same as those that affect extreme diagnostic categories. The basic method of analysis involves a type of regression analysis commonly known as the DeFries and Fulker method after the authors who first published it (DeFries & Fulker, 1988). The findings have shown that ADHD and dyslexia appear to lie on continua, with high scores being as highly heritable as scores within the normal range, although the power to detect differences at the extreme end using this method is low. In contrast, high adolescent depression symptom scores, at least when self-rated, tend to be predominantly influenced by shared environmental factors, whereas the rest of the continuum is more highly heritable (Eley, 1997; Rende, Plomin, Reiss *et al.*, 1993; Rice, Harold, & Thapar, 2002). This suggests etiological discontinuity for adolescent-reported depression symptoms.

The other phenotypic issue that has been examined using twin study designs is informant (e.g., parent and teacher) agreement and disagreement (for discussion of informant issues see chapter 20). These methods have also been used to test ways of integrating information from different informants informed by different patterns of genetic and environmental contribution. Here, the twin strategy used is the same as that outlined for examining comorbidity. The aim is to examine the extent to which covariation between raters is a result of shared genetic and environmental risk factors. The findings of such studies have suggested that while parents and teachers rate a construct of ADHD that is influenced by a common set of genetic factors, there are also informant-specific genetic and environmental contributions. Twin studies have also been used to examine rater biases. For example, there is evidence that mothers, but not teachers, may contrast twins when rating ADHD symptom scores (see chapter 34), with a tendency to increase twin differences. This results in near zero or negative DZ twin correlations, which are biologically implausible.

Potential Clinical Implications

Genetics research is of enormous scientific relevance but what is the current and likely future clinical relevance in child psychiatry? The answer does not lie in any supposed deterministic influence of genes. As Kendler (1995, 2005) has noted, the effects of all known susceptibility genes in psychiatry are quite low (with odds ratios in the region of 1.4). As a result, it is seriously misleading to refer to genes "for" schizophrenia, autism or indeed any other form of mental disorder. Accordingly, there is a very limited scope for genetic testing in the case of complex multifactorial disorders; this applies to almost all forms of psychiatric disorder. On the other hand, genes are involved in one way or another in the causal processes leading to all forms of disorder and it is imperative that clinicians understand how these operate (Kendler, 2005).

Supposed Dichotomy Between Genetic and Environmental Disorders

Traditionally, many clinicians and researchers have sought to make a main subdivision between disorders that are mainly genetic and those that are mainly environmental. A key message from genetics is that this dichotomy is largely false. Gene–environment correlations and interactions mean that, even with strongly environmental disorders such as post-traumatic stress disorder (PTSD), individuals vary greatly in their response to stress and adversity, and that this variation is genetically influenced in part. However, it is not just a question of individual differences in "constitutional" susceptibility to environmental hazards, it is also a matter of genetically influenced differences in exposure to such hazards. Clinicians, like researchers, need to pay attention to the origins of risk factors and to differential susceptibility to them. Moreover, it may be misleading to view the genetic influences as applying just to vulnerability. Thus, it has been suggested (Boyce & Jemerin, 1990) that evolutionary considerations mean that they may concern responsivity, with such responsivity working in both positive and negative directions.

Primacy of the Environment or Genetic Determinism

In the past, many clinicians assumed the primacy of the environment in contributing to child psychopathology and sometimes this view led to blaming parents for their children's problems (see chapter 1). This style of blame was unacceptable on many different grounds – ethical and clinical, as well as scientific. However, genetic research (along with other research strategies) has been helpful in showing that parental behavior may be influenced by psychopathology and in indicating that this is subject to genetic and environmental influences and the interplay between them (Kendler & Prescott, 2006; Rutter, Moffitt, & Caspi, 2006). Far from implying genetic determinism, the findings point to the need to understand the complex mixture of influences on individual behavior. As we have sought to emphasize here, exactly the same applies with respect to children's behavior. The additional message from findings on gene–environment correlations is that just as child-rearing experiences influence children's behavior, so also children's behavior influences how parents respond to them. Both genetic and environmental research are at one in pointing to the evidence that bidirectional influences are the rule rather than the exception.

Conceptualization of Disorders, Diagnostic Boundaries and Subtypes

Some genetic enthusiasts expect that genetic findings will form the basis of new classificatory systems for psychiatric disorders. We disagree. The disagreement is primarily because most classificatory schemes that concern multifactorial disorders are best based on pathophysiology rather than any single basic causal factor (because there is not one). Nevertheless, it is likely that genetic advances will indirectly influence and support both diagnosis and classification because they will (through associated biological studies) lead to a better understanding of pathophysiology and because they will be informative on the commonalities and differences among different disorders (Kendler, 2006). Already it is clear that genetic findings have forced a broadening of the concept of both autism and schizophrenia and have shown the importance of considering dimensional risk and phenotypic features (with respect, for example, to ADHD, antisocial behavior and depression).

Prediction

Families with a family history of disorder (e.g., schizophrenia or depression) may well wish to know what the risk of disorder is for offspring or siblings. At present, clinicians are reliant on global risk scores derived from family studies (e.g., informing the family that the child is four times more likely than the average child to show the condition in question). Unfortunately, such information – which deals with population risks – is of very limited value for individual prediction. Identified susceptibility genes will help personalize risks but it is important to appreciate that the risks will still be probabilistic, rather than determinative, because the actual outcome will depend on the presence of other (as yet to be identified) susceptibility genes, contributory genetic background factors and exposure to relevant environmental hazards. Genetic counseling in the case of multifactorial disorder is a much more uncertain enterprise than in the case of wholly genetic Mendelian disorders (see chapter 73).

Nevertheless, genetic findings on G × E can be helpful in personalizing the nature of risks. For example, where there is a familial risk of schizophrenia, the use of cannabis may be more risky. Moreover, there is now evidence to indicate that those carrying a specific *COMT* gene variant are more likely to be unusually sensitive to the adverse effects of cannabis smoking on psychotic symptoms (Caspi, Moffitt, Cannon *et al.*, 2005). These findings suggest that there are increased risks of using cannabis in this specific group.

For obvious reasons, the comparable genetic influences on susceptibility to child maltreatment and to life stressors do not have such a straightforward preventive implication. It would not be very helpful to recommend that children should avoid being physically abused and should avoid life stressors! Nevertheless, in the longer term there is a clinical implication. Once we understand why and how genetic factors influence susceptibility to risk environments, there will be implications for prevention and interventions. Also, pharmacogenetic findings may, in time, be helpful in indicating which individuals are likely to be responsive to particular mediations and which have an unusually high risk of side-effects. The research findings, so far, do not provide such guidance (other than at a rather rudimentary level) but it is likely that they will be more helpful in the future.

Finally, genetic findings may be helpful in identifying individuals for whom interventions may be especially needed. Traditionally, it has often been assumed that these individuals will be those with disorders that are least influenced by genetic factors. The findings on G × E and rGE suggest that often the reverse may be the reality. The need for environmental interventions may be greatest in those who are genetically most vulnerable. Once more, the findings are not yet at a point at which they have a direct implication for action but they do challenge the traditional assumptions.

Nature of Environmental Interventions

Potentially, an understanding of genetic mechanisms should lead to important guidelines on what sort of environmental intervention is likely to be effective. The most striking example is provided by the Mendelian disorder of phenylketonuria. It is in a real sense a wholly genetic disorder because the resulting metabolic defect (leading to profound intellectual disability) is entirely brought about by the genetic anomaly. However, because the clinical effects are brought about by the body's inability to deal with the normal dietary component of phenylalanine, the effective treatment is provided by a radical change in diet. In an equally real sense, the resulting handicap is entirely environmentally determined (albeit entirely dependent on the presence of the genetic anomaly). We have no idea whether there will be any other equivalent in the field of multifactorial psychiatric disorders. Nevertheless, genetic knowledge indicates that we should not necessarily assume that the pathophysiological mechanisms will necessarily involve neurotransmitters. We may ask, for example, why it is that a disorder such as autism is so remarkably unresponsive to the medications used so far. The answer may lie in our having used the wrong drugs but, equally, it might be because the underlying pathophysiological mechanisms involve the immune system rather than neurotransmitters. That is, genetics can point the way to novel treatment targets for the development of specific pharmacological agents. The basic point is that we need to be aware that the brain is part of the body and of broader bodily systems and the underlying causal processes could involve these rather than (or in addition to) brain systems.

Conclusions

Genetics research into complex disorders, including psychiatric disorders, is at an exciting stage. This is not purely because susceptibility genes are beginning to be found, although this often captures most media and public interest, but because genetics is now moving into an era in which it is being integrated with epidemiological and psychosocial research whereby environment and genes are being examined together. Now that susceptibility genes are being identified, genetics is being increasingly embraced by other areas of neuroscience, notably molecular biology, imaging and neurocognitive science as well as mainstream epidemiology. The clinical implications are important and it is crucial not only that genetics research is informed by clinical practice, but equally that findings from these studies are recognized by clinicians and put into practice.

Further reading

Institute of Medicine Board on Health Sciences Policy. (2006). *Genes, behavior and the social environment: moving beyond the nature nurture debate*. Washington DC: National Academies Press. (http://www.nap.edu)

Kendler, K. S., & Prescott, C. A. (2006). *Genes, environment and psychopathology: Understanding the causes of psychiatric and substance use disorders*. New York, NY/London: Guilford Press.

Rutter, M. (2006). *Genes and behavior: Nature–nurture interplay explained*. Blackwell: Oxford.

Rutter, M., Moffitt, T. E., & Caspi, A. (2006). Gene–environment interplay and psychopathology: multiple varieties but real effects. *Journal of Child Psychology and Psychiatry*, *47*, 226–261.

References

Abiola, O., Angel, J. M., Avner, P., Bachmanov, A. A., Belknap, J. K., Bennett, B., *et al.* (2003). The nature and identification of quantitative trait loci: a community's view. *Nature Reviews. Genetics*, *4*, 911–916.

Altshuler, D., & Clark, A. G. (2005). Genetics: Harvesting medical information from the human family tree. *Science*, *307*, 1052–1053.

Autism Genome Project Consortium, Szatmari, P., Paterson, A. D., Zwaigenbaum, L., *et al.* (2007). Mapping autism risk loci using genetic linkage and chromosomal rearrangements. *Nature Genetics*, *39*, 319–328.

Bell, R. Q. (1968). A reinterpretation of the direction of effects in studies of socialization. *Psychological Review*, *75*, 81–95.

Bergeman, C. S., Plomin, R., Pedersen, N. L., & McClearn, G. E. (1991). Genetic mediation of the relationship between social support and psychological well-being. *Psychology and Aging*, *6*, 640–646.

Boyce, W. T., & Jemerin, J. M. (1990). Psychobiological differences in childhood stress response. I. Patterns of illness and susceptibility. *Journal of Developmental and Behavioral Pediatrics*, *11*, 86–94.

Bray, N. J., Buckland, P. R., Williams, N. M., Williams, H. J., Norton, N., Owen, M. J., *et al.* (2003). A haplotype implicated in schizophrenia susceptibility is associated with reduced COMT expression in human brain. *American Journal of Human Genetics*, *73*, 152–161.

Brunner, H. G., Nelen, M. R., van Zandvoort, P., Abeling, N. G., van Gennip, A. H., Wolters, E. C., *et al.* (1993). X-linked borderline mental retardation with prominent behavioral disturbance: phenotype, genetic localization, and evidence for disturbed monoamine metabolism. *American Journal of Human Genetics*, *52*, 1032–1039.

Cannon, T. D. (2005). The inheritance of intermediate phenotypes for schizophrenia. *Current Opinion in Psychiatry*, *18*, 135–140.

Carlson, C. S., Eberle, M. A., Kruglyak, L., & Nickerson, D. A. (2004). Mapping complex disease loci in whole-genome association studies. *Nature*, *429*, 446–452.

Caron, C., & Rutter, M. (1991). Comorbidity in child psychopathology: Concepts, issues and research strategies. *Journal of Child Psychology and Psychiatry*, *32*, 1063–1080.

Caspi, A., Langley, K., Milne B., Moffitt, T. E., O'Donovan, M., Owen, M. J., *et al.* (2008). A replicated molecular-genetic basis for subtyping antisocial behaviour in children with ADHD. *Archives of General Psychiatry*, *65*, 203–10.

Caspi, A., McClay, J., Moffitt, T. E., Mill, J., Martin, J., Craig, I. W., *et al.* (2002). Role of genotype in the cycle of violence in maltreated children. *Science*, *297*, 851–854.

Caspi, A., Moffitt, T. E., Cannon, M., McClay, J., Murray, R., Harrington, H., *et al.* (2005). Moderation of the effect of adolescent-onset cannabis use on adult psychosis by a functional polymorphism in the catechol-O-methyltransferase gene: Longitudinal evidence of a gene × environment interaction. *Biological Psychiatry*, *57*, 1117–1127.

Caspi, A., Moffitt, T. E., Morgan, J., Rutter, M., Taylor, A., Arseneault, L., *et al.* (2004). Maternal expressed emotion predicts children's antisocial behavior problems: Using monozygotic-twin differences to identify environmental effects on behavioral development. *Developmental Psychology*, *40*, 149–161.

Castillo-Davis, C. I. (2005). The evolution of noncoding DNA: How much junk, how much func? *Trends in Genetics*, *21*, 533–536.

Cope, N., Harold, D., Hill, G., Moskvina, V., Stevenson, J., Holmans, P., *et al.* (2005). Strong evidence that KIAA0319 on chromosome 6p is a susceptibility gene for developmental dyslexia. *American Journal of Human Genetics*, *76*, 581–591.

Craddock, N., O'Donovan, M. C., & Owen, M. J. (2006). Genes for schizophrenia and bipolar disorder? Implications for psychiatric nosology. *Schizophrenia Bulletin*, *32*, 9–16.

DeFries, J. C., & Fulker, D. W. (1988). Multiple regression analysis of twin data: etiology of deviant scores versus individual differences. *Acta Geneticae Medicae et Gemellologiae*, *37*, 205–216.

D'Onofrio, B. M., Turkheimer, E. N., Eaves, L. J., Corey, L. A., Berg, K., Solaas, M. H., *et al.* (2003). The role of the children of twins design in elucidating causal relations between parent characteristics and child outcomes. *Journal of Child Psychology and Psychiatry*, *44*, 1130–1144.

Dunn, J., Deater-Deckard, K., Pickering, K., O'Connor, T. G., & Golding, J. (1998). Children's adjustment and prosocial behaviour in step-, single-parent, and non-stepfamily settings: Findings from a community study. ALSPAC Study Team. Avon Longitudinal Study of Pregnancy and Childhood. *Journal of Child Psychology and Psychiatry*, *39*, 1083–1095.

Eaves, L., Silberg, J., & Erkanli, A. (2003). Resolving multiple epigenetic pathways to adolescent depression. *Journal of Child Psychology and Psychiatry*, *44*, 1006–1014.

Eley, T. C. (1997). Depressive symptoms in children and adolescents: Etiological links between normality and abnormality – a research note. *Journal of Child Psychology and Psychiatry*, *38*, 861–865.

Faraone, S. V., Perlis, R. H., Doyle, A. E., Smoller, J. W., Goralnick, J. J., Holmgren, M. A., *et al.* (2005). Molecular genetics of attention-deficit/hyperactivity disorder. *Biological Psychiatry*, *57*, 1313–1323.

Fullerton, J., Cubin, M., Tiwari, H., Wang, C., Bomhra, A., Davidson, S., *et al.* (2003). Linkage analysis of extremely discordant and concordant sibling pairs identifies quantitative-trait loci that influence variation in the human personality trait neuroticism. *American Journal of Human Genetics*, *72*, 879–890.

Ge, X. (1996). The developmental interface between nature and nurture: A mutual influence model of child antisocial behavior and parent behaviors. *Developmental Psychology*, *32*, 574–589.

Goodman, R., & Stevenson, J. (1991). Parental criticism and warmth towards unrecognized monozygotic twins. *Behavioral and Brain Sciences*, *14*, 394–395.

Goody, A., Rice, F., Boivin, J., Harold, G. T., Hay, D. F., & Thapar, A. (2005). Twins born following fertility treatment: implications for quantitative genetic studies. *Twin Research and Human Genetics*, *8*, 337–345.

Goring, H. H., Terwilliger, J. D., & Blangero, J. (2001). Large upward bias in estimation of locus-specific effects from genome-wide scans. *American Journal of Human Genetics*, *69*, 1357–1369.

Gosden, R., Trasler, J., Lucifero, D., & Faddy, M. (2003). Rare congenital disorders, imprinted genes, and assisted reproductive technology. *Lancet*, *361*, 1975–1977.

Gottesman, II, & Gould, T. D. (2003). The endophenotype concept in psychiatry: Etymology and strategic intentions. *American Journal of Psychiatry*, *160*, 636–645.

Hamshere, M. L., Williams, N., Norton, N., Williams, H., Cardno, A., Zammit, S., *et al.* (2005). Genome-wide significant linkage in schizophrenia conditioning on occurrence of depressive episodes. *Journal of Medical Genetics*, *43*, 563–567.

Hariri, A. R., Drabant, E. M., Munoz, K. E., Kolachana, B. S., Mattay, V. S., Egan, M. F., *et al.* (2005). A susceptibility gene for affective disorders and the response of the human amygdala. *Archives of General Psychiatry*, *62*, 146–152.

Hariri, A. R., Drabant, E. M., & Weinberger, D. R. (2006). Imaging genetics: perspectives from studies of genetically driven variation in serotonin function and corticolimbic affective processing. *Biological Psychiatry*, *59*, 888–897.

Heinz, A., Braus, D. F., Smolka, M. N., Wrase, J., Puls, I., Hermann, D., *et al.* (2005). Amygdala–prefrontal coupling depends on a genetic variation of the serotonin transporter. *Nature Neuroscience*, *8*, 20–21.

Jacobs, N., Van Gestel, S., Derom, C., Thiery, E., Vernon, P., Derom, R., *et al.* (2001). Heritability estimates of intelligence in twins: effect of chorion type. *Behavior Genetics*, *31*, 209–217.

Jaffee, S. R., Caspi, A., Moffitt, T. E., Dodge, K. A., Rutter, M., Taylor, A., *et al.* (2005). Nature × nurture: Genetic vulnerabilities interact with physical maltreatment to promote conduct problems. *Development and Psychopathology*, *17*, 67–84.

Jaffee, S. R., Caspi, A., Moffitt, T. E., Polo-Tomas, M., Price, T. S., & Taylor, A. (2004). The limits of child effects: Evidence for genetically mediated child effects on corporal punishment but not on physical maltreatment. *Developmental Psychology*, *40*, 1047–1058.

Kendler, K. S. (1995). Genetic epidemiology in psychiatry. Taking both genes and environment seriously. *Archives of General Psychiatry*, *52*, 895–899.

Kendler, K. S. (2005). "A gene for . . .": The nature of gene action in psychiatric disorders. *American Journal of Psychiatry*, *162*, 1243–1252.

Kendler, K. S. (2006). Reflections on the relationship between psychiatric genetics and psychiatric nosology. *American Journal of Psychiatry*, *163*, 1138–1146.

Kendler, K. S., Kessler, R. C., Walters, E. E., MacLean, C., Neale, M. C., Heath, A. C., *et al.* (1995). Stressful life events, genetic liability, and onset of an episode of major depression in women. *American Journal of Psychiatry*, *152*, 833–842.

Kendler, K., Kuhn, J., Vittum, J., Prescott, C., & Riley, B. (2005). The interaction of stressful life events and a serotonin transporter polymorphism in the prediction of episodes of major depression: A replication. *Archives of General Psychiatry*, *62*, 529–535.

Kendler, K. S., Masterson, C. C., Ungaro, R., & Davis, K. L. (1984). A family history study of schizophrenia-related personality disorders. *American Journal of Psychiatry*, *141*, 424–427.

Kendler, K. S., Neale, M. C., Prescott, C. A., Kessler, R. C., Heath, A. C., Corey, L. A., *et al.* (1996). Childhood parental loss and alcoholism in women: A causal analysis using a twin-family design. *Psychological Medicine*, *26*, 79–95.

Kendler, K. S., & Prescott, C. A. (2006). *Genes, environment and psychopathology: Understanding the causes of psychiatric and substance use disorders*. Guilford Press.

Kim-Cohen, J., Caspi, A., Taylor, A., Williams, B., Newcombe, R., Craig, I. W., *et al.* (2006). MAOA, maltreatment, and gene–environment interaction predicting children's mental health: New evidence and a meta-analysis. *Molecular Psychiatry*, *11*, 903–913.

Klein, R. J., Zeiss, C., Chew, E. Y., Tsai, J. Y., Sackler, R. S., Haynes, C., *et al.* (2005). Complement factor H polymorphism in age-related macular degeneration. *Science*, *308*, 385–389.

Lander, E., & Kruglyak, L. (1995). Genetic dissection of complex traits: Guidelines for interpreting and reporting linkage results. *Nature Genetics*, *11*, 241–247.

Le Couteur, A., Bailey, A., Goode, S., Pickles, A., Robertson, S., Gottesman, I., *et al.* (1996). A broader phenotype of autism: The clinical spectrum in twins. *Journal of Child Psychology and Psychiatry*, *37*, 785–801.

Malhotra, A. K., Murphy, G. M. Jr., & Kennedy, J. L. (2004). Pharmacogenetics of psychotropic drug response. *American Journal of Psychiatry*, *161*, 780–796.

McGuffin, P., Owen, M. J., & Gottesman, I. I. (Eds.). (2002). *Psychiatric Genetics and Genomics*. Oxford: Oxford University Press.

Meaney, M. J., & Szyf, M. (2005). Environmental programming of stress responses through DNA methylation: life at the interface between a dynamic environment and a fixed genome. *Dialogues in Clinical Neuroscience*, *7*, 103–123.

Meyer, J. M., Rutter, M., Silberg, J. L., Maes, H. H., Simonoff, E., Shillady, L. L., *et al.* (2000). Familial aggregation for conduct disorder symptomatology: The role of genes, marital discord and family adaptability. *Psychological Medicine*, *30*, 759–774.

Meyer-Lindenberg, A., Buckholtz, J. W., Kolachana, B. R., Hariri, A., Pezawas, L., Blasi, G., *et al.* (2006). From the cover: Neural mechanisms of genetic risk for impulsivity and violence in humans. *Proceedings of the National Academy of Sciences of the USA*, *103*, 6269–6274.

Meyer-Lindenberg, A., & Weinberger, D. R. (2006). Intermediate phenotypes and genetic mechanisms of psychiatric disorders. *Nature Reviews. Neuroscience*, *7*, 818–827.

Mill, J., Xu, X., Ronald, A., Curran, S., Price, T., Knight, J., *et al.* (2005). Quantitative trait locus analysis of candidate gene alleles associated with attention deficit hyperactivity disorder (ADHD) in five genes: DRD4, DAT1, DRD5, SNAP-25, and 5HT1B. *American Journal of Medical Genetics. Part B, Neuropsychiatric Genetics*, *133*, 68–73.

Millar, J. K., Pickard, B. S., Mackie, S., James, R., Christie, S., Buchanan, S. R., *et al.* (2005). DISC1 and PDE4B are interacting genetic factors in schizophrenia that regulate cAMP signaling. *Science*, *310*, 1187–1191.

Moffitt, T. E., Caspi, A., & Rutter, M. (2005). Strategy for investigating interactions between measured genes and measured environments. *Archives of General Psychiatry*, *62*, 473–481.

Newman, T. K., Syagailo, Y. V., Barr, C. S., Wendland, J. R., Champoux, M., Graessle, M., *et al.* (2005). Monoamine oxidase A gene promoter variation and rearing experience influences aggressive behavior in rhesus monkeys. *Biological Psychiatry*, *57*, 167–172.

Nuffield Council on Bioethics. (1998). *Mental disorders and genetics: The ethical context*. London.

O'Connor, T. G. (1998). Genotype–environmental correlations in late childhood and early adolescence: Antisocial behavioral problems and coercive parenting. *Developmental Psychology*, *34*, 970–981.

Owen, M. J., Craddock, N., & O'Donovan, M. C. (2005). Schizophrenia: genes at last? *Trends in Genetics*, *21*, 518–525.

Pezawas, L., Meyer-Lindenberg, A., Drabant, E. M., Verchinski, B. A., Munoz, K. E., Kolachana, B. S., *et al.* (2005). 5-HTTLPR polymorphism impacts human cingulate–amygdala interactions: A genetic susceptibility mechanism for depression. *Nature Neuroscience*, *8*, 828–834.

Pickles, A., & Angold, A. (2003). Natural categories or fundamental dimensions: on carving nature at the joints and the rearticulation of psychopathology. *Development and Psychopathology*, *15*, 529–551.

Pike, A., & Plomin, R. (1996). Importance of non-shared environmental factors for childhood and adolescent psychopathology. *Journal of the American Academy of Child and Adolescent Psychiatry*, *35*, 560–570.

Pike, A., Reiss, D., Hetherington, E. M., & Plomin, R. (1996). Using MZ differences in the search for non-shared environmental effects. *Journal of Child Psychology and Psychiatry*, *37*, 695–704.

Plomin, R. (1994). *Genetics and experience: The interplay to nature and nurture*. Thousand Oaks, CA: Sage.

Purcell, S., & Koenen, K. C. (2005). Environmental mediation and the twin design. *Behavior Genetics*, *35*, 491–498.

Reiss D. J. J., Hetherington E. M., & Plomin R. (2000). *The relationship code: Deciphering genetic and social influences on adolescence*. London: Harvard University Press.

Rende, R. D., Plomin, R., Reiss, D., & Hetherington, E. M. (1993). Genetic and environmental influences on depressive symptomatology in adolescence: individual differences and extreme scores. *Journal of Child Psychology and Psychiatry*, *34*, 1387–1398.

Rice, F., van den Bree, M. B., Thapar, A. (2004). A population-based study of anxiety as a precursor for depression in childhood and adolescence. *BMC Psychiatry*, *4*, 43.

Rice, F., Harold, G. T., & Thapar, A. (2003). Negative life events as an account of age-related differences in the genetic aetiology of depression in childhood and adolescence. *Journal of Child Psychology and Psychiatry*, *44*, 977–987.

Rice, F., Harold, G. T., Thapar, A. (2002). Assessing the effects of age, sex and shared environment on the genetic aetiology of depression in childhood and adolescence. *Journal of Child Psychology & Psychiatry*, *43*, 1039–1051.

Roche, A. F. (1979). Secular trends in human growth, maturation, and development. *Monographs of the Society for Research in Child Devopment*, *44*, 1–120.

Rowe, D. C., Jacobson, K. C., & Van den Oord, E. J. (1999). Genetic and environmental influences on vocabulary IQ: Parental education level as moderator. *Child Development*, *70*, 1151–1162.

Rutter, M. (1989). Pathways from childhood to adult life. *Journal of Child Psychology and Psychiatry*, *30*, 23–51.

Rutter, M. (2003). Categories, dimensions and the mental health of children and adolescents. In: J. A. King, C. F. Ferris & I. I. Lederhendler (Eds). *Roots of mental illness*. New York: The New York Academy of Sciences (pp. 11–21).

Rutter, M. (2005). Autism research: Lessons from the past and prospects for the future. *Journal of Autism and Developmental Disorders*, *35*, 241–257.

Rutter, M. (2006). *Genes and behaviour: Nature–nurture interplay explained*. Oxford: Blackwell Publishing.

Rutter, M. (2007). Proceedings from observed correlation to causal inference: The use of natural experiments. *Perspectives on Psychological Sciences*, *2*, 377–395.

Rutter, M., Caspi, A., & Moffitt, T. E. (2003). Using sex differences in psychopathology to study causal mechanisms: Unifying issues and research strategies. *Journal of Child Psychology and Psychiatry*, *44*, 1092–1115.

Rutter, M., Moffitt, T. E., & Caspi, A. (2006). Gene–environment interplay and psychopathology: Multiple varieties but real effects. *Journal of Child Psychology and Psychiatry*, *47*, 226–261.

Rutter, M., Silberg, J., O'Connor, T., & Simonoff, E. (1999a). Genetics and child psychiatry. I. Advances in quantitative and molecular genetics. *Journal of Child Psychology and Psychiatry*, *40*, 3–18.

Rutter, M., Silberg, J., O'Connor, T., & Simonoff, E. (1999b). Genetics and child psychiatry. II. Empirical research findings. *Journal of Child Psychology and Psychiatry*, *40*, 19–55.

Sadee, W., & Dai, Z. (2005). Pharmacogenetics/genomics and personalized medicine. *Human Molecular Genetics*, *14* (Spec No. 2), R207–R214.

Schiffman, S., Bronstein, M., Sternfeld, M., Pisante-Shalom, A., Lev-Lehman, E., Weizman, A., *et al.* (2002). A highly significant association between a COMT haplotype and schizophrenia. *American Journal of Human Genetics*, *71*, 1296–1302.

Shao, Y., Cuccaro, M. L., Hauser, E. R., Raiford, K. L., Menold, M. M., Wolpert, C. M., *et al.* (2003). Fine mapping of autistic disorder to chromosome 15q11-q13 by use of phenotypic subtypes. *American Journal of Human Genetics*, *72*, 539–548.

Silberg, J., & Eaves, L. (2004). Analysing the contributions of genes and parent–child interaction to childhood behavioural and emotional problems: A model for the children of twins. *Psychological Medicine*, *34*, 347–356.

Silberg, J., Pickles, A., Rutter, M., Hewitt, J., Simonoff, E., Maes, H., *et al.* (1999). The influence of genetic factors and life stress on depression among adolescent girls. *Archives of General Psychiatry*, *56*, 225–232.

Silberg, J., Rutter, M., Meyer, J., Maes, H., Hewitt, J., Simonoff, E., *et al.* (1996). Genetic and environmental influences on the covariation between hyperactivity and conduct disturbance in juvenile twins. *Journal of Child Psychology and Psychiatry*, *37*, 803–816.

Silberg, J., Rutter, M., Neale, M., & Eaves, L. (2001). Genetic moderation of environmental risk for depression and anxiety in adolescent girls. *British Journal of Psychiatry*, *179*, 116–121.

Smalley, S. L., Kustanovich, V., Minassian, S. L., Stone, J. L., Ogdie, M. N., McGough, J. J., *et al.* (2002). Genetic linkage of attention-deficit/hyperactivity disorder on chromosome 16p13, in a region implicated in autism. *American Journal of Human Genetics*, *71*, 959–963.

Stranger, B. E., Forrest, M. S., Dunning, M., Ingle, C. E., Beazley, C., Thorne, N., *et al.* (2007). Relative impact of nucleotide and copy number variation on gene expression phenotypes. *Science*, *315*, 848–853.

Thapar, A., Langley, K., O'Donovan, M., & Owen, M. (2006). Refining the attention deficit hyperactivity disorder phenotype for molecular genetic studies. *Molecular Psychiatry*, *11*, 714–720.

Thapar, A., Langley, K., Fowler, T., Rice, F., Turic, D., Whittinger, N., *et al.* (2005a). Catechol-O-methyltransferase gene variant and birth weight predict early-onset antisocial behavior in children with attention-deficit/hyperactivity disorder. *Archives of General Psychiatry*, *62*, 1275–1278.

Thapar, A., O'Donovan, M., & Owen, M. J. (2005b). The genetics of attention deficit hyperactivity disorder. *Human Molecular Genetics*, *14* (Spec No. 2), R275–R282.

Thapar, A., & Rice, F. (2006). Twin studies in pediatric depression. *Child and Adolescent Psychiatric Clinics of North America*, *15*, 869–881.

Thorpe, K., Rutter, M., & Greenwood, R. (2003). Twins as a natural experiment to study the causes of mild language delay: II. Family interaction risk factors. *Journal of Child Psychology and Psychiatry*, *44*, 342–355.

Tully, L. A., Moffitt, T. B., & Caspi, A. (2003). Maternal adjustment, parenting and child behaviour in families of school-aged twins conceived after IVF and ovulation induction. *Journal of Child Psychology and Psychiatry*, *44*, 316–325.

Tunbridge, E. M., Harrison, P. J., & Weinberger, D. R. (2006). Catechol-O-methyltransferase, cognition, and psychosis: Val(158)Met and beyond. *Biological Psychiatry*, *60*, 141–151.

Turkheimer, E., Haley, A., Waldron, M., D'Onofrio, B., & Gottesman, II. (2003). Socioeconomic status modifies heritability of IQ in young children. *Psychological Science*, *14*, 623–628.

Van Eerdewegh, P., Little, R. D., Dupuis, J., Del Mastro, R. G., Falls, K., Simon, J., *et al.* (2002). Association of the *ADAM33* gene with asthma and bronchial hyperresponsiveness. *Nature*, *418*, 426–430.

van Os, J., Pedersen, C. B., & Mortensen, P. B. (2004). Confirmation of synergy between urbanicity and familial liability in the causation of psychosis. *American Journal of Psychiatry*, *161*, 2312–2314.

Weaver, I. C., Champagne, F. A., Brown, S. E., Dymov, S., Sharma, S., Meaney, M. J., *et al.* (2005). Reversal of maternal programming of stress responses in adult offspring through methyl supplementation: altering epigenetic marking later in life. *Journal of Neuroscience*, *25*, 11045–11054.

Wellcome Trust Case Control Consortium (2007). Genome-wide association study of 14,000 cases of seven common diseases and 3,000 shared controls. *Nature*, *447*, 661–678.

Zammit, S., & Owen, M. J. (2006). Stressful life events, 5-HTT genotype and risk of depression. *British Journal of Psychiatry*, *188*, 199–201.

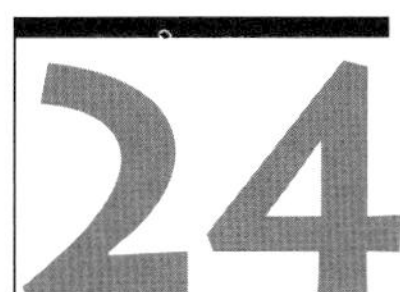

Behavioral Phenotypes and Chromosomal Disorders

David H. Skuse and Anna Seigal

The term "behavioral" or "cognitive" phenotype is used to describe a typical style of behavior or cognition that occurs in association with developmental disorders, in which a genetic anomaly has been demonstrated. Behavioral or cognitive phenotypes reflect the maldevelopment of neural systems that are dysfunctional. Some such characteristics are common to many disorders, such as inattention. Others are found in association with specific genetic substrates. Behavioral phenotypes range from self-injury, hyperphagia and impulsivity to peculiar motor stereotypies. Cognitive deficits can affect visuospatial skills, language, social understanding and mathematical abilities. Occasionally, a particular genetic mutation, or deletion, is associated with a behavioral phenotype that looks like a known disease, such as autism or schizophrenia. The finding does not imply the genetic locus has any direct part to play in idiopathic cases of the syndrome. Major psychiatric disorders have a multigenic etiology; complex mental disorders are not caused by mutations in single genes, but we may get a clue about the neural systems involved in the etiology of idiopathic psychiatric illness by studying "phenocopies" that result from a known genetic etiology.

Genetic Mechanisms Leading to Behavioral Phenotypes

Mutations and Polymorphisms

Any germ-line alteration in the nucleotide sequence of cells that produce gametes (sperm or eggs) will be inherited by the cells of subsequent generations. Most changes are neutral, with no effect on the phenotype, because the genetic code-reading machinery does not transcribe much of the human genome. Transcribed genes are not all translated into protein products. Nucleotide changes within coding regions may simply substitute one synonymous codon for another. Neutral substitutions lead to DNA polymorphisms, or alternative forms of DNA sequence. Such polymorphisms (which may subtly affect the function of the gene, such as the speed of its translation) are important for tracking down genes in families or populations. The term "mutation" implies that the change in nucleotide sequence leads to an alteration in gene product that affects the phenotype. Evidence for such change will depend on the sensitivity of the measures used to detect it. In complex disorders, such as psychiatric conditions, the phenotype results from the interaction of several polymorphisms, interacting epistatically. One such mutation may be necessary but not sufficient to produce a phenotype. Others may be neither necessary nor sufficient in their own right. The genotype at any given locus may affect the probability of disease, but does not fully determine the outcome. Environmental factors also have a crucial part to play, for example, influencing the timing of onset of the phenotype and its severity.

Mendelian Inheritance

The term Mendelian inheritance is used to describe conditions in which single mutant genes are inherited that have a major impact upon the phenotype. Homozygotes have mutant alleles at the same genetic locus, on each of the pair of chromosomes that was inherited, one from mother and one from father. Recessive conditions, in the clinical sense, are seen only in homozygotes. Heterozygotes have two different alleles at the same locus, one of which is mutant. If the mutation is associated with a phenotype, that phenotype is dominant. Even though Mendelian mechanisms are conceptually simple, phenotypic manifestations are variable and multisystemic, because mutations of single genes do not always occur in exactly the same place. We have an excellent model of this mechanism in the Mendelian recessive condition cystic fibrosis. Whereas there is one common genotypic abnormality, more than 1300 mutations have been described in the *CGTR* gene (Haston & Hudson, 2005). Other anomalies comprise not only single-nucleotide, but also large deletions within the gene. Even among patients who are homozygous for the most common ΔF508 mutation, there is a wide variation in phenotype (e.g., in terms of pulmonary function), and now genetic modifiers are being discovered too (Drumm, Konstan, Schluchter *et al.*, 2005). The degree to which the varying aspects of the phenotype manifest in affected individuals will depend crucially on the rest of their genetic make-up, as well as upon environmental influences. Currently, we know little about the role of genetic modifiers (elsewhere in the genome) in any disease, let alone psychiatric disorders, but they may directly influence the metabolic and cellular pathways involved in the primary pathophysiology of a susceptibility gene (Haston & Hudson, 2005) or they may act in secondary pathways that have a role

Rutter's Child and Adolescent Psychiatry, 5th edition. Edited by M. Rutter, D. Bishop, D. Pine, S. Scott, J. Stevenson, E. Taylor and A. Thapar. © 2008 Blackwell Publishing, ISBN: 978-1-4051-4549-7.

in influencing the course of the disorder, especially one that is neurodevelopmental in origin.

Chromosomal Anomalies

Some behavioral phenotypes are brought about by abnormalities in chromosomal structure or in the total complement of material. The expression of several or even many genes is affected. Chromosomal abnormalities can be numerical or structural. *Numerical* abnormalities are associated with either the loss of one of a pair of chromosomes, or with the aberrant formation of more than one copy of a chromosome (as in trisomy 21, 45,X or 47,XXY). *Structural* anomalies are more subtle, and usually involve microdeletions of a few thousand nucleotide bases, or more rarely the loss of a substantial part of a chromosome. Such anomalies may occur during the formation of the sperm or egg, during formation of the zygote at the time the egg and sperm fuse, or after cell division begins in early embryonic development. In the former situation, the abnormality is going to be represented in every somatic cell. If the structural problem occurred later, in just a proportion of developing cells, the individual will be a mosaic for the abnormality. Some cells will show it and others will not. The distribution of the affected cells will be clonal, reflecting the original population of normal or abnormal cells from which they were derived. We should not expect the distribution of those clones to be random. It depends on whether the abnormal cells in question are able to function sufficiently adequately to contribute to the development of the particular tissue. If they are not capable of functioning to a certain minimal degree of efficiency, they could be selected against as the tissue develops over time, and would not then be represented.

Structural Chromosomal Anomalies

Small deleted regions, known as microdeletions, comprise just a few megabases (Mb) of DNA, affecting maybe 20 or 30 genes. Examples include 22q11.2 deletion syndrome, Smith–Magenis syndrome and Williams syndrome. Many genes, but not all, are required in two complete copies for normal function. If one copy is missing, there will be haploinsufficiency (insufficiency because the gene is haploid rather than diploid) for that gene product. In the past couple of years, submicroscopic deletions and other rearrangements of large chunks of DNA have been described. These are known collectively as structural variations, and include deletions of DNA (which may occur within a gene), insertions of DNA sequences, inversions and multiple copies of genomic DNA (Redon, Ishikawa, Fitch *et al.*, 2006). Major aberrations in the gene sequences of people who otherwise seem healthy had not been expected, but now we know that each of us is likely to have some such variants in our genome. Their significance is still being determined, and clinical significance may be linked to whether they are inherited or whether they occur *de novo*. Those that are inherited are more likely to be benign. There is hope that structural variation may shed new light on complex diseases, such as neurodevelopmental psychiatric disorders in which the phenotype is caused by the interaction of many different genes, such as autism (Check, 2005).

Epigenetic Mechanisms

The study of epigenetics is relatively recent, and encompasses processes such as methylation or chromatin remodeling which leads to the silencing of genes, on one or other copy, early in development. While strictly speaking heritable, because such modifications occur during the formation of eggs or sperm, they do not change the structure of DNA and can be undone in the germ cells of the next generation. However, we have recently seen evidence that such epigenetically mediated changes in the phenotype could potentially be stable over many generations (Richards, 2006). Concerns have recently been expressed that epigenetic mechanisms could have a role in the disruption of patterns of DNA methylation in the embryo, which may lead to developmental alteration in the offspring with persistent changes in the germ-line (Crews & McLachlan, 2006).

Some hormonally active chemicals can have devastating effects on subsequent generations. For example, treatment with diethylstilbestrol (DES) during pregnancy results in vaginal cancer in the female offspring of humans, and mice. In mice, when mated to control males, female offspring who were not themselves exposed produce females who themselves develop the same rare cancer. There are equivalent transgenerational effects upon males, which have been described in rats treated with certain pesticides. The chemicals responsible for these plausibly epigenetically transmitted changes seem to act by mimicking or blocking endogenous hormones. They behave as biological signals that are misinterpreted by the organism. To date, most affect estrogen activity (and are misinterpreted by the organism as endogenous estrogens), hence they influence sexual reproduction directly or indirectly.

Crews and McLachlan (2006) suggested that the significant gender differences in relative risk of many psychiatric disorders (e.g., ADHD, autism, eating disorders) could imply that phenotypic manifestations are modulated by sex steroids (hormones). Endocrine disruptors could therefore indirectly influence manifestations of psychiatric disease, through this mechanism or even through an influence on maternal care. The work of Szyf, Weaver, Champagne *et al.* (2005) has shown that the quality of maternal care provided during the early postnatal period (by rats) is influenced by the stress that the mother was exposed to during her pregnancy. Furthermore, the quality of care she provides has an epigenetic effect on specific genes, concerned with neuronal growth in the hippocampus of her offspring. Many genes are potentially regulated by maternal care, and they can influence the behavior of that offspring in adulthood (Weaver, Meaney, & Szyf, 2006). Because the genomic changes are epigenetic, they are also potentially reversible. To date, psychiatrists have not often discussed epigenetic influences on the risk of mental illness, but this is likely to change quite soon as evidence accumulates in human as well as animal models implying specific mechanisms of dysfunction (Persico & Bourgeron, 2006; Rutter, Moffit, & Caspi, 2006).

Imprinted Genes

A small proportion of genes are systematically different in activity, depending on whether they have been inherited from mother or from father. This phenomenon is known as genomic imprinting. There is expression of the gene in question from only one of the pair of alleles. Imprinting may only be detected in certain tissues, or at certain periods of development. There is no alteration in the underlying DNA sequence. The existence of imprinted genes in a region may be revealed when the only active copy is mutated and ceases to function, or is lost because of a structural abnormality of the chromosome containing it. Occasionally, the chromosome, or a region of the chromosome bearing the gene, undergoes uniparental disomy. Both copies of the gene (and part of the surrounding genome) are inherited from just one parent.

In general, the clinical phenotypes that result from abnormalities involving imprinted loci tend to be severe. To date, most imprinted genes have been described on the autosomes but Skuse, James, Bishop *et al.* (1997) proposed that imprinting of genes on the X chromosome could be associated with sexually dimorphic characteristics. Although we have yet to demonstrate the mechanism in humans, there is now evidence for imprinting on the mouse X chromosome having an impact upon a sexually dimorphic behavioral characteristic – anxiety in a novel and potentially threatening situation, which affects males to a greater degree than females (Davies, Isles, Smith *et al.*, 2005).

Trinucleotide Expansion Repeats and Anticipation

Some dominant conditions result in phenotypes that become more severe in successive generations. A mechanism associated with this phenomenon is known as "anticipation," and is exemplified by the Fragile X syndrome and by Huntington disease. Trinucleotide repeat expansions have been proposed as the biological basis of this phenomenon (Pearson, Edamura, & Cleary, 2005). Trinucleotide repeats are triplets of nucleotides, and those associated with anticipation usually comprise some combination of cytosine, guanine and arginine. These are designated CGG, CAG and so on. The repeats may occur within genes, or they may be found in regions of DNA that lie between genes. If they lie actually within genes they may be in transcribed sequences (exons), or within DNA sequences that are excised by the RNA-making machinery (introns). Expansions occur in the course of DNA replication. The repeats grow in length as they are passed from one generation to the next, and indicate germ-line instability. Paternal and maternal expansions could be driven by processes that are specific to sperm or eggs, but we do not know for certain why they occur. For reasons that we do not understand, there are proportionately more neurological than other diseases caused by expansion of CTG, CGG, CAG or GAA repeats. The conditions caused by the expansion are associated with considerable phenotypic heterogeneity, for there is variability in the length of the repeat sequences, and in the degree to which they disrupt transcription and function of the genes with which they are associated. Conditions associated with this phenomenon that have a characteristic cognitive or behavioral phenotype include Fragile X syndrome and Huntington disease.

Fragile X syndrome is caused by disruption to the *FMR1* gene on the X chromosome; within an untranslated region of the gene the fragile site normally has between 6 and 53 copies of CGG but in people with the disorder there are over 230 copies. Expansion of the repeated sequence only occurs when the unstable gene is transmitted by a female (Van Esch, 2006).

The distribution of CAG repeats in the coding region of the Huntington disease gene may be divided into four categories (Myers, 2004). Repeats of 26 or fewer are normal. Repeats between 27 and 35 are rare and are not associated with the expression of the disease, but occasionally fathers with repeats in this range will transmit a repeat to descendants that is expanded to the range for expression of the illness. Repeats between 36 and 39 are associated with reduced penetrance, and some affected individuals will develop the disease but others will not. Repeats of 40 or larger are associated with the phenotypic expression of Huntington disease eventually, although this may be late in adulthood.

Eight of the trinucleotide repeat disorders have the same repeated triplet, CAG, which codes for the amino acid glutamine. Consequently, they are commonly referred to as polyglutamine diseases (e.g., Huntington disease). Another six disorders do not have similar repeats and are classified as non-polyglutamine diseases (e.g., Fragile X syndrome). Polyglutamine (PolyQ) diseases are characterized by a progressive degeneration of nerve cells usually affecting people later in life. Although these diseases share the same repeated codon (CAG) and some symptoms, the repeats for the different polyglutamine diseases occur on different chromosomes. The non-polyglutamine diseases do not share any specific symptoms.

Behavioral Phenotypes Associated with Single-Gene Mutations

Duchenne Muscular Dystrophy

This X-linked recessive condition, the most common neuromuscular disease of childhood, occurs in about 1 in 3500 male births. There is an inexorable course, with proximal muscle weakness increasing through early adulthood, and death usually occurring before the third decade from chronic respiratory insufficiency.

The myopathy manifests fully only in boys. It results from microdeletions (60%), duplications (10%) or point mutations within the *DMD* gene (Xp21.2), which is the largest in the human genome (>2.0 Mb), and produces the protein dystrophin. A specific isoform of dystrophin is expressed in the brain. Becker muscular dystrophy is a milder form with the same underlying etiology, but with a much better prognosis.

The condition is associated with a mild to moderate degree of intellectual disability, affecting verbal skills in particular. Mean IQ is 80 and about one-third of children have IQs below 70. Behavioral characteristics include limited social skills, depression and a remarkably high incidence of autistic behaviors (social and communication deficits) in one-third or more of individuals (Hinton & Goldstein, 2007). There is a limited verbal working memory (Hinton, De Vivo, Nereo *et al.*, 2001). The intellectual deficits are non-progressive and may even improve over time.

There is no simple correlation between the size or location of the deletion and the severity or prognosis of the muscular disorder (Prior & Bridgeman, 2005); however, mutations located at the 5′ end of the gene are not generally associated with intellectual disability. Inherited cases are invariably associated with maternal carrier status. No study has yet investigated the association with a behavioral–cognitive phenotype in mothers of probands, which would be influenced by random X inactivation. Dystrophin could play an important part in the function of $GABA_A$ receptors, especially in cerebral cortex, hippocampus and cerebellum (Muntoni, Torelli, & Ferlini, 2003).

Tuberous Sclerosis

Tuberous sclerosis (incidence 1 in 6000 neonates) is both genetically and phenotypically heterogenous (de Vries, Humphrey, McCartney *et al.*, 2005). Males and females are equally affected; the heritable form is autosomal dominant. There are structural neural abnormalities including cortical tubers, cortical dysphasia, subcortical heterotopias, white matter abnormalities, subependymal nodules and subependymal giant cell astrocytomas (Zaroff & Isaacs, 2005). Affected systems include renal, cardiac, pulmonary and dermatological, as well as the brain. The brain lesions develop in early fetal life. The syndrome has considerable phenotypic heterogeneity, probably partly because of the seemingly random distribution of the areas of abnormal cell proliferation; even monozygotic twins can have quite different phenotypes. Symptoms may take years to become apparent, and the condition often goes unrecognized or misdiagnosed.

Inheritance is autosomal dominant, but two-thirds of cases arise from a spontaneous *de novo* mutation. Either of two genes is responsible, both of which encode tumor suppressors: *TSC1* on chromosome 9 (9q34) and *TSC2* on chromosome 16 (16p13). Their protein products are hamartin and tuberin, respectively: intracellularly they form a dimer that prevents uncontrolled cellular proliferation, so if either one is dysfunctional there is a danger of tuber formation, and both genetic mutations are sufficient to produce the syndrome.

Epileptic seizures usually presage other problems, typically infantile spasms. Fewer than 50% of affected individuals have an intellectual disability, but there is probably a bimodal distribution of ability because nearly one-third have severe to profound deficits. Risk factors include the number, size and location of tubers and the type and age of onset of epilepsy, especially uncontrolled infantile spasms.

Cognitive deficits include dyspraxia, speech delay, dyscalculia and visuomotor disturbance. In childhood, behavioral complications include temper tantrums, aggression and attention deficit/hyperactivity disorder (ADHD; 50%). In adulthood, there is an increased incidence of emotional lability, including anxiety (60%) and depression (15–20%). Specific impairments in executive function skills, such as attention switching and planning, are particularly handicapping in adult life.

There is an association between tuberous sclerosis and pervasive developmental disorders (Bolton, Park, Higgins *et al.*, 2002). *TSC2* mutations are more likely to be associated with autism spectrum conditions. The risk of clinically significant autistic features is up to 50%, being highest if there is associated intellectual disability, early onset epilepsy and bilateral tubers of the temporal lobes. Chronic uncontrolled epileptiform activity may interfere with the normal development of social reciprocal functions.

Poor attention skills occur in up to 90%, with impaired vigilance, sustained attention, selective attention and response inhibition, even in those whose cognitive abilities are within the normal range. Their severity is correlated with the pattern of tuberous anomalies in the frontal, parietal and subcortical regions of the brain.

Behavioral and cognitive characteristics of tuberous sclerosis do progress. Educational difficulties are more pronounced as children move into secondary school, and demands on attention and other executive skills such as planning and organization become more complex and sustained. Emotional disorders can arise in adolescence, because of increasing self-awareness and the impact of subtle deficits in social reciprocity skills, reflected in limited or maladaptive peer relationships.

Fragile X Syndrome

Fragile X syndrome is the most common cause of inherited intellectual disability, affecting 1 in 4000 males (Pembrey, Barnicoat, Carmichael *et al.*, 2001). A partial phenotype is seen in females, with a prevalence of 1 in 8000. Most mothers of boys with the syndrome have no knowledge of their potential risk for delivering an affected child, and have not been investigated for behavioral anomalies or cognitive deficits. Affected males have fairly distinctive physical features and behavioral characteristics. The most striking deficit is moderate to severe intellectual impairment, with most having IQs under 50.

Fragile X syndrome is caused by the deficiency or absence of the fragile X mental retardation protein 1 (FMR1). In well over 99% of cases, the molecular defect is an expansion of cytosine–guanine–guanine (CGG) repeats in the 5′ untranslated region of the *FMR1* gene, which lies on the long arm of the X chromosome at Xq27.3. Large expansions in this region, known as *full* mutations (more than 200 repeats), inhibit transcription and lead to silencing of the gene (Musci & Caughey, 2005).

Fragile X syndrome is associated with a complex pattern of cognitive disabilities. Despite global intellectual disability, skills that require face and emotion processing, and theory of mind, may be spared (Cornish, Turk, Wilding *et al.*, 2004). There is poor sequential on-line processing, short-term visuospatial memory deficits, impaired motor planning and a repetitive impulsive style of interaction. A characteristic form of repetitive and impulsive speech is found, together with an autistic style of conversation, including concrete understanding and use of language, and turn-taking difficulties. Inattentiveness, restlessness and fidgetiness are more severe than in equivalent intellectual level. Psychiatric problems include anxiety, mood lability, social communication problems and selective mutism (Hagerman, Ono, & Hagerman, 2005).

The association between Fragile X syndrome and autism has intrigued researchers and clinicians for many years. Social anxiety and withdrawal, hyperarousal, peer relationship problems, stereotypic behaviors, gaze aversion and other anomalies of social reciprocity as well as language of an autistic type are found (Hessl, Glaser, Dyer-Friedman *et al.*, 2006). Increased risk could be associated with the premutation as well as the full mutation (Hagerman, Ono, & Hagerman, 2005). It is rare to find the mutation among autistic children of normal range IQ. Just over 2% of autistic children overall will have the *FMR1* full mutation (Reddy, 2005).

Rett Syndrome

Rett syndrome is a progressive neurodevelopmental X-linked disorder, occurring in 1 in 10,000–15,000 female neonates. Affected boys usually die soon after birth. Although devastating in its consequences upon normal development, the progression of the disease is variable. Progressive hypotonia, loss of speech and diminished eye contact occur, together with some autistic symptoms. Intellectual disability is almost invariable, together with seizures. Other features, thought to be peculiar to this syndrome, include compulsive hand movements that simulate wringing or washing, and hyperventilation. Following a period of early regression, affected girls may remain in a state where no further deterioration takes place for many years, so affected women can live at least to middle age.

The condition is caused by a mutation in the gene that encodes methyl-CpG-binding protein 2 (*MECP2*), which has widespread actions within the central nervous system; it lies at Xq28. *MECP2* is required for the formation or maintenance of mature neurons and dendrites, and may have a critical role in the development of the monoaminergic system (Segawa & Nomura, 2005). It binds to other genes that play a critical part in brain development such as *BDNF*. Mutations may lead to erroneous amino acid production (hence an abnormal protein) or to premature truncation of the protein product. There are many different mutations (over 200 have been described), and variants may be sporadic or inherited. Despite having the classic features of the syndrome, up to one-quarter of clinical cases do not seem to have any mutation in *MECP2*, suggesting another gene may also be involved.

There are several stages in the development of the disorder. The earliest occurs 6–18 months after birth, and is associated with a general slowing of developmental progress. There is less eye contact, and diminished interest in the environment. Gross motor skills are delayed. After a few months there is rapid regression. The second phase, which comes on between 1 and 4 years typically, is associated with loss of spoken language and attempts to communicate, hand-wringing, together with other compulsive movements including clapping or tapping, and moving the hands back and forth to the mouth. Periods of hyperventilation and apnea disappear during sleep. In the third stage there is no further deterioration. Some autistic features can develop during the second stage, including indifference to people and poor eye contact (Mount, Hastings, Reilly *et al.*, 2001) to a degree that is greater than in comparably profoundly retarded girls (Charman, Neilson, Mash *et al.*, 2005). Finally, motor deterioration occurs, characterized by muscle weakness, scoliosis and loss of previously acquired skills such as walking, but no further cognitive deterioration. Sudden death can occur due to cardiac arrhythmias.

Attempts to find mutations within the *MECP2* gene that could predispose to autism among males have not been productive. Few autistic girls have the mutation. Despite the theoretical implication that this X-inactivated gene's pattern of inactivation in females will correlate with the phenotype, there is no clear evidence, although patterns of X inactivation in human brain cannot be determined *in vivo* (Weaving, Williamson, Bennetts *et al.*, 2003). Some argue that in Rett syndrome and autism there are similar neuropathological changes, with a decrease in neuronal size and increased neuronal packing, together with a reduction in the arborization of dendrites (Segawa & Nomura, 2005; Shibayama, Cook, Feng *et al.*, 2004). Both Rett syndrome and some cases of autism show abnormalities of the sleep–wake cycle, suggesting a possible common underlying pathology, involving abnormalities of brainstem aminergic neurons.

Microdeletion and Duplication Syndromes

Williams Syndrome

Williams syndrome (also known as Williams–Beuren syndrome) is a rare sporadic disorder with an incidence of about 1 in 7500 live births (Stromme, Bjornstad, & Ramstad, 2002). It is associated with a distinctive cognitive and behavioral profile, a superficial facility with language, sociability, good facial recognition and very poor visuospatial skills.

In over 90% of clinically diagnosed cases, there is a submicroscopic deletion on the long arm of chromosome 7 at 7q11.2 (Bayes, Magano, Rivera *et al.*, 2003). This microdeletion contains several genes of possible relevance to the phenotype including:

1 Elastin (*ELN*), responsible for connective tissue problems including cardiac anomalies;

2 Lim kinase 1 (*LIMK1*), expressed in the brain, and linked to the visuospatial deficits of the syndrome by several authors (Hoogenraad, Akhmanova, Galjart *et al.*, 2004);

3 General transcription factor II (*GTF2I*), linked to the intellectual disability associated with Williams syndrome;

4 Syntaxin1A (*STX1A*), a transcription factor involved in neurotransmitter release;

5 Bromodomain adjacent to leucine zipper 1B (*BAZ1B*), which may have metabolic influences;

6 Cytoplamic linker 2 (*CYLN2*), which is strongly expressed in the brain, and may be associated with cerebellar abnormalities (Hoogenraad *et al.*, 2004);

7 Another transcription factor (*GTF2IRD1*), which is implicated in the craniofacial and visuospatial anomalies (Tassabehji, Hammond, Karmiloff-Smith *et al.*, 2005); and

8 Neutrophil cystolic factor 1 (*NCF1*), associated with hypertension.

Up to 20 genes may be deleted; the extent of the deletion is variable but the classic Williams syndrome phenotype is always associated with deletion of *ELN*, and usually *LIMK1*. Inversion of the segment of chromosome 7 occurs in about 7% of the general population, and in up to one-third of the parents of probands who transmitted the deleted chromosome 7.

Because of the considerable discrepancy between verbal and non-verbal abilities, the computation of an overall or Full Scale IQ is inappropriate (Meyer-Lindenberg, Mervis, & Faith, 2006). Verbal IQ averages about 70. Visuospatial skills are generally about 2.5 standard deviations below population norms. There is relatively preserved verbal short-term memory and verbal fluency, although it is qualitatively abnormal. Claims about the cognitive strengths of children with Williams syndrome (e.g., their innate musical ability) are based on massive ascertainment bias, a situation that applies equally to many other neurodevelopmental syndromes. Language acquisition in the syndrome is delayed, and the progression of language development may follow an unusual path (Scerif & Karmiloff-Smith, 2005). Grammatical abilities are consonant with verbal IQ. There is no unusual and sophisticated language as was once claimed. In general, pragmatic skills (language used for social communication) are weak.

The social interactions of children with the disease are not unimpaired; they are unusual and lack social reciprocity. Eye contact is sometimes good, and they possess empathic skills from infancy onwards. They are interested in faces – their technique for performing relatively well on tests of face recognition memory shows a cognitive style based on the sum of parts, rather than a gestalt of the face. The children are often uninhibited, and relate indiscriminately to unfamiliar children and adults, which may put them at social risk. They perform poorly on standard tests of attention. Tager-Flusberg and Sullivan (2000) describe poor social–cognitive skills including theory of mind, and an ability to interpret other people's facial expressions, especially negative facial expressions.

At this stage, there is no incontestable link between any single gene in the critical region and an aspect of the cognitive or behavioral phenotype. Some progress has been made by studying individuals who are lacking a smaller critical region than is usual (thereby apparently ruling out a few genes) and by the construction of animal models in which putative contributory genes have been knocked out. The greatest interest to date has focused on genes *LIMK1* and *GTF2IRD1*, together with *CYLN2*. All are thought to have some role in the visuoconstructional deficits associated with the syndrome. While there is no doubt that *ELN* has an important role in many features of the syndrome, the gene is not expressed in brain and therefore it is not a candidate for cognitive aspects of the phenotype.

Prader–Willi Syndrome

Prader–Willi syndrome is a distinctive disorder, associated with a genetic anomaly on the long arm of chromosome 15, in which hyperphagia, mild to moderate intellectual disability and obesity combine with a typical developmental history. In the great majority of cases there is no inherited predisposition, but a sporadic event leads to the failure to express the paternal copy of the critical region. The estimated prevalence is 1 in 10,000–25,000.

This disorder is associated with structural rearrangements of a critical region about 4 Mb DNA in length, on the long arm of chromosome 15, at 15q11.2–3. The anomalies include deletions, translocations, inversions and supernumerary marker chromosomes, as well as uniparental disomy. Approximately 70% of individuals with the syndrome have a deleted segment of the paternally inherited copy of the chromosome. The critical finding is that the paternally inherited region is absent, and the maternally inherited region is silent (imprinted). In about 25% of cases both copies of chromosome 15 are inherited from the mother.

The most characteristic behavioral feature is hyperphagia (80–90% of cases), with an onset at 2 years (always before 6 years). Food-seeking behavior, hoarding and foraging, pica and consequent obesity occur, associated with elevated levels of ghrelin, a hormone produced by P/D1 cells lining the fundus of the human stomach that stimulate appetite (Butler, Bittel, & Talebizadeh, 2004). Sweet foods are often preferred, small amounts may be used as a reward to shape behavior. Temper tantrums, impulsivity, mood fluctuations, stubbornness and aggression and a variety of other characteristics including skin picking, repetitive speech, obsessive and ritualistic behaviors are reported (Milner, Craig, Thompson *et al.*, 2005).

Children and adults with Prader–Willi syndrome are hypoactive and lethargic, in part because of co-ordination problems, resulting from hypotonia. Obesity following excessive eating will be increased by inactivity (Davies & Joughin, 1992; Nardella, Sulzbacher, & Worthington-Roberts, 1983). Sleep architecture studies show abnormalities too (Helbing-Zwanenburg, Kamphuisen, & Mourtazaev, 1993), with excessive day-time sleepiness. During the night, Prader–Willi syndrome is associated with limited rapid eye movement (REM) and slow wave sleep.

Average IQ is 60 and motor milestones are seriously delayed. Speech difficulties occur in around 80–90% (Cassidy, 1992). Deficits in attention, perceptual–motor integration are found, and sequential processing is weak. Just under half of children with Prader–Willi syndrome attend a mainstream elementary school, fewer attend a mainstream secondary school. There is no relationship between IQ and maladaptive behaviors.

There could be phenotypic differences according to the genetic anomaly, depending on whether chromosome 15 has been deleted, or both chromosomes are intact. Rare instances of point mutations in the imprinting center within the critical region might be different again. Patients with uniparental disomy could be less severely affected than those with deletions, with fewer facial characteristics, obsessive-compulsive symptoms and self-injurious behaviors, plus a higher verbal IQ. Hyperphagia is unaltered.

Within the past few years, interest has developed in the idea that 15q11 constitutes a region that could contain susceptibility genes for autistic disorders (Veenstra-Vanderweele & Cook, 2004). Duplications of the Prader–Willi syndrome critical region have been associated with autistic features of behavior, associated with presumed overexpression of maternally derived genes (Veltman, Craig, & Bolton, 2005). In deletion cases, there are two main classes described depending on the size of the deletion (Butler, Bittel, Kibiryeva *et al.*, 2004). In one variant there are four non-imprinted genes deleted, one of which (*NIPA1*) is widely expressed in the central nervous system. It is possible that those with the larger breakpoint have a more severe phenotype in terms of performance on multiple psychological and behavioral tests. Adaptive behavior and specific obsessive-compulsive behaviors are worse in those with larger deletions, as are reading, maths and visuomotor integration skills (Milner *et al.*, 2005).

There is uncertainty about which genes in the Prader–Willi syndrome critical region are associated with the greatest risk of cognitive or behavioral abnormalities. Some assistance has come from the development of animal models, showing, for instance, that the small nuclear ribonucleoprotein N (*SNRPN*) is a prime candidate. This is expressed from the paternally inherited chromosome only, and is functional in the brain as well as other tissues. Other imprinted genes in the region include *MKRB3*, *NDN* and *MAGEL2*. The only identified protein products are for the *SNRPN* and *MKRN3* genes, the latter being a zinc finger protein expressed from the paternal chromosome and presumably involved in transcriptional regulation.

Angelman Syndrome

Angelman syndrome is characterized by severe developmental delay, associated communication defects (little speech, nonverbal skills somewhat better) and gait ataxia (Williams, Beaudet, Clayton-Smith *et al.*, 2006). All have excitability, apparent happiness, laughter and smiling with hand flapping, or waving. Most have microcephaly by the age of 2 years, and seizures before 3 years of age. The electroencephalogram (EEG) is characteristic, and associated with seizures. The prevalence is 1 in 15,000 live births.

There are imprinting defects in the same critical region as Prader–Willi syndrome, involving genes that are maternally expressed. Most (70%) have a 4–6 Mb deletion at 15q11.2–3. Uniparental disomy for parental chromosomes is rare (7%). A specific imprinting defect accounts for about 3% of affected individuals; 10–20% are microdeletions and in the other 80–90% there is an epigenetic mutation. Unlike the complex genetic etiology of Prader–Willi syndrome, Angelman syndrome is known to be caused by failure of expression of the gene *UBE3A*, a maternally expressed gene that is paternally imprinted. Molecular genetic testing identifies *UBE3A* anomalies in about 90%. It is unknown why the other 10% of phenotypically classic cases have no detectable genetic anomaly.

Abnormal sleep–wake cycles and a diminished need for sleep are common, together with a strange attraction to water and a fascination with plastics and paper that crinkles. The smiling and laughing, which are so characteristic of the syndrome, are dependent on contextual cues, and Horsler and Oliver (2006) warn against the concluding behavioral phenotypes being determined by the underlying genetic anomaly independent of environmental and developmental considerations.

Severe developmental delay is the rule, and a ceiling for psychomotor development occurs at about 24–30 months (Thompson & Bolton, 2003). Very few individuals develop even the simplest language for social communication. Visual skills and a social style based on non-verbal rather than verbal interactions are strengths.

There are differences in phenotype depending on whether the condition is associated with deletion, an imprinting deficit or uniparental disomy. In general, those with the deletion have the most severe phenotype (Williams *et al.*, 2006).

Smith–Magenis Syndrome

Smith–Magenis syndrome is usually caused by (in 90% of cases) a microdeletion of the short arm of chromosome 17, at 17p11.2 (Potocki, Shaw, Stankiewicz *et al.*, 2003), including the retinoic acid-induced protein 1 (*RAI1*) gene, which is probably both necessary and sufficient to cause the condition. Larger deletions may be associated with the deletion of *PMP22*, which carries with it a risk of a neuropathy in addition to Smith–Magenis syndrome. Virtually all cases are *de novo*. Incidence is about 1 in 25,000 births. Mutation screening of the gene is not routinely available. The most prominent clinical features of the syndrome are a distinctive facies, short stature, an increased risk of a range of health problems involving cardiac, renal and ophthalmic systems, and cognitive impairments together with a range of severe maladaptive behaviors that persist throughout the lifespan (Madduri, Peters, Voigt *et al.*, 2006; Martin, Wolters, & Smith, 2006).

Infancy is characterized by feeding difficulties, failure to thrive, hypotonia, prolonged napping or need to awaken for feeds, and generalized lethargy. Significant sleep disturbance, stereotypies, and maladaptive and self-injurious behaviors are rarely apparent before 18 months of age. The sleep–wake cycle is inverted, associated with an inverted melatonin circadian rhythm and is a chronic lifelong problem. Individuals are awake at night and sleepy during the day. Whether this can be successfully treated with melatonin or beta-adrenergic blockers is as yet undetermined (Shelley & Robertson, 2005). Adaptive behavior skills are worse as children grow into adolescence (Martin, Wolters, & Smith, 2006). Social skills are relatively preserved; patients are friendly, sociable and outgoing.

Neurobehavioral features of the syndrome are amongst its most striking features. They are severe, and include hyperactivity, distractibility, temper tantrums and attention-seeking, impulsivity, disobedience, aggression and toileting difficulties. Amongst the most unusual and disturbing behaviors are inserting foreign objects into body orifices including ears, nose, rectum and vagina (polyemoilokomania, up to 50%); pulling out of finger nails and/or toenails (onchyotillomania, 15–30%);

stereotypic behavior including "spasmodic upper body squeeze" or "self-hug" evoked by happiness (60%), which seems to be specific to Smith–Magenis syndrome (Madduri *et al.*, 2006). Additional stereotypies include covering eyes or ears (~70%); mouthing objects; insertion of hand in mouth (~90%); teeth grinding (~90%); body rocking (~50%); spinning or twirling objects (~50%); self-injurious behavior (Martin, Wolters, & Smith, 2006; Shelley & Robertson, 2005); hand and wrist biting (up to 90%); head-banging, skin picking and slapping of self (>50%). Gross motor skills are impaired in about two-thirds of patients.

Cognitive and adaptive functioning do not vary much; the majority of individuals with Smith–Magenis syndrome function in the mild to moderate range of intellectual disability. Verbal and non-verbal IQ are consonant with one another, with a mean of about 50–55. Daily living skills are relatively severely impaired compared to communication and socialization skills.

The size of the deletion at 17p11.2 varies; the larger the deletion, the greater the intellectual impairment. Larger deletion size is also associated with poorer adaptive function skills in terms of day-to-day living. This suggests that the phenotype cannot wholly be caused by anomalies in the *RAI1* gene. There has been no study of individuals with a point mutation in the gene, compared with those who have a deletion. It is presumed, but has never been assessed systematically, that many of the severe behavioral problems associated with the syndrome are worse than might be expected, given the degree of intellectual disability.

Velocardiofacial Syndrome, 22q11.2 Deletion Syndrome

Velocardiofacial syndrome (VCFS; Shprintzen, Goldberg, Young *et al.*, 1981) is characterized by cardiac defects (~75%), cleft palate, intellectual impairment and a characteristic facial appearance, together with a genetic anomaly on chromosome 22 at 22q11.2. The incidence is estimated to be 1 in 3000–5000 live births. Most cases are sporadic but, when inherited, it has an autosomal dominant pattern of transmission. There is an increased risk of severe behavioral problems in children with the condition, and of major psychiatric illness in adulthood including mood disorders and psychosis (Murphy, 2002).

Up to 30% of adults with VCFS will develop a major psychiatric illness, the majority fulfilling diagnostic criteria for schizophrenia (Murphy, Jones, & Owen, 1999). The risk of mental health problems increases with age. ADHD and bipolar affective disorder are the most common diagnoses in childhood, but cognitive and behavioral phenotypes have been poorly described and are largely based on clinical observation rather than systematic assessment.

About four out of five patients with VCFS have a deletion at 22q11.2, with a proximal breakpoint that is similar in most cases (Weksberg, Stachon, Squire *et al.*, 2007). Usually, about 40 genes are affected by the most common deletions.

During infancy there are serious feeding difficulties, independent of cardiac or palatal complications, with motor dysfunction in the oropharynx. Difficulty swallowing and nasopharyngeal reflux can be severe. Gross motor skills are poor, walking is usually not achieved until around 18 months. In a minority, symptoms similar to those of ADHD persist into adulthood.

By adolescence, people with 22q11.2 deletion syndrome express diverse psychiatric symptoms, the most prevalent of which are mood disruptions, attention deficits and psychotic phenomena (Baker & Skuse, 2005). Social and occupational functioning are significantly impaired. Some symptoms (psychotic experiences and frequent angry outbursts) are not found in most equivalently retarded children. Within the syndrome, there is no relationship between psychopathology and IQ. The majority report schizotypal symptoms, correlating with poor social functioning and few interests, and greater functional impairment as the individuals approach early adulthood.

Schizophrenia is a late manifestation in around 30% of cases, on a par with the risk to offspring of two schizophrenic parents (Murphy, Jones, & Owen, 1999). People with schizophrenia have an 80-fold increased prevalence of the microdeletion relative to the general population (Karayiorgou, Morris, Morrow *et al.*, 1995). Individuals with schizophrenia and a 22q11.2 microdeletion are similar in age of onset, symptom profiles or medication responses (Bassett, Chow, AbdelMalik *et al.*, 2003). Linkage and association findings also suggest schizophrenia susceptibility loci at 22q (Harrison & Owen, 2003). Proportionately more young people with the syndrome describe psychotic symptoms than the 25–30% who are predicted to go on to develop a psychotic illness (Baker, Baldeweg, Sivagnanasundaram *et al.*, 2005), implying there is a continuum of psychotic disorder within the 22q11.2 deletion syndrome group from mild to severe, with no clear division between "affected" and "unaffected" categories.

The observed association in 22q11.2 deletion syndrome between older age and poorer functional adjustment reflects a process of intraindividual functional decline. Genetic high-risk studies have not as yet collected sufficiently fine-grained data in an adequate sample to observe such a decline in individuals who develop idiopathic adult-onset psychosis. However, recent clinical research aiming to facilitate early identification and preventive intervention for schizophrenia has identified high-risk groups of young people presenting to psychiatric services with prodromal symptoms. Recent reports from the largest such cohort indicate that, although attenuated psychotic symptoms are moderately predictive of risk of illness within a 12-month period, detection rates are greatly increased when measures of functional capacity and, crucially, recent functional decline are taken into account (Yung, Stanford, Cosgrave *et al.*, 2006).

Psychopathological decline may be mirroring a process of neuropsychological (IQ and memory) and anatomical (medial temporal lobe) deterioration in already at-risk individuals (Pantelis, Yucel, Wood *et al.*, 2003). Longitudinal follow-up of adolescents with 22q11.2 deletion syndrome will determine whether a similar trajectory characterizes the emergence of debilitating psychotic illness in syndromal cases. Several small randomized controlled trials have now been carried out within clinically high-risk samples, to determine whether it is possible to prevent or delay deterioration in idiopathic schizophrenia by pharmacological or psychotherapeutic intervention. Findings from these trials have been mixed so far, limited by small sample size and short follow-up periods, but ongoing development of detection criteria and treatment protocols may yield results of clinical benefit. We do not know whether such intervention would benefit children with 22q11.2 deletion syndrome. It is also worth noting that autistic symptoms have recently been reported in close association with the syndrome, an observation that appears to have been formerly overlooked (Vorstman, Morcus, Duijff *et al.*, 2006). Their clinical significance is at this juncture uncertain, and it is not known whether the subgroup with autistic spectrum disorders comprises the same children who are at risk of psychosis.

Intellectual impairment is usual, but not invariable. There is no significant difference between impairment of verbal and non-verbal skills in early childhood, but some verbal abilities become relatively poorer over time. Mean IQ is about 75. Standardized neuropsychological tests have identified a specific cognitive profile in 22q11.2 (Zinkstok & van Amelsvoort, 2005) with poor visuospatial memory (Simon, Bish, Bearden *et al.*, 2005; Woodin, Wang, Aleman *et al.*, 2001) and low arithmetic attainment (Swillen, Devriendt, Legius *et al.*, 1999). Deficits in executive function include poor cognitive flexibility (Woodin *et al.*, 2001) and attentional focus (Bish, Ferrante, Donald-McGinn *et al.*, 2005). By adulthood, verbal comprehension is about two standard deviations below the population mean, but vocabulary and the ability to detect verbal similarities are less severely affected, being on average about the 10th population centile. Non-verbal skills such as picture arrangement and block design are between the 5th and the 10th population centile. Executive function deficits, such as the Wisconsin Card Sort, are also moderately impaired (Chow, Watson, Young *et al.*, 2006).

Children with VCFS have speech and language problems secondary to the cleft palate abnormalities, so speech sounds are hypernasal. Language development is often delayed and impoverished in content, with poor expressive skills, immature grammar, poor syntax and low utterance length. Concept formation is very limited, confined to concrete operations. Sight reading ability may be markedly superior to reading comprehension skills.

At least 40 genes are encoded in the commonly deleted segment in 22q11.2, the region containing a locus that may have a role in idiopathic schizophrenia (Norton, Williams, & Owen, 2006). There are at least three genes of interest (Karayiorgou & Gogos, 2004): *PRODH*, *TBX1* and *COMT*. Paterlini, Zakharenko, Lai *et al.* (2005) have recently demonstrated epistatic interaction between the *PRODH* and *COMT* genes in mouse models, perhaps providing a basis for understanding the high risk of schizophrenia. Baker, Baldeweg, Sivagnanasundaram *et al.* (2005) proposed that allelic variants of the *COMT* gene in 22q11.2 could modulate performance on an evoked response potential task relevant to psychosis risk. The *COMT* gene contains a variant substitution of A for G at codon 108/158, which results in a triplet coding for either methionine (*met*) or valine (*val*). Baker, Baldeweg, Sivagnanasundaram *et al.* (2005) found that the *met* allele was associated with reduced fronto-temporal functional connectivity compared to *val*. In other studies, prepulse inhibition of the startle response was measured. Normally, we do not startle as much to a sudden loud noise if it is preceded by a softer noise within a critical time window, but response is abnormal in schizophrenia and schizotypal personality disorder (Braff, Geyer, Light *et al.*, 2001). In the mouse model of 22q11.2 deletion syndrome, the genes that are critically needed for a normal prepulse inhibition response are *TBX1* and *GNB1l* (Paylor, Glaser, Mupo *et al.*, 2006). There are a few identified human patients with *TBX1* mutations, and they may have behavioral phenotypes but their prepulse inhibition is not known. Mutations of *TBX1* are associated with some of the physical deficits of the syndrome in humans (Yagi, Furutani, Hamada *et al.*, 2003) as well as in mice.

Chromosomal Aneuploidies

Turner Syndrome

About 50% of clinically identified cases of Turner syndrome are associated with a single X chromosome (X monosomy), and affected females therefore have 45 rather than the usual 46 intact chromosomes (Jacobs, Dalton, James *et al.*, 1997). Most lose the paternal sex chromosome. In 50%, there is tissue mosaicism for a complex variation. The prevalence is 4 per 10,000 live female births, the most common chromosomal aneuploidy.

All affected females will be short relative to their parents in adulthood. They have only one copy of a gene (*SHOX*) that is important for normal growth in stature and is required in two working copies (Rao, Weiss, Fukami *et al.*, 1997). Turner syndrome is usually associated with degeneration of the ovaries soon after birth ("streak ovaries") so there are absent secondary sexual characteristics without estrogen replacement therapy. Verbal intelligence is normal, but there are associated deficits in non-verbal skills and in arithmetical abilities. Autistic traits, found in over 30%, are mainly in the domains of social reciprocity and communication.

In humans, partial or complete loss of one of the sex chromosomes, either the second X chromosome or the Y chromosome, results in the condition. It is associated with a phenotype because of two main influences. First, because there is insufficient dosage of genes that are normally expressed from both X chromosomes in females (Carrel & Willard, 2005). Second, hormonal factors secondary to degeneration of the ovaries leads to estrogen insufficiency. Genetic influences are probably the more important for cognitive and some aspects of social development.

Because males invariably inherit their single X chromosome from their mother, X-linked imprinted genes could theoretically have sexually dimorphic expression. Expression exclusively from the paternally inherited X chromosome can only occur in females (Skuse *et al.*, 1997). Recent work with a mouse model of the syndrome has identified a paternally imprinted maternally expressed gene as having a circumscribed impact on a cognitive–behavioral phenotype (Davies, Isles, Smith *et al.*, 2005), but no human equivalent has been found.

Adolescence is a time of difficulty for a number of different reasons: short stature, sexual immaturity and specific deficits in social cognitive competence. As adults, many women experience difficulties with social and partner relationships, and cannot fit into a normal work environment with adults. Consequently, many choose to work primarily with children and a disproportionate number find employment as nursery nurses. Social deficits are more severe among those who inherited their single X chromosome from their mother (Skuse *et al.*, 1997).

Deficits in non-verbal IQ are typical, affecting 80%, and typified by poor ability to copy or recognize complex designs, visuospatial memory defects, and impaired motor task skills that are linked to visuospatial demands (Bishop, Canning, Elgar *et al.*, 2000).

Deficits in socioperceptual processing are usual, affecting memory for faces, facial expressions of emotion (Lawrence, Kuntsi, Coleman *et al.*, 2003b) and interpretation of direction of gaze (Elgar, Campbell, & Skuse, 2002). The risk of autism is increased at least 500-fold (Creswell & Skuse, 1999). "Theory of mind" skills are poor (Baron-Cohen, Wheel-wright, Hill *et al.*, 2001; Lawrence *et al.*, 2003b) to a degree that is *more* severe than in people with autism. A relatively specific deficit in recognizing "fear" from faces is as profound in women with Turner syndrome as in high functioning people with autism (Lawrence, Campbell, Swettenham *et al.*, 2003a; Lawrence *et al.*, 2003b). These claims of relative difference must, however, be taken as indicative rather than authoritative, because the tasks are sensitive to verbal and non-verbal intelligence, and show age-related differences (Campbell, Lawrence, Mandy *et al.*, 2006).

Many phenotypic features of Turner syndrome are caused by insufficient dosage for a gene, or several genes, that are expressed from both X chromosomes in normal females (i.e., are not subject to X inactivation; Skuse, 2006). With the publication of the genetic sequence of the X chromosome (Ross, Grafham, Coffey *et al.*, 2005) it has become possible to map susceptibility genes more accurately. Using the technique of deletion-mapping, which localized the only "Turner" gene identified to date (*SHOX*), we searched for a gene that influences social cognitive competence (Good, Lawrence, Thomas *et al.*, 2003). We discovered that *EFHC2*, a brain-expressed gene important for the modulation of calcium-related neurotransmission mechanisms, is probably responsible for some of the social–cognitive deficits associated with the syndrome (Weiss, Purcell, Waggoner *et al.*, 2007).

Klinefelter Syndrome (XXY Syndrome)

Klinefelter syndrome is a sex chromosome aneuploidy of males, occurring with remarkable frequency, perhaps as many as 1 in 500 male live births. It is associated with an additional X chromosome, which can be either maternal or paternal in origin (each is equally common). The physical phenotype is often not apparent until after puberty, and it is very variable. Tall stature is usual, with long limbs. Testis development is characteristically inadequate, and the majority of affected men are infertile. If the condition is not picked up in childhood, it may go unnoticed until adulthood, when it is revealed by investigations of infertility. However, the majority of cases are never identified clinically (Lanfranco, Kamischke, Zitzmann *et al.*, 2004).

There is considerable variability in the cognitive and behavioral phenotype, but this is not because of tissue mosaicism, which is very unusual in Klinefelter syndrome. There is no clear relationship with parental age. The behavioral phenotype of Klinefelter syndrome may be associated with an increased risk of schizophrenia or affective disorder with psychotic features (Bojesen, Juul, Birkebaek *et al.*, 2006; Delisi, 2005). There is autistic-like behavior in a proportion of 47,XXY males, who find social interactions difficult and who are introverted, anxious, impulsive, quiet, unassertive and socially withdrawn (Geschwind, Boone, Miller *et al.*, 2000). Socially inappropriate and antisocial behaviors were once thought to characterize the syndrome, but this is probably because of an ascertainment bias (Bojesen, Juul, & Gravholt, 2003).

There are often poor verbal skills, particularly those used for reading and language comprehension (Bender, Linden, & Harmon, 2001; Delisi, Maurizio, Svetina *et al.*, 2005). Verbal working memory is impaired (Fales, Knowlton, Holyoak *et al.*, 2003) but non-verbal abilities tend to be unaffected.

As with Turner syndrome, where for years the social problems associated with the syndrome were attributed entirely to short stature and sexual immaturity, social difficulties in Klinefelter syndrome may also arise from deficits in social cognitive processing. Social cognitive deficits probably contribute to some of the behavioral characteristics of the syndrome (van Rijn, Swaab, Aleman *et al.*, 2006). These include disturbances in perception, experience and expression of social cognitive information, executive functions, including response inhibition, but spared concept formation, problem-solving, task-switching and speeded response (Temple & Sanfilippo, 2003). Affected men may have increased emotional arousal in response to emotion-inducing events, they are excessively influenced by their emotions in strategic decision-making and they also find it difficult to perceive their own emotions, a state of mind reminiscent of alexythymia.

The parental origin of the additional X chromosome in Klinefelter syndrome has no obvious effect, but an additional paternal X chromosome might be associated with more impairments of fine and gross motor skills, and speech and language problems (Stemkens, Roza, Verrij *et al.*, 2006). This finding is consistent with the Skuse, James, Bishop *et al.* (1997) hypothesis concerning X-linked imprinting because males would never normally inherit a paternal X chromosome; the implication is that by so doing one would expect a more severe phenotype. Lopes, Ross, Close *et al.* (2006) have suggested that the non-imprinted gene *PCDH11X* could be a candidate for other symptoms. It has a homolog on the Y chromosome and is strongly expressed in the brain. Because current indications suggest it is likely to escape X inactivation (Ross, Wadekar, Lopes *et al.*, 2006), the gene could be overexpressed in men with the syndrome.

Another contributory influence on the physical, but not necessarily the cognitive or behavioral phenotype, is the X-linked androgen receptor gene. This carries a nucleotide repeat polymorphism, the length of which is inversely associated with the somatic influence of androgens. XXY men with longer repeats within the gene on their active X chromosome have more feminizing traits, such as gynecomastia. Shorter repeats are associated with masculine traits such as greater adult penile length (Zinn, Ramos, Elder *et al.*, 2005).

XYY syndrome

XYY syndrome is a sex chromosome aneuploidy of males, occurring in up to 1 in 1000 male live births (Ratcliffe, 1994). It is associated with an additional Y chromosome, which is invariably paternal in origin. The aneuploidy is not selected against before birth, presumably because the Y chromosome contains relatively few expressed genes (Robinson & Jacobs, 1999). Most boys with XYY syndrome are never diagnosed (Abramsky & Chapple, 1997). The physical phenotype is apparent before puberty, because of increased linear growth from around 2 years of age. Tall stature is usual, with a final height of nearly 190 cm, which is above the 95th male adult centile according to current norms (Ogden, Kuczmarski, Flegal *et al.*, 2002). Testicular development is normal, and the majority of affected men are believed to be fertile. Apart from the excessively tall stature, and a possible associated acneiform disorder, there are no characteristic physical features.

There are occasional males who have XYY syndrome with mosaicism for a normal XY cell-line, and in them the physical phenotype is less marked. There is no greater risk of men, with either variant of the syndrome, producing children who have chromosomal anomalies. The various mechanisms by which the extra Y chromosome can be generated are discussed in Robinson and Jacobs (1999).

The behavioral phenotype of XYY syndrome was once thought to be strongly associated with criminality, resulting from observations at the time it was first discovered in the mid-1960s that suggested that an excessive proportion of affected males could be found in prison. Although early reports suggested males with the syndrome were more likely to commit criminal acts against people, there were concerns about ascertainment bias. A follow-up of an unbiased population sample (Gotz, Johnstone, & Ratcliffe, 1999) found a small but significant increase in the overall rate of offences, when compared with controls who had a similar number of years at risk. The causal mechanism could not be ascertained with any certainty, but one possible contributory factor was IQ, which tended to be lower in the XYY than in males from the general population. Interestingly, this group of investigators has reported a consistently higher social class distribution among XYY males' families of origin than would be expected by chance, indicating that family background is biased against the emergence of criminal behavior. Pooled analysis of three population-based studies (Rutter, Giller, & Hagell, 1998) yielded a much larger unbiased sample and this showed a substantial increase in antisocial behavior (37.5% versus 13.0%) that could not simply be accounted for by lower IQ. In summary, there does appear to be an enhanced risk of antisocial personality traits, coupled with increased antisocial behavior, especially during adolescence.

Autistic-like symptoms have been observed in a proportion of 47,XYY males, but this association has not been investigated in any detail, and may simply be a coincidence (Geerts, Steyaert, & Fryns, 2003; Nicolson, Bhalerao, & Sloman, 1998).

Cognitive abilities of males with XYY syndrome are within the normal range, but may be overall about one standard deviation below expected values in terms of both verbal and performance skills (Ratcliffe, 1999). There are reports of delayed onset of language, which may affect up to half (Geerts, Steyaert, & Fryns, 2003; Ratcliffe, 1999). Many have difficulty learning to read, to a degree that is disproportionate with their verbal intelligence, although they do not have comparable difficulties in numerical and arithmetical attainments.

Males with XYY syndrome are likely to be relatively clumsy, with especially poor fine motor skills. Few studies have looked at brain development by means of neuroimaging, but if there is any impact on structural features it must be subtle; to date, none has been reported. There is no evidence of anomalies that are equivalent in magnitude to those found among individuals with aneuploidies of the X chromosome. There is no increased risk of specific psychiatric disorders in childhood or adulthood, apart from a possible influence upon a combined schizophreniform–bipolar phenotype. However, psychiatric difficulties in general may be more common among both children with the disorder (who are reported to be more disruptive at school) and in adults (who are more likely to face marital breakdown, although not unemployment; Ratcliffe, 1999).

Down syndrome

The phenotype of Down syndrome (or trisomy 21 syndrome as some would prefer) is caused by a triple copy of the genes on chromosome 21, hence overexpression of genes that are normally tightly regulated. About 130 are expressed in the brain. As this chromosome was the first to be sequenced, it was hoped that genes that are primarily responsible for the phenotypic manifestations of the syndrome would soon be identified. Unfortunately, this has not proved to be the case (Gardiner, Davisson, Pritchard *et al.*, 2005; Patterson & Costa, 2005; Roubertoux & Kerdelhue, 2006).

The most striking features of Down syndrome include intellectual impairment. All individuals with the condition have a low IQ, although there is great interindividual variability. In a very small proportion of cases, not more than 2–3%, there is mosaicism for a normal cell-line; such children are likely to be less severely affected. Developmental delay from the outset is the rule, with late acquisition of motor skills – some children do not walk until 6 years of age. However, the pattern of motor skill acquisition is normal. Intellectual abilities are low, with an average IQ of about 45 and progressive deterioration with age, between early childhood and late adolescence (Vicari, 2006). In adults with the condition there is an increased risk of early onset dementia, which has many features of Alzheimer disease. The ability of children with Down syndrome to use language is very poor, and may be compounded by the hearing loss found in up to 80%. Comprehension of language is rather better, but it has been argued that linguistic skills in the condition follow an abnormal trajectory rather than simply being developmentally retarded. There may be preserved islets of ability (e.g., in terms of spatial processing), although visual perceptual skills are poor (Vicari, 2006).

The behavioral profile of children with Down syndrome varies with age – there is a degree of developmental progression (Capone, Goyal, Ares *et al.*, 2006). During the preschool period, children may have sensory sensitivities (e.g., to sounds), which are associated with anxiety. In most other respects their behavior is unremarkable, but they show little interest in peers and play is rudimentary. By the time they reach school-age, hyperactivity and impulsivity are marked and can lead to management problems, especially if combined with oppositional and defiant behaviors. In recent years, it has become clearer that a substantial proportion of children with the syndrome have an autistic profile, including regression in cognitive, language and social skills (Capone, Goyal, Ares *et al.*, 2006). The associated autistic symptoms include abnormalities in social reciprocity and interest in people, social withdrawal and stereotyped repetitive behaviors with sensory sensitivities. Adolescents and adults are at risk of emotional disorders, including depression and obsessive-compulsive behavior. Occasionally, very severe depressive symptoms are associated with psychotic phenomena.

There has been little progress made in understanding the relationship between abnormal gene expression in the region of trisomy on chromosome 21 and the human characteristics of Down syndrome. An alternative approach to investigating this issue entails using the mouse as a model of the syndrome, and the Ts65Dn mouse seems to be working well (Patterson & Costa, 2005). They have many of the features of Down syndrome in humans, including learning and memory deficits that imply abnormal hippocampal function, deteriorating cognition with age and several neural indicators of abnormal brain development. Aging in Down syndrome is accompanied by amyloid and neurofibrillary pathology, the regional and laminar distribution of which resembles pathological changes seen in Alzheimer disease (Teipel, Schapiro, Alexander *et al.*, 2005). There is atrophy of the corpus callosum and hippocampus in non-demented subjects with age, and corpus callosum size (especially posteriorly) seems to be correlated with cognitive performance deterioration. To date, there has been little progress in discovering the genetic basis of systems that affect the phenotype, because of the immense complexity of those systems and the number of plausible candidates.

Conclusions

A major challenge in developing a truly scientific nosology of child psychopathology for the new millennium is to bring together expertise from multiple complementary disciplines. Such a plea has already been expressed in respect of adult psychiatry. Some years ago, many thought we would soon understand the biological basis of major psychiatric disorders in terms of anomalies in neural circuitry. Andreasen, Nopoulos, O'Leary *et al.* (1999) suggested that the clinical phenotypes of schizophrenia could be caused by a common pathophysiology (a neurodevelopmental mechanism), associated with misconnections in a cortical–thalamic–cerebellar–cortical circuit. Frith (2004) proposed that schizophrenia, dyslexia and autism, conditions strongly influenced by genetic susceptibility, could all result from functional disconnections between key neural processing centers. Over the past few years, we have seen the publication of the Human Genome Project and an explosion of work on psychiatric genetics. It is arguable that much of what we have learned about the pathophysiology of neurodevelopmental disorders has come from the intensive study of people with anomalous genomes, rather than from genomic linkage studies of affected relative pairs.

If there was any specificity between the genetic basis of the conditions described here and distinctive psychiatric disorders, we might be able to identify candidate genes that have a part to play (albeit perhaps indirectly) in the etiology of otherwise idiopathic conditions. However, we suspect the genes responsible for those idiopathic conditions in the general population are of small effect and individually they increase risk by only a marginal amount. Consequently, we should be cautious in concluding that there is any simple connection between, say, the mutation found in Fragile X syndrome or Rett syndrome and idiopathic autism. Both conditions are associated with gross maldevelopment of neural systems that affect general intelligence, as well as social intelligence. Within the last few years, one of the most striking discoveries in behavioral phenotype research is how many syndromes are associated with some features of autism. This lack of specificity could reflect, in part, the fact that many of them are also associated with moderate to severe intellectual disability.

We have known for many years that certain "single gene" conditions often have distinct autistic-like features, especially Fragile X (Brown, Friedman, Jenkins *et al.*, 1982) and Rett syndrome (Hagberg, Aicardi, Dias *et al.*, 1983), in which their prevalence is 30–40%. Theories have evolved to explain why such associations could lead to a revealing of idiopathic autism's neural substrate (Belmonte & Bourgeron, 2006; LaSalle, Hogart, & Thatcher, 2005). When only a handful of genetic syndromes had been studied systematically this explanation seemed plausible. Now, given the diversity of conditions with a similar prevalence of autistic traits, the time has come to reappraise earlier optimistic conjectures. Duchenne muscular dystrophy is associated with autistic behaviors (social and communication deficits) in one-third or more of individuals (Hinton, Nereo, Fee *et al.*, 2006). Tuberous sclerosis (especially *TSC2* mutations) is associated with clinically significant autistic features in up to 50% (Bolton, 2004). Williams syndrome children have poor theory of mind skills, and lack social reciprocity (Tager-Flusberg & Sullivan, 2000). Prader–Willi syndrome critical region duplications and overexpression of maternally derived genes are associated with autistic spectrum disorders in up to 25% (Veltman, Craig, & Bolton 2005). Over one-third of children with velocardiofacial syndrome have autistic spectrum disorders (Antshel, Aneja, Strunge *et al.*, 2007; Vorstman, Morcus, Duijff *et al.*, 2006). Down syndrome children frequently display social withdrawal and stereotypies of an autistic nature (Carter, Capone, Gray *et al.*, 2007). All the sex chromosome aneuploidies have autistic behavior at a rate far in excess of that expected by chance, including Turner syndrome (Creswell & Skuse, 1999), Klinefelter syndrome (Geschwind, Boone, Miller *et al.*, 2000) and possibly 47,XYY and 47,XXX syndromes (Geerts, Steyaert, & Fryns, 2003; Patwardhan, Brown, Bender *et al.*, 2002). Autistic traits are often found in genetically mediated metabolic disorders, such as Smith–Lemli–Opitz syndrome (e.g., Sikora, Pettit-Kekel, Penfield *et al.*, 2006), but have not been widely investigated yet. Specificity between syndrome manifestations has not been established and it is premature to conclude that such metabolic conditions could share neurobiological mechanisms with idiopathic autism. The more closely we look for autistic traits, the more often they are discovered.

If neural connectivity is indeed disrupted as a consequence of the genetic anomaly in many syndromes, and neural connectivity problems probably lie at the heart of much major psychiatric illness, why then do we more commonly discover autistic traits in the syndromes that have been discussed here than in, for example, psychotic phenomena? One possibility is that the neural pathways for the integrity of social intelligence are just far more vulnerable to disruption than those that protect us from psychosis. Every one of the syndromes described is associated with intellectual impairments of one sort or another – both verbal and visuospatial pathways are liable to be affected, as well as executive and other higher cognitive functions. The range and complexity of neural connectivity associated with our ability to perform cognitive functions such as verbal comprehension or visuospatial design are probably so far-reaching that most neurodevelopmental anomalies are going to disrupt its efficient functioning to some extent. A second possibility is that we have not sufficiently investigated the presence of psychotic phenomena among individuals with the syndromes during the period of maximal risk (i.e., in adulthood). Bearing in mind the poor verbal abilities of many subjects, and the difficulties of asking about psychotic phenomena in such a way that one elicits reliable and valid responses, the proposal would not be easy to implement. Psychotic phenomena may be much more prevalent than we suspect, as was found by Baker and Skuse (2005) when they interviewed adolescents with 22q11.2 deletion syndrome, none of whom had yet developed any schizophreniform disorder.

Perhaps, rather than focusing on the symptoms of psychiatric disorder as reported by others, or identified by self-report, we could move closer to an understanding of etiological mechanisms underlying major mental disorders by examining the cognitive consequences of neural processes that might be disrupted by the genetic anomaly in these conditions associated with "behavioral phenotypes." Studying those phenotypes at the level of cognitive processing, brain structure or neural function, by means of neuroimaging, is becoming increasingly popular among scientists who want to discover how vulnerability to mental illness arises. Genetic influences on endophenotypes or intermediate phenotypes sometimes seem easier to identify and replicate than the impact of genetic variation on behavior at the level of symptoms (Gottesman & Hanson, 2005; Prathikanti & Weinberger, 2005). Whether the two levels of investigation into genetic influence comprising, on the one hand, studies of symptoms/syndromes and, on the other, specific cognitive traits, can ever be reconciled to provide a unifying diagnostic framework is debatable. The idea that we could derive a rational diagnostic system for psychiatric disorders by means of identifying genes that increase susceptibility to them is discussed with considerable skepticism by Kendler (2006).

Some of the problems are exemplified by the history of research into behavioral and cognitive phenotypes. First, even single-gene disorders (such as Fragile X or Rett syndrome) have pleiotropic effects and are not invariably associated with any clearly identifiable set of characteristics, in the sense of predictive validity for either cognitive or behavioral dysfunction. In both cases, there is a substantial body of people with the syndrome but no demonstrable genetic anomaly, or who have an anomaly of the candidate gene but lack the classic symptomatic phenotype. Second, it has proved extraordinarily difficult to identify a clear relationship between the influence of a single gene (out of several potential candidates) and any aspect of the phenotype in conditions such as velocardiofacial syndrome or Williams syndrome, where the "risk region" of the genome is clearly defined by a microdeletion and every nucleotide/gene in that region has been mapped. Third, the intensive study of syndromes described in this review has revealed a worrying lack of specificity about clusters of symptoms that were thought to represent coherent disorders, in the sense that they were likely to have a common etiology. Most of the disorders described are to a greater or lesser degree associated with a substantially increased risk of autistic spectrum disorders. In each case, the discovery of what appeared to be a clue to the etiology of "autism" was greeted with great excitement and sponsored new research efforts. If only we understood why there was such a risk in tuberous sclerosis or Rett syndrome, we would – so the argument went – gain insights into the pathophysiology of autism itself. But then we find a similar risk in Fragile X syndrome, velocardiofacial syndrome, Prader–Willi syndrome, Turner syndrome, even Duchenne muscular dystrophy (in each case the proportion affected seems to be about 30%). These discoveries must call into question the hypothesis that there is a specific genetic susceptibility (in each case) in common with idiopathic autistic disorders. In all the examples given above, formal evaluation of autistic symptoms using standardized measures demonstrates an enormously increased risk compared with the accepted population prevalence for autistic spectrum disorders of 0.6%.

Cognitive psychology aims to understand the adult mind by dividing it into component domains such as perception, language and executive functions, often employing evidence from lesions to determine localization by observing the absence of function after injury. It is arguable that the very plasticity and flexibility of the developing child's central nervous system make it less susceptible to study by that approach (Scerif & Karmiloff-Smith, 2005). We hoped to identify genetic mechanisms that influence adaptive behavior by a similar approach to that used by cognitive psychology. Observe individuals with genetic anomalies, identify in what domains they differ from normal, and thereby link genes to processes that are associated with mental disorders. We believed that by so doing we could begin to understand the origins of the cognitive dysfunction that underlies much child psychiatric disorder. In a discipline for which there are few if any clear boundaries between "disease" and "normal" states of mind, a starting point that relies upon categorical disease (or disorder) models may not be appropriate for the investigation of putative genetic etiological mechanisms, even in highly heritable conditions.

Interestingly, since the last edition of this book there has been remarkably little progress made in identifying susceptibility genes for common childhood psychiatric disorders, although some promising findings are emerging with respect to ADHD, at the level of gene variant–symptom relationships (Faraone, Perlis, Doyle *et al.*, 2005) by means of association studies. An alternative approach has also proved successful, albeit in a limited contextual framework. Here, the aim is first to identify plausible candidate genes from intensive studies of people with genetic anomalies (e.g., 22q11.2 microdeletions) and a heightened risk of psychiatric disorder. Second, to discover whether these genes have common variants with different functional activity (e.g., the 108/158 *val* and *met* variants of *COMT* which lie within the deleted region). Third, to genotype individuals from the general population (without psychiatric disorder) in order to investigate the variant's influence on the neural structure and cognitive–behavioral characteristics of asymptomatic typical individuals. The approach is providing potentially valuable insights into genetic variants that do influence neural functions, and under what circumstances they do so (Meyer-Lindenberg & Weinberger, 2006), although deficiencies in experimental design and the optimistic interpretation of ambiguous results often characterize this line of work. To date, few candidate genes have been studied intensively by these means, and their role in susceptibility to major mental disorder is uncertain.

Arguably, in the search for genes that predispose to the development of symptomatically defined child psychiatric disorders it is both inefficient and conceptually muddled to seek the genetic components of relatively amorphous diseases (still less "comorbid" disorders). As Kendler (2006) reflected, it is highly unlikely that we will discover any direct relationship between gene variation and conventional categories of psychiatric disorder. Rather, we should look for evidence that functional variation in candidate genes influences neural functions that may be common to a number of diseases or disorders. We need to learn how genes control neurobiological development and, in so doing, increasing use will be made of animal studies (Gould & Gottesman, 2006). Creating a heuristic cognitive model of neurodevelopmental disorders will in due course lead to the integration of disciplines, as we seek the biological roots during childhood of psychiatric conditions whose clinical onset is in adulthood. Genetic influences (in the form of quantitative trait loci) on our predisposition to develop psychiatric disorders act throughout the lifespan. The proportion of variance in a trait that is explained by the candidate measured at a particular point in time may be small, just a few percent, yet even genes of such minor effect upon a measured state may be associated with a substantially greater cumulative risk because they have shaped developmental trajectories from embryonic beginnings. It behooves us to remember that stochastic and environmental events often play a critical part in translating a genetic predisposition, measured in terms of cognitive or other vulnerability, into the symptoms and behaviors that are characteristic of a defined syndrome.

To summarize, we agree with Scerif and Karmiloff-Smith (2005) that optimistic statements such as Pinker's (2001) proclamation that we are now experiencing the "dawn of cognitive genetics" are premature. It is extraordinarily difficult to find any specific links between the functions of individual genes and circumscribed cognitive-level processes, although there are exceptions (Weiss *et al.*, 2007). Reasons to be skeptical include the following issues. When we consider the impact of a genetic anomaly on cognitive or behavioral outcomes, we must first take account of the developmental processes and the possibility that the manifestations of that anomaly may differ along the trajectory from childhood to adulthood. When we choose to study those manifestations will strongly influence our conclusions about their impact. Second, we should be aware that it is very unlikely that the genetic anomaly (whether monogenic or not) affects just one cognitive system, even though that may be the most obvious manifestation. For example, it is notable that the majority of syndromes discussed in the chapter have non-specific effects upon generalized cognitive abilities quite apart from their more characteristic manifestations. To what extent more specific manifestations are a consequence of genetic variation quite remote from the genetic anomaly of interest is not clear, but the difficulty in finding any direct link between the (polygenic) anomaly in 22q11.2 microdeletion and the symptoms of psychosis despite over a decade of research should serve as a cautionary tale.

Although the overt manifestations of these conditions, in terms of their behavioral and cognitive characteristics, superficially imply that the genetic anomaly directly causes them, we need to be aware that there is very unlikely to be developmental independence between the mechanisms leading to the phenotype. Scerif and Karmiloff-Smith (2005) give, as an example of this interdependence, the difficulty children with Williams syndrome have in understanding spatial language. They also have a fundamental problem with the concept of cardinality, and their verbal abilities predict their competence in that domain (unlike typical children for whom the predictor is visuospatial skills). They propose that a fundamental difficulty in abstracting the relational characteristics of the surrounding perceptual environment could account not only for that language deficit, but also for the problems with number development and configural interpretation of facial characteristics. Genetic anomalies are generally likely to operate at the level of such fundamental impairments, rather than at the refined level of "symptoms" or higher cognitive skills such as language (Marcus & Rabagliati, 2006).

In practical terms, the knowledge that genetic anomalies such as those described here are often associated with characteristic patterns of behavior and cognitive deficits can be of great significance for the appropriate management of the condition. That knowledge can be reassuring to parents, and can lead to a rational basis for educational support. We must remember not to be seduced by our knowledge of the genotype into a state of genetic determinism – whatever the nature of the anomaly, there are usually potential compensatory mechanisms. Our role, as clinicians, is to find them, implement them and support the family until they are firmly embedded in the child's social or educational repertoire.

References

Abramsky, L., & Chapple, J. (1997). 47,XXY (Klinefelter syndrome) and 47,XYY: Estimated rates of and indication for postnatal diagnosis with implications for prenatal counseling. *Prenatal Diagnosis*, *17*, 363–368.

Andreasen, N. C., Nopoulos, P., O'Leary, D. S., Miller, D. D., Wassink, T., & Flaum, M. (1999). Defining the phenotype of schizophrenia: Cognitive dysmetria and its neural mechanisms. *Biological Psychiatry*, *46*, 908–920.

Antshel, K. M., Aneja, A., Strunge, L., Peebles, J., Fremont, W. P., Stallone, K., *et al.* (2007). Autistic spectrum disorders in velo-cardio facial syndrome (22q11.2 deletion). *Journal of Autism and Developmental Disorders*, *37*, 1776–1786.

Baker, K., Baldeweg, T., Sivagnanasundaram, S., Scambler, P., & Skuse, D. (2005). COMT Val108/158 Met modifies mismatch negativity and cognitive function in 22q11 deletion syndrome. *Biological Psychiatry*, *58*, 23–31.

Baker, K. D., & Skuse, D. H. (2005). Adolescents and young adults with 22q11 deletion syndrome: Psychopathology in an at-risk group. *British Journal of Psychiatry*, *186*, 115–120.

Baron-Cohen, S., Wheelwright, S., Hill, J., Raste, Y., & Plumb, I. (2001). The "Reading the Mind in the Eyes" Test revised version: a study with normal adults, and adults with Asperger syndrome or high-functioning autism. *Journal of Child Psychology and Psychiatry*, *42*, 241–251.

Bassett, A. S., Chow, E. W., AbdelMalik, P., Gheorghiu, M., Husted, J., & Weksberg, R. (2003). The schizophrenia phenotype in 22q11 deletion syndrome. *American Journal of Psychiatry*, *160*, 1580–1586.

Bayes, M., Magano, L. F., Rivera, N., Flores, R., & Perez Jurado, L. A. (2003). Mutational mechanisms of Williams–Beuren syndrome deletions. *American Journal of Human Genetics*, *73*, 131–151.

Belmonte, M. K., & Bourgeron, T. (2006). Fragile X syndrome and autism at the intersection of genetic and neural networks. *Nature Neuroscience*, *9*, 1221–1225.

Bender, B. G., Linden, M. G., & Harmon, R. J. (2001). Neuropsychological and functional cognitive skills of 35 unselected adults with sex chromosome abnormalities. *American Journal of Medical Genetics*, *102*, 309–313.

Bish, J. P., Ferrante, S. M., Donald-McGinn, D., Zackai, E., & Simon, T. J. (2005). Maladaptive conflict monitoring as evidence for executive dysfunction in children with chromosome 22q11.2 deletion syndrome. *Developmental Science*, *8*, 36–43.

Bishop, D. V., Canning, E., Elgar, K., Morris, E., Jacobs, P. A., & Skuse, D. H. (2000). Distinctive patterns of memory function in subgroups of females with Turner syndrome: Evidence for imprinted loci on the X-chromosome affecting neurodevelopment. *Neuropsychologia*, *38*, 712–721.

Bojesen, A., Juul, S., Birkebaek, N. H., & Gravholt, C. H. (2006). Morbidity in Klinefelter syndrome: A Danish register study based on hospital discharge diagnoses. *Journal of Clinical Endocrinology and Metabolism*, *91*, 1254–1260.

Bojesen, A., Juul, S., & Gravholt, C. H. (2003). Prenatal and postnatal prevalence of Klinefelter syndrome: A national registry study. *Journal of Clinical Endocrinology and Metabolism*, *88*, 622–626.

Bolton, P. F. (2004). Neuroepileptic correlates of autistic symptomatology in tuberous sclerosis. *Mental Retardation and Developmental Disabilities Research Reviews*, *10*, 126–131.

Bolton, P. F., Park, R. J., Higgins, J. N., Griffiths, P. D., & Pickles, A. (2002). Neuro-epileptic determinants of autism spectrum disorders in tuberous sclerosis complex. *Brain*, *125*, 1247–1255.

Braff, D. L., Geyer, M. A., Light, G. A., Sprock, J., Perry, W., Cadenhead, K. S., *et al.* (2001). Impact of prepulse characteristics on the detection of sensorimotor gating deficits in schizophrenia. *Schizophrenia Research*, *49*, 171–178.

Brown, W. T., Friedman, E., Jenkins, E. C., Brooks, J., Wisniewski, K., Raguthu, S., *et al.* (1982). Association of fragile X syndrome with autism. *Lancet*, *8263*, 100.

Butler, M. G., Bittel, D. C., Kibiryeva, N., Talebizadeh, Z., & Thompson, T. (2004). Behavioral differences among subjects with Prader–Willi syndrome and type I or type II deletion and maternal disomy. *Pediatrics*, *113*, 565–573.

Butler, M. G., Bittel, D. C., & Talebizadeh, Z. (2004). Plasma peptide YY and ghrelin levels in infants and children with Prader–Willi syndrome. *Journal of Pediatric Endocrinology and Metabolism*, *17*, 1177–1184.

Campbell, R., Lawrence, K., Mandy, W., Mitra, C., Jeyakuma, L., & Skuse, D. (2006). Meanings in motion and faces: Developmental associations between the processing of intention from geometrical animations and gaze detection accuracy. *Development and Psychopathology*, *18*, 99–118.

Capone, G., Goyal, P., Ares, W., & Lannigan, E. (2006). Neurobehavioral disorders in children, adolescents, and young adults with Down syndrome. *American Journal of Medical Genetics. Part C, Semininars in Medical Genetics*, *142*, 158–172.

Carrel, L., & Willard, H. F. (2005). X-inactivation profile reveals extensive variability in X-linked gene expression in females. *Nature*, *434*, 400–404.

Carter, J. C., Capone, G. T., Gray, R. M., Cox, C. S., & Kaufmann, W. E. (2007). Autistic-spectrum disorders in Down syndrome: Further delineation and distinction from other behavioral abnormalities. *American Journal of Medical Genetics. Part B, Neuropsychiatriatric Genetics*, *144*, 87–94.

Cassidy, S. B. (1992). Introduction and overview of Prader–Willi syndrome. In S. B. Cassidy (Ed.), *Prader–Willi syndrome and other chromosome 15q deletion disorders. NATO Advanced Research Workshop* (pp. 1–11). Berlin: Springer.

Charman, T., Neilson, T. C., Mash, V., Archer, H., Gardiner, M. T., Knudsen, G. P., *et al.* (2005). Dimensional phenotypic analysis and functional categorisation of mutations reveal novel genotype–phenotype associations in Rett syndrome. *European Journal of Human Genetics*, *13*, 1121–1130.

Check, E. (2005). Human genome: Patchwork people. *Nature*, *437*, 1084–1086.

Chow, E. W., Watson, M., Young, D. A., & Bassett, A. S. (2006). Neurocognitive profile in 22q11 deletion syndrome and schizophrenia. *Schizophrenia Research*, *87*, 270–278.

Cornish, K. M., Turk, J., Wilding, J., Sudhalter, V., Munir, F., Kooy, F., *et al.* (2004). Annotation. Deconstructing the attention deficit in fragile X syndrome: A developmental neuropsychological approach. *Journal of Child Psychology and Psychiatry*, *45*, 1042–1053.

Creswell, C. S., & Skuse, D. H. (1999). Autism in association with Turner syndrome: Genetic implications for male vulnerability to pervasive developmental disorders. *Neurocase*, *5*, 101–108.

Crews, D., & McLachlan, J. A. (2006). Epigenetics, evolution, endocrine disruption, health, and disease. *Endocrinology*, *147*, S4–10.

Davies, P. S., & Joughin, C. (1992). Assessment of body composition in the Prader–Willi syndrome using bioelectrical impedance. *American Journal of Medical Genetics*, *44*, 75–78.

Davies, W., Isles, A., Smith, R., Karunadasa, D., Burrmann, D., Humby, T., *et al.* (2005). Xlr3b is a new imprinted candidate for X-linked parent-of-origin effects on cognitive function in mice. *Nature Genetics*, *37*, 625–629.

De Vries, V. P., Humphrey, A., McCartney, D., Prather, P., Bolton, P., & Hunt, A. (2005). Consensus clinical guidelines for the assessment of cognitive and behavioural problems in tuberous sclerosis. *European Child and Adolescent Psychiatry*, *14*, 183–190.

Delisi, L. E. (2005). Current concepts in schizophrenia research: Advancing progress towards understanding etiology and new treatments in year 2004. *Current Opinion in Psychiatry*, *18*, 109–110.

Delisi, L. E., Maurizio, A. M., Svetina, C., Ardekani, B., Szulc, K., Nierenberg, J., *et al.* (2005). Klinefelter's syndrome (XXY) as a genetic model for psychotic disorders. *American Journal of Medical Genetics. Part B, Neuropsychiatric Genetics*, *135B*, 15–23.

Drumm, M. L., Konstan, M. W., Schluchter, M. D., Handler, A., Pace, R., Zou, F., *et al.* (2005). Genetic modifiers of lung disease in cystic fibrosis. *New England Journal of Medicine*, *353*, 1443–1453.

Elgar, K., Campbell, R., & Skuse, D. (2002). Are you looking at me? Accuracy in processing line-of-sight in Turner syndrome. *Proceedings. Biological Sciences*, *269*, 2415–2422.

Fales, C. L., Knowlton, B. J., Holyoak, K. J., Geschwind, D. H., Swerdloff, R. S., & Gonzalo, I. G. (2003). Working memory and relational reasoning in Klinefelter syndrome. *Journal of the International Neuropsychological Society*, *9*, 839–846.

Faraone, S. V., Perlis, R. H., Doyle, A. E., Smoller, J. W., Goralnick, J. J., Holmgren, M. A., *et al.* (2005). Molecular genetics of attention-deficit/hyperactivity disorder. *Biological Psychiatry*, *57*, 1313–1323.

Frith, C. (2004). Is autism a disconnection disorder? *Lancet Neurology*, *3*, 577.

Gardiner, K., Davisson, M. T., Pritchard, M., Patterson, D., Groner, Y., Crnic, L. S., *et al.* (2005). Report on the Expert Workshop on the Biology of Chromosome 21: Towards gene–phenotype correlations in Down syndrome, held June 11–14, 2004, Washington D.C. *Cytogenetic and Genome Research*, *108*, 269–277.

Geerts, M., Steyaert, J., & Fryns, J. P. (2003). The XYY syndrome: A follow-up study on 38 boys. *Genetic Counseling*, *14*, 267–279.

Geschwind, D. H., Boone, K. B., Miller, B. L., & Swerdloff, R. S. (2000). Neurobehavioral phenotype of Klinefelter syndrome. *Mental Retardation and Developmental Disabilities Research Reviews*, *6*, 107–116.

Good, C. D., Lawrence, K., Thomas, N. S., Price, C. J., Ashburner, J., Friston, K. J., *et al.* (2003). Dosage-sensitive X-linked locus influences the development of amygdala and orbitofrontal cortex, and fear recognition in humans. *Brain*, *126*, 2431–2446.

Gottesman, I. I., & Hanson, D. R. (2005). Human development: Biological and genetic processes. *Annual Review of Psychology*, *56*, 263–286.

Gotz, M. J., Johnstone, E. C., & Ratcliffe, S. G. (1999). Criminality and antisocial behaviour in unselected men with sex chromosome abnormalities. *Psychological Medicine*, *29*, 953–962.

Gould, T. D., & Gottesman, I. I. (2006). Psychiatric endophenotypes and the development of valid animal models. *Genes, Brain and Behavior*, *5*, 113–119.

Hagberg, B., Aicardi, J., Dias, K., & Ramos, O. (1983). A progressive syndrome of autism, dementia, ataxia, and loss of purposeful hand use in girls: Rett's syndrome. Report of 35 cases. *Annals of Neurology*, *14*, 471–479.

Hagerman, R. J., Ono, M. Y., & Hagerman, P. J. (2005). Recent advances in fragile X: A model for autism and neurodegeneration. *Current Opinion in Psychiatry*, *18*, 490–496.

Harrison, P. J., & Owen, M. J. (2003). Genes for schizophrenia? Recent findings and their pathophysiological implications. *Lancet*, *361*, 417–419.

Haston, C. K., & Hudson, T. J. (2005). Finding genetic modifiers of cystic fibrosis. *New England Journal of Medicine*, 353, 1509–1511.

Helbing-Zwanenburg, B., Kamphuisen, H. A. C., & Mourtazev, M. S. (1993). The origin of excessive day-time sleepiness in the Prader–Willi syndrome. *Journal of Intellectual Disability*, *37*, 533–541.

Hessl, D., Glaser, B., Dyer-Friedman, J., & Reiss, A. L. (2006). Social behavior and cortisol reactivity in children with fragile X syndrome. *Journal of Child Psychology and Psychiatry*, *47*, 602–610.

Hinton, V., & Goldstein, E. (2007). Duchenne muscular dystrophy. In M. Mazzocco, & J. Ross (Eds.), *Neurogenetic developmental disorders: Identification and Manifestation in Childhood.* MIT Press.

Hinton, V. J., De Vivo, V., Nereo, N. E., Goldstein, E., & Stern, Y. (2001). Selective deficits in verbal working memory associated with a known genetic etiology: The neuropsychological profile of Duchenne muscular dystrophy. *Journal of the International Neuropsychological Society*, *7*, 45–54.

Hinton, V. J., Nereo, N. E., Fee, R. J., & Cyrulnik, S. E. (2006). Social behavior problems in boys with Duchenne muscular dystrophy. *Journal of Developmental and Behavioral Pediatrics*, *27*, 470–476.

Hoogenraad, C. C., Akhmanova, A., Galjart, N., & De Zeeuw, C. I. (2004). LIMK1 and CLIP-115: Linking cytoskeletal defects to Williams syndrome. *Bioessays*, *26*, 141–150.

Horsler, K., & Oliver, C. (2006). The behavioural phenotype of Angelman syndrome. *Journal of Intellectual Disability Research*, *50*, 33–53.

Jacobs, P., Dalton, P., James, R., Mosse, K., Power, M., Robinson, D., *et al.* (1997). Turner syndrome: A cytogenetic and molecular study. *Annals of Human Genetics*, *61*, 471–483.

Karayiorgou, M., & Gogos, J. A. (2004). The molecular genetics of the 22q11-associated schizophrenia. *Brain Research. Molecular Brain Research*, *132*, 95–104.

Karayiorgou, M., Morris, M. A., Morrow, B., Shprintzen, R. J., Goldberg, R., Borrow, J., *et al.* (1995). Schizophrenia susceptibility associated with interstitial deletions of chromosome 22q11. *Proceedings of the National Academy of Sciences of the USA*, *92*, 7612–7616.

Kendler, K. S. (2006). Reflections on the relationship between psychiatric genetics and psychiatric nosology. *American Journal of Psychiatry*, *163*, 1138–1146.

Lanfranco, F., Kamischke, A., Zitzmann, M., & Nieschlag, E. (2004). Klinefelter's syndrome. *Lancet*, *364*, 273–283.

LaSalle, J. M., Hogart, A., & Thatcher, K. N. (2005). Rett syndrome: A Rosetta stone for understanding the molecular pathogenesis of autism. *International Review of Neurobiology*, *71*, 131–165.

Lawrence, K., Campbell, R., Swettenham, J., Terstegge, J., Akers, R., Coleman, M., *et al.* (2003a). Interpreting gaze in Turner syndrome: Impaired sensitivity to intention and emotion, but preservation of social cueing. *Neuropsychologia*, *41*, 894–905.

Lawrence, K., Kuntsi, J., Coleman, M., Campbell, R., & Skuse, D. (2003b). Face and emotion recognition deficits in Turner syndrome: A possible role for X-linked genes in amygdala development. *Neuropsychology*, *17*, 39–49.

Lopes, A. M., Ross, N., Close, J., Dagnall, A., Amorim, A., & Crow, T. J. (2006). Inactivation status of PCDH11X: Sexual dimorphisms in gene expression levels in brain. *Human Genetics*, *119*, 267–275.

Madduri, N., Peters, S. U., Voigt, R. G., Llorente, A. M., Lupski, J. R., & Potocki, L. (2006). Cognitive and adaptive behavior profiles in Smith–Magenis syndrome. *Journal of Developmental and Behavioral Pediatrics*, *27*, 188–192.

Marcus, G., & Rabagliati, H. (2006). What developmental disorders can tell us about the nature and origins of language. *Nature Neuroscience*, *10*, 1226–1229.

Martin, S. C., Wolters, P. L., & Smith, A. C. (2006). Adaptive and maladaptive behavior in children with Smith–Magenis syndrome. *Journal of Autism and Developmental Disorders*, *36*, 541–552.

Meyer-Lindenberg, A., Mervis, C. B., & Faith, B. K. (2006). Neural mechanisms in Williams syndrome: A unique window to genetic influences on cognition and behaviour. *Nature Reviews. Neuroscience*, *7*, 380–393.

Meyer-Lindenberg, A., Weinberger, D. R. (2006). Intermediate phenotypes and genetic mechanisms of psychiatric disorders. *Nature Reviews Neuroscience*, *7*, 818–827.

Milner, K. M., Craig, E. E., Thompson, R. J., Veltman, M. W., Thomas, N. S., Roberts, S., *et al.* (2005). Prader–Willi syndrome: Intellectual abilities and behavioural features by genetic subtype. *Journal of Child Psychology and Psychiatry*, *46*, 1089–1096.

Mount, R. H., Hastings, R. P., Reilly, S., Cass, H., & Charman, T. (2001). Behavioural and emotional features in Rett syndrome. *Disability and Rehabilitation*, *23*, 129–138.

Muntoni, F., Torelli, S., & Ferlini, A. (2003). Dystrophin and mutations: one gene, several proteins, multiple phenotypes. *Lancet Neurology*, *2*, 731–740.

Murphy, K. C. (2002). Schizophrenia and velo-cardio-facial syndrome. *Lancet*, *359*, 426–430.

Murphy, K. C., Jones, L. A., & Owen, M. J. (1999). High rates of schizophrenia in adults with velo-cardio-facial syndrome. *Archives of General Psychiatry*, *56*, 940–945.

Musci, T. J., & Caughey, A. B. (2005). Cost-effectiveness analysis of prenatal population-based fragile X carrier screening. *American Journal of Obstetrics and Gynecology*, *192*, 1905–1912.

Myers, R. H. (2004). Huntingdon's disease genetics. *Journal of the American Society for Experimental NeuroTherapeutics*, *1*, 255–262.

Nardella, M. T., Sulzbacher, S. I., & Worthington-Roberts, B. S. (1983). Activity levels of persons with Prader–Willi syndrome. *American Journal of Mental Deficiency*, *87*, 498–505.

Nicolson, R., Bhalerao, S., & Sloman, L. (1998). 47,XYY karyotypes and pervasive developmental disorders. *Canadian Journal of Psychiatry*, *43*, 619–622.

Norton, N., Williams, H. J., & Owen, M. J. (2006). An update on the genetics of schizophrenia. *Current Opinion in Psychiatry*, *19*, 158–164.

Ogden, C. L., Kuczmarski, R. J., Flegal, K. M., Mei, Z., Guo, S., Wei R., *et al.* (2002). Centers for Disease Control and Prevention 2000 growth charts for the United States: Improvements to the 1977 National Center for Health Statistics version. *Pediatrics*, *109*, 45–60.

Pantelis, C., Yucel, M., Wood, S. J., McGorry, P. D., & Velakoulis, D. (2003). Early and late neurodevelopmental disturbances in schizophrenia and their functional consequences. *Australian and New Zealand Journal of Psychiatry*, *37*, 399–406.

Paterlini, M., Zakharenko, S. S., Lai, W. S., Qin, J., Zhang, H., Mukai, J., *et al.* (2005). Transcriptional and behavioral interaction between 22q11.2 orthologs modulates schizophrenia-related phenotypes in mice. *Nature Neuroscience*, *8*, 1586–1594.

Patterson, D., & Costa, A. C. (2005). Down syndrome and genetics: A case of linked histories. *Nature Review Genetics*, *6*, 137–147.

Patwardhan, A. J., Brown, W. E., Bender, B. G., Linden, M. G., Eliez, S., Reiss, A. L. (2002). Reduced size of the amygdala in individuals with 47, XXY and 47, XXX karyotypes. *American Journal of Medical Genetics*, *114*, 93–98.

Paylor, R., Glaser, B., Mupo, A., Ataliotis, P., Spencer, C., Sobotka, A., *et al.* (2006). Tbx1 haploinsufficiency is linked to behavioral disorders in mice and humans: Implications for 22q11 deletion syndrome. *Proceedings of the National Academy of Sciences of the USA*, *103*, 7729–7734.

Pearson, C. E., Edamura, K. N., & Cleary, J. D. (2005). Repeat instability: mechanisms of dynamic mutations. *Nature Reviews. Genetics*, *6*, 729–742.

Pembrey, M. E., Barnicoat, A. J., Carmichael, B., Bobrow, M., & Turner, G. (2001). An assessment of screening strategies for fragile X syndrome in the UK. *Health Technology Assessment*, *5*, 1–95.

Persico, A. M., & Bourgeron, T. (2006). Searching for ways out of the autism maze: Genetic, epigenetic and environmental clues. *Trends in Neuroscience*, *29*, 349–358.

Pinker, S. (2001). Talk of genetics and vice versa. *Nature*, *413*, 465–466.

Potocki, L., Shaw, C. J., Stankiewicz, P., & Lupski, J. R. (2003). Variability in clinical phenotype despite common chromosomal deletion in Smith–Magenis syndrome [del(17)(p11.2p11.2)]. *Genetics in Medicine*, *5*, 430–434.

Prathikanti, S., & Weinberger, D. R. (2005). Psychiatric genetics – the new era: genetic research and some clinical implications. *British Medical Bulletin*, *73–74*, 107–122.

Prior, T. W., & Bridgeman, S. J. (2005). Experience and strategy for the molecular testing of Duchenne muscular dystrophy. *Journal of Molecular Diagnosis*, *7*, 317–326.

Rao, E., Weiss, B., Fukami, M., Rump, A., Niesler, B., Mertz, A., *et al.* (1997). Pseudoautosomal deletions encompassing a novel homeobox gene cause growth failure in idiopathic short stature and Turner syndrome. *Nature Genetics*, *16*, 54–63.

Ratcliffe, S. G. (1994). The psychological and psychiatric consequences of sex chromosome abnormalities in children, based on population studies. In F. Poustka (Ed.), *Basic approaches to genetic and molecular biological developmental psychiatry* (pp. 99–122). Berlin: Quintessenz.

Ratcliffe, S. (1999). Long-term outcome in children of sex chromosome abnormalities. *Archives of Disease in Childhood*, *80*, 192–195.

Reddy, K. S. (2005). Cytogenetic abnormalities and fragile-X syndrome in autism spectrum disorder. *BMC Medical Genetics*, *6*, 3.

Redon, R., Ishikawa, S., Fitch, K., Feuk, L., Perry, G. H., Andrews, T. D, *et al.* (2006). Global variation in copy number in the human genome. *Nature*, *444*, 444–454.

Richards, E. J. (2006). Inherited epigenetic variation? Revisiting soft inheritance. *Nature Reviews Genetics*, *7*, 395–401.

Robinson, D. O., & Jacobs, P. A. (1999). The origin of the extra Y chromosome in males with a 47,XYY karyotype. *Human Molecular Genetics*, *8*, 2205–2209.

Ross, M. T., Grafham, D. V., Coffey, A. J., Scherer, S., McLay, K., Muzny, D., *et al.* (2005). The DNA sequence of the human X chromosome. *Nature*, *434*, 325–337.

Ross, N. L., Wadekar, R., Lopes, A., Dagnall, A., Close, J., Delisi, L. E., *et al.* (2006). Methylation of two *Homo sapiens*-specific X-Y homologous genes in Klinefelter's syndrome (XXY). *American Journal of Medical Genetics. Part B, Neuropsychiatric Genetics*, *141*, 544–548.

Roubertoux, P. L., & Kerdelhue, B. (2006). Trisomy 21: From chromosomes to mental retardation. *Behavioral Genetics*, *36*, 346–354.

Rutter, M., Moffitt, T. E., & Caspi, A. (2006). Gene–environment interplay and psychopathology: Multiple varieties but real effects. *Journal of Child Psychology and Psychiatry*, *47*, 226–261.

Rutter, M., Giller, H., & Hagell, A. (1998). *Antisocial behaviour by young people* (p. 132). Cambridge: Cambridge University Press.

Scerif, G., & Karmiloff-Smith, A. (2005). The dawn of cognitive genetics? Crucial developmental caveats. *Trends in Cognitive Sciences*, *9*, 126–135.

Segawa, M., & Nomura, Y. (2005). Rett syndrome. *Current Opinion in Neurology*, *18*, 97–104.

Shelley, B. P., & Robertson, M. M. (2005). The neuropsychiatry and multisystem features of the Smith–Magenis syndrome: A review. *Journal of Neuropsychiatry and Clinical Neurosciences*, *17*, 91–97.

Shibayama, A., Cook, E. H. Jr., Feng, J., Glanzmann, C., Yan, J., Craddock, N., *et al.* (2004). MECP2 structural and 3′-UTR variants in schizophrenia, autism and other psychiatric diseases: A possible association with autism. *American Journal of Medical Genetics. Part B, Neuropsychiatric Genetics*, *128*, 50–53.

Shprintzen, R. J., Goldberg, R. B., Young, D., & Wolford, L. (1981). The velo-cardio-facial syndrome: A clinical and genetic analysis. *Pediatrics*, *67*, 167–172.

Sikora, D. M., Pettit-Kekel, K., Penfield, J., Merkens, L. S., & Steiner, R. D. (2006). The near universal presence of autism spectrum disorders in children with Smith–Lemli–Opitz syndrome. *American Journal of Medical Genetics, A*. *140*, 1511–1518.

Simon, T. J., Bish, J. P., Bearden, C. E., Ding, L., Ferrante, S., Nguyen, V., *et al.* (2005). A multilevel analysis of cognitive dysfunction and psychopathology associated with chromosome 22q11.2 deletion syndrome in children. *Developmental Psychopathology*, *17*, 753–784.

Skuse, D. H. (2006). Sexual dimorphism in cognition and behaviour: The role of X-linked genes. *European Journal of Endocrinology*, *155* (Supplement 1), S99–S106.

Skuse, D. H., James, R. S., Bishop, D. V., Coppin, B., Dalton, P., Amodt-Leeper, G., *et al.* (1997). Evidence from Turner's syndrome of an imprinted X-linked locus affecting cognitive function. *Nature*, *387*, 705–708.

Stemkens, D., Roza, T., Verrij, L., Swaab, H., van, W. M., Alizadeh, B., *et al.* (2006). Is there an influence of X-chromosomal imprinting on the phenotype in Klinefelter syndrome? A clinical and molecular genetic study of 61 cases. *Clinical Genetics*, *70*, 43–48.

Stromme, P., Bjornstad, P. G., & Ramstad, K. (2002). Prevalence estimation of Williams syndrome. *Journal of Child Neurology*, *17*, 269–271.

Swillen, A., Devriendt, K., Legius, E., Prinzie, P., Vogels, A., Ghesquiere, P., *et al.* (1999). The behavioural phenotype in velo-cardio-facial syndrome (VCFS): From infancy to adolescence. *Genetic Counseling*, *10*, 79–88.

Szyf, M., Weaver, I. C., Champagne, F. A., Diorio, J., & Meaney, M. J. (2005). Maternal programming of steroid receptor expression and phenotype through DNA methylation in the rat. *Frontiers in Neuroendocrinology*, *26*, 139–162.

Tager-Flusberg, H., & Sullivan, K. (2000). A componential view of theory of mind: Evidence from Williams syndrome. *Cognition*, *76*, 59–90.

Tassabehji, M., Hammond, P., Karmiloff-Smith, A., Thompson, P., Thorgeirsson, S. S., Durkin, M. E., *et al.* (2005). GTF2IRD1 in craniofacial development of humans and mice. *Science*, *310*, 1184–1187.

Teipel, S. J., Schapiro, M. B., Alexander, G. E., Krasuski, J. S., Horwitz, B., Hoehne, C., *et al.* (2003). Relation of corpus callosum and hippocampal size to age in nondemented adults with Down's syndrome. *American Journal of Psychiatry*, *160*, 1870–1878.

Temple, C. M., & Sanfilippo, P. M. (2003). Executive skills in Klinefelter's syndrome. *Neuropsychologia*, *41*, 1547–1559.

Thompson, R. J., & Bolton, P. F. (2003). Case report. Angelman syndrome in an individual with a small SMC(15) and paternal uniparental disomy: A case report with reference to the assessment of cognitive functioning and autistic symptomatology. *Journal of Autism and Developmnetal Disorders*, *33*, 171–176.

van Esch, H. (2006). The Fragile X premutation: New insights and clinical consequences. *European Journal of Medical Genetics*, *49*, 1–8.

van Rijn, S., Swaab, H., Aleman, A., & Kahn, R. S. (2006). X chromosomal effects on social cognitive processing and emotion regulation: A study with Klinefelter men (47,XXY). *Schizophrenia Research*, *84*, 194–203.

Veenstra-Vanderweele, J., & Cook, E. H. Jr. (2004). Molecular genetics of autism spectrum disorder. *Molecular Psychiatry*, *9*, 819–832.

Veltman, M. W., Craig, E. E., & Bolton, P. F. (2005). Autism spectrum disorders in Prader–Willi and Angelman syndromes: A systematic review. *Psychiatric Genetics*, *15*, 243–254.

Vicari, S. (2006). Motor development and neuropsychological patterns in persons with Down syndrome. *Behavioral Genetics*, *36*, 355–364.

Vorstman, J. A., Morcus, M. E., Duijff, S. N., Klaassen, P. W., Heineman-de Boer, J. A., Beemer, F. A., *et al.* (2006). The 22q11.2 deletion in children: High rate of autistic disorders and early onset of psychotic symptoms. *Journal of the American Academy of Child and Adolescent Psychiatry*, *45*, 1104–1113.

Weaver, I. C., Meaney, M. J., & Szyf, M. (2006). Maternal care effects on the hippocampal transcriptome and anxiety-mediated behaviors in the offspring that are reversible in adulthood. *Proceedings of the National Academy of Sciences of the USA*, *103*, 3480–3485.

Weaving, L. S., Williamson, S. L., Bennetts, B., Davis, M., Ellaway, C. J., Leonard, H., *et al.* (2003). Effects of MECP2 mutation type, location and X-inactivation in modulating Rett syndrome phenotype. *American Journal of Medical Genetics, A*, *118*, 103–114.

Weiss, L. A., Purcell, S., Waggoner, S., Lawrence, K., Spektor, D., Daly, M. J., *et al.* (2007). Identification of *EFHC2* as a quantitative trait locus for fear recognition in Turner syndrome. *Human Molecular Genetics*, *16*, 107–113.

Weksberg, R., Stachon, A. C., Squire, J. A., Moldovan, L., Bayani, J., Meyn, S., *et al.* (2007). Molecular characterization of deletion breakpoints in adults with 22q11 deletion syndrome. *Human Genetics*, *120*, 837–845.

Williams, C. A., Beaudet, A. L., Clayton-Smith, J., Knoll, J. H., Kyllerman, M., Laan, L. A., *et al.* (2006). Angelman syndrome 2005: Updated consensus for diagnostic criteria. *American Journal of Medical Genetics, A*, *140*, 413–418.

Woodin, M., Wang, P. P., Aleman, D., Donald-McGinn, D., Zackai, E., & Moss, E. (2001). Neuropsychological profile of children and adolescents with the 22q11.2 microdeletion. *Genetics in Medicine*, *3*, 34–39.

Yagi, H., Furutani, Y., Hamada, H., Sasaki, T., Asakawa, S., Minoshima, S., *et al.* (2003). Role of TBX1 in human del22q11.2 syndrome. *Lancet*, *362*, 1366–1373.

Yung, A. R., Stanford, C., Cosgrave, E., Killackey, E., Phillips, L., Nelson, B., *et al.* (2006). Testing the ultra high risk (prodromal) criteria for the prediction of psychosis in a clinical sample of young people. *Schizophrenia Research*, *84*, 57–66.

Zaroff, C. M., & Isaacs, K. (2005). Neurocutaneous syndromes: Behavioral features. *Epilepsy and Behavior*, *7*, 133–142.

Zinkstok, J., & van Amelsvoort, T. (2005). Neuropsychological profile and neuroimaging in patients with 22Q11.2 deletion syndrome: A review. *Child Neuropsychology*, *11*, 21–37.

Zinn, A. R., Ramos, P., Elder, F. F., Kowal, K., Samango-Sprouse, C., & Ross, J. L. (2005). Androgen receptor CAGn repeat length influences phenotype of 47,XXY (Klinefelter) syndrome. *Journal of Clinical Endocrinology and Metabolism*, *90*, 5041–5046.

25 Psychosocial Adversity and Resilience

Jennifer Jenkins[1]

Human development is the process of individual adaptation to a complex and ever-changing environment. At times the adaptation is smooth; the environment provides support to the individual and the individual is able to use their own skills in a successful adaptation to their circumstance. At other times, however, the adaptation of the individual fails. This may be because the challenges in the environment are too great, the individual's abilities in adapting to their environment are insufficient or both individual and environmental factors combine together, such that the failure of adaptation can only be explained by understanding the ways in which both sets of processes operate together. This is called the study of risk and resilience. In this chapter we examine the environmental circumstances that pose challenges for children's development. We also consider why some children seem to manage better than others under similar degrees of environmental stress.

Much of our knowledge about processes of risk and resilience in children come from epidemiology. Population studies carried out from the 1960s onwards (Offord, Boyle, Szatmari *et al.*, 1987; Rutter, Tizard, & Whitmore, 1970) examined the ways in which mental health problems correlate with environmental adversity. Children have been found to show differential levels of aggression and violence as a function of countries, neighborhoods, schools and families (Boyle & Lipman, 2002; Jenkins, Simpson, Dunn *et al.*, 2005; Rutter, Maughan, Mortimore *et al.*, 1979). By studying characteristics of the environment and relating it to rates of disorder we have learned much about which children are likely to show problems. The bulk of the research that we present deals with findings from correlational studies (see chapter 5). Children are observed in their natural environment and patterns of correlation between their mental health and their environment are examined. Understanding patterns of correlation, although an important step in understanding causal process, is not equivalent to it. In order to understand the very specific mechanisms that are likely to explain why some children are more vulnerable than others, we need to draw on results from studies based on other designs.

In illustration of this problem we present the results from a study carried out by the author and colleagues to investigate protective factors of children exposed to marital conflict (Jenkins & Smith, 1990). This was a cross-sectional interview study with children and parents. First, we found that children being raised in high-conflict homes showed more disruptive behavior than children being raised in low-conflict homes. Second, we found that children living in high-conflict homes who had very close relationships with siblings or grandparents showed much lower levels of disturbance than children without a close relationship with a sibling or grandparent. Two conclusions suggested themselves. First, a process in the environment (exposure to parental conflict), either through modeling or some other learning mechanism, caused children to be aggressive. Second, social support from siblings and grandparents helped children in high-risk circumstances to withstand the adverse effects of those circumstances.

However, on the basis of the design it was impossible to rule out other explanations. The association between marital conflict and child adjustment might have been entirely genetically mediated. Biological parents pass on both genes and environments to children. Without some means of disentangling these two sets of influences we cannot conclude that environmental mediation operated.

The interpretation of social support as a protective influence was also questionable. A "child effect" (O'Connor, 2002) may have been operating such that characteristics of the child elicited social support from others. In other words, aspects of children's personalities may contribute to the environments that they shape around themselves. The critical point is that the mechanism is unclear.

Fortunately, data from different kinds of designs can help disambiguate such findings. Before presenting evidence on psychosocial adversity and resilience we describe the contributions that design innovations have made to this field.

Research Designs that Disambiguate Effects in Risk and Resilience Research

Experimental Design

The essence of experimental design is the random assignment of individuals to conditions. If we could:

Rutter's Child and Adolescent Psychiatry, 5th edition. Edited by M. Rutter, D. Bishop, D. Pine, S. Scott, J. Stevenson, E. Taylor and A. Thapar. © 2008 Blackwell Publishing, ISBN: 978-1-4051-4549-7.

[1] Written with Rossana Bisceglia, Connie Cheung, Kristen Frampton, Krista Gass, Andrea Gonzales, Anna Simpson, Rocio Valencia and Bing Yu.

1 Randomly assign children to homes in which they either experienced a lot of marital conflict or a little;
2 Ensure that both groups were equivalent on children's mental health at the start of the study; and
3 Hold all other aspects of the environment constant, then any changes in mental health could only be attributable to their exposure to marital conflict.

Because of the nature of the factors in risk research, however, random assignment to experimental conditions would never be allowed in children. Animal models are extremely valuable in this regard. Both rodents and non-human primates have been exposed to extreme environmental conditions that provide analogs to environmental risk that humans experience. Such studies have shown that environmental stress does change the neurobiology, physiology and behavior of the developing organism (Sanchez, Ladd, & Plotsky, 2001). Experimental paradigms offer the only incontrovertible method for establishing a causal effect. Of course, the problem with these models is one of generalization. Can the meaning of stressors be equated for humans and animals? How do we know whether humans respond in the same way as the species under investigation?

A second source of experimental data, also helpful in showing that environmental stress has a causal role in children's outcomes, comes from intervention studies that aim to reduce environmental adversity. Children showing disturbance and their families have been randomly assigned to treatment conditions in which the goal is to reduce one of the following environmental adversities: problematic parenting (DeGarmo & Forgatch, 2005; Olds, 1989), marital conflict (Stanley, Amato, Johnson *et al.*, 2006), neighborhood adversity (Leventhal & Brooks-Gunn, 2004); or a combination of high-risk circumstances including negative peer influence and parenting (Chamberlain & Reid, 1998). Results show that reducing environmental adversities does result in reduced psychopathology for children, lending support to the proposition that environmental adversity has a causal influence on behavior.

Disentangling Genetic from Environmental Influence

Genetically sensitive designs have been developed to tease apart genetic and environmental influence. As parents provide children with both genes and the environment in which children are raised, normal epidemiological designs confound these two influences. Details of behavioral genetic designs, including a critique of their strengths and weaknesses, can be found elsewhere (Rutter, 2002; also see chapter 23). Here we briefly describe the logic of the design and its importance for interpreting findings from risk and resilience research. The twin design teases apart genetic and environmental influences by comparing siblings who share 100% of their genes (monozygotic [MZ] twins) with those who share only half of their genes (dizygotic [DZ] twins). Knowing the degree of *genetic similarity* between the two types of twin and comparing their *behavioral similarity* allows one to make an inference about the relative importance of genes and the environment. The same estimates can be made utilizing samples of full, half, unrelated siblings and cousins (Guo & Wang, 2002). Results from genetically sensitive designs show that genetic influences are considerable, that siblings are more dissimilar than similar on behavior and personality once genetic effects have been controlled, and that environmental influences are considerable given that genetic influence rarely explains more than half the variance in behavior (Plomin, 1994; Rutter, Silberg, O'Connor *et al.*, 1999).

Three other genetically sensitive designs also provide evidence for environmental effects. The first type of design attempts to explain differences between MZ twins through exposure to adversity in the environment. As MZ twins are genetically identical, any differences in their behavior cannot be attributed to genetic influences. Investigators have found that differences in the child-rearing environment between two siblings have explained differences between the twins in their behavior (Caspi, Moffitt, Morgan *et al.*, 2004). A second genetically sensitive design involves an examination of the association between adversity and child outcome when parents and children are not genetically related. An association between parental divorce and disturbed child behavior was found amongst unrelated parents and their children (O'Connor, Caspi, DeFries *et al.*, 2000), suggesting that an environmental mechanism explained the association between divorce and child behavior.

The advent of molecular genetics has allowed for the investigation of gene–environment interaction in behavior: individual children may be more susceptible to the influence of negative environments if they carry specific polymorphisms on specific genes. Recent work in this area has shown evidence for this hypothesis in children (Caspi, McClay, Moffitt *et al.*, 2002; Caspi, Sugden, Moffitt *et al.*, 2003). Candidate genes are identified on the basis of animal work as well as case–control studies in humans. Levels of psychopathology amongst individuals in the population are examined as a function of environmental stress, polymorphisms of the gene under investigation and their combined effects that constitute the gene–environment interaction.

Longitudinal Models

Time has an important role in the attribution of causality when correlational data are examined. One criterion for arguing causation is that cause must precede effect. In a cross-sectional design this condition cannot be met. By utilizing longitudinal data we can examine whether an adverse environmental condition existed prior to a behavioral outcome and whether the condition predicts *change* in the behavioral outcome (see chapter 9). An autoregressive design deals with this issue: effects on behavior at time 2 are predicted by time 1 environmental adversities, while controlling for time 1 behavior. A cross-lagged design enables us to examine reciprocal effects: what effect do two factors have on one another over time? In these designs two processes that covary (e.g., parental harshness and difficult child behavior) are examined over time and the goal is to examine which of the two processes predicts change in the other more strongly (e.g., marital conflict predicts change in child behavior or child behavior predicts change in marital conflict). Examples of such designs can be seen in Hetherington, Henderson, Reiss *et al.* (1999) and Jenkins *et al.* (2005). Examining reciprocal effects is particularly important when family relationships are postulated as the psychosocial adversity. Family members are so proximal to one another, with so many occasions for mutual influence, that we need a design that will help differentiate between influences of different members in order to attribute causality correctly. Autoregressive and cross-lagged analyses investigate general patterns of association between measures in groups of children.

Growth curve modeling (Singer & Willett, 2003) investigates changes for individual children. In this, the behavioral trajectory of individual children can be modeled over time. Circumstances that vary in children's lives such as moving in and out of poverty, or changes in parents' marital circumstances (called time-varying predictors), can be used to explain changes in children's functioning. As we are using *changes* in the environment to predict *changes* in the child, the likelihood that associations are spurious is reduced. With such data it is still possible that a third variable, associated with both changes in the environment and changes in the child, is responsible for the correlation, which is why covariates are always entered into such models (see chapter 9).

Natural Experiments

One of the difficulties with correlational designs is that risks co-occur such that we have problems isolating the causal mechanism. Several investigators have capitalized on naturally occurring changes in environments to simulate a "natural experiment." The goal is to hold everything constant while one thing, the causal mechanism of interest, changes (Rutter, Pickles, Murray *et al.*, 2001). This method has been used to examine the impact of maternal anxiety on the developing fetus (King & Laplante, 2005), as well as the effects of poverty (Costello, Compton, Keeler *et al.*, 2003) and maternal deprivation on children (Rutter & O'Connor, 2004). Experiments are most closely simulated when the "condition effect" occurs randomly. Thus, when maternally deprived and non-deprived children are compared, the assumption is that the children in the two groups would have been indistinguishable before exposure to the stress and none of their characteristics influenced their membership in either group (referred to as a selection effect). When examining results from "natural" experiments it is important to evaluate the extent to which this condition has been met.

Testing Competing Models of Mechanism

In testing causality, the importance of working with competing models, not just disconfirming the null hypothesis, is well documented (Cochran & Chambers, 1965). In this type of study, several causal explanations of behavior are compared on the extent to which the different explanations explain the data. Jenkins, Shapka, & Sorenson (2006) examined the indirect effects, over a 12-year period, of maternal anger on children in a sample of women who had given birth when they were teenagers. Two potential mechanisms through which maternal anger prior to the birth of the child could lead to increased child opposition 12 years later were contrasted: exposure to partner conflict or partner relationship transitions. They found stronger support for the mechanism of partner conflict than relationship transitions.

Effects of Psychosocial Adversity on Children

Conceptual Issues

Before turning to empirical results on psychosocial adversity it is important to consider conceptual issues that must frame our interpretation of existing findings. We do this by considering the role of distal and proximal influences, the extent to which psychosocial adversities are shared by all members of a family or are child-specific, and the mechanisms through which environments affect behavior.

Multilevel Effects: Distal and Proximal Influences

Bronfenbrenner (1979) proposed a model for understanding context effects on children. He suggested that development occurred within embedded "layers" of context. The first layer involves relationships in which the child takes part: relationships with parents, siblings and peers. These interactions are embedded within structures that have a bearing on how the relationships develop. Thus, the pattern of interaction that occurs in a stepfamily is different from that in an intact family (Hetherington, Henderson, Reiss *et al.*, 1999). Bullying in a peer group is a function of the number and proximity of teachers supervising in the playground (Stephens, 1997). More distal influences such as the economics of the community in which school and family structures are embedded will have a further impact on their functioning. Cultures, cultural values, customs and laws represent yet another layer. Such distal influences can be significant, for instance in national differences in homicide (Krug, Powell, & Dahlberg, 1998) related to laws surrounding gun control.

It is necessary to distinguish proximal and distal influences on children. These are relative terms to connote the proximity of the influence on the child. For instance, a friendship with a deviant peer is a more proximal influence than the child being raised in a high-crime neighborhood. Although distal and proximal are simply descriptive terms, they are most commonly used within the framework of mediation. Within this framework, proximal influences have a direct influence on children's functioning, and distal influences have a direct influence on the proximal process but an indirect influence on the child. Poverty leading to an increase in harsh parenting, which in turn has an influence on children's antisocial behavior, are examples of distal and proximal risks within a mediation model (Baron & Kenny, 1986). A mediational model requires that a direct effect is established between the distal process and both the mediator (proximal process) and the outcome, when bivariate correlations are examined. When both the distal and mediator variables are in the model, the mediator should explain some of the variance in the outcome which was initially explained by the distal variable.

Mediational models are often considered to be "causal" models: the mediator is conceptualized as the active agent that is causally responsible for the relationship between two other variables. It is important to note, however, that theories of causation are very discipline-based and influenced by our current scientific knowledge. For example, although "modeling" offers a causal mechanism for behavioral scientists, for neuroscientists causal mechanisms occur at synapses. For a neuroscientist, a parent's aggressive displays towards a child will always be an indirect effect, explained by the more proximal mechanism of the change in neurotransmitters that influences behavior. One of the challenges in developmental science is to link up explanatory mechanisms at different levels of description.

Family Level and Child-Specific Risks within Families

One of the most intriguing findings from behavioral genetic research is that children who are raised in the same family and thus share a common environment are more dissimilar than similar after controlling for genetic effects (Plomin & Daniels, 1987). How can environmental influences operate if children develop so differently from one another while exposed to similar influences? We need to distinguish between two aspects of environmental influence: the objective and effective environments (Turkheimer & Waldron, 2000). The *objective environment* refers to the measured environment that children experience: the amount of parental conflict in their home, the parenting that they receive and the income level of parents. The *effective environment* is not directly measured but refers instead to the extent of sibling similarity (given that siblings are raised in a similar environment). The concept comes from behavioral genetics. In this field, inferences about the operation of the environment are made on the basis of the similarity and differences between siblings on behavior and personality (after accounting for genetic effects; see chapter 23). Findings about sibling dissimilarity, once genetic effects have been accounted for (the effective environment), have led environmental researchers to develop more sophisticated ways of thinking about how objective environments affect children.

The objective environment can be divided into the family and the child-specific. Environmental risks that are held in common by all siblings in a family can be thought of as family level risks (e.g., parental divorce). Experiences such as the way that a parent relates to a child, or the child's peer relationships, will vary across children in the same family and are therefore child-specific. Risks that we might think of as family level, such as parental conflict, depending on the way in which the construct is measured and the way that it is expressed in a family, may be child-specific. Jenkins *et al.* (2005) found that siblings had more similar experiences of exposure to parental conflict than they had about the amount that parents argued about them. Thus, exposure to parental conflict is more of a family level risk than amount of parental argument about children.

As siblings are more dissimilar than similar once genetic effects have been taken into account, some have argued that family level environmental influences cannot have a large causal role in disturbance (Harris, 1998). This is not the case. It may be that family level risks are important influences on behavior but they operate by increasing dissimilarity between siblings. Jenkins *et al.* (2005) found that marital conflict at time 1 increased the dissimilarity between siblings on disruptive behavior from time 1 to time 2. This is likely to be because of endogenous factors already operating within children at the time of the stress. One sibling may react to parental conflict with increased aggression, but in a child without such a behavioral tendency, increased aggression will not occur.

A second source of sibling difference is the set of risk factors unique to individual children (e.g., hostile parenting and negative peer relationships). Although child-specific experiences are certainly important in understanding sibling differences, they have not been found to explain as much variance (1–5%) in sibling differences as was once hoped (Turkheimer & Waldron, 2000). By differentiating between family level and child-specific risks and utilizing research designs that allow us to look at both the objective and effective environments, we can gain some clarity on the ways in which adverse environments influence children.

Mechanisms Involved in Stress Causing Emotional and Behavioral Disturbance in Children

Probably the best way to think about the adverse effects of stress on humans is to think about the way in which environmental adversity affects the emotion system. Emotions involve many component processes with manifestations that can be biological, behavioral, cognitive or relational. The emotion system refers to all these component parts that make up emotional experience. Thus, the experience of anger is associated with characteristic muscle movements of the face, cognitions about the intent of other people in their actions towards the self, as well as behaviors such as raising the voice and aggression towards others. There are also characteristic interpersonal consequences from the expression of anger (for a review of all of these areas see Oatley, Keltner, & Jenkins, 2006). Although connections across components of the emotion system have been established (Oatley, Keltner, & Jenkins, 2006; Panksepp, 1998), there is enormous complexity in how experiences in one part of the system affect another. Thus, associations have been shown between biology and behavior; cognitions and behavior; behavior, cognition and relationships. However, the direction of causality is not well understood, and bidirectional influences are likely. Thus, depression is thought to involve a perturbation of the neurotransmitter serotonin. Cognitive therapy, shown to be effective in the treatment of depression, involves changing cognitions with a consequent change in behavior and mood. Have cognitions changed neurotransmitters?

Stressful environments have been shown to affect all levels of the emotion system. Experiments with rodents and non-human primates show that multiple biological systems are affected including the hypothalamic–pituitary–adrenal (HPA) axis, neurotransmitter systems and brain cytoarchitecture (Fleming, 2006; Kraemer, 1992; Repetti, Taylor, & Seeman, 2002; Sanchez, Ladd, & Plotsky, 2001). In humans, environmental stressors have been shown to influence the functioning of the HPA axis, patterns of cognitive appraisal, emotion understanding, perception of others' emotions and psychopathology (Bugenthal, Martorell, & Barraza, 2003; Cole, Teti, & Zahn-Waxler, 2003; Dodge, Bates, & Pettit, 1990; Fries & Pollak, 2004).

Empirical Findings on Distal Risk Factors

Distal risk factors are those associated with behavioral problems in children, which increase the risk of proximal stresses and play an indirect part in children's disturbance.

Deprived Neighborhoods

Deprived neighborhoods have impoverished conditions characterized by high unemployment rates, predominate minority populations, dense public housing, crime and violence, as well as social isolation (e.g., Massey & Kanaiaupuni, 1993). Effects of deprived neighborhoods account for 5–10% of the variance observed in developmental outcomes (Leventhal & Brooks-Gunn, 2000).

Boyle and Lipman (2002), in a Canadian sample, found that 4–5% of the variance in teacher reported emotional and conduct problems was attributable to neighborhood. Xue, Leventhal, Brooks-Gunn *et al.* (2005), in Chicago, found that 11% of the variance in emotional disturbance was attributable to the neighborhood. Further, using an autoregressive design, they showed that characteristics of neighborhoods predicted a *change* in emotional disturbance over 2 years. This provides more compelling evidence than a cross-sectional study for a causal effect. However, methodological problems of a correlational design remain. Although many individual and family level characteristics are included in models examining the effect of neighborhoods on children, it remains possible that uncontrolled effects at the individual and family levels contribute to the neighborhood effect (poor families end up in poor neighborhoods; Duncan, Connell, & Klebanov, 1997).

Results from an experimental study (Leventhal & Brooks-Gunn, 2004), the Move to Opportunity (MTO) program, provide more compelling causal data. Families recruited from high-poverty neighborhoods in the USA were randomly assigned to the experimental or control condition. The experimental group was given vouchers to move to a low-poverty area. Control families were not offered the option of moving. Children's achievement was tested on standardized reading and math tests 2.5 years after their families had entered into the program. Approximately 40% of families in the experimental condition took up the option of moving and effects were calculated for all families (intention to treat). Positive effects were most evident for adolescent boys, who showed significantly higher scores on reading and math than boys in the control group. Children who moved to low-poverty neighborhoods were found to engage in more homework, which was identified as a partial mediator of the program effect. Some caution must be exercised about the long-term benefits, as a subsequent follow-up (Leventhal, Fauth, & Brooks-Gunn, 2005) did not reveal significant program effects (thought to be the result of selective attrition in the control group).

One component of the neighborhood effect may be exposure to violence, with most relevant studies sampling in deprived US cities. Gorman-Smith and Tolan (1998) interviewed African-American and Latino adolescents in public high schools in deprived neighborhoods in the Chicago area, with the majority of the sample living in poverty. They found that 16.5% reported that a family member had been robbed or attacked and 15.6% had seen someone shot or killed in the previous year. These rates are consistent with those reported by others working with samples drawn from deprived US neighborhoods (Aisenberg & Ell, 2005). With respect to possible causal effects on emotional and behavioral problems, Gorman-Smith and Tolan (1998) found that exposure to violence in the community at time 1 predicted an increase in adolescents' disruptive behavior over a 1-year period. The use of the autoregressive design strengthened the conclusion that violence exposure was causally related to the development of disturbance rather than simply an association.

Deprived neighborhoods have negative effects on parents. In poor neighborhoods parents show higher levels of depression, less positive parenting and more negative parenting (Klebanov, Brooks-Gunn, & Duncan, 1994; Pinderhughes, Nix, Foster *et al.*, 2001). Effects on parents partially mediate the negative influence of poor neighborhoods on negative child outcomes (Gutman, McLoyd, & Tokoyawa, 2005).

Exposure to War

Children in war-torn countries can be exposed to extremely high levels of violence. Three thousand and thirty children 8–19 years old living in 11 prefectures were interviewed in the year following the Rwandan genocide (Dyregrov, Gupta, Gjestad *et al.*, 2000). Seventy-eight percent of those interviewed experienced a death in the family, while 70% saw someone being killed or injured and 15% reported hiding under a dead body to escape detection during the massacre. Rates of disturbance among refugee children are substantially higher than amongst non-refugee populations (Hodes, 2000). Rates vary as a function of direct exposure to violence and trauma (Sack, McSharry, Clarke *et al.*, 1994). The most common form of psychopathology found in children and youth exposed to war violence is post-traumatic stress disorder (PTSD), but the full range of childhood disorder is also seen (Howard & Hodes, 2000; see chapters 31 & 42). In a random sample of 209 youth who were living in Cambodia during the Pol Pot regime who subsequently emigrated to the USA, the prevalence of PTSD was 18%. Fifty-three percent of their mothers had PTSD. It is important to note that there is marked heterogeneity in levels of disturbance amongst children exposed to violence. Factors that account for such heterogeneity are discussed on p. 386 (see also chapter 31).

Poverty

Many studies have shown that living in poverty is associated with increased risk of mental health problems in children. Here we describe four studies that use methodologies that suggest a causal influence of poverty on children's behavior. Costello *et al.* (2003) took advantage of a natural experiment in order to investigate the impact on children of an acute infusion of money into a previously poor community. Fortuitously, a longitudinal study was ongoing on a Native American reserve that later housed a new casino. The casino provided every Native American family with an income supplement. Children's behavior was compared pre- and post-casino. When children were able to move out of poverty, a reduction in conduct problems was observed. Emotional problems did not, however, show a similar reduction.

Two other studies use longitudinal data and growth curve modeling to examine changes in children's well-being as a function of changes in their environment. Macmillan, McMorris, & Kruttschnitt (2004) examined whether changes in mothers' lives on poverty, marital status, education and employment predicted antisocial behavior of children using four waves of child data from the 1979 National Longitudinal Survey of Youth (NLSY79). Investigators coded families for changes in poverty, and formed groups who had experienced poverty for varying lengths of time and at different times in the children's lives. Years living in poverty had a large effect on initial levels of antisocial behavior. Further, children exposed to persistent poverty, those who only moved out of poverty for a short time and those who moved into poverty showed faster *rates of change* on antisocial behavior than children who had never lived in poverty. One methodological advantage of this study was that many other time-varying demographic predictors such as periods of unemployment, changes in marital status and changes in maternal education were included in the models. Effects of poverty were stronger than any other demographic factors and persisted after all such effects were accounted for. The NICHD Early Child Care Research Network (2005) reported similar findings.

Similar to the research on neighborhoods, parenting has been found to have a mediating role in the relationship between poverty and children's well-being. Several researchers have shown that the psychological stress associated with poverty increases parents' use of harsh and unsupportive parenting, which subsequently leads to adverse mental health outcomes in children and adolescents (Grant, Compas, Stuhlmacher *et al.*, 2003).

In addition to harsh inconsistent parenting, poverty also affects parental abilities to monitor their children. In the natural experiment described above (Costello *et al.*, 2003), when parents moved out of poverty their supervision of children increased. This in turn explained the relationship between poverty and children's antisocial behavior. Differential parenting refers to the extent of difference in parental behavior to different children in the family. Higher levels of differential parenting predict more negative outcomes in children (Dunn, Stocker, & Plomin, 1991). Jenkins, Rasbash, & O'Connor (2003) found that differential parenting was greater in families experiencing socioeconomic deprivation.

There are experimental data from animal work on foraging that may have some relevance for the effects of poverty on parenting. Champoux, Zanker, & Levine (1993) randomly assigned squirrel monkeys to conditions that varied on how easy it was to find food. When it took more effort to find food, monkeys showed more inactivity and chronically elevated cortisol than when food was more easily available. Extending this design, Lyons, Kim, Schatzberg *et al.* (1998) looked at the effect on mothers and their offspring. They found that when it was harder to find food, parenting became less optimal: mothers pushed their offspring towards less contact, while infants demanded more contact. As in the Champoux, Zanker, & Levine (1993) study, there was a negative impact of the experimental condition on maternal physiology (elevated cortisol) although the same effect on the infants' physiology was not seen. Results suggest that exposing mothers to scarce resources may have a negative effect on their own stress reactivity as well as their parental behavior. Although we cannot directly equate foraging for food in squirrel monkeys with exposure to poverty in humans, it may be that there is commonality in the experience of not having ready access to the basics that support existence and the effect on physiological systems in animals and humans.

Empirical Findings on Proximal Risk Factors

Parenting

Failures of parenting represent the best-documented proximal risks in childhood. We deal with two types of parenting risk: attachment failures and parenting quality.

Parenting in early infancy centers on attachment processes. Bowlby (1971) proposed that the attachment system is a biobehavioral system developed for the protection of young. He suggested that the parent provides the infant with a secure base from which to explore the world. When the infant experiences fear he or she signals distress to the parent and the parent responds by providing protection. The core mechanism of this theory relates to parental responsivity to distress (Goldberg, Grusec, & Jenkins, 1999). As the infant enters the second year of life, and representational abilities including linguistic skills become more advanced, physical proximity is no longer necessary to provide this sense of protection to the infant. It has been suggested that mental representations, based on the infant's experiences with the caregivers at times of distress, form the basis for the development of subsequent close relationships built on trust.

The best evidence that failures of the attachment system affect infants comes from a series of studies beginning in the 1950s examining the outcomes of children who were raised without primary attachment figures (see chapter 55). Deficits in cognitive and socioemotional development have been noted

(Rutter & O'Connor, 2004). This experience is associated with relationship anomalies in childhood, such as indiscriminant friendliness and poor peer relationships (Chisholm, 1999). In adulthood, women institutionalized as children are more likely to have difficulties parenting their infants and likely to experience more relationship transitions with partners. Depression and other mental health problems are more likely (Quinton & Rutter, 1988). Similarly detrimental outcomes have been noted for children who are raised in the family home but experience high levels of parental neglect (Trickett & McBride-Chang, 1995). It is notable that there is enormous heterogeneity amongst individuals who have been exposed to institutional care, with some showing no adverse outcomes and others showing very compromised development, an issue that we return to later.

Results from experimental studies in animals support the findings for humans and suggest some of the physiological systems that are involved in the relationship between psychosocial adversities and negative outcomes. Rodent models involve offspring being raised without their mothers. These separations lead to marked behavioral abnormalities in adulthood. Maternally deprived rats show reduced consumption of sweetened solution (perhaps indicative of anhedonia), as well as increased freezing, decreased exploration in an open field test and of novel environments, increased acoustic startle response as well as increased hyperactivity and inattention (Caldji, Francis, Sharma *et al.*, 2000; Fleming, 2006; Fleming & Li, 2002; Ladd, Huot, Thrivikraman *et al.*, 2000).

These behavioral changes are accompanied by a myriad of physiological and neurobiological alterations that last into adulthood. Maternally separated rats exhibit differences in HPA axis response to stressors, such as increased adrenocorticotropic hormone (ACTH) and corticosterone (Ladd *et al.*, 2000), alterations in corticosterone releasing factor system (CRF; Ladd *et al.*, 2000; Plotsky & Meaney, 1993) and serotonergic and GABA dysfunction (Caldji *et al.*, 2000). These studies suggest that maternal separation during critical periods of development produce enduring neurobiological changes.

Similar studies have been carried out with non-human primates raised without mothers. In one study, infant rhesus monkeys were separated from their mothers within 2 days of birth, and were either mother-deprived or raised with a terry-cloth surrogate mother for the first 30 days of life (Kraemer, Ebert, Schmidt *et al.*, 1991). Both groups of maternally separated monkeys developed depression symptoms and lower CNS concentrations of norephinephrine (Kraemer *et al.*, 1991). Other studies have found increased pituitary–adrenal and behavioral responses to stress in adulthood in monkeys that were maternally deprived during infancy (Suomi, 1991). This evidence across humans and animals, both correlational and experimental, suggests that deprivation in care for infants has a causal role in the development of disturbance.

Non-attachment-based aspects of parenting become important beyond infancy. The study of parenting quality is extensive and diverse (Bornstein, 1995). Here we concentrate only on those aspects of parenting that have been shown to increase the risk of psychopathology in children. The aspect of parenting most consistently linked to psychopathology is parental harshness. Harsh parenting can be viewed dimensionally with physical abuse as the endpoint. Effects, however, are evident all along the continuum and long before physical abuse is an issue. Harsh parenting involves verbal aggression, hostility and criticism towards children. It has been shown to predict *change* in child behavior using a longitudinal design that controls for previous behavior, lending support to the idea that harsh parenting has a causal role in childhood disturbance (Ge, Conger, Cadoret *et al.*, 1996; Kim, Conger, Lorenz *et al.*, 2001). Physical abuse is associated with an increased risk of both disruptive and emotional psychopathology in children (Cicchetti & Toth, 2005), as well as antisocial personality disorder (Caspi *et al.*, 2002), depression and anxiety in adulthood (Brown, Harris, & Eales, 1996).

It should be remembered that aversive interactions between parents and children are partially child-driven effects. Children who are hyperactive, impulsive and negative in their mood (Bates, Pettit, Dodge *et al.*, 1998; Shaw, Owens, Giovannelli *et al.*, 2001) are harder for parents to manage. Patterson, Capaldi, & Bank (1991) have proposed a social learning mechanism to explain how ineffective parenting of temperamentally difficult children can result in later disruptive behavior problems for children, based on longitudinal observations of parent–child behavior.

Differential parenting is another aspect of parenting found to increase the risk of psychopathology. Caspi *et al.* (2004) investigated the longitudinal effects of differential parenting on MZ twins. They found that differential harsh parenting did predict increased disruptive behavior in the twin who was treated more negatively. It is also interesting to note that higher average differential parenting in a family is associated with more negative adjustment amongst all children, after accounting for individual level effects (Boyle, Jenkins, Georgiades *et al.*, 2004). This suggests that not only is differential parenting more negative for the individual who experiences most harshness, but there is also a spillover element such that all siblings are worse off when treatment across children is more differential.

Another dimension of parenting that is associated with psychopathology, particularly disruptive behavior and particularly in adolescence, is lack of parental monitoring. Parental knowledge about where children are, who they are with and what they are doing, has been found to be a strong predictor of youth crime; interventions that increase parental monitoring by tracking children and doing random checks on their whereabouts have reduced antisocial behavior (Dishion & Kavanagh, 2003). However, see Kerr and Stattin (2000) for evidence that, at least in part, this reflects what children choose to tell parents about their activities.

Siblings

Another proximal process shown to affect the development of disorder in children is aggression in the sibling relationship.

Patterson (1984) has suggested that siblings train one another towards higher levels of aggression through escalating coercive behavior that results in the other sibling backing down. Sibling interactions in the home have been observed over time. Using an autoregressive design, the aggression of one child has been shown to predict a change in the aggression of the other child for preschool (Garcia, Shaw, Winslow *et al.*, 2000) and adolescent boys (Bank, Burraston, & Snyder, 2004).

Peers

A similar risk mechanism to that described for siblings is likely to operate for peers. Several studies, including one involving an experimental design, have shown that peers may train one another to increased levels of deviant disruptive behavior. The most convincing demonstration of the negative impact of deviant peers comes from a group treatment study (Dishion, McCord, & Poulin, 1999). The experimental group was offered treatment for their delinquency in a group setting. The treatment for the comparison group was individually administered. Boys were randomly assigned to treatments and the two groups were indistinguishable at the start of treatment. The investigators were surprised to find on follow-up that adolescents who were treated in group settings showed a major rise in delinquency over time. Through group treatment the investigators had inadvertently facilitated introductions to other delinquent youth. The boys formed groups outside of the sessions. They reinforced one another, exchanged techniques and encouraged further delinquent activities. Other studies have produced somewhat inconsistent findings on peer group deviancy amplifying effects (Dodge, Dishion & Lansford, 2006). That they can occur is not in doubt, but uncertainties remain on their generality.

Exposure to deviant peers is not only a problem in adolescence. Boys in grade 1 were assessed and followed up into their early adolescence (Kellam, Ling, Merisca *et al.*, 1998). After taking account of the boys' own aggression in grade 1, the average level of aggression in the classroom predicted an increase in target boys' aggression over the next 7 years. Howes (2000) assessed levels of aggression in preschool classes in childcare settings. When the proportion of aggressive children was higher in the preschool daycare, this resulted in children being more aggressive themselves when they entered grade 2, after taking account of children's own aggression in preschool.

Marital Conflict

The following three risks – marital conflict, separation and parental depression – show both distal (indirect) and proximal (direct) properties with respect to children's outcomes.

Marital conflict has been found to be associated with a wide range of emotional and disruptive behavior outcomes, with the association between the latter and marital conflict being particularly robust. A number of studies provide convincing longitudinal evidence that marital conflict influences child behavior, in designs whereby marital conflict at time 1 predicted child behavior at time 2, controlling for child behavior at time 1 (Davies, Harold, Goeke-Morey *et al.*, 2002; Grych, Harold, & Miles, 2003; Jenkins *et al.*, 2005).

The aspect of marital conflict found to be most harmful for children is openly expressed, interparental hostility or aggression. Silence, ignoring or other unexpressed modes of unhappiness in marriage do not have the same negative impact on children, at least in the short term (Jenkins & Smith, 1991). Children rate themselves as feeling more upset by conflict that remains unresolved between parents than conflict that is resolved (Cummings & Davies, 1994). Conflict that is about children has been found to be more distressing than conflict that is about non-child-related issues (Grych & Fincham, 1993).

There is enormous variability in the extent to which children are negatively affected by marital conflict. Children's attributional processes concerning the conflict explain some of this variability. Those who perceive the conflict as threatening to family well-being (Davies, Harold, Goeke-Morey *et al.*, 2002) or who blame themselves for it are more adversely affected (Grych, Harold, & Miles, 2003). Attributional processes change as children mature cognitively. When children are around 5 years of age their understanding of parental conflict tends to be more self-focused, behavioral and unidimensional. By 9 years old they show a more complex understanding that involves understanding how two parents can have different goals and the implication of triangulation for family relationships (Jenkins & Buccioni, 2000). The quality of the parent–child relationship has been found to be a partial mediator of the relationship between marital conflict and children's well-being (Buehler & Gerard, 2002).

Separation and Divorce

Parental divorce is associated with an increased risk of psychopathology (Amato, 2001; Cherlin, Furstenberg, Chase-Landale *et al.*, 1991) which continues into adulthood (Amato & Sobolewski, 2001). Several reasons for this association including father absence, decreased access to financial resources for the custodial parent and undermined parenting have been examined. The strongest factors, however, appear to be the presence of interparental conflict (Amato, 2001) and disruptions to parenting (Amato & Sobolewski, 2001). These usually precede and follow separation. There is also some evidence to suggest that marital quality prior to divorce affects how divorce is experienced: children react more adversely when there has been low parental conflict prior to divorce. When conflict is high it may be that divorce is more welcome (Morrison & Coiro, 1999).

Parental Mental Illness

Children are at risk who have a parent with depression (Dowdney & Coyne, 1990), schizophrenia (Niemi, Survisaari, & Huakka, 2004), alcoholism (Lewis, 2000) or personality disorder (Jaffee, Moffitt, Caspi *et al.*, 2003; see chapter 25). The transmission of the risk is both genetic and environmental. Significant genetic influence has been described for the most common emotional and disruptive behavior disorders for children (Rutter *et al.*, 1999). The environmental effect is explained by a disturbance in parenting as well as concomitant exposure to other risks such as parental conflict (Dowdney & Coyne, 1990). Risks have been shown to potentiate one another (Rutter, 1979) such that children exposed to multiple family adversities are more likely to demonstrate disturbance than children exposed to single risks. Parental depression has been shown to be associated with more problematic attachment processes (Lyons-Ruth, Connell, Grunebaum *et al.*, 1990), lower levels of warmth, monitoring and discipline (Cummings, Keller, & Davies, 2005) and less verbalization to children with later effects on vocabulary (Pan, Rowe, Singer *et al.*, 2005). Maternal depression and anxiety during pregnancy may have negative effects on the developing fetus (Van den Bergh & Marcoen, 2004), as prenatal exposure has been shown to predict disturbance in later childhood after accounting for any periods of postnatal exposure.

Summary of Effects of Psychosocial Adversity on Children

In summary, the evidence suggests that exposure to a range of environmental adversities increases the risk of disorder in children. However, there is enormous heterogeneity in children's response to stressful environments. Although some children react to stress with the development of psychopathology, other children show no adverse behavioral reaction. One type of environmental adversity does not cause one type of disturbance; most of the risks outlined above have been shown to result in an increase in both emotional and disruptive behavior disturbances. The relationship between the type of risk to which a child is exposed and the outcome that results is non-specific. One reason for heterogeneity in response to stress relates to individual vulnerability, both genetic and non-genetic, as well as the complex ways that factors across different levels of children's environments operate together. These issues are discussed next.

Resilience

Conceptual Issues

Resilience is the study of individual differences in response to stress. The interest in resilience research lies in understanding why certain children are more vulnerable to the adverse effects of negative environments than other children. The study of this issue should not be confused with the study of why some children show better functioning than other children. When children across the population are compared with one another there are large differences in adjustment that can be accounted for simply by the presence and severity of risks in their lives. This difference in functioning amongst children is sometimes referred to by researchers as resilience (Luthar, Cicchetti, & Becker, 2000; Masten, Hubbard, Gest *et al.*, 1999). However, this is not how the term is used in this chapter. Here we use it to refer only to children who do well despite the fact that they are exposed to high levels of environmental adversity. We want to know that the same factor does not operate to confer advantage to all children (both children exposed and not exposed to adversity), but rather that it operates specifically to confer protection on children that need protection. Demonstrating that a factor operates differently for children in high- and low-risk circumstances requires the investigation of contingencies, an issue that we return to shortly. The study of resilience is explicitly inferential (Riley & Masten, 2005). Judgments are made regarding the exposure of individuals to experiences that have the *potential* to disrupt normative functioning, but this potential is not realized in a minority of individuals, who are resilient.

Resilience is best understood from the perspective of developmental processes and transactional models. Individuals are in continual interaction with other social and physical systems (Sameroff & Mackenzie, 2003). Accordingly, resilience is a dynamic process that involves adaptations that occur prior to, during and after stress exposure (Rutter, 1999). Individual adaptation arises from many dynamic processes occurring *within* the organism at the biological (e.g., genetic, hormonal) and behavioral levels (e.g., attention, capacity for learning) as well as *between* the organism and the various levels of the different systems in which the individual is embedded (close relationships with caregivers and peers, influences from school and community). This complex process of adaptation can function to alter the impact of adverse events on the organism, increasing or decreasing individual susceptibility (Masten & Powell, 2003).

Contingencies occur within and across developmental periods. Most of the literature on resilience deals with contingencies that involve predictors moderating one another within a developmental period. But contingencies are also evident across time that depend on the way in which events are sequenced or when they occur. Connor, Morrison, & Petrella (2004) have shown that certain types of reading instruction only benefit the child when preceded by other types of instruction. The formation of good peer relationships in middle childhood is in part dependent on attachment relationships during infancy (Sroufe, Egeland, & Carlson, 1999). Events at one point in a life can have more of an impact than at another point. Elder and Clipp (1988) found that friendships developed during war combat were experienced as more significant (and presumably more protective) than those developed under less traumatic circumstances.

The demonstration of contingent effects in human research is somewhat crude as it relies on statistical interactions between two influences. These can be hard to identify (McClelland & Judd, 1993; Rutter & Pickles, 1991), even when contingent influences are almost certainly occurring. In order to demonstrate contingent relationships the design needs to include children in high- and low-stress environments. If a significant interaction is present, a second factor has a different effect on the outcome in high- and low-risk circumstances. When referring to beneficial outcomes under high-risk circumstances this second factor is called protective, when referring to negative outcomes it is called a vulnerability factor. These are simply two ways of discussing the same contingent effect. Different kinds of contingencies, with slightly different meanings, have been outlined (Luthar, Cicchetti, & Becker, 2000). Examining contingent relationships gives us unique insight into the ways in which factors combine to moderate the influence of one another.

Empirical Findings on Child-Specific Attributes: Biological, Cognitive and Behavioral as Moderators of Stress

We begin by considering child-specific characteristics at the biological, behavioral and cognitive levels that have been shown to moderate the impact of psychosocial adversity. These factors describe vulnerabilities about individual children that result in certain children being more susceptible to the adverse effects of stress. The results we describe are based on single-child-per-family designs; there have been few sibling studies of resilience. The factors to be discussed, however, as assessed at the child-specific level, should also explain within-family differences in development. Future research will examine whether these child-specific factors explain why siblings react to family level environmental adversities so differently.

Biological Moderators

Biological vulnerabilities may be endogenous (e.g., genetic effects) or they may arise from environmental adversities that affect the developing brain (Repetti, Taylor, & Seeman, 2002). Thus, smoking (Fergusson, 1999) during pregnancy has been found to be associated with an increased risk of emotional and behavioral problems later in child development, as is poor nutrition in early childhood (Liu, Raine, Venables *et al.*, 2004). These biological vulnerabilities may in turn alter the individual's susceptibility to subsequent stressors. This process is referred to as the diathesis–stress model: the vulnerabilities of some individuals (diatheses) increase susceptibility to the adverse effects of stress (Davidson & Neale, 2001). Here we review a range of individual diatheses that demonstrate such patterns.

Polymorphisms of genes that affect neurotransmitters have been found to increase vulnerability to stress for certain types of disturbance. The MAOA enzyme is involved in the metabolism of mono-amine neurotransmitters, and one form of a *MAOA* gene has been found in animal and human studies to be associated with increased aggression. Following this research, Caspi *et al.* (2002) found that males with this form of the *MAOA* gene were at very high risk for conduct disorder when they had also been exposed to maltreatment during childhood. The presence of either risk – this particular form of the gene or exposure to maltreatment – did not raise the risk of disorder if present on its own. In a second study on the same sample, Caspi *et al.* (2003) found that individuals exposed to life events were more likely to develop depression if they had a short, rather than a long form of a gene involved in the production of serotonin. Experimental work with rhesus monkeys gives a further indication of mechanism (Kraemer, 1992; Suomi, 2005). Bennett, Lesch, Heils *et al.* (2002) found lower concentrations of a serotonin metabolite in the cerebrospinal fluid of monkeys who were peer reared (stress condition) and had the short rather than the long form variant of the serotonin gene. The gene was not associated with concentrations of the serotonin metabolite in mother-reared animals. These studies show first that genetic diatheses exist that increase individual vulnerability to disorders in the presence of particular kinds of life stresses and, second, that neurotransmitters are likely to be important mediators in this process.

Vagal tone is another biological factor that has been shown to moderate the effects of stressful environments. It represents a measure of emotion regulation as it represents an individual's ability to maintain homeostasis and regulate physiologically (Porges, 1995). Low vagal tone has been found to be associated with behavioural problems. El-Sheikh (2005) found that for children with high vagal tone, exposure to parental alcohol abuse did not predict an increase in externalizing or internalizing problems. For children with low vagal tone, however, exposure to parental alcohol abuse was a predictor of an increase in both types of symptomatology over time.

Cognitive Moderators

Masten, Hubbard, Gest *et al.* (1999) predicted change in positive behavioral functioning from childhood to adolescence as a function of life events and children's IQ in a 10-year longitudinal study. They found that IQ protected children from *developing* conduct problems when they were exposed to significant life events. When children experienced few life events, IQ was a weaker predictor of change in conduct problems. The use of the autoregressive design made for a stronger argument with respect to causal processes.

The ways that children and adults appraise or give meaning to events in their world have also been found to be important contingencies in how individuals react to stress. Negative appraisals of the self (Hammen, 1988) and events in the world (Mazur, Wolchik, Virdin *et al.*, 1999) have been shown to increase individual vulnerability to adverse environments. A similar moderating effect has been shown for children's social problem-solving skills (Dubow & Tisak, 1989).

Coping Moderators

Individuals differ in their sense of personal agency and the repertoire of coping mechanisms they can utilize when faced with adversity (Rutter, 2006). Although research evidence is lacking to show that such factors *moderate* the relationship between risk and adjustment, such factors have been shown to differentiate between the outcomes of high-risk children. Hauser, Allen, & Golden (2006) interviewed adults admitted to a psychiatric institution as adolescents. They found that adolescents with a sense of personal agency, a self-reflective style and a commitment to relationships experienced far better outcomes than adolescents who did not possess these characteristics.

Temperament Moderators

Temperament refers to stable individual differences in emotionality and self-regulation that are thought to have a biological basis (Goldsmith, 1993; see chapter 14). Positive mood has been shown to buffer the negative effects of family stress on drug abuse (Wills, Sandy, Yaeger *et al.*, 2001). Inhibitory control and attention regulation have been shown to moderate the impact of stressful family and neighborhood environments (Lengua, 2002; Lynam, Caspi, Moffit *et al.*, 2000).

Empirical Findings on Relationships as Moderators of Stress

Social support is the most consistent "external" factor found to moderate psychosocial adversity. Beneficial effects of social support have been shown for adults and children and across a wide variety of stresses. Social support has been operationalized in many ways, but basically indicates whether a person is accepted, loved and involved in social relationships where communication is open (Sarason, Shearin, Pierce *et al.*, 1987).

Warm and nurturant parent–child relationships have been found to moderate the effects of psychosocial adversity on children (Masten, Hubbard, Gest *et al.*, 1999). Wyman, Cowen, Work *et al.* (1999) found that parenting practices that emphasized the emotional and instrumental needs of the child and that managed behavior with minimal coercive tactics and threats were associated with lower levels of aggression amongst families living in poverty. Moderating effects of social support have been shown for emotional and behavioral problems (Youngstrom, Weist, & Albus, 2003), school performance (Cauce, Hannan, & Sargeant, 1992) and substance abuse (Wills, Sandy, Yaeger *et al.*, 2001). The quality of the parent–child relationship during childhood has been found to act as a buffer for life events during adult life (Dougherty, Klein, & Davila, 2004).

Affectionate sibling relationships have also been found to decrease the risk of emotional disorders in response to life events in a longitudinal study (Gass, Jenkins, & Dunn, 2007). Kempton, Armistead, Wierson *et al.* (1991) found that simply the presence of a sibling was protective for children exposed to parental divorce. Relationships with grandparents appear to function in a similar way (Jenkins & Smith, 1990).

Children derive positive and compensatory effects from their relationships with peers. In a 2-year longitudinal study involving 5-year-old children, Criss, Pettit, Bates *et al.* (2002) found that children who experienced higher levels of family adversity (ecological disadvantage, violent marital conflict and harsh discipline) benefited from having greater peer acceptance and friendship at time 1 (kindergarten and grade 1). These positive peer experiences also protected them against later victimization (Schwartz, Dodge, Pettit *et al.*, 2000).

There is some suggestion that for maximum efficacy the source of social support may need to be from within the domain of the stress. Thus, social support from friends is more protective for stresses occurring within the peer domain than that occurring within the family domain (Gore & Aseltine, 1995).

However, it is important not to overinterpret the role of social support as a purely environmental effect. Children who are easier temperamentally elicit more positive reactions from those in their environment (Lengua & Kovacs, 2005). Further, more physically attractive babies elicit more positivity and attachment behaviors than less attractive infants (Langlois, Ritter, Casey *et al.*, 1995). Such findings suggest that characteristics of children contribute to the supportiveness of the environment that forms around them. This is referred to as an evocative gene–environment correlation.

Future Directions

We have shown that understanding the effects of adversity and the processes of resilience depends on an integration of findings from different methods in developmental science. As we move forward, certain kinds of studies hold particular promise. First, for researchers examining the effects of stress on children, animal models are extremely important. They will provide an understanding of the way in which stress affects brain development as well as providing an understanding of the reversibility of such effects, once therapeutic interventions are applied. Second, within-family designs will be central to the next decade of research on risk and resilience. Such designs will allow us to differentiate between child-specific and family-wide risks, to distinguish between the objective and the effective environment and to understand why siblings exposed to similar environments develop so differently. It is important that such studies collect high-quality observational longitudinal data that allow us to examine reciprocal influences of parents, children and siblings. Third, studies that combine molecular genetic data with measures of environmental risk will allow for the examination of gene–environment interaction. This will be a key focus of research over the next decade. Fourth, emotion processes in humans occur within biological, cognitive, behavioral and relational levels of analysis. It is important that we understand the ways in which these different levels of experience operate together. Finally, limiting the definition of resilience to factors that operate differentially in high- and low-risk environments will enable us to gain a better understanding of compensatory processes in development.

Further Reading

http://www.excellence-earlychildhood.ca/home.asp?lang=EN

Kraemer, G. W. (1992). A psychobiological theory of attachment. *Behavioral and Brain Sciences*, *15*, 493–541.

Luthar, S. (2006). Resilience in development: A synthesis of research across five decades. In D. Cicchetti, & D. Cohen (Eds.), *Developmental psychopathology*. Vol. 3. *Risk, disorder, and adaptation* (2nd ed., pp. 739–795). Hoboken, NJ: John Wiley & Sons.

Oatley, K., Keltner, D., & Jenkins, J. M. (2006). *Understanding emotions: In psychology, psychiatry, and social science* (2nd edn.). Cambridge, MA: Blackwell.

Pennington, B. (2002). *The development of psychopathology: Nature and nurture*. New York: Guilford Press.

References

Aisenberg, E., & Ell, K. (2005). Contextualizing community violence and its effects. An ecological model of parent–child interdependent coping. *Journal of Interpersonal Violence*, *20*, 855–871.

Amato, P. R. (2001). Children of divorce in the 1990s: An update of the Amato and Keith (1991) meta-analysis. *Journal of Family Psychology*, *15*, 355–370.

Amato, P. R., & Sobolewski, J. M. (2001). The effects of divorce and marital discord on adult children's psychological well-being. *American Sociological Review*, *66*, 900–921.

Bank, L., Burraston, B., & Snyder, J. (2004). Sibling conflict and ineffective parenting as predictors of adolescent boys' antisocial behavior and peer difficulties: Additive and interactional effects. *Journal of Research on Adolescence*, *14*, 99–125.

Baron, R. M., & Kenny, D. A. (1986). The moderator-mediator variable distinction in social psychological research: Conceptual, strategic, and statistical considerations. *Journal of Personality and Social Psychology*, *51*, 1173–1182.

Bates, J. E., Pettit, G. S., Dodge, K. A., & Ridge, B. (1998). Interaction of temperamental resistance to control and restrictive parenting in the development of externalizing behavior. *Developmental Psychology*, *34*, 982–995.

Bennett, A. J., Lesch, K. P., Heils, A., Long, J. C., Lorenz, J. G., Shoaf, S. E., *et al.* (2002). Early experience and serotonin transporter gene variation interact to influence primate CNS function. *Molecular Psychiatry*, *7*, 118–122.

Bornstein, M. (1995). *Handbook of parenting*. Mahweh, NJ: Erlbaum.

Bowlby, J. (1971). *Attachment and loss*. Vol. 1. *Attachment*. London: Hogarth Press.

Boyle, M. H., Jenkins, J. M., Georgiades, K., Cairney, J., Duku, E., & Racine, Y. (2004). Differential-maternal parenting behavior: Estimating within- and between-family effects on children. *Child Development*, *75*, 1457–1476.

Boyle, M. H., & Lipman, E. L. (2002). Do places matter? Socio-economic disadvantage and behavioral problems of children in Canada. *Journal of Consulting and Clinical Psychology*, *70*, 378–389.

Bronfenbrenner, U. (1979). Contexts of child rearing: Problems and prospects. *American Psychologist*, *34*, 844–850.

Brown, G. W., Harris, T. O., & Eales, M. J. (1996). Social factors and comorbidity of depressive and anxiety disorders. *British Journal of Psychiatry*, *168* (Supplement 30), 50–57.

Buehler, C., & Gerard, J. M. (2002). Marital conflict, ineffective parenting, and children's and adolescents' maladjustment. *Journal of Marriage and Family*, *64*, 78–92.

Bugental, D. B., Martorell, G. A., & Barraza, V. (2003). The hormonal costs of subtle forms of infant maltreatment. *Hormones and Behavior*, *43*, 237–244.

Caldji, C., Francis, D., Sharma, S., Plotsky, P. M., & Meaney, M. J. (2000). The effects of early rearing environment on the development of GABAA and central benzodiazepine receptor levels and novelty-induced fearfulness in the rat. *Neuropsychopharmacology*, *22*, 219–229.

Caspi, A., McClay, J., Moffitt, T., Mill, J., Martin, J., Craig, I. W., *et al.* (2002). Role of genotype in the cycle of violence in maltreated children. *Science*, *297*, 851–854.

Caspi, A., Moffitt, T. E., Morgan, J., Rutter, M., Taylor, A., Arseneault, L., *et al.* (2004). Maternal expressed emotion predicts children's antisocial behavior problems: Using monozygotic-twin differences to identify environmental effects on behavioral development. *Developmental Psychology*, *40*, 149–161.

Caspi, A., Sugden, K., Moffitt, T. E., Taylor, A., Craig, I. W., Harrington, H., *et al.* (2003). Influence of life stress on depression: Moderation by a polymorphism in the 5-HTT gene. *Science*, *301*, 386–389.

Cauce, A. M., Hannan, K., & Sargeant, M. (1992). Life stress, social support, and locus of control during early adolescence: Interactive effects. *American Journal of Community Psychology*, *20*, 787–798.

Chamberlain, P., & Reid, J. B. (1998). Comparison of two community alternatives to incarceration for chronic juvenile offenders. *Journal of Consulting and Clinical Psychology*, *66*, 624–633.

Champoux, M., Zanker, D., & Levine, S. (1993). Food search demand effort effects on behavior and cortisol in adult female squirrel monkeys. *Physiology & Behavior*, *54*, 1091–1097.

Cherlin, A. J., Furstenberg, F. F., Chase-Lansdale, P. L., & Kiernan, K. E. (1991). Longitudinal studies of effects of divorce on children in Great Britain and the United States. *Science*, *252*, 1386–1389.

Chisholm, K. (1999). A three year follow-up of attachment and indiscriminate friendliness in children adopted from Romanian orphanages. *Child Development*, *69*, 1092–1106.

Cicchetti, D., & Toth, S. L. (2005). Child maltreatment. *Annual Review of Clinical Psychology*, *1*, 409–438.

Cochran, W. G., & Chambers, S. P. (1965). The planning of observational studies of human populations. *Journal of Royal Statistical Society. Series A (General)*, *128*, 234–266.

Cole, P. M., Teti, L. O., & Zahn-Waxler, C. (2003). Mutual emotion regulation and the stability of conduct problems between preschool and early school age. *Development and Psychopathology*, *15*, 1–18.

Connor, C. M., Morrison, F. J., & Petrella, J. N. (2004). Effective reading comprehension instruction: Examining child × instruction interactions. *Journal of Educational Psychology*, *96*, 682–698.

Costello, E. J., Compton, S. N., Keeler, G. & Angold, A. (2003). Relationships between poverty and psychopathology. *Journal of the American Medical Association*, *290*, 2023–2029.

Criss, M. M., Pettit, G. S., Bates, J. E., Dodge, K. A., & Lapp, A. L. (2002). Family adversity, positive peer relationships, and children's externalizing behavior: A longitudinal perspective on risk and resilience. *Child Development*, *73*, 1220–1237.

Cummings, E. M., & Davies, P. (1994). *Children and marital conflict: The impact of family dispute and resolution*. New York: Guilford Press.

Cummings, E. M., Keller, P. S., & Davies, P. T. (2005). Towards a family process model of maternal and paternal depressive symptoms: Exploring multiple relations with child and family functioning. *Journal of Child Psychology and Psychiatry*, *46*, 479–489.

Davidson, G. C., & Neale, J. M. (2001). *Abnormal psychology* (8th edn.). New York: Wiley.

Davies, P. T., Harold, G. T., Goeke-Morey, M. C., & Cummings, E. M. (2002). Child emotional security and interparental conflict. *Monographs of the Society for Research in Child Development*, *67*, vii–viii.

DeGarmo, D. S., & Forgatch, M. S. (2005). Early development of delinquency within divorced families: Evaluating a randomized preventive intervention trial. *Developmental Science*, *8*, 229–239.

Dishion, T. J., & Kavanagh, K. (2003). *Intervening in adolescent problem behavior: A family-centered approach*. New York, NY: Guilford Press.

Dishion, T. J., McCord, J., & Poulin, F. (1999). When interventions harm: Peer groups and problem behavior. *American Psychologist*, *54*, 755–764.

Dodge, K. A., Bates, J. E., & Pettit, G. S. (1990). Mechanisms in the cycle of violence. *Science*, *250*, 1678–1683.

Dodge, K. A., Dishion, T. J., & Lansford, J. E. (Eds.). (2006). *Deviant peer influences in programs for youth: problems and solutions*. New York and London: Guilford Press.

Dougherty, L. R., Klein, D. N., & Davila, J. (2004). A growth curve analysis of the course of dysthymic disorder: The effects of chronic stress and moderation by adverse parent–child relationships and family history. *Journal of Consulting and Clinical Psychology*, *72*, 1012–1021.

Dowdney, G., & Coyne, J. C. (1990). Children of depressed parents. *Psychological Bulletin*, *108*, 50–76.

Dubow, E. F., & Tisak, J. (1989). The relation between stressful life events and adjustment in elementary school children: The role of social support and social problem-solving skills. *Child Development*, *60*, 1412–1423.

Duncan, G. J., Connell, J. P., & Klebanov, P. K. (1997). Conceptual and methodological issues in estimating causal effects of neighborhood and family conditions on individual development. In J. Brooks-Gunn, G. J. Duncan, & J. L. Aber (Eds.), *Neighborhood poverty*. Vol. 1. *Context and consequences for children* (pp. 219–250). New York, NY: Russell Sage Foundation.

Dunn, J., Stocker, C., & Plomin, R. (1991). Nonshared experiences within the family: Correlates of behavior problems in middle childhood. *Development and Psychopathology*, *2*, 113–126.

Dyregrov, A., Gupta, L., Gjestad, R., & Mukanoheli, E. (2000). Trauma exposure and psychological reactions to genocide among Rwandan children. *Journal of Traumatic Stress*, *13*, 3–21.

Elder, G. H., & Clipp, E. C. (1988). Wartime losses and social bonding: Influences across 40 years in men's lives. *Psychiatry: Journal for the Study of Interpersonal Processes*, *51*, 177–198.

El-Sheikh, M. (2005). Does poor vagal tone exacerbate child maladjustment in the context of parental problem drinking? A longitudinal examination. *Journal of Abnormal Psychology. Special Issue: Toward a Dimensionally Based Taxonomy of Psychopathology*, *114*, 735–741.

Fergusson, D. M. (1999). Prenatal smoking and antisocial behavior. *Archives of General Psychiatry*, *56*, 223–224.

Fleming, A. S. (2006). Plasticity of innate behavior. In C. S. Carter, L. Ahnert, K. E. Grossman, S. B. Hrdy, M. E. Lamb, S. W. Porges, *et al.* (Eds.), *Attachment and bonding: A new synthesis*. Cambridge, MA: MIT Press.

Fleming, A. S., & Li, M. (2002). Psychobiology of maternal behavior and its early determinants in nonhuman mammals. In M. H. Bornstein (Ed.), *Handbook of parenting* (pp. 61–97). Mahwah, NJ: Erlbaum.

Fries, A. B. W., & Pollak, S. D. (2004). Emotion understanding in postinstitutionalized Eastern European children. *Development and Psychopathology*, *16*, 355–369.

Garcia, M. M., Shaw, D. S., Winslow, E. B., & Yaggi, K. E. (2000). Destructive sibling conflict and the development of conduct problems in young boys. *Developmental Psychology*, *36*, 44–53.

Gass, K. R., Jenkins, J. M., Dunn, J. (2007). Are sibling relationships protective? A longitudinal study. *Journal of Child Psychology and Psychiatry*, *48*, 167–175.

Ge, X., Conger, R. D., Cadoret, R. J., Neiderhiser, J. M., Yates, W., Troughton, E., *et al.* (1996). The developmental interface between nature and nurture: A mutual influence model of child antisocial behavior and parent behaviors. *Developmental Psychology*, *32*, 574–589.

Goldberg, S., Grusec, J. E., & Jenkins, J. M. (1999). Confidence in protection: Arguments for a narrow definition of attachment. *Journal of Family Psychology*, *13*, 475–483.

Goldsmith, H. H. (1993). Temperament: Variability in developing emotion systems. In M. Lewis & J. M. Haviland (Eds.), *Handbook of emotions* (pp. 353–364). New York, NY: Guilford Press.

Gore, S., & Aseltine, R. H. (1995). Protective processes in adolescence: Matching stressors with social resources. *American Journal of Community Psychology*, *23*, 301–327.

Gorman-Smith, D., & Tolan, P. (1998). The role of exposure to community violence and developmental problems among inner-city youth. *Development and Psychopathology*, *10*, 101–116.

Grant, K. E., Compas, B. E., Stuhlmacher, A. F., Thurm, A. E., McMahon, S. D., & Halpert, J. A. (2003). Stressors and child and adolescent psychopathology: Moving from markers to mechanisms of risk. *Psychological Bulletin*, *129*, 447–466.

Grych, J. H., & Fincham, F. D. (1993). Children's appraisals of marital conflict: Initial investigations of the cognitive-contextual framework. *Child Development*, *64*, 215–230.

Grych, J. H., Harold, G. T., & Miles, C. J. (2003). A prospective investigation of appraisals as mediators of the link between interparental conflict and child adjustment. *Child Development*, *74*, 1176–1193.

Guo, G., & Wang, J. (2002). The mixed or multilevel model for behavior genetic analysis. *Behavior Genetics*, *32*, 37–49.

Gutman, L. M., McLoyd, V. C., & Tokoyawa, T. (2005). Financial strain, neighborhood stress, parenting behaviors and adolescent adjustment in urban African American families. *Journal of Research on Adolescence*, 15, 425–449.

Hammen, C. (1988). Self-cognitions, stressful events, and the prediction of depression in children of depressed mothers. *Journal of Abnormal Child Psychology*, *16*, 347–360.

Harris, J. R. (1998). *The nurture assumption: Why children turn out the way they do*. New York: Free Press.

Hauser, S., Allen, J., & Golden, E. (2006). *Out of the woods: Tales of resilient teens*. Cambridge, MA: Harvard University Press.

Hetherington, E. M., Henderson, S. H., Reiss, D., Anderson, E. R., Bridges, M., Chan, R. W., *et al.* (1999). Adolescent siblings in stepfamilies: Family functioning and adolescent adjustment. *Monographs of the Society for Research in Child Development*, *64*, 222.

Hodes, M. (2000). Psychologically distressed refugee children in the United Kingdom. *Child Psychology and Psychiatry Review*, *5*, 57–68.

Howard, M., & Hodes, M. (2000). Psychopathology, adversity, and service utilization of young refugees. *Journal of the American Academy of Child and Adolescent Psychiatry*, *39*, 368–377.

Howes, C. (2000). Social-emotional classroom climate in child care, child–teacher relationships and children's second grade peer relations. *Social Development*, *9*, 191–204.

Jaffee, S. R., Moffitt, T. E., Caspi, A., & Taylor, A. (2003). Life with (or without) father: The benefits of living with two biological parents depend on the father's antisocial behavior. *Child Development*, *74*, 109–126.

Jenkins, J. M., & Buccioni, J. M. (2000). Children's understanding of marital conflict and the marital relationship. *Journal of Child Psychology and Psychiatry*, *41*, 161–168.

Jenkins, J. M., Rasbash, J., & O'Connor, T. G. (2003). The role of the shared family context in differential parenting. *Developmental Psychology*, *39*, 99–113.

Jenkins, J. M., Shapka, J., & Sorenson, A. (2006). Teenage mothers' anger over twelve years: partner conflict, partner transitions and children's anger. *Journal of Child Psychology and Psychiatry*, *47*, 775–782.

Jenkins, J., Simpson, A., Dunn, J., Rasbash, J., & O'Connor, T. G. (2005). Mutual influence of marital conflict and children's behavior problems: Shared and nonshared family risks. *Child Development*, *76*, 24–39.

Jenkins, J. M., & Smith, M. A. (1990). Factors protecting children living in disharmonious homes: Maternal reports. *Journal of the American Academy of Child and Adolescent Psychiatry*, *29*, 60–69.

Jenkins, J. M., & Smith, M. A. (1991). Marital disharmony and children's behaviour problems: Aspects of a poor marriage that affect children adversely. *Journal of Child Psychology and Psychiatry*, *32*, 793–810.

Kellam, S. G., Ling, X., Merisca, R., Brown, C. H., & Ialongo, N. (1998). The effect of the level of aggression in the first grade classroom on the course and malleability of aggressive behavior into middle school. *Development and Psychopathology*, *10*, 165–185.

Kempton, T., Armistead, L., Wierson, M., & Forehand, R. (1991). Presence of a sibling as a potential buffer following parental divorce: An examination of young adolescents. *Journal of Clinical Child Psychology*, *20*, 434–438.

Kerr, M., & Stattin, H. (2000). What parents know, how they know it and several forms of adolescent adjustment: further support for a reinterpretation of monitoring. *Developmental Psychology*, *36*, 366–380.

Kim, K. J., Conger, R. D., Lorenz, F. O., & Elder, G. H. J. (2001). Parent–adolescent reciprocity in negative affect and its relation to early adult social development. *Developmental Psychology*, *37*, 775–790.

King, S., & Laplante, D. P. (2005). The effects of prenatal maternal stress on children's cognitive development: Project Ice Storm. *International Journal on the Biology of Stress*, *8*, 35–45.

Klebanov, P. K., Brooks-Gunn, J., & Duncan, G. J. (1994). Does neighborhood and family poverty affect mother's parenting, mental health, and social support? *Journal of Marriage and the Family*, *56*, 441–455.

Kraemer, G. W. (1992). A psychobiological theory of attachment. *Behavioral and Brain Sciences*, *15*, 493–541.

Kraemer, G. W., Ebert, M. H., Schmidt, D. E., & McKinney, W. T. (1991). Strangers in a strange land: A psychobiological study of infant monkeys before and after separation from real or inanimate mothers. *Child Development*, *62*, 548–566.

Krug, E., Powell, K., & Dahlberg, L. (1998). Firearm-related deaths in the United States and 35 other high and upper-middle income countries. *International Journal of Epidemiology*, *27*, 214–221.

Ladd, C. O., Huot, R. L., Thrivikraman, K. V., Nemeroff, C. B., Meaney, M. J., & Plotsky, P. M. (2000). Long-term behavioral and neuroendocrine adaptations to adverse early experience. *Progress in Brain Research*, *122*, 81–103.

Langlois, J. H., Ritter, J. M., Casey, R. J., & Sawin, D. B. (1995). Infant attractiveness predicts maternal behaviors and attitudes. *Developmental Psychology*, *31*, 464–472.

Lengua, L. J. (2002). The contribution of emotionality and self-regulation to the understanding of children's response to multiple risk. *Child Development*, *73*, 144–161.

Lengua, L. J., & Kovacs, E. A. (2005). Bidirectional associations between temperament and parenting and the prediction of adjustment problems in middle childhood. *Journal of Applied Developmental Psychology*, *26*, 21–38.

Leventhal, T., & Brooks-Gunn, J. (2000). The neighborhoods they live in: The effects of neighborhood residence on child and adolescent outcomes. *Psychological Bulletin*, *126*, 309–337.

Leventhal, T., & Brooks-Gunn, J. (2004). A randomized study of neighborhood effects on low-income children's educational outcomes. *Developmental Psychology*, *40*, 488–507.

Leventhal, T., Fauth, R. C., & Brooks-Gunn, J. (2005). Neighborhood poverty and public policy: A 5-year follow-up of children's educational outcomes in the New York City Moving to Opportunity demonstration. *Developmental Psychology*, *41*, 933–952.

Lewis, H. S. (2000). Psychosocial adjustment of adult children of alcoholics: A review of the recent empirical literature. *Clinical Psychology Review*, *20*, 311–337.

Liu, J., Raine, A., Venables, P. H., & Mednick, S. A. (2004). Malnutrition at age 3 years and externalizing behavior problems at ages 8, 11, and 17 years. *American Journal of Psychiatry*, *161*, 2005–2013.

Luthar, S. S., Cicchetti, D., & Becker, B. (2000). The construct of resilience: A critical evaluation and guidelines for future work. *Child Development*, *71*, 543–562.

Lynam, D. R., Caspi, A., Moffit, T. E., Wikström, P., Loeber, R., & Novak, S. (2000). The interaction between impulsivity and neighborhood context on offending: The effects of impulsivity are stronger in poorer neighborhoods. *Journal of Abnormal Psychology*, *109*, 563–574.

Lyons, D. M., Kim, S., Schatzberg, A. F., & Levine, S. (1998). Postnatal foraging demands alter adrenocortical activity and psychosocial development. *Developmental Psychobiology*, *32*, 285–291.

Lyons-Ruth, K., Connell, D. B., Grunebaum, H. U., & Botein, S. (1990). Infants at social risk: Maternal depression and family support services as mediators of infant development and security of attachment. *Child Development*, *61*, 85–98.

Macmillan, R., McMorris, B. J., & Kruttschnitt, C. (2004). Linked lives: Stability and change in maternal circumstances and trajectories of antisocial behavior in children. *Child Development*, *75*, 205–220.

Massey, D. S., & Kanaiaupuni, S. M. (1993). Public housing and the concentration of poverty. *Social Science Quarterly*, *74*, 109–122.

Masten, A. S., & Powell, J. L. (2003). A resilience framework for research, policy, and practice. In S. S. Luthar (Ed.), *Resilience and vulnerability: Adaptation in the context of childhood adversities* (pp. 1–25). New York, NY: Cambridge University Press.

Masten, A. S., Hubbard, J. J., Gest, S. D., Tellegen, A., Garmezy, N., & Ramirez, M. (1999). Competence in the context of adversity: Pathways to resilience and maladaptation from childhood to late adolescence. *Development and Psychopathology*, *11*, 143–169.

Mazur, E., Wolchik, S. A., Virdin, L., Sandler, I. N., & West, S. G. (1999). Cognitive moderators of children's adjustment to stressful divorce events: The role of negative cognitive errors and positive illusions. *Child Development*, *70*, 231–245.

McClelland, G. H., & Judd, C. M. (1993). Statistical difficulties of detecting interactions and moderator effects. *Psychological Bulletin*, *114*, 376–390.

Morrison, D. R., & Coiro, M. J. (1999). Parental conflict and marital disruption: Do children benefit when high-conflict marriages are dissolved? *Journal of Marriage and the Family*, *61*, 626–637.

NICHD Early Child Care Research Network. (2005). Duration and developmental timing of poverty on children's cognitive and social development from birth to third grade. *Child Development*, *76*, 795–810.

Niemi, L. T., Survisaari, H., & Huakka, J. K. (2004). Cumulative incidence of mental disorder among offspring of mothers with psychotic disorder: Results from the Helsinki High-Risk Study. *British Journal of Psychiatry*, *185*, 11–17.

Oatley, K., Keltner, D., & Jenkins, J. M. (2006). *Understanding emotions: In psychology, psychiatry, and social science* (2nd edn.). Cambridge, MA: Blackwell.

O'Connor, T. G. (2002). Annotation: The "effects" of parenting reconsidered: Findings, challenges, and applications. *Journal of Child Psychology and Psychiatry*, *43*, 555–572.

O'Connor, T. G., Caspi, A., DeFries, J. C., & Plomin, R. (2000). Are associations between parental divorce and children's adjustment genetically mediated? An adoption study. *Developmental Psychology*, *36*, 429–437.

Offord, D. R., Boyle, M. H., Szatmari, P., & Rae-Grant, N. I. (1987). Ontario child health study. II. Six-month prevalence of disorder and rates of service utilization. *Archives of General Psychiatry*, *44*, 832–836.

Olds, D. (1989). The prenatal/early infancy project: A strategy for responding to the needs of high risk mothers and their children. *Prevention in Human Services*, *7*, 58–97.

Pan, B. A., Rowe, M. L., Singer, J. D., & Snow, C. E. (2005). Maternal correlates of growth in toddler vocabulary production in low-income families. *Child Development*, *76*, 763–782.

Panksepp, J. (1998). *Affective neuroscience*. Oxford: Oxford University Press.

Patterson, G. R. (1984). Siblings: Fellow travelers in coercive family processes. In R. J. Blancard, & D. C. Blanchard (Eds.), *Advances in the study of aggression*. Vol. 1. (pp. 174–215). New York, NY: Academic Press.

Patterson, G. R., Capaldi, D., & Bank, L. (1991). The early starter model for predicting delinquency. In D. J. Pepler & K. H. Rubin (Eds.), *The development and treatment of childhood aggression*. Hillsdale, NJ: Lawrence Erlbaum.

Pinderhughes, E. E., Nix, R., Foster, E. M. & Jones, D. (2001). Parenting in context: Impact of neighborhood poverty, residential stability, public services, social networks, and danger on parental behaviors. *Journal of Marriage and Family*, *63*, 941–953.

Plomin, R. (1994). *Genetics and experience: The interplay between nature and nurture*. Thousand Oaks, CA: Sage Publications.

Plomin, R., & Daniels, D. (1987). Why are children in the same family so different from one another? *Behavioral and Brain Sciences*, *10*, 1–16.

Plotsky, P. M., & Meaney, M. J. (1993). Early, postnatal experience alters hypothalamic corticotropin-releasing factor (CRF) mRNA, median eminence CRF content and stress-induced release in adult rats. *Brain research. Molecular Brain Research*, *18*, 195–200.

Porges, S. W. (1995). Cardiac vagal tone: A physiological index of stress. *Neuroscience and Biobehavioral Reviews*, *19*, 225–233.

Quinton, D., & Rutter, M. (1988). *Parenting breakdown: The making and breaking of inter-generational links.* Aldershot, Hants: Avebury.

Repetti, R. L., Taylor, S.E., & Seeman, T. E. (2002). Risky families: Family social environments and the mental and physical health of offspring. *Psychological Bulletin*, *128*, 330–366.

Riley, J. R., & Masten, A. S. (2005). Resilience in context. In R. D. Peters, B. Leadbeater & R. J. McMahon (Eds.), *Resilience in children, families, and communities: Linking context to practice and policy* (pp. 13–25). New York, NY: Kluwer Academic/Plenum Publishers.

Rutter, M. (1979). Protective factors in children's responses to stress and disadvantage. In M. W. Kent & J. E. Rolf (Eds.), *Primary prevention in psychopathology*, Vol. 3. *Social competence in children* (pp. 49–74). Hanover, NH: University Press of New England.

Rutter, M. (1999). Resilience concepts and findings: Implications for family therapy. *Journal of Family Therapy*, *21*, 119–144.

Rutter, M. (2002). Nature, nurture, and development: From evangelism through science toward policy and practice. *Child Development*, *73*, 1–21.

Rutter, M. (2006). Implications of resilience concepts for scientific understanding. *Annals of the New York Academy of Sciences, 1094*, 1–12.

Rutter, M., Maughan, B., Mortimore, P., & Ouston, J. (1979). *Fifteen thousand hours: Secondary schools and their effects on children.* London: Open Books.

Rutter, M., & O'Connor, T. G. (2004). Are there biological programming effects for psychological development? Findings from a study of Romanian adoptees. *Developmental Psychology*, *40*, 81–94.

Rutter, M., & Pickles, A. (1991). Person–environment interactions: Concepts, mechanisms, and implications for data analysis. In T. D. Wachs, & R. Plomin (Eds.), *Conceptualization and measurement of organism–environment interaction* (pp. 105–141). Washington, DC: American Psychological Association.

Rutter, M., Pickles, A., Murray, R., & Eaves, L. (2001). Testing hypotheses on specific environmental causal effects on behavior. *Psychological Bulletin*, *127*, 291–324.

Rutter, M., Silberg, J., O'Connor, T., & Simonoff, E. (1999). Genetics and child psychiatry: II. Empirical research findings. *Journal of Child Psychology and Psychiatry and Allied Disciplines*, *40*, 19–55.

Rutter, M., Tizard, K., & Whitmore, K. (1970). *Education, health and behavior*. London: Kriegar, FL: Longman.

Sack, W. H., McSharry, S., Clarke, G. N., Kinney, R. *et al.* (1994). The Khmer adolescent project: I. Epidemiologic findings in two generations of Cambodian refugees. *Journal of Nervous and Mental Disease*, *182*, 387–395.

Sameroff, A. J., & Mackenzie, M. (2003). Research strategies for capturing transactional models of development: The limit of the possible. *Development and Psychopathology*, *15*, 613–640.

Sanchez, M. M., Ladd., C.O., & Plotsky, P. M. (2001). Early adverse experience as a developmental risk factor for later psychopathology: Evidence from rodent and primate models. *Development and Psychopathology*, *13*, 419–449.

Sarason, B. R., Shearin, E. N., Pierce, G. R., & Sarason, I. G. (1987). Interrelations of social support measures: Theoretical and practical implications. *Journal of Personality and Social Psychology*, *52*, 813–832.

Schwartz, D., Dodge, K. A., Pettit, G. S., Bates, J. E., & The Conduct Problems Prevention Research Group. (2000). Friendship as a moderating factor in the pathway between early harsh home environment and later victimization in the peer group. *Developmental Psychology*, *36*, 646–662.

Shaw, D. S., Owens, E. B., Giovannelli, J., & Winslow, E. B. (2001). Infant and toddler pathways leading to early externalizing disorders. *Journal of the American Academy of Child and Adolescent Psychiatry*, *40*, 36–43.

Singer, J. D., & Willett, J. B. (2003). *Applied longitudinal data analysis: Modeling change and event occurrence.* New York: Oxford University Press.

Sroufe, L. A., Egeland, B., & Carlson, E. A. (1999). One social world: The integrated development of parent–child and peer relationships. In W. A. Collins, & B. Laursen (Eds.), *Relationships as developmental contexts: Minnesota Symposium on Child Psychology* (Vol. 30). Hillsdale, NJ: Erlbaum.

Stanley, S. M., Amato, P. R., Johnson, C. A., & Markman, H. J. (2006). Premarital education, marital quality, and marital stability: Findings from a large, random household survey. *Journal of Family Psychology*, *20*, 117–126.

Stephens, R. D. (1997). National trends in school violence: Statistics and prevention strategies. In A. P. Goldstein, & J. C. Conoley (Eds.), *School violence intervention: A practical handbook* (pp. 72–90). New York, NY: Guilford Press.

Suomi, S. J. (1991). Early stress and adult emotional reactivity in rhesus monkeys. *Ciba Foundation symposium*, *156*, 171–188.

Suomi, S. (2005). How gene–environment interactions shape the development of impulsive aggression in rhesus monkeys. In D. Stoff, & E. Susman (Eds.), *Developmental psychobiology of aggression.* New York, NY: Cambridge University Press.

Trickett, P. K., & McBride-Chang, C. (1995). The developmental impact of different forms of child abuse and neglect. *Developmental Review*, *15*, 311–337.

Turkheimer, E., & Waldron, M. (2000). Nonshared environment: A theoretical, methodological, and quantitative review. *Psychological Bulletin*, *126*, 78–108.

Van den Bergh, B., & Marcoen, A. (2004). High antenatal maternal anxiety is related to ADHD symptoms, externalizing problems and anxiety in 8- and 9-year-olds. *Child Development*, *75*, 1085–1097.

Wills, T. A., Sandy, J. M., Yaeger, A., & Shinar, O. (2001). Family risk factors and adolescent substance use: Moderation effects for temperament dimensions. *Developmental Psychology*, *37*, 283–297.

Wyman, P. A., Cowen, E. L., Work, W. C., Hoyt-Meyers, L., Magnus, K. B., & Fagen, D. B. (1999). Caregiving and developmental factors differentiating young at-risk urban children showing resilient versus stress-affected outcomes: A replication and extension. *Child Development*, *70*, 645–659.

Xue, Y., Leventhal, T., Brooks-Gunn, J., & Earls, F. J. (2005). Neighborhood residence and mental health problems of 5- to 11-year-olds. *Archives of General Psychiatry*, *62*, 554–563.

Youngstrom, E., Weist, M. D., & Albus, K. E. (2003). Exploring violence exposure, stress, protective factors and behavioral problems among inner-city youth. *American Journal of Community Psychology*, *32*, 115–129.

26 Acute Life Stresses

Seija Sandberg and Michael Rutter

Historical Background

It has long been generally recognized that stressful life experiences may have an adverse effect on health and predispose to physical and psychiatric illness (Haavet & Grünfeld, 1997; Rutter, 2005). Through experimental and clinical studies, Cannon (1929) laid the groundwork for psychophysiological research by demonstrating that external stimuli associated with emotional arousal caused changes in basic physiological processes. Some three decades later, a bridge to psychiatry was firmly laid out. Meyer (1957), a physician and psychiatrist, argued that to be pathogenic, life events need not be catastrophic or particularly unusual. He advocated the value of life charts to bring out temporal links between happenings such as change of habitat, school entrance, graduation, marriage, divorce and bereavement, and the onset of psychiatric disorder.

This proposition was further developed in the 1960s by Holmes and Rahe (1967) through their production of questionnaires to provide overall scores of degree of life change in adults – the assumption then being that it was the extent of life change that was stressful and not necessarily the unpleasant nature of the experiences. In addition, there were numerous studies of specific life events affecting all age groups – such as family break-up, bereavement, and disasters such as floods, earthquakes or hijacking. The realization that it was necessary to take into account the social context of life events in order to assess their meaning and hence their stressful quality constituted perhaps the most significant conceptual advance that followed (Brown & Harris, 1978).

Two main approaches have been applied in the assessment of life events in children. First, questionnaires have been used to ask about the occurrence of specified life events during a particular time period (Allen & Rapee, 2006; Johnson, 1982), most commonly the previous year. The main advantage of questionnaires is their low cost and ease of administration to a large number of individuals, making them readily applicable for large-scale epidemiological enquiries (Silberg, Pickles, Rutter *et al.*, 1999). However, they have the considerable disadvantage that they cannot readily deal with the personal meaning or social context of events and they are limited in their ability to obtain accurate timing. As a result, there is substantial variability in what broad categories of "events" (e.g., divorce or illness) actually reflect in terms of personal experiences (Dohrenwend, 2006).

Second, interviews have been employed to obtain detailed descriptions of life events, and of their surrounding circumstances, during a defined time period (Goodyer, 1990; Monck & Dobbs, 1985; Sandberg, Rutter, Giles *et al.*, 1993; Sandberg, Paton, Ahola *et al.*, 2000; Williamson, Birmaher, Ryan *et al.*, 2003). Accurate timing is facilitated by using personalized time points such as birthdays, family holidays, school terms and the like. The notion of *contextual threat* (i.e., psychological threat to the individual as viewed in the light of that person's personal social context), first introduced by Brown and Harris (1978), has been incorporated as a cornerstone measure in all these interview-based life event assessments with children. The level of contextual threat is commonly assessed in terms of enduring effects. In the Psychosocial Assessment of Childhood Experiences (PACE; Glen, Simpson, Drinnan *et al.*, 1993; Sandberg & Zimmer, 2002; Sandberg *et al.*, 1993) the threats include the following:

- Loss of an attachment figure (e.g., parent or close friend);
- Threat of loss of an attachment figure (e.g., parent threatening to abandon child);
- Loss of a valued idea (major disappointment/humiliation);
- Physical jeopardy (e.g., being in physical danger because of an accident);
- Trauma as witness (being witness to a frightening incident involving someone else); and
- Psychological challenge (taking on a new role or new responsibilities).

Brown & Harris (1978) were also the first to emphasize the need to differentiate between *independent* and *dependent* life events (i.e., those that could and could not have been brought about by the person's own behavior) – a distinction included similarly in the interview-based assessments with children. Thus, bereavement would fall in the former category and rejection by a close friend in the latter (with it probably being to some extent related to the child's own behavior). In addition, in the PACE (Sandberg & Zimmer, 2002; Sandberg *et al.*, 1993) there is the further distinction between independence from the child's behavior and independence from the behavior of the parent(s). Parental divorce and abuse of the child are examples of life events dependent on the parents' behavior.

Rutter's Child and Adolescent Psychiatry, 5th edition. Edited by M. Rutter, D. Bishop, D. Pine, S. Scott, J. Stevenson, E. Taylor and A. Thapar. © 2008 Blackwell Publishing, ISBN: 978-1-4051-4549-7.

Some life events rate high on contextual threat because they cause a major alteration in life circumstances (e.g., death of a parent). In other events the threat is primarily cognitive. That is, the event drastically changes the child's perception of an aspect of themselves, or of other people or things in a way that presents a threat to the child's self-esteem (e.g., severe humiliation) or reduces his or her perceived sense of security (e.g., parent threatening to abandon the child). Life events may also involve a combination of real life change and cognitively mediated threat (e.g., the parents' marital separation).

Most life events occurring to children involve important social relationships, whereas far fewer can be seen as being largely unpredictable "acts of fate." The latter mainly include major traumatic experiences such as being kidnapped or sudden losses of close persons.

Risk Effects of Life Events

Life events may carry risk either because they tend to provoke the onset of psychiatric disorder, or because they increase the overall liability to recurrent or chronic disorders. The former risk has mainly been studied through case–control studies focusing on the timing of the life events, and the latter risk through population studies measuring the overall burden of life stresses over time.

The causal effect on the onset of disorder has mainly been tested through showing that, in comparison with controls, there is a major provoking life event in the 2 months preceding onset, whereas this occurs less often in other time periods, life events in controls being distributed in a more random fashion. Alternatively, a few longitudinal studies have shown an increased likelihood of onset of disorder in the weeks or months immediately following a major life event. Most of this research has concerned adults (Brown & Harris, 1978, 1986; Brown, Harris, & Eales, 1996). The findings in children have been much less consistent. Only one study (Goodyer, Herbert, Tamplin *et al.*, 2000) has shown a strong timing effect, with a significant increase of negative life events shortly before onset. Others have tended to show an increase in negative events over a more extended period of time (Jensen, Richters, Ussery *et al.*, 1991; Olsson, Nordström, Arinell *et al.*, 1999; Sandberg *et al.*, 1993; Williamson, Birmaher, Ryan *et al.*, 2003). Even in the Goodyer *et al.* (2000) study, only half of the adolescents with an onset of depressive disorder during the 12-month prospective follow-up period had experienced a high-threat life event in the month preceding the onset. Furthermore, in many cases the life event ("personal disappointment") was not classified as independent of the individual's behavior and hence, could conceivably have been related to symptoms of depression.

Although case–control comparison on timing constitutes the standard life events method, it involves several important methodological limitations with respect to the causal inference (Goodyer, Herbert, Tamplin *et al.*, 2000; Sandberg, Rutter, Pickles *et al.*, 2001). First, the case–control comparison for a specific time period will be affected by any general (non-time-specific) difference in life events as brought about by either genetic liability or other environmental factors (e.g., chronic psychosocial adversity). A more rigorous test is provided by within-individual comparisons of the pre-onset time period with other time periods. The only study so far to use this method gave rise to weak inconclusive time effects, although showing the usual case–control difference (Sandberg *et al.*, 2001). Second, with very few exceptions (Sandberg *et al.*, 2001; Silberg, Rutter, Neale *et al.*, 2001), studies with both adults and children have used the same informant for data on life events and data on the onset of disorder. The possibility of reporting bias is clear. Third, the timing method presupposes that each episode of disorder has a simple unambiguous time point when it began. The available evidence suggests that this is an exception rather than the rule. Some onsets are gradual, some symptoms begin before others, and often there is a different point when symptoms lead to social impairment (Rutter & Sandberg, 1992; Sandberg *et al.*, 2001). Moreover, inter-informant and retest reliability on the timing of children's psychiatric onsets is weak (Angold, Erkanlis, Costello *et al.*, 1996). Fourth, many psychiatric disorders are recurrent or chronic; this is so in both childhood and adult life. Accordingly, a more basic question with respect to the causal role of life events is whether they affect liability to psychopathology over time, rather than just having a provoking role with respect to the timing of onset.

The causal effect of life events in relation to the overall liability to disorder has been most rigorously tested through twin designs, which can take account of possible genetic mediation (Kendler, Karkowski, & Prescott, 1999). Studies with adults show a clear environmentally mediated risk effect. Findings in children show the same (Rutter, 2005). It should be noted, however, that the risk is only indexed by the life events. It could be that the main risk derives from chronic psychosocial adversities associated with the acute stresses, rather than from the acute stresses themselves. There is abundant evidence that, in psychiatric samples, acute life events are very frequently associated with chronic adversities and that it is the longer-lasting psychosocial hazards that constitute the greater risk (Rojo, Conesa, Bermudez *et al.*, 2006; Sandberg *et al.*, 1993; Sandberg, McGuinness, Hilary *et al.*, 1998). Nevertheless, acute stressful life events, especially those carrying long-term threat to the psychological security of the child, may add to the risk provided by chronic adversities and, in some circumstances, constitute a sufficient risk in their own right (Sandberg *et al.*, 2001).

The distinction between independent and dependent life events constituted an important methodological innovation that helped in testing the causal connection with psychopathology. Nevertheless, the fact that a person brought about a particular experience through their own behavior does not mean that the experience cannot then influence his or her later behavior or predispose to disorder (Rutter, Silberg, & Simonoff,1993). Thus, for example, people choose whether or not to smoke cigarettes but that does not mean that smoking cannot have a carcinogenic risk effect on lung cancer. Similarly, the fact that a person behaves in a way that leads to rebuffs or rejections from peers, or predisposes them to being scapegoated in the family, does not mean that the rejection or scapegoating will not constitute a significant stress experience for them. It is essential to use research designs and data analyses that can provide a rigorous test of the postulated stress effect, but at the same time it is important to appreciate that the implication is for the choice of research strategy and not for an automatic ruling out of a stress effect. That is pertinent to the findings that children and adolescents with psychiatric disorder differ from community controls in their exposure to both independent and dependent life events, as well as chronic adversities (Allen & Rapee, 2006; Allen, Rapee, & Sandberg, unpublished data; Olsson *et al.*, 1999; Sandberg *et al.*, 1993; Williamson, Birmaher, Anderson *et al.*, 1995; Williamson *et al.*, 2003). They have also been shown to experience more of such acute and chronic stresses than children with physical illnesses such as asthma (Sandberg *et al.*, 1998).

Some life events carry both a negative and positive affective valence. The contextually positive features usually refer to hedonic qualities, enhancement of self-esteem or favorable effect on life circumstances. So far, research on positive aspects of life events has been limited, and the findings with respect to psychiatric disorder have been inconclusive (Brown, Lemyre, Bifulco, 1992; Jensen *et al.*, 1991; Leenstra, Ormel, & Giel, 1995; Sandberg *et al.*, 1993). The only study to have demonstrated a protective function of positive life events against the increased risk relating to negative life events is that by Sandberg, McCann, Ahola *et al.* (2002). In a prospective study of children with asthma, positive life events, provided they occurred in close proximity to the negative ones, significantly reduced the risk of a new asthma attack following a severely negative life event. However, this protective function was not observed among those children who lived in conditions characterized by high chronic stress. Once again, the significant role of chronic psychosocial adversities was highlighted.

Individual Differences in Exposure to Stressful Life Events

Children, like adults, vary enormously in the extent to which they experience stressful life events. Accordingly, it is necessary to consider the origin of these individual differences. First, a few stressful life events represent chance or an act of fate. That applies to natural and man-made disasters such as war, floods, earthquakes and shipping accidents. Second, stressful life events may reflect structural factors in society that make negative experiences much more likely as a result of racial (or other) discrimination, poverty, social disorganization or dangerous life circumstances (such as in areas of high violence). Third, dependent life events may come about because a person's own behavior shapes their experiences to a considerable extent (Sandberg *et al.*, 1993, 1998). The recognition of the importance of individual differences in exposure to risk experiences, together with an appreciation of the multiplicity of influences on this individual variation led to an increase in the study of the possible causal processes involved (Adams & Adams, 1993, 1996; King, Schwab-Stone, Flisher *et al.*, 2001; Rutter, Champion, Quinton *et al.*, 1995; Wals, Hillegers, Reichart *et al.*, 2005; Williamson *et al.*, 1995; Williamson, Birmaher, Frank *et al.*, 1998).

Longitudinal studies have shown the important extent to which a person's own behavior predicts their later experiences. Thus, Robins' (1966) classic follow-up of child guidance clinic attendees into mid-adult life found that antisocial behavior in childhood was associated with a major increase in negative life experiences many years later. These included multiple divorces, unemployment, frequent job changes, lack of friends and lack of social support. Similarly, Champion, Goodall, & Rutter's (1995) 20-year follow-up of London school children demonstrated that psychopathology at age 10 years (especially conduct problems but, to a lesser extent, emotional disturbance) was associated with a more than doubling in the risk of both acute negative life events and chronic stressful experiences in adult life. Both studies suggested that the sequelae frequently depended on chain events that involved links reflecting separate psychological processes – including learned maladaptive emotional responses, self-perpetuating behavior patterns or habits, lowered self-esteem influencing the ability to deal with future experiences, and getting into situations that generated severely negative life events.

The Christchurch longitudinal study (Fergusson, Woodward, & Horwood, 2000) confirmed these cumulative chain effects and indicated that stressful life events in the 15–21-year age period were associated with a several-fold increase in suicidal ideation and suicidal acts, with the effects of childhood risk factors largely mediated through mental health problems in the intervening years. Somewhat similarly, in their prospective study of children of parents with a bipolar disorder, Wals *et al.* (2005) found that sub-threshold anxiety and depressive symptoms both increased the rate of behavior-dependent stressful life events and the onset and/or recurrence of a mood disorder.

Similarly, Daley, Hammen, Burge *et al.*'s (1997) 2-year longitudinal study of late adolescent women found that depression that was comorbid with other problems was associated with more stress experiences later, even after controlling for chronic adversity. They concluded that stresses arose, not just from individual behavior, but also from their broader social world, in turn shaped by interpersonal and intrapersonal factors.

Through gene–environment correlations (see chapter 23), genetically influenced child and parent behaviors have a role in the shaping and selecting of environments, and in the responses evoked in other people. For these reasons, twin studies have shown significant genetic effects on people's likelihood of experiencing negative life events (Kendler, Neale, Kessler *et al.*, 1993; Silberg *et al.*, 1999; Thapar, Harold, & McGuffin, 1998). It is important to note, however, that the effect of children's genetically influenced behavior in eliciting negative reactions from other people to some extent depends on social context. Thus, Riggins-Caspers, Cadoret, Knutson *et al.* (2003) found that the effect of children's disruptive behavior in eliciting negative reactions from their adoptive parents mainly applied when the parents themselves were distressed or impaired in some way.

To an important extent, parents who pass on risky genes are more likely also to create risky rearing environments. Thus, Rutter and Quinton (1984) found that parental personality disorder was associated with a much higher rate of marital discord and of hostility focused on the children than in a comparable general population sample. Parental mental disorders of varied types have been found to be associated with adverse rearing features in a range of other studies (Adrian & Hammen, 1993; Minde, Eakin, Hechtman *et al.*, 2003; Murray & Cooper, 1997; Rutter, 1989).

Acute Life Stresses and Chronic Adversity

Much research has shown that negative life events are more common in individuals who also have chronic psychosocial adversities (Brown & Harris, 1986; Rojo, Conesa, Bermudez *et al.*, 2006; Sandberg *et al.*, 1993, 2000). That raises several rather different issues. It highlights the fact that many of the stressful life events impinging on children are influenced in one way or another by their parents' behavior. This is the case, for example, with divorce, abuse, domestic violence, crime, substance abuse and neglect.

It is not just parental mental disorder that predisposes to the generation of stressors; personality features may do the same. Ellenbogen & Hodgins (2004) in a cross-sectional study of children whose parents had a bipolar disorder, major depression or no disorder found that high parental neuroticism was associated with less good psychosocial functioning, more poor parenting, more dependent stressful life events and less good coping than other parents. The implication (with the caveat that the association was cross-sectional) was that a substantial part of the risk effects on the children derived from the neuroticism-generated stresses and adversities.

Societal influences outside the family can also generate stress. Thus, in the case of sexual abuse it is not just the acts of abuse that are traumatic, but also repeatedly having to testify in court is associated with an increased risk of long-term sequelae, especially if there is a lack of maternal support and a lack of corroborating evidence so that doubt is cast on the child's account (Goodman, Batterman-Fraunce, & Kenny, 1992; Quas, Goodman, Ghetti *et al.*, 2005; see also chapters 28 & 29).

Broader living conditions are also influential. Geographical areas characterized by social disorganization not only predispose to crime (Brooks-Gunn, Duncan, & Aber, 1997; Sampson, Raudenbush, & Earls, 1997), but also provide environments in which young people are more likely to be the targets of violence and the witnesses of the shootings of friends and family. Similarly, poverty and poor life circumstances are likely to predispose to family ill health and interparental conflicts, which in turn increase the likelihood of acute negative events (Sandberg *et al.*, 1993, 2000), as well as make harmonious effective parenting more difficult (Beck & Shaw, 2005; Brody, Murry, Gerrard *et al.*, 2004; Conger, Ge, Elder *et al.*, 1994).

The well-documented association between acute negative life events and chronic adversity raises the question of the extent to which the psychopathological risks derive from the event itself or from the chronic adversities with which it is associated. One of the crucial advances was the appreciation by Brown and Harris (1978) that the main risk in adults was provided by the long-term contextual threat, and not by the acute unpleasantness of the event or the degree of life change involved. The same seems to apply in childhood. By long-term threat, what is meant is not just the practical consequences such as the effects on parenting or on intimate relationships, but also the possible long-term effects on self-esteem and self-image. Because of this, public humiliation is usually more of a stressor than, say, being bitten by a dog. In adults, especially in the case of depression, a single high-threat event in the 6–9 weeks preceding onset was sufficient to provoke a major affective disorder (Brown & Harris, 1978; Surtees & Wainwright, 1999). As noted, this clear-cut timing effect has been less evident in most studies of children.

That does not necessarily mean that a single high-threat event cannot provoke the onset of disorder. That it can has, perhaps, been most clearly shown in the case of sexual or physical abuse (see chapters 28 & 29). Nevertheless, even in these cases, the sequelae are most striking when the abuse has been recurrent, as well as severe, and when it has implications that involve a breach of trust. What is important, however, is that the sequelae can persist for many years after the abuse came to an end (see chapter 13).

Three issues need to be considered. First, can acute life stresses create an increased ongoing liability to disorder that extends beyond any onset-provoking effect? Second, is any such increased liability a function of the multiplicity of acute events, rather than the overwhelming effect of a single stress event carrying a long-term threat? Third, is any overall increase in liability really a function of chronic adversity, rather than acute stress, with the latter no more than an index of the longer-lasting life difficulties or hazards? No clear-cut answers to these questions are available. Nevertheless, it is evident that life events carrying long-term psychological threat to children nearly always involve social interaction, and derive from, or lead to, chronic psychosocial adversities ranging from being the victim of bullying to illness and discordant relationships within the family (Essex, Klein, Cho *et al.*, 2003; Goodyer, Wright, Altham, 1988; Goodyer, Herbert, Tamplin *et al.*, 1997; Jensen *et al.*, 1991; Sandberg *et al.*, 1993, 1998, 2000; Tiet, Bird, Davies *et al.*, 1998). Also, it is evident from epidemiological and clinical studies that the main psychopathological risk associated with family break-up derives from the associated family conflict rather than from family separations or changes (Cuffe, McKeown, Addy *et al.*, 2005; Fergusson, Horwood, & Lynskey, 1992; McMahon, Grant, Compas *et al.*, 2003). It is for this reason that, on the whole, parental divorce carries a greater psychopathological risk than the loss of a parent through death (Rutter, 1971).

Sandberg *et al.* (1993, 1998) showed that the main risk for children derived from the acute stresses that stemmed from, or were otherwise associated with, chronic adversity. It may be concluded that, although single severe stress events may carry risk, it is multiple events and events associated with chronic adversity that carry the greatest risk.

Specificity of Stress Effects

It is conceivable that specific associations between particular stressors and particular outcomes could be mediated by psychological, biological or social processes, and the specific nature of the stressor. In adults, some findings have suggested a degree of specificity, with "loss" events more important in the provocation of depression, and "danger" events in the onset of anxiety disorders (Brown, Harris, & Eales, 1996; Finlay-Jones & Brown, 1981; Miller & Ingham, 1985). In contrast, little evidence that this is so in children exists so far, and even this is inconsistent (Allen, Rapee, Sandberg, unpublished data, Eley & Stevenson, 2000; Goodyer, Wright, & Altham, 1990a,b; Williamson, Birmaher, Dahl *et al.*, 2005). This may be because, up to now, very few studies testing full specificity designs (i.e., specific stressors linked to specific outcomes, via specific mediators, in the context of specific moderators) have been carried out in children.

The general lack of specificity (for review see McMahon *et al.*, 2003) may have several explanations. Particular claims have been made with respect to possibly specific effects of sexual abuse (with respect to later sexual difficulties) but non-specific effects of both physical and sexual abuse outweigh specific sequelae (see chapters 28 & 29). The one relatively specific stress effect (applying to overwhelming unusual stresses) concerns post-traumatic stress disorder (PTSD) but it should be noted that PTSD is by no means the only response to overwhelming stress (see chapter 42).

Most crucially, many stressors include several rather different components involving loss, conflict, humiliation and danger. It is possible – although not yet demonstrated – that these components when they occur separately do have more specific effects. In addition, most studies have failed to differentiate between acute stresses occurring outside the context of chronic adversity and those occurring in association with ongoing lasting hazards of various kinds.

Individual Differences in Response to Stressful Life Events

Some of the earlier clinical reports on the effects of stress tended to assume that negative life events necessarily increased psychopathological risk. However, both human and animal studies have been consistent in showing that, in some circumstances, stress experiences may be protective, exerting "steeling" effects (Rutter, 1983). For example, prospective studies by Parker, Buckmaster, Schatzberg *et al.* (2004) and Parker, Buckmaster, Sundlass *et al.* (2006) in non-human primates have demonstrated that moderately stressful early experiences strengthened socioemotional and neuroendocrine resistance to subsequent stressors. Brief separations from mother, at an age when biologically but not socially independent, led to diminished anxiety and enhanced exploratory and play behavior backed up by neurohormonal evidence indicating less biological stress response. It was also established that stress inoculation, rather than increased levels of maternal care following stress exposure, was the important factor. These results therefore suggest that a combination of mild stress causing acute anxiety and hypothalamic–pituitary–adrenal (HPA) axis activation is necessary for the development of subsequent stress resistance. The possible neural mediation of "steeling" effects has been investigated by Maier and colleagues in a series of rat studies (Amat, Paul, Zarza *et al.*, 2006). Earlier experiments had shown that controllable stress provided some form of "immunizing" protection against later stress. Amat *et al.* found that behavioral immunization was blocked by inactivation of the ventral medial prefrontal cortex (mPFCv) by the administration of muscimol. The same effect was produced by anisomycin at the time of the initial controllable stress, but this was not found if it was only given later at the time of uncontrollable stress. The implication seems to be that the mPFCv is needed both to process information about the controllability of stress and to use this information to regulate responses to subsequent stressors. Replication is awaited.

"Steeling" effects reflect the fact that negative experiences, as well as challenges and transitions, are a normal part of life that all people have to learn to cope with. Successful physiological and/or psychological coping may be strengthening rather than weakening. This recognition has led to the concept of resilience, meaning the phenomenon that, whereas some individuals succumb following stress, others survive relatively unscathed, or even strengthened, following severely adverse experiences (Rutter, 2005, 2006c).

Resilience

Traditionally, clinicians and researchers have tended to view this marked individual variation in people's responses to stressful life experiences in terms of the overall balance between risk and protective factors. This has meant a focus on variables – asking, for example, whether the risks are mitigated, or compensated for, by compensatory positive experiences. That does indeed constitute an important consideration. However, Rutter (2006b,c) has argued for the need to go beyond the concepts of risk and protection that carry the implicit assumption that effects will apply similarly to everyone (see chapter 25). Instead, he suggested the value of examining the mechanisms and processes involved in individual differences in response. It is implicit in this concept of resilience that it does not refer to an individual trait, and it does not assume that the same processes will apply to all individuals, all stresses and all outcomes, or indeed to all phases in a person's life. The focus, therefore, is not on fixed variables but rather on coping processes – coping incorporating both physiological and psychological mechanisms. This means that resilience cannot be measured directly as an observed trait, for it is not a single quality.

Several different implications follow from what is known as resilience. First, there is good evidence of the importance of gene–environment interactions (Kramer, 2005; Rutter, 2006a; Rutter, Moffitt, & Caspi, 2006b; see chapter 23). Thus, Caspi, McLay, Moffitt *et al.* (2002) and Caspi, Sugden, Moffitt *et al.* (2003) showed that allelic variants of the *MAOA* gene and the serotonin transporter promoter gene moderated the effects of child abuse and recurrent negative life events on the liability to antisocial disorder and to depression. There was no main effect of the genetic variant on the psychopathological outcome as such, but there was a substantial and significant effect in influencing the susceptibility to the environmental stressors. Structural and functioning imaging studies in human adult volunteers without psychopathology showed that the allelic variation was associated with a substantial measurable neural response to fearful stimuli or challenging situations (Hariri, Mattay, Tessitore *et al.*, 2002; Hariri, Drabant, Munoz *et al.*, 2005; Meyer-Lindenberg, Buckholtz, Kolachana *et al.*, 2006; Pezawas, Meyer-Lindenberg, Drabant *et al.*, 2005). The importance of these (and other related findings) is that it provides pointers to the biological basis of the stress response, it suggests that the causal chain for the genetic effects and the stress effects may be the same and it indicates that the processes apply not just to people with a disorder but also to those without psychopathology.

A second resilience consideration derives from the evidence (albeit still limited) that protection may be fostered by controlled exposure to risk rather than by avoidance of risk. The parallel here is the protection against infectious disease afforded by either naturally acquired immunity or immunization. The psychological parallel, perhaps, is the evidence that the elimination of phobias is better achieved through controlled exposure than by avoidance.

A third consideration is the recognition that protection may be afforded by features or circumstances that are neutral (or even risky) in the absence of stress. For example, Quinton and Rutter (1988) found that a planning tendency (fostered by good school experiences) was protective for girls reared in institutions but not for girls in the general population. The point was that the latter did not need to plan because their environments were generally benign and supportive whereas that was far from the case with the girls returning to discordant dysfunctional families on discharge from institutions.

A fourth consideration is that it matters how people deal with the stresses and challenges they face. Adverse sequelae are much more likely if maladaptive responses (such as reliance on drugs or alcohol) are employed than if more adaptive practical or emotional coping strategies are used. Finally, it is clear that resilience may come about by experiences both preceding and following the stress events or chronic adversities (Laub & Sampson, 2003; Rutter, 1996).

Brown, Lemyre, & Bifulco (1992) have suggested that, in adults, positive experiences that directly counter the negative effects of the stressful event may be protective. Thus, a happy occasion is not likely to help much but a new loving relationship may do much to make up for a lost relationship. Whether or not the same applies in childhood is not known. On the whole, little effect (apart from one study of new asthma exacerbations; Sandberg *et al.*, 2002) has been found for hedonically positive events. However, there is evidence that a good close confiding relationship may partially mitigate the effect of family discord and conflict (Jenkins & Smith, 1990), and that a lack of such a relationship may increase the adverse effects of severely negative life events (Sandberg *et al.*, 1993).

Sensitizing Effects

Clinicians have long recognized the possibility of sensitizing effects of stress experiences. Thus, experience suggests that someone who has experienced the death of a much-loved person (either within the family or a close friend) may be more vulnerable to the psychopathological effects of a later second bereavement. Likewise, studies in adults have highlighted the role of early loss events (especially if leading to lack of care) in sensitizing to later stressors (life events involving loss, in particular), and thus paving the way to depression (Brown & Harris 1986; Hammen, Henry, & Daley, 2000). Similarly, one major humiliation may increase sensitization to further humiliations, or even predispose the person to interpret minor rebuffs as humiliating rejection. Abuse (physical or sexual) in the context of a trusting or dependent relationship may also give rise to a more pervasive reluctance to trust people even when they give no indication that a lack of trust is warranted. This was evidenced, for example, in a Canadian study of high school students (Wolfe, Scott, Wekerle *et al.*, 2001). Boys with a childhood history of maltreatment were three times more likely to engage in violence towards their dating partners compared with youngsters who had not been abused. So far, however, little sound empirical research in children exists that could document the strength or importance of sensitizing effects, or indicate when such effects are likely to arise.

An exception here is a longitudinal study by Essex, Klein, Cho *et al.* (2002) starting with an unselected sample of expectant mothers recruited from antenatal clinics. When assessed at 4.5 years, the children whose mothers had experienced high levels of stress both during the child's infancy (three assessments in the first year of life) and at the time of assessment, had significantly higher cortisol levels compared with the rest of the sample. Furthermore, exposure to maternal depression beginning in infancy was the strongest predictor of the children's high cortisol level. The same study also showed that the children with high cortisol levels exhibited significantly more problems in their emotional and behavioral adjustment.

Research on adults has also clarified the biological basis of the sensitization phenomenon by showing that trauma experience can interact with a pre-existing biological abnormality. This was demonstrated by a twin study of adult trauma patients by Gilbertson, Shenton, Ciszewski *et al.* (2002), who showed that smaller hippocampal volumes in those with PTSD represent a preexisting familial vulnerability factor rather than being a neurotoxic product of trauma per se. The design, however, did not allow any assessment of whether the vulnerability factor was in any way related to earlier stresses.

Anniversary reactions in which there is the recurrence of psychopathology on the anniversary of some major stress event or loss represent another example of past experience sensitizing to a later one. In adults, the majority of evidence on this stems from studies of war veterans (Morgan, Hill, Fox *et al.*, 1999), but attention has also been drawn to anniversary reactions possibly constituting a subgroup of seasonal mood disorders and bipolar disorder (Beratis, Gourzis, & Gabriel, 1996). Once more, as far as children are concerned there is clinical evidence of the reality of the phenomenon but a paucity of research that might be informative on its frequency or importance. In the psychoanalytic literature, however, the topic of anniversary reactions has been more extensively dealt with regarding both children (Azarian, Miller, Palumbo *et al.*, 1997) and adults (Taylor, 2002).

A cognitive vulnerability–transactional stress theory proposed by Hankin and Abrahamson (2001) to explain the development of gender differences in depression in adolescence is worth noting here. This transactional model involving bidirectional effects among biological changes, negative affect, pubertal timing and "social" life events posits a causal chain leading to a higher rate of depression in girls. It argues that in girls, negative affect resulting from a negative life event is more likely to be perpetuated by their negative cognitive style (possibly related to pre-existing vulnerability resulting from early abuse, for example), thus leading to clinical depression, which once established promotes self-generated negative interpersonal life events, and these in turn help to keep the chain going.

The concept of sensitization can also be utilized in the context of treatment. Thus, there is evidence that cognitive–behavioral treatment programs involving desensitization, in the form of careful graded exposure to traumatic memories, are helpful for children with PTSD (Stein, Jaycox, Kataoka *et al.*, 2003).

The Concept of Adjustment Disorder

For many years, the diagnosis of "adjustment disorder" was extremely popular in child and adolescent psychiatry (for a systematic review see Hill, 2002). Its prime use seems to have been the apparent value of avoiding stigmatizing diagnostic terms that implied a poor prognosis. At that time, many clinicians assumed a substantial discontinuity between child and adult psychopathology, with the former more benign and more normative. The relationship with a putative stressor constituted the "peg" on which to hang this diagnostic notion.

Research findings have cast doubt on virtually all of these assumptions. Acute stress experiences are associated with a wide range of psychopathological disorders and there is nothing particularly distinctive about those provoked by stress. Moreover, although some stress reactions are quite brief in duration, others are long-lasting. Moreover, mild disorders that fall short of the symptom criteria specified for other diagnoses may not be associated with stress events and may nevertheless involve significant social impairment (Angold, Costello, Farmer *et al.*, 1999). Finally, the continuities between child and adult psychopathology are strong rather than weak (Rutter, 2005; Rutter, Maughan, & Kim-Cohen, 2006a; see also chapter 13).

Both the major classification schemes – ICD-10 (World Health Organization, 1996) and DSM-IV (American Psychiatric Association, 2000) – still include the diagnostic category of adjustment disorder, but it is noteworthy in being the only diagnosis without a characteristic clinical picture. Rules are specified to indicate when the diagnosis may be made but they are essentially arbitrary and lacking empirical research support. The category probably retains some utility in providing a means of recording mild non-specific disorders that do not meet the criteria for other specific diagnostic categories and yet involve significantly impaired social functioning, but its use should not be misleadingly tied to the association with a life stressor. Accordingly, the concept is best regarded as an historical anachronism rather than a solid diagnostic category and it will not be considered further here (for a review of the evidence see Hill, 2002).

Bereavement as a Specific Kind of Life Stress

Traditionally, bereavement has been given special attention as a stress reaction. DSM-IV excludes bereavement reactions lasting less than 3 months from psychiatric disorders on the grounds that these are normal expected reactions. However, pathological grief reactions are considered disorders if they last longer than 3 months and if they include specified symptoms (the symptoms being ones that are more appropriate for adults than for children). ICD–10, on the other hand, does not have a specific pathological grief diagnosis and does not exclude bereavement reactions just because they last less than 3 months, provided that they are associated with significant social impairment. Unlike DSM-IV, it also recognizes that the disorders that follow bereavement may take many different forms. The literature on bereavement was well reviewed by Black (2002) and only the key findings are noted here.

First, the notion that, in the general population, normal grief reactions do not last longer than 3 months is simply wrong. To the contrary, most follow-up studies indicate that sequelae often last up to 2 years (perhaps more clearly shown in adults than in children). For example, in a longitudinal study of parent-bereaved children and adolescents (Cerel, Fristad, Verducci *et al.*, 2006) an increased rate of impairing psychiatric symptoms, especially depression, was still present at the 2-year follow-up.

Second, with children, the long-term sequelae depend more on the consequences of the bereavement than the parental loss as such. Thus, the long-term risks are particularly influenced by the effects on the quality of parental care and on the psychopathology of the surviving parent, as well as by the child's own psychiatric problems predating the bereavement (Cerel *et al.*, 2006; Dowdney, 2000; Harris, Brown, & Bifulco, 1986). Accordingly, childhood bereavement as such is not a major risk factor for later psychopathology (Harrington & Harrison,

1999) with the risks substantially less than those associated with parental divorce or family break-up (Rutter, 1971).

Third, this conclusion applies to bereavements arising from illness or accidents. The sequelae of bereavements deriving from sudden, unexpected, violent or mutilating deaths, particularly if witnessed by the child – especially those of family members – produce more serious psychopathology. Children can get caught up in war and civil conflict, and may witness the murder of parents, siblings and other familiar people (Newman, Black, & Harris-Hendriks, 1997; Osofsky, 1997). Of the children who experience death of a loved one, those who witness a sudden, horrific and unexpected death and those who perceive a threat to their own life are more likely to develop PTSD (Harris-Hendricks, Black, & Kaplan, 1993; Pynoos, Frederick, Nader *et al.*, 1987; Stoppelbein & Greening, 2000). Family survivors of homicide are at high risk of developing dysfunctional symptoms such as PTSD that tend to persist longer than in other bereavements (Amick-McMullan, Kilpatrick, & Resnick, 1991; Masters, Friedman, & Getzel, 1988). These features are considered more fully in chapter 31.

Fourth, it is important to recognize that children's responses to bereavement are not identical to those seen in adults. Young children are more likely than older ones to have difficulty comprehending death and in enduring feelings of grief and mourning. For example, according to the review of children's reactions to death (Cuddy-Casey & Orvaschel, 1997) the concepts of irreversibility and universality were found to be understood before causality, and external events, such as moving and speaking, were believed by children to cease before internal ones, such as thinking and feeling. Children younger than 5 years generally appear unable to give a narrative account of the sequence of events around bereavement. Likewise, children's capacity to sustain sad affects increases gradually with age and maturity. Thus, young children do not sustain affects for long periods and their apparent lack of sadness may deceive their caregivers into believing that they are unaffected by the loss.

The reactions of young children often take an immature form and therefore appear different. It is also not unusual for young children to develop pathological mourning reactions (Goodyer, 1990). At a preverbal age, for example, children react to loss with bodily responses. They may lose their recently acquired control over urination or defecation, lose their appetites, fail to settle to sleep or become restless. Motility or speech may be temporarily lost. Lowered resistance to infections and other illnesses has also been noted in young children following the loss of a parent (for a broader review of the effects of stress and adversity on immunological responses see Institute of Medicine of the National Academies, 2006). As children may not understand the source of emotions of grief they often suffer alone without seeking support from carers or other adults. The misconstruing of emotions can lead to hypochondriasis or other psychosomatic symptoms and these in turn may bind the surviving parent to the child, thus reinforcing the symptoms. Children may also hide their own grief in order to protect their parent and avoid upsetting them. Disruption of attachment because of the death of a caregiver – usually a mother – during early childhood increases the risk of an attachment disorder, a separation anxiety disorder, anxiety, depression or other emotional disorder during childhood or adolescence. Adolescents in the process of separating from parents may either take a step back by becoming more involved with the family, especially if they are the eldest or the same sex as the deceased parent, or react by rejecting the family and moving into a premature adult role.

The effects on children of a sibling death have been less well studied than that of a parent. The available studies indicate a mixed picture, with some (Pettle Michael & Lansdown, 1986) reporting high levels of both emotional and behavioral disturbance up to 3 years following sibling bereavement, while others (Brent, Moritz, Bridge *et al.*, 1997), although detecting a several-fold increase of major depression in the first 6 months, found the risk disappearing by the 3-year follow-up.

According to Black (2002), the assessment of children and adolescents who have been bereaved, especially by a traumatic death, must involve not only evaluation for the presence of psychiatric disorders, but also their attachment needs, where they should live (if it is not possible or desirable to live with the parents) and what contact they should have with a perpetrator parent (if the death has been brought about by homicide). The assessment must also include an evaluation of the effect of the bereavement on their carers' parenting capabilities. Likewise, it is essential to interview each affected child (and adult) individually. The specific assessment of post-traumatic reactions is necessary in traumatic bereavements, and is desirable in the case of all bereaved children.

The majority of bereaved children will not require psychiatric treatment, but most will benefit from contact with a concerned adult outside the family to help the child understand and come to terms with their loss. Such help may be provided by a school counselor, health visitor or counselor attached to a GP's surgery, or volunteer bereavement counseling services. Child and adolescent mental health services can provide useful support, training and consultation to such services. Black (2002) recommended that in an effort to prevent morbidity and focus resources, psychiatric assessment should be made available to the following high-risk groups: children under 10 years; those with learning difficulties; those who have suffered previous losses; where there is a family or personal history of psychiatric disorder; where the death is sudden or otherwise traumatic; children caught up in witnessing violent deaths of those known to them (homicide, accident, suicide); where there is perceived threat to their own life; those with multiple psychosocial adversities; and those where the surviving parent(s) are failing in their care of the child.

Mechanisms Moderating and Mediating Stress Responses

In so far as negative life experiences have enduring effects on mental health, it is necessary to consider the mediating mechanisms by which the sequelae are carried forward in time, and what factors have a moderating role in this process (Rutter, 2000a,b). First, persistence may come about because the initial adverse experiences led to altered patterns of interpersonal interaction (Moss, Cyr, & Dubois-Comtois, 2004) which, in turn, brought about further negative experiences (Rutter *et al.*, 1995; Rutter, Giller, & Hagell, 1998). Alternatively, as suggested by the findings relating to physical abuse, the experience may result in altered cognitive sets or styles of emotional and cognitive processing (Dodge, Pettit, Bates *et al.*, 1995; Overmier & Murison, 2005). A third possibility is that the stress affects neurobiological structure and function, as suggested first by animal studies and subsequently by a growing body of research on humans (for reviews see Dickerson & Kemeny 2004; Grossman, Churchill, McKinney *et al.*, 2003; Levine, 2005; Shea, Walsh, MacMillan *et al.*, 2004). In their meta-analytic review of 208 laboratory studies with adults, Dickerson and Kemeny (2004) concluded that it is particularly tasks containing both uncontrollable and social-evaluative elements that are associated with the largest cortisol and adrenocorticotropin hormone changes and with the longest times for recovery. The implication (as yet untested) is that it is these elements that may be most important in more naturally occurring stress events in childhood, as well as adulthood.

The mechanism with respect to severe and lasting early adversities could also lie in the developmental programming of the brain (for reviews see Bremner & Vermetten, 2001; Granger, Hood, Dreschel *et al.*, 2001; Kaufman, Plotsky, Nemeroff *et al.*, 2000; Ladd, Huot, Thrivikraman *et al.*, 2000; LeDoux, 2002; Pine, 2003). Evidence from preclinical studies has been most consistent in demonstrating the effects of early adverse experiences on brain structure and function. Thus, it has been established that stress effects on the development of hippocampus are mediated by at least three forms of structural plasticity: neuronal atrophy, neurotoxicity and neurogenesis. Of these, neuronal atrophy can be caused by exposure to stress leading to a cascade of glucocorticoids; however, it is a reversible effect. Prolonged stress, on the other hand, leads to a neurotoxic effect with a permanent effect. Stress may also inhibit the normal neurogenesis leading to reduced hippocampal volume. Studies of maternal depression and postnatal handling have highlighted the importance of early experience on the development of the brain and the multiple neurotransmitter systems (Kaufman *et al.*, 2000).

Similarly, research in rodents and non-human primates has led to greater understanding of the brain areas and brain functions, including neurochemical responses, involved in threat perception (Pine, 2003). Thus, stress during key stages of development has been shown to produce long-term alterations in the threat response. These comprise a neuroanatomical circuit involving two major cortical pathways (pre-frontal cortex and components of temporal lobes), two key subcortical structures (amygdala and hippocampus) and a neurochemical pathway consisting of ascending brainstem monoamine neurons. Regulation of this circuit can be shaped through experiences during development.

There is also evidence of experience-related developmental plasticity (Pine, 2003; Yehuda & McEwen, 2004), with experience having a direct role in organizing stress regulatory systems during development. Here, the key factors are the level and nature of early maternal care, which can affect behavior, as well as the hormonal and neural systems related to stress regulation. These maternal influences, beginning soon after birth and appearing to operate within a critical window in the early postpartum phase, can also permanently alter the HPA axis in adulthood (Yehuda & McEwen, 2004).

Animal studies have also shown that the subsequent caregiving environment can moderate the adverse effects of early stress on neurobiological systems (Kaufman *et al.*, 2000), and "adoption with optimal parenting" ("cross-fostering") has been found to reverse maladaptive HPA axis alterations. Furthermore, there is evidence to suggest that comparable effects could occur in humans and therefore have therapeutic implications.

Clinical studies of adults with a childhood history of abuse have implicated long-term dysfunction of the stress response systems (HPA axis, noradrenergic and hippocampal systems) and it has been proposed that these effects underlie the symptoms of PTSD and other stress-related disorders (Delahanty, Nugent, Christopher *et al.*, 2005; McEwen, 2000; Olff, Langeland, & Gersons, 2005). Likewise, dysregulation of the HPA axis has been suggested as the possible link between exposure to major traumatic events such as sexual abuse and subsequent psychiatric disorder in children (Carrion, Weems, Ray *et al.*, 2002). An association between abnormal cortisol levels and emotional problems accompanied by extreme behavioral inhibition, social wariness and withdrawal has also been reported in studies with children (Ashman, Dawson, Panagiotides *et al.*, 2002; Essex *et al.*, 2002; Smider, Essex, Kalin *et al.*, 2002). The findings have, however, by no means been consistent with regard to the nature of the dysregulation and the patterns of association (for review see Gunnar & Donzella, 2002; Gunnar & Vazquez, 2006).

A more consistent, but complex, picture has emerged from neurochemical studies in adults (Yehuda & McEwen, 2004). These have established with some certainty that stress should no longer be defined by glucocorticoid excess any more than glucocorticoid excess be taken as evidence of stress. Here, a study by Yehuda, Halligan, Golier *et al.* (2004) on the effects of trauma exposure on cortisol response to dexamethasone administration has been especially informative. It has helped to clarify the likely reasons for previous conflicting findings regarding cortisol levels in major depressive disorder (MDD). The study was able to establish the important role of major traumatic experiences in enhancing cortisol suppression (i.e., lower cortisol levels in PTSD patients), in contrast to higher cortisol levels in persons with MDD. However, in individuals with both PTSD and MDD, those with a trauma experience predating that causing PTSD, cortisol levels resembled those found in PTSD. Heim, Newport, Bonsall *et al.* (2001) reported similar findings and concluded that a history of early abuse may explain why only about half of MDD patients show reduced suppression, thus indicating that neurobiological sensitization of HPA axis is a prominent neuroendocrine response in MDD in the presence of PTSD.

There is also evidence that vulnerability to later emotional and behavioral dysregulation extends to include prenatal stress in both animals (Coe & Lubach, 2000; Kofman, 2002; Schneider, Moore, Roberts *et al.*, 2001; Yehuda & McEwen, 2004) and humans (Gutteling, de Werth, & Buitelaar, 2005; Kraemer & Clarke, 1996; Phillips & Jones, 2006; Wadhwa, 2005). A neurobiological model of prenatal stress proposes that maternal stress exerts a negative influence on fetal developmental outcome that is mediated by the HPA system. Central to an understanding of how high levels of glucocorticoids in maternal circulation may alter fetal development is the knowledge that maternal–fetal communication during gestation is endocrine rather than neural, and cortisol levels in the fetus correlate with those in the maternal circulation. This has important implications, because excess levels of cortisol inhibit intrauterine growth, may accelerate the onset of parturition indirectly and may alter the regulation of glucocorticoid receptors in the brain of the developing fetus. It has been suggested that intrauterine exposure to high levels of cortisol could permanently increase the "set point" for HPA axis deactivation in relevant brain areas, resulting in stress responses and behavioral alterations consistent with depressive illness. Glucocorticoid exposure in the third trimester appears to be the critical period for stress programming.

Primate research has also presented evidence that chronic unpredictable stress during pregnancy may have long-lasting effects on brain activity and behavior of the offspring (Coe & Lubach, 2000; Schneider *et al.*, 2001). Prenatal stress appears to affect the neurobiology of the neonate so that its responses to common events and stimuli are markedly altered. These effects on brain mechanisms are more likely to be diffuse, rather than specific. As a consequence, the neonate may, for example, be more fussy and difficult, affecting how the caregiver is able to cope. Thus, prenatal stress appears to set the infant's neurobiology into a state in which vital attachments are hard to achieve and adverse experiences more likely. The adverse experiences can in turn result in further neurobiological deflection of development. Prenatal effects on fetal neurobiological development may also be easily confused with genetic predisposition. Prospective studies of prenatal maternal stress on children's neuroendocrine and behavioral functioning have shown significant associations with both (Gutteling, de Weerth, & Buitelaar, 2005; Phillips & Jones, 2006; Wadhwa, 2005). The effects are best demonstrated in relation to birth weight but they extend more widely. Up to now the inferences about mediation are limited by a lack of tests of genetic mediation and by limited contrasts with postnatal stresses. Nevertheless, some prenatal effects seem probable.

In children and in adults, not only have negative life events been associated with a wide range of psychopathology (Gowers, North, & Byram, 1996; Sandberg *et al.*, 1993), but they have also been shown to precede the onset of many somatic illnesses and to relate to their reoccurrence (Haavet & Grünfeld, 1997). The role of stress in viral infections has been the focus of research in more recent years. Thus, it has been shown that stressful experiences have adverse effects on the body's immunological responses (for review see Segerstrom & Miller, 2004), this possibly providing the mediating factor in relation to the demonstrated effects of adverse life events in increasing susceptibility to infections. It is also well acknowledged that the immune system and the central nervous system form a bidirectional communication network. In this network pro-inflammatory cytokines have a critical role (see chapter 57).

Implications for Clinical Practice

Most children presenting with the common forms of psychopathology have experienced, and may continue to be experiencing, acute life events carrying long-term threat. Such events are clinically important for a variety of different reasons and it is necessary that any adequate diagnostic assessment includes enquiring about them. Thus, they may have had a role in precipitating the sudden onset or exacerbation of acute emotional disorders or of suicidal acts or ideation. The key events might include bullying at school, humiliating experiences, rejection by friends, unexpected or supposedly unwarranted punishment at school or home, or episodes of physical or sexual abuse. Clearly, a key consideration in all instances is whether the events are ongoing, whether they should be preventable, and how the child (and family) are coping with them.

The events may also serve as an important index of ongoing chronic adversities – at home, at school, or in the family. In that connection, a key question is whether parents or teachers are responding to the child's behavior in ways that create stress. Are misdemeanors being dealt with through humiliating or stigmatizing the child or by outbursts of uncontrolled anger? The main point here lies in the identification of the coping responses used by the child and the child's family (or teachers). The focus in this instance is less on the causal impact of the life events than on the ways in which patterns of interpersonal interactions may be working in positive or negative ways.

In that connection, equal attention needs to be paid to how the child is responding to stresses and challenges. That is where resilience concepts come into their own. What are the ways in which the child is coping effectively and how may they be used in planning effective therapeutic interventions? A particular issue concerns comparisons among siblings. If, apparently, other children in the family are coping successfully with comparable stresses, but the child-patient is not, what are the factors that seem to be making a difference? Do the differences among siblings reflect variations in the ways parents are treating the children or do they reflect differences in the children's coping strategies? In other words, the main importance of stressful life events does not lie in the causal attributes given to particular events but rather to the implications for coping strategies. By the same token, the focus needs to be as much on the mechanisms involved in the *creation* of negative life events as in their effects.

Looking into the Future

A major growth area in stress research concerns the mediating mechanisms that underlie both the development of psychopathology and the development of resilience. Much of the research has focused on the HPA axis but we lack a good understanding of whether the neuroendocrine changes mediate (i.e., account for) the psychopathological sequelae. Evidence is beginning to accumulate on the differences in response to acute negative events and to chronic adversities but the findings so far are rather inconclusive. We know even less about what it is that leads to "steeling" rather than "sensitizing" effects. It is evident that both occur but why and how? The findings on gene–environment interaction (G × E) are particularly promising in providing leads on both the genetic and environmental causal pathways and, most especially, on the ways in which they come together. However, it would be a mistake to focus exclusively on neuroendocrine effects. Negative life events may have effects on self-esteem, cognitive sets and internal working models. There is a general acceptance that they are likely to be important in mediating both positive and negative consequences but research into their role is in its infancy. What is particularly needed is research that seeks to contrast competing alternative mediating mechanisms in G × E, neuroendocrine responses, cognitive mechanisms, coping responses and effects on interpersonal interactions, to mention but a few possibilities. These issues apply as much to anniversary reactions as to sensitizing effects. Do these reflect the same or different phenomena?

Although there is now evidence that the mother's anxiety during the pregnancy can have effects on the fetus, little is known about the psychopathological consequences after birth. There have been speculative suggestions about biological programming effects but, so far, these remain as just one possibility. Systematic research into mechanisms (using animal models as well as human studies) is required and this will have to examine competing possible processes, including the mediators for the psychopathological consequences when they occur.

Finally, we need to turn to a topic not considered in this chapter. Our focus has been on definable negative life events. As we have shown, they are important. In addition, however, we need to draw attention to the fact that many of the more common psychopathological disorders in young people (but not in older age groups) have tended to rise over the last 50 years (Collishaw, Maughan, Goodman *et al.*, 2004; Rutter & Smith, 1995). Why? Could this be because there have been changes in the pattern of life challenges as they face young people? That remains an almost wholly under-researched topic, but clearly it is one of huge policy and practical importance.

Further Reading

McEwan, B., & Lasley, E. N. (2002). *The end of stress as we know it.* Co-published with the Dana Press Washington DC: Joseph Henry Press.

References

Adams, J., & Adams, M. (1993). Effects of a negative life event and negative perceived problem-solving alternatives on depression in adolescents: a prospective study. *Journal of Child Psychology and Psychiatry*, *34*, 743–747.

Adams, J., & Adams, M. (1996). The association among negative life events, perceived problem solving alternatives, depression, and suicidal ideation in adolescent psychiatric patients. *Journal of Child Psychology and Psychiatry*, *37*, 715–720.

Adrian, C., & Hammen, C. (1993). Stress exposure and stress generation in children of depressed mothers. *Journal of Consulting and Clinical Psychology*, *61*, 354–359.

Allen, J. L., & Rapee, R. M. (2006). *Child and Adolescent Survey of Experiences (CASE): Parent and child versions.* Sydney: Macquarie University.

Amat, J., Paul, E., Zarza, C., Watkins, L. R., & Maier, S. F. (2006). Previous experience with behavioral control over stress blocks the behavioral and dorsal raphe nucleus activating effects of later uncontrollable stress: Role of the ventral medial prefrontal cortex. *Journal of Neuroscience*, *26*, 13264–13272.

American Psychiatric Association. (2000). *Diagnostic and statistical manual of mental disorders* (4th edn.) Text Revision. Washington, DC: American Psychiatric Press.

Amick-McMullan, A., Kilpatrick, D. G., & Resnick, H. S. (1991). Homicide as a risk factor for PTSD among surviving family members. *Behaviour Modification*, *15*, 545–559.

Angold, A., Costello, E. J., Farmer, E. M., Burns, B. J., & Erkanli, A. (1999). Impaired but undiagnosed. *Journal of the American Academy of Child and Adolescent Psychiatry*, *38*, 129–137.

Angold, A., Erkanli, A., Costello, E. J., & Rutter, M. (1996). Precision, reliability and accuracy in the dating of symptom onsets in child and adolescent psychopathology. *Journal of Child Psychology and Psychiatry*, *37*, 657–664.

Ashman, S. B., Dawson, G., Panagiotides, H., Yamada, E., & Wilkinson, C. W. (2002). Stress hormone levels in children of depressed mothers. *Development and Psychopathology*, *14*, 333–349.

Azarian, A., Miller, T. W., Palumbo, A. J., & Skriptchenko-Gregorian, V. (1997). Anniversary reactions in a five-year-old boy: Unresolved conflict, guilt, and self-identification. *Psychoanalytic Study of the Child*, *52*, 214–226.

Beck, J. E., & Shaw, D. S. (2005). The influence of perinatal complications and environmental adversity on boys' antisocial behavior. *Journal of Child Psychology and Psychiatry*, *46*, 35–46.

Beratis, S., Gourzis, P., & Gabriel, J. (1996). Psychological factors in the development of mood disorders with a seasonal pattern. *Psychopathology*, *29*, 331–339.

Black, D. (2002). Bereavement. In M. Rutter, & E. Taylor (Eds.), *Child and adolescent psychiatry* (pp. 299–308). Oxford: Blackwell.

Bremner, J. D., & Vermetten, E. (2001). Stress and development: Behavioral and biological consequences. *Development and Psychopathology*, *13*, 473–489.

Brent, D. A., Moritz, G., Bridge, J., & Perper, J. (1997). The impact of adolescent suicide on siblings and parents: A longitudinal follow-up. *Suicide and Life-Threatening Behaviour*, *26*, 253–259.

Brody, G. H., Murry, V. M., Gerrard, M., Gibbons, F. X., Molgaard, V., McNair, L., *et al.* (2004). The Strong African American Families Program: Translating research into prevention programming. *Child Development*, *75*, 900–917.

Brooks-Gunn, J., Duncan, G. J., & Aber, J. L. (1997). *Neighborhood poverty*. Vol. 1. *Context and consequences for children*. New York: Russell Sage Foundation.

Brown, G. W., & Harris, T. O. (1978). *The social origins of depression: A study of psychiatric disorder in women*. London: Tavistock.

Brown, G. W., & Harris, T. O. (1986). Establishing causal links: The Bedford College studies of depression. In H. Katschnig (Ed.), *Life events and psychiatric disorders: Controversial issues* (pp. 107–187). London: Cambridge University Press.

Brown, G. W., Harris, T. O., & Eales, M. J. (1996). Social factors and comorbidity of depressive and anxiety disorders. *British Journal of Psychiatry*, *168* (Supplement 30), 50–57.

Brown, G. W., Lemyre, L., & Bifulco, A. (1992). Social factors and recovery from anxiety and depressive disorders: A test of specificity. *British Journal of Psychiatry*, *161*, 44–54.

Cannon, W. B. (1929). *Bodily changes in pain, hunger, fear and rage*. New York: Appleton.

Carrion, V. G., Weems, C. F., Ray, R. D., Glaser, B., Hessl, D., & Reiss, A. L. (2002). Diurnal salivary cortisol in pediatric posttraumatic stress disorder. *Biological Psychiatry*, *51*, 575–582.

Caspi, A., McLay, J., Moffitt, T. E., Mill, J., Marin, J., Craig, I. W., *et al.* (2002). Role of genotype in the cycle of violence in maltreated children. *Science*, *297*, 851–854.

Caspi, A., Sugden, K., Moffitt, T. E., Taylor, A., Craig, I. W., Harrington, H., *et al.* (2003). Influence of life stress on depression: Moderation by a polymorphism in the 5-HTT gene. *Science*, *301*, 386–389.

Cerel, J., Fristad, M. A., Verducci, J., Weller, R. A., & Weller, E. B. (2006). Childhood bereavement: Psychopathology in the 2 years post-parental death. *Journal of the American Academy of Child and Adolescent Psychiatry*, *45*, 681–690.

Champion, L. A., Goodall, G. M., & Rutter, M. (1995). Behavioural problems in childhood and stressors in early adult life: A 20-year follow-up of London school children. *Psychological Medicine*, *25*, 231–246.

Coe, S. L., & Lubach, G. R. (2000). Prenatal influences on neuroimmune set points in infancy. *Annals of the New York Academy of Sciences*, *917*, 468–477.

Collishaw, S., Maughan, B., Goodman, R., & Pickles, A. (2004). Time trends in adolescent mental health. *Journal of Child Psychology and Psychiatry*, *45*, 1350–1362.

Conger, R., Ge, X., Elder, G. H., Lorenz, F. O., & Simons, R. (1994). Economic stress, coercive family processes and developmental problems of adolescents. *Child Development*, *65*, 541–561.

Cuddy-Casey, M., & Orvaschel, H. (1997). Children's understanding of death in relation to child suicidality and homicidality. *Clinical Psychology Review*, *17*, 33–45.

Cuffe, S. P., McKeown, R. E., Addy, C. L., & Garrison, C. Z. (2005). Family and psychosocial risk factors in a longitudinal epidemiological study of adolescents. *Journal of the American Academy of Child and Adolescent Psychiatry*, *44*, 121–129.

Daley, S. E., Hammen, C., Burge, D., Davila, J., Paley, B., Lindberg, N., *et al.* (1997). Predictors of the generation of episodic stress: A longitudinal study of late adolescent women. *Journal of Abnormal Psychology*, *106*, 251–259.

Delahanty, D. L., Nugent, N. R., Christopher, N. C., & Walsh, M. (2005). Initial urinary epinephrine and cortisol levels predict acute PTSD symptoms in child trauma victims. *Psychoneuroendocrinology*, *30*, 121–128.

Dickerson, S. S., & Kemeny, M. E. (2004). Acute stressors and cortisol responses: A theoretical integration and synthesis of laboratory research. *Psychological Bulletin*, *130*, 355–391.

Dodge, K. A., Pettit, G. S., Bates, J. E., & Valente, E. (1995). Social information-processing patterns partially mediate the effects of early physical abuse on later conduct problems. *Journal of Abnormal Psychology*, *104*, 632–643.

Dohrenwend, B. P. (2006). Inventorying stressful life events as risk factors for psychopathology: Toward resolution of the problem of intracategory variability. *Psychology Bulletin*, *132*, 477–495.

Dowdney, L. (2000). Childhood bereavement following parental death. *Journal of Child Psychology and Psychiatry*, *41*, 819–830.

Eley, T. C., & Stevenson, J. (2000). Specific life events and chronic experiences differentially associated with depression and anxiety in young twins. *Journal of Abnormal Child Psychology*, *28*, 383–394.

Ellenbogen, M. A., & Hodgins, S. (2004). The impact of high neuroticism in parents on children's psychosocial functioning in a population at high risk for major affective disorder: A family–environmental pathway of intergenerational risk. *Development and Psychopathology*, *16*, 113–136.

Essex, M. J., Klein, M. H., Cho, E., & Kalin, N. H. (2002). Maternal stress beginning in infancy may sensitize children to later stress exposure: Effects on cortisol and behavior. *Biological Psychiatry*, *52*, 776–784.

Essex, M. J., Klein, M. H., Cho, E., & Kraemer, H. C. (2003). Exposure to maternal depression and marital conflict: Gender differences in children's later mental health symptoms. *Journal of the American Academy of Child and Adolescent Psychiatry*, *42*, 728–737.

Fergusson, D. M., Horwood, L. J., & Lynskey, M. T. (1992). Family change, parental discord and early offending. *Journal of Child Psychology and Psychiatry*, *33*, 1059–1075.

Fergusson, D. M., Woodward, L. J., & Horwood, L. J. (2000). Risk factors and life processes associated with the onset of suicidal behaviour during adolescence and early adulthood. *Psychological Medicine*, *30*, 23–39.

Finlay-Jones, R., & Brown, G. W. (1981). Types of stressful life event and the onset of anxiety and depressive disorders. *Psychological Medicine*, *11*, 803–815.

Gilbertson, M. W., Shenton, M. E., Ciszewski, A., Kasai, K., Lasko, N. B., Orr, S. P., *et al.* (2002). Smaller hippocampal volume predicts pathologic vulnerability to psychological trauma. *Nature Neuroscience*, *5*, 1242–1247.

Glen, S., Simpson, A., Drinnan, D., McGuinness, D., & Sandberg, S. (1993). Testing the reliability of a new measure of life events and experiences in childhood: The psychosocial assessment of childhood experiences (PACE). *European Child and Adolescent Psychiatry*, *2*, 98–110.

Goodman, G. S., Batterman-Faunce, J. M., & Kenny, R. (1992). Optimizing children's testimony: Research and social policy issues concerning allegations of child sexual abuse. In D. Cicchetti, & S. Toth (Eds.), *Child abuse, child development and social policy*. Norwood, NJ: Ablex.

Goodyer, I. M. (1990). *Life experiences, development and childhood psychopathology*. Chichester: Wiley.

Goodyer, I. M., Herbert, J., Tamplin, A., & Altham, P. M. E. (2000). Recent life events, cortisol, dehydroepiandrosterone and the onset of major depression in high-risk adolescents. *British Journal of Psychiatry*, *177*, 499–504.

Goodyer, I. M., Herbert, J., Tamplin, A., Secher, S. M., & Pearson, J. (1997). Short-term outcome of major depression II: Life events, family dysfunction, and friendship difficulties as predictors of persistent disorder. *Journal of the American Academy of Child and Adolescent Psychiatry*, *36*, 474–480.

Goodyer, I. M., Wright, C., & Altham, P. M. E. (1988). Maternal adversity and recent life events in anxious and depressed children. *Journal of Child Psychology and Psychiatry*, *29*, 651–667.

Goodyer, I., Wright, C., & Altham, P. (1990a). The friendships and recent life events of anxious and depressed school-age children. *British Journal of Psychiatry*, *156*, 689–698.

Goodyer, I. M., Wright, C., & Altham, P. (1990b). Recent achievements and adversities in anxious and depressed school-age children. *Journal of Child Psychology and Psychiatry*, *31*, 1063–1077.

Gowers, S. G., North, C. D., & Byram, V. (1996). Life event precipitants of adolescent anorexia nervosa. *Journal of Child Psychology and Psychiatry*, *37*, 469–477.

Granger, D. A., Hood, K. E., Dreschel, N. A., Sergeant, E., & Likos, A. (2001). Developmental effects of early immune stress on aggressive, socially reactive, and inhibited behaviors. *Development and Psychopathology*, *13*, 599–610.

Grossman, A. W., Churchill, J. D., McKinney, B. C., Kodish, I. M., Otte, S. L., & Greenough, W. T. (2003). Experience effects on brain development: possible contributions to psychopathology. *Journal of Child Psychology and Psychiatry*, *44*, 33–63.

Gunnar, M. R., & Donzella, B. (2002). Social regulation of the cortisol levels in early human development. *Psychoneuroendocrinology*, *27*, 199–220.

Gunnar, M. R., & Vazquez, M. (2006). Stress neurobiology and development psychopathology. In D. Cicchetti, & D. J. Cohen (Eds.), *Developmental psychopathology* (2nd edn.). *Developmental neuroscience*, Vol. 2 (pp. 533–577). NY: Wiley.

Gutteling, B. M., de Weerth, C., & Buitelaar, J. K. (2005). Prenatal stress and children's cortisol reaction to the first day of school. *Psychoneuroendocrinology*, *30*, 541–549.

Haavet, O. R., & Grünfeld, B. (1997). Are life experiences of children significant for the development of somatic disease? A literature review. *Tidsskrift főr den Norske Laegefőre*, *117*, 3644–3647.

Hammen, C., Henry, R., & Daley, S. E. (2000). Depression and sensitization to stressors among young women as a function of childhood adversity. *Journal of Consulting and Clinical Psychology*, *68*, 782–787.

Hankin, B. J., & Abramson, L. Y. (2001). Development of gender differences in depression: an elaborated cognitive vulnerability-transactional stress theory. *Psychological Bulletin*, *127*, 773–796.

Hariri, A., Drabant, E., Munoz, K., Kolachana, B., Venkata, S., Egan, M., *et al.* (2005). A susceptibility gene for affective disorders and the response of the human amygdala. *Archives of General Psychiatry*, *62*, 146–152.

Hariri, A., Mattay, V., Tessitore, A., Kolachana, B., Fera, F., Goldman, D., *et al.* (2002). Serotonin transporter genetic variation and the response of the human amygdala. *Science*, *297*, 400–403.

Harrington, R., & Harrison, L. (1999). Unproven assumptions about the impact of bereavement on children. *Journal of the Royal Society of Medicine*, *92*, 230–233.

Harris, T., Brown, G. W., & Bifulco, A. (1986). Loss of parent in childhood and adult psychiatric disorder: The role of lack of adequate parental care. *Psychological Medicine*, *16*, 641–659.

Harris-Hendriks, J., Black, D., & Kaplan, T. (1993). (2nd edn., 2000). *When father kills mother: Guiding children through trauma and grief.* London: Routledge.

Heim, C., Newport, D. J., Bonsall, R., Miller, A. H., & Nemeroff, C. B. (2001). Altered pituitary–adrenal axis responses to provocative challenge tests in adult survivors of childhood abuse. *American Journal of Psychiatry*, *158*, 575–581.

Hill, P. (2002). Adjustment disorders. In M. Rutter, & E. Taylor (Eds.), *Child and adolescent psychiatry* (pp. 510–519). Oxford: Blackwell.

Holmes, T. H., & Rahe, R. H. (1967). The social readjustment rating scale. *Journal of Psychosomatic Research*, *11*, 213–218.

Institute of Medicine of the National Academies. (2006). *Genes, behavior and the social environment: Moving beyond the nature/nurture debate.* L. Hernandez & D. Blazer (Eds.). Committee on Assessing Interactions, Among Social, Behavioral and Genetic Factors in Health, Board on Health Sciences Policy. Washington, DC: National Academies Press.

Jenkins, J. M., & Smith, M. A. (1990). Factors protecting children living in disharmonious homes: Maternal reports. *Journal of the American Academy of Child and Adolescent Psychiatry*, *29*, 60–69.

Jensen, P. S., Richters, J., Ussery, T., Bloedau, L., & Davis, H. (1991). Child psychopathology and environmental influences: discrete life events versus ongoing adversity. *Journal of the American Academy of Child and Adolescent Psychiatry*, *30*, 303–309.

Johnson, J. H. (1982). Life events as stressors in childhood and adolescence. In B. B. Lahey, & A. E. Kazdin (Eds.), *Advances in clinical child psychology* (pp. 213–253). New York: Plenum Press.

Kaufman, J., Plotsky, P. M., Nemeroff, C. B., & Charney, D. S. (2000). Effects of early adverse experiences on brain structure and function: clinical implications. *Biological Psychiatry*, *48*, 778–790.

Kendler, K. S., Karkowski, L. M., & Prescott, C. A. (1999). Causal relationship between stressful life events and the onset of major depression. *American Journal of Psychiatry*, *156*, 837–841.

Kendler, K. S., Neale, M., Kessler, R., Heath, A., & Eaves, L. (1993). A twin study of recent life events and difficulties. *Archives of General Psychiatry*, *50*, 789–796.

King, R. A., Schwab-Stone, M., Flisher, A. J., Greenwald, S., Kramer, R. A., Goodman, S. H., *et al.* (2001). Psychosocial and risk behavior correlates of youth suicide attempts and suicidal ideation. *Journal of the American Academy of Child and Adolescent Psychiatry*, *40*, 837–846.

Kofman, O. (2002). The role of prenatal stress in the etiology of developmental behavioral disorders. *Neuroscience Biobehavioral Review*, *26*, 457–470.

Kraemer, G. W., & Clarke, A. S. (1996). Social attachment, brain function, and aggression. *Annals of the New York Academy of Sciences*, *794*, 121–135.

Kramer, D. A. (2005). Commentary: Gene–environment interplay in the context of genetics, epigenetics, and gene expression. *Journal of the American Academy of Child and Adolescent Psychiatry*, *44*, 19–27.

Ladd, C. O., Huot, R. L., Thrivikraman, K. V., Nemeroff, C. B., Meaney, M. J., & Plotsky, P. M. (2000). Long-term behavioral and endocrine adaptations to adverse early experience. *Progress in Brain Research*, *122*, 81–103.

Laub, J. H., & Sampson, R. J. (2003). *Shared beginnings, divergent lives: Delinquent boys to age 70.* Cambridge, MA: Harvard University Press.

LeDoux, J. E. (2002). *Synaptic self: How our brains become who we are.* New York: Viking Press.

Leenstra, A. S., Ormel, J., & Giel, R. (1995). Positive life change and recovery from depression and anxiety: A three-stage longitudinal study of primary care attenders. *British Journal of Psychiatry*, *166*, 333–343.

Levine, S. (2005). Developmental determinants of sensitivity and resistance to stress. *Psychoneuroendocrinology*, *30*, 939–946.

McEwen, B. S. (2000). The neurobiology of stress: From serendipity to clinical relevance. *Brain Research*, *886*, 172–189.

McMahon, S. D., Grant, K. E., Compas, B. E., Thurm, A. E., & Ey, S. (2003). Stress and psychopathology in children and adolescents: Is there evidence of specificity? *Journal of Child Psychology and Psychiatry*, *44*, 107–133.

Masters, R., Friedman, L. N., & Getzel, G. (1988). Helping families of homicide victims: A multidimensional approach. *Journal of Traumatic Stress*, *1*, 109–125.

Meyer, A. (1957). *Psychobiology: A science of man.* Springfield, IL: Charles C. Thomas.

Meyer-Lindenberg, A., Buckholtz, J. W., Kolachana, B., Hariri, A., Pezawas, L., Blasi, G., *et al.* (2006). Neural mechanisms of genetic risk for impulsivity and violence in humans. *Proceedings of the National Academy of Sciences USA*, *103*, 6269–6274.

Miller, P. M., & Ingham, J. G. (1985). Dimensions of experience and symptomatology. *Journal of Psychosomatic Research*, *29*, 475–488.

Minde, K., Eakin, L., Hechtman, L., Ochs, E., Bouffard, R., Greenfield, B., *et al.* (2003). The psychosocial functioning of children and spouses of adults with ADHD. *Journal of Child Psychology and Psychiatry*, *44*, 637–646.

Monck, E., & Dobbs, R. (1985). Measuring life events in an adolescent population: Methodological issues and related findings. *Psychological Medicine*, *15*, 841–850.

Morgan, C. A. 3rd, Hill, S., Fox, P., Kingham, P., & Southwick, S. M. (1999). Anniversary reactions in Gulf War veterans: A follow-up inquiry 6 years after the war. *American Journal of Psychiatry*, *156*, 1075–1079.

Moss, E., Cyr, C., & Dubois-Comtois, K. (2004). Attachment at early school age and developmental risk: Examining family contexts and behavior problems of controlling-caregiving, controlling-punitive, and behaviorally disorganized children. *Developmental Psychology*, *40*, 519–532.

Murray, L., & Cooper, P. J. (1997). *Postpartum depression and child development*. New York: Guilford Press.

Newman, M., Black, D., & Harris-Hendriks, J. (1997). Victims of disaster, war, violence or homicide: psychological effects on siblings. *Child Psychology and Psychiatry Review*, 2, 140–149.

Olff, M., Langeland, W., & Gersons, B. P. R. (2005). The psychobiology of PTSD: coping with trauma. *Psychoneuroendocrinology*, *30*, 974–982.

Olsson, I. G., Nordström, M.-L., Arinell, H., & Von Knorring, A.-L. (1999). Adolescent depression and stressful life events: A case–control study within diagnostic subgroups. *Nordic Journal of Psychiatry*, *53*, 339–346.

Osofsky, J. D. (1997). *Children in a violent society*. New York: Guilford Press.

Overmier, J. B., & Murison, R. (2005). Trauma and resulting sensitization effects are modulated by psychological factors. *Psychoneuroendocrinology*, *30*, 965–973.

Parker, K. J., Buckmaster, C. L., Schatzberg, A. F., & Lyons, D. M. (2004). Prospective investigation of stress inoculation in young monkeys. *Archives of General Psychiatry*, *61*, 933–941.

Parker, K. J., Buckmaster, C. L., Sundlass, K., Schatzberg, A. F., & Lyons, D. M. (2006). Maternal mediation, stress inoculation, and the development of neuroendocrine stress resistance in primates. *Proceedings of the National Academy of Sciences of the USA*, *103*, 3000–3005.

Pettle Michael, S. A., & Lansdown, R. G. (1986). Adjustment to the death of a sibling. *Archives of Disease in Childhood*, *61*, 278–283.

Pezawas, L., Meyer-Lindenberg, A., Drabant, E. M., Verchinski, B. A., Munoz, K. E., Kolachana, B. S., *et al.* (2005). 5-HTTLPR polymorphism impacts human cingulated-amygdala interactions: A genetic susceptibility mechanism for depression. *Nature Neuroscience*, *8*, 828–834.

Phillips, D. I. W., & Jones, A. (2006). Fetal programming of autonomic and HPA function: Do people who were small babies have enhanced stress responses? *Journal of Physiology*, *572*, 45–50.

Pine, D. S. (2003). Developmental psychobiology and response to threats: Relevance to trauma in children and adolescents. *Biological Psychiatry*, *53*, 796–808.

Pynoos, R. S., Frederick, C., Nader, K., Arroyo, W., Steinberg, A., Eth, S., *et al.* (1987). Life threat and post-traumatic stress in school-age children. *Archives of General Psychiatry*, *44*, 1057–1063.

Quas, J. A., Goodman, G. S., Ghetti, S., Alexander, K. W., Edelstein, R., Redlich, A. D., *et al.* (2005). Childhood sexual assault victims: Long-term outcomes after testifying in criminal court. *Monographs of the Society of Research in Child Development*, *70*, 1–128.

Quinton, D., & Rutter, M. (1988). *Parenting breakdown: The making and breaking of inter-generational links*. Aldershot: Avebury.

Riggins-Caspers, K. M., Cadoret, R. J., Knutson, J. F., & Langbehn, D. (2003). Biology–environment interaction and evocative biology–environment correlation: Contributions of harsh discipline and parental psychopathology to problem adolescent behaviors. *Behavior Genetics*, *33*, 205–220.

Robins, L. (1966). *Deviant children grown up: A sociological and psychiatric study of sociopathic personality*. Baltimore: Williams & Wilkins.

Rojo, L., Conesa, L., Bermudez, O., & Livianos, L. (2006). Influence of stress in the onset of eating disorders: Data from a two-stage epidemiological controlled study. *Psychosomatic Medicine*, *68*, 628–635.

Rutter, M. (1971). Parent–child separation: Psychological effects on the children. *Journal of Child Psychology and Psychiatry*, *12*, 233–260.

Rutter, M. (1983). Stress, coping and development: Some issues and some questions. In: R. Garmezy, & M. Rutter (Eds.), *Stress, coping and development in children* (pp. 1–41). New York: McGraw-Hill.

Rutter, M. (1989). Pathways from childhood to adult life. *Journal of Child Psychology and Psychiatry*, *30*, 23–51.

Rutter, M. (1996). Transitions and turning points in developmental psychopathology: As applied to the age span between childhood and mid-adulthood. *International Journal of Behavioural Development*, *19*, 603–626.

Rutter, M. (2000a). Negative life events and family negativity: Accomplishments and challenges. In T. Harris (Ed.), *Where inner and outer worlds meet: Essays in honour of George W. Brown* (pp. 123–149). London: Routledge.

Rutter, M. (2000b). Resilience reconsidered: Conceptual considerations, empirical findings, and policy implications. In J. P. Shonkoff, & S. J. Meisels (Eds.), *Handbook of early childhood interventions* (2nd edn., pp. 651–682). New York: Cambridge University Press.

Rutter, M. (2005). Environmentally mediated risks for psychopathology: Research strategies and findings. *Journal of the American Academy of Child and Adolescent Psychiatry*, *44*, 3–18.

Rutter, M. (2006a). *Genes and behavior: Nature–nurture interplay explained*. Oxford: Blackwell Publishing.

Rutter, M. (2006b). The promotion of resilience in the face of adversity. In A. Clarke-Stewart, & J. Dunn (Eds.), *Families count: Effects on child and adolescent development* (pp. 26–52). New York & Cambridge: Cambridge University Press.

Rutter, M. (2006c). Implications of resilience concepts for scientific understanding. *Annals of the New York Academy of Sciences*, *1094*, 1–12.

Rutter, M., Champion, L., Quinton, D., Maughan, B., & Pickles, A. (1995). Understanding individual differences in environmental risk exposure. In P. Moen, G. H. Elder Jr., & K. Lüscher (Eds.), *Examining lives in context: Perspectives on the ecology of human development* (pp. 61–93). Washington DC: American Psychological Association.

Rutter, M., Giller, H., & Hagell, A. (1998). *Antisocial behavior by young people: The main messages from a major new review of the research*. New York: Cambridge University Press.

Rutter, M., Maughan, B., & Kim-Cohen, J. (2006a). Continuities and discontinuities in psychopathology between childhood and adult life. *Journal of Child Psychology and Psychiatry*, *47*, 276–295.

Rutter, M., Moffitt, T. E., & Caspi, A. (2006b). Gene–environment interplay and psychopathology: Multiple varieties but real effects. *Journal of Child Psychology and Psychiatry*, *47*, 226–261.

Rutter, M., & Quinton, D. (1984). Parental psychiatric disorder: Effects on children. *Psychological Medicine*, *14*, 853–880.

Rutter, M., & Sandberg, S. (1992). Psychosocial stressors: Concepts, causes and effects. *European Journal of Child and Adolescent Psychiatry*, *1*, 3–13.

Rutter, M., Silberg, J., & Simonoff, E. (1993). Whither behavioral genetics? A developmental psychopathological perspective. In R. Plomin, & G. E. McClearn (Eds.), *Nature, nurture, and psychology* (pp. 433–456). Washington DC: APA Books.

Rutter, M., & Smith, D. (1995). *Psychosocial disorders in young people: Time trends and their causes*. Chichester: Wiley.

Sampson, R. J., Raudenbush, S. W., & Earls, F. W. (1997). Neighborhoods and violent crime: A multilevel study of collective efficacy. *Science*, *27*, 918–924.

Sandberg, S., McCann, D. C., Ahola, S., Oja, H., Paton, J. Y., & McGuinness, D. (2002). Positive experiences and the relationship between stress and asthma in children. *Acta Paediatrica*, *91*, 152–158.

Sandberg, S., McGuinness, D., Hillary, C., & Rutter, M. (1998). Independence of childhood life events and chronic adversities: A comparison of two patient groups and controls. *Journal of the American Academy of Child and Adolescent Psychiatry*, *37*, 728–735.

Sandberg, S., Paton, J. Y., Ahola, S., McCann, D. C., McGuinness, D., Hillary, C. R., *et al.* (2000). The role of acute and chronic stress in asthma attacks in children. *Lancet*, *356*, 982–987.

Sandberg, S., Rutter, M., Giles, S., Owen, A., Champion, L., Nicholls, J., *et al.* (1993). Assessment of psychosocial experiences in childhood: Methodological issues and some illustrative findings. *Journal of Child Psychology and Psychiatry*, *34*, 879–897.

Sandberg, S., Rutter, M., Pickles, A., McGuinness, D., & Angold, A. (2001). Do high-threat life events really provoke the onset of psychiatric disorder in children? *Journal of Child Psychology and Psychiatry*, *42*, 523–532.

Sandberg, S., & Zimmer, R. (2002). *Manual for PACE-R: Coverage, guidelines on questioning, interviewer ratings and panel ratings on life events and long-term psychosocial experiences.* University College London: Department of Psychiatry and Behavioural Sciences.

Schneider, M. L., Moore, C. F., Roberts, A. D., & Dejesus, O. (2001). Prenatal stress alters early neurobehavior, stress reactivity and learning in non-human primates: A brief review. *Stress*, *4*, 183–193.

Segerstrom, S. C., & Miller, G. E. (2004). Psychological stress and the human immune system: a meta-analytic study of 30 years of inquiry. *Psychological Bulletin*, *130*, 601–630.

Shea, A., Walsh, C., MacMillan, H., & Steiner, M. (2004). Child maltreatment and HPA axis dysregulation: Relationship to major depressive disorder and post traumatic stress disorder in females. *Psychoneuroendocrinology*, *30*, 162–178.

Silberg, J., Pickles, A., Rutter, M., Hewitt, J., Simonoff, E., Maes, H., *et al.* (1999). The influence of genetic factors and life stress on depression among adolescent girls. *Archives of General Psychiatry*, *56*, 225–232.

Silberg, J., Rutter, M., Neale, M., & Eaves, L. (2001). Genetic moderation of environmental risk for depression and anxiety in adolescent girls. *British Journal of Psychiatry*, *179*, 116–121.

Smider, N. A., Essex, M. J., Kalin, N. H., Buss, K. A., Klein, M. H., Davidson, R. J., *et al.* (2002). Salivary cortisol as a predictor of socioemotional adjustment during kindergarten: A prospective study. *Child Development*, *73*, 75–92.

Stein, B., Jaycox, L. H., Kataoka, S. H., Wong, M., Tu, W., Elliott, M. N., *et al.* (2003). A mental health intervention for schoolchildren exposed to violence: A randomized controlled trial. *Journal of the American Medical Association*, *290*, 603–611.

Stoppelbein, L., & Greening, L. (2000). Posttraumatic stress symptoms in parentally bereaved children and adolescents. *Journal of the American Academy of Child and Adolescent Psychiatry*, *39*, 1112–1119.

Surtees, P. G., & Wainwright, N. W. J. (1999). Surviving adversity: Event decay, vulnerability and the onset of anxiety and depressive disorder. *European Archives of Psychiatry and Clinical Neuroscience*, *249*, 86–95.

Taylor, G. J. (2002). Mind–body–environment: George Engel's psychoanalytic approach to psychosomatic medicine. *Australian and New Zealand Journal of Psychiatry*, *36*, 449–457.

Thapar, A., Harold, G., & McGuffin, P. (1998). Life events and depressive symptoms in childhood: Shared genes or shared adversity? A research note. *Journal of Child Psychology and Psychiatry*, *39*, 1153–1158.

Tiet, Q. Q., Bird, H. R., Davies, M., Hoven, C., Cohen, P., Jensen, P. S., *et al.* (1998). Adverse life events and resilience. *Journal of the American Academy of Child and Adolescent Psychiatry*, *37*, 1191–1200.

Wadhwa, P. D. (2005). Psychoneuroendocrine processes in human pregnancy influence fetal development and health. *Psychoneuroendocrinology*, *30*, 724–743.

Wals, M., Hillegers, M. H. J., Reichart, C. G., Verhulst, F. C., Nolen, W. A., & Ormel, J. (2005). Stressful life events and onset of mood disorders in children of bipolar parents during 14-month follow-up. *Journal of Affective Disorders*, *87*, 253–263.

Williamson, D. E., Birmaher, B., Anderson, B., Al-Shabbout, M., & Ryan, N. (1995). Stressful life events in depressed adolescents: the role of dependent events during the depressive episode. *Journal of the American Academy of Child and Adolescent Psychiatry*, *34*, 591–598.

Williamson, D. E., Birmaher, B., Dahl, R. E., & Ryan, N. D. (2005). Stressful life events in anxious and depressed children. *Journal of Child and Adolescent Psychopharmacology*, *15*, 571–580.

Williamson, D. E., Birmaher, B., Frank, E., Anderson, B. P., Matty, M. K., & Kupfer, D. J. (1998). Nature of life events and difficulties in depressed adolescents. *Journal of the American Academy of Child and Adolescent Psychiatry*, *37*, 1049–1057.

Williamson, D. E., Birmaher, B., Ryan, N. D., Shiffrin, T. P., Lusky, J. A., Protopapa, J., *et al.* (2003). The stressful life events schedule for children and adolescents: development and validation. *Psychiatry Research*, *119*, 225–241.

Wolfe, D. A., Scott, K., Wekerle, C., & Pittman, A.-L. (2001). Child maltreatment: Risk of adjustment problems and dating violence in adolescence. *Journal of the American Academy of Child and Adolescent Psychiatry*, *40*, 282–289.

World Health Organization (WHO). (1996). *Multiaxial classification of child and adolescent psychiatric disorders: ICD-10 Classification of Mental and Behavioural Disorders in children and adolescents.* Cambridge, UK: Cambridge University Press.

Yehuda, R., Halligan, S. L., Golier, J. A., Grossman, R., & Bierer, L. M. (2004). Effects of trauma exposure on the cortisol response to dexamethasone administration in PTSD and major depressive disorder. *Psychoneuroendocrinology*, *29*, 389–404.

Yehuda, R., & McEwen, B. S. (2004). Protective and damaging effects of the biobehavioral stress response: Cognitive, systemic and clinical aspects. ISPNE XXXIV meeting summary. *Psychoneuroendocrinology*, *29*, 1212–1222.

Impact of Parental Psychiatric Disorder and Physical Illness

Alan Stein, Paul Ramchandani and Lynne Murray

Brief Review of Main Disorders Considered

There is now a substantial body of evidence that psychiatric and physical disorders in parents are associated with an increase in a range of psychological disturbances in children. For many parental psychiatric disorders the rates of transmission to the child are substantial. This is particularly important because, even after remission of the disorder in the parents, disturbance in children may persist. There is therefore a need for clinical measures to reduce risk to the offspring, and for the introduction of policies to prevent difficulties arising. In addition, the elucidation of the processes involved in intergenerational transmission of disorder is scientifically important in that it will provide insight into the understanding of the pathways involved in both disturbances in child development and the evolution of disorders, as well as healthy development and resilience.

What is the Scale of the Problem?

The issue of the effects of parental disorder on children applies both to mothers and fathers; most of this chapter will concentrate on parental *psychiatric* disorders, as that is where most research has been carried out. However, we also provide a brief review of the evidence in relation to physical disorders. Some disorders are especially common in the childbearing years, such as depression, anxiety, eating disorders and alcoholism. In the following section we primarily focus on the psychiatric or psychosocial outcomes for children. Alongside these, other difficulties, such as the impact on normal family functioning, must also be considered. These are summarized in the section on clinical implications.

Parental Psychiatric Disorders

Depression is the most common psychiatric condition amongst women of childbearing age and has a point prevalence of over 8% (Weissman, Leaf, Tischler *et al.*, 1988). A significant proportion of the research conducted on parental depression has focused on the postnatal period, and this is considered separately below (see p. 408). However, depression affecting parents of older children has also revealed consistent associations with difficulties in their children. These include an increased risk of insecure attachment to the depressed parent (Martins & Gaffan, 2000), an increased risk of behavioral problems, such as conduct disorder in school-aged children, and, in adolescence, an increased risk of psychiatric disorder. This is most noticeable for depression, but also includes an increased risk of anxiety disorders (Beardslee, Versage, & Gladstone, 1998). An increased risk of psychiatric disorder persists into adulthood. In a 20-year longitudinal study, Weissman, Pilowsky, Wickramaratne *et al.* (2006) found that the offspring of depressed parents had a three-fold increase in major depressive disorder, anxiety disorders and substance dependence, as well as an increased risk of physical health problems and greater social impairment. There is evidence that the more severe and chronic the parental depression, the greater the impact on risk for offspring disorder (Hammen & Brennan, 2003).

Anxiety disorders in parents are also common, the lifetime rate for the most prevalent of the anxiety disorders, social phobia, being 13% (Kessler, McGonagle, Zhao *et al.*, 1994). Studies of children of parents with anxiety disorders show them to be at high risk for anxiety themselves (Biederman, Petty, Faraone *et al.*, 2006). In one study, children of parents with anxiety disorders were seven times more likely to be diagnosed with an anxiety disorder compared with normal control groups, and twice as likely as children of parents with dysthymia (Turner, Beidel, & Costello, 1987). One well-controlled study found that there was a two-fold increased risk of anxiety disorders among offspring of anxious parent probands, compared with offspring of substance abusing parents or controls (Merikangas, Dierker, & Szatmari, 1998). Social phobia has been reported in almost one-quarter of the children of patients with social phobia (Mancini, Van-Ameringen, Szatmari *et al.*, 1996).

In a 5-year prospective study of the adolescent children of parents with bipolar disorder (Hillegers, Reichart, Wals *et al.*, 2005), lifetime prevalence was found to be 10% for bipolar disorder, with prevalence for mood disorders of 40% and psychopathology in general of 59%. Seven percent of offspring showed current mood disorder, with 28% displaying current psychopathology. Other studies have found even higher rates of disorder, with much higher risks for both bipolar disorder (morbidity risk 33.0 versus 2.8) and earlier onset depression (by age 12 years, morbidity risk 34.2 versus 7.5) in children of parents with bipolar disorder compared to children of adults without mood disorder (Henin, Biederman, Mick *et al.*, 2005).

Rutter's Child and Adolescent Psychiatry, 5th edition. Edited by M. Rutter, D. Bishop, D. Pine, S. Scott, J. Stevenson, E. Taylor and A. Thapar. © 2008 Blackwell Publishing, ISBN: 978-1-4051-4549-7.

Eating disorders have also been shown to occur commonly among women of childbearing age (Fairburn & Harrison, 2003), and the prevalence may be rising. Most affected women with eating disorders have bulimia nervosa or eating disorder not otherwise specified (EDNOS; see chapter 41). A small minority have anorexia nervosa and their low weight (and the fact that they are not ovulating) means that this last group are less likely to conceive. Underweight women required an average of 29 months to conceive, compared to 6.8 months in normal weight women (Hassan & Killick, 2004). Nonetheless, potential eating disorders involve psychopathological risks for the offspring, particularly during infancy and adolescence (Patel, Wheatcroft, Park *et al.*, 2002). A large Scandinavian study (Brinch, Isager, & Tolstrup, 1988), using retrospective reports, found that 17% of children of women with a history of anorexia nervosa failed to thrive in the first year of life. Two longitudinal studies have shown some adverse outcomes for children of mothers with eating psychopathology in the postnatal year. Stein, Woolley, Cooper *et al.* (2006) showed that, compared with controls, children whose mothers had experienced an eating disorder in the postnatal year were more likely to have conflictual mealtimes at 5 years of age. At 10 years they were more likely to have concerns about body shape and weight and to use dietary restraint. Stice, Agras, & Hammer (1999) found that childhood eating disturbance at 5 years of age was predicted by a range of maternal variables such as body dissatisfaction and the internalization of the thin ideal. Furthermore, at 8 years of age, higher maternal restraint scores predicted worries about being too fat in girls but not in boys, while maternal disinhibition scores predicted weight control behaviors in daughters (Jacobi, Agras, & Hammer, 2001).

Alcoholism and substance abuse are conditions that are easily overlooked. However, they are not uncommon amongst adults of childbearing age, and are certainly associated with higher risks amongst the children (Lieberman, 2000). For example, a large Dutch study (Cuijpers, Langendoen, & Bijl, 1999) found that adult children of alcoholics had a significantly higher 1-month, 12-month and lifetime prevalence of mood, anxiety and abuse and/or dependence disorders than offspring of non-alcoholic parents (lifetime risk for any disorder 57.7% versus 39.5%). Sons of problem drinkers had a higher occurrence of eating disorders (2.0% versus 0.1%) and schizophrenia (1.6% versus 0.3%). Rates were especially high for the children of fathers with drinking problems. The authors concluded that, relative to other parental problem behaviors, parental problem drinking is a strong predictor of psychiatric disorders, especially abuse and/or dependence disorders. One particular hazard of alcoholism is drinking during pregnancy, which has been shown to be associated with fetal alcohol syndrome (FAS). For example, Von Knorring (1991) reported that FAS appears in 5.9% of births of alcoholic women, compared to a rate of 0.01–0.03% in the general population (but see chapter 30 for a discussion of uncertainties about the boundaries of FAS).

Some severe psychiatric disorders such as schizophrenia are associated with lowered birth rates, but a good proportion of affected adults do have children. Similarly, those with personality disorders, while having difficulties in forming intimate relationships, are still likely to have children. Compared with the general population, parents with a diagnosis of schizophrenia have a greatly increased risk of having a child who later develops schizophrenia themselves (Gottesman & Shields, 1976). In addition, although most of the study samples have been relatively small, they do suggest that children of affected parents have a raised risk of a range of other mental disorders, including attention deficit/hyperactivity disorder, anxiety disorders and depressive disorder.

Postnatal Psychiatric Disorders

The postnatal period has been much studied in recent years. This is in part because of the relative vulnerability of the developing infant at this time, who is entirely dependent on carers for his or her health and successful development. There has also been a recognition of the significant morbidity and distress caused by postnatal psychiatric disorder, in particular postnatal depression. Other important psychiatric disorders can occur in the postnatal period and have significant effects on the mother and her family, including anxiety, schizophrenia, substance abuse and some eating disorders. However, in this section we focus on depression and, to a lesser degree, affective psychosis, as mood disorders are the most prevalent and the most studied.

Estimates of depression occurring specifically in the postnatal period appear to be somewhat higher than at other times, at 13% (O'Hara & Swain, 1996). Most research has been conducted in the developed world; more recent studies of developing world populations have often shown rates to be substantially higher, although there is significant variability (Halbreich & Karkun, 2006). The symptoms of depression occurring at this time are largely the same as at other times, with low mood and loss of interest and enjoyment usually prominent. Those at particular risk of developing postnatal depression include women with a past history of depression and those without good confiding relationships. Other factors can include relative socioeconomic deprivation and social isolation (Boyce, 2003).

An increasing number of longitudinal studies have identified associations between maternal postnatal depression and adverse child outcomes. The potential mechanisms by which any risk may be transmitted from parents to children are considered on p. 411, but the difficulties reported include more difficulties managing the babies' crying (Seeley, Murray, & Cooper, 1996); characteristic impairments in mother–infant interaction (Murray, Fiori-Cowley, Hooper *et al.*, 1996a); and higher rates of emotional (Lyons-Ruth, Alpern, & Repacholi, 1993) and behavioral problems as the children approach school age (Sinclair & Murray, 1998). A number of studies have also found an association between postnatal depression and poorer cognitive development (Hay, Pawlby, Sharp *et al.*, 2001; Murray, Kempton, Woolgar *et al.*, 1993; Murray *et al.*, 1996a) although this has not been confirmed by all studies (e.g., Murray, Hipwell, Hooper *et al.*, 1996b). There are few longer-term studies that have followed up children into adolescence, but one identified a higher risk of both mood and anxiety disorders for the offspring of mothers who were postnatally depressed (Halligan, Murray, Martins *et al.*, 2007).

Postpartum psychosis is far less common, affecting 1–2 women per 1000. Episodes are frequently affective in nature and the most notable risk factor is a past or family history of affective psychosis. These disorders can have a devastating effect on the mother, infant and family. The impact on an infant can be manifest both in terms of a mother's ability to care for herself and her infant (poorer quality caregiving), and by the infant becoming the focus of a mother's delusional beliefs. Fortunately, this latter problem is a relatively rare occurrence; nevertheless, when it does occur, provision of a high level of treatment, supervision and support becomes necessary. This will often require in-patient care, ideally in a specialist mother and baby unit, where the baby can remain with the mother in all but the most extreme of presentations, and where experienced skilled staff can provide the level of care and supervision necessary. It is in these circumstances in particular where the clinician also has to be aware of potential danger to the child's well-being, either through direct risk from a mother with delusional beliefs and/or hallucinations, or through neglect of the child. The need to balance the risk (to mother and child) with the desire to keep parent and child together to promote the development of a positive relationship and facilitate the mother's recovery requires experienced clinical judgment. These concerns regarding the protection of the child's well-being are not confined to the occurrence of psychotic illness in the mother, although they are more often to the fore here. These should also be considerations when severe parental depression may lead to neglect of their infant's care.

Similar issues also arise with other disorders. There has been little study of the longer-term outcome of children whose mothers suffered a postnatal psychotic episode. The few small studies that there have been (McNeil & Kaij, 1987) tend to suggest an absence of ill effects, possibly because episodes are of limited duration, and recovery is generally good. For a fuller discussion of how to assess a range of psychiatric disorders and the risk of infanticide in the immediate puerperium, and the role of mother and baby psychiatric units, see Marks, Hipwell, & Kumar (2002).

Alcohol and drug problems can often coexist with depressive disorder. Some of the risks and potential effects of these disorders are considered elsewhere (see chapter 36), but of particular relevance to the early postpartum period is the problem of the withdrawal syndrome. Newborn babies of mothers who are drug-dependent are already at higher risk than non-exposed infants for perinatal complications such as prematurity and low birth weight. A withdrawal syndrome can develop in some cases, particularly where the mother has been using opiates, but this can also occur with other drugs such as benzodiazepines. The symptoms and signs seen in the infant depend on the drug used, and the risk and severity of these symptoms are diminished significantly if the mother has been abstinent from drug use for more than a few days (American Academy of Pediatrics: Committee on Drugs, 1998). In circumstances where a child exhibits a withdrawal reaction, the issue of child protection will also require careful consideration and, where parents have a continuing substance addiction, child protection will be a continuing concern for the professionals involved.

Parental Physical Disorders

The association between physical illnesses and child disturbance and development has been less-well studied than that with parental psychiatric disorder. Nonetheless, some physical illnesses are relatively common in adults of parenting age, and a number of chronic conditions have been shown to affect women of childbearing age; indeed, almost 10% of women aged 18–44 years report some restriction of activity caused by chronic disease (Misra, Grason, & Weisman, 2000). In this relatively limited research field, much of the work has focused on cancers that affect parents. Breast cancer alone affects 1 in 9 women in the Western world. Over one-quarter of those affected have children living with them and, consequently, this has tended to be the most frequently studied condition. Reviews of the effects of parental cancer on children's development have, unsurprisingly, revealed a relatively complex story (Visser, Huizinga, van der Graaf *et al.*, 2004). There is a relatively consistent increase in emotional problems seen in adolescent offspring of parents with cancer. However, there is less evidence regarding emotional problems in younger children, and it is inconsistent. That is not to say that they are unaffected, as qualitative interview studies have highlighted common feelings of guilt and distress, but these may not always translate to changes in measured scores on psychological questionnaires. The effects on children appear to be moderated by a number of the same factors that moderate the effects of parental psychiatric illness on children (see p. 411). These include the degree to which the cancer affects parental, family and marital functioning, and the pre-existing relationship between parent and child. Pre-existing family structure has been shown to significantly predict child outcome, with children from single-parent families more at risk (Visser, Huizinga, Hoekstra *et al.*, 2006).

HIV/AIDS has become the largest pandemic ever, and in sub-Saharan Africa in particular it has reached catastrophic proportions. Young people of childbearing age, particularly women, are most affected with, for example, 10 million people in sub-Saharan Africa aged 15–24 being infected – the next generation of parents. There is now substantial evidence that the offspring of mothers with HIV are at increased risk in terms of their development, growth and survival (Stein, Krebs, Richter *et al.*, 2005). In parts of sub-Saharan Africa, up to 40% of women attending antenatal clinics are HIV-positive. Untreated, transmission to the infant (during pregnancy, labor, delivery, or through breastfeeding) can occur in up to 40% of cases. However, this can be dramatically reduced to 10% by the provision of a single dose of nevirapine to the mother as she goes into labor and to the infant within the first few days of birth. The transmission can be reduced to well below 10% with the addition of Cesarean section and formula feeding. However, both infected and uninfected children show increased levels of developmental problems. Surprisingly, relatively little research has been carried out into this. Nonetheless, the research that has been carried out suggests that uninfected children born to mothers with HIV are at increased risk of a range of problems including attentional difficulties, behavioral problems, difficulties with social adjustment and language development (see chapter 58). One of the most important mechanisms is likely to be through compromised maternal care, especially in the context of maternal depression. Maternal depression has been shown to be relatively common amongst women following the diagnosis of HIV/AIDS during pregnancy (Rochat, Richter, Doll *et al.*, 2006), which is when most women in Africa receive their diagnosis.

Studies of parents with other illnesses have used diverse groups of physical health problems, including diabetes and multiple sclerosis (Korneluk & Lee, 1998). Some studies have compared children of these parents with children from "healthy" families, and some with families where a parent has a psychiatric disorder. Overall, children in families where a parent has a physical illness have higher rates of anxiety and depression than children in "healthy" families, but broadly similar rates to those seen in families where a parent has a psychiatric disorder. It should be stressed that most of the studies were relatively small, and had limited scope to investigate the mechanisms by which any increased risk may occur. Similar moderating influences, such as those apparent in the literature on parental cancer outlined above, are likely to operate (Pederson & Revenson, 2005), although there is a lack of research addressing this at present. Given the high prevalence of chronic physical illnesses in adults of parenting age, further research to understand the way in which increased risk to the child occurs is important, particularly as it may point the way towards the development of effective interventions. Anxiety and depression are clearly only two areas of child functioning that may be affected by parental ill-health. They are the most studied, but some studies of functional disorders (e.g., irritable bowel syndrome) have also examined responses to illness in the children themselves. This research has shown the way in which the adult's disorder is linked to a change in parental behavior in seeking medical help when their young child exhibits common symptoms of illness (Crane & Martin, 2004). These studies suggest that a lower parental threshold for seeking help may potentially affect children's interpretations of symptoms as they grow up to take increasing responsibility for their own health.

Studies of the Parents of Children with Disorders

Another way in which researchers have attempted to illuminate some of the associations between disorders in children and parents is to conduct "bottom-up" studies. In these studies, the psychiatric states of parents of children who are known to have disorders are examined in an attempt to illuminate the nature of the risk. These types of study complement those that begin with parents as the index, and are of particular use when a relatively rare child disorder is being studied. They can also provide additional information in relation to more common child disorders such as anxiety. For example, Martin, Cabrol, Bouvard *et al.* (1999) found an increased prevalence of both anxiety and depressive disorders in mothers and fathers of anxious school-refusing children. Increased prevalences of simple phobia and/or social phobia were found among the fathers and mothers of phobic disordered school refusers, and increased prevalences of panic disorder and/or agoraphobia were found among the parents of separation anxiety disordered school refusers. Similarly, Cooper and Eke (1999), in a community sample, found raised rates of social phobia among the parents of shy children. A recent study, using a clinic sample, found that social phobia and separation anxiety in the child were each associated with an increase in these same disorders in their mothers (Cooper, Fearn, Willetts *et al.*, 2006). Similar patterns have been seen in eating disorders, where raised rates of eating psychopathology have been found among the mothers of children with feeding problems (Cooper, Whelan, Woolgar *et al.*, 2004; Stein, Stein, Walters *et al.*, 1995).

Such patterns of association suggest a degree of specificity in some of the links between the disorders in parents and offspring, particularly for social phobia and separation anxiety, and possibly eating disorders, while other parental disorders (e.g., depression and general anxiety disorder) appear to be more general in their intergenerational association.

Summary of Findings

In summary, although the evidence is relatively limited, there do appear to be increased risks of anxiety and depression in children when a parent has a chronic physical illness. The exact extent of these risks is clearly dependent on a number of family factors such as the family's structure and current social situation, functioning, and also the developmental stage of the child.

It can be seen from the above that a wide range of common disorders that affect parents are associated with an increased risk of adverse outcomes for their children. Parents can, of course, be affected by more than one illness, and the risks to children's development associated with multiple disorders can be greater than those associated with a single disorder. In the following section we consider some of the mechanisms by which this increased risk might operate; of particular note is the fact that the symptoms of many of these disorders will impact on parents' psychosocial functioning and interfere with the demands of parenting (i.e., positive, sensitive and responsive parenting to facilitate child development). Examples of such symptoms include:

1 *Depression* – sadness, withdrawal and focus on negative aspects of life;

2 *Anxiety* – focus on the perception of threat in the environment;

3 *Schizophrenia and other psychotic disorders* – delusions, abnormal beliefs about a range of issues especially paranoid ones; and

4 *Alcoholism* – unpredictability and the potential impact as well on socioeconomic circumstances.

It is not difficult to see how some of these patterns of behavior can interfere with optimal parenting. The recurrent hospital admissions and separations associated with severe illness further affect normal parenting functioning. However, it is worth stressing two further points. First, many children manage well in the face of these adversities and so there is also need to consider this in any model of mechanisms and risk indicators. Second, there are other mechanisms by which these disorders exert their influence through the generations. We move now to consider these.

Overview and Introduction to Mechanisms

The previous section has outlined the increased risks (of psychopathology and other social, cognitive, emotional and behavioral disturbances) experienced by the children of parents with a range of psychiatric and physical disorders. The nature of transmission of this increased risk is clearly complex and multifactorial. The fact that many children of parents with disorders do not develop problems themselves is testimony to the fact that the associations seen are not deterministic, but rely on a number of risk factors coming together. There is strong evidence that as the number of risk factors accumulate for children, the likelihood that they will develop psychological disturbance dramatically increases. Rutter (1999) has shown the synergistic effects of multiple risk factors on adverse child outcome. Nonetheless, it is important, both clinically and scientifically, to elucidate as precisely as we are able the exact mechanisms underlying intergenerational transmission of risk. This allows us to better identify potential points of intervention, as well as increasing our understanding of the disorders themselves. Recent years have seen significant advances in our understanding of how genetic risks operate in different circumstances and interact with environmental factors (Rutter, Moffitt, & Caspi, 2006) and also in our understanding of how important environmental factors such as disturbances in parenting and marital conflict mediate the pathway between parental mental illness and child developmental disturbance (Cummings, Keller, & Davies, 2005).

The following sections attempt to disentangle a number of these potential mechanisms while recognizing that, in reality, they frequently co-occur and interact with one another (Rutter, 1989). Although genetic mechanisms are referred to first, the focus is predominantly on environmental mechanisms as, although they may not always be the strongest influence in absolute terms (depending on the condition in question and the developmental stage of the child or adolescent), they are the factors that are more amenable to intervention in the current clinical context.

Genetic Mechanisms

Decades of research have shown that children of parents with severe psychiatric disorders such as schizophrenia, bipolar disorder and depression are at increased risk for those disorders. This is not unique to psychiatric disorders, as many physical illnesses such as asthma and heart disease also show familial transmission. Twin studies and adoption studies have consistently demonstrated this increased risk and pointed to a significant genetic component, but have also shown that the risk is variable. For example, not all children with a parent with schizophrenia will develop schizophrenia. Recent developments in research have begun to explain why some of this variability occurs, including research on epigenetic effects, whereby other factors, both genetic and environmental, moderate the expression of genes (for a fuller description see chapter 23). In addition, the variability is different for different disorders. For example, bipolar disorder has a relatively high genetic risk for the offspring of affected parents (Henin *et al.*, 2005), while anxiety disorders carry a smaller genetic risk (Gordon & Hen, 2004). Earlier attempts to identify individual genes for psychiatric disorder, and thereby account for the apparent increased genetic risk to children of parents with psychiatric disorder, proved disappointing, with the realization that effects of multiple genes are likely to be involved in the majority of cases. In recent years there has also been an increased recognition of the complex interplay of genetic and environmental effects. These facets of gene–environment interplay are addressed later in this chapter (see p. 413).

Environmental Mechanisms

Many of the environmental mechanisms of transmission of risk from parents with disorder to their children have been most clearly elucidated in the field of mood and anxiety disorders, and so examples will be used from this field of research. However, many of the same mechanisms may operate in other conditions, and while these will not be exhaustively referred to here, other studies are available (Patel, Wheatcroft, Park *et al.*, 2002; Rutter, 1989). Here, antenatal effects are considered first, followed by the associations of parental psychiatric disorder with parent–child interaction, and with marital functioning. The direct involvement of children in the symptoms of the parent's psychopathology is considered, followed by some of the methodological complexities of elucidating these mechanisms. Finally, both gender-specific and age-dependent associations are briefly considered.

Antenatal Effects

It has been apparent for many years that alcohol and drugs (including some prescribed drugs) can have a dramatic and enduring effect on fetal development. High levels of alcohol consumption by pregnant women are associated with an outcome for a newborn child characterized as fetal alcohol syndrome (Mukherjee, Hollins, & Turk, 2006). It has been more difficult to demonstrate whether lower levels of alcohol consumption lead to increased risks for the developing fetus. Other drugs, such as opiates and cocaine, can also have a significant effect on fetal development in the short and longer term (Bennett, Bendersky, & Lewis, 2002). Exposure in the form of maternal smoking is also associated with adverse outcomes, including low birth weight. These risk factors are likely to exert their influence by a variety of mechanisms. Animal research suggests that this may include direct brain effects of the substance and other effects; for example, fetal hypoxia in the case of smoking (Chiriboga, 2003).

Over a decade ago the Barker hypothesis (that a substantial proportion of the risk for adult disorders such as coronary heart disease was determined by the *in utero* environment and antenatal development) had a dramatic effect on the way in which risk for these disorders, and their etiology, was considered (Barker, Osmond, Rodin *et al.*, 1995). This did not have a major impact on thinking about psychiatric disorders at the time, although animal models began to demonstrate that stress in pregnancy had potentially lasting effects on the developing infant. More recently, epidemiological evidence has demonstrated an association between high levels of anxiety in pregnancy and an increased risk of behavioral problems in children (O'Connor, Heron, Golding *et al.*, 2003). It seems likely that the mechanism of risk operates through an effect in pregnancy on the hypothalamic–pituitary–adrenal (HPA) axis of the developing fetus. The finding of high levels of cortisol in these children at older ages lends some support to this notion (O'Connor, Ben-Shlomo, Heron *et al.*, 2005), although other mechanisms, such as reduced placental blood flow in response to stress, are also possible. This had led to some enthusiastic calls for antenatal intervention although, given the relatively small size of the associations, it is probably too early to be advocating widespread interventions aimed at reducing anxiety in pregnant women. It may be that the identification of women with particularly high levels of anxiety in pregnancy becomes warranted, especially given that this is also a clear risk marker for postnatal depression. It is less clear whether depression occurring in the antenatal period is also associated with increased risks for the developing child. One study found that, while maternal depression occurring postnatally was associated with an increased risk of conduct disorder in children, depression in the antenatal period was not (Kim-Cohen, Moffitt, Taylor *et al.*, 2005). Further studies using similar designs are likely to prove informative.

Postnatal Psychiatric Disorder and Parent–Child Interaction

Depression in mothers occurring in the postnatal period has become one of the most studied psychiatric phenomena in recent years, and a substantial body of work has now examined the links between postnatal depression and child development (see for example Murray & Cooper, 2003). It should come as no surprise that the cardinal features of depression (i.e., low mood, low energy and loss of interest or enjoyment in activities) have the potential to have an important impact on a mother's parenting abilities. Postnatal depression is associated with significant changes in the patterns of interaction between mothers and their infants. Most notable are a decrease in positive parenting behaviors by mothers, and an increase in negative and intrusive interactions (Field, Healy, Goldstein *et al.*, 1988; Murray *et al.*, 1996a; Stein, Gath, Bucher *et al.*, 1991). These alterations in maternal sensitivity and responsiveness are associated with adverse subsequent cognitive development in the children (Murray *et al.*, 1996a). The exact mechanisms remain somewhat uncertain, but it seems likely that the decrease in parental stimulation and appropriate contingent response decreases learning opportunities for the infant at a crucial stage of development early in life. A lack of appropriate emotional responsiveness, and particularly the occurrence of negative or hostile interactions, may similarly interfere with the development of child emotion regulation, and affect subsequent peer interactions and other emotional development, including vulnerability to depression (Murray, Woolgar, Cooper *et al.*, 2001).

Although other psychiatric disorders affecting mothers in the postnatal period have been less extensively studied, the links between eating disorders and mothers' interactions with their infants at mealtimes have been characterized (Stein, Woolley, & McPherson, 1999). Mothers with eating disorders have been shown to be less facilitating and more intrusive than control mothers when interacting with their infants at mealtimes. Finally, research is emerging on the links between maternal anxiety disorder and potentially adverse mother–infant interactions; for example, mothers with social phobia show particular difficulties in supporting their infant's interactions with other people, partly by "modeling" their fearful responses to unfamiliar people, and also by being less actively facilitating of the infant's contact with them. Such responses in turn affect the development of infant social responsiveness (Murray, Cooper, Creswell *et al.*, 2007). In a community sample, mothers with higher anxiety were found to be less responsive to their infants during interaction than mothers with lower anxiety (Nicol-Harper, Harvey, & Stein, 2007).

There has been far less research examining the associations between psychiatric disorder in fathers and their children's early development (Ramchandani, Stein, Evans *et al.*, 2005), and less still on any effects of disorder on their interactions with their infants (Field, Hossain, & Malphurs, 1999). Most of these studies have been small and so it is difficult to draw any firm conclusions. The wider literature on paternal influences suggests that there may be specific differences between the effects of psychiatric disorder in mothers and fathers, both in terms of the areas of functioning affected and relative gender specificity. However, the precise nature of the operation of these effects has yet to be elucidated.

Psychiatric Disorder and Parental Relationships

The effects of psychiatric disorder on a parent's functioning are pervasive, so it is no surprise that parents' own relationships are affected by disorders such as depression occurring in either parent. Indeed, depression is clearly associated with an increased risk of marital problems (Cummings, Keller, & Davies, 2005), and can have a direct effect on the mood and functioning of the other parent. This has importance as a mechanism by which parental disorder impacts upon children in two ways. First, where one parent is depressed, having a second parent who is well can have a protective effect upon the child. In contrast, having a second depressed parent can have a double-dosing effect on a child, as well as depriving them of a potentially "protective" well parent (Goodman & Gotlib, 1999). Second, exposure to marital conflict is a clear risk factor for an increased risk of behavioral problems in children (perhaps particularly in boys), and so this is another pathway by which the effects of parental depression can affect children's development. Although less well studied, the effects of parental alcohol and drug misuse, as well as antisocial personality traits, may also operate strongly through a deleterious effect on the marital relationship. In addition, many psychiatric disorders are associated with an increased risk of marital breakdown, leading in many cases to dislocated relationships for the child, and exposure to other risk factors such as increased socioeconomic adversity.

Direct Involvement of the Child in the Parental Psychopathology

This refers to the situation where a child becomes a role-player in the parent's own psychopathology. At its most extreme, it might mean the child becoming involuntarily involved in a homicide/suicide where a severely depressed parent includes the child in their own death because of extreme hopelessness about the future. Children can also become the focus of other parental delusional beliefs, or incorporated into other parental psychopathology such as obsessions.

Bidirectional Effects and Confounding Effects

All of the mechanisms outlined above assume a single direction of causality. That is, the parental psychiatric disorder leads to the marital dysfunction or the eventual disturbance in the child. In reality, of course, the picture is more complex than this. Clearly, just as parents can influence their children, so children can also affect their parents (Yarrow, Campbell, & Burton, 1968). For example, children with severe disabilities place greater demands upon the parenting capacity of any parent, and so higher rates of some disorders such as depression might be expected in parents in these circumstances. A second example is that more difficult temperamental characteristics in infants are associated with a higher risk of depression for their mothers (Murray, Stanley, Hooper *et al.*, 1996c). So, these effects can be bidirectional. In addition, other factors, such as socioeconomic deprivation, may confound the relationships seen between parental illness and child development problems, as both the parental and the child problems may be more common in situations of socioeconomic stress. These confounding factors may be very important to consider; nonetheless, there remains a substantial body of research pointing to a very real influence of parental illness on the various domains of child development, as outlined above.

Gene–Environment Interplay

The complex area of gene–environment interplay has become one of the most exciting areas of developmental science and, while there are few implications of direct clinical relevance from this work at present, it is likely to be influential in the thinking about the development of psychiatric disorder in children and adolescents in the years ahead (see chapter 23). Rutter, Moffitt, & Caspi (2006) have provided an extensive review of the current state of the research area. There are three mechanisms of interplay between genetic and environmental factors that seem particularly promising.

The first is the process whereby genes can affect the types of environments in which children (and adults) find themselves. This is known as gene–environment *correlation*, and can refer to both child and parental genes. For example, twin studies have shown that genes are implicated in individual differences in exposure to a wide range of environments having important associations with psychopathology (Rutter, 2007; Rutter, Moffitt, & Caspi, 2006).

The second mechanism is that of gene–environment *interactions* (see chapter 23). Recent examples of this include the finding of an interaction between a polymorphism of the serotonin transporter gene and stressful life events, leading to increased risk of depression. Carriers of the shorter alleles of the serotonin transporter gene (conferring increased risk) are only at higher risk of subsequent depression in the presence of stressful life events (Caspi, Sugden, Moffitt *et al.*, 2003). These findings have been confirmed in some, but not all, subsequent studies to examine this question. Gene–environment interactions have been described in other areas of psychopathology. The gene encoding for higher levels of monoamine oxidase A (*MAOA*) is found to moderate the strong association between exposure to maltreatment as a child and subsequent antisocial behavior (Caspi, McClay, Moffitt *et al.*, 2002). In addition, a variant of the catechol-O-methyltransferase (*COMT*) gene is found to interact with low birth weight to predict conduct problems in a high-risk group of children (Thapar, Langley, Fowler *et al.*, 2005).

The third area of gene–environmental interplay is that of *epigenetic* effects, which is where environmental factors exert a clear influence on the expression of genes. So, without altering the DNA itself, they nonetheless affect how genes then code for specific proteins, and so effectively alter the function of the genes. The mechanisms are described in chapter 23. Most of the current research of relevance to child psychosocial development is occurring with animals, with Canadian researchers identifying early maternal nurturing (licking and grooming behavior) in rodents as having a direct impact on the genetic expression of genes related to the HPA axis (Weaver, Cervoni, Champagne *et al.*, 2004). Although it is not yet clear how directly applicable to early nurturant behavior in humans this research is, it does point the way to potentially promising avenues of research in understanding the effects of adverse early experience in increasing the risk of mood disorders in developing children and adolescents. Our understanding of these important areas of interplay between genes and environmental risk factors is likely to grow hugely in the years ahead.

Gender

There are three types of gender effects to consider here, at a parental level (mother versus father), at a child level (boy versus girl vulnerability) and the interaction between the two (e.g., mother–daughter versus mother–son associations, or similar father–child associations). There is an increasing literature on the role of the father in normative child development (Tamis-LeMonda, Shannon, Cabrera *et al.*, 2004); however, the quantity of research addressing the role of paternal psychopathology is far more limited. The range of psychopathology experienced by fathers differs from that of mothers (the higher rates of alcohol and antisocial disorders in fathers compare with the higher rates of anxiety and depression in mothers). It follows that the types of psychopathology that a child is exposed to in different parents will thus differ at the population level. This may account for some of the difference in associations seen with maternal versus paternal psychopathology. But what of exposure to the same disorder in mothers or fathers? Limited work suggests that this may result in differing effects for the child. For example, depression in fathers is more specifically linked with behavioral problems in children, whereas exposure to maternal depression has more diffuse associations with child psychopathology (Ramchandani, Stein, Evans *et al.*, 2005). This raises the question of potentially differing mechanisms by which maternal and paternal psychopathology might impact on children. Two particular candidates are direct parent–child interaction and the effects of psychopathology on the parents' own relationship. Mothers and fathers have different amounts and types of direct interaction with their children (with fathers typically less involved, but spending more of their limited time with their children in play; Tamis-LeMonda *et al.*, 2004). This may moderate the exposure that children have to psychopathology. Work on antisocial behavior in fathers suggests that this may well be the case (Jaffee, Moffitt, Caspi *et al.*, 2003). In addition to these direct links with parent–child interaction, less direct mechanisms may operate. For example, depression is strongly associated with an increase in marital conflict, and exposure to this conflict is linked, in turn, to increased rates of child behavioral problems.

There are conflicting results regarding the differences seen in boys and girls. Some, but by no means all, research on postnatal depression in mothers has shown an increased risk for boys compared with girls, in terms of their cognitive performance (Hay *et al.*, 2001; Murray *et al.*, 1993). Whether this is because of the increased vulnerability of boys to a range of risks for their neurocognitive development, or whether there is a degree of specificity in the risk from factors like parental depression is as yet unclear. Although there is little research comparing specific risk pathways from mothers to daughters versus mothers to sons and father–son versus father–daughter risks, there are suggestions that boys may be more particularly at risk to paternal de-pression and other paternal psychopathology (Ramchandani *et al.*, 2005).

Developmental or Age-Specific Effects

There is an assumption that children and adolescents will be more vulnerable to the potential impact of parental depression at two particular points in their life: the postnatal period and adolescence. During the immediate postnatal period, infants are rapidly developing, with enormous brain growth (Gale, O'Callaghan, Godfrey *et al.*, 2004), and, in spite of their immaturity, young infants are highly sensitive to the quality of other people's interactions with them. Infants are therefore extremely vulnerable to the effects of any factor, such as depression, that impairs the ability of their caregiver to give optimum care. During adolescence, a large number of crucial developmental changes occur, both physiological and psychosocial. This is also the time when the common emotional disorders, such as depression, begin to significantly increase in prevalence. Research has confirmed the association between parental depression and increased risk to children and adolescents in both the postnatal period (Murray & Cooper, 2003) and adolescence (Beardslee, Versage, & Gladstone, 1998; Halligan, Murray, Martins *et al.*, 2007). It is apparent that children present with different symptoms and disorders at different ages, despite exposure to the same parental disorder (Radke-Yarrow, 1998). It remains somewhat unclear whether this is a result of the naturally changing patterns of psychopathology seen as children develop, or whether there are different effects because the exposure to a similar parental psychopathology has a differential impact itself at different ages.

Clinical Implications

There is a substantial research literature on the treatment of children who are themselves diagnosed with a disorder. However, the question of treatment in the case of offspring who may be *at risk* for developmental problems by virtue of psychiatric disorder in their parents has received relatively little attention. Nevertheless, this is an important topic for research, not only because of the clinical implications, but also because treatment research can help scientifically in elucidating the factors that explain the process of development in these populations.

The few studies there are have principally addressed the question in relation to parental depression. One study of 7- to 17-year-old children whose mothers were simply treated with antidepressant medication found that maternal remission within 3 months (occurring in approximately one-third of women) was associated with a significant decrease in child and adolescent disorder and symptoms, particularly of the emotional variety (Weissman, Pilowsky, Wickramaratne *et al.*, 2006). A similar association of symptom reduction in the parent with better child outcome in this age group was found in a study conducted by Beardslee and colleagues (Beardslee & Gladstone, 2001; Beardslee, Gladstone, Wright *et al.*, 2003), where psycho-educational support was directed to the whole family. An intervention with somewhat older children (13- to

18-year-olds) found, by contrast, that the involvement of parents in a psycho-educational group program that was principally directed at the adolescents themselves was of no additional benefit (Clarke, Hornbrook, Lynch *et al.*, 2002). Together these studies suggest that involvement of the affected parent in treatment might be more important when children are younger, and become less critical as they reach later adolescence.

With regard to infants and toddlers of depressed mothers, some benefits of treatment in terms of maternal reports of problem behavior in the children have been found. In one trial, maternal reports of child attachment security improved with an attachment-oriented toddler–parent psychotherapy delivered over a 1-year period (Cicchetti, Toth, & Rogosch, 1999). Similarly, brief (2 month) psychological treatments for postnatally depressed mothers, whether counseling, cognitive–behavioral therapy (CBT) or a dynamic therapy, were associated with maternal reports of a reduction of problems in the relationship with the infant immediately after treatment, and at 18-month follow-up there were benefits in terms of reported infant behavior problems (Murray, Cooper, Wilson *et al.*, 2003a). Nevertheless, other outcomes in this study showed no benefit of the interventions, and there was no long-term benefit (5 year) on any measure, including the recurrence of maternal depression.

A number of imaginative interventions have been designed by Field and colleagues to target infants of depressed mothers in high-risk groups; these have included infant massage (Field, 1995), giving support to mothers in observing infant responses (Hart, Field, & Nearing, 1998), and coaching in relation to specific aspects of problematic mother–infant interactions (Malphurs, Field, Larraine *et al.*, 1996). While all appeared to result in improvements at the time they were delivered, whether they can bring about longer-term benefits is still unclear. Infant massage has subsequently been shown to be associated with improved mother–child interaction and infant sleeping in studies of non-depressed parents (Underdown, Barlow, Chung *et al.*, 2006). Long-term monitoring and treatment may be necessary, however, because postnatal depression is associated with recurrent episodes (Cooper & Murray, 1995; Halligan, Murray, Martins *et al.*, 2007), even if successfully treated at the time (Cooper, Murray, Wilson *et al.*, 2003), and because chronicity is an important predictor of several child outcomes.

Treatment aimed at reducing risk to offspring in the context of maternal eating disorder has been examined in only one study. Stein *et al.* (2006) evaluated a treatment delivered over 13 sessions which used video feedback to help mothers with an eating disorder become more aware of, and responsive to, their infant's behavior during feeding. Post-treatment assessments showed benefits in terms of reduced rates of mother–child conflict, enhanced maternal facilitation of infant behavior and increased infant autonomy compared to a counseling control group. Both groups maintained good infant weight with no differences between them.

With regard to parental anxiety disorder, no direct evidence is available concerning the implications for the children of treatment. The facts that risk for disorder in the offspring of affected parents is substantial, and that a number of parenting dimensions are implicated in intergenerational transmission of disorder, make it important to conduct treatment research in this area.

A considerable practical challenge when considering treatment from the point of view of the offspring of parents affected by psychiatric disorder is that secondary adult clinical services are often not sufficiently well co-ordinated with child and adolescent mental health teams to take on board the issue of risk to offspring. With regard to community, as opposed to clinic, populations, somewhat different problems are posed, the most notable being that depressed parents may not be motivated to seek treatment, either for themselves or their children. With regard to treatment in the postpartum period, although good tools have been developed for primary health care workers to screen for depression, such as the Edinburgh Postnatal Depression Scale (Cox, Holden, & Sagovsky, 1987), the detection and identification of the disorder have been quite poor, especially in the early postpartum weeks. Furthermore, those who are likely to be at greatest risk for parenting difficulties associated with depression may be the least willing to take up interventions (Murray, Woolgar, Murray *et al.*, 2003b).

A helpful overall framework for assessing the potential risks to children where a parent has a psychiatric disorder is provided by Rutter (1989). It is wise not to assume risk to children purely because their parent has a psychiatric disorder. Careful assessment should include the areas most likely to be affected by the parental disorder. These are outlined above, but include specific deficits in parental interaction with their children, the quality and type of care the parent is able to provide, and the presence of family and marital discord. The specific feelings that an affected parent has towards their child (or children) can be discussed. Review of these factors over the past history, as well as at the present time, can give useful insight into any potential areas of difficulty that may exist. A thorough and individualized assessment of this kind will be the best guide to the areas where intervention (if required) is most likely to be of benefit.

Clinicians can also have a practical, positive role in providing support, information and, if necessary, treatment to parents affected by psychiatric disorder. The establishment of close collaborative links with adult psychiatric services is likely to lead to the most positive outcomes for families where a parent has chronic severe psychiatric difficulties, but this is not always possible, either because such services are not readily available, or because of differences in thresholds for accepting referrals. Nevertheless, there is sufficient clinical knowledge, and an evidence base (Cobham, Dadds, & Spence, 1998; Sonuga-Barke, Daley, & Thompson, 2002; Weissman *et al.*, 2006) to suggest that treating parental psychiatric difficulties will, in many cases, lead to better outcomes for the child and family, even when it is a child in the family who is presenting to health services. This is now being recognized in treatment guidelines; for example, the UK guidelines for the treatment of depression in children and young people specifically identify the assessment of parental mood as part of the clinical assessment (NICE, 2005). Indeed, in some circumstances, this is a critical part of case management and, without it, children's recovery may be hampered (Cooper, Fearn, Willetts *et al.*, 2006). What then to do in terms of treatment is sometimes a difficult clinical judgment. When the ideal circumstance of close joint management with adult services is not available, a clinician might be able to liaise with the parent's general practitioner, but in some circumstances provision of treatment directly to the parent within the child and adolescent mental health setting may be the best course of action. The crucial point is to remember to assess, recognize and arrange appropriate management of parental difficulties, as well as the child's presenting problem.

There has been very little research examining how to mitigate the potential impact of a serious parental physical disorder on children's development. However, a number of studies have focused on the nature of the communication between parents and children in the context of maternal breast cancer and provide pointers to intervention (Barnes, Kroll, Burke *et al.*, 2000; Forrest, Plumb, Ziebland *et al.*, 2006). These studies indicate that many children will have picked up that something is seriously wrong from changes in their parent's mood or behavior well before they are told of the diagnosis. From as young as 7 years children may associate the diagnosis of cancer with the threat of dying, and therefore not talking about this connection does not protect children. Children's reactions to bad news may belie their feelings. Thus, withdrawal, lack of upset, or else angry challenging behavior does not necessarily indicate indifference, a lack of distress or lack of sympathy or empathy. Parents and clinicians often underestimate children's needs for information and try and protect them, and children may not ask about emotionally charged subjects. However, the more children are prepared and informed (as appropriate for their age and development), the more it seems to help them to cope. Individual differences, as well as age, developmental stage and previous experience need to be taken into account. Parents diagnosed with cancer or other serious illnesses should be offered help to think about whether, what and how to tell their children about their illness, and about what the children can understand, especially as the parents may well be struggling themselves to come to terms with their illness. In the first instance, this is probably best done by clinicians involved with the illness, but guidance or even direct involvement of mental health professionals may be of particular benefit. Mental health professionals can have a key role in the training of other clinicians undertaking this work.

Among the many children who live with a parent who has some chronic physical or psychiatric illness, a small proportion (perhaps 4%) will have acted regularly as a carer for a parent or other relative during their childhood. The extent to which a carer role is undertaken will depend on many factors, including the severity and chronicity of the parent's illness, the input of the second parent, other family and social supports, the age of the child and siblings, and pre-existing family relationships (including that between parent and child). A number of recent reports (Aldridge & Becker, 2003) rightly stress that each family and presentation is different, and that the carer role is not always detrimental to the child's well-being. Nonetheless, there are important possible difficulties and risks for a child required to take on a caring role which must be considered by clinicians. These include potentially missing out on some normal activities such as school and meeting with friends, lacking or inconsistently experiencing parental support and discipline, as well as experiencing anxiety about their parent's health and fearing possible separations for episodes of hospital admission. In relation to maternal depression, it has been hypothesized that caring for the mother may be particularly burdensome for the child (Radke-Yarrow, Zahn-Waxler, Richardson *et al.*, 1994), and may form part of the process whereby the offspring of depressed parents come to be at increased risk for depression themselves (Zahn-Waxler, Cole, & Barrett, 1991; Zahn-Waxler, Kochanska, Krupnick *et al.*, 1990). While these will not all be issues for many children, they are important to consider, as professionals may be able to assist children and parents in accessing supportive services as well as those services to help effectively treat the parental illness.

Future Considerations

It seems very likely that there will be a number of exciting developments in both clinical and research domains within the next few years of direct relevance to our understanding of parental psychiatric disorder, and its effects on children. Research is likely to lead to clearer elucidation of the early developmental risks for children, including parental psychopathology, and to an increased understanding of the mechanisms by which risk is transmitted from parents to their children. There are three main areas of research that we highlight as being particularly promising.

First is the study of the early developmental origins of mental disorder, and of parental psychiatric illness as a key measurable risk in this endeavor. There are two specific time periods whose study seems most likely to lead to advances that will affect our understanding and practice. These are the antenatal (prenatal) period and the early postnatal period. The rapid advances in knowledge regarding the early developmental origins of health, in both animal research and in the study of other human diseases such as diabetes (Gluckman, Hanson, Spencer *et al.*, 2005), are likely to extend increasingly into the study of early effects on behavioral and emotional development. We have already alluded to some of the research on maternal postnatal depression that has given some insight into the effects of disturbances in early care on child development, and other work has demonstrated an independent association between maternal stress or anxiety in pregnancy with children's subsequent behavioral development, and also with the longer-term setting of their HPA axis. These strands of work are likely to advance with scientific developments in psychoendocrinology and also scanning technologies, with implications for early preventative work.

Second is the area of epigenetic effects. These are likely to lead to an increased understanding of the complex mechanisms by which parental psychopathology affects children. Relatively recent work (Weaver, Cervoni, Champagne *et al.*, 2004) has begun to point to the ways in which early environmental exposures might impact upon the genetic expression in the HPA axis. This is likely to have particular significance for our scientific understanding of the intergenerational transmission of mood and anxiety disorders.

The third area where we anticipate significant advance is in our understanding of those factors that predict resilience and more positive outcome in the face of adversity. Once risk factors such as parental depression are identified, an important, and often neglected, next step is the study of those children who do well despite exposure to the risk factor. Through these means we can anticipate further improvements in our understanding of the way in which risks exert their effects. This has particular significance for clinical practice, and it is to this arena that we now turn our attention.

There are two particular areas of clinical advance for the coming years that we wish to highlight: the further development of early-years interventions, and the internationalizing of these clinical interventions. Recent years have seen a significant focus on early child development. This has included the development and implementation of a number of early-years interventions. Coupled with some of the research advances we anticipate above, these should become more sophisticated both in terms of the intervention components, and in their targeting. There are already developments in the targeting of specific interventions for key clinical groups in research studies (e.g., the use of video feedback for parents; Velderman, Bakermans-Kranenburg, Juffer *et al.*, 2006) and specifically mothers with eating disorders (Stein *et al.*, 2006). The next stage is the translation of these findings to clinical populations in a strategic and efficient manner.

The second clinical area is the importance of this work in the international context, especially in relation to developing countries. Very little research has been conducted in this context, and this omission needs to be rectified. It is becoming increasingly clear that the bulk of the burden of impact of parental psychiatric disorder falls not in the developed world, where most of the interventions are developed and used, but on the developing world. Depression is already one of the leading causes of disability worldwide (Murray & Lopez, 1997) and its impact is set to increase. Much of the study of parental psychiatric disorder has been conducted in developed country settings, with uncertainty about the applicability of these findings across different developed country settings, let alone their extrapolation to developing nations. However, the impact of maternal depression in particular on children's physical as well as psychological health is becoming clear in developing countries, including India and Pakistan (Patel, DeSouza, & Rodrigues, 2003; Patel, Rahman, Jacob *et al.*, 2004; Tomlinson, Cooper, & Murray, 2005). The identification of high levels of depression in association with HIV, in particular, argues for urgent research into the impact of depression on children's development in this area. We hope to see increasing development of interventions that are adapted to the setting in which people find themselves, where individual-specific components are developed with the context in mind, so that this vulnerable group of children and their families can be helped across far more of the world than at present.

References

Aldridge, J., & Becker, S. (2003). *Children caring for parents with mental illness*. Bristol: Policy Press.

American Academy of Pediatrics: Committee on Drugs. (1998). Neonatal drug withdrawal. *Pediatrics*, *101*, 1079–1088.

Barker, D. J. P., Osmond, C., Rodin, I., Fall, C. H. D., & Winter, P. D. (1995). Low weight gain in infancy and suicide in adult life. *British Medical Journal*, *311*, 1203.

Barnes, J., Kroll, L., Burke, O., Lee, J., Jones, A., Stein, A., *et al.* (2000). Qualitative interview study of communication between parents and children about maternal breast cancer. *British Medical Journal*, *321*, 479–482.

Beardslee, W. R., & Gladstone, T. R. (2001). Prevention of childhood depression: Recent findings and future prospects. *Biological Psychiatry*, *49*, 1101–1110.

Beardslee, W. R., Gladstone, T. R., Wright, E. J., & Cooper, A. B. (2003). A family-based approach to the prevention of depressive symptoms in children at risk: Evidence of parental and child change. *Pediatrics*, *112*, e119–131.

Beardslee, W. R., Versage, E. M., & Gladstone, T. R. (1998). Children of affectively ill parents: A review of the past 10 years. *Journal of the American Academy of Child and Adolescent Psychiatry*, *37*, 1134–1141.

Bennett, D. S., Bendersky, M., & Lewis, M. (2002). Children's intellectual and emotional–behavioral adjustment at 4 years as a function of cocaine exposure, maternal characteristics, and environmental risk. *Developmental Psychology*, *38*, 648–658.

Biederman, J., Petty, C., Faraone, S. V., Henin, A., Hirshfeld-Becker, D., Pollack, M. H., *et al.* (2006). Effects of parental anxiety disorders in children at high risk for panic disorder: A controlled study. *Journal of Affective Disorders*, *94*, 191–197.

Boyce, P. M. (2003). Risk factors for postnatal depression: a review and risk factors in Australian populations. *Archives of Women's Mental Health*, *6* (Supplement 2), S43–50.

Brinch, M., Isager, T. & Tolstrup, K. (1988). Anorexia nervosa and motherhood: Reproduction pattern and mothering behavior of 50 women. *Acta Psychiatrica Scandinavica*, *77*, 611–617.

Caspi, A., McClay, J., Moffitt, T. E., Mill, J., Martin, J., Craig, I. W., *et al.* (2002). Role of genotype in the cycle of violence in maltreated children. *Science*, *297*, 851–854.

Caspi, A., Sugden, K., Moffitt, T. E., Taylor, A., Craig, I. W., Harrington, H., *et al.* (2003). Influence of life stress on depression: moderation by a polymorphism in the S-HTT gene. *Science*, *301*, 386–389.

Chiriboga, C. A. (2003). Fetal alcohol and drug effects. *Neurologist*, *9*, 267–279.

Cicchetti, D., Toth, S. L., & Rogosch, F. A. (1999). The efficacy of toddler–parent psychotherapy to increase attachment security in offspring of depressed mothers. *Attachment and Human Devopment*, *1*, 34–66.

Clarke, G. N., Hornbrook, M., Lynch, F., Polen, M., Gale, J., O'Connor, E., *et al.* (2002). Group cognitive–behavioral treatment for depressed adolescent offspring of depressed parents in a health maintenance organization. *Journal of the American Academy of Child and Adolescent Psychiatry*, *41*, 305–313.

Cobham, V. E., Dadds, M. R., & Spence, S. H. (1998). The role of parental anxiety in the treatment of childhood anxiety. *Journal of Consulting and Clinical Psychology*, *66*, 893–905.

Cooper, P. J., & Eke, M. (1999). Childhood shyness and maternal social phobia: A community study. *British Journal of Psychiatry*, *174*, 439–443.

Cooper, P. J., Fearn, V., Willetts, L., Seabrook, H., & Parkinson, M. (2006). Affective disorder in the parents of a clinic sample of children with anxiety disorders. *Journal of Affective Disorders*, *93*, 205–212.

Cooper, P. J., & Murray, L. (1995). Course and recurrence of postnatal depression: Evidence for the specificity of the diagnostic concept. *British Journal of Psychiatry*, *166*, 191–195.

Cooper, P. J., Murray, L., Wilson, A., & Romaniuk, H. (2003). Controlled trial of the short- and long-term effect of psychological treatment of post-partum depression. I. Impact on maternal mood. *British Journal of Psychiatry*, *182*, 412–419.

Cooper, P. J., Whelan, E., Woolgar, M., Morrell, J., & Murray, L. (2004). Association between childhood feeding problems and maternal eating disorder: Role of the family environment. *British Journal of Psychiatry*, *184*, 210–215.

Cox, J. L., Holden, J. M., & Sagovsky, R. (1987). Detection of postnatal depression: Development of the 10-item Edinburgh Postnatal Depression Scale. *British Journal of Psychiatry*, *150*, 782–786.

Crane, C., & Martin, M. (2004). Illness-related parenting in mothers with functional gastrointestinal symptoms. *American Journal of Gastroenterology*, *99*, 694–702.

Cuijpers, P., Langendoen, Y., & Bijl, R. V. (1999). Psychiatric disorders in adult children of problem drinkers: Prevalence, first onset and comparison with other risk factors. *Addiction*, *94*, 1489–1498.

Cummings, E. M., Keller, P. S., & Davies, P. T. (2005). Towards a family process model of maternal and paternal depressive symptoms: Exploring multiple relations with child and family functioning. *Journal of Child Psychology and Psychiatry*, *46*, 479–489.

Fairburn, C. G., & Harrison, P. J. (2003). Eating disorders. *Lancet*, *361*, 407–416.

Field, T. (1995). Massage therapy for infants and children. *Journal of Developmental and Behavioral Pediatrics*, *16*, 105–111.

Field, T., Healy, B., Goldstein, S., Perry, S., Bendell, D., Schanberg, S., *et al.* (1988). Infants of depressed mothers show "depressed" behavior even with nondepressed adults. *Child Development*, *59*, 1569–1579.

Field, T., Hossain, Z., & Malphurs, J. (1999). "Depressed" fathers' interactions with their infants. *Infant Mental Health Journal*, *20*, 322–332.

Forrest, G., Plumb, C., Ziebland, S., & Stein A. (2006). Breast cancer in the family: Children's perceptions of their mother's cancer and its initial treatment: qualitative study. *British Medical Journal*, *332*, 998–1003.

Gale, C. R., O'Callaghan, F. J., Godfrey, K. M., Law, C. M., & Martyn, C. N. (2004). Critical periods of brain growth and cognitive function in children. *Brain*, *127*, 321–329.

Gluckman, P. D., Hanson, M. A., Spencer, H. G., & Bateson, P. (2005). Environmental influences during development and their later consequences for health and disease: Implications for the interpretation of empirical studies. *Proceedings. Biological Sciences*, *272*, 671–677.

Goodman, S. H., & Gotlib, I. H. (1999). Risk for psychopathology in the children of depressed mothers: A developmental model for understanding mechanisms of transmission. *Psychological Review*, *106*, 458–490.

Gordon, J. A., & Hen, R. (2004). Genetic approaches to the study of anxiety. *Annual Review of Neurosciences*, *27*, 193–222.

Gottesman, I. I., & Shields, J. (1976). A critical review of recent adoption, twin, and family studies of schizophrenia: Behavioral genetics perspectives. *Schizophrenia Bulletin*, 2, 360–401.

Halbreich, U., & Karkun, S. (2006). Cross-cultural and social diversity of prevalence of postpartum depression and depressive symptoms. *Journal of Affective Disorders*, *91*, 97–111.

Halligan, S. L., Murray, L., Martins, C., & Cooper P. J. (2007). Maternal depression and psychiatric outcomes in adolescent offspring: A 13-year longitudinal study. *Journal of Affective Disorders*, *97*, 145–154.

Hammen, C., & Brennan, P. A. (2003). Severity, chronicity, and timing of maternal depression and risk for adolescent offspring diagnoses in a community sample. *Archives of General Psychiatry*, *60*, 253–258.

Hart, S., Field, T., & Nearing, G. (1998). Depressed mothers' neonates improve following the MABI and a Brazelton demonstration. *Journal of Pediatric Psychology*, *23*, 351–356.

Hassan, M. A., & Killick, S. R. (2004). Negative lifestyle is associated with a significant reduction in fecundity. *Fertility and Sterility*, *81*, 384–392.

Hay, D. F., Pawlby, S., Sharp, D., Asten, P., Mills, A., & Kumar, R. (2001). Intellectual problems shown by 11-year-old children whose mothers had postnatal depression. *Journal of Child Psychology and Psychiatry*, *42*, 871–889.

Henin, A., Biederman, J., Mick, E., Sachs, G. S., Hirshfeld-Becker, D. R., Siegel, R. S., *et al.* (2005). Psychopathology in the offspring of parents with bipolar disorder: A controlled study. *Biological Psychiatry*, *58*, 554–561.

Hillegers, M. H., Reichart, C. G., Wals, M., Verhulst, F. C., Ormel, J., & Nolen, W. A. (2005). Five-year prospective outcome of psychopathology in the adolescent offspring of bipolar parents. *Bipolar Disorders*, *7*, 344–350.

Jacobi, C., Agras, W. S., & Hammer, L. (2001). Predicting children's reported eating disturbances at 8 years of age. *Journal of the American Academy of Child and Adolescent Psychiatry*, *40*, 364–372.

Jaffee, S. R., Moffitt, T. E., Caspi, A., & Taylor, A. (2003). Life with (or without) father: The benefits of living with two biological parents depend on the father's antisocial behavior. *Child Development*, *74*, 109–126.

Kessler, R. C., McGonagle, K. A., Zhao, S., Nelson C. B., Hughes, M., Swartz, M., *et al.* (1994). Lifetime and 12-month prevalence of DSM-III-R psychiatric disorders in the United States. Results from the National Comorbidity Survey. *Archives of General Psychiatry*, *51*, 8–19.

Kim-Cohen, J., Moffitt, T. E., Taylor, A., Pawlby, S. J., & Caspi, A. (2005). Maternal depression and children's antisocial behavior: Nature and nurture effects. *Archives of General Psychiatry*, 62, 173–181.

Korneluk, Y. G., & Lee, C. M. (1998). Children's adjustment to parental physical illness. *Clinical Child and Family Psychology Review*, *1*, 179–193.

Lieberman, D. (2000). Children of alcoholics: An update. *Current Opinion in Pediatrics*, *12*, 336–340.

Lyons-Ruth, K., Alpern, L., & Repacholi, B. (1993). Disorganized infant attachment classification and maternal psychosocial problems as predictors of hostile-aggressive behavior in the preschool classroom. *Child Development*, *64*, 572–585.

Malphurs, J., Field, T., Larraine, C., Pickens, J., Pelaez-Noqueras, M., Yando, R., *et al.* (1996). Altering withdrawn and intrusive interaction behaviors of depressed mothers. *Infant Mental Health Journal*, *17*, 152–160.

Mancini, C., Van-Ameringen, M., Szatmari, P., & Fugere, C. (1996). A high-risk pilot study of the children of adults with social phobia. *Journal of the American Academy of Child and Adolescent Psychiatry*, *35*, 1511–1517.

Marks, M., Hipwell, A., & Kumar, C. (2002). Implications for the infant of maternal puerperal psychiatric disorders. In M. Rutter, & E. Taylor (Eds.), *Child and adolescent psychiatry* (4th edn., pp. 858–880). Oxford: Blackwell Publishing.

Martin, C., Cabrol, S., Bouvard, M. P., Lepine, J. P., & Mouren-Simeoni, M. C. (1999). Anxiety and depressive disorders in fathers and mothers of anxious school-refusing children. *Journal of the American Academy of Child and Adolescent Psychiatry*, *38*, 916–922.

Martins, C., & Gaffan, E. A. (2000). Effects of early maternal depression on patterns of infant–mother attachment: A meta-analytic investigation. *Journal of Child Psychology and Psychiatry*, *41*, 737–746.

McNeil, T. F. & Kaij, L. (1987). Swedish high-risk study: Sample characteristics at age 6. *Schizophrenia Bulletin*, *13*, 373–381.

Merikangas, K. R., Dierker, L. C., & Szatmari, P. (1998). Psychopathology among offspring of parents with substance abuse and/or anxiety disorders: A high-risk study. *Journal of Child Psychology and Psychiatry*, *39*, 711–720.

Misra, D. P., Grason, H., & Weisman, C. (2000). An intersection of women's and perinatal health: The role of chronic conditions. *Women's Health Issues*, *10*, 256–267.

Mukherjee, R. A., Hollins, S. & Turk, J. (2006). Fetal alcohol spectrum disorder: An overview. *Journal of the Royal Society of Medicine*, *99*, 298–302.

Murray, C. J., & Lopez, A. D. (1997). Alternative projections of mortality and disability by cause 1990–2020: Global Burden of Disease Study. *Lancet*, *349*, 1498–1504.

Murray, L., & Cooper, P. (2003). Intergenerational transmission of affective and cognitive processes associated with depression: Infancy and the preschool years. In I. Goodyer (Ed.), *Unipolar depression: A lifespan perspective* (pp. 17–46). Oxford: Oxford University Press.

Murray, L., Cooper, P. J., Wilson, A., & Romaniuk, H. (2003a). A controlled trial of the short- and long-term effect of psychological treatment of postpartum depression: II. Impact on the mother child relationship and child outcome. *British Journal of Psychiatry*, *182*, 420–427.

Murray, L., Woolgar, M., Murray, J., & Cooper, P. J. (2003b). Self-exclusion from health care in women at high risk for post-partum depression. *Journal of Public Health Medicine*, *25*, 2, 131–137.

Murray, L., Cooper, P., Creswell, C., Schofield, E., & Sack, C. (2007). The effects of maternal social phobia on mother–infant interactions and infant social responsiveness. *Journal of Child Psychology and Psychiatry*, *48*, 45–52.

Murray, L., Fiori-Cowley, A., Hooper, R., & Cooper, P. (1996a). The impact of postnatal depression and associated adversity on early mother–infant interactions and later infant outcome. *Child Development*, *67*, 2512–2526.

Murray, L., Hipwell, A., Hooper, R., Stein, A., & Cooper, P. (1996b). The cognitive development of 5-year-old children of postnatally depressed mothers. *Journal of Child Psychology and Psychiatry*, *37*, 927–935.

Murray, L., Kempton, C., Woolgar, M., & Hooper, R. (1993). Depressed mothers' speech to their infants and its relation to infant gender and cognitive development. *Journal of Child Psychology and Psychiatry*, *34*, 1083–1101.

Murray, L., Stanley, C., Hooper, R., King, F., & Fiori-Cowley, A. (1996c). The role of infant factors in postnatal depression and mother–infant interactions. *Developmental Medicine and Child Neurology*, *38*, 109–119.

Murray, L., Woolgar, M., Cooper, P., & Hipwell, A. (2001). Cognitive vulnerability to depression in 5-year-old children of depressed mothers. *Journal of Child Psychology and Psychiatry*, *42*, 891–899.

National Institute for Health and Clinical Excellence (NICE). (2005). *Depression in children and young people: Identification and management in primary, community and secondary care*. London: National Institute for Health and Clinical Excellence.

Nicol-Harper, R., Harvey, A. G., & Stein, A. (2007). Interactions between mothers and infants: Impact of maternal anxiety. *Infant Behavior and Development*, *30*, 161–167.

O'Connor, T. G., Heron, J., Golding, J., & Glover, V. (2003). Maternal anxiety and behavioural/emotional problems in children: a test of a programming hypothesis. *Journal of Child Psychology and Psychiatry*, *44*, 1025–1036.

O'Connor, T. G., Ben-Shlomo, Y., Heron, J., Golding, J., Adams, D., & Glover, V. (2005). Prenatal anxiety predicts individual differences in cortisol in pre-adolescent children. *Biological Psychiatry*, *58*, 211–217.

O'Hara, M., & Swain, A. (1996). Rates and risk of postpartum depression: A meta-analysis. *International Review of Psychiatry*, *8*, 37–54.

Patel, P., Wheatcroft, R., Park, R. J., & Stein, A. (2002). The children of mothers with eating disorders. *Clinical Child and Family Psychology Review*, *5*, 1–19.

Patel, V., DeSouza, N., & Rodrigues, M. (2003). Postnatal depression and infant growth and development in low income countries: A cohort study from Goa, India. *Archives of Disease in Childhood*, *88*, 34–37.

Patel, V., Rahman, A., Jacob, K. S., & Hughes, M. (2004). Effect of maternal mental health on infant growth in low income countries: New evidence from South Asia. *British Medical Journal*, *328*, 820–823.

Pederson, S., & Revenson, T. A. (2005). Parental illness, family functioning, and adolescent well-being: A family ecology framework to guide research. *Journal of Family Psychology*, *19*, 404–419.

Radke-Yarrow, M. (1998). *Children of depressed mothers: from early childhood to maturity*. Cambridge: Cambridge University Press.

Radke-Yarrow, M., Zahn-Waxler, C., Richardson, D. T., & Susman, A. (1994). Caring behavior in children of clinically depressed and well mothers. *Child Development*, *65*, 1405–1414.

Ramchandani, P., Stein, A., Evans, J., & O'Connor, T. G. (2005). Paternal depression in the postnatal period and child development: A prospective population study. *Lancet*, *365*, 2201–2205.

Rochat, T., Richter, L., Doll, H., Buthelezi, N., Tomkins, A., & Stein, A. (2006). Depression among pregnant rural South African women undergoing HIV testing. *Journal of the American Medical Association*, *295*, 1376–1378.

Rutter, M. (1989). Psychiatric disorder in parents as a risk factor for children. In D. Schaffer, I. Phillips, & N. B. Enger (Eds.), *Prevention of mental disorder, alcohol and other drug use in children and adolescents* (pp. 157–189). Rockville, MD: Office for Substance Abuse, USDHHS.

Rutter, M. L. (1999). Psychosocial adversity and child psychopathology. *British Journal of Psychiatry*, 174, 480–493.

Rutter, M. (2007). Gene–environment interdependence. *Developmental Science*, *10*, 12–18.

Rutter, M., Moffitt, T. E., & Caspi, A. (2006). Gene–environment interplay and psychopathology: Multiple varieties but real effects. *Journal of Child Psychology and Psychiatry*, *47*, 226–261.

Seeley, S., Murray, L., & Cooper, P. J. (1996). The outcome for mothers and babies of health visitor intervention. *Health Visitor*, *69*, 4.

Sinclair, D., & Murray, L. (1998). Effects of postnatal depression on children's adjustment to school: Teacher's reports. *British Journal of Psychiatry*, *172*, 58–63.

Sonuga-Barke, E. J., Daley, D., & Thompson, M. (2002). Does maternal ADHD reduce the effectiveness of parent training for preschool children's ADHD? *Journal of the American Academy of Child and Adolescent Psychiatry*, *41*, 696–702.

Stein, A., Gath, D. H., Bucher, J., Bond, A., Day, A., & Cooper, P. J. (1991). The relationship between post-natal depression and mother–child interaction. *British Journal of Psychiatry*, *158*, 46–52.

Stein, A., Krebs, G., Richter, L., Tomkins, A., Rochat, T., & Bennish, M. L. (2005). Babies of a pandemic. *Archives of Diseases in Childhood*, *90*, 116–118.

Stein, A., Stein, J., Walters, E. A., & Fairburn, C. G. (1995). Eating habits and attitudes among mothers of children with feeding disorders. *British Medical Journal*, *310*, 228.

Stein, A., Woolley, H., Cooper, S., Winterbottom, J., Fairburn, C. G., & Cortina-Borja, M. (2006). Eating habits and attitudes among 10-year-old children of mothers with eating disorders: A longitudinal study. *British Journal of Psychiatry*, *189*, 324–329.

Stein, A., Woolley, H., & McPherson, K. (1999). Conflict between mothers with eating disorders and their infants during mealtimes. *British Journal of Psychiatry*, *175*, 455–461.

Stice, E., Agras, W. S., & Hammer, L. D. (1999). Risk factors for the emergence of childhood eating disturbances: A five-year prospective study. *International Journal of Eating Disorders*, *25*, 375–387.

Tamis-LeMonda, C. S., Shannon, J. D., Cabrera, N. J., & Lamb, M. E. (2004). Fathers and mothers at play with their 2- and 3-year-olds: Contributions to language and cognitive development. *Child Development*, *75*, 1806–1820.

Thapar, A., Langley, K., Fowler, T., Rice, F., Turic, D., Whittinger, N., *et al.* (2005). Catechol o-methyltransferase gene variant and birth weight predict early-onset antisocial behavior in children with attention-deficit/hyperactivity disorder. *Archives of General Psychiatry*, *62*, 1275–1278.

Tomlinson, M., Cooper, P., & Murray, L. (2005). The mother–infant relationship and infant attachment in a South African peri-urban settlement. *Child Development*, *76*, 1044–1054.

Turner, S. M., Beidel, D. C., & Costello, A. (1987). Psychopathology in the offspring of anxiety disorders patients. *Journal of Consulting and Clinical Psychology*, *55*, 229–235.

Underdown, A., Barlow, J., Chung, V., & Stewart-Brown, S. (2006). Massage intervention for promoting mental and physical health in infants aged under six months. *Cochrane Database System Review*, CD005038.

Velderman, M. K., Bakermans-Kranenburg, M. J., Juffer, F., & van IJzendoorn, M. H. (2006). Effects of attachment-based interventions on maternal sensitivity and infant attachment: differential susceptibility of highly reactive infants. *Journal of Family Psychology*, *20*, 266–274.

Visser, A., Huizinga, G. A., Hoekstra, H. J., van der Graaf, W. T., & Hoekstra-Weebers, J. E. (2006). Parental cancer: Characteristics of parents as predictors for child functioning. *Cancer*, *106*, 1178–1187.

Visser, A., Huizinga, G. A., van der Graaf, W. T., Hoekstra, H. J., & Hoekstra-Weebers, J. E. (2004). The impact of parental cancer on children and the family: A review of the literature. *Cancer Treatment Reviews*, *30*, 683–694.

Von Knorring, A. L. (1991). Annotation: Children of alcoholics. *Journal of Child Psychology and Psychiatry and Allied Disciplines*, *32*, 411–421.

Weaver, I. C., Cervoni, N., Champagne, F. A., D'Alessio, A. C., Sharma, S., Seckl, J. R., *et al.* (2004). Epigenetic programming by maternal behavior. *Nature Neuroscience*, *7*, 847–854.

Weissman, M., Pilowsky, D. J., Wickramaratne, P. J., Talati, A., Wisniewski, S. R., Fava, M., *et al.* (2006). Remissions in maternal depression and child psychopathology: A STAR*D-Child Report. *Journal of the American Medical Association*, *295*, 1389–1398.

Weissman, M. M., Leaf, P. J., Tischler, G. L., Blazer, D. G., Karno, M., Bruce, M. L., *et al.* (1988). Affective disorders in five United States communities. *Psychological Medicine*, *18*, 141–153.

Yarrow, M. R., Campbell, J. D., & Burton, R. V. (1968). *Child rearing: An inquiry in research and methods*. San Francisco, CA: Jossey-Bass.

Zahn-Waxler, C., Cole, P. M., & Barrett, K. C. (1991). Guilt and empathy: Sex differences and implications for the development of depression. In J. Garber, & K. A. Dodge (Eds.), *The development of emotion regulation and dysregulation* (pp. 243–272). New York: Cambridge University Press.

Zahn-Waxler, C., Kochanska, G., Krupnick, J., & McKnew, D. (1990). Patterns of guilt in children of depressed and well mothers. *Developmental Psychology*, *26*, 51–59.

28 Child Maltreatment

David P. H. Jones

Child Maltreatment and Mental Health

The abuse and neglect of children and young people are issues of grave social concern, internationally (World Health Organization [WHO], 2002). They involve fundamental human rights for children and adults; children having the right to be free from abuse and neglect; and parents the right to family life. Child maltreatment is the antithesis of adequate caregiving and parenting (Wolfe, 1991). Not surprisingly, maltreatment of children is associated with significantly increased risk for psychopathology throughout life. Hence, child maltreatment is of major importance to those working in child and adolescent mental health services, research, social welfare, policy-making and legal systems.

Maltreatment incorporates a variety of acts, and deprivation of care, by those who look after children. It involves parents, carers and those who care for children within settings such as schools, hospitals and residential units. The concept has expanded over the past 40 years from physical assault to incorporate neglect, sexual and emotional abuse of all severities. The exponential rise in referrals in North America, the UK and Australasia has led to efforts to reformulate the notion of child abuse and neglect, to distinguish situations where the child's primary need is for added services and support in order to facilitate the child's development, from those who need protection from overt harm. In England and Wales this has been achieved through amending the guidance linked to the Children Act, 1989, so that two streams, support and protection, are distinguished in policy and practice guidelines (Department of Health, the Department of Education & Employment and the Home Office [DOH, DOEE & HO], 2000).

Child maltreatment is not a psychiatric diagnosis; rather a description of a phenomenon affecting children and young people. It may or may not lead to discernible harm, physically or psychologically. There are no specific syndromes of physical or sexual abuse, instead child maltreatment is a major environmental risk factor for non-optimal development, both physically and psychologically. The influence of maltreatment on development and psychopathology, and implications for child mental health practitioners, are now examined further.

Rutter's Child and Adolescent Psychiatry, 5th edition. Edited by M. Rutter, D. Bishop, D. Pine, S. Scott, J. Stevenson, E. Taylor and A. Thapar. © 2008 Blackwell Publishing, ISBN: 978-1-4051-4549-7.

International Perspective

WHO (2002) defines child abuse and neglect, or child maltreatment, as all forms of physical and/or emotional ill-treatment, sexual abuse, neglect or negligent treatment, or commercial or other exploitation resulting in actual or potential harm to the child's health, survival, development or dignity in the context of a relationship of responsibility, trust or power.

Definitions in North America, the UK and Australasia all center on the notion of harm caused to children as a consequence of care provided to them. Definitions vary at the operational level, including the degree to which intention and detectable harm are included.

Reporting practices differ between countries. Some countries have followed the American policy of mandatory, legally required, reporting of potential cases, while in others a voluntary system is in place. The UK has no legal requirement to report suspected cases, but professional regulation and government guidance emphasize requirement to report, resulting in the UK being closer to mandatory than voluntary reporting. In some western European countries, such as Belgium and the Netherlands, the approach is more voluntary, with greater emphasis on social support and intervention.

The focus of each country's concern will vary according to the most numerically pressing problem that it faces. For some countries the emphasis is on child labor or prostitution, while in others the focus is on intrafamilial abuse. Nonetheless, all countries need to attend to the full range of maltreatment of children within their boundaries. Additionally, each country should consider how it may make a contribution on a worldwide basis (e.g., the UK's initiative to curb child "sex tourism").

A Major Public Health Issue

WHO's (1999) initiative on violence and human health stressed that children are vulnerable to violence from war and natural disaster, and maltreatment in the context of a relationship of responsibility, and sometimes both. The response plan recommended includes national action plans for violence prevention; data collection; research on causes, consequences and prevention of maltreatment; strengthening victim responses; and better collation and information exchange (Mian, 2004).

Public health principles shift the emphasis from a reaction to violence to a focus on underlying social, behavioral and environmental factors (Mercy, Rosenberg, Powell *et al.*, 1993). To this may be added genetic factors (Rutter, 2005; Rutter, Moffitt, & Caspi, 2006a). The health burden of child maltreatment on human health has also been evaluated (Andrews, Corry, Slade *et al.*, 2004). These initiatives have placed violence and child maltreatment in the forefront of international public health concern, forcing the agenda toward prevention, with integration of different disciplines, organizations and communities (Mercy, Rosenberg, Powell *et al.*, 1993).

Types of Maltreatment

WHO (2002) distinguishes five subtypes: physical, sexual, and emotional abuse, neglect, and exploitation. The focus of this chapter is neglect, physical and emotional abuse. Exploitation refers to children used in work or other activities for the benefit of others (e.g., child labor, prostitution and child soldiers; WHO, 2002). In England and Wales the Government's definitions (HM Government, 2006) are similar to WHO's, but differ through being more operationally defined, and to varying degrees incorporating harm caused to the child. As this distinction is similar to that in other countries, England and Wales definitions are utilized in the sections below.

Physical abuse involves "hitting, shaking, throwing, poisoning, burning or scalding, drowning, suffocating, or otherwise causing physical harm to a child. Physical harm may also be caused when a parent or carer fabricates symptoms of, or deliberately induces, illness in a child" (HM Government, 2006). The "battered child syndrome" refers to younger children presenting with multiple bruises, skeletal and head injuries, frequently accompanied by visceral trauma or neglect and fearfulness, whose parents deny responsibility (Kempe, Silverman, Steele *et al.*, 1962). It represents the severe end of the continuum of physical abuse.

Physical abuse is normally diagnosed by pediatricians, on the basis of the discrepancy between physical findings and history, in the absence of a non-abusive explanation. Occasionally, the child makes a direct account, or there is a witness, or confession by a carer. There may have been previous similar, less severe episodes. Explanations, imputed or proffered, include developmental challenges, persistent crying, toileting, feeding problems or issues of discipline and independence in later childhood. Delay in presentation and parental absence of concern or unreasonable behavior described by Kempe, Silverman, Steele *et al.* (1962) are not reliably present.

Fabricated or induced illness (FII) is where a parent or carer feigns an impression or induces a state of ill health in a child whom they are looking after. The child is harmed either through the fabrication of symptoms, signs, reports or specimens, through directly inducing ill health (HM Government, 2006; Jones & Bools, 1999) or through combinations thereof. A wide variety of presentations have been described (Rosenberg, 1987), but common forms include fabricated epilepsy, non-accidental poisoning or life-threatening events in infancy (either fabricated or directly induced).

FII is best considered a form of child maltreatment than a type of parental psychopathology, notwithstanding the observation that personality disorder is common amongst perpetrators. DSM-IV tends to emphasize the latter rather than the former. This is unfortunate, because much controversy has emanated from assumptions being made about parental motivation when children have been harmed in this way.

The phenomenon involves the coalescence of three elements: health professionals being misled; a child harmed (directly or through unnecessary investigation or treatment); and parental need for involving health-care systems is met through apparent, or actual, ill health in the child (Jones & Bools, 1999).

The concept has had utility in pediatrics, enabling the possibility of harm to be considered in the differential diagnosis of unusual presentations; much as in the 1960s the use of the emotive term Battered Child Syndrome drew professional attention to previously unrecognized harm caused by carers. The concept should remain confined to health consultations, and not expanded to disparate situations where parents deceive professionals (Jones, 1996a).

Covert video surveillance has been successfully employed to identify serious cases (Southall, Plunkett, Banks *et al.*, 1997). However, the practice remains highly controversial. The practice brings a child's right to be protected from harm and parental right to privacy into conflict. Clearly, covert surveillance is highly intrusive and therefore the threshold for its use must be very high. Normally it is only employed when all alternative sources of assessment have been exhausted but where high levels of suspicion remain. Even then, in England and Wales, the practice only occurs with the involvement of police and high-level prior strategic planning, when all aspects, including ethical dimensions, are thoroughly explored. It may be more acceptable ethically, and fruitful diagnostically, to require a period of enforced separation of child and parent in order to see whether symptoms recede in the absence of the suspected fabricator. Nonetheless, many would agree that an unpleasant degree of professional secrecy is acceptable in order to prevent a child continuing to be seriously harmed, provided no other, less intrusive, means can be employed. It is therefore important that the possibility of its use is retained, albeit uncommonly used.

Sexual abuse is considered in chapter 29. It involves "forcing or enticing a child or young person to take part in sexual activities, including prostitution, whether or not the child is aware of what is happening" (HM Government, 2006).

Neglect is defined as "the persistent failure to meet a child's basic physical and/or psychological needs, likely to result in the serious impairment of the child's health or development." (HM Government, 2006). Neglect comprises four principal domains: physical, supervision, cognitive and emotional neglect (Straus & Kantor, 2005). Prenatal neglect and abuse may occur through maternal substance abuse. Physical neglect includes failing to provide adequate food, clothing, shelter, or exclusion or abandonment. Supervision also includes the use of unsafe caretakers and failure to utilize health care. Emotional neglect involves inattention to the child's emotional cues and insufficient parental love and affection. Some authors have termed this "psychological unavailability," describing parents/carers who ignore their children's cues and signals, despite clear indication of the child's needs for warmth and comfort (Erikson & Egeland, 1996). Cognitive neglect ranges from inadequate parental speech and responsiveness, leading to speech and language delay (Thorpe, Rutter, & Greenwood, 2003), through to denying access to education.

Neglect must be linked to the developmental needs of the child and distinguished from the effects of poverty. Recognition is assisted by utilizing multiple sources of information, including the children themselves, caregivers, examination of longitudinal case records, observation and standardized measures. Recognition is often delayed because of its chronic insidious nature, absence of crises requiring immediate social services or health responses, problems with definition and high thresholds for social services intervention (Gibbons, Conroy, & Bell, 1995; Smith & Fong, 2004). Despite these difficulties, neglect is the most common form of child maltreatment.

Emotional abuse is "the persistent emotional maltreatment of a child such as to cause severe and persistent adverse effects on the child's emotional development." The definition proceeds to incorporate the following: conveying to children they are worthless, unloved, inadequate or only valued to meet the needs of another person; developmentally inappropriate expectations, including overprotection, limitation of exploration and learning, or preventing normal social interaction; witnessing the ill-treatment of another; serious bullying and terrifying, exploitation or corruption (HM Government, 2006).

It is evident from the above that in England and Wales there is considerable overlap between definitions of neglect and emotional abuse, particularly with respect to the omission of affection, care and parental psychological availability. This confusion is reflected internationally. Schneider, Ross, Graham *et al.* (2005) found only four cases of "pure" emotional maltreatment in a sample of 250 where this was recorded, despite emotional maltreatment being recorded in half of the children suffering other forms. They found that neglect of psychological safety and security (including exposure to domestic violence, threats of injury, suicide and abandonment), or acceptance and self-esteem (included verbal and non-verbal negativity, or active rejection) were the most common categories of emotional maltreatment, with neglect of age-appropriate autonomy or restriction being uncommon. Glaser (2002) also found that children living with a parent with physical or mental illness, disability or marked impairment or those who were exposed to interparental violence were also increasingly identified as suffering emotional abuse. Clearly, other psychological dimensions to parenting are omitted from the above approaches, including guidance, limit-setting, promoting socialization and supporting children's relationships (Jones, 2001; Sroufe, 2005). Emotional abuse would probably be better termed "psychological maltreatment" in order to encompass all impairments to psychological aspects of parenting (Jones, 2001).

While there is little disagreement that protection is necessary for serious neglect of physical and/or emotional needs that threaten a child's safety or health, for many, extra services for the child are required rather than safeguarding (see p. 429; Emery & Laumann-Billings, 2002).

Child abuse and neglect are not clinical conditions but terms arising from social consensus concerning the care of children. While there is little debate about overt physical abuse and sexual abuse between and within cultures, it is nevertheless important to retain cultural sensitivity in relation to practices that do not necessarily cause major harm to children and young people. For example, Korbin (1997) has drawn attention to the fact that leaving an infant all day in the care of a 7- or 8-year-old sibling is relatively usual in parts of the Far East, but considered neglectful in contemporary North American society. Conversely, parents in some parts of South-East Asia consider the western European practice of young children sleeping separately from their parents as neglectful (Korbin, 1997). Difficulties arise where there is disagreement about harm caused (e.g., female circumcision) or where strongly held belief systems lead to child welfare considerations being held secondary to religious certainties (e.g., animist beliefs and practices, which were one thread in the events that led to Victoria Climbié's death; Department of Health, 2003). Anthropologists traditionally eschew taking a moral stance on such issues, yet an international public health perspective requires just such a moral position and legal stance, as has been adopted with female genital mutilation (UNICEF, 2006, p. 64). In an individual case, the laws of the respective country dictate responses to controversial practices affecting children's health and development (see chapters 8 & 15).

Family Violence

The importance of family violence is underlined by strong associations between child maltreatment and intimate partner violence (IPV), and possibly also elder violence, within the same household (Slep & O'Leary, 2005). The traditional stereotype of one aggressor to both partner and children has been overtaken, through community-based studies, by a picture of violence within a family characterized by verbal and physical violence occurring in multiple directions (Krueger, Moffitt, Caspi *et al.*, 1998). Slep and O'Leary (2005) found that 60% of families exhibiting significant violence were characterized by violence occurring between the parents in both directions and between each parent and each child. Furthermore, the predominant pattern of aggression changed over time in one longitudinal study (Sternberg, Lamb, Guterman *et al.*, 2006). Studies using multiple informants reveal higher rates of IPV (Slep & O'Leary, 2005; Sternberg, Lamb, Guterman *et al.*, 2006).

IPV shows a weak to moderate effect on emotional and behavior disturbance in children in meta-analyses (Kitzmann, Gaylord, Holt *et al.*, 2003; Wolfe, Crooks, Lee *et al.*, 2003).

Effects include emotional and disruptive symptoms, particularly anxiety, depression, post-traumatic stress and aggressiveness. Physical health outcomes of childhood exposure to IPV are likely to be seen in terms of risk-taking behaviors, including substance use, early and multiple sexual partners (Bair-Merritt, Blackstone, & Feudtner, 2006).

However, these effects lose significance once persisting child abuse and other adverse events are accounted for (Fergusson, Boden, & Horwood, 2006; Wolfe, Crooks, Lee *et al.*, 2003). Sturge-Apple, Davies, & Cummings (2006) found that the effect of interparental hostility was indirect, and mediated via parental emotional unavailability.

Nonetheless, despite an absence of convincing evidence of long-term effects of IPV, unless accompanied by child abuse and other adversity, effects are evident in the short term. Children under the age of 2 years are most at risk of physical injury, through being caught in the cross-fire of partner violence (Casanueva, Foshee, & Barth, 2005). Additionally, initial as yet unreplicated findings suggest that infants of 1 year may be more irritable and become developmentally regressed when exposed to IPV (Bogat, DeJonghe, Levendosky *et al.*, 2006).

IPV is therefore an important aspect of family violence, causing significant distress, and part of a common constellation of adversity and violence, which occurs in multiple directions in aggressive families. It appears to be only relatively weakly causatively linked to emotional and behavior disturbances in children and adolescents when considered in isolation, but much more significant when combined with child maltreatment, emotional unavailability and other family adversity, when the combined effects have the potential to cause significant mental health problems during childhood and into adult life. Clinically, IPV can also be considered an important marker for child abuse and other co-occurring risk factors for poor mental health outcome in children. Lastly, and most importantly, the most severe forms of intimate partner violence sometimes end in homicide of adult partners and/or children, together with accompanying bereavement.

Epidemiology

It has always proved difficult to obtain accurate figures for child maltreatment incidence and prevalence because of variations in methods of ascertainment and recording. Maltreatment is so frequently kept private by individuals, families and communities. One consequence is the wide gulf between incidence and prevalence figures for all kinds of maltreatment.

The incidence of significant violence to children has been assessed using the Conflict Tactics Scales on representative community samples. This revealed rates of 49 per 1000 children in the USA in 1995 (Strauss, Hamby, Finkelhor *et al.*, 1998); 83 per 1000 in Italian children (Bardi & Borgogni-Tarli, 2001); and 90 per 1000 British children, using a slightly expanded verson (Ghate, Hazel, Creighton *et al.*, 2003).

The USA National Incidence Studies have used child health, education and social care professionals to record incidents of maltreatment. The third national study provided a maltreatment rate of 23 per 1000 children (Sedlak & Broadhurst, 1996). This study surveyed over 5500 professionals, and distinguished between maltreatment causing harm (36%) and significant risk thereof. Girls were three times more likely than boys to be maltreated, but when boys were maltreated the harm was more serious. There were no significant race differences. Risk was significantly elevated among single parents, those with large families and, overwhelmingly, families living in poverty. Social services departments were only involved with a minority of cases, even among the most serious.

Officially reported child abuse and neglect incidence rates are substantially lower, ranging from 2 to 12 per 1000 child population (Australian Institute of Health and Welfare [AIHW], 2004; Department for Education and Skills [DFES], 2005; Department of Health and Human Services [DHHS], 2003; Trocmé, MacLaurin, Fallon *et al.*, 2005). Neglect was the largest category. Children with a disability are three times more likely to be maltreated than the non-impaired (Westcott & Jones, 1999). Physical abuse comprised 15–28%; sexual abuse 10–28%, emotional abuse 7–34% and neglect 34–59%. The incidence of maltreatment increases from cases reported through to cases known about by professionals working with children, to incidence rates obtained from representative samples of the general public.

Prevalence rates of physical abuse in childhood range from 3% to 28%, with most studies reporting in the 5–10% range (Berger, Knutson, Mehm *et al.*, 1988; Stevenson, 1999; Straus & Gelles, 1986). May-Chahal and Cawson (2005) report a rate of 7% in their representative sample of 2869 18- to 24-year-olds recalling childhood experiences. Longitudinal studies have been especially useful in elucidating both prevalence rates and associated risk factors and effects. Fergusson and Lynskey (1997), reporting on the Christchurch birth cohort of 1265 children followed-up into young adult life, reported a prevalence rate of 3.9% of children overly frequently harshly punished or abused. Brown, Cohen, Johnson *et al.*'s (1998) longitudinal study of 644 families revealed a prevalence of 3–24% dependent upon whether, and how many, psychosocial risk factors were also present. Silverman, Reinherz, & Giaconia (1996), in another longitudinal study, found 5.3% of boys and 6.4% of girls suffering physical abuse during childhood. Mullen, Martin, Anderson *et al.* (1996), reporting on their New Zealand sample, found that 7.8% of women reported serious physical abuse during their childhood. Brown, Cohen, Johnson *et al.* (1998) drew data from both self-reported and officially recorded maltreatment and revealed an important lack of correspondence between the two, with substantial proportions of cases missing from each data source.

Neglect and emotional abuse are especially problematic to ascertain in prevalence studies. Estimates range between 5% and 12% (Hussey, Chang, & Kotch, 2006; May-Chahal & Cawson, 2005), but rise much higher when supervisory neglect is added. Emotional abuse estimates have ranged from 6% to 12% (Hussey, Chang, & Kotch, 2006; May-Chahal & Cawson, 2005).

Overall, it is clear that child maltreatment of all kinds is common across cultures, social and economic groups, and in both genders (Strauss, Hamby, Finkelhor *et al.*, 1998; WHO, 2002). Substantial variation between studies and across time probably reflect ascertainment and reporting difficulties largely, but nonetheless it is clear that official rates of reported child abuse represent but the tip of the iceberg of maltreatment experienced by children across cultures.

Serious Abuse and Death

The indications are that rates of serious and life-threatening maltreatment have not decreased in industrialized societies, despite their child protection systems (Emery & Laumann-Billings, 2002; Sedlak & Broadhurst, 1996). Existing figures for maltreatment-related child fatalities underestimate maltreatment as a cause by at least 50% (Jenny & Isaac, 2006). Mortality rates range from 0.1 to 2.2 per 100,000 children in industrialized societies, rising to 2–3 times more than this in low- to mid-income countries (Jenny & Isaac, 2006). The WHO estimates that 57,000 children die each year from maltreatment (Krug, Dahlberg, Mercy *et al.*, 2002). The majority are during infancy, with the neonatal period proving the most common time for maltreatment fatality (Brockington, 1996, 2004; Jenny & Isaac, 2006). Neonates and infants under 2 months are more commonly killed by their mothers, whereas unrelated males more commonly kill older children. Head trauma is the most common cause of death, followed by neglect, suffocation and poisoning (Jenny & Isaac, 2006).

Conceptual Framework

There is consensus that the developmental–ecological perspective offers a comprehensive framework for researchers and practitioners to understand the occurrence and consequences of child maltreatment (National Research Council, 1993). This approach allows for integration of risk and protective factors for maltreatment, and levels of social complexity surrounding the individual (Bronfenbrenner, 1977) to be integrated with principles of developmental psychopathology, especially those that emphasize transactions between disparate factors over time (Belsky & Vondra, 1989). Besides the integrative value of this framework for researchers, it has also informed the Assessment Framework for practitioners, advanced by the Government in England and Wales (DOH, DOEE & HO, 2000).

Factors Associated with the Occurrence of Maltreatment

A range of factors are associated with the risk of maltreatment occurring. Factors that contribute to physical abuse, neglect and psychological maltreatment are organized below, using the domains that emerge from the eco-developmental framework, above.

First, however, it is necessary to note some inherent difficulties raised by discussing factors that are associated with a raised or lowered risk of child maltreatment occurring, in addition to well-established methodological problems (for summary see Ammerman, 1998). Distinguishing statistical association from causal influence is crucial (see chapter 5). Whereas longitudinal studies have helped considerably, there remains the difficulty that if a particular factor was not examined, or if the research design did not necessarily permit its impact to be elucidated (e.g., genetic factors; Moffitt, 2005; Rutter, Moffitt, & Caspi, 2006a), then its influence on maltreatment would not necessarily be evident. Certain factors, or combinations thereof, may be more salient for the occurrence of one type of maltreatment than another. Where such combinations are known they are indicated below, but otherwise risk factors are reviewed here that apply to physical abuse, neglect and psychological abuse. A further difficulty is that the factors themselves depend upon different processes for ascertainment. For example, assessments of quality of interaction and attachment require a different level of observation and recording than, say, family income. In addition, a factor-based approach tends to conflate those operating at a very general level (e.g., neighborhood toxicity or poverty) with intra- and interpersonal factors. Further, transactions between different factors are all important (Cicchetti & Toth, 1995). Some factors may be enduring in nature, while others are present only briefly. Even longitudinal studies have difficulty detecting direction of effect, especially when young adults are being asked to recall whether they were abused in childhood, bearing in mind that abuse in the early years may be impossible to recall accurately, quite apart from the difficulty in articulating experiences of neglect or emotional unavailability retrospectively.

At this point, consideration of risk mediating factors can be viewed through a lens that integrates non-linearity of linkages between risk mediators and maltreatment; acknowledges multiple influences and complexity of processes involved (Sroufe, 2005), while accepting that no one comprehensive model of development is available (Rutter, Kim-Cohen, & Maughan, 2006b). However, mediating processes are capable of being identified (Rutter, Kim-Cohen, & Maughan, 2006b; see chapter 25).

Individual Factors

Both child and parent factors are associated with risk and resilience for child maltreatment. Child factors include children under 3 years (Emery & Laumann-Billings, 2002), those with physical or mental health and behavioral difficulties and difficult temperaments (Belsky & Vondra, 1989; Brown, Cohen, Johnson *et al.*, 1998). Higher intelligence, easier temperament and sociability, social competence and having peer relationships all appear to reduce the risk of a child being maltreated (Stevenson, 1999; but see also Jaffee, Caspi, Moffitt *et al.*, 2004a).

Parents with maladaptive personality characteristics such as poor impulse control, negative affectivity, heightened reactivity to stress and those with substance abuse problems are at greater risk of maltreating their children (Dixon, Browne, & Hamilton-Giachritsis, 2005a; National Research Council, 1993). Parental personality difficulties emerge as a significant risk factor for the occurrence of maltreatment in several longitudinal studies (e.g., Brown, Cohen, Johnson *et al.*, 1998; Mullen, Martin, Anderson *et al.*, 1996). Emery and Laumann-Billings (2002) summarized evidence that suggests child abusers differ from non-abusers in how they perceive their children, ascribing greater negativity to their acts than do non-abusing parents; bearing unrealistic expectations concerning their development and generally finding their child's behavior more stressful. Parental age under 19 years is also associated with a raised risk of maltreatment (Brown, Cohen, Johnson *et al.*, 1998; Egeland, Bosquet, & Chung, 2002).

Parents who themselves suffered maltreatment during childhood are less likely to show sensitivity in caregiving towards their own children, and are more likely to maltreat, or become associated with partners who maltreat their children (Belsky & Vondra, 1989; Egeland, Bosquet, & Chung, 2002; Kaufman & Zigler, 1989). However, it is important to stress that such continuity of parenting difficulty occurs in a minority, around one-third (Emery & Laumann-Billings, 2002). It is also likely that genetic and environmental effects contribute to the continuity observed (Emery & Laumann-Billings, 2002). Such genetic effects may be individual but may also occur through assortative mating (Krueger, Moffitt, Caspi *et al.*, 1998).

Dixon, Browne, & Hamilton-Giachritsis (2005a) examined intergenerational continuity by comparing 135 families where one parent had a childhood history of maltreatment with the remaining 4216 who did not. The authors then explored the mediational properties of risk factors for maltreatment prospectively after birth. By 13 months, 6.7% of the prior childhood maltreatment parents had maltreated their own children, compared with 0.4% of comparison families. Three risk factors stood out in the mediational analysis: parents under 21 years of age, a history of mental illness and having a violent adult partner. However, while these three factors explained 53% of the total effect, explanation was improved to 62% once parenting style (a measure of parental attributions and behavior) was also taken into account (Dixon, Hamilton-Giachritis, & Browne, 2005b).

Family Factors

Poverty and low income are associated with child maltreatment, probably as risk indicators and distal markers for the factors listed below. Family-based factors associated with maltreatment include low parental involvement with the child, early separation, low parental warmth, unwanted pregnancy and maternal dissatisfaction with her child (Brown, Cohen, Johnson *et al.*, 1998; Egeland, Bosquet, & Chung, 2002). Abusive parents are also more likely to use severe physical punishments, employ them for everyday social transgressions and to exercise power and control more frequently than non-abusive parents (Brown *et al.*, 1998).

A further set of factors involve conflict and violence between the adult partners, together with parent–child hostility and a greater use of physical punishment, power and control (Brown, Cohen, Johnson *et al.*, 1998; Dixon, Browne, & Hamilton-Giachritsis, 2005a). Co-parenting difficulties may accompany these features (McHale & Rasmussen, 1998). Linked with these factors are a group of parent–child relationship factors, including poor quality interaction, minimal speech, play and responsiveness when combined with unrealistic developmental expectations, negative perceptions, and low sensitivity and acceptance (Dixon, Browne, & Hamilton-Giachritsis, 2005a). These features are likely to be associated with disorganized and avoidant patterns of attachment (Sroufe, 2005). Such families are also likely to be socially isolated (Egeland, Bosquet, & Chung, 2002). By contrast, families with supportive relationships, with an extended family and friends, and containing positive relationships between siblings may be protective (Stevenson, 1999). Equally, where young adults report recalling positive interparental relationships with expressions of warmth, maltreatment was significantly less likely to occur (Mullen, Martin, Anderson *et al.*, 1996). Parental warmth and support and acceptance of a child are also protective of future abuse (Dixon, Hamilton-Giachritsis, & Browne, 2005b; Stevenson, 1999). Families in which there was strong religious affiliation were less likely to maltreat their children (Brown, Cohen, Johnson *et al.*, 1998; Mullen, Martin, Anderson *et al.*, 1996). Thus, there is a group of factors, which is associated with family violence, parental lack of involvement and warmth, combined with social isolation and high parenting stress, which is linked to negative parent–child perceptions, attributions and relationships, that sets the context within which maltreatment occurs.

Community and Social Influences

Community factors also raise the risk of maltreatment occurring. "Socially toxic neighborhoods" (Garbarino, 1997) that lack social support networks and opportunities (Brown, Cohen, Johnson *et al.*, 1998; Coulton, Korbin, Su *et al.*, 1995) are associated with higher levels of maltreatment. Such neighborhoods contain greater social disorganization, lack of community identity, and higher rates of violent crime and substance abuse. By contrast, socially supportive neighborhoods with better education, health care, neighborhood friendship and support, watchfulness for harm to others and environmental safety, benefit from improved cohesive community identity and have lower rates of maltreatment, notwithstanding comparable poverty levels (Coulton, Korbin, Su *et al.*, 1995; Garbarino, 1997).

Broader social influences also appear to affect rates of violence towards children. The WHO (2002) points to factors that create an acceptable climate for violence and also reduce inhibitions against violence. Although intuitively feasible, finding evidence to support these contentions is more elusive. However, high rates of physical abuse can be linked to areas of the world where there are high levels of conflict and war (WHO, 2002). It is also of interest that maltreatment death rates in industrialized countries are linked with homicide rates (Jenny & Isaac, 2006). These findings provide some support for the proposition that societal influences create a context within which family violence is more common.

Outcomes and Effects

The sequelae of child maltreatment have been reviewed by Cicchetti and Toth (1995), Emery and Laumann-Billings (2002) and Stevenson (1999). These authors draw attention to methodological difficulties, yet conclude that child maltreatment is linked with a range of long-term negative psychological outcomes, which persist when other, frequently co-occurring adversities, are controlled for. A variety of symptoms are reported, and no effects specific to maltreatment, but a possible link of symptoms to types of abuse. Physical abuse and neglect have been noted to be as harmful as sexual abuse. They also note that a substantial minority of children remain resilient in the face of adversity (see chapter 25; Rutter, 2006b). Resilience is associated with dispositional aspects of the child's behavior, including sociability, intelligence and social and/or academic competencies, family factors such as supportive emotional ties, and support from significant others outside the family (Stevenson, 1999). External potential sources of resilience include school experiences, quality alternative care and therapeutic assistance (Egeland, 1997).

For brevity, and following Cicchetti and Toth (1995), outcomes have been organized in Table 28.1 according to themes of major developmental importance: affective and self development, socialization (including attachment), cognitive and physical development. Outcomes frequently involve more than one area of developmental salience.

Child maltreatment behaves like many other adversities that children experience: many different outcomes stem from the same adversity; and many risk factors can result in similar outcomes (Cicchetti & Blender, 2004). Further, maltreatment does not operate as an isolated factor, but normally occurs in concert with other adversities. These other adversities may potentiate, or lower, the risk of poor psychological outcome and, possibly, physical health outcomes too. For instance, the context within which maltreatment occurs, particularly poverty, family stress, poor family functioning, chaotic and disorganized home environments, plus the impact of subsequent life changes upon the child who has already suffered maltreatment, all affect subsequent outcome (Egeland, 1997; Fergusson & Horwood, 2001; Lansford, Dodge, Pettit *et al.*, 2002). Egeland (1997), reporting on the Minnesota longitudinal study, noted that early neglect, including parental emotional unavailability, with its chronic and unremitting nature, had a particularly severe impact on social adjustment and future self-harm behaviors in adolescence.

A cumulative conceptualization of risk fits the data best, in terms of accounting for the mediating effects of factors in addition to maltreatment that pre-exist, accompany and operate subsequently to abuse and neglect experiences, and their combined effect upon outcome.

However, maltreatment is not like any other risk factor. It represents the antithesis of an expectable environment of caretaking (Cicchetti, 1989): a fundamental insult to the developing child's need for care and nurturance. Hence, it is not surprising that consequences are observable throughout all domains of development, and remain significant even when other adversities are accounted for, in the longitudinal studies.

Severe maltreatment (degree of abuse, duration, frequency) and the occurrence of multiple types are associated with more psychological ill effects and social adjustment difficulties. Abuse starting at a young age is also associated with more severe psychological sequelae, in keeping with developmental theory.

In addition, evidence exists for a dose–response relationship for certain outcomes, such as alcohol and drug misuse, and some physical health outcomes (Felitti, Anda, Nordenberg *et al.*, 1998), and mental health outcomes such as suicidality, depression and antisocial behavior (Brown, Cohen, Johnson *et al.*, 1998; Dube, Anda, Felitti *et al.*, 2001; Edwards, Holden, Felitti *et al.*, 2003; Evans, Hawton, & Rodham, 2005; Jaffee, Caspi, Moffitt *et al.*, 2004b). Furthermore, in the multisite Adverse Childhood Events studies, the more adverse events, the greater the number of comorbid physical and psychological health problems in adult life (Anda, Felitti, Bremner *et al.*, 2006).

The effect of physical maltreatment is moderated by genetic risk. Caspi, McClay, Moffitt *et al.* (2002) provided evidence that a functional polymorphism in the *MAOA* gene moderated the impact of early childhood maltreatment on the development of antisocial behavior in adult males, utilizing the Dunedin birth cohort. Those who were maltreated as children but who had high levels of *MAOA* expression were less likely to develop antisocial problems, compared with those with low levels.

A study of over 1000 British 5-year-old twin pairs demonstrated that physical maltreatment was only weakly associated with the probability of a conduct disorder diagnosis among those children at low genetic risk for conduct disorder, but significantly increased among those at high genetic risk. Genetic risk was assessed as a function of zygosity and the cotwin's conduct disorder status (Jaffee, Caspi, Moffitt *et al.*, 2005). Thus, there is genetic sensitivity, both in terms of risk and protection for antisocial behavior outcomes related to physical abuse.

Jaffee, Caspi, Moffitt *et al.* (2004b), using the same twin sample, examined whether physical maltreatment is an environmental risk factor that is causally related to future antisocial behavior. They demonstrated that physical maltreatment predicted antisocial outcome; bore a dose–response relationship to antisocial outcome; new antisocial behavior arose subsequent to abuse; the children's victimization experiences were not influenced by genetic factors; effects of maltreatment remained significant after controlling for the parents' history of antisocial behavior; and that the effect of physical maltreatment was significant even after controlling for any genetic transmission of antisocial behavior risk. This study underlines the causal nature of the link between physical maltreatment and

Table 28.1 Consequences of child maltreatment.

	Child	Adolescent	Adult
Physical	Death Direct injury Disability Brain; HPA axis Corpus callosum [PA, NEG] [boys] Pituitary volume increase Endocrine: Glucocorticoid receptor sensitivity Early menarche [CSA] Growth reduction Underimmunization	Risk-taking behaviors Early first sex partner Multiple partners Pregnancy before age 19 Drug and/or alcohol use	Ischemic heart disease [CSA] Cancer COPD [PA] IBS Arthritis Fibromyalgia Peptic ulcer Diabetes Autoimmune disorders Chronic pelvic pain [CSA, IPV] Dyspareunia [CSA] Thyroid disorder [CSA, women] Stroke
Affective	Emotional disorders Depression [PA] Aggression [NEG] Decreased emotional regulation [PA] Anger, fear PTSD Paucity of positive affect [NEG] Decreased empathy [NEG] Hypervigilance Hyperactivity Lack of self-control	Depression Panic disorder [CSA] PTSD [CSA]	Depression Anxiety disorders
Relationships (including attachment)	Insecure attachment Disorganized attachment Attachment disorders	Maladaptive internal working models Violence in romantic relationships Victimization in romantic relationships	Relationship disruption and dissatisfaction Insecure attachments with children Intimate partner violence
Socialization (including peer relationship)	Withdrawal [NEG] Poor social interactions [NEG, PA] Aggression [NEG] Social information processing deficit	Social withdrawal	
Personal/self-system	Delayed theory of mind Dissociation Shame [CSA] Reduced self-esteem Reduced symbolic play Impaired self-recognition Impoverished internal state language	Reduced self-esteem Impaired perceived competence Continuing shame [CSA] Recklessness and risk-taking behaviors Self-harm External locus of control	Pregnancy before age 19 Personality disorder Substance misuse Deliberate self-harm
Cognitive	Language delay Educational difficulties Cognitive delay [PA, NEG]	Educational dropout Educational underachievement	Illiteracy Reduced employment opportunity
Behavior/ psychopathology	Aggression Conduct disorder ADHD Oppositional disorder	Antisocial behavior Conduct disorder Heavy substance misuse School exclusion Aggression Bullying Depression	Substance abuse Personality disorder Eating disorder [CSA] Somatization Major affective disorder Sleep disorders PTSD

ADHD, attention deficit/hyperactivity disorder; COPD, chronic obstructive pulmonary disease; CSA, child sexual abuse; HPA, hypothalamic–pituitary–adrenal; IBS, irritable bowel syndrome; IPV, intimate partner violence; NEG, neglect; PA, physical abuse; PTSD, post-traumatic stress disorder.

antisocial behavior outcome, itself a crucial component of intergenerational transmission of violence.

Altogether, these findings indicate a causal link between child maltreatment and a range of psychosocial and physical effects in childhood and adult life. Normally, maltreatment is embedded within, and rendered more severe by, accompanying family adversity and violence. It is clear that genetic factors have the capacity to mediate the sensitivity of individual children to maltreatment, at least in terms of antisocial outcomes, and possibly affective ones too (Cicchetti & Blender, 2004).

There has been considerable debate about whether different types of maltreatment can be linked with particular outcomes. Physical abuse has been linked with aggressive and resistant behavior, and conduct disorder and depression; whereas neglect has been considered more closely linked with lower intellectual functioning, language delay, attachment problems, social withdrawal and internalizing problems (Hildyard & Wolfe, 2002; Wolfe, 1994). However, physical abuse has also been linked with language delay and poor social competence. Sexual abuse is linked with disruptive behavior difficulties and post-traumatic stress disorder.

There are a number of problems with this approach. Maltreatment is normally coded, at least in social services organizations, by predominant type. However, repeated studies have indicated that pure types of maltreatment rarely exist in isolation (Manly, 2005). Two or more subtypes of maltreatment normally occur within the same report. Furthermore, over time, the relative contribution of different subtypes changes (Sternberg, Lamb, Guterman *et al.*, 2006). Also, within each subtype there is a wide range of caregiver omissions or commissions. Thus, the category neglect may incorporate lack of supervision and/or physical neglect. From the perspective of outcome, the relative influence of severity, frequency, duration, chronicity and co-occurrence probably differs dependent upon predominant subtype at any one time. For example, cases involving chronic low-level child physical neglect have been demonstrated to have a severe impact on later psychological adjustment (Manly, Cicchetti, & Barnett, 1994; Manly, Kim, Rogosch *et al.*, 2001). However, a single episode of physical abuse can result in death.

The LONGSCAN multisite project in the USA has the benefit of detailed coding of a large number of child protection service reports, which have now been followed-up from infancy to age 8, with psychological and social adjustment measures of outcome. The analyses conducted so far have elucidated many of the issues connected with the type of abuse and relationship to outcome. The main weakness of the studies has been that they are based on reports to child protection services, and outcome measures do not include teacher or third-party assessments. Nonetheless, a number of useful insights emerged. In the first place, social work department categorization related poorly to that of researchers. For example, 10% of neglect cases were thought by the researchers to have physical or sexual abuse as predominant categories (Runyan, Cox, Dubowitz *et al.*, 2005).

Interestingly, neglect alone was not found to have the severe outcome expected. This was probably because effects were masked by a frequency measure, combined with absence of teacher reports (Dubowitz, Pitts, Litrownik *et al.*, 2005). However, when neglect was associated with physical, sexual or emotional abuse, effects were more striking. Interestingly, lack of supervision was not associated with poor outcome, whereas physical neglect and failure to provide were associated with poor behavioral outcomes and impoverished socialization.

The emotional abuse analyses suffered from the fact that only four cases of "pure" emotional abuse were found amongst 250 cases. However, in 246 where emotional abuse was conjoined with neglect, physical or sexual abuse, there were significant effects on psychological and social adjustment (Schneider, Ross, Graham *et al.*, 2005). Overall, the most severe psychological outcomes were, unsurprisingly, associated with severe abuse, of whatever type, multiple types co-occurring, early onset and of chronic nature. The authors confirmed that abuse that crossed developmental stages had more severe effects. Type of abuse per se was not the determining factor.

Overall, the type of maltreatment is less important for poor psychosocial outcomes than variations within type: early age of onset, chronicity, frequency, multiple subtypes and severity.

Assessment

Health care professionals have several different functions, depending upon the nature of their working relationship with the maltreated child and family (Jones, 1996b). Professionals must clarify whether they are undertaking a forensic assessment, or clinical, or a combination. Assessment is complex because of the number of professionals and systems involved, yet it is the cornerstone for effective case planning and intervention. It needs to be ongoing, not merely initial because of the effect of established changes in the interplay of factors over time on the developing child, with the potential to raise or lower the likelihood of better outcome. In this overview of assessment some background issues are considered first, before considering what comprises assessment.

Child Mental Health Practitioners

Child mental health practitioners can operate at different systemic levels in relation to child maltreatment (Jones, 1996b). They can have an important role in overall planning and integration of services locally or nationally, ensuring that a developmental perspective and mental health contribution are made in the most expedient way. They can contribute to the imperative for services to remain culturally sensitive, and responsive to impairment and disability. Child mental health practitioners can also bring a scientific perspective to planning services and research initiatives, and apply messages from research to planning and practice.

Child mental health practitioners have a role in teaching and training at all systemic levels, and direct practice with respect to investigation, assessment, treatment and liaison with other health services. Their training should also allow a contribution at different systemic levels with regard to the personal impact of maltreatment work upon all practitioners; a role requiring both personal self-awareness and awareness of the ethos and working practices of other professionals from different disciplines.

Recognition

Child mental health practitioners' major contribution is in being sufficiently aware of the possibility of maltreatment to ask the necessary questions. When one clinic's practice changed to routinely asking questions about the possibility of child sexual abuse, the proportion of children who reported this went up from 7% before its introduction to 31% following training (Lanktree, Briere, & Zaidi, 1991). How such questions are put to children and young people is critical in order to avoid the possibility of leading questions (see chapter 7). Some mental health practitioners may develop a specific role in relation to interviewing children suspected of being harmed, perhaps helping other professionals communicate with mentally disordered or disabled children (Jones, 2003).

Child mental health practitioners also identify maltreatment directly when working with children. They deal regularly with cases involving apparent deficits in psychological aspects of parenting, as well as psychologically unavailable parenting and sometimes frank neglect. Deciding whether to involve child protection services can be complex where there are no clear cut-off points to guide practitioners. Assessment of severity, persistence, balance of maltreatment with positive parenting, combined with a thorough assessment of the child's mental health and developmental status and a family assessment enables conclusions to be drawn in most cases. Discussion with an informed colleague may be helpful if in doubt. Cases involving hostility, rejection and unavailability will need to be assessed for the possibility of coexisting physical or sexual abuse, or physical neglect. Subtler deficits in the psychological aspects of parenting will not need a child protection response, but it may prove helpful to consider whether psychological or other forms of maltreatment are present at review, bearing in mind that physical and sexual abuse may well not be apparent or revealed at first assessment.

Neglect has a major association with poverty. Clinically, it may be hard to distinguish neglect cases within very impoverished neighborhoods. Under-recognition can result because serious neglect becomes explained away by practitioners, overwhelmed by neighborhood deprivation in their local areas. However, here especially, decision-making can be helped by maintaining a central focus from the child's developmental needs, mental health and physical and cognitive status, combined with using standardized measures, to encourage objectivity (HM Government, 2006; Strauss & Kantor, 2005). It is important to emphasize that the majority of the poor do not abuse or neglect their children, even if the task of parenting is rendered more stressful and difficult within disadvantaged neighborhoods (Coulton, Korbin, Su *et al.*, 1995).

Some specialized teams will also identify maltreatment in the context of fabricated or induced illness, perhaps through non-epileptic seizure presentations (Jones & Newbold, 2001). More commonly, however, practitioners encounter presentations that are commonly linked with prior maltreatment, such as sexual behavior problems, or deliberate self-harm (Evans, Hawton, & Rodham, 2005), when exploratory questions about maltreatment are necessary (Jones, 2003).

Decision-making

If dangerous cases are not identified, serious consequences, or even death, may ensue (Department of Health, 1995, 2003). Equally, overzealous evaluations of the potential for harm can lead to false positives and severe disruption to children and families (Butler-Sloss, 1988; Jones, 2003). Maltreatment is an emotive area for public and professional alike (Cicchetti & Toth, 1995; Rushton & Nathan, 1996), yet it is known that professionals' affective responses have an impact on the decisions they make. Similarly, emotional containment is a key factor for accurate interviewing with vulnerable children (for review see Jones, 2003). These issues may be further compounded by a lack of mutual understanding or respect between different professionals at the multidisciplinary level of decision-making (Jones, Hindley, & Ramchandani, 2006).

Galanter and Patel (2005) reviewed the sources of error and bias affecting experts and novices alike. They noted that experienced practitioners generally utilize more shortcuts and come to conclusions earlier. In the maltreatment field it is critical that practitioners suspend these tendencies and keep alternative explanations in mind and continually attend to potential sources of error in decision-making (Galanter & Patel, 2005; Jones, 2003).

Structured risk assessment schemas have been introduced in order to try to overcome variations in decision-making. There has been no proven benefit from their introduction in terms of the quality of decisions made, despite practitioners generally welcoming them (for review see Knoke & Trocmé, 2005). It is probable that a greater emphasis on how assessment data are utilized and applied will be more fruitful. Additionally, the content of assessments may be lacking in direct assessment of children, involvement of men and reviews of past history. A greater emphasis on decision-making process, rather than outcome, may be more fruitful in the long term, in order to expose the root causes and sequences of decision-making (Jones, Hindley, & Ramchandani, 2006).

Legal Work

Working with maltreated children and their families often leads to subsequent family court work, where practitioners make highly valued contributions to case plans. Practitioners' major responsibility is to maintain neutrality when different systems come together in the court arena, rather than adopting the position of advocate (David, 2004). The discipline of distinguishing history and observation from interpretation and opinion, as well as making transparent how decisions and proposals are reasoned, are all emphasized in court work (see chapter 8).

Recent concerns about expert opinions in legal settings underline the importance of court experts obtaining feedback and working within a context of continuing professional development. Written and oral legal opinions should be proffered within the same ethos of expectation of peer review and constructive criticism as presentation of work for publication or conference proceedings. Novel perspectives or opinions should be subject to peer review before being floated within a legal context, in order to avoid distorting processes of justice (Wall, 2000).

Interdisciplinary Working

Maltreatment is multifaceted in nature and therefore several professional systems have a stake in its detection, prevention and response (HM Government, 2006). A central tenet of child protection has been that a multiagency perspective is superior to a single-agency one, because otherwise the full situation of child and family will not be appreciated (DHSS, 1974; HM Government, 2006). However, there are significant challenges in bringing disparate professionals together, with different frames of reference, professional responsibilities, ethos and style as well as status levels within society (Hudson, 2000). The sensitive area of information sharing, particularly if one agency has confidential information, has brought these difficulties into relief. Nevertheless, principles to guide information sharing have been published in England and Wales in order to assist practitioners (HM Government, 2006). In England and Wales, both government guidance and advice from professional organizations emphasize the requirement to reveal confidentially obtained information if a child is suffering or at risk of suffering significant harm (GMC, 2004). Provided the professional acts reasonably, he or she cannot be found wanting in law if those suspicions in fact turn out to be unfounded.

It is important that child mental health practitioners contribute in written or oral form to interdisciplinary planning forums, because this is the best way to appreciate the full range of concerns raised by others as well as to influence decision-making and case planning. The Assessment Framework introduced in England and Wales (2000) provides a useful means of overcoming the varied perspectives of different professionals. It is grounded in an ecological perspective on child maltreatment, and incorporates principles of developmental psychopathology, rendering it sympathetic to mental health practitioners. Nonetheless, mental health professionals need a basic understanding of the law and procedure relating to child protection in order to operate within their particular country (e.g., for England, HM Government, 2006).

Assessment by Child Mental Health Professionals

Child maltreatment is not a psychiatric entity, and therefore assessments of children where this has occurred will need to consider children's safety from future harm, the child's future living arrangements, physical health and education, including special educational needs, as well as mental health status. The mental health component is therefore part of the whole assessment (DOH, DOEE & HO, 2000). The approach to assessment will depend on the purpose or aims; is the assessment to evaluate the child and family for the possibility of mental health disorder and/or psychiatric treatment; or is the assessment being requested for court purposes? In either situation it is assumed that all will receive a comprehensive mental health assessment; however, certain aspects will receive greater emphasis when maltreatment is present. Normally, child mental health practitioners are not involved in determining whether a child has been maltreated (although see exceptions on p. 430).

Particular aspects of child and family functioning that will need assessment where child maltreatment has occurred include the following. First, practitioners will need to have information about all types of maltreatment that the child may have experienced and any other form of family violence he or she has witnessed or experienced. This information may be obtained directly from the family, or involve review of case files (health and social work files often have rich information on parenting capacity and family functioning, recorded over time, which is particularly relevant when assessing neglect or emotional abuse).

Confidentiality constraints will need to be made explicit with both children and parents. The child's perspective on maltreatment is an important subject of evaluation, along with how he or she has coped with or responded to the experience. Assessment of child–parent interaction is a key ingredient, including both parental caregiving and child attachment elements (Cassidy & Shaver, 1999). Collateral sources of information and different perspectives can be of particular value in maltreatment cases. History from the child's parents will usually involve more forensic aspects than is usual for child mental health evaluations. Family relationships are also important to assess, including the quality of interparental relationships and co-parenting capacity.

Assessments undertaken for family courts will generally follow the same principles but with a greater emphasis on and awareness of forensic requirements (Budd, 2005; Jones, 2006). Budd (2005) has emphasized that family court assessments should be centered firmly on parenting capacity (rather than parental mental health per se); have a functional emphasis (assessing beliefs, knowledge, actions and capacity, in relation to an individual child), which should emphasize strengths and weaknesses, and be contextualized and consider the likelihood of remediation. Assessments should rest on an assessment of the minimal parenting standard, not the optimal. Jones (2006) emphasized the need to link data-gathering with a structured approach to decision-making in order to place relative weight on the many factors, both positive and negative, that will be derived from a comprehensive assessment (see p. 433; Jones, Hindley, & Ramchandani, 2006).

Treatment and Intervention

Psychological treatments have been developed for specific types of maltreatment, despite "pure" forms of maltreatment being the rarity rather than the norm (Manly, 2005). Hence, it is important to identify treatment models that can target specific symptom clusters, accommodate different levels of severity and chronicity of maltreatment experience, and which are focused at the appropriate developmental level, rather than design treatments for specific maltreatment types (Cohen, Mannarino, Murray *et al.*, 2006).

Intervention will have a different focus where a child has been removed, contrasted with treatment aimed at family preservation or reunification. Cicchetti and Toth (1995) emphasized that interventions should address the fundamental challenges to development that maltreatment brings; in particular, affect regulation, attachment, the evolving self-system and peer relationships. The overall aim of intervention is to avert subsequent problems with self-esteem, interpersonal relationships and social adjustment which occur when maltreatment derails developmental stage-salient progress (Cicchetti & Toth, 1995). In this section, general principles and approaches to intervention are outlined first, before considering effective interventions.

First, interventions have to address the question of safety. This requires interdisciplinary coordination and, in many cases, care planning to ensure that the child or young person is not harmed again (Azar & Wolfe, 1989; Jones, 1996b; Stevenson, 1999). There is consensus that intervention should be organized around the welfare of the child as the primary guiding principle (rather than family preservation, primarily); should emphasize the child's physical and emotional safety; should address the child's specific range of problems from a developmental perspective; and address parenting and caretaking deficits, simultaneously (Azar & Wolfe, 1989; Jones, 1996b, 1997; National Research Council, 1993; Saunders, Berliner, & Hanson, 2004; Stevenson, 1999). To these may be added the importance of acknowledging the children's experience of abuse and the need to characterize it as wrong, unlawful or harmful (Jones, 1997; Jones & Ramchandani, 1999; Saunders, Berliner, & Hanson, 2004); intervention should be both abuse-informed as well as addressing general mental health issues; supportive, non-abusing carers should be included in the treatment; and treatments with the highest level of empirical support should be first-choice interventions. Parental acknowledgement of maltreatment should comprise part of the intervention (Jones, 1997; Saunders, Berliner, & Hanson, 2004); treatment goals should include prevention of likely problems associated with maltreatment, as well as relief of the current ones (Saunders, Berliner, & Hanson, 2004).

Saunders, Berliner, & Hanson (2004) review of available interventions for physical and sexual abuse assessed 24 treatment protocols, some for children alone and others that were family or parent–child focused, as well as two offenders' treatments, rating the degree of empirical support for each. Of the 24, 16 had some degree of empirical support for efficacy with child abuse cases. These were principally behavioral and cognitive–behavioral interventions. They were characterized by being goal directed (addressing specific measurable problems within children and their families); were structured in their approach (often with sequential staging of treatment components toward therapeutic goals); and emphasized skill building to manage emotional distress and behavioral disturbance in children and parents. They note that while other treatments were commonly in use and had strong theoretical bases they lacked empirical support for claimed effects; trauma-focused play therapy being one such example. They also noted that one treatment protocol, corrective attachment therapy, was associated with an unacceptably high level of risk of harm, even being associated with deaths of children, such that the authors discouraged its use (see also Chaffin, Saunders, Nichols *et al.*, 2006).

Trauma-focused cognitive–behavioral therapies have been shown to be significantly superior to family and general psychotherapeutic treatments with both physical and sexual abuse (Cohen, Mannarino, Murray *et al.*, 2006; Jones & Ramchandani, 1999; Kolko, 2002; Saunders, Berliner, & Hanson, 2004). In these programs combinations of psychoeducation, exposure therapy, cognitive procedures and restructuring, as well as behavior management techniques are all employed. Techniques involve practicing skills and active therapist feedback. Children are assisted with emotion recognition and regulation, specific anxiety management skills, attention to maladaptive cognitions (e.g., that the child was not responsible for his or her victimization) and problem-solving skills. Concurrently, parents are taught to use effective behavior management skills with their children, emphasizing positive reward and curbing harsh, sometimes violent consequences or isolation (Cohen, Mannarino, Murray *et al.*, 2006; Saunders, Berliner, & Hanson, 2004). Sometimes, additional specific treatments for parents include anger management, mental health or substance use difficulties and interparental violence.

Child–parent psychotherapy has shown significant benefit for children and their mothers, compared with individual psychotherapy among multiply maltreated preschoolers. It comprises a blend of psychodynamic and cognitive–behavioral components, delivered intensively with both children and parents over a 1-year period (Lieberman, Ippen, & Van Horn, 2006).

Parent–child interaction therapy (PCIT) has shown promise with physically abusing parents, reducing the frequency of recurrence from 49% among cases assigned to the standard community group treatment to 19% in the PCIT group, in a randomized trial (Chaffin, Silovsky, Funderburk *et al.*, 2004). However, the impact on children's symptoms was not assessed.

There have been fewer studies evaluating the effectiveness of treatment when neglect or emotional abuse is the predominant issue. A systematic review of treatment in neglect revealed tentative support for specific programs of play therapy (group play training and resilient peer treatment) and for a therapeutic day treatment program (Allin, Wathen, & MacMillan, 2005). There was also some support for multisystemic therapy, and a day treatment program focusing on enhancing self-esteem. However, numerous methodological problems beset the studies, reducing confidence in these conclusions. Empirical studies of treatment efficacy for emotional abuse and neglect are not yet available.

Reviewers have emphasized that first-line interventions should comprise those for which there is the best empirical support. In the field of maltreatment, cognitive and behavioral approaches have led the way (Jones & Ramchandani, 1999; Saunders, Berliner, & Hanson, 2004). This is not to imply that other well-respected treatments may not be very helpful for abused children and their families, but at this point firm evidence of such is lacking (Cohen, Mannarino, Murray *et al.*, 2006; Saunders, Berliner, & Hanson, 2004).

The above intervention programs have tended to focus on child and immediate family factors with minimal attention to surrounding ecological influences, despite strong calls for programs to do so (Cicchetti & Toth, 1995; NRC, 1993). Specifically, interventions could actively involve school and the local network of child protection personnel in a systemic fashion (Swenson & Chaffin, 2006). It must be stressed, however, that most maltreated children receive no treatment (Cohen, Mannarino, Murray *et al.*, 2006; Saunders, Berliner, & Hanson, 2004).

When treatment interventions such as those listed above are employed in the context of family preservation, or reunification, practitioners are faced with significant problems in assessing the risk of reabuse and/or poor child outcomes, versus the likelihood of an improved outcome if the child is removed into substitute care. These decisions are further complicated by difficulties facing maltreated children when placed in substitute care. The principal factors associated with reabuse or poor outcomes for children in the wake of significant harm have been reviewed, to evaluate the rate of recurrence and other outcomes (Jones, 1991, 1998). He reported that once child maltreatment had occurred, rates of recurrence were 20–30%; however, it was not necessarily the same type of abuse that recurred. Recurrence rates for neglect were higher than for other forms of maltreatment, were more difficult to work with and had poorer outcomes, compared with other forms of maltreatment. Poor outcome in terms of behavior and educational adjustment befell up to half of the children on follow-up, but better outcome was associated with provision of services, especially where those contained an outreach component and where partnerships with parents could be forged. Follow-up studies indicated little value for prolonged assistance being offered to resistant families. Focused treatments were generally better than nonspecific support.

Factors associated with a better outcome for the child versus possibility of future harm, derived from these reviews, were tabulated utilizing an eco-developmental framework. A subsequent systematic review of studies relating to outcome following identification of maltreatment (Hindley, Ramchandani, & Jones, 2006) permitted factors with the strongest association with recurrence to be italicized in Table 28.2. Remaining factors have support from other studies but less strongly than the italicized ones (Jones, Hindley, & Ramchandani, 2006).

As can be seen, the factors with the strongest association with recurrence of maltreatment were a prior history of maltreatment before the indexed case, neglect cases, cases involving family violence and interparental conflict, and parental mental health problems. There was a strong but less powerful link with parental substance or alcohol abuse, continuing high family stress, lack of social support and family isolation, families with younger children and where parents had histories of personal abuse during their own childhood. Jones, Hindley, & Ramchandani (2006) suggested a staged approach to decision-making based upon the following:

1 Data gathering
2 Weighing relative significance of multiple factors
3 Formulating and/or diagnostic stage
4 Identifying circumstances that might alter the child's future welfare status
5 Identifying prospects for change
6 Establishing criteria through which to gauge effectiveness of intervention and desired outcomes
7 Outlining a timetable that is developmentally appropriate
8 Formulating a plan for the child, incorporating needs and protection, as well as the roles and responsibilities of different professionals and agencies, and a timescale for review.

They also emphasized that not all families can achieve change (Jones, Hindley, & Ramchandani, 2006), and that some families may be "untreatable." Bringing efforts at family preservation to a halt may be stressful for professionals, but essential for children's welfare (Saunders, Berliner, & Hanson, 2004). This concept is central to concurrent planning (Wigfall, Monck, & Reynolds, 2006), in which the possibility of substitute care is held in the minds of family members and professionals, while in parallel providing specific psychological treatments from the outset of the intervention process. If treatment is unsuccessful in achieving its goals and the child's welfare continues to be compromised, temporary foster care is converted into permanent substitute care. In this way the child's welfare and safety are held paramount above all other considerations.

Prevention

This section addresses primary and secondary prevention of child maltreatment; that is, programs aimed at the whole population (see chapter 60), and ones focused on those deemed at risk (see chapter 61). Primary prevention efforts include public awareness campaigns relating to family violence, encouraging non-violent approaches to discipline and raising awareness about childhood maltreatment; and at the community level, positive parenting programs and school-based programs aimed at reducing violence in adolescence (Wolfe, 2006). In addition, primary heath care by nurses, health visitors and developmental child health services has a role in primary prevention. Primary prevention should also focus on social institutions for children, including training, awareness raising and overcoming myths and barriers to reporting concerns raised by children

Table 28.2 Factors associated with future harm. After Jones *et al.* (2006).

Factors	Future significant harm more likely	Future significant harm less likely
Abuse	Severe physical abuse including burns/scalds *Neglect* Severe growth failure Mixed abuse *Previous maltreatment* Sexual abuse with penetration or over long duration Fabricated/induced illness Sadistic abuse	Less severe forms of abuse If severe, yet compliance and lack of denial, success still possible
Child	Developmental delay with special needs Mental health problems Very young – requiring rapid parental change	Healthy child Attributions (in sexual abuse) Later age of onset One good corrective relationship
Parent	*Personality* – Antisocial – Sadism – Aggressive Lack of compliance Denial of problems Learning difficulties plus *mental illness* Substance abuse *Paranoid psychosis* Abuse in childhood – not recognized as a problem	Non-abusive partner Willingness to engage with services Recognition of problem Responsibility taken Mental disorder, responsive to treatment Adaptation to childhood abuse
Parenting and parent–child interaction	Disordered attachment Lack of empathy for child Poor parenting competency Own needs before child's	Normal attachment Empathy for child Competence in some areas
Family	*Interparental conflict and violence* Family stress Power problems: poor negotiation, autonomy and affect expression	Absence of domestic violence Non-abusive partner Capacity for change Supportive extended family
Professional	Lack of resources Ineptitude	Therapeutic relationship with child Outreach to family Partnership with parents
Social setting	Social isolation Lack of social support Violent, unsupportive neighborhood	Social support More local child care facilities Volunteer networks

or staff members. The overall approach is health promotion rather than surveillance (Blair & Hall, 2006).

At the secondary prevention level, the most common approaches are home visiting and parent education for identified high-risk parents (Leventhal, 2005). A different approach aims to strengthen local communities through networks of voluntary and professional organizations, based on research linking maltreatment to neighborhood impoverishment (Daro & Cohn Donnelly, 2002; Korbin, 2002; Melton & Barry, 1994).

Home visiting programs for at-risk families have been well researched and have shown small to moderate reductions in maltreatment rates among the group receiving home intervention from trained nurses antenatally and postnatally, especially with young first-time mothers who have other risk factors for maltreatment (Fergusson, Grant, Horwood *et al.*, 2006; MacMillan, MacMillan, Offord *et al.*, 1994; Olds, Eckenrode, Henderson *et al.*, 1997). Trained nurses or social workers appear more successful than paraprofessionals (Duggan, Fuddy, Burrell *et al.*, 2004a,b; Windham, Rosenberg, Fuddy *et al.*, 2004). However, not all programs have demonstrated benefit (see Chaffin, 2004, 2005; and special issue edited by Leventhal, 2005). Some programs have revealed an increase in maltreatment among intervention compared with comparison groups (Barlow, Davis, McIntosh *et al.*, 2007; Rutter, 2006a). While this may represent a surveillance effect, and increased recognition of maltreatment seen as a positive outcome, the precise reasons for this paradoxical finding remain unanswered. Currently, prevention services incorporate many disparate elements, and it is necessary to tease apart those aspects that may benefit children from those that may increase the chances of maltreatment among some parents (Rutter, 2006a,b).

Parent education programs are similarly diverse. They reveal modest and promising improvements from educational and support efforts, taken overall (Wolfe, 1994). Daro and Cohn Donnelly (2002) identified key aspects of successful programs. They should start prior to, or close to, the birth of the first child; be tied to the child's specific developmental level; provide opportunities for parents to model positive interactions and discipline methods; extend for several months in order to change attitudes and strengthen parenting and personal skills, as opposed to simply imparting knowledge; emphasize social supports available in the community; and be sensitive to cultural differences. Interestingly, programs that also contained individual support for those especially needy and at-risk families, in addition to the group-based parenting program, were most effective (Wolfe, 1994; Barlow & Stewart-Brown, 2005).

It is probable that existing programs need to be more adaptable to individual difference (Leventhal, 2005). For example, a menu of additional services needs to be available to add on to home visitation programs, dependent on the specific needs of the family, e.g. interventions for maternal depression, domestic violence, parental mental illness, substance abuse, or severe learning difficulties, rather than uniformity.

At this point, a universal health promotion approach for all families, plus carefully supervised and monitored home visiting for high-risk parents (young, poor, parental mental health problems) focusing on increasing parenting sensitivity and competence directly, and which can flexibly adapt and draw in other services for particular subgroups, appears the most promising approach. But programs for high-risk parents need to overcome barriers in engaging the hard-to-reach (Barlow, Kirkpatrick, Stewart-Brown *et al.*, 2005; Blair & Hall, 2006). A good example of an integrated approach across an area is provided by North Carolina (Hughes, Earls, Odom *et al.*, 2005). Here, primary, secondary and tertiary (intervention) services at different ecological levels are fully co-ordinated through a state-wide interdepartmental leadership team. The newly integrated children's services in England and Wales should provide a suitable vehicle for similar initiatives. This would be a crucial antidote to uneven provision and development of individual programs, which merely focus on one aspect. The public health approach to tackling maltreatment, at the primary or secondary level of prevention, offers the best hope for a genuine reduction in the prevalence of maltreatment.

Conclusions

Child maltreatment is a major public health problem internationally, with established threat to human health, throughout the lifespan. Although maltreatment is seen as an environmental risk factor, as a phenomenon it illustrates the complex interactions between genes and environment. The key tasks now are to make further progress elucidating effective interventions and management of risk of serious harm to children. Additionally, to understand better why prevention, universally and with high-risk individuals, has not measured up to its initial hope and promise.

References

Allin, H., Wathen, C. N., & MacMillan, H. (2005). Treatment of child neglect: A systematic review. *Canadian Journal of Psychiatry, 50*, 497–504.

Ammerman, R. T. (1998). Methodological issues in child maltreatment research. In J. R. Lutzker (Ed.), *Handbook of child abuse research and treatment* (pp. 117–132). New York, London: Plenum.

Anda, R. F., Felitti, V. J., Bremner, J. D., Walker, J. D., Whitfield, C., Perry, B. D., *et al.* (2006). The enduring effects of abuse and related adverse experiences in childhood. *European Archives of Psychiatry and Clinical Neuroscience, 256*, 174–186.

Andrews, G., Corry, J., Slade, T., Issakidis, C., & Swanston, H. (2004). Child sexual abuse. In M. Ezzati, A. Lopez, A. Rodgers, & C. Murray (Eds.), *Comparative quantification in health risks: Global and regional burden of disease attributable to selected major risk factors* (pp. 1851–1940). Geneva: World Health Organization.

Australian Institute of Health and Welfare (AIHW). (2004). *Child protection Australia, 2002–2003*. Canberra: AIHW (Child Welfare Series No.34).

Azar, S. T., & Wolfe, D. (1998). Child abuse and neglect. In E. Mash, & J Berkley (Eds.), *Treatment of childhood disorders*. New York: Guilford.

Bair-Merritt, M. H., Blackstone, M., & Feudtner, C. (2006). Physical health outcomes of childhood exposure to intimate partner violence: Systematic review. *Pediatrics, 117*, 278–290.

Bardi, M., & Borgogni-Tarli, S. M. (2001). A survey on parent–child conflict resolution: Intrafamily violence in Italy. *Child Abuse and Neglect, 25*, 839–853.

Barlow, J., Davis, H., McIntosh, E., Jarrett, P., Mockford, C., & Stewart-Brown, S. (2007). The role of home visiting in improving parenting and health in families at risk of abuse and neglect: results of a multicentre randomised controlled trial and economic evaluation. *Archives of Disease in Childhood*, 92, 229–233.

Barlow, J., Kirkpatrick, S., Stewart-Brown, S., & Davis, H. (2005). Hard to reach or out of reach? Reasons why women refuse to take part in early interventions. *Children and Society, 19*, 199–210.

Barlow, J., & Stewart-Brown, S. (2005). Child abuse and neglect. *Lancet, 365*, 1750–1752.

Belsky, J., & Vondra, J. (1989). Lessons from child abuse: The determinants of parenting. In D. Cicchetti, & V. Carlson (Eds.), *Child maltreatment: Theory and research on the causes and consequences of child abuse and neglect* (pp. 153–202). Cambridge: Cambridge University Press.

Berger, A. M., Knutson, J. G., Mehm, J. G., & Perkins, K. A. (1988). The self-report of punitive childhood experiences of young adults and adolescents. *Child Abuse and Neglect, 12*, 251–262.

Blair, M., & Hall, D. (2006). From health surveillance to health promotion: The changing focus in preventive children's services. *Archives of Disease in Childhood, 91*, 730–735.

Bogat, G. A., DeJonghe, E., Levendosky, A. A., Davidson, W. S., & von Ewe, A. (2006). Trauma symptoms among infants exposed to intimate partner violence. *Child Abuse and Neglect, 30*, 109–125.

Brockington, I. (1996). *Motherhood and mental health*. Oxford: Oxford University Press.

Brockington, I. (2004). Post-partum psychiatric disorders. *Lancet, 363*, 303–310.

Bronfenbrenner, U. (1977). Towards an experimental ecology of human development. *American Psychologist, 52*, 513–531.

Brown, J., Cohen, P., Johnson, J. G., & Salzinger, S. (1998). A longitudinal analysis of risk factors for child maltreatment: findings of a seventeen year prospective study of officially recorded and self-reported child abuse and neglect. *Child Abuse and Neglect, 22*, 1065–1078.

Budd, K. S. (2005). Assessing parenting capacity in a child welfare context. *Children and Youth Services Review, 27*, 429–444.

Butler-Sloss, E. (1988). *Report of the inquiry into child abuse in Cleveland in 1987*. London: HMSO.

Casanueva, C., Foshee, V. A., & Barth, R. P. (2005). Intimate partner violence as a risk factor for children's use of the emergency room and injuries. *Children and Youth Services Review, 27*, 1223–1242.

Caspi, A., McClay, J., Moffitt, T. E., Mill, J., Martin, J., Craig, I., *et al.* (2002). Role of the genotype in the cycle of violence in maltreated children. *Science, 297*, 851–854.

Cassidy, J. & Shaver, P. (1999). *Handbook of attachment*. London: Guilford Press.

Chaffin, M. (2004). Invited commentary. Is it time to re-think healthy start/healthy families? *Child Abuse and Neglect, 28*, 589–595.

Chaffin, M. (2005). Response to letters. *Child Abuse and Neglect, 29*, 241–249.

Chaffin, M., Saunders, R. H. B. E., Nichols, T., Barnett, D., Zeanah, C., Berliner, L., *et al.* (2006). Report of the APSAC task force on attachment therapy, reactive attachment disorder, and attachment problems. *Child Maltreatment, 11*, 76–89.

Chaffin, M., Silovsky, J., Funderburk, B., Valle, L. A., Brestan, E. V., Balachova, T., *et al.* (2004). Parent–child interaction therapy with physically abusive parents: Efficacy for reducing future abuse reports. *Journal of Consulting and Clinical Psychology*, *72*, 491–499.

Cicchetti, D. (1989). How research on child maltreatment has informed the study of child development: Perspectives from developmental psychopathology. In D. Cicchetti, & V. Carlson (Eds.), *Child maltreatment: Theory and research on the causes and consequences of child abuse and neglect* (pp. 377–431). Cambridge: Cambridge University Press.

Cicchetti, D., & Blender, J. A. (2004). A multiple-levels-of-analysis approach to the study of developmental processes in maltreated children. *Proceedings of the National Academy of Sciences USA, 101*, 17325–17326.

Cicchetti, D., & Toth, S. L. (1995). A developmental psychopathology perspective on child abuse and neglect. *Journal of the American Academy of Child and Adolescent Psychiatry, 34*, 541–565.

Cohen, J. A., Mannarino, A, P., Murray, L. K., & Igelman, R. (2006). Psychosocial interventions for maltreated and violence-exposed children. *Journal of Social Issues*, *62*, 737–766.

Coulton, C. J., Korbin, J. E., Su, M., & Chow, J. (1995). Community level factors and child maltreatment rates. *Child Development*, *66*, 1162–1176.

Daro, D., & Cohn Donnelly, A. (2002). Child abuse prevention: accomplishments and challenges. In J. Myers, L. Berliner, J. Briere, C. T. Hendrix, C. Jenny, & T. A. Reid (Eds.), *The APSAC handbook on child maltreatment* (pp. 431–448). London: Sage.

David, T. (2004). Avoidable pitfalls when writing medical reports for Court proceedings in cases of suspected child abuse. *Archives of Disease in Childhood, 89*, 799–804.

Department for Education and Skills (DFES). (2005). *Referrals, assessments and children and young people on child protection registers, year ending 31 March 2005*. London: The Stationery Office.

Department of Health. (1995). *Child protection: messages from research*. London: HMSO.

Department of Health. (2003). *The Victoria Climbié Inquiry*. London: The Stationery Office.

Department of Health, Department of Education and Employment and the Home Office (DOH, DOEE & HO). (2000). *Framework for the assessment of children in need and their families*. London: The Stationery Office.

Department of Health and Human Services. (2003). *Child maltreatment 2001*. Washington, DC: US Government Printing Office.

Department of Health and Social Security (DHSS). (1974). *Report of the Committee of inquiry into the care and supervision provided in relation to Maria Colwell*. London: HMSO.

Dixon, L., Browne, K., & Hamilton-Giachritsis, C. (2005a). Risk factors of parents abused as children: A mediational analysis of the intergenerational continuity of child maltreatment (Part 1). *Journal of Child Psychology and Psychiatry*, *46*, 47–57.

Dixon, L., Hamilton-Giachritsis, C., & Browne, K. (2005b). Attributions and behaviours of parents abused as children: A mediational analysis of the intergenerational continuity of child maltreatment (Part 2). *Journal of Child Psychology and Child Psychiatry*, *46*, 58–68.

Dubowitz, H., Pitts, S. C., Litrownik, A. J., Cox, C. E., Runyan, D. K., & Black, M. M. (2005). Defining child neglect based on child protective services data. *Child Abuse and Neglect*, *29*, 493–511.

Dube, S. R., Anda, R. F., Felitti, V. J., Chapman, D. P., Williamson, D. F., & Giles, W. H. (2001). Childhood abuse, household dysfunction, and the risk of attempted suicide throughout the lifespan: Findings from the adverse childhood experiences study. *Journal of the American Medical Association*, *286*, 3089–3096.

Duggan, A., Fuddy, L., Burrell, L., Higman, S. M., McFarlane, E., Windham, A. L., *et al.* (2004a). Randomized trial of a state-wide home visiting program to prevent child abuse: Impact in reducing parental risk factors. *Child Abuse and Neglect*, *28*, 623–643.

Duggan, A., McFarlane, E., Fuddy, L., Burrell L., Higman, S. M., Windham, A., *et al.* (2004b). Randomized trial of a state-wide home visiting program: Impact in preventing child abuse and neglect. *Child Abuse and Neglect*, *28*, 597–622.

Edwards, V. J., Holden, G. W., Felitti, V. J., & Anda, R. F. (2003). Relationship between multiple forms of childhood maltreatment and adult mental health in community respondence: Results from the adverse childhood experiences study. *American Journal of Psychiatry*, *160*, 1453–1460.

Egeland, B. (1997). Mediators of the effects of child maltreatment on developmental adaptation in adolescence. In D. Cicchetti, & S. Toth (Eds.), *Rochester symposium on developmental psychopathology. 8. Developmental perspectives on trauma; theory, research and intervention* (pp. 403–434). New York: University of Rochester Press.

Egeland, B., Bosquet, M., & Chung A. L. (2002). Continuities and discontinuities in the inter-generational transmission of child maltreatment: Implications for breaking the cycle of abuse. In K. D. Brown, H. Hanks, P. Stratton, & C. E. Hamilton (Eds.), *Early prediction and prevention of child abuse: A handbook* (pp. 217–232). Chichester: Wiley.

Emery, R. E., & Laumann-Billings, L. (2002). Child abuse. In M. Rutter, & E. Taylor (Eds.), *Child and adolescent psychiatry* (4th edn., pp. 325–339). Oxford: Blackwell.

Erickson, M., & Egeland, B. (1996). Child neglect. In L. Berliner, J. Briere, J. Bulkley, C. Jenny, & T. Reid (Eds.), *The APSAC handbook on child abuse and neglect* (pp. 4–20). London: Sage.

Evans, E., Hawton, K., & Rodham, K. (2005). Suicidal phenomena and abuse in adolescence: A review of epidemiological studies. *Child Abuse and Neglect*, *29*, 45–58.

Felitti, V. J., Anda, R. F., Nordenberg, D., Williamson, D. F., Spitz, A. M., Edwards, V., *et al.* (1998). Relationship of childhood abuse and household dysfunction to many of the leading causes of death in adults. The adverse childhood experiences (ACE) study. *American Journal of Preventive Medicine*, *14*, 245–258.

Fergusson, D. M., & Horwood, L. J. (2001). The Christchurch Health and Development Study: Review of findings on child and adolescent mental health. *Australian and New Zealand Journal of Psychiatry*, *35*, 287–296.

Fergusson, D. M., & Lynskey, M. T. (1997). Physical punishment/maltreatment during childhood, and adjustment in young adulthood. *Child Abuse and Neglect*, *21*, 617–630.

Fergusson, D. M., Boden, J. M., & Horwood, L. J. (2006). Examining the intergenerational transmission of violence in a New Zealand birth cohort. *Child Abuse and Neglect*, *30*, 89–108.

Fergusson, D. M., Grant, H., Horwood, L. J., & Ridder, E. M. (2006). Randomized trial of the early start program of home visitation: Parent and family outcomes. *Pediatrics*, *117*, 781–786.

Galanter, C. A., & Patel, V. L. (2005). Medical decision making: A selective review for child psychiatrists and psychologists. *Journal of Child Psychology and Psychiatry*, *46*, 675–689.

Garbarino, J. (1997). Growing up in a socially toxic environment. In D. Cicchetti, & S. L. Toth (Eds.), *Developmental perspectives on trauma: Theory, research, and intervention* (pp. 141–154). New York: University of Rochester Press.

General Medical Council (GMC). (2004). *Confidentiality: Protecting and providing information*. London: GMC.

Ghate, D., Hazel, N., Creighton, S., & Finch, S. (2003). Parents, children and discipline: A national study of families in Britain. http://www.nspcc.org.uk/Inform/Publications/Downloads/ParentsChildrenAndDisciplineSummary_pdf_gf25464.pdf

Gibbons, J. Conroy, S., & Bell, C. (1995). *Operating the child protection system*. London: HMSO.

Glaser, D. (2002). Emotional abuse and neglect (psychological maltreatment): A conceptual framework. *Child Abuse and Neglect*, *26*, 697–714.

Hildyard, K., & Wolfe, D. (2002). Child neglect: Developmental issues and outcomes. *Child Abuse and Neglect*, *26*, 679–695.

Hindley, N., Ramchandani, P., & Jones, D. P. H. (2006). Risk factors for recurrence of maltreatment: a systematic review. *Archives of Disease in Childhood*, *91*, 744–752.

HM Government. (2006). *Working together to safeguard children: a guide to interagency working to safeguard and promote the welfare of children*. London: The Stationery Office.

Hudson, B. L. (2000). Inter-agency collaboration: A sceptical view. In A. Brechin, H. Browne, & M. Eby (Eds.), *Critical practice in health and social care*. London: Sage.

Hughes, M., Earls, M. F., Odom, C. H., Dubay, K. L., Sayers, A. R., Whiteside, J. T., *et al.* (2005). Preventing child maltreatment in North Carolina: New directions for supporting families and children. *North Carolina Medical Journal*, *66*, 343–355.

Hussey, J. M., Chang, J. J., & Kotch, J. B. (2006). Child maltreatment in the United States: Prevalence, risk factors, and adolescent health consequences. *Pediatrics*, *118*, 933–942.

Jaffee, S. R., Caspi, A., Moffitt, T. E., Polo-Thomas, M., Price, T.S., & Taylor, A. (2004a). The limits of child effects: Evidence for genetically mediated child effects on corporal punishment but not on physical maltreatment. *Developmental Psychology*, *40*, 1047–1058.

Jaffee, S. R., Caspi, A., Moffitt, T. E., & Taylor, A. (2004b). Physical maltreatment victim to antisocial child: Evidence of an environmentally mediated process. *Journal of Abnormal Psychology*, *113*, 44–55.

Jaffee, S. R., Caspi, A., Moffitt, T. E., Dodge, K. A., Rutter, M., Taylor, A., *et al.* (2005). Nature × nurture: Genetic vulnerabilities interact with physical maltreatment to promote conduct problems. *Development and Psychopathology*, *17*, 67–84.

Jenny, C., & Isaac, R. (2006). The relation between child death and child maltreatment. *Archives of Disease in Childhood*, *91*, 265–269.

Jones, D. P. H. (1991). The effectiveness of intervention and the significant harm criteria. In M. Adcock, R. White, & A. Hollows (Eds.), *Significant harm*. Croydon: Significant Publications Ltd.

Jones, D. P. H. (1996a). Commentary: Munchausen syndrome by proxy – is expansion justified? *Child Abuse and Neglect*, *20*, 983–984.

Jones, D. P. H. (1996b). Management of the sexually abused child. *Advances in Psychiatric Treatment*, *2*, 39–45.

Jones, D. P. H. (1997). Treatment of the child and the family where child abuse or neglect has occurred. In R. Helfer, R. Kempe, & R. Krugman (Eds.), *The battered child* (5th edn., pp. 521–542). Chicago: University of Chicago Press.

Jones, D. P. H. (1998). The effectiveness of intervention. In M. Adcock, & R. White (Eds.), *Significant harm: Its management and outcome* (2nd edn., pp. 91–119). Croydon: Significant Publications Ltd.

Jones, D. P. H. (2001). Assessment of parenting capacity. In J. Horwath (Ed.), *The child's world: Assessing children in need* (pp. 255–272). London: Jessica Kingsley.

Jones, D. P. H. (2003). *Communicating with vulnerable children: A guide for practitioners*. London: Gaskell.

Jones, D. P. H. (2006). Assessment of parenting for the family court. *Psychiatry*, *5*, 29–32.

Jones, D. P. H. & Bools, C. N. (1999). Facititious illness by proxy. In T. David (Ed.), *Recent advances in paediatrics*, Vol. 17 (pp. 57–71). Edinburgh: Churchill Livingstone.

Jones, D. P. H., & Newbold, C. (2001). Assessment of abusing families. In G. Adshead, & D. Brooke (Eds.), *Munchausen's syndrome by proxy: Current issues in assessment, treatment and research* (pp. 109–119). London: Imperial College Press.

Jones, D. P. H., & Ramchandani, P. (1999). *Child sexual abuse: Informing practice from research*. Abingdon: Radcliffe Medical Press.

Jones, D. P. H., Hindley, N., & Ramchandani, P. (2006). Making plans: Assessment, intervention and evaluating outcomes. In J. Aldgate, D. Jones, W. Rose, & C. Jeffery (Eds.), *The Developing world of the child* (pp. 267–286). London: Jessica Kingsley.

Kaufman, J., & Zigler, E. (1989). The intergenerational transmission of child abuse. In D. Cicchetti, & V. Carlson (Eds.), *Child maltreatment: Theory and research on the causes and consequences of child abuse and neglect* (pp. 129–150). Cambridge: Cambridge University Press.

Kempe, C. H., Silverman, F., Steele, B., Droegemueller, W., & Silver, H. (1962). The battered child syndrome. *Journal of the American Medical Association*, *181*, 4–11.

Kitzmann, K. M., Gaylord, N. K., Holt, A. R., & Kenny, E. D. (2003). Child witnesses to domestic violence: A meta-analytic review. *Journal of Consulting and Clinical Psychology*, *71*, 339–352.

Knoke, D., & Trocmé, N. (2005). Reviewing the evidence on assessing risk for child abuse and neglect. *Brief Treatment and Crisis Intervention*, *5*, 310–327.

Kolko, D. J. (2002). Child physical abuse. In J. Myers, L. Berliner, J. Briere, C. Hendrix, C. Jenny, & T. Reid (Eds.), *The APSAC handbook on child maltreatment* (pp. 21–54). London: Sage.

Korbin, J. E. (1997). Culture and child maltreatment. In M. Helfer, R. Kempe, & R. Krugman (Eds.), *The battered child* (pp. 29–48). London: University of Chicago Press.

Korbin, J. E. (2002). Culture and child maltreatment: Cultural competence and beyond. *Child Abuse and Neglect*, *26*, 637–644.

Krueger, R. F., Moffitt, T. E., Caspi, A., Bleske, A., & Silva, P. A. (1998). Assortative mating for antisocial behaviour: developmental and methodological implications. *Behaviour Genetics*, *28*, 173–186.

Krug, E. G., Dahlberg, L. L., Mercy, J. A., Zwi, A. B., & Lozano, R. (2002). *World report on violence and health*. Geneva: World Health Organization.

Lanktree, C., Briere, J., & Zaidi, L. (1991). Incidence and impact of sexual abuse in a child outpatient sample: The role of direct inquiry. *Child Abuse and Neglect*, *15*, 447–454.

Lansford, J. E., Dodge, K. A., Pettit, G. S., Bates, J. E., Crozier, J., & Kaplow, J. (2002). Long-term effects of early child physical maltreatment on psychological, behavioural and academic problems in adolescence: A twelve year prospective study. *Archives of Pediatrics and Adolescent Medicine*, *156*, 824–830.

Leventhal, J. (2005). Getting prevention right: Maintaining the status quo is not an option. *Child Abuse and Neglect*, *29*, 209–213.

Lieberman, A. F., Ippen, C. G., & Van Horn, P. (2006). Child–parent psychotherapy: Six-month follow-up of a randomized controlled trial. *Journal of the American Academy of Child and Adolescent Psychiatry*, *45*, 913–918.

MacMillan, H. L., MacMillan, J. H., Offord, D. R., Griffith, L., & MacMillan, A. (1994). Primary prevention of child physical abuse and neglect: A critical review. Part I. *Journal of Child Psychology and Psychiatry*, *35*, 835–856.

Manly, J. T. (2005). Advances in research definitions of child maltreatment. *Child Abuse and Neglect*, 29, 425–439.

Manly, J., Kim, J., Rogosch, F., & Cicchetti, D. (2001). Dimensions of child maltreatment and children's adjustment: Contributions of developmental timing and sub-type. *Development and Psychopathology*, *13*, 759–782.

Manly, J. T., Cicchetti, D., & Barnett, D. (1994). The impact of subtype, frequency, chronicity, and severity of maltreatment on social competence and behaviour problems. *Development and Psychopathology*, 6, 121–143.

May-Chahal, C., & Cawson, P. (2005). Measuring child maltreatment in the United Kingdom: A study of the prevalence of child abuse and neglect. *Child Abuse and Neglect*, *29*, 969–984.

McHale, J., & Rasmussen, J. (1998). Coparental and family group level dynamics during infancy: Early family precursors of child and family functioning during pre-school. *Development and Psychopathology*, *10*, 39–59.

Melton, G. B., & Barry, F. D. (1994). *Protecting children from abuse and neglect: Foundations for a new national strategy*. London: Guilford Press.

Mercy, J. A., Rosenberg, M. L., Powell, K. E., Broome, C.V., & Roper, W. L. (1993). Public health policy for preventing violence. *Health Affairs*, *12*(4), 7–29.

Mian, M. (2004). World report on violence and health: What it means for children and pediatricians. *Journal of Pediatrics*, *145*, 14–19.

Moffitt, T. E. (2005). The new look of behavioral genetics in developmental psychopathology: Gene–environment interplay in anti-social behaviors. *Psychological Bulletin*, *131*, 533–554.

Mullen, P. E., Martin, J. L., Anderson, J.C., Romans, S. E., & Herbison, G. P. (1996). The long-term impact of the physical, emotional, and sexual abuse of children: A community study. *Child Abuse and Neglect*, *20*, 7–21.

National Research Council (NRC). (1993). Etiology of child maltreatment. In National Research Council (Ed.), *Understanding child abuse and neglect* (pp. 106–160). Washington DC: National Academy Press.

Olds, D. L., Eckenrode, J., Henderson, C. Jr., Kitzman, H., Powers, J., Cole, R., *et al.* (1997). Long-term effects of home visitation on maternal life course and child abuse and neglect: Fifteen-year follow-up of a randomized trial. *Journal of the American Medical Association*, *278*, 637–643.

Rosenberg, D. (1987). Web of deceit: A literature review of Munchausen syndrome by proxy. *Child Abuse and Neglect*, *11*, 547–563.

Runyan, D. K., Cox, C. E., Dubowitz, H., Newton, R. R., Upadhyaya, M., Kotch, J. B., *et al.* (2005). Describing maltreatment: Do child protective service reports and service definitions agree? *Child Abuse and Neglect*, *29*, 461–478.

Rushton, A., & Nathan, J. (1996). The supervision of child protection work. *British Journal of Social Work*, *26*, 357–374.

Rutter, M. (2005). How the environment affects mental health. *British Journal of Psychiatry*, *186*, 4–6.

Rutter, M. (2006a). Is Sure Start an effective preventive intervention? *Child and Adolescent Mental Health*, *11*, 135–141.

Rutter, M. (2006b). Implications of resilience concepts for scientific understanding. *Annals of the New York Academy of Sciences*, *1094*, 1–12.

Rutter, M., Moffitt, T. E., & Caspi, A. (2006a). Gene–environment interplay and psychopathology: Multiple varieties but real effects. *Journal of Child Psychology and Psychiatry*, *47*, 226–261.

Rutter, M., Kim-Cohen, J., & Maughan, B. (2006b). Continuities and discontinuities in psychopathology between childhood and adult life. *Journal of Child Psychology and Psychiatry*, *47*, 276–295.

Saunders, B. E., Berliner, L., & Hanson, R. F. (Eds.). (2004). *Child physical and sexual abuse: Guidelines for treatment (Final Report: January 15, 2003)*. Charleston, SC: National Crimes Victims Research and Treatment Center.

Sedlak, A. J., & Broadhurst, D. D. (1996). *Executive summary of the third national incidence study of child abuse and neglect*. Washington DC: US Department of Health and Human Services.

Schneider, M. W., Ross, A., Graham, J. C., & Zielinski, A. (2005). Do allegations of emotional maltreatment predict developmental outcome beyond that of other forms of maltreatment? *Child Abuse and Neglect*, *29*, 513–532.

Silverman, A. B., Reinherz, H. Z., & Gianconia, R. M. (1996). The long-term sequelae of child and adolescent abuse: A longitudinal community study. *Child Abuse and Neglect*, *20*, 709–723.

Slep, A. M. S., & O'Leary, S. G. (2005). Parent and partner violence in families with young children: Rates, patterns, and connections. *Journal of Consulting and Clinical Psychology*, *73*, 435–444.

Smith, M. G., & Fong, R. (2004). *The children of neglect: When no one cares*. NY & Hove: Brunner-Routledge.

Southall, D. P., Plunkett, M. C., Banks, M. W., Falkov, A. F., & Samuels, M. P. (1997). Covert video recordings of life-threatening child abuse: Lessons for child protection. *Pediatrics*, *100*, 735–760.

Sroufe, L. A. (2005). Attachment and development: A prospective, longitudinal study from birth to adulthood. *Attachment and Human Development*, *7*, 349–367.

Sternberg, K., Lamb, M., Guterman, E., & Abbott, C. (2006). Effects of early and later family violence on children's behavior problems and depression: A longitudinal, multi-informant perspective. *Child Abuse and Neglect*, *30*, 283–306.

Stevenson, J. (1999). The treatment of the long-term sequelae of child abuse. *Journal of Child Psychology and Psychiatry*, *40*, 89–111.

Straus, M., & Gelles, R. (1986). Societal change and change in family violence from 1975 to 1985 as revealed by two national surveys. *Journal of Marriage and Family*, *48*, 465–479.

Straus, M. A., & Kantor, G. K. (2005). Definition and measurement of neglectful behavior: Some principles and guidelines. *Child Abuse and Neglect*, *29*, 19–29.

Straus, M. A., Hamby, S. L., Finkelhor, D., Moore, D. W., & Runyan, D. K. (1998). Identification of child maltreatment with the parent–child conflict tactics scales: Development and psychometric data for a national sample for American parents. *Child Abuse and Neglect*, *22*, 249–270.

Sturge-Apple, M. L., Davies, P. T., & Cummings, E. M. (2006). Impact of hostility and withdrawal in inter-parental conflict on parental emotional unavailability and children's adjustment difficulties. *Child Development*, *77*, 1623–1641.

Swenson, C. C., & Chaffin, M. (2006). Beyond psychotherapy: Treating abused children by changing their social ecology. *Aggression and Violent Behavior*, *11*, 120–137.

Thorpe, K., Rutter, M., & Greenwood, R. (2003). Twins as a natural experiment to study the causes of mild language delay. II. Family interaction risk factors. *Journal of Child Psychology and Psychiatry*, *44*, 342–355.

Trocmé, N., MacLaurin, B., Fallon B., Black, T., & Lajoie, J. (2005). *Child abuse and neglect investigations in Canada: Comparing 1998 and 2003 data*. CECW Information Sheet, No.26E. Montreal, QC: McGill University School of Social Work. Retrieved May 5, 2006 from: HTTP://www.CECW-CEPB.ca/docseng/cis comparisons 26E PDF.

UNICEF. (2006). *The state of the world's children, 2006*. New York: UNICEF.

Wall, N. (2000). *A handbook for expert witnesses in Children Act cases*. Bristol: Jordan.

Westcott, H. L., & Jones, D. P. H. (1999). The abuse of disabled children. *Journal of Child Psychology and Psychiatry*, *40*, 497–506.

Wigfall, V., Monck, E., & Reynolds, J. (2006). Putting programme into practice: The introduction of concurrent planning into mainstream adoption and fostering services. *British Journal of Social Work*, *36*, 41–55.

Windham, A. M., Rosenberg, L., Fuddy, L., McFarlane, E., Sia, C., & Duggan, A. K. (2004). Risk of mother-reported child abuse in the first three years of life. *Child Abuse and Neglect*, *28*, 645–667.

Wolfe, D. A. (1991). *Preventing physical and emotional abuse of children*. London: Guilford Press.

Wolfe, D. A. (1994). The role of intervention and treatment services in the prevention of child abuse and neglect. In G. Melton, & F. Barry (Eds.), *Protecting children from abuse and neglect: Foundations for a new national strategy* (pp. 224–303). London: Guilford Press.

Wolfe, D. A. (2006). Preventing violence in relationships: Psychological science addressing complex social issues. *Canadian Psychology*, *47*, 44–50.

Wolfe, D. A., Crooks, C. V., Lee, V., McIntyre-Smith, A., & Jaffe, P. G. (2003). The effects of children's exposure to domestic violence: a meta-analysis and critique. *Clinical Child and Family Psychology Review*, 6, 171–187.

World Health Organization (WHO). (1999). *Report of the consultation on child abuse prevention*. Geneva: World Health Organization.

World Health Organization (WHO). (2002). *World report on violence and health*. Geneva: World Health Organization.

Websites

California Evidence-based Clearinghouse for Child Welfare. http://www.cachildwelfareclearinghouse.org/

Every Child Matters. http://www.everychildmatters.gov.uk/

International Society for the Prevention of Child Abuse and Neglect http://www.ispcan.org/

National Society for the Prevention of Cruelty to Children http://www.nspcc.org.uk/

29 Child Sexual Abuse

Danya Glaser

Sexual abuse is a significant risk factor for the development of psychopathology in childhood, adolescence and adulthood. Familiarity with the phenomenon (including its presentation and treatment) is therefore of particular importance to the practice of child and adolescent psychiatry. The hallmarks of child sexual abuse are its secret nature and the very frequent denial of the abuse by the abuser, once it is alleged to have happened. These two factors play a central part in the process of the abuse and in its aftermath. Sexual abuse includes a far wider spectrum than incest, occurs both within the family and outside it but, in either circumstance, the abuser is frequently already known to the child. Indeed, this acquaintance may be based on a deliberate befriending or "grooming" of the child by the abuser for the purposes of preplanned abuse. Because it involves sexuality, this form of abuse is particularly emotive.

Child sexual abuse is not a new phenomenon. The incest taboo has been in existence for over 4000 years, first records being in the Babylonian code of Hammurabi (*c.*2150 BC), which referred to "a man be known to his daughter" (Handcock, 1932) where "known" has been translated as "to conceive a child" (ten Bensel, Rheinberger, & Radbill, 1997). The laws of Moses (*c.*3000 BC) describe incest as a sin (Leviticus 18:6). General Booth, founder of the Salvation Army, wrote in 1890: "I understand that the Society for the Protection of Children prosecuted last year a fabulous number of fathers for unnatural sins with their children" (Booth, 1890). Despite sporadic earlier pronouncements, child sexual abuse only began to be noted as a significant form of child abuse in the 1970s. Increasing recognition came with the development of the women's movement, reports by adult women survivors of their childhood abuse and a greater openness regarding sexuality. This pattern of increasing recognition has swept through successive countries, with reports appearing in the scientific press, in particular in *Child Abuse and Neglect, the International Journal.*

The universal disapproval of child sexual abuse is exemplified in the UN Convention on the Rights of the Child. In the UK, this disapproval is expressed by the legal prohibition of incest and sexual contact between an adult and a child, and its inclusion as various offences under criminal law. However, some of the harmful effects of child sexual abuse such as the denial of the abuse by the abuser, and guilt and self-blame by the victim, are largely consequent on this expressed disapproval by society. Moreover, the fact that child sexual abuse is a relatively common experience for children and young persons implies a lack of protection of, and care for, these vulnerable members of society. Despite the now repeated findings of very high reported rates of child sexual abuse (see p. 442), most suspicions of sexual abuse continue to be met with caution, and disclosures are often regarded with suspicion. The fact that an apparently common phenomenon is so often doubted or disbelieved is probably explained by the social taboo surrounding adult sexual contact with children and by at least two further factors. First, the absence of non-involved witnesses to this (secret) activity helps to support the frequent denial of the abuse by the alleged abuser. Second, the potentially serious consequences for the alleged abuser, if found guilty, govern the attitude to investigation. Alongside the high rate of reports of sexual abuse of children and adolescents, the rates of prosecution and conviction are low. In an English sample of 188 cases of contact abuse, the rate of prosecution was 36% with 17% convictions. A further 5% received a caution (Prior, Glaser, & Lynch, 1997). Two independent studies from the USA found that less than one in five cases of alleged abuse reached the stage of prosecution (Martone, Jaudes, & Cavins, 1996; Tjaden & Thoennes, 1992). The stringent test of the evidence in criminal law, "beyond reasonable doubt," which is higher than "on balance of probabilities" required in civil law, may help to explain this low rate. Many children who have been abused find difficulty in comprehending the lack of more frequent criminal convictions, especially when they have been prepared to testify in court.

Heated controversy has surrounded memories recovered in adulthood, of childhood sexual abuse, the veracity of which is disputed by the alleged abusers (Davies & Dalgleish, 2001). Some memories have returned spontaneously whereas others have been triggered by reminders or recalled in response to enquiry that included leading questions and other forms of suggestion (Loftus, Garry, & Feldman, 1994; see also chapter 7). A few have been induced by overzealous therapists. This debate has (inappropriately) rekindled doubts about the general truth of allegations made by children.

Rutter's Child and Adolescent Psychiatry, 5th edition. Edited by M. Rutter, D. Bishop, D. Pine, S. Scott, J. Stevenson, E. Taylor and A. Thapar. © 2008 Blackwell Publishing, ISBN: 978-1-4051-4549-7.

Definitions

A myriad of definitions for legal, research and other purposes continue to be developed and used. A recent definition guiding child protection work in England states: Sexual abuse involves forcing or enticing a child or young person to take part in sexual activities, including prostitution, whether or not the child is aware of what is happening. The activities may involve physical contact, including penetrative (e.g., rape, buggery or oral sex) or non-penetrative acts. They may include non-contact activities, such as involving children in looking at, or in the production of, pornographic material or watching sexual activities, or encouraging children to behave in sexually inappropriate ways (Department for Education and Skills, 2006). It is important to note that the abuser's intentions or motivations are not considered necessary to be included in many definitions. The term pedophilia applies to a sexual attraction to, and arousal by prepubertal children, of either gender. It is clear that many sexual abusers are therefore not pedophiles.

Cultural Practices

Some definitions refer to social or cultural norms, making it necessary to consider what is a culture-specific practice. This is particularly relevant where ethnic minority groups are living in a majority host culture whose norms differ. Cultural practices are expected to alter with time and context, and the dominant culture tends to set prevailing childrearing standards (Korbin, 1997). However, Ahn and Gilbert (1992), for example, found that among Koreans living in the USA, a grandfather touching the genitalia of his preschool grandson was seen as expressing pride in the fact that this child would continue the family line. Cultural practices may not be benign and culturally sanctioned, and normative practices may affect adversely the well-being of children (McKee, 1984). A particular case is the issue of female genital mutilation (Powell, Leye, Jayakody *et al.*, 2004). There is clearly also individual deviation in child care and other practices within cultures (Korbin, 1981). Whereas it is important to avoid misidentifying culture as abuse and vice versa (Abney & Gunn, 1993), this can be quite difficult in practice.

Legal Considerations

Under English civil law, child sexual abuse is recognized in the Children Act, 1989 as a form of Significant Harm. In criminal law, child sexual abuse is subsumed under a number of different offences. They include incest, which applies to vaginal intercourse between a male and a female whom the offender knows to be his (legal) daughter, granddaughter, sister or mother. Incest is thus not necessarily child sexual abuse. Under English law (Home Office, 2004) the child is defined as under 16 years of age. Offences include rape, assault by penetration, sexual assault, causing or inciting a child to engage in sexual activity, engaging in sexual activity in the presence of a child, causing a child to watch a sexual act, abuse of children through prostitution and pornography, arranging or facilitating commission of a child sex offence and meeting a child following sexual grooming. It also includes child sex offences committed by children or young persons.

In some jurisdictions, such as in England and the USA, civil and criminal proceedings can continue in parallel and independently of each other. This means that, in theory although not always in practice, a child may be protected from an abuser by being moved from their care under civil law, when there has been no criminal trial and potentially even if a criminal trial failed to convict the alleged abuser. In other jurisdictions, child protective procedures will only be undertaken following the criminal conviction of the abuser. This confers considerably less protection on children, especially as the rate of convictions worldwide is low relative to the number of allegations.

Nature of the Abuse

Within the spectrum of sexual abuse, an early distinction was made between non-contact and contact abuse (Wyatt & Peters, 1986a). However, with the advent of new technologies, this distinction is becoming more blurred.

Contact Abuse

Broadly, in western societies, any physical contact between the breasts and genitalia of a child or adult and a part of the other's body, with the exception of isolated accidental touch (e.g., in the bath or in bed), and for developmentally and age-appropriate cleaning or for applying medication or ointment, is considered to be sexual abuse. Abusive contact includes fondling, masturbation, oral–genital contact or penetration, attempted or actual digital and penal penetration of, and the insertion of objects into, the vagina or anus. Active abuse is often preceded by an insidious process of "grooming" in which the abuser, having identified a particular child or children, finds ways of befriending the child or increasing the opportunities for being with the child unobserved. Given the addictive nature of much child sexual abuse, it is in the abuser's interest to be able to continue to abuse a child. Therefore, there is typically a gradual progression from touching to more penetrative abuse (Berliner & Conte, 1990), so as to avoid causing initial pain or injury, which would be more likely to lead the child to complain about or report the abuse. Anal abuse is understandably more common in boys, although younger girls are not infrequently anally abused (Hobbs & Wynne, 1989). In a small proportion of cases, actual physical violence is used, either as a way of intimidating or coercing the child, or as an integral aspect of the abuse (30% in the study reported by Gomes-Schwartz, Horowitz, & Cardarelli, 1990).

Non-contact Abuse and the Use of the Internet and Mobile Phone Technology

This includes deliberate exposure of children to adult genitalia or sexual activity, either live or depicted in photographs or film. It also includes intrusive looking at the young person's body, inducing children to interact sexually with each other and the taking of photographs for pornographic purposes. There has been debate about the point at which the threshold for Significant Harm or actual abuse is reached when the concerns are about non-contact sexual interaction. It is important to ascertain whether the interaction was deliberate and the extent of coercion used, with greater coercion increasing the harm. Although the most serious effects of sexual abuse are associated with contact, and especially penetrative, abuse, many young persons report the experience of being intrusively observed as humiliating and intimidating.

The Internet and mobile phone technology have become a source of sexual abuse of children (Taylor & Quayle, 2003). Children may view pornographic images by encountering them inadvertently or by deliberately searching for them. This exposure is increasing (Wolak, Mitchell, & Finkelhor, 2006). Children report being very disturbed by unwanted exposure to such material (Finkelhor, Mitchell, & Wolak, 2000). The Internet is also a means by which adults may ask for children's pictures of themselves or groom adolescents with the intention of luring them into sexual activity (O'Connell, 2003). In addition, children are being made the subjects of abuse images (Palmer, 2005). Lastly, child pornography may act as a motivator or reinforcer of sexually abusive activity by adolescents (Quayle & Taylor, 2006). Some of this activity involves adolescent peers acting together and includes distributing images of other children, which may have been taken on mobile phones. This activity is likely to be enhanced by the normalizing effect of pornographic imagery on the Internet. As with other forms of sexual abuse, children and adolescents may be reluctant to tell about this abuse, which may be discovered rather than disclosed. Children may thus become involved in criminal investigations.

Commercial Sexual Exploitation of Children

Commercial sexual exploitation takes the inter-related forms of trafficking and prostitution. Trafficking includes movement of children for financial gain, usually across borders and largely for sexually exploitation. Abuse through pornography may also be included (Chase & Statham, 2005). Prostitution is found both in girls and boys and is now clearly recognized as a form of sexual exploitation and abuse. There is a complex relationship between sexual exploitation and drug abuse, the sexual exploitation either providing a source of money to support drug dependency or introducing the young person to addictive drugs as a means of gaining control over the child for subsequent sexual exploitation.

Epidemiology

For mental health care planning (and other services), sufficient provision needs to be made for the treatment of the consequences of a common problem. Unfortunately, the published figures for incidence and prevalence of child sexual abuse vary considerably according to the definition used, the source of data and the population studied. Whereas broad definitions point to the extent of the problem, they are less helpful in indicating severity and the kind of therapeutic services required.

Although annual reports of child sexual abuse could, in theory, indicate prevalence, such figures are inaccurate underestimates. Many occurrences of child sexual abuse are not reported at the time of the abuse (Finkelhor, Hotaling, Lewis *et al.*, 1990) and some are not reported at all.

Prevalence

The most accurate figures are from population studies. Even here, responses to interviews or questionnaires may be underestimates, because of reluctance to report or a lack of recall of previous abuse, even when this had been documented at the time (Williams, 1994). It has been suggested that interviews, which tend to yield higher rates of reported abuse, may be more specific in their questions and more likely to prompt recall of abuse (Wyatt & Peters, 1986b).

In population, as opposed to victim samples, non-penetrative contact abuse is the form most commonly described (Haugaard & Reppucci, 1988). Russell (1983), in her urban community study of 930 women, found that 38% had suffered contact abuse under the age of 18 years, and very serious sexual abuse (forced vaginal or anal intercourse and oral–genital abuse) in 27% of intrafamilial cases. In a British study of students (Kelly, Regan, & Burton, 1991), 27% female and 11% male respondents reported contact abuse. Four per cent of female and 2% of male respondents respectively reported serious penetrative or coercive abuse, with an age difference between abuser and victim of more than 5 years. In a recent study using a questionnaire with a random probability sample of 18- to 24-years-olds in the UK (May-Chahal & Cawson, 2005), 10% reported experiencing contact sexual abuse while under 16 years of age (15% girls and 6% boys). By contrast, the rate for the most serious forms of abuse in clinical samples rose to 65% (Gomes-Schwartz, Horowitz, & Cardarelli, 1990).

Rates of reporting increased over the 20 years after 1970, both in the UK (Markowe, 1988) and in the USA (Finkelhor, 1991) probably because of increased awareness, but there had been little evidence to suggest that the actual incidence had been changing significantly (Feldman, Feldman, Goodman *et al.*, 1991). Indeed, the number of substantiated cases of child sexual abuse in the USA decreased by an estimated 49% between 1990 and 2004 (Finkelhor & Jones, 2006). The findings in Australia (Dunne, Purdie, Cook *et al.*, 2003) and England are broadly similar. The fall could be brought about by:

1 An actual decline (Finkelhor & Jones, 2004) which might signal a positive effect of interventions for reported child sexual abuse; growing awareness of children's rights or greater vigilance and child-focused parenting;

2 A decline in reporting caused, for instance, by fear of legal repercussions; or

3 Changes in agency responses to reported abuse, such as increased cautiousness and acting on allegations with a raised threshold for an active professional response.

The fall in rate parallels the decline in substantiated cases of physical abuse and improvements in other aspects of child welfare, at least in the USA, and it is likely that, to some extent, the fall is real (Finkelhor & Jones, 2006).

Frequency and Duration of Abuse for an Individual Child

Whereas population studies have shown a majority for whom sexual abuse is a single episode, in clinical samples the majority of children have been abused more than once by the same abuser. It appears that single episodes of abuse are less likely to be reported and subsequently referred to helping agencies. There is evidence that a child who has been sexually abused is vulnerable to further abuse by others, 14% in the Baker and Duncan (1985) study. This is likely to be because of a combination of the original vulnerability of the child and the added vulnerability conferred by the experience of having been abused. A distinction needs to be made between repeat victimization by the same abuser and revictimization by different abusers (Hamilton & Browne, 1999). Children subjected to organized abuse (see p. 444) are often multiply abused. Repeated abuse often continues for several years (Gomes-Schwartz, Horowitz, & Cardarelli, 1990). Duration, frequency and severity, including penetration, are thus linked factors.

Age of Victims

Children may be abused from infancy onwards. Children who experience intercourse tend to be older, with an average age of 11.4 years in the Gomes-Schwartz, Horowitz, & Cardarelli (1990) study, compared with 9.1 years for other forms of significant contact abuse.

Gender of Victims

Girls are more commonly victims of sexual abuse than boys. There is a tendency for sexual abuse of boys to be under-reported (Holmes & Slap, 1998), in part because of shame and the fear of homosexuality. Adolescent boys are increasingly reluctant to talk about their abuse, even in therapy (Nasjleti, 1980). This may explain some reports that boys are abused at a younger mean age than girls (e.g., Singer, 1989). Younger boys are not infrequently abused alongside their sisters rather than in isolation (Vander Mey, 1988). Extra-familial abuse more commonly involves boys although there is no agreement about whether boys are more commonly abused by strangers (Watkins & Bentovim, 1992).

Disability

National statistics on child abuse do not contain data on abused children's disabilities (Kelly, 1992). However, in studies of children with disabilities the rate of sexual abuse is two or three times that in "normal" children (Sullivan & Knutson, 2000). The reasons for this greater prevalence include: the children's difficulties in communicating about abuse (Morris, 1999); their dependency on intimate physical care; social isolation in institutional care (Utting, Baines, Stuart *et al.*, 1997); and care by staff rather than parents (Westcott & Jones, 1999). Kendall-Tackett, Lyion, Taliaferro *et al.* (2005) urge professionals to include disability as a variable in studies of abused children so as to increase awareness of their existence among abused children.

Abusers

The majority of abusers (85–95%) are male. Whereas male abusers who abuse prepubertal children may well target both boys and girls, there is some gender specificity in relation to adolescent girl victims. By the time a sexual abuser is identified, his pattern of abusing has often been well established. A small proportion of child sexual abuse is carried out by female abusers (Saradjian, 1996), often in conjunction with a man. Women abusers on their own are more likely to abuse boys (Faller, 1989). Age is no bar to sexually abusive interactions and older men may well continue to abuse children.

There has been much debate about a possible psychological profile of abusers or about a commonality of childhood experiences that might have led them to abuse children. Whereas many will have experienced disruption and physical abuse in their formative years (Seghorn, Prensky, & Boucher, 1987), a person's own sexual abuse is one predisposing factor to sexually abusing children (summarized in Watkins & Bentovim, 1992) but it is not a prerequisite. A study sought differences between the previous experiences of four comparison samples each consisting of 15 boys aged 11–15 who had, respectively: (i) been sexually abused; (ii) abused other children; (iii) been abused as well as abused other children; and (iv) had a conduct disorder (Skuse, Bentovim, Hodges *et al.*, 1998). Factors predating the sexually abusive activity by the boys included discontinuity of care, exposure to or experience of physical violence and emotional abuse. Such findings help to explain why, in practice, sexual abusers constitute a heterogeneous group in terms of personal, social and demographic factors.

Juvenile Abusers

Sexual abuse by both children and adolescents, mostly boys, has become widely recognized (Abel, Becker, Mittelman *et al.*, 1987) and is no longer considered an acceptable variant of childhood or adolescent sexual development. A significant proportion of adolescent abusers are of low intellectual ability. Most children and adolescents who sexually abuse other children have experienced psychosocial adversity. A recent study has found that for boys who had been sexually abused, predisposing risk factors to becoming a sexual abuser included material neglect, lack of supervision, sexual abuse by a female person and witnessing intrafamilial violence (Salter, McMillan, Richards *et al.*, 2003). Adolescent abusers show heterogeneous maladaptive mental schemata regarding social interaction and abuse (Richardson, 2005). Many adult abusers report the onset of their abusive activities in adolescence and abuse by an adolescent cannot necessarily be considered safely to "burn out" in adulthood (Vizard, Monck, & Misch, 1995).

Abuser–Child Relationship

The majority of children know their abuser before commencement of the abuse. This acquaintance may have been deliberately fostered by the abuser as part of a grooming process, or the abuser and child may be part of the same family or social network. In community studies, the most common relationship is stepfather–stepdaughter (Finkelhor, 1984). The same abuser may abuse children both within and outside the family, and include biological as well as stepchildren. Risk to other children in the family and in contact with the abuser is therefore difficult to predict and an assumption must be made that the proven capacity to actually abuse children renders all children in contact with that abuser at risk.

Organized Abuse

Many abusers abuse in isolation. Nevertheless, there are also organized forms of abuse involving more than one abuser and multiple children, some of whom are recruited in sex rings (Wild & Wynne, 1986). It is said that organized abuse may include formalized rituals (Frude, 1996). There are, in these cases, serious questions about the reliability, verifiability and credibility of the reports (Young, Sachs, Braun *et al.*, 1991). Organized abuse also includes the use of children and young persons for the production of child pornography; this constitutes a more serious problem. Children in residential settings in particular may be subject to sexual abuse. These children, who are already vulnerable, are dependent on staff and often isolated from confiding contact with adults outside the residential setting (Utting *et al.*, 1997).

Abuse by Clergy

Widespread occurrence of sexual abuse by Catholic clergy has come to light over the last few years in a number of countries including the UK, Ireland and the USA. Some of the clergy abused one or two children whereas others had multiple victims. The abuse included pedophilia as well as the abuse of adolescents, of both genders (Haywood, Kravitz, Grossman *et al.*, 1996). This form of sexual abuse arose in an opportunistic setting which brought together potential abusers and potential victims, with clergy's own possible sexual difficulties linked both with the choice and consequences of enforced celibacy.

Finkelhor (2003) pointed out that this discovery led to a number of consequences to the field of child sexual abuse, some of which can be regarded as positive. It has increased public belief in the existence of child sexual abuse, has reinforced the recognition of the need to enable children to talk about possible abuse and has enabled more children and adolescents to come forward with accounts of their own abuse. It has lessened the stigmatization of sexual abuse for boys. There has also been recognition of the increased need for corporate or organizational responsibility for employees' behavior.

Ethnicity, Culture and Socioeconomic Status

Both in the UK and the USA, population-based studies have shown no ethnic differences in the rates of child sexual abuse (Fontes, 1995; Kelly, Regan, & Burton, 1991; Korbin, 1997). However, data on ethnic and cultural variations are weak, partly because details on racial and ethnic background are inadequate, and partly because shame and denial about sexual abuse within some cultures conspire against reporting.

Socioeconomic status is unrelated to the incidence of child sexual abuse in population studies (Berliner & Elliott, 1996) but there is an overrepresentation of lower socioeconomic groups in clinic samples (Bentovim, Boston, & van Elburg, 1987). This may be because these groups are more likely to come to the attention of child protective agencies than middle class families, who may find ways of hiding the abuse or avoiding its reporting (Gomes-Schwartz, Horowitz, & Cardarelli, 1990). Different forms of child abuse and neglect are not infrequently found in the same family and the same child (Mullen, Martin, Anderson *et al.*, 1994), especially among the socially disadvantaged. Child sexual abuse is associated with troubled family life including family disruption (Russell, 1986), reconstituted families, intrafamilial violence (Bifulco, Brown, & Adler, 1991) and parents who are perceived as emotionally distant and uncaring (Alexander & Lupfer, 1987).

Risk and Causation, and Maintaining Factors for Child Sexual Abuse

There is no unitary theory of causation to explain child sexual abuse (Glaser & Frosh, 1993). Although it involves an interaction between the abuser and the child, or the perpetrator and the victim, intention and responsibility rest with the abuser. The abuser's wish for power and sexual gratification are the two main aspects. Sexual arousal to prepubertal children or pedophilia is likely to be a strong motivating force for abusers of prepubertal children.

Finkelhor (1984) has brought together several factors in a systemic model of four preconditions that, he postulates, are necessary for child sexual abuse to occur:

1. Motivation to sexually abuse children;
2. Absence of internal inhibitors;
3. Absence of external inhibitors;
4. Absence of child's resistance (or a child's vulnerability).

Preconditions for Potential Abusers

Motivations refer to the abuser's sexuality and sexual development and include pedophilia, fear and/or avoidance of peer sexual relationships and sadism. They also address interpersonal motivators such as a need to overpower or gain mastery over more vulnerable persons, arising as a result of one's own past abuse and low self-esteem. It is noteworthy that in a survey of male undergraduates, 5–9% expressed sexual interest in children (Briere & Runtz, 1989). This suggests that the predisposition to sexual abuse is far more common than the action, supporting the postulated need for other factors to exist before abuse will actually occur. Some of the motivations for female abusers are discussed by Welldon (1988) who described incestuous mothers as simultaneously attacking and emotionally engulfing or possessing their children.

Absence of internal inhibitors includes the effects of alcohol and stress. It also refers particularly to the cognitive distortions or rationalizations that abusers employ in continuing to perpetrate abuse and which have been studied by those treating sexual abusers. These cognitive distortions include minimization of the harmful effect of the abuse on the child; conceptualizing the abuse as "love" or "education"; and placing responsibility on the child or adolescent, who is described as inviting or requesting the abuse.

Child Risk Factors

External inhibitors of sexual abuse include protective family structures and relationships surrounding the child, in particular a secure attachment to primary caregiver(s), good monitoring of the child's whereabouts and the existence of confiding relationships for the child. Their lack provides a risk for sexual abuse. The child's vulnerability by virtue of age, disability, neglect or social isolation increases the likelihood of sexual abuse. Indeed, abusers recognize these factors as rendering a child suitable for abuse (Conte, Wolfe, & Smith, 1989). This explanatory schema does not remove the abuser's responsibility for the abuse, whatever the nature of contributory risk factors.

Maintaining Factors

Summit (1983, 1992) used his clinical experience to hypothesize a Child Sexual Abuse Accommodation Syndrome or Pattern to explain how children progressively adjust to sexual abuse by a trusted person, by accommodating psychologically to the inherent contradictions, confusions and enforced secrecy accompanying the experience, and the way in which many children come to disclose sexual abuse. He postulated five stages:

1 Secrecy;
2 Helplessness;
3 Entrapment and accommodation;
4 Delayed, unconvincing disclosure; and
5 Retraction.

This conceptualization carries plausibility in social contexts in which child sexual abuse is a secret and unwitnessed activity, in which children are told not to talk about it and in which they are often not believed (but see chapter 7 for strong reservations). It may constitute a coping strategy, enabling some children to remain asymptomatic during the abuse and leaving the abuse undiscovered. The abuser's own pattern of denial of the abuse through cognitive distortions lessens his potential discomfort and enables him to continue the abuse. By the time sexual abuse is discovered in childhood, it has usually occurred many times. Not all disclosures are unconvincing and they are not necessarily retracted. Moreover, in some societies, there is now a growing recognition and acceptance of the fact of child sexual abuse. This may counteract the need for psychological accommodation by the child and may be contributing to the decreasing rate of substantiated sexual abuse, by allowing for earlier disclosure.

Effects of Child Sexual Abuse

A majority of children who have suffered sexual abuse experience a variety of problems (Beitchman, Zucker, Hood *et al.*, 1991; Kendall-Tackett, Williams, & Finkelhor, 1993), some of which extend into adulthood (Wyatt & Powell, 1988); there is no specific post child sexual abuse syndrome (Kendall-Tackett, Williams, & Finkelhor, 1993; Paolucci, Genuis, & Violato, 2001). Some effects are direct consequences of the sexual experience, such as age-inappropriate sexualized behavior. Others develop as a response to the abusive nature of what happened. The actual effects are shaped by the child's gender, age, family circumstances, ethnicity and social class. In non-clinical samples, adolescents report higher levels of depression and anxiety than younger children (Gidycz & Koss, 1989), suggesting that with increasing maturity, the adolescent more fully comprehends the implications of having been abused sexually. This is also supported by the finding that distress following child sexual abuse is greater in girls with higher cognitive functioning (Shapiro, Leifer, Martone *et al.*, 1992). This is despite the fact that, in general, higher innate ability and the capacity to understand are considered to be protective factors in overcoming adverse life experiences.

Effects in Childhood and Adolescence

Sexual abuse may lead to unwanted pregnancy or sexually transmitted disease. Rarely, it may cause genital injuries. However, less than 50% of children with documented sexual abuse have physical findings (Muram, 1989). Deleterious psychological effects constitute the starting points for suspecting sexual abuse, but often they are recognized only retrospectively, because many are non-specific. About 1 in 3 young people show no outward indicators (Kendall-Tackett, Williams, & Finkelhor, 1993), allowing abuse to be undetected over prolonged periods. This is particularly likely with children compared to adolescents (McLeer, Dixon, Henry *et al.*, 1998). Although most findings derive from clinical samples, studies of non-clinical adolescents also show raised rates of emotional and/or behavioral difficulties (McLeer *et al.*, 1998).

Sexualized Behavior

A majority of children include in their activity and play some aspects of exploration of their body and its functions including genitalia, pregnancy, "mummies and daddies" and "doctors and nurses," peaking at age 5. Friedrich, Fisher, Broughton *et al.* (1998) developed the Child Sexual Behavior Inventory (CSBI) based on parent reports. Observations of preschool children have also shown that masturbation in preschool children is a part of normal development, many preschool children touch women's breasts, look at or touch each other's genitalia and some simulate sexual intercourse while remaining fully clothed (Lindblat, Gustafsson, & Larson, 1995). A significant proportion add genitalia to their figure drawings at some point in their early years. Sexual talk and some preoccupation with sexual touching can be found within the autism spectrum.

Age-inappropriate sexualized behavior is found significantly more commonly in, although not in most, sexually abused children (Cosentino, Meyer-Bahlburg, Alpert *et al.*, 1995; Friedrich, 1993) and is an important unwanted outcome of child sexual abuse. It refers to genitally orientated and sexual behavior, often involving another child, a doll or sometimes an adult. These inappropriate behaviors include inserting fingers, objects or a penis into the vagina or anus, and oral–genital contact (Lloyd Davies, Glaser, & Kossoff, 2000). It also includes more commonly seen genitally oriented behaviors such as looking at, touching or drawing genitalia or simulating sexual intercourse fully clothed, and when these are repeated they become a preoccupation for the child, or are accompanied by coercion of another child in the activity. This troubling behavior is particularly likely to follow abuse at an early age (McClellan, McCurry, Ronnei *et al.*, 1996). In boys, it may be regarded as a way of reasserting their masculinity (Rogers & Terry, 1984). It may also be a form of re-experiencing the abuse as part of a post-traumatic response (Kiser, Ackerman, Brown *et al.*, 1988). It is often intractable, a challenge to treatment (see p. 451) and leads to serious difficulties in finding alternative placements for these children, who are considered to pose a risk to other children and who may become socially excluded as a result. In some children, this behavior comes to be regarded as actual sexual abuse of another child.

Unplanned Pregnancy

In adolescence, there is an association between early pregnancy and a history of sexual abuse (Mullen *et al.*, 1994). This reflects the sexual vulnerability of these girls to sexual abuse, which is expressed in a number of ways including: low self-esteem, which leads to a lowered threshold to, or welcoming of, sexual approaches; a confusion between affectionate approaches and sexual attention towards the girls; and actual behavior that is perceived by others as inviting sexual approaches. A history of child sexual abuse is also frequently found in both boy and girl child prostitutes.

Psychological Sequelae

Despite clinical experience, Tremblay, Herbert, and Piche (1999) among others, have found that a majority of 7- to 12-year-old children who had been sexually abused maintained a relatively high sense of global worth. Post-traumatic stress disorder (PTSD) has been found as a sequel of child sexual abuse, the frequency varying from 44% in an abused group being evaluated for psychiatric disorders and treatment needs (McLeer, Deblinger, Henry *et al.*, 1992) to 71% in a clinical symptomatic sample (Trowell, Ugarte, Kolvin *et al.*, 1999). Depression is found more commonly among sexually abused than non-abused children (Wozencraft, Wagner, & Pellegrin, 1991). Whereas depression is found in all age groups, suicidal ideation and self-injurious behavior are mainly confined to adolescence (Lanktree, Briere, & Zaidi, 1991), where they are found to be associated significantly with a history of child sexual abuse in boys (Oates, 2004). Anxiety is encountered in both sexually abused boys and girls, and in both clinical and non-clinically referred children post abuse.

Children with a history of sexual abuse have subsequently been found to show more bulimic symptoms and a significant proportion of children with eating disorders report a history of child sexual abuse. This more commonly takes the form of bulimia (binging and purging) than the more calorie restrictive form of anorexia nervosa (Carter, Bewell, Blackmore *et al.*, 2006). Aggression and disruptive behavior may also follow sexual abuse (Kendall-Tackett, Williams, & Finkelhor, 1993). Difficulties with peer relationships may arise due to sexualized behavior, low self-esteem, shame and lack of trust (Mannarino, Cohen, & Berman, 1994). Running away, substance abuse usage and involvement in prostitution are found in boy and girl adolescents following sexual abuse.

Patterns and Continuities

Charting the "natural history" of sexual abuse-related symptomatology is difficult, because prognosis depends not only on the child's coping and adaptation (Friedrich, Beilke, & Urquiza, 1988), but also on the nature of the response that the child encounters. This includes treatment which, if successful, will modify outcomes. Moreover, some difficulties are related to age and developmental stage so that new difficulties may arise with maturation. Some children become more symptomatic than when initially seen (Kendall-Tackett, Williams, & Finkelhor, 1993). Some symptoms resolve more rapidly than others; dissociation, post-traumatic phenomena and sexualized behavior all attenuate only slowly (Beitchman *et al.*, 1991), even with treatment (Lanktree & Briere, 1995). Improvement in family functioning, particularly in the domain of problem-solving, correlates with improvement in children's behavior while maternal coping through avoidance strategies correlates with deterioration in behavior (Oates, O'Toole, Lynch *et al.*, 1994). If the abuser is a close family member, and especially if he is denying the fact of the abuse, the family will be more troubled. Whereas there is an overall trend towards improvement in children's functioning, the path is neither smooth nor is its direction straight or entirely predictable. There has been little systematic study of the effects of child sexual abuse on people with learning disability. Findings suggest that the effects are similar to those in the general population (Sequeira & Hollins, 2003).

Effects in Adulthood

Studies of male and female adult survivors of child sexual abuse show a clear pattern of interpersonal and intrapsychic difficulties (Nelson, Heath, Madden *et al.*, 2002) although this does not constitute a syndrome (Fontes, 1995; Stein, Golding, Siegel *et al.*, 1988). A longitudinal study of a birth cohort of more than 1000 children in New Zealand has shown a significant association between childhood sexual abuse in both boys and girls and psychiatric disorders in young adulthood, which held when possible confounding variables were allowed for (Fergusson, Horwood, & Lynskey, 1996).

The most commonly reported symptom is depression; deliberate self-harm is significantly higher in women abused in childhood than in non-abused women (e.g., 16% versus 6%) even in community samples (Saunders, Villeponeaux, Lipovsky *et al.*, 1992). Anxiety is also reported but less commonly. Drug and alcohol abuse are important long-term sequelae (Mullen, Martin, Anderson *et al.*, 1993), found more commonly in men survivors (Stein *et al.*, 1988). An adult female twin study has concluded that the significant association found between a history of child sexual abuse and major depression, anxiety, drug and alcohol abuse is a causal and direct one, rather than being confounded by genetic factors or mediated by common environmental factors (Kendler, Bulik, Silberg *et al.*, 2000).

A history of child sexual abuse has been found significantly more often in adults with PTSD, dissociation and psychotic symptoms, including hallucinations and delusions, particularly as part of a diagnosis of schizophrenia (Read, van Os, Morrison *et al.*, 2005; see also chapter 42). With respect to the claimed specific risk for schizophrenia see Morgan and Fisher (2007) for a balanced critique. A dose effect appears to operate, relating the severity of adult psychopathology to the severity of the child sexual abuse.

Mullen *et al.* (1994) have also found difficulties in the sexual functioning and intimate interpersonal relationships, and distrust of men in women who had been abused, and all the deleterious effects were exacerbated by abuse that had included intercourse. Less disturbance of sexual functioning has been found in men survivors (Stein *et al.*, 1988). Only a minority of homosexual men has been sexually abused in childhood, and they have no greater sexual interest in children than heterosexual men.

One study that tested the validity of Finkelhor and Browne's traumagenic model (see p. 448) in a sample of 192 adult women survivors, found that stigma and self-blame, but not betrayal and powerlessness, mediated the effects of sexual abuse on adult psychological functioning (Coffey, Leitenberg, Henning *et al.*, 1996). Some of these difficulties, including low self-esteem, impact on the parenting functions of adult survivors and contribute to the explanation of intergenerational continuities of child abuse. Continuing low self-esteem is also reflected in higher rates of unskilled or semiskilled work among women sexually abused in childhood (Mullen *et al.*, 1994). Eating disorders have been reported as occurring more commonly in women survivors of childhood sexual abuse (Mullen *et al.*, 1993).

Factors Contributing to the Effects of Sexual Abuse

Tremblay, Herbert, & Piche (1999) found that abuse variables, parental support and the child's coping strategies contributed independently to the psychological outcome for a group of 50, 7- to 12-year-old children. Pre-abuse circumstances, child characteristics and post-abuse responses were also relevant.

Abuse Variables

Abuse variables include the nature, duration and severity of the abuse, and the relationship between the abuser and the child. Abuse factors that are associated with more severe psychological sequelae include prolonged duration and greater frequency of abuse (Caffaro-Rouget, Lang, & van Santen, 1989), penetration of mouth, anus or vagina and abuse accompanied by threats or force (Gomes-Schwartz, Horowitz, & Cardarelli, 1990).

Closeness in the relationship between the abuser and the child adversely affects prognosis. Clinical impression suggests a worse prognosis when there have been several abusers, although empirical findings are equivocal on this point (Kendall-Tackett, Williams, & Finkelhor, 1993). Abuse by mothers of their boy neonates (e.g., by sucking their penises) has shown a powerful sexualizing effect on the boys at a very young age (Chasnoff, Burns, Schnoll *et al.*, 1986). There are few available data about the specific effects on girls of abuse by women.

Child Variables

There is no consistent difference in the magnitude or severity of response between boys and girls. Contrary to expectations, there is no conclusive empirical evidence indicating that boys who have been sexually abused show more disruptive behavior than girls. However, boys experience more anxiety about becoming homosexual or about latent homosexuality within them that, they sometimes believe, had been detected by the abuser (Watkins & Bentovim, 1992). The evidence on effects of age at onset of abuse is inconclusive when studied independently of duration of abuse. However, many studies indicate that older children are more symptomatic at the time of presentation. Early sexual abuse, before the age of 7 years, appears to be a risk factor for later inappropriate sexualized behavior (Mian, Marton, & LeBaron, 1996).

Interestingly, the child's coping strategies and cognitive evaluation of the abusive experiences have been shown to contribute less to the child's later functioning than severity of the abuse and the support of the non-abusing carer (Spaccarelli & Kim, 1995). On the other hand, Bal, Van Oost, De Bourdeaudhuij *et al.* (2003) suggest that for adolescents, avoidant coping strategies following sexual abuse are associated with more distress.

Pre-abuse and Family Circumstances

The child's family and the nature of caregiving experienced by the child influence the outcome for the child (Waterman, Kelly, McCord *et al.*, 1993). Pre-existing adverse family relationships and circumstances may have increased the child's prior vulnerability to abuse as well as contributing to the adverse impact of the abuse on the child (Conte & Schuerman, 1988). This includes neglect of supervision; lack of provision for basic needs, which renders the child more vulnerable to predatory abusers; the formation of insecure attachments by the child, which lessens the likelihood of the child talking about worrying experiences such as sexual abuse; and social isolation. In some cases, sexual abuse can be regarded as a marker for other detrimental factors in the family which in themselves contribute significantly to later psychopathology (Mullen *et al.*, 1993; Mullen, Martin, Anderson *et al.*, 1996).

Post-abuse Response

The post-abuse response includes the investigation, the response of the non-abusing caregiver(s) and the abuser, as well as protective steps taken to ensure the child's future safety. Denial of the allegation by the alleged abuser naturally leads to a stringent testing and even discrediting of the child's verbal descriptions (Summit, 1992). Child protective steps, which may include removing the child from their home, are often necessary because of the denial of the abuse by the abuser (Glaser, 1991).

Many mothers remain supportive of their child following discovery of sexual abuse (Sirles & Franke, 1989). The non-abusing carer's belief, support and active protection of the child are significant determinants of a good outcome for the child regardless of the nature of the sexual abuse (e.g., Everson, Hunter, Runyan *et al.*, 1989). Conversely, the mother's emotional distress adversely affects outcome for the child (Cohen & Mannarino, 1998). This points to the need to ensure that at the time of discovery of sexual abuse, help and support are directed at the non-abusing caregiver(s) who are often faced with a conflict of interests, between the abuser and the child. The closer the relationship between the abuser and the non-abusing caregiver, the less supported will the child be by the family (Berliner & Elliott, 1996) and the worse the adjustment of the child (Spaccarelli & Kim, 1995). Abuse by a stepfather or a mother's current boyfriend is a particularly risky circumstance, compromising support of the child by the mother (Elliot & Briere, 1994).

Belief in the child's account of abuse is the first step towards support for the child. It is not, however, synonymous with consistent protection of the child; this requires the primary carer(s) to distance themselves and the child from the abuser, both emotionally and physically. This is particularly difficult when the abuser is the mother's partner (Heriot, 1996).

Model for the Effects of Child Sexual Abuse

Finkelhor and Browne (1985) developed a model to explain the effects of child sexual abuse. This eclectic and comprehensive model reflects the complexity, and consequently the heterogeneous nature of the effects of child sexual abuse. It comprises traumatic sexualization, betrayal, stigmatization and powerlessness.

Traumatic sexualization refers to the abuse experience and combines the trauma and the developmentally inappropriate sexual aspects of the abuse. Finkelhor (1988) postulated that the process of the abuse fetishizes children's genitalia in a developmentally inappropriate way, rewards children for, and confuses children about the meaning and involvement of their sexual behavior, and leads to an association of sexuality with trauma. These aspects are considered to be unique to child sexual abuse.

A sense of betrayal refers to aspects of the child–abuser and child–caregiver relationships. It reflects the fact that abusers have usually been trusted by the child, either inherently by the nature of the relationship, or by the relationship that has been created by the abuser, sometimes deliberately, prior to the abuse. The sense of betrayal also extends to the experience of not being believed by their non-abusing caregivers, especially mothers (Herman, 1981). Young children, who believe in the power of their parents to protect them from harm, lose this sense of safety and protection when they become abused.

Stigmatization concerns the child's emotional response and self-view. It includes the sense of shame, blame and guilt and worthlessness which are both communicated to the child in the process of the abuse and by the way sexual abuse is regarded. Children often seek to "explain" why they were targeted and ascribe self-denigrating meanings. Boys sometimes believe that they must have been recognized as homosexual in order to have been "chosen." Many girls express feelings of having become "spoilt goods" (Rogers & Terry, 1984).

Powerlessness refers to the child's experience of threat or overwhelming fear sometimes associated with sexual abuse and the origin of post-traumatic stress responses. Less traumatically, it also encompasses the child's experience of being overruled and their body invaded and spoiled.

Shapiro (1989) discussed a reciprocal relationship between self-blame and helplessness or powerlessness in sexually abused children. If the child's perception of helplessness is confined to the abuse situation, this may mitigate against self-blame for the abuse. Conversely, if the child blames themself, this may help to overcome the perception of themself as powerless.

Role of Child and Adolescent Mental Health Services in Child Sexual Abuse

Child sexual abuse is sometimes part of the referral presentations and sometimes its occurrence is discovered incidentally during assessment or treatment. Also, some troubled parents will have been sexually abused in childhood. The possibility of abuse in family members therefore always needs to be considered; familiarity with its effects as well as with its investigation, and with protection and legal aspects, is important. Sexual abuse needs to be considered especially in children showing age-inappropriate sexualized behavior and in depressed or suicidal adolescents. At times, an unsolicited disclosure is made by a child during therapeutic work. Child psychologists, psychiatrists and psychotherapists may contribute to investigations of child sexual abuse, particularly in assessment interviews of young or very traumatized children, or in children with communication difficulties. Consultation to social services in case management and to carers of children who have been sexually abused is often requested. A particular role is the provision of individually appropriate treatment for abused children and their families.

Child sexual abuse may also call for forensic work. This includes assessments for Children Act, 1989 proceedings, providing expert reports and oral evidence (Wall, 2000). Comments are usually requested on the presence or absence of Significant Harm and on the nature of the Care Plan, which includes the future care and residence of the child, contact with family members including the abuser, and the child's and family's therapeutic needs. Risk assessments on adolescent abusers may also be required. In the UK, children who have been sexually abused are eligible for Criminal Injury Compensation Authority awards, and child mental health professionals may be requested to provide reports about the nature and extent of the harm to the child and their treatment needs.

Initial Professional Encounters With Child Sexual Abuse – Suspicion, Recognition, Investigation, Validation and Protection

Principles

Whenever sexual abuse is suspected or presented explicitly to a professional, including child mental health practitioners, multidisciplinary professional involvement follows inevitably. Its broad aims are to ascertain what, if anything, has happened to the child and to gain an understanding of the child's development and family context and needs. If the child has been abused, the child's needs will include:

1 The immediate and long-term protection of the child from sexual abuse.

2 The amelioration of the effects of the abuse including:

(i) reduction of distress and the resolution of internal conflicts for the child;

(ii) resolution of interpersonal conflicts surrounding the child;

(iii) treating physical consequences of the abuse.

3 Ensuring optimal development for the child following cessation of abuse.

Although these aims are clear, their achievement in practice is fraught with difficulties. Suspicions need to be verified and a child's account tested, because protection comes at a cost and therapy can only follow protection. Because there are rarely witnesses to the abuse, establishing whether it has occurred will rest heavily on the child's verbal description, which may be retracted even if it was true. Discovery of abuse is often accompanied by denial by the alleged abuser, and some doubt or disbelief, and usually constitutes a crisis for the family and a challenge to the professional system. The child's ultimate well-being will, to a significant extent, be determined by the support given by the family. The nature of the early intervention by professionals and their consideration of the position and needs of the mother or non-abusing caregivers will have long-lasting effects on the child's and the family's subsequent expectations and attitudes towards professionals with whom they may need to continue to work (Sharland, Seal, Croucher *et al.*, 1996).

In some countries, including the UK, the responsibility for child protection rests with social services to whom suspicions of, or actual abuse are reported. The subsequent multidisciplinary and multiagency process involves, in addition, the police, health and education and the courts. In other countries, the responsibility for child protection remains with the courts. A number of well-established steps in the process have been identified (Department for Education and Skills, 2006), each step depending on the outcome of the previous one:

1 Suspicion or recognition leading to referral to (child protection) social services.

2 Establishing whether there is a need for immediate protection.

3 Planning the investigation, including:

interagency discussion;

interviewing the child;

medical examination of the child;

initial assessment of the family.

4 Validation and initial child protection meeting (conference).

5 Protection plan and a more comprehensive assessment.

6 Implementation of plans and review.

7 Prosecution.

8 Therapy.

Different combinations of agencies are involved in the many stages.

Suspicion, Recognition and Disclosure

Suspicion is based on one or more indicators, both specific and non-specific (Glaser & Frosh, 1993). Specific indicators include: inappropriate sexualized behavior (see p. 445), genital physical signs (Hobbs & Wynne, 1989) including sexually transmitted diseases, and pregnancy in a young girl or when the identity of the father is unclear, running away and deliberate self-harm in adolescence, sexual abuse of other children in the family, and known contact with a sexual abuser. Non-specific indicators include a variety of behavioral, emotional and educational difficulties. Sexual abuse needs to be considered especially when there is a sudden onset of difficulties in a previously untroubled child and when no other obvious explanations are available. These difficulties include inability to sustain attention, deterioration in educational progress, social isolation or aggressiveness, indicators of low self-esteem, marked unhappiness or depression, disturbed sleep and nightmares, fearfulness and separation anxiety, and eating disorders.

In child and adolescent psychiatric practice, it is important to consider the possibility of sexual abuse as one explanation for those difficulties that are recognized as effects of sexual abuse. This includes, for instance, sexualized behavior and talk for which a source of exposure needs to be sought. Rather than an initial direct enquiry about sexual abuse, it is preferable to enquire about upsetting and unwanted experiences and previous contact with social services. With adolescents, a direct enquiry could be made, especially following deliberate self-harm. Careful notes should be made of such assessment interviews (Jones, Hopkins, Godfrey *et al.*, 1993) and it is always advisable to discuss one's concerns and suspicions with a colleague. It is also possible to request an "anonymous consultation" with a social worker, in which the child's identity is not divulged. As a result of such assessments, sexual abuse may come to light that may or may not already be known about by child protection agencies. If it is a new disclosure, the child needs to be listened to, avoiding interruptions and questions and the conversation needs to be carefully recorded in writing. Talking about an event enables a child to organize the experience in a more coherent way and enhances the laying down of a more coherent account and memory of the experience (Haden, Haine, & Fivush, 1997). Although the fact of a conversation will distort the memory to some extent, talking improves the later capacity to recall an experience as well as to make sense of it, especially when the experience is stressful or traumatic (Goodman & Quas, 1997).

Although in the UK, unlike in the USA, there is no *mandatory* reporting of seriously suspected or actual sexual abuse, it is considered to be good professional practice to report serious suspicions or disclosures to child protective or social services (Department for Education and Skills, 2006). This overrides the usual rules of confidentiality. A child may not wish for their disclosure to be divulged to another agency. When it is not possible to accede to the child's wishes, the child's misgivings need to be explored, the reasons given for the need to report the abuse, and the child needs to be involved in the process of notifying social services. Referral is usually made with the knowledge of the family, unless there are indicators that this will place the child at increased risk, including pressure on the child to retract an allegation. Abuse more usually comes to light when a child talks about it to a relative, friend or teacher (Bradley & Wood, 1996). Children who spontaneously describe sexual abuse and who make an intentional disclosure are likely to be accurate in their account.

The need for immediate protection is a decision of social services in consultation with other professionals and agencies and might require an emergency protection order in respect of the child (Children Act, 1989).

Investigation and Formal Interview

The next step in the investigative and protection process is a professionals (or strategy) meeting, which is convened by the statutory agencies – police and social services. It will also include any professionals with immediate relevant knowledge about the concerns and about the child and the family, including a professional to whom an allegation or disclosure has been made. This could therefore be a child psychiatrist or other mental health professional. The purpose of the strategy discussion is to plan the investigation, the approach to the family, the formal interview with the child and the medical examination (Heger & Emans, 2000). Children will be interviewed formally if there are clear suspicions of abuse or if the child has already disclosed the abuse informally. Both clinical experience and empirical evidence (Keary & Fitzpatrick, 1994) show that children (especially younger ones) will not usually describe sexual abuse during a formal interview, unless they have previously spoken about it. (However, the converse is not true.) Submitting a child who has not yet actually disclosed abuse to a formal interview may not yield a description of abuse which may, nevertheless, have occurred.

The formal interview is video recorded and may be used both as prosecution evidence in a subsequent criminal trial, and in civil child protection legal proceedings. It is therefore carried out by police and social services according to strictly specified guidelines. Rarely, children are encountered whose distressed or traumatized mental state, or whose difficulties in communication, indicate the need for the interviewing skills of a child mental health professional. Some people have used facilitated communication with autistic children who are suspected of having been abused, but systematic studies have made it clear that what is communicated usually does *not* derive from the child (Howlin & Jones, 1996). This is an unsafe procedure.

In chapter 7 Bruck, Ceci, Kulkovsky *et al.* discuss what is known about children's memory and their reliability as witnesses. Among many other factors not associated with memory but which may, nevertheless, be misinterpreted as poor recall is the extent to which the child is motivated to talk about past events. The child may well continue to be cared for by, or be in close contact with an abuser, and may therefore consider disclosure of the abuse to be a betrayal of the abuser. Silence may be one way of dealing with this dilemma (Freyd, 1996). Children who are interviewed some time after the abuse and who may be suffering from PTSD may find difficulty in talking about the abuse.

The child's responses are by no means related only to the strength of memories or the power of recall. As well as challenging the child's capacity to recall, the child's truthfulness, clarity of thought as opposed to confusion and the child's capacity to withstand misleading suggestions are all often questioned. There is now much research evidence to show that the circumstances in which the child's account is sought and obtained, and the power differential in the relationship between the interviewer and the child, have a significant bearing on the child's "performance" (for a review see Lamb, Sternberg, Esplin *et al.*, 1997). Interviewing styles and forms of questioning are capable of significantly distorting children's accounts which do not then reflect what the child had previously recalled. For instance, when the rapport-building stage of the interview consists of open questions, children's response to the first, open question regarding a past experience yields 2.5 times more details and words than following a closed question. Moreover, this initial pattern continues in response to open questions throughout the interview. Repeated occasions per se, in which the child is simply invited to describe past experiences, without pressure or suggestion, do not compromise accuracy of recall (Fivush & Schwarzmueller, 1995) but there are concerns regarding repeated interviews (see chapter 7). By contrast, closed questions requiring a forced choice, yes or no answers (and not infrequently used by advocates in court) yield far less accurate information. However, in order to obtain optimal information and verify certain facts, closed questions can be alternated with open ones. There are now evidence-based guidelines for obtaining information which is optimal in terms of accuracy and amount of detail (Hershkowitz, Horowitz, Lamb *et al.*, 2004; Orbach, Hershkowitz, Lamb *et al.*, 2000).

There has been much debate about the use of anatomically correct dolls in interviewing of children. There is little evidence that young non-abused children proceed beyond exploration of the dolls' genitalia to enact sexualized behavior (Glaser & Collins, 1989). Nevertheless, the dolls should not be used as a screening tool (Boat & Everson, 1994) or cue (Everson & Boat, 1994), but rather to enable young children to illustrate what they have conveyed verbally.

Validation

Validation of child sexual abuse requires assessment of the evolution of suspicions, and the circumstances as well as the content of the child's first description or disclosure of abuse. The outcome of a formal interview and the findings in a medical examination receive obvious scrutiny, particularly in legal proceedings, both civil and criminal. Other factors include family circumstances; the child's relationship with the alleged abuser; and the responses to the allegation by the mother or the non-abusing caregivers, and by the alleged abuser. In a retrospective review of 551 case notes of reported concerns about possible child sexual abuse, 43% were substantiated, 21% were inconclusive and 34% were not considered to be abuse cases. Only 2.5% were erroneous concerns emanating from children, and included only eight (1.5%) of false allegations originating from the child, and three made in collusion with a parent (Oates, Jones, Denson *et al.*, 2000). In other studies, false allegations are found to be most commonly made by a parent in the context of contact or residence disputes between warring parents, or rarely under the influence of a parent in the context of interparental disputes (Faller, 2005).

The Nature of Protection

A child who is believed to have been abused is deemed to be protected providing all contact with the alleged abuser is either fully supervised or stopped. A child can only be protected in a context in which there is belief in the child's allegations, without explicit blame of the child and where there is a commitment by the child's non-abusing caregiver to protect the child. Children abused by persons outside the family tend to be excluded from child protective services on the, sometimes erroneous (Tebbutt, Swanston, Oates *et al.*, 1997), assumption that they will be protected by their families. If protection is achieved, and if no legal proceedings ensue, there may never be a formal record of the validated fact of the abuse.

Child Protection Conference and Planning

A multidisciplinary child protection conference is convened if there is a reasonable likelihood that a child has been abused *and* remains unprotected. The purpose of a conference is to determine, on the basis of information gathered, whether the child continues to be at risk of Significant Harm and, if so, the nature of the protection plan that will ensure the child's safety. This plan will include a comprehensive assessment of the child's and the family's needs and commencement of therapeutic work, to both of which child mental health services are often required to contribute.

Legal Proceedings

There are both civil and criminal proceedings in which the question of child sexual abuse is at issue (see chapter 8). Civil proceedings concern the future safety of the child. In England under the Children Act (1989) the child's welfare is paramount. The child does not attend court or give evidence; hearsay and expert evidence are allowed. Civil proceedings include:

1 Public law care proceedings in which Significant Harm is determined and a finding may be made about sexual abuse having occurred. The court may grant an order (care or supervision) to ensure the child's well-being and a care plan is required, for which the local authority is responsible.

2 Private law family proceedings in which residence and contact disputes between parents are sometimes based on allegations of sexual abuse of the child while in the care of one of the parents.

In criminal proceedings, the child is an accessory to the court process, whose interest is the determination of the guilt or innocence of the alleged abuser. Unless the alleged abuser pleads guilty, both the child's account of the abuse (which may have previously been video recorded) and cross-examination of the child are required. Expert evidence and opinion regarding the child's credibility is not permitted in English courts, that being an issue for the jury and the judge to decide.

Therapeutic Work

A systematic treatment approach to the effects of child sexual abuse requires consideration of the child's needs, both individually and in the context of the family, but no single programmatic universal treatment is appropriate. Each case needs individual consideration. A starting point is consideration of the individual needs of, and relationships between the three participants in the "abuse triangle" – the abuser, the child and the non-abusive caregiver (Glaser, 1991).

The fulfillment of the child's and family members' needs often requires social work support as well as more formal psychological therapy and psychiatric treatment. An integrated multidisciplinary and multiagency approach is required (Furniss, 1991) in which therapy both deals with needs as they arise and according to their severity, and is offered at appropriate points in the post-abuse process (Jones, 1996). For instance, it is not appropriate for a child to receive group or individual therapy for the effects of the abuse while the child remains unprotected; children in transition from one family to a new permanent home are often more preoccupied with their impermanence and their family's response than with the sexual abuse; it may be inadvisable for a child to join a therapeutic group before testifying in impending criminal proceedings; therapy might need to await the outcome of criminal proceedings if a child has retracted allegations and the alleged abuser denies the abuse. Furthermore, work with the child is most beneficial when undertaken in parallel with work with the parent(s) or carers and family (Monck, Bentovim, Goodall *et al.*, 1996). Some of the child's needs can only be addressed by work with the non-abusing carers alone or with the child and mother/parents together (Celano, Hazard, Webb *et al.*, 1996). For other difficulties, it is appropriate to work with the child alone or in a peer-group setting.

Children's Therapeutic Needs

Not all children who have been sexually abused require prolonged or even systematic therapy. However, as a minimum requirement it is important to ascertain that the child is able to talk about their experiences to a parent or other identified person, who believes the child and is able to listen to the child supportively and uncritically. Coping by avoidance, which includes not talking about the abuse, is a predisposing factor for the later development of PTSD (Kaplow, Dodge, Amaya-Jackson *et al.*, 2005). Children who have been sexually abused also require age-appropriate education about sexuality and the nature and risks of sexual abuse. Many children are symptomatic and therefore require treatment. Whereas some symptoms such as sexualized behavior are readily apparent, others such as PTSD or depression may need to be actively sought. Specific instruments such as the Children's Impact of Traumatic Events Scale – Revised (CITES-R; Wolfe, Gentile, Michienzi *et al.*, 1991), the Trauma Symptom Checklist for Children (Briere, Johnson, Bissada *et al.*, 2001) and measures of depression such as the Childhood Depression Inventory (Kovacs, 1983) are of particular help. It is important to include children who have been abused by strangers or by someone outside the family (Grosz, Kempe, & Kelly, 2000; Van Scoyk, Gray, & Jones, 1988), whose therapeutic needs may be overlooked when protection from reabuse is not considered to be an issue (Sharland *et al.*, 1996).

Overall, treatments that are directed at specific difficulties have been shown to be more effective than no treatment (Finkelhor & Berliner, 1995), or the mere passage of time (Deblinger & Heflin, 1996), and length of treatment has been found to be predictive of outcome for depression (Lanktree & Briere, 1995). There are some findings of no effect (Oates *et al.*, 1994; Tebbutt *et al.*, 1997) or some deterioration for a minority of children during therapy (Jones & Ramchandani, 1999). It is not clear what the relative contribution of intercurrent developments in the child's life or the therapy itself made to the reported deterioration. In the light of the mostly positive outcome for therapy, it would not be appropriate to withhold treatment from symptomatic children. However, these findings point to the importance of monitoring the child's psychological state during treatment and a preparedness to halt therapy if necessary.

There are several ways by which treatment approaches for children can be categorized. Children may be treated individually or in groups; treatment may be directed at specific symptoms; and specific therapeutic approaches such as psychodynamic or cognitive–behavioral therapy (CBT) (Deblinger & Heflin, 1996) may be selected.

Group and Individual Therapy

The shared membership of a group offers an alternative to the secretiveness, isolation and shame experienced by most sexually abused children; this may explain findings from a small sample of children who expressed a preference for group over individual therapy (Prior, Lynch, & Glaser, 1994). The group setting is appropriate for learning about sexuality and for developing a socially appropriate "story" about one's own abuse. The observation of children in groups enables professionals to assess children's further therapeutic needs, which may include longer-term individual psychotherapy.

It is preferable for a group to have more than one child with a particular attribute such as minority ethnicity, abuse by a stranger or living away from home. Groups for children aged over 7 are more appropriately offered separately for boys and girls, and broadly age-banded (Nelki & Watters, 1989). Groups require two therapists of whom one should be a woman. Groups for pre-adolescent children are usually activity-based and follow a program that addresses issues commonly encountered by children who have been abused. These include a range of distressing feelings such as shame, guilt, anger and low self-esteem; sexuality; confiding and secrets (Berliner, 1997). Adolescents are able to use groups for a more reflective exploration of their feelings (Furniss, Bingley-Miller, & Van Elburg, 1988).

Children's attendance in therapy, whether group or individual, is dependent on their parents' psychological and physical support. The provision of support or therapy for the accompanying parent or carer in conjunction with the child's therapy is therefore useful in addressing both emotional and practical issues of the parents (Damon & Waterman, 1986). This can be offered individually or in a group. It also enables the parents to remain involved in, and informed about relevant aspects of the child's therapy, in order to support that process (Rushton & Miles, 2000).

Whereas groups are widely used and their process well documented (e.g., Berman, 1990), a review of published outcome studies of therapy for sexually abused children (Jones & Ramchandani, 1999) found overall little difference in effect between group and individual treatments in improving children's symptoms. In one of the studies reviewed (Trowell, Kolvin, Weeramanthri *et al.*, 2002), the outcome for very troubled girls randomly assigned to individual psychodynamic psychotherapy or group therapy showed significant improvement in a number of symptoms including depression and PTSD of a comparable extent at 1 and 2 year follow-up after both forms of therapy. The only significant difference was a greater decrease in PTSD re-experiencing of trauma, and persistent avoidance of stimuli dimensions, for girls receiving individual therapy.

Specific Symptoms: Sexualized Behavior, PTSD, Anxiety and Depression

Sexualized behavior (e.g., Trowell *et al.*, 1999) and PTSD had been found to be particularly difficult to alleviate. However, CBT directed at particular difficulties has now been shown in a number of randomized treatment studies to be significantly more efficacious than non-directive supportive therapy in improving outcome for sexually abused children. This has included a significant decrease in sexualized behavior (Cohen & Mannarino, 1997), where the effects of therapy have been shown to be enduring for at least a year after completion of treatment (Cohen, Mannarino, & Knudsen, 2005), anxiety and depression. CBT offered to the mother as well as to the child is overall more beneficial and including the family in the CBT has been shown to decrease anxiety in sexually abused children (King, Tonge, Mullen *et al.*, 2000).

An extension of CBT has been shown to be very effective in treating PTSD (Cohen, Mannarino, & Deblinger, 2006). This programmatic, trauma-focused work involves the child and parent. It includes psychoeducation, parenting skills and relaxation for the child. It moves on to recognition of feelings and learning to master and modulate affect, followed by cognitive coping. A narrative about the trauma is then created and leads to the beginning of reprocessing of the traumatic experience, while correcting inaccurate recollections and unhelpful cognitions, and mastering traumatic reminders.

Therapeutic Work with Caregivers and Family

Mothers and Non-abusing Caregivers

The mental health of the non-abusing mother or caregiver, as well as her belief in and support of the child are important factors determining the outcome for a sexually abused child. In the absence of parental support, children may not remain living with their biological family, because of both blame and lack of protection. There are many obstacles to maternal or parental support following the discovery of abuse, which are amenable to change through specific therapeutic work, either individually or in a group. The obstacles include the nature of the relationship between the carer and the abuser and the need for an imposed distance or termination of that relationship; the mother's or carer's guilt about not protecting the child; anger towards the child; and memories of some mothers' own abuse. The discovery of sexual abuse and its aftermath also offer opportunities for helping parents with parenting issues (Celano *et al.*, 1996).

Siblings and the Family

Siblings are sometimes the silent witnesses of abuse and their needs and feelings may be overlooked in the process of attending to the sexually abused child and the mother. Meetings with the whole family can redress this balance, also enabling the family to talk openly about the fact of the abuse, whose mention is often avoided despite the fact that family members are acutely aware of it. However, family meetings would not include the abuser unless they have taken responsibility for the abuse and are receiving treatment. Family work is important when there is indication of blaming or scapegoating of the abused child. Other dysfunctional aspects of family interactions that are associated with child sexual abuse include, in particular, inappropriate intergenerational boundaries, disorganization, parental neglect and unavailability (Bentovim, 1992; Madonna, Van Scoyk, & Jones, 1991). They require more formal family therapy (Elton, 1988).

Work with Abusers

Child and Adolescent Abusers

The treatment of child and adolescent abusers is important in order to prevent progression of abuse into adulthood. The prognosis may be more encouraging than with adult abusers because the adolescent may be less defensive and at a developmental stage when he or she is emotionally vulnerable and responsive to change. Moreover, the child protective and youth justice systems can be instrumental in encouraging attendance at therapy. A particularly important factor is the support, by the young abuser's parents, for the adolescent to own up to the abuse. Without this, it is difficult to offer therapy. Because of the heterogeneous nature of maladaptive cognitions found in adolescent abusers, a number of issues will need addressing in therapy. An approach is required that encompasses both the young abuser's responsibility for the abuse and his likely past emotional, physical or sexual victimization. The indicated therapeutic approach for the abusive behavior is CBT (Kolko, Noel, Thomas *et al.*, 2004), which may be offered individually (Woods, 1997) or in groups (Smets & Cebula, 1987). Using activities as well as words, a group can offer peer support, challenging denial and minimization of the abuse and responsibility for it, sex education, development of social skills, victim awareness, recognition of cognitive distortions concerning the abuse, mapping the abuse cycle (Hawkes, 1999) and learning to halt its progression.

Adult Abusers

The issue of treatment for adult abusers is important for those children who are closely related to their abuser and who wish to resume a meaningful relationship with them. Central to treatment, often carried out in group settings, is reduction of denial by the abuser (Salter, 1988). Initial denial of their involvement is encountered in the majority of abusers. There is commonly also denial of the extent of the abuse, responsibility for the abuse, the harm caused to the child or the inappropriate nature of the sexual contact. CBT has been shown to reduce recidivism in sex offenders (Hanson, Gordon, Harris *et al.*, 2002). Therapy needs to recognize the emotional comfort that denial offers and to acknowledge the cost of assuming responsibility. A metaanalysis of treatment for sex offenders has shown significant reductions in recidivism using CBT (Hanson *et al.*, 2002). The issues described above in adolescent abuser groups also apply to adult abusers. Common to both is the recognition that the risk for returning to child sexual abuse remains a possibility.

Conclusions

Child sexual abuse is a discrete, definable and often repeated event that is embedded in a complex web of contextual factors, both historical and relational. Its antecedents and consequences are manifold and not necessarily specific. For these reasons, specific prevention is particularly difficult and alertness to the possibility and early recognition offer the best hope for damage limitation. Children cannot be relied upon to protect themselves. Secrecy, denial and disbelief are integrally related to sexual abuse and exert a very significant influence on the professional response and outcome for the children and their families.

References

Abel, G., Becker, J., Mittelman, M., Cunningham-Rathier, J., Rouleau, J., & Murphy, W. (1987). Self reported sex crimes in noninarcerated paraphiliacs. *Journal of Interpersonal Violence*, *2*, 3–25.

Abney, V., & Gunn, K. (1993). Culture: A rationale for cultural competency. *APSAC Advisor*, *6*, 19–22.

Ahn, H., & Gilbert, N. (1992). Cultural diversity and sexual abuse prevention. *Social Service Review*, *66*, 410–427.

Alexander, P., & Lupfer, S. (1987). Family characteristics and long-term consequences associated with sexual abuse. *Archives of Sexual Behaviour*, *16*, 235–245.

Baker, A., & Duncan, S. (1985). Child sexual abuse: A study of prevalence in Great Britain. *Child Abuse and Neglect*, *9*, 457–467.

Bal, S., Van Oost, P., De Bourdeaudhuij, I., & Crombez, G. (2003). Avoidant coping as a mediator between self-reported sexual abuse and stress-related symptoms in adolescents. *Child Abuse and Neglect*, *27*, 883–897.

Beitchman, J., Zucker, K., Hood, J., da Costa, G., & Akman, D. (1991). A review of the short-term effects of child sexual abuse. *Child Abuse and Neglect*, *15*, 537–556.

Bentovim, A. (1992). *Trauma organised systems: Physical and sexual abuse in families*. London: Karnac.

Bentovim, A., Boston, P., & van Elburg, A. (1987). Child sexual abuse: Children and families referred to a treatment project and the effects of intervention. *British Medical Journal*, *295*, 1453–1457.

Berliner, L. (1997). Intervention with children who experienced trauma. In D. Cicchetti, & S. Toth (Eds.), *Developmental perspectives on trauma: Theory, research and intervention* (pp. 491–514). Rochester, NY: University of Rochester Press.

Berliner, L., & Conte, J. (1990). The process of victimization: The victim's perspective. *Child Abuse and Neglect*, *14*, 29–40.

Berliner, L., & Elliott, D. (1996). Sexual abuse of children. In J. Briere, L. Berliner, J. Bulkley, C. Jenny, & T. Reid (Eds.), *The APSAC handbook on child maltreatment* (pp. 51–71). London: Sage.

Berman, P. (1990). Group therapy techniques for sexually abused preteen girls. *Child Welfare*, *69*, 239–252.

Bifulco, A., Brown, G., & Adler, Z. (1991). Early sexual abuse and clinical depression in adult life. *British Journal of Psychiatry*, *159*, 115–122.

Boat, B., & Everson, M. (1994). Exploration of anatomical dolls by nonreferred preschool-aged children: Comparisons by age, gender, race, and socioeconomic status. *Child Abuse and Neglect*, *18*, 139–153.

Booth, W. (1890). A preventive home for unfallen girls when in danger. In *Darkest England and the Way Out* (pp. 192–193). London: International Headquarters of the Salvation Army.

Bradley, A., & Wood, J. (1996). How do children tell? The disclosure process in child sexual abuse. *Child Abuse and Neglect*, *20*, 881–891.

Briere, J., Johnson, K., Bissada, A., Damon, L., Crouch, J., Gil, E., *et al.* (2001). The Trauma Symptom Checklist for Young Children (TSCYC): Reliability and association with abuse exposure in a multisite study. *Child Abuse and Neglect*, *25*, 1001–1014.

Briere, J., & Runtz, M. (1989). University males' sexual interest in children predicting potential indices of "paedophilia" in a nonforensic sample. *Child Abuse and Neglect*, *13*, 65–75.

Caffaro-Rouget, A., Lang, R., & van Santen, V. (1989). The impact of child sexual abuse. *Annals of Sex Research*, *2*, 29–47.

Carter, J., Bewell, C., Blackmore, E., & Woodside, D. (2006). The impact of childhood sexual abuse in anorexia nervosa. *Child Abuse and Neglect*, *30*, 257–269.

Celano, M., Hazard, A., Webb, C., & McCall, C. (1996). Treatment of traumagenic beliefs among sexually abused girls and their mothers: An evaluation study. *Journal of Abnormal Child Psychology*, *24*, 1–17.

Chase, E., & Statham, J. (2005). Commercial and sexual exploitation of children and young people in the UK: A review. *Child Abuse Review*, *14*, 4–25.

Chasnoff, M., Burns, W., Schnoll, S., Burns, K., Chisum, G., & Kyle-Spore, L. (1986). Maternal–neonatal incest. *American Journal of Orthopsychiatry*, *56*, 577–580.

Children Act, 1989. (1989). London: HMSO.

Coffey, P., Leitenberg, H., Henning, K., Turner, T., & Bennett, R. (1996). Mediators of the long-term impact of child sexual abuse: Perceived stigma, betrayal, powerlessness, and self-blame. *Child Abuse and Neglect*, *20*, 447–455.

Cohen, J., & Mannarino, A. (1997). A treatment study for sexually abused preschool children: Outcome during a one-year follow-up. *Journal of the American Academy of Child and Adolescent Psychiatry*, *36*, 1228–1235.

Cohen, J., & Mannarino, A. (1998). Factors that mediate treatment outcome of sexually abused preschool children: six and 12 month follow-up. *Journal of the American Academy of Child and Adolescent Psychiatry*, *37*, 44–51.

Cohen, J., Mannarino, A., & Deblinger, E. (2006). *Treating trauma and traumatic grief in children and adolescents*. London: Guilford.

Cohen, J., Mannarino, A., & Knudsen, K. (2005). Treating sexually abused children: 1 year follow-up of a randomized controlled trial. *Child Abuse and Neglect*, *29*, 135–145.

Conte, J., & Schuerman, J. (1988). The effects of sexual abuse on children: A multidimensional view. In G. Wyatt, & G. Powell (Eds.), *The lasting effects of child sexual abuse* (pp. 157–170). CA: Sage.

Conte, J., Wolfe, S., & Smith, T. (1989). What sexual offenders tell us about prevention strategies. *Child Abuse and Neglect*, *13*, 293–302.

Cosentino, S., Meyer-Bahlburg, H., Alpert, J., Weinberg, S., & Gaines, R. (1995). Sexual behavior problems and psychopathology symptoms in sexually abused girls. *Journal of the American Academy of Child and Adolescent Psychiatry*, *34*, 1033–1042.

Damon, L., & Waterman, J. (1986). Parallel group treatment of children and their mothers. In K. MacFarlane, & J. Waterman (Eds.), *Sexual abuse of young children* (pp. 244–298). New York: Guilford.

Davies, G., & Dalgleish, T. (2001). *Recovered memories: Seeking the middle ground*. Chichester: Wiley.

Deblinger, E., & Heflin, A. (1996). *Treating sexually abused children and their non-offending parents: A cognitive behavioural approach*. London: Sage.

Department for Education and Skills. (2006). Department of Health, Home Office. *Working together to safeguard children*. London: The Stationery Office.

Dunne, M., Purdie, D., Cook, M., Boyle, F., & Najman, J. (2003). Is child sexual abuse declining? Evidence from a population-based survey of men and women in Australia. *Child Abuse and Neglect*, *27*, 141–152.

Elliott, D., & Briere, J. (1994). Forensic sexual abuse evaluations: Disclosures and symptomatology. *Behavioural Sciences and the Law*, *12*, 261–277.

Elton, A. (1988). Working with substitute carers. In A. Bentovim, A. Elton, J. Hildebrand, M. Tranter, & E. Vizard (Eds.), *Child sexual abuse within the family: Assessment and treatment* (pp. 238–251). London: John Wright.

Everson, M., & Boat, B. (1994). Putting the anatomical doll controversy in perspective: An examination of major uses of the dolls in child sexual abuse evaluations. *Child Abuse and Neglect*, *18*, 113–129.

Everson, M., Hunter, W., Runyan, D., Edelsohn, G., & Coulter, M. (1989). Maternal support following disclosure of incest. *American Journal of Orthopsychiatry*, *59*, 198–207.

Faller, K. (1989). Characteristics of a clinical sample of sexually abused children: How boy and girl victims differ. *Child Abuse and Neglect*, *13*, 281–291.

Faller, K. (2005). False accusations of child maltreatment: A contested issue. *Child Abuse and Neglect*, *29*, 1327–1331.

Feldman, W., Feldman, E., Goodman, J. T., McGrath, P. J., Pless, R. P., Corsini, L., *et al.* (1991). Is child sexual abuse really increasing in prevalence? Analysis of the evidence. *Pediatrics*, *88*, 29–33.

Fergusson, D., Horwood, J., & Lynskey, M. (1996). Childhood sexual abuse and psychiatric disorder in young adulthood. II. Psychiatric outcomes of childhood sexual abuse. *Journal of the American Academy of Child and Adolescent Psychiatry*, *35*, 1365–1374.

Finkelhor, D. (1984). *Child sexual abuse*. New York: Free Press.

Finkelhor, D. (1988). The trauma of child sexual abuse. In G. Wyatt, & G. Powell (Eds.), *The lasting effects of child sexual abuse* (pp. 61–82). CA: Sage.

Finkelhor, D. (1991). The scope of the problem. In K. Murray, & D. Gough (Eds.), *Intervening in child sexual abuse* (pp. 9–17). Glasgow: Scottish Academic Press.

Finkelhor, D. (2003). The legacy of the clergy abuse scandal. *Child Abuse and Neglect*, *27*, 1225–1229.

Finkelhor, D., & Berliner, L. (1995). Research on the treatment of sexually abused children: A review and recommendations. *Journal of the American Academy of Child and Adolescent Psychiatry*, *34*, 1408–1423.

Finkelhor, D., & Browne, A. (1985). The traumatic impact of child sexual abuse: A conceptualization. *American Journal of Orthopsychiatry*, *55*, 530–541.

Finkelhor, D., Hotaling, G., Lewis, L., & Smith, C. (1990). Sexual abuse in a national survey of adult men and women: Prevalence, characteristics and risk factors. *Child Abuse and Neglect*, *14*, 19–28.

Finkelhor, D., & Jones, L. (2004). *Explanations for the decline in child sexual abuse cases*. Juvenile Justice Bulletin No. NC199298. Washington, DC: Office of Juvenile Justice and Delinquency Prevention.

Finkelhor, D., & Jones, L. (2006). Why have child maltreatment and child victimization declined? *Journal of Social Issues*, *62*, 685–716.

Finkelhor, D., Mitchell, K., & Wolak, J. (2000). Online victimization: A report on the nation's youth. Alexandria, VA: National Center for Missing and Exploited Children.

Fivush, R., & Schwarzmueller, A. (1995). Say it once again: effects of repeated questions on children's event recall. *Journal of Traumatic Stress*, *8*, 555–580.

Fontes, L. (Ed.). (1995). *Sexual abuse in nine North American cultures*. CA: Sage.

Freyd, J. (1996). *Betrayal trauma: The logic of forgetting childhood abuse*. Cambridge, MA: Harvard University Press.

Friedrich, W. (1993). Sexual victimization and sexual behavior in children: A review of recent literature. *Child Abuse and Neglect*, *17*, 59–66.

Friedrich, W., Beilke, R., & Urquiza, A. (1988). Behavior problems in young sexually abused boys: A comparison study. *Journal of Interpersonal Violence*, *3*, 21–28.

Friedrich, W., Fisher, J., Broughton, D., Houston, M., & Shafran, C. (1998). Normative sexual behavior in children: A contemporary sample. *Pediatrics*, *101*, e9.

Frude, N. (1996). Ritual abuse: Conceptions and reality. *Clinical Child Psychology and Psychiatry*, *1*, 59–77.

Furniss, T. (1991). *The multiprofessional handbook of child sexual abuse*. London: Routledge.

Furniss, T., Bingley-Miller, I., & Van Elburg, A. (1988). Goal-oriented group treatment for sexually abused adolescent girls. *British Journal of Psychiatry*, *152*, 97–106.

Gidycz, C., & Koss, M. (1989). The impact of adolescent sexual victimization. Standardized measures of anxiety, depression and behavioral deviancy. *Violence and Victims*, *4*, 139–149.

Glaser, D. (1991). Treatment issues in child sexual abuse. *British Journal of Psychiatry*, *159*, 769–782.

Glaser, D., & Collins, C. (1989). The response of young nonsexually abused children to anatomically correct dolls. *Journal of Child Psychology and Psychiatry*, *30*, 547–560.

Glaser, D., & Frosh, S. (1993). *Child sexual abuse*. London: Macmillan.

Gomes-Schwartz, B., Horowitz, J., & Cardarelli, A. (1990). *Child sexual abuse: The initial effects*. CA: Sage.

Goodman, G., & Quas, J. (1997). Trauma and memory: Individual differences in children's recounting of a stressful experience. In L. Stein, P. Ornstein, B. Tversky, & C. Brainerd (Eds.), *Memory for everyday and emotional events* (pp. 267–294). Mahwah, NJ: Lawrence Erlbaum.

Grosz, C., Kempe, R., & Kelly, M. (2000). Extrafamilial sexual abuse: Treatment for child victims and their families. *Child Abuse and Neglect*, *24*, 9–23.

Haden, C., Haine, R., & Fivush, R. (1997). Developing narrative structure in parent–child conversations about the past. *Developmental Psychology*, *33*, 295–307.

Hamilton, C., & Browne, K. (1999). Recurrent maltreatment during childhood: A survey of referrals to police child protection units in England. *Child Maltreatment*, *4*, 275–286.

Handcock, P. (Ed.). (1932). *The code of Hammurabi*. New York: Macmillan.

Hanson, R., Gordon, A., Harris, A., Marques, J., Murphy, W., Quinsey, V., *et al.* (2002). First report of the collaborative outcome data project on the effectiveness of psychological treatment for sex offenders. *Sexual Abuse*, *14*, 169–194.

Haugaard, J., & Reppucci, N. (1988). *The sexual abuse of children*. San Francisco, CA: Jossey-Bass.

Hawkes, C. (1999). Linking thoughts to actions: Using the integrated abuse cycle. In H. Kemshall, & J. Pritchard (Eds.), *Good practice in working with violence* (pp. 149–167). London: Jessica Kingsley.

Haywood, T., Kravitz, H., Grossman, L., Wasyliw, O., & Hardy, D. (1996). Psychological aspects of sexual functioning among cleric and noncleric alleged sex offenders. *Child Abuse and Neglect*, *20*, 527–536.

Heger, A., & Emans, J. (2000). *Evaluation of the sexually abused child* (2nd edn). Oxford: Oxford University Press.

Heriot, J. (1996). Maternal protectiveness following the disclosure of intrafamilial child sexual abuse. *Journal of Interpersonal Violence*, *11*, 181–194.

Herman, J. (1981). *Father–daughter incest*. Cambridge, MA: Harvard University Press.

Hershkowitz, I., Horowitz, D., Lamb, M., Orbach, Y., & Sternberg, K. (2004). Interviewing youthful suspects in alleged sex crimes: A descriptive analysis. *Child Abuse and Neglect*, *28*, 423–438.

Hobbs, C., & Wynne, J. (1989). Sexual abuse of English boys and girls: The importance of anal examination. *Child Abuse and Neglect*, *13*, 195–210.

Holmes, W., & Slap, G. (1998). Sexual abuse of boys: Definition, prevalence, correlates, sequelae and management. *Journal of the American Medical Association*, *280*, 1855–1862.

Home Office. (2004). *The Sexual Offences Act*. London: The Stationery Office.

Howlin, P., & Jones, D. P. H. (1996). An assessment approach to abuse allegations made through facilitated communication. *Child Abuse and Neglect*, *20*, 103–110.

Jones, D. P. H. (1996). Management of the sexually abused child. *Advances in Psychiatric Treatment*, *2*, 39–45.

Jones, D. P. H., Hopkins, C., Godfrey, M., & Glaser, D. (1993). The investigative process. In W. Stainton-Rogers, & M. Worrel (Eds.), *Investigative interviewing with children* (pp. 12–18). Milton Keynes: Open University Press.

Jones, D. P. H., & Ramchandani, P. (1999). *Child sexual abuse: Informing practice from research*. Abingdon: Radcliffe Medical Press.

Kaplow, J., Dodge, K., Amaya-Jackson, L., & Saxe, G. (2005). Pathways to PTSD. II. Sexually abused children. *American Journal of Psychiatry*, *162*, 1305–1310.

Keary, K., & Fitzpatrick, C. (1994). Children's disclosure of sexual abuse during formal investigations. *Child Abuse and Neglect*, *18*, 543–548.

Kelly, L. (1992). The connections between disability and child abuse: A review of the research evidence. *Child Abuse Review*, *1*, 157–167.

Kelly, L., Regan, L., & Burton, S. (1991). *An exploratory study of the prevalence of sexual abuse in a sample of 16–21 year olds*. London: Polytechnic of North London.

Kendall-Tackett, K., Williams, L., & Finkelhor, D. (1993). Impact of sexual abuse on children: A review and synthesis of recent empirical studies. *Psychological Bulletin*, *113*, 164–180.

Kendall-Tackett, K., Lyion, T., Taliaferro, G. & Little, L. (2005). Why child maltreatment researchers should include children's disability status in their maltreatment studies. *Child Abuse and Neglect*, *29*, 147–151.

Kendler, K., Bulik, C., Silberg, J., Hettema, J., Myers, J., & Prescott, C. (2000). Childhood sexual abuse and adult psychiatric and substance use disorders in women. *Archives of General Psychiatry*, *57*, 953–959.

Kiser, L., Ackerman, B., Brown, E., Edwards, N. B., McColgan, E., Pugh, R., *et al.* (1988). Post traumatic stress disorder in young children: A reaction to purported sexual abuse. *Journal of the American Academy of Child and Adolescent Psychiatry*, *27*, 258–264.

King, N., Tonge, B., Mullen, P., Myerson, N., Heyne, D., Rollings, S., *et al.* (2000). Treating sexually abused children with posttraumatic stress symptoms: A randomized clinical trial. *Journal of the American Academy of Child and Adolescent Psychiatry*, *39*, 1347–1355.

Korbin, J. (Ed.). (1981). *Child abuse and neglect: Cross-cultural perspectives*. Berkeley and Los Angeles, CA: University of California Press.

Korbin, J. (1997). Culture and child maltreatment. In M. Helfer, R. Kempe, & R. Krugman (Eds.), *The battered child* (pp. 29–48). Chicago: University of Chicago Press.

Kolko, D., Noel, C., Thomas, G., & Torres, E. (2004). Cognitive–behavioral treatment for adolescents who sexually offend and their families: Individual and family applications in a collaborative outpatient program. *Journal of Child Sexual Abuse*, *13*, 157–192.

Kovacs, M. (1983). *The Children's Depression Inventory: A self-rated depression scale for school-aged youngsters*. Pittsburgh, PA: University of Pittsburgh School of Medicine.

Lamb, M., Sternberg, J., Esplin, P., Hershkowitz, I., & Orbach, Y. (1997). Assessing the credibility of children's allegations of sexual abuse: A survey of recent research. *Learning and Individual Differences*, *9*, 175–194.

Lanktree, C., & Briere, J. (1995). Outcome of therapy for sexually abused children: A repeated measures study. *Child Abuse and Neglect*, *19*, 1145–1156.

Lanktree, C., Briere, J., & Zaidi, L. (1991). Incidence and impact of sexual abuse in a child outpatient sample: The role of direct inquiry. *Child Abuse and Neglect*, *15*, 447–453.

Lindblad, F., Gustafsson, P., Larson, I., & Lundig, B. (1995). Preschoolers' sexual behavior at day care centers: An epidemiological study. *Child Abuse and Neglect*, *19*, 569–577.

Lloyd Davies, S., Glaser, D., & Kossoff, R. (2000). Children's sexual play and behavior in pre-school settings: Staff's perceptions, reports, and responses. *Child Abuse and Neglect*, *24*, 1329–1343.

Loftus, E. F., Garry, M., & Feldman, J. (1994). Forgetting sexual trauma: What does it mean when 38% forget? *Journal of Consulting and Clinical Psychology*, *62*, 1177–1181.

Madonna, P., Van Scoyk, S., & Jones, D. P. H. (1991). Family interactions within incest and non-incest families. *American Journal of Psychiatry*, *148*, 46–49.

Mannarino, A., Cohen, J., & Berman, S. (1994). The Children's Attributions and Perceptions Scale: A new measure of sexual abuse-related factors. *Journal of Clinical Child Psychology*, *23*, 204–211.

Markowe, H. (1988). The frequency of child sexual abuse in the UK. *Health Trends*, *20*, 2–6.

Martone, M., Jaudes, P., & Cavins, M. (1996). Criminal prosecution of child sexual abuse cases. *Child Abuse and Neglect*, *20*, 457–464.

May-Chahal, C., & Cawson, P. (2005). Measuring child maltreatment in the United Kingdom: A study of the prevalence of child abuse and neglect. *Child Abuse and Neglect*, *29*, 969–984.

McClellan, J., McCurry, C., Ronnei, M., Adams, J., Eisner, A., & Storck, M. (1996). Age of onset of sexual abuse: Relationship to sexually inappropriate behaviours. *Journal of the American Academy of Child and Adolescent Psychiatry*, *35*, 1375–1383.

McKee, L. (1984). Sex differentials in survivorship and customary treatment of infants and children. *Medical Anthropology*, *8*, 91–108.

McLeer, S., Deblinger, E., Henry, D., & Orvaschel, H. (1992). Sexually abused children at high risk for post-traumatic stress disorder. *Journal of the American Academy of Child and Adolescent Psychiatry*, *31*, 875–879.

McLeer, S., Dixon, J., Henry, D., Ruggiero, K., Escovitz, K., Niedda, T., *et al.* (1998). Psychopathology in non-clinically referred sexually abused children. *Journal of the American Academy of Child and Adolescent Psychiatry*, *37*, 1326–1333.

Mian, M., Marton, P., & LeBaron, D. (1996). The effects of sexual abuse on 3- to 5-year-old girls. *Child Abuse and Neglect*, *20*, 731–745.

Monck, E., Bentovim, A., Goodall, G., Lwin, R., & Sharland, E. (1996). *Child sexual abuse: A descriptive and treatment study*. London: HMSO.

Morgan, C., & Fisher, H. (2007). Environmental factors in schizophrenia: Childhood trauma. *Schizophrenia Bulletin*, 33, 3–10.

Morris, J. (1999). Disabled children, child protection systems and the Children Act 1989. *Child Abuse Review*, *8*, 91–108.

Mullen, P., Martin, J., Anderson, J., Romans, S., & Herbison, G. (1993). Childhood sexual abuse and mental health in adult life. *British Journal of Psychiatry*, *163*, 721–732.

Mullen, P., Martin, J., Anderson, J., Romans, S., & Herbison, G. (1994). The effect of child sexual abuse on social, interpersonal and sexual function in adult life. *British Journal of Psychiatry*, *165*, 35–47.

Mullen, P., Martin, J., Anderson, J., Romans, S., & Herbison, G. (1996). The long-term impact of the physical, emotional, and sexual abuse of children: A community study. *Child Abuse and Neglect*, *20*, 7–21.

Muram, D. (1989). Child sexual abuse: Relationship between sexual acts and genital findings. *Child Abuse and Neglect*, *13*, 211–216.

Nasjileti, M. (1980). Suffering in silence: The male incest victim. *Child Welfare*, *59*, 269–275.

Nelki, J., & Watters, J. (1989). A group for sexually abused young children: Unravelling the web. *Child Abuse and Neglect*, *13*, 369–377.

Nelson, E., Heath, A., Madden, P., Cooper, M., Dinwiddie, S., Bucholz, K., *et al.* (2002). Association between self-reported childhood sexual abuse and adverse psychosocial outcomes: Results from a twin study. *Archives of General Psychiatry*, *59*, 139–145.

Oates, R., O'Toole, B., Lynch, D., Stern, A., & Cooney, G. (1994). Stability and change in outcomes for sexually abused children. *Journal of the American Academy of Child and Adolescent Psychiatry*, *33*, 945–953.

Oates, R., Jones, D. P. H., Denson, D., Sirotnak, A., Gary, N., & Krugman, R. (2000). Erroneous concerns about child sexual abuse. *Child Abuse and Neglect*, *24*, 149–157.

Oates, R. (2004). Sexual abuse and suicidal behavior. *Child Abuse and Neglect*, 28, 487–489.

O'Connell, R. (2003). *A typology of cybersexploitation and on-line grooming practices*. University of Central Lancashire: Cyberspace Research Unit.

Orbach, Y., Hershkowitz, I., Lamb, M. E., Esplin, P. W., & Horowitz, D. (2000). Assessing the value of structured protocols for forensic interviews of alleged child abuse victims. *Child Abuse and Neglect*, *24*, 733–752.

Palmer, T. (2005). Behind the screen: Children who are the subjects of abuse images. In E. Quayle, & M. Taylor (Eds.), *Viewing child pornography on the Internet. Understanding the offence, managing the offender, helping the victims* (pp. 61–74). Lyme Regis: Russell House.

Paolucci, E., Genuis, M., & Violato, C. (2001). A meta-analysis of the published research on the effects of child sexual abuse. *Journal of Psychology*, *135*, 17–36.

Powell, R., Leye, E., Jayakody, A., Mwangi-Powell, F., & Morison, L. (2004). Female genital mutilation, asylum seekers and refugees: The need for an integrated European Union agenda. *Health Policy*, *70*, 151–162.

Prior, V., Glaser, D., & Lynch, M. A. (1997). Responding to child sexual abuse: The criminal justice system. *Child Abuse Review*, *6*, 128–140.

Prior, V., Lynch, M. A., & Glaser, D. (1994). *Messages from children: Children's evaluations of the professional response to child sexual abuse*. London: NCH Action For Children.

Quayle, E., & Taylor, M. (2006). Young people who sexually abuse: The role of the new technologies. In M. Erooga, & H. Masson (Eds.), *People who sexually abuse others* (pp. 115–128). London: Routledge.

Read, J., van Os, J., Morrison, A., & Ross, C. (2005). Childhood trauma, psychosis and schizophrenia: A literature review with theoretical and clinical implications. *Acta Psychiatrica Scandinavica*, *112*, 330–350.

Richardson, G. (2005). Early maladaptive schemas in a sample of British adolescent sexual abusers: implications for therapy. *Journal of Sexual Aggression*, *11*, 259–276.

Rogers, C., & Terry, T. (1984). Clinical interventions with boy victims of sexual abuse. In I. Stuart, & J. Greer (Eds.), *Victims of sexual aggression: Treatment of children, women and men* (pp. 91–104). New York: Van Nostrand Reinhold.

Rushton, A., & Miles, G. (2000). A study of a support service for the current carers of sexually abused girls. *Clinical Child Psychology and Psychiatry*, *5*, 411–426.

Russell, D. (1983). The incidence and prevalence of intrafamilial and extrafamilial sexual abuse of female children. *Child Abuse and Neglect*, *7*, 133–146.

Russell, D. (1986). *The secret trauma: Incest in the lives of girls and women*. New York: Basic Books.

Salter, A. (1988). *Treating child sex offenders and victims*. CA: Sage.

Salter, D., McMillan, D., Richards, M., Talbot, T., Hodges, J., Bentovim, A., *et al.* (2003). Development of sexually abusive behaviour in sexually victimized males: A longitudinal study. *Lancet*, *361*, 471–476.

Saradjian, J. (1996). *Women who sexually abuse children*. Chichester: Wiley.

Saunders, B., Villeponeaux, L., Lipovsky, J., & Kilpatrick, D. (1992). Child sexual assault as a risk factor for mental disorder among women: A community survey. *Journal of Interpersonal Violence*, *7*, 189–204.

Seghorn, T., Prensky, R., & Boucher, R. (1987). Childhood sexual abuse in the lives of sexually aggressive offenders. *Journal of the American Academy of Child and Adolescent Psychiatry*, *26*, 262–267.

Sequeira, H., & Hollins, S. (2003). Clinical effects of sexual abuse on people with learning disability. *British Journal of Psychiatry*, *182*, 13–19.

Shapiro, J. (1989). Self-blame versus helplessness in sexually abused children: An attributional analysis with treatment recommendations. *Journal of Social and Clinical Psychology*, *8*, 442–455.

Shapiro, J., Leifer, M., Martone, M., & Kassem, L. (1992). Cognitive functioning and social competence as predictors of maladjustment in sexually abused girls. *Journal of Interpersonal Violence*, *7*, 156–164.

Sharland, E., Seal, H., Croucher, M., Aldgate, J., & Jones, D. P. H. (1996). *Professional intervention in child sexual abuse*. London: HMSO.

Singer, K. (1989). Group work with men who experienced incest in childhood. *American Journal of Orthopsychiatry*, *59*, 468–472.

Sirles, E., & Franke, P. (1989). Factors influencing mothers' reactions to intrafamilial sexual abuse. *Child Abuse and Neglect*, *13*, 131–139.

Skuse, D., Bentovim, A., Hodges, J., Stevenson, J., Andreou, C., Lanyado, M., *et al.* (1998). Risk factors for the development of sexually abusive behaviour in sexually victimised adolescent males: Cross-sectional study. *British Medical Journal*, *317*, 175–179.

Smets, A., & Cebula, C. (1987). A group treatment program for adolescent sex offenders: Five steps towards resolution. *Child Abuse and Neglect*, *11*, 247–254.

Spaccarelli, S., & Kim, S. (1995). Resilience criteria and factors associated with resilience in sexually abused girls. *Child Abuse and Neglect*, *19*, 1171–1182.

Stein, J., Golding, J., Siegel, J., Burnam, M., & Sorensen, S. (1988). Long-term psychological sequelae of child sexual abuse. *Journal of the American Academy of Child and Adolescent Psychiatry*, *27*, 650–654.

Sullivan, P., & Knutson, J. (2000). Maltreatment and disabilities: A population-based epidemiological study. *Child Abuse and Neglect*, *10*, 1257–1273.

Summit, R. (1983). The child sexual abuse accommodation syndrome. *Child Abuse and Neglect*, *7*, 177–193.

Summit, R. (1992). Abuse of the child sexual accommodation syndrome. *Journal of Child Sexual Abuse*, *1*, 153–163.

Taylor, M., & Quayle, E. (2003). *Child pornography: An Internet crime*. London: Bruner Routledge.

Tebbutt, J., Swanston, H., Oates, R., & O'Toole, B. (1997). Five years after child sexual abuse: Persisting dysfunction and problems of prediction. *Journal of the American Academy of Child and Adolescent Psychiatry*, *36*, 330–339.

ten Bensel, R., Rheinberger, M., & Radbill, S. (1997). Children in a world of violence: The roots of child maltreatment. In M. Helfer, R. Kempe, & R. Krugman (Eds.), *The battered child* (pp. 3–28). Chicago: University of Chicago Press.

Tjaden, P., & Thoennes, N. (1992). Predictors of legal intervention in child maltreatment cases. *Child Abuse and Neglect*, *16*, 807–821.

Tremblay, C., Herbert, M., & Piche, C. (1999). Coping strategies and social support as mediators of consequences in child sexual abuse victims. *Child Abuse and Neglect*, *23*, 929–945.

Trowell, J., Kolvin, I., Weeramanthri, T., Sadowski, H., Berelowitz, M., Glaser, D., *et al.* (2002). Psychotherapy for sexually abused girls: Psychopathological outcome findings and patterns of change. *British Journal of Psychiatry*, *180*, 234–247.

Trowell, J., Ugarte, B., Kolvin, I., Berelowitz, M., Sadowski, J., & Le Couteur, A. (1999). Behavioural psychopathology of child sexual abuse in schoolgirls referred to a tertiary centre: A North London study. *European Child and Adolescent Psychiatry*, *8*, 107–116.

Utting, W., Baines, C., Stuart, M., Rolands, J., & Vialva, R. (1997). *People like us. The report of the review of the safeguards for children living away from home*. London: The Stationery Office.

Vander Mey, B. J. (1988). The sexual victimization of male children: a review of previous research. *Child Abuse and Neglect*, *12*, 61–72.

Van Scoyk, S., Gray, J., & Jones, D. P. H. (1988). A theoretical framework for evaluation and treatment of the victims of child sexual assault by a nonfamily member. *Family Process*, *27*, 105–113.

Vizard, E., Monck, E., & Misch, P. (1995). Child and adolescent sex abuse perpetrators: a review of the research literature. *Journal of Child Psychology and Psychiatry*, *36*, 731–756.

Wall, N. (2000). *Handbook for expert witnesses in Children Act cases*. Bristol: Family Law.

Waterman, J., Kelly, R., McCord, J., & Oliveri, M. (1993). *Behind the playground walls: Sexual abuse in preschools*. New York: Guilford Press.

Watkins, B., & Bentovim, A. (1992). The sexual abuse of male children and adolescents: A review of current research. *Journal of Child Psychology and Psychiatry*, *33*, 197–248.

Welldon, E. (1988). *Mother, madonna, whore*. London: Free Association Books.

Westcott, H., & Jones, D. P. H. (1999). The abuse of disabled children. *Journal of Child Psychology and Psychiatry*, *40*, 497–506.

Wild, N., & Wynne, J. (1986). Child sex rings. *British Medical Journal*, *293*, 183–185.

Williams, L. (1994). Recall of childhood trauma: A prospective study of women's memories of child sexual abuse. *Journal of Consulting Clinical Psychology*, *62*, 1167–1176.

Wolak, J., Mitchell, K., & Finkelhor, D. (2006). *Online victimization of youth: Five years later*. Alexandria, VA: National Center for Missing and Exploited Children.

Wolfe, V., Gentile, C., Michienzi, T., Sas, L., & Wolfe, D. (1991). The children's impact of traumatic events scale: A measure of post-sexual abuse PTSD symptoms. *Behavioral Assessment*, *13*, 359–383.

Woods, J. (1997). Breaking the cycle of abuse and abusing: Individual psychotherapy for juvenile sex offenders. *Clinical Child Psychology and Psychiatry*, *2*, 379–392.

Wozencraft, T., Wagner, W., & Pellegrin, A. (1991). Depression and suicidal ideation in sexually abused children. *Child Abuse and Neglect*, *15*, 505–510.

Wyatt, G., & Peters, S. (1986a). Issues in the definition of child sexual abuse in prevalence research. *Child Abuse and Neglect*, *10*, 231–240.

Wyatt, G., & Peters, S. (1986b). Methodological considerations in research on the prevalence of child sexual abuse. *Child Abuse and Neglect*, *10*, 241–251.

Wyatt, G., & Powell, G. (1988). Identifying the lasting effects of child sexual abuse. In G. Wyatt, & G. Powell (Eds.), *The lasting effects of child sexual abuse* (pp. 11–17). CA: Sage.

Young, W., Sachs, R., Braun, B., & Watkins, R. (1991). Patients reporting ritual abuse in childhood: A clinical syndrome. *Child Abuse and Neglect*, *15*, 181–189.

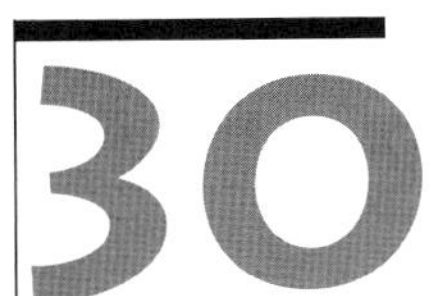

Brain Disorders and their Effect on Psychopathology

James Harris

At one time, major mental disorders were subdivided into those that were "organic" and those that were "functional." This subdivision has been dropped from official classifications because of the evidence that the supposedly "functional" disorders (e.g., schizophrenia) involved major neural dysfunction (see chapter 45). The same applies to neurodevelopmental disorders such as specific language impairment (SLI), dyslexia, autism and attention deficit/hyperactivity disorder (ADHD; see chapter 3). Moreover, empirical findings also showed that disorders that involve a strong environmental influence (such as post-traumatic stress disorder [PTSD], see chapter 42; stress reactions, see chapter 26; or attachment disorders, see chapter 55) included neural effects. The old fashioned dichotomy between brain and mind provides a most misleading simplification (see chapter 12). Nevertheless, there are conditions in which the brain dysfunction effects on psychopathology are more obviously direct (Harris, 1998a,b). It is these disorders that are discussed in this chapter – taking as exemplars acute confusional states (delirium or acute organic reactions), degenerative disorders and fetal alcohol syndrome (FAS), together with the psychopathological effects of cerebral palsy, epilepsy and head injury. Before considering these in turn, it is necessary to discuss the epidemiological evidence on the possible role of brain disorders, considered as a group, in the causation of psychiatric disorders in childhood and adolescence. The psychopathology associated with medical disorders resulting from a chromosomal anomaly or a Mendelian condition is discussed in chapter 24 and will not be dealt with here.

Psychopathology in Young People with Overt Brain Disorders

The first solid epidemiological evidence was provided by the Isle of Wight neuropsychiatric study, which involved total population coverage (Rutter, Graham, & Yule, 1970a). The rates of psychiatric disorder were compared across four groups:

1 those without any form of physical disability (of whom 7% had a psychiatric disorder);
2 those with a physical disability not involving the brain (rate of 12%);
3 those with uncomplicated epilepsy (rate of 29%); and
4 those with cerebral palsy or some other form of structural brain disorder (rate of 44%).

Children with a severe intellectual disability were excluded from all four groups. The findings were clear-cut in showing that the major psychopathological risk was associated specifically with brain dysfunction and not just with a physical disability. However, this risk applies almost as strongly to uncomplicated epilepsy as to structural brain disorders. A further separate study (Seidel, Chadwick, & Rutter, 1975) confirmed the specific risk effect associated with cerebral dysfunction by comparing children with disorders above and below the brainstem. Similar conclusions derived from Breslau's (1985) study of psychiatric disorder in children with physical disabilities.

There can be no doubt that overt brain disorders provide a major risk for psychopathology but, equally, the Isle of Wight studies showed that such disorders were found in less than 10% of the children with psychiatric disorders (Rutter, Graham, & Yule, 1970a; Rutter, Tizard, & Whitmore, 1970b). The latter finding has relevance with respect to the medical study of children presenting with some psychiatric disorders (see chapter 22). Detailed neurological study or investigations should not be a routine. Nevertheless, clinicians need to be alert to the psychopathological effects of key brain conditions that they are likely to encounter – particularly in pediatric liaison work (see chapter 70).

Developmental Perspective

Three elements must be considered in development from infancy to old age: the maturation of the brain (see chapter 12); everyday life experiences at home, at school, and at work (the facilitating environment); and the capacity to master developmental challenges and tasks. Brain disorders may disrupt the consecutive series of reorganizations of brain connections from one developmental stage to the next, and constrain the interplay between nature and nurture (Rutter, 2006).

Changes in the brain are accompanied by changes in the capacity to make sense of the world, to speak and to learn. The prefrontal cortex is one of the last parts of the brain to develop and is particularly vulnerable to environmental insult. Damage or disrupted development of the prefrontal cortex impacts on executive function: planning, anticipating change, regulating emotion and behavior over time. Although brain disorders may be non-progressive, the effects are unlikely to be static because the brain continues to develop right into early adult life.

Rutter's Child and Adolescent Psychiatry, 5th edition. Edited by M. Rutter, D. Bishop, D. Pine, S. Scott, J. Stevenson, E. Taylor and A. Thapar. © 2008 Blackwell Publishing, ISBN: 978-1-4051-4549-7.

Brain disorders may also have a psychopathological impact through effects on life experiences and on the capacity for emotional and cognitive coping and mastery. In typical brain development, the capacity to plan, self-regulate and adapt emerges during the preschool years and continues into adolescence. Working memory, behavioral inhibition and cognitive flexibility are essential components of executive functioning. Through working memory, one holds information in mind, manipulates it mentally and decides what actions to take. Thus, action can take place based on choice and not impulse. The capacity to inhibit allows self-control and self-regulation to resist inappropriate behaviors and urges. Cognitive flexibility results in quick and effective adaptive responses (Davidson, Amso, Anderson *et al.*, 2006; Rubia, Smith, Woolley *et al.*, 2006). In brain disorders, problems with inhibitory brain processes that are important in task mastery are common and may be linked to inattention and hyperactivity (Floden & Stuss, 2006).

The richness of environmental experience facilitates the maturation of the brain. As the brain develops, the individual makes use of new-found capacities to master developmental tasks. The term mastery motivation refers to goal orientation and persistence in completing a task. Task completion, solving a problem or engaging a person is, in itself, intrinsically rewarding and motivates new behavior. In brain disorders, persistence in task mastery is commonly affected and may be delayed or disrupted. A person with a brain disorder may become frustrated by restrictions imposed by others concerned about their safety and by their own difficulty in controlling their impulses, emotions and behavior.

Associations between brain disorders and behavior may be direct; for example, brain systems involved in attention, emotion regulation and inhibition are dysfunctional in children with traumatic brain injury or FAS disorder. Other associations are more indirect, involving psychological effects on self-image such as unrealistic expectations at home and school, family cohesion, parental overprotection and rejection, peer discrimination, inadequate educational programming, and overt physical or sexual abuse. Other stresses relate to medical procedures and repeated hospitalizations that disrupt family life. Both direct and indirect effects must be considered in clinical care; attention also needs to be paid to the ways in which the young person is tackling key developmental tasks and to the manner in which these may be influenced by stigma as well as brain pathology.

Acute Confusional States: Delirium

Young children are especially vulnerable to changes in mental state during medical illness and may be confused by unexpected and unpredictable experiences related to medical care. The most severe change in mental state linked to illness and hospitalization is delirium.

Delirium is a disturbance of consciousness with an acute onset and fluctuating course. It is characterized by disorientation, impaired attention, distortions in language and visuospatial functioning and deterioration in cognition not explained by an underlying dementia (Turkel & Tavare, 2003). Infections and medication use are the most frequent causes but it may result from toxic exposures, metabolic disorder, acute brain injury or fever of any cause.

Clinical Presentation

Developmental factors that make young children vulnerable to confusional states include a poorly established sense of self and of time, and limited verbal ability and narrative capacity to discuss their experiences. Because, with delirium, there are fluctuations in consciousness with lucid intervals alternating with periods of confusion, the time of assessment is critical and repeated interviews may be needed. Children and adults may differ in their presentation (Turkel, Trzepacz, & Tavare, 2006). Children more often are confused, agitated, emotionally labile, oppositional, socially withdrawn, unduly suspicious and have disturbed sleep. In adults, impaired memory, speech problems and depressed mood receive greater emphasis. Impaired alertness, apathy and hallucinations are common to both children and adults. Without careful evaluation, symptoms in children with delirium may be confused with depression (non-verbal, irritable and withdrawn), oppositional defiant behavior (agitation, non-compliance) or paranoia (suspiciousness). Delirium may occur in children, especially in young children, as they emerge from anesthesia; it is more likely to occur when there is excessive anxiety before medical or surgical procedures requiring anesthesia. Delirium is a risk in intensive care units where social isolation (restricted visiting by family members), immobilization, excessive noise and sleep deprivation may occur. Finally, the use of anticholinergic drugs may elicit delirium.

Treatment

Medical treatment of the underlying illness, controlling fever and adequate hydration are essential. The management of delirium involves restoring orientation, providing comfort, soothing the child and helping to make daily experiences more predictable, and restoring the normal day–night rhythm. Familiar toys and photographs of home and family may facilitate orientation. Although low doses of neuroleptic medications used in adults are also used for treatment in children, there are no prospective or retrospective studies regarding their use for this indication in childhood. Delirium rating scales may be used to monitor response to treatment (Turkel, Braslow, Tavare *et al.*, 2003). To prevent emergent delirium following anesthesia, special attention must be paid to reducing preoperative anxiety, providing treatment for postoperative pain and offering a quiet environment for postanesthesia recovery.

Dementia and Other Neurodegenerative Disorders

Clinical psychiatrists and psychologists may encounter dementing conditions as part of pediatric liaison work, when the key issue is how to deal with the psychopathological disturbance. However, when there has been a loss of skills without, as yet, an identifiable neurological disorder, the presentation may lead to an assumption that it is a hysterical conversion disorder (see chapter 57). A loss of skills may also constitute a prominent aspect of certain autism spectrum disorders (see chapter 46). Clinicians therefore need to be aware of how to respond in these various circumstances.

Childhood dementia is characterized by an overall deterioration in mental functioning – with progressive loss of established language, social, self-care and cognitive skills following a period of normal development. Unlike acute confusional states (in which complete recovery tends to follow resolution of the acute medical condition giving rise to the state), dementia is progressive, although the course may involve ups and downs in the level of functioning. The diagnosis of dementia needs to be particularly considered when there are other features suggestive of a brain disorder (e.g., epileptic seizures, visual impairment, tremor and postural disturbance) or when there are relevant risk factors (e.g., a close relative with Huntington disease, a mother with AIDS, recent severe brain trauma or an attack of measles).

The degenerative disorders are fortunately rare; psychiatric or psychological involvement with them ordinarily occurs most commonly on consultation services to help families cope with the diagnosis and ongoing care for the affected child. It is also relevant that dealing with degenerative disorders provides stress for the clinicians. In most circumstances, those working in child and adolescent mental health services do not need to be concerned with the details of specific disorders but, because these are helpful in providing a context, these are provided at the end of this chapter (see p. 469).

Pervasive Developmental Disorder–Autism Spectrum Disorder

The possibility of a neurodegenerative disorder arises in pervasive developmental disorder (PDD) in four main circumstances. First, about one-third of children with autism show a temporary loss of language skills – usually at about 18–24 months (Lainhart, Ozonoff, Coon *et al.*, 2002; see also chapter 46). This phase of regression seems to be particularly characteristic of autism, but there are no published systematic comparisons with other conditions involving language delay. This regression is not dementia because ordinarily it is not progressive and its occurrence neither differentiates it from other cases of autism nor indicates any form of neurodegenerative disorder. The neural basis of the regression is not known, but it might reflect a change in the neural underpinning of language in that age period.

Second, there is a disorder involving a marked decline in cognitive, language and social functioning – usually after age 3 years (but certainly after age 2 years), following a prior period of apparently normal development (Volkmar, Koenig, & Slate, 2005). This was first described by Heller a century ago, using the term "dementia infantilis," but it is now usually called childhood disintegrative disorder. At first sight, this appears to be a neurodegenerative disorder and numerous cases have been investigated for the possibility of some underlying neurological condition. Very occasionally that has been found, but the usual experience is that investigations are non-contributory. Once established, the clinical picture and course is that of other cases of autism spectrum disorder (ASD). Whether or not the disintegrative disorder is an unusual variant of autism (it is far less common), or something different, remains uncertain but despite surface impressions to the contrary, it does not appear to represent any known kind of dementia.

Third, Rett syndrome is a phenotypically distinctive progressive X-linked dominant disorder that almost exclusively affects females (for a detailed description see chapter 24). What is most distinctive clinically is that, following an apparently normal development in the first 6 months of life (and a normal head circumference at birth), there is a slowing or cessation of acquisition of developmental milestones, associated with a failure in head growth and a loss of purposive hand movements. Later there is kyphosis/scoliosis, epilepsy and severe intellectual disability. The great majority of cases are caused by mutation in the *MECP2* gene (Moretti & Zoghbi, 2006).

Finally, there may be occasional confusion with the Landau–Kleffner syndrome (see chapter 47), in which there is loss of language associated with electroencephalogram (EEG) abnormalities and/or epilepsy, but the maintenance of non-verbal IQ.

These disorders involving developmental regressions are clinically important but they do not follow the pattern of childhood dementia.

Fetal Alcohol Spectrum Disorder

For more than a century, clinicians have been concerned over the possible damage to the fetus associated with the mother's very heavy drinking. The turning point, however, came with the observation by Jones, Smith, Ulleland *et al.* (1973) of a characteristic pattern of dysmorphic facial features. The causal role of prenatal alcohol exposure was supported a few years later by the reproduction of similar dysmorphic features and behavioral sequelae in an animal model (Becker, Diaz-Granados, & Randall, 1996). The importance of FAS disorder was that it represented identification of a prenatal risk factor giving rise to an apparently distinctive anthropomorphic and behavioral pattern. The three main criteria for the diagnosis of the full FAS syndrome are:

1 prenatal and postnatal growth retardation with short stature;
2 a triad of facial features: flat philtrum and flat midface, thin upper lip and small palpebral fissures; and
3 evidence of central nervous system dysfunction (behavioral, neurological and/or cognitive disabilities); (American Academy of Pediatrics, 2000; Chudley, Conry, Cook *et al.*, 2005; Hoyme, May, Kalberg *et al.*, 2005).

Since the early reports, a range of studies has shown somewhat similar associations between prenatal alcohol exposure and developmental impairment and psychopathology in individuals without the diagnostic dysmorphic features (Henderson,

Gray, & Brocklehurst, 2007; Stratton, Howe, & Battaglia, 1996; Streissguth & O'Malley, 2000; Streissguth, Bookstein, Barr *et al.*, 2004). Animal studies have clearly shown the neurotoxic effect of prenatal alcohol exposure and have also indicated that there is no clear threshold above which there are sequelae and below which there are not. Human studies too indicate the high likelihood of adverse psychological sequelae even in the absence of dysmorphic features. This recognition led to the subclassification of effects in terms of the full syndrome, a partial syndrome and alcohol-related effects – collectively referred to as fetal alcohol spectrum disorder (Stratton, Howe, & Battaglia, 1996).

The problem is how to recognize this spectrum when the dysmorphic features are absent. Obviously, there must be a history of prenatal alcohol exposure – but how heavy must the exposure be? The full FAS syndrome is most likely with exposure in the first trimester, but there might be risk later in the pregnancy. Does the damage come from cumulative alcohol exposure or from short episodes of very high exposure (as with binge drinking)? We do not know; this remains a matter needing further research.

A normal birth weight would tend to argue against FAS disorder but how much notice should be paid to a low birth weight and impaired postnatal growth? Similarly, cognitive deficits would be in keeping with the possibility of FAS disorder but most instances of cognitive deficit are not caused by alcohol exposure and the pattern of deficits is not clearly distinctive. The deficits may particularly involve executive functioning (Rasmussen, 2005), but this is very broad. There is an ongoing effort to define a cognitive–behavioral phenotype (Nash, Rovet, Greenbaum *et al.*, 2006) but, at least as yet, there is nothing diagnostic at an individual level. Brain imaging findings showing a disproportionate reduction in the size of the corpus callosum have been suggested as a possible biological marker (Bookstein, Connor, Covell *et al.*, 2005), but it is not yet useful at an individual level. The same applies to psychopathology. ADHD, disruptive behavior and poor psychosocial adaptation are all particularly common in children born to women who drank heavily during the pregnancy, but these are common in any group of children. Most critically, if the women continue drinking heavily (as will often be the case with alcoholism), it is extremely problematic to separate the prenatal risks from the postnatal risks associated with an adverse rearing environment. Studies of alcohol-exposed children who have been adopted or fostered (Moe, 2002) point to the reality of prenatal effects (as do animal studies), but in ordinary clinical practice the importance of the postnatal environment has to be assessed.

Given the huge problems in defining the limits of the FAS disorder, it is scarcely surprising that there are equally huge differences in clinicians' willingness to make the diagnosis. In the USA, Sampson, Streissguth, Bookstein *et al.* (1997) estimated a prevalence of 1 per 1000 for the full FAS and nine times that for the partial syndrome. The figures in the UK are a tiny proportion of those in the USA. It is scarcely likely that, given the rates of alcohol consumption in the two countries, these reflect true variations in incidence. It is much more likely that they represent diagnostic practice. It would seem that UK physicians require a lot of evidence before being willing to diagnose FAS disorder, whereas US physicians are willing to make the diagnosis when the probability of a disorder being truly part of the spectrum is much weaker, and are inclined to view the situation in Europe as underdiagnosis. Nevertheless, it has to be agreed that, at present, there are no satisfactory data from which to decide what prevalence figure for the spectrum is correct, or what criteria should be sufficient to diagnose disorders on the spectrum. The concern in the two countries is much the same (Mukherjee, Hollins, & Turk, 2006) and regardless of the diagnostic uncertainties, the preventive needs are great.

Cerebral Palsy

Definition and Classification

Cerebral palsy is the term applied to a non-progressive, but not unchanging, group of disorders of movement and posture that are the consequence of insult to, or anomaly of, the immature nervous system (Neville & Goodman, 2000; Stanley, Blair, & Alberman, 2000). Symptoms usually become apparent in the first months of life when the cerebral palsy is severe, but they are not apparent until after the age of 1 year in about half of mild cases (Stanley, Blair, & Alberman, 2000). Although it is described as a static rather than progressive motoric disability, there are changes that occur as the brain continues to develop. For example, a hypotonic infant may develop spasticity or rigidity and a child who was initially diagnosed as choreoathetoid may subsequently become increasingly dystonic and develop contractures. Such musculoskeletal problems are pervasive and affect the quality of life. With intervention there can be gradual improvement; however, some children reach a plateau. Some may require bracing and surgery. Cognitive functioning ranges from severe intellectual disability to above average intelligence with comparable academic achievement. Epilepsy is common, occurring in about one-quarter to one-third of cases, especially in the more severe varieties of cerebral palsy.

Spastic hemiplegia (one side of body affected, upper extremity involvement greater than lower) is the most common variety of cerebral palsy – followed by the other spastic forms involving both sides of the body and sometimes all four limbs. Less commonly, ataxia and dyskinesia are the main features.

Epidemiology

The incidence of cerebral palsy is estimated to be 1–2 per 1000 live births (Neville & Goodman, 2000; Stanley, Blair, & Alberman, 2000). The overall rate has not changed greatly over time but over the last three decades there has been an increase in the proportion with severe cerebral palsy.

Etiology

One of the striking findings with cerebral palsy is that it

is very rare to find both twins affected, whether the pair is monozygotic (MZ) or dizygotic (DZ). Family studies too find that it is uncommon for cerebral palsy to run in families (Neville & Goodman, 2000). The implication is that genetic influences have a negligible role in causation and the same applies to environmental factors that affect siblings equally. There are recorded cases of cerebral palsy affecting all four limbs that appear to be genetic in origin, but they constitute rare exceptions.

The one clearly established risk factor for cerebral palsy is extreme prematurity. Infants born before 32 weeks' gestation have a risk of cerebral palsy that is up to 13 times higher than that for a term infant. The risk for bilateral spastic cerebral palsy is even greater than that. At one time, birth complications were thought to have a major role but both epidemiological findings (Nelson & Ellenberg, 1986) and brain imaging findings (Neville & Goodman, 2000) have made it clear that they have a very minor role. About 5–15% of cases arise from a central malformation reflecting neuronal migration defects – probably arising in the second trimester. Periventricular pathology accounts for 40–50% of cases; periventricular leukomalacia (a white matter abnormality) is typical (Kuban & Leviton, 1994). In term infants this probably arises preterm, but in very preterm infants the damage may arise in the first weeks of life. About 10–15% of hemiplegic cerebral palsy cases have had a vascular catastrophe in the third trimester. In addition, in about one-third of cases there is no obvious clinical antecedent and the imaging findings are normal. Nevertheless, a variety of neuroimaging techniques are valuable to understand structural and functional brain abnormalities in prematurity (Hoon, 2005), and it is recommended (Bax, Tydeman, & Flodmark, 2006) that children with cerebral palsy should always have magnetic resonance imaging (MRI) to establish the timing and extent of lesions. In medico-legal cases, scans can be reviewed regarding the relationship of pathological findings to prenatal events and those occurring at the time of delivery.

Psychopathology

Both questionnaires and clinical assessments of epidemiological samples have been consistent in showing that psychiatric disorders are found in about half of all individuals with cerebral palsy (Goodman & Yude, 2000). They take a varied form, including both emotional and disruptive disorders to an equal extent. Within a hemiplegic cerebral palsy group, the strongest predictive factor is a lower IQ, but some evidence of bilateral brain involvement and the occurrence of epilepsy also both add to the risk. Various studies have investigated the associations, within a cerebral palsy group, between family functioning and psychopathology. Findings have shown that disorder is associated with higher rates of parental anxiety and depression, more parental criticism of the child (Goodman & Graham, 1996) and a lack of family cohesion (Breslau, 1990).

Two main uncertainties remain. First, do the associations reflect the impact of the family on the child or the other way round? Goodman and Yude (2000) concluded from longitudinal observation that the main explanation was that the parental distress reflected a reaction to the child's problems, and Raina, O'Donnell, Rosenbaum *et al.* (2005) made much the same inference, but evidence on causal direction remains extremely limited. Second, does the presence of cerebral palsy render children more vulnerable to psychosocial adversity? Breslau (1985, 1990), on the basis of a case–control study, concluded not. There was a risk effect from cerebral palsy and from family adversity but there was no evidence of synergism between the two. Again, more evidence is needed to resolve the issue.

It would be a mistake, however, to assume that psychosocial risks always involve the family. Goodman's studies of children with hemiplegic cerebral palsy (and controls) in ordinary schools (Goodman & Yude, 2000; Yude & Goodman, 1999; Yude, Goodman, & McConachie, 1998) found that those with cerebral palsy were more often rejected by their peers, had fewer friends and were more often victimized. Studied over time, lower IQ, disruptiveness and hyperactivity were risk factors for continuing difficulties with peer relationships. Parents also described some of the children with cerebral palsy as naïve in their interpersonal relationships, and as having difficulty understanding social situations. Sorting out cause and effect from epidemiological findings of this kind is difficult, but the implication would seem to be that the brain disorder both increased the likelihood of peer difficulties and decreased the children's ability to understand their meaning and, thereby, to cope with them successfully. It may be, too, that the educational difficulties experienced by some children with cerebral palsy add to the children's stresses.

The conclusions on the origins of the increased rate of psychopathology in children with cerebral palsy are that the main risk usually arises from the brain disorder itself and from the associated cognitive impairment and epilepsy. These features also much increase the risk of peer relationship problems which, in turn, may have a contributory role in the risk for psychopathology. Family dysfunction, when present, doubtless adds to the risk, as it does in all groups of children, but family problems are not exceptionally frequent and probably, at most, play a minor part only in causation. On the other hand, the children's behavior is likely to create stresses for the family (Raina *et al.*, 2005) and a key therapeutic challenge is helping the family function well as a unit.

Goodman and Yude (2000) argued that, in most respects, the treatment of psychiatric disorders in children with cerebral palsy needed to use the same principles and same techniques as those found to be effective in children without the disorder. Nevertheless, there were three differences. First, it is important to help parents realize that it is the child's brain disorder that has created the main reason for the psychiatric problem. Equally, the fact that the brain disorder cannot be removed definitely does not mean that the psychological complications cannot be alleviated. Second, the frequent co-occurrence with epilepsy means that an important need is to ensure proper control of the epileptic attacks and to ensure that the anticonvulsant medication being used does not have an adverse effect on behavior. Third, attention may need to be paid explicitly to the young person's attitude to and method of responding to their disability. This attention should also include ensuring that inappropriate or excessive help from professionals or family is not adding to the child's burden. Clinical experience suggests that parental overprotection can sometimes be an issue.

Epilepsy

The term epileptic attack (or seizure) is applied to an episode of altered brain functioning that is associated with an excessive self-limited neuronal discharge. The diagnosis of epilepsy applies when repeated episodes of this type occur without a detectable extracerebral cause (e.g., diabetic hypoglycemia or anoxia resulting from breath-holding attacks). This definition also excludes the 3% of preschool children who have one or more convulsions provoked by fever. That is because nearly all such febrile convulsions (about 98%) do *not* develop into true epilepsy.

Epilepsy is necessarily of major interest to child psychiatrists for several different reasons. First, it is a common occurrence in both intellectual disability (see chapter 49) and autism (see chapter 46), both of which result in referral to child and adolescent mental health services (CAMHS). Some psychotropic drugs (particularly chlorpromazine, olanzapine and clozapine) lower the seizure threshold, making the occurrence of epileptic seizures slightly more likely (Besag & Berry, 2006). Also, some have risks in pregnancy because of their teratogenic effects. Psychiatrists may be asked to help differentiate between true seizures and pseudoseizures. Young people with epilepsy have a much increased rate of psychopathology. In most societies, epilepsy is a source of stigma and those working in CAMHS may be asked to advise on its prevention or the alleviation of the consequences. Finally, in some countries, psychiatrists are expected to be responsible for the diagnosis and treatment of epilepsy. This chapter is not intended to provide what is needed for those clinicians, who should consult more specialized texts.

Varieties of Epileptic Seizure

The official classification of epileptic seizures (Commission on Classification and Terminology of the International League Against Epilepsy, 1989) uses a scheme that combines clinical features, EEG ictal pattern and EEG interictal pattern. It has a logic but, for present purposes, a strictly clinical classification is used because it focuses attention on the features that clinicians need to be able to recognize.

1 Generalized tonic–clonic seizures ("grand mal"), in which there is loss of consciousness and a characteristic type of convulsion which most people know about.

2 "Petit mal", the much briefer absence attacks, in which mental functioning is interrupted so that the individual seems to "lose touch" but neither falls nor passes out. It is important to appreciate that, uncommonly, these may recur repeatedly in what used to be termed petit mal status. When this happens, there will be a more prolonged episode of impaired and altered mental functioning, which initially may not be recognized as epileptic in origin.

3 Partial seizures, involving localized clonic phenomena not associated with loss of consciousness, but which may proceed to a full generalized tonic–clonic seizure.

4 Atonic "drop attack" seizures that, again, may not initially be recognized as epileptic.

5 Temporal lobe epilepsy (TLE) attacks, in which the onset may involve a rising epigastric feeling of fear. Other complex distortions of higher cognitive functioning follow. There is associated EEG evidence of a temporal lobe origin. The TLE complex partial seizures are usually, but not always, accompanied at other times by generalized seizures. The particular importance of temporal lobe epilepsy is that it is a risk factor for a schizophrenia-like psychosis in adult life (Davison & Bagley, 1969; Ounsted, Lindsay, & Richards, 1987). The evidence is contradictory on whether or not there is also a particularly high risk of psychopathology in childhood.

6 Rarer complex partial seizures deriving from a frontal lobe focus, which tend to be brief (less than a minute) but which are associated with odd movements, postures and vocalizations that may be particularly difficult to differentiate from pseudoseizures (Stores, Zaiwalla, & Bergel, 1991).

There are other varieties of seizure (e.g., myoclonic) but the one that is of most psychiatric interest involves "infantile spasms" in which there are runs of brief jack-knife spasms beginning in infancy, accompanied by a loss of acquired skills, the presence of a hypsarrhythmic EEG and a high rate of psychopathological sequelae (Riikonen & Amnell, 1981). In most cases, a clear cause, such as a major brain malfunction, can be identified. The most important cause to recognize is tuberous sclerosis (Hunt & Dennis, 1987). Where such a cause is absent, the prognosis may be better.

With respect to epilepsy as a diagnosis, a key differentiation is between uncomplicated epilepsy and epilepsy that is associated with some overt brain disorder such as cerebral palsy or severe intellectual disability. The psychopathological consequences are more frequent with complicated epilepsy and cognitive deficits are much greater.

Pseudoseizures

Stores (1999) suggested the following criteria be considered in the diagnosis of pseudoseizures:

1 The attack follows a non-physiological progression or pattern with variable involvement of parts of the body; unusual visual and sensory complaints must arouse suspicion.

2 There is prompt recovery following what is apparently a generalized convulsion.

3 There is disorientation "in person" after the attack.

4 Attacks are never witnessed by others.

5 Attacks are easily induced by verbal suggestion.

6 There is similarity to seizures witnessed in other people.

7 Changes in the nature of the attack are in keeping with differences in attacks witnessed in other people.
8 There is a previous history of somatic responses to stress.
9 Goodman (2002) added a gradual rather than sudden onset.
10 Quivering or uncontrolled flailing.
11 Theatrical semipurposive movements with screaming.
12 The avoidance of painful stimuli and the absence of injury.
13 No EEG change during the attack.

Combined EEG and video monitoring (see chapter 17) should be helpful. What makes differentiation particularly difficult is that pseudoseizures often occur in children who also have true epileptic seizures. Frontal lobe attacks are the ones most easily mistaken for pseudoseizures but it is helpful that these (unlike pseudoseizures) frequently arise during sleep.

Epidemiology and Psychopathology

The prevalence of epilepsy in the general population is about 1%, or slightly less. The peak age of onset is early childhood, but the epilepsy associated with autism is different in having its peak in late adolescence or early adult life (see chapter 46). It is highly likely that this difference has an important pathophysiological meaning, but what that might be remains unknown.

The Isle of Wight survey (Rutter, Graham, & Yule, 1970a) showed that children with epilepsy had a rate of psychiatric disorder (29%) that was four-fold that in children without a physical disorder, and twice that in children with a physical disorder not involving the brain. The findings of the much more recent British Child and Adolescent Mental Health Survey (Davies, Heyman, & Goodman, 2003) were similar. They canvassed over 10,000 children and adolescents and identified 0.7% of 5- to 15-year-olds with a diagnosis of epilepsy. Rates of psychiatric disorder were 37% in persons with epilepsy, 11% in a comparison group with diabetes and 9% in another control group. Clinic studies provide similar findings on the whole (Jalava, Sillanpaa, Camfield *et al.*, 1997; Ott, Siddarth, Gurbani *et al.*, 2003; Pellock, 2004). Claims have been made for particular associations with depression (Baker, 2006) and psychosis (Kanner & Dunn, 2004) but the epidemiological findings are consistent in showing that what is distinctive about epilepsy is the high rate of psychopathology, and *not* an association with any particular psychiatric disorder (other than with rare exceptions).

Most studies have found that children with uncomplicated epilepsy have a mean IQ that is slightly, but only slightly, below 100. However, the meaning of this association remains uncertain. The National Collaborative Perinatal Project, which followed a large general population sample from before birth to 7 years (Ellenberg, Hirtz, & Nelson, 1986), found an overall 10-point IQ deficit, but this dropped to 4 points when comparison was made with sibs rather than population norms. It seems that much of the deficit is probably a result of family factors of some kind rather than the epilepsy as such. In so far as there is minor cognitive impairment, it could reflect the adverse effects of anticonvulsant medication or, very occasionally, the effects of subclinical seizure activity. There does not seem to be a particular pattern of cognition associated with uncomplicated epilepsy but, not surprisingly, there are differences in the cognitive pattern associated with frontal lobe and temporal lobe epilepsy (Culhane-Shelbourne, Chapieski, Hiscock *et al.*, 2002). What is clear from the epidemiological evidence is that, even after taking IQ into account, children with uncomplicated epilepsy have a much increased rate of reading difficulties (Rutter, Graham, & Yule, 1970a).

Etiology of Epilepsy

Twin studies (Berkovic, Mulley, Scheffer *et al.*, 2006; Prasad & Prasad, 2007) have shown a major genetic influence on all varieties of epilepsy – both generalized and focal, plus febrile seizures. EEG patterns, similarly, show a much greater concordance in MZ than DZ pairs. What seems to be different with both focal and febrile seizures is that the DZ concordance rate is much less than half the MZ rate. This points to the likelihood of some kind of synergistic interaction among genes or among allelic variations. Family studies, together with the twin findings, make clear that most cases of uncomplicated epilepsy reflect multifactorial causation, with genetic effects probabilistic rather than determinative (Tan, Mulley, & Scheffer, 2006). Nevertheless, there are rare families showing epilepsy that follows a Mendelian pattern and, in several cases, genes affecting ion channels have been identified (as they have in animal models). The channels are diverse, including those concerned with potassium or sodium and those concerned with glutamate metabolism. Appropriately, but speculatively, the findings have led to suggestions that channelopathies may also be involved in the causation of idiopathic multifactorial varieties of epilepsy (Scott & Neville, 1998; Wong, 2005).

Etiology of the Psychopathology Associated with Epilepsy

The main risk factor involves the brain disorder itself. The finding underlines the reality of the risks associated with abnormal neurophysiological functioning of the brain, although the precise mechanisms involved remain unclear. The rate of psychiatric disorder is twice as high in epilepsy associated with manifest neurological problems (Rutter, Graham, & Yule, 1970a) but it is nevertheless much raised even when these are absent. The evidence is contradictory on whether either high frequency of seizures, or particular types of seizures, increase the risk (Goodman, 2002), as it is too with respect to the adverse effects of inappropriate multiple anticonvulsant use (Hermann, Whitman, & Dell, 1989). Cognitive impairment and associated reading difficulties add to the risk (Rutter, Graham, & Yule, 1970a) and family adversity does too (Grunberg & Pond, 1957; Hermann, Whitman, & Dell, 1989). Social stigma is common too (Gordon & Sillanpaa, 1997); its role in psychopathological risk is unclear but probably it is both a consequence and a cause. Finally, witnessing a seizure is a frightening experience for family members, who also have to cope with the stigma and the effects on them of the child's disturbed behavior (Ellis, Upton, & Thompson, 2000; Hoare, 1984). It must be expected

– although it has not been systematically evaluated – that such impact on the family may also have implications for the development, or course, of psychopathology in the child.

It follows that the handling of psychiatric disorders in young people with epilepsy requires the same broad-based approach as with any other child. Nevertheless, there are several key differences. First, clinicians will need to help families understand the nature of epilepsy and appreciate the psychiatric risks that stem from the disorder itself. Second, it is necessary to be aware of the ways in which some forms of epilepsy (especially frontal lobe and temporal lobe seizures and petit mal status) may not at first sight be recognized as epileptic in nature. Third, careful attention needs to be paid to both adequate seizure control and possible adverse behavioral effects of anticonvulsant medication. Both are well reviewed by Guerrini (2006), Guerrini & Parmiggiani (2006) and Besag (2004a,b). In addition, it will be crucial to ensure an effective liaison and coordination with the neurologist or pediatrician primarily dealing with the epilepsy, and with the psychologist mainly concerned with educational issues.

Traumatic Brain Injury

Traumatic brain injury (TBI) is the most common neurological cause of death and disability in childhood. It has been estimated that in the USA, 185 children per 100,000 under the age of 14 are hospitalized each year for TBI (Kraus & Nourjah, 1988). The comparable figure for the 15–19 age group is 550 per 100,000. The UK figures are probably broadly similar (Middleton, 2001). The assessment of TBI needs to encompass three rather different sets of risk factors. First, there are the features of the TBI itself with respect to both type and severity. The measurement of the duration of both coma and post-traumatic amnesia are well-validated indices, and scales are available for quantification. In recent times, brain imaging is taking over as a more direct index of neural consequences of the injury and of compensatory reorganization of the brain during the recovery process (Munson, Schroth, & Ernst, 2006; Wilde, Chu, Bigler *et al.*, 2006).

Second, there is the cause of the TBI, where the key distinction is between those resulting from physical abuse and those not (Keenan, Runyan, Marshall *et al.*, 2003). The children whose TBI has been inflicted as part of abuse have been found to have more sequelae (Keenan, Hooper, Wetherington *et al.*, 2007). This is likely to reflect both the greater likelihood of previous TBI when the injury has been inflicted (Ewing-Cobbs, Kramer, Prasad *et al.*, 1998) and also the associated psychosocial adversity and the abuse and/or neglect that has not resulted in TBI.

Third, there are the pre-injury circumstances – meaning both the child's own behavior and his or her psychosocial situation. The TBI may result from impulsive risk-taking behavior (more common in boys) leading to falling out of trees or off garage roofs. In some cases the risk-taking may be part of a psychiatric disorder such as ADHD. A severe closed head injury may result in a secondary ADHD (Gerring, Brady, & Chen, 1998; Schachar, Levin, Max *et al.*, 2004) but the ADHD that is evident post-injury may have been present before (Brown, Cladwick, Shaffer *et al.*, 1981) and pre-injury behavioral problems have been found to predict a worse outcome post TBI (Schachar *et al.*, 2004). Also, Max, Schachar, Levin *et al.* (2005) found that psychosocial adversity before the TBI was an independent predictor of secondary ADHD in the second year after injury. The adversity may encompass family dysfunction, parental mental disorder and socioeconomic disadvantage. In summary, the clinical assessment of psychiatric disorder post TBI needs to cover all of these features.

Concussion

A concussion is an alteration in mental status following trauma that may or may not involve a loss of consciousness (Quality Standards Subcommittee, 1997). The term refers to a mild head injury generally occurring after blunt head injury or from whiplash if there is sufficient force applied to the brain. The force of the injury is not sufficient to fracture the skull. In children aged 7–13 years, brain injuries, primarily concussions, are reported in 1–2% of sporting events. Concussions make up approximately 1% of 300,000 sports injuries per year in the USA. Around 3–8% of US high school and collegiate football players experience a concussion each season (Guskiewicz, McCrea, Marshall *et al.*, 2003; McCrea, Guskiewicz, Marshall *et al.*, 2003). There may be no loss of consciousness or a brief loss of consciousness.

Concussion is characterized by transient headache, altered sensorium (dizziness, confusion), fatigue, somnolence, nausea and vomiting that occurs immediately after the injury. The altered mental state results from shear strain on the upper brainstem although no morphological abnormality may be demonstrated in the brain with neuroimaging. There is functional neuronal impairment that is thought to result from abrupt neuronal depolarization, release of excitatory neurotransmitters, ionic shifts, altered glucose metabolism and cerebral blood flow, and impairment in axonal function culminating in axonal injury and neuronal dysfunction (Kelly, 1999).

Children with mild head injury tend to recover without sequelae but problems may ensue with repeated concussions, even if separated over time from one another. Second-impact syndrome refers to a second blow to the head that takes place while still symptomatic from an earlier concussion. The second-impact syndrome may affect the autoregulation of the brain's blood supply. The immature brain may be more vulnerable to diffuse injury with second impact than the adult brain. Considerable caution is required in regard to when an athlete may return to play after a head injury; guidelines are available (Kirkwood, Yeates, & Wilson, 2006; McCrea *et al.*, 2003). Generally postconcussive symptoms will resolve quickly without treatment. Still, there are no accurate neurobiological markers, so recovery must be monitored by repeated physical examination along with standardized behavioral ratings. McCrea *et al.* (2003) prospectively studied the natural recovery from concussion in 1631 football players in 15 US colleges and found that several days may be needed for recovery from symptoms, cognitive dysfunction and postural instability. If there is loss of consciousness, amnesia may occur; it may be temporary and retrograde antedating the injury. Permanent retrograde amnesia for the few seconds or minutes prior to the injury may occur. Moreover, temporary post-traumatic memory loss (anterograde), linked to the ability to form new memories, may last for hours after the injury. With loss of consciousness, late symptoms may occur, so monitoring over time is necessary. Brown *et al.* (1981), in a 2¼-year prospective study, reported that head injuries resulting in a post-traumatic amnesia of less than 1 week did not appreciably increase the long-term psychiatric risk.

Severe traumatic brain injury

TBI is classified as open or closed; the types differ in the pattern of injury and neurobehavioral outcome. Closed head injury results from acceleration, deceleration or rotation of the brain within the skull. Different parts of the brain have different densities and therefore shearing stresses arising during rapid brain movement cause injury. Moreover, compression of blood vessels against the falx cerebri or tentorium may result in infarction of the areas that these blood vessels supply. Open head injury refers to penetration of the skull (e.g., a depressed skull fracture or bullet wound); the extent of damage depends on the specific brain regions damaged. Penetrating traumatic brain injury causes specific and direct loss of neural tissue.

Direct brain injury results in bruising or contusion or tearing (i.e., a laceration of brain tissue). There may be loss of consciousness and post-traumatic amnesia lasting over 24 hours. The damage occurs at the site of impact or more remotely under the skull surface opposite the area of impact (contrecoup injury). Brain laceration in the mediotemporal, posterofrontal and anteroparietal areas is associated with focal signs including post-traumatic seizures; there may be hemorrhage into the brain. Neuroimaging techniques such as computed tomography (CT) or MRI are used in the evaluation.

The most important landmarks for recovery are related to the time of emergence from coma and the time of emergence from post-traumatic amnesia. Immediately after emergence from coma, the child will not be able to form new memories. The time from the accident to the time when new memories emerge is referred to as post-traumatic amnesia. The frequency of post-traumatic amnesia is most likely related to concurrent injury to the temporal lobes. Children with severe head trauma will rarely have specific memories of the accident itself.

Cerebral edema, hematoma formation both inside and outside the brain, and infection are complications of traumatic brain injury that may result in neurological deficits and their effects may be widespread. Moreover, compensatory mechanisms involved in the recovery process itself may alter brain function. Traumatic brain injury is likely to have both neurological and psychiatric complications. Both psychosocial and physiological factors are involved.

Children are more likely than adults to develop early seizures and status epilepticus. Post-traumatic seizures do not necessarily increase the risk of later epilepsy. They are most likely to occur in the first 2 years after injury; approximately 80% occur in the first year and 90% by the second year. For those with penetrating head trauma, up to 50% may develop seizures (Agrawal, Timothy, Pandit *et al.*, 2006). Hydrocephalus may be a late neurological complication, particularly when there is subarachnoid or intraventricular bleeding. Spasticity occurs only in severe brain injury. Post-traumatic hypothalamic dysfunction with endocrine dysfunction can be associated with appetite disturbance, precocious puberty and short stature.

Cognitive and Behavioral Sequelae

Cognitive and behavioral sequelae are common. The length of coma and the duration of post-traumatic amnesia are major factors. Early studies (Brink, Garrett, Hale *et al.*, 1970) that found a strong inverse relationship between duration of coma and subsequent IQ have been confirmed. Psychiatric sequelae may be divided into those that occur during early and late phases of recovery. In the acute phase, behavioral and affective symptoms are related to the neurological presentation. The earliest sequelae appear before the termination of post-traumatic amnesia. Those associated with mild injury include transient symptoms of dizziness, headaches, confusion and fatigue. The most common psychiatric diagnosis is delirium with agitation, loss of orientation and limited attention span. Symptoms commonly noted with more serious injury are transient short-term psychopathological symptoms such as loss of initiative, forgetfulness, emotional lability and irritability. More severe symptoms include extended periods of amnesia, psychotic symptoms, including hallucinations and delusions, and disturbances in the sleep–wake cycle.

In the chronic phase, specific impairments include agnosia, apraxia and aphasia. Persistent symptoms may result in a diagnosis of dementia, with behaviors similar to a frontal lobe syndrome in adults or a post-traumatic change in personality. Social disinhibition, poor impulse control, hyperactivity, attention deficits, disinhibited talk and forgetfulness are among the chronic sequelae. Rutter, Chadwick, and Shaffer (1984) reported that children showed behavioral disinhibition after severe closed traumatic brain injury, with overtalkativeness, ignoring social conventions, impulsiveness and poor personal hygiene. After severe head injury, new psychiatric disorders may be seen in children who were without disorder before the accident. Essentially, there is a dose–response relationship that depends on the severity of brain injury; this suggests a causal relationship. The development of psychiatric disorders in children with severe head injuries is also influenced by pre-accident behavior, intellectual level and psychosocial background. With the exception of social disinhibition and a tendency to show greater persistence of behavioral disturbance over time, psychiatric disorders attributable to head injury do not show specific features (Brown *et al.*, 1981). Max, Levin, Schachar *et al.*s' (2006) detailed follow-up study of children who suffered TBI showed that MRI-diagnosed superior frontal lobe damage was the strongest predictor of personality change but pre-injury poor adaptation also had some predictive value.

Injuries involving focal frontal lobe dysfunction are associated with impulsive aggression and behavioral dyscontrol (Brower & Price, 2001), most often focal orbitofrontal injury. However, the rate of actual aggression is less than often assumed. When forensic issues are raised regarding violent behavior each case should be studied individually, taking into account the type of head injury along with other risk factors, especially a history of physical abuse.

Transient psychotic features may occur occasionally. Hallucinations tend to be less bizarre and more concrete than the typical hallucination in schizophrenia. Nevertheless, post-traumatic psychosis and mania do occur. Moreover, head injury in childhood may accelerate the expression of schizophrenia in families where there is strong genetic predisposition (AbdelMalik, Husted, Chow *et al.*, 2003).

Chadwick, Rutter, Brown *et al.* (1981) correlated the persistence of cognitive deficits with the duration of post-traumatic amnesia. The more persistent deficits were found if there were more than 2 weeks of post-traumatic amnesia. However, when post-traumatic amnesia lasted less than 24 hours, no cognitive sequelae – either transient or persistent – were documented. In the 1-day to 2-week range, the threshold for impairment was associated with the severity of injury. The extent of impairment in intellectual functions depended on the degree of brain damage. Non-verbal test measures (visuospatial and visuomotor) were more highly correlated with the extent of injury than verbal scores. There may be a loss of skills and slower rate of learning with reduced speed of information processing that affect other cognitive skills following the injury. This may be particularly noticeable in school where rapid processing of complex information is required. Recovery was most rapid in the early months following the injury; however, substantial recovery continued for 1 year and into the second year in some children who were severely injured. Age, sex and social class did not significantly affect the course of recovery.

Communication impairments include problems in expressive and written language, naming and deficits in verbal fluency. Persistent verbal memory impairment has been reported as long as 10 years after injury in one-quarter of those studied (Gaidolfi & Vignolo, 1980). Slowed speech, articulation difficulties and lack of prosody may be noted. Preschool children may have problems in syntax and grammar, and older children with more complex language tasks. In school, failure to remember instructions, absentmindedness, attention problems and limited on-task behavior are common complaints. Following moderate to severe TBI, clinical neuropsychological assessment should be used to assess executive functions and their impact on everyday life (see chapter 21). Executive functions may be disturbed because of effects on frontally guided neuronal networks that affect environmental adaptation to changing demands. Slowing of information processing seems to be specifically linked to brain trauma (Levin & Hanten, 2005). Of particular concern in school are deficits in attention and orientation, working memory, semantic representation and self-regulation. These deficits affect educational achievement and are associated with reading problems, difficulty with written language and/or deficits in arithmetic skills.

There is increasing recognition that executive function is frequently impaired by traumatic brain injury in children and may be important in mediating the neurobehavioral sequelae (Levin & Hanten, 2005). Children injured at a younger age may be at greatest risk for impairment. Performance on tests of executive function does not depend only on the frontal lobes. Damage to parietal or temporal lobes can disrupt visuospatial or verbal processing, leading to impaired performance on executive function tests. Finally, the association between total number of lesions and executive function may be linked to disconnections and disruption of frontal–subcortical systems (Slomine, Gerring, Grados *et al.*, 2002).

Family Adjustment and Support

One study of long-term adjustment (Ponsford, Olver, Ponsford *et al.*, 2003) measured family functioning, anxiety and depression, anger control and psychosocial functioning 2–5 years after the injury. Most families were functioning normally. However, anxiety and depression were commonly found in those responsible for the care of their injured relative. The presence of cognitive, behavioral and emotional sequelae was the strongest predictor of anxiety and depression and of unhealthy family functioning. Long-term support and care should be particularly targeted on families whose children have emotional and behavioral problems. Long-term intervention is particularly important when there has been traumatic brain injury induced by child abuse.

Treatment of Traumatic Head Injury and its Consequences

Multidisciplinary cognitive rehabilitation teams (Broman & Michael, 1995; Levin & Hanten, 2005) include physicians (pediatricians, psychiatrists, neurologists), occupational, speech and physical therapists, neuropsychologists and social workers. Although controlled trials are lacking, there are reports of successful interventions for executive function deficits and the teaching of adaptive thinking strategies (Limond & Leeke, 2005). Intervention through retraining and the use of cognitive memory aids is targeted to improve areas of cognitive functioning such as memory, attention, language and perception (Limond & Leeke, 2005).

Behavioral management focuses on skills training and contingency management. Family intervention focuses on helping family members, including siblings (for a meta-analysis of sibling effects see Sharpe & Rossiter, 2002), to accept the nature of the illness, understand the prognosis and to live with uncertainty. Educational interventions are best based on neuropsychological assessment and may require adaptation of the school curriculum. Psychopharmacological interventions for attention disorder, mood lability, anxiety disorders, depression and psychosis may be indicated. However, such interventions are provided with the understanding that children with brain injury may be more sensitive to side-effects of these drugs.

Conclusions and Future Prospects

The importance of brain disorders for clinicians working in CAMHS stems from both the frequency with which they have a role in some of the conditions encountered in CAMHS (such as intellectual disability or autism), and from the more general messages about how the abnormal functioning of brain systems may predispose to psychopathology of the same types seen in young people without a manifest brain disorder. As yet, we have a very limited understanding of the mechanisms involved in the interconnections between brain and mind (but see chapter 12), but important progress is being made. A better understanding will require research on groups with brain disorders (as considered in this chapter), those with somewhat distinctive behavioral phenotypes associated with chromosomal anomalies or genetic disorders (see chapter 24), those with psychopathology that has no manifest connection with a diagnosable brain disorder but which may nevertheless prove to have a neural underpinning that has some role in liability, and in young people without psychopathology – because we need to learn much more about normal development if we are to understand the mechanisms involved in age-related (or age-specific) psychopathological features. Genetic advances (see chapter 23) and advances in imaging (see chapter 11) constitute two vital technologies but, particularly with respect to epilepsy, neurophysiological advances (see chapter 17) and gains in an understanding of basic neuropsychopharmacology (see chapter 16) will also be important. Precisely where such research advances will lead is unclear but what is apparent is that developmental neuropsychiatry is relevant for all practicing clinicians in CAMHS and not just those working in specialized tertiary referral centers.

Appendix

Key Details of Individual Neurodegenerative Disorders Arising in Childhood

HIV Encephalopathy

Considered worldwide, it may well be that human immunodeficiency virus (HIV) is now the most common cause of dementia in childhood (see chapter 58). The extent of the neurotoxic effects of HIV depend on the viral load, the age of the child at the time of the infection, and associated risk features such as malnutrition (Willen, 2006). Some infected children make slow developmental progress; others reach a plateau and fail to advance; and still others have a progressive encephalopathy with gradual and insidious loss of cognitive and motor skills. With improvements in treatment, many children are surviving into adolescence and young adulthood. The young people need to cope with the implications of the diagnosis as well as with the adolescent developmental tasks in coping with a chronic illness (see chapter 57). Adaptation may also be influenced by family stress associated with the death or illness of the primary caregiver.

Subacute Sclerosing Panencephalitis

Subacute sclerosing panencephalitis (SSPE) is a progressive brain disease caused by an infection of the brain by a mutant measles virus (Campbell, Levin, Humphreys *et al.*, 2005). The onset (generally 5–15 years) usually starts with an insidious intellectual deterioration and personality change. The behavior varies markedly from irritability to withdrawal, and from oppositional defiant behavior to inappropriate affection. Myoclonic epilepsy without interruption of consciousness usually follows some months later – the jerking often progresses to frequent gross movements (accompanied by characteristic EEG changes). High titers of measles antibodies are found in the cerebrospinal fluid. In industrialized countries with routine measles immunization programs, SSPE is exceedingly rare, but it is much more common in developing countries that lack such immunization. Even in countries with good immunization procedures, the existence of SSPE is a reminder that measles can be a very serious disease, and that there are significant dangers associated with any reduced take-up of immunization stemming from real or supposed risks.

Batten Disease (Juvenile Onset Neuronal Ceroid Lipofuscinosis)

This diagnosis is applied to a group of neurodegenerative disorders, usually inherited as an autosomal recessive. Its incidence is about 1 per 25,000, making it the most common of the childhood neurodegenerative disorders (Elmslie, Gardiner, & Lehesjoki, 2002). Usually it presents first with visual failure in middle childhood, but obvious dementia follows some years later. The greatest diagnostic difficulty arises at the predementia phase, when "hysterical" blindness may be wrongly identified. Epilepsy usually develops but hard neurological signs are a late event. Because the mutated gene has been identified, DNA tests can confirm the diagnosis.

Wilson Disease

Wilson disease is an autosomal recessive disorder occurring in about 1 person per 30,000 (Packman, 2007). It involves defective copper metabolism (giving rise to reduced copper and caeruloplasmin in the blood and increased copper in the urine). The Kayser–Fleisher ring on the iris is diagnostic. Liver damage is characteristic in the early school years but, after about age 10, neurological features, cognitive decline and non-specific changes in emotional responsiveness and behavior become apparent. Dystonic movements and posturing may be misdiagnosed as conversion hysteria. Early diagnosis is important because administration of the copper bonding agent D-penicillamine may succeed in halting the disease, although side-effects of this treatment can be serious. A mutant gene on chromosome 13 has been identified.

Childhood-Onset X-linked Adrenoleukodystrophy

This X-linked recessive metabolic disorder results from the accumulation of very long chain fatty acids (Moser, Mahmood, & Raymond, 2007). It has a very variable pattern of manifestation in which either adrenal failure or dementia may predominate. Restlessness, inattention, poor concentration and cognitive perplexity are common – very occasionally giving rise to confusion with ADHD (if the adrenal failure is not recognized). Early identification is important because of the possibility of therapies being developed (Moser, Raymond, & Dubey, 2005).

Huntington Disease

Huntington disease is a rare autosomal dominant disease with an incidence of about 3–7 per 100,000 (Hayden, Pouladi, & Kremer, 2007). The typical age of onset is about 40 years, but some 5–10% of cases begin in childhood (Gonzalez-Alegre & Afifi, 2006). The first manifestation in adults usually involves minor motor abnormalities, proceeding to gross chorea, but rigidity tends to be more common in childhood, as do oropharyngeal motor abnormalities. Epilepsy occurs in some 30–50% of children with Huntington disease. Mental deterioration is usually first evident in declining school performance but this goes on to a severe progressive dementia. Various forms of disruptive behavior are common. The gene contains a trinucleotide CAG repeat (see chapter 23), with some tendency for a high number of repeats to be associated with an earlier age of onset. The diagnosis is usually signaled by the family history, of which most members of the family are likely to be aware.

Sanfilippo Syndrome

This is a rare mucopolysaccharidosis – almost always inherited as an autosomal recessive (Spranger, 2007). The syndrome is the only mucopolysaccharidosis that commonly presents with cognitive decline and behavioral problems in childhood. It is clinically suspected on the basis of abundant coarse head hair (often with slightly coarse facial features and mild skeletal changes; see chapter 22). Loss of speech and a severe progressive dementia follow – usually with epilepsy. The diagnosis can be confirmed by measuring urinary mucopolysaccharides.

References

AbdelMalik, P., Husted, J., Chow, E. W., & Bassett, A. S. (2003). Childhood head injury and expression of schizophrenia in multiply affected families. *Archives of General Psychiatry*, *60*, 231–236.

Agrawal, A., Timothy, J., Pandit, L., & Manju, M. (2006). Post-traumatic epilepsy: An overview. *Clinical Neurology and Neurosurgery*, *108*, 433–439.

American Academy of Pediatrics. (2000). Committee on Substance Abuse and Committee on Children With Disabilities. Fetal alcohol syndrome and alcohol-related neurodevelopmental disorders. *Pediatrics*, *106* (2 Part 1), 358–361.

Baker, G. A. (2006). Depression and suicide in adolescents with epilepsy. *Neurology*, *66*, S5–S12.

Bax, M., Tydeman, C., & Flodmark, O. (2006). Clinical and MRI correlates of cerebral palsy: The European Cerebral Palsy Study. *Journal of the American Medical Association*, *296*, 1602–1608.

Becker, H. C., Diaz-Granados, J. L., & Randall, C. L. (1996). Teratogenic actions of ethanol in the mouse: A mini-review. *Pharmacology Biochemistry and Behavior*, *55*, 501–513.

Berkovic, S. F., Mulley, J. C., Scheffer, I. E., & Petrou, S. (2006). Human epilepsies: Interaction of genetic and acquired factors. *Trends in Neuroscience*, *29*, 391–397.

Besag, F. M. (2004a). Behavioral aspects of pediatric epilepsy syndromes. *Epilepsy & Behavior*, *5*, 3–13.

Besag, F. M. (2004b). Behavioural effects of the newer antiepileptic drugs: An update. *Expert Opinion on Drug Safety*, *3*, 1–8.

Besag, F. M., & Berry, D. (2006). Interactions between antiepileptic and antipsychotic drugs. *Drug Safety*, *29*, 95–118.

Bookstein, F. L., Connor, P. D., Covell, K. D., Barr, H. M., & Gleason C. A. (2005). Preliminary evidence that prenatal alcohol damage may be visible in averaged ultrasound images of the neonatal human corpus callosum. *Alcohol*, *36*, 151–160.

Breslau, N. (1985). Psychiatric disorder in children with physical disabilities. *Journal of the American Academy of Child and Adolescent Psychiatry*, *24*, 87–94.

Breslau, N. (1990). Does brain dysfunction increase children's vulnerability to environmental stress? *Archives of General Psychiatry*, *47*, 15–20.

Brink, J. D., Garrett, A. L., Hale, W. R., Nickel, V. L., & Woo-Sam, J. (1970). Recovery of motor and intellectual function in children sustaining severe head injuries. *Developmental Medicine and Child Neurology*, *12*, 565–571.

Broman, S. H., & Michel, M. E. (1995). *Traumatic head injury in children*. Oxford: Oxford University Press.

Brower, M. C., & Price, B. H. (2001). Neuropsychiatry of frontal lobe dysfunction in violent and criminal behaviour: A critical review. *Journal of Neurology, Neurosurgery and Psychiatry*, *7*, 720–726.

Brown, G., Chadwick, O., Shaffer, D., Rutter M., & Traub, M. (1981). A prospective study of children with head injuries. III. Psychiatric sequelae. *Psychological Medicine*, *11*, 63–78.

Campbell, C., Levin, S., Humphreys, P., Walop, W., & Brannan, R. (2005). Subacute sclerosing panencephalitis: Results of the Canadian Paediatric Surveillance Program and review of the literature. *BMC Pediatrics*, *5*, 47–57.

Chadwick, O., Rutter, M., Brown, G., Shaffer, D., & Traub, M. U. (1981). A prospective study of children with head injuries. II. Cognitive sequelae. *Psychological Medicine*, *11*, 49–61.

Chudley, A. E., Conry, J., Cook, J. L., Loock, C., Rosales, T., & LeBlanc, N. (2005). Public Health Agency of Canada's National Advisory Committee on Fetal Alcohol Spectrum Disorder. Fetal alcohol spectrum disorder: Canadian guidelines for diagnosis. *Canadian Medical Association Journal*, *172* (5 Supplement), S1–S21.

Commission on Classification and Terminology of the International League Against Epilepsy. (1989). Proposal for revised classification of epilepsies and epileptic syndromes. *Epilepsia*, *30*, 389–399.

Culhane-Shelburne, K., Chapieski, L., Hiscock, M., & Glaze, D. (2002). Executive functions in children with frontal and temporal lobe epilepsy. *Journal of the International Neuropsychological Society*, *8*, 623–632.

Davidson, M. C., Amso, D., Anderson, L. C., & Diamond, A. (2006). Development of cognitive control and executive functions from 4 to 13 years: Evidence from manipulations of memory, inhibition, and task switching. *Neuropsychologia*, *44*, 2037–2078.

Davies, S., Heyman, I., & Goodman, R. (2003). A population survey of mental health problems in children with epilepsy. *Developmental Medicine and Child Neurology*, *45*, 292–295.

Davison, K., & Bagley, C. R. (1969). Schizophrenia-like psychoses associated with organic disorders of the central nervous system: A review of the literature. *British Journal of Psychiatry, Special Publication*, *4*, 113–118.

Ellenberg, J. H., Hirtz, D. G., & Nelson, D. B. (1986). Do seizures in children cause intellectual deterioration? *New England Journal of Medicine*, *314*, 1085–1088.

Ellis, N., Upton, D., & Thompson, P. (2000). Epilepsy and the family: A review of current literature. *Seizure*, *9*, 22–30.

Elmslie, F., Gardiner M., & Lehesjoki, A. E. (2002). The epilepsies. In D. L. Rimoin, J. M. Connor, R. E. Pyeritz, & B. R. Korf (Eds.), *Emery and Rimoin's Principles and Practice of Medical Genetics* (4th edn., pp. 3036–3075). Philadelphia, PA & London: Churchill Livingstone.

Ewing-Cobbs, L., Kramer, L., Prasad, M., Canales, D. N., Louis, P. T., Fletcher, J. M., *et al.* (1998). Neuroimaging, physical, and developmental findings after inflicted and noninflicted traumatic brain injury in young children. *Pediatrics*, *10*, 300–307.

Floden, D., & Stuss, D. T. (2006). Inhibitory control is slowed in patients with right superior medial frontal damage. *Journal of Cognitive Neuroscience*, *18*, 1843–1849.

Gaidolfi, E., & Vignolo, L. A. (1980). Closed head injuries of school-age children: Neuropsychological sequelae in early adulthood. *Italian Journal of Neurological Science*, *1*, 65–73.

Gerring, J. P., Brady, K. D., & Chen, A. (1998). Premorbid prevalence of ADHD and development of secondary ADHD after closed head injury. *Journal of the American Academy of Child and Adolescent Psychiatry*, *37*, 647–654.

Gonzalez-Alegre, P., & Afifi, A. K. (2006). Clinical characteristics of childhood-onset (juvenile) Huntington disease: Report of 12 patients and review of the literature. *Journal of Child Neurology*, *21*, 223–229.

Goodman, R. (2002). Brain disorders. In M. Rutter, & E. Taylor (Eds.), *Child and adolescent psychiatry* (4th edn., pp. 241–260). Oxford: Blackwell Publishing.

Goodman R., & Graham, P. (1996). Psychiatric problems in children with hemiplegia: Cross-sectional epidemiological survey. *British Medical Journal*, *312*, 1065–1069.

Goodman, R., & Yude, C. (2000). Emotional, behavioral and social consequences. In B. Neville, & R. Goodman (Eds.), *Congenital hemiplegia: Clinics in developmental medicine, No. 150* (pp. 166–178). London: MacKeith Press.

Gordon, N., & Sillanpaa, M. (1997). Epilepsy and prejudice with particular relevance to childhood. *Developmental Medicine and Child Neurology*, *39*, 777–781.

Grunberg, F., & Pond, D. A. (1957). Conduct disorders in epileptic children. *Journal of Neurology, Neurosurgery and Psychiatry*, *20*, 65–68.

Guerrini, R. (2006). Epilepsy in children. *Lancet*, *367*, 499–524.

Guerrini, R., & Parmeggiani, L. (2006). Practitioner review: Use of antiepileptic drugs in children. *Journal of Child Psychology and Psychiatry*, *47*, 115–126.

Guskiewicz, K. M., McCrea, M., Marshall, S. W., Cantu, R. C., Randolph, C., Barr, W., *et al.* (2003). Cumulative effects associated with recurrent concussion in collegiate football players: The NCAA Concussion Study. *Journal of the American Medical Association*, *290*, 2549–2555.

Harris, J. (1998a). *Developmental neuropsychiatry: The fundamentals.* New York: Oxford University Press.

Harris, J. (1998b). *Developmental neuropsychiatry: Assessment, diagnosis and treatment of the developmental disorders.* New York: Oxford University Press.

Hayden, M. R., Pouladi, M. A., & Kremer, B. (2007). Basal ganglia disorders. In D. L. Rimoin, J. M. Connor, R. E. Pyeritz, & B. R. Korf (Eds.), *Emery and Rimoin's principles and practice of medical genetics* (5th edn., pp. 2703–2736). Philadelphia, PA: Churchill Livingstone Elsevier.

Henderson, J., Gray, R., & Brocklehurst, P. (2007). Systematic review of effects of low–moderate prenatal alcohol exposure on pregnancy outcome. *British Journal of Obstetrics and Gynaecology*, *114*, 243–252.

Hermann, B. P., Whitman, S., & Dell, J. (1989). Correlates of behaviour problems and social competence in children with epilepsy, aged 6–11. In B. P. Hermann, & M. Seidenberg (Eds.), *Childhood epilepsies: Neuropsychological, psychosocial and interventions aspects* (pp. 143–157). Chichester: John Wiley.

Hoare, P. (1984). The development of psychiatric disorder among school children with epilepsy. *Developmental Medicine and Child Neurology*, *26*, 3–13.

Hoon, A. H. Jr. (2005). Neuroimaging in cerebral palsy: Patterns of brain dysgenesis and injury. *Journal of Child Neurology*, *12*, 936–939.

Hoyme, H. E., May, P. A., Kalberg, W. O., Kodituwakku, P., Gossage, J. P., Trujillo, P. M., *et al.* (2005). A practical clinical approach to diagnosis of fetal alcohol spectrum disorders: Clarification of the 1996 Institute of Medicine criteria. *Pediatrics*, *115*, 39–47.

Hunt, A., & Dennis, J. (1987). Psychiatric disorder among children with tuberous sclerosis. *Developmental Medicine and Child Neurology*, *29*, 190–198.

Jalava, M., Sillanpaa, M., Camfield, C., & Camfield, P. (1997). Social adjustment and competence 35 years after onset of childhood epilepsy: A prospective controlled study. *Epilepsia*, *38*, 708–715.

Jones, K. L., Smith, D. W., Ulleland, C. H., & Streissguth, A. P. (1973). Pattern of malformation in offspring of chronic alcoholic mothers. *Lancet*, *1*, 1267–1271.

Kanner, A. M., & Dunn, D. W. (2004). Diagnosis and management of depression and psychosis in children and adolescents with epilepsy. *Journal of Child Neurology*, *19* (Supplement 1), S65–S72.

Keenan, H. T., Hooper, S. R., Wetherington, C. E., Nocera, M., & Runyan, D. K. (2007). Neurodevelopmental consequences of early traumatic brain injury in 3-year-old children. *Pediatrics*, *119*, e616–623.

Keenan, H. T., Runyan, D. K., Marshall, S. W., Nocera, M. A., Merten, D. F., & Sinal, S. H. (2003). A population-based study of inflicted traumatic brain injury in young children. *Journal of the American Medical Association*, *290*, 621–626.

Kelly, J. (1999). Traumatic brain injury and concussion in sports. *Journal of the American Medical Association*, *282*, 2283–2285.

Kirkwood, M. W., Yeates, K. O., & Wilson, P. E. (2006). Pediatric sport-related concussion: A review of the clinical management of an oft-neglected population. *Pediatrics*, *117*, 1359–1371.

Kraus, J. F., & Nourjah P. (1988). The epidemiology of mild, uncomplicated brain injury. *Journal of Trauma*, *28*, 1637–1643.

Kuban, K. C., & Leviton, A. (1994). Cerebral palsy. *New England Journal of Medicine*, *330*, 188–195.

Lainhart, J. E., Ozonoff, S., Coon, H., Krasny, L., Dinh, E., Nie, J., *et al.* (2002). Autism, regression, and the broader autism phenotype. *American Journal of Medical Genetics*, *113*, 231–237.

Levin, H. S., & Hanten, G. (2005). Executive functions after traumatic brain injury in children. *Pediatric Neurology*, *33*, 79–93.

Limond, J., & Leeke, R. (2005). Practitioner review: Cognitive rehabilitation for children with acquired brain injury. *Journal of Child Psychology and Psychiatry*, *46*, 339–352.

Max, J. E., Levin, H. S., Schachar, R. J., Landis, J., Saunders, A. E., Ewing-Cobbs, L., *et al.* (2006). Predictors of personality change due to traumatic brain injury in children and adolescents six to twenty-four months after injury. *Journal of Neuropsychiatry and Clinical Neurosciences*, *18*, 21–32.

Max, J. E., Schachar, R. J., Levin, H. S., Ewing-Cobbs, L., Chapman, S. B., Dennis, M., *et al.* (2005). Predictors of secondary attention-deficit/hyperactivity disorder in children and adolescents 6 to 24 months after traumatic brain injury. *Journal of the American Academy of Child and Adolescent Psychiatry*, *44*, 1041–1049.

McCrea, M., Guskiewicz, K. M., Marshall, S. W., Barr, W., Randolph, C., Cantu R. C., *et al.* (2003). Acute effects and recovery time following concussion in collegiate football players: The NCAA Concussion Study. *Journal of the American Medical Association*, *290*, 2556–2563.

Middleton, J. A. (2001). Practitioner review: Psychological sequelae of head injury in children and adolescents. *Journal of Child Psychology and Psychiatry*, *42*, 165–180.

Moe, V. (2002). Foster-placed and adopted children exposed *in utero* to opiates and other substances: Prediction and outcome at four and a half years. *Journal of Developmental and Behavioural Pediatrics*, *23*, 330–339.

Moretti, P., & Zoghbi, H. Y. (2006). MeCP2 dysfunction in Rett syndrome and related disorders. *Current Opinion in Genetics and Development*, *16*, 276–281.

Moser, H. W., Mahmood, A., & Raymond, G. V. (2007). X-linked adrenoleukodystrophy. *Nature Clinical Practice Neurology*, *3*, 140–151.

Moser, H. W., Raymond, G. V., & Dubey, P. (2005). Adrenoleukodystrophy: New approaches to a neurodegenerative disease. *Journal of the American Medical Association*, *294*, 3131–3134.

Mukherjee, R. A., Hollins, S., & Turk, J. (2006). Fetal alcohol spectrum disorder: An overview. *Journal of the Royal Society of Medicine*, *99*, 298–302.

Munson, S., Schroth, E., & Ernst, M. (2006). The role of functional neuroimaging in pediatric brain injury. *Pediatrics*, *117*, 1372–1381.

Nash, K., Rovet, J., Greenbaum, R., Fantus, E., Nulman, I., & Koren, G. (2006). Identifying the behavioural phenotype in fetal alcohol spectrum disorder: Sensitivity, specificity and screening potential. *Archives of Women's Mental Health*, *9*, 181–186.

Nelson, K. B., & Ellenberg, J. H. (1986). Antecedents of cerebral palsy: Multivariate analysis of risk. *New England Journal of Medicine*, *315*, 81–86.

Neville, B., & Goodman, R. (Eds.). (2000). *Congenital hemiplegia*. Cambridge: MacKeith Press.

Ott, D., Siddarth, P., Gurbani, S., Koh, S., Tournay, A., Shields, W. D., *et al.* (2003). Behavioral disorders in pediatric epilepsy: Unmet psychiatric need. *Epilepsia*, *44*, 591–597.

Ounsted, C., Lindsay, J., & Richards, P. (1987). *Temporal lobe epilepsy, 1948–86: A biographical study. Clinics in Developmental Medicine No. 103*. Oxford: MacKeith Press/Blackwell Scientific Publications.

Packman, S. (2007). Copper metabolism. In D. L. Rimoin, J. M. Connor, R. E. Pyeritz, & B. R. Korf (Eds.), *Emery and Rimoin's principles and practice of medical genetics* (5th edn., pp. 2359–2371). Philadelphia, PA: Churchill Livingstone Elsevier.

Pellock, J. M. (2004). The challenge of neuropsychiatric issues in pediatric epilepsy. *Journal of Child Neurology*, *19* (Supplement 1), S1–S5.

Ponsford, J., Olver, J., Ponsford, M., & Nelms, R. (2003). Long-term adjustment of families following traumatic brain injury where comprehensive rehabilitation has been provided. *Brain Injury*, *17*, 453–468.

Prasad, A. N., & Prasad, C. (2007). Genetic aspects of human epilepsy. In D. L. Rimoin, J. M. Connor, R. E. Pyeritz, & B. R. Korf (Eds.), *Emery and Rimoin's principles and practice of medical genetics* (5th edn., pp. 2676–2702). Philadelphia, PA: Churchill Livingstone Elsevier.

Quality Standards Subcommittee. (1997). Practice parameter: The management of concussion in sports (summary statement). *Neurology*, *48*, 581–585.

Raina, P., O'Donnell, M., Rosenbaum, P., Brehaut, J., Walter, S. D., Russell, D., *et al.* (2005). The health and well-being of caregivers of children with cerebral palsy. *Pediatrics*, *115*, 626–636.

Rasmussen, C. (2005). Executive functioning and working memory in fetal alcohol spectrum disorder. *Alcoholism, Clinical and Experimental Research*, *29*, 1359–1367.

Riikonen, R., & Amnell, G. (1981). Psychiatric disorders in children with earlier infantile spasms. *Developmental Medicine and Child Neurology*, *23*, 747–760.

Rubia, K., Smith, A. B., Woolley, J., Nosarti, C., Heyman, I., Taylor, E., *et al.* (2006). Progressive increase of frontostriatal brain activation from childhood to adulthood during event-related tasks of cognitive control. *Human Brain Mapping*, *27*, 973–993.

Rutter, M. (2006). *Genes and behavior: Nature–nurture interplay explained*. Oxford: Blackwell Publishing.

Rutter, M., Chadwick, O., & Shaffer, D. (1984). Head injury. In M. Rutter (Ed.), *Developmental neuropsychiatry* (pp. 83–111). Edinburgh: Churchill Livingstone.

Rutter, M., Graham, P., & Yule, W. (1970a). A neuropsychiatric study in childhood. *Clinics in Developmental Medicine, Nos. 35/36*. London: S.I.M.P./Heinemann.

Rutter, M., Tizard, J., & Whitmore, K. (1970b). *Education, health and behaviour*. London: Longmans.

Sampson, P. D., Streissguth, A. P., Bookstein, F. L., Little, R. E., Clarren, S. K., Dehaene, P., *et al.* (1997). Incidence of fetal alcohol syndrome and prevalence of alcohol-related neurodevelopmental disorder. *Teratology*, *56*, 317–326.

Schachar, R., Levin, H. S., Max, J. E., Purvis, K., & Chen, S. (2004). Attention deficit hyperactivity disorder symptoms and response inhibition after closed head injury in children: Do preinjury behavior and injury severity predict outcome? *Developmental Neuropsychology*, *25*, 179–198.

Scott, R. C., & Neville, G. R. (1998). Developmental perspectives on epilepsy. *Current Opinion in Neurology*, *11*, 115–118.

Seidel, U. P., Chadwick, O. F. D., & Rutter, M. (1975). Psychological disorders in crippled children: A comparative study of children with and without brain damage. *Developmental Medicine and Child Neurology*, *17*, 563–573.

Sharpe, D., & Rossiter, L. (2002). Siblings of children with a chronic illness: A meta-analysis. *Journal of Pediatric Psychology*, *27*, 699–710.

Slomine, B. S., Gerring, J. P., Grados, M. A., Vasa, R., Brady, K. D., Christensen, J. R., *et al.* (2002). Performance on measures of executive function following pediatric traumatic brain injury. *Brain Injury*, *16*, 759–772.

Spranger, J. (2007). Mucopolysaccharidoses. In D. L. Rimoin, J. M. Connor, R. E. Pyeritz, & B. R. Korf (Eds.), *Emery and Rimoin's principles and practice of medical genetics* (5th edn., pp. 2403–2412). Philadelphia, PA: Churchill Livingstone Elsevier.

Stanley, F., Blair, E., & Alberman, E. (2000). Cerebral palsies: Epidemiology and causal pathways. *Clinics in Developmental Medicine, No. 151*. London: McKeith Press.

Stores, G. (1999). Practitioner review: Recognition of pseudoseizures in children and adolescents. *Journal of Child Psychology and Psychiatry*, *40*, 851–857.

Stores, G., Zaiwalla, Z., & Bergel, N. (1991). Frontal lobe complex partial seizures in children: A form of epilepsy at particular risk of misdiagnosis. *Developmental Medicine and Child Neurology*, *33*, 998–1009.

Stratton, K., Howe, C., & Battaglia, F. (1996). *Fetal alcohol syndrome diagnosis, epidemiology, prevention and treatment*. Washington, DC: Institute of Medicine, National Academy Press.

Streissguth, A. P., Bookstein, F. L., Barr, H. M., Sampson, P. D., O'Malley, K., & Young J. K. (2004). Risk factors for adverse life outcomes in fetal alcohol syndrome and fetal alcohol effects. *Journal of Developmental and Behavioral Pediatrics*, *25*, 228–238.

Streissguth, A. P., & O'Malley, K. (2000). Neuropsychiatric implications and long-term consequences of fetal alcohol spectrum disorders. *Seminars in Clinical Neuropsychiatry*, *5*, 177–190.

Tan, N. C., Mulley, J. C., & Scheffer, I. E. (2006). Genetic dissection of the common epilepsies. *Current Opinion in Neurology*, *19*, 157–163.

Turkel S. B., Braslow K., Tavare C. J., & Trzepacz P. T. (2003). The delirium rating scale in children and adolescents. *Psychosomatics*, *44*, 126–129.

Turkel, S. B., & Tavare, C. J. (2003). Delirium in children and adolescents. *Journal of Neuropsychiatry & Clinical Neuroscience*, *15*, 431–435.

Turkel S. B., Trzepacz P. T., & Tavare C. J. (2006). Comparing symptoms of delirium in adults and children. *Psychosomatics*, *47*, 320–324.

Volkmar, F. R., Koenig, K., & Slate, M. (2005). Childhood disintegrative disorder. In F. R. Volkmar, R. Paul, A. Klin, & D. Cohen (Eds.), *Handbook of autism and pervasive developmental disorders* (3rd edn., Vol. 1, pp. 70–87). Hoboken, NJ: Wiley.

Wilde, E. A., Chu, Z., Bigler, E. D., Hunter, J. V., Fearing, M. A., Hanten, G., *et al.* (2006). Diffusion tensor imaging in the corpus callosum in children after moderate to severe traumatic brain injury. *Journal of Neurotrauma*, *23*, 1412–1426.

Willen, E. J. (2006). Neurocognitive outcomes in pediatric HIV. *Mental Retardation and Developmental Disability Research Reviews*, *12*, 223–228.

Wong, M. (2005). Advances in the pathophysiology of developmental epilepsies. *Seminars in Pediatric Neurology*, *12*, 72–87.

Yude, C., & Goodman, R. (1999). Peer problems of 9- to 11-year-old children with hemiplegia in mainstream schools: Can these be predicted? *Developmental Medicine and Child Neurology*, *41*, 4–8.

Yude, C., Goodman, R., & McConachie, H. (1998). Peer problems of children with hemiplegia in mainstream primary schools. *Journal of Child Psychology and Psychiatry*, *39*, 533–541.

31 Psychopathology in Refugee and Asylum Seeking Children

Matthew Hodes

War and organized violence bring death and misery to combatants and civilian populations, especially those who are most vulnerable, such as women and children. Direct attacks may have devastating physical effects, including death and injury, and fear of further violence may cause the flight of surviving communities, with resulting disruption to family and cultural life. It is self-evident that such adversities bring great psychological distress. The massive scale of these events makes this an important topic in understanding international child and adolescent mental health (UNHCR, 2000, 2006).

This chapter reviews some of the major trends in population movements and the backgrounds of asylum seekers and refugees, and then focuses on psychopathology that may occur in young refugees. Factors associated with increased risk and continuity of disorder, as well as those that enhance resilience, are considered. Finally, there is a brief overview of some key issues and implications for mental health service and psychiatric treatment provision.

Population Movements

Population movements to escape persecution, organized violence and economic hardship that may be severe enough to cause famine are long-standing phenomena in human history. However, the 20th century witnessed migrations of far greater numbers of people (Kushner & Knox, 1999). The number of international migrants (defined as those who live outside their country for at least a year) has increased from 75.9 million in 1960 to 174.9 million in 2000 (United Nations Department of Economic and Social Affairs, 2004). Most of the migration is within regions.

War and organized violence have been important causes of migration. It has been estimated that since 1945 there have been at least 160 wars and 24 million war-related deaths (Pedersen, 2002). During the 1970s and 1980s there were proxy wars of the Cold War conflict in South-East Asia, the Horn of Africa, Afghanistan and Central America (UNHCR, 2000). In the 14-year period after the Cold War ended, 1990–2003, there have been 59 major armed conflicts in 48 locations, although only four have involved war between countries (UNICEF, 2004). The collapse of Soviet communism was associated with a reduction of power of many states, and the 1990s saw the destruction of Yugoslavia, an increase in wars in Central Asian areas such as Afghanistan, Chechnya, Tajikistan and Georgia, as well as war and genocide in central Africa including Rwanda (UNHCR, 2000). Since 1991 there has been increased war in the Middle East, especially in Iraq, and continuation of conflict in Gaza and the West Bank involving Israelis and Palestinians.

The United Nations, created in the aftermath of World War II, has had an important global role in monitoring and supporting populations. It defines a refugee as a person who "Owing to well-founded fear of being persecuted for reasons of race, religion, nationality, membership of a particular social group or political opinion, is outside the country of his/her nationality and is unable or, owing to such fear, is unwilling to avail him/herself of the protection of that country; or who, not having a nationality and being outside that country of his/her former habitual residence as a result of such events, is unable or, owing to such fear, is unwilling to return to it" (UNHCR, 2000). A displaced person may experience the same kinds of threat but remains within his or her national borders.

People of concern to the UNHCR include those who leave their own countries (refugees, whose legal rights are recognized, and asylum seekers who are applying for refugee status) as well as those who are displaced within their national borders, or are returning refugees. From 1995 to 2005, the overall number had been fluctuating at around 20 million. In 2006 32.9 million people were of concern, of whom 9.7 million were in Africa, 14.9 million in Asia, 3.4 million in Europe, and 3.5 million in Latin American and the Caribbean (UNHCR, 2007). From 2000 to 2004, the numbers of asylum applications submitted to the top five European countries were: UK 393,800; Germany 324,100; France 270,300; Austria 144,800; and Sweden 127,300. The main countries of origin of asylum applicants in the top 10 European receiving countries were Serbia and Montenegro, Iraq, Turkey, Afghanistan and the Russian Federation (UNHCR, 2006).

Over the 15 years until 1998 it was estimated that approximately 300,000 refugees and asylum seekers came to the UK (Bardsley & Storkey, 2000). In 2004, there were 33,960 asylum applications in the UK. Most of the applicants were from Iran, Somalia, China, Zimbabwe and Pakistan (Home Office, 2005). In the same year, 54,310 people, including

Rutter's Child and Adolescent Psychiatry, 5th edition. Edited by M. Rutter, D. Bishop, D. Pine, S. Scott, J. Stevenson, E. Taylor and A. Thapar. © 2008 Blackwell Publishing, ISBN: 978-1-4051-4549-7.

dependants, were accepted for permanent settlement (reflecting the fact that some people sought asylum before 2004).

For a variety of reasons it is difficult to obtain accurate figures on the numbers of people who are asylum seekers and have obtained refugee status in any one country. A high proportion of asylum seekers may not obtain the right to remain in a resettlement country, and leave that country after a short period. Years may elapse until applications are processed, and there may be many legal steps to obtain the legal right to remain. Some asylum seekers may reside in a country illegally. Others will obtain the right to remain and may then move between countries.

A further issue is that there may be many motives for migrating in the aftermath of war or organized violence. Wars result in loss of life to combatants and civilians, and destruction of property, but also contribute to many other difficulties such as economic collapse, poor food supplies and famine (Southall & O'Hare, 2002). Displacement will disrupt the continuation of important community activities including provision of health care and education (UNICEF, 2004). Thus, people categorized as "immigrants," whose expressed reason for resettlement is to improve economic standing and life chances, may have experienced some of the same war events as asylum seekers or refugees, even if they were less frequent (Silove, Steel, McGorry *et al.*, 1998).

Methodological Considerations

Refugees are a heterogeneous group, and this has major implications for research. In addition to the usual demographic variables, age and sex, the refugee population may also be ethnically and linguistically diverse. This introduces considerable complexity for carrying out research as instruments need to be selected according to the age of the subjects and translated. There are standard procedures for translating instruments used in psychiatric research, and these are generally applicable to work with young people (Westermeyer & Janca, 1997). The legal status of the subjects may be an important issue, as this is associated with different rights and will influence economic status and housing provision (e.g., asylum seekers in the UK are unable to work, while those with the legal right to remain have this entitlement, and also have access to permanent housing). A further factor is the duration of settlement. Over time, asylum seekers, some of whom will acquire legal rights to settlement, will build up social networks and acquire greater linguistic ability in the language of the host country (Hauff & Vaglum, 1997).

Asylum seekers and refugees generally have a high level of mobility, although there are exceptions (e.g., people who are displaced but forcibly settled). This means that care is needed over sampling for studies. While random sampling may be the ideal for epidemiological studies (Mollica, Poole, Son *et al.*, 1997), the sample may need to be derived from municipality (local government) lists or areas (Thabet, Abed, & Vostanis, 2002). Research with children and adolescents is facilitated as children who are asylum seekers, as well as refugees, have entitlement to many welfare services including education. Many studies have used school registers as a way of defining the sample (Fazel & Stein, 2003; Leavey, Hollins, King *et al.*, 2004; Smith, Perrin, Yule *et al.*, 2002; Tousignant, Habimana, Biron *et al.*, 1999). Other studies have selected children on the basis of agency support, such as social services that have responsibilities for unaccompanied asylum seeking children (Wade, Mitchell, & Baylis, 2005). Other techniques may be needed to access refugees, such as targeted sampling (e.g., recruiting from ethnic or religious centers), convenience sampling and snowball sampling. Interestingly, in one of the few studies that has looked at these methods, the sample characteristics were only slightly different according to method of recruitment, probably because of the care with which the study was carried out, including adequate sample size (Spring, Westermeyer, Halcon *et al.*, 2003).

Refugees will be heterogeneous with respect to the kinds of war events and other adversities they have experienced (see chapter 25), and so consideration needs to be given to the way these are assessed. A number of instruments have been developed for the assessment of exposure to war and torture, initially developed for use with adults but since widely used for the investigation of adolescents (Hollifield, Warner, Lian *et al.*, 2002). Some instruments such as the Harvard Trauma Scale (Mollica, Caspi-Yavin, Bollini *et al.*, 1992) have been widely used, their brevity makes them accessible, and they show statistically significant associations with health status (Hollifield *et al.*, 2002; Willis & Gonzalez, 1998). Interview methods of assessments of past traumatic events and adversities may be preferable (Rutter & Sandberg, 1992; Sandberg, Rutter, Giles *et al.*, 1993), but their benefit with this population which has often experienced very high levels of trauma has not yet been established. One particular issue is that memories of past events may be unstable (Herlihy, Scragg, & Turner, 2002; Spinhoven, Bean & Eurelings-Bontekoe, 2006).

There are a number of ethical considerations for research with refugees, who are a vulnerable population (Leaning, 2001). Asylum seekers in particular may have fears regarding disclosure of information, in view of their insecure legal position, and so assurances of confidentiality are important. Specific care is needed in research with unaccompanied children seeking asylum, especially with regard to consent (Thomas & Byford, 2003). Nevertheless, refugees may regard participation in research as a positive experience (Dyregrov, Dyregrov, & Raundalen, 2000). Furthermore, it has been argued that research may be used to challenge the oppression and inequalities experienced by refugees (Kirmayer, Rousseau, & Crepeau, 2004).

Conceptual Issues in Refugee Mental Health

A number of controversies, mostly focused on post-traumatic stress disorder (PTSD), in view of its association with exposure to violent events, have arisen in the refugee mental health field (see chapter 42). These partly relate to issues in psychiatric research with culturally diverse populations. It has been argued that PTSD is a culturally constructed psychiatric disorder that does not have validity in non-western cultures (Bracken, Giller, & Summerfield, 1995; Eisenbruch, 1991; Summerfield, 2000, 2001). Rather, it is suggested that suffering and psychiatric symptoms should be described on the basis of local meanings, to produce a more culturally "embedded" understanding (Eisenbruch, 1991; Kleinman, Das, & Lock, 1997). The social use, and indeed abuse of the concept of PTSD has been blamed as a contributory factor for the poor organization and inappropriate development of psychological trauma services in the aftermath of disasters (Summerfield, 1999, 2000).

There are numerous reasons for rejecting this critique (Hodes, 2002a). PTSD has been found in all cultures in which people have been exposed to violent events, and there have been no reports of a "culture-specific illness associated with mass violence and torture experienced by refugees" (Mollica, 2000). Numerous studies attest to the validity of the disorder (e.g., the recognition of symptoms across cultures and feasibility of translating instruments; de Jong, Komproe, van Ommeren *et al.*, 2001; Elsass, 2001; Sack, Seeley, & Clarke, 1997), the association of PTSD with the degree of exposure to past war events (rather than all adversities; Heptinstall, Sethna, & Taylor, 2004; Sack, Clarke, & Seeley, 1996), the stability of the disorder and a trajectory different to that of other comorbid disorders such as depression (Sack, Him, & Dickason, 1999). It is important to bear in mind that an approach that includes psychopathology, such as recognition of PTSD, does not determine the kind of mental health service provision, which should be influenced by many social factors such as the level of infrastructure development and human resources, and cultural influences regarding treatment appropriateness (see p. 481; de Jong, 2002; van Ommeren, Saxena, & Saracena, 2005).

Epidemiological Findings

Community Studies

The studies in this section are described according to the sequence of refugee experiences: before flight from the home community, in-flight and on arrival in resettlement countries (Hodes, 2000; Lustig, Kia-Keating, Knight *et al.*, 2004). There have been an increasing number of community-based studies regarding the pre-flight and in-flight phases (e.g., those in refugee camps) with young people in recent years, especially those from Vietnam (Felsman, Leong, Johnson *et al.*, 1990) and Cambodia (Mollica *et al.*, 1997; Savin, Sack, Clarke *et al.*, 1996), the former Yugoslavia, mainly Croatia (Zivcic, 1993; Kuterovac-Jagodic, 2003) and Bosnia-Herzogovina (Jones & Kafetsios, 2005; Smith, Perrin, Yule *et al.*, 2001; Smith *et al.*, 2002), and also the Middle East, focusing on Palestinians (Garbarino & Kostelny, 1996; Punamaki, 1996; Quota, Punamaki, & El Sarraj, 2003, 2005; Thabet, Abed, & Vostanis, 2002, 2004; Thabet, Karin, & Vostanis, 2006) and people from Iraq (Ahmad, Sofi, Sundelin-Wahlsten *et al.*, 2000), and other countries such as Afghanistan (Mghir, Freed, Raskin *et al.*, 1995) and regions in Africa (Paardekooper, de Jong, & Hermanns, 1999). They have assessed psychopathology mainly using questionnaires, with report by parents and sometimes self-report by older children (but there are rare interview-based studies, e.g., Ahmad *et al.*, 2000). The studies described here are selected on the basis of methodological quality.

There are a number of considerations in interpreting epidemiological studies of young refugees. Many have been designed to investigate post-traumatic stress, anxiety and depressive symptoms following exposure to traumatic events and most have confirmed high levels of these symptoms. These studies do not reflect the psychiatric heterogeneity that occurs amongst this population. For example, high levels of disruptive behavior have been found amongst populations exposed to ongoing war events and hardship (Quota, Punamaki, & El Sarraj, 2005). Other symptoms such as nocturnal enuresis which might arise from stress are often not assessed. Severe disorders such as psychoses that may occur at higher prevalence amongst some refugee populations such as those from Africa have not been systematically investigated (Fearon, Kirkbride, Morgan *et al.*, 2006). Many studies have relied on questionnaire measures that identify symptom levels rather than psychiatric disorder. While high levels of symptoms indicate high risk of disorder, the questionnaires are rarely calibrated against interview-based measures in the populations under investigation, so that estimates of prevalence are somewhat inaccurate. Another consideration relates to the frequent absence of measures of psychosocial impairment, which may elevate estimated rates of disorder. The studies are varied with respect to duration of exposure to war events and also time delay until participation in the studies (Table 31.1). Thus, the study of Bosnian children (Smith *et al.*, 2002) did not find elevated rates of depressive symptoms, perhaps because the study was carried out years after the cessation of hostilities. By contrast, investigation of Palestinian children living in a situation of ongoing conflict showed a strong association between post-traumatic and depressive symptoms (Thabet, Abed, & Vostanis, 2004).

The high-quality interview-based studies carried out in western resettlement countries add to the findings regarding pre-flight and displaced populations, and reveal high rates of psychiatric disorder and comorbidity. A systematic review of interview-based studies carried out in resettlement countries identified five surveys of 260 children and adolescents younger than 18 years (Fazel, Wheeler, & Danesh, 2005). The prevalence rate for PTSD was 11%, approximately 10 times the rate in non-refugee peers.

Numerous surveys have been carried out in resettlement countries using questionnaire methods of assessment, investigating ethnically diverse refugee populations (Espino, 1991; Leavey *et al.*, 2004; Montgomery, 1998; Rousseau, Drapeau, & Corin, 1996). Some surveys of ethnically mixed refugees

Table 31.1 Selected community studies of prevalence of psychopathology amongst young refugees.

Stage of refugee experiences	Ethnicity/culture of subjects	Sample characteristics	Instruments	Main findings	References
Pre-flight	Bosnian 98% Muslim	$n = 2976$. Mean age 12.1 years (range 9–14). Exposed to bombing over 2 years. Data collected 2 years later	RIES; DSRS; RCMAS	On RIES 52% high-risk PTSD; DSRS low, but higher than UK normative data; RCMAS not elevated. War exposure explained most of variance	Smith *et al.* (2002)
	* Palestinian, in Gaza	$n = 309$ aged 3–6 years. Exposed to regular bombardment, displacement, economic deprivation	Strengths & Difficulties Questionnaire; BCL	War exposure predicted symptoms; BCL symptoms (e.g., faddy eating, settling at night) overactivity much higher than UK comparison	Thabet *et al.* (2006)
	* Palestinian, in Gaza	$n = 91$ exposed to bombardment & home demolition; $n = 89$ not exposed Age 9–18 years	Child post-traumatic stress reaction index; RCMAS; Children fears checklist	Severe PTSD reaction in 59% exposed, 25% non-exposed ($P = 0.0009$); high-risk anxiety disorders less amongst those not exposed. Bombardment predicted PTSD symptoms and fears	Thabet *et al.* (2002)
In-flight	Kurdish in Iraq	$n = 45$. Mean age 12.4 years (range 7–17). Exposed to "Anfal," many killed, moved to displacement camps	Post-traumatic stress symptoms in children	87% children had PTSD. Duration of captivity and war exposure predictors of symptoms	Ahmad *et al.* (2000)
	Cambodia	$n = 182$, in refugee camp. Aged 12–13, parents included as informants	CBCL Youth self-report	CBCL: 54% had total problem scores in clinical range, 26% by self-report. Most common symptoms somatic, withdrawal, social problems. Less than 10% significant functional impairment. Cumulative trauma associated with increased functional impairment	Mollica *et al.*, (1997)
In resettlement countries	Cambodia	$n = 46$; 40 exposed to Pol Pot regime aged 8–12 years; Mean age 17 years (range 14–20) when assessed in USA	SADS using Research diagnostic criteria CGAS	20 had PTSD and 21 had some type of depression (5 major depression). CGAS 43–75 for those exposed to Pol Pot regime, CGAS 84 for those not exposed. Impairment visible in school settings	Kinzie *et al.* (1986) Sack *et al.* (1986)
	Cambodia	$n = 209$ living in USA. Age 13–25 years. As children, many witnessed atrocities including killing of family	SADS GAF	18% had PTSD (GAF 72); 11% depression (GAF 68). GAF 82 in those without PTSD or depression	Sack *et al.* (1994, 1995b)
	Iranian	$n = 50$ living in Sweden. Experienced attacks in war, family separation. Mean age 5 years 10 months	Semistructured interview parents and child	19 (38%) preoccupied with violence; only 13 (26%) good emotional well-being	Almquist & Brandell-Forsberg (1995)
	From 35 nations (29% South-East Asia; 27% Central America)	$n = 203$ Age 13–19 years 70% migrated to Canada before age 6 years; most not war exposed	DISC – 2.25	Rate psychiatric disorder 21% refugee group vs. 11% non-refugee peers. Over-anxious disorder in 13% in refugee group. Psychiatric diagnosis associated with family status (single/reconstituted family) and parental unemployment for 6 months after arrival in Canada	Tousignant *et al.* (1999)

BCL, Behavior Checklist; CBCL, children's behavior checklist; CGAS, children's global assessment scale; DISC, Diagnostic interview schedule for children; DSRS, depression self-rating scale; GAF, global assessment of functioning; SADS, Schedule for Affective Disorder and Schizophrenia; RCMAS, revised childrens' manifest anxiety scale; RIES, revised impact of events scale.

* These studies included some children living in refugee camps so overlap with the "in-flight" section of table.

have been carried out in the UK. A survey of primary school children found that the refugee children were more distressed than their peer group (Fazel & Stein, 2003). Another study of refugee children, mean age 11 years, mainly non-referred, used self-report measures of post-traumatic stress and depressive symptoms (Heptinstall, Sethna, & Taylor, 2004). A high level of post-traumatic and depressive symptoms was found, with more than half of the children being at risk of PTSD and depression.

A different picture emerges of multiethnic refugee adolescents who were living in Montreal, most of whom had not been exposed to war (Table 31.1; Tousignant *et al.*, 1999). The greatest differences occurred amongst females, who had elevated rates of over-anxious disorder and phobias compared with non-refugee peers. Psychosocial impairment was greatest amongst those with conduct disorder.

Clinic- and Service-Based Studies

It is well known that only a small proportion of children and adolescents in the community with psychiatric disorders are attending mental health services (Ford, Sayal, Meltzer *et al.*, 2005; Verhulst & van der Ende, 1997). A number of factors influence who gets help, including the severity of the disorder and level of social impairment. Only a small number of studies of young refugees who have accessed mental health services have been published.

Young refugees often present with disorders that reflect exposure to past violence and disruptions of relationships such as PTSD, adjustment disorders and depression (Arroyo & Eth, 1985; Howard & Hodes, 2000). Interestingly, a report from Kosovo of child mental health service users soon after the war (1998–99) found that in addition to stress-related disorders such as PTSD and adjustment disorder, enuresis was a frequent problem (Jones, Rrustemi, Shahini *et al.*, 2003). Psychosocial impairment of the refugee children may be similar to that of other children in the same service, and certainly much greater than would be expected in a community comparison group (Howard & Hodes, 2000).

Young refugees using services may have disorders that have multifactorial causation, but may be precipitated by experience of adversities and cultural change. Eating disorders, anorexia nervosa (Kope & Sack, 1987) or bulimia nervosa (Stein, Chalhoub, & Hodes, 1998) have been reported, as well as rarer severe problems such as somatoform disorders associated with depression, in which children become withdrawn and lose the ability to eat and talk (Bodegard, 2005). High levels of stressful events including intrafamilial abuse may also precipitate violent deliberate self-harm (Patel & Hodes, 2006). Young refugees were highly represented in a survey of adolescent psychiatric in-patients in London, largely because of psychosis (Tolmac & Hodes, 2004). This group were predominantly African adolescents who had experienced a high level of war exposure, including witnessing the killing of family members, and had low social support, reflected in the fact that they were less likely to be living with a parent than other in-patients (Hodes & Tolmac, 2005).

It should be remembered that young refugees could have psychiatric and developmental difficulties (e.g., learning difficulties, pervasive developmental disorders, obsessive compulsive disorder and hyperkinetic disorder), which can occur independently of adverse experiences and displacement (Howard & Hodes, 2000; Williams & Westermeyer, 1983).

Risk and Resilience for Psychopathology

Some theoretical considerations are important in considering the variation in children's psychological response to organized violence and associated adversities. First, in relation to risk events, as can be seen from the account already given, isolated events in "refugee" experiences are relatively unusual, and adversities typically cluster, occurring in close temporal proximity and perhaps also as a protracted process. Available evidence suggests that greater psychological harm comes from an accumulation of risk factors. This refers both to the type of event and duration of exposure, with increasing risk associated with increasing personal threat (Espino, 1991; Garbarino & Kostelny, 1996; Kinzie, Sack, Angell *et al.*, 1986; Mollica *et al.*, 1997; Sack, Clarke, & Seeley, 1996; Sack, Seely, & Clarke, 1997). Second, with regard to resilience, it has been cogently explained that "Resilience does not constitute an individual trait or characteristic. . . . Resilience involves a range of processes that bring together quite diverse mechanisms operating before, during or after the encounter with the stress experience or adversity that is being considered . . ." (Rutter, 1999). The succinct account that follows, which cannot bring out all the subtleties of the findings, might appear to be organized as if risk and resilience are characteristics of events or individuals, but a tendency to interpret the data this way should be resisted (see chapter 25). Some of the main influences on mental health that have been investigated in young refugees are shown in Table 31.2.

Many of the risk factors described here are also considered in chapter 42 with regards to PTSD. Individual attributes such as age and gender may influence psychological adjustment in complex ways. Age and developmental level influence cognitive function, including appraisal of events, as well as biological processes such as responses to stress. Gender may be associated with differing war exposure (Ahmad *et al.*, 2000; Derluyn, Broekaert, Schuyten *et al.*, 2004; Montgomery, 1998; Somasundaram, 2002). Research investigating associations between war events and psychological distress has often controlled for number of events, rather than looking at the links between types of events and gender (Smith *et al.*, 2002; Vizek-Vidovic, Kuterovac-Jagodic, & Aarambasic, 2000). Some reports have found greater levels of post-traumatic and anxiety symptoms among girls than boys (Jones & Kafetsios, 2005; Smith *et al.*, 2001; Vizek-Vidovic, Kuterovac-Jagodic, & Aarambasic, 2000), but other studies did not find this (Thabet, Abed, & Vostanis, 2002).

Table 31.2 Risk and protective factors for psychopathology.

	Risk factors	Protective factors
Individual experience of war events	Proximity to events: range from witnessing at distance, to direct involvement in violent events Repetition of events Degree of personal threat, including witnessing maltreatment of family Appraisal of events that involve hopelessness and despair	Low-level exposure to distant war events might increase resilience Appraisal of events that reflects ideological commitment in conflict Cultural and religious influences on appraisal of events
Individual factors	Gender: **1** Gender differences in exposure to war events: females more likely to be victims of sexual assault; males more likely to become combatants **2** Females probably more vulnerable to internalizing symptoms; males more vulnerable to externalizing symptoms Temperament: anxious or vulnerable temperament increases risk Past psychopathology	
Family factors	Separation from family Parental psychological distress (mostly investigated for mothers) Family conflict	Greater family cohesion Appropriate family expectations of resettlement country Parental fluency in language of host country
Social factors	Uncertainty regarding asylum application and legal status Detention and restrictive living arrangements Financial hardship Parental unemployment High mobility and poor housing Social isolation Hostility and discrimination in host country	Greater social support including links with same ethnic/language group

The individual's understanding of events is also important. This will be shaped by beliefs and ideologies that may be shared with the social or cultural group, including specific attitudes to preparedness for war events (Jones & Kafetsios, 2005; Punamaki, 1996). Realistic expectations are associated with better adjustment (McKelvey & Webb, 1996).

Positive effects of the family were observed during World War II, when it was noted that the presence of parents protected against psychological distress during bombing (Freud & Burlingham, 1943). Investigation of unaccompanied asylum seeking children suggest that they may be more distressed than those who are accompanied (see p. 480; McKelvey & Webb, 1995). Large surveys have shown that children's distress is related to parental distress, although the studies have largely focused on mothers rather than fathers (Smith *et al.*, 2001). There may be an interaction between a child's gender and the effect of maternal distress. A study of Palestinian children in Gaza found that boys were at special risk for post-traumatic and emotional symptoms when the mothers and the boys themselves were exposed to a high level of war, whereas for girls these symptoms were more associated with mothers' exposure (Quota, Punamaki, & El Sarraj, 2005). The quality of family relationships is also important, as children in cohesive well-functioning families experience less distress from external war events (Garbarino & Kostleny, 1996; Laor, Wolmer, Mayes *et al.*, 1996).

Societal response to those who have experienced organized violence and displacement can influence psychological adjustment. In societies where there have been abductions and suspected but not confirmed killings, grieving is not possible, and this heightens distress for children (Quirk & Casco, 1994). Those who have fled their own communities and live in refugee camps may experience very difficult conditions with regard to the physical environment, such as overcrowding and inadequate facilities for children. For asylum seekers in resettlement countries, detention policies (Fazel & Silove, 2006; Reijneveld, De Boer, Bean *et al.*, 2005) and long delays and uncertainties regarding their application for refugee status may increase psychiatric disorders such as anxiety, depression and somatoform disorders (Laban, Gernaat, Komproe *et al.*, 2004). Ongoing daily hassles, or resettlement stressors have been shown to increase depressive symptoms in children (Heptinstall, Sethna, & Taylor, 2004; Sack, Clarke, & Seeley, 1996). Greater resilience for parents and well-being of children is seen amongst those who have stronger social networks, usually associated with greater ethnic density, more opportunities for work and greater residential stability (Ahearn, 2000).

Course and Intergenerational Effects

The persistence of psychopathology has been identified from studies with children with diverse cultural backgrounds. A cohort of 46 children from Cambodia, 40 of whom had experienced the Pol Pot regime in primary school years, were followed up while living in the USA (Sack, Clarke, Him *et al.*, 1993; Sack, Him, & Dickason, 1999). Six years after the initial assessment, 48% had PTSD and the figure was 35% at 12 years. Regarding depression, the figures at the same time points were 7% and 14%, respectively. Other studies have found the persistence of PTSD but lower levels of depression with resettlement (Hubbard, Realmuto, Northwood *et al.*, 1995). The persistence was also found in a report of Kurdish children who had PTSD years after experiencing a military campaign against their communities and experiencing displacement at a later time (Ahmad, Sofi, Sundelin-Wahlsten *et al.*, 2000). Many of the young people in the studies had quite good social function with respect to school attendance and attainment despite the presence of psychopathology.

Very long-term psychiatric outcomes have been described in survivors of the Holocaust, experienced in adolescence or early adulthood. Emotional distress, including anxiety symptoms, lower mood and psychiatric service use were much higher in middle-aged Holocaust survivors than immigrant controls (Carmil & Carel, 1986). In old age, the Holocaust survivors continued to have more distress with regard to post-traumatic symptoms and general psychopathology (Joffe, Brodaty, Luscombe *et al.*, 2003). The Holocaust survivors were also more likely to experience further post-traumatic symptoms when retraumatized by bombing (Robinson, Hemmendinger, Netanel *et al.*, 1994).

The catastrophic losses and abuse experienced by survivors of the Holocaust will often have long-term effects on feelings of safety or insecurity, self-esteem and development and maintenance of relationships. For this reason, attention has been given to the children of Holocaust survivors, as many reports suggested that they were at increased risk of psychopathology (Felsen, 1998). However, a meta-analysis has found that children of Holocaust survivors are no less well-adjusted than their peers, and had not experienced secondary traumatization (van IJzendoorn, Bakermans-Kraneberg, & Sagi-Schwartz, 2003).

Aggregation of disorders in families has been investigated with regard to the association between child and adult psychopathology, especially PTSD and war trauma (see above). A report regarding PTSD across two generations of Cambodian refugees living in the USA found a significant relationship between parent–child PTSD, but not depression (Sack, Clarke, & Seeley, 1995a). Clustering of disorders in families may occur because of genetic factors, but these have not been investigated amongst refugee populations.

The changes associated with migration, adaptation to new cultures and communities will affect generations in different ways. Adult asylum seekers may have limited rights, be unable to work, their acquisition of the language of the resettlement country may be slow and they may be socially isolated. By contrast, their children will attend school, will rapidly have a peer group and opportunity to learn the new language. Thus, the children will assimilate and adapt much more quickly than their parents. They may take on tasks to support the family, and in some case they may become carers of parents who are unwell (e.g., because of torture or psychiatric impairment). These changes can also create tensions, in part because of the burden for the children, but also because the usual family organization and parental authority may diminish (Tobin & Friedman, 1984). This may result in poor boundaries and containment for younger children, and reduced surveillance and advice for adolescent offspring (Westermeyer, 1991). These factors might in part explain the higher level of psychiatric disorders including conduct disorder amongst the refugee adolescents in Canada who had largely not been exposed to war experiences (Table 31.1; Tousignant *et al.*, 1999).

Unaccompanied Asylum Seeking Children

During the course of war and organized violence, family members may become separated and children orphaned. Some children are sent away from imminent danger, and may experience harrowing journeys, with further risk of abuse or illness. In some regions of the world, such as Sri Lanka and North Uganda, abduction of children has been common, and many of them are then forced to become soldiers (Derluyn *et al.*, 2004; Somasundaram, 2002). It has been estimated that there are 300,000 child soldiers worldwide (Human Rights Watch, 2006). It is unclear how many unaccompanied asylum seeking children there are globally. Estimates of the numbers in the UK suggest the number has increased since 1990, and over the first part of the decade, 2000–2005, has been around 5500.

Unaccompanied asylum seeking children can be regarded as at special risk. They have experienced high levels of war events and separations (McKelvey & Webb, 1995; Thomas, Thomas, Nafees *et al.*, 2004). Journeys may have been harrowing, and their arrival in resettlement countries may be associated with great uncertainties. It is expected that child asylum seekers will be offered special protection (UNHCR, 1994). In the UK they are entitled to care under the Children Act 1989, and so are supported by local authorities (Wade, Mitchell, & Baylis, 2005). However, the initial assessment and level of support, including accommodation, may be poor (Wade, Mitchell, & Baylis, 2005).

Available evidence suggests that unaccompanied asylum seeking children and young adults have high levels of psychological distress even after controlling for traumatic events (Bean, Eurelings-Bontekoe, Mooijaart *et al.*, 2006; McKelvey & Webb, 1995). A study from Finland of 46 adolescents mainly from Somali background, found that on the basis of the Child

Behavior Checklist, nearly half were in the clinical or borderline range (Sourander, 1998). Younger children were significantly more distressed than the older ones. Studies of child soldiers from Uganda and Sri Lanka who had experienced very high levels of war events, including killing someone themselves, found high levels of post-traumatic stress, anxiety and somatization (Derluyn *et al.*, 2004; Somasundaram, 2002).

Agencies that provide care for these children have considered the importance of foster care or group homes that might mitigate the effects of losses and increase resilience, by increasing social links with an ethnically and linguistically similar peer group and community (Geltman, Grant-Knight, Mehta *et al.*, 2005; Porte & Tomey-Purta, 1987; Wade, Mitchell, & Baylis, 2005). Same ethnic group foster families, or perhaps group homes, are much preferred to fostering with culturally different families (Geltman *et al.*, 2005; Wade, Mitchell, & Baylis, 2005). The preferred arrangement has been found to be associated with significantly less risk of depression, in the case of South-East Asian youngsters (Porte & Tomey-Purta, 1987), and PTSD, in the case of Sudanese adolescents (Geltman *et al.*, 2005).

Implications for Services and Interventions

There has been debate regarding the best means of intervening and promoting the welfare of displaced people. Primary prevention of conflict sadly seems to be unattainable, but concerted international efforts have been made over years to regulate the treatment of prisoners and detained people (UNHCR, 2006). Children's special needs and rights have been identified (UNHCR, 1994). Recruiting children into armies has been condemned by the United Nations, but that organization has been criticized for not being adequately effective (Editorial, *Lancet*, 2004).

When it is feasible after cessation of hostilities, there is a need for general welfare provision which should include schools and other services (Inter-agency Standing Committee 2007; van Ommeren, Saxena, & Saraceno, 2005). In this tiered approach to the provision of services, community support will benefit large populations. Services that might specifically help children include family reunification programs, adequate protection and care – including medical care – for orphans or unaccompanied asylum seeking children. In the more affluent countries such as the UK, general services that target excluded communities with children may include refugees within their remit (Hodes, 2002b). Strengthening families is likely to promote the mental health of parents and children. Initiatives in Kosovo that promote family strengths, using psychoeducation and multifamily groups (Griffiths, Agani, Weine *et al.*, 2005), have been reported. Other useful approaches may focus on maintaining continuities in family life, and coping with change including reunification with separated family members (Rousseau, Rufagari, Bagilishya *et al.*, 2004; Weine, Dheeraj, Merita *et al.*, 2003). A well-designed study from Bosnia offered weekly group meetings with mothers over 5 months, with the provision of psychoeducation regarding their children's needs and helping the children to describe traumatic experiences, in addition to medical care, which was the only intervention for the control group (Dybdahl, 2001). Those who received the psychosocial intervention made greater progress: mothers had better mental health, children gained more weight and had better psychosocial functioning.

Controversies have arisen regarding the extent to which mental health services in disaster zones, including areas where there are refugees, should be established to focus on post-traumatic psychopathology. Trauma services have been criticized for focusing on psychological distress outside of a context that considers the whole infrastructure and resource provision, and may neglect cultural factors and other disorders (Eisenbruch, de Jong, & van de Prut, 2004; Summerfield, 1999; van Ommeren, Saxena, & Saraceno, 2005). The criticism is especially cogent in view of the absence of evidence of effectiveness in support of primary prevention of post-traumatic stress symptoms for those exposed to traumatic events, and failure to show benefit for non-refugee populations suggest this would be an inappropriate use of resources.

A preferred option is to integrate trauma-based care into general mental health care (Eisenbruch, de Jong, & van de Prut, 2004; Inter-agency Standing Committee 2007; Summerfield, 1999; van Ommeren, Saxena, & Saraceno, 2005). The benefit of this is apparent from the report from Kosovo described previously, in which by the second year after the war ended, frequent reasons for attending were learning difficulties (intellectual disability) and enuresis (Jones *et al.*, 2003). However, even in affluent countries, mainstream services including primary care may have organizational difficulties meeting the mental health needs of refugees. Access should be facilitated by using interpreters, and consider the fact that asylum seekers may live in homeless accommodation and experience high mobility (Lamb & Cunningham, 2003).

More targeted services can be established for special populations such as unaccompanied asylum seeking children. This group will have health screening and ideally this should include screening assessment of mental health difficulties (Geltman *et al.*, 2005; Wade, Mitchell, & Baylis, 2005). Preschool children may be prioritized by health visitors and others working with this age group.

In view of the difficulties that might arise for young refugees in gaining access to clinic-based child and adolescent services, outreach programs in schools have been described, with some encouraging data available from evaluations (Ehntholt, Smith, & Yule, 2005; Hodes, 2002b; O'Shea, Hodes, Down *et al.*, 2000; Stein, Jaycox, Kataoka *et al.*, 2003). Such services have been provided in communities such as Bosnia following the war, with the involvement of teachers as therapists, in view of the dearth of child mental health professionals there (Udwin, 1995). One advantage of school-based work is that all refugee children, regardless of legal status, are expected to attend. Teachers can identify those who are psychologically distressed and make referral to the school-based mental health service, so bypassing reliance on primary care which may be difficult for refugees to access. Families may also experience school-based services as less stigmatizing than clinic-based services. A further advantage is that child mental health practitioners working in the schools will establish good liaison with teachers, and can also provide a consultation model to reach more children. Given resource limitations, it may only be feasible to provide child mental health outreach to schools that have significant numbers of refugee pupils, and adequate infrastructure including effective school referral systems and support from interpreters.

The psychiatric heterogeneity of young impaired refugees, including some with high levels of distress and poor social function, means that some will need referral to specialist child and adolescents mental health services. Despite the difficulties the young refugees and families may have had in accessing services, and the very frequent need for interpreters, they may not have a higher dropout that non-refugees in the same service (Howard & Hodes, 2000). Impressions are that newly arrived asylum seekers are more likely to be seen because of post-traumatic stress, anxiety and mood disorders but, as the communities become more settled, children will be increasingly referred because of disruptive behaviors. The clinical assessment may be complex as it is necessary to consider development in environments that may have been very abnormal (e.g., absence of schooling, prison, multiple moves between countries, homes and carers). The high level of background stressors may have contributed to behavioral, conduct and attentional problems, making the differential diagnosis among hyperkinetic, conduct disorders and adjustment disorders difficult. For some children a symptomatic treatment approach and regular reassessments may identify stable specific symptom clusters, and clarify diagnostic difficulties. In these situations, psychometric testing for intellectual ability and physical examination to assess in particular coordination disorder, which is commonly comorbid with hyperkinetic disorder (Gillberg & Kadesjo, 2003), may point towards a neurodevelopmental basis for the attentional and conduct problems.

Some children will require psychiatric admission for further assessment and treatment. This group may have experienced high levels of past war traumatic events and current low family support. This combination may in part explain the high rate of involuntary admission for adolescents with severe psychopathology including psychosis (Tolmac & Hodes, 2004).

Clinical work may require an expanded role for child and adolescent mental health professionals. Requests may be made for reports to access housing and school, and legal reports to support asylum applications (Tufnell, 2003). Attention needs to be given to parental mental health difficulties (Ahearn & Athey, 1991; Howard & Hodes, 2000). Intervention often needs to be multiagency, and draw on the range of services from social services as well as other heath services such as child health (Geltman *et al.*, 2005; Wade, Mitchell, & Baylis, 2005; Westermeyer, 1991).

There are specific skills in working with interpreters, and key points are given here (Farooq & Fear, 2003; Raval, 2005). First, it is generally not appropriate to involve a child as an interpreter, in part because of the responsibility this gives to the child, and also because of the effect on family relationships, as parents become dependent on their child's skills and integrity for accurate interpreting. If an interpreter is needed, it is necessary to consider their gender and ethnicity, and their suitability for the particular family. Discussion with the family, perhaps involving the interpreter (e.g., over the telephone), might be useful. There are techniques for interviewing with the interpreter. During the session, eye contact and questions should be directed to the person who is being addressed, not the interpreter. Speech should be at an appropriate speed, and technical words and terms that elicit feelings or particular psychological experiences may require discussion with the interpreter. Following the session it is often useful to speak to the interpreter to identify any difficulties that might have arisen.

Asylum seeking families in particular may have fears regarding the "assessment" process, which may be reminiscent of interrogations. Furthermore, there may be unease, perhaps not voiced, regarding the degree of confidentiality in the clinic setting. A further feature of work with refugees is that many things may be "unknown" for the clinician. Families may find it hard, or unthinkable, to disclose background adversities (e.g., the rape of females in the family).

Regarding treatments, given the heterogeneity of psychiatric disorders and problems, it is not possible to provide an adequate account here, but summary accounts are available elsewhere for specific disorders such as PTSD (see chapter 42; Hodes & Diaz-Caneja, 2006). A number of general points can be made (Hodes, 2000). Culturally shaped attitudes may influence the way parents explain their children's adjustment and responses to the changes they have encountered, and this may affect attitudes to specific treatments. One aspect of this is the wish to look forward, rather than back. This may be manifest as a preference to deal with current difficulties (e.g., school problems) rather than look back and address past traumatic events, which would be required for cognitive–behavioral work. Another related feature is the extent to which evidence-based treatments can be provided for this culturally heterogeneous population. Evidence available for PTSD is that existing treatments are effective (see chapter 41; Neuner, Schauer, Klaschik *et al.*, 2004; NCCMH, 2005; Onyut, Neurer, Schauer *et al.*, 2005; Paunovic & Ost, 2001; Stein, Jaycox, Kataoka *et al.*, 2003). However, treatment needs to be adapted to be culturally congruent with families' understanding and beliefs.

Conclusions

The scale of war and organized violence globally has had a major impact on child and adolescent mental health. In recent years, increasing attention has been paid to this area but there are still significant gaps in knowledge. From a research perspective, there is a need to investigate further young peoples' risk and resilience for psychopathology, as well as the effectiveness of available interventions. It continues to be important to plan services for this vulnerable population.

Further Reading

Hodes, M. (Ed.). (2005). Special issue: Children and war. *Clinical Child Psychology and Psychiatry*, *10* (2).

Medical Foundation for the Care of Victims of Torture http://www.torturecare.org.uk/

Refugee Council http://www.refugeecouncil.org.uk/

United Nations High Commission for Refugees (UNHCR). http://www.unhcr.org/home.html

Wilson, J. P., & Drozdek, B. (2004). *Broken spirits: The treatment of traumatized asylum seekers, refugees, war and torture victims*. New York, Hove: Brunner-Routledge.

References

Ahearn, F. L. (2000). *Psychosocial wellness of refugees: Issues in qualitative and quantitative research*. New York & Oxford: Berghahn Books.

Ahearn, F., & Athey, J. L. (Eds.). (1991). *Refugee children: Theory, research and services*. Baltimore and London: Johns Hopkins University Press.

Ahmad, A., Sofi, M. A., Sundelin-Wahlsten, V., & von Knorring, A. L. (2000). Posttraumatic stress disorder in children after the military operation "Anfal" in Iraqi Kurdistan. *European Child and Adolescent Psychiatry*, *9*, 235–243.

Almquist, K., & Brandell-Forsberg, M. (1995). Iranian refugee children in Sweden: Effects of oganized violence and forced migration on preschool children. *American Journal of Orthopsychiatry*, *65*, 225–237.

Arroyo, W., & Eth, S. (1985). Children traumatized by Central American warfare. In S. Eth, & R. S. Pynoos (Eds.), *Post-traumatic stress in children*. Washington, DC: American Psychiatric Press.

Bardsley, M., & Storkey, M. (2000). Estimating the numbers of refugees in London. *Journal of Public Health Medicine*, *22*, 406–412.

Bean, T., Eurelings-Bontekoe, E., Mooijaart, A., & Spinhoven, P. (2006). Factors associated with mental health service need and utilization among unaccompanied refugee adolescents. *Administration and Policy in Mental Health and Mental Health Services Research*, *33*, 342–355.

Bodegard, G. (2005). Life-threatening loss of function in refugee children: Another expression of pervasive refusal syndrome? *Clinical Child Psychology and Psychiatry*, *10*, 337–350.

Bracken, P. J., Giller, J. E., & Summerfield, D. (1995). Psychological responses to war and atrocity: The limitations of current concepts. *Social Science and Medicine*, *40*, 1073–1082.

Carmil, D., & Carel, R. S. (1986). Emotional distress and satisfaction in life among Holocaust survivors: A community study of survivors and controls. *Psychological Medicine*, *16*, 141–149.

de Jong, J. T. V. M. (2002). Public mental health, traumatic stress and human rights violations in low-income countries: A culturally appropriate model in times of conflict, disaster and peace. In J. T. V. M. de Jong (Ed.), *Trauma, war and violence: Public mental health in socio-cultural context* (pp. 1–91). New York: Plenum/Kluver.

de Jong, J. T. V. M., Komproe, I. H., van Ommeren, M., El-Masri, M., Mesfin, A., Khaled, N., *et al.* (2001). Lifetime events and post-traumatic stress disorder in four post-conflict settings. *Journal of the American Medical Association*, *286*, 555–562.

Derluyn, I., Broekaert, E., Schuyten, G., & de Temmerman, E. (2004). Post-traumatic stress in former Ugandan child soldiers. *Lancet*, *363*, 861–863.

Dybdahl, R. (2001). Children and mothers in war: An outcome study of a psychosocial intervention program. *Child Development*, *72*, 1214–1230.

Dyregrov, K., Dyregrov, A., & Raundalen, M. (2000). Refugee families' experience of research participation. *Journal of Traumatic Stress*, *13*, 413–426.

Editorial, *Lancet*. (2004). The hidden health trauma of child soldiers. *Lancet*, *363*, 831.

Ehntholt, K., Smith, P., & Yule, W. (2005). School-based cognitive–behavioural therapy group intervention for refugee children who have experienced war-related trauma. *Clinical Child Psychology and Psychiatry*, *10*, 235–250.

Eisenbruch, M. (1991). From post-traumatic stress disorder to cultural bereavement: Diagnosis of Southeast Asian refugees. *Social Science and Medicine*, *33*, 673–680.

Eisenbruch, M., de Jong, J. T. V. M., & van de Prut, W. (2004). Bringing order out of chaos: A culturally competent approach to managing the problems of refugees and victims of organized violence. *Journal of Traumatic Stress*, *17*, 123–131.

Elsass, P. (2001). Individual and collective traumatic memories: A qualitative study of post-traumatic stress disorder symptoms in two Latin American localities. *Transcultural Psychiatry*, *38*, 306–316.

Espino, C. M. (1991). Trauma and adaptation: The case of Central American children. In F. Ahearn, & J. L. Athey (Eds.), *Refugee children: Theory, research and services* (pp. 106–124). Baltimore and London: Johns Hopkins University Press.

Farooq, S., & Fear, C. (2003). Working through interpreters. *Advances in Psychiatric Treatment*, *9*, 104–109.

Fazel, M., & Silove, D. (2006). Detention of refugees. *British Medical Journal*, *332*, 251–252.

Fazel, M., & Stein, A. (2003). Mental health of refugee children: Comparative study. *British Medical Journal*, *327*, 134.

Fazel, M., Wheeler, J., & Danesh, J. (2005). Prevalence of serious mental disorder in 7000 refugees resettled in western countries: A systematic review. *Lancet*, *365*, 1309–1314.

Fearon, P., Kirkbride, J. B., Morgan, C., Dazan, P., Morgan, K., Lloyd, T., *et al.*, AESOP Study Group. (2006). Incidence of schizophrenia and other psychoses in ethnic minority groups: results from the MRC AESOP Study. *Psychological Medicine*, *36*, 1541–1550.

Felsen, I. (1998). Transgenerational transmission of effects of the Holocaust. The North American Perspective. In Y. Danieli (Ed.), *International Handbook of Multigenerational Legacies of Trauma* (pp. 43–68). New York & London: Plenum Press.

Felsman, J. K., Leong, F. T. L., Johnson, M. C., & Felsman, I. C. (1990). Estimates of psychological distress among Vietnamese refugees: Adolescents, unaccompanied minors and young adults. *Social Science and Medicine*, *31*, 1251–1256.

Ford, T., Sayal, K., Meltzer, H., & Goodman, R. (2005). Parental concerns about their child's emotions and behaviour and referral to specialist services: General population survey. *British Medical Journal*, *331*, 1435–1436.

Freud, A., & Burlingham, D. T. (1943). *War and children*. London: Medical War Books.

Garbarino, J., & Kostelny, K. (1996). The effects of political violence on Palestinian children's behavior problems: A risk accumulation model. *Child Development*, *67*, 33–45.

Geltman, P. L., Grant-Knight, W., Mehta, S. D., Lloyd-Travaglini, C., Lustig, S., Lindgraf, J. M., *et al.* (2005). The "Lost boys of Sudan". Functional and behavioral health of unaccompanied refugee minors resettled in the United States. *Archives of Pediatrics and Adolescent Medicine*, *159*, 585–591.

Gillberg, C., & Kadesjo, B. (2003). Why bother about clumsiness? The implications of having developmental coordination disorder (DCD). *Neural Plasticity*, *10*, 59–68.

Griffiths, J. L., Agani, F., Weine, S., Ukshini, S., Pulleyblank-Cofey, E., Ulaj, J., *et al.* (2005). A family-based mental health program of recovery from state terror in Kosova. *Behavioral Sciences and the Law*, *23*, 547–558.

Hauff, E., & Vaglum, P. (1997). Establishing social contact in exile: A prospective community cohort study of Vietnamese refugees in Norway. *Social Psychiatry and Psychiatric Epidemiology*, *32*, 408–415.

Herlihy, J., Scragg, P., & Turner, S. (2002). Discrepancies in autobiographical memories. Implications for the assessment of asylum seekers: Repeated interviews study. *British Medical Journal*, *324*, 324–327.

Heptinstall, E., Sethna, V., & Taylor, E. (2004). PTSD and depression in refugee children: associations with pre-migration trauma and post-migration stress. *European Child and Adolescent Psychiatry*, *13*, 373–380.

Hodes, M. (2000). Psychologically distressed refugee children in the United Kingdom. *Child Psychology and Psychiatry Review*, *5*, 57–68.

Hodes, M. (2002a). Three key issues for young refugees' mental health. *Transcultural Psychiatry*, *39*, 196–213.

Hodes, M. (2002b). Implications for psychiatric services of chronic civilian strife or war: Young refugees in the UK. *Advances in Psychiatric Treatment*, *8*, 366–376.

Hodes, M., & Diaz-Caneja, A. (2006). Treatment options for young people and refugees with posttraumatic stress disorder. In A. Hosin (Ed.), *Children, families and refugees of multiple traumas: Contemporary issues in mental health*. Basingstoke, Hampshire: Palgrave.

Hodes, M., & Tolmac, J. (2005). Severely impaired young refugees. *Clinical Child Psychology and Psychiatry*, *10*, 251–261.

Hollifield, M., Warner, T. D., Lian, N., Krakow, B., Jenkins, J. H., Kesler, J., *et al.* (2002). Measuring trauma and health status in refugees: a critical review. *Journal of the American Medical Association*, *288*, 611–621.

Home Office. (2005). *Asylum Statistics. United Kingdom 2004*. 13/05. London: Home Office. Website: http://www.homeoffice.gov.uk/rds/pdfs05/hosb1305.pdf Accessed May 12, 2006.

Howard, M., & Hodes, M. (2000). Psychopathology, adversity and service utilization of young refugees. *Journal of the American Academy of Child and Adolescent Psychiatry*, *39*, 368–377.

Hubbard, J., Realmuto, G., Northwood, A., & Masten, A. (1995). Comorbidity of psychiatric diagnoses with posttraumatic stress disorder in survivors of childhood trauma. *Journal of the American Academy of Child and Adolescent Psychiatry*, *34*, 1167–1173.

Human Rights Watch. (2006). http://www.humanrightswatch.org/wr2k6/ Accessed June 9, 2006.

Inter-agency Standing Committee (IASC) (2007). *IASC Guidelines on Mental Health and Psychosocial Support in Emergency Settings*. Geneva: IASC.

Joffe, C., Brodaty, H., Luscombe, G., & Ehrlich, F. (2003). The Sydney Holocaust study: Posttraumatic stress disorder and other psychosocial morbidity in an aged community sample. *Journal of Traumatic Stress*, *16*, 39–47.

Jones, L., & Kafetsios, K. (2005). Exposure to political violence and psychological well-being in Bosnian adolescents: A mixed method approach. *Clinical Child Psychology and Psychiatry*, *10*, 157–176.

Jones, L., Rrustemi, A., Shahini, M., & Uka, A. (2003). Mental health services for war affected children: Report of a survey in Kosovo. *British Journal of Psychiatry*, *183*, 540–546.

Kinzie, J. D., Sack, W. H., Angell, R. H., Manson, S., & Rath, B. (1986). The psychiatric effects of massive trauma on Cambodian children. I. The children. *Journal of the American Academy of Child Psychiatry*, *25*, 370–376.

Kirmayer, L., Rousseau, C., & Crepeau, F. (2004). Research ethics and the plight of refugees in detention. *Monash Bioethics Review*, *23*, 85–92.

Kleinman, A., Das, V., & Lock, M. (1997). *Social suffering*. Berkeley, CA: University of California.

Kope, T. M., & Sack, W. H. (1987). Anorexia nervosa in Southeast Asians: a report on three cases. *Journal of the American Academy of Child and Adolescent Psychiatry*, *26*, 795–797.

Kushner, T., & Knox, K. (1999). *Refugees in an age of genocide: Global, national and local perspectives during the twentieth century*. London: Frank Cass.

Kuterovac-Jagodie, G. (2003). Posttraumatic stress symptoms in Croatian children exposed to war: A prospective study. *Journal of Clinical Psychology*, *59*, 9–25.

Laban, C. J., Gernaat, H. B., Komproe, I. H., Schreuders, B. A., & de Jong, T. (2004). Impact of a long asylum procedure on the prevalence of psychiatric disorders in Iraqi asylum seekers in the Netherlands. *Journal of Nervous and Mental Disorders*, *192*, 843–851.

Lamb, C. F., & Cunningham, M. (2003). Dichotomy or decision making: Specialisation and mainstreaming in health service design for refugees. In P. Allotey (Ed.), *The health of refugees: Public health perspectives from crisis to settlement* (pp. 123–138). Oxford: Oxford University Press.

Laor, N., Wolmer, L., Mayes, L. C., Golomb, A., Silverberg, D. S., Weizman, R., *et al.* (1996). Israeli preschoolers under Scud missile attack. *Archives of General Psychiatry*, *53*, 416–423.

Leaning, J. (2001). Ethics of research in refugee populations. *Lancet*, *357*, 1432–1433.

Leavey, G., Hollins, K., King, M., Barnes, J., Papadopoulos, C., & Grayson, K. (2004). Psychological disorder amongst refugee and migrant schoolchildren in London. *Social Psychiatry and Epidemiological Psychiatry*, *39*, 191–195.

Lustig, S. L., Kia-Keating, M., Knight, W. G., Geltman, P., Ellis, H., Kinzie, J. D., *et al.* (2004). Review of child and adolescent refugee mental health. *Journal of the American Academy of Child and Adolescent Psychiatry*, *43*, 24–36.

McKelvey R. S., & Webb, J. A. (1995). Unaccompanied status as a risk factor in Vietnamese Amerasians. *Social Science and Medicine*, *41*, 261–266.

McKelvey, R. S., & Webb, J. A. (1996). Premigratory expectations and postmigratory mental health symptoms in Vietnamese Amerasians. *Journal of the American Academy of Child and Adolescent Psychiatry*, *35*, 240–245.

Mghir, R., Freed, W., Raskin, A., & Katon, W. (1995). Depression and post-traumatic stress disorder among a community sample of adolescent and young adult Afghan refugees. *Journal of Nervous and Mental Disease*, *183*, 24–30.

Mollica, R. F. (2000). The special psychiatric problems of refugees. In M. G. Gelder, J. J. Lopez-Ibor, N. Andreasen (Eds.), *New Oxford textbook of psychiatry* (pp. 1595–1601). Oxford: Oxford University Press.

Mollica, R. F., Caspi-Yavin, M. A. R., Bollini, P., Truong, T., Tor, S., & Lavelle, J. (1992). The Harvard Trauma Questionnaire: Validating a cross-cultural instrument for measuring torture, trauma, and posttraumatic stress disorder in Indochinese refugees. *Journal of Nervous and Mental Disease*, *180*, 111–116.

Mollica, R. F., Poole, C., Son, L., Murray, C. C., & Tor, S. (1997). Effects of war trauma on Cambodian refugee adolescents' functional health and mental health status. *Journal of the American Academy of Child and Adolescent Psychiatry*, *36*, 1098–1106.

Montgomery, E. (1998). Refugee children from the Middle East. *Scandinavian Journal of Social Medicine*, Supplementum 54.

National Collaborating Centre for Mental Health (NCCMH). (2005). *Post-traumatic stress disorder: The management of PTSD in adults and children in primary and secondary care*. London: Royal College of Psychiatrists and British Psychological Society.

Neuner, F., Schauer, M., Klaschik, C., Karunakara, U., & Elbert, T. (2004). A comparison of narrative exposure therapy, supportive counselling and psychoeducation for treating posttraumatic stress disorder in an African refugee settlement. *Journal of Consulting Clinical Psychology*, *72*, 579–587.

Onyut, L. P., Neurer, F., Schauer, E., Ertl, V., Odenwald, M., Shauer, M., *et al.* (2005). Narrative exposure therapy as a treatment for child war survivors with posttraumatic stress disorder: Two case reports and a pilot study in an African refugee settlement. *BMC Psychiatry*, *5*, 7 (www.biomedcentral.com/1471-244X/5/7)

O'Shea, B., Hodes, M., Down, G., & Bramley, J. (2000). A school-based mental health service for refugee children. *Clinical Child Psychology and Psychiatry*, *5*, 189–201.

Paardekooper, B., de Jong, J. T. V. M., & Hermanns, J. M. A. (1999). The psychological impact of war and the refugee situation on South Sudanese children in refugee camps in Northern Uganda: An exploratory study. *Journal of Child Psychology and Psychiatry*, *40*, 529–536.

Patel, N., & Hodes, M. (2006). Violent deliberate self harm amongst adolescent refugees. *European Child and Adolescent Psychiatry*, *15*, 367–370.

Paunovic, N., & Ost, L. G. (2001). Cognitive–behaviour therapy vs. exposure therapy in the treatment of PTSD in refugees. *Behaviour Research and Therapy*, *39*, 1183–1197.

Pedersen, D. (2002). Political violence, ethnic conflict, and contemporary wars: Broad implications for health and social well-being. *Social Science and Medicine*, *55*, 175–190.

Porte, Z., & Tomey-Purta, J. (1987). Depression and academic achievement among Indochinese refugee unaccompanied minors in ethnic and nonethnic placements. *American Journal of Orthopsychiatry*, *57*, 536–547.

Punamaki, R-L. (1996). Can dialogical commitment protect children's psychosocial well-being in situations of political violence? *Child Development*, *67*, 55–69.

Quirk, G. J., & Casco, L. (1994). Stress disorders of families of the disappeared: A controlled study in Honduras. *Social Science and Medicine*, *39*, 1675–1679.

Quota, S., Punamaki, R-L., & El Sarraj, E. (2003). Prevalence and determinants of PTSD among Palestinian children exposed to military violence. *European Child and Adolescent Psychiatry*, *12*, 265–272.

Quota, S., Punamaki, R-L., & El Sarraj, E. E. (2005). Mother–child expression of psychological distress in war trauma. *Clinical Child Psychology and Psychiatry*, *10*, 135–156.

Raval, H. (2005). Being heard and understood in the context of seeking asylum and refuge: Communicating with the help of bilingual co-workers. *Clinical Child Psychology and Psychiatry*, *10*, 197–216.

Reijneveld, S. A., De Boer, J. B., Bean, T., & Korfker, D. G. (2005). Unaccompanied adolescents seeking asylum: Poorer mental health under a restrictive reception. *Journal of Nervous and Mental Disease*, *193*, 759–761.

Robinson, S., Hemmendinger, J., Netanel, R., Rapaport, M., Zilberman, L., & Gal, A. (1994). Retraumatization of Holocaust survivors during the Gulf War and SCUD missile attacks on Israel. *British Journal of Medical Psychology*, *67*, 353–362.

Rousseau, C., Drapeau, A., & Corin, E. (1996). School performance and emotional problems in refugee children. *American Journal of Orthopsychiatry*, *66*, 239–251.

Rousseau, C., Rufagari, M-C., Bagilishya, D., & Measham, T. (2004). Remaking family life: strategies for re-establishing continuity among Congolese refugees during the family reunification process. *Social Science and Medicine*, *59*, 1095–1108.

Rutter, M. (1999). Resilience concepts and findings: Implications for family therapy. *Journal of Family Therapy*, *21*, 119–144.

Rutter, M., & Sandberg, S. (1992). Psychosocial stressors: Concepts, causes and effects. *European Child and Adolescent Psychiatry*, *1*, 3–13.

Sack, W. H., Angell, R. H., Kinzie, J. D., & Rath, B. (1986). The psychiatric effects of massive trauma on Cambodian children. II. The family, home, and the school. *Journal of the American Academy of Child Psychiatry*, *25*, 377–383.

Sack, W. H., Clarke, G., Him, C., Dickason, D., Goff, B., Lanham, K., *et al.* (1993). A six year follow-up study of Cambodian refugee adolescents traumatized as children. *Journal of the American Academy of Child and Adolescent Psychiatry*, *32*, 431–437.

Sack, W. H., Clarke, G., & Seeley, J. (1995a). Posttraumatic stress disorder across two generations of Cambodian refugees. *Journal of the American Academy of Child and Adolescent Psychiatry*, *34*, 1160–1166.

Sack, W. H., Clarke, G. N., Kinney, R., Belestos, G., Him, C., & Seeley, J. (1995b). The Khmer Adolescent Project. II. Functional capacities in two generations of Cambodian refugees. *Journal of Nervous and Mental Disease*, *183*, 177–181.

Sack, W. H., Clarke, G. N., & Seeley, J. R. (1996). Multiple forms of stress in Cambodian adolescent refugees. *Child Development*, *67*, 107–116.

Sack, W. H., Him, C., & Dickason, D. (1999). Twelve-year follow-up study of Khmer youths who suffered massive war trauma as children. *Journal of the American Academy of Child and Adolescent Psychiatry*, *38*, 1173–1179.

Sack, W. H., McSharry, S., Clarke, G. N., Kinney, R., Seeley, J., & Lewinsohn, P. (1994). The Khmer Adolescent Project. I. Epidemiologic findings in two generations of Cambodian refugees. *Journal of Nervous and Mental Disease*, *182*, 387–395.

Sack, W. H., Seeley, J. R., & Clarke, G. N. (1997). Does PTSD transcend cultural barriers? A study from the Khmer adolescent refugee project. *Journal of the American Academy of Child and Adolescent Psychiatry*, *36*, 49–54.

Sandberg, S., Rutter, M., Giles, S., Owen, A., Champion, L., Nicholls, J., *et al.* (1993). Assessment of psychosocial experiences in childhood: Methodological issues and some illustrative findings. *Journal of Child Psychology and Psychiatry*, *34*, 879–897.

Savin, D., Sack, W. H., Clarke, G. N., Meas, N., & Richart, I. (1996). The Khmer adolescent project. III. A study of trauma from Thailand's Site II refuge camp. *Journal of the American Academy of Child and Adolescent Psychiatry*, *35*, 384–391.

Silove, D., Steel, Z., McGorry, P., & Mohan, P. (1998). Trauma exposure, postmigration stressors, and symptoms of anxiety, depression and post-traumatic stress in Tamil asylum seekers: Comparison with refugees and immigrants. *Acta Psychiatrica Scandinavica*, *97*, 175–181.

Smith, P., Perrin, S., Yule, W., Hacam, B., & Stuvland, R. (2002). War exposure among children from Bosnia-Hercegovina: psychological adjustment in a community setting. *Journal of Traumatic Stress*, *15*, 147–156.

Smith, P., Perrin, S., Yule, W., & Rabe-Hesketh, S. (2001). War exposure and maternal reactions in the psychological adjustment of children from Bosnia-Hercegovina. *Journal of Child Psychology and Psychiatry*, *42*, 395–404.

Somasundaram, D. (2002). Child soldiers: Understanding the context. *British Medical Journal*, *324*, 1268–1271.

Sourander, A. (1998). Behaviour problems and traumatic events of unaccompanied refugee minors. *Child Abuse and Neglect*, *22*, 719–727.

Southall, D. P., & O'Hare, B. A. M. (2002). Empty arms: The effect of the arms trade on mothers and children. *British Medical Journal*, *325*, 1457–1461.

Spinhoven, P., Bean, T., & Eurelings-Bontekoe, L. (2006). Inconsistencies in the self-report of traumatic experiences by unaccompanied refugee minors. *Journal of Traumatic Stress*, *19*, 663–673.

Spring, M., Westermeyer, J., Halcon, L., Savik, K., Robertson, C., Johnson, D. R., *et al.* (2003). Sampling in difficult to access refugee and immigrant communities. *Journal of Nervous and Mental Disease*, *191*, 813–819.

Stein, B. D., Jaycox, L. H., Kataoka, S. S. H., Wong, M., Tu, W., Elliott, M. N., *et al.* (2003). A mental health intervention for schoolchildren exposed to violence: A randomized controlled trial. *Journal of the American Medical Association*, *290*, 603–611.

Stein, S., Chalhoub, N., & Hodes, M. (1998). Very early-onset bulimia nervosa: report of two cases. *International Journal of Eating Disorders*, *24*, 323–327.

Summerfield, D. (1999). A critique of seven assumptions behind psychological trauma programmes in war-affected areas. *Social Science and Medicine*, *48*, 1449–1462.

Summerfield, D. (2000). Childhood, war, refugeedom and "trauma": Three core questions for mental health professionals. *Transcultural Psychiatry*, *37*, 417–433.

Summerfield, D. (2001). The invention of post-traumatic stress disorder and the social usefulness of a psychiatric category. *British Medical Journal*, *322*, 95–98.

Thabet, A. A. M., Abed, Y., & Vostanis, P. (2002). Emotional problems in Palestinian children living in a war zone: A cross-sectional study. *Lancet*, *359*, 1801–1804.

Thabet, A. A., Abed, Y., & Vostanis, P. (2004). Comorbidity of PTSD and depression among refugee children during war conflict. *Journal of Child Psychology and Psychiatry*, *45*, 533–542.

Thabet, A. A. M., Karim, K., & Vostanis, P. (2006). Trauma exposure in re-school children in a war zone. *British Journal of Psychiatry*, *188*, 154–158.

Thomas, S., & Byford, S. (2003). Research with unaccompanied children seeking asylum. *British Medical Journal*, *327*, 1400–1402.

Thomas, S., Thomas, S., Nafees, B., & Bhugra, D. (2004). "I was running away from death": The pre-flight experiences of unaccompanied asylum seeking children in the UK. *Child: Care, Health & Development*, *30*, 113–122.

Tobin, J., & Friedman, J. (1984). Intercultural and developmental stresses confronting Southeast Asian refugee adolescents. *Journal of Operational Psychiatry*, *15*, 39–45.

Tolmac, J., & Hodes, M. (2004). Ethnic variation amongst adolescent psychiatric inpatients with psychotic disorders. *British Journal of Psychiatry*, *184*, 428–431.

Tousignant, M., Habimana, E., Biron, C., Malo, C., Sidoli-LeBlanc, E., & Bendris, N. (1999). The Quebec adolescent refugee project: Psychopathology and family variables in a sample from 35 nations. *Journal of the American Academy of Child and Adolescent Psychiatry*, *38*, 1426–1432.

Tufnell, G. (2003). Refugee children, trauma and the law. *Clinical Child Psychology and Psychiatry*, *8*, 431–443.

Udwin, O. (1995). Psychological intervention with war-traumatised children: A consultation model. *ACPP Review and Newsletter*, *17*, 195–200.

UNICEF. (2004). *The state of the world's children 2005*. New York: UNICEF.

United Nations Department of Economic and Social Affairs. (2004). *World economic and social survey 2004: International migration*. New York: United Nations.

UNHCR. (1994). *Refugee children: Guidelines on protection and care*. Geneva: UNHCR.

UNHCR. (2000). *The state of the world's refugees. Fifty years of humanitarian action*. Oxford: Oxford University Press.

UNHCR. (2006). *The state of the world's refugees. Human displacement in the new Millennium*. Oxford: Oxford University Press.

UNHCR. (2007). *2006 Global Trends: Refugees, Asylum seekers, Returnees, Internally Displaced and Stateless Persons*. Geneva: UNHCR. Revised 16 July 2007. http://www.unhcr.org/statistics/STATISTICS/4676a71d4.pdf

Van IJzendoorn, M. H., Bakermans-Kraneberg, M. J., & Sagi-Schwartz, A. (2003). Are children of Holocaust survivors less well-adapted? A meta-analytic investigation of secondary traumatization. *Journal of Traumatic Stress*, *16*, 459–469.

Van Ommeren, M., Saxena, S., & Saraceno, B. (2005). Mental and social health during and after acute emergencies: Emerging consensus? *Bulletin of the World Health Organization*, *83*, 71–76.

Verhulst, F. C., & van der Ende, J. (1997). Factors associated with child mental health service use in the community. *Journal of the American Academy of Child and Adolescent Psychiatry*, *36*, 901–909.

Vizek-Vidovic, V., Kuterovac-Jagodic, G., & Aarambasic, L. (2000). Posttraumatic symptomatology in children exposed to war. *Scandinavian Journal of Psychology*, *41*, 297–306.

Wade, J., Mitchell, F., & Baylis, G. (2005). *Unaccompanied asylum seeking children: The response of the social work services*. London: British Association of Adoption and Fostering.

Weine, S. M., Raina, D., Zhubi, M., Delesi, M., Huseni, D., Feetham, S., *et al.* (2003). The TAFES multi-family group intervention for Kosovar refugees: A feasibility study. *Journal of Nervous and Mental Disease*, *191*, 100–107.

Westermeyer, J. (1991). Psychiatric services for refugee children. In F. Ahearn, & J. L. Athey (Eds.), *Refugee children: Theory, research and services* (pp. 127–162). Baltimore and London: Johns Hopkins University Press.

Westermeyer, J., & Janca, A. (1997). Language, culture and psychopathology: Conceptual and methodological issues. *Transcultural Psychiatry*, *34*, 291–311.

Williams, C. L., & Westermeyer, J. (1983). Psychiatric problems among adolescent Southeast Asian refugees. *Journal of Nervous and Mental Disease*, *171*, 79–85.

Willis, G. B., & Gonzalez, A. (1998). Methodological issues in the use of survey questionnaires to assess the health effects of torture. *Journal of Nervous and Mental Disease*, *186*, 283–289.

Zivcic, I. (1993). Emotional reactions of children to war stress in Croatia. *Journal of the American Academy of Child and Adolescent Psychiatry*, *32*, 709–713.

32 Residential and Foster Family Care

Alan Rushton and Helen Minnis

All societies need to decide how to respond when children lose or are abandoned by their parents, when parenting breaks down, or when serious abuse, neglect or family dysfunction means that children need to be safeguarded by removal from their biological families. At one time, extensive use was made of orphanages but, for good reasons, most countries have sought greatly to reduce or eliminate the use of residential care for very young children. Countries differ in their approaches to child welfare and major variations exist in policy and practice among countries. The threshold at which intervention in family life is justified by the child welfare agencies differs. The length of time spent in care away from home, the type of placement that is favored and the extent of moves between placements vary. Children enter public care for a variety of reasons in the UK but the majority do so because of abuse, neglect and family dysfunction. Sixty-eight percent are placed in foster care, 13% in residential care and about 9% are placed with their birth families. The remainder are placed for adoption or in more specialist placements (DfES, 2006).

This chapter focuses on mental health aspects of residential and foster family care. It deals with the mental health of children in residential and foster family care in countries with modern child welfare systems and considers assessment and intervention in both settings. It covers the effects of orphanage care where it still exists and recent attempts to improve its quality. Finally, it deals with comparisons of residential and foster family outcomes, cost-effectiveness and future directions.

Much of the published research on residential care and foster family care concerns the provision and management of children's placements. Research funds are largely raised to answer policy and economic questions rather than developmental ones and studies often resemble audits of the local child welfare agency's activities. This kind of research is crucial to the provision of good quality care but less illuminating regarding children's mental health. We will therefore only be attending in passing to issues of recruitment, assessment, retention and remuneration of foster and residential care staff; policies to raise standards and eradicate abuse in care settings and the growing attention to children's rights. Kinship care will not be dealt with here (see chapter 33) and only brief mention will be made of short-term foster placements with a view to return home.

Rutter's Child and Adolescent Psychiatry, 5th edition. Edited by M. Rutter, D. Bishop, D. Pine, S. Scott, J. Stevenson, E. Taylor and A. Thapar. © 2008 Blackwell Publishing, ISBN: 978-1-4051-4549-7.

Institutional Care in Early Life: Assessing Effects and Improving Environments

Effects of Institutional Care in Early Life

It is over 50 years since the first studies drew attention to the negative effects on children raised in institutions (Goldfarb, 1945; Spitz, 1945) and since Bowlby (1951) published *Maternal care and mental health*, where he voiced his concerns about the importance of secure early attachment relationships. Subsequent empirical investigations have refined our understanding of what kind of effects, including disorders of attachment, are produced by what kinds of environment.

Two influential studies have been conducted in the UK on children with different amounts of exposure to residential care. Tizard and colleagues studied infants who had experienced residential nursery care for the first 2 years of life, involving high turnover of caregivers, and compared those who went home with those who were adopted or who remained in institutions. When they were assessed at 4½ years (Tizard & Rees, 1975), those who remained in institutions had higher mean behavior problem scores and had not formed deep attachments. A substantial proportion of the sample, when followed up to adolescence, showed social difficulties, especially in peer relationships (Hodges & Tizard, 1989). This study suggested that early institutional care can have enduring effects.

Quinton and Rutter (1988) studied outcomes of children who had disrupted early years, were taken into public care and then spent prolonged periods in group homes in the 1960s. The regimes were not harsh, but multiple changes of staff resulted in little consistent affection. The adult follow up of this ex-care sample (Rutter, Quinton, & Hill, 1990) showed that one-third were faring poorly. With regard to the ex-care women, 30% had a poor general psychosocial outcome and 40% had a rating of poor parenting, much higher than in the general population comparison group. However, it was evident that many did not show poor parenting and a minority, surprisingly, showed good parenting. These studies indicate that an institutional environment, when involving lack of consistent personalized care, can contribute to harmful effects on development but also that later positive experiences can divert some from negative outcomes.

Continued Use of Institutional Care for Very Young Children

Despite recognition of the significance of the caregiver–child relationship and the known ill effects and costs of prolonged residential care, the lessons have not been equally absorbed in all countries. Browne, Hamilton-Giachritsis, Johnson *et al.* (2006) have recently conducted a survey on the use of institutional care for children under 3 years in 46 countries in the European region. The data were all based on official government figures, with the usual limitations, but the overall rate of institutional care was estimated at 14.4 per 10,000 children under 3 years. This amounts to nearly 44,000 very young children. The countries with the highest use of institutional care in proportion to the population under 3 years were Bulgaria (69 per 10,000), Latvia, Belgium, Romania and Serbia and Montenegro. These data provide a useful benchmark figure with which to compare the highest use with countries with no institutional care for very young children and in order to compare future efforts at replacing institutional with family-based care for this group. It was suggested that low spending on health and social care was related to a higher proportion of institutionalized children.

As understaffed poor-quality group residential care still exists in many countries, this has afforded the possibility of conducting studies on the development of children raised in extremely depriving circumstances. Chisholm's (1998) follow-up study revealed more insecure attachment and indiscriminately friendly behavior in children adopted from Romanian orphanages than among never-institutionalized and early adopted comparison groups. Vorria, Papaligoura, Dunn *et al.* (2004), in a study based in the Metera babies' center in Greece, showed much higher rates of disorganized attachment in residential care infants compared with infants living in birth families. Follow-up in adoptive placements at age 4 showed that the institutionalized children continued to have poorer cognitive development, were less secure and had poorer understanding of emotions compared to family controls (Vorria, Papaligoura, Sarafidou *et al.*, 2006). The Bucharest early intervention project group (Zeanah, Smyke, Koga *et al.*, 2005) has also shown that an institutionalized Romanian group exhibited serious disturbances of attachment (see chapter 55) compared with a never-institutionalized community group. Furthermore, variation in the quality of caregiving was related to the attachment status of children in the institutional group.

Other researchers have begun to investigate the effect of early maltreatment and institutionalization on the hypothalamic–pituitary axis and results suggest that deficiencies in early care may be associated with abnormal patterns of diurnal cortisol production (Dozier, Manni, Gordon *et al.*, 2006). The neuroendocrine system appears susceptible to relationship disturbance and periods of long-term exposure to stressors may result in damage to areas of the brain and this may confer vulnerability for later disorder. Low levels of cortisol seen in older foster children may result from a system that has been downregulated through continuous response to stress (Dozier & Rutter, in press).

A major question is whether these are enduring effects, or whether a radical change of circumstances following institutional care, especially by means of adoption, can erase the effects of early adversity. The English Romanian Adoptees (ERA) Study Team have followed up children ($n = 144$) who were placed in institutions, mostly in the first month of life, and who had very poor early experience with little stimulation or interaction with caregivers and with inadequate nutrition. It was shown that these children can achieve significant developmental catch-up, depending on their age at adoptive placement (O'Connor & Rutter, 2000; Rutter *et al.*, 1998). In terms of psychological functioning assessed at 6 years of age, 70% of those entering the UK at less than 6 months showed no impairment, but of those entering later, 24–42 months, only one-quarter had no impairment. However, when compared with a UK adoption sample who had not experienced institutional care, they exhibited cognitive impairment, quasi-autistic patterns, inattention/overactivity, disinhibited attachment disorder symptoms and poorer peer relations. It was concluded that psychological deficits persist in a substantial minority. Cognitive functioning and disinhibited attachment disorder symptoms were strongly related to poor quality institutional care that persisted beyond the age of 6 months (Rutter, Beckett, Castle *et al.*, 2007). It was suggested that disinhibited attachment disorder symptoms were related to a relative failure to develop selective attachment, whereas cognitive impairment was more likely to be related to neural impairment. However, both outcomes could reflect some form of programming effect on brain development (see chapter 12; Rutter *et al.*, 2007).

Further follow-ups are planned for many of these early institution-reared samples. Catch-up appears to be more possible with regard to physical development and cognitive ability, but with an enduring impact for some children on behavioral and social development. Questions remain as to what contribution is made to longer-term differential outcome by genetic inheritance, mother's physical and mental health during pregnancy, perinatal factors, child temperament and the benefit of subsequent high-quality environments.

Longer-Term Consequences of Institutional Care on Young Children

So far, few follow-up studies have been undertaken to see how early privation affects development into later phases of the adult years. However, follow-up studies of children who remained in, or were adopted out of, orphanages in the 1950s and 1960s offer the prospect of lifespan studies to examine group outcomes. Although tracking representative samples may be problematic, this could reveal whether subsequent favorable experience can modify or remove the risks, or whether there are subgroups with poor adjustment, in particular having continuing social relationship problems.

There appears to be only one very long-term study of orphanage infants followed up into later adulthood and compared with a matched community group (Sigal, Perry, Rossigol *et al.*, 2003). The ex-institutional adults were found to be more isolated and had more stress-related physical illness. However, the study was based on a convenience sample of litigants in a self-help group and this may have contributed to sample bias.

Improving the Environments of Young Children in Institutional Care

As the pattern of short- and long-term negative effects continues to be worked out, so policies on what is best for children are being developed. In those countries where institutional rearing continues to be the main form of care for unwanted or relinquished babies and children, efforts are now being made to reduce the carer–infant ratio in order to provide greater contact time and continuity of relationships. Better training for staff will emphasize the importance of more individualized care.

One experiment is evaluating the outcomes of such efforts. Groark, Muhamedrahimov, Palmov *et al.* (2005) have developed interventions in baby homes in St. Petersburg to see if the stability and social responsiveness of caregivers can be improved and whether the developmental progress of the infants can be promoted. The homes prior to the intervention were orderly but impersonal and the physical care sufficient but mechanical. They compared two active interventions with a no-intervention group. In the first experimental group, carers were helped to replace detached caregiving with more warmth and sensitive responsiveness. In the second group, structural changes only were made to increase the stability of caregivers to provide more continuity of relationships. Initial data (see www.education.pitt.edu/ocd/projects/russiaproject.pdf) have shown that significant changes were observed in the carers' behavior and in children's development (physical growth, psychological development and positive affect), but the full analysis comparing outcomes across groups is ongoing.

In a Romanian intervention study, Sparling, Dragomir, Ramey *et al.* (2005) established small groups with a familiar adult, stressing enriched educational activities. Significant developmental progress was demonstrated compared with usual institutional care controls. Zeanah, Nelson, Fox *et al.* (2003) are conducting a randomized controlled trial into foster family care as an alternative to institutionalization in Bucharest. Institutional children are being randomly selected into a newly set up foster care system and compared with those who remained in the institutions.

It is important to consider which features of early institutional care affect outcomes across a range of developmental domains. The specific contributions of inadequate nutrition, physical and sexual abuse, lack of play and stimulation, of opportunity for selective attachments and lack of personalized care need to be investigated. Further research, based on follow-ups from differing early care environments is needed in order to tease apart these influences.

Clearly, those families willing to take on the care of ex-institutional children need good evidence-based information on their likely life course plus relevant preparation and long-term support services (Groze & Ileana, 1996). Those families facing continuing difficulties should be encouraged to seek help from specialist child and adolescent mental health services for the assessment and treatment of complex developmental and social problems. There remains a great amount of institutional care internationally and warnings have been sounded that the AIDS epidemic will produce many more orphans where the family and community are not able to absorb them (Levine, 2000).

Modern Residential Care and Children's and Adolescents' Mental Health

Residential provision for children and young people, when defined most broadly, can embrace care settings with a variety of titles. In this chapter we deal with non-family settings that aim to provide care, protection and control, variously known as children's homes, community homes or group homes. We will also deal with residential treatment centers that aim to provide therapeutic care for mental health needs and are specifically staffed and resourced to do so. However, severe problems can be found in each setting, because examples of major mental illness that have been missed can be found in social care settings (McCann, James, Wilson *et al.*, 1996). Child and adolescent psychiatric units (see chapter 69), special residential schools (often for older disabled children; see chapter 74), young offender institutions (see chapter 68) and independent fee-paying boarding schools may all be seen as forms of residential care but are beyond the scope of this review.

Defining types of residential care can be problematic and even services carrying the same name (e.g., "residential group home") will differ widely within and across countries, especially with regard to the size and characteristics of the resident population, the staffing ratio, typical length of stay, objectives and culture: all of which make for difficulties in making meaningful comparisons of "residential" outcomes. Residential care is clearly not a single entity, as the physical and psychological environment for the child is capable of considerable variation, with the quality of care likely to be the most important aspect. Furthermore, it is hard to judge the validity of classic studies conducted several decades ago when practices and attitudes may have been very different.

Reviews of residential care outcome studies have generally lamented both the small volume and modest quality of evaluative research (Bates, English, & Kouidou-Giles, 1997; Foltz, 2004; Whittaker, 2000). Few studies have been conducted at Level One, that is employing experimental evaluation (see the York Centre for Reviews and Dissemination hierarchy of research designs), and most research is at Level 3, that is cohort studies without controls. The research requirements to answer "what works" questions are similar to those for other psychosocial interventions; namely, adequate sample size, random allocation to the intervention, appropriate and reliable multiple outcome measures across time, detailed identification of the intervention and fidelity in its application, appropriate statistical analysis and economic costing. The fact that such studies are rare is partly because of the ethical and logistical obstacles to be surmounted in randomly allocating children in "real world" settings to residential care or to alternatives. Most studies are therefore of single children's homes, or study samples combining children from several homes, and employing within-group analysis of outcomes. Single sample designs do not, of course, permit conclusions about the effectiveness of residential care, but can be used to see which factors predict differential outcomes. However, even where controlled studies have been conducted in related areas, namely on young offenders and child and adolescent psychiatric inpatients, few differences in outcome have been shown on key measures. When benefits have been shown, the effect sizes have been small (Lyman & Campbell, 1996).

Unfortunately, experimental studies comparing different models of residential care would necessitate large cluster randomized trials and the cost may not fall within the budgets of the child welfare research funding agencies. In the near-absence of randomized controlled comparisons, the residential field has had to rely on culling the best information from existing studies, despite their limitations. The following studies have been selected because they have been conducted recently, thus reflecting current practice, and on relatively large samples.

Group Homes for Children Designed to Offer Care, Protection and Control

This section deals with the population of children in countries where residential care is no longer used for younger children, but continues to be used for young people without available families or those who cannot live with, or be managed within, their own or a foster family. In the UK, the residential care population constitutes a relatively small, but high-risk and resource-consuming aspect of child welfare.

In the UK, most residents will be young adolescents showing very raised levels of social and emotional problems, and dysfunctional coping strategies (Meltzer, 2003). They are likely to have experienced abuse and/or neglect, to have been in previous failed placements, to have an ethnic minority background and may have been placed by virtue of being unaccompanied asylum seekers or refugees. Young people in residential care are also more likely to have physical or intellectual disabilities that may raise the risk for attendant mental health problems (Sinclair, 2005).

Given these problematic backgrounds, the staff of children's homes are therefore confronted with numerous problems in managing the young people in their care. The home must carefully judge its protective response to the young people in relation to sexual exploitation, bullying, drug-taking and exposure to health risks. Conflicts are likely to arise in controlling disruptive behavior or threats against staff and in the application of restrictions, forms of punishment and physical restraint. Sometimes, these "care" and "control" principles are in conflict (e.g., when the "right" of a young person to abscond conflicts with the aims of the home to protect the young person from risk).

The heavy criticism of the quality of residential child care evidenced both by abuse inquiries (Utting, 1997; Waterhouse, 2000) and studies of the psychological needs and problems of residents has led many to the conclusion that residential care is ineffective, or at worst positively harmful, and resulted in a swing to a "family is best" ideology. This, combined with the cost, has made residential care a disfavored option and in many countries has led to the rapid run down of residential care places. However, the current literature reveals a spectrum of views on the future of residential care including advocates of high-quality selectively used facilities (Hellinckk, 2002; Pecora, Whittaker, Maluccio *et al.*, 2000). Arguments in favor of residential care are that it is often the young person's preference, that it can provide better support for educational progress for some and may remove the residents from the influence of delinquent peers in the community. Countries that have tried to do without residential care have had to pull back and recognize that family-based care can have its limits, may similarly result in abuse and that specialized and selective residential facilities are still needed (Ainsworth & Hansen, 2005). Further efforts need to be made to ensure that residential care provides a good quality, safe environment (Stein, 2006). This will include improving the vetting, selection, training and support of residential staff, guidelines on best practices and effective complaints procedures to expose institutional abuse.

Two recent studies have examined the outcomes of group home care. Sinclair and Gibbs (1998), in their study of 48 children's homes in the UK, assessed the outcome of former residents against the effect of having been in what was characterized as a "good home." This rating was an attempt to develop an overall measure of the social climate or culture by which the homes could be differentiated. Reports by staff and residents of high morale, friendliness and resident involvement were defined as a "good home." However, having been in a "good home" was found to be unrelated to the outcome measures, particularly when the residents had moved from the home. They concluded that the beneficial experience was true only for their time as residents and did not relate to subsequent outcome. The lack of impact may have been because of the negative effect of the new environment they then entered and may argue for greater continuity of support and mental health intervention.

Scholte and van der Ploeg (2000) monitored the outcomes of 200 young people 2 years after admission to residential care. This was a social care setting in the Netherlands that employed some use of specialist psychological interventions. Those who left as planned had reasonable outcomes, whereas those who left prematurely had further developmental difficulties including problems of aggression and antisocial behavior as severe as before their admission. Factors predicting good outcome included the therapeutic climate of the home, use of cognitive–behavioral therapy, emotional support and "home centeredness." Subsequent negative post-care factors may undo the benefits of good quality residential care while a longer period in good quality care may lead to greater benefit. Better post-care support may help to sustain the positive changes.

Residential Treatment Centers

Several recent studies have examined the post-residential outcomes of specialized treatment programs for children. A US study (Connor, Miller, Cunningham *et al.*, 2002) examined a psycho-educational program using individual and group therapy and medication for seriously emotionally disturbed children. One-third of the children showed improvement or stayed the same, but the remainder showed deterioration. Children with a high level of psychopathology at admission and children with abuse histories were more likely to be in the deteriorated group. Gorske, Sreabus, and Walls (2003) investigated the outcomes for 150 adolescents in residential treatment centers in Pennsylvania which employed a combination of psychological interventions. Most cases resulted in successful discharge. Those more likely to succeed exhibited less antisocial behavior, lived with family members prior to placement and were given a combination of treatments. Another psycho-educational program (Hooper, Murphy, Devaney *et al.*, 2000), with a longer prospective design than most, found that 6 months after discharge, performance was rated as satisfactory for 68% but reduced to 29% by 24 months. This implies that, in future studies, the effect of the post-care environment will need to be evaluated.

Only limited conclusions can be drawn from follow-up from single settings. Studies that show positive outcomes may at first appear encouraging, but leave open the possibility of several explanations. The improvements could have occurred simply through maturation and development. Children in settings that were not studied could have benefited from other more cost-effective interventions. However, it can reasonably be concluded from within-group analysis that those with more adverse histories and more severe problems generally do worse; that continued involvement with a reasonably well-functioning birth family is a positive factor and that the post-discharge period is critical for positive development or for the re-emergence of problems. Where the outcomes were poor, it is possible that the residential care environment was not specialized enough to meet their needs.

Interest has recently turned to German and Scandinavian models in the search for improved quality of residential care (Cameron, 2004). The "social pedagogy" model, which emphasizes careworkers sharing the everyday lives of young people in residential services, placing educational aims more centrally and working with their families and the community in order to achieve effective integration into society, is likely to become more influential in the UK (Boddy, Cameron, & Petrie, 2005). This model is not directly comparable with UK services, however, as it has much better staffed and trained workers with higher remuneration. Rigorous evaluations of its effectiveness do not seem to have been conducted, or planned.

What is the Quality of the Evidence on Residential Care Environments?

Several points need to be made about conceptualization and methodological concerns in residential care research. First, it is evident that the terms institutional and residential care cover a broad range of environments in terms of severity and types of deprivation. It is misleading therefore to refer to the effects of residential care per se. The environment needs to be clearly examined as to the potentially negative and beneficial physical and psychological elements. Second, reliable data are often lacking about events and circumstances prior to admission to residential care. In building a comprehensive model of the factors leading to outcomes subsequent to residential care it is necessary to take into account not simply the degree of exposure to an institutional experience, but genetic inheritance, risk exposure during the pregnancy, perinatal and other pre-residential factors. These may all contribute, in combination with the residential care experience, to long-term development.

In addition to these prior factors, it is important to consider how long-term outcomes are mediated by subsequent events and how residential care experiences may have different types of adverse effect depending on the developmental age of the child. If the negative effects are reversible, or at least reducible, what is the capacity for adaptability of the individual, or constraints on making flexible responses to a changed environment?

Finally, is it possible to have a form of residential care that comes without the usual disadvantages? If resources allowed for the quality of the physical environment, nutrition and medical care to be raised to the highest standard, could paid non-related carers replicate, or approximate, the level of investment and involvement provided by most birth parents? The key test would be whether the quality of staff would be such as to provide consistent individualized care capable of promoting selective attachments.

Guidance for Practitioners on the Use of Residential Care

Evidence is often lacking to support clear-cut placement choices. However, children with repeated failed foster placements, high-risk behavior or strong opposition to family placement might well be better placed in appropriate residential care. Contact with attachment figures should be maintained where possible, while bearing in mind that children can have very powerful attachments to parents who are abusive and that further rejection, or re-involvement in the negative circumstances that led to care, might result from contact. Careful assessment of risk factors, and of the quality of current relationships with attachment figures, is necessary to counterbalance the presumption that contact is beneficial.

Providing Foster Family Care

Many children spend only a matter of weeks in public care. Such short-stay foster care placements are known to be a helpful response at times of crisis or to provide a valuable short break during family hardship and stress. These placements commonly meet their aims, may prevent family breakdown and need not lead to serious distress for the children depending, of course, on how well the move and return are handled and the quality of the alternative care (Aldgate & Bradley, 1999). However, when a safe return home then becomes hard to achieve, the children may drift into becoming part of the longer-stay group.

Foster care is considered to be the preferred placement for children who have experienced family breakdown or maltreatment (Roy, Rutter, & Pickles, 2000), but of those so placed a significant proportion disrupts; that is, the child has to leave the placement in a manner that is not in accordance with the plans of the foster care agency or department. This is seen as one of the major flaws of foster family care. Rates of breakdown range from 20% to 50% and differ considerably according to the national context and placing agency (Minty, 1999). Ward and Skuse (2001) found that in the first year of care less than half of the children remained in the same placement although half of these moves were regarded as "planned transitions." We know virtually nothing about the effect of these planned moves on children's mental health. A recent meta-analysis suggests that the first 6 months of placement pose the greatest risk of breakdown (Oosterman, Schuengel, Slot *et al.*, 2007). For all concerned, a *precipitate placement* ending is traumatic, not least for the child who then faces changes of school, community and friendships and is left with an uncertain future. When a child has experienced a series of placement disruptions, residential care may be seen as either the "end of the road" or as a relief from the pain of forming relationships that may fail again. Alternatively, the child may drift back to the birth family in the late teenage years, often with unsatisfactory results.

Efforts are currently being made to convert stable foster placements into adoption, but little is known about the proportion for whom this legal change is being achieved and with what outcome. It is likely that these placements will be more stable than stranger adoptive placements as positive relationships will largely have been established when the application to adopt is made (Barth, Berry, Yoshikami *et al.*, 1988).

What are the factors associated with foster care stability? These are difficult to collate as studies use different samples, definitions of placement endings and different follow-up periods, but meta-analysis has demonstrated significant associations with behavior problems in the child, older age of the child at placement and a history of residential care (Oosterman, Schuengel, Slot *et al.*, 2007). It has been alleged that transracial foster placements have negative effects on the children, especially in relation to identity and self-esteem. However, in the 1990s, Tizard and Phoenix's (1995) UK study of mixed parentage adolescents suggested that social class, school and peer groups exerted greater effects on racial identity than the ethnicity of their parents. Rushton and Minnis (1997) reviewed the comparative outcome literature on transracial placement and, although they did not find worse outcomes on standard measures, they did highlight the difficulties that may arise for the children of being separated from the community of origin. In the UK, ethnically matched placements are sought as far as this is feasible and within reasonable time limits.

Sinclair and Wilson (2003) found significant associations with outcome for the child wanting to stay in the placement, having high prosocial scores and low disturbance scores. Foster carer characteristics such as warmth and child-oriented foster carers were significantly associated with success. Further multivariate analysis attempted to examine the interactions between child and foster carer characteristics. They found that where foster carers are committed to the child, despite child disturbance, outcomes can be good, at least in the short term. In placements where the foster carers are less committed and the child has a high level of difficulties, outcomes are likely to be less successful. Reinforcing commitment as well as promoting parenting skills should both, in the light of this, be targets for support services. Clearly, policy needs to be directed towards greater recruitment of carefully selected foster families permitting more placement choice, more effective training, more intensive support for foster carers, promoting a skilled and committed children's social care workforce. Increased financial rewards for foster parents have been shown to be related to retention rates and outcomes for the children and campaigns have been mounted to increase remuneration for foster carers (Chamberlain, Moreland, & Reid, 1992). The impact of such changes has not been subject to recent evaluation.

What do we Know About the Mental Health of Children in Residential and Foster Family Care in Modern Child Welfare Systems?

All studies have consistently demonstrated a high level of mental health problems in children in public care (Blower, Addo, Hodgson *et al.*, 2004; Curtis McMillen, Zima, Scott *et al.*, 2005; Dimigen, Del Priore, Butler *et al.*, 1999; Halfon, Mendonca, & Berkowitz, 1995; McCann *et al.*, 1996; Meltzer, 2003; Meltzer, Gatward, Goodman *et al.*, 1999). Recent estimates suggest an approximately five-fold prevalence compared to the general population (Meltzer, 2003). These problems include some previously unrecognized major psychiatric disorders (McCann *et al.*, 1996) and a high prevalence of both disruptive behavioral and emotional problems (Meltzer, 2003).

Recent work in the USA has demonstrated that nearly 90% of young children entering an episode of care, regardless of placement type, have physical, developmental or mental health needs, with more than half demonstrating more than one problem (Leslie, Gordon, Meneken *et al.*, 2005). A key question here is whether the mental health difficulties of children in public care are a cause or consequence of that care. Harsh parenting and a tendency toward emotional overarousal (which may be inherited) interact in very early life to increase the risk of conduct disorder (Scaramella & Leve, 2004). Disruptive behavioral disorders are particularly linked with foster family breakdown (James, 2004; Leathers, 2002, 2006) and these disorders may test carers beyond their capabilities.

Child and adolescent psychiatrists are well aware of the phenomenon of children "testing" their parental figures with disruptive behavior, sometimes resulting in a cycle of increasingly coercive parenting. If this style of child–carer interaction actually results in the foster carer relinquishing the child, a vicious cycle of distrust of parental figures may result.

It is well established that factors prior to coming into a current placement, such as maltreatment and frequent changes of caregiver, are important contributing factors towards poor mental health (Dimigen *et al.*, 1999; St. Claire & Osborne, 1987), but problems with emotion understanding and theory of mind (Pears & Fisher, 2005) and post-traumatic stress disorder (PTSD; Dubner & Motta, 1999) may also be obstacles to relationship development. Mental health difficulties of children in public care may be brought about by prior adversity, but these problems may also be compounded by unstable placements and poorly matched substitute care. Comparisons in rates of mental health problems simply across placement types can be uninformative without taking into account prior care histories and child characteristics.

Scholastic difficulties and poor educational attainment constitute a major aspect of the problems presented by looked after children to child psychiatric services. Abundant evidence exists that poor attainment is extremely common, resulting in a low level of qualifications on leaving care. The percentage of looked after children in England achieving 5 GCSEs has risen slightly, but remains very low, at about 10%, compared with 56% for the non-looked after population (DfES, 2005). It is not clear why this is so. One possibility is to do with the educational environment. However, studies in Europe and the USA indicate similar educational problems. A high-quality French study of young adults who had spent at least 5 years in foster care showed that two-thirds obtained no general educational diploma (a rate more than double the national norm). Poor educational outcome was particularly associated with learning difficulties before going into care (Dumaret, Coppel-Batsch, & Couraud, 1997). It may be that the stability of these long-term placements was important for children to achieve better educational outcomes, which suggests that poor educational outcomes may be associated with frequent changes of placement. One US study compared educational outcomes of high school and post-high school foster care youth matched with those living with their birth families (Blome, 1997). More educational disruption was evident for the foster care youth, a higher rate of school dropout, behavioral problems in school and less financial assistance from their carers for education support. Other factors worth considering in influencing poor progress are the effects of adverse experiences on cognitive development, broken relationships with peers and adults in the school setting associated with placement changes and breakdown, foster carers' level of engagement with the child's education and the young person's feelings of self-worth and ambition. Securing the stability of the foster care placement should therefore be a major aim, as well as striving for better collaboration between education and social services. Adults need to guard against having lower expectations of young people in foster care and to promote opportunities to remain in education. Research is needed to identify promising socio-educational interventions and to evaluate their impact. Improving academic achievement will be central to future employment prospects, to economic status, to life satisfaction and indeed to the mental health of the ex-care population.

Comprehensive Assessment of Psychosocial Problems of Children in Public Care

The current agenda is to understand how to achieve comprehensive assessments leading to effective interventions. No generally accepted, evidence-based model exists for assessing these children. Recent US research has shown that nearly 90% of children newly entering care placements have complex difficulties including mental health, academic and language problems (Evans, Scott, & Schultz, 2004) and other US evidence suggests that specialists are more successful than community practitioners at recognizing these multiple problems (Horwitz, Owens, & Simms, 2000). Despite this evidence, a recent US survey of national guidelines for the assessment of children entering foster care found that, in less than half of the areas studied, was there a requirement for comprehensive physical, mental health and developmental examinations of all children (Leslie, Hurlburt, Landsverk *et al.*, 2003).

Achieving comprehensive assessment of children entering foster family and residential care is complex. Full assessment of child psychopathology usually depends both on current symptomatology and on developmental history and acquiring this information can be difficult, especially for a child who has recently been placed in a new foster or residential placement (Garwood & Close, 2001). Foster carers or residential workers may be able to report on current symptoms, if they have had time to get to know the child, but may have little information on early developmental milestones. Timing of assessment is also important. Many commonly used measures of psychosocial functioning have been normed in the general population and are designed neither to detect problems in recently traumatized children nor to discriminate between ongoing psychopathology and adjustment reactions.

In addition to the assessment of conventionally recognized mental health problems, the child's current relationship functioning needs to be considered. In an innovative project in Louisiana, every child coming into foster care under the age of 4 years has a comprehensive assessment by a specialist Infant Mental Health Team (Zeanah, Larrieu, Heller *et al.*, 2001). The assessment consists of face-to-face contact with the child and each important caregiver such as birth parents, foster carers and child care providers. It includes home- and clinic-based observations, interviews and self-report measures designed to identify strengths and weaknesses in children and families. In a quasi-experimental design, this group has shown that the assessment package, plus an intervention designed to help parents accept responsibility for their maltreatment, significantly reduces the recurrence of maltreatment of children who return home and significantly reduces maltreatment of subsequent children by the same parent. Interestingly, the rate of freeing for adoption was also increased in the group receiving intensive assessment and treatment, suggesting that the assessment allows a clear decision to be made regarding the viability of the child–birth family relationship.

In the UK, many new specialist mental health teams for children in foster and residential care have been developed over the last few years, but models of assessment and treatment vary from teams that offer mainly consultation, to those that offer detailed assessment of the child in the family context. Although studies comparing different models of assessment are rare in this population, there is evidence that problems are commonly missed in this group (Evans, 2004; Horowitz, Bell, Trybulski *et al.*, 2001; McCann *et al.*, 1996). This, and our clinical experience, would lead us to recommend that there should be a thorough assessment of the child's strengths, interests and potential protective factors that could be built on, all areas of psychopathology, speech and language functioning and the quality of attachment relationships. Because educational difficulties are so common in this group, we would strongly recommend full cognitive and educational assessment even when problems are not suspected.

Interventions to Improve the Mental Health of Children in Public Care

Interventions in Residential Settings

Long-standing problems exist in recognizing mental health problems in the residents of children's homes, and despite the call for greater involvement of specialist child mental health services, few projects have been evaluated. Many problems are potentially treatable by a range of psychological interventions. The efficacy of such interventions has been reviewed by Fonagy, Targey, Cottrell *et al.* (2002) but there is a lack of evidence on the extent to which modifications may be needed when applied in the context of residential care. In considering how to achieve greater access to evidence-based interventions, residential care managers and practitioners will need to assess which staff members with what levels of experience and skill might use these interventions. Many aspects of the children's and young peoples' lives will be different in the residential care context so that individual, group- and family-based approaches may need to be thoughtfully adapted.

The quality of the relationships between staff and young people is likely to be a major factor in promoting positive mental health. The rationale is that supportive and containing relationships between young people and staff can contribute to ameliorating past negative relationships (Berridge, 2002; Moses, 2000). The residential careworkers may be the best target for providing training, support and mental health consultation because they are likely to have the greatest influence in helping the young person to develop self-understanding and prospects for change (Wilson, Petrie, & Sinclair, 2003). Careworkers need skills in managing oppositional behavior and aggression, containing the expression of powerful feelings as well as understanding the underlying problems in order to shape their response more appropriately. However, little evidence has so far emerged to show that improving the skills and knowledge of the staff can have a beneficial impact on the resident, both during and after residential care. The external residential consultant will need to respect the stresses that fall on, frequently young, residential staff providing 24-hour care. The mental health consultants can help the staff of a residential home to have a greater understanding of the possible origins of a young person's current difficulties and to help staff to adopt rational management strategies. They can identify the type and severity of disorders and recommend appropriate treatment, based either in the home or in the clinic.

Interventions in Foster Family Care

There has been a sea change, at least in the UK and USA, in attempts to intervene with the psychosocial difficulties of children in public care. The accumulating evidence regarding placements themselves (Sinclair, 2005) and about these children's difficulties, along with a realization of the need for co-ordination between different agencies (Callaghan, Young, Pace *et al.*, 2004; Racusin, Maerlender, Sengupta *et al.*, 2005), has stimulated the development of teams whose remit is to provide specialist intervention for these children. Interventions tend to fall into two main categories: symptom focused or systemic (Racusin *et al.*, 2005).

However, considerable variation still exists in the provision of child and adolescent mental health services for such children (Callaghan *et al.*, 2004; Leslie, Gordon, Meneken *et al.*, 2005; Minnis & Del Priore, 2001). Some of the most vulnerable children do not access child and adolescent mental health services (CAMHS) because of their mobility through placements, a tendency for social workers and foster carers not to refer on despite recognition of problems or, once referred, their mental health profile not fitting with conventional diagnostic criteria used in CAMHS (Callaghan, Young, Pace *et al.*, 2004).

Because almost all children in public care have suffered disruption of attachments and been maltreated, an obvious focus for intervention is attachment relationships. Maltreatment (Carlson, Cicchetti, Barnett *et al.*, 1989) and institutional care (Vorria *et al.*, 2004) are both strongly associated with disorganized attachment but, in addition, unusual attachment patterns are common in children adopted from institutions (Chisholm, 1998; Marcovitch, Goldberg, Gold *et al.*, 1997; O'Connor & Zeanah, 2003a). Reactive attachment disorder (RAD) describes a constellation of social behavioral abnormalities, including: (i) disinhibition with strangers; or (ii) inhibited, hypervigilant or highly ambivalent reactions (American Psychiatric Association, 2000) and, although the research database is scant, there is now research on both institutionalized (Boris, Zeanah, Larrieu *et al.*, 1998; Boris, Hinshaw-Fuselier, Smyke *et al.*, 2004; Chisholm, 1998; O'Connor &

Zeanah, 2003b; Smyke, Dumitrescu, & Zeanah, 2002) and otherwise maltreated groups of young children (see chapter 55; Boris *et al.*, 2004). RAD and insecure attachment patterns are different entities and it is possible to have RAD yet an apparently secure attachment with the current caregiver.

Placement in a stable family environment is a major intervention in itself (van IJzendoorn & Juffer, 2006) and there is evidence of the development of attachments between children adopted from institutions and their adoptive parents (Chisholm, 1998; O'Connor & Zeanah, 2003a). A study of children placed in foster care in Romania from institutions showed a reduction in RAD symptoms, compared to controls. After around 18 months, there was no difference between foster care and never-institutionalized comparisons for emotionally withdrawn/inhibited symptoms whereas disinhibited symptoms persisted, albeit in a reduced form (Zeanah & Smyke, 2005). Conversely, the development of secure attachment in foster care seems to depend more on the foster carer's "state of mind" with respect to attachment than on the child's history (Dozier, Lindhiem, & Ackerman, 2005), so the story is far from simple.

Zeanah's group in New Orleans (Zeanah & Smyke, 2005), and Dozier's group in Delaware have developed intervention packages to help children and new foster carers develop attachments. Barriers to attachment in the child can include regulatory, psychosocial and developmental problems, an internal working model of relationships as being inconsistent and conflicting loyalties between birth parents and foster carers (Zeanah & Smyke, 2005). Foster carers may present their own barriers related to their own experience of parenting and child care and to their experience of, and attitudes towards, fostering. Dozier, Lindhiem, & Ackerman (2005) found that foster mothers with dismissing and unresolved states of mind with respect to attachment were likely to have infants with disorganized patterns. They conclude that it is easier for a child in foster care to organize his or her attachment system if the caregiver is nurturing and is autonomous with respect to his or her own attachment history. A key goal of treatment therefore is to assist foster carers to become the person the child goes to when distressed. In order to achieve this, both the New Orleans and Delaware teams aim to support foster families to provide a safe and predictable environment, help the child regulate emotions, understand the child's (often confusing) signals and provide nurturance even in the face of avoidance from the infant (Dozier, Lindhiem, & Ackerman, 2005; Zeanah & Smyke, 2005).

More intrusive therapies, previously called "holding therapies," have been used in an attempt to treat RAD and great concern has been raised because of certain particularly coercive forms that resulted in child deaths (O'Connor & Zeanah, 2003a). Some therapists who came from this tradition have now explicitly stated that they no longer use coercive techniques and small-scale research suggests clinical benefits from what is now called dyadic developmental psychotherapy (Becker-Weidman, 2006; Hughes, 2003). These methods require adequate evaluation for both effectiveness and safety.

There have now been a number of randomized controlled trials (RCTs) evaluating training of foster carers to be agents of therapeutic change for the child. For example, two UK studies have used the RCT design to evaluate group-based interventions with foster carers aimed at improving parenting and, hence, children's emotional and behavioral functioning. One used an attachment-based model (Minnis & Del Priore, 2001) while the other used a cognitive–behavioral model (Macdonald & Turner, 2005). Overall effect sizes were small and non-significant with respect to changes in the children, despite carers reporting benefits from the interventions in both cases. The interventions may not have been intensive enough, or insufficiently targeted on the specific problems or not followed through tenaciously enough with the carers to produce significant change in the children, although all changes were in a positive direction. It seems counterintuitive that group interventions should be effective in vulnerable populations (Scott, Spender, Doolan *et al.*, 2001) yet apparently less effective in foster care. One possible explanation may be that foster carers are already engaging in effective parenting practices so that effect sizes will inevitably be small compared to families in which there is greater scope for change. Furthermore, foster care training, while important, is a minimal intervention when the complexity of children's lives and difficulties is considered and should be seen as part of a comprehensive package of support to foster families.

A number of promising developments in the UK include the Coram Family adaptation of Webster-Stratton's Incredible Years program for the fostering population (Henderson & Sargent, 2005), publication of the comprehensive Fostering Changes manual (Pallett, Blackeby, Yule *et al.*, 2005) and pre-post study (Pallett, Scott, & Blackeby *et al.*, 2002) and Rushton, Monck, Upright *et al.*s' (2006) RCT comparing behavioral and educational parenting interventions with social work support service as usual.

Treatment Foster Care

Treatment Foster Care (TFC) is not just a more specialized form of foster care but a treatment in itself and an alternative to psychiatric inpatient treatment or incarceration (Meadowcroft & Thomlison, 1994). Although there are various treatment foster care models, the best known and best evaluated is multidimensional treatment foster care (MTFC; www.mtfc.com). MTFC is a multimodal approach in which foster carers receive extensive pre-service training and ongoing consultation and support from program staff. Children receive individual therapy and birth parents or other permanent placement resources receive parent training.

RCTs from the Oregon Social Learning Center indicate that MTFC, when delivered to antisocial children who then return to their birth families, had a modest positive effect on behavior problems and on other psychological outcomes such as self-esteem and had large positive effects on social skills (Reddy, Hay, Murray *et al.*, 1997). MTFC is currently being evaluated in 20 local authorities in the UK.

Although MTFC initially developed to provide an alternative to secure accommodation/incarceration for delinquent adolescents (Chamberlain, Price, Reid *et al.*, 2006; Clark, Prange, Lee *et al.*, 1994), more recent modifications for preschool children have also demonstrated success, particularly in terms of securing permanent placements (Fisher, Burraston, & Pears, 2005).

In the Oregon MTFC model, for both adolescents and preschoolers, key elements of the program include foster carers having daily telephone contacts in which the child's progress is reviewed systematically, weekly foster parent support group meetings and 24-hour on-call crisis intervention. Children have services of behavioral specialists who work in preschool or daycare and at home, and children attend a weekly therapeutic playgroup. A consulting psychiatrist provides medication management. When the child enters a permanent placement, a family therapist works to train the parents in the same parenting skills as foster carers, whether the birth parent, relative or non-relative adopter. The training, for both foster carers and permanent carers/parents, emphasizes encouragement for pro-social behavior, consistency, non-abusive limit setting and close supervision of the child. The preschool program also follows a developmental framework of helping carers understand delayed maturation and the program attempts to create optimal environmental conditions to facilitate developmental progress including a responsive and consistent caregiver and a predictable daily routine with preparation for transitions between activities (Chamberlain, 1995).

The apparent success of TFC has prompted recent calls, in the USA, for an end to the use of "shelters" or "safe houses" where group care is used for crisis management, assessment and planning for children requiring substitute placements (Barth, 2005). Recent research has shown that ordinary foster care is superior to such group care (DeSena, Murphy, Douglas-Palumberi *et al.*, 2005) and that TFC is superior for the most vulnerable children to ordinary foster care (Chamberlain & Reid, 1998), although this has not yet been proven for maltreated children who do not have serious mental health problems or risky behavior.

Despite the evidence for TFC, its implementation in practice is not always easy, especially if placement goals are unclear. It requires a high level of co-ordination of services and success may depend on the ability of the model to span the multiple systems involved in these children's lives (Meadowcroft & Thomlison, 1994). There has been considerable focus on risk behaviors, such as violence, as an outcome measure of TFC (Chamberlain & Reid, 1998; Hahn, Lowy, Bilukha *et al.*, 2004), but this may not always be in the best interests of the child. In an evaluation of an intensive foster care scheme in Scotland, tensions were evident between social services' desire to use the scheme for the reduction of risk behaviors before moving on to less intensive (and less costly) placements, and the desire by social workers, foster carers and young people themselves to allow young people to develop stable relationships rather than move on quickly (Walker, Hill, & Triseliotis, 2002).

Leaving Residential and Foster Family Care

Although this chapter might strictly concern the period children spend in residential or foster family care, the importance of the transition out of care and into independence must be recognized and will be referred to briefly in relation to recent UK studies. Clearly, the nature of childhood experiences prior to and during care will affect progress after care. As most young people leave care at around 16–17 years, they have to face the challenges of independent living earlier than their peers. Although a proportion of care leavers do well, those with worse outcomes are likely to have unstable living arrangements, difficulties in personal relationships, poor social networks, lack of involvement in education and training opportunities, unemployment and poverty. Coping with early pregnancy and parenthood is a common challenge. Black and mixed heritage children leaving care may have more difficulties in contact with family and community and difficulties are compounded for disabled children. Biehal and Wade (1996) showed that older ex-care young people rarely return to their birth families, at least not in the short term. Good relationships with them are often irretrievable following histories of abuse, neglect and rejection. Some young people, but by no means all, maintain continuing relationships with their foster parents, but this is less so with residential care staff.

Leaving care schemes, mentoring and personal adviser projects designed to help in the transition to adulthood and independence have been developing and are beginning to be researched, but specified interventions to improve post-care life chances have not yet been rigorously evaluated (Dixon, Wade, Byford *et al.*, 2006). Prospective studies are needed comparing matched groups receiving contrasting leaving care services and followed up at multiple time points.

An important part of post-care services should be to attend to mental health needs by more intensive psychological interventions with special concern for problems of identity and self-esteem, establishing and sustaining social relationships, developing interpersonal problem-solving skills, managing emotional problems and controlling drug and alcohol use. Problems in providing accessible, acceptable mental health services to this group have been highlighted (Broad, 2005) and more progress is needed in promoting links between care leaving projects and specialist child and adolescent mental health services.

Comparative Outcomes and Costs and Future Directions

Studies Comparing Residential and Foster Family Care Outcomes

It has not been possible to provide definitive answers as to the differential effectiveness of residential and foster family care. The review of studies by Curtis, Alexander, and Lunghofer (2001) highlighted the methodological weaknesses in studies that have attempted to compare out-of-home care outcomes. The study by Chamberlain and Reid (1998) of adolescent delinquent boys is one of the very few to compare TFC with community-based group care using randomized allocation. It was established that the groups were equivalent on key variables, although the foster care group received more therapeutic help. More positive outcomes were recorded for the TFC group, including less criminality a year after discharge.

The study by Roy, Rutter, & Pickles (2000) has helped to tease out the effects of prior problems from the effects of being in care by studying children from similar social environments who experienced two contrasting "in care" child rearing environments: either residential or family foster care. Both groups were compared with classroom controls and although both were more prone to hyperactivity/inattention, such a problem was substantially more marked in the group who had experienced residential care. The same applied to scholastic achievement (Roy & Rutter, 2006). A picture is emerging that genetic risk, early environment (both pre-care and state care environments) and poor educational provision may interact to compromise educational progress (Roy, Rutter, & Pickles, 2000). This in turn may have a negative effect on self-esteem and life chances.

The Odyssey Project (Drais-Parillo, 2006) examined a large sample of over 2000 children and young people in either residential group care (RGC) or TFC on assessment, at admission, at discharge and 6, 12 and 24 months post-discharge. The RCG group was found to be older, more likely to be male, more ethnically diverse, with more psychiatric and criminal history. Although fairly good outcomes were reported for both groups, major sample attrition compromised the ability of the study to make valid post-discharge statistical comparisons.

When definitive evidence is lacking, practitioners involved in making placement choices for young people will need to apply flexible decision-making, sensitive to the needs of the individuals. The quality of the care environment and the population residing in each placement type will need to be taken into account in making these choices.

One recent study examined placement alternatives for children orphaned as a consequence of violence in Iraqi Kurdistan (Ahmad, Qahar, Siddiq *et al.*, 2005). Those placed in traditional foster care ($n = 94$), indicating integration of the child into the family, mostly kin, were compared with orphanage children ($n = 48$) living in impersonal and regimented group care, but where contact with birth family members could occur. Efforts were made to achieve comparability of the groups on other factors. The mean age of the children was 11 years and 1 and 2 year follow-ups were conducted. Similar outcomes were found on many measures, including some deterioration, but improvement in problem profiles and traumatic stress scores after 2 years were found to be more significant in the foster care than the orphanage sample. The authors concluded that foster care provided more suitable conditions ("a natural family atmosphere") and that the best policy was to support foster families rather than to build more orphanages.

Cost-Effectiveness

Considering estimates of costs alongside evaluations of effectiveness of psychosocial interventions is becoming more common and will deliver more useful evidence for service providers. (DeSena *et al.*, 2005; Knapp, 1997; Minnis, Everett, Pelosi *et al.*, 2006). In a recent study of costs in foster care, a tiny minority of children were found to be attracting a disproportionately high level of services and costs (Barth, 2005; Minnis *et al.*, 2006). It may therefore be necessary to accept that the few most vulnerable children will require very expensive services.

A recent cost-effectiveness comparison of placing children in group care versus family foster care placements in the USA has shown that family foster care is both more effective in terms of placement stability and considerably cheaper (Barth, 2005; DeSena *et al.*, 2005). Residential care in the UK has been claimed to be seven times more costly than comparable foster care (Polnay, Glaser, & Dewhurt, 1997), but when full comparative costing is undertaken, including education, a smaller, four-fold difference has been reported (Curtis & Netten, 2005). Current average costs for statutory and non-statutory residential care are in the region of £118,000–121,000 per resident per year. TFC has been shown to be expensive, but cost-effective for very disturbed adolescents (Chamberlain & Weinrott, 1990). Foster family care may be cheaper and produce better outcomes in general, but where family-based care is not tenable, high-quality expensive well-targeted residential care may be the best option for some young people (Barber, Delfabbrol, & Cooper, 2001).

Future Directions

The evidence base is often lacking in order to support specific practice guidelines for out-of-home care. As little assessment has been made of the long-term adaptation of children once placed in out-of-home care, this hampers the ability to select the most promising placement according to the characteristics and history of the individual young person. Future studies, rather than simply comparing residential care with foster family care, could be conducted on appropriate *sequences* of residential and family foster care used flexibly and as required.

However, we have sufficient findings about the mental health problems of this group of children to push forward with high-quality assessment linked to appropriate interventions. In the past, children in public care have had their mental health needs neglected and a major task is to ensure that these children have proportionate access to services. Interventions need to be evaluated using gold standard research techniques. At present, the gold standard is considered to be the RCT with health economic evaluation and, despite the logistical and ethical challenges of such research, attempts must be made to achieve this. Promising practices and service developments need to be defined more precisely and the specific characteristics and intensity of the approaches identified. Without this, effectiveness trials will be uninformative.

In addition to intervention studies, more information is needed on how outcomes of foster and residential care compare with matched cases living in birth families with similar pre-care backgrounds. More research is needed to reveal the complex interactions of factors that predict placement outcome. More needs to be known about how long it takes, and to what extent, children with disadvantaged or abusive circumstances can catch up with their peers once placed in good quality out-of-home care. Further research is needed to reveal what principles and procedures should be followed for matching carers and children in order to produce the best outcomes.

Despite efforts to keep children out of care, keep their families together, intervene early on when there are signs of poor quality or abusive parenting and conduct a wider search for possible placements with extended family and friends, some children will need to be cared for by the state and looked after by strangers. An expanding research base is needed on what kinds of placements produce what kinds of outcomes and for which children. This should strengthen the capacity for practitioners to make rational placement decisions and service providers and policy makes to extend the range of good quality placements.

References

Ahmad, A., Qahar, J., Siddiq, A., Majeed, A., Raheed, J., Jabar, F., *et al.* (2005). A 2-year follow-up of orphans' competence, socio-emotional problems and post-traumatic stress symptoms in traditional foster care and orphanages in Iraqi Kurdistan. *Childcare, Health and Development*, *31*, 203–215.

Ainsworth, F., & Hansen, P. (2005). A dream come true: No more residential care – a corrective note. *International Journal of Social Welfare*, *14*, 195–199.

Aldgate, J., & Bradley, M. (1999). *Supporting families through short term fostering*. London: The Stationery Office.

American Psychiatric Association. (2000). *Diagnostic and statistical manual of mental disorders* (4th edn.). Text revision. Washington, DC: American Psychiatric Association.

Barber, J. G., Delfabbrol, P. H., & Cooper, L. (2001). Predictors of the unsuccessful transition to foster care. *Journal of Child Psychiatry and Psychology*, *42*, 785–790.

Barth, R. (2005). Foster home care is more cost-effective than shelter care: Serious questions continue to be raised about the utility of group care in child welfare services. *Child Abuse and Neglect*, *29*, 623–625.

Barth, R., Berry, M., Yoshikami, R., Goodfield, R. K., & Carson, M. L. (1988). Predicting adoption disruption. *Social Work*, *33*, 227–233.

Bates, B., English, D., & Kouidou-Giles, S. (1997). Residential treatment and its alternatives: A review of the literature. *Child and Youth Care Forum*, *26*, 7–51.

Becker-Weidman, A. (2006). Treatment for children with trauma-attachment disorders: Dyadic developmental psychotherapy. *Child and Adolescent Social Work Journal*, *23*, 147–171.

Berridge, D. (2002). *What works for children? Effective services for children and families*. Open University Press.

Biehal, N., & Wade, J. (1996). Looking back, looking forward: Care leavers, families and change. *Children and Youth Services Review*, *18*, 425–445.

Blome, W. W. (1997). What happens to foster kids: Educational experiences of a random sample of foster care youth and a matched group of non-foster care youth. *Child and Adolescent Social Work Journal*, *14*, 41–53.

Blower, A., Addo, A., Hodgson, J., Lamington, L., & Towlson, K. (2004). Mental health of "looked after" children: A needs assessment. *Clinical Child Psychology and Psychiatry*, *9*, 117–129.

Boddy, J., Cameron, C., & Petrie, P. (2005). The professional care worker: The social pedagogue in Northern Europe. In C. Boddy (Ed.), *Care Work: Present and Future*. London: Routledge.

Boris, N. W., Zeanah, C. H., Larrieu, J. A., Scheeringa, M. S., & Heller, S. S. (1998). Attachment disorders in infancy and early childhood: A preliminary investigation of diagnostic criteria. *American Journal of Psychiatry*, *155*, 295–297.

Boris, N. W., Hinshaw-Fuselier, S. S., Smyke, A. T., Scheeringa, M. S., Heller, S. S., & Zeanah, C. H. (2004). Comparing criteria for attachment disorders: Establishing reliability and validity in high-risk samples. *Journal of the American Academcy of Child and Adolescent Psychiatry*, *43*, 568–577.

Bowlby, J. (1951). *Maternal care and mental health*. Geneva: World Health Organization.

Broad, B. (2005). Young people leaving care: Implementing the Children (Leaving Care) Act 2000. *Children and Society*, *19*, 371–384.

Browne, K., Hamilton-Giachritsis, C., Johnson, R., & Oestergren, M. (2006). Overuse of institutional care for children in Europe. *British Medical Journal*, *332*, 485–487.

Callaghan, J., Young, B., Pace, F., & Vostanis, P. (2004). Evaluation of a new mental health service for looked after children. *Clinical Child Psychology and Psychiatry*, *9*, 130–148.

Cameron, C. (2004). Social pedagogy and care: Danish and German practice in young people's residential care. *Journal of Social Work*, *4*, 133–151.

Carlson, V., Cicchetti, D., Barnett, D., & Braunwald, K. (1989). Disorganized/disorientated attachment relationships in maltreated infants. *Developmental Psychology*, *25*, 525–531.

Chamberlain, P. (1995). *Family connections: A treatment foster care model for adolescents with delinquency*. Eugene, OR: Castalia Publishing.

Chamberlain, P., Moreland, S., & Reid, K. (1992). Enhanced services and stipends for foster parents: effects on retention rates and outcomes for children. *Child Welfare*, *71*, 387–401.

Chamberlain, P., Price, J. M., Reid, J. B., Landsverk, J., Fisher, P. A., & Stoolmiller, M. (2006). Who disrupts from placement in foster and kinship care? *Child Abuse and Neglect*, *30*, 409–424.

Chamberlain, P., & Reid, J. B. (1998). Comparison of two community alternatives to incarceration for chronic juvenile offenders. *Journal of Consulting and Clinical Psychology*, *66*, 624–633.

Chamberlain, P., & Weinrott, M. (1990). Specialized foster care: treating seriously emotionally disturbed children. *Children Today*, *19*, 24–27.

Chisholm, K. (1998). A three year follow-up of attachment and indiscriminate friendliness in children adopted from Romanian orphanages. *Child Development*, *69*, 1092–1106.

Clark, H. B., Prange, M. E., Lee, B., Boyd, L. A., McDonald, B. A., & Stewart, E. S. (1994). Improving adjustment outcomes for foster children with emotional and behavioral disorders: Early findings from a controlled study on individualized services. *Journal of Emotional and Behavioral Disorders*, *2*, 207–218.

Connor, D., Miller, K., Cunningham, J., & Melloni, R. (2002). What does getting better mean? Child improvement and measures of outcome in residential treatment. *American Journal of Orthopsychiatry*, *72*, 110–117.

Curtis McMillen, J., Zima, B. T., Scott, L. D., Auslander, W. F., Munson, M. R., Ollie, M. T., *et al.* (2005). Prevalence of psychiatric disorder among older youths in the foster care system. *Journal of the American Academy of Child and Adolescent Psychiatry*, *44*, 88–95.

Curtis, L., & Netten, A. (2005). *Unit costs of health and social care*. Canterbury: PSSU.

Curtis, P., Alexander, G., & Lunghofer, L. (2001). A literature review comparing the outcomes of residential group care and therapeutic foster care. *Child and Adolescent Social Work Journal*, *18*, 377–392.

DeSena, A., Murphy, R., Douglas-Palumberi, H., Blau, G., Kelly, B., Horwitz, S., *et al.* (2005). Safe homes: Is it worth the cost? An evaluation of a group home permanent planning program for children who first enter out-of-home care. *Child Abuse and Neglect*, *29*, 627–643.

Department for Education and Skills (DfES). (2005). *Children looked after by local authorities*. London: Her Majesty's Stationery Office.

Department for Education and Skills (DfES). (2006). *Care matters: Transforming the lives of children and young people in care*. London: Her Majesty's Stationery Office.

Dimigen, G., Del Priore, C., Butler, S., Evans, S., Ferguson, L., & Swan, M. (1999). Psychiatric disorder among children at time of entering local authority care: questionnaire survey. *British Medical Journal*, *319*, 675.

Dixon, J., Wade, J., Byford, S., Wetherley, H., & Lee, J. (2006). *Young people leaving care: A study of costs and outcomes*. Report to the Department of Education and Skills.

Dozier, M., Lindhiem, O., & Ackerman, J. P. (2005). Attachment and biobehavioral catch-up. In L. J. Berlin, *et al.* (Eds.), *Enhancing early attachments. Theory, research, intervention, and policy* (pp. 178–194). New York, London: Guilford Press.

Dozier, M., Manni, M., Gordon, M. K., Peloso, E., Gunnar, M. R., Stovall-McClough, K. C., *et al.* (2006). Foster children's diurnal production of cortisol: An exploratory study. *Child Maltreatment*, *11*, 189–197.

Dozier, M., & Rutter, M. (in press). Challenges to the development of attachment relationships faced by young children in foster and adoptive care. In J. Cassidy, & P. Shaver (Eds.), *Handbook of attachment*. New York, London: Guilford Press.

Drais-Parillo, A. A. (2006). *The Odyssey Project: A descriptive and prospective study of children and youth in residential group care and therapeutic foster care. Final Report*. Child Welfare League of America. Atlanta, Georgia, USA.

Dubner, A., & Motta, R. (1999). Sexually and physically abused foster care children and post traumatic stress disorder. *Journal of Consulting and Clinical Psychology*, *67*, 367–373.

Dumaret, A.-C., Coppel-Batsch, M., & Couraud, S. (1997). Adult outcome of children for long-term periods in foster families. *Child Abuse and Neglect*, *21*, 911–927.

Evans, L. D., Scott, S. S., & Schulz, E. G. (2004). The need for educational assessment of children entering foster care. *Child Welfare*, *83*, 565–580.

Evans, R. (2004). Ethnic differences in ADHD and the mad/bad debate. [Comment]. *American Journal of Psychiatry*, *161*, 932; author reply 932.

Fisher, P. A., Burraston, B., & Pears, K. (2005). The Early Intervention Foster Care Program: permanent placement outcomes from a randomized trial. *Child Maltreatment*, *10*, 61–71.

Foltz, R. (2004). The efficacy of residential treatment: An overview of the evidence. *Residential Treatment for Children and Youth*, *22*, 1–19.

Fonagy, P., Target, M., Cottrell, D., Phillips, J., & Kurtz, Z. (2002). What works for whom? *A cricial review of treatments for children and adolescents*. New York: Guilford.

Garwood, M. M., & Close, W. (2001). Identifying the psychological needs of foster children. *Child Psychology and Human Development*, *32*, 125–135.

Goldfarb, W. (1945). Effects of psychological deprivation in infancy and subsequent stimulation. *American Journal of Psychiatry*, *102*, 18–33.

Gorske, T., Sreabus, D., & Walls, R. (2003). Adolescents in residential treatment centers: Characteristics and treatment outcome. *Children and Youth Services Review*, *25*, 317–326.

Groark, C. J., Muhamedrahimov, R. J., Palmov, O. I., Nikiforova, N. V., & McCall, R. B. (2005). Improvements in early care in Russian orphanages and their relationship to observed behaviors. *Infant Mental Health Journal*, *26*, 96–109.

Groze, V., & Ileana, D. (1996). A follow-up study of adopted children from Romania. *Child and Adolescent Social Work Journal*, *13*, 541–565.

Hahn, R. A., Lowy, J., Bilukha, O., Snyder, S., Briss, P., Crosby, A., *et al.* (2004). Therapeutic foster care for the prevention of violence: A report on recommendations of the task force on community preventive services. *Mortality and Morality Weekly Report*, *53*, 1–10.

Halfon, N., Mendonca, A., & Berkowitz, G. (1995). Health status of children in foster care. The experience of the Center for the Vulnerable Child. *Archives of Pediatric and Adolescent Medicine*, *149*, 386–392.

Hellinckk, W. (2002). Last resort or vital link? *International Journal of Child and Family Welfare. Special Issue*, *5*, no. 3.

Henderson, K., & Sargent, N. (2005). Developing the Incredible Years Webster-Stratton parenting skills training programme for use with adoptive families. *Adoption and Fostering*, *29*, no. 4.

Hodges, J., & Tizard, B. (1989). Social and family relationships of ex-institutional adolescents. *Journal of Child Psychology and Psychiatry*, *30*, 77–97.

Hooper, S., Murphy, J., Devaney, A., & Hultman, T. (2000). Ecological outcomes of adolescents in a psychoeducational residential treatment facility. *American Journal of Orthopsychiatry*, *70*, 491–500.

Horowitz, J. A., Bell, M., Trybulski, J., Munro, B. H., Moser, D., Hartz, S. A., *et al.* (2001). Promoting responsiveness between mothers with depressive symptoms and their infants. *Journal of Nursing Scholarship*, *33*, 323–329.

Horwitz, M. S., Owens, P., & Simms, M. D. (2000). Specialized assessments for children in foster care. *Pediatrics*, *106*, 59–66.

Hughes, D. A. (2003). Psychological interventions for the spectrum of attachment disorders and intrafamilial trauma. *Attachment and Human Development*, *5*, 271–277.

James, S. (2004). Why do foster placements disrupt? An investigation of reasons for placement changes in foster care. *Social Service Review*, *78*, 601–627.

Knapp, M. (1997). Economic evaluations and interventions for children and adolescents with mental health problems. *Journal of Child Psychology and Psychiatry*, *38*, 3–25.

Leathers, S. (2006). Placement disruption and negative placement outcomes among adolescents in long-term foster care: the role of behavior problems. *Child Abuse and Neglect*, *30*, 307–324.

Leathers, S. J. (2002). Foster children's behavioural disturbance and detachment from caregivers and community institutions. *Children and Youth Services Review*, *24*, 239–268.

Leslie, L. K., Hurlburt, M. S., Landsverk, J., Rolls, J. A., Wood, P. A., & Kelleher, K. J. (2003). Comprehensive assessments for children entering foster care: A national perspective. *Pediatrics*, *112*, 134–142.

Leslie, L. K., Gordon, J. N., Meneken, L., Premji, K., Michelmore, K. L., & Ganger, W. (2005). The physical, developmental, and mental health needs of young children in child welfare by initial placement type. *Developmental and Behavioral Pediatrics*, *26*, 177–185.

Levine, C. (2000). AIDS and a new generation of orphans. *Residential Treatment for Children and Youth*, *17*, 105–120.

Lyman, R. D., & Campbell, N. R. (1996). *Treating children and adolescents in residential and inpatient settings*. Thousand Oaks, CA: Sage.

Macdonald, G., & Turner, W. (2005). An experiment in helping foster-carers manage challenging behaviour. *British Journal of Social Work*, *35*, 1265–1282.

Marcovitch, S., Goldberg, S., Gold, A., Washington, J., Wasson, C., Krekewich, K., *et al.* (1997). Determinants of behavioral problems in Romanian children adopted in Ontario. *International Journal of Behavioral Development*, *20*, 17–31.

McCann, J., James, A., Wilson, S., & Dunn, G. (1996). Prevalence of psychiatric disorders in young people in the care system. *British Medical Journal*, *313*, 1529–1530.

Meadowcroft, P., & Thomlison, B. (1994). Treatment foster care services: a research agenda for child welfare. *Child Welfare*, *73*, 565–581.

Meltzer, H. (2003). *The mental health of young people looked after by local authorities in England*. London: HMSO.

Meltzer, H., Gatward, R., Goodman, R., & Ford, T. (1999). *The mental health of children and adolescents in Great Britain: Report of a survey carried out by the Social Survey Division of the Office for National Statistics*. Chapter 6. London: Stationery Office.

Minnis, H., & Del Priore, C. (2001). Mental health services for looked after children: implications from two studies. *Adoption and Fostering*, *25*, 27–38.

Minnis, H., Everett, K., Pelosi, A. J., Dunn, J., & Knapp, M. (2006). Children in foster care: Mental health, service use and costs. *European Child and Adolescent Psychiatry*, *15*, 63–70.

Minty, B. (1999). Annotation: Outcomes in long-term foster family care. *Journal of Child Psychology and Psychiatry*, *40*, 991–999.

Moses, T. (2000). Attachment theory and residential treatment: A study of staff–client relationships. *American Journal of Orthopsychiatry*, *70*, 474–490.

O'Connor, T., & Rutter, M. and the English and Romanian Adoptees Study Team. (2000). Attachment disorder behavior following early severe deprivation: Extension and longitudinal follow-up. *Journal of the American Academy of Child and Adolescent Psychiatry*, *39*, 703–712.

O'Connor, T. G., & Zeanah, C. H. (2003a). Attachment disorders: assessment strategies and treatment approaches. *Attachment and Human Development*, *5*, 223–244.

O'Connor, T. G., & Zeanah, C. H. (2003b). Introduction to the special issue: Current perspectives on assessment and treatment of attachment disorders. *Attachment and Human Development*, *5*, 221–222.

Oosterman, M., Schuengel, C., Slot, N. W., Bullens, R. A. R., & Doreleijers, T. A. H. (2007). Disruptions in foster care: A review and meta-analysis. *Children and Youth Services Review*, *29*, 53–76.

Pallett, C., Blackeby, K., Yule, W., Weissman, R., & Scott, S. (2005). Fostering changes: How to improve relationships and manage difficult behaviour – a training programme for foster carers. *British Agencies for Adoption and Fostering*. London.

Pallett, C., Scott, S., Blackeby, K., Yule, W., & Weissman, R. (2002). Fostering changes: A cognitive–behavioural approach to help foster carers manage children. *Adoption and Fostering*, *26*, 39–47.

Pears, K., & Fisher, P. (2005). Emotion understanding and theory of mind among maltreated children in foster care: Evidence of deficits. *Development and Psychopathology*, *17*, 47–65.

Pecora, P., Whittaker, J., Maluccio, A., & Barth, R. (2000). Residential group care services. In P. Pecora, J. Whittaker, A. Maluccio, & R. Barth. (Eds.), *The Child Welfare Challenge: Policy Practice and Research* (2nd edn.). New York: Aldine De Gruyter.

Polnay, L., Glaser, D., & Dewhurt, T. (1997). Children in residential care: What cost? *Archives of Disease in Childhood*, *77*, 394–395.

Quinton, D., & Rutter, M. (1988). *Parenting breakdown: The making and breaking of inter-generational links*. Aldershot, Hants: Avebury.

Racusin, R., Maerlender, A., Sengupta, A., Isquith, P., & Straus, M. (2005). Psychosocial treatment of children in foster care: A review. *Community Mental Health Journal*, *341*, 199–221.

Reddy, V., Hay, D., Murray, L., & Trevarthen, C. (1997). Communication in infancy: Mutual regulation of affect and attention. In G. Bremner, & A. Slater (Eds.), *Infant Development: Recent Advances* (pp. 247–273). Hove: Psychology Press/Erlbaum.

Roy, P., & Rutter, M. (2006). Institutional care: Associations between inattention and early reading performance. *Journal of Child Psychology and Psychiatry*, *47*, 480–487.

Roy, P., Rutter, M., & Pickles, A. (2000). Institutional care: Risk from family background or pattern of rearing? *Journal of Child Psychology and Psychiatry*, *41*, 139–149.

Rushton, A., Monck, E., Upright, H., & Davidson, M. (2006). Enhancing adoptive parenting: devising promising interventions. *Child and Adolescent Mental Health*, *11*, 25–31.

Rushton, A., & Minnis, H. (1997). Annotation: Transracial family placements. *Journal of Child Psychology and Psychiatry*, *38*, 147–159.

Rutter, M. & the English and Romanian Adoptees (ERA) Study Team. (1998). Developmental catch-up, and deficit, following adoption after severe global early privation. *Journal of Child Psychology and Psychiatry*, *39*, 465–476.

Rutter, M., Beckett, C., Castle, J., Colvert, E., Kreppner, J., Mehta, M., *et al.* (2007). Effects of profound early institutional deprivation: An overview of findings from a UK longitudinal study of Romanian adoptees. *European Journal of Developmental Psychology*, *4*, *3*, 332–350.

Rutter, M., Quinton, D., & Hill, J. (1990). Adult outcomes of institution reared children: Males and females compared. In L. N. Robins, & M. Rutter (Eds.), *Straight and devious pathways from childhood to adulthood*. Cambridge: Cambridge University Press.

Scaramella, L. V., & Leve Leslie, D. (2004). Clarifying parent–child reciprocities during early childhood: The early childhood coercion model. *Clinical Child and Family Psychology Review*, *7*, 89–107.

Scholte, E., & van der Ploeg, J. (2000). Exploring factors governing successful residential treatment of youngsters with serious behavioural difficulties: Findings from a longitudinal study in Holland. *Childhood*, *7*, 129–153.

Scott, S., Spender, Q., Doolan, M., Jacobs, B., Aspland, H., & Webster-Stratton, C. (2001). Multicentre controlled trial of parenting groups for childhood antisocial behaviour in clinical practice. *British Medical Journal*, *323*, 194–198.

Sigal, J., Perry, C., Rossigol, M., & Ouimet, M. (2003). Unwanted infants: Psychological and physical consequences of inadequate orphanage care 50 years later. *American Journal of Orthopsychiatry*, *73*, 3–12.

Sinclair, I. (2005). *Fostering Now: Messages from Research*. Department for Education and Skills. London: Jessica Kingsley.

Sinclair, I., & Gibbs, I. (1998). *Children's homes: A study in diversity*. Chichester: Wiley.

Sinclair, I., & Wilson, K. (2003). Matches and mismatches: The contribution of carers and children to the success of foster placements. *British Journal of Social Work*, *33*, 871–884.

Smyke, A. T., Dumitrescu, A., & Zeanah, C. H. (2002). Attachment disturbances in young children. I. The continuum of caretaking casualty. *Journal of the American Academy of Child and Adolescent Psychiatry*, *41*, 972–982.

Sparling, J., Dragomir, C., Ramey, S., & Florescu, L. (2005). Intervention in Romanian orphanages. *Infant Mental Health Journal*, *26*, 127–142.

Spitz, R. R. (1945). Hospitalism: An inquiry into the genesis of psychiatric conditions in early childhood. *Psychoanalytic Study of the Child*, *1*, 53–74.

St. Claire, L., & Osborne, A. F. (1987). The ability and behaviour of children who have been "in care" or separated from their parents. *Early Development and Care*, *28*, no. 3, Special issue.

Stein, M. (2006). Missing years of abuse in children's homes. *Child and Family Social Work*, *11*, 11–22.

Tizard, B., & Phoenix, A. (1995). The identity of mixed parentage adolescents. *Journal of Child Psychology and Psychiatry*, *36*, 1399–1410.

Tizard, B., & Rees, J. (1975). The effect of early institutional rearing on the behaviour problems and affectional relationships of four-year-old children. *Journal of Child Psychology and Psychiatry*, *16*, 61–73.

Utting, W. (1997). *People like us: The report of the review of the safeguards for children living away from home*. London: HMSO.

van IJzendoorn, M. H., & Juffer, F. (2006). The Emanuel Miller Memorial Lecture 2006: Adoption as intervention. Meta-analytic evidence for massive catch-up and plasticity in physical, socio-emotional, and cognitive development. *Journal of Child Psychology and Psychiatry*, *47*, 1228–1245.

Vorria, P., Papaligoura, Z., Dunn, J., van IJzendoorn, M., Steele, H., Kontopolou, A., *et al.* (2004). Early experiences and attachment relationships of Greek infants raised in residential group care. *Journal of Child Psychology and Psychiatry*, *44*, 1208–1220.

Vorria, P., Papaligoura, Z., Sarafidou, J., Kopakaki, M., Dunn, J., van IJzendoorn, M. H., *et al.* (2006). The development of adopted children after institutional care: A follow-up study. *Journal of Child Psychology and Psychiatry*, *47*, 1246–1254.

Walker, M., Hill, M., & Triseliotis, J. (2002). *Testing the limits of foster care: Fostering as an alternative to secure accommodation.* Nottingham: Russel Press.

Ward, H., & Skuse, T. (2001). Performance targets and stability of placements for children long looked after away from home. *Children and Society*, *15*, 333–346.

Waterhouse, R. (2000). *Lost in care: Report of the Tribunal of Inquiry into the abuse of children in care in the former county council areas of Gwynedd and Clwyd since 1974.* London: The Stationery Office.

Whittaker, J. (2000). The future of residential group care. *Child Welfare*, *29*, 59–74.

Wilson, K., Petrie, S., & Sinclair, I. (2003). A kind of loving: A model of effective foster care. *British Journal of Social Work*, 33, 991–1004.

Zeanah, C. H., Nelson, C. A., Fox, N. A., Smyke, A. T., Marshall, P., Parker, S. W., *et al.* (2003). Designing research to study the effects of institutionalization on brain and behavioural development: the Bucharest Early Intervention Project. *Development and Psychopathology*, *15*, 885–907.

Zeanah, C. H., Larrieu, J. A., Heller, S. S., Valliere, M. S. W., Hinshaw-Fuselier, S., Aoki, Y., *et al.* (2001). Evaluation of a preventive intervention for maltreated infants and toddlers in foster care. *Journal of the American Academy of Child and Adolescent Psychiatry*, *40*, 214–221.

Zeanah, C. H., & Smyke, A. T. (2005). Building attachment relationships following maltreatment and severe deprivation. In L. J. Berlin *et al.*, (Eds.), *Enhancing Early Attachments. Theory, Research, Intervention, and Policy* (pp. 195–216). New York, London: Guilford Press.

Zeanah, C. H., Smyke, A. T., Koga, S. F., & Carlson, E. (2005). Attachment in institutionalized and community children in Romania. *Child Development*, *76*, 1015–1028.

33 Adoption

Nancy J. Cohen

Adoption is an increasingly common means of forming a family. Most broadly, it has contributed to a redefinition of the essential features of the nuclear biological family and come to be intertwined with other trends in family formation such as step-parenting, kinship care, parenting by gay and lesbian couples, and use of assisted reproductive technologies. These trends have raised some of the same issues as confronted by adoptive families such as the relative contribution of genetic, biological, social and psychological factors to child development. They also have translated the definition of family from a biological and ethnocultural concept to one that emphasizes family as psychological parenting of a child. Moreover, with the increase in open adoptions and the more rapid movement of children from foster care to adoption, many adoptive families are, in essence, multiple families with birth parents and sometimes extended birth families, maintaining contact with adopted children and their families over time. Searches for birth parents and reunions of adopted adolescents and adults are also increasingly common and represent another way that birth and adoptive families connect.

The chapter begins with an update of these trends in adoption practices and families created with the help of assisted reproductive technologies. It then goes on to discuss the outcomes of domestic and intercountry adoption. Finally, both post-adoption and clinical services are discussed, highlighting the increasing attention paid by the professional community to adoption-related issues.

Contemporary Trends in Adoptive Family Formation

Sources of Children for Adoption

For some time there has been a decline in the number of infants available for adoption domestically, accounted for by greater prevalence of single motherhood and legal avenues to control reproduction through birth control and abortion. This is coupled with a greater demand for children related to infertility associated with delayed childbearing and greater acceptance of non-traditional parents who are single, gay or lesbian.

Rutter's Child and Adolescent Psychiatry, 5th edition. Edited by M. Rutter, D. Bishop, D. Pine, S. Scott, J. Stevenson, E. Taylor and A. Thapar. © 2008 Blackwell Publishing, ISBN: 978-1-4051-4549-7.

In comparison with domestic adoption, intercountry adoption continues to grow worldwide. Intercountry adoption originated with efforts to rescue children victimized by epidemics and other calamities such as war. More recently, intercountry adoption includes children abandoned because of poverty and population control policies and is now motivated by preference for adopting infants and/or children without apparent special needs and children who are not observably racially different, and for adoptions that are fully closed.

The most recent estimates indicate that more than 40,000 children are adopted worldwide each year from over 100 countries (Selman, 2002). An important historical event was the establishment of the Hague Convention in 1993, which set out minimum rights and procedures for intercountry adoption. Thus, whereas the earlier years of intercountry adoption were clouded by irregularities in procedures and shady practices such as child abduction and trafficking of infants, procedures have become more regularized and integrated with those of the agencies or governments in countries where adoptive parents reside.

The needs of children being adopted have also changed. Prior to the 1990s, most intercountry adoptees came from Korea, which had a high standard of living and health care, and where children were cared for in foster homes (Johnson & Dole, 1999). Subsequent sending countries have not had such high standards. Typically, children have lived in institutions and experienced some degree of deprivation, which affects all areas of functioning (Gunnar, Bruce, & Grotevant, 2000). Currently, most international adoptions to the USA are from China, Russia, Guatemala, South Korea and Kazakhstan whereas most international adoptions in Europe are from China, Russia, Colombia, Ukraine and Bulgaria. To counteract the effects of deprivation, there has been a move toward increasing opportunities for foster care and implementing programs to improve the caregiving and environmental conditions within orphanages (Groark, Muhamedrahimov, Palmov *et al.*, 2005).

Open Adoption

Up until 35 years ago, severing ties with the birth family was a natural prerequisite for forming an adoptive family. In this way, the genetic and psychological heritage of the adoptee was minimized in favor of adoption kinship. This practice also meant that members of the adoption triad (i.e., the birth parents, adopting parents and adopted child) were protected from the perceived stigma of adoption by the confidentiality of the adoption process. The intention was to create a situation in which all members of the adoption triad could get on with their lives. The reality proved to be otherwise and since the 1970s a gradual movement toward greater openness emerged, largely spearheaded by birth mothers. Some degree of openness in domestic adoptions is now becoming the norm rather than the exception (Grotevant & McRoy, 1997).

The term "open adoption" typically applies to adoption of infants and refers to a continuum of contact and communication among members of the child's adoptive and birth families (Grotevant, 2000). Openness became increasingly more possible once fewer infants were available for adoption and birth mothers could have a say in choosing the adoptive parents. Openness has been allowed to take various forms, although laws related to openness vary in different jurisdictions. At one end of the continuum are fully open adoptions that allow contact and communication directly between birth and adopted children and their families. There are also mediated arrangements where contact occurs through a third party, such as an adoption agency, without identifying information. At the other end of the continuum are fully closed adoptions where there is no contact, communication or shared identifying information. Once established, these arrangements are not carved in stone and it may be necessary to change contact arrangements over time (Berry, Cavazos Dylla, Barth *et al.*, 1998). It is important to acknowledge that openness has been a negative experience for some adoptive parents who prefer closed adoption or who are repeatedly not chosen by the birth mother to parent her child.

In order for openness to work, commitment, communication, flexibility and mutual respect on the part of both adoptive and birth parents are necessary (Grotevant, 2000). The best outcomes ensue when adoptive parents demonstrate high levels of empathy and sensitivity towards the child and the birth parent and are motivated to help the child integrate past and present experiences (Neil, Beek, & Schofield, 2003). This seems obvious but may be more difficult to keep in mind if rough spots in the relationship emerge. Ultimately, the arrangements must benefit and support the child. Mediated open adoption remains the most predominant arrangement (Henney, McRoy, Ayers-Lopez *et al.*, 2003). There are practical implications for adoption agencies in that supports for educating birth and adoptive parents, mediating openness arrangements (e.g., amount and schedule of contact), and providing ongoing services to both birth and adoptive parents must be established (Maynard, 2005).

It is still not clear what factors need to be taken into account and how to decide the best level of openness for a particular triad (Fravel, McRoy, & Grotevant, 2000). In a follow-up study of adolescents, Mendenhall, Berge, Wrobel *et al.* (2004) found that adolescents involved in adoptive arrangements in which there was contact with birth parents maintained higher satisfaction with contact status than those who did not have contact. Moreover, although many adolescents did not have contact with their birth fathers, when they did it was a positive experience. The benefits of openness, however, have not been fully established. Much of the research on openness has been carried out with infants who are relinquished voluntarily and there is little information on contact among groups of children and adoptive parents who were involuntarily removed because of abuse or neglect. Openness can be detrimental when birth parents make unrealistic promises or continue to perpetrate the physical and psychological abuse that led to the child's removal in the first place. Although not specific to adoption, it has been shown that outcomes are worse when children continue having contact with violent fathers (Jaffee, Moffitt, Caspi *et al.*, 2003).

In a recent review, Rushton (2004) summarized the limited studies indicating that contact can be managed by adoptive families if they feel that they have control over the situation. Research on openness in older children in foster care who are adopted also suggests some benefits in promoting the child's ability to accept the adoptive family and resolve the child's loyalty conflicts. Given the increasing move from foster care to adoption, which is discussed next, more research is clearly needed.

It is also important to acknowledge that there are many children for whom openness is not possible, most obviously, children adopted from other countries, and domestically adopted children whose birth parents have chosen closed adoption or where contact has been lost because the birth parent has died or disappeared (Sullivan & Lathrop, 2004). Brodzinsky (2005) has suggested that, in these cases, openness can be conceptualized in a different way as a state of mind rather than a concrete event. It is important to all adopted children to know that there is an openness in their adoptive families to actively consider the impact of adoption in their lives and on their emotions and affective attunement (Brodzinsky, 2005; Leon, 2002).

Moving from Foster Care to Adoption: Adoption with Contact

Current trends show an increase in the number of both infants and older children entering the foster care system and the length of time they spend there (see chapter 32; Shapiro, Shapiro, & Paret, 2001). These children often have been abused, neglected or otherwise stressed and traumatized. Some children are in and out of foster care and their birth family home numerous times before permanent plans are made. The numbers of children in foster care are of tremendous concern because they are more likely to exhibit behavioral and emotional problems (Simmel, Brooks, Barth *et al.*, 2001). Historically, the policy for permanency planning was to return children to their family after steps were taken to ensure the child's safety. Often this means that children remained in the limbo of foster care for years, sometimes growing to maturity in that environment or making repeated moves from their birth family to foster care. More recently, at least in the USA, the best interests of the child have begun to take priority such that permanency planning has been hastened toward adoption. About two-thirds of children are adopted by their unrelated foster parents, which means that they experience continuity in relationships, 15% by relatives and 23% by families they have never known (Shapiro, Shapiro, & Paret, 2001).

Because openness in adoption is generally more accepted, older children may have some limited contact with birth parents or information that can flow both ways. Approximately 15 years ago, Triseliotis (1991) made a strong case for adoption with contact with birth parents, drawing a parallel with findings indicating that children's adjustment following divorce is related to consistent and ongoing relationships with both parents who are able to cooperate. When children lack contact, they also may continue to worry about their birth family. Opposing arguments usually claim that continuing contact will interfere with the child's bonding to the new family. Where children have suffered severe abuse within the birth family, the question remains as to whether contact eases or is disruptive to adjustment in the adoptive home (Freundlich, 2002). There is some evidence that the time in foster care is shortened and the number of different placements reduced when a child advocate or caseworker oversees the child until permanency planning is achieved (Calkins & Millar, 1999).

Kinship Care

Care by family members is a long-standing tradition for children whose parents have died or could not meet their children's needs. Use of kinship care has increased and is now used more frequently to reduce or eliminate a child's stay in foster care. It has become part of the formal child welfare system associated with permanency planning (Brooks, 2002; O'Brien, Massat, & Gleeson, 2001). Kinship care has come about with changes in laws that permit family members to become foster parents and thereby gain financial support for care, the push toward rapid permanency planning, and the desire to keep children within their extended family and in the same ethnic and cultural community. For all of these reasons, on the surface, kinship care seems like an optimal solution. In the USA, children of color are most likely to be living in this situation with a single parent, usually a grandmother (Burnette, 1999), whereas in the UK kin carers are more likely to be white couples (Farmer, 2006).

There are potential problems, however. For instance, children's physical health and mental health are at risk if early experiences have been traumatic. Sometimes, family members have contributed to abuse directly or as part of an intergenerational pattern that may be repeated. There also is a risk that standards for placement are lower for kinship placements and that monitoring and services are not as complete as for foster care (Farmer, 2006). Furthermore, kin carers may have multiple stresses of their own that will impact directly on the child, and especially the capacity to cope with grieving and vulnerable children who may have a history of mistrust. Some kin carers do not even know the children who are suddenly thrust into their lives.

Intervention with intergenerational families is often complex because individual, family and societal factors are at play. Both professional and financial supports are frequently necessary to stabilize the household (Burnette, 1999). Just as in any adoptive or foster situation, the quality of earlier experiences influences those that follow. The kin carers and the child must deal with loss while taking into account that the relationship with the birth parent may continue in some way and be an ongoing source of distress and disruption. Establishing an alliance with kin carers can be difficult for professionals because of issues of trust related to fears about loss of children into public care, especially in ethnic or poor families. Research has identified poverty, isolation, mental and physical health problems and high stress to be related to the degree of kin caregiving burden (Burnette, 1999). Generally, there is less support for kinship carers than for foster and adoptive families so that development of outreach services is an important undertaking.

Transracial Adoption

Transracial adoption is a long-standing controversial issue that remains salient in the public eye, and within some racial groups, despite research showing little reason for concern from the child's or family's perspective. Earlier research on this topic was largely focused on White family adoption of Black children but the racial mix in most countries has expanded, partly as a result of intercountry adoption. In a review of the literature, Lee (2003) noted that ethnic minority adoptees are portrayed as passive rather than active participants. Research typically asks about the impact of racial and ethnic experiences rather than the more important question of how adoptees act on their environment to negotiate identities and their place in society which, in the long run, is more important. Four patterns or strategies emerged from the literature that adopted children and their families pursue:

1 Cultural assimilation, in which adoptive parents reject or downplay differences;

2 Enculturation, which involves adoptive parents acknowledging differences within the family which promote children's learning about their birth culture and heritage;

3 Racial inculcation, which involves adoptive parents teaching coping skills to facilitate their children's capacity to deal effectively with racism and discrimination; and

4 Child choice, wherein adoptive parents provide their children with cultural opportunities but ultimately abide by their children's interests (Lee, 2003).

Longitudinal research has shown that, based on parent report, adjustment problems are no more common in adulthood among transracial than inracial adoptees (Burrow & Finley, 2004; Tizard & Phoenix, 1995). In the USA, a 19-year follow-up study of transracial adoptees as young adults indicated that females were better adjusted than males, and individuals adopted from Asia adjusted better than either African-Americans or Caucasian domestic adoptees. When international and domestic adoptions were combined, African-American males were most prone to adjustment problems but inracial adopted Caucasian males had the worst outcomes (Brooks & Barth, 1999). Meta-analytic studies of intercountry adoption indicate that most transracial adoptees, domestic or international, do not have serious behavioral or emotional problems (Bimmel, Juffer, van IJzendoorn *et al.*, 2003; Juffer & van IJzendoorn, 2005). Bimmel *et al.* wisely point out that there is heterogeneity across samples and differences in conditions in various countries, adoption procedures and age at arrival. Thus, there may be subgroups of youngsters at greater or lesser risk for development of adjustment problems, making report of overall percentages unhelpful.

Racial and ethnic identity development also varies according to children's age and social and emotional development. Transracially adopted pre-adolescents tend to identify with birth cultures. For adolescents and adults, sense of race and ethnicity generally diminish but may become more ambivalent in some cases and more salient in others (Lee, 2003). When racial and ethnic experiences are positive, they contribute to good psychosocial adjustment (DeBerry, Scarr, & Weinberg, 1996). This is especially so when adoptive parents actively promote their children's ethnic culture (Yoon, 2001). Some benefits also accrue to adoptive families living in racially heterogeneous communities (Feigelman, 2000).

Contrasting results have been reported by Cederblad, Hook, Irhammar *et al.* (1999), who found that self-perceived negative racial and ethnic experiences were related to behavior problems, emotional distress and low self-esteem among transracially adopted youth in Sweden when family functioning and structure and support from friends were taken into account. Consistent with this, Hjern, Lindblad, and Vinnerljung (2002) found that rates of psychiatric disorder and social maladjustment were higher among transracial adoptees and immigrants than domestic adoptees and the general population. In Holland, Juffer, Stams, and van IJzendoorn (2004) found that adopted children's wish to be White uniquely predicted mother-reported behavior problems. Such findings raise the question of whether there are national differences dependent not only on a history of racism, but also attitudes toward immigrants.

From a clinical perspective, the takeaway message is that there is considerable variability in the psychological experiences and psychological adjustment of transracial adoptees which are dependent on the child, family and social milieu. In other words, it is prudent not to make assumptions but to ask questions; that is, to understand adoptive identity through narrative in both research and clinical practice (Grotevant, Dunbar, Kohler *et al.*, 2000).

Adoption by Non-Traditional Families

Assisted Reproductive Technology

Almost 30 years ago, science opened the door to a new opportunity for family formation through application of various forms of assisted reproductive technology (ART). The separation of conception from intimate sexuality, and the possibility of collaborative parenthood, have raised many questions similar to those regarding open adoption. There are some issues that differ between families who adopt and those who use ART although, in both cases, parents must confront feelings of loss and grief.

The forms of ART have different implications for parents and children. Both *in vitro* fertilization (IVF) and intracytoplasmic sperm injection (ICSI) involve fertilization of an egg with the father's sperm so that both parents are genetically related to the child. Donor insemination (DI) has been used in couples with an infertile male partner and by single or lesbian women or couples and involves insemination of banked sperm from an anonymous donor.

Citing statistics from the Institute for Science, Law, and Technology Working Group (1998), Shapiro, Shapiro, & Paret, (2001) reported that as of that date approximately 75,000 babies were born annually through the use of ART, with 60,000 of these births resulting from DI and 15,000 resulting from the use of IVF in the laboratory. A further 1000 births per year occur through surrogate or gestational parenthood. According to these authors, twice the number of infants are born using ART than there are infants available for adoption at birth. The number has likely increased since these statistics were published.

In these latter forms of ART, only the mother is related. In egg donation, there is a genetic tie with the father and not the mother. However, unlike DI where the donor is typically anonymous, egg donors are often relatives or friends of the parents and thus may have contact with the child over time. The final form of ART, artificial insemination surrogacy, also involves a situation where the father but not the mother is genetically related to the child. Again, the surrogate may be someone in the family or a friend who will have ongoing contact with the child.

Both adoption and some forms of ART give a chance for parents to be selective about preferred child traits by reading physical descriptions and the donor's family health history. In general, birth mothers pursue donors they believe to have positive inheritable characteristics such as good health, desirable physical and personal attributes, and intellectual abilities. Character also is thought to be important but birth mothers tend to believe that character is more a product of environment than genetics (Scheib, Kristiansen, & Wara, 1997), an assumption that genetic research would suggest is naive.

To date, there is no evidence of problematic cognitive or socioemotional outcomes or that parent–child relationships are affected based on research on any of these forms of ART (Golombok, 2006; Golombok & MacCallum, 2003). However, a recent review concluded that there is heightened risk of birth defects following IVF or ICSI compared with spontaneously conceived infants (Hansen, Bower, Milne *et al.*, 2005).

A basic difference between adoption and ART is that in some forms of ART there is a genetic link with the child (with the exception of DI). Although the child is biologically linked with one parent, there may be some tension and feelings of loss within the marriage or between partners. There is an assumption that the emotional connection to the child will diminish any feelings of loss that may emerge. Couples do not only have to confront issues that arise between them, but also must decide what to tell their children. In fact, one of the main concerns is that parents using DI tend to keep the means of conception secret from their child (Golombok & MacCallum, 2003). This is very much the opposite of common practice with adopted children, where the benefits of open discussion with children about their origins and feelings are widely acknowledged (Feast, 2003).

Single, Gay and Lesbian Families

Single women are choosing parenthood to an increasing extent. Some have an agreement with a known partner to conceive a child, others use ART and others adopt. A number of factors contribute to the choice including feelings about having a genetically related child, attitudes about an unknown sperm donor, comfort in undertaking infertility treatment if needed, carrying a child to term without the support of a partner, and a host of financial, religious and cultural issues. Research has shown that single-parent adoptions are successful and should not be compared critically to two-parent homes (Shireman, 1996). Brooks and Goldberg (2001) outlined strengths that facilitate adoption success, such as having support from family and friends, psychological stability, resourcefulness, sensitivity, educational success and financial security. Organizations such as Single Mothers by Choice also provide information and support. A small but growing number of single men are also choosing to adopt.

Gay and lesbian adoption has expanded but is not universally accepted and varies even within regions of countries. Brodzinsky, Patterson, and Vaziri (2003) estimated that 2.9% of public and private adoptions in the USA involve children placed with self-identified gay and lesbian individuals and couples. However, this is likely to be an underestimate because not all individuals and couples identify themselves as gay or lesbian in their applications. For both single and gay or lesbian parents, establishing a close supportive relationship with their child or children will help the children cope with the special nature of their family and the questions and issues that emerge as they mature.

There are a number of routes to gay and lesbian adoption. In some jurisdictions only older and other special needs children are available for adoption by gay and lesbian families. While international adoption from some countries is open to single parents, it is not consistently open to gay and lesbian parents, meaning that one parent often adopts as a single parent. This places the co-parent at a disadvantage in terms of legal parental status and accompanying practical matters in relation to health benefits and inheritance. Should the couple separate, the co-parent is also at a disadvantage in terms of custody, visitation rights and continuation of a relationship with the child (Horowitz & Maruyama, 1995).

Similarly, when a child is born using ART, a decision must be made as to who carries the child, which may stimulate reactions in the couple and their extended families. As in heterosexual families, changes arising from pregnancy and childbirth may also upset the relationship. Particularly in lesbian relationships, both partners may feel equal in the mothering role but physiological changes in the mother giving birth, and the child's possible preferential reaction to her, can disturb this sense of equality. Thus, parents in lesbian families may need guidance and support in negotiating their early relationship with their child at different developmental turning points.

There are more lesbian than gay parents. Some gay couples also choose to form their families through adopting older and other special needs children or through ART with the use of surrogate birth mothers. Much the same as for lesbian mothers, gay fathers' parenting compares well with that of single heterosexual fathers (Patterson, 2002). In this context, parenting includes encouraging children's sexual identity as well as sharing child care and engaging in cohesive and affectionate family interactions. Again, a complicating factor is prejudice in the broader community. Gay and lesbian families likely benefit from becoming part of their community and known as individuals and as a couple before bringing a child into their home. In urban areas there are also likely to be support networks for gay and lesbian parents.

Research on single and gay and lesbian families has focused on the impact of growing up in these non-traditional families on the children's development and on the nature of the relationship between parents and children. There are often important psychosocial factors to take into account outside of the family constellation in such studies. These include the acceptance of neighbors, schools and religious institutions in the community where children can potentially encounter bias toward themselves or their parent(s), which complicates the developmental process. By and large, however, studies indicate that there are no significant differences in gender identity or gender role behavior, self-esteem or health of social relationships of children raised by gay or lesbian parents compared to children raised in heterosexual families. Moreover, they have not found the children to be vulnerable to psychopathology (Patterson, 2002). Furthermore, findings from a longitudinal study have shown that mental health and work status of adults raised by lesbian parents compared well with adults from heterosexual families (Tasker & Golombok, 1997).

While these are generally positive findings, clinicians must be sensitive to the psychological health of parents and to the prejudice that single, gay and lesbian families may experience and support the family's strengths. Clinicians also must become aware of their own biases.

Opening the Birth Records: Search for Birth Parents and Birth Children

Just as openness in infant adoption has become more normative, so too has the search for birth parents by adolescent and adult adoptees. Factors motivating a search include curiosity, looking for a sense of belonging, seeking medical information, developing a sense of personal identity, wanting more information about physical similarities, having an interest in what happened to a birth relative (Howe & Feast, 2000) and being at a life cycle transition point (Campbell, Silverman, & Patti, 1991). In some cases, only non-identifying information is exchanged while in other cases there is ongoing personal contact. Interviews with adoptees who reunited with birth parents indicate that various types of relationships evolve following reunion (Gladstone & Westhues, 1998). However, in general, early contact usually diminishes in frequency and intensity over time and continues through letters or by telephone.

A number of factors predict the outcome of reunions. Howe and Feast (2001) found that the emotional stability and security of either the adopted or the birth relative are paramount. While feelings of emotional closeness are important, other factors mediate the outcome of reunion including geography, perceived response of birth relatives or adoptive family members, sexual attraction and expectations that each party has of the others (Gladstone & Westhues, 1998). In a follow-up of adult adoptees 5 and 8 years post-reunion, regardless of the outcome of the reunion, most adult adoptees say that the search and contact experience was satisfying and worthwhile and that it helped to answer questions about their origins, background and the reason for being placed (Howe & Feast, 2001; Triseliotis, Feast, & Kyle, 2005; Wrobel, Grotevant, & McRoy, 2004). Of those who met their birth mother, 63% were still in some form of contact 8 years or more after their reunion (Howe & Feast, 2001). From the perspective of the birth mother, 94% were pleased that the adopted adult had contacted them (Howe & Feast, 2001). When asked to identify the hardest parts of the reunion process, all parties indicated that the waiting period prior to reunion and the adjustment period that accompanied the negotiation of the relationships afterward were the most difficult (Sullivan & Lathrop, 2004). For adoptive parents, fear of the potential loss associated with sharing their child with someone who they did not know was most threatening. It is also important to realize that choosing not to search can be positive (Wrobel, Grotevant, & McRoy, 2004).

A widely held belief has been that only individuals who have an unsatisfactory relationship with adoptive parents want to reunite with a birth parent. Although a negative evaluation of adoption made it more likely that an individual would remain in contact with their birth mother, a positive evaluation of the adoption had no effect. Howe and Feast (2001) concluded that whereas many adopted people feel a need to know their genetic and genealogical background in and of itself, this does not imply a need, or even wish, for a relational connection that will supersede those formed in early childhood.

Many individuals who are searching for birth parents or a birth child do not want interference from the public system, whereas some seek help. Gladstone and Westhues (1998) suggested that clinicians should become knowledgeable about the search process so that they can be a resource. It may be necessary for the adoptee to deal with guilt feelings regarding disloyalty towards their adoptive family. Aspects of a reunion experience may underlie other issues which an adopted person presents within therapy or counseling. Help may be needed to resolve conflicts associated with expectations, inappropriate behavior, role ambiguity and differences in attitudes or values. There are few social guidelines indicating the ways that these family members should behave towards one another and clinicians may be requested to help in negotiating the relationship. Finally, clinicians can help the adoptee to deal with the reality of post-reunion relationships and their outcomes.

Children born through ART will likely be interested in their heritage for the same reasons adoptees are (Feast, 2003; Howe & Feast, 2000). There is no legislation at this time to protect children's right to search in the way that adoptees can (Golombok, 2006). There are also legal issues with ART, with the donor legally absolved of all parental responsibility and assured that identity is safeguarded. The rights of donor-conceived individuals to access to information regarding their genealogical heritage is increasingly being voiced and some donors do agree to be contacted when the child reaches 18 years of age. In England, the Human Fertilization and Embryology Act, 1990 allows inquiry regarding whether an individual is genetically related to the person they plan to marry but information on heritage or genetic history is not available. However, there are websites designed to unite children who share a donor and therefore a genetic link (http://www.donorsiblingregistry.com). This has also become the practice in families adopting internationally, some of whom search for siblings of abandoned children through DNA matching (e.g., http://www.kinsearchregistry.com/index.html). Thus, although a direct link with parents may not be possible, families are looking at alternative ways of acknowledging other biological connections for their child.

Outcomes of Adoption: Factors Contributing to Risk and Resilience

It is recognized that there are various pathways to development and adjustment. These are determined by an ongoing transaction between genetically influenced strengths and vulnerabilities, prenatal factors, premature birth and associated complications, and early growth promoting and traumatic experiences such as abuse or neglect. These are critical, especially in children adopted late (Haugaard, 1998; Howe, 1997).

Studies of adopted children have been used to understand that genetic factors are important but do not fully explain heightened risk. For instance, although children born to parents with psychiatric and antisocial disorders are at higher risk for psychopathology, this is most likely if such disorders and/or associated psychosocial adversity are also present in the adoptive family (Peters, Atkins, Marc *et al.*, 1999), a situation that is relatively uncommon (because of the screening of people wishing to adopt). A more plausible explanation is that adopted children who are at genetic risk for antisocial behavior exhibit some characteristics that draw more negative control from parents than those children not at risk (O'Connor, Deater-Deckard, Fulker *et al.*, 1998). Furthermore, longitudinal research suggests that genetic influences increase and shared environmental influences decrease in terms of cognitive ability. More specifically, although the cognitive and behavioral style of young adopted children is congruent with that of adoptive parents, by adolescence these styles diverge (O'Connor *et al.*, 1998) and children make choices and select opportunities that may suit their genetic disposition (Scarr & McCartney, 1983). Adoptive parents typically put high value on achievement and the power of the environment and of their capacity to shape their children's future. This may lead to frustration and conflict later in development as it has been a long-standing finding that one of the most important predictors of adjustment of adopted children is the capacity of parents to set realistic expectations for their child (Barth & Berry, 1988).

Biological factors such as nutrition, limited medical care for the child and birth parent, and prenatal exposure to drugs and alcohol are documented risks (Barth & Brooks, 2000; Moe, 2000). Even if children experience adequate caregiving, biomedical risks associated with prenatal drug exposure are still a potential determinant of specific developmental problems (Moe, 2000). Early disruptive life experiences, including a history of multiple placements prior to adoption, and a history of abuse or neglect also have serious consequences for developing adjustment problems (Dance & Rushton, 2005; Howe & Fearnley, 2003). Findings regarding the specific prevalence of adjustment problems vary across studies but, for instance, Dance and Rushton (2005) report that of domestically late placed adoptees, 49% had a positive outcome, 28% were difficult but continuing and 23% disrupted.

We now know that some children facing negative life circumstances are more resilient than others. Genetically shaped characteristics such as intelligence and easy temperament are protective factors as well as having a sense of curiosity, a feeling of personal control and prior experience in establishing a close interpersonal relationship (Masten, 2001). Another protective factor, of course, is adoption into a positive family environment.

Outcomes of Domestic Adoption

The positive outcomes for domestically adopted infants have been well documented in relation to both development and attachment security (e.g., Singer, Brodzinsky, Ramsay *et al.*, 1985). However, there is a shortage of healthy infants for adoption. Older children coming into care continue to be available for adoption in large numbers. These children have been identified as "special needs" adoptions, not only because they are older but because they often have cognitive, physical, emotional or behavioral problems that can make adoptive parenting more challenging. The preponderance of research indicates that, despite inauspicious beginnings, the majority of adopted children with special needs and their families have a positive outcome. For instance, analysis of data from the National Longitudinal Study of Adolescent Health indicated that background characteristics, early maltreatment, peer and family relations were associated with antisocial behavior but that adoption status contributed little or no additional predictive power (Grotevant, van Dulmen, Dunbar *et al.*, 2006). There is also accumulating evidence that satisfying attachment relationships do develop among late placed children and their adoptive parents within the first years of adoption, which supports the resilience of children when offered experiences that promote social–emotional growth (Rushton & Mayes, 1997).

Two meta-analytic reviews of both domestically and internationally adopted children's cognitive, behavioral and emotional outcomes put these findings into clearer perspective. Van IJzendoorn, Juffer, and Poelhuis (2005) concluded that adopted children performed better than left-behind non-adopted siblings and peers but lagged behind non-adopted environmental peers and siblings. Although adopted children's cognitive skills were in the average range and similar to current peers, there was a two-fold increase in special education referrals for learning problems for the adopted children. In a meta-analysis of emotional and behavioral problems, Juffer and van IJzendoorn (2005) showed that adoptees exhibited more behavioral and emotional problems. For both cognitive development and behavioral and emotional problems the effect sizes were small. However, adoptees were overrepresented in mental health referrals. Thus, adoption is an effective intervention that improves behavioral, emotional and cognitive development. Adoptive families likely seek help because they have a lower threshold for referral for mental health services both because of their expectations of their children and because they tend to be people who utilize services (van IJzendoorn, Juffer, & Poelhuis, 2005).

At the extreme, disruption of adoptive placements has been associated with the child's age at placement, length of time in care, the number of moves and returns to the birth home, the child's level of behavior problems and inattention/overactivity, preferential rejection by birth parents, and the child's ability to show signs of attachment to their new family (Dance & Rushton, 2005; Rushton & Dance, 2003). In contrast, children with identifiable developmental or physical disabilities have fared well (Glidden, 1991).

Haugaard (1998) strongly advised clinicians not to generalize the risk of adjustment problems to the entire adopted population, as it is applicable only to a small subset of adopted children. Similarly, Hodges, Steele, Hillman *et al.* (2003) found that, during their first year of adoption, children who had been maltreated showed an increase in mental representations of adults helping and limit-setting and being aware when children needed them. When older children do have behavioral and emotional problems, it is important to recognize the unique histories that they bring to their adoptive families. When raised in environments of abuse, neglect and rejection, children develop strategies to ensure survival that make them ill-equipped for loving and responsive care. Many of these children are unable either to elicit sensitive care or to respond to it, which raises the risk that the adoptive family will feel rejected or punished by the child. Such findings reinforce the need for parents adopting older children to receive help to set realistic expectations, to understand their children's needs, and to appraise both their own and their child's contribution to the relationship (Stovall & Dozier, 1998). Rushton, Mayes, Dance *et al.* (2003) followed the development of new relationships and the presence of behavioral and emotional problems in domestically adopted 5- to 9-year-old children placed with adoptive families. A relatively small proportion failed to form an attachment relationship with one or both parents by the end of their first year in placement (27%) but they were more likely to exhibit behavioral problems. Some of the ways that these children interact and show their emotions (e.g., false affection, superficiality and distancing behavior) may be misperceived by parents, who take the behavior at face value rather than as defensive actions.

Outcomes of Intercountry Adoption

Reports from a number of countries confirm the positive outcome of intercountry adoption. Most intercountry adoptees have lived in institutions of varying quality prior to adoption, deprived of health care, optimal cognitive and social stimulation, and individualized attention which may have observable effects for months or years following adoption (Kreppner, Rutter, Beckett, *et al.*, 2007; Rutter, 2005).

Intercountry adoptees are at risk for infectious diseases and other health and neurological problems, often not diagnosed until parents bring their child home (Johnson, 2000). Malnutrition and inadequate stimulation are also common, leading to children weighing less, being shorter and having a smaller head circumference than children raised in birth families or adopted domestically (Mason & Narad, 2005). Fortunately, most of these problems can be managed with appropriate medical and dietary intervention (Johnson, 2002; Mason & Narad, 2005). The rate of catch-up growth depends on the quality of early experience and the age at adoption. Thus, children adopted younger, and from presumably less depriving conditions, such as those in institutions in East Asia and China, grow rapidly within the first 6 months after adoption (Cohen, Lojkasek, Yaghoub Zadeh *et al.*, in press; Miller & Hendrie, 2000; Pomerleau, Malcuit, Chicoine *et al.*, 2005) whereas for children adopted later from more depriving environments catch-up growth takes longer (Rutter, O'Connor, & the ERA Study Team, 2004). It is important to note, however, that two years after adoption, at approximately 3 years of age, the physical measurements of children adopted from China were still lower than those of non-adopted comparison children (Cohen *et al.*, in press).

Problems with cognitive, motor and language development are common in children who have experienced institutional care and are dependent on the length of institutionalization (Ames, 1997; Cohen *et al.*, in press; Marcovitch, Goldberg, Gold *et al.*, 1997; Miller & Hendrie, 2000; Pomerleau *et al.*, 2005; Rutter, O'Connor and the ERA, 2004). At one extreme are children adopted from Romania at the fall of the Ceausescu regime in 1989. Whereas some children adopted later than 6 months of age made remarkable gains, most showed marked delays that persisted, even up to 7.5 years post-adoption (Beckett, Maughan, Rutter *et al.*, 2006; Croft, Beckett, Rutter *et al.*, 2007). In fact, by the age of 11 years, outcomes for children deprived for 6–12 months were similar to those who had been deprived longer. These findings for children who had been profoundly deprived suggest both a sensitive period for development and limits on the effects of exposure to a stimulating environment as there were no differences in adoptive family characteristics.

At the other end of the continuum are children adopted from China and other East Asian countries who experienced less severe deprivation. For instance, when Cohen *et al.* (in press) followed children who were, on average, 13 months of age at adoption, from the time of their arrival to Canada and then 6, 12 and 24 months later, rapid gains were made within 6 months. By this time children were functioning within the average range in cognitive, motor and language development, a pattern also observed at 6-month follow-up by Pomerleau, Malcuit, Chicoine *et al.* (2005) in children adopted between 6 and 18 months from China, East Asia and Russia. Although there were rapid changes, Cohen *et al.* (in press) found that the children adopted from China did not catch up to non-adopted peers from similar family backgrounds until 2 years post-adoption.

Taking a broad view of the literature on intercountry adoption, the meta-analysis carried out by van IJzendoorn, Juffer, & Poelhuis (2005) on cognitive development and achievement of adopted children also included intercountry adoptees. That review showed positive outcomes for children adopted younger than 1 year of age.

The importance of establishing secure attachment relationships is widely recognized. Similar to infants adopted domestically, intercountry infants adopted before focused attachment occurs do not exhibit difficulties (Juffer & Rosenboom, 1997; Stams, Juffer, & van IJzendoorn, 2002). Moreover, even children previously institutionalized in Romania were able to form a secure or insecure attachment relationship with adoptive parents within a few years after adoption, and there was no evidence of children being unattached (Chisholm, 1998; O'Connor, Marvin, Rutter *et al.*, 2003).

At the same time, there is agreement that in institutional settings children rarely have the sort of individualized positive interactions with caregivers required to meet emotional needs. Some older placed children who were adopted from Romanian institutions were at increased risk for atypical maladaptive behaviors such as indiscriminate social behavior, characterized by affectionate or friendly behavior towards all new adults, including strangers, with lack of the caution exhibited by non-adopted family reared children (Gunnar, Bruce, & Grotevant, 2000; MacLean, 2003; Rutter, Colvert, Kreppner *et al.*, 2007). Surprisingly, neither age at adoption nor the length of time in institutional care was related to the quality of attachment insecurity (Chisholm, 1998; Judge, 2004).

Rather, insecure attachment was associated with lower child IQ scores (Chisholm, 1998; Judge, 2004), a higher degree of behavioral problems (Chisholm, 1998; Marcovitch *et al.*, 1997), adopting more than one child at a time (Ames & Chisholm, 2001) and high levels of parenting stress (Chisholm, 1998).

The few studies of attachment in intercountry adoptees have considered outcomes 1 year or more after adoption. One study has examined the process of attachment formation from arrival among infants adopted from China. Among the children who were, on average, 13 months of age at the time of adoption, Pugliese (2006) found that within weeks of being adopted there were signs of forming an attachment, based on mother-completed questionnaires, interviews and mother–infant observation. Interviews at bi-weekly intervals showed a gradual increase in attachment behaviors over time. Although in the first month with their adoptive parents, some infants showed atypical or extreme patterns of behavior (e.g., showing attachment behavior in nonstressful situations), for the most part these disappeared by 6 months post-adoption.

Like their domestically adopted counterparts, intercountry adoptees who experienced poor institutional care are at greater risk for behavioral and emotional problems than those who experienced less extreme early care (Ellis, Fisher, & Zaharie, 2004; Hoksbergen, Rijk, van Dijkum *et al.*, 2004; Verhulst, 2000a,b). Some different patterns of symptoms were observed among children adopted from Romania, a form of inattentiveness/overactivity and autistic-like symptoms (6%), which were qualitatively different from attention deficit/hyperactivity disorder (ADHD) or autism observed in western clinical settings and which might have been an outcome of institutional care (Kreppner, O'Connor, Rutter & the ERA Study Team Group, 2001). The latter symptoms, along with disinhibited attachment and cognitive impairment, were associated with social and emotional difficulties at the age of 11 years only in children who had experienced institutional deprivation for longer than their first 6 months of life. There was also an increase in emotional, but not behavioral, problems when children were followed from age 6 to age 11 years with evidence that difficulties with emotion recognition might have a role in the emergence of these problems (Colvert, Rutter, Beckett *et al.*, in press), something that would not have been easily observed when the children were younger.

Again, using meta-analysis to examine intercountry adoptees, whereas adoptees from a wide range of countries had more behavioral and emotional problems compared to domestically adopted children, the effect sizes were small (Bimmel *et al.*, 2003; Juffer & van IJzendoorn, 2005). Thus, most children were well adjusted despite many having experienced poor institutional care. Moreover, intercountry adoptees had less severe emotional and behavioral problems and were less likely to be referred for mental health services than domestic adoptees. Juffer and van IJzendoorn (2005) speculate that the sources of emotional and behavioral disturbance among intercountry adoptees may be different than for domestic adoptees. Intercountry adoption comes about because children are given over to institutions for economic or political reasons rather than genetic or prenatally determined risk factors or removal from birth parents because of abuse or neglect.

Intercountry adoptees also exhibit other types of behavior problems such as problems with eating (Ames, 1997; Beckett, Bredenkamp, Castle *et al.*, 2002; Johnson, 2002), stereotyped and self-stimulating behaviors, pain agnosia and tactile defensiveness with hyper- or hyposensitivity to touch, light, sound, smell and taste (Ames, 1997; Beckett *et al.*, 2002; Fisher, Ames, Chisholm *et al.*, 1997; Groze & Ileana, 1996). It has been presumed that these atypical behaviors arose as a response to experiencing a depriving environment in institutional care and were adaptive within that context (e.g., self-soothing in times of distress). Such problems tend to be transitional and decline during the post-adoption period (Ames, 1997; Fisher *et al.*, 1997; Johnson, 2002). Nevertheless, 40% of previously institutionalized Romanian children continued to display some of the stereotyped behaviors 3 years post-adoption, 18% continued to rock at 6 years of age (Ames, 1997; Beckett *et al.*, 2002) and 15% still had difficulties with eating solid foods at 6 years of age (Beckett *et al.*, 2002). Moreover, among adoptees who had experienced institutional deprivation, about 1 in 10 show a pattern of autistic-like behavior in the British study of adoptees from Romania (Rutter, Anderson-Wood, Beckett *et al.*, 1999; Rutter, Kreppner, Croft *et al.*, 2007).

There is little known about adjustment in intercountry adoptees in adulthood. In a survey of a mixed group of intercountry adoptees, Tieman, van der Ende, and Verhulst (2005) found that although the majority of adults, ranging in age from 22 to 32 years, did not show serious mental health problems, there was increased risk among children raised in high socioeconomic class families, possibly because of the unrealistic demands and expectations set by these parents. They also noted that those adoptees who could not be contacted or who dropped out of the study earlier had initially higher problem behavior scores. Thus, the study may have underestimated the risk for mental health problems in adult intercountry adoptees.

Selection, Preparation and Assessment of Adopted Children and Adoptive Families

Whether a child is adopted from a public, private or independent agency, attention is paid to assessing adopters to ensure that children will be safe and that relational support and educational opportunities will be provided. In parents, personal qualities such as warmth, mental health and parenting capacity and style are taken into account. Parents' own attachment histories are not systematically assessed but Steele, Hodges, Kaniuk *et al.* (2003) found that 3 months after adoption, children whose adoptive mothers showed signs of insecure attachment exhibited aggressiveness in their themes to a story completion task relative to children adopted by mothers with secure attachment responses. In older children, a rather ill-defined criterion regarding whether a child wants and feels ready to be adopted is also considered.

The process of adoption is especially complex for children who are older at adoption, have a history of abuse, and birth parent history of drug and alcohol use. In domestic adoption, the needs of both child and family are addressed through arranging multiple visits of increasing length so that the prospective parents and children can get to know one another, gain comfort and make a gradual transition to adoptive family life. Group meetings for prospective adoptive parents are arranged to provide information, talk with experienced adoptive parents and air potential risks in the adoption process. These have gone some way to challenge unrealistic expectations. Moreover, in some cases information is targeted for particular subgroups, something that is common in agencies arranging special needs and intercountry adoptions.

Families of both domestic and intercountry adoptees are generally dissatisfied with the amount of information provided prior to adoption and some feel that they were not fully aware of the difficulties they would face. Showing parents of domestically adopted children videos of children available for adoption is becoming a common practice. Some internationally adopted children also have a pre-adoption video for prospective adoptive parents to review with a physician before making their commitment to adoption (Boone, Hostetter, & Weitzman, 2003). The value of this review is that the clinician can help parents to understand the consequences of prolonged institutional care and other risk factors. For instance, a video can help to identify dysmorphic features associated with fetal alcohol syndrome and genetic or neurological disorders. Boone, Hostetter, & Weitzman (2003) found that estimates of development from the video were correlated with direct assessment of child development post-adoption. However, this procedure cannot estimate relational differences between children.

It is important to highlight that assessment of some critically important adoptive parent qualities may be difficult prior to adoption. These qualities include flexibility in setting realistic expectations and understanding not only the importance of attachment relationships but also that some of the children's behavior problems may actually be an indirect way of getting closer. Dance, Rushton, and Quinton (2002) found that adoptive parent characteristics such as warmth, the ability to deal with both the facts and the effects of children's early experiences, and the competence to manage child behaviors, assessed immediately after placement, were related to outcome one year post-adoption. Even more important was the nature of the relationship that emerged over this period. Among children aged 5–11 years who had been preferentially rejected by their birth parents, an important predictor of maladjustment in the first year post-adoption was false display of affection by the child early in placement and not the level of behavioral difficulties. Moreover, lack of warmth and sensitivity in parent interactions was heightened when the adoptee had problems with attention and affect regulation (Rushton, Dance, & Quinton, 2000). It was recommended that these children should be flagged for more intensive work in the preparation of parents and in post-adoption services. Mistrust of relationships, low self-esteem, anger and fear of abandonment all contribute to the likelihood of significant child psychopathology during the transition to adoption and unresponsiveness to parents' bids for closeness. Parents may need guidance in evaluating their child's behavior and finding the right level of interaction to sensitively read their child's signals and to pace their efforts in forming a relationship. This is notable because in their sample Rushton and Dance (2006) found that more than one-third of children had ongoing difficulties 6 years later. Such findings heighten the need for post-adoption services as a routine part of the adoption process.

Post-adoption Services

It is not possible to prepare parents for everything that they will encounter once a child joins their family. Parents often minimize genetic and prenatal physiological conditions in favor of a family systems explanation for maladaptive behaviors and do not acknowledge the potential limitations of the post-adoption environment (Barth, 2002). Pinderhughes (1996) has described four stages through which families move in the process of including a child with special needs: anticipation when the family looks forward to the child's placement with the accompanying expectations and fantasies; accommodation to a child who may test limits and, in doing so, disappoint parents' expectations; resistance when family members experience ambivalence; and restabilization when the family achieves a new equilibrium where expectations and reality are more closely matched. Parents adopting children internationally, although prepared by adoption agencies, may not be fully aware of the long-term effects of institutional rearing and go through their own adjustment stages. Moreover, parents need to be made aware that they should limit contact with other adults in favor of maximizing opportunities for parent–child interaction and generally avoid overstimulating the child with too many toys and outings. As well, toys should be purchased that fit the child's developmental level rather than age.

For both domestic and intercountry adoptions, a comprehensive assessment should be carried out once children join their adoptive families, and include a thorough medical examination, a developmental assessment of cognitive, motor and language ability, and observation of the child in structured and unstructured situations. Observations should consider the child's predominant affective tone, curiosity, involvement in particular situations, sharing of activities with others and reaction to transitions (Weitzman, 2003). Functional rather than standardized evaluations are preferred, and interpreters should be available for children over the age of 3 years in order to evaluate language competence. Behavior problems, including unusual behaviors (e.g., rocking and other self-stimulating behaviors) and, for older children, aggressive behavior and inattention should be recorded. Parents should be encouraged to seek help when it is needed (Johnson & Dole, 1999).

There is a long-standing awareness of the need to provide health focused post-adoption services early in the adoption process with a view toward easing the transition and preventing difficulties down the road, especially in families adopting children with special needs. It is not possible to talk about post-adoption services in a unitary fashion. The expanding variety and needs of adoptive families call for multiple forms of support and co-ordination of services. In the UK, a survey of local authority adoption services in the year 2000 led to the development of new adoption support services (Rushton & Dance, 2003). In the USA, this happened as a result of the President's Adoption 2000 initiative (cited by Shapiro, Shapiro, & Paret, 2001).

For example, Juffer, Hoksbergen, Riksen-Walraven *et al.* (1997) compared two short-term programs directed at promoting maternal sensitive responsiveness in international infant adoptions. One involved giving participants a book that focused on sensitive parenting and a second that involved using the book in conjunction with three video-feedback sessions. Intervention effects were observed in relation to an untreated comparison group in maternal sensitive responsiveness, infant competence and infant–mother attachment in the group receiving both the book and video feedback (Juffer *et al.*, 1997) and a lower rate of disorganized attachment in infancy (Juffer, Bakermans-Kranenburg, & van IJzendoorn, 2005). When the children were followed at the age of 7 years, both boys and girls who had received the intervention showed less internalizing behavior problems and girls showed greater ego-resiliency (Stams, Juffer, van IJzendoorn *et al.*, 2001).

Other programs have been directed at dealing with the transition to adoption (Cohen & Duvall, 1996) and with behavior problems in older adopted children, especially those who have experienced trauma associated with an early family history of abuse, neglect and multiple moves (e.g., Dozier, Albus, Fisher *et al.*, 2002; Rushton, Monck, Upright *et al.*, 2006).

Some systematic post-adoption services for these children are currently being tested. For instance, Rushton *et al.* (2006) are comparing two manualized interventions for parents adopting older children in relation to routine support services. One is based on cognitive behavior modification that focuses on dealing with understanding the current meaning of challenging behaviors and ways of dealing with these. The second is an educational model based on understanding the meaning of children's behavior from a historical point of view, focusing on broken or distorted attachments and the child's coping mechanisms. Unfortunately, there are not yet empirical data on the outcome of these services.

In a survey of post-adoption service use, Brooks, Allen, and Barth (2002) found that less than 30% of adoptive families used post-adoption services although a higher percentage read books and articles on adoption (82%) and attended lectures or seminars (43%). These latter activities were the most accessible as families could pursue them on their own, something that may be most appealing to the educated parents likely to adopt. Although books and lectures can be helpful, they are neither geared to the families' individual needs nor are they experiential. Independent adopters made the least use of post-adoption services, most likely because they involve fewer children with special needs. Nevertheless, given findings that adoptive parents are more likely to use services, a potential need for specialized post-adoption consultation and intervention continues to be valid.

Families involved in kinship adoptions and in various open adoption arrangements have different post-adoption needs to those involved in extrafamilial adoptions. Moreover, the increase in open adoptions and various other forms of adoption with ongoing contact with the birth family has accelerated a need for continued mediation between adoptive and birth parents. This raises a need for systematic study of programs for these families.

Picking up the thread of openness in adoption as a state of mind as well as a set of actions, an important health focused post-adoption activity that contributes to promoting mental health for all adopted children, but is often overlooked, is preparation of a Life Book. This provides children with a sense of their own personal histories and an acknowledgement of the positive value that adoptive parents place on that history. Optimally, child protection workers who take domestically adopted children into care collect background information and mementoes for children from birth or foster families, but this is sometimes overlooked. One might assume that children adopted as infants or adopted internationally, some of whom were abandoned with no clues as to birth parenthood or history, cannot have a Life Book. However, there are creative suggestions in both books and websites that provide ideas of how to construct a history for the child. For instance, information about the town where the child was born, where the institution was located, current events on the day of the child's birth obtained from a newspaper archive, photos, a narrative about the transition to adoptive family life, and older children's drawings of what they imagine about their birth family are examples of what can be included (http://www.lifebooks@earthlink.net).

There is also need for health focused post-adoption services at later points in the post-adoption life cycle. Brodzinsky (1987) has suggested that for children adopted as infants there are key turning points related to shifts in cognitive development and consequent understanding of the meaning and implications of adoption. One turning point comes in the early school years, around the ages of 6–7, when children first truly understand the meaning of adoption. Another turning point is in adolescence when thoughts about their own reproductive future and life choices give rise to adolescents' questions about their identity. Sometimes they decide to meet or know more about the birth family or, in the case of ART, the donor. Changing needs with respect to provision of and discussion about different types of information (Wrobel,

Kohler, Grotevant *et al.*, 2003), response to emotions evoked at life transition points (Brodzinsky, 2005) and styles of coping with birth parent loss (Smith & Brodzinsky, 2002) are important content for post-adoption services for these children and youths. It is impossible to prepare parents for these possible reactions when children are very young or at the beginning of the adoption process. Consequently, it is essential that mental health professionals be aware of these turning points so that they can provide resources to meet the changing needs of adoptive families.

Clinical Services

Adoptive parents are more likely to seek services some time after adoption has occurred when they encounter difficulties within their families, in relation to their children's behavior or in attachment relationships. These problems have been conceptualized in different ways relating to behavior management, family systems and attachment theory, and parenting style, which have been used to shape clinical as well as post-adoption services (Cohen & Duvall, 1996; Juffer *et al.*, 1997; Rushton *et al.*, 2006).

Attachment research has been influential in providing advice to parents about how attachment behaviors can sometimes be displayed in unexpected ways. For instance, from reviewing 83 clinical referrals of parents and their adopted foster care children, Lieberman (2003) found that parents often missed subtle attachment cues and misinterpreted defiance and temper tantrums as signs that the child did not care for them. It is a difficult task for parents both to acknowledge their children's displays of attachment behavior and provide appropriate warmth and support while, at the same time, being able to set limits in a non-rejecting firm way. Thus, the adoptive parent must consciously teach attachment skills to the child, as the feeling of being wanted does not come automatically to a child who has never known love and care. Clinical services need to educate adoptive parents on the psychological and emotional challenges of children deprived of a consistent and reliable attachment figure during their formative years. They also need to provide guidance and experience with interpreting and appropriately responding to children's emotional needs.

For the most part, post-adoption and clinical services are focused on helping children to develop selective attachment relationships. This is achieved by facilitating sensitive responsive and pleasurable interactions between parent and child and increasing parents' ability to be good observers of their child's behavior. However, these services have not been specific to adoption (e.g., Cohen, Muir, Lojkasek *et al.*, 1999; Juffer *et al.*, 1997; Lanyado, 2003; Lieberman, Silverman, & Pawl, 2000). It is also important to note that these interventions were developed for young children. It remains a challenge to devise parallel interventions for older children and adolescents (Cohen & Duvall, 1996). Moreover, in any intervention, some individuals are likely to benefit more than others. Thus, it is notable that outside of the adoption literature it has been observed that mothers' own attachment style is related to their response to particular forms of therapy; something that should be taken into consideration in therapy with adoptive families and in research (Bakermans-Kranenburg, Juffer, & van IJzendoorn, 1998).

Even when children develop attachment relationships with parents, they continue to have problems in peer relationships that extend into the school years (Hodges & Tizard, 1989; LeMare, 2004). O'Connor and Zeanah (2003) suggest that symptoms of attachment disorder that extend beyond primary caregivers to peer relationships should be a focus of treatment. For instance, group therapy for adopted children is becoming more common (Nickman, Rosenfeld, Fine *et al.*, 2005). For children with severe attachment problems (e.g., reactive attachment disorder) there is little by way of systematic study of treatment outcomes. A dual focus on attachment promoting and behavioral management interventions may be needed over a long period of time, recognizing that such attachments may not form at all or that they may not be achieved until adulthood (Howe, 1996). For children with severe attachment disorder, support groups for adoptive parents may be of benefit (O'Connor & Zeanah, 2003).

Unfortunately, untested and potentially damaging forms of therapy continue to be used, many of which are touted on the Internet as providing certain cure. The most contentious of these is holding therapy, an intervention that involves close physical contact of a child with a therapist and/or parent. The rationale behind this is that it provides the child with the experience of touching and holding that is essential in the normative attachment process and helps to contain children prone to extreme distress or rage. Tragically, there have been at least six deaths from various forms of holding therapy. According to Hughes (1999), most therapists have now modified holding therapies by seeking the child's consent to being touched or held and always including the parent in therapy. In any event, there are no empirical data suggesting that any form of holding therapy is effective. While parents need help in controlling children's uncontrollable outbursts, this should not be confused with attachment and can be addressed with more conventional treatments for behavioral and emotional problems (Webster-Stratton, 2005).

There is not a "one size fits all" intervention. As in any clinical service, it is essential to make a thorough assessment of factors within the child, parents and environment before proceeding. For the most part, the kinds of interventions that have been applied to birth families have been used with adoptive families, hopefully with sensitivity to particular issues that adoptive families may bring to the fore. Moreover, while helping parents set realistic expectations may be important in any therapy, this may be an especially salient issue with adoptive families. Finally, it must be recognized that in some cases therapeutic interventions need to be long-term and multimodal without promise of a desired outcome. Adoptive parents who are used to finding effective solutions to problems may be frustrated with the apparently impervious nature of their children's problems.

Adoption and the Professional Community

In the past, the professional community was criticized for being insensitive to the needs of post-adoptive families (Nickman & Lewis, 1994). There has been a welcome growth in the private sector in attending to the specialized needs of post-adoptive families. Professionals working in the adoption field also are increasingly involved in setting a curriculum and developing training models, and training a range of other professionals engaging with adopted children (American Academy of Child and Adolescent Psychiatry, 2005; Chamberlin, 2005; Dozier *et al.*, 2002; Palacios & Sanchez-Sandoval, 2005). Some specialized medical clinics for intercountry adoptees have been established that provide thorough medical and developmental examination, review records to identify potential risk factors, and observe the child to determine affective tone, involvement in testing, quality of relationship with the examiner and adoptive parents, and atypical behaviors. It is important to follow closely intercountry adoptees on all of these fronts. While these clinics assess and monitor children, they typically do not offer mental health services.

Conclusions and Future Challenges

Adoption has come to have an increasingly prominent role in the fabric of family life worldwide. The research base for many adoption-specific issues accordingly has broadened. Moreover, since the last edition of this book, there has been significant growth in the understanding of specific issues relevant to adoptive families by professionals. It is heartening to know that many prejudices surrounding adoption have been overcome although some remain around gay and lesbian adoption, for instance. Moreover, while there is greater acceptance of openness in adoption, for the most part, this has applied to children adopted as infants. One of the challenges in years to come will be to test forms of openness for children adopted under less benign conditions to determine whether there is value in contact with birth families who, for one reason or another, have not been able to provide proper direct care for their children. Furthermore, new issues will come to the fore as children conceived through ART (and especially DI) mature into adolescence and adulthood and consider searching for a biological parent. Given the large number of children available for domestic adoption who are older and have other special needs, there is a continuing challenge in moving children into a permanent arrangement and providing supports that will facilitate positive adjustment. There is also a challenge in testing the effectiveness of various practices.

More research on the impact of intercountry adoption on children is also needed. There have been active efforts to improve the early lives of children in institutional care and there is now a fuller range of pre-adoption experiences to consider. Longitudinal studies are especially important to track the progress of children and families over time. It is essential not only to describe the outcomes for children adopted internationally, but also to provide information about the process of development and adjustment that will contribute to better preparation of families and establishment of post-adoption services. Finally, the systematic implementation and study of both post-adoption and clinical services tailored to the needs of adoptive families have been a long time in coming. There are now signs that these important tasks are under way. Until there is solid ground for recommending post-adoption and clinical services, the lure of a quick cure will continue to appeal to some families who are experiencing serious problems in their relationships with their adopted children.

References

American Academy of Child and Adolescent Psychiatry. (2005). Practice parameter for the assessment and treatment of children and adolescents with reactive attachment disorder of infancy and early childhood. *Journal of the American Academy of Child and Adolescent Psychiatry*, *44*, 1206–1219.

Ames, E. W. (1997). *The development of Romanian orphanage children adopted to Canada.* Final Report to Human Resources Development Canada, 1997.

Ames, E. W., & Chisholm, K. (2001). Social and emotional development in children adopted from institutions. In D. Bailey Jr., J. T. Bruer, F. J. Symons, & J. W. Lichtman (Eds.), *Critical thinking about critical periods* (pp. 129–148). Baltimore: MD Brookes.

Bakermans-Kranenburg, M. J., Juffer, F., & van IJzendoorn, M. H. (1998). Interventions with video feedback and attachment discussions: Does type of maternal insecurity make a difference? *Infant Mental Health Journal*, *19*, 202–219.

Barth, R. P. (2002). Outcomes of adoption and what they tell us about designing adoption services. *Adoption Quarterly*, *6*, 45–60.

Barth, R. P., & Berry, M. (1988). *Adoption and disruption: Rates, risks, and responses.* New York: Aldine De Gruyter.

Barth, R. P., & Brooks, D. (2000). Outcomes of drug-exposed children eight years post adoption. In R. Barth, M. Freundlich, & D. Brodzinsky (Eds.), *Adoption and prenatal alcohol and drug exposure: Research, policy and practice* (pp. 23–58). Washington, DC: Child Welfare League of America.

Beckett, C., Bredenkamp, D., Castle, J., Groothues, C., O'Connor, T. G., & Rutter, M. (2002). Behavior patterns associated with institutionalized deprivation: A study of children adopted from Romania. *Journal of Developmental and Behavioral Pediatrics*, *23*, 297–303.

Beckett, C., Maughan, B., Rutter, M., Castle, J., Colvert, E., Groothues, C., *et al.* (2006). Do the effects of early severe deprivation on cognition persist into early adolescence? Findings from the English and Romanian Adoptees Study. *Child Development*, *77*, 696–711.

Berry, M., Cavazos Dylla, D. J., Barth, R. P., & Needell, B. (1998). The role of open adoption in the adjustment of adopted children and their families. *Children and Youth Services Review*, *20*, 151–171.

Bimmel, N., Juffer, F., van IJzendoorn, M. H., & Bakermans-Kranenburg, M. J. (2003). Problem behavior of internationally adopted adolescents: A review and meta-analysis. *Harvard Review of Psychiatry*, *11*, 64–77.

Boone, J. L., Hostetter, M. K., & Weitzman, C. C. (2003). The predictive accuracy of pre-adoption video review in adoptees from Russian and Eastern European orphanages. *Clinical Pediatrics*, *42*, 585–590.

Brodzinsky, D. M. (1987). Adjustment to adoption: A psychosocial perspective. *Clinical Psychology Review*, *7*, 25–47.

Brodzinsky, D. M. (2005). Reconceptualizing openness in adoption: Implications for theory, research, and practice. In D. M.

Brodzinsky, & J. Palacios (Eds.), *Psychological issues in adoption: Research and Practice* (pp. 145–166). Westport, CT: Praeger.

Brodzinsky, D. M., Patterson, C. J., & Vaziri, M. (2003). Adoption agency perspectives on lesbian and gay prospective parents: A national study. *Adoption Quarterly*, *5*, 5–23.

Brooks, S. L. (2002). Kinship and adoption. *Adoption Quarterly*, *5*, 55–66.

Brooks, D., Allen, J., & Barth, R. P. (2002). Adoption services use, helpfulness, and need: A comparison of public and private agency and independent adoptive families. *Children and Youth Services Review*, *24*, 213–238.

Brooks, D., & Barth R. P. (1999). Adjustment outcomes of adult transracial and inracial adoptees: Effects of race, gender, adoptive family structure, and placement history. *American Journal of Orthopsychiatry*, *69*, 87–102.

Brooks, D., & Goldberg, S. (2001). Gay and lesbian adoptive and foster care placements: Can they meet the needs of waiting children? *Social Work*, *46*, 147–157.

Burnette, D. (1999). Custodial grandparents in Latino families: Patterns of service use and predictors of unmet needs. *Social Work*, *44*, 22–34.

Burrow, A. L., & Finley, G. E. (2004). Transracial, same-race adoptions, and the need for multiple measures of adolescent adjustment. *American Journal of Orthopsychiatry*, *74*, 577–583.

Calkins, C. A., & Millar, M. (1999). The effectiveness of court appointed special advocates to assist in permanency planning. *Child and Adolescent Social Work Journal*, *16*, 37–47.

Campbell, L. H., Silverman, P. R., & Patti, P. B. (1991). Reunions between adoptees and birth parents: The adoptees' experience. *Social Work*, *36*(4), 329–335.

Cederblad, M., Hook, B., Irhammar, M., & Mercke, A. M. (1999). Mental health in international adoptees as teenagers and young adults: An epidemiological study. *Journal of Child Psychology and Psychiatry*, *40*, 239–248.

Chamberlin, J. (2005). Adopting a new American family. *Monitor on Psychology*, *36*, 70–71.

Chisholm, K. (1998). A three year follow-up of attachment and indiscriminate friendliness in children adopted from Romanian orphanages. *Child Development*, *69*, 1092–1106.

Cohen, N. J., & Duvall, J. D. (1996). *Manual for the family attachment program: An innovative program for working with families adopting older children*. Toronto, ON: Hincks-Dellcrest Institute.

Cohen, N. J., Lojkasek, M., Yaghoub Zadeh, Z., Pugliese, M., & Kiefer, H. (in press). Children adopted from China: A prospective study of their growth and development. *Journal of Child Psychology & Psychiatry*.

Cohen, N. J., Muir, E., Lojkasek, M., Muir, R., Parker, C-J., Barwick, M., *et al.* (1999). Watch, wait, and wonder: Testing the effectiveness of a new approach to mother–infant psychotherapy. *Infant Mental Health Journal*, 20, 429–451.

Colvert, E., Rutter, M., Beckett, C., Castle, J., Groothues, C., Hawkins, A., *et al.* (in press). Emotional difficulties in early adolescence following severe early deprivation: Findings from the English and Romanian Adoptees Study. *Development and Psychopathology*.

Croft, C., Beckett, C., Rutter, M., Castle, J., Colvert, E., Groothues, C., *et al.* (2007). Early adolescent outcomes of institutionally deprived and non-deprived adoptees. II. Language as a protective factor and a vulnerable outcome. *Journal of Child Psychology and Psychiatry*, *48*, 31–44.

Dance, C., & Rushton, A. (2005). Predictors of outcome for unrelated adoptive placements made during middle childhood. *Child and Family Social Work*, *10*, 269–280.

Dance, C., Rushton, A., & Quinton, D. (2002). Emotional abuse in early childhood: Relationships with progress in subsequent family placement. *Journal of Child Psychology and Psychiatry*, *43*, 395–409.

DeBerry, K. M., Scarr, S., & Weinberg, R. (1996). Family racial socialization and ecological competence: Longitudinal assessments of African-American transracial adoptees. *Child Development*, *67*, 2375–2399.

Dozier, M., Albus, K., Fisher, P. A., & Sepulveda, S. (2002). Interventions for foster parents: Implications for developmental theory. *Development and Psychopathology*, *14*, 843–860.

Ellis, H. B., Fisher, P. A., & Zaharie, M. S. (2004). Predictors of disruptive behavior, developmental delays, anxiety, and affective symptomatology among institutionally reared Romanian children. *Journal of the American Academy of Child and Adolescent Psychiatry*, *43*, 1283–1292.

Farmer, F. (2006). Fostering, adoption and alternative care. Presentation made at the Emanuel Miller Lecture and Day Conference, March 16, 2006, London, UK.

Feast, J. (2003). Using and not losing the messages from the adoption experience for donor-assisted conception. *Human Fertility*, *6*, 41–45.

Feigelman, W. (2000). Adjustment of transracially and inracially adopted young adults. *Child and Adolescent Social Work*, *17*, 165–183.

Fisher, L., Ames, E. W., Chisholm, K., & Savoie, L. (1997). Problems reported by parents of Romanian orphans adopted to British Columbia. *International Journal of Behavioral Development*, 20, 67–82.

Fravel, D. L., McRoy, R. G., & Grotevant, H. D. (2000). Birthmother perceptions of the psychologically present adopted child: Adoption openness and boundary ambiguity. *Family Relations*, *49*, 425–433.

Freundlich, M. (2002). Adoption research: An assessment of empirical contributions to the advancement of adoption practice. *Journal of Social Distress and the Homeless*, *11*, 143–166.

Gladstone, J., & Westhues, A. (1998). Adopted reunions: A new side to intergenerational family relationships. *Family Relations. Interdisciplinary Journal of Applied Family Studies*, *47*, 177–184.

Glidden, L. M. (1991). Adopted children with developmental disabilities: Post-placement family functioning. *Children and Youth Services Review*, *13*, 363–377.

Golombok, S. (2006). New family forms. In A. Clarke-Stewart, & J. Dunn (Eds.), *Families Count: Effects on child and adolescent development* (pp. 273–298). Cambridge: Cambridge University Press.

Golombok, S., & MacCallum, F. (2003). Practitioner review. Outcomes for parents and children following non-traditional conception: what do clinicians need to know? *Journal of Child Psychology and Psychiatry*, *44*, 303–315.

Groark, C. J., Muhamedrahimov, R. J., Palmov, O. I., Nikiforova, N. V., & McCall, R. B. (2005). Improvements in early care in Russian orphanages and their relationship to observed behaviors. *Infant Mental Health Journal*, *26*, 96–109.

Grotevant, H. D. (2000). Openness in adoption: Research with the adoption kinship network. *Adoption Quarterly*, *4*, 45–65.

Grotevant, H. D., Dunbar, N., Kohler, J. K., & Esau, A. L. (2000). Adoptive identity: How contexts within and beyond the family shape developmental pathways. *Family Relations*, *49*, 379–387.

Grotevant, H. D., & McRoy, R. G. (1997). The Minnesota/Texas adoption research project: Implications of openness in adoption for development and relationships. *Applied Developmental Science*, *1*, 168–186.

Grotevant, H. D., van Dulmen, M. H., Dunbar, N., Nelson-Christinedaughter, J., Christensen, M., Fan, X., *et al.* (2006). Antisocial behavior of adoptees and nonadoptees: Prediction from early history and adolescent relationships. *Journal of Research on Adolescence*, *16*, 105–131.

Groze, V., & Ileana, D. (1996). A follow-up study of adopted children from Romania. *Child and Adolescent Social Work Journal*, *13*, 541–565.

Gunnar, M. R., Bruce, J., & Grotevant, H. D. (2000). International adoption of institutionally reared children: Research and policy. *Development and Psychopathology*, *12*, 677–693.

Hansen, M., Bower, C., Milne, E., de Klerk, N., & Kurinczuk, J. J. (2005). Assisted reproductive technologies and the risk of birth defects: A systematic review. *Human Reproduction*, *20*, 328–338.

Haugaard, J. J. (1998). Is adoption a risk factor for the development of adjustment problems? *Clinical Psychology Review*, *18*, 47–69.

Henney, S., McRoy, R. G., Ayers-Lopez, S., & Grotevant, H. D. (2003). The impact of openness on adoption agency practices: A longitudinal perspective. *Adoption Quarterly*, *6*, 31–51.

Hjern, A., Lindblad, F., & Vinnerljung, B. (2002). Suicide, psychiatric illness, and social maladjustment in intercountry adoptees in Sweden: A cohort study. *Lancet*, *360*, 443–448.

Hodges, J., Steele, M., Hillman, S., Henderson, K., & Kaniuk, J. (2003). Changes in attachment representations over the first year of adoptive placement: Narratives of maltreated children. *Clinical Child Psychology and Psychiatry*, *8*, 351–367.

Hodges, J., & Tizard, B. (1989). Social and family relationships of ex-institutional adolescents. *Journal of Child Psychology and Psychiatry*, *30*, 77–97.

Hoksbergen, R., Rijk, K., van Dijkum, C., & ter Laak, J. (2004). Adoption of Romanian children in the Netherlands: Behavior problems and parenting burden of upbringing for adoptive parents. *Developmental and Behavioral Pediatrics*, *25*, 175–180.

Horowitz, R. M., & Maruyama, H. (1995). Legal issues: In A. Sullivan (Ed.), *Proceedings of the Fourth annual Peirce-Warwick Adoption Symposium* (pp. 11–21). Washington, DC: Child Welfare League of America.

Howe, D. (1996). Adopters' relationships with their adopted children from adolescence to early adulthood. *Adoption and Fostering*, *20*, 35–43.

Howe, D. (1997). Parent-reported problems in 211 adopted children: Some risk and protective factors. *Journal of Child Psychology and Psychiatry*, *38*, 401–411.

Howe, D., & Fearnley, S. (2003). Disorders of attachment in adopted and fostered children: Recognition and treatment. *Clinical Child Psychology and Psychiatry*, *8*, 369–387.

Howe, D., & Feast, J. (2000). *Adoption, search and reunion: The long term experience of adopted adults*. London: The Children's Society.

Howe, D., & Feast, J. (2001). The long-term outcome of reunions between adult adopted people and their birth mothers. *British Journal of Social Work*, *31*, 351–368.

Hughes, D. A. (1999). Adopting children with attachment problems. *Child Welfare*, *78*, 541–560.

Jaffee, S. R., Moffitt, T. E., Caspi, A., & Taylor, A. (2003). Life with (or without) father: The benefits of living with two biological parents depend on the father's antisocial behavior. *Child Development*, *74*, 109–126.

Johnson, D. E. (2000). Long-term medical issues in international adoptees [Special issue]. *Pediatric Annals*, *29*, 234–241.

Johnson, D. E. (2002). Adoption and the effect on children's development. *Early Human Development*, *68*, 39–54.

Johnson, D. E., & Dole, K. (1999). International adoptions: Implications for early intervention. *Infants and Young Children*, *11*, 34–44.

Judge, S. (2004). Adoptive families: The effects of early relational deprivation in children adopted from Eastern European orphanages. *Journal of Family Nursing*, *10*, 338–356.

Juffer, F., Bakermans-Kranenburg, M. J., & van IJzendoorn, M. H. (2005). The importance of parenting in the development of disorganized attachment: Evidence from a preventive intervention study in adoptive families. *Journal of Child Psychology and Psychiatry*, *46*, 263–274.

Juffer, F., Hoksbergen, R. A. C., Riksen-Walraven, J. M., & Kohnstamm, G. A. (1997). Early intervention in adoptive families: Supporting maternal sensitive responsiveness, infant–mother attachment and infant competence. *Journal of Child Psychology and Psychiatry*, *38*, 1039–1050.

Juffer, F., & Rosenboom, L. G. (1997). Infant–mother attachment of internationally adopted children in the Netherlands. *International Journal of Behavioral Development*, *20*, 93–107.

Juffer, F., Stams, G-J. J. M., & van IJzendoorn, M. H. (2004). Adopted children's problem behavior is significantly related to their ego resiliency, ego control, and sociometric status. *Journal of Child Psychology and Psychiatry*, *45*, 697–706.

Juffer, F., & van IJzendoorn, M. H. (2005). Behavior problems and mental health referrals of international adoptees. A meta-analysis. *Journal of the American Medical Association*, *293*, 2501–2515.

Kreppner, J. M., O'Connor, T. G., Rutter, M., & the ERA Research Team. (2001). Can inattention/overactivity be an institutional deprivation syndrome? *Journal of Abnormal Child Psychology*, *29*, 513–528.

Kreppner, J. M., Rutter, M., Beckett, J., Castle, E., Colvert, C., Groothues, A., *et al.* (2007). Normality and impairment following profound early institutional deprevation: A longitudinal follow-up into early adolescence. *Developmental Psychology*, *43*, 931–946.

Lanyado, M. (2003). The emotional tasks of moving from fostering to adoption: Transitions, attachment, separation and loss. *Clinical Child Psychology and Psychiatry*, *8*, 337–349.

Lee, R. M. (2003). The transracial adoption paradox: History, research and counseling implications of cultural socialization. *Counseling Psychologist*, *31*, 711–744.

LeMare, L. (2004). Development of children adopted to Canada from Romanian orphanages ten years later. Paper presented to the Intercountry Adoption Policy Roundtable, organized by Intercountry Adoption Services, Social Development Canada.

Leon, I. G. (2002). Adoption losses: Naturally occurring socially or constructed? *Child Development*, *73*, 652–653.

Lieberman, A. F. (2003). The treatment of attachment disorder in infancy and early childhood: Reflections from clinical intervention with later-adopted foster care children. *Attachment and Human Development*, *5*, 279–282.

Lieberman, A. F., Silverman, R., & Pawl, J. (2000). Infant–parent psychotherapy: Core concepts and current approaches. In C. H. Zeanah (Ed.), *Handbook of infant mental health* (pp. 472–485). New York: Basic Books.

MacLean, K. (2003). The impact of institutionalization on child development. *Development and Psychopathology*, *15*, 853–884.

Marcovitch, S., Goldberg, S., Gold, A., Washington, J., Wasson, C., Krekewich, K., *et al.* (1997). Determinants of behavioral problems in Romanian children adopted in Ontario. *International Journal of Behavioral Development*, *20*, 17–31.

Mason, P., & Narad, C. (2005). International adoption: A health and developmental prospective. *Seminars in Speech and Language*, *26*, 1–9.

Masten, A. S. (2001). Ordinary magic: Resilience processes in development. *American Psychologist*, *56*, 227–238.

Maynard, J. (2005). Permanency mediation: A path to open adoption for children in out-of-home care. *Child Welfare*, *84*, 507–526.

Mendenhall, T. J., Berge, J. M., Wrobel, G. M., Grotevant, H. D., & McRoy, R. G. (2004). Adolescents' satisfaction with contact in adoption. *Child and Adolescent Social Work Journal*, *21*, 175–190.

Miller, L. C., & Hendrie, N. W. (2000). Health of children adopted from China. *Pediatrics*, *105*, 1–6.

Moe, V. (2000). Foster-placed and adopted children exposed *in utero* to opiates and other substances: Prediction and outcomes at four and a half years. *Journal of Developmental and Behavioral Pediatrics*, *24*, 330–339.

Neil, E., Beek, M., & Schofield, G. (2003). Thinking about and managing contacts in permanent placements: The differences and similarities between adoptive parents and foster care. *Clinical Child Psychology and Psychiatry*, *8*, 401–418.

Nickman, S. L., & Lewis, R. G. (1994). Adoptive families and professionals: When the experts make things worse. *Journal of the American Academy of Child and Adolescent Psychiatry*, *33*, 753–755.

Nickman, S. L., Rosenfeld, A. A., Fine, P., MacIntyre, J. C., Pilowsky, D. J., Howe, R. A., *et al.* (2005). Children in adoptive families: Overview and update. *Journal of the American Academy of Child and Adolescent Psychiatry*, *44*, 987–995.

O'Brien, P., Massat, C. R., & Gleeson, J. P. (2001). Upping the ante: Relative caregivers' perceptions of changes in child welfare policies. *Child Welfare*, *80*, 719–748.

O'Connor, T. G., Deater-Deckard, K., Fulker, D., Rutter, M., & Plomin, R. (1998). Genotype–environment correlations in late childhood and early adolescence: Antisocial behavioral problems and coercive parenting. *Developmental Psychology*, *34*, 970–981.

O'Connor, T. G., Marvin, R. S., Rutter, M., Olrick, J. T., Britner, P. A., & the English and Romanian Adoptees Study Team. (2003). Child–parent attachment following early institutional deprivation. *Developmental Psychopathology*, *15*, 19–38.

O'Connor, T., & Zeanah, C. (2003). Attachment disorders: Assessment strategies and treatment approaches. *Attachment and Human Development*, *5*, 223–244.

Palacios, J., & Sanchez-Sandoval, Y. (2005). Beyond adopted/nonadpted comparisons. In D. M. Brodzinsky, & J. Palacios (Eds.), *Psychological issues in adoption: Theory, research and application* (pp. 117–144). Westport, CT: Praeger.

Patterson, C. J. (2002). Lesbian and gay parenthood. In M. Bornstein (Ed.), *Handbook of parenting*. Vol. 3. *Being and becoming a parent* (2nd edn., pp. 317–338). Hillsdale, NJ: Lawrence Erlbaum Associates.

Peters, B. R., Atkins, M. S., Marc, S., & McKay, M. M. (1999). Adopted children's behavior problems: A review of five explanatory models. *Clinical Psychology Review*, *19*, 297–328.

Pinderhughes, E. E. (1996). Toward understanding family readjustment following older child adoptions: The interplay between theory generation and empirical research. *Children and Youth Services Review*, *18*, 115–138.

Pomerleau, A., Malcuit, G., Chicoine, J.-F., Seguin, R., Belhumeur, C., Germain, P., *et al.* (2005). Health status, cognitive and motor development of young children adopted from China, East Asia and Russia across the first six months after adoption. *Journal of Applied Developmental Psychology*, *29*, 445–457.

Pugliese, M. (2006). Becoming attached: The emerging attachment relationship between newly adopted previously institutionalized Chinese infant girls and their adoptive mothers. Unpublished Doctoral Dissertation, University of Toronto, Toronto, Canada.

Rushton, A. (2004). A scoping and scanning review of research on the adoption of children placed from public care. *Clinical Child Psychology and Psychiatry*, *9*, 89–106.

Rushton, A., & Dance, C. (2003). Preferentially rejected children and their development in permanent family placements. *Child and Family Social Work*, *8*, 257–267.

Rushton, A., & Dance, C. (2006). The adoption of children from public care: A prospective study of outcome in adolescence. *Journal of the American Academy of Child and Adolescent Psychiatry*, *45*, 877–883.

Rushton, A., Dance, C., & Quinton, D. (2000). Findings from a UK based study of late permanent placements. *Adoption Quarterly*, *3*, 51–72.

Rushton, A., & Mayes, D. (1997). Forming fresh attachments in childhood: A research update. *Child and Family Social Work*, *2*, 121–127.

Rushton, A., Mayes, D., Dance, C., & Quinton, D. (2003). Parenting late-placed children: The development of new relationships and the challenge of behavioral problems. *Clinical Child Psychology and Psychiatry*, *8*, 389–400.

Rushton, A., Monck, E., Upright, H., & Davidson, M. (2006). Enhancing adoptive parenting: Devising promising interventions. *Child and Adolescent Mental Health*, *11*, 25–31.

Rutter, M. (2005). Adverse preadoption experiences and psychological outcomes. In D. M. Brodzinsky, & J. Palacios (Eds.), *Psychological issues in adoption: Research and Practice* (pp. 67–92). Westport, CT: Praeger.

Rutter, M., Anderson-Wood, L., Beckett, C., Bredenkamp, D., Castle, J., Groothues, C., *et al.* (1999). Quasi-autistic patterns following severe early global privation. *Journal of Child Psychology and Psychiatry*, *40*, 537–549.

Rutter, M., Colvert, E., Kreppner, J., Beckett, C., Castle, J., Groothues, C., *et al.* (2007). Early adolescent outcomes for institutionally deprived and non-deprived adoptees. I. Disinhibited attachment. *Journal of Child Psychology and Psychiatry*, *48*, 17–30.

Rutter, M., Kreppner, J., Croft, C., Murin, M., Colvert, E., Beckett, C., *et al.* (2007). Early adolescent outcomes of institutionally deprived and non-deprived adoptees. III. Quasi-autism. *Journal of Child Psychology and Psychiatry*, *48*, 1200–1207.

Rutter, M., O'Connor, T., and the English and Romania Adoptees Study Team. (2004). Are there biological programming effects for psychological development: Findings from a study of Romanian adoptees. *Developmental Psychology*, *40*, 81–94.

Scarr, S., & McCartney, K. (1983). How people make their own environments: A theory of genotype → environments effects. *Child Development*, *54*, 424–435.

Scheib, J. E., Kristiansen, A., & Wara, A. (1997). A Norwegian note on sperm donor selection and the psychology of female mate choice. *Evolution and Human Behavior*, *18*, 143–149.

Selman, P. (2002). Intercountry adoption in the new millennium; the "quiet migration" revisited. *Population Research Policy Review*, *21*, 205–225.

Shapiro, V. B., Shapiro, J. R., & Paret, I. (Eds.). (2001). *Complex adoption and assisted reproductive technology: A developmental approach to clinical practice*. New York: Guilford Press.

Shireman, J. (1996). Single parent adoptive homes. *Child and Youth Services Review*, *18*, 23–36.

Simmel, C., Brooks, D., Barth, R. P., & Hinshaw, S. P. (2001). Externalizing symptomatology among adoptive youth: Prevalence and preadoption risk factors. *Journal of Abnormal Child Psychology*, *29*, 57–71.

Singer, M. L., Brodzinsky, D. M., Ramsay, D., Steir, M., & Waters, E. (1985). Mother–infant attachment in adoptive families. *Child Development*, *56*, 1543–1551.

Smith, D. W., & Brodzinsky, D. M. (2002). Coping with birth-parent loss in adopted children. *Journal of Child Psychology and Psychiatry*, *43*, 213–223.

Stams, G-J. J. M., Juffer, F., & van IJzendoorn, M. H. (2002). Maternal sensitivity, infant attachment, and temperament in early childhood predict adjustment in middle childhood: The case of adopted children and their biologically unrelated parents. *Developmental Psychology*, *38*, 806–821.

Stams, G-J. J. M., Juffer, F., van IJzendoorn, M. H., & Hoksbergen, R. A. (2001). Attachment-based intervention in adoptive families in infancy and children's development at age 7: Two follow-up studies. *British Journal of Developmental Psychology*, *19*, 159–180.

Steele, M., Hodges, J., Kaniuk, J., Hillman, S., & Henderson, K. (2003). Attachment representation and adoption: Associations between maternal states of mind and emotion narratives in previously maltreated children. *Journal of Child Psychotherapy*, *29*, 187–205.

Stovall, K. C., & Dozier, M. (1998). Infants in foster care: An attachment theory perspective. *Adoption Quarterly*, *2*, 55–58.

Sullivan, R., & Lathrop, E. (2004). Openness in adoption: Retrospective lessons and prospective choices. *Children and Youth Services*, *26*, 393–411.

Tasker, F. L., & Golombok, S. (1997). Adults raised as children in lesbian families. *American Journal of Orthopsychiatry*, *65*, 205–215.

Tieman, W., van der Ende, J., & Verhulst, F. C. (2005). Psychiatric disorders in young adult intercountry adoptees: An epidemiological study. *American Journal of Psychiatry*, *162*, 592–598.

Tizard, B., & Phoenix, A. (1995). The identity of mixed parentage adolescents. *Journal of Child Psychology and Psychiatry*, *36*, 1399–1410.

Triseliotis, J. (1991). Maintaining the links in adoption. *British Journal of Social Work*, *21*, 401–414.

Triseliotis, J., Feast, J., & Kyle, F. (2005). *The adoption triangle revisited: A study of adoption, search and reunion experiences.* London: British Association for Adoption & Fostering. (BAAF).

van IJzendoorn, M. H., Juffer, F., & Poelhuis, C. W. (2005). Adoption and cognitive development: A meta-analytic comparison of adopted and nonadopted children's IQ and school performance. *Psychological Bulletin*, *131*, 301–316.

Verhulst, F. C. (2000a). The development of internationally adopted children. In P. Selman (Ed.), *Intercountry adoption: Developments, trends and perspectives* (pp. 126–142). London: British Agencies for Adoption and Fostering.

Verhulst, F. C. (2000b). Internationally adopted children: The Dutch longitudinal adoption study. *Adoption Quarterly*, *4*, 27–44.

Webster-Stratton, C. (2005). The incredible years: A training series for the prevention and treatment of conduct problems in young children. In E. D. Hibbs, & P. Jensen (Eds.), *Psychosocial treatments for children and adolescent disorders: Empirically based strategies for clinical practice* (2nd edn., pp. 507–555). Washington, DC: American Psychological Association.

Weitzman, C. C. (2003). Developmental assessment of the international adopted child: Challenges and rewards. *Clinical Child Psychology and Psychiatry*, *8*, 303–313.

Wrobel, G. M., Grotevant, H. D., & McRoy, R. G. (2004). Adolescent search for birthparents: Who moves forward? *Journal of Adolescent Research*, *19*, 132–151.

Wrobel, G. M., Kohler, J. K., Grotevant, H. D., & McRoy, R. G. (2003). The family adoption communication (FAC) model: Identifying pathways of adoption-related communication. *Adoption Quarterly*, *7*, 53–83.

Yoon, D. P. (2001). Causal modeling predicting psychological adjustment of Korean-born adoptees. *Journal of Human Behavior in the Social Environment*, *3*, 65–82.

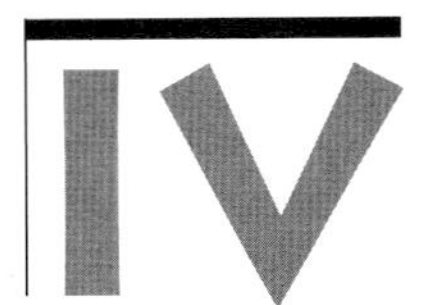

Clinical Syndromes

34 Disorders of Attention and Activity

Eric Taylor and Edmund Sonuga-Barke

Many children show a persistent style of behaving in an impulsive, inattentive and restless fashion. The style can endure for many years, but tends to manifest in somewhat different ways at different ages. When the behaviors are severe they carry considerable importance for clinicians; most importantly, because extreme levels put children at risk for later antisocial adjustment, educational failure and aspects of personality dysfunction in later adolescence and adult life. Impulsiveness, inattentiveness and restlessness can also be very unpleasant for the caregivers, and for this reason constitute some of the most common reasons for clinical referral during the school years.

This chapter treats these behaviors as a lifespan condition rather than one restricted to middle childhood and early adolescence.

Clinical Presentations

Inattentiveness refers to a style of behavior, involving disorganization and lack of persistence, rather than to the psychological processes that are indexed by tests of attention. The presentation is naturally in different forms at different ages, as summarized in Table 34.1, and the impact varies with the demands for attention that the environment makes. The behaviors can be seen by direct observation (at least in childhood) if the setting is appropriate (Taylor, 1998). Motivation improves attention, as for everybody else; and some children's activities (such as playing computer games with very frequent and insistent rewards) provide so many and so rapid incentives that they are not good ways of assessing function in the ordinary world. As people enter adult life, poor attention often becomes the most salient aspect of the condition (Kessler, Adler, Barkley *et al.*, 2006; Millstein, Wilens, Biederman *et al.*, 1998).

Overactivity refers simply to an excess of movements; it is often the most salient problem in early childhood but the least important in adult life. Its features are statistically closely allied to impulsiveness and they are often combined into one construct of "hyperactivity."

Impulsiveness means acting without reflecting. This is often the aspect that gets young people into trouble, or irritates other people. However, in early childhood, and to some extent later, these features of impulsiveness can be difficult to distinguish from other types of oppositional behavior. Lack of clarity about social rules or angry resistance to adults can be other causes of rule-breaking, so it is important, but often difficult, to go beyond the description of unacceptable conduct to determine whether thoughtless impulsiveness underlies it (see chapter 35).

Subjectively, adults often come to recognize these problems in themselves, and either describe themselves as confused or overreactive, with their thoughts in a whirl and their actions often half-considered and unwise. Children do not often do so, but some will describe the subjective difference when medication is effective, and say that they are now able to think things through more clearly without the intrusion of other thoughts. The subjective experience of children with hyperactivity is more often one of being unfairly punished or discriminated against: they experience the reactions of others to the condition rather than the condition itself.

Some degrees of inattentiveness, high activity and impulsiveness are of course shown by ordinary children. Diagnostic identification needs to be based on the extent, severity and consistency of the behaviors and on their impact on social adjustment. It is quite possible for inexperienced parents or teachers to regard ordinary childish high spirits as evidence of hyperactive behavior. The tolerance of parents varies a good deal, and in community surveys it, and the degree of financial loss suffered because of the child's problems, are strong predictors of which hyperactive children will be referred for professional attention (Sayal, Taylor, Beecham *et al.*, 2002).

Diagnostic Definitions

There are two main approaches to defining disorders of inattentiveness, hyperactivity and impulsiveness: DSM-IV-TR (American Psychiatric Association, 2000), which recognizes "Attention Deficit/Hyperactivity Disorder" (ADHD), and ICD-10 (World Health Organization, 1992), which uses the category of "Hyperkinetic Disorder." They are based on essentially the same descriptions of behavior, but weight the different items differently (Swanson, Sergeant, Taylor *et al.*, 1998). In brief, hyperkinetic disorder requires all three components to be present, while ADHD is divided into cases where this is so ("Combined type") and those where only inattentiveness, or only overactivity and impulsiveness, are present.

Rutter's Child and Adolescent Psychiatry, 5th edition. Edited by M. Rutter, D. Bishop, D. Pine, S. Scott, J. Stevenson, E. Taylor and A. Thapar. © 2008 Blackwell Publishing, ISBN: 978-1-4051-4549-7.

Table 34.1 Typical presentations at different ages.

	Preschool	Primary school	Adolescence	Adulthood
Inattentive	Short play sequences (<3 min); leaving activities incomplete; not listening	Brief activities (<10 min); premature changes of activity; forgetful; disorganized; distracted by environment	Persistence less than peers (<30 min); lack of focus on details of a task; poor planning ahead	Details not completed; appointments forgotten; lack of foresight
Overactive	"Whirlwind"	Restless when calm expected	Fidgety	Subjective sense of restlessness
Impulsive	Does not listen; no sense of danger (hard to distinguish from oppositionality)	Acting out of turn, interrupting other children and blurting out an answer; thoughtless rule-breaking; intrusions on peers; accidents	Poor self-control; reckless risk-taking	Motor and other accidents; premature and unwise decision-making; impatience

However, hyperkinetic disorder cannot be simply identified as the combined type of ADHD; the definition is even more exacting. The diagnostic criteria must be met in more than one situation (e.g., both home and school), while ADHD requires only that there should be some impairment in more than one setting. Hyperkinetic disorder is excluded by the presence of other disorders such as autism and anxiety states, while ADHD is only excluded if its signs are better explained by a coexistent disorder. Both schemes require that the level of behaviors should be out of keeping with the person's developmental age, and that they should be impairing to social adjustment.

The practical consequence of these differences in definitions is that the ICD-10 category of hyperkinetic disorder is a subgroup of ADHD (Santosh, Taylor, Swanson *et al.*, 2005). Evidence on which definition is more useful does not give clear answers. Researchers often do not make very clear distinctions. Indeed, research papers on ADHD very often require convergent identification by parents and schoolteachers, often focus on the combined type (or contain a predominance of combined type cases) and usually exclude cases with coexistent autism or affective disorders – although anxiety is not necessarily an exclusion. This not only achieves a refined phenotype of ADHD, but also entails that hyperkinetic disorder criteria are usually met. Much of the neurodevelopmental validation of ADHD, reviewed below, therefore leaves open the possibility that findings are confined to the hyperkinetic subgroup. When the hyperkinetic subgroup has been systematically compared with other forms of ADHD, it appears that it is particularly likely to be associated with a marked response to stimulant medication and a poor response to behavioral treatment alone (Santosh *et al.*, 2005), and a high clustering of other neurodevelopmental anomalies such as delays in language and motor development (Taylor, Sandberg, Thorley *et al.*, 1991). Some latent class analyses of family and twin data suggest that one of the classes that breed true is a severe and pervasive form of hyperactivity and inattentiveness (e.g., Rasmussen, Neuman, Heath *et al.*, 2004).

On the other hand, the genetic evidence of large twin studies has suggested that the degree of heritability is very similar at all levels of hyperactive behavior (Gjone, Stevenson, & Sundet, 1996), so that genetic findings would validate a dimension of hyperactivity rather than either diagnostic category. No separate etiological pathway has yet been established at any level of severity. Membership of the hyperkinetic disorder subtype does not seem to determine the course over time: persistence is not greater than in a wider ADHD phenotype (Lahey, Pelham, Chronis *et al.*, 2006). Responsiveness to stimulant medication is not confined to a subgroup (although it differs in degree); indeed, ordinary people without ADHD show some enhancement in attention when they receive stimulants (Elliot, Sahakian, Matthews *et al.*, 1997; Mehta, Owen, Sahakian *et al.*, 2000; Rapoport, Buchsbaum, Weingartner *et al.*, 1980).

Clinicians may find it useful to use the concepts of both schemes, recognizing their strengths and weaknesses. A broad notion of ADHD is helpful in the screening and initial detection of cases, and marks a group at risk. However, it may encourage an inappropriately wide identification of cases, and blur some important differences of presentation within the category. The narrower concept of hyperkinetic disorder may mark a group where medication is particularly useful and neurobiological changes particularly relevant, but if it were the only category it would exclude children in need of intervention. Furthermore, the exclusion criteria in ICD-10 would, if applied too literally, rule out the diagnosis for children who deserve it in all respects except that they have other problems too.

Subtypes of Disorder

Apart from the distinction between "broad" ADHD and "narrow" hyperkinetic disorder, other subtypes have been suggested within the broad grouping of ADHD, even though current scientific evidence does not allow for clear conclusions about whether biologically valid subtypes are present or whether the clinical heterogeneity should be conceptualized as variation of expression within a single broader disorder.

Attention deficit without hyperactivity can be identified as a separate group in community surveys (Taylor *et al.*, 1991). It is not often seen in psychiatric clinics, but often presents as a failure of academic progress. Children are not disruptive or overactive; they may be dreamy and even somewhat inert, but they are often muddled and disorganized in the classroom and find it hard to persist. Cognitive deficits are usually present, but they are both wider and less specific than in children who also show impulsiveness. They include working memory problems, poor spatial skills and delays of language development; motor coordination is often poor; and the IQ is often lowered (Warner-Rogers, Taylor, Taylor *et al.*, 2000; Weiss, Worling, & Wasdell, 2003).

Evidence on the scientific validity of the inattentive subtype is inconclusive so far. On the one hand, it has emerged from some latent class analyses as a distinct group (Todd, Sitdhiraksa, Reich *et al.*, 2002); Stawicki, Nigg, & von Eye (2006) have provided a meta-analysis of six studies that included informative family history information, with the conclusion that there is indeed evidence for specific subtype transmission in families. On the other hand, Geurts, Verte, Oosterlaan *et al.* (2005) argued against the validity of an inattentive subtype on the basis that executive dysfunction was similarly impaired in that and the combined subtype. Perhaps one should conclude that inattentiveness is a separable component from hyperactivity-impulsivity, and that it is responsible for much of the cognitive impairment (but little of the oppositionality) of the combined subtype. The DSM-IV definition may be responsible for some confusion: the inattentive subtype (ADHD-I) requires only that the diagnostic criteria for hyperactivity-impulsivity are not met, so many apparent cases of ADHD-I may be better considered as showing mild ADHD-C. Furthermore, the behavioral descriptions of inattentiveness are not necessarily factorially pure; they include descriptions, such as failing to follow through on instructions that are very easy to confuse with non-compliance.

For clinical practice we suggest that "pure" inattentiveness deserves recognition, and distinction from other subtypes. It is particularly important to detect whether the inattentive behaviors are secondary to intellectual disability or specific academic disability; and to expect the absence of hyperactive-impulsive behaviors and not just a subdiagnostic level. The risk it carries is for educational and occupational underachievement rather than for psychiatric disorders.

An overactive/impulsive type without inattention has been harder to identify, and is decidedly uncommon in clinical series. In epidemiological studies it is probably less common than the other forms of ADHD (Taylor *et al.*, 1991). It can be hard to distinguish from oppositional disorder. A recent population survey of teacher ratings of children did not identify an attentive-but-hyperactive subgroup (de Nijs, Ferdinand, & Verhulst, 2007); and indeed it is ordinarily a feature of parental rather than teacher descriptions. In our developmental perspective, it is consistent with a notion that the relevant problems in the first 3 years of life are a rather diffuse set of difficulties in emotional, cognitive and behavioral self-regulation, and that at school entry the attentional component becomes particularly significant because of the scholastic difficulties it brings (see p. 532). In this account, a subtype without inattentiveness persists in problems at home rather than at school.

Situationality (i.e., children whose hyperactivity presents only at home or only at school) may also be worth distinguishing. Some evidence from twin studies suggests that this is not caused only by misidentification by one or the other party, but that to some extent there may be different genetic influences on behavior in the two settings (Nadder, Rutter, Silberg *et al.*, 2002). Ho, Luk, Leung *et al.* (1996) surveyed a Chinese school population in Hong Kong with parent and teacher questionnaires, and selected those who showed hyperactive behavior at home only, at school only, or pervasively across both situations. The home-specific group showed less evidence of cognitive problems and more evidence of family conflict and adversity; perhaps they reacted with misbehavior that in turn was poorly controlled. The school-specific group showed more evidence of academic learning difficulties; perhaps some of their off-task behavior was a result of inability to cope with the lessons. In keeping with this, a cluster analytic study of subgroups in a clinically referred population in the UK found that the behavior problems in a school-situational group tended to appear later, only after school entry (Taylor, Everitt, Thorley *et al.*, 1986).

The diagnostic and assessment work should not stop at the point where ADHD is recognized, but go on to a wider range of strengths and weaknesses.

Overactivity with stereotyped movements is a rather different pattern seen in clinical practice, especially in young people with severe intellectual disability. The activity can be extreme, but its repetitive quality distinguishes it from the disorganized and unpredictable activity of ADHD. ICD-10 recognizes it as a distinct category – "Overactive disorder associated with intellectual disability and stereotyped movements" – and places it as a type of pervasive developmental disorder, distinct from autism. The ICD-10 description includes the comment that stimulant medication is often unhelpful.

Such a disorder has not been validated – in fact, the idea has led to virtually no research. A key question is whether it is useful to separate it from autism and other brain disorders. Several predictions could test this: the pattern of activity and attention will not be the same as that of ADHD when it coexists with autism (see p. 524); it will not be brought about only by akithisia and dyskinesias caused by neuroleptic medication; it will be a persistent trait (rather than the episodes of catatonic overactivity sometimes seen in complex brain disorders); and it will not be accompanied by the characteristic social impairments of autism. All these can be tested; in the meantime the concept is of uncertain validity.

There are two useful current implications: the first is to emphasize a subgroup of overactive and handicapped children whose condition may actually be worsened by stimulants. The second is more theoretical: the idea relates to a distinction that can be made in animal experiments between hyper- and hypodopaminergic states. Some experiments can cause reduced dopamine transport activity in the brains of animals such as mice, and these lead to overactivity and changes in learning (Gainetdinov, Wetsel, Jones *et al.*, 1999). Some forms of environmental stress on animals can also lead to overactivity and cognitive alterations, and these are mediated by excess of dopamine (Arnsten & Goldman-Rakic, 1998). These states are probably not identical to that of the overactivity associated with hypodopaminergic states (see p. 529): they are often accompanied by stereotypic behaviors, made worse by novelty and improved by serotonin reuptake inhibitors or dopamine blockers rather than by stimulants (Gainetdinov *et al.*, 1999). It is not impossible that such a heterogeneity might exist also in humans.

Coexistent Disorders

Clinical cases are often dominated by the coexistence of other problems alongside ADHD. The reasons for these associations need to be understood in the formulation of individual cases. There are three main sorts of associated psychiatric condition: neurodevelopmental disorders, disorders of childhood onset and adult type mental illnesses.

Neurodevelopmental Disorders

ADHD behaves in many ways like other neurodevelopmental disorders (see chapter 49). The male sex predominance, the course of persisting disability, research findings about altered brain structure and function, and associations with motor and language delays all parallel the findings in other conditions such as autism and other pervasive developmental disorders, learning disability, and Tourette disorder. Each of these conditions raises the probability of others being found in the same person. The likely reasons are that enhanced assessment leads to the discovery of other conditions, that the risk factors overlap and are of diffuse effect upon brain development and that the associated conditions all represent different aspects of neurological compromise with a range of expression.

In the case of *autism and allied disorders*, there is a clear clinical distinction to be made, and ADHD does not by itself produce the characteristic behaviors of autism (see chapter 46). The brain changes and neuropsychological alterations of autism are so different from those of ADHD that it seems unhelpful to regard them as a single condition. The small size of the brain in hyperkinetic disorder contrasts with the increased size in some cases of autism; the family histories do not overlap much; at the neuropsychological level both show difficulties in executive function, but inhibitory dysfunction is characteristic of ADHD while the more autistic problems of central coherence and theory of mind deficits are not (Banaschewski, Hollis, Oosterlaan *et al.*, 2005). The comorbid state tends to have the associations of both conditions. It seems likely therefore that the two disorders are independent but often associated.

It is too soon to be clear about genetic similarities or differences. It is noteworthy that genome scans for autism and those for ADHD have both identified chromosomal loci that appear to be similar (Faraone, Perlis, Doyle *et al.*, 2005). It is possible that there will prove to be both genetic influences of general effect, acting as susceptibility for a range of neurodevelopmental problems, and others of more specific influence on individual disorders. At present, however, the results of molecular mapping of the chromosomes are too unstable for firm conclusions to be drawn. Some conditions known to have diffuse brain effects – notably congenital rubella and tuberous sclerosis – also raise the probability of showing both hyperkinetic disorder and autism.

It is sometimes possible for autism and hyperactivity to be associated in a different way: autism can produce a different sort of motor restlessness, to be distinguished from ADHD by its stereotyped nature and the perseveration upon idiosyncratic concerns. The distinction is made by the type of overactivity, which contrasts with the impulsive and frequently changing behaviors seen in hyperkinetic disorder. Conversely, children with ADHD may become very unpopular. Their social isolation and unreserved approaches to other children can then be mistaken for the social obliviousness of young people in the spectrum of autism. These conditions can often be distinguished on the basis of: (i) the presence of good social understanding that is shown by children with ADHD only, when they are given time to reflect about their social relationships; and (ii) direct observation of children interacting with their peers for the nature of the difficulties that they are showing.

When both problems are present together, detailed assessment is often needed. Sometimes the specific features of autism can be masked by the chaotic presentation of ADHD, so persistent observation over time is needed and the diagnosis should be reviewed when overactivity and impulsiveness have been reduced (e.g., by medication). It can be important to recognize the presence of ADHD in children with autism, even though the diagnostic schemes of ICD-10 and DSM-IV regard them as exclusive categories. Stimulant medication can be valuable for the control of overactive impulsiveness even in people who have clear autistic syndromes (Aman, Smedt, Derivan *et al.*, 2002; Research Units on Pediatric Psychopharmacology Autism Network, 2005).

Intellectual disability can also both simulate and coexist with hyperactive syndromes (Willcutt, Pennington, & DeFries, 2000). For this reason, assessment of generalized and specific learning difficulties should be included in the evaluation of children presenting with hyperactivity and inattention syndromes. Attention problems can be secondary to cognitive impairment, and this may contribute to the finding of a late-onset and school-specific version in some cases (see p. 523). Problems in learning, however, can be secondary to poor attention and it is wise to re-evaluate the severity of academic difficulties after medication has been given. The widespread difficulties of children with intellectual disability (see chapter 49) usually include poor concentration, but it is only sensible to make the additional diagnosis of ADHD when the impairment of attention and activity control is out of proportion to developmental level. The way to allow for developmental delay has not been rigorously established, and it would be helpful to develop norms for different levels of disability. Until that is done, a useful clinical rule of thumb is to judge the patient's attentiveness with reference to that which would be expected in a child of chronological age equivalent to the patient's mental age.

Tourette disorder can either simulate ADHD or be an association of it. Evidence at this time is not conclusive about the reasons for the association of the two disorders. Some analyses of whether other family members are affected have indicated that the two are unlikely to be related genetically (Pauls, Hurst, Kruger *et al.*, 1986), others that there is a genetic link (Comings, 2001). Occasionally, the presentation of overactivity proves on close analysis to be attributable to a large quantity of different tics, making it difficult to appreciate the repetitiveness involved unless and until prolonged observation is undertaken, perhaps with videotaping for detailed analysis. More commonly, ADHD and Tourette symptoms pursue different courses in the same individual, with the waxing and waning of tics being in some contrast to the persisting difficulties imposed by the ADHD. Stimulants will sometimes (but not necessarily) make the tics worse and improve the ADHD. Careful delineation of the target problems in the individual child and monitoring of treatment effects are then required.

Associations with Childhood Onset Problems

The most common overlap of symptomatology is between ADHD and *oppositional/defiant* or *conduct disorders*. Statistical analysis of symptoms, such as the latent dimension modeling by Ferguson and Horwood (1995), have suggested that they can be seen as independent dimensions, but that they are highly intercorrelated. A major diagnostic trap is to regard ADHD as present when the evidence is only that of oppositional misbehavior. It is also possible to make the opposite error and attribute uncontrolled and impulsive behavior to deliberate defiance. There is considerable scope for misunderstanding among parents, teachers and health professionals.

In general, studies of children with both hyperactive and defiant behavior have suggested that they show the associations of both conditions. Associations with other neurodevelopmental delays are present as strongly in the combined group as in those with hyperactivity alone; indeed, family histories may be even more likely in the comorbid group (Thapar, Harrington, & McGuffin, 2001). The group with both problems is also more likely than those with ADHD alone to show adverse factors in family life, including high levels of critical expressed emotion (Taylor *et al.*, 1991). Cross-twin cross-trait analyses have suggested that a good deal of the genetic influence on oppositional and conduct disorders is the same as that influencing hyperactivity. When both problems are present, the history usually suggests that hyperactivity came first; and follow-up of community ascertained children who showed hyperactivity but not oppositionality indicated that oppositionality could develop in people who had originally shown hyperactivity only, but that the reverse pathway was uncommon and that children with oppositional disorders did not develop hyperactivity later (Taylor, Chadwick, Heptinstall *et al.*, 1996). The drug treatment of hyperactivity is no less effective in those who have conduct problems too than in those who do not (MTA Cooperative Group, 1999).

Putting all these sources of evidence together, the suggestion is that hyperactivity represents either a risk factor for later oppositional and conduct disorders, or that it is an early-onset form of conduct problem, with the longitudinal evidence favoring the former hypothesis. The clinical implications are important; it is worth detecting and treating hyperactivity even before conduct problems have appeared. When conduct problems do appear, the most useful diagnostic approach is not whether they or hyperactivity predominate in the picture, but whether hyperactivity and inattention are in fact present – in which case a mixed disorder is recognized.

There is also an association with *anxiety disorders*: about 25% of children with ADHD also have an anxiety disorder (Pliszka, 2000). These cases may represent a separate condition, as implied by the ICD-10 rules in which anxiety excludes the diagnosis of hyperkinetic disorder; may represent an independent problem, as in DSM-IV's conceptualization of multiple diagnoses; or could represent a developmental change in which some children with ADHD are at risk for the development of anxiety as a complication. Research has not yet distinguished these possibilities securely.

Adult Type Mental Disorders

In adolescence and adult life, ADHD starts to show an association with other diagnoses that are seldom made in childhood. Adolescent *substance misuse*, in particular, seems to be much more common in people with the diagnosis of ADHD (Wilens, Faraone, Biederman *et al.*, 2003), although it is not yet clear whether it is the ADHD per se that generates the risk or the coexistent presence of antisocial activities and peer groups. ADHD is common in personality-disordered offenders (Young, Gudjonsson, Ball *et al.*, 2003). Surveys in prison populations have suggested that many incarcerated young adults also show both previous histories and currently high levels of hyperactive behaviors (45% in a survey by Rosler, Retz, Retz-Junginger *et al.*, 2004).

It has become increasingly popular to diagnose *bipolar disorder*, even in prepubertal children (see chapter 38). Traditionally, the distinction has been fairly easy to make. Bipolar disorder has been associated with euphoria, grandiosity and a cycling course, with each episode lasting for at least several days. ADHD, by contrast, has been regarded as a persisting disability in which euphoria is not particularly a feature. The goal-directed overactivity of mania is usually seen as in some contrast with the disorganized and off-task activity of ADHD. However, there has been a broadening of the concept of bipolar disorder to include cases where the mood change is not euphoria but irritability, and where the cyclical nature consists of many changes within a single day. This leads to a very considerable similarity in formal definitions between this so-called ultradian version of bipolar disorder and ADHD. An unstable and overreactive mood is very common in ADHD, even though it is not part of the diagnostic definitions, and the development of an oppositional disorder, in which frequent tantrums are common, can be described as an "irritable" state and therefore contribute to a bipolar diagnosis. For this chapter, it is important chiefly to note that the assessment of ADHD needs to include the recognition of rapid and volatile mood changes when they are present, and that they sometimes deserve intervention in their own right and monitoring as an outcome measure. Many assessment measures, such as the Conners' scales, do indeed include such symptoms.

Possible associations with *schizophrenia* are raised because both groups can show erratic behavior and inattentiveness in childhood. Follow-up studies of ADHD into adult life (summarized below) have not shown an increased rate of psychosis, but the numbers involved have not yet been large enough to detect a modest increase in the rate. The clinical question sometimes arises of whether stimulant medication is unacceptably hazardous for the children of a schizophrenic parent. The strongest concern is usually to promote the best possible social adjustment for the child, so stimulants should not be ruled out lightly.

Etiology and Pathophysiology

A Complex and Multifaceted Condition

Metaphors are often used in science to communicate complex and subtle ideas with clarity, coherence and power (Bradie, 1999). There are three metaphors commonly used in relation to ADHD: a *genetic disorder* (Comings, Chen, Blum *et al.*, 2005), a *frontostriatal/executive dysfunction disorder* (Loge, Staton, & Beatty, 1990; Wasserstein & Lynn, 2001) and a *catecholamine disorder* (Levy & Swanson, 2001). In contrast to these simple metaphors, research suggests that ADHD is a heterogeneous and multifaceted condition involving interplay between diverse systems across multiple levels within the individual (Asherson, Kuntsi, & Taylor, 2005; Nigg, Willcutt, Doyle *et al.*, 2005). In what follows, to help convey this complexity and sharpen the focus, existing empirical evidence will be set against the three simple metaphors mentioned.

Is ADHD a Genetic Disorder?

Heritability

Genetic factors are clearly important in ADHD (Thapar, Harrington, & McGuffin, 2005a) but little is known about the mechanisms by which their influence is exerted (Asherson, Kuntsi, & Taylor, 2005). Family, adoption and twin studies suggest ADHD is familial and highly heritable (Rietveld, Hudziak, Bartels *et al.*, 2003). Parents and siblings of cases display up to an eight-fold increased risk for ADHD (Faraone & Biederman, 2000) and biological relatives are more at risk than adoptive family members (Sprich, Biederman, Crawford *et al.*, 2000). According to twin studies, ADHD is amongst the most heritable conditions with estimates between 60 and 90% (Thapar, Harrington, Ross *et al.*, 2000).

Specific Genes

Candidate gene studies have produced a number of replicated associations (Faraone *et al.*, 2005). The monoamines (especially dopamine, norepinephrine and serotonin) have been a major focus because of their hypothesized role in ADHD pathophysiology. In meta-analysis, significant pooled effects have been reported for three polymorphisms of dopamine genes; the D4 and D5 receptors (*DRD4* and *DRD5*) and the dopamine transporter (*DAT1*; e.g., Faraone *et al.*, 2005; Thapar, O'Donovan, & Owen, 2005a). Of these, the *DRD4* and *DAT1* are most likely to have functional significance. However, the *DAT1* association has been challenged in recent meta-analysis (Wohl, Purper-Ouakil, Mouren *et al.*, 2005). Given its claimed role in ADHD pathophysiology, it is surprising that there is as yet no evidence that norepinephrine gene variants are associated with ADHD (although it may be forthcoming). Based on animal knockout models, tests of potentially functional polymorphisms of the serotonin transporter and receptor genes (*SLC6A4* and *HTR1B*) suggest an association with ADHD (Faraone *et al.*, 2005). Genes coding for other neurotransmitter systems are actively being pursued.

Interpreting Genetic Effects

In contrast to the high heritability estimates, the effects of specific genes are small. When aggregated, they account for only a fraction of variance in symptom expression. How can this gap be explained? First, twin studies, although a potentially powerful tool for dissecting genetic and environmental effects, need to be interpreted with caution for a number of reasons, as they may overestimate genetic main effects (Rutter, 2002). For instance, heritability estimates subsume the effects of gene × environment interactions so that subtler environmental effects can be missed.

Second, it remains possible that a large number of genes, some of at least moderate effect, exist but have yet to be identified. The results from linkage studies, if further replicated, provide support for this although genes of major effect are unlikely (Arcos-Burgos, Castellanos, Pineda *et al.*, 2004; Bakker, van der Meulen, Buitelaar *et al.*, 2003; Hebebrand, Dempfle, Saar *et al.*, 2006; Smalley, Kustanovich, Minassian *et al.*, 2002).

Third, genes may interact with each other (Carrasco, Rothhammer, Moraga *et al.*, 2006) and with environmental risk factors (see below) to increase the risk of ADHD in a non-linear manner so that genes of small main effect have disproportionate power when acting together or with environmental factors (Rutter, Moffitt, & Caspi, 2006).

Fourth, ADHD may be an etiologically heterogeneous condition with different combinations of genes (and environments) producing ADHD in different groups of ADHD children (Buitelaar, 2005; Todd, 2000). To combat this, researchers are attempting to create genetically more homogenous groupings by partitioning heterogeneity using clinical phenotypes (Faraone, Chen, Warburton *et al.*, 1995) or by identifying pathophysiological intermediates that are more likely to be linked to specific genes than is the clinical disorder: so-called endophenotypes (Doyle, Faraone, Seidman *et al.*, 2005).

Candidate Environments

The growing realization of the limitations of the study of genes in isolation from environments has led to renewed interest in environmental risk in ADHD.

Prenatal Factors

Maternal lifestyle during pregnancy (e.g., smoking and drinking) has been linked to ADHD (Linnet, Dalsgaard, Obel *et al.*, 2003). The evidence is strongest for maternal smoking, for which a dose–response relationship with ADHD appears to exist (Thapar, Fowler, Rice *et al.*, 2003). The findings for alcohol consumption are less clear-cut if fetal alcohol syndrome is not implicated (Linnet *et al.*, 2003). Exposure to cocaine has a range of harmful effects *in utero*, of which an increased risk of ADHD might be one (Linares, Singer, Kirchner *et al.*, 2006). Maternal stress during pregnancy and associated oversecretion of cortisol have been implicated in ADHD (Kapoor, Dunn, Kostaki *et al.*, 2006; O'Connor, Heron, Golding *et al.*, 2003; Rodriguez & Bohlin, 2005). Exposure to medication (e.g., benzodiazepines; anticonvulsants) may represent a risk although these effects are difficult to disentangle from the effects of the maternal mental illness (Steinhausen, Losche, Koch *et al.*, 1994).

Perinatal Factors

Bhutta, Cleves, Casey *et al.* (2002) reported a two-fold increase in ADHD in children born with a very low birth weight; an effect possibly mediated by small and subtle lesions in fronto-striatal brain circuits (Carmody, Bendersky, Dunn *et al.*, 2006). ADHD children are more likely to have experienced pregnancy and birth complications (Ben Amor, Grizenko, Schwartz *et al.*, 2005) but these effects are difficult to disentangle from low birth weight and the increased risk that vulnerable children may be at for a difficult birth.

Postnatal Physical Factors

Social and biological factors appear to have a role in the postnatal period. The role of artificial food additives remains controversial but a randomized controlled trial (McCann, Barrett, Cooper *et al.*, 2007) showed important effects. Idiosyncratic allergies and intolerances of specific food stuffs are often identified by parents (Aardoom, Hirasing, Rona *et al.*, 1997), and a recent meta-analysis and a large well-designed trial both suggested small but significant effects in exclusion and challenge trials (Bateman, Warner, Hutchinson *et al.*, 2004; Schab & Trinh, 2004). Exposure to lead and related neurotoxins may be associated with a substantially increased risk of inattentive and hyperactive behavior – but these exposures are both linked to social disadvantage and cause other non-specific neurodevelopmental difficulties (Levitt, 1999). Animal models implicate exposure to insecticides, such as DDT, although a clinical link has yet to be confirmed (Mariussen & Fonnum, 2006). Suggestions of the role of dietary deficiencies (e.g., omega-3 fatty acids, Richardson & Montgomery, 2005; iron, Konofal, Lecendreux, Arnulf *et al.*, 2004) require further examination in large-scale trials.

Postnatal Social Environment

Chronic exposure to exceptional social environments early on during development can increase the risk for ADHD-like patterns. In the English and Romanian Adoptees study, for example, children who experienced extreme physical, cognitive and social deprivation in infancy were at an increased risk of pervasive and persistent overactivity and inattention (Kreppner, O'Connor, & Rutter, 2001; Stevens, Sonuga-Barke, Kreppner *et al.*, in press) despite being adopted into well-resourced and committed homes before the age of 4 years. Claims that parenting is implicated in the causes of ADHD are controversial. Whereas children suffering extreme neglect and abuse may be at increased risk for ADHD (Glod & Teicher, 1996), variation in parenting style within the normal range has been assumed not to play a part (but see Morrell & Murray, 2003). Child ADHD can evoke negative and hostile responses from parents (Seipp & Johnston, 2005), while parental characteristics (including adult ADHD symptoms) can moderate these responses and exacerbate co-ercive cycles (Murray & Johnston, 2006). However, the very limited evidence from good longitudinal studies does not support the idea that this increases the likelihood of ADHD onset or persistence; rather, it predicts the onset of later comorbid conduct disorder (Taylor, 1999) and depression (Ostrander & Herman, 2006). However, the fact that parent training can significantly reduce core ADHD symptoms in preschoolers highlights the potential power of the social environment to influence the course of ADHD (Sonuga-Barke, Daley, Thompson *et al.*, 2001).

Interpreting Environmental Effects

As with genetic effects, the literature suggests a role for multiple environmental influences of small effect. However, one must be cautious when interpreting these findings because specific environmental risks are embedded in a network of other factors relating to lifestyle, social class/economic adversity and maternal personality (Taylor & Warner Rogers, 2005). Furthermore, interpreting these associations is complicated by the fact that environmental risks may be markers of genetic risk (Dick, Viken, Kaprio *et al.*, 2005). These sorts of effects can be because environments experienced by the child are correlated with genes shared with parents (passive gene–environment correlation; Kendler & Baker, 2007). Knopik, Heath, Jacob *et al.* (2006) found evidence in support of this by exploring levels of ADHD in the children of identical twins with or without a history of alcohol abuse: ADHD was common both in the children of twins with a history of alcohol abuse and of the monozygotic cotwins who had no such history themselves. Environmental associations could also be evoked by genetically based characteristics in the child – as when ADHD symptoms elicit maternal hostility (active gene–environment correlations). Although these gene–environment correlations are assumed to exist and account for a proportion of environmental risk in ADHD, little evidence exists for their role.

Because of the limited size of effects of genes and environments when each is considered in isolation, attention has turned to gene–environment interactions. A gene–environment interaction occurs when the phenotypic effects of a gene vary as a function of the physical or social environment (Caspi, Sugden, Moffitt *et al.*, 2003) and the two risks are combined in a nonlinear way to account for a disproportionate amount of variance in ADHD. Gene–environment interactions have been reported for ADHD involving both maternal smoking (Kahn, Khoury, Nichols *et al.*, 2003) and alcohol consumption during pregnancy (Brookes, Mill, Guindalini *et al.*, 2006) and *DAT1* as well as for *DRD4* and season of birth (Seeger, Schloss, Schmidt *et al.*, 2004). These findings, although potentially important, require replication before their ultimate significance can be assessed.

In summary, ADHD is not a genetic disorder in a simple sense. A reasonable working hypothesis is that genetic and environmental influences of small effect, while correlated to some extent, likely act together (both additively and multiplicatively) to create a spectrum of neurobiological risk.

Is ADHD a Fronto-striatal/Executive Function Disorder?

The Fronto-striatal/Executive Function Disorder Hypothesis

Evidence for the role of alterations in brain structure and function in ADHD is compelling. Debate continues as to which specific brain circuits are most important. The search for the biological basis of ADHD has been motivated by the assumption that a common core of neurobiological dysfunction is responsible for the condition (Sonuga-Barke, 1998). Following the reconceptualization of hyperactivity disorders in DSM-IIIR, the role of attention was highlighted, placing neurocognitive deficits at the core of the disorder (Castellanos, Sonuga-Barke, Tannock *et al.*, 2006). Subsequent attempts to "fine-map" deficits in terms of more refined attentional concepts from cognitive psychology have mostly been unsuccessful (Huang-Pollack, Nigg, & Carr, 2005).

The fronto-striatal/executive function disorder (FS/ED) hypothesis involves a broader conception of cognitive deficits based on the observation of similarities between people with ADHD and those with disorders caused by frontal lobe lesion or disease (Denckla, 2002). The publication of Barkley's model, in which early established inhibitory processes are a developmental precursor to the emergence of executive competence, has been extremely influential (Barkley, 1997). FS/ED focuses on higher order intentional cognitive processes including response inhibition, planning, working memory, attentional flexibility and speech fluency: constructs grouped loosely under the umbrella of executive function; a concept, although criticized for its lack of specificity, that continues to be used widely in the psychological literature. Neuroanatomically, these functions are linked to activity within the "cognitive" thalamo-cortico-striatal loop (Alexander & Crutcher, 1990). Projections from the prefrontal cortex (specifically the dorsolateral region) to the neostriatum (specifically the caudate nucleus) pass via a complex set of direct and indirect basal ganglia pathways through the thalamus and back to the prefrontal cortex. Although anatomically and functionally segregated, this network has strong connections to other more posterior regions including the frontal motor cortices, the parietal cortex and the cerebellum (Timmann, Richter, Schoch *et al.*, 2006). Activity within this circuit is mediated by GABA and glutamate and modulated by the catecholamines – dopamine and norepinephrine.

Evidence Supporting the FS/ED Hypothesis

Neuropsychology

Recent quantitative reviews support the association between ADHD and executive dysfunction across a wide range of domains and measures within domains (Huang-Pollock & Nigg, 2003; Lijffijt, Kenemans, Verbated *et al.*, 2005; Oosterlaan, Logan, & Sergeant, 1998; Willcutt, Doyle, Nigg *et al.*, 2005). A comprehensive review is outside the scope of this chapter but a brief survey provides robust and convincing evidence that children with ADHD perform worse than controls in domains such as response inhibition and interference control, planning and working memory. Pooled effect sizes from a meta-analysis of nearly 7000 children are only in the moderate range (0.4–0.6; Willcutt *et al.*, 2005). Furthermore, in a very large study using an extensive battery of tasks only about half of the children with ADHD displayed a deficit on any one executive task and very few subjects showed a pervasive pattern of EF deficits (Nigg *et al.*, 2005). This is in keeping with the idea that neuropsychological tests are of limited value diagnostically, in and of themselves.

Structural Neuroanatomy

Total brain volumes of children with ADHD are reduced by up to 5% with effects on both gray and white matter and larger reductions apparent in the right hemisphere (Seidman, Valera, & Makris, 2005). Reductions in intracranial volume have been reported (Durston, Pol, Schnack *et al.*, 2004). Unsurprisingly, given the dominance of the FS/ED hypothesis, work has concentrated on two regions in particular – the prefrontal cortex and the striatum, especially the caudate nucleus. Region of interest (ROI) analyses provide good evidence of alterations within the dorsolateral prefrontal cortex and the neostriatum (caudate/putamen; Castellanos, Lee, Sharp *et al.*, 2002). Cortical thinning may be especially marked in prefrontal regions implicated in executive control (Shaw, Lerch, Greenstein *et al.*, 2006). While these effects persist after controlling for medication status and comorbidity, most are lost if total brain volume is taken into account (Castellanos *et al.*, 2002).

Functional Neuroanatomy

Functional magnetic resonance imaging (fMRI) case–control studies report reduced activation within both the ventrolateral and dorso-lateral prefrontal cortex (Durston, Tottenham, Thomas *et al.*, 2003; Rubia, Overmeyer, Taylor *et al.*, 1999, 2005) as well as the neostriatum (i.e., caudate and putamen; Rubia *et al.*, 1999; Vaidya, Bunge, Dudukovic *et al.*, 2005), with the most consistent findings relating to the caudate nucleus. Positron emission tomography (PET) and single photon emission computed tomography (SPECT) report reduced glucose metabolism in frontal regions (Ernst, Kimes, London *et al.*, 2003; Schweitzer, Lee, Hanford *et al.*, 2003). Studies using event-related potentials (ERPs) and other electrophysiological paradigms provide further evidence for the FS/ED hypothesis (Fallgatter, Ehlis, Rosler *et al.*, 2005).

Beyond Fronto-striatal/Executive Dysfunction

Despite this focus on the FS/ED circuit there is strong evidence for the involvement of other brain circuits and related psychological functions. At the neuropsychological level, a very broad range of extra-executive domains has been implicated, including timing and temporal synchrony (likely implicating thalamo-cerebellar circuits; Toplak, Dockstader, & Tannock, 2006); reward and motivation (likely implicating orbito-frontal-ventral-striatal circuitry; Sagvolden, Johansen, Aase *et al.*, 2005; Sonuga-Barke, 2005); attentional orienting and alerting (likely implicating posterior parietal networks; Banaschewski, Brandeis, Heinrich *et al.*, 2004) and more broadly based difficulties in the regulation of arousal and alertness (Sergeant, 2005) and heightened stimulation seeking (Antrop, Roeyers, Van Oost *et al.*, 2004). In these studies, effect sizes are in the range reported for executive deficits; again suggesting that only a subgroup of ADHD children are affected by each pattern of difficulty. Structural alterations are also widespread affecting temporal, occipital and parietal lobes, the corpus callosum and cingulum (for a review see Seidman, Valera, & Makris, 2005). Effects in relation to the cerebellum are perhaps most striking (Castellanos *et al.*, 2002). There is emerging evidence of alterations in key foci such as the amygdala (Plessen, Bansal, Zhu *et al.*, 2006). In terms of functional imaging studies, two types of evidence for extra-executive circuitry involvement come from imaging studies. First, there are those studies that have specifically probed executive circuits but found evidence for the role of other brain regions. For instance, response conflict studies using Stroop-like tasks have reported reduced activation in widely distributed networks with loci not normally conceptualized within the executive loops (i.e., anterior cingulate cortex; Bush, Frazier, Rauch *et al.*, 1999; Rubia *et al.*, 1999; Tamm, Menon, Ringel *et al.*, 2004), the parietal and temporal lobes and cerebellum (Tian, Jiang, Wang *et al.*, 2006; Vaidya *et al.*, 2005). There are also those studies that have purposefully probed other regions and processes in an attempt to explore the neurobiological basis of the diverse neuropsychological processes implicated in ADHD. Although currently less common these studies have started to delineate the functional neuroanatomy of alerting and reorienting and reward anticipation (Scheres, Dijkstra, Ainslie *et al.*, 2006).

Interpreting the Neuroscience Evidence

Although, at the group level, FS/ED is associated with ADHD, a closer examination of the evidence does not support a strong version of the FS/ED hypothesis – that FS/ED is the common core dysfunction of ADHD. In fact, FS/ED may be sufficient for ADHD but it is not necessary. It seems increasingly clear that: (i) at the group level, ADHD is associated with a diverse range of non-executive deficits; and (ii) at an individual level, many children with ADHD appear not be affected by executive dysfunction to any significant degree. Recent models have emphasized this psychopathophysiological heterogeneity (Sonuga-Barke, 2005) and developed the idea that ADHD is an umbrella construct which, while clinically useful, subsumes multiple groups of patients with distinctive etiological and pathophysiological profiles. Studies with measures from multiple domains and large samples sufficient to test this multiple pathway hypothesis are currently rare and limited to the neuropsychological domain. Solanto, Abikoff, Sonuga-Barke *et al.* (2001) found that executive dysfunction (measured using the stop signal paradigm – a measure of the ability to inhibit an already initiated response when requested) and delay aversion (measured using the choice delay task – a preference between a small immediate and a large delayed reward) were both deficient in ADHD, despite being uncorrelated with each other – suggesting two dissociable bases for the disorder. Similar results were found in samples of preschoolers (Dalen, Sonuga-Barke, Hall *et al.*, 2004) and children with hydrocephalus and spina bifida (Stevenson & Cate, 2004). Research extending this account to other areas of deficit and levels of analysis is currently under way.

In summary, ADHD is not an FS/ED disorder in any simple sense. A reasonable working hypothesis is that ADHD is an umbrella construct that subsumes multiple subgroups of patients each with their own distinctive psychopathophysiological signature, of which fronto-striatal/executive dysfunction is just one.

Is ADHD a Catecholamine Disorder?

Four observations provide indirect evidence for the role of catecholamine dysregulation in ADHD. First, ADHD symptoms are reduced by dopamine (DA) and norepinephrine (NE) agonists such as methylphenidate, amphetamine and atomoxetine, which act via different mechanisms to increase extracellular DA and NE but have similar clinical effects (Pliszka, 2005). Second, as reported above, there are a number of associated polymorphisms in genes affecting catecholamines, especially DA (Faraone *et al.*, 2005). Third, within animal models pharmacological lesions and gene knockout of catecholamine systems produce behaviors that mimic ADHD (Arnsten & Li, 2005; Madras, Miller, & Fischman, 2005). Fourth, NE and DA, although widely distributed within the brain, have core branches that heavily innervate regions implicated in the neuropsychological underpinnings of ADHD. There are two main dopamine branches: the meso-cortico-limbic branch with cells projecting from the midbrain ventral tegmental area to the limbic regions including the amygdala, the ventral striatum and the frontal cortex and the nigro-striatal branch projecting from the substantia nigra to the striatum. The norepinephrine system has major projections from the locus ceruleus throughout the cortex (anterior and posterior) and into the cerebellum.

More direct evidence for the role of catecholamines in ADHD comes from several sources, with the literature being largely limited to DA. SPECT and PET studies have found increased dopamine binding in the striatum in ADHD (reviewed by Spencer, Biederman, Madras *et al.*, 2005), a finding that fits well with the clinical action of methylphenidate (Volkow, Wang, Fowler *et al.*, 2005). Methylphenidate (MPH) has remedial effects on neuropsychological deficits in the domains of inhibition (Boonstra, Kooij, Oosterlaan *et al.*, 2005; Klein, Fischer, Fischer, *et al.*, 2002; Turner, Blackwell, Dowson *et al.*, 2005), sustained attention (Boonstra *et al.*, 2005), working memory (Mehta, Goodyer, & Sahakian, 2004; Turner *et al.*, 2005), set shifting and planning (Kempton, Vance, Maruff *et al.*, 1999). MPH appears to have beneficial effects on other areas of functioning not traditionally linked to the fronto-striatal cognitive loop, such as visual memory (Rhodes, Coghill, & Matthews, 2004), timing (Baldwin, Chelonis, Flake *et al.*, 2004) and the motivational salience of a task (Volkow, Wang, Fowler *et al.*, 2004), but whether these effects are related to the treatment of ADHD is not known.

Interpreting Neuropsychopharmacology of ADHD

Although the evidence implicating the catecholamines is persuasive, much of it is circumstantial and indirect in nature and therefore difficult to interpret. Even if one can demonstrate that dopamine agonists reduce symptoms and improve functioning, and that this varies as a function of genotype, it does not necessarily implicate DA in the pathophysiology of the disorder. There are a number of reasons for caution. Case–control studies suggest that the effects of MPH are similar in nature for both clinical cases and controls. In keeping with this, recent reports have suggested that MPH has a broad-based generic effect on arousal and the motivational salience of tasks rather than specific effects on the neural circuits shown to be affected in ADHD (Volkow *et al.*, 2005). Interpreting these effects vis-à-vis the role of DA in ADHD is further complicated by observation that MPH can have effects on both the phasic and tonic aspect of the DA response. Volkow and Swanson (2003) have argued that the therapeutic effects of DA occur following slow and stable increases in DA (i.e., increased DA tone), while its abuse potential is related to short and rapid changes that mimic phasic firing. The significance of these effects for understanding the specificity of the "dopamine deficit" (in phase or tone) in ADHD is as yet unclear. The most direct evidence for DA deficits comes from those PET imaging studies showing increased dopamine transporter (DAT) density in ADHD (although there have been a number of non-replications of this effect). However, the adaptive quality of neural systems means that DAT up-regulation is likely to be a consequence of a complex set of neuroanatomic alterations (Russell, 2002). While lower densities could represent a relatively permanent trait closely linked to the fundamental neurobiological causes of ADHD, they could equally be a consequence of the condition or a marker of some more fundamental neurobiological process (Madras, Miller, & Fischman, 2002). Animal models suggest that DA and NE systems interact (Liprando, Miner, Blakely *et al.*, 2004) with each other and with other neurotransmitters such as serotonin and acetylcholine (Olijslagers, Werkman, McCreary *et al.*, 2006), and future models of both the pathophysiology of the disorder and its treatment need to take account of this.

In summary, a sensible working hypothesis is that catecholamine function appears to be implicated in ADHD but the issues of cause and effect are difficult to disentangle and the particular mechanisms are likely to be complex and involve interactions between NE and DA as well as other neurotransmitters.

An Integrative Framework for ADHD Etiology and Pathophysiology

Figure 34.1 illustrates a framework that integrates the working hypotheses set out above with the aim of communicating the key themes set out in this section. Multiple early genetic and environmental influences of small effect act together to create a spectrum of neurobiological risk by altering brain structure and function and associated cognitive processes that mediate the emergence of ADHD. The postnatal environment also has an important role within the model, both as secondary direct influences on brain processes (e.g., diet, environmental toxins) and as mediators/moderators of outcome through reciprocal coercive cycles of interaction (e.g., negative parenting). The framework also makes explicit the heterogeneity in ADHD by including multiple pathways to ADHD, each potentially associated with a different set of primary influences, and mediating and moderating processes. In this particular model, three different pathways are hypothesized but this is for illustrative purposes only. Exploring these different pathways by examining the way that neuroanatomic and neurofunctional and psychological processes mediate the effects of genes and environments on ADHD represents a major research priority (Castellanos & Tannock, 2002). From a clinical point of view, this sort of model highlights the need for broad-based assessments of multiple impairments across diverse regions of functioning as well as tailoring of treatment to a child's particular areas of difficulty rather than generic or formulaic approaches.

The assumption behind most of the research on pathophysiology has been that the basis for ADHD is similar during all developmental periods. This means that there are few comparative data across different stages. Studying developmental changes in the pathophysiology of ADHD is an important priority for future studies.

Epidemiology

Several studies converge on a point prevalence for hyperkinetic disorder of about 1.5% in the primary school age population, and about 5% for ADHD (Swanson *et al.*, 1998).

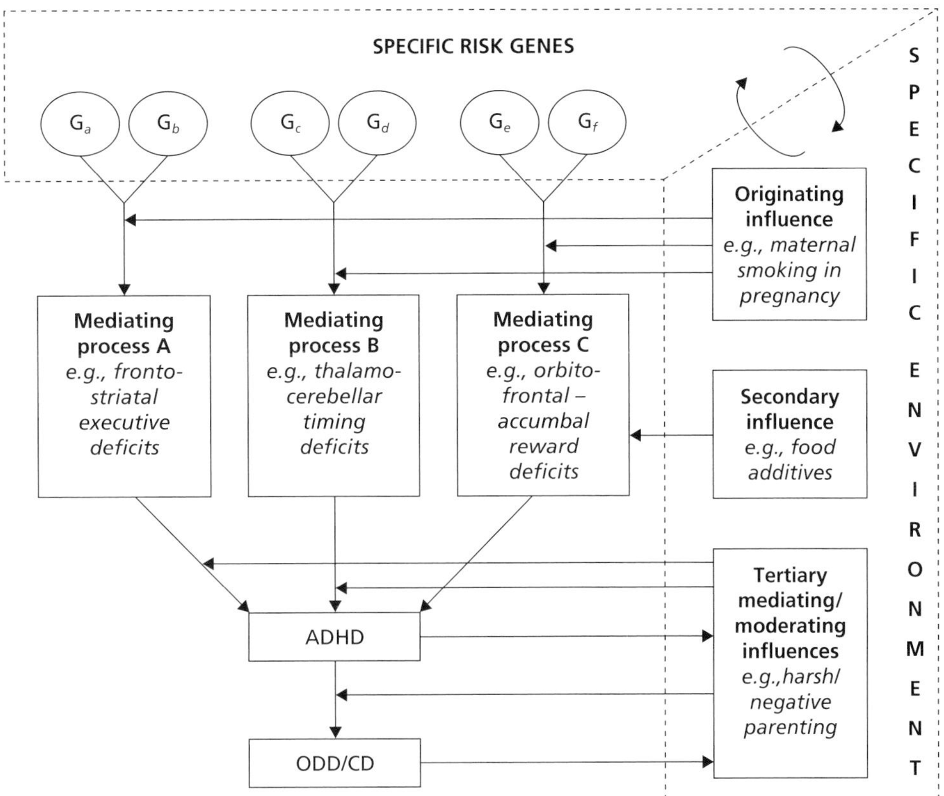

Fig. 34.1 A simplified generic framework of the pathophysiology of ADHD designed to communicate the key themes in the *pathophysiology and etiology* section: multiple pathways between originating genetic–environmental influences are mediated by alternations in the neurocognitive processes. Genes and environments are correlated. Tertiary social environmental factors influence outcome through reciprocal relationships in which a child's difficult behavior evokes negative parental behavior that in turn exacerbates/escalates behavior problems. ODD/CD: oppositional defiant disorder/conduct disorder.

A recent National Morbidity Survey in the UK was based on a nationally representative sample of more than 10,000 children studied with rating scales and structured interviews given by non-clinical researchers, after which clinicians made diagnoses on the basis of the information gathered (Meltzer & Gatward, 2000). The rate for hyperkinetic disorder was about 14 per 1000 children, with the rate substantially lower for girls than for boys (the usual ratio in the population being around 1 : 3; Heptinstall & Taylor, 2002).

The use of health services was quite high in the hyperkinetic group, with nearly half of the children receiving some sort of intervention – but this did not necessarily imply that their hyperactivity had been identified as a problem. Indeed, an epidemiological study in a London borough found that only about 1 child in 10, out of those identified by high scores on rating scales from teacher and parent, were in practice receiving a diagnosis of ADHD (Sayal *et al.*, 2002). National UK figures suggest that stimulant medication is given for only about 3 children per 1000 (NICE, 2005), and most other European nations are lower still. By contrast, surveys in the USA indicate about 3% of all school-age children being diagnosed and treated (Olfson, Gameroff, Marcus *et al.*, 2003; Safer & Zito, 2000) – although with considerable variation in different parts of the nation.

A child whose behavior is hyperactive has a complex journey to becoming a diagnosed case. The knowledge, tolerance and attitudes of parents, teachers and health practitioners will all affect the apparent prevalence. The great international differences in the prevalence of diagnosed conditions appear to reflect the criteria used more than the behavior of children (Swanson *et al.*, 1998). ADHD point prevalence estimates internationally cluster around 5–10%; hyperkinetic disorder around 1–2%; screening questionnaire ratings of those at risk around 10–20%. Attention deficit without hyperactivity has received less research attention, but is troublesome for something like another 1% of the school-age population.

In countries where there is a large difference between population rates and the numbers diagnosed in practice, there can be considerable fluctuations over time in the apparent prevalence. The numbers treated in the UK appear to have risen some five-fold in a 10-year period (NICE, 2005), but the point prevalence in the UK's National Morbidity Survey was very similar to that of estimates made more than 10 years previously (Meltzer & Gatward, 2000; Taylor *et al.*, 1991).

Hyperactive behavior seems to have been relatively stable over decades at a time when other types of mental health problem in young people have been rising (Collishaw, Maughan, Goodman *et al.*, 2004). One implication is that changes in society – such as the rise of television viewing and eating processed food – are unlikely to be critical factors, but that recognition of problems can change dramatically in a short time.

Longitudinal course

The course from early childhood into the school years is variable. From infancy to the age of about 3 years there is a great deal of variation, and indeed the early stage may be a rather wide set of temperamental problems in self-regulation, but by the age of 4 years a diagnosis of ADHD is very likely to persist into school age (Lahey, Pelham, Loney *et al.*, 2004). A population study comparing monozygotic with dizygotic twins has concluded that there are genetic influences on the course of hyperactive behavior over the early years, not only on the initial appearance of the problem (Asherson, 2005). The transitions into nursery and school life bring different kinds of challenge to children with less well-developed control of impulse and attention than their peers.

From childhood into adolescence, there is a risk for the core behaviors to continue and about half of previously diagnosed cases will still meet diagnostic criteria (Klein & Mannuzza, 1991). Indeed, unreferred cases in the community, and those with high levels of behavior problems that fall short of the diagnosis, continue to show impaired social development: impulsiveness declines in absolute terms, but remains deviant relative to age-matched peers (Taylor *et al.*, 1996). Lack of friends, work and constructive leisure activities are prominent in adolescence, motor accidents become a considerable risk, and there is academic underachievement. A major possible outcome for those who show impulsiveness and overactivity (as opposed to inattentiveness alone) is the development of aggressive and antisocial behavior and delinquency (Farrington, 1995).

Substance misuse deserves particular mention because of its importance in young people's development (see chapter 36). A review and meta-analysis by Wilens *et al.* (2003) has indicated both that ADHD is associated with (and precedes) substance misuse, and that the association is not caused by prescribed medication, for those taking stimulants show lower rates of substance misuse. There is some evidence from longitudinal research (Taylor *et al.*, 1996) that the pathway from ADHD into misuse is dependent upon the appearance of conduct disorder.

Several prospective studies have followed patients through adolescence into adulthood (Barkley, Fischer, Edelbrock *et al.*, 1990; Biederman, Faraone, Milberger *et al.*, 1996a,b; Faraone, Biederman, Mennin *et al.*, 1996; Faraone, Biederman, & Mick, 2006; Hechtman & Weiss, 1983; Mannuzza, Klein, Bessler *et al.*, 1998; Mick, Faraone, & Biederman, 2004; Weiss & Hechtman, 1993). These studies taken together suggest that a majority of diagnosed young people no longer meet criteria for ADHD in adult life, but that nevertheless many will still show above-average levels of inattentiveness and impulsivity (estimated variously at 10–40%: Barkley, 2002; Biederman, Mick, & Faraone, 2000; Faraone *et al.*, 1996; Faraone, Biederman, & Mick, 2006; Hill & Schoener, 1996; Spencer, Biederman, Wilens *et al.*, 1996). There is something of a puzzle in that ADHD diagnosed using strict DSM-IV criteria ought to be substantially less common in adults according to the longitudinal studies, yet cross-sectional surveys in adult life come up with surprisingly high prevalence rates of about 4% (Kessler *et al.*, 2006). Adult surveys also indicate a very high degree of comorbidity, so it may be that ADHD criteria can be met because of the presence of adult mental disorders or that persistence of ADHD is a strong cause of other adult disorders.

The functional importance in adults is variable. Antisocial behavior tends to persist (Hechtman & Weiss, 1986), and sometimes the overall impact may worsen because of the increased demands of an adult environment and manifest as: educational, organizational or occupational failures; substance use disorders and other dependent, risky, antisocial or illegal behaviors; or emotional and relationship difficulties (Millstein *et al.*, 1998). Nevertheless, for some, adult life can also bring opportunities for better social adjustment. People can choose occupational niches, such as sales and trading, in which good skills in immediate problem-solving are more important than longer drawn out planning and foresight.

It is also quite possible for ADHD to present for the first time in adult life. There will then be a story of symptoms having been present in childhood but having been unrecognized, or misattributed or not impairing. Protective factors, such as high intelligence or capable upbringing, may have meant that there was in effect no problem. Some of these protections may have been left behind, or more difficult challenges may have appeared. Sometimes, life changes, such as embarking on higher education or promotion to increasingly responsible positions, may be the first occasions for ADHD to cause failure and presentation to a health service.

The influences determining persistence or remission of ADHD into adolescence and adult life should be very important: they ought to be key targets for intervention. More research is needed to determine this. Environmental childhood factors did not turn out to influence the persistence of inattention and impulsiveness into early adult life in a prospective longitudinal study of untreated and non-comorbid hyperactivity (Taylor *et al.*, 1996). However, factors such as hostile attitudes from parents and non-acceptance by peers did predict whether aggressive and other antisocial complications would develop (Rutter, Maughan, Meyer *et al.*, 1997); and a *val-val* genotype in a *COMT* gene polymorphism together with a low birth weight predicted the development of antisocial symptoms in those with ADHD (Caspi, Langley, Milne *et al.*, in press; Thapar, Langley, Fowler *et al.*, 2005b). Polymorphisms in the dopamine genes (*DAT1* and *DRD4*) have predicted persistence to poor social outcome later (Mill, Caspi, Williams *et al.*, 2006). Persistent cases of ADHD tend to have stronger histories of ADHD in other family members (Faraone, 2004), suggesting that genetic factors influence course at this stage of development too; that family relationships help to determine the course; or that one family member's behavior makes others act in the same way. The implications for practice are that from childhood to early adult life, and perhaps longer, severe levels of hyperactivity and inattentiveness should be seen as potentially chronic disability, and that intervention should target not only the core symptoms but also the surrounding tangle of adverse personal relationships and educational failure.

Clinical Assessment

At all ages there is a need for information from multiple sources. Clinical recognition needs to be based upon experience of what is expected of children at different ages and at different developmental levels.

In *preschool*, observational approaches are often required. There is a wide range of variation of parental tolerance, and considerable overlap with other aspects of a "difficult" temperament. It may be possible to witness directly the overactivity, the disinclination to wait and the choice of immediate rather than delayed gratification – for example, by setting up a waiting situation in which the children will have a larger reward if they refrain from grabbing an immediate one. Parental interview accounts are especially useful if they are based on observable behaviors rather than global descriptions such as "irritable."

By *school age*, a wide variety of parent and teacher rating scales are available and have been reviewed (Stein & Perrin, 2003; Taylor, Dopfner, Sergeant *et al.*, 2004) with conclusions that instruments developed for the specific purpose of assessing ADHD are usually more accurate than general purpose psychopathological instruments (Miller, Lee, & Raina, 1998). The sensitivity and specificity of such instruments often appear to be very good, yet even then the classification obtained can be inadequate. Measures such as Conners' rating scales show an effect size for children with ADHD, compared to normal controls, of around 3 standard deviations (SD), and this level of discrimination should correspond roughly to 80% levels of sensitivity and specificity, or even better.

While this sounds very impressive, the difference in base rates implies that non-hyperactive children will still be wrongly identified as ADHD so often that they may outnumber the true cases. (In the above example, and assuming a 5% prevalence, the 20% wrongly identified come from about 95% of the children, resulting in 18% false positives; while correctly detected true cases will be about 4% of the population.) Causes of false positives include raters without sufficient appreciation of the developmental norms for that age, raters who bring qualities of their relationship with the child to bear on making their rating of behavior, and contrast effects in which children are implicitly rated against other members of the family or other members of the subculture.

Detailed clinical interview with the parent (or other caregiver) is usually the most valuable single measure. In this context it is possible to go beyond the request for a rating of whether a child's impulsiveness is abnormal, to a description of the behavior on which that rating was based. The interviewer can then apply a clinically informed judgment as to whether that level of behavior is in fact abnormal for the child. Every effort should be made to obtain and discuss ratings by schoolteachers.

Observations of the child's behavior are also valuable, especially when there is diagnostic doubt. By the time of school entry, however, much of the overt behavior will be modified – at least in the artificial circumstances of clinic assessment. The novelty of the situation, the focused adult attention and the structured nature of the situation all militate against hyperactivity being readily observable. The diagnosis should therefore not be dismissed for the sole reason that the child appears well controlled during assessment. Nevertheless, when abnormality is seen, then direct observation is invaluable for detecting its pattern, its antecedents and its consequences.

For *adults* who seek services for the first time, their own account of themselves is often the main presentation. However, self-report is of limited value by itself. There was less continuity between childhood hyperactivity at age 7 and self-reports at age 17 than there was for ratings made by people who knew the young person well (Danckaerts, Heptinstall, Chadwick *et al.*, 2000). Genetic influences are less strong for self-report than for ratings by others. Whenever possible, diagnostic assessments should include the accounts of parents, partners or other good informants, and the differential needs to include hypomania and personality disorder.

Various rating scales have been developed for adults. The Wender Utah Rating Scale focuses on retrospective symptoms in childhood plus current hyperactivity, inattention and other symptoms: the recall of childhood has been validated against parent report and found to be reasonably reliable (Ward, Wender, & Reimherr, 1993). The Adult Self Report Scale (Adler, Kessler, & Spencer, 2004; Kessler, Adler, Ames *et al.*, 2005), Conners' Adult ADHD Rating Scale (Conners, Erhardt, Sparrow *et al.*, 1998) and Brown Adult Attention Deficit Disorder Scale (Brown, 1996) are also available.

Assessment should not stop at the recognition (or exclusion) of a syndrome of hyperactivity and inattentiveness, but go on to consider the subtypes, any coexistent disorder and the likely causal pathways as sketched in this chapter. The strengths and weaknesses of the family and school are important for their ability to cope and for what kinds of intervention will be most appropriate.

Physical examination should be close enough to uncover any evidence of neurological disease and assess coordination; to exclude hearing impairment; and to note any evidence of underlying chromosomal disorder or thyroid disease. Physical investigations are not routinely needed, but should be guided by history and examination. Psychological testing does not normally give the diagnosis (which is behavioral) but is valuable for several other purposes: analyzing reasons for poor learning, providing suggestions for classroom education, detecting coexistent cognitive impairments, and establishing an approximate estimation of mental age, against which the specificity of attention impairment should be measured. The research tests reviewed earlier in the chapter have not in general been developed to the point that their test–retest reliability is known and they have not been standardized to the point where normal values are known, so they are not yet recommended for clinical practice. There are several commercial versions of Continuous Performance Tests (which are not necessary for following the response to medication but can be useful in cases where the response is unclear), and a convenient set of tests of sustaining, focusing and dividing attention and inhibition is available as the TEACH (Test of Everyday Attention for Children; Manly, Anderson, Nimmo-Smith *et al.*, 2001).

Treatment

Intervention begins with an explanation of the disorder and its nature, directed to the child, family and teachers. Sometimes this is enough in itself. The alleviation of adult guilt and irritation with the child may benefit the child considerably. Advice and assessment should try to ensure that the parenting context includes positive contacts between parent(s) and child together with clear expectations for appropriate, and sanctions for inappropriate, behavior. Simple advice to schools on managing hyperactivity was helpful in reducing hyperactivity ratings of the children in a large-scale randomized non-blind trial (Tymms & Merrell, 2005).

Trial evidence has appeared for some more specific interventions – especially medication, behavior therapy and dietary treatments.

Stimulant medication – usually methylphenidate or dexamfetamine – is widely given and licensed for children in many countries. Atomoxetine has a license in the USA for children and adults and is licensed in Europe for children and for adults if their treatment has started in childhood. These three medicines have received extensive trials and systematic reviews (that by NICE, 2005, is particularly comprehensive). All three are efficacious in comparisons with placebo: effect sizes of MPH on hyperactivity symptoms in randomized controlled trials are between 0.8 and 1.1 SD; and those of atomoxetine around 0.6 SD (Banaschewski, Coghill, Santosh *et al.*, 2006).

Behavior therapy has received several trials, but no very satisfactory systematic review. Miller, Lee, & Raina (1998) excluded most trials on methodological grounds, and from the two trials remaining thought there was no evidence of superiority to standard clinical care. One large-scale random allocation non-blind trial in the USA focused on the comparison between careful medication management, intensive behaviorally oriented psychosocial therapy, a combination of the two, or a simple referral back to community agencies (which usually resulted in medication) (MTA Cooperative Group, 1999). The main conclusions after 14 months' treatment were that careful medication was more powerful than behavior treatment, and considerably more effective than routine medication in the community. There were many advantages in adding medication to behavior therapy, but relatively few to adding behavior therapy to medication. The superiority of careful medication to behavior therapy was all the more striking in that the behavior therapy provision was much more intensive and prolonged than could be achieved by a community service. The combination of behavior therapy and medication did have some benefits: better control of aggressive behavior at home; improving the overall sense of satisfaction of parents; possibly reducing the medication dosage; and increasing the rate of achieving "normalization" (the reduction of problems to a level where none was rated as more than minor). These improvements were real but modest, and would probably not justify the very high costs of the full treatment package in this research-based form. Follow-up 2 years after the end of the trial suggested that the differences between therapies had lessened or disappeared.

It does not follow from the power of medication that it is always the first choice treatment. Behavioral therapy may be less effective, but it is still helpful for many children. The costs of a short course of parent training are comparable to those of medication; the outcome may be somewhat less favorable in terms of symptom reduction, but it has the advantage of carrying very little physical hazard.

A re-analysis of the MTA study has found that the superiority of medication to behavior therapy is greater in hyperkinetic disorder than in other types of ADHD (Santosh *et al.*, 2005). The trial suggests that most children whose problems are severe enough to get a diagnosis of hyperkinetic disorder will need medication. Family attitudes should of course be respected, and often a trial of psychological treatment will be attempted, but medication should be advised if there has been no substantial improvement after a few weeks.

For children at lesser degrees of severity – those who show ADHD but not hyperkinetic disorder – the choice of initial therapy is more evenly balanced. In these milder cases there are options about which treatment to start with. Decisions will depend on the analysis of the individual child, the strengths and weaknesses of their school and classroom environment, the severity of disturbance of peer relationships, and the preferences of the families. It is quite reasonable to start with either therapy, in the knowledge that one will proceed to the other should the response be suboptimal.

The details of treatments have been spelled out in guidelines (e.g., Taylor *et al.*, 2004) and textbooks (e.g., Barkley, 2000). The principles of behavioral intervention do not differ greatly from those used in therapy of other behavioral problems in childhood. Specifically and operationally described problems should be identified, the contingencies that affect them established, and a monitored approach taken to enhancement of adult attention to the child and effective instruction (see chapters 62 & 64). Particular attention should be paid to speed in the delivery of rewards or response cost; explaining to the child which of their behaviors has earned the reward, or loss of reward; varying rewards frequently; and ensuring that there is variety and novelty in the management system. These aspects of therapy have particular relevance to overcoming the attention problems that often compromise the response to behavior therapy. Novel non-pharmacological approaches that target core ADHD deficits (e.g., working memory training; Klingberg, Fernell, Olesen *et al.*, 2005) have been developed but lack sufficient empirical support to recommend them at present.

Medication usually starts with immediate-release MPH given three times a day in doses starting with 5–5–2.5 mg or 10–10–5 mg (depending on the size of the child), and should be monitored by parents and teachers (and if possible by the child) using a simple scale such as the abbreviated Conners. The initial monitoring scale focuses on the key target of hyperactivity and a checklist of possible adverse effects; it can be helpful to add to the scale other items that are of particular relevance to the individual child. In the first stage of titrating dosage, monitoring should be frequent – ideally daily but, more realistically, weekly. The dose is then titrated upwards – often weekly, but a daily variation in dosage can also be reliable – until there is a good response, adverse effects become troublesome or the ceiling of 0.7 mg/kg/dose is reached – whichever comes first. Monitoring should include growth in height and weight plotted on developmental charts, pulse and blood pressure, and observation of mental state in case adverse effects such as depression, lack of spontaneity, or perseveration should appear. Blood tests are not routinely required (but the manufacturer recommends them, for unknown reasons).

Treatment with a long-acting medicine is helpful for some children, and can be considered from the start. The advantages over repeated doses of immediate-release medication are for the child, whose treatment can be more private if not delivered in school; and for the school, which does not have to store and administer controlled drugs. Preparations of MPH vary in the physics of their delivery system and the proportion of immediate-release to extended-release that is present. Concerta XL has an action lasting about 12 hours, Equasym XL and Ritalin LA about 8 hours, and a skin patch is also available in the USA. Surveillance of millions of children treated has led to a few reports of sudden death, epileptic seizures, liver failure and electrocardiogram (ECG) abnormality – especially, prolongation of Q-Tc interval. They are too rare to know whether they are in fact associated with the medications or represent coincident disease, or whether they are more common in one drug than another. We suggest that a preceding heart problem – structural, or suggested by a history of breathlessness or exercise syncope or a history of sudden death in youthful family members – should be a signal for a cardiological examination before therapy, including ECG.

Stimulants are not contraindicated in coexistent disorders, but caution is needed in the presence of autism or Tourette disorder, both of which can be worsened by stimulants and need careful monitoring. There is some contradiction about the effect of stimulant drugs on those who show high anxiety as well as ADHD. Placebo-controlled trials have indicated that stimulants are of less effect on hyperactivity in children where there is anxiety too (Buitelaar, Van der Gaag, Swaab-Barneveld *et al.*, 1995; Taylor, Schachar, Thorley *et al.*, 1987). By contrast, the MTA study found that the general superiority of medication to behavior therapy was not affected by the coexistent presence of high anxiety (MTA Cooperative Group, 1999). Inspection of the MTA data suggests that medication was substantially less effective in the group that received stimulants as part of community treatment; the benefits of stimulants were essentially in the group treated with the careful monitoring of the research group. It may be that particularly close attention to monitoring and dosage is required for successful treatment of comorbid states.

Atomoxetine has been introduced more recently; it is an inhibitor of the norepinephrine transporter, and raises synaptic levels of both norepinephrine and (at least in frontal cortex) dopamine. The action will usually last throughout the day if it is given in the morning. Onset of clinical effectiveness is slower than for stimulants; some action is often seen after 2 weeks of administration, but may still be increasing at the 6-week point. There have been case reports of suicidal ideation, liver failure and epileptic seizures. These adverse effects are so rare that it is hard to know whether they are more common in those who take the drug than those who do not, but they deserve vigilance in monitoring and parents should therefore be informed of what to watch for. The choice between atomoxetine and an extended-release stimulant will be made on the basis of effect size and speed of action (favoring MPH or dexamfetamine), freedom from risk of abuse (favoring atomoxetine), balance of adverse effects (insomnia, growth retardation and tics being more common with stimulants, nausea and sedation with atomoxetine), user preferences, and cost. If stimulants are ineffective, atomoxetine may nevertheless be helpful.

Medication is usually effective. If it is not, then the reasons should be sought. Is it being swallowed? If not, careful and sympathetic exploration of the reasons for refusal may help. Has the dose been titrated carefully to the child? The range of effective doses is great, and attention both to this and the timing of doses can correct non-response. Have adverse effects appeared? If so, they can often be managed symptomatically – e.g., with dose adjustment and sleep hygiene measures for insomnia, or rescheduled meals for loss of appetite. If one of the licensed medications has failed, has another one been tried? Has the diagnosis been reviewed (refractoriness to therapy may be associated with an underlying disorder such as autism)? Only after such a process should the disorder be seen as refractory and an unlicensed therapy attempted. Second-line drugs include some with reasonable controlled trial evidence for superiority to placebo (clonidine, modafinil, imipramine, pemoline) and some with limited trial evidence or anecdotal tributes or randomized controlled trial evidence in specific groups (e.g., tiapride, nicotine patches, guanfacine). They should all be used with specialist guidance.

If medication has been effective, then a review of the case should be conducted. What coexistent problems still need intervention, and of what kind? What is the child's and family's attitude to the success of treatment? Will they rely on it to the exclusion of educational adjustment or other kinds of help?

Will they now attribute all the child's successes to the drug rather than their efforts? Do they have an understanding of the limits within which dosage can be varied in response to changing circumstances? A good response to medication is sometimes taken as a proof that the diagnosis of ADHD was correct: this is not logical, because of the evidence that ordinary people respond in qualitatively similar ways (see p. 522). At most, a substantial reduction in hyperactive behavior can be partially helpful in making inferences about how much functional impairment was attributable to that problem.

The question of the length of time for which medication should be continued has not been answered scientifically. Accordingly, an individual approach needs to be taken. At agreed intervals (e.g., once a year) the medicine should be discontinued for a trial period, preferably lasting 2 weeks, to determine whether it is still required.

For preschool children, there has been a beginning of randomized controlled trials of psychological and pharmacological therapies. The most promising intervention is parent training – but this recommendation is based on practice, for there have been few comparative trials. Sonuga-Barke *et al.* (2001) made a comparison between this, a program of parent counseling and support, and a waiting list control. Parent training was more effective than the other interventions in reducing the symptoms of ADHD and of oppositional defiant disorder, and it also increased the mother's sense of general well-being. The gains in the parent training group were not entirely transient: they were still present at a 15-week follow-up. The investigators in another trial compared behavioral family intervention (in both standard and enhanced forms) with a waiting list control and again found that the experimental groups showed reduced levels of behavior problems and greater competence by the parents (Bor, Sanders, & Markie-Dodds, 2002). In this study also, gains were maintained at follow-up, and this time the follow-up period was 1 year.

Compared with the school-aged years there has been little published systematic research about drug treatment in preschool children. The few studies of the stimulants in this age group suggest that they can indeed reduce impulsiveness and improve general social adjustment more effectively than a placebo (Kratochvil, Egger, Greenhill *et al.*, 2006). They may also improve the quality of mother–child relationships. To set against this, the short-term safety and longer term side-effects of medication for children less than 4 years old is uncertain. This does not seem to have deterred many US physicians from using it in this age group, but risks would need much more understanding before medication in this age group could be considered rational.

Dietary treatments, if effective, would be of particular relevance in this age group, while it is still feasible to control what children are eating. Schab and Trinh (2004) have reviewed the evidence about artificial colors from randomized controlled trials, and suggest a small but positive effect size around 0.2 SD. The most promising avenues have been those excluding any of a range of foodstuffs to which a child may have an idiosyncratic response; all four controlled trials addressing the issue have found significant effect sizes, either by comparing a restricted with an ordinary diet or by crossover studies of the reintroduction of incriminated foodstuffs by comparison with harmless items. However, care should be taken to avoid a progressive round of arduous restriction in the absence of clear evidence of benefit.

For adults, meta-analysis indicates that stimulants and atomoxetine are more effective than placebo (Banaschewski *et al.*, 2006; Faraone, Spencer, Aleardi *et al.*, 2004). Child and adolescent psychiatrists are increasingly asked to manage adult cases because of their understanding of the disorder from experience with young people, and the increasing recognition by adults and society that conditions of inattentiveness and impulsive overactivity can be persistently impairing and usefully treatable. Consensus guidelines have been developed by Baldwin, Anderson, Nutt *et al.* (2005).

The future should bring advances from research to clinical practice. Understanding the neuropsychological basis should make psychological intervention programs more rational, and monitoring medication more effective. New medications should appear from molecular research, with enhanced safety and acceptability or with clearer indications, such as in comorbid situations. More fundamentally, the controversies over how broadly to recognize and when to treat should be susceptible to research on the nosology, later outcomes and influences on course for children whose inattention and impulsivity present as a problem for themselves and those around them.

References

Aardoom, H. A., Hirasing, R. A., Rona, R. J., Sanavro, F. L., vandenHeuvel, E. W., & Leeuwenburg, J. (1997). Food intolerance (food hypersensitivity) and chronic complaints in children: The parents' perception. *European Journal of Pediatrics*, *156*, 110–112.

Adler, L. A., Kessler, R. C., & Spencer, T. (2004). *Adult ADHD Self-Report Scale-V1.1 (ASRS-v1.1) Symptom Checklist.* New York, NY. Retrieved from www.med.nyu.edu/psych/assets/adhdscreen18.pdf. 27/09/07

Alexander, G. E., & Crutcher, M. D. (1990). Functional architecture of basal ganglia circuits: Neural substrates of parallel processing. *Trends in Neurosciences*, *13*, 266–271.

Aman, M. G., Smedt, G. D., Derivan, A., Lyons, B., & Findling, R. L. (2002). Double-blind, placebo-controlled study of risperidone for the treatment of disruptive behaviours in children with sub-average intelligence. *American Journal of Psychiatry*, *159*, 1337–1346.

American Psychiatric Association (APA). (2000). *Diagnostic and Statistical Manual of Mental Disorders, version IV, text revision.* Washington, DC: American Psychiatric Association.

Antrop, I., Roeyers, H., Van Oost, P., & Buysse, A. (2004). Stimulation seeking and hyperactivity in children with ADHD. *Journal of Child Psychology and Psychiatry*, *41*, 225–231.

Arcos-Burgos, M., Castellanos, F. X., Pineda, D., Lopera, F., Palacio, J. D., Palacio, L.G., *et al.* (2004). Attention-deficit/hyperactivity disorder in a population isolate: Linkage to loci at 4q13.2, 5q33.3, 11q22, and 17p11. *American Journal of Human Genetics*, *75*, 998–1014.

Arnsten, A. F. T., & Goldman-Rakic, P. S. (1998). Noise stress impairs prefrontal cortical cognitive function in monkeys: Evidence for a hyperdopaminergic mechanism. *Archives of General Psychiatry*, *55*, 362–368.

Arnsten, A. F. T., & Li, B. M. (2005). Neurobiology of executive functions: Catecholamine influences on prefrontal cortical functions. *Biological Psychiatry*, *57*, 1377–1384.

Asherson, P. (2005). Clinical assessment and treatment of attention deficit hyperactivity disorder in adults. *Expert Review of Neurotherapeutics*, *5*, 525–539.

Asherson, P., Kuntsi, J., & Taylor, E. (2005). Unravelling the complexity of attention-deficit hyperactivity disorder: A behavioural genomic approach. *British Journal of Psychiatry*, *187*, 103–105.

Bakker, S. C., van der Meulen, E. M., Buitelaar, J. K., Sandkuijl, L. A., Pauls, D. L., Monsuur, A. J., *et al.* (2003). A whole-genome scan in 164 Dutch sib pairs with attention-deficit/hyperactivity disorder: Suggestive evidence for linkage on chromosomes 7p and 15q. *American Journal of Human Genetics*, *72*, 1251–1260.

Baldwin, D. S., Anderson, I. M., Nutt, D. J., Bandelow, B., Bond, A., Davidson, J. R. T., *et al.* (2005). Evidence-based guidelines for the pharmacological treatment of anxiety disorders: Recommendations from the British Association of Psychopharmacology. *Journal of Psychopharmacology*, *19*, 567–596.

Baldwin, R. L., Chelonis, J. J., Flake, R. A., Edwards, M. C., Field, C. R., Meaux, J. B., *et al.* (2004). Effect of methylphenidate on time perception in children with attention-deficit/hyperactivity disorder. *Experimental and Clinical Psychopharmacology*, *12*, 57–64.

Banaschewski, T., Brandeis, D., Heinrich, H., Albrecht, B., Brunner, E., & Rothenberger, A. (2004). Questioning inhibitory control as the specific deficit of ADHD: Evidence from brain electrical activity. *Journal of Neural Transmission*, *111*, 841–864.

Banaschewski, T., Coghill, D., Santosh, P., Zuddas, A., Asherson, P., Buitelaar, J., *et al.* (2006). Long-acting medications for the hyperkinetic disorders: A systematic review and European treatment guideline. *European Child and Adolescent Psychiatry*, *15*, 476–495.

Banaschewski, T., Hollis, C., Oosterlaan, J., Roeyers, H., Rubia, K., Willcutt, E., *et al.* (2005). Towards an understanding of unique and shared pathways in the psychopathophysiology of ADHD. *Developmental Science*, *8*, 132–140.

Barkley, R. A. (1997). Behavioral inhibition, sustained attention, and executive functions: Constructing a unifying theory of ADHD. *Psychological Bulletin*, *121*, 65–94.

Barkley, R. A. (2000). *Taking charge of ADHD*. New York: Guilford Press.

Barkley, R. A. (2002). Major life activity and health outcomes associated with attention-deficit/hyperactivity disorder. *Journal of Clinical Psychiatry*, *63* (Supplement 12), 10–15.

Barkley, R. A., Fischer, M., Edelbrock, C. S., & Smallish, L. (1990). The adolescent outcome of hyperactive children diagnosed by research criteria. I. An 8-year prospective follow-up study. *Journal of the American Academy of Child and Adolescent Psychiatry*, *29*, 546–557.

Bateman, B., Warner, J. O., Hutchinson, E., Dean, T., Rowlandson, P., Gant, C., *et al.* (2004). The effects of a double blind, placebo controlled, artificial food colourings and benzoate preservative challenge on hyperactivity in a general population sample of preschool children. *Archives of Disease in Childhood*, *89*, 506–511.

Ben Amor, L., Grizenko, N., Schwartz, G., Lageix, P., Baron, C., Ter-Stepanian, M., *et al.* (2005). Perinatal complications in children with attention-deficit hyperactivity disorder and their unaffected siblings. *Journal of Psychiatry and Neuroscience*, *30*, 120–126.

Bhutta, A. T., Cleves, M. A., Casey, P. H., Cradock, M. M., & Anand, K. J. S. (2002). Cognitive and behavioral outcomes of school-aged children who were born preterm: A meta-analysis. *Journal of the American Medical Association*, *288*, 728–737.

Biederman, J., Faraone, S., Milberger, S., Guite, J., Mick, E., Chen, L., *et al.* (1996b). A prospective 4-year follow-up study of attention-deficit hyperactivity and related disorders. *Archives of General Psychiatry*, *53*, 437–446.

Biederman, J., Faraone, S. V., Milberger, S., Jetton, J. G., Chen, L., Mick, E., *et al.* (1996a). Is childhood oppositional defiant disorder a precursor to adolescent conduct disorder? Findings from a four-year follow-up study of children with ADHD. *Journal of the American Academy of Child and Adolescent Psychiatry*, *35*, 1193–1204.

Biederman, J., Mick, E., & Faraone, S. V. (2000). Age-dependent decline of symptoms of attention deficit hyperactivity disorder: Impact of remission definition and symptom type. *American Journal of Psychiatry*, *157*, 816–818.

Boonstra, A. M., Kooij, J. S. S., Oosterlaan, J., Sergeant, J. A., & Buitelaar, J. K. (2005). Does methylphenidate improve inhibition and other cognitive abilities in adults with childhood-onset ADHD? *Journal of Clinical and Experimental Neuropsychology*, *27*, 278–298.

Bor, W., Sanders, M. R., & Markie-Dadds, C. (2002). The effects of the Triple P-Positive Parenting Program on preschool children with co-occurring disruptive behavior and attentional/hyperactive difficulties. *Journal of Abnormal Child Psychology*, *30*, 571–587.

Bradie, M. (1999). Science and metaphor. *Biology and Philosophy*, *14*, 159–166.

Brookes, K. J., Mill, J., Guindalini, C., Curran, S., Xu, X. H., Knight, J., *et al.* (2006). A common haplotype of the dopamine transporter gene associated with attention-deficit/hyperactivity disorder and interacting with maternal use of alcohol during pregnancy. *Archives of General Psychiatry*, *63*, 74–81.

Brown, T. E. (1996). *Brown Attention-Deficit Disorder Scales*. San Antonio: Psychological Corporation.

Buitelaar, J. K. (2005). ADHD: Strategies to unravel its genetic architecture. *Journal of Neural Transmission*, Supplement, 1–17.

Buitelaar, J. K., Van der Gaag, R. J., Swaab-Barneveld, H., & Kuiper, M. (1995). Prediction of clinical response to methylphenidate in children with attention-deficit hyperactivity disorder. *Journal of the American Academy of Child and Adolescent Psychiatry*, *34*, 1025–1032.

Bush, G., Frazier, J. A., Rauch, S. L., Seidman, L. J., Whalen, P. J., Jenike, M. A., *et al.* (1999). Anterior cingulate cortex dysfunction in attention-deficit/hyperactivity disorder revealed by fMRI and the counting stroop. *Biological Psychiatry*, *45*, 1542–1552.

Carmody, D. P., Bendersky, M., Dunn, S. M., DeMarco, J. K., Hegyi, T., Hiatt, M., *et al.* (2006). Early risk, attention, and brain activation in adolescents born preterm. *Child Development*, *77*, 384–394.

Carrasco, X., Rothhammer, P., Moraga, M., Henriquez, H., Chakraborty, R., Aboitiz, F., *et al.* (2006). Genotypic interaction between DRD4 and DAT1 loci is a high risk factor for attention-deficit/hyperactivity disorder in Chilean families. *American Journal of Medical Genetics, Part B. Neuropsychiatric Genetics*, *141B*, 51–54.

Caspi, A., Langley, K., Milne, B., Moffitt, T. E., O' Donovan, M., Owen, M. J., *et al.* (in press). A replicated molecular genetic basis for subtyping antisocial behavior in ADHD. *Archives of General Psychiatry*.

Caspi, A., Sugden, K., Moffitt, T. E., Taylor, A., Craig, I. W., Harrington, H., *et al.* (2003). Influence of life stress on depression: Moderation by a polymorphism in the 5-HTT gene. *Science*, *301*, 386–389.

Castellanos, F. X., Lee, P. P., Sharp, W., Jeffries, N. O., Greenstein, D. K., Clasen, L. S., *et al.* (2002). Developmental trajectories of brain volume abnormalities in children and adolescents with attention-deficit/hyperactivity disorder. *Journal of the American Medical Association*, *288*, 1740–1748.

Castellanos, F. X., & Tannock, R. (2002). Neuroscience of attention-deficit/hyperactivity disorder: The search for endophenotypes. *Nature Reviews Neuroscience*, *3*, 617–628.

Castellanos, X., Sonuga-Barke, E. J. S., Tannock, R., & Milham, M. (2006). Characterizing cognition in ADHD: Beyond executive dysfunction. *Trends in Cognitive Science*, *10*, 117–123.

Collishaw, S., Maughan, B., Goodman, R., & Pickles, A. (2004). Time trends in adolescent mental health. *Journal of Child Psychology and Psychiatry*, *45*, 1350–1362.

Comings, D. E. (2001). Clinical and molecular genetics of ADHD and Tourette syndrome: Two related polygenic disorders. *Annals of the New York Academy of Sciences*, *931*, 50–83.

Comings, D. E., Chen, T. J., Blum, K., Mengucci, J. F., Blum, S. H., & Meshkin, B. (2005). Neurogenetic interactions and aberrant behavioral co-morbidity of attention deficit hyperactivity disorder (ADHD): Dispelling myths. *Theoretical Biology and Medical Modelling*, *2*, 50.

Conners, C. K., Erhardt, D., Sparrow, E., & Conners, M. A. (1998). *CAARS Adult ADHD Rating Scales*. New York, NY: Multi Health Systems.

Dalen, L., Sonuga-Barke, E. J., Hall, M., & Remington, B. (2004). Inhibitory deficits, delay aversion and preschool AD/HD: Implications for the dual pathway model. *Neural Plasticity*, *11*, 1–11.

Danckaerts, M., Heptinstall, E., Chadwick, O., & Taylor, E. (2000). A natural history of hyperactivity and conduct problems: Self-reported outcome. *European Child and Adolescent Psychiatry*, *9*, 26–38.

de Nijs, P. F., Ferdinand, R. F., & Verhulst, F. C. (2007). No hyperactive-impulsive subtype in teacher-rated attention-deficit/hyperactivity problems. *European Child and Adolescent Psychiatry*, *16*, 25–32.

Denckla, M. B. (2002). Attention Deficit Hyperactivity Disorder: Spectrum and mechanisms. In A. K. Asbury, G. M. McKhann, W. I. McDonald, P. J. Goadsby, & J. C. McArthur (Eds.), *Diseases of the Nervous System: Clinical Neuroscience and Therapeutic Principles* (3rd edn., Volume 1, pp. 422–430). New York: Cambridge University Press.

Dick, D. M., Viken, R. J., Kaprio, J., Pulkkinen, L., & Rose, R. J. (2005). Understanding the covariation among childhood externalizing symptoms: Genetic and environmental influences on conduct disorder, attention deficit hyperactivity disorder, and oppositional defiant disorder symptoms. *Journal of Abnormal Child Psychology*, *33*, 219–229.

Doyle, A. E., Faraone, S. V., Seidman, L. J., Willcutt, E. G., Nigg, J. T., Waldman, I. D., *et al.* (2005). Are endophenotypes based on measures of executive functions useful for molecular genetic studies of ADHD? *Journal of Child Psychology and Psychiatry*, *46*, 774–803.

Durston, S., Pol, H. E. H., Schnack, H. G., Buitelaar, J. K., Steenhuis, M. P., Minderaa, R. B., *et al.* (2004). Magnetic resonance imaging of boys with attention-deficit/hyperactivity disorder and their unaffected siblings. *Journal of the American Academy of Child and Adolescent Psychiatry*, *43*, 332–340.

Durston, S., Tottenham, N. T., Thomas, K. M., Davidson, M. C., Eigsti, I. M., Yang, Y. H., *et al.* (2003). Differential patterns of striatal activation in young children with and without ADHD. *Biological Psychiatry*, *53*, 871–878.

Elliott, R., Sahakian, B. J., Matthews, K., Bannerjea, A., Rimmer, J., & Robbins, T. W. (1997). Effects of methylphenidate on spatial working memory and planning in healthy young adults. *Psychopharmacology*, *131*, 196–206.

Ernst, M., Kimes, A. S., London, E. D., Matochik, J. A., Eldreth, D., Tata, S., *et al.* (2003). Neural substrates of decision making in adults with attention deficit hyperactivity disorder. *American Journal of Psychiatry*, *160*, 1061–1070.

Fallgatter, A. J., Ehlis, A. C., Rosler, M., Strik, W. K., Blocher, D., & Herrmann, M. J. (2005). Diminished prefrontal brain function in adults with psychopathology in childhood related to attention deficit hyperactivity disorder. *Psychiatry Research*, *138*, 157–169.

Faraone, S., Chen, W., Warburton, R., Biederman, J., Milberger, S., & Tsuang, M. (1995). Genetic heterogeneity in attention-deficit hyperactivity disorder (ADHD): Gender, psychiatric comorbidity, and maternal ADHD. *Journal of Abnormal Psychology*, *104*, 334–345.

Faraone, S. V. (2004). Genetics of adult attention-deficit/hyperactivity disorder. *Psychiatric Clinics of North America*, *27*, 303–321.

Faraone, S. V., & Biederman, J. (2000). Nature, nurture, and attention deficit hyperactivity disorder. *Developmental Review*, *20*, 568–581.

Faraone, S. V., Biederman, J., Mennin, D., Gershon, J., & Tsuang, M. T. (1996). A prospective four-year follow-up study of children at risk for ADHD: Psychiatric, neuropsychological, and psychosocial outcome. *Journal of the American Academy of Child and Adolescent Psychiatry*, *35*, 1449–1459.

Faraone, S. V., Biederman, J., & Mick, E. (2006). The age-dependent decline of attention deficit hyperactivity disorder: A meta-analysis of follow-up studies. *Psychological Medicine*, *36*, 159–165.

Faraone, S. V., Perlis, R. H., Doyle, A. E., Smoller, J. W., Goralnick, J. J., Holmgren, M. A., *et al.* (2005). Molecular genetics of attention-deficit/hyperactivity disorder. *Biological Psychiatry*, *57*, 1313–1323.

Faraone, S. V., Spencer, T., Aleardi, M., Pagano, C., & Biederman, J. (2004). Meta-analysis of the efficacy of methylphenidate for treating adult attention-deficit/hyperactivity disorder. *Journal of Clinical Psychopharmacology*, *24*, 24–29.

Farrington, D. P. (1995). The Twelfth Jack Tizard Memorial Lecture. The development of offending and antisocial behaviour from childhood: Key findings from the Cambridge Study in Delinquent Development. *Journal of Child Psychology and Psychiatry*, *36*, 929–964.

Fergusson, D. M., & Horwood, L. J. (1995). Predictive validity of categorically and dimensionally scored measures of disruptive childhood behaviors. *Journal of the American Academy of Child and Adolescent Psychiatry*, *34*, 477–485.

Gainetdinov, R. R., Wetsel, W. C., Jones, S. R., Levin, E. D., Jaber, M., & Caron, M. G. (1999). Role of serotonin in the paradoxical calming effect of psychostimulants on hyperactivity. *Science*, *283*, 397–401.

Geurts, H. M., Verte, S., Oosterlaan, J., Roeyers, H., & Sergeant, J. A. (2005). ADHD subtypes: Do they differ in their executive functioning profile? *Archives of Clinical Neuropsychology*, *20*, 457–477.

Gjone, H., Stevenson, J., & Sundet, J. M. (1996). Genetic influence on parent-reported attention-related problems in a Norwegian general population twin sample. *Journal of the American Academy of Child and Adolescent Psychiatry*, *35*, 588–596.

Glod, C. A., & Teicher, M. H. (1996). Relationship between early abuse, posttraumatic stress disorder, and activity levels in prepubertal children. *Journal of the American Academy of Child and Adolescent Psychiatry*, *35*, 1384–1393.

Hebebrand, J., Dempfle, A., Saar, K., Thiele, H., Herpertz-Dahlmann, B., Linder, M., *et al.* (2006). A genome-wide scan for attention-deficit/hyperactivity disorder in 155 German sib-pairs. *Molecular Psychiatry*, *11*, 196–205.

Hechtman, L., & Weiss, G. (1983). Long-term outcome of hyperactive children. *American Journal of Orthopsychiatry*, *53*, 532–541.

Hechtman, L., & Weiss, G. (1986). Controlled prospective fifteen-year follow-up of hyperactives as adults: Non-medical drug and alcohol use and anti-social behaviour. *American Journal of Orthopsychiatry*, *54*, 415–425.

Heptinstall, E., & Taylor, E. (2002). Sex differences and their significance. In S. Sandberg (Ed.), *Hyperactivity and attention disorders of childhood*. Cambridge: Cambridge University Press.

Hill, J. C., & Schoener, E. P. (1996). Age-dependent decline of attention deficit hyperactivity disorder. *American Journal of Psychiatry*, *153*, 1143–1146.

Ho, T. P., Luk, E. S. L., Leung, P. W. L., Taylor, E., Mak, F. L. & Bacon-Shone, J. (1996). Situational versus pervasive hyperactivity in a community sample. *Psychological Medicine*, *26*, 309–321.

Huang-Pollock, C. L., & Nigg, J. T. (2003). Searching for the attention deficit in attention deficit hyperactivity disorder: The case of visuospatial orienting. *Clinical Psychology Review*, *23*, 801–830.

Huang-Pollock, C. L., Nigg, J. T., & Carr, T. H. (2005). Deficient attention is hard to find: Applying the perceptual load model of selective attention to attention deficit hyperactivity disorder subtypes. *Journal of Child Psychology and Psychiatry*, *46*, 1211–1218.

Kahn, R. S., Khoury, J., Nichols, W. C., & Lanphear, B. P. (2003). Role of dopamine transporter genotype and maternal prenatal smoking in childhood hyperactive-impulsive, inattentive, and oppositional behaviors. *Journal of Pediatrics*, *143*, 104–110.

Kapoor, A., Dunn, E., Kostaki, A., Andrews, M. H., & Matthews, S. G. (2006). Fetal programming of hypothalamo-pituitary-adrenal function: Prenatal stress and glucocorticoids. *Journal of Physiology*, *572*, 31–44.

Kempton, S., Vance, A., Maruff, P., Luk, E., Costin, J., & Pantelis, C. (1999). Executive function and attention deficit hyperactivity disorder: Stimulant medication and better executive function performance in children. *Psychological Medicine*, *29*, 527–538.

Kendler, K. S., & Baker, J. H. (2007). Genetic influences on measures of the environment: A systematic review. *Psychological Medicine*, *37*, 615–626.

Kessler, R. C., Adler, L., Ames, M., Demler, O., Faraone, S., Hiripi, E., *et al.* (2005). The World Health Organization Adult ADHD Self-Report Scale (ASRS): A short screening scale for use in the general population. *Psychological Medicine*, *35*, 245–256.

Kessler, R. C., Adler, L., Barkley, R., Biederman, J., Conners, C. K., Demler, O., *et al.* (2006). Prevalence of adult ADHD in the United States: Results from the National Comorbidity Survey Replication (NCS-R). *American Journal of Psychiatry*, *163*, 716–723.

Klein, C., Fischer, B., Fischer, B., & Hartnegg, K. (2002). Effects of methylphenidate on saccadic responses in patients with ADHD. *Experimental Brain Research*, *145*, 121–125.

Klein, R. G., & Mannuzza, S. (1991). Long-term outcome of hyperactive children: A review. *Journal of the American Academy of Child and Adolescent Psychiatry*, *30*, 383–387.

Klingberg, T., Fernell, E., Olesen, P. J., Johnson, M., Gustafsson, P., Dahlstrom, K., *et al.* (2005). Computerized training of working memory in children with ADHD: A randomized, controlled trial. *Journal of the American Academy of Child and Adolescent Psychiatry*, *44*, 177–186.

Knopik, V. S., Heath, A. C., Jacob, T., Slutske, W. S., Bucholz, K. K., Madden, P. A., *et al.* (2006). Maternal alcohol use disorder and offspring ADHD: Disentangling genetic and environmental effects using a children-of-twins design. *Psychological Medicine*, *36*, 1461–1471.

Konofal, E., Lecendreux, M., Arnulf, I., & Mouren, M. C. (2004). Iron deficiency in children with attention-deficit/hyperactivity disorder. *Archives of Pediatrics and Adolescent Medicine*, *158*, 1113–1115.

Kratochvil, C. J., Egger, H., Greenhill, L. L., & McGough, J. J. (2006). Pharmacological management of preschool ADHD. *Journal of the American Academy of Child and Adolescent Psychiatry*, *45*, 115–118.

Kreppner, J. M., O'Connor, T. G., & Rutter, M. (2001). Can inattention/overactivity be an institutional deprivation syndrome? *Journal of Abnormal Child Psychology*, *29*, 513–528.

Lahey, B. B., Pelham, W. E., Chronis, A., Massetti, G., Kipp, H., Ehrhardt, A., *et al.* (2006). Predictive validity of ICD-10 hyperkinetic disorder relative to DSM-IV attention-deficit/hyperactivity disorder among younger children. *Journal of Child Psychology and Psychiatry*, *47*, 472–479.

Lahey, B. B., Pelham, W. E., Loney, J., Kipp, H., Ehrhardt, A., Lee, S. S., *et al.* (2004). Three-year predictive validity of DSM-IV attention deficit hyperactivity disorder in children diagnosed at 4–6 years of age. *American Journal of Psychiatry*, *161*, 2014–2020.

Levitt, M. (1999). Toxic metals, preconception and early childhood development. *Social Science Information*, *38*, 179–201.

Levy, F., & Swanson, J. M. (2001). Timing, space and ADHD: The dopamine theory revisited. *Australian and New Zealand Journal of Psychiatry*, *35*, 504–511.

Lijffijt, M., Kenemans, J. L., Verbaten, M. N., & van Engeland, H. (2005). A meta-analytic review of stopping performance in attention-deficit/hyperactivity disorder: Deficient inhibitory motor control? *Journal of Abnormal Psychology*, *114*, 216–222.

Linares, T. J., Singer, L. T., Kirchner, H. L., Short, E. J., Min, M. O., Hussey, P., *et al.* (2006). Mental health outcomes of cocaine-exposed children at 6 years of age. *Journal of Pediatric Psychology*, *31*, 85–97.

Linnet, K. M., Dalsgaard, S., Obel, C., Wisborg, K., Henriksen, T. B., Rodriguez, A., *et al.* (2003). Maternal lifestyle factors in pregnancy risk of attention deficit hyperactivity disorder and associated behaviors: Review of the current evidence. *American Journal of Psychiatry*, *160*, 1028–1040.

Liprando, L. A., Miner, L. H., Blakely, R. D., Lewis, D. A., & Sesack, S. R. (2004). Ultrastructural interactions between terminals expressing the norepinephrine transporter and dopamine neurons in the rat and monkey ventral tegmental area. *Synapse*, *52*, 233–244.

Loge, D., Staton, R., & Beatty, W. (1990). Performance of children with ADHD on tests sensitive to frontal-lobe dysfunction. *Journal of the American Academy of Child and Adolescent Psychiatry*, *29*, 540–545.

Madras, B. K., Miller, G. M., & Fischman, A. J. (2002). The dopamine transporter: Relevance to attention deficit hyperactivity disorder (ADHD). *Behavioural Brain Research*, *130*, 57–63.

Madras, B. K., Miller, G. M., & Fischman, A. I. (2005). The dopamine transporter and attention-deficit/hyperactivity disorder. *Biological Psychiatry*, *57*, 1397–1409.

Manly, T., Anderson, V., Nimmo-Smith, I., Turner, A., Watson, P., & Robertson, I. H. (2001). The differential assessment of children's attention: The Test of Everyday Attention for Children (TEA-Ch), normative sample and ADHD performance. *Journal of Child Psychology and Psychiatry*, *42*, 1065–1081.

Mannuzza, S., Klein, R. G., Bessler, A., Malloy, P., & LaPadula, M. (1998). Adult psychiatric status of hyperactive boys grown up. *American Journal of Psychiatry*, *155*, 493–498.

Mariussen, E., & Fonnum, F. (2006). Neurochernical targets and behavioral effects of organohalogen compounds: An update. *Critical Reviews in Toxicology*, *36*, 253–289.

McCann, D., Barrett, A., Cooper, A., Crumpler, D., Dalen, L., Grimshaw, H. *et al.*, (2007). Food additives and hyperactive behaviour in 3-year-old and 8/9-year-old children in the community: a randomized, double-blinded, placebo controlled trial. *The Lancet*, *370(9598)*, 1560–1567.

Mehta, M. A., Goodyer, I. M., & Sahakian, B. J. (2004). Methylphenidate improves working memory and set-shifting in AD/HD: Relationships to baseline memory capacity. *Journal of Child Psychology and Psychiatry*, *45*, 293–305.

Mehta, M. A., Owen, A. M., Sahakian, B. J., Mavaddat, N., Pickard, J. D., & Robbins, T. W. (2000). Methylphenidate enhances working memory by modulating discrete frontal and parietal lobe regions in the human brain. *Journal of Neuroscience*, *20*, RC65.

Meltzer, H., & Gatward, R. (with Goodman, R., & Ford, T.). (2000). *Mental health of children and adolesdents in Great Britain*. London: The Stationery Office.

Mick, E., Faraone, S. V., & Biederman, J. (2004). Age-dependent expression of attention-deficit/hyperactivity disorder symptoms. *Psychiatric Clinics of North America*, *27*, 215–224.

Mill, J., Caspi, A., Williams, B. S., Craig, I., Taylor, A., Polo-Tomas, M., *et al.* (2006). Prediction of heterogeneity in intelligence and adult prognosis by genetic polymorphisms in the dopamine system among children with attention-deficit/hyperactivity disorder: Evidence from 2 birth cohorts. *Archives of General Psychiatry*, *63*, 462–469.

Miller, A., Lee, S. K., Raina, P., *et al.* (1998). *A review of therapies for attention-deficit/hyperactivity disorder*. Ottawa, ON: Canadian Coordinating Office for Health Technology Assessment.

Millstein, R., Wilens, T., Biederman, J., & Spencer, T. (1998). Presenting ADHD symptoms and subtypes in clinically referred adults with ADHD. *Attention*, *2*, 159–166.

Morrell, J., & Murray, L. (2003). Parenting and the development of conduct disorder and hyperactive symptoms in childhood: a prospective longitudinal study from 2 months to 8 years. *Journal of Child Psychology and Psychiatry*, *44*, 489–508.

MTA Cooperative Group. (1999). A 14-month randomized clinical trial of treatment strategies for attention-deficit/hyperactivity disorder. Multimodal Treatment Study of Children with ADHD. *Archives of General Psychiatry*, *56*, 1073–1086.

Murray, C., & Johnston, C. (2006). Parenting in mothers with and without attention-deficit/hyperactivity disorder. *Journal of Abnormal Psychology*, *115*, 52–61.

Nadder, T. S., Rutter, M., Silberg, J. L., Maes, H. H., & Eaves, L. J. (2002). Genetic effects on the variation and covariation of attention deficit-hyperactivity disorder (ADHD) and oppositional-defiant disorder/conduct disorder (ODD/CD) symptomatologies across informant and occasion of measurement. *Psychological Medicine*, *32*, 39–53.

National Institute for Health and Clinical Excellence (NICE). (2005). *Methylphenidate, atomoxetine and dexamfetamine for the treatment of attention deficit hyperactivity disorder in children and adolescents*. Retrieved from http://guidance.nice.org.uk/TA98 27/09/07.

Nigg, J. T., Willcutt, E. G., Doyle, A. E., & Sonuga-Barke, E. J. S. (2005). Causal heterogeneity in attention-deficit/hyperactivity disorder: Do we need neuropsychologically impaired subtypes? *Biological Psychiatry*, *57*, 1224–1230.

O'Connor, T. G., Heron, J., Golding, J., & Glover, V. (2003). Maternal antenatal anxiety and behavioural/emotional problems in children: A test of a programming hypothesis. *Journal of Child Psychology and Psychiatry*, *44*, 1025–1036.

Olfson, M., Gameroff, M. J., Marcus, S. C., & Jensen, P. S. (2003). National trends in the treatment of attention deficit hyperactivity disorder. *American Journal of Psychiatry*, *160*, 1071–1077.

Olijslagers, J. E., Werkman, T. R., McCreary, A. C., Kruse, C. G., & Wadman, W. J. (2006). Modulation of midbrain dopamine neurotransmission by serotonin, a versatile interaction between neurotransmitters and significance for antipsychotic drug action. *Current Neuropharmacology*, *4*, 59–68.

Oosterlaan, J., Logan, G. D., & Sergeant, J. A. (1998). Response inhibition in AD/HD, CD, comorbid AD/HD + CD, anxious, and control children: A meta-analysis of studies with the stop task. *Journal of Child Psychology and Psychiatry*, *39*, 411–425.

Ostrander, R., & Herman, K. C. (2006). Potential cognitive, parenting, and developmental mediators of the relationship between ADHD and depression. *Journal of Consulting and Clinical Psychology*, *74*, 89–98.

Pauls, D. L., Hurst, C. R., Kruger, S. D., Leckman, J. F., Kidd, K. K., & Cohen, D. J. (1986). Gilles de la Tourette's syndrome and attention deficit disorder with hyperactivity. Evidence against a genetic relationship. *Archives of General Psychiatry*, *43*, 1177–1179.

Plessen, K. J., Bansal, R., Zhu, H. T., Whiteman, R., Amat, J., Quackenbush, G. A., *et al.* (2006). Hippocampus and amygdala morphology in attention-deficit/hyperactivity disorder. *Archives of General Psychiatry*, *63*, 795–807.

Pliszka, S. R. (2000). Patterns of psychiatric comorbidity with attention-deficit/hyperactivity disorder. *Child and Adolescent Psychiatric Clinics of North America*, *9*, 525–540.

Pliszka, S. R. (2005). The neuropsychopharmacology of attention-deficit/hyperactivity disorder. *Biological Psychiatry*, *57*, 1385–1390.

Rapoport, J. L., Buchsbaum, M. S., Weingartner, H., Zahn, T. P., Ludlow, C., & Mikkelsen, E. J. (1980). Dextroamphetamine: Its cognitive and behavioral effects in normal and hyperactive boys and normal men. *Archives of General Psychiatry*, *37*, 933–943.

Rasmussen, E. R., Neuman, R. J., Heath, A. C., Levy, F., Hay, D. A., & Todd, R. D. (2004). Familial clustering of latent class and DSM-IV defined attention-deficit/hyperactivity disorder (ADHD) subtypes. *Journal of Child Psychology and Psychiatry*, *45*, 589–598.

Research Units on Pediatric Psychopharmacology Autism Network. (2005). Randomized, controlled, crossover trial of methylphenidate in pervasive developmental disorders with hyperactivity. *Archives of General Psychiatry*, *62*, 1266–1274.

Rhodes, S. M., Coghill, D. R., & Matthews, K. (2004). Methylphenidate restores visual memory, but not working memory function in attention deficit-hyperkinetic disorder. *Psychopharmacology*, *175*, 319–330.

Richardson, A. J., & Montgomery, P. (2005). The Oxford–Durham study: A randomized, controlled trial of dietary supplementation with fatty acids in children with developmental coordination disorder. *Pediatrics*, *115*, 1360–1366.

Rietveld, M. J. H., Hudziak, J. J., Bartels, M., van Beijsterveldt, C. E. M., & Boomsma, D. I. (2003). Heritability of attention problems in children. I. Cross-sectional results from a study of twins, age 3–12 years. *American Journal of Medical Genetics, Part B. Neuropsychiatric Genetics*, *117B*, 102–113.

Rodriguez, A., & Bohlin, G. (2005). Are maternal smoking and stress during pregnancy related to ADHD symptoms in children? *Journal of Child Psychology and Psychiatry*, *46*, 246–254.

Rosler, M., Retz, W., Retz-Junginger, P., Hengesch, G., Schneider, M., Supprian, T., *et al.* (2004). Prevalence of attention-deficit/hyperactivity disorder (ADHD) and comorbid disorders in young male prison inmates. *European Archives of Psychiatry and Clinical Neuroscience*, *254*, 365–371.

Rubia, K., Overmeyer, S., Taylor, E., Brammer, M., Williams, S. C. R., Simmons, A., *et al.* (1999). Hypofrontality in attention deficit hyperactivity disorder during higher-order motor control: A study with functional MRI. *American Journal of Psychiatry*, *156*, 891–896.

Rubia, K., Smith, A. B., Brammer, M. J., Toone, B., & Taylor, E. (2005). Abnormal brain activation during inhibition and error detection in medication-naive adolescents with ADHD. *American Journal of Psychiatry*, *162*, 1067–1075.

Russell, V. A. (2002). Hypodopaminergic and hypernoradrenergic activity in prefrontal cortex slices of an animal model for attention-deficit hyperactivity disorder: The spontaneously hypertensive rat. *Behavioural Brain Research*, *130*, 191–196.

Rutter, M. (2002). The interplay of nature, nurture, and developmental influences: The challenge ahead for mental health. *Archives of General Psychiatry*, *59*, 996–1000.

Rutter, M., Moffitt, T. E., & Caspi, A. (2006). Gene–environment interplay and psychopathology: Multiple varieties but real effects. *Journal of Child Psychology and Psychiatry*, *47*, 226–261.

Rutter, M., Maughan, B., Meyer, J., Pickles, A., Silberg, J., Simonoff, E., *et al.* (1997). Heterogeneity of antisocial behavior: Causes, continuities, and consequences. In D. W. Osgood (Ed.), *Motivation and delinquency* (pp. 45–118). Lincoln, NE: University of Nebraska Press; and *Nebraska Symposium on Motivation*, *44*, 45–118.

Safer, D. J., & Zito, J. M. (2000). Pharmacoepidemiology of methylphenidate and other stimulants for the treatment of ADHD. In L. L. Greenhill, & B. B. Osman (Eds.), *Ritalin: Theory and practice* (pp. 7–26). Larchmont, NY: MA Liebert.

Sagvolden, T., Johansen, E. B., Aase, H., & Russell, V. A. (2005). A dynamic developmental theory of attention-deficit/hyperactivity disorder (ADHD) predominantly hyperactive/impulsive and combined subtypes. *Behavioral Brain Science*, *28*, 397–419.

Santosh, P. J., Taylor, E., Swanson, J., Wigal, T., Chuang, S., Davies, M., *et al.* (2005). Refining the diagnoses of inattention and overactivity syndromes: A reanalysis of the Multimodal Treatment study of attention deficit hyperactivity disorder (ADHD) based on

ICD-10 criteria for hyperkinetic disorder. *Clinical Neuroscience Research*, *5*, 307–314.

Sayal, K., Taylor, E., Beecham, J., & Byrne, P. (2002). Pathways to care in children at risk of attention-deficit hyperactivity disorder. *British Journal of Psychiatry*, *181*, 43–48.

Schab, D. W., & Trinh, N. H. T. (2004). Do artificial food colors promote hyperactivity in children with hyperactive syndromes? A meta-analysis of double-blind placebo-controlled trials. *Journal of Developmental and Behavioral Pediatrics*, *25*, 423–434.

Scheres, A., Dijkstra, M., Ainslie, E., Balkan, J., Reynolds, B., Sonuga-Barke, E., *et al.* (2006). Temporal and probabilistic discounting of rewards in children and adolescents: Effects of age and ADHD symptoms. *Neuropsychologia*, *44*, 2092–2103.

Schweitzer, J. B., Lee, D. O., Hanford, R. B., Tagamets, M. A., Hoffman, J. M., Grafton, S. T., *et al.* (2003). A positron emission tomography study of methylphenidate in adults with ADHD: Alterations in resting blood flow and predicting treatment response. *Neuropsychopharmacology*, *28*, 967–973.

Seeger, G., Schloss, P., Schmidt, M. H., Ruter-Jungfleisch, A., & Henn, F. A. (2004). Gene–environment interaction in hyperkinetic conduct disorder (HD + CD) as indicated by season of birth variations in dopamine receptor (DRD4) gene polymorphism. *Neuroscience Letters*, *366*, 282–286.

Seidman, L. J., Valera, E. M., & Makris, N. (2005). Structural brain imaging of attention-deficit/hyperactivity disorder. *Biological Psychiatry*, *57*, 1263–1272.

Seipp, C. M., & Johnston, C. (2005). Mother–son interactions in families of boys with attention-deficit/hyperactivity disorder with and without oppositional behavior. *Journal of Abnormal Child Psychology*, *33*, 87–98.

Sergeant, J. A. (2005). Modeling attention-deficit/hyperactivity disorder: A critical appraisal of the cognitive-energetic model. *Biological Psychiatry*, *57*, 1248–1255.

Shaw, P., Lerch, J., Greenstein, D., Sharp, W., Clasen, L., Evans, A., *et al.* (2006). Longitudinal mapping of cortical thickness and clinical outcome in children and adolescents with attention-deficit/hyperactivity disorder. *Archives of General Psychiatry*, *63*, 540–549.

Smalley, S. L., Kustanovich, V., Minassian, S. L., Stone, J. L., Ogdie, M. N., McGough, J. J., McCracken, J. T., *et al.* (2002). Genetic linkage of attention-deficit/hyperactivity disorder on chromosome 16p13, in a region implicated in autism. *American Journal of Human Genetics*, *71*, 959–963.

Solanto, M. V., Abikoff, H., Sonuga-Barke, E. J. S., Schachar, R., Logan, G. D., Wigal, T., *et al.* (2001). The ecological validity of measures related to impulsiveness in AD/HD. *Journal of Abnormal Child Psychology*, *29*, 215–228.

Sonuga-Barke, E. J. (2005). Causal models of attention-deficit/hyperactivity disorder: From common simple deficits to multiple developmental pathways. *Biological Psychiatry*, *57*, 1231–1238.

Sonuga-Barke, E. J. S. (1998). Categorical model in child psychopathology: A conceptual and empirical analysis. *Journal of Child Psychology and Psychiatry*, *39*, 115–133.

Sonuga-Barke, E. J. S., Daley, D., Thompson, M., Laver-Bradbury, C., & Weeks, A. (2001). Parent-based therapies for preschool attention-deficit/hyperactivity disorder: A randomized, controlled trial with a community sample. *Journal of the American Academy of Child and Adolescent Psychiatry*, *40*, 402–408.

Spencer, T. J., Biederman, J., Madras, B. K., Faraone, S. V., Dougherty, D. D., Bonab, A. A., *et al.* (2005). *In vivo* neuroreceptor imaging in attention-deficit/hyperactivity disorder: A focus on the dopamine transporter. *Biological Psychiatry*, *57*, 1293–1300.

Spencer, T., Biederman, J., Wilens, T., Harding, M., O'Donnell, D., & Griffin, S. (1996). Pharmacotherapy of attention-deficit/hyperactivity disorder across the life cycle. *Journal of the American Academy of Child and Adolescent Psychiatry*, *35*, 409–432.

Sprich, S., Biederman, J., Crawford, M. H., Mundy, E., & Faraone, S. V. (2000). Adoptive and biological families of children and adolescents with ADHD. *Journal of the American Academy of Child and Adolescent Psychiatry*, *39*, 1432–1437.

Stawicki, J. A., Nigg, J. T., & von Eye, A. (2006). Family psychiatric history evidence on the nosological relations of DSM-IV ADHD combined and inattentive subtypes: New data and meta-analysis. *Journal of Child Psychology and Psychiatry*, *47*, 935–945.

Stein, M. T., & Perrin, J. M. (2003). Diagnosis and treatment of ADHD in school-age children in primary care settings: A synopsis of the AAP Practice Guidelines. *Pediatrics in Review*, *24*, 92–98.

Steinhausen, H. C., Losche, G., Koch, S., & Helge, H. (1994). The psychological development of children of epileptic parents. I. Study design and comparative findings. *Acta Paediatrica*, *83*, 955–960.

Stevens, S., Sonuga-Barke, E. J. S., Kreppner, J., Beckett, C., Castle, J., Colvert, E., *et al.* (in press). Inattention/overactivity following early severe institutional deprivation: Presentations and associations in early adolescence. *Journal Abnormal Child Psychology*.

Stevenson, J., & Cate, I. P. (2004). The nature of hyperactivity in children and adolescents with hydrocephalus: A test of the dual pathway model. *Neural Plasticity*, *11*, 13–21.

Swanson, J. M., Sergeant, J., Taylor, E., Sonuga-Barke, E., Jensen, P. S., & Cantwell, D. (1998). Attention deficit hyperactivity disorder and hyperkinetic disorder. *Lancet*, *351*, 429–433.

Tamm, L., Menon, V., Ringel, J., & Reiss, A. L. (2004). Event-related fMRI evidence of frontotemporal involvement in aberrant response inhibition and task switching in attention-deficit/hyperactivity disorder. *Journal of the American Academy of Child and Adolescent Psychiatry*, *43*, 1430–1440.

Taylor, E. (1998). Clinical foundations of hyperactivity research. *Behavioural Brain Research*, *94*, 11–24.

Taylor, E. (1999). Developmental neuropsychopathology of attention deficit and impulsiveness. *Development and Psychopathology*, *11*, 607–628.

Taylor, E., Chadwick, O., Heptinstall, E., & Danckaerts, M. (1996). Hyperactivity and conduct problems as risk factors for adolescent development. *Journal of the American Academy of Child and Adolescent Psychiatry*, *35*, 1213–1226.

Taylor, E., Dopfner, M., Sergeant, J., Asherson, P., Banaschewski, T., Buitelaar, J., *et al.* (2004). European clinical guidelines for hyperkinetic disorder: First upgrade. *European Child and Adolescent Psychiatry*, *13* (Supplement 1), 17–30.

Taylor, E., Sandberg, S., Thorley, G., & Giles, S. (1991). *The epidemiology of childhood hyperactivity*. Maudsley Monograph No. 33. Oxford: Oxford University Press.

Taylor, E., & Warner-Rogers, J. (2005). Practitioner review: Early adversity and developmental disorders. *Journal of Child Psychology and Psychiatry*, *46*, 451–467.

Taylor, E. A., Everitt, B., Thorley, G., Schachar, R., Rutter, M., & Wieselberg, M. (1986). Conduct disorder and hyperactivity. II. A cluster analytic approach to the identification of a behavioural syndrome. *British Journal of Psychiatry*, *149*, 768–777.

Taylor, E. A., Schachar, R., Thorley, G., Wieselberg, H. M., Everitt, B., & Rutter, M. (1987). Which boys respond to stimulant medication? A controlled trial of methylphenidate in boys with disruptive behaviour. *Psychological Medicine*, *17*, 121–143.

Thapar, A., Fowler, T., Rice, F., Scourfield, J., van den Bree, M., Thomas, H., *et al.* (2003). Maternal smoking during pregnancy and attention deficit hyperactivity disorder symptoms in offspring. *American Journal of Psychiatry*, *160*, 1985–1989.

Thapar, A., Harrington, R., Ross, K., & McGuffin, P. (2000). Does the definition of ADHD affect heritability? *Journal of the American Academy of Child and Adolescent Psychiatry*, *39*, 1528–1536.

Thapar, A., Langley, K., Fowler, T., Rice, F., Turic, D., Whittinger, N., *et al.* (2005b). Catechol O-methyltransferase gene variant and birth weight predict early-onset antisocial behavior in children with attention-deficit/hyperactivity disorder. *Archives of General Psychiatry*, *62*, 1275–1278.

Thapar, A., O'Donovan, M., & Owen, M. J. (2005a). The genetics of attention deficit hyperactivity disorder. *Human Molecular Genetics*, *14*, R275–R282.

Thapar, A., Harrington, R., & McGuffin, P. (2001). Examining the comorbidity of ADHD related behaviours and conduct problems using a twin study design. *British Journal of Psychiatry*, *179*, 224–229.

Tian, L., Jiang, T., Wang, Y., Zang, Y., He, Y., Liang, M., *et al.* (2006). Altered resting-state functional connectivity patterns of anterior cingulated cortex in adolescents with attention deficit hyperactivity disorder. *Neuroscience Letters*, *400*, 39–43.

Timmann, D., Richter, S., Schoch, B., & Frings, M. (2006). Cerebellum and cognition: A review of the literature. *Aktuelle Neurologie*, *33*, 70–80.

Todd, R. D. (2000). Genetics of attention deficit/hyperactivity disorder: Are we ready for molecular genetic studies? *American Journal of Medical Genetics*, *96*, 241–243.

Todd, R. D., Sitdhiraksa, N., Reich, W., Ji, T. H., Joyner, C. A., Heath, A. C., *et al.* (2002). Discrimination of DSM-IV and latent class attention-deficit/hyperactivity disorder subtypes by educational and cognitive performance in a population based sample of child and adolescent twins. *Journal of the American Academy of Child and Adolescent Psychiatry*, *41*, 820–828.

Toplak, M. E., Dockstader, C., & Tannock, R. (2006). Temporal information processing in ADHD: Findings to date and new methods. *Journal of Neuroscience Methods*, *151*, 15–29.

Turner, D. C., Blackwell, A. D., Dowson, J. H., McLean, A., & Sahakian, B. J. (2005). Neurocognitive effects of methylphenidate in adult attention-deficit/hyperactivity disorder. *Psychopharmacology*, *178*, 286–295.

Tymms, P., & Merrell, C. (2005). *Screening and interventions for inattentive, hyperactive and impulsive young children.* Research report to the Economic and Social Research Council (ESRC).

Vaidya, C. J., Bunge, S. A., Dudukovic, N. M., & Zalecki, C. A. (2005). Altered neural substrates of cognitive control in childhood ADHD: Evidence from functional magnetic resonance imaging. *American Journal of Psychiatry*, *162*, 1605–1613.

Volkow, N. D., & Swanson, J. M. (2003). Variables that affect the clinical use and abuse of methylphenidate in the treatment of ADHD. *American Journal of Psychiatry*, *160*, 1909–1918.

Volkow, N. D., Wang, G. J., Fowler, J. S., & Ding, Y. S. (2005). Imaging the effect of methylphenidate on brain dopamine: New model on its therapeutic actions for attention-deficit/hyperactivity disorder. *Biological Psychiatry*, *57*, 1410–1415.

Volkow, N. D., Wang, G. J., Fowler, J. S., Telang, F., Maynard, L., Logan, J., *et al.* (2004). Evidence that methylphenidate enhances the saliency of a mathematical task by increasing dopamine in the human brain. *American Journal of Psychiatry*, *161*, 1173–1180.

Ward, M. F., Wender, P. H., & Reimherr, F. W. (1993). The Wender Utah Rating Scale: An aid in the retrospective diagnosis of childhood attention deficit hyperactivity disorder. *American Journal of Psychiatry*, *150*, 885–890. Erratum in: *150*, 1280.

Warner-Rogers, J., Taylor, A., Taylor, E., & Sandberg, S. (2000). Inattentive behavior in childhood: Epidemiology and implications for development. *Journal of Learning Disabilities*, *33*, 520–536.

Wasserstein, J., & Lynn, A. (2001). Metacognitive remediation in adult ADHD: Treating executive function deficits via executive functions. *Annals of the New York Academy of Sciences*, *931*, 376–384.

Weiss, G., & Hechtman, L. T. (1993). *Hyperactive children grown up* (2nd edn). New York, NY: Guilford.

Weiss, M., Worling, D., & Wasdell, M. (2003). A chart review study of the inattentive and combined types of ADHD. *Journal of Attention Disorders*, *7*, 1–9.

Wilens, T. E., Faraone, S. V., Biederman, J., & Gunawardene, S. (2003). Does stimulant therapy of attention-deficit/hyperactivity disorder beget later substance abuse? A meta-analytic review of the literature. *Pediatrics*, *111*, 179–185.

Willcutt, E. G., Doyle, A. E., Nigg, J. T., Faraone, S. V., & Pennington, B. F. (2005). Validity of the executive function theory of attention-deficit/hyperactivity disorder: A meta-analytic review. *Biological Psychiatry*, *57*, 1336–1346.

Willcutt, E. G., Pennington, B. F., & DeFries, J. C. (2000). Twin study of the etiology of comorbidity between reading disability and attention-deficit/hyperactivity disorder. *American Journal of Medical Genetics*, *96*, 293–301.

Wohl, M., Purper-Ouakil, D., Mouren, M. C., Ades, J., & Gorwood, P. (2005). Meta-analysis of candidate genes in attention-deficit hyperactivity disorder. *Encephale-Revue de Psychiatrie Clinique Biologique et Therapeutique*, *31*, 437–447.

World Health Organization (WHO). (1992). *The ICD-10 classification of mental and behavioural disorders: Clinical descriptions and diagnostic guidelines.* Geneva: World Health Organization.

Young, S., Gudjonsson, G., Ball, S., & Lam, J. (2003). Attention Deficit Hyperactivity Disorder in personality disordered offenders and the association with disruptive behavioural problems. *Journal of Forensic Psychiatry and Psychology*, *14*, 491–505.

Conduct Disorders of Childhood and Adolescence

Terrie E. Moffitt and Stephen Scott

Children with conduct disorders (persistent disruptive, deceptive and aggressive behaviors) are highly likely to require clinical intervention. Furthermore, such children constitute an important opportunity to prevent a future burden of poor adult health and social maladjustment. During childhood, conduct problems cause considerable distress for children, their families and their schools, and conduct problems are associated with consequential social and educational impairments for the child (Lahey, Loeber, Quay *et al.*, 1997).

Later, during adolescence and adulthood, children with conduct problems are at substantially increased risk of poor prognosis. This increased risk involves adulthood antisocial outcomes such as antisocial personality disorder, criminal and violent offending, and potential incarceration. Moreover, childhood conduct problems further predict adulthood risk for serious difficulties in education, work and finances, homelessness, abuse and dependence on tobacco, alcohol and drugs, and even compromised physical health including injuries, sexually transmitted infections, compromised immune function, dental health and respiratory health, as well as a variety of mental disorders and suicide attempts (Moffitt, Caspi, Harrington *et al.*, 2002; Odgers, Caspi, Poulton *et al.*, 2007a; Robins 1991). An excess of conduct disorders characterizes the juvenile psychiatric histories of adult patients with substance, affective, anxiety and eating disorders, and even patients with schizophrenia spectrum disorders and mania (Kim-Cohen, Caspi, Moffitt *et al.*, 2003).

As adolescents and young adults, children with conduct problems are more likely to enter and contribute to cohabitations and marriages with domestic violence, and to engage in early childbearing and poor parenting practices, hence putting the next generation at risk (Jaffee, Belsky, Sligo *et al.*, 2006; Moffitt & Caspi, 1998). This breadth of compromised long-term outcomes highlights the prevention opportunity afforded when children with conduct problems are successfully treated.

The conduct disorders are distinctive among mental disorders in that they are embedded in the patient's social context and have consequences for victims, apart from conferring harm on the individual patient. Many of the features are seen in social interactions, notably verbal and physical aggression, bullying, oppositional behavior and lying. This means that the symptoms of the disorders are also social behaviors that arise in the context of family, peer, educational and wider social relationships, and which in turn have a detrimental impact on these relationships. The origins, maintenance and cessation of the symptoms cannot be understood independently of these contexts. Equally, the symptoms are not simply the product of social processes, in that individual vulnerabilities are known to play a prominent part. Biological, psychological and social processes are all implicated in the etiology and treatment of the conduct disorders, through additive and interactive effects (Hill, 2002; Rutter, Giller, & Hagell, 1998).

This chapter aims to introduce clinicians and researchers to major issues involved in conduct disorders of childhood and adolescence. It covers classification, prevalence, subtypes, associated co-occurring disorders and complicating conditions. Risk factors are examined at the levels of the individual child, the family and the extra-familial social context. Issues in clinical assessment and diagnosis are covered, as are intervention approaches. An exhaustive citation bibliography of all studies of conduct problems is far beyond the scope of this chapter. Thus, only key individual studies with strong methods are cited as examples, and the reader is directed to reviews of the literature when those are available.

Classification of Juvenile Antisocial Disorders

Conduct Disorder and Oppositional Defiant Disorder in DSM-IV and ICD-10

Two principal classification systems, DSM-IV (American Psychiatric Association, 2000) and ICD-10 (World Health Organization, 1996) are quite similar in that both specify behaviors required for diagnosis. Both emphasize the persistent duration of the symptom behaviors for some months. The principal difference is that, in DSM-IV, Oppositional Defiant Disorder (ODD) and Conduct Disorder (CD) are separated, whereas in ICD-10 the criterion set of items required for CD is very close to what would be obtained by combining the DSM-IV ODD and CD items (Angold & Costello, 2001). ODD is defined as a recurrent pattern of negativistic, defiant, disobedient and hostile behaviors leading to impairment of day to day activities,

Rutter's Child and Adolescent Psychiatry, 5th edition. Edited by M. Rutter, D. Bishop, D. Pine, S. Scott, J. Stevenson, E. Taylor and A. Thapar. © 2008 Blackwell Publishing, ISBN: 978-1-4051-4549-7.

and CD as the repetitive and persistent violation of the basic rights of others and societal norms.

Are ODD and CD distinct conditions? It is not clear how valid the distinction is between ODD and CD, because the items in each are clearly age-related (Angold & Costello, 2001). Although some studies have found evidence that CD and ODD symptoms have independent associations with certain clinical correlates, it is commonly accepted that ODD and CD may be different age-related manifestations of the same condition, in which early ODD often develops into eventual CD (Lahey *et al.*, 1997; Loeber, Burke, Lahey *et al.*, 2000; Maughan, Rowe, Messer *et al.*, 2004).

Category, or Continuum?

Although the principal classification systems, DSM-IV and ICD-10, take a categorical approach, this has disadvantages. Unless there is good evidence that the problems operate in a categorical fashion, the cut-off point will inevitably be arbitrary; studies searching for such evidence have not found it (e.g., Moffitt, Caspi, Rutter *et al.*, 2001). One study has systematically examined the predictive validity of categorical diagnoses versus dimensional measures of ODD and CD (Fergusson & Horwood, 1995). The dimensional variables were better predictors of outcome, and there appeared to be a dose–response relationship of increasing risk for juvenile offending and school dropout associated with increasing severity of disruptive behaviors. Genetic influences appear to operate in a similar manner in relation to conduct problems whether they are assessed as dimensions or categories (Eaves, Silver, Meyer *et al.*, 1997). Although diagnoses are expected in clinical settings, using a categorical approach entails the risk that important differences of severity or type of dysfunction below and above the cut-off will be lost (Hinshaw, Lahey, & Hart, 1993).

Other Conceptualizations

There has been immense variation in the ways that conduct problems have been conceptualized and measured in the research consulted for this chapter. Many studies have used the DSM diagnoses, but a range of measures such as aggressive personality traits, antisocial behaviors, psychopathic traits and juvenile delinquent offending have also been employed. The terms "conduct problems" and "antisocial behaviors" will be used here to refer broadly to children's aggressive and disruptive behaviors, measured in a range of ways.

Descriptive Epidemiology

Overall Prevalence

Estimates of the prevalence of conduct problems vary according to the criteria used (Angold & Costello, 2001; Green, McGinnity, Meltzer *et al.*, 2005). However, on the basis of the majority of epidemiological studies from the industrialized west, 5–10% of children and adolescents have significant persistent oppositional, disruptive or aggressive behavior problems.

Prevalence by Historical Period, Social Class and Ethnicity

With respect to historical period, both short-term changes and longer-term changes in youth antisocial behavior have been examined. One example of short-term change was observed in the USA during the 1990s when rates of youth violence, particularly homicide, increased dramatically and then decreased again, a change attributable to short-term alterations in local drug and firearm markets, and to altered policies in policing and sentencing (Blumstein & Wallman, 2005). A longer-term modest rise in diagnosable conduct disorder over the second half of the 20th century has also been observed in a study comparing assessments of three successive birth cohorts in Britain (Collishaw, Maughan, Goodman *et al.*, 2004). Presumably, this increase arises from some societal level factor that has also been characterized by gradual change during the same time period, such as changing family structure.

With respect to socioeconomic class, measured class differences in juvenile antisocial behavior are not as wide as might be expected. Research has consistently failed to find the expected relationship between low family social class and individual youth's conduct problems or offending, particularly when this behavior is assessed through youth self-reports (Tittle & Meier, 1990). One study found that among low social class adolescents, offending was associated with attitudes of alienation, whereas among high social class, offending was associated with attitudes of unconventionality, suggesting that social class may condition motivation for antisocial conduct (Wright, Caspi, Moffitt *et al.*, 1999).

With respect to ethnicity, the over-representation of offenders of Black African ancestry in US and UK jails and prisons has focused much debate, and some research, on the thorny question of ethnic group differences in antisocial behavior (Morenoff, 2005; Smith, 2005). Research into ethnic differences has not really studied childhood conduct problems, but rather is limited to studies of adolescent and adult offending. Recognizing that the over-representation of Black African-ancestry offenders in official statistics could arise from race bias among police and courts, researchers also consult sources of data such as youth self-reports of antisocial behaviors and crime victim survey reports of perpetrators' ethnicity. These data, although influenced by their own serious sources of ethnicity-related bias, also tend to show an excess of offenders of Black African ancestry, although the Black–White difference is generally somewhat narrower than in official data. Importantly, Hispanic Americans in the USA and British Asians in the UK do not tend to show an excess of offending when compared to their white counterparts. Hypothesized explanations for a Black–White difference in offending include poverty, prejudice, family structure, subculture, neighborhood context and individual characteristics such as intelligence, but research is insufficient to support conclusions (Morenoff, 2005; Smith, 2005).

Sex Differences in Prevalence

Where studies have included males and females with conduct

problems, the sex ratio is approximately 2.5 males for each female overall, with males further exceeding females in the frequency and severity of behaviors (Costello, Angold, Burns *et al.*, 1996; Moffitt *et al.*, 2001). In the light of the gender difference the question arises as to whether the sexes have different risk mechanisms. One study found that the individual and family factors associated with self-reported delinquency were the same for males and females, but were more common in males (Rowe, Vazsonyi, & Flannery, 1995). This same conclusion was reached in a systematic analysis of a wide variety of risk factors comparing the males and females of the Dunedin longitudinal study (Moffitt *et al.*, 2001). Reviews of twin studies have revealed no systematic differences between the sexes in the contributions of genetic and environmental factors (Rhee & Waldman, 2002). On balance, research suggests that the causes of conduct problems are the same for the sexes, but males have more conduct disorder because they experience more of its individual-level risk factors (e.g., hyperactivity, neurodevelopmental delays). However, recent years have seen increasing concern among clinicians about treating antisocial behavior among girls, and this is currently the topic of intense research (Pullatz & Bierman, 2004).

Developmental Subtypes

Life-Course-Persistent Versus Adolescence-Limited

There has been considerable attention paid to the distinction between aggressive and disruptive behaviors that are first seen in early childhood versus those that start in adolescence (Moffitt, 1993a; Patterson & Yoerger, 1993), and these two subtypes are encoded in the DSM-IV diagnostic system for CD. Early onset is a strong predictor of persistence through childhood, and early-onset delinquency is more likely to persist into adult life. Findings from the Dunedin longitudinal study following a 1972–73 birth cohort have shown that those with early onset differ from those with later onset in that they have lower IQ, more attentional and impulsivity problems, poorer scores on neuropsychological tests, greater peer difficulties and they are more likely to come from adverse family circumstances (Moffitt *et al.*, 2001). Those with later onset, by contrast, are thought to become delinquent predominantly as a result of social influences such as association with other delinquent youths, or seeking social status through delinquent behaviors. Moffitt (1993a) termed the early-onset group "life-course-persistent" and the later-onset group "adolescence-limited," thus linking developmental course to the differences in underlying deficits. The distinction between the two groups has been broadly supported in longitudinal studies of several cohorts from a dozen countries (Moffitt, 2006). Findings from the follow-up of the Dunedin cohort support relatively poorer adult outcomes for the early-onset group in domains of violence, mental health, substance abuse, work and family life (Moffitt, Caspi, Harrington *et al.*, 2002). Follow-up to age 32 revealed that the early-onset life-course-persistent group had compromised physical health relative to other cohort men, as shown by increased injuries, primary care physician and hospital visits, and clinical tests of sexually transmitted infections, systemic inflammation, periodontal disease, decayed teeth and chronic bronchitis (Odgers *et al.*, 2007a).

However, the "adolescence-limited" group was not without adult difficulties (Moffitt *et al.*, 2002; Odgers *et al.*, 2007a). As adults they still engaged in self-reported offending, and they also had problems with alcohol and drugs. The Cambridge Study in Delinquent Development, a longitudinal study of 411 London males from age 8 to 46 years, also found that those with antisocial behaviors starting in adolescence were likely to continue to commit undetected crimes in adult life, although their work performance and close relationships were not impaired (Nagin, Farrington, & Moffitt, 1995). Thus, the age-of-onset subtype distinction has strong predictive validity, but adolescent-onset antisocial behaviors may have more long-lasting consequences than previously supposed, and thus both childhood onset and adolescent onset conduct problems warrant clinical attention.

Childhood-Limited Conduct Problems

Robins (1966) first pointed out that half of children with conduct problems do not grow up to have antisocial personalities. Longitudinal studies aiming to document the continuity of antisocial behavior from childhood through adolescence to adulthood have repeatedly revealed the existence of an exceptional group of children who lack such continuity. These are often termed "childhood-limited" conduct problems (Moffitt, 2006). Some studies define this childhood-limited group broadly (as a large group of children having any elevated disruptive behavior), and these draw our attention to the ubiquity of temporary conduct problems in the healthy population of children, and show that so long as mild conduct problems do not persist they need not portend poor prognosis (Odgers, Milne, Caspi *et al.*, 2007b; Tremblay, 2003). In contrast, other studies define this childhood-limited group more narrowly (as a small group of children exhibiting extreme, pervasive and persistent antisocial behavior problems only during childhood). These studies report that such childhood-limited antisocial boys develop into adult men who are depressed, anxious, socially isolated and have low-paid jobs (Farrington, Gallagher, Morley *et al.*, 1988; Moffitt *et al.*, 2002). Thus, boys whose conduct problems are severe and persistent enough to warrant a clinical diagnosis may not later develop antisocial personality, but they will suffer other forms of maladjustment as adults. Thus, all children with conduct disorders warrant clinical attention.

When a young child presents for assessment, the clinician's task is to make a differential diagnosis between childhood-onset CD that will be only childhood-limited, versus childhood-onset CD that will in future have a life-course-persistent course and pathological prognosis. DSM-IV's age-of-onset distinction cannot help with this task because all child patients, by definition, have childhood onset. Researchers have tried to distinguish life-course-persistent versus childhood-limited trajectory groups by using childhood risk factors, without much success (Moffitt, 2006). However, initial evidence indicates that comorbid attention deficit/hyperactivity disorder (ADHD), as well as family psychiatric history, characterize the persistent subtype but not the childhood-limited subtype. Alcohol problems in the child's parents and grandparents seem particularly prognostic (Odgers *et al.*, 2007b).

Associated Disorders and Conditions

Co-occurring Mental Disorders

Epidemiological studies concur that more than 90% of individuals having conduct or antisocial personality disorder also meet diagnostic criteria for other disorders (Moffitt *et al.*, 2001; Robins & Regier, 1991), and conduct disorder has been shown to feature prominently in the developmental history of virtually every adult psychiatric disorder, including schizophrenia and eating disorders (Kim-Cohen *et al.*, 2003). Particularly striking is the frequent overlap between antisocial behaviors and hyperactive-impulsive-inattentive behaviors in the young population (Waschbusch, 2002). A meta-analysis of associations among child psychiatric disorders estimated the odds ratio for ADHD in the presence of conduct disorder is 10.7 (7.7–14.8) (Angold, Costello, & Erkanli, 1999). Children who have both ODD/CD and ADHD have more varied and severe ODD/CD symptoms, greater levels of parental psychopathology, more conflictual interactions with parents, greater peer problems, school difficulties and psychosocial adversity, worse neuropsychological deficits and poorer prognosis into adulthood than those with either condition alone (Angold, Costello, & Erkanli, 1999; Lynam, 1996). Twin studies suggest a common genetic component underlying ADHD and conduct disorder (Moffitt, 2005a). Lynam (1996) reviewed literature suggesting that children with the combination of conduct problems and hyperactivity-attentional difficulties are likely to be "fledgling psychopaths," who warrant especial clinical attention and may be particularly difficult to treat.

Apart from ADHD, young people with conduct problems have also been shown to have other associated disorders at markedly elevated rates (Vermeiren, Jespers, & Moffitt, 2006). The disorders most consistently implicated are adolescent depression and substance abuse. In each case, comorbidity between conduct problems and the co-occurring disorder grows stronger with age, becoming more marked in adolescence. Diagnoses of learning disabilities and reading impairment are also highly prevalent among children with conduct problems (Carroll, Maughan, Goodman *et al.*, 2005). When conduct disorder is diagnosed, any co-occuring behavioral or learning disorders should also be ascertained, as these may afford an opportunity for prevention.

Complicating Conditions

In addition to the aforementioned diagnosable disorders that often co-occur with conduct problems, certain conditions that are not diagnosable disorders also tend to complicate the clinical picture of children with conduct disorder. This section reviews four such conditions: psychopathy, autistic traits, victimization by others and violence between adolescent romantic partners.

Psychopathy

The characteristics of the psychopath include grandiosity, callousness, deceitfulness, shallow affect and lack of remorse (see chapter 51). These traits, as assessed by the Hare Psychopathy Checklist, have been shown to predict which individuals will engage in the most serious and violent crime careers, even among prison inmates (Hare, Hart, & Harpur, 1991). Can the "fledgling psychopath" be identified in childhood, as a high priority target for prevention? Contrasting approaches to this question have been taken. One approach has suggested that children showing hyperactivity/attentional problems and conduct problems are at risk for subsequent psychopathy (Lynam, 1996; Lynam & Gudonis, 2005). Another approach emphasizes callous unemotional traits such as lack of guilt, absence of empathy and shallow constricted emotions in children (Barry, Frick, DeShazo *et al.*, 2000). A third approach proposes that psychopathy is associated with a failure to inhibit aggression in response to signs of distress in others, arising from a deficit in processing victims' distress cues, and reduced ability to recognize fear and sadness (Blair, Mitchell, & Blair, 2005). A number of reliable instruments are now available for the clinical assessment and diagnosis of psychopathic traits in juvenile patients (Farrington, 2005). If childhood psychopathy proves a useful clinical concept, it will be crucial that this provides a more refined background to improved treatments, and not a means of writing off some children.

Autistic Traits

A very recent development connects conduct disorders with symptoms formerly thought to be key features of autism and limited to patients with autism (Gilmour, Hill, Place *et al.*, 2004). Children with autism, children referred for clinical evaluation of conduct problems and children excluded from school for disruptive behaviors were compared, and all three groups were found to have similar high prevalence of pragmatic language skill deficits and social communication difficulties. Some of the difficulties measured might be secondary to externalizing disorder, such as disrupted social relationships with peers. However, other difficulties such as speech articulation and fluency deficits, misunderstanding of context cues, misuse of gesture and eye contact, and unusual rigid interests have not been previously identified as part of conduct disorder. The importance of this finding is as yet not established, but it may point to new modes of therapy for conduct problems.

Bullying

The past decade has witnessed growing concerns from parents and schools about young children involved in bullying at or after school (Spivak, 2003; Tolan, 2004). Surveys indicate that nearly half of children are involved in bullying at some time in childhood, although chronic involvement as a victim is somewhat less common (Nansel, Craig, Overpeck *et al.*, 2004). Bullying and cruelty toward other children are key symptom criteria for diagnosing conduct disorder. Risk factors for becoming a bully are thus the same as risk factors for conduct disorder in general (Olweus, 1993). Risk factors that invite victimization by a bully are somewhat different, including emotional problems, low self-regard and poor social skills, as well as physical characteristics such as obesity. Because such risk factors pre-exist involvement in bullying, researchers must control for them in order to determine whether involvement in bullying has any consequences. One longitudinal study was able to control for pre-existing risk factors at age 5 school entry. This study reported that children who were victims in the intervening 2 years before follow-up at age 7 developed more emotional problems, more disruptive behavior problems, fewer prosocial behaviors and were less happy at school (Arseneault, Walsh, Trzesniewski *et al.*, 2006). Thus, being targeted by bullies appears to lead to wide-ranging maladjustment in children, and should be a clinical concern.

Crime Victimization

Whereas most attention is focused on the potential of youth with conduct problems to harm others, such youth are often victims of violence committed by other people in their communities. Much research has documented that adult psychiatric patients are frequent targets of violence. Although children and adolescents are less often studied as victims, conduct disorder and its co-occurring disorders also place young people in harm's way (Smith & Ecob, 2007; Snyder & Sickmund, 2006). In the US national Addhealth cohort study, the advent of puberty brought increased victimization risk to adolescents (Haynie & Piquero, 2006). In another cohort study, young people who were regular alcohol and cannabis abusers were twice as likely than healthy young people to become the victim of threatened, attempted or completed physical and sexual assaults in their community, even after controlling for their own prior perpetration of antisocial behaviors (Silver, Arseneault, Langley *et al.*, 2005). Clinicians and researchers should be alert to the potential that their patients will become crime victims, with ensuing symptoms of post-traumatic stress disorder (PTSD).

Adolescent Partner Violence

The terms "marital violence" and "domestic abuse" generate the impression that partner abuse takes place primarily among adults, but recent research exposes high rates of aggression in the romantic or sexual relationships of teenagers (Halpern, Oslak, Young *et al.*, 2001). Indeed, the peak age for partner aggression is between ages 15 and 25, and early-onset participation in relationship aggression is ominous because it predicts continued high risk for more injurious violence in later adult relationships (Capaldi & Gorman-Smith, 2003). One of the strongest predictors that a teenager will become involved in partner aggression is his or her prior childhood history of conduct problems, suggesting that partner aggression is part of a pre-established long-standing tendency to use violence to solve interpersonal disagreements (Ehrensaft, Moffitt, & Caspi, 2004). Both boys and girls engage in aggression toward partners, but qualitative research with high-school pupils suggests the aggression has shared meaning for the sexes (Tolman, Spencer, Rosen-Reynoso *et al.*, 2003). Boys attributed their partner aggression to the need to appear sexually dominant to peers, aiming to establish their heterosexual credentials beyond doubt. Girls believed boys were sexual predators who exploit girls, but girls were willing to stay in an aggressive relationship rather than to be seen by peers to have no boyfriend. Thus, the almost compulsory pressure among adolescents to prove one can have and keep a heterosexual relationship seems an important context for relationship violence, which warrants attention from clinicians who see adolescents.

Etiology

Risk Factors

Risk factors for conduct problems have been extensively reviewed in many reference sources (Hawkins, Herrenkohl, Farrington *et al.*, 1998; Hill, 2002; Hill & Maughan, 2001; Lahey, Moffitt, & Caspi, 2003; Rutter, Giller, & Hagell, 1998). Here we briefly consider primary risk factors that are present in early childhood before the onset of conduct problems.

Individual Level Characteristics

Identified Genotypes

The search for specific genetic polymorphisms associated with conduct problems is a very new scientific initiative, and little has yet been accomplished. One genome-wide linkage study identified chromosomal regions that are good bets for harboring conduct problem-related polymorphisms, but the polymorphisms have not been specified and the regions have not been replicated (Stallings, Corley, Dennehey *et al.*, 2005). The most-studied candidate gene in relation to conduct problems is the *MAOA* promoter polymorphism. The gene encodes the MAOA enzyme, which metabolizes neurotransmitters linked to aggressive behavior by previous research in mice, and among men in a Dutch family pedigree. Thus, *MAOA* was selected as the candidate gene to test a hypothesis that genetic vulnerability might moderate the effect of child maltreatment on later conduct problems in the cycle of violence (Caspi, McClay, Moffitt *et al.*, 2002).

Maltreatment history and genotype interacted to predict four different measures of antisocial outcome: diagnosed adolescent conduct disorder; a personality assessment of aggression; symptoms of adult antisocial personality disorder reported by informants who knew the study member well; and adult court conviction for violent crime. Replication of this study was of utmost importance because reports of associations between measured genes and disorders are notorious for their poor replication record. Positive and negative replication studies have appeared, and a meta-analysis of these studies showed the association between *MAOA* genotype and conduct problems is modest but statistically significant (Kim-Cohen, Caspi, Taylor *et al.*, 2006). Findings of specific genetic polymorphisms associated with antisocial behavior will probably not be applied for genetic diagnosis purposes, because of the inherent complexity of gene–behavior connections. Rather, gene–environment research will benefit efforts to understand how brain mechanisms connect external risk factors and genomic variation to the conduct disorders (Meyer-Lindenberg, Buckholtz, Kolachana *et al.*, 2006).

Perinatal Complications

Birth complications might be a contributory factor to neuropsychological deficits that are associated with conduct problems (Moffitt, 1993b). The evidence regarding this was mixed but recent reports from large-scale general population studies have found associations between life-course-persistent type conduct problems and perinatal complications, minor physical anomalies and low birth weight (Brennan, Grekin, & Mednick, 2003). Most studies support a biosocial model in which obstetric complications might confer vulnerability to other co-ocurring risks such as hostile or inconsistent parenting (Arseneault, Tremblay, Boulerice *et al.*, 2002; Kratzer & Hodgins, 1999; Raine, Brennan & Mednick, 1997; Tibbetts & Piquero, 1999). Studies have further indicated that smoking in pregnancy is a statistical risk predictor of offspring conduct problems (Brennan, Grekin, & Mednick, 2003), but a causal link between smoking and conduct problems has not been established (Fergusson, 1999).

Temperament

Individual differences in infancy that might contribute to subsequent risk of psychopathology were conceptualized by Thomas, Chess, and Birch (1968) in terms of temperament, which they viewed as inherited and not significantly influenced by experience. Several prospective studies have shown associations between temperament and conduct problems (Keenan & Shaw, 2003), and also predicted antisocial personality disorder and criminal offending into adulthood (Caspi, Moffitt, Newman *et al.*, 1996). Temperament, as originally conceived, should be strongly heritable and experience-free. However, measures of temperament are only moderately heritable, and a child's engagement with the social world from birth means that temperament measures inevitably assess the outcome of social processes. It may be that the contributions of temperament will be seen most consistently in combination with environmental risk factors (Nigg, 2006).

Neurotransmitters

Neurotransmitters have been linked to antisocial behavior in adult samples, and in non-human animal models (Nelson, 2006). It would be a major advance if it were possible to link neurotransmitter levels and activity to conduct problems in children. However, in general, the findings with children have not been consistent (Hill, 2002). For example, in the Pittsburgh youth cohort, boys with long-standing conduct problems showed downward changes in urinary epinephrine level following a stressful challenge task, whereas prosocial boys showed upward epinephrine responses to the challenge (McBurnett, Raine, Stouthamer-Loeber *et al.*, 2005). However, other studies have failed to find an association between conduct disorder and measures of norepinephrine in children (Hill, 2002). Some limited evidence supports the view that, as in adults, serotonin is linked with aggression in children, but findings for indices of serotonin function in children are also markedly inconsistent (Pine, Coplan, Wasserman *et al.*, 1997). It should be borne in mind that neurotransmitters in the brain are only indirectly measured, most measures of neurotransmitter levels are crude indicators of activity and little is known about neurotransmitters in the juvenile brain.

Verbal Deficits

Children with conduct problems have been shown consistently to have increased rates of deficits in language-based verbal skills (Lynam & Henry, 2001; Nigg & Huang-Pollock, 2003). Conduct-disordered children, delinquent adolescents and adult antisocial individuals show poor performance on standardized tests of verbal ability, and in tests of IQ, poor verbal and performance scores. These associations hold after controlling for potential confounds such as race, socioeconomic status, academic attainment and test motivation (Lynam, Moffitt, & Stouthamer-Loeber, 1993). Longitudinal studies show that persistence in antisocial behavior over periods of years is predicted by low verbal IQ in childhood (Farrington & Hawkins, 1991; Lahey, Loeber, Hart *et al.*, 1995; Lynam & Henry, 2001). Deficits in verbal capacities are found also with oppositional defiant disorder among preschool-aged clinic-referred boys (Speltz, McClellan, DeKlyen *et al.*, 1999). Several possible ways in which poor verbal ability might influence behavior can be drawn from Luria's theory of the role of verbal memory and verbal abstract reasoning in the development of self-control (Luria, 1961). The abilities to recall oral instructions and to use language to think through the consequences of actions contribute to the effective control of actions. Children who cannot reason or assert themselves verbally may attempt to gain control of social exchanges using aggression (Dodge, 1993). It is likely that there are also indirect effects in which low verbal IQ contributes to academic difficulties which in turn mean that the child's experience of school becomes unrewarding, rather than a source of self-esteem and support.

Executive Dysfunction

Children and adolescents with conduct problems have been shown consistently to have poor tested executive functions (Ishikawa & Raine, 2003; Lynam & Henry, 2001; Moffitt, 1993b; Nigg & Huang-Pollock, 2003). Executive functions comprise those abilities implicated in successfully achieving goals through appropriate effective actions. Specific skills include learning and applying contingency rules, abstract reasoning, problem-solving, self-monitoring, sustained attention and concentration, relating previous actions to future goals and inhibiting inappropriate responses. These mental functions are largely, although not exclusively, associated with frontal lobes (Pennington & Ozonoff, 1996). Important data come from a Montreal cohort studied from the age of 6 years (Séguin, Boulerice, Harden *et al.*, 1999). The study used executive function tests that have been shown to be associated with different anatomical structures in the brain, on the basis of lesion and functional imaging studies. Chronic aggression was associated with lower scores on tests tapping executive functions of the frontal brain region, and the findings held after controlling for general memory, IQ and ADHD. Although most studies of executive deficit involve adolescents, such deficits have also been linked with disruptive behaviors in very young preschool children (Hughes, Dunn, & White, 1998; Speltz, DeKlyen, Calderon *et al.*, 1999).

Autonomic Reactivity

A low resting pulse rate or slow heart rate has been found consistently to be associated with antisocial behavior, and a meta-analysis of 40 studies suggested it is the best replicated biological correlate of antisocial behavior (Ortiz & Raine, 2004). For example, in the longitudinal Cambridge Study in Delinquent Development, slow heart rate was associated with convictions for violence after controlling for all other risk variables (Farrington, 1997). Other psychophysiological indicators of slow autonomic system reactivity have also been examined. For example, in a longitudinal study of Pittsburgh boys, those most antisocial and psychopathic were also slowest to show a skin-conductance response to aversive blasts of noise (Fung, Raine, Loeber *et al.*, 2005). The explanation for the link between slow autonomic activity and antisocial behavior remains unclear.

Information Processing and Social Cognition

Dodge (1993) proposed the leading information-processing model for the genesis of aggressive behaviors within social interactions. The model hypothesizes that children who are prone to aggression focus on threatening aspects of others' actions, interpret hostile intent in the neutral actions of others and are more likely to select and to favor aggressive solutions to social challenges. Several studies have demonstrated that aggressive children make such errors of social cognition. An extensive review of the many studies of social cognition among children with conduct problems has been presented elsewhere (Dodge, Coie, & Lynam, 2006). Dodge (1993) hypothesized that the tendencies to encode hostile aspects of situations and to attribute hostile intent to ambiguous social cues, and to access and favor aggressive responses to social challenges, are the result of repeated exposure to physical maltreatment. This prediction was tested prospectively (Dodge, Petit, Bates *et al.*, 1995). Physical abuse documented in kindergarten was strongly associated with conduct problems in primary school; 28% of the abused group developed conduct problems compared to 6% of the non-abused. Encoding errors, hostile attributions and biases toward accessing and favoring aggressive responses were each associated with conduct problem outcome, and with having experienced physical abuse. Encoding errors and accessing aggressive responses mediated the link between physical abuse and conduct problems, but hostile attributions and positive evaluation of aggressive responses did not. This prospective study thus provided some support for the social cognition model.

Risks Outside the Family

Risks in the Neighborhood

It has long been assumed that bad neighborhoods have the effect of encouraging children to develop conduct problems. Parents strive to secure the best neighborhood and school for their child that they can afford. Although it is obvious that some local areas have higher crime rates than others, it has been difficult to document any direct link between neighborhood characteristics and child behavior, for a number of reasons. For example, neighborhood characteristics were conceptualized in overly simple structural demographic terms such as percentage of non-White residents or percentage of single-parent households. Moreover, research designs could not rule out the alternative possibility that families whose members are antisocial tend to selectively move into bad neighborhoods. A new generation of neighborhood research is addressing these challenges (Beyers, Bates, Petit *et al.*, 2003; Caspi, Taylor, Moffitt *et al.*, 2000; Sampson, Raudenbusch, & Earls, 1997). New research suggests that the neighborhood factors that are important go beyond structural demographic characteristics. Neighborhood-level social processes such as "collective efficacy" and "social control" do influence young children's conduct problems, probably by supporting or failing to support parents in their efforts to rear children.

Peer Influences

Children with conduct problems have poorer peer relationships than non-disordered children in that they tend to associate with children with similar antisocial behaviors, they have discordant interactions with other children and experience rejection by non-deviant peers (Vitaro, Tremblay, & Bukowski, 2001). Three principal explanations have been tested, and evidence found for all three. Either children's antisocial behaviors lead them to have peer problems, or deviant peer relationships lead to antisocial behaviors, or some common factor leads to both.

Peer Rejection in Childhood

Regarding the possibility that conduct problems lead to peer difficulties, there is ample evidence that children with established conduct problems are more likely to have more conflict with peers, and to be rejected by non-deviant peers (Coie, 2004). This peer rejection has been shown to contribute to declines in academic achievement and increases in aggression across the first year of primary schooling (Coie, 2004). One consequence of rejection by healthy peers is that from as young as 5 years aggressive-antisocial children are obliged to associate with other deviant children (Farver, 1996; Fergusson, Woodward, & Horwood, 1999).

Peer Groups Promote Conduct Problems in Adolescence

In the light of the limited evidence that peer difficulties prompt the onset of childhood conduct problems, and the rather more substantial evidence that children's peer difficulties are a consequence of their conduct problems, is there any reason to think that peer processes influence the long-term course of conduct problems? Regarding the possibility that peers lead to conduct problems, this has been shown to come about in several ways. Youth who are aggressive are attracted to each other, and deviant youth reinforce each others' antisocial behaviors and attitudes (Boivin & Vitaro, 1995). Evidence that peer influences do increase antisocial behaviors applies primarily to the adolescent developmental stage (Warr, 2002). Strong evidence comes from treatment experiments: in two controlled clinical trials, boys treated in groups did worse than untreated controls; treatment was followed by increased adolescent problem behaviors and poorer outcomes (Dishion, McCord, & Poulin, 1999). After group-level treatment brought the boys together they mutually reinforced each others' antisocial activities, a finding that argues for individual treatment approaches. A natural experiment study tracked change in antisocial behavior among boys who joined a gang, to reveal that joining a gang increased each adolescent's individual offending over his pre-gang baseline, whereas leaving the gang decreased each individual's personal offending rate (Thornberry, Krohn, Lizotte *et al.*, 1993). Overall, we must consider the dynamic and reciprocal manner in which children's conduct problems influence who their friends are, and in which those friends later promote the young person's conduct problems (Vitaro, Tremblay, & Bukowski, 2001).

Family Level Influences

Concentration of Crime in Families

Fewer than 10% of the families in any community account for more than 50% of that community's criminal offenses (Farrington, Jolliffe, Loeber *et al.*, 2001; Rowe & Farrington, 1997). This familial concentration of crime most certainly reflects the co-incidence of genetic and environmental risks, directing researchers who wish to understand the origins of conduct problems to look for interactions between both types of risk.

Familial Genetic Liability

There is now solid evidence from twin and adoption studies that conduct problems assessed both dimensionally and categorically are substantially heritable (Moffitt, 2005a; Rhee & Waldman, 2002). However, knowing that conduct problems are under some genetic influence is less useful clinically than knowing that this genetic influence appears to be reduced, or enhanced, depending on interaction with circumstances in the child's environment.

Several genetically sensitive studies have allowed interactions between family genetic liability and rearing environment to be examined. Adoption studies have reported an interaction between antisocial behavior in the biological parent and adverse conditions in the adoptive home that predicted the adopted child's antisocial outcome (Bohman, 1996; Cadoret, Yates, Troughton *et al.*, 1995). The genetic risk was modified by the rearing environment. A twin study also yielded evidence that family genetic liability and environmental risks interact (Jaffee, Caspi, Moffitt *et al.*, 2005). In this study, the experience of maltreatment was associated with an increase of 24% in the probability of diagnosable conduct disorder among children at high genetic risk, but an increase of only 2% among children at low genetic risk. Thus, awareness of a familial liability toward psychopathology increases the urgency to intervene to improve a child's social environment (Odgers *et al.*, 2007b).

Family Poverty

There is an association between severe poverty and early childhood conduct problems (Farrington & Loeber, 1998). Early theories proposed direct effects of poverty related to strains arising from the gap between aspirations and realities, and from lacking opportunity to acquire social status and prestige. Subsequent research has indicated that the association between low income and childhood conduct problems is indirect, mediated via family processes such as marital discord and parenting deficits (Maughan, 2001).

As one example of this research, the Iowa longitudinal study of 378 rural families found that family economic stress was associated with adolescent conduct problems, but this was mediated via parental depression, marital conflict and parental hostility (Conger, Ge, Elder *et al.*, 1994). Another study took advantage of a naturally occurring experiment (Costello, Compton, Keeler *et al.*, 2003). Native American families in North Carolina, formerly living below the poverty line, benefitted from increased income from newly opened casinos. In many families, the children's behavior problems decreased markedly as a result. However, the effect of increased income was mediated through better parent–child relationships. This mediation is not limited to poverty in recent times. Glueck's study of delinquency from the historical period of economic depression also found that harsh discipline, low supervision and weak parent–child attachments accounted for the effects of poverty on children's antisocial behaviors in the 1930s (Sampson & Laub, 1984).

Parent–Child Attachment

Parent–child relationships provide the setting for the development of later social functioning, and disruption of these attachment relationships (e.g., through institutional care) is associated with subsequent difficulties in relating (Robins, 1966; Rutter, Quinton, & Hill, 1990). Thus, conduct problems might be expected to arise from infant attachment difficulties. Indeed, attachment theory had its origins in Bowlby's (1944) study of adolescent thieves.

However, the evidence is rather mixed (Vondra, Shaw, Swearingen *et al.*, 2001). One study found an increased rate of each of the categories of insecure attachment (avoidant, ambivalent, controlling) in preschool boys referred with ODD (Speltz, DeKlyen, & Greenberg, 1999). However, in a follow-up of the clinic boys, attachment did not predict the severity of conduct problems. By contrast, another study found that ambivalent and controlling attachment predicted disruptive behaviors after controlling for baseline differences (Moss, Smolla, Cyr *et al.*, 2006). Early studies of low-risk samples, using the secure–insecure classification, failed to find robust associations with disruptive behavior problems, but subsequent studies of higher risk samples using the disorganized classification report that disorganized attachment can predict conduct problems (Van IJzendoorn, Schuengel, & Bakermans-Kranenburg, 1999). Disorganization is identified in Ainsworth's Strange Situation Test if the child shows bizarre or contradictory behaviors with the caregiver when reunited after separation (Main & Solomon, 1986). However, low rates of infants with disorganized attachment in study samples mean that findings should be viewed with caution. Although it seems obvious that poor parent–child relations in general predict conduct problems, it has yet to be established whether attachment difficulties as measured by observational paradigms have an independent causal role in the development of behavior problems. Attachment classifications could be markers for other relevant family risks.

Discipline and Parenting

Patterns of parenting associated with conduct problems were delineated by Patterson (1982) in his seminal work *Coercive Family Process* and subsequent publications. In brief, parents of antisocial children were found to be more inconsistent in their use of rules; to issue more, and unclear, commands; to be more likely to respond to their children on the basis of mood rather than the characteristics of the child's behavior; to be less likely to monitor their children's whereabouts; and to be unresponsive to their children's prosocial behavior. Patterson proposed a specific mechanism for the promotion of oppositional and aggressive behaviors in children. A parent responds to mild oppositional behavior by a child with a prohibition to which the child responds by escalating his or her behavior, and mutual escalation continues until the parent backs off, thus negatively reinforcing the child's behavior. The parent's inconsistent behavior increases the likelihood of the child showing further oppositional or aggressive behavior. In addition to specific tests of Patterson's reinforcement model (Gardner, 1989; Snyder & Patterson, 1995) there is ample evidence that conduct problems are associated with hostile, critical, punitive and coercive parenting (Rutter, Giller, & Hagell, 1998).

In considering the role of coercive processes in the origins or maintenance of conduct problems, we need to consider possible alternative explanations: (i) that the associations reflect familial genetic liability toward children's psychopathology and parents' coercive discipline; (ii) that they represent effects of children's behaviors on parents; and (iii) that coercive parenting may be a correlate of other features of the parent–child relationship or family functioning that influence child behaviors. There is considerable evidence that children's difficult behaviors do evoke parental negativity. One experiment observed the interactions of normal and conduct disordered children when with their own parents, the parents of normal children and the parents of other conduct disordered children (Anderson, Lytton & Romney, 1986). Conduct disordered children elicited more negative reactions from all groups of parents than did non-conduct disordered children.

Adoption studies (Ge, Conger, Cadoret *et al.*, 1996; O'Connor, Deater-Deckard, Fulker *et al.*, 1998) have shown that adoptees at genetic risk of antisocial disorders are more likely than low-risk children to evoke negative parenting in the adoptive home. The role of the child in influencing parental monitoring has also received attention. Stattin and Kerr (2000) pointed out that studies of parental monitoring have generally assessed how much knowledge parents have of their children's whereabouts, but not how parents acquired it. They showed, in a study of 14-year-olds, that the majority of this knowledge came from what the child chose to tell the parent, and conduct-problem adolescents told their parents less about what they were doing.

The fact that children's behaviors can evoke negative parenting does not, however, mean that negative parenting has no impact on children's behavior. One study reported that negative maternal control at age 4 was significantly associated with conduct problems at age 9, after controlling for children's initial behavior problems at age 4 (Campbell, Pierce, Moore *et al.*, 1996). The Environmental-Risk longitudinal twin study of British families examined the effects of fathers' parenting on young children's aggression (Jaffee, Moffitt, Caspi *et al.*, 2003). As expected, a prosocial father's *absence* predicted more aggression by his children. But, in contrast, an antisocial father's *presence* predicted more aggression by his children, and his harmful effect was exacerbated the more time each week he spent taking care of the children.

In another report, the E-Risk study evaluated the hypothesis that because depressed mothers provide inept parenting, maternal depression promotes children's aggression (Kim-Cohen, Moffitt, Taylor *et al.*, 2005). Children of depressed mothers often develop conduct problems, but it has not been clear that this correlation represents environmental transmission. Although the connection between mothers' depression and children's conduct problems decreased somewhat after stringent control for familial liability to psychopathology, it remained statistically significant. Further, depressed women might exaggerate their ratings of their children's problem behaviors, but the pattern of findings remained the same when teachers rated the children's behavior. A temporal analysis showed that if E-Risk mothers experienced depression only before their children's birth, the children were not unusually aggressive. In contrast, only if mothers suffered depression while rearing their children were the children likely to develop aggression. Finally, the possibility that the association was spurious because children's aggression provoked their mothers' depression was ruled out by documenting that children exposed to an episode of maternal depression between ages 5 and 7 became even more aggressive by age 7 than they had been at age 5. Taken together, these and other findings provide good evidence for the role of discipline in conduct problems (Moffitt, 2005b).

Exposure to Adult Marital Conflict and Domestic Violence
It is likely that family processes other than parenting skills and quality of parent–child attachment relationships have a role. Many studies have shown that children exposed to domestic violence between adults are subsequently more likely to become aggressive themselves (Moffitt & Caspi, 1998). Davies and Cummings (1994) proposed that marital conflict influences children's behavior because of its effect on their regulation of emotion. For example, a child may respond to frightening emotion arising from marital conflict by down-regulating his or her own emotion through denial of the situation. This in turn may lead to inaccurate appraisal of other social situations and ineffective problem-solving. Repeated exposure to family conflict is thought to lower children's thresholds for psychological dysregulation, resulting in greater behavioral reactivity to stress (Cummings & Davies, 2002). Children's aggression may also be increased by marital discord because children are likely to imitate aggressive behavior modeled by their parents (Bandura, 1977). Through parental aggression, children may learn that aggression is a normative part of family relationships, that it is an effective way of controlling others and that aggression is sanctioned, not punished (Osofsky, 1995).

Maltreatment
Physical punishment is widely used, and parents of children with conduct problems frequently resort to it out of desperation. However, links with conduct problems are not straightforward. One study found that physical punishment was clearly associated with behavior problems in White American children, but not in African-American children (Deater-Deckard, Dodge, Bates *et al.*, 1996). Furthermore, the risk for conduct problems does not apply equally to all forms of physical punishment. The E-Risk longitudinal twin study was able to compare the effects of corporal punishment (smacking, spanking) versus injurious physical maltreatment using twin-specific reports of both experiences (Jaffee, Caspi, Moffitt *et al.*, 2004). Results showed that children's genetic endowment accounted for virtually all of the association between their corporal punishment and their conduct problems. This indicated a "child effect," in which children's bad conduct provokes their parents to use more corporal punishment, rather than the reverse. Findings about injurious physical maltreatment were the opposite. There was no child effect provoking maltreatment and, moreover, significant effects of maltreatment on child aggression remained after controlling for any genetic transmission of liability to aggression from antisocial parents.

Overall, associations between physical abuse and conduct problems are well established (Hill, 2002). In the Christchurch cohort, child sexual abuse predicted conduct problems, after controlling for other childhood adversities (Ferguson, Horwood, & Lynskey, 1996). In a large prospective study of court substantiated cases of abuse and neglect, 26% of abused and neglected adolescents were antisocial, contrasted with 17% in a well-matched comparison group, implying a modest but long-lasting effect of abuse and neglect (Widom, 1997). Investigating the relationship of child maltreatment to psychopathology is particularly difficult for ethical reasons. Little is known about the possible mechanisms linking maltreatment to conduct problems, although threats to security of attachment, difficulties in affect regulation, distortions of information processing and self-concept reviewed elsewhere in this chapter are likely to be relevant.

From Risk Predictor to Evidence for Causation

Associations have been documented between conduct problems and a wide range of risk factors. A variable is called a "risk factor" if it has a documented predictive relation with antisocial outcomes, whether or not the association is causal. The causal status of most of these risk factors is unknown; we know what statistically predicts conduct problem outcomes, but not how or why (Kraemer, 2003). Establishing a causal role for a risk factor is by no means straightforward, particularly as it is unethical to experimentally expose healthy children to risk factors to observe whether those factors can generate new conduct problems. There is no one solution to the problem, although the use of genetically sensitive designs and the study of within-individual change in natural experiments and treatment studies have considerable methodological advantages for suggesting causal influences on conduct problems (Moffitt, 2005b; Rutter, 2000; Rutter, Moffitt, & Caspi, 2006).

This chapter has emphasized risk factors that have research evidence to support a causal role in conduct problems. For example, above we have cited research that supports causation by depressed mothers' poor discipline (Kim-Cohen, Arseneault, Caspi *et al.*, 2005), child maltreatment (Dodge *et al.*, 1995; Jaffee *et al.*, 2004), family poverty (Costello *et al.*, 2003), familial genetic liability (Moffitt, 2005a) and affiliating with delinquent peers (Dishion, McCord, & Poulin, 1999; Thornberry *et al.*, 1993). These studies' designs either took advantage of natural experiments or otherwise were able to rule out alternative explanations to causation (Moffitt, 2005b). Other risk factors described here have not been decisively tested for causation yet, but they do have evidence that they are robust predictors of conduct problems across many studies carried out in different contexts (e.g., perinatal complications, temperament, verbal and executive deficits, slow heart rate, social cognitions, exposure to parental conflict). Still other risk factors benefit from strong causal theory, warranting inclusion in this chapter, but the evidence base to show reliable association with conduct problems is not yet strong (e.g., attachment, neurotransmitters, *MAOA* genotype, pregnancy smoking, neighborhood context).

Contemporary Issues in Clinical Assessment and Diagnosis

How Young Can a Diagnosis of Conduct Disorder be Made?

One controversy about the diagnosis of conduct disorders is particularly current: How young can and should a child be diagnosed? Evidence suggests that conduct problems emerge in preschoolers, that the youngest age of onset is associated with the poorest long-term prognosis and that long-established conduct problems are difficult to treat. This evidence base has resulted in calls for intervention at preschool ages to prevent conduct problems from becoming chronic. However, to intervene early in individual cases, valid methods must be available to diagnose conduct disorders in young children. Whether valid diagnoses of conduct disorders can, or should, be made in very young children has been a focus of controversy (Campbell, 2002; Keenan & Wakschlag, 2002). Some argue that disruptive behaviors in young children should not be pathologized, because aggressive, disruptive and defiant behaviors are thought to be common and developmentally normative in the preschool period, and most children will outgrow them. Others believe that children falsely identified as having conduct disorder will be stigmatized, and unnecessary referral for treatment will waste health care resources. Some argue that the predictive accuracy of conduct problems for prognosis improves only when children are older, and applying diagnostic criteria meant for older children may promote overdiagnosis.

One study tested the validity of the DSM-IV conduct disorder diagnosis for preschoolers, by applying it to screen a birth cohort of 2200 4- to 5-year-olds (Kim-Cohen *et al.*, 2005). The diagnosis successfully identified the children in the cohort who most needed treatment: they were aggressive and antisocial, had co-occurring cognitive deficits and ADHD symptoms, came from adverse family backgrounds, and were likely to have experienced harsh parenting and physical maltreatment. Followed up 2 years later, at age 7, over half of the diagnosed children still met diagnostic criteria for conduct disorder, but even the apparently remitted children continued to evidence clinically significant behavioral and academic difficulties at school, suggesting preschool intervention with them would not have been wasted.

The study indicated that clinicians wishing to minimize false positives can adopt a conservative approach by requiring the more stringent number of criteria specified by DSM-IV for moderate conduct disorder (five symptoms) as opposed to mild conduct disorder (three symptoms). Even better, standardized interview, checklist, and observational methods and guidelines for diagnosing preschool children have been developed (Egger & Angold, 2006). Thus, when necessary to support intervention, the conduct disorder diagnosis can be made for a very young child, albeit with very careful attention to developmental considerations.

Resource Instruments and Multiple Informants to Enhance Diagnostic Validity

There are many different measurement instruments for assessing conduct problems for research and clinical practice; systematic evaluation of their strengths and weaknesses is beyond the scope of this chapter. Earlier we mentioned that juvenile antisocial behavior can be defined in terms of diagnostic categories or continuous distributions of symptom behaviors. Assessment tools reflect these two options. Structured interviews aim to operationalize the specific DSM and ICD criteria to achieve a categorical diagnosis (Costello *et al.*, 1996; Goodman, Ford, Richards *et al.*, 2000; Shaffer, Fisher, Lucas *et al.*, 2000). Symptom checklists aim to broadly cover a variety of conduct and oppositional behavior problems, operating on the evidence-based principle that variety of antisocial behaviors is the best predictor of poor prognosis (Achenbach & Rescorla, 2000; Elander & Rutter, 1996; Goodman, 1997). Whatever instruments are applied, the field has reached consensus that information must be obtained from multiple informants, including if possible parents, teachers, police, clinicians and the child (Arseneault, Kim-Cohen, Taylor *et al.*, 2005; Koot, Crijnen, & Ferdinand, 1999). Multiple informants are an essential part of assessment because no single reporter can have the opportunity to observe all manifestations of antisocial conduct and thus they provide complementary information. In addition, poor prognosis characterizes children who show conduct problems pervasively across multiple different settings such as home, school and neighborhood (Loeber, Green, Lahey *et al.*, 1991).

Risk Assessment and Treatment Planning Approaches

A recent approach to diagnosis and assessment of children with conduct problems may prove especially useful for clinicians. In this approach, assessment is guided by a manual. Examples of such manuals are the SAVRY (*Structured Assessment of Violence Risk in Youth*; Borum, Bartel, & Forth, 2002), the EARL-20B (*Early Assessment Risk List for Boys*; Augimeri, Koegl, Webster *et al.*, 2001) and the EARL-21G (*Early Assessment Risk List for Girls*; Levene, Augimeri, Pepler *et al.*, 2001). These easy-to-use manuals are grounded in the scientific literature, providing operational definitions to assist clinicians in assessing risk factors that are the most valid predictors of a child's poor antisocial prognosis. Scales are included for rating the severity of each risk factor, resulting in a risk profile that points to key intervention targets in a particular child's life. Each child's specific areas of strength are highlighted to exploit in treatment planning, as are specific factors known to predict engagement in treatment versus resistance to treatment. Risk and protective factors can then be linked to approaches for case management, tailored for each juvenile patient and their family members. Formal evaluation of these manual-guided assessments has not been reported, and their long-term predictive validity is unknown, but they are evidence-based and they have strong inherent appeal to many clinicians.

Interventions

The following sections cover treatment of children aged 2–12 years. (For prevention see chapter 61. For treatment of teenagers with conduct disorder, and of delinquents, including functional family therapy and multisystemic therapy, see chapter 68. For further reviews of treatments see Farmer, Compton, Burns *et al.*, 2002; Bloomquist & Schnell, 2002.)

Principles of Intervention

Basing Treatment on the Assessment

The intervention needs to fit the particular needs of the child and family. Many risk factors have been delineated in this chapter, but usually not all occur in the same child. Intervention needs to be tailored according to the needs and strengths of the family revealed by the assessment, which should include all aspects of the child's environment and functioning – the multiaxial framework of ICD-10 provides a helpful framework for doing this (World Health Organization, 1996).

Choosing Which Treatment Modality to Use

The behavior may predominantly occur in the home, at school, with peers, in the community, or it may be pervasive. If possible, interventions need to address each context specifically, rather than assuming that successful treatment in one area will generalize to another. Thus, improvements in the home arising from a successful parent training program will not necessarily lead to less antisocial behavior at school (Scott, 2002). Therefore, for cases with difficulties that are mainly at home, where the child is doing reasonably at school and has a friend or two, parent training would be the first line of treatment. If classroom behavior is a problem and a school visit shows that the teacher is not using effective methods, then advice to the teacher and other school staff can be very effective. Where there are pervasive problems including fights with peers, then individual work on anger management and social skills should be added; on it own, anger management is unlikely to be nearly as successful as when it is combined with other approaches. Medication is controversial and generally best avoided; possible indications are discussed below.

Developing Strengths

Identifying strengths of the young person and the family is crucial. This helps engagement, and increases the chances of effective treatment. Encouragement of abilities helps the child spend more time behaving constructively rather than destructively (e.g., more time spent playing football is less time spent hanging round the streets looking for trouble). Encouragement of prosocial activities (e.g., to complete a good drawing, or to play a musical instrument well) also increases achievements and self-esteem and hope for the future. Stattin and Magnusson (1995) found that for children with antisocial behavior living in high-risk areas (which the majority do), those with strengths or skills ended up with far lower rates of criminality than those without.

Engaging the Family

Any family coming to a mental health service is likely to have some fears about being judged as bad and possibly mad. Families of children with conduct problems are more likely to be disadvantaged and disorganized, to have had arguments with official agencies such as schools and welfare officers and to be suspicious of officialdom. Dropout rates in treatment for conduct problem families are high – often up to 60% (Kazdin, 1996a). Practical measures, such as assisting with transportation, providing child care and holding sessions in the evening or at other times to suit the family are all likely to facilitate retention. Forming a good alliance with the family is especially important, and Prinz and Miller (1994) showed that adding engagement strategies during the assessment such as showing parents that the therapist clearly understood their viewpoint led to increased attendance at treatment sessions. Once engaged, the quality of the therapist's alliance with the family affects treatment success, accounting for 15% of the variance in outcome in the meta-analysis by Shirk and Carver (2003).

Treating Comorbid Conditions

Child antisocial behavior often affects others so strongly that comorbid conditions can easily be missed. Yet, in clinical referrals, comorbidity is the rule rather than the exception. Common accompaniments are depression and ADHD; a number will have PTSD (e.g., in the context of violence inflicted on them by a father, or witnessing beatings received by their mother from a partner). In recent years there has been increasing recognition of the overlap with autistic spectrum disorders (Gilmour *et al.*, 2004), and that a minority will have psychopathic traits (see chapter 51). Each of these conditions requires appropriate management in its own right.

Promoting Social and Scholastic Learning

Treatment involves more than the reduction of antisocial behavior – for example, stopping tantrums and aggressive outbursts, while helpful, will not lead to good functioning if the child lacks the skills to make friends or to negotiate: positive behaviors need to be taught too. Specific learning disabilities such as reading retardation, which is particularly common in these children, need treatment, as do more general difficulties such as planning homework.

Making Use of Guidelines

The American Academy of Child and Adolescent Psychiatry (AACAP) has published sensible practice parameters for the assessment and treatment of conduct disorder (AACAP, 1997), and the UK National Institute for Health and Clinical Excellence (NICE, 2006) has published a "technology appraisal" of the clinical and cost effectiveness of parent-training programs. This sets out criteria for choosing parent-training programs, such as being backed by evidence from randomized controlled trials. NICE guidelines are strongly influential on service commissioners and should help improve practice considerably.

Treating the Child in their Natural Environment

Most of the interventions described below are intended for out-patient or community settings. Psychiatric hospitalization is very rarely necessary; there is no evidence that in-patient admissions lead to gains that are maintained after the child is returned to their family. The objective of treatment is to enable the child to cope with the environment he or she lives in, and alter the environment where necessary. Where there is parenting breakdown or total inability to manage the child, then foster care may be necessary.

Family Interventions

Several studies have repeatedly found that family factors are strongly associated with antisocial behavior and, as reviewed above, these appear to have a causal role in many cases. Even where the antisocial behavior appears to have arisen "in a clear blue sky" without adverse family risk factors, living with a child with marked antisocial behavior can itself lead to coercive parenting styles, which in turn may exacerbate the problems (O'Connor *et al.*, 1998). Therefore, improving family risk factors such as coercive parenting is likely to be beneficial, whether or not they were originally implicated as a cause. Family interventions can be divided into two main types, those derived from family systems theory, which tend to be more broadly based, and those derived from social learning theory, which tend to be more specifically focused on training parents to improve moment-to-moment interactions with their children.

Family Systemic Therapies

Typically, family systemic therapies involve all family members attending. Their goals differ according to the style and underlying theory of the particular variant of therapy. For example, structural family therapy as pioneered by leaders such as Minuchin (1974) would try to restore clear boundaries of authority of the parents over the child, because often antisocial children have become domineering in their own homes. Other forms of family therapy try to improve patterns of communication that have gone wrong, and "systemic" variants try to reveal and address relevant factors that impinge on the family system from both within and outside the family. There have been rather few good quality evaluations of family or systemic therapies for childhood antisocial behavior; for a fuller discussion see chapter 65. One exception is functional family therapy pioneered by Jim Alexander (Barton & Alexander, 1985), which is particularly focused on antisocial children and has several trials to support it (see chapter 68).

Parent Management Training

Parent management training programs are designed to improve parents' behavior management skills and the quality of the parent–child relationship. Most target skills such as promoting play and developing a positive parent–child relationship, using praise and rewards to increase desirable social behavior, giving of clear directions and rules, using consistent and calm consequences for unwanted behavior, and reorganizing the child's day to prevent problems. Parenting interventions may also address distal factors likely to inhibit change (e.g., parental drug or alcohol abuse, maternal depression and relational violence between parents). Treatment can be delivered in individual parent–child appointments, or in a parenting group. Individual approaches offer the advantages of *in vivo* observation of the parent–child dyad and therapist coaching and feedback regarding progress.

Examples of Good Practice

Helping the non-compliant child (McMahon & Forehand, 2003) and *Parent Child Interaction Therapy* (PCIT; Eyberg, 1988) are two examples of well-validated individual programs. Group treatment has been shown to be equally effective, and offers opportunities for parents to share their experience with others who are struggling with a disruptive child. Group treatments emphasize discussion among group leaders and parents, and may use videotaped vignettes of parent–child interactions that illustrate the "right" and "wrong" ways to handle situations. Two well-known group treatments are the Incredible Years Program (IY; Webster-Stratton, 1981) and the Positive Parenting Program (Triple P; Sanders & Markie-Dadds, 1996; Sanders, Markie-Dadds, & Turner, 2000).

Effectiveness

Behavioral parent training is the most extensively studied treatment for conduct problems, and there is considerable empirical support for its effectiveness (Weisz, Hawley, & Doss, 2004). Several of the programs are considered "well-established," according to American Psychological Association criteria, with multiple randomized trials (e.g., Patterson, Chamberlain, & Reid, 1982; Webster-Stratton, Reid, & Hammond, 2001a) and replications by independent research groups (e.g., Scott, Spencer, Doolan *et al.*, 2001). There have also been randomized trials showing the effectiveness of PCIT and Triple P (e.g., Bor, Sanders, & Markie-Dadds, 2002; Sanders, Markie-Dadds, Tully *et al.*, 2000), and there is at least one independent replication of the PCIT model (Nixon, Sweeney, Erickson *et al.*, 2003). Studies suggest that behavioral parent training leads to short-term reductions in antisocial behavior, with moderate to large effect sizes of $d = 0.5$–0.8. Follow-up studies suggest enduring effects at up to 6 years post-treatment (Hood & Eyberg, 2003; Reid, Webster-Stratton, & Hammond, 2003).

Recently, some programs have included an element training parents to read with their children in addition to behavior management, with the idea of targeting multiple risk factors for antisocial behavior. Although teaching parents to read with their children has not always proved successful, Scott, Sylva, Doolan *et al.* (in press) combined a 12-week behavior management program with a relatively intense, detailed reading program (10 2-hour sessions) for 5- and 6-year-olds. In a randomized controlled trial, this combination reduced the rate of ODD by half and increased reading age by 6 months; ADHD symptoms were also reduced. This kind of approach is promising because it is relatively inexpensive, using parents as the only vehicle for treatment, yet hits multiple risk factors for poor outcomes in antisocial behavior (parenting, ODD, ADHD symptoms, reading ability; for more details of parenting programs see chapter 64).

Child Therapies

Cognitive–behavioral therapy (CBT) and social skills therapies can have several targets:

1 To reduce children's aggressive behavior such as shouting, pushing and arguing.

2 To increase prosocial interactions such as entering a group, starting a conversation, participating in group activities, sharing, cooperating, asking questions politely, listening and negotiating.

3 To correct the cognitive deficiencies, distortions and inaccurate self-evaluation exhibited by many of these children.

4 To ameliorate emotional regulation and self-control problems so as to reduce emotional lability, impulsivity and explosiveness, enabling the child to be more reflective and able to consider how best to respond in provoking situations.

In practice, most programs cover all four target areas to a greater or lesser extent. While child CBT was originally mainly used with school-age children and older, more recently it has been successfully adapted for preschoolers. These interventions may be delivered in individual or group therapy formats. Although groups offer several advantages (e.g., opportunities to practice peer interactions), there is some research documenting iatrogenic effects (Dishion, McCord, & Poulin, 1999). This appears to be particularly problematic in larger groups and those with inadequate therapist supervision, where children may learn deviant behavior from their peers and encourage each other to act in antisocial ways. A lower patient : therapist ratio is therefore recommended for group work.

Examples of Good Practice

Two of the more popular treatment models for conduct disorder are Kazdin's *Problem Solving Skills Training with in vivo Practice* (PSST-P; for a review see Kazdin, 1996b) and Lochman and Wells' (1996) *Coping Power Program*. In PSST-P, which is used from the age of 7 upwards, the child receives individual training in interpersonal cognitive problem-solving techniques for 12–20 1-hour sessions. The focus is on identifying problem situations, learning a series of problem-solving steps and applying the steps first to hypothetical situations, then in role plays and finally in real-life situations. Therapeutic strategies include games, therapist modeling and role play with therapist feedback. A token system is used in session to reinforce children's efforts to practice target skills. Parents are involved periodically for conjoint sessions, and may receive behavioral parent training as an adjunctive treatment. The Coping Power program is for children aged 8 years upwards, and is fairly lengthy, comprising 33 one-to-one and half-hour group sessions, with periodic (at least monthly) individual meetings. Training focuses on interpretation of social cues, generating prosocial solutions to problems and anger management with arousal reduction strategies. Treatment is delivered in groups of 5–7 children by a therapist and co-therapist. Sessions include imagined scenarios, therapist modeling, role plays with corrective feedback and assignments to practice outside of sessions. Parent and teacher training components have also been developed as adjunctive treatments.

Specifically targeting younger children with conduct problems aged 4–8, Webster-Stratton, Reid, and Hammond (2001b, 2004) have added a group child social skills training component to their IY program, called Dinosaur School. The program lasts for 20–22 2-hour sessions, during which parents usually attend a parallel parenting group. It covers interpersonal problem-solving for young children in a group format with about six children at a time. Sessions include discussion of hypothetical situations and possible solutions, therapist modeling of prosocial responses and practice role playing with therapist feedback. Videotaped vignettes are used to present situations for discussion. Puppets are used for interactive role plays, as well as child-friendly cue cards, coloring books and cartoons. The Dinosaur School program dovetails with other interventions in the IY program, including parent training and a curriculum to train teachers in classroom management skills.

Effectiveness

In two randomized controlled trials, Kazdin, Esveldt-Dawson, French *et al.* (1987) and Kazdin, Bass, Siegel *et al.* (1989) found that PSST results in significant decreases in deviant behavior and increases in prosocial behavior. Outcomes were superior to a client-centered relationship-based treatment and were maintained at 1-year follow-up. The addition of *in vivo* practice and a parent training component were both found to enhance outcomes. Evaluations of the Coping Power program demonstrate reductions in aggression and substance use, and improved social competence (e.g., Lochman & Wells, 2002). Treatment effects were maintained at 1-year follow-up, particularly for those who also received parent training components (Lochman & Wells, 2004). Now replications by independent research groups are needed. In studies by Webster-Stratton, Reid, & Hammond (2001b, 2004), Dinosaur School has been found to result in significant decreases in behavior problems and increased prosocial behavior; treatment gains appeared to be maintained after 1 year. These findings have been independently replicated (Hutchings, Lane, Owen *et al.*, 2004).

The literature is generally not supportive of the effectiveness of individual psychodynamic psychotherapies, art and drama therapies in this population, especially when used as a sole treatment modality, although decisive studies are yet to be undertaken. One or two studies, although methodologically limited, suggest that an attachment-based approach (Moretti, Holland, & Peterson, 1994) or a classic exploratory approach (Fonagy & Target, 1993) might possibly be helpful, at least for a subset of antisocial children; again, properly conducted randomized controlled trials are needed.

Interventions in School

Interventions to Promote Positive Behavior

Typically, teachers are taught techniques that they can apply to all children in their class as well as to those exhibiting the most antisocial behavior. Successful approaches use proactive strategies and include a focus on positive behavior and group interventions, and combine effective instructional strategies with effective behavioral management. Typically, they target four areas of functioning:

1 Promote positive behaviors such as compliance and following established classroom rules and procedures.
2 Prevent problem behaviors such as talking at inappropriate times and fighting.
3 Teach social and emotional skills such as conflict resolution and problem-solving.
4 Prevent the escalation of angry, acting out behavior.

A number of these targets can be met by training teachers in similar methods as parents, as described above. However, other techniques are classroom specific. For example, establishing and teaching rules and procedures involves setting rules such as "use a quiet voice," "listen when others are speaking," "keep your hands and feet to yourself" and "use respectful words." Note that these rules are all expressed positively, describing what the child should do, rather than as prohibitions stating what they should not do. Streipling (1997) offers six "rules for making rules":

1 Make few rules (3–6).
2 Negotiate them with the children.
3 State them behaviorally and positively.
4 Make a contract with the children to adhere to them.
5 Post them in the classroom.
6 Send a copy home to parents.

Crucial to all this is a systematic and consistent response to children following or not following the rules. Rewards can be social (teacher praise, peer recognition, notes home to parents), material (stickers, certificates, tokens to exchange for food, etc.), or privileges (e.g., extra breaktime, games, parties, computer time). Mild punishments include reprimands, response-costs procedures (losing privileges or points) and time out (being sent to the corner of the room or to another boring place).

Interventions to Promote Academic Engagement and Learning

These include self-management and self-reinforcement training programs, for example, to help children spend more time on task and to complete written work more quickly and accurately. An older review of 16 studies found moderate to large effects of such programs (Nelson, Smith, Young *et al.*, 1991), and subsequent trials uphold this (e.g., Levendoski & Cartledge, 2000).

A number of programs build on the evidence that antisocial failing children often have parents who do not get involved in their academic schoolwork, and indeed may not value it highly. They do not read with their children, encourage homework or attend school meetings. Approaches include removing barriers to home–school cooperation through training parents to approach teachers positively (often their own memories of school and teachers will be negative and discouraging) and, equally, training teachers to be constructive in solving children's difficulties and helping parents engage in academic activities with their children. Although there are good descriptions of programs (e.g., Christenson & Buerkle, 1999), to date rigorous evaluations are lacking. For more details of special education programs see chapter 74.

Medication

At present, there are no pharmacological interventions approved specifically for conduct disorder. Nonetheless, in the USA, medications are used relatively frequently and increasingly in this population (Steiner, Saxena, & Chang, 2003; Turgay, 2004). Primary care physicians are often placed in the position of managing such medications. Concerns have been raised because primary care clinicians often lack adequate training in developmental psychopathology, and adequate time for thorough assessment and monitoring (Vitiello, 2001). In the UK, medication would not generally be supported as good practice because, as discussed below, well-replicated trials of effectiveness are limited, particularly for children without ADHD.

The best-studied pharmacological interventions for youth with conduct problems are psychostimulants (methylphenidate and dexamfetamine), as used with children with comorbid ADHD and conduct disorder. In these circumstances, there is evidence that reduction in hyperactivity-impulsivity will also result in reduced conduct problems (Connor, Glatt, Lopez *et al.*, 2002; Gerardin, Cohen, Mazet *et al.*, 2002). There is insufficient reliable evidence to decide whether stimulants reduce aggression in the absence of ADHD; one study by Klein, Abikoff, Klass *et al.* (1997) found that improvements in conduct disorder symptoms were independent of ADHD symptom reduction, but this needs replication.

Other pharmacological approaches for antisocial behavior have tended to target reactive aggression and overarousal, primarily in highly aggressive and psychiatrically hospitalized youth. Medications used in these conditions include those purported to target affect dysregulation (e.g., buspirone, clonidine), mood stabilizers (e.g., lithium, carbamazepine). Whereas Campbell *et al.* found that lithium reduced aggression and hostility in psychiatrically hospitalized youth (Campbell, Adams, Small *et al.*, 1995; Malone, Delaney, Luebbert *et al.*, 2000), others have failed to show effectiveness in out-patient samples (e.g., Klein, 1991) and in studies of shorter treatment intervals (i.e., 2 weeks or less; Rifkin, Karajgi, Dicker *et al.*, 1997). Carbamazepine failed to out-perform placebo in a double-blind placebo controlled study (Cueva, Overall, Small *et al.*, 1996). In children with aggression and hyperactivity, Hazell and Stuart (2003) in a placebo controlled randomized trial of stimulants plus placebo versus stimulants plus clonidine found the latter was more effective. However, it should be noted that the use of polypharmacy treatment also carries the risk of increased side-effects (Impicciatore, Choonara, Clarkson *et al.*, 2001).

In the last few years, the use of antipsychotics such as risperidone, clonidine and others in out-patient settings has been increasing. However, there is only modest evidence for their effectiveness in conduct disorder in normal IQ children without ADHD. The review by Pappadopoulos, Woolston, Chait *et al.* (2006) found that effect sizes were larger where ADHD or intellectual disability were present. Findling, McNamara, Branicky *et al.* (2000), in a small ($n = 10$ per group), double-blind placebo controlled study, found significant short-term reductions in aggression. The Risperidone Disruptive Behavior Study Group used a placebo controlled double-blind design to study the effects of risperidone in 110 children with sub-average IQ and conduct problems. Results suggested that risperidone leads to significant improvements in behavior versus placebo (Aman, De Smedt, Derivan *et al.*, 2002; Snyder, Turgay, Aman *et al.*, 2002), but it remains unclear whether the same findings would apply to normal IQ children. Even newer antipsychotics, while not especially sedating, have substantial side-effects (e.g., risperidone typically leads to considerable weight gain) and the prevalence of movement disorders in the long term is unknown. When might they be contemplated? Clinical experience suggests they can lead to dramatic reductions in aggression in some cases, especially where there is poor emotional regulation characterized by prolonged rages. Prescribing antipsychotics for relatively short periods (say, up to 4 months) in lower doses (say, no more than 1–1.5 mg/day risperidone) can help families cope; during this time it is crucial to introduce more effective psychological management.

Conclusions and the Way Forward

Conduct disorder is a common disorder among children, and intervention is essential because most children with conduct disorder show poor health and social outcomes for many years, ultimately accounting for a substantial proportion of the adulthood health burden. In coming years we expect to see new research into the following unanswered questions. First, given the plethora of statistical risk factors for conduct problems at the levels of individual, family and community, which among them are causal and which are the best candidates for intervention? Second, what factors can help clinicians predict long-term prognosis and select which youth with conduct problems most warrant scarce treatment resources? Third, given that preschool-onset conduct problems and psychopathic traits are good predictors of prognosis in research settings, how can these features be safely used in clinical settings without the iatrogenic effects of assigning derogatory labels to young children? Fourth, do girls with conduct problems need a different causal theory from boys, and perhaps different interventions? Fifth, what biomarkers are reliably associated with conduct problems, and do any of these suggest new treatment possibilities?

As our review of treatments demonstrated, psychological therapies are the mainstay of treatment for conduct problems. However, despite this strong evidence base, in both the USA and the UK only a minority of children receive any treatment, and even fewer receive empirically supported interventions. Further, the "effectiveness" of these interventions as practiced in community settings tends to lag behind documented "efficacy" in controlled trials (e.g., Curtis, Ronan, & Borduin, 2004). As can already be seen in recent efforts with many of the interventions described here, the next generation of evidence-based treatments for conduct problems will likely include much greater attention to dissemination, including strategies for ongoing training and supervision of practitioners to ensure treatment fidelity. The ultimate goal, of course, is to ensure that children with these disorders have access to high-quality empirically based care.

Acknowledgments

We are indebted to Jonathan Hill, who assisted us with this chapter.

Resource Websites for Ongoing Intervention Program Evaluations

University of Colorado Blueprints for Violence Prevention: http://www.colorado.edu/cspv/blueprints

Center for Disease Control National Youth Violence Prevention Resource Center: http://www.safeyouth.org/scripts/index.asp

Preventing violence and related health-risking behaviors in adolescents, an NIH State of the Science Consensus report: http://consensus.nih.gov/PREVIOUSSTATEMENTS.htm#2004YouthViolence

University of Maryland, Treating juvenile delinquency, what works? http://www.preventingcrime.org

Further Reading

Bowlby, J. (1944). Forty-four juvenile thieves: Their characters and home-life. *International Journal of Psycho-Analysis*, *25*, 19–52, 107–127.

Cleckley, H. (1976). *The mask of sanity*. St. Louis, MO: Mosby.

Hill, J., & Maughan, B. (2001). *Conduct disorder in context*. Cambridge, UK: Cambridge University Press.

Lahey, B., Moffitt, T. E., & Caspi, A. (2003). *Causes of conduct disorder and juvenile delinquency*. NY: Guilford Press.

Moffitt, T. E., Caspi, A., Rutter, M., & Silva, P. A. (2001). *Sex differences in antisocial behavior*. Cambridge, UK: Cambridge University Press.

Patterson, G. (1982). *Coercive family process*. Eugene, OR: Castalia.

Robins, L. N. (1966). *Deviant children grown-up: A sociological and psychiatric study of sociopathic personalities*. Baltimore: Williams and Wilkins.

Rutter, M., Giller, H., & Hagell, A. (1998). *Antisocial behaviour by young people*. Cambridge: Cambridge University Press.

References

Achenbach, T. M., & Rescorla, L. A. (2000). *Manual for the ASEBA preschool forms and profiles: An integrated system of multi-informant assessment*. Burlington, VT: University of Vermont Department of Psychiatry.

Aman, M. G., De Smedt, G., Derivan, A., Lyons, B., Findling, R. L., Risperidone Disruptive Behavior Study Group. (2002). Double-blind, placebo-controlled study of risperidone for the treatment of disruptive behaviors in children with subaverage intelligence. *American Journal of Psychiatry*, *159*, 1337–1346.

American Academy of Child and Adolescent Psychiatry (AACAP). (1997). Practice parameters for the assessment and treatment of children and adolescents with conduct disorder. *Journal of the American Academy of Child and Adolescent Psychiatry*, *36*, 122S–139S.

American Psychiatric Association. (2000). *Diagnostic and statistical manual of mental disorders* (4th edn.). Text revision. Washington, DC: American Psychiatric Association.

Anderson, K. E., Lytton, H., & Romney, D. M. (1986). Mothers' interactions with normal and conduct-disordered boys: Who affects whom? *Developmental Psychology*, *22*, 604–609.

Angold, A., & Costello, E. J. (2001). The epidemiology of disorders of conduct: Nosological issues and comorbidity. In J. Hill, & B. Maughan (Eds.), *Conduct disorders in childhood and adolescence* (pp. 1–31). Cambridge: Cambridge University Press.

Angold, A., Costello, E. J., & Erkanli, A. (1999). Comorbidity. *Journal of Child Psychology and Psychiatry*, *40*, 57–87.

Arseneault, L., Kim-Cohen, J., Taylor, A., Caspi, A., & Moffitt, T. E. (2005). Psychometric evaluation of 5- and 7-year-old children's self-reports of conduct problems. *Journal of Abnormal Child Psychology*, *33*, 537–550.

Arseneault, L., Tremblay, R. E., Boulerice, B., & Saucier, J.-F. (2002). Obstetric complications and adolescent violent behaviors: Testing two developmental pathways. *Child Development*, *73*, 496–508.

Arseneault, L., Walsh, E., Trzesniewski, K., Newcombe, R., Caspi, A., & Moffitt, T. E. (2006). Bullying victimization uniquely contributes to adjustment problems in young children: A nationally representative cohort study. *Pediatrics*, *118*, 130–138.

Augimeri, L. K., Koegl, C. J., Webster, C. D., & Levene, K. S. (2001). *Early Assessment Risk List for Boys (EARL-20B)*. Toronto, Ontario: Earlscourt Child and Family Centre.

Bandura, A. (1997). *Social learning theory*. Englewood Cliffs, NJ: Prentice-Hall.

Barry, C. T., Frick, P. J., DeShazo, T. M., McCoy, M. G., Ellis, M., & Loney, B. R. (2000). The importance of callous-unemotional traits for extending the concept of psychopathy to children. *Journal of Abnormal Psychology*, *109*, 335–340.

Barton, C., & Alexander, J. F. (1981). Functional family therapy. In A. S. Gurman, & D. P. Kniskern (Eds.), *Handbook of family therapy* (pp. 403–443). New York: Brunner/Mazel.

Beyers, J. M., Bates, J. E., Pettit, G. S., & Dodge, K. A. (2003). Neighborhood structure, parenting processes, and the development of youths' externalizing behaviors: A multi-level analysis. *American Journal of Community Psychology*, *31*, 35–53.

Blair, R. J. R., Mitchell, D., & Blair, K. (2005). *The psychopath*. London: Blackwell.

Bloomquist, M. L., & Schnell, S. V. (2002). *Helping children with aggression and conduct problems: Best practices for intervention*. New York: Guilford Press.

Blumstein, A., & Wallman, J. (2005). *The crime drop in America*. Cambridge, UK: Cambridge University Press.

Bohman, M. (1996). Predisposition to criminality: Swedish adoption studies in retrospect. In G. R. Bock, & J. A. Goode (Eds.), *Genetics of criminal and antisocial behaviour*. Ciba Foundation Symposium no. 194 (pp. 99–114). Chichester: Wiley.

Boivin, N., & Vitaro, F. (1995). The impact of peer relationships on aggression in childhood: Inhibition through coercion or promotion through peer support. In J. McCord (Ed.), *Coercion and punishment in long-term perspectives* (pp. 183–197). Cambridge, UK. Cambridge University Press.

Bor, W., Sanders, M. R., & Markie-Dadds, C. (2002). The effects of the Triple P-Positive Parenting Program on preschool children with co-occurring disruptive behavior and attentional/hyperactive difficulties. *Journal of Abnormal Child Psychology*, *30*, 571–587.

Borum, R., Bartel, P., & Forth, A. (2002). *Manual for the structured assessment of violence risk in youth (SAVRY)*. Tampa, FL: University of South Florida.

Bowlby, J. (1944). Forty-four juvenile thieves: their characters and home-life. *International Journal of Psycho-Analysis*, *25*, 19–52, 107–127.

Brennan, P. A., Grekin, E. R., & Mednick, S. A. (2003). In B. Lahey, T. E. Moffitt, & A. Caspi (Eds.), *Causes of conduct disorder and delinquency* (pp. 319–344). NY: Guilford Press.

Cadoret, R. J., Yates, W. R., Troughton, E., Woodworth, G., & Stewart, M. A. (1995). Genetic–environmental interaction in the genesis of aggressivity and conduct disorders. *Archives of General Psychiatry*, *52*, 916–924.

Campbell, M., Adams, P. B., Small, A. M., Kafantaris, V., Silva, R. R., Shell, J., *et al.* (1995). Lithium in hospitalized aggressive children with conduct disorder: A double-blind and placebo-controlled study. *Journal of the American Academy of Child & Adolescent Psychiatry*, *34*, 445–453.

Campbell, S. B. (2002). *Behavior problems in preschool children: Clinical and developmental issues* (2nd edn.). NY: Guilford Press.

Campbell, S. B., Pierce, E. W., Moore, G., Marakovitz, S., & Newby, K. (1996). Boys' externalising problems at elementary school age: Pathways from early behaviour problems, maternal control, and family stress. *Development and Psychopathology*, *8*, 701–719.

Capaldi, D., & Gorman-Smith, D. (2003). The development of aggression in young male/female couples. In P. Florsheim (Ed.), *Adolescent romantic relationships and sexual behavior* (pp. 243–278). Mahwah, NJ: Lawrence Erlbaum Associates.

Carroll, J. M., Maughan, B., Goodman, R., & Meltzer, H. (2005). Literacy difficulties and psychiatric disorders: Evidence for comorbidity. *Journal of Child Psychology and Psychiatry*, *46*, 524–532.

Caspi, A., McClay, J., Moffitt, T., Mill, J., Martin, J., Craig, I., *et al.* (2002). Evidence that the cycle of violence in maltreated children depends on genotype. *Science*, *297*, 851–854.

Caspi, A., Moffitt, T. E., Newman, D. L., & Silva, P. A. (1996). Behavioural observations at age 3 predict adult psychiatric disorders: Longitudinal evidence from a birth cohort. *Archives of General Psychiatry*, *53*, 1033–1039.

Caspi, A., Taylor, A., Moffitt, T. E., & Plomin, R. (2000). Neighborhood deprivation affects children's mental health: Environmental risks identified using a genetic design. *Psychological Science*, *11*, 338–342.

Christenson, S. L., & Buerkle, K. (1999). Families as educational partners for childrens' school success: Suggestions for school psychologists. In C. R. Reynolds, & T. B. Gutkin (Eds.), *The handbook of school psychology* (3rd edn., pp. 709–744). New York: Wiley.

Coie, J. D. (2004). The impact of negative social experiences on the development of antisocial behavior. In J. B. Kupersmidt, & K. A. Dodge (Eds.), *Children's peer relations: From development to intervention* (pp. 243–267). Washington, DC: American Psychological Association.

Collishaw, S., Maughan, B., Goodman, R., & Pickles, A. (2004). Time trends in adolescent mental health. *Journal of Child Psychology and Psychiatry*, *45*, 1350–1362.

Conger, R. D., Ge, X., Elder, G. H., Lorenz, F. O., & Simmons, R. L. (1994). Economic stress, coercive family process and developmental problems of adolescents. *Child Development*, *65*, 541–561.

Connor, D. F., Glatt, S. J., Lopez, I. D., Jackson, D., & Melloni, R. H. (2002). Psychopharmacology and aggression. I. A meta-analysis of stimulant effects on overt/covert aggression-related behaviors in ADHD. *Journal of the American Academy of Child and Adolescent Psychiatry*, *41*, 253–261.

Costello, E. J., Angold, A., Burns, B., Stangl, D., Tweed, D., & Erkanli, A. (1996). The Great Smoky Mountain Study of Youth. I. Prevalence and correlates of DSM-III-R disorders. *Archives of General Psychiatry*, *53*, 1137–1143.

Costello, E. J., Compton, S. N., Keeler, G., & Angold, A. (2003). Relationships between poverty and psychopathology: A natural experiment. *Journal of the American Medical Association*, *290*, 2023–2029.

Cueva, J. E., Overall, J. E. Small, A. M., Armenteros, J. L., Perry, R., & Campbell, M. (1996). Carbamazepine in aggressive children with conduct disorder: A double-blind and placebo-controlled study. *Journal of the American Academy of Child and Adolescent Psychiatry*, *35*, 480–490.

Cummings, E. M., & Davies, P. (2002). Effects of marital conflict on children: Recent advances and emerging themes in process-oriented research. *Journal of Child Psychology and Psychiatry*, *43*, 31–64.

Curtis, N. M., Ronan, K. R., & Borduin, C. M. (2004). Multisystemic therapy: A meta-analysis of outcome studies. *Journal of Family Psychology*, *18*, 411–419.

Davies, P. T., & Cummings, E. M. (1994). Marital conflict and child adjustment: An emotional security hypothesis. *Psychological Bulletin*, *116*, 387–411.

Deater-Deckard, K., Dodge, K. A., Bates, J. E., & Pettit, G. S. (1996). Physical discipline among African American and European American mothers: Links to children's externalizing behaviors. *Developmental Psychology*, *32*, 1065–1072.

Dishion, T. J., McCord, J., & Poulin, F. (1999). When interventions harm: Peer groups and problem behavior. *American Psychologist*, *54*, 755–764.

Dodge, K. A. (1993). Social-cognitive mechanisms in the development of conduct disorder and depression. In L. W. Porter, & M. R. Rosenweig (Eds.), *Annual Review of Psychology* (Volume 44, pp. 559–584).

Dodge, K. A., Coie, J. D., & Lynam, D. R. (2006). Aggression and antisocial behavior in youth. In W. Damon, & R. A. Lerner (Editors in Chief) & N. Eisenberg (Volume Editor), *Handbook of Child Psychology* (6th edn., Volume 3), *Social, emotional and personality development* (pp. 719–788). New York: J. Wiley.

Dodge, K. A., Pettit, G. S., Bates, J. E., & Valente, E. (1995). Social information: Processing patterns partially mediate the effect of early physical abuse on later conduct problems. *Journal of Abnormal Psychology*, *104*, 632–643.

Eaves, L. J., Silver, J. L., Meyer, J. M., Maes, H. H., Simonoff, E., Pickles, A., *et al.* (1997). Genetics and developmental psychopathology. 2. The main effects of genes and environmental behavioral problems in the Virginia Twin Study of Adolescent Behavioral Development. *Journal of Child Psychology and Psychiatry*, *38*, 965–980.

Egger, H. L., & Angold, A. (2006). Common emotional and behavioural disorders in preschool children: Presentation, nosology, and epidemiology. *Journal of Child and Adolescent Psychiatry*, *47*, 313–337.

Ehrensaft, M., Moffitt, T. E., & Caspi, A. (2004). Clinically abusive relationships and their developmental antecedents in an unselected birth cohort. *Journal of Abnormal Psychology*, *113*, 258–270.

Elander, J., & Rutter, M. (1996). Use and development of the Rutter parents' and teachers' scale. *International Journal of Methods in Psychiatric Research*, *6*, 63–78.

Eyberg, S. M. (1988). Parent–Child Interaction Therapy: Integration of traditional and behavioral concerns. *Child and Family Behavior Therapy*, *10*, 33–48.

Farmer, E. M., Compton, S. N., Burns, B. J., & Robertson, E. (2002). Review of the evidence base for treatment of childhood psychopathology: externalizing disorders. *Journal of Consulting and Clinical Psychology*, *70*, 1267–1302.

Farrington, D. P. (1997). The relationship between low resting heart rate and violence. In A. Raine, P. A. Brennan, D. P. Farrington, & S. A. Mednick (Eds.), *Biosocial bases of violence* (pp. 89–105). New York: Plenum Press.

Farrington, D. P. (2005). The importance of child and adolescent psychopathy. *Journal of Abnormal Child Psychology*, *33*, 489–497.

Farrington, D. P., Gallagher, B., Morley, L., St. Ledger, R. J., & West, D. (1988). Are there any successful men from criminogenic backgrounds? *Psychiatry*, *51*, 116–130.

Farrington, D. P., & Hawkins, J. D. (1991). Predicting participation, early onset, and later persistence in officially recorded offending. *Criminal behaviour and mental health*, *1*, 1–33.

Farrington, D. P., & Loeber, R. (1998). Transatlantic replicability of risk factors in the development of delinquency. In P. Cohen, C. Slomkowski, & L. M. Robins (Eds.), *Where and when: The influence of history and geography on aspects of psychopathology* (pp. 299–329). Hillsdale, NJ: Lawrence Erlbaum Assoc.

Farrington, D. P., Jolliffe, D., Loeber, R., Stouthamer-Loeber, M., & Kalb, L. (2001). The concentration of offenders in families, and family criminality in the prediction of boys' delinquency. *Journal of Adolescence*, *24*, 579–596.

Farver, J. A. M. (1996). Aggressive behaviour in pre-schoolers' social networks: Do birds of a feather flock together? *Early Childhood Research Quarterly*, *11*, 333–350.

Fergusson, D. M. (1999). Prenatal smoking and antisocial behaviour: Commentary. *Archives of General Psychiatry*, *56*, 223–224.

Fergusson, D. M., & Horwood, L. J. (1995). Predictive validity of categorically and dimensionally scored measures of disruptive childhood behaviors. *Journal of the American Academy of Child and Adolescent Psychiatry*, *34*, 477–487.

Fergusson, D. M., Horwood, L. J., & Lynskey, M. T. (1996). Childhood sexual abuse and psychiatric disorder in young adulthood. II. Psychiatric outcomes of childhood sexual abuse. *Journal of the American Academy of Child and Adolescent Psychiatry*, *35*, 1365–1374.

Fergusson, D. M., Woodward, L. J., & Horwood, L. J. (1999). Childhood peer relationship problems and young people's involvement with deviant peers in adolescence. *Journal of Abnormal Child Psychology*, *27*, 357–370.

Findling, R. L., McNamara, N. K., Branicky, L. A., Schluchter, M. D., Lemon, E., & Blumer, J. L. (2000). A double-blind pilot study of risperidone in the treatment of conduct disorder. *Journal of the American Academy of Child and Adolescent Psychiatry*, *39*, 509–516.

Fonagy, P., & Target, M. (1993). The efficacy of psychoanalysis for children with disruptive disorders. *Journal of the American Academy of Child and Adolescent Psychiatry*, *33*, 45–55.

Fung, M. T., Raine, A., Loeber, R., Lynam, D., Steinhauer, S. R., Venables, P. H., *et al.* (2005). Reduced electrodermal activity in psychopathy-prone adolescents. *Journal of Abnormal Psychology*, *114*, 187–196.

Gardner, F. E. M. (1989). Inconsistent parenting: is there evidence for a link with children's conduct problems? *Journal of Abnormal Child Psychology*, *17*, 223–233.

Ge, X., Conger, R., Cadoret, R. J., Neiderhiser, J. M., Yates, W., Troughton, E., *et al.* (1996). The developmental interface between nature and nurture: A mutual influence model of child antisocial behaviour and parent behaviours. *Developmental Psychology*, *32*, 574–589.

Gerardin, P., Cohen, D., Mazet, P., & Flament, M. F. (2002). Drug treatment of conduct disorder in young people. *European Neuropsychopharmacology*, *12*, 361–370.

Gilmour, J., Hill, B., Place, M., & Skuse, D. (2004). Social communication deficits in conduct disorder. *Journal of Child Psychology and Psychiatry*, *45*, 967–978.

Goodman, R. (1997). The Strengths and Difficulties Questionnaire (SDQ). *Journal of Child Psychology and Psychiatry*, *38*, 581–586.

Goodman, R., Ford, T., Richards, H. Gatward, R., & Meltzer, H. (2000). The Development & Well-Being Assessment (DAWBA). *Journal of Child Psychology and Psychiatry*, *41*, 645–655.

Green, H., McGinnity, A., Meltzer, H., Ford, T., & Goodman, R. (2005). *Mental health of children and young people in Great Britain*. London: The Stationery Office.

Halpern, C. T., Oslak, S. G., Young, M. L., Martin, S. L., & Kupper, L. L. (2001). Partner violence among adolescents in opposite-sex relationships: National Longitudinal Study of Adolescent Health. *American Journal of Public Health*, *91*, 1679–1685.

Hare R. D., Hart S. D., & Harpur T. J. (1991). Psychopathy and the DSM-IV criteria for antisocial personality disorder. *Journal of Abnormal Psychology*, *100*, 391–398.

Hawkins, J. D., Herrenkohl, T., Farrington, D. P., Brewer, D., Catalano, R. F., & Harachi, T. W. (1998). A review of predictors of youth violence. In R. Loeber, & D. P. Farrington (Eds.), *Serious and violent juvenile offenders: risk factors and successful interventions*. Thousand Oaks: Sage.

Haynie, D. L., & Piquero, A. (2006). Pubertal development and physical victimization in adolescence. *Journal of Research in Crime and Delinquency*, *43*, 3–35.

Hazell, P. L., & Stuart, J. E. (2003). A randomized controlled trial of clonidine added to psychostimulant medication for hyperactive and aggressive children. *Journal of the American Academy of Child and Adolescent Psychiatry*, *42*, 886–894.

Hill, J. (2002). Biological, psychological and social processes in the conduct disorders. *Journal of Child Psychology and Psychiatry*, *43*, 133–164.

Hill, J., & Maughan, B. (Eds.). (2001). *Conduct disorders in childhood and adolescence*. Cambridge, UK: Cambridge University Press.

Hinshaw, S. P., Lahey, B. B., & Hart, E. L. (1993). Issues of taxonomy and comorbidity in the development of conduct disorder. *Development and Psychopathology*, *5*, 31–40.

Hood, K., & Eyberg, S. M. (2003). Outcomes of parent–child interaction therapy: Mothers' reports on maintenance 3 to 6 years after treatment. *Journal of Clinical Child and Adolescent Psychology*, *32*, 419–429.

Hughes, C., Dunn, J., & White, A. (1998). Trick or treat? Patterns of cognitive performance and executive dysfunction among hard to manage preschoolers. *Journal of Child Psychology and Psychiatry*, *39*, 981–994.

Hutchings, J., Lane, E., Owen, R. E., & Gwyn, R. (2004). The introduction of the Webster-Stratton Incredible Years Classroom Dinosaur School Programme in Gwynedd, North Wales: A pilot study. *Educational and Child Psychology*, *21*, 4–15.

Impicciatore, P., Choonara, I., Clarkson, A., Provasi, D., Pandolfini, C., & Bonati, M. (2001). Incidence of adverse drug reactions in paediatric in/out-patients: A systematic review and meta-analysis of prospective studies. *British Journal of Clinical Pharmacology*, *52*, 77–83.

Ishikawa, S. S., & Raine, A. (2003). Prefrontal deficits and antisocial behavior: A causal model. In B. Lahey, T. E. Moffitt, & A. Caspi (Eds.), *Causes of conduct disorder and delinquency* (pp. 277–304). NY: Guilford Press.

Jaffee, S. R., Belsky, J., Sligo, J., Harrington, H. L., Caspi, A., & Moffitt, T. E. (2006). When parents have a history of adolescent conduct disorder: Parenting, offspring behavior, and the caregiving environment. *Journal of Abnormal Psychology*, *115*, 309–319.

Jaffee, S. R., Caspi, A., Moffitt, T. E., Dodge, K. A., Rutter, M., Taylor, A., *et al.* (2005). Nature × nurture: Genetic vulnerabilities interact with physical maltreatment to promote conduct problems. *Development and Psychopathology*, *17*, 67–84.

Jaffee, S. R., Caspi, A., Moffitt, T. E., Polo-Tomas, M., Price, T. S., & Taylor, A. (2004). The limits of child effects: Evidence for genetically mediated child effects on corporal punishment, but not on physical maltreatment. *Developmental Psychology*, *40*, 1047–1058.

Jaffee, S. R., Moffitt, T. E., Caspi, A., & Taylor, A. (2003). Life with (or without) father: The benefits of living with two biological parents depend on the father's antisocial behavior. *Child Development*, *74*, 109–126.

Kazdin, A. E. (1996a). Dropping out of child therapy: Issues for research and implications for practice. *Clinical Child Psychology and Psychiatry*, *1*, 133–156.

Kazdin, A. E. (1996b). Problem solving and parent management in treating aggressive and antisocial behavior. In E. S. Hibbs, & P. S. Jensen (Eds.), *Psychosocial treatments for child and adolescent disorders: Empirically-based strategies for clinical practice* (pp. 377–408). Washington, DC: American Psychological Association.

Kazdin, A. E., Bass, D., Siegel, T., & Thomas, C. (1989). Cognitive–behavioural treatment and relationship therapy in the treatment of children referred for antisocial behaviour. *Journal of Consulting and Clinical Psychology*, *57*, 522–535.

Kazdin, A. E., Esveldt-Dawson, K., French, N. H., & Unis, A. S. (1987). Problem-solving skills training and relationship therapy in the treatment of antisocial child behavior. *Journal of Consulting and Clinical Psychology*, *55*, 76–85.

Keenan, K., & Shaw, D. S. (2003). Starting at the beginning: Exploring the etiology of antisocial behavior in the first years of life. In B. Lahey, T. E. Moffitt, & A. Caspi (Eds.), *Causes of conduct disorder and delinquency* (pp. 153–181). NY: Guilford Press.

Keenan, K., & Wakschlag, L. S. (2002). Can a valid diagnosis of disruptive behavior disorder be made in preschool children? *American Journal of Psychiatry*, *159*, 351–358.

Kim-Cohen, J., Arseneault, L., Caspi, A., Polo Tomas, M., Taylor, A., & Moffitt, T. E. (2005). Validity of *DSM-IV* Conduct Disorder in 4½–5-year-old children: A longitudinal epidemiological study. *American Journal of Psychiatry*, *162*, 1108–1117.

Kim-Cohen, J., Caspi, A., Moffitt, T. E., Harrington, H., Milne, B. J., & Poulton, R. (2003). Prior juvenile diagnoses in adults with mental disorder: Developmental follow-back of a prospective-longitudinal cohort. *Archives of General Psychiatry*, *60*, 709–717.

Kim-Cohen, J., Caspi, A., Taylor, A., Williams, B., Newcombe, R., Craig, I. W., *et al.* (2006). MAOA, early adversity, and gene–environment interaction predicting children's mental health: New evidence and a meta-analysis. *Molecular Psychiatry*, *11*, 903–913.

Kim-Cohen, J., Moffitt, T. E., Taylor, A., Pawlby, S. J., & Caspi, A. (2005). Maternal depression and child antisocial behavior: Nature and nurture effects. *Archives of General Psychiatry*, *62*, 173–181.

Klein, R. (1991). *Preliminary results: lithium effects in conduct disorders*. In: CME Syllabus and Proceedings Summary, 144th Annual Meeting of the American Psychiatric Association, New Orleans (pp. 119–120).

Klein, R. G., Abikoff, H., Klass, E., Ganeles, D., Seese, L. M., & Pollack, S. (1997). Clinical efficacy of methylphenidate in conduct disorder with and without attention deficit hyperactivity disorder. *Archives of General Psychiatry*, *54*, 1073–1080.

Koot, H., Crijnen, A., & Ferdinand, R. (1999). *Child psychiatric epidemiology*. The Netherlands: van Gorcum.

Kraemer, H. C. (2003). Current concepts of risk in psychiatric disorders. *Current Opinion in Psychiatry*, *16*, 421–430.

Kratzer, L., & Hodgins, S. (1999). A typology of offenders: A test of Moffitt's theory among males and females from childhood to age 30. *Criminal Behaviour and Mental Health*, *9*, 57–73.

Lahey, B. B., Loeber, R., Hart, E. L., Frick, P. J., Applegate, B., Zhang, Q., *et al.* (1995). Four-year longitudinal study of conduct disorder in boys: Patterns and predictors of persistence. *Journal of Abnormal Psychology*, *104*, 83–93.

Lahey, B. B., Loeber, R., Quay, H. C., Frick, P. J., & Grimm, J. (1997). Oppositional defiant disorder and conduct disorder. In T. A. Widiger, A. J. Frances, H. A. Pincus, R. Ross, M. B. First, & W. Davis (Eds.), *DSM-IV sourcebook* (Volume 3, pp. 189–209.). Washington, DC: American Psychiatric Association.

Lahey, B., Moffitt, T. E., & Caspi, A. (Eds.). (2003). *Causes of conduct disorder and delinquency*. NY: Guilford Press.

Levendoski, L. S., &. Cartledge, G. (2000). Self-monitoring for elementary school children with serious emotional disturbances: Classroom applications for increased academic responding. *Behavioral Disorders*, *25*, 211–224.

Levene, K. S., Augimeri, L. K., Pepler, D. J., Walsh, M. M., Webster, C. D., & Koegl, C. J. (2001). *Early Assessment Risk List for Girls (EARL-21G)*. Toronto, Ontario: Earlscourt Child and Family Centre.

Lochman, J. E., & Wells, K. C. (1996). A social–cognitive intervention with aggressive children: Prevention effects and contextual implementation issues. In R. Peters, & R. J. McMahon (Eds.), *Prevention and early intervention: Childhood disorders, substance use and delinquency* (pp. 111–143). Thousand Oaks, CA: Sage.

Lochman, J. E., & Wells, K. C. (2002). The Coping Power Program at the middle school transition: Universal and indicated prevention effects. *Psychology of Addictive Behaviors*, *16*, 540–554.

Lochman, J. E., & Wells, K. C. (2004). The coping power program for preadolescent aggressive boys and their parents: outcome effects at the 1-year follow-up. *Journal of Consulting and Clinical Psychology*, *72*, 571–578.

Loeber, R., Burke, J. D., Lahey, B. B., Winters, A., & Zera, M. (2000). Oppositional defiant and conduct disorder: a review of the past 10 years, Part I. *Journal of the American Academy of Child and Adolescent Psychiatry*, *39*, 1468–1484.

Loeber, R., Green, S. M., Lahey, B. B., & Stouthamer-Loeber, M. (1991). Differences and similarities between children, mothers, and teachers as informants on disruptive child behavior. *Journal of Abnormal Child Psychology*, *19*, 75–95.

Luria, A. R. (1961). *The role of speech in the regulation of normal and abnormal behavior*. New York: Basic Books.

Lynam, D. R. (1996). The early identification of chronic offenders: Who is the fledgling psychopath? *Psychological Bulletin*, *120*, 209–234.

Lynam, D. R., & Gudonis, L. (2005). The development of psychopathy. *Annual Reviews of Clinical Psychology*, 1, 381–407.

Lynam, D. R., & Henry, W. (2001). The role of neuropsychological deficits in conduct disorders. In J. Hill, & B. Maughan (Eds.), *Conduct disorders in childhood and adolescence* (pp. 235–263). Cambridge, UK: Cambridge University Press.

Lynam, D. R., Moffitt, T., & Stouthamer-Loeber, M. (1993). Explaining the relationship between IQ and delinquency: Class, race, test motivation, school failure or self-control? *Journal of Abnormal Psychology*, *102*, 187–196.

Malone, R. P., Delaney, M. A., Luebbert, J. F., Cater, J., & Campbell M. (2000). A double-blind placebo-controlled study of lithium in hospitalized aggressive children and adolescents with conduct disorder. *Archives of General Psychiatry*, *57*, 649–654.

Main, M., & Solomon, J. (1986). Discovery of a new, insecure-disorganized/disoriented attachment pattern. In T. B. Brazelton, & M. W. Yogman (Eds.), *Affective Development in Infancy* (pp. 95–124). Norwood, NJ: Ablex.

Maughan, B. (2001). Conduct disorder in context. In J. Hill, & B. Maughan (Eds.), *Conduct disorders in childhood and adolescence* (pp. 169–201). Cambridge, UK: Cambridge University Press.

Maughan, B., Rowe, R, Messer, J., Goodman, R., & Meltzer, H. (2004). Conduct disorder and oppositional defiant disorder in a national sample: developmental epidemiology. *Journal of Child Psychology and Psychiatry*, *45*, 609–621.

McBurnett, K., Raine, A., Stouthamer-Loeber, M., Loeber, R., Kumar, A. M., Kumar, M., *et al.* (2005). Mood and hormone responses to psychological challenge in adolescent males with conduct problems. *Biological Psychiatry*, *57*, 1109–1116.

McMahon R. J., & Forehand R. L. (2003). *Helping the noncompliant child: family-based treatment for oppositional behavior* (2nd edn.). New York: Guilford Press.

Meyer-Lindenberg, A., Buckholtz, J. W., Kolachana, B., Hariri, A., Pezawas, L., Blasi, G., *et al.* (2006). Neural mechanisms of genetic risk for impulsivity in violence in humans. *Proceedings of the National Academy of Sciences*, *103*, 6269–6274.

Minuchin, S. (1974). *Families and family therapy*, Cambridge, MA: Harvard University Press.

Moffitt, T. E. (1993a). "Life-course-persistent" and "adolescence-limited" antisocial behavior: A developmental taxonomy. *Psychological Review*, *100*, 674–701.

Moffitt, T. E. (1993b). The neuropsychology of conduct disorder. *Development and Psychopathology*, *5*, 135–151.

Moffitt, T. E. (2005a). Genetic and environmental influences on antisocial behaviors: Evidence from behavioral-genetic research. *Advances in Genetics*, *55*, 41–104.

Moffitt, T. E. (2005b). The new look of behavioral genetics in developmental psychopathology: Gene–environment interplay in antisocial behavior. *Psychological Bulletin*, *131*, 533–554.

Moffitt, T. E. (2006). Life-course persistent versus adolescence-limited antisocial behavior. In D. Cicchetti, & D. Cohen (Eds.), *Developmental psychopathology* (2nd edn.). NY: Wiley.

Moffitt, T. E., & Caspi, A. (1998). Annotation: Implications of violence between intimate partners for child psychologists and psychiatrists. *Journal of Child Psychology and Psychiatry*, *39*, 137–144.

Moffitt, T. E., Caspi, A., Harrington, H., & Milne, B. J. (2002). Males on the life-course persistent and adolescence-limited antisocial pathways: Follow-up at age 26. *Development and Psychopathology*, *14*, 179–206.

Moffitt, T. E., Caspi, A., Rutter, M., & Silva, P. A. (2001). Sex differences in antisocial behavior: *Conduct disorder, delinquency and violence in the Dunedin Longitudinal Study*. Cambridge, UK: Cambridge University Press.

Morenoff, J. D. (2005). Racial and ethnic disparities in crime and delinquency in the United States. In M. Rutter, & M. Tienda (Eds.), *Ethnicity and causal mechanisms* (pp. 139–173). Cambridge, UK: Cambridge University Press.

Moretti, M., Holland R., & Peterson, S. (1994). Long-term outcome of an attachment-based program for conduct disorder. *Canadian Journal of Psychiatry*, *39*, 360–370.

Moss, E., Smolla, N., Cyr, C., Dubois-Comtois, K., Mazzarello, T., & Berthiaume, C. (2006). Attachment and behaviour problems in middle childhood as reported by adult and child informants. *Development and Psychopathology*, *18*, 425–444.

Nagin, D. S., Farrington, D. P., & Moffitt, T. (1995). Life-course trajectories of different types of offenders. *Criminology*, *29*, 163–190.

Nansel, T. R., Craig, W., Overpeck, M. D., Saluja, G., & Ruan, J. (2004). Cross-national consistency in the relationship between bullying behaviours and psychosocial adjustment. *Archives of Pediatric and Adolescent Medicine*, *158*, 730–736.

National Institute of Health and Clinical Excellence (NICE). (2006). *Heath Technology Appraisal: Parent training and education programmes for childhood conduct disorder*. London: NICE.

Nelson, J. R., Smith, D. J., Young, R. K., & Dodd, J. M. (1991). A review of self-management outcome research conducted with students who exhibit behavioral disorders. *Behavioral Disorders*, *16*, 168–179.

Nelson, R. J. (2006). *Biology of aggression*. Oxford: Oxford University Press.

Nigg, J. T. (2006). Temperament and developmental psychopathology. *Journal of Child Psychology and Psychiatry*, *47*, 395–422.

Nigg, J. T., & Huang-Pollock, C. (2003). An early-onset model of the role of executive functions and intelligence in conduct disorder/delinquency. In B. Lahey, T. E. Moffitt, & A. Caspi (Eds.), *Causes of conduct disorder and delinquency* (pp. 227–253). NY: Guilford Press.

Nixon, R. D., Sweeney, L., Erickson, D. B., & Touyz, S. W. (2003). Parent–child interaction therapy: A comparison of standard and abbreviated treatments for oppositional defiant preschoolers. *Journal of Consulting & Clinical Psychology*, *71*, 251–260.

Odgers, C., Caspi, A., Poulton, R., Harrington, H. L., Thomson, M., Broadbent, J., Dickson, N., & Moffitt, T. E. (2007a). Conduct problem subtypes predict differential adult health burden. *Archives of General Psychiatry*, *64*, 476–484.

Odgers, C., Milne, B., Caspi, A., Crump, R., Poulton, R., & Moffitt, T. E. (2007b). Projecting prognosis for the conduct-problem boy: Can family history help? *Journal of American Academy of Child and Adolescent Psychiatry*, *46*, 1240–1249.

O'Connor, T. G., Deater-Deckard, K., Fulker, D., Rutter, M., & Plomin, R. (1998). Genotype–environment correlations in late childhood and early adolescence: Antisocial behavioural problems and coercive parenting. *Developmental Psychology*, *34*, 970–981.

Olweus, D. (1993). *Bullying at school*. Oxford, UK: Blackwell.

Ortiz, J., & Raine, A. (2004). Heart rate level and antisocial behavior in children and adolescents: A meta-analysis. *Journal of the*

American Academy of Child and Adolescent Psychiatry, *43*, 154–162.

Osofsky, J. D. (1995). The effects of exposure to violence on young children. *American Psychologist*, *50*, 782–788.

Pappadopulos, E., Woolston, S., Chait, A., Perkins, M., Connor, D. F., & Jensen, P. S. (2006). Pharmacotherapy of aggression in children and adolescents: Efficacy and effect size. *Journal of the Canadian Academy of Child and Adolescent Psychiatry*, *15*, 27–39.

Patterson, G. R. (1982). *Coercive family process*. Eugene, OR: Castalia.

Patterson, G. R., Chamberlain, P., & Reid, J. B. (1982). A comparative evaluation of a parent training program. *Behavior Therapy*, *13*, 638–650.

Patterson, G. R., & Yoerger, K. (1993). Developmental models for delinquent behaviour. In S. Hodgins (Ed.), *Mental disorder and crime* (pp. 140–172). Newbury Park: Sage.

Pennington, B. F., & Ozonoff, S. (1996). Executive functions and developmental psychopathology. *Journal of Child Psychology and Psychiatry*, *37*, 51–88.

Pine, D. S., Coplan, J. D., Wasserman, G. A., Miller, L. S., Fried, J. E., Davies, M., *et al.* (1997). Neuroendocrine response to fenfluramine challenge in boys. Associations with aggressive behavior and adverse rearing. *Archives of General Psychiatry*, *54*, 839–846.

Prinz, R. J., & Miller, G. E. (1994). Family-based treatment for childhood antisocial behavior: Experimental influences on dropout and engagement. *Journal of Consulting and Clinical Psychology*, *62*, 645–650.

Pullatz, M., & Bierman, K. L. (2004). *Aggression, antisocial behaviour, and violence among girls: A developmental perspective*. New York: Guilford Publications.

Raine, A., Brennan, P., & Mednick, S. A. (1997). Interaction between birth complications and early maternal rejection in predisposing individuals to adult violence: Specificity to serious, early onset violence. *American Journal of Psychiatry*, *154*, 1265–1271.

Reid, M. J., Webster-Stratton, C., & Hammond, M. (2003). Follow-up of children who received the Incredible Years intervention for oppositional-defiant disorder: Maintenance and prediction of 2-year outcome. *Behavior Therapy*, *34*, 471–491.

Rhee, S. H., & Waldman, I. D. (2002). Genetic and environmental influences on antisocial behavior: A meta-analysis of twin and adoption studies. *Psychological Bulletin*, *128*, 490–529.

Rifkin, A., Karajgi, B., Dicker, R., Perl, E., Boppana, V., Hasan, N., *et al.* (1997). Lithium treatment of conduct disorders in adolescents. *American Journal of Psychiatry*, *154*, 554–555.

Robins, L. N. (1966). *Deviant children grown-up: A sociological and psychiatric study of sociopathic personalities*. Baltimore: Williams and Wilkins.

Robins, L. N. (1991). Conduct disorder. *Journal of Child Psychology and Psychiatry*, *32*, 193–212.

Robins, L. N., & Regier, D. A. (1991). *Psychiatric disorders in America*. NY: Free Press.

Rowe, D. C., & Farrington, D. P. (1997). The familial transmission of criminal convictions. *Criminology*, *35*, 177–201.

Rowe, D. C., Vazsonyi, A. T., & Flannery, D. J. (1995). Sex differences in crime: Do means and within-sex variation have similar causes? *Journal of Research in Crime and Delinquency*, *32*, 84–100.

Rutter, M. (2000). Psychosocial influences: critiques, findings and research tools. *Development and Psychopathology*, *12*, 375–406.

Rutter, M., Giller, H., & Hagell, A. (1998). *Antisocial behaviour by young people*. Cambridge: Cambridge University Press.

Rutter, M., Moffitt, T. E., & Caspi, A. (2006). Gene–environment interplay and psychopathology: Multiple varieties but real effects. *Journal of Child Psychiatry and Psychology Annual Review*, *47*, 226–261.

Rutter, M., Quinton, D., & Hill, J. (1990). Adult outcome of institution-reared children. In L. M. Robins, & M. Rutter (Eds.), *Straight and devious pathways from childhood to adulthood*. Cambridge: Cambridge University Press.

Sampson, R. J., & Laub, J. H. (1984). Urban poverty and the family context of delinquency: A new look at structure and process in a classic study. *Child Development*, *65*, 523–540.

Sampson, R. J., Raudenbush, S. W., & Earls, F. (1997). Neighborhoods and violent crime: A multi-level study of collective efficacy. *Science*, *277*, 918–924.

Sanders, M. R., & Markie-Dadds, C. (1996). Triple P: A multi-level family intervention program for children with disruptive behavior disorders. In P. Cotton, & H. Jackson (Eds.), *Early intervention and prevention in mental health* (pp. 59–85). Melbourne: Australian Psychological Society.

Sanders, M. R., Markie-Dadds, C., Tully, L. A., & Bor, W. (2000). The Triple P-Positive Parenting Program: A comparison of enhanced, standard, and self-directed behavioral family intervention for parents of children with early onset conduct problems. *Journal of Consulting and Clinical Psychology*, *68*, 624–640.

Sanders, M. R., Markie-Dadds, C., & Turner, K. M. T. (2000). Theoretical, scientific, and clinical foundations of the Triple P-Positive Parenting Program: A population approach to the promotion of parenting competence. *Parenting Research and Practice Monograph*, *1*, 1–21.

Scott, S. (2002). Parent training programmes. In M. Rutter, & E. Taylor (Eds.), *Child and adolescent psychiatry* (4th edn.). Oxford: Blackwell.

Scott, S., Spender, Q., Doolan, M., Jacobs, B., & Aspland, H. (2001). Multicentre controlled trial of parenting groups for childhood antisocial behaviour in clinical practice. *British Medical Journal*, *323*, 1–7.

Scott, S., Sylva, K., Doolan, M., Jacobs, B, Price, J, Crook, C., & Landau, S. (in press). Randomized controlled trial of parenting groups for child antisocial behaviour targeting multiple risk factors: the SPOKES project. *Journal of the American Academy of Child and Adolescent Psychiatry*,

Séguin, J. R., Boulerice, B., Harden, P. W., Tremblay, R. E., & Pihl, R. O. (1999). Executive functions and physical aggression after controlling for Attention Deficit Hyperactivity Disorder, general memory, and IQ. *Journal of Child Psychology and Psychiatry*, *40*, 1197–1208.

Shaffer, D., Fisher, P., Lucas, C. P., Dulcan, M. K., & Schwab-Stone, M. E. (2000). NIMH Diagnostic Interview Schedule for Children Version IV (NIMH DISC-IV): description, differences from previous versions, and reliability of some common diagnoses. *Journal of the American Academy of Child and Adolescent Psychiatry*, *39*, 28–38.

Shirk, S. R., & Karver, M. (2003). Prediction of treatment outcome from relationship variables in child and adolescent therapy: A meta-analytic review. *Journal of Consulting & Clinical Psychology*, *71*, 452–464.

Silver, E., Arseneault, L., Langley, J., Caspi, A., & Moffitt, T. E. (2005). Mental disorder and violent victimization in a total birth cohort. *American Journal of Public Health*, *95*, 2015–2021.

Smith, D. J. (2005). Explaining ethnic variations in crime and antisocial behaviour in the United Kingdom. In M. Rutter, & M. Tienda (Eds.), *Ethnicity and Causal Mechanisms* (pp. 174–205). Cambridge, UK: Cambridge University Press.

Smith, D. J., & Ecob, R. (2007). An investigation of causal links between victimization and offending in adolescents. *British Journal of Sociology*, *58*, 633–659.

Snyder, H., & Sickmund, M. (2006). *Juvenile offenders and victims: 2006 national report, NCJ212906*. Washington, DC: Office of Juvenile Justice and Delinquency Prevention.

Snyder, J., & Patterson, G. R. (1995). Individual differences in social aggression: A test of a reinforcement model of socialisation in the natural environment. *Behaviour Therapy*, *26*, 371–391.

Snyder, R., Turgay, A., Aman, M., Binder, C., Fisman, S., Carroll, A., & Risperidone Conduct Study Group. (2002). Effects of risperidone on conduct and disruptive behavior disorders in children with subaverage IQs. *Journal of the American Academy of Child and Adolescent Psychiatry*, *41*, 1026–1036.

Speltz, M. L., DeKlyen, M., Calderon, R., Greenberg, M. T., & Fisher, P. A. (1999). Neuropsychological characteristics and test behaviours of boys with early onset conduct problems. *Journal of Abnormal Psychology*, *108*, 315–325.

Speltz, M. L., DeKlyen, M., & Greenberg, M. T. (1999). Attachment in boys with early onset conduct problems. *Development and Psychopathology*, *11*, 269–286.

Speltz, M. L., McClellan, J., DeKlyen, M., & Jones, K. (1999). Preschool boys with oppositional defiant disorder: Clinical presentation and diagnostic change. *Journal of the American Academy of Child and Adolescent Psychiatry*, *38*, 838–845.

Spivak, H. (2003). Bullying: Why all the fuss? *Pediatrics*, *112*, 1421–1422.

Stallings, M. C., Corley, R. P., Dennehey, B., Hewitt, J. K., Krauter, K. S., Lessem, J. M., *et al.* (2005). A genome-wide search for quantitative trait loci that influence antisocial drug dependence in adolescence. *Archives of General Psychiatry*, *62*, 1042–1051.

Stattin, H., & Kerr, M. (2000). Parental monitoring: A reinterpretation. *Child Development*, *71*, 1072–1085.

Stattin, H., & Magnusson, D. (1995). Onset of official delinquency: Its co-occurence in time with educational, behavioural, and interpersonal problems. *British Journal of Criminology*, *35*, 417–449.

Steiner, H., Saxena, K., & Chang, K. (2003). Psychopharmacologic strategies for the treatment of aggression in juveniles. *CNS Spectrums*, *8*, 298–308.

Striepling, S. H. (1997). The low-aggression classroom: A teacher's view. In A. P. Goldstein, & J. C. Conoley (Eds.), *School violence intervention: A practical handbook* (pp. 23–45). New York: Guilford Press.

Thomas, A., Chess, S., & Birch, H. G. (1968). *Temperament and behavior disorders in children*. New York: New York University Press.

Thornberry, T. P., Krohn, M. D., Lizotte, A. J., & Chard-Wierschem, D. (1993). The role of juvenile gangs in facilitating delinquent behavior. *Journal of Research in Crime and Delinquency*, *30*, 55–87.

Tibbetts, S., & Piquero, A. (1999). The influence of gender, low birth weight and disadvantaged environment on predicting early onset of offending: A test of Moffitt's interactional hypothesis. *Criminology*, *37*, 843–878.

Tittle, C. R., & Meier, R. F. (1990). Specifying the SES–delinquency relationship. *Criminology*, *28*, 271–299.

Tolan, P. H. (2004). International trends in bullying and children's health: giving them due consideration. *Archives of Pediatric and Adolescent Medicine*, *158*, 831–832.

Tolman, D. L., Spencer, R., Rosen-Reynoso, M., & Porche, M. V. (2003). Sowing the seeds of violence in heterosexual relationships: Early adolescents narrate compulsory heterosexuality. *Journal of Social Issues*, *59*, 159–178.

Tremblay, R. E. (2003). Why socialization fails. In B. Lahey, T. E. Moffitt, & A. Caspi (Eds.), *Causes of conduct disorder and delinquency* (pp. 182–226). NY: Guilford Press.

Turgay, A. (2004). Aggression and disruptive behavior disorders in children and adolescents. *Expert Review of Neurotherapeutics*, *4*, 623–632.

Van IJzendoorn, M. H., Schuengel, C., & Bakermans-Kranenburg, M. J. (1999). Disorganized attachment in early childhood: Meta-analysis of precursors, concomitants, and sequelae. *Development & Psychopathology*, *11*, 225–249.

Vermieren, R., Jespers, I., & Moffitt, T. E. (2006). Mental health problems in juvenile justice populations. *Child and Adolescent Psychiatric Clinics of North America*, *15*, 333–351.

Vitaro, F., Tremblay, R. E., & Bukowski, W. M. (2001). Friends, friendships and conduct disorders. In J. Hill, & B. Maughan (Eds.), *Conduct disorders in childhood and adolescence* (pp. 346–376). Cambridge: Cambridge University Press.

Vitiello, B. (2001). Psychopharmacology for young children: clinical needs and research opportunities. *Pediatrics*, *108*, 983–989.

Vondra, J. I., Shaw, D. S., Swearingen, L., Cohen, M., & Owens, E. B. (2001). Attachment stability and emotional and behavioral regulation from infancy to preschool age. *Development and Psychopathology*, *13*, 13–33.

Warr, M. (2002). *Companions in crime*. Cambridge, UK: Cambridge University Press.

Waschbusch, D. A. (2002). A meta-analytic examination of comorbid hyperactive-impulsive-inattention problems and conduct problems. *Psychological Bulletin*, *128*, 118–150.

Webster-Stratton, C. (1981). Modification of mothers' behaviors and attitudes through a videotape modeling group discussion program. *Behavior Therapy*, *12*, 634–642.

Webster-Stratton, C., Reid, J., & Hammond, M. (2001a). Preventing conduct problems, promoting social competence: a parent and teacher training partnership in head start. *Journal of Clinical Child Psychology*, *30*, 283–302.

Webster-Stratton, C., Reid, J., & Hammond, M. (2001b). Social skills and problem-solving training for children with early-onset conduct problems: Who benefits? *Journal of Child Psychology and Psychiatry*, *42*, 943–952.

Webster-Stratton, C., Reid, M.J., & Hammond, M. (2004). Treating children with early-onset conduct problems: Intervention outcomes for parent, child, and teacher training. *Journal of Clinical Child and Adolescent Psychology*, *33*, 105–124.

Weisz, J. R., Hawley, K. M., & Doss, A. J. (2004). Empirically tested psychotherapies for youth internalizing and externalizing problems and disorders. *Child and Adolescent Psychiatric Clinics of North America*, *13*, 729–815.

Widom, C. S. (1997). Child abuse, neglect and witnessing violence. In D. Stoff, J. Breiling, & J. D. Maser (Eds.), *Handbook of antisocial behavior* (pp. 159–170). New York: John Wiley and Sons.

World Health Organization (WHO). (1996). *Multiaxial classification of child and adolescent psychiatry disorders*. Cambridge, UK: Cambridge University Press.

Wright, B. R. E., Caspi, A., Moffitt, T. E., & Silva, P. A. (1999). Reconsidering the relationship between SES and delinquency: Causation but not correlation. *Criminology*, *37*, 175–194.

36 Substance Use and Substance Use Disorder

Andrew C. Heath, Michael T. Lynskey and Mary Waldron

Adolescent and pre-adolescent substance use and substance use disorder bring immediate risks of harm. The acute effects of intoxication can be devastating: alcohol-related motor vehicle accidents remain one of the leading causes of mortality among youth; sharing needles and related injecting paraphernalia has emerged as a leading vector for the transmission of blood borne viruses; and acute intoxication has also been associated with sexual risk taking, sexual victimization and unintentional injury (Hingson & Kenkel, 2004). In treatment samples, excessive alcohol use has been reported to be associated with neurocognitive deficits (Brown & Tappert, 2004) which, if confirmed to be a consequence of alcohol misuse rather than predisposing deficits, would raise the possibility of longer-term disadvantages as a consequence of misuse. Adverse health effects of smoking have been shown in adolescent smokers, including adverse effects on lung function (Gold, Wang, Wipij *et al.*, 1996). Despite these risks, and despite the high rates of co-occurrence of substance use or substance use disorders with other childhood disorders seen in clinical practice (Abrantes, Strong, Ramsey *et al.*, 2005; Wilens, Biederman, Abrantes *et al.*, 1997), adolescent substance use has been relatively neglected in clinical practice and in research studies.

The societal costs of this neglect of adolescent substance use are high. The Global Burden of Disease project identified tobacco, alcohol and illicit drugs as, respectively the 2nd, 9th and 20th leading causes of mortality globally (Ezzati, Lopez, Rodgers *et al.*, 2003). If current trends continue, tobacco smoking alone is projected to lead to 1 billion premature deaths globally during the 21st century (Mackey, Eriksen, & Shafey, 2006). Continued and heavy use of these substances has a spectrum of adverse outcomes including physical, social and legal consequences. While many of these conditions, and particularly those relating to physical ill health, develop only after chronic use spanning several decades, and are therefore rare in children and adolescents, an understanding of substance use and substance use problems during adolescence is critical to any approach aimed at lessening these consequences, as it is during childhood and adolescence that the use of these substances typically first occurs. Some studies suggest that, if substance use has not been initiated by age 21, it is unlikely to ever be initiated (Chen & Kandel, 1995). Further, age at initiation to substance use has consistently been shown to be associated with higher lifetime consumption, more risky patterns of use, and with the onset, duration and severity of dependence (see p. 570). While the interpretation of these associations remains controversial, it is clearly the case that early-onset use is a robust indicator of risk for future substance-related problems.

In this chapter we first outline research characterizing patterns of adolescent substance use, the assessment of substance use and substance use problems in adolescents, and diagnostic criteria for substance use disorders, including issues relating to the extent to which such criteria may be applicable to adolescents. We also examine outcomes associated with adolescent substance use. We next consider research findings on the etiology of substance use disorders, and their comorbidity with other disorders. Finally, we review treatment approaches and prevention strategies.

Epidemiology

Much of the literature on the prevalence of substance use in children and adolescents is hampered by methodological challenges including small and unrepresentative samples and varying definitions of substance involvement. We limit our consideration to a relatively small number of studies using large and representative samples that have examined prevalence of substance use. We attempt where possible to provide accurate estimates of the ages at which substance use has been assessed, because childhood and adolescence is a time of very rapid escalation in the prevalence of lifetime use and escalation in involvement and thus even relatively small age differences may be associated with quite large changes in the extent of substance use.

Tobacco Use

Tobacco, principally but not exclusively in the form of smoked cigarettes, is widely used among children and adolescents. Perhaps the most comprehensive information on patterns of licit and illicit drug use among children and adolescents comes from the USA Monitoring the Future project, which has conducted large surveys of the school-aged population at annual intervals since 1975 (Johnston, O'Malley, Bachman *et al.*, 2006). The most recent data available from this study are for the year 2005, which indicate that about 50% of 12th grade

Rutter's Child and Adolescent Psychiatry, 5th edition. Edited by M. Rutter, D. Bishop, D. Pine, S. Scott, J. Stevenson, E. Taylor and A. Thapar. ISBN: 978-1-4051-4549-7.

students (ages 17–18) and 25.9% of 8th grade students (ages 13–14) have smoked cigarettes while 17.5% and 10.1%, respectively, have used smokeless tobacco products. Further, 13.7% of 12th graders and 4.1% of 8th graders reported smoking cigarettes daily during the 30 days preceding the survey while about 2.5% and 0.7% reported using smokeless tobacco products about once a day or more often.

While international comparisons show considerable variability in the prevalence of tobacco smoking and the use of smokeless tobacco products, the use of these products among youth is widespread. For example, the Global Youth Tobacco Survey, which surveyed 13- to 15-year-old school students from 131 countries, reported that rates of past 30-day tobacco use ranged from 11.4% to 22.2% of students (Warren, Jones, Eriksen *et al.*, 2006).

Alcohol Consumption

In the 2005 Monitoring the Future study, by 12th grade, 75.1% of all students had used alcohol at least once and 57.5% reported having been drunk at least once, with corresponding percentages of 41% and 19.5% in 8th grade. By 12th grade, rates of lifetime alcohol use were approximately equal across genders (75.7% in males and 74.5% in females), although more males (60.5%) than females (54.4%) reported lifetime drunkenness. There was also evidence of a relatively small subgroup of students who were drinking heavily regularly: 18.1% of students in their final year at high school, and 18.1% of 8th graders, reported having five or more drinks in a row on at least two occasions in the preceding 2 weeks.

There is also information available on patterns of alcohol use internationally. Schmid, Ter Bogt, Godeau *et al.* (2003) reported on patterns of consumption among 15-year-olds in 22 countries: the prevalence of lifetime alcohol use across these countries ranged from 66% (in the USA and Norway) to 92.2% (in Greece and Denmark) among males and from 66% (in the USA) to 91% (in Denmark) among females. Among students who had drunk alcohol, the prevalence of ever having been drunk was 47–85% of males and 42–93% of females.

Illicit Drug Use

Prevalence estimates derived from the Monitoring the Future Survey lead to several important conclusions. First, at least some lifetime use of illicit drugs is widespread – 21.4% of 8th graders reported using illicit drugs on at least one occasion, and by the final year of high school in excess of 50% of school attendees report some illicit drug use. Second, cannabis is by far the most widely used illicit drug, with 44.8% of 12th graders and 16.5% of 8th graders reporting having used this drug. Relatively few individuals reporting lifetime use of illicit drugs have not used cannabis (22.9% of 8th graders and 11.1% of 12th graders who report any illicit drug use). The lifetime use of other illicit drugs is less prevalent but substantial minorities report some experience with amphetamines (13.1% of 12th graders, 7.4% of 8th graders), inhalants (11.4%, 17.1%, suggesting younger respondents are considering a wider range of experiences as inhalant use, or older respondents are forgetting), sedatives (10.5%, no data for 8th graders), tranquilizers (9.9%, 4.1%), hallucinogens (8.8%, 3.8%), cocaine (8.0%, 3.7%), MDMA (ecstasy; 5.4%, 2.8%) and heroin (1.5%, 1.5%). In addition, there are marked gender differences with the prevalence of use of all drugs being higher among males than among females (e.g., 49.1% versus 40.2% for cannabis use among 12th graders). However, gender differences in the prevalence of illicit drug use appear to have declined in more recent years, with rates of use among females converging on rates among males, a trend that mirrors similar findings in the tobacco and alcohol literatures (Johnson & Gerstein, 1998). Finally, rapid escalation in use occurs over the high school years: rates of ever use of cannabis rose from 16.5% among 8th graders to 44.8% among 12th graders.

While these estimates of the prevalence of illicit drug use may appear high, it is worth noting that, because of the sampling frame of this study (school attendees) it is likely, in fact, to underestimate the true prevalence of illicit drug use among youth. School surveys such as this exclude individuals who no longer attend school as well as those who, for whatever reason (e.g., habitual truancy), are unavailable on the day of testing, a group likely to have higher rates of illicit drug use (Johnston *et al.*, 2006).

Finally, the figures cited above are for any lifetime use and it is also important to consider the frequency and progression of illicit drug use among youth. While the Monitoring the Future Survey does not provide good information on the frequency or extent of illicit drug use, it appears that the majority of those reporting any lifetime illicit drug use have used the drug on relatively few occasions. For example, while 44.8% of 12th grade high school students in the Monitoring the Future Survey reported lifetime cannabis use, 22.3% of these (10.0% of the entire sample) reported using cannabis on only one or two occasions in their life. Nonetheless, there is a smaller minority of youth who report relatively frequent illicit drug use: 4.9% of these students reported using cannabis on 10 or more occasions in the previous 30 days.

Substance Use Disorders

There is generally less information on the prevalence of substance use disorders (e.g., abuse, dependence as operationalized in DSM-IV [American Psychiatric Association, 2000]) in youth. This likely reflects a convergence of factors: potential difficulties in the application of standard abuse/dependence criteria to samples of youth (see p. 569); the need for exceptionally large and representative samples given the relatively low base rate of these disorders within the general population; and the fact that they are likely to be concentrated in subgroups of the population (e.g., homeless, those who have left school) who are difficult to capture using traditional survey methodologies. Although there have been a number of relatively large-scale epidemiological surveys of psychiatric disorders among children and adolescents, surprisingly few of these have yielded estimates of the prevalence of substance use disorders. Published studies have either not reported any information on the prevalence of substance abuse/dependence or have adopted the convention of combining all (typically non-tobacco) diagnoses to form a single category of substance use disorder. For example, in a representative sample of approximately 1000 New Zealand children studied at age 15 years, Fergusson, Horwood, and Lynskey (1993) reported that 7.7% of this sample met criteria for a substance use disorder, defined as nicotine dependence, or alcohol or other substance abuse or dependence. Such studies were reviewed by Costello, Egger, and Angold (2005), who reported that the median estimate from studies of substance use disorders was in the region of 5%, although there was wide variation among studies in these estimates.

An alternative strategy for estimating the prevalence of substance use disorders among youth is to consider retrospective reports of the age of onset of substance use disorders from large and representative samples of the general population. For example, in the NCS Replication survey of adults aged 18 years and older, Kessler, Berglund, Demler *et al.* (2005) reported, for 50% of all those meeting lifetime criteria for a substance use disorder (not including nicotine dependence), the onset of these disorders occurred before age 21 for alcohol abuse, before age 23 for alcohol dependence, before age 19 for drug abuse, before age 21 for drug dependence and before age 20 for any substance use disorder.

Implications for the Assessment of Adolescent Substance Use and Problems

Research suggests that face-to-face interview assessment leads to underreporting of substance use by adolescents. In the USA, the discrepancy between rates of self-reported substance use in early national household surveys of drug use that used traditional interview methods, and self-reports based on responses to questionnaires administered in schools, led to several changes in strategy: first to using a self-administered questionnaire, during an interview, to obtain drug use history information; and then to using a computer self-administered interview to obtain this same information (Gfroerer, Eyerman, & Chromy, 2006). Self-report data obtained by questionnaire (e.g., Rutgers Alcohol Problem Index: White & Labouvie, 1989; Drug Use Screening Inventory: Kirisci, Mezzich, & Tartar, 1995) or computer self-administered interview (Turner, Ku, Rogers *et al.*, 1998), particularly where this can be supplemented by toxicology screens, are likely to become the norm for adolescent research assessment. We know of no research comparing the accuracy of information gathered by a standard clinician interview with supplementation by self-report checklist or computer-based assessment, but would anticipate that substantial underreporting at interview would also occur in this clinical context, suggesting that supplementation by checklist or computer-based assessment be used. Brief screens for use and problem use should be utilized across a spectrum of clinical settings as such use and/or problems are common – and elevated – in youth accessing treatment.

Diagnosis

At the time of writing, the development of the next generation of diagnostic criteria for drug use disorders by the American Psychiatric Association (DSM-V) remains a work in progress. However, while important innovations have been proposed (e.g., use of semicontinuous ratings for each dependence criterion, to permit a more nearly continuous assessment of level of problems), the need to preserve continuity of clinical and research practice, and lack of the necessary empirical base to support more radical change, are expected to limit changes from DSM-IV to DSM-V. The application of diagnostic criteria developed for drug use problems in adults to adolescents remains controversial, with many areas of difficulty (Crowley, 2006), but some of these difficulties highlight shortcomings in the existing diagnostic criteria. In discussions of the assessment and diagnosis of substance use problems in children and adolescents, four important shortcomings of existing evidence are faced.

1 The lack of large general population psychiatric surveys of children and adolescents of the magnitude (minimally, tens of thousands of participants) that is necessary to give confidence in attempts to use advanced statistical methods (e.g., Muthen, 2006) to refine diagnostic criteria for specific drug use disorders in general community samples. This has the implication that much of what we can guess about the applicability of diagnostic criteria sets to adolescent substance use disorders derives from retrospective recall of adults about their past history of drug use and problems. While such "back-testing" of diagnostic schema to determine their applicability to adolescents has been underutilized by researchers, the pitfalls associated with reliance on retrospective reports are considerable.

2 The lack of large-scale follow-up studies of clinically treated adolescents with drug use disorders with sample sizes of the magnitude (500–1000 or more participants) available for adults. This makes prospective validation of proposed diagnostic criteria sets, by comparing prediction of future course, treatment–response and other outcomes, a special challenge for pediatric substance use disorders.

3 The narrow focus of most contemporary research assessments of substance use disorders on existing (and in some cases earlier) diagnostic criteria sets, which leaves a weak evidence base for modifying existing criteria.

4 The predominant focus of much research on the nosology of substance use disorders on one drug, alcohol, because of its widespread use and the recognition by psychiatrists of the clinical significance of alcohol use disorders. Tobacco dependence, although widespread and associated with severe long-term physical health risks, is widely neglected in psychiatry. Cannabis use disorders, also increasingly prevalent, have likewise tended to be neglected, perhaps because viewed by many psychiatrists as benign.

The Dependence Syndrome

Current operationalizations of substance dependence, in both DSM-IV and ICD-10, derive ultimately from the formulation of the "dependence syndrome" by Edwards (1986), developed initially with respect to alcohol dependence and then generalized to other drug classes, which represented an attempt to define a physiological syndrome of dependence. Primacy was given to:

1 The experiencing of repeated symptoms of withdrawal, with other defining symptoms being;
2 Relief or avoidance of withdrawal symptoms by further drug use;
3 Increased tolerance;
4 Subjective awareness of compulsion to use the drug, including loss of control;
5 Rapid reinstatement after abstinence;
6 Narrowing of the drug use repertoire; and
7 Salience of drug-seeking behavior.

Withdrawal, Withdrawal Relief; Tolerance

Both DSM-IV (American Psychiatric Association [APA], 2000) and ICD-10 (World Health Organization, 1996) specify withdrawal syndromes separately for each drug, but using the same criterion for each drug – namely, that the syndrome is due to the cessation or reduction in substance use that has been heavy or prolonged. In DSM-IV no cannabis withdrawal syndrome was recognized, but subsequent laboratory-based studies (Budney, Hughes, Moore *et al.*, 2004), supported by psychometric data (Budney, 2006), make it likely that a cannabis withdrawal syndrome will be included in DSM-V, leaving hallucinogens as the main drug class with no known withdrawal syndrome. Tolerance is defined in DSM by a need for markedly increased amounts of a drug to achieve intoxication or a desired effect or (as may occur after a history of chronic heavy use) by a markedly diminished effect with continued use of the same amount (APA, 2000).

At least two schools of thought exist concerning the assessment of drug withdrawal, and of tolerance. One, in its most extreme form, emphasizes the severe and sometimes life-threatening withdrawal syndromes seen with very long-term opiate, alcohol or sedative dependence that may include grand mal convulsions and delirium tremens. Caetano and Babor (2006) emphasized the development of withdrawal after 25–30 years of heavy drinking, and contrasted this with the problems reported by young adults, arguing that the latter are not truly describing withdrawal symptoms. Likewise, it is possible to operationalize tolerance in such a way that it describes individuals with prolonged histories of excessive substance use (Caetano & Babor, 2006) whose acquired tolerance enables them to function at levels of consumption that would cause severe impairment in most of the population. From this perspective, the alcohol withdrawal syndrome will almost never be encountered in adolescents, and the tolerance reported by adolescents is the acquired behavioral tolerance (Vogel-Sprott, 1997) that comes from learning to adapt to intoxicating levels of alcohol or other drugs, rather than the chronic adaptations that occur after a prolonged history of substance use. However, a consequence of this approach is that the alcohol dependence syndrome as originally conceptualized (with withdrawal as a cardinal feature) becomes a severe but rare disorder, with the majority of individuals who experience problems with alcohol needing to be covered by a residual alcohol use disorder category, an unfortunate consequence given the desirability of providing clinical help before individuals reach the stage of such severe dependence. Alternatively, if a broader conceptualization of dependence is used, drug withdrawal and tolerance defined this stringently become essentially irrelevant to diagnosis, because most individuals reporting drug withdrawal or tolerance will also report many other less severe symptoms. While retention of stringent criteria for a severe withdrawal syndrome requiring careful medical management is clearly essential, this, together with stringently defined tolerance, will usually be irrelevant in pediatric practice.

The second school of thought considers withdrawal and tolerance as symptoms arising relatively early in the course of drug use, that may indeed impact the development of other symptoms of dependence. Tolerance may be defined more broadly, so that it is endorsed by many individuals with few or no other dependence symptoms (Muthen, 2006). For alcohol withdrawal, support for a broader operationalization (Muthen, 2006) derives primarily from research using structured diagnostic assessments with quite non-specific wordings to assess withdrawal, which may indeed be endorsed by youngsters who are confusing effects of alcohol intoxication with effects of alcohol withdrawal (Caetano & Babor, 2006). Other research studies that have used a more stringent operationalization of alcohol withdrawal find it to be a relatively severe symptom (e.g., Bucholz, Heath, Reich *et al.*, 2006) that would be quite rare in adolescents.

We do not have good empirical data to support preference for either narrower or broader definitions, and need to be sensitive to the possibility that we are arbitrarily dichotomizing continuums of tolerance or withdrawal severity and thereby sacrificing diagnostic precision. Basic science studies have shown *acute* alcohol withdrawal effects after a single high dose (e.g., handling-induced seizures in mice; Metten *et al.*, 1998) with evidence for genetic overlap of vulnerability to chronic versus acute withdrawal effects (Metten *et al.*, 1998). It has been speculated that hangover in humans may represent such an acute alcohol withdrawal effect, and rates of reported hangover are certainly elevated in those at high risk of alcohol dependence by virtue of a positive family history of alcoholism (Piasecki, Sher, Slutske *et al.*, 2005). Such acute withdrawal effects may be not uncommon in adolescent heavy drinkers, because many have a typical pattern of intermittent heavy consumption; they simply have not been usually assessed, because not a part of the DSM-IV criteria, and their prognostic significance is therefore unknown.

Consideration of tobacco dependence suggests that tolerance and withdrawal *can* be important in adolescence. Koob (2006) cited evidence that "measures of brain reward function during acute abstinence from all major drugs with dependence potential have revealed increases in brain reward thresholds as measured by brain stimulation reward," suggesting that withdrawal symptoms involving dysphoria may be a common feature, across drug classes, of drug withdrawal. Nicotine withdrawal symptoms, which in DSM-IV predominantly involve affective symptoms, are reported by adolescents relatively early in their smoking careers, as well as by adults (Prokhovov, Hudmon, de Moor *et al.*, 2001), and it is plausible that this pattern for affective symptoms of withdrawal will be confirmed across drug classes. In contrast with alcohol, nicotine is not a drug used for intoxication (hence the more severe operationalizations of tolerance are irrelevant for this drug), and most smokers would not describe their smoking in terms of achieving a "desired effect" (Hughes, 2006). Nicotine in doses smoked by some heavy smoking adolescents (e.g., 20 cigarettes per day; Hurt, Croghan, Beede *et al.*, 2000), however, would be extremely toxic in someone with no prior smoking history: by this example, tolerance is clearly acquired by many adolescent smokers.

In the absence of careful laboratory-based studies of adolescent withdrawal, and of real-time field assessments of adolescent withdrawal and tolerance (such as are now possible using palm-pilot based ecological momentary assessment techniques), the present state of the science must be to assess both broadly and stringently and determine whether either or both measures have predictive value for adolescent substance use disorders.

Compulsive Use – Loss of Control; Difficulty Quitting/Cutting Down

The notion of "loss of control," as experienced by an individual with alcohol problems who, across repeated drinking sessions, intends to limit his or her drinking but drinks to intoxication, has little relevance to tobacco dependence, where the smoker typically maintains a very stable pattern of smoking from day to day. If defined broadly (the language of DSM-IV includes "often taken in larger amounts . . . than intended," relaxing the requirement for intoxication), it does not discriminate very well in heavy-drinking cohorts (Bucholz *et al.*, 1996). Loss of control is more likely to be experienced by a smoker as difficulty quitting, despite a persistent desire to quit. Concern has been expressed about whether adolescents understand questions about such experiences in the same way as adults, and thus may overreport dependence symptoms because of difficulty distinguishing symptoms from the normal fluctuations of adolescence (Prokhovov, Hudmon, Cinciripini *et al.*, 2005). It may also be the case that an adolescent who has progressed from occasional experimentation to more regular use of a drug is actually a better informant about the experience of compulsion to use than, say, an adult chronic heavy smoker who has adapted to drug use over a period of many years. DSM-IV defines as a separate dependence symptom (also considered an indicator of compulsive use) spending a great deal of time obtaining, using or recovering from the effects of the substance, which applies in quite different ways to illicit drug use (seeking out drugs from a dealer), drinking (recovering from effects of hangover) and also is made to apply to smoking (by giving chain-smoking as an example of spending a great deal of time using), but the connection with compulsive use appears far more remote in these cases.

Continued Use Despite Negative Consequences

Hasin, Hatzenbuehler, Keyes *et al.* (2006) correctly drew attention to the rather idiosyncratic ways in which continued use despite substance-related problems is handled in current diagnostic criteria. In DSM-IV, continued use despite knowledge that this is causing physical or emotional problems is considered a symptom of dependence. Giving up important social, occupational or recreational activities because of substance use is considered a separate symptom of dependence. Both are inferred to be manifestations of loss of control, although the evidence to support the implicit assertion that it is the compulsion to use that leads ultimately to the pattern of continued use despite negative consequences is not supplied.

In contrast, continued use despite interference with major role responsibilities (e.g., schooling, parenting, work); continued use despite social problems (e.g., disruption of relationships) or legal problems; or continued use in situations that are physically hazardous (e.g., drunk driving), are considered manifestations of "abuse," a residual category whose survival or demise in DSM-V remains controversial (Schuckit & Saunders, 2006). DSM-IV uses the phrase "recurrent" to describe these latter problems (although continued use is clearly implied). It is precisely the latter types of problem that adolescents are more likely to encounter through substance use. Continued use despite being aware of other negative consequences that do not involve immediate physical hazard (e.g., heavy drinking leading to inappropriate sexual behavior by an adolescent) is discounted. Continued smoking that is increasing an individual's long-term risk of cancer is also discounted. The adolescent who is continuing to use at medically unsafe levels, or the adolescent who is experiencing distress because their substance use is leading to inappropriate sexual behavior or sexual risk-taking, may be experiencing symptoms of comparable importance to the older adult who is already experiencing physical problems associated with their substance use, but these problems are classified quite differently.

Clinically Significant Distress/Impairment

DSM-IV includes a requirement, for a diagnosis of substance abuse or dependence, that there be evidence of clinically significant distress or impairment, thereby excluding all those cases whose significance lies purely in the realm of physical medicine (e.g., alcohol-related liver damage; smoking-related health risks), or where individuals' behavior puts themselves or others in danger (e.g., recurrent driving under the influence) without personal remorse or impairment in daily life. Reliance on subjective evaluations of distress or impairment may be particularly problematic for adolescents whose social milieu discourages recognition of impairment. The wisdom of such exclusions must be questioned.

Reconceptualizing Adolescent Substance Use Disorder

There remains debate about how well criteria for substance use disorders developed for adults apply to adolescents, and whether indeed separate criteria should be developed for adolescents or young adults (Crowley, 2006; Martin, Chung, Kirisci *et al.*, 2006). We argue that consideration of: (i) heaviness of use (indexed by tolerance); (ii) loss of control (including difficulty quitting); (iii) continued use despite awareness of negative consequences of use; and in some cases, (iv) problems associated with cessation of use (withdrawal) will identify significant numbers of adolescents experiencing substance-related problems; and that the same profile of problems occurring in a 17-year-old and a 47-year-old would not be an indicator that the 47-year-old does not have problems.

There is accumulating evidence in support of a "dimensional" conceptualization of alcohol dependence symptoms (which have been more extensively studied than is the case for other substance use disorders), with individuals with more severe problems more likely to endorse particular symptoms, individuals with less severe problems less likely to endorse the same symptoms, but with no unique symptom profiles identifying particular subclasses of dependent patients (e.g., Bucholz *et al.*, 1996). Under these conditions, defining diagnostic criteria sets that correctly classify severely affected chronic substance dependent individuals is easy; the real challenge is posed by ensuring that individuals with milder problems are correctly classified, a group in which an increased proportion of adolescents will be represented. From this perspective, difficulties identified in the application of diagnostic criteria to adolescents are highlighting broader limitations of these criteria.

Risks Associated With Early Use

A consistent – albeit controversial – finding is that age of initiation to substance use is strongly associated with later risks of problems. For example, using data from a diagnostic interview survey of a representative sample of US adults (the NESARC study), Hingson, Heeren, and Winter (2006) reported that age of onset of alcohol use was inversely related not only to lifetime risks of alcohol dependence, but also to the severity and duration of dependence. Specifically, individuals who commenced drinking before age 14, compared to those who commenced after age 21, were more likely to meet the criteria for alcohol dependence in the 10 years immediately following drinking initiation, in the 12 months prior to the interview and ever in their lifetimes. They were also more likely to experience multiple distinct episodes of alcohol dependence. Comparisons restricted to those experiencing lifetime alcohol dependence indicated that early-onset alcohol dependence was also associated with higher rates of long duration episodes and with meeting six or more dependence criteria.

Hingson, Heeren, Zakocs *et al.* (2003) reported a 3.5-fold increased risk of being involved in an alcohol-related accident among individuals who began drinking at age 14 relative to those who started drinking after age 21. Importantly, these associations persisted after control for a range of covariates including alcohol dependence and length of drinking career, and when consideration was limited to alcohol-related accidents in the 12 months prior to the interview. These results parallel findings from other studies that an earlier age of alcohol initiation is associated with heavy and more prolonged drinking (Fergusson, Horwood, & Lynskey, 1995; Pitkanen, Lyyra, & Pulkkinen, 2005), alcohol dependence (Hingson, Heeren, & Winter, 2006) and unsafe sexual practices (Hingson *et al.*, 2003). Analogous, although less striking, results have also been reported for tobacco use, with early-onset tobacco use being associated with heightened risks for the development of nicotine dependence (Hu, Davies, & Kandel, 2006) and also for illicit drug use (Lynskey, Heath, Bucholz *et al.*, 2003).

Some commentators have implied that these associations are causal and therefore advocated delaying the onset of alcohol use as a potential means of reducing longer-term exposure to alcohol-related harm (Pitkanen, Lyyra, & Pulkkinen, 2005). Alternatively, it has been argued that these associations are likely to be non-causal and arise from the effects of social, family and related (including genetic) factors preceding the onset of alcohol consumption that increase risks both of early initiation of alcohol use and of subsequent alcohol-related harm, for which there may have been inadequate statistical control (Prescott & Kendler, 1999). Prescott and Kendler (1999), using a genetically informative research design, reported that apparent associations between age of onset of alcohol consumption and lifetime alcohol dependence could largely be attributed to shared genetic vulnerabilities. An alternative possibility, not excluded by those analyses, is that genetic differences in dependence risk and early-onset alcohol use are combining interactively (a genotype × early-onset use interaction effect) to determine dependence risk, so the controversy remains unresolved.

The Gateway Hypothesis

A highly controversial theory concerns whether early-onset cannabis use may act as a risk factor that increases risks for the initiation and escalation in use of other drugs such as heroin and cocaine. This theory, sometimes referred to as the stage or gateway theory, is largely based on findings that, among those reporting the use of drugs such as heroin or cocaine, nearly all people report having also used cannabis and also, among these individuals, use of cannabis is almost always initiated before the use of these other drugs. These findings, and the interpretation placed on them, have been described as one of the most influential research findings in drug policy and have been used as a major rationale for sustaining legal prohibitions against cannabis in the USA and other countries where cannabis use and possession remain illegal. However, temporal sequence alone does not imply causality and it is equally possible that the observed patterns of association between cannabis use and other drug use could be explained by a model assuming no causal associations between cannabis use and subsequent use of illicit drugs (Morral, McCaffrey, & Paddock, 2002).

Nonetheless, a number of studies that have attempted to control for observed covariates have reported that, even after such control, significant associations remain between early-onset cannabis use and subsequent illicit drug use (Fergusson,

Boden, & Horwood, 2006). Using a cotwin methodology to control for both genetic and shared environmental risk factors that may be associated both with early-onset cannabis use and with subsequent use of other illicit drugs, Lynskey *et al.* (2003) reported that early-onset cannabis users had odds of sedative, hallucinogen, cocaine/other stimulants and opioid use that were 2.6–5.2 times higher than those of their non-early using cotwin. Subsequent studies using a variety of genetically informative research strategies have also failed to discount the possibility that the use of cannabis may influence subsequent risks for the development of illicit drug use (Agrawal, Neale, Prescott *et al.*, 2004; Lynskey, Vink, & Boomsma, 2006).

There are a number of different possible explanations for the mechanisms underlying the observed associations. First, it remains possible that the associations are wholly non-causal and arise both from the joint influence of shared risk factors (including genetic and shared environmental risk factors that were controlled for in the genetically informed research studies mentioned above), and from non-shared risk factors – such as peer affiliations – that were not controlled. While popular interpretations of the "gateway" properties of cannabis imply pharmacological effects of adolescent exposure to cannabis, such mechanisms seem unlikely; the levels of exposure typically employed in animal models are often many times higher than is typical in early-onset cannabis users. An alternative explanation of the observed associations is that they arise because use of and access to cannabis increase exposure and opportunity to use other drugs (Wagner & Anthony, 2002).

Psychosocial and Genetic Risk Factors

In evaluating pertinent literature on the etiology of substance use disorders, ideally one would wish to know about at least four dimensions of risk:

1 Predictors of early onset, because early initiation of substance use will itself predict increased risk of later problems (see p. 570);

2 Predictors of heaviness of use (or other aspects of substance use patterning that may be associated with increased risks of problems);

3 Predictors of dependence vulnerability, conditional upon duration and heaviness of use; and

4 Predictors of desistance (i.e., protective factors that may facilitate quitting or overcoming substance use-related problems).

It is rare to find that these different dimensions of risk have been considered in a single study.

Genetic Research

We know relatively little about the genetics of adolescent substance use and substance use disorder, with the limited information deriving from a small number of studies (McGue, Iacono, Legrand *et al.*, 2001; Rose, Dick, Viken *et al.*, 2004; Slutske, Cronk, Sher *et al.*, 2002a) that are mostly ongoing at the time of writing but should eventually provide important information about how genetic influences on adolescent substance use and substance use disorder overlap with genetic influences on adult substance use disorder. For the time being, what we may anticipate in adolescents is largely guided by information about genetic contributions to risk of *adult* substance dependence, which derives from multiple sources.

Family, Including Prospective High-Risk Studies

From the 1950s onwards, a growing literature acknowledged the strong familiality of alcoholism, with some families having large numbers of alcohol-dependent cases. In the recent multisite US COGA study, rates of alcohol dependence in the relatives of an index case ascertained through treatment sources were increased three- to eight-fold, varying by gender (Reich, Edenberg, Goate *et al.*, 1998). This work has been extended to examine outcomes associated with index case illicit drug dependence (Merikangas, Stolar, Stevens *et al.*, 1998; Rounsaville, Kosten, Weissman *et al.*, 1991), with research finding support for at least partial drug specificity of familial risks. Intergenerational transmission of smoking has been surprisingly weak in many studies (Avenevoli & Merikangas, 2003), although this may in part reflect generational change in the determinants of smoking associated with pronounced secular changes in rates of smoking and recognition of the health hazards of smoking: sibling and twin correlations typically have been much higher (Avenovoli & Merikangas, 2003; Heath & Madden, 1995).

Increasingly, family studies have been implemented for the purposes of discovering genetic linkage (i.e., co-segregation of a genetic marker and a "trait" locus that influences risk of a disorder) in order to identify individual genes that contribute to risk, with some positive findings reported initially for alcohol dependence (Prescott, Sullivan, Kuo *et al.*, 2006; Reich *et al.*, 1998) and more recently for other substance use disorders including cocaine dependence (Gelernter, Panhuysen, Weiss *et al.*, 2005), opiate dependence (Gelernter, Panhuysen, Wilcox *et al.*, 2006) and tobacco dependence (Li, Payne, Ma *et al.*, 2006). Specific features of the design of a study (e.g., an emphasis on ascertainment of large extended pedigrees; Reich *et al.*, 1998) may also define the types of genes that are more or less likely to be discovered in that study (in this case, making it less likely that genetic risk factors associated with antisocial alcoholism will be discovered, because of the decreased likelihood of large full sibships in the case of an antisocial personality disordered father).

The evidence for significant parent–offspring and sibling correlations from family studies establishes the importance of familial factors, but of course does not exclude non-genetic causes for family resemblance. Family studies also provide evidence for significant spousal concordance for substance use and substance use disorder which, at least some studies suggest (Agrawal, Heath, Grant *et al.*, 2006) may be explained by assortative mating, the tendency for like to marry like, and which may vary over time. Any increased tendency for an alcoholic to marry another alcoholic (or, more broadly, substance abusing) partner will increase genetic risk to the offspring generation, compared to random mating. Thus, while the genes that are segregating in a population will not change over time, and thus cannot account for secular changes in rates of disorder, changes in the intensity of assortative mating (e.g., in periods of disruption such as war) do have the potential to impact on the distribution of risk in the next generation.

Recognition of the strong familiality of alcoholism has in turn produced a large literature of high-risk research studies contrasting outcomes in offspring of alcohol-dependent parents (typically fathers) and controls (Sher, Walitzer, Wood *et al.*, 1991), with some important prospective studies beginning either in early childhood (Zucker, Wong, Puttler *et al.*, 2003) or in adolescence (Chassin, Rogosch, & Barrera, 1991). Such studies can provide important information about early precursors of substance use disorders, but at the cost of lengthy delays before early outcomes can be conclusively linked to adolescent or adult substance use. Because of the extensive psychiatric comorbidity of substance use with other psychiatric disorders, and the extensive environmental risk-exposures of offspring of a parent with a substance use disorder history (which typically will be associated with risks that are not specific to offspring substance use disorder), it is only by the time that offspring are mostly through their period of risk for substance use disorder onset that the connection of early behaviors with later substance use disorder can be confirmed. The sampling strategy used to ascertain high-risk families incurs important limitations to the generalizability of findings from a particular study: for example, the work of Chassin (Chassin, Rogosch, Barrera, 1991) is unusual in requiring that a custodial parent be alcoholic at the time a family was entered into the study but, in the general population, a relatively high proportion of families with parental alcoholism will have experienced parental divorce by the time the offspring reach early adolescence (see p. 575).

Of particular note have been the prospective high-risk studies of Schuckit (e.g., Schuckit, Smith, Pierson *et al.*, 2006), using an alcohol challenge paradigm, with administration of a standardized dose of alcohol under the controlled conditions of the research laboratory, to compare level of response to alcohol in young adult offspring from high-risk with control families. While the precise interpretation of Schuckit's findings remains controversial, because the adult offspring that he was testing were not alcohol-naïve, it is clear that level of response to alcohol, indexed by such measures as self-reported intoxication, differentiates high-risk from control offspring, and is prospectively predictive of alcohol dependence risk, with low level of response associated with familial alcoholism history and independently predictive of increased risk of dependence, findings that emphasize that individual differences in drug response may themselves be important (and heritable; Heath, Madden, Dinwiddie *et al.*, 1999) determinants of risk. A similar association is also seen in a (non-genetic) prospective study of marijuana reactions and subsequent dependence risk (Fergusson, Horwood, Lynskey *et al.*, 2003).

The high-risk paradigm has been relatively fruitful in alcohol research, but underutilized for illicit drug dependence (but see e.g., Tarter, Kirisci, Mezzich *et al.*, 2003). A new generation of studies is emerging as the children and adolescent offspring of adult linkage samples are followed prospectively, which should allow prospective characterization of the behavioral effects of genes identified as associated with alcohol dependence risk in the parental generation.

Adoption, Twin and Children-of-Twins Studies

Detailed reviews of individual studies are available elsewhere for alcoholism (Heath, Slutske, & Madden, 1997), smoking (Heath & Madden, 1995) and marijuana dependence (Agrawal & Lynskey, 2006). Here we emphasize overall findings and conceptual issues concerning the interpretation of research from these studies, noting that most have been based on adult samples from older twin cohorts (typically born in the 1970s or earlier), but that a new generation of prospective studies including studies of international adoptees (McGue, Sharma, & Benson, 1996) and of open adoptions (where the biological mother remains in contact with the adoptive family), and prospective twin studies (cited earlier), as well as the emerging children-of-twins studies (Jacob, Waterman, Heath *et al.*, 2003) are characterizing adolescent substance use and its adult outcomes.

From the *adoption study* literature, there is very consistent evidence that alcoholism or more broadly defined substance dependence (which will be chiefly alcohol or marijuana dependence) in adoptees is significantly correlated with alcoholism or antisociality in biological fathers, and uncorrelated, or only weakly correlated, with alcoholism in adoptive parents. A similar pattern is seen for antisocial traits (Langbehn, Cadoret, Yates *et al.*, 1998). This consistency of evidence is seen despite considerable variability in how biological parent alcoholism was assessed: by direct interview in the original Danish adoption study (Goodwin, Schulsinger, Hermansen *et al.*, 1973); by a record review that would have classified as positive individuals with a single drunk-driving conviction (i.e., defining a relatively mild, high-prevalence phenotype) in the case of the Scandinavian adoption studies (Cloninger, Bohman, & Sigvardsson, 1981); and by a record review that disproportionately identified alcoholic fathers through the prison and hospital systems, defining a low-prevalence severe antisocial alcoholic/substance abusing paternal phenotype, in the case of the Iowa adoption studies (Cadoret, Troughton, & Woodworth, 1994). However, the adoption study literature is less consistent with the hypothesis that the comorbidity of depression and alcoholism is largely determined by genetic factors (Cadoret, Winokur, Langbehn *et al.*, 1996).

The adoption study literature must be interpreted with recognition of certain important limitations. Because of the much higher prevalence of alcoholism in males than females, particularly for the older birth cohorts from which the older adoption studies were based, the studies have mainly been informative about outcomes associated with paternal alcoholism, although the Swedish studies do provide some data about associations with maternal alcoholism. Selective placement (i.e., the possibility that individuals from high-risk genetic backgrounds will be more likely to be placed with high-risk adoptive parents) is probably an overstated problem, given the typically quite limited sophistication, from a psychiatric perspective, of the evaluations conducted in the adoption process, and random placement a closer approximation to reality. On the other hand, it is clear that by selecting children given up for adoption, there is overrepresentation of biological parent antisociality, and, conversely, adoptive home environments may not represent the full range of environmental adversity encountered in non-adoptive families (because adoptive parents will include fewer young parents with active substance use disorder at the time of their parenting). (However, rates of prenatal substance exposure may be more elevated in adoptees, given higher rates of maternal antisociality, and mothers who were not planning to keep their offspring: certainly prenatal effects appear more pronounced than would be anticipated for general population samples; Yates, Cadoret, Troughton *et al.*, 1998.) Thus, the early adoption studies are most likely to be informative about genetic influences on alcoholism occurring in the context of a history of antisocial traits, and while the adoption study design may provide useful insights into pertinent environmental risk mechanisms, it is information that cannot easily be generalized, in terms of magnitude of effects or their importance relative to other environmental risk mechanisms, to non-adoptive families. A new generation of studies is emerging that takes advantage of international adoptions (McGue, Sharma, & Benson, 1996) and open adoptions (where adoptive and biological parents remain in contact with one another) in the USA that may overcome some of the limitations of the earlier studies.

Twin Studies

A series of diagnostic interview and record-linkage twin studies provide additional support for the importance of genetic factors in the familial transmission of alcohol dependence risk (Heath, Slutske, & Madden, 1997; Knopik, Heath, Madden *et al.*, 2004). A smaller number of diagnostic interview studies have provided evidence for genetic influences on nicotine dependence (Lessov, Martin, Statham *et al.*, 2004) and illicit drug dependence (Agrawal, Lynskey, Bucholz *et al.*, 2007; Kendler, Jacobson, Prescott *et al.*, 2003), although many questionnaire studies have documented genetic effects on various non-diagnostic aspects of smoking behavior including heaviness of smoking and persistence versus successful desistance (Heath & Madden, 1995). As far as concerns alcoholism, studies have ranged from analyses of medical record or hospital discharge data in the Swedish and US World War II twin panels – which will have defined a relatively severe alcoholism phenotype – to diagnostic interview surveys which typically will have defined a much broader phenotype.

In general, these studies have confirmed the inference of important genetic effects on substance use disorder inferred from adoption studies, and provided evidence for important genetic influences in women (where assessed) as well as men, and for severe phenotypes as well as milder phenotypes. If one twin has a history of substance use disorder, it is much more likely that the cotwin will also have a history if the cotwin is monozygotic (genetically identical) than if the cotwin is dizygotic (an ordinary full sibling). Quantity of alcohol consumed also appears to be influenced by genetic factors (Heath & Martin, 1994), emphasizing that genetic effects on dependence risk may be at least partially, or substantially, mediated through effects on consumption patterns (Whitfield, Zhu, Madden *et al.*, 2004). Multivariate genetic analyses have also documented high genetic correlation between substance use disorder (principally alcohol dependence) and traits that might be broadly characterized as indicators of behavioral disinhibition (Iacono, Malone, & McGue, 2003; Slutske, Heath, Madden *et al.*, 2002b), but also moderately strong genetic correlation between history of major depression and alcohol dependence risk (Kendler, Heath, Neale *et al.*, 1993).

As with adoption studies, limitations of the traditional twin study design must be considered carefully. Foremost is the question of whether the assumption of equally correlated environmental exposures in monozygotic compared to dizygotic pairs is justified for drug use. While investigations of this question for a broad range of behavioral and psychiatric phenotypes have generally found support for this assumption (Hettema, Neale, & Kendler, 1995; Kendler, Neale, Kessler *et al.*, 1994), the very low proportion of monozygotic pairs who are discordant for use of some drug classes (e.g., tobacco) must make us suspect that frequently once one twin uses, he or she initiates his or her cotwin. Where investigated, it has not been found that this biases inferences about the later outcomes of substance use: for example, conditioning upon whether or not a twin pair start smoking at the same time still leads to consistent estimates for the importance of genetic effects on later smoking outcomes (Pergadia, Heath, Agrawal *et al.*, 2006).

Additional limitations to consider in the interpretation of twin data are: (i) the confounding of shared environmental and non-additive genetic effects, which can lead to the underestimation of the importance of shared environmental influences on risk; and (ii) the confounding of genetic and genotype × shared environment interaction effects, which leads to reported genetic variances or heritabilities (or, in the multivariate case, genetic correlations) combining both the main effects of genes on risk, and the effects of genotype × shared environment interaction (Heath, Todorov, Nelson *et al.*, 2002). It is possible to model explicitly the interaction of latent genotype with a measured environmental modifier; however, power to detect such interaction effects will be low, particularly if a low-prevalence binary environmental modifier is used for analysis, and published reports have not always excluded the full range of alternative explanations before claiming such interaction effects (e.g., variance differences between exposure conditions can lead to erroneous inference of G × E effects, unless appropriately modeled). Thus, while convincing demonstration of the importance of G × E interaction effects in the substance use disorder literature have been relatively few, we shall see in our review of environmental risks (see p. 574) that it is probably quite unsafe to assume the absence of such effects.

An informative extension of the classic twin design examines outcomes of children of twins who are concordant or discordant for history of substance use disorder (Jacob *et al.*, 2003). Assuming adequate statistical control for psychopathology in the coparent (Jacob *et al.*, 2003), the children-of-twins design allows contrasts of outcomes in children at high genetic and high environmental risk (twin parent has a history of substance use disorder); high genetic but reduced environmental risk (twin parent is unaffected but parent's monzygotic [MZ] cotwin has a history of substance use disorder); intermediate genetic but reduced environmental risk (twin parent is unaffected but parent's dizygotic [DZ] cotwin has a history of substance use disorder); and low genetic and low environmental risk (twin parent, and parent's cotwin, both have no history of substance use disorder).

Unexpectedly, the one study for which results have been published to date found increased offspring risk of alcohol use disorder only in the presence of both genetic risk (parent or MZ cotwin alcohol dependent) and environmental exposure (the parent, if not alcohol dependent, had a history of alcohol abuse; Jacob *et al.*, 2003). However, these are results for a single study, whose offspring were relatively early in their period of risk for the onset of alcohol use disorder, so it remains to be determined whether this pattern (for which one interpretation is important genotype × shared environment interaction effects) is confirmed.

Genetic Association Studies: Effects of Metabolism Genes

We shall not attempt to review the early case–control literature on genetic association studies of substance use disorders: by contemporary standards, most early research was severely underpowered, lacked correction for multiple testing of the very many plausible candidate genes that can be identified for substance use disorders, and thus had high probability of generating false positive findings. More systematic approaches guided by linkage findings are now beginning to identify and replicate genetic associations (Edenberg & Faroud, 2006), and the new era of Genome-Wide Association Studies and high-throughput candidate gene studies (Bierut, Madden, Breslau *et al.*, 2007; Saccone, Hinrichs, Saccone *et al.*, 2007), provided studies are adequately powered, is likely to lead to rapid advances in this literature. Some of the same studies that have been used to identify genetic linkage have also been obtaining prospective data from the pre-adolescent and adolescent offspring in their families, so findings of more direct relevance to adolescent substance use disorder are to be anticipated.

We use a concrete example to illustrate some of the issues raised, for clinical practice as well as research, by the identification of a gene with (in this example) important effects on risk. Arguably the best example of how a polymorphism at a single genetic locus may affect a major psychiatric phenotype is provided by the example of alcoholism, and its associations with ALDH2 (aldehyde dehydrogenase) genotype in individuals of Asian ancestry. Ethanol is converted by the enzyme alcohol dehydrogenase to the toxic metabolite acetaldehyde, which in turn is converted by the enzyme acetaldehyde dehydrogenase to acetic acid. A single point mutation in the gene for ALDH2 leads to an inactive enzyme, so that those who are heterozygotes (ALDH2*1/*2) have substantially elevated blood acetaldehyde concentrations after ingestion of alcohol and experience a characteristic flushing response (Wall, Peterson, Peterson *et al.*, 1997). Individuals who are homozygous for the null allele but develop alcohol problems are extraordinarily rare, reflecting their typically very low consumption of alcohol (a 10-fold difference in average consumption in males between the normal and null homozygotes in one community sample; Higuchi, Matsushita, Muramatsu *et al.*, 1996).

In the Japanese context where much of this research was conducted, pronounced genotype × gender effects are also seen, with women with the high-risk genotype drinking at the same level as men with the lowest risk genotype (Higuchi *et al.*, 1996). Heterozygotes are also rarer in alcoholic patient series than in control series, although at least among Japanese this difference appears to be declining over time (Higuchi, Matsushita, Imazeki *et al.*, 1994), a trend that the authors attributed to increased social pressures on Japanese males to drink after work. At the same time, those heterozygotes who progress to heavier drinking appear to be at increased risk of adverse medical consequences, including increased frequency of alcohol-related cancers (e.g., Hori, Kawano, Endo *et al.*, 1997), presumably because of impaired metabolism of alcohol. Among Asian American youth, however, genotype effects on consumption levels have not been found (Hendershot, MacPherson, Myers *et al.*, 2005). Thus, in considering this single example we find evidence for: (i) an important single gene effect on alcohol dependence risk, which may at least in part be mediated through heaviness of consumption; (ii) important modifiers of this effect, including gender, age-cohort and/or society, and secular change in drinking practices; and (iii) evidence for increased vulnerability (to adverse medical outcomes) in the heterozygote group that were at low risk of becoming heavy drinkers. This example also raises the interesting issue of whether genetic information should be used in counseling adolescents (or adults) about their substance use. In this case, a subset of youth, of Asian ancestry, are at substantially increased risk of adverse medical consequences from alcohol misuse, but they and their families may be unaware of this (particularly in the case of international adoptions by European ancestry parents).

Environmental Risks

The existing research literature has identified a range of environmental risk factors that are associated with increased rates of adolescent substance use and substance use problems. These risk factors are not specific to substance use problems, being also associated with increased risk of conduct disorder (see chapter 35) and in many cases other disorders (e.g., major depression and attention deficit/hyperactivity disorder [ADHD]; see chapters 37 and 34), but their associations with substance use are not, in general, limited to those with co-occurrence of these other disorders. A brief summary of key domains of putative risk is provided below, with comment on methodological considerations pertinent to each domain. We conclude with a discussion of significant clustering observed among environmental risks and between environmental risks and parental substance use disorder history.

Prenatal Alcohol and Other Drug Exposure

Maternal heavy alcohol use during pregnancy is now rare in most contemporary western cultures. Its association with fetal alcohol syndrome is well documented and characterized in clinical follow-up studies, with an extensive supporting basic science literature (see chapter 30). Broader literatures have also developed examining possible consequences of milder levels of prenatal alcohol exposure (fetal alcohol effects) as well as effects of other prenatal drug exposures, and in particular tobacco and cocaine.

Parental history of substance use disorder is associated with increased risk of offspring prenatal alcohol and other substance exposure (Yates *et al.*, 1998), which in turn predicts cognitive and behavioral self-regulation difficulties (Knopik, Sparrow, Madden *et al.*, 2005; Weissman, Warner, Wickramaratne *et al.*, 1999), which also increase risk of adolescent substance use and abuse (Biederman, Monuteaux, Mick *et al.*, 2006). However, it is by no means clear that these associations are causal. Higher rates of substance use disorders and antisocial traits in both the pregnant woman who smokes or uses other drugs during pregnancy, and her partner (Knopik *et al.*, 2005), will predict increased risk of externalizing problems for her offspring, quite apart from any prenatal exposure effect. In the Iowa adoption study (Yates *et al.*, 1998), maternal alcohol use during pregnancy, as abstracted from adoption records (and therefore most probably limited to cases of heavy alcohol use) was predictive of increased risk of offspring drug involvement. However, because biological mothers' psychopathology could be inferred only indirectly from records, it is quite possible that reported maternal alcohol use during pregnancy is functioning merely as an index of greater maternal antisociality, so the possibility of genetic confounding cannot be excluded. This possibility will become clearer with a new generation of studies taking advantage of open adoptions, where the biological mothers can be directly evaluated.

While basic science literatures have developed that indicate that deficits associated with prenatal exposure might be anticipated (for reviews see Ernst, Moolchan, & Robinson, 2001; Slawecki, Thomas, Riley *et al.*, 2004), imperfect control for parental and situational risk factors is likely to make identification of such effects in clinical research challenging. More convincing characterization of such prenatal exposure effects will arise only when systematic within-mother between-pregnancy comparisons are made of full sibling offspring born to mothers who used during one pregnancy but not during a second pregnancy, so that heritable traits in the biological parents can be controlled for. Even these comparisons will have important limitations, because the most severely dependent mothers are the least likely to have refrained from substance use during at least one pregnancy.

Child Maltreatment and Abuse

Childhood neglect, physical abuse (PA), sexual abuse (CSA) and other forms of childhood maltreatment are predictive of early onset tobacco, alcohol, marijuana and other illicit drug use (Anda, Croft, Felitti *et al.*, 1999; Dube, Felitti, Dong *et al.*, 2003; Dube, Miller, Brown *et al.*, 2006), and alcohol or other drug problems during adolescence (Fergusson, Horwood, & Lynskey, 1996) and into adulthood (Molnar, Buka, & Kessler, 2001; Nelson, Heath, Lynskey *et al.*, 2006), especially among women (Widom, Ireland, & Glynn, 1995). Whereas the association between childhood trauma (CSA, in particular) and early and escalating substance involvement observed during adolescence is well documented, debate continues regarding the magnitude of reported effects, and importantly, the causal role of maltreatment in the development of problem substance use. Methodological differences, such as use of retrospective versus prospective assessments and recruitment of study participants from individuals in treatment for substance use disorder or other psychiatric disorders versus large-scale community or population-based sampling, contribute to continued debate. In addition, abuse during childhood is variously defined in terms of age of onset and severity, with some researchers limiting analysis to abuse occurring during younger childhood years (e.g., before age 12 or 16) or to more severe forms of abuse, such as CSA involving penetration or intercourse, or court documented cases of abuse.

Researchers also differ in whether or not, and to what extent, potential third variable confounds are controlled. Rates of maltreatment are higher for children raised in families characterized by a host of other risks, including parental substance use disorder, which might directly impact on vulnerability to early and problem substance use during adolescence. Thus, parental substance use disorder and correlating risks that pre-date both maltreatment and substance initiation may account for at least some of the reported effects. Many recent studies of childhood maltreatment and later outcome include statistical controls for a variety of potentially confounding risk factors; however, few include prospective assessment of offspring outcomes and/or confounded risks. Work by Fergusson, Horwood, and Lynskey (1996) on CSA is an exception, and one of few population-based longitudinal studies in which adolescent substance use disorder is examined.

With growing interest in identifying causal mechanisms underlying the association between childhood maltreatment and early and problem substance involvement, genetically informed methodologies have been increasingly employed to rule out heritable third variables that might independently contribute to substance use disorder risk in adolescence and adulthood. To date, genetically informed research is limited to the examination of substance use disorder in adults. In several studies employing a discordant twin design, higher rates of substance use and substance use disorder among individuals reporting CSA have been observed (Kendler, Bulik, Silberg *et al.*, 2000;

Nelson *et al.*, 2006). However, even in discordant twin comparisons it is not clear to what extent substance use outcomes are secondary to other deficits and early disadvantages that are not shared by members of the twin pair.

Marital Conflict, Parental Divorce and Repartnering

Parental divorce, subsequent repartnering and marital conflict often preceding separation, are associated with increased rates of offspring alcohol, tobacco, marijuana and other illicit drug use initiation (Hoffman & Johnson, 1998), heavier use of these substances (Doherty & Needle, 1991; Hoffman, 1995; Needle, Su, & Doherty, 1990) and greater risk of problem use (Fergusson, Horwood, & Lynskey, 1994; Hoffman & Johnson, 1998; Needle, Su, & Doherty, 1990). However, interpretation of these associations is complicated by confounded risks associated with family disruption that might independently contribute to offspring substance involvement, including parental substance use disorder. Results from a handful of studies that assess prospectively offspring outcomes and/or confounded risks that pre-date family disruption suggest small but significant effects of family disruption on adolescent substance use and substance use problems (Fergusson, Horwood, & Lynskey, 1994; Doherty & Needle, 1991).

In addition, behavioral genetic studies have noted genetic effects on the risk of divorce (McGue & Lykken, 1992), a not unexpected finding given the importance of genetic effects on parental characteristics such as substance use disorder history that are associated with increased divorce risk. Thus, it may be questioned to what extent risks associated with parental divorce are mediated environmentally, rather than by genetic transmission.

This issue has been the focus of a number of recent genetically informed studies of substance use disorder in adults. For example, Kendler, Neale, Prescott *et al.* (1996) examined environmental mediation of parental loss effects on risk for alcoholism in a large sample of adult female twins. Kendler reported parental loss through separation (but not death) had both causal and non-causal effects. Specifically, associations between alcoholism risk and parental separation were mediated by environmental factors specific to parental separation as well as genetic factors associated with susceptibility to alcoholism. In a recent study of adolescent and young adult offspring of Australian twins discordant for divorce, D'Onofrio, Turkheimer, Emery *et al.* (2005) report divorce-specific environmental mediation of associations between parental divorce prior to age 16 and marijuana use. However, mediation by environmental factors specific to divorce either before or after age 16 was not observed for ever use of alcohol or cigarettes, age at first use of alcohol, cigarettes or marijuana, having experienced alcohol intoxication, or age at first alcohol intoxication. In both studies, inferences about environmental mediation are model-dependent, so that unmeasured genetic confounders in the parental generation would potentially lead to false positive (or false negative) inference. Additional, more robust support for environmental mediation of divorce effects (and parental psychopathology) on offspring substance involvement is provided by Cadoret, Troughton, O'Gorman *et al.* (1986), who in an early report on a cohort of Iowa adoptees found an increased risk for drug abuse among adoptees whose adoptive parents divorced or had a history of psychiatric difficulties compared to adoptees whose adoptive parents remained together and had no history of psychiatric difficulties. Similar results were reported in a separate study of male adoptees (Cadoret, Yates, Troughton *et al.*, 1995), with marital and psychiatric problems in adoptive parents contributing to adoptee risk of drug abuse independently of genetic influences.

Overall, it is clear that children in disrupted families show increased risk of early substance involvement and abuse and/or dependence, but the underlying mechanisms remain uncertain. It remains unclear whether, and certainly cannot be assumed that, removal of a parent with a history of substance use disorder from the home produces better outcomes for offspring: indeed, one study using a children-of-twins design failed to find any significant effect of duration of paternal presence in the home as a moderator of paternal alcoholism effects (Duncan, Scherrer, Fu *et al.*, 2006).

Parenting Influences

Results from cross-sectional and an increasing number of prospective longitudinal studies of adolescent substance involvement support the importance of a range of parenting influences. Inconsistent, ineffective discipline and poor supervision and monitoring (Chilcoat & Anthony, 1996), parent–child conflict (Brook, Brook, Gordon *et al.*, 1990; Sokol-Katz, Dunham, & Zimmerman, 1997), low levels of parent support and parent–child attachment (Allen, Hauser, & Borman-Spurell, 1996) and permissive or tolerant attitudes about substance use (Ary, Tildesley, Hops *et al.*, 1993; Brook, Whiteman, Gordon *et al.*, 1986) are among parenting behaviors predictive of both early and problem alcohol, tobacco, marijuana and other illicit drug use during adolescence.

Identification of mediating and moderating effects of parenting on adolescent substance involvement is the focus of much recent research on parenting influences. In addition to parsing direct from indirect effects of parental substance use disorder (Urberg, Goldstein, & Toro, 2005), this work has documented significant moderation by parenting of associations between parental substance use disorder and adolescent substance use and misuse (Doherty & Allen, 1994). Consistent with results from cross-sectional studies (Brook *et al.*, 1990; Kung & Farrell, 2000), there is now longitudinal evidence that some parenting behaviors, particularly monitoring, work to moderate peer influences on adolescent substance use and substance use problems (Ary, Duncan, Duncan *et al.*, 1999; Barnes, Hoffman, Welte *et al.*, 2006; Marshal & Chassin, 2000).

Peer Influences

Whereas deviant peer affiliation continues to be one of the best predictors of early and problem substance use during the adolescent years (Fergusson, Swain-Campbell, & Horwood, 2002), mechanisms underlying this association remain largely unknown. Among competing explanations is the possibility that deviant peers have a direct influence through peer pressure and socialization, both modeling and providing reinforcement of alcohol and other drug use. However, selective processes are also likely; for example, parental substance use disorder increases risk for both substance involvement and affiliation with deviant peers, and might thereby account for their association. In addition, substance-using adolescents may seek out peers who also use substances, a form of social homophily (Bauman & Ennett, 1994).

To disentangle direct and indirect effects of deviant peer affiliation on early and problem use of alcohol and other substances, an increasing number of researchers are capitalizing on the strengths of prospective longitudinal designs in attempts to rule out third variable confounds. Results from this work largely support both socialization and selection explanations, together suggesting parental substance use disorder, along with impairments in parenting, increase the likelihood of affiliating with substance-using peers (Fergusson & Horwood, 1999; Larzelere & Patterson, 1990) which, in turn, has direct effects on adolescent substance involvement.

Conclusions: Clustering of Risks

In interpreting the literature on putative risk factors, it is important to note the high degree of overlap or clustering of these risk factors, and their associations with conduct disorder and other disorders. For example, prenatal drug exposure is more common among children of parents with substance use disorder. These offspring are also at heightened risks for experiencing family disruption, childhood abuse, neglect and otherwise compromised parenting that together increase the likelihood of affiliations with delinquent or substance-using peers. Despite the high degree of overlap and clustering of risk factors, most of the accumulated literature on potential risk factors in fact derives from research that has considered relatively few risk factors, ignoring others, and that may have imperfect or no characterization of parental psychopathology. However, these challenges do not reduce the importance of considering the total effects, both direct and through correlated environmental risks, in so far as they help identify particular groups of individuals (e.g., children of divorced parents; children with a history of abuse) at increased risk of early substance involvement and problems.

A further issue concerns the interplay between genetic and environmental risks. Despite the extensive evidence for genetic effects on risks of substance use disorders, it must be remembered that most of this evidence derives from non-adopted families, so that genetic effects are occurring in these same contexts of environmental risks such as prenatal substance exposures, early trauma and parental conflict and separation/divorce. While there has been only limited characterization of gene–environment interaction effects at the time of writing, the likely importance of such effects should not be ignored.

Behavioral and Pharmacotherapies

The efficacy of pharmacotherapies for adolescent drug use disorders has not been established, although some promising pharmacotherapies are emerging for use with adults. Clinical trials with adolescents have been few in number and underpowered. Whereas some studies using complex combination cognitive–behavioral interventions have been able to demonstrate improved adolescent desistance rates, there is at this time limited understanding of the mechanisms by which adolescent desistance or reduction in use is achieved, and of the risk or protective factors that influence these outcomes, whether in or out of the context of treatment. Thus, while appealing treatment programs have been developed for therapy with adolescent substance abusers (MacPherson, Frissell, Brown *et al.*, 2006), the evidentiary base for identifying particular components of therapy as critical for successful outcome, or particularly efficacious with particular adolescents, does not yet exist. This is further complicated by substantial comorbidity between substance use disorders and the range of psychiatric disorders, particularly disruptive behavior disorders, and mood disorders. Despite high rates of comorbidity, there is relatively little research evidence addressing the extent to which specific treatment approaches may be best suited for specific patterns of co-occurring substance use and psychiatric disorders.

In summary, randomized clinical trials focused on adolescent substance abusers have been rare and typically single-site (therefore of uncertain generalizability to patient populations across diverse clinical settings), underpowered and with little attention to the potential influence of comorbid conditions on clinical outcomes.

Some insights can be obtained from randomized clinical trials with adult patient populations; however, such trials have the advantage of adult participants who have usually volunteered to participate precisely because they are at a point in their life where they are motivated to change their pattern of drug use; the challenge with adolescents, who commonly are referred to treatment through parental, school or legal influences, is much greater. Furthermore, the specific ethical challenges of clinical research with minors (requirement to obtain parental consent for participation; potential for confidentiality breach in obtaining parental consent) raise additional (but not insurmountable) difficulties.

Tobacco

It is common in psychiatric practice for smoking and tobacco dependence to be ignored, a peculiar oversight given that smoking accounts for a substantial proportion of early deaths in most western societies. This relative neglect of tobacco use has been no less the case for children and adolescents. While nicotine replacement therapy (NRT) has been used successfully for adult smoking cessation, an early open-label trial using nicotine patch with adolescent smokers desiring to quit reported no benefit (5% abstinence rate at 6 months; Hurt, Croghan, Beede *et al.*, 2000), and a single underpowered clinical trial failed to find a significant improvement in abstinence rates at 6 months using the nicotine patch (Grimshaw & Stanton, 2006; Moolchan, Robinson, Ernst *et al.*, 2005). Use of amfebutamone, in combination with NRT patch, for adolescent smoking cessation has also not been found to be useful (Grimshaw & Stanton, 2006).

In adults, there is a substantial clinical trial literature documenting improved smoking cessation rates with NRT (1.5- to two-fold, across a range of different modalities for nicotine administration, compared with placebo or other control group; Silagy, Lancaster, Stead *et al.*, 2006), and some antidepressants (amfebutamone, nortriptyline; a doubling of the odds of cessation) but not selective serotonin reuptake inhibitors (Hughes, Stead, & Lancaster, 2004). There have also been promising developments using a selective $\alpha_4\beta_2$-nicotinic receptor partial agonist, with a phase II trial reporting, at the 1 mg twice daily dose, increased long-term success rates compared to sustained-release amfebutamone and to placebo, with 48% reporting 4 or more weeks without smoking during the 6-week treatment phase (versus 33%, 17%) and continuous quit rates at 12-month follow-up also higher (approximately a three-fold increase: 14.4% versus 6.3%, 4.9%; Nides, Oncken, Gonzales *et al.*, 2006). A phase III trial with a 12-week treatment phase has confirmed increased rates of continuous abstinence, compared with both placebo and amfebutamone, during the final month of treatment, and at follow-up at up to 52 weeks (Jorenby, Hays, Rigotti *et al.*, 2006).

Given the weak evidentiary basis for assessing pharmacotherapy effects for adolescent smokers, and the fact that NRT products in many countries are available over-the-counter, it seems premature to conclude that pharmacotherapies for smoking cessation by adolescents will not be successful. Despite shorter smoking histories, a significant number of adolescents are smoking at levels similar to those of adults being entered into clinical trials (e.g., 20 cigarettes per day, scores on the Fagerstrom Test of Nicotine Dependence of 5 or more; Hurt, Croghan, Beede *et al.*, 2000). However, the case for efficacy for pharmacological treatment of adolescent smokers remains to be established.

Some evidence from controlled trials for efficacy of behavioral interventions for smoking cessation in adolescents has been obtained (Grimshaw & Stanton, 2006). Some of this has been generated within the theoretical framework of the Transtheoretical Model (TTM; DiClemente, Prochaska, Fairhurst *et al.*, 1991) and, despite the considerable limitations of the TTM framework (Sutton, 2001), these studies have achieved reasonable increases in rates of adolescent smoking cessation (pooled odds ratio of 1.70 at 12 months), a testament to the loose coupling between theoretical perspective and behavioral intervention results. Cognitive–behavioral therapy (CBT) interventions (pooled odds ratio 1.87) and interventions including a motivational interviewing component (pooled odds ratio 2.05) have also shown some success. These effect sizes are generally consistent with those obtained using non-pharmacological individual or group-based treatments in adult smoking cessation (Lancaster & Stead, 2005; Stead & Lancaster, 2005).

Alcoholism and Illicit Drug Use Disorders

The treatment of adult alcoholism has shifted from in-patient to out-patient-based treatments. While this change occurred largely because of economic factors, it appears that the effectiveness of out-patient-based treatment is comparable to in-patient treatment, except in cases of serious comorbid medical or psychiatric conditions (Finney, Hahn, & Moos, 1996). Large-scale multisite randomized clinical trials of alcoholism have been limited to samples of adults. In the 1990s, the US Project MATCH (Project MATCH Research Group, 1997a,b) investigated matching client characteristics to treatments, but found approximate comparability of outcomes with the three contrasted approaches: motivational enhancement therapy (MET), which uses structured feedback to motivate the client to utilize his or her resources to change behavior; 12-step facilitation, an approach popular in the USA which makes use of the 12-step framework developed by Alcoholics Anonymous (AA) and makes attendance at and participation in AA meetings an important component of recovery; and a CBT-based approach. There is only limited evidence for the value of patient–treatment matching.

There have been no multisite randomized clinical trials of pharmacotherapies for alcoholism in adolescents, and in the absence of such data, the most recent findings from large US multisite trials with adults suggest that behavioral interventions should remain the treatment of choice for adolescents with alcohol problems. In a multisite trial involving almost exclusively males, with chronic severe alcohol dependence ($n = 627$, median age approximately 50), supplementation of 12-step facilitation counseling with short-term (3 month) or long-term (12 month) administration of naltrexone (50 mg/day), an opioid receptor antagonist, compared with placebo, produced no differences in time to relapse at 13 weeks, nor in percentage drinking days or drinks per drinking day, at 12-month follow-up. Substantial decreases in percent days abstinent were achieved across all conditions (from approximately 35% at baseline to 82% at 12-month follow-up), with more modest reductions in number of drinks per drinking day (from 13–14 at baseline to 9–10 at 12-month follow-up; Krystal, Cramer, Krol *et al.*, 2001). Other studies using naltrexone have reported modest short-term and medium-term improvements in time to first drink and diminished craving, compared with placebo, with some evidence for improved outcome when combined with an intensive psychosocial treatment (Srisurapanont & Jarusuraisin, 2005).

More recently, Project COMBINE (Anton, O'Malley, Ciraulo *et al.*, 2006), using a 16-week treatment period ($n = 1383$, two-thirds male, median age 44), found no improvements in outcome associated with use of acamprosate (a medication that had been reported to be efficacious in some European trials; 3 g/day), either alone or in combination with naltrexone or a combined behavioral intervention (CBI); a modest increase in abstinence days (versus 25% at baseline) compared with placebo plus medical monitoring (75%) under conditions of naltrexone administration (100 mg/day) plus medical monitoring (81%), or the combined behavioral intervention plus medical monitoring (79%), but not both (77%), these differences being rather modest and no longer significant (but with trends in the same direction) at 12 months. While Project COMBINE was in very many respects a model for its quality control procedures, one unfortunate aspect of its design complicates interpretation of findings: a CBI-only group was included that showed worse outcomes (67% days abstinent) compared to the CBI plus placebo plus medical monitoring group. However, medical management involved an initial baseline 45-minute session with 20-minute follow-ups at 1, 2, 4, 6, 8, 10, 12 and 16 weeks, conducted by a nurse, physician, pharmacist or physician assistant, and included a focus on the alcohol dependence diagnosis and negative consequences of drinking, and the importance of medications compliance, at baseline, with review of medication compliance, adverse effects, and drinking and overall functioning, at subsequent follow-ups. The medical practitioner contact under the CBI-only condition was more limited, leaving open the possibility that it was the intermittent nurse/physician contact, combined with CBI, rather than taking of pills, that explained the improved success under the CBI plus placebo condition.

From these studies of older adults one may conclude that in adults wishing to overcome problems with alcohol, substantial harm reduction may be achieved through behavioral interventions in terms of reduction in drinking days, even without the use of pharmacotherapy, as other have noted (Miller, Walters, & Bennett, 2001). Given the absence of adolescent pharmacotherapy trial data, reliance on behavioral interventions seems the preferred strategy at this time. Unfortunately, rigorous clinical trial data on the components of behavioral interventions that are effective with adolescents, and the mechanisms by which changes in drinking are achieved, are lacking: thus, the clinician is left to select from a menu of strategies that have been found to give improved outcome (e.g., motivational enhancement; cognitive–behavioral skills training), sometimes packaged as an esthetically pleasing package (MacPherson *et al.*, 2006) but nonetheless having relatively weak empirical support to justify the necessity of individual components of the package.

Although there is now considerable evidence that methadone maintenance – and other opioid agonist maintenance agents such as buprenorphine – are effective at reducing illicit opioid use (Ward, Hall, & Mattick, 1999), relatively little research has been conducted on the effectiveness of these treatments in children and adolescents. This may be a reflection of a number of factors including the lower rate of heroin dependence (relative to tobacco or alcohol) in the general population, the later mean age of onset of this disorder and a widespread belief among clinicians that maintenance therapies are better suited to older individuals with a long-term history of chronic heavy opioid use. Nonetheless, findings from the limited adolescent-focused research converge on those from larger, more carefully controlled studies with adult samples to suggest that methadone (and, by extension, other maintenance therapies) is likely to be effective in reducing long-term use of heroin and other illicit opioids in those adolescents who have developed severe dependence (Kellogg, Melia, Khuri *et al.*, 2006).

There is considerably less research on pharmacotherapies for cannabis or other illicit drugs, although there are a number of possible therapies being considered for use. These include the use of antidepressant medication, particularly among those with comorbid substance use disorders and major depressive disorder (Cornelius, Clark, Bukstein *et al.*, 2005), the use of CBI agonists specifically for tobacco dependence (Cohen, Kodas, & Griebel, 2005), and maintenance stimulant prescription for treatment of cocaine and other illicit stimulant dependence (Grabowski, Shearer, Merrill *et al.*, 2004). There is little research evaluating these treatments empirically, what literature is available is based almost entirely on adult, rather than adolescent samples and evaluations of the efficacy of these alternative pharmacotherapies have produced, at best, equivocal results regarding their efficacy (DeLima, Soares, Reisser *et al.*, 2002).

Coerced Treatment

Largely in the area of illicit drug use and related problems, there has been ongoing interest in the extent to which mandated or coerced treatment, either as an adjunct to, or in replacement of, criminal justice interventions (e.g., imprisonment), may be efficacious in reducing the use of illicit drugs and related problems (Harrison & Scarpitti, 2002). While such interventions, including so-called drug courts, have been most popular in the USA (Turner, Longshore, Wenzel *et al.*, 2002), there is increasing interest in implementing them in other countries (Bean, 2002). Evaluations of such programs have generally shown them to be both effective and cost effective (relative to alternatives), suggesting that, provided the myriad ethical issues involved in such mandated treatment (Caplan, 2006) can be addressed, they may have a role in the treatment of drug use problems, particularly among those more severely afflicted.

Similarly, diversion from the criminal justice system for more minor drug offences (principally possession of small amounts of cannabis) may be an effective strategy to continue discouraging illicit drugs while avoiding imposing the potentially heavy individual consequences of a drug conviction for what may be relatively minor drug use (Barratt, Chanteloup, Lenton *et al.*, 2005). As with many issues surrounding the legal status of illicit drugs and legal approaches to limiting the use of licit drugs (e.g., taxation, licensing hours), consideration of such interventions raises a number of social, political and ethical issues, the resolution of which may be only slightly influenced by empirical evidence of effectiveness.

Brief Interventions

Spanning the intersection of treatment and public health interventions, there has also been considerable interest in the extent to which brief interventions, targeted at individuals who may be using substances heavily but who are not seeking treatment nor necessarily meet criteria for a substance use disorder, may reduce substance use and/or prevent escalation to heavier, problematic or dependent use. Evaluations of such interventions have been conducted in a number of settings including general medical practices, hospital emergency departments and other health care providers and have generally been positive. For example, in a sample of 152 13- to 17-years-olds presenting at an emergency department after an alcohol-related event, Spirito, Monti, Barnett *et al.* (2004) reported that a brief intervention involving motivational interviewing reduced the average number of drinking days per month and frequency of heavy drinking at 12-month follow-up, relative to those receiving standard care. Similarly, Colby, Monti, O'Leary Tevyaw *et al.* (2005) reported 6-month follow-up in a group of 85 14- to 19-year-olds randomized to receive a brief intervention or no intervention for tobacco use, delivered in medical settings (hospital out-patient or emergency departments). Results indicated some reductions in smoking among those treated, but overall reductions were small. Whereas the bulk of brief interventions with adolescents have been targeted at either tobacco or alcohol use, there is emerging evidence of their feasibility for use with cannabis use (Martin, Copeland, & Swift, 2005) and across multiple substances, including illicit drugs (McCambridge & Strang, 2004).

Prevention

Legislative Approaches Aimed at Limiting Availability of and Access to Substances Among Youth

These include policies regulating the sale and availability of alcohol (Chikritzhs & Stockwell, 2006; Stockwell & Grunewald, 2004), restrictions on the sale of alcohol and tobacco to youth (Ahmad & Billimek, 2007; Wagenaar & Toomey, 2002), as well as legal prohibitions against the supply and possession of cannabis and other illicit drugs (MacCoun & Reuter, 2001). In terms of the licit drugs – tobacco and alcohol – there seems to be considerable evidence supporting the efficacy of legal and policy approaches limiting access to these substances among youth.

Research indicates that raising the minimum legal age for purchasing alcohol results not only in a reduction in use, but also a reduction in alcohol-related harm among youth (Wagenaar & Toomey, 2002), while demonstrated price elasticity of cigarettes indicates that raising prices through the imposition of taxation is likely to decrease both the prevalence of smoking among youth and the frequency of smoking among youthful smokers (Hopkins, Briss, Ricard *et al.*, 2001; Zhang, Cohen, Ferrence *et al.*, 2006). Evidence in favor of legal sanctions for reducing illicit drug – and especially cannabis – use appears more mixed (MacCoun & Reuter, 2001) with cross-national comparisons indicating that lifetime prevalence of cannabis use is lower in some countries that have relatively liberal legal approaches (e.g., the Netherlands) compared to countries with more restrictive legal approaches (e.g., the USA; Vega, Aguilar-Gaxiola, Andrade *et al.*, 2002) highlighting that differences in legal approach alone cannot explain the often quite large differences between countries in rates of substance use and substance use disorders.

Community and Mass Media Campaigns

There have also been a variety of media campaigns or interventions including both laws to limit or eliminate tobacco or alcohol advertising and mass media campaigns designed to limit or reduce licit and illicit drug use. Within the tobacco field there is evidence that such campaigns can be successful (Farrelly, Niederdeppe, & Yarsevich, 2003), although it is uncertain what specific components of these campaigns are likely to be most effective. Similarly, some alcohol-related campaigns, focused primarily on reducing alcohol-related harm rather than alcohol use per se, have been shown to be effective in reducing such behaviors (Elder, Shults, Sleet *et al.*, 2004), although, to the extent that these have often be implemented in the context of a comprehensive array of interventions, it is often difficult to isolate the impact of a specific intervention. Within the illicit drug field, it has also been recently suggested that there may be a synergistic effect between media and school-based interventions aimed at reducing the uptake of illicit drugs. Thus, the greatest benefit of these programs may be in helping to provide a milieu that is supportive of and conducive to other more intensive interventions by helping to create a social milieu that is generally supportive of drug abstinence.

School and Educational Interventions

A variety of school-based interventions – including both knowledge-based educational programs and others focused more broadly on social skills, assertiveness and related training – have been widely adopted. Nonetheless, the enthusiasm with which such programs are adopted appears to be unmatched by empirical evidence of efficacy or effectiveness. Indeed, there is controversy surrounding the extent to which some such interventions – and particularly those focused on imparting knowledge about drugs – may actually increase experimentation and use of these substances. Nonetheless, there is some evidence that well-conducted interventions *not* focusing on drug knowledge but instead focusing on social skills training may lead to consistent, yet modest, reductions in drug use uptake (Faggiano, Vigna-Taglianti, Versino *et al.*, 2005).

Increasingly in the USA there has been interest in implementing drug-testing procedures whereby students are tested on a regular basis. Comprehensive assessments of the efficacy of such programs appear lacking and, whereas a study indicated that rates of self-reported drug use did not differ between schools with drug testing programs and those without (Yamaguchi, Johnston, & O'Malley, 2003), problems with the interpretation of such findings (in particular, the fact that there are likely to be pre-existing differences in rates of drug use between schools that adopt such measures and those that do not), mean that it is difficult to draw any firm conclusions regarding the utility of such programs.

Parenting Programs

Interventions aimed at parents include broad community-based interventions, such as media campaigns discussed above, more family focused interventions aimed at delaying or preventing substance use in adolescents (Gerrard, Gibbons, Brody *et al.*, 2006; Komro, Perry, Veblen-Mortenson *et al.*, 2006) and highly intensive interventions, typically targeted at families identified as "high risk" (Fergusson, Grant, Horwood *et al.*, 2005; Olds, Robinson, Pettitt *et al.*, 2004). Such interventions often address a range of risk factors and, while not targeted specifically at substance use, likely have the advantage of limiting risk across a range of adverse outcomes including substance use, delinquency and psychiatric disorder.

Harm Reduction Initiatives

Whereas a major focus of many prevention efforts involves the delay or avoidance of substance use onset and/or cessation of use (particularly for tobacco and the illicit drugs), there are also a number of interventions aimed at limiting or reducing the harm caused by substance use, even if substance use itself continues. These include campaigns that aim to reduce alcohol-related harm not necessarily by reducing alcohol consumption but by reducing driving under the influence (Elder, Shults, Sleet *et al.*, 2004). Similarly, needle and syringe exchange programs have been successful in reducing transmission of blood-borne viruses without reducing drug use per se (Lurie & Drucker, 1997; Wodak & Cooney, 2006), although it is also important to note that, despite claims by critics of these programs, there is no evidence indicating that such programs increase either the prevalence of drug use or the frequency of drug use among users (Fisher, Fenaughty, Cagle *et al.*, 2003).

Conclusions

Throughout this chapter we have emphasized the need for greater attention to be paid to adolescent substance use and dependence, both in clinical practice and in research. We have tried to draw attention to areas of uncertainty in the literature on adolescent substance use disorders, including uncertainty concerning classification and diagnosis, etiology, consequences of adolescent substance use and substance use disorder, and treatment, prevention and intervention strategies. We have also attempted to encourage critical awareness of the limitations of many existing research strategies. We have done so because we see this area of research as being extraordinarily rich in opportunities for rapid research advances, but currently underserved by the research community. Given the long-term economic costs of substance use disorders in most western societies and their origins in adolescence, and the immediate personal, family and societal costs of adolescent substance use disorder, the relative neglect of this area of research cannot be justified. The problem of adolescent substance use and substance use disorders, more than most areas of child and adolescent psychiatry, also has a strong societal component. As the substantial reductions in rates of smoking that were achieved in California illustrate (Fichtenberg & Glantz, 2000), much can be achieved through local and national policies to reduce rates of adolescent (and adult) substance use. We differ from some (Merikangas & Risch, 2003), however, in believing that whereas social change can reduce rates of substance use and substance use disorder, there will always remain a core group of individuals requiring clinical assistance, who merit our best research efforts at understanding the causes and consequences of adolescent substance use disorder.

References

Abrantes, A. M., Strong, D. R., Ramsey, S. E., Lewinsohn, P. M., & Brown, R. A. (2005). Substance use disorder characteristics and externalizing problems among inpatient adolescent smokers. *Journal of Psychoactive Drugs*, *37*, 391–399.

Agrawal, A., Heath, A. C., Grant, J. D., Pergadia, M. L., Statham, D. J., Bucholz, K. K., *et al.* (2006). Assortative mating for cigarette smoking and for alcohol consumption in female Australian twins and their spouses. *Behavior Genetics*, *36*, 553–566.

Agrawal, A., & Lynskey, M. T. (2006). The genetic epidemiology of cannabis use, abuse and dependence. *Addiction*, *101*, 801–812.

Agrawal, A., Lynskey, M. T., Bucholz, K. K., Martin N. G., Madden, P. A., & Heath, A. C. (2007). Contrasting models of genetic co-morbidity for cannabis and other illicit drugs in adult Australian twins. *Psychological Medicine*, *37*, 49–60.

Agrawal, A., Neale, M. C., Prescott, C. A., & Kendler, K. S. (2004). A twin study of early cannabis use and subsequent use and abuse/dependence of other illicit drugs. *Psychological Medicine*, *34*, 1227–1237.

Ahmad, S., & Billimek, J. (2007). Limiting youth access to tobacco: Comparing the long-term health impacts of increasing cigarette excise taxes and raising the legal smoking age to 21 in the United States. *Health Policy*, *80*, 378–391.

Allen, J. P., Hauser, S. T., & Borman-Spurell, E. (1996). Attachment theory as a framework for understanding sequelae of sever adolescent psychopathology: An 11-year follow-up study. *Journal of Consulting and Clinical Psychology*, *64*, 254–263.

American Psychiatric Association. (2000). *Diagnostic and Statistical Manual of Mental Disorders* (4th edn.) Text revision. Washington, DC: American Psychiatric Association.

Anda, R. F., Croft, J. B., Felitti, V. J., Nordenberg, D., Giles, W. H., Williamson, D. F., *et al.* (1999). Adverse childhood experiences and smoking during adolescence and adulthood. *Journal of the American Medical Association*, *282*, 1652–1658.

Anton, R. F., O'Malley, S. S., Ciraulo, D. A., Cisler, R. A., Couper, D., Donovan, D. M., *et al.*, COMBINE Study Research Group. (2006). Combined pharmacotherapies and behavioral interventions for alcohol dependence: The COMBINE study: A randomized controlled trial. *Journal of the American Medical Association*, *295*, 2003–2017.

Ary, D., Duncan, T. E., Duncan, S. C., & Hops, H. (1999). Adolescent problem behavior: The influence of parents and peers. *Behavior Research and Therapy Incorporating Behavioral Assessment*, *37*, 217–230.

Ary, D., Tildesley, E., Hops, H., & Andrews, J. A. (1993). The influence of parent, sibling, and peer modeling and attitudes on adolescent use of alcohol. *International Journal of the Addictions*, *28*, 853–880.

Avenevoli, S., & Merikangas, K. R. (2003). Familial influences on adolescent smoking. *Addiction*, *98*, 1–20.

Barnes, G. M., Hoffman, J. H., Welte, J. W., Farrell, M. P., & Dintcheff, B. A. (2006). Effects of parental monitoring and peer deviance on substance use and delinquency. *Journal of Marriage and the Family*, *68*, 1084–1104.

Barratt, M. J., Chanteloup, F., Lenton, S., & Marsh, A. (2005). Cannabis law reform in Western Australia: An opportunity to test theories of marginal deterrence and legitimacy. *Drug and Alcohol Review*, *24*, 321–330.

Bauman, K. E., & Ennett, S. T. (1994). Peer influence on adolescent drug use. *American Psychology*, *49*, 820–822.

Bean, P. (2002). Drug treatment courts, British style: the drug treatment court movement in Britain. *Substance Use and Misuse*, *37*, 1595–1614.

Biederman, J., Monuteaux, M. C., Mick, E., Spencer, T., Wilens, T. E., Silva, J. M., *et al.* (2006). Young adult outcome of attention deficit hyperactivity disorder: A controlled 10-year follow-up study. *Psychological Medicine*, *36*, 167–179.

Bierut, L. J., Madden, P. A. F., Breslau, N., Johnson, E. O., Hatsukami, D., Pomerleau, O. F., *et al.* (2007). Novel genes identified in a high-density genome wide association study for nicotine dependence. *Human Molecular Genetics*, *16*, 24–35.

Brook, J. S., Brook, D. W., Gordon, A. S., Whiteman, M., & Cohen, P. (1990). The psychosocial etiology of adolescent drug use: a family interactional approach. *Genetic, Social, and General Psychology Monographs*, *116*, 111–267.

Brook, J. S., Whiteman, M., Gordon, A. S., & Cohen, P. (1986). Dynamics of childhood and adolescent personality traits and adolescent drug use. *Developmental Psychology*, *22*, 403–414.

Brown, S. A., & Tapert, S. F. (2004). Health consequences of adolescent alcohol involvement. In National Research Council and Institute of Medicine, *Reducing Underage Drinking: A Collective Responsibility*. Washington, DC: National Academies Press.

Bucholz, K. K., Heath, A. C., Reich, T., Hesselbrock, V. M., Kramer, J. R., Nurnberger, J. I. Jr., *et al.* (1996). *Alcoholism: Clinical and Experimental Research*, *20*, 1462–1471.

Budney, A. J. (2006). Are specific dependence criteria necessary for different substances: How can research on cannabis inform this issue? *Addiction*, *101*, 125–133.

Budney, A. J., Hughes, J. R., Moore B. A., & Vandrey R. (2004). Review of the validity and significance of cannabis withdrawal syndrome. *American Journal of Psychiatry*, *161*, 1967–1977.

Cadoret, R. J., Troughton, E., O'Gorman, T. W., & Heywood, E. (1986). An adoption study of genetic and environmental factors in drug abuse. *Archives of General Psychiatry*, *43*, 1131–1136.

Cadoret R. J., Troughton, E., & Woodworth, G. (1994). Evidence of heterogeneity of genetic effect in Iowa adoption studies. *Annals of the New York Academy of Sciences*, *708*, 59–71.

Cadoret, R. J., Winokur, G., Langbehn, D., Troughton, E., Yates, W. R., & Stewart, M. A. (1996). Depression spectrum disease. I. The role of gene–environment interaction. *American Journal of Psychiatry*, *153*, 892–899.

Cadoret, R. J., Yates, W. R., Troughton, E., Woodworth, G., & Stewart, M. A. (1995). Adoption study demonstrating two genetic pathways to drug abuse. *Archives of General Psychiatry*, *52*, 42–52.

Caetano, R., & Babor, T. F. (2006). Diagnosis of alcohol dependence in epidemiological surveys: An epidemic of youthful alcohol dependence or a case of measurement error? *Addiction*, *101*, 111–114.

Caplan, A. L. (2006). Ethical issues surrounding forced, mandated, or coerced treatment. *Journal of Substance Abuse Treatment*, *31*, 117–120.

Chassin, L., Rogosch, F., & Barrera, M. (1991). Substance use and symptomatology among adolescent children of alcoholics. *Journal of Abnormal Psychology*, *100*, 449–463.

Chen, K., & Kandel, D. B. (1995). The natural history of drug use from adolescence to the mid-thirties in a general population sample. *American Journal of Public Health*, *85*, 41–47.

Chikritzhs, T., & Stockwell, T. (2006). The impact of later trading hours for hotels on levels of impaired driver road crashes and driver breath alcohol levels. *Addiction*, *101*, 1254–1264.

Chilcoat, H. D., & Anthony, J. C. (1996). Impact of parent monitoring on initiation of drug use through late childhood. *Journal of the American Academy of Child and Adolescent Psychiatry*, *35*, 91–100.

Cloninger, C. R., Bohman, M., & Sigvardsson, S. (1981). Inheritance of alcohol abuse: Cross-fostering analysis of adopted men. *Archives of General Psychiatry*, *38*, 861–868.

Cohen, C., Kodas, E., & Griebel, G. (2005). CB1 receptor antagonists for the treatment of nicotine addiction. *Pharmacology, Biochemistry and Behavior*, *81*, 387–395.

Colby, S. M., Monti, P. M., O'Leary Tevyaw, T., Barnett, N. P., Spirito, A., Rohsenow, D. J., *et al.* (2005). Brief motivational intervention for adolescent smokers in medical settings. *Addictive Behaviors*, *30*, 865–874.

Cornelius, J. R., Clark, D. B., Bukstein, O. G., Birmaher, B., Salloum, I. M., & Brown, S. A. (2005). Acute phase and five-year follow-up study of fluoxetine in adolescents with major depression and a comorbid substance use disorder: A review. *Addictive Behaviors*, *30*, 1824–1833.

Costello, E. J., Egger, H., & Angold, A. (2005). 10-year research update review: the epidemiology of child and adolescent psychiatric disorders. I. Methods and public health burden. *Journal of the American Academy of Child and Adolescent Psychiatry*, *44*, 972–986.

Crowley, T. J. (2006). Adolescents and substance-related disorders: research agenda to guide decisions on *Diagnostic and Statistical Manual of Mental Disorders, 5th edition (DSM-V)*. *Addiction*, *101*, 115–124.

DeLima, M. S., Soares, G. D., Reisser, A. A. P., & Farrell, M. (2002). Pharmacological treatment of cocaine dependence: a systematic review. *Addiction*, *97*, 931–949.

DiClemente, C. C., Prochaska, J. O., Fairhurst, S. K., Velicer, W. F., Velasquez, M. M., & Rossi, J. S. (1991). The process of smoking cessation: An analysis of precontemplation, contemplation, and preparation stages of change. *Journal of Consulting and Clinical Psychology*, *59*, 295–304.

Doherty, W. J., & Allen, W. (1994). Family functioning and parental smoking as predictors of adolescent cigarette use: A six-year prospective study. *Journal of Family Psychology*, *8*, 347–353.

Doherty, W. J., & Needle, R. H. (1991). Psychological adjustment and substance use among adolescents before and after a parental divorce. *Child Development*, *62*, 328–337.

D'Onofrio, B. M., Turkheimer, E., Emery, R. E., Slutske, W. S., Heath, A. C., Madden, P. A. *et al.* (2005). A genetically informed study of marital instability and its association with offspring psychopathology. *Journal of Abnormal Psychology*, *114*, 570–586.

Dube, S. R., Felitti, V. J., Dong, M., Chapman, D. P., Giles, W. H., & Anda, R. F. (2003). Childhood abuse, neglect and household dysfunction and the risk of illicit drug use: The Adverse Childhood Experience Study. *Pediatrics*, *111*, 564–572.

Dube, S. R., Miller, J. W., Brown, D. W., Giles, W. H., Felitti, V. J., Dong, M., *et al.* (2006). Adverse childhood experiences and the association with ever using alcohol and initiating alcohol use during adolescence. *Journal of Adolescent Health*, *38*, 444.e1–444.e10.

Duncan, A. E., Scherrer, J., Fu, Q., Bucholz, K. K., Heath, A. C., True, W. R., *et al.* (2006). Exposure to paternal alcoholism does not predict development of alcohol-use disorders in offspring: Evidence from an offspring-of-twins study. *Journal of Studies on Alcohol*, *67*, 649–656.

Edenberg, H. J., & Foroud, T. (2006). The genetics of alcoholism: Identifying specific genes ghrough family studies. *Addiction Biology*, *11*, 386–396.

Edwards, G. (1986). The alcohol dependence syndrome: A concept as stimulus to enquiry. *British Journal of Addiction*, *81*, 171–183.

Elder, R. W., Shults, R. A., Sleet, D. A., Nichols, J. L., Thompson, R. S., & Rajab, W., Task Force on Community Preventive Services. (2004). Effectiveness of mass media campaigns for reducing drinking and driving and alcohol-involved crashes: A systematic review. *American Journal of Preventive Medicine*, *27*, 57–65.

Ernst, M., Moolchan, E. T., & Robinson, M. L. (2001). Behavioral and neural consequences of prenatal exposure to nicotine. *Journal of the American Academy of Child and Adolescent Psychiatry*, *40*, 630–641.

Ezzati, M., Lopez, A. D., Rodgers, A., Vander Hoorn, S., Murray, C. J., Comparative Risk Assessment Collaborating Group. (2003). Selected major risk factors and global and regional burden of disease. *Lancet*, *360*, 1347–1360.

Faggiano, F., Vigna-Taglianti, F. D., Versino, E., Zambon, A., Borraccino, A., & Lemma, P. (2005). School-based prevention for illicit drugs' use. *Cochrane Database of Systematic Reviews*, Apr 18 (2), CD003020.

Farrelly, M. C., Niederdeppe, J., & Yarsevich, J. (2003). Youth tobacco prevention mass media campaigns: Past, present, and future directions. *Tobacco Control*, *12*, 35–47.

Fergusson, D. M., Boden, J. M., & Horwood, L. J. (2006). Cannabis use and other illicit drug use: Testing the cannabis gateway hypothesis. *Addiction*, *101*, 556–569.

Fergusson, D. M., Grant, H., Horwood, L. J., & Ridder, E. M. (2005). Randomized trial of the Early Start program of home visitation. *Pediatrics*, *116*, 803–809.

Fergusson, D. M., & Horwood, L. J. (1999). Prospective childhood predictors of deviant peer affiliations in adolescence. *Journal of Child Psychology and Psychiatry*, *40*, 581–592.

Fergusson, D. M., Horwood, L. J., & Lynskey, M. T. (1993). Prevalence and comorbidity of DSM-III-R diagnoses in a birth cohort of 15 year olds. *Journal of the American Academy of Child and Adolescent Psychiatry*, *32*, 1127–1234.

Fergusson, D. M., Horwood, L. J., & Lynskey, M. T. (1994). Parental separation, adolescent psychopathology and problem behaviors. *Journal of the American Academy of Child and Adolescent Psychiatry*, *33*, 1122–1133.

Fergusson, D. M., Horwood, L. J., & Lynskey, M. T. (1995). The prevalence and risk factors associated with abusive or hazardous alcohol consumption in 16-year-olds. *Addiction*, *90*, 935–946.

Fergusson, D. M., Horwood, L. J., & Lynskey, M. T. (1996). Childhood sexual abuse and psychiatric disorder in young adulthood. II. Psychiatric outcomes of childhood sexual abuse. *Journal of the American Academy of Child and Adolescent Psychiatry*, *35*, 1365–1374.

Fergusson, D. M., Horwood, L. J., Lynskey, M. T., & Madden, P. A. (2003). Early reactions to cannabis predict later dependence. *Archives of General Psychiatry*, *60*, 1033–1039.

Fergusson, D. M., Swain-Campbell, N. R., & Horwood, L. J. (2002). Deviant peer affiliations, crime and substance use: A fixed effects regression analysis. *Journal of Abnormal Child Psychology*, *30*, 419–430.

Fichtenberg, C. M., & Glantz, S. A. (2000). Association of the California Tobacco Control Program with declines in cigarette consumption and mortality from heart disease. *New England Journal of Medicine*, *343*, 1772–1777.

Finney, J. W., Hahn, A. C., & Moos, R. H. (1996). The effectiveness of inpatient and outpatient treatment for alcohol abuse: The need to focus on mediators and moderators of setting effects. *Addiction*, *91*, 1773–1796.

Fisher, D. G., Fenaughty, A. M., Cagle, H. H., & Wells, R. S. (2003). Needle exchange and injection drug use frequency: a randomized clinical trial. *Journal of Acquired Immune Deficiency Syndromes*, *33*, 199–205.

Gelernter, J., Panhuysen, C., Weiss, R., Brady, K., Hesselbrock, V., Rounsaville, B., *et al.* (2005). Genomewide linkage scan for cocaine dependence and related traits: Significant linkages for a cocaine-related trait and cocaine-induced paranoia. *American Journal of Medical Genetics Part B: Neuropsychiatric Genetics*, *136*, 45–52.

Gelernter, J., Panhuysen, C., Wilcox, M., Hesselbrock, V., Rounsaville, B., Poling, J., *et al.* (2006). Genomewide linkage scan for opioid dependence and related traits. *American Journal of Human Genetics*, *78*, 759–769.

Gerrard, M., Gibbons, F. X., Brody, G. H., Murry, V. M., Cleveland, M. J., & Wills, T. A. (2006). A theory-based dual-focus alcohol intervention for preadolescents: The Strong African American Families Program. *Psychology of Addictive Behaviors*, *20*, 185–195.

Gfroerer, J., Eyerman, J., & Chromy, J. (2002). *Redesigning an ongoing national household survey: Methodological issues.* DHSS Publication No. SMA 03-3768. Rockville, MD: Substance Abuse and Mental Health Services Administration, Office of Applied Statistics.

Gold, D. R., Wang, X., Wypij, D., Speizer, F. E., Ware, J. H., & Dockery, D. W. (1996). Effects of cigarette smoking on lung function in adolescent boys and girls. *New England Journal of Medicine*, *335*, 931–937.

Goodwin, D. W., Schulsinger, F., Hermansen, L., Guze, S. B., & Winokur, G. (1973). Alcohol problems in adoptees raised apart from alcoholic biological parents. *Archives of General Psychiatry*, *28*, 238–243.

Grabowski, J., Shearer, J., Merrill, J., & Negus, S. S. (2004). Agonist-like, replacement pharmacotherapy for stimulant abuse and dependence. *Addictive Behaviors*, *29*, 1439–1464.

Grimshaw, G. M., & Stanton, A. (2006). Tobacco cessation interventions for young people. *Cochrane Database of Systematic Reviews*, Oct 18 (4).

Harrison, L. D., & Scarpitti, F. R. (2002). Introduction: Progress and issues in drug treatment courts. *Substance Use and Misuse*, *37*, 1441–1467.

Hasin, D. S., Hatzenbuehler, M. L., Keyes, K., & Ogburn, E. (2006). Substance use disorders: Diagnostic and Statistical Manual of Mental Disorders, 4th edition (DSM-IV) and International Classification of Diseases, 10th edition (ICD-10). *Addiction*, *101*, 59–75.

Heath, A. C., Todorov, A. A., Nelson, E. C., Madden, P. A. F., Bucholz, K. K., & Martin, N. G. (2002). Gene–environment interaction effects on behavioral variation and risk of complex disorders: The example of alcoholism and other psychiatric disorders. *Twin Research*, *5*, 30–37.

Heath, A. C., & Madden, P. A. F. (1995). Genetic influences on smoking behavior. In J. R. Turner, L. R. Cardon, & J. K. Hewitt (Eds.), *Behavior genetic approaches in behavioral medicine*. New York: Plenum Press.

Heath, A. C., Madden, P. A. F., Dinwiddie, S. H., Slutske, W. S., Bierut, L. J., Statham, D. J., *et al.* (1999). Genetic differences in alcohol sensitivity and the inheritance of alcoholism risk. *Psychological Medicine*, *29*, 1069–1081.

Heath, A. C., & Martin, N. G. (1994). Genetic influences on alcohol consumption patterns and problem drinking: Results from the Australian NH&MRC Twin Panel follow-up survey. *Annals of the New York Academy of Sciences*, *708*, 72–85.

Heath, A. C., Slutske, W. S., & Madden, P. A. F. (1997). Gender differences in the genetic contribution to alcoholism risk and to alcohol consumption patterns. In R. W. Wilsnack, & S. C. Wilsnack (Eds.), *Gender and alcohol* (pp. 114–119). Rutgers: Rutgers University Press.

Hendershot, C. S., MacPherson, L., Myers, M. G., Carr, L. G., & Wall, T. L. (2005). Psychosocial, cultural and genetic influences on alcohol use in Asian American youth. *Journal of Studies on Alcohol*, *66*, 185–195.

Hettema, J. M., Neale, M. D., & Kendler, K. S. (1995). Physical similarity and the equal-environment assumption in twin studies of psychiatric disorders. *Behavior Genetics*, *25*, 327–335.

Higuchi, S., Matsushita, S., Imazeki, H., Kinoshita, T., Takagi, S., & Kono, H. (1994). Aldehyde dehydrogenase genotypes in Japanese alcoholics. *Lancet*, *343*, 741–742.

Higuchi, S., Matsushita, S., Muramatsu, T., Murayama, M., & Hayashida, M. (1996). Alcohol and aldehyde dehydrogenase genotypes and drinking behavior in Japanese. *Alcoholism: Clinical and Experimental Research*, *20*, 493–497.

Hingson, R. W., Heeren, T., & Winter, M. R. (2006). Age at drinking onset and alcohol dependence: Age at onset, duration, and severity. *Archives of Pediatrics and Adolescent Medicine, 160*, 739–746.

Hingson, R., Heeren, T., Zakocs, R., Winter, M., & Wechsler, H. (2003). Age of first intoxication, heavy drinking, driving after drinking and risk of unintentional injury among U.S. college students. *Journal of Studies on Alcohol, 64*, 23–31.

Hingson, R., & Kenkel, D. (2004). Social, health and economic consequences of underage drinking. In National Research Council and Institute of Medicine, *Reducing Underage Drinking: A Collective Responsibility*. Washington, DC: National Academies Press.

Hoffman, J. P. (1995). The effects of family structure and family relations on adolescent marijuana use. *International Journal of the Addictions, 30*, 1207–1241.

Hoffman, J. P., & Johnson, R. A. (1998). A National Portrait of Family Structure and Adolescent Drug Use. *Journal of Marriage and the Family, 60*, 633–645.

Hopkins, D. P., Briss , P. A., Ricard, C. J., Husten, C. G., Carande-Kulis, V. G., Fielding, J. E., *et al.*, Task Force on Community Preventive Services. (2001). Reviews of evidence regarding interventions to reduce tobacco use and exposure to environmental tobacco smoke. *American Journal of Preventive Medicine, 20*, 16–66.

Hori, H., Kawano, T., Endo, M., & Yuasa, Y. (1997). Genetic polymorphisms of tobacco- and alcohol-related metabolizing enzymes and human esophageal squamous cell carcinoma susceptibility. *Journal of Clinical Gastroenterology, 25*, 568–575.

Hu, M. C., Davies, M., & Kandel, D. B. (2006). Epidemiology and correlates of daily smoking and nicotine dependence among young adults in the United States. *American Journal of Public Health, 96*, 299–308.

Hughes, J., Stead, L., & Lancaster, T. (2004). Antidepressants for smoking cessation. *Cochrane Database of Systematic Reviews*, Oct 19 (4).

Hughes, J. R. (2006). Should criteria for drug dependence differ across drugs? *Addiction, 101*, 134–141.

Hurt, R. D., Croghan, G. A., Beede, S. D., Wolter, T. D., Croghan, I. T., & Patten, C. A. (2000). Nicotine patch therapy in 101 adolescent smokers: Efficacy, withdrawal symptom relief, and carbon monoxide and plasma cotinine levels. *Archives of Pediatrics and Adolescent Medicine, 154*, 31–37.

Iacono, W. G., Malone, S. M., & McGue, M. (2003). Substance use disorders, externalizing psychopathology, and P300 event-related potential amplitude. *International Journal of Psychophysiology, 48*, 147–178.

Jacob, T., Waterman, B., Heath, A., True, W., Bucholz, K. K., Haber, R., *et al.* (2003). Genetic and environmental effects on offspring alcoholism: New insights using an offspring-of-twins design. *Archives of General Psychiatry, 60*, 1265–1272.

Johnson, R. A., & Gerstein, D. R. (1998). Initiation of use of alcohol, cigarettes, marijuana, cocaine, and other substances in US birth cohorts since 1919. *American Journal of Public Health, 88*, 27–33.

Johnston, L. D., O'Malley, P. M., Bachman, J. G., & Schulenberg, J. E. (2006). *Monitoring the Future National Survey Results on Drug Use, 1975–2005. Volume I: Secondary School Students* (NIH Publication No. 06-5883). Bethesda, MD: National Institute on Drug Abuse.

Jorenby, D. E., Hays, J. T., Rigotti, N. A., Azoulay, S., Watsky, E. J., Williams, K. E., *et al.*, Varenicline Phase 3 Study Group. (2006). Efficacy of varenicline, an $\alpha_4\beta_2$ nicotinic acetylcholine receptor partial agonist, vs placebo or sustained-release bupropion for smoking cessation: A randomized controlled trial. *Journal of the American Medical Association, 296*, 56–63.

Kellogg, S., Melia, D., Khuri, E., Lin, A., Ho, A., & Kreek, M. J. (2006). Adolescent and young adult heroin patients: Drug use and success in methadone maintenance treatment. *Journal of Addictive Diseases, 25*, 15–25.

Kendler, K. S., Bulik, C. M., Silberg, J., Hettema, J. M., Myers, J., & Prescott, C. A. (2000). Childhood sexual abuse and adult psychiatric and substance use disorders in women: An epidemiological and cotwin control analysis. *Archives of General Psychiatry, 57*, 953–959.

Kendler, K. S., Heath, A. C., Neale, M. C., Kessler, R. C., & Eaves, L. J. (1993). Alcoholism and major depression in women. A twin study of the causes of comorbidity. *Archives of General Psychiatry, 50*, 690–698.

Kendler, K. S., Jacobson, K. C., Prescott, C. A., & Neale, M. C. (2003). Specificity of genetic and environmental risk factors for use and abuse/dependence of cannabis, cocaine, hallucinogens, sedatives, stimulants, and opiates in male twins. *American Journal of Psychiatry, 160*, 687–695.

Kendler, K. S., Neale, M. C., Kessler, R. C., Heath, A. C., & Eaves, L. J. (1994). Parental treatment and the equal environment assumption in twin studies of psychiatric illness. *Psychological Medicine, 24*, 579–590.

Kendler, K. S., Neale, M. C., Prescott, C. A.., Kessler, R. C., Heath, A. C., Corey, L. A., *et al.* (1996). Childhood parental loss and alcoholism in women: A causal analysis using a twin-family design. *Psychological Medicine, 26*, 79–95.

Kessler, R. C., Berglund, P., Demler, O., Jin, R., Merikangas, K. R., & Walters, E. E. (2005). Lifetime prevalence and age-of-onset distributions of DSM-IV disorders in the National Comorbidity Survey Replication. *Archives of General Psychiatry, 62*, 593–602.

Kirisci, L., Mezzich, A., & Tarter, R. (1995). Norms and sensitivity of the adolescent version of the drug use screening inventory. *Addictive Behaviors, 20*, 149–157.

Knopik, V. S., Heath, A. C., Madden, P. A. F., Bucholz, K. K., Slutske, W. S., Nelson, E. C., *et al.* (2004). Genetic effects on alcohol dependence risk: Re-evaluating the importance of psychiatric and other heritable risk factors. *Psychological Medicine, 34*, 1519–1530.

Knopik, V. S., Sparrow, E. P., Madden, P. A. F., Bucholz, K. K., Hudziak, J. J., Reich, W., *et al.* (2005). Contributions of parental alcoholism, prenatal substance exposure, and genetic transmission to child ADHD risk: A female twin study. *Psychological Medicine, 35*, 625–635.

Komro, K. A., Perry, C. L., Veblen-Mortenson, S., Farbakhsh, K., Kugler, K. C., Alfano, K. A., *et al.* (2006). Cross-cultural adaptation and evaluation of a home-based program for alcohol use prevention among urban youth: The "Slick Tracy Home Team Program". *Journal of Primary Prevention, 27*, 135–154.

Koob, G. F. (2006). The neurobiology of addiction: A neuroadaptational view relevant for diagnosis. *Addiction, 101*, 23–30.

Krystal, J. H., Cramer, J. A., Krol, W. F., Kirk, G. F., Rosenheck, R. A., Veterans Affairs Naltrexone Cooperative Study 425 Group. (2001). Naltrexone in the treatment of alcohol dependence. *New England Journal of Medicine, 345*, 1734–1739.

Kung, E. M., & Farrell, A. D. (2000). The role of parents and peers in early adolescent substance use: An examination of mediating and moderating effects. *Journal of Children and Family Studies, 9*, 509–528.

Lancaster T., & Stead, L. F. (2005). Individual behavioural counseling for smoking cessation. *Cochrane Database of Systematic Reviews*, Apr 18 (2).

Langbehn, D. R., Cadoret, R. J., Yates, W. R., Troughton, E. P., & Stewart, M. A. (1998). Distinct contributions of conduct and oppositional defiant symptoms to adult antisocial behavior: Evidence from an adoption study. *Archives of General Psychiatry, 55*, 821–829.

Larzelere, R. E., & Patterson, G. R. (1990). Parental management: Mediator of the effect of socioeconomic status on early delinquency. *Criminology, 28*, 301–324.

Lessov, C. N., Martin, N. G., Statham, D. J., Todorov, A. A., Slutske, W. S., Bucholz, K. K., *et al.* (2004). Defining nicotine dependence for genetic research: Evidence from Australian twins. *Psychological Medicine, 34*, 865–879.

Li, M. D., Payne, T. J., Ma, J. Z., Lou, X. Y., Zhang, D., Dupont, R. T., *et al.* (2006). A genomewide search finds major susceptibility loci for nicotine dependence on chromosome 10 in African Americans. *American Journal of Human Genetics*, *79*, 745–751.

Lurie, P., & Drucker, E. (1997). An opportunity lost: HIV infections associated with lack of a national needle-exchange programme in the USA. *Lancet*, *349*, 604–608.

Lynskey, M. T., Heath, A. C., Bucholz, K. K., Slutske, W. S., Madden, P. A. F., Nelson, E. C., *et al.* (2003). Escalation of drug use in early-onset cannabis users versus co-twin controls. *Journal of the American Medical Association*, *289*, 427–433.

Lynskey, M. T., Vink, J. M., & Boomsma, D. I. (2006). Early onset cannabis use and progression to other drug use in a sample of Dutch twins. *Behavior Genetics*, *36*, 195–200.

MacCoun, R., & Reuter, P. (2001). Evaluating alternative cannabis regimes. *British Journal of Psychiatry*, *178*, 123–128.

Mackey, J., Eriksen, M., & Shafey, O. (2006). *The tobacco atlas* (2nd edn.). Atlanta, GA: American Cancer Society.

MacPherson, L., Frissell, K., Brown, S. A. & Myers, M. G. (2006). Adolescent substance use problems. In E. J. Mash, & R. A. Barkley (Eds.), *Treatment of childhood disorders* (pp. 731–777). New York: Guilford.

Marshal, M. P., & Chassin, L. (2000). Peer influence on adolescent alcohol use: The moderating role of parental support and discipline. *Applied Developmental Science*, *42*, 80–88.

Martin, C. S., Chung, T., Kirisci, L., & Langenbucher, J. W. (2006). Item response theory analysis of diagnostic criteria for alcohol and cannabis use disorders in adolescents: Implications for DSM-V. *Journal of Abnormal Psychology*, *115*, 807–814.

Martin, G., Copeland, J., & Swift, W. (2005). The Adolescent Cannabis Check-Up: Feasibility of a brief intervention for young cannabis users. *Journal of Substance Abuse Treatment*, *29*, 207–213.

McCambridge, J., & Strang, J. (2004). The efficacy of single-session motivational interviewing in reducing drug consumption and perceptions of drug-related risk and harm among young people: results from a multi-site cluster randomized trial. *Addiction*, *99*, 39–52.

McGue, M., Iacono, W. G., Legrand, L. N., Malone, S., & Elkins, I. (2001). Origins and consequences of age at first drink. I. Associations with substance-use disorders, disinhibitory behavior and psychopathology, and P3 amplitude. *Alcoholism: Clinical and Experimental Research*, *25*, 1156–1165.

McGue, M., & Lykken, D. T. (1992). Genetic influence on risk of divorce. *Psychological Science*, *6*, 368–373.

McGue, M., Sharma, A., & Benson, P. (1996). Parent and sibling influences on adolescent alcohol use and misuse: Evidence from a US adoption cohort. *Journal of Studies on Alcohol*, *57*, 8–18.

Merikangas, K. R., & Risch, N. (2003). Genomic priorities and public health. *Science*, *302*, 599–601.

Merikangas, K. R., Stolar, M., Stevens, D. E., Goulet, J., Preisig, M. A., Fenton, B., *et al.* (1998). Familial transmission of substance use disorders. *Archives of General Psychiatry*, *55*, 973–979.

Metten, P., Phillips, T. J., Crabbe, J. C., Tarantino, L. M., CcClearn, G. E., Plomin, R., *et al.* (1998). High genetic susceptibility to ethanol withdrawal predicts low ethanol consumption. *Mammalian Genome*, *9*, 983–990.

Miller, W. R., Walters, S. T., & Bennett, M. E. (2001). How effective is alcoholism treatment in the United States? *Journal of Studies on Alcohol*, *62*, 211–220.

Molnar, B. E., Buka, S. L., & Kessler, R. C. (2001). Child sexual abuse and subsequent psychopathology: Results from the National Comorbidity Survey. *American Journal of Public Health*, *9*, 753–760.

Moolchan, E. T., Robinson, M. L., Ernst, M., Cadet, J. L., Pickworth, W. B., Heishman, S. J., *et al.* (2005). Safety and efficacy of the nicotine patch and gum for the treatment of adolescent tobacco addiction. *Pediatrics*, *115*, e407–414.

Morral, A. R., McCaffrey, D. F., & Paddock, S. M. (2002). Reassessing the marijuana gateway effect. *Addiction*, *97*, 1493–1504.

Muthen, B. (2006). Should substance use disorders be considered as categorical or dimensional? *Addiction*, *101*, 6–16.

Needle, R. H., Su, S., & Doherty, W. J. (1990). Divorce, remarriage, and adolescent drug involvement: A longitudinal study. *Journal of Marriage and the Family*, *52*, 157–169.

Nelson, E. C., Heath, A. C., Lynskey, M., Bucholz, K. K., Madden, P. A., Statham, D. J., *et al.* (2006). Childhood sexual abuse and risks for licit and illicit drug use: A twin study. *Psychological Medicine*, *36*, 1473–1483.

Nides, M., Oncken, C., Gonzales, D., Rennard, S., Watsky, E. J., Anziano, R., *et al.* (2006). Smoking cessation with varenicline, a selective $\alpha_4\beta_2$ nicotinic receptor partial agonist: results from a 7-week, randomized, placebo- and bupropion-controlled trial with 1-year follow-up. *Archives of Internal Medicine*, *166*, 1561–1568.

Olds, D. L., Robinson, J., Pettitt, L., Luckey, D. W., Holmberg, J., Ng, R. K., *et al.* (2004). Effects of home visits by paraprofessionals and by nurses: age 4 follow-up results of a randomized trial. *Pediatrics*, *114*, 1560–1568.

Pergadia, M. L., Heath, A. C., Agrawal, A., Bucholz, K. K., Martin, N. G., & Madden, P. A. F. (2006). The implications of simultaneous smoking initiation for inferences about the genetics of smoking behavior from twin data. *Behavior Genetics*, *36*, 567–576.

Piasecki, T. M., Sher, K. J., Slutske, W. S., & Jackson, K. M. (2005). Hangover frequency and risk for alcohol use disorders: Evidence from a longitudinal high-risk study. *Journal of Abnormal Psychology*, *114*, 223–234.

Pitkanen, T., Lyyra, A. L., & Pulkkinen, L. (2005). Age of onset of drinking and the use of alcohol in adulthood: A follow-up study from age 8–42 for females and males. *Addiction*, *100*, 652–661.

Prescott, C. A., & Kendler, K. S. (1999). Age at first drink and risk for alcoholism: A non-causal association. *Alcoholism: Clinical and Experimental Research*, *23*, 101–107.

Prescott, C. A., Sullivan, P. F., Kuo, P. H., Webb, B. T., Vittum, J., Patterson, D. G., *et al.* (2006). Genomewide linkage study in the Irish affected sib pair study of alcohol dependence: Evidence for a susceptibility region for symptoms of alcohol dependence on chromosome 4. *Molecular Psychiatry*, *11*, 603–611.

Project MATCH Research Group. (1997a). Matching alcoholism treatments to client heterogeneity: Project MATCH posttreatment drinking outcomes. *Journal of Studies on Alcohol*, *58*, 7–29.

Project MATCH Research Group. (1997b). Project MATCH secondary a priori hypotheses. *Addiction*, *92*, 1671–1698.

Prokhovov, A. V., Hudmon, K. S., Cinciripini, P. M., & Marani, S. (2005). "Withdrawal symptoms" in adolescents: A comparison of former smokers and never-smokers. *Nicotine and Tobacco Research*, *7*, 909–913.

Prokhovov, A. V., Hudmon, K. S., de Moor, C. A., Kelder, S. H., Conroy, J. L., & Ordway, N. (2001). Nicotine dependence, withdrawal symptoms, and adolescents' readiness to quit smoking. *Nicotine and Tobacco Research*, *3*, 151–155.

Reich, T., Edenberg, H., Goate, A., Williaims, T. J., Rice, J., Van Eerdwegh, P., *et al.* (1998). A genome-wide search for genes affecting the risk for alcohol dependence. *American Journal of Medical Genetics*, *81*, 207–215.

Rose, R. J., Dick, D. M., Viken, R. J., Pulkkinen, L., & Kaprio, J. (2004). Genetic and environmental effects on conduct disorder and alcohol dependence symptoms and their covariation at age 14. *Alcoholism: Clinical and Experimental Research*, *28*, 1541–1548.

Rounsaville, B. J., Kosten, T. R., Weissman, M. M., Prusoff, B., Pauls, D., Anton, S. F., *et al.* (1991). Psychiatric disorders in relatives of probands with opiate addiction. *Archives of General Psychiatry*, *48*, 33–42.

Saccone, S. F., Hinrichs, A. L., Saccone, N. L., Chase, G. A., Konvicka, K., Madden, P. A., *et al.* (2007). Cholinergic nicotinic receptor genes implicated in a nicotine dependence association study targeting 348 candidate genes with 3713 SNPs. *Human Molecular Genetics*, *16*, 36–49.

Schmid, H., Ter Bogt, T., Godeau, E., Hublet, A., Dias, S. F., & Fotiou A. (2003). Drunkenness among young people: A cross-national comparison. *Journal of Studies on Alcohol*, *64*, 650–661.

Schuckit, M. A., & Saunders, J. B. (2006). The empirical basis of substance use disorders diagnosis: Research recommendations for the *Diagnostic and Statistical Manual of Mental Disorders*, 5th edition (DSM-V). *Addiction*, *101*, 170–173.

Schuckit, M., Smith, T., Pierson, J., Danko, G., & Beltran, I. A. (2006). Relationships among the level of response to alcohol and the number of alcoholic relatives in predicting alcohol-related outcomes. *Alcoholism: Clinical and Experimental Research*, *30*, 1308–1314.

Sher, K. J., Walitzer, K. S., Wood, P. K., & Brent, E. E. (1991). Characteristics of children of alcoholics: Putative risk factors, substance use and abuse, and psychopathology. *Journal of Abnormal Psychology*, *100*, 427–448.

Silagy, C., Lancaster, T., Stead, L., Mant, D., & Fowler, G. (2006). Nicotine replacement therapy for smoking cessation. *Cochrane Database of Systematic Reviews*, *3*, CD000146.

Slawecki, C. J., Thomas, J. D., Riley, E. P., & Ehlers, C. L. (2004). Neurophysiologic consequences of neonatal ethanol exposure in the rat. *Alcohol*, *34*, 187–196.

Slutske, W. S., Cronk, N. J., Sher, K. J., Madden, P. A., Bucholz, K. K., & Heath, A. C. (2002a). Genes, environment, and individual differences in alcohol expectancies among female adolescents and young adults. *Psychology of Addictive Behaviors*, *16*, 308–317.

Slutske, W. S., Heath, A. C., Madden, P. A., Bucholz, K. K., Statham, D. J., & Martin, N. G. (2002b). Personality and the genetic risk for alcohol dependence. *Journal of Abnormal Psychology*, *111*, 124–133.

Sokol-Katz, J., Dunham, R., & Zimmerman, R. (1997). Family structure versus parental attachment in controlling adolescent deviant behavior: A social control model. *Adolescence*, *32*, 199–215.

Spirito, A., Monti, P. M., Barnett, N. P., Colby, S. M., Sindelar, H., Rohsenow, D. J., *et al.* (2004). A randomized clinical trial of a brief motivational intervention for alcohol-positive adolescents treated in an emergency department. *Journal of Pediatrics*, *145*, 396–402.

Srisurapanont, M., & Jarusuraisin, N. (2005). Opioid antagonists for alcohol dependence. *Cochrane Database of Systematic Reviews*, *1*, CD001867.

Stead, L. F., & Lancaster, T. (2005). Group behaviour therapy programmes for smoking cessation. *Cochrane Database of Systematic Reviews*, April 18 (2).

Stockwell, T., & Gruenewald, P. (2004). Controls on physical availability of alcohol. In N. Heather, & T. Stockwell (Eds.), *The essential handbook of treatment and prevention of alcohol problems.* Chichester: Wiley and Sons.

Sutton, S. (2001). Back to the drawing board? A review of applications of the transtheoretical model to substance use. *Addiction*, *96*, 175–186.

Tarter, R. E., Kirisci, L., Mezzich, A., Cornelius, J. R., Pajer, K., Vanyukov, M., *et al.* (2003). Neurobehavioral disinhibition in childhood predicts early age at onset of substance use disorder. *American Journal of Psychiatry*, *160*, 1078–1085.

Turner, C. F., Ku, L., Rogers, S. M., Lindberg, L. D., Pleck, J. H., & Sonenstein, F. L. (1998). Adolescent sexual behavior, drug use, and violence: Increased reporting with computer survey technology. *Science*, *280*, 867–873.

Turner, S., Longshore, D., Wenzel, S., Deschenes, E., Greenwood, P., Fain, T., *et al.* (2002). A decade of drug treatment court research. *Substance Use and Misuse*, *37*, 1489–1527.

Urberg, K., Goldstein, M. S., & Toro, P. A. (2005). Supportive relationships as a moderator of the effects of parent and peer drinking on adolescent drinking. *Journal of Research on Adolescence*, *15*, 1–19.

Vega, W. A., Aguilar-Gaxiola, S., Andrade, L., Bijl, R., Borges, G., Caraveo-Anduaga, J. J., *et al.* (2002). Prevalence and age of onset for drug use in seven international sites: Results from the international consortium of psychiatric epidemiology. *Drug and Alcohol Dependence*, *68*, 285–297.

Vogel-Sprott, M. (1997). Is behavioral tolerance learned? *Alcohol Health and Research World*, 21, 161–168.

Wagenaar, A. C., & Toomey, T. L. (2002). Effects of minimum drinking age laws: review and analyses of the literature from 1960 to 2000. *Journal of Studies on Alcohol*, Suppl. (14), 206–225.

Wagner, F. A., & Anthony, J. C. (2002). Into the world of illegal drug use: Exposure opportunity and other mechanisms linking the use of alcohol, tobacco, marijuana, and cocaine. *American Journal of Epidemiology*, *155*, 918–925.

Wall, T. L., Peterson, C. M., Peterson, K. P., Johnson, M. L., Thomasson, H., Cole, M., *et al.* (1997). Alcohol metabolism in Asian-American men with genetic polymorphisms of aldehyde dehydrogenase. *Annals of Internal Medicine*, *127*, 376–379.

Ward, J., Hall, W., & Mattick, R. P. (1999). Role of maintenance treatment in opioid dependence. *Lancet*, *353*, 221–226.

Warren, C. W., Jones, N. R., Eriksen, M. P., Asma, S., Global Tobacco Surveillance System (GTSS) Collaborative Group. (2006). Patterns of global tobacco use in young people and implications for future chronic disease burden in adults. *Lancet*, *367*, 749–753.

Weissman, M. M., Warner, V., Wickramaratne, P. J., & Kandel, D. B. (1999). Maternal smoking during pregnancy and psychopathology in offspring followed to adulthood. *Journal of the American Academy of Child and Adolescent Psychiatry*, *38*, 892–899.

White, H. R., & Labouvie, E. W. (1989). Towards the assessment of adolescent problem drinking. *Journal of Studies on Alcohol*, *50*, 30–37.

Whitfield, J. B., Zhu, G., Madden, P. A., Neale, M. C., Heath, A. C., & Martin, N. G. (2004). The genetics of alcohol intake and of alcohol dependence. *Alcoholism: Clinical and Experimental Research*, *28*, 1153–1160.

Widom, C. S., Ireland, T., & Glynn, P. J. (1995). Alcohol abuse in abused and neglected children followed up: Are they at increased risk? *Journal of Studies on Alcohol*, *56*, 207–217.

Wilens, T. E., Biederman, J., Abrantes, A. M., & Spencer, T. J. (1997). Clinical characteristics of psychiatrically referred adolescent outpatients with substance use disorder. *Journal of the American Academy of Child and Adolescent Psychiatry*, *36*, 941–947.

Wodak, A., & Cooney, A. (2006). Do needle syringe programs reduce HIV infection among injecting drug users: A comprehensive review of the international evidence. *Substance Use and Misuse*, *41*, 777–813.

World Health Organization (WHO). (1996). *Multiaxial classification of child and adolescent psychiatric disorders: The ICD-10 classification of mental and behavioral disorders in children and adolescents.* Cambridge, UK: Cambridge University Press.

Yamaguchi, R., Johnston, L. D., & O'Malley, P. M. (2003). Relationship between student illicit drug use and school drug-testing policies. *Journal of School Health*, *73*, 159–164.

Yates, W. R., Cadoret, R. J., Troughton, E. P., Stewart, M., & Giunta, T. S. (1998). Effect of fetal alcohol exposure on adult symptoms of nicotine, alcohol, and drug dependence. *Alcoholism: Clinical and Experimental Research*, *22*, 914–920.

Zhang, B., Cohen, J., Ferrence, R., & Rehm, J. (2006). The impact of tobacco tax cuts on smoking initiation among Canadian young adults. *American Journal of Preventive Medicine*, *30*, 474–479.

Zucker, R. A., Wong, M. M., Puttler, L. I., & Fitzgerald, H. E. (2003). Resilience and vulnerability among sons of alcoholics: Relationship to developmental outcomes between early childhood and adolescence. In S. S. Luthar (Ed.), *Resilience and vulnerability: Adaptation in the context of childhood adversities.* New York: Cambridge University Press.

Depressive Disorders in Childhood and Adolescence

David Brent and V. Robin Weersing

In this chapter we describe the clinical picture of unipolar depressive disorders, diagnostic subcategories, differential diagnosis and common comorbidities. The descriptive epidemiology, onset, course, sequelae and predictors are discussed. Evidence-based psychopharmacological and psychosocial acute and continuation treatments of depression are presented, along with current controversies. More general issues of clinical management such as determination of intensity of care and the role of hospitalization are also reviewed.

Clinical Picture

Clinical Presentation and Classification

Depressive disorders in childhood and adolescence are characterized by persistent and pervasive sadness, anhedonia, boredom or irritability that is functionally impairing, and relatively unresponsive to pleasurable activities, interactions and attention from other people. In one of the first studies of the clinical picture of depression in preschoolers, anhedonia was found to be characteristic of depression in these children (Luby, Heffelfinger, Mrakotsky, *et al.*, 2003). Functional impairment is most salient in distinguishing depression from the "normal ups and downs" of childhood and adolescence.

Depressive disorders exist on a continuum, and are classified on the basis of severity, pervasiveness and presence or absence of mania. At the mildest end of the spectrum are adjustment disorders with depressed mood, which are mild, self-limited and occur in response to a clear stressor. Depression not otherwise specified (NOS), also referred to as "minor" or subsyndromal depression, is diagnosed in the presence of depressed mood, anhedonia or irritability, and up to three symptoms of major depression. This term "minor" depression is misleading in so far as depression NOS is associated with functional impairment and increased risk of major depression (Fergusson, Horwood, Ridder *et al.*, 2005). Dysthymic disorder also has fewer symptoms than major depression, but its most notable characteristic is its chronicity, lasting a minimum of a year. In explaining this condition to parents and children, it may be helpful to describe major depression as a "cloudy sky," and dysthymia as "partly cloudy" (Birmaher, Ryan, Williamson *et al.*, 1996b). The co-occurrence of dysthymic disorder and major depression, termed "double depression," is associated with a chronic course. Major depression is the "full-blown" condition, with either sad or irritable mood, or anhedonia, along with at least five other symptoms, such as social withdrawal, worthlessness, guilt, suicidal thoughts or behavior, increased or decreased sleep, decreased motivation and/or concentration, and increased or decreased appetite (American Psychiatric Association, 2000). Rarely, depressed patients also have psychotic symptoms such as auditory hallucinations or delusions, usually with some self-derogatory, paranoid or depressive content.

Rutter's Child and Adolescent Psychiatry, 5th edition. Edited by M. Rutter, D. Bishop, D. Pine, S. Scott, J. Stevenson, E. Taylor and A. Thapar. © 2008 Blackwell Publishing, ISBN: 978-1-4051-4549-7.

Differential Diagnosis

The most important differential diagnosis is between unipolar and bipolar depression (see chapter 38), the latter being characterized by past or current mania or hypomania (e.g., expansive mood, hypersexuality, grandiosity, decreased need for sleep). Often, young bipolar patients present with either rapid cycling or a mixed state (an admixture of depressive and manic symptoms), so that detection of bipolarity requires care, persistence and longitudinal follow-up (Birmaher, Axelson, Strober *et al.*, 2006).

Anxiety disorders are often associated with significant dysphoria that is relieved if the anxiogenic situation, such as that of separation or social situations, is eliminated. The social withdrawal of depression should be differentiated from the avoidance of social situations because of anxiety.

Altered concentration is not only a symptom of depression, but is also a key feature of attention deficit/hyperactivity disorder (ADHD; see chapter 34). Concentration difficulties in ADHD are not associated with changes in mood-related symptoms. Moreover, ADHD usually has a much earlier onset. Children with ADHD often become demoralized because of peer rejection and difficulties at school. This demoralization can be ascribed to ADHD in absence of other depressive symptoms.

Irritability is a prominent symptom of conduct and oppositional disorders (see chapter 35), and, in the absence of other mood symptoms, this symptom is more likely to be caused by the behavioral disorder than depression. Substance abuse (see chapter 36) can mimic mood disorder by disrupting sleep, concentration, motivation and appetite; moreover, these conditions frequently co-occur with mood disorders in clinical practice. A careful history and, when warranted, a drug toxicology screen is often the only way to detect this important and serious condition. Patients with eating disorders (see chapter 41) often show lassitude and dysphoria, which can in part be attributed to poor nutritional status. A diagnosis of current depression in an eating disordered patient should not be made until adequate nutritional status has been restored.

Comorbidity

Differential diagnosis notwithstanding, comorbidity is the rule rather than the exception in depressed children and adolescents, especially in clinical samples (Angold, Costello, & Erkanli, 1999; see also chapter 2). Comorbidity may result from shared etiology, or as a cause or consequence of depression. Comorbid conditions affect both the course and outcome of depression. Anxiety is frequently a precursor of mood disorder. Anxiety and depression may be comorbid because of a shared genetic diathesis (Middeldorp, Cath, van Dyck *et al.*, 2005). ADHD and depression are also often comorbid. Comorbidity between depression and behavioral disorders and substance abuse may be attributable to shared family risk factors, such as abuse, exposure to family violence and discord, and parental substance abuse (Fergusson & Woodward, 2002). Alcohol, drug and tobacco abuse are associated with depression, and longitudinal studies suggest a bidirectional causality, with substance abuse both leading to, and occurring as a consequence of depression. Depression increases the likelihood of initiation and development of substance abuse problems, but substance abuse problems lead to life events that increase the likelihood of depression (Kuo, Gardner, Kendler *et al.*, 2006; Libby, Orton, Stover *et al.*, 2005). Conduct disorder is frequently comorbid with depression, particularly in prepubertal samples (Harrington, 2000).

Assessment

The psychiatric interview is the "gold standard" for assessment of depressive diagnoses (Myers & Winters, 2002). The main advantages of psychiatric interview over self- or parent-report are that interviews can determine the temporal sequence, course and functional significance of different symptoms, determine to what extent these symptoms should be attributed to a depressive disorder or to another condition, and facilitate the integration and resolve discrepancies between parent and child sources of information. The main disadvantages of direct interviews are cost and time, and for semistructured interviews a high level of training and ongoing quality monitoring. Interviews are conducted with both the parent and the child. Parents are usually better informants about past history treatment and symptoms that are tied to external behavior, such as social withdrawal, decline in school performance and agitation. Children are better reporters about internal experiences and thoughts, such as suicidal ideation, anhedonia, guilt, psychosis and lack of motivation. Epidemiological studies have found fairly consistent results using both fully structured (Diagnostic Interview Schedule for Children [DISC] and Composite International Diagnostic Interview [CIDI], the latter just in adolescents; Shaffer, Fisher, & Lucas, 2004) and semi-structured interviews (Schedule for Affective Disorders and Schizophrenia–Epidemiological version [K-SADS-E], Schedule for Affective Disorders and Schizophrenia for School-Age Children–Present and Lifetime version [K-SADS-PL], Child and Adolescent Psychiatric Assessment [CAPA]; Angold, Prendergast, Cox *et al.*, 1995; Kaufman, Birmaher, Brent *et al.*, 1997a). The Preschool Age Psychiatric Assessment (PAPA), a downward extension of the CAPA, shows good reliability and internal consistency with regard to assessment of preschool psychopathology, including depression (Egger, Erkanli, Keeler *et al.*, 2006). The advantages, disadvantages and psychometric properties of each of these instruments are reviewed in more detail in chapter 19.

The most commonly used continuous interview-based measure of depressive symptomatology is the Children's Depression Rating Scale–Revised (CDRS-R), a 17-item assessment that is analogous to the Hamilton Depression Rating Scale (Poznanski, Freeman, & Mokros, 1985). The measure ranges from 17 to 113, with 40 or above associated with clinically significant depression, and less than 29 with symptomatic remission. Discriminant and convergent validity, as well as sensitivity to treatment effects, have been demonstrated (Emslie, Rush, Weinberg *et al.*, 1997). Among its limitations are that the CDRS-R emphasizes neurovegetative rather than cognitive symptoms and has less than straightforward anchor points for the suicide ideation item.

The Mood and Feelings Questionnaire (MFQ) is the only self-report scale validated for both children and adolescents and comes in a 37-item and 13-item form; the latter is useful for screening for depressive disorders (Thapar & McGuffin, 1998). This measure also has a parent report version. Internal consistency, convergent and discriminant validity have been reported, with the ability to discriminate depression from anxiety and from conduct disorder.

The Children's Depression Inventory (CDI) was developed as a downward extension of the Beck Depression Inventory (BDI), and has a self, parent and teacher report form, although usually the former is used in the literature (Kovacs, 1985). The CDI is highly correlated with other measures of depression, but does not discriminate well from anxiety disorders and so is better used as a measure of emotional disturbance rather than depression per se.

The Center for Epidemiological Studies–Depression Scale (CES-D) has been used in several epidemiological and treatment studies of adolescents of diverse ethnic origin, works well as a screen for depression, has good discriminant validity and is sensitive to treatment effects (Dierker, Albano, Clarke *et al.*, 2001; Lewinsohn, Rohde, & Seeley, 1998). One weakness is that it does not have a suicide ideation item. The Beck Depression Inventory (BDI) is very widely used in studies of adolescents, is a good screen for depressive disorders, is sensitive to treatment effects and may be a more effective screen for major depression than the CES-D (Dierker, Albano, Clarke *et al.*, 2001; Roberts, Lewinsohn, & Seeley, 1991). It has strong psychometric properties of the adolescent instruments but emphasizes the cognitive component of depressive disorders.

The Reynolds Adolescent Depression Scale (RADS) is another scale with very good psychometric properties that is sensitive to treatment effects (March, Silva, Petrycki *et al.*, 2004; Reynolds & Mazza, 1998). The Preschool Feelings Checklist is a 16-item parent report measure that, in a preliminary report, appears to have high sensitivity and specificity for preschool depressive disorders (Luby, Heffelfinger, Koenig-McNaught *et al.*, 2004). Studies of adults in primary care have shown that a two-item screen (about low mood and anhedonia) is as efficient as longer self-report inventories, but no studies in children or adolescents have yet been published (Whooley, Avins, Miranda *et al.*, 1997).

Descriptive Epidemiology

The point prevalence of depressive disorders is 1–2% in prepubertal children and 3–8% in adolescents, with a lifetime prevalence by the end of adolescence of around 20% (Costello, Mustillo, Erkanli *et al.*, 2003; Fergusson, Horwood, Ridder *et al.*, 2005; Lewinsohn, Rohde, & Seeley, 1998). The point prevalence of clinically significant depressive symptomatology in multinational studies is even higher (10–13% in boys and 12–18% for girls; Ruchkin, Sukhodolsky, Vermeiren *et al.*, 2006). The prevalence of depression in preschoolers is unknown. The rate of depressive disorders may be increasing in subsequent birth cohorts, with the age of onset becoming earlier (Kovacs & Gatsonis, 1994; Ryan, Williamson, Iyengar *et al.*, 1992b). Whereas some or even most of this apparent effect might be attributable to recall bias, a cohort effect is consistent with a concomitant rise in the youth suicide rate from the 1950s to the early 1990s (Costello, Erkanli, & Angold, 2006).

Age and Gender

There is an upsurge in the rate of depression that accompanies the onset of puberty, at which point the dramatic female predominance in mood disorders first emerges (Angold, Costello, & Worthman, 1998), perhaps mediated by increases in estradiol and testosterone. The higher female than male rate of depression may also be a result of higher rates of anxiety disorder in females, greater tendency to engage in ruminative thinking, greater total cortisol excretion after the corticotropin-releasing hormone challenge and increased interpersonal sensitivity, all of which may increase vulnerability for depression (Breslau, Schultz, & Peterson, 1995; Nolen-Hoeksema, Larson, & Grayson, 1999; Stroud, Papandonatos, Williamson *et al.*, 2004).

Prepubertal depression appears to be of two types. The first, more common presentation of pre-pubertal depression is with comorbid behavioral problems, parental criminality, parental substance abuse and family discord. The course of these children resembles those with conduct disorder much more than those with mood disorders, without an increased risk for recurrence of depression into adult life (Harrington, Rutter, Weissman *et al.*, 1997; Weissman, Wolk, Wickramaratne *et al.*, 1999a). The second, less common, form is highly familial, with multigenerational loading for depression, with high rates of anxiety and bipolar disorder, and recurrences of depression in adolescence and adulthood. Adolescent onset depressive disorder has a high risk of recurrent mood disorder into adulthood (Harrington, 2000; Harrington, Rutter, Weissman *et al.*, 1997; Weissman, Wolk, Goldstein *et al.*, 1999b). Twin studies suggest a greater genetic component in adolescent versus pre-pubertal onset depression, supportive of the view that child and adolescent onset depression may differ in etiology (Scourfield, Rice, Thapar *et al.*, 2003). In clinical samples, depressed adolescents, compared to depressed children, showed more hopelessness, decreased energy, and fatigue, hypersomnia, suicidality and substance abuse, whereas depressed children showed more comorbid separation anxiety and ADHD (Yorbik, Birmaher, Axelson *et al.*, 2004).

Developmental Factors

Girls with earlier onset of puberty may be at increased risk for depression and other disorders (Graber, Seeley, Brooks-Gunn *et al.*, 2004). The relationship between early onset of puberty and depressive symptoms is complex, because early onset of puberty is related to factors that are also related to risk for depression onset, including maternal depression, mother–child discord and child–step-parent discord (Ellis & Garber, 2000). As girls undergo the transition to adolescence, there is also an increase in child-generated parent–child and peer–peer interpersonal conflict, which may increase the likelihood of depressive disorder (Rudolph & Hammen, 1999). A greater physiological need for sleep, along with a tendency to actually obtain less sleep may also increase vulnerability to depression (Dahl, 2004).

Course and Outcome

Episode Length and Recovery

Depression is a chronic and recurrent condition. The duration for depressive episodes is 3–6 months for community samples and 5–8 months for referred samples (Birmaher, Arbelaez, & Brent, 2002). Greater episode length is associated with comorbid dysthymic disorder, comorbidity with anxiety disorder or substance abuse, greater initial severity of the depressive condition, current or past suicidal ideation or behavior, chronicity and number of episodes of parental depression and other disorders and family discord (Birmaher, Brent, Kolko *et al.*, 2000a; Kovacs, Feinberg, Crouse-Novak *et al.*, 1984a; Warner, Weissman, Fendrich *et al.*, 1992). In both clinical and community samples, around 20% of adolescents with a lifetime history of depression have a persistent depression of 2 years or greater (Birmaher, Arbelaez, & Brent, 2002; Lewinsohn, Rohde, & Seeley, 1998).

Risk for Recurrence

In one meticulously conducted study that examined the course of depressive disorder in 8- to 13-year-olds, the risk of recurrence was 40% in 2 years, and 72% in 5 years (Kovacs, 1996; Kovacs, Feinberg, Crouse-Novak *et al.*, 1984b). Other longitudinal studies have shown that the risk for recurrent depression in adolescent depression followed forward is extremely high, with the rate of relapse or recurrence ranging 30–70% in 1–2 years of follow-up in clinical samples, and 16–33% in 2–4 year follow-up in community samples (Birmaher, Arbelaez, & Brent, 2002; Lewinsohn, Rohde, & Seeley, 1998). Prepubertal depressed children with a family history of depression have a similar risk of recurrence (Birmaher, Williamson, Dahl *et al.*, 2004; Harrington, Rutter, Weissman *et al.*, 1997). Risk factors for recurrence include early onset of mood disorder in a parent, lack of complete recovery (defined as either subsyndromal depression or return to a dysthymic baseline), pre-existing social dysfunction, history of sexual abuse and family discord (Birmaher, Arbelaez, & Brent, 2002; Lewinsohn, Rohde, & Seeley, 1998).

Other Sequelae

Both depressed children and adolescents are at increased risk for conduct disorder, personality disorders, alcohol, tobacco and drug abuse, and suicidal behavior (Fergusson & Woodward, 2002; Lewinsohn, Rohde, Seeley *et al.*, 2003). They also are at increased risk for obesity, risky sexual behavior, unfulfilling and problematic social relationships, and educational and occupational underachievement (Fergusson & Woodward, 2002; Pine, Goldstein, Wolk *et al.*, 2001). Whereas some studies conclude that most negative sequelae are the residue of incomplete depressive symptom resolution (Lewinsohn, Rohde, Seeley *et al.*, 2003), others find that these "sequelae" may result from common factors that contribute to risk for depression, and for other problems, namely, parental criminality, parental substance abuse, physical or sexual abuse and family discord (Fergusson & Woodward, 2002).

Alcohol and Substance Abuse

Whereas alcohol and substance abuse are more likely to occur in depressed adolescents, many predictors of alcohol and substance abuse are also risk factors for depression, including comorbid behavior disorder, neuroticism, parental history of substance abuse, parental criminality, history of sexual abuse, low parental education, family discord and association with a deviant peer group (Fergusson & Woodward, 2002; Rao, Ryan, Dahl *et al.*, 1999). Alcohol and substance use appears to be a consequence of depression, but can also lead to negative life events that precipitate depression (Libby, Orton, Stover *et al.*, 2005; Kuo, Gardner, Kendler *et al.*, 2006).

Suicidal Behavior

Depression is a strong predictor of suicide attempts and completion (Brent, Baugher, Bridge, *et al.*, 1999; Gould, King, Greenwald, *et al.*, 1998; Shaffer, Gould, Fisher, *et al.*, 1996). Among depressed children and adolescents, greater severity and chronicity of depression, current ideation with a plan or a history of a suicide attempt, comorbid conduct disorder, substance abuse, or impulsive-aggressive personality traits, greater hopelessness, a family history of suicidal behavior, a history of abuse, family conflict and lack of support, distinguish depressed suicide attempters and non-attempters both cross-sectionally and prospectively (Bridge, Goldstein, & Brent, 2006; and see chapter 40).

Risk for Bipolar Disorder

The risk of bipolar disorder in early onset depression is estimated to be around 10–20% (Geller, Zimerman, Williams *et al.*, 2001), with elevated risk in patients who present with hypomania in response to treatment, psychotic features, hypersomnia (in some studies) and a family history of bipolar disorder (Geller, Zimerman, Williams *et al.*, 2001; Strober & Carlson, 1982). Children and younger adolescents exposed to antidepressants, according to one pharmaco-epidemiological study, are at particularly high risk for manic switch (Martin, Young, Leckman *et al.*, 2004).

Risk Factors

Genetic

Twin studies demonstrate that depressive symptoms have a greater concordance among monozygotic than among dizygotic twins, with a heritability of around 40% (Glowinski, Madden, Bucholz *et al.*, 2003; Todd & Botteron, 2002). If cases are defined by longitudinal, rather than just cross-sectional data, the heritability of depression is higher, around 65% (O'Connor, Neiderhiser, Reiss *et al.*, 1998; Todd & Botteron, 2002). Thus, 35–60% of variance is explained by non-genetic factors, such as family adversity and protective factors described below. Adolescent onset depression symptomatology has a greater heritable component than does child onset depressive symptomatology (Scourfield, Rice, Thapar *et al.*, 2003). However, this finding of developmentally mediated differential heritability of depression may be because of the relatively low number of younger children in these twin samples, or due to an increase in the number of behavior-dependent life events that emerge in adolescence (Rice, Harold, & Thapar, 2003; Todd & Botteron, 2002). There is evidence that liability to depression is co-transmitted along with anxiety symptoms, with heritability of co-transmission estimated to be 61–65% (Hudziak, Rudiger, Neale *et al.*, 2000; Thapar & McGuffin, 1997). The genetic relationship between anxiety and depression, according to one series of twin studies, is as follows:

1 Genes that affect liability to anxiety also lead to an increased sensitivity to life events; and

2 Genes that increase risk for anxiety also increase the likelihood of exposure to depressogenic life events (Eaves, Silberg, & Erkanli, 2003).

This formulation is consistent with several longitudinal studies that show an association between child characteristics, child-generated life events and eventual depression (Daley, Hammen, Davila *et al.*, 1998).

The first-degree relatives of depressed children or adolescents have a two- to four-fold increased risk of depression (Kovacs

& Devlin, 1998). Family studies of prepubertal depressives find increased parental rates of criminality, abuse, antisocial disorder and mania (Harrington, Rutter, Weissman *et al.*, 1997; Wickramaratne, Warner, & Weissman, 2000b). In contrast, family studies of adolescent depression have more consistently found an increased rate of mood disorders in first-degree relatives (Harrington, Rutter, Weissman *et al.*, 1997; Wickramaratne, Warner & Weissman, 2000).

"Top-down" studies have also shown an increased risk of depressive disorder in the offspring of depressed parents (Klein, Lewinsohn, Rohde *et al.*, 2005). Greater family loading, such as depression in two generations and increased rates of parental anxiety disorders, was associated with an increased risk and earlier onset of depression, and an increased rate of anxiety disorders, further supporting the view that the liability to depression and that to anxiety are co-transmitted (Weissman, Pilowsky, Wickramaratne *et al.*, 2006; Williamson, Birmaher, Axelson *et al.*, 2004).

There are ongoing genetic studies of recurrent depression that suggest linkage, but none has focused particularly on childhood and adolescent depression (McGuffin, Knight, Breen *et al.*, 2005). The risk of depression, in the presence of stressful life events, is higher in those who had a shorter allele variant of the serotonin transporter (*SLC6A4*), which results in less vigorous transcription of this gene (Caspi, Sugden, Moffitt *et al.*, 2003). A polymorphism of the gene encoding brain-derived neurotrophic factor (*BDNF*) has been reported to be associated with early-onset depression, both alone and in interaction with early childhood adversity (Kaufman, Yang, Douglas-Palumberi *et al.*, 2006; Strauss *et al.*, 2005).

Cognitive Bias and Emotional Regulation

Depressed individuals have been shown to have a cognitive bias towards a negative view of self, future and the world. Prospective studies have found that in non-depressed individuals, especially those at risk for depression, these biases predispose to depressive symptomatology when confronted with stressful life events (Garber, Keiley, & Martin, 2002; Hammen, 1988; Lewinsohn, Joiner, & Rohde, 2001). Moreover, the relationship between negative mood and self-critical cognitions appears to be bidirectional (Kelvin, Goodyer, Teasdale *et al.*, 1999; Park, Goodyer, & Teasdale, 2005; Rudolph, Hammen, & Burge, 1997; Stewart, Kennard, Lee *et al.*, 2004). Depressive symptoms are correlated positively with experimental increases in rumination and negatively with distraction (Lyubomirsky, Caldwell, & Nolen-Hoeksema, 1998).

Neurocognitive studies of depressed adolescents and youth at risk for depression are consistent with the cognitive theory of depression. Both currently and previously depressed youth show greater attention to negative affect, sad words and other negative emotional distractors, whereas youth at low risk for depression show greater attention to positive distractors (Kyte, Goodyer, & Sahakian, 2006; Ladouceur, Dahl, Williamson *et al.*, 2005). Other probes of emotional regulation in children and adolescents at risk for depression, compared to those at low risk, show greater difficulty in inhibition of negative affect, less use of active distraction and less ability to generate positive affect in the face of distraction (Forbes, Fox, Cohn *et al.*, 2006a; Goodyer, 2002; Silk, Shaw, Skuban *et al.*, 2006). It is unclear if these deficits in inhibition are affectively specific, or reflect more global executive function difficulties, consistent with deficits in categorical autobiographic memory and poorer decision-making on gambling tasks associated with adolescent depression (Kyte, Goodyer, & Sahakian, 2006; Park, Goodyer, & Teasdale, 2002). For example, children with a past depression showed deficits in memory for fearful faces (Pine, 2004).

Comorbid Diagnoses

The trait of fearfulness, as well as anxiety disorder per se, and especially social phobia, are associated with increased risk of depression (Goodwin, Fergusson, & Horwood, 2004b; Pine, Cohen, & Brook, 2001; Pine, Cohen, Gurley *et al.*, 1998). The rates of depression are increased both in patients with ADHD and their parents (Faraone & Biederman, 1997). Early symptoms of impulsivity and hyperactivity have been reported as precursors of depression (Jaffee, Moffitt, Caspi *et al.*, 2002). The rates of depression are elevated in children with conduct disorder, perhaps because of shared risk factors (Fergusson & Woodward, 2002). Furthermore, conduct-disordered individuals tend to associate with like-minded peers, which leads to further conduct difficulties, resultant stressful life events (e.g., getting arrested) and more depressive episodes (Fergusson, Wanner, Vitaro *et al.*, 2003).

Family Environmental Factors

Twin studies show a greater role for shared environment in explaining concordance of depressive symptoms in prepubertal children by comparison with adolescents, for whom non-shared environment has a much larger role than shared environment (Scourfield, Rice, Thapar *et al.*, 2003). Family discord and expressed emotion directed towards the child predicted onset or recurrence in at-risk subjects (Asarnow, Goldstein, Tompson *et al.*, 1993; Frye & Garber, 2005). Greater chronicity and severity of maternal depression have been related to greater liability for parent–child conflict, and for cognitive distortions, both of which increase liability for and persistence of child depressive symptoms (Garber & Flynn, 2001). Longitudinal studies show reciprocal interrelationships between maternal and child interpersonal and emotional difficulties, child cognitive distortions and child depressive outcome (Frye & Garber, 2005; Garber & Robinson, 1997; Garber, Keiley, & Martin, 2002; Hammen, Burge, & Stansbury, 1990).

Physical and sexual abuse are among the most potent family–environmental risk factors for the onset and recurrence of depression, and also increase risk for comorbid post-traumatic stress disorder, substance abuse, conduct disorder and suicidal behavior (Barbe, Bridge, Birmaher *et al.*, 2004; Fergusson, Horwood, & Lynskey, 1996; and see chapters 28 and 29). These effects are strongest for more severe and chronic abuse, such as sexual abuse resulting in intercourse (Fergusson, Horwood, & Lynskey, 1996). However, it is difficult to isolate the effects of abuse from the other adverse aspects of parental functioning and home environment that are associated with it: parental mood disorder, substance abuse, criminality, lower parental education and income, and marital discord. The relationship between depression and abuse is much stronger in the presence of other family–genetic risk factors such as a family history of depression and a specific genotype of an *SLC6A4* polymorphism (Caspi, Sugden, Moffitt *et al.*, 2003; Kaufman, Birmaher, Brent *et al.*, 1998a).

Bullying and Same Sex Attraction

Both bulliers and the bullied have higher rates of depression than controls (Ivarsson, Broberg, Arvidsson *et al.*, 2005; Kaltiala-Heino, Rimpela, Rantanen *et al.*, 2000). Same sex attraction, activity, and bisexual or homosexual identification have been related to increased rates of depression, as well as substance abuse and suicidal behavior (Fergusson, Horwood, & Beautrais, 1999). The relationship between sexual attraction/activity/orientation and depression may be mediated by gender atypical behavior, peer rejection, bullying and parental rejection (D'Augelli, Grossman, Salter *et al.*, 2005).

Bereavement and Other Stressful Life Events

Most generally, there is a relationship between stressful life events and depressive disorder in children and adolescents, observed both prospectively and concurrently (Brent, Perper, Moritz *et al.*, 1993; Lewinsohn, Rohde, & Seeley, 1998; Williamson, Birmaher, Ryan *et al.*, 2003), and experience of stress is more likely to result in depression in those with a diathesis as determined by family history or presence of certain genotypes (Brent, Perper, Moritz *et al.*, 1993; Caspi, Sugden, Moffitt *et al.*, 2003; Kaufman, Birmaher, Brent *et al.*, 1998a, 2006). Studies of bereaved children and adolescents find rates of diagnosable depression around 30% within a year of the death, but these occur almost exclusively among those who are at risk because of other factors such as a previous personal or family history of depression (Brent, Perper, Moritz *et al.*, 1993). The impact of parent loss may be mediated by a cascade of other factors, such as a drop in living standard, geographic dislocation and mental health of the surviving parent (Tremblay & Israel, 1998).

Protective Factors

A positive connection to parents and to school may protect against depression and associated health risk behaviors such as suicidal behavior, substance use, binge eating and binge drinking, tobacco use and lack of exercise (Resnick, Bearman, Blum *et al.*, 1997). More specifically, these protective factors include a positive connection between parent and child, active parental supervision and clear behavioral and academic expectations on the part of the parent for the child, parents and children spending leisure and meal time together, academic success, a positive connection between child and school, and a pro-social peer group (Conrad & Hammen, 1993; Fergusson & Lynskey, 1996; King, Schwab-Stone, Flisher *et al.*, 2001). Surprisingly few of these findings have found their way into the intervention literature, with some notable exceptions (Thompson, Eggert, Randell *et al.*, 2001).

Comorbid Medical Illness

A relationship between less than ideal physical health and depression has been reported in community studies of adolescents (Lewinsohn, Rohde, & Seeley, 1998). Lewinsohn, Rohde, & Seeley (1998) posit that illness interferes with activities that are likely to be enjoyable or enhance a sense of mastery, which in turn predisposes to depression. There may also be systemic effects of some chronic illnesses or their treatments in diseases such as epilepsy (Jones, Hermann, Barry *et al.*, 2003; Plioplys, 2003), juvenile onset diabetes (Kovacs, Goldston, Obrosky *et al.*, 1997), inflammatory bowel disease (Addolorato, Capristo, Stefanini *et al.*, 1997) and asthma (Goodwin, Fergusson, & Horwood, 2004a). Twin studies suggest co-transmission of liability to eczema and mood disorder (Wamboldt, Hewitt, Schmitz *et al.*, 2000). There is also an increased risk of medical problems in depressed offspring of depressed parents, suggesting that factors associated with risk for depression may also increase risk for ill health, an observation also made in a genetic linkage study of early-onset recurrent depression (Kramer, Warner, Olfson *et al.*, 1998; Zubenko, Zubenko, Spiker *et al.*, 2001).

Neuroendocrine

Direct measures of cortisol secretion have not distinguished between early-onset depressives and controls (Feder, Coplan, Goetz *et al.*, 2004; Puig-Antich, Dahl, Ryan *et al.*, 1989). There were no differences between depressed children and controls with regard to adrenocorticotropin hormone (ACTH) release, after stimulation with corticotropin releasing hormone (CRH), although a small subgroup of melancholic children showed a blunted response (Birmaher, Dahl, Perel *et al.*, 1996a), and ACTH release was *increased* in depressed children who had a history of abuse (Kaufman, Birmaher, Perel *et al.*, 1997b). Increased cortisol secretion around sleep onset is associated with adolescent depression and predicts depressive recurrence and substance abuse in young adults who were studied during adolescence (Dahl, Ryan, Puig-Antich *et al.*, 1991; Rao, Ryan, Dahl *et al.*, 1999). Goodyer *et al.* found that in adolescents at high risk for depression, increased morning dehydroepiandrosterone (DHEA) was associated with onset of depression, and high morning cortisol : DHEA ratio at intake was related to persistence of depressive symptoms (Goodyer, Herbert, & Tamplin, 2003; Goodyer, Herbert, Tamplin *et al.*, 2000). A decrease in growth hormone (GH) release in response to a provocative challenge of growth hormone releasing hormone (GHRH), which may be related to central norepinephrine neurotransmission, has been reported in depressed children versus controls during both episode and recovery, and in never-depressed children of depressed parents (Birmaher, Dahl, Williamson *et al.*, 2000b; Dahl, Birmaher, Williamson *et al.*, 2000). In a longitudinal study of depressed children grown up, increased amount of GH release in the first 4 hours of sleep was related to recurrence of depression and suicide attempt (Pine, Coplan, Wasserman *et al.*, 1997).

A blunted cortisol and exaggerated prolactin response (the latter in girls only) to L-5 hydroxytryptophan (L-5HT) has been found in both depressed children and never-depressed children at risk for depression due to parental depression, compared to controls (Birmaher, Kaufman, Brent *et al.*, 1997; Ryan, Birmaher, Perel *et al.*, 1992a), consistent with central dysregulation of serotonin neurotransmission. Increased gastrointestinal distress in response to this challenge predicted an increased risk of anxiety or depression over time (Campo, Dahl, Williamson *et al.*, 2003). However, similar neuroendocrine responses to provocative challenge may be found in those with adverse home environments, and with high levels of aggression (Kaufman, Birmaher, Perel *et al.*, 1998b; Pine, Coplan, Wasserman *et al.*, 1997).

Sleep

Subjective sleep complaints are a very prominent component of early-onset depression, although subjective complaints and objective observations of sleep in a sleep laboratory are not closely correlated (Bertocci, Dahl, Williamson *et al.*, 2005). Decreased rapid eye movement (REM) latency and increased latency of sleep-onset are not frequently observed in prepubertal depression, although the presence of these markers was associated with greater depressive severity (Dahl, Ryan, Puig-Antich *et al.*, 1991). Decreased REM latency and increased latency of sleep-onset is observed in depressed adolescents, but only after a strict sleep–wake schedule was imposed. Decreased REM latency, increased REM density and decreased sleep efficiency have been reported to be associated with depressive onset, recurrence and persistence more consistently in older adolescents (Dahl & Lewin, 2002).

Studies of Hemispheric Lateralization

Studies of infants and children at high risk for depression have found evidence of decreased left hemisphere electroencephalogram (EEG) activity (Dawson, Frey, Panagiotides *et al.*, 1997; Tomarken, Dichter, Garber *et al.*, 2004). Low left frontal EEG activity was also related to greater negative affect and less positive affiliative behavior in babies of depressed mothers (Bruder, Tenke, Warner *et al.*, 2005; Forbes, Shaw, Fox *et al.*, 2006b). In adolescent and adult offspring of depressed and non-depressed parents, those at risk for depression had less activity over right central and parietal regions, whereas those offspring with a history of depression had less left frontal activity (Bruder, Tenke, Warner *et al.*, 2005; Kentgen, Tenke, Pine *et al.*, 2000; Shankman, Tenke, Bruder *et al.*, 2005).

Neuroimaging Studies

Structural imaging studies of adult subjects with early-onset familial depression as well as in adolescents with depression have found reduced volume of the left subgenual prefrontal cortex, with others finding more global differences between familial and non-familial pediatric depression (Botteron, Raichle, Drevets *et al.*, 2002; Drevets, Price, Simpson *et al.*, 1997; Lyoo, Kyu Lee, Hyun Jung *et al.*, 2002; Nolan, Moore, Madden *et al.*, 2002). Preliminary studies of female adolescent depressed twins suggest that this structural difference is genetically transmitted and may mediate the heritability of depression (Todd & Botteron, 2002). Decreased amygdala size has been reported in depressed children and adolescents (Rosso, Cintron, Steingard *et al.*, 2005). Steingard, Renshaw, Hennen *et al.* (2002) reported decreased prefrontal cortex and increased third and fourth ventricular volume in depressed adolescents, although these findings have now been reported in a variety of neuropsychiatric disorders and may be a marker for the effects of chronicity. Other findings, such as altered hippocampal size, may be attributable to early trauma (Kaufman & Charney, 2001; Vythilingam, Heim, Newport *et al.*, 2002).

In studies using magnetic resonance imaging (MRI) spectroscopy, lower glutamate concentrations have been reported in the anterior cingulate cortex in depressed children and adolescents versus non-depressed controls (Mirza, Tang, Russell *et al.*, 2004). The degree of functional impairment was inversely correlated with glutamate concentration. However, this finding is not specific to major depression, as lower anterior cingulate glutamate is also found in children with obsessive-compulsive disorder (Rosenberg, Mirza, Russell *et al.*, 2004). Increased choline concentrations in the left dorso-lateral and in orbito-frontal prefrontal cortex of depressed children and adolescents have also been reported (Farchione, Moore, & Rosenberg, 2002; Steingard, Yurgelun-Todd, Hennen *et al.*, 2000).

Thomas, Drevets, Dahl *et al.* (2001) evaluated responses of depressed and anxious children and control children to fearful faces, and found increased amygdala activation in anxious children and decreased amygdala activation in depressed children. In contrast, increased amygdala activation has been found in depressed adolescents during recall of fearful faces. Increased amygdala activation was also found in depressed adolescents, relative to controls, during participation in reward-related decision-making and response to outcome (Forbes, May, Siegle *et al.*, 2006c; Roberson-Nay, McClure, Monk *et al.*, 2006).

Clinical Management

Risk Assessment and Treatment Planning

The first determination in the assessment of a depressed child or adolescent is whether the child can safely be treated as an out-patient. A patient with suicide ideation with a plan and intent, or who has made a recent suicide attempt with continued intent, should initially be hospitalized or treated in a more acute setting than out-patient unless the patient, clinician and family can develop a safety plan for coping with future suicidal urges upon which all can mutually agree (Birmaher & Brent, 2007; National Institute for Health and Clinical Excellence [NICE], 2005; Shaffer & Pfeffer, 2001; see also chapter 40). In addition, patients who are acutely psychotic, in a bipolar mixed state or are substance dependent may not be able to be treated as out-patients. Patients who are being abused at home should be removed from the home temporarily, although not necessarily to hospital. Whereas most US standards of care recommend psychiatric hospitalization for greater acuity and safety concerns, there has been almost no empirical assessment of the value of psychiatric hospitalization versus other types of treatment. Therefore, if a patient and family refuse hospital admission, unless there appears to be an obvious clinical counterindication (e.g., patient psychotic and refusing to eat), it may be preferable to preserve an alliance with the patient and family and schedule out-patient visits several times per week in the initial stabilization phase. As a general framework, clinicians need to consider the following hierarchy of priorities:

1 Life-threatening issues (e.g., suicidality, homicidality, exposure to domestic violence, intravenous drug use);
2 Therapy-threatening issues (hopelessness about treatment, chronically depressed parent who is unable to bring the child for treatment); and
3 Symptom and functionally oriented treatment.

Patient and Family Education

Because depression is often a chronic and recurrent illness, it is vital to establish a long-term partnership with the patient and family with regard to its management. This can be achieved by providing the patient and family with all the requisite information about depression and its treatment, and then making treatment decisions collaboratively (Brent, Poling, McKain *et al.*, 1993). As described in Table 37.1, education focuses on depression as an illness, recognition and monitoring of depressive symptomatology, knowing risks and benefits of different treatments, and, if symptom relief is achieved, development of a plan to prevent relapse and recurrence.

Family, Social and Individual Context

The treatment plan for depressed children and adolescents should consider four levels of contextual factors: parents, peers, school and individual. Depressed children and adolescents who are clinically referred often have parents who have active psychiatric difficulties, most commonly depression, anxiety and substance abuse (Hammen, Rudolph, Weisz *et al.*, 1999). These difficulties may make it very difficult for the family to comply with treatment recommendations, and may also create stressors that make it less likely for the patient to respond to treatment. For example, three different research groups have reported that current parental depressive symptoms make it less likely that a child will respond to cognitive–behavioral therapy (CBT) for depression or anxiety (Brent, Kolko, Birmaher *et al.*, 1998; Lewinsohn, Rohde, & Seeley, 1998; Southam-Gerow, Kendall, & Weersing, 2001). Treatment of maternal depression is associated with amelioration of child symptomatology (Weissman, Pilowsky, Wickramaratne *et al.*, 2006). Therefore, facilitation of a treatment referral for the depressed parent should be part of the child's treatment plan. Abuse, exposure to family violence or high levels of criticism or discord must be addressed because of safety issues for the child as well as the negative impact of these factors on duration and recurrence of depressive episodes. When parents are unable to provide the necessary support for treatment, they sometimes are willing to allow involvement of adult surrogates, such as older siblings, other relatives or close friends who may temporarily step in and help with transportation and even monitoring of treatment response.

Table 37.1 Psychoeducation: key elements for parents and patients.

Depression is an illness and not the fault of the patient or family
How to recognize and monitor depressive symptoms, detect early relapse and recurrence
Modal course, in order to have reasonable expectations for pace and extent of recovery
Risks and benefits of different treatment options, in order to make an informed decision
How to collaborate in development of a plan for relapse prevention, continuation and maintenance treatment

Depressed adolescents, particularly those with comorbid behavioral traits and substance use, often are involved in friendships with similarly depressed, substance abusing and disaffected youth, which tend to reinforce depressive attitudes and also encourage antisocial acts that in turn lead to depressogenic life events (Fergusson, Wanner, Vitaro *et al.*, 2003). Therefore, the possibility of developing more prosocial relationships should be on the treatment agenda.

As a result of decreased energy and concentration and motivational difficulties, depressed children and adolescents often fall behind in school, which in turn leads to a sense of failure, increased anxiety and a tendency to give up and disconnect from school. There also may be specific school-related stressors that contribute to depressive symptomatology, such as being the target of bullying, or teasing by students or teachers. Conversely, cross-sectional data and one intervention study suggest that a positive connection between school and student, as well as high parental academic expectations appropriate to the child, are protective against depression (Resnick, Bearman, Blum *et al.*, 1997; Thompson, Eggert, Randell *et al.*, 2001). Therefore, the clinician should assess the depressed child's current school function, identify any school-related stressors, and, if the patient has fallen behind academically, develop a plan, in conjunction with the school, for a reduced workload and a plan for catching up that is mutually acceptable to school, family and student.

With regard to individual context, it is important to identify comorbid health risk behaviors or psychiatric disorders that are likely to be life-threatening or disruptive to therapy, in which case, they should be attended to first. Life-threatening behavior, like intravenous drug use, aggressive criminal behavior or non-compliance with a serious chronic illness, should be addressed prior to treatment of depression, even recognizing that depression may be contributing to this problem. Higher priority to targeting comorbid conditions should be given if these symptoms are causing the greatest functional impairment and if the treatment of depression is likely not to be successful unless the other condition is addressed first. For example, the treatment of a patient with both depression and ADHD whose main difficulties are decrease in motivation, suicidal ideation and hopelessness should probably initially focus on the depression, whereas a patient with similar comorbidity whose depression emerges secondary to school and peer failure due to impulsivity and inattention should probably have the ADHD addressed first.

Treatment

There are currently three treatments for adolescent depression with some empirical support: antidepressant treatment, CBT and interpersonal therapy. Meta-analyses show support for the efficacy of fluoxetine in prepubertal depression but, because of small numbers and a smaller effect size, not for other agents (Bridge, Iyengar, Salary *et al.*, 2007). There has been considerably less research on treatment of prepubertal children with depression, although there is some support for the efficacy of antidepressants. Each of these three approaches will be discussed, followed by a recommendation for "best practice" which is based on both empirical support and expert consensus (Brent, 2004; Brent & Birmaher, 2002; Birmaher & Brent, 2007; NICE, 2005). Because of the controversies surrounding the efficacy of antidepressants and of psychotherapy for pediatric depression, we provide a synopsis of the effect sizes of the extant clinical trials in Tables 37.2–37.4.

Antidepressant Medication

Evidence of Efficacy

Both the single largest placebo-controlled comparison study of tricyclic antidepressants (TCAs) and placebo, and a subsequent meta-analysis showed no difference between drug and placebo (Hazell, O'Connell, Heathcote *et al.*, 1995; Keller, Ryan, Strober *et al.*, 2001), whereas several studies have demonstrated efficacy with selective serotonin reuptake inhibitor (SSRI) antidepressants, especially using fluoxetine (Bridge, Iyengar, Salary *et al.*, 2007). This may be reflective of an overall developmental difference in so far as adolescents and younger adults may respond better to serotonergic agents, whereas older adults respond equally as well to serotonergic and to noradrenergic agents (Mulder, Watkins, Joyce *et al.*, 2003).

Fluoxetine is the best-studied antidepressant with the strongest efficacy data, and consequently is the only antidepressant to receive US Food and Drug Administration (FDA) and Medicine and Healthcare Products Regulatory Agency (MHRA) approval for the treatment of depression in children and adolescents (Emslie, Rush, Weinberg *et al.*, 1997, 2002; March, Silva, Petrycki *et al.*, 2004). In the three published studies of fluoxetine, a higher proportion of those treated with fluoxetine were "much or very much improved" compared to those treated with placebo (52–61% versus 33–37%), with a number needed to treat (NNT) = 5. In the Treatment of

Table 37.2 Differences in efficacy outcomes for antidepressant-treated and placebo-treated groups. (Table provided by Jeffrey Bridge, PhD.)

Drug	Study	n	Response rate %*		Risk difference (95% CI)	NNT (95% CI)	Primary scalar measure of efficacy Hedges's g (95% CI)
			Medication Group	Placebo Group			
Fluoxetine	Simeon *et al.* (1990)	–	–	–	–	–	0.21
Fluoxetine	Emslie *et al.* (1997)	96	56	33	23		0.60
Fluoxetine	Emslie *et al.* (2002)	210	65	54	12	9	0.50
Fluoxetine	TADS Study Team 2004	221	61	35	26	4	0.040
Fluoxetine	*Pooled estimates*	*527*	*62*	*42*	*20 (11 to 29)*	*6 (4 to 10)*	*0.46 (0.29 to 0.62)*
Paroxetine	Keller *et al.* (2001)	177	67	55	12	9	0.22
Paroxetine	Berard *et al.* (2006)	268	61	58	2	46	0.07
Paroxetine	Emslie *et al.* (2006)	201	49	46	3	40	−0.06
Paroxetine	*Pooled estimates*	*646*	*59*	*53*	*5 (−3 to 13)*	*20 (8 to ∞ to NNH 38)*	*0.07 (−0.09 to 0.23)*
Sertraline	Wagner *et al.* (2004)	364	69	59	10	10	–
Citalopram	Wagner *et al.* (2004)	174	36	24	12	9	0.32
Escitalopram	Wagner *et al.* (2006)	261	63	52	11	10	0.13
Venlafaxine	Study 382	141	50	41	9	12	0.16
Venlafaxine	Study 394	193	68	61	7	14	0.13
Venlafaxine	*Pooled estimates*	*334*	*61*	*52*	*8 (−2 to 18)*	*13 (6 to ∞ to NNH 42)*	*0.14 (−0.07 to 0.35)*
Nefazadone	CN104-141	195	62	42	20	6 (3 to 17)	0.28
Mirtazapine	003-045	249	57	49	7	14 (5 to ∞ to NNH 18)	0.20
	Overall	*2750*	*60*	*48*	*11*	*9 (7 to 14)*	*0.23*

CI, confidence interval; NNH, number needed to treat to harm; NNT, number needed to treat to benefit.

* Clinical Global Impression-Improvement Score (CGI-I) <2.

Adolescent Depression Study (TADS), fluoxetine was more efficacious than both cognitive–behavior therapy and placebo (proportion "significantly improved," 61% versus 43% versus 35%; March *et al.*, 2004). However, combined treatment (fluoxetine plus CBT) resulted with the highest rate of symptomatic remission (37% versus 20% on fluoxetine alone; Kennard, Silva, Vitiello *et al.*, 2006).

A meta-analysis of all available clinical trials, both published and unpublished, shows that SSRIs are superior to placebo, with the average response rate for drug versus placebo for antidepressants 60% versus 49%, with NNT = 9, with a comparable effect size on scalar measures (Hedges's G = 0.23; Bridge, Iyengar, Salary *et al.*, 2007; see Table 37.2). The relatively low effect size in SSRIs versus placebo in child and adolescent depression is caused in part by the high placebo response rate. The drug–placebo difference was inversely proportional to the number of study sites involved in the trial, suggesting that some studies with large numbers of sites may have been less selective in recruitment (Bridge, Iyengar, Salary *et al.*, 2007). Duration was also inversely proportional to response. Other explanations for the relative modest effects of antidepressants include use of inadequate dosage, duration of treatment too short to achieve the full effect, and aggregation of results of children and adolescents when, in some studies, there were significant effects for adolescents but not for children.

Besides fluoxetine, other drugs with published efficacy data include citalopram, paroxetine and sertraline (Keller, Ryan, Strober *et al.*, 2001; Wagner, Ambrosini, Rynn *et al.*, 2003, 2004), although the effect sizes were relatively small and there are other negative studies for these agents (Emslie, Kratochvil, Vitiello *et al.*, 2006; von Knorring, Olsson, Thomsen *et al.*, 2006). A review of the published and unpublished studies indicates that, for paroxetine and for venlafaxine, the response to medication was superior to placebo for adolescents, but not for children (Emslie, Yeung, Kunz *et al.*, 2007). In some studies, such as those for venlafaxine, the doses appeared to be substantially below those recommended for clinical practice (Emslie, Kratochvil, Vitiello *et al.*, 2006).

Amfebutamone, a monocyclic aminoketone that inhibits the reuptake of dopamine and norepinephrine, has been found in open trials to improve depressive symptoms and ADHD symptoms in patients comorbid for both conditions (Daviss, Bentivoglio, Racusin *et al.*, 2001), but this agent has not been studied in randomized trials in depressed children or adolescents. Antidepressant efficacy is correlated with concentration of amfebutamone and metabolites, most significantly, hydroxyamfebutamone (Daviss, Perel, Brent *et al.*, 2006).

Adverse Events in Antidepressant Treatment

The US FDA conducted a meta-analysis that found a higher rate of spontaneously reported suicide-related adverse events on drug than on placebo (4% versus 2%; Hammad, Laughren, & Racoosin, 2006). There were relatively few suicide attempts, no completions and most suicidal events occurred early in treatment. The increased risk for suicidality was found in subjects treated for depression, obsessive compulsive disorder (OCD) and anxiety. Another meta-analysis that included additional studies not reported on in the FDA meta-analysis and using random rather than fixed effects models reported rates of suicidal adverse events for drug and placebo of 2.5% versus 1.7%, respectively, for a risk difference of 0.8%, and a number needed to harm (NNH) of 125. Thus, the number of those who benefit from SSRIs (NNT = 10) compared to those who become suicidal (NNH = 125) is around 14 : 1. (Bridge, Iyengar, Salary *et al.*, 2007).

Baseline predictors of spontaneously reported events in all pooled studies using paroxetine identified suicidal ideation at intake, agitation at baseline and female gender as risk factors (Apter, Lipschitz, Fong *et al.*, 2006). No mechanism has been established that explains the relationship between SSRI use and suicidality, although some speculate that it could be a result of rapid metabolism, non-compliance and/or withdrawal symptoms, induction of a mixed state (combination of manic and depressed symptoms), akathisia or SSRI-induced disinhibition (Brent, 2004).

The clinical significance of these spontaneously reported suicide-related adverse events is unclear. Almost all are increased suicidal ideation or suicidal threats, with very few attempts and no completions in over 4300 subjects (Hammad, Laughren, & Racoosin, 2006). Moreover, no difference between drug and placebo has been detected in the subset of studies that also assessed for suicidality using standard measures, although there was an effect of medication on suicidality on the Suicide Ideation Questionnaire in the TADS study (Emslie, Kratochvil, Vitiello *et al.*, 2006). If SSRIs significantly increased suicidal risk, one would expect to see a recent increase in the rate of adolescent suicide, given the dramatic increase in the use of SSRIs in adolescents. However, the adolescent suicide rate has declined over the past decade, and some pharmaco-epidemiological studies find a relationship between increased prescription and sales of SSRIs and a decline in completed suicide, which is particularly notable among the young (Brent, 2004; Gibbons, Hur, Bhaumik *et al.*, 2006; Olfson, Shaffer, Marcus *et al.*, 2003). In one record linkage study, the rate of attempted suicide in both adults and adolescents started on SSRIs was highest in the month before initiation of medication (Simon, Savarino, Operskalski *et al.*, 2006). Nonetheless, caution and close monitoring for increased suicidality are warranted in mood-disordered patients treated with SSRIs.

In addition to the concern over suicide and self-injurious behavior, antidepressants are associated with increased incidence of sleep disruption, vivid dreams, nausea and gastrointestinal distress, increase in agitation, akathisia, anxiety, headache, serotonin syndrome (particularly in combination with other serotonergic agents) and bruising (caused by a prolongation of clotting time; Goldstein & Goodnick, 1998). The last side-effect is usually not clinically significant, but can become so in patients with intrinsic coagulation disorders or who are undergoing surgery. One pharmaco-epidemiological study found that the risk of SSRI-treatment-associated mania was greatest in patients under the age of 14 (Martin, Young, Leckman *et al.*, 2004).

Predictors of Antidepressant Response

One naturalistic study found that comorbid attentional problems predicted poorer response to an SSRI in depressed adolescents (Hamilton & Bridge, 1999). A naturalistic follow-up after a clinical trial found that poorer outcome was predicted by family discord, comorbidity and greater severity at intake (Emslie, Rush, Weinberg *et al.*, 1998). In the TADS study, predictors of poor outcome, regardless of treatment assignment, were severity (depressive symptoms and functional impairment), complexity (comorbidity) and chronicity (Curry, Rohde, Simons *et al.*, 2006).

A higher dose may lead to better outcome in those patients who fail to respond to a lower dose of SSRI (Heiligenstein, Hoog, Wagner *et al.*, 2006). There is evidence that adolescents metabolize sertraline, citalopram and paroxetine (but not fluvoxamine) faster than do adults, so that higher doses than typically recommended for adults may be needed (Axelson, Perel, Birmaher *et al.*, 2002; Findling, McNamara, Stansbrey *et al.*, 2006; Labellarte *et al.*, 2004).

Biological Predictors of Response

Two small studies found a correlation between percent reuptake of serotonin in platelet receptors and clinical response (Axelson *et al.*, 2005; Sallee, Hilal, Dougherty *et al.*, 1998). One study found an association between up-regulation of glucocorticoid type II receptors and response to sertraline (Sallee, Nesbitt, Dougherty *et al.*, 1995). Several studies found that the short allelic variant of the serotonin transporter gene (*SLC6A4*) is associated with a poorer response to SSRIs in adults (Lerer & Macciardi, 2002), and preliminary data in depressed children and adolescents are consistent with these findings. Depressed adults who responded to CBT showed high amygdala and low subgenual cingulate cortex response to sustained emotional processing. Depressed adults who responded to fluoxetine showed greater left versus right hemisphere activation to dichotic listening, whereas the reverse predicted poor outcome (Bruder, Stewart, Tenke *et al.*, 2001; Siegle, Carter, & Thase, 2006).

Role in Continuation

In patients who have been successfully treated with fluoxetine for the acute phase, a 32-week double-blind comparison of continuation treatment with fluoxetine versus placebo showed a relapse rate of 30% on continuation versus 60% on placebo, with a median time to relapse of 6 versus 2.3 months (Emslie, Heiligenstein, Hoog *et al.*, 2004).

Cognitive–Behavior Therapy

Theory and Techniques

CBT is based on the theory of depression that holds that depressed individuals show "distortions" in their thinking and information processing, tending to emphasize the negative aspects of a situation and to underemphasize the positive, as has been demonstrated in self-report and neurocognitive evaluations (see p. 604; Beck, Rush, Shaw *et al.*, 1979). This tendency to focus differentially on the negative appears to have a role in the genesis and maintenance of depressive episodes and negative mood states during times of stress (Garber & Robinson, 1997; Garber, Keiley, & Martin, 2002; Lewinsohn, Joiner, & Rohde, 2001).

CBT treatments for depression focus on interrupting this cycle of negative thinking, depressed mood and maladaptive behavior, through a variety of cognitive techniques and behavioral skill-building exercises. Central to CBT is *cognitive restructuring*, that is, making the patient aware of negative "distortions" and teaching the individual how to counteract them, with subsequent relief of depression. Another key component of CBT is *behavioral activation*; for example, encouraging patients to normalize their routine and engage in rewarding activities, even if they do not feel like it at the time. This component of CBT is derived from the observation that depressed mood has been shown to fluctuate proportionally to the degree of involvement in potentially reinforcing activities (Lewinsohn, Rohde, & Seeley, 1998).

However, the content of CBT treatment manuals, tested in clinical trials, varies greatly in the emphasis on each of these techniques (behavior activation, cognitive restructuring) and the inclusion of other adjunctive skill-building elements (e.g., problem-solving, emotion regulation, relaxation, social skills training). In addition, CBT approaches vary with regard to the length, structure and emphasis format (e.g., group or individual), which makes differences in outcome across studies difficult to interpret.

Efficacy of CBT

Many pioneering studies of CBT for child depression involved symptomatic volunteers (Weisz, McCarty, & Valeri, 2006). However, in order to allow comparability to the above-noted medication trials, we focus our review on studies enrolling samples that meet formal diagnostic criteria for a depressive disorder (Table 37.3). All of these investigations are in depressed adolescents; as yet there are no published CBT efficacy trials in diagnosed samples composed primarily of prepubertal youth, although an open trial of a psychosocial treatment with a focus on emotional regulation with some cognitive elements, described below, has been reported (Kovacs, Sherril, George *et al.*, 2006). A comprehensive meta-analysis of child psychotherapy studies found an overall effect size for CBT treatment of depression of 0.34, although in the absence of the large, and essentially negative contrast between CBT and placebo in the TADS study, the overall effect size was 0.48 (Weisz, McCarty, & Valeri, 2006).

The most commonly studied intervention for depressed adolescents is the CBT-based course Coping with Depression for Adolescents (CWD-A), a group-administered structured program that includes psychoeducation, pleasant activity scheduling, social skills training, problem-solving and cognitive

Table 37.3 Cognitive–behavioral therapy (CBT) for adolescents with clinically diagnosed depression. (After Weersing *et al.*, 2006.)

Study	*n*	Treatment and control conditions	Mean sessions	Source of sample	Definition of clinical response	Responding at post-treatment (%)	NNT	Primary symptom measure	CBT effect size
Brent *et al.* (1997)	107	CBT Family Supportive	12.1 10.7 11.2	Clinic, diagnosed depression	No mood diagnosed and normal BDI	60 38 39	5	BDI	CBT: 0.40
Clarke *et al.* (1999)	123	CBT CBTP Waitlist	16 16 + 9 –	Community, screened for diagnosis	No mood diagnosed	65 69 48	5–6	BDI	CBT: 0.58 CBTP: 0.24
Clarke *et al.* (2002)	88	CBT+TAU TAU	16 CBT 8 week	Community, offspring of depressed parents, screened for diagnosis	No mood diagnosed	58 53	20	CES-D	0.20
Lewinsohn *et al.* (1990)	69	CBT CBTP Waitlist	14 14 + 7 –	Community, screened for diagnosis	No mood diagnosed	43 47 5	3	BDI	CBT: 0.92 CBTP: 1.45
Rosello & Bernal (1999)	71	CBT IPT-A Waitlist	12 12 –	Community, screened for diagnosis	Normal CDI	59 82 –	–	CDI	0.34
Treatment of Adolescent Depression Study (TADS) (2004)	223	Placebo	11	Clinic, diagnosed depression	CGI-I ≤ 2	43 35	12	CDRS-R	−0.03
Vostanis *et al.* (1996)	63	CBT Supportive	6 6	Clinic, diagnosed depression	No mood diagnosed	86 75	9	MFQ-P	0.51
Wood *et al.* (1996)	53	CBT Relaxation	6.4 6.2	Clinic, diagnosed depression	"Clinical remission"	54 21	4	MFQ-P	0.40

BDI, Beck Depression Inventory; CBT, Cognitive–behavioral therapy; CBTP, CBT – parent design; CDI, Children's Depression Inventory; CDRS-R, Children's Depression Rating Scale – Revised; CES-D, Center for Epidemiological Studies, Depression; CGI-I, Clinical Global Impression-Improvement; IPT-A, Interpersonal psychotherapy for depressed adolescents; MFQ-P, Mood and Feelings Questionnaire, Parent; NNT, Number needed to treat; School TAU, school counseling services.

restructuring. Two studies compared CWD-A, with or without a multisession parent curriculum, and a waitlist control group (Clarke, Lewinsohn, Rohde *et al.*, 1999; Lewinsohn, Clarke, Hops *et al.*, 1990). In both of these investigations, CWD-A was superior to waitlist at the end of treatment, with regard to diagnosed depression and dimensional measures of depression. However, the addition of the parent group had no additive effect to the group CBT alone. In the second study, one to two booster sessions were provided, which did not reduce the rate of depressive recurrence, but did seem to be helpful to those who had not yet recovered from their depressive episode (Clarke, Lewinsohn, Rohde *et al.*, 1999).

Subsequently, the program has been employed with depressed conduct-disordered youth, and has been adapted for depressed incarcerated youth (Rohde, Clarke, Mace *et al.*, 2004a; Rohde, Jorgensen, Seeley *et al.*, 2004b). The success rate was more modest for these more clinically complex youth, but the effect sizes for reduction in rates and severity of depression between the experimental treatment and waitlist controls were comparable to the initial studies.

To date, there have been four studies to test the efficacy of CBT in clinically referred depressed adolescents. Vostanis, Feehan, Grattan *et al.* (1996) compared CBT to supportive treatment and found no difference between treatment groups (86% versus 75% no longer depressed). Treatment was very brief (around six sessions) and was offered over an extended time frame (1–5 months). In contrast, Wood, Harrington, and Moore (1996), who used a similar but more concentrated treatment model (5–8 sessions of CBT over 12 weeks), found that brief CBT was superior to relaxation therapy in depressed adolescents; improvements were also noted in functional impairment, anxiety and dimensional measures of depression. Upon follow-up, there was a tendency for those treated with CBT to relapse so that differences were no longer statistically significant.

Brent, Holder, Kolko *et al.* (1997) compared 12–16 sessions of CBT that was an adaptation of Beck's approach (Beck *et al.*, 1979) with family therapy and with supportive treatment, all delivered by therapists who were trained in and adherents of their treatment model. At post-treatment, CBT produced outcomes superior to the alternative intervention, with regard to decline in depressive symptoms, achievement of remission and speed of response. Upon 2-year follow-up, there were no statistically significant differences among the three randomized groups (Birmaher, Brent, Kolko *et al.*, 2000a).

The final CBT efficacy trial in a diagnosed sample is the Treatment of Adolescents with Depression Study (TADS; March, Silva, Petrycki *et al.*, 2004). TADS is the only published study to compare CBT, fluoxetine, their combination and placebo. In this large well-powered investigation, CBT (43% significantly improved) was not superior to placebo (35%), whereas both combination of CBT and fluoxetine (71%) and fluoxetine alone (61%) were markedly superior to both CBT and to placebo.

Given the generally positive effects of CBT in other investigations, why did CBT fail to outperform placebo in TADS? The authors posit that CBT was less efficacious because of severity, comorbidity and economic disadvantage of the sample. However, other studies found stronger effects for CBT in poorer samples that had comparable severity and comorbidity, with comorbid anxiety actually being a positive prognosticator (Brent, Holder, Kolko *et al.*, 1997, 1998; Rohde, Clarke, Lewinsohn *et al.*, 2001). TADS subjects did have greater duration of depression than was reported in other studies, which, in turn, was associated with poorer response to treatment in the TADS study and one meta-analysis of all antidepressant trials for depression (Bridge, Iyengar, Salary *et al.*, 2007; Curry, Rohde, Simons *et al.*, 2006). Another possible explanation for the relatively weak performance of CBT in this study could be the type of treatment delivered. The TADS treatment package attempted to deliver, in a relatively brief treatment, a large number of accepted approaches: problem-solving, behavior activation, cognitive restructuring, emotion regulation, relaxation training and parent–child sessions, whereas some of the more successful interventions have mainly focused on cognitive restructuring or on behavior activation and problem-solving. It is possible that in the TADS manual's attempt to be inclusive of a variety of successful techniques, subjects never received an adequate "dose" of any one of these specific CBT techniques (Hollon, Garber, & Shelton, 2005).

Combined CBT and Medication

In TADS the combination of CBT and fluoxetine was superior to drug alone in the overall sample, and also for the subgroup with mild to moderate depression, with regard to speed and completeness of response (Curry, Rohde, Simons *et al.*, 2006; Kennard, Silva, Vitiello *et al.*, 2006; Vitiello, Rohde, Silva *et al.*, 2006). Overall combination treatment resulted in the best functional outcomes and highest rates of remission (37% versus 20% for placebo). However, the combination treatment was not superior to medication alone for more severely depressed subjects, although the trends favored combination (effect size [ES] 0.84 for combination versus 0.69 for fluoxetine alone; Curry, Rohde, Simons *et al.*, 2006). In addition to the TADS study, there have been two other investigations of the impact of combined CBT and antidepressant management compared with antidepressant alone, which, in aggregate, do not make a strong case for the use of combined treatment, counterintuitive as this seems. Clarke, Debar, Lynch *et al.* (2005) studied the addition of the CWD-A treatment to antidepressant management in primary care. This combined treatment resulted in some modest improvement in quality of life, but improvement in depressive symptoms never reached statistical significance; moreover, patients in the combined treatment were more likely to stop their antidepressants. A study conducted in the UK compared combination treatment, using the CBT model that had been used successfully by Wood, Harrington, & Moore (1996), with fluoxetine alone, for moderate to severely ill depressed adolescents. CBT did not add to medication alone with regard to global functioning, quality of life or depressive symptomatology (Goodyer, 2006).

Effectiveness

Three published investigations have produced findings relevant to the effectiveness of CBT in practice. As noted above, Clarke, Debar, Lynch *et al.* (2005) found in their primary care investigation that adding CBT to high-quality medication management provided only modest benefits on measures of symptoms and functioning. However, these very small improvements occurred as youths significantly reduced their use of psychotropic medication in the CBT plus SSRI arm. In another study based in primary care, depressed adolescents were randomized to either clinical monitoring and usual care or clinical monitoring plus on-site specialty mental health care, with the latter consisting of the patient's choice of CBT, medication, or both (Asarnow, Jaycox, Duan *et al.*, 2005). The quality improvement (QI) arm, which most often consisted of CBT, was superior to treatment as usual in increasing teens' access to depression care (i.e., number of sessions) and on improving depression symptoms and quality of life, similar to parallel studies in adults (Wells, Sherbourne, Schoenbaum *et al.*, 2000). One benchmarking study compared CBT to an unselected, clinically complicated sample of depressed adolescents with the results of CBT delivered in a research study at the same site (Weersing, Iyengar, Kolko *et al.*, 2006). Results of clinic-based CBT were quite similar to the published effects of CBT, once symptom trajectories in the research subjects were adjusted for the difference in the proportion of subjects who came by advertisement, as the latter tended to respond more favorably to treatment (Brent, Kolko, Birmaher *et al.*, 1998; Weersing, Iyengar, Kolko *et al.*, 2006).

Predictors of Outcome

Greater intake severity, older age of onset, low involvement in pleasurable activities, greater hopelessness and other cognitive distortions, history of sexual abuse and parental depression were found to be predictive of less positive response in CBT clinical trials (Barbe *et al.*, 2004; Brent, Kolko, Birmaher *et al.*, 1998; Clarke, Hops, Lewinsohn *et al.*, 1992;

Clarke, Hornbrook, Lynch *et al.*, 2001; Lewinsohn, Rohde, & Seeley, 1998; Rohde, Clarke, Lewinsohn *et al.*, 2001). Parental depressive symptoms moderated treatment response to CBT in so far as in the absence of maternal depression CBT was superior to alternative treatments whereas in its presence, CBT was no better than the alternatives (Brent, Kolko, Birmaher *et al.*, 1998; Lewinsohn, Rohde, & Seeley, 1998). Family discord and comorbid substance abuse predicted a slower response to treatment overall (Birmaher, Brent, Kolko *et al.*, 2000a; Rohde, Clarke, Lewinsohn *et al.*, 2001). In contrast, referral by advertisement as compared to clinical referral predicted a good response in all conditions, and comorbid anxiety disorder predicted a particularly positive response to CBT (Brent, Kolko, Birmaher *et al.*, 1998; Rohde, Clarke, Lewinsohn *et al.*, 2001). In some studies, changes in cognitive distortions or improvements in involvement in pleasurable activities are associated with improvement (Ackerson, Scogin, McKendree-Smith *et al.*, 1998; Kaufman, Rohde, Seeley *et al.*, 2005; Kolko, Brent, Baugher *et al.*, 2000). Findings from the TADS study were mostly but not completely consistent with the above-noted results. In contradistinction, greater cognitive distortion predicted *better* response, at least in the combination cell, and source of referral was unrelated to outcome. Higher family income (≥$75,000/year) also predicted better response to CBT, both alone and in combination with medication (Curry, Rohde, Simons *et al.*, 2006).

Prevention of Onset, Relapse or Recurrence

An adaptation of the CWD-A program reduced the risk of onset of major depression in two groups of at-risk adolescents, those with subsyndromal depression (15% in CBT versus 26% control; Clarke, Hawkins, Murphy *et al.*, 1995) and in at-risk adolescent offspring with either subsyndromal depression or a past history of depression or depressed parents (9% CBT versus 28% control; Clarke, Hornbrook, Lynch *et al.*, 2001). A meta-analysis of CBT prevention packages has found that selected or indicated interventions that focus on youth with subsyndromal symptoms show more positive effects than universal programs both at the end of the intervention (ES 0.30 versus 0.12) and upon follow-up (ES 0.31–0.34 versus 0.02), in part because at-risk youth continue to become more symptomatic over time (Horowitz & Garber, 2006).

With regard to the prevention of relapse, CBT does not appear to produce significantly greater benefit than other interventions at intermediate or long-term follow-up after brief acute treatment of depression (Birmaher, Brent, Kolko *et al.*, 2000a; Wood, Harrington, & Moore, 1996). While the addition of up to six individual CBT monthly booster sessions reduced the rate of relapse from 50% to 20%, the addition of 1–2 group or individual booster sessions did not, suggesting a dose effect (Birmaher, Brent, Kolko *et al.*, 2000a; Clarke, Lewinsohn, Rohde *et al.*, 1999; Kroll, Harrington, Jayson *et al.*, 1996). Although several studies highlight the role of family conflict in onset, duration of episode and risk of recurrence, family interventions have not yet been studied with regard to these outcomes.

Interpersonal Therapy (Table 37.4)

Theory and Techniques

Interpersonal psychotherapy for adolescents (IPT-A) is an adaptation of interpersonal therapy (IPT), a well-established efficacious treatment for adult unipolar depression (Mufson, Weissman, Moreau *et al.*, 1999). IPT-A conceptualizes depression as occurring within an interpersonal matrix, and targets resolution of interpersonal stress that seems to be associated with the adolescent's depression. IPT-A begins by taking an interpersonal inventory of important relationships in order to determine appropriate treatment targets. The types of problems typically targeted by IPT-A are loss, role disputes, role transitions, interpersonal skills deficits or adjustment to a single-parent family. The goal of treatment is to replace conflictual, unfulfilling relationships with meaningful lower-conflict relationships.

Evidence of IPT Efficacy

Mufson, Weissman, Moreau *et al.* (1999) conducted the first efficacy trial of IPT-A in a patient population of depressed adolescents. Forty-eight adolescents were randomized to either IPT-A or monthly clinical management. A much higher proportion of adolescents met recovery criteria (Hamilton Depression Scale-Depression ≤6) in the IPT-A group (75% versus 46%). There was a much higher attrition rate in the clinical monitoring group. Analyses of dimensional measures of depressive symptomatology, functional status and social adaptation also favored IPT-A.

In an independent investigation, Rossello and Bernal (1999) compared the efficacy of IPT, "culturally adapted" CBT, with a waitlist control condition in a sample of depressed Puerto Rican adolescents. There was a high rate of attrition, as only 68% and 52% of IPT and CBT-treated subjects completed the 12-session intervention. Using a clinical cut-off on the CDI in completer analyses, 59% of those in the CBT condition and 82% of those treated with IPT achieved a clinically significant improvement by post-treatment. Thus, on some measures of depression and functional status, IPT was superior to CBT.

Effectiveness

Mufson, Dorta, Wickramaratne *et al.* (2004) tested IPT-A versus usual care in school-based mental health clinics with school social workers delivering both interventions. Those in the IPT-A arm had a brief training in IPT-A and weekly supervision. IPT-A was superior to usual care on dimensional measures of depression, global function, social adjustment and global clinical status (50% versus 33% symptomatically improved). This strongly supports the transportability of IPT-A into community sites.

Predictors of Response and Adverse Events

Mufson, Weissman, Moreau *et al.* (1999) found that IPT-A was differentiated from clinical monitoring only in those sub-

Table 37.4 Interpersonal, family treatments for adolescents with depression. (After Weersing *et al.*, 2006.)

Study	*n*	Treatment and control conditions	Mean sessions	Source of sample	Definition of clinical response	Responding at post-treatment (%)	NNT	Primary symptom measure	Target treatment effect size (symptoms)
Brent *et al.* (1997)	107	Family Supportive CBT	10.7 11.2 12.1	Clinic diagnosed depression	No mood diagnosed and normal BDI	38 39 60	99	BDI	0.07
Diamond *et al.* (2002)	32	Family Waitlist	12 6 week	Unclear, screened for diagnosis	No mood diagnosed	81 47		BDI	0.75
Mufson *et al.* (1999)	48	Family Waitlist	9.8 2.8	Clinic diagnosed depression	Normal HAM-D	75 46	3	BDI	0.57
Mufson *et al.* (2004)	63	IPT-A School TAU	10.5 7.9	Community screened for diagnosis	Normal HAM-D	50 34	6	BDI	0.40
Rosello & Bernal (1999)	71	IPT-A CBT Waitlist	12 12	Community screened for diagnosis	Normal CDI	82 59	–	CDI	0.74
Young *et al.* (2006)	31	Family psychoeducation + TAU TAU	9.9 –	Clinic diagnosed depression	No MDD	79 50	4	RADS SSAI-A SSAI-P	0.52–0.64* 0.93–1.14 0.96–1.17

BDI, Beck Depression Inventory; CBT, Cognitive–behavior therapy; CDI, Children's Depression Inventory; Ham-D, Hamilton Rating Scale for Depression; IPT-A, Interpersonal psychotherapy for depressed adolescents; MDD, major depressive disorder; NNT, Number needed to treat; RADS, Reynolds Adolescent Depression Scale; SSAI, Structured Social Adjustment Interview (A, Adolescent, P, Parent); School TAU, school counseling services.

* At 6 and 9 months after intake.

jects who had moderate or severe depression. Improvements in depression were also associated with improvements in social functioning and problem-solving in IPT-A treatment (Mufson, Weissman, Moreau *et al.*, 1999, 2004). In a follow-up analysis of the school-based effectiveness study, comorbid anxiety was found to result in a poorer overall outcome with regard to depression. In the subgroup with comorbid anxiety, the effect size for IPT-A did appear to be larger than the effect size for usual care, although this escaped statistical significance (Young, Mufson, & Davies, 2006), similar to CBT trial results (Brent, Kolko, Birmaher *et al.*, 1998; Rohde, Clarke, Lewinsohn *et al.*, 2001). In one trial, the rate of suicidal events was similar in IPT-A and clinical management (Mufson, Weissman, Moreau *et al.*, 1999).

Prevention of Onset, Relapse or Recurrence

Thus far, there have been no prevention or continuation studies conducted, but one open study showed a high rate of sustained recovery 1 year after receipt of IPT-A (Mufson & Fairbanks, 1996).

Other Available Interventions

The involvement of family factors in the pathogenesis and recurrence of early-onset depression suggests that targeted family interventions aimed at reducing criticism, facilitating treatment of parental depression and increasing protective factors such as support and time spent together may prove to be efficacious. One study did not demonstrate superior efficacy of a systemic behavioral family therapy over supportive therapy (Brent, Holder, Kolko *et al.*, 1997). One small randomized treatment study found that a family intervention that focused on interpersonal attachment, when compared with a minimal contact waitlist control, resulted in a reduction in both depression and anxiety, with sustained improvement on 6-month follow-up (Diamond, Reis, Diamond *et al.*, 2002). One study piloted the additive benefit of "family psychoeducation" to treatment as usual for depressed adolescents (Sanford, Boyle, McCleary *et al.*, 2006). The treatment consisted of 12 90-minute sessions, and provided education about depression and its treatment, enhanced communication skills, family problem-solving, increasing support and decreased unproductive interactions. The family treatment resulted in improved social functioning in the adolescent, improved quality of parent–child relationship and a trend towards greater improvement in adolescent depressive symptoms.

An open trial of a new psychosocial treatment, Contextual Emotion-Regulation Therapy (CERT) was reported in 20 chronically depressed prepubertal children (Kovacs, Sherril, George *et al.*, 2006). CERT focuses on improving the depressed child's emotion regulation and coping skills, helping the child to identify triggers for mood dysregulation, and development of adaptive coping and problem-solving strategies to improve mood and overall functioning. Parents are involved as an "assistant coach," which also serves to strengthen the parent–child relationship. In open treatment, which consisted of 30 sessions delivered over 10 months, a very high proportion of children achieved remission of their depression (80%) and dysthymia (92%).

Beardslee, Gladstone, Wright *et al.* (2003) compared clinician-facilitated 6–11-session family psychoeducation with a didactic intervention for families with a depressed parent and non-depressed children aged 8–15. Both interventions aimed at demystifying depression, decreasing guilt and blame, and building resilience, with the clinician-facilitated intervention individualizing the intervention to the particular circumstances of each family. The children in both groups had a decrease in emotional disturbance, although there were no between-group differences (Beardslee *et al.*, 2003).

With regard to non-medication somatic treatments, light therapy has been shown to be beneficial for pediatric seasonal affective disorder (Swedo, Allen, Glod *et al.*, 1997). One small randomized trial of depressed children aged 6–12 found that treatment with omega-3 fatty acids (eicosapentanoic acid and docosahexanenoic acid) resulted in significant improvement in depressive symptoms, with effects comparable to those for SSRIs (Nemets, Nemets, Apter *et al.*, 2006). Although electroconvulsive therapy (ECT) has not been rigorously studied in adolescent depression, there is general clinical consensus that it has a role in the management of early-onset depression that is refractory to pharmacological and psychosocial management, particularly for adolescents without significant personality disorder traits (Walter & Rey, 2003).

Recommendations for Current Best Practice Treatment

Because there is a relatively high response rate to placebo or brief supportive treatment and education in many of the published treatment studies, the first approach for mild depression should be family education, supportive counseling, case management and problem-solving (Birmaher & Brent, 2007; Bridge, Iyengar, Salary *et al.*, 2007; Goodyer, 2006; NICE, 2005; Renaud, Brent, Baugher *et al.*, 1998). For more persistent or severe depression, one of the three empirically validated treatments, SSRI medication, CBT or IPT, is indicated. Current US guidelines recommend initial treatment with any of the three treatments for moderate depression, with the choice informed primarily by patient preference and the availability of local expertise. The British guidelines vary slightly in so far as they recommend use of an indicated psychotherapy for moderate to severe depression for 3 months prior to initiation of an antidepressant medication. They also emphasize that medication should not be given without concomitant psychotherapy.

Both sets of guidelines recommend continuing a given treatment for at least 6–8 weeks, assessing response to treatment and, if the patient is not responding, consider combination of psychotherapy and medication, a dose adjustment or switch in medication, or a medication augmentation strategy (Birmaher & Brent, 2007; NICE, 2005).

The extant evidence suggests that more generic psychotherapies practiced in the community may not be helpful in the treatment of youth depression (Brent, Holder, Kolko *et al.*, 1997; Weersing & Weisz, 2002; Weisz, McCarty, & Valeri, 2006; Wood, Harrington, & Moore, 1996). In the absence of available specialized psychotherapy, or in the face of a patient's disinclination to engage in psychotherapy, use of an antidepressant as a first-line intervention is indicated. Some evidence suggests that for more severely depressed adolescents, particularly those with difficulties with motivation, concentration, sleep and appetite, medication should be a first-line treatment (Curry, Rohde, Simons *et al.*, 2006; Goodyer, 2006). In adults, combination of psychotherapy and medication is superior to either monotherapy in chronic and severe depression, although the support for the use of combined treatment in younger populations is more modest (Clarke, Debar, Lynch *et al.*, 2005; Goodyer, 2006; Keller, McCullough, Klein *et al.*, 2000; March, Silva, Petrycki *et al.*, 2004; Thase, Greenhouse, Frank *et al.*, 1997). Relative contraindications for use of antidepressant medication are a history of mania or hypomania, when mood stabilization should be undertaken prior to the use of antidepressants, and for those with a strong family history of bipolar disorder, for whom it may be safer to begin with psychotherapy for the same reasons.

Given that the most evidence for efficacy exists for fluoxetine, this should be a first-line medication. For those who have failed to respond to fluoxetine, cannot tolerate it or for some reason do not wish to take it, use of one of the other SSRIs for which there is some evidence of efficacy is warranted. Current clinical recommendations are to begin with half the usual initial target dose (e.g., 10 mg fluoxetine) for 1 week, to determine if the patient can tolerate the medication, and then increase to 20 mg for the next 3 weeks. If the patient is still depressed, then one can continue to increase the dosage around every 4 weeks because it takes around that amount of time to tell if an increase is going to be helpful (Nierenberg, McLean, Alpert *et al.*, 1995). Most patients who respond to fluoxetine achieve symptomatic relief at 20–80 mg fluoxetine. Once symptomatic relief has been achieved, treatment should continue for a minimum of 6–12 months in order to prevent relapse.

If a patient fails to respond to a fluoxetine at an adequate dose and duration (i.e., around 40–80 mg), then it is reasonable to switch to another SSRI. However, it is important to rule out reasons for continued depression such as rapid drug metabolism, non-compliance, severe family conflict, parental depression, covert substance abuse or the influence of other comorbid conditions, such as OCD, ADHD or anxiety, an undiagnosed mixed state, psychosis, or medical illness, such as hypothyroidism. There are no empirical studies in adolescents to guide clinicians for patients who have failed to respond to an SSRI, although clinical guidelines based upon expert consensus exist (Birmaher & Brent, 2007; Hughes, Emslie, Crismon *et al.*, 1999). However, based on clinical consensus and some studies in adults, if one has obtained a partial response, it is reasonable to augment with lithium, another antidepressant such as amfebutamone, or one of the empirically supported psychotherapies. If one has obtained no response, a reasonable second step is to switch to a second SSRI, or to add psychotherapy. If after treatment with a second SSRI there is still complete non-response, most clinicians recommend using a different class of medication, such as venlafaxine, amfebutamone or lamotrigine (Birmaher & Brent, 2007).

Future Clinical and Research Challenges

Depression in childhood and adolescence is a complex and debilitating disease that frequently has a lifelong chronic recurrent course. In this concluding section, we focus on the unknowns of youth depression and suggest several key areas for future investigation.

Genetic and Environmental Determinants of Unipolar Depression

Adolescent depressive symptomatology is highly familial, with genetic and non-shared environmental factors each contributing half of the variance for familial occurrence. Future work should focus on identification of clinical endophenotypes (chronic depression, anxiety plus depression, "neuroticism") and those determined by laboratory measures (e.g., neurocognitive measures of emotional information processing and brain correlates thereof) that may help to more precisely map genes onto behavior. Moreover, it is critical that future research recognizes the importance of gene × environmental interactions, including seemingly environmental factors (e.g., life events) that in fact are genetically influenced. With a greater understanding of genetics, we can identify youth at risk, and use our knowledge of environment and gene × environment interaction to attenuate familial transmission.

Neurobiology of Depression

Functional neuroimaging shows promise of being able to delineate brain regions and circuitry most closely implicated in depressive onset and recovery, thereby helping to clarify both the clinical phenotype and potential targets for prevention and treatment. Neuroimaging studies of youth at high risk for depression may help to better identify the biological and genetic factors involved in the onset of depressive illness. Genetic neuroimaging, in which functional MRI (fMRI) tests the effects of genotype in moderating response to a specific probe, may be a particularly promising approach (Hariri, Mattay, Tessitore *et al.*, 2002). Moreover, neurobiological effects may not only be genetic, but be caused by early adversity or continued stress, including continued depression.

Matching Patients to Treatments

The approach to the treatment of pediatric depression is currently determined more by the comfort and expertise of the clinician than the patient profile, in part because of the lack of knowledge about how patient characteristics should inform treatment approach. Future studies should attempt to take what is known about treatment response to see if addressing those issues (e.g., comorbidity, parental depression) can actually improve treatment outcome. Remarkably, no studies have examined the relationship of drug level and metabolites to treatment outcome in any pharmacological clinical trial, which means that non-response and non-compliance cannot be distinguished. One possible promising measure for SSRI action is a measurement of platelet receptor serotonin reuptake inhibition. Moreover, future investigations should harness advances in genetics and neuroscience to predict individual differences in treatment response. More specifically, future studies should examine the relationship between candidate gene polymorphisms and treatment response, controlling for pharmacokinetic factors. Both pharmacological and psychotherapy studies should examine the impact of treatment on neurocognitive and neuroimaging measures, which may help elucidate mechanisms of action and also provide some clues as to how to further boost outcome.

Incomplete Symptomatic and Functional Recovery

In the TADS study, as is true in other pharmacological and psychotherapy trials, a very high rate of continued depressive symptoms and functional impairment was reported at the end of 12 weeks of treatment across treatments (Brent, Holder, Kolko *et al.*, 1997; Emslie, Rush, Weinberg *et al.*, 1997; Kennard, Silva, Vitiello *et al.*, 2006; Vitiello, Rohde, Silva *et al.*, 2006). While patients may continue to improve with time, the rate of incomplete recovery is high, which in turn increases the risk for another depressive episode, as well as interpersonal difficulties, educational underachievement, substance abuse, suicidal behavior and other health risk behaviors. There appear to be some common family and social factors that protect against most of these outcomes. Can a parsimonious treatment package such as "Well-Being Therapy" used by Fava in adults, be developed to improve overall functional outcome for depressed youth that increases these protective factors (Fava, Ruini, Rafanelli *et al.*, 2005)?

Management and Prevention of Suicidal Behavior

The most serious correlates of depressive disorder are suicidal ideation and behavior, which in depressed patients are associated with greater severity, chronicity and comorbidity (Lewinsohn, Rohde, & Seeley, 1996, 1998). It is an open question as to whether treatment of depression is sufficient to prevent suicidality or whether additional types of interventions are required, because reductions in depression and in suicidality do not always occur together (Harrington, Kerfoot, Dyer *et al.*, 1998b; Wood, Trainor, Rothwell, Moore *et al.*, 2001). However, patients with serious suicidality are often excluded from clinical trials, and suicidal outcomes are not often reported. Interventions, including those that involve the treatment of depression, can only be evaluated with regard to their impact on suicidal risk if patients at high suicidal risk are admitted to such studies. The design of studies that meet human subject standards is an important step to addressing this pressing issue. Our ability to predict and influence suicidality is particularly salient, given current concerns about suicidal adverse events in SSRI treatment. It is important to better understand the clinical, pharmacokinetic, pharmacogenetic and neurocognitive predictors of suicidal adverse events in youth treated with SSRIs.

Treatment of Prepubertal Depression

Currently, there are no established psychological approaches to prepubertal depression. Moreover, because in some studies the response to medication in pre-adolescent children was less vigorous than in adolescents, the role of antidepressants and psychological treatments needs focused evaluation in younger children.

Treatment of Bipolar Depression, and Youth At Risk for Bipolar Disorder

The pharmacological management of depression in youth at risk for bipolar disorder carries with it a risk for inducing a mixed or manic state, yet, at the same time, depressive symptoms are a considerable source of the morbidity of this condition. Research should address pharmacological and psychosocial approaches to the management of depression in those at risk for bipolar disorder, including identification of clinical, genetic and neurocognitive predictors of manic switch.

Early Intervention and Public Health Interventions

Convergent evidence supports the view that the more chronic the depression, the more difficult it becomes to treat. Yet tertiary care mental health is not equipped to facilitate early identification and intervention, because of inadequate capacity and other barriers to access such as stigma. Consequently, capacity for treatment of children at earlier stages of risk and disorder needs to be developed in other sectors, such as primary care and school-based mental health services. The cost-effectiveness of interventions delivered in alternative settings should be studied.

Another key factor in reducing the public health burden of depression likely will be the efficient dissemination of our best practice models to the youth health and education systems. As discussed on p. 593, there are still very few data on the effectiveness of SSRIs, CBT and IPT when delivered in actual practice settings. The data that are available on CBT and IPT are promising, suggesting that bringing these research-based psychosocial interventions to the community may substantially improve on current models of depression care. Similar data are not available for the SSRIs, despite the fact that SSRI prescriptions are dramatically more prevalent and are more available in community settings than either of the empirically based psychosocial interventions. In the adult literature, there is a growing evidence base on the efficacy and cost-effectiveness of relatively brief psychosocial, antidepressant and combined treatments for mild to moderate depression, delivered in settings such as primary care, that may serve as models for future investigations in younger populations (Katon, Unutzer, & Simon, 2004).

Decreasing the Public Burden of Depression

Two extreme views with regard to decreasing the public health burden of early-onset depression are well articulated by Harrington and Clarke (1998): on the one hand, focus the bulk of resources on the relatively small number with moderate to severe disease, or, alternatively, provide preventive intervention to those who are at risk or mildly depressed. From a public health point of view, the impairment burden on the population is mostly from "subsyndromal depression," so that a small reduction in depressive symptoms in a large number of people may indeed benefit more people. Horowitz and Garber (2006), in their meta-analysis, found much greater effect sizes for indicated and selective interventions, but acknowledged that the appropriate metric is really the cost per effect, which may be comparable with a cheaper, less selective intervention that does not involve the costs of screening. Harrington and Clarke (1998) argued that a universal approach that enhances protective factors such as problem-solving, interpersonal skills, family connection and school connection may be more acceptable and have broader impact. Research on the relative utility of these different approaches to prevention on the overall public mental health of youth is warranted.

References

Ackerson, J., Scogin, F., McKendree-Smith, N., & Lyman, R. D. (1998). Cognitive bibliotherapy for mild and moderate adolescent depressive symptomatology. *Journal of Consulting and Clinical Psychology*, *66*, 685–690.

Addolorato, G., Capristo, E., Stefanini, G., & Gasbarrini, G. (1997). Inflammatory bowel disease: A study of the association between anxiety and depression, physical morbidity, and nutritional status. *Scandinavian Journal of Gastroenterology*, *31*, 1013–1021.

American Psychiatric Association. (2000). *Diagnostic and Statistical Manual of Mental Disorders: DSM-IV-TR*. (4th edn.). Text revision. Washington, DC: American Psychiatric Association.

Angold, A., Costello, E. J., & Erkanli, A. (1999). Comorbidity. *Journal of Child Psychology and Psychiatry*, *40*, 57–87.

Angold, A., Costello, E. J., & Worthman, C. M. (1998). Puberty and depression: The roles of age, pubertal status and pubertal timing. *Psychological Medicine*, *28*, 51–61.

Angold, A., Prendergast, M., Cox, A., Rutter, M., & Harrington, R. (1995). The Child and Adolescent Psychiatric Assessment (CAPA). *Psychological Medicine*, *25*, 739–753.

Apter, A., Lipschitz, A., Fong, R., Carpenter, D. J., Krulewicz, S., Davies, J. T., *et al.* (2006). Evaluation of suicidal thoughts and behaviors in children and adolescents taking paroxetine. *Journal of Child and Adolescent Psychopharmacology*, *16*, 77–90.

Asarnow, J. R., Goldstein, M. J., Tompson, M., & Guthrie, D. (1993). One-year outcomes of depressive disorders in child psychiatric in-patients: Evaluation of the prognostic power of a brief measure of expressed emotion. *Journal of Child Psychology and Psychiatry*, *34*, 129–137.

Asarnow, J. R., Jaycox, L. H., Duan, N., LaBorde, A. P., Rea, M. M., Murray, P., *et al.* (2005). Effectiveness of a quality improvement intervention for adolescent depression in primary care clinics: a randomized controlled trial. *Journal of the American Medical Association*, *293*, 311–319.

Axelson, D., Perel, J., Birmaher, B., Rudolph, G., Nuss, S., & Brent, D. (2002). Sertraline pharmacokinetics and dynamics in adolescents. *Journal of the American Academy of Child and Adolescent Psychiatry*, *41*, 1037–1044.

Axelson, D. A., Perel, J. M., Birmaher, B., Rudolph, G., Nuss, S., Yurasits, L., *et al.* (2005). Platelet serotonin reuptake inhibition and response to SSRIs in depressed adolescents. *American Journal of Psychiatry*, *162*, 802–804.

Barbe, R. P., Bridge, J., Birmaher, B., Kolko, D. J., & Brent, D. A. (2004). Lifetime history of sexual abuse, clinical presentation, and outcome in a clinical trial for adolescent depression. *Journal of Clinical Psychiatry*, *65*, 77–83.

Beardslee, W., Gladstone, T. R. G., Wright, E. J., & Cooper, A. B. (2003). A family-based approached to the prevention of depressive symptoms in children at risk: Evidence of parental and child change. *Pediatrics*, *112*, e119–e131.

Beck, A. T., Rush, A. J., Shaw, B. F., & Emery, G. (1979). *Cognitive therapy of depression*. New York: Guilford Press.

Berard, R., Fong, R., Carpenter, D. J., Thomason, C., & Wilkinson, C. (2006). An international, multicenter, placebo-controlled trial of paroxetine in adolescents with Major Depressive Disorder. *Journal of Child and Adolescent Psychopharmacology*, *16*, 59–75.

Bertocci, M. A., Dah, R. E., Williamson, D. E., Isof, A. M., Birmaher, B., Axelson, D. A., *et al.* (2005). Subjective sleep complaints in pediatric depression: A controlled study and comparison with EEG measures of sleep and waking. *Journal of the American Academy of Child and Adolescent Psychiatry*, *44*, 1158–1166.

Birmaher, B., Arbelaez, C., & Brent, D. (2002). Course and outcome of child and adolescent major depressive disorder. *Child and Adolescent Psychiatric Clinics of North America*, *11*, 619–637.

Birmaher, B., Axelson, D., Strober, M., Gill, M. K., Valeri, S., Chiappetta, L., *et al.* (2006). Clinical course of children and adolescents with bipolar spectrum disorders. *Archives of General Psychiatry*, *63*, 175–183.

Birmaher, B., & Brent, D. (2007). Practice parameters for the assessment and treatment of children and adolescents with depressive disorders. *Journal of the American Academy of Child and Adolescent Psychiatry*, *46*, 1503–1526.

Birmaher, B., Brent, D. A., Kolko, D., Baugher, M., Bridge, J., Iyengar, S., *et al.* (2000a). Clinical outcome after short-term psychotherapy for adolescents with major depressive disorder. *Archives of General Psychiatry*, *57*, 29–36.

Birmaher, B., Dahl, R. E., Perel, J., Williamson, D. E., Nelson, B., Stull, S., *et al.* (1996a). Corticotropin-releasing hormone challenge in prepubertal major depression. *Biological Psychiatry*, *39*, 267–277.

Birmaher, B., Dahl, R. E., Williamson, D. E., Perel, J. M., Brent, D. A., Axelson, D. A., *et al.* (2000b). Growth hormone secretion in children and adolescents at high risk for major depressive disorder. *Archives of General Psychiatry*, *57*, 867–872.

Birmaher, B., Kaufman, J., Brent, D. A., Dahl, R. E., Perel, J. M., Al-Shabbout, M., *et al.* (1997). Neuroendocrine response to L-5-hydroxytryptophan in prepubertal children at high risk for major depressive disorder. *Archives of General Psychiatry*, *54*, 1113–1119.

Birmaher, B., Ryan, N. D., Williamson, D. E., Brent, D. A., Kaufman, J., Dahl, R. E., *et al.* (1996b). Child and adolescent depression: A review of the past 10 years. Part 1. *Journal of the American Academy of Child and Adolescent Psychiatry*, *35*, 1427–1439.

Birmaher, B., Williamson, D. E., Dahl, R. E., Axelson, D. A., Kaufman, J., Dorn, L., *et al.* (2004). Clinical presentation and course of depression in youth: Does onset in childhood differ from onset in adolescence? *Journal of the American Academy of Child and Adolescent Psychiatry*, *43*, 63–70.

Botteron, K. N., Raichle, M. E., Drevets, W. C., Heath, A. C., & Todd, R. D. (2002). Volumetric reduction in left subgenual prefrontal cortex in early onset depression. *Biological Psychiatry*, *51*, 342–344.

Brent, D. A. (2004). Antidepressants and pediatric depression: The risk of doing nothing. *New England Journal of Medicine*, *351*, 1598–1601.

Brent, D. A., Baugher, M., Bridge, J., Chen, J., & Beery, L. (1999). Age and sex-related risk factors for adolescent suicide. *Journal of the American Academy of Child and Adolescent Psychiatry*, *38*, 1497–1505.

Brent, D. A., & Birmaher, B. (2002). Adolescent depression. *New England Journal of Medicine*, *347*, 667–671.

Brent, D. A., Holder, D., Kolko, D., Birmaher, B., Baugher, M., Roth, C., *et al.* (1997). A clinical psychotherapy trial for adolescent depression comparing cognitive, family, and supportive treatments. *Archives of General Psychiatry*, *54*, 877–885.

Brent, D. A., Kolko, D., Birmaher, B., Baugher, M., Bridge, J., Roth, C., *et al.* (1998). Predictors of treatment efficacy in a clinical trial of three psychosocial treatments for adolescent depression. *Journal of the American Academy of Child and Adolescent Psychiatry*, *37*, 906–914.

Brent, D. A., Perper, J. A., Moritz, G., Allman, C., Schweers, J., Roth, C., *et al.* (1993). Psychiatric sequelae to the loss of an adolescent to suicide. *Journal of the American Academy of Child and Adolescent Psychiatry*, *32*, 509–517.

Brent, D. A., Poling, K., McKain, B., & Baugher, M. (1993). A psychoeducational program for families of affectively ill children and adolescents. *Journal of the American Academy of Child and Adolescent Psychiatry*, *32*, 770–774.

Breslau, N., Schultz, L., & Peterson, E. (1995). Sex differences in depression: A role for preexisting anxiety. *Psychiatry Research*, *58*, 1–12.

Bridge, J., Iyengar, S., Salary, C. B., Barbe, R. P., Birmaher, B., Pincus, H., *et al.* (2007). Clinical response and risk of reported suicidal ideation and suicide attempts in pediatric antidepressant treatment: A meta-analysis of randomized controlled trials. *Journal of the American Medical Association*, *297*, 1683–1696.

Bridge, J. A., Goldstein, T. R., & Brent, D. A. (2006). Adolescent suicide and suicidal behavior. *Journal of Child Psychology and Psychiatry*, *47*, 372–394.

Bruder, G. E., Stewart, J. W., Tenke, C. E., McGrath, P. J., Leite, P., Bhattacharya, N., *et al.* (2001). Electroencephalographic and perceptual asymmetry differences between responders and nonresponders to an SSRI antidepressant. *Biological Psychiatry*, *49*, 416–425.

Bruder, G. E., Tenke, C. E., Warner, V., Nomura, Y., Grillon, C., Hille, J., *et al.* (2005). Electroencephalographic measures of regional hemispheric activity in offspring at risk for depressive disorders. *Biological Psychiatry*, *57*, 328–335.

Campo, J. V., Dahl, R. E., Williamson, D. E., Birmaher, B., Perel, J. M., & Ryan, N. D. (2003). Gastrointestinal distress to serotonergic challenge: A risk marker for emotional disorder? *Journal of the American Academy of Child and Adolescent Psychiatry*, *42*, 1221–1226.

Caspi, A., Sugden, K., Moffitt, T. E., Taylor, A., Craig, I. W., Harrington, H., *et al.* (2003). Influence of life stress on depression: Moderation by a polymorphism in the 5-HT gene. *Science*, *301*, 386–389.

Clarke, G., Hops, H., Lewinsohn, P. M., Andrew, J., & Williams, J. (1992). Cognitive–behavioral group treatment of adolescent depression: Prediction of outcome. *Behavioral Therapy*, *23*, 341–354.

Clarke, G. C., Debar, L., Lynch, F., Powell, J., Gale, J., O'Connor, E., *et al.* (2005). A randomized effectiveness trial of brief cognitive-behavior therapy for depressed adolescents receiving antidepressant medication. *Journal of the American Academy of Child and Adolescent Psychiatry*, *44*, 888–898.

Clarke, G. N., Hawkins, W., Murphy, M., Sheeber, L. B., Lewinsohn, P. M., & Seeley, J. R. (1995). Targeted prevention of unipolar depressive disorder in an at-risk sample of high school adolescents: A randomized trial of group cognitive intervention. *Journal of the American Academy of Child and Adolescent Psychiatry*, *34*, 312–321.

Clarke, G. N., Hornbrook, M., Lynch, F., Polen, M., Gale, J., Beardslee, W., *et al.* (2001). A randomized trial of a group cognitive intervention for preventing depression in adolescent offspring of depressed parents. *Archives of General Psychiatry*, *58*, 1127–1134.

Clarke, G. N., Lewinsohn, P. M., Rohde, P., Hops, H., & Seeley, J. R. (1999). Cognitive–behavioral group treatment of adolescent depression: Efficacy of acute group treatment and booster sessions. *Journal of the American Academy of Child and Adolescent Psychiatry*, *38*, 272–279.

Conrad, M., & Hammen, C. (1993). Protective and resource factors in high- and low-risk children: A comparison of children with unipolar, bipolar, medically ill and normal mothers. *Development and Psychopathology*, *5*, 593–607.

Costello, E. J., Mustillo, S., Erkanli, A., Keeler, G., & Angold, A. (2003). Prevalence and development of psychiatric disorders in childhood and adolescence. *Archives of General Psychiatry*, *60*, 837–844.

Costello, E. J., Erkanli, A., & Angold, A. (2006). Is there an epidemic of child or adolescent depression? *Journal of Child Psychology and Psychiatry*, *47*, 1263–1271.

Curry, J., Rohde, P., Simons, S., Silva, S., Vitiello, B., Kratochvil, C., *et al.* (2006). Predictors and moderators of acute outcome in the Treatment for Adolescents with Depression Study (TADS). *Journal of the American Academy of Child and Adolescent Psychiatry*, *45*, 1427–1439.

Dahl, R. E. (2004). Regulation of sleep and arousal: Comments on Part VII. In R. E. Dahl, & L. P. Spear (Eds.), *Adolescent brain development: Vulerabilities and opportunities* (pp. 292–293). New York: New York Academy of Sciences.

Dahl, R. E., Birmaher, B., Williamson, D. E., Dorn, L., Perel, J., Kaufman, J., *et al.* (2000). Low growth hormone response to growth hormone-releasing hormone in child depression. *Biological Psychiatry*, *48*, 981–988.

Dahl, R. E., & Lewin, D. S. (2002). Pathways to adolescent health: Sleep regulation and behavior. *Journal of Adolescent Health*, *31*, 175–184.

Dahl, R. E., Ryan, N. D., Puig-Antich, J., Nguyen, N. A., Al-Shabbout, M., Meyer, V. A., *et al.* (1991). 24-hour cortisol measures in adolescents with major depression: A controlled study. *Biological Psychiatry*, *30*, 25–36.

Daley, S. E., Hammen, C., Davila, J., & Burge, D. (1998). Axis II symptomatology, depression, and life stress during the transition from adolescence to adulthood. *Journal of Consulting and Clinical Psychology*, *66*, 595–603.

D'Augelli, A. R., Grossman, A. H., Salter, N. P., Vasey, J. J., Starks, M. T., & Sinclair, K. O. (2005). Predicting the suicide attempts of lesbian, gay, and bisexual youth. *Suicide and Life-threatening Behavior*, *35*, 646–660.

Daviss, W. B., Bentivoglio, P., Racusin, R., Brown, K. M., Bostic, J. Q., & Wiley, L. (2001). Bupropion sustained release in adolescents with comorbid attention deficit hyperactivity disorder and depression. *Journal of the American Academy of Child and Adolescent Psychiatry*, *40*, 307–314.

Daviss, W. B., Perel, J. M., Brent, D. A., Axelson, D. A., Rudolph, G. R., Gilchrist, R., *et al.* (2006). Acute antidepressant response and plasma levels of bupropion and metabolites in a pediatric-aged sample: An exploratory study. *Therapeutic Drug Monitoring*, *28*, 190–198.

Dawson, G., Frey, K., Panagiotides, H., Osterling, J., & Hessl, D. (1997). Infants of depressed mothers exhibit atypical frontal brain activity: A replication and extension of previous findings. *Journal of Child Psychology and Psychiatry*, *38*, 179–186.

Diamond, G. S., Reis, B. F., Diamond, G. M., Siqueland, L., & Isaacs, L. (2002). Attachment based family therapy for depressed adolescents: A treatment development study. *Journal of the American Academy of Child and Adolescent Psychiatry*, *41*, 1190–1196.

Dierker, L., Albano, A. M., Clarke, G. N., Heimberg, R. G., Kendall, P. C., Merikangas, K. R., *et al.* (2001). Screening for anxiety and depression in early adolescence. *Journal of the American Academy of Child and Adolescent Psychiatry*, *40*, 929–936.

Drevets, W. C., Price, J. L., Simpson Jr, J. R., Todd, R. D., Reich, T., Vannier, M., *et al.* (1997). Subgenual prefrontal cortex abnormalities in mood disorders. *Nature*, *386*, 824–827.

Eaves, L., Silberg, J., & Erkanli, A. (2003). Resolving multiple epigenetic pathways to adolescent depression. *Journal of Child Psychology and Psychiatry*, *44*, 1006–1014.

Egger, H. L., Erkanli, A., Keeler, G., Potts, E., Walter, B. K., & Angold, A. (2006). Test–retest reliability of the Preschool Age Psychiatric Assessment (PAPA). *Journal of the American Academy of Child and Adolescent Psychiatry*, *45*, 538–549.

Ellis, B. J., & Garber, J. (2000). Psychosocial antecedents of variation in girls' pubertal timing: Maternal depression, stepfather presence, and marital and family stress. *Child Development*, *71*, 485–501.

Emslie, G., Heiligenstein, J. H., Wagner, K. D., Hoog, S. L., Ernest, D. E., Brown, E., *et al.* (2002). Fluoxetine for acute treatment of depression in children and adolescents: A placebo-controlled, randomized clinical trial. *Journal of the American Academy of Child and Adolescent Psychiatry*, *41*, 1205–1215.

Emslie, G., Kratochvil, C., Vitiello, B., Silva, S., Mayes, T., McNulty, S., *et al.* (2006). Treatment for Adolescents with Depression Study (TADS): Safety results. *Journal of the American Academy of Child and Adolescent Psychiatry*, *45*, 1440–1455.

Emslie, G., Rush, J. A., Weinberg, W. A., Kowatch, R. A., Hughes, C. W., Carmody, T., *et al.* (1997). A double-blind, randomized placebo-controlled trial of fluoxetine in children and adolescents with depression. *Archives of General Psychiatry*, *54*, 1031–1037.

Emslie, G. J., Heiligenstein, J. H., Hoog, S. L., Wagner, K. D., Findling, R. L., McCracken, J. T., *et al.* (2004). Fluoxetine treatment for prevention of relapse of depression in children and adolescents: A double-blind, placebo-controlled study. *Journal of the American Academy of Child and Adolescent Psychiatry*, *43*, 1397–1405.

Emslie, G. J., Rush, A. J., Weinberg, W. A., Kowatch, R. A., Carmody, T., & Mayes, T. L. (1998). Fluoxetine in child and adolescent depression: Acute and maintenance treatment. *Depression and Anxiety*, *7*, 32–39.

Emslie, G. J., Wagner, K. D., Kutcher, S., Krulewicz, S., Fong, R., Carpenter, D. J., *et al.* (2006). Paroxetine treatment in children and adolescents with major depressive disorder: A randomized, multicenter, double-blind, placebo-controlled trial. *Journal of the American Academy of Child and Adolescent Psychiatry*, *45*, 709–719.

Emslie, G. J., Yeung, P. P., Kunz, N. R., & Li, Y. (2007). Venlafaxine ER for the treatment of pediatric subjects with de-pression: Results of two placebo-controlled trials. *Journal of the American Academy of Child and Adolescent Psychiatry*, *46*, 479–488.

Faraone, S. V., & Biederman, J. (1997). Do attention deficit hyperactivity disorder and major depression share familial risk factors? *Journal of Nervous and Mental Disease*, *185*, 533–541.

Farchione, T. R., Moore, G. T., & Rosenberg, D. R. (2002). Proton magnetic resonance spectroscopic imaging in pediatric major depression. *Biological Psychiatry*, *52*, 86–92.

Fava, G. A., Ruini, C., Rafanelli, C., Finos, L., Salmaso, L., Mangelli, L., *et al.* (2005). Well-being therapy of generalized anxiety disorder. *Psychotherapy and Psychosomatics*, *74*, 26–30.

Feder, A., Coplan, J. D., Goetz, R. R., Mathew, S. J., Pine, D. S., Dahl, R. E., *et al.* (2004). Twenty-four-hour cortisol secretion patterns in prepubertal children with anxiety or depressive disorders. *Biological Psychiatry*, *56*, 198–204.

Fergusson, D. M., Horwood, J., & Beautrais, A. L. (1999). Is sexual orientation related to mental health problems and suicidality in young people? *Archives of General Psychiatry*, *56*, 876–880.

Fergusson, D. M., Horwood, L., & Lynskey, M. T. (1996). Childhood sexual abuse and psychiatric disorder in young adulthood. II. Psychiatric outcomes of childhood sexual abuse. *Journal of the American Academy of Child and Adolescent Psychiatry*, *35*, 1365–1374.

Fergusson, D. M., Horwood, L. J., Ridder, E. M., & Beautrais, A. L. (2005). Subthreshold depression in adolescence and mental health outcomes in adulthood. *Archives of General Psychiatry*, *62*, 66–72.

Fergusson, D. M., & Lynskey, M. T. (1996). Adolescent resiliency to family adversity. *Journal of Child Psychology and Psychiatry*, *37*, 281–292.

Fergusson, D. M., Wanner, B., Vitaro, F., Horwood, L. J., & Swain-Campbell, N. (2003). Deviant peer affiliations and depression: confounding or causation? *Journal of Abnormal Child Psychology*, *31*, 605–618.

Fergusson, D. M., & Woodward, L. J. (2002). Mental health, educational, and social role outcomes of adolescents with depression. *Archives of General Psychiatry*, *59*, 225–231.

Findling, R. L., McNamara, N. K., Stansbrey, R. J., Feeny, N. C., Young, C. M., Peric, F. V., *et al.* (2006). The relevance of pharmacokinetic studies in designing efficacy trials in juvenile major depression. *Journal of Child and Adolescent Psychopharmacology*, *16*, 131–145.

Forbes, E. E., Fox, N. A., Cohn, J., Galles, S., & Kovacs, M. (2006a). Children's affect regulation during a disappointment: Psychophysiological responses and relation to parent history of depression. *Biological Psychiatry*, *71*, 264–277.

Forbes, E. E., Shaw, D. S., Fox, N. A., Cohn, J. F., Silk, J. S., & Kovacs, M. (2006b). Maternal depression, child frontal asymmetry, and child affective behavior as factors in child behavior problems. *Journal of Child Psychology and Psychiatry*, *47*, 79–87.

Forbes, E. E., May, C., Siegle, G. J., Ladouceur, C. D., Ryan, N. D., Carter, C. S., *et al.* (2006c). Reward-related decision-making in pediatric major depressive disorder: An fMRI study. *Journal of Child Psychology and Psychiatry*, *47*, 1031–1040.

Frye, A. A., & Garber, J. (2005). The relations among maternal depression, maternal criticism, and adolescents' externalizing and internalizing symptoms. *Journal of Abnormal Child Psychology*, *33*, 1–11.

Garber, J., & Flynn, C. (2001). Predictors of depressive cognitions in young adolescents. *Cognitive Therapy and Research*, *25*, 353–376.

Garber, J., Keiley, M. K., & Martin, N. C. (2002). Developmental trajectories of adolescents' depressive symptoms: Predictors of change. *Journal of Consulting and Clinical Psychology*, *70*, 79–95.

Garber, J., & Robinson, N. S. (1997). Cognitive vulnerability in children at risk for depression. *Cognition and Emotion*, *11*, 619–635.

Geller, B., Zimerman, B., Williams, M., Bolhofner, K., & Craney, J. L. (2001). Bipolar disorder at prospective follow-up of adults who had prepubertal major depression disorder. *American Journal of Psychiatry*, *158*, 125–127.

Gibbons, R. D., Hur, K., Bhaumik, D. K., & Mann, J. J. (2006). The relationship between antidepressant medication use and rate of early adolescent suicide. *American Journal of Psychiatry*, *163*, 1898–1904.

Glowinski, A. L., Madden, P. A. F., Bucholz, K. K., Lynskey, M. T., & Heath, A. C. (2003). Genetic epidemiology of self-reported lifetime DSM-IV major depressive disorder in a population-based twin sample of female adolescents. *Journal of Child Psychology and Psychiatry and Allied Disciplines*, *44*, 988–996.

Goldstein, B. J., & Goodnick, P. J. (1998). Selective serotonin reuptake inhibitors in the treatment of affectives disorders. III. Tolerability, safety and pharmacoeconomics. *Journal of Psychopharmacology*, *12*, S55–S87.

Goodwin, R. D., Fergusson, D. M., & Horwood, L. J. (2004a). Asthma and depressive and anxiety disorders among young persons in the community. *Psychological Medicine*, *34*, 1465–1474.

Goodwin, R. D., Fergusson, D. M., & Horwood, L. J. (2004b). Early anxious/withdrawn behaviours predict later internalising disorders. *Journal of Child Psychology and Psychiatry*, *45*, 874–883.

Goodyer, I. M. (2002). Social adversity and mental functions in adolescents at high risk of psychopathology. *British Journal of Psychiatry*, *181*, 383–386.

Goodyer, I. M. (2006). *A randomised controlled trial of SSRIs with and without cognitive behaviour therapy in adolescents with major depression*. Cambridge, UK: NHS Research and Development Co-ordinating Centre for Health Technology Assessment (HTA).

Goodyer, I. M., Herbert, J., & Tamplin, A. (2003). Psychoendocrine antecedents of persistent first-episode major depression in adolescents: A community-based longitudinal enquiry. *Psychological Medicine*, *33*, 601–610.

Goodyer, I. M., Herbert, J., Tamplin, A., & Altham, P. M. (2000). First-episode major depression in adolescents. Affective, cognitive and endocrine characteristics of risk status and predictors of onset. *British Journal of Psychiatry*, *176*, 142–149.

Gould, M. S., King, R., Greenwald, S., Fisher, P., Schwab-Stone, M., Kramer, R., *et al.* (1998). Psychopathology associated with suicidal ideation and attempts among children and adolescents. *Journal of the American Academy of Child and Adolescent Psychiatry*, *37*, 915–923.

Graber, J. A., Seeley, J. R., Brooks-Gunn, J., & Lewinsohn, P. M. (2004). Is pubertal timing associated with psychopathology in young adulthood? *Journal of the American Academy of Child and Adolescent Psychiatry*, *43*, 718–726.

Hamilton, J. A., & Bridge, J. (1999). Outcome at 6 months for 50 adolescents with major depression treated in a health maintenance organization. *Journal of the American Academy of Child and Adolescent Psychiatry*, *38*, 1340–1346.

Hammad, T. A., Laughren, T., & Racoosin, J. (2006). Suicidality in pediatric patients treated with antidepressant drugs. *Archives of General Psychiatry*, *63*, 332–339.

Hammen, C. (1988). Self-cognitions, stressful events, and the prediction of depression in children of depressed mothers. *Journal of Abnormal Child Psychology*, *16* (3), 347–360.

Hammen, C., Burge, D., & Stansbury, K. (1990). Relationship of mother and child variables to child outcomes in a high-risk sample: A causal modeling analysis. *Developmental Psychology*, *26*, 24–30.

Hammen, C., Rudolph, K., Weisz, J., Rao, U., & Burge, D. (1999). The context of depression in clinic-referred youth: Neglected areas in treatment. *Journal of the American Academy of Child and Adolescent Psychiatry*, *38*, 64–71.

Hariri, A. R., Mattay, V. S., Tessitore, A., Kolachana, B., Fera, F., Goldman, D., *et al.* (2002). Serotonin transporter genetic variation and the response of the human amygdala. *Science*, *297*, 400–403.

Harrington, R. (2000). Childhood depression: Is is the same disorder? In J. Rapoport (Ed.), *Childhood onset of "adult" psychopathology: Clinical and research advances* (pp. 223–243). Washington: American Psychiatric Publishing.

Harrington, R., & Clark, A. (1998). Prevention and early intervention for depression in adolescence and early adult life. *European Archives of Psychiatry and Clinical Neuroscience*, *248*, 32–45.

Harrington, R., Kerfoot, M., Dyer, E., McNiven, F., Gill, J., Harrington, V., *et al.* (1998). Randomized trial of a home-based family intervention for children who have deliberately poisoned themselves. *Journal of the American Academy of Child and Adolescent Psychiatry*, *37*, 512–518.

Harrington, R., Rutter, M., Weissman, M., Fudge, H., Groothues, C., Bredenkamp, D., *et al.* (1997). Psychiatric disorders in the relatives of depressed probands. I. Comparison of prepubertal, adolescent and early adult onset cases. *Journal of Affective Disorders*, *42*, 9–22.

Hazell, P., O'Connell, D., Heathcote, D., Robertson, J., & Henry, D. (1995). Efficacy of tricyclic drugs in treating child and adolescent depression: A meta-analysis. *British Medical Journal*, *310*, 897–901.

Heiligenstein, J., Hoog, S. L., Wagner, K. D., Findling, R. L., Galil, N., Kaplan, S., *et al.* (2006). Fluoxetine 40–60 mg versus fluoxetine 20 mg in the treatment of children and adolescents with a less-than-complete response to nine-week treatment with fluoxeting 10–20 mg: A pilot study. *Journal of Child and Adolescent Psychopharmacology*, *16*, 207–217.

Hollon, S. D., Garber, J., & Shelton, R. C. (2005). Treatment of depression in adolescents with cognitive behavior therapy and medications: A commentary on the TADS project. *Cognitive and Behavioral Practice*, *12*, 149–155.

Horowitz, J. L., & Garber, J. (2006). The prevention of depressive symptoms in children and adolescents: A meta-analytic review. *Journal of Consulting and Clinical Psychology*, *74*, 401–415.

Hudziak, J. J., Rudiger, L. P., Neale, M. C., Heath, A. C., & Todd, R. D. (2000). A twin study of inattentive, aggressive, and anxious/depressed behaviors. *Journal of the American Academy of Child and Adolescent Psychiatry*, *39*, 469–476.

Hughes, C. W., Emslie, G. J., Crismon, L., Wagner, K. D., Birmaher, B., Geller, B., *et al.* (1999). The Texas children's medication algorithm project: Report of the Texas consensus conference panel on medication treatment of childhood major depressive disorder. *Journal of the American Academy of Child and Adolescent Psychiatry*, *38*, 1442–1454.

Ivarsson, T., Broberg, A. G., Arvidsson, T., & Gillberg, C. (2005). Bullying in adolescence: Psychiatric problems in victims and bullies as measured by the youth self report (YSR) and the depression self-rating scale (DSRS). *Nordic Journal of Psychiatry*, *59*, 365–373.

Jaffee, S. R., Moffitt, T. E., Caspi, A., Fombonne, E., Poulton, R., & Martin, J. (2002). Differences in early childhood risk factors for juvenile-onset and adult-onset depression. *Archives of General Psychiatry*, *59*, 215–222.

Jones, J. E., Hermann, B. P., Barry, J. J., Gilliam, F. G., Kanner, A. M., & Meador, K. J. (2003). Rates and risk factors for suicide, suicidal ideation, and suicide attempts in chronic epilepsy. *Epilepsy and Behavior*, *4* (Supplement 3), S31–S38.

Kaltiala-Heino, R., Rimpela, M., Rantanen, P., & Rimpela, A. (2000). Bullying at school: An indicator of adolescents at risk for mental disorders. *Journal of Adolescence*, *23*, 661–674.

Katon, W. J., Unutzer, J., & Simon, G. (2004). Treatment of depression in primary care: Where we are, where we can go. *Medical Care*, *42*, 1153–1157.

Kaufman, J., Birmaher, B., Brent, D., Dahl, R., Bridge, J., & Ryan, N. D. (1998a). Psychopathology in the relatives of depressed-abused children. *Child Abuse and Neglect*, *22*, 171–181.

Kaufman, J., Birmaher, B., Brent, D., Rao, U., Flynn, C., Moreci, P., *et al.* (1997a). Schedule for Affective Disorders and Schizophrenia for School-Age Children-Present and Lifetime version (K-SADS-PL): Initial reliability and validity data. *Journal of the American Academy of Child and Adolescent Psychiatry*, *36*, 980–988.

Kaufman, J., Birmaher, B., Perel, J., Dahl, R., Stull, S., Brent, D., *et al.* (1998b). Serotonergic functioning in depressed abused children: Clinical and familial correlates. *Biological Psychiatry*, *44*, 973–981.

Kaufman, J., Birmaher, B., Perel, J., Dahl, R. E., Moreci, P., Nelson, B., *et al.* (1997b). The corticotropin-releasing hormone challenge in depressed abused, depressed nonabused, and normal control children. *Biological Psychiatry*, *42*, 669–679.

Kaufman, J., & Charney, D. (2001). Effects of early stress on brain structure and function: Implications for understanding the relationship between child maltreatment and depression. *Development and Psychopathology*, *13*, 451–471.

Kaufman, J., Yang, B. Z., Douglas-Palumberi, H., Grasso, D., Lipschitz, D., Houshyar, S., *et al.* (2006). Brain-derived neurotrophic factor-5-HHTLPR gene interactions and environmental modifiers of depression in children. *Biological Psychiatry*, *59*, 673–680.

Kaufman, N. K., Rohde, P., Seeley, J. R., Clarke, G. N., & Stice, E. (2005). Potential mediators of cognitive–behavioral therapy for adolescents with comorbid major depression and conduct disorder. *Journal of Consulting and Clinical Psychology*, *73*, 38–46.

Keller, M., Ryan, N. D., Strober, M., Klein, R. G., Kutcher, S. P., Birmaher, B., *et al.* (2001). Efficacy of paroxetine in the treatment of adolescent major depression: A randomized, controlled study. *Journal of the American Academy of Child and Adolescent Psychiatry*, *40*, 762–772.

Keller, M. B., McCullough, J. P., Klein, D. N., Arnow, B., Dunner, D. L., Gelenberg, A. J., *et al.* (2000). A comparison of nefazodone, the cognitive behavioral-analysis system of psychotherapy, and their combination for the treatment of chronic depression. *New England Journal of Medicine*, *342*, 1462–1470.

Kelvin, R. G., Goodyer, I. M., Teasdale, J. D., & Brechin, D. (1999). Latent negative self-schema and high emotionality in well adolescents at risk for psychopathology. *Journal of Child Psychology and Psychiatry*, *40*, 959–968.

Kennard, B., Silva, S., Vitiello, B., Curry, J., Kratochvil, C., Simons, A., *et al.* (2006). Remission and residual symptoms after acute treatment of adolescents with major depressive disorder. *Journal of the American Academy of Child and Adolescent Psychiatry*, *45*, 1404–1411.

Kentgen, L. M., Tenke, C. E., Pine, D. S., Fong, R., Klein, R. G., & Bruder, G. E. (2000). Electroencephalographic asymmetries in adolescents with major depression: Influence of comorbidity with anxiety disorders. *Journal of Abnormal Psychology*, *109*, 797–802.

King, R. A., Schwab-Stone, M., Flisher, A. J., Greenwald, S., Kramer, R. A., Goodman, S. H., *et al.* (2001). Psychosocial and risk behavior correlates of youth suicide attempts and suicidal ideation. *Journal of the American Academy of Child and Adolescent Psychiatry*, *40*, 837–846.

Klein, D. N., Lewinsohn, P. M., Rohde, P., Seeley, J. R., & Olino, T. M. (2005). Psychopathology in the adolescent and young adult offspring of a community sample of mothers and fathers with major depression. *Psychological Medicine*, *35*, 353–365.

Kolko, D. J., Brent, D. A., Baugher, M., Bridge, J., & Birmaher, B. (2000). Cognitive and family therapies for adolescent depression: Treatment specificity, mediation, and moderation. *Journal of Consulting and Clinical Psychology*, *68*, 603–614.

Kovacs, M. (1985). The children's depression inventory (CDI). *Psychopharmacology Bulletin*, *21*, 995–998.

Kovacs, M. (1996). Presentation and course of major depressive disorder during childhood and later years of the life span. *Journal of the American Academy of Child and Adolescent Psychiatry*, *35*, 705–715.

Kovacs, M., & Devlin, B. (1998). Internalizing disorders in childhood. *Journal of Child Psychology and Psychiatry*, *39*, 47–63.

Kovacs, M., Feinberg, T., Crouse-Novak, M., Paulauskas, S., Pollock, M., & Finkelstein, R. (1984a). Depressive disorders in childhood. I. A longitudinal study of characteristics and recovery. *Archives of General Psychiatry*, *41*, 229–237.

Kovacs, M., Feinberg, T., Crouse-Novak, M., Paulauskas, S., Pollock, M., & Finkelstein, R. (1984b). Depressive disorders in childhood. II. A longitudinal study of the risk for a subsequent major depression. *Archives of General Psychiatry*, *41*, 643–649.

Kovacs, M., & Gatsonis, C. (1994). Secular trends in age at onset of major depressive disorder in a clinical sample of children. *Journal of Psychiatric Research*, *28*, 319–329.

Kovacs, M., Goldston, D., Obrosky, D. S., & Bonar, L. K. (1997). Psychiatric disorders in youths with IDDM: Rates and risk factors. *Diabetes Care*, *20*, 36–44.

Kovacs, M., Sherril, J., George, C. J., Pollock, M., Tumuluru, R. V., & Ho, V. (2006). Contextual emotion-regulation therapy for childhood depression: Description and pilot testing of a new intervention. *Journal of the American Academy of Child and Adolescent Psychiatry*, *45*, 892–903.

Kramer, R. A., Warner, V., Olfson, M., Ebanks, C. M., Chaput, F., & Weissman, M. M. (1998). General medical problems among the offspring of depressed parents: A 10-year follow-up. *Journal of the American Academy of Child and Adolescent Psychiatry*, *37*, 602–611.

Kroll, L., Harrington, R., Jayson, D., & Fraser, J. (1996). Pilot study of continuation cognitive-behavioral therapy for major depression in adolescent psychiatric patients. *Journal of the American Academy of Child and Adolescent Psychiatry*, *35*, 1156–1161.

Kuo, P. H., Gardner, C. O., Kendler, K. S., & Prescott, C. A. (2006). The temporal relationship of the onsets of alcohol dependence and major depression: Using a genetically informative study design. *Psychological Medicine*, *36*, 1153–1162.

Kyte, Z. A., Goodyer, I. M., & Sahakian, B. J. (2006). Selected executive skills in adolescents with recent first episode major depression. *Journal of Child Psychology and Psychiatry*, *46*, 995–1005.

Labellarte, M. J., Biederman, J., Emslie, G., Ferguson, J., Khan, A., Ruckle, J., *et al.* (2004). Multiple-dose pharmacokinetics of fluvoxamine in children and adolescents. *Journal of the American Academy of Child and Adolescent Psychiatry*, *43*, 1497–1505.

Ladouceur, C. D., Dahl, R. E., Williamson, D. E., Birmaher, B., Ryan, N. D., & Casey, B. J. (2005). Altered emotional processing in pediatric anxiety, depression and comorbid anxiety-depression. *Journal of Abnormal Child Psychology*, *33*, 165–177.

Lerer, B., & Macciardi, F. (2002). Pharmacogenetics of antidepressant and mood-stabilizing drugs: A review of candidate-gene studies and future research. *International Journal of Neuropsychopharmacology*, *5*, 255–275.

Lewinsohn, P. M., Clarke, G. N., Hops, H., & Andrews, J. (1990). Cognitive–behavioral treatment for depressed adolescents. *Behavior Therapy*, *21*, 385–401.

Lewinsohn, P. M., Joiner, T. E., & Rohde, P. (2001). Evaluation of cognitive diathesis–stress models in predicting major depressive disorder in adolescents. *Journal of Abnormal Psychology*, *110*, 203–215.

Lewinsohn, P. M., Rohde, P., & Seeley, J. R. (1996). Adolescent suicidal ideation and attempts: Prevalence, risk factors, and clinical implications. *Clinical Psychology: Science and Practice*, *3*, 25–46.

Lewinsohn, P. M., Rohde, P., & Seeley, J. R. (1998). Major depressive disorder in older adolescents: Prevalence, risk factors, and clinical implications. *Clinical Psychology Review*, *18*, 765–794.

Lewinsohn, P. M., Rohde, P., Seeley, J. R., Klein, D. N., & Gotlib, I. H. (2003). Psychosocial functioning of young adults who have experienced and recovered from major depressive disorder during adolescence. *Journal of Abnormal Psychology*, *112*, 353–363.

Libby, A. M., Orton, H. D., Stover, S. K., & Riggs, P. D. (2005). What came first, major depression or substance use disorder? Clinical characteristics and substance use comparing teens in a treatment cohort. *Addictive Behaviors*, *30*, 1649–1662.

Luby, J. L., Heffelfinger, A. K., Mrakotsky, C., Brown, K. M., Hessler, M. J., Wallis, J. M., *et al.* (2003). The clinical picture of depression in preschool children. *Journal of the American Academy of Child and Adolescent Psychiatry*, *42*, 340–348.

Luby, J. L., Heffelfinger, A., Koenig-McNaught, A. L., Brown, K., & Spitznagel, E. (2004). The Preschool Feelings Checklist: A brief and sensitive screening measure for depression in young children. *Journal of the American Academy of Child and Adolescent Psychiatry*, *43*, 708–717.

Lyoo, I. K., Kyu Lee, H., Hyun Jung, J., Noam, G. G., & Renshaw, P. F. (2002). White matter hyperintensities on magnetic resonance imaging of the brain in children with psychiatric disorders. *Comprehensive Psychiatry*, *43*, 361–368.

Lyubomirsky, S., Caldwell, N. D., & Nolen-Hoeksema, S. (1998). Effects of ruminative and distracting responses to depressed mood on retrieval of autobiographical memories. *Journal of Personality and Social Psychology*, *75*, 166–177.

March, J. S., Silva, S., Petrycki, S., Curry, J., Wells, K., Fairbank, J., *et al.* (2004). Fluoxetine, cognitive–behavioral therapy, and their combination for adolescents with depression. Treatment for Adolescent Depression Study (TADS) randomized controlled trial. *Journal of the American Medical Association*, *292*, 807–820.

Martin, A., Young, C., Leckman, J. F., Mukonoweshuro, C., Rosenheck, R., & Leslie, D. (2004). Age effects on antidepressant-induced manic conversion. *Archives of Pediatrics and Adolescent Medicine*, *158*, 773–780.

McGuffin, P., Knight, J., Breen, G., Brewster, S., Boyd, P. R., Craddock, N., *et al.* (2005). Whole genome linkage scan of recurrent depressive disorder from the depression network. *Human Molecular Genetics*, *14*, 3337–3345.

Middeldorp, C. M., Cath, D. C., van Dyck, R., & Boomsma, D. I. (2005). The co-morbidity of anxiety and depression in the perspective of genetic epidemiology: A review of twin and family studies. *Psychological Medicine*, *35*, 611–624.

Mirza, Y., Tang, J., Russell, A., Banerjee, P., Bhandari, R., Ivey, J., *et al.* (2004). Reduced anterior cingulate cortex glutamatergic concentrations in childhood major depression. *Journal of the American Academy of Child and Adolescent Psychiatry*, *43*, 341–348.

Mufson, L., Dorta, K. P., Wickramaratne, P., Nomura, Y., Olfson, M., & Weissman, M. M. (2004). A randomized effectiveness trial of interpersonal psychotherapy for depressed adolescents. *Archives of General Psychiatry*, *61*, 577–584.

Mufson, L., & Fairbanks, J. (1996). Interpersonal psychotherapy for depressed adolescents: A one-year naturalistic follow-study. *Journal of the American Academy of Child and Adolescent Psychiatry*, *35*, 1145–1155.

Mufson, L., Weissman, M. M., Moreau, D., & Garfinkel, R. (1999). Efficacy of interpersonal psychotherapy for depressed adolescents. *Archives of General Psychiatry*, *56*, 573–579.

Mulder, R. T., Watkins, W. G. A., Joyce, P. R., & Luty, S. E. (2003). Age may affect response to antidepressants with serotonergic and noradrenergic actions. *Journal of Affective Disorders*, *76*, 143–149.

Myers, K., & Winters, N. C. (2002). Ten-year review of rating scales. II. Scales for internalizing disorders. *Journal of the American Academy of Child and Adolescent Psychiatry*, *41*, 634–659.

National Institute for Health and Clinical Excellence (NICE). (2005). *Depression in children and young people. Identification and management in primary, community, and secondary care*. Developed by the National Collaborating Centre for Mental Health.

Nemets, H., Nemets, B., Apter, A., Bracha, Z., & Belmaker, R. H. (2006). Omega-3 treatment of childhood depression: A controlled, double-blind pilot study. *American Journal of Psychiatry*, *163*, 1098–1100.

Nierenberg, A. A., McLean, N. E., Alpert, J. E., Worthington, J. J., Rosenbaum, J. F., & Fava, M. (1995). Early nonresponse to fluoxetine as a predictor of poor 8-week outcome. *American Journal of Psychiatry*, *152*, 1500–1503.

Nolan, C. L., Moore, G. J., Madden, R., Farchione, T., Bartoi, M., Lorch, E., *et al.* (2002). Prefrontal cortical volume in childhood-onset major depression. *Archives of General Psychiatry*, *59*, 173–179.

Nolen-Hoeksema, S., Larson, J., & Grayson, C. (1999). Explaining the gender difference in depressive symptoms. *Journal of Personality and Social Psychology*, *77*, 1061–1072.

O'Connor, T. G., Neiderhiser, J. M., Reiss, D., Hetherington, E. M., & Plomin, R. (1998). Genetic contributions to continuity, change, and co-occurrence of antisocial and depressive symptoms in adolescence. *Journal of Child Psychology and Psychiatry*, *39*, 323–336.

Olfson, M., Shaffer, D., Marcus, S. C., & Greenberg, T. (2003). Relationship between antidepressant medication treatment and suicide in adolescents. *Archives of General Psychiatry*, *60*, 978–982.

Park, R. J., Goodyer, I. M., & Teasdale, J. D. (2005). Self-devaluative dysphoric experience and the prediction of persistent first-episode major depressive disorder in adolescents. *Psychological Medicine*, *35*, 539–548.

Park, R. J., Goodyer, I. M., & Teasdale, J. D. (2002). Categoric overgeneral autobiographical memory in adolescents with major depressive disorder. *Psychological Medicine*, *32*, 267–276.

Pine, D., Coplan, J., Wasserman, G. A., Miller, L. S., Fried, J. E., Davies, M., *et al.* (1997). Neuroendocrine response to fenfluramine challenge in boys: Associations with aggressive behavior and adverse rearing. *Archives of General Psychiatry*, *54*, 839–846.

Pine, D. S. (2004). Face-memory and emotion: Associations with major depression in children and adolescents. *Journal of Child Psychology and Psychiatry*, *45*, 1199–1208.

Pine, D. S., Cohen, P., & Brook, J. (2001). Adolescent fears as predictors of depression. *Biological Psychiatry*, *50*, 721–724.

Pine, D. S., Cohen, P., Gurley, D., Brook, J., & May, Y. (1998). The risk for early-adulthood anxiety and depressive disorders in adolescents with anxiety and depressive disorders. *Archives of General Psychiatry*, *55*, 56–64.

Pine, D. S., Goldstein, R. B., Wolk, S., & Weissman, M. M. (2001). The association between childhood depression and adulthood body mass index. *Pediatrics*, *107*, 1049–1056.

Plioplys, S. (2003). Depression in children and adolescents with epilepsy. *Epilepsy and Behavior*, *4*, S39–S45.

Poznanski, E. O., Freeman, L. N., & Mokros, H. B. (1985). Children's Depression Rating Scale – Revised. *Psychopharmacology Bulletin*, *21*, 979–989.

Puig-Antich, J., Dahl, R., Ryan, N., Novacenko, H., Goetz, D., Goetz, R., *et al.* (1989). Cortisol secretion in prepubertal children with major depressive disorder. Episode and recovery. *Archives of General Psychiatry*, *46*, 801–809.

Rao, U., Ryan, N. D., Dahl, R. E., Birmaher, B., Rao, R., Williamson, D. E., *et al.* (1999). Factors associated with the development of substance use disorder in depressed adolescents. *Journal of the American Academy of Child and Adolescent Psychiatry*, *38*, 1109–1117.

Renaud, J., Brent, D. A., Baugher, M., Birmaher, B., Kolko, D. J., & Bridge, J. (1998). Rapid response to psychosocial treatment for adolescent depression: A two-year follow-up. *Journal of the American Academy of Child and Adolescent Psychiatry*, *37*, 1184–1190.

Resnick, M. D., Bearman, P. S., Blum, R. W., Bauman, K. E., Harris, K. M., Jones, J., *et al.* (1997). Protecting adolescents from harm: Findings from the National Longitudinal Study on Adolescent Health. *Journal of the American Medical Association*, *278*, 823–832.

Reynolds, W. M., & Mazza, J. J. (1998). Reliability and validity of the Reynolds Adolescent Depression Scale with young adolescents. *Journal of School Psychology*, *36*, 295–312.

Rice, F., Harold, G. T., & Thapar, A. (2003). Negative life events as an account of age-related differences in the genetic aetiology of depression in childhood and adolescence. *Journal of Child Psychology and Psychiatry*, *44*, 977–987.

Roberts, R. E., Lewinsohn, P. M., & Seeley, J. R. (1991). Screening for adolescent depression: a comparison of depression scales. *Journal of the American Academy of Child & Adolescent Psychiatry*, *30*, 58–66.

Roberson-Nay, R., McClure, E. B., Monk, C. S., Nelson, E. E., Guyer, A. E., Fromm, S. J., *et al.* (2006). Increased amygdala activity during successful memory encoding in adolescent major depressive disorder: An fMRI Study. *Biological Psychiatry*, *60*, 966–973.

Rohde, P., Clarke, G. N., Lewinsohn, P. M., Seeley, J. R., & Kaufman, N. K. (2001). Impact of comorbidity on a cognitive–behavioral group treatment for adolescent depression. *Journal of the American Academy of Child and Adolescent Psychiatry*, *40*, 795–802.

Rohde, P., Clarke, G. N., Mace, D. E., Jorgensen, J. S., & Seeley, J. R. (2004a). An efficacy/effectiveness study of cognitive–behavioral treatment for adolescents with comorbid major depression and conduct disorder. *Journal of the American Academy of Child and Adolescent Psychiatry*, *43*, 660–668.

Rohde, P., Jorgensen, J. S., Seeley, J. R., & Mace, D. E. (2004b). Pilot evaluation of the Coping Course: A cognitive–behavioral intervention to enhance coping skills in incarcerated youth. *Journal of the American Academy of Child and Adolescent Psychiatry*, *43*, 669–676.

Rosenberg, D. R., Mirza, Y., Russell, A., Tang, J., Smith, J. M., Banerjee, S. P., *et al.* (2004). Reduced anterior cingulate glutamatergic concentrations in childhood OCD and major depression versus healthy controls. *Journal of the American Academy of Child and Adolescent Psychiatry*, *43*, 1146–1153.

Rossello, J., & Bernal, G. (1999). The efficacy of cognitive-behavioral and interpersonal treatments for depression in Puerto Rican adolescents. *Journal of Consulting and Clinical Psychology*, *67*, 734–745.

Rosso, I. M., Cintron, C. M., Steingard, R. J., Renshaw, P. F., Young, A. D., & Yurgelun-Todd, D. (2005). Amygdala and hippocampus volumes in pediatric major depression. *Biological Psychiatry*, *57*, 21–26.

Ruchkin, V., Sukhodolsky, D. G., Vermeiren, R., Koposov, R. A., & Schwab-Stone, M. (2006). Depressive symptoms and associated psychopathology in urban adolescents: A cross-cultural study of three countries. *Journal of Nervous and Mental Disease*, *194*, 106–113.

Rudolph, K. D., & Hammen, C. (1999). Age and gender as determinants of stress exposure, generation, and reactions in youngsters: A transactional perspective. *Child Development*, *70*, 660–677.

Rudolph, K. D., Hammen, C., & Burge, D. (1997). A cognitive-interpersonal approach to depressive symptoms in preadolescent children. *Journal of Abnormal Child Psychology*, *25*, 33–45.

Ryan, N. D., Birmaher, B., Perel, J. M., Dahl, R. E., Meyer, V., Al-Shabbout, M., *et al.* (1992a). Neuroendocrine response to L-5-hydroxytryptophan challenge in prepubertal major depression. *Archives of General Psychiatry*, *49*, 843–851.

Ryan, N. D., Williamson, D. E., Iyengar, S., Orvaschel, H., Reich, T., Dahl, R. E., *et al.* (1992b). A secular increase in child and adolescent onset affective disorder. *Journal of the American Academy of Child and Adolescent Psychiatry*, *31*, 600–605.

Sallee, F. R., Hilal, R., Dougherty, D., Beach, K., & Nesbitt, L. (1998). Platelet serotonin transporter in depressed children and adolescents: 3H-paroxetine platelet binding before and after sertraline. *Journal of the American Academy of Child and Adolescent Psychiatry*, *37*, 777–784.

Sallee, F. R., Nesbitt, L., Dougherty, D., Hilal, R., Nandagopal, V. S., & Sethuraman, G. (1995). Lymphocyte glucocorticoid receptor: Predictor of sertraline response in adolescent major depressive disorder. *Psychopharmacology Bulletin*, *31*, 339–345.

Sanford, M., Boyle, M., McCleary, L., Miller, J., Steele, M., Duku, E., *et al.* (2006). A pilot study of adjunctive family psychoeducation in adolecent major depression: Feasibility and treatment effect. *Journal of the American Academy of Child and Adolescent Psychiatry*, *45*, 386–395.

Scourfield, J., Rice, F., Thapar, A., Harold, G. T., Martin, N., & McGuffin, P. (2003). Depressive symptoms in children and adolescents: Changing aetiological influences with development. *Journal of Child Psychology and Psychiatry*, *44*, 968–976.

Shaffer, D., Fisher, P., & Lucas, C. (2004). The Diagnostic Interview Schedule for Children (DISC). In M. J. Hilsenroth, & D. L. Segal (Eds.), *Comprehensive handbook of psychological assessment*, Volume 2: *Personality assessment* (pp. 256–270). Hoboken, NJ: John Wiley & Sons.

Shaffer, D., Gould, M. S., Fisher, P., Trautman, P., Moreau, D., Kleinman, M., *et al.* (1996). Psychiatric diagnosis in child and adolescent suicide. *Archives of General Psychiatry*, *53*, 339–348.

Shaffer, D., & Pfeffer, C. (2001). Summary of the practice parameters for the assessment and treatment of children and adolescents with suicidal behavior. *Journal of the American Academy of Child and Adolescent Psychiatry*, *40*, 24S–51S.

Shankman, S. A., Tenke, C. E., Bruder, G. E., Durbin, C. E., Hayden, E. P., & Klein, D. N. (2005). Low positive emotionality in young children: Association with EEG asymmetry. *Development and Psychopathology*, *17*, 85–98.

Siegle, G. J., Carter, C. S., & Thase, M. E. (2006). Use of fMRI predicts recovery from unipolar depression with cognitive behavior therapy. *American Journal of Psychiatry*, *163*, 735–738.

Silk, J. S., Shaw, D. S., Skuban, E. M., Oland, A. A., & Kovacs, M. (2006). Emotion regulation strategies in offspring of childhood-onset depressed mothers. *Journal of Child Psychology and Psychiatry*, *47*, 69–78.

Simeon, J. G., Dinicola, V. F., Ferguson, B., & Copping, W. (1990). Adolescent depression: A placebo-controlled fluoxetine treatment study and follow-up. *Progress in Neuro-Psychopharmacology and Biological Psychiatry*, *14*, 791–795.

Simon, G. E., Savarino, J., Operskalski, B., & Wang, P. S. (2006). Suicide risk during antidepressant treatment. *American Journal of Psychiatry*, *163*, 41–47.

Southam-Gerow, M. A., Kendall, P. C., & Weersing, V. R. (2001). Examining outcome variability: Correlates of treatment response in a child and adolescent anxiety clinic. *Journal of Clinical Child Psychology*, *30*, 422–436.

Steingard, R., Renshaw, P. F., Hennen, J., Lenox, M., Bonella Cintron, C., Young, A. D., *et al.* (2002). Smaller frontal lobe white matter volumes in depressed adolescents. *Biological Psychiatry*, *52*, 413–417.

Steingard, R. J., Yurgelun-Todd, D., Hennen, J., Moore, J. C., Moore, C. M., Vakili, K., *et al.* (2000). Increased orbitofrontal cortex levels of choline in depressed adolescents as detected by *in vivo* proton magnetic resonance spectroscopy. *Biological Psychiatry*, *48*, 1053–1061.

Stewart, S., Kennard, B. D., Lee, P. W. H., Hughes, C. W., Mayes, T. L., Emslie, G. J., *et al.* (2004). A cross-cultural investigation of cognitions and depressive symptoms in adolescents. *Journal of Abnormal Psychology*, *113*, 248–257.

Strauss, J., Barr, C. L., George, C. J., Devlin, B., Vetro, A., Kiss, E., *et al.* (2005). Brain-derived neurotrophic factor variants are associated with childhood-onset mood disorder: Confirmation in a Hungarian sample. *Molecular Psychiatry*, *10*, 861–867.

Strober, M., & Carlson, G. (1982). Bipolar illness in adolescents with major depression: Clinical, genetic, and psychopharmacologic predictors in a three- to four-year prospective follow-up investigation. *Archives of General Psychiatry*, *39*, 549–555.

Stroud, L. R., Papandonatos, G. D., Williamson, D. E., & Dahl, R. E. (2004). Sex differences in the effects of pubertal development on responses to a corticotropin-releasing hormone challenge: The Pittsburgh psychobiologic studies. *Annals of the New York Academy of Sciences*, *1021*, 348–351.

Swedo, S. E., Allen, A. J., Glod, C. A., Clark, C. H., Teicher, M. H., Richter, D., *et al.* (1997). A controlled trial of light therapy for the treatment of pediatric seasonal affective disorder. *Journal of the American Academy of Child and Adolescent Psychiatry*, *36*, 816–821.

Thapar, A., & McGuffin, P. (1997). Anxiety and depressive symptoms in childhood: A genetic study of comorbidity. *Journal of Child Psychology and Psychiatry*, *38*, 651–656.

Thapar, A., & McGuffin, P. (1998). Validity of the shortened Mood and Feelings Questionnaire in a community sample of children and adolescents: A preliminary research note. *Psychiatry Research*, *81*, 259–268.

Thase, M. E., Greenhouse, J. B., Frank, E., Reynolds, C. F. III, Pilkonis, P. A., Hurley, K., *et al.* (1997). Treatment of major depression with psychotherapy or psychotherapy–pharmacotherapy combinations. *Archives of General Psychiatry*, *54*, 1009–1015.

Thomas, K. M., Drevets, W. C., Dahl, R. E., Ryan, N. D., Birmaher, B., Eccard, C. H., *et al.* (2001). Amydgala response to fearful faces in anxious and depressed children. *Archives of General Psychiatry*, *58*, 1057–1063.

Thompson, E. A., Eggert, L. L., Randell, B. P., & Pike, K. C. (2001). Evaluation of indicated suicide risk prevention approaches for potential high school dropouts. *American Journal of Public Health*, *91*, 742–752.

Todd, R. D., & Botteron, K. N. (2002). Etiology and genetics of early-onset mood disorders. *Child and Adolescent Psychiatric Clinics of North America*, *11*, 499–518.

Tomarken, A. J., Dichter, G. S., Garber, J., & Simien, C. (2004). Resting frontal brain activity: Linkages to maternal depression and socio-economic status among adolescents. *Biological Psychiatry*, *67*, 77–102.

Tremblay, G. C., & Israel, A. C. (1998). Children's adjustment to parental death. *Clinical Psychology: Science and Practice*, *5*, 424–438.

Vitiello, B., Rohde, P., Silva, S., Wells, K., Casat, C., Waslick, B., *et al.* (2006). Effects of treatment on level of functioning, global health, and quality of life in depressed adolescents. *Journal of the American Academy of Child and Adolescent Psychiatry*, *45*, 1427–1429.

von Knorring A. L., Olsson, G. I., Thomsen, P. H., Lemming, O. M., & Hulten, A. (2006). A randomized, double-blind, placebo-controlled study of citalopram in adolescents with major depressive disorder. *Journal of Clinical Pharmacology*, *26*, 311–315.

Vostanis, P., Feehan, C., Grattan, E., & Bickerton, W. (1996). A randomised controlled out-patient trial of cognitive-behavioural treatment for children and adolescents with depression: 9-month follow-up. *Journal of Affective Disorders*, *40*, 105–116.

Vythilingam, M., Heim, C., Newport, J., Miller, A. H., Anderson, E., Bronen, R., *et al.* (2002). Childhood trauma associated with smaller hippocampal volume in women with major depression. *American Journal of Psychiatry*, *159*, 2072–2080.

Wagner, K. D., Ambrosini, P., Rynn, M., Wohlberg, C., Yang, R., Greenbaum, M. S., *et al.* (2003). Efficacy of sertraline in the treatment of children and adolescents with major depressive disorder: two randomized controlled trials. *Journal of the American Medical Association*, *290*, 1033–1041.

Wagner, K. D., Jonas, J., Findling, R. L., Ventura, D., & Saikali, K. (2006). A double-blind, randomized, placebo-controlled trial of escitalopram in the treatment of piedatric depression. *Journal of the American Academy of Child and Adolescent Psychiatry*, *45*, 280–288.

Wagner, K. D., Robb, A. S., Findling, R. L., Jin, J., Gutierrez, M. M., & Heydorn, W. E. (2004). A randomized, placebo-controlled trial of citalopram for the treatment of major depression in children and adolescents. *American Journal of Psychiatry*, *161*, 1079–1083.

Walter, G., & Rey, J. M. (2003). Has the practice and outcome of ECT in adolescents changed? Findings from a whole-population study. *Journal of ECT*, *19*, 84–87.

Wamboldt, M. Z., Hewitt, J. K., Schmitz, S., Wamboldt, F. S., Rasanen, M., Koskenvuo, M., *et al.* (2000). Familial association between allergic disorders and depression in adult Finnish twins. *American Journal of Medical Genetics*, *96*, 146–153.

Warner, V., Weissman, M. M., Fendrich, M., Wickramaratne, P., & Moreau, D. (1992). The course of major depression in the offspring of depressed parents: Incidence, recurrence and recovery. *Archives of General Psychiatry*, *49*, 795–801.

Weersing, V. R., Iyengar, S., Kolko, D., Birmaher, B., & Brent, D. A. (2006). Effectiveness of cognitive–behavioral therapy for adolescent depression: A benchmarking investigation. *Behavior Therapy*, *37*, 36–48.

Weersing, V. R., & Weisz, J. R. (2002). Community clinic treatment of depressed youth: Benchmarking usual care against CBT clinical trials. *Journal of Consulting and Clinical Psychology*, *70*, 299–310.

Weissman, M. M., Wolk, S., Wickramaratne, P., Goldstein, R. B., Adams, P., Greenwald, S., *et al.* (1999a). Children with prepubertal-onset major depressive disorder and anxiety grown up. *Archives of General Psychiatry*, *56*, 794–801.

Weissman, M. M., Pilowsky, D. J., Wickramaratne, P. J., Talati, A., Wisniewski, S. R., Fava, M., *et al.* (2006). Remissions in maternal depression and child psychopathology: A STAR*D child report. *Journal of American Medical Association*, *295*, 1389–1398.

Weissman, M. M., Wolk, S., Goldstein, R. B., Moreau, D., Adams, P., Greenwald, S., *et al.* (1999b). Depressed adolescents grown up. *Journal of American Medical Association*, *281*, 1707–1713.

Weisz, J. R., McCarty, C. A., & Valeri, S. M. (2006). Effects of psychotherapy for depresssion in children and adolescents: A meta-analysis. *Psychological Bulletin*, *132*, 132–149.

Wells, K. B., Sherbourne, C. D., Schoenbaum, M., Duan, N., Meredith, L., Unutzer, J., *et al.* (2000). Impact of disseminating quality improvement programs for depression in managed primary care: A randomized controlled trial. *Journal of the American Medical Association*, *283*, 212–220.

Whooley, M. A., Avins, A. L., Miranda, J., & Browner, W. S. (1997). Case-finding instruments for depression: Two questions are as good as many. *Journal of General Internal Medicine*, *12*, 439–445.

Wickramaratne, P., Warner, V., & Weissman, M. M. (2000). Selecting early-onset MDD probands for genetic studies: Results from a longitudinal high-risk study. *American Journal of Medical Genetics*, *96*, 93–101.

Williamson, D. E., Birmaher, B., Axelson, D. A., Ryan, N. D., & Dahl, R. E. (2004). First episode of depression in children at low and high familial risk for depression. *Journal of the American Academy of Child and Adolescent Psychiatry*, *43*, 291–297.

Williamson, D. E., Birmaher, B., Ryan, N. D., Shiffrin, T. P., Lusky, J. A., Protopapa, J., *et al.* (2003). The Stressful Life Events Schedule for children and adolescents: Development and validation. *Psychiatry Research*, *119*, 225–241.

Wood, A., Harrington, R., & Moore, A. (1996). Controlled trial of a brief cognitive–behavioural intervention in adolescent patients with depressive disorders. *Journal of Child Psychology and Psychiatry*, *37*, 737–746.

Wood, A., Trainor, G., Rothwell, J., Moore, A., & Harrington, R. (2001). Randomized trial of a group therapy for repeated deliberate self-harm in adolescents. *Journal of the American Academy of Child and Adolescent Psychiatry*, *40*, 1246–1253.

Yorbik, O., Birmaher, B., Axelson, D., Williamson, D., & Ryan, N. D. (2004). Clinical characteristics of depressive symptoms in children and adolescents with major depressive disorder. *Journal of Clinical Psychiatry*, *65*, 1654–1659.

Young, J. F., Mufson, L., & Davies, M. (2006). Impact of cormorbid anxiety in an effectiveness study of interpersonal psychotherapy for depressed adolescents. *Journal of the American Academy of Child and Adolescent Psychiatry*, *45*, 904–912.

Zubenko, G. S., Zubenko, W. N., Spiker, D. G., Giles, D. E., & Kaplan, B. B. (2001). Malignancy of recurrent, early-onset major depression: A family study. *American Journal of Medical Genetics*, *105*, 690–699.

38 Bipolar Disorder in Children and Adolescents

Ellen Leibenluft and Daniel P. Dickstein

There has been a recent marked upsurge in interest in pediatric bipolar disorder (PBD), with almost twice as many articles published on the subject in the past 5 years as in the entire previous decade. Several factors may be contributing to this trend. First, while it is clear that relatively few children have a classic adult-like presentation of bipolar disorder (BD), the number of US children being considered for the diagnosis has expanded as prominent researchers have suggested that BD presents differently in children than adults. Specifically, in a view that remains controversial, US researchers have suggested that children with severe irritability, hyperactivity and distractibility are exhibiting a "broad phenotype" of PBD (Leibenluft, Charney, Towbin *et al.*, 2003; NIMH, 2001).

Second, studies of children with either classic BD symptoms or the "broad phenotype" suggest that PBD is both markedly impairing and treatment-resistant, increasing the demand for relevant information and research (Biederman, Faraone, Wozniak *et al.*, 2005a; Geller, Tillman, Craney *et al.*, 2004b; Kowatch, Youngstrom, Danielyan *et al.*, 2005b). Finally, because of increased interest in developmental psychopathology research generally, and the advent of safe and non-invasive techniques for studying brain function in children, PBD is one of several illnesses that have become the focus of pathophysiological research (Rich, Vinton, Roberson-Nay *et al.*, 2006).

We begin by reviewing the available data concerning the *clinical presentation* of PBD, including its phenomenology and course, and by providing guidelines for the assessment of children who may have PBD. We then describe research on associated illnesses, prodromes and age of onset. Next, we describe *pathophysiological studies*, including those using behavioral testing, neuroimaging and genetic/familial techniques. Finally, we conclude with a review of the *pharmacological and psychotherapeutic treatment* of PBD.

Clinical Presentation

Diagnosis, Phenomenology and Course

Most investigators outside the USA, and some inside, use unmodified DSM-IV-TR diagnostic criteria and assessment techniques to assess bipolar disorder in children. These techniques ascertain whether distinct well-defined episodes of mania or hypomania are present. Using such techniques, researchers in Britain find that pre-adolescent mania is exceptionally rare (Harrington & Myatt, 2003). In the USA, researchers have recruited sizable samples of children meeting strict DSM-IV-TR criteria. For example, the Course of Bipolar Youth (COBY) study in the USA recruited 263 children with clearly episodic bipolar illness (Axelson, Birmaher, Strober *et al.*, 2006; Birmaher, Axelson, Strober *et al.*, 2006). Of the children in the COBY study, 92% had euphoria and 84% had irritability, indicating that most youth with PBD have *both* symptoms. Over 2-year follow-up, patients ($n = 152$) had mixed mania or rapid cycling 29% of weeks, significantly more than BD adults (Birmaher, Axelson, Strober *et al.*, 2006). In another sample of 90 children with clearly episodic BD, 86% had elevated mood, while 92% had irritability; also, 50% had a rapid cycling course, and periods of euthymia were identifiable but brief (Findling, Gracious, McNamara *et al.*, 2001).

However, in the USA, some recent PBD research has been shaped by case descriptions suggesting that BD presents differently in children than in adults. For example, in response to reports that children with PBD may have very rapid and complex mood cycles, Geller *et al.* developed a new semistructured interview for PBD (WASH-U-KSADS; Geller, Warner, Williams *et al.*, 1998b; Geller, Williams, Zimerman *et al.*, 1998c), and new conventions for describing cycling patterns. The WASH-U KSADS defines an episode as the entire duration of illness (rather than, as in DSM-IV-TR, a distinct symptomatic period) and defines cycles as mood changes lasting a minimum of 4 hours (Geller, Tillman, Craney *et al.*, 2004b; Tillman & Geller, 2003). Also, given the overlap between symptoms of mania and attention deficit/hyperactivity disorder (ADHD), Geller *et al.* require that children with mania exhibit either elevated mood or grandiosity (Geller, Warner, Williams *et al.*, 1998b,c). Using these techniques, Geller *et al.* described a BD sample ($n = 86$) in which most had mixed mania (88%), irritability (98%), elated mood (90%) and grandiosity (86%) as well as daily cycling (78%) and a mean of 3.5 ± 2.0 cycles/day.

Similarly, Biederman and collaborators were influenced by case series suggesting that children with BD have irritability rather than euphoria, and that the severity of the irritability in PBD differentiates it from other illnesses. Thus, when assessing irritability, these investigators inquire about extremely

Rutter's Child and Adolescent Psychiatry, 5th edition. Edited by M. Rutter, D. Bishop, D. Pine, S. Scott, J. Stevenson, E. Taylor and A. Thapar. ISBN: 978-1-4051-4549-7.

impairing and severe irritability ("super angry, grouchy, or cranky"). If such irritability is endorsed, then they consider the DSM-IV-TR episodicity criterion to be met, even if the irritability does not represent a distinct change from the patient's usual level of function (Mick, Spencer, Wozniak *et al.*, 2005). Using these techniques, Biederman *et al.* found that only 33% of children ($n = 129$) had euphoria while manic (considerably fewer than in the COBY study or Findling, Gracious, McNamara *et al.*, 2001), while 92% had irritability (Biederman, Faraone, Wozniak *et al.*, 2005a).

Overall, four conclusions can be drawn from the literature on the phenomenology and course of PBD. First, descriptions of the "typical" bipolar child vary markedly across studies (Kowatch, Youngstrom, Danielyan *et al.*, 2005b), probably because of different assessment techniques. The adoption of standard diagnostic procedures would facilitate future research, allowing comparisons among pediatric studies and, if adult procedures are used, with the rich clinical literature on adult BD. Second, data from the COBY study and Findling, Gracious, McNamara *et al.* (2001), obtained using diagnostic techniques comparable to those used in adults, contradict frequent statements in the literature that children with BD do not have euphoria, because almost all patients in these studies experienced euphoria, in addition to irritability (Axelson, Birmaher, Strober *et al.*, 2006; Findling, Gracious, McNamara *et al.*, 2001). On the other hand, several studies indicate that mixed states may be more common in youth versus adults with BD (Birmaher, Axelson, Strober *et al.*, 2006; McElroy, Strakowski, West *et al.*, 1997; Patel, DelBello, Keck *et al.*, 2006). This developmental difference may reflect reporting bias (i.e., when assessing children, parents are also interviewed; irritability is more salient to others than to the patient themself), or the fact that children are unable to use coping strategies that hypomanic or manic adults often employ to avoid having their manic goals thwarted (e.g., skipping work/school, not going to bed).

Third, studies support the contention that early-onset BD is associated with high episode frequency (Birmaher, Axelson, Strober *et al.*, 2006; Findling, Gracious, McNamara *et al.*, 2001; Lin, McInnis, Potash *et al.*, 2006; Perlis, Miyahara, Marangell *et al.*, 2004). However, the data do not indicate that children with BD have a non-episodic illness, because several investigators have recruited sizable samples of children with clearly defined episodes meeting DSM-IV duration criteria (Birmaher, Axelson, Strober *et al.*, 2006; Dickstein, Nelson, McClure *et al.*, 2007; Findling, Gracious, McNamara *et al.*, 2001). Finally, consistent with the observation that children tend to cycle more frequently than adults with BD, all studies agree that PBD is a very impairing illness, leaving affected children symptomatic most of the time.

Assessment and Differential Diagnosis

Whereas investigators use a variety of techniques to diagnose PBD, there are advantages to using those that parallel the adult literature, albeit with developmentally appropriate thresholds. Thus, the interviewer should ask child and parent to identify episodes, lasting at least several days, during which the child had a distinct change in mood and became either euphoric, markedly irritable or depressed. Importantly, even an adult with classic euphoric mania is not euphoric 24 hours a day; therefore, symptoms present most of the day should be considered to be at threshold.

Once episodes are identified, the interviewer should inquire whether the DSM-IV-TR "B" symptoms of mania or depression (e.g., sleep and activity changes, increased distractibility) occurred concurrent with mood changes. If the family cannot identify distinct episodes, then the appropriateness of the diagnosis of BD is called into question. Euphoria should exceed that which a typically developing child would experience in a very exciting situation, such as going to Disneyland, and true grandiosity should be distinguished from developmentally appropriate fantasy or oppositional behavior. Grandiosity or euphoria should represent a distinct change from the child's usual level of function, and should occur at the same time as other symptoms of mania (e.g., decreased need for sleep, increased goal-directed activity). Decreased need for sleep should be differentiated from more typical insomnia, in which youth would prefer to sleep and may nap during the day.

When manic symptoms are occurring, it is best for caretakers to bring the child to the clinic, to allow clinicians to observe behaviors first-hand. While the DSM-IV-TR diagnosis of Bipolar Disorder Not Otherwise Specified (BP-NOS) has been used in a number of clinical situations, it is best reserved for children who have distinct episodes that fail to meet the criteria for a manic episode because they are shorter than 4 days (see p. 615; Birmaher, Axelson, Strober *et al.*, 2006).

When assessing associated illnesses, clinicians should diagnose such illnesses only if symptoms are present when the patient is not in an acute mood episode (Axelson, Birmaher, Strober *et al.*, 2006; Dickstein, Rich, Binstock *et al.*, 2005b). For example, a child with BD should be diagnosed with ADHD only if ADHD symptoms are present when he or she is euthymic or subsyndromally ill. Conversely, for a symptom such as distractibility to count toward the diagnosis of mania in a child with ADHD, the distractibility must worsen significantly during the putative manic episode.

Attempting to differentiate unipolar from bipolar depression is extremely important, because the treatment for the two conditions in adults differs. Careful interviewing to ascertain possible past hypomanic or manic symptoms is therefore essential. While a family history of BD is contributory, children should be treated on the basis of their own clinical presentation, not solely on the basis of family history. ADHD can be distinguished from mania in that children with ADHD alone do not have distinct episodes of mood change accompanied by DSM-IV-TR "B" criteria of mania. Similarly, BD youth with associated ADHD and oppositional defiant disorder (ODD) may have severe irritability, but irritability resulting from ADHD or ODD is distinct from manic irritability in that only the latter occurs, or worsens, during distinct time periods that last days or weeks and during which "B" mania criteria also occur. Therefore, using these techniques, the differentiation of ADHD, or ADHD and ODD, from BD is relatively straightforward. Whereas children with mania may have psychosis, it occurs concurrently with mood symptoms; psychosis in the absence of such symptoms suggests schizophrenia or schizoaffective disorder. Finally, adolescents should be assessed for substance abuse, because cocaine, amphetamine and a number of other illicit substances can cause symptoms resembling those of mania.

Bipolar Spectrum Disorders

Several investigators have suggested classification systems separating children who clearly meet DSM-IV criteria for BD from those whose nosological status is murky. For example, in addition to recruiting youth with DSM-IV-TR-defined BP-I (i.e., a disorder involving one or more definite manic or mixed episodes) and BP-II (i.e., recurrent major depressive episodes with hypomania episodes), the COBY study also recruited patients meeting criteria for BP-NOS, defined as having shorter episodes or fewer symptoms than required for BP-I or II (Birmaher, Axelson, Strober *et al.*, 2006). Over 2-year follow-up, 25% of BP-NOS ($n = 92$) subjects, most of whom had episodes shorter than 4 days, converted to BP-I or II, and the BP-NOS subjects were ill (syndromally or subsyndromally) 65% of weeks.

At the National Institute of Mental Health (NIMH) we have defined a phenotypic categorization system to facilitate research on the boundaries of PBD (Leibenluft, Charney, Towbin *et al.*, 2003). The broad phenotype, or severe mood and behavioral dysregulation (SMD), operationalizes criteria for the children whose diagnosis is most controversial. Specifically, children with SMD have severe impairing irritability, characterized by baseline abnormal mood, noticeable to others, and developmentally inappropriate reactivity to negative emotional stimuli at least three times weekly. The irritability is persistent, rather than occurring in clearly defined episodes. Finally, children with SMD have ADHD-like symptoms (e.g., hyperactivity, distractibility, intrusiveness; Leibenluft, Charney, Towbin *et al.*, 2003). Preliminary data indicate that SMD or severe chronic irritability in childhood is associated with major depressive disorder (MDD) in early adulthood (Leibenluft, Cohen, Gorrindo *et al.*, 2006) and that the pathophysiology of narrow and broad phenotypes of PBD may differ (Rich, Schmajuk, Perez-Edgar *et al.*, 2005, 2007).

Associated Illnesses

In all studies of PBD, associated illnesses are common, especially ADHD, anxiety disorders and ODD. Distractibility, hyperactivity and restlessness are symptoms of both ADHD and mania, and investigators consistently report that more than 70% of children with PBD also have ADHD (Axelson, Birmaher, Strober *et al.*, 2006; Dickstein, Rich, Binstock *et al.*, 2005b; Findling, Gracious, McNamara *et al.*, 2001; Geller, Tillman, Craney *et al.*, 2004b; Wozniak, Biederman, Kiely *et al.*, 1995). It has been suggested that there is a familial association between ADHD and early-onset BD (Faraone, Biederman, Mennin *et al.*, 1997).

Rates of other associated illnesses in PBD vary widely. Those of ODD range from 46% (Axelson, Birmaher, Strober *et al.*, 2006) to over 80% (Biederman, Faraone, Wozniak *et al.*, 2005a), while those of conduct disorder (CD) range from 12% (Axelson, Birmaher, Strober *et al.*, 2006) to 41% (Biederman, Faraone, Chu *et al.*, 1999); higher rates are reported by investigators who view irritability as particularly characteristic of PBD. Rates of anxiety disorders range from 14% (Findling, Gracious, McNamara *et al.*, 2001) to 76% (Harpold, Wozniak, Kwon *et al.*, 2005). Substance abuse disorders have received little attention, although one study found that 32% of adolescents with BD ($n = 57$) also had a substance use disorder (Wilens, Biederman, Kwon *et al.*, 2004).

Age of Onset

Two large epidemiological studies of BD adults report a median onset age of 18 (Christie, Burke, Regier *et al.*, 1988) or 25 years (Kessler, Chiu, Demler *et al.*, 2005). However, studies indicate that BD age of onset is not distributed normally, with two recent studies (Bellivier, Golmard, Rietschel *et al.*, 2003; Lin, McInnis, Potash *et al.*, 2006) each reporting three peaks of onset age. Early onset may be familial (Leboyer, Bellivier, McKeon *et al.*, 1998; Lin, McInnis, Potash *et al.*, 2006) and/or associated with a strong family history of BD (Bellivier, Golmard, Henry *et al.*, 2001; Chengappa, Kupter, Frank *et al.*, 2003; Johnson, Cohen, & Brook, 2000; Kennedy, Everitt, Boydell *et al.*, 2005).

Clinical Prodromes/Risk Factors

Several longitudinal community-based studies have queried which childhood or adolescent diagnoses are associated with increased risk for later BD. One found that anxiety disorder at age 14 or 16 was associated with BD at age 22 (odds ratio [OR] 5.76; 95% confidence interval [CI], 1.44–22.95; Johnson, Cohen, Brook *et al.*, 2000). Another found that mania at age 26 was associated with depression (OR 3.3; 95% CI, 1.2–9.2) and CD/ODD (OR 2.5; 95% CI, 1.1–5.4) at age 11–15, but not with ADHD (Kim-Cohen, Caspi, Moffitt *et al.*, 2003); the association between adult mania and childhood anxiety was a statistical trend (OR 2.1; 95% CI, 0.9–4.8). Thus, epidemiological samples do not support the contention that ADHD is a risk factor for subsequent BD, although anxiety, depression and CD/ODD may be. Clinic-based follow-up studies of children with ADHD give somewhat more mixed results, although the bulk of the evidence is consistent with the epidemiological data (Biederman, Monuteaux, Mick *et al.*, 2006; Hazell, Carr, Lewin *et al.*, 2003; Mannuzza, Klein, Bessler *et al.*, 1998).

All eight clinical studies ($n = 28–83$) that followed depressed children into late adolescence or early adulthood find that prepubertal MDD is associated with increased risk for BD (Geller, Zimerman, Williams *et al.*, 2001; Harrington, Fudge, Rutter *et al.*, 1990; Kovacs, Akiskal, Gatsonis *et al.*, 1994; McCauley, Myers, Mitchell *et al.*, 1993; Rao, Ryan, Birmaher *et al.*, 1995; Strober & Carlson, 1982; Strober, Lampert, Schmidt *et al.*, 1993; Weissman, Wolk, Wickramaratne *et al.*,

1999). However, the prevalence of BD ranged widely, perhaps because of small sample sizes. Positive family history, psychosis and rapid symptom onset may predict BD (Akiskal, Walker, Puzantian *et al.*, 1983; Geller, Fox, & Clark, 1994; Strober & Carlson, 1982; Strober, Lampert, Schmidt *et al.*, 1993).

Preschoolers

Controversy has surrounded recent American reports suggesting that BD may occur in preschool children (Dilsaver & Akiskal, 2004; Scheffer & Niskala Apps, 2004; Tumuluru, Weller, Fristad *et al.*, 2003; Wilens, Biederman, Brown *et al.*, 2002, 2003). These reports are of particular interest given data indicating a rapid rise in the percentage of US preschoolers receiving psychotropic medication (Zito, Safer, dosReis *et al.*, 2000).

The two largest samples of preschoolers diagnosed with BD ($n = 44$, Wilens, Biederman, Forkner *et al.*, 2003; $n = 31$, Scheffer & Niskala Apps, 2004) report very high rates of ADHD (80–95%) and mixed states (i.e., co-occurring manic and depressive symptoms) in approximately 80%. Severe, impairing irritability is ubiquitous in preschoolers diagnosed with BD, and elated mood and grandiosity are also reported, with the caveat that the boundaries of these symptoms in controls or typical preschoolers with ADHD are not well defined, and many case descriptions of preschool mania do not identify the presence of distinct mood episodes. Preschoolers diagnosed with BD tend to have strongly positive family histories (e.g., 70%). Longitudinal follow-up of these children is essential to ascertain the extent to which they meet DSM-IV-TR criteria for BD in adolescence and adulthood.

Clinical Presentation: Summary

The burgeoning research on BD in youth permits some preliminary conclusions about clinical presentation. Research groups who use adult assessment techniques find that children with BD have definable (albeit frequent) episodes that are typically characterized by euphoria mixed with irritability. Research groups using other techniques find either that euphoria is relatively rare, or that distinct episodes cannot be identified. Longitudinal studies will determine whether children ascertained using these alternative techniques develop into adults who fit neatly into the DSM-IV-TR category of BD, have bipolar spectrum illness, exhibit symptoms of another psychiatric illness or have a healthy outcome. As the number of genetic studies of PBD increase, it will be particularly important for investigators to specify precisely their phenotyping methods.

Prevalence

Cross-national epidemiological studies of adults find a lifetime prevalence rate of 1–3% for BD (Kessler, Chiu, Demler *et al.*, 2005; Lasch, Weissman, Wickramaratne *et al.*, 1990; ten Have, Vollebergh, Bijl *et al.*, 2002; Weissman, Bland, Canino *et al.*, 1996). In youth, community-based studies find low rates of BD. Lewinsohn *et al.* found that 1.1% of adolescents ($n = 1507$) met the criteria for BD, while 2.1% of a subset reassessed at age 24 ($n = 893$) did so (Lewinsohn, Klein, & Seeley, 1995, 2000; Lewinsohn, Seeley, Buckley *et al.*, 2002). A second study ($n = 1015$, 9–13 years) found no manic cases and a 3-month prevalence of $0.10 \pm 0.06\%$ for hypomania (Costello, Angold, Burns *et al.*, 1996), while a third ($n = 717$) found that the 12-month prevalence of BD was 1.9% in patients assessed at ages 14 ± 3 years and 16 ± 3 years (Johnson, Cohen, & Brook, 2000). Finally, a twin sample enriched for ADHD ($n = 1610$, 7–18 years), found a BD prevalence of 0.2% (Reich, Neuman, Volk *et al.*, 2005).

Pathophysiology

Behavioral Data

Some behavioral paradigms assess traditional neuropsychological domains to determine a patient's level of cognitive function or gain clues to pathophysiology. Such data indicate that youth with BD, like BD adults, have trait-related deficits in verbal memory and sustained attention (Doyle, Wilens, Kwon *et al.*, 2005; McCarthy, Arrese, McGlashan *et al.*, 2004; McClure, Treland, Snow *et al.*, 2005a,b; Pavuluri, Schenkel, Aryal *et al.*, 2006), although there are some negative studies of sustained attention (DelBello, Zimmerman, Mills *et al.*, 2004b; McCarthy, Arrese, McGlashan *et al.*, 2004; Robertson, Kutcher, & Lagace, 2003). Deficits have also been identified in working memory (Doyle, Wilens, Kwon *et al.*, 2005; Pavuluri, Schenkel, Aryal *et al.*, 2006) and mathematical skill (Lagace, Kutcher, & Robertson, 2003).

Other behavioral studies are aimed at elucidating the neural circuitry mediating PBD. These paradigms assess emotional function (e.g., by measuring responses to reward, punishment or emotional faces) and find three specific deficits in BD youth. First, they have difficulty adapting their behavior to changes in reward contingencies (i.e., selecting a novel stimulus when the previously rewarded one begins to lose, rather than win, points; Dickstein, Treland, Snow *et al.*, 2004; Gorrindo, Blair, Budhani *et al.*, 2005; McClure, Treland, Snow *et al.*, 2005b). This deficit is reminiscent of parents' complaints that patients will not stop one activity and switch to another when appropriate. Deficits in response flexibility may be relevant to the pathophysiology of BD in that response inflexibility, present during euthymia, may be a *forme fruste* of the more marked response inflexibility seen when bipolar patients are acutely ill. That is, when patients with BD are depressed or manic, they have marked deficits in their ability to respond appropriately to emotional rewarding stimuli, as evidenced by the anhedonia present during depression and the hyperhedonia characteristic of mania.

Second, youth with BD have difficulty labeling the emotion displayed on faces (McClure, Pope, Hoberman *et al.*, 2003; McClure, Treland, Snow *et al.*, 2005b). Deficits in face emotionly recognition may in turn be associated with these patients' third abnormality (i.e., an inability to focus their attention when experiencing strong emotions; Rich, Schmajuk, Perez-Edgar *et al.*, 2005). In patients with BD, the adverse impact of emotion on attention may contribute to their inability to label emotions properly. Future study will elucidate the neural circuitry of these deficits and possible associations between abnormal processing of emotional stimuli and core features of BD, such as switching mood states.

Neuroimaging

Structural Magnetic Resonance Imaging

By far the most replicated structural magnetic resonance imaging (MRI) finding in PBD is significantly decreased amygdala volume compared to controls (Blumberg, Kaufman, Martin *et al.*, 2003; Chang, Karchemskiy, Barnea-Goraly *et al.*, 2005; DelBello, Zimmerman, Mills *et al.*, 2004b; Dickstein, Milham, Nugent *et al.*, 2005a). Because structural MRI studies of BD adults have reported both increased and unchanged amygdala volume (Altshuler, Bartzokis, Grieder *et al.*, 1998; Altshuler, Bartzokis, Grieder *et al.*, 2000; Brambilla, Harenski, Nicoletti *et al.*, 2003; Pearlson, Barta, Powers *et al.*, 1997; Strakowski, DelBello, Sax *et al.*, 1999), decreased amygdala volume may represent a marker of childhood-onset BD, although further work is needed to determine the effects of development, gender, medications and comorbidity on amygdala size. Individual studies suggest possible differences between patients with PBD and controls in other brain regions (e.g., prefrontal cortex and striatum), but the literature is less consistent (for reviews see Blumberg, Charney, & Krystal, 2002; DelBello, Adler, & Strakowski, 2006a).

Functional Magnetic Resonance Imaging

Functional MRI (fMRI) allows investigators to quantify neural activation while subjects perform tasks engaging specific psychological processes. For example, investigators study the neural mechanisms mediating patients' impulsivity and inattention by using fMRI tasks requiring motor inhibition or the ability to direct one's attention away from distracting stimuli. These studies indicate striatal dysfunction in PBD. For example, Blumberg, Kaufman, Martin *et al.* (2003) found increased striatal activation in BD adolescents, compared to controls, during a Stroop paradigm of cognitive interference. Using a motor inhibition task, Leibenluft, Rich, Vinton *et al.* (2007) found that, compared to controls, PBD subjects had a reduced striatal "error signal" during failed motor inhibition (Leibenluft, Rich, Vinton *et al.*, 2007), a deficit that might contribute to the patients' inability to inhibit effectively.

In an fMRI study building on the finding that children with PBD have face emotion identification deficits (McClure, Treland, Snow *et al.*, 2005a), Rich, Vinton, Roberson-Nay *et al.* (2006) found that PBD subjects viewed neutral faces as more hostile and feared these faces more than did controls, and that these between-group differences in ratings were associated with increased amygdala and striatal activation in PBD versus control youth (Rich, Vinton, Roberson-Nay *et al.*, 2006). Interestingly, whereas both children with PBD and those with anxiety disorders exhibit amygdala dysfunction during this fMRI task (relative to controls), the precise nature of that dysfunction varies among diagnoses (McClure, Monk, Nelson *et al.*, 2007). It will be important for future work to compare the pathophysiology of PBD with that of other mood disorders, as well as with ADHD.

Magnetic Resonance Spectroscopy

Magnetic resonance spectroscopy (MRS) research in BD has focused on *N*-acetyl aspartate (NAA), an intraneuronal marker whose levels are decreased in neuropathology, and myoinositol (mI), an intracellular second messenger, thought to be overabundant in mania, whose levels are decreased by lithium (Moore, Bebchuk, Parrish *et al.*, 1999; Silverstone, Wu, O'Donnell *et al.*, 2002).

Youth with familial BD (Chang, Adleman, Dienes *et al.*, 2003), and adults with BD (Winsberg, Sachs, Tate *et al.*, 2000), have significantly decreased NAA in the dorsolateral prefrontal cortex compared to controls and, in one study, lithium treatment was associated with increased NAA in a sample of adult controls and BP patients (Manji, Moore, & Chen, 2000; Moore, Bebchuk, Hasanat *et al.*, 2000). In BD youth, olanzapine treatment resulted in significantly greater medial ventral prefrontal cortex NAA in remitters ($n = 11$, 58%) versus non-remitters ($n = 8$, 42%; DelBello, Cecil, Adler *et al.*, 2006). Studies also indicate that PBD subjects have increased anterior cingulate coretex (ACC) mI compared to healthy controls or youth with intermittent explosive disorder (Davanzo, Yue, Thomas *et al.*, 2003). Moreover, 7 days of lithium treatment significantly decreased mI in the ACC, and this decrease was more prominent in lithium responders than in non-responders (Davanzo, Thomas, Yue *et al.*, 2001). Together, these MRS studies suggest that PBD may be characterized by specific neurochemical alterations that respond to psychopharmacological treatment; future work in this area may ultimately inform such treatment.

Diffusion Tensor Imaging

Diffusion tensor imaging (DTI) is an emerging neuroimaging technique used to study the integrity of white matter tracts. A DTI study found that adolescents experiencing their first manic episode have less fractional anisotropy in the prefrontal cortex than controls, indicating disruption of white matter tracts (Adler, Adams, DelBello *et al.*, 2006). Future DTI studies, in combination with MRS and structural and functional MRI studies, may allow investigators to define more precisely the causes of neural dysfunction in youth with PBD.

Familial Risk and Genetics

Children At Risk for Bipolar Disorder

Compared to children without a first-degree relative with BD, those with such a relative are at an approximately 10-fold increased risk for BD (Hodgins, Faucher, Zarac *et al.*, 2003; Kelsoe, 2003; Smoller & Finn, 2003). Twin studies suggest that the heritability of BD in adults is greater than 60%, with greater concordance for BD in monozygotic (60–70%) than dizygotic twins (20–30%) (Bertelsen, Harvald, & Hauge, 1977; Smoller & Finn, 2003).

The clinical status and neurocognitive function of children with a first-degree relative with BD are of considerable interest. Six studies with $n > 50$ have assessed children recruited through their parents with BD (Carlson & Weintraub, 1993; Chang, Steiner, & Ketter, 2000; Grigoroiu-Serbanescu, Christodorescu, Jipescu *et al.*, 1989; Henin, Biederman, Mick *et al.*, 2005; Hillegers, Reichart, Wals *et al.*, 2005; Wals, Hillegers, Reichart *et al.*, 2001). All find very high rates of psychopathology in these youth, with 44–63% meeting criteria for at least one DSM-IV-TR diagnosis, including ADHD, anxiety disorder, MDD and/or PBD.

Molecular Genetics

Currently, much research aims to identify genetic mechanisms underlying the increased familial risk for BD. Studies implicate a number of genetic regions in the transmission of adult BD (Hayden & Nurnberger, 2006; Kelsoe, 2003), with a locus on 6q21–q25 having perhaps the strongest evidence (McQueen, Devlin, Faraone *et al.*, 2005). Candidate gene studies implicate the genes coding for brain-derived neurotrophic factor (*BDNF*) perhaps especially in rapid-cycling BD (Green, Raybould, Macgregor *et al.*, 2006) and *DAOA*(G72)/G30. However, it is clear that all conclusions must be considered tentative in the absence of replication, because the genetics of BD are complex, with multiple genes involved and no one gene of main effect (Kelsoe, 2003). In addition, recent research indicates that there may be significant overlap between the genes conferring risk for BD and those implicated in schizophrenia (Craddock & Forty, 2006; Kelsoe, Spence, Loetscher *et al.*, 2001). Other studies implicating dopaminergic genes (e.g., the dopamine transporter gene [*DAT*] on chromosome 5p; Keikhaee, Fadai, Sargolzaee *et al.*, 2005) in both ADHD and BD may be of particular interest in PBD, given the strong association between ADHD and early-onset BD (Geller, Williams, Zimerman *et al.*, 1998c; Wilens, Biederman, Forkner *et al.*, 2003). In PBD, three genetic studies have been conducted, with one finding that the val66 allele of the *BDNF* gene on chromosome 11p was preferentially transmitted in PBD ($n = 53$ trios; Geller, Badner, Tillman *et al.*, 2004a).

Treatment

Clinicians attempting to prescribe evidence-based treatment for PBD are confronted by a dearth of randomized placebo-controlled trials (RCTs) that precludes designating any psychopharmacological or psychotherapeutic treatment as having "strong" evidentiary support. RCTs are essential because placebo response rates range 10–50% in both acute and maintenance treatment trials of adult mania (Keck, Welge, McElroy *et al.*, 2000a,b). In fact, fewer than 10 published placebo-controlled RCTs have been conducted in pediatric BD. Given the paucity of pediatric data, clinicians often rely on data from adult BD; hence, we summarize briefly the most relevant adult data. However, caution is urged in basing treatment on adult data, because youth sometimes respond differently from adults, as in major depression (Hazell, O'Connell, Heathcote *et al.*, 1995).

We discuss both psychopharmacological and psychotherapeutic approaches to PBD. Again, the lack of systematic data precludes firm recommendations as to how these two modalities should be prioritized, although it is likely that both modalities will ultimately prove to be important in the treatment of PBD. Our discussion focuses on children clearly meeting DSM-IV-TR criteria for bipolar disorder who, like adults with the illness, are typically too severely impaired to benefit from psychotherapeutic approaches without initial stabilization with pharmacotherapy. This is the population that is generally targeted in RCTs of medications. In children exhibiting the "broad phenotype" of PBD (see p. 615), whose major presenting problem is non-episodic irritability, psychosocial approaches, including interventions with the child, family and school environment, may be particularly important.

Generally, clinicians should focus treatment on the most acute and disabling aspects of BD (e.g., acute mania, depression, psychosis, substance abuse, suicidality; Fig. 38.1). Later treatment addresses other problems (e.g., comorbid anxiety, ADHD, substance abuse, deficient social skills). Treatment decisions require collaboration among physicians, patients and families to identify target symptoms, educate about side-effects, and evaluate each treatment's efficacy. Daily ratings of target symptoms by parents and/or patients allow treatment to be based upon prospective, rather than retrospective, data.

Ideally, medication trials should be at least 6–8 weeks long, with only one new agent added at a time. However, this approach may not be feasible in acutely manic or psychotic patients. Physicians should assess continuously the need for each medication to determine whether any can be discontinued. Moreover, as noted above, symptoms do not typically resolve on medication alone; rather, comprehensive treatment usually requires both psychopharmacology and psychotherapy. Finally, treatment must develop in synchrony with a child's illness, because acute and maintenance interventions differ.

Psychopharmacology for Pediatric Bipolar Disorder

Pharmacotherapy of Mania

Mania should be the initial treatment focus in BD, because antimanic medications not only reduce manic symptoms but may also prevent activation secondary to antidepressants or psychostimulants. Currently available antimanic medications include:

1 Lithium;

2 Antiepileptic medications (AEDs, e.g. valproate and carbamazepine); and

3 Atypical antipsychotic medications (Fig. 38.1).

In general, relatively weak support exists concerning the efficacy of any of these agents in PBD. This complicates efforts to select any one agent as a first-line treatment and again emphasizes the importance of thorough discussions with patients and their families concerning the available data on each agent's efficacy and safety. In our discussion of each medication, we focus

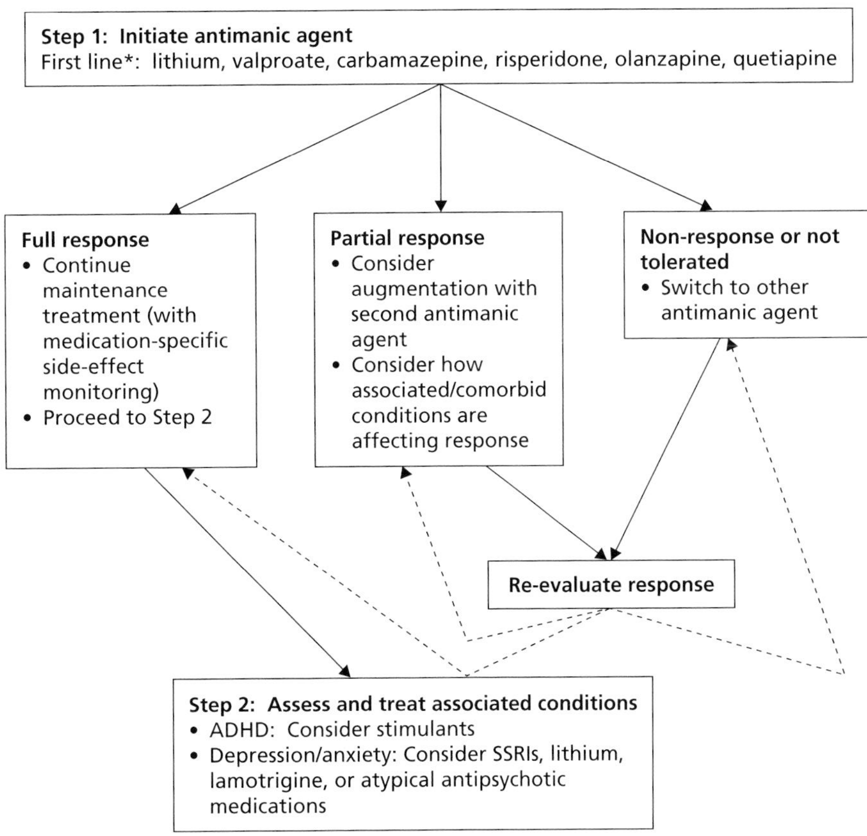
Step 1: Initiate antimanic agent
First line*: lithium, valproate, carbamazepine, risperidone, olanzapine, quetiapine
Full response
• Continue maintenance treatment (with medication-specific side-effect monitoring)
• Proceed to Step 2
Partial response
• Consider augmentation with second antimanic agent
• Consider how associated/comorbid conditions are affecting response
Non-response or not tolerated
• Switch to other antimanic agent
Re-evaluate response
Step 2: Assess and treat associated conditions
• ADHD: Consider stimulants
• Depression/anxiety: Consider SSRIs, lithium, lamotrigine, or atypical antipsychotic medications
* 1st line agents based upon present data in pediatrican BD.

Fig. 38.1 Pediatric bipolar disorder psychopharmacology algorithm. After Kowatch *et al.* (2005a).

on efficacy in BD, and only mention side-effects of particular interest; readers are also referred to other references for dosing guidelines and a more thorough discussion of side-effects (Correll, Penzner, Parikh *et al.*, 2006; Kowatch, Fristad, Birmaher *et al.*, 2005a).

Lithium

Support for lithium's utility in PBD is mixed. Among the three categories of medications typically used in PBD, efficacy data are stronger for lithium than for the AEDs but weaker than for the atypical antipsychotics. Similarly, in terms of safety data, lithium should probably also be placed in an intermediate category relative to these two other treatments.

While lithium is the only medication with a US Food and Drug Administration (FDA) indication for the treatment of mania in patients as young as 12 years, this indication was granted at a time when FDA decisions for children were based largely on adult data. If lithium efficacy data were reviewed today, an FDA indication would not be granted because of the lack of two large placebo-controlled RCTs to demonstrate efficacy. Nevertheless, given the data from open trials, small studies, etc., and the extensive efficacy data in adults with BD, it is reasonable to prescribe lithium for youth with PBD.

One small parallel-group placebo-controlled RCT examined the use of lithium in a heterogeneous group of 25 patients with substance abuse and either DSM-III-R BD, or MDD plus at least one feature associated with elevated risk for BD (e.g., BD in a first-degree relative; Geller, Cooper, Sun *et al.*, 1998a). On global response ratings, 46.2% of patients responded to lithium versus 8.3% to placebo, but lithium had no specific benefit for mood symptoms (Geller, Cooper, Sun *et al.*, 1998a). Another study (Kafantaris, Coletti, Dicker *et al.*, 2004) used a discontinuation design, whereby acutely manic adolescents ($n = 108$) were treated with lithium openly before randomization to either continued lithium treatment or placebo. Consistent with other trials (Findling, Gracious, McNamara *et al.*, 2001; Kafantaris, Coletti, Dicker *et al.*, 2003; Kowatch, Suppes, Carmody *et al.*, 2000), 42% of patients responded to open lithium treatment. However, the blinded discontinuation trial found no difference between lithium and placebo, with a relapse rate greater than 50% in both groups.

In adults, there is robust evidence for the efficacy of lithium in adult acute mania (Bowden, Brugger, Swann *et al.*, 1994, 2005; Small, Klapper, Milstein *et al.*, 1991) and long-term prophylaxis (Bowden, Calabrese, Sachs *et al.*, 2003). Longterm lithium treatment also appears to reduce suicide risk in adult BD (Cipriani, Pretty, Hawton *et al.*, 2005; Goodwin, Fireman, Simon *et al.*, 2003).

Adult studies suggest that optimal lithium levels are between 0.6 and 1.0 mEq/L for acute mania and down to 0.4 mEq/L for maintenance treatment, but this has not been tested rigorously in youth (Gelenberg, Kane, Keller *et al.*, 1989; Keller, Lavori, Kane *et al.*, 1992; Stokes, Shamoian, Stoll *et al.*, 1971). Of note, an MRS study showed that PBD youth ($n = 9$) had lower brain/serum lithium concentrations than BD adults ($n = 18$; Moore, Demopulos, Henry *et al.*, 2002), suggesting that PBD patients, compared to adults with the illness, may require higher doses of lithium to achieve the same brain concentration of lithium. However, the clinical implications of this finding have not been studied systematically.

Antiepileptic Drugs

Relative to lithium or atypical antipsychotic medication, support for the therapeutic efficacy of the AEDs in PBD is weakest. However, because many AEDs are used in pediatric epilepsy, considerable data exist concerning long-term effects in children (de Silva, MacArdle, McGowan *et al.*, 1996). The safety data for AEDs is generally strong, with the exception of questions regarding acute hepatic or pancreatic failure and possible adverse effects on female gonadal function (see below).

Data from RCTs fail to demonstrate the benefits of AEDs in pediatric BPD. First, DelBello, Findling, Kushner *et al.* (2005) found no difference in reduction of manic symptoms in patients treated with topiramate ($n = 29$) versus placebo ($n = 27$), although secondary measures provided some suggestion of greater benefit from topiramate. Second, Wagner, Weller, Carlson *et al.* (2002) found no difference in efficacy between oxacarbazepine and placebo in more than 300 youth with PBD. While open-label trials, most of them small, document some evidence of benefit for carbamazepine, valproate or lamotrigine, in the absence of a placebo control these studies can provide only weak support for efficacy (Chang, Saxena, & Howe, 2006; Findling, McNamara, Youngstrom *et al.*, 2005; Kowatch, Suppes, Carmody *et al.*, 2000; Wagner, Weller, Carlson *et al.*, 2002).

In adult BD, acute antimanic efficacy has been demonstrated for valproate and a long-acting form of carbamazepine, leading to FDA indications for both in BD (Pope, McElroy, Keck *et al.*, 1991, Weisler, Keck, Swann *et al.*, 2005). Lamotrigine is another AED with an FDA indication for BD, although data suggest that it is more effective as a maintenance treatment, preventing depressive and manic relapse, than for acute mania (Bowden, Calabrese, Sachs *et al.*, 2003; Bowden & Karren, 2006; Goodwin, Bowden, Calabrese *et al.*, 2004; Ichim, Berk, & Brook, 2000).

Valproate has a black-box FDA warning because of the possibility of acute life-threatening hepatic failure and pancreatitis (Grauso-Eby, Goldfarb, Feldman-Winter *et al.*, 2003). Therefore, any patient taking valproate who develops the acute onset of nausea, vomiting or acute abdominal pain should have a prompt medical evaluation. In addition, irregular menses and polycystic ovary syndrome (i.e., polycystic ovarian morphology, increased serum testosterone or leutenizing hormone and irregular menses) may be associated with valproate use (McIntyre, Mancini, McCann *et al.*, 2003).

Regarding lamotrigine, the FDA issued a black-box warning for use in children younger than 16 because of the association between lamotrigine use and the development of two potentially life-threatening rashes, Stephens–Johnson syndrome and toxic epidermal necrolysis (TEN). More benign rashes are common, and a meta-analysis found that increased risk for such rashes was associated with patient age less than 12 years or co-administration of medications that inhibit hepatic metabolism (e.g., valproate; Calabrese, Sullivan, Bowden *et al.*, 2002). Experts suggest that the risk of rash can be minimized by increasing the dose extremely slowly. If a rash occurs, the patient should be seen urgently by a physician to rule out Stephens–Johnson syndrome or TEN.

Antipsychotic Medications

Atypical antipsychotic agents have the strongest efficacy data in PBD; however, given the small number of trials, even here the evidence is moderate at best. Moreover, there are more safety concerns regarding this class of medications versus AEDs and probably also versus lithium.

At present, two RCTs evaluate efficacy of quetiapine in PBD. First, a small 6-week double-blind placebo-controlled RCT in manic/mixed BD adolescents found that valproate plus quetiapine ($n = 15$) was significantly more effective than valproate plus placebo ($n = 15$) (DelBello, Schwiers, Rosenberg *et al.*, 2002). The second showed similar efficacy for quetiapine ($n = 25$) versus valproate monotherapy ($n = 25$) (DelBello, Kowatch, Adler *et al.*, 2006c), although quetiapine had advantages on secondary outcome measures. Additional open trials of atypical antipsychotics, including olanzapine, risperidone and aripiprazole, suggest efficacy (Barzman DelBello, Kowatch *et al.*, 2004; Biederman, Mick, Hammerness *et al.*, 2005b,c; Frazier, Meyer, Biederman *et al.*, 1999, 2001; Pavuluri, Henry, Carbray *et al.*, 2004b). Atypical antipsychotic medications that are FDA approved for the treatment of mania in adults include aripiprazole, olanzapine, quetiapine, risperidone and ziprasidone (Bowden, Grunze, Mullen *et al.*, 2005; Calabrese, Keck, Macfadden *et al.*, 2005; Hirschfeld, Keck, Kramer *et al.*, 2004; Keck, Marcus, Tourkodimitris *et al.*, 2003a,b; Khanna, Vieta, Lyons *et al.*, 2005; McIntyre, Brecher, Paulsson *et al.*, 2005; Tohen, Greil, Calabrese *et al.*, 2005; Vieta, Bourin, Sanchez *et al.*, 2005).

A particular concern is the association of atypical antipsychotic medication with "metabolic syndrome" (i.e., extreme and rapid weight gain and endocrine abnormalities, including diabetes mellitus; Caballero, 2003). For example, BD youth gained an average of 5 kg in 8 weeks in an open-label study of olanzapine (Frazier, Biederman, Tohen *et al.*, 2001). Patients should be monitored routinely for weight, height and body mass index, and possibly every 6 months for fasting glucose and lipid panel (Correll, Penzner, Parikh *et al.*, 2006; Straker, Correll, Kramer-Ginsberg *et al.*, 2005). Finally, for atypical antipsychotics, firm conclusions on the risk of tardive dyskinesia are not possible because of the lack of long-term data (Ghaemi, Hsu, Rosenquist *et al.*, 2006).

Pharmacotherapy of Depression or ADHD in PBD

No RCT has targeted bipolar depression in children or adolescents. RCTs in adult bipolar depression demonstrate efficacy for lamotrigine, quetiapine and the combination of olanzapine plus fluoxetine (Altshuler, Suppes, Black *et al.*, 2003; Calabrese, Bowden, Sachs *et al.*, 1999, 2005; Tohen, Greil, Calabrese *et al.*, 2005; Zornberg & Pope, 1993). Studies give conflicting results as to whether selective serotonin reuptake inhibitor (SSRI) antidepressants or lithium are preferable in the treatment of adult bipolar depression (Amsterdam, Garcia-Espana, Fawcett *et al.*, 1998; Nemeroff, Evans, Gyulai *et al.*, 2001). No RCTs address this issue in youth. Of note, some evidence suggests that the risk of antidepressant-induced mania is higher in pre-pubertal children than in older adolescents or adults (Martin, Young, Leckman *et al.*, 2004; Rey & Martin, 2006).

One double-blind crossover RCT in children with PBD and ADHD found that, once mania remitted on valproate, the addition of amphetamine salts to valproate was more effective in reducing ADHD symptoms than was placebo plus valproate, and amphetamine salts did not exacerbate manic symptoms ($n = 30$) (Scheffer, Kowatch, Carmody *et al.*, 2005). Thus, clinicians treating youth with BD and comorbid ADHD should treat the patient's mania, and then consider psychostimulant treatment.

Psychotherapy for Pediatric Bipolar Disorder

While there are few trials of psychotherapy in youth or adults with BD, preliminary data suggest that any one of three types of psychotherapy, in combination with psychopharmacology, may reduce morbidity in BD. First, in families with BD offspring ($n = 35$), multifamily psycho-educational groups are associated with increased knowledge about BD and ability to obtain appropriate services (Fristad, Gavazzi, & Mackinaw-Koons, 2003). Second, in BD youth, open cognitive–behavioral therapy ($n = 34$) with family involvement was associated with significant symptom reduction (Pavuluri, Graczyk, Henry *et al.*, 2004a). Third, in family-focused psycho-educational therapy (FFT), families participate in psycho-education, communication enhancement and problem-solving skills training. In PBD adolescents ($n = 20$), FFT resulted in a 12-month reduction of depression (38% improvement) and mania (46% improvement) ratings (Miklowitz, George, Axelson *et al.*, 2004).

In sum, these data suggest that the combination of psychotherapy plus psycho-pharmacotherapy may reduce the morbidity of BD in youth. However, there is a clear need for RCTs to document efficacy definitively.

Conclusions

We now know much more about PBD than we did as recently as a decade ago. Several conclusions can be drawn. BD occurs in children and adolescents, and when it does it tends to be severely impairing. Several studies implicate depression and anxiety as risk factors for PBD. The prevalence of BD in children and adolescents is 1% or less. PBD is associated with several neurocognitive deficits, consistent with functional and structural neuroimaging data implicating prefrontal cortex–amygdala–striatal circuitry in its pathophysiology. BD is clearly heritable, with high rates of psychopathology in the offspring of adults with BD. The hunt for susceptibility genes for BD is on, although the clearest findings at this time are that the genetics of the illness are likely to be complex, and there are likely to be susceptibility genes involved in the pathogenesis of both BD and schizophrenia.

Finally, interest in the clinical presentation and pathophysiology of PBD has been accompanied by similar interest in its treatment. However, the rarity of the disease, the fact that the children tend to be severely impaired and the scarcity of trained investigators conspire to create a paucity of double-blind placebo-controlled treatment trials. Because of the woefully limited data, strong recommendations cannot be made for any treatment. In the meantime, clinicians must strive to stay current with the literature while also extrapolating from the latest treatment research in adults with BD, bearing in mind that PBD patients do not respond to therapeutic interventions as "little adults." Furthermore, the applicability of the adult treatment data is greatest to those children who have been assessed using techniques similar to those used in adults. It is to be hoped that the near future will bring great advances in the knowledge base about the treatment of PBD, just as the recent past has brought significant advances in the literature about the phenomenology and short-term course of the illness.

References

Adler, C. M., Adams, J., DelBello, M. P., Holland, S. K., Schmithorst, V., Levine, A., *et al.* (2006). Evidence of white matter pathology in bipolar disorder adolescents experiencing their first episode of mania: a diffusion tensor imaging study. *American Journal of Psychiatry*, *163*, 322–324.

Akiskal, H. S., Walker, P., Puzantian, V. R., King, D., Rosenthal, T. L., & Dranon, M. (1983). Bipolar outcome in the course of depressive illness. Phenomenologic, familial, and pharmacologic predictors. *Journal of Affective Disorders*, *5*, 115–128.

Altshuler, L., Suppes, T., Black, D., Nolen, W. A., Keck, P. E. Jr., Frye, M. A., *et al.* (2003). Impact of antidepressant discontinuation after acute bipolar depression remission on rates of depressive relapse at 1-year follow-up. *American Journal of Psychiatry*, *160*, 1252–1262.

Altshuler, L. L., Bartzokis, G., Grieder, T., Curran, J., Jimenez, T., Leight, K., *et al.* (2000). An MRI study of temporal lobe structures in men with bipolar disorder or schizophrenia. *Biological Psychiatry*, *48*, 147–162.

Altshuler, L. L., Bartzokis, G., Grieder, T., Curran, J., & Mintz, J. (1998). Amygdala enlargement in bipolar disorder and hippocampal reduction in schizophrenia: An MRI study demonstrating neuro-anatomic specificity. *Archives of General Psychiatry*, *55*, 663–664.

Amsterdam, J. D., Garcia-Espana, F., Fawcett, J., Quitkin, F. M., Reimherr, F. W., Rosenbaum, J. F., *et al.* (1998). Efficacy and safety of fluoxetine in treating bipolar II major depressive episode. *Journal of Clinical Psychopharmacology*, *18*, 435–440.

Axelson, D., Birmaher, B., Strober, M., Gill, M. K., Valeri, S., Chiappetta, L., *et al.* (2006). Phenomenology of children and adolescents with bipolar spectrum disorders. *Archives of General Psychiatry*, *63*, 1139–1148.

Barzman, D. H., DelBello, M. P., Kowatch, R. A., Gernert, B., Fleck, D. E., Pathak, S., *et al.* (2004). The effectiveness and tolerability of aripiprazole for pediatric bipolar disorders: A retrospective chart review. *Journal of Child and Adolescent Psychopharmacology*, *14*, 593–600.

Bellivier, F., Golmard, J. L., Henry, C., Leboyer, M., & Schurhoff, F. (2001). Admixture analysis of age at onset in bipolar I affective disorder. *Archives of General Psychiatry*, *58*, 510–512.

Bellivier, F., Golmard, J. L., Rietschel, M., Schulze, T. G., Malafosse, A., Preisig, M., *et al.* (2003). Age at onset in bipolar I affective disorder: further evidence for three subgroups. *American Journal of Psychiatry*, *160*, 999–1001.

Bertelsen, A., Harvald, B., & Hauge, M. (1977). A Danish twin study of manic-depressive disorders. *British Journal of Psychiatry*, *130*, 330–351.

Biederman, J., Faraone, S. V., Chu, M. P., & Wozniak, J. (1999). Further evidence of a bidirectional overlap between juvenile mania and conduct disorder in children. *Journal of the American Academy of Child and Adolescent Psychiatry*, *38*, 468–476.

Biederman, J., Faraone, S. V., Wozniak, J., Mick, E., Kwon, A., Cayton, G. A., *et al.* (2005a). Clinical correlates of bipolar disorder in a large, referred sample of children and adolescents. *Journal of Psychiatric Research*, *39*, 611–622.

Biederman, J., Mick, E., Hammerness, P., Harpold, T., Aleardi, M., Dougherty, M., *et al.* (2005b). Open-label, 8-week trial of olanzapine and risperidone for the treatment of bipolar disorder in preschool-age children. *Biological Psychiatry*, *58*, 589–594.

Biederman, J., Mick, E., Wozniak, J., Aleardi, M., Spencer, T., & Faraone, S. V. (2005c). An open-label trial of risperidone in children and adolescents with bipolar disorder. *Journal of Child and Adolescent Psychopharmacology*, *15*, 311–317.

Biederman, J., Monuteaux, M. C., Mick, E., Spencer, T., Wilens, T. E., Silva, J. M., *et al.* (2006). Young adult outcome of attention deficit hyperactivity disorder: a controlled 10-year follow-up study. *Psychological Medicine*, *36*, 167–179.

Birmaher, B., Axelson, D., Strober, M., Gill, M. K., Valeri, S., Chiappetta, L., *et al.* (2006). Clinical course of children and adolescents with bipolar spectrum disorders. *Archives of General Psychiatry*, *63*, 175–183.

Blumberg, H. P., Charney, D. S., & Krystal, J. H. (2002). Frontotemporal neural systems in bipolar disorder. *Seminars in Clinical Neuropsychiatry*, *7*, 243–254.

Blumberg, H. P., Kaufman, J., Martin, A., Whiteman, R., Zhang, J. H., Gore, J. C., *et al.* (2003). Amygdala and hippocampal volumes in adolescents and adults with bipolar disorder. *Archives of General Psychiatry*, *60*, 1201–1208.

Bowden, C. L., Brugger, A. M., Swann, A. C., Calabrese, J. R., Janicak, P. G., Petty, F., *et al.* (1994). Efficacy of divalproex vs lithium and placebo in the treatment of mania. The Depakote Mania Study Group. *Journal of the American Medical Association*, *271*, 918–924.

Bowden, C. L., Calabrese, J. R., Sachs, G., Yatham, L. N., Asghar, S. A., Hompland, M., *et al.* (2003). A placebo-controlled 18-month trial of lamotrigine and lithium maintenance treatment in recently manic or hypomanic patients with bipolar I disorder. *Archives of General Psychiatry*, *60*, 392–400.

Bowden, C. L., Grunze, H., Mullen, J., Brecher, M., Paulsson, B., Jones, M., *et al.* (2005). A randomized, double-blind, placebo-controlled efficacy and safety study of quetiapine or lithium as monotherapy for mania in bipolar disorder. *Journal of Clinical Psychiatry*, *66*, 111–121.

Bowden, C. L., & Karren, N. U. (2006). Anticonvulsants in bipolar disorder. *Australian and New Zealand Journal of Psychiatry*, *40*, 386–393.

Brambilla, P., Harenski, K., Nicoletti, M., Sassi, R. B., Mallinger, A. G., Frank, E., *et al.* (2003). MRI investigation of temporal lobe structures in bipolar patients. *Journal of Psychiatric Research*, *37*, 287–295.

Caballero, E. (2003). Obesity, diabetes, and the metabolic syndrome: new challenges in antipsychotic drug therapy. *CNS Spectrums*, *8*, 19–22.

Calabrese, J. R., Bowden, C. L., Sachs, G. S., Ascher, J. A., Monaghan, E., & Rudd, G. D. (1999). A double-blind placebo-controlled study of lamotrigine monotherapy in outpatients with bipolar I depression. Lamictal 602 Study Group. *Journal of Clinical Psychiatry*, *60*, 79–88.

Calabrese, J. R., Keck, P. E. Jr., Macfadden, W., Minkwitz, M., Ketter, T. A., Weisler, R. H., *et al.* (2005). A randomized, double-blind, placebo-controlled trial of quetiapine in the treatment of bipolar I or II depression. *American Journal of Psychiatry*, *162*, 1351–1360.

Calabrese, J. R., Sullivan, J. R., Bowden, C. L., Suppes, T., Goldberg, J. F., Sachs, G. S., *et al.* (2002). Rash in multicenter trials of lamotrigine in mood disorders: Clinical relevance and management. *Journal of Clinical Psychiatry*, *63*, 1012–1019.

Carlson, G. A., & Weintraub, S. (1993). Childhood behavior problems and bipolar disorder – relationship or coincidence? *Journal of Affective Disorders*, *28*, 143–153.

Chang, K., Adleman, N., Dienes, K., Barnea-Goraly, N., Reiss, A., & Ketter, T. (2003). Decreased *N*-acetylaspartate in children with familial bipolar disorder. *Biological Psychiatry*, *53*, 1059–1065.

Chang, K., Karchemskiy, A., Barnea-Goraly, N., Garrett, A., Simeonova, D. I., & Reiss, A. (2005). Reduced amygdalar gray matter volume in familial pediatric bipolar disorder. *Journal of the American Academy of Child and Adolescent Psychiatry*, *44*, 565–573.

Chang, K., Saxena, K., & Howe, M. (2006). An open-label study of lamotrigine adjunct or monotherapy for the treatment of adolescents with bipolar depression. *Journal of the American Academy of Child and Adolescent Psychiatry*, *45*, 298–304.

Chang, K. D., Steiner, H., & Ketter, T. A. (2000). Psychiatric phenomenology of child and adolescent bipolar offspring. *Journal of the American Academy of Child and Adolescent Psychiatry*, *39*, 453–460.

Chengappa, K. N., Kupfer, D. J., Frank, E., Houck, P. R., Grochocinski, V. J., Cluss, P. A., *et al.* (2003). Relationship of birth cohort and early age at onset of illness in a bipolar disorder case registry. *American Journal of Psychiatry*, *160*, 1636–1642.

Christie, K. A., Burke, J. D. Jr., Regier, D. A., Rae, D. S., Boyd, J. H., & Locke, B. Z. (1988). Epidemiologic evidence for early onset of mental disorders and higher risk of drug abuse in young adults. *American Journal of Psychiatry*, *145*, 971–975.

Cipriani, A., Pretty, H., Hawton, K., & Geddes, J. R. (2005). Lithium in the prevention of suicidal behavior and all-cause mortality in patients with mood disorders: A systematic review of randomized trials. *American Journal of Psychiatry*, *162*, 1805–1819.

Correll, C. U., Penzner, J. B., Parikh, U. H., Mughal, T., Javed, T., Carbon, M., *et al.* (2006). Recognizing and monitoring adverse events of second-generation antipsychotics in children and adolescents. *Child and Adolescent Psychiatric Clinics of North America*, *15*, 177–206.

Costello, E. J., Angold, A., Burns, B. J., Erkanli, A., Stangl, D. K., & Tweed, D. L. (1996). The Great Smoky Mountains Study of Youth. Functional impairment and serious emotional disturbance. *Archives of General Psychiatry*, *53*, 1137–1143.

Craddock, N., & Forty, L. (2006). Genetics of affective (mood) disorders. *European Journal of Human Genetics*, *14*, 660–668.

Davanzo, P., Thomas, M. A., Yue, K., Oshiro, T., Belin, T., Strober, M., *et al.* (2001). Decreased anterior cingulate myo-inositol/creatine spectroscopy resonance with lithium treatment in children with bipolar disorder. *Neuropsychopharmacology*, *24*, 359–369.

Davanzo, P., Yue, K., Thomas, M. A., Belin, T., Mintz, J., Venkatraman, T. N., *et al.* (2003). Proton magnetic resonance spectroscopy of bipolar disorder versus intermittent explosive disorder in children and adolescents. *American Journal of Psychiatry*, *160*, 1442–1452.

de Silva, M., MacArdle, B., McGowan, M., Hughes, E., Stewart, J., Neville, B. G., *et al.* (1996). Randomised comparative monotherapy trial of phenobarbitone, phenytoin, carbamazepine, or sodium valproate for newly diagnosed childhood epilepsy. *Lancet*, *347*, 709–713.

DelBello, M. P., Adler, C. M., Amicone, J., Mills, N. P., Shear, P. K., Warner, J., *et al.* (2004a). Parametric neurocognitive task design:

a pilot study of sustained attention in adolescents with bipolar disorder. *Journal of Affective Disorders*, *82* (Supplement 1), S79–S88.

DelBello, M. P., Adler, C. M., & Strakowski, S. M. (2006a). The neurophysiology of childhood and adolescent bipolar disorder. *CNS Spectrums*, *11*, 298–311.

DelBello, M. P., Cecil, K. M., Adler, C. M., Daniels, J. P., & Strakowski, S. M. (2006b). Neurochemical effects of olanzapine in first-hospitalization manic adolescents: A proton magnetic resonance spectroscopy study. *Neuropsychopharmacology*, *31*, 1264–1273.

DelBello, M. P., Findling, R. L., Kushner, S., Wang, D., Olson, W. H., Capece, J. A., Fazzio, L., Rosenthal, N. R. (2005). A pilot controlled trial of topiramate for mania in children and adolescents with bipolar disorder. *Journal of the American Academy of Child & Adolescent Psychiatry*, *44*, 539–547.

DelBello, M. P., Kowatch, R. A., Adler, C. M., Stanford, K. E., Welge, J. A., Barzman, D. H., *et al.* (2006c). A double-blind randomized pilot study comparing quetiapine and divalproex for adolescent mania. *Journal of the American Academy of Child and Adolescent Psychiatry*, *45*, 305–313.

DelBello, M. P., Schwiers, M. L., Rosenberg, H. L., & Strakowski, S. M. (2002). A double-blind, randomized, placebo-controlled study of quetiapine as adjunctive treatment for adolescent mania. *Journal of the American Academy of Child and Adolescent Psychiatry*, *41*, 1216–1223.

DelBello, M. P., Zimmerman, M. E., Mills, N. P., Getz, G. E., & Strakowski, S. M. (2004b). Magnetic resonance imaging analysis of amygdala and other subcortical brain regions in adolescents with bipolar disorder. *Bipolar Disorders*, *6*, 43–52.

Dickstein, D. P., Milham, M. P., Nugent, A. C., Drevets, W. C., Charney, D. S., Pine, D. S., *et al.* (2005a). Frontotemporal alterations in pediatric bipolar disorder: results of a voxel-based morphometry study. *Archives of General Psychiatry*, *62*, 734–741.

Dickstein, D. P., Nelson, E. E., McClure, E. B., Grimley, M. E., Knopf, L., Brotman, M. A., *et al.* (2007). Cognitive flexibility in phenotypes of pediatric bipolar disorder. *Journal of the American Academy of Child and Adolescent Psychiatry*, *46*, 341–355.

Dickstein, D. P., Rich, B. A., Binstock, A. B., Pradella, A. G., Towbin, K. E., Pine, D. S., *et al.* (2005b). Comorbid anxiety in phenotypes of pediatric bipolar disorder. *Journal of Child and Adolescent Psychopharmacology*, *15*, 534–548.

Dickstein, D. P., Treland, J. E., Snow, J., McClure, E. B., Mehta, M. S., Towbin, K. E., *et al.* (2004). Neuropsychological performance in pediatric bipolar disorder. *Biological Psychiatry*, *55*, 32–39.

Dilsaver, S. C., & Akiskal, H. S. (2004). Preschool-onset mania: Incidence, phenomenology and family history. *Journal of Affective Disorders*, *82* (Supplement 1), S35–S43.

Doyle, A. E., Wilens, T. E., Kwon, A., Seidman, L. J., Faraone, S. V., Fried, R., *et al.* (2005). Neuropsychological functioning in youth with bipolar disorder. *Biological Psychiatry*, *58*, 540–548.

Faraone, S. V., Biederman, J., Mennin, D., Wozniak, J., & Spencer, T. (1997). Attention-deficit hyperactivity disorder with bipolar disorder: A familial subtype? *Journal of the American Academy of Child and Adolescent Psychiatry*, *36*, 1378–1387.

Findling, R. L., Gracious, B. L., McNamara, N. K., Youngstrom, E. A., Demeter, C. A., Branicky, L. A., *et al.* (2001). Rapid, continuous cycling and psychiatric co-morbidity in pediatric bipolar I disorder. *Bipolar Disorders*, *3*, 202–210.

Findling, R. L., McNamara, N. K., Youngstrom, E. A., Stansbrey, R., Gracious, B. L., Reed, M. D., *et al.* (2005). Double-blind 18-month trial of lithium versus divalproex maintenance treatment in pediatric bipolar disorder. *Journal of the American Academy of Child and Adolescent Psychiatry*, *44*, 409–417.

Frazier, J. A., Biederman, J., Tohen, M., Feldman, P. D., Jacobs, T. G., Toma, V., *et al.* (2001). A prospective open-label treatment trial of olanzapine monotherapy in children and adolescents with bipolar disorder. *Journal of Child and Adolescent Psychopharmacology*, *11*, 239–250.

Frazier, J. A., Meyer, M. C., Biederman, J., Wozniak, J., Wilens, T. E., Spencer, T. J., *et al.* (1999). Risperidone treatment for juvenile bipolar disorder: A retrospective chart review. *Journal of the American Academy of Child and Adolescent Psychiatry*, *38*, 960–965.

Fristad, M. A., Gavazzi, S. M., & Mackinaw-Koons, B. (2003). Family psychoeducation: An adjunctive intervention for children with bipolar disorder. *Biological Psychiatry*, *53*, 1000–1008.

Gelenberg, A. J., Kane, J. M., Keller, M. B., Lavori, P., Rosenbaum, J. F., Cole, K., *et al.* (1989). Comparison of standard and low serum levels of lithium for maintenance treatment of bipolar disorder. *New England Journal of Medicine*, *321*, 1489–1493.

Geller, B., Badner, J. A., Tillman, R., Christian, S. L., Bolhofner, K., & Cook, E. H. Jr. (2004a). Linkage disequilibrium of the brain-derived neurotrophic factor Val66Met polymorphism in children with a prepubertal and early adolescent bipolar disorder phenotype. *American Journal of Psychiatry*, *161*, 1698–1700.

Geller, B., Cooper, T. B., Sun, K., Zimerman, B., Frazier, J., Williams, M., *et al.* (1998a). Double-blind and placebo-controlled study of lithium for adolescent bipolar disorders with secondary substance dependency. *Journal of the American Academy of Child and Adolescent Psychiatry*, *37*, 171–178.

Geller, B., Fox, L. W., & Clark, K. A. (1994). Rate and predictors of prepubertal bipolarity during follow-up of 6- to 12-year-old depressed children. *Journal of the American Academy of Child and Adolescent Psychiatry*, *33*, 461–468.

Geller, B., Tillman, R., Craney, J. L., & Bolhofner, K. (2004b). Four-year prospective outcome and natural history of mania in children with a prepubertal and early adolescent bipolar disorder phenotype. *Archives of General Psychiatry*, *61*, 459–467.

Geller, B., Warner, K., Williams, M., & Zimerman, B. (1998b). Prepubertal and young adolescent bipolarity versus ADHD: Assessment and validity using the WASH-U-KSADS, CBCL and TRF. *Journal of Affective Disorders*, *51*, 93–100.

Geller, B., Williams, M., Zimerman, B., Frazier, J., Beringer, L., & Warner, K. L. (1998c). Prepubertal and early adolescent bipolarity differentiate from ADHD by manic symptoms, grandiose delusions, ultra-rapid or ultradian cycling. *Journal of Affective Disorders*, *51*, 81–91.

Geller, B., Zimerman, B., Williams, M., Bolhofner, K., & Craney, J. L. (2001). Bipolar disorder at prospective follow-up of adults who had prepubertal major depressive disorder. *American Journal of Psychiatry*, *158*, 125–127.

Ghaemi, S. N., Hsu, D. J., Rosenquist, K. J., Pardo, T. B., & Goodwin, F. K. (2006). Extrapyramidal side effects with atypical neuroleptics in bipolar disorder. *Progress in Neuro-Psychopharmacology and Biological Psychiatry*, *30*, 209–213.

Goodwin, F. K., Fireman, B., Simon, G. E., Hunkeler, E. M., Lee, J., & Revicki, D. (2003). Suicide risk in bipolar disorder during treatment with lithium and divalproex. *JAMA*, *290*, 1467–1473.

Goodwin, G. M., Bowden, C. L., Calabrese, J. R., Grunze, H., Kasper, S., White, R., *et al.* (2004). A pooled analysis of 2 placebo-controlled 18-month trials of lamotrigine and lithium maintenance in bipolar I disorder. *Journal of Clinical Psychiatry*, *65*, 432–441.

Gorrindo, T., Blair, R. J., Budhani, S., Dickstein, D. P., Pine, D. S., & Leibenluft, E. (2005). Deficits on a probabilistic response-reversal task in patients with pediatric bipolar disorder. *American Journal of Psychiatry*, *162*, 1975–1977.

Grauso-Eby, N. L., Goldfarb, O., Feldman-Winter, L. B., & McAbee, G. N. (2003). Acute pancreatitis in children from valproic acid: Case series and review. *Pediatric Neurology*, *28*, 145–148.

Green, E. K., Raybould, R., Macgregor, S., Hyde, S., Young, A. H., O'Donovan, M. C., *et al.* (2006). Genetic variation of brain-derived neurotrophic factor (BDNF) in bipolar disorder: Case–control study of over 3000 individuals from the UK. *British Journal of Psychiatry*, *188*, 21–25.

Grigoroiu-Serbanescu, M., Christodorescu, D., Jipescu, I., Totoescu, A., Marinescu, E., & Ardelean, V. (1989). Psychopathology in children aged 10–17 of bipolar parents: psychopathology rate and correlates of the severity of the psychopathology. *Journal of Affective Disorders*, *16*, 167–179.

Harpold, T. L., Wozniak, J., Kwon, A., Gilbert, J., Wood, J., Smith, L., *et al.* (2005). Examining the association between pediatric bipolar disorder and anxiety disorders in psychiatrically referred children and adolescents. *Journal of Affective Disorders*, *88*, 19–26.

Harrington, R., Fudge, H., Rutter, M., Pickles, A., & Hill, J. (1990). Adult outcomes of childhood and adolescent depression. I. Psychiatric status. *Archives of General Psychiatry*, *47*, 465–473.

Harrington, R. & Myatt, T. (2003). Is preadolescent mania the same condition as adult mania? A British perspective. *Biological Psychiatry*, *53*, 961–969.

Hayden, E. P., & Nurnberger, J. I. Jr. (2006). Molecular genetics of bipolar disorder. *Genes, Brain, and Behavior*, *5*, 85–95.

Hazell, P., O'Connell, D., Heathcote, D., Robertson, J., & Henry, D. (1995). Efficacy of tricyclic drugs in treating child and adolescent depression: a meta-analysis. *British Medical Journal*, *310*, 897–901.

Hazell, P. L., Carr, V., Lewin, T. J., & Sly, K. (2003). Manic symptoms in young males with ADHD predict functioning but not diagnosis after 6 years. *Journal of the American Academy of Child and Adolescent Psychiatry*, *42*, 552–560.

Henin, A., Biederman, J., Mick, E., Sachs, G. S., Hirshfeld-Becker, D. R., Siegel, R. S., *et al.* (2005). Psychopathology in the offspring of parents with bipolar disorder: A controlled study. *Biological Psychiatry*, *58*, 554–561.

Hillegers, M. H., Reichart, C. G., Wals, M., Verhulst, F. C., Ormel, J., & Nolen, W. A. (2005). Five-year prospective outcome of psychopathology in the adolescent offspring of bipolar parents. *Bipolar Disorders*, *7*, 344–350.

Hirschfeld, R. M., Keck, P. E. Jr., Kramer, M., Karcher, K., Canuso, C., Eerdekens, M., *et al.* (2004). Rapid antimanic effect of risperidone monotherapy: A 3-week multicenter, double-blind, placebo-controlled trial. *American Journal of Psychiatry*, *161*, 1057–1065.

Hodgins, S., Faucher, B., Zarac, A., & Ellenbogen, M. (2002). Children of parents with bipolar disorder. A population at high risk for major affective disorders. *Child and Adolescent Psychiatric Clinics of North America*, *11*, 533–553, ix.

Ichim, L., Berk, M., & Brook, S. (2000). Lamotrigine compared with lithium in mania: a double-blind randomized controlled trial. *Annals of Clinical Psychiatry*, *12*, 5–10.

Johnson, J. G., Cohen, P., & Brook, J. S. (2000). Associations between bipolar disorder and other psychiatric disorders during adolescence and early adulthood: A community-based longitudinal investigation. *American Journal of Psychiatry*, *157*, 1679–1681.

Kafantaris, V., Coletti, D. J., Dicker, R., Padula, G., Kane, J. M. (2003). Lithium treatment of acute mania in adolescents: a large open trial. *Journal of the American Academy of Child & Adolescent Psychiatry*, *42*, 1038–1045.

Kafantaris, V., Coletti, D. J., Dicker, R., Padula, G., Pleak, R. R., Alvir, J. M. (2004). Lithium treatment of acute mania in adolescents: a placebo-controlled discontinuation study. *Journal of the American Academy of Child & Adolescent Psychiatry*, 43, 984–993.

Keck, P. E. Jr., Marcus, R., Tourkodimitris, S., Ali, M., Liebeskind, A., Saha, A., *et al.* (2003a). A placebo-controlled, double-blind study of the efficacy and safety of aripiprazole in patients with acute bipolar mania. *American Journal of Psychiatry*, *160*, 1651–1658.

Keck, P. E. Jr., Versiani, M., Potkin, S., West, S. A., Giller, E., & Ice, K. (2003b). Ziprasidone in the treatment of acute bipolar mania: A three-week, placebo-controlled, double-blind, randomized trial. *American Journal of Psychiatry*, *160*, 741–748.

Keck, P. E. Jr., Welge, J. A., McElroy, S. L., Arnold, L. M., & Strakowski, S. M. (2000a). Placebo effect in randomized, controlled studies of acute bipolar mania and depression. *Biological Psychiatry*, *47*, 748–755.

Keck, P. E. Jr., Welge, J. A., Strakowski, S. M., Arnold, L. M., & McElroy, S. L. (2000b). Placebo effect in randomized, controlled maintenance studies of patients with bipolar disorder. *Biological Psychiatry*, *47*, 756–761.

Keikhaee, M. R., Fadai, F., Sargolzaee, M. R., Javanbakht, A., Najmabadi, H., & Ohadi, M. (2005). Association analysis of the dopamine transporter (DAT1)-67A/T polymorphism in bipolar disorder. *American Journal of Medical Genetics. B Neuropsychiatric Genetics*, *135*, 47–49.

Keller, M. B., Lavori, P. W., Kane, J. M., Gelenberg, A. J., Rosenbaum, J. F., Walzer, E. A., *et al.* (1992). Subsyndromal symptoms in bipolar disorder: A comparison of standard and low serum levels of lithium. *Archives of General Psychiatry*, *49*, 371–376.

Kelsoe, J. R. (2003). Arguments for the genetic basis of the bipolar spectrum. *Journal of Affective Disorders*, *73*, 183–197.

Kelsoe, J. R., Spence, M. A., Loetscher, E., Foguet, M., Sadovnick, A. D., Remick, R. A., *et al.* (2001). A genome survey indicates a possible susceptibility locus for bipolar disorder on chromosome 22. *Proceedings of the National Academy of Sciences of the USA*, *98*, 585–590.

Kennedy, N., Everitt, B., Boydell, J., Van Os, J., Jones, P. B., & Murray, R. M. (2005). Incidence and distribution of first-episode mania by age: Results from a 35-year study. *Psychological Medicine*, *35*, 855–863.

Kessler, R. C., Chiu, W. T., Demler, O., Merikangas, K. R., & Walters, E. E. (2005). Prevalence, severity, and comorbidity of 12-month DSM-IV disorders in the National Comorbidity Survey Replication. *Archives of General Psychiatry*, *62*, 617–627.

Khanna, S., Vieta, E., Lyons, B., Grossman, F., Eerdekens, M., & Kramer, M. (2005). Risperidone in the treatment of acute mania: Double-blind, placebo-controlled study. *British Journal of Psychiatry*, *187*, 229–234.

Kim-Cohen, J., Caspi, A., Moffitt, T. E., Harrington, H., Milne, B. J., & Poulton, R. (2003). Prior juvenile diagnoses in adults with mental disorder: developmental follow-back of a prospective-longitudinal cohort. *Archives of General Psychiatry*, *60*, 709–717.

Kovacs, M., Akiskal, H. S., Gatsonis, C., & Parrone, P. L. (1994). Childhood-onset dysthymic disorder: Clinical features and prospective naturalistic outcome. *Archives of General Psychiatry*, *51*, 365–374.

Kowatch, R. A., Fristad, M., Birmaher, B., Wagner, K. D., Findling, R. L., & Hellander, M. (2005a). Treatment guidelines for children and adolescents with bipolar disorder. *Journal of the American Academy of Child and Adolescent Psychiatry*, *44*, 213–235.

Kowatch, R. A., Suppes, T., Carmody, T. J., Bucci, J. P., Hume, J. H., Kromelis, M., *et al.* (2000). Effect size of lithium, divalproex sodium, and carbamazepine in children and adolescents with bipolar disorder. *Journal of the American Academy of Child and Adolescent Psychiatry*, *39*, 713–720.

Kowatch, R. A., Youngstrom, E. A., Danielyan, A., & Findling, R. L. (2005b). Review and meta-analysis of the phenomenology and clinical characteristics of mania in children and adolescents. *Bipolar Disorders*, *7*, 483–496.

Lagace, D. C., Kutcher, S. P., & Robertson, H. A. (2003). Mathematics deficits in adolescents with bipolar I disorder. *American Journal of Psychiatry*, *160*, 100–104.

Lasch, K., Weissman, M., Wickramaratne, P., & Bruce, M. L. (1990). Birth-cohort changes in the rates of mania. *Psychiatry Research*, *33*, 31–37.

Leboyer, M., Bellivier, F., McKeon, P., Albus, M., Borrman, M., Perez-Diaz, F., *et al.* (1998). Age at onset and gender resemblance in bipolar siblings. *Psychiatry Research*, *81*, 125–131.

Leibenluft, E., Charney, D. S., Towbin, K. E., Bhangoo, R. K., & Pine, D. S. (2003). Defining clinical phenotypes of juvenile mania. *American Journal of Psychiatry*, *160*, 430–437.

Leibenluft, E., Cohen, P., Gorrindo, T., Brook, J. S., & Pine, D. S. (2006). Chronic vs. episodic irritability in youth: A community-based, longitudinal study of clinical and diagnostic associations. *Journal of Child and Adolescent Psychopharmacology*, *16*, 456–466.

Leibenluft, E., Rich, B. A., Vinton, D. T., Nelson, E. E., Fromm, S. J., Berghorst, L. H., *et al.* (2007). Neural circuitry engaged during unsuccessful motor inhibition in pediatric bipolar disorder. *American Journal of Psychiatry*, *164*, 52–60.

Lewinsohn, P. M., Klein, D. N., & Seeley, J. R. (1995). Bipolar disorders in a community sample of older adolescents: Prevalence, phenomenology, comorbidity, and course. *Journal of the American Academy of Child and Adolescent Psychiatry*, *34*, 454–463.

Lewinsohn, P. M., Klein, D. N., & Seeley, J. R. (2000). Bipolar disorder during adolescence and young adulthood in a community sample. *Bipolar Disorders*, *2*, 281–293.

Lewinsohn, P. M., Seeley, J. R., Buckley, M. E., & Klein, D. N. (2002). Bipolar disorder in adolescence and young adulthood. *Child and Adolescent Psychiatric Clinics of North America*, *11*, 461–75, vii.

Lin, P. I., McInnis, M. G., Potash, J. B., Willour, V., MacKinnon, D. F., DePaulo, J. R., *et al.* (2006). Clinical correlates and familial aggregation of age at onset in bipolar disorder. *American Journal of Psychiatry*, *163*, 240–246.

Manji, H. K., Moore, G. J., & Chen, G. (2000). Lithium up-regulates the cytoprotective protein Bcl-2 in the CNS *in vivo*: A role for neurotrophic and neuroprotective effects in manic depressive illness. *Journal of Clinical Psychiatry*, *61*, 82–96.

Mannuzza, S., Klein, R. G., Bessler, A., Malloy, P., & LaPadula, M. (1998). Adult psychiatric status of hyperactive boys grown up. *American Journal of Psychiatry*, *155*, 493–498.

Martin, A., Young, C., Leckman, J. F., Mukonoweshuro, C., Rosenheck, R., & Leslie, D. (2004). Age effects on antidepressant-induced manic conversion. *Archives of Pediatrics and Adolescent Medicine*, *158*, 773–780.

McCarthy, J., Arrese, D., McGlashan, A., Rappaport, B., Kraseski, K., Conway, F., *et al.* (2004). Sustained attention and visual processing speed in children and adolescents with bipolar disorder and other psychiatric disorders. *Psychological Reports*, *95*, 39–47.

McCauley, E., Myers, K., Mitchell, J., Calderon, R., Schloredt, K., & Treder, R. (1993). Depression in young people: initial presentation and clinical course. *Journal of the American Academy of Child and Adolescent Psychiatry*, *32*, 714–722.

McClure, E. B., Monk, C. S., Nelson, E. E., Parrish, J. M., Adler, A., Blair, R. J. R., *et al.* (2007). Abnormal attention modulation of fear circuit function in pediatric generalized anxiety disorder. *Archives of General Psychiatry*, *64*, 97–106.

McClure, E. B., Pope, K., Hoberman, A. J., Pine, D. S., & Leibenluft, E. (2003). Facial expression recognition in adolescents with mood and anxiety disorders. *American Journal of Psychiatry*, *160*, 1172–1174.

McClure, E. B., Treland, J. E., Snow, J., Dickstein, D. P., Towbin, K. E., Charney, D. S., *et al.* (2005a). Memory and learning in pediatric bipolar disorder. *Journal of the American Academy of Child and Adolescent Psychiatry*, *44*, 461–469.

McClure, E. B., Treland, J. E., Snow, J., Schmajuk, M., Dickstein, D. P., Towbin, K. E., *et al.* (2005b). Deficits in social cognition and response flexibility in pediatric bipolar disorder. *American Journal of Psychiatry*, *162*, 1644–1651.

McElroy, S. L., Strakowski, S. M., West, S. A., Keck, P. E. Jr., & McConville, B. J. (1997). Phenomenology of adolescent and adult mania in hospitalized patients with bipolar disorder. *American Journal of Psychiatry*, *154*, 44–49.

McIntyre, R. S., Brecher, M., Paulsson, B., Huizar, K., & Mullen, J. (2005). Quetiapine or haloperidol as monotherapy for bipolar mania: A 12-week, double-blind, randomised, parallel-group, placebo-controlled trial. *European Neuropsychopharmacology*, *15*, 573–585.

McIntyre, R. S., Mancini, D. A., McCann, S., Srinivasan, J., & Kennedy, S. H. (2003). Valproate, bipolar disorder and polycystic ovarian syndrome. *Bipolar Disorders*, *5*, 28–35.

McQueen, M. B., Devlin, B., Faraone, S. V., Nimgaonkar, V. L., Sklar, P., Smoller, J. W., *et al.* (2005). Combined analysis from eleven linkage studies of bipolar disorder provides strong evidence of susceptibility loci on chromosomes 6q and 8q. *American Journal of Human Genetics*, *77*, 582–595.

Mick, E., Spencer, T., Wozniak, J., & Biederman, J. (2005). Heterogeneity of irritability in attention-deficit/hyperactivity disorder subjects with and without mood disorders. *Biological Psychiatry*, *58*, 576–582.

Miklowitz, D. J., George, E. L., Axelson, D. A., Kim, E. Y., Birmaher, B., Schneck, C., *et al.* (2004). Family-focused treatment for adolescents with bipolar disorder. *Journal of Affective Disorders*, *82* (Supplement 1), S113–S128.

Moore, C. M., Demopulos, C. M., Henry, M. E., Steingard, R. J., Zamvil, L., Katic, A., *et al.* (2002). Brain-to-serum lithium ratio and age: An *in vivo* magnetic resonance spectroscopy study. *American Journal of Psychiatry*, *159*, 1240–1242.

Moore, G. J., Bebchuk, J. M., Hasanat, K., Chen, G., Seraji-Bozorgzad, N., Wilds, I. B., *et al.* (2000). Lithium increases *N*-acetyl-aspartate in the human brain: *in vivo* evidence in support of bcl-2's neurotrophic effects? *Biological Psychiatry*, *48*, 1–8.

Moore, G. J., Bebchuk, J. M., Parrish, J. K., Faulk, M. W., Arfken, C. L., Strahl-Bevacqua, J., *et al.* (1999). Temporal dissociation between lithium-induced changes in frontal lobe myo-inositol and clinical response in manic-depressive illness. *American Journal of Psychiatry*, *156*, 1902–1908.

Nemeroff, C. B., Evans, D. L., Gyulai, L., Sachs, G. S., Bowden, C. L., Gergel, I. P., *et al.* (2001). Double-blind, placebo-controlled comparison of imipramine and paroxetine in the treatment of bipolar depression. *American Journal of Psychiatry*, *158*, 906–912.

National Institute of Mental Health (NIMH). (2001). National Institute of Mental Health research roundtable on prepubertal bipolar disorder. *Journal of the American Academy of Child and Adolescent Psychiatry*, *40*, 871–878.

Patel, N. C., DelBello, M. P., Keck, P. E. Jr., & Strakowski, S. M. (2006). Phenomenology associated with age at onset in patients with bipolar disorder at their first psychiatric hospitalization. *Bipolar Disorders*, *8*, 91–94.

Pavuluri, M. N., Graczyk, P. A., Henry, D. B., Carbray, J. A., Heidenreich, J., & Miklowitz, D. J. (2004a). Child- and family-focused cognitive-behavioral therapy for pediatric bipolar disorder: Development and preliminary results. *Journal of the American Academy of Child and Adolescent Psychiatry*, *43*, 528–537.

Pavuluri, M. N., Henry, D. B., Carbray, J. A., Sampson, G., Naylor, M. W., & Janicak, P. G. (2004b). Open-label prospective trial of risperidone in combination with lithium or divalproex sodium in pediatric mania. *Journal of Affective Disorders*, *82* (Supplement 1), S103–S111.

Pavuluri, M. N., Schenkel, L. S., Aryal, S., Harral, E. M., Hill, S. K., Herbener, E. S., *et al.* (2006). Neurocognitive function in unmedicated manic and medicated euthymic pediatric bipolar patients. *American Journal of Psychiatry*, *163*, 286–293.

Pearlson, G. D., Barta, P. E., Powers, R. E., Menon, R. R., Richards, S. S., Aylward, E. H., *et al.* (1997). Ziskind–Somerfeld Research Award 1996. Medial and superior temporal gyral volumes and cerebral asymmetry in schizophrenia versus bipolar disorder. *Biological Psychiatry*, *41*, 1–14.

Perlis, R. H., Miyahara, S., Marangell, L. B., Wisniewski, S. R., Ostacher, M., DelBello, M. P., *et al.* (2004). Long-term implications of early onset in bipolar disorder: Data from the first 1000 participants in the systematic treatment enhancement program for bipolar disorder (STEP-BD). *Biological Psychiatry*, *55*, 875–881.

Pope, H. G. Jr., McElroy, S. L., Keck, P. E. Jr., & Hudson, J. I. (1991). Valproate in the treatment of acute mania. A placebo-controlled study. *Archives of General Psychiatry*, *48*, 62–68.

Rao, U., Ryan, N. D., Birmaher, B., Dahl, R. E., Williamson, D. E., Kaufman, J., *et al.* (1995). Unipolar depression in adolescents: clinical outcome in adulthood. *Journal of the American Academy of Child and Adolescent Psychiatry*, *34*, 566–578.

Reich, W., Neuman, R. J., Volk, H. E., Joyner, C. A., & Todd, R. D. (2005). Comorbidity between ADHD and symptoms of bipolar disorder in a community sample of children and adolescents. *Twin Research and Human Genetics*, *8*, 459–466.

Rey, J. M., & Martin, A. (2006). Selective serotonin reuptake inhibitors and suicidality in juveniles: Review of the evidence and implications for clinical practice. *Child and Adolescent Psychiatric Clinics of North America*, *15*, 221–237.

Rich, B. A., Schmajuk, M., Perez-Edgar, K., Pine, D. S., Fox, N. A., & Leibenluft, E. (2007). Different psychophysiological and behavioral responses elicited by frustration in pediatric bipolar disorder and severe mood dysregulation. *American Journal of Psychiatry*, *164*, 309–317.

Rich, B. A., Schmajuk, M., Perez-Edgar, K. E., Pine, D. S., Fox, N. A., & Leibenluft, E. (2005). The impact of reward, punishment, and frustration on attention in pediatric bipolar disorder. *Biological Psychiatry*, *58*, 532–539.

Rich, B. A., Vinton, D. T., Roberson-Nay, R., Hommer, R. E., Berghorst, L. H., McClure, E. B., *et al.* (2006). Limbic hyperactivation during processing of neutral facial expressions in children with bipolar disorder. *Proceedings of the National Academy of Sciences of the USA*, *103*, 8900–8905.

Robertson, H. A., Kutcher, S. P., & Lagace, D. C. (2003). No evidence of attentional deficits in stabilized bipolar youth relative to unipolar and control comparators. *Bipolar Disorders*, *5*, 330–339.

Scheffer, R. E., Kowatch, R. A., Carmody, T., & Rush, A. J. (2005). Randomized, placebo-controlled trial of mixed amphetamine salts for symptoms of comorbid ADHD in pediatric bipolar disorder after mood stabilization with divalproex sodium. *American Journal of Psychiatry*, *162*, 58–64.

Scheffer, R. E. & Niskala Apps, J. A. (2004). The diagnosis of preschool bipolar disorder presenting with mania: open pharmacological treatment. *Journal of Affective Disorders*, *82* (Supplement 1), S25–S34.

Silverstone, P. H., Wu, R. H., O'Donnell, T., Ulrich, M., Asghar, S. J., & Hanstock, C. C. (2002). Chronic treatment with both lithium and sodium valproate may normalize phosphoinositol cycle activity in bipolar patients. *Human Psychopharmacology*, *17*, 321–327.

Small, J. G., Klapper, M. H., Milstein, V., Kellams, J. J., Miller, M. J., Marhenke, J. D., *et al.* (1991). Carbamazepine compared with lithium in the treatment of mania. *Archives of General Psychiatry*, *48*, 915–921.

Smoller, J. W., & Finn, C. T. (2003). Family, twin, and adoption studies of bipolar disorder. *American Journal of Medical Genetics. C. Seminars in Medical Genetics*, *123*, 48–58.

Stokes, P. E., Shamoian, C. A., Stoll, P. M., & Patton, M. J. (1971). Efficacy of lithium as acute treatment of manic-depressive illness. *Lancet*, *1*, 1319–1325.

Straker, D., Correll, C. U., Kramer-Ginsberg, E., Abdulhamid, N., Koshy, F., Rubens, E., *et al.* (2005). Cost-effective screening for the metabolic syndrome in patients treated with second-generation antipsychotic medications. *American Journal of Psychiatry*, *162*, 1217–1221.

Strakowski, S. M., DelBello, M. P., Sax, K. W., Zimmerman, M. E., Shear, P. K., Hawkins, J. M., *et al.* (1999). Brain magnetic resonance imaging of structural abnormalities in bipolar disorder. *Archives of General Psychiatry*, *56*, 254–260.

Strober, M., & Carlson, G. (1982). Bipolar illness in adolescents with major depression: Clinical, genetic, and psychopharmacologic predictors in a three- to four-year prospective follow-up investigation. *Archives of General Psychiatry*, *39*, 549–555.

Strober, M., Lampert, C., Schmidt, S., & Morrell, W. (1993). The course of major depressive disorder in adolescents. I. Recovery and risk of manic switching in a follow-up of psychotic and nonpsychotic subtypes. *Journal of the American Academy of Child and Adolescent Psychiatry*, *32*, 34–42.

ten Have, M., Vollebergh, W., Bijl, R., & Nolen, W. A. (2002). Bipolar disorder in the general population in The Netherlands (prevalence, consequences and care utilisation): results from The Netherlands Mental Health Survey and Incidence Study (NEMESIS). *Journal of Affective Disorders*, *68*, 203–213.

Tillman, R., & Geller, B. (2003). Definitions of rapid, ultrarapid, and ultradian cycling and of episode duration in pediatric and adult bipolar disorders: a proposal to distinguish episodes from cycles. *Journal of Child and Adolescent Psychopharmacology*, *13*, 267–271.

Tohen, M., Greil, W., Calabrese, J. R., Sachs, G. S., Yatham, L. N., Oerlinghausen, B. M., *et al.* (2005). Olanzapine versus lithium in the maintenance treatment of bipolar disorder: A 12-month, randomized, double-blind, controlled clinical trial. *American Journal of Psychiatry*, *162*, 1281–1290.

Tumuluru, R. V., Weller, E. B., Fristad, M. A., & Weller, R. A. (2003). Mania in six preschool children. *Journal of Child and Adolescent Psychopharmacology*, *13*, 489–494.

Vieta, E., Bourin, M., Sanchez, R., Marcus, R., Stock, E., McQuade, R., *et al.* (2005). Effectiveness of aripiprazole v. haloperidol in acute bipolar mania: double-blind, randomised, comparative 12-week trial. *British Journal of Psychiatry*, *187*, 235–242.

Wagner, K. D., Weller, E. B., Carlson, G. A., Sachs, G., Biederman, J., Frazier, J. A., *et al.* (2002). An open-label trial of divalproex in children and adolescents with bipolar disorder. *Journal of the American Academy of Child and Adolescent Psychiatry*, *41*, 1224–1230.

Wals, M., Hillegers, M. H., Reichart, C. G., Ormel, J., Nolen, W. A., & Verhulst, F. C. (2001). Prevalence of psychopathology in children of a bipolar parent. *Journal of the American Academy of Child and Adolescent Psychiatry*, *40*, 1094–1102.

Weisler, R. H., Keck, P. E., Jr, Swann, A. C., Cutler, A. J., Ketter, T. A., Kalali, A. H. for the SPD417 Study Group. (2005). Extended-release carbamazepine capsules as monotherapy for acute mania in bipolar disorder: A multicenter, randomized, double-blind, placebo-controlled trial. *Journal of Clinical Psychiatry*, *66*, 323–330.

Weissman, M. M., Bland, R. C., Canino, G. J., Faravelli, C., Greenwald, S., Hwu, H. G., *et al.* (1996). Cross-national epidemiology of major depression and bipolar disorder. *Journal of the American Medical Association*, *276*, 293–299.

Weissman, M. M., Wolk, S., Wickramaratne, P., Goldstein, R. B., Adams, P., Greenwald, S., *et al.* (1999). Children with prepubertal-onset major depressive disorder and anxiety grown up. *Archives of General Psychiatry*, *56*, 794–801.

Wilens, T. E., Biederman, J., Brown, S., Tanguay, S., Monuteaux, M. C., Blake, C., *et al.* (2002). Psychiatric comorbidity and functioning in clinically referred preschool children and school-age youths with ADHD. *Journal of the American Academy of Child and Adolescent Psychiatry*, *41*, 262–268.

Wilens, T. E., Biederman, J., Forkner, P., Ditterline, J., Morris, M., Moore, H., *et al.* (2003). Patterns of comorbidity and dysfunction in clinically referred preschool and school-age children with bipolar disorder. *Journal of Child and Adolescent Psychopharmacology*, *13*, 495–505.

Wilens, T. E., Biederman, J., Kwon, A., Ditterline, J., Forkner, P., Moore, H., *et al.* (2004). Risk of substance use disorders in adolescents with bipolar disorder. *Journal of the American Academy of Child and Adolescent Psychiatry*, *43*, 1380–1386.

Winsberg, M. E., Sachs, N., Tate, D. L., Adalsteinsson, E., Spielman, D., & Ketter, T. A. (2000). Decreased dorsolateral prefrontal *N*-acetyl aspartate in bipolar disorder. *Biological Psychiatry*, *47*, 475–481.

Wozniak, J., Biederman, J., Kiely, K., Ablon, J. S., Faraone, S. V., Mundy, E., *et al.* (1995). Mania-like symptoms suggestive of childhood-onset bipolar disorder in clinically referred children. *Journal of the American Academy of Child and Adolescent Psychiatry*, *34*, 867–876.

Zito, J. M., Safer, D. J., dosReis, S., Gardner, J. F., Boles, M., & Lynch, F. (2000). Trends in the prescribing of psychotropic medications to preschoolers. *Journal of the American Medical Association*, *283*, 1025–1030.

Zornberg, G. L., & Pope, H. G. Jr. (1993). Treatment of depression in bipolar disorder: New directions for research. *Journal of Clinical Psychopharmacology*, *13*, 397–408.

39 Anxiety Disorders

Daniel S. Pine and Rachel G. Klein

The current chapter reviews five anxiety disorders: phobic disorders, separation anxiety disorder, social anxiety disorder, generalized anxiety disorder and panic disorder. It is organized around four themes. The first section focuses on diagnosis, nosology and assessment. The second summarizes data on prevalence, risk factors and outcome. The third reviews research on family genetics and psychobiology. Treatment is summarized in the final section.

Clinical Presentation of Childhood Anxiety Disorders

Diagnosis

For phenomena that fall on a continuum, extremes have been viewed alternatively as severe expressions of continuously distributed traits or as distinct pathological entities. Controversy remains regarding the relative advantages and disadvantages in conceptualizing pediatric anxiety as a continuous or categorical phenomenon. A key reason for categorizing children presenting in the clinic as affected by anxiety disorders is to allocate services for those anxious children most in need. However, categorization of one or another group of children does not imply distinct etiology.

Distinguishing normal anxiety from pathological anxiety can be problematic because childhood anxieties are not only common, but may be adaptive. Diagnostically, anxiety may be considered pathological at any age if it limits developmentally appropriate behavior and thus causes functional limitation. However, anxiety may be considered pathological even when the child's activities are not affected if there is significant distress. Classification of disorders with little or no manifest impairment and only distress is often difficult, because the threshold for considering distress as clinically significant varies according to many factors, such as the child's age, life circumstances or cultural background. Another guide for diagnosis is the child's ability to recover from anxiety. As such, failure to adapt represents a hallmark of pathology.

Disagreements on definitional boundaries between normal and pathological anxiety are likely to persist as long as clinical descriptors remain the exclusive basis for diagnosis. Other data may shed light, leading to nosological changes by identifying which syndromes carry long-term significance. As with definitions of hypertension, the definition of "abnormal" anxiety could change as longitudinal data identify factors that contribute to excessive long-term risk (Pine, Cohen, Gurley *et al.*, 1998; Pine, Cohen, & Brook, 2001). Eventually, advances in genetics or neuroscience also may impact on nosology. However, considerable progress is needed before such approaches can provide clinical utility.

Nosology of Childhood Anxiety Disorders

Delimitating specific syndromes that facilitate communication among professionals is not a trivial accomplishment, but it represents a minimal standard for a useful nomenclature. While DSM-IV and ICD-10 meet this minimal goal, questions concerning the distinctiveness of anxiety disorders persist. These questions emerge as a result of comorbidity among anxiety disorders, coupled with inconsistent findings of distinct natural histories and factors used to validate diagnosis. The ICD-10 and DSM-IV have similar diagnoses for childhood anxiety disorders. The major difference concerns the handling of comorbidity: ICD-10 provides a single diagnosis for co-occurring anxiety and behavior disorders, whereas the DSM-IV requires separate diagnoses for each condition. In addition, obsessive compulsive disorder (OCD) and post-traumatic stress disorder (PTSD) are classified as anxiety disorders in the DSM-IV, but not in ICD-10 (these are not considered in this chapter because they are clinically distinct from the disorders examined here). Finally, some differences exist in the definitions of childhood anxiety disorders between ICD-10 and DSM-IV (Klein, 1994); however, this chapter focuses on common clinical features.

Presentation of Specific Anxiety Disorders

Phobic Disorder

Phobic disorder is defined by marked unreasonable fear of a specific object that is not intrinsically dangerous, such as animals, or a situation, such as heights. The level of fear is considered extreme, and exposure invariably elicits extreme fear. In addition, the phobia must either cause clinically significant distress or impair the person's well-being by leading to interference with ordinary activities because of avoidance. Phobic disorders may begin at any age, but typical onset is in childhood (Fyer, 1998; Pine, Cohen, Gurley *et al.*, 1998).

Rutter's Child and Adolescent Psychiatry, 5th edition. Edited by M. Rutter, D. Bishop, D. Pine, S. Scott, J. Stevenson, E. Taylor and A. Thapar. © 2008 Blackwell Publishing, ISBN: 978-1-4051-4549-7.

Phobias can be classified based on the nature of the feared object: animals, natural environments, blood infection; or specific situations, such as elevators. Most children with phobic disorders share a limited number of feared situations. Attempts to differentiate among phobias on pathophysiological grounds have not yielded divergent features, except for blood injury phobia (Fyer, 1998), whose distinct physiological signature consists of a sudden drop in blood pressure and heart rate, and fainting.

Separation Anxiety Disorder

Separation anxiety disorder represents the only anxiety diagnosis that must begin in childhood. In ICD-10, onset must be in early childhood, whereas in the DSM-IV, onset must occur any time before age 18. The onset is frequently in late childhood, before adolescence, and decreases as children mature into adolescence. As the name connotes, the disorder reflects anxiety at separation from home or caretakers that causes impairment by leading to avoidance. The terms "school phobia" and "school refusal" have been used to describe a pattern of school avoidance (Egger, Costello, & Angold, 2003). In preadolescents, refusal to attend school because of fears is most often related to separation anxiety disorder. Feared separations situations often seem illogical. For example, a child may have no difficulty going to school, but be highly anxious while visiting familiar friends' homes. Difficulty sleeping alone is especially salient in children with separation anxiety disorder. As reviewed below, some evidence suggests relationships between childhood separation anxiety disorder and adult panic disorder.

Social Phobia/Social Anxiety Disorder

Social anxiety disorder is characterized by anxiety in a range of social situations because of fear of scrutiny, ridicule, humiliation or embarrassment. Some children may not articulate these concerns but feel uncomfortable in social settings. Children must experience discomfort with peers, not only with adults, and anxiety cannot be caused by impaired capacity for socialization, as evidenced by the fact that the children interact satisfactorily with those who are familiar to them. The diagnostic distinction between severe social anxiety disorder and mild pervasive developmental disorder can be problematic. Chronic avoidance of social interactions might limit development of social competence, contributing to similarities with mild pervasive developmental disorder. However, in general, children and adolescents with social anxiety desire social contacts, whereas those with pervasive developmental disorder typically lack interest in reciprocal relationships.

The diagnostic qualifier, generalized social phobia, denotes anxiety in multiple social settings. There are no standard definitions for distinguishing it from the non-generalized form, leading to divergent interpretations. Some apply the non-generalized label to individuals who experience social anxiety in only one or two situations, such as parties; others use the diagnosis for individuals who experience only performance anxiety, such as public speaking, eating in front of people, as well as test anxiety, but who do not have anxiety during social interactions. Performance anxiety may occur without significant anxiety in social situations, but the reverse is unusual.

Epidemiological evidence supports the distinction between generalized and non-generalized social anxiety disorder. The generalized form has been reported to have earlier onsets, more chronicity, more comorbidity and more psychopathology in relatives (Wittchen, Stein, & Kessler, 1999). This work exemplifies how epidemiological studies can inform diagnostic validity.

Generalized Anxiety Disorder

Generalized anxiety disorder encompasses multiple worries about a variety of life circumstances, such as school work, one's appearance or future. The age of onset is poorly understood, but typically it is not in early childhood. Prior to the DSM-IV, "overanxious disorder" was used for children and adolescents with multiple worries. It remains unclear to what degree the outdated diagnosis of overanxious disorder overlaps with generalized anxiety disorder (Pine, Cohen, Gurley *et al.*, 1998). Generalized anxiety disorder is the only anxiety disorder that requires somatic symptoms. However, there is no documentation that these occur preferentially in this anxiety disorder.

Relative to other anxiety disorders, generalized anxiety disorder has very high rates of comorbidity, and it rarely presents on its own in clinic patients. Beyond comorbidity with other anxiety disorders, it has a strong relationship with major depressive disorder (Costello, Pine, Hammen *et al.*, 2002; Kessler, Andrade, Bijl *et al.*, 2002). This high comorbidity raises questions about whether the diagnosis identifies a unique syndrome as opposed to a complication of other associated disorders. Because the symptoms consist mostly of worries, the disorder is not usually characterized by avoidant behavior, although there are exceptions. For example, children with extreme worries about academic performance may miss school on testing days.

Panic Disorder

The essential clinical feature of panic disorder is the repeated experience of unprovoked spontaneous panic attacks, which may lead to limited independent travel or agoraphobia. The panic attacks are characterized by intense fear of impending doom, accompanied by physical symptoms, such as rapid heartbeat, shortness of breath, choking sensation, sweating, depersonalization or derealization. To some extent, these symptoms identify meaningful subtypes of panic disorder patients. Thus, patients who present with respiratory symptoms have been reported to differ from other panic disorder patients in treatment response and familial aggregation (Briggs, Stretch, & Brandon, 1993; Horwath, Adams, Wickramaratne *et al.*, 1997). Usual onset begins with spontaneous panic attacks, typically during adolescence. Progression to full-blown panic disorder occurs in a minority, typically during early adulthood (Pine, Cohen, Gurley *et al.*, 1998).

Diagnostic confusion arises concerning panic disorder because panic reactions can occur in many anxiety states, including in various phobias during exposure to feared situations. The key distinction is that, in panic disorder, panic attacks occur without cues, as prototypically exemplified by nocturnal panic attacks. Moreover, young children may display panic reactions, but whether they experience spontaneous, unprovoked panic attacks, the hallmark of panic disorder, remains controversial. Whether panic disorder occurs in pre-adolescents is still an unresolved issue, but if it does, it must be very rare (Costello, Egger, & Angold, 2004). This scarcity has limited systematic study.

It has been suggested that, in keeping with the cognitive model of anxiety, children lack the cognitive resources for misinterpreting somatic experiences in a catastrophic fashion, and therefore do not have panic attacks. This conjecture seems unlikely, because panic reactions associated with terror occur in children. It is the sudden unprovoked aspect of panic that seems to be missing in childhood, not the catastrophic reaction. At the same time, it is possible that true panic attacks have age-related clinical variants.

Comorbidity of Childhood Anxiety Disorders

Comorbidity is an important clinical feature because it entails greater dysfunction than either condition alone. Two forms of diagnostic overlap are considered: comorbidity among anxiety disorders, and anxiety disorders with other disorders.

Anxiety Comorbidity

Children referred for treatment exhibit especially high comorbidity among anxiety disorders (Costello, Egger, & Angold, 2004). Such patterns likely reflect ascertainment biases. In a large treatment study, social anxiety, separation anxiety and generalized anxiety disorders were each diagnosed in about 60% of children (RUPP, 2001). Comorbidity was particularly elevated in children with generalized anxiety disorder who, in 90% of cases, also had another anxiety disorder. Clearly, comorbidity is less marked in community than clinical samples, but strong comorbidity across anxiety disorders, especially for generalized anxiety or overanxious disorder, is also found in population studies (Anderson, Williams, McGee *et al.*, 1987; Bird, Canino, Rubio-Stipec *et al.*, 1988; Essau, Conradt, & Petermann, 1999; Fergusson, Horwood, & Lynskey, 1993; McGee, Feehan, Williams *et al.*, 1990; Verhulst, van der Ende, Ferdin-and *et al.*, 1997). This high comorbidity has raised questions regarding the diagnostic separation of these three disorders.

Non-Anxiety Disorders

There is unanimous agreement that major depression is highly comorbid with anxiety disorders. The strength of this relationship rivals virtually all others in developmental psychopathology (Angold, Costello, & Erkanli, 1999; Costello, 2004; Costello, Pine, Hammen *et al.*, 2002). Because depression is rarer than anxiety disorders, especially in pre-adolescents, it follows that among those with anxiety the overlap with depression is not as striking as when one selects those with depression, and that this comorbidity increases with age. Although some clinical reports indicate comorbidity between anxiety and attention deficit hyperactivity disorder (ADHD), population-based studies find weak relationships (Angold, Costello, & Erkanli, 1999). There is some evidence of comorbidity between anxiety disorders and substance abuse or conduct disorder (Kaplow, Curran, Angold *et al.*, 2001; Rutter, Maughan, & Kim-Cohen, 2006).

Assessment

The assessment of pediatric anxiety has benefitted from a proliferation of instruments. They include paper-and-pencil rating scales for children, parents and teachers, clinician-rated scales, as well as child and parent interviews. Several reviews have appeared of self, parent and teacher rated anxiety scales for children (Brooks & Kutcher, 2003; Seligman, Ollendick, Langley *et al.*, 2004; Silverman & Ollendick, 2005). Therefore, only an overview is provided.

Rating Scales

Rating scales serve diverse purposes. They may screen large groups to identify children most in need of assistance or to implement prevention programs. Scales may be used for economic reasons, as they provide an economical way for assessments in epidemiological or behavioral genetic studies (Topolski, Hewitt, Eaves *et al.*, 1999). In clinical studies, scales may serve as indices of severity (RUPP, 2003).

Rating scales that anteceded DSM-III and ICD-10 were not designed to reflect the current classification. They comprised factors such as worry, physiological anxiety and fear of bodily harm, as in the Revised Children's Manifest Anxiety Scale (RCMA; Reynolds & Richmond, 1985), the State-Trait Anxiety Inventory for Children (STAIC; Speielberger, 1973) and the Revised Fear Survey Schedule for Children (FSSC-R; Ollendick, Yang, King *et al.*, 1996). The widely used Children's Behaviour Checklist (CBCL; Achenbach, 1991) generates a non-specific factor of emotional disturbance, called "internalizing" factor. In general, these scales assess constructs distinct from those generated by newer scales.

An important clinical challenge is to differentiate between anxiety and depression, a challenge reflected by the fact that a single unitary factor of the CBCL encompasses both dysfunctions. Many other scales that purport to differentiate anxiety from depression fail to do so (Klein, 1994). The meaning of scale ratings of anxiety is further complicated by the poor agreement between parent or child ratings with information obtained from clinical interviews (RUPP, 2003). It is beyond the purview of this chapter to provide comprehensive discussion of psychometric requirements for diagnostic indices.

Growing interest spurred the development of more diagnostically relevant measures of childhood anxiety. Recent efforts reflect shifts in the classification of anxiety disorders, with greater relevance given to diagnostic groupings. Standardized scales include the Multidimensional Anxiety Scale for Children (MASC; March, Parker, Sullivan *et al.*, 1997; March & Sullivan, 1999) and the Self Report for Child Anxiety Related Disorders (SCARED; Birmaher, Khetarpal, Brent *et al.*, 1997). The MASC and SCARED stand out as promising clinically relevant indices. Both measures demonstrate adequate test–retest reliability, divergent validity from depression measures, reasonable correlations with clinical ratings of anxiety severity, and sensitivity to treatment effects.

Several anxiety scales are designed for clinicians. The Hamilton Anxiety Scale (HAS; Hamilton, 1969) developed for adults has had limited application in younger populations. In a controlled treatment study, it performed less well than another clinician-rated index, the Pediatric Anxiety Rating Scale (PARS), which taps diagnostic criteria and has good psychometric properties (RUPP, 2003).

Diagnostic Interviews

Diagnostic interviews serve different purposes. The highly structured DISC was developed for epidemiological studies, to be administered by individuals without clinical training or by computer (Shaffer, Fisher, Lucas *et al.*, 2000). Support for the clinical utility of the DISC is mixed. Fair agreement between DISC diagnoses and clinical interviews conducted by the same clinicians led to the claim that the DISC had a role in clinical settings (Schwab-Stone, Shaffer, Dulcan *et al.*, 1996). However, other data do not support the claim. For example, diagnostic rates are high in epidemiological studies using the DISC (Table 39.1). Moreover, other findings question the validity of anxiety diagnoses generated by the DISC (March, Swanson, Arnold *et al.*, 2000).

The Child and Adolescent Psychiatric Assessment (CAPA; Angold & Costello, 2000), highly structured and administered by non-clinicians, is also used in epidemiological studies. Relative to the DISC, the CAPA requires more training and more closely resembles the clinical interview. While CAPA appears promising, the unavailability of data concerning treatment sensitivity precludes endorsement of clinical relevance.

The key issue is whether anxiety disorders generated by structured interviews are valid. Some evidence from longitudinal, family-based and imaging studies points towards validity. However, inconsistent findings concerning the predictive significance of childhood anxiety disorders among girls and boys studied epidemiologically (Costello, Angold, & Keeler, 1999; McGee, Feehan, Williams *et al.*, 1992; Pine, Cohen, Gurley *et al.*, 1998) raise questions about the validity of anxiety diagnoses in community samples.

The Kiddie-Schedule for Affective Disorder and Schizophrenia (K-SADS) was developed for use by clinicians and allows full latitude of inquiry. Multiple versions exist, including a highly structured version administered by lay interviewers (Kaufman, Birmaher, Brent *et al.*, 1997, 2000). The Diagnostic Interview for Children and Adolescents (DICA; Reich, 2000), also highly structured, has been used in semistructured format. The Anxiety Disorders Interview Schedule for Children (ADIS) allows full clinical inquiry (Silverman, Saavedra, & Pina, 2001). As with other clinically based semistructured interviews, the quality of data depends highly on interviewers' training and qualifications.

There is little to guide the selection of one instrument over another, in terms of better reliability or validity. All have demonstrated modest to adequate test–retest reliability, with anxiety disorders faring no better than mood disorders and slightly worse than behavioral disorders. The major factor informing selection concerns the availability of skilled clinicians for implementation. Although conceived for research purposes, diagnostic interviews may be useful to clinicians because they provide comprehensive coverage of symptomatic status (see chapter 19), and represent excellent teaching tools for training in clinical diagnosis.

Epidemiology of Pediatric Anxiety Disorders

Across several continents, well-executed epidemiological studies delineate key features of anxiety disorders, including prevalence, risk factors and longitudinal outcomes. These studies have the great advantage of avoiding clinical biases introduced by clinical samples.

Prevalence of Childhood Anxiety Disorders

Prevalence studies that have relied on interviews with parents and/or children are presented in Table 39.1. Most report the prevalence of broadly conceptualized anxiety disorders. Ongoing epidemiological studies are obtaining DSM-IV and ICD-10 diagnoses. However, most anxiety diagnoses have remained virtually unchanged, so that previous studies are relevant to the current nomenclature.

Most epidemiological studies at all ages find anxiety disorders to be the most common mental disorders. The few population-based studies of panic disorder have found very low rates in children and adolescents, below 1% for lifetime and lower frequencies for the past 6 or 12 months (Pine, Cohen, Gurley *et al.*, 1998; Reed & Wittchen, 1998; Verhulst, van der Ende, Ferdinand *et al.*, 1997; Whitaker, Johnson, Shaffer *et al.*, 1990). In pre-adolescents, separation anxiety disorder is probably the most prevalent diagnosis (Anderson, Williams, McGee *et al.*, 1987; Costello, Angold, Burns *et al.*, 1996, 1999; Costello, Egger, & Angold, 2005; Pine, Cohen, Brook *et al.*, 1998), whereas social anxiety disorder, generalized anxiety disorder and what was previously termed overanxious disorder, increase in adolescence (Fergusson, Horwood, & Lynskey, 1993; McGee, Feehan, Williams *et al.*, 1990; Pine, Cohen, Gurley *et al.*, 1998; Verhulst, van der Ende, Ferdinand *et al.*, 1997). All longitudinal epidemiological studies (Anderson, Williams, McGee *et al.*, 1987; Costello, Angold & Keeler 1999; Kim-Cohen, Caspi, Moffitt *et al.*, 2003; McGee, Feehan, Williams *et al.*, 1992; Pine, Cohen, Gurley *et al.*, 1998) find an increment in social phobia during adolescence, confirming that the disorder often emerges in adolescence.

Rates of any anxiety disorder within the past 6 or 12 months range widely, from 1.8% in New Zealand (Anderson, Williams, McGee *et al.*, 1987) to 23.5% in Holland (Verhulst, van der Ende, Ferdinand *et al.*, 1997). Variation may reflect true differences as a result of cultural influences. However, disparate rates emerge even when site differences seem minimal. For

Table 39.1 Prevalence (%) of anxiety disorders in children, adolescents, and adults followed prospectively.

Location	Authors	*n*	Age (years)	Interview	Time frame (months)	Rates (%)					
						Any	SiPh	SAD	OAD	SoPh	PD
New Zealand											
Dunedin	Anderson *et al.* (1987)[a]	785	11	DISC-C[b]	12[c]	1.8–7.5	0–2.4	0.06–3.5	0.05–2.9	0–0.9	–
					12[d]	3.6*	1.7	1.9	2.5	0.4	
	McGee *et al.* (1990)[a]	943	15	DISC-C	12[e]	10.7*	3.6	2.0	5.9	1.1	–
	Kim-Cohen *et al.* (2003)[a]	976	26	DIS	12[e]	26.1*	7.1	–	5.5 (GAD)	10.7	3.9
Christchurch	Fergusson *et al.* (1993)	986	15	DISC-P	12[e]	3.9	1.3	0.1	0.6	0.7	
		965		DISC-C	12[e]	10.8	5.1	0.5	2.1	1.7	
	Goodwin *et al.* (2004)	969	16–18	M-CIDI[i,o]	12[e]	18.4	9.6	–	2.7 (GAD)	7.5	–
		957	18–21	M-CIDI[i,o]	12[e]	14.6	6.5	–	1.8 (GAD)	6.7	–
Germany											
Manheim	Essau *et al.* (1999)	191	13	Graham/Rutter P/C[f,g,m]	6	5.8	–	–	–	–	–
Munich	Reed & Wittchen (1998)[a]	3021	14–24	M-CIDI[h,i]	12	–	–	–	–	–	0.6
					Lifetime	–	–	–	–	–	0.8
	Wittchen *et al.* (1999)[a]	925	14–17	M-CIDI[h,i]	12	–	–	–	–	3.0	–
					Lifetime	–	–	–	–	4.0	–
Bremen	Essau *et al.* (1999)	1035	12–17	M-CIDI[h,i]	Lifetime	–	–	–	–	1.6	–
UK											
London‡	Kramer & Garralda (1998)	131	13–17	K-SADS[i,j]	12	5.3	–	–	3.1	1.5	0.8
Holland	Verhulst *et al.* (1997)	312/780[k]	13–18	DISC-C	6	10.5	4.5	1.4	1.8	3.7	0.2
				DISC-P		16.5	9.2	0.6	1.5	6.3	0.3
				DISC[l]		23.5	12.7	1.8	3.1	9.2	0.4
				DISC[m]		5.3	–	–	–	–	–
						4.4					
Puerto Rico	Bird *et al.* (1988)	386/777[h]	4–16	DISC[m]	6	7.0	2.6	4.7	–	–	–
							1.3	2.1	–	–	–
USA											
Missouri	Kashani *et al.* (1987)	150	14–16	DICA[i,n]	12	8.7	–	–	–	–	–
Pennsylvania	Costello *et al.* (1988)[a]	300/789[k]	7–11	DISC-C	12	10.5	6.7	4.1	2.0	1.0	–
				DISC-P	12	6.5	3.0	0.4	2.8	0	–
	Benjamin *et al.* (1990)[a]	300/789[k]	7–11	DISC[e]	12	15.4	9.1	4.1	4.6	1.0	–
New York State	Pine *et al.* (1998)	776	9–18	DISC[e]	12	–	11.6	8.6	14.3	8.4	0.0
		760	11–20	DISC[e]	12	–	5.9	3.7	8.0	9.9	0.0
		716	17–26	DISC[e]	12	–	22.1	–	5.0 (GAD)	5.6	0.1

New Jersey	Whittaker *et al.* (1990)	356/5596[k]	13–18	Study interview[l]	Lifetime	–	–	–	3.7	–	0.6
Nationwide	Magee *et al.* (1996)	1765	15–24	CIDI[i,o]	Lifetime	–	10.8	–	–	14.9	–
North Carolina	Costello *et al.* (1996)	1015	9, 11, 13	CAPA[i,p]	3	5.7	0.3	3.5	1.4	0.6	0.03
	Costello *et al.* (2003)	1420	9–16	CAPA[i,p]	3	2.4	–	–	–	–	–
Georgia, New Haven New York Puerto Rico	Shaffer *et al.* (1996)	1285	9–17	DISC-P[q,r]	6	21.0	11.7	2.5	4.3	7.9	–
				DISC-C[r]		23.7	11.2	3.1	5.4	8.5	
				DISC[m]		18.5	9.5	4.1	8.0	8.2	–
						13.9	6.8	3.5	6.5	6.6	
				DISC		20.5	3.3	5.8	7.7	7.6	–
Oregon	Lewinsohn *et al.* (1998)	1709	15.5	K-SADS	12	2.8	1.3	0.2	0.5	0.9	0.3
Virginia	Simonoff *et al.* (1997)	2762 (twins)	8–16	CAPA[p,t]	3	–	21.2	7.2	10.8	8.4	–
							4.4	1.5	4.4	2.5	

C-GAS, children's global assessment scale; GAD, generalized anxiety disorder; OAD, overanxious disorder; P/C, parent/child; PD, panic disorder; SAD, separation anxiety disorder; SiPh, simple phobia; SoPh, social phobia.
* Rates calculated from papers.
‡ Adolescents in primary care clinics.
[a] Same cohort within site.
[b] DISC-C and DISC-P, Diagnostic Interview Schedule for Children, Child and Parent Versions (Costello *et al.*, 1984).
[c] Rates vary depending on diagnostic criteria based on DISC-C, and parent and teacher ratings, e.g., diagnostic criteria met: (1) by two of three sources or by one source and symptoms confirmed by at least one other source; (2) by one source but no other source confirms symptoms; (3) by combining symptoms from all three sources.
[d] Percentage meeting diagnostic criteria applying same standards as at age 15 in McGee *et al.* (1992).
[e] Percent meeting criteria based on DISC-C plus parent ratings.
[f] Interview by Graham & Rutter (1968).
[g] Includes anxiety and mood disorders.
[h] M-CIDI, Munich modification of CIDI (Wittchen *et al.*, 1999).
[i] Diagnosis based on interview with adolescent.
[j] K-SADS, Kiddie Schedule for Affective Disorders and Schizophrenia (Ambrosini *et al.*, 1989).
[k] Two stage study: N in stage 2/N in Stage 1.
[l] Percent meeting diagnostic criteria based on interview with parent *or* child.
[m] *Top line:* percentage meeting diagnostic criteria on parent *or* child interview *and* had a C-GAS <61 (Shaffer *et al.*, 1983).
Bottom line: percentage meeting diagnostic criteria on parent *or* child interview *and* had a C-GAS of 61–70.
[n] DICA, Diagnostic Interview for Children and Adolescents (Herjanic & Reich, 1982).
[o] CIDI, Composite International Diagnostic Interview (Wittchen, 1994).
[p] CAPA, Child and Adolescent Psychiatric Assessment (Angold & Costello, 2000).
[q] DISC Version 2.3 (Shaffer *et al.*, 1996).
[r] Percentage meeting diagnostic criteria only for symptom number, age of onset and duration.
[s] Percentage meeting diagnostic criteria and impairment linked to the specific disorder.
[t] *Top line:* percentage meeting diagnostic criteria.
Bottom line: percentage meeting diagnostic criteria *and* impairment criteria.

example, two well-executed studies of adolescents, using similar interviews and both conducted in urban sites in Germany, Bremen (Essau, Conradt, & Petermann, 1999) and Munich (Wittchen, Stein, & Kessler, 1999), report lifetime rates for social phobia of 1.6% and 4%, respectively. As is evident in Table 39.1, another case in point are the New Zealand studies from Dunedin (McGee, Feehan, Williams *et al.*, 1990) and Christchurch (Fergusson, Horwood, & Lynskey, 1993). No anxiety disorder is spared discrepancies in prevalence, even when diagnostic definitions are identical and sites appear indistinguishable.

Table 39.1 illustrates clearly that diagnostic rates are reduced sharply if diagnoses are made irrespective of the "extreme distress" criterion, when only impairment is present. Not surprisingly, the one study that compared prevalence as a function of impairment (Shaffer, Fisher, Dulcan *et al.*, 1996) found that applying an impairment criterion led to a dramatic lowering of prevalence estimates.

Could secular changes affect rates of anxiety disorders? This possibility cannot be ruled out, but does not seem to account for discrepancies across studies, because results do not suggest time-dependent rates of anxiety disorders (Table 39.1). Similarly, could methods for combining informant information contribute to cross-study differences? The low rate of informant agreement in most studies makes this a reasonable possibility. Depending on their age, children contribute varyingly valuable levels of information, and prevalence of anxiety disorders varies as a function of the reporting source (Table 39.1).

It is generally agreed that the answer regarding optimal approach to diagnosis will come from studies that examine the relative accuracy of diagnostic conventions in predicting course, as well as other features such as genetics and biological markers. One study reported that childhood anxiety disorders without impairment are not predictive of difficulties in adolescence, whereas the same is not true for disorders with impairment (Costello, Angold, & Keeler, 1999). However, these findings were not supported by another study (Pine, Cohen, & Brook, 2001). Further complicating diagnosis, impairment may occur in subthreshold syndromes (Reed & Wittchen, 1998).

In conclusion, a fair estimate of current prevalence for any pediatric anxiety disorder accompanied by impairment appears to be 5–10%. Additionally, epidemiological studies have been important in confirming that child and adolescent anxiety disorders are associated with significant impairment in multiple functional domains.

Risk Factors

As a result of the impact of referral biases in clinical samples, epidemiological studies provide more precise identification of risk factors. The current section reviews a range of potential risk factors, including demographic factors, various forms of environmental insult or stress, pre-diagnostic manifestations and medical conditions. Because of inconsistent findings and very small numbers of anxiety disorder cases in epidemiological samples, we also review data from clinically based studies.

Gender emerges as the most consistent risk factor for anxiety. Higher rates of most anxiety disorders have been found in females relative to males as early as age 6 (Lewinsohn, Gotlib, Lewinsohn *et al.*, 1998). Anxiety in girls may also have greater predictive impact than in boys for later anxiety (Costello, Angold, & Keeler, 1999; McGee, Feehan, Williams *et al.*, 1992), but findings are not unanimous (Pine, Cohen, Gurley *et al.*, 1998).

Little consensus exists regarding socio-environmental risk factors. Anxiety has been linked to various features, including economic disadvantage, school failure, stressful life events, family dysfunction, single home households, parental emotional problems and low parental education, but no consistent pattern has emerged. Using a quasi-experimental design, Costello, Compton, Keeler *et al.* (2003) did not find that changes in social welfare were associated with changes in rates of anxiety. Negative findings may reflect limitations of epidemiological studies. Although they have the advantage of minimizing referral biases, they typically study relatively small numbers of affected children, often with relatively mild disorders. For example, among 1035 adolescents in one study (Essau, Conradt, & Petermann, 1999), only 17 had social phobia.

Inconsistent associations for socio-environmental risk factors also emerge in clinical or family-based studies. For example, a recent meta-analysis identified an association between pediatric anxiety and parenting behaviors (Wood, McLeod, Sigman *et al.*, 2003). However, these are non-specific correlates of psychopathology that occur in multiple childhood disorders. Interest in the relationship between pediatric anxiety disorders and adverse social experiences emerges from at least two sets of findings. First, as reviewed below, rodents and non-human primates display developmental plasticity in behavioral and neural responses to threats (Gross & Hen, 2004), as shown by findings that alterations in social experiences produce long-term alterations in stress responses. These data generate questions concerning the degree to which adverse social experiences might shape humans' responses to threats during childhood. Second, children who experienced trauma exhibited marked increases in various anxiety disorders, not exclusively PTSD (Pine & Cohen, 2002; Steinberg & Avenevoli, 2000).

Associations between adverse life events and pediatric anxiety have not been found consistently (Eley & Stevenson, 2000; Hankin & Abramson, 2001; Williamson, Birmaher, Dahl *et al.*, 2005). Because most studies are cross-sectional, it remains unclear whether life events represent correlates, as opposed to causes, of anxiety. However, in a longitudinal study, adverse life events in adolescence predicted incidence of future anxiety, with a particularly strong risk in females for generalized anxiety disorder (Pine, Cohen, Johnson *et al.*, 2002). Similar associations have been found among adults, in that the same varieties of psychosocial risk exhibit associations with pediatric and adult anxiety disorders.

Subclinical elevations on anxiety rating scales and personality style questionnaires, such as the Children's Anxiety Sensitivity Index (CASI), have been considered risk factors for anxiety disorders (Pine, Cohen, & Brook, 2001). Whether such measures reflect current anxiety, as opposed to risk factors, remains controversial (Mannuzza, Klein, Moulton *et al.*, 2002). So far, no data document an association between such scale ratings and future anxiety.

Finally, risks associated with medical conditions have been reported. In the perinatal period, various adversities have been linked to risk for anxiety. These include neurological injury, febrile seizures, low birth weight, exposure to toxins and minor neurological findings (Breslau, 1995; Breslau & Chilcoat, 2000; Breslau, Chilcoat, Johnson *et al.*, 2000; Shaffer, Schonfeld, O'Connor *et al.*, 1985; Vasa, Gerring, Grados *et al.*, 2002; Whitaker, Van Rossem, Feldman *et al.*, 1997). However, as with other risk factors, no consistent findings emerge.

The strongest medical risk factor appears to be respiratory dysregulation. Circumstances that produce recurrent dyspnea predict risk for pediatric anxiety disorders (Goodwin, Pine, & Hoven, 2003; Slattery, Klein, Pine *et al.*, 2002); associations are particularly strong with asthma, which confers risk for separation anxiety disorder and panic attacks. Cigarette smoking during adolescence also incurs risk for future panic attacks, but not for social anxiety disorder (Johnson, Cohen, Pine *et al.*, 2000). Similar associations have not been found for illicit substances (Rutter, Maughan, & Kim-Cohen, 2006). Findings are consistent with other work implicating respiratory dysfunction in separation anxiety disorder and panic disorder.

Kagan, Snidman, McManis *et al.* (2001) noted a relationship between what has been designated as inhibited childhood temperament and later anxiety disorders. Children with inhibited temperament are defined as high reactive during infancy, behaviorally inhibited and reacting with apprehension to novelty during toddlerhood. They are defined as in the top 15% in delay to speak and smile in novel settings.

Altogether, associations between inhibition and psychopathology have been examined in thousands of children. Findings by Kagan (1994) suggest an association between behavioral inhibition and later anxiety, with distinct associations at different developmental periods. During school-age years, increased risk occurs for various anxiety disorders, including separation anxiety disorder and phobias. Others find that inhibition at age 3 predicts risk for depression but not anxiety at age 21 (Caspi, Moffitt, Newman *et al.*, 1996).

Associations with anxiety vary in strength, and correlations between inhibition and anxiety ratings cross-sectionally, let alone over time, are rarely greater than 0.20–0.40. Hence, the magnitude of associations is at best moderate. However, some evidence suggests particularly strong associations for measures of social anxiety in adolescence (Hayward, Killen, Kraemer *et al.*, 1998; Schwartz, Snidman, & Kagan, 1999). Comparable associations also emerge with shyness in early childhood, and with anxiety in early adolescence, with odds ratios in the moderate range (Prior, Smart, Sanson *et al.*, 2000), as well as for teacher or parent measures of anxious/withdrawn behavior in childhood and anxiety disorders in adulthood (Goodwin, Fergusson, & Horwood, 2004).

Longitudinal Outcome

The long-term consequences of childhood anxiety disorders take on special importance given the high proportion of affected children. The study of diagnostic stability has used community cases, high-risk children and clinic patients, using retrospective and prospective designs.

Seven community-based studies have examined the course of specific anxiety disorders. The first, from Dunedin (Anderson, Williams, McGee *et al.*, 1987), provides indirect evidence on outcome for individual anxiety disorders (Feehan, McGee, & Williams, 1993; Kim-Cohen, Caspi, Moffitt *et al.*, 2003; McGee, Feehan, Williams *et al.*, 1992; Poulton, Pine, & Harrington, in press). In the initial follow-up, from age 11 to 15, a composite index of any mood or anxiety disorder predicted later anxiety for girls, but not boys (McGee, Feehan, Williams *et al.*, 1992). This sex difference was obtained in two other prospective studies (Costello, Angold, & Keeler, 1999; Rueter, Scaramella, Wallace *et al.*, 1999). The latter also found that emotional symptoms predicted major depression. Further follow-up documents longitudinal associations in anxiety disorders, with little relationship between specific child and adult anxiety disorders. The results from two other community-based studies provide similar evidence of non-specific risk for adult anxiety disorders among adolescents with a range of anxiety disorders (Bittner, Goodwin, Wittchen *et al.*, 2004; Lewinsohn, Zinbarg, Seeley *et al.*, 1997).

Thus, five studies found that anxiety disorders during childhood or adolescence predicted risk for an array of mood or anxiety disorders during adulthood. None documented diagnostic specificity in outcome. Two other studies found evidence of specificity. A school-based study found specificity in the course of social phobia but not separation anxiety disorder across adolescence (Hayward, Killen, Kraemer *et al.*, 1998). Perhaps the strongest evidence of longitudinal specificity derives from the New York longitudinal study (Pine, Cohen, Gurley *et al.*, 1998). From childhood or adolescence to adulthood, specific phobias predicted specific phobias exclusively. Similarly, social phobia was predictive of social phobia exclusively. Separation anxiety disorder predicted no specific disorder, but tended to predict panic attacks, and overanxious disorder was associated with an array of adult disorders including anxiety disorders, but not overanxious disorder, and major depression.

Beyond these community-based studies, evidence of specificity in course also emerged from a prospective high-risk study that followed children of parents with either major depression or panic disorder. Phobias and overanxious disorder, but not separation anxiety disorder, carried a two- to four-fold increase of major depression at follow-up (Weissman, Warner, Wickramaratne *et al.*, 1997). The course of childhood anxiety disorders has also been reported for clinic samples. Two studies ascertained children with school refusal and prominent anxiety symptoms prior to the nosological system introduced in the early 1980s (Berg & Jackson, 1985; Flakerska-Praquin, Lindstoem, & Gillberg, 1997). The majority of children experienced relatively benign clinical courses into adulthood. Three other clinical studies (Aschenbrand, Kendall, Webb *et al.*, 2003; Klein, 1995; Last, Hansen, & Franco, 1997) confirm a relatively low rate of later anxiety disorders in children with anxiety disorders. In the study by Klein (1995), separation anxiety disorder coupled with school phobia predicted panic disorder, as well as major depression, although panic disorder was not a frequent outcome (7% versus 0% in non-anxious comparisons). Another short-term follow-up found an elevated rate of panic disorder only among clinic children with "primary" separation anxiety disorder (Aschenbrand, Kendall, Webb *et al.*, 2003).

In conclusion, data from outcome studies support several observations. Although childhood anxiety disorders show considerable stability, most children with anxiety disorders do not have anxiety disorders or depression in adulthood. However, most adults with anxiety or mood disorders are likely to have a childhood history of anxiety. Evidence of specific risk for adult mood and anxiety disorders is not strong.

Pathophysiology

Family Genetics

Familial aggregation studies have relied on multiple designs, summarized below.

Family Studies

During the past 25 years, more than 20 studies have reported an association between various forms of parental psychopathology and childhood anxiety (Beidel & Turner, 1997; McClure, Brennan, Hammen *et al.*, 2001; Merikangas, Avenevoli, Dierker *et al.*, 1999; Middeldorp, Cath, Van Dyke *et al.*, 2005; Rende, Wickramaratne, Warner *et al.*, 1995; Turner, Beidel, & Costello, 1987; Warner, Mufson, & Weissman, 1995; Weissman, Leckman, Merikangas *et al.*, 1984). These studies include so-called "top-down" studies, which evaluate children of parents with anxiety or depressive disorders, as well as a handful of so-called "bottom-up" studies, which ascertain parents of children with anxiety disorders. Multiple studies reported higher rates of anxiety disorders in children of parents with anxiety disorders, relative to children of non-ill parents, as shown in Table 39.2. Questions arising from these studies concern the specificity of parent–child concordance for anxiety disorders versus depression, and specificity of aggregation for distinct anxiety disorders (Middeldorp, Cath, Van Dyck *et al.*, 2005). The weight of evidence from the studies in Table 39.2 suggests non-specificity in the associations between offspring anxiety disorders and parental anxiety and depression. Some work provides evidence of specificity for parent–child anxiety disorders aggregation. An association between panic disorder in parents and separation anxiety disorder in offspring is the most consistent finding (Biederman, Faraone, Hirshfeld-Becker *et al.*, 2001, 2004; Capps, Sigman, Sena *et al.*, 1996). Coupled with data implicating respiratory dysfunction in the two conditions, these data suggest that panic disorder and separation anxiety disorder share an underlying diathesis (Klein, 1993). An association between parental depression and separation anxiety disorder in offspring has also been noted (Biederman, Monuteaux, Faraone *et al.*, 2004). Other data suggest that parental depression is associated with offspring social anxiety disorder, phobias and generalized anxiety disorder, but not separation anxiety disorder (Lieb, Isensee, Höfler *et al.* 2002; Merikangas, Avenevoli, Dierker *et al.*, 1999). Finally, late adolescent rather than adult onset panic disorder may be particularly heritable (Goldstein, Wickram-aratne, Horwath *et al.*, 1997).

Genetic Studies

In the light of consistent cross-generational transmission, attempts have been made to decompose familial transmission into environmental and genetic components. Few studies have been conducted in pediatric anxiety, none using an adoption design and most relying on symptom scales.

Among adults, a growing literature suggests that genetic factors account for approximately 40% of the variability in risk for anxiety, with most of the remaining variance attributed to non-shared environmental factors (Hettema, Neale, & Kendler, 2001; Hettema, Prescott, Myers *et al.*, 2005). These studies provide evidence of both unique and shared liabilities across distinct adult disorders. Generalized anxiety disorder and major depressive disorder appear to share a genetic substrate, and differ largely in contributions from non-shared environmental factors (Hettema, Neale, & Kendler, 2001). Studies in adolescents suggest similar genetic patterns, with common genes predisposing towards anxiety before puberty and depression after puberty (Silberg, Pickles, Rutter *et al.*, 1999; Silberg, Rutter, & Eaves, 2001). Other anxiety disorders appear to have more disorder-specific genetic risk. For example, genetic risk for panic disorder appears distinct from the risk for phobias, generalized anxiety disorder and major depression (Hettema, Prescott, Myers *et al.*, 2005). While not all twin data support specificity, the weight of evidence indicates that adult anxiety disorders are influenced by both disorder-specific and disorder-unique liability factors (Middeldorp, Cath, Van Dyck *et al.*, 2005).

Genetic influences on anxiety comorbidity have been examined in a large twin study (Hettema, Prescott, Myers *et al.*, 2005). The study found genetic influences to separate two groups of anxiety disorders. One consisted of panic disorder and generalized anxiety disorder, the other of specific phobias. Based on these genetic findings, comorbidity between panic disorder and generalized anxiety disorder is to be expected. Other work in this sample suggests that shared liability to a range of anxiety states may be expressed through underlying personality factors, such as neuroticism (Hettema, Neale, Myers *et al.*, 2006). Extending the search for possible explanations of comorbidity across anxiety disorders, the twin sample was used to test the contribution of neuroticism to the genetic variance in anxiety disorders (Hettema, Neale, Myers *et al.*, 2006).

In children, divergent estimates of heritability emerge from studies using scale scores (Bolton, Eley, O'Connor *et al.*, 2006; Eley, Bolton, O'Connor *et al.*, 2003; Eley & Stevenson, 1999; Eley, Stirling, Ehlers *et al.*, 2004; Topolski, Hewitt, Eaves *et al.*, 1999). Similar assessment methods have yielded divergent estimates for parent and child rated anxiety scales. Twin data in children are consistent in suggesting a modest genetic component to most forms of childhood anxiety, with heritabilities generally accounting for less than 40% of the variance. These relatively low heritabilities across the age range have led to the suggestion that genes confer a broad diathesis towards anxiety as opposed to a predilection for one or another specific disorder. Consistent with this possibility, heritabilities for temperamental factors, such as behavioral inhibition, have been somewhat higher than those for specific anxiety symptoms or disorders (Goldsmith & Lemery, 2000). Non-shared environmental factors account for much of the remaining variance in child-based twin studies of anxiety symptoms, much as they do in adults. Results in children show variability in genetic and environmental contributions to anxiety. This variability, which may reflect distinct genetic and environmental effects across age, sex and specific forms

Table 39.2 Anxiety in children as a function of parental psychopathology.

Author Top-down studies	Parental diagnosis (No of offspring)	Odds ratio between parental psychopathology and anxiety disorders in offspring vs. normal controls
Weissman *et al.* (1984)	MDD and PD (19) (mothers)	10.4*
	MDD (23) (mothers)	2.3
Turner *et al.* (1987)	OCD or AGO (16)	7.2*
	Dysthymia (14)	5.5*
Rende *et al.* (1995)	MDD (164)	2.2 T1*; 2.9 T2*
	No MDD (68)	0.92 T1; 0.92 T2
Warner *et al.* (1995)	MDD (32)	2.5*
	MDD and PD (60)	1.1
	PD (17)	2.3*
Capps *et al.* (1996)	AGO (16)	3.9*
Beidel & Turner (1997)	AD (28)	5.4*
	MDD (24)	5.7*
	AD and MDD (29)	5.4*
Merikangas *et al.* (1999)	AD, AGO and OAD (36)	2.5
Biederman *et al.* (2001)		(≤2 anxiety disorders)
	PD and MDD (141)	8.2*
	MDD (46)	4.3
	PD (26)	8.8*
	No PD or MDD (99)	–
McClure *et al.* (2001)	Anxiety, no MDD (40 in mother)	3.1* (anxiety in child)
	MDD, no Anxiety (248 in mother)	1.6 (anxiety in child)
	Anxiety and MDD (110 in mother)	3.6* (anxiety in child)
Biederman *et al.* (2004)		(≤2 anxiety disorders)
	PD and MDD (56)	2.3* (anxiety in child, PD in parent)
	MDD (132)	1.3 (anxiety in child, MDD in parent)
	PD (55)	
	No PD or MDD (491)	
Pine *et al.* (2005a)	PD and MDD (41)	4.9* (anxiety in child, PD in parent)
	MDD (53)	4.8* (anxiety in child, MDD in parent)
	PD (24)	
	No PD or MDD (26)	

Author Bottom-up studies	Children's diagnoses (No of mothers)	Odds ratio between parental psychopathology and anxiety disorders in offspring vs. normal controls
Last *et al.* (1991)	SAD (19)	With PD in Parents 1.4 (SAD in child)
	OAD (22)	4.2* (OAD in child)
	OAD and SAD (17)	10.7* (OAD & SAD in child)
Lieb *et al.* (2000)	SoPh ($n = 58$)	With SoPh in child 4.7* (parent SoPh)
		3.5* (parent other anxiety)
		3.6* (parent depression)

Parental diagnoses: AGO, agoraphobia; MDD, major depression; OCD, obsessive compulsive disorder; PD, panic disorder.

Offspring diagnoses: AD, anxiety disorder including PD, OCD or social phobia; GAD, generalized anxiety disorder; OAD, overanxious disorder; SAD, separation anxiety disorder. T1, time one; T2, 2-year follow-up.

* 95% Confidence interval of odds ratio excludes 1.0 (i.e., statistically significant at $P \le 0.05$).

of anxiety, complicates clear interpretation of the nature of transmission.

As noted in chapter 23, the identification of genes will contribute greatly to our understanding of causal factors. No genomic studies have been conducted in childhood anxiety disorder. In adults, panic disorder, which has been shown to be familial, has been examined for influential genes. Replications have failed. Some suggest that it is futile to expect nosological clarity in psychiatry from genetic findings (Kendler & Greenspan, 2006). It is unlikely that the search for genes in childhood anxiety disorders will fare better than it has for adult anxiety disorders. This failure will limit definitive statements regarding the exact nature of genetic influences, but it will not alter the need to rely on other informative clinical and biological strategies to determine the nosological validity of childhood anxiety disorders.

Endophenotypes

Research has begun to move beyond examination of familial aggregation in anxiety symptoms to the study of underlying mechanisms. Anxiety is viewed as a downstream manifestation of genetically based perturbations in neural function that do not directly map on to diagnostic categories. Rather, they cause abnormalities in information processing that lead to psychopathology.

The term "endophenotype" has been used to describe heritable abnormalities in neural function and associated information-processing capacities (Gottesman & Gould, 2003). Endophenotypes show independent associations with psychiatric disorders and with their risk factors. Strong evidence for potential endophenotypes is scarce; working memory abnormalities in schizophrenia probably represent the most compelling example in psychiatry.

Three lines of work provide preliminary data on potential endophenotypes in pediatric anxiety disorders. First, behavioral inhibition has been conceptualized as an endophenotype. Longitudinal studies note associations with anxiety disorders, and family studies with parental panic disorder (Kagan, Snidman, McManis *et al.*, 2001). This work views temperament and anxiety as alternative manifestations of perturbations in the brain's fear circuit. However, because behavioral inhibition may also be associated with parental depression, there may not be diagnostic specificity in this relationship (Caspi, Moffitt, Newman *et al.*, 1996; Rosenbaum, Biederman, Hirshfeld-Becker *et al.*, 2000). In addition, some suggest that behavioral inhibition represents manifest psychopathology, as opposed to a risk factor or endophenotype. An intervention study found stronger treatment effects on anxiety symptoms than on behavioral inhibition (Rapee, Kennedy, Ingram *et al.*, 2005), supporting the endophenotype perspective for behavioral inhibition.

Second, some work implicates enhanced autonomic reactivity in risk for anxiety (Grillon, Dierker, & Merikangas, 1997; Merikangas, Avenevoli, Dierker *et al.*, 1999). As with behavioral inhibition, reactivity-based endophenotypes are presumed to result from perturbations in fear-circuit function. Particular interest has focused on measures of hypothalamic–pituitary–adrenal (HPA) axis activity, although such findings in pediatric anxiety disorders are inconsistent (Terleph, Klein, Roberson-Nay *et al.*, 2006). Third, information-based approaches suggest that abnormal attention regulation during threat exposure may represent an endophenotype (Pine, Klein, Roberson-Nay *et al.*, 2005b). Attention-processing abnormality to threat, also presumed to result from fear-circuit dysfunction, has been linked to both pediatric anxiety disorders and parental panic disorder.

Molecular Genetics

Studies of molecular genetic correlates have extended the modern view of psychopathology as the result of circuitry-based perturbations in information processing. Perspectives on psychiatric genetics have advanced considerably in the past 10 years, to the point where most common forms of psychopathology, including pediatric anxiety disorders, are viewed as so-called "complex disorders." Such conditions are caused by panoplies of genetic and non-genetic factors, each making relatively small contributions to the phenotype.

In anxiety disorders, the most productive research has attempted to link specific genetic polymorphisms to neural and cognitive dysfunction. Virtually all work on anxiety is of adults. Current findings implicate a polymorphism of the serotonin transporter gene in fear-circuitry dysfunction (Hariri, Mattay, Tessitore *et al.*, 2002). Other work, again largely in adults, suggests that such genetically based perturbations predispose to psychopathology through interactions with environmental risk (Caspi, Sugden, Moffitt *et al.*, 2003). Although much of this work examines associations with adult depression, it is relevant to pediatric anxiety disorders, given their associations with adult depression. Two studies have reported a gene–environment interaction with the serotonin transporter in pediatric depression (Eley, Stirling, Ehlers *et al.*, 2004; Kaufman, Douglas-Palumberi, Houshyar *et al.*, 2004), and another found such an interaction for behavioral inhibition (Fox, Nichols, Henderson *et al.*, 2005). Behavioral inhibition also has been linked to a polymorphism in the gene for corticotropin-releasing factor (CRF), a key regulator of HPA function (Smoller, Yamaki, Fagerness *et al.*, 2005). Such an association is consistent with data implicating HPA axis function in fear-circuit activity (see p. 639).

Psychobiology

Neural Circuitry in Animals

Advances in basic science have altered theories of anxiety disorders. They are viewed as reflecting individual differences in neural function: pediatric anxiety disorders are hypothesized, by some, to result from abnormalities in physiological systems implicated in animal models of anxiety (Gross & Hen, 2004). This view has led investigators to target various physiological systems in an effort to document psychobiological substrates of anxiety.

Animal models of anxiety benefit from strong cross-species conservation in brain circuitry and pharmacology. Distinct forms of fear are regulated by inter-related brain systems involving the prefrontal and medial temporal lobes. Perhaps the best understood phenomena are learned fears, which can be modeled by "fear conditioning" experiments, where an aversive stimulus, such as a shock, is paired with a neutral stimulus, such as a light. Following such pairings, an organism exhibits fear of the formerly neutral stimulus. Learned fear depends upon a neural circuit involving the amygdala, a bilateral collection of individual nuclei located within the brain's medial temporal lobes (LeDoux, 2000). Learning to fear a previously harmless stimulus involves changes in neural function within the basolateral nucleus of the amygdala, and expression of this learning involves output through the central nucleus. Similarly, the process of extinction, whereby a feared stimulus no longer elicits a fear response, requires communication between the amygdala and frontal cortex, and perturbations in extinction reflect aberrant communication between these regions (Quirk & Gehlert, 2003).

Other forms of fear develop without prior learning and are regulated by distinct but related neural circuits. For example, nocturnal organisms such as rodents fear well-lit environments (Davis, 1998). Unlike learned fears, this fear does not extinguish and may actually increase with repeated exposure. Unlearned fear involves the basolateral but not the central nucleus of the amygdala; the two circuits are regulated by distinct neurochemical systems. For example, infusions with CRF may potentiate unlearned fear, but not conditioned fear.

Neural Development and Fear

The mature fear circuit reflects long-term influences of early-life rearing environment. A wealth of investigations with rodents shows that alterations in maternal care produce long-term changes in the threshold for engaging the medial temporal lobe and prefrontal components of the fear circuit (Meaney, 2001). These effects arise through non-genomic influences, involving DNA methylation. Specifically, functional aspects are altered for genes involved in regulation of the medial temporal lobe and frontal cortex. Work in non-human primates demonstrates comparable associations between rearing and threat responses (Suomi, 2003). These influences appear also for indices of HPA axis function, generating interest in the relationship between HPA axis function and pediatric anxiety disorders. Much of the scientific interest in rearing effects was based on the implicit assumption of permanent scarring. However, the influence of early life experiences is complicated. For example, over 900 genes are regulated by maternal care (Weaver, Meaney, & Szyf, 2006). Moreover, some effects of rearing on genes are reversible. Further complicating an understanding of effects of early rearing, Mathew, Coplan, Smith *et al.* (2002) not only failed to replicate increased cerebrospinal fluid (CSF) corticotropin releasing factor (CRF) in primates raised under stress, but obtained diametrically opposite results (Mathew, Coplan, Smith *et al.*, 2002). In sum, the effects of early maternal behavior and stress on later functions are highly complex, indirect and not regularly irreversible.

Another approach uses anatomic, neurochemical and genetic manipulation to demonstrate developmental plasticity in the fear circuit. Lesion studies in non-human primates find distinct effects of amygdala lesions on fear-related behaviors in mature relative to immature primates (Amaral, 2002). Genetic and chemical manipulations in rodents produce long-term alterations in fear-related behaviors and associated neural circuitry among immature mice, but not in mature mice exposed to the same manipulations (Gross & Hen, 2004). Altogether, animal data suggest that function of the mature fear circuit reflects influences during childhood on fear-circuit development, but the nature of these influences is likely to be highly complex.

Human Physiology and Neural Circuitry

Functional aspects of brain circuits that regulate learned and innate fears can be elicited reliably in lower mammals as well as humans, through changes in physiological indices; of these, the startle reflex has the best understood neuroanatomic circuit. The reflex is augmented by presentations of mildly stressful stimuli. The neural circuit involved in fear conditioning in rodents is thought to mediate augmentation of this reflex in humans.

Adults with various forms of anxiety exhibit startle abnormalities (Grillon, 2002; Grillon & Baas, 2003). Asymptomatic children of parents with anxiety disorders also have been found to have abnormalities in startle regulation (Grillon, Dierker, & Merikangas, 1997, 1998). Problematically, startle abnormalities reported in at-risk offspring have not been found in youth with anxiety disorders. In addition, startle abnormalities occur in offspring at risk for anxiety and for depression as well, raising questions about the specificity of associations between abnormal startle and anxiety (Grillon, Warner, Hille *et al.*, 2005).

Kagan, Snidman, McManis *et al.* (2001) suggested that behavioral inhibition, a marker of risk, results from abnormalities in the same brain circuits implicated in startle potentiation, based on peripheral physiological profiles, using indices influenced by circuits that regulate fear in mammals. In spite of parallels in neural circuits of fear regulation in humans and animals, there are crucial pharmacological inconsistencies. For example, medications effective in panic disorder do not affect fear conditioning, although they appear to affect certain forms of unlearned fear (Blanchard, Griebel, Henrie *et al.*, 1997; Cassella & Davis, 1985). Moreover, associations between fear conditioning and clinical anxiety disorders are marginal at best (Lissek, Powers, McClure *et al.*, 2005). Accordingly, risk for anxiety disorders has been hypothesized to relate to failures in extinction, or to inherited tendencies to respond to innate unlearned fearful stimuli, rather than to abnormalities in fear-learning per se.

The most developed line of research examines respiratory dysregulation in panic disorder (Klein, 1993, 1996). Much like a well-lit room for a rodent, respiratory stimulants represent unlearned fear-inducing stimuli for air-breathing organisms, including humans. A wealth of evidence suggests that sensitivity to respiratory stimulants identifies individuals with a diathesis for types of anxiety closely related to spontaneous panic attacks. For example, adults with panic disorder have enhanced responses to respiratory stimulants, such as CO_2, sodium lactate, cholecystokinin or doxapram. Sensitivity to CO_2 has also been found in children with anxiety disorders, specifically separation anxiety disorder, but not those with social anxiety disorder (Pine, Klein, Roberson-Nay *et al.*, 2005a). Syndromes such as subclinical panic disorder that have strong familial associations with panic disorder are also characterized by enhanced responses to respiratory stimulants. Moreover, in adults, signs of respiratory abnormalities, such as enhanced sensitivity to CO_2, occur especially among panic patients with high familial loading (Horwath, Adams, Wickramaratne *et al.*, 1997). In addition, healthy adult first-degree relatives of panic patients also exhibit enhanced responses to respiratory stimuli (Coryell, Fyer, Pine *et al.*, 2001); however, CO_2 sensitivity was not found among offspring at risk for panic disorder (Pine, Klein, Roberson-Nay *et al.*, 2005a).

Cognition and Anxiety

Cognitive processing, specifically memory and attention, is preferentially mobilized by perceived threats, presumably due to the responses' adaptive value. Brain imaging which has been used to delineate fear-circuit dysfunction in anxiety susceptibility has focused on threats' abilities to disrupt strategic control of attention or attention orienting (Davis & Whalen, 2001). Two procedures have been common to probe threat-related effects on cognitive processes in humans. One relies on the "emotional Stroop test," which taps disruption of strategic attention control. Latencies increase when naming colors of "threat" words as opposed to "neutral" words (Williams, Mathews, & McLeod, 1996). Adults with various anxiety disorders show relatively prolonged latencies to name the color of "threat" words, such as "panic," presumably because of enhanced vigilance to them. The second procedure uses the dot-probe test, which measures attention orienting. Reaction time to a spatial probe is quantified as a function of the proximity of the probe to "threat" words or pictures (Bar-Haim, Lamy, & Pergamin, 2007; Mogg & Bradley 1998). Adults with anxiety show faster reaction times to probes proximal to threatening stimuli, an effect attributed to enhanced vigilance to threats. In both procedures, there are relatively subtle but consistent positive associations between adult anxiety and reaction times to threat presentations. Some evidence suggests similar effects in childhood anxiety disorders (Monk, Nelson, McClure *et al.*, 2006; Pine, Mogg, Bradley *et al.*, 2005c).

Beyond these two procedures, other less frequently used indices quantify attentional resources during self-monitoring of attention states. In adolescents an association has been reported between aberrant anxiety-state monitoring with anxiety disorders as well as panic disorder in their parents (Pine, Klein, Roberson-Nay *et al.*, 2005b). Finally, diagnostic specificity of cognitive biases is in question, because biases have also been found in depression. In addition, cognitive bias for threat does not appear to be a marker of risk because it occurs primarily in symptomatic adults and disappears with treatment (Williams, Mathews, & MacLeod, 1996). Nevertheless, manipulating bias experimentally has been shown to alter adults' stress responses (MacLeod, Rutherford, Campbell *et al.*, 2002).

Brain Imaging

Two imaging procedures have been used in pediatric anxiety disorders, neuromorphometry, which examines brain structure, and functional magnetic resonance imaging (fMRI), which reflects blood flow changes during cognitive processes.

Two sets of studies have compared brain structure in pediatric anxiety disorders with healthy comparisons. The first, which examined 10 adolescents with generalized anxiety and healthy comparisons (De Bellis, Casey, Dahl *et al.*, 2000a, 2002), found larger volumes in patients' amygdala and superior temporal gyrus. The second study involved 15 adolescents with mixed anxiety disorders (Millham, Nugent, Drevets *et al.*, 2005). Consistent with findings in adults, this study found reduced amygdala volume in pediatric anxiety disorders, particularly in generalized anxiety disorder. The difference disappeared after successful treatment. Three fMRI studies report amygdala activity in pediatric anxiety disorders or related states in response to facial photographs. One study found enhanced amygdala activation during the viewing of evocative face-emotion displays (Thomas, Drevets, Dahl *et al.*, 2001). These findings, consistent with those in adults, implicate amygdala hypersensitivity in some forms of anxiety. The second study found no increased amygdala activation in anxious adolescents but observed enhanced activation in the ventral prefrontal cortex, a region implicated in extinction (Monk, Nelson, McClure *et al.*, 2006). Moreover, prefrontal cortex activity correlated negatively with anxiety severity in patients, suggesting that anxiety reflects perturbed functioning in a distributed neural circuit regulated, in part, by the prefrontal cortex. A final study compared amygdala activity in adults classified as inhibited or not inhibited in childhood (Schwartz, Wright, Shin *et al.*, 2003). Enhanced amygdala activity was found in the formerly inhibited individuals, implicating amygdala function in risk for anxiety.

Treatment

Distress and impairment engendered by anxiety disorders and their long-term liability highlight the need for effective treatments. Some interventions, such as cognitive–behavior therapy (CBT), are based on a theoretical model of anxiety; others, such as selective serotonin reuptake inhibitor (SSRI) medications, follow from demonstrated efficacy in adult anxiety disorders. The literature is replete with case studies reporting efficacy of treatments. The review is of systematic controlled trials.

Psychotherapy

CBT is the best-studied intervention. Because CBT is based on the notion that distorted cognitions underlie anxiety symptoms, aspects of many CBT treatments focus on the child's thought processes, aiming to replace negative beliefs with more realistic neutral cognitions. Some CBT treatments recruit the family's active involvement to facilitate exposure. The contribution that parents can make in treatment is likely to vary as a function of the child's disorder and age.

A major positive feature of CBT is the availability of treatment manuals. CBT has been compared with no-treatment waitlist controls (Kendall, 1994; Kendall, Flannery-Schroeder, Panichelli-Mindel *et al.*, 1997) or a non-specific control intervention (Beidel, Turner, & Morris, 2000; Last, Hansen, & Franco, 1998; Silverman, Kurtines, Ginsburg *et al.*, 1999). While often used in psychotherapy trials, the use of waitlist controls is methodologically problematic when applied to clinic patients. This disposition confirms to patients that they require treatment but it is withheld. Not only might such an intervention fail to help anxiety, it may have a deleterious impact. The most informative studies are those that have relied on a credible comparison treatment. Finally, it is essential that treatment outcome be evaluated by individuals who are not aware of the treatment delivered, rather than by the therapist. In this fashion, one ensures that biases introduced by treatment allegiances do not influence estimates of outcome. These design features are very infrequently met in current studies of psychotherapy in anxiety disorders.

CBT was examined in two systematic studies by Kendall (1994) and Kendall, Flannery-Schroeder, Panichelli-Mindel *et al.* (1997). Children received CBT for 16 weeks, or were on a waitlist for 8 weeks before then receiving CBT. In both trials, relative to the waitlist, CBT was significantly superior. Moreover, sustained reductions in anxiety continued over several years. Waitlist controls have been used in other studies of CBT; only three studies used "attention" controls (Beidel, Turner, & Morris, 2000; Last, Hansen, & Franco, 1998; Silverman, Kurtines, Ginsburg *et al.*, 1999), with one finding efficacy for CBT in social phobia (Beidel, Turner, & Morris, 2000). Other studies have examined variations in treatment, providing preliminary evidence that either parental involvement (Mendlowitz, Manassis, Bradley *et al.*, 1999) or a group-based format (Barrett, Dadds, & Rapee, 1996) may lead to particularly high rates of response. Finally, on the basis of a systematic trial of group CBT, group family CBT and waitlist control, one study concluded that CBT could be implemented effectively in a group format (Barrett, Duffy, Dadds *et al.*, 2001). While results show that CBT produces significant gains in children with anxiety disorders, considerably more work is needed, particularly with credible control conditions.

A recent comparative efficacy study raises major unanticipated questions on the comparative efficacy of CBT, relative to pill-placebo and SSRI medication, in the treatment of adolescent depression (March, Silva, Petrycki *et al.*, 2004). These findings emphasize the need for a comparable large-scale CBT/SSRI study in anxiety disorders. Such a study in child anxiety disorders is ongoing.

The success of CBT in the treatment of impairing anxiety disorders has raised questions on the role of this treatment for prevention. Attempts to use CBT preventatively have typically relied on what is termed "secondary" prevention, whereby children with mild anxiety receive CBT. While results generally suggest that CBT reduces anxiety symptoms in such groups (Rapee, Kennedy, Ingram *et al.*, 2005), whether results apply to primary prevention is unclear. These interventions have been shown to work in children in the preschool years and onwards. Because children with symptoms are targeted in this work, such interventions might be characterized as therapeutic rather than preventive. Far less work has used alternative approaches, targeting broader portions of the population independently of those with mild symptoms or other risk factors.

Pharmacotherapy

SSRIs have documented efficacy in virtually all adult anxiety disorders. Four placebo-controlled trials have been published for SSRIs in pediatric anxiety disorders. The first large multisite 8-week study found that fluvoxamine was superior to placebo in children with either social anxiety, separation anxiety or generalized anxiety disorders (RUPP, 2001). Another large study demonstrated comparable benefit for paroxetine over placebo, in children and adolescents with social anxiety disorder (Wagner, Berard, Stein *et al.*, 2004). Finally, two modest-sized studies demonstrated efficacy for fluoxetine and sertraline, each relative to placebo (Birmaher, Axelson, Monk *et al.*, 2003; Rynn, Siqueland, & Rickels, 2001).

Concern about SSRIs emerged in 2002–2004, following reports that SSRIs were associated with a two-fold increase in suicidal ideation or behavior, relative to placebo treatment (approximately 4% versus approximately 2%). This observation led to cautionary statements from regulatory officials in Europe and the USA, although debate continues concerning the significance of these data (Vasa, Carlino, & Pine, 2006). Diagnosis did not moderate this association, suggesting that concerns might apply equally to anxiety and mood disorders. A previous literature review (Klein & Pine, 2002) indicated that there was inconsistent support for the efficacy of tricyclic antidepressants in children with separation anxiety. Finally, although there have been some reports on the use of benzodiazepines in anxious children (Klein & Pine, 2002), the efficacy and safety profile of the SSRIs weaken consideration of benzodiazepines.

Conclusions

Multiple findings have documented the importance of childhood anxiety disorders. These include their elevated prevalence, their associated impairment, the fact that they put children at risk for later depression and their moderate but significant continuity with anxiety disorders in adulthood.

Epidemiological studies have generated divergent rates of current anxiety disorders. The evidence suggests 5–10% point prevalence in the general population, with girls over-represented. Some have found greater stability of anxiety in girls than boys. Childhood anxiety disorders predict adult anxiety and depression, but no other psychopathology.

Knowledge of antecedents would enable identification of children at risk and the development of preventive efforts. Few antecedents have been established. Early inhibited temperament is weakly related to later anxiety, especially social phobia. A modest influence for genetic transmission has been found, with non-shared environmental factors having a greater role. The non-genetic factors in childhood anxiety disorders are poorly understood. As a result, they make little contribution to the clinical management of children with anxiety disorders.

Models of brain circuits that regulate fear in animals, also studied in adults, are being applied to children. Early studies suggest that children show abnormalities in underlying fear circuitry, as measured by startle responses to unconditioned fear stimuli, and information processing of fear-related stimuli. However, it is difficult to determine which is cause and which is effect. Neuroimaging studies have focused on the hypothesis of amygdala involvement in anxiety. At this time, the best-documented biological feature of childhood anxiety is respiratory dysregulation, as indexed by hypersensitivity to CO_2 exposure in children with separation anxiety disorder.

Treatment of anxiety disorders encompasses psychotherapeutic and psychopharmacological interventions. Most treatment studies have included a mixture of anxiety disorders. Most behavioral treatment studies have methodological limitations, but there is evidence of short-term and sustained improvement. SSRIs have been shown to be effective in childhood anxiety disorders. Treatments based on empirical evidence can now be offered to children with anxiety disorders.

References

Achenbach, T. M. (1991). *Manual for the child behavior checklist and 1991 child behavior profile*. Burlington, VT: University of Vermont, Department of Psychiatry.

Amaral, D. G. (2002). The primate amygdala and the neurobiology of social behavior: Implications for understanding social anxiety. *Biological Psychiatry*, *51*, 11–17.

Ambrosini, P. J., Metz, C., Prabucki, K., Lee, J. C. (1989). Videotape reliability of the third revised edition of the K-SADS. *Journal of the American Academy of Child & Adolescent Psychiatry*, *28*, 723–728.

Anderson, J., Williams, S., McGee, R., & Silva, P. A. (1987). DSM-III disorders in preadolescent children: Prevalence in a large sample from the general population. *Archives of General Psychiatry*, *44*, 69–76.

Angold, A., & Costello, E. J. (2000). The Child and Adolescent Psychiatric Assessment (CAPA). *Journal of the American Academy of Child and Adolescent Psychiatry*, *39*, 39–48.

Angold, A., Costello, E. J., & Erkanli, A. (1999). Comorbidity. *Journal of Child Psychology and Psychiatry*, *40*, 57–87.

Aschenbrand, S. G., Kendall, P. C., Webb, A., Safford, S. M., & Flannery-Schroeder, E. (2003). Is childhood separation anxiety disorder a predictor of adult panic disorder and agoraphobia? A seven-year longitudinal study. *Journal of the American Academy of Child and Adolescent Psychiatry*, *42*, 1478–1485.

Bar-Haim, Y., Lamy, D., Pergamin, L., Bakermans-Kranenburg, M. J., & van IJzendoorn, M. H. (2007). Threat-related attentional bias in anxious and non-anxious individuals: A meta-analytic study. *Psychological Bulletin*, *133*, 1–24.

Barrett, P. M., Dadds, M. R., & Rapee, R. M. (1996). Family treatment of childhood anxiety: A controlled trial. *Journal of Consulting and Clinical Psychology*, *64*, 333–342.

Barrett, P. M., Duffy, A. L., Dadds, M. R., & Rapee, R. M. (2001). Cognitive–behavioral treatment of anxiety disorders in children: Long-term (6-year) follow-up. *Journal of Consulting and Clinical Psychology*, *69*, 135–141.

Beidel, D. C., & Turner, S. M. (1997). At risk for anxiety. I. Psychopathology in the offspring of anxious parents. *Journal of the American Academy of Child and Adolescent Psychiatry*, *36*, 918–924.

Beidel, D. C., Turner, S. M., & Morris, T. L. (2000). Behavioral treatment of childhood social phobia. *Journal of Consulting and Clinical Psychology*, *68*, 1072–1080.

Benjamin, R. S., Costello, E. J., Warren, M. (1990). Anxiety disorders in a pediatric sample. *Journal of Anxiety Disorders*, *4*, 293–316.

Berg, I., & Jackson, A. (1985). Teenage school refusers grow up: A follow-up study of 168 subjects, ten years on average after in-patient treatment. *British Journal of Psychiatry*, *147*, 366–370.

Biederman, J., Faraone, S. V., Hirshfeld-Becker, D. R., Friedman, D., Robin, J. A., & Rosenbaum, J. F. (2001). Patterns of psychopathology and dysfunction in high-risk children of parents with panic disorder and major depression. *American Journal of Psychiatry*, *158*, 49–57.

Biederman, J., Monuteaux, M. C., Faraone, S. V., Hirshfeld-Becker, D. R., Henin, A., Gilbert, J., *et al.* (2004). Does referral bias impact findings in high-risk offspring for anxiety disorders? A controlled study of high-risk children of non-referred parents with panic disorder/agoraphobia and major depression. *Journal of Affective Disorders*, *82*, 209–216.

Bird, H. R., Canino, G., Rubio-Stipec, M., Gould, M. S., Ribera, J., Sesman, M., *et al.* (1988). Estimates of the prevalence of childhood maladjustment in a community survey in Puerto Rico. The use of combined measures. *Archives of General Psychiatry*, *45*, 1120–1126.

Birmaher, B., Axelson, D. A., Monk, K., Kalas, C., Clark, D. B., Ehmann, M., *et al.* (2003). Fluoxetine for the treatment of childhood anxiety disorders. *Journal of the American Academy of Child and Adolescent Psychiatry*, *42*, 415–423.

Birmaher, B., Khetarpal, S., Brent, D., Cully, M., Balach, L., Kaufman, J., *et al.* (1997). The Screen for Child Anxiety Related Emotional Disorders (SCARED): Scale construction and psychometric characteristics. *Journal of the American Academy of Child and Adolescent Psychiatry*, *36*, 545–553.

Bittner, A., Goodwin, R. D., Wittchen, H. U., Beesdo, K., Höfler, M., & Lieb, R. (2004). What characteristics of primary anxiety disorders predict subsequent major depressive disorder? *Journal of Clinical Psychiatry*, *65*, 618–626, quiz 730.

Blanchard, R. J., Griebel, G., Henrie, J. A., & Blanchard, D. C. (1997). Differentiation of anxiolytic and panicolytic drugs by effects on rat and mouse defense test batteries. *Neuroscience and Biobehavioral Reviews*, *21*, 783–789.

Bolton, D., Eley, T. C., O'Connor, T. G., Perrin, S., Rabe-Hesketh, S., Rijsdijk, F., *et al.* (2006). Prevalence and genetic and environmental influences on anxiety disorders in 6-year-old twins. *Psychological Medicine*, *36*, 335–344.

Breslau, N. (1995). Psychiatric sequelae of low birth weight. *Epidemiology Review*, *17*, 96–106.

Breslau, N., & Chilcoat, H. D. (2000). Psychiatric sequelae of low birth weight at 11 years of age. *Biological Psychiatry*, *47*, 1005–1011.

Breslau, N., Chilcoat, H. D., Johnson, E. O., Andreski, P., & Lucia, V. C. (2000). Neurologic soft signs and low birthweight: Their association and neuropsychiatric implications. *Biological Psychiatry*, *47*, 71–79.

Briggs, A. C., Stretch, D. D., & Brandon, S. (1993). Subtyping of panic disorder by symptom profile. *British Journal of Psychiatry*, *163*, 201–209.

Brooks, S. J., & Kutcher, S. (2003). Diagnosis and measurement of anxiety disorder in adolescents: A review of commonly used instruments. *Journal of Child and Adolescent Psychopharmacology*, *13*, 351–400.

Capps, L., Sigman, M., Sena, R., Henker, B., & Whalen, C. (1996). Fear, anxiety and perceived control in children of agoraphobic parents. *Journal of Child Psychology and Psychiatry*, *37*, 445–452.

Caspi, A., Moffitt, T. E., Newman, D. L., & Silvam P. (1996). Behavioral observations at age 3 years predict adult psychiatric disorders. Longitudinal evidence from a birth cohort. *Archives of General Psychiatry*, *53*, 1033–1039.

Caspi, A., Sugden, K., Moffitt, T. E., Taylor, A., Craig, I. W., Harrington, H., *et al.* (2003). Influence of life stress on depression: moderation by a polymorphism in the 5-HTT gene. *Science*, *301*, 386–389.

Cassella, J. V., & Davis, M. (1985). Fear-enhanced acoustic startle is not attentuated by acute or chronic imipramine. *Psychopharmacology*, *87*, 278–282.

Coryell, W., Fyer, A., Pine, D., Martinez, J., & Arndt, S. (2001). Aberrant respiratory sensitivity to CO_2 as a trait of familial panic disorder. *Biological Psychiatry*, *49*, 582–587.

Costello, E., Pine, D. S., Hammen, C., March, J. S., Plotsky, P. M., Weissman, M. M., *et al.* (2002). Development and natural history of mood disorders. *Biological Psychiatry*, *52*, 529–542.

Costello, E. J., Angold, A., Burns, B. J., Stangl, D. K., Tweed, D. L., Erkanli, A., *et al.* (1996). The Great Smoky Mountains Study of Youth. Goals, design, methods, and the prevalence of DSM-III-R disorders. *Archives of General Psychiatry*, *53*, 1129–1136.

Costello, E. J., Angold, A., & Keeler, G. P. (1999). Adolescent outcomes of childhood disorders: The consequences of severity and impairment. *Journal of the American Academy of Child and Adolescent Psychiatry*, *38*, 121–128.

Costello, E. J., Compton, F. N., Keeler, G., & Angold, A. (2003). Relationships between poverty and psychopathology: A natural experiment. *Journal of the American Medical Association*, *290*, 2023–2029.

Costello, E. J., Costello, A. J., Edelbrock, C., Burns, B. J., Dulcan, M. K., Brent, D., Janiszewski, S. (1988). Psychiatric disorders in pediatric primary care. Prevalence and risk factors. *Archives of General Psychiatry*, *45*, 1107–1116.

Costello, E. J., Egger, H. L., & Angold, A. (2004). Developmental epidemiology of anxiety disorders. In M. J. Ollendick (Ed.), *Phobic and Anxiety Disorders in Children and Adolescents* (pp. 61–91). New York, NY: Oxford University Press.

Costello, E. J., Egger, H. L., & Angold, A. (2005). The developmental epidemiology of anxiety disorders: Phenomenology, prevalence, and comorbidity. *Child and Adolescent Psychiatric Clinics of North America*, *14*, 631–648, vii.

Davis, M. (1998). Are different parts of the extended amygdala involved in fear versus anxiety? *Biological Psychiatry*, *44*, 1239–1247.

Davis, M., & Whalen, P. J. (2001). The amygdala: Vigilance and emotion. *Molecular Psychiatry*, *6*, 13–34.

De Bellis, M. D., Casey, B. J., Dahl, R. E., Birmaher, B., Williamson, D. E., Thomas, K. M., *et al.* (2000a). A pilot study of amygdala volumes in pediatric generalized anxiety disorder. *Biological Psychiatry*, *48*, 51–57.

De Bellis, M. D., Keshavan, M. S., Frustaci, K., Shifflett, H., Iyengar, S., Beers, S. R., *et al.* (2002). Superior temporal gyrus volumes in pediatric generalized anxiety disorder. *Biological Psychiatry*, *51*, 553–562.

Egger, H. L., Costello, E. J., & Angold, A. (2003). School refusal and psychiatric disorders: A community study. *Journal of the American Academy of Child and Adolescent Psychiatry*, *42*, 797–807.

Eley, T. C., Bolton, D., O'Connor, T. G., Perrin, S., Smith, P., & Plomin, R. (2003). A twin study of anxiety-related behaviours in pre-school children. *Journal of Child Psychology and Psychiatry*, *44*, 945–960.

Eley, T. C., & Stevenson, J. (1999). Exploring the covariation between anxiety and depression symptoms: A genetic analysis of the effects of age and sex. *Journal of Child Psychology and Psychiatry*, *40*, 1273–1282.

Eley, T. C., & Stevenson, J. (2000). Specific life events and chronic experiences differentially associated with depression and anxiety in young twins. *Journal of Abnormal Child Psychology*, *28*, 383–394.

Eley, T. C., Stirling, L., Ehlers, A., Gregory, A. M., & Clark, D. M. (2004). Heart-beat perception, panic/somatic symptoms and anxiety sensitivity in children. *Behavior Research and Therapy*, *42*, 439–448.

Eley, T. C., Sugden, K., Corsico, A., Gregory, A. M., Sham, P., McGuffin, P., *et al.* (2004). Gene–environment interaction analysis of serotonin system markers with adolescent depression. *Molecular Psychiatry*, *9*, 908–915.

Essau, C., Conradt, J., & Petermann, F. (1999). Frequency and comorbidity of social phobia and social fears in adolescents. *Behavior Research and Therapy*, *37*, 831–843.

Feehan, M., McGee, R., & Williams, S. M. (1993). Mental health disorders from age 15 to age 18 years. *Journal of the American Academy of Child and Adolescent Psychiatry*, *32*, 1118–1126.

Fergusson, D. M., Horwood, L. J., & Lynskey, M. T. (1993). Prevlance and comorbidity of DSM-III-R diagnoses in a birth cohort of 15 year olds. *Journal of the American Academy of Child and Adolescent Psychiatry*, *32*, 1172–1134.

Flakerska-Praquin, N., Lindstroem, M., & Gillberg, C. (1997). School phobia with separation anxiety disorder: A comparative 20- to 29-year follow-up study of 35 school refusers. *Comprehensive Psychiatry*, *38*, 17–22.

Fox, N. A., Nichols, K., Henderson, H., Rubin, K., Schmidt, C., Hamer, D., *et al.* (2005). Evidence for a gene–environment interaction in predicting behavioral inhibition in middle childhood. *Psychological Science*, *16*, 921–926.

Fyer, A. J. (1998). Current approaches to etiology and pathophysiology of specific phobia. *Biological Psychiatry*, *44*, 1295–1304.

Goldsmith, H. H., & Lemery, K. S. (2000). Linking temperamental fearfulness and anxiety symptoms: A behavior-genetic perspective. *Biological Psychiatry*, *48*, 1199–1209.

Goldstein, R. B., Wickramaratne, P. J., Horwath, E., & Weissman, M. M. (1997). Familial aggregation and phenomenology of 'early'-onset (at or before age 20 years) panic disorder. *Archives of General Psychiatry*, *54*, 271–278.

Goodwin, R. D., Fergusson, D. M., & Horwood, L. J. (2004). Early anxious/withdrawn behaviours predict later internalising disorders. *Journal of Child Psychology and Psychiatry*, *45*, 874–883.

Goodwin, R. D., Pine, D. S., & Hoven, C. W. (2003). Asthma and panic attacks among youth in the community. *Journal of Asthma*, *40*, 139–145.

Gottesman, I. I., & Gould, T. D. (2003). The endophenotype concept in psychiatry: Etymology and strategic intentions. *American Journal of Psychiatry*, *160*, 636–645.

Graham, P., Rutter, M. (1968). The reliability and validity of the psychiatric assessment of the child. II. Interview with the parents. *British Journal of Psychiatry*, *114*, 581–592.

Grillon, C. (2002). Associative learning deficits increase symptoms of anxiety in humans. *Biological Psychiatry*, *51*, 851–858.

Grillon, C., & Baas, J. (2003). A review of the modulation of the startle reflex by affective states and its application in psychiatry. *Clinical Neurophysiology*, *114*, 1557–1579.

Grillon, C., Dierker, L., & Merikangas, K. R. (1997). Startle modulation in children at risk for anxiety disorders and/or alcoholism. *Journal of the American Academy of Child and Adolescent Psychiatry*, *36*, 925–932.

Grillon, C., Dierker, L., & Merikangas, K. R. (1998). Fear-potentiated startle in adolescent offspring of parents with anxiety disorders. *Biological Psychiatry*, *44*, 990–997.

Grillon, C., Warner, V., Hille, J., Merikangas, K. R., Bruder, G. E., Tenke, C. E., *et al.* (2005). Families at high and low risk for depression: A three-generation startle study. *Biological Psychiatry*, *57*, 953–960.

Gross, C., & Hen, R. (2004). The developmental origins of anxiety. *Nature Reviews. Neuroscience*, *5*, 545–552.

Hamilton, M. (1969). Diagnosis and rating of anxiety. *British Journal of Psychiatry*, *Special Publication*, *3*, 76–79.

Hankin, B. L., & Abramson, L. Y. (2001). Development of gender differences in depression: An elaborated cognitive vulnerability–transactional stress theory. *Psychological Bulletin*, *127*, 773–796.

Hariri, A. R., Mattay, V. S., Tessitore, A., Kolachana, B. S., Fera, F., Goldman, D., *et al.* (2002). Serotonin transporter genetic variation and the response of the human amygdala. *Science*, *297*, 400–403.

Hayward, C., Killen, J. D., Kraemer, H. C., & Taylor, C. B. (1998). Linking self-reported childhood behavioral inhibition to adolescent social phobia. *Journal of the American Academy of Child and Adolescent Psychiatry*, *37*, 1308–1316.

Herjanic, B., Reich, W. (1982). Development of a structured psychiatric interview for children: agreement between child and parent on individual symptoms. *Journal of Abnormal Child Psychology*, *10*, 307–324.

Hettema, J. M., Neale, M. C., & Kendler, K. S. (2001). A review and meta-analysis of the genetic epidemiology of anxiety disorders. *American Journal of Psychiatry*, *158*, 1568–1578.

Hettema, J. M., Neale, M. C., Myers, J. M., Prescott, C. A., & Kendler, K. S. (2006). A population-based twin study of the relationship between neuroticism and internalizing disorders. *American Journal of Psychiatry*, *163*, 857–864.

Hettema, J. M., Prescott, C. A., Myers, J. M., Neale, M. C., & Kendler, K. S. (2005). The structure of genetic and environmental risk factors for anxiety disorders in men and women. *Archives of General Psychiatry*, *62*, 182–189.

Horwath, E., Adams, P., Wickramaratne, P., Pine, D., & Weissman, M. M. (1997). Panic disorder with smothering symptoms: Evidence for increased risk in first-degree relatives. *Depression and Anxiety*, *6*, 147–153.

Johnson, J. G., Cohen, P., Pine D. S., Klein, D. F., Kasen, S., & Brook, J. S. (2000). Association between cigarette smoking and anxiety disorders during adolescence and early adulthood. *Journal of the American Medical Association*, *284*, 2348–2351.

Kagan, J. (1994). *Galen's Prophecy*. New York, NY: Basic Books.

Kagan, J., & Snidman, N. (1999). Early childhood predictors of adult anxiety disorders. *Biological Psychiatry*, *46*, 1536–1541.

Kagan, J., Snidman, N., McManis, M., & Woodward, S. (2001). Temperamental contributions to the affect family of anxiety. *Psychiatric Clinics of North America*, *24*, 677–688.

Kaplow, J. B., Curran, P. J., Angold, A., & Costello, E. J. (2001). The prospective relation between dimensions of anxiety and the initiation of adolescent alcohol use. *Journal of Clinical Child Psychology*, *30*, 316–326.

Kashani, J. H., Beck, N. C., Hoeper, E. W., Fallahi, C., Corcoran, C. M., McAllister, J. A., Rosenberg, T. K., Reid, J. C. (1987). Psychiatric disorders in a community sample of adolescents. *American Journal of Psychiatry*, *144*, 584–589.

Kaufman, J., Birmaher, B., Brent, D., Rao, U., Flynn, C., Moreci, P., *et al.* (1997). Schedule for Affective Disorders and Schizophrenia for School-Age Children-Present and Lifetime Version (K-SADS-PL): Initial reliability and validity data. *Journal of the American Academy of Child and Adolescent Psychiatry*, *36*, 980–988.

Kaufman, J., Birmaher, B., Brent, D. A., Ryan, N. D., & Rao, U. (2000). K-SADS-PL. *Journal of the American Academy of Child and Adolescent Psychiatry*, *39*, 1208.

Kaufman, J., Yang, B. Z., Douglas-Palumberi, H., Houshyar, S., Lipschitz, D., Krystal, J. H., & Gelernter, J. (2004). Social supports and serotonin transporter gene moderate depression in maltreated children. *Proceedings of the National Academy of Sciences of the USA*, *101*, 17316–17321.

Kendall, P. C. (1994). Treating anxiety disorders in children: Results of a randomized clinical trial. *Journal of Consulting and Clinical Psychology*, *62*, 100–110.

Kendall, P. C., Flannery-Schroeder, E., Panichelli-Mindel, S. M., Southam-Gerow, M., Henin, A., & Warman, M. (1997). Therapy for youths with anxiety disorders: a second randomized clinical trial. *Journal of Consulting and Clinical Psychology*, *65*, 366–380.

Kendler, K. S., & Greenspan, R. J. (2006). The nature of genetic influences on behavior: lessons from "simpler" organisms. *American Journal of Psychiatry*, *163*, 1683–1694.

Kessler, R. C., Andrade, L. H., Bijl, R. V., Offord, D. R., Demler, O. V., & Stein, D. J. (2002). The effects of co-morbidity on the onset and persistence of generalized anxiety disorder in the ICPE surveys. International Consortium in Psychiatric Epidemiology. *Psychological Medicine*, *32*, 1213–1225.

Kim-Cohen, J., Caspi, A., Moffitt, T. E., Harrington, H. L., Milne, B. S., & Poulton, R. (2003). Prior juvenile diagnoses in adults with mental disorder: Developmental follow-back of a prospective-longitudinal cohort. *Archives of General Psychiatry*, *60*, 709–717.

Klein, D. F. (1993). False suffocation alarms, spontaneous panics, and related conditions. An integrative hypothesis. *Archives of General Psychiatry*, *50*, 306–317.

Klein, D. F. (1996). Panic disorder and agoraphobia: hypothesis hothouse. *Journal of Clinical Psychiatry*, *57*, 21–27.

Klein, R. G. (1994). Anxiety disorders. In M. Rutter, L. Hersov, & E. Taylor (Eds.), *Child and Adolescent Psychiatry: Modern Approaches* (pp. 351–373). Oxford: Blackwell Scientific Publications.

Klein, R. G. (1995). Is panic disorder associated with childhood separation anxiety disorder? *Clinical Neuropharmacology*, *18*, S7–S14.

Klein, R. G., & Pine, D. S. (2002). Anxiety disorders. In M. Rutter, & E. Taylor (Eds.) *Child and Adolescent Psychiatry* (4th edn., pp. 486–509). New York, Elsevier.

Kramer, T., Garralda, E. (1998). Psychiatric disorders in adolescents in primary care. *British Journal of Psychiatry*, *173*, 508–513.

Last, C. G., Hansen, C., & Franco, N. (1997). Anxious children in adulthood: A prospective study of adjustment. *Journal of the American Academy of Child and Adolescent Psychiatry*, *36*, 645–652.

Last, C. G., Hansen, C., & Franco, N. (1998). Cognitive–behavioral treatment of school phobia. *Journal of the American Academy of Child and Adolescent Psychiatry*, *37*, 404–411.

Last, C. G., Hersen, M., Kazdin, A., Orvaschel, H., Perrin, S. (1991). Anxiety disorders in children and their families. *Archives of General Psychiatry*, *48*, 928–934.

LeDoux, J. E. (2000). Emotion circuits in the brain. *Annual Review of Neuroscience*, *23*, 155–184.

Lewinsohn, P. M., Gotlib, I. H., Lewinsohn, M., Seeley, J. R., & Allen, N. B. (1998). Gender differences in anxiety disorders and anxiety symptoms in adolescents. *Journal of Abnormal Psychology*, *107*, 109–117.

Lewinsohn, P. M., Zinbarg, R., Seeley, J. R., Lewinsohn, M., & Sack, W. H. (1997). Lifetime comorbidity among anxiety disorders and between anxiety disorders and other mental disorders in adolescents. *Journal of Anxiety Disorders*, *11*, 377–394.

Lieb, R., Isensee, B., Höfler, M., Pfister, H., & Wittchen, H. U. (2002). Parental major depression and the risk of depression and other mental disorders in offspring: A prospective-longitudinal community study. *Archives of General Psychiatry*, *59*, 365–374.

Lieb, R., Wittchen, H. U., Hofler, M., Fuetsch, M., Stein, M. B., Merikangas, K. R. (2000). Parental psychopathology, parenting styles, and the risk of social phobia in offspring: a prospective-longitudinal community study. *Archives of General Psychiatry*, *57*, 859–866.

Lissek, S., Powers, A. S., McClure, E. B., Phelps, E. A., Woldehawariat, G., Grillon C., *et al.* (2005). Classical fear conditioning in the anxiety disorders: A meta-analysis. *Behavior Research and Therapy*, *43*, 1391–1424.

MacLeod, C., Rutherford, E., Campbell, L., Ebsworthy, G., & Holker, L. (2002). Selective attention and emotional vulnerability: assessing the causal basis of their association through the experimental manipulation of attentional bias. *Journal of Abnormal Psychology*, *111*, 107–123.

Magee, W. J., Eaton, W. W., Wittchen, H. U., McGonagle, K. A., Kessler, R. C. (1996). Agoraphobia, simple phobia, and social phobia in the National Comorbidity Survey. *Archives of General Psychiatry*, *53*, 159–168.

Mannuzza, S., Klein, R. G., Moulton, J. L., Scarfone, N., Malloy, P., Vosburg, S. K., *et al.* (2002). Anxiety sensitivity among children of parents with anxiety disorders: A controlled high-risk study. *Journal of Anxiety Disorders*, *16*, 135–148.

March, J., Silva, S., Petrycki, S., Curry, J., Wells, K., Fairbank, J., *et al.*, & the Treatment for Adolescents With Depression Study (TADS) Team. (2004). Fluoxetine, cognitive–behavioral therapy, and their combination for adolescents with depression: Treatment for Adolescents with Depression Study (TADS) randomized controlled trial. *Journal of the American Medical Association*, *292*, 807–820.

March, J. S., Parker, J. D., Sullivan, K., Stallings, P., & Conners, C. K. (1997). The Multidimensional Anxiety Scale for Children (MASC): Factor structure, reliability, and validity. *Journal of the American Academy of Child and Adolescent Psychiatry*, *36*, 554–565.

March, J. S., & Sullivan, K. (1999). Test–retest reliability of the Multidimensional Anxiety Scale for Children. *Journal of Anxiety Disorders*, *13*, 349–358.

March, J. S., Swanson, J. M., Arnold, L. E., Hoza, B., Conners, C. K., Hinshaw, S. P., *et al.* (2000). Anxiety as a predictor and outcome variable in the multimodal treatment study of children with ADHD (MTA). *Journal of Abnormal Child Psychology*, *28*, 527–541.

Mathew, S. J., Coplan, J. D., Smith, E. L., Scharf, B. A., Owens, M. J., Nemeroff, C. B., *et al.* (2002). Cerebrospinal fluid concentrations of biogenic amines and corticotropin-releasing factor in adolescent non-human primates as a function of the timing of adverse early rearing. *Stress*, *5*, 185–193.

McClure, E. B., Brennan, P. A., Hammen, C., & Le Brocque, R. M. (2001). Parental anxiety disorders, child anxiety disorders, and the perceived parent–child relationship in an Australian high-risk sample. *Journal of Abnormal Child Psychology*, *29*, 1–10.

McGee, R., Feehan, M., Williams, S. & Anderson, J. (1992). DSM-III disorders from age 11 to age 15 years. *Journal of the American Academy of Child and Adolescent Psychiatry*, *31*, 50–59.

McGee, R., Feehan, M., Williams, S., Partridge, F., Silva, P. A., & Kelly, J. (1990). DSM-III disorders in a large sample of adolescents. *Journal of the American Academy of Child and Adolescent Psychiatry*, *29*, 611–619.

Meaney, M. J. (2001). Maternal care, gene expression, and the transmission of individual differences in stress reactivity across generations. *Annual Review of Neurosciences*, *24*, 1161–1192.

Mendlowitz, S. L., Manassis, K., Bradley, S., Scapillato, D., Miezitis, S., & Shaw, B. F. (1999). Cognitive–behavioral group treatments in childhood anxiety disorders: The role of parental involvement. *Journal of the American Academy of Child and Adolescent Psychiatry*, *38*, 1223–1229.

Merikangas, K. R., Avenevoli, S., Dierker, L., & Grillon, C. (1999). Vulnerability factors among children at risk for anxiety disorders. *Biological Psychiatry*, *46*, 1523–1535.

Middeldorp, C. M., Cath, D. C., Van Dyck, R., & Boomsma, D. I. (2005). The co-morbidity of anxiety and depression in the perspective of genetic epidemiology. A review of twin and family studies. *Psychological Medicine*, *35*, 611–624.

Millham, M. P., Nugent, A. C., Drevets, W. C., Leibenluft, E., Ernst, M., Charney, D. S., *et al.* (2005). Selective reduction in amygdala volume in pediatric generalized anxiety disorder: A voxel-based morphometry investigation. *Biological Psychiatry*, *57*, 961–966.

Mogg, K., & Bradley, P. P. (1998). A cognitive–motivational analysis of anxiety. *Behavior Research and Therapy*, *36*, 809–848.

Monk, C. S., Nelson, E. E., McClure, E. B., Mogg, K., Bradley, B. P., Leibenluft, E., *et al.* (2006). Ventrolateral prefrontal cortex activation and attentional bias in response to angry faces in adolescents with generalized anxiety disorder. *American Journal of Psychiatry*, *163*, 1091–1097.

Ollendick, T. H., Yang, B., King, N. J., Dong, Q., & Akande, A. (1996). Fears in American, Australian, Chinese, and Nigerian children and adolescents: A cross-cultural study. *Journal of Child Psychology and Psychiatry*, *37*, 213–220.

Pine, D. S., & Cohen, J. A. (2002). Trauma in children and adolescents: Risk and treatment of psychiatric sequelae. *Biological Psychiatry*, *51*, 519–531.

Pine, D. S., Cohen, P., & Brook, J. (2001). Adolescent fears as predictors of depression. *Biological Psychiatry*, *50*, 721–724.

Pine, D. S., Cohen, P., Gurley, D., Brook, J., & Ma, Y. (1998). The risk for early-adulthood anxiety and depressive disorders in adolescents with anxiety and depressive disorders. *Archives of General Psychiatry*, *55*, 56–64.

Pine, D. S., Cohen, P., Johnson, J. G., & Brook, J. S. (2002). Adolescent life events as predictors of adult depression. *Journal of Affective Disorders*, *68*, 49–57.

Pine, D. S., Klein, R. G., Roberson-Nay, R., Mannuzza, S., Moulton, J. L. 3rd, Woldehawariat, G., *et al.* (2005a). Response to 5% carbon dioxide in children and adolescents: Relationship to panic disorder in parents and anxiety disorders in subjects. *Archives of General Psychiatry*, *62*, 73–80.

Pine, D. S., Klein, R. G., Roberson-Nay, R., Mannuzza, S., Moutlon, J. L., Woldehawariat, G., *et al.* (2005b). Face emotion processing and risk for panic disorder in youth. *Journal of the American Academy of Child and Adolescent Psychiatry*, *44*, 664–672.

Pine, D. S., Mogg, K., Bradley, B. P., Montgomery, L., Monk, C. S., McClure, E., *et al.* (2005c). Attention bias to threat in maltreated children: Implications for vulnerability to stress-related psychopathology. *American Journal of Psychiatry*, *162*, 291–296.

Prior, M., Smart, D., Sanson, A., & Oberklaid, F. (2000). Does shy-inhibited temperament in childhood lead to anxiety problems in adolescence? *Journal of the American Academy of Child and Adolescent Psychiatry*, *39*, 461–468.

Poulton, R., Pine, D. S., & Harrington, H. (in press). Are anxiety disorders and their etiologies stable across the lifecourse? In D. A. Regier (Ed.), *DSM-V Workgroups on Fear and Stress Disorders*. Washington, DC: American Psychiatric Association.

Quirk, G. J., & Gehlert, D. R. (2003). Inhibition of the amygdala: Key to pathological states? *Annals of the New York Academy of Sciences*, *985*, 263–272.

Rapee, R. M., Kennedy, S., Ingram, M., Edwards, S., & Sweeney, L. (2005). Prevention and early intervention of anxiety disorders in inhibited preschool children. *Journal of Consulting and Clinical Psychology*, *73*, 488–497.

Reed, V., & Wittchen, H. U. (1998). DSM-IV panic attacks and panic disorder in a community sample of adolescents and young adults: How specific are panic attacks? *Journal of Psychiatric Research*, *32*, 335–345.

Reich, W. (2000). Diagnostic Interview for Children and Adolescents (DICA). *Journal of the American Academy of Child and Adolescent Psychiatry*, *39*, 59–66.

Rende, R., Wickramaratne, P., Warner, V., & Weissman, M. M. (1995). Sibling resemblance for psychiatric disorders in offspring at high and low risk for depression. *Journal of Child Psychology and Psychiatry*, *36*, 1353–1363.

Research Unit on Pediatric Psychopharmacology Anxiety Study Group (RUPP). (2001). Fluvoxamine for the treatment of anxiety disorders in children and adolescents. The Research Unit on Pediatric Psychopharmacology Anxiety Study Group. *New England Journal of Medicine*, *344*, 1279–1285.

Research Unit on Pediatric Psychopharmacology Anxiety Study Group (RUPP). (2003). The Pediatric Anxiety Rating Scale (PARS): Development and psychometric properties. *Journal of the American Academy of Child and Adolescent Psychiatry*, *42*, 13–21.

Reynolds, C. R., & Richmond, B. O. (1985). *Revised Children's Manifest Anxiety Scale: Manual*. Los Angeles, CA: Western Psychological Services.

Rosenbaum, J. F., Biederman, J., Hirshfeld-Becker, D. R., Kagan, J., Snidman, N., Friedman, D., *et al.* (2000). A controlled study of behavioral inhibition in children of parents with panic disorder and depression. *American Journal of Psychiatry*, *157*, 2002–2010.

Rueter, M. A., Scaramella, L., Wallace, L. E., & Conger, R. D. (1999). First onset of depressive or anxiety disorders predicted by the longitudinal course of internalizing symptoms and parent–adolescent disagreements. *Archives of General Psychiatry*, *56*, 726–732.

Rutter, M., Maughan, B., & Kim-Cohen, J. (2006). Continuities and discontinuities in psychopathology between childhood and adult life. *Journal of Child Psychology and Psychiatry*, *47*, 276–295.

Rynn, M. A., Siqueland, L., & Rickels, K. (2001). Placebo-controlled trial of sertraline in the treatment of children with generalized anxiety disorder. *American Journal of Psychiatry*, *158*, 2008–2014.

Schwab-Stone, M. E., Shaffer, D., Dulcan, M. K., & Jensen, P. S. (1996). Criterion validity of the NIMH Diagnostic Interview Schedule for Children, Version 2.3 (DISC-2.3). *Journal of the American Academy of Child and Adolescent Psychiatry*, *35*, 878–888.

Schwartz, C. E., Snidman, N., & Kagan, J. (1999). Adolescent social anxiety as an outcome of inhibited temperament in childhood. *Journal of the American Academy of Child and Adolescent Psychiatry*, *38*, 1008–1015.

Schwartz, C. E., Wright, C. I., Shin, L. M., Kagan, J., & Rauch, S. L. (2003). Inhibited and uninhibited infants "grown up": Adult amygdalar response to novelty. *Science*, *300*, 1952–1953.

Seligman, L. D., Ollendick, T. H., Langley, A. K., & Baldacci, H. B. (2004). The utility of measures of child and adolescent anxiety: A meta-analytic review of the Revised Children's Manifest Anxiety Scale, the State-Trait Anxiety Inventory for Children, and the Child Behavior Checklist. *Journal of Clinical Child and Adolescent Psychology*, *33*, 557–565.

Shaffer, D., Fisher, P., Dulcan, M. K., Davies, M., Piacentini, J., Schwab-Stone, M. E., *et al.* (1996). The NIMH Diagnostic Interview Schedule for Children Version 2.3 (DISC-2.3): Description, acceptability, prevalence rates, and performance in the MECA Study. Methods for the Epidemiology of Child and Adolescent Mental Disorders Study. *Journal of the American Academy of Child and Adolescent Psychiatry*, *35*, 865–877.

Shaffer, D., Fisher, P., Lucas, C. P., Dulcan, M. K., & Schwab-Stone, M. E. (2000). NIMH Diagnostic Interview Schedule for Children Version IV (NIMH DISC-IV): Description, differences from previous versions, and reliability of some common diagnoses. *Journal of the American Academy of Child and Adolescent Psychiatry*, *39*, 28–38.

Shaffer, D., Gould, M. S., Brasic, J., Ambrosini, P., Fisher, P., Bird, H., Aluwahlia, S. (1983). A children's global assessment scale (CGAS). *Archives of General Psychiatry*, *40*, 1228–1231.

Shaffer, D., Schonfeld, I., O'Connor, P. A., Stokman, C., Trautman, P., Shafer, S., *et al.* (1985). Neurological soft signs. Their relationship to psychiatric disorder and intelligence in childhood and adolescence. *Archives of General Psychiatry*, *42*, 342–351.

Silberg, J., Pickles, A., Rutter, M., Hewitt, J., Simonoff, E., Maes, H., *et al.* (1999). The influence of genetic factors and life stress on depression among adolescent girls. *Archives of General Psychiatry*, *56*, 225–232.

Silberg, J. L., Rutter, M., & Eaves, L. (2001). Genetic and environmental influences on the temporal association between earlier anxiety and later depression in girls. *Biological Psychiatry*, *49*, 1040–1049.

Silverman, W. K., Kurtines, W. M., Ginsburg, G. S., Weems, C. F., Rabian, B., & Serafini, L. T. (1999). Contingency management, self-control, and education support in the treatment of childhood phobic disorders: A randomized clinical trial. *Journal of Consulting and Clinical Psychology*, *67*, 675–687.

Silverman, W. K., & Ollendick, T. H. (2005). Evidence-based assessment of anxiety and its disorders in children and adolescents. *Journal of Clinical Child and Adolescent Psychology*, *34*, 380–411.

Silverman, W. K., Saavedra, L. M., & Pina, A. A. (2001). Test–retest reliability of anxiety symptoms and diagnoses with the Anxiety Disorders Interview Schedule for DSM-IV: Child and parent versions. *Journal of the American Academy of Child and Adolescent Psychiatry*, *40*, 937–944.

Simonoff, E., Pickles, A., Meyer, J. M. Silberg, J. L., Maes, H. H., Loeber, R., *et al.* (1997). The Virginia Twin Study of Adolescent Behavioral Development. Influences of age, sex, and impairment on rates of disorder. *Archives of General Psychiatry*, *54*, 801–808.

Slattery, M. J., Klein, D. F., Pine, D. S., & Klein, R. G., Mannuzza, S., Moulton, J. L. 3rd (2002). Relationship between separation anxiety disorder, parental panic disorder, and atopic disorders in children: A controlled high-risk study. *Journal of the American Academy of Child and Adolescent Psychiatry*, *41*, 947–954.

Smoller, J. W., Yamaki, L. H., Fagerness, J. A., Biederman, J., Racette, S., Laird, N. M., *et al.* (2005). The corticotropin-releasing hormone gene and behavioral inhibition in children at risk for panic disorder. *Biological Psychiatry*, *57*, 1485–1492.

Speielberger, C. D. (1973). *State-Trait Anxiety Inventory for Children*. Palo Alto, CA: Consulting Psychologists Press.

Steinberg, L., & Avenevoli, S. (2000). The role of context in the development of psychopathology: A conceptual framework and some speculative propositions. *Child Development*, *71*, 66–74.

Suomi, S. J. (2003). Gene–environment interactions and the neurobiology of social conflict. *Annals of the New York Academy of Sciences*, *1008*, 132–139.

Terleph, T. A., Klein, R. G., Roberson-Nay, R., Mannuzza, S., Moulton, J. L. 3rd, Woldehawariat, G., *et al.* (2006). Stress responsivity and HPA axis activity in juveniles: Results from a home-based CO_2 inhalation study. *American Journal of Psychiatry*, *163*, 738–740.

Thomas, K. M., Drevets, W. C., Dahl, R. E., Ryan, N. D., Birmaher, B., Eccard, C. H., *et al.* (2001). Amygdala response to fearful faces in anxious and depressed children. *Archives of General Psychiatry*, *58*, 1057–1063.

Topolski, T. D., Hewitt, J. K., Eaves, L., Meyer, J. M., Silberg, J. L., Simonoff, E., *et al.* (1999). Genetic and environmental influences on ratings of manifest anxiety by parents and children. *Journal of Anxiety Disorders*, *13*, 371–397.

Turner, S. M., Beidel, D. C., & Costello, A. (1987). Psychopathology in the offspring of anxiety disorders patients. *Journal of Consulting and Clinical Psychology*, *55*, 229–235.

Vasa, R. A., Carlino, A. R., & Pine, D. S. (2006). Pharmacotherapy of depressed children and adolescents: Current issues and potential directions. *Biological Psychiatry*, *59*, 1021–1028.

Vasa, R. A., Gerring, J. P., Grados, M., Slomine, B., Christensen, J. R., Rising, W., *et al.* (2002). Anxiety after severe pediatric closed head injury. *Journal of the American Academy of Child and Adolescent Psychiatry*, *41*, 148–156.

Verhulst, F. C., van der Ende, J., Ferdinand, R. F., & Kasius, M. C. (1997). The prevalence of DSM-III-R diagnoses in a national sample of Dutch adolescents. *Archives of General Psychiatry*, *54*, 329–336.

Wagner, K. D., Berard, R., Stein, M. B., Wetherhold, E., Carpenter, D. J., Perera, P., *et al.* (2004). A multicenter, randomized, double-blind, placebo-controlled trial of paroxetine in children and adolescents with social anxiety disorder. *Archives of General Psychiatry*, *61*, 1153–1162.

Warner, V., Mufson, L., & Weissman, M. M. (1995). Offspring at high and low risk for depression and anxiety: Mechanisms of psychiatric disorder. *Journal of the American Academy of Child and Adolescent Psychiatry*, *34*, 786–797.

Weaver, I. C., Meaney, M. J., & Szyf, M. (2006). Maternal care effects on the hippocampal transcriptome and anxiety-mediated behaviors in the offspring that are reversible in adulthood. *Proceedings of the National Academy of Sciences of the USA*, *103*, 3480–3485.

Weissman, M. M., Leckman, J. F., Merikangas, K. R., Gammon, G. D., & Prusoff, B. A. (1984). Depression and anxiety disorders in parents and children. Results from the Yale family study. *Archives of General Psychiatry*, *41*, 845–852.

Weissman, M. M., Warner, V., Wickramaratne, P., Moreau, D., & Olfson, M. (1997). Offspring of depressed parents: 10 years later. *Archives of General Psychiatry*, *54*, 932–940.

Whitaker, A., Johnson, J., Shaffer, D., Rapoport, J. L., Kalikow, K., Walsh, B. T., *et al.* (1990). Uncommon troubles in young people: Prevalence estimates of selected psychiatric disorders in a non-referred adolescent population. *Archives of General Psychiatry*, *47*, 487–496.

Whitaker, A. H., Van Rossem, R., Feldman, J. F., Schonfeld, I. S., Pinto-Martin, J. A., Tore, C., *et al.* (1997). Psychiatric outcomes in low-birth-weight children at age 6 years: Relation to neonatal cranial ultrasound abnormalities. *Archives of General Psychiatry*, *54*, 847–856.

Williams, J. M., Mathews, A., & MacLeod, C. (1996). The emotional Stroop task and psychopathology. *Psychological Bulletin*, *120*, 3–24.

Williamson, D. E., Birmaher, B., Dahl, R. E., & Ryan, N. D. (2005). Stressful life events in anxious and depressed children. *Journal of Child and Adolescent Psychopharmacology*, *15*, 571–580.

Wittchen, H.-U. (1994). Reliability and validity studies of the WHO–Composite International Diagnostic Interview (CIDI): a critical review. *J Psychiatr Res*, *28*, 57–84.

Wittchen, H. U., Stein, M. B., & Kessler, R. C. (1999). Social fears and social phobia in a community sample of adolescents and young adults: Prevalence, risk factors and co-morbidity. *Psychological Medicine*, *29*, 309–323.

Wood, J. J., McLeod, B. D., Sigman, M., Hwang, W. C., & Chu, B. C. (2003). Parenting and childhood anxiety: Theory, empirical findings, and future directions. *Journal of Child Psychology and Psychiatry*, *44*, 134–151.

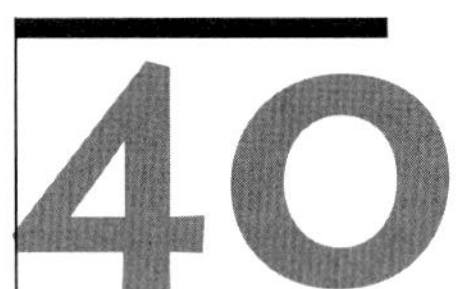

Suicidal Behavior and Deliberate Self-Harm

Keith Hawton and Sarah Fortune

In this chapter we first address the issue of operational definitions of suicidal phenomena in research and clinical practice, followed by consideration of the variety of motives and intentions associated with acts of self-harm in young people. The rates of suicidal behaviors are presented, in conjunction with a summary of research on risk and protective factors. Clinical assessment issues and possible outcomes following an episode of self-harm are described. Treatment options, including psychological interventions and medication, are reviewed, with particular consideration of the issue of engagement in treatment with young people and their families. Finally, we consider factors that influence help-seeking and outline prevention initiatives.

Range of Suicidal Behaviors Including Suicide Ideation, Deliberate Self-Harm and Suicide

Many young people consider suicide or self-harm at some point in their lives. Some carry out non-suicidal acts of self-injury, while fewer make suicide attempts. A small minority will die, either intentionally or unintentionally. There is a continuum of suicidality but there are also two main points at which discontinuity exists. First, of those who have suicidal ideas only a small proportion engage in some form of deliberate self-harm (DSH). This represents an important behavioral threshold. Second, some people engage in DSH once, never to repeat, while others carry out repeated acts of DSH.

Definitions of Terms

Suicide *ideation* is defined as thoughts about an act of DSH or suicide, including wishing to kill oneself, making plans of when, where and how to carry out the act, and having thoughts about the impact of one's self-harm or suicide on others. *DSH* is defined as any form of non-fatal self-poisoning or self-injury (such as cutting, taking an overdose, hanging, self-strangulation and running into traffic), regardless of motivation or the degree of intention to die. *Suicide* includes deaths resulting directly from acts of deliberate self-harm. Official verdicts in the UK, and many other countries, are determined by the coroner and are classified using ICD-10 (World Health Organization, 1996). To reach a verdict of suicide a coroner needs to be satisfied that the act was self-inflicted and that death was the intended outcome. However, strict adherence to these criteria may result in underestimation of the true extent of suicide. Operational definitions are the subject of much debate in both suicide research and clinical practice (Beck, Davis, Frederick *et al.*, 1973; Maris, Berman, Maltsberger *et al.*, 1992; O'Carroll, Berman, Maris *et al.*, 1998).

Motives for Suicidal Behaviors and DSH

Acts of self-harm may have a variety of motives or intentions, such as finding one's thoughts or one's situation unbearable, wanting to die or needing to communicate to others the extent of current distress (Bancroft & Hawton, 1983; Hjelmeland, Stiles, Bille-Brahe *et al.*, 1998). The patterns of motives for DSH described by people who have self-harmed are relatively consistent across the lifespan (Hjelmeland & Groholt, 2005) and across countries (Hjelmeland, Hawton, Nordvik *et al.*, 2002). There are differences according to the method of DSH. In a school-based survey, adolescents who took overdoses often said they wanted to die, whereas those who cut themselves more often reported self-punishment and escape from a terrible state of mind as motives for their DSH (Rodham, Hawton, & Evans, 2004). Escape from a difficult state of mind is a common motive for DSH in adolescents (Hawton, Cole, O'Grady *et al.*, 1982; Kienhorst, de Wilde, Diekstra, & Wolters, 1995). Depression and hopelessness are related to an expressed desire to die as a reason for DSH (Boergers, Spirito, & Donaldson, 1998).

Some clinicians and researchers have distinguished self-mutilation as having distinctly different motivations compared with other types of deliberate self-harm. Self-mutilation is defined by Favazza (1992) as the deliberate destruction or alteration of body tissue without conscious suicidal intent, most often by cutting. This behavior is thought to reduce anger, tension or dissociative numbness. This definition suggests habitual cutting among adolescents who lack suicidal intent. However, studies of older individuals who had engaged in self-mutilation behavior indicated a significant risk of subsequent suicide (Stanley, Gameroff, Michalson *et al.*, 2001) and several recent studies have identified high rates of psychiatric morbidity and other risk-taking behaviors among this group of young people (Guertin, Lloyd-Richardson, Spirito *et al.*, 2001; Muehlenkamp & Gutierrez, 2004). On balance it is probably best to consider self-mutilation as part of the continuum of suicidal

Rutter's Child and Adolescent Psychiatry, 5th edition. Edited by M. Rutter, D. Bishop, D. Pine, S. Scott, J. Stevenson, E. Taylor and A. Thapar. © 2008 Blackwell Publishing, ISBN: 978-1-4051-4549-7.

phenomena, given that sometimes it can lead on to both suicide attempts and death by suicide.

Establishing the intent or motives for an episode of DSH can be complicated as adolescents are often ambivalent about their possible suicidality. In addition, fluctuating mood states can make it difficult to get clear information from adolescents, particularly retrospectively. Self-reported intent may also be influenced by the aftermath of the DSH act. The method of DSH is often taken as a proxy measure of intent. This may be problematic for three reasons. First, young people are known to underestimate risks and habitually engage in behaviors that carry high risk (Millstein & Halpern-Felsher, 2002). Thus, they may not intend to die but nevertheless select a method of DSH that is lethal or, conversely, they do intend to die but select a method that is relatively benign. Second, many young people have poor knowledge about the potential lethality of substances taken in overdose (Harris & Myers, 1997). Third, young people may switch between different methods of deliberate self-harm. Presentation with a relatively low lethality method may follow past acts involving more dangerous methods or may be followed by future episodes in which a more lethal method is used (Fortune, 2006).

Introduction to the "Suicidal Process"

Among adolescents, suicidal thinking is relatively common in the community, deliberate self-harm is less common and suicide is a rare event (Evans, Hawton, & Rodham, 2005a). To date there has been little research on the extent to which the spectrum of suicidal behaviors may appear or disappear in the lives of young people. Runeson, Beskow, & Waern (1996) have described the "suicidal process," which they define as an interaction between the individual and their environment that accumulates in such a way that suicidal ideas become plans, and plans are acted upon. They argue that the suicidal process operates at both conscious and unconscious levels. The person's experience of the process may or may not be communicated to others, but represents increasing vulnerability to acts of DSH and possibly suicide.

Broader Developmental Processes

The development of suicidal phenomena must be considered in the context of the broader developmental challenges faced by children and adolescents in which emerging physical, cognitive and personality characteristics transform the individual from a child to a young adult. Children pass through a series of stages in intellectual development. Some time after the age of 11 years the child begins to break away from tangible objects towards abstract principles and hypothetical possibilities (Piaget, 1968) and become increasingly able to consider abstract ideas such as the meaning of life. Conceptualizations of death reflect these cognitive changes and start with an early realization, around 8 years of age, that everyone dies (Mishara, 2003), through to an existential "choice to live" during adolescence. Erikson (1968) argued that the key developmental task of adolescence is development of identity versus role confusion, with the peer group assuming primacy over the family as part of this process. The exploration of intimate relationships during this developmental phase makes adolescents particularly vulnerable to rejection. At the same time, the desire to fit in with peers makes adolescents vulnerable to the risk of taking on the behaviors of deviant peers. Youth culture may also have impact on the likelihood of suicide. Adolescents in western cultures appear to be less judgmental about suicide compared with their parents and modern youth culture may portray suicide in positive terms (Cantor, 2000). Youth culture has also de-emphasized the religious–moral dimension of suicide while simultaneously emphasizing an individual's right to suicide (Bagley & Ramsay, 1997).

Population Prevalence of Suicide, Suicidal Ideation and DSH

Suicide

Reported rates of suicide deaths among children and adolescents around the world vary considerably as can be seen in Table 40.1. Some of this diversity may reflect differences in definition as outlined above, and the cultural and legal mores that surround this issue. Generally, more males than females die by suicide in all countries for which data are published, with the exception of China (Cantor & Neulinger, 2000). In a recent large population-based study in India suicide rates were also found to be higher among adolescent females compared to adolescent males (Aaron, Joseph, Abraham *et al.*, 2004). These findings are the reverse of those in adolescents who have died by suicide in other countries.

In several countries rates of suicide are higher in indigenous or aboriginal populations, particularly among young people. For example, First Nations people in the USA (US Department of Health and Human Services, Centers for Disease Control and Prevention, & National Center for Health Statistics, 2004), Metis and Inuit in Canada (Kirmayer, Malus, & Boothroyd, 1996), Australian Aborigines (Tatz, 2001) and New Zealand Māori (Ministry of Health, 2005). Historically, the rate of suicide among Black people in the USA has been considerably lower than White people (Bingham, Bennion, Openshaw *et al.*, 1994); however, from 1980 to 1995 there was a dramatic increase in suicide deaths among Black youth (Joe & Kaplan, 2001).

Youth suicide rates in the UK are declining following a period in which rates in young males had been rising alarmingly. It should be noted that official statistics markedly underestimate the true rates of suicide, especially in children and adolescents, with some apparent suicide deaths being recorded as open verdicts, accidents or misadventure (Madge & Harvey, 1999). In the UK, the rate of suicide and undetermined deaths for adolescent males 15–19 years old in 2003 was 6.58 per 100,000 and 2.24 per 100,000 for females of the same age. The rate of suicide and undetermined deaths among children aged 10–14 years was much lower, at 0.62 per 100,000 for males and 0.42 per 100,000 for females (Office of National Statistics, 2004).

Country	Year	Male age-specific rate per 100,000 population		Female age-specific rate per 100,000 population	
		5–14 years	15–24 years	5–14 years	15–24 years
Australia	2002	0.3	17.9	0.3	4.4
Austria	2004	0.4	21.6	0.0	4.3
Belgium	1997	1.0	19.2	0.0	5.4
Canada	2002	0.9	17.5	0.9	5.2
China	1999	0.9	5.4	0.8	8.6
Denmark	2001	0.6	12.5	0.0	2.4
Finland	2004	1.2	33.1	0.3	9.7
France	2002	0.6	11.9	0.4	3.1
Germany	2004	0.4	10.5	0.2	2.7
Ireland	2002	0.4	27.3	0.7	4.4
Italy	2002	0.2	6.5	0.2	1.5
Japan	2003	0.5	15.5	0.6	7.8
Lithuania	2004	2.7	42.9	0.5	7.4
Netherlands	2004	0.7	7.3	0.2	2.6
New Zealand	2002	0.0	22.8	0.0	11.0
Norway	2003	1.9	20.6	1.0	6.3
Russian Federation	2004	3.6	47.4	1.0	8.2
Spain	2003	0.1	6.8	0.1	2.1
Sweden	2002	0.7	14.6	0.5	4.5
UK	2002	0.1	8.2	0.1	2.4
USA	2002	0.9	16.5	0.3	2.9

Table 40.1 Male and female suicide rates for children, adolescents and young adults for selected countries (World Health Organization, 2006). Note: Comparison years vary by country because of availability of data.

Suicidal Ideation and DSH

A recent systematic review on the prevalence of suicidal phenomena in adolescents based on community or school-based studies in several countries demonstrated that suicidal ideation is more common than DSH, which is in turn more common than attempted suicide. Nearly 1 in 5 adolescents had thought about suicide in the previous year. The mean lifetime prevalence of deliberate self-harm was 13%, with 26% reporting deliberate self-harm in the previous year. The mean proportion of adolescents who had attempted suicide was 10%, with 6% making a suicide attempt in the previous 12 months. Rates of suicidal phenomena were higher among females than males (Evans, Hawton, Rodham *et al.*, 2005b).

In the UK, relatively few studies have been conducted on the prevalence of suicidal ideation and self-harm in the community. In a school-based study of 6020 students, 15% reported thoughts of deliberate self-harm (which had not been acted on) in the preceding year. This was much more common among females (22%) than males (9%). DSH in the past year occurred in 7% and was also much more frequent among females (11%) than males (3%; Hawton, Rodham, Evans *et al.*, 2002a). In contrast, in a large national study of suicidal phenomena among children and adolescents 5–15 years old, based on parental report, 1% of 5- to 10-year-olds had ever tried to harm, hurt or kill themselves, rising to 2% among those aged 11–15 years (Meltzer, Harrington, Goodman *et al.*, 2001). Parents are often unaware of DSH acts by their offspring (Huey, Henggeler, Rowland *et al.*, 2004; Meltzer, Harrington, Goodman *et al.*, 2001; Sourander, Aromaa, Pihlakoski *et al.*, 2006), especially where self-cutting is involved.

Two studies that used a similar methodology to Hawton, Rodham, Evans *et al.* (2002a) were conducted in Australia (De Leo & Heller, 2004) and Norway (Ystgaard, Reinholdt, Husby *et al.*, 2003); these suggested that rates of DSH in adolescents in the UK, Australia and Norway are similar. In a comparative study, again using equivalent methodology, rates of DSH were also similar in Belgium, but considerably lower in the Netherlands (Hawton, Rodham, & Evans, 2006).

There appear to be some differences between rates of non-fatal suicidal behavior in children and adolescents of different ethnic groups. In the USA, for example, several studies have indicated that Hispanic youth, particularly females, experience higher rates of suicide ideation, DSH and hopelessness than their White and Black peers (for review see Canino & Roberts, 2001). In New Zealand, a large national health study found that Māori youth reported significantly higher rates of depression, suicide ideation and suicide attempts in the last year than European/Pakeha students (Adolescent Health Research Group, 2005).

There have been a small number of studies of DSH among ethnic minority children and adolescents in the UK which have produced somewhat conflicting results. The most robust data come from the school-based study described above, in which DSH was less common among Asian (7%) and Black (7%)

girls than White girls (12%). Rates of DSH were similar among Asian and White males (3%; Hawton, Rodham, Evans *et al.*, 2002a). More recent studies have reported similar (Bhugra, Thompson, Singh *et al.*, 2003) or lower rates of DSH among Asian youth (Bhugra, Thompson, Singh *et al.*, 2004). This issue is reviewed in Bhugra and Bhui (2007).

Methods of Suicide and DSH by Gender and International Differences

There is significant variation among cultures in the methods most commonly used for suicide. The preferred methods of suicide in any given country may have an impact on suicide rates, given that some methods are potentially more lethal than others. In addition, deaths involving a certain method may increase or decrease depending on the availability of that method (Grossman & Kruesi, 2000; Hawton, 2005). For example, in the USA firearms are the most common method of suicide among both Black and White young people, but account for a relatively small number of deaths in the UK, New Zealand and Australia. The substitution of method relies on both the acceptability and availability of alternative methods; the increasing rate of hanging in young people suggests that it has become an increasingly acceptable method of suicide (Centers for Disease Control, 2004). It is also extremely accessible as well as having a high rate of lethality. The reason for the spread in acceptability of hanging as a method of suicide is not known.

The globalization of information has already resulted in rapid transmission of previously unknown and very lethal methods of suicide; for example, the spread of the use of charcoal burning from Hong Kong to Taiwan and Japan and the rapid rise in the popularity of this method. The mechanisms underlying the apparent increased acceptability, cultural meaning and preference for methods of suicide such as this require further research, including the likely role of the media, including the Internet, in influencing this trend.

In India, in contrast with other countries, hanging is a slightly more frequent method of suicide in girls (57%) than boys (50%), whereas poisoning is slightly more common in boys (50%) than girls (37%; Lalwani, Sharma, Kabra *et al.*, 2004). The use of toxic pesticides in agrarian communities such as in China, India (Prasad, Abraham, Minz *et al.*, 2006) and Sri Lanka (Eddleston, Gunnell, Karunaratne *et al.*, 2005b) means that a similar method (self-poisoning) is associated with much higher mortality in these countries than in countries where analgesics and other medications are the most frequently used substances for self-poisoning. The medical management of organophosphate poisoning is difficult and a lack of adequate medical services and distances to hospitals in developing countries may elevate death rates (Eddleston, Eyer, Worek *et al.*, 2005a).

At the community level the most common methods of DSH in the UK and many other countries are cutting and overdose. Hawton, Rodham, Evans *et al.* (2002a) found that cutting (65%) and overdose (31%) were the main methods of DSH among adolescents in the community. Studies using the same methodology showed similar rates of cutting in Australia (59%; De Leo & Heller, 2004) but higher rates in Norway (74%; Ystgaard, Reinholdt, Husby *et al.*, 2003). However, only a minority of young people engaging in DSH in the community go to hospital, with those taking overdoses most likely to do so (Hawton, Rodham, Evans *et al.*, 2002a). In studies based on presentations to general hospitals in the UK, the majority of adolescents had harmed themselves by taking an overdose, self-poisoning with analgesics being particularly common (Hawton, Hall, Simkin *et al.*, 2003).

Risk Factors Associated with Suicidal Phenomena in Children and Adolescents

An overall model of suicide behavior can help the clinician or researcher conceptualize the main contributory factors identified in a wide range of research studies. This can also provide a framework to support formulations and treatment planning. In such a model (Beautrais, 2000) suicidal behaviors are viewed as the endpoint of adverse life events in which multiple risk factors combine to encourage the development of suicidal behaviors (Fig. 40.1). This essentially represents a stress–diathesis model (Schotte & Clum, 1982), which suggests that temperamental and genetic factors and early experiences may make some young people particularly vulnerable to subsequent internal or external stressors.

There are a number of comprehensive reviews of the research literature on risk factors associated with fatal and non-fatal suicide behaviors among children and adolescents to which the reader is directed (Beautrais, 2000; Brent, 1995; Bridge, Goldstein, & Brent, 2006; Evans, Hawton, & Rodham, 2004; Gould, Greenberg, Velting *et al.*, 2003). Below we highlight contributory factors for which there is at least reasonably strong evidence.

Genetic and Neurobiological Aspects of Suicidal Behavior in Young People

Suicidal behavior runs in families (Brent, Bridge, Johnson *et al.*, 1996a). However, the risk in these families is not entirely accounted for by the increased rates of psychiatric disorder. The heritability of impulsive aggression also appears to be important (for a review see Brent & Mann, 2005). Twin studies have shown that the concordance for fatal and non-fatal suicidal behavior is higher among monozygotic than dyzygotic twins (Roy, 1993). The clustering of suicidal behavior in families cannot be explained entirely by behavioral imitation (Brent & Mann, 2005). Importantly, adoption studies have shown elevated rates of suicide among the biological relatives of adoptees who die by suicide compared with those of non-suicidal adoptees (Roy, Rylander, & Sarchiapone, 1997).

Genetic factors may affect the risk of suicide behaviors by their influence on neurobiology and much of this work

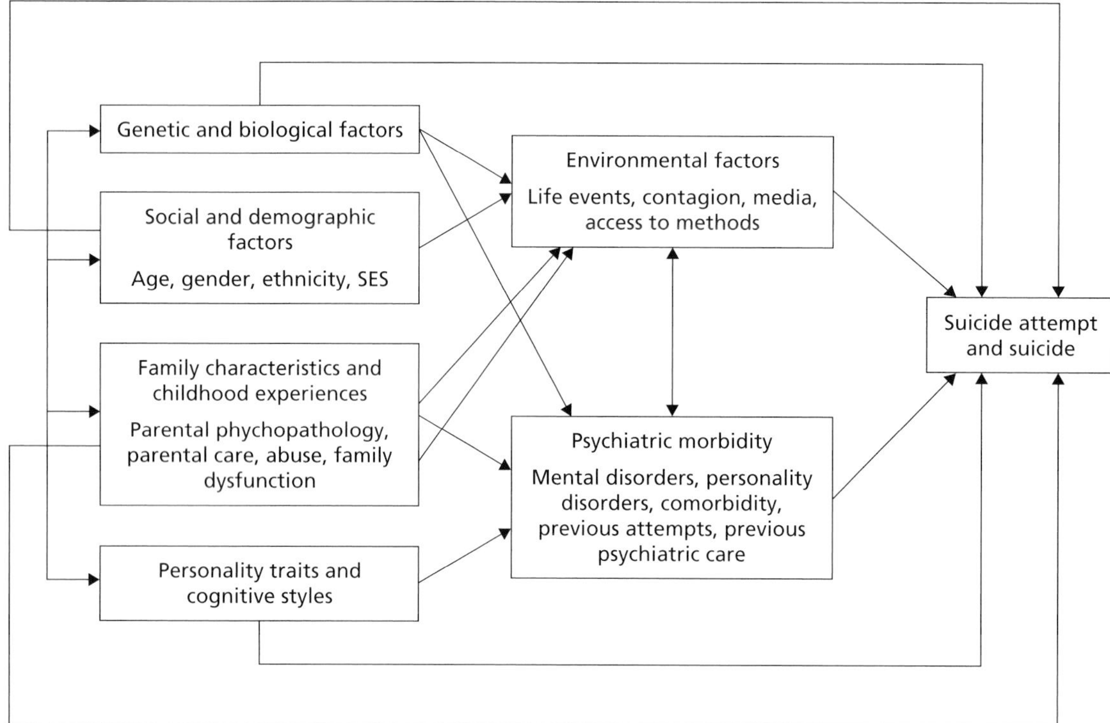

Fig. 40.1 Conceptual model of domains of risk factors for suicide and attempted suicide. SES, socio-economic status (After Beautrais, 2000, p. 429, with permission from the publisher.)

has arisen from the investigation of genetic factors in depression (for review see Levinson, 2006). The relationship between genetics and depression is dealt with in more detail in chapter 37. Deviations in the serotonin system are one of the most robust neurobiological findings associated with suicidal behavior (Asberg & Forslund, 2000). The relationship between serotonin dysregulation and suicide behavior may reflect poor impulse control, which is observed in suicidal, violent and impulsive behaviors. Earlier studies examined serotonin metabolites in cerebrospinal fluid and found lower than average levels of 5-hydroxytryptamine (serotonin 5-HT) and the metabolite 5-hydoxyindoleacetic acid (5-HIAA) in suicide victims (Arango, Underwood, Gubbi *et al.*, 1995), and people at risk of repetition of suicide attempts and suicide (Nordstrom, Samuelsson, Asberg *et al.*, 1994). More sophisticated neuroanatomical studies have identified a reduced density of serotonin 1A receptors and serotonin transporter receptors in the prefrontal cortex and brainstem of those who have died by suicide (Arango, Underwood, Boldrini *et al.*, 2001; Mann, Huang, Underwood *et al.*, 2000). Dysregulation of serotonin function may predispose a person experiencing stressful events to react impulsively (Mann, Brent, & Arango, 2001). There is less evidence for other neurobiological markers for suicidal behaviors such as dopamine, noradrenaline, cortisol and serum cholesterol (Asberg & Forslund, 2000; Bondy, Buettner, & Zill, 2006).

The main focus of interest in the genetic studies of suicidal behavior has been on three gene types: trytophan hydroxylase (TPH), serotonin transporter (SERT), located on chromosome 17, and serotonin A receptor genes (Arango, Underwood, Boldrini *et al.*, 2001). Serotonin transporter polymorphisms, particularly the "short" allele of the 5HTTLPR genotype, are associated with suicidal behavior in adults with psychiatric disorder and in particular violent attempts (Lin & Tsai, 2004). More recent studies in adults have explored the role of cannabinoids in the model of anxiety and stress responses underpinning suicidal behavior, in particular cannabinoid receptors (CB1), corticotropin-releasing hormone (CRH) and γ-aminobutyric acid (GABA) (Bondy, Buettner, & Zill, 2006). Despite the interest in this area to date, there are relatively few replicated findings or meta-analyses, particularly in children and adolescents.

Psychological and Cognitive Characteristics

Psychological characteristics associated with suicidal behavior include hopelessness (Evans, Hawton, & Rodham, 2004), dichotomous (all or nothing) thinking, negative biases in future judgment (Pfeffer, 2000; Williams & Pollock, 2000) and an external locus of control, or the belief that "things happen to you" because of forces outside your own control (Kienhorst, de Wilde, Diekstra *et al.*, 1992). Impaired problem-solving may be another contributory factor (Speckens & Hawton, 2005). This appears to be related to overgeneralized autobiographical memory (Williams & Pollock, 2000), although this phenomenon is not specific to suicidal behavior (Evans, Hawton, & Rodham, 2004).

Certain personality characteristics such as impulsivity, aggression, neuroticism and trait anxiety may act as intermediate factors that are relatively independent from major psychiatric disorders (Bridge, Goldstein, & Brent, 2006). Irritability and impulsivity have also been strongly associated with suicide in young men (Conner, Meldrum, Wieczorek *et al.*, 2004) and non-fatal acts in both genders (Bridge, Goldstein, & Brent, 2006). Aggression is also associated with DSH (Sourander, Aromaa, Pihlakoski *et al.*, 2006). A review of the associations between attention deficit/hyperactivity disorder (ADHD) and suicidal behavior concluded that they are modest, with elevated risk for fatal and non-fatal suicidal behavior, particularly in males, mediated by comorbid conditions, notably depression, conduct disorder and substance abuse, with the risk considerably elevated in young people with all three conditions (James, Lai, & Dahl, 2004).

Psychiatric Disorders Associated with DSH and Suicide

Many studies have demonstrated high rates of mental illness in adolescents engaging in both fatal and non-fatal suicidal behavior (for review see Evans, Hawton, & Rodham, 2004). In this section we highlight strong and recent findings about the relationship between mental illness and suicidal phenomena which have been investigated prospectively through longitudinal studies, retrospectively through psychological autopsy studies, and smaller cross-sectional and clinical population studies (which often provide less robust findings). Although mental illness is present in many children and adolescents who engage in suicidal behaviors, clearly not all people who experience mental illness engage in suicidal behavior, so it may be a strong precursor but not a complete explanation.

In a systematic review of psychological autopsy studies (Cavanagh, Carson, Sharpe *et al.*, 2003, p. 400) results of seven studies of adolescents or young adults suggested that 47–74% of suicides examined were attributable to a mental disorder, of which affective disorders made the greatest contribution. This review also highlighted that comorbidity, particularly comorbidity of mental disorder and substance abuse, made a strong contribution to the risk of suicide. An earlier review (Marttunen, Aro, & Lonnqvist, 1993) indicated that antisocial behavior was present in 43–73% of suicide deaths in adolescents, often in combination with depressive symptoms and/or substance abuse. Several more recent psychological autopsy studies (Fortune, Stewart, Yadav *et al.*, 2007; Houston, Hawton, & Sheppard, 2001; Portzky, Audenaert, & van Heeringen, 2005) point towards an interaction among mental illness, substance abuse and interpersonal problems (and, for some, antisocial behaviors). In a case–control study of young people who had died by suicide, serious suicide attempters and a non-suicidal control group, the same risk factors of mood disorder, requirement for psychiatric care, educational disadvantage and stressful life events were associated with both death by suicide and serious attempts, although the relative weighting of the factors was different. Mood disorders had a higher odds ratio for attempts than for death by suicide, and stressful life events had a higher odds ratio for suicide than attempts (Beautrais, 2003). However, it must also be borne in mind that 5–10% of young people who die by suicide have no mental health disorder. This group tend to include those with less disturbed families, who have no previous history of suicide behavior (Marttunen, Henriksson, Isometsae *et al.*, 1998).

Multiple co-occuring mental disorders are common among children and adolescents presenting with suicidal behaviors and those who have died by suicide. There is evidence to suggest that a greater number of diagnoses is associated with worse psychosocial outcomes generally, and more specifically risk of DSH (Beautrais, Joyce, Mulder *et al.*, 1996b; Fergusson & Lynskey, 1996; Miller & Taylor, 2005; Sansone, Gaither, Songer *et al.*, 2005) and suicide (Brent, Baugher, Bridge *et al.*, 1999; Reith, Whyte, Carter *et al.*, 2004).

Mood Disorders

Depression is the most prevalent mental health disorder reported in psychological autopsy studies (Brent, Baugher, Bridge *et al.*, 1999; Houston, Hawton, & Sheppard, 2001; Portzky, Audenaert, & van Heeringen, 2005; Shaffer, Gould, Fisher *et al.*, 1996) and non-fatal suicidal behaviors (Evans, Hawton, & Rodham, 2004). Hopelessness is an important mediating variable between depression and suicidal behavior (Thompson, Mazza, Herting *et al.*, 2005). There is also a link between suicide ideation and depression, with increasing severity of depression associated with increasing likelihood of suicide ideation (Allison, Roeger, Martin *et al.*, 2001). The course of depression across adolescence also appears to influence suicidality. In a longitudinal study of 193 children and adolescents, persistent depression was associated with significantly higher rates of suicidal ideation and suicide attempts. Depressed females were more likely to experience recurrent episodes, while males tended to experience persistent mental illness (Dunn & Goodyer, 2006).

Whereas most studies have concerned adolescents with an overt mood disorder, in a recent longitudinal study of 10- to 17-year-olds from a birth cohort, those presenting with subthreshold mood disorders (i.e., those with some symptoms but not meeting the criteria for a diagnosis) had an increased risk of later development of depression, anxiety, suicidal ideation and DSH. The risk, in terms of suicide ideation, associated with subthreshold depression was similar to that of major depressive disorder (Fergusson, Horwood, Ridder *et al.*, 2005).

Bipolar disorder has also been associated with elevated rates of suicide attempts, with the lifetime prevalence ranging from 20% (Strober, Schmidtlackner, Freeman *et al.*, 1995) to 44% (Lewinsohn, Seeley, & Klein, 2003). Case–control studies suggest that bipolar disorder in young people is associated with elevated risk of suicide (Brent, Perper, & Moritz, 1993).

Anxiety

Anxiety, particularly when comorbid with depression, has

been identified as increasing the risk of fatal and non-fatal acts, although this does not appear to be a direct association (Bridge, Goldstein, & Brent, 2006; Evans, Hawton, & Rodham, 2004). In a case–control study anxiety was more strongly associated with suicide attempts than suicide deaths (Beautrais, 2001). Panic attacks have been associated with increased risk of suicidal ideation and DSH (Gould, King, Greenwald *et al.*, 1998). Young adult females who reported multiple suicide attempts had higher rates of childhood anxiety disorders than ideators and those who had made a single suicide attempt (Rudd, Joiner, & Rumzek, 2004).

Substance Abuse

Substance abuse disorders, including cigarette smoking, are associated with increased risk of suicide attempts (Evans, Hawton, & Rodham, 2004) and suicide deaths (Beautrais, 2000). Several reviews (Esposito-Smythers & Spirito, 2004; Gould, King, Greenwald *et al.*, 1998; Gould, Greenberg, Velting *et al.*, 2003) have shown that substance abuse is more strongly correlated with suicide attempts than ideation and that the relationship is likely to be direct (Evans, Hawton, & Rodham, 2004). Suicide risk is highest among young men and older adolescents with substance abuse (Bridge, Goldstein, & Brent, 2006). Clinically, it can be difficult to establish if substance abuse precedes or follows the mental health difficulties and suicidal phenomena. Up to one-third of young people presenting to hospital following an episode of deliberate self-harm have consumed alcohol around the time of the act (Hawton, Hall, Simkin *et al.*, 2003), and alcohol abuse is associated with increased rates of repetition (Vajda & Steinbeck, 2000).

Psychosis

Approximately 5% of patients of all ages diagnosed with schizophrenia die by suicide, with young people and those early in the course of illness being most likely to kill themselves (Palmer, Pankratz, & Bostwick, 2005). However, psychotic disorders make a relatively small contribution to the overall youth suicide rate (Beautrais, 2000). Suicide risk is increased among young people with psychotic disorders where there were higher levels of premorbid functioning, better insight, higher intelligence and preservation of cognitive function (Apter & Freudenstein, 2000; Pompili, Mancinelli, Girardi *et al.*, 2004). A recent systematic review of risk factors for suicide among those with schizophrenia identified depression, previous suicide attempts, drug abuse, agitation, fear of mental disintegration, poor engagement with treatment and recent loss as important, whereas specific psychotic symptoms had less predictive value than the factors associated with general psychosocial functioning and affective disturbance (Hawton, Sutton, Haw *et al.*, 2005). Many adolescents with schizophrenia also abuse drugs and alcohol, thus exacerbating the risk for DSH and death by suicide (Apter & Freudenstein, 2000).

Conduct Disorder/Antisocial Behavior

Antisocial behavior is a risk factor for DSH among females although, perhaps surprisingly, the relationship is less clear for males (Evans, Hawton, & Rodham, 2004). Many of the risk factors for conduct disorder are also risk factors for DSH, including family disruption, childhood abuse, personal and familial substance abuse and negative life events (Apter & Freudenstein, 2000). There are higher than average rates of DSH (Coffey, Wolfe, Lovett *et al.*, 2004; Morgan & Hawton, 2004) and suicide among imprisoned youth (Coffey, Wolfe, Lovett *et al.*, 2004; Shaw, Baker, Hunt *et al.*, 2004). Antisocial behaviors are prominent among young men who die by suicide (Gould, Greenberg, Velting *et al.*, 2003; Marttunen, Aro, & Lonnqvist, 1993) and those with comorbid antisocial and substance abuse disorders (Bridge, Goldstein, & Brent, 2006).

Eating Disorders

Poor body image and disordered eating are associated with suicidal phenomena and some consider starvation to be a form of suicidal behavior that obviates the need for other methods of DSH. Suicide risk in anorexia nervosa has been estimated to be 2–15% and 0.4–2% for bulimia nervosa, with higher rates among adolescent males than females with eating disorders (Dancyger & Fornari, 2005).

Poor Physical Health Related to Psychological Problems

The relationship between physical illness and suicide in young people has received less attention than in adult populations. However, psychosomatic and physical presentations among suicidal children and adolescents are important for two reasons. First, although some adolescents with depression may present with similar symptoms to adults, they also commonly present with psychosomatic complaints such as headaches, loss of energy, chest pain, abdominal pain or other physical symptoms (McPherson, 2005). Second, poor physical health and many chronic illnesses are associated with increased risk for suicide ideation (Suris, Parera, & Puig, 1996) and DSH (Evans, Hawton, & Rodham, 2005a), independent of psychiatric disorder (Goodwin, Marusic, & Hoven, 2003; Vajda & Steinbeck, 2000).

Environmental Factors Including Biopsychosocial Stressors

Family Factors Including Parental Psychiatric Disorders, Violence, Abuse

Longitudinal community studies have shown that difficulties in parent–child relationships, including those related to early attachment problems, perceived low levels of parental caring and communication are related to increased risk of suicide and suicide attempts among children and adolescents (Ackard, Neumark-Sztainer, Story *et al.*, 2006; Fergusson & Lynskey, 1995b; Fergusson, Woodward, & Horwood, 2000); similar observations have been made in clinical samples (Lessard & Moretti, 1998; Pfeffer, 2000).

Several reviews have concluded that adolescents from families that have experienced parental separation or divorce are at increased risk of suicide behavior, particularly among females (e.g., Beautrais, 2000; Brent, Perper, Moritz *et al.*, 1994a; Gould, Fisher, Parides *et al.*, 1996). It seems that conflict between parents, both before and after their relationship ends, has a detrimental impact on children.

Family History of Suicide Behavior

Research consistently indicates that a family history of suicidal behavior is associated with increased risk for suicide deaths (Agerbo, Nordentoft, & Mortensen, 2002; Brent, Perper, Moritz *et al.*, 1994a; Brent, Perper, Goldstein *et al.*, 1988; Gould, Fisher, Parides *et al.*, 1996) and non-fatal DSH behavior by adolescents (Hawton, Rodham, Evans *et al.*, 2002a; Johnson, Brent, Bridge *et al.*, 1998; Roy, Rylander, & Sarchiapone, 1997). Similarly, exposure to fatal and non-fatal suicidal behavior in the family increases suicidal ideation in adolescents (Cerel & Roberts, 2005) and has been associated with more violent suicide attempts (Bridge, Goldstein, & Brent, 2006; Roy, Rylander, & Sarchiapone, 1997).

Having a suicidal family member may model to adolescents that suicide is a possible solution to overwhelming psychological pain (Roy, Rylander, & Sarchiapone, 1997), although the detrimental effects of living with a parent who has undiagnosed or undertreated mental health problems are also significant (Agerbo, Nordentoft, & Mortensen, 2002). More work is required to clarify the extent to which suicidal behavior can be considered as a construct that is transmitted through families independently of the established association with familial risk of depression, impulsivity and other psychopathology (Brent & Mann, 2005).

Parental Mental Health Disorders

Parental mental health disorders are associated with increased risk of their children dying by suicide, particularly parental depression and substance abuse (Brent, Perper, Moritz *et al.*, 1994a). Several authors have found an association between poor parental mental health and both suicide ideation and non-fatal suicide behavior (Fergusson & Lynskey, 1995a; Meltzer, Harrington, Goodman *et al.*, 2001; Sourander, Aromaa, Pihlakoski *et al.*, 2006).

Childhood Physical and Sexual Abuse

A strong and direct association exists between suicide attempts and both childhood sexual abuse and physical abuse (Beautrais, 2000; Evans, Hawton, & Rodham, 2005a). Parental history of childhood sexual abuse is also associated with an increased risk of suicide attempts among offspring (Brent, Oquendo, Birmaher *et al.*, 2002). Bullying is associated with poor mental health, suicide ideation and attempts (Coggan, Bennett, Hooper *et al.*, 2003; Kaltiala-Heino, Rimpela, Marttunen *et al.*, 1999; Sourander, Aromaa, Pihlakoski *et al.*, 2006). There has been recent concern about suicides by young people allegedly bullied by peers using mobile telephones and via the Internet (Smith, 2004).

Peers, Including the Influence of Peer Suicidal Behaviors and Suicide Clusters

The importance of peer relationships and suicidal behaviors among groups of friends is becoming increasingly apparent. Having a friend who attempted suicide in the previous year increased rates of suicide ideation and attempts among both girls and boys (Evans, Hawton, & Rodham, 2004). The relative risk of suicide among those exposed to an index suicide has been shown to be 2–4 times higher in 15- to 19-year-olds, with contagion less salient among those aged over 25 years (Gould, Greenberg, Velting *et al.*, 2003). In a large study in the USA, socially isolated girls were more likely to experience suicide ideation and both boys and girls with dense social networks were less likely to attempt suicide (Bearman & Moody, 2004).

Clusters of suicidal acts in adolescents sometimes occur, particularly in institutional settings such as schools and inpatient psychiatric units. This may reflect modeling of the behavior and exposure to similar stressors (Gould, Wallenstein, & Davidson, 1989). Suicide clusters are relatively unusual and account for only 5% of all youth suicides. Subsequent suicide behavior is more likely among young people who were already experiencing mental health difficulties (Beautrais, 2000).

Sexual Orientation

Gay, lesbian and bisexual young people are at increased risk of engaging in DSH (Remafedi, French, Story *et al.*, 1998; Russell & Joyner, 2001), with estimates of risk ranging 2–6 times that of heterosexual young people (Gould, Greenberg, Velting *et al.*, 2003). In one of the relatively few studies in this area, 59% of males in New York who had made a suicide attempt reported it was related to their sexual orientation and 38% of females who had made an attempt attributed this to issues relating to their sexuality (D'Augeli, Grossman, Salter *et al.*, 2005). No study has yet documented increased rates of death by suicide related to sexual orientation (Gould, Greenberg, Velting *et al.*, 2003). However, gay, lesbian and bisexual youth are more likely to experience risk factors associated with suicide (Shaffer & Pfeffer, 2001), particularly mental health difficulties (Fergusson, Horwood, & Beautrais, 1999).

School

Several reviews of studies of young suicide attempters (Beautrais, Joyce, & Mulder, 1996a; Evans, Hawton, & Rodham, 2004) and those who die by suicide (Gould, Fisher, Parides *et al.*, 1996) have indicated that more have had school-based difficulties and/or have dropped out of school than have non-suicidal adolescents. Dropping out of school has been shown to be a risk factor for medically serious suicide attempts, in addition to the socio-economic disadvantages that are associated with having few educational qualifications (Donald, Dower, Correa-Velez *et al.*, 2006). Children and adolescents who remain in school but have special educational needs appear to have higher rates of suicidal phenomena than their peers without such needs (Denny, Clark, & Watson, 2003; Meltzer, Harrington, Goodman *et al.*, 2001).

Proximal Risk Factors/Life Stressors

Both psychological autopsy (Marttunen, Aro, & Lonnqvist, 1993) and case–controlled studies (Beautrais, 2000) suggest that, compared with controls, young people who die by suicide experience higher rates of exposure to recent stressful life events such as rejection, conflict or loss following the break-up of a relationship (Brent, Moritz, & Liotus, 1996d; Donald, Dower, Correa-Velez *et al.*, 2006), disciplinary or legal crises (Marttunen, Henriksson, Isometsae *et al.*, 1998). Life stressors are also associated with DSH (Hawton, Hall, Simkin *et al.*, 2003). The nature of the stressors seems to vary according to age. For example, children and younger adolescents describe familial stress, whereas older adolescents typically describe peer-related stressors (Gould, Greenberg, Velting *et al.*, 2003; Hawton, Hall, Simkin *et al.*, 2003). Becoming intoxicated is a short-term solution that many adolescents engage in following crises. Intoxication leads to impaired judgment and decreased inhibition, and can facilitate suicidal behavior (Apter & Freudenstein, 2000).

Refugees and asylum seekers face particular psychosocial stressors that are likely to have an impact on young people and their families. Unemployment, social isolation and the difficulties involved in applying for asylum experienced by parents are factors that, together with the high rates of depression, anxiety and post-traumatic stress disorder (PTSD) in this population, may lead to suicidal behavior (Fazel, Wheeler, & Danesh, 2005; Keller, Rosenfeld, Trinh-Shevrin *et al.*, 2003; Sultan & O'Sullivan, 2001).

Exposure to Suicide in the Media, Music and the Internet

The accumulated evidence suggests that certain types of media reports and portrayals of suicide and attempted suicide can increase the risk of suicidal behavior (for reviews see Hawton & Williams, 2005; Pirkis & Blood, 2001; Pirkis, Francis, Blood *et al.*, 2002; Schmidtke & Schaller, 2000). The greatest influence is probably on methods used for suicide and deliberate self-harm and seems to be particularly marked in young people (Phillips & Carstensen, 1988; Stack, 1991). It appears that such effects are more likely where media reporting or portrayal is dramatic, features details of a specific method of suicide, is on television and is repeated (Pirkis & Blood, 2001; Pirkis, Burgess, Francis *et al.*, 2006b; Stack, 2003).

Many children appear to learn about suicide from television (Mishara, 1999; Pirkis & Blood, 2001). Some people may respond quickly to media presentations of suicide, acting impulsively or putting previous thoughts about suicide into action, while others may make a more considered response (Schmidtke & Häfner, 1988). Thus, in addition to potential immediate changes in suicidal behavior, media influences may also have longer-term effects, by changing attitudes, providing information about methods of suicidal behavior or planting the idea that suicide is an appropriate response to problems.

While concern has been raised about the possible influence of music (especially certain types of popular music) on suicidal phenomena among children and adolescents, this has received very limited attention in the research literature (Martin, Clarke, & Pearce, 1993).

Recently, concern has been raised about Internet sites dealing with suicide and their potential negative influence on adolescent suicidal behavior (Gould, Munfakh, Lubell *et al.*, 2002). The provision of interactive experiences and the development of "online communities" mean that the Internet may have a unique role in influencing suicidal behavior and/or providing peer support and possibly helping prevent suicidal behavior. It is not known if technology-based communication has implications for the consideration of contagion in young people, or what role cyber-bullying (i.e., bullying via Internet, email and text messaging) is a stressor among young people who engage in suicide behaviors.

Few studies have been conducted in this area. In a large community study, depressed young people, especially boys, were heavier users of the Internet, more likely to access the Internet at school and more likely to use chat-rooms and interact with peers they saw infrequently in person, and also strangers (Ybarra, Alexander, & Mitchell, 2005). A study of online postings to message boards focusing on self-injurious behavior by young people aged 12–20 years suggested that online interactions provide important social support to users, but that these interactions may also normalize or encourage self-injurious behavior (Whitlock, Powers, & Eckenrode, 2006). The Internet may also provide opportunities for suicide prevention. For example, 6 months after a school-based presentation promoting the use of a website for young people experiencing emotional difficulties, 45% of students said they had visited the website (Nicholas, Oliver, Lee *et al.*, 2004).

Availability of Means for DSH/Suicide

The preferred method of DSH has an impact on suicide rates, given that some methods are potentially more lethal than others. In the UK, self-laceration and overdose are the most commonly used methods of DSH among children and adolescents (Hawton, Rodham, & Evans, 2006). Children and adolescents who die by suicide in the UK are most likely to have used hanging, self-poisoning, carbon monoxide poisoning or drowning (Hawton, Houston, & Sheppard, 1999a).

Deaths involving a certain method may increase or decrease depending on the availability of that method (Grossman & Kruesi, 2000; Hawton, 2005). For example, in the USA firearms are the most common method of suicide (Stack & Wasserman, 2005), but account for a relatively small number of deaths in the UK, New Zealand and Australia. The substitution of one method for another relies on both the acceptability and availability of alternative methods. For example, a decrease in the use of firearms and self-poisoning among young people in the USA was accompanied by an increase in deaths by suffocation, mostly hanging (Centers for Disease Control, 2004). Rates of hanging have also increased among young people of both genders in the UK (Gunnell, Bennewith, Hawton *et al.*, 2005). The increasing rate of hanging suggests that this has become an increasingly acceptable method of suicide (Centers for Disease Control, 2004). Hanging is also extremely accessible as well as having a high rate of lethality. The reasons for the spread in acceptability of hanging and the increased use of this method among young females as a method of suicide are not known.

The ready availability of pesticides in agrarian communities such as in China and Sri Lanka is associated with the use of these for self-poisoning. Because of their high lethality, suicide rates in young people are relatively high compared with those in developed countries (Eddleston, Gunnell, Karunaratne *et al.*, 2005b).

Protective Factors

Compared with the volume of research on risk factors, relatively little work has been conducted on factors that protect against the development of suicide behavior in adolescents. The concepts of adversity and resilience are dealt with in chapters 25 and 26. In summary, factors that protect against mental illness associated with suicidal phenomena include good social skills, problem-solving abilities and an internal locus of control (Merry, McDowell, Hetrick *et al.*, 2002). Factors thought to protect against the risk of suicide include enjoyment and involvement with school (Dexheimer Pharris, Resnick, & Blum, 1997), playing sports (Tomori & Zalar, 2000), family cohesiveness (Rubenstein, Halton, Kasten *et al.*, 1998), religious affiliation and a commitment to life-affirming beliefs (Neeleman, Halpern, Leon *et al.*, 1997; Stack, 2000).

Impact of Suicide on Peers, School and Relatives

Suicide by a peer has a significant impact on their friends, family, school and community. In a series of studies on peers of children and adolescents who died by suicide, Brent, Perper, Moritz *et al.* (1994b) found worsening of depression among those who were already depressed at the time of their peer's death and elevated overall rates of depression (Brent, Perper, Moritz *et al.*, 1992), anxiety and PTSD, particularly in the first 6 months after the death (Brent, Moritz, Bridge *et al.*, 1996b).

The siblings and parents of adolescents who died by suicide showed elevated levels of grief over a prolonged period of time, with an increased risk of recurrence of maternal depression (Brent, Moritz, Bridge *et al.*, 1996a). Traumatic grief reactions, distinct from depression or PTSD, have also been identified in friends (Melhem, Day, Shear *et al.*, 2004a,b).

A small group of adolescents who have lost a peer by suicide may witness the effects of the suicide on the community and "may find themselves wishing that they too could create the same effects" (Rivers, 1995, p. 15). This issue is a particular challenge for postvention among school peers. However, as noted earlier, clusters of suicides do occur in adolescents, they are relatively unusual (Beautrais, 2000).

There has been little research into the effects of DSH on parents. In the USA, Wagner, Aiken, Mullaley *et al.* (2000) showed that parental reactions to suicidal behavior may include anger, fear, sadness and frustration. Parents may be intimidated by the intensity of the suicidal behavior. They may adopt greater restrictiveness in their parenting style, or alternatively retreat to a position of minimal limit setting or try to transfer responsibility for their child to someone else (Hazell, 2000). How parents react to DSH may be influenced by factors such as the nature of the previous relationship with their son or daughter, the degree of suicidal intent involved in the act and whether the DSH act was a first episode or a repeat (Wagner, Aiken, Mullaley *et al.*, 2000). The types of motives attributed to the act by parents, including whether the parents interpret the DSH as an act of manipulation, a sign of distress or a definite attempt to die, may also be important (James & Hawton, 1985).

Outcome Following DSH

Single Episode of DSH Compared With Those Who Repeat

Some young people who harm themselves do so on only one occasion, whereas others repeat the behavior. Conceptually, the first act of self-harm is different from all those that follow it, and each act falls somewhere on the spectrum of suicidality in so far as many acts of self-harm have death as a possible outcome (either psychologically or medically). A history of previous suicidal behavior increases the risk of future attempts in both clinical and general populations (Evans, Hawton, & Rodham, 2004; Gould, Greenberg, Velting *et al.*, 2003). The greatest risk of repetition is in the first year following DSH.

The estimates of risk of repetition are 5–15% per year (Bridge, Goldstein, & Brent, 2006), although this may be much higher where repetition that does not come to clinical attention is considered (Hawton, Rodham, & Evans, 2006). The risk of repetition remains high for many years after an episode of DSH. For example, in a 10-year follow-up, Gibb, Beautrais, and Fergusson (2005) reported that 28% of those admitted for a suicide attempt had been readmitted, with the highest risk in the first 2 years. In a study of 450 adolescents who had taken overdoses, 12% re-presented to hospital with further overdoses within 5 years. Repetition is associated with substance abuse, psychotic illness and personality disorder (Reith, Whyte, & Carter, 2003). There are mixed findings on whether repetition rates are higher in one gender or the other (Gibb, Beautrais, & Fergusson, 2005; Goldacre & Hawton, 1985).

Once an adolescent has actually engaged in DSH they cross a behavioral threshold. Repeat DSH may be more likely if the act resulted in the adolescent receiving relief from undesirable affect or if an earlier attempt prompted a desirable change in their lives as a result of the responses of others. These factors plus further exposure to stressful life events and problems combine to place them at increased risk for engaging in DSH when facing similar situations; following the initial episode DSH becomes an additional tool in their behavioral repertoire where it did not exist previously (Goldston, Sergent Daniel, Reboussin *et al.*, 1999). Depression is a key factor associated with repetition of DSH in adolescents (Hawton, Kingsbury, Steinhardt *et al.*, 1999b).

Similarly, self-reported DSH at age 12 years predicts suicidal ideation and DSH at 15 years (Sourander, Aromaa, Pihlakoski *et al.*, 2006). A recent study by Harrington, Pickles, Aglan *et al.* (2006) showed that in most cases deliberate self-harm by adolescents ceased within 3 years. However, those who continued to self-harm into adulthood were characterized by higher rates of psychopathology and adversity in both childhood and adulthood; and, in another study, by anxiety, at least for females (Rudd, Joiner, & Rumzek, 2004).

Emergence of Personality Disorders

To date there has been little research on the prevalence and morbidity associated with personality disorders among adolescents. Borderline personality disorder (BPD) has long been associated with non-fatal DSH among adults, and some argue it takes a similar form in adolescents as seen with adults (Bradley, Conklin, & Westen, 2005). The use of this diagnosis in those under the age of 18 years is somewhat contentious (Vito, Ladame, & Orlandini, 1999).

Worthlessness, guilt, hopelessness and anger are associated with both BPD and suicide (Apter & Freudenstein, 2000; Brodsky, Malone, Ellis *et al.*, 1997) and may place young people at risk of poor psychosocial outcomes. In a community-based longitudinal study, adolescents with personality disorders had significantly higher rates of major psychiatric disorder and suicidal ideation in early adulthood, after controlling for comorbid mental disorders and suicidality during adolescence (Johnson, Cohen, Skodol *et al.*, 1999). Rudd, Joiner, & Rumzek (2004) suggested that the frequency and chronicity of suicide attempts in adulthood are related to childhood anxiety disorders through the emergence of personality psychopathology, with different patterns for males and females. The authors highlighted histrionic and paranoid traits in females and schizoid, avoidant, dependent, aggressive and borderline traits in males.

Suicide Following DSH: Risk and Timing

A history of past suicide attempts is one of the most powerful and clinically relevant predictors of eventual suicide. Most studies find elevated risk of overall mortality following DSH (Carter, Reith, Whyte *et al.*, 2005; Gibb, Beautrais, & Fergusson, 2005; Goldacre & Hawton, 1985; Suominen, Isometsa, Suokas *et al.*, 2004). In one follow-up study of 15- to 24-year-olds who had presented to hospital following an episode of DSH, the overall number of deaths from all causes was 3%, four times higher than expected. This was mainly because of an excess number of suicides (2%), which were 10 times more frequent than expected. The main risk factors for suicide were male gender, previous DSH, prior psychiatric history and high suicide intent (Hawton & Harriss, 2007).

Clinical Assessment

Clinicians should conduct risk assessments when young people express suicidal thoughts or behaviors. Both the purpose and the process of such assessments need to be given careful consideration. A significant issue is establishing the purpose of the assessment, particularly suicide prediction compared with risk assessment (Bryan & Rudd, 2006). It is extremely difficult for clinicians to predict accurately the risk of their patient dying by suicide or of engaging in non-fatal suicidal behavior. An assessment should form the basis of future clinical management and establishing treatment goals. In adults, having a psychosocial assessment has been associated with reduced rates of repetition (Kapur, House, Dodgson *et al.*, 2002). The fact that many adolescents spend very little, if any, time planning their deliberate self-harm (Rodham, Hawton, & Evans, 2004), and that being intoxicated is often associated with many such acts, compounds this issue (Esposito-Smythers & Spirito, 2004). A core task of a risk assessment is to establish an interactive and dynamic relationship; to be part of a response to the young person's distress that offers some hope for a better future.

Assessment following DSH

Improved assessment and management of deliberate self-harm are highlighted in a number of published guidelines (American Academy of Child and Adolescent Psychiatry, 1999; National Institute for Clinical Excellence, 2004; Royal Australian and New Zealand College of Psychiatrists, 2004). The assessment of children and adolescents following DSH is influenced by a range of process and service issues. At a process level, the assessment of adolescents can present particular challenges, as young people are often ambivalent about their suicidality and fluctuating mood states can make it difficult to get clear information, particularly retrospectively. Current guidelines emphasize standards of care and note that several studies have suggested that some staff responsible for medical care have, or are perceived by DSH patients as having, negative attitudes towards those who deliberately harm themselves (Herron, Tichehurst, Appleby *et al.*, 2001; Hopkins, 2002) and may not recognize the complex relationships between DSH and mental illness (Friedman, Newton, Coggan *et al.*, 2006). Poor continuity of care requiring frequent repetition of their "story" (Dower, Donald, Kelly *et al.*, 2000) and negative expectations about post-discharge therapy (Rotheram-Borus, Piacentini, Van Rossem *et al.*, 1996) contribute to dissatisfaction among some adolescents who have self-harmed. In a study of adolescent DSH patients, those who were more satisfied with hospital management and subsequent therapy appeared to have better therapeutic outcomes (Burgess, Hawton, & Loveday, 1998).

Screening and Case Identification Procedures

Some schools have tried to detect young people at high risk of suicide through screening programs. Case-finding strategies have been employed in schools in an effort to reduce suicide by early detection of young people at high risk. This approach has particularly been pursued in the USA (Gould, Greenberg, Velting *et al.*, 2003). Although these methods are increasingly sensitive to detecting young people with problems, engagement in treatment following identification remains a significant issue (Shaffer & Craft, 1999; Shaffer & Pfeffer, 2001; Shaffer, Scott, Wilcox *et al.*, 2004). Data from the Colombia Teen Screen program indicates that 19% of "at risk" young people refused a referral, 25% did not attend the first appointment and 17% attended one session only (Shaffer, 2003).

There are also difficulties with some schools accepting this approach for various reasons, including lack of staff resources and concerns that asking students about suicide will give them ideas about harming themselves. However, in a recent randomized controlled trial, depressed adolescents and previous attempters reported lower levels of distress and suicidality following a screening questionnaire that included specific questions about suicidal behaviors compared with their counterparts who were not asked those questions. This study also demonstrated that asking about suicide does not "put the idea into a young person's head" for those who would not ordinarily be thinking about this issue (Gould, Marrocco, Kleinman *et al.*, 2005).

Treatment Following DSH

A range of treatment studies have been conducted with adults following DSH, but few interventions with children and adolescents who have harmed themselves have been evaluated.

Cognitive–Behavior Therapy and Problem-Solving

Cognitive–behavior therapy (CBT) is the principal treatment for adolescent depression and affective disorders (Harrington, Whittaker, & Shoebridge, 1998; Merry, McDowell, Hetrick *et al.*, 2002) and targets depressive thoughts and behavior patterns (see chapter 63). In a large randomized controlled trial, 439 patients aged 12–17 years with major depressive disorder (MDD) were randomly allocated to one of four treatment conditions, each lasting 12 weeks:

1 Fluoxetine alone;
2 CBT alone;
3 CBT with fluoxetine; or
4 Placebo.

The CBT treatment consisted of 15 1-hour sessions. Patients treated in all conditions showed a reduction in suicide ideation across the trial, those treated with CBT plus fluoxetine showing the greatest improvement (Treatment of Adolescent Depression Study Team, 2004).

Problem-solving therapy, in which patients are assisted to identify problems and enhance their strategies for addressing them, has been noted in three recent systematic reviews of treatments for DSH to offer a promising area for further investigation (Gaynes, West, Ford *et al.*, 2004; Hawton, Townsend, Arensman *et al.*, 2000; Townsend, Hawton, Altman *et al.*, 2001). However, there have been no evaluations of problem-solving therapy with younger patients.

Family Therapy

Family therapy is a mechanism of intervening with suicide behavior among adolescents, given that family issues are implicated in the etiology of suicide behavior (Spirito & Boergers, 1997). Family therapy focuses on the relationships, roles and communication patterns between family members (see chapter 65). In a treatment study of depressed adolescents who were randomly allocated to CBT, systemic behavioral family therapy (SBFT) or non-directive supportive therapy (NST), those who were currently or previously suicidal were more depressed at the start of therapy and were significantly less likely to complete it. In addition, NST did not appear to ameliorate the MDD of these adolescents (Barbe, Bridge, Birmaher *et al.*, 2004).

Rotheram-Borus, Piacentini, Miller *et al.* (1994) developed brief CBT in a family context. Kerfoot, Harrington, and Dyer (1995) implemented a brief structured home-based intervention with suicidal adolescents and their families. Non-depressed adolescents in the home-based group had less suicidal ideation than controls, but the home-based intervention was no more effective for depressed adolescents (Harrington, Kerfoot, Dyer *et al.*, 2000).

Group Therapy

Group therapy approaches are often used in child and adolescent mental health services, although there are few well-designed studies of this approach with suicidal adolescents. Wood, Trainor, Rothwell *et al.* (2001) randomly assigned 63 adolescents with a history of repeated self-harm to group therapy plus treatment as usual (TAU) or TAU only. Although there was no apparent effect on depression, group attendees were less likely to repeat DSH, used fewer routine services and had better school attendance than those who received TAU.

Dialectical Behavior Therapy

Dialectical behavior therapy (DBT) is a therapeutic approach that focuses on the management of emotional states and interpersonal relationships. DBT has been researched as a psychotherapeutic intervention with suicidal adults (Linehan, Rizvi, Welch *et al.*, 2000) and is being investigated with adolescents (Rathus & Miller, 2002).

Multisystemic Therapy

Multisystemic therapy (MST) was developed to treat delinquent youth, targeting the systems in which the young people live. MST includes parenting skills, family therapy and educational attainment. In a randomized controlled trial, young people aged 10–17 years were assigned to MST or hospitalization following a psychiatric emergency. MST was significantly more effective in reducing youth-reported repetition of suicide attempts (Huey, Henggeler, Rowland *et al.*, 2004).

Medication

There has been considerable recent debate about the use of antidepressant medications in the treatment of children and adolescents with depression, with a specific focus on whether selective serotonin reuptake inhibitors (SSRIs) increase the risk of suicidal behaviors in some young people (for summary see Ryan, 2005; see also chapters 37 and 67). A recent meta-analysis indicates a modest increased risk of suicidality among those prescribed antidepressant medication (Hammad, Laughren, & Racoosin, 2006). This may be related to the agitation that can occur shortly after starting the drug. In contrast, some researchers have suggested that increased prescribing of SSRIs has resulted in decreased suicide rates (Gibbons, Hur, Bhaumik *et al.*, 2006; Olfson, Shaffer, Marcus *et al.*, 2003). Conversely, based on data from both published and unpublished randomized controlled trials, the British Medicines and Healthcare Products Regulatory Agency has stated that sertraline, citalopram, paroxetine and venlafaxine are contraindicated in those under 18 years with MDD (Medicines and Healthcare Products Regulatory Agency, 2004). These medications are required to carry a "black box" warning label in the USA (US Food and Drug Administration, 2004). Also, fluoxetine for treating depression in adolescents is supported by the European Medicines Agency only where psychological interventions alone have failed (Eaton, 2006). The Society for Adolescent Medicine recommended the prudent use of antidepressant medication for adolescents, under close clinical supervision and as part of an overall therapeutic approach (Lock, Walker, Rickert *et al.*, 2005; see also chapter 37).

Hospitalization

The decision to treat adolescents following DSH in an in-patient setting is usually based on risk of further self-harm and suicide, and severity of psychiatric disorder (Olfson, Gameroff, Marcus *et al.*, 2005). It may also be influenced by other factors including concerns about litigation, characteristics of the individual and their family (Spooren, Jannes, & van Heeringen, 1997), the experience and training of the mental health clinician (Morrissey, Dicker, Abikoff *et al.*, 1995) and the availability of in-patient beds.

However, there is no evidence to suggest that hospitalization prevents young people, particularly those with prior attempts, mood disorder and substance abuse, from making another attempt or dying by suicide (Gould, Greenberg, Velting *et al.*, 2003; Greenhill & Waslick, 1997). Furthermore, prior hospitalization for any injury, not just DSH, is associated with increased risk of suicidal behaviors (Agerbo, Nordentoft, & Mortensen, 2002; Bridge, Goldstein, & Brent, 2006), although this may be related to severity of psychopathology and other risk factors.

Two recent studies have attempted to address these issues. In the first, conducted in the USA, 289 adolescents were randomly allocated to receive social network intervention plus TAU, or TAU alone, following psychiatric hospitalization. There was a reduction in suicidal ideation and parent-reported functional impairment at 6 months follow-up in those assigned to social network intervention, but no effects on repetition of DSH or emotional symptoms (King, Kramer, Preuss *et al.*, 2006). In the second study, 286 adolescents were assigned to rapid response out-patient follow-up or TAU following presentation to an emergency department in Canada. The results showed psychiatric hospitalizations can be prevented using the rapid response model of care (Greenfield, Larson, Hechtman *et al.*, 2002).

Issues of Access to Treatment and Engagement in Treatment

Whereas many adolescents may be offered care following an episode of DSH, only a small proportion are successfully engaged in ongoing treatment. Treatment retention for non-hospitalized adolescents is generally below 50% (Brent, 1997; Swedo, 1989; van Heeringen, Jannes, Buylaert *et al.*, 1995), and can be as low as 20%, with significant and rapid drop-out from treatment (King, Hovey, Brand *et al.*, 1997).

Several studies have investigated mechanisms to improve engagement with treatment, including green-card passes (Cotgrove, Zirinsky, Black *et al.*, 1995), enhanced emergency department protocols (Rotheram-Borus, Piacentini, Cantwell *et al.*, 2000; Spirito, Boergers, Donaldson *et al.*, 2002), enhanced CBT interventions (Rotheram-Borus, Piacentini, Miller *et al.*, 1994) and skills-based interventions (Donaldson, Spirito, & Esposito-Smythers, 2005). However, to date such efforts have largely been unsuccessful and new strategies must be developed to address this important issue (Burns, Dudley, Hazell *et al.*, 2005).

Many young people who engage in DSH do not seek help for their problems. If they do, it is most likely to be from friends and family rather than professionals (De Leo & Heller, 2004; Hawton, Rodham, & Evans, 2006). There are also gender differences, with distressed young men being less likely to seek help of any kind and those who seek help from their GP showing more severe symptoms than their female counterparts when they do (Biddle, Gunnell, Sharp *et al.*, 2004). High school students at highest risk of suicide were found to be more likely to endorse isolative coping strategies such as believing you should be able to sort out your problems on your own and less likely to endorse strategies such as getting advice from friends (Gould, Velting, Kleinman *et al.*, 2004).

Prevention of DSH and Suicide by Children and Adolescents

Suicide prevention strategies include both specific interventions for individuals at risk and population-level interventions aimed at reducing overall risk in the general population. Specific interventions include, for example, treatment and care of suicidal children or adolescents to help families and communities where a suicide death has occurred to cope with the aftermath (Leenaars & Wenckstern, 1999). Given the complicated nature of the lives of many people who engage in suicidal behavior, no single strategy is likely to provide all the answers (Centers for Disease Control and Prevention, 1992; Evans, 2000).

School-based Interventions

Prevention programs that are aimed at students as helpers, not as victims, are based on evidence that adolescents turn to their peers for support rather than discussing their problems with adults (Beautrais, Joyce, & Mulder, 1998; Hawton, Rodham, & Evans, 2006; Hazell & King, 1996). This approach often raises concerns that not all peer confidants communicate with adults about friends whose problems cause them particular concern (Bennett, Coggan, Lee *et al.*, 2003) and that young men in particular do not respond to troubled peers in helping ways (Hazell & King, 1996; Kalafat, Elias, & Gara, 1993). Skills-based programs in schools, targeting the development of problem-solving, coping and cognitive skills appear to have a positive impact on suicide behavior and coping with distress (Gould, Greenberg, Velting *et al.*, 2003). A school-based intervention in the USA called Signs of Suicide showed fewer suicide attempts in the intervention group compared with controls, and a modest improvement in knowledge and attitudes about depression and suicide. However, no improvement in help-seeking was observed (Aseltine & DeMartino, 2004). A randomized controlled trial of a school-based depression prevention program also showed positive results (Merry, McDowell, Wild *et al.*, 2004).

Reviews of older school-based programs (Garland, Shaffer, & Whittle, 1989) and their effect on suicidal adolescents (Shaffer, Vieland, Garland *et al.*, 1990) raised serious concerns about these programs, in particular the message that suicide is a reaction to stressful life events that could happen to anyone and the minimization of the importance of mental illness, and gave rise to the establishment of the Columbia Teen Screen program. One obvious difficulty with any school-based program is the fact that high-risk individuals, particularly school drop-outs and those with high rates of absenteeism, will not be reached using this approach (Burns & Patton, 2000).

Reducing Access to Methods of Suicide

The strategy of restricting access by the general population to certain methods of suicide is a widely practized public health initiative and an effective method of preventing suicide. Research suggests that restricting access to particular methods reduces deaths by that method. Most studies show a reduction in overall suicide deaths, while others do not because of substitution of method (for a review see Mann, Apter, Bertolote *et al.*, 2005). Methods of suicide used by young people vary significantly across different countries. Restricting access to firearms has been a significant focus of suicide prevention in North America because of the high number of deaths resulting from firearms (Brent, Perper, Goldstein *et al.*, 1988; Brent, Baugher, Bridge *et al.*, 1999; Gould, Greenberg, Velting *et al.*, 2003). The number of firearms suicides in the UK is small so this does not form a major thrust of suicide prevention (Haw, Sutton, Simkin *et al.*, 2004).

Much suicidal behavior in young people involves intentional overdoses (Bennett, Coggan, Hooper *et al.*, 2002; Hawton, Fagg, Simkin *et al.*, 2000). Preventative approaches include safety packaging, limiting tablet quantity for high-risk drugs such as tricyclic antidepressants, education of practitioners regarding safer practices, disposal of out-of-date and unwanted drugs and limiting advertising (Cantor & Neulinger, 2000; Commonwealth Department of Health and Aged Care, 1999). Acetaminophen (paracetamol) is a drug widely used for self-poisoning among young people in several western countries (Bennett, Coggan, Hooper *et al.*, 2002; Hawton, Fagg, Simkin *et al.*, 2000). Legislation was introduced in the UK in 1998 reducing pack sizes and the number of packs that can be purchased at one time. This was followed by a decrease in the rates of deaths, liver transplants and the average number of tablets ingested in overdose (Hawton, Simkin, Deeks *et al.*, 2004).

Hanging is an increasingly popular method of suicide and attempted suicide in several countries but it is difficult to reduce access to the means of hanging, except in institutional settings such as psychiatric in-patient units and prisons. Carbon monoxide poisoning from car exhaust gases was a common method of suicide. However, the introduction of catalytic converters in cars has had a significant impact in reducing deaths by this method (Amos, Appleby, & Kiernan, 2001).

Crisis Centers and Hot Lines

Crisis centers and hot lines offering direct counseling or links to mental health services are conceptually popular. Overall, research suggests that such services tend to be used by young White females, with less impact on young men (de Anda & Smith, 1993). Beautrais, Joyce, & Mulder, (1998) reported that 14% of serious suicide attempters had used a telephone crisis line in the year prior to their attempt. There is little evidence of beneficial effects on rates of suicide (Burns & Paton, 2000), although this would be difficult to demonstrate.

Guidelines on Media Reporting of Suicides

Media coverage of suicide has been shown to encourage imitative suicides (Gould, 2001; Hawton & Williams, 2005; Pirkis & Blood, 2001). It appears that in the short term, media reporting can lead to an increase in suicidal behavior and in the long term it may model suicide as common and acceptable. Many countries now have voluntary guidelines for media reporting (Pirkis, Blood, Beautrais *et al.*, 2006a). Compliance with guidelines is variable although guidelines leading to reduced reporting of specific types of suicide have been associated with reduced rates of suicide by these methods in

Austria (Etzersdorfer, Sonneck, & Nagel-Kuess, 1992) and Canada (Littmann, 1983).

Conclusions, Future Clinical and Research Directions

Suicidal behavior exists on a continuum. Nearly 1 in 6 adolescents have considered self-harm or suicide in the previous year and 1 in 10 have harmed themselves in the previous year (Evans, Hawton, Rodham *et al.*, 2005b). Death by suicide is relatively infrequent in adolescents. However, in most countries, more males than females die by suicide, although this may not be the case in India and China. In contrast, more females engage in non-fatal suicidal behavior. These differences are thought to reflect differences in the methods of deliberate self-harm utilized by males and females, although there is evidence that more violent methods, especially hanging, may be increasing in females.

Acts of DSH are associated with a variety of motives or intentions. Wanting relief from unbearable feelings or situations, to die and to communicate distress are commonly endorsed motives in both hospital and community samples. Establishing the intent or motives associated with an episode of DSH by adolescents can be difficult. Using the method of DSH as a proxy for intent can be misleading; self-cutting and other methods of self-mutilation do not always involve suicidal intent, but some studies have found that young people who engage in cutting behaviors are at high risk of poor psychosocial outcomes and death by suicide. Community-based studies of adolescents indicate that cutting is the most frequently used method of DSH, whereas adolescents presenting to hospitals are most likely to have taken an overdose. Few differences exist, including in psychiatric symptomatology, between those who engage in self-harm by various methods.

It is now clear that depression, sexual and physical abuse, substance abuse, hopelessness, family breakdown, poor coping, and suicidal behavior by family and friends and in the media increase the risk of suicidal phenomena among children and adolescents. Impulsivity and aggression are vulnerability factors that require further investigation. The role of emergent media forms such as cell phones and the Internet in suicide prevention and contagion is also an area in which one can expect research in the next few years. Relatively little research work has been conducted on factors that protect against the development of suicide behavior. Relevant factors appear to be social connectedness, problem-solving skills, an internal locus of control, involvement with school and recreational activities, life affirming beliefs and religious affiliation.

Whereas many young people who harm themselves do so on only one occasion, others repeat the behavior. A history of previous suicidal behavior increases the risk of future attempts and suicide. The greatest risk of repetition is in the first year following DSH. The reasons why some young people, even those who experience multiple risk factors, stop self-harming require investigation.

The core task of a risk assessment when young people express suicidal thoughts or behaviors is to establish an interactive and dynamic relationship and to be part of a response to the young person's distress that offers some hope for a better future. Improved assessment and management of deliberate self-harm are highlighted in published guidelines.

A number of key studies have evaluated treatment approaches, including CBT (with or without fluoxetine), MST and DBT. There has been considerable debate about the use of antidepressant medications in the treatment of children and adolescents with depression, with a specific focus on whether SSRIs increase the risk of suicidal behaviors in some young people. Antidepressants should only be used in adolescents when combined with psychological treatment. Further efforts are needed to improve engagement in treatment by children, adolescents and their families.

Many young people who engage in DSH do not seek help for their problems. If they do it is most likely to be from friends and family in preference to formal helping agencies or professionals. There are also gender differences, with distressed young males being less likely to seek help of any kind.

Suicide prevention strategies include specific interventions focused on high-risk groups, such as the management of suicide attempts, and population-level interventions such as restricting access to certain methods of suicide, school-based interventions targeted at the prevention of depression and equipping adolescents who are approached by a distressed peer to respond appropriately. Further refinement of these and other strategies to address the gender differences in help-seeking behavior and the isolation of those who are already experiencing mental health difficulties are required.

References

Aaron, R., Joseph, A., Abraham, S., Muliyil, J., George, K., Prasad, J., *et al.* (2004). Suicides in young people in Southern India. *Lancet*, *363*, 1117–1118.

Ackard, D. M., Neumark-Sztainer, D., Story, M., & Perry, C. (2006). Parent–child connectedness and behavioral and emotional health among adolescents. *American Journal of Preventative Medicine*, *30*, 59–66.

Adolescent Health Research Group. (2005). *New Zealand Youth: A profile of their health and wellbeing: Māori report*. Auckland: University of Auckland.

Agerbo, E., Nordentoft, M., & Mortensen, P. B. (2002). Familial, psychiatric and socioeconomic risk factors for suicide in young people: A nested case control study. *British Medical Journal*, *325*, 74–77.

Allison, S., Roeger, L., Martin, G., & Keeves, J. (2001). Gender differences in the relationship between depression and suicidal ideation in young adolescents. *Australian and New Zealand Journal of Psychiatry*, *35*, 498–503.

American Academy of Child and Adolescent Psychiatry. (1999). *Practice parameters for the assessment and treatment of children and adolescents with suicidal behavior*. Washington, DC: American Academy of Child and Adolescent Psychiatry.

Amos, T., Appleby, L., & Kiernan, K. (2001). Changes in rates of suicide by car exhaust asphyxiation in England and Wales. *Psychological Medicine*, *31*, 935–939.

Apter, A., & Freudenstein, O. (2000). Adolescent suicidal behaviour: Psychiatric populations. In K. Hawton, & K. van Heeringen (Eds.), *The international handbook of suicide and attempted suicide* (pp. 261–273). Chichester: Wiley.

Arango, V., Underwood, M., Boldrini, M., Tamir, H., Kassir, S. A., Hsiung, S., *et al.* (2001). Serotonin 1A receptors, serotonin transporter binding and serotonin transporter mRNA expression in the brainstem of depressed suicide victims. *Neuropsychopharmacology, 25*, 892–903.

Arango, V., Underwood, M. D., Gubbi, A. V., & Mann, J. J. (1995). Localized alterations in pre and post-synaptic serotonin binding sites in the ventrolateral prefrontal cortex of suicide victims. *Brain Research, 688*, 121–133.

Asberg, M., & Forslund, K. (2000). Neurobiological aspects of suicide behavior. *International Review of Psychiatry, 12*, 62–74.

Aseltine, R. H., & DeMartino, R. (2004). An outcome evaluation of the SOS Suicide Prevention Program. *American Journal of Public Health, 94*, 446–451.

Bagley, C., & Ramsay, R. (1997). Attitudes to suicide and suicidal behaviours. In C. Bagley, & R. Ramsay (Eds.), *Suicidal behaviour in adolescents and adults* (p. 267). Aldershot: Ashgate.

Bancroft, J., & Hawton, K. (1983). Why people take overdoses: A study of psychiatrists' judgements. *British Journal of Medical Psychology, 56*, 197–204.

Barbe, R. P., Bridge, J., Birmaher, B., Kolko, D., & Brent, D. A. (2004). Suicidality and its relationship to treatment outcome in depressed adolescents. *Suicide and Life-Threatening Behavior, 34*, 44–55.

Bearman, P. S., & Moody, J. (2004). Suicide and friendships among American adolescents. *American Journal of Public Health, 94*, 89–95.

Beautrais, A. (2000). Risk factors for suicide and attempted suicide among young people. *Australian and New Zealand Journal of Psychiatry, 34*, 420–436.

Beautrais, A. (2001). Suicides and serious suicide attempts: Two populations or one? *Psychological Medicine, 31*, 837–845.

Beautrais, A. (2003). Suicide and serious suicide attempts in youth: A multiple group comparison study. *American Journal of Psychiatry, 160*, 1093–1099.

Beautrais, A., Joyce, P. R., & Mulder, R. T. (1996a). Risk factors for serious suicide attempts among youths aged 13 through 24 years. *Journal of the American Academy of Child and Adolescent Psychiatry, 35*, 1174–1182.

Beautrais, A., Joyce, P. R., & Mulder, R. T. (1998). Psychiatric contacts among youths aged 13 through 24 years who have made serious suicide attempts. *Journal of the American Academy of Child and Adolescent Psychiatry, 37*, 504–511.

Beautrais, A., Joyce, P. R., Mulder, R. T., Fergusson, D. M., Deavoll, B. J., & Nightingale, S. K. (1996b). Prevalence and comorbidity of mental disorders in persons making serious suicide attempts: A case–control study. *American Journal of Psychiatry, 153*, 1009–1014.

Beck, A. T., Davis, J. H., Frederick, C. J., Perlin, S., Pokorny, A. D., Schulman, R. E., *et al.* (1973). Classification and nomenclature. In H. L. P. Resnick, & B. C. Hathorne (Eds.), *Suicide prevention in the seventies* (pp. 7–12). Washington, DC: US Government Printing Office.

Bennett, S., Coggan, C., Hooper, R., Lovell, C., & Adams, P. (2002). Presentations by youth to Auckland Emergency Departments following a suicide attempt. *International Journal of Mental Health Nursing, 11*, 144–153.

Bennett, S., Coggan, C., Lee, M., & Fill, J. (2003). *Yellow Ribbon Ambassadors Survey.* Auckland: Injury Prevention Research Centre, School of Population Health, University of Auckland.

Bhugra, D., & Bhui, K. (Eds.). (2007). *Textbook of Cultural Psychiatry.* Cambridge: Cambridge University Press.

Bhugra, D., Thompson, N., Singh, J., & Fellow Smith, E. (2003). Inception rates of deliberate self-harm among adolescents in West London. *International Journal of Social Psychiatry, 49*, 247–250.

Bhugra, D., Thompson, N., Singh, J., & Fellow-Smith, E. (2004). Deliberate self-harm in adolescents in West London: Socio-cultural factors. *European Journal of Psychiatry, 18*, 91–98.

Biddle, L., Gunnell, D., Sharp, D., & Donovan, J. L. (2004). Factors influencing help seeking in mentally distressed young adults: A cross-sectional survey. *British Journal of General Practice, 54*, 248–253.

Bingham, C. R., Bennion, L. D., Openshaw, D. K., & Adams, G. P. (1994). An analysis of age, gender and racial differences in recent national trends of youth suicide. *Journal of Adolescence, 17*, 53–71.

Boergers, J., Spirito, A., & Donaldson, D. (1998). Reasons for adolescent suicide attempts: Associations with psychological functioning. *Journal of the American Academy of Child and Adolescent Psychiatry, 37*, 1287–1293.

Bondy, B., Buettner, A., & Zill, P. (2006). Genetics of suicide. *Molecular Psychiatry, 11*, 336–351.

Bradley, R., Conklin, C. Z., & Westen, D. (2005). The borderline personality diagnosis in adolescents: Gender differences and subtypes. *Journal of Child Psychology and Psychiatry, 46*, 1006–1019.

Brent, D. (1997). The aftercare of adolescents with deliberate self-harm. *Journal of Child Psychology & Psychiatry & Allied Disciplines, 38*, 277–286.

Brent, D., Perper, J. A., & Moritz, G. (1993). Psychiatric risk factors for adolescent suicide: a case-control study. *Journal of the American Academy of Child and Adolescent Psychiatry, 32*, 521–529.

Brent, D., Perper, J. A., Moritz, G., & Liotus, L. (1994a). Familial risk factors for adolescent suicide: a case-controlled study. *Acta Psychiatrica Scandinavica, 89*, 52–58.

Brent, D. A. (1995). Risk factors for adolescent suicide and suicidal behavior: Mental and substance abuse disorders, family environmental factors, and life stress. *Suicide & Life-Threatening Behavior, 25*, 52–63.

Brent, D. A., Baugher, M., Bridge, J., Chen, T., & Chiappetta, L. (1999). Age and sex-related risk factors for adolescent suicide. *Journal of the American Academy of Child & Adolescent Psychiatry, 38*, 1497–1505.

Brent, D. A., Bridge, J., Johnson, B. A., & Connolly, J. (1996). Suicidal behavior runs in families: A controlled family study of adolescent suicide victims. *Archives of General Psychiatry, 53*, 1145–1152.

Brent, D. A., & Mann, J. J. (2005). Family genetic studies, suicide, and suicidal behavior. *American Journal of Medical Genetics Part C: Seminars in Medical Genetics, 133C*, 13–24.

Brent, D. A., Moritz, G., Bridge, J., Perper, J., & Canobbio, R. (1996a). The impact of adolescent suicide on siblings and parents: A longitudinal follow-up. *Suicide & Life-Threatening Behavior, 26*, 253–259.

Brent, D. A., Moritz, G., Bridge, J., Perper, J., & Canobbio, R. (1996b). Long-term impact of exposure to suicide: A three-year controlled follow-up. *Journal of the American Academy of Child & Adolescent Psychiatry, 35*, 646–653.

Brent, D. A., Mortiz, G., & Liotus, L. (1996). A test of the diathesis-stress model of adolescent depression in friends and acquaintances of adolescent suicide victims. In C. R. Pfeffer (Ed.), *Severe stress and mental disturbance in children.* (pp. 347–360). Washington: American Psychiatric Press, Inc.

Brent, D. A., Oquendo, M., Birmaher, B., Greenhill, L., Kolko, D., Stanley, B., Zelazny, J., Brodsky, B., Bridge, J., Ellis, S., Salazar, J. O., & Mann, J. J. (2002). Familial pathways to early-onset suicide attempt: Risk for suicidal behavior in offspring of mood-disordered suicide attempters. *Archives of General Psychiatry, 59*, 801–807.

Brent, D. A., Perper, J., Moritz, G., Allman, C., Friend, A., Schweers, J., Roth, C., Balach, L., & Harrington, K. (1992). Psychiatric effects of exposure to suicide among the friends and acquaintances of adolescent suicide victims. *Journal of the American Academy of Child & Adolescent Psychiatry, 31*, 629–639.

Brent, D. A., Perper, J. A., Goldstein, C. E., Kolko, D. J., *et al.* (1988). Risk factors for adolescent suicide: A comparison of adolescent suicide victims with suicidal inpatients. *Archives of General Psychiatry, 45*, 581–588.

Brent, D. A., Perper, J. A., Moritz, G., & Liotus, L. (1994b). Major depression or uncomplicated bereavement? A follow-up of youth exposed to suicide. *Journal of the American Academy of Child & Adolescent Psychiatry*, *33*, 231–239.

Bridge, J. A., Goldstein, T. R., & Brent, D. A. (2006). Adolescent suicide and suicidal behaviour. *Journal of Child Psychology and Psychiatry*, *47*, 372–394.

Brodsky, B. S., Malone, K. M., Ellis, S. P., Dulit, R., & Mann, J. J. (1997). Characteristics of borderline personality disorder associated with suicidal behavior. *American Journal of Psychiatry*, *154*, 1715–1719.

Bryan, C. J., & Rudd, M. D. (2006). Advances in the assessment of suicide risk. *Journal of Clinical Psychology*, *62*, 185–200.

Burgess, S., Hawton, K., & Loveday, G. (1998). Adolescents who take overdoses: Outcome in terms of changes in psychopathology and the adolescents' attitudes to care and to their overdose. *Journal of Adolescence*, *21*, 209–219.

Burns, J., Dudley, M., Hazell, P., & Patton, G. (2005). Clinical management of deliberate self-harm in young people: The need for evidence-based approaches to reduce repetition. *Australian and New Zealand Journal of Psychiatry*, *39*, 121–128.

Burns, J. M., & Patton, G. C. (2000). Preventative interventions for youth suicide: A risk factor-based approach. *Australian and New Zealand Journal of Psychiatry*, *34*, 388–407.

Canino, G., & Roberts, R. E. (2001). Suicidal behavior among Latino youth. *Suicide and Life-Threatening Behavior*, *31*, 122–131.

Cantor, C. H. (2000). Suicide in the Western World. In K. Hawton, & K. van Heeringen (Eds.), *The international handbook of suicide and attempted suicide* (pp. 9–28). Chichester: John Wiley and Sons.

Cantor, C. H., & Neulinger, K. (2000). The epidemiology of suicide and attempted suicide. *Australian and New Zealand Journal of Psychiatry*, *34*, 370–387.

Carter, G., Reith, D. M., Whyte, I. M., & McPherson, M. (2005). Repeated self-poisoning: Increasing severity of self-harm as a predictor of subsequent suicide. *British Journal of Psychiatry*, *186*, 253–257.

Cavanagh, J. T. O., Carson, A. J., Sharpe, M., & Lawrie, S. M. (2003). Psychological autopsy studies of suicide: A systematic review. *Psychological Medicine*, *33*, 395–405.

Centers for Disease Control. (2004). Methods of suicide among persons aged 10–19 years, United States, 1992–2001. *Morbidity and Mortality Weekly Report*, *53*, 471–474.

Centres for Disease Control and Prevention. (1992). *Youth suicide prevention programs: A resource guide*. Atlanta: US Department of Health and Human Services.

Cerel, J., & Roberts, T. A. (2005). Suicidal behavior in the family and adolescent risk behavior. *Journal of Adolescent Health*, *36*, 352, e9–16.

Coffey, C., Wolfe, R., Lovett, A. W., Moran, P., Cini, E., & Patton, G. C. (2004). Predicting death in young offenders: a retrospective cohort study. *Medical Journal of Australia*, *181*, 473–477.

Coggan, C., Bennett, S., Hooper, R., & Dickinson, P. (2003). Association between bullying and mental health status in New Zealand adolescents. *International Journal of Mental Health Promotion*, *5*, 16–22.

Commonwealth Department of Health and Aged Care. (1999). *National youth suicide prevention strategy: Setting the evidence based research agenda for Australia. A literature review*. Canberra: Commonwealth of Australia.

Conner, K. R., Meldrum, S., Wieczorek, W. F., Duberstein, P. R., & Welte, J. W. (2004). The association of irritability and impulsivity with suicidal ideation among 15- to 20-year-old males. *Suicide and Life-Threatening Behavior*, *34*, 363–373.

Cotgrove, A., Zirinsky, L., Black, D., & Weston, D. (1995). Secondary prevention of attempted suicide in adolescence. *Journal of Adolescence*, *18*, 569–577.

D'Augeli, A. R., Grossman, A. H., Salter, N. P., Vasey, J. J., Starks, M. T., & Sinclair, K. O. (2005). Predicting the suicide attempts of lesbian, gay and bisexual youth. *Suicide and Life-Threatening Behavior*, *35*, 646–660.

Dancyger, I. F., & Fornari, V. M. (2005). A review of eating disorders and suicide risk in adolescents. *The Scientific World Journal*, *28*, 803–811.

de Anda, D., & Smith, M. A. (1993). Differences among adolescent, young adult, and adult callers of suicide help lines. *Social Work*, *38*, 421–428.

De Leo, D., & Heller, T. S. (2004). Who are the kids who self-harm? An Australian self-report school survey. *Medical Journal of Australia*, *181*, 140–144.

Denny, S. J., Clark, T. C., & Watson, P. D. (2003). Comparison of health-risk behaviors among students in alternative high schools from New Zealand and the USA. *Journal of Pediatrics and Child Health*, *39*, 33–39.

Dexheimer Pharris, M., Resnick, M., & Blum, R. (1997). Protecting against hopelessness and suicidality in sexually abused American Indian adolescents. *Journal of Adolescent Health*, *21*, 400–406.

Donald, M., Dower, J., Correa-Velez, I., & Jones, M. (2006). Risk and protective factors for medically serious suicide attempts: A comparison of hospital-based with population-based samples of young adults. *Australian and New Zealand Journal of Psychiatry*, *40*, 87–96.

Donaldson, D., Spirito, A., & Esposito-Smythers, C. (2005). Treatment for adolescents following suicide attempt: results of a pilot trial. *Journal of the American Academy of Child & Adolescent Psychiatry*, *44*, 113–120.

Dower, J., Donald, M., Kelly, B., & Raphael, B. (2000). *Pathways to care for young people who present for non-fatal deliberate self-harm*. Queensland: School of Population Health, University of Queensland.

Dunn, V., & Goodyer, I. M. (2006). Longitudinal investigation into childhood- and adolescence-onset depression: Psychiatric outcome in early adulthood. *British Journal of Psychiatry*, *188*, 216–222.

Eaton, L. (2006). European agency approves use of fluoxetine for children and teens. *British Medical Journal*, *332*, 1407.

Eddleston, M., Eyer, P., Worek, F., Mohamed, F., Senarathna, L., von Meyer, L., *et al.* (2005a). Differences between organophosphorus insecticides in human self-poisoning: a prospective cohort study. *Lancet*, *366*, 1452–1459.

Eddleston, M., Gunnell, D., Karunaratne, A., de Silva, D., Sheriff, M. H. R., & Buckley, N. A. (2005b). Epidemiology of intentional self-poisoning in rural Sri Lanka. *British Journal of Psychiatry*, *187*, 583–584.

Erikson, E. (1968). *Identity: youth and crisis*. New York: W.W. Norton.

Esposito-Smythers, C., & Spirito, A. (2004). Adolescent substance use and suicidal behavior: A review with implications for treatment research. *Alcoholism, Clinical and Experimental Research*, *28*, 77S–88S.

Etzersdorfer, E., Sonneck, G., & Nagel-Kuess, S. (1992). Newspaper reports and suicide. *New England Journal of Medicine*, *327*, 502–503.

Evans, E., Hawton, K., & Rodham, K. (2004). Factors associated with suicidal phenomena in adolescents: A systematic review of population-based studies. *Clinical Psychology Review*, *24*, 957–979.

Evans, E., Hawton, K., & Rodham, K. (2005a). Suicidal phenomena and abuse in adolescents: A review of epidemiological studies. *Child Abuse and Neglect*, *29*, 45–48.

Evans, E., Hawton, K., Rodham, K., & Deeks, J. (2005b). The prevalence of suicidal phenomena in adolescents: A systematic review of population-based studies. *Suicide and Life-Threatening Behavior*, *35*, 239–250.

Evans, J. (2000). Interventions to reduce repetition of deliberate self-harm. *International Review of Psychiatry*, *12*, 44–47.

Favazza, A. R. (1992). Repetitive self mutilation. *Psychiatric Annals*, *22*, 60–63.

Fazel, M., Wheeler, J., & Danesh, J. (2005). Prevalence of serious mental disorder in 7000 refugees resettled in western countries: a systematic review. *Lancet*, *365*, 1309–1314.

Fergusson, D. M., Horwood, L. J., & Beautrais, A. L. (1999). Is sexual orientation related to mental health problems and suicidality in young people? *Archives of General Psychiatry*, *56*, 876–880.

Fergusson, D. M., Horwood, L. J., Ridder, E. M., & Beautrais, A. L. (2005). Subthreshold depression in adolescence and mental health outcomes in adulthood. *Archives of General Psychiatry*, *62*, 66–72.

Fergusson, D. M., & Lynskey, M. T. (1995a). Childhood circumstances, adolescent adjustment, and suicide attempts in a New Zealand birth cohort. *Journal of the American Academy of Child and Adolescent Psychiatry*, *34*, 612–622.

Fergusson, D. M., & Lynskey, M. T. (1995b). Suicide attempts and suicidal ideation in a birth cohort of 16-year-old New Zealanders. *Journal of the American Academy of Child and Adolescent Psychiatry*, *34*, 1308–1317.

Fergusson, D. M., & Lynskey, M. T. (1996). Adolescent resiliency to family adversity. *Journal of Child Psychology and Psychiatry and Allied Disciplines*, *37*, 281–292.

Fergusson, D. M., Woodward, L., & Horwood, L. J. (2000). Risk factors and life processes associated with the onset of suicidal behaviour during adolescence and early adulthood. *Psychological Medicine*, *30*, 23–39.

Fortune, S. A. (2006). An examination of cutting and other methods of DSH among children and adolescents presenting to an outpatient psychiatric clinic in New Zealand. *Clinical Child Psychology and Psychiatry*, *11*, 407–416.

Fortune, S. A., Stewart, A., Yadav, V., & Hawton, K. (2007). Suicide in adolescents: using life charts to understand the suicidal process. *Journal of Affective Disorders*, *100*, 199–210.

Friedman, T., Newton, C., Coggan, C., Hooley, S., Patel, R., Pickard, M., *et al.* (2006). Predictors of A&E staff attitudes to self-harm patients who use self-laceration: influence of previous training and experience. *Journal of Psychosomatic Research*, *60*, 273–277.

Garland, A., Shaffer, D., & Whittle, B. (1989). A national survey of school-based, adolescent suicide prevention programs. *Journal of the American Academy of Child and Adolescent Psychiatry*, *28*, 931–934.

Gaynes, B. N., West, S. L., Ford, C., Frame, P., Klein, J., & Lohr, K. N. (2004). *Screening for suicide risk: a systematic evidence review for the US Preventative Services Task Force*. Rockville: Agency for Healthcare Research and Quality.

Gibb, S. L., Beautrais, A. L., & Fergusson, D. M. (2005). Mortality and further suicidal behaviour after index suicide attempt: A 10-year study. *Australian and New Zealand Journal of Psychiatry*, *39*, 95–100.

Gibbons, R. D., Hur, K., Bhaumik, D. K., & Mann, J. J. (2006). The relationship between antidepressant prescription rates and rate of early adolescent suicide. *American Journal of Psychiatry*, *163*, 1898–1904.

Goldacre, M., & Hawton, K. (1985). Repetition of self-poisoning and subsequent death in adolescents who take overdoses. *British Journal of Psychiatry*, *146*, 395–398.

Goldston, D. B., Sergent Daniel, S., Reboussin, D. M., Reboussin, B. A., Frazier, P. H., & Kelley, A. E. (1999). Suicide attempts among formerly hospitalized adolescents: A prospective naturalistic study of risk during the first 5 years after discharge. *Journal of the American Academy of Child and Adolescent Psychiatry*, *38*, 660–671.

Goodwin, R. D., Marusic, A., & Hoven, C. W. (2003). Suicide attempts in the United States: the role of physical illness. *Social Science and Medicine*, *56*, 1783–1788.

Gould, M., Fisher, P., Parides, M., Flory, M., & Shaffer, D. (1996). Psychosocial risk factors of child and adolescent completed suicide. *Archives of General Psychiatry*, *53*, 1155–1162.

Gould, M., Greenberg, T., Velting, D. M., & Shaffer, D. (2003). Youth suicide risk and preventative interventions: A review of the past 10 years. *Journal of the American Academy of Child and Adolescent Psychiatry*, *42*, 386–405.

Gould, M. S. (2001). Suicide and the media. In H. Hendin, & J. J. Mann (Eds.), *The clinical science of suicide prevention* (Volume 932, pp. 200–224). New York: New York Academy of Sciences.

Gould, M. S., King, R., Greenwald, S., Fisher, P., Schwab-Stone, M., Kramer, R., *et al.* (1998). Psychopathology associated with suicidal ideation and attempts among children and adolescents. *Journal of the American Academy of Child and Adolescent Psychiatry*, *37*, 915–923.

Gould, M. S., Marrocco, F. A., Kleinman, M., Graham Thomas, J., Mostkoff, K., Cote, J., *et al.* (2005). Evaluating iatrogenic risk of youth suicide screening programs. *Journal of the American Medical Association*, *293*, 1635–1643.

Gould, M. S., Munfakh, J. L. H., Lubell, K., Kleinman, M., & Parker, S. (2002). Seeking help from the Internet during adolescence. *Journal of the American Academy of Child and Adolescent Psychiatry*, *41*, 1182–1189.

Gould, M. S., Velting, D., Kleinman, M., Lucas, C., Thomas, J. G., & Chung, M. (2004). Teenagers' attitudes about coping strategies and help-seeking behavior for suicidality. *Journal of the American Academy of Child and Adolescent Psychiatry*, *43*, 1124–1133.

Gould, M. S., Wallenstein, S., & Davidson, L. (1989). Suicide clusters: A critical review. In I. S. Lann, & E. K. Moscicki (Eds.), *Strategies for studying suicide and suicidal behavior* (pp. 17–29). New York: Guilford Press.

Greenfield, B., Larson, C., Hechtman, L., Rousseau, C., & Platt, R. (2002). A rapid-response outpatient model for reducing hospitalization rates among suicidal adolescents. *Psychiatric Services*, *53*, 1574–1579.

Greenhill, L. L., & Waslick, B. (1997). Management of suicidal behavior in children and adolescents. *Psychiatric Clinics of North America*, *20*, 641–665.

Grossman, J. A., & Kruesi, M. J. P. (2000). Innovative approaches to youth suicide prevention: An update of issues and research findings. In R. W. Maris, & S. S. Canetto (Eds.). *Review of suicidology* (pp. 170–201). New York: Guilford Press.

Guertin, T., Lloyd-Richardson, E., Spirito, A., Donaldson, D., & Boergers, J. (2001). Self-mutilative behavior in adolescents who attempt suicide by overdose. *Journal of the American Academy of Child and Adolescent Psychiatry*, *40*, 1062–1069.

Gunnell, D., Bennewith, O., Hawton, K., Simkin, S., & Kapur, N. (2005). The epidemiology and prevention of suicide by hanging: a systematic review. *International Journal of Epidemiology*, *34*, 433–442.

Hammad, T. A., Laughren, T., & Racoosin, J. (2006). Suicidality in pediatric patients treated with antidepressant drugs. *Archives of General Psychiatry*, *63*, 332–339.

Harrington, R., Kerfoot, M., Dyer, E., McNiven, F., Gill, J., Harrington, V., *et al.* (2000). Deliberate self-poisoning in adolescence: Why does a brief family intervention work in some cases and not others? *Journal of Adolescence*, *23*, 13–20.

Harrington, R., Pickles, A., Aglan, A., Harrington, V., Burroughs, H., & Kerfoot, M. (2006). Early adult outcomes of adolescents who deliberately poison themselves. *Journal of the American Academy of Child and Adolescent Psychiatry*, *45*, 337–345.

Harrington, R., Whittaker, J., & Shoebridge, P. (1998). Psychological treatment of depression in children and adolescents: A review of the treatment research. *The British Journal of Psychiatry*, *173*, 291–298.

Harris, H. E., & Myers, W. C. (1997). Adolescents' misperceptions of the dangerousness of acetaminophen in overdose. *Suicide and Life-Threatening Behavior*, *27*, 274–277.

Haw, C., Sutton, L., Simkin, S., Gunnell, D., Kapur, N., Nowers, M., *et al.* (2004). Suicide by gunshot in the United Kingdom: A review of the literature. *Medicine, Science and the Law*, *44*, 295–310.

Hawton, K. (Ed.). (2005). *Prevention and treatment of suicidal behaviour: From science to practice*. Oxford: Oxford University Press.

Hawton, K., Cole, D., O'Grady, J., & Osborn, M. (1982). Motivational aspects of deliberate self-poisoning in adolescents. *British Journal of Psychiatry*, *141*, 286–291.

Hawton, K., Fagg, J., Simkin, S., Bale, E., & Bond, A. (2000). Deliberate self-harm in adolescents in Oxford, 1985–1995. *Journal of Adolescence*, *23*, 47–55.

Hawton, K., Hall, S., Simkin, S., Bale, E., Bond, A., Codd, S., *et al.* (2003). Deliberate self-harm in adolescents: A study of characteristics and trends in Oxford, 1990–2000. *Journal of Child Psychology and Psychiatry and Allied Disciplines*, *44*, 1191–1198.

Hawton, K., & Harriss, L. (2007). Deliberate self-harm in young people: characteristics and subsequent mortality in a 20-year cohort of patients presenting to hospital. *Journal of Clinical Psychiatry*, *68*, 1574–1583.

Hawton, K., Houston, K., & Sheppard, R. (1999a). Suicide in young people. Study of 174 cases, aged under 25 years, based on coroners' and medical records. *British Journal of Psychiatry*, *175*, 271–276.

Hawton, K., Kingsbury, S., Steinhardt, K., James, A., & Fagg, J. (1999b). Repetition of deliberate self-harm by adolescents: The role of psychological factors. *Journal of Adolescence*, *22*, 369–378.

Hawton, K., Rodham, K., & Evans, E. (2006). *By their own young hand: Deliberate self-harm and suicidal ideas*. London: Jessica Kingsley.

Hawton, K., Rodham, K., Evans, E., & Weatherall, R. (2002a). Deliberate self harm in adolescents: Self report survey in schools in England. *British Medical Journal*, *325*, 1207–1211.

Hawton, K., Simkin, S., Deeks, J., Cooper, J., Johnston, A., Waters, K., *et al.* (2004). UK legislation on analgesic packs: Before and after study of long term effect on poisonings. *British Medical Journal*, *329*, 1076–1080.

Hawton, K., Sutton, L., Haw, C., Sinclair, J., & Deeks, J. J. (2005). Schizophrenia and suicide: Systematic review of risk factors. *British Journal of Psychiatry*, *187*, 9–20.

Hawton, K., Townsend, E., Arensman, E., Gunnell, D., Hazell, P., House, A., *et al.* (2000). Psychosocial and pharmacological treatments for deliberate self harm. *Cochrane Database of Systematic Reviews*, 2: CD001764.

Hawton, K., & Williams, K. (2005). Media influences on suicidal behaviour: Evidence and prevention. In K. Hawton (Ed.), *Prevention and treatment of suicidal behaviour: From science to practice*. Oxford: Oxford University Press (pp. 293–306).

Hazell, L., & King, R. (1996). Arguments for and against teaching suicide prevention in schools. *Australian and New Zealand Journal of Psychiatry*, *30*, 633–642.

Hazell, P. (2000). Treatment strategies for adolescent suicide attempters. In K. Hawton, & K. van Heeringen (Eds.), *The international handbook of suicide and attempted suicide* (pp. 519–538). Chichester: Wiley.

Herron, J., Tichehurst, H., Appleby, L., Perry, A., & Cordingly, L. (2001). Attitudes toward suicide prevention in front-line health staff. *Suicide and Life-Threatening Behavior*, *31*, 342–347.

Hjelmeland, H., Hawton, K., Nordvik, H., Bille Brahe, U., De Leo, D., Fekete, S., *et al.* (2002). Why people engage in parasuicide: A cross-cultural study of intentions. *Suicide and Life-Threatening Behavior*, *32*, 380–393.

Hjelmeland, H., & Groholt, B. (2005). A comparative study of young and adult deliberate self-harm patients. *Crisis*, *26*, 64–72.

Hjelmeland, H., Stiles, T. C., Bille-Brahe, U., Ostapowicz, G., Salander-Renberg, E., & Wasserman, D. (1998). Parasuicide: The value of suicidal intent and various motives as predictors of future suicidal behaviour. *Archives of Suicide Research*, *4*, 209–225.

Hopkins, C. (2002). 'But what about the really ill, poorly people'. An ethnographic study into what it means to nurses on medical admission units to have people who have harmed themselves as their patients. *Journal of Psychiatric and Mental Health Nursing*, *9*, 147–154.

Houston, K., Hawton, K., & Sheppard, R. (2001). Suicide in young people aged 15–24: A psychological autopsy study. *Journal of Affective Disorders*, *63*, 159–170.

Huey, S. J., Henggeler, S. W., Rowland, M. D., Halliday-Boykins, C. A., Cunningham, P. N., Pickrel, S. G., *et al.* (2004). Multisystemic therapy effects on attempted suicide by youths presenting psychiatric emergencies. *Journal of the American Academy of Child and Adolescent Psychiatry*, *43*, 183–190.

James, A., Lai, F. H., & Dahl, C. (2004). Attention deficit hyperactivity disorder and suicide: A review of possible associations. *Acta Psychiatrica Scandinavica*, *110*, 408–415.

James, D., & Hawton, K. (1985). Overdoses: Explanations and attitudes in self-poisoners and significant others. *British Journal of Psychiatry*, *146*, 481–485.

Joe, S., & Kaplan, M. S. (2001). Suicide among African American men. *Suicide and Life-Threatening Behavior*, *31*, 106–121.

Johnson, B. A., Brent, D., Bridge, J., & Connolly, J. (1998). The familial aggregation of adolescent suicide attempts. *Acta Psychiatrica Scandinavica*, *97*, 18–24.

Johnson, J. G., Cohen, P., Skodol, A. E., Oldham, J. M., Kasen, S., & Brook, J. S. (1999). Personality disorders in adolescence and risk of major mental disorders and suicidality during adulthood. *Archives of General Psychiatry*, *56*, 805–811.

Kalafat, J., Elias, M., & Gara, J. (1993). The relationship of bystander intervention variables to adolescents' responses to suicidal peers. *Journal of Primary Prevention*, *13*, 231–244.

Kaltiala-Heino, R., Rimpela, M., Marttunen, M., Rimpela, A., & Rantanen, P. (1999). Bullying, depression, and suicidal ideation in Finnish adolescents: School survey. *British Medical Journal*, *319*, 348–351.

Kapur, N., House, A., Dodgson, K., May, C., & Creed, F. (2002). Effect of general hospital management on repeat episodes of deliberate self poisoning: Cohort study. *British Medical Journal*, *325*, 866–867.

Keller, A. S., Rosenfeld, B., Trinh-Shevrin, C., Meserve, C., Sachs, E., Leviss, J. A., *et al.* (2003). Mental health of detained asylum seekers. *Lancet*, *362*, 1721–1723.

Kerfoot, M., Harrington, R., & Dyer, E. (1995). Brief home-based intervention with young suicide attempters and their families. *Journal of Adolescence*, *18*, 557–568.

Kienhorst, I. C. W. M., de Wilde, E. J., Diekstra, R. F. W., & Wolters, W. H. G. (1992). Differences between adolescent suicide attempters and depressed adolescents. *Acta Psychiatrica Scandinavica*, *85*, 222–228.

Kienhorst, I. C. W. M., de Wilde, E. J., Diekstra, R. F. W., & Wolters, W. H. G. (1995). Adolescents' image of their suicide attempt. *Journal of the American Academy of Child and Adolescent Psychiatry*, *34*, 623–628.

King, C. A., Hovey, J. D., Brand, E., & Wilson, R. (1997). Suicidal adolescents after hospitalization: Parent and family impacts on treatment follow-through. *Journal of the American Academy of Child and Adolescent Psychiatry*, *36*, 85–93.

King, C. A., Kramer, A., Preuss, L., Kerr, D. C. R., Weisse, L., & Venkataraman, S. (2006). Youth-nominated support team for suicidal adolescents (Version 1): A randomized controlled trial. *Journal of Consulting and Clinical Psychology*, *74*, 199–206.

Kirmayer, L. J., Malus, M., & Boothroyd, L. J. (1996). Suicide attempts among Inuit youth: A community survey of prevalence and risk factors. *Acta Psychiatrica Scandinavica*, *94*, 8–17.

Lalwani, S., Sharma, G. A., Kabra, S. K., Girdhar, S., & Dogra, T. D. (2004). Suicide among children and adolescents in South Delhi (1991–2000). *Indian Journal of Paediatrics*, *71*, 701–703.

Leenaars, A., & Wenckstern, S. (1999). Suicide prevention in schools: The art, the issues and the pitfalls. *Crisis: Journal of Crisis Intervention & Suicide*, *20*, 132–142.

Lessard, J. C., & Moretti, M. M. (1998). Suicidal ideation in an adolescent clinical sample: Attachment patterns and clinical implications. *Journal of Adolescence*, *21*, 383–395.

Levinson, D. F. (2006). The genetics of depression: A review. *Biological Psychiatry*, *60*, 84–92.

Lewinsohn, P. M., Seeley, J. R., & Klein, D. N. (2003). Bipolar disorder in adolescents: epidemiology and suicidal behavior. In B. Geller, & M. P. Del Bello (Eds.), *Bipolar Disorder in Childhood and Early Adolescence* (pp. 7–24). New York: Guilford Press.

Lin, P.-Y., & Tsai, G. (2004). Association between serotonin transporter gene promoter polymorphism and suicide: Results of a meta-analysis. *Biological Psychiatry*, *55*, 1023–1030.

Linehan, M. M., Rizvi, S. L., Welch, S. S., & Page, B. (2000). Psychiatric aspects of suicidal behaviour: Personality disorders. In K. Hawton, & K. van Heeringen (Eds.), *The international handbook of suicide and attempted suicide* (pp. 147–178). Chichester: Wiley.

Littmann, S. K. (1983). *The role of the press in the control of suicide epidemics.* Paper presented at the International Association for Suicide Prevention and Crisis Intervention, Paris.

Lock, J., Walker, L. R., Rickert, V. I., & Katzman, D. K. (2005). Suicidality in adolescents being treated with antidepressant medications and the black box label: Position paper of the Society for Adolescent Medicine. *Journal of Adolescent Health*, *36*, 92–93.

Madge, N., & Harvey, J. G. (1999). Suicide among the young: The size of the problem. *Journal of Adolescence*, *22*, 145–155.

Mann, J. J., Apter, A., Bertolote, J., Beautrais, A., Currier, D., Haas, A., *et al.* (2005). Suicide prevention strategies: A systematic review. *Journal of the American Medical Association*, *294*, 2064–2074.

Mann, J. J., Brent, D. A., & Arango, V. (2001). The neurobiology and genetics of suicide and attempted suicide: A focus on the serotonergic system. *Neuropsychopharmacology*, *24*, 467–477.

Mann, J. J., Huang, Y., Underwood, M., Kassir, S. A., Oppenheim, S., Kelly, T. M., *et al.* (2000). A serotonin transporter gene promoter polymorphism (5-HTTLPR) and prefrontal cortical binding in major depression and suicide. *Archives of General Psychiatry*, *57*, 729–738.

Maris, R. W., Berman, A. L., Maltsberger, J. T., & Yuffit, R. I. (1992). *Assessment and prediction of suicide.* New York: Guilford Press.

Martin, G., Clarke, M., & Pearce, C. (1993). Adolescent suicide: Music preferences as an indicator of vulnerability. *Journal of the American Academy of Child and Adolescent Psychiatry*, *32*, 530–535.

Marttunen, M. J., Aro, H. M., & Lonnqvist, J., K. (1993). Adolescence and suicide: A review of psychological autopsy studies. *European Child and Adolescent Psychiatry*, *2*, 10–18.

Marttunen, M. J., Henriksson, M. M., Isometsae, E. T., Heikkinen, M. E., Aro, H. M., & Lonnqvist, J. K. (1998). Completed suicide among adolescents with no diagnosable psychiatric disorder. *Adolescence*, *33*, 669–681.

McPherson, A. (2005). Adolescents in primary care. *British Medical Journal*, *330*, 465–467.

Medicines and Healthcare Products Regulatory Agency. (2004). Safety of selective serotonin reuptake inhibitor antidepressants. Retrieved March 1, 2005, from http://medicines.mhra.gov.uk/ourwork/monitorsafequalmed/safetymessages/ssri_letter_061204.pdf

Melhem, N. M., Day, N., Shear, M., Day, R., Reynolds, C. F., & Brent, D. (2004a). Traumatic grief among adolescents exposed to a peer's suicide. *American Journal of Psychiatry*, *161*, 1411–1416.

Melhem, N. M., Day, N., Shear, M., Day, R., Reynolds, C. F. III, & Brent, D. (2004b). Predictors of complicated grief among adolescents exposed to a peer's suicide. *Journal of Loss and Trauma*, *9*, 21–34.

Meltzer, H., Harrington, R., Goodman, R., & Jenkins, R. (2001). *Children who try to harm, hurt or kill themselves.* London: Office for National Statistics.

Merry, S., McDowell, H., Hetrick, S., Bir, J., Muller, N., Hawton, K., *et al.* (2002). Psychological and/or educational interventions for the prevention of depression in children and adolescents. *Cochrane Database of Systematic Reviews*, 2.

Merry, S., McDowell, H., Wild, C. J., Bir, J., & Cunliffe, R. (2004). A randomized placebo-controlled trial of a school-based depression prevention program. *Journal of the American Academy of Child and Adolescent Psychiatry*, *43*, 538–547.

Miller, T. R., & Taylor, D. M. (2005). Adolescent suicidality: Who will ideate, who will act. *Suicide and Life-Threatening Behavior*, *35*, 425–435.

Millstein, S. G., & Halpern-Felsher, B. L. (2002). Perceptions of risk and vulnerability. *Journal of Adolescent Health*, *31*, 10–27.

Ministry of Health. (2005). *Suicide facts: provisional 2002 all-ages statistics.* Wellington: Ministry of Health.

Mishara, B. L. (1999). Conceptions of death and suicide in children ages 6–12 and their implications for suicide prevention. *Suicide and Life-Threatening Behavior*, *29*, 105–118.

Mishara, B. L. (2003). How the media influences children's conceptions of suicide. *Crisis: Journal of Crisis Intervention & Suicide*, *24*, 128–130.

Morgan, J., & Hawton, K. (2004). Self-reported suicidal behavior in juvenile offenders in custody: prevalence and associated factors. *Crisis*, *25*, 8–11.

Morrissey, R. F., Dicker, R., Abikoff, H., Alvir, J. M., De Marco, A., & Koplewicz, H. S. (1995). Hospitalizing the suicidal adolescent: An empirical investigation of decision-making criteria. *Journal of the American Academy of Child and Adolescent Psychiatry*, *34*, 902–911.

Muehlenkamp, J. J., & Gutierrez, P. M. (2004). An investigation of differences between self-injurious behavior and suicide attempts in a sample of adolescents. *Suicide and Life-Threatening Behavior*, *34*, 12–23.

National Institute for Clinical Excellence (NICE). (2004). *Self-harm: the short-term physical and psychological management and secondary prevention of self-harm in primary and secondary care.* London: NICE.

Neeleman, J., Halpern, D., Leon, D., & Lewis, G. (1997). Tolerance of suicide, religion and suicide rates: an ecological and individual study of 19 Western countries. *Psychological Medicine*, *27*, 1165–1171.

Nicholas, J., Oliver, K., Lee, K., & O'Brien, M. (2004). Help-seeking behaviour and the Internet: An investigation among Australian adolescents. *Australian e-Journal for the Advancement of Mental Health* Vol, 3. www.auseinet.com/journal/vol3iss1/nicholas.pdf

Nordstrom, P., Samuelsson, M., Asberg, M., Traskman-Bendz, L., Aberg-Wistedt, A., Nordin, C., & Bertilsson, L. (1994). CSF 5-HIAA predicts suicide risk after attempted suicide. *Suicide and Life-Threatening Behavior*, *24*, 1–9.

O'Carroll, P., W, Berman, A. L., Maris, R., Moscicki, E. K., Tanney, B., & Silverman, M. (1998). Beyond the Tower of Babel: A nomenclature for suicidology. In R. Kosky, H. S. Eskevari, R. D. Goldney, & R. Hassan (Eds.). *Suicide prevention: The global context.* New York: Plenum (pp. 23–39).

Office of National Statistics. (2004). *Mortality statistics: Review of the Registrar General of deaths by cause, sex and age in England and Wales 2003.* London: Office of National Statistics.

Olfson, M., Gameroff, M. J., Marcus, S. C., Greenberg, T., & Shaffer, D. (2005). National trends in hospitalization of youth with intentional self-inflicted injuries. *American Journal of Psychiatry*, *162*, 1328–1335.

Olfson, M., Shaffer, D., Marcus, S., & Greenberg, T. (2003). Relationship between antidepressant medication treatment and suicide in adolescents. *Archives of General Psychiatry*, *60*, 978–982.

Palmer, B. A., Pankratz, V. S., & Bostwick, J. M. (2005). The lifetime risk of suicide in schizophrenia: A re-examination. *Archives of General Psychiatry*, *62*, 247–253.

Pfeffer, C. R. (2000). Suicidal behaviour in children: An emphasis on developmental influences. In K. Hawton, & K. van Heeringen (Eds.). *The international handbook of suicide and attempted suicide* (pp. 237–248). Chichester: Wiley.

Phillips, D. P., & Carstensen, L. L. (1988). The effect of suicide stories on various demographic groups. *Suicide and Life-Threatening Behavior*, *18*, 100–114.

Piaget, J. (1968). *Judgement and reasoning in the child*. London: Routledge.

Pirkis, J., & Blood, R. W. (2001). *Suicide and the media: A critical review*. Canberra: Commonwealth Department of Health and Aged Care.

Pirkis, J., Francis, C., Blood, R. W., Burgess, P., Morley, B., Stewart, A., *et al.* (2002). Reporting of suicide in the Australian media. *Australian and New Zealand Journal of Psychiatry*, *36*, 190–197.

Pirkis, J. E., Blood, R. W., Beautrais, A. L., Burgess, P. M., & Skehan, J. (2006a). Media guidelines on the reporting of suicide. *Crisis*, *27*, 82–87.

Pirkis, J. E., Burgess, P. M., Francis, C., Blood, R. W., & Jolley, D. J. (2006b). The relationship between media reporting of suicide and actual suicide in Australia. *Social Science and Medicine*, *62*, 2874–2886.

Pompili, M., Mancinelli, I., Girardi, P., & Tatarelli, R. (2004). Preventing suicide in young schizophrenics who are substance "abusers". *Substance Use and Misuse*, *39*, 1435–1439.

Portzky, G., Audenaert, K., & van Heeringen, K. (2005). Suicide among adolescents: A psychological autopsy study of psychiatric, psychosocial and personality-related risk factors. *Social Psychiatry and Psychiatric Epidemiology*, *40*, 922–930.

Prasad, J., Abraham, V. J., Minz, S., Abraham, S., Joseph, A., Muliyil, J. P., *et al.* (2006). Rates and factors associated with suicide in Kaniyambadi Block, Tamil Nadu, South India 2000–2002. *International Journal of Social Psychiatry*, *52*, 65–71.

Rathus, J. H, & Miller, A., L. (2002). Dialectical behaviour therapy adapted for suicidal adolescents. *Suicide and Life-Threatening Behavior*, *32*, 146–157.

Reith, D. M., Whyte, I., & Carter, G. (2003). Repetition risk for adolescent self-poisoning: a multiple event survival analysis. *Australian and New Zealand Journal of Psychiatry*, *37*, 212–218.

Reith, D. M., Whyte, I., Carter, G., McPherson, M., & Carter, N. (2004). Risk factors for suicide and other deaths following hospital treated self-poisoning in Australia. *Australian and New Zealand Journal of Psychiatry*, *38*, 520–525.

Remafedi, G., French, S., Story, M., Resnick, M. D., & Blum, R. (1998). The relationship between suicide risk and sexual orientation: Results of a population-based study. *American Journal of Public Health*, *88*, 57–60.

Rivers, L. (1995). *Young person suicide. Guidelines to understanding, preventing and dealing with the aftermath*. Wellington: Special Education Service.

Rodham, K., Hawton, K., & Evans, E. (2004). Reasons for deliberate self-harm: Comparison of self-poisoners and self-cutters in a community sample of adolescents. *Journal of the American Academy of Child and Adolescent Psychiatry*, *43*, 80–87.

Rotheram-Borus, M. J., Piacentini, J., Cantwell, C., Belin, T. R., & Song, J. (2000). The 18-month impact of an emergency room intervention for adolescent female suicide attempters. *Journal of Consulting and Clinical Psychology*, *68*, 1081–1093.

Rotheram-Borus, M. J., Piacentini, J., Miller, S., Graae, F., & Castro-Blanco, D. (1994). Brief cognitive behavioral treatment for adolescent suicide attempters and their families. *Journal of the American Academy of Child and Adolescent Psychiatry*, *33*, 508–517.

Rotheram-Borus, M. J., Piacentini, J., Van Rossem, R., Graae, F., Cantwell, C., Castro-Blanco, D., *et al.* (1996). Enhancing treatment adherence with a specialized emergency room program for adolescent suicide attempters. *Journal of the American Academy of Child and Adolescent Psychiatry*, *35*, 654–663.

Roy, A. (1993). Genetic and biological risk factors for suicide in depressive disorders. *Psychiatric Quarterly*, *64*, 345–358.

Roy, A., Rylander, G., & Sarchiapone, M. (1997). Genetic studies of suicidal behavior. *Psychiatric Clinics of North America*, *20*, 595–611.

Royal Australian and New Zealand College of Psychiatrists. (2004). Australian and New Zealand clinical practice guidelines for the management of adult deliberate self-harm. *Australian and New Zealand Journal of Psychiatry*, *38*, 868–884.

Rubenstein, J. L., Halton, A., Kasten, L., Rubin, C., & Stechler, G. (1998). Suicidal behavior in adolescents: Stress and protection in different family contexts. *American Journal of Orthopsychiatry*, *68*, 274–284.

Rudd, M., Joiner, T. E. Jr., & Rumzek, H. (2004). Childhood diagnoses and later risk for multiple suicide attempts. *Suicide and Life-Threatening Behavior*, *34*, 113–125.

Runeson, B. S., Beskow, J., & Waern, M. (1996). The suicidal process in suicides among young people. *Acta Psychiatrica Scandinavica*, *93*, 35–42.

Russell, S. T., & Joyner, K. (2001). Adolescent sexual orientation and suicide risk: Evidence from a national study. *American Journal of Public Health*, *91*, 1276–1281.

Ryan, N. D. (2005). Treatment of depression in children and adolescents. *Lancet*, *366*, 933–940.

Sansone, R. A., Gaither, G. A., Songer, D. A., & Allen, J. A. (2005). Multiple psychiatric diagnoses and self-harm behavior. *International Journal of Psychiatry in Clinical Practice*, *9*, 41–44.

Schmidtke, A., & Häfner, N. (1988). The Werther effect after television films: New evidence for an old hypothesis. *Psychological Medicine*, *18*, 665–676.

Schmidtke, A., & Schaller, S. (2000). The role of mass media in suicide prevention. In K. Hawton, & K. Van Heeringen (Eds.), *The international handbook of suicide and attempted suicide*. Chichester: Wiley (pp. 675–697).

Schotte, D. E., & Clum, G. A. (1982). Suicide ideation in a college population: A test of a model. *Journal of Consulting and Clinical Psychology*, *50*, 690–696.

Shaffer, D. (2003). *Screening of children at risk in schools*. Paper presented at the XXII World Congress of the International Association for Suicide Prevention, Stockholm, Sweden.

Shaffer, D., & Craft, L. (1999). Methods of adolescent suicide prevention. *Journal of Clinical Psychiatry*, *60*, 70–74.

Shaffer, D., Gould, M. S., Fisher, P., & Trautman, P. (1996). Psychiatric diagnosis in child and adolescent suicide. *Archives of General Psychiatry*, *53*, 339–348.

Shaffer, D., & Pfeffer, C. R. (2001). Practice parameter for the assessment and treatment of children and adolescents with suicidal behavior. *Journal of the American Academy of Child and Adolescent Psychiatry*, *40*, 495–499.

Shaffer, D., Scott, M., Wilcox, H., Maslow, C., Hicks, R., Lucas, C. P., *et al.* (2004). The Columbia Suicide Screen: Validity and reliability of a screen for youth suicide and depression. *Journal of the American Academy of Child and Adolescent Psychiatry*, *43*, 71–79.

Shaffer, D., Vieland, C., Garland, A., Rojas, M., Underwood, M., & Busner, C. (1990). Adolescent suicide attempters: response to suicide-prevention programs. *Journal of the American Medical Association*, *264*, 3151–3155.

Shaw, J., Baker, D., Hunt, I. M., Moloney, A., & Appleby, L. (2004). Suicide by prisoners. National clinical survey. *British Journal of Psychiatry*, *184*, 263–267.

Smith, P. K. (2004). Bullying: Recent developments. *Child and Adolescent Mental Health*, *9*, 98–103.

Sourander, A., Aromaa, M., Pihlakoski, L., Haavisto, A., Rautava, P., Helenius, H., *et al.* (2006). Early predictors of deliberate self-harm among adolescents: A prospective follow-up study from age 3 to age 15. *Journal of Affective Disorders*, *93*, 87–96.

Speckens, A. E. M., & Hawton, K. (2005). Social problem-solving in adolescents with suicidal behaviour: A systematic review. *Suicide and Life-Threatening Behavior*, *35*, 365–387.

Spirito, A., & Boergers, J. (1997). Family therapy techniques with adolescent suicide attempters. *Crisis: Journal of Crisis Intervention and Suicide*, *18*, 106–108.

Spirito, A., Boergers, J., Donaldson, D., Bishop, D., & Lewander, W. (2002). An intervention trial to improve adherence to community treatment by adolescents after a suicide attempt. *Journal of the American Academy of Child and Adolescent Psychiatry*, *41*, 435–442.

Spooren, D. J., Jannes, C., & van Heeringen, K. (1997). Factors influencing the decision for further hospitalisation or in-patient crisis intervention at the psychiatric emergency department of civil hospitals in Belgium. *Journal of Mental Health*, *6*, 399–407.

Stack, S. (1991). Social correlates of suicide by age: media impacts. In A. Leenars (Ed.), *Life span perspectives of suicide: Time-lines in the suicide process* (pp. 187–213). New York: Plenum Press.

Stack, S. (2000). Suicide: a 15-year review of the sociological literature. II. Modernization and social integration perspectives. *Suicide and Life-Threatening Behavior*, *30*, 163–176.

Stack, S. (2003). Media coverage as a risk factor in suicide. *Journal of Epidemiology and Community Health*, *57*, 238–240.

Stack, S., & Wasserman, I. (2005). Race and method of suicide: Culture and opportunity. *Archives of Suicide Research*, *9*, 57–68.

Stanley, B., Gameroff, M. J., Michalson, V., & Mann, J. J. (2001). Are suicide attempters who self-mutilate a unique population? *American Journal of Psychiatry*, *158*, 427–432.

Strober, M., Schmidt-Lackner, S., Freeman, R., Bower, S., Lampert, C., & de Antonio, M. (1995). Recovery and relapse in adolescents with bipolar affective illness: A five year naturalistic, prospective follow-up. *Journal of the American Academy of Child and Adolescent Psychiatry*, *34*, 724–731.

Sultan, A., & O'Sullivan, K. (2001). Psychological disturbances in asylum seekers held in long term detention: A participant observer account. *Medical Journal of Australia*, *175*, 593–596.

Suominen, K., Isometsa, E., Suokas, J., Haukka, J., Achte, K., & Lonnqvist, J. (2004). Completed suicide after a suicide attempt: A 37-year follow-up study. *American Journal of Psychiatry*, *161*, 562–563.

Suris, J. C., Parera, N., & Puig, C. (1996). Chronic illness and emotional distress in adolescence. *Journal of Adolescent Health*, *19*, 153–156.

Swedo, S. E. (1989). Post discharge therapy of hospitalized adolescent suicide attempters. *Journal of Adolescent Health Care*, *10*, 541–544.

Tatz, C. (2001). *Aboriginal suicide is different. A portrait of life and self-destruction.* Canberra: Australian Institute of Aboriginal and Torres Strait Islander Studies.

Thompson, E. A., Mazza, J. J., Herting, J. R., Randell, B. P., & Eggert, L. L. (2005). The mediating roles of anxiety, depression, and hopelessness on adolescent suicidal behaviors. *Suicide and Life-Threatening Behavior*, *35*, 14–34.

Tomori, M., & Zalar, B. (2000). Sport and physical activity as possible protective factors in relation to adolescent suicide attempts. *International Journal of Sport Psychology*, *31*, 405–413.

Townsend, E., Hawton, K., Altman, D. G., Arensman, E., Gunnell, D., Hazell, P., *et al.* (2001). The efficacy of problem-solving treatments after deliberate self-harm: Meta-analysis of randomized controlled trials with respect to depression, hopelessness and improvement in problems. *Psychological Medicine*, *31*, 979–988.

Treatment of Adolescent Depression Study Team. (2004). Fluoxetine, cognitive-behavioral therapy, and their combination for adolescents with depression: Treatment for Adolescents With Depression Study (TADS) randomized controlled trial. *Journal of The American Medical Association*, *292*, 807–820.

US Department of Health and Human Services, Centers for Disease Control and Prevention, & National Center for Health Statistics. (2004). *Health, United States, 2004*. Washington, DC: US Department of Health and Human Services, Centers for Disease Control and Prevention, National Center for Health Statistics.

US Food and Drug Administration. (2004). Suicidality in children and adolescents being treated with antidepressant medications. Retrieved March 23, 2005, from http://www.fda.gov/cder/drug/antidepressants/SSRIPHA200410.htm

Vajda, J., & Steinbeck, K. (2000). Factors associated with repeat suicide attempts among adolescents. *Australian and New Zealand Journal of Psychiatry*, *34*, 437–445.

van Heeringen, K., Jannes, S., Buylaert, W. D. H., de Bacquer, D., & van Remoortel, J. (1995). The management of non-compliance with referral to out-patient and after-care among attempted suicide patients: A controlled intervention study. *Psychological Medicine*, *25*, 963–970.

Vito, E. D., Ladame, F., & Orlandini, A. (1999). Adolescence and personality disorders: Current perspectives on a controversial problem. In J. Derksen, & C. Maffei (Eds.), *Treatment of personality disorders* (pp. 77–95). Milan: Centre for Study of Adolescence.

Wagner, B. M., Aiken, C., Mullaley, P. M., & Tobin, J. J. (2000). Parents' reactions to adolescents' suicide attempts. *Journal of the American Academy of Child and Adolescent Psychiatry*, *39*, 429–436.

Whitlock, J., Powers, J. L., & Eckenrode, J. (2006). The virtual cutting edge: The Internet and adolescent self-injury. *Developmental Psychology*, *42*, 407–417.

Williams, J. M. G., & Pollock, L. R. (2000). The psychology of suicidal behaviour. In K. Hawton, & K. van Heeringen (Eds.), *The international handbook of suicide and attempted suicide* (pp. 79–94). Chichester: Wiley.

Wood, A., Trainor, G., Rothwell, J., Moore, A., & Harrington, R. (2001). Randomized trial of group therapy for repeated deliberate self-harm in adolescents. *Journal of the American Academy of Child and Adolescent Psychiatry*, *40*, 1246–1253.

World Health Organization. (1996). *Multiaxial classification of child and adolescent psychiatric disorders: ICD-10 classification of mental and behavioural disorders in children and adolescents.* New York: Cambridge University Press.

World Health Organization. (2006). Suicide rates per 100 000 per country, year and sex. Retrieved December 15, 2006, from http://www.who.int/mental_health/prevention/suicide_rates/en/print.html

Ybarra, M. L., Alexander, C., & Mitchell, K. J. (2005). Depressive symptomatology, youth Internet use, and online interactions: A national survey. *Journal of Adolescent Health*, *36*, 9–18.

Ystgaard, M., Reinholdt, N. P., Husby, J., & Mehlum, L. (2003). Deliberate self harm in adolescents. *Tidsskr Nor Laegeforen*, *123*, 2241–2245.

41 Eating Disorders

Christopher G. Fairburn and Simon G. Gowers

The term "eating disorders" refers to anorexia nervosa and bulimia nervosa and their variants. These disorders typically develop in adolescence or early adulthood but in some cases they start earlier. They are not distinct conditions; they share much the same psychopathology and many patients migrate between them. The etiology of the eating disorders is complex and ill-understood and, with the exception of bulimia nervosa, there has been limited research on their treatment. Cases that present in childhood or adolescence have a fairly good prognosis, but those that persist into adulthood are generally self-perpetuating and difficult to treat. The prompt detection and treatment of childhood and adolescent cases are of paramount importance.

Classification of Eating Disorders in Childhood and Adolescence

The ICD and DSM schemes for classifying and diagnosing eating disorders are similar and recognize two main conditions: anorexia nervosa and bulimia nervosa. Where the schemes differ is in their classification of eating disorders other than anorexia nervosa and bulimia nervosa. In DSM-IV these states are placed in a single category termed "eating disorder not otherwise specified" (eating disorder NOS), whereas in ICD-10 a number of different eating disorder variants are recognized. In this chapter, the DSM-IV scheme is followed because it is more empirically based than ICD-10 and it is the one generally used in research.

Eating disorders need to be distinguished from the DSM-IV diagnosis "feeding disorder of infancy or early childhood." This refers to a persistent failure to eat adequately resulting in significant failure to gain weight or significant weight loss. The disturbance in eating should not be secondary to a general medical disorder or any other psychiatric condition, and its onset should be before the age of 6 years although typically it is much earlier (see chapter 53). More minor problems with feeding are common, especially in infancy, and faddy eating occurs in over 20% of preschool children. Some of the eating problems seen in late childhood or early adolescence are extensions of these earlier difficulties or variants on them. Various subtypes have been recognized including "food avoidance emotional disorder," "selective eating," "restrictive eating," "food refusal" and "pervasive refusal" (Bryant-Waugh, 2000). In none of these states is there the overevaluation of shape and weight that characterizes anorexia nervosa and bulimia nervosa.

Rutter's Child and Adolescent Psychiatry, 5th edition. Edited by M. Rutter, D. Bishop, D. Pine, S. Scott, J. Stevenson, E. Taylor and A. Thapar. ISBN: 978-1-4051-4549-7.

Diagnostic Criteria

In essence, three features need to be present to make a diagnosis of anorexia nervosa:

1 The overevaluation of shape and weight; that is, judging self-worth largely, or even exclusively, in terms of shape and weight. This is often expressed as an intense fear of becoming fat.

2 The active maintenance of an unduly low body weight (e.g., maintaining a body weight less than 85% of that expected, or a body mass index below the 2nd percentile for age).

3 Amenorrhea (in postpubertal females). The value of the amenorrhea criterion is questionable because the majority of female patients who meet the other two diagnostic criteria are amenorrheic, and those who do menstruate closely resemble those who do not.

Three features also need to be present to make a diagnosis of bulimia nervosa:

1 The overevaluation of shape and weight, as in anorexia nervosa.

2 The presence of recurrent binge eating. A "binge" is an episode of eating during which there is a sense of loss of control and an objectively large amount of food is eaten.

3 The presence of extreme weight-control behavior, such as strict dietary restriction, recurrent self-induced vomiting or marked laxative misuse.

It is also specified that the diagnostic criteria for anorexia nervosa should not be met because otherwise some patients would be eligible to receive both eating disorder diagnoses.

There are no specific diagnostic criteria for eating disorder NOS. Instead, it is a residual category for eating disorders of clinical severity that do not meet the diagnostic criteria for anorexia nervosa or bulimia nervosa. Although neglected until recently, these states are common, both in adults and in children and adolescents. The relationship between the diagnoses anorexia nervosa, bulimia nervosa and eating disorder NOS is illustrated schematically in Fig. 41.1.

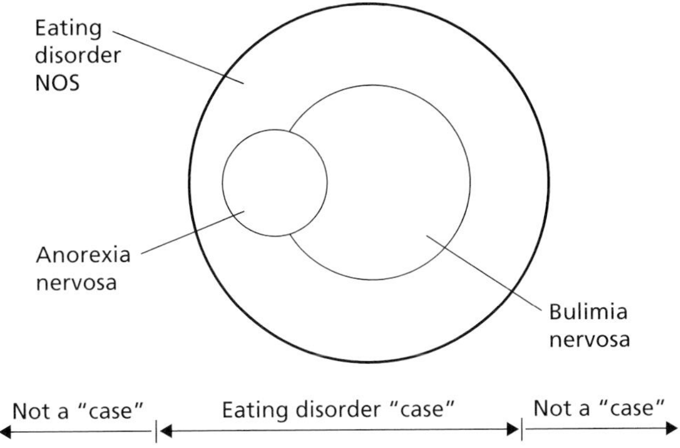

Fig. 41.1 A schematic representation of the relationship between the diagnoses anorexia nervosa, bulimia nervosa and eating disorder not otherwise specified (NOS). From Fairburn and Bohn (2005) with permission.

It has recently been proposed that an additional eating disorder be recognized, termed "binge eating disorder." Because it is somewhat different in character to the other three eating disorders and mainly affects middle-aged adults, it will be discussed separately later in the chapter. Technically, binge eating disorder comes under the rubric of eating disorder NOS.

Applying the diagnostic criteria for anorexia nervosa and bulimia nervosa to the clinical problems seen in children and adolescents poses certain problems. For example, some common clinical presentations do not fit the adult-oriented diagnostic criteria for eating disorders, this being particularly true of "anorexia nervosa" in children and younger adolescents. In this age group a significant number of those who are underweight because of purposeful undereating show no evidence of overconcern about shape or weight: rather, their dietary restriction appears to stem from an overevaluation of controlling eating per se. Strictly speaking, such patients should not be given the diagnosis of anorexia nervosa because a central diagnostic feature is not present. Instead, they should be given the diagnosis eating disorder NOS. Of course, it can be problematic identifying this psychopathology in younger patients because of the difficulty children have describing their thoughts, attitudes and behavior, combined sometimes with a reluctance to do so. Obtaining supplementary information from parents and other informants is essential and can be illuminating. The psychopathology of anorexia nervosa should never be inferred.

Another problem centers on the weight criterion of anorexia nervosa because it is difficult to use with children and younger adolescents. This is for two main reasons: first, adult body mass index thresholds do not apply to younger age groups; and, second, growth may have been stunted. To address these problems it is advisable to compare the patient's current centile for age, gender, weight and height with earlier ones if possible.

The amenorrhea criterion also poses problems in premenarcheal cases who might be expected to have completed their puberty after the disturbance of eating began. In such cases it is best to ignore this feature.

Clinical Features

Anorexia nervosa and bulimia nervosa, and most cases of eating disorder NOS, share a distinctive "core psychopathology" which is essentially the same in females and males, adults and adolescents. This is the overevaluation of shape and weight. Whereas most people evaluate themselves on the basis of their perceived performance in a variety of domains of life (such as the quality of their relationships with their family and friends, their work, their sporting prowess), patients with anorexia nervosa or bulimia nervosa judge their self-worth largely, or even exclusively, in terms of their shape and weight and their ability to control them. This overevaluation of shape and weight results in a pursuit of weight loss – note it is weight loss that is sought, not a specific weight – and an intense fear of weight gain and fatness. Most of the other features of these disorders are secondary to this psychopathology and its consequences (e.g., undereating and being severely underweight). Thus, in anorexia nervosa there is a sustained and determined pursuit of weight loss and, to the extent that this pursuit is successful, this behavior is not seen as a problem. Indeed, it tends to be viewed as an accomplishment and, as a consequence, patients have a limited desire to change. In bulimia nervosa equivalent attempts to restrict food intake are punctuated by repeated episodes of binge eating with the result that patients may describe themselves as "failed anorexics." The great majority of these patients are distressed by their loss of control over eating which makes them easier to engage in treatment, although because of the associated shame and secrecy there is typically a delay of many years before they seek help.

This core psychopathology of anorexia nervosa and bulimia nervosa has other expressions too. Many patients mislabel adverse physical and emotional states as "feeling fat" and equate this with actually being fat. In addition, most repeatedly scrutinize aspects of their shape, focusing on parts that they dislike. This may contribute to them overestimating their size. Others actively avoid seeing their bodies, assuming that they look fat and disgusting. Equivalent behavior is seen with respect to weighing (weight checking) with most patients weighing themselves frequently and as a result becoming preoccupied with trivial day-to-day fluctuations, whereas others actively avoid knowing their weight while nevertheless being highly concerned about it.

Anorexia Nervosa

In anorexia nervosa the pursuit of weight loss is successful in that a very low weight is attained. This is primarily the result of a severe and selective restriction of food intake with foods viewed as fattening being excluded. Generally, there is no true "anorexia" as such. The undereating may also be an expression of other motives including asceticism and competitiveness with others. Some young people engage in a driven type of exercising which also contributes to their weight loss. Self-induced vomiting and other forms of weight-control behavior (such as the misuse of laxatives or diuretics) are practiced by a subgroup, and an overlapping group have episodes of loss of control over eating although the amount eaten is often not objectively large (subjective binge eating). Depressive and anxiety features, irritability, lability of mood, impaired concentration, loss of sexual appetite and obsessional symptoms are frequently present. Typically, these features get worse as weight is lost and improve with weight regain. Interest in the outside world also declines as patients become underweight with the result that most become socially withdrawn and isolated. This too tends to reverse with weight regain.

Bulimia Nervosa

The eating habits of young people with bulimia nervosa resemble those seen in anorexia nervosa. The main distinguishing feature is that the attempts to restrict food intake are punctuated by repeated episodes of binge eating. The amount consumed in these binges varies but is typically 1000–2000 kcal per episode, and their frequency ranges from once or twice a week (the diagnostic threshold) to many times a day. In most cases, each binge is followed by compensatory self-induced vomiting or laxative misuse but there is a subgroup who do not "purge." The weight of most of these patients is in the healthy range (equivalent to a body mass index of 20–25 in an adult) because the effects of the undereating and overeating cancel each other out. As a result, patients with bulimia nervosa do not experience the secondary psychosocial and physical effects of maintaining a very low weight. Depressive and anxiety symptoms are prominent in bulimia nervosa – indeed, more so than in anorexia nervosa – and there is a subgroup who engage in substance misuse or self-injury or both. This subgroup, which is also present among those anorexia nervosa patients who binge eat, is probably overrepresented in specialist treatment centers.

Eating Disorder NOS

The psychopathology of eating disorder NOS closely resembles that seen in anorexia nervosa and bulimia nervosa, albeit the various clinical features are present at somewhat different levels or in different combinations (Fairburn & Bohn, 2005). Many adult cases of eating disorder NOS have had frank anorexia nervosa or bulimia nervosa in the past, their present state being simply the latest expression of an evolving eating disorder. Equivalent information on course has yet to be reported in adolescents.

It is helpful to distinguish two subgroups within eating disorder NOS, although there is no sharp boundary between them. The first comprises cases that closely resemble anorexia nervosa or bulimia nervosa but just fail to meet their diagnostic thresholds (e.g., body weight may be marginally above the limit for anorexia nervosa or the frequency of binge eating may be just too low for a diagnosis of bulimia nervosa). These cases may be classed as "subthreshold" forms of anorexia nervosa or bulimia nervosa, respectively, and should generally be managed as such. In the second group are cases in which the clinical features of anorexia nervosa and bulimia nervosa are combined in a different way to that seen in these two disorders. Such states may be described as "mixed" in character. Other terms have been used to describe the clinical presentations seen in eating disorder NOS including "subclinical" for the former subgroup, a term that is inappropriate given that these states are of clinical severity; and "atypical" or "partial" for the second subgroup. Both the latter terms are problematic; the first because these states are common and the second because of the implication that they are less severe than the full syndromes.

Distribution

There is limited reliable information on the distribution of eating disorders and the data that do exist come from studies of western samples. Virtually nothing is known about the distribution of eating disorders in non-western countries. Within western samples, most is known about the distribution of eating disorders among young adults. There have been few studies of children and adolescents, and the findings to date must therefore be regarded as tentative and imprecise (Commission on Adolescent Eating Disorders, 2005).

What is clear is that anorexia nervosa is rare. Most estimates of the point prevalence of anorexia nervosa come from studies of adolescent girls or young adult women, the group thought to be at greatest risk. Even within this group, the prevalence figures obtained are low at 0–0.9% (Hoek, 2006). Outside this age group, and in boys and men, anorexia nervosa is likely to be even less common. Figures for the incidence of anorexia nervosa are particularly suspect as most are based on cases detected medically. They suggest that anorexia nervosa has become more common over recent decades, and especially so in adolescent females, but the apparent increase could well be because of greater help-seeking, better detection and changes in diagnostic practice rather than any true increase in the incidence of the disorder (van Son, van Hoeken, Bartelds,van Furth, & Hoek, 2006). In clinical samples, anorexia nervosa is the least common of the three eating disorder diagnoses, comprising 10–15% of adult cases. In adolescent samples the proportion is higher (Nicholls, Chater, & Lask, 2000). The ratio of females : males is about 10:1 in adults but it appears to be somewhat lower in adolescents (Doyle & Bryant-Waugh, 2000).

Unlike anorexia nervosa, epidemiological data indicate that bulimia nervosa is more a disorder of early adulthood than adolescence, with most patients being in their twenties (Fairburn, Welch, Doll, Davies, & O'Connor, 1997; Hoek & van Hoeken, 2006). It is more common than anorexia nervosa, in part because the age group at risk is broader (18- to 40-year-old women) and in part because the point prevalence rate is higher (1.0–2.0%). There are no reliable data on the prevalence of bulimia nervosa in boys or men. Clinical experience suggests that bulimia nervosa became considerably more common in the 1970s and 1980s, and limited epidemiological data support this, although there is evidence that the rise has now ceased (van Son, van Hoeken, Bartelds *et al.*, 2006). The explanation for these changes is not clear. What is known is that most cases of bulimia nervosa are not in treatment and the subgroup that is receiving help is atypical in that the eating disorder is more severe and there is greater psychiatric comorbidity (Fairburn, Welch, Norman *et al.*, 1996). Within clinical samples male cases are unusual. Bulimia nervosa comprises about 30–40% of adult eating disorder cases.

The most glaring gap in knowledge about the epidemiology of eating disorders is the total absence of reliable data on the prevalence and incidence of eating disorder NOS in community samples (Hoek, 2006). Studies of adolescents and young adults often report detecting large numbers of people with "partial" or "atypical" syndromes but the status of these cases is unclear in the absence of an agreed definition of eating disorder NOS. What is now well-established is that eating disorder NOS is the most common eating disorder diagnosis among adults, comprising 50–60% of cases (Fairburn & Bohn, 2005) and the same is true of adolescents (Nicholls, Chater, & Lask, 2000). As with anorexia nervosa and bulimia nervosa, it is females who are primarily affected.

Development and Subsequent Course

Eating disorders typically develop in adolescence and therefore in the context of "normative" concerns about shape, weight and eating. Physical self-consciousness is common as adolescents come to terms with the changes in their shape that occur at puberty; early pubertal development in girls being associated with especially high rates of body dissatisfaction. Many children, particularly girls, believe that thinness is important to attractiveness, and academic and social success. Even small children believe that fat is undesirable, and girls have been found to prefer thin rather than fat girls as friends. It is therefore not surprising that dieting is common among adolescent girls. This said, there are distinct differences between the behavior and concerns of teenage girls and the psychopathology of people with eating disorders. For example, teenage dieting tends to be intermittent, flexible and not particularly strict, whereas the dietary restraint and restriction of people with eating disorders are persistent, rigid and extreme. While many teenage girls are dissatisfied with their appearance, few show the core psychopathology of eating disorders (i.e., the judging of their self-worth largely, or even exclusively, in terms of their shape and weight). Also, behaviors such as binge eating (as technically defined), self-induced vomiting, laxative misuse and driven exercising are unusual outside those with a frank eating disorder.

The relationship between normative dieting and the development of an eating disorder is ill-understood (for further consideration of this topic see chapter 13). Whereas many adolescent girls diet, few develop an eating disorder of clinical severity. Controlled community-based risk-factor studies have shown that those who develop anorexia nervosa or bulimia nervosa have not only been exposed to circumstances that are likely to increase their risk of dieting (e.g., presence of dieting and weight concern in the family, and a history of childhood obesity in the case of bulimia nervosa), but they have also raised rates of exposure to risk factors for other psychiatric disorders (e.g., family history of depression, adverse childhood experiences including sexual abuse). In addition, premorbid negative self-evaluation and perfectionism are common (Fairburn, Welch, Dou *et al.*, 1997; Fairburn, Cooper, Doll *et al.*, 1999; Fairburn, Cowen, & Harrison, 1999). Thus, it is thought that dieting and shape concern, together with other general psychiatric vulnerability factors, put people at risk of developing an eating disorder. As yet, there have been no satisfactory prospective studies of the development of eating disorders so the findings of the risk-factor research have not been corroborated (Jacobi, 2005). Longitudinal studies such as the Dunedin multidisciplinary health and development study (Arsenault, Moffitt, Caspi *et al.*, 2000; Silva & Stanton, 1997) have the potential to do this and indeed 1.4% of the females in this large cohort had developed an eating disorder by the age of 21 years. However, such studies have been unable to differentiate between risk factors for dieting (e.g., body dissatisfaction), which is an extremely common behavior of no psychopathological significance, and those for clinical eating disorders, which are uncommon. Fairburn, Cooper, Doll *et al.* (2005) followed almost 3000 16- to 23-year-old dieters over 2 years to determine the characteristics of those who would go on to develop an eating disorder. As expected, only a small proportion of the dieters developed an eating disorder. Not surprisingly, the dieters who developed an eating disorder had more disturbed eating habits and attitudes at baseline than those who did not. Also unsurprising was the fact that several of the features that best identified future cases were features seen in people with eating disorders albeit to a much greater extent (e.g., binge eating, purging and being underweight). Other ominous features were less predictable: eating in secret; preoccupation with food, eating, shape, or weight; fear of losing control over eating; and wanting to have a completely empty stomach.

There are data that suggest that eating disorders are more common than would be expected among models and ballet dancers. It is debatable whether this is as a result of the occupational pressure to be thin, because clinical experience suggests that people who are already concerned about their appearance may be particularly attracted to such careers.

Anorexia Nervosa

Anorexia nervosa generally starts as teenage dieting which becomes progressively more extreme and out of control. Often the disorder is short-lived and self-limiting, or it only requires a brief intervention. This is most typical of young cases with a short history. In other cases, it becomes entrenched and may require intensive treatment. Recent outcome studies in which adolescents have been followed-up after 10 years or more report a good outcome in 49–76% of cases, an intermediate outcome in 11–41%, and a poor outcome in 8–14% (Råstam, Gillberg, & Wentz, 2003; Strober, Freeman, & Morrell, 1997). In adults, less than half of cases have a good outcome (Steinhausen, 2002). This heterogeneity in outcome is often neglected in accounts of the disorder.

Even after successful treatment, some residual features are common, particularly a degree of over concern about shape, weight and eating. In cases that persist a frequent occurrence is the development of binge eating and frank bulimia nervosa. Most prominent among the favorable prognostic factors are an early age of onset and a short history, whereas unfavorable factors include a long history, severe weight loss and vomiting. This said, the prognostic significance of age of onset is inconsistent (Steinhausen, 2002), possibly because the early-onset cases comprise two groups with different outcomes; the prepubertal cases having a poor prognosis whereas the others have a relatively good outcome (Russell, 1992). Anorexia nervosa is the one eating disorder to be associated with a raised mortality rate, anorexia nervosa patients being 12 times more likely to die than women of a similar age in the general population (Keel, Dorer, Eddy *et al.*, 2003). The mortality rate among adolescents is low. Most deaths are either a direct result of medical complications or from suicide.

The outcome in terms of the presence of other psychiatric disorders generally fails to distinguish between those present at the time of diagnosis, which may influence outcome, from those that develop later on. A systematic review of 119 outcome studies found high rates of anxiety disorders and affective disorders at follow-up (Steinhausen, 2002). Difficulties with social and personality functioning are often reported, as are negative physical outcomes such as failure to reach expected height, stunted breast development and reduced bone density. Whereas a range of Axis 1 psychiatric disorders and personality disorders have been reported at long-term follow-up, these appear to be largely absent in those whose eating disorder has fully remitted.

In the longer term, eating disorders may have an impact on pregnancy and motherhood. In those recovering from anorexia nervosa, fertility problems, spontaneous abortion, prematurity and small-for-dates babies are regularly reported, as are elevated rates of infant mortality (Key, Mason, & Bolton, 2000; Zipfel, Lowe, & Herzog, 2003). In bulimia nervosa, symptoms often improve during pregnancy and in the period after birth, because of the mother's attempts to exert behavioral control over her eating for the good of the child. Nevertheless, women with bulimia nervosa are at risk of having small babies and higher rates of Cesarean section.

Concerns have been expressed about the parenting abilities of mothers with eating disorders, particularly with respect to difficulties managing infants' meal times and play. A number have been shown to be intrusive and controlling, and they may have difficulty tolerating messy foods and activities resulting in a strained emotional atmosphere around meal times (Stein, Woolley, & Murray, 2001).

Bulimia Nervosa

Both community and clinic-based studies indicate that bulimia nervosa has a somewhat later age of onset than anorexia nervosa although it usually starts in much the same way: indeed, in about one-quarter of cases the diagnostic criteria for anorexia nervosa are met for a time. Eventually, however, episodes of binge eating begin to interrupt the dietary restriction and as a result body weight rises to normal or near normal levels. The disorder is remarkably self-perpetuating once established. Adult patients generally present with a 5–10-year history of unremitting symptoms, and even 5–10 years after presentation between one-third and half still have an eating disorder of clinical severity although in many cases it has evolved into a form of eating disorder NOS (Keel, Mitchell, Miller, Davis, & Crow, 1999). A large-scale prospective study of cases in the community indicated that they have a similarly poor prognosis (Fairburn, Cooper, Doll, Norman, & O'Connor, 2000). Mortality rate does not appear to be raised in bulimia nervosa (Keel Dorer, Eddy *et al.*, 2003). No consistent predictors of outcome have been identified, although childhood obesity, low self-esteem and personality disturbance are often associated with a worse prognosis. The course of bulimia nervosa in adolescence has not been studied.

Eating Disorder NOS

The course of eating disorder NOS has barely been studied. As with bulimia nervosa, a 5–10-year history of unremitting symptoms is the norm among adult cases with many patients having a history of anorexia nervosa or bulimia nervosa.

When a longitudinal perspective is taken, the distinctiveness of the three eating disorder diagnoses begins to break down. Most patients with an eating disorder migrate between these diagnoses, and from their perspective they have had one evolving eating problem. This temporal movement, together with the fact that anorexia nervosa, bulimia nervosa and eating disorder NOS share much the same distinctive psychopathology, suggests that common mechanisms are involved in the persistence of these disorders (Fairburn, Cooper, & Shafran, 2003). However, the fact that eating disorders do not evolve into other conditions supports the distinctiveness of the diagnostic category as a whole.

Etiology

Research on the etiology of the eating disorders has focused almost exclusively on anorexia nervosa and bulimia nervosa. It is clear that there is a genetic predisposition and a range of environmental risk factors, and there is some information regarding the identity and relative importance of these contributions. However, virtually nothing is known about the individual causal processes involved or how they interact and vary across the development and maintenance of these disorders.

Genetic Factors

Eating disorders and certain associated traits run in families with there being cross-transmission between anorexia nervosa, bulimia nervosa and eating disorder NOS (Strober, Freeman, Lampert, Diamond, & Kaye, 2000). This suggests that there is a shared familial liability. There is a raised prevalence of depression in these families, the pattern of familial transmission being unclear (Lilenfeld, Kaye, Greeno *et al.*, 1998). The prevalence of substance abuse is also increased, especially among the relatives of bulimic probands, but in this case there seems to be no cross-transmission (Lilenfeld, Kaye, Greeno *et al.*, 1998). In addition, there is evidence of familial coaggregation of anorexia nervosa and obsessional and perfectionist traits (Lilenfeld, Kaye, Greeno *et al.*, 1998).

In the absence of adoption studies, twin designs have been used to establish the extent of the genetic contribution to the familiality of eating disorders (Slof-Op 't Landt, van Furth, Meulenbelt *et al.*, 2005). Clinic samples show concordance for anorexia nervosa of around 55% in monozygotic twins and 5% in dizygotic twins, with the corresponding figures for bulimia nervosa being 35% and 30%, respectively (Bulik, Sullivan, Wade, & Kendler, 2000; Fairburn, Cowen, & Harrison, 1999). These findings suggest a significant heritability of anorexia nervosa but not bulimia nervosa. Because clinic-based samples are potentially biased, population-based studies have also been conducted. These have used broader phenotypes because of the relative rarity of these disorders, and varied findings have emerged. As a result there is still uncertainty as to the extent of the genetic contribution to anorexia nervosa and bulimia nervosa, with there being differing point estimates and wide confidence intervals. The same applies to the contributions of individual-specific and shared (common) environmental factors. There is some evidence that the magnitude of the genetic contribution may increase during adolescence (Klump, McGue, & Iacono, 2003).

Given the clear and possibly substantial genetic contribution to both anorexia nervosa and bulimia nervosa, molecular genetic studies have been conducted to identify the underlying loci and genes. Genetic association studies have focused in particular on polymorphisms in 5-HT (serotonin) related genes because this neurotransmitter system is important in the regulation of eating and mood, but a range of other polymorphisms have also been investigated. Despite this, no associations with eating disorders have been clearly replicated or confirmed in a family study or by meta-analysis. There has been one multicenter genome-wide linkage study. It found linkage peaks for anorexia nervosa and bulimia nervosa on chromosomes 1, 4, 10 and 14. A further analysis, which covaried for related behavioral traits, identified a different locus on chromosome 1, as well as loci on chromosomes 2 and 13. All these findings await replication.

Other Risk Factors

Many other risk factors have been implicated in clinic and community-based case–control studies (Commission on Adolescent Eating Disorders, 2005; Jacobi, Hayward, de Zwaan, Kraemer, & Agras, 2004). Satisfactory prospective studies are lacking, in part because of the rarity of these disorders. The main putative risk factors are listed in Table 41.1. These differ in the nature, strength and specificity of their association with individual eating disorders. Some are adverse premorbid experiences of the type associated with many psychiatric disorders (e.g., childhood sexual abuse), there being no specific association with eating disorders. Others are common to anorexia nervosa and bulimia nervosa (e.g., parental concerns about shape and weight; a family history of a frank eating disorder; see chapter 27), whereas others appear to predispose especially to bulimia nervosa (e.g., childhood and parental obesity, early menarche, parental alcoholism). Certain of these factors are likely to operate by sensitizing the person to her or his shape thereby encouraging dieting, an effect that is most likely to be seen in women in western societies in view of the social pressure on them to be slim. Yet other risk factors are character traits, the two most prominent being low self-esteem and perfectionism, the latter being a particularly common antecedent of anorexia nervosa. There have been no studies of protective factors.

Table 41.1 Main putative risk factors for anorexia nervosa and bulimia nervosa. After Fairburn and Harrison (2003).

General factors
Female
Adolescence and early adulthood
Living in a western society

Individual-specific factors
Family history
- Eating disorder of any type
- Depression
- Substance abuse, especially alcoholism (bulimia nervosa)
- Obesity (bulimia nervosa)

Premorbid experiences
- Adverse parenting (especially low contact, high expectations, parental discord)
- Sexual and physical abuse
- Family dieting
- Critical comments about eating, shape or weight from family and others
- Occupational and recreational pressure to be slim (e.g., ballet dancing)

Premorbid characteristics
- Low self-esteem
- Perfectionism (anorexia nervosa and to a lesser extent bulimia nervosa)
- Anxiety disorders (especially social phobia and obsessive-compulsive disorder)
- Obesity (bulimia nervosa)
- Early menarche (bulimia nervosa)

There is limited information on the distribution and form of eating disorders in non-western societies (Becker & Fay, 2006). There is no doubt that eating disorders occur in most societies, but their relative prevalence is not known. Within western societies there is evidence that some ethnic minority groups may be equally at risk of developing an eating disorder as their White peers. Aspects of the psychopathology of eating disorders may differ in non-western cases. For example, it has been noted that Chinese patients with "anorexia nervosa" often do not show the pathognomonic overevaluation of shape and weight; rather, their purposeful weight loss appears to result from other motives. Similarly, there is evidence that British Asian patients have less marked shape concerns than their

British White counterparts. It has been proposed that bulimia nervosa may be more culturally determined than anorexia nervosa and that heritability estimates for bulimia nervosa may therefore show greater cross-cultural variability than those for anorexia nervosa (Keel & Klump, 2003).

Neurobiological Findings

There has been extensive research on the neurobiology of eating disorders. This has mainly focused on the neuropeptide and monoamine (especially 5-HT) systems thought to be central to the physiology of eating and weight regulation (Kaye, Frank, Bailer *et al.*, 2005). Of the various central and peripheral abnormalities reported, many are likely to be secondary to the disturbance of eating and associated weight loss. However, some aspects of 5-HT function remain abnormal after recovery, leading to speculation that there is a trait monoamine abnormality that may predispose to the development of eating disorders or to associated characteristics such as perfectionism. Furthermore, normal dieting in healthy women alters central 5-HT function, providing a potential mechanism by which eating disorders might be precipitated in women vulnerable for other reasons.

Brain imaging studies have identified altered activity in the frontal, cingulate, temporal and parietal cortical regions in both anorexia nervosa and bulimia nervosa, and there is some evidence that these alterations persist after recovery (Kaye, Wagner, Frank, & Bailer, 2006). Whether they are a consequence of the eating disorder (i.e., a "scar") or have somehow contributed to it is not known. It is important to stress that the findings to date have not been consistent. The eating disorder field has somewhat lagged behind others in terms of brain imaging research.

Postulated Psychological Processes

Specific psychological theories have been proposed to account for the development and maintenance of eating disorders. Most influential in terms of treatment have been cognitive–behavioral theories. In brief, these propose that the restriction of food intake that characterizes the onset of many eating disorders has two main origins, both of which may operate in an individual case. The first is a need to feel "in control" of life which gets displaced on to controlling eating. This need for control may be greatest in those who are constitutionally anxious, perfectionist or lacking in self-esteem. The second is an overevaluation of shape and weight in those who have been sensitized to their appearance, either by prior experiences (e.g., childhood obesity, parental concerns about eating) or by the changes in shape that occur during puberty. In both instances, the resulting dietary restriction and weight loss are highly reinforcing. Subsequently, other processes begin to operate and serve to maintain the eating disorder. These differ according to the form of the eating disorder. In patients who are severely underweight certain of the so-called "starvation symptoms" have this effect, particularly the preoccupation with food and eating, heightened fullness because of delayed gastric emptying, and social withdrawal. In patients who are binge eating and vomiting, other maintaining mechanisms operate. For example, rigid dietary restraint increases the likelihood of binge eating which in turn encourages further dietary restraint. Self-induced vomiting, while used to compensate for binge eating, results in the binges becoming larger and more frequent. External processes are important too. In those who are primarily restricting their eating, interpersonal conflict (e.g., family arguments) and other forms of stress (e.g., school examinations) tend to lead to an intensification of the dietary restriction thereby bolstering the person's sense of self-control. In those prone to binge eat, adverse events and negative moods may trigger episodes of binge eating, the binges tending to modulate the negative mood and distract the person from the problem at hand. These processes are described in more detail in cognitive–behavioral accounts of eating disorders (Fairburn, 2006).

Binge Eating Disorder

In comparison to anorexia nervosa and bulimia nervosa, little is known about binge eating disorder. Although it shares with bulimia nervosa the phenomenon of binge eating, its overlap with the other eating disorders is limited: most patients are middle-aged, the gender ratio is less uneven, and the binge eating occurs against the background of a general tendency to overeat rather than dietary restraint (which probably accounts for its strong association with obesity). Furthermore, findings from natural history studies and drug trials suggest that there is a high spontaneous remission rate, unlike the other eating disorders seen in adults. Binge eating disorder does occur in adolescence, generally in combination with obesity, and it is likely to be a risk factor for weight gain. Table 41.2 summarizes current knowledge about the disorder.

Medical Complications and their Management

Most of the physical abnormalities seen in anorexia nervosa are thought to be caused by these patients' disturbed eating habits and the resulting low weight. Hence, the great majority are reversed by treatment focused on establishing healthy eating habits and a normal weight. The principal physical features are listed in Table 41.3. The physical abnormalities found in bulimia nervosa are usually minor unless purging (vomiting or laxative or diuretic misuse) is frequent, in which case there is risk of fluid and electrolyte disturbance. Those patients who vomit frequently are also at risk of dental damage. The physical abnormalities found in eating disorder NOS depend on the nature of the eating disturbance and the patient's weight. There are no established medical complications of binge eating disorder per se (other than those secondary to comorbid obesity).

Most of the medical complications occur with equal frequency in adults and adolescents. Some points need to be stressed,

Table 41.2 Current knowledge about binge eating disorder. After Fairburn and Harrison (2003).

Definition
Recurrent episodes of binge eating in the absence of extreme weight-control behavior. Binge eating disorder is subsumed under the diagnosis eating disorder NOS

Clinical features
Frequent binge eating, much as in bulimia nervosa, but against the background of a general tendency to overeat. Strong association with obesity. By definition, self-induced vomiting and laxative misuse are not present or only occasional. Depressive features and dissatisfaction with shape are present, although they tend to be less severe than in bulimia nervosa

Distribution
Patients typically present in their forties and as many as one-third are male. Prevalence in the community has not been satisfactorily established. Present in 5–10% of adults seeking treatment for obesity

Pathogenesis
Barely studied. Lower exposure to "eating disorder risk factors" than in anorexia nervosa and bulimia nervosa. Nature of relationship with obesity unclear

Course
Little known. Patients typically give long histories of being prone to binge eat, particularly at times of stress, but many also report extended periods free from binge eating. Spontaneous remission rate appears high

Medical complications
None established other than those secondary to comorbid obesity

Response to treatment
In the short term, binge eating disorder appears more treatment-responsive than anorexia nervosa and bulimia nervosa. Notable placebo response rate. Frequency of binge eating declines in response to a variety of pharmacological and psychological treatments, including cognitive–behavior therapy, interpersonal psychotherapy, behavioral weight loss programs and self-help but with little accompanying weight change. No studies of long-term course or outcome

however, when considering adolescents (Commission on Adolescent Eating Disorders, 2005). First, young adolescents have incomplete stores of body fat and other substrates and as a result experience major medical complications after relatively small amounts of weight loss. Second, when anorexia nervosa develops prior to the completion of growth it can result in growth retardation and short stature. This is especially likely in boys because boys grow, on average, for 2 years longer than girls. Catch-up growth can occur with nutritional rehabilitation but nevertheless these adolescents may never reach their height potential. Third, pubertal delay frequently occurs among those who develop the disorder prior to the completion of puberty. Weight gain and the establishment of healthy eating habits usually result in the resumption of spontaneous menstruation but in some cases the amenorrhea may be prolonged. Fourth, the osteopenia and osteoporosis of anorexia nervosa are especially relevant to this age group because adolescence is a critical time for bone mass acquisition. Those who develop anorexia nervosa during adolescence are unlikely to reach their optimal peak bone mass with the consequence that they may be at heightened fracture risk for many years even if they recover from the eating disorder. The underlying pathophysiology is ill-understood and there is uncertainty over the best form of treatment. Restoration of healthy eating habits and weight, and an adequate diet, and with them the resumption of spontaneous menstruation, are of central importance. It is also usual to prescribe calcium supplements, generally given as a multimineral preparation. Hormone replacement therapy is not recommended because there is no evidence that it is effective and there is a risk that it might cause premature closure of the epiphyses.

The panoply of physical abnormalities seen in the eating disorders can cloud thinking about diagnosis and management. The diagnosis of an eating disorder is made on positive grounds by using the history and mental state examination to detect the characteristic behavioral and attitudinal features, not by simply ruling out possible physical causes. No laboratory tests are required to make the diagnosis and, unless there are positive reasons to suspect the presence of physical disease, no tests are required to exclude other medical disorders. In general, the management of any physical abnormalities should focus on the correction of the eating disorder. However, life-threatening complications must be addressed and the patient's nutritional state needs to be optimized.

Table 41.3 Principal physical features of anorexia nervosa. After Fairburn and Harrison (2003).

Physical symptoms
Heightened sensitivity to cold
Gastrointestinal symptoms (e.g., constipation, fullness after eating, bloatedness)
Dizziness and syncope
Amenorrhea (in females not taking an oral contraceptive); low sexual appetite; infertility
Poor sleep with early morning wakening

Physical signs
Emaciation; stunted growth and failure of breast development (if prepubertal onset)
Dry skin; fine downy hair (lanugo) on the back, forearms and side of the face; in patients with hypercarotenemia, orange discoloration of the skin of the palms and soles
Swelling of parotid and submandibular glands (especially in bulimic patients)
Erosion of inner surface of front teeth (perimylolysis) in those who vomit frequently
Cold hands and feet; hypothermia
Bradycardia; orthostatic hypotension; cardiac arrhythmias (especially in underweight patients and those with electrolyte abnormalities)
Dependent edema (complicating the evaluation of body weight)
Weak proximal muscles (elicited as difficulty rising from a squatting position)

Abnormalities on physical investigation
Endocrine
Low LH, FSH and estradiol
Low T3, T4 in low normal range, normal TSH ("low T3 syndrome")
Mild elevation of plasma cortisol
Elevated growth hormone
Severe hypoglycemia (rare)
Low leptin (but possibly higher than would be expected for body weight)

Cardiovascular
ECG abnormalities (especially in those with electrolyte disturbance): conduction defects, especially prolongation of the Q-T interval, of major concern

Gastrointestinal
Delayed gastric emptying
Decreased colonic motility (secondary to chronic laxative misuse)
Acute gastric dilatation (rare, secondary to binge eating or excessive refeeding)

Hematological
Moderate normocytic normochromic anemia
Mild leucopenia with relative lymphocytosis
Thrombocytopenia

Other metabolic abnormalities
Hypercholesterolemia
Increased serum carotene
Hypophosphatemia (exaggerated during refeeding)
Dehydration
Electrolyte disturbance (varied in form; present in those who vomit frequently or misuse large quantities of laxatives or diuretics): vomiting – metabolic alkalosis and hypokalemia; laxative misuse – metabolic acidosis, hyponatremia, hypokalemia

Other abnormalities
Osteopenia and osteoporosis (with heightened fracture risk)
Enlarged cerebral ventricles and external cerebrospinal fluid spaces (pseudoatrophy)

ECG, electrocardiogram; FSH, follicle-stimulating hormone; LH, luteinizing hormone; TSH, thyroid-stimulating hormone.

Management of Eating Disorders

Research Evidence

There has been very little research on the treatment of anorexia nervosa but most of the work that has been carried out has concerned adolescents. There has been much more research on the treatment of bulimia nervosa but so far it has focused exclusively on adults (Commission on Adolescent Eating Disorders, 2005; National Institute for Clinical Excellence, 2004).

One general point is worth stressing at the outset. Treatment outcome among adolescents with anorexia nervosa is generally good, in marked contrast with that amongst adults (Deter, Schellberg, Köpp, Friederich, & Herzog, 2005). This is probably an inherent property of the disorder in these two age groups rather than a reflection of the potency of the treatments used. Adolescents with anorexia nervosa tend to have had the disorder for a very short time – often little more than a year – whereas adults generally have a history of 5 or more years of unremitting symptoms. Thus, many of the maintaining mechanisms that obstruct change in the more enduring cases may not yet be operating in younger patients with the result that they are more responsive to treatment. The same is likely to be true of adolescent cases of bulimia nervosa and eating disorder NOS. Accordingly, priority should be given to the detection and treatment of eating disorders in adolescence in order to prevent them becoming established and progressively more treatment-resistant.

Anorexia Nervosa

There is a range of treatment options for anorexia nervosa. There are various treatment settings, the main ones being out-patient, day patient (partial hospitalization) and in-patient treatment; and within these settings a variety of interventions may be provided, pharmacological or psychological or both. To complicate matters, patients may move from one setting to another, and within any one setting often more than one treatment is employed.

There is no empirical evidence to support the use of any one treatment setting over any other in terms of treatment outcome. There has been just one attempt to randomize patients to different treatment settings and, unfortunately, the comparison was compromised by the unsurprising finding that many patients randomized to in-patient treatment did not want it.

In-patient treatment is used differently in different places; for example, it is common in some countries but unusual in others, and length of stay also varies markedly. Such differences are not evidence-based as in-patient treatment has received scant research attention. Even the most basic questions about in-patient treatment have not been adequately formulated, let alone addressed. For example, not only are the indications for hospitalization not established, but the specific goals are not agreed nor is it known how best to achieve them. Also, it is not clear whether the indications, goals and treatments should differ for adolescents and adults. At best, there is modest evidence from cohort studies to support a focus on eating and an emphasis on weight regain. Comparisons of flexible behavioral programs with more rigid ones have either yielded no significant differences in the rate of weight regain or have favored the more flexible regimes. There is no evidence that drug treatment significantly enhances weight regain.

Even less is known about day patient treatment. Again, the indications are not agreed and the goals not established. It is not clear whether day patient treatment is best viewed as a less expensive alternative to in-patient treatment, as an intensive form of out-patient treatment, or as a distinct modality with particular strengths and weaknesses.

Whatever the place of in-patient and day patient treatment, out-patient treatment is the mainstay of the treatment of anorexia nervosa. Out-patient treatment is the sole treatment for many patients, and even if patients receive in-patient or day patient treatment, it is usually followed by out-patient treatment.

Turning to the form of treatment provided, there is no evidence to support the use of drugs in the treatment of anorexia nervosa. An initial report on young adults suggested that fluoxetine reduced the rate of relapse following in-patient treatment but a subsequent well-conducted two-center study, again on young adults, failed to replicate the finding (Walsh, Kaplan, Attia *et al.*, 2006). Nor is there evidence to support any specific psychological treatment. It is widely thought that there is good evidence to support the use of family therapy to treat adolescents with the disorder. This is not the case.

There have been two comparisons of family therapy with another form of treatment. In the first, Russell, Szmukler, Dare, & Eisler (1987) compared 1 year of an eating disorder-focused form of family therapy with 1 year of supportive psychotherapy in patients who had just been discharged from a specialist in-patient unit (mean age 16.6 years, mean duration of eating disorder 1.2 years). The family therapy studied has since come to be known as the "Maudsley method" (Lock, le Grange, Agras, & Dare, 2001). The results favored the family therapy, both at the end of treatment and 5 years later (Eisler, Dare, Russell *et al.*, 1997; Russell, Szmukler, Dare *et al.*, 1987). The first study involved a comparison of a treatment similar to the Maudsley method with a psychodynamically oriented treatment in which the adolescent patients were seen individually with occasional supportive sessions for their parents (Robin, Siegel, Moye *et al.*, 1999). The outcome of both groups was good, both at the end of treatment and 1 year later. There was one statistically significant difference between them; in terms of increase in body mass index the patients in the family therapy condition did better. However, it is not possible to attribute this finding to the family therapy as many of the patients were hospitalized during their treatment and this was especially common among those who received family therapy.

In summary, only two studies have compared family therapy with another form of treatment and the findings of the second are uninterpretable. Thus, the case for favoring family therapy over other forms of treatment rests on a single study (Russell, Szmukler, Dare *et al.*, 1987) which involved just 21 patients – 10 of whom received family therapy – all of whom had recently been discharged from a specialist in-patient unit. This is a very modest body of data and one of questionable relevance to routine out-patient treatment. It must also be noted that the superiority of the family therapy over the supportive psychotherapy condition might not have been because of the involvement of the patient's family because there was another important difference between the two treatments: the family therapy placed great emphasis on getting patients to eat well and maintain a healthy weight, whereas there was nothing like the same focus on eating and weight in the supportive psychotherapy condition.

In addition to these two studies, there have been comparisons of different ways of administering the Maudsley method. Their findings are also inconclusive, in part because the studies have been small in size and therefore underpowered. Interestingly, there is no evidence that seeing the family together is superior to seeing them separately from the young person (Eisler, Dare, Hodes *et al.*, 2000). There has also been a larger-scale comparison of a 6-month 10-session version of the treatment with a 12-month 20-session version (Lock, Agras, Bryson, & Kraemer, 2005). They were equally effective.

Clearly, what are needed are adequately powered comparisons of the Maudsley method of family therapy with other forms of treatment, both individual and family-based. It is plausible that family therapy might best suit younger adolescents while a more individually focused form of treatment (such as cognitive–behavior therapy), but one nevertheless involving the family, might be a better option for older patients.

Bulimia Nervosa

There have been no studies of the treatment of adolescents with bulimia nervosa. However, there have been over 50 randomized controlled trials evaluating treatments for adults and the main findings are reasonably consistent (National Institute for Clinical Excellence, 2004). Although almost all the trials have been efficacy rather than effectiveness studies, there are good reasons to think that their findings are relevant to most psychiatric settings. Three main findings have emerged. First, the great majority of patients can be managed on an out-patient basis. Second, the most effective treatment is a specific type of cognitive–behavior therapy that focuses on modifying the behavior and ways of thinking that are thought to maintain these patients' eating disorder (Fairburn, 2006; Fairburn, Marcus, & Wilson, 1993). The treatment typically involves about 20 individual treatment sessions over 5 months. The third finding is that antidepressant drugs have an "antibulimic" effect. They often result in a rapid decline in the frequency of binge eating and purging, and an improvement in mood, but meta-analysis indicates that the effect is not as great as that obtained with cognitive–behavior therapy (National Institute for Clinical Excellence, 2004) and, more importantly, clinical experience and the limited research evidence suggest that it is often not sustained (Walsh, Hadigan, Devlin, Gladis, & Roose, 1991). None of these data have come from studies of adolescents.

Three less robust findings have also emerged. First, combining cognitive–behavior therapy with antidepressant drugs results in few consistent benefits over cognitive–behavior therapy alone. Second, data from two trials suggest that "interpersonal psychotherapy" (IPT), a well-known focal psychotherapy (Weissman, Markowitz, & Klerman, 2000), may be as effective as cognitive–behavior therapy but it takes considerably longer to work. Third, simple, largely behavioral treatments (including forms of self-help) that include elements of cognitive–behavior therapy may help a subset of patients although they are unlikely to be sufficient for the majority.

In the absence of research focused on adolescents, the assumption is that cognitive–behavior therapy, suitably modified (Wilson & Sysko, 2006), is likely to be the most effective form of treatment. A possible alternative is interpersonal psychotherapy, an adolescent version of which exists (Mufson, Dorta, Moreau, & Weissman, 2004). For younger adolescents eating disorder-focused family therapy is the other obvious treatment option.

Eating Disorder NOS

There have been no studies of the treatment of eating disorder NOS, either in adults or adolescents. This is a remarkable omission given that this is the most common eating disorder diagnosis.

Clinical Recommendations

Assessment

While the general principles of assessment in child and adolescent psychiatry apply to patients with eating disorders, it is worth emphasizing the importance of certain aspects of the assessment.

Frequently, young people with eating disorders are at a developmental stage when they are negotiating independence from their parents. A significant proportion will be having difficulty with this developmental stage, either attempting to exert their independence and rule parents out of having a role in their lives or else behaving in an immature dependent fashion. It is generally helpful to take an approach that is respectful and age-appropriate but recognizes the role of parents in providing a developmental history, their perspective on the problem and their potential role in treatment. At the same time, whatever the age of the patient, it is important to acknowledge overtly their own perspective. Within any assessment, time should be set aside to enable a sympathetic understanding of the young person's point of view and a full assessment of their mental state including cognition and risk. This can only be conducted with the young person alone. Thus, there needs to be an individual assessment in addition to a joint interview with the parents. Some advocate a separate parental interview but the gains in terms of information gathering may be offset by the alienation of the young person and potential breaches of confidentiality. Attention to the young person's physical state is also important if there is a risk that it might be affected.

Management of Anorexia Nervosa

Effective management comprises interventions for both the psychological and physical aspects of the disorder. The relative importance of each will depend on the degree of physical ill health, but it is important to keep in mind that the physical features are merely consequences of the underlying illness and that restoration of physical health alone cannot be expected to cure the disorder. When anorexia nervosa has been present for any length of time, adverse social and educational consequences generally follow and so a rehabilitative component will also need to be added to the treatment plan. The psychological features include specific abnormal cognitions related to weight and shape and, commonly, non-specific negative cognitions of ineffectiveness, low mood, guilt and worthlessness. Many young people also have regressed to an immature developmental stage in which they have relinquished age-appropriate responsibility and autonomy. Therefore there is a danger in addressing the physical aspects of the condition that steps by parents and clinicians to take behavioral control will exacerbate the psychological disturbance.

Generally, treatment should be planned to span at least 6 months and only a minority will have fully recovered in 1 year. In other than the mildest cases, treatment should be offered by services experienced in the management of eating disorders. Two important early considerations are when to admit to hospital and the relative importance of family versus individual therapies.

A distinction should be drawn between medical admission to address physical complications and psychiatric admission to treat the underlying disorder. The former is clearly indicated in situations of medical instability, when short-term pediatric management usually benefits from a degree of psychiatric liaison. Although lengthy psychiatric admission is offered in many countries other than the USA, combining psychological therapies with full weight restoration, evidence for the effectiveness of this very expensive approach is lacking.

Education is an essential element of treatment. The young person and his or her parents need to be educated about eating disorders and their management. Often, efforts to give the young person an understanding of the disorder, particularly if the young person is seen alone, make it possible to effectively engage them as a patient. It is often useful if the clinician attempts to empathize with the young person's experience and how it has led to the eating disorder.

When outlining the treatment plan, it is important to highlight the role of the patient and generally the family in bringing about change. At one end of the spectrum, the parents' role may be merely to support the young person and encourage their out-patient attendance. At the other extreme (as in the Maudsley method; Lock, le Grange, Agras *et al.*, 2001), their involvement in meal production and supervision may be crucial. Obtaining the young person's motivation and co-operation can be extremely difficult and it may be necessary to address this continually during treatment. An approach that aims to work with, rather than against the young person, empathizes with their predicament and fears, and instills hope that change will lead to benefits while acknowledging the costs, is generally most productive. In all but the mildest cases, a multidisciplinary approach is recommended. The treating team will usually comprise a psychiatrist, an individual psychotherapist (of whatever discipline), a family therapist, a physician and a nutritionist/dietitian. Specialist in-patient and day patient services may include a physiotherapist, occupational or creative therapists, and teachers.

The management plan will vary for younger children and also for boys. Talking therapies must be age-appropriate and will often use art and other non-verbal approaches with younger patients. Parents of younger children will have a greater role in supporting treatment, particularly in meal planning and supervised eating. In older adolescents, recovery generally implies restoration to a premorbid state of physical health (i.e., return of weight and hormonal functioning against a background of completed growth). In pubescent girls, treatment-imposed weight gain may precipitate the menarche, with all that that implies experientially. A recovering prepubertal child will face the uncertainty of a physical and social identity that has not been experienced before. In a number of respects this will mean "growing up," and addressing the attendant anxieties that may have played a part in the original development of the condition. A related issue concerns the need to ensure that the "recovered" child or adolescent does not "stand still" – that is to say a 13-year-old restored to a healthy weight might be considered recovered but their health will decline if they are unable to keep pace with the expected trajectories of healthy physical and social development.

The presentation and management of boys are essentially similar to those of girls. However, boys will be expected to continue growth into their late teenage years and ongoing supervision should ensure that their growth potential is maintained. Some boys are uncertain about their sexual identity and such anxieties may be exacerbated by attending a service that predominantly caters for girls. Services should include staff who are familiar with, and comfortable discussing, the common developmental concerns of pubertal boys.

Physical Management

Because of the potentially irreversible effect of anorexia nervosa on adolescent growth and development, the threshold for medical intervention should be lower in children and adolescents than adults. Furthermore, medical complications can occur early in younger subjects before evidence of significant weight loss. Prepubertal children are at particular risk of physical complications of starvation because of their relative lack of body fat and a tendency to dehydrate quickly. Routine blood count, electrolyte levels and liver and thyroid function should be measured. Assessment of serum calcium, phosphate, vitamin B_{12} and folate is indicated in severe starvation and during refeeding.

Height and weight should be plotted on centile charts and if possible related to premorbid values. Heart rate and blood pressure should be measured and an electrocardiogram performed if cardiac function is compromised or antidepressant treatment proposed. Pubertal status may be assessed by Tanner staging, which provides mean ages and ranges for the development of secondary sexual characteristics. Concerns arise if this staging is more than two standard deviations behind the mean. Ultrasonography can confirm (and enable monitoring of) ovarian function, although an overemphasis on physical progress should be avoided.

When treating the malnourished young person, care should be taken to avoid the refeeding syndrome, a potentially life-threatening disturbance of fluid and electrolyte balance which can follow sudden increases in nutritional intake in those who have been in a state of starvation. This can be achieved by regular monitoring of heart rate, orthostatic vital signs and serum electrolytes including phosphorus, glucose, magnesium and potassium, although total body electrolytes may be depleted even in the presence of normal serum levels. Note that the refeeding syndrome occurs more commonly with parenteral than enteral feeding. There is a lack of consensus regarding oral feeding requirements. A weight gain of around 1 kg per week is generally recommended for in-patients and 0.5 kg per week for out-patients. After an initial safe weight has been achieved, the young person's food intake should be adjusted to ensure that growth is in keeping with normal weight and height trajectories.

Weight restoration should utilize the least invasive procedures possible and should be provided within a caring age-appropriate setting. Nasogastric feeding should only be resorted to in the face of persistent refusal to eat normally. Strict behavioral regimes in which young people have to earn privileges through eating and weight gain are not desirable or acceptable as they militate against the therapeutic alliance and there is no evidence that these approaches work, other than by achieving short-term weight gain. In the long term, undue coercion either may be perceived by the young person as a recapitulation of abuse or neglect that they may have suffered previously or it may reinforce low self-esteem and feelings of ineffectiveness, both of which are common antecedents of anorexia nervosa.

Psychological Treatment

All young people should have individual psychological therapies to address their specific and non-specific psychopathology. Such features as clinical perfectionism, mood disorder and peer relationship difficulties can usefully be addressed. The behavioral aspects of treatment should also be tackled, hence a cognitive–behavioral approach rather than a supportive or insight-orientated one is to be preferred. The practical aspects of treatment are often ineffective unless the parents are also involved in establishing behavioral control. Parental responsibility for the behavioral aspects of treatment (e.g., dietary planning, involvement in sports), should be age-appropriate and therefore greater with younger patients. Family interventions may also be useful in tackling family communication and relationship problems but it should be noted that the outcomes of family interventions for families with high expressed emotion have to date been poor.

Pharmacological Treatment

There is no evidence to support the use of medication in the treatment of eating disorders. Medication may be indicated to treat comorbid disorders, especially depression and obsessive-compulsive disorder. Depressive symptoms are a feature of starvation and so are common in anorexia nervosa. This said, there is a subgroup of adult patients who have a true comorbid clinical depression as indicated by a broad range of depressive features (e.g., hopelessness, thoughts of death and dying, pathological guilt, decreased energy and drive). With such patients, antidepressant medication is indicated. In adolescents in whom "biological" symptoms are less common, the role of antidepressants is less clear and major concerns exist about unwanted effects. Fluoxetine is currently the only antidepressant recommended for first-line use in adolescents in most countries and is sometimes used on empirical grounds. Minor tranquillizers are sometimes used symptomatically to reduce high levels of anxiety, particularly around eating.

Management of Bulimia Nervosa

As in the treatment of anorexia nervosa, treatment should include motivational aspects, attention to physical complications, and cognitive and behavioral elements. Young people may benefit from their parents' involvement, both to assist in meal planning and other practical issues, and also to enable parents to better understand the condition and the treatment plan. As young people rarely present with bulimia nervosa before 16 years of age, the involvement of parents will usually be at the young person's discretion.

Psychological Treatment

Although there have been no adequate studies of psychological treatments for adolescents with bulimia nervosa, it seems appropriate to offer them the empirically supported treatments developed for adults, specifically cognitive–behavior therapy, with appropriate modifications for adolescents (Wilson & Sysko, 2006). The main modifications are the use of age-appropriate written material, the involvement of the family (chiefly the parents), and the addressing of the developmental challenges faced by this age group (e.g., peer relationships, education, use of alcohol, rebellion and conformity). Parents may benefit from psychoeducation delivered either face-to-face, through reading material or by attending a parental support group. Group parental meetings are particularly helpful when the young person declines to involve the parents in their treatment.

Pharmacological Treatment

Arguably, this is not indicated because the research on adults indicates that the beneficial effects are less than those obtained with cognitive–behavior therapy and they tend not to be maintained. They could be used as an initial step in management. Recent findings suggest that if patients do not show an early response (within 2 weeks), they are unlikely to benefit (Walsh, Kaplan, Attia *et al.*, 2006).

Physical Management

The main physical complications of bulimia nervosa are disturbances of fluid and electrolyte balance resulting from vomiting and laxative misuse. Hypokalemia should be treated with oral potassium supplements. Advice on dental hygiene should be offered to avoid the effects of acid erosion. Psychiatric admission to hospital is not recommended, but on rare occasions medical admission may be required to correct physical complications (e.g., when bulimia nervosa coexists with diabetes mellitus).

Management of Eating Disorder NOS

The UK NICE guidelines addressed the absence of any research on the treatment of eating disorder NOS by recommending that clinicians follow bulimia nervosa treatment guidelines with cases resembling bulimia nervosa and anorexia nervosa guidelines with cases resembling anorexia nervosa (National Institute for Clinical Excellence, 2004). The trouble with this recommendation is that most cases within eating disorder NOS are of the "mixed" variety rather than subthreshold forms of anorexia nervosa or bulimia nervosa. Of relevance to this gap in knowledge is the development of a new "transdiagnostic" form of cognitive–behavior therapy designed to be suitable for the full range of clinical eating disorders seen in clinical practice including eating disorder NOS (Fairburn, 2006; Fairburn, Cooper, & Shafran, 2003). Emerging evidence suggests that it is as effective as a treatment for eating disorder NOS as it is for bulimia nervosa. This treatment is beginning to be used with adolescents incorporating modifications of the type outlined above.

Ethical and Legal Issues

Eating disorders are unusual amongst presentations in Child and Adolescent Psychiatry in that they are potentially life-threatening and may have very serious physical and psychosocial consequences if effective treatment is not provided. Given that young people with eating disorders are often reluctant to seek or accept treatment, practitioners need effective ethical and legal guidelines in order to make treatment decisions (Foreman, 2006).

Where at all possible attempts should be made to establish a therapeutic alliance with the young person, both in order to achieve consent to treatment on ethical grounds and also because effectiveness of treatment depends in large part on the patient's cooperation. In the former case, many countries permit parents or those with parental authority to consent to treatment on their child's behalf even in the face of the child's opposition. In England and Wales, parents may consent on their children's behalf up to the age of 18 but different countries operate different age limits. In considering the desirability of obtaining the young person's consent, a distinction should be drawn between treatment directed at reducing risk from the physical consequences of the eating disorder and treatment of the disorder itself. Physical aspects of treatment (e.g., refeeding) may be provided in extreme situations without the young person's consent and may on occasion be life-saving. However, the psychological and behavioral aspects of the disorder require psychological interventions. While family interventions can proceed to some extent without the young person's agreement, individual psychotherapy requires the active participation of the patient if it is to be effective.

On occasion young people with anorexia nervosa decline treatment and clinicians have to decide whether to proceed with treatment against the patient's will. Rarely, similar considerations apply to extreme cases of bulimia nervosa (e.g., when it is combined with diabetes mellitus). In general, the decision surrounds the desirability of admission to hospital. Given the relatively poor outcome of in-patient treatment for anorexia nervosa in terms of producing full and lasting recovery and the probable poorer outcome in those opposed to treatment, this step should probably only be taken in cases where the child is in acute medical danger. In the UK, there are three potential approaches to the compulsory treatment of young people under the age of 18:

1 Treatment on the basis of parental consent;
2 Treatment under the Mental Health Act (1983); and
3 Treatment under the Children Act (1989; see chapter 8).

Legislation differs between countries but a number of principles underlying the choice apply. Parental consent is often the appropriate framework to employ, particularly in younger patients and in the short term. In many cases, the young person's opposition will diminish in the early days of an admission once attempts have been made to engage them and they feel safe within the treatment setting. Nevertheless, in these cases the young person's lack of initial agreement to treatment should be recorded, along with the legal basis for proceeding. Where the young person's opposition is not readily overcome, is persistent, leads to absconding or requires active treatment against his or her wishes (e.g., nasogastric feeding), consideration should be given to using mental health legislation to provide the basis for treatment.

Prevention of Eating Disorders

From conceptual and methodological points of view there are many difficulties to overcome when considering how to develop and test means of preventing eating disorders (Commission on Adolescent Eating Disorders, 2005; Piran, Levine, & Steiner-Adair, 1999). First, there are no substantiated modifiable risk factors. As a result there are no clear targets for preventive interventions. Second, eating disorders are uncommon, with the consequence that to demonstrate that an intervention was effective would require a study on a huge scale. To get round this problem researchers have focused on modifying dieting and concerns about shape and weight. The trouble with this strategy is that these phenomena, while of interest and possible concern, have only a loose relationship to eating disorders of clinical severity. The studies themselves have had other shortcomings. Sample sizes have been relatively small, assessment measures weak and follow-up periods short. As a result of these and other problems, little is known.

The interventions tested so far have mostly been "universal" interventions rather than "targeted" ones, and they have generally taken place in schools. To an extent some have had limited success in that they have increased knowledge about eating disorders and healthy weight regulation, but few have altered attitudes or actual behavior even in the short term. An unmet challenge is how to integrate eating disorder-focused preventive interventions – which generally aim to reduce dieting and concerns about shape and weight – with those targeted at the prevention of obesity, a more pressing health problem.

Acknowledgments

CGF is supported by a Principal Research Fellowship (046386) from the Wellcome Trust.

References

Arsenault, L., Moffitt, T. E., Caspi, A., Taylor, P. J., Silva, P. A. (2000). Mental disorders and violence in a total birth cohort: Results from the Dunedin Study. *Archives of General Psychiatry*, *57*, 979–986.

Becker, A. E., & Fay, K. (2006). Sociocultural issues and eating disorders. In S. Wonderlich, J. E. Mitchell, M. de Zwaan, & H. Steiger (Eds.), *Annual review of eating disorders*, Part 2 (pp. 35–63). Oxford: Radcliffe.

Bryant-Waugh, R. (2000). Overview of the eating disorders. In B. Lask & R. Bryant-Waugh (Eds.), *Anorexia nervosa and related eating disorders in childhood and adolescence* (2nd edn., pp. 27–40). Hove: Psychology Press.

Bulik, C. M., Sullivan, P. F., Wade, T. D., & Kendler, K. S. (2000). Twin studies of eating disorders: A review. *International Journal of Eating Disorders*, *27*, 1–20.

Commission on Adolescent Eating Disorders. (2005). Eating disorders. In D. L. Evans, E. B. Foa, R. E. Gur, H. Hendin, C. P. O'Brien, M. E. P. Seligman, *et al.* (Eds.), *Treating and preventing adolescent mental health disorders* (pp. 257–332). New York: Oxford University Press.

Deter, H. C., Schellberg, D., Köpp, W., Friederich, H. C., & Herzog, W. (2005). Predictability of a favourable outcome in anorexia nervosa. *European Psychiatry*, *20*, 165–172.

Doyle, J., & Bryant-Waugh, R. (2000). Epidemiology. In B. Lask, & R. Bryant-Waugh (Eds.), *Anorexia nervosa and related eating disorders in childhood and adolescence* (2nd edn., pp. 41–61). Hove: Psychology Press.

Eisler, I., Dare, C., Hodes, M., Russell, G., Dodge, E., & le Grange, D. (2000). Family therapy for adolescent anorexia nervosa: The results of a controlled comparison of two family interventions. *Journal of Child Psychology and Psychiatry and Allied Disciplines*, *41*, 727–736.

Eisler, I., Dare, C., Russell, G. F. M., Szmukler, G., leGrange, D., & Dodge, E. (1997). Family and individual therapy in anorexia nervosa: A 5-year follow-up. *Archives of General Psychiatry*, *54*, 1025–1030.

Fairburn, C. G. (2006). *Cognitive behavior therapy for eating disorders*. New York: Guilford Press.

Fairburn, C. G., & Bohn, K. (2005). Eating disorder NOS (EDNOS): an example of the troublesome "not otherwise specified" (NOS) category in DSM-IV. *Behaviour Research and Therapy*, *43*, 691–701.

Fairburn, C. G., Cooper, Z., Doll, H. A., & Davies, B. A. (2005). Identifying dieters who will develop an eating disorder: A prospective population-based study. *American Journal of Psychiatry*, *162*, 2249–2255.

Fairburn, C. G., Cooper, Z., Doll, H. A., Norman, P., & O'Connor, M. (2000). The natural course of bulimia nervosa and binge eating disorder in young women. *Archives of General Psychiatry*, *57*, 659–665.

Fairburn, C. G., Cooper, Z., Doll, H. A., & Welch, S. L. (1999). Risk factors for anorexia nervosa: Three integrated case–control comparisons. *Archives of General Psychiatry*, *56*, 468–476.

Fairburn, C. G., Cooper, Z., & Shafran, R. (2003). Cognitive behaviour therapy for eating disorders: a "transdiagnostic" theory and treatment. *Behaviour Research and Therapy*, *41*, 509–528.

Fairburn, C. G., Cowen, P. J., & Harrison, P. J. (1999). Twin studies and aetiology of eating disorders. *International Journal of Eating Disorders*, *26*, 349–358.

Fairburn, C. G., Marcus, M. D., & Wilson, G. T. (1993). Cognitive–behavioral therapy for binge eating and bulimia nervosa: A comprehensive treatment manual. In C. G. Fairburn, & G. T. Wilson (Eds.), *Binge eating: Nature, assessment and treatment* (pp. 361–404). New York: Guilford Press.

Fairburn, C. G., Welch, S. L., Doll, H. A., Davies, B. A., & O'Connor, M. E. (1997). Risk factors for bulimia nervosa: A community-based case–control study. *Archives of General Psychiatry*, *54*, 509–517.

Fairburn, C. G., Welch, S. L., Norman, P. A., O'Connor, M. E., & Doll, H. A. (1996). Bias and bulimia nervosa: How typical are clinic cases? *American Journal of Psychiatry*, *153*, 386–391.

Foreman, D. (2006). The law in relation to children. In S. G. Gowers (Ed.), *Seminars in child and adolescent psychiatry* (2nd edn., pp. 90–101). London: Gaskell.

Hoek, H. W. (2006). Incidence, prevalence and mortality of anorexia nervosa and other eating disorders. *Current Opinion in Psychiatry*, *19*, 389–394.

Hoek, H. W., & van Hoeken, D. (2006). Review of the prevalence and incidence of eating disorders. *International Journal of Eating Disorders*, *34*, 383–396.

Jacobi, C. (2005). Psychosocial risk factors for eating disorders. In S. Wonderlich, J. Mitchell, M. de Zwaan, & H. Steiger (Eds.), *Eating disorders review*, Part 1 (pp. 59–85). Oxford: Radcliffe.

Jacobi, C., Hayward, C., de Zwaan, M., Kraemer, H. C., & Agras, W. S. (2004). Coming to terms with risk factors for eating disorders: Application of risk terminology and suggestions for a general taxonomy. *Psychological Bulletin*, *130*, 19–65.

Kaye, W. H., Frank, G. K., Bailer, U. F., Henry, S. E., Meltzer, C. C., Price, J. C., *et al.* (2005). Serotonin alterations in anorexia and bulimia nervosa: New insights from imaging studies. *Physiology & Behavior*, *85*, 73–81.

Kaye, W. H., Wagner, A., Frank, G., & Bailer, U. F. (2006). Review of brain imaging in anorexia and bulimia nervosa. In S. Wonderlich, J. E. Mitchel, M. de Zwaan, & H. Steiger (Eds.), *Annual review of eating disorders*, Part 2 (pp. 113–129). Oxford: Radcliffe.

Keel, P. K., Mitchell, J. E., Miller, K. B., Davis, T. L., & Crow, S. J. (1999). Long-term outcome of bulimia nervosa. *Archives of General Psychiatry*, *56*, 63–69.

Keel, P. K., Dorer, D. J., Eddy, K. T., Franko, D., Charatan, D. L., & Herzog, D. B. (2003). Predictors of mortality in eating disorders. *Archives of General Psychiatry*, *60*, 179–183.

Keel, P. K., & Klump, K. L. (2003). Are eating disorders culture-bound syndromes? Implications for conceptualizing their etiology. *Psychological Bulletin*, *129*, 747–769.

Key, A., Mason, H., & Bolton, J. (2000). Reproduction and eating disorders: A fruitless union. *European Eating Disorders Review*, *8*, 98–107.

Klump, K. L., McGue, M., & Iacono, W. G. (2003). Differential heritability of eating attitudes and behaviors in prepubertal versus pubertal twins. *International Journal of Eating Disorders*, *33*, 287–292.

Lilenfeld, L. R., Kaye, W. H., Greeno, C. G., Merikangas, K. R., Plotnicov, K., Pollice, C., *et al.* (1998). A controlled family study of anorexia nervosa and bulimia nervosa: Psychiatric disorders in first-degree relatives and effects of proband comorbidity. *Archives of General Psychiatry*, *55*, 603–610.

Lock, J., Agras, W. S., Bryson, S., & Kraemer, H. C. (2005). A comparison of short- and long-term family therapy for adolescent anorexia nervosa. *Journal of the American Academy of Child and Adolescent Psychiatry*, *44*, 632–639.

Lock, J., le Grange, D., Agras, W. S., & Dare, C. (2001). *Treatment manual for anorexia nervosa: A family-based approach*. New York: Guilford Press.

Mufson, L., Dorta, K. P., Moreau, D., & Weissman, M. M. (2004). *Interpersonal psychotherapy for depressed adolescents* (2nd edn.) New York: Guilford Press.

National Institute for Clinical Excellence. (2004). *Eating disorders: Core interventions in the treatment and management of eating disorders in primary and secondary care*. London: National Institute for Clinical Excellence.

Nicholls, D., Chater, R., & Lask, B. (2000). Children into DSM don't go: A comparison of classification systems for eating disorders in childhood and early adolescence. *International Journal of Eating Disorders*, *28*, 317–324.

Piran, N., Levine, M. P., & Steiner-Adair, C. (1999). *Preventing eating disorders*. New York: Brunner/Mazel.

Råstam, M., Gillberg, C., & Wentz, E. (2003). Outcome of teenage-onset anorexia nervosa in a Swedish community-based sample. *European Child and Adolescent Psychiatry*, *12*, 78–90.

Robin, A. L., Siegel, P. T., Moye, A. W., Gilroy, M., Dennis, A. B., & Sikand, A. (1999). A controlled comparison of family versus individual therapy for adolescents with anorexia nervosa. *Journal of the American Academy of Child and Adolescent Psychiatry*, *38*, 1482–1489.

Russell, G. F. M. (1992). Anorexia nervosa of early onset and its impact on puberty. In P. Cooper (Ed.), *Feeding problems and eating disorders in children and adolescents* (pp. 85–112). Chur: Harwood Academic.

Russell, G. F. M., Szmukler, G. I., Dare, C., & Eisler, I. (1987). An evaluation of family therapy in anorexia nervosa and bulimia nervosa. *Archives of General Psychiatry*, *44*, 1047–1056.

Silva, P. A., & Stanton, W. R. (1997). *From Child to Adult: The Dunnedin Multidisciplinary Health and Development Study*. New York, NY: Oxford University Press.

Slof-Op 't Landt, M., van Furth, E. F., Meulenbelt, I., Slagboom, R. E., Bartels, M., Boomsma, D. I., *et al.* (2005). Eating disorders: From twin studies to candidate genes and beyond. *Twin Research and Human Genetics*, *8*, 467–482.

Stein, A., Woolley, H., Murray, L., *et al.* (2001). Influence of psychiatric disorder on the controlling behaviour of mothers with 1-year-old infants. A study of women with maternal eating disorder, post-natal depression and a healthy comparison group. *British Journal of Psychiatry*, *179*, 157–162.

Steinhausen, H-C. (2002). The outcome of anorexia nervosa in the twentieth century. *American Journal of Psychiatry*, *159*, 1284–1293.

Strober, M., Freeman, R., Lampert, C., Diamond, J., & Kaye, W. (2000). Controlled family study of anorexia nervosa and bulimia nervosa: Evidence of shared liability and transmission of partial syndromes. *American Journal of Psychiatry*, *157*, 393–401.

Strober, M., Freeman, R., & Morrell, W. (1997). The long-term course of severe anorexia nervosa in adolescents: Survival analysis of recovery, relapse, and outcome predictors over 10–15 years in a prospective study. *International Journal of Eating Disorders*, *22*, 339–360.

van Son, G. E., van Hoeken, D., Bartelds, A. I. M., van Furth, E. F., & Hoek, H. W. (2006). Time trends in the incidence of eating disorders: A primary care study in the Netherlands. *International Journal of Eating Disorders*, *39*, 565–569.

Walsh, B. T., Hadigan, C. M., Devlin, M. J., Gladis, M., & Roose, S. P. (1991). Long-term outcome of antidepressant treatments for bulimia nervosa. *American Journal of Psychiatry*, *148*, 1206–1212.

Walsh, B. T., Kaplan, A. S., Attia, E., Olmsted, M., Parides, M., Carter, J. C., *et al.* (2006). Fluoxetine after weight restoration in anorexia nervosa: A randomized controlled trial. *Journal of the American Medical Association*, *295*, 2605–2612.

Weissman, M. M., Markowitz, J. C., & Klerman, G. L. (2000). *Comprehensive guide to interpersonal psychotherapy*. New York: Basic Books.

Wilson, G. T., & Sysko, R. (2006). Cognitive–behavioural therapy for adolescents with bulimia nervosa. *European Eating Disorders Review*, *14*, 8–16.

Zipfel, S., Lowe, B., & Herzog, W. (2003). Medical complications. In J. Treasure, U. Schmidt, & E. Van Furth (Eds.), *Handbook of eating disorders* (2nd edn., pp. 169–90). Chichester: Wiley.

42 Post-Traumatic Stress Disorder

William Yule and Patrick Smith

Both ICD-10 (WHO, 1996) and DSM-IV (APA, 2000) diagnostic systems now acknowledge that major stressors can cause serious morbidity and that children may suffer from post-traumatic stress disorder (PTSD). The past 15 years have seen a great increase in studies of the effects of major stresses, as encountered in disasters, war and other life-threatening experiences. However, the question for child psychiatry remains whether severe acute stresses (see chapter 26), as opposed to chronic ones linked to social adversity (see chapter 25), carry a substantial increased risk of psychiatric sequelae. If so, what sort of stressors carry such increased risk? What are the most common psychological sequelae? Do these vary according to stressor, according to developmental level? What is the role of the family in moderating the reactions? Are there other known risk and protective factors? Indeed, is PTSD a truly separate disorder or is it merely a variant of other well-recognized disorders such as anxiety, phobias and depression? Finally, what is currently known about intervention?

Concept of Post-Traumatic Stress Disorder

The diagnosis of PTSD was first conceptualized in response to observations of Vietnam war veterans presenting with what came to be recognized as a particular pattern of symptoms in three clusters: intrusive recollections of a traumatic event; emotional numbing and avoidance of reminders of that event; and physiological hyperarousal. In retrospect, similar patterns were noted as reactions in earlier wars and in prospect, the criteria were adapted, partly operationalized and applied to adult civilians. Next, the diagnosis was applied to children who had experienced an "event outside the range of usual human experience . . . that would be markedly distressing to almost anyone" (DSM-III-R, 1987).

Thus, it was argued that there were certain types of stressful experiences that were very severe and/or unusual and that there was a distinctive form of stress reaction to these. PTSD was classified as an anxiety disorder, but many argued that it should be included as a dissociative disorder. It was increasingly described as "a normal reaction to an abnormal situation," and so, logically, it was queried whether it should be regarded as a psychiatric disorder at all (O'Donohue & Eliot, 1992). Even if it were regarded as a normal reaction, it causes substantial impairment in sufficient cases to be regarded as a disorder.

Results from studies of adults have reasonably established that PTSD, while being predominantly an anxiety disorder, differs from other anxiety disorders in important ways. Thus, Foa, Steketee, & Olasov-Rothbaum (1989) showed that the trauma suffered violated more of the patient's safety assumptions than did events giving rise to other forms of anxiety. There was a much greater generalization of fear responses in the PTSD groups, and, unlike other anxious patients, they reported far more frequent re-experiencing of the traumatic event. Indeed, it is this internal, subjective experience that seems most to mark out PTSD from other disorders (Jones & Barlow, 1992). Epidemiological investigations in adults suggest that exposure to traumatic events is common (Kessler, Sonnega, Bromet *et al.*, 1995), and that only a minority of exposed individuals go on to develop the disorder (McFarlane, 2005). The argument is therefore made that PTSD is an "abnormal reaction" that involves a complex interaction of biological, psychological and social causes (Yehuda & McFarlane, 1995); exposure to trauma is insufficient to explain development of the disorder. Current biopsychosocial and cognitive models (see p. 689) are paying increasing attention to factors underlying individual differences in response to traumatic events. Concern has been expressed that there are other forms of stress reactions to chronic stressors as experienced in repeated physical or sexual abuse (see chapters 28 and 29). Terr (1991), for example, draws a distinction between type I and II traumas, roughly the distinction between acute and chronic. While these are important debates that will alter the views taken on PTSD, here we concentrate on acute conditions as manifested in children and adolescents.

With its roots in studies of adult psychopathology, the concept has been uneasily extended to apply to stress reactions in children and adolescents. The major difficulty from the outset has been that some of the symptoms are developmentally inappropriate for younger people. Indeed, the younger the child, the less appropriate the criteria. Many writers agree that it is very difficult to elicit evidence of emotional numbing in children (Frederick, 1985). Some children do show loss of interest in activities and hobbies that previously gave them pleasure. Preschool children show much more regressive behavior as

Rutter's Child and Adolescent Psychiatry, 5th edition. Edited by M. Rutter, D. Bishop, D. Pine, S. Scott, J. Stevenson, E. Taylor and A. Thapar. © 2008 Blackwell Publishing, ISBN: 978-1-4051-4549-7.

well as more antisocial, aggressive and destructive behavior. There are many anecdotal accounts of preschool children showing repetitive drawing and play involving themes about the trauma they experienced. Although parents and teachers initially report that young children do not easily talk about the trauma, recent experience has been that many young children easily give very graphic accounts of their experiences and were also able to report how distressing the re-experiencing in thoughts and images was (Misch, Phillips, Evans, & Berelowitz, 1993; Sullivan, Saylor, & Foster, 1991).

All clinicians and researchers need to have a good understanding of children's development to be able to assist them express their inner distress.

Manifestations of Stress Reactions in Children and Adolescents

Immediately following a very frightening experience, children are likely to be very distressed, tearful, frightened and in shock. They need protection and safety. They need to be reunited with their families wherever possible. Clinical experience, surveys and clinical descriptive studies quoted below show that the main manifestations of stress reactions are as follows.

Starting almost immediately, most children are troubled by *repetitive, intrusive thoughts* about the accident. Such thoughts can occur at any time, but particularly when the children are otherwise quiet, as when they are trying to drop off to sleep. At other times, the thoughts and vivid recollections are triggered off by reminders in their environment. Vivid, dissociative *flashbacks* are uncommon. In a flashback, the child reports that he or she is re-experiencing the event, as if it were happening all over again. It is almost a dissociated experience. *Sleep disturbances* are very common, particularly in the first few weeks. *Fears* of the dark and bad dreams, *nightmares*, and waking through the night are widespread (and often manifest outside the developmental age range in which they normally occur).

Separation difficulties are frequent, even among teenagers. For the first few days, children may not want to let their parents out of their sight, even reverting to sleeping in the parental bed. Many children become much more *irritable and angry* than previously, both with parents and peers.

Although child survivors experience a *pressure to talk* about their experiences, paradoxically they also find it very *difficult to talk with their parents and peers*. Often they do not want to upset the adults, and so parents may not be aware of the full extent of their children's suffering. Peers may hold back from asking what happened in case they upset the child further; the survivor often feels this as a rejection.

Children report a number of *cognitive changes*. Many experience *difficulties in concentration*, especially in school work. Others report *memory problems*, both in mastering new material and in remembering old skills such as reading music. They become very *alert to danger* in their environment, being adversely affected by reports of other disasters.

Survivors have learned that life is very fragile. This can lead to a loss of faith in the future or a *sense of foreshortened future*, or a *premature awareness of their own mortality*. Their priorities change. Some feel they should live each day to the full and not plan far ahead. Others realize they have been overconcerned with materialistic or petty matters and resolve to rethink their values. Their "assumptive world" has been challenged (Janoff-Bulman, 1985).

Not surprisingly, many develop *fears* associated with specific aspects of their experiences. They avoid situations they associate with the disaster. Many experience "*survivor guilt*" – about surviving when others died; about thinking they should have done more to help others; about what they themselves did to survive.

Adolescent survivors report significantly high rates of *depression*, some becoming clinically depressed, having suicidal thoughts and taking overdoses in the year after a disaster. A significant number become very *anxious* after accidents, although the appearance of *panic attacks* is sometimes considerably delayed. Some children may have been bereaved and may develop traumatic grief reactions.

In summary, children and adolescents surviving a traumatic event may show a wide range of symptoms which tend to cluster around signs of re-experiencing the traumatic event, trying to avoid dealing with the emotions that this gives rise to, and a range of signs of increased physiological arousal. In a substantial minority, this cluster of symptoms will amount to a diagnosable PTSD. Just as in adults, a broad range of adverse outcomes is common (Bolton, O'Ryan, Udwun, Boyle, & Yule, 2000; Pine & Cohen, 2002): there may be considerable overlap of symptoms with depression, generalized anxiety or pathological grief reactions, although whether this indicates the presence of mixed disorders or comorbidity of separate disorders remains to be clarified.

However, this has implications for assessment. It is not sufficient to enquire solely about symptoms of PTSD. Symptoms of anxiety, depression and grief need also to be formally investigated. Nor are self-completed questionnaires measuring these aspects sufficient to make a diagnosis. They have an important role, but sensitive clinical interviews with the child and separately with the parents remain the cornerstone of good assessment.

Developmental Aspects

Considerable debate remains as to whether the very young child's limited cognitive development is protective against developing a chronic post-traumatic stress reaction. Certainly, the diagnostic criteria in both of the major classification schemes are not appropriate for preschool children.

In a series of studies, Scheeringa, Zeanah, Drell *et al.* (1995); Scheeringa, Peebles, Cook *et al.* (2001); Scheeringa, Zeanah, Myers *et al.* (2003); Scheeringa, Wright, Hunt *et al.* (2006) examined the phenomenology reported in published cases of trauma in infants and young children and evolved an alternative set of criteria for diagnosing PTSD in very young children. Re-experiencing was seen as being manifested in post-traumatic play; re-enactment of the trauma; recurrent recollection of the traumatic event; nightmares; flashbacks or distress at exposure to reminders of the event. Only one positive item was needed. Numbing was present if one of the following was manifested: constriction of play; socially more withdrawn; restricted range of affect; or loss of previously acquired developmental skill. Increased arousal was noted if one of the following was present: night terrors; difficulty getting off to sleep; night waking; decreased concentration; hypervigilance; or exaggerated startle response. A new subset of new fears and aggression was suggested and is said to be present if one of the following is recorded: new aggression; new separation anxiety; fear of toileting alone; fear of the dark or any other unrelated new fear.

Prospective 2-year follow-up studies have demonstrated good concurrent and predictive validity for this alternative method of diagnosing PTSD in young children. Almqvist & Brandell-Forsberg (1997) provided evidence on how a standard set of play materials can be used to obtain objective data on traumatic stress reactions from preschool children. Thus, one can anticipate further refining of criteria and methods of assessment of PTSD in preschool children in the next few years.

Incidence and Prevalence

Estimates of the incidence of PTSD in trauma-exposed children vary enormously, partly as a result of differing methodologies, and partly as a result of different types of traumatic event. Studies of the mental health of child refugees from war-torn countries find the incidence to be close to 67%. Sexual abuse results in high rates of PTSD (Salmon & Bryant, 2002), as does witnessing violence (Margolin & Gordis, 2000). In various studies of the effects of traffic accidents (that did not result in an overnight stay in hospital), rates of 25–30% are reported (Stallard, Salter, & Velleman, 2004). A study of 200 adolescent survivors of the sinking of the cruise ship *Jupiter* (Yule, Bolton, Udwin *et al.*, 2000) reported an incidence of PTSD of 51%. Most cases manifested within the first few weeks with delayed onset being rare. Following a nightclub fire in Gothenburg, 25% of the 275 adolescent survivors met DSM-IV criteria for PTSD 18 months after the fire (Broberg, Dyregrov, & Lilled, 2005). Overall, it has been estimated that 36% of children will meet criteria for PTSD following a range of traumas (Fletcher, 1996). This appears fairly constant across developmental levels. In other words, significantly increased demands will be made at all levels of primary and secondary child and adolescent mental health services following traumatic events.

Most epidemiological studies have been of older adolescents and adults. Giaconia, Reinherz, Silverman *et al.* (1995) reported a lifetime prevalence of 6% in a community sample of older adolescents. Kessler, Sonnega, Bromet *et al.* (1995) reported a lifetime prevalence of 10% using data collected from older adolescents and adults in the (USA) National Comorbidity Survey. A national sample of eighth grade Danish students estimated a 9% lifetime prevalence (Elklit, 2002). By contrast, the British National Survey of Mental health of over 10,000 children and adolescents (Meltzer, Gatward, Goodman, 2003) reported that only 0.4% of 11- to 15-year-olds were diagnosed with PTSD, with girls showing twice the rate of boys. Below age 10, it was scarcely registered. This lower rate is a point prevalence estimate and is bound to be lower than a lifetime prevalence estimate. Moreover, the screening instrument was not specifically developed to screen for PTSD. The implication is that while the numbers of children and adolescents experiencing PTSD at any one point in time may be as low as 1%, this is still a significant level of morbidity in any community.

Prospective Longitudinal Studies

Data from numerous adult studies show that there is substantial natural recovery from PTSD in the initial months after the trauma. Many individuals recover from PTSD without treatment, and the steepest decline in rates of PTSD is usually seen in the first year. Of course, this still leaves a substantial minority – roughly one-third – who are likely to develop a chronic disorder which may persist for years if left untreated (NICE, 2005).

A similar picture is emerging from recent prospective follow-up studies of children. For example, Meiser-Stedman, Yule, Smith *et al.* (2005) found that among young survivors of assaults and traffic accidents, nearly one in five met criteria for Acute Stress Disorder 2–4 weeks after the event. When re-interviewed at 6 months post-trauma, the rate of PTSD was 12%. The question remains: what factors distinguish those children who will recover spontaneously from those who will go on to develop a chronic reaction requiring treatment (see p. 690)?

There have been very few long-term follow-up studies of children who developed PTSD. The 5–7 year follow-up study of adolescents who survived the sinking of the cruise ship *Jupiter* found that 15% still met criteria for PTSD that long after the event (Yule, Bolton, Udwin *et al.*, 2000). More recently, a 33 year follow-up of the children who survived the Aberfan landslide disaster found that 29% of those traced and interviewed still met criteria for PTSD (Morgan, Scourfield, Williams *et al.*, 2003). Thus, the long-term effects of life-threatening traumatic events in childhood can be severe and long-lasting.

Risk, Protective and Maintaining Factors

Not all children exposed to trauma will develop PTSD, and of those who do, many will recover without treatment. From this it follows that factors other than exposure to trauma must influence the onset and maintenance of the disorder. Recent research efforts have attempted to characterize these factors in order to better understand chronic stress reactions, and inform treatment approaches.

Exposure–Response Relationship

One of the key concepts in PTSD is that anyone can develop the disorder, irrespective of prior vulnerabilities, provided the stressor is sufficiently great. There is therefore considerable interest in whether there is any evidence for an exposure–response relationship between stressor and pathology. A number of studies bear on this point in relation to children.

In an early study of a sniper attack on a Californian school, Pynoos and colleagues (Pynoos & Eth, 1986; Pynoos & Nader, 1988; Pynoos, Frederick, Nader *et al.*, 1987) reported that approximately 1 month after the event, nearly 40% of the children had moderate to severe PTSD on their Post Traumatic Stress Reaction Index. There was a very strong relationship between exposure and later effects in that those children who were trapped in the playground scored much higher than those who had left the vicinity of the school before the attack or were not in school that day.

Evidence for an exposure–response relationship has also emerged in studies of young people exposed to disasters and war. For example, among children affected by the Armenian earthquake of 1988, there was a clear exposure–response relationship, with the most exposed children at the epicenter reporting highest scores (Goenjian, Pynoos, Steinberg *et al.*, 1995). In a large sample of Rwandese children, Gupta, Dyregrov, Gjestad, & Mukanoheli (1996) found a significant relationship between the number of traumatic events children had been exposed to during the genocide and later stress reactions. In a systematic study of nearly 3000 9- to 14-year-old children following the Bosnian war in Mostar, a very strong relationship between exposure to war trauma and self-reported psychopathology was found (Smith, Perrin, Yule, Hacam, & Stuvland, 2002).

Whereas studies of adults have shown that some types of traumatic event are consistently associated with higher rates of PTSD, data are lacking in this regard with respect to children. Findings from the child studies above strongly suggest that given the same type of exposure, there is a relationship between level of exposure to the stressor and subsequent adjustment. Nevertheless, in most studies, the "objective" level of trauma exposure accounts for a surprisingly small proportion of variance in later adjustment.

Family Influences

Various aspects of children's family environment have been found to be associated with children's reports of post-traumatic symptoms. These include maternal post-traumatic stress symptoms in cases where mother and child have been exposed to the same trauma (Smith, Perrin, Yule, & Rabe-Hesketh, 2001). Maternal depression (Smith, Perrin, Yule *et al.*, 2002; Wolmer, Laor, Gershon, Mayes, & Cohen, 2000) and general family functioning or emotional atmosphere (Green, Korol, Grace *et al.*, 1991; McFarlane, 1987) have also been implicated. In a recent prospective study of child and adolescent attendees at Accident and Emergency Departments, Meiser-Stedman, Yule, Dalgleish, Smith, & Glucksman (2006) found that parental depression was related to child post-traumatic symptoms at both 2–4 weeks post-accident and again at 6 months after the trauma. Parental worry mediated the relationship between parental depression and child symptoms of stress, but general family functioning appeared less important.

The mechanisms underlying these familial associations remain unclear. In part, they may derive from a complex interaction between parents and children, who can become locked into cycles of not talking about the event for fear of upsetting each other. That is, parents and children may negatively reinforce each other for avoiding processing their traumatic memories, and this is likely to maintain the symptoms of both.

Cognitive Aspects and Cognitive Models

Early work recognized that objective measures of exposure were insufficient to explain the variability in children's post-traumatic stress reactions; subjective appraisal also has a key role. For example, among children exposed to war (Nader, Pynoos, Fairbanks, Al-Ajeel, & al-Asfoir, 1993; Smith, Perrin, Yule *et al.*, 2002) or genocide (Gupta, Dyregrov, Gjestad *et al.*, 1996), perceived direct life threat is strongly related to later PTSD. Similarly, among adolescents involved in a shipping accident, those who made guilt or shame-inducing attributions showed higher levels of PTSD symptoms (Joseph, Brewin, Yule, & Williams, 1993).

More recent work has investigated the applicability to children of adult cognitive models of the disorder (Brewin, 2001; Ehlers & Clark, 2000; Meiser-Stedman, 2002; Salmon & Bryant, 2002). For example, under Ehlers and Clark's (2000) model, PTSD is maintained by: the disjointed nature of the memory; misappraisals of the trauma and its sequelae; and maladaptive (i.e., avoidant) coping strategies. Retrospective analyses (Stallard, 2003) and well-designed prospective studies (Ehlers, Mayou, & Bryant, 2003; Meiser-Stedman, Yule, Smith *et al.*, 2005) provide evidence that such models do indeed apply to children, at least from the age of about 8 years old. That is, characteristic cognitive distortions and misappraisals appear to have a central role in maintaining PTSD in older children and adolescents, and this has clear implications for treatment (see p. 692).

However, dissociation, which was initially thought to be a key cognitive aspect of the trauma response, appears to be unrelated to the maintenance of PTSD symptoms. Acute stress disorder (ASD) is explicitly conceived as a dissociative response to trauma, requiring three of a possible five dissociation symptoms (APA, 2000). Two recent studies with children show that although acute stress disorder in the first 4 weeks post-trauma is a good predictor of later PTSD, dissociation symptoms do not have a significant role (Kassam-Adams & Winston, 2004; Meiser-Stedman, Yule, Smith *et al.*, 2005). These findings require replication, but are in line with recent adult work which showed that the dissociation criteria do not enhance the ability of ASD to predict later PTSD (Brewin, Andrews, & Rose, 2003).

Finally, there is a small but growing literature on cognitive biases in memory and attention in children with PTSD (for an overview see Dalgleish, Meiser-Stedman, & Smith, 2005). This approach seeks to examine how basic cognitive processes are affected by trauma exposure, and how such changes may in turn function to maintain post-traumatic stress reactions. An intriguing set of findings has emerged from a handful of experimental studies using the emotional Stroop task, the dotprobe paradigm, and recall tasks. Some studies report evidence for an "avoidant" bias with respect to traumarelated material (Pine, Mogg, Bradley *et al.*, 2005), whereas other studies find a bias in favor of trauma or threat-related material (Moradi, Taghavi, Neshat-Doost, Yule, & Dalgleish, 2000), consistent with the adult literature. In terms of memory, there is evidence for a memory bias for negative material in children with PTSD compared with non-traumatized controls (Moradi, Taghavi, Neshat-Doost *et al.*, 2000). Given the small number of studies, and the mixed set of findings, further research is called for.

Protective Factors

There have been few studies that have set out to identify protective factors properly and so inferences have had to be drawn from the general literature on psychopathology and some cross-sectional studies. The main factors commented on have been age, gender, ability and attainment, family factors and coping strategies. In brief, developmental level acts in two opposing ways: younger children may not fully appreciate the extent of the danger facing them, but also immature cognitions may produce more distorted memories. There is generally good agreement from a number of studies that developing PTSD following a traumatic experience is more common in females than in males. Prior poor adjustment and difficult family relationships, including domestic violence, are all associated with a higher risk of developing PTSD and so the opposite, positive attributes are seen as protective. Perceived and actual social support, especially from the family, are noted as being protective, as is possessing a range of effective coping strategies. Where there has been material loss – of home or other possessions – following a natural disaster, then higher income in the family is a protective factor (for reviews see Udwin, Boyle, Yule, Bolton, & O'Ryan, 2000; Yule, Perrin, & Smith, 1999).

Summary

In addition to objective exposure severity, subjective appraisals, maladaptive coping strategies and family influences, a number of other factors are implicated in risk for onset and maintenance of PTSD in children. Findings on the role of individual child characteristics such as age, sex and ethnicity have been inconsistent (Vernberg, La Greca, Silverman, & Prinstein, 1996), although there is an emerging consensus that, as with other emotional disorders, girls are more at risk than boys. Udwin, Boyle, Yule *et al.* (2000) reported that a history of previous exposure to violence and a psychiatric history prior to the trauma increased risk of developing PTSD. In line with adult work (Brewin, Andrews, & Valentine, 2000), the availability of social support in the aftermath of a trauma appears to be import-ant in the subsequent duration and severity of the disorder (Udwin, Boyle, Yule *et al.*, 2000; Vernberg, La Greca, Silverman *et al.*, 1996). Further work is needed to clarify these sets of risk factors.

The implications for intervention remain to be worked out in detail. The successful trials of Narrative Exposure Therapy and of Trauma Focused cognitive–behavioral therapy (CBT) indicate that active CBT therapies must pay close attention both to the trauma narrative and to correcting cognitive distortions in memory. Simple exposure is not enough. The findings from the protective function of social support again indicate that therapists must pay attention to sources of support for the child both within the family and at school.

Physiological Reactions

Children's exposure to trauma can result in biological as well as psychological changes. Recent investigations of a variety of physiological changes in traumatized children have been driven by contemporary neuroscience accounts of fear and stress. These accounts draw on animal models, and have been tested most thoroughly in trauma-exposed adults. In broad summary, traumatic stress activates the locus ceruleus and the sympathetic nervous system (SNS), leading to increased catecholamine turnover, and resulting in increased heart rate, blood pressure, metabolic rate, alertness and circulating catecholamines (adrenaline, noradrenaline and dopamine) – a classic "flight or flight" reaction. During stress, the locus ceruleus also stimulates the hypothalamic–pituitary–adrenal (HPA) axis. The resulting release of corticotropin-releasing factor (CRF) from the hypothalamus stimulates the pituitary to secrete adrenocorticotropin, which in turn promotes cortisol release from the adrenal gland, further stimulating the SNS, and causing intense arousal. Cortisol then suppresses the HPA axis, acting via negative feedback inhibition on the hypothalamus, pituitary and hippocampus, leading to homeostasis. In animals, these neurophysiological processes lead to behaviors consistent with anxiety, hyperarousal and hypervigilance – core symptoms of PTSD. In adults and children, investigation of these two major stress systems – the catecholamine system and the HPA axis – and associated brain structures has therefore been the focus of recent research (for reviews see Cohen, Perel, DeBellis, Friedman, & Putnam, 2002; De Bellis, 2001; Pine, 2003).

There is evidence that the catecholamine system is disrupted in traumatized children with and without full-blown PTSD. De Bellis, Chrousos, Dorn *et al.* (1994); De Bellis, Baum, Birmaher *et al.* (1999a); De Bellis, Keshavan, Clark *et al.* (1999b) reported significantly increased dopamine in the urine of sexually abused girls, and of maltreated boys and girls with PTSD, which was correlated with the severity of PTSD symptoms. It is hypothesized that excessive dopamine results in under-functioning of the prefrontal cortex, which normally acts to extinguish conditioned fear responses. These same studies (De Bellis, Chrousos, Dorn *et al.*, 1994; De Bellis, Baum, Birmaher *et al.*, 1999a; De Bellis, Keshavan, Clark *et al.*, 1999b) also found that children with abuse-related PTSD showed increased 24-h urinary adrenaline and noradrenaline and/or their metabolites. Consistent with a malfunctioning adrenergic response, Perry (1994) found that abused children with PTSD had greater increases in heart rate when exposed to a physiological challenge, compared with non-PTSD control children. In line with this work, Scheeringa, Zeanah, Myers *et al.* (2004) have more recently shown that even very young (preschool) children with PTSD resulting from exposure to violence or highly invasive medical procedures show increased heart rate in response to trauma reminders, compared to non-traumatized controls. Importantly, it appears that early changes in peripheral physiology may predict later symptoms of PTSD in children. Kassam-Adams, Garcia-España, Fein *et al.* (2005) reported that among children involved in a road traffic accident, acute heart rate (measured in hospital within hours of the accident) was significantly associated with severity of PTSD symptoms some 6 months later.

In contrast to this relatively straightforward sensitization of the catecholamine system, investigations of HPA axis functioning in traumatized children show that this system works in a rather complex manner. Different patterns of dysregulation may arise, related to time since trauma exposure, and to whether the child has subsequently been exposed to further stress or trauma. In acutely traumatized children, there is evidence for *hypersecretion* of cortisol (Carrion, Weems, Ray *et al.*, 2002). In contrast, investigations of young samples with chronic PTSD reveal *lower* resting baseline levels of cortisol (Goenjian, Yehuda, Pynoos *et al.*, 1996) and a blunted corticotropin response (De Bellis, Chrousos, Dorn *et al.*, 1994). The suggestion is that compensatory downregulation of the HPA axis occurs in children with chronic PTSD, leading to an increasingly maladaptive response over time. Furthermore, children with a history of severe maltreatment plus concurrent exposure to new stressors showed an *increased* corticotropin response and high levels CRF in one study (Kaufman, Birmaher, Perel *et al.*, 1997). De Bellis (2001) suggests that individuals with a history of chronic PTSD may demonstrate a hyperresponding of the HPA axis when encountering new stressors. Evidence for disruption to the HPA axis has led to the administration of low-dose cortisol to treat symptoms of PTSD in adults (Aerni, Traber, Hock *et al.*, 2004), but similar treatments have not been tested in children.

In addition to the study of neurotransmitter systems and neuroendocrine axes, a small number of studies have examined related brain morphology. Of particular interest is the hippocampus, which has a central role in memory processing. High levels of cortisol are toxic to the hippocampus, and studies of adults with chronic PTSD have found the predicted decreased hippocampal volume (Bremner, Randall, Scott *et al.*, 1995; Bremner, Randall, Vermetten *et al.*, 1997).

However, studies with young children have not found this expected damage to the hippocampus (De Bellis, Keshavan, Clark *et al.*, 1999b). It is possible that the adult findings were confounded by alcohol misuse among those with chronic PTSD (because alcohol is also toxic to the hippocampus). Alternatively, the absence of decreased volume in young samples may be because hippocampal damage depends on chronicity of PTSD, occurs at a later developmental stage, or is masked by the normal increase in volume seen during adolescence. Although the expected specific changes to the hippocampus have not been found, it appears that children with PTSD show global adverse brain development: De Bellis, Keshavan, Clark *et al.* (1999b) found children with PTSD to have smaller intracranial volume and a smaller corpus callosum than controls.

Finally, a number of other psychobiological systems are activated during acute stress. In adults, evidence exists for disruption to the endogenous opiate system, the serotonin system, and to the amygdala and prefrontal cortex, but studies of children are lacking.

In summary, there is growing evidence that children with symptoms of PTSD may show alterations to a number of interrelated neurophysiological systems. Further work will help to develop a better understanding of the complex interplay between physiological and psychological responses to traumatic events. Nevertheless, the need for early identification and treatment of PTSD is already highlighted by studies that have shown that an abnormal neurophysiological response in trauma-exposed children may persist for many years (Goenjian, Yehuda, Pynoos *et al.*, 1996; Ornitz & Pynoos, 1989).

Evidence-based Intervention

There are very few randomized controlled trials of any therapy with children, let alone therapies specifically for PTSD. One has therefore to be cautious in drawing conclusions solely by downward extension of results from work with adults. There have been a number of recent reviews that summarize the published evidence, and they agree to a substantial extent on which studies are included in their reviews (Feeny, Foa, Treadwell *et al.*, 2004; NICE, 2005; Stallard, 2006).

Early Interventions

Whereas prevention is seen as better than cure, in respect of PTSD this has to be seen as preventing the occurrence of traumatic events or children's exposure to them. Early intervention would be attractive if it could be shown that it prevented later development of PTSD or other disorders, but, as with adult studies, there have been few properly controlled trials of any early intervention. The only one known is that of Stallard Velleman, Salter *et al.* (2006), in which a trauma-focused discussion on an individual basis was compared with a generally supportive talk. At follow-up, both groups of road traffic accident (RTA) survivors had made good progress and both reported how helpful it had been to talk about the accident (presumably when establishing what happened and inadvertently validating reactions by asking about them systematically).

A later development of this study was to examine a group of survivors of RTAs only at the equivalent time the follow-up interviews were undertaken (i.e., without the baseline interview). This group was also doing well. The study had been designed when single, brief interventions were considered as possible ways of providing early intervention. It is now widely agreed that such one-off, brief, individually administered interventions do not help reduce later PTSD, but this follow-on study demonstrated that children were not upset by talking about their traumatic accident, and this alone should help adults when uncertain about whether to talk to affected children or not.

Cognitive–Behavioral Therapies

PTSD and Single Event Traumas

Few studies have examined the efficacy of psychological treatments for children who have developed PTSD following single event traumas. Goenjian, Karayan, Pynoos *et al.* (1997) reported that a 7-session schools-based CBT intervention for young people with PTSD some 1.5 years after an earthquake resulted in symptom reduction, whereas an untreated control group showed no such improvement. March, Amaya-Jackson, Murray *et al.*, (1998) used a single-case design to evaluate an 18-session group CBT intervention for 17 young people who had developed PTSD following a variety of trauma (RTAs, accidental injury, gunshot injury and fires). After treatment, there were significant reductions in PTSD symptoms and associated psychopathology (anxiety, depression and anger). This methodologically strong study (using reliable and valid self-report instruments, and a semi-structured interview to evaluate the effect of a manualized treatment protocol) laid the groundwork for subsequent randomized controlled trials (RCTs).

To date, three RCTs of psychological interventions with children who developed PTSD symptoms as a result of single event traumas have been reported (Chemtob, Nakashima, & Hamada, 2002; Smith, Yule, Perrin *et al.*, 2007; Stein, Jaycox, Kataoka *et al.*, 2003).

After Hurricane Iniki hit Hawaii, all elementary school children were screened for serious stress reactions and the high-risk group of 248 children were randomly assigned to one of three treatments (Chemtob, Nakashima, & Hamada, 2002). This comprised four sessions delivered either individually or in groups. The specially developed, manualized treatment had many elements in common with other CBT approaches. Both individual and group treatment had equally good results compared with controls and achieved an effect size of 0.50 on the Kauai Recovery Index (Hamada, Kameoka, & Yanagida, 1996). On the better known Child PTSD Reaction Index (Pynoos, Frederick, Nader *et al.*, 1987) completed on a sample of children by clinicians, the effect size was 0.76. More children dropped out of individual than group treatment.

Stein, Jaycox, Kataoka *et al.* (2003) report an RCT in which 61 children who had been exposed to violence were given 10 sessions of group CBT and compared with 65 children who were allocated to a delayed intervention condition. At 3 months post treatment, the treated group had significantly lower scores on the Child PTSD Symptom Scale (Foa, Johnson, Feeney *et al.*, 2000). Significant differences were also found on measures of depression and psychosocial dysfunction. Teacher-rated behavioral difficulties did not reflect improvement. The delayed treatment group then made significant PTSD improvement following treatment.

In both of these studies, children were recruited from school-based screening rather than from clinic-referred children. Not all participants had diagnoses of PTSD. The first RCT to report the effects of an individual Trauma Focused Cognitive Behavioural Therapy (TF-CBT) intervention for children following a single event trauma avoided many of the design problems noted above and used a flexible manualized approach to treating 12 children who developed clinician-validated PTSD following assault or RTA (Smith, Yule, Perrin *et al.*, 2007). Treatment was based on Ehlers and Clark's (2000) model of PTSD, and included a variety of components aimed at reducing known maintaining factors (see p. 689). Post treatment, 11 of the 12 young people who received CBT no longer met criteria for PTSD compared to 5 of the 12 on the waitlist. Treated children also showed significant reductions in symptoms of depression and anxiety. The effect size was 2.20 on the self-report measure and 1.59 on the CAPS-CA (the clinician rated severity on standardized interview). The differences remained at 6 month follow-up. As predicted, therapeutic gains in the CBT group were mediated via changes in maladaptive cognitions.

PTSD and Child Sexual Abuse

In recent years, many of the reactions children develop to sexual abuse have been formulated as part of a spectrum of post-traumatic stress reactions. This has resulted in a number of therapeutic trials of CBT to treat these reactions, including full PTSD.

Ramchandani and Jones (2003) report a systematic review of RCTs treating a range of psychological symptoms in sexually abused children. They identified 12 RCTs: three investigating group CBT; six investigating individual CBT; one of adding group therapy to a family therapy intervention; and two comparing individual (non-CBT) therapy with group therapy. However, the dependent (outcome) measures were very varied, and only four studies looked at recognized specific measures of PTSD.

Celano, Hazzard, Webb *et al.* (1996) compared 15 girls in an abuse-specific program with 17 given a parallel set of 8 non-directive supportive sessions. There were no differences on child scores including on the Child Impact of Traumatic Events Scale Revised (CITES-R). Deblinger, Stauffer, Steer (2001) enrolled 67 children aged 2–8 years. Although only 44 completed all 11 sessions of treatment, 21 completed group CBT and 23 completed a support group. There was significantly better outcome for CBT, but that group had had higher scores to start with. King, Tonge, Mullen *et al.* (2000) studied 36 sexually abused children aged 5–17 years who met criteria for PTSD. There were 12 children in each of three conditions:

CBT with child and family; CBT with child alone; and wait-list control. Both treatment conditions consisted of 20 sessions. Using Anxiety Disorders Interview Schedule for Children and Adolescents (ADIS-C) to assess PTSD, there was a significant improvement on PTSD, as well as on self-reported anxiety scales. Both ways of delivering CBT were equally effective. Cohen, Deblinger, Mannarino *et al.*'s (2004) more recent multisite RCT provides further convincing evidence in favor of CBT.

The immediate and long-term psychological effects of childhood sexual abuse are many, varied and serious (see chapter 29). The studies reviewed by Ramchandani and Jones strongly indicate that CBT is currently the treatment of choice, although there is clearly a great need for better RCTs. As Feeny, Foa, Treadwell *et al.* (2004) noted, child survivors of sexual abuse may present a different symptom picture to that of children exposed to single incident traumas and so generalization of findings to those may be problematic (see also American Academy of Child and Adolescent Psychiatry, 1998).

Eye Movement Desensitization and Reprocessing

Eye Movement Desensitization and Reprocessing (EMDR) was discovered by chance by Shapiro (2001) and has been applied with good results in adults (NICE, 2005). Again, there are a number of case reports claiming effectiveness of EMDR in treating PTSD in children, but a dearth of published RCTs or even other group studies. EMDR is an empirical treatment with little theoretical underpinning. The detailed protocols for treatment include a careful history and ensuring that the patient can have a break if the intrusions during treatment prove too frightening. Essentially, the child is asked to focus on a bad memory while simultaneously following the moving fingers of the therapist. This "dual attention" task is thought to help the child confront the frightening memory and so "process" the emotional reaction to that memory. There is some controversy about the active components of treatment in EMDR. For example, dismantling studies (Pitman, Orr, Altman *et al.*, 1996) have not provided evidence for a cardinal role for saccadic eye movements. The overlap between treatment components of CBT and EMDR (e.g., therapeutic exposure) have led some to suggest that the mechanisms of change may be broadly similar in both approaches.

Chemtob, Nakashima, & Hamada (2002) identified 32 children who still met criteria for PTSD after other attempts at treatment. They achieved significant drops in children's PTSD symptoms following three sessions of EMDR, with significant but lower drops on depression and anxiety. DeRoos, Greenwald, de Jongh *et al.* (2004) reported an RCT involving 52 children following the 2000 Enschede (Netherlands) fireworks disaster. Both EMDR and CBT produced significant lowering of stress symptoms, with EMDR doing slightly better in fewer sessions.

Whereas the NICE report (2005) found good evidence from RCTs with adults that allowed a firm recommendation that it be available to patients in the UK NHS, the evidence base with children is far less robust. Even despite the lack of a theoretical basis for EMDR, it appears that it can work very quickly and so should be considered as a possible treatment with children.

Narrative Exposure Therapy

Arising in part from South American methods of helping victims of torture and in part from a thoroughgoing analysis of the neurobiology of autobiographical memory and ways of completing fragmented memories, Schauer, Neuner, & Elbert (2004) have developed Narrative Exposure Therapy (NET) and used it in RCTs with adult refugees in the Sudan (Neuner, Schauer, Klascik, Karynakara, & Elbert, 2004) and war-affected children in Sri Lanka (Schauer, Neuner, Elbert *et al.*, 2004). Pennebaker (1995) has long demonstrated that writing about emotional events in structured ways can have very positive effects, and so one can anticipate that structured writing therapies and NET will develop more in the near future.

Medication

Despite the paucity of proper trials on children by pharmaceutical companies in developing psychotropic drugs, many children are indeed prescribed such medication following traumas (often by general practitioners rather than child specialists). Given the recent disclosures that trials of selective serotonin reuptake inhibitors (SSRIs) increased suicidal ideation in depressed adolescents, one's confidence in the use of medication with children is not great. Indeed, the NICE Guideline Development Group (2005) found no study that met its stringent criteria. Medication is not recommended as a treatment for PTSD in children.

Contingency Planning

When trauma affects a large number of children at once, as in an accident at school, then a public health approach to dealing with the emergency is required (Pynoos, Goenjian, & Steinberg, 1995). Schools need to plan ahead, not only to deal with large-scale disasters, but also to respond to the needs of children after threatening incidents that affect only a few of them. There are now a number of texts written especially for schools to help them develop contingency plans to deal with the effects of a disaster (Johnson, 1993; Klingman, 1993; Yule & Gold, 1993).

Most developed countries have well-established plans to deal with major civil emergencies. Increasingly, these include a psychosocial or mental health component and it is advisable for child and adolescent mental health services to be involved in the planning (Canterbury & Yule, 1999). UN agencies are increasingly prepared to meet the mental health needs of children after war and major disasters (Machel, 2001) and again mental health services need to collaborate with other agencies to meet such needs.

In considering the need to plan for "Mental Health in Complex Emergencies," Mollica, Lopes Cardoza *et al.* (2004) argued that all countries should develop plans to meet mental health sequelae of disasters. Because most disasters occur in developing countries, it is vital that appropriate assessment and intervention tools are developed that are culturally appropriate. It is also essential that such interventions are properly evaluated. Research is essential, not a luxury; that message needs to be accepted by non-governmental officers responding to disasters. Given that disasters happen with great frequency, then by planning ahead, proper consideration can be given to the ethical aspects of intervening soon after a crisis. Unless early interventions are evaluated responsibly, significant resources are wasted and survivors suffer unnecessarily.

Conclusions and Recommendations

Since its formulation in 1980, the diagnosis of PTSD has become widely used in child mental health practice. Using standard criteria and measures, significant minorities of children and adolescents have been diagnosed with PTSD following a variety of major stressors, from transport accidents, natural disasters such as hurricanes or earthquakes, and war. These reactions have now been shown to be long-lasting and disabling in many cases. Most research to date has concerned children of school age, and further work is needed in more closely delineating the stress reactions of very young children.

While it is comforting to children who develop PTSD to be told that their frightening symptoms are "normal," not all children do react this way, and so greater emphasis is needed on attempts to discover why some children are more vulnerable than others. The recent research focus on identifying risk and maintaining factors in carefully designed prospective studies has been fruitful, and has led to effective interventions which aim to reverse those maintaining factors. Further work in identifying modifiable maintaining factors is still required, especially with regard to parent–child interactions in trauma-affected families.

There is considerable overlap in disorders that present after a major traumatic event (Bolton, O'Ryan, Udwin *et al.*, 2000). However, there seems to be more than heuristic value in regarding PTSD to be separate from both other anxiety disorders and from depression. For example, available evidence suggests that PTSD and depression in children are associated with different risks post trauma (Smith, Perrin, Yule *et al.*, 2001), and show a different course and treatment response (Goenjian, Yehuda, Pynoos *et al.*, 1996). Further attention to multiple outcomes following trauma would enhance our understanding of the broad range of reactions that children may show, and may lead to more effective treatments for them.

The treatment outcome literature is small but growing. It remains the case that the most solid evidence relates to children traumatized by sexual abuse: here, the evidence is strong for TF-CBT as an effective treatment (NICE, 2005). In contrast, there is a paucity of well-controlled treatment studies for children with PTSD following relatively common single incident stressors such as RTAs and assaults. Published studies support TF-CBT as the treatment of choice for these young people too, but further RCTs are clearly needed. A range of treatments is now available, including EMDR and NET in addition to CBT, and it is expected that RCTs involving more than one active treatment will shed further light on what works for whom.

Studying PTSD has proved a remarkably rich, fertile ground for studying child psychopathology. It is a diagnostic category that helps focus mental health professionals on the needs of children – always providing that they ask the children themselves about their inner experiences and reactions.

References

Aerni, A., Traber, R., Hock, C., Roozendaal, B., Schelling, G., Papassotiropoulos, A., *et al.* (2004). Low-dose cortisol for symptoms of posttraumatic stress disorder. *American Journal of Psychiatry*, *161*, 1488–1490.

Almqvist, K., & Brandell-Forsberg, M. (1997). Refugee children in Sweden: Post-traumatic stress disorder in Iranian preschool children exposed to organized violence. *Child Abuse and Neglect*, *21*, 351–366.

American Academy of Child and Adolescent Psychiatry. (1998). Practice parameters for the assessment and treatment of children and adolescents with post traumatic stress disorder. *Journal of the American Academy of Child and Adolescent Psychiatry*, *37*, 4–26.

American Psychiatric Association (APA). (2000). *Diagnostic and Statistical Manual of Mental Disorders* (4th edn.). Text Revision. Washington, DC: American Psychiatric Association.

Bolton, D., O'Ryan, D., Udwin, O., Boyle, S., & Yule, W. (2000). The long-term psychological effects of a disaster experienced in adolescence. II. General psychopathology. *Journal of Child Psychology and Psychiatry*, *41*, 513–523.

Bremner, J. D., Randall, P., Scott, T. M., Bronen, R. A., Seibyl, J. P., Southwick, S. M., *et al.* (1995). MRI-based measurement of hippocampal volume in patients with combat-related posttraumatic stress disorder. *American Journal of Psychiatry*, *152*, 973–981.

Bremner, J. D., Randall, P., Vermetten, E., Staib, L., Bronen, R. A., Capelli, S., *et al.* (1997). MRI-based measurement of hippocampal volume in posttraumatic stress disorder related to childhood physical and sexual abuse: A preliminary report. *Biological Psychiatry*, *41*, 23–32.

Brewin, C., Andrews, B., & Valentine, J. (2000). Meta-analysis of risk factors for posttraumatic stress disorder in trauma-exposed adults. *Journal of Consulting and Clinical Psychology*, *68*, 748–766.

Brewin, C. R. (2001). A cognitive neuroscience account of posttraumatic stress disorder and its treatment. *Behaviour Research and Therapy*, *39*, 373–393.

Brewin, C. R., Andrews, B., & Rose, S. (2003). Overlap between acute stress disorder and PTSD in victims of violent crime. *American Journal of Psychiatry*, *160*, 783–785.

Broberg, A., Dyregrov, A., & Lilled, L. (2005). The Goteborg discotheque fire: Posttraumatic stress, and school adjustment as reported by the primary victims 18 months later. *Journal of Child Psychology and Psychiatry*, *46*, 1279–1286.

Canterbury, R., & Yule, W. (1999). Debriefing and crisis intervention. In W. Yule (Ed.), *Post Traumatic Stress Disorder* (pp. 221–238). Chichester: Wiley.

Carrion, V. G., Weems, C. F., Ray, R. D., Glaser, B. H., Hessl, D., & Reiss, A. L. (2002). Diurnal salivary cortisol in pediatric posttraumatic stress disorder. *Biological Psychiatry*, *51*, 575–582.

Celano, M., Hazzard, A., Webb, C., & McCall, C. (1996). Treatment of traumagenic beliefs among sexually abused girls and their mothers: An evaluation study. *Journal of Abnormal Child Psychology*, *24*, 1–17.

Chemtob, C. M., Nakashima, J. P., & Hamada, R. S. (2002). Psychosocial intervention for postdisaster trauma symptoms in elementary school children: A controlled community field study. *Archives of Pediatrics and Adolescent Medicine*, *156*, 211–216.

Cohen, J. A., Deblinger, E., Mannarino, A. P., & Steer, R. A. (2004). A multisite, randomized controlled trial for children with sexual abuse-related PTSD symptoms. *Journal of the American Academy of Child and Adolescent Psychiatry*, *43*, 393–402.

Cohen, J. A., Perel, J. M., DeBellis, M., Friedman, M., & Putnam, F. W. (2002). Treating traumatized children: Clinical implications of the psychobiology of posttraumatic stress disorder. *Trauma, Violence, & Abuse*, *3*, 91–108.

Dalgleish, T., Meiser-Stedman, R., & Smith, P. (2005). Cognitive aspects of posttraumatic stress reactions and their treatment in children and adolescents: an empirical review and some recommendations. *Behavioural and Cognitive Psychotherapy*, *33*, 459–486.

De Bellis, M. D. (2001). Developmental traumatology: The psychobiological development of maltreated children and its implications for research, treatment, and policy. *Development and Psychopathology*, *13*, 539–564.

De Bellis, M. D., Chrousos, G. P., Dorn L. D., Burke, L., Helmers, K., Kling, M. A., *et al.* (1994). Hypothalamic–pituitary–adrenal axis dysregulation in sexually abused girls. *Journal of Clinical Endocrinology and Metabolism*, *78*, 249–255.

De Bellis, M. D., Baum, A. S., Birmaher, B., Keshavan, M. S., Eccard, C. H., Boring, A. M., *et al.* (1999a). A. E. Bennett Research Award Developmental traumatology. 1. Biological stress systems. *Biological Psychiatry*, *45*, 1259–1270.

De Bellis, M. D., Keshavan, M. S., Clark, D. B., Casey, B. J., Giedd, J. N., Boring, A. M., *et al.* (1999b). A. E. Bennett Research Award Developmental traumatology. 2. Brain development. *Biological Psychiatry*, *45*, 1271–1284.

Deblinger, E., Stauffer, L. B., & Steer, R. A. (2001). Comparative efficacies of supportive and cognitive behavioral group therapies for young children who have been sexually abused and their non-offending mothers. *Child Maltreatment: Journal of the American Professional Society on the Abuse of Children*, *6*, 332–343.

de Roos, C., Greenwald, R., de Jongh, A., & Noorthoorn, E. E. (2004). EMDR versus CBT for disaster-exposed children: A controlled study. Poster presented at ISTSS 20th Annual Meeting, New Orleans, November.

Ehlers, A., & Clark, D. M. (2000). A cognitive model of posttraumatic stress disorder. *Behaviour Research and Therapy*, *38*, 319–345.

Ehlers, A., Mayou, R. A., & Bryant, B. (2003). Cognitive predictors of posttraumatic stress disorder in children: Results of a prospective longitudinal study. *Behaviour Research and Therapy*, *41*, 1–10.

Elkit, A. (2002). Victimization and PTSD in a Danish national youth probability sample. *Journal of the American Academy of Child and Adolescent Psychiatry*, *41*, 174–181.

Feeny, N. C., Foa, E. B., Treadwell, K. R., & March, J. (2004). Posttraumatic stress disorder in youth: A critical review of the cognitive and behavioral treatment outcome literature. *Professional Psychology: Research and Practice*, *35*, 466–476.

Fletcher, K. E. (1996). Childhood posttraumatic stress disorder. In E. J. Mash, & R. A. Barkley (Eds.), *Child psychopathology* (pp. 242–276). New York: Guilford.

Foa, E. B., Johnson, K., Feeney, N. C., & Treadwell, K. (2000). The child PTSD symptom scale: A preliminary examination of its psychometric properties. *Journal of Clinical Child Psychology*, *30*, 376–384.

Foa, E. B., Steketee, G., & Olasov-Rothbaum, B. (1989). Behavioral/cognitive conceptualizations of post-traumatic stress disorder. *Behavior Therapy*, *20*, 155–176.

Frederick, C. J. (1985). Children traumatized by catastrophic situations. In S. Eth, & R. Pynoos (Eds.), *Post-traumatic stress disorder in children* (pp. 73–99). Washington: American Psychiatric Press.

Giaconia, R. M., Reinherz, H. Z., Silverman, A. B., Pakiz, B., Frost, A. K., & Cohen, E. (1995). Traumas and posttraumatic stress disorder in a community population of older adolescents. *Journal of the American Academy of Child and Adolescent Psychiatry*, *34*, 1369–1380.

Goenjian, A. K., Karayan, I., Pynoos, R. S., Minassian, D., Najarian, L. M., Steinberg, A. M., *et al.* (1997). Outcome of psychotherapy among early adolescents after trauma. *American Journal of Psychiatry*, *154*, 536–542.

Goenjian, A. K., Pynoos, R. S., Steinberg, A. M., Najarian, L. M., Asarnow, J. R., Karayan, I., *et al.* (1995). Psychiatric comorbidity in children after the 1988 earthquake in Armenia. *Journal of the American Academy of Child and Adolescent Psychiatry*, *34*, 1174–1184.

Goenjian, A. K., Yehuda, R., Pynoos, R. S., Steinberg, A. M., Tashjian, M., Yang, R. K., *et al.* (1996). Basal cortisol, dexamethasone suppression of cortisol, and MHPG in adolescents after the 1988 earthquake in Armenia. *American Journal of Psychiatry*, *153*, 929–934.

Green, B., Korol, M., Grace, M., Vary, M., Leonard, A. C., Gleser, G. C., *et al.* (1991). Children and disaster: Age, gender, and parental effects on PTSD symptoms. *Journal of the American Academy of Child and Adolescent Psychiatry*, *30*, 945–951.

Gupta, L., Dyregrov, A., Gjestad, R., & Mukanoheli, X. (1996). Trauma, exposure, and psychological reactions to genocide among Rwandan refugees. Paper presented at the 12th Annual Convention of the International Society for Traumatic Stress Studies (November), San Francisco, CA.

Hamada, R. S., Kameoka, V., & Yanagida, E. (1996). The Kauai recovery inventory; screening for posttraumatic stress symptoms in children. Paper presented at the 12th Annual meeting of the International Society for Traumatic Stress Studies (November), San Francisco, CA.

Janoff-Bulman, R. (1985). The aftermath of victimization: Rebuilding shattered assumptions. In C. R. Figley (Ed.), *Trauma and its wake*. New York: Brunner/Mazel.

Johnson, K. (1993). *School crisis management: A team training guide*. Alameda, CA: Hunter House.

Jones, J. C., & Barlow, D. H. (1992). A new model of posttraumatic stress disorder. In P. A. Saigh (Ed.), *Posttraumatic stress disorder: A behavioral approach to assessment and treatment* (pp. 147–165). New York: Macmillan.

Joseph, S., Brewin C. R., Yule, W., & Williams, R. (1993). Causal attributions and post-traumatic stress in adolescents. *Journal of Child Psychology and Psychiatry*, *34*, 247–253.

Kassam-Adams, N., & Winston, F. K. (2004). Predicting child PTSD: The relationship between acute stress disorder and PTSD in injured children. *Journal of the American Academy of Child and Adolescent Psychiatry*, *43*, 403–411.

Kassam-Adams, N., Garcia-España, F., Fein, J. A., & Winston, S. K. (2005). Heart rate and posttraumatic stress in injured children. *Archives of General Psychiatry*, *62*, 335–340.

Kaufman, J., Birmaher, B., Perel, J., Dahl, R. E., Moreci, P., Nelson, B., Wells, W., & Ryan, N. D. (1997). The corticotropin-releasing hormone challenge in depressed abused, depressed non-abused, and normal control children. *Biological Psychiatry*, *42*, 669–679.

Kessler, R. C., Sonnega, A., Bromet, E., Hughes, M., & Nelson, C. B. (1995). Post-traumatic stress disorder in the National Comorbidity Survey. *Archives of General Psychiatry*, *52*, 1048–1060.

King, N. J., Tonge, B. J., Mullen, P., Myerson, N., Heyne, D., Rollings, S., *et al.* (2000). Treating sexually abused children with posttraumatic stress symptoms: A randomized clinical trial. *Journal of the American Academy of Child and Adolescent Psychiatry*, *39*, 1347–1355.

Klingman, A. (1993). School-based intervention following a disaster. In C. F. Saylor (Ed.), *Children and disasters* (pp. 187–210). New York: Plenum.

McFarlane, A. C. (1987). Family functioning and overprotection following a natural disaster: The longitudinal effects of post-traumatic morbidity. *Australia and New Zealand Journal of Psychiatry*, *21*, 210–218.

McFarlane, A. (2005). Psychiatric morbidity following disasters: Epidemiology, risk and protective factors. In J. Lopez-Ibor, G. Christodoulou, M. Maj, N. Sartorius, & A. Okasha (Eds.), *Disasters and mental health* (pp. 37–63). New York, NY: John Wiley & Sons.

Machel, G. (2001). *The impact of war on children: A review of progress since the 1996 United Nations report on the impact of armed conflict on children*. London, UK: Hurst & Co.

March, J. S., Amaya-Jackson, L., Murray, M. C., & Schulte, A. (1998). Cognitive–behavioral psychotherapy for children and adolescents with post-traumatic stress disorder after a single incident stressor. *Journal of the American Academy of Child and Adolescent Psychiatry*, *37*, 585–593.

Margolin, G., & Gordis, E. B. (2000). The effects of family and community violence on children. *Annual Review of Psychology*, *51*, 445–479.

Meiser-Stedman, R. (2002). Towards a cognitive–behavioral model of PTSD in children and adolescents. *Clinical Child and Family Psychology Review*, *5*, 217–232.

Meiser-Stedman, R., Yule, W., Dalgleish, T., Smith P., & Glucksman E. (2006). The role of the family in child and adolescent posttraumatic stress following attendance at an emergency department. *Journal of Pediatric Psychology*, *31*, 397–402.

Meiser-Stedman, R., Yule, W., Smith, P., Glucksman, E., & Dalgleish, T. (2005). Acute stress disorder and posttraumatic stress disorder in children and adolescents involved in assaults or motor vehicle accidents. *American Journal of Psychiatry*, *162*, 1381–1383.

Meltzer, H., Gatward, R., Goodman, R., & Ford, T. (2003). Mental health of children and adolescents in Great Britain. *International Review of Psychiatry*, *15*, 185–187.

Misch, P., Phillips, M., Evans, P., & Berelowitz, M. (1993). Trauma in pre-school children: A clinical account. In G. Forrest (Ed.), *Trauma and crisis management*. ACPP Occasional Paper.

Mollica, R. F., Lopes Cardoza, B., Osofsky, H. J., Raphael, B., Ager, A., & Salama, P. (2004). Mental health in complex emergencies. *Lancet*, *364*, 2058–2067.

Morgan, L., Scourfield, J., Williams, D., Jasper, A., & Lewis, G. (2003). The Aberfan disaster: 33-year follow-up of survivors. *British Journal of Psychiatry*, *182*, 532–536.

Moradi, A., Taghavi, M. R., Neshat-Doost, H., Yule, W., & Dalgleish, T. (2000). Memory bias for emotional information in children and adolescents with posttraumatic stress disorder. *Journal of Anxiety Disorders*, *14*, 521–534.

Nader, K., Pynoos, R., Fairbanks, L., Al-Ajeel, M., & al-Asfour, A. (1993). A preliminary study of PTSD and grief among the children of Kuwait following the Gulf crisis. *British Journal of Clinical Psychology*, *32*, 407–416.

Neuner, F., Schauer, M., Klaschik, C., Karunakara, U., & Elbert, T. (2004). A comparison of narrative exposure therapy, supportive counseling, and psychoeducation for treating posttraumatic stress disorder in an African refugee settlement. *Journal of Consulting and Clinical Psychology*, *72*, 579–587.

National Institute for Clinical Excellence (NICE). (2005). *Post traumatic stress disorder: The management of PTSD in adults and children in primary and secondary care* (Clinical Guideline 26). London: Gaskell and the British Psychological Society.

O'Donohue, W., & Eliot, A. (1992). The current status of post-traumatic stress disorder as a diagnostic category: Problems and proposals. *Journal of Traumatic Stress*, *5*, 421–439.

Ornitz, E. M., & Pynoos, R. S. (1989). Startle modulation in children with post-traumatic stress disorder. *American Journal of Psychiatry*, *146*, 866–870.

Pennebaker, J. W. (Ed.). (1995). *Emotion, disclosure, and health*. Washington, DC: American Psychological Association.

Perry, B. D. (1994). Neurobiological sequelae of childhood trauma: Post-traumatic stress disorder in children. In M. M. Murburg (Ed.), *Catecholamine function in posttraumatic stress disorder: Emerging concepts* (pp. 233–255). Washington, DC: American Psychiatric Press.

Pine, D. S. (2003). Developmental psychobiology and response to threats: Relevance to trauma in children and adolescents. *Biological Psychiatry*, *53*, 796–808.

Pine, D. S., & Cohen, J. (2002). Trauma in children and adolescents: risk and treatment of psychiatric sequelae. *Biological Psychiatry*, *51*, 519–531.

Pine, D. S., Mogg, K., Bradley, B. P., Montgomery, L., Monk, C. S., McClure, E., *et al.* (2005). Attention bias to threat in maltreated children: Implications for vulnerability to stress-related psychopathology. *American Journal of Psychiatry*, *162*, 291–296.

Pitman, R. K., Orr, S. P., Altman, B., Longpre, R. E., Poiré, R. E., & Macklin, M. L. (1996). Emotional processing during eye movement desensitization and reprocessing therapy of Vietnam veterans with chronic posttraumatic stress disorder. *Comprehensive Psychiatry*, *37*, 419–429.

Pynoos, R. S., & Eth, S. (1986). Witness to violence: The child interview. *Journal of the American Academy of Child Psychiatry*, *25*, 306–319.

Pynoos, R. S., Frederick, C., Nader, K., Arroyo, W., Steinberg, A., Eth, S., *et al.* (1987). Life threat and posttraumatic stress in school-age children. *Archives of General Psychiatry*, *44*, 1057–1063.

Pynoos, R. S., Goenjian, A., & Steinberg, A. M. (1995). Strategies of disaster interventions for children and adolesacents. In S. E. Hobfoll, & M. deVries (Eds.), *Extreme stress and communities: Impact and intervention*. Dordrecht, Netherlands: Kluwer.

Pynoos, R. S., & Nader, K. (1988). Psychological first aid and treatment approach for children exposed to community violence: research implications. *Journal of Traumatic Stress*, *1*, 243–267.

Ramchandani, P., & Jones, D. P. H. (2003). Treating psychological symptoms in sexually abused children: From research findings to service provision. *British Journal of Psychiatry*, *183*, 484–490.

Salmon, K., & Bryant, R. (2002). Posttraumatic stress disorder in children: The influence of developmental factors. *Clinical Psychology Review*, *22*, 163–188.

Schauer, M., Neuner, F., & Elbert, T. (2005). *Narrative exposure therapy: A short-term intervention for traumatic stress disorders after war, terror, or torture*. OH, USA: Hogrefe & Huber Publishers.

Schauer, E., Neuner, F., Elbert, T., Ertl, V., Onyut, L. P., Odenwald, M., *et al.* (2004). Narrative exposure therapy in children: A case study. *Intervention: International Journal of Mental Health, Psychosocial Work and Counselling in Areas of Armed Conflict*, *2*, 18–32.

Scheeringa, M., Peebles, C. D., Cook, C., & Zeanah C. H. (2001). Toward establishing procedural, criterion, and discriminant validity for PTSD in early childhood. *Journal of the American Academy of Child and Adolescent Psychiatry*, *40*, 52–60.

Scheeringa, M., Wright, M., Hunt, J. P., & Zeanah, C. H. (2006). Factors affecting the diagnosis and prediction of PTSD symptomatology in children and adolescents. *American Journal of Psychiatry*, *163*, 644–651.

Scheeringa, M. S., Zeanah, C. H., Drell, M. J., & Larrieu, J. A. (1995). Two approaches to the diagnosis of posttraumatic stress disorder in infancy and early childhood. *Journal of the American Academy of Child and Adolescent Psychiatry*, *34*, 191–200.

Scheeringa, M., Zeanah, C. H., Myers, L., & Putnam, F. (2003). New findings on alternative criteria for PTSD in preschool children. *Journal of the American Academy of Child and Adolescent Psychiatry*, *42*, 561–570.

Scheeringa, M. S., Zeanah, C. H., Myers, L., & Putnam, F. (2004). Heart period and variability findings in preschool children with posttraumatic stress symptoms. *Biological Psychiatry*, *55*, 685–691.

Shapiro, F. (2001). *Eye movment desensitization and reprocessing: Basic principles, protocols and procedures* (2nd edn.). New York: Guilford Press.

Smith, P., Perrin, S., Yule, W., & Rabe-Hesketh, S. (2001). War exposure and maternal reactions in the psychological adjustment of children from Bosnia-Hercegovina. *Journal of Child Psychology and Psychiatry*, *42*, 395–404.

Smith, P., Perrin, S. G., Yule, W., Hacam, B., & Stuvland, R. (2002). War exposure among children from Bosnia-Hercegovina: Psychological adjustment in a community sample. *Journal of Traumatic Stress*, *15*, 147–156.

Smith, P., Yule, W., Perrin, S., Tranah, T., Dalgleish, T., & Clark, D. M. (2007). A randomized controlled trial of cognitive behavior therapy for PTSD in children and adolescents. *Journal of the American Academy of Child and Adolescent Psychiatry*, *46*, 1051–1061.

Stallard, P. (2003). A retrospective analysis to explore the applicability of the Ehlers and Clark (2000) cognitive model to explain PTSD in children. *Behavioural and Cognitive Psychotherapy*, *31*, 337–345.

Stallard, P. (2006). Psychological interventions for post-traumatic stress reactions in children and young people: A review of randomised controlled trials. *Clinical Psychology Review*, *26*, 895–911.

Stallard, P., Salter, E., & Velleman, R. (2004). Posttraumatic stress disorder following road traffic accidents: A second prospective study. *European Child and Adolescent Psychiatry*, *13*, 172–178.

Stallard, P., Velleman, R., Salter, E., Howse, I., Yule, W., & Taylor, G. (2006). A randomised controlled trial to determine the effectiveness of an early psychological intervention with children involved in road traffic accidents. *Journal of Child Psychology and Psychiatry*, *47*, 127–134.

Stein, B. D., Jaycox, L. H., Kataoka, S. H., Wong, M., Tu, W., Elliott, M. N., *et al.* (2003). A mental health intervention for schoolchildren exposed to violence: A randomized controlled trial. *Journal of the American Medical Association*, *290*, 603–611.

Sullivan, M. A., Saylor, C. F., & Foster, K. Y. (1991). Post-hurricane adjustment of preschoolers and their families. *Advances in Behaviour Research and Therapy*, *13*, 163–171.

Terr, L. C. (1991). Childhood traumas: An outline and overview. *American Journal of Psychiatry*, *148*, 10–20.

Udwin, O., Boyle, S., Yule, W., Bolton, D., & O'Ryan, D. (2000). Risk factors for long-term psychological effects of a disaster experienced in adolescence: Predictors of post traumatic stress disorder. *Journal of Child Psychology and Psychiatry*, *41*, 969–979.

Vernberg, E. M., La Greca, A., Silverman, W. K., & Prinstein, M. J. (1996). Prediction of posttraumatic stress symptoms in children after hurricane Andrew. *Journal of Abnormal Psychology*, *105*, 237–248.

Wolmer, L., Laor, N., Gershon, A., Mayes, L. C., & Cohen, D. J. (2000). The mother–child dyad facing trauma: A developmental outlook. *Journal of Nervous and Mental Disease*, *188*, 409–415.

World Health Organization (WHO). (1996). *Multiaxial classification of child and adolescent psychiatric disorders: The ICD-10 classification of mental and behavioural disorders in children and adolescents*. Cambridge, UK: Cambridge University Press.

Yehuda, R., & McFarlane, A.C. (1995). Conflict between current knowledge about posttraumatic stress disorder and its original conceptual basis. *American Journal of Psychiatry*, *152*, 1705– 1713.

Yule, W., Bolton, D., Udwin, O., Boyle, S., O'Ryan, D., & Nurrish, J. (2000). The long-term psychological effects of a disaster experienced in adolescence. I. The incidence and course of post traumatic stress disorder. *Journal of Child Psychology and Psychiatry*, *41*, 503–511.

Yule, W., & Gold, A. (1993). *Wise before the event: Coping with crises in schools*. London: Calouste Gulbenkian Foundation.

Yule, W., Perrin, S., & Smith, P. (1999). Post-traumatic stress disorders in children and adolescents. In W. Yule (Ed.), *Post traumatic stress disorder* (pp. 25–50). Chichester: Wiley.

43 Obsessive-Compulsive Disorder

Judith L. Rapoport and Philip Shaw

Definition: the Concept and Current Issues

Obsessive-compulsive disorder was once considered rare in childhood, but recent advances in diagnosis and treatment have led to recognition that the disorder is a common cause of distress for children and adolescents. It is characterized by the presence of obsessions (unwanted, repetitive or intrusive thoughts) and compulsions (unnecessary repetitive behaviors or mental activities). Because the obsessive-compulsive thoughts and rituals are usually recognized by the child as nonsensical, they are often kept hidden for as long as possible – from both parents and practitioners. This secrecy may have contributed to the fact that until the 1980s OCD was unfamiliar to most child psychiatrists, even though classic descriptions of the disorder featured cases with childhood presentation (Janet, 1903). The recognition that OCD was more common in adults than previously believed, and retrospective reports that one-half to one-third of adult subjects had their onset in childhood or adolescence, focused the attention of the child psychiatric community on this chronic and often disabling disorder (Karno & Golding, 1991; Karno, Golding, Sorenson *et al.*, 1988).

Until the mid-nineteenth century, obsessive-compulsive phenomena were considered to be a variant of insanity. However, as the disorder was better defined, it came into focus as one of the neuroses. The descriptions of repetitive unwanted thoughts or rituals, often characterized by magical thinking and usually kept private by the sufferer, were relatively constant observations in those early reports. Debate about core deficits and the relative importance of volitional, intellectual and emotional impairments (all of which are in some way abnormal in OCD) have flourished for over 100 years (Berrios, 1989).

Freud (1906; 1958) speculated about the similarity between obsessive-compulsive phenomena, children's games and religious rites. Although psychoanalytic theory is empirically unproved and has not been shown to be effective in the treatment of OCD, the broad questions raised by Freud about continuity and discontinuity within individual development and OCD, as well as with regard to secular and religious rituals, remain fascinating issues. In addition, the association between certain neurological disorders, such as Tourette's disorder (see chapter 44), and OCD, supported by current imaging research, has led to possible localization of brain circuits mediating obsessive-compulsive behaviors as well as mechanisms for behavioral encoding. Over the past decade, interest in these general questions, as well as the possibility of unique pediatric subgroups of OCD, has generated a wealth of clinical and translational research (Apter, Fallon, Jr., King *et al.*, 1996; Fitzgerald, MacMaster, Paulson *et al.*, 1999; Graybiel & Rauch, 2000; Rapoport & Inoff-Germain, 2007). Key issues which appear throughout this chapter are the degree to which at least some cases with childhood onset represent a distinct subtype (e.g., patients with Tourette's/tics and/or patients with a possible infectious trigger or Pediatric Autoimmune Neuropsychiatric Disorders Associated with Streptococcal infections – PANDAS) and the extent to which there is continuity with normal development. Another important topic is how to optimize treatment for this often chronic condition.

Epidemiology

The Epidemiological Catchment Area (ECA) study of over 18,500 individuals in five different sites in the USA included OCD as a separate category and provided the first large-scale information on the prevalence of this disorder in adults (Karno & Golding, 1991; Karno, Golding, Sorenson *et al.*, 1988) (see page 699). Using the Diagnostic Interview Schedule, a structured interview designed for lay interviewers, lifetime prevalence rates without DSM-III exclusions ranged from 1.9 to 3.3% across sites. Even with DSM-III exclusions, the rates were 1.2–2.4%. These rates were 25–60 times greater than had been estimated on the basis of clinical populations. The mean age of onset across the sites ranged from 20 to 25 years with 50% developing symptoms in childhood or adolescence (Karno & Golding, 1991), providing further support for the retrospective accounts of the frequent pediatric onset of this disorder (Black, 1974). More recent cross-cultural studies with adults have been supportive of similar rates of between 1.9 and 2.5 percent prevalence across widely differing cultures (Horwath & Weissman, 2000). Higher rates are found using DSM-IV than with ICD-10, with only 64% agreement between the two systems (Andrews, Slade, & Peters, 1999). As about a half of adult patients report onset after adolescence or childhood, the similar rates for adult and child populations suggest that

Rutter's Child and Adolescent Psychiatry, 5th edition. Edited by M. Rutter, D. Bishop, D. Pine, S. Scott, J. Stevenson, E. Taylor and A. Thapar. © 2008 Blackwell Publishing, ISBN: 978-1-4051-4549-7.

Table 43.1 Community studies of OCD prevalence in children & adolescents.

Study	Sample, age of	Ascertainment & evaluation	Prevalence (%)
Flament *et al.* (1988)	5596 students grades 9–12 (USA)	Initial screening with Leyton, epidemiological version; 356 subject meeting screening criteria for OCD were then evaluated using semi-structured interview by clinicians	1.0 & 1.9 (current & lifetime, respectively)
Zohar *et al.* (1992)	562 consecutive army recruits, ages 16–17 yrs (Israel)	Short semi-structured interview by a child psychiatrist	3.6 (point)
Reinherz *et al.* (1993)	384 mostly 18 yr olds (USA)	Structured interview by trained interviewers with research or clinical experience	1.3, 1.3, 2.1 (1-mo, 6-mo, & lifetime, respectively)
Lewinsohn *et al.* (1993)	1,710 14–18 yr olds (USA)	Semi-structured interview mostly by trained, clinically experienced interviewers	0.06, 0.53 (current & lifetime, respectively)
Valleni-Basile *et al.* (1994)	3,283 (mostly) 12–15 yr olds (USA)	3,283 screened; 488 mother–child pairs then given semi-structured interview by psychiatric nurses	2.95 (wt. current)
Douglas *et al.* (1995)	930 18 yr olds from a birth cohort followed since birth (New Zealand)	Structured interview by trained mental health interviewers	4.0 (1-yr)
Apter *et al.* (1996)	861 consecutive army recruits, years 16–17 (Israel)	Initial screening by an OCD self-report questionnaire followed by a structured interview by a child psychiatrist	2.3 (lifetime)
Wittchen *et al.* (1998)	3,021 14–24 yrs (Germany)	Semi-structured interview by clinical interviewers & trained professional health research interviewers	0.6 & 0.7 (1-yr & lifetime, respectively)
Rapoport *et al.* (2000)	NIMH MECA four-site sample of caretaker-child dyads of 1,285 9–17 yr olds (USA)	Structured interview by trained interviewers	0.3, 2.5, 2.7 (parent-report, child-report, & total, respectively)

some pediatric patients must remit. This apparent discrepancy from the chronic nature of most pediatric OCD studied clinically has not been resolved (see discussion below), but may reflect in part that adult cases are typically identified using only one informant, whereas childhood cases are frequently diagnosed on the basis of two informants (the child and parent).

A number of early epidemiological studies of OCD focused on children and adolescents [see review by Zohar (1999)]. One recent additional study examined the results of a large four-site community survey in the USA (the National Institute of Mental Health [NIMH] Methods for the Epidemiology of Child and Adolescent Mental Disorders [MECA] Study) (Rapoport, Inoff-Germain, Weissman *et al.*, 2000). The lifetime prevalence across eight studies (from these two articles combined) indicates relative consistency with a lifetime prevalence from 0.7 to 2.9%. (Also see Table 43.1). Males have an earlier onset than females, contributing to a striking preponderance of males in most pediatric samples (Geller, Biederman, Jones *et al.*, 1998). The variance in prevalence rates is likely to reflect differences in study design, particularly whether clinicians or non-clinicians conducted interviews. Additionally, prevalence estimates may also be sensitive to the diagnostic tools employed. Structured interviews in particular may yield false positives when given to children, who are apt to misinterpret the questions (Breslau, 1987).

There is increasing reliance on standardized interviews and rating scales for both the study and clinical management of OCD. Structured interviews are covered in detail in chapter 19. The most commonly used tools, the Diagnostic Interview for Children and Adolescents (Herjanic & Campbell, 1977; Herjanic & Reich, 1982) and the Schedule for Affective Disorder and Schizophrenia for School-Age Children (Kaufman, Birmaher, Brent *et al.*, 1997), have sections on OCD. In addition, there are several rating scales in general use, including the child version of the Leyton Obsessional Inventory (Berg, Rapoport, Whitaker *et al.*, 1989) and the Yale-Brown Obsessive Compulsive Scale (Y-BOCS) (Goodman, Price, Rasmussen, Mazure, Delgado *et al.*, 1989; Goodman, Price, Rasmussen, Mazure, Fleischmann *et al.*, 1989).

Diagnostic Issues

Continuity with Normal Development

The boundaries of diagnosis are complex in any disorder, and this is clearly the case with OCD. Individual "habits" that are typical of OCD are extremely common across populations. For example, in one Israeli study, only 18% of the sample endorsed no obsessive-compulsive symptoms at all. Moreover, many ritualistic and "magical" behaviors are part of normal development (Leonard, 1989). As is the case with many disorders, family genetic studies seem to indicate that familiarity of obsessive-compulsive symptoms may extend across the entire range of severity, and similarly twin studies support the model of OCD as the extreme of a continuously distributed trait with biological continuity between normal and abnormal behaviors (Jonnal, Gardner, Prescott, & Kendler, 2000). However, there is evidence from a pediatric sample that symptom levels below the level needed for a categorical diagnosis of OCD do not predict the disorder at follow-up, although interestingly there was some prediction of depression (Berg, Rapoport, Whitaker *et al.*, 1989).

The Importance of Informant History

Secrecy appears to be a hallmark of childhood onset OCD. The children recognize that their symptoms are nonsensical and are embarrassed by them, so they go to great lengths to hide them. Hand-washing might be disguised as more frequent voiding and rituals are carried out in private, so that children are often symptomatic for months before their parents are aware of a problem. Teachers and peers typically are aware only for cases with greater severity. As with Tourette's disorder, children may expend effort controlling their behaviors in public and "let go" when at home. This partial voluntary control of symptoms often baffles and angers parents. Because of the variable degree and timing of the control of symptoms, the nature of the informant has a particularly important influence on recognition and diagnosis of OCD. As shown for the MECA data (Rapoport, Inoff-Germain, Weissman *et al.*, 2000), only 0.3% were identified by parents while 2.5% were identified through self-report from the child, with only one overlapping case.

Issues with DSM-IV Diagnosis

OCD is defined in both ICD-10 and DSM-IV as repetitive intrusive thoughts and/or rituals that are unwanted and which interfere significantly with function or cause marked distress. The severity criteria avoid confusion of OCD with many childhood habits that are part of normal development. Both the content and relative insight into the unreasonableness of the thoughts/behaviors differentiate OCD from other disorders.

Whereas clinical experience suggests that the adult criteria can be applied to childhood cases, there are several important caveats. Both DSM-IV and ICD-10 state that compulsions are designed to neutralize or prevent some dreaded event. This may not always be the case, at least for childhood OCD. While some children may not be willing or able to verbalize their obsessive thoughts, long-term contact has demonstrated that about 40% of children with OCD do not have obsessive thoughts; they steadfastly report the presence of only compulsive rituals accompanied by a vague sense of discomfort if the rituals are not carried out (Swedo, Rapoport, Leonard, Lenane, & Cheslow, 1989). At least a third of pediatric patients report that certain stimuli trigger their rituals and that avoidance of the trigger "protects" them from the obsessive-compulsive symptoms (Karno, Golding, Sorenson, & Burnam, 1988). The degree of insight needed for the diagnosis is also in dispute as some patients, at least some of the time, "believe" their obsessive thoughts. It is probable that for both children and adolescents and particularly in severe cases, diagnostic criteria should allow some partial "belief" in the necessity for these thoughts/behaviors.

Changes in diagnostic systems have an obvious impact on estimates of the prevalence of a disorder. In the case of OCD, the most recent version of DSM includes impairment and distress as criteria, as opposed to the earlier version, which included these features only as modifiers. Thus, because of exclusion of either false positives or milder cases, rates of OCD tend to be lower with DSM-IV, with a 12-month prevalence rate of 0.6% being reported in a recent study (Crino, Slade, & Andrews, 2005). Estimates of lifetime prevalence appear to be less affected by the change in diagnostic criteria (Angst, Gamma, Endrass *et al.*, 2004; Swedo, Leonard, & Rapoport, 2004). There are several important differences between the ICD-10 and DSM-IV criteria, such as whether exclusions are made based on comorbid psychotic disorders, such as schizophrenia. DSM-IV (and DSM III-R) allow patients to receive a diagnosis of OCD even in the presence of schizophrenia (APA, 2000) in light of convincing evidence of coexistence with schizophrenia (Byerly, Goodman, Acholonu, Bugno, & Rush, 2005; Poyurovsky & Koran, 2005).

Continuity with Obsessive-Compulsive Spectrum Disorders

Another diagnostic issue involves potential "obsessive-compulsive spectrum disorders." These proposed "spectrum" disorders represent a range of candidates, such as body dysmorphic disorder, hypochondriasis and trichotillomania (involving tension-related, recurrent pulling out of one's hair). The phenomenological similarities are often striking. For example, similarly to OCD, body dysmorphic disorder and hypochondriasis are characterized by anxiety-arousing concerns and anxiety-reducing rituals, and several impulse control disorders have very prominent compulsive aspects, particularly the repetitive and typically anxiety-relieving motor behavior of trichotillomania. A neurobiological overlap with OCD is suggested by the increased rate of subclinical OCD features in relatives of those with spectrum disorder (Bienvenu, Samuels, Riddle *et al.*, 2000). There are also many studies that have suggested some efficacy for serotonin reuptake inhibiting drugs in the treatment of these disorders, although there are also several notable negative treatment trials (Christenson, Mackenzie, Mitchell, & Callies, 1991; Hollander, 1996; Hollander, King, Delaney, Smith, & Silverman, 2003; Hollander & Wong, 1995; Karno, Golding, Sorenson, & Burnam, 1988). We will consider later the overlap between the neural substrates of OCD and the spectrum disorders.

Children with disorders that are less obviously related to OCD, such as pervasive developmental disorder, frequently exhibit a compulsive need for sameness but lack other features such as ego-dystonicity (the individual's sense that the contents of his symptoms are alien and unlike his normal self). Several other disorders exhibit a high comorbidity with OCD but share few of the cardinal symptoms of OCD itself. Thus, disorders such as pyromania, pathological gambling disorder and anorexia nervosa overlap with OCD principally in that their symptoms involve over-focused ideation. There continues to be debate about classification of OCD as an anxiety disorder. Whereas both involve intense internal preoccupation, depression rather than anxiety is the major comorbidity with OCD, and there is evidence from family studies that OCD does not segregate with other anxiety disorders and may have a different pattern of genetic transmission (for a review of this issue, see Bartz & Hollander, 2006).

Unique Childhood Onset Subtypes

This leads to a related question as to whether OCD with very early onset represents an important subtype of the disorder or possibly a different disorder altogether. There is growing evidence that at the very least, early age of onset represents a more familial form of the disorder, particularly for pediatric cases with ordering compulsions (Pauls, Alsobrook, Goodman, Rasmussen, & Leckman, 1995). In one study, no patient with adult onset of OCD had a first-degree relative with OCD (Nestadt, Samuels, Riddle *et al.*, 2000). Additionally, very early onset OCD appears to be more frequently associated with tics and/or Tourette's disorder (Chabane, Delorme, Millet *et al.*, 2004; Grados, Riddle, Samuels *et al.*, 2001). Moreover, family studies have found that tic disorders are more likely to occur in patients who have relatives with OCD than in patients who lack a familial loading for OCD (Pauls, Alsobrook, Goodman, Rasmussen, & Leckman, 1995).

The postulation of a post-infectious subgroup of pediatric OCD came about as a result of early reports of the association of OCD with Sydenham's chorea (Freeman *et al.*, 1965; Osler, 1894). This supported converging evidence of basal ganglia involvement in the etiology and/or maintenance of OCD (Wise & Rapoport, 1989). One example of a possible post-infectious subgroup has been identified by research at the NIMH which identified a group of pediatric patients in whom symptom onset or exacerbations are triggered by streptococcal infections; the subgroup is identified by the acronym PANDAS (Pediatric Autoimmune Neuropsychiatric Disorders Associated with Streptococcal infections) (Swedo, Leonard, & Rapoport, 2004). This group of patients appears to have a relatively sudden onset of symptoms, typically has an abnormal neurological examination during exacerbations (particularly tic or choreiform movements – see chapter 44) and tends to have a better outcome. The disorder is thought to arise through a process of molecular mimicry, with the group A ß-hemolytic streptococcus (*Streptococcus pyogenes*) (GABHS) evoking antibodies that are capable of cross-reacting with specific areas of the human brain (e.g., the basal ganglia) to produce neuropsychiatric and behavioral symptoms. However, there remains considerable controversy around the diagnosis, particularly in view of some studies failing to detect elevated levels of autoantibodies in those otherwise meeting criteria for PANDAS (Singer, Hong, Yoon, & Williams, 2005).

Clinical Presentation

Childhood onset OCD has been documented as early as age 2 but more typically begins later in childhood or early adolescence (APA, 1994). In general, the symptoms of OCD in children mirror those in adult patients. Thus, obsessions on the themes of contamination, danger to self or others (such as fears that parents will be harmed), symmetry or moral issues are common; and typical compulsions include washing, checking and repeating – particularly until the child experiences a feeling of "getting it just right" (Despert, 1955; Masi, Millepiedi, Mucci *et al.*, 2005; Thomsen, 1991). Most children have a combination of obsessions and rituals, and pure obsessives are rare compared with the more frequent pure ritualizers. Children with an early age at onset (below age 6) usually begin their rituals or obsessions in an easily recognizable fashion, such as excessive hand-washing or ritualized checking and repeating. In some cases, however, the clinical presentation is altered by the child's developmental immaturity. For example, one 6-year-old boy, who was compelled to draw zeros repetitively, had started at age 3 to circle manhole covers on city streets. His tantrums when the circling was interrupted, his subjective distress during the behavior and his lack of other psychosocial abnormalities or disorders (such as autism or pervasive developmental disorder) led to the diagnosis of OCD. Another child, who presented at age 7 with clinically significant checking compulsions, had been evaluated previously at 3 years of age when he developed a "compulsion" to walk only on the edges of the floor tiles. Cleaning rituals in children too young to reach the water faucet can present as excessive hand-wiping or licking.

A large community-based study of young adolescents found females more frequently reported compulsions and males more commonly reported obsessions (Valleni-Basile, Garrison, Jackson *et al.*, 1994). The most common compulsions were arranging (56%), counting (41%), washing (17%) and checking (12%). The presenting symptoms of 70 children and adolescents consecutively evaluated at the NIMH are summarized in Table 43.2 (Swedo, Rapoport, Leonard, Lenane, & Cheslow, 1989), which gives greater detail on the content of obsessions. While there is considerable overlap in the symptom profile between the community and clinic samples' symptom profile, washing compulsions were the most common symptom in the NIMH sample, occurring at some time during the course of the illness in over half of the patients. Hand washing and showering were the most common, and the use of chemicals such as alcohol or detergents provoked eczematoid dermatitis in several cases.

A cluster analysis of symptoms in 213 children with OCD produced five clusters: mental rituals/touching/ordering; cleaning/contamination; superstitions; obsessions/checking/confessing;

Table 43.2 Presenting symptoms in 70 consecutive children and adolescents with primary obsessive-compulsive disorder.

Reported symptoms at initial interview	N	%
Obsessions		
Concerns with dirt, germs, environmental toxins	28	40
Something terrible happening (e.g., death of loved one)	17	24
Symmetry, order or exactness	12	17
Scrupulosity (religious obsessions)	9	13
Concern or disgust with bodily waste or secretions	6	8
Lucky or unlucky numbers	6	8
Forbidden, aggressive or perverse sexual thoughts, images or impulses	3	4
Fear of harming others or self	3	4
Concern with household items	2	3
Intrusive nonsense sounds, words or music	1	1
Compulsions		
Excessive or ritualized hand-washing, showering, bathing or grooming	60	86
Repeating rituals (e.g., going in and out of the door)	36	51
Checking (e.g., doors, locks, stoves)	32	46
Miscellaneous rituals (e.g., writing, moving, speaking)	18	26
Rituals to remove contact with contaminants	16	23
Touching	14	20
Measures to prevent harm to self or others	11	16
Ordering or arranging	12	17
Counting	13	18
Hoarding/collecting rituals	8	11
Rituals of cleaning household or inanimate objects	4	6

Note: As multiple obsessions and compulsions are possible, the total thus exceeds 70.
Based on Swedo *et al.* (1989).

and somatic concerns (Ivarsson & Valderhaug, 2006). A similar factor structure of OCD symptoms in children and adolescents was found in an independent analysis (McKay, Piacentini, Greisberg *et al.*, 2006). This shows some overlap with factor analytic studies of symptoms in adult OCD, which have consistently indicated four main symptom clusters in OCD: symmetry/ordering, contamination/cleaning, hoarding and obsessions/checking (Mataix-Cols, Rosario-Campos, & Leckman, 2005). The symptom profiles differ, however, in the absence of a hoarding subgroup in children as well as the prominence of a "superstition" symptom cluster in children with magical thinking and acts as central features. The usefulness of these factors in treatment prediction and genetic studies is being explored (see below).

Approximately one third of pediatric patients report that certain stimuli trigger their rituals and that avoidance of the trigger "protects" them from the obsessive-compulsive symptoms (Swedo, Rapoport, Leonard, Lenane, & Cheslow, 1989). For example, a 16-year-old girl with elaborate front door touching and stepping rituals would "sneak" into her house by a side door, avoiding the sight of the front door and successfully averting the compulsion. Several children avoided looking at certain parts of a room (e.g., "corners of the ceiling") which set off various gaze rituals. These phenomena have been viewed from an ethological perspective, with the compulsions conceptualized as "fixed action patterns" released by key environmental stimuli (Modell, Mountz, Curtis, & Greden, 1989; Wise & Rapoport, 1989). These triggers are of particular interest for treatment as they often determine the key approach during behavioral desensitization, namely, exposure with response prevention (see below).

Course and Natural History

Epidemiological studies indicate that over 50% of adults with OCD report that their symptoms started during childhood or adolescence, with males generally having earlier onset than females (Rasmussen & Tsuang, 1984). A single epidemiological study of OCD in a group of 18-year-olds suggested that past depression and substance abuse were predictive of onset of OCD (Douglass, Moffitt, Dar, McGee, & Silva, 1995). There may also be a prodromal phase: parents of nearly half of the NIMH sample revealed that their children had displayed "micro episodes of OCD" years before developing full-blown symptoms. During these episodes, excessive rigidity and repetitive rituals (e.g., wearing the same clothes for a month, refusal to take a different path through the house) were a source of concern, albeit briefly.

A prospective epidemiological survey of 976 children, initially assessed between the ages of 1 and 10 years and then 8, 10, and 15 years later, delineated predictors of OCD symptoms

(Peterson, Pine, Cohen, & Brook, 2001). In prospective analyses, tics in childhood and early adolescence predicted an increase in OCD symptoms in late adolescence and early adulthood, whereas ADHD symptoms in adolescence predicted more OCD symptoms in early adulthood.

The clinical course of the disorder indicates some developmental influence on symptoms over time. In a clinic sample, this sensitivity to developmental stage was found firstly in symptom profile, with the presenting obsessions and compulsions changing over time in 90% of the NIMH pediatric patients (Rettew, Swedo, Leonard, Lenane, & Rapoport, 1992). Most children began with a single obsession or compulsion and continued with this for months to years, and then gradually acquired different obsessions or rituals. Although the primary symptom would change (e.g., from counting to washing and then checking), some earlier symptoms often remained problematic, although to a lesser degree. The nature of the compulsive rituals also changed over time. A study of adolescents demonstrated that counting and symmetry were most prominent during grade school years, but were replaced by washing rituals during early and mid adolescence (Maina, Albert, Bogetto, & Ravizza, 1999).

The outcome of OCD may also have a similar relationship to developmental stage. In their longitudinal epidemiological study of tics, OCD, and ADHD described above, Peterson and colleagues found in prospective analyses that both younger and older adolescents with OCD were more likely to develop depressive and ADHD symptoms. Early adolescents with OCD, however, were especially likely to develop more anxiety and simple phobias in later adolescence. Epidemiological studies of adults suggest that spontaneous remissions occur in as many as one-third of patients (Karno & Golding, 1990). A recent prospective study of 591 adult subjects assessed patients at six time points between ages 20 and 40 (Angst, Gamma, Endrass *et al.*, 2004). While OCD was chronic in 60% of the cases, there was considerable improvement over time, even in those who continued to meet diagnostic criteria. It is often argued that pediatric cases will have a more chronic course, and a recent meta-analysis of studies based on sixteen independent samples (521 OCD participants) followed for a mean of 11.2 years indicated earlier age of onset to be a poor prognosis factor, along with comorbid psychiatric illness and poor initial treatment response (Stewart, Geller, Jenike *et al.*, 2004). Overall, there was a 41% persistence for full and 60% for full or sub-threshold OCD. However, the pathways determining clinical outcome are complex, and any one single developmental variable, such as age of onset, is likely to account for only a modest amount of the overall variance in final outcome.

OCD patients with comorbid tics or Tourette's have a waxing and waning course (Bloch, Peterson, Scahill *et al.*, 2006). In patients with comorbid Tourette's and OCD, tics generally start to improve around age 10, while the obsessive-compulsive symptoms typically continue for several more years. PANDAS are also characterized as relapsing/remitting in relation to streptococcal infection (Leonard, Swedo, Garvey *et al.*, 1999).

Associated Disorders

Both epidemiological (Karno & Golding, 1991) and clinical (LaSalle, Cromer, Nelson *et al.*, 2004) studies indicate broad and complex comorbidity for OCD similar to that seen for other major Axis I disorders. The patterns of comorbidity among childhood onset cases are generally comparable with those of adult samples, but with tic disorders and specific developmental disorders appearing more frequently in the pediatric population. In the NIMH sample, only 25% of the pediatric subjects had OCD as a single diagnosis (Swedo, Rapoport, Leonard, Lenane, & Cheslow, 1989). Tic disorders (30%), major depression (26%) and specific developmental disabilities (17%) were the most common comorbidities, and there were also high rates of simple phobias (17%), over-anxious disorder (16%), adjustment disorder (11%), attention deficit disorder (10%), conduct disorder (7%), separation anxiety disorder (7%), and enuresis/encopresis (4%). While our own experience with comorbid bipolar disorder is limited, other groups find increased bipolar comorbidity in severely affected pediatric OCD cases (Masi, Perugi, Toni *et al.*, 2004). This broad comorbidity remains to be explained (for this and other disorders) and is not accounted for by any of the etiological models discussed below. An interesting exception to the broad comorbidity is the lack of association between obsessive-compulsive or anankastic personality disorder and OCD in adults, although the rates (or even the definition, in childhood) of this personality disorder are not known in children and adolescents (Albert, Maina, Forner, & Bogetto, 2004; Masi, Perugi, Toni *et al.*, 2004).

Case Illustrations

Case 1

A 14-year-old boy, whose symptoms had begun gradually, recalls at a very early age having to wash his hands repetitively. He was unable to associate an obsessive thought with this ritual, but he felt compelled to perform it. By age 6, he had developed an obsessive fear of tornadoes. He would repeatedly check the sky for clouds, listen to all weather reports and query his mother about approaching storms. The tornado obsession faded over time and was replaced by a generalized fear of harm coming to himself or his family. He responded with extensive rituals to protect himself and his family. Particularly at times of separating, such as bedtime or leaving for school, the patient would be compelled to repeat actions perfectly or to check repetitively. When asked how many times he would have to repeat an action, he replied, "It depends. The number isn't always the same, I just have to do it right." When asked how he knew when it was right, he said, "I don't know, it just feels right." As the patient entered puberty, he became obsessed with acquired immunodeficiency syndrome (AIDS) and was convinced he would acquire it through his mouth. He began spitting in an effort to cleanse his mouth and would spit every 15–20 seconds. In addition, he began extensive washing rituals. Despite these cleansing and washing compulsions, his personal appearance was slovenly and dirty. He never tied his shoelaces because they had touched the ground and were "contaminated"; if he tied them, his hands would be "dirty" and he would have to wash until they were "clean" again. Remarkably, although his family was aware that "something had been wrong for a long time," most of the content of his obsessions was kept secret. This case illustrates the contamination concerns common to adolescents as well as the variety and evolution of obsessive-compulsive symptoms during development.

Case 2

A 16-year-old girl had symptoms that began abruptly, shortly after the onset of menses. She called herself "a prisoner of my own mind." Her obsessions centered around a fear of harm to her parents. She was plagued by recurrent thoughts of her mother dying in a car accident, her father being killed by an intruder, or both her parents dying of burns received in a house fire. Always a light sleeper, she began to get up during the night to check. She spent hours checking that the doors were locked, that the coffee pot was unplugged, and that the family dog was safely ensconced in the garage. Despite her obsessions about fire, however, she did not check the smoke detector, an excellent example of the irrationality of this superficially rational disorder. This patient involved her family in her rituals. Her mother made a checklist that the daughter carried to school, and both parents had to check the twenty-four items on the list, signing that they had done so. At night she would wake her father to help her check. The family involvement was so profound that behavioral treatment could only take place after a period of family counseling in which the parents were helped to separate from their daughter's illness.

The Differential Diagnosis: Distinguishing OCD from Other Disorders

The broad comorbidity of OCD and an array of associated features make the diagnosis in theory seem difficult; in practice, however, it is usually more straightforward. The diagnosis of OCD must be made only if the "obsessive worries" are true obsessions, rather than symptoms of another disorder such as depressive ruminations or phobic avoidance. For example, when OCD is comorbid with bulimia or anorexia, the content of the obsessions or compulsions must be typical for OCD, e.g., washing, arranging, counting and repeating, and not be solely over-focused ideas about food or diet. Depressive ruminations and psychotic preoccupations are also distinguished by the negative content (e.g., everyone dislikes me, I fail at everything). Phobic disorders are distinguished not only by the content of the preoccupation (more often heights, spiders, the dark, etc.), but also by the absence of discomfort when the patient is not confronted with the phobic object. It may be more difficult to separate the obsessional concerns of OCD from the fears and worries of generalized anxiety disorder (Brown, Moras, Zinbarg, & Barlow, 1993). Comorbidity of OCD and anxiety disorders is common, so assigning specific symptoms to a specific disorder may be less important than identifying the presence of OCD in a child presenting with generalized anxiety or separation anxiety disorder.

Asperger syndrome can be differentiated from OCD by its lack of ego-dystonicity and, in addition, by the content of the preoccupations. For example, in Asperger's disorder, concerns about danger or contamination occur only rarely, while these are common among children with OCD. Autistic patients also may exhibit obsessive-compulsive symptoms, but these occur within the context of cognitive and psychosocial abnormalities and should not be confused with symptoms of OCD.

The differential diagnosis from Tourette's disorder is problematic, and the relationship between the two disorders remains obscure. Distinguishing between a compulsion and a tic may be difficult, given the presence of premonitory urges before tics and the complexity of some motor tics (Miguel, do Rosário-Campos, Prado *et al.*, 2000). Some 20–80% of patients with clear Tourette's disorder have been reported to have obsessive-compulsive symptoms or OCD, while 24–67% of children with primary OCD have been observed to have comorbid tics (Leonard, Lenane, Swedo *et al.*, 1992; Zohar, Ratzoni, Pauls *et al.*, 1992). Tics are seen often in younger patients, those with acute illness and in males. Preliminary impressions are that compulsions associated with Tourette's disorder may be more likely to involve symmetry, rubbing, touching, or staring and blinking rituals than washing and cleaning (Baer, 1994; Leckman, Grice, Barr *et al.*, 1994). Additionally, aggressive and/or sexual thoughts or rituals have been reported as more frequent in patients with tics and OCD than in those with OCD alone (Despert, 1955; Masi, Millepiedi, Mucci *et al.*, 2005; Thomsen, 1991). However, although some features distinguish the two disorders, the overlapping clinical profiles and family studies provide partial support for the speculation that some cases of OCD and Tourette's may be alternative forms of the same disorder. Any Tourette/OCD formulation, however, is likely to be oversimplified, as both tic disorders and OCD may be symptoms of basal ganglia-frontal circuitry dysfunction for which genetic, toxic, traumatic and infectious agents can be etiological. In particular, the working model of PANDAS involves the origin of both the tics and OCD through an autoimmune response to group A beta-hemolytic streptococcus.

Theories of Etiology

Over the past thirty years, it has become increasingly clear that OCD is not caused solely by psychological factors as had been posited by Kanner when he cited "an 'overdose' of parental perfectionism" as the source of obsessional neuroses (Kanner, 1962). Instead, accumulated evidence suggests that OCD is caused by a combination of biological and psychological factors, with both genetic and environmental influence.

Biological Factors

OCD is remarkable in the consistency of support for a conceptual model which links a disorder characterized by endless, repetitive thoughts and actions with uncontrolled activity of parallel, discrete loops within the brain. These loops connect the basal ganglia, prefrontal cortex – particularly the orbitofrontal and anterior cingulate regions – and thalamus, the so-called cortico-striato-thalamocortical (CSTC) loops (Alexander, DeLong, & Strick, 1986; Kopell, Greenberg, & Rezai, 2004; Modell, Mountz, Curtis, & Greden, 1989; Rapoport & Wise, 1988; Saxena, Bota, & Brody, 2001).

Several CSTCs have been assumed to be of particular importance in OCD, based on clinical, imaging and lesion studies. The first "direct" pathway is in essence a positive feedback loop that results in the initiation and continuation of thought and action. It is counterbalanced by an "indirect" pathway that acts as a check on the activation of the direct pathway (Fig. 43.1). The direct pathway starts with a glutamatergic signal to the striatum, which in turn sends an inhibitory GABA-ergic signal to the globus pallidus. This results in a disinhibition of the thalamus which is fed forward to the prefrontal cortex, particularly orbitofrontal regions. The indirect pathway differs in that the striatum projects an inhibitory signal to the globus pallidus, which increases inhibition on the thalamus and thus decreases prefrontal cortical activation. While there are multiple neurotransmitters involved in this circuit, including substance P and GABA, there are also serotonergic projections to this component from the dorsal raphe to the ventral striatum. These projections are speculated to be inhibitory. OCD symptoms could arise when an aberrant positive feedback loop develops in the first circuit, which is inadequately modulated by the output from the second circuit. Finally, some have recently argued for the need to incorporate limbic structures to account for the strong anxiety component of OCD.

Neuroanatomical Anomalies

The implication of abnormal activity in CSTCs is supported by consistent findings of structural and functional anomalies within these circuits in children with OCD. For example, a host of neurological disorders that affect the basal ganglia, including Huntington's chorea, post-encephalitic Parkinsonism and acquired lesions of the caudate and putamen, have been linked with the development of OCD in adulthood (Chacko, Corbin, & Harper, 2000). The autoimmune sequelae of streptococcal infection, which may target the caudate, have long been recognized in the pathogenesis of Sydenham's chorea, and may be of particular importance in the etiology of obsessions in a subgroup of children (PANDAS) (Swedo, Leonard, & Rapoport, 2004). All the components of the basal ganglia (caudate, putamen and globus pallidus) have been reported as abnormal in children with OCD – see Table 43.3. Volumetric studies of the caudate are typical for the field in the inconsistency of findings, with reports of increase, decrease and no change in caudate volume in children with OCD (Giedd, Rapoport, Garvey, Perlmutter, & Swedo, 2000; Luxenberg, Swedo, Flament *et al.*, 1988; Rosenberg, Averbach, O'Hearn *et al.*, 1997; Szeszko, MacMillan, McMeniman *et al.*, 2004). The marked variability in findings may reflect not only technical aspects relating to heterogeneity of definitions of regions of interest, but also comorbidities such as tic disorder and

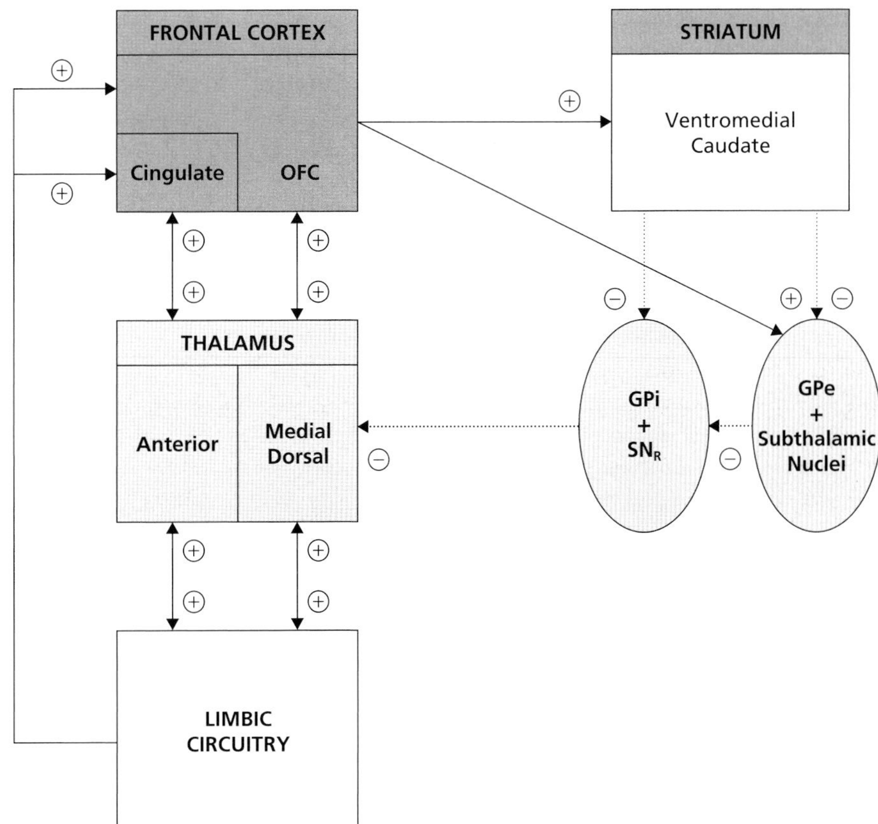

Fig. 43.1 The direct and indirect circuitry thought to underlie the pathogenesis of OCD. OFC=orbitofrontal cortex; GPi=globus pallidus pars interna, GPe=globus pallidus pars externa; SNr=substantia nigra pars reticulata. Excitatory links are shown in thick black lines and inhibitory connections in dashed black lines. In the DIRECT pathway the frontal cortex projects to the striatum and then to the GPi/SN complex which provides the main output of the basal ganglia. This in turn projects to the thalamus and finally back to the frontal cortex. The pathway has two excitatory and two inhibitory projections and thus is a net positive feedback loop. This circuit is balanced by the INDIRECT pathway which has a net inhibitory effect. This differs in the projection from the striatum to the GPe and subthalamic nuclei (which also receive direct frontal input) before relaying onto the output station of the basal ganglia. Interactions with the limbic system have been increasingly recognized in view of deficits in emotional processing and the anxiety prominent in OCD.

Table 43.3 Anatomic brain MRI studies of OCD in children and adolescents.

	Subjects	Technique	Findings	Comments
Basal ganglia				
Szeszko *et al.* (2004)	Childhood study: 23 patients with OCD and 27 controls	Manual tracing of regions of interest	Decreased volume of L globus pallidus: caudate and putamen did not differ	Medication naïve. Conflicts with earlier reports from this center of decreased volume in putamen (Rosenberg, Keshavan *et al.*, 1997). Attributed to sample differences
Giedd *et al.* (2000)	18 children with OCD arising in context of streptococcal infection	Manual tracing of regions of interest	Increased volume of caudate, putamen and globus pallidus	Increased volume similar to that reported in Sydenham's chorea. Included 16 children with tics – also showed similar enlargement
Luxenberg *et al.* (1988)	Childhood onset OCD; 10 males with OCD and 10 healthy controls	Manual tracing of region of interest on CT scans	Decreased volume of caudate bilaterally	Patients were heavily comorbid with tic disorder, which may have contributed independently to the volume reduction
Rosenberg *et al.* (1997)	Childhood study: 19 children with OCD and 19 healthy controls	Manual tracing of region of interest	Decreased volume of caudate and putamen	
Thalamus				
Gilbert *et al.* (2000)	Childhood study: 21 children with OCD and 21 matched healthy controls	Manual tracing of region of interest	Increased volume of thalamus in OCD	Successful treatment with paroxetine in 10 of the subjects was associated with a partial normalization of the volume of the thalamus
Frontal lobes				
Szeszko *et al.* (2004)	See above	Separately measured gray and white matter in frontal regions	Increase in gray matter in left anterior cingulate cortex	No reduction noted in the gray matter of the superior frontal gyrus, in line with predictions
Szeszko *et al.* (1999)	Childhood study: 26 children with OCD and 26 matched controls	Manual tracing of region of interest	Reduction in total volume of orbitofrontal cortex	No reduction in total anterior cingulate cortex as this study did not separately measure gray and white matter
Rosenberg *et al.* (1998)	Childhood study: 21 treatment naïve	Manual tracing of region of interest	Increase of volume in anterior cingulate only (not posterior cingulate/ dorsolateral prefrontal cortex)	Positive correlation between volume of anterior cingulate and obsessive symptoms scores
Rosenberg *et al.* (1997)	See above	Measured entire frontal lobes	No difference in volume of gray or white matter in prefrontal lobes	

the possible contribution of post-infectious inflammatory processes contributing to volume enlargement, as is proposed in PANDAS (Swedo & Grant, 2005). Importantly, some structural changes normalize as symptoms resolve, suggesting that they may be epiphenomenal and do reflect underlying neurobiological vulnerability. Prompted partly by the inconsistent volumetric findings in the basal ganglia, Bartha and colleagues (1998) examined ultrastructural features of the caudate nucleus using magnetic resonance spectroscopy (MRS) in adults with OCD. They reported no gross structural changes in the volume of the caudate but found a reduced amount of N-acteylaspartate (NAA) in the left caudate. The exact physiological function of NAA is unclear, but appears to relate to the regulation of metabolic processes within neurons and may thus reflect subtle neuronal dysfunction within the caudate, not usually detectable by gross anatomic techniques.

Turning to the frontal lobes, acquired lesions of the ventromedial and polar frontal cortex have also been linked with the *de novo* onset of OCD and some of its cardinal symptoms, such as hoarding (Anderson, Damasio, & Damasio,

2005). In children with OCD, specific reduction in the volume of the orbitofrontal cortex has been reported, a finding congruent with our preliminary reports of a highly localized thinning of the cortex in right orbitofrontal and polar frontal regions in early onset OCD (Shaw & Rapoport, unpublished data; Szeszko, Robinson, Alvir *et al.*, 1999). Expansion of gray matter in the left anterior cingulate cortex in an unmedicated pediatric OCD population, which was not found in other prefrontal regions, was found to be positively correlated with obsessive symptoms scores and has been consistently reported by several groups (Rosenberg & Keshavan, 1998; Szeszko, MacMillan, McMeniman *et al.*, 2004). Positive correlations between expansion of the anterior cingulate and the putamen were also reported, compatible with the postulation of abnormal cingulate-striatal circuitry. Reports of anomalies in the dorsolateral prefrontal cortex are less common, although magnetic resonance spectroscopy has demonstrated anomalies in the level of the putative neuronal marker NAA in the dorsolateral prefrontal cortex of unmediated children with OCD (Russell, Cortese, Lorch *et al.*, 2003).

Thalamic hyperactivation, which is fed forward to the frontal cortex, is the final component of the pathophysiological circuit in OCD, and might be predicted to have trophic effects. Indeed, thalamic enlargement which resolves following successful treatment with paroxetine has been reported in pediatric OCD (Gilbert, Moore, Keshavan *et al.*, 2000). This is complemented by reports of abnormal thalamic NAA and choline levels in pediatric OCD (Fitzgerald, Moore, Paulson, Stewart, & Rosenberg, 2000). One interpretation is that the NAA levels reflect neuronal perturbations and the abnormal choline levels reflect anomalous myelination in childhood; both factors could contribute to volume change in the thalamus.

Turning to white matter, Rosenberg and colleagues have demonstrated a positive correlation between increased surface area of the corpus callosum and symptoms scores in children with OCD. They also found abnormal signal intensity (which might reflect anomalous myelination) in the portion of the corpus callosum that connects the ventral prefrontal cortex with the striatum (MacMaster, Keshavan, Dick, & Rosenberg, 1999; Rosenberg, Averbach, O'Hearn *et al.*, 1997; Rosenberg, Keshavan, O'Hearn *et al.*, 1997). More recent developments in white matter imaging such as the use of diffusion tensors to assess the integrity and coherence of white matter tracts have been reported in adults only and similarly show anomalies in the region of the anterior cingulate (Russell, Cortese, Lorch *et al.*, 2003). The white matter changes may represent a possible neuroanatomical substrate for aberrant connectivity between these regions.

Functional neuroimaging studies also support the fronto-striatal model. Both functional MRI (fMRI, measuring change in blood flow) and positron emission tomography (PET, measuring glucose utilization as an index of brain activity) studies have demonstrated symptom-provoked hyperactivation (fMRI) and resting hypermetabolism (PET) in the orbitofrontal cortex, cingulate gyrus and the caudate in patients with OCD (Szeszko, Ardekani, Ashtari *et al.*, 2005). The specificity of these regional anomalies is demonstrated by the partial normalization following effective treatment (Saxena, Brody, Maidment *et al.*, 1999). Functional imaging studies using the OCD symptom-provocation paradigm report additional hyperactivation of many of the same regions, with some recent work suggesting that different components of the fronto-striato-thalamic circuit may mediate the anxiety associated with different symptom clusters (Mataix-Cols, Cullen, Lange *et al.*, 2003; Mataix-Cols, Wooderson, Lawrence *et al.*, 2004; Perani, Colombo, Bressi *et al.*, 1995).

Neurochemistry

Monoaminergic neurotransmitters which extensively project from the brain stem to regions within the fronto-striato-thalamic circuitry may contribute to the pathogenesis of OCD. OCD symptoms are frequently exacerbated by serotonin agonists (such as meta-chlorophenylpiperazine), and the serotonin reuptake inhibitors are the most effective therapeutic agents (Gross-Isseroff, Cohen, Sasson, Voet, & Zohar, 2004). Abnormalities of serotonergic transmission in OCD are suggested by imaging studies of central serotonin receptors using specific ligands, which have demonstrated a reduction in 5-HT synthesis in the ventral prefrontal cortex and caudate in eleven treatment-naïve pediatric subjects, which partially normalized following successful treatment (Simpson, Lombardo, Slifstein *et al.*, 2003). Inconsistent findings on the levels of central serotonin transporter availability may be partly attributable to developmental effects, as an increase in central serotonin transporter availability (indexed by the binding profiles of a ligand thought to bind to the transporter) was reported only for those with child- but not adult-onset OCD (Pogarell, Hamann, Popperl *et al.*, 2003; Simpson, Lombardo, Slifstein *et al.*, 2003; Stengler-Wenzke, Muller, Angermeyer, Sabri, & Hesse, 2004). There are less consistent findings for the dopaminergic system, with mixed results concerning changes in peripheral dopaminergic markers and the provocation of obsessive symptoms by dopamine agonists (Denys, Zohar, & Westenberg, 2004). PET neuroimaging studies, however, have demonstrated higher caudate dopamine transporter densities in tandem with lower concentrations of the dopamine D2 receptor, consistent with receptor down-regulation resulting from higher synaptic concentrations of striatal dopamine in adults with OCD (Denys, van der Wee, Janssen, De Geus, & Westenberg, 2004; van der Wee, Stevens, Hardeman *et al.*, 2004). Glutamate is the major excitatory neurotransmitter in the fronto-striatal circuitry, and magnetic resonance spectroscopy has demonstrated elevation in levels of glutamate and glutamine in the thalamus of treatment-naïve children with OCD, with a reduction in symptoms occurring in tandem with normalization of the glutamatergic marker (Rosenberg, MacMaster, Keshavan *et al.*, 2000). A decrease in glutamate levels in the anterior cingulate has also been found, although this may not be specific to OCD as it was also seen in children with major depression (Rosenberg, Mirza, Russell *et al.*, 2004). There is, thus, some direct support for anomalous serotonergic neurotransmission and more indirect and somewhat inconsistent evidence of abnormal dopaminergic and glutamatergic signaling.

Neuroendocrinology

Several lines of evidence suggest that endocrine perturbations may play an etiological role in OCD. Obsessive symptoms frequently worsen around the time of menses and during the post-partum period, and there are case reports of improvement with anti-androgen therapy (Brandes, Soares, & Cohen, 2004; Casas, Alvarez, Duro *et al.*, 1986; Rasmussen & Eisen, 1992). The finding of short stature in children with OCD (Hamburger, Swedo, Whitaker, Davies, & Rapoport, 1989) implicates the growth hormone (GH) axis and is supported by evidence of a lower bone age in OCD (Katz, Gothelf, Hermesh *et al.*, 1998). However, assaying the growth hormone axis using a clonidine challenge (which acts at the alpha 2 adrenergic receptor to cause GH release) found an enhanced GH response in children with OCD and comorbid anxiety, suggesting an intact growth axis (Sallee, Richman, Sethuraman *et al.*, 1998). Additionally, the only direct study of growth hormone in OCD found no difference from healthy controls in baseline levels, but did find reduced sensitivity for the OCD group following stimulation of growth hormone with growth hormone releasing hormone (Brambilla, Bellodi, Perna, Arancio, & Bertani, 1998).

Neuropsychological Models

Failure to resist obsessions and compulsions has been conceptualized as a failure of cognitive control in childhood OCD (Chamberlain, Blackwell, Fineberg, Robbins, & Sahakian, 2005). Deficits in suppressing prepotent motor responses in children with OCD have been reported, which in turn have been linked to reduced amplitude of evoked potentials in the orbitofrontal cortex (Malloy, 1987). Similarly, children with OCD have deficits in suppressing oculomotor reflexive responses to external cues, suggesting compromise in prefrontal cortical circuitry (Rosenberg, Dick, O'Hearn, & Sweeney, 1997). Using a probe designed to assess cognitive control (requiring the monitoring of repeated or conflicting information), anomalous activation in the anterior cingulate was found in a group of young adult OCD subjects, with much more extensive anomalous activation of posterior brain regions in those subjects who reported little resistance to their obsessions (Viard, Flament, Artiges *et al.*, 2005). Similarly, deficits in the inhibition of irrelevant information have been demonstrated using variants of the Stroop task (Nakao, Nakagawa, Yoshiura *et al.*, 2005).

A related model of OCD views the disorder as the result of over-activation of a system designed to monitor performance completion, leading to a constant feeling that an action is "not just right", which thus creates a need to correct perceived mistakes. A range of tasks assessing aspects of performance monitoring, error detection and response to conflicts have converged to show hyperactivity in the anterior cingulate in patients with OCD (Fitzgerald, Welsh, Gehring *et al.*, 2005; Maltby, Tolin, Worhunsky, O'Keefe, & Kiehl, 2005; Ursu, Stenger, Shear, Jones, & Carter, 2003; van Veen & Carter, 2002).

Other fMRI studies have delineated aberrant processing of affectively charged material in OCD, by both the amygdala (for frightening stimuli) and the insula (for disgust) in OCD (Cannistraro, Wright, Wedig *et al.*, 2004; Shapira, Liu, He *et al.*, 2003; van den Heuvel, Veltman, Groenewegen *et al.*, 2004). These data provide the basis for the incorporation of the rich structural and functional interactions between these components of the limbic system with the fronto-striato-thalamic loops in current models of OCD (for such a model see Figure 43.1).

A wide range of deficits on standard neuropsychological tasks has been reported, particularly in visuospatial ability and non-verbal memory (reviewed in Kuelz, Hohagen, & Voderholzer, 2004). Some of these deficits can be related to dysfunction in frontostriatal circuitry. For example, implicit learning (knowledge acquired through repetition or exposure and expressed without conscious reference to the learning experience) is thought to rely on the striatum, in contrast to explicit learning (learning with conscious coding and retrieval), which relies on fronto-temporal cortical integrity. Subjects with OCD show normal implicit learning, but unlike healthy controls do not recruit the striatum during this learning, but rather show possible compensatory activation of the medial temporal lobes (Rauch, Whalen, Curran *et al.*, 2001). Planning abilities have been inconsistently reported as impaired in OCD (Chamberlain, Blackwell, Fineberg, Robbins, & Sahakian, 2005; Veale, Sahakian, Owen, & Marks, 1996) and, in one functional imaging study, such dysfunction was accompanied by abnormal activation of the dorsal prefrontal cortex and caudate in patients with OCD (van den Heuvel, Veltman, Groenewegen *et al.*, 2005). However, many of these neuropsychological deficits are not specific to OCD, their causal relationship with the symptoms of OCD is unclear, and the deficits are more consistently reported in adults rather than children with OCD (Douglass, Moffitt, Dar, McGee, & Silva, 1995; Thomsen & Jensen, 1991).

Behavioral formulations of compulsions have formed the mainstay of psychological treatments and view compulsive behaviors as a form of avoidance that maintains obsessive fears through reducing anxiety (negative reinforcement) and by blocking opportunities for habituation to feared situations. Cognitive psychologists emphasize elements such as the interaction of intrusive thoughts with dysfunctional underlying assumptions (e.g., having an over-inflated sense of personal responsibility) in maintaining symptoms (for a review, see Salkovskis, Shafran, Rachman, & Freeston, 1999).

How specific is this neural substrate to OCD? Similar anomalous interaction between the striatum and prefrontal cortex is also held to be important in ADHD (see Castellanos & Tannock, 2002; see also chapter 33). Additionally, the neural circuitry underpinning several anxiety disorders, particularly social phobia and post-traumatic stress disorder, includes the limbic regions implicated in more recent refinements of models of OCD (Shin, Wright, Cannistraro *et al.*, 2005; Stein, 2002). Some degree of overlap is perhaps inevitable, but there are several unique features in the OCD model outlined above, most importantly, the emphasis on an imbalance of the direct and indirect pathways in OCD and the prominence given to glutaminergic neurotransmission.

The overlap between the neural substrates for OCD and the spectrum disorders is harder to disentangle, as only a few studies have attempted a direct comparison of the neural circuitry. For example, specific attentional biases to specific OCD-related stimuli, underpinned by anomalous fronto-striatal activation, were found in an fMRI study of adults with OCD, which was distinct from a more pervasive attentional bias to all affectively arousing material found in patients with panic disorder and hypochondriasis (van den Heuvel, Veltman, Groenewegen, Witter *et al.*, 2005).

Genetics

There is now little doubt that OCD is a highly heritable neuropsychiatric disorder. Twin studies show a much higher concordance rate in monozygotic (~80–90%) over dizygotic twins (~50%), and family studies report an increased prevalence of 7–15% in first-degree relatives of children with OCD (reviewed in Grados, Walkup, & Walford, 2003). In a study of over 4,000 child twin pairs, Hudziak and colleagues used structural equation modeling (see chapter 9) to estimate that genetic (~50%) and unique environmental (~50%) factors both equally influence parental ratings of obsessive and compulsive symptoms in children (Hudziak, Van Beijsterveldt, Althoff *et al.*, 2004). Most studies have focused on the heritability of the DSM-IV diagnosis of the disorder. Others, however, have looked at other aspects of the OCD endophenotype which may be more meaningful for genetic studies, such as symptom dimensions, or have tried to fractionate the disorder into subcategories (e.g., by age of onset or by association with common comorbidities).

Candidate gene studies have examined the monoaminergic and glutamatergic neurotransmitters in OCD, and more recently there has been interest in the trophic factors which regulate brain development. One of the most promising genes lies on the small arm of chromosome 9 (9p24), a region which has been linked with OCD in two independent genomewide scans on different families with multiply-affected individuals (Hanna, Veenstra-VanderWeele, Cox *et al.*, 2002; Willour, Yao Shugart, Samuels *et al.*, 2004). This region contains the gene SLC1A1 which codes for the neural glutamate transporter excitatory amino acid carrier 1. While one initial study failed to show biased transmission in a family-based associated analysis of two single nucleotide polymorphisms (Veenstra-VanderWeele, Kim, Gonen *et al.*, 2001), two more recent comprehensive and independent analyses, including more polymorphisms within the gene, found a positive association between the gene and OCD in males (Arnold, Sicard, Burroughs, Richter, & Kennedy, 2006; Dickel, Veenstra-VanderWeele, Cox *et al.*, 2006). The functional significance of these findings is unclear, but SLC1A1 is a strong candidate for OCD given the evidence for altered glutamate neurotransmission in the disorder.

Most of the remaining genetic findings are more typical for the field, with few being replicated and even fewer polymorphisms having been shown to have clear functional effects that can be linked plausibly to the pathogenesis of the disorder. Association studies of functional variants of a promter region variant in the serotonergic transporter (l and s variants of the SLC6A4 gene on chromosome 17) (Bengel, Greenberg, Cora-Locatelli *et al.*, 1999; Billett, Richter, King *et al.*, 1997) and one receptor gene ($5\text{-HT}1_{D\beta}$) have given inconsistent evidence for linkage with OCD (Di Bella, Cavallini, & Bellodi, 2002; Mundo, Richter, Zai *et al.*, 2002). Polymorphisms of genes encoding the monoaminergic system enzymes, monoamine oxidase A, and catechol-O-methyl-transferase (COMT) have also been linked to OCD, particularly in males (Karayiorgou, Sobin, Blundell *et al.*, 1999). Moves to examine associations between risk genes and specific symptom dimensions have proved promising, with reports of links between the serotonin transporter polymorphisms and clusters of religious and somatic concerns (Camarena, Aguilar, Loyzaga, & Nicolini, 2004; Kim, Lee, & Kim, 2005) and between polymorphisms of COMT and compulsive hoarding (Lochner, Kinnear, Hemmings *et al.*, 2005). Association with the dopaminergic DRD4 receptor gene emerges, particularly when probands who have comorbid tic disorder are studied, demonstrating the promise of phenotypic definitions which may cut across traditional diagnostic boundaries (Cruz, Camarena, King *et al.*, 1997; Millet, Chabane, Delorme *et al.*, 2003). Within the glutamatergic neurotransmitter system, positive associations have been reported for N-methyl D-aspartate (NMDA) receptors (GRIN2B) and for GRIK2 (a kainate receptor) recently also associated with autism (Arnold, Rosenberg, Mundo *et al.*, 2004; Delorme, Krebs, Chabane *et al.*, 2004). As some cases of pediatric OCD may represent an impaired immune response to streptococcal infection, the association between alleles of the myelin oligodendrocyte glycoprotein (MOG) gene, which plays an important role in mediating the complement cascade in the immune response, and OCD is of interest (Zai, Bezchlibnyk, Richter *et al.*, 2004).

Neurodevelopmental models of OCD emphasize anomalies of the neurotrophic factors which regulate cell survival, differentiation and death, particularly in early development. Animal models show that deficiencies of brain-derived neurotrophic factor (BDNF) in early development lead to a loss of serotonergic transmission in adulthood. Interestingly, different sequence variants of this gene in humans are associated with not only the risk for OCD, but also its age of onset (Hall, Dhilla, Charalambous, Gogos, & Karayiorgou, 2003).

Treatment Approaches

Psychological Treatment

The cornerstone of psychological therapies for children is exposure and response prevention (ERP), and its efficacy has been demonstrated in multiple open studies and two randomized controlled trials (Barrett, Healy-Farrell, & March, 2004; POTS, 2004). A hierarchy of increasingly intense anxiety-provoking situations that trigger obsessional thinking is constructed, and subjects are exposed gradually to these situations and encouraged to refrain from engaging in compulsive behaviors (March & Mulle, 1998). Gradually, the patient progresses through the hierarchy so that situations can be tolerated with minimal anxiety, thus attaining an ever-decreasing urge to engage in compulsions. In clinical practice, and in all controlled studies, ERP is usually combined with other behavioral techniques, such as anxiety management training and extinction (e.g., instructing parents not to give reassurance when a child compulsively seeks it). This makes it difficult to disentangle the relative therapeutic importance of each element. Frequently, cognitive components are added, such as normalizing intrusive thoughts and reappraising notions of personal responsibility. Again, the necessity of these cognitive components is unclear in children as there are no controlled trials comparing these approaches. Tailoring therapy to the symptom profile of the child may be helpful. For example, ERP may be ideal for younger children as it has been shown to be effective in those under 11 and may be particularly helpful for symptoms such as contamination fears and symmetry rituals (Barrett, Healy, & March, 2003). By contrast, cognitive approaches may be more suited to the child with obsessional moral guilt or pathological doubt.

The involvement of the family in treatment is essential. Psycho-education can help the family to avoid both punitive responses and the alternative "enabling" that can occur if the family becomes enmeshed in rituals. A randomized controlled study demonstrated that such family-based cognitive behavioral therapy may be equally efficacious when conducted either with individual families or in a group setting (Barrett, Healy-Farrell, & March, 2004).

While the efficacy of behavior therapy (BT) with ERP as a core component is accepted, the most efficient and efficacious method of providing this treatment is less clear. At one extreme lies computer-based delivery systems with minimal therapist contact time (Kenwright, Marks, Graham, Franses, & Mataix-Cols, 2005); at the other extreme are highly intensive day or in-patient treatment programs. Only one trial has directly compared once weekly with daily therapy; no significant differences in outcome were found, although this study was not randomized and thus limited conclusions can be drawn (Franklin, Kozak, Cashman *et al.*, 1998). A meta-analysis suggested that while more therapist-intensive approaches were more efficacious, even those involving relatively little therapist contact time (less than 10 hours) were also effective (NICE, 2005). In practice, the severity of the symptom profile, the complexity of comorbidity, and resources available within the family and local health care services are likely to determine the treatment intensity. Many countries also have self-help groups which provide a valuable source of support and information, as well as act as advocates for those living with the disorder.

Pharmacotherapy

There is a relative abundance of randomized controlled trials demonstrating the efficacy of clomipramine and of selective serotonin re-uptake inhibitors – SSRIs (sertraline, fluoxetine, paroxetine and fluvoxamine) in the acute phase treatment of childhood OCD, reviewed in Table 43.4.

A meta-analysis of 12 studies of SSRIs and clomipramine (an SRI) found all medications to be superior to placebo and found that clomipramine showed superiority over all the SSRIs, which did not differ from one another (Geller, Biederman, Stewart *et al.*, 2003). However, clomipramine is associated with several adverse side effects, including potential arrhythmogenic effects.

Although generally well tolerated, SSRIs are associated with a range of side effects, with nausea, headache and agitation being common to all in this class. Of greatest concern are reports of increased suicidal ideation and behavior, which have led to recommendations that treatment should be closely monitored with regular follow-up, perhaps ideally in conjunction with BT. As a result of these concerns, the pharmacological options have become limited in several countries.

Depression is highly comorbid with OCD, and the treatment of this combination is often challenging. Two studies have found that adding imipramine (Foa, Kozak, Steketee, & McCarthy, 1992) or SSRIs (Abramowitz, Franklin, Street, Kozak, & Foa, 2000) either before or during ERP may be effective for alleviating depressive symptoms but did not potentiate ERP. There are case reports supporting the use of cognitive therapeutic techniques to increase motivation and compliance in the depressed patient to help them engage with difficult exposure assignments (Abramowitz, 2004).

In children, low initial doses with slow upward titration is the rule. Patients should be made aware of the common side effects and the need for a 12-week treatment trial. Partial or complete failure to respond to the first SSRI should prompt treatment with BT and consideration of another SSRI. The use of augmenting agents for youths with treatment-resistant OCD is discussed below.

Combination Treatment

How do pharmacological and psychological treatments compare? The best current evidence comes from the Pediatric OCD Treatment (POTS) multi-center study, which randomized 112 children to either sertraline, cognitive behavioral therapy (CBT), the treatments combined or pill placebo for 12 weeks (POTS, 2004). All active treatments were superior to pill placebo. Combined treatment also proved superior to CBT alone and to sertraline alone, which did not differ from each other. Site differences emerged for CBT and sertraline but not for combined treatment, suggesting that combined treatment is less susceptible to setting-specific variations, and, given this generalizability, combined treatment may be the option of choice. Notably, there was no evidence of treatment-emergent suicidality. Much smaller studies similarly found that a combination of behavior therapy (based on ERP) and fluvoxamine was superior to medication alone, both in short-term response and at a follow-up period of one year (Neziroglu, Yaryura-Tobias, Walz, & McKay, 2000). A direct comparison of behavior therapy with clomipramine in 22 children found a non-significant superiority for psychotherapy (de Haan,

Table 43.4 Controlled studies of medication in the treatment of pediatric OCD.

Study	Design	Participants	Interventions	Outcomes
Clomipramine				
DeVeaugh-Geiss *et al.* (1992)	RCT, 8 weeks	N=60, mean age=14	Clomipramine vs placebo	Mean reduction in Children's Yale-Brown Obsessive Compulsive Scale (CY-Bocs) score of 37% compared to 8% in the placebo group. Sustained at 1 year
Greist *et al.* (1990)	RCT, 8 weeks	N=32, mean age=15	Clomipramine vs placebo	Of 15 patients who received at least 3wks of CMI, 11 (73%) improved, 5 (33%) improved by more than 50%, and none worsened. Only 2 (12.5%) of the 16 placebo-treated patients improved, 1 (6%) by more than 50%; two (12.5%) worsened
Flament *et al.* (1985)	Cross-over, 5 weeks in each treatment	N=27, mean age=14	Clomipramine vs placebo	Clomipramine significantly more effective than placebo in reduction on all symptom scores
Leonard *et al.* (1989)	Cross-over, 5 weeks in each treatment (double bind) and 2 weeks on placebo (single bind)	N=49, mean age=14	Clomipramine vs desipramine vs placebo	Clomipramine significantly more effective than desipramine in symptom reduction. Higher rate of relapse when desipramine was substituted for clomipramine
SSRIs				
POTS (2004)	RCT, DB 12 weeks	N=112, mean age =12	CBT vs CBT+sertraline vs sertraline	Combined treatment proved superior to CBT alone and to sertraline alone, which did not differ from each other. CBT alone was associated with (non-significantly) higher rates of remission than sertraline
March *et al.* (1998)	RCT, DB 10 weeks	N=189, mean age=13	Sertraline vs placebo	Sertraline produced significantly greater improvement in CY-BOCS. Based on CGI-I ratings at end point, 42% of patients receiving sertraline and 26% of patients receiving placebo were very much or much improved. Neither age nor sex predicted response to treatment
Geller *et al.* (2001)	RCT, DB 13 weeks	N=103, mean age=11.4	Fluoxetine vs placebo	Fluoxetine produced significantly greater improvement in CY-BOCS (fall of 9.5 points compared to 5.2 for placebo)
Liebowitz *et al.* (2002)	RCT, DB 12 weeks	N=43, mean age=13	Fluoxetine vs placebo	No significant difference at 8 weeks; but by 16 weeks, fluoxetine was associated with greater reduction in CY-BOCS (9.74 points) than was placebo (4.14 points)
Riddle *et al.* (1992)	Cross-over DB 16 weeks	N=14, mean age=12	Fluoxetine vs placebo	CY-BOCS total score decreased 44% (N = 7, p = 0.003) after the initial 8 weeks of fluoxetine treatment, compared with a 27% decrease (N = 6, p = 0.13) after placebo
Geller *et al.* (2004)	RCT, BD 10 weeks	N=207, mean age=11	Paroxetine vs placebo	Paroxetine produced significantly greater improvement in CY-BOCS (fall of 8.78 points compared to 5.34 points in placebo group)
Riddle *et al.* (2001)	RCT, DB 10 weeks followed by 1 year open label extension	N=120, mean age=13	Fluvoxamine vs placebo	The CY-BOCS total score decreased 44% after the initial 8 weeks of fluoxetine treatment, compared with a 27% decrease after placebo

Hoogduin, Buitelaar, & Keijsers, 1998). Overall, it is clear that while medication alone is effective and generally safe and well tolerated, CBT may have the edge in terms of a first-line treatment, particularly when combined with an SSRI or clomipramine.

Augmenting Strategies for Partial Responders

Up to 50% of children will show only a partial response to initial SSRI treatment (Geller, Biederman, Jones *et al.*, 1998). For adults showing such sub-optimal response to an SSRI, several trials have shown a significant reduction of obsessive symptoms in patients with either adjunctive haloperidol or risperidone (Li, May, Tolbert *et al.*, 2005; McDougle, Epperson, Pelton, Wasylink, & Price, 2000). Other treatment strategies in adults include augmentation with clonazepam or oral morphine or combining two SSRIs (for a review see Walsh & McDougle, 2004). There are some case reports demonstrating the potential for the use of each of these strategies in children, although there are no controlled studies to guide the clinician in this complex field (Figueroa, Rosenberg, Birmaher, & Keshavan, 1998; Leonard, Topol, Bukstein *et al.*, 1994; Lombroso, Scahill, King *et al.*, 1995). Clearly, the side effects of each augmenting agent need to be considered, particularly the risk of tardive dyskinesia with haloperidol, metabolic side effects of risperidone, and risk of tolerance and dependence with clonazepam.

In spite of the major advances in drug treatment, at least 10% of the OCD population remains severely affected. In adults, for extreme cases there is an option for neurosurgical procedures, which are aimed at disrupting the CSTC loops either through creating a permanent lesion through excision or through repetitive deep brain stimulation (Greenberg, Price, Rauch *et al.*, 2003). Such physical therapies are not appropriate for children, and less invasive alternatives such as transcranial magnetic stimulation, while giving insight into the abnormal responsivity of the motor cortex in OCD (Gilbert, Bansal, Sethuraman *et al.*, 2004; Greenberg, Murphy, & Swedo, 1998) have not proved effective in the treatment of adults and remain untested in children (Martin, Barbanoj, Perez, & Sacristan, 2003).

Maintenance treatment

OCD is frequently a chronic disorder and long-term maintenance therapy should be anticipated, with the current recommendation being a minimum treatment period of six months following full remission. The need for such maintenance was illustrated by an 8-month study of 26 children and adolescents with severe OCD who had received clomipramine for a mean of 17 months; a 2-month double-blind desipramine-substitution phase resulted in 89% of the substituted (versus 18% of the non-substituted) subjects relapsing during the substitution phase (Leonard, Swedo, Lenane *et al.*, 1991).

Immunomodulatory treatments

Based on the observation that some childhood-onset OCD patients had onset apparently related to infection with group A beta-hemolytic streptococcus (GABHS), a subgroup of children were proposed who were hypothesized to have an autoimmune based form of the disorder – PANDAS (Swedo, Leonard, & Rapoport, 2004). As a partial test of this model, two treatments were examined. A controlled treatment trial of intravenous immunoglobulin was carried out, together with an open trial of plasmaphoresis (Perlmutter, Leitman, Garvey *et al.*, 1999). Both treatments were effective in lessening of symptom severity for children with infection-triggered OCD and tic disorders. Penicillin or arithromycin prophylaxis of sufficient intensity to decrease streptococcal infections was also found to decrease neuropsychiatric symptom exacerbations among children in the PANDAS subgroup (Snider, Lougee, Slattery, Grant, & Swedo, 2005). This study is limited by the absence of a placebo control, particularly as a previous placebo-controlled trial using penicillin prophylaxis was negative (Garvey, Perlmutter, Allen *et al.*, 1999). These fascinating findings have yet to be replicated but raise the possibility of the prevention of OCD in at least a subset of children with the disorder.

Conclusions

Public awareness of OCD has increased greatly over recent years, allowing this once "secret" disorder to be more readily recognized by both families and mental health professionals. Functional neuroimaging studies increasingly inform and refine models of the pathogenesis of the disorder, and are being matched by neuroanatomical imaging studies which allow a delineation of structural change at an ever-increasing level of resolution. Whereas candidate gene studies have provided some validation of the implication of monoaminergic anomalies in the disorder, the application of new technologies to scan the entire genome is likely to provide novel insights into the genetics of OCD. Of most practical importance, though, are the strengthening of the evidence base for treatment through recent large-scale double-blind trials and the renewed interest in the management of those with treatment-resistant symptoms. The strides in understanding the neurobiology of the disorder are thus matched by definitive demonstrations of treatment efficacy in children, and make it all the more important that children, parents and health care professionals remain aware of the disorder and the availability of effective help.

References

Abramowitz, J. S. (2004). Treatment of obsessive-compulsive disorder in patients who have comorbid major depression. *Journal of Clinical Psychology*, *60*, 1133–1141.

Abramowitz, J. S., Franklin, M. E., Street, G. P., Kozak, M. J., & Foa, E. B. (2000). Effects of comorbid depression on response to treatment for obsessive-compulsive disorder. *Behavior Therapy*, *31*, 517–528.

Albert, U., Maina, G., Forner, F., & Bogetto, F. (2004). DSM-IV obsessive-compulsive personality disorder: prevalence in patients with anxiety disorders and in healthy comparison subjects. *Comprehensive Psychiatry*, *45*, 325–332.

Alexander, G., DeLong, M., & Strick, P. (1986). Parallel organization of functionally segregated circuits linking basal ganglia and cortex. *Annual Review of Neuroscience*, *9*, 357–381.

Anderson, S. W., Damasio, H., & Damasio, A. R. (2005). A neural basis for collecting behaviour in humans. *Brain*, *128*, 201–212.

Andrews, G., Slade, T., & Peters, J. L. (1999). Classification in psychiatry: ICD-10 versus DSM-IV. *British Journal of Psychiatry*, *174*, 3–5.

Angst, J., Gamma, A., Endrass, J., Goodwin, R., Ajdacic, V., Eich, D., *et al.* (2004). Obsessive-compulsive severity spectrum in the community: prevalence, comorbidity, and course. *European Archives of Psychiatry & Clinical Neuroscience*, *254*, 156–164.

American Psychiatric Association. (2000). *Diagnostic and Statistical Manual of Mental Disorders* (4th ed.). Text Revision. Washington DC: American Psychiatric Press.

Apter, A., Fallon, T. J., Jr., King, R. A., Ratzoni, G., Zohar, A. H., Binder, M., *et al.* (1996). Obsessive-compulsive characteristics: from symptoms to syndrome. *Journal of the American Academy of Child & Adolescent Psychiatry*, *35*, 907–912.

Arnold, P. D., Rosenberg, D. R., Mundo, E., Tharmalingam, S., Kennedy, J. L., & Richter, M. A. (2004). Association of a glutamate (NMDA) subunit receptor gene (GRIN2B) with obsessive-compulsive disorder: a preliminary study. *Psychopharmacology*, *174*, 530–538.

Arnold, P. D., Sicard, T., Burroughs, E., Richter, M. A., & Kennedy, J. L. (2006). Glutamate transporter gene SLC1A1 associated with obsessive-compulsive disorder. *Archives of General Psychiatry*, *63*, 769–776.

Baer, L. (1994). Factor analysis of symptom subtypes of obsessive compulsive disorder and their relation to personality and tic disorders. *Journal of Clinical Psychiatry*, *55*, 18–23.

Barrett, P., Healy-Farrell, L., & March, J. S. (2004). Cognitive-behavioral family treatment of childhood obsessive-compulsive disorder: a controlled trial. *Journal of the American Academy of Child & Adolescent Psychiatry*, *43*, 46–62.

Barrett, P., Healy, L., & March, J. S. (2003). Behavioral avoidance test for childhood obsessive-compulsive disorder: a home-based observation. *American Journal of Psychotherapy*, *57*, 80–100.

Bartha, R., Stein, M. B., Williamson, P. C., Drost, D. J., Neufeld, R. W. J., Carr, T. J., *et al.* (1998). A short echo 1H spectroscopy and volumetric MRI study of the corpus striatum in patients with obsessive-compulsive disorder and comparison subjects. *American Journal of Psychiatry*, *155*, 1584–1591.

Bartz, J. A., & Hollander, E. (2006). Is obsessive-compulsive disorder an anxiety disorder? *Progress in Neuro-Psychopharmacology & Biological Psychiatry*, *30*, 338–352.

Bengel, D., Greenberg, B. D., Cora-Locatelli, G., Altemus, M., Heils, A., Li, Q., *et al.* (1999). Association of the serotonin transporter promoter regulatory region polymorphism and obsessive-compulsive disorder. *Molecular Psychiatry*, *4*, 463–466.

Berg, C. Z., Rapoport, J. L., Whitaker, A., Davies, M., Leonard, H., Swedo, S. E., *et al.* (1989). Childhood obsessive compulsive disorder: a two-year prospective follow-up of a community sample. *Journal of the American Academy of Child & Adolescent Psychiatry*, *28*, 528–533.

Berrios, G. E. (1989). Obsessive-compulsive disorder: its conceptual history in France during the 19th century. *Comprehensive Psychiatry*, *30*, 283–295.

Bienvenu, O. J., Samuels, J. F., Riddle, M. A., Hoehn-Saric, R., Liang, K. Y., Cullen, B. A., *et al.* (2000). The relationship of obsessive-compulsive disorder to possible spectrum disorders: results from a family study. *Biological Psychiatry*, *48*, 287–293.

Billett, E. A., Richter, M. A., King, N., Heils, A., Lesch, K. P., & Kennedy, J. L. (1997). Obsessive compulsive disorder, response to serotonin reuptake inhibitors and the serotonin transporter gene. *Molecular Psychiatry*, *2*, 403–406.

Black, A. (1974). The natural history of obsessional neurosis. In H. Beech (Ed.), *Obsessional States* (pp. 19–54). London: Methuen.

Bloch, M., Peterson, B. S., Scahill, L., Otka, J., Katsovich, L., Zhang, H., *et al.* (2006). Adult outcome of tic and obsessive-compulsive severity in children with Tourette syndrome. *Archives of Pedatric and Adolescent Medicine*, *160*, 65–69.

Brambilla, F., Bellodi, L., Perna, G., Arancio, C., & Bertani, A. (1998). Growth hormone response to growth hormone-releasing hormone stimulation in obsessive-compulsive disorder. *Psychiatry Research*, *81*, 293–299.

Brandes, M., Soares, C. N., & Cohen, L. S. (2004). Postpartum onset obsessive-compulsive disorder: diagnosis and management. *Archives of Women's Mental Health*, *7*, 99–110.

Breslau, N. (1987). Inquiring about the bizarre: false positives in Diagnostic Interview Schedule for Children (DISC) ascertainment of obsessions, compulsions, and psychotic symptoms. *Journal of the American Academy of Child & Adolescent Psychiatry*, 26, 639–644.

Brown, T. A., Moras, K., Zinbarg, R., & Barlow, D. (1993). Diagnostic and symptom distinguishability of genralized anxiety disorder and obsessive-compulsive disorder. *Behavior Therapy*, *24*, 227–240.

Byerly, M., Goodman, W., Acholonu, W., Bugno, R., & Rush, A. J. (2005). Obsessive compulsive symptoms in schizophrenia: frequency and clinical features. *Schizophrenia Research*, *76*, 309–316.

Camarena, B., Aguilar, A., Loyzaga, C., & Nicolini, H. (2004). A family-based association study of the 5-HT-1D beta receptor gene in obsessive-compulsive disorder. *International Journal of Neuropsychopharmacology*, *7*, 49–53.

Cannistraro, P. A., Wright, C. I., Wedig, M. M., Martis, B., Shin, L. M., Wilhelm, S., *et al.* (2004). Amygdala responses to human faces in obsessive-compulsive disorder. *Biological Psychiatry*, *56*, 916–920.

Casas, M., Alvarez, E., Duro, P., Garcia-Ribera, C., Udina, C., Velat, A., *et al.* (1986). Antiandrogenic treatment of obsessive-compulsive neurosis. *Acta Psychiatrica Scandinavica*, *73*, 221–222.

Castellanos, F. X., & Tannock, R. (2002). Neuroscience of attention-deficit/hyperactivity disorder: the search for endophenotypes. *Nature Reviews. Neuroscience*, *3*, 617–628.

Chabane, N., Delorme, R., Millet, B., Moureau, M., Leboyer, M., & Pauls, D. (2004). Early-onset obsessive-compulsive disorder: a subgroup with a specific clinical and familial pattern? *Journal of Child Psychology and Psychiatry*, *46*, 881–887.

Chacko, R. C., Corbin, M. A., & Harper, R. G. (2000). Acquired obsessive-compulsive disorder associated with basal ganglia lesions. *Journal of Neuropsychiatry & Clinical Neurosciences*, *12*, 269–272.

Chamberlain, S. R., Blackwell, A. D., Fineberg, N. A., Robbins, T. W., & Sahakian, B. J. (2005). The neuropsychology of obsessive compulsive disorder: the importance of failures in cognitive and behavioural inhibition as candidate endophenotypic markers. *Neuroscience & Biobehavioral Reviews*, *29*, 399–419.

Christenson, G. A., Mackenzie, T. B., Mitchell, J. E., & Callies, A. L. (1991). A placebo-controlled, double-blind crossover study of fluoxetine in trichotillomania. *American Journal of Psychiatry*, *148*, 1566–1571.

Crespo-Facorro, B., Cabranes, J. A., Lopez-Ibor Alcocer, M. I., Paya, B., Fernandez Perez, C., Encinas, M., *et al.* (1999). Regional cerebral blood flow in obsessive-compulsive patients with and without a chronic tic disorder. A SPECT study. *European Archives of Psychiatry & Clinical Neuroscience*, *249*, 156–161.

Crino, R., Slade, T., & Andrews, G. (2005). The changing prevalence and severity of obsessive-compulsive disorder criteria from DSM-III to DSM-IV. *American Journal of Psychiatry*, *162*, 876–882.

Cruz, C., Camarena, B., King, N., Paez, F., Sidenberg, D., de la Fuente, J. R., *et al.* (1997). Increased prevalence of the seven-repeat variant of the dopamine D4 receptor gene in patients with obsessive-compulsive disorder with tics. *Neuroscience Letters*, *231*, 1–4.

de Haan, E., Hoogduin, K. A., Buitelaar, J. K., & Keijsers, G. P. (1998). Behavior therapy versus clomipramine for the treatment of obsessive-compulsive disorder in children and adolescents. *Journal of the American Academy of Child & Adolescent Psychiatry*, *37*, 1022–1029.

Delorme, R., Krebs, M. O., Chabane, N., Roy, I., Millet, B., Mouren-Simeoni, M. C., *et al.* (2004). Frequency and transmission of glutamate receptors GRIK2 and GRIK3 polymorphisms in patients with obsessive compulsive disorder. *Neuroreport*, *15*, 699–702.

Denys, D., van der Wee, N., Janssen, J., De Geus, F., & Westenberg, H. G. (2004). Low level of dopaminergic D2 receptor binding in obsessive-compulsive disorder. *Biological Psychiatry*, *55*, 1041–1045.

Denys, D., Zohar, J., & Westenberg, H. G. (2004). The role of dopamine in obsessive-compulsive disorder: preclinical and clinical evidence. *Journal of Clinical Psychiatry*, *65*, 11–17.

Despert, J. L. (1955). Differential diagnosis between obsessive-compulsive neurosis and schizophrenia in children. In P. H. Hoch & J. Zubin (Eds.), *Psychopathology of Childhood* (pp. 240–253). New York: Grune and Stratton.

DeVeaugh-Geiss, J., Moroz, G., Biederman, J., Cantwell, D., Fontaine, R., Greist, J. H., *et al.* (1992). Clomipramine hydrochloride in childhood and adolescent obsessive-compulsive disorder – a multicenter trial. *Journal of the American Academy of Child & Adolescent Psychiatry*, *31*, 45–49.

Di Bella, D., Cavallini, M. C., & Bellodi, L. (2002). No association between obsessive-compulsive disorder and the 5-HT(1Dbeta) receptor gene. *American Journal of Psychiatry*, *159*, 1783–1785.

Dickel, D. E., Veenstra-VanderWeele, J., Cox, N. J., Wu, X., Fischer, D. J., Van Etten-Lee, M., *et al.* (2006). Association testing of the positional and functional candidate gene SLC1A1/EAAC1 in early-onset obsessive-compulsive disorder. *Archives of General Psychiatry*, *63*, 778–785.

Douglass, H. M., Moffitt, T. E., Dar, R., McGee, R., & Silva, P. (1995). Obsessive-compulsive disorder in a birth cohort of 18-year-olds: prevalence and predictors. *Journal of the American Academy of Child & Adolescent Psychiatry*, *34*, 1424–1431.

Figueroa, Y., Rosenberg, D. R., Birmaher, B., & Keshavan, M. S. (1998). Combination treatment with clomipramine and selective serotonin reuptake inhibitors for obsessive-compulsive disorder in children and adolescents. *Journal of Child & Adolescent Psychopharmacology*, *8*, 61–67.

Fitzgerald, K. D., MacMaster, F. P., Paulson, L. D., & Rosenberg, D. R. (1999). Neurobiology of childhood obsessive-compulsive disorder. *Child and Adolescent Psychiatric Clinics of North America*, *8*, 533–575, ix.

Fitzgerald, K. D., Moore, G. J., Paulson, L. A., Stewart, C. M., & Rosenberg, D. R. (2000). Proton spectroscopic imaging of the thalamus in treatment-naive pediatric obsessive-compulsive disorder.[see comment]. *Biological Psychiatry*, *47*, 174–182.

Fitzgerald, K. D., Welsh, R. C., Gehring, W. J., Abelson, J. L., Himle, J. A., Liberzon, I., *et al.* (2005). Error-related hyperactivity of the anterior cingulate cortex in obsessive-compulsive disorder. *Biological Psychiatry*, *57*, 287–294.

Flament, M. F., Rapoport, J. L., Berg, C. J., Sceery, W., Kilts, C., Mellstrom, B., *et al.* (1985). Clomipramine treatment of childhood obsessive-compulsive disorder. A double-blind controlled study. *Archives of General Psychiatry*, *42*, 977–983.

Flament, M. F., Whitaker, A., Rapoport, J. L., Davies, M., *et al.* (1988). Obsessive compulsive disorder in adolescence: An epidemiological study. *Journal of the American Academy of Child & Adolescent Psychiatry*, *27*, 764–771.

Foa, E. B., Kozak, M. J., Steketee, G. S., & McCarthy, P. R. (1992). Treatment of depressive and obsessive-compulsive symptoms in OCD by imipramine and behaviour therapy. *British Journal of Clinical Psychology*, *31*, 279–292.

Franklin, M. E., Kozak, M. J., Cashman, L. A., Coles, M. E., Rheingold, A. A., & Foa, E. B. (1998). Cognitive-behavioral treatment of pediatric obsessive-compulsive disorder: an open clinical trial. *Journal of the American Academy of Child & Adolescent Psychiatry*, *37*, 412–419.

Freud, S. (1906). Obsessive actions and religious practices. In J. A. Strachey (Ed.), *The Standard Edition of the Complete Psychological Works of Sigmund Freud* (Vol. 9, pp. 117–127). London: Hogarth Press.

Freud, S. (1958). The disposition to obsessional neurosis (1913). In J. A. Strachey (Ed.), *The Standard Edition of the Complete Psychological Works of Sigmund Freud* (Vol. 12, pp. 311–326). London: Hogarth Press.

Garvey, M. A., Perlmutter, S. J., Allen, A. J., Hamburger, S., Lougee, L., Leonard, H. L., *et al.* (1999). A pilot study of penicillin prophylaxis for neuropsychiatric exacerbations triggered by streptococcal infections. *Biological Psychiatry*, *45*, 1564–1571.

Geller, D. A., Biederman, J., Jones, J., Shapiro, S., Schwartz, S., & Park, K. S. (1998). Obsessive-compulsive disorder in children and adolescents: a review. *Harvard Review of Psychiatry*, *5*, 260–273.

Geller, D. A., Biederman, J., Stewart, S. E., Mullin, B., Martin, A., Spencer, T., *et al.* (2003). Which SSRI? A meta-analysis of pharmacotherapy trials in pediatric obsessive-compulsive disorder [see comment]. *American Journal of Psychiatry*, *160*, 1919–1928.

Geller, D. A., Hoog, S. L., Heiligenstein, J. H., Ricardi, R. K., Tamura, R., Kluszynski, S., *et al.* (2001). Fluoxetine treatment for obsessive-compulsive disorder in children and adolescents: a placebo-controlled clinical trial [see comment]. *Journal of the American Academy of Child & Adolescent Psychiatry*, *40*, 773–779.

Geller, D. A., Wagner, K. D., Emslie, G., Murphy, T., Carpenter, D. J., Wetherhold, E., *et al.* (2004). Paroxetine treatment in children and adolescents with obsessive-compulsive disorder: a randomized, multicenter, double-blind, placebo-controlled trial. *Journal of the American Academy of Child & Adolescent Psychiatry*, *43*, 1387–1396.

Giedd, J. N., Rapoport, J. L., Garvey, M. A., Perlmutter, S., & Swedo, S. E. (2000). MRI assessment of children with obsessive-compulsive disorder or tics associated with streptococcal infection. *American Journal of Psychiatry*, *157*, 281–283.

Gilbert, A. R., Moore, G. J., Keshavan, M. S., Paulson, L. A., Narula, V., Mac Master, F. P., *et al.* (2000). Decrease in thalamic volumes of pediatric patients with obsessive-compulsive disorder who are taking paroxetine. *Archives of General Psychiatry*, *57*, 449–456.

Gilbert, D. L., Bansal, A. S., Sethuraman, G., Sallee, F. R., Zhang, J., Lipps, T., *et al.* (2004). Association of cortical disinhibition with tic, ADHD, and OCD severity in Tourette syndrome. *Movement Disorders*, *19*, 416–425.

Goodman, W. K., Price, L. H., Rasmussen, S. A., Mazure, C., Delgado, P., Heninger, G. R., *et al.* (1989). The Yale-Brown Obsessive Compulsive Scale. II. Validity. *Archives of General Psychiatry*, *46*, 1012–1016.

Goodman, W. K., Price, L. H., Rasmussen, S. A., Mazure, C., Fleischmann, R. L., Hill, C. L., *et al.* (1989). The Yale-Brown Obsessive Compulsive Scale. I. Development, use, and reliability. *Archives of General Psychiatry*, *46*, 1006–1011.

Grados, M. A., Riddle, M. A., Samuels, J. F., Liang, K. Y., Hoehn-Saric, R., Bienvenu, O. J., *et al.* (2001). The familial phenotype of obsessive-compulsive disorder in relation to tic disorders: the Hopkins OCD family study. *Biological Psychiatry*, *50*, 559–565.

Grados, M. A., Walkup, J., & Walford, S. (2003). Genetics of obsessive-compulsive disorders: new findings and challenges. *Brain & Development*, *25* (Suppl), S55–S61.

Graybiel, A. M., & Rauch, S. L. (2000). Toward a neurobiology of obsessive-compulsive disorder. *Neuron*, *28*, 343–347.

Greenberg, B. D., Murphy, D. L., & Swedo, S. E. (1998). Symptom exacerbation of vocal tics and other symptoms associated with streptococcal pharyngitis in a patient with obsessive-compulsive disorder and tics. *American Journal of Psychiatry*, *155*, 1459–1460.

Greenberg, B. D., Price, L. H., Rauch, S. L., Friehs, G., Noren, G., Malone, D., *et al.* (2003). Neurosurgery for intractable obsessive-compulsive disorder and depression: critical issues. *Neurosurgery Clinics of North America*, *14*, 199–212.

Greist, J. H., Jefferson, J. W., Rosenfeld, R., Gutzmann, L. D., March, J. S., & Barklage, N. E. (1990). Clomipramine and obsessive compulsive disorder: a placebo-controlled double-blind study of 32 patients.[see comment]. *Journal of Clinical Psychiatry*, *51*, 292–297.

Gross-Isseroff, R., Cohen, R., Sasson, Y., Voet, H., & Zohar, J. (2004). Serotonergic dissection of obsessive compulsive symptoms: a challenge study with m-chlorophenylpiperazine and sumatriptan. *Neuropsychobiology*, *50*, 200–205.

Hall, D., Dhilla, A., Charalambous, A., Gogos, J. A., & Karayiorgou, M. (2003). Sequence variants of the brain-derived neurotrophic factor (BDNF) gene are strongly associated with obsessive-compulsive disorder. *American Journal of Human Genetics*, *73*, 370–376.

Hamburger, S. D., Swedo, S., Whitaker, A., Davies, M., & Rapoport, J. L. (1989). Growth rate in adolescents with obsessive-compulsive disorder. *American Journal of Psychiatry*, *146*, 652–655.

Hanna, G. L., Veenstra-VanderWeele, J., Cox, N. J., Boehnke, M., Himle, J. A., Curtis, G. C., *et al.* (2002). Genome-wide linkage analysis of families with obsessive-compulsive disorder ascertained through pediatric probands. *American Journal of Medical Genetics*, *114*, 541–552.

Herjanic, B., & Campbell, W. (1977). Differentiating psychiatrically disturbed children on the basis of a structured interview. *Journal of Abnormal Child Psychology*, *5*, 127–134.

Herjanic, B., & Reich, W. (1982). Development of a structured psychiatric interview for children: agreement between child and parent on various symptoms. *Journal of Abnormal Child Psychology*, *10*, 307–324.

Hollander, E. (1996). Obsessive-compulsive disorder-related disorders: the role of selective serotonergic reuptake inhibitors. *International Clinical Psychopharmacology*, *11*, 75–87.

Hollander, E., King, A., Delaney, K., Smith, C. J., & Silverman, J. M. (2003). Obsessive-compulsive behaviors in parents of multiplex autism families. *Psychiatry Research*, *117*, 11–16.

Hollander, E., & Wong, C. M. (1995). Body dysmorphic disorder, pathological gambling, and sexual compulsions. *Journal of Clinical Psychiatry*, *56*, 7–12; discussion 13.

Horwath, E., & Weissman, M. M. (2000). The epidemiology and cross-national presentation of obsessive-compulsive disorder. *Psychiatric Clinics of North America*, *23*, 493–507.

Hudziak, J. J., Van Beijsterveldt, C. E., Althoff, R. R., Stanger, C., Rettew, D. C., Nelson, E. C., *et al.* (2004). Genetic and environmental contributions to the Child Behavior Checklist Obsessive-Compulsive Scale: a cross-cultural twin study. *Archives of General Psychiatry*, *61*, 608–616.

Ivarsson, T., & Valderhaug, R. (2006). Symptom patterns in children and adolescents with obsessive-compulsive disorder (OCD). *Behaviour Research and Therapy*, *44*, 1105–1116.

Janet, P. (1903). *Les Obsessions et la Psychiatrie. Vol. 1.* Paris: Felix Alan.

Jonnal, A. H., Gardner, C. O., Prescott, C. A., & Kendler, K. S. (2000). Obsessive and compulsive symptoms in a general population sample of female twins. *American Journal of Medical Genetics*, *96*, 791–796.

Kanner, L. (1962). *Chld Psychiatry* (3rd ed.). Springfield, IL: Charles C. Thomas.

Karayiorgou, M., Sobin, C., Blundell, M. L., Galke, B. L., Malinova, L., Goldberg, P., *et al.* (1999). Family-based association studies support a sexually dimorphic effect of COMT and MAOA on genetic susceptibility to obsessive-compulsive disorder. *Biological Psychiatry*, *45*, 1178–1189.

Karno, M., & Golding, J. (1990). Obsessive-compulsive disorder. In L. Robins & D. A. Regier (Eds.), *Psychiatric Disorders in America: the Epidemiological Catchment Area Study* (pp. 207–229). New York: Free Press.

Karno, M., & Golding, J. M. (1991). Obsessive compulsive disorder. In L. N. Robins & D. A. Regier (Eds.), *Psychiatry Disorders in America* (pp. 204–219). New York: The Free Press.

Karno, M., Golding, J. M., Sorenson, S. B., & Burnam, M. A. (1988). The epidemiology of obsessive-compulsive disorder in five US communities. *Archives of General Psychiatry*, *45*, 1094–1099.

Katz, N., Gothelf, D., Hermesh, H., Weizman, A., Apter, A., & Horev, G. (1998). Bone age in adolescents with schizophrenia and obsessive-compulsive disorder. *Schizophrenia Research*, *33*, 119–122.

Kaufman, J., Birmaher, B., Brent, D., Rao, U., Flynn, C., Moreci, P., *et al.* (1997). Schedule for Affective Disorders and Schizophrenia for School-Age Children-Present and Lifetime Version (K-SADS-PL): initial reliability and validity data. *Journal of the American Academy of Child & Adolescent Psychiatry*, *36*, 980–988.

Kenwright, M., Marks, I., Graham, C., Franses, A., & Mataix-Cols, D. (2005). Brief scheduled phone support from a clinician to enhance computer-aided self-help for obsessive-compulsive disorder: randomized controlled trial. *Journal of Clinical Psychology*, *61*, 1499–1508.

Kim, S. J., Lee, H. S., & Kim, C. H. (2005). Obsessive-compulsive disorder, factor-analyzed symptom dimensions and serotonin transporter polymorphism. *Neuropsychobiology*, *52*, 176–182.

Kopell, B. H., Greenberg, B., & Rezai, A. R. (2004). Deep brain stimulation for psychiatric disorders. *Journal of Clinical Neurophysiology*, *21*, 51–67.

Kuelz, A. K., Hohagen, F., & Voderholzer, U. (2004). Neuropsychological performance in obsessive-compulsive disorder: a critical review. *Biological Psychology*, *65*, 185–236.

LaSalle, V. H., Cromer, K. R., Nelson, K. N., Kazuba, D., Justement, L., & Murphy, D. L. (2004). Diagnostic interview assessed neuropsychiatric disorder comorbidity in 334 individuals with obsessive-compulsive disorder. *Depression and Anxiety*, *19*, 163–173.

Leckman, J. F., Grice, D. E., Barr, L. C., de Vries, A. L., Martin, C., Cohen, D. J., *et al.* (1994). Tic-related vs. non-tic-related obsessive compulsive disorder. *Anxiety*, *1*, 208–215.

Leonard, H. L. (1989). Childhood rituals and superstitions: developmental and cultural perspective. In J. L. Rapoport (Ed.), *Obsessive-Compulsive Disorder in Children & Adolescents* (pp. 289–309). Washington DC: American Psychiatric Press.

Leonard, H. L., Swedo, S. E., Garvey, M., Beer, D., Perlmutter, S., Lougee, L., *et al.* (1999). Postinfectious and other forms of obsessive-compulsive disorder. *Child & Adolescent Psychiatric Clinics of North America*, *8*, 497–511.

Leonard, H. L., Lenane, M. C., Swedo, S. E., Rettew, D. C., Gershon, E. S., & Rapoport, J. L. (1992). Tics and Tourette's disorder: a 2- to 7-year follow-up of 54 obsessive-compulsive children. *American Journal of Psychiatry*, *149*, 1244–1251.

Leonard, H. L., Swedo, S. E., Lenane, M. C., Rettew, D. C., Cheslow, D. L., Hamburger, S. D., *et al.* (1991). A double-blind desipramine substitution during long-term clomipramine treatment in children and adolescents with obsessive-compulsive disorder. *Archives of General Psychiatry*, *48*, 922–927.

Leonard, H. L., Swedo, S. E., Rapoport, J. L., Koby, E. V., Lenane, M. C., Cheslow, D. L., *et al.* (1989). Treatment of obsessive-compulsive disorder with clomipramine and desipramine in children and adolescents. A double-blind crossover comparison. *Archives of General Psychiatry*, *46*, 1088–1092.

Leonard, H. L., Topol, D., Bukstein, O., Hindmarsh, D., Allen, A. J., & Swedo, S. E. (1994). Clonazepam as an augmenting agent in the treatment of childhood-onset obsessive-compulsive disorder. *Journal of the American Academy of Child & Adolescent Psychiatry*, *33*, 792–794.

Lewinsohn, P. M., Hops, H., Roberts, R. E., Seeley, J. R., & Andrews, J. A. (1993). Adolescent psychopathology: I. Prevalence and incidence of depression and other DSM-III-R disorders in high school students. *Journal of Abnormal Psychology*, *102*, 133–144.

Li, X., May, R. S., Tolbert, L. C., Jackson, W. T., Flournoy, J. M., & Baxter, L. R. (2005). Risperidone and haloperidol augmentation of serotonin reuptake inhibitors in refractory obsessive-compulsive disorder: a crossover study. *Journal of Clinical Psychiatry*, *66*, 736–743.

Liebowitz, M. R., Turner, S. M., Piacentini, J., Beidel, D. C., Clarvit, S. R., Davies, S. O., *et al.* (2002). Fluoxetine in children and adolescents with OCD: a placebo-controlled trial. *Journal of the American Academy of Child & Adolescent Psychiatry*, *41*, 1431–1438.

Lochner, C., Kinnear, C. J., Hemmings, S. M., Seller, C., Niehaus, D. J., Knowles, J. A., *et al.* (2005). Hoarding in obsessive-compulsive disorder: clinical and genetic correlates. *Journal of Clinical Psychiatry*, *66*, 1155–1160.

Lombroso, P. J., Scahill, L., King, R. A., Lynch, K. A., Chappell, P. B., Peterson, B. S., *et al.* (1995). Risperidone treatment of children and adolescents with chronic tic disorders: a preliminary report. *Journal of the American Academy of Child & Adolescent Psychiatry, 34*, 1147–1152.

Luxenberg, J. S., Swedo, S. E., Flament, M. F., Friedland, R. P., Rapoport, J., & Rapoport, S. I. (1988). Neuroanatomical abnormalities in obsessive-compulsive disorder detected with quantitative X-ray computed tomography. *American Journal of Psychiatry, 145*, 1089–1093.

MacMaster, F. P., Keshavan, M. S., Dick, E. L., & Rosenberg, D. R. (1999). Corpus callosal signal intensity in treatment-naive pediatric obsessive compulsive disorders. *Progress in Neuro-Psychopharmacology & Biological Psychiatry, 23*, 601–612.

Maina, G., Albert, U., Bogetto, F., & Ravizza, L. (1999). Obsessive-compulsive syndromes in older adolescents. *Acta Psychiatrica Scandinavica, 100*, 447–450.

Malloy, P. (1987). Frontal lobe dysfunction in OCD. In E. Perecman (Ed.), *The Frontal Lobes Revisited* (pp. 207). New York: IRBN Press.

Maltby, N., Tolin, D. F., Worhunsky, P., O'Keefe, T. M., & Kiehl, K. A. (2005). Dysfunctional action monitoring hyperactivates frontal-striatal circuits in obsessive-compulsive disorder: an event-related fMRI study. *Neuroimage, 24*, 495–503.

March, J. S., Biederman, J., Wolkow, R., Safferman, A., Mardekian, J., Cook, E. H., *et al.* (1998). Sertraline in children and adolescents with obsessive-compulsive disorder: a multicenter randomized controlled trial.[see comment][erratum appears in *Journal of the American Medical Association* 2000 Mar 8;283(10):1293]. *JAMA, 280*, 1752–1756.

March, J. S., & Mulle, K. (1998). *OCD in children and adolescents: A cognitive-behavioral treatment manual* (No. 1-57230-242-9 (hardcover)).

Martin, J. L., Barbanoj, M. J., Perez, V., & Sacristan, M. (2003). Transcranial magnetic stimulation for the treatment of obsessive-compulsive disorder. *Cochrane Database of Systematic Reviews* (3), CD003387.

Masi, G., Millepiedi, S., Mucci, M., Bertini, N., Milantoni, L., & Arcangeli, F. (2005). A naturalistic study of referred children and adolescents with obsessive-compulsive disorder. *Journal of the American Academy of Child & Adolescent Psychiatry, 44*, 673–681.

Masi, G., Perugi, G., Toni, C., Millepiedi, S., Mucci, M., Bertini, N., *et al.* (2004). Obsessive-compulsive bipolar comorbidity: focus on children and adolescents. *Journal of Affective Disorders, 78*, 175–183.

Mataix-Cols, D., Cullen, S., Lange, K., Zelaya, F., Andrew, C., Amaro, E., *et al.* (2003). Neural correlates of anxiety associated with obsessive-compulsive symptom dimensions in normal volunteers. *Biological Psychiatry, 53*, 482–493.

Mataix-Cols, D., Rosario-Campos, M. C., & Leckman, J. F. (2005). A multidimensional model of obsessive-compulsive disorder. *American Journal of Psychiatry, 162*, 228–238.

Mataix-Cols, D., Wooderson, S., Lawrence, N., Brammer, M. J., Speckens, A., & Phillips, M. L. (2004). Distinct neural correlates of washing, checking, and hoarding symptom dimensions in obsessive-compulsive disorder. *Archives of General Psychiatry, 61*, 564–576.

McDougle, C. J., Epperson, C. N., Pelton, G. H., Wasylink, S., & Price, L. H. (2000). A double-blind, placebo-controlled study of risperidone addition in serotonin reuptake inhibitor-refractory obsessive-compulsive disorder [see comment]. *Archives of General Psychiatry, 57*, 794–801.

McKay, D., Piacentini, J., Greisberg, S., Graae, F., Jaffer, M., & Miller, J. (2006). The structure of childhood obsessions and compulsions: dimensions in an outpatient sample. *Behaviour Research and Therapy, 44*, 137–146.

Miguel, E. C., do Rosário-Campos, M. C., Prado, H. S., do Valle, R., Rauch, S. L., Coffey, B. J., *et al.* (2000). Sensory phenomena in obsessive-compulsive disorder and Tourette's disorder. *Journal of Clinical Psychiatry, 61*, 150–156; quiz 157.

Millet, B., Chabane, N., Delorme, R., Leboyer, M., Leroy, S., Poirier, M. F., *et al.* (2003). Association between the dopamine receptor D4 (DRD4) gene and obsessive-compulsive disorder. *American Journal of Medical Genetics. Part B, Neuropsychiatric Genetics: the Official Publication of the International Society of Psychiatric Genetics, 116*, 55–59.

Modell, J. G., Mountz, J. M., Curtis, G. C., & Greden, J. F. (1989). Neurophysiologic dysfunction in basal ganglia/limbic striatal and thalamocortical circuits as a pathogenetic mechanism of obsessive-compulsive disorder [see comments]. *Journal of Neuropsychiatry & Clinical Neurosciences, 1*, 27–36.

Mundo, E., Richter, M. A., Zai, G., Sam, F., McBride, J., Macciardi, F., *et al.* (2002). 5HT1Dbeta receptor gene implicated in the pathogenesis of obsessive-compulsive disorder: further evidence from a family-based association study. *Molecular Psychiatry, 7*, 805–809.

National Institute for Health and Clinical Excellence: Core interventions in the treatment of OCD and BDD: National clinical Practice Guideline Number 31. Published by the British Psychological Society and The Royal College of Psychiatrists (2006). Office of Public Sector Information, London.

Nakao, T., Nakagawa, A., Yoshiura, T., Nakatani, E., Nabeyama, M., Yoshizato, C., *et al.* (2005). A functional MRI comparison of patients with obsessive-compulsive disorder and normal controls during a Chinese character Stroop task. *Psychiatry Research, 139*, 101–114.

Nestadt, G., Samuels, J., Riddle, M., Bienvenu, O. J., 3rd, Liang, K. Y., LaBuda, M., *et al.* (2000). A family study of obsessive-compulsive disorder. *Archives of General Psychiatry, 57*, 358–363.

Neziroglu, F., Yaryura-Tobias, J. A., Walz, J., & McKay, D. (2000). The effect of fluvoxamine and behavior therapy on children and adolescents with obsessive-compulsive disorder. *Journal of Child & Adolescent Psychopharmacology, 10*, 295–306.

Osler, W. (1894). On Chorea and Choreiform Affections. Philadelphia: Blakiston & Sons.

Pauls, D. L., Alsobrook, J. P., 2nd, Goodman, W., Rasmussen, S., & Leckman, J. F. (1995). A family study of obsessive-compulsive disorder. *American Journal of Psychiatry, 152*, 76–84.

Perani, D., Colombo, C., Bressi, S., Bonfanti, A., Grassi, F., Scarone, S., *et al.* (1995). [18F]FDG PET study in obsessive-compulsive disorder. A clinical/metabolic correlation study after treatment. *British Journal of Psychiatry, 166*, 244–250.

Perlmutter, S. J., Leitman, S. F., Garvey, M. A., Hamburger, S., Feldman, E., Leonard, H. L., *et al.* (1999). Therapeutic plasma exchange and intravenous immunoglobulin for obsessive-compulsive disorder and tic disorders in childhood. *Lancet, 354*, 1153–1158.

Peterson, B. S., Pine, D. S., Cohen, P., & Brook, J. S. (2001). Prospective, longitudinal study of tic, obsessive-compulsive, and attention-deficit/hyperactivity disorders in an epidemiological sample. *Journal of the American Academy of Child & Adolescent Psychiatry, 40*, 685–695.

Pogarell, O., Hamann, C., Popperl, G., Juckel, G., Chouker, M., Zaudig, M., *et al.* (2003). Elevated brain serotonin transporter availability in patients with obsessive-compulsive disorder. *Biological Psychiatry, 54*, 1406–1413.

POTS Team. (2004). Cognitive-behavior therapy, sertraline, and their combination for children and adolescents with obsessive-compulsive disorder: the Pediatric OCD Treatment Study (POTS) randomized controlled trial. *JAMA, 292*, 1969–1976.

Poyurovsky, M., & Koran, L. M. (2005). Obsessive-compulsive disorder (OCD) with schizotypy vs. schizophrenia with OCD: diagnostic dilemmas and therapeutic implications. *Journal of Psychiatric Research, 39*, 399–408.

Rapoport, & Wise. (1988). Obsessive-compulsive disorder: evidence for basal ganglia dysfunction. *Psychopharmacology Bulletin*, *24*, 380–384.

Rapoport, J. L., & Inoff-Germain, G. (2007). Neurobiology and pharmacotherapy of obsessive-compulsive disorder. In D. Sibley (Ed.), *Handbook of Contemporary Neuropharmacology*. Hoboken, NJ: Wiley and Sons. pp. 215–247.

Rapoport, J. L., Inoff-Germain, G., Weissman, M. M., Greenwald, S., Narrow, W. E., Jensen, P. S., *et al.* (2000). Childhood obsessive-compulsive disorder in the NIMH MECA study: parent versus child identification of cases. Methods for the Epidemiology of Child and Adolescent Mental Disorders. *Journal of Anxiety Disorders*, *14*, 535–548.

Rasmussen, S. A., & Eisen, J. L. (1992). The epidemiology and differential diagnosis of obsessive compulsive disorder. *Journal of Clinical Psychiatry*, *53 Suppl*, 4–10.

Rasmussen, S. A., & Tsuang, M. T. (1984). The epidemiology of obsessive compulsive disorder. *Journal of Clinical Psychiatry*, *45*, 450–457.

Rauch, S. L., Whalen, P. J., Curran, T., Shin, L. M., Coffey, B. J., Savage, C. R., *et al.* (2001). Probing striato-thalamic function in obsessive-compulsive disorder and Tourette syndrome using neuroimaging methods. *Advances in Neurology*, *85*, 207–224.

Reinherz, H. H. Z., Giaconia, R. R. M., Lefkowitz, E. E. S., Pakiz, B. B., & Frost, A. A. K. (1993). Prevalence of psychiatric disorders in a community population of older adolescents. *Journal of the American Academy of Child & Adolescent Psychiatry*, *32*, 369–377.

Rettew, D. C., Swedo, S. E., Leonard, H. L., Lenane, M. C., & Rapoport, J. L. (1992). Obsessions and compulsions across time in 79 children and adolescents with obsessive-compulsive disorder. *Journal of the American Academy of Child & Adolescent Psychiatry*, *31*, 1050–1056.

Riddle, M. A., Reeve, E. A., Yaryura-Tobias, J. A., Yang, H. M., Claghorn, J. L., Gaffney, G., *et al.* (2001). Fluvoxamine for children and adolescents with obsessive-compulsive disorder: a randomized, controlled, multicenter trial. *Journal of the American Academy of Child & Adolescent Psychiatry*, *40*, 222–229.

Riddle, M. A., Scahill, L., King, R. A., Hardin, M. T., Anderson, G. M., Ort, S. I., *et al.* (1992). Double-blind, crossover trial of fluoxetine and placebo in children and adolescents with obsessive-compulsive disorder. *Journal of the American Academy of Child & Adolescent Psychiatry*, *31*, 1062–1069.

Rosenberg, D. R., Averbach, D. H., O'Hearn, K. M., Seymour, A. B., Birmaher, B., & Sweeney, J. A. (1997). Oculomotor response inhibition abnormalities in pediatric obsessive-compulsive disorder. *Archives of General Psychiatry*, *54*, 831–838.

Rosenberg, D. R., Dick, E. L., O'Hearn, K. M., & Sweeney, J. A. (1997). Response-inhibition deficits in obsessive-compulsive disorder: an indicator of dysfunction in frontostriatal circuits. *Journal of Psychiatry & Neuroscience*, *22*, 29–38.

Rosenberg, D. R., & Keshavan, M. S. (1998). A. E. Bennett Research Award. Toward a neurodevelopmental model of obsessive-compulsive disorder. *Biological Psychiatry*, *43*, 623–640.

Rosenberg, D. R., Keshavan, M. S., O'Hearn, K. M., Dick, E. L., Bagwell, W. W., Seymour, A. B., *et al.* (1997). Frontostriatal measurement in treatment-naive children with obsessive-compulsive disorder [see comment]. *Archives of General Psychiatry*, *54*, 824–830.

Rosenberg, D. R., MacMaster, F. P., Keshavan, M. S., Fitzgerald, K. D., Stewart, C. M., & Moore, G. J. (2000). Decrease in caudate glutamatergic concentrations in pediatric obsessive-compulsive disorder patients taking paroxetine. *Journal of the American Academy of Child & Adolescent Psychiatry*, *39*, 1096–1103.

Rosenberg, D. R., Mirza, Y., Russell, A., Tang, J., Smith, J. M., Banerjee, S. P., *et al.* (2004). Reduced anterior cingulate glutamatergic concentrations in childhood OCD and major depression versus healthy controls. *Journal of the American Academy of Child & Adolescent Psychiatry*, *43*, 1146–1153.

Russell, A., Cortese, B., Lorch, E., Ivey, J., Banerjee, S. P., Moore, G. J., *et al.* (2003). Localized functional neurochemical marker abnormalities in dorsolateral prefrontal cortex in pediatric obsessive-compulsive disorder. *Journal of Child & Adolescent Psychopharmacology*, *13* (Suppl), S31–S38.

Salkovskis, P., Shafran, R., Rachman, S., & Freeston, M. H. (1999). Multiple pathways to inflated responsibility beliefs in obsessional problems: possible origins and implications for therapy and research. *Behaviour Research & Therapy*, *37*, 1055–1072.

Sallee, F. R., Richman, H., Sethuraman, G., Dougherty, D., Sine, L., & Altman-Hamamdzic, S. (1998). Clonidine challenge in childhood anxiety disorder. *Journal of the American Academy of Child & Adolescent Psychiatry*, *37*, 655–662.

Saxena, S., Bota, R. G., & Brody, A. L. (2001). Brain-behavior relationships in obsessive-compulsive disorder. *Seminars in Clinical Neuropsychiatry*, *6*, 82–101.

Saxena, S., Brody, A. L., Maidment, K. M., Dunkin, J. J., Colgan, M., Alborzian, S., *et al.* (1999). Localized orbitofrontal and subcortical metabolic changes and predictors of response to paroxetine treatment in obsessive-compulsive disorder. *Neuropsychopharmacology*, *21*, 683–693.

Shapira, N. A., Liu, Y., He, A. G., Bradley, M. M., Lessig, M. C., James, G. A., *et al.* (2003). Brain activation by disgust-inducing pictures in obsessive-compulsive disorder. *Biological Psychiatry*, *54*, 751–756.

Shin, L. M., Wright, C. I., Cannistraro, P. A., Wedig, M. M., McMullin, K., Martis, B., *et al.* (2005). A functional magnetic resonance imaging study of amygdala and medial prefrontal cortex responses to overtly presented fearful faces in posttraumatic stress disorder. *Archives of General Psychiatry*, *62*, 273–281.

Simpson, H. B., Lombardo, I., Slifstein, M., Huang, H. Y., Hwang, D. R., Abi-Dargham, A., *et al.* (2003). Serotonin transporters in obsessive-compulsive disorder: a positron emission tomography study with [(11)C]McN 5652. *Biological Psychiatry*, *54*, 1414–1421.

Singer, H. S., Hong, J. J., Yoon, D. Y., & Williams, P. N. (2005). Serum autoantibodies do not differentiate PANDAS and Tourette syndrome from controls [see comment]. *Neurology*, *65*, 1701–1707.

Snider, L. A., Lougee, L., Slattery, M., Grant, P., & Swedo, S. E. (2005). Antibiotic prophylaxis with arithromycin or penicillin for childhood-onset neuropsychiatric disorders. *Biological Psychiatry*, *57*, 788–792.

Stein, D. J. (2002). Obsessive-compulsive disorder. *Lancet*, *360*(9330), 397–405.

Stengler-Wenzke, K., Muller, U., Angermeyer, M. C., Sabri, O., & Hesse, S. (2004). Reduced serotonin transporter availability in obsessive-compulsive disorder (OCD). *European Archives of Psychiatry & Clinical Neuroscience*, *254*, 252–255.

Stewart, S. E., Geller, D. A., Jenike, M., Pauls, D., Shaw, D., Mullin, B., *et al.* (2004). Long-term outcome of pediatric obsessive-compulsive disorder: a meta-analysis and qualitative review of the literature [see comment]. *Acta Psychiatrica Scandinavica*, *110*, 4–13.

Swedo, S. E., & Grant, P. J. (2005). Annotation: PANDAS: a model for human autoimmune disease. *Journal of Child Psychology & Psychiatry & Allied Disciplines*, *46*, 227–234.

Swedo, S., Leonard, H., & Rapoport, J. (2004). The pediatric autoimmune neuropsychiatric disorders associated with streptococcal infection (PANDAS) subgroup: Separating fact from fiction. *Pediatrics*, *113*, 907–911.

Swedo, S., Rapoport, J., Leonard, H., Lenane, M., & Cheslow, D. (1989). Obsessive-compulsive disorder in children and adolescents. Clinical phenomenology of 70 consecutive cases. *Archives of General Psychiatry*, *46*, 335–341.

Szeszko, P. R., Ardekani, B. A., Ashtari, M., Malhotra, A. K., Robinson, D., Bilder, R. M., *et al.* (2005). White matter abnormalities in OCD. *Archives of General Psychiatry*, *62*, 782–790.

Szeszko, P. R., MacMillan, S., McMeniman, M., Chen, S., Baribault, K., Lim, K. O., *et al.* (2004). Brain structural abnormalities in psychotropic drug-naive pediatric patients with obsessive-compulsive disorder. *American Journal of Psychiatry*, *161*, 1049–1056.

Szeszko, P. R., Robinson, D., Alvir, J. M., Bilder, R. M., Lencz, T., Ashtari, M., *et al.* (1999). Orbital frontal and amygdala volume reductions in obsessive-compulsive disorder. *Archives of General Psychiatry*, *56*, 913–919.

Thomsen, P. H. (1991). Obsessive-compulsive symptoms in children and adolescents. A phenomenological analysis of 61 Danish cases. *Psychopathology*, *24*, 12–18.

Thomsen, P. H., & Jensen, J. (1991). Latent class analysis of organic aspects of obsessive-compulsive disorder in children and adolescents. *Acta Psychiatrica Scandinavica*, *84*, 391–395.

Ursu, S., Stenger, V. A., Shear, M. K., Jones, M. R., & Carter, C. S. (2003). Overactive action monitoring in obsessive-compulsive disorder: evidence from functional magnetic resonance imaging. *Psychological Science*, *14*, 347–353.

Valleni-Basile, L. A., Garrison, C. Z., Jackson, K. L., Waller, J. L., McKeown, R. E., Addy, C. L., *et al.* (1994). Frequency of obsessive-compulsive disorder in a community sample of young adolescents. *Journal of the American Academy of Child & Adolescent Psychiatry*, *33*, 782–791.

van den Heuvel, O. A., Veltman, D. J., Groenewegen, H. J., Cath, D. C., van Balkom, A. J., van Hartskamp, J., *et al.* (2005). Frontal-striatal dysfunction during planning in obsessive-compulsive disorder. *Archives of General Psychiatry*, *62*, 301–309.

van den Heuvel, O. A., Veltman, D. J., Groenewegen, H. J., Dolan, R. J., Cath, D. C., Boellaard, R., *et al.* (2004). Amygdala activity in obsessive-compulsive disorder with contamination fear: a study with oxygen-15 water positron emission tomography. *Psychiatry Research*, *132*, 225–237.

van den Heuvel, O. A., Veltman, D. J., Groenewegen, H. J., Witter, M. P., Merkelbach, J., Cath, D. C., *et al.* (2005). Disorder-specific neuroanatomical correlates of attentional bias in obsessive-compulsive disorder, panic disorder, and hypochondriasis. *Archives of General Psychiatry*, *62*, 922–933.

van der Wee, N. J., Stevens, H., Hardeman, J. A., Mandl, R. C., Denys, D. A., van Megen, H. J., *et al.* (2004). Enhanced dopamine transporter density in psychotropic-naive patients with obsessive-compulsive disorder shown by [123I]beta-CIT SPECT. *American Journal of Psychiatry*, *161*, 2201–2206.

van Veen, V., & Carter, C. S. (2002). The anterior cingulate as a conflict monitor: fMRI and ERP studies. *Physiology & Behavior*, *77*, 477–482.

Veale, D. M., Sahakian, B. J., Owen, A. M., & Marks, I. M. (1996). Specific cognitive deficits in tests sensitive to frontal lobe dysfunction in obsessive-compulsive disorder. *Psychological Medicine*, *26*, 1261–1269.

Veenstra-VanderWeele, J., Kim, S. J., Gonen, D., Hanna, G. L., Leventhal, B. L., & Cook, E. H., Jr. (2001). Genomic organization of the SLC1A1/EAAC1 gene and mutation screening in early-onset obsessive-compulsive disorder. *Molecular Psychiatry*, 6,160–167.

Viard, A., Flament, M. F., Artiges, E., Dehaene, S., Naccache, L., Cohen, D., *et al.* (2005). Cognitive control in childhood-onset obsessive-compulsive disorder: a functional MRI study. *Psychological Medicine*, *35*, 1007–1017.

Walsh, K. H., & McDougle, C. J. (2004). Pharmacological augmentation strategies for treatment-resistant obsessive-compulsive disorder. *Expert Opinion on Pharmacotherapy*, *5*, 2059–2067.

Willour, V. L., Yao Shugart, Y., Samuels, J., Grados, M., Cullen, B., Bienvenu, O. J., 3rd, *et al.* (2004). Replication study supports evidence for linkage to 9p24 in obsessive-compulsive disorder. *American Journal of Human Genetics*, *75*, 508–513.

Wise, S. P., & Rapoport, J. L. (1989). Obsessive compulsive disorder: is it a basal ganglia dysfunction? In J. L. Rapoport (Ed.), *Obsessive-compulsive disorder in Children and Adolescents* (pp. 327–344). New York, USA: American Psychiatric Press.

Wittchen, H. U., Nelson, C. B., & Lachner, G. (1998). Prevalence of mental disorders and psychosocial impairments in adolescents and young adults. *Psychological Medicine*, *28*, 109–126.

Zai, G., Bezchlibnyk, Y. B., Richter, M. A., Arnold, P., Burroughs, E., Barr, C. L., *et al.* (2004). Myelin oligodendrocyte glycoprotein (MOG) gene is associated with obsessive-compulsive disorder. *American Journal of Medical Genetics. Part B, Neuropsychiatric Genetics: the Official Publication of the International Society of Psychiatric Genetics*, *129*, 64–68.

Zohar, A. H. (1999). The epidemiology of obsessive-compulsive disorder in children and adolescents. *Child & Adolescent Psychiatric Clinics of North America*, *8*, 445–460.

Zohar, A. H., Ratzoni, G., Pauls, D. L., Apter, A., Bleich, A., Kron, S., *et al.* (1992). An epidemiological study of obsessive-compulsive disorder and related disorders in Israeli adolescents. *Journal of the American Academy of Child & Adolescent Psychiatry*, *31*, 1057–1061.

44 Tic Disorders

James F. Leckman and Michael H. Bloch

Tic disorders are transient or chronic conditions associated with difficulties in self-esteem, family life, social acceptance or school or job performance that are directly related to the presence of motor and/or phonic tics. Although tic symptoms have been reported since antiquity, systematic study of individuals with tic disorders dates only from the 19th century with the reports of Itard (1825) and Gilles de la Tourette (1885). Gilles de la Tourette described nine cases characterized by motor "incoordinations" or tics, "inarticulate shouts accompanied by articulated words with echolalia and coprolalia." In addition to identifying the cardinal features of severe tic disorders, his report noted an association between tic disorders and obsessive-compulsive symptoms as well as the hereditary nature of the syndrome in some families.

In addition to tics, individuals with tic disorders may present with a broad array of behavioral difficulties including disinhibited speech or conduct, impulsivity, distractibility, motoric hyperactivity, and obsessive-compulsive symptoms (Leckman & Cohen, 1998). Scientific opinion has been divided on how broadly to conceive the spectrum of maladaptive behaviors associated with Tourette syndrome (TS) (Comings, 1988; Shapiro, Shapiro, Young, & Freinberg, 1988). This controversy is fueled in part by the frustration that parents and educators encounter when they attempt to divide an individual child's repertoire of problem behaviors into those that are "Tourette-related" and those that are not. Population-based epidemiological studies and family-genetic studies have begun to clarify these issues, but much work remains to be done.

In this chapter, a presentation of the phenomenology and classification of tic disorders precedes a review of the etiology, neurobiological substrates, assessment and management of these conditions. The general perspective presented is that TS and related disorders are model neurobiological disorders in which to study multiple genetic and environmental (epigenetic) mechanisms that interact over the course of development to produce a distinctive range of complex syndromes of varying severity.

Rutter's Child and Adolescent Psychiatry, 5th edition. Edited by M. Rutter, D. Bishop, D. Pine, S. Scott, J. Stevenson, E. Taylor and A. Thapar. © 2008 Blackwell Publishing, ISBN: 978-1-4051-4549-7.

Definitions and Classifications

Phenomenology of Tics

A *tic* is a sudden repetitive movement, gesture or utterance that typically mimics some aspect or fragment of normal behavior. Individual tics rarely last more than a second. Many tics occur in bouts with brief inter-tic intervals (Peterson & Leckman, 1998). Individual tics can occur singly or together in an orchestrated pattern. They vary in their intensity or forcefulness. Motor tics vary from simple abrupt movements such as eye blinking, head jerks or shoulder shrugs to more complex, apparently purposive behaviors such as facial expressions or gestures of the arms or head. In extreme cases, these movements can be obscene (copropraxia) or self-injurious (e.g., hitting or biting). Phonic or vocal tics can range from simple throat clearing sounds to more complex vocalizations and speech. In severe cases, coprolalia (obscene or socially unacceptable speech) is present.

By the age of 10 years, most individuals with tics are aware of premonitory urges that may be experienced either as a focal perception in a particular body region where the tic is about to occur (like an itch or a tickling sensation) or as a mental awareness (Leckman, Walker, & Cohen, 1993). Most patients also report a fleeting sense of relief after a bout of tics has occurred. These premonitory and consummatory phenomena contribute to an individual's sense that tics are a habitual yet partially intentional response to unpleasant stimuli. Indeed, most adolescent and adult subjects describe their tics as either "voluntary" or as having both voluntary and involuntary aspects. In contrast, many young children are oblivious to their tics and experience them as wholly involuntary movements or sounds. Most tics can also be suppressed for brief periods of time. The warning given by premonitory urges may contribute to this phenomenon.

Clinicians characterize tics by their anatomical location, number, frequency and duration. The intensity or "forcefulness" of the tic can also be an important characteristic. Finally, tics vary in terms of their "complexity." Complexity usually refers to how simple or involved a movement or sound is, ranging from brief meaningless abrupt fragments (simple tics) to ones that are longer, more involved and seemingly more goal-directed in character (complex tics). Each of these elements has been incorporated into clinician rating scales, which have proven to be useful in monitoring tic severity (Leckman, Riddle, Hardin *et al.*, 1989).

Diagnostic Categories

Diagnostic categories provide a common basis for discussion and are an essential tool in epidemiological and clinical research. Several widely used diagnostic classifications currently include sections on tic disorders. These include both the DSM-IV classification system published by the American Psychiatric Association (1994), and the ICD-10 criteria by the World Health Organization (1996). Although differences exist, these classification schemes are broadly congruent, with each containing three major categories: TS or its equivalent; chronic motor or vocal tic disorder (CMT or CVT) or its equivalent; and transient tic disorder or its equivalent.

To minimize error in case ascertainment and produce an instrument measuring lifetime likelihood of having had TS, clinical members of the American Tourette Syndrome Association International Genetic Collaboration have developed the Diagnostic Confidence Index (DCI) (Robertson, Banerjee, Kurlan *et al.*, 1999). The DCI produces a score from 0 to 100 that is a measure of the likelihood of having or ever having had TS. However, the DCI along with the ICD-10 and DSM-IV diagnostic groupings suffer from uncertainties on how best to categorize conditions that potentially encompass a broad range of symptoms that wax and wane in severity. Because the current nosological boundaries are set by convention and clinical practice, they may not reflect true etiological differences.

Prevalence

Children are 5–12 times more likely to be identified as having a tic disorder than adults (Burd, Kerbeshian, Wikenheiser, & Fisher, 1986a,b). Although boys are more commonly affected with tic behaviors than girls, the male : female ratio in most community surveys is less than 2:1. For example, in the Isle of Wight study of 10- to 11-year-olds, approximately 6% of boys and 3% of girls were reported by their parents to have "twitches, mannerisms, tics of face or body" (Rutter, Tizard, & Whitmore, 1970).

Once thought to be rare, current estimates of the prevalence of TS vary 100-fold, from 2.9 per 10,000 (Caine, McBride, Chiverton *et al.*, 1988) to 299 per 10,000 (Mason, Banerjee, Eapen, Zeitlin, & Robertson, 1998). In the largest study to date, Apter, Pauls, Bleich *et al.* (1993) have reported a prevalence rate of 4.5 per 10,000 for full-blown TS among 16- to 17-year-olds in Israel. More recently, Khalifa and von Knorring (2003, 2005) studied a total population of 4479 Swedish children aged 7–15 years. Twenty-five were identified as having TS, yielding a prevalence estimate of 5.6 per 1000 pupils.

Clinical Descriptions and Natural History

With the exception of TS (Bloch, Landeros-Weisenberger, Kelmendi *et al.*, 2006b; Leckman, Zhang, Vitale *et al.*, 1998b), relatively few cross-sectional or longitudinal studies of tic disorders have been performed so that most of the information provided below is based on clinical experience and anecdotal reports.

Transient Tic Disorder

Almost invariably a disorder of childhood, transient tic disorder is usually characterized by one or more simple motor tics that wax and wane in severity over weeks to months. The anatomical distribution of these tics is usually confined to the eyes, face, neck or upper extremities. Transient phonic tics, in the absence of motor tics, can also occur, although more rarely. The age of onset is typically 3–10 years. Boys are at greater risk. The initial presentation may be unnoticed. Family practitioners, pediatricians, allergists and ophthalmologists are typically the first to see the child. Missed diagnoses are common, particularly as the symptoms may have completely disappeared by the time of the consultation. To meet diagnostic criteria for transient tic disorder, there must be fewer than 12 consecutive months of active symptomatology. This is therefore often a retrospective diagnosis as the clinician is unable to know with certainty which children will show progression of their symptoms and which children will display a self-limiting course.

Chronic Motor or Vocal Tic Disorder

This chronic condition can be observed among children and adults. As with other tic disorders, chronic motor tic disorder (CMTD) is characterized by a waxing and waning course and a broad range of symptom severity. Chronic simple and complex motor tics are the most common manifestations. A majority of tics involve the eyes, face, head, neck and upper extremities. Although some children may display other developmental difficulties such as attention deficit/hyperactivity disorder (ADHD), the disorder is not incompatible with an otherwise normal course of childhood. This condition can also appear as a residual state, where a predictable repertoire of tic symptoms may be seen only during periods of heightened stress or fatigue.

Tourette Syndrome (Combined Vocal and Multiple Motor Tic Disorder)

The most severe tic disorder is best known by the eponym Gilles de la Tourette's syndrome. Typically, the disorder begins in early childhood with transient bouts of simple motor tics such as eye blinking or head jerks. These tics may initially come and go, but eventually they become persistent and begin to have adverse effects on the child and the family. The repertoire of motor tics can be vast, incorporating virtually any voluntary movement by any portion of the body. Although some patients have a "rostral–caudal" progression of motor tics (head, neck, shoulders, arms, torso), this course is not predictable. As the syndrome develops, complex motor tics may appear. Typically, they accompany simple motor tics. Often they have a "camouflaged" or purposive appearance (e.g., brushing hair away from the face with an arm), and can only be distinguished as tics by their repetitive character.

They can involve dystonic movements. In a small fraction of cases (<5%), complex motor tics have the potential to be self-injurious. These self-injurious symptoms may be relatively mild (e.g., slapping or tapping) or quite dangerous (e.g., punching one side of the face, biting a wrist or gouging eyes to the point of blindness).

On average, phonic tics begin 1–2 years after the onset of motor symptoms and are usually simple in character (e.g., throat clearing, grunting and squeaks). More complex vocal symptoms such as echolalia (repeating another's speech), palilalia (repeating one's own speech) and coprolalia occur in a minority of cases. Other complex phonic symptoms include dramatic and abrupt changes in rhythm, rate and volume of speech.

Motor and phonic tics tend to occur in bouts. Their frequency ranges from non-stop bursts that are virtually uncountable (>100 tics per minute) to rare events that occur only a few times a week. Single tics may occur in isolation or there may be orchestrated combinations of motor and phonic tics that involve multiple muscle groups. The forcefulness of motor tics and the volume of phonic tics can also vary from behaviors that are not noticeable (a slight shrug or a hushed guttural noise) to strenuous displays (arm thrusts or loud barking) that are frightening and exhausting. During periods of waxing tic symptoms, clinicians may find themselves under extreme pressure to intervene medically. While such interventions may be warranted, it is often the case that the tic symptoms will wane substantially within a few weeks.

By the age of 10 years, most children and adolescents have some awareness of the premonitory urges that frequently precede both motor and vocal tics. These urges add to the subjective discomfort associated with having a tic disorder. They may also contribute to an individual's ability to suppress their tics for longer periods of time.

The factors that determine the degree of disability and handicap versus resiliency are largely unknown. They are likely to include the presence of additional developmental, mental and behavioral disorders; the level of support and understanding from parents, peers and educators; and the presence of special abilities (as in sports) or personal attributes (intelligence, social abilities and personality traits). The behavioral and emotional problems that frequently complicate TS range from impulsive, "disinhibited" and immature behavior to compulsive touching or sniffing. At present, there are no clear dividing lines between these disruptive behaviors and complex tics on the one hand and comorbid conditions of ADHD and obsessive-compulsive disorder (OCD) on the other. Some investigators believe that the "spectrum" of TS includes attentional deficits, impulsivity, hyperactivity, disruptive behavior, learning disabilities, pervasive developmental disorders and affective and anxiety disorders, as well as tics and OCD (Comings, 1988).

Although children with TS can be loving and affectionate, maintaining age-appropriate social skills is a particularly difficult area for many of them (Bawden, Stokes, Camfield, Camfield, & Salisbury, 1998; Dykens, Leckman, Riddle *et al.*, 1990; Stokes, Bawden, Camfield, Backman, & Dooley, 1991). Whether this is because of the stigmatizing effects of the tics, the patient's own uneasiness or some more fundamental difficulty linked to the neurobiology of this disorder is unknown.

Tic disorders tend to improve in late adolescence and early adulthood. In many instances, the phonic symptoms become increasingly rare or may disappear altogether, and the motor tics may be reduced in number and frequency. Complete remission of both motor and phonic symptoms has also been reported (Shapiro, Shapiro, Young *et al.*, 1988). In contrast, adulthood is also the period when the most severe and debilitating forms of tic disorder can be seen. The factors that influence the continuity of tic disorders from childhood to adolescence to adulthood are not well understood but likely involve the interaction of normal maturational processes occurring in the CNS with the neurobiological mechanisms responsible for TS, the exposure to cocaine, other CNS stimulants, androgenic steroids and the amount of intramorbid emotional trauma and distress experienced by affected individuals during childhood and adolescence. In addition, tic disorders may be etiologically separable so that some of these factors, such as activation of the immune system or exposure to heat stress, may influence the pathogenesis and intramorbid course for some tic disorders but not others. Other factors, such as psychological stress, may have a more uniform impact.

Coexisting Conditions

The past decade has seen a renewed emphasis on the range of neurological and psychiatric symptoms seen in patients with TS (Leckman & Cohen, 1998). In both clinical and epidemiological samples, TS alone is the exception rather than the rule (Khalifa & von Knorring, 2005, 2006). Symptoms associated with ADHD and OCD have received the most attention. It is also becoming clear that the more severe the tic disorder, the greater the likelihood of detecting coexisting conditions, even in representative population-based samples (Khalifa & von Knorring, 2005).

Coexisting Attention Deficit Hyperactivity Disorder

Both clinical and epidemiological studies vary according to setting and established referral patterns, but it is not uncommon to see reports of 30–50% of children with TS diagnosed with comorbid ADHD (Khalifa & von Knorring, 2006). TS has the highest rate of ADHD relative to the other lesser variants of tic disorders. Although the etiological relationship between TS and ADHD is in dispute, it is clear that those individuals with both TS and ADHD are at a much greater risk for a variety of untoward outcomes (Carter, O'Donnell, Schultz *et al.*, 2000; Peterson, Pine, Cohen, & Brook, 2001a; Sukhodolsky, Scahill, Zhang *et al.*, 2003, Sukhodolsky, do Rosario-Campos, Scahill *et al.*, 2005). They are often regarded as less likeable, more aggressive and more withdrawn than their classmates (Stokes, Bawden, Camfield *et al.*, 1991). These social difficulties are amplified in a child with TS who also has ADHD (Bawden, Stokes, Camfield *et al.*, 1998; Dykens, Leckman, Riddle *et al.*, 1990; Sukhodolsky, Scahill, Zhang *et al.*, 2003, Sukhodolsky, do Rosario-Campos, Scahill *et al.*, 2005). Surprisingly, levels of tic severity are less predictive of peer acceptance than is the presence of ADHD (Bawden, Stokes, Camfield *et al.*, 1998).

Obsessive-Compulsive Symptoms

More than 40% of individuals with TS experience recurrent obsessive-compulsive (OC) symptoms (Hounie, do Rosario-Campos, Diniz *et al.*, 2006; Khalifa & von Knorring, 2005; Leckman, Walker, Goodman *et al.*, 1994, Leckman, Grice, Boardman *et al.*, 1997). Genetic, neurobiological and treatment response studies suggest that there may be qualitative differences between tic-related forms of OCD and cases of OCD in which there is no personal or family history of tics. Specifically, tic-related OCD has a male preponderance, an earlier age of onset, a poorer level of response to standard anti-obsessional medications and a greater likelihood of first-degree family members with a tic disorder (Hounie, do Rosario-Campos, Diniz *et al.*, 2006). Symptomatically, the most common OC symptoms encountered in TS patients are obsessions concerning a need for symmetry or exactness, repeating rituals, counting compulsions and ordering/arranging compulsions (Leckman, Grice, Boardman *et al.*, 1997). Also, OC symptoms, when present in children with TS, appear more likely to persist into adulthood than the tics themselves (Bloch, Landeros-Weisenberger, Kelmendi *et al.*, 2006b).

Coexisting Depression and Anxiety Disorders

The co-occurrence of depression and anxiety symptoms with TS is commonplace and may reflect the cumulative psychosocial burden of having tics or shared biological diatheses or both (Robertson & Orth, 2006; Robertson, Williamson, & Eapen, 2006). Antecedent depressive symptoms do predict modest increases in tic severity (Lin, Katsovich, Ghebremichael *et al.*, 2007). However, this study also documented that future depression severity is more closely associated with antecedent worsening of psychosocial stress and OC symptoms than it is with future measures of tic severity.

Other Developmental and Neurological Disorders

Children with a range of developmental disorders are at increased risk for tic disorders. Kurlan, Whitmore, Irvine, McDermott, and Como (1994) reported a four-fold increase in the prevalence of tic disorders among children in special educational settings in a single school district in upstate New York. These children were not intellectually impaired but did have significant learning disabilities or other speech or physical impairments. Children with autism and other pervasive developmental disorders are also at higher risk for developing TS (Baron-Cohen, Mortimore, Moriarty, Izaguirre, & Robertson, 1999).

Neurophysiological Findings

Although motor and phonic tics constitute the core elements of the diagnostic criteria for TS, perceptual and cognitive difficulties are also common. These neuropsychological symptoms are potentially informative about the pathobiology of the disorder. Moreover, these associated difficulties can be more problematic for school and social adjustment than the primary motor symptoms.

Review of the literature suggests that the most consistently observed deficits occur on tasks requiring the accurate copying of geometric designs (i.e., "visual–motor integration" or "visual–graphic" ability; Schultz, Carter, Gladstone *et al.*, 1998). Even after controlling statistically for visual–perceptual skill, intelligence and fine motor control, children with TS performed worse than controls on the visual–motor tasks, suggesting that the integration of visual inputs and organized motor output is a specific area of weakness. Poorer performance with the dominant hand on the Purdue Pegboard test during childhood is associated with worse adulthood tic severity (Bloch, Sukhodolsky, Leckman *et al.*, 2006c).

In studies of procedural memory (habit learning), children with severe tic symptoms had a higher level of impairment than those with less severe symptoms. In contrast, no deficits were seen in declarative memory functioning (Keri, Szlobodnyik, Benedek, Jenka, & Gadoros, 2002; Marsh, Alexander, Packard *et al.*, 2004, Marsh, Alexander, Packard *et al.*, 2005).

Etiology and Pathogenesis

Genetic Factors

Twin and family studies provide evidence that genetic factors are involved in the vulnerability to TS and related disorders (Pauls & Leckman, 1986). The concordance rate for TS among monozygotic twin pairs is greater than 50% while the concordance of dizygotic twin pairs is about 10% (Price, Kidd, Cohen, Pauls, & Leckman, 1985). If cotwins with chronic motor tic disorder are included, these concordance figures increase to 77% for monozygotic and 30% for dizygotic twin pairs. These differences in the concordance of monozygotic and dizygotic twin pairs indicate that genetic factors have an important role in the etiology, but the fact that concordance for monozygotic twins is less than 100% also indicates that non-genetic factors are critical in determining the nature and severity of the clinical syndrome.

Other studies indicate that first-degree family members of probands with TS are at substantially higher risk for developing TS, chronic motor tic disorder and OCD than unrelated individuals (Pauls, Raymond, Stevenson, & Leckman, 1991). The rates are substantially higher than might be expected by chance in the general population, and greatly exceed the rates for these disorders among the relatives of individuals with other psychiatric disorders except OCD.

The pattern of vertical transmission among family members has led several groups of investigators to test specific genetic hypotheses. While not definitive, segregation analyses could not rule out autosomal transmission (Pauls & Leckman, 1986). However, subsequent efforts to identify susceptibility genes within large multigenerational families or using affected sibling pair designs have met with limited success (Tourette Syndrome Association International Consortium for Genetics, 1999, 2007).

In addition, a number of cytogenetic abnormalities have been reported in TS families (Cuker, State, King, Davis, & Ward, 2004; State, Greally, Cuker *et al.*, 2003). Among the more recent findings, Verkerk, Mathews, Joosse *et al.* (2003) reported the disruption of the contactin-associated protein 2 gene on chromosome 7. This gene encodes a membrane protein located at nodes of Ranvier of axons that may be important for the distribution of the K^+ channels, which would affect signal conduction along myelinated neurons. In addition, using a candidate gene approach identified by chromosomal anomalies, Abelson, Kwan, O'Roak *et al.* (2005) identified and mapped a *de novo* chromosome 13 inversion in a patient with TS. The gene *SLITRK1* was identified as a brain-expressed candidate gene mapping approximately 350 kb from the 13q31 breakpoint. Mutation screening of 174 patients was undertaken with the resulting identification of a truncating frameshift mutation in a second family affected with TS. In addition, two examples of a rare variant were identified in a highly conserved region of the 3′ untranslated region of the gene corresponding to a brain-expressed micro-RNA binding domain. None of these anomalies was demonstrated in 3600 controls. *In vitro* studies showed that both the frameshift and the micro-RNA binding site variant had functional potential and were consistent with a loss-of-function mechanism. Studies of both *SLITRK1* and the micro-RNA predicted to bind in the variant-containing 3′ region showed expression in multiple neuroanatomical areas implicated in TS neuropathology, including the cortical plate, striatum, globus pallidus, thalamus and subthalamic nucleus.

Neural Circuits

Neuroanatomy

Investigators interested in procedural learning, habit formation and internally and externally guided motor control have focused their attention on multisynaptic cortico-striato-thalamo-cortical (CSTC) circuits or loops that link the cerebral cortex with several subcortical regions (Graybiel & Canales, 2001; Middleton & Strick, 2000). As a result the most widely accepted neuroanatomical model of TS proposes a regional imbalance of the direct vs. the indirect pathway within one of more of these CSTCs (Albin & Mink, 2006). In the direct pathway, an excitatory glutamatergic signal projects to the striatum, sending an inhibitory gamma-aminobutyric acid (GABA)-ergic signal to the internal part of the globus pallidus. This signal results in a decreased inhibition (disinhibition) of the thalamus and thus an increased excitatory effect on the prefrontal cortex. In the indirect pathway, the striatum projects an inhibitory signal to the external part of the globus pallidus and the subthalamic nucleus, sending an excitatory signal to the internal part of the globus pallidus. The net effect is an increased inhibition of the thalamus and decreased excitation of the prefrontal cortex. It is hypothesized that the direct pathway functions as a self-reinforcing positive feedback loop and contributes to the initiation and continuation of behaviors, whereas the indirect pathway provides a mechanism of negative feedback which is important for the inhibition of behaviors and in switching between behaviors. Based on postmortem studies, as well as structural and functional neuroimaging studies, it appears that an imbalance between these frontal–striatal circuits might mediate tic symptomatology as well as that of related disorders.

Neuropathological Data

Although neuropathological studies of postmortem TS brains are few in number, a recent stereological study indicates that there is a marked alteration in the number and density of GABA-ergic parvalbumin-positive cells in basal ganglia structures (Kalanithi, Zheng, Kataoka *et al.*, 2005). In the caudate there was a greater than 50% reduction in the GABA-ergic fast spiking interneurons and a 30–40% reduction of these same cells in the putamen. This same study found a reduction of the GABA-ergic parvalbumin-positive projection neurons in the external segment globus pallidus (GPe) as well as a dramatic increase (>120%) in the number and proportion of GABA-ergic projection neurons of the internal segment of the globus pallidus. These alterations are consistent with a developmental defect in tangential migration of some GABA-ergic neurons. Further studies are needed to confirm and extend these findings, such as toward a more complete understanding of how the different striatal interneurons are affected, and to determine how alterations in GABA-ergic interneurons and globus pallidus projection neurons could lead to a form of thalamocortical dysrhythmia (Leckman, Vaccarino, Kalanithi, & Rothenberger, 2006; Llinas, Urbano, Leznik, Ramirez, & van Marle, 2005).

Structural Brain Imaging

Volumetric magnetic resonance imaging (MRI) studies of basal ganglia in individuals with TS are largely consistent with these postmortem results – with the finding of a slight reduction in caudate volume (Hyde, Stacey, Coppola *et al.*, 1995; Peterson, Thomas, Kane *et al.*, 2003). For example, in a study of 154 subjects with TS and 130 healthy controls, Peterson, Thomas, Kane *et al.* (2003) found a significant decrease in the volume of the caudate nucleus in both children and adults. Although there was no correlation between symptom severity and caudate volumes in this cross-sectional study, Bloch, Leckman, Zhu, and Peterson (2005) found an inverse correlation between caudate volumes measured in childhood and tic severity rated in early adulthood.

The same group of individuals with TS had larger volumes in dorsal prefrontal regions, larger volumes in parieto-occipital regions, and smaller inferior occipital volumes (Peterson, Staib, Scahill *et al.*, 2001b). Regional cerebral volumes were significantly associated with the severity of tic symptoms in orbitofrontal, midtemporal and parieto-occipital regions. This may reflect the natural history of the disorder, or brain compensations, or may yet be explained by other subtle confounding variables, such as the manner in which brain volumes are determined in different studies. In addition, Lee, Yoo, Cho *et al.* (2006) used volumetric MRI methods to compare thalamic volume in 18 treatment-naïve boys with 16 healthy control subjects, finding larger left thalamic volume in the TS cases. More volumetric studies using comparable methods across all implicated brain regions are needed to clarify the brain morphology of TS.

Functional Brain Imaging

Thus far, there have only been a few published studies of TS using functional magnetic resonance imaging (fMRI), which takes advantage of state-dependent blood oxygenation as a measure of brain activity. In adults with TS, Peterson, Skudlarski, Anderson *et al.* (1998a) compared brain activity during blocks of time during which tics were voluntarily suppressed or not suppressed. During tic suppression, prefrontal cortical, thalamic and basal ganglia areas were activated. These activations were inversely correlated with tic severity (i.e., lower activation was associated with higher tic severity). This suggests that a greater ability of basal ganglia to suppress cortical activity might be linked with decreased tic severity, and is in agreement with single photon emission computed tomography (SPECT) and positron emission tomography (PET) studies that suggest involvement of the basal ganglia in TS (Braun, Randolph, Stoetter *et al.*, 1995). More recently, Bohlhalter, Goldfine, Matteson *et al.* (2006) studied the neural correlates of tics and associated urges using an event-related fMRI protocol. On the basis of synchronized video/audio recordings, fMRI activities were analyzed 2 s before and at tic onset. A brain network of paralimbic areas including the anterior cingulate and insular cortex, supplementary motor area and parietal operculum was found to be activated before tic onset. In contrast, at the beginning of tic action, significant fMRI activities were found in sensorimotor areas including superior parietal lobule bilaterally and cerebellum. The results of this study indicate that paralimbic and sensory association areas are critically implicated in tic generation.

Changes in the coupling of the putamen and ventral striatum with a number of other brain regions also differentiate patients with TS from controls. For example in PET studies, Jeffries, Schooler, Schoenbach *et al.* (2002) noted a reversal in the pattern of CSTC circuit interactions in motor and lateral orbitofrontal cortices. Similarly, Stern, Silbersweig, Chee *et al.* (2000) found that increased activity in a set of neocortical, paralimbic and subcortical regions (including supplementary motor, premotor, anterior cingulate, dorsolateral–rostral prefrontal and primary motor cortices, Broca's area, insula, claustrum, putamen and caudate) were highly correlated with tic behavior. Perhaps not surprisingly, in the one patient with prominent coprolalia the vocal tics were associated with increased activity in prerolandic and postrolandic language regions, insula, caudate, thalamus and cerebellum.

Neurophysiology

Non-invasive *in vivo* neurophysiological research in TS has led to several areas of significant progress. The first concerns the use of a startle paradigm to measure inhibitory deficits by monitoring the reduction in startle reflex magnitude. Swerdlow, Karban, Ploum *et al.* (2001) have confirmed and extended earlier findings indicating that patients with TS have deficits in sensory gating across a number of sensory modalities. Prepulse inhibition abnormalities have been observed across a variety of neuropsychiatric populations including schizophrenia, OCD, Huntington's disease, nocturnal enuresis, ADHD, Asperger syndrome and TS, suggesting that some final common pathways mediate abnormal prepulse inhibition in all of these conditions. With respect to TS, these deficits are consistent with the idea that there is diminished ability to appropriately manage or "gate" sensory inputs to motor programs, which are released as tics (Swerdlow & Sutherland, 2006).

A second advance has been the investigation of motor system excitability by means of single and paired pulse transcranial magnetic stimulation. Studies of groups of patients with TS have indicated that the cortical silent period (a period of decreased excitability following stimulation) is shortened. This intracortical excitability is frequently seen in children with ADHD comorbid with a tic disorder (Moll, Wischer, Heinrich *et al.*, 1999; Ziemann, Paulus, & Rothenberger, 1997). This heightened level of cortical excitability may be related to a reduction in the number of GABA-ergic interneurons in the cortex.

Serrien, Orth, Evans, Lees, & Brown (2005) recently identified similar sensorimotor–frontal connections involved in the acute suppression of involuntary tics as evidenced by increased EEG coherence in the alpha frequency band (8–12 Hz) during suppression of voluntary movements in individuals with TS and healthy subjects during a Go–NoGo task. This finding, taken with the functional findings from Peterson, Skudlarski, Anderson *et al.* (1998a), suggests that the frontal lobes may have a key role in tic suppression, and coherence in the alpha band may be part of this process.

The preliminary findings that ablation (or high-frequency stimulation using deep brain electrodes) in regions of the globus pallidus and/or the midline thalamic nuclei can ameliorate tics in severe persistent cases of TS (Hassler & Dieckmann, 1973; Vandewalle, Van der Linden, Groenwegen, & Caemaert, 1999) powerfully support the view that electrophysiological studies and interventions hold promise just as they do for disorders such as Parkinson's disease.

Prospective longitudinal studies with higher resolution will be needed to examine fully the developmental processes, sexual dimorphisms and possible effects of medication on critical cell compartments. It will also be important to confirm if any of these volumetric and functional findings in childhood are predictive of later clinical outcomes. The combination of imaging techniques with real-time neurophysiological techniques, such as electroencephalography or magnetoencephalography, may help to determine whether any abnormalities seen on brain imaging contribute to the production of tics or whether they constitute a compensatory response (Leckman, Vaccarino, Kalanithi *et al.*, 2006; Llinas, Urbano, Leznik *et al.*, 2005).

Neurochemical and Neuropharmacological Data

Extensive immunohistochemical studies of the basal ganglia have demonstrated the presence of a wide spectrum of classic neurotransmitters, neuromodulators and neuropeptides. The most compelling data have implicated central dopaminergic systems in the pathobiology of TS (Albin & Mink, 2006).

Dopaminergic Systems

Explicit "dopamine" hypotheses for TS posit either an excess of dopamine release or an increased sensitivity of D2 dopamine receptors. These hypotheses are consistent with multiple lines of empirical evidence as well as emerging data from animal models of habit formation. Data implicating central dopaminergic mechanisms include the results of double-blind clinical trials in which haloperidol, pimozide, tiapride and other neuroleptics that preferentially block dopaminergic D2 receptors have been found to be effective in the temporary suppression of tics for a majority of patients (Scahill, Erenberg, Berlin *et al.*, 2006). Tic suppression has also been reported following administration of agents such as tetrabenazine that reduce dopamine synthesis (Kenney & Jankovic, 2006). Increased tics have been reported following withdrawal of neuroleptics or following exposure to agents that increase central dopaminergic activity such as L-dopa and CNS stimulants, including cocaine. Using these imaging techniques, a number of investigators have also found increased levels of dopaminergic innervation of the striatum in TS subjects compared with controls (Albin, Koeppe, Bohne *et al.*, 2003; Cheon, Ryu, Namkoong *et al.*, 2004; Malison, McDougle, van Dyck *et al.*, 1995; Singer, Szymanski, Giuliano *et al.*, 2002; Wolf, Jones, Knable *et al.*, 1996). Although not all studies agree, the strongest evidence suggests an increased density of dopaminergic terminals in the ventral striatum (Albin, Koeppe, Bohne *et al.*, 2003). Postmortem brain studies have reported alterations in the number or affinity of presynaptic dopamine carrier sites in the striatum (Singer, Hahn, & Moran, 1991). In summary, while the evidence that dopaminergic pathways are intimately involved in the pathobiology of TS is compelling, the exact nature of the abnormality remains to be elucidated but likely involves the potentiation of limbic inputs to the striatum.

Amino Acid Systems

The excitatory neurotransmitter glutamate is released upon depolarization by the corticostratial, corticosubthalamic, subthalamic and thalamocortical projection neurons. These excitatory neurons are key players in the functional anatomy of the basal ganglia and the CSTC loops and likely have a crucial role in the emergence of tics as well as related normal behaviors.

Neurons containing inhibitory amino acid neurotransmitters, particularly GABA, also form major portions of CSTC loops and are also present in key sets of interneurons in the cortex, striatum and thalamus. If the initial reports of a reduced number of GABA-ergic fast-spiking interneurons in the caudate and an increased number of GABA-ergic projection neurons in the globus pallidus are confirmed, this may provide a basis for understanding the anatomical and neurophysiological origins of some cases of severe TS (Kalanithi, Zheng, Kataoka *et al.*, 2005; Leckman, Vaccarino, Kalanithi *et al.*, 2006).

Cholinergic Systems

Cholinergic projections from the basal forebrain are found throughout the cortex and within key structures of the basal ganglia and mesencephalon, including the internal segment of the globus pallidos (GP), the pars reticulata of the substantia nigra, and the locus ceruleus. Evidence of cholinergic involvement in the pathobiology of TS comes from the reported potentiation of D2 dopamine receptor blocking agents through the use of transdermal nicotine or nicotine gum (Sanberg, Silver, Shytle *et al.*, 1997).

Noradrenergic Systems

Noradrenergic projections from the locus ceruleus project innervate the prefrontal and other cortical regions. Noradrenergic pathways are also likely to indirectly influence central dopaminergic pathways via projections to areas near the ventral tegmental area (Grenhoff & Svensson, 1989). Speculation that noradrenergic mechanisms might be relevant to the pathobiology of TS was based initially on the beneficial effects of α_2-adrenergic agonists including clonidine and guanfacine. The involvement of the noradrenergic pathways may be one mechanism by which stressors influence tic severity. For example, a series of adults with TS had elevated levels of cerebrospinal fluid (CSF) norepinephrine (Leckman, Goodman, Anderson *et al.*, 1995) and excreted high levels of urinary norepinephrine in response to the stress of the lumbar puncture (Chappell, Riddle, Anderson *et al.*, 1994). These elevated levels of CSF norepinephrine may also contribute to the elevation in levels of CSF corticotopin-releasing factor seen in some patients with TS (Chappell, Leckman, Goodman *et al.*, 1996).

Serotonergic Systems

Ascending serotonergic projections from the dorsal raphe have been invoked as playing a part in the pathophysiology of both TS and OCD. The most compelling evidence relates to OCD and is based largely on the well-established efficacy of potent serotonin reuptake inhibitors such as clomipramine and fluvoxamine in the treatment of OCD. However, some investigators have reported that the serotonin reuptake inhibitors are less effective in treating tic-related OCD than other forms of OCD (McDougle, Goodman, Leckman *et al.*, 1993).

Gender-Specific Endocrine Factors

Males are more frequently affected with TS than females (Shapiro, Shapiro, Young *et al.*, 1988), but male–male transmission within families rules out the presence of an X-linked vulnerability gene. This observation has led us to hypothesize that androgenic steroids act at key developmental periods to influence the natural history of TS and related disorders

(Peterson, Leckman, Scahill *et al.*, 1992). These developmental periods include the prenatal period when the brain is being formed, adrenarche when adrenal androgens first appear at age 5–7 years, and puberty. Androgenic steroids may be responsible for these effects or they may act indirectly through estrogens formed in key brain regions by the aromatization of testosterone.

The importance of gender differences in expression of associated phenotypes is also clear given the observation that women are more likely than men to develop OC symptoms without concomitant tics (Pauls, Raymond, Stevenson *et al.*, 1991) and that boys with TS are much more likely than girls to display ADHD disruptive behaviors.

Surges in testosterone and other androgenic steroids during critical periods in fetal development are involved in the production of long-term functional augmentation of subsequent hormonal challenges (as in adrenarche and during puberty) and in the formation of structural CNS dimorphisms (Sikich & Todd, 1988). Sexually dimorphic brain regions include portions of the amygdala (and related limbic areas) and the hypothalamus (including the medial preoptic area, which mediates the body's response to thermal stress; Boulant, 1981). These regions contain high levels of androgen and estrogen receptors and influence activity in the basal ganglia both directly and indirectly. Indeed, a proportion of patients with TS appear to be uniquely sensitive to thermal stress such that when their core body temperature increases and they begin to sweat their tics increase (Lombroso, Mack, Scahill, King, & Leckman, 1991). It is also of note that some of the neurochemical and neuropeptidergic systems implicated in TS and related disorders, such as dopamine, serotonin and the opioids, are involved with these regions and appear to be regulated by sex-specific factors.

Further support for a role for androgens comes from anecdotal reports of tic exacerbation following androgen use (Leckman & Scahill, 1990) and from trials of antiandrogens in patients with severe TS and/or OCD (Peterson, Zhang, Anderson, & Leckman, 1998b). In the most rigorous study to date, Peterson, Zhang, Anderson *et al.* (1998b) found that the therapeutic effects of the antiandrogen flutamide were modest in magnitude and these effects were short-lived, possibly because of physiological compensation for androgen receptor blockade.

The view that sex steroids of gonadal origin organize the neural circuits of the developing brain has recently been challenged by the finding that, independent of the masculinizing effects of gonadal secretions, XY and XX brain cells have different patterns of gene expression that influence their differentiation and function. Remarkably, one of the male-specific genes, *Sry*, is specifically expressed in the dopamine-containing cells of the substantia nigra (Dewing, Chiang, Sinchak *et al.*, 2006). It appears that *Sry* directly affects the function of these dopaminergic neurons and the specific motor behaviors they control. Because these results demonstrate a direct male-specific effect on the brain by a gene encoded only in the male genome, without any mediation by gonadal hormones, it is possible that allelic variation or epigenetic effects at this locus may be important in the pathophysiology of TS.

Perinatal Risk Factors

The search for non-genetic factors that mediate the expression of a genetic vulnerability to TS and related disorders has also focused on the role of adverse perinatal events. This interest dates from the report of Pasamanick and Kawi (1956) who found that mothers of children with tics were 1.5 times more likely to have experienced a complication during pregnancy than the mothers of children without tics. Further, among monozygotic twins discordant for TS, the index twins with TS had lower birth weights than their unaffected cotwins (Hyde, Stacey, Coppola *et al.*, 1995; Leckman, Price, Walkup *et al.*, 1987). Low Apgar scores, severity of maternal life stress during pregnancy, maternal smoking, and severe nausea and/or vomiting during the first trimester have also emerged as potential risk factors in the development of tic disorders (Burd, Severud, Klug, & Kerbeshian, 1999; Leckman, Dolnansky, Hardin *et al.*, 1990; Mathews, Bimson, Lowe *et al.*, 2006). Finally, there is limited evidence that smoking and alcohol use, as well as forceps delivery, can predispose individuals with a vulnerability to TS to develop comorbid OCD (Santangelo, Pauls, Goldstein *et al.*, 1994). The only nested case–control study to date, which examined TS cases arising in a Swedish community sample, found that the mothers of children with TS were two times more likely to have had complications during pregnancy (Khalifa & von Knorring, 2005).

Post-Infectious Autoimmune Mechanisms

It is well established that group A β hemolytic streptococci (GABHS) can trigger immune-mediated disease in genetically predisposed individuals (Bisno, 1991). Speculation concerning a post-infectious (or at least a post-rheumatic fever) etiology for tic disorder symptoms dates from the late 1800s (Kushner, 1999). Acute rheumatic fever is a delayed sequela of GABHS, occurring approximately 3 weeks following an inadequately treated upper respiratory tract infection. Rheumatic fever is characterized by inflammatory lesions involving the heart (rheumatic carditis), joints (polymigratory arthritis) and/or central nervous system (Sydenham's chorea). The immune response in the CNS of patients with Sydenham's chorea appears to involve molecular mimicry between streptococcal antigens and self-antigens (Kirvan, Swedo, Heuser, & Cunningham, 2003). Sydenham's chorea and TS, OCD and ADHD share common anatomical targets – the basal ganglia of the brain and the related cortical and thalamic sites (Husby, van de Rijn, Zabriskie, Abdin, & Williams, 1976). Furthermore, people with Sydenham's chorea frequently display motor and vocal tics, OC and ADHD symptoms, suggesting the possibility that at least in some instances these disorders share a common etiology (Swedo, Rapoport, Cheslow *et al.*, 1989).

It has been proposed that pediatric autoimmune neuropsychiatric disorder associated with streptococcal infection (PANDAS) represents a distinct clinical entity, and includes Sydenham's chorea and some cases of TS and OCD (see chapter 43; Swedo, Leonard, Garvey *et al.*, 1998). The most compelling evidence of an etiological link between these disorders and GABHS infection comes from a study that found an increased proportion of GABHS infections (odds ratio 13.6) within the preceding 12 months in children newly diagnosed with TS compared with well-matched controls (Mell, Davis, & Owens, 2005). The PANDAS hypothesis is indirectly supported by the presence of high levels of antistreptococcal antibodies in some patients with TS (Cardona & Orefici, 2001; Church, Dale, Lees, Giovannoni, & Robertson, 2003). Thus far, however, prospective longitudinal studies have provided little support for the idea that GABHS infections induce future tic exacerbations (Luo, Leckman, Katsovich *et al.*, 2004; Perrin, Murphy, Casey *et al.*, 2004).

A number of studies have been designed to detect and characterize the putative cross-reactive epitopes. Patients with TS may have higher levels of circulating antineural antibodies (Church, Dale, Lees *et al.*, 2003; Morshed, Parveen, Leckman *et al.*, 2001; Singer, Giuliano, Hansen *et al.*, 1998), but no specific epitopes have been unequivocally identified (Dale, Candler, Church, & Pocock, 2004; Kirvan, Swedo, Heuser, & Cunningham, 2006; Singer, Hong, Yoon, & Williams, 2005a). Animal models that involve the injection of patient sera high in levels of antineural antibodies into tic-related basal ganglia areas have also led to equivocal results (Singer, Mink, Loiselle *et al.*, 2005b). However, there is evidence that tic and OC symptoms may improve following plasma exchange in selected patients with the PANDAS phenotype (Perlmutter, Leitman, Garvey *et al.*, 1999).

Additional evidence that acute exacerbations of TS and OCD could also be triggered by GABHS comes from four independent reports demonstrating that the majority of patients with childhood-onset TS or OCD have elevated expression of a stable B-cell marker (Hoekstra, Bijzet, Limburg *et al.*, 2001; Luo, Leckman, Katsovich *et al.*, 2004; Swedo, Leonard, Mittleman *et al.*, 1997). The D8/17 marker identifies close to 100% of rheumatic fever patients (with or without Sydenham's chorea) but is present at low levels of expression in healthy control populations.

The bias for studies addressing the role of B-cell immunity in TS pathogenesis has been driven by the common view that GABHS is an extracellular bacterium and that its clearance is mediated primarily by antibodies. However, GABHS can be internalized in human cells with the same frequency as the classic intracellular pathogens *Listeria* and *Salmonella* species and activates human T lymphocytes (Degnan, Kehoe, & Goodacre, 1997). This topic is just beginning to be addressed with the finding that there may be a reduced number of regulatory T cells in selected patients with TS (Kawikova, Leckman, Kronig *et al.*, 2007). There is also a single report that suggests that individuals with TS may have elevated levels of proinflammatory cytokines under baseline conditions and a further increase during periods of tic exacerbations (Leckman, Katsovich, Kawikova *et al.*, 2005).

In summary, a substantial body of circumstantial evidence links post-infectious autoimmune phenomena with TS, OCD and ADHD. However, these data are not compelling with regard to specific immunological mechanisms, nor do they establish where in the sequence of causal events these immune changes occur. These potentially important findings require replication in independent samples and warrant more intensive investigation using prospective longitudinal designs.

Psychological Factors

Tic disorders have long been identified as "stress-sensitive" conditions. Typically, symptom exacerbations follow in the wake of stressful life events. As noted by Shapiro, Shapiro, Young *et al.* (1988), these events need not be adverse in character. Clinical experience suggests that in some instances a vicious cycle is initiated in which attempts to suppress the symptoms by punishment and humiliation lead to a further exacerbation of symptoms and further increase in stress in the child's interpersonal environment. Unchecked, this vicious cycle can lead to the most severe manifestations of TS. Prospective longitudinal studies have shown that patients with TS experience more stress than matched healthy controls (Findley, Leckman, Katsovich *et al.*, 2003) and that antecedent stress may have a role in subsequent tic exacerbation (Lin, Katsovich, Ghebremichael *et al.*, 2007). Increases in depressive symptoms have also emerged as a significant predictor of future tic severity (Lin, Katsovich, Ghebremichael *et al.*, 2007).

In addition to the intramorbid effects of stress, anxiety and depression, premorbid stress may also act as a sensitizing agent in the pathogenesis of TS among vulnerable individuals (Leckman, Cohen, Price *et al.*, 1984). It is likely that the immediate family environment (e.g., parental discord) and the coping abilities of family members have some role (Leckman, Dolnansky, Hardin *et al.*, 1990), and this may lead to a sensitization of stress responsive biological systems such as the hypothalamic–pituitary–adrenal axis (Chappell, Riddle, Anderson *et al.*, 1994, Chappell, Leckman, Goodman *et al.*, 1996; Leckman, Goodman, Anderson *et al.*, 1995).

Differential Diagnosis

The differential diagnosis of simple motor tics includes a variety of hyperkinetic movements: myoclonus, tremors, chorea, athetosis, dystonias, akathitic movements, paroxysmal dyskinesias, ballistic movements and hyperekplexia (Jankovic & Mejia, 2006). These movements may be associated with genetic conditions such as Huntington's chorea or Wilson's disease; structural lesions, as in hemiballismus (associated with lesions to the contralateral subthalamic nucleus); infectious processes as in Sydenham's chorea; idiopathic functional instability of neuronal circuits, as in myoclonic epilepsy; and pharmacological treatments such as acute akathisia and dystonias associated with the use of neuroleptic agents. Differentiation between these conditions and tic disorders is usually based on the presentation of the disorder and its natural history. Although aspects of tics such as their abruptness, their paroxysmal timing or their suppressible nature may be similar to symptoms seen in other conditions, it is rare for all of these features to be combined in the absence of a *bona fide* tic disorder. Occasionally, diagnostic tests are needed to exclude alternative diagnoses.

Complex motor tics can be confused with other complex repetitive behaviors such as stereotypies or compulsive rituals. Differentiation among these behaviors may be difficult, particularly among retarded individuals with limited verbal skills. In other settings where these symptoms are closely intertwined, as in individuals with both TS and OCD, efforts to distinguish between complex motor tics and compulsive behaviors may be futile. In cases of a tic disorder, it is unusual to see complex motor tics in the absence of simple tics. Involuntary vocal utterances are uncommon neurological signs in the absence of a tic disorder. Examples include sniffing and uttering brief sounds in Huntington's disease and involuntary moaning in Parkinson's disease, particularly as a result of L-dopa toxicity. Complex phonic tics characterized by articulate speech typically can be distinguished from other conditions including voluntary coprolalia. Because of their rarity in other syndromes, phonic tics can have an important role in differential diagnosis.

Anamnesis, family history, observation and neurological examination are usually sufficient to establish the diagnosis of a tic disorder. There are no confirmatory diagnostic tests. Neuroimaging studies, electroencephalography (EEG) based studies and laboratory tests are usually non-contributory except in atypical cases.

Assessment

Once the diagnosis has been established, care should be taken to focus on the overall course of an individual's development, not simply on his or her tic symptoms. This may be a particular problem in the case of TS, where the symptoms can be dramatic and there is the temptation to organize all of an individual's behavioral and emotional difficulties under a single all-encompassing rubric.

The principal goal of an initial assessment is to determine the individual's overall level of adaptive functioning and to identify areas of impairment and distress (Leckman, King, Scahill *et al.*, 1998a). Close attention to the strengths and weaknesses of the individual and his or her family is crucial. Relevant dimensions include the presence of comorbid mental, behavioral, developmental or physical disorders; family history of psychiatric and/or neurological disease; relationships with family and peers; school and/or occupational performance; and the history of important life events. Medication history is important, particularly if the disorder is long-standing or if medications have been prescribed for physical disorders. It may be necessary to evaluate the adequacy of the prior trials with pharmacological agents used to treat tic disorders. Inventories such as the Yale Child Study Center: Tourette's Syndrome Obsessive-Compulsive Disorder Symptom Questionnaire (Leckman & Cohen, 1998, Appendix 1) completed by the family prior to their initial consultation can help gain a long-term perspective of the child's developmental course and the natural history. In addition, several valid and reliable clinical rating instruments have been developed to quantify recent tic symptoms including the Yale Global Tic Severity Scale (YGTSS; Leckman, Riddle, Hardin *et al.*, 1989), the Shapiro Tourette Syndrome Severity Scale (Shapiro, Shapiro, Young *et al.*, 1988) and the Hopkins Motor and Vocal Tic Scale (Walkup, Rosenberg, Brown, & Singer, 1992).

The YGTSS is a state-of-the-art, clinician-rated, semi-structured scale that begins with a systematic inventory of tic symptoms that the clinician rates as present or absent over the past week. Current motor and phonic tics are then rated separately according to number, frequency, intensity, complexity and interference on a 6-point ordinal scale (0 = absent; 1–5 for severity) yielding three scores.

Direct observational methods include videotaping tic-counting procedures or *in vivo* evaluation of tic symptoms (Chappell, Riddle, Anderson *et al.*, 1994; Goetz, Pappert, Louis, Raman, & Leurgans, 1999). These direct observational methods are objective, but the frequency of tics varies according to setting and activity. In addition, many individuals with TS can suppress their symptoms for brief periods of time. In practice, videotaped tic counting appears to be most useful for acute research procedures that take place over several hours. Clinically, videotaping can be valuable when the diagnosis is in doubt or when tics are not observed in the consultation room.

Treatment

Tic disorders are frequently chronic, if not lifelong, conditions. Continuity of care is desirable and should be considered before embarking on a course of treatment. Usual clinical practice focuses initially on the educational and supportive interventions. Pharmacological treatments are typically held in reserve. Given the waxing and waning course of the disorders, it is likely that whatever is done (or not done) will lead in the short term to some improvement in tic severity. The decision to employ psychoactive medications is usually made after the educational and supportive interventions have been in place for a period of months and it is clear that the tic symptoms are persistently severe and are themselves a source of impairment in terms of self-esteem, relationships with the family or peers, or school performance.

Educational and Supportive Interventions

Educational activities are among the most important interventions available to the clinician. They should be undertaken first, not only with children with TS but also with those with milder presentations. Although the efficacy of these educational and supportive interventions has not been rigorously assessed, they appear to have positive effects by reshaping familial expectations and relationships (Cohen, Ort, Leckman, Riddle, & Hardin, 1988). This is particularly true when the family and others have misconstrued the tic symptoms as being intentionally provocative. Families also find descriptions of the natural history comforting in that the disorders tend not to be relentlessly progressive and usually improve during adulthood. This information often contradicts the impressions gained from the available lay literature on TS, which typically focuses on the most extreme cases. Armed with this knowledge, patients and family members and others can begin to understand why waiting before beginning medical treatment makes sense. If a child is in the midst of a bad period of tics it is likely that, whether or not a new medication is prescribed, the tics will improve in the near future. This insight will also help children and their families realize why at times in the past their medications have suddenly stopped working. These dialogs can be relieving and can interrupt a vicious cycle of recrimination that leads to further tic exacerbation, and it can help parents shift the focus from blame to problem-solving.

For children, contact with their teachers can be enormously valuable. By educating the educators, clinicians can make significant progress towards securing for the child a positive and supportive environment in the classroom. If possible, teachers need to respond to outbursts of tics with grace and understanding. Repeatedly scolding a child for his or her tics can be counterproductive. The child may develop a negative attitude to authority figures and may be reluctant to attend school, and classmates may feel freer to tease the child. If tics interfere with a student's ability to receive information in the classroom, it is imperative to find alternative ways to present the material. By helping the student find a way to function even during periods of severe tics, teachers model problem-solving skills that will foster future self-esteem. It is also important for teachers to know that in unstructured settings such as the cafeteria, gym, playground and school bus, peers who tease or taunt tend to take advantage of the lack of adult supervision. The assignment of a paraprofessional aide to accompany the student can be remarkably beneficial – particularly in situations where there is a history of teasing. Other useful strategies that teachers may consider include providing short breaks out of the classroom to let the tics out in private, allowing students with severe tics to take tests in private so that a child does not have the pressure to suppress tics during the test period, and being flexible with regard to scheduling so that the child is not expected to make an oral presentation at a point when the tics are severe (Bronheim, 1991). A compendium of educational accommodations is available at http://www.tourettesyndrome.net/.

Educated peers are equally important. Many clinicians actively encourage children, families and teachers to help educate peers and classmates about TS. It is remarkable what can be tolerated in the classroom and playground when teachers and peers simply know what the problem is and learn to disregard it.

Finally, it is important for clinicians to determine the family's awareness of and potential interest in advocacy organizations such as the Tourette Syndrome Association (www.tsa-usa.org/), Obsessive Compulsive Foundation (http://www.ocfoundation.org/) and the Children and Adults with Attention Deficit Disorder (http://www.chadd.org/). In the USA, these organizations have made a positive contribution to the lives of many patients and their families by providing support and information. They can also be a valuable outlet for families – to advance research and raise the general level of awareness among health care professionals, educators and the public at large.

Behavioral, Cognitive and Other Psychotherapeutic Treatments

The presence of premonitory urges and the characteristic suppressibility of tic symptoms may have broad implications for behavioral interventions and treatment. Prior to seeking professional consultation, many families will have experimented with a variety of *ad hoc* behavioral approaches on their own. It is useful to elicit information concerning these efforts and their sequelae.

A variety of cognitive and behavioral approaches have been used with TS (King, Scahill, Findley, & Cohen, 1998). Although success with various techniques such as assertiveness training, biofeedback, massed practice, time-out, hypnosis and differential reinforcement has been reported, most of these studies have involved small numbers of poorly characterized participants with no replication (Piacentini & Chang, 2006). To date, only *habit reversal training* has been shown to be efficacious in two randomized clinical trials with moderately to severely affected adults with TS (Deckersbach, Raunch, Buhlmann, & Wilhelm, 2005; Wilhelm, Deckersbach, Coffey *et al.*, 2003). This intervention includes a number of techniques: awareness training, self-monitoring, contingency management, inconvenience review, relaxation and competing responses. For example, awareness training includes:

1 Response description (i.e., the patient is trained to describe tic occurrences in detail and to re-enact tic movements while looking in a mirror);

2 Response detection, where the therapist helps the patient's ability to detect tics;

3 An early warning procedure, in which the patient is taught to become aware of the earliest signs of tic occurrence (such as the premonitory urge); and

4 Situation awareness training, in which situations that make tics more likely are identified.

When the patient is able to detect the tic and related urges, he or she is instructed to invoke a Competing Response at each occurrence of the tic or the urge and to hold it until the urge passes. Azrin and Nunn (1973) proposed that the Competing Response should be opposite to the tic movement, be able to be maintained for several minutes, produce heightened awareness of the tic movements by contraction of involved muscles, be socially inconspicuous and compatible with normal activities. Patients using habit reversal training are taught to design their own Competing Response to ensure that the responses are acceptable to them and to prepare them for potential changes in tic repertoire.

Although not indicated for the treatment of tics, individual and family counseling may alleviate secondary symptoms such as low self-esteem, defiant and disruptive behavior as well as family conflict. These interventions may also serve to reduce a significant source of psychological stress.

Pharmacological Treatments

The decision whether or not to use medication is based on the level of symptoms and the clinical presentation of the individual case. Given the waxing and waning of tic symptoms, it is best to withhold psychotropic medications until the tics, even at their best, are a significant source of impairment. Many cases of TS can be successfully managed without medication. When patients present with coexisting ADHD, OCD, depression or bipolar illness it is often better to treat these comorbid conditions first, as successful treatment of these disorders often will diminish tic severity.

Pharmacotherapy of Tics

A variety of therapeutic agents are now available to treat tics (Scahill, Erenberg, Berlin *et al.*, 2006). Each medication should be selected on the basis of expected efficacy and potential side effects. Clonidine and guanfacine are potent α_2-receptor agonists that are thought to reduce central noradrenergic activity. Initial randomized trials of clonidine had mixed results (Goetz, Tanner, Wilson *et al.*, 1987; Leckman, Hardin, Riddle *et al.*, 1991). However, a subsequent trial involving 136 subjects with chronic tics or TS confirmed the efficiacy of clonidine in the treatment of tics (Tourette's Syndrome Study Group, 2002). Clinical trials indicate that subjects can expect on average a 25–35% reduction in their symptoms over an 8–12-week period. Motor tics may show greater improvement than phonic symptoms. The usual starting dose is 0.05 mg on arising. Further 0.05-mg increments at 3–4-h intervals are added weekly until a dosage of 5 μg·kg^{-1} is reached or the total daily dose exceeds 0.25 mg. Although clonidine is clearly less effective than haloperidol and pimozide for immediate tic suppression, it is considerably safer. The principal side effect associated with its use is sedation, which occurs in 10–20% of subjects and usually abates with continued use. Other side effects include dry mouth, transient hypotension and rare episodes of worsening behavior. Clonidine should be tapered and not withdrawn abruptly, to reduce the likelihood of symptom or blood pressure rebound (Leckman, Ort, Caruso *et al.*, 1986). Guanfacine is another α_2-receptor agonist that has been demonstrated in double-blind studies to be effective in the treatment of TS and TS with comorbid ADHD (Scahill, Chappell, Kim *et al.*, 2001). Guanfacine is generally preferred to clonidine because it is less sedating and not associated with rebound hypertension following withdrawal. Guanfacine is generally started at a dose of 0.5 mg at night and then gradually increased by approximately 0.5 mg weekly to three times daily dosing with a maximum dose of 4 mg·day^{-1} (Scahill, Chappell, Kim *et al.*, 2001).

Dopamine D2 receptor antagonists remain the most predictably effective tic-suppressing agents in the short term. Documentation of the effectiveness of haloperidol in the early 1960s was a landmark in the history of TS as it called into question the prevailing view that tics were psychogenic in nature. The most widely used typical D2 receptor antagonists are haloperidol, pimozide, fluphenazine and tiapride (not currently available in the USA). Favorable data from double-blind clinical trials are available for haloperidol, pimozide and tiapride (Eggers, Rothenberger, & Berghaus, 1988; Sallee, Nesbitt, Jackson, Sine, & Sethuraman, 1997; Shapiro, Shapiro, Fulop *et al.*, 1989; Tourette's Syndrome Study Group, 1999). The US Food and Drug Administration has approved TS as an indication for haloperidol and pimozide use. Long-term experience has been less favorable, and the "reflexive" use of these agents should be avoided. Typically, treatment is initiated with a low dose (0.25 mg haloperidol or 1 mg pimozide) given before sleep. Further increments (0.5 mg haloperidol or 1 mg pimozide) may be added at 7–14-day intervals if the tic behaviors remain severe. In most instances, 0.5–6.0 mg·day^{-1} haloperidol or 1.0–10.0 mg·day^{-1} pimozide administered over a period of 4–8 weeks is sufficient to achieve adequate control of tic symptoms. Common potential side effects include tardive dyskinesia, acute dystonic reactions, sedation, depression, school and social phobias and/or weight gain. In many instances, by starting at low doses and adjusting the dosage upwards slowly, clinicians can avoid these side effects. The goal should be to use as little of these medications as possible to render the tics "tolerable." Efforts to stop the tics completely risk overmedication.

To avoid the extrapyramidal side effects associated with typical neuroleptics, atypical neuroleptics (e.g., risperidone, olanzapine and ziprasidone) have been used to treat tic symptoms. These agents have potent 5-HT2 blocking effects as well as more modest blocking effects on dopamine D2. Four randomized controlled trials have shown that risperidone was superior to placebo (Bruggeman, van der Linden, Buitelaar *et al.*, 2001; Dion, Annable, Sandor, & Choinard, 2002; Gaffney, Perry, Lund *et al.*, 2002; Scahill, Leckman, Schultz, Katsovich, & Peterson, 2003). Dosage in the range 1.5–3.5 mg·day^{-1} was effective and neurological side effects were rare. The most common adverse effects were weight gain, lipid metabolism abnormalities, sedation and sleep disturbance; social phobia and erectile dysfunction occurred in a few patients.

Pergolide is a mixed dopamine agonist used in Parkinson's disease which, in lower doses, is thought to have a greater effect on presynaptic autoreceptors, and lead to decreased dopamine release. Pergolide has been evaluated in two placebo-controlled trials (Gilbert, Sethuraman, Sine, Peters, & Sallee, 2000), which suggest that it has a positive, but moderate effect on tics. Adverse effects include nausea, syncope, sedation and dizziness. This agent may be especially useful if a child presents with comorbid restless legs syndrome.

Only small open-label pilot studies are available for medications such as tetrabenazine and benzodiazepines. Tetrabenazine is a non-antipsychotic dopamine antagonist, approved as an investigational drug; it may be useful but more study is needed (Scahill, Erenberg, Berlin *et al.*, 2006). The benzodiazepines (e.g., clonazepam) are used as anxiolytics and occasionally as an adjunctive treatment for tics, although it has not been well studied (Scahill, Erenberg, Berlin *et al.*, 2006). Common side effects with benzodiazepine use include sedation, ataxia, short-term memory problems, disinhibition, depression and addiction. Given these drawbacks, clonazepam is not used widely in TS.

The use of botulinum toxin injections to weaken temporarily muscles associated with severe motor or vocal tics also appears effective (Jankovic, 1994; Kwak, Hanna, & Jankovic, 2000), and also appears to significantly reduce the premonitory urges associated with both motor and vocal tics in the regions injected.

Pharmacotherapy of Coexisting ADHD

The stimulants methylphenidate, D-amphetamine, and mixtures of D- and L-amphetamine are first-line agents for the medical management of ADHD (Brown, Amler, Freeman *et al.*, 2005). However, the use of stimulants in ADHD associated with a tic disorder is controversial. While many patients with both ADHD and a pre-existing tic disorder will do well on stimulants, data from clinical case reports and controlled studies indicate that some children with ADHD will exhibit tics *de novo* when exposed to a stimulant. In other cases, tics may increase to a level that warrants discontinuation of the stimulant. To address this question, a multicenter randomized double-blind clinical trial was conducted with 136 children with ADHD and a chronic tic disorder (Tourette's Syndrome Study Group, 2002). Subjects were randomly administered clonidine alone, methylphenidate alone, or the combination in a 2×2 factorial design. Significant improvements in ADHD symptoms occurred for subjects assigned to clonidine alone and those assigned to methylphenidate alone. Compared with placebo, the greatest benefit occurred with combination regimens. Clonidine appeared to be most helpful for impulsivity and hyperactivity, while methylphenidate appeared to be most helpful for inattention. The proportion of individuals reporting a worsening of tics was no higher in those treated with methylphenidate (20%) than those being administered clonidine alone (26%) or placebo (22%). Sedation was common with clonidine treatment (28% reported moderate or severe sedation), but otherwise the drugs were tolerated well, with no evidence of cardiac toxicity. This trial did not support prior recommendations to avoid methylphenidate in these children because of concerns of worsening tics. Commonly used non-stimulants for the treatment of ADHD include the tricyclic antidepressants desipramine and nortriptyline, atypical antidepressants such as bupropion, and α_2-agonists clonidine and guanfacine (Brown, Amler, Freeman *et al.*, 2005). The latter has been demonstrated to be effective in subjects with both ADHD and coexisting tics (Scahill, Chappell, Kim *et al.*, 2001).

Pharmacotherapy of Coexisting OCD

Unfortunately, many patients with OCD and a coexisting tic disorder do not respond well to cognitive–behavioral therapies, which are the standard interventions for OCD (McDougle, Goodman, Leckman *et al.*, 1993). Controlled clinical trials have shown that addition of small doses of the neuroleptic haloperidol, or the atypical neuroleptic risperidone increases the response to serotonin reuptake inhibitors (Bloch, Peterson, Scahill *et al.*, 2006a; McDougle, Goodman, Leckman *et al.*, 1994).

Special Populations – PANDAS

Although initial results from immunomodulatory treatments, including plasma exchange, are promising, caution is warranted (Perlmutter, Leitman, Garvey *et al.*, 1999). It is also premature to recommend prophylactic antibiotic treatment (King, 2006).

Neurosurgical Interventions

Neurosurgical interventions for TS have been appropriately reserved for adults with intractable tics that severely affect social functioning. Many neurosurgical sites have been targeted for tics in previous lesioning studies: frontal cortex, limbic cortex, thalamus, infrathalamic area and cerebellum (Rauch, Baer, Cosgrove, & Jenike, 1995). Deep brain stimulation (DBS) is a relatively reversible, stereotactic technique, which has been looked to as the preferred method of neurosurgical treatment for medically intractable tics. The original electrode placement for DBS surgery was in the medial part of the thalamus, based on the results of previous lesioning studies (Hassler & Dieckmann, 1973). All four patients who received bilateral medial thalamic DBS surgery experienced a substantial improvement in tic severity (Ackermans, Temel, Cath *et al.*, 2006; Visser-Vandewalle, Temel, Boon *et al.*, 2003). Subsequent case reports demonstrated comparable efficacy in bilateral palladial stimulation compared with bilateral medial thalamic stimulation (Mink, Walkup, Frey *et al.*, 2006). However, currently in DBS for tics, the site of electrode placement and the electrode stimulation parameters have not been examined in carefully controlled clinical studies and differ markedly in the few sites willing to engage in this procedure. Therefore DBS is currently not advisable for all but the most severe and treatment-refractory adults with TS (Mink, Walkup, Frey *et al.*, 2006).

Future Directions

Along with a deepening appreciation of the clinical phenomenology of TS and related disorders, recent progress in genetics, neuroanatomy, systems neuroscience and functional *in vivo* neuroimaging has set the stage for a major advance in our understanding of TS and related disorders. Success in this area will lead to the targeting of specific brain circuits for more intensive study. Diagnostic and prognostic advances can also be anticipated (e.g., which circuits are involved and to what degree?). How does that degree of involvement affect the patient's symptomatic course and outcome?

Given this potential, TS can be considered a model disorder to study the dynamic interplay of neurobiological systems during development. It is likely that the research paradigms utilized in these studies and many of the empirical findings resulting from them will be relevant to other disorders of childhood onset and will enhance our understanding of normal development.

Acknowledgments

We are indebted to the Yale Tourette's Syndrome and Obsessive-Compulsive Disorder Research Group. Portions of the research described in this review were supported by grants from the National Institutes of Health: MH18268, MH49351, MH30929, HD03008, NS16648 and RR00125, as well as by the Tourette Syndrome Association.

References

Abelson, J. F., Kwan, K. Y., O'Roak, B. J., Baek, D. Y., Stillman, A. A., Morgan, T. M., *et al.* (2005). Sequence variants in SLITRK1 are associated with Tourette's syndrome. *Science*, *310*, 317–320.

Ackermans, L., Temel, Y., Cath, D. C., van der Linden, C., Bruggeman, R., Kleijer, M., *et al.* (2006). Deep brain stimulation in Tourette's syndrome: Two targets? *Movement Disorders*, *21*, 709–713.

Albin, R. L., Koeppe, R. A., Bohne, A., Nichols, T. E., Meyer, P., Wernette, K., *et al.* (2003). Increased ventral striatal monoaminergic innervation in Tourette syndrome. *Neurology*, *61*, 310–315.

Albin, R. L., & Mink, J. W. (2006). Recent advances in Tourette syndrome research. *Trends in Neurosciences*, *29*, 175–182.

American Psychiatric Association (APA). (2000). *Diagnostic and Statistical Manual of Mental Disorders* (4th edn.). Text Revision. Washington, DC: American Psychiatric Association.

Apter, A., Pauls, D. L., Bleich, A., Zohar, A. H., Kron, S., Ratzoni, G., *et al.* (1993). An epidemiologic study of Gilles de la Tourette's syndrome in Israel. *Archives of General Psychiatry*, *50*, 734–738.

Azrin, N. H., & Nunn, R. G. (1973). Habit-reversal: A method of eliminating nervous habits and tics. *Behavior Research and Therapy*, *11*, 619–628.

Baron-Cohen, S., Mortimore, C., Moriarty, J., Izaguirre, J., & Robertson, M. (1999). The prevalence of Gilles de la Tourette's syndrome in children and adolescents with autism. *Journal of Child Psychology and Psychiatry*, *40*, 213–218.

Bawden, H. N., Stokes, A., Camfield, C. S., Camfield, P. R., & Salisbury, S. (1998). Peer relationship problems in children with Tourette's disorder or diabetes mellitus. *Journal of Child Psychology and Psychiatry*, *39*, 663–668.

Bisno, A. L. (1991). Group A streptococcal infections and acute rheumatic fever. *New England Journal of Medicine*, *325*, 783–793.

Bloch, M. H., Landeros-Weisenberger, A., Kelmendi, B., Coric, V., Bracken, M. B., & Leckman, J. F. (2006b). A systematic review: antipsychotic augmentation with treatment refractory obsessive-compulsive disorder. *Molecular Psychiatry*, *11*, 622–632.

Bloch, M. H., Leckman, J. F., Zhu, H., & Peterson, B. S. (2005). Caudate volumes in childhood predict symptom severity in adults with Tourette syndrome. *Neurology*, *65*, 1253–1258.

Bloch, M. H., Peterson, B. S., Scahill, L., Otka, J., Katsovich, L., Zhang, H., *et al.* (2006a). Adulthood outcome of tic and obsessive-compulsive symptom severity in children with Tourette syndrome. *Archives of Pediatric and Adolescent Medicine*, *160*, 65–69.

Bloch, M. H., Sukhodolsky, D. G., Leckman, J. F., Schultz, R. T. (2006c). Fine-motor skill deficits in childhood predict adulthood tic severity and global psychosocial functioning in Tourette's syndrome. *Journal of Child Psychology and Psychiatry*, *47*, 551–559.

Bohlhalter, S., Goldfine, A., Matteson, S., Garraux, G., Hanakawa, T., Kansaku, K., *et al.* (2006). Neural correlates of tic generation in Tourette syndrome: An event-related functional MRI study. *Brain*, *129*, 2029–2037.

Boulant, J. A. (1981). Hypothalamic mechanisms in thermoregulation. *Federation Proceedings*, *40*, 2843–2850.

Braun, A. R., Randolph, C., Stoetter, B., Mohr, E., Cox, C., Vladar, K., *et al.* (1995). The functional neuroanatomy of Tourette's syndrome: An FDG-PET Study. II. Relationships between regional cerebral metabolism and associated behavioral and cognitive features of the illness. *Neuropsychopharmacology*, *13*, 151–168.

Bronheim, S. (1991). An educator's guide to Tourette syndrome. *Journal of Learning Disabilities*, *24*, 17–22.

Brown, R. T., Amler, R. W., Freeman, W. S., Perrin, J. M., Stein, M. T., Feldman, H. M., *et al.* (2005). Treatment of attention-deficit/hyperactivity disorder: Overview of the evidence. *Pediatrics*, *115*, e749–757.

Bruggeman, R., van der Linden, C., Buitelaar, J. K., Gericke, G. S., Hawkridge, S. M., & Temlett, J. A. (2001). Risperidone versus pimozide in Tourette's disorder: A comparative double-blind parallel-group study. *Journal of Clinical Psychiatry*, *62*, 50–56.

Burd, L., Kerbeshian, J., Wikenheiser, M., & Fisher, W. (1986a). Prevalence of Gilles de la Tourette's syndrome in North Dakota adults. *American Journal of Psychiatry*, *143*, 787–788.

Burd, L., Kerbeshian, J., Wikenheiser, M., & Fisher, W. (1986b). A prevalence study of Gilles de la Tourette syndrome in North Dakota school-age children. *Journal of the American Academy of Child Psychiatry*, *25*, 552–553.

Burd, L., Severud, R., Klug, M. G., & Kerbeshian, J. (1999). Prenatal and perinatal risk factors for Tourette disorder. *Journal of Perinatal Medicine*, *27*, 295–302.

Caine, E. D., McBride, M. C., Chiverton, P., Bamford, K. A., Rediess, S., & Shiao, J. (1988). Tourette's syndrome in Monroe County school children. *Neurology*, *38*, 472–475.

Cardona, F., & Orefici, G. (2001). Group A streptococcal infections and tic disorders in an Italian pediatric population. *Journal of Pediatrics*, *138*, 71–75.

Carter, A. S., O'Donnell, D. A., Schultz, R. T., Scahill, L., Leckman, J. F., & Pauls, D. L. (2000). Social and emotional adjustment in children affected with Gilles de la Tourette's syndrome: Associations with ADHD and family functioning. Attention Deficit Hyperactivity Disorder. *Journal of Child Psychology and Psychiatry*, *41*, 215–223.

Chappell, P., Leckman, J., Goodman, W., Bissette, G., Pauls, D., Anderson, G., *et al.* (1996). Elevated cerebrospinal fluid corticotropin-releasing factor in Tourette's syndrome: Comparison to obsessive compulsive disorder and normal controls. *Biological Psychiatry*, *39*, 776–783.

Chappell, P. B., Riddle, M., Anderson, G., Scahill, L., Hardin, M., Walker, D., *et al.* (1994). Enhanced stress responsivity of Tourette syndrome patients undergoing lumbar puncture. *Biological Psychiatry*, *36*, 35–43.

Cheon, K. A., Ryu, Y. H., Namkoong, K., Kim, C. H., Kim, J. J., & Lee, J. D. (2004). Dopamine transporter density of the basal ganglia assessed with [123I] IPT SPECT in drug-naive children with Tourette's disorder. *Psychiatry Reseach*, *130*, 85–95.

Church, A. J., Dale, R. C., Lees, A. J., Giovannoni, G., & Robertson, M. M. (2003). Tourette's syndrome: A cross sectional study to examine the PANDAS hypothesis. *Journal of Neurology, Neurosurgery and Psychiatry*, *74*, 602–607.

Cohen, D. J., Ort, S. I., Leckman, J. F., Riddle, M. A., & Hardin, M. T. (1988). Family functioning and Tourette's syndrome. In D. J. Cohen, R. D. Bruun, & J. F. Leckman (Eds.), *Tourette's syndrome and tic disorders* (p. 179). New York: John Wiley and Sons.

Comings, D. E. (1988). *Tourette syndrome and human behavior*. Daurte, CA: Hope Press.

Cuker, A., State, M. W., King, R. A., Davis, N., & Ward, D. C. (2004). Candidate locus for Gilles de la Tourette syndrome/obsessive compulsive disorder/chronic tic disorder at 18q22. *American Journal of Medical Genetics A*, *130*, 37–39.

Dale, R. C., Candler, P., Church, A. R., & Pocock, J. G. (2004). Glycolytic enzymes on neuronal membranes are candidate auto-antigens in post-streptococcal neuropsychiatric disorders. *Movement Disorders*, *9*, 19.

Deckersbach, T., Rauch, S., Buhlmann, U., & Wilhelm, S. (2005). Habit reversal versus supportive psychotherapy in Tourette's disorder: A randomized controlled trial and predictors of treatment response. *Behavior Research and Therapy*, *44*, 1079–1090.

Degnan, B. A., Kehoe, M. A., & Goodacre, J. A. (1997). Analysis of human T cell responses to group A streptococci using fractionated *Streptococcus pyogenes* proteins. *FEMS Immunology and Medical Microbiology*, *17*, 161–170.

Dewing, P., Chiang, C. W., Sinchak, K., Sim, H., Fernagut, P. O., Kelly, S., *et al.* (2006). Direct regulation of adult brain function by the male-specific factor SRY. *Current Biology*, *16*, 415–420.

Dion, Y., Annable, L., Sandor, P., & Chouinard, G. (2002). Risperidone in the treatment of Tourette syndrome: A double-blind, placebo-controlled trial. *Journal of Clinical Psychopharmacology*, *22*, 31–39.

Dykens, E., Leckman, J., Riddle, M., Hardin, M., Schwartz, S., & Cohen, D. (1990). Intellectual, academic, and adaptive functioning of Tourette syndrome children with and without attention deficit disorder. *Journal of Abnormal Child Psychology*, *18*, 607–615.

Eggers, C., Rothenberger, A., & Berghaus, U. (1988). Clinical and neurobiological findings in children suffering from tic disease following treatment with tiapride. *European Archives of Psychiatry and Neurological Sciences*, *237*, 223–229.

Findley, D. B., Leckman, J. F., Katsovich, L., Lin, H., Zhang, H., Grantz, H., *et al.* (2003). Development of the Yale Children's Global Stress Index (YCGSI) and its application in children and adolescents with Tourette's syndrome and obsessive-compulsive disorder. *Journal of the American Academy of Child and Adolescent Psychiatry*, *42*, 450–457.

Gaffney, G. R., Perry, P. J., Lund, B. C., Bever-Stille, K. A., Arndt, S., & Kuperman, S. (2002). Risperidone versus clonidine in the treatment of children and adolescents with Tourette's syndrome. *Journal of the American Academy of Child and Adolescent Psychiatry*, *41*, 330–336.

Gilbert, D. L., Sethuraman, G., Sine, L., Peters, S., & Sallee, F. R. (2000). Tourette's syndrome improvement with pergolide in a randomized, double-blind, crossover trial. *Neurology*, *54*, 1310–1315.

Gilles de la Tourette, G. (1885). Étude sur une affection nerveuse caractérisée par l'incoordination motrice, accompagnée d'écholalie et de coprolalie. *Archive Neurologie*, *9*, 19–42, 158–200.

Goetz, C. G., Pappert, E. J., Louis, E. D., Raman, R., & Leurgans, S. (1999). Advantages of a modified scoring method for the Rush Video-Based Tic Rating Scale. *Movement Disorders*, *14*, 502–506.

Goetz, C. G., Tanner, C. M., Wilson, R. S., Carroll, V. S., Como, P. G., & Shannon, K. M. (1987). Clonidine and Gilles de la Tourette's syndrome: Double-blind study using objective rating methods. *Annals of Neurology*, *21*, 307–310.

Graybiel, A. M., & Canales, J. J. (2001). The neurobiology of repetitive behaviors: Clues to the neurobiology of Tourette syndrome. *Advances in Neurology*, *85*, 123–131.

Grenhoff, J., & Svensson, T. H. (1989). Clonidine modulates dopamine cell firing in rat ventral tegmental area. *European Journal of Pharmacology*, *165*, 11–18.

Hassler, R., & Dieckmann, G. (1973). Relief of obsessive-compulsive disorders, phobias and tics by stereotactic coagulations of the rostral intralaminar and medial-thalamic nuclei. In L. Laitinen, & K. Livingston (Eds.), *Surgical approaches in psychiatry: Proceedings of the Third International Congress of Psychosurgery* (pp. 206–212). Cambridge: Garden City Press.

Hoekstra, P. J., Bijzet, J., Limburg, P. C., Steenhuis, M. P., Troost, P. W., Oosterhoff, M. D., *et al.* (2001). Elevated D8/17 expression on B lymphocytes, a marker of rheumatic fever, measured with flow cytometry in tic disorder patients. *American Journal of Psychiatry*, *158*, 605–610.

Hounie, A. G., do Rosario-Campos, M. C., Diniz, J. B., Shavitt, R. G., Ferrao, Y. A., Lopes, A. C., *et al.* (2006). Obsessive-compulsive disorder in Tourette syndrome. *Advances in Neurology*, *99*, 22–38.

Husby, G., van de Rijn, I., Zabriskie, J. B., Abdin, Z. H., & Williams, R. C. Jr. (1976). Antibodies reacting with cytoplasm of subthalamic and caudate nuclei neurons in chorea and acute rheumatic fever. *Journal of Experimental Medicine*, *144*, 1094–1110.

Hyde, T. M., Stacey, M. E., Coppola, R., Handel, S. F., Rickler, K. C., & Weinberger, D. R. (1995). Cerebral morphometric abnormalities in Tourette's syndrome: A quantitative MRI study of monozygotic twins. *Neurology*, *45*, 1176–1182.

Itard, J. M. G. (1825). Memoire sur quelques fonctions involontaries ses appareils de la locomotion de la prehension et de la voix. *Archives Générales de Médecine*, *8*, 385–407.

Jankovic, J. (1994). Botulinum toxin in the treatment of dystonic tics. *Movement Disorders*, *9*, 347–349.

Jankovic, J., & Mejia, N. I. (2006). Tics associated with other disorders. *Advances in Neurology*, *99*, 61–68.

Jeffries, K. J., Schooler, C., Schoenbach, C., Herscovitch, P., Chase, T. N., & Braun, A. R. (2002). The functional neuroanatomy of Tourette's syndrome: an FDG PET study. III. Functional coupling of regional cerebral metabolic rates. *Neuropsychopharmacology*, *27*, 92–104.

Kalanithi, P. S., Zheng, W., Kataoka, Y., DiFiglia, M., Grantz, H., Saper, C. B., *et al.* (2005). Altered parvalbumin-positive neuron distribution in basal ganglia of individuals with Tourette syndrome. *Proceedings of the National Academy of Sciences of the USA*, *102*, 13307–13312.

Kawikova, I., Leckman, J. F., Kronig, H., Katsovich, L., Bessen, D. E., Ghebremichael, M., *et al.* (2007). Decreased number of regulatory T cells suggests impaired immune tolerance in children with Tourette's syndrome. *Biological Psychiatry*, *61*, 273–278.

Kenney, C., & Jankovic, J. (2006). Tetrabenazine in the treatment of hyperkinetic movement disorders. *Expert Review of Neurotherapeutics*, *6*, 7–17.

Kéri, S., Szlobodnyik, C., Benedek, G., Janka, Z., & Gádoros, J. (2002). Probabilistic classification learning in Tourette syndrome. *Neuropsychologia*, *40*, 1356–1362.

Khalifa, N., & von Knorring, A. L. (2003). Prevalence of tic disorders and Tourette syndrome in a Swedish school population. *Developmental Medicine and Child Neurology*, *45*, 315–319.

Khalifa, N., & von Knorring, A. L. (2005). Tourette syndrome and other tic disorders in a total population of children: Clinical assessment and background. *Acta Paediatrica*, *94*, 1608–1614.

Khalifa, N., & von Knorring, A. L. (2006). Psychopathology in a Swedish population of school children with tic disorders. *Journal of the American Academy of Child and Adolescent Psychiatry*, *45*, 1346–1353.

King, R. A. (2006). PANDAS: to treat or not to treat? *Advances in Neurology*, *99*, 179–183.

King, R. A., Scahill, L., Findley, D., & Cohen, D. J. (1998). Psychosocial and behavioral treatments. In J. F. Leckman, & D. J. Cohen (Eds.), *Tourette's syndrome tics, obsessions, compulsions: Developmental psychopathology and clinical care* (pp. 338–359). New York: John Wiley and Sons.

Kirvan, C. A., Swedo, S. E., Heuser, J. S., & Cunningham, M. W. (2003). Mimicry and autoantibody-mediated neuronal cell signaling in Sydenham chorea. *Nature Medicine*, *9*, 914–920.

Kirvan, C. A., Swedo, S. E., Kurahara, D., & Cunningham, M. W. (2006). Streptococcal mimicry and antibody-mediated cell signaling in the pathogenesis of Sydenham's chorea. *Autoimmunity*, *39*, 21–29.

Kurlan, R., Whitmore, D., Irvine, C., McDermott, M. P., & Como, P. G. (1994). Tourette's syndrome in a special education population: A pilot study involving a single school district. *Neurology*, *44*, 699–702.

Kushner, H. I. (1999). *A cursing brain? The histories of Tourette syndrome.* Cambridge, MA: Harvard University Press.

Kwak, C. H., Hanna, P. A., & Jankovic, J. (2000). Botulinum toxin in the treatment of tics. *Archives of Neurology*, *57*, 1190–1193.

Leckman, J. F., & Cohen, D. J. (1998). *Tourette's syndrome tics, obsessions, compulsions: Developmental psychopathology and clinical care.* New York, NY: John Wiley and Sons.

Leckman, J. F., Cohen, D. J., Price, R. A., Minderaa, R. B., Anderson, G. M., & Pauls, D. L. (1984). The pathogenesis of Gilles de la Tourette's syndrome: A review of data and hypothesis. In A. B. Shah, N. S. Shah, & A. G. Donald (Eds.), *Movement disorders.* New York: Plenum.

Leckman, J. F., Dolnansky, E. S., Hardin, M. T., Clubb, M., Walkup, J. T., Stevenson, J., *et al.* (1990). Perinatal factors in the expression of Tourette's syndrome: An exploratory study. *Journal of the American Academy of Child and Adolescent Psychiatry*, *29*, 220–226.

Leckman, J. F., Goodman, W. K., Anderson, G. M., Riddle, M. A., Chappell, P. B., McSwiggan-Hardin, M. T., *et al.* (1995). Cerebrospinal fluid biogenic amines in obsessive compulsive disorder, Tourette's syndrome, and healthy controls. *Neuropsychopharmacology*, *12*, 73–86.

Leckman, J. F., Grice, D. E., Boardman, J., Zhang, H., Vitale, A., Bondi, C., *et al.* (1997). Symptoms of obsessive-compulsive disorder. *American Journal of Psychiatry*, *154*, 911–917.

Leckman, J. F., Hardin, M. T., Riddle, M. A., Stevenson, J. Ort, S. I., Cohen, D. J. (1991). Clonidine treatment of Gilles de la Tourette's syndrome. *Archives of General Psychiatry*, *48*, 324–328.

Leckman, J. F., Katsovich, L., Kawikova, I., Lin, H., Zhang, H., Kronig, H., *et al.* (2005). Increased serum levels of interleukin-12 and tumor necrosis factor-alpha in Tourette's syndrome. *Biological Psychiatry*, *57*, 667–673.

Leckman, J. F., King, R. A., Scahill, L., Findley, D., Ort, S., & Cohen, D. J. (1998a). Yale approach to assessment and treatment. In J. F. Leckman, & D. J. Cohen (Eds.), *Tourette's syndrome tics, obsessions, compulsions: Developmental psychopathology and clinical care* (pp. 285–309). New York: John Wiley and Sons.

Leckman, J. F., Ort, S., Caruso, K. A., Anderson, G. M., Riddle, M. A., Cohen, D. J. (1986). Rebound phenomena in Tourette's syndrome after abrupt withdrawal of clonidine. Behavioral, cardiovascular, and neurochemical effects. *Archives of General Psychiatry*, *43*, 1168–1176.

Leckman, J. F., Price, R. A., Walkup, J. T., Ort, S., Pauls, D. L., & Cohen, D. J. (1987). Nongenetic factors in Gilles de la Tourette's syndrome. *Archives of General Psychiatry*, *44*, 100.

Leckman, J. F., Riddle, M. A., Hardin, M. T., Ort, S. I., Swartz, K. L., Stevenson, J., *et al.* (1989). The Yale Global Tic Severity Scale: Initial testing of a clinician-rated scale of tic severity. *Journal of the American Academy of Child and Adolescent Psychiatry*, *28*, 566–573.

Leckman, J. F., & Scahill, L. (1990). Possible exacerbation of tics by androgenic steroids. *New England Journal of Medicine*, *322*, 1674.

Leckman, J. F., Vaccarino, F. M., Kalanithi, P. S., & Rothenberger, A. (2006). Tourette syndrome: A relentless drumbeat. *Journal of Child Psychology and Psychiatry*, *47*, 537–550.

Leckman, J. F., Walker, D. E., & Cohen, D. J. (1993). Premonitory urges in Tourette's syndrome. *American Journal of Psychiatry*, *150*, 98–102.

Leckman, J. F., Walker, D. E., Goodman, W. K., Pauls, D. L., & Cohen, D. J. (1994). "Just right" perceptions associated with compulsive behavior in Tourette's syndrome. *American Journal of Psychiatry*, *151*, 675–680.

Leckman, J. F., Zhang, H., Vitale, A., Lahnin, F., Lynch, K., Bondi, C., *et al.* (1998b). Course of tic severity in Tourette syndrome: The first two decades. *Pediatrics*, *102*, 14–19.

Lee, J. S., Yoo, S. S., Cho, S. Y., Ock, S. M., Lim, M. K., & Panych, L. P. (2006). Abnormal thalamic volume in treatment-naive boys with Tourette syndrome. *Acta Psychiatrica Scandinavica*, *113*, 64–67.

Lin, H., Katsovich, L., Ghebremichael, M., Findley, D., Grantz, H., Lombroso, P. J., *et al.* (2007). Psychosocial stress predicts future symptom severities in children and adolescents with Tourette syndrome and/or obsessive-compulsive disorder. *Journal of Child Psychology and Psychiatry*, *48*, 157–166.

Llinas, R., Urbano, F. J., Leznik, E., Ramirez, R. R., & van Marle, H. J. (2005). Rhythmic and dysrhythmic thalamocortical dynamics: GABA systems and the edge effect. *Trends in Neurosciences*, *28*, 325–333.

Lombroso, P. J., Mack, G., Scahill, L., King, R. A., & Leckman, J. F. (1991). Exacerbation of Gilles de la Tourette's syndrome associated with thermal stress: A family study. *Neurology*, *41*, 1984–1987.

Luo, F., Leckman, J. F., Katsovich, L., Findley, D., Grantz, H., Tucker, D. M., *et al.* (2004). Prospective longitudinal study of children with tic disorders and/or obsessive-compulsive disorder: Relationship of symptom exacerbations to newly acquired streptococcal infections. *Pediatrics*, *113*, e578–585.

Malison, R. T., McDougle, C. J., van Dyck, C. H., Scahill, L., Baldwin, R. M., Seibyl, J. P., *et al.* (1995). [123I] β-CIT SPECT imaging of striatal dopamine transporter binding in Tourette's disorder. *American Journal of Psychiatry*, *152*, 1359–1361.

Marsh, R., Alexander, G. M., Packard, M. G., Zhu, H., & Peterson, B. S. (2005). Perceptual-motor skill learning in Gilles de la Tourette syndrome: Evidence for multiple procedural learning and memory systems. *Neuropsychologia*, *43*, 1456–1465.

Marsh, R., Alexander, G. M., Packard, M. G., Zhu, H., Wingard, J. C., Quackenbush, G., *et al.* (2004). Habit learning in Tourette syndrome: A translational neuroscience approach to a developmental psychopathology. *Archives of General Psychiatry*, *61*, 1259–1268.

Mason, A., Banerjee, S., Eapen, V., Zeitlin, H., & Robertson, M. M. (1998). The prevalence of Tourette syndrome in a mainstream school population. *Developmental Medicine and Child Neurology*, *40*, 292–296.

Mathews, C. A., Bimson, B., Lowe, T. L., Herrera, L. D., Budman, C. L., Erenberg, G., *et al.* (2006). Association between maternal smoking and increased symptom severity in Tourette's syndrome. *American Journal of Psychiatry*, *163*, 1066–1073.

McDougle, C. J., Goodman, W. K., Leckman, J. F., Barr, L. C., Heninger, G. R., & Price, L. H. (1993). The efficacy of fluvoxamine in obsessive-compulsive disorder: Effects of comorbid chronic tic disorder. *Journal of Clinical Psychopharmacology*, *13*, 354–358.

McDougle, C. J., Goodman, W. K., Leckman, J. F., Lee, N. C., Heninger, G. R., & Price, L. H. (1994). Haloperidol addition in fluvoxamine-refractory obsessive-compulsive disorder: A double-blind, placebo-controlled study in patients with and without tics. *Archives of General Psychiatry*, *51*, 302–308.

Mell, L. K., Davis, R. L., & Owens, D. (2005). Association between streptococcal infection and obsessive-compulsive disorder, Tourette's syndrome, and tic disorder. *Pediatrics*, *116*, 56–60.

Middleton, F. A., & Strick, P. L. (2000). Basal ganglia and cerebellar loops: Motor and cognitive circuits. *Brain Research. Brain Research Reviews*, *31*, 236–250.

Mink, J. W., Walkup, J., Frey, K. A., Como, P., Cath, D., Delong, M. R., Erenberg, G., Jankovic, J., Juncos, J., Leckman, J. F., Swerdlow, N., Visser-Vandewalle, V., Vitek, J. L; Tourette Syndrome Association, Inc. (2006). Patient selection and assessment recommendations for deep brain stimulation in Tourette syndrome. *Movement Disorders*, *21*, 1831–1838.

Moll, G. H., Wischer, S., Heinrich, H., Tergau, F., Paulus, W., & Rothenberger, A. (1999). Deficient motor control in children with tic disorder: Evidence from transcranial magnetic stimulation. *Neuroscience Letters*, *272*, 37–40.

Morshed, S. A., Parveen, S., Leckman, J. F., Mercadante, M. T., Bittencourt Kiss, M. H., Miguel, E. C., *et al.* (2001). Antibodies against neural, nuclear, cytoskeletal, and streptococcal epitopes in children and adults with Tourette's syndrome, Sydenham's chorea, and autoimmune disorders. *Biological Psychiatry*, *50*, 566–577.

Pasamanick, B., & Kawi, A. (1956). A study of the association of prenatal and paranatal factors with the development of tics in children: A preliminary investigation. *Journal of Pediatrics*, *48*, 596–601.

Pauls, D. L., & Leckman, J. F. (1986). The inheritance of Gilles de la Tourette's syndrome and associated behaviors: Evidence for autosomal dominant transmission. *New England Journal of Medicine*, *315*, 993–997.

Pauls, D. L., Raymond, C. L., Stevenson, J. M., & Leckman, J. F. (1991). A family study of Gilles de la Tourette syndrome. *American Journal of Human Genetics*, *48*, 154–163.

Perlmutter, S. J., Leitman, S. F., Garvey, M. A., Hamburger, S., Feldman, E., Leonard, H. L., *et al.* (1999). Therapeutic plasma exchange and intravenous immunoglobulin for obsessive-compulsive disorder and tic disorders in childhood. *Lancet*, *354*, 1153–1158.

Perrin, E. M., Murphy, M. L., Casey, J. R., Pichichero, M. E., Runyan, D. K., Miller, W. C., *et al.* (2004). Does group A beta-hemolytic streptococcal infection increase risk for behavioral and neuropsychiatric symptoms in children? *Archives of Pediatric and Adolescent Medicine*, *158*, 848–856.

Peterson, B. S., & Leckman, J. F. (1998). The temporal dynamics of tics in Gilles de la Tourette syndrome. *Biological Psychiatry*, *44*, 1337–1348.

Peterson, B. S., Leckman, J. F., Scahill, L., Naftolin, F., Keefe, D., Charest, N. J., *et al.* (1992). Steroid hormones and CNS sexual dimorphisms modulate symptom expression in Tourette's syndrome. *Psychoneuroendocrinology*, *17*, 553–563.

Peterson, B. S., Pine, D. S., Cohen, P., & Brook, J. S. (2001a). Prospective, longitudinal study of tic, obsessive-compulsive, and attention-deficit/hyperactivity disorders in an epidemiological sample. *Journal of the American Academy of Child and Adolescent Psychiatry*, *40*, 685–695.

Peterson, B. S., Skudlarski, P., Anderson, A. W., Zhang, H., Gatenby, J. C., Lacadie, C. M., *et al.* (1998a). A functional magnetic resonance imaging study of tic suppression in Tourette syndrome. *Archives of General Psychiatry*, *55*, 326–333.

Peterson, B. S., Staib, L., Scahill, L., Zhang, H., Anderson, C., Leckman, J. F., *et al.* (2001b). Regional brain and ventricular volumes in Tourette syndrome. *Archives of General Psychiatry*, *58*, 427–440.

Peterson, B. S., Thomas, P., Kane, M. J., Scahill, L., Zhang, H., Bronen, R., *et al.* (2003). Basal ganglia volumes in patients with Gilles de la Tourette syndrome. *Archives of General Psychiatry*, *60*, 415–424.

Peterson, B. S., Zhang, H., Anderson, G. M., & Leckman, J. F. (1998b). A double-blind, placebo-controlled, crossover trial of an antiandrogen in the treatment of Tourette's syndrome. *Journal of Clinical Psychopharmacology*, *18*, 324–331.

Piacentini, J. C., & Chang, S. W. (2006). Behavioral treatments for tic suppression: Habit reversal training. *Advances in Neurology*, *99*, 227–233.

Price, R. A., Kidd, K. K., Cohen, D. J., Pauls, D. L., & Leckman, J. F. (1985). A twin study of Tourette syndrome. *Archives of General Psychiatry*, *42*, 815–820.

Rauch, S. L., Baer, L., Cosgrove, G. R., & Jenike, M. A. (1995). Neurosurgical treatment of Tourette's syndrome: A critical review. *Comprehensive Psychiatry*, *36*, 141–156.

Robertson, M. M., Banerjee, S., Kurlan, R., Cohen, D. J., Leckman, J. F., McMahon, W., *et al.* (1999). The Tourette syndrome diagnostic confidence index: Development and clinical associations. *Neurology*, *53*, 2108–2112.

Robertson, M. M., & Orth, M. (2006). Behavioral and affective disorders in Tourette syndrome. *Advances in Neurology*, *99*, 39–60.

Robertson, M. M., Williamson, F., & Eapen, V. (2006). Depressive symptomatology in young people with Gilles de la Tourette Syndrome: A comparison of self-report scales. *Journal of Affective Disorders*, *91*, 265–268.

Rutter, M., Tizard, J., & Whitmore, K. (1970). *Education, health, and behaviour*. Longman, London.

Sallee, F. R., Nesbitt, L., Jackson, C., Sine, L., & Sethuraman, G. (1997). Relative efficacy of haloperidol and pimozide in children and adolescents with Tourette's disorder. *American Journal of Psychiatry*, *154*, 1057–1062.

Sanberg, P. R., Silver, A. A., Shytle, R. D., Philipp, M. K., Cahill, D. W., Fogelson, H. M., *et al.* (1997). Nicotine for the treatment of Tourette's syndrome. *Pharmacology and Therapeutics*, *74*, 21–25.

Santangelo, S. L., Pauls, D. L., Goldstein, J. M., Faraone, S. V., Tsuang, M. T., & Leckman, J. F. (1994). Tourette's syndrome: What are the influences of gender and comorbid obsessive-compulsive disorder? *Journal of the American Academy of Child and Adolescent Psychiatry*, *33*, 795–804.

Scahill, L., Chappell, P. B., Kim, Y. S., Schultz, R. T., Katsovich, L., Shepherd, E., *et al.* (2001). A placebo-controlled study of guanfacine in the treatment of children with tic disorders and attention deficit hyperactivity disorder. *American Journal of Psychiatry*, *158*, 1067–1074.

Scahill, L., Erenberg, G., Berlin, C. M. Jr., Budman, C., Coffey, B. J., Jankovic, J., *et al.* (2006). Contemporary assessment and pharmacotherapy of Tourette syndrome. *NeuroRx*, *3*, 192–206.

Scahill, L., Leckman, J. F., Schultz, R. T., Katsovich, L., & Peterson, B. S. (2003). A placebo-controlled trial of risperidone in Tourette syndrome. *Neurology*, *60*, 1130–1135.

Schultz, R. T., Carter, A. S., Gladstone, M., Scahill, L., Leckman, J. F., Peterson, B. S., *et al.* (1998). Visual-motor integration functioning in children with Tourette syndrome. *Neuropsychology*, *12*, 134–145.

Serrien, D. J., Orth, M., Evans, A. H., Lees, A. J., & Brown, P. (2005). Motor inhibition in patients with Gilles de la Tourette syndrome: Functional activation patterns as revealed by EEG coherence. *Brain*, *128*, 116–125.

Shapiro, A. K., Shapiro, E. S., Young, J. G., & Freinberg, T. E. (1988). *Gilles de la Tourette syndrome* (2nd edn.). New York: Raven Press.

Shapiro, E., Shapiro, A. K., Fulop, G., Hubbard, M., Mandeli, J., Nordlie, J., *et al.* (1989). Controlled study of haloperidol, pimozide and placebo for the treatment of Gilles de la Tourette's syndrome. *Archives of General Psychiatry*, *46*, 722–730.

Sikich, L., & Todd, R. D. (1988). Are the neurodevelopmental effects of gonadal hormones related to sex differences in psychiatric illnesses? *Psychiatric Developments*, *6*, 277–309.

Singer, H. S., Giuliano, J. D., Hansen, B. H., Hallett, J. J., Laurino, J. P., Benson, M., *et al.* (1998). Antibodies against human putamen in children with Tourette syndrome. *Neurology*, *50*, 1618–1624.

Singer, H. S., Hahn, I. H., & Moran, T. H. (1991). Abnormal dopamine uptake sites in postmortem striatum from patients with Tourette's syndrome. *Annals of Neurology*, *30*, 558–562.

Singer, H. S., Hong, J. J., Yoon, D. Y., & Williams, P. N. (2005a). Serum autoantibodies do not differentiate PANDAS and Tourette syndrome from controls. *Neurology*, *65*, 1701–1707.

Singer, H. S., Mink, J. W., Loiselle, C. R., Burke, K. A., Ruchkina, I., Morshed, S., *et al.* (2005b). Microinfusion of antineuronal antibodies into rodent striatum: Failure to differentiate between elevated and low titers. *Journal of Neuroimmunology*, *163*, 8–14.

Singer, H. S., Szymanski, S., Giuliano, J., Yokoi, F., Dogan, A. S., Brasic, J. R., *et al.* (2002). Elevated intrasynaptic dopamine release in Tourette's syndrome measured by PET. *American Journal of Psychiatry*, *159*, 1329–1336.

State, M. W., Greally, J. M., Cuker, A., Bowers, P. N., Henegariu, O., Morgan, T. M., *et al.* (2003). Epigenetic abnormalities associated with a chromosome 18(q21–q22) inversion and a Gilles de la Tourette syndrome phenotype. *Proceedings of the National Academy of Sciences of the USA*, *100*, 4684–4689.

Stern, E., Silbersweig, D. A., Chee, K. Y., Holmes, A., Robertson, M. M., Trimble, M., *et al.* (2000). A functional neuroanatomy of tics in Tourette syndrome. *Archives of General Psychiatry*, *57*, 741–748.

Stokes, A., Bawden, H. N., Camfield, P. R., Backman, J. E., & Dooley, J. M. (1991). Peer problems in Tourette's disorder. *Pediatrics*, *87*, 936–942.

Sukhodolsky, D. G., do Rosario-Campos, M. C., Scahill, L., Katsovich, L., Pauls, D. L., Peterson, B. S., *et al.* (2005). Adaptive, emotional, and family functioning of children with obsessive-compulsive disorder and comorbid attention deficit hyperactivity disorder. *American Journal of Psychiatry*, *162*, 1125–1132.

Sukhodolsky, D. G., Scahill, L., Zhang, H., Peterson, B. S., King, R. A., Lombroso, P. J., *et al.* (2003). Disruptive behavior in children with Tourette's syndrome: Association with ADHD comorbidity, tic severity, and functional impairment. *Journal of the American Academy of Child and Adolescent Psychiatry*, *42*, 98–105.

Swedo, S. E., Leonard, H. L., Garvey, M., Mittleman, B., Allen, A. J., Perlmutter, S., *et al.* (1998). Pediatric autoimmune neuropsychiatric disorders associated with streptococcal infections: Clinical description of the first 50 cases. *American Journal of Psychiatry*, *155*, 264–271.

Swedo, S. E., Leonard, H. L., Mittleman, B. B., Allen, A. J., Rapoport, J. L., Dow, S. P., *et al.* (1997). Identification of children with pediatric autoimmune neuropsychiatric disorders associated with streptococcal infections by a marker associated with rheumatic fever. *American Journal of Psychiatry*, *154*, 110–112.

Swedo, S. E., Rapoport, J. L., Cheslow, D. L., Leonard, H. L., Ayoub, E. M., Hosier, D. M., *et al.* (1989). High prevalence of obsessive-compulsive symptoms in patients with Sydenham's chorea. *American Journal of Psychiatry*, *146*, 246–249.

Swerdlow, N. R., Karban, B., Ploum, Y., Sharp, R., Geyer, M. A., & Eastvold, A. (2001). Tactile prepuff inhibition of startle in children with Tourette's syndrome: In search of an "fMRI-friendly" startle paradigm. *Biological Psychiatry*, *50*, 578–585.

Swerdlow, N. R., & Sutherland, A. N. (2006). Preclinical models relevant to Tourette syndrome. *Advances in Neurology*, 99, 69–88.

Tourette Syndrome Association International Consortium for Genetics, Centre National de Génotypage. (2007). Genome scan for Tourette's disorder in affected sib-pair and multigenerational families. *American Journal of Human Genetics*, *80*, 265–272.

Tourette Syndrome Association International Consortium for Genetics. (1999). A complete genome screen in sib pairs affected by Gilles de la Tourette syndrome. The Tourette Syndrome Association International Consortium for Genetics. *American Journal of Human Genetics*, *65*, 1428–1436.

Tourette's Syndrome Study Group. (1999). Short-term versus longer-term pimozide therapy in Tourette's syndrome: A preliminary study. *Neurology*, *52*, 874–877.

Tourette's Syndrome Study Group. (2002). Treatment of ADHD in children with tics: A randomized controlled trial. *Neurology*, *58*, 527–536.

Vandewalle, V., Van der Linden, C., Groenewegen, H. J., & Caemaert, J. (1999). Stereotactic treatment of Gilles de la Tourette syndrome by high frequency stimulation of thalamus. *Lancet*, 353, 724.

Verkerk, A. J., Mathews, C. A., Joosse, M., Eussen, B. H., Heutink, P., & Oostra, B. A. (2003). CNTNAP2 is disrupted in a family with Gilles de la Tourette syndrome and obsessive compulsive disorder. *Genomics*, *82*, 1–9.

Visser-Vandewalle, V., Temel, Y., Boon, P., Vreeling, F., Colle, H., Hoogland, G., *et al.* (2003). Chronic bilateral thalamic stimulation: A new therapeutic approach in intractable Tourette syndrome. Report of three cases. *Journal of Neurosurgery*, *99*, 1094–1100.

Walkup, J. T., Rosenberg, L. A., Brown, J., & Singer, H. S. (1992). The validity of instruments measuring tic severity in Tourette's syndrome. *Journal of the American Academy of Child and Adolescent Psychiatry*, *31*, 472–477.

Wilhelm, S., Deckersbach, T., Coffey, B. J., Bohne, A., Peterson, A. L., & Baer, L. (2003). Habit reversal versus supportive psychotherapy for Tourette's disorder: A randomized controlled trial. *American Journal of Psychiatry*, *160*, 1175–1177.

Wolf, S. S., Jones, D. W., Knable, M. B., Gorey, J. G., Lee, K. S., Hyde, T. M., *et al.* (1996). Tourette syndrome: Prediction of phenotypic variation in monozygotic twins by caudate nucleus D2 receptor binding. *Science*, *273*, 1225–1227.

World Health Organization (WHO). (1996). *Multiaxial classification of child and adolescent disorders: The ICD-10 classification of mental and behavioural disorders in children and adolescents* (pp. 43–45). Cambridge: World Health Organization, Cambridge University Press.

Ziemann, U., Paulus, W., & Rothenberger, A. (1997). Decreased motor inhibition in Tourette's disorder: Evidence from transcranial magnetic stimulation. *American Journal of Psychiatry*, *154*, 1277–1284.

45 Schizophrenia and Allied Disorders

Chris Hollis

Schizophrenia is one of the most devastating psychiatric disorders to affect children and adolescents. Although extremely rare before the age of 10, the incidence of schizophrenia rises steadily though adolescence to reach its peak in early adult life. The clinical severity, impact on development and poor prognosis of child- and adolescent-onset schizophrenia reinforce the need for early detection, prompt diagnosis and effective treatment.

The current concept of schizophrenia in children and adolescents evolved from a different perspective held during much of the 20th century. Until the early 1970s, the term childhood schizophrenia was applied to children who would now be diagnosed with autism. Until the 1990s, there was doubt about the validity of diagnosing schizophrenia in children and younger adolescents. However, in DSM-III and ICD-9 the separate category of childhood schizophrenia was removed, and the same diagnostic criteria for schizophrenia were applied across the age range. Good evidence for the validity of the diagnosis of schizophrenia in childhood and adolescence comes from the Maudsley Child and Adolescent Psychosis Follow-up Study (Hollis, 2000). First, a DSM-III-R diagnosis of schizophrenia in childhood and adolescence predicted a significantly poorer adult outcome compared to other non-schizophrenic psychosis. Second, the diagnosis of schizophrenia showed a high level of stability, with 80% having the same diagnosis recorded at adult follow-up (Jarbin, Ott, & Van Knorring, 2003).

Clinical Features

Schizophrenia is characterized by psychotic symptoms as follows.

1 *Hallucinations* These are sensory perceptions in the absence of external stimuli. Auditory hallucinations (hearing voices) are by far the most common type of hallucination in schizophrenia. Typically, their content is threatening, derogatory or commanding. Auditory hallucinations are classified according to their form: voices addressing the patient directly (second person); voices discussing or commenting on the patient's actions in the third person (third person or running commentary); and voices speaking the patient's thoughts aloud (thought echo).

2 *Delusions* These are false beliefs, incompatible with the patient's social, religious and educational background, arising from an incorrect inference about external reality and not amenable to reason. Paranoid delusions (belief that one is persecuted), delusions of reference (belief that events or people's behavior refer to oneself) or delusions of control (belief that one's own thoughts, emotions or movements are controlled by external forces) are particularly common in schizophrenia.

3 *Passivity phenomena* These include the experience of one's own thoughts becoming automatically available to others (thought broadcast); alien thoughts being inserted into one's mind (thought insertion); and the experience of one's thoughts being removed from one's mind (thought withdrawal).

4 *Disordered thought and speech* This may present as incoherent speech (loosening of associations), neologisms or a paucity of content and ideas (poverty of speech).

5 *Reduced or inappropriate emotional reactivity and lack of volition* People with schizophrenia may demonstrate reduced emotional expression (flattened affect) or incongruous emotional reactions, lack of drive and initiative, and social withdrawal.

6 *Motor abnormalities* These phenomena may include posturing, mannerisms, stereotopies and catatonic immobility or excitement.

Symptoms in schizophrenia can be seen as representing either an excess or distortion of normal function (positive symptoms) or a reduction or loss of normal function (negative symptoms). Positive symptoms include hallucinations, delusions, passivity phenomena, thought disorder, disorganized behavior and inappropriate affect. Negative symptoms include poverty of thought and speech, blunted affect, impaired volition and social withdrawal. Liddle (1987) showed that symptoms in chronic schizophrenia cluster into three syndromes: psychomotor poverty (negative symptoms); reality distortion (hallucinations and delusions); and disorganization (bizarre behavior, inappropriate affect and disorganized thought). The relationship between these different groups of symptoms and underlying brain function in schizophrenia is considered in more detail below.

A wide variety of anomalous perceptual experiences may occur at the onset of an episode of schizophrenia, leading to a sense of fear or puzzlement which may constitute a delusional mood and herald a full psychotic episode. These anomalous experiences may include the sense that familiar places and

Rutter's Child and Adolescent Psychiatry, 5th edition. Edited by M. Rutter, D. Bishop, D. Pine, S. Scott, J. Stevenson, E. Taylor and A. Thapar. © 2008 Blackwell Publishing, ISBN: 978-1-4051-4549-7.

people and their reactions have changed in some subtle way. These experiences can result from a breakdown between perception and memory (for familiar places and people) and associated affective responses (salience given to these perceptions). For example, a young person at the onset of illness may study their reflection in the mirror for hours because it looks strangely unfamiliar, misattribute threatening intent to an innocuous comment or experience family members or friends as being unfamiliar, leading to a secondary delusional belief that they have been replaced by doubles or aliens. In summary, some clinical phenomena in schizophrenia can be understood in terms of a loss of normal contextualization and co-ordination of cognitive and emotional processing.

Clinical Phases of Schizophrenia

Premorbid Social and Developmental Impairments

Child- and adolescent-onset schizophrenia is associated with poor premorbid functioning and early developmental delays (Alaghband-Rad, McKenna, Gordon *et al.*, 1995; Hollis, 1995, 2003). Similar developmental and social impairments in childhood have been reported in adult-onset schizophrenia, but premorbid impairments appear to be more common and severe in the child- and adolescent-onset forms of the disorder. In the Maudsley study (Hollis, 2003), significant early delays were particularly common in the areas of language (20%), reading (30%) and bladder control (36%). Just over 20% of cases of adolescent schizophrenia had significant early delays in either language or motor development. In contrast, language and motor developmental delays have been reported in only about 10% of individuals who develop schizophrenia in adult life (Jones, Rogers, Murray, & Marmot, 1994). A consistent characteristic in the premorbid phenotype is impaired sociability. For example, in the Maudsley study of child- and adolescent-onset psychoses (Hollis, 2003), about one-third of cases with schizophrenia had significant difficulties in social development affecting the ability to make and keep friends.

Premorbid IQ in child- and adolescent-onset schizophrenia is in the mid to low 80s, some 10–15 points lower than in the adult form of the disorder (Alaghband-Rad, McKenna, Gordon *et al.*, 1995; Asarnow, Thompson, Hamilton, Goldstein, & Guthrie, 1994; Hollis, 2000). In the Maudsley study (Hollis, 2000), one-third of child- and adolescent-onset cases had an IQ below 70, with the whole distribution of IQ shifted down compared to both adolescent affective psychoses and adult schizophrenia.

Cannon, Caspi, Moffitt *et al.* (2002) reported a specific association between adult schizophreniform disorder and an antecedent pattern of childhood pan-developmental impairments involving motor development, receptive language and IQ. These findings are consistent with the view that premorbid impairments are manifestations of a genetic and/or developmental liability to schizophrenia. It seems clear that the premorbid phenotype does not just represent non-specific psychiatric disturbance. Looking backward from schizophrenia to early impairment, subtle problems of language, attention and social relationships are typical, whereas, in contrast, conduct problems are rare. However, looking forward from childhood impairments to later schizophrenia, prediction is much weaker. In addition, premorbid social and behavioral difficulties are not unique to schizophrenia and occur in other psychoses.

Are Premorbid Impairments a Risk or Precursor of Psychosis?

Premorbid impairments could lie on a causal pathway for psychosis or, alternatively, they could be markers of an underlying neuropathological process, such as aberrant neural connectivity, which may be the cause of both premorbid social impairment and psychosis. Frith (1994) has speculated on the possible cognitive mechanisms that might link deficits in social cognition or "theory of mind" in a causal pathway to both positive and negative psychotic symptoms. If these characteristics are causally related then modifying the "primary" cognitive or social deficits may reduce the risk of psychosis. Alternatively, cognitive and social deficits, although often present, may not be necessary in the pathogenesis. The fact that individuals may develop schizophrenia without obvious premorbid impairments supports this view. In these circumstances, an intervention aimed at the neurobiological level (e.g., antipsychotic medication) may be necessary. Only a high-risk longitudinal intervention study can adequately address the issue of causality, and this would require an intervention that had benefits for individuals who had the premorbid phenotype but did not develop psychosis.

Premorbid Psychopathology

A diverse range of clinical diagnoses, including attention deficit/hyperactivity disorder (ADHD), conduct disorder, anxiety, depression and autism spectrum disorders, may precede the diagnosis of schizophrenia in children and adolescents (Schaeffer & Ross, 2002) and in adults (Kim-Cohen, Caspi, Moffitt *et al.*, 2003). However, there is a lack of any specific premorbid diagnosis that could practically aid early clinical identification of those at high risk for schizophrenia. A more promising line of research has demonstrated a strong link between self-reported psychotic symptoms in childhood and later schizophrenia (Poulton, Caspi, Moffitt *et al.*, 2000).

In the Dunedin cohort, psychotic symptoms at age 11 increased the risk of schizophreniform disorder at age 26 but not other psychiatric diagnoses. Relative to the rest of the cohort, those identified at age 11 with "strong" psychotic symptoms also had significant impairments in motor development, receptive language and IQ (Cannon, Caspi, Moffitt *et al.*, 2002). Whereas none of these cases met criteria for a diagnosis of schizophrenia during adolescence, it appears that isolated or attenuated psychotic symptoms, in combination with pan-developmental impairment, constitute a significant high-risk premorbid phenotype.

Prodromal Symptoms and Onset of Psychosis

People who develop schizophrenia typically enter a prodromal phase characterized by a gradual but marked decline in social and academic functioning that precedes the onset of active psychotic symptoms. An insidious deterioration prior to the onset of psychosis is typical of the presentation of schizophrenia in children and adolescents (Werry, McClellan, Andrews, & Ham, 1994), and is more common in schizophrenia than in affective psychoses (Hollis, 1999). Non-specific behavioral changes including social withdrawal, declining school performance and uncharacteristic and odd behavior began, on average, over a year before the onset of positive psychotic symptoms. In retrospect, non-specific behavioral changes were frequently early negative symptoms, which had their onset well before positive symptoms such as hallucinations and delusions.

Early recognition of disorder is difficult, as premorbid cognitive and social impairments gradually shade into prodromal symptoms before the onset of active psychotic symptoms (Hafner & Nowotny, 1995). Prodromal symptoms can include odd ideas, eccentric interests, changes in affect, unusual experiences and bizarre perceptual experiences. Whereas these are also characteristic features of schizotypal personality disorder, in a schizophrenic prodrome there is usually progression to more severe dysfunction.

Diagnosis of Schizophrenia in Childhood and Adolescence

Diagnostic Criteria for Schizophrenia

The two dominant diagnostic systems (DSM and ICD) have slightly different definitions for schizophrenia, although both require the clear evidence of psychosis (in the absence of predominant affective symptoms) with minimum duration criteria. The reader should refer to the original manuals (DSM-IV and ICD-10) when making diagnoses in clinical or research practice.

ICD-10 criteria are closer to the Schneiderian concept of schizophrenia and place more reliance than DSM-IV on the presence of first-rank symptoms. In contrast, the DSM-IV definition reflects Kraepelin's concept of a psychotic disorder with a chronic and deteriorating course (Maj, 1998). In addition, DSM-IV stipulates a 6-month duration of disturbance, which makes it more restrictive than the 1-month duration criterion of ICD-10. The DSM-IV category of schizophreniform disorder is used for cases with the same symptoms but an overall duration of disturbance of less than 6 months. As a result, the DSM-III-R/DSM-IV definition of schizophrenia has greater specificity but lower sensitivity than ICD-10 in first-episode psychoses (Mason, Harrison, Croudace, Glazebrook, & Medley, 1997). Not surprisingly, cases of schizophrenia defined using DSM-IV have a worse prognosis than those defined using ICD-10.

DSM-IV also describes various subtypes of schizophrenia defined by the most prominent symptomatology:

1 *Paranoid type* characterized by delusions and hallucinations;
2 *Disorganized type* characterized by disorganization of speech, behavior and negative symptoms (i.e., flat or inappropriate affect);
3 *Catatonic type* characterized by motor abnormalities; and
4 *Residual type.*

Clinical Characteristics of Schizophrenia in Childhood and Adolescence

Even if strict adult definitions of schizophrenia (DSM-III-R/DSM-IV or ICD-10) are applied, there are age-dependent variations in phenomenology. Child- and adolescent-onset cases are characterized by a more insidious onset, negative symptoms, hallucinations in different modalities and fewer systematized or persecutory delusions (Green, Padron-Gayol, Hardesty *et al.*, 1992; Werry, McClellan, Andrews *et al.*, 1994). Early-onset schizophrenia is characterized by greater disorganization (incoherence of thought and disordered sense of self) and more negative symptoms, while in later-onset cases there is a higher frequency of systematized and paranoid delusions (Hafner & Nowotny, 1995).

Course and Outcome

Short-Term Course

Child- and adolescent-onset schizophrenia characteristically runs a chronic course, with only a minority of cases making a full symptomatic recovery from the first psychotic episode. Hollis (1999) found that only 12% of schizophrenic cases were in full remission at discharge compared to 50% of cases with affective psychoses. The short-term outcome for schizophrenia presenting in early life appears to be worse than that of first-episode adult patients (Robinson, Woerner, Alvir *et al.*, 1999). If full recovery does occur then it is most likely within the first 3 months of the onset of psychosis. In the Maudsley study, those adolescent-onset patients who were still psychotic after 6 months had only a 15% chance of achieving full remission, whereas over half of all cases that made a full recovery had active psychotic symptoms for less than 3 months (Hollis, 1999). The clinical implication is that the early course over the first 6 months is the best predictor of remission and that longer observation over 6 months adds relatively little new information.

Long-Term Outcome

A number of long-term follow-up studies of child- and adolescent-onset schizophrenia describe a typically chronic unremitting long-term course with severely impaired functioning in adult life (Eggers & Bunk, 1997; Fleischhaker, Schulz, Tepper *et al.*, 2005; Hollis, 2000; Jarbin, Ott, & Von Knorring, 2003; Lay, Blanz, Hartmann, & Schmidt, 2000; Schmidt, Blanz, Dippe, Koppe, & Lay, 1995; Werry, McClellan, & Chard, 1991). Referral bias towards selecting more severe cases is a potential problem in clinical follow-up studies. However, population-based studies have yielded similar results (Hollis, 2000). Several common themes emerge from these studies. First, the generally poor outcome of early onset schizophrenia conceals considerable heterogeneity. About one-fifth of patients in most studies have a good outcome with only mild impairment, whereas at the other extreme about one-third of patients are severely impaired, requiring intensive social and psychiatric support. Second, after the first few years of illness there is little evidence of further progressive decline. Third, child- and adolescent-onset schizophrenia has a worse outcome than either adolescent-onset affective psychoses or adult-onset schizophrenia. Fourth, social functioning, in particular the ability to form friendships and love relationships, appears to be very impaired in early-onset schizophrenia. Taken together, these findings confirm that schizophrenia presenting in childhood and adolescence lies at the extreme end of a continuum of phenotypic severity.

Prognostic Factors

The predictors of poor outcome in adolescent-onset affective psychoses include premorbid social and cognitive impairments (Fleischhaker, Schulz, Tepper *et al.*, 2005; Hollis, 1999), a prolonged first psychotic episode (Schmidt, Blanz, Dippe *et al.*, 1995), extended duration of untreated psychosis and the presence of negative symptoms (Hollis, 1999). Premorbid functioning and negative symptoms at onset provide better prediction of long-term outcome than categorical diagnosis (Fleischhaker, Schulz, Tepper *et al.*, 2005; Hollis, 1999).

Mortality

The risk of premature death is increased in child- and adolescent-onset psychoses. In the Maudsley study (Hollis, 1999), there were nine deaths out of the 106 cases followed-up (8.5%), corresponding to a 12-fold increase in the risk of death compared to an age and sex matched general UK population over the same period. Of the nine deaths in the cohort, seven were male and seven had a diagnosis of schizophrenia. Three subjects suffered violent deaths, two died from self-poisoning and three had unexpected deaths from previously undetected physical causes (cardiomyopathy and status epilepticus) and were possibly associated with high-dose antipsychotic medication.

Epidemiology

Incidence and Prevalence

Good population-based incidence figures for child- and adolescent-onset schizophrenia are lacking, although there are data for broader categories of psychosis, with diagnoses made without the benefit of standardized assessments. Gillberg, Wahlstrom, Forsman, Hellgren, and Gillberg (1986) calculated age-specific prevalence for all psychoses (including schizophrenia, schizophreniform psychosis, affective psychosis, atypical psychosis and drug psychoses) in the age range 13–18 years using case-register data from Goteborg, Sweden. Of the cases, 41% had a diagnosis of schizophrenia. At age 13 years, the prevalence for all psychoses was 0.9 in 10,000, showing a steady increase during adolescence, reaching a prevalence of 17.6 in 10,000 at age 18 years.

Sex Ratio

Males are overrepresented in many clinical studies of childhood-onset schizophrenia (Russell, Bott, & Sammons, 1989; Spencer & Campbell, 1994). However, other studies of predominantly adolescent-onset schizophrenia have described an equal sex ratio (Gordon, Frazier, McKenna *et al.*, 1994; Hollis, 2000; Werry, McClellan, Andrews *et al.*, 1994). The interpretation of these studies is complicated by the possibility of referral biases to clinical centers. In an epidemiological study of first admissions for schizophrenia and paranoia in children and adolescents there was an equal sex ratio for patients under the age of 15 (Galdos, van Os, & Murray, 1993). The finding of an equal sex distribution with adolescent-onset is intriguing as it differs from the consistent male predominance (ratio 2:1) reported in incident samples of early adult-onset schizophrenia (Castle & Murray, 1991). Clearly, future studies require population-based samples free from potential referral biases.

Etiology and Risk Factors

Pregnancy and Birth Complications

Pregnancy and birth complications (PBC) have long been implicated as a risk factor in schizophrenia, although the evidence is mixed (Geddes & Lawrie, 1995; Kendall, McInneny, Juszczak, & Bain, 2000). In two independent case–control studies of childhood-onset schizophrenia, Matsumoto, Takei, Saito *et al.* 1999; Matsumoto, Takei, Saito *et al.*, 2001 reported an odds ratio of 3.2–3.5 for PBC, suggesting a greater risk in very early-onset cases. However, in the National Institute of Mental Health (NIMH) study of childhood-onset schizophrenia, PBCs were no more common in cases than in sibling controls (Nicolson, Giedd, Lenane *et al.*, 1999). Insofar as there is a significant association, it seems likely that PBCs are *consequences* rather than *causes* of abnormal neurodevelopment (Goodman, 1988). This view is supported by the finding that people with schizophrenia have smaller head size at birth than controls (McGrath & Murray, 1995), which is likely to be a consequence of either defects in genetic control of neurodevelopment or earlier environmental factors such as viral exposure.

Prenatal Famine

Severe maternal intrauterine nutritional deficiency may increase the risk for schizophrenia in adult life. Evidence of a two-fold increase for schizophrenia in children born to the most malnourished mothers comes from studies of the 1944–1945 Dutch Hunger Winter (Susser & Lin, 1992) and the Chinese famine of 1959–1961 (St. Clair, Xu, Wang *et al.*, 2005).

Cannabis and Schizophrenia

There is little doubt that acute intoxication with cannabis and other illicit substances such as stimulants and hallucinogens can precipitate psychotic symptoms or exacerbations of existing psychotic illness. However, there is controversy whether cannabis use in particular is a risk factor for the development of schizophrenia. A meta-analysis of four well-conducted longitudinal population-based studies from Sweden (Swedish conscript cohort), the Netherlands (NEMESIS) and New Zealand

(Dunedin and Christchurch cohorts) concluded that, at an individual level, cannabis confers an overall two-fold increased risk for later schizophrenia (Arseneault, Cannon, Witton, & Murray, 2004). In the Dunedin cohort, Arseneault, Cannon, Poulton *et al.* (2002) showed that the association was strongest for the youngest cannabis users (after controlling for prior psychotic symptoms), with 10.3% of the cannabis users at age 15 developing schizophreniform disorder at age 26. So far, cannabis use has not been directly implicated in child- and adolescent-onset schizophrenia – possibly because of the relatively lower prevalence of cannabis use in younger adolescents and a short duration between exposure and psychotic outcome. However, cannabis use is associated with earlier age of onset of schizophrenia in adults (Arendt, Rosenberg, Foldager, Perto, & Munk-Jorgensen, 2005).

The mechanism and causal direction for this association remain unclear. It is possible that subtle social and developmental impairments that precede schizophrenia are also risk factors for cannabis use (reverse causality or a third factor). Perhaps a more plausible explanation is a gene × environment interaction effect whereby cannabis exposure causes schizophrenia only in those with a pre-existing susceptibility. Caspi, Moffitt, Cannon *et al.* (2005) provided evidence for such a gene × environment interaction specific to adolescent cannabis exposure: The COMT val^{158}met polymorphism moderated the link between psychosis and adolescent-onset cannabis use, but not adult-onset cannabis use. The COMT val allele is associated with greater COMT activity (relative to the COMT met allele) and reduced dopamine transmission in the prefrontal cortex. These results, taken together with human (Dean, Bradbury, & Copolov, 2003) and animal (Pistis, Perra, Pillolla *et al.*, 2004) neuropharmacological studies suggest that cannabis may enhance the risk of schizophrenia in vulnerable individuals during a critical period of adolescent brain development.

Psychosocial Risks

Expressed Emotion

High levels of expressed emotion (EE) among relatives of adults with schizophrenia predict psychotic relapse and poor outcome (Leff & Vaughn, 1985), raising the question of whether high EE might act to "bring forward" the onset of the disorder in a vulnerable individual. Goldstein (1987) reported that measures of parental criticism and overinvolvement taken during adolescence were associated with an increased risk of schizophrenia spectrum disorders in young adulthood. However, a causal link was not proven, and the association may reflect either an expression of some common underlying trait or a parental response to premorbid disturbance in the preschizophrenic adolescent. More direct comparisons between the parents of adult- and childhood-onset cases of schizophrenia fail to support the hypothesis of higher parental EE in childhood-onset cases. Asarnow, Thompson, Hamilton *et al.* (1994) used the Five Minute Speech Sample to measure parental EE and found that people with childhood-onset schizophrenia were no more likely to have "high EE" parents than normal controls. It appears that, on average, the parents of children with schizophrenia generally express *lower* levels of criticism and hostility than parents of adult-onset patients, because of a greater tendency to attribute their children's behavior to an illness that is beyond their control (Hooley, 1987).

Migration and Social Class

Two variables, migration and social class, are associated with significant variation in the incidence of schizophrenia. First and second generation migrants have a 2–4-times greater risk of schizophrenia (Cantor-Graae & Selten, 2005). The relative risk is highest in migrants from developing countries and where the majority population is Black. Adjustment for social class reduces, but does not eliminate, the effects of migration. Migrants living in deprived inner cities are exposed to a range of psychosocial adversities including increased exposure to drugs, violence and crime. The mechanisms linking social adversity to psychosis are unclear – but one suggestion is that experience of social defeat and isolation increases liability to dopamine dysregulation and cognitive distortions (Broome, Woolley, Tabraham *et al.*, 2005).

Childhood Abuse and Neglect

A causal link between child abuse and psychosis, in particular hallucinations, in adult life has been proposed (Read, van Os, Morrison, & Ross, 2005). While strong claims have been made for this link, the evidence to date remains inconclusive, with most studies supporting the link having serious methodological weaknesses (Morgan & Fisher, 2007).

Concepts of Schizophrenia

Neurodevelopmental Model

Over the last two decades, the concept of schizophrenia as a neurodevelopmental disorder has been the dominant explanatory model with a tension between "early" and "late" versions of the model. However, more recently these positions have converged as it has been recognized that both early events (during pre- and perinatal brain development) and late events (during adolescent brain maturation) contribute to schizophrenia (Hollis & Taylor, 1997; Rapoport, Addington, & Frangou, 2005).

The "early" neurodevelopmental model views the primary cause of schizophrenia as a static "lesion," either neurogenetic or environmental in origin, occurring during fetal brain development (Weinberger, 1987). Two main lines of evidence support this model. First, Roberts, Colter, Lofthouse *et al.* (1986) reported an absence of gliosis, suggesting aberrant neurodevelopment rather than neurodegeneration. Second, schizophrenia is associated with premorbid social and cognitive impairments (Jones, Rogers, Murray *et al.*, 1994), pregnancy and birth complications (Lewis & Murray, 1987) and minor physical anomalies (Gualtieri, Adams, & Chen, 1982). According to this "early" model, during childhood this lesion is relatively silent, giving rise only to subtle social and cognitive impairments. However, in adolescence, or early adult life, the lesion interacts with the process of *normal* brain maturation (e.g., myelination of cortico-limbic circuits, and/or synaptic pruning and remodeling) and leads to psychotic symptoms.

A limitation of the "early" model is that a neurodevelopmental insult on its own cannot account for the finding of increased extracerebral (sulcal) cerebrospinal fluid (CSF) space in schizophrenia. Diffuse loss of brain tissue limited to the pre- or perinatal periods would result in enlargement of the lateral ventricles but not increased extracerebral CSF space (Woods, 1998).

The "late" neurodevelopmental model, first proposed by Feinberg (1983), argues that the key neuropathological events in schizophrenia occur as a result of *abnormal* brain development during adolescence. The current formulation of the "late" neurodevelopmental model proposes that *excessive* synaptic and/or dentritic elimination occuring during adolescence produces aberrant neural connectivity (McGlashan & Hoffman, 2000; Woods, 1998). This "late" model characterizes schizophrenia as a *progressive* late-onset neurodevelopmental disorder and predicts that progressive structural brain changes and cognitive decline will be seen in adolescence around the onset of psychosis. Excessive synaptic pruning is regarded as an amplification of the normal process of progressive pruning and elimination of synapses that begins in early childhood and extends through late adolescence (Purves & Lichtmen, 1980). In the "late" model, premorbid abnormalities in early childhood are viewed as non-specific risk factors rather than early manifestations of an underlying schizophrenic neuropathology.

Both the "early" and "late" models suppose that there is a direct and specific expression of the eventual brain pathology as schizophrenic disorder. A third viewpoint, the neurodevelopmental "risk" model, proposes that early and/or late brain pathology acts as a risk factor rather than a sufficient cause, so that its effects can only be understood in the light of an individual's exposure to other risk and protective factors (Hollis & Taylor, 1997). This latter formulation provides a probabilistic model of the onset of schizophrenia in which aberrant brain development is expressed as neurocognitive impairments that interact with environmental risk factors to produce psychotic symptoms.

Over the last decade, further evidence has emerged to refine the neurodevelopmental model of schizophrenia. Data from premorbid social and developmental impairments, brain morphology, neuropsychology and genetics all suggest an aberrant neurodevelopmental process resulting from an interplay of genetic and environmental factors that is set in train before the onset of psychotic symptoms and continues into late adolescence.

Neurobiology of Schizophrenia

Neuropathology

In the postmortem brains of people with schizophrenia there is an absence of gliosis, which is the necessary hallmark of neurodegeneration (Roberts, Colter, Lofthouse *et al.*, 1986). The prominent neuropathology in schizophrenia is not the classic form involving neuronal cell death, but instead a loss or reduction in dendritic spines and synapses, which are the elements of neural connectivity (Glantz & Lewis, 2000). As a result, the brain in schizophrenia is characterized by increased neuronal density, decreased intraneuronal space and reduced overall brain volume. Furthermore, the decrease in dentritic spine density appears to be both region- and disease-specific, being found in the dorsolateral prefrontal cortex (layer 3 pyramidal cells), but not in the visual cortex (Glantz & Lewis, 2000). These findings are compatible with the hypothesis of reduced cortical and/or thalamic excitatory inputs to the dorsolateral prefrontal cortex in schizophrenia. However, early postmortem findings of aberrant neuronal migration have not been replicated. Hence, while there is a broad consensus that reduced dendritic arborization and synaptic density are core neuropathological features in schizophrenia, there is much less certainty regarding the timing of these changes during development.

Structural Brain Abnormalities

Neuroimaging and postmortem studies have shown that the brain as a whole and the frontal and temporal cortices in particular are smaller than normal in people with schizophrenia (Nopoulos, Torres, Flaum *et al.*, 1995). Brain volume reductions are specific to gray matter (Gur, Turetsky, Cowell *et al.*, 2000b), which supports neuropathological findings of increased neuronal density and reduced intraneuronal neuropil rather than neuronal loss (Selemon, Rajkowska, & Goldman-Rakic, 1995).

The volume of the hippocampus and amygdala is reduced bilaterally by 4.5–10% (Gur, Turetsky, Cowell *et al.*, 2000b; Nelson, Saykin, Flashman, & Riodan, 1998), and prefrontal gray matter volume is reduced by about 10% (Gur, Cowell, Latshaw *et al.*, 2000a). Enlargement of the third and lateral ventricles is a consistent finding, with ventricular volume increased by about 40% bilaterally (Lawrie & Abukmeil, 1998). Ventricular enlargement and frontal gray matter abnormalities are associated with neuropsychological impairment and negative symptoms (Vita, Dieci, Giobbio *et al.*, 1991).

The brain changes reported in childhood-onset schizophrenia appear to be very similar to those described in adult schizophrenia, supporting the idea of an underlying neurobiological continuity. In the NIMH study of childhood-onset schizophrenia (onset less than 13 years of age), subjects had smaller brains than controls, with larger lateral ventricles and reduced prefrontal lobe volume (Jacobsen & Rapoport, 1998). As in adult studies, reduced total cerebral volume is associated with negative symptoms (Alaghband-Rad, Hamburger, Giedd, Frazier, & Rapoport, 1997). Midsagittal thalamic area is decreased while midsagittal area of the corpus callosum is increased (Giedd, Castellanos, Rajapaske, Vaituzis, & Rapoport, 1996) suggesting that the reduction in total cerebral volume in childhood-onset schizophrenia is caused by relative reduction in gray matter with relative sparing of white matter. Childhood-onset patients have a higher rate of developmental brain abnormalities than controls, including an increased frequency of an enlarged cavum septum pellucidum (Nopoulos, Giedd, Andreasen, & Rapoport, 1998). Abnormalities of the cerebellum have also been found, including reduced volume of the vermis, midsagittal area and inferior posterior lobe (Jacobsen, Giedd, Berquin *et al.*, 1997a). Associated with reports of reduced cortical thickness are gyrification abnormalities including more flattened curvature in the sulci and more peaked or steep curvature in the gyri (White, Andreasen, Nopoulos, & Magnotta, 2003), consistent with a neurodevelopmental origin of cortical abnormalities. In adolescent-onset schizophrenia patients, there is evidence of ventricular enlargement and reduced volume of the prefrontal cortex and reduced thalamic volume (Dasari, Friedman, Jesberger *et al.*, 1999; James, Smith, & Jayaloes, 2004).

Progressive Brain Changes

Two different types of progressive brain change have been described in schizophrenia. First, treatment with traditional antipsychotics appears to cause progressive enlargement of the basal ganglia, with these structures returning to their original size when patients are transferred to the atypical antipsychotic clozapine (Frazier, Giedd, Kaysen *et al.*, 1996). Second, there is evidence of progressive volume reductions in the temporal and frontal lobes during the first 2–3 years after the onset of schizophrenia (Gur, Cowell, Turetsky *et al.*, 1998). In the NIMH study of childhood-onset schizophrenia, longitudinal repeated magnetic resonance imaging (MRI) scans through adolescence revealed a progressive increase in ventricular volume and progressive decrease in cortical volume with frontal (11% decrease), parietal (8.5% decrease) and temporal lobes (7% decrease) disproportionately affected (Rapoport, Giedd, Blumenthal *et al.*, 1999; Sporn, Greenstein, Gogtay *et al.*, 2003). Overall, this represents a four-fold greater reduction in cortical volume than in healthy adolescents. A similar progressive loss in cerebellar volume has been reported in the same NIMH childhood-onset schizophrenia sample (Keller, Castellanos, Vaituzis *et al.*, 2003). Age-related volume reduction across adolescence has also been reported for the anterior cingulate gyrus (Marquardt, Levitt, Blanton *et al.*, 2005). Progressive changes appear to be time-limited to adolescence, with the rate of volume reduction in frontal and temporal structures associated with premorbid developmental impairment and baseline symptom severity (Sporn, Greenstein, Gogtay *et al.*, 2003) and declining as subjects reach adult life (Giedd, Jeffries, Blumenthal *et al.*, 1999). The pattern of progressive cortical volume reduction described in the NIMH childhood-onset schizophrenia sample appears to be an exaggeration of the normal "back to front" pattern of cortical volume reduction seen during adolescence (Gogtay, Sporn, Clasen *et al.*, 2004). At present, it is unclear whether the dramatic findings from the NIMH childhood-onset schizophrenia sample, which is atypical in terms of very early onset (<13 years) and neuroleptic treatment resistance, can be generalized to other samples of children and adolescents with schizophrenia (cf. James, Javaloyes, James, & Smith, 2002).

Because progressive brain changes have been described *after* the onset of psychosis, it is possible that they are a consequence of neurotoxic effects of psychosis. Evidence that progressive brain changes precede the onset of psychosis is very limited. Pantelis, Velakoulis, McGorry *et al.* (2003) have reported brain MRI findings in high-risk subjects scanned before and after the transition into psychosis. The baseline cross-sectional comparison found that those about to develop psychosis had reduced cortical gray matter in the right temporal, inferior frontal cortex and cingulate bilaterally. When rescanned, those subjects who developed psychosis had further volume reductions in gray matter in the left parahippocampal, fusiform, orbitofrontal and cerebellar cortices and cingulate gyri. The only significant longitudinal changes in cases who remained non-psychotic were in the cerebellum. These are important findings, and if replicated would provide strong support for the idea that excessive developmental reductions in gray matter both predate and accompany the onset of psychotic symptoms.

Functional Brain Imaging

The emergence of functional brain imaging technology has provided a unique opportunity to link symptoms and cognitive deficits in schizophrenia to underlying brain activity. In studies of adults with schizophrenia, there are associations between:

1 Negative symptoms, cognitive executive function deficits and abnormal frontal activity;

2 Disorganization symptoms (thought disorder and inappropriate affect) and anterior cingulate activity; and

3 Thought disorder/hallucinations and activity in the superior temporal gyrus (Liddle & Pantellis, 2003).

Reduced activity of the anterior cingulate cortex in schizophrenia is associated with impaired ability to monitor response errors and response to conflict (Kerns, Cohen, MacDonald *et al.*, 2005), which may underlie psychotic symptoms (Frith, 1994). Reduced activity in the right dorsolateral prefrontal cortex has also been associated with working memory impairments and disorganization symptoms (Perlstein, Carter, Noll, & Cohen, 2001).

The notion of "hypofrontality" has been proposed to account for schizophrenia, but is certainly an oversimplification. Evidence suggests that frontal activation is diminished only when processing load is high and task performance diminishes (Perlstein, Carter, Noll *et al.*, 2001). In contrast, baseline resting frontal activation may be increased in acute schizophrenia relative to healthy subjects as a result of abnormal self-generated mental activity associated with psychotic symptoms. When an external task places an increased processing load on an individual with psychosis, the prefrontal cortex may be unable to meet the demand, resulting in reduced performance and activation (Liddle & Pantellis, 2003).

In a positron emission tomography (PET) study in childhood-onset schizophrenia using the Continuous Performance Test (CPT), Jacobsen, Hamburger, Van Horn *et al.* (1997b) reported reduced activation compared to healthy controls in the mid and superior frontal gyrus, and increased activation in the inferior frontal, supramarginal gyrus and insula. Clearly, a simple description of "hypofrontality" does not capture the complex pattern of changes involving interconnected frontal areas. Older, localizationist, models based on focal cerebral dysfunction in schizophrenia have tended to give way to models of cerebral disconnectivity (Bullmore, O'Connell, Frangou *et al.*, 1997) that fit well with both neuropathological and functional neuroimaging findings. This may be one reason for inconsistent neuroanatomical findings in schizophrenia, as "lesions" in different areas of a widely distributed neural system could produce similar functional disturbance.

Magnetic Resonance Spectroscopy: Abnormal Neuronal Metabolism

Magnetic resonance spectroscopy (MRS) is an imaging technique that can be used to extract *in vivo* information on dynamic biochemical processes at a neuronal level. Proton (^{1}H) MRS focuses on changes in the neuronal marker *N*-acetylaspartate (NAA). Studies in adult schizophrenic patients have shown reductions in NAA in the hippocampal area and dorsolateral prefrontal cortex (DLPFC). Similar reductions in NAA ratios specific to the hippocampus and DLPFC (Bertolino, Kumra, Callicott *et al.*, 1988) and frontal gray matter (Thomas, Ke, Levitt *et al.*, 1998) have been reported in childhood-onset schizophrenia, suggesting neuronal damage or malfunction in these regions.

Pettegrew, Keshavan, Panchalingam *et al.* (1991) used ^{31}P MRS with non-medicated patients during a first episode of schizophrenia and found reduced phosphomonoester (PME) resonance and increased phosphodiester (PDE) resonance in the prefrontal cortex. This result is compatible with reduced synthesis and increased breakdown of connective processes in the prefrontal cortex. A similar finding of reduced PME and increased PDE resonance has been reported in adults with autism, although they showed increased prefrontal metabolic activity, which was not seen in people with schizophrenia (Pettegrew, Keshavan, Panchalingam *et al.*, 1991). Keshavan, Stanley, Montrose *et al.* (2003) reported reduced PME moieties (e.g., synaptic vesicles and phosphorylated proteins) in the prefrontal cortex using ^{31}P MRS in a sample of children and adolescents at genetic high risk for schizophrenia. These findings suggest that abnormal synaptic structure and function in the prefrontal cortex is a marker of schizophrenia risk. Further follow-up is required to determine if these findings have predictive value.

Implications for Neurodevelopmental Models of Schizophrenia

Taken together, the neuropathological and brain imaging findings provide considerable support for the idea of progressive neurodevelopmental changes in schizophrenia including excessive synaptic elimination resulting in aberrant neural connectivity. The progressive nature of brain volume reductions in adolescence, and the fact that reduced brain volume is not accompanied by reduced intracranial volume, suggests that a static pre- or perinatal brain insult is insufficient to account for this process. While early random events in fetal neurodevelopment (e.g., hypoxia, viruses) may affect baseline synaptic density, genetically determined excessive synaptic elimination as proposed by the "late" neurodevelopmental model may be the neurobiological process underlying disorders in the schizophrenia spectrum (McGlashan & Hoffman, 2000). What is unclear is whether excessive synaptic elimination in the prefrontal cortex (and possibly other brain regions) is a sufficient cause for psychosis to occur, or whether it provides a vulnerable neurocognitive substrate that must interact with environmental stressors (e.g., cannabis exposure or cognitive or social stressors) to produce psychotic symptoms.

Genetics of Schizophrenia

Multigene Models of Risk

Twin studies have suggested the heritability of schizophrenia to be as high as 83% (Cannon, Kaprio, Lonnqvist, Huttunen, & Koskenvuo, 1998). However, one of the most significant implications of twin, adoption and family studies in schizophrenia has been the challenge the results pose to traditional qualitatively distinct categories of disorder (Rutter & Plomin, 1997). Quantitative genetic studies have shown that the genetic liability to schizophrenia extends to schizoptypal personality disorders and other conditions viewed as lying on the broader schizophrenia spectrum (Erlenmeyer-Kimling, Squires-Wheeler, Adamo *et al.*, 1995; Kendler, Neale, & Walsh, 1995). These results suggest that what is inherited in schizophrenia is likely to be quantitative traits that determine liability to disorder.

While the mode of inheritance in schizophrenia remains unknown, most evidence supports a multilocus or multifactorial threshold model. This model proposes that schizophrenia results from the combined action of multiple genes of small effect that confer susceptibility to the schizophrenic phenotype, with the disorder being expressed above a particular liability threshold. Susceptibility to the disorder is expressed as a dimension in the population (i.e., the risk of schizophrenia in the population is distributed normally, not bimodally). Because there are likely to be multiple genes involved, the genetics of schizophrenia is moving away from the rather simplistic notion of finding a single major gene for the disorder, towards a search for genes that confer susceptibility traits. Susceptibility alleles may be quite common in the population and hence the predictive value of any individual allele alone will be low.

It is commonly assumed that genes affecting brain development in schizophrenia are only expressed during fetal neurodevelopment. However, it is quite possible that while some susceptibility genes for schizophrenia may affect fetal brain development, other genes do not exert their effect until adolescence, possibly causing excessive or aberrant synaptic pruning with reduction in temporal and frontal lobe volume (Feinberg, 1997).

Linkage Studies

Two meta-analyses of schizophrenia linkage studies have supported a multilocus model with several chromosomal regions implicated. Lewis, Levinson, Wise *et al.* (2003) found the strongest evidence for linkage on 2q, with weaker support obtained for regions on chromosomes 5q, 3p, 11q, 6p, 1q, 22q, 8p, 20q and 14p. Meanwhile, Badner and Gershon (2002) found evidence supporting susceptibility genes on chromosomes 8p, 13q and 22q. Hence, both studies converged on two regions: 8p and 22q, with nine other regions being supported by only one metaanalysis. While failure to replicate genetic findings has plagued schizophrenia research, this is to be expected if schizophrenia is an etiologically (and genetically) heterogeneous disorder.

Positional Candidate Genes and Neurobiology

Convergent findings from linkage studies have led to mapping of implicated regions and identification of putative susceptibility genes. A number of replicated associations have recently been reported between DNA polymorphisms of various positional candidate genes and schizophrenia. The positional candidate genes most clearly implicated impact on either synaptogenesis or glutamate neurotransmission (Harrison & Owen, 2003). The strongest evidence favors dysbindin (*DTNBP1*) (6p22.3) and neuroregulin (*NRG1*) (8p21–p22). There is also promising but less compelling evidence for catecholamine-O-methyltransferase (*COMT*), D-amino-acid oxidase (*DAO*), its activator *DAOA* (previously known as *G72*) and regulator G protein signaling 4 (*RGS4*). The high-risk *COMT* val allele associated with schizophrenia is hypothesized to have its effect by reducing dopaminergic transmission in the prefrontal cortex. Dysbindin may affect the uptake of glutamate into synaptic vesicles, *NRG1* is released from glutamate terminals and regulates *N*-methyl-D-aspartate (NMDA) glutamate receptors and *DAO*, activated by *DAOA*, is an indirect modulator of NMDA receptors. The actions of many of these genes converge on a shared pathophysiological process that suggests that abnormalities of synaptic signaling, in particular at the glutamatergic synapse, may be a primary abnormality in schizophrenia (Harrison & Weinberger, 2005; Mirnics, Middleton, Lewis, & Levitt, 2001). At a simple conceptual level, these genes are all thought to influence information processing (via synaptic signaling) in cortical circuits. The clinical correlates of these candidate genes are more likely to be neurodevelopmental and cognitive impairments than fluctuating positive symptoms of schizophrenia.

Candidate Genes in Childhood-Onset Schizophrenia

The *DAOA* polymorphism (13q33.2) was associated with childhood-onset schizophrenia (COS) in the NIMH sample (Addington, Gornick, Sporn *et al.*, 2004). Interestingly, in the same NIMH sample *DAOA* was associated with *later* age of onset and *lower* scores for premorbid autism symptoms. Another intriguing finding in the NIMH COS sample is an association between dysbindin (*DTNBP1*) (6p22.3) and poor premorbid social and academic adjustment (Rapoport, Addington, & Frangou, 2005). Finally, a polymorphism of the *GAD1* (glutamic acid decarboxylase) gene has been associated with both childhood-onset schizophrenia and abnormal frontal gray matter loss (Addington, Gornick, Duckworth *et al.*, 2005).

Cytogenetic Abnormalities

The association between schizophrenia and chromosomal deletions offers another possible route to locating candidate genes (Hennah, Thompson, Peltonen, & Porteous, 2006). The velocardiofacial syndrome (VCFS) microdeletion on chromosome 22q11 (which includes the *COMT* gene plus two candidates, *PRODH* and *ZDHHC8*) is associated with adult schizophrenia, occurring at a rate of 2% compared to 0.02% in the normal population (see chapter 24; Karayiogou, Morris, Morrow *et al.*, 1995). The association with schizophrenia is not specific, as the VCFS microdeletion is also linked with higher rates of other psychiatric disorders (e.g., affective disorder, ADHD). In the NIMH COS study, a high rate of previously undetected cytogenetic abnormalities was found, including 4 of 80 (5%) with *VCFS* (Sporn, Addington, Reiss *et al.*, 2004b). The 22q11DS is associated with progressive cortical gray matter loss in children and adolescents who are not yet psychotic, suggesting that a gene or genes mapping to 22q11 is responsible for a high-risk phenotype (Sporn, Addington, Reiss *et al.*, 2004b).

Another major finding based on a chromosomal abnormality comes from an extended Scottish pedigree where a balanced translocation (1:11)(q42;q14.3) showed linkage with a phenotype including schizophrenia, bipolar disorder and depression (Hennah, Thompson, Peltonen *et al.*, 2006). The translocation disrupts two genes on chromosome 1: *DISC1* and *DISC2*. There is some evidence that *DISC1* is linked to the regulation of neural migration, which may have a role in the pathogenesis of schizophrenia. Two studies found mutations or polymorphisms of *DISC1* associated with schizophrenia, while two other studies have failed to find an association (Owen, Craddock, & O'Donovan, 2005).

Overlap with Bipolar Disorder

Several genes influence susceptibility to both schizophrenia and bipolar disorder, including *NRG1*, *DISC1* and *G72* (*DAOA*; Owen, Craddock, & O'Donovan, 2005). These findings suggest that the two disorders share pathogenic mechanisms and challenge the long-held Kraepelinian dichotomy that views schizophrenia and bipolar disorder as separate diagnostic entities. Prototypic schizophrenia and bipolar disorder can be seen as lying at the extreme ends of a spectrum of psychosis with mixed or intermediate phenotypes lying in between. Within this spectrum of psychosis, dysbindin (*DTNBP1*) predisposes predominantly to schizophrenia with negative symptoms, *DAOA* and *BDNF* predispose predominantly to mood disorder, and *NRG1* and *DISC1* predispose to both prototypic forms of disorder (Craddock, O'Donovan, & Owen, 2005).

Neuropsychology of Schizophrenia

Pattern of Cognitive Deficits

There is growing awareness that cognitive deficits in schizophrenia are a core feature of the disorder and cannot simply be dismissed as secondary consequences of psychotic symptoms (Breier, 1999). The degree of cognitive impairment is greater in child- and adolescent-onset than in adult-onset patients. These findings raise several important questions.

1 Are the cognitive deficits specific or general (i.e., are some aspects of cognitive functioning affected more than others?)?
2 Which deficits precede the onset of psychosis and could be causal, and which are consequences of psychosis?
3 Is the pattern of deficits specific to schizophrenia or shared with other developmental and psychotic disorders?
4 Are cognitive impairments progressive or static after the onset of psychosis?

Children with schizophrenia have specific difficulties with cognitive tasks that make demands on short-term working memory and selective and sustained attention and speed of processing (Asarnow, Brown, & Stranberg, 1995). These deficits are similar to the deficits reported in adult schizophrenia (Saykin, Shtasel, Gur *et al.*, 1994). Deficits of attention, short-term and recent long-term memory have also been reported in adolescents with schizophrenia (Friedman, Findling, Buch *et al.*, 1996). In contrast, well-established "over learned" rote language and simple perceptual skills are unimpaired in child- and adolescent-onset schizophrenia. Asarnow, Granholm, & Sherman (1991), Asarnow, Brown, & Stranberg (1995) have shown that children with schizophrenia have impairments on the span of apprehension task (a target stimulus has to be identified from an array of other figures when displayed for 50 ms). Performance on the task deteriorates markedly when increasing demands are made on information processing capacity (e.g., increasing the number of letters in the display from 3 to 10). Furthermore, event-related potential (ERP) studies using the span of apprehension task in both children and adults with schizophrenia, when compared with age-matched controls, show less negative endogenous activity measured 100–300 ms after the stimulus. Similar findings of reduced ERPs (processing negativity Np, and P2 components) have been found during the CPT in both childhood- and adult-onset schizophrenia (Strandburg, Marsh, & Brown, 1999). These findings indicate a deficit in the allocation of attentional resources to a stimulus (Asarnow, Brown, & Stranberg, 1995). As with adults, children and adolescents with schizophrenia show high basal autonomic activity and less autonomic responsivity than controls (Gordon, Frazier, McKenna *et al.*, 1994), with attenuated increases in skin conductance following the presentation of neutral sounds (Zahn, Jacobsen, Gordon *et al.*, 1997). Childhood-onset patients, like adults, show increased reaction times with a loss of ipsimodal advantage compared to healthy controls (Zahn, Jacobsen, Gordon *et al.*, 1998). Eye tracking dysfunction (ETD) – a proxy of frontal lobe dysfunction – as indexed by abnorm-alities in smooth pursuit eye movements (SPEM) has also been found in childhood-onset schizophrenia (Kumra, Sporn, Hommer *et al.*, 2001). Similar ETD has been reported in adult schizophrenia (Iacono & Koenig, 1983). ETD is also a potential genetic endophenotype trait marker for schizophrenia that has been detected in healthy siblings of COS and parents of adult-onset schizophrenia patients (Sporn, Greenstein, Gogtay *et al.*, 2005). Non-psychotic relatives of schizophrenic patients also show eye-tracking deficits that correlate with subtle frontal lobe dysfunction (O'Driscoll, Benkelfat, Florencio *et al.*, 1999). Finally, children with schizophrenia also show similar impairments to adult patients on tests of frontal lobe executive function such as the Wisconsin Card Sorting Test (WCST; Asarnow, Thompson, Hamilton *et al.*, 1994). Hence, reduced prefrontal activation may be one expression of a genetic susceptibility to schizophrenia.

In summary, while basic sensorimotor skills, associative memory and simple language abilities tend to be preserved in children with schizophrenia, deficits are most marked on tasks that require focused and sustained attention, flexible switching of cognitive set, high information processing speed and suppression of prepotent responses (Asarnow, Brown, & Stranberg, 1995). The diverse cognitive processes described here have been integrated under the cognitive domain of "executive functions", which are presumed to be mediated by the prefrontal cortical system. Executive function skills are necessary to generate and execute goal-directed behavior, especially in novel situations. Goalorientated actions require that information in the form of plans and expectations are held "online" in working memory, and flexibly changed in response to feedback. Similar deficits have also been found in children genetically at "high risk" for schizophrenia (Erlenmeyer-Kimling & Cornblatt, 1978) and non-psychotic relatives of schizophrenic probands (Park, Holzman, & Goldman-Rakic, 1995). This strengthens the argument that cognitive deficits cannot be simply dismissed as non-specific consequences of schizophrenic symptoms, but rather are likely to be indicators of underlying genetic and neurobiological risk. Several candidate susceptibility genes (dysbindin-1 and *COMT*) have been linked to impaired working memory and may provide molecular mechanisms underlying this intermediate (endo)phenotype of schizophrenia (Egan, Goldberg, Kolachana *et al.*, 2001). However, executive functions deficits are probably not a primary or sufficient cause of schizophrenia given that they also occur in other neurodevelopmental disorders including autism and ADHD (Pennington, 1997).

Course of Cognitive Deficits

Kraepelin's term "dementia praecox" implied a progressive cognitive decline as part of the disease process. Jones, Rogers, Murray *et al.* (1994) described how academic performance becomes progressively more deviant during adolescence in those individuals destined to developed schizophrenia in adult life. A similar finding of IQ decline from childhood through adolescence which precedes the onset of schizophrenia in adult life has been reported from a large Israeli population-based cohort (Reichenberg, Weiser, Rapp *et al.*, 2005). There is some tentative evidence for a small decline in IQ following the onset of psychosis in childhood-onset schizophrenia (Alaghband-Rad, McKenna, Gordon *et al.*, 1995), followed by a stabilization of cognitive function despite progressive cortical gray matter loss during adolescence (Gochman, Greenstein, Sporn *et al.*, 2005). However, without longitudinal control data this is difficult to evaluate, given that, in typically developing samples, most IQ tests will show improved scores with repeated administration. Furthermore, the small drop in IQ after the onset of psychosis could possibly be caused by the effect of psychotic symptoms on performance. In so far as there is an effect, it looks like premature arrest, or slowing, of normal cognitive development in child- and adolescent-onset schizophrenia, rather than a progressive dementia.

Assessment

The assessment of a child or adolescent with possible schizophrenia should include a detailed history, mental state and physical examination. In addition, a baseline psychometric assessment is desirable. A detailed understanding of specific cognitive deficits in individual cases of adolescent schizophrenia can be particularly helpful in guiding education and rehabilitation. In the physical examination, particular attention should be given to detecting dysmorphic features that may betray an underlying genetic syndrome. The neurological examination should focus on abnormal involuntary movements and other signs of extrapyramidal dysfunction. Spontaneous abnormal involuntary movements have been detected in a proportion of drug-naïve first-episode schizophrenic or schizophreniform patients as well as in those receiving typical antipsychotics (Gervin, Browne, Lane *et al.*, 1998).

Developmental Issues

The cognitive level of the child will influence their ability to understand and express complex psychotic symptoms such as passivity phenomena, thought alienation and hallucinations. In younger children, careful distinctions have to be made between developmental immaturity and psychopathology. For example, distinguishing true hallucinations from normal subjective phenomena such as dreams and communication with imaginary friends may be difficult for young children. Developmental maturation can also affect the localization of hallucinations in space. Internal localization of hallucinations is more common in younger children and makes these experiences more difficult to differentiate subjectively from inner speech or thoughts (Garralda, 1984). Formal thought disorder may also appear very similar to the pattern of illogical thinking and loose associations seen in children with immature language development. Negative symptoms can appear very similar to non-psychotic language and social impairments and can also be easily confused with anhedonia and depression.

Differential Diagnosis

Psychotic symptoms in children and adolescents are diagnostically non-specific, occurring in a wide range of functional psychiatric and organic brain disorders. A summary of physical investigations in children and adolescents with suspected schizophrenia is listed in Table 45.1. Referral for a neurological opinion is recommended if neurodegenerative disorder is suspected (see chapter 30).

Affective, Schizoaffective and "Atypical" Psychoses

The high rate of positive psychotic symptoms found in adolescent-onset major depression and mania can lead to diagnostic confusion (Joyce, 1984). Affective psychoses are most likely to be misdiagnosed as schizophrenia if a Schneiderian concept of schizophrenia is applied with its emphasis on first-rank symptoms. Because significant affective symptoms also occur in about one-third of first-episode patients with schizophrenia, it may be impossible to make a definitive diagnosis on the basis of a single cross-sectional assessment. In DSM-IV the distinction between schizophrenia, schizoaffective disorder

Table 45.1 Physical investigations in child- and adolescent-onset psychoses.

Investigation	Target disorder
Urine drug screen	Drug-related psychosis (amphetamines, ecstasy, cocaine, LSD and other psychoactive compounds)
EEG	Complex partial seizures/TLE
MRI brain scan	Ventricular enlargement, structural brain anomalies (e.g. cavum septum pellucidum) Enlarged caudate (typical antipsychotics) Demyelination (metachromatic leukodystrophy) Hypodense basal ganglia (Wilson's disease)
Serum copper and ceruloplasmin	Wilson's disease
Urinary copper	
Arylsulfatase A (white blood cell)	Metachromatic leukodystrophy
Karyotype/cytogentics (FISH)	Sex chromosome aneuploidies, velocardiofacial syndrome (22q11 microdeletion)

EEG, electroencephalogram; FISH, fluorescent *in situ* hybridization; LSD, lysergic acid diethylamide; MRI, magnetic resonance imaging; TLE, temporal lobe epilepsy.

and affective psychoses is determined by the relative predominance and temporal overlap of psychotic symptoms (hallucinations and delusions) and affective symptoms (elevated or depressed mood). Given the difficulty in applying these rules with any precision, there is a need to identify other features to distinguish between schizophrenia and affective psychoses. Irrespective of the presence of affective symptoms, the most discriminating symptoms of schizophrenia are an insidious onset and the presence of negative symptoms (Hollis, 1999). Similarly, complete remission from a first psychotic episode within 6 months of onset is the best predictor of a diagnosis of affective psychosis (Hollis, 1999). Schizoaffective and atypical psychoses are diagnostic categories with low predictive validity and little longitudinal stability (Hollis, 2000).

Autistic Spectrum and Developmental Language Disorders

Some children on the autistic spectrum or with Asperger syndrome have social and cognitive impairments that overlap closely with the premorbid phenotype described in schizophrenia. Furthermore, children on the autistic spectrum can also develop psychotic symptoms in adolescence (Volkmar & Cohen, 1991). Towbin, Dykens, Pearson, and Cohen (1993) have labeled another group of children who seem to belong within the autistic spectrum as having "multiplex developmental disorder." An increased risk for psychosis has also been noted in the adult follow-up of childhood developmental receptive language disorders (Clegg, Hollis, & Rutter, 2005). In the NIMH COS sample, 19 cases (25%) had a lifetime diagnosis of autism spectrum disorder (ASD), one had autism, two had Asperger syndrome and 16 had pervasive develomental disorder not otherwise specified (PDD-NOS; Sporn, Addington, Gogtay *et al.*, 2004a). The COS-ASD subgroup did not differ from the rest of the COS sample on a range of measures including age of onset, IQ, response to medications and familial schizotypy. However, the rate of cortical gray matter loss was greater in the ASD group. While the authors concluded that ASD was more likely to be a severe form of premorbid social impairment rather than true comorbidity, an unexplained finding was the occurrence of two cases of autism in the siblings of the COS-ASD subgroup. While some children on the autistic spectrum can show a clear progression into classic schizophrenia, others show a more episodic pattern of psychotic symptoms without the progressive decline in social functioning and negative symptoms characteristic of child- and adolescent-onset schizophrenia.

Often it is only possible to distinguish between schizophrenia and disorders on the autistic spectrum by taking a careful developmental history that details the age of onset and pattern of autistic impairments in communication, social reciprocity and interests/behaviors. According to DSM-IV, schizophrenia cannot be diagnosed in a child with autism/PDD unless hallucinations/delusions are present for at least 1 month. DSM-IV does not rank the active phase symptoms of thought disorder, disorganization or negative symptoms as sufficient to make a diagnosis of schizophrenia in the presence of autism. In contrast, ICD-10 does not include autism/PDD as exclusion criteria for diagnosing schizophrenia.

"Multidimensionally Impaired Syndrome" and Schizotypal Personality Disorder

Multidimensionally impaired syndrome (MDI) is a label applied to children who have brief transient psychotic symptoms, emotional lability, poor interpersonal skills, normal social skills and multiple deficits in information processing (Kumra, Jacobsen, Lenane *et al.*, 1998c). The diagnostic status of this group remains to be fully resolved. Short-term follow-up suggests that they do not develop full-blown schizophrenic psychosis. However, they have an increased risk of schizophrenia spectrum disorders among first-degree relatives and the neurobiological findings (e.g., brain morphology) are similar to those in childhood onset schizophrenia (Kumra, Jacobsen, Lenane *et al.*, 1998c). At 11 year follow-up, 38% (12 of 32) of patients met criteria for bipolar 1 disorder, 12% (4 of 32) for major depressive disorder (MDD), and 3% (1 of 32) for schizoaffective disorder. The remaining 47% of patients (15 of 32) were divided into two groups on the basis of whether they were in remission and neuroleptic-free ("good outcome," $n = 5$) or still severely impaired and/or psychotic regardless of pharmacotherapy ("poor outcome," $n = 10$; Stayer, Sporn, Gogtay *et al.*, 2005).

Children with schizotypal personality disorder (SPD) lie on a phenotypic continuum with schizophrenia and have similar cognitive and social impairments and are prone to magical thinking, mood disturbances and non-psychotic perceptual disturbances. Distinction from the prodromal phase of schizophrenia is particularly difficult when there is a history of social and academic decline without clear-cut, or persisting, psychotic symptoms. A follow-up of children with SPD found that 25% developed schizophrenia spectrum disorders (schizophrenia and schizoaffective disorder), suggesting that SPD may be a precursor of schizophrenia (Asarnow, 2005). It has been reported that negative symptoms and attention in SPD improve with a low dose of risperidone (0.25–2.0 mg; Rossi, Mancini, Stratta *et al.*, 1997).

Epilepsy

Psychotic symptoms can occur in temporal and frontal lobe partial seizures (for a description of these seizures see chapter 30). A careful history is usually sufficient to reveal an aura followed by clouding of consciousness and the sudden onset of brief ictal psychotic phenomena accompanied often by anxiety, fear, derealization or depersonalization. However, longer-lasting psychoses associated with epilepsy can occur in clear consciousness during postictal or interictal periods (Sachdev, 1998). In epileptic psychoses, hallucinations, disorganized behavior and persecutory delusions predominate, while negative symptoms are rare. Children with complex partial seizures also have increased illogical thinking and use fewer linguistic-cohesive devices which can resemble formal thought disorder (Caplan, Guthrie, Shields, & Mori, 1992). A PET study showed hypoperfusion in the frontal, temporal and basal ganglia in psychotic patients with epilepsy compared with non-psychotic epileptic patients (Gallhofer, Trimble, Frackowiak, Gibbs, & Jones, 1985).

Epilepsy and schizophrenia may co-occur in the same individual, so that the diagnoses are not mutually exclusive. The onset of epilepsy almost always precedes psychosis unless seizures are secondary to antipsychotic medication. In a long-term follow-up of 100 children with temporal lobe epilepsy, 10% developed schizophrenia in adult life (Lindsay, Ounstead, & Richards, 1979).

An electroencephalogram (EEG) should be performed if a seizure disorder is considered in the differential diagnosis or arises as a side effect of antipsychotic treatment. Ambulatory EEG monitoring and telemetry with event recording may be required if the diagnosis remains in doubt.

Neurodegenerative Disorders

Rare neurodegenerative disorders with onset in late childhood and adolescence (see chapter 30) can mimic schizophrenia. The most important examples are Wilson's disease (hepatolenticular degeneration), and metachromatic leukodystrophy. These disorders usually involve significant extrapyramidal symptoms (e.g., tremor, dystonia and bradykinesia) or other motor abnormalities (e.g., unsteady gait) and a progressive loss of skills (dementia), which can aid the distinction from schizophrenia. Suspicion of a neurodegenerative disorder is one of the clearest indications for brain MRI in adolescent psychoses. Adolescents with schizophrenia show relative gray matter reduction with white matter sparing. In contrast, metachromatic leukodystrophy is characterized by frontal and occipital white matter destruction and demyelination. In Wilson's disease, hypodense areas are seen in the basal ganglia, together with cortical atrophy and ventricular dilatation. The pathognomonic Kayser–Fleisher ring in Wilson's disease begins as a greenish-brown crescent-shaped deposit in the cornea above the pupil (this is most easily seen during slit lamp examination). In Wilson's disease there is increased urinary copper excretion, and reduced serum copper and serum ceruloplasmin levels. The biochemical marker for metachromatic leukodystrophy is reduced arylsulfatase-A (ASA) activity in white blood cells. This enzyme deficiency results in a deposition of excess sulfatides in many tissues including the CNS.

Drug Psychoses

Illicit drug use is increasingly common among young people (see chapter 36), so the frequent co-occurrence of drug use and psychosis is to be expected. Psychotic symptoms can occur as a direct pharmacological effect of intoxication with stimulants (amphetamine, ecstasy and cocaine), hallucinogens (lysergic acid diethylamide "LSD," phencyclidine, psilocybin "magic mushrooms" and mescaline), cannabis (Poole & Brabbins, 1996) and ketamine, an NMDA receptor antagonist and anesthetic (Krystal, Perry, Gueorguieva *et al.*, 2006). The psychotic symptoms associated with drug intoxication are usually short-lived and resolve within a few days of abstinence from the drug. These drugs can have surprisingly long half-lives, with cannabinoids still measurable up to 6 weeks after a single dose. Psychotic symptoms in the form of "flashbacks" can also occur after cessation from chronic cannabis and LSD abuse. These phenomena are similar to alcoholic hallucinosis and typically involve transient vivid auditory hallucinations occurring in clear consciousness.

It is often assumed that there is a simple causal relationship between drug use and psychosis, with any evidence of drug use excluding the diagnosis of a functional psychosis. However, this is a naïve approach, as drug use can be either a consequence of psychosis with patients using drugs to "treat" their symptoms in the early stages of a psychotic relapse or, with cannabis, a cause of schizophrenia in susceptible individuals (Arseneault, Cannon, Witton *et al.*, 2004). Overall, there is very little evidence to invoke a separate entity of "drug-induced" psychosis in cases where psychotic symptoms arise during intoxication but then persist after the drug is withdrawn (Poole & Brabbins, 1996). Patients whose so-called "drug-induced" psychoses last for more than 6 months appear to have more clear-cut schizophrenic symptoms, a greater familial risk for psychosis and greater premorbid dysfunction (Tsuang, Simpson, & Kronfold, 1982). DSM-IV takes the sensible position that a functional psychosis should not be excluded unless there is compelling evidence that symptoms are uniquely associated with drug use.

Other Investigations

Whether any physical investigations should be viewed as routine is debatable (see chapter 22). However, it is usual to obtain a full blood count and biochemistry including liver and thyroid function and a drug screen (urine or hair analysis). The high yield of cytogenetic abnormalities reported in childhood-onset schizophrenia (Nicolson, Giedd, Lenane *et al.*, 1999) suggests the value of cytogenetic testing including karyotyping for sex chromosome aneuploidies and fluorescent *in situ* hybridization (FISH) for 22q11DS (velocardiofacial syndrome). The evidence of progressive structural brain changes (Rapoport, Giedd, Blumenthal *et al.*, 1999) indicates the value of obtaining a baseline and annual follow-up brain MRI scans, although this is not a diagnostic test.

Assessment Interviews and Rating Scales

Structured diagnostic investigator-based interviews that cover child and adolescent psychotic disorders include the Schedule for Affective Disorders and Schizophrenia for School-Age Children (K-SADS; Ambrosini, 2000), the Child and Adolescent Psychiatric Assessment (CAPA; Angold & Costello, 2000) and the Diagnostic Interview for Children and Adolescents (DICA; Reich, 2000). The DSM and ICD definitions of schizophrenia do not provide symptom definitions so the detailed glossaries that accompany these interviews are particularly useful.

Rating scales give quantitative measures of psychopathology and functional impairment. Scales to assess psychotic symptoms include the Scale for Assessment of Positive Symptoms (SAPS;

Andreasen, 1984), the Scale for Assessment of Negative Symptoms (SANS; Andreasen, 1983) and the Positive and Negative Syndrome Scale (PANSS; Kay, Opler, & Lindenmayer, 1987). The 30-item Kiddie-PANSS has been developed for use in children and adolescents, and contains three subscales: positive syndrome, negative syndrome and general psychopathology (Fields, Grochowski, Lindenmayer *et al.*, 1994). The Children's Global Assessment Scale (C-GAS) provides a rating of functional impairment on a 0–100 scale (Shaffer, Gould, Brasic *et al.*, 1983). These scales can be used to record the longitudinal course of illness and treatment response. The Kiddie Formal Thought Disorder Story Game and Kiddie Formal Thought Disorder Scale (Caplan, Guthrie, Tanguay, Fish, & David-Lando, 1989) are research instruments produced for the assessment of thought disorder in children. Assessments of extrapyramidal symptoms and involuntary movements can be made using the Abnormal Involuntary Movements Scale (AIMS; Rapoport, Conners, & Reatig, 1985) and the Simpson–Angus Neurological Rating Scale (Simpson & Angus, 1970).

Treatment Approaches

General Principles

While antipsychotic drugs remain the cornerstone of treatment in child and adolescent schizophrenia, all young patients with schizophrenia require a multimodal treatment package that includes pharmacotherapy, family and individual counseling, education about the illness, and provision to meet social and educational needs (AACAP, 2001; Clark & Lewis, 1998).

Prevention and Early Detection

In theory at least, the onset of schizophrenia could be prevented if an intervention reduced the premorbid "risk" status or exposure to causative risk factors. The difficulty with the premorbid phenotype as currently conceived (i.e., subtle social and developmental impairments) is its extremely low specificity and positive predictive value for schizophrenia in the general population. The premorbid psychopathology in childhood-onset schizophrenia is equally non-specific with a range of diagnoses (e.g., conduct disorder, ADHD, anxiety states, depression and ASD preceding schizophrenia; Schaeffer & Ross, 2002). Future refinement of the premorbid phenotype is likely to move from the traditional phenomenological approach to include genetic and neurocognitive markers in order to achieve greater sensitivity and specificity.

An alternative approach is to target putative environmental risk factors such as cannabis exposure. If a direct causal relationship between cannabis and schizophrenia is assumed, then the population attributable fraction for the Dunedin cohort is 8% (Arseneault, Cannon, Witton *et al.*, 2004). Put another way, removal of cannabis use from 15-year-olds in the Dunedin cohort would have resulted in an 8% reduction in the incidence of schizophrenia. Given the rising prevalence of cannabis use in younger adolescents – a group who may be particularly sensitive to its effects – an important public policy intervention would be to delay the onset of cannabis use in young people.

In contrast to primary prevention, the aim of early detection is to identify the onset of deterioration in vulnerable individuals with a high predictive validity. Follow-up of the Australian Early Psychosis Prevention and Intervention Centre (EPPIC) "ultra high risk" sample over 12 months found 40.8% developed a psychotic disorder. Significant predictors of transition to psychosis included long duration of prodromal symptoms, poor functioning at intake, low-grade psychotic symptoms, depression and disorganization (Yung, Phillips, Yuen *et al.*, 2003). A key question is whether early intervention in an "ultra high risk" or prodromal group can prevent the transition to psychosis. The EPPIC group conducted a randomized controlled trial of combined low-dose risperidone (mean 1.3 $mg.day^{-1}$) and cognitive–behavioral therapy (CBT) compared to standard needs-based intervention in the "ultra high risk" group (McGorry, Yung, Phillips *et al.*, 2002). The risperidone/CBT intervention significantly reduced transition to psychosis at 6 months (3 of 31 vs. 10 of 28 developed psychosis) but there was no significant difference by 12 months. These findings suggest that aggressive early intervention in a population presenting with high-risk mental states and attenuated psychotic symptoms may delay the onset of frank psychosis (prevalence reduction) but may not necessarily reduce the incidence of psychosis. A pragmatic stance would be to monitor children and adolescents with a strong family history and/or suggestive prodromal symptoms to ensure prompt treatment of psychosis.

A key argument used to support early intervention in psychosis has been the finding that a long duration of untreated psychosis is associated with poor long-term outcome in schizophrenia (Loebel, Lieberman, Alvir *et al.*, 1992; Wyatt, 1995). A similar association has been found in child- and adolescent-onset psychoses (Hollis, 1999). While the association between duration of untreated psychosis and poor outcome seems secure, the causal connection is far less certain. A long duration of untreated psychosis is also associated with insidious onset and negative symptoms, which could confound links with poor outcome. While there are good a priori clinical reasons for the early treatment of symptoms to relieve distress and prevent secondary impairments, as yet it remains unproven whether early intervention actually alters the long-term course of schizophrenia.

Pharmacological Treatments

Because of the very small number of trials of antipsychotics conducted with child and adolescent patients, it is necessary to extrapolate most evidence on drug efficacy from studies in adults. This seems a reasonable approach given that schizophrenia is essentially the same disorder whether it has onset in childhood or adult life. However, it should be noted that children and adolescents show a greater sensitivity to a range of antipsychotic-related adverse events including extrapyramidal side effects (EPS) and treatment resistance with traditional antipsychotics (Kumra, Jacobsen, Lenane *et al.*, 1998b) and weight gain, obesity and metabolic syndrome with the newer atypical antipsychotics (Ratzoni, Gothelf, Brand-Gothelf *et al.*, 2002).

Antipsychotics can be broadly divided into the traditional "typical" and newer "atypical" drugs. The typical drugs include haloperidol, chlorpromazine and trifluoperazine, which block D2 receptors, produce catalepsy in rats, raise plasma prolactin and induce EPS. The newer atypical drugs are effective antipsychotics that are "atypical" in the sense that they do not produce catalepsy, do not raise prolactin levels and produce significantly fewer EPS. Not all atypicals neatly fit this definition; for example, risperidone raises prolactin levels and may cause EPS at higher doses (>4 mg·day^{-1}) with "atypicality" resulting from antagonism of 5HT receptors rather than reduced D2 receptor blockade. The atypicals were introduced during the 1990s and currently include clozapine, risperidone, olanzapine, quetiapine, zotepine and amisulpride. More recently, aripiprazole, a partial dopamine agonist, has been introduced. The pharmacological profile of the atypicals is diverse, involving various combinations of 5HT and dopamine receptor blockade. Aripiprazole acts as a dopamine antagonist at hyperdopaminergic sites (e.g., mesolimibic system in schizophrenia) and as a dopamine agonist at hypodopaminergic sites (e.g., prefrontal cortex in schizophrenia). Interestingly, the therapeutic effects of clozapine (potent affinity for D4 and $5HT_{1,2,3}$ receptors) is independent of D2 receptor occupancy, previously thought to be essential for antipsychotic action.

The typical antipsychotic haloperidol has been shown to be superior to placebo in two double-blind controlled trials of children and adolescents with schizophrenia (Pool, Bloom, Miekle, Roniger, & Gallant, 1976; Spencer & Campbell, 1994). It is estimated that about 70% of patients show good or partial response to antipsychotic treatment although this may take 6–8 weeks to become apparent (AACAP, 2001; Clark & Lewis, 1998). The main drawbacks concerning the use of high-potency typicals such as haloperidol in children and adolescents is the high risk of EPS (produced by D2 blockade of the nigrostriatal pathway), tardive dyskinesia and the lack of effect against negative symptoms and cognitive impairment. Clozapine (the prototypic atypical) has been shown to be superior to haloperidol in a double-blind trial of 21 cases of childhood-onset schizophrenia (Kumra, Frazier, Jacobsen *et al.*, 1996). Larger open clinical trials of clozapine confirm its effectiveness in child- and adolescent-onset schizophrenia (Remschmidt, Schultz, & Martin, 1994). Similar, although less marked, benefits of olanzapine over typical antipsychotics in childhood-onset schizophrenia have been reported (Kumra, Jacobsen, Lenane *et al.*, 1998a).

Recent head-to-head comparisons of atypicals (risperidone and olanzapine) vs. typicals (haloperidol) in adolescents with schizophrenia have reported broadly similar efficacy against psychotic symptoms (with a non-significant trend in favor of atypicals) but a differing profile of adverse effects (Gothelf, Apter, Reidman *et al.*, 2003; Sikich, Hamer, Bashford, Sheitman, & Lieberman, 2004). These finding broadly replicate results from the large NIMH-CATIE pragmatic trial that found no overall difference in effectiveness between typical and atypical antipsychotics in adults, whereas there were differences in tolerability and side effect profiles (Lieberman, Stroup, McEvoy *et al.*, 2005). The UK CUtLASS study compared effects after randomization to either typical or atypical antipsychotics following a clinical decision to change medication in adults with chronic schizophrenia (Jones, Barnes, Davies *et al.*, 2006). There were no differences in outcome (quality of life, symptoms and adverse events) measured at 1 year when comparing the broad classes of typical and atypical antipsychotic. While similar pragmatic clinical effectiveness studies are needed in children and adolescents with schizophrenia, we know that younger and first-episode patients are more sensitive to both therapeutic and adverse effects of antipsychotics. Furthermore, individual drugs within both classes differ importantly in terms of tolerability and side effect profiles when prescribed to children and adolescents. In younger patients (children and adolescents), EPS are more common with haloperidol and high-dose risperidone than olanzapine. Weight gain and obesity are more common with olanzapine (most), then risperidone and least with haloperidol. Sedation is greater with olanzapine and haloperiol than risperidone (Toren, Ratner, Laor, & Weizman, 2004). Further evidence is emerging that children and adolescents experience more rapid and serious weight gain on olanzapine and risperidone than do adults (Ratzoni, Gothelf, Brand-Gothelf *et al.*, 2002). Morbid obesity (body mass index [BMI] >90th percentile) is found in up to 50% of adolescents and young people chronically treated with atypical antipsychotics (Theisen, Linden, Geller *et al.*, 2001). Complications of obesity include hyperglycemia (type 2 diabetes), hyperlipidemia and hypercholesterolemia. It is recommended that dietary advice (reducing carbohydrate intake) combined with regular exercise should be prescribed before initiating atypicals in children and adolescents.

Drawing this evidence together, a strong case can be made for the first-line use of atypicals in child and adolescent schizophrenia (clozapine is licensed in the UK only for treatment-resistant schizophrenia). Treatment resistance in child and adolescent patients should be defined as follows:

1 Non-response with at least two antipsychotics (drawn from different classes and at least one being an atypical), each used for at least 4–6 weeks; and/or

2 Significant adverse effects with conventional antipsychotics.

The recommended order of treatment for first-episode schizophrenia in children and adolescents is as follows: atypical as first line, if inadequate response change to a different atypical or conventional antispyschotic, if response is still inadequate or side effects are intolerable then initiate clozapine.

While atypicals reduce the risk of EPS, they can produce other troublesome side effects (usually dose-related) including weight gain (olanzapine, clozapine, risperidone), hyperlipidemia (olanzapine), sedation, hypersalivation and seizures (clozapine, olanzapine, quetiapine) and hyperprolactinemia (risperidone, amisulpride). The risk of blood dyscrasias on clozapine is effectively managed by mandatory routine blood monitoring.

However, knowledge about potential adverse reactions with the newest atypicals is still limited in child and adolescent patients. Baseline investigations and follow-up monitoring every 6 months are recommended when prescribing antipsychotics. Baseline monitoring should include height, weight, blood pressure, full blood count, liver function and creatine kinase, fasting glucose, prolactin (risperidone, amisulpride), lipids (olanzapine, clozapine) and electrocardiogram (ECG) (zotapine). A further consideration is the greater cost of newer atypicals compared to traditional antipsychotics. Although economic studies of cost-effectiveness have suggested that the costs of the atypicals are recouped in reduced in-patient stays and indirect social costs (Aitcheson & Kerwin, 1997), the high cost of these drugs may limit availability, particularly in developing countries.

The UK National Institute for Health and Clinical Excellence (NICE, 2002) has recommended the use of atypicals (risperidone, olanzapine, quetiapine, amisulpride and zotapine) in all first-episode, newly diagnosed patients with schizophrenia and those on established therapy showing resistance to typical antipsychotics. Clinical trial evidence suggests that clozapine is the most effective antipsychotic in child- and adolescent-onset schizophrenia, although its use is restricted to treatment-resistant cases. In summary, atypicals such as olanzapine or risperidone should be used as a first-line treatment given that child- and adolescent-onset schizophrenia is characterized by negative symptoms, cognitive impairments, sensitivity to EPS and relative resistance to traditional antipsychotics. However, a growing awareness of adverse effect profiles of different drugs and greater sensitivity to these effects in children and adolescents means drug choice should be a collaborative exercise, tailored to the needs and preferences of the young person and their family.

Psychosocial Interventions

Psychosocial interventions range from CBT targeted at symptoms, problem-solving skills and stress reduction, to patient and family psychoeducation, family therapy, counseling and support, social skills training and remedial education.

Psychoeducation and Family Interventions

The rationale for psychosocial family interventions follows from the association between high EE and the risk of relapse in schizophrenia (Dixon & Lehman, 1995). The overall aim is to prevent relapse (secondary prevention) and improve the patient's level of functioning by modifying the family atmosphere. Psychosocial family interventions have a number of principles in common (Lam, 1991). First, it is assumed that it is useful to regard schizophrenia as an illness as patients are less likely to be seen as responsible for their symptoms and behavior. Second, the family is not implicated in the etiology of the illness. Instead, the burden borne by the family in caring for a disturbed or severely impaired young person is acknowledged. Third, the intervention is offered as part of a broader multimodal package including drug treatment and out-patient clinical management.

An important issue when working with parents of children and adolescents with schizophrenia is to recognize that the illness typically results in a bereavement process for the loss of their "normal" child. Parents will often value a clear diagnosis of schizophrenia as it can provide an explanation for previously unexplained perplexing and disturbed behavior. Understanding schizophrenia as a disorder of the developing brain can also relieve commonly expressed feelings of guilt among parents and carers.

Lam (1991) conducted a systematic review of published trials of psychoeducation and more intensive family interventions in schizophrenia and drew the following conclusions. First, education packages on their own increase knowledge about the illness but do not reduce the risk of relapse. Second, more intensive family intervention studies with high EE relatives have shown a reduction in relapse rates linked to a lowering of EE. Third, family interventions tend to be costly and time-consuming with most clinical trials employing highly skilled research teams. Whether these interventions can be transferred into routine clinical practice is uncertain. Fourth, interventions have focused on the reduction of EE in "high-risk" families. Whether low EE families would also benefit from these interventions is less clear. This is particularly relevant to the families of children and adolescents with schizophrenia as, on average, these parents express *lower* levels of criticism and hostility than parents of adult-onset patients (Asarnow, Thompson, Hamilton *et al.*, 1994).

Cognitive–Behavioral Therapy

In adult patients, cognitive-behavioral therapy (CBT) has been used to reduce the impact of treatment-resistant positive symptoms (Tarrier, Beckett, Harwood *et al.*, 1993). CBT has been shown to improve the shortterm (6 month) outcome of adult schizophrenic patients with neuroleptic-resistant positive symptoms (Turkington & Kingdon, 2000). Whether CBT is equally effective with younger patients, or those with predominantly negative symptoms, remains to be established.

Cognitive Remediation

Cognitive remediation is a relatively new psychological treatment that aims to arrest or reverse the cognitive impairments in attention, concentration and working memory associated with negative symptoms and poor functional outcome in schizophrenia (Greenwood, Landau, & Wykes, 2005). The results of an early controlled trial in adults are promising, with gains found in the areas of memory and social functioning (Wykes, Reeder, Williams *et al.*, 2000). The severity of cognitive executive impairments in child and adolescent patients suggests that early remediation strategies may be a particularly important intervention in younger patients. Helpful advice can also be offered to parents, teachers and professionals such as breaking down information and tasks into small manageable parts to reduce demands on working memory and speed of processing.

Organization of Treatment Services

It is a paradox that patients with very early-onset schizophrenia have the most severe form of the disorder yet they often receive inadequate and poorly co-ordinated services. Possibly, this is because the responsibility for schizophrenia is seen to lie with adult psychiatric services with a remit that typically does not extend to patients under age 18. In the UK, community-based child and adolescent mental health services (CAMHS) provide the first-line assessment and care for child and young adolescent psychoses, with only about half of these cases referred to in-patient units (Slaveska, Hollis, & Bramble, 1998). Whereas adolescent in-patient admission is often inappropriate, generic CAMHS services are usually unable to provide the mix of assertive outreach, early intervention and crisis resolution services that have developed over the last decade in UK adult mental health services for psychoses and severe mental illness. Young people with schizophrenia are not generally well served by a separation of services and professional responsibilities at age 16 or 18 (see chapter 13). An alternative model is a community-based young person's psychosis service spanning ages 14–25 with access to dedicated adolescent and young adult beds. Such a service would provide early intervention, assertive outreach, intensive home treatment and crisis resolution. It would integrate professional expertise from CAMHS (in particular, addressing family, developmental and educational issues) and adult mental health services.

Conclusions

The last decade has seen a dramatic growth in our understanding of the clinical course and neurobiological underpinnings of schizophrenia presenting in childhood and adolescence. It is now clear that adult-based diagnostic criteria have validity in this age group and the disorder has clinical and neurobiological continuity with schizophrenia in adults. Childhood-onset schizophrenia is a severe variant of the adult disorder associated with greater premorbid impairment, a higher familial risk, more severe clinical course and poorer outcome. The poor outcome of children and adolescents with schizophrenia has highlighted the need to target early and effective treatments and develop specialist services for this high-risk group. Unraveling neurocognitive and clinical heterogeneity should lead to improvements in our ability to deliver individually targeted treatments, as well as the ability to identify those "at risk" in order to prevent the onset of psychosis.

Further Reading

Harrison, P. J., & Owen, M. J. (2003). Genes for schizophrenia? Recent findings and their pathophysiological implications. *Lancet*, *361*, 417–419.

Hirsch, S. R., & Weinberger, D. (Eds.). (2003). *Schizophrenia* (2nd edn.). Oxford: Blackwell.

Rapoport, J. L., Addington, A. M., & Frangou, S. (2005). The neurodevelopmental model of schizophrenia: update, 2005. *Molecular Psychiatry*, *10*, 434–449.

References

Addington, A. M., Gornick, M., Duckworth, J. Sporn, A., Gogtay, N., Bobb, A., *et al.* (2005). GAD1 (2q31.1), which encodes glutamic acid decarboxylase (GAD67), is associated with childhood-onset schizophrenia and cortical gray matter loss. *Molecular Psychiatry*, *10*, 581–588.

Addington, A. M., Gornick, M., Sporn, A. L. Gogtay, N., Greenstein, D., Lenane, M. C., *et al.* (2004). Polymorphisms in the 13q33.2 gene G72/G30 are associated with childhood-onset schizophrenia and psychosis not otherwise specified. *Biological Psychiatry*, *55*, 976–980.

Aitchison, K. J., & Kerwin, R. W. (1997). The cost effectiveness of clozapine. *British Journal of Psychiatry*, *171*, 125–130.

Alaghband-Rad, J., McKenna, K., Gordon, C. T., Albus, K. E., Hamburger, S. D., Rumsey, J. M., *et al.* (1995). Childhood-onset schizophrenia: The severity of premorbid course. *Journal of the American Academy of Child and Adolescent Psychiatry*, *34*, 1273–1283.

Alaghband-Rad, J., Hamburger, S. D., Giedd, J., Frazier, J. A., & Rapoport, J. L. (1997). Childhood-onset schizophrenia: Biological markers in relation to clinical characteristics. *American Journal of Psychiatry*, *154*, 64–68.

Ambrosini, P. J. (2000). Historical development and present status of the Schedule for Affective Disorders and Schizophrenia for School-Age Children (K-SADS). *Journal of the American Academy of Child and Adolescent Psychiatry*, *39*, 49–58.

American Academy of Child and Adolescent Psychiatry (AACAP). (2001). Practice parameter for the assessment and treatment of children and adolescents with schizophrenia. *Journal of the American Academy of Child and Adolescent Psychiatry*, *40*, 4S–23S.

Andreasen, N. C. (1983). *Scale for the Assessment of Negative Symptoms (SANS)*. University of Iowa: Iowa City.

Andreasen, N. C. (1984). *Scale for the Assessment of Positive Symptoms (SAPS)*. University of Iowa: Iowa City.

Angold, A., & Costello, J. E. (2000). The Child and Adolescent Psychiatric Assessment (CAPA). *Journal of the American Academy of Child and Adolescent Psychiatry*, *39*, 39–48.

American Psychiatric Association. (2000). *Diagnostic and Statistical Manual of Mental Disorders* (4th en.). Text revision. Washington, DC: American Psychiatric Association.

Arendt, M., Rosenberg, R., Foldager, L., Perto, G., & Munk-Jorgensen, P. (2005). Cannabis-induced psychosis and subsequent schizophrenia-spectrum disorders: follow-up study of 535 incident cases. *British Journal of Psychiatry*, *187*, 510–515.

Arseneault, L., Cannon, M., Poulton, R., Murray, R., Caspi, A., & Moffitt, T. E. (2002). Cannabis use in adolescence and risk for adult psychosis: Longitudinal prospective study. *British Medical Journal*, *325*, 1212–1213.

Arseneault, L., Cannon, M., Witton, J., & Murray, R. (2004). Causal association between cannabis and psychosis: Examination of the evidence. *British Journal of Psychiatry*, *184*, 110–117.

Asarnow, J. R. (2005). Childhood-onset schizotypal disorder: A follow-up study and comparison with childhood-onset schizophrenia. *Journal of Child and Adolescent Psychopharmacology*, *15*, 395–402.

Asarnow, R., Granholm, E., & Sherman, T. (1991). Span of apprehension in schizophrenia. In: S. R. Steinhauer, J. H. Gruzelier, & J. Zubin (Eds.), *Handbook of Schizophrenia*, Vol. 5. *Neuropsychology, Psychophysiology and Information Processing* (pp. 335–370). Amsterdam: Elsevier.

Asarnow, J. R., Thompson, M. C., Hamilton, E. B., Goldstein, M. J., & Guthrie, D. (1994). Family-expressed emotion, childhood-onset depression, and childhood-onset schizophrenia spectrum disorders: Is expressed emotion a nonspecific correlate of child psychopathology or a specific risk factor for depression? *Journal of Abnormal Child Psychology*, *22*, 129–146.

Asarnow, R., Brown, W., & Stranberg, R. (1995). Children with schizophrenic disorder: Neurobehavioural studies. *Neuroscience European Archives of Psychiatry and Clinical Neuroscience*, *245*, 70–79.

Badner, J. A., & Gershon, E. S. (2002). Meta-analysis of whole-genome linkage scans of bipolar disorder and schizophrenia. *Molecular Psychiatry*, *7*, 405–411.

Bertolino, A., Kumra, S., Callicott, J. H., Muttay, V. S., Lestz, R. M., Jacobsen, L., *et al.* (1998). Common pattern of cortical pathology in childhood-onset and adult-onset schizophrenia as identified by proton magnetic resonance spectroscopic imaging. *American Journal of Psychiatry*, *155*, 1376–1383.

Breier, A. (1999). Cognitive deficit in schizophrenia and its neurochemical basis. *British Journal of Psychiatry*, *174*, 16–18.

Broome, M. R., Woolley, J. B., Tabraham, P., Johns, L. C., Bramon E., Murray, G. K., *et al.* (2005). What causes the onset of psychosis? *Schizophrenia Research*, *79*, 23–34.

Bullmore, E. T., O'Connell, P., Frangou, S., & Murray, R. M. (1997). Schizophrenia as a developmental disorder or neural network integrity: The dysplastic net hypothesis. In M. S. Keshavan, & R. M. Murray (Eds.), *Neurodevelopment and adult psychopathology* (pp. 253–266). Cambridge: Cambridge University Press.

Cannon, M., Caspi, A., Moffitt, T. E., Harrington, H., Taylor, A., Murray, R. M., *et al.* (2002). Evidence for early childhood, pan-developmental impairment specific to schizophreniform disorder: Results from a longitudinal birth cohort. *Archives of General Psychiatry*, *59*, 449–456.

Cannon, T. D., Kaprio, J., Lonnqvist, J., Huttunen, M., & Koskenvuo, M. (1998). The genetic epidemiology of schizophrenia in a Finnish twin cohort: A population-based modeling study. *Archives of General Psychiatry*, *55*, 67–74.

Cantor-Graae, E., & Selten, J. P. (2005). Schizophrenia and migration: A meta-analysis and review. *American Journal of Psychiatry*, *162*, 12–24.

Caplan, R., Guthrie, D., Tanguay, P. E., Fish, B., & David-Lando, G. (1989). The Kiddie Formal Thought Disorder Scale (K-FTDS): Clinical assessment reliability and validity. *Journal of the American Academy of Child and Adolescent Psychiatry*, *28*, 408–416.

Caplan, R., Guthrie, D., Shields, W. D., & Mori, L. (1992). Formal thought disorder in pediatric complex partial seizure disorder. *Journal of Child Psychology and Psychiatry*, *33*, 1399–1412.

Caspi, A., Moffitt, T. E., Cannon, M., McClay, J., Murray, R., Harrington, H., *et al.* (2005). Moderation of the effect of adolescent-onset cannabis use on adult psychosis by a functional polymorphism in the catechol-O-methyltransferase gene: Longitudinal evidence of a gene × environment interaction. *Biological Psychiatry*, *57*, 1117–1127.

Castle, D., & Murray, R. (1991). The neurodevelopmental basis of sex differences in schizophrenia. *Psychological Medicine*, *21*, 565–575.

Clark, A., & Lewis, S. (1998). Treatment of schizophrenia in childhood and adolescence. *Journal of Child Psychology and Psychiatry*, *39*, 1071–1081.

Clegg, J., Hollis, C., & Rutter, M. (2005). Developmental language disorders: A follow-up in later adult life. Cognitive, language and psychosocial outcomes. *Journal of Child Psychology and Psychiatry*, *46*, 128–149.

Craddock, N., O'Donovan, M. C., & Owen, M. J. (2005). Genes for schizophrenia and bipolar disorder? Implications for psychiatric nosology. *Schizophrenia Bulletin*, *32*, 9–16.

Dasari, M., Friedman, L., Jesberger, J., Stuve, T. A., Findling, R. L., Swales, T. P., *et al.* (1999). A magnetic resonance study of thalamic area in adolescent patients with either schizophrenia or bipolar disorder as compared to healthy controls. *Psychiatry Research*, *91*, 155–162.

Dean, B., Bradbury, R., & Copolov, D. L. (2003). Cannabis-sensitive dopaminergic markers in postmortem central nervous system: changes in schizophrenia. *Biological Psychiatry*, *53*, 585–592.

Dixon, L. B., & Lehman, A. F. (1995). Family interventions for schizophrenia. *Schizophrenia Bulletin*, *21*, 631–643.

Egan, M. F., Goldberg, T. E., Kolachana, B. S., Callicott, J. H., Mazzanti, C. M., Straub, R. E., *et al.* (2001). Effect of COMT Val108/158Met genotype on frontal lobe function and risk for schizophrenia. *Proceedings of the National Academy of Sciences of the USA*, *98*, 6917–6922.

Eggers, C., & Bunk, D. (1997). The long-term course of childhood-onset schizophrenia: A 42-year follow-up. *Schizophrenia Bulletin*, *23*, 105–117.

Erlenmeyer-Kimling, L., & Cornblatt, B. (1978). Attentional measures in a study of children at high risk for schizophrenia. In L. C. Wynne, R. L. Cromwell, & S. Matthysse (Eds.), *The Nature of Schizophrenia: New approaches to research and treatment* (pp. 359–365). New York: Wiley.

Erlenmeyer-Kimling, L., Squires-Wheeler, E., Adamo, U. H., Rock, D., Roberts, S. A., Bassett, A. S., *et al.* (1995). The New York High Risk Project: Psychoses and Cluster A personality disorders in offspring of schizophrenic parents at 23 years of follow-up. *Archives of General Psychiatry*, *52*, 857–865.

Feinberg, I. (1983). Schizophrenia: Caused by a fault in programmed synaptic elimination during adolescence. *Journal of Psychiatric Research*, *17*, 319–344.

Fields, J. H., Grochowski, S., Lindenmayer, J. P., Kay, S. R., Grosz, D., Hyman, R. B., *et al.* (1994). Assessing positive and negative symptoms in children and adolescents. *American Journal of Psychiatry*, *151*, 249–253.

Fleischhacker, C., Schulz, R., Tepper, K., Martin, M., Hennighausen, K., & Remschmidt, H. (2005). Long-term course of adolescent schizophrenia. *Schizophrenia Bulletin*, *31*, 769–780.

Frazier, J. A., Giedd, J. N., Kaysen, D., Albus, K., Hamburger, S., Alaghband-Rad, J., *et al.* (1996). Childhood-onset schizophrenia: Brain magnetic resonance imaging rescan after two years of clozapine maintenance. *American Journal of Psychiatry*, *153*, 564–566.

Friedman, L., Findling, R. L., Buch, J., Cola, D. M., Swales, T. P., Kenny, J. T., *et al.* (1996). Structural MRI and neuropsychological assesments in adolescent patients with either schizophrenia or affective disorders. *Schizophrenia Research*, *18*, 189–190.

Feinberg, I. (1997). Schizophrenia as an emergent disorder of late brain maturation. In: M. S. Keshervan, & R. M. Murray (Eds), Neurodevelopment and Adult Psychopathology. Cambridge University Press: Cambridge (pp. 237–252).

Frith, C. D. (1994). Theory of mind in schizophrenia. In A. David, & J. S. Cutting (Eds.), *The Neuropsychology of Schizophrenia* (pp. 147–161). Hove: Lawrence Erlbaum.

Galdos, P. M., van Os, J., & Murray, R. (1993). Puberty and the onset of psychosis. *Schizophrenia Research*, *10*, 7–14.

Gallhofer, B., Trimble, M. R., Frackowiak, R., Gibbs, J., & Jones, T. (1985). A study of cerebral blood flow and metabolism in epileptic psychosis using positron emission tomography and oxygen. *Journal of Neurology Neurosurgery and Psychiatry*, *48*, 201–206.

Garralda, M. E. (1984). Hallucinations in children with conduct and emotional disorders. I. The clinical phenomena. *Psychological Medicine*, *14*, 589–596.

Geddes, J. R., & Lawrie, S. M. (1995). Obstetric complications and schizophrenia: A meta-analysis. *British Journal of Psychiatry*, *167*, 786–793.

Gervin, M., Browne, S., Lane, A., Clarke, M., Waddington, J. L., Larkin, C., *et al.* (1998). Spontaneous abnormal involuntary movements in first-episode schizophrenia and schizophreniform disorder: Baseline rate in a group of patients from an Irish catchment area. *American Journal of Psychiatry*, *155*, 1202–1206.

Giedd, J. N., Castellanos, F. X., Rajapakse, J. C., Vaituzis, A. C., & Rapoport, J. L. (1996). Quantitative analysis of grey matter volumes in childhood-onset schizophrenia and attention deficit/hyperactivity disorder. *Society for Neuroscience Abstracts*, *22*, 1166.

Giedd, J. N., Jeffries, N. O., Blumenthal, J., Castellanos, F. X., Vaituzis, A. C., Fernandez, T., *et al.* (1999). Childhood-onset schizophrenia: Progressive brain changes during adolescence. *Biological Psychiatry*, *46*, 892–898.

Gillberg, C., Wahlstrom, J., Forsman, A., Hellgren, L., & Gillberg, J. C. (1986). Teenage psychoses: Epidemiology, classification and reduced optimality in the pre-, peri- and neonatal periods. *Journal of Child Psychology and Psychiatry*, *27*, 87–98.

Glantz, L. A., & Lewis, D. A. (2000). Decreased dendritic spine density on prefrontal cortical pyramidal neurons in schizophrenia. *Archives of General Psychiatry*, *57*, 65–73.

Gochman, P. A., Greenstein, D., Sporn, A., Gogtay, N., Keller, B., Shaw, P., *et al.* (2005). IQ stabilization in childhood-onset schizophrenia. *Schizophrenia Research*, *77*, 271–277.

Goldstein, M. J. (1987). The UCLA High-Risk Project. *Schizophrenia Bulletin*, *13*, 505–514.

Goodman, R. (1988). Are complications of pregnancy and birth causes of schizophrenia? *Developmental Medicine and Child Neurology*, *30*, 391–406.

Gogtay, N., Sporn, A., Clasen, L. S., Nugent, T. F. 3rd., Greenstein, D., Nicholson, R., *et al.* (2004). Comparison of progressive cortical gray matter loss in childhood-onset schizophrenia and that in childhood-onset atypical psychoses. *Archives of General Psychiatry*, *61*, 17–22.

Gordon, C. T., Frazier, J. A., McKenna, K., Giedd, J., Zametkin, A., Zahn, T., *et al.* (1994). Childhood-onset schizophrenia: A NIMH study in progress. *Schizophrenia Bulletin*, *20*, 697–712.

Gothelf, D., Apter, A., Reidman, J., Brand-Gothelf, A., Bloch, Y., Gal, G., *et al.* (2003). Olanzapine, risperidone and haloperidol in the treatment of adolescent patients with schizophrenia. *Journal of Neural Transmission*, *110*, 545–560.

Green, W., Padron-Gayol, M., Hardesty, A., & Bassiri, M. (1992). Schizophrenia with childhood onset: a phenomenological study of 38 cases. *Journal of the American Academy of Child and Adolescent Psychiatry*, *31*, 968–976.

Greenwood, K. E., Landau, S., & Wykes, T. (2005). Negative symptoms and specific cognitive impairments as combined targets for improved functional outcome within cognitive remediation therapy. *Schizophrenia Bulletin*, *31*, 910–921.

Gualtieri, C. T., Adams, A., & Chen, C. D. (1982). Minor physical abnormalities in alcoholic and schizophrenic adults and hyperactive and autistic children. *American Journal of Psychiatry*, *139*, 640–643.

Gur, R. E., Cowell, P., Turetsky, B. I., Gallacher, F., Cannon, T., Bilker, W., *et al.* (1998). A follow-up magnetic resonance imaging study of schizophrenia: Relationship of neuroanatomical changes to clinical and neurobehavioral measures. *Archives of General Psychiatry*, *55*, 145–152.

Gur, R. E., Cowell, P., Latshaw, A., Turetsky, B. I., Grossmand, R. I., Arnold, S. E., *et al.* (2000a). Reduced dorsal and orbital prefrontal gray matter volumes in schizophrenia. *Archives of General Psychiatry*, *57*, 761–768.

Gur, R. E., Turetsky, B. I., Cowell, P., Finkelman, C., Maany, V., Grossman, R. I., *et al.* (2000b). Temporolimbic volume reductions in schizophrenia. *Archives of General Psychiatry*, *57*, 769–775.

Hafner, H., & Nowotny, B. (1995). Epidemiology of early-onset schizophrenia. *European Archives of Psychiatry and Clinical Neuroscience*, *245*, 80–92.

Harrison, P. J., & Owen, M. J. (2003). Genes for schizophrenia? Recent findings and their pathophysiological implications. *Lancet*, *361*, 417–419.

Harrison, P. J., & Weinberger, D. R. (2005). Schizophrenia genes, gene expression, and neuropathology: On the matter of their convergence. *Molecular Psychiatry*, *10*, 40–68.

Hennah, W., Thompson, P., Peltonen, L., & Porteous, D. (2006). Genes and schizoprenia: Beyond schizophrenia: The role of DISC1 in major mental illness. *Schizophrenia Bulletin*, *32*, 409–416.

Hollis, C. (1995). Child and adolescent (juvenile onset) schizophrenia: A case–control study of premorbid developmental impairments. *British Journal of Psychiatry*, *166*, 489–495.

Hollis, C. (1999). *A study of the course and adult outcomes of child and adolescent-onset psychoses*. PhD Thesis, University of London.

Hollis, C. (2000). The adult outcomes of child and adolescent-onset schizophrenia: Diagnostic stability and predictive validity. *American Journal of Psychiatry*, *157*, 1652–1659.

Hollis, C. (2003). Developmental precursors of child- and adolescent-onset schizophrenia and affective psychoses: Diagnostic specificity and continuity with symptom dimensions. *British Journal of Psychiatry*, *182*, 37–44.

Hollis, C., & Taylor, E. (1997). Schizophrenia: A critique from the developmental psychopathology perspective. In M. S. Keshavan, & R. M. Murray (Eds.), *Neurodevelopment and adult psychopathology* (pp. 213–233). Cambridge: Cambridge University Press.

Hooley, J. M. (1987). The nature and origins of expressed emotion. In K. Hahlweg, & M. J. Goldstein (Eds.), *Understanding major mental disorder: The contribution of family interaction research* (pp. 176–194). New York: Family Process.

Iacono, W. G., & Koenig, W. G. R. (1983). Features that distinguish smooth the pursuit eye-tracking performance of schizophrenic, affective-disorder, and normal individuals. *Journal of Abnormal Psychology*, *92*, 29–41.

Jacobsen, L., Giedd, J. N., Berquin, P. C., Krain, A. L., Hamburger, S. D., Kumra, S., *et al.* (1997a). Quantitative morphology of the cerebellum and fourth ventricle in childhood-onset schizophrenia. *American Journal of Psychiatry*, *154*, 1663–1669.

Jacobsen, L., Hamburger, S. D., Van Horn, J. D., Vaituzis, A. C., McKenna, K., Frazier, J. A., *et al.* (1997b). Cerebral glucose metabolism in childhood-onset schizophrenia. *Psychiatry Research*, *75*, 131–144.

Jacobsen, L., & Rapoport, J. (1998). Research update: Childhood-onset schizophrenia: Implications for clinical and neurobiological research. *Journal of Child Psychology and Psychiatry*, *39*, 101–113.

James, A. C. D., Javaloyes, A., James, S., & Smith, D. M. (2002). Evidence for non-progressive changes in adolescent-onset schizophrenia: Follow-up magnetic resonance imaging study. *British Journal of Psychiatry*, *180*, 339–344.

James, A. C. D., Smith, D. M., & Jayaloes, J. S. (2004). Cerebellar, prefrontal cortex, and thalamic volumes over two time points in adolescent-onset schizophrenia. *American Journal of Psychiatry*, *161*, 1023–1029.

Jarbin, H., Ott, Y., & Von Knorring, A. L. (2003). Adult outcome of social function in adolescent-onset schizophrenia and affective psychosis. *Journal of the American Academy of Child and Adolescent Psychiatry*, *42*, 176–183.

Jones, P., Rogers, B., Murray, R., & Marmot, M. (1994). Child development risk factors for adult schizophrenia in the British, 1946 birth cohort. *Lancet*, *344*, 1398–1402.

Jones, P. B., Barnes, T. R., Davies, L., Dunn, G., Lloyd, H., Hayhurst, K. P., *et al.* (2006). Randomized controlled trial of the effect on Quality of Life of second- vs. first-generation antipsychotic drugs in schizophrenia: Cost Utility of the Latest Antipsychotic Drugs in Schizophrenia Study (CUTLASS 1). *Archives of General Psychiatry*, *63*, 1079–1087.

Joyce, P. R. (1984). Age of onset in bipolar affective disorder and misdiagnosis of schizophrenia. *Psychological Medicine*, *14*, 145–149.

Karayiorgou, M., Morris, M. A., Morrow, B., Shprintzen, R. J., Goldberg, R., Borrow, J., *et al.* (1995). Schizophrenia susceptibility associated with interstitial deletions of chromosome 22q11. *Proceedings of the National Academy of Sciences of the USA*, *92*, 7612–7616.

Kay, S. R., Opler, L. A., & Lindenmayer, J. P. (1987). The Positive and Negative Syndrome Scale (PANSS) for schizophrenia. *Schizophrenia Bulletin*, *13*, 261–276.

Keller, A., Castellanos, F., Vaituzis, C. A., Jefferies, N. O., Giedd, J. N., & Rapoport, J. L. (2003). Progressive loss of cerebellar volume in childhood-onset schizophrenia. *American Journal of Psychiatry*, *160*, 128–133.

Kendall, R. E., McInneny, K., Juszczak, E., & Bain, M. (2000). Obstetric complications and schizophrenia: Two case–control studies based on structured obstetric records. *British Journal of Psychiatry*, *176*, 516–522.

Kendler, K. C., Neale, M. C., & Walsh, D. (1995). Evaluating the spectrum concept of schizophrenia in the Roscommon Family Study. *American Journal of Psychiatry*, *152*, 749–754.

Kerns, J. G., Cohen, J. D., MacDonald, A. W., Johnson, M. K., Stenger, V. A., Aizenstein, H., *et al.* (2005). Decreased conflict- and error-related activity in the anterior cingulate cortex in subjects with schizophrenia. *American Journal of Psychiatry*, *162*, 1833–1839.

Keshavan, M. S., Stanley, J. A., Montrose, D. M., Minshew, N. J., & Pettegrew, J. W. (2003). Prefrontal membrane phospholipid metabolism of child and adolescent offspring at risk for schizophrenia or schizoaffective disorder: An *in vivo* 31p MRS study. *Molecular Psychiatry*, *8*, 316–323, 251.

Kim-Cohen, J., Caspi, A., Moffitt, T. E., Harrington, H., Milne, B. J., & Poulton, R. (2003). Prior juvenile diagnosis in adults with mental disorder: Developmental follow-back of a prospective longitudinal cohort. *Archives of General Psychiatry*, *60*, 709–717.

Krystal, J. H., Perry, E. B., Gueorguieva, R., Belger, A., Madonick, S. H., Abi-Dargham, A., *et al.* (2006). Comparative and interactive human psychopharmacologic effects of ketamine and amphetamine: Implications for glutamatergic and dopaminergic model psychoses and cognitive function. *Archives of General Psychiatry*, *62*, 985–995.

Kumra, S., Frazier, J. A., Jacobsen, L. K., McKenna, K., Gordon, C. T., Lenane, M. C., *et al.* (1996). Childhood-onset schizophrenia: A double blind clozapine–haloperidol comparison. *Archives of General Psychiatry*, *53*, 1090–1097.

Kumra, S., Jacobsen, L. K., Lenane, M., Karp, B. I., Frazier, J. A., Smith, A. K., *et al.* (1998a). Childhood-onset schizophrenia: An open-label study of olanzapine in adolescents. *Journal of the American Academy of Child and Adolescent Psychiatry*, *37*, 360–363.

Kumra, S., Jacobsen, L. K., Lenane, M., Smith, A., Lee, P., Malanga, C. J., *et al.* (1998b). Case series: Spectrum of neuroleptic-induced movement disorders and extrapyramidal side-effects in childhood-onset schizophrenia. *Journal of the American Academy of Child and Adolescent Psychiatry*, *37*, 221–227.

Kumra, S., Jacobsen, L. K., Lenane, M., Zahn, T. P., Wiggs, E., Alaghband-Rad, J., *et al.* (1998c). "Multidimensionally impaired disorder": Is it a variant of very early-onset schizophrenia? *Journal of the American Academy of Child and Adolescent Psychiatry*, *37*, 91–99.

Kumra, S., Sporn, A., Hommer, D. W., Nicholson, R., Thaker, G., Israel, E., *et al.* (2001). Smooth pursuit eye-tracking impairment in childhood-onset psychotic disorders. *American Journal of Psychiatry*, *158*, 1291–1298.

Lam, D. H. (1991). Psychosocial family intervention in schizophrenia: A review of empirical studies. *Psychological Medicine*, *21*, 423–441.

Lawrie, S. M., & Abukmeil, S. S. (1998). Brain abnormalities in schizophrenia: A systematic and quantitative review of volumetric magnetic resonance imaging studies. *British Journal of Psychiatry*, *172*, 110–120.

Lay, B., Blanz, B., Hartmann, M., & Schmidt, M. H. (2000). The psychosocial outcome of adolescent-onset schizophrenia: A 12-year follow-up. *Schizophrenia Bulletin*, *26*, 801–816.

Leff, J., & Vaughn, C. (1985). *Expressed emotion in families: Its significance for mental illness*. Guilford Press: London.

Lewis, C. M., Levinson, D. F., Wise, L. H., DeLisi, L. E., Straub, R. E., Hovatta, I., *et al.* (2003). Genome scan meta-analysis of schizophrenia and bipolar disorder. II. Schizophrenia. *American Journal of Human Genetics*, *73*, 34–48.

Lewis, S. W., & Murray, R. M. (1987). Obstetric complications, neurodevelopmental deviance and risk of schizophrenia. *Journal of Psychiatric Research*, *21*, 414–421.

Liddle, P. (1987). The symptoms of chronic schizophrenia: A re-examination of the positive–negative dichotomy. *British Journal of Psychiatry*, *151*, 145–151.

Liddle, P., & Pantelis, C. (2003). Brain imaging in schizophrenia. In S. R. Hirsch, & D. R. Weinberger (Eds.), *Schizophrenia* (2nd edn.). Oxford: Blackwell.

Lieberman, J. A., Stroup, T. S., McEvoy, J. P., Swartz, M. S., Rosenheck, R. A., Perkins, D. O., *et al.* (2005). Effectiveness of antipsychotic drugs in patients with chronic schizophrenia. *New England Journal of Medicine*, *353*, 1209–1223.

Lindsay, J., Ounsted, C., & Richards, P. (1979). Long-term outcome of children with temporal lobe seizures. II. Marriage, parenthood and sexual indifference. *Developmental Medicine and Child Neurology*, *21*, 433–440.

Loebel, A. D., Lieberman, J. A., Alvir, J. M., Mayerhoff, D. I., Geisler, S. H., & Szymanski, S. R. (1992). Duration of psychosis and outcome in first-episode schizophrenia. *American Journal of Psychiatry*, *149*, 1183–1188.

Maj, M. (1998). Critique of the DSM-IV operational diagnostic criteria for schizophrenia. *British Journal of Psychiatry*, *172*, 458–460.

Marquardt, R. K., Levitt, J. G., Blanton, R. E., Caplan, R., Asarnow, R., Siddarth, P., *et al.* (2005). Abnormal development of the anterior cingulate in childhood-onset schizophrenia: A preliminary quantitative MRI study. *Psychiatry Research*, *138*, 221–233.

Mason, P., Harrison, G., Croudace, T., Glazebrook, C., & Medley, I. (1997). The predictive validity of a diagnosis of schizophrenia. *British Journal of Psychiatry*, *170*, 321–327.

Matsumoto, H., Takei, N., Saito, H., Kachi, K., & Mori, N. (1999). Childhood-onset schizophrenia and obstretic complications: A case–control study. *Schizophrenia Research*, *38*, 93–99.

Matsumoto, H., Takei, N., Saito, H., Kachi, K., & Mori, N. (2001). The association between obstretric complications and childhood-onset schizophrenia: A replication study. *Psychological Medicine*, *31*, 907–914.

McGlashan, T. H., & Hoffman, R. E. (2000). Schizophrenia as a disorder of developmentally reduced synaptic connectivity. *Archives of General Psychiatry*, *57*, 637–648.

McGrath, J., & Murray, R. (1995). Risk factors for schizophrenia: from conception to birth. In S. R. Hirsch, & D. R. Weinberger (Eds.), *Schizophrenia* (pp. 187–205). Oxford: Blackwell Science.

McGorry, P. D., Yung, A. R., Phillips, L. J., Yuen, H. P., Francey, S., Cosgrave, E. M., *et al.* (2002). Randomized controlled trial of interventions designed to reduce the risk of progression to first-episode psychosis in a clinical sample with subthreshold symptoms. *Archives of General Psychiatry*, *59*, 921–928.

Mirnics, K., Middleton, F. A., Lewis, D. A., & Levitt, P. (2001). Analysis of complex brain disorders with gene expression microarrays: Schizophrenia as a disease of the synapse. *Trends in Neuroscience*, *24*, 479–486.

Morgan, C., & Fisher, H. (2007). Environmental factors in schizophrenia: Childhood trauma. *Schizophrenia Bulletin*, *33*, 3–10.

National Institute for Clinical Excellence (NICE). (2002). Guidance on the use of newer (atypical) antipsychotic drugs for the treatment of schizophrenia. *NICE Technology Appraisal Guidance No. 43*. London: NICE.

Nelson, M. D., Saykin, A. J., Flashman, L. A., & Riodan, H. J. (1998). Hippocampal volume reduction in schizophrenia assessed by magnetic resonance imaging: A meta-analytic study. *Archives of General Psychiatry*, *55*, 433–440.

Nicolson, R. M., Giedd, J. N., Lenane, M., Hamburger, S., Singaracharlu, S., Bedwell, J., *et al.* (1999). Clinical and neurobiological correlates of cytogenetic abnormalities in childhood-onset schizophrenia. *American Journal of Psychiatry*, *156*, 1575–1579.

Nopoulos, P., Torres, I., Flaum, M., Andreasen, N. C., Ehrhaerdt, J. C., & Yuh, W. T. C. (1995). Brain morphology in first-episode schizophrenia. *American Journal of Psychiatry*, *152*, 1721–1723.

Nopoulos, P. C., Giedd, J. N., Andreasen, N. C., & Rapoport, J. L. (1998). Frequency and severity of enlarged septi pellucidi in childhood-onset schizophrenia. *American Journal of Psychiatry*, *155*, 1074–1079.

O'Driscoll, G. A., Benkelfat, C., Florencio, P. S., Wolff, A. L., Joober, R., Lal, S., *et al.* (1999). Neural correlates of eye tracking deficits in first-degree relatives of schizophrenic patients: A positron emission tomography study. *Archives of General Psychiatry*, *56*, 1127–1134.

Owen, M. J, Craddock, N., & O'Donovan, M. C. (2005). Schizophrenia: Genes at last? *Trends in Genetics*, *21*, 518–525.

Pantelis, C., Velakoulis, D., McGorry, P. D., Wood, S. J., Suckling, J., Phillips, L. J., *et al.* (2003). Neuroanatomical abnormalities before and after onset of psychosis: a cross-sectional and longitudinal MRI comparison. *Lancet*, *361*, 281–288.

Park, S., Holzman, P. S., & Goldman-Rakic, P. S. (1995). Spatial working memory deficits in the relatives of schizophrenic patients. *Archives of General Psychiatry*, *52*, 821–828.

Perlstein, W. M., Carter, C. S., Noll, D. C., & Cohen, J. D. (2001). Relation of prefrontal cortex dysfunction to working memory and symptoms in schizophrenia. *American Journal of Psychiatry*, *158*, 1105–1113.

Pennington, B. F. (1997). Dimensions of executive functions in normal and abnormal velopment. In N. Krasnegor, G. R. Lyon, & P. S. Goldman-Rakic (Eds.), *Prefrontal cortex: Evolution, development, and behavioral neuroscience* (pp. 265–281). Baltimore: Brooke Publishing.

Pettegrew, J. W., Keshavan, M. S., Panchalingam, K., Strychor, S., Kaplan, D. B., Tretta, M. G., *et al.* (1991). Alterations in brain high-energy phosphate and membrane phospholipid metabolism in first-episode, drug-naive schizophrenics: A pilot study of the dorsal prefrontal cortex by *in vivo* phosphorus 31 nuclear magnetic resonance spectroscopy. *Archives of General Psychiatry*, *48*, 563–568.

Pistis, M., Perra, S., Pillolla, G., Melia, M., Muntoni, A. L., & Gessa, G. L. (2004). Adolescent exposure to cannabinoids induces long-lasting changes in the response to drugs of abuse of rat midbrain dopamine neurons. *Biological Psychiatry*, *56*, 86–94.

Pool, D., Bloom, W., Miekle, D. H., Roniger, J. J., & Gallant, D. M. (1976). A controlled trial of loxapine in 75 adolescent schizophrenic patients. *Current Therapeutic Research*, *19*, 99–104.

Poole, R., & Brabbins, C. (1996). Drug induced psychosis. *British Journal of Psychiatry*, *168*, 135–138.

Poulton, R., Caspi, A., Moffitt, T. E., Cannon, M., Murray, R., & Harrington, H. (2000). Children's self-reported psychotic symptoms and adult schizophreniform disorder: A 15-year longitudinal study. *Archives of General Psychiatry*, *57*, 1053–1058.

Purves, D. L., & Lichtmen, J. W. (1980). Elimination of synapses in the developing nervous system. *Science*, *210*, 153–157.

Rapoport, J. L., Addington, A. M., & Frangou, S. (2005). The neurodevelopmental model of schizophrenia: Update, 2005. *Molecular Psychiatry*, *10*, 434–449.

Rapoport, J. L., Conners, C., & Reatig, N. (1985). Rating scales and assessment instruments for use in paediatric psychopharmacology research. *Psychopharmacology Bulletin*, *21*, 1077–1080.

Rapoport, J. L., Giedd, J., Blumenthal, J., Hamburger, S., Jeffries, N., Fernandez, T., *et al.* (1999). Progressive cortical change during adolescence in childhood-onset schizophrenia: A longitudinal magnetic resonance imaging study. *Archives of General Psychiatry*, *56*, 649–654.

Ratzoni, G., Gothelf, D., Brand-Gothelf, A., Reidman, J., Kikinzon, L., Gal, G., *et al.* (2002). Weight gain associated with olanzapine and risperidone in adolescent patients: A comparative prospective study. *Journal of the American Academy of Child and Adolescent Psychiatry*, *41*, 337–343.

Read, J., van Os, J., Morrison, A. P., & Ross, C. A. (2005). Childhood trauma, psychosis and schizophrenia: A literature review with theoretical implications. *Acta Psychiatrica Scandinavica*, *112*, 330–350.

Reich, W. (2000). Diagnostic Interview for Children and Adolescents (DICA). *Journal of the American Academy of Child and Adolescent Psychiatry*. *39*, 59–66.

Reichenberg, A., Weiser, M., Rapp, M. A., Rabinowitz, J., Caspi, A., Schmeidler, J., *et al.* (2005). Elaboration on Premorbid Intellectual Performance in Schizophrenia: Premorbid Intellectual Decline and Risk for Schizophrenia. *Arch Gren Psychiatry*, *62*, 1297–1304.

Remschmidt, H., Schultz, E., & Martin, M. (1994). An open trial of clozapine with thirty-six adolescents with schizophrenia. *Journal of Child and Adolescent Psychopharmacology*, *4*, 31–41.

Roberts, G. W., Colter, N., Lofthouse, R., Bogerts, B., Zech, M., & Crow, T. J. (1986). Gliosis in schizophrenia: A survey. *Biological Psychiatry*, *21*, 1043–1050.

Robinson, D., Woerner, M. G., Alvir, J. M., Bilder, R., Goldman, R., Geisler, S., *et al.* (1999). Predictors of relapse following a first episode of schizophrenia or schizoaffective disorder. *Archives of General Psychiatry*, *56*, 241–247.

Rossi, A., Mancini, F., Stratta, P., Mattei, P., Gismondi, R., Pozzi, F., *et al.* (1997). Risperidone, negative symptoms and cognitive deficit in schizophrenia: An open study. *Acta Psychiatrica Scandinavica*, *95*, 40–43.

Russell, A. T., Bott, L., & Sammons, C. (1989). The phenomena of schizophrenia occurring in childhood. *Journal of the American Academy of Child and Adolescent Psychiatry*, *28*, 399–407.

Rutter, M., & Plomin, R. (1997). Opportunities for psychiatry from genetic findings. *British Journal of Psychiatry*, *171*, 209–219.

Sachdev, P. (1998). Schizophrenia-like psychosis and epilepsy: The status of the association. *American Journal of Psychiatry*, *155*, 325–336.

Saykin, A. J., Shtasel, D. L., Gur, R. E., Kester, D. B., Mozley, L. H., Stafiniak, P., *et al.* (1994). Neuropsychological deficits in neuroleptic-naive patients with first-episode schizophrenia. *Archives of General Psychiatry*, *51*, 124–131.

Schaeffer, J. L., & Ross, R. G. (2002). Childhood-onset schizophrenia: Premorbid and prodromal diagnostic and treatment histories. *Journal of the American Academy of Child and Adolescent Psychiatry*, *41*, 538–545.

Schmidt, M., Blanz, B., Dippe, A., Koppe, T., & Lay, B. (1995). Course of patients diagnosed as having schizophrenia during first episode occurring under age 18 years. *European Archives of Psychiatry and Clinical Neuroscience*, *245*, 93–100.

Selemon, L. D., Rajkowska, G., & Goldman-Rakic, P. S. (1995). Abnormally high neuronal density in the schizophrenic cortex: A morphometric analysis of prefrontal area 9 and occipital area 17. *Archives of General Psychiatry*, *52*, 805–818.

Shaffer, D., Gould, M. S., Brasic, J., Ambrosini, P., Fisher, P., Bird, H., *et al.* (1983). The Children's Global Assessment Scale (CGAS). *Archives of General Psychiatry*, *40*, 1228–1231.

Sikich, L., Hamer, R. M., Bashford, R. A., Sheitman, B. B., & Lieberman, J. A. (2004). A pilot study of risperidone, olanzapine, and haloperidol in psychotic youth: A double-blind, randomized, 8-week trial. *Neuropsychopharmacology*, *29*, 133–145.

Simpson, G., & Angus, J. S. W. (1970). A rating scale for extrapyramidal side effects. *Acta Psychiatrica Scandinavica*, *212*, 9–11.

Slaveska, K., Hollis, C. P., & Bramble, D. (1998). The use of antipsychotics by the child and adolescent psychiatrists of Trent region. *Psychiatric Bulletin*, *22*, 685–687.

Spencer, E. K., & Campbell, M. (1994). Children with schizophrenia: Diagnosis, phenomenology and pharmacotherapy. *Schizophrenia Bulletin*, *20*, 713–725.

Sporn, A. L., Addington, A. M., Gogtay, N., Ordonez, A. E., Gornick, M., Clasen, L., *et al.* (2004a). Pervasive developmental disorder and childhood-onset schizophrenia: Co-morbid disorder or phenotypic variant of a very early onset illness? *Biological Psychiatry*, *55*, 989–994.

Sporn, A. L., Addington, A. M., Reiss, A. L., Dean, M., Gogtay, N., Potocnik, U., *et al.* (2004b). 22q11 deletion syndrome in childhood-onset schizophrenia: An update. *Molecular Psychiatry*, *9*, 225–226.

Sporn, A. L., Greenstein, D., Gogtay, N., Jeffries, N. O., Lenane, M., Gochman, P., *et al.* (2003). Progressive brain volume loss during adolescence in childhood-onset schizophrenia. *American Journal of Psychiatry*, *160*, 1281–1289.

Sporn, A. L., Greenstein, D., Gogtay, N., Sailer, F., Hommer, D. W., Rawlings, R., *et al.* (2005). Childhood-onset schizophrenia: Smooth pursuit eye-tracking dysfunction in family members. *Schizophrenia Research*, *73*, 243–252.

St. Clair, D., Xu, M., Wang, P., Yu, Y., Fang, Y., Zhang, F., *et al.* (2005). Rates of adult schizophrenia following prenatal exposure to the Chinese Famine of 1959–1961. *Journal of the American Medical Association*, *294*, 557–562.

Stayer, C., Sporn, A., Gogtay, N., Tossell, J. W., Lenane, M., Gochman, P., *et al.* (2005). Multidimensionally impaired: The good news. *Journal of Child and Adolescent Psychopharmacology*, *15*, 510–519.

Strandburg, R. J., Marsh, J. T., Brown, W. S., *et al.* (1999). Continuous-processing ERPS in adult schizophrenia: Continuity with childhood-onset schizophrenia. *Biological Psychiatry*, *45*, 1356–1369.

Susser, E., & Lin, S. P. (1992). Schizophrenia after prenatal exposure to the Dutch Hunger Winter of 1944–1945. *Archives of General Psychiatry*, *49*, 983–988.

Tarrier, N., Beckett, R., Harwood, S., Baker, A., Yusupoff, L., & Ugarteburu, I. (1993). A trial of two cognitive–behavioural methods of treating drug-resistant residual psychotic symptoms in schizophrenic patients. I. Outcome. *British Journal of Psychiatry*, *162*, 524–532.

Thomas, M. A., Ke, Y., Levitt, J., Caplan, R., Curran, J., Asarnow, R., *et al.* (1998). Preliminary study of frontal lobe ^{1}H MR spectroscopy in childhood-onset schizophrenia. *Journal of Magnetic Resonance Imaging*, *8*, 841–846.

Theisen, F. M., Linden, A., Geller, F., Schafer, H., Martin, M., Remschmidt, H., *et al.* (2001). Prevalence of obesity in adolescent and young adult patients with and without schizophrenia and in relationship to antipsychotic medication. *Journal of Psychiatric Research*, *35*, 339–345.

Toren, P., Ratner, S., Laor, N., & Weizman, A. (2004). Benefit–risk assessment of atypical antipsychotics in the treatment of schizophrenia and comorbid disorders in children and adolescents. *Drug Safety*, *27*, 1135–1156.

Towbin, K. R., Dykens, E. M., Pearson, G. S., & Cohen, D. J. (1993). Conceptualizing "borderline syndrome of childhood" and "childhood schizophrenia" as a developmental disorder. *Journal of the American Academy of Child and Adolescent Psychiatry*, *32*, 775–782.

Tsuang, M. T., Simpson, J. C., & Kronfold, Z. (1982). Subtypes of drug abuse with psychosis. *Archives of General Psychiatry*, *39*, 141–147.

Turkington, D., & Kingdon, D. (2000). Cognitive–behavioural techniques for general psychiatrists in the management of patients with psychoses. *British Journal of Psychiatry*, *177*, 101–106.

Vita, A., Dieci, M., Giobbio, G. M., Azzone, P., Garbarini, M., Sacchetti, E., *et al.* (1991). CT scan abnormalities and outcome of chronic schizophrenia. *American Journal of Psychiatry*, *148*, 1577–1579.

Volkmar, F. R., & Cohen, D. J. (1991). Comorbid association of autism and schizophrenia. *American Journal of Psychiatry*, *148*, 1705–1707.

Weinberger, D. R. (1987). Implications of normal brain development for the pathogenesis of schizophrenia. *Archives of General Psychiatry*, *44*, 660–669.

Werry, J. S., McClellan, J. M., & Chard, L. (1991). Childhood and adolescent schizophrenia, bipolar and schizoaffective disorders: A clinical and outcome study. *Journal of the American Academy of Child and Adolescent Psychiatry*, *30*, 457–465.

Werry, J. S., McClellan, J. M., Andrews, L., & Ham, M. (1994). Clinical features and outcome of child and adolescent schizophrenia. *Schizophrenia Bulletin*, *20*, 619–630.

White, T., Andreasen, N. C., Nopoulos, P., & Magnotta, V. (2003). Gyrification abnormalities in childhood-onset schizophrenia. *Biological Psychiatry*, *54*, 418–426.

Woods, B. T. (1998). Is schizophrenia a progressive neurodevelopmental disorder? Toward a unitary pathogenetic mechanism. *American Journal of Psychiatry*, *155*, 1661–1670.

World Health Organization. (1996). *Multiaxial classification of child and adolescent psychiatric disorders: The ICD-10 classification of mental and behavioural disorders in children and adolescents.* Cambridge, UK: Cambridge University Press.

Wyatt, R. J. (1995). Early intervention in schizophrenia: can the course be altered? *Biological Psychiatry*, *38*, 1–3.

Wykes, T., Reeder, C., Williams, C., Corner, J., Rice, C., & Everitt, B. (2000). Cognitive remediation: Predictors of success and durability of improvements (Abstract). *Schizophrenia Research*, *41*, 221.

Yung, A. R., Phillips, L. J., Yuen, H. P., Francey, S. M., McFarlane, C. A., Hallgren, M., *et al.* (2003). Psychosis prediction: 12-month follow up of a high-risk ("prodromal") group. *Schizophrenia Research*, *60*, 21–32.

Zahn, T. P., Jacobsen, L. K., Gordon, C. T., McKenna, K., Frazier, K., & Rapoport, J. L. (1997). Autonomic nervous system markers of psychopathology in childhood-onset schizophrenia. *Archives of General Psychiatry*, *54*, 904–912.

Zahn, T. P., Jacobsen, L. K., Gordon, C. T., McKenna, K., Frazier, K., & Rapoport, J. L. (1998). Attention deficits in childhood-onset schizophrenia: Reaction time studies. *Journal of Abnormal Psychology*, *107*, 97–108.

46 Autism Spectrum Disorders

Herman van Engeland and Jan K. Buitelaar

Autism spectrum disorders (ASD; or Pervasive Developmental Disorders, PDD) are a group of conditions characterized by three cardinal clinical features: qualitative impairments in social interactions; qualitatively impaired verbal and non-verbal communication; and restricted range of interests. Additional characteristics include onset early in life, delay and/or deviance of development of key psychological functions, multifactorial etiology in which several as yet unknown genetic risk factors interact with each other and with environmental factors, change and mitigation of symptomatic expression by age and, despite this, a chronic course with strong persistence of handicaps over time. However, it is equally true that ASD are clinically very heterogeneous conditions. A main factor that determines diversity is variation in level of cognitive functioning and language skills. There is a large difference between a severely intellectually impaired person with autism who is unable to speak and who engages in motor stereotypies and self-injury, and a highly skilled computer engineer with Asperger disorder or with high functioning autism who is fluent in his one-sided exchange of excessive and obsessive preoccupations about, for example, the constellation of the planets and stars. Other aspects of diversity concern age, severity of cardinal features, coexisting somatic conditions including epilepsy, and coexisting psychiatric conditions.

Over the past decades, clinical and research interest has moved from a focus on a more narrowly defined group of subjects with severe manifestations of the three cardinal features (i.e., "typical autism") to a broader and more prevalent category with more subtle and less severe symptoms, usually classified as atypical autism or pervasive developmental disorder not otherwise specified (PDD-NOS). Although most of our knowledge about ASD is still derived from research in typical autism, this chapter takes a perspective on the whole range of severity of ASD.

Recent findings indicate that ASD can be conceptualized as disorders of early brain development. Functional and morphological abnormalities of the brain, induced by both static persistent processes that started *in utero* and dynamic processes that change over time and continue to change in postnatal life, underlie the complex behavioral and cognitive manifestations of ASD.

Rutter's Child and Adolescent Psychiatry, 5th edition. Edited by M. Rutter, D. Bishop, D. Pine, S. Scott, J. Stevenson, E. Taylor and A. Thapar. ISBN: 978-1-4051-4549-7.

History

Kanner (1943) first described a syndrome of "autistic disturbances" with case histories of 11 children who presented between the ages of 2 and 8 years and who shared unique and previously unreported patterns of behavior including social remoteness, obsessiveness, stereotypy and echolalia. After its initial description, autism was poorly ascertained during the middle decades of the 20th century. In DSM-I, autism was classified as a childhood type of schizophrenia. Despite this early view of autism as a psychosis, several prominent research groups had formulated the first set of diagnostic criteria for this disorder by the 1970s (Ritvo & Freeman, 1978; Rutter & Hersov, 1977). With DSM-III, the term Pervasive Developmental Disorders (PDD) was first used to describe disorders characterized by distortions in the development of multiple basic psychological functions that are involved in the development of social skills and language, such as attention, perception, reality testing and motor movement. The term PDD was selected because it described most accurately that many basic areas of psychological development are severely affected at the same time. This new PDD umbrella included, for the first time, the term Infantile Autism (with onset prior to age 30 months) as well as Childhood Onset Pervasive Developmental Disorder (with onset after age 30 months). In DSM-III, autism was also clearly differentiated from childhood schizophrenia and other psychoses for the first time, and the absence of psychotic symptoms, such as delusions and hallucinations, became one of the six diagnostic criteria.

In 1944, Asperger wrote the first paper (in German), on what has come to be known as his disorder (translated into English in Frith, 1991). He outlined the clinical picture of four children with normal IQ who were socially odd, naïve and inappropriate, had good grammar and extensive vocabularies, poor non-verbal communication, circumscribed interests and poor motor coordination. However, this paper was virtually unnoticed until it was extensively discussed in an English publication (Wing, 1981). Asperger syndrome was first included as a diagnostic category in DSM-IV (American Psychiatric Association, 2000) and ICD-10 (World Health Organization, 1996).

Clinical Characteristics

The diagnostic frameworks currently used, DSM-IV and ICD-10, include a very similar list of disorders under ASD or PDD.

Qualitative Impairment in Social Interactions

The emphasis is on the qualitative impairment in reciprocal social interactions and not on the absolute lack of social behaviors. There is wide variation in social symptoms, which range from a total lack of awareness of another person to intrusive social approaches that are inappropriate to context. In the first year of life, some children with autism do not lift up their arms or change posture in anticipation of being held. Some children do make eye contact, often only in brief glances, but the eye contact is usually not used to direct attention to objects or events of interest. Other children make inappropriate eye contact, by turning someone else's head to gaze into their eyes, or tend to stare at other people's faces. Some children make indiscriminate approaches to strangers (e.g., may climb into the examiner's lap before the parent has even entered the room).

The capacity to make social connections and engage in relationships appropriate to age level is limited. Young children may demonstrate lack of interestin, or even lack of awareness of other children. Older children with autism have no age-appropriate friends, are socially isolated and may be teased or bullied. Nonetheless, they may express social interest by saying they want "friends." Tragically, they do not understand the principles of the reciprocity and sharing of interests inherent in friendship and they lack the pragmatics of "how socially to do what, when and where." More verbally able children may have one "friend" but the relationship is usually very limited and based on a similar circumscribed interest, such as dinosaurs or a particular computer game. They often do not point things out or use eye contact to share the pleasure of seeing something with another person, which is called joint attention. There are often deficits in reading social cues in body language and facial expressions of others. Some children tend to have a more passive type of social interaction characterized by a lack of social initiative and an observing and compliant style of simply following the directions of others.

Qualitative Impairment in Communication

In a similar way, the communication impairments seen in ASD are diverse, and vary from simple speech delay to muteness, to fluency with subtle peculiarities of intonation and inability to adjust vocabulary and conversational style to social context. As a result, fluency is often accompanied by many semantic (word meaning) and verbal pragmatic errors. Young autistic children, even if verbal, almost universally have comprehension deficits, in particular deficits in understanding higher order complex questions. Some children with autism do not respond to their names when called by a parent or other favored caretaker, and often they are initially presumed to be severely hearing-impaired. A characteristic behavior of many children with autism is mechanically to use another person's hand to indicate the desired object, often called "hand over hand pointing." Other "independent" children make no demands or requests of the parents, but rather learn to climb at a young age and acquire the desired object for themselves. When language is present, children with autism seem unable or unwilling to initiate or sustain conversation in a give-and-take fashion. Speech tends to be in a monotone without the usual emphasis to support meaning of phrases. The autistic child may also use neologisms, echoing or pronoun reversal. Remember that immediate echolalia is a crucial aspect of normal language development under the age of 2 years. It becomes pathological when it is still present as the sole and predominant expressive language after the age of about 24 months, and can often be present throughout the preschool or school-age years in children with autism. ASD are also associated with deficits in nonverbal communication, including the use of gestures such as pointing, showing and nodding. Some children with autism do not use miniature objects, animals or dolls appropriately in pretend play. Others use the materials in a repetitive mechanical fashion without evidence of flexible representational play. Some highly verbal children may invent a fantasy world which becomes the sole focus of repetitive play. Imitation skills are weak or absent, as is the ability to engage in social play, such as peek-a-boo or hide and seek.

Restricted, Repetitive and Stereotypic Patterns of Behaviors, Interests and Activities

Some children show an unusual and intense preoccupation with a topic of private interest such as washing machines, trains or railway schedules. Other children are absorbed in fixed daily routines and rituals. Many children with autism are so preoccupied with "sameness" in their home and school environments, or with routines, that little can be changed without prompting a tantrum or other emotional disturbance. For example, some insist on taking only a certain route to school, entering the supermarket only by one specific door, or never stopping or turning around once the car starts moving. Repetitive behaviors commonly observed in children with autism may include motor mannerisms such as hand-flapping, rocking, flipping objects or lining up toys in a fixed fashion. Some display sensory abnormalities, and are preoccupied by auditory, visual, tactile, haptic or kinesthetic stimuli and apparently are hypo- or hyper-responsive to these. These repetitive and sensory abnormalities can be a source of pleasure or self-stimulation, which differentiates these behaviors from those seen in obsessive-compulsive disorder.

Classification

The prototype of ASD, autistic disorder, is defined by the presence of marked symptoms in all three of the key domains of qualitative impairments in social interactions, qualitatively impaired communication and restricted range of interests. In addition, at least some of these features must have been manifest by the age of 3 years (APA, 2000; WHO, 1996).

Asperger syndrome is defined by the presence of social impairment and repetitive behaviors and restricted interests, as in autism. However, in contrast to autism, there is no overall delay in language development, as indexed from the use of single words by age 2 and communicative phrases by age 3 years. Normal or near-normal IQ is also the rule. The lack of clear language deviance usually leads to later clinical recognition than with other ASD, which is presumably a result of the normal or near-normal adaptive behavior early in life (Volkmar & Cohen, 1991). Yet the language in Asperger disorder is clearly not typical or normal. Individuals usually have pedantic and poorly modulated speech, poor non-verbal pragmatic or communication skills, and intense preoccupations with circumscribed topics such as the weather or railway timetables. They often have both fine and gross motor deficits, including clumsy and uncoordinated movements and odd postures.

In spite of the consensus definition of Asperger disorder in DSM-IV and ICD-10, the validity of Asperger disorder as a discrete diagnostic entity distinct from high-functioning (verbal) autism has remained controversial (Klin, McPartland, & Volkmar, 2005a; Schopler, Mesibov, & Kunce, 1998). Researchers have adopted various diagnostic schemes which differ by whether the focus was on onset of any concerns before age 3, on the presence of speech delay by age 2–3 or by the application of unique investigator-based criteria (Klin, Pauls, Schultz *et al.*, 2005b).

The diagnosis of PDD-NOS (or atypical autism) is appropriate when a subject exhibits impairments in social interactions, impaired communication or restricted range of interests, but does not meet the full criteria for autistic disorder or Asperger disorder. This would apply when the number of criteria met is subthreshold, age of onset is after age 3 years, atypical symptoms are present or more than one of these are present. Balancing sensitivity and specificity in differentiating PDD-NOS from both autism and non-ASD conditions, diagnostic algorithms have been proposed that describe PDD-NOS as a lesser variant of autism, requiring that at least 4 of the 12 DSM-IV criteria of autism are met, including at least one of the social interaction criteria (Buitelaar & van der Gaag, 1998; Buitelaar, van der Gaag, Klin, & Volkmar, 1999a).

Epidemiology

Whereas the first epidemiological studies of autism reported the population prevalence at around 4 per 10,000 (Lotter, 1966), recent large systematic surveys indicate a much higher rate. The current estimates are 30–100 per 10,000 for all ASD, including 13–30 per 10,000 for autism and 3 per 10,000 for Asperger disorder (Baird, Simonoff, Pickles *et al.*, 2006; Fombonne, 1999, 2003). Estimates from single studies vary widely, because of differences in screening and ascertainment procedures, sample size, publication year and geographic location. The increase in reported rates of ASD is largely a consequence of two factors (Rutter, 2005). First, recent studies used systematic standardized and often multiple screenings of total populations or birth cohorts, and by consequence have missed fewer children with ASD than older studies that were more focused on special populations or case registries. Second, over the years the diagnostic concept of ASD has broadened considerably and has included a much better recognition of the expression of autistic symptoms in individuals with near-normal or normal non-verbal intelligence, along with insights from family genetic and twin studies that the genetic liability of autism extends well beyond the traditional categories into more subtle social and communicative abnormalities (Bolton, Macdonald, Pickles *et al.*, 1994; Le Couteur, Bailey, Goode *et al.*, 1996).

However, it is unclear whether there is also a rise in the true incidence of ASD, and whether – if so – this is a result of some as yet unknown environmental factor. The increase, particularly since the early 1980s, has led to claims that specific environmental factors such as the use of mumps–measles–rubella (MMR) triple vaccine are a major factor (Roger, 2000; Wakefield, Murch, Anthony *et al.*, 1998). However, empirical evidence for these claims is absent (Rutter, 2005). For example, a total population study in the Yokohama district, Japan, was able to examine the cumulative incidence of ASD before the introduction of the MMR vaccination and after its withdrawal (Honda, Shimizu, & Rutter, 2005). The findings indicated a continuing rise in incidence of ASD even after the withdrawal of the vaccination. Further, the incidence pattern of ASD associated with regression was similar to that of ASD as a whole. It is also relevant that an independent study of Wakefield's claims on finding the measles virus in body tissues has not confirmed the findings (D'Souza, Fombonne, & Ward, 2006). Finally, in particular the incidence of ASD with high IQ showed a significant increase. The use of thimerosal, a vaccine preservative that contains ethyl mercury, has in a somewhat similar way been linked to a rise in incidence of ASD. Because mercury, in high dosage, can cause neurodevelopmental sequelae, there is greater biological plausibility in this argument. However, discontinuation of the thimerosal-containing vaccines in Denmark was followed by an increase in the incidence of ASD and not by the predicted decrease (Atladóttir, Parner, Schendel *et al.*, 2007; Madsen, Lauritsen, Pedersen *et al.*, 2003).

Recent surveys continue to indicate associations of ASD with gender, IQ and other medical disorders (Fombonne, 2003). Males are about four times more often affected than females, with gender differences even more pronounced in the normal range of intellectual functioning, up to a male : female ratio of 6:1. The gender difference in ASD is poorly understood. Although Baron-Cohen, Knickmeyer, and Belmonte (2005) have speculated that autism may represent an extreme male brain, there is a paucity of supporting evidence and the suggestion side-steps the important finding that most early-onset neurodevelopmental disorders (such as attention deficit/hyperactivity disorder [ADHD] and dyslexia) show a marked male preponderance (see chapter 3; Rutter, Caspi, & Moffitt, 2003a). It may be more profitable to ask why males are more vulnerable to this range of disorders, rather than to view autism as a special case.

The rate of coexisting severe to profound intellectual impairment is about 40%, mild to moderate cognitive impairments are found in 30% and normal intellectual functioning in another 30%. Potentially causal medical associations are found in about 5–10% of the cases. The strongest connection is found for tuberous sclerosis (Smalley, 1998); approximately 20% of patients with tuberous sclerosis also have autism, although, in contrast, tuberous sclerosis is found only in a small percentage of cases with autism. Other medical conditions that may be associated with autism are cerebral palsy, fragile X, phenylketonuria, neurofibromatosis, congenital rubella and Down's syndrome (Fombonne, 2003). These associations with intellectual impairment and known medical conditions are much stronger for typical autism than more broadly defined ASD.

Course of Autism

Most children with autism are identified by their parents as showing abnormalities or delays in the second year of life, and many parents suspect problems long before this (Zwaigenbaum, Bryson, Rogers *et al.*, 2005). Parents who have already had a child tend to recognize social deficits earlier than parents of firstborns, and social deficits are often less recognizable in very young children than when they are older (De Giacomo & Fombonne, 1998).

Often, the problems noticed are not specific autistic features, but rather concerns that the child is less socially responsive and has difficulties in settling, eating and sleeping (Dahlgren & Gillberg, 1989). Home videos similarly show that by the age of 12–18 months (or even earlier) there may be manifestations of abnormal development, but often the indications are quite subtle (Rutter, 2005). Many autistic children under the age of 3 years do not yet show clear examples of restricted or repetitive behaviors (Cox, Klein, Charman *et al.*, 1999).

It has long been noted that about one-quarter to one-third of all children with ASD appear to lose previously acquired language skills (usually between 18 and 24 months; Rogers & DiLalla, 1990; Rutter, 2005). Surprisingly, the phenomenon has been subject to remarkably little systematic study. Some of these apparent developmental regressions are minor and probably of little significance but there is no doubt that a marked loss of skills does occur in a substantial minority of children with ASD. In one well-documented study (Pickles, Simonoff, Conti-Ramsden *et al.*, submitted), the phenomenon was shown to be common in children with ASD but did not occur in those with specific language impairment (SLI). If confirmed, this would suggest that developmental regression is of some diagnostic significance. However, its meaning remains obscure. Despite claims to the contrary (in relation to MMR), it does not imply any environmental cause and there is no evidence that ASD with regression is becoming more frequent (Rutter, 2005).

When children with ASD enter school, many of them are described as more flexible and socially directed. Data from 13 follow-up studies extending into adult life show a general pattern of modest improvement over time (Howlin, 2005). Some adults with ASD experience real behavioral and social improvements in their late 20s and early 30s (Mesibov, 1984). However, autism is a lifelong disorder, and the likelihood of complete independence is low. Individuals with both autism and intellectual disability require supervised living and working situations throughout their lives. Opportunities within communities, rather than in institutions, have increased in the last decades. Most adults with ASD, even those with average or greater intelligence, require some help in finding and keeping jobs and coping with responsibilities and social demands. Comparisons of outcome studies over the last 30 years suggest that among those of intelligence within the normal range, there has been some increase in the proportion obtaining employment. Admissions with institutional care have also fallen. Nevertheless, even in individuals with an IQ above 70, only about one-quarter show good social functioning. Early reports commented on apparent cognitive deterioration in adolescence in some individuals, but true cognitive decline seems uncommon.

In a recent large follow-up study with a low attrition rate and using systematic interviews to obtain clinical information, Hutton, Goode, Murphy *et al.* (in press) found that 16% of the autistic participants developed a definite new psychiatric disorder that was not just a worsening of pre-existing autistic features. Five out of 135 developed an obsessive-compulsive disorder and/or catatonia; a further eight developed affective disorders with marked obsessional features; and seven developed complex or straightforward affective disorders. There was no case of schizophrenia in this study, indicating a lack of continuity between autism and schizophrenia (Volkmar & Cohen, 1991). However, there are reports of autistic individuals who show isolated psychotic symptoms, including hallucinations and delusional thoughts (Clarke, Littlejohns, Corbett, & Joseph, 1989; Szatmari, Bartolucci, & Bremmer, 1989; Vorstman, Staal, van Daalen *et al.*, 2006; Wing & Shah, 2000). Hutton, Goode, Murphy *et al.* (in press) found that one-fifth of individuals with ASD followed into adult life experience one or more epileptic attacks and that about two-thirds of these had their onset in adolescence or adult life.

There are a number of largely anecdotal reports of offending by people with autism or Asperger syndrome. Inappropriate social responses, especially to strangers, may result in police involvement and crimes may also be linked to obsessional interests. Because of this, offending may well be of an unusual or even bizarre nature (Baron-Cohen, 1988; Chesterman & Rutter, 1994). Scragg and Shah (1994) assessed the entire male population of Broadmoor Special Hospital and identified three cases of autism and six with Asperger syndrome out of a total of 392 (just over 2%), clearly a much higher figure than the rates for autism or Asperger syndrome in the general population. In their review of offending by people with Asperger syndrome, Ghaziuddin, Tsai, and Ghaziuddin (1991) found that only 3 out of a total of 132 cases had a clear history of violent behavior. Estimates on the prevalence of violence in people with ASD can only be made on the basis of community studies; these are lacking so far.

Predictors of Outcome

Predictors of outcome from preschool to later childhood and adolescence have included joint attention (Sigman, Ruskin,

Arbeile *et al.*, 1999), verbal imitation (Smith & Bryson, 1994) and social communicative aspects of adaptive skills (Lord & Schopler, 1989). However, non-verbal IQ and language are the most powerful predictors. A non-verbal IQ below 50 in preschool years is associated with a reduced likelihood that the child will acquire a useful level of spoken language and a very low probability of good social functioning in adolescence or adulthood (Lockyer & Rutter, 1969). Variations in non-verbal IQ in the range of 50–70 have a somewhat similar effect, but those within the normal range do not.

In children with autism but without severe intellectual disability, language skills (and verbal IQ) are the strongest predictors of social outcome. A child who does not have fluent speech by the age of 5 years will make significant gains, but the later these gains come, the less likely the child's language will be flexible and complex, and the more likely language delays of some sort will reduce his or her level of independence (Szatmari, Bryson, Streiner *et al.*, 2000). Although intrinsic factors such as high IQ and good language abilities are important for outcome, these alone are not enough to ensure a positive outcome. External factors, including appropriate junior and secondary school provision, improved transitional programs for entry into college and supported employment schemes, are also crucial (Howlin, Alcock, & Burkin, 2005; Keel, Mesibov, & Woods, 1997; Smith, Belcher, & Juhrs, 1995).

It is clear that a considerable minority of individuals with ASD, although continuing to be affected by their condition, can find work, live independently and maintain relationships with others. However, such achievements do not come easily. While some individuals have access to specialist support systems, in many cases jobs are found only with the support of families, and opportunities to live independently depend heavily on local provision – and often too on parental determination and persistence.

Differential Diagnosis

In daily practice it is often not simple to distinguish autistic syndrome from other pervasive developmental disorders, developmental language disorder, intellectual impairment, sensory defects and severe emotional neglect. Each of these syndromes is briefly described below, and possible differential diagnostic characteristics mentioned.

Atypical Autism/Pervasive Developmental Disorder Not Otherwise Specified

These terms refer to non-specific patterns that seem to involve the same deficits as those associated with autism, although they do not fulfill all the accepted diagnostic criteria (Buitelaar, van der Gaag, Klin *et al.*, 1999a). The atypicality may lie in the symptom pattern, its severity or age of first manifestation. Epidemiological analyses (Wing & Gould, 1979) and clinical investigations indicate the frequency of these atypical patterns but they have been subject to little systematic research. It is likely that they reflect variations in the ways in which ASD may present, rather than a separate category (Rapin, 1997; Wing, 1997). The service needs are similar to those for autism, and it remains unknown whether the apparent atypicality has any implications for etiology.

Asperger Syndrome

In the last two decades, the concept of Asperger syndrome as used by researchers (Frith, 1991; Gillberg, 1989; Klin, Volkmar, & Sparrow, 2000) and clinicians (Attwood, 1997; Wing, 1981) has served to highlight the occurrence of ASD in individuals who are intellectually able and verbally fluent (Grandin & Sciarino, 1986). It has not proved easy to produce satisfactory diagnostic criteria, and differences in both definition and sampling have led to conflicting findings (Green, Gilchrist, Burton, & Cox, 2000; Klin, Volkmar, & Sparrow, 2000; Szatmari, Bryson, Streiner *et al.*, 2000). In keeping with the lack of language delay, the diagnosis tends to be made substantially later than in autism as such, and the diagnosis of Asperger syndrome tends to be associated with a higher verbal than non-verbal IQ (Klin, Volkmar, Sparrow, Cicchetti, & Rourke, 1995). It remains uncertain whether Asperger syndrome and autism differ in pattern of neuropsychological deficits (Ozonoff, Pennington, & Rogers, 1991a,b) and outcome (Howlin, 2003).

Rett Syndrome

Rett syndrome is a progressive developmental disorder that affects 1 in 10,000–15,000 girls (Kozinetz, Skender, MacNaughton *et al.*, 1993) and is the only pervasive developmental disorder with a known genetic cause (see chapter 24). Rett syndrome is brought about by mutations in the X-linked gene encoding methyl-CpG-binding protein 2 (MECP2; Moretti & Zoghbi, 2006). It is characterized by a relatively normal general and psychomotor development through the first 6–18 months of life, followed by stagnation of developmental acquisitions and a rapid deterioration of behavior and mental status, resulting in dementia with apparently autistic-like features within less than 18 months; loss of purposeful use of the hands following the earlier acquisition of normal grasp function; jerky ataxia of the trunk and limbs, awkward, unsteady gait and acquired microcephaly; followed by a protracted period with a relatively stable mental status, marked by the emergence over years of other neurological abnormalities – especially spasticity of the lower limbs and epilepsy (Hagberg, Aicardi, Dias, & Ramos, 1983). Because of its crucial prognostic significance, its diagnosis is most important. The acquired microcephaly (after a normal head circumference at birth), associated with the loss of purposive hand movement and often a midline "handwashing" stereotypy, may be most crucial. There are no specific treatments currently available, although recent animal studies suggest that, potentially, the neural degeneration might ultimately prove to be reversible (Guy, Gan, Selfridge, Cobb, & Bird, 2007).

Childhood Disintegrative Disorder

Childhood disintegrative disorder (previously termed Heller

syndrome) is a very rare disorder (prevalence rate 0.2 per 10,000; Fombonne, 2002) that manifests after an apparently normal development for the first 2 years of life. Receptive and expressive language functions are lost, and there is often a loss of coordination and the development of fecal and urine incontinence (Volkmar & Rutter, 1995). The child withdraws from social engagement and develops hand and finger stereotypies and simple rituals similar to those seen in autism. The deterioration continues for several months before reaching a plateau that is often difficult to distinguish from autism combined with intellectual impairment (Mouridsen, Rich, & Isager, 1999). In some cases the deterioration progresses and motor dysfunction, epileptic attacks and localized neurological deficits can occur (Corbett, Harris, Taylor, & Trible, 1977). While a very few cases of childhood disintegrative disorder are caused by cerebral lipoidosis or leukodystrophy, in most cases a cause cannot be established (see chapter 30). It remains quite unknown whether it constitutes an atypical variant of ASD or some meaningfully different syndrome.

Receptive-Expressive Language Disorders

Language delay is a common reason for initial referral of children with autistic disorder (Siegel, Pliner, Eschler, & Elliot, 1988); autistic spectrum disorders differ from the more common varieties of developmental language disorder in the severity of receptive language impairment (Fischel, Whitehurst, Caulfield, & DeBaryshe, 1989; Kjelgaard & Tager-Flusberg, 2001).

There are non-autistic children of normal non-verbal intelligence who have a severe receptive-expressive language disorder (see chapter 47). Many have some symptoms that overlap with ASD, and some may fit descriptions of "semantic-pragmatic disorder" (Bishop, 1989; Boucher, 1998), meaning problems with the social communicative aspects of conversational interchange. These children with receptive-expressive language disorder may have immediate echolalia, substantial social impairment and limited imaginative play; in contrast to children with autism they seldom show stereotyped behavior or preoccupations and their non-verbal behavior (looking at people; facial expressions and gestures) is not really impaired.

Landau–Kleffner Syndrome

Landau–Kleffner syndrome or acquired aphasia with epilepsy (Miller, Campbell, Chapman, & Weismer, 1984; Mouridsen, 1995) may mimic autism, although the differentiation is usually straightforward. Children with this disorder have normal development and then lose receptive and expressive language in conjunction with epileptic seizures or transient electroencephalogram (EEG) abnormalities. The regression may be associated with some social withdrawal and behavioral abnormalities, while non-verbal cognitive and motor functioning remain intact. Sometimes language is regained.

Intellectual Disability

More than two-thirds of children with autism are also intellectually impaired. Wing and Gould (1979), studying children with an intellectual disability, found that half of all children with an IQ lower than 50 also had disturbances of social communication, stereotyped behavior and/or disorders of language development. These three symptoms are similar to the diagnostic core criteria of autism, and these children are usually classified as having PDD-NOS. In daily practice it is not always easy to determine whether a child has a "pure" intellectual disability or intellectual impairment that is part of ASD (see chapter 49).

Sensory Deficits

The parents of a child with autism often approach their general practitioner with the suspicion that their child is deaf, because the child does not react to his or her name or to doors slamming shut, etc. A careful history should clarify the situation, but this does not obviate the need to carry out auditory testing, if necessary supplemented with monitoring of brainstem-evoked responses. As babies, children with autism are often noticeable for not making eye contact – they stare into space or fixedly gaze at something, such as a lamp. This sometimes makes parents think that their child is blind. Extensive ophthalmological investigations may provide information regarding the differential diagnosis.

Emotional Neglect

Children who have experienced very severe institutional deprivation can show language delay, abnormal social behavior and marked circumscribed interests and preoccupations (Rutter, Anderson-Wood, Beckett *et al.*, 1999). In early childhood the clinical picture is rather like autism, although there is usually more social reciprocity than typical with autism, and the course is different, so that by middle childhood it is social disinhibition and circumscribed interests that tend to predominate.

Assessment

Because no single symptom is pathognomonic for ASD, the essence of the diagnostic process is to recognize a particular pattern of social and communicative symptoms and of rigidity that was first manifest early in life, is rather stable over development and cannot better be attributed to other conditions. Assessment requires sufficient expertise with the wide range of expression of the symptoms of ASD by age and level of cognitive and language skills, and is best performed systematically and in a stepwise fashion. Extensive information about assessment of ASD can be found in recent practice parameters (American Academy of Pediatrics, 2000; Volkmar, Cook, Pomeroy, Realmuto, & Tanguay, 1999).

The interview with the parents or caregivers should cover both the core features of ASD as well as comorbid symptoms such as aggression, tantrums, hyperactivity, inattention, impulsivity, sleep problems and self-injury. In older children and adolescents, it is often helpful to focus on age 4–5 years, when the expression of symptoms of ASD is most typical. Necessary components of the interview are a family history with probes for ASD, intellectual disability, fragile X syndrome, tuberous sclerosis, and more subtle language, learning and communication problems (see chapter 22). The child's medical history-taking should explore signs of deterioration, seizure activity, brain injury, gastrointestinal disease, pica and other medical conditions. The observation or interview of the child is best conducted in conditions of both high-structure and low-structure, and by using several strategies varying from direct and intrusive approach and probes for engagement to passive observation while the child wanders around or is with others. It allows the clinician to document behaviors reported in the interview and explore the responses of the child to intrusiveness and structure.

Diagnostic Instruments

Several standardized diagnostic instruments are available to facilitate the assessment of ASD. These instruments are commonly used in research and also increasingly in clinical practice. The Autism Diagnostic Interview–Revised (ADI-R) is a comprehensive diagnostic interview conducted by a trained clinical interviewer (Le Couteur, Lord, & Rutter, 2003; Rutter, Le Couteur, & Lord, 2003b). It focuses both on the period between 4 and 5 years of age and on current symptoms, encompasses 92 questions and takes about 120 min to administer. The ADI-R is reliable and valid, and has a scoring algorithm for DSM-IV and ICD-10 diagnoses of autism, but not for PDD-NOS or Asperger disorder.

Less often used is the Diagnostic Interview for Social and Communicative Disorders (DISCO) which also provides a broad base of information on developmental and behavioral issues (Leekam, Libby, Wing, Gould, & Taylor, 2002; Wing, Leekam, Libby, Gould, & Larcombe, 2002). The Vineland Adaptive Behavior Scale is a semi-structured interview with parents or caregivers to measure functional ability in everyday life on three domains: communication, daily living and socialization (Sparrow, Balla, & Cicchetti, 1984). The interview has US norms for age and gender. Individuals with autism often have Vineland scores that are 2 standard deviations below their measured IQ. Rating scales that can be used to assess a broader spectrum of behavioral problems in ASD are the Aberrant Behavior Checklist (ABC; Aman, Singh, Stewart, & Field, 1985) and the Developmental Behavior Checklist (DBC; Einfeld & Tonge, 1995).

Rating scales that have been developed to measure the core symptoms of autism but also more subtle manifestations that characterize subjects with the broad autism phenotype are the Social Responsiveness Scale (SRS; Constantino, Gruber, Davis *et al.*, 2004) and the Child Social Behavior Questionnaire (CSBQ; Hartman, Luteijn, Serra, & Minderaa, 2006). A rating scale to be completed by parents, based on items from the ADI-R and developed to be used as a screening instrument, is the Social Communication Questionnaire (SCQ; Berument, Rutter, Lord, Pickles, & Bailey, 1999). The scale has good validity in differentiating ASD from non-ASD in children of 4 years and older, relatively independently from IQ, but has not been studied sufficiently below age 4 years.

The most often used standardized observation schedule is the Autism Diagnostic Observation Schedule (ADOS; Lord, Rutter, DiLavore, & Risi, 2001). It is built on a series of structured and semi-structured scenarios for interaction with the child by a well-trained interviewer. The presentation of the modules varies according to the child's verbal skills and the modules have been developed to optimally elicit the core symptoms of ASD. The ADOS takes about 40 min to administer, after which the scoring sheet should be completed.

The selection of specific IQ tests depends on the chronological age, mental age, verbal skills and level of cooperation, and should be carried out by an experienced psychologist. The same applies to the selection of language tests. A summary of available tests can be found elsewhere (Howlin, 1998).

A comprehensive physical examination is an indispensable component of the assessment. Particular attention should be paid to the presence of identifiable clinical syndromes, such as tuberous sclerosis (including the use of Wood's light to assess any skin lesions) or neurofibromatosis, dysmorphic features and any localizing neurological impairments (see chapter 22). Most experts agree that there is no indication in the clinical setting for routine magnetic resonance imaging (MRI) of the brain or lumbar punctures or metabolic screens, except when neurological abnormalities or clear major regression are present (Filipek, Accardo, Ashwal *et al.*, 2000). Given the increased rate of chromosomal anomalies in ASD, there is a need for routine DNA testing, including high-resolution chromosome testing, fluorescent *in situ* hybridization testing for Williams syndrome and subtelomeric deletions, and testing for the fragile X anomaly. There is a possibility that the premutation status (with an increase in trinucleotide repeats compared to the general population but below the full mutation expansion) has an increased risk for either ASD or other cognitive or behavioral problems (Hagerman, 2006). Lead levels should be obtained for children with developmental delays, even in the absence of a clear history of pica. About 30% of subjects with autism develop seizures, with a first manifestation either before age 5 years or in adolescence (Volkmar & Nelson, 1990). Sudden unexplained behavioral changes that are outside of the context of autistic symptoms should alert the clinician to this possibility. Assessment procedures that cannot be recommended as a routine are allergy testing, hair analysis, chelation challenge testing, gut permeability studies and stool analysis (Filipek, 2005).

Early Detection

Early identification of ASD is now considered to be clinical best practice, because it enables avoidance of unnecessary medical shopping for parents with clinical concerns, provides for early guidance and genetic counseling and starting early interventions (Charman & Baird, 2002; Rutter, 2006). A large proportion of subjects with ASD will nowadays be diagnosed around age 3–4 years, but somewhat later when early cognitive and language development are intact (Howlin & Moore, 1997).

Systematic analysis of video home movies of children in the first 2 years of their life and later diagnosed with ASD has shown that manifestation of ASD as early as 9–12 months may include difficulties orienting to social stimuli (e.g., less looking at people or faces and less responsiveness to name). This tends to be accompanied by less babbling, a limited understanding of spoken language and a paucity of gestures to express social interest or to draw attention to some object of interest in the environment (as distinct from gestures pointing to an object that the child wants). These difficulties tend to become more obvious in the second year of life, and extend to differences in joint attention and verbal communication. Prospective studies in high-risk siblings report consistent results (Zwaigenbaum, Bryson, Rogers *et al.*, 2005). The frequent association with intellectual impairment makes the early differentiation between ASD and intellectual disability problematic, and only a reduced frequency of looking at people and responding to name appears to differentiate ASD. The discriminative value of other behaviors is less clear, such as increased frequency of unusual visual inspection of objects, abnormal sensory reactions, and decreased flexibility and variety of play (Swinkels, Dietz, van Daalen *et al.*, 2006).

In contrast to this early-onset type of autism, 20–40% of children with ASD manifest an early regression of language and behavior, most often between 18 and 24 months (Werner & Dawson, 2005). Although there is no accepted definition of regression, parents report loss of using words or phrases, together with the loss of sociability and loss of interest in playing with toys, and in some cases the appearance of stereotypies and rigid behavior patterns. Home movies have confirmed the reality of developmental regression and shown that children who regress in the second year of life nonetheless tend to show subtle pre-existent social and regulatory problems (Werner & Dawson, 2005). It is unknown whether early regression represents a specific genetic or neurobiological subtype of ASD. The clinical and prognostic meaning of early regression is also unclear.

At this stage, the wide range of individual differences in both typical and atypical development in the first years of life makes effective screening for ASD below 18 months in normal populations not useful when parents have no clinical concerns (Dietz, Swinkels, van Daalen, van Engeland, & Buitelaar, 2006). Screening is possible and worthwhile after 18 months, particularly in cases of high-risk status or clinical concerns by parents or health care professionals, and is recommended as part of more comprehensive surveillance programs to identify children in need of further assessment. In addition to parental concerns about poor communication, socialization or other behavioral problems, absolute indications for further specialist referral are the absence of babbling by 12 months, the absence of gesturing (pointing, waving bye-bye, etc.) by 12 months, no single words by 16 months, no two-word spontaneous (not just echolalic) phrases by 24 months, and any loss of any language or social skills at any age (Filipek, Accardo, Baranek *et al.*, 1999). A number of instruments are available to be used around 18–30 months such as the Checklist for Autism in Toddlers (CHAT; Baron-Cohen, Allen, & Gillberg, 1992, Baron-Cohen, Wheelwright, Cox *et al.*, 2000), Modified Checklist for Autism in Toddlers (M-CHAT; Robins, Fein, Barton, & Green, 2001) and Early Screening for Autistic Traits (ESAT; Swinkels, Dietz, van Daalen *et al.*, 2006).

Cognitive Theories

Cognitive models have been developed in an attempt to explain the heterogeneous clinical manifestations of ASD by a so-called core deficit (i.e., a basic impairment that is primary and underived from other cognitive factors in development, and underlies the clinical social symptoms).

Mentalizing Ability

The theory of mind hypothesis proposes that individuals with ASD have a fundamental problem in attributing mental states such as feelings, desires, intentions, fantasies, dreams and beliefs to others and oneself. This leads to "mind-blindness," a failure to perceive others as social agents, and therefore results in deficient social, emotional and communicative actions and responses, and a failure of imagination. This hypothesis has stimulated a body of experimental psychological work in individuals with ASD that has revealed widespread problems in mentalizing and empathizing ability (Baron-Cohen, 1995; Baron-Cohen, Tager-Flusberg, & Cohen, 1993; Frith, 2003). The spin-off has also been studies into the neural substrate of mentalizing skills in normal subjects and in ASD (Baron-Cohen, Ring, Wheelwright *et al.*, 1999; Castelli, Frith, Happe, & Frith, 2002). Important components of the so-called "social brain" are the amygdala, the orbitofrontal and medial frontal cortex, and the superior temporal sulcus and gyrus in these regions have shown abnormalities in autism.

However, there are several arguments against a core deficit in theory of mind in autism. Social dysfunction in autism is typically present prior to the time at which even the earliest precursors of a theory of mind emerge (Klin, Volkmar, & Sparrow, 1992). The theory of mind hypothesis is less able to explain the lack of spontaneous and original activity of persons with autism, their repetitive behavior, their impairment in understanding conversation (Yirmiya, Sigman, Kasari, & Mundy, 1992) and their executive dysfunctioning (Hughes, Russell, & Robbins, 1994). Impairments in theory of mind do not seem to be specific, nor are they universally present in ASD (Buitelaar, van der Wees, Swaab Barneveld, & van der Gaag, 1999b). Relatively able individuals with ASD, such as those with Asperger disorder, can solve theory of mind problems, albeit often by idiosyncratic and alternative strategies, and still present with major social handicaps in everyday life (Bowler, 1992; Ozonoff & McEvoy, 1994; Ziatas, Durkin, & Pratt, 1998).

The mentalizing account of ASD was later extended to the empathizing–systemizing (E-S) theory (Baron-Cohen, 2002). In addition to weak mentalizing–empathizing skills, systemizing is either intact or superior. Systemizing is the drive to analyze systems in terms of their underlying rules and regularities. Good systemizing skills would explain islets of abilities, the content of obsessional symptoms and repetitive behavior. Such predictions have yet to be adequately tested.

Central Coherence Theory

The central coherence theory originally suggested that a core deficit in processing information for meaning and for global (gestalt) form would explain the social symptoms in ASD (Frith, 1991). Weak central coherence, with an undue focus on details, would lead to a disregard to contextual issues, and to fragmented perceptions of the external world. This was illustrated remarkably well by performances on the Block Design test of the Wechler's Intelligence Scales and on the Embedded Figures test. Both tests require "field independence," that is, the ability to disregard context (Frith & Happé, 1994). However, later work has challenged this view in the following ways (for review see Happé & Frith, 2006). Weak global extraction of information may be the result of a superior performance in local processing of details, rather than vice versa. Further, many individuals with ASD seem able to pay sufficient attention to global information when specifically directed to do so. This means that the strong preference for local detailed information is a cognitive style or processing bias rather than a cognitive deficit. Weak central coherence characterizes a subsample of the ASD population and seems to be an aspect of their cognitive set-up of ASD, but does not serve as the all-explaining core deficit.

Executive Functioning

Executive functions (EFs) are mental control processes that enable the self-control necessary for the attainment of a future goal (Pennington & Ozonoff, 1996). EF refers to cognitive functions mediated by the prefrontal cortex (Fuster, 1997), such as inhibition, working memory, cognitive flexibility or set-shifting, planning and verbal fluency (Pennington & Ozonoff, 1996). The EF account of ASD assumes that the weak performance of one or more of these cognitive functions (poor attentional regulation, inability to shift attention) on the basis of some form of neurological abnormality of the prefrontal cortex, leads to the perseverative inflexible problem-solving strategies commonly observed in ASD and ultimately to the other social and communicative symptoms. Multiple studies have identified EF deficits in preschoolers, children and adolescents as well as adults with autism (Geurts, Verte, Oosterlaan, Roeyers, & Sergeant, 2004; Williams, Goldstein, Carpenter, & Minshew, 2005), although inconsistent findings have also been reported (Griffith, Pennington, Wehner, & Rogers, 1999; Ozonoff & Strayer, 1997; Russell, Jarrold, & Hood, 1999).

However, it would be simplistic to assume that autism can be explained by poor EF, because:

1 Poor EF is also found in other disorders such as ADHD, although EF deficits were much more widespread in ASD than in ADHD in a direct comparison (Geurts, Verte, Oosterlaan *et al.*, 2004);

2 EF deficits are not always seen in ASD;

3 Children with early frontal lesions do not all appear to be autistic (Ozonoff, Pennington, & Rogers, 1991a,b); and

4 The correlation between EF deficits and social impairment is not very strong (Dawson & Osterling, 1997).

Treatment

The main aims of the treatment of ASD are (Rutter, 1985):

1 As much as possible to facilitate and stimulate the normal development of cognition, language and socialization;

2 To decrease autism-bound maladaptive behaviors such as rigidity, stereotypy, and inflexibility;

3 To reduce or even eliminate non-specific maladaptive behaviors such as hyperactivity, irritability and impulsivity; and

4 To alleviate stress and burden for the family.

Further information about treatment of ASD is available in recent US practice parameters (American Academy of Pediatrics, 2000; Volkmar, Cook, Pomeroy *et al.*, 1999). The treatment of individuals with ASD should be multimodal, with a combination of family counseling, structured and special educational techniques, individual behavior modification, home training, and placement in special schools or daycare centers. So far, ASD are chronically disabling conditions for which no effective evidence-based cure exists. This does not detract from the great benefits that can be brought by a comprehensive and intensive treatment plan to patients and their families in terms of improvement in quality of life. Recent research suggests that the most effective results stem from early intensive behavioral interventions. Medication treatment has not been shown to influence the core symptoms of ASD, but may be considered when troublesome target and comorbid symptoms such as aggression, temper tantrums, irritability, hyperactivity, self-injurious behavior, rigidity, anxiety and sleeping problems do not respond to behavioral interventions or seriously interfere with the application of these interventions.

There are some general principles of treatment of ASD that are important. Individuals with ASD reach a higher level of social functioning in highly structured than in unstructured situations. For example, the daily routines of a classroom provide structure, whereas anxiety, social isolation and rigidities may emerge rapidly during free time and lunch breaks. In relation to this, the social functioning of those with ASD is usually better in an environment with moderate levels of expression of emotions and symbolic meanings. For example, the difficulty for individuals with ASD to grasp the symbolic meaning of special events and ceremonies such as a birthday party or Christmas can easily make them anxious or lead to aggressive reactions when pushed too much. The intensity of social stimulation offered should be adjusted to the level that can be handled. When a child has reached an equilibrium in interacting with one or two other children as buddies at school, this should first be consolidated before other classmates are to be involved. Every treatment plan should accommodate for the often profound limitations in communication of individuals with ASD. This could be addressed by some form of speech and language therapy, and for very young or nonverbal subjects by the Picture Exchange Communication System

(Bondy & Frost, 1998, 2001), Social Stories, which is the use of cartoon-type illustrations to help children understand how to respond in social situations, or peer-mediated intervention (Roeyers, 1996). Training and interventions should be performed as much as possible in daily-life situations, in an attempt to overcome the problems of the transfer of skills mastered in one setting to another.

Counseling for Parents and Family Support

It is very important to inform parents about the diagnosis and implications for the future of the child. Parents may have difficulty in accepting the diagnosis. Once a family has a child with ASD, the risk of recurrence of ASD in subsequent children rises to 3–7%. Therefore, parents need appropriate counseling on genetic issues. During the different stages of development, the child and parents have different needs. For example, placement in a school that provides a specialized education can be enough for the first years, but when behavior management problems occur, more intensive counseling, behavioral therapy and/or medication may be an option. In some countries, patients and their families are organized into National Autistic Societies which hold information evenings where parents can meet each other and where "non-professional" support is given. Most parents benefit from training courses aimed at skills building and reduction of problematic behavior. In adolescence, attention should be paid to sexuality issues that may be relevant to ASD – such as masturbation, inappropriate touching, privacy issues and public exposure.

Early Intervention

There are great expectations in the field from the benefits of intensive early interventions for children with ASD (Butter, Wynn, & Mulick, 2003). Typically, these interventions would be started shortly after diagnosis and continued up to kindergarten or primary school, depending on the child's progress and areas of handicap. Work on early intensive treatment has started with claims about significant gains in IQ and outcome in a sample of 19 young autistic children (Lovaas, 1987). However, this promising result and that of a related study (McEachin, Smith, & Lovaas, 1993) have been questioned because of methodological problems (Campbell, Schopler, Cueva, & Hallin, 1996). There are now a number of positive studies of intensive early intervention which indicate that a subsample of children with ASD make considerable progress and nearly all children show some benefits (Medical Research Council, 2001; National Research Council, 2001). However, observations also indicate that some young children with ASD improve rapidly with relatively little intervention, and others show very little progress despite very intensive and comprehensive multimodal treatments. It is claimed that effective early interventions include the following important components (Kabot, Masi, & Segal, 2003):

1 Provision at the earliest possible age;
2 High intensity, with the suggestion of a threshold of at least 20 h per week spent one-to-one with the child;
3 Strongly based on parent involvement, training and support;
4 Various modules and training schemes to stimulate social and communicative functioning of the child in a developmentally oriented way;
5 Systematic instruction with individual goals, based on applied-behavioral analysis (ABA) and stepwise approach; and
6 Investment in attempts to generalize acquired skills to other settings of daily life.

Further research is needed to test these claims.

Education

Opportunities for adequate education are essential, as follow-up studies have indicated that children who complete some form of education have a better outcome (van der Gaag, 1993). It is necessary for the teacher to be informed about the nature of autism and the child's needs. An autistic child at school needs extra individual attention, a very structured approach and special education programs, such as the Treatment and Education of Autistic and related Communication-handicapped CHildren program (TEACCH; Mesibov, Shea, & Schopler, 2004). This program emphasizes extensive collaboration with and training of the parents, so that they become knowledgeable about their child's disorder and needs. This program provides a highly structured approach for autistic children at school. Based on principles from cognitive–behavioral theory, a system is developed with stepwise visualization of the actions needed to fulfill a task. Through this system the life-environment can be structured, and parents can act as co-therapists and continue with the principles of TEACCH at home.

Skills Training and Behavioral Therapy

Depending on clinical needs, a number of specific treatment modalities may be helpful. In cases of clumsiness or delays in motor development, there is an indication for sensorimotor training. Language and communication skills can be facilitated by means of language training. Occupational therapy and play therapy may be of use in some cases. For high-functioning autistic children, individual therapy can be an option, for instance when the child is suffering from the awareness of being different. Social skills training programs, delivered on an individual or on a group basis, are being offered to children and adolescents with ASD at an increasing rate (Bauminger, 2002; Koegel & Frea, 1993). Recently, social skills training programs have been nurtured with ideas from research on theory of mind and emotion recognition deficits in autism (Howlin, Baron-Cohen, & Hadwin, 1999). Although the benefits may be an improvement of social awareness and the acquisition of routine social skills, the merits on a long-term basis are often disappointing because of a lack of generalization of skills.

Behavioral treatment based on classic and operant conditioning is the most studied and publicized form of non-medical treatment. There is a clear indication for specific behavioral interventions in cases of severely interfering and maladaptive behaviors such as stereotypies, self-injury and negativism. Also, the acquisition of normal behaviors, such as toileting, may benefit from behavioral interventions. These interventions should be based on a detailed analysis of the functional relationship between the child and the environment (Campbell, Schopler, Cueva *et al.*, 1996), which can then give rise to an individual treatment plan designed for the child.

Vocational Training

ASD are lifelong disorders that impact on the ability of individuals to obtain employment, care for themselves and live independently. As a result, many individuals with autism require some form of community support. Projects have been established that involve autistic people living with more or less intensive supervision by a professional. Specialist-supported employment services have been designed for high-ability adults with autism; approximately 68% of clients found employment (Howlin, Alcock, & Burkin, 2005; Mawhood & Howlin, 1999).

Medication

There is no drug that has been shown to have a consistent and worthwhile effect on the core symptoms of autism. Accordingly, treatment plans should not involve any presupposition that medication should be used. Nevertheless, drugs can be useful in modifying some specific behaviors and hence we review the findings accordingly. When using medication, it is important to select appropriate targets of treatment and to monitor efficacy and side effects on a regular basis. Potential benefits of any medication should be weighed against side effects and risks.

Concern over side effects such as tardive dyskinesia and extrapyramidal symptoms (EPS) of conventional antipsychotics has led to increased use of the newer atypical antipsychotics. Risperidone, the best studied and most often used atypical antipsychotic, has shown superiority to placebo in short-term randomized controlled trials in children and adolescents with ASD (McCracken, McGough, Shah *et al.*, 2002; Shea, Turgay, Carroll *et al.*, 2004) and in adults (McDougle, Holmes, Carlson *et al.*, 1998). Maintenance of effect of risperidone over a period of 6 months has been established in placebo-controlled discontinuation studies (RUPP, 2005b; Troost, Lahuis, Steenhuis *et al.*, 2005). Risperidone in low daily doses (0.5–1.5 mg for most subjects) appears to be effective in decreasing irritability, temper tantrums, hyperactivity, aggression and self-injurious behavior in ASD, but without convincing positive effects on the core symptoms. Although risperidone is usually well tolerated, except for mild initial sedation, and the risk of EPS is low, a serious limitation of the use of risperidone is the risk of significant weight gain. Weight gain should be monitored each week, and an increase of 3 kg or more in the first month of treatment should lead to discontinuation. Less well studied in ASD are other atypical antipsychotics such as olanzapine, quetiapine, ziprasidone and aripiprazole.

Fluoxetine treatment has been studied in children and adults with ASD and was shown to be effective in reducing compulsive and repetitive behaviors, stereotypies and rituals (DeLong, Teague, & McSwain, 1998; Hollander, Phillips, Chaplin *et al.*, 2005). Fluoxetine was generally well tolerated; adverse effects included agitation, hyperactivity, hypomania and disinhibition. Similar treatment effects were obtained with fluvoxamine in a controlled trial in adults with autism (McDougle, Naylor, Cohen *et al.*, 1996b). However, a trial with fluvoxamine in children and adolescents with autism was unable to establish a significant treatment response but documented a high rate of side effects and adverse behavioral activation (McDougle, personal communication).

A recent large controlled trial with methylphenidate in children with ASD and symptoms of ADHD found that the clinical response was lower and that the risk for adverse effects such as irritability was increased, compared to that in children with typical ADHD. When using low dosages (0.125–0.5 $mg{\cdot}kg^{-1}$ per day) and careful clinical monitoring, treatment with stimulants none the less may be of substantial clinical value in individuals with ASD and symptoms of ADHD (RUPP, 2005a).

Mood stabilizers such as lithium and valproic acid have been used to treat affective instability, impulsivity and aggression in individuals with ASD (Hollander, Dolgoff-Kaspar, Cartwright, Rawitt, & Novotny, 2001; Kerbeshian, Burd, & Fisher, 1987; Plioplys, 1994). Anticonvulsants are important in the management of the seizure disorders in ASD.

Buspirone, an agonist of the serotonin $5T_{1a}$ receptor, may be useful in improving anxiety, temper tantrums, and aggression associated with ASD in regimens of 10–45 $mg{\cdot}day^{-1}$ (Buitelaar, van der Gaag, & van der Hoeven, 1998). Propranolol, a lipophilic beta-blocker, may be used to treat aggression, self-injury and impulsivity in developmental disorders (Ratey, Bemporad, Sorgi *et al.*, 1987a; Ratey, Mikkelsen, Sorgi *et al.*, 1987b). It is necessary to obtain an electrocardiogram (ECG) before treatment starts and to monitor pulse rate and blood pressure regularly because of the risk of bradycardia and hypotension.

Ineffective or Unproven Treatments

Probably more often than in any other psychiatric condition of childhood and adolescence, parents of children with ASD tend to seek out complementary and alternative medical (CAM) treatments both for the core symptoms and for comorbid symptoms (Levy & Hyman, 2003). It is important to respect parents' views, critically discuss the merits and risk–benefit ratio of these treatments and advise the family on treatments with and without supporting evidence, and for families choosing CAM treatments, assisting to determine if the treatment is helpful by gathering clinical outcome data (Aman, 2005). Among the ineffective or unproven treatments are facilitated communication, administration of secretin (a gastrointestinal peptide hormone with putative effects on the brain), auditory integration training, treatment with vitamin B_6 and magnesium, gluten- and casein-free diets, essential fatty acid treatment, Son-Rise Program and cranial osteopathy (Aman, 2005; Howlin, 2005).

Etiology

Environmental Risk Factors

Although the high heritability of ASD might seem to imply that environmental risk factors will be unimportant, this does not necessarily follow (Rutter, 2006; Rutter, Moffitt, & Caspi, 2006). If the rise in the rate of diagnosed ASD represents a true rise in incidence (which remains quite uncertain), there would be the implication that some new (or increased) environmental risk factor was operative. If so, it is likely that the risks would stem from some prenatal or early postnatal factor, most likely of a physical nature. The large-scale Norwegian prospective longitudinal study of a cohort of some 100,000 being followed from pregnancy provides the possibility of identifying any such risks (Magnus, Irgens, Haug *et al.*, 2006; Rønningen, Paltiel, Meltzer *et al.*, 2006). They could be in toxins, pollutants, diet or immunological abnormalities.

An area of uncertainty includes the possibility of abnormalities in the immune system in ASD. Studies of immunological function reveal a wide range of abnormalities, including decreased cellular immune capacity, decreased plasma complement component C4b, and increased humoral immune and autoantibody responses (Hornig & Lipkin, 2001). These abnormalities of the peripheral immune system have been linked to the hypothesis that children with ASD are predisposed to abnormal responses to viral infections either through the establishment of persistent infections or a virally triggered autoimmune diathesis. However, immune dysfunction in ASD has not been established or corroborated by measures more directly related to the brain, such as by studies of cerebrospinal fluid (CSF) or at autopsy. Thus, it is unclear whether systemic immune dysfunction is truly common in ASD (Murch, 2005). With respect to possible environmental risk factors, it will also be necessary to consider the possible role of gene–environment interaction (Hornig, Chian, & Lipkin, 2004; Rutter, 2006; Rutter, Moffitt, & Caspi, 2006).

There is a long-standing interest in obstetric risk factors, and recent studies have confirmed that individuals with autism have more obstetric risk factors than controls, as evidenced, for example, by the presence of fetal distress, being delivered by elective or emergency Cesarean section, more frequent breech presentations, and lower Apgar scores at 1 or 5 min (Glasson, Bower, Petterson *et al.*, 2004; Larsson, Eaton, Madsen *et al.*, 2005). Cases with PDD-NOS or Asperger disorder had lower risk scores than subjects with typical autism, and higher than controls (Glasson, Bower, Petterson *et al.*, 2004). However, because unaffected siblings of cases were more similar to cases than to control subjects in their profile of complications, the higher rate of obstetric complications may reflect underlying genetic vulnerability or an interaction between genetic factors and the environment. Other data support the view that obstetric hazards are, at least in part, consequences of genetically influenced abnormal prenatal development rather than independent etiological factors (Bolton, Murphy, Macdonald *et al.*, 1997). For example, postmortem studies of autism have not detected lesions typical of perinatal brain damage, and studies of autistic singletons have found that the number of minor congenital anomalies is higher in probands than in siblings or normal controls, which suggests that the early *in utero* development of autistic individuals may be suboptimal (Bailey, Phillips, & Rutter, 1996).

Developmental Perturbations

Traditionally, studies of non-genetic influences on causal pathways for disorders have focused on specific environmental hazards of some kind. However, as Molenaar, Boomsma, and Dolan (1993) pointed out, it is also necessary to consider the possibility of chance causing developmental perturbations that increase the risk of some maladaptive outcomes. Three sets of findings suggest that such perturbations may contribute to the liability to autism. First, surveys indicate that 5–10% of individuals with ASD have some form of chromosomal anomaly (Autism Genome Project Consortium, 2007). However, apart from duplications of 15q11–q13, typically of maternal origin (which occur in 1–3% of cases), the anomalies span virtually all chromosomes and offer no good leads for the location of susceptibility genes. Nevertheless, the raised rate of anomalies relative to the general population does suggest some type of developmental perturbation. Perhaps the significant feature lies in the suggestion that development has gone awry, rather than the specific form of the anomaly. The parallel would be in the increased rate of minor congenital anomalies associated with an increased risk for many types of psychopathology. Second, the large-scale Autism Genome Project Consortium (2007) study found an increased rate of copy number abnormalities (CNAs) – such as exemplified by the chromosome 15 duplication. For a variety of conceptual and technical reasons, it is difficult to provide a confident quantitative estimate of their frequency, but a figure of about 10% seems likely for families in which all affected individuals share the same possibly detrimental abnormality. Third, a recent large-scale study of Israeli army conscripts found an association between autism and raised paternal age (Reichenberg, Gross, Weiser *et al.*, 2006). The finding has yet to be replicated, but it too suggests that a focus on developmental perturbations might prove profitable.

Neural Basis of Autism

The last decade has seen an enormous proliferation of studies seeking to identify the neural basis of autism (for reviews see DiCicco-Bloom, Lord, Zwaigenbaum *et al.*, 2006; Moldin & Rubenstein, 2006; Moldin, Rubenstein, & Hyman, 2006). Attention has been drawn to the possible role of mirror neuron dysfunction because these neurons respond to perceived mental states (Dapretto, Davies, Pfeifer *et al.*, 2006). A range of animal models has been proposed but, at least so far, their relevance to autism seems quite uncertain. Thus, there was excitement over the social differences between montane and prairie moles, with findings pointing to the role of oxytocin and vasopressin (Young & Wang, 2004) but knockout mice display social amnesia, which is not what is found in autism. Numerous leads are worth following up but they have yet to deliver; accordingly, we focus primarily on human studies.

Head Circumference

One of the most consistent anatomical findings in autism research is an enlarged head circumference (Bailey, Phillips, & Rutter, 1996; DiCicco-Bloom, Lord, Zwaigenbaum *et al.*, 2006;

Fombonne, Rogé, Claverie, Courty, & Frémolle, 1999). Brain size is approximately normal at birth but increases in the preschool years so that by 3–4 years of age, the average brain size in individuals with autism in increased by about 10%. The evidence with respect to older ages is more limited but it seems that brain size remains increased to some extent (Palmen, Hulshoff Pol, Kemner *et al.*, 2005) but probably to a lesser degree. The available evidence suggests that the increased brain growth affects both gray and white matter, but the findings are inconsistent and inconclusive (Palmen, Hulshoff Pol, Kemner *et al.*, 2005). Whether or not it reflects an excess of neurons, and/or reduced synaptic pruning, remains uncertain (Keller & Persico, 2003). It also remains uncertain how far the macrocephaly is proportionate or disproportionate to overall body growth (Torrey, Dhavale, Lawlor, & Yolken, 2004). Accordingly, it remains unclear what role the increased rate of brain growth in early life plays in the pathogenesis of autism.

Neuroimaging

Structural neuroimaging studies in individuals with autism converge to show that the brain is abnormally large in some, but not all children with autism (Lainhart, 2006; Palmen & van Engeland, 2004). Advances in structural brain mapping have been used to investigate morphological connectivity. Structures in the brain whose functions are tightly coupled grow and develop in unison. Children with autism show evidence of marked disruption in relationships between cortical–subcortical and cortical–cortical gray matter volumes (McAlonan, Cheung, Cheung *et al.*, 2005). Correlations between frontal lobe gray matter volume and temporal lobe, parietal lobe and subcortical gray matter have been found to be aberrant in autistic children.

Functional MRI (fMRI) studies examine functional connectivity in the brain by measuring the correlation between the amount of activation of two brain areas during task performance measuring social attribution, sentence comprehension and working memory (Castelli, Frith, Happe *et al.*, 2002; Just, Cherkassky, Keller, & Minshew, 2004; Koshino, Carpenter, Minshew *et al.*, 2005). Aberrant or reduced connectivity patterns have been found. Other fMRI studies of brain function during tasks or in response to visual and auditory stimuli show evidence that individuals with autism appear to be using different cognitive strategies and some different brain areas to process information (Gervais, Belin, Boddaert *et al.*, 2004; Hadjiklani, Joseph, Snyder *et al.*, 2004; Muller, Kleinhans, Kemnotsu, Pierce, & Courchesne, 2003; Pierce, Haist, Sedaghar, & Courchesne, 2004; Piggot, Kwon, Mobbs *et al.*, 2004; Schultz, Gauthier, Klein *et al.*, 2000; Wang, Ting, Dapretto *et al.*, 2004; Williams, Goldstein, Carpenter *et al.*, 2005).

Neuropathology

A review of postmortem studies in autism revealed that approximately 40 brains have been studied (Palmen & van Engeland, 2004) with an emerging pattern of increased cell packing in the limbic system, reduced numbers of Purkinje cells in the cerebellum, age-related changes in cerebellar nuclei and inferior olives, cortical dysgenesis and increased brain weight. However, all reported studies had to contend with the problem of small sample sizes, the use of quantification techniques not free of bias and assumptions, and high percentages of autistic subjects with co-occurring intellectual impairment and epilepsy (at least 70% and 40%, respectively).

Cortical minicolumns have been measured in postmortem brains of autistic persons and compared with non-affected controls. Minicolumns consist of approximately 80–100 neurons arranged radially like beads on a string and are believed to comprise the smallest level of functional organization in the cortex cerebri (Mountcastle, 1997). Minicolumnar width, interneuronal distance, peripheral neuropil space and compactness were evaluated and it was found that minicolumns in the brains of autistic persons were more numerous, "narrower" with less peripheral neuropil space and increased spacing among the constituent cells (Casanova, 2004; Casanova, Buxhoeveden, Switala *et al.*, 2002; Casanova, van Kooten, Switala *et al.*, 2006). The authors conjecture that these micro-architectural abnormalities originate during prenatal development and reflect progressive encephalization, defined as a disproportionate increase in white matter relative to gray matter.

Neurophysiology

Along with epilepsy (Rutter, 1970), one of the first indications of abnormal brain function in autism came from EEG studies. With repeated or extensive testing, EEG abnormalities are found in about 50% of individuals with autism (Minshew, 1991). Although regional differences in EEG power have been reported, there is no evidence of regional localization of abnormalities (Dawson & Osterling, 1997).

For many years event-related potentials (ERPs) were the only means available to investigate brain function during specific cognitive tasks (Burack, Enns, Stauder, Mottron, & Randolphe, 1997). Event-related evoked potentials and magneto-electro-encephalography provide information about temporal and spatial aspects of brain functioning in autism. Studies using these methods show that individuals with autism have slowed face processing, decreased sensitivity to whether a face is upright or inverted, less effect to repeated presentation of a face, abnormal brain response to eye-gaze detection, abnormal hemispheric lateralization and different localization of processing within the cortex (Bailey, Braeutigam, Jousmäki, & Swithenby, 2005; Grice, Halit, Farroni *et al.*, 2005; McPartland, Dawson, Webb, Panagiotides, & Carver, 2004).

Behavioral studies have shown subjects with ASD to have a variety of abnormalities in attentional processing (Allen & Courchesne, 2001). Several ERP studies focused on attentional and perceptual processing of visual stimuli in persons with autism. Although some studies reported that subjects with ASD show less long-latency activity (mostly reflected in P3 peak) in response to infrequently occurring stimuli within an oddball paradigm, these findings are not consistent (Kemner & van Engeland, 2006). A serious problem in the interpretation of these studies is that subjects were not matched for IQ and age, and there is evidence that the P3 peak is sensitive to these variables (Polich & Herbst, 2000; Wahlovd & Fjell, 2003). The only study in which subjects were age and IQ matched (Kemner, Verbaten, Cuperus, Camfferman, & van Engeland, 2004) did not find differences between persons with autism and control groups in this respect. Additionally, there are no indications that individuals with autism have a decreased processing capacity (Hoeksma, Kenemans, Kemner, & van Engeland, 2005). ERP studies of the ability to focus attention on a specific channel of information (selective attention) failed to find consistent evidence of abnormal attentional processing in subjects with autism (Ciesielski, Courchesne, & Elmasian, 1990; Hoeksma, Kenemans, Kemner *et al.*, 2005).

Recently, several studies have indicated that the atypical processing of visual stimuli in autistic children and adolescents might occur at a perceptual level, because ERP studies have provided evidence that activity over the modality-specific cortex is already abnormal at an early stage of processing (Boeschoten, Kemner, Kenemans, & van Engeland, 2007; Hoeksma, Kenemans, Kemner *et al.*, 2005; Kemner, Verbaten, Cuperus *et al.*, 2004; Verbaten, Roelofs, van Engeland, Kenemans, & Slangen, 1991). The authors conjecture that this abnormal brain activation might be related to the spatial frequency content of the visual stimuli and a decreased specialization of the visual brain pathways for spatial frequency processing (Kemner & van Engeland, 2006).

Other studies have examined the processing of auditory stimuli in autism. These studies found evidence that children with autism have neural-based impairments in automatically orienting to speech-like sounds but not to non-speech sounds (Ceponiene, Lepistö, Shestakova *et al.*, 2003). Adults with autism may have impairments in one of the earliest levels of cortical speech processing, automatic detection of change in speech (Kasai, Hashimoto, Kawakubo *et al.*, 2005). In noisy environments, individuals with autism appear to have neural-based deficits in recognizing and understanding speech and attending to socially relevant sounds (Alcantara, Weisblatt, Moore, & Bolton, 2004; Teder-Salajarri, Pierce, Courchesne, & Hillyard, 2005). Involuntary orienting to sound depends on neural communication in a widely distributed network, involving auditory cortex, multimodal sensory areas in the parietal lobe, and dorsolateral prefrontal cortex.

Neurochemistry

The most robust and well-replicated biological finding is the 25–50% increase in levels of serotonin in blood platelets in subjects with autism (for reviews see Lam, Aman, & Arnold, 2006; McDougle, Erickson, Stigler, & Posey, 2005) and the broader phenotype (Mulder, Anderson, Kema *et al.*, 2004). The mechanism of the alteration remains unknown. Additional factors that may determine serotonin levels in blood are pubertal status, race and use of medication (McBride, Anderson, Hertzig *et al.*, 1998). Abnormalities of central rather than peripheral serotonin systems matter when considering the pathophysiology of ASD. Acute depletion of dietary tryptophan (the dietary precursor of serotonin) leads to a forced lowering of serotonin in the brain and worsening of autistic symptomatology (McDougle, Naylor, Cohen *et al.*, 1996a; McDougle, Naylor, Cohen *et al.*, 1996b), underlining the role of central serotonin in the expression of the syndrome. Further, positron emission tomography (PET) using a tracer for the synthesis of serotonin in the brain found indications for an abnormal serotonin synthesis capacity over time in autism (Chugani, Muzik, Rothermel *et al.*, 1997). Because serotonin acts as a growth factor and regulator of early neuronal development before assuming its role as a neurotransmitter in the mature brain, this suggests that developmental dysregulation of serotonin synthesis may be involved in the pathogenesis of ASD (Whitaker-Azimitia, 2001).

Research into the dopamine neurotransmitter system by measuring levels of dopamine's major metabolite homovanillic acid (HVA) in blood, urine and CSF did not reveal significant differences (McDougle , Erickson, Stigler *et al.*, 2005). A PET scan study showed reduced accumulation of dopamine in the prefrontal cortex of subjects with autism (Ernst, Zametkin, Matochik, Pascualvaca, & Cohen, 1997). There are no notable abnormalities in neurochemical indices of the norepinephrine transmitter system in ASD.

Little research has been performed examining the role of glutamate and gamma-aminobutyric acid (GABA) in ASD. Glutamate is the primary excitatory transmitter and is crucially involved in neuronal plasticity and higher cognitive functions (Purcell, Jeon, Zimmerman, Blue, & Pevsner, 2001), whereas GABA is the primary inhibitory transmitter in the brain. Measuring peripheral levels of these transmitters has produced conflicting findings, but postmortem studies found indirect evidence for altered status of glutamate and GABA receptors in the hippocampus (Fatemi, Halt, Stary *et al.*, 2002).

Animal work has led to interest in the role of neuropeptides such as endogenous opioids, oxytocin and vasopressin in regulating social behavior. Nevertheless, neither evaluations of levels of opioids in body fluids nor clinical trials investigating the effects of opioid receptor antagonists lend support for a key role of opioids in the pathophysiology of ASD (Tordjman, Anderson, McBride *et al.*, 1997; Willemsen-Swinkels, Buitelaar, Nijhof, & van Engeland, 1995). Children with autism were shown to have lower plasma levels of oxytocin (Green, Fein, Modahl *et al.*, 2001) but intravenous administration of oxytocin did not lead to changes in the core symptoms of ASD (Hollander, Novotny, Hanratty *et al.*, 2003). Research on melatonin and secretin does not support a role of these neuropeptides in the pathophysiology of ASD (Esch & Carr, 2004; Nir, Meir, Zilber *et al.*, 1995).

Findings of early abnormalities in the development of the brain in ASD, and a potential contribution therein of neuropeptides and/or neurotrophins, led to an analysis of peptide concentrations in frozen blood samples of neonates subsequently diagnosed with ASD and contrast and control samples (Nelson, Grether, Croen *et al.*, 2001; Nelson, Kuddo, Song *et al.*, 2006). Concentrations of some neurotrophic factors were higher in subjects with ASD and with intellectual disability but they did not differentiate these two groups; these results await replication and extension.

Genetics

Data from several epidemiological twin and family studies provide substantial evidence that ASD are amongst the most heritable complex disorders (Rutter, 2000). The concordance rate in monozygotic (MZ) twins is 60–90% and the autism rate in siblings is about 5% (Bailey, Palferman, Heavey *et al.*, 1998b; Szatmari, Jones, Zwaigenbaum, & MacLean, 1998). Folstein and Rutter's (1977) twin study was remarkable for indicating that the phenotype associated with a genetic predisposition to autistic disorder included cognitive and social difficulties extending beyond autism as traditionally diagnosed. In a follow-up into adulthood of this original sample, the majority of non-autistic MZ cotwins showed social and/or cognitive abnormalities, with the most severely affected individuals having more well-defined ASD (Bailey, Le Couteur, Gottesman *et al.*, 1995). A parallel family history study found similar social and/or cognitive abnormalities at a higher rate in relatives of probands with autism compared to relatives of probands with Down syndrome (Bolton, Macdonald, Pickles *et al.*, 1994). In fact, individuals with autism represented only a small proportion of all the individuals showing phenotypic expression.

Since then numerous family studies have reported mild autism-related behavioral phenotypes manifesting as social, communicative and repetitive impairments, either alone or in combination in first-, second- or third-degree family members of autistic probands (for a review Bailey, Palferman, Heavey *et al.*, 1998b). Some relatives of autistic individuals show a lack of interest in others, or a lack of socioemotional responsiveness, whereas others may show socially odd behavior, a history of language delay, circumscribed interests, rigidity, obsessive-compulsive and repetitive behavior and a lack of seeking change (Bailey, Palferman, Heavey *et al.*, 1998b; Lainhart, 1999; Piven, Palmer, Jacobi, Childress, & Arndt, 1997; Starr, Berument, Pickles *et al.*, 2001). It is estimated that this "broader phenotype" or "milder variant" can be found in 20–30% of the relatives of autistic individuals (de Jonge, 2006; Fombonne, Bolton, Prior, Jordan, & Rutter, 1997). The highest rates of "broader phenotype" characteristics were found in multi-incidence families (Lainhart, 1999; Piven, Palmer, Jacobi *et al.*, 1997; Szatmari, Bryson, Streiner *et al.*, 2000).

Clearly, genetic risk ASD is not conferred in a simple Mendelian fashion. Statistical modeling of the data derived from twin and family studies has implicated the involvement of several genes interacting with one another to produce the clinical phenotype that is a multilocal model with epistasis. Latent class analysis of twin and family data has suggested that as few as 3–4 predisposing genes may be involved (Pickles, Bolton, Macdonald *et al.*, 1995), although the presence of as many as 15 loci has been proposed (Risch, 1999). The clinical complexity and heterogeneity of the autism phenotype are also likely to reflect the presence of genetic heterogeneity (different genes or combination of genes may be involved in different families). Other factors, such as sex and environmental influences, may also affect phenotypic expression. Moreover, epigenetic mechanisms such as DNA methylation defects or abnormal imprinting have also been proposed as possible factors in the etiology of autism (Abdolmaleky, Smith, Faraone *et al.*, 2004; Lamb, Barnby, Bonora *et al.*, 2005).

Although autism and ASD exhibit high heritability, the identification of susceptibility genes has so far been elusive. The major challenges are represented by the complex inheritance pattern, the likely involvement of multiple genes each having a moderate effect on disease risk, the high degree of heterogeneity and the lack of clear pathophysiological clues that could suggest particularly strong candidate genes. Therefore, the typical approach adopted by many research groups has been to perform genome-wide scans for linkage. This entails screening large samples of affected sib pair (ASP) or affected relative pair (ARP) families using microsatellite markers, in order to identify chromosomal regions that co-segregate with the phenotype within families.

During the last decade at least a dozen genome scan studies of ASD have been published (for reviews see Autism Genome Project Consortium, 2007; Bachelli & Maestrini, 2006; Coon, 2006; Trikalinos, Karvouni, Zintzaras *et al.*, 2006), each identifying several chromosomal regions of suggestive linkage. Although no region of strong evidence of linkage has been consistently replicated, the overlap in linkage findings from these international family collections points to a few regions that are likely to harbor autism susceptibility genes. A region on chromosome 7q, designated as AUTs 1, stands out as the region with the greatest concordance of findings (Bachelli & Maestrini, 2006; IMGSAC, 1998; Lamb, Barnby, Bonora *et al.*, 2005). Another region of interest is on chromosome 2q, representing the strongest linkage finding obtained in the expanded IMGSAC data set of 219 ASP (IMGSAC, 2001; Lamb, Barnby, Bonora *et al.*, 2005), which overlaps with linkage results reported by three additional studies (Buxbaum, Silverman, Smith *et al.*, 2001; Philippe, Martinez, Guilloud-Bataille *et al.*, 1999; Shao, Raiford, Wolpert *et al.*, 2002). Similarly, overlapping linkage findings have been reported for a region on chromosome 17q, although these were not confirmed in the large-scale consortium study. However, it did produce suggestive evidence of linkage in the vicinity of 11q12–13 (Autism Genome Project Consortium, 2007).

The overlaps in findings of these scans are somewhat encouraging, providing a first step towards the identification of autism susceptibility loci. However, there are some limitations in the interpretation of these results. Each genome scan has shown little evidence for strong linkage signals, the loci found so far are rather broad, containing many genes, and most of the linkage results do not converge on the same linkage peaks (Bachelli & Maestrini, 2006). The lack of reproducibility between linkage studies suggests that autism may involve extensive genetic heterogeneity and/or many interacting genes of weak effect. The identification of many potential susceptibility loci and the failure to narrow down the chromosomal intervals using linkage or cytogenetic approaches have prompted many groups to undertake association studies of candidate genes.

Candidate genes are genes thought to be involved in relevant pathophysiological processes (functional candidates), or genes within the chromosomal interval identified by linkage analysis or close to cytogenetic rearrangements associated with autism (positional candidates). In the last decade, over 100 positional and functional candidate genes have been studied, such as the neuroligin genes, the serotonin transporter gene, the Reelin gene and several GABA-ergic genes (for a review see Bachelli & Maestrini, 2006). Up until now the candidate gene studies are characterized by a lack of reproducibility because of similar problems to those encountered in linkage analysis. A clear involvement of any gene in autism has not yet been conclusively identified (Bachelli & Maestrini, 2006).

Future Directions

Autism is a disorder with a strong genetic basis. It is unclear whether the 10% variance that is not genetic is due to stochastic factors, measurement error, environmental influence, mitochondrial genomic variation or other non-Mendelian genetic influences. There is no doubt that a feeling of disappointment in the field of autism genetics because definitive answers have not come more easily. However, there are several reasons to put this aside and push forward:

1 Autism remains strongly genetic, and even – if possible – more complex than originally estimated.

2 The development of novel, and more accurate high-throughput approaches, together with access to data from large international patient samples and bioinformatics resources is now providing the opportunity to generate an unprecedented amount of information.

3 Identification of susceptibility genes will lead directly to studies of protein function in single cell systems, and might possibly lead to the development of animal models of autism.

4 These cell systems seen in animal models may provide an opportunity to study the neuropathological and neurophysiological consequences of gene activity in the developing organism and to develop novel psychopharmacological strategies.

There have been significant advances in our understanding of some central aspects of developmental psychopathology in ASD. Nevertheless, there is still a need to identify more accurately those abnormalities that are potentially specific as well as to understand the possible interactions among different processes early in development.

Functional imaging and evoked electrocortical response techniques provide a means to move beyond localization of abnormal brain activity to an understanding of underlying mechanisms such as functional coherence in neuronal networks and connectivity.

There is growing evidence that early detection of ASD at 2 years of age is feasible and there are great expectations from the benefits of intensive early interventions for children with ASD. The available evidence on the effectiveness of early intervention approaches is not conclusive, and further randomized and large-scale studies and follow-up measurements are required. Questions to be answered are about intensity and dosage (is there really a threshold at 20 h per week one-to-one contact with the child?; does this apply to all children, or is there a subgroup for which lower-intensity treatment is sufficient?), timing, cost-effectiveness, feasibility and availability of high-intensity treatment, the specific behavioral domains improved, and the magnitude and persistence of change induced.

In clinical work, difficulties in dissemination and availability of services and facilities are often more limiting than the absence of knowledge. Continued parent and professional advocacy for clinical, educational and vocational services remains necessary, and service models should be modified to address the needs of individuals, from younger children to older adults and their families. The importance of multifaceted individual treatment plans, specific to a particular child and family and supported by knowledgeable clinicians and educators, must continue to be recognized, as models for evidence-based and manualized interventions are disseminated.

Further Reading

Moldin, S. O., & Rubenstein, J. L. R. (Eds.). (2006). *Understanding autism: From basic neuroscience to treatment.* Boca Raton, FL: CRC Press, Taylor & Francis Group.

Volkmar, F. R., Paul, R., Klin, A., & Cohen, D. (Eds.). (2005). *Handbook of autism and pervasive developmental disorders.* (3rd edn., Vols 1 & 2). New Jersey: John Wiley & Sons.

References

Abdolmaleky, H. M., Smith, C. L., Faraone, S. W., Shafe, R., Stone, W., Glatt, S. S., *et al.* (2004). Methylomics in psychiatry: Modulation of gene–environment interactions may be through DNA methylation. *American Journal of Medical Genetics. B. Neuropsychiatric Genetics*, *127*, 51–59.

Alcantara, J. I., Weisblatt, E., Moore, B., & Bolton, P. (2004). Speech-in-noise perception in high-functioning individuals with autism or Asperger syndrome. *Journal of Child Psychology and Psychiatry*, *45*, 1107–1114.

Allen, G., & Courchesne, E. (2001). Attention function and dysfunction in autism. *Frontiers in Bioscence*, *6*, D105–D119.

Aman, M. G. (2005). Treatment planning for patients with autism spectrum disorders. *Journal of Clinical Psychiatry*, *66*, 38–45.

Aman, M. G., Singh, N. N., Stewart A. W., & Field C. J. (1985). Psychometric characteristics of the Aberrant Behavior Checklist. *American Journal of Mental Deficiency*, *89*, 492–502.

American Academy of Pediatrics. (2000). Clinical practice guideline: diagnosis and evaluation of the child with attention-deficit/hyperactivity disorder. *Pediatrics*, *105*, 1158–1170.

American Psychiatric Association (APA). (2000). *Diagnostic and statistical manual of mental disorders* (4th edn.). Text revision. Washington, DC: American Psychiatric Association.

Atladóttir, H. O., Parner, E. T., Schendel, D., Dalsgaard, S., Thomsen, P. H., & Thorsen, P. (2007). Time trends in reported diagnoses of childhood neuropsychiatric disorders: A Danish cohort study. *Archives of Pediatrics and Adolescent Medicine*, *161*, 193–198.

Attwood, T. (1997). *Asperger syndrome: A guide for parents and professionals.* London: Jessica Kingsley.

Autism Genome Project Consortium. (2007). Mapping autism risk loci using genetic linkage and chromosomal rearrangements. *Nature Genetics*, *39*, 319–328.

Bacchelli, E., & Maestrini, E. (2006). Autism spectrum disorders: Molecular genetic advances. *American Journal of Medical Genetics. C. Seminars in Medical Genetics*, *142*, 13–23.

Bailey, A. J., Braeutigam, S., Jousmäki, V., & Swithenby, S. J. (2005). Abnormal activation of face processing systems at early and intermediate latency in individuals with autism spectrum disorder: A magnetoencephalographic study. *European Journal of Neuroscience*, *21*, 2575–2585.

Bailey, A., Le Couteur, A., Gottesman, I., Bolton, P., Simonoff, E., Yuzda, E., *et al.* (1995). Autism as a strongly genetic disorder: Evidence from a British twin study. *Psychological Medicine*, *25*, 63–77.

Bailey, A., Luthert, P., Dean, A., Harding, B., Janota, I., Montgomery, M., *et al.* (1998a). A clinicopathological study of autism. *Brain*, *121*, 889–905.

Bailey, A., Palferman, S., Heavey, L., & Le Couteur, A. (1998b). Autism: The phenotype in relatives. *Journal of Autism and Developmental Disorders*, *28*, 369–392.

Bailey, A., Phillips, W., & Rutter, M. (1996). Autism: Towards an integration of clinical, genetic, neuropsychological, and neurobiological perspectives. *Journal of Child Psychology and Psychiatry and Allied Disciplines*, *37*, 89–126.

Baird, G., Simonoff, E., Pickles, A., Chandler, S., Loucas, T., Meldrum, D., *et al.* (2006). Prevalence of disorders of the autism spectrum in a population cohort of children in South Thames: The Special Needs and Autism Project (SNAP). *Lancet*, *368*, 210–215.

Baron-Cohen, S. (1988). An assessment of violence in a young man with Asperger syndrome. *Journal of Child Psychology and Psychiatry*, *29*, 351–360.

Baron-Cohen, S. (1995). *Mindblindness: An essay on autism and theory of mind*. Boston, MA: MIT Press/Bradford Books.

Baron-Cohen, S. (2002). The extreme male brain theory of autism. *Trends in Cognitive Sciences*, *6*, 248–254.

Baron-Cohen, S., Allen, J., & Gillberg, C. (1992). Can autism be detected at 18 months? The needle, the haystack, and the CHAT. *British Journal of Psychiatry*, *161*, 839–843.

Baron-Cohen, S., Knickmeyer, R. C., & Belmonte, M. K. (2005). Sex differences in the brain: Implications for explaining autism. *Science*, *310*, 819–823.

Baron-Cohen, S., Ring, H. A., Wheelwright, S., Bullmore, E. T., Brammer, M. J., Simmons, A., *et al.* (1999). Social intelligence in the normal and autistic brain: An fMRI study. *European Journal of Neuroscience*, *11*, 1891–1898.

Baron-Cohen, S., Tager-Flusberg, H., & Cohen, D. (1993). *Understanding other minds: Perspectives from autism*. Oxford: Oxford University Press.

Baron-Cohen, S., Wheelwright, S., Cox, A., Baird, G., Charman, T., Swettenham, J., *et al.* (2000). Early identification of autism by the Checklist for Autism in Toddlers (CHAT*)*. *Journal of the Royal Society of Medicine*, *93*, 521–525.

Bauminger, N. (2002). The facilitation of social-emotional understanding and social interaction in high-functioning children with autism: Intervention outcomes. *Journal of Autism and Developmental Disorders*, *32*, 283–298.

Berument, S. K., Rutter, M., Lord, C., Pickles, A., & Bailey, A. (1999). Autism screening questionnaire: Diagnostic validity. *British Journal of Psychiatry*, *175*, 444–451.

Bishop, D. V. (1989). Autism, Asperger syndrome and semantic-pragmatic disorder: Where are the boundaries? *British Journal of Disorders of Communication*, *24*, 107–121.

Boeschoten, M. A., Kemner, C., Kenemans, J. L., & van Engeland, H. (2007). Abnormal spatial frequency processing in children with Pervasive Developmental Disorder (PDD). *Clinical Neurophysiology*, *118*, 2076–2088.

Bolton, P., Macdonald, H., Pickles, A., Rios, P., Goode, S., Crowson, M., *et al.* (1994). A case–control family history study of autism. *Journal of Child Psychology and Psychiatry*, *35*, 877–900.

Bolton, P. F., Murphy, M., Macdonald, H., Whitlock, B., Pickles, A., & Rutter, M. (1997). Obstetric complications in autism: Consequences or causes of the condition? *Journal of the American Academy of Child and Adolescent Psychiatry*, *36*, 272–281.

Bondy, A. S., & Frost, L. A. (1998). The picture exchange communication system. *Seminars in Speech and Language*, *19*, 373–388.

Bondy, A., & Frost, L. (2001). The Picture Exchange Communication System. *Behavior Modification*, *25*, 725–744.

Boucher, J. (1998). SPD as a distinct diagnostic entity: Logical considerations and directions for future research. *International Journal of Language and Communication Disorders*, *33*, 71–108.

Bowler, D. M. (1992). Theory of mind in Asperger syndrome. *Journal of Child Psychology and Psychiatry*, *33*, 877–893.

Buitelaar, J. K., & van der Gaag, R. J. (1998). Diagnostic rules for children with PDD-NOS and multiple complex developmental disorder. *Journal of Child Psychology and Psychiatry*, *39*, 911–920.

Buitelaar, J. K., van der Gaag, R. G., Klin, A., & Volkmar, F. (1999a). Exploring the boundaries of Pervasive Developmental Disorder Not Otherwise Specified: Analyses of data from the DSM-IV autistic disorder field trial. *Journal of Autism and Developmental Disorders*, *29*, 33–43.

Buitelaar, J. K., van der Gaag, R. J., & van der Hoeven, J. (1998). Buspirone in the management of anxiety and irritability in children with pervasive developmental disorders: results of an open-label study. *Journal of Clinical Psychiatry*, *59*, 56–59.

Buitelaar, J. K., van der Wees M., Swaab-Barneveld, H., & van der Gaag, R. J. (1999b). Theory of mind and emotion-recognition functioning in autistic spectrum disorders and in psychiatric control and normal children. *Development and Psychopathology*, *11*, 39–58.

Burack, J. A., Enns, J. T., Stauder, J. E., Mottron, L., & Randolph, B. (1997). Attention and autism: Behavioral and electrophysiological evidence. In D. J. Cohen, & F. R. Volkmar (Eds.), *Handbook of autism and pervasive developmental disorder* (2nd edn., pp. 226–242). New York: John Wiley & Sons.

Butter, E. M., Wynn, J., & Mulick, J. A. (2003). Early intervention critical to autism treatment. *Pediatric Annals*, *32*, 677–684.

Buxbaum, J. D., Silverman, J. M., Smith, J. C., Kilifarski, M., Reichert, J., Hollander, E., *et al.* (2001). Evidence for a susceptibility gene for autism on chromosome 2 and for genetic heterogeneity. *American Journal of Human Genetics*, *68*, 1514–1520.

Campbell, M., Schopler, E., Cueva, J. E., & Hallin, A. (1996). Treatment of autistic disorder. *Journal of the American Academy of Child and Adolescent Psychiatry*, *35*, 134–143.

Casanova, M. F. (2004). White matter volume increase and minicolums in autism. *Annals of Neurology*, *56*, 453.

Casanova, M. F., Buxhoeveden, D. P., Switala, A. E., & Roy, E. (2002). Minicolumnar pathology in autism. *Neurology*, *58*, 428–432.

Casanova, M. F., van Kooten, I., Switala, A. E., van Engeland, H., Heinsen, H., Steinbusch, H. W., *et al.* (2006). Minicolumnar abnormalities in autism. *Acta Neuropathologica (Berlin)*, *112*, 287–303.

Castelli, F., Frith, C., Happe, F., & Frith, U. (2002). Autism, Asperger syndrome and brain mechanisms for the attribution of mental states to animated shapes. *Brain*, *125*, 1839–1849.

Ceponiene, R., Lepistö, T., Shestakova, A., Vanhala, R., Alku, P., Näätänen, R., *et al.* (2003). Speech-sound-selective auditory impairment in children with autism: They can perceive but do not attend. *Proceedings of the National Academy of Sciences of the USA*, *100*, 5567–5572.

Charman, T., & Baird, G. (2002). Practitioner review: Diagnosis of autism spectrum disorder in 2- and 3-year-old children. *Journal of Child Psychology and Psychiatry and Allied Disciplines*, *43*, 289–305.

Chesterman, P., & Rutter, S. C. (1994). A case report: Asperger syndrome and sexual offending. *Journal of Forensic Psychiatry*, *4*, 555–562.

Chugani, D. C., Muzik, O., Rothermel, R., Behen, M., Chakraborty, P., Mangner, T., *et al.* (1997). Altered serotonin synthesis in the dentatothalamocortical pathway in autistic boys. *Annals of Neurology*, *42*, 666–669.

Ciesielski, K. T., Courchesne, E., & Elmasian, R. (1990). Effects of focused selective attention tasks on event-related potentials in autistic and normal individuals. *Electroencephalography and Clinical Neurophysiology*, *75*, 207–220.

Clarke, D. J., Littlejohns, C. S., Corbett, J. A., & Joseph, S. (1989). Pervasive developmental disorders and psychoses in adult life. *British Journal of Psychiatry*, *155*, 692–699.

Constantino, J. N., Gruber, C. P., Davis, S., Hayes, S., Passanante, N., & Przybeck, T. (2004). The factor structure of autistic traits. *Journal of Child Psychology and Psychiatry and Allied Disciplines*, *45*, 719–726.

Coon, H. (2006). Current perspectives on the genetic analysis of autism. *American Journal of Medical Genetics. C. Seminars in Medical Genetics*, *142*, 24–32.

Corbett, J., Harris, R., Taylor, E., & Trible, M. (1977). Progressive integrative psychosis of childhood. *Journal of Child Psychology and Psychiatry*, *18*, 211–219.

Cox, A., Klein, K., Charman, T., Baird, G., Baron-Cohen, S., Swettenham, J., *et al.* (1999). Autism spectrum disorders at 20 and 42 months of age: Stability of clinical and ADI-R diagnosis. *Journal of Child Psychology and Psychiatry*, *40*, 719–732.

Dahlgren, S. O., & Gillberg, C. (1989). Symptoms in the first two years of life: A preliminary population study of infantile autism. *European Archives of Psychiatry and Neurological Science*, *238*, 169–174.

Dapretto, M., Davies, M. S., Pfeifer, J. H., Scott, A. A., Sigman, M., Bookheimer, S. Y., *et al.* (2006). Understanding emotions in others: Mirror neuron dysfunction in children with autism spectrum disorder. *Nature Neuroscience*, *9*, 28–30.

Dawson, G., & Osterling, J. (1997). Early intervention in autism: Effectiveness and common elements of current approaches. In M. Guralnick (Ed.), *The effectiveness of early intervention: Second generation research* (pp. 307–326). Baltimore: Brookes.

de Jonge, M. V. (2006). *The search for endophenotypic markers of autism spectrum disorders*. Unpublished dissertation, Utrecht University.

De Giacomo, A., & Fombonne, E. (1998). Parental recognition of developmental abnormalities in autism. *European Child and Adolescent Psychiatry*, *7*, 131–136.

DeLong, G. R., Teague, L. A., & McSwain, K. M. (1998). Effects of fluoxetine treatment in young children with idiopathic autism. *Developmental Medicine and Child Neurology*, *40*, 551–562.

D'Souza, Y., Fombonne, E., & Ward, B. J. (2006). No evidence of persisting measles virus in peripheral blood mononuclear cells from children with autism spectrum disorder. *Pediatrics*, *118*, 1664–1675.

DiCicco-Bloom, E., Lord, C., Zwaigenbaum, L., Courchesne, E., Dager, S. R., Schmitz, C., *et al.* (2006). The developmental neurobiology of autism spectrum disorder. *Journal of Neuroscience*, *26*, 6897–6906.

Dietz, C., Swinkels, S., van Daalen, E., van Engeland, H., & Buitelaar, J. K. (2006). Screening for Autistic Spectrum Disorder in children aged 14–15 months. II. Population screening with the Early Screening of Autistic Traits questionnaire (ESAT). Design and general findings. *Journal of Autism and Developmental Disorders*, *36*, 713–722.

Einfeld, S. L., & Tonge, B. J. (1995). The Developmental Behavior Checklist: The development and validation of an instrument to assess behavioral and emotional disturbance in children and adolescents with mental retardation. *Journal of Autism and Developmental Disorders*, *25*, 81–104.

Ernst, M., Zametkin, A. J., Matochik, J. A., Pascualvaca, D., & Cohen, R. M. (1997). Low medial prefrontal dopaminergic activity in autistic children [letter]. *Lancet*, *350*, 638.

Esch, B. E., & Carr, J. E. (2004). Secretin as a treatment for autism: A review of the evidence. *Journal of Autism and Developmental Disorders*, *34*, 543–556.

Fatemi, S. H., Halt, A. R., Stary, J. M., Kanodia, R., Schulz, S. C., & Realmuto, G. R. (2002). Glutamic acid decarboxylase 65 and 67 kDa proteins are reduced in autistic parietal and cerebellar cortices. *Biological Psychiatry*, *52*, 805–810.

Filipek, P. A. (2005). Medical aspects of autism. In F. R. Volkmar, R. Paul, A. Klin, & D. Cohen (Eds.), *Handbook of autism and pervasive developmental disorders* (3rd edn., Vols 1 & 2, pp. 534–581). Hoboken, NJ: John Wiley & Sons.

Filipek, P. A., Accardo, P. J., Ashwal, S., Baranek, G. T., Cook, E. H. Jr., Dawson, G., *et al.* (2000). Practice parameter: Screening and diagnosis of autism. Report of the Quality Standards Subcommittee of the American Academy of Neurology and the Child Neurology Society. *Neurology*, *55*, 468–479.

Filipek, P. A., Accardo, P. J., Baranek, G. T., Cook, E. H. Jr., Dawson, G., Gordon, B., *et al.* (1999). The screening and diagnosis of autistic spectrum disorders. *Journal of Autism and Developmental Disorders*, *29*, 439–484.

Fischel, J. E., Whitehurst, G. J., Caulfield, M. B., & DeBaryshe, B. (1989). Language growth in children with expressive language delay. *Pediatrics*, *83*, 218–227.

Folstein, S., & Rutter, M. (1977). Infantile autism: A genetic study of 21 twin pairs. *Journal of Child Psychology and Psychiatry*, *18*, 297–321.

Fombonne, E. (1999). The epidemiology of autism: A review. *Psychological Medicine*, *29*, 769–786.

Fombonne, E. (2002). Epidemiological trends in rates of autism. *Molecular Psychiatry*, *7*, S4–S6.

Fombonne, E. (2003). The prevalence of autism. *Journal of the American Medical Association*, *289*, 87–89.

Fombonne, E., Bolton, P., Prior, J., Jordan, H., & Rutter, M. (1997). A family study of autism: Cognitive patterns and levels in parents and siblings. *Journal of Child Psychology and Psychiatry*, *38*, 667–683.

Fombonne, E., Rogé, B., Claverie, J., Courty, S., & Frémolle, J. (1999). Microcephaly and macrocephaly in autism. *Journal of Autism and Developmental Disorders*, *29*, 113–119.

Frith, U. (1991). *Autism and Asperger Syndrome* (pp. 37–92). Cambridge, UK: Cambridge University Press. [Translation of Asperger, H. (1944). Die autistischen Psychopathen im Kindesalter. *Archiv fur Psychiatrie und Nervenkrankheitan*, *117*, 76–136.]

Frith, U. (2003). *Autism: Explaining the enigma* (2nd edn.). Oxford, UK: Blackwell Publishing.

Frith, U., & Happé, F. (1994). Autism: Beyond "theory of mind". *Cognition*, *50*, 115–132.

Fuster, J. M. (1997). *The prefrontal cortex: Anatomy, physiology, and neuropsychology of the frontal lobe* (3rd edn.). Philadelphia: Lippincott-Raven.

Gervais, H., Belin, P., Boddaert, N., Leboyer, M., Coez, A., Sfaello, I., *et al.* (2004). Abnormal cortical voice processing in autism. *Nature Neuroscience*, *7*, 801–802.

Geurts, H. M., Verte, S., Oosterlaan, J., Roeyers, H., & Sergeant, J. A. (2004). How specific are executive functioning deficits in attention deficit hyperactivity disorder and autism? *Journal of Child Psychology and Psychiatry and Allied Disciplines*, *45*, 836–854.

Ghaziuddin, M., Tsai, L., & Ghaziuddin, N. (1991). Brief report: Violence in Asperger syndrome: A critique. *Journal of Autism and Developmental Disorders*, *21*, 349–354.

Gillberg, C. (1989). Asperger syndrome in 23 Swedish children. *Developmental Medicine and Child Neurology*, *31*, 520–531.

Glasson, E. J., Bower, C., Petterson, B., de Klerk, N., Chaney, G., & Hallmayer, J. F. (2004). Perinatal factors and the development of autism: A population study. *Archives of General Psychiatry*, *61*, 618–627.

Grandin, T., & Scariano, M. (1986). *Emergence: Labeled autistic*. New York: Warner Books.

Green, J., Gilchrist, A., Burton, D., & Cox, A. (2000). Social and psychiatric functioning in adolescents with Asperger syndrome compared with conduct disorder. *Journal of Autism and Developmental Disorders*, *30*, 279–293.

Green, L., Fein, D., Modahl, C., Feinstein, C., Waterhouse, L., & Morris, M. (2001). Oxytocin and autistic disorder: Alterations in peptide forms. *Biological Psychiatry*, *50*, 609–613.

Grice, S. J., Halit, H., Farroni, T., Baron-Cohen, S., Bolton, P., & Johnson, M. H. (2005). Neural correlates of eye-gaze detection in young children with autism. *Cortex*, *41*, 342–353.

Griffith, E. M., Pennington, B. F., Wehner, E. A., & Rogers, S. J. (1999). Executive functions in young children with autism. *Child Development*, *70*, 817–832.

Guy, J., Gan, J., Selfridge, J., Cobb, S., & Bird, A. (2007). Reversal of neurological defects in a mouse model of Rett syndrome. *Science*, *315*, 1143–1147.

Hadjikhani, N., Joseph, R. M., Snyder, J., Chabris, C. F., Clark, J., Steele, S., *et al.* (2004). Activation of the fusiform gyrus when individuals with autism spectrum disorder view faces. *Neuroimage*, *22*, 1141–1150.

Hagberg, B., Aicardi, J., Dias, K., & Ramos, O. (1983). A progressive syndrome of autism, dementia, ataxia, and loss of purposeful hand use in girls: Rett syndrome. Report of 35 cases. *Annals of Neurology*, *14*, 471–479.

Hagerman, R. J. (2006). Lessons from fragile X regarding neurobiology, autism and neurodegeneration. *Journal of Developmental and Behavioral Pediatrics*, *27*, 63–74.

Happé, F., & Frith, U. (2006). The weak coherence account: Detail-focused cognitive style in autism spectrum disorders. *Journal of Autism and Developmental Disorders*, *36*, 5–25.

Hartman, C. A., Luteijn, E., Serra, M., & Minderaa, R. (2006). Refinement of the Children's Social Behavior Questionnaire (CSBQ): An instrument that describes the diverse problems seen in milder forms of PDD. *Journal of Autism and Developmental Disorders*, *36*, 325–342.

Hoeksma, M. R., Kenemans, J. L., Kemner, C., & van Engeland, H. (2005). Variability in spatial normalization of pediatric and adult brain images. *Clinical Neurophysiology*, *116*, 1188–1194.

Hollander, E., Dolgoff-Kaspar, R., Cartwright, C., Rawitt, R., & Novotny, S. (2001). An open trial of divalproex sodium in autism spectrum disorders. *Journal of Clinical Psychiatry*, *62*, 530–534.

Hollander, E., Novotny, S., Hanratty, M., Yaffe, R., DeCaria, C. M., Aronowitz, B. R., *et al.* (2003). Oxytocin infusion reduces repetitive behaviors in adults with autistic and Asperger disorders. *Neuropsychopharmacology*, *28*, 193–198.

Hollander, E., Phillips, A., Chaplin, W., Zagursky, K., Novotny, S., Wasserman, S., *et al.* (2005). A placebo controlled crossover trial of liquid fluoxetine on repetitive behaviors in childhood and adolescent autism. *Neuropsychopharmacology*, *30*, 582–589.

Honda, H., Shimizu, Y., & Rutter, M. (2005). No effect of MMR withdrawal on the incidence of autism: A total population study. *Journal of Child Psychology and Psychiatry and Allied Disciplines*, *46*, 572–579.

Hornig, M., & Lipkin, W. I. (2001). Infectious and immune factors in the pathogenesis of neurodevelopmental disorders: Epidemiology, hypotheses, and animal models. *Mental Retardation and Developmental Disabilities Research Reviews*, *7*, 200–210.

Hornig, M., Chian, D., & Lipkin W. I. (2004). Neurotoxic effects of postnatal thimerosal are mouse strain dependent. *Molecular Psychiatry*, *9*, 833–845.

Howlin, P. (1998). Practitioner review: Psychological and educational treatments for autism. *Journal of Child Psychology and Psychiatry*, *39*, 307–322.

Howlin, P. (2003). Outcome in high-functioning adults with autism with and without early language delays: Implications for the differentiation between autism and Asperger syndrome. *Journal of Autism and Developmental Disorders*, *33*, 3–13.

Howlin, P. (2005). Outcomes in autism spectrum disorders. In F. R. Volkmar, R. Paul, A. Klin, & D. Cohen (Eds.), *Handbook of autism and pervasive developmental disorders* (3rd edn), (pp. 201–220). Hoboken, NJ: John Wiley & Sons.

Howlin, P. (2005). The effectiveness of interventions for children with autism. *Journal of Neural Transmission Supplementum*, *69*, 101–119.

Howlin, P., Alcock, J., & Burkin, C. (2005). An 8 year follow-up of a specialist supported employment service for high-ability adults with autism or Asperger syndrome. *Autism: the International Journal of Research and Practice*, *9*, 533–549.

Howlin, P., Baron-Cohen, S., & Hadwin, J. (1999). *Teaching children with autism to mind-read: A practical guide for teachers and parents.* New York/London: Wiley & Son.

Howlin, P., & Moore, A. (1997). Diagnosis of autism: a survey of over 1200 patients in the UK. *Autism*, *1*, 135–162.

Hughes, C., Russell, J., & Robbins, T. W. (1994). Evidence for executive dysfunction in autism. *Neuropsychologia*, *32*, 477–492.

Hutton, J., Goode, S., Murphy, M., Le Couteur, A., & Rutter, M. (in press). New-onset psychiatric disorders in individuals with autism. *Autism*.

International Molecular Genetic Study of Autism Consortium (IMGSAC). (1998). A full genome screen for autism with evidence for linkage to a region on chromosome 7q. *Human Molecular Genetics*, *7*, 571–578.

International Molecular Genetic Study of Autism Consortium (IMGSAC). (2001). A genomewide screen for autism: Strong evidence for linkage to chromosomes 2q, 7q, and 16p. *American Journal of Human Genetics*, *69*, 570–581.

Just, M. A., Cherkassky, V. L., Keller, T. A., & Minshew, N. J. (2004). Cortical activation and synchronization during sentence comprehension in high-functioning autism: Evidence of underconnectivity. *Brain*, *127*, 1811–1821.

Kasai, K., Hashimoto, O., Kawakubo, Y., Yumoto, M., Kamio, S., Itoh, K., *et al.* (2005). Delayed automatic detection of change in speech sounds in adults with autism: A magnetoencephalographic study. *Clinical Neurophysiology*, *116*, 1655–1664.

Kabot, S., Masi, W., & Segal, M. (2003). Advances in the diagnosis and treatment of autism spectrum disorders. *Professional Psychology*, *34*, 26–33.

Kanner, L. (1943). Autistic disturbances of affective contact. *Nervous Child*, *2*, 217–250.

Keel, J. H., Mesibov, G. B., & Woods, A. V. (1997). TEACCH-supported employment program. *Journal of Autism and Developmental Disorders*, *27*, 3–9.

Keller, F., &. Persico, A. M. (2003). The neurobiological context of autism. *Molecular Neurobiology*, *28*, 1–22.

Kemner, C., & van Engeland, H. (2006). ERPs and eye movements reflect atypical visual perception in pervasive developmental disorder. *Journal of Autism and Developmental Disorders*, *36*, 45–54.

Kemner, C., Verbaten, M. N., Cuperus, J. M., Camfferman, G., & van Engeland, H. (2004). Visual and somatosensory event-related brain potentials in autistic children and three different control groups. *Electroencephalography and Clinical Neurophysiology*, *92*, 225–237.

Kerbeshian, J., Burd, L., & Fisher, W. (1987). Lithium carbonate in the treatment of two patients with infantile autism and atypical bipolar symptomatology. *Journal of Clinical Psychopharmacology*, *7*, 401–405.

Kjelgaard, M. M., & Tager-Flusberg, H. (2001). An investigation of language impairment in autism: Implications for genetic subgroups. *Language and Cognitive Processes*, *16*, 287–308.

Klin, A., McPartland, J., & Volkmar F. R. (2005a). Asperger syndrome. In F. R. Volkmar, R. Paul, A. Klin, & D. Cohen (Eds.), *Handbook of autism and pervasive developmental disorders* (3rd edn., pp. 88–125). Hoboken, NJ: John Wiley & Sons.

Klin, A., Pauls, D., Schultz, R., & Volkmar, F. (2005b). Three diagnostic approaches to Asperger syndrome: Implications for research. *Journal of Autism and Developmental Disorders*, *35*, 221–234.

Klin, A., Volkmar, F. R., & Sparrow, S. S. (1992). Autistic social dysfunction: Some limitations of the theory of mind hypothesis. *Journal of Child Psychology and Psychiatry*, *33*, 861–876.

Klin, A., Volkmar, F. R., & Sparrow, S. S. (Eds.). (2000). *Asperger syndrome*. New York: Guilford Press.

Klin, A., Volkmar, F. R., Sparrow, S. S., Cicchetti, D. V., & Rourke, B. P. (1995). Validity and neuropsychological characterization of Asperger syndrome: Convergence with nonverbal learning disabilities syndrome. *Journal of Child Psychology and Psychiatry*, *36*, 1127–1140.

Koegel, R. L., & Frea, W. D. (1993). Treatment of social behavior in autism through the modification of pivotal social skills. *Journal of Applied Behavior Analysis*, *26*, 369–377.

Koshino, H., Carpenter, P. A., Minshew, N. J., Cherkassky, V. L., Keller, T. A., & Just, M. A. (2005). Functional connectivity in an fMRI working memory task in high-functioning autism. *Neuroimage*, *24*, 810–821.

Kozinetz, C. A., Skender, M. L., MacNaughton, N., Almes, M. J., Schultz, R. J., Percy, A. K., *et al.* (1993). Epidemiology of Rett syndrome: A population-based registry. *Pediatrics*, *91*, 445–450.

Lainhart, J. E. (1999). Psychiatric problems in individuals with autism, their parents and siblings. *International Review of Psychiatry*, *11*, 278–298.

Lainhart, J. E. (2006). Advances in autism neuroimaging research for the clinician and geneticist. *American Journal of Medical Genetics. C. Seminars in Medical Genetics*, *142*, 33–39.

Lam, K. S. L., Aman, M. G., & Arnold, L. E. (2006). Neurochemical correlates of autistic disorder: A review of the literature. *Research in Developmental Disabilities*, *27*, 254–289.

Lamb, J. A., Barnby, G., Bonora, E., Sykes, N., Bachelli, E., Blasi, F., *et al.* (2005). Analysis of IMGSAC autism susceptibility loci: Evidence for sex limited and parent of origin specific effects. *Journal of Medical Genetics*, *42*, 132–137.

Larsson, H. J., Eaton, W. W., Madsen, K. M., Vestergaard, M., Olesen, A. V., Agerbo, E., *et al.* (2005). Risk factors for autism: Perinatal factors, parental psychiatric history, and socioeconomic status. *American Journal of Epidemiology*, *161*, 916–925.

Le Couteur, A. C., Bailey, A., Goode, S., Pickles, A., Robertson, S., Gottesman, I., *et al.* (1996). A broader phenotype of autism: The clinical spectrum in twins. *Journal of Child Psychology and Psychiatry*, *37*, 785–801.

Le Couteur, A., Lord, C., & Rutter, M. (2003). *The Autism Diagnostic Interview: Revised (ADI-R)*. Los Angeles, CA: Western Psychological Services.

Leekam, S. R., Libby, S. J., Wing, L., Gould, J., & Taylor, C. (2002). The Diagnostic Interview for Social and Communication Disorders: Algorithms for ICD-10 childhood autism and Wing and Gould autistic spectrum disorder. *Journal of Child Psychology and Psychiatry and Allied Disciplines*, *43*, 327–342.

Levy, S. E., & Hyman, S. L. (2003). Use of complementary and alternative treatments for children with autistic spectrum disorders is increasing. *Pediatric Annals*, *32*, 685–691.

Lockyer, L., & Rutter M. (1969). A five- to fifteen-year follow-up study of infantile psychosis. III. Psychological aspects. *British Journal of Psychiatry*, *115*, 865–882.

Lord, C., & Schopler, E. (1989). Stability of assessment results of autistic and non-autistic language-impaired children from preschool years to early school age. *Journal of Child Psychology and Psychiatry*, *30*, 575–590.

Lord, C., Rutter, M., DiLavore, P. C., & Risi, S. (2001). Autism Diagnostic Observation Schedule (ADOS manual). Los Angeles, CA: Western Psychological Services.

Lotter, V. (1966). Epidemiology of autistic conditions in young children. I. Prevalence. *Social Psychiatry*, *1*, 124–137.

Lovaas, O. I. (1987). Behavioral treatment and normal educational and intellectual functioning in young autistic children. *Journal of Consulting and Clinical Psychology*, *55*, 3–9.

Madsen, K. M., Lauritsen, M. B., Pedersen, C. B., Thorsen, P., Plesner, A. M., Andersen, P. H., *et al.* (2003). Thimerosal and the occurrence of autism: Negative ecological evidence from Danish population-based data. *Pediatrics*, *112*, 604–606.

Magnus, P., Irgens, L. M., Haug, K., Nystad, W., Skjaerven, R., Stoltenberg, C., & the MoBa Study Group. (2006). Cohort profile: The Norwegian mother and child cohort study (MoBa). *International Journal of Epidemiology*, *35*, 1146–1150.

Mawhood, L. M., & Howlin, P. (1999). The outcome of a supported employment scheme for high functioning adults with autism of Asperger syndrome. *Autism: International Journal of Research and Practice*, *3*, 229–253.

McAlonan, G. M., Cheung, V., Cheung, C., Suckling, J., Lam, G. Y., Tai, K. S., *et al.* (2005). Mapping the brain in autism: A voxel-based MRI study of volumetric differences and intercorrelations in autism. *Brain*, *128*, 268–276.

McBride, P. A., Anderson, G. M., Hertzig, M. E., Snow, M. E., Thompson, S. M., Khait, V. D., *et al.* (1998). Effects of diagnosis, race, and puberty on platelet serotonin levels in autism and mental retardation. *Journal of the American Academy of Child and Adolescent Psychiatry*, *37*, 767–776.

McCracken J. T., McGough, J., Shah, B., Cronin, P., Hong, D., Aman, M. G., *et al.* (2002). Risperidone in children with autism and serious behavioral problems. *New England Journal of Medicine*, *5*, 314–321.

McDougle, C. J., Erickson, C. A., Stigler, K. A., & Posey, D. J. (2005). Neurochemistry in the pathophysiology of autism. *Journal of Clinical Psychiatry*, *66*, 9–18.

McDougle, C. J., Holmes, J. P., Carlson, D. C., Pelton, G. H., Cohen, D. J., & Price, L. H. (1998). A double-blind, placebo-controlled study of risperidone in adults with autistic disorder and other pervasive developmental disorders [see comments]. *Archives of General Psychiatry*, *55*, 633–641.

McDougle, C. J., Naylor, S. T., Cohen, D. J., Aghajanian, G. K., Heninger, G. R., & Price, L. H. (1996a). Effects of tryptophan depletion in drug-free adults with autistic disorder. *Archives of General Psychiatry*, *53*, 993–1000.

McDougle, C.J., Naylor, S.T., Cohen, D.J., Volkmar, F.R., Heninger, G.R., & Price L.H. (1996b). A double-blind placebo-controlled study of fluvoxamine in adults with autistic disorder. *Archives of General Psychiatry*, *53*, 1001–1008.

McEachin, J. J., Smith, T., & Lovaas, O. I. (1993). Long-term outcome for children with autism who received early intensive behavioral treatment. *American Journal of Mental Retardation*, *97*, 359–372.

McPartland, J., Dawson G., Webb, S. J., Panagiotides, H., & Carver, L. J. (2004). Event-related brain potentials reveal anomalies in temporal processing of faces in autism spectrum disorder. *Journal of Child Psychology and Psychiatry*, *45*, 1235–1245.

Medical Research Council. (2001). *MRC review of autism research: Epidemiology and causes*. London: Medical Research Council.

Mesibov, G. B. (1984). Social skills training with verbal autistic adolescents and adults: A program model. *Journal of Autism and Developmental Disorders*, *14*, 395–404.

Mesibov, G., Shea, V., & Schopler, E. (2004). *The TEACCH approach to autism spectrum disorders*. New York: Plenum Press.

Miller, J. F., Campbell, T. F., Chapman, R. S., & Weismer S. E. (1984). Language behaviour in acquired childhood aphasia. In A. Holland (Ed.), *Language disorders in children* (pp. 57–99). Cambridge: College-Hill.

Minshew, N. J. (1991). Indices of neural function in autism: Clinical and biologic implications. *Pediatrics*, *87*, 774–780.

Moldin, S. O., & Rubenstein, J. L. R. (Eds.). (2006). *Understanding autism: From basic neuroscience to treatment*. Boca Raton, FL: CRC Press, Taylor & Francis Group.

Moldin, S. O., Rubenstein, J. L., & Hyman, S. E. (2006). Can autism speak to neuroscience? *Journal of Neuroscience*, 26, 6893–6896.

Molenaar, P. C. M., Boomsma, D. I., & Dolan, C. V. (1993). A third source of developmental differences. *Behavior Genetics*, *23*, 519–524.

Moretti, P., & Zoghbi, H. Y. (2006). MeCP2 dysfunction in Rett syndrome and related disorders. *Current Opinion in Genetics and Development*, *16*, 276–281.

Mountcastle, V. B. (1997). The columnar organization of the neocortex. *Brain*, *120*, 701–722.

Mouridsen, S. E. (1995). The Landau–Kleffner syndrome: A review. *European Child and Adolescent Psychiatry*, *4*, 223–228.

Mouridsen, S. E., Rich, B., & Isager, T. (1999). Psychiatric morbidity in disintegrative psychosis and infantile autism: A long-term follow-up study. *Psychopathology*, *32*, 177–183.

Mulder, E. J., Anderson, G. M., Kema, I. P., de Bildt, J. A., van Lang, N. D., Den Boer, J. A., *et al.* (2004). Platelet serotonin levels in pervasive developmental disorders and mental retardation: Diagnostic group differences, within-group distribution, and behavioral correlates. *Journal of the American Academy of Child and Adolescent Psychiatry*, *43*, 491–499.

Müller, R. A., Kleinhans, N., Kemnotsu, N., Pierce, K., & Courchesne, E. (2003). Abnormal variability and distribution of functional maps in autism: An FMRI study of visuomotor learning. *American Journal of Psychiatry*, *160*, 1847–1862.

Murch, S. (2005). Diet, immunity, and autistic spectrum disorders. *Journal of Pediatrics*, *146*, 582–584.

National Research Council. (2001). *Educating children with autism*. Committee on Educational Interventions for Children with Autism. Washington, DC: National Academy Press.

Nelson, K. B., Grether, J. K., Croen, L. A., Dambrosia, J. M., Dickens, B. F., Jelliffe, L. L., *et al.* (2001). Neuropeptides and neurotrophins in neonatal blood of children with autism or mental retardation. *Annals of Neurology*, *49*, 597–606.

Nelson, P. G., Kuddo, T., Song, E. Y., Dambrosia, J. M., Kohler, S., Satyanarayana, G., *et al.* (2006). Selected neurotrophins, neuropeptides, and cytokines: Developmental trajectory and concentrations in neonatal blood of children with autism or Down syndrome. *International Journal of Developmental Neuroscience*, *24*, 73–80.

Nir, I., Meir, D., Zilber, N., Knobler, H., Hadjez, J., & Lerner, Y. (1995). Brief report: Circadian melatonin, thyroid-stimulating hormone, prolactin, and cortisol levels in serum of young adults with autism. *Journal of Autism and Developmental Disorders*, *25*, 641–654.

Ozonoff, S., & McEvoy, R. E. (1994). A longitudinal study of executive function and theory of mind development in autism. *Development and Psychopathology*, *6*, 415–431.

Ozonoff, S., Pennington, B., & Rogers, S. (1991a). Executive function deficits in high-functioning autistic children: Relationship to theory of mind. *Journal of Child Psychology and Psychiatry*, *31*, 1081–1105.

Ozonoff, S., Rogers, S. J., & Pennington, B. F. (1991b). Asperger syndrome: Evidence of an empirical distinction from high-functioning autism. *Journal of Child Psychology and Psychiatry*, *32*, 1107–1122.

Ozonoff, S., & Strayer, D. L. (1997). Inhibitory function in non-retarded children with autism. *Journal of Autism and Developmental Disorders*, *27*, 59–77.

Palmen, S. J., & van Engeland, H. (2004). Review on structural neuroimaging findings in autism. *Journal of Neural Transmission*, *111*, 903–929.

Palmen, S. J., Hulshoff Pol, H. E., Kemner, C., Schnack, H. G., Sitskoorn, M. M., Appels, M. C., *et al.* (2005). Brain anatomy in non-affected parents of autistic probands: An MRI study. *Psychological Medicine*, *35*, 1411–1420.

Pennington, B. F., & Ozonoff, S. (1996). Executive functions and developmental psychopathology. *Journal of Child Psychology and Psychiatry*, *37*, 51–87.

Philippe, A., Martinez, M., Guilloud-Bataille M., Gillberg, C., Rastam Sponheim E., Coleman, M., *et al.* (1999). Genome-wide scan for autism susceptibility genes. Paris Autism Research International Sibpair Study. *Human Molecular Genetics*, *8*, 805–812.

Pickles, A., Bolton, P., Macdonald, H., Bailey, A., Le Couteur, A., Sim, C. H., *et al.* (1995). Latent-class analysis of recurrence risks for complex phenotypes with selection and measurement error: A twin and family history study of autism. *American Journal of Human Genetics*, *57*, 717–726.

Pickles, A., Simonoff, E., Conti-Ramsden, G., Falcaro, M., Simkin, Z., Charman, T., *et al.* (submitted). Loss of language in early development of autism and specific language impairment.

Pierce, K., Haist, F., Sedaghar, F., & Courchesne, E. (2004). The brain response to personally familiar faces in autism: Findings of fusiform activity and beyond. *Brain*, *127*, 2703–2716.

Piggot, J., Kwon, H., Mobbs, D., Blasey, C., Lotspeich, L., Menon, V., *et al.* (2004). Emotional attribution in high-functioning individuals with autistic spectrum disorder: A functional imaging study. *Journal of the American Academy of Child and Adolescent Psychiatry*, *43*, 473–480.

Piven, J., Palmer, P., Jacobi, D., Childress, D., & Arndt, S. (1997). Broader autism phenotype: evidence from a family history study of multiple-incidence autism families. *American Journal of Psychiatry*, *154*, 185–190.

Plioplys, A. V. (1994). Autism: Electroencephalogram abnormalities and clinical improvement with valproic acid. *Archives of Pediatric and Adolescent Medicine*, *148*, 220–222.

Polich, J., & Herbst K. L. (2000). P300 as a clinical assay: Rationale, evaluation, and findings. *International Journal of Psychophysiology*, *38*, 3–19.

Purcell, A. E., Jeon, O. H., Zimmerman, A. W., Blue, M. E., & Pevsner, J. (2001). Postmortem brain abnormalities of the glutamate neurotransmitter system in autism. *Neurology*, *57*, 1618–1628.

Rapin, I. (1997). Autism. *New England Journal of Medicine*, *337*, 97–104.

Ratey, J. J., Bemporad, J., Sorgi, P., Bick, P., Polakoff, S., O'Driscoll, G., *et al.* (1987a). Brief report: Open trial effects of beta-blockers on speech and social behaviors in 8 autistic adults. *Journal of Autism and Developmental Disorders*, *17*, 439–446.

Ratey, J. J., Mikkelsen, E., Sorgi, P., Zuckerman, S., Polakoff, S., Bemporad, J., *et al.* (1987b). Autism: The treatment of aggressive behaviors. *Journal of Clinical Psychopharmacology*, *7*, 35–41.

Reichenberg, A., Gross, R., Weiser, M., Bresnahan, M., Silverman, J., Harlap, S., *et al.* (2006). Advancing paternal age and autism. *Archive of General Psychiatry*, *63*, 1026–1032.

Research Units on Pediatric Psychopharmacology (RUPP). (2005a). Randomized, controlled, crossover trial of methylphenidate in pervasive developmental disorders with hyperactivity. *Archives of General Psychiatry*, *62*, 1266–1274.

Research Units on Pediatric Psychopharmacology (RUPP). (2005b). Risperidone treatment of autistic disorder: Longer-term benefits and blinded discontinuation after 6 months. *American Journal of Psychiatry*, *162*, 1361–1369.

Risch, N. (1999). Linkage strategies for genetically complex traits. *American Journal of Human Genetics*, *46*, 222–253.

Ritvo, E. R., & Freeman, B. J. (1978). Current research on the syndrome of autism: introduction. The National Society for Autistic Children's definition of the syndrome of autism. *Journal of the American Academy of Child Psychiatry*, *17*, 565–575.

Robins, D. L., Fein, D., Barton, M. L., & Green, J. A. (2001). The Modified Checklist for Autism in Toddlers: An initial study investigating the early detection of autism and pervasive developmental disorders. *Journal of Autism and Developmental Disorders*, *31*, 131–144.

Roeyers, H. (1996). The influence of nonhandicapped peers on the social interactions of children with a pervasive development disorder. *Journal of Autism and Developmental Disorders*, *26*, 303–320.

Roger, J. H. (2000). The MMR question. *Lancet*, *356*, 160–161.

Rogers, S. J., & DiLalla, D. L. (1990). Age of symptom onset in young children with pervasive developmental disorders. *Journal of the American Academy of Child and Adolescent Psychiatry*, *29*, 863–872.

Rønningen, K. S., Paltiel, L., Meltzer, H. M., Nordhagen, R., Lie, K. K., Hovengen, R., *et al.* (2006). The biobank of the Norwegian Mother and Child Cohort Study: A resource for the next 100 years. *European Journal of Epidemiology*, *21*, 619–625.

Russell, J., Jarrold, C., & Hood, B. (1999). Two intact executive capacities in children with autism: Implications for the core executive dysfunctions in the disorder. *Journal of Autism and Developmental Disorders*, *29*, 103–112.

Rutter, M. (1970). Autistic children: Infancy to adulthood. *Seminars in Psychiatry*, *2*, 435–450.

Rutter, M. (1985). The treatment of autistic children. *Journal of Child Psychology and Psychiatry*, *26*, 193–214.

Rutter, M. (2000). Genetic studies of autism: From the 1970s into the millennium. *Journal of Abnormal Child Psychology*, *28*, 3–14.

Rutter, M. (2005). Incidence of autism spectrum disorders: Changes over time and their meaning. *Acta Paediatrica*, *94*, 2–15.

Rutter, M. (2006). Autism: Its recognition, early diagnosis, and service implications. *Journal of Developmental and Behavioral Pediatrics*, *27*, S54–S58.

Rutter, M., & Hersov, L. (1977). *Child psychiatry: Modern approaches*. Oxford: Blackwell Publishing.

Rutter, M., Anderson-Wood L., Beckett, C., Bredenkamp, D., Castle, J., Groothues C., *et al.* (1999). Quasi-autistic patterns following severe early global privation. English and Romanian Adoptees (ERA) Study Team. *Journal of Child Psychology and Psychiatry*, *40*, 537–549.

Rutter, M., Caspi, A., & Moffitt, T. E. (2003a). Using sex differences in psychopathology to study causal mechanisms: Unifying issues and research strategies. *Journal of Child Psychology and Psychiatry*, *44*, 1092–1115.

Rutter, M., Le Couteur, A., & Lord, C. (2003b). *Autism Diagnostic Interview revised (ADI-R)*. Los Angeles, CA: Western Psychological Services.

Rutter, M., Moffitt, T. E., & Caspi, A. (2006). Gene–environment interplay and psychopathology: Multiple varieties but real effects. *Journal of Child Psychology and Psychiatry*, *47*, 226–261.

Schopler, E., Mesibov, G. B., & Kunce, L. J. (1998). *Asperger syndrome or high-functioning autism?* New York/London: Plenum Press.

Schultz, R. T., Gauthier, I., Klein, A., Fulbright, R. K., Anderson A. W., Volkmar, F., *et al.* (2000). Abnormal ventral temporal cortical activity during face discrimination among individuals with autism and Asperger syndrome. *Archives of General Psychiatry*, *57*, 331–340.

Scragg, P., & Shah, A. (1994). Prevalence of Asperger syndrome in a secure hospital. *British Journal of Psychiatry*, *161*, 679–682.

Shao, Y., Raiford, K. L., Wolpert, C. M., Cope, H. A., Ravan, S. A., Ashley-Koch A. A., *et al.* (2002). Phenotypic homogeneity provides increased support for linkage on chromosome 2 in autistic disorder. *American Journal of Human Genetics*, *70*, 1058–1061.

Shea, S., Turgay, A., Carroll, A., Schulz, M., Orlik, H., Smith, I., *et al.* (2004). Risperidone in the treatment of disruptive behavioral symptoms in children with autistic and other pervasive developmental disorders. *Pediatrics*, *114*, 634–641.

Siegel, B., Pliner, C., Eschler, J., & Elliott, G. R. (1988). How children with autism are diagnosed: Difficulties in identification of children with multiple developmental delays. *Journal of Developmental and Behavioral Pediatrics*, *9*, 199–204.

Sigman, M., Ruskin, E., Arbeile, S., Corona, R., Dissanayake, C., Espinosa, M., *et al.* (1999). Continuity and change in the social competence of children with autism, Down syndrome, and developmental delays. *Monographs of the Society for Research in Child Development*, *64*, 1–114.

Smalley, S. L. (1998). Autism and tuberous sclerosis. *Journal of Autism and Developmental Disorders*, *28*, 407–414.

Smith, I. M., & Bryson, S. E. (1994). Imitation and action in autism: A critical review. *Psychological Bulletin*, *116*, 259–273.

Smith, M. D., Belcher, R. G., & Juhrs, P. D. (1995). *A guide to successful employment for individuals with autism*. Baltimore: Paul H. Brookes.

Sparrow, S. S., Balla, D., & Cicchetti, D. V. (1984). *Vineland Adaptive Behavior Scales: Manual*. Circle Pines, MN: American Guidance Service.

Starr, E., Berument, S. K., Pickles, A., Tomlins, M., Bailey, A., Papanikolaou, K., *et al.* (2001). A family genetic study of autism associated with profound mental retardation. *Journal of Autism and Developmental Disorders*, *31*, 89–96.

Swinkels, S. H. N., Dietz, C., van Daalen, E., Kerkhof, I. H., van Engeland, H., & Buitelaar, J. K. (2006). Screening for autistic spectrum in children aged 14 to 15 months. I. The development of the Early Screening of Autistic Traits Questionnaire (ESAT). *Journal of Autism and Developmental Disorders*, *36*, 723–732.

Szatmari, P., Bartolucci, G., & Bremner, R. (1989). Asperger syndrome and autism: comparison of early history and outcome. *Developmental Medicine and Child Neurology*, *31*, 709–720.

Szatmari, P., Bryson, S. E., Streiner D. L., Wilson, F. B. A., Archer, L., & Ryerse, C. (2000). Two-year outcome of preschool children with autism or Asperger syndrome. *American Journal of Psychiatry*, *157*, 1980–1987.

Szatmari, P., Jones, M. B., Zwaigenbaum, L., & MacLean, J. E. (1998). Genetics of autism: Overview and new directions. *Journal of Autism and Developmental Disorders*, *28*, 351–368.

Teder-Sälejärvi, W. A., Pierce, K. L., Courchesne, E., & Hillyard, S. A. (2005). Auditory spatial localization and attention deficits in autistic adults. *Brain Research. Cognitive Brain Research*, *23*, 221–234.

Tordjman, S., Anderson, G. M., McBride, P. A., Hertzig, M. E., Snow, M. E., Hall, L. M., *et al.* (1997). Plasma beta-endorphin, adrenocorticotropic hormone, and cortisol in autism. *Journal of Child Psychology and Psychiatry*, *38*, 705–715.

Torrey, E. F., Dhavale, D., Lawlor, J. P., & Yolken, R. H. (2004). Autism and head circumference in the first year of life. *Biological Psychiatry*, *56*, 892–894.

Trikalinos, T. A., Karvouni, A., Zintzaras, E., Ylisaukko-oja, T., Peltonen, L., Jarvela, I., *et al.* (2006). A heterogeneity-based genome search meta-analysis for autism-spectrum disorders. *Molecular Psychiatry*, *11*, 29–36.

Troost, P. W., Lahuis, B. E., Steenhuis, M. P., Ketelaars, C. E., Buitelaar, J. K., van Engeland, H., *et al.* (2005). Long-term effects of risperidone in children with autism spectrum disorders: A placebo discontinuation study. *Journal of the American Academy of Child and Adolescent Psychiatry*, *44*, 1137–1144.

Van der Gaag, R. J. (1993). *Multiplex developmental disorder: An exploration of borderlines on the autistic spectrum*. Utrecht: Unpublished thesis, Utrecht University.

Verbaten, M. N., Roelofs, J. W., van Engeland, H., Kenemans, J. K., & Slangen, J. L. (1991). Abnormal visual event-related potentials of autistic children. *Journal of Autism and Developmental Disorders*, *21*, 449–470.

Volkmar, F., Cook, E. H. Jr., Pomeroy, J., Realmuto, G., & Tanguay, P. (1999). Practice parameters for the assessment and treatment of children, adolescents, and adults with autism and other pervasive developmental disorders. American Academy of Child and Adolescent Psychiatry Working Group on Quality Issues. *Journal of the American Academy of Child and Adolescent Psychiatry*, *38*, 32S–54S.

Volkmar, F. R., & Cohen, D. J. (1991). Comorbid association of autism and schizophrenia. *American Journal of Psychiatry*, *148*, 1705–1707.

Volkmar, F. R., & Nelson, D. S. (1990). Seizure disorders in autism. *Journal of the American Academy of Child and Adolescent Psychiatry*, *29*, 127–129.

Volkmar, F. R., & Rutter, M. (1995). Childhood disintegrative disorder: Results of the DSM-IV autism field trial. *Journal of the American Academy of Child and Adolescent Psychiatry*, *34*, 1092–1095.

Vorstman, J. A., Staal, W. G., van Daalen, E., van Engeland, H., Hochstenbach, P. F. R., & Franke, L. (2006). Identification of novel autism candidate regions through analysis of reported cytogenetic abnormalities associated with autism. *Molecular Psychiatry*, *11*, 18–28.

Wakefield, A. J., Murch, S. H., Anthony, A., Linnell, J., Casson, D. M., Malik, M., *et al.* (1998). Ileal-lymphoid-nodular hyperplasia, non-specific colitis, and pervasive developmental disorder in children [see comments]. *Lancet*, *351*, 637–641.

Walhovd, K. B., & Fjell, A. M. (2003). The relationship between P3 and neuropsychological function in an adult life span sample. *Biological Psychology*, *62*, 65–87.

Wang, A. T., Ting, M. A., Dapretto, M., Hariri, A. R., Sigman, M., & Bookheimer, S. Y. (2004). Neural correlates of facial affect processing in children and adolescents with autism spectrum disorder. *Journal of the American Academy of Child and Adolescent Psychiatry*, *43*, 481–490.

Werner, E., & Dawson, G. (2005). Validation of the phenomenon of autistic regression using home videotapes. *Archives of General Psychiatry*, *62*, 889–895.

Whitaker-Azmitia, P. M. (2001). Serotonin and brain development: Role in human developmental diseases. *Brain Research Bulletin*, *56*, 479–485.

Willemsen-Swinkels, S. H., Buitelaar, J. K., Nijhof, G. J., & van Engeland, H. (1995). Failure of naltrexone hydrochloride to reduce self-injurious and autistic behavior in mentally retarded adults: Double-blind placebo-controlled studies. *Archives of General Psychiatry*, *52*, 766–773.

Williams, D. L., Goldstein, G., Carpenter, P. A., & Minshew, N. J. (2005). Verbal and spatial working memory in autism. *Journal of Autism and Developmental Disorders*, *35*, 747–756.

Wing, L. (1997). The autistic spectrum. *Lancet*, *350*, 1761–1766.

Wing, L. (1981). Asperger syndrome: A clinical account. *Psychological Medicine*, *11*, 115–129.

Wing, L., Leekam, S. R., Libby, S. J., Gould, J., & Larcombe, M. (2002). The Diagnostic Interview for Social and Communication Disorders: Background, inter-rater reliability and clinical use. *Journal of Child Psychology and Psychiatry and Allied Disciplines*, *43*, 307–325.

Wing, L., & Gould, J. (1979). Severe impairments of social interaction and associated abnormalities in children: Epidemiology and classification. *Journal of Autism and Developmental Disorders*, *9*, 11–29.

Wing, L., & Shah, A. (2000). Catatonia in autistic spectrum disorders. *British Journal of Psychiatry*, *176*, 357–362.

World Health Organization (WHO). (1996). *Multiaxial classification of child and adolescent psychiatric disorders: The ICD-10 classification of mental and behavioural disorders in children and adolescents*. Cambridge, UK: Cambridge University Press.

Yirmiya, N., Sigman, M. D., Kasari, C., & Mundy, P. (1992). Empathy and cognition in high-functioning children with autism. *Child Development*, *63*, 150–160.

Young, L. J., & Wang, Z. (2004). The neurobiology of pair bonding. *Nature Neuroscience*, *7*, 1048–1054.

Ziatas, K., Durkin, K., & Pratt, C. (1998). Belief term development in children with autism, Asperger syndrome, specific language impairment, and normal development: Links to theory of mind development. *Journal of Child Psychology and Psychiatry*, *39*, 755–763.

Zwaigenbaum, L., Bryson, S., Rogers, T., Roberts, W., Brian, J., & Szatmari, P. (2005). Behavioral manifestations of autism in the first year of life. *International Journal of Developmental Neuroscience*, *23*, 143–152.

47

Speech and Language Disorders

Dorothy V. M. Bishop and Courtenay Frazier Norbury

Speech, Language and Communication

The distinction between speech, language and communication may be illustrated by three child cases. Emma is a lively and engaging 9-year-old who has difficulty making herself understood because her production of speech sounds is very unclear. However, she demonstrates normal *language* skills: she understands what others say to her, and can express herself in writing using long and complex sentences. Her ability to communicate is hampered by her speech difficulties, but she enjoys interacting with others, and when people fail to understand her, she supplements her utterances with gesture and facial expression to get her message across.

Thomas is a 6-year-old who has no difficulty in producing speech sounds clearly, but his language skills are limited, as evidenced by his use of simple and immature sentence construction. Instead of saying "I'd like a drink" he says "Me want drink." However, although his language is far more simple than that of other 6-year-olds, he does use it to communicate with other children and adults. In contrast, 4-year-old Jack produces a great deal of complex, fluent and clearly articulated language, but he does not use it to communicate effectively. Thus, his opening gambit to a stranger might be to say: "In Deep Space Nine you can't get to level 6 until you have killed all the foot soldiers, but if you get to level 6, you have to first destroy the klingons before you can enter the palace of death."

One way of depicting the relationship between speech, language and communication is shown in Fig. 47.1, where language is a subset of communication and speech is a subset of language. Communication is defined by McArthur (1992, p. 238) as "the transmission of information (a message) between a source and a receiver, using a signaling system." The primary means of communication between humans is through language, but communication also encompasses other means of signaling meaning, such as facial expression, bodily gesture and non-verbal sounds. Language differs from these other communicative modes; it is a complex formal system in which a small number of elements are combined in a rule-based manner to generate an infinite number of possible meanings. Most human language is expressed in speech (i.e., meanings are represented by words that are composed of a small set of speech sounds, or phonemes). Where learning of oral language is compromised because a child is deaf, manual (sign) languages have evolved, showing similar structural characteristics to spoken languages. In addition, oral language can be expressed in written form. Language involves more than speech, and communication involves more than language. However, it is possible for someone to speak without producing language (e.g., when a person utters meaningless gobbledegook), and it is possible for someone to produce utterances that obey the formal rules of language, yet communication is not achieved, as in the case of Jack. In evaluating children with impairments, it is important to keep these three levels in mind, and to recognize that a problem at one level does not necessarily entail a problem at another.

In this chapter we make a broad division between disorders affecting speech, and those affecting language and communication. This distinction has some similarity with the distinction made in DSM-IV-TR (American Psychiatric Association, 2000) between phonological disorder (315.39) and language disorder (315.31), but the coverage is broader. Among speech disorders, we cover disorders affecting fluency, voice and prosody as well as problems of speech sound production that may have a neurological basis. For language and communication disorders, we focus heavily on specific language impairment (SLI), which is analogous to the DSM language disorder category, but we also consider other conditions required for a differential

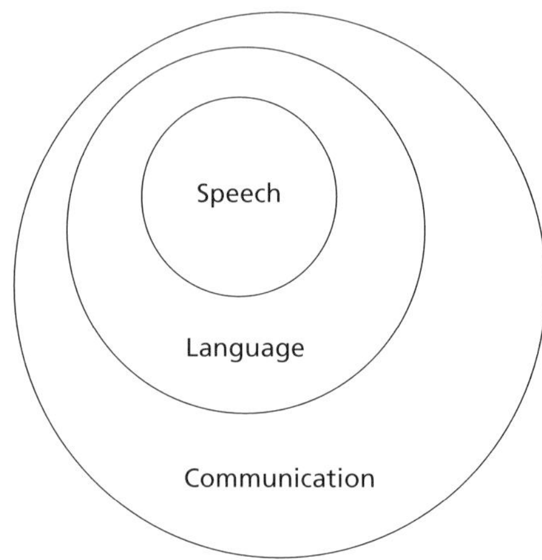

Fig. 47.1 Relationship between speech, language and communication.

Rutter's Child and Adolescent Psychiatry, 5th edition. Edited by M. Rutter, D. Bishop, D. Pine, S. Scott, J. Stevenson, E. Taylor and A. Thapar. © 2008 Blackwell Publishing, ISBN: 978-1-4051-4549-7.

diagnosis, including acquired epileptic aphasia, autistic disorder and selective mutism.

General Principles of Assessment

In most instances, detailed assessment of the speech and language system will be carried out by a specialist speech-language therapist, who will have extensive knowledge of linguistics and language development, the anatomy and physiology that support the language system, and access to a variety of assessment and intervention techniques. With regard to communication, the primary decisions for the practitioner to make at initial assessment are:

1 Is the child's communication development delayed or disordered?

2 What aspects of communication are causing the most concern?

3 Is referral to speech-language therapy warranted?

The first port of call in the assessment process is the case history. This will give the practitioner an opportunity to explore with the child's parents *who* is concerned about communication, and precisely *what* they are concerned about. Although many parents will be concerned about their child's language development, others may not be aware of difficulties with communication. These parents may not see language as the central problem, but will voice concerns about behavior, social skills and learning that may be related to underlying language difficulties.

As part of the case history, it is essential to obtain from parents clear examples of what motivates the child to communicate and how the child achieves communication. For example, does the child communicate only to get his or her basic needs met? Does the child communicate to show others things that interest him or her? Does the child use words or phrases? If not, does the child gesture, vocalize and/or point in an effort to get the message across? In addition to concrete examples of the types of communication the child produces, it is also important to ascertain the types of communication the child can understand. Does the child follow an adult's point or eye gaze? Can he or she follow simple verbal instructions out of context? For more able children this may not pose a problem, but they may have difficulty following a story or getting the point of a joke.

Once the practitioner has gained an impression of the child from the parents, it will be necessary to determine directly the child's current level of functioning. Throughout the rest of this chapter, we give specific signposts to impairment in speech, language and broader communication, and suggest standardized assessments in each of these domains that can assist in the diagnostic process (Table 47.1). However, it is usually preferable to start by observing the child's communication in a less structured setting. This can be achieved by videoing the child playing with his or her parents or siblings in the clinic. If the child has some verbal language, this play session can be supplemented by asking the child to recall a favorite story, computer game or television program.

During these informal tasks, the practitioner can make a number of important observations. The first concerns the child's expressive language output. How long and grammatically complex are the child's utterances? How rich is the child's vocabulary? Does he or she struggle to find the words for common objects? Does he or she use gestures and facial expression? Is the speech fluent, or is the child's speech peppered with hesitations and repetitions? What is the child's voice quality like? Is he or she shouting and hoarse, or whispering inappropriately? Is the child intelligible, or are there numerous speech errors that impede understanding? Does the child tell a story as a coherent sequence of events, or does he or she get muddled and leave important events out?

The next set of observations concerns the child's understanding, which may be more difficult to gauge in this setting. Nevertheless, it can be revealing to observe how the child responds to the questions and comments of others. Are the answers appropriate to the questions? Does the child follow adult directions? Does the child understand the premise of a story or does he or she misinterpret key events? Does the child appear to understand the gestures and facial expressions of others? Can the child listen while engaged with something else, or must the adult focus his or her attention before speaking?

Finally, these informal interactions enable the practitioner to observe other important behaviors. How and why does the child engage with the other people in the room? Does he or she look up when called? Is the child's play creative and imaginative, or destructive and repetitive? Can the child stick with an activity, or is his or her attention span unduly short? Is the child frustrated when he or she is not understood? Does he or she try again? Does the child recognize when he or she has not understood something and ask for clarification? Is the child anxious, or does he or she quickly adjust to the new situation?

In combination with the case history, this set of observations should provide the practitioner with a working hypothesis of the child's strengths and weaknesses, which will guide the assessment process (see chapters 19 and 21).

Speech Disorders

Speech refers to the production of oral language, which is achieved by modifications to the vocal tract while a stream of air is breathed out from the lungs. Speech difficulties in children are not difficult to detect, but accurate diagnosis requires specialist assessment by a speech and language therapist. The main types of difficulty that are encountered are those affecting the distinctive production of speech sounds, fluency of connected speech, voice, and prosody (i.e., speech melody and intonation).

Differential Diagnosis of Speech Sound Disorders

All spoken languages encode meaning in terms of a small set of vowels and consonants: in standard British English there are 24 consonants and 20 vowels that can be combined to yield thousands of words. When a child's speech is difficult

Table 47.1 Language assessments in common use in the UK.

Assessment	Age range	Description
Phonology		
Goldman–Fristoe Test of Articulation–2 (Goldman & Fristoe, 2000)	2–21 years	Naming task which samples all consonants and clusters of English in initial, medial and final word positions. Assesses spontaneous and imitated speech
Diagnostic Evaluation of Articulation and Phonology (DEAP) (Dodd *et al.*, 2002)	3–6 years	Picture materials elicit speech with goal of differentiating between articulation problems, delayed phonology and consistent versus inconsistent phonological disorder
Phonological Assessment Battery (PhAB) (Frederickson *et al.*, 1997)	6–14 years	Tests of phonological processing: alliteration, naming speed, rhyme, spoonerisms, fluency and non-word reading
Children's Test of Non-word Repetition (Gathercole & Baddeley, 1996)	4–8 years	A measure of phonological short-term memory; the child listens to non-words and repeats them
Semantics		
MacArthur–Bates Communicative Development Inventories (Fenson *et al.*, 2003)	8–30 months	Parent reports of words child understands and produces early communicative gestures and early word combinations
British Picture Vocabulary Scales–2 (Dunn *et al.*, 1998)	3–15 years	Understanding of single words. Child matches spoken word to one of four pictures
Expressive/Receptive One Word Picture Vocabulary Tests (Gardner, 2000)	2–12 years	Child either names a picture (expressive) or matches a spoken word to one of four pictures
Test of Word Knowledge (ToWK) (Wiig & Secord, 1992)	5–17 years	Expressive and receptive semantics including definitions, antonyms, synonyms, multiple meanings
Syntax		
Renfrew Action Picture Test (RAPT) (Renfrew, 1988)	3–8 years	Sentence elicitation task in which children describe what is happening in 10 different pictures. Scored for information content and syntactic complexity
Test for Reception of Grammar–2 (TROG-2) (Bishop, 2003b)	4 years–adult	Child matches spoken sentence to one of four pictures. Assesses range of grammatical structures
Narrative		
The Bus Story (Renfrew, 1988)	3–8 years	Provides age equivalent scores for story information and sentence complexity
Expression, Reception and Recall of Narrative Instrument (ERRNI) (Bishop, 2004)	6 years–adult	Narrative assessment that provides standard scores for information content, complexity of grammatical structure, comprehension of pictured story, recall of narrative
Pragmatics		
Children's Communication Checklist–2 (CCC-2) (Bishop, 2003a)	4–16 years	Parental report of language and pragmatic behaviors in everyday situations. Provides standard scores
Omnibus tests		
Assessment of Comprehension and Expression (ACE) (Adams *et al.*, 2001)	6–11 years	Assesses sentence comprehension, inferencing, naming, formulating sentences, semantics, non-literal language comprehension, narrative
Clinical Evaluation of Language Fundamentals–Preschool (Wiig *et al.*, 1992) and Clinical Evaluation of Language Fundamentals (Semel *et al.*, 2003)	3–6 years; 5 years–adult	Assesses basic concepts, syntax, morphology, semantics, verbal memory. Provides receptive and expressive as well as total language score
Pre-school Language Scales–3 (Zimmerman *et al.*, 1997)	Birth–6 years	Assesses listening comprehension, expressive communication and provides a total language score
Reynell Developmental Language Scales–3 (Edwards *et al.*, 1997)	1–7 years	Measures receptive language (verbal and non-verbal) and expressive language, including structure and vocabulary
Test of Language Competence (Wiig & Secord, 1989)	9–18 years	Assesses higher level language skills such as inferencing, multiple meanings, figurative language, sentence production in conversational contexts
Test of Language Development–3 (TOLD-3) (Newcomer & Hammill, 1997)	4–12 years	Subtests measure both semantic knowledge and grammar

to understand, analysis of the pattern of errors will be helpful in distinguishing whether the difficulty is the result of a structural or motor impairment affecting the articulatory apparatus (i.e., a dysarthria) or whether other explanations need to be sought (Dodd, 2005). Usually, dysarthria will be accompanied by other evidence of physical or neurological impairment, and the production of speech sounds will be distorted or labored.

Phonological Disorder

Contrary to popular belief, most childhood problems with speech production do not have a physical basis. For many years there was a belief that children's speech difficulties could be caused by "tongue tie," which could be cured by cutting the frenum. However, surgery is seldom effective in improving speech and it is now recognized that interventions that train children to perceive and produce sounds accurately are more effective. The key point to note is that speech production involves more than articulation: in learning a language, the child has to integrate speech perception with production, and work out which sounds in the language are used to signal contrasts in meaning (i.e., correspond to *phonemes*). To illustrate the difference between articulation and phonology, consider the following: many native English-speakers have great difficulty in correctly learning to produce the French words "rue" and "roux" distinctively. This is because the vowel contrast in these words does not match the phonemes in English, where there is just one "oo" sound. This has nothing to do with the structure of the articulatory apparatus, and everything to do with perceptual experience of a language, which leads English-speakers to treat all instances of "oo" as one phoneme, where French-speakers divide the vowel space into two phonemes. Most cases of childhood speech production difficulties appear analogous to the problems of the second language-learner: they arise because the child has not learned to categorize speech sounds appropriately, and so may fail to differentiate sounds that are important for signaling contrasts in meaning. Over the years, a variety of terminology has been used to describe such difficulties, including functional articulation disorder and phonological disorder/impairment.

Developmental Verbal Dyspraxia

Sitting somewhat uneasily between dysarthria on the one hand, and phonological disorder on the other is the category of developmental verbal dyspraxia, also known as developmental apraxia of speech. An early use of the term was by Morley (1957), who applied it to children in whom the neuromuscular control of the articulators seemed adequate for all purposes except the rapid integrated movements used in speech. Such children might be able to imitate accurately a simple syllable or word, but would make errors if asked to produce longer words or connected sentences. Stackhouse and Wells (1997) noted that production of longer words may be inconsistent as well as inaccurate, so that "caterpillar" could be produced as "capertillar," "taperkiller" or "takerpillar." The term "dyspraxia" is taken from adult neurology where it describes a disorder of planning movement sequences that is not accounted for in terms of lower-level difficulties in executing individual movements. However, it is unclear whether motor programing is at the root of the inconsistent speech difficulties seen in children. Individuals with the clinical picture of developmental verbal dyspraxia often have major problems in perception as well as production of speech sounds, doing poorly on tests that require them to discriminate or classify sounds (Stackhouse & Wells, 1997). Some experts argue that developmental verbal dyspraxia is simply an unusually severe kind of phonological disorder in children, reflecting an underlying difficulty learning the categorization of speech sounds, rather than having motor origins. The jury is still out on this question, not least because different experts use different diagnostic criteria (Forrest, 2003).

One way of bypassing diagnostic difficulties has been to use the more general term "speech sound disorder" (SSD) to encompass all difficulties of speech sound production in children that do not have a physical basis, without needing to specify whether they are motor-based or phonological in origin. Although such "lumping" of disorders might seem likely to obscure important differences between phenotypes, Lewis, Freebairn, Hansen *et al.* (2004) argued in its favor. They compared family pedigrees of children with verbal dyspraxia and children with other forms of SSD. Verbal dyspraxia showed very high familiality, but the disorder did not "breed true," and affected relatives were more likely to have other forms of SSD or language impairment than to have verbal dyspraxia themselves. Lewis, Freebairn, Hansen *et al.* (2004) concluded that the principal difference between children with verbal dyspraxia and those with other SSD was in the degree of genetic loading for disorder.

Assessment of Speech Sound Disorders

Coplan and Gleason (1988) provided guidelines to help health professionals decide when to refer a child for speech assessment, based on a parent's response to the question, "How much of your child's speech can a stranger understand?" By 2 years, it should be possible to understand at least 50% of what the child says, by 3 years, 75%, and by 4 years the child's speech should be completely intelligible. Referral should be considered if these cut offs are not met (see p. 786).

Assessment by the speech-language therapist will involve examination of the articulatory apparatus. A history of difficulty with sucking, chewing, dribbling, licking or blowing should alert the clinician to the possibility of physical impairment, such as submucous cleft palate, or neurological impairment. Where there is facial dysmorphology or evidence of neurological dysfunction, referral to specialist medical services (pediatric neurology, otolaryngology or clinical genetics) is warranted.

The speech-language therapist will construct a phonemic inventory of sounds the child is able to produce and will look for inconsistency of word pronunciations and the presence of "phonological processes" (i.e., consistent error patterns), such as replacing /k/ with /t/ so that "cat" becomes "tat" and "take" becomes "tate." Many of these processes are seen in the course of normal phonological development; however, an SSD is diagnosed when such processes continue beyond the normal age, or when there are numerous inconsistencies and atypical phonological processes.

"Phonological processing" is a general term used to cover more subtle difficulties in using phonological information. Phonological awareness in particular is nowadays often targeted in assessment as research has demonstrated links with later literacy difficulties (Snowling & Stackhouse, 2006). This refers to the ability to manipulate the sound segments in the language and includes tasks such as rhyming, segmenting syllables and phonemes in words, identifying initial and final word sounds, and deleting, adding or transposing phonemes in words. Such problems can been seen in children with normal speech sound production but are often also seen in children with SSD, suggesting their difficulties do not involve the physical act of articulating speech, but rather the ability to perceive and categorize different exemplars of the same phoneme (Bird, Bishop, & Freeman, 1995; Stackhouse & Wells, 1997).

An important point to stress is that although speech and language difficulties are not the same thing, they do often co-occur. We therefore recommend that any child who presents with a speech difficulty should have a full assessment of both speech and language.

Prevalence, Causes and Correlates of Speech Sound Disorders

Estimates of prevalence of SSD are hampered by inconsistencies in diagnostic criteria. Gierut (1998) cited a 1994 report from the US National Institute on Deafness and Other Communication Disorders which estimated that phonological disorders affected approximately 10% of preschool and school-aged children, and that in 80% of cases the disorder was severe enough to merit clinical treatment. At 6 years of age, the prevalence of "speech delay" was estimated at 3.8% in a US epidemiological study (Shriberg, Tomblin, & McSweeny, 1999).

Campbell, Dollaghan, Rockette *et al.* (2003) identified a number of factors that greatly increased the risk of speech sound disorders in preschool children. These included male gender, limited maternal education and a positive family history of speech and language disorder. These authors also suggested that an accumulation of risk factors exerted a greater threat to developmental outcome than individual risks. Children with only one risk factor were 1.7–2.6 times more likely than children who had none of these characteristics to have speech delay at 3 years; children with all three risk factors present were almost eight times more likely to have speech delay at 3 years.

Both family (Lewis, Freebairn, Hansen *et al.*, 2004) and twin studies (Bishop, 2002; DeThorne, Petrill, Deater-Deckard *et al.*, 2006) suggest a strong genetic etiology for SSD. Although verbal dyspraxia can follow an autosomal dominant pattern of inheritance in some families (Hurst, Baraitser, Auger, Graham, & Norell, 1990), in most cases there are numerous genes that contribute to risk of poor speech and language skills, rather than a single genetic mutation. To date, progress in the search for a molecular basis has been limited to one report of linkage to a site on chromosome 3 (Stein, Schick, Taylor *et al.*, 2004).

Intervention and Prognosis for Speech Sound Disorders

A variety of techniques may be employed to improve speech intelligibility, and research to date suggests that no single treatment approach is appropriate for all children with SSD (Dodd & Bradford, 2000). Techniques might include using tactile and visual cues to enable children to produce the target sound accurately. This will be combined with repeated practice at producing the target sound in words with corrective feedback. More meta-linguistic approaches involve games and exercises to develop the child's awareness of meaningful phonemic contrasts (Gierut, 1998).

In a recent meta-analysis of the literature, Law, Garrett, and Nye (2004) found that phonological interventions were generally effective when compared with no treatment. The most effective treatments were those carried out by speech-language therapists, rather than parent-administered treatments, and those that lasted for longer than 8 weeks. Therapist-led treatments may incorporate a variety of techniques, such as "articulation drills" in which the child learns and practices correct production of speech sounds with visual aids such as cued articulation (hand gestures that illustrate the place and manner of articulation) or symbols (pictures of place and manner of articulation). Other techniques (e.g., Metaphon) emphasize a meta-linguistic approach to improving speech production (Howell & Dean, 1994). This treatment teaches sound "concepts" so that children learn, for example, the differences between "short" sounds (/t/ and /d/) and "long" sounds (/s/ and /f/). The therapy also utilizes "meaningful minimal contrasts," in which the child is required to alter speech production to avoid ambiguity. For instance, if the child is "fronting" (producing /k/ sounds as /t/ sounds), the therapist might construct a game in which the child has to ask for "key" or "tea." If the child intends to ask for the "key" but the therapist responds with the "tea," the child is forced to adapt his pronunciation to convey his or her intended meaning. Many therapists will use a combination of techniques depending on the needs of the child, as there is currently no evidence that one method of treatment is more effective than any other method.

The longer-term prognosis for children with isolated phonological impairments is much better than that of language impairment, especially if the phonological difficulties resolve by the time the child starts school. However, the child who starts school with phonological difficulties is at increased risk of long-lasting literacy deficits (Stothard, Snowling, Bishop, Chipchase, & Kaplan, 1998).

Other Types of Speech Disorder

Fluency Disorders

Stuttering and stammering are two popular terms for dysfluent speech. Developmental dysfluency is characterized by involuntary repetitions, blocks or prolongations of sounds, syllables and words in discourse. These may be accompanied by secondary behaviors such as physical tension in the speech musculature, eye blinking or breaking of eye contact, movements of the head and limbs, and emotional reactions to the dysfluency, including anxiety and avoidance of speaking.

Persistent dysfluency is estimated to affect 1% of the population (Yairi & Ambrose, 1999), although many more children produce normal dysfluencies during the preschool years. Like many speech, language and communication disorders, it appears to be strongly familial, and more boys are affected more often than girls (ratio of 1.65:1; Mansson, 2000). Campbell, Dollaghan, and Yaruss (2002) suggest referral to a speech-language therapist if parents report:

1 Frequent part-word dysfluencies;
2 Noticeable physical tension or struggle;
3 Any sign that the child is frustrated or concerned about talking; or
4 Concerns about any other aspect of speech and language development.

The etiology of childhood stuttering appears to be multifactorial, with a significant genetic component (Yairi, Ambrose, & Cox, 1996). An international study by Suresh, Ambrose, Roe *et al.* (2006) suggested a complex etiology, with the strongest linkages being found when separate analyses were conducted for males (linkage to chromosome 7, LOD score 2.99) and females (linkage to chromosome 21, LOD score 4.5), and when interactions between sites on different chromosomes were considered.

Stuttering has been associated with early difficulties in language formulation (Bloodstein, 2006) and atypical development of the auditory temporal cortex (Foundas, Bollich, Feldman *et al.*, 2004). Furthermore, comorbidity with speech sound disorders is 30% (Yairi & Ambrose, 1999). Therefore, assessment of broader speech and language abilities is warranted.

Approximately 75% of preschoolers will recover from dysfluency without professional involvement (Yairi & Ambrose, 1999). However, prognosis is poor for those who continue to stutter beyond the age of 7 years (Campbell, Dollaghan, & Yaruss, 2002). There is considerable debate regarding the most appropriate form of intervention. One approach, exemplified by the Michael Palin Centre for stammering in London (www.stammeringcentre.org), focuses on modifying the environment to reduce speaking pressure and working with children and families to reduce anxiety about speaking (for a full description see Rustin, Cook, Botterill, Hughes, & Kelman, 2001). An alternative approach, exemplified by the Lidcombe Programme (http://www3.fhs.usyd.edu.au/asrcwww/treatment/lidcombe.htm), provides direct behavioral modification to reinforce fluent speech. There are few, if any, methodologically sound investigations of treatment efficacy and no studies that we are aware of that explicitly compare the two treatment approaches. However, there is some preliminary evidence that behavioral approaches are effective in reducing dysfluent speech in the preschool years (Jones, Onslow, Packman *et al.*, 2005).

Voice Disorders

A voice disorder, dysphonia, should be suspected when a child speaks with abnormal pitch, loudness and/or hoarseness. These features can have profound effects on how a child is perceived by others and adversely affect socialization.

Recent prevalence estimates from a population-based study suggest 6–11% of school-aged children present with dysphonia (Carding, Roulsone, Northstone, & Team, 2006). This is considerably higher than would be predicted from clinical referrals, but this probably reflects widespread lack of recognition of the problem (Boyle, 2000). Gender (male) and older siblings were the most significant risk factors in the Carding, Roulstone, Northstone *et al.* study. Campbell, Dollaghan, & Yaruss (2002) reported unpublished data from their own sample of 427 clinical referrals to a specialist clinic; 93% of these children had abnormal voice quality associated with laryngeal pathology. The most common pathology was vocal nodules (i.e., mechanical trauma caused by one vocal fold making excessive contact with the other). Surgical treatment is not recommended in such cases, as nodules are likely to return if damaging vocal behavior is not altered. Behavioral treatments can be effective and center on modifying the environment (i.e., reducing competing noise) and training the child to use the voice more appropriately.

Prosodic Disorders

Prosody may be defined as the suprasegmental properties of the speech signal that modulate and enhance its meaning (Paul, Shriberg, McSweeny *et al.*, 2005a). Prosody includes variations in pitch, loudness, duration, rhythm, tempo and pausing, and serves a wide range of grammatical, pragmatic and affective functions. For example, variations in stress and intonation may signal the difference between a noun (*con* vict) and a verb (con *vict*), highlight elements within the sentence for attentional focus (the *blue* book, as opposed to the red one), and convey a speaker's emotional state.

It is frequently reported that impaired prosody is characteristic of verbal individuals with autistic spectrum disorder (ASD), although it may not be universal. Paul, Shriberg, McSweeny *et al.* (2005a) reported that 47% of the 30 adolescent and adult speakers with ASD they investigated had prosodic abnormalities. Such abnormalities have a negative effect on how listeners perceive social and communicative competence and pose significant obstacles to social integration and employment (Paul, Augustyn, Klin *et al.*, 2005b).

Disorders of Language and Communication

Components of Language

Competent adults produce language so effortlessly that it is easy to forget just what a complex system it is. All spoken languages can be studied in terms of four levels of description: phonology (speech sounds); semantics (meaning); grammar (formal ways of using word order and inflection); and pragmatics (use of language to communicate). However, there is considerable variation from one language to another at all of these levels. For instance, Chinese does not have word inflections, whereas Turkish has numerous inflections that are appended to word stems in an agglutinative fashion. Clearly, the task confronting the young language learner is going to be very different in these two languages, and in English, which uses inflections, but much more sparsely than many other languages. As well as the different levels of linguistic representation, language can be divided into expressive (production) and receptive (comprehension) aspects. To be a competent communicator, the child must learn to recognize and produce the distinctive speech sounds in the language (the phonology), establish a "mental lexicon" containing representations of words as phoneme sequences linked to meanings, master the grammatical structure of the ambient language, and learn how to select a message to convey meanings economically and effectively to others (pragmatics). Furthermore, language processing has to be carried out at speed.

Differential Diagnosis of Specific Language Impairment

When a child presents with language impairment, the clinician needs to establish whether there is any causal factor present that could explain the language difficulty, or whether the language impairment is part of a recognized syndrome. The majority of cases of language impairment in children have no obvious cause (Shevell, Majnemer, Rosenbaum, & Abrhamowicz, 2000), and occur in the context of otherwise normal development. This is known as specific language impairment (SLI) and also as primary language impairment, developmental language disorder or developmental dysphasia. Before considering the characteristics of SLI we briefly discuss other conditions that need to be considered when making a differential diagnosis.

Low Non-verbal Ability

An early step in the assessment of a language-impaired child is administration of a non-verbal IQ test. Cases of intellectual disability (non-verbal IQ more than 2 SD below average) are usually straightforward enough to identify (see chapter 49). However, there are many children with slow language development who do not have a syndrome of intellectual disability, but nevertheless have below-average non-verbal IQ. Traditional definitions of SLI usually require that non-verbal IQ is broadly within normal limits. More stringent definitions also require that there should be a significant mismatch between language ability and non-verbal IQ (equivalent to 1 SD in ICD-10). However, there is increasing disquiet about the use of IQ discrepancy criteria, because these exclude large numbers of children who are not intellectually impaired and yet have evident language difficulties. For instance, if we require there to be a 1 SD difference between a language and non-verbal index, then we would exclude a child with a language level 2 SD below the mean and a non-verbal score 1.3 SD below the mean. This child would not meet criteria for intellectual disability and so would be left in a diagnostic limbo and may be denied access to intervention, even though the profile and severity of language difficulty may be similar to those seen in a child who does meet the discrepancy criterion (Tomblin & Zhang, 1999). Furthermore, twin studies suggest the same genetic risk factors operate for children with language difficulties regardless of their non-verbal IQ (Bishop, 1994). Thus, the logic of distinguishing between children who do and do not meet strict IQ discrepancy criteria is questionable.

Auditory Problems

Hearing should always be assessed by an audiologist in a child who presents with language impairment. As neonatal screening programs become more widespread, it is unusual to find an undetected sensorineural hearing loss in a language-impaired child, but one needs to be alert to the possibility of screening errors or a progressive hearing loss. Hearing loss restricted to a specific frequency range is easy to miss, because the child appears responsive to sound, yet crucial information may be lost from the speech signal, leading to a profile of impaired language development that may look similar to SLI (Stelmachowicz, Pittman, Hoover, Lewis, & Moeller, 2004).

It is much more common to find conductive losses in young children with language impairments. However, it is not easy to know how to interpret these. Early studies suggested unusually high rates of language and literacy problems in children who had otitis media with effusion (OME; Holm & Kunze, 1969). OME typically causes a conductive loss of up to 40 dB, and it seems plausible that such a loss might assume significance in a child in the early stages of language learning. However, more recent epidemiological studies have questioned whether OME is a major etiological factor in language impairment (Feldman, Dollaghan, Campbell *et al.*, 2003). A substantial number of children under 5 years of age have undetected and asymptomatic middle ear disease, particularly in the winter months. Prospective studies of children with and without prolonged episodes of OME have found little or no impact on verbal skills, suggesting that language development is resilient in the face of the mild associated hearing losses. OME may assume more importance if it is chronic and persistent (Feldman, Dollaghan, Campbell *et al.*, 2003). However, we would recommend caution in assuming that OME is the main causal factor if it is detected in a child with language impairment.

There is a large body of knowledge on assessment of the integrity of the peripheral auditory pathways in children, but much less agreement concerning diagnosis of central auditory processing deficits. In some countries, notably the USA and Australia, the diagnosis of auditory processing disorder (APD – sometimes prefixed with C for central) is frequently made. However, it is far less common in the UK. The principal difficulty with the APD concept is that it is typically diagnosed using tests that use verbal materials (e.g., listening to speech in noise) or being presented with two streams of speech in different ears (Moore, 2006). These tests have demonstrated validity when used to identify central auditory lesions in adults with acquired brain damage, who can be assumed to have normal language abilities. However, their interpretation is complicated in children, because it is difficult to distinguish poor performance resulting from a primary language problem from a genuine auditory difficulty (Rosen, 2005). To illustrate this point, consider how you would fare if you were asked to carry out a range of listening tests presented in a language with which you had limited competence. It is likely that under optimal listening conditions you would do much better than when words were presented in noise or in a competing speech situation. This is because a competent speaker of a language does not simply decode speech by bottom-up analysis of the speech signal; he or she also employs top-down processing to predict and fill in information. If one uses speech-based tests in diagnosis, then one is likely to end up finding numerous cases of language impairment that appear to be caused by APD, but where the problem may in fact arise for quite different reasons. In our experience, many children who receive a diagnosis of APD from an audiologist would be given a diagnosis of SLI, dyslexia, attention deficit/hyperactivity disorder (ADHD) or autistic disorder if seen by a speech and language therapist, psychologist or child psychiatrist.

In emphasizing these assessment difficulties, we do not wish to imply that APD is not a valid category; it is plausible that some children have immature or dysfunctional development of the central auditory pathways and this might well impact on language development. However, our concern is that APD is often diagnosed using instruments of questionable validity, leading to implementation of auditory-based interventions that may not be justified. It is vital to adopt an interdisciplinary approach, whereby audiologists work together with other professionals to ensure that children receive appropriate diagnoses and intervention. It is hoped that as research on APD advances, better assessment methods, using more objective electrophysiological as well as non-verbal behavioral tests (Liasis, Bamiou, Campbell *et al.*, 2003) will give a clearer picture.

Acquired Epileptic Aphasia

Acquired epileptic aphasia (AEA), also known as Landau–Kleffner syndrome, is a rare cause of childhood language impairment which is often misdiagnosed. The typical presentation is one of deterioration in language skills in the preschool years after a period of normal development. Because the child previously spoke normally, the disorder may be misdiagnosed as selective mutism (see p. 791); however, in AEA, there is genuine loss of language skills, with comprehension problems predominating. Deafness is usually suspected but ruled out on the basis of a hearing test. Many children with AEA have relatively selective problems with language in the context of preserved non-verbal ability, but in some children there are associated behavioral disturbances, which further complicate the diagnosis (Deonna & Roulet-Perez, 2005). The epileptic manifestations of AEA are not obvious, because overt seizures are uncommon, and it may be necessary to carry out a sleep electroencephalogram (EEG) to demonstrate EEG abnormalities. These can be marked, and there has been debate as to how far this disorder overlaps with slow wave status epilepticus in sleep (SWSS). Some children, particularly those with onset after 6 years of age, can make a good recovery, but the prognosis for those with preschool onset is often poor and substantial receptive language deficits may persist to adulthood. Our recommendation is that any child with language regression accompanied by comprehension problems should be referred to a pediatric neurologist for an evaluation of AEA. Deonna and Roulet-Perez (2005) note that pharmacological interventions can be effective, but there is wide variation in responsiveness to treatment, and in the absence of controlled clinical trials it is difficult to give precise guidelines. Deonna (2000) recommended that when receptive language difficulties persist for more than a few weeks or months, it is crucial to provide the child with an alternative mode of communication. Sign language can be effective and does not interfere with attempts to retrain comprehension of auditory language (Roulet-Perez, Davidoff, Prélaz *et al.*, 2001).

Delayed Language Development: Late-Talkers

When diagnosing SLI, it is important to determine when a young child's language delay represents a significant departure from normal variation, which can be difficult when the child is younger than 3 years old. Late-talkers are identified as having severely restricted vocabulary at age 2 years (fewer than 50 words). It is unclear how many late-talkers have similarly impaired receptive language skills, because many studies include only children with normal comprehension (Rescorla, 2005). Many late-talkers meet typical exclusionary criteria for SLI such as normal non-verbal ability and no hearing loss; however, most late-talking 2-year-olds will normalize language function by the time they enter school (Rescorla, 2005), whereas the long-term prognosis for school-aged children with SLI is less optimistic (Stothard, Snowling, Bishop *et al.*, 1998).

Dale, Price, Bishop, and Plomin (2003) followed a large sample of twins from 2 to 4 years of age. Late-talkers were identified as those 2-year-olds with expressive vocabulary scores in the bottom 10th centile (15 words or fewer on a modified version of the MacArthur Communicative Development Inventory). By age 4, 60% had age-appropriate scores on parent-report measures of vocabulary, grammar and use of abstract language.

It appears that gains in language skill are maintained over time. Paul (2000) reported that 84% of late-talkers in her cohort had language scores within the normal range at age 7. Rescorla (2005) followed 28 late-talkers from preschool to age 13 and found that, at this age, all of the children scored within the normal range on standard measures of language and literacy. However, their scores were significantly lower than a comparison group of typically developing children matched for socioeconomic status (cf. Stothard, Snowling, Bishop *et al.*, 1998). Rescorla argued that late-talkers represent a subgroup of SLI characterized by less severe language weakness.

Although 60–85% of late-talking children will improve without direct intervention, a minority will not (Paul, 2000; Dale, Price, Bishop *et al.*, 2003). It is not currently possible to distinguish reliably between those children with transient and persistent impairments. Dale, Price, Bishop *et al.* (2003) found that severity of language delay at age 2 did not predict language status at age 4. In addition, neither gender nor level of maternal education significantly predicted group outcome. Paul (2000) reported that children with persistent language difficulties tended to have lower non-verbal abilities, although scores on non-verbal assessments were still within the normal range and there was considerable overlap between groups with good and poor outcome. In addition, high socioeconomic status and prosocial adaptive communicative behaviors were associated with good outcome at age 7. A much smaller-scale study by Thal, Tobias, and Morrison (1991) indicated that poor receptive language skills and failure to use gesture were associated with persisting language difficulties.

Given these findings, a dilemma facing practitioners is what to do when language delay is identified during the preschool years. Conventional wisdom posits that early intervention is desirable, but Paul (2000) questioned the ethics of treating children who are otherwise developing normally, have normal language comprehension and do not present with any additional risk factors for a language "disorder" that they may overcome naturally without any professional help. Instead, she advocates initial parent training to optimize language input in conjunction with careful monitoring of language development.

Even though good language outcomes are often seen in late-talkers, there is evidence to suggest they should be monitored because such children may be at risk for other developmental difficulties. In a survey of over 1000 children, Horwitz, Irwin, Briggs-Gowan *et al.* (2003) found that late-talkers tended to show poor social interaction, which was in turn associated with an increased risk of emotional and behavioral disorders. Furthermore, it would seem prudent to give the child support in the early stages of reading and writing, given a suggestion that there is a risk of weak literacy skills in children who were late-talkers (Rescorla, 2005).

Autism and Pragmatic Language Impairments

Delayed language development and poor communication skills are hallmarks of autistic disorder, and the issue of differential diagnosis between autistic disorder and specific developmental language disorder frequently crops up in the clinical setting. Diagnosis of autistic disorder is covered in detail in chapter 46, so in this chapter we focus on areas of diagnostic difficulty.

Autistic disorder should be considered when the child's language difficulties are accompanied by more pervasive difficulties affecting social interaction, non-verbal communication and play, or if the child shows unusual repetitive or ritualistic behaviors or restricted interests. The clinician needs to consider whether language development is merely delayed, or whether there are deviant features that would not be regarded as normal at any age, such as repetitive use of stereotyped catchphrases, unusual and exaggerated intonation, pronoun reversal or a frequent failure to respond when the parent attempts to attract the child's attention.

Some higher-functioning children with autistic disorder (i.e., those children with non-verbal IQs within the normal range) resemble our illustrative child Jack in having superficially complex language; they may appear verbose and achieve age-appropriate scores on tests of expressive language or simple vocabulary measures. However, such measures may overestimate true language ability (Mottron, 2004) and the same children usually have significant comprehension deficits in less structured and more naturalistic discourse settings (Adams, Green, Gilchrist, & Cox, 2002).

Textbook cases of autistic disorder and SLI are relatively easy to differentiate, but many children present with a pattern of symptoms that does not fit unambiguously in either category, while showing some features of both. Thus, their difficulties extend beyond the characteristic grammatical deficits seen in SLI, but they do not have the full triad of impairments in severe enough form to warrant a diagnosis of autism. Differentiation between the two disorders may be hampered by a changing clinical picture over time (Charman, Taylor, Drew *et al.*, 2005; Mawhood, Howlin, & Rutter, 2000). Conti-Ramsden, Simkin, and Botting (2006) applied standard diagnostic instruments (Autism Diagnostic Interview – Revised; Lord, Rutter, & Le Couteur, 1994; Autism Diagnostic Observation Schedule – Generic; Lord, Risi, Lambrecht *et al.*, 2000) to 76 adolescents with a history of SLI, none of whom had been regarded as autistic in middle childhood. The majority of individuals did not meet criteria on either measure, but 3.9% met criteria for autistic disorder on both assessments, a prevalence rate more than three times greater than would be expected from the general population (Baird, Simonoff, Pickles *et al.*, 2006). A further 26% met criteria on one or other measure but not both. Similar results were obtained by Bishop and Norbury (2002), who noted that many children with language impairment displayed difficulties with broader aspects of communication and social interaction, although restricted interests and rigid behaviors were less characteristic of this population.

In cases where a child meets criteria in one or two domains of the autistic triad or exhibits subthreshold symptomatology across domains, a diagnosis of "pervasive developmental disorder not otherwise specified" or "atypical autism" is frequently applied. However, there is concern that these terms may be overused, and do not provide helpful information about symptom profile, nor do they facilitate decisions about educational placement. Bishop (2000) suggested that the term "pragmatic language impairment" (formerly "semantic-pragmatic disorder") might be useful for describing children who do not meet full diagnostic criteria for autistic disorder, but whose language difficulties affect social interaction and the use of language in context. The use of this term was not intended to imply a new and discrete disorder; rather, "pragmatic language impairment" is seen as a variable correlate of both SLI and milder forms of autistic spectrum disorder (Norbury, Nash, Bishop, & Baird, 2004).

In reality, the diagnostic label chosen may reflect the practitioner's theoretical stance and the practical implications a particular diagnosis brings with regard to accessing appropriate educational and remedial provision. The important point to recognize is that rather than attempting to draw a discrete diagnostic line between SLI and autistic disorder, it is more helpful to think in terms of multidimensional space, with children varying in terms of the severity of impairments in language, social interaction and range of interests.

Selective Mutism

Occasionally, the clinician will encounter a child who is extremely reticent in the clinic setting. In these instances, it is important to establish that the child does speak with others in more familiar situations such as school and home. However, if the child's communication varies significantly in different settings, the practitioner should consider the possibility of selective mutism.

Selective mutism (SM) is diagnosed in the child who consistently does not speak in certain situations in which there is an expectation for speaking (e.g., school), but can and does speak normally in some situations (e.g., at home; Steinhausen, Wachter, Laimbock *et al.*, 2006). The disorder was previously known as "elective" mutism, but the terminology has been revised to avoid implying that children are being obstinate or oppositional when they remain silent (Cline & Baldwin, 2004; Cohan, Chavira, & Stein, 2006a).

DSM-IV-TR (American Psychiatric Association, 2000) and ICD–10 (World Health Organization, 1996) criteria stipulate that in order to receive a diagnosis, the mutism must persist for more than 1 month (not including the first month of school), and cannot be accounted for by a communication disorder or a lack of familiarity with the ambient language of the social situation. Toppelberg, Tabors, Coggins, Lum, and Burger (2005) further recommend that bilingual children are not diagnosed with SM unless the mutism persists for longer than 6 months and is apparent in both languages.

Prevalence estimates vary depending on the criteria used and the population studied, with higher rates of transient mutism associated with starting school. Cline and Baldwin (2004) estimate 6–8 cases of selective mutism per 1000 throughout childhood, with a preponderance of girls (55–65% of cases), consistent with the results of recent community studies, which have found rates of approximately 75% (Cohan, Chavira, & Stein, 2006a).

The precise cause(s) of SM is unknown; although trauma may precipitate mutism, it is not implicated in the majority of cases (Steinhausen & Juzi, 1996). SM is generally regarded as a variant of anxiety disorder (Steinhausen, Wachter, Laimbock *et al.*, 2006; Vecchio & Kearney, 2005), rather than being categorized with speech and language disorders. Rates of comorbid anxiety and phobic disorders are high, both in affected children and their first-degree relatives, and some success in treatment has been reported using drugs that effectively reduce anxiety (for a review see Cline & Baldwin, 2004). However, it would be wrong to imply that social anxiety is the only problem; other factors are also often implicated, including bilingualism and speech and language impairment, suggesting that self-consciousness about inadequate communication plays a part in maintaining the disorder (Manassis, Fung, Tannock *et al.*, 2003). The consensus of opinion is that SM is the culmination of multiple predisposing, precipitating and perpetuating factors (Cohan, Price, & Stein, 2006b; Johnson & Wintgens, 2001).

Assessment of the child with SM may be particularly challenging, as the assessment process itself might further increase anxiety and reluctance to speak. At first meeting, it is most important to create a relaxed atmosphere in which the child feels little pressure to communicate with an unfamiliar adult. In this session, the clinician may take a detailed case history from the parents, focusing on where, when and with whom the child does speak and obtaining detailed examples of how the child communicates in different settings. During conversation with the parents, the clinician may unobtrusively observe the child playing and, if possible, interacting with parents or siblings.

Direct assessment of expressive language may not be possible at this point, although many children with SM will cooperate with receptive language testing if this just involves carrying out commands or pointing to pictures, and this can give valuable information about general language level (Manassis, Fung, Tannock *et al.*, 2003). Formal assessment may be supplemented by asking parents to record the child's language skills in a more comfortable arena, perhaps telling a story at home, or keep a diary of what the child says and the contexts in which language occurs. Johnson and Wintgens (2001) provide further examples of techniques for gaining the child's confidence to enable assessment to proceed.

The most successful treatments are thought to combine behavioral and psychopharmacological interventions, but there appears to be no systematic research on the efficacy of this approach (Cline & Baldwin, 2004). Cohan, Chavira, & Stein (2006a) conducted a critical review of psychosocial treatments published over a 15-year period. The techniques used in these studies included positive reinforcement for speaking to classmates, systematic desensitization to anxiety-provoking situations, language training, family therapy and self-modeling techniques, in which the child with SM listens to recordings of him or herself speaking in situations in which he or she is usually mute. Although the majority of these studies report increases in speaking behavior, the findings are limited by very small participant numbers and a lack of suitable control groups.

A recent longitudinal study demonstrated considerable improvement in symptoms of SM over time, but rates of psychiatric disorder, especially social phobia, remained high (Steinhausen, Wachter, Laimbock *et al.*, 2006). Prognosis is especially poor when a family history of SM is present.

Assessment of Language and Communication

Approximately 50% of children referred for psychiatric evaluation have clinically significant language impairments that are frequently unsuspected (Cohen, 2001). In many clinical contexts it is not possible to offer the time and expertise necessary for every referral to receive an in-depth assessment of language. However, it can be informative to gain an overview of the child's language development and current communicative functioning by taking a detailed case history and asking caregivers to complete a screening checklist.

The Children's Communication Checklist-2 (CCC-2; Bishop, 2003a) is a 70-item checklist for children aged 4 years and over that asks parents to rate the frequency of communicative behaviors in everyday situations, thus providing a naturalistic assessment of functioning. One advantage of this assessment is that it covers both structural aspects of language (phonology and syntax) as well as pragmatic aspects of communication, which are more difficult to measure on face-to-face assessment. The CCC-2 reliably distinguishes children with communication impairment from typically developing children (Norbury, Nash, Bishop *et al.*, 2004) and an earlier version of the checklist identified children at genetic risk for language impairment as effectively as standardized tests (Bishop, Laws, Adams, & Norbury, 2006b). However, it should be noted that CCC-2 is not suitable for children who are not yet speaking in sentences.

More detailed evaluation of language and communicative functioning will typically be undertaken by a speech-language therapist or specialist psychologist. A number of standardized assessments tapping all domains of language are available in English, but this is not necessarily so in other languages. The application of English language assessments to children from non-English speaking backgrounds is not recommended, as test scores may not accurately reflect the child's competence in his or her native language.

There is evidence that "knowledge-dependent" measures, such as vocabulary tests, exaggerate cultural and socioeconomic differences between children, whereas "processing" measures that vary difficulty by manipulating the amount of material that has to be processed (e.g., nonsense word repetition), provide a culturally unbiased estimate of language ability (Campbell, Dollaghan, Needleman, & Janosky, 1997). Table 47.1 provides a list of commonly used language assessments in the UK, including the domain of language targeted and the age range appropriate for testing.

There is currently no clear consensus on what degree of impairment on standardized assessment constitutes a significant difficulty. A score of –1 SD (equivalent to 16th centile) on a single assessment may not interfere with the child's educational or social development, whereas consistently low scores across a number of language domains or an extremely low score on one measure (–2 SD or 3rd centile) may be more problematic. Tomblin, Records, and Zhang (1996) used a battery of language tests covering different aspects of receptive and expressive processing, and combined these into five composites: expressive language, comprehension, vocabulary, grammar and narrative. SLI was diagnosed if two or more of these composites fell more than 1.25 SD below age level (10th centile), non-verbal IQ was 87 or more, and no exclusionary conditions were present. In a population sample, this resulted in 0.85 sensitivity (identifying true cases of impairment) and 0.99 specificity (correctly identifying unimpaired cases). Note that the definition of SLI used by Tomblin *et al.* was considerably less stringent than that of ICD-10 (World Health Organization, 1996), which requires that language test scores must be 2 SD or more below age level. Application of this criterion would give a lower prevalence rate.

In DSM-IV-TR (American Psychiatric Association, 2000) a distinction is drawn between expressive vs. mixed receptive-expressive subtypes of language disorder. The importance of establishing the level of receptive language should not be underestimated: poor comprehension is an important predictor of outcome in a language-impaired child (Stothard, Snowling, Bishop *et al.*, 1998). However, if strictly interpreted, the DSM-IV system is unworkable. This is because it defines Expressive Language Disorder as having an expressive language score that is "substantially below" *both* non-verbal IQ and receptive language, whereas in Mixed Receptive-Expressive Language Disorder, both expressive and receptive language are "substantially below" non-verbal IQ. This creates a problem of how to categorize a child with average non-verbal IQ and a mild receptive language impairment and a more severe expressive impairment (e.g., receptive language score is 0.8 SD below average and expressive language score is 1.2 SD below average). If we interpret "substantially below" in terms of a 1-SD discrepancy, such a child would not meet criteria for either DSM subtype. Furthermore, the distinction between the two subtypes seems artificial; both genetic and developmental data suggest that they correspond to points on a continuum of severity (Bishop, North, & Donlan, 1995).

Prevalence, Causes and Correlates of Specific Language Impairment

Research on SLI is complicated by the variety of diagnostic criteria that have been employed. It is rather unusual to find research that focuses on "pure" SLI in which there is a substantial discrepancy with non-verbal IQ. More commonly, an IQ cut-off is used to establish that children are within broadly normal limits. In addition, as noted in chapter 3, SLI is often accompanied by other neurodevelopmental disorders: rates of co-occurrence of ADHD, developmental coordination disorder and academic difficulties are all high. Studies vary in how far they explicitly include or exclude children with these comorbid conditions, with speech problems or with autistic features. It is likely that estimates of prevalence, comorbidity and etiology will depend on the phenotype that is studied.

Prevalence

The most frequently cited prevalence figure for SLI comes from an epidemiological study by Tomblin, Records, Buckwalter *et al.* (1997), who estimated that 7.4% (95% confidence interval [CI] 6.3–8.5%) of 5- to 6-year-old children in an Iowa sample met diagnostic criteria as defined above. Intriguingly, of those who did meet criteria for SLI, only 29% had previously been identified as having language difficulties. If the criteria were made more stringent, to include only those with composite language scores more than 2 SD below average, it was still the case that only a minority of affected children (39%) had been identified clinically. This result suggests that the features that lead to a child being identified as having an SLI are different from those that are picked up by standardized tests (Bishop, Laws, Adams *et al.*, 2006b). In general, teachers and parents will notice a child whose speech is unclear or whose language structure is so immature as to sound ungrammatical, but poor verbal memory, limited understanding, weak vocabulary and lack of complex grammar are easier to miss.

As with many other neurodevelopmental disorders, more males than females are affected with SLI, although the male preponderance was far less in the epidemiological study of Tomblin, Records, Buckwalter *et al.* (1997), who reported 1.33:1 boys to girls, than in samples recruited from clinical sources (e.g., Robinson, 1991, reported a ratio of 3.8:1). There is no evidence that different genetic influences are implicated in causing language impairment in males and females; a comparison of same-sex and opposite-sex twin pairs found a similar magnitude of genetic and environmental influences in both sexes (Viding, Spinath, Price *et al.*, 2004).

As Tomblin, Records, Buckwalter *et al.* (1997) pointed out, there is an intrinsic difficulty in attempting to compare prevalence in different racial groups, because even if the core language is the same across races, there are likely to be cultural differences in language use that will lead to biased test results. Campbell, Dollaghan, Needleman *et al.* (1997) suggested such bias could be eliminated by avoiding language tests that were affected by prior knowledge or experience, but we are not aware of any epidemiological studies that used such measures to compare different rates of SLI in different races or cultures.

Correlates of SLI

Although SLI is "specific" insofar as the language disorder is not accompanied by low non-verbal ability, there are frequently accompanying impairments in other aspects of functioning. Literacy problems are found in most but not all children with SLI. The question of what characterizes those children who learn to read and write despite SLI is intriguing but as yet not fully understood; however, poor phonological processing appears a key factor (Bishop & Snowling, 2004; Catts, Adlof, Hogan, & Weismer, 2005). Another frequent accompaniment to SLI is motor impairment, which may not be evident in everyday interactions, but becomes so on formal testing (Hill, 2001; Webster, Majnemer, Platt, & Shevell, 2005).

Comorbidity with Psychiatric Disorder

Early research by Cantwell and Baker (1991) demonstrated a high rate of psychiatric disorder, including but not limited to ADHD, in children referred for speech and language disorders. In one of the few epidemiological studies to address this issue, the Ottowa Longitudinal Study, it was found that language impairment in 5-year-olds was one of the strongest predictors of psychiatric outcome at 12 years of age, even after measures of social background were taken into account (for review see Beitchman, Brownlie, & Wilson, 1996). In this study, ADHD and emotional disorders were the most common psychiatric diagnoses. A series of studies by Cohen, Hodson, O'Hare *et al.* demonstrated that the converse also applied. Of children referred for psychiatric assessment solely for socioemotional disturbances, 33% were found to have previously undiagnosed language impairment. When combined with those whose language impairments had already been identified, some 50% of school-aged children referred to out-patient mental health clinics had clinically significant language impairments (for review see Cohen, 2001).

Such co-occurrences raise a host of questions about causation. An obvious possibility is that inability to express one's needs and ideas leads to a sense of frustration and impotence, and subsequent acting-out behavior. However, if this were the principal route to psychiatric disorder, we would expect the greatest evidence of psychopathology to be seen in children with expressive difficulties, whereas most studies find receptive language difficulties pose substantially greater risk. Failure to comprehend language can lead to inappropriate accusations in the classroom of laziness, willfulness or inattention, and it will also limit the opportunities to form close relationships that would normally exert a protective effect. Redmond and Rice (1998) contrasted this latter type of "social adaptation" account with a "social deviance" model that regards both behavior and language problems as indicators of an underlying trait of disturbed psychosocial development. They argued that parent and teacher ratings of socioemotional status in children with SLI showed little congruence or temporal stability, supporting the idea that behavioral problems were consequences of specific communicative experiences rather than reflecting intrinsic deficits in the child. However, rates of behavior disorder were relatively low in their sample, and the possibility remains that more severely affected children have socioemotional deficits that go beyond what could be reasonably regarded as adaptations to poor communication (see also Bishop, 2000).

Another route from language impairment to psychiatric disorder is through the experience of school failure. Both Beitchman, Brownlie, & Wilson (1996) and Tomblin, Zhang, Buckwalter, and Catts (2000) found that the risk of psychiatric disorder was substantially raised in those children whose language impairment was accompanied by reading disability, and was much lower in those who were experiencing academic success. In both these studies, this association was less evident when the same children's behavior problems were assessed before they learned to read; this suggests that it is experience of school failure that exacerbates psychiatric risk.

One further mechanism whereby language could affect psychiatric status is through its role in inner speech and self-regulation. Language is a tool for thought as well as a means of communication, and it affects how we structure our experiences, plan for the future and reflect on the past. A child with limited language understanding is anchored more firmly in the here and now, and may find it hard to delay gratification, think through another person's motivations or appreciate chains of causality. In the case of autistic disorder, verbal ability is strongly linked to the development of understanding of other minds, which is thought to mediate social understanding and interaction (Happé, 1995), and those children with significantly lower verbal ability in relation to non-verbal ability demonstrate the most severe deficits in social interaction (Joseph, Tager-Flusberg, & Lord, 2002).

We need more research relating specific aspects of language skill to cognitive processes and behavioral outcomes in SLI to evaluate the plausibility of different causal pathways to disorder, compared with other accounts such as one that would regard language impairment and psychiatric disorder as independent consequences of some third factor such as poor parenting or social disadvantage. In addition, we need research on how best to help children whose psychiatric problems are associated with language difficulties. The role of language in thinking has implications for intervention: some children have language problems that could make it difficult to use methods such as cognitive–behavioral therapy. For instance, if the child does not understand what is meant by "if . . . then", and has difficulty thinking about events beyond the here and now, then it may be counterproductive to try to use social problem-solving approaches that involve thinking about solutions to hypothetical situations.

Genetic Factors

Twin studies have converged in finding that SLI is a highly heritable disorder (for review see Bishop, 2001). In 1990, excitement was generated by the discovery of a three-generation family, the K.E. family, in which a speech and language disorder appeared to be inherited in an autosomal dominant fashion. The earliest account of this family focused on their verbal dyspraxia (Hurst, Baraitser, Auger *et al.*, 1990), but subsequent reports have drawn attention to coexisting problems with broader oral language skills (Watkins, Dronkers, & Vargha-Khadem, 2002). The mutation responsible for the disorder has since been identified as affecting the function of a transcription factor, the *FOXP2* gene, which influences the development of the brain as well as other organs (for an overview see Fisher, 2005). Although other cases of speech and language impairment linked to *FOXP2* have been reported (Feuk, Kalervo, Lipsanen-Nyman *et al.*, 2006; Macdermot, Bonora, Sykes *et al.*, 2005), it is evident that this is a rare mutation that cannot account for the majority of cases of SLI. Although it is possible that other single major genes may be involved in the etiology of some cases of SLI (Bishop, 2005), it is likely that for many children the etiology will involve the combined influence of several genes and environmental factors, each of small effect.

Research on the genetics of SLI is moving ahead on three fronts. First, there are molecular studies that have made progress in identifying linkages to sites on chromosomes 3, 16 and 19 (Newbury & Monaco, in press). Second, there are behavioral genetic studies that attempt to refine the phenotype of heritable SLI. In general, these suggest that we will make better progress in molecular genetic studies if we abandon the conventional clinical criteria for SLI and move instead to define the phenotype in terms of measures of underlying cognitive and linguistic processes (Bishop, 2006). One important clinical message to emerge from genetic studies is that genes can increase a child's risk of SLI, but they do not act in a deterministic fashion. Whether or not a genetic risk is manifest as a language disorder may depend on environmental factors (Bishop, 2001). Finally, there is a recognition that we need to move away from focusing on individual neurodevelopmental disorders, to consider whether there are genetic risks for SLI that also affect related conditions such as developmental dyslexia or autistic disorder. In the case of dyslexia, it is clear that there are some genetic variants that increase the risk for both SLI and reading problems but, nevertheless, there is little overlap in the sites of significant linkage found in whole-genome scans for these two conditions (Fisher, 2006). There has been considerable interest in the idea that a common genetic locus might be found that increases the risk for both SLI and autism (Folstein & Mankoski, 2000), but this has yet to be validated, and behavioral studies suggest that phenotypic similarities between the two disorders may be only superficial (Bishop, Maybery, Wong *et al.*, 2004; Whitehouse, Barry, & Bishop, 2007).

Environmental Factors

There is little evidence that environmental factors alone are sufficient to cause the *selective* deficits in grammar and phonology that characterize SLI. However, environmental factors may be implicated in early language delay and can have a role in mediating the developmental course of language disorders and the impact of language impairment on the child's well-being.

Family socioeconomic status (SES) has long been associated with child language development, with children from lower SES environments experiencing protracted rates of language development in relation to peers from more affluent homes. It is suggested that the relationship between SES and language impairment is mediated by maternal education, via the quantity and quality of mothers' communicative interactions with their children (Hoff & Tian, 2005). However, other studies have found that SES (as measured by income or maternal education) is not a reliable predictor of long-term language impairment (Dale, Price, Bishop *et al.*, 2003; Paul, 2000). Furthermore, even when SES is implicated in language or literacy impairment, one must consider that environments are at least partially genetically influenced (Oliver, Dale, & Plomin, 2005). In other words, a mother may have a limited educational experience and poor career prospects because of her own language limitations. Nevertheless, early language delay in the presence of low SES should alert the clinician of the need to monitor linguistic progress carefully.

In a multicultural society, one must establish whether a child is presenting with a language disorder or a language difference. Two questions must be addressed:

1 Is the child impaired only in his or her ability to learn the ambient language, or are language impairments evident in the child's home language as well?

2 If the child does have language impairment, does exposure to more than one language exacerbate the child's language learning difficulties?

Studies of SLI in bilingual language learners are in their infancy, and there is a dearth of longitudinal data with which to answer these important questions. For some languages, such as Spanish in the USA, there now exists a range of culturally appropriate, well-standardized assessments with which to assess bilingual children, but the situation is far less satisfactory for many other language communities. It is not safe to assume that a straightforward translation of an English test into the child's home language will provide an accurate picture of the child's language ability. In these instances, it will be important to obtain a picture of the child's communicative competence from the primary caregiver. It may be particularly beneficial to ascertain whether the caregiver is concerned about the child's communication and how this child's development compares with other children in the family or community.

The limited research available suggests that experience with two or more languages does *not* cause or compound SLI (Paradis, Crago, Genesee, & Rice, 2003). Thus, most speech-language clinicians recommend that families continue to provide rich input in the child's home language and that, where possible, intervention should target both languages. However, there is a no systematic research comparing monolingual vs. bilingual therapy in such cases, and it could be argued that the child with SLI may be particularly handicapped by the challenge of mastering two or more languages simultaneously. One recent study by Cheuk, Wong, and Leung (2005) endorsed this view, but focused on preschool children; thus, it is likely that many would achieve normal language outcomes. Longitudinal studies of bilingual children with SLI are clearly needed.

Neurobiology

Most children with SLI show no gross abnormalities of the brain on structural imaging. More fine-grained analyses have revealed evidence for four kinds of developmental brain anomaly associated with SLI:

1 Abnormalities in the organization of different kinds of brain cell (ectopias and microgyri; Galaburda, Sherman, Rosen, Aboitiz, & Geschwind, 1985);

2 Additional gyri in frontal or temporal regions (Clark & Plante, 1998; Plante & Jackson, 1997);

3 Unusual proportions of different brain regions (Herbert, Ziegler, Makris *et al.*, 2003; Jernigan, Hesselink, Sowell, & Tallal, 1991; Leonard, Lombardino, Walsh *et al.*, 2002); and

4 Anomalous cerebral lateralization (De Fossé, Hodge, Makris *et al.*, 2004; Gauger, Lombardino, & Leonard, 1997; Herbert, Ziegler, Makris *et al.*, 2003). However, the field is plagued by inconsistent findings: for instance, whereas SLI was associated with small cerebral volume in studies by Jernigan, Hesselink, Sowell *et al.* (1991) and Leonard, Lombardino, Walsh *et al.* (2002), it was associated with large cerebral volume in the study by Herbert, Ziegler, Makris *et al.* (2003). Leonard (1997) noted that such associations as are found are weak and probabilistic, and abnormalities that are more frequent in SLI than in typically developing children may also be seen in other disorders. In her own research, she has had some success in showing clearer relationships between disorder and brain anomaly by distinguishing between cases with language comprehension impairments and those with more restricted phonological deficits (Leonard, Lombardino, Walsh *et al.*, 2002, Leonard, Eckert, Given *et al.*, 2006).

Overall, the picture from structural brain imaging has been confusing and contradictory. The one thing we can conclude is that such anomalies as are found in SLI appear to arise early in neurodevelopment, rather than being brought about by early acquired lesions. This fits with the view of SLI as a disorder in which genetic influences lead to a brain that is wired up in a non-optimal fashion. From a clinical perspective, it is unlikely that brain imaging will provide information of diagnostic or prognostic utility in a child with SLI (Shevell, Majnemer, Rosenbaum *et al.*, 2000).

Few functional imaging studies have been conducted with SLI, and those that have been performed are difficult to interpret. Thus, if one shows underactivation of regions implicated in language processing, it is unclear if this is cause or consequence of the language disorder. Functional imaging can nevertheless be useful in providing evidence for unusual localization of specific functions (e.g., studies of the affected members of the K.E. family have shown that when they perform a verb generation task they have diffuse bilateral brain activation), in contrast to unaffected individuals, who show more focal activation of traditional language regions in the left hemisphere (Vargha-Khadem, Gadian, Copp, & Mishkin, 2005).

Electrophysiological methods have been used to study brain–behavior relationships in children with SLI, but results are characterized by the same level of inconsistency as is seen in the structural imaging studies (see chapter 17; Bishop & McArthur, 2005; Bishop, 2007). Furthermore, research in this field is handicapped by a lack of normative data on typically developing children.

Cognitive Factors

Theoretical accounts of SLI have traditionally attempted to explain the disproportionate difficulties with grammar that characterize the disorder. Many of these theories are grounded in a linguistic tradition and propose that SLI results from a delay or disruption of the development of a specialized brain system that serves grammatical computations (Rice, 2004; van der Lely, 2005). Tasks tapping grammatical marking of tense and agreement, as well as comprehension of complex grammatical relations, discriminate children with SLI and typically developing peers (Conti-Ramsden, 2003) and poor performance on grammatical tasks has been put forward as a behavioral marker of heritable forms of SLI (Rice, 2004).

However, a number of researchers have criticized the notion of an innate modular language faculty and suggest that specialized language function is the developmental outcome of a number of domain-general endowments acting in concert (Bates, 2004). Children with SLI are impaired not only on grammatical tasks, but also on measures of phonological short-term memory. These tasks require children to repeat strings of unfamiliar speech sounds (e.g., "blonterstaping"), an ability that is seen to facilitate the learning of new words (Baddeley, Gathercole, & Papagno, 1998). Attention has also been focused on the abilities of children with SLI to process rapid brief auditory signals (Tallal, 2000); an ability that is argued to underpin the recognition and learning of grammatical contrasts in English (Joanisse & Seidenberg, 2003).

A recent study confirmed that deficits in nonsense word repetition, like deficits in grammatical inflection, are highly heritable and sensitive markers of SLI (Bishop, Adams, & Norbury, 2006a). Intriguingly, there appeared to be little etiological overlap between the two deficits, indicating that different risk genes may be involved in these different aspects of language difficulty. However, auditory processing deficits showed no genetic influence (Bishop, Bishop, Bright *et al.*, 1999) and cannot fully account for the linguistic deficits seen in SLI (Norbury, Bishop, & Briscoe, 2001; van der Lely, Rosen & Adlard, 2004). Thus, auditory impairment may be seen as an environmentally based risk factor that comes into play in those children at genetic risk of the disorder.

The conclusions that we draw from theoretical studies of SLI are that there is unlikely to be a single cognitive or biological factor that can cause the variety of language profiles captured by a diagnosis of SLI. Instead, multiple risk factors in the child's genetic and biological make-up are likely to interact with factors in the child's environment to determine the severity and course of language impairment (Bishop, 2006).

Intervention and Prognosis for Specific Language Impairment

Intervention is usually determined by speech and language therapists, who use a wide range of techniques to stimulate language learning. In preschool, intervention may involve working with parents and caregivers to provide optimal language input for the child. Such approaches often involve videotaping parent–child interactions and using these videos constructively to foster better communication techniques (e.g., The Hanen program; Girolametto & Weitzman, 2006; see www.hanen.org for details). The advice given focuses on following the child's lead in play, talking about what the child is doing rather than asking questions, recasting what the child says in a grammatically correct form, and increasing communication opportunities by giving children choices rather than anticipating their needs.

In a meta-analysis of intervention, Law, Garrett, & Nye (2004) found that treatment for preschool children with expressive language delays was successful when compared with no treatment, and treatments lasting longer than 8 weeks produced the most favorable outcomes. Parent-led interventions were as successful as direct intervention by a speech-language therapist in developing young children's language; such interventions are cost-effective and encourage generalization of language gains into everyday environments. With such methods, speech-language therapists are instrumental in identifying communicative targets for parents to work on, and supporting parents throughout the intervention program. Nevertheless, as noted by Nelson, Nygren, Walker, and Panoscha (2006), there is a dearth of good-quality research on long-term efficacy of interventions for preschool children, a problem that is compounded by the fact that existing studies are small and heterogeneous.

There is even less research on intervention for children with receptive language difficulties or school-aged children. In general, randomized controlled studies are rare and studies that explicitly compare different treatment approaches for the same language problem simply do not exist. The field is plagued by studies in which the participant numbers are small, the interventions poorly described and methodological problems abound. The studies outlined below are pilot studies in nature, but offer promise for larger-scale investigations of treatment efficacy.

Ebbels (2007) reported preliminary data for a school-based intervention that focuses on grammar. This intervention uses visual cues such as shapes and colors to teach children with language impairment different parts of speech, and how these parts of speech may combine in different grammatical constructions. By situating the intervention in a school setting, classroom materials can be used in therapy to promote generalization. Other approaches advocate developing the child's linguistic repertoire in more naturalistic settings. Fey, Long, and Finestack (2003) presented 10 principles for facilitating grammar development. Although the authors recognize the need to teach specific grammatical forms, they argue that these forms should rarely be taught in isolation. Instead, the targeted forms should be embedded in natural contexts such as play or story-telling. The role of the therapist in this approach is to manipulate the environment so that the targeted form is salient and frequently occurring, providing ample opportunity for modeling and shaping the child's production.

Adams (2005) reported a series of case studies detailing treatment for children with pragmatic language impairments. Standardized assessments often lack the sensitivity to detect subtle improvements in social communication and interaction, but using detailed conversational analysis, Adams was able to demonstrate improvement in discourse functioning in school-aged children. These studies lacked a suitable control group necessary to evaluate specific treatment effects, but hold promise for larger-scale studies with school-aged populations with pragmatic deficits.

A radically different approach to treatment was developed by Tallal, Miller, Bedi *et al.* (1996), who devised a computer-based intervention, FastForWord, which involves prolonged and intensive training on specific components of language and auditory processing. The advantage of computerized presentation is that children may be persuaded to participate in thousands of training trials in a way that would not be possible in standard therapist-based interventions. Unfortunately, after initially promising results using the FastForWord program (Merzenich, Jenkins, Johnston *et al.*, 1996), randomized controlled studies have failed to demonstrate a significant advantage of this approach over other methods in improving children's language or literacy skills (Cohen, Hodson, O'Hare *et al.*, 2005; Pokorni, Worthington, & Jamison, 2004; Rouse & Krueger, 2004). Children in these studies had receptive as well as expressive language impairments, which appear particularly resistant to treatment (Law, Garrett, & Nye, 2004).

The limited intervention studies available suggest that there is no cure for SLI. Despite years of intensive specialist training, many children will continue to have language deficits. However, one should bear in mind the broader aims of therapeutic intervention for SLI. One cannot "cure" a sensorineural hearing loss or a physical impairment; in these instances intervention will seek to maximize potential and lessen the impact of the child's impairment on his or her social well-being and educational experiences.

In the absence of a "quick-fix," many children with SLI will present with long-term special educational needs. There is a lack of consensus on the most suitable type of provision for children with SLI. Experience in the UK suggests that some children will benefit from a special school or language unit placement where there is access to regular speech and language therapy and where the curriculum may be supported by using signed English or a visual symbol system. Others will benefit from a mainstream placement. Unfortunately, specialist support for children within mainstream settings is limited and almost non-existent by secondary school (Lindsay, Dockrell, Mackie, & Letchford, 2005).

A number of longitudinal studies have shed light on the developmental course of SLI. There is general agreement that the child with severely impaired understanding of language has a poor prognosis, even if the diagnosis is made early. Comprehension problems do not resolve spontaneously and, as they grow older, children with such problems experience increasing difficulties with social cognition and interaction (Clegg, Hollis, Mawhood, & Rutter, 2005; Howlin, Mawhood, & Rutter, 2000), non-verbal reasoning (Botting, 2005; Stothard, Snowling, Bishop *et al.*, 1998) and an increased risk of psychiatric disturbance (Howlin, Mawhood, & Rutter, 2000; Snowling, Bishop, Chipchase, & Kaplan, 2006).

For children with normal non-verbal abilities and expressive language impairments, the outlook is much more positive, particularly if expressive deficits have resolved by school entry (Stothard, Snowling, Bishop *et al.*, 1998). However, there is evidence that literacy skills may remain an area of weakness for these children (Botting, Simkin, & Conti-Ramsden, 2006; Rescorla, 2005); although these "resolved" cases may score within the normal range on standardized assessment, their scores are frequently lower than those of an IQ-matched peer group.

Conclusions

This chapter has considered various factors designed to facilitate clinical decision-making in this complex and difficult area. It is important to realize that cases of "pure" SLI are rare in clinical practice. Rather, children present with a range of co-occurring deficits and challenges that may cloud diagnostic decisions. The most important message for clinicians to remember is that speech, language and communication skills are critical to the cognitive and social development of children, whatever their primary diagnosis. Thus, attention to these aspects of development is fundamental for children presenting to psychiatric clinics.

Further Reading

Beitchman, J. H., Cohen, N. J., Konstantareas, M. M., & Tannock, R. (Eds.). (1996). *Language, learning, and behavior disorders*. Cambridge: Cambridge University Press.

Bishop, D. V. M. (1997). *Uncommon understanding: Development and disorders of language comprehension in children*. Hove: Psychology Press.

McCauley, R. J., & Fey, M. E. (Eds.). (2006). *Treatment of language disorders in children*. Baltimore: Paul H. Brookes. [Includes examples on DVD.]

Paul, R. (2006). *Language disorders from infancy through adolescence: Assessment and intervention* (3rd edn.). St. Louis: Mosby-Year Book.

References

Adams, C. (2005). Pragmatic language impairment: case studies of social and pragmatic language therapy. *Child Language Teaching and Therapy*, *21*, 227–250.

Adams, C., Cooke, R., Crutchley, A., Hesketh, A., & Reeves, D. (2001). *Assessment of comprehension and expression (6–11)*. Windsor: NFER-Nelson.

Adams, C., Green, J., Gilchrist, A., & Cox, A. (2002). Conversational behaviour of children with Asperger syndrome and conduct disorder. *Journal of Child Psychology and Psychiatry*, *43*, 679–690.

American Psychiatric Association. (2000). *Diagnostic and statistical manual of mental disorders* (4th edn.). Text revision. Washington, DC: American Psychiatric Association.

Baddeley, A., Gathercole, S., & Papagno, C. (1998). The phonological loop as a language learning device. *Psychological Review*, *105*, 158–173.

Baird, G., Simonoff, E., Pickles, A., Chandler, S., Loucas, T., Meldrum, D., *et al.* (2006). Prevalence of disorders of the autism spectrum in a population cohort of children in South Thames: The Special Needs and Autism Project (SNAP). *Lancet*, *368*, 210–215.

Bates, E. A. (2004). Commentary: Explaining and interpreting deficits in language development across clinical groups: Where do we go from here? *Brain and Language*, *88*, 248–253.

Beitchman, J. H., Brownlie, E. B., & Wilson, B. (1996). Linguistic impairment and psychiatric disorder: Pathways to outcome. In J. Beitchman, N. J. Cohen, M. M. Konstantareas, & R. Tannock (Eds.), *Language, learning and behavior disorders: Developmental, biological and clinical perspectives* (pp. 493–514). New York: Cambridge University Press.

Bird, J., Bishop, D. V. M., & Freeman, N. (1995). Phonological awareness and literacy development in children with expressive phonological impairments. *Journal of Speech and Hearing Research*, *38*, 446–462.

Bishop, D. V. M. (1994). Is specific language impairment a valid diagnostic category? Genetic and psycholinguistic evidence. *Philosophical Transactions of the Royal Society, Series B*, *346*, 105–111.

Bishop, D. V. M. (2000). Pragmatic language impairment: A correlate of SLI, a distinct subgroup, or part of the autistic continuum? In D. V. M. Bishop, & L. B. Leonard (Eds.), *Speech and language impairments in children: Causes, characteristics, intervention and outcome* (pp. 99–114). Hove: Psychology Press.

Bishop, D. V. M. (2001). Genetic and environmental risks for specific language impairment in children. *Philosophical Transactions of the Royal Society, Series B*, *356*, 369–380.

Bishop, D. V. M. (2002). Motor immaturity and specific speech and language impairment: Evidence for a common genetic basis. *American Journal of Medical Genetics: Neuropsychiatric Genetics*, *114*, 56–63.

Bishop, D. V. M. (2003a). *The Children's Communication Checklist – 2*. London: Harcourt Assessment.

Bishop, D. V. M. (2003b). *The Test for Reception of Grammar, version 2 (TROG-2)*. London: Harcourt Assessment.

Bishop, D. V. M. (2004). *Expression, Reception and Recall of Narrative Instrument (ERRNI)*. London: Harcourt Assessment.

Bishop, D. V. M. (2005). DeFries–Fulker analysis of twin data with skewed distributions: Cautions and recommendations from a study of children's use of verb inflections. *Behavior Genetics*, *35*, 479–490.

Bishop, D. V. M. (2006). Developmental cognitive genetics: How psychology can inform genetics and vice versa. *Quarterly Journal of Experimental Psychology*, *59*, 1153–1168.

Bishop, D. V. M. (2007). Using mismatch negativity to study central auditory processing in developmental language and literacy impairments: Where are we, and where should we be going? *Psychological Bulletin*, *133*, 651–672.

Bishop, D. V. M., Adams, C. V., & Norbury, C. F. (2006a). Distinct genetic influences on grammar and phonological short-term memory deficits: Evidence from 6-year-old twins. *Genes, Brain and Behavior*, *5*, 158–169.

Bishop, D. V. M., Bishop, S. J., Bright, P., James, C., Delaney, T., & Tallal, P. (1999). Different origin of auditory and phonological processing problems in children with language impairment: Evidence from a twin study. *Journal of Speech, Language and Hearing Research*, *42*, 155–168.

Bishop, D. V. M., Laws, G., Adams, C., & Norbury, C. F. (2006b). High heritability of speech and language impairments in 6-year-old twins demonstrated using parent and teacher report. *Behavior Genetics*, *36*, 173–184.

Bishop, D. V. M., & McArthur, G. M. (2005). Individual differences in auditory processing in specific language impairment: A follow-up study using event-related potentials and behavioural thresholds. *Cortex*, *41*, 327–341.

Bishop, D. V. M., Maybery, M., Wong, D., Maley, A., Hill, W., & Hallmayer, J. (2004). Are phonological processing deficits part of the broad autism phenotype? *American Journal of Medical Genetics. Part B, Neuropsychiatric Genetics*, *128*, 54–60.

Bishop, D. V. M., & Norbury, C. F. (2002). Exploring the borderlands of autistic disorder and specific language impairment: A study using standardised diagnostic instruments. *Journal of Child Psychology and Psychiatry*, *43*, 917–929.

Bishop, D. V. M., North, T., & Donlan, C. (1995). Genetic basis of specific language impairment: Evidence from a twin study. *Developmental Medicine and Child Neurology*, *37*, 56–71.

Bishop, D. V. M., & Snowling, M. J. (2004). Developmental dyslexia and specific language impairment: Same or different? *Psychological Bulletin*, *130*, 858–886.

Bloodstein, O. (2006). Some empirical observations about early stuttering: A possible link to language development. *Journal of Communication Disorders*, *39*, 185–191.

Botting, N. (2005). Non-verbal cognitive development and language impairment. *Journal of Child Psychology and Psychiatry*, *46*, 317–326.

Botting, N., Simkin, Z., & Conti-Ramsden, G. (2006). Associated reading skills in children with a history of specific language impairment. *Reading and Writing (special issue)*, *19*, 77–98.

Boyle, B. (2000). Voice disorders in children. *Support for Learning*, *15*, 71–75.

Campbell, T., Dollaghan, C., Needleman, H., & Janosky, J. (1997). Reducing bias in language assessment: Processing-dependent measures. *Journal of Speech, Language and Hearing Research*, *40*, 519–525.

Campbell, T. F., Dollaghan, C., & Yaruss, J. S. (2002). Disorders of language, phonology, fluency and voice in children: Indicators for referral. In C. Bluestone, S. Stool, C. Alper, E. Arjmand, M. Casselbrant, J. Dohar, *et al.* (Eds.), *Pediatric otolaryngology* (4th edn., Vol. 2, pp. 1773–1788). Philadelphia: Saunders.

Campbell, T. F., Dollaghan, C. A., Rockette, H. E., Paradise, J. L., Feldman, H. M., Shriberg, L. D., *et al.* (2003). Risk factors for speech delay of unknown origin in 3-year-old children. *Child Development*, *74*, 346–357.

Cantwell, D. P., & Baker, L. (1991). *Psychiatric and developmental disorders in children with communication disorder*. Washington, DC: American Psychiatric Press.

Carding, P. N., Roulstone, S., Northstone, K., & Team, A. S. (2006). The prevalence of childhood dysphonia: A cross-sectional study. *Journal of Voice*, *20*, 623–630.

Catts, H. W., Adlof, S. M., Hogan, T. P., & Weismer, S. E. (2005). Are specific language impairment and dyslexia distinct disorders? *Journal of Speech, Language, and Hearing Research*, *48*, 1378–1396.

Charman, T., Taylor, E., Drew, A., Cockerill, H., Brown, J.-A., & Baird, G. (2005). Outcome at 7 years of children diagnosed with autism at age 2: Predictive validity of assessments conducted at 2 and 3 years of age and pattern of symptom change over time. *Journal of Child Psychology and Psychiatry*, *46*, 500–513.

Cheuk, D. K. L., Wong, V., & Leung, G. M. (2005). Multilingual home environment and specific language impairment: A case–control study in Chinese children. *Paediatric and Perinatal Epidemiology*, *19*, 303–314.

Clark, M. M., & Plante, E. (1998). Morphology of the inferior frontal gyrus in developmentally language-disordered adults. *Brain and Language*, *61*, 288–303.

Clegg, J., Hollis, C., Mawhood, L., & Rutter, M. (2005). Developmental language disorders: A follow-up in later adult life. Cognitive, language and psychosocial outcomes. *Journal of Child Psychology and Psychiatry*, *46*, 128–149.

Cline, T., & Baldwin, S. (2004). *Selective mutism in children* (2nd edn.). Hoboken, NJ: Wiley.

Cohan, S. L., Chavira, D. A., & Stein, M. B. (2006a). Psychosocial interventions for children with selective mutism: A critical evaluation of the literature from 1990–2005. *Journal of Child Psychology and Psychiatry*, *47*, 1085–1097.

Cohan, S. L., Price, J. M., & Stein, M. B. (2006b). Suffering in silence: Why a developmental psychopathology perspective on selective mutism is needed. *Journal of Developmental and Behavioral Pediatrics*, *27*, 341–355.

Cohen, N. J. (2001). *Language impairment and psychopathology in infants, children and adolescents*. London: Sage Publications.

Cohen, W., Hodson, A., O'Hare, A., Boyle, J., Durrani, T., McCartney, E., *et al.* (2005). Effects of computer-based intervention through acoustically modified speech (Fast ForWord) in severe mixed receptive-expressive language impairment: Outcomes from a randomized controlled trial. *Journal of Speech, Language, and Hearing Research*, *48*, 715–729.

Conti-Ramsden, G. (2003). Processing and linguistic markers in young children with specific language impairment. *Journal of Speech, Language, and Hearing Research*, *46*, 1029–1037.

Conti-Ramsden, G., Simkin, Z., & Botting, N. (2006). The prevalence of autistic spectrum disorders in adolescents with a history of specific language impairment (SLI). *Journal of Child Psychology and Psychiatry*, *47*, 621–628.

Coplan, J., & Gleason, J. R. (1988). Unclear speech: Recognition and significance of unintelligible speech in preschool children. *Pediatrics*, *82*, 447–452.

Dale, P. S., Price, T. S., Bishop, D. V. M., & Plomin, R. (2003). Outcomes of early language delay. I. Predicting persistent and transient delay at 3 and 4 years. *Journal of Speech, Language, and Hearing Research*, *46*, 544–560.

De Fossé, L., Hodge, S., Makris, N., Kennedy, D., Caviness, V., McGrath, L., *et al.* (2004). Language-association cortex asymmetry in autism and specific language impairment. *Annals of Neurology*, *56*, 757–766.

Deonna, T. (2000). Acquired epileptic aphasia (AEA) or Landau-Kleffner Syndrome: from childhood to adulthood. In D. V. M. Bishop & L. B. Leonard (Eds), *Speech and Language Impairments in Children: Causes, Characteristics, Intervention and Outcome* (pp. 261–272). Hove, UK: Psychology Press.

Deonna, T., & Roulet-Perez, E. (2005). *Cognitive and behavioural disorders of epileptic origin in children*. London: Mac Keith Press/ Cambridge University Press.

DeThorne, L. S., Petrill, S. A., Deater-Deckard, K., Thompson, L. A., Schatschneider, C., Hart, S. A., *et al.* (2006). Children's history of speech-language difficulties: Genetic influences and associations with reading-related measures. *Journal of Speech, Language, and Hearing Research*, *49*, 1280–1293.

Dodd, B. (2005). *Differential diagnosis and treatment of children with speech disorder* (2nd edn.). London: Whurr Publishers.

Dodd, B., & Bradford, A. (2000). A comparison of three therapy methods for children with different types of developmental phonological disorder. *International Journal of Language and Communication Disorders*, *35*, 189–209.

Dodd, B., Hua, Z., Crosbie, S., Holm, A., & Ozanne, A. (2002). *Diagnostic Evaluation of Articulation and Phonology (DEAP)*. London: Harcourt Assessment.

Dunn, L., Dunn, L., Whetton, C., & Burley, J. (1998). *British Picture Vocabulary Scales–II*. Windsor, UK: NFER-Nelson.

Ebbels, S. H. (2007). Teaching grammar to school-aged children with specific language impairment using shape coding. *Child Language Teaching and Therapy*, *23*, 67–93.

Edwards, S., Fletcher, P., Garman, M., Hughes, A., Letts, C., & Sinka, I. (1997). *Reynell Developmental Language Scales III*. Windsor: NFER-Nelson.

Feldman, H. M., Dollaghan, C. A., Campbell, T. F., Colborn, D. K., Janosky, J., Kurs-Lasky, M., *et al.* (2003). Parent-reported language skills in relation to otitis media during the first 3 years of life. *Journal of Speech, Language, and Hearing Research*, *46*, 273–287.

Fenson, L., Dale, P. S., Reznick, J. S., Thal, D., Bates, E., Hartung, J. P., *et al.* (2003). *MacArthur–Bates Communicative Development Inventories*. Baltimore, MD: Brookes Publishing.

Feuk, L., Kalervo, A., Lipsanen-Nyman, M., Skaug, J., Nakabayashi, K., Finucane, B., *et al.* (2006). Absence of a paternally inherited *FOXP2* gene in developmental verbal dyspraxia. *American Journal of Human Genetics*, *79*, 965–972.

Fey, M. E., Long, S. H., & Finestack, L. H. (2003). Ten principles of grammar facilitation for children with specific language impairments. *American Journal of Speech-Language Pathology*, *12*, 3–15.

Fisher, S. E. (2005). Dissection of molecular mechanisms underlying speech and language disorders. *Applied Psycholinguistics*, *26*, 111–128.

Fisher, S. E. (2006). Tangled webs: Tracing the connections between genes and cognition. *Cognition*, *10*, 270–297.

Folstein, S. E., & Mankoski, R. E. (2000). Chromosome 7q: Where autism meets language disorder. *American Journal of Human Genetics*, *67*, 278–281.

Forrest, K. (2003). Diagnostic criteria of developmental apraxia of speech used by clinical speech-language pathologists. *American Journal of Speech-Language Pathology*, *12*, 376–380.

Foundas, A. L., Bollich, A. M., Feldman, J., Corey, D. M., Hurley, M., Lemen, L. C., *et al.* (2004). Aberrant auditory processing and atypical planum temporale in developmental stuttering. *Neurology*, *63*, 1640–1646.

Frederickson, N., Frith, U., & Reason, R. (1997). *Phonological Assessment Battery (PhAB)*. Windsor: NFER-Nelson.

Galaburda, A. M., Sherman, G. F., Rosen, G. D., Aboitiz, F., & Geschwind, N. (1985). Developmental dyslexia: Four consecutive cases with cortical anomalies. *Annals of Neurology*, *18*, 222–233.

Gardner, M. (2000). *Expressive and Receptive One-Word Picture Vocabulary Tests*. Austin, TX: Pro-Ed.

Gathercole, S., & Baddeley, A. (1996). *Children's Test of Nonword Repetition (CN REP)*. London: Harcourt Assessment.

Gauger, L. M., Lombardino, L. J., & Leonard, C. M. (1997). Brain morphology in children with specific language impairment. *Journal of Speech, Language, and Hearing Research*, *40*, 1272–1284.

Gierut, J. A. (1998). Treatment efficacy: Functional phonological disorders in children. *Journal of Speech, Language, and Hearing Research*, *41*, S85–S100.

Girolametto, L., & Weitzman, E. (2006). It takes two to talk: The Hanen program for parents. In R. J. McCauley, & M. E. Fey (Eds.), *Treatment of language disorders in children* (pp. 77–103). Baltimore: Paul H. Brookes.

Goldman, R., & Fristoe, M. (2000). *Goldman–Fristoe Test of Articulation – 2*. Eagan, MN: Pearson Assessments.

Happé, F. (1995). The role of age and verbal ability in the theory of mind task performance of subjects with autism. *Child Development*, *66*, 843–855.

Herbert, M. R., Ziegler, D. A., Makris, N., Bakardjiev, A., Hodgson, J., Adrien, K. T., *et al.* (2003). Larger brain and white matter volumes in children with developmental language disorder. *Developmental Science*, *6*, F11–F22.

Hill, E. L. (2001). Non-specific nature of specific language impairment: A review of the literature with regard to concomitant motor impairments. *International Journal of Language and Communication Disorders*, *36*, 149–171.

Hoff, E., & Tian, C. (2005). Socioeconomic status and cultural influences on language. *Journal of Communication Disorders*, 38, 271–278.

Holm, V. A., & Kunze, L. H. (1969). Effect of chronic otitis media on language and speech development. *Pediatrics*, *43*, 833–839.

Horwitz, S. M., Irwin, J. R., Briggs-Gowan, M. J., Bosson Heenan, J. M., Mendoza, J., & Carter, A. S. (2003). Language delay in a community cohort of young children. *Journal of the American Academy of Child and Adolescent Psychiatry*, *42*, 932–940.

Howell, J., & Dean, E. (1994). *Treating Phonological Disorders in Children. Metaphon: Theory to Practice* (2nd edn.). Chichester: John Wiley & Sons.

Howlin, P., Mawhood, L., & Rutter, M. (2000). Autism and developmental receptive language disorder: A follow-up comparison in early adult life. II. Social, behavioural, and psychiatric outcomes. *Journal of Child Psychology and Psychiatry*, *41*, 561–578.

Hurst, J. A., Baraitser, M., Auger, E., Graham, F., & Norell, S. (1990). An extended family with a dominantly inherited speech disorder. *Developmental Medicine and Child Neurology*, *32*, 352–355.

Jernigan, T., Hesselink, J. R., Sowell, E., & Tallal, P. (1991). Cerebral structure on magnetic resonance imaging in language- and learning-impaired children. *Archives of Neurology*, *48*, 539–545.

Joanisse, M. F., & Seidenberg, M. S. (2003). Phonology and syntax in specific language impairment: Evidence from a connectionist model. *Brain and Language*, *86*, 40–56.

Johnson, M., & Wittgens, A. (2001). *The selective mutism resource manual*. Bicester, Oxon: Speechmark Publishing.

Jones, M., Onslow, M., Packman, A., Williams, S., Ormond, T., Schwarz, I. E., *et al.* (2005). Randomised controlled trial of the Lidcombe programme of early stuttering intervention. *British Medical Journal*, *331*, 659.

Joseph, R. M., Tager-Flusberg, H., & Lord, C. (2002). Cognitive profiles and social-communicative functioning in children with autism spectrum disorder. *Journal of Child Psychology and Psychiatry*, *43*, 807–821.

Law, J., Garrett, Z., & Nye, C. (2004). The efficacy of treatment for children with developmental speech and language delay/disorder: A meta-analysis. *Journal of Speech, Language, and Hearing Research*, *47*, 924–943.

Leonard, C. M. (1997). Language and the prefrontal cortex. In N. Krasnegor, G. R. Lyon, & P. S. Goldman-Rakic (Eds.), *Prefrontal cortex: Evolution, development, and behavioral neuroscience* (pp. 141–166). Baltimore: Paul H. Brookes.

Leonard, C. M., Lombardino, L. J., Walsh, K., Eckert, M. A., Mockler, J. L., Rowe, L. A., *et al.* (2002). Anatomical risk factors that distinguish dyslexia from SLI predict reading skill in normal children. *Journal of Communication Disorders*, *35*, 501–531.

Leonard, C., Eckert, M., Given, B., Virginia, B., & Eden, G. (2006). Individual differences in anatomy predict reading and oral language impairments in children. *Brain*, *129*, 3329–3342.

Lewis, B. A., Freebairn, L. A., Hansen, A., Taylor, H. G., Iyengar, S., & Shriberg, L. D. (2004). Family pedigrees of children with suspected childhood apraxia of speech. *Journal of Communication Disorders*, *37*, 157–175.

Liasis, A., Bamiou, D., Campbell, P., Sirimanna, T., Boyd, S., & Towell, A. (2003). Auditory event-related potentials in the assessment of auditory processing disorders: A pilot study. *Neuropediatrics*, *34*, 23–29.

Lindsay, G., Dockrell, J. E., Mackie, C., & Letchford, B. (2005). Local education authorities' approaches to provision for children with specific speech and language difficulties in England and Wales. *European Journal of Special Needs Education*, *20*, 329–345.

Lord, C., Rutter, M., & Le Couteur, A. (1994). Autism Diagnostic Interview–Revised: A revised version of a diagnostic interview for caregivers of individuals with possible pervasive developmental disorders. *Journal of Autism and Developmental Disorders*, *24*, 659–685.

Lord, C., Risi, S., Lambrecht, L., Cook, E. H., Leventhal, B. L., Dilavore, P., *et al.* (2000). The Autism Diagnostic Observation Schedule–Generic: A standard measure of social and communication deficits associated with the spectrum of autism. *Journal of Autism and Developmental Disorders*, *30*, 205–223.

Macdermot, K. D., Bonora, E., Sykes, N., Coupe, A. M., Lai, C. S., Vernes, S. C., *et al.* (2005). Identification of *FOXP2* truncation as a novel cause of developmental speech and language deficits. *American Journal of Human Genetics*, *76*, 1074–1080.

Manassis, K., Fung, D., Tannock, R., Sloman, L., Fiksenbaum, L., & McInnes, A. (2003). Characterizing selective mutism: Is it more than social anxiety? *Depression and Anxiety*, *18*, 153–161.

Mansson, H. (2000). Childhood stuttering: Incidence and development. *Journal of Fluency Disorders*, *25*, 47–57.

Mawhood, L., Howlin, P., & Rutter, M. (2000). Autism and developmental receptive language disorder: A follow-up in early adult life. I. Cognitive and language outcomes. *Journal of Child Psychology and Psychiatry*, *41*, 547–559.

McArthur, T. (Ed.). (1992). *The Oxford companion to the English language*. Oxford: Oxford University Press.

Merzenich, M. M., Jenkins, W. M., Johnston, P., Schreiner, C., Miller, S. L., & Tallal, P. (1996). Temporal processing deficits of language-learning impaired children ameliorated by training. *Science*, *271*, 77–81.

Moore, D. R. (2006). Auditory processing disorder (APD): Definition, diagnosis, neural basis, and intervention. *Audiological Medicine*, *4*, 4–11.

Morley, M. E. (1957). *The development and disorders of speech in childhood*. Edinburgh: Churchill Livingstone.

Mottron, L. (2004). Matching strategies in cognitive research with individuals with high-functioning autism: Current practices, instrument biases and recommendations. *Journal of Autism and Developmental Disorders*, *34*, 19–27.

Nelson, H. D., Nygren, P., Walker, M., & Panoscha, R. (2006). Screening for speech and language delay in preschool children: Systematic evidence review for the US Preventive Services Task Force. *Pediatrics*, *117*, e298–319.

Newbury, D. F., & Monaco, A. P. (in press). The application of molecular genetics to the study of language impairments. In C. F. Norbury & J. B. Tomblin & D. V. M. Bishop (Eds.), *Understanding Developmental Language Disorders*. Hove: Psychology Press.

Newcomer, P., & Hammill, D. D. (1997). *Test of Language Development – Primary* (3rd edn.). Austin, TX: Pro-Ed.

Norbury, C. F., Bishop, D. V. M., & Briscoe, J. (2001). Production of English finite verb morphology: A comparison of SLI and mild–moderate hearing impairment. *Journal of Speech, Language, and Hearing Research*, *44*, 165–178.

Norbury, C. F., Nash, M., Bishop, D. V. M., & Baird, G. (2004). Using parental checklists to identify diagnostic groups in children with communication impairment: A validation of the Children's Communication Checklist–2. *International Journal of Language and Communication Disorders*, *39*, 345–364.

Oliver, B., Dale, P. S., & Plomin, R. (2005). Predicting literacy at age 7 from preliteracy at age 4. *Psychological Science*, *16*, 861–865.

Paradis, M., Crago, M., Genesee, F., & Rice, M. (2003). French–English bilingual children with SLI: How do they compare with their monolingual peers? *Journal of Speech, Language, and Hearing Research*, *46*, 113–127.

Paul, R. (2000). Predicting outcomes of early expressive language delay: Ethical implications. In D. V. M. Bishop, & L. B. Leonard (Eds.), *Speech and language impairments in children: Causes, characteristics, intervention and outcome* (pp. 195–209). Hove, UK: Psychology Press.

Paul, R., Shriberg, L., McSweeny, J., Cicchetti, D., Klin, A., & Volkmar, F. (2005a). Brief report: relations between prosodic performance and communication and socialization ratings in high functioning speakers with autism spectrum disorders. *Journal of Autism and Developmental Disorders*, *35*, 861–869.

Paul, R., Augustyn, A., Klin, A., & Volkmar, F. R. (2005b). Perception and production of prosody by speakers with autism spectrum disorders. *Journal of Autism and Developmental Disorders*, *35*, 205–220.

Plante, E., & Jackson, T. (1997). Gyral morphology in the posterior Sylvian region in families affected by developmental language disorder. *Neuropsychology Review*, *6*, 81–94.

Pokorni, J. L., Worthington, C. K., & Jamison, P. J. (2004). Phonological awareness intervention: A comparison of three programs – Fast ForWord, Earobics, and LiPS. *Journal of Educational Research*, *97*, 147–157.

Redmond, S. M., & Rice, M. L. (1998). The socioemotional behaviors of children with SLI: Social adaptation or social deviance? *Journal of Speech, Language, and Hearing Research*, *41*, 688–700.

Renfrew, C. E. (1988). *Renfrew language scales*. Bicester, Oxon: Winslow Press.

Rescorla, L. (2005). Age 13 language and reading outcomes in late-talking toddlers. *Journal of Speech, Language, and Hearing Research*, *48*, 459–472.

Rice, M. (2004). Growth models of developmental language disorders. In M. Rice, & S. F. Warren (Eds.), *Developmental language disorders: From phenotypes to etiologies* (pp. 207–240). Mahwah, NJ: Lawrence Erlbaum Associates.

Robinson, R. J. (1991). Causes and associations of severe and persistent specific speech and language disorders in children. *Developmental Medicine and Child Neurology*, *33*, 943–962.

Rosen, S. (2005). A riddle wrapped in mystery inside an enigma: Defining Central Auditory Processing Disorder (CAPD). *American Journal of Audiology*, *14*, 139–142.

Roulet-Perez, E., Davidoff, V., Prélaz, A., Morel, B., Rickli, F., Metz-Lutz, M., *et al.* (2001). Sign language in childhood epileptic aphasia (Landau–Kleffner syndrome). *Developmental Medicine and Child Neurology*, *43*, 739–744.

Rouse, C., & Krueger, A. (2004). Putting computerized instruction to the test: A randomized evaluation of a "scientifically based" reading program. *Economics of Education Review*, *23*, 323–338.

Rustin, L., Cook, F., Botterill, W., Hughes, C., & Kelman, E. (2001). *Stammering: A practical guide for teachers and other professionals*. London: David Foulton.

Semel, E., Wiig, E. H., & Secord, W. A. (2003). *Clinical Evaluation of Language Fundamentals®, fourth edition (CELF®-4)*. London: Harcourt Assessment.

Shevell, M. I., Majnemer, A., Rosenbaum, P., & Abrahamowicz, M. (2000). Etiologic yield in single domain developmental delay: A prospective study. *Journal of Pediatrics*, *137*, 633–637.

Shriberg, L. D., Tomblin, J. B., & McSweeny, J. L. (1999). Prevalence of speech delay in 6-year-old children and comorbidity with language impairment. *Journal of Speech, Language, and Hearing Research*, *42*, 1461–1481.

Snowling, M. J., Bishop, D. V. M., Stothard, S. E., Chipchase, B., & Kaplan, C. (2006). Psychosocial outcomes at 15 years of children with a preschool history of speech-language impairment. *Journal of Child Psychology and Psychiatry*, *47*, 759–765.

Snowling, M. J., & Stackhouse, J. (2006). *Dyslexia, speech and language* (2nd edn.). London: Whurr Publishers.

Stackhouse, J., & Wells, B. (1997). *Children's speech and literacy difficulties: A psycholinguistic framework*. London: Whurr Publishers.

Stein, C. M., Schick, J. H., Taylor, H. G., Shriberg, L. D., Millard, C., Kundtz-Kluge, A., *et al.* (2004). Pleiotropic effects of a chromosome 3 locus on speech-sound disorder and reading. *American Journal of Human Genetics*, *74*, 283–297.

Steinhausen, H. C., & Juzi, C. (1996). Elective mutism: An analysis of 100 cases. *Journal of the American Academy of Child and Adolescent Psychiatry*, *35*, 606–614.

Steinhausen, H. C., Wachter, M., Laimbock, K., & Winkler Metzke, C. (2006). A long-term outcome of selective mutism in childhood. *Journal of Child Psychology and Psychiatry*, *47*, 751–756.

Stelmachowicz, P. G., Pittman, A. L., Hoover, B. M., Lewis, D. E., & Moeller, M. P. (2004). The importance of high-frequency audibility in the speech and language development of children with hearing loss. *Archives of Otolaryngology: Head and Neck Surgery*, *130*, 556–562.

Stothard, S. E., Snowling, M. J., Bishop, D. V. M., Chipchase, B. B., & Kaplan, C. A. (1998). Language-impaired preschoolers: A follow-up into adolescence. *Journal of Speech, Language, and Hearing Research*, *41*, 407–418.

Suresh, R., Ambrose, N., Roe, C., Pluzhnikov, A., Wittke-Thompson, J. K., Ng, M. C. Y., *et al.* (2006). New complexities in the genetics of stuttering: Significant sex-specific linkage signals. *American Journal of Human Genetics*, *78*, 554–563.

Tallal, P. (2000). Experimental studies of language learning impairments: From research to remediation. In D. V. M. Bishop, & L. B. Leonard (Eds.), *Speech and language impairments in children: Causes, characteristics, intervention and outcome* (pp. 131–155). Hove, UK: Psychology Press.

Tallal, P., Miller, S. L., Bedi, G., Byma, G., Wang, X., Nagarajan, S. S., *et al.* (1996). Language comprehension in language-learning impaired children improved with acoustically modified speech. *Science*, *271*, 81–84.

Thal, D. J., Tobias, S., & Morrison, D. (1991). Language and gesture in late talkers: A one-year follow-up. *Journal of Speech and Hearing Research*, *34*, 604–612.

Tomblin, J. B., Records, N. L., Buckwalter, P., Zhang, X., Smith, E., & O'Brien, M. (1997). Prevalence of specific language impairment in kindergarten children. *Journal of Speech and Hearing Research*, *40*, 1245–1260.

Tomblin, J. B., Records, N., & Zhang, X. (1996). A system for the diagnosis of specific language impairment in kindergarten children. *Journal of Speech and Hearing Research*, *39*, 1284–1294.

Tomblin, J. B., & Zhang, X. (1999). Language patterns and etiology in children with specific language impairment. In H. Tager-Flusberg (Ed.), *Neurodevelopmental disorders: Developmental cognitive neuroscience* (pp. 361–382). Cambridge, MA: MIT Press.

Tomblin, J. B., Zhang, X., Buckwalter, P., & Catts, H. (2000). The association of reading disability, behavioral disorders, and language impairment among second-grade children. *Journal of Child Psychology and Psychiatry*, *41*, 473–482.

Toppelberg, C. O., Tabors, P., Coggins, A., Lum, K., & Burger, C. (2005). Differential diagnosis of selective mutism in bilingual children. *Journal of the American Academy of Child and Adolescent Psychiatry*, *44*, 592–595.

Van der Lely, H. K. J. (2005). Domain-specific cognitive systems: Insight from Grammatical-SLI. *Trends in Cognitive Sciences*, *9*, 53–59.

Van der Lely, H. K. J., Rosen, S., & Adlard, A. (2004). Grammatical language impairment and the specificity of cognitive domains: Relations between auditory and language abilities. *Cognition*, *94*, 167–183.

Vargha-Khadem, F., Gadian, D., Copp, A., & Mishkin, M. (2005). *FOXP2* and the neuroanatomy of speech and language. *Nature Reviews. Neuroscience*, *6*, 131–138.

Vecchio, J. L., & Kearney, C. A. (2005). Selective mutism in children: Comparison to youths with and without anxiety disorders. *Journal of Psychopathology and Behavioral Assessment*, *27*, 31–37.

Viding, E., Spinath, F. M., Price, T. S., Bishop, D. V. M., Dale, P. S., & Plomin, R. (2004). Genetic and environmental influence on language impairment in 4-year-old same-sex and opposite-sex twins. *Journal of Child Psychology and Psychiatry*, *45*, 315–325.

Watkins, K. E., Dronkers, N. F., & Vargha-Khadem, F. (2002). Behavioural analysis of an inherited speech and language disorder: Comparison with acquired aphasia. *Brain*, *125*, 452–464.

Webster, R. L., Majnemer, A., Platt, R. W., & Shevell, M. I. (2005). Motor function at school age in children with a preschool diagnosis of developmental language impairment. *Journal of Pediatrics*, *146*, 80–85.

Whitehouse, A., Barry, J. G., & Bishop, D. V. M. (2007). The broader language phenotype of autism: A comparison with specific language impairment. *Journal of Child Psychology and Psychiatry*, *48*, 822–830.

Wiig, E. H., & Secord, W. (1989). *Test of language competence: Expanded edition*. London: Harcourt Assessment.

Wiig, E. H., & Secord, W. (1992). *Test of word knowledge*. New York: Harcourt Assessment.

Wiig, E. H., Secord, W., & Semel, E. (1992). *Clinical Evaluation of Language Fundamentals: Preschool (CELF-Preschool)*. San Antonio: Harcourt Assessment.

World Health Organization (WHO). (1996). *Multiaxial classification of child and adolescent psychiatric disorders: The ICD-10 classification of mental and behavioural disorders in children and adolescents*. Cambridge, UK: Cambridge University Press.

Yairi, E. & Ambrose, N. G. (1999). Early childhood stuttering I: persistency and recovery rates. *Journal of Speech, Language, and Hearing Research*, *42*, 1097–1112.

Yairi, E., Ambrose, N., & Cox, N. (1996). Genetics of stuttering: A critical review. *Journal of Speech and Hearing Research*, *39*, 771–784.

Zimmerman, I. L., Steiner, V., & Pond, R. (1997). *Preschool Language Scale-UK*. London: Harcourt Assessment.

48 Reading and Other Specific Learning Difficulties

Margaret J. Snowling and Charles Hulme

Learning difficulties can occur in the context of global delays in development or where there are circumscribed deficits in specific cognitive processes. It has proven productive in theory and in practice to differentiate these two forms of learning difficulties (Rutter & Maughan, 2005). The term specific learning difficulties is used to refer to poor educational attainment in the absence of general cognitive deficits, whereas the term general learning difficulties (now more appropriately termed intellectual disability; see chapter 49) is used to refer to problems associated with low IQ.

This chapter deals with specific learning difficulties, the major focus being on reading difficulties. More research has been conducted on the nature and causes of reading difficulties than on other learning difficulties, and interventions to ameliorate reading impairments have been evaluated. The chapter also considers specific difficulties in arithmetic and non-verbal learning disabilities including motor impairments; much less is known about the causes and treatments of these other learning disorders.

The assessment of specific learning difficulties is more often the domain of psychologists and educators than of psychiatrists and hence, the term "difficulties" is usually used rather than "disorders" or "disabilities," which derive from the medical model. According to diagnostic manuals, there is a variety of such difficulties, viz, reading disorder, spelling disorder, mathematical disorder, disorder of written expression and mixed disorder of scholastic skills (DSM-IV, American Psychiatric Association, 2000). However, there is not a one-to-one correspondence between the classifications specified in the diagnostic manuals and those typically used by school systems or researchers in the field. Importantly, "discrepancy definitions" (that prescribe that attainments should be low relative to age and *intelligence*) are seldom strictly adhered to; in particular, the measurement of IQ is no longer considered central to the diagnosis of reading disorders. The main reason for this is that there are few cognitive differences relevant to reading between poor readers of high and low IQ. Given targeted support, children with specific reading difficulties make similar progress in reading (as measured by decoding) to those with general reading difficulties (Hatcher & Hulme, 1999; Shaywitz, Fletcher, Holahan, & Shaywitz, 1992a). However, in the absence of such intervention, outcomes for reading and spelling have been reported to differ, children with intellectual disability faring better in literacy although less well in arithmetic (Rutter & Maughan, 2005).

Rutter's Child and Adolescent Psychiatry, 5th edition. Edited by M. Rutter, D. Bishop, D. Pine, S. Scott, J. Stevenson, E. Taylor and A. Thapar. © 2008 Blackwell Publishing, ISBN: 978-1-4051-4549-7.

Disorders of Reading and Spelling

Definition, Classification and Incidence

Difficulties in reading accuracy (measured by tasks requiring decoding of single words) are distinct from difficulties with reading comprehension (measured by tasks tapping understanding of text). Whereas problems with decoding inevitably limit reading comprehension, there are a substantial minority of children (perhaps as many as 10%; Nation, 2005) who have difficulties with reading comprehension in the absence of problems with reading accuracy. In English-speaking countries, reading difficulties have been reported to affect 4–8% of school-aged children. Epidemiological studies in England reported prevalence rates of just over 3% (3.1% on tests of reading accuracy and 3.6% on tests of reading comprehension) among 9- and 10-year-olds in a non-metropolitan area using a stringent IQ-discrepancy criterion of 2 standard errors of prediction below expected performance (Rutter & Yule, 1975). Using exactly comparable assessment procedures, rates were more than doubled (6.3% for reading accuracy and 9.3% for reading comprehension) in an inner city area, suggesting that social factors have a key role in risk for reading disability (Rutter & Maughan, 2005; Yule, Rutter, Berger, & Thompson, 1974). Boys are more likely to be referred for reading difficulties than girls (Shaywitz, Shaywitz, Fletcher, & Escobar, 1990) but this is not simply a matter of referral bias because sex ratios of between 1.5:1 and 3:1 boys to girls have been reported in large-scale community studies (Rutter, Caspi, Fergusson *et al.*, 2004). However, rates of reading difficulties vary with age (Shaywitz, Escobar, Shaywitz, Fletcher, & Makugh, 1992b) with some children falling just below a chosen threshold at one age and just above at another. Problems with word decoding are likely to predominate in the earliest years of schooling, whereas a later-emerging group of poor readers who cope with the initial stages of learning to read fare less well when the school curriculum places heavier emphasis on comprehension. Later still, through into adulthood, individuals may face persisting problems with spelling or written expression (Maughan, Messer, Collishaw *et al.*, submitted).

The language in which children learn to read also affects the likelihood of reading difficulties, although data do not exist to allow fair comparison of prevalence rates. European languages vary in the consistency of their writing systems. Languages such as Italian, German and Greek are regular in the way they map speech sounds onto written forms, whereas others – most notably English (and to a lesser extent Danish and French) are more irregular or opaque. Regular orthographies present children with fewer challenges in learning to read than do opaque writing systems (Seymour, 2005). However, differences in diagnostic practice may have overemphasized the differences between reading difficulties in different languages and played down the similarities (Caravolas, 2005). In both the irregular English and the regular Czech language, the correlates of reading skill and the predictors of reading difficulties have been reported to be similar (Caravolas, Volin, & Hulme, 2005). In line with this, a recent survey of 150,000 Dutch children reported a 9% prevalence of reading and spelling problems among 11- to 12-year-olds, and further assessment revealed that these were specific to literacy (and not more general) for 3.6% of children (Blomert, 2005). The case might be thought different when considering reading difficulties in non-alphabetic languages, such as Chinese, but there is little direct evidence that supports this view (Hanley, 2005).

Normal Literacy Development: A Framework

In an alphabetic language such as English, the foundation of literacy is a system of mappings between orthography (the letters of printed words) and phonology (the speech sounds of spoken words). Learning to read requires the child to abstract the idea that the letters of printed words represent phonemes in spoken words (Byrne, 1998).

More formally, the relationship between oral and written language skills has been simulated in computational models. According to the Triangle model of Plaut, McClelland, Seidenberg *et al.* (1996; after Seidenberg & McClelland, 1989) depicted in Fig. 48.1, reading involves the interaction of a phonological pathway (mapping from letters to sounds) and a semantic pathway (mapping from letters to meanings and then to sounds). It is thought that beginning readers place most reliance on the phonological pathway (*phonics*) and then gradually start to use the semantic pathway to gain fluency in their reading. This use of the semantic pathway is important in English for reading exception words that do not conform to English letter-sound rules (e.g. *yacht* and *pint*). When children read words they usually occur in a sentence context; context exerts its influence on reading via activation through the semantic pathway.

The Triangle model makes predictions about the cognitive resources that children require in order to learn to read. It is now agreed that early reading development depends on phoneme awareness (the ability to reflect on and manipulate speech sounds in words) and letter knowledge (Bowey, 2005). Later in development, broader language skills (such as vocabulary and grammar) predict gains in reading fluency and are critical foundations for reading comprehension (Catts,

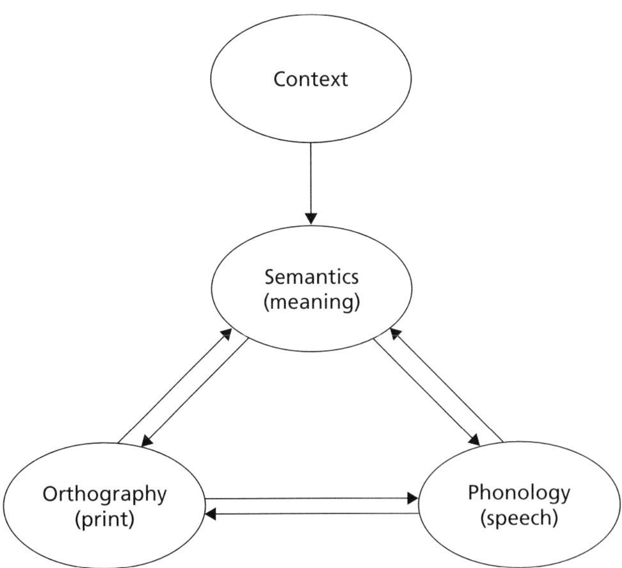

Fig. 48.1 The Triangle framework. [After Seidenberg & McClelland, 1989.]

Fey, Zhang, & Tomblin, 1999; Muter, Hulme, Snowling, & Stevenson, 2004; Share, 1995). In addition, higher-level skills, such as inference making, are important for some aspects of text comprehension (Yuill & Oakhill, 1991). Thus, reading difficulties can occur for different reasons.

Problems of Decoding

Problems that specifically affect a child's ability to decode text are commonly referred to as "dyslexia." Although the term has had a chequered history, international voluntary agencies concerned with children's specific reading difficulties now provide definitions of the "disorder" that are informed by research (International Dyslexia Association, 2002) and national initiatives (Riddick, 2006) have lent credence to the judicious use of the term.

Theories of Dyslexia

Phonological Deficit Theory

The majority of children with specific reading difficulties have phonological (speech processing) difficulties that affect their decoding skill to some extent (Vellutino, Fletcher, Snowling, & Scanlon, 2004). The predominant theoretical account views the primary cognitive cause of dyslexia as a phonological (speech) processing impairment (Harm & Seidenberg 1999; Ramus, Rosen, Dakin *et al.*, 2003). According to this hypothesis, children with dyslexia have difficulty establishing the phonological reading pathway (Snowling, 2000); the development of the semantic pathway is affected less because the mappings in this pathway do not depend upon identifying the phonemes of speech.

Aside from reading, phonological deficits explain why people with dyslexia typically have difficulties with a wide range of cognitive tasks that engage phonological processes such as limitations of verbal short-term memory, long-term verbal (phonological) learning, slow naming of letters, digits, color and objects and word finding difficulties. Together, this evidence led Stanovich and colleagues to propose the *phonological-core variable-difference* model of dyslexia (Stanovich & Siegel, 1994); according to this model poor phonology is related to poor reading performance, irrespective of IQ. It is now believed that this model holds irrespective of language background (Caravolas, 2005; Goulandris, 2003).

Rate Deficits and Double Deficits

Some have argued that the phonological deficit theory does not fully account for the reading problems found in children with dyslexia. Lovett, Ransby, and Barron (1988) differentiated accuracy-impaired and rate-impaired poor readers, and Wolf and Bowers (1999) distinguished between disabled readers with single deficits in either phonological awareness or in naming speed (measured by the speed to retrieve names of digits or letters; Wimmer, Mayringer, & Landerl, 2000) and a subgroup with deficits in both processes.

An alternative to the phonological deficit hypothesis is the automatization hypothesis (Nicolson & Fawcett, 1990). According to this theory, people with dyslexia have difficulty learning skills to the point at which they become completely automatic, and, although they can learn to read, they have difficulty developing reading fluency. This model conceptualizes the phonological deficit in dyslexia as a consequence of problems with speech-articulation. A feature that marks this hypothesis out from the phonological deficit hypothesis is that it places the deficit in dyslexia at a domain-general level – that is, the automatization deficit places similar constraints on the learning of all skills, including basic motor skills, and is associated with cerebellar dysfunction (Nicolson, Fawcett, & Dean, 2001). The theory does not account well for the finding that dyslexia can occur in the absence of motor deficits.

Perceptual Theories of Dyslexia

A large body of research has assessed whether reading difficulties are associated with low-level perceptual processing impairments. Investigations have examined putative impairments in visual, auditory and motor domains as explanations for different manifestations of dyslexia.

Visual Deficits Although most people with reading difficulties have normal visual acuity, there is a raised incidence of abnormalities on psychophysical tasks assessing motion processing and contrast sensitivity (Skoyles & Skottun, 2004). These impairments have been related to a deficit within the magnocellular division of the visual system, which responds to rapid changes in visual stimulation and to moving stimuli (Lovegrove, Martin, & Slaghuis, 1986; Stein & Talcott, 1999). However, some studies have found no evidence of abnormal sensitivity, whereas others have suggested that group differences may be related to uncontrolled differences in IQ (Hulslander, Talcott, Witton *et al.*, 2004). Problems of visual attention have also been considered a putative cause of dyslexia (Facoetti, Turatto, Lorusso, & Mascetti, 2001; Hari, Renvall, & Tanskanen, 2001; Roach & Hogben, 2004) but again the evidence is inconsistent. It has therefore been proposed that phonological and visual attention could be dissociable causes of dyslexia that may co-occur (Valdois, Bosse, & Tainturier, 2004).

Although scientific understanding of how visual deficits might affect reading is limited, the use of colored lenses or filters to reduce visual stress and improve reading performance is recommended by some practitioners. To date, there is no evidence for the effectiveness of such interventions as a treatment for reading impairments in dyslexia.

Auditory Deficits A hypothesis that has attracted considerable research is that the phonological deficit in dyslexia stems from a deficit in basic auditory processing (Tallal, 1980); specifically, an auditory processing deficit affects the perception of consonants, which in turn affects the development of phonological skills (cf. Mody, 2003). The plausibility of this hypothesis is supported by evidence that infants at family risk of dyslexia or language impairment are less sensitive to the speech sounds that signal meaning changes than typically developing children (Leppänen, Eklund, & Lyytinen, 1997), and that behavioral and brain responses to speech sounds in the first year of life correlate with later language and reading development (Guttorm, Leppänen, Poikkeus *et al.*, 2005).

Investigation of auditory deficits has extended to tasks tapping frequency discrimination, frequency modulation, binaural processing, backward masking (for review see Bailey & Snowling, 2002) and amplitude onset sensitivity (Goswami, Thomson, Richardson *et al.*, 2002). However, the findings are inconsistent and typically only 30–40% of people with dyslexia show auditory impairments.

The direct investigation of speech perception in dyslexia has produced some positive findings (Manis, McBride-Chang, Seidenberg *et al.*, 1997). Current evidence comes primarily from performance on categorical perception tasks (e.g., identifying synthetic speech tokens as [ka] or [ga]). As a group, children with dyslexia show fuzzy boundaries between different phonemes, constituting a categorical speech perception deficit (it should be noted that such difficulties are more marked if children have concomitant language impairments; see chapter 47; Joanisse, Mains, Keating, & Seidenberg, 2000). Serniclaes, Van Heghe, Mousty, Carré, & Sprenger-Charolles (2004) showed that not only did children with dyslexia show reduced between-category discrimination, but also they were more sensitive to (within category) variations in the acoustic characteristics of individual phonemes than age-matched controls. Such hypersensitivity implies that phoneme categories are not well-defined and this in turn may pose important problems for learning to read in all alphabetic systems that depend on knowledge of how phonemes are related to letters.

Overall, evidence for the involvement of perceptual problems in dyslexia is equivocal; findings suggest that neither auditory nor visual (nor cerebellar) deficits are necessary or sufficient causes of dyslexia (Ramus, Rosen, Dakin *et al.*, 2003; White, Milne, Rosen *et al.*, 2006). However, in the absence of longitudinal data it remains possible that a sensory deficit early in development (which may resolve by the time children are diagnosed as having reading problems) may still have had a causal role in the etiology of the disorder.

Spelling Difficulties

Typically, the spelling difficulties of people with dyslexia are more severe and more resistant to remediation than their reading difficulties (Romani, Olson, & DiBetta, 2005). Such problems may be seen as a direct consequence of difficulties in mastering the mappings between orthography (spelling patterns) and sound within the phonological pathway (Fig. 48.1). The spelling errors made by people with dyslexia include both phonetic spelling errors, where the sound pattern of the word is represented accurately (e.g., biscuit → biskit; chaos → kaos), and phonetically unacceptable spelling errors (e.g., umbrella → unbrl; adventure → afveorl).

The term dyslexia has sometimes been applied to individuals who have spelling difficulties in the absence of reading problems. These children (called "dysgraphic"; Frith, 1980) tend to have higher verbal than performance IQ and they make phonetically accurate spelling errors (Nelson & Warrington, 1974; Romani, Olson, & Di Betta, 2005). Evidence from single-case studies suggests they may have subtle visual memory impairments (Goulandris & Snowling, 1991; Romani, Ward, & Olson, 1999). This cognitive profile has also been observed in "unaffected" offspring of parents with dyslexia, suggesting that it may represent a broader phenotype of dyslexia in which good oral language skills have mitigated the risk of reading problems (Snowling, Muter, & Carroll, 2007).

Reading Comprehension Impairments

In contrast to children with dyslexia, "poor comprehenders" decode well but have problems understanding what they read. Their difficulties often go unnoticed in the classroom because they can read aloud competently. Poor comprehenders typically have normal non-verbal abilities and good phonology; they do well on phoneme awareness tasks and on simple memory tests (Nation, 2005). However, they have cognitive impairments that encompass poor working memory, problems making inferences and deficits in metacognitive processes, such as comprehension monitoring (Cain, Oakhill, Barnes, & Bryant, 2001; Cain, Oakhill, & Bryant, 2004). Clinically, the profile is often seen in combination with attention deficit/hyperactivity disorder (ADHD).

Within the Triangle model, poor comprehenders have problems both within the semantic pathway and in grammatical processes that feed it. The consequences are a tendency to rely heavily on a "phonic" approach, leading to the tendency to regularize words (e.g., to read *broad* as "brode" or *bread* as "breed"), a reduction in the benefit of context (i.e., limited semantic facilitation of word reading) and problems of reading comprehension – their defining characteristic. The reading comprehension impairments shown by these children are related to a range of oral language processing weaknesses (see chapter 47; Nation, Clarke, Marshall, & Durand, 2004).

Etiology of Reading Difficulties

Genetic Influences on Dyslexia

Prospective studies following the development of children born to parents with dyslexia confirm a heightened risk of literacy impairment in "dyslexic" families (Lyytinen, Erskine, Tolvanen *et al.*, 2006; Scarborough, 1990; Snowling, Gallagher, & Frith, 2003). However, families share environments as well as genes, and twin studies can be helpful in disentangling genetic and environmental influences on reading behavior (see chapter 23).

Twin studies of dyslexia find that the proportion of variance attributable to genetic factors (heritability) is significant (Pennington & Olson, 2005), and heritability appears to be higher among more severely disabled readers (Bishop, 2001) and among those with higher IQ (Olson, Datta, & DeFries, 1999). Two relatively small-scale British twin studies have reported that shared environment accounted for most of the variance in reading, once IQ had been controlled for (Bishop, 2001; Stevenson, Graham, Fredman, & McLoughlin, 1987), perhaps reflecting more diverse educational experiences in these samples. Moreover, it is important to bear in mind that some of the shared genetic variance between twins may be caused by gene–environment correlation (Rutter, 2006). For example, the home literacy background provided by more literate parents may foster reading skills, and better readers may themselves actively seek out more literary experiences.

Studies of the molecular basis of genetic influences on reading have used a variety of methods (for reviews see Fisher & DeFries, 2002; Grigorenko, 2005). To date, the strongest evidence for linkage with dyslexia (in terms of number of replications) is a site on the short arm of chromosome 6. Other linkages that have been replicated although less frequently are on chromosomes 1, 2, 3, 11, 15 and 18 (Grigorenko, 2005). Recently, some candidate susceptibility genes have been identified within these chromosomal regions, including *K1AA0319* on 6p (Cope, Harold, Hill *et al.*, 2005) and *DYX1C1* in the 15q21 region (Taipale, Kaminen, Nopola-Hemmi *et al.*, 2003). However, it is important to remember that genetic influences are probabilistic; complex disorders depend on the combined influence of many genes of small effect, as well as on environmental influences. Moreover, the findings of linkage studies depend upon the behavioral phenotype, such that the use of different definitions of dyslexia by different groups will affect the genotypes that are identified (particularly when data are taken from children learning to read in different languages).

To date, there is no comparable analysis of the genetic bases of reading comprehension difficulties. However, work on the genetic basis of specific language impairments is likely to be relevant here (SLI Consortium, 2002, 2004).

Brain Bases of Dyslexia

The majority of children with specific reading difficulties do not show any gross structural brain abnormalities, but early neurodevelopmental abnormalities appear to be involved (Galaburda, 1994; Galaburda & Kemper, 1978). It has been reported that there are a wide range of structural brain differences between people with dyslexia and controls (Eckert, 2004) and an "anatomical risk index" comprising measurements taken from the brain regions implicated in dyslexia has been reported to distinguish between people with specific decoding difficulties and those with poor reading comprehension (Leonard, Eckert, Lombardino *et al.*, 2001, Leonard, Eckert, Given *et al.*, 2006).

Functional brain imaging studies have contributed to understanding of the brain bases of dyslexia (see chapter 11). Findings indicate that children and adults with dyslexia typically show less activity than controls in left hemisphere temporo-parietal cortex when reading (Price & McCrory, 2005; Shaywitz, Shaywitz, Blachman *et al.*, 2004), and preliminary evidence suggests that intervention may reduce this underactivation (Simos, Fletcher, Bergman *et al.*, 2002). The causal status of brain differences in dyslexia is debatable because brain development shows considerable plasticity and both its structure and function are shaped by use (Johnson, 2005). A reasonable conclusion is that the brain differences between dyslexic and normal readers reflect the interplay of genetic influences and environmental experiences on brain development.

Social and Environmental Influences on Reading Development and Disorder

Home and School Background

It is important not to overlook the critical role of the environment in shaping a child's reading development (Phillips & Lonigan, 2005). Evidence indicates that reading disorders show a strong social gradient that is not entirely attributable to differences in phonological skills or general intellectual abilities (Hecht, Burgess, Togesen, Wagner, & Rashotte, 2000), and poor readers often come from large families, where later-born children may face delays in language development (see chapter 47). One aspect of delayed language development is poor vocabulary, a mediator of deficits in phoneme awareness (Carroll, Snowling, Hulme, & Stevenson, 2003). Direct literacy-related activities in the home are also important (Whitehurst & Lonigan, 1998), although these primarily affect reading comprehension, via vocabulary growth (Stevenson & Fredman, 1990).

Traditional definitions of dyslexia excluded children whose reading failure was caused by "inadequate opportunity to learn," but how to interpret this is unclear. Comparisons of children from the same catchment area attending different schools have emphasized that schooling can make a substantial difference to reading achievement (Rutter & Maughan, 2002). Equally, school experience can differ markedly between good and poor readers.

Cross-linguistic Manifestations of Reading Disorders

Aside from the home and school environment, an important macro-environmental influence on reading development is the language in which a child learns (Harris & Hatano, 2000). The reading and spelling symptoms of dyslexia vary across orthographies; in languages such as German or Italian, reading difficulties are identified by slow rates of reading (few reading errors occur), whereas in English poor reading accuracy is the primary behavioral marker (Landerl, Wimmer, & Frith, 1997). However, reading universally is a process involving the mapping of visual characters on to phonological forms; it follows that children with phonological impairments are at risk of reading difficulties in all languages.

Gene–Environment Correlation and Reading Practice

Aside from the above, being a poor reader affects the motivation to read. From very early in development, children differ in their interest in books, and children at risk of dyslexia may well be among those who are more difficult to engage. Where parents themselves have literacy problems, this might also set the stage for less than optimal reading-related experiences in the home (cf. Petrill, Deater-Deckard, Schatsneider, & Davis, 2005).

One variable that can have a significant impact on the behavioral manifestation of a reading disorder is reading practice. Measures of "print exposure" (assessed by questionnaires that require participants to differentiate real book titles or real authors' names from distracter items, and which document reading habits) account for variance in reading skills when other critical variables such as IQ and phonological awareness have been controlled (Cunningham & Stanovich, 1990). Print exposure measures are simply a proxy for the amount of reading done and it is likely that the effects of low exposure are cumulative, causing reader-differences in reading competence to become magnified over time.

In summary, as might be expected for a complex trait such as reading, the etiology of reading disorders is varied and depends on both genetic and environmental factors. It is critical to distinguish between problems with decoding and problems of reading comprehension. Some children carry a genetic risk of dyslexia but whether or not they are classified as dyslexic depends upon the particular language and school context in which they learn and the other skills (or deficits) they bring to the task of reading. In keeping with this, there is currently a move away from single-deficit toward multifactorial models that explain the nature and causes of dyslexia (Pennington, 2006).

Language-Learning Impairments

In recent years, there has been a growing tendency to collapse together disorders of reading (primarily dyslexia) with disorders of speech and language development, reflecting the clinical impression of considerable behavioral overlap between these disorders and their effects on academic performance. However, this is a retrograde step. Children with speech and language impairments are at high risk of reading problems be they children at family risk of dyslexia (Lyytinen, Erskine, Tolvanen *et al.*, 2006; Pennington & Lefly, 2001; Scarborough, 1990; Snowling, Gallagher, & Frith, 2003), children with specific language impairment (Bishop & Adams, 1990; Catts, Adlof, Hogan, & Weismer, 2005; Snowling, Bishop, & Stothard, 2000) or children with speech sound disorders (see chapter 47; Bird, Bishop, & Freeman, 1995; Nathan,

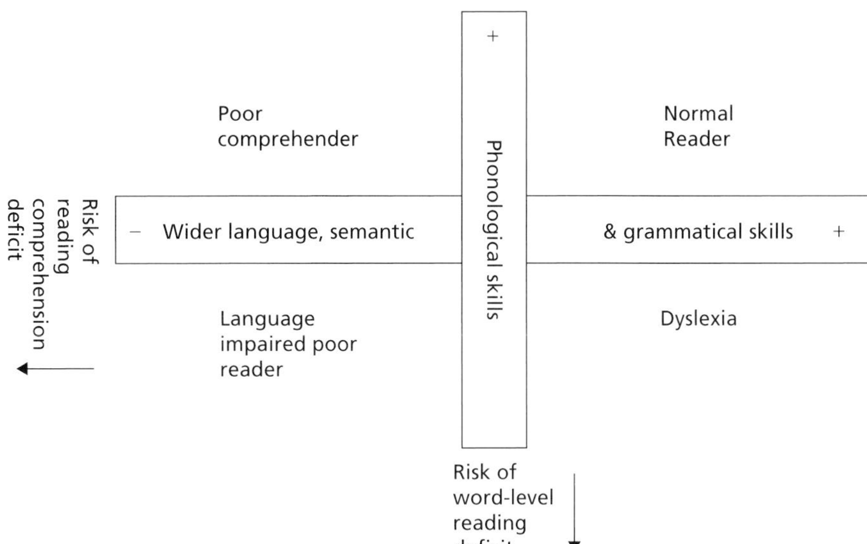

Fig. 48.2 A two-dimensional model of the relationship between dyslexia and language impairment. [After Bishop & Snowling, 2004, with permission.]

Stackhouse, Goulandris, & Snowling, 2004; Raitano, Pennington, Tunick, & Broada, 2004). The nature of the risk depends on a number of factors including the pervasiveness and persistence of the speech-language impairment.

In order to understand the relationship between the different disorders, Bishop and Snowling (2004) proposed a two-dimensional model (Fig. 48.2). Within this model, the risk of word-level decoding deficits is related to phonological skills (that vary from good to poor) and the risk of reading comprehension deficits is related to language skills beyond phonology (grammar and vocabulary, again varying from good to poor). This two-dimensional model has direct implications for the assessment and management of children's reading difficulties and suggests that concerns over whether a particular child fulfills the diagnostic criteria for a specific reading disorder may be of little importance – there are continuous variations in reading skills in the general population and children with either decoding or reading comprehension problems will benefit from appropriate educational interventions which need to be tailored to individual children's needs.

Problems of Numeracy

Definition, Classification and Incidence

Children experience different kinds of difficulty with numeracy skills. Some affect arithmetic (computation) whereas others affect more conceptual aspects of mathematics that require problem-solving. However, these are not well differentiated either in diagnostic manuals or in practice; tests of number skills differ in the extent to which they assess basic arithmetic as opposed to mathematical concepts (e.g., numerosity, magnitude, commutativity or geometry) and this leads to an unhelpful tendency to categorize all mathematical difficulties together. It is also important to note that mathematical learning is a cumulative process and therefore a basic deficit in computation will have downstream effects: addition, subtraction and multiplication processes are involved in higher-level mathematics, such as geometry, algebra and calculus. In addition, high levels of anxiety are often associated with mathematics and these can pose obstacles to learning for children who find basic arithmetical tasks difficult (Ashcraft & Kirk, 2001).

Individual differences in the manifestation of number problems have been reported in the cognitive–neuropsychological literature using a framework developed by McCloskey, Caramazza, and Basili (1985). Within this framework, the calculation system can be dissociated from the number processing system. Temple (1994) has reported single-case evidence for the existence in childhood of "digit dyslexia," in which there is a specific difficulty in the acquisition of lexical processes within the number processing system (i.e., problems in encoding the meaning of numerals such as 34, 8483), "procedural dyscalculia," in which there is difficulty in learning procedures and algorithms and "number fact dyscalculia," in which there is specific difficulty in acquiring numerical facts.

The manifestations of arithmetic difficulty depend on the age and stage of the child. Children with arithmetic difficulties initially experience problems with the count sequence, as they grow older they may tend to rely on the "count-on" strategy in simple addition for longer than typically developing children, albeit error-prone, and they have difficulty in learning number facts. With more complex addition problems, they tend to guess more and less accurately than their peers (Geary, Hoard, Byrd-Craven & DeSoto, 2004). Geary (1990) suggested that mathematically disabled children use the same strategies as age-matched controls but differ in the speed and skill of strategy execution, they can retrieve fewer number facts, they are poor at monitoring their counting and they are poor at detecting computational errors (Geary, Bow-Thomas, & Yao, 1992).

The incidence of mathematics difficulties is less well documented than for reading difficulties. In the UK, Lewis, Hitch, and Walker (1994) used a simple cut-off approach to defining difficulties among 9- to 10-year-old children and reported that only 1.3% of children showed a specific difficulty in maths (standard score less than 85) in the presence of normal nonverbal ability and reading (at or above a standard score of 90 on both). However, another 2.3% had both reading and maths problems defined in an analogous way. This study reported an equal incidence of maths difficulties in boys and girls, in contrast to the higher incidence of reading difficulties among boys that they (and other studies) reported. Other large-scale studies have reported incidence rates of 6–7% for mathematics difficulties (Baker & Cantwell 1985; Gross-Tsur, Manor, & Shalev, 1996) while Share, Moffit, and Silva, (1988) using laxer criteria (a standard score of 92, the bottom 30% of the population) found combined rates of mathematics difficulties (with and without reading problems) of 11.2%. Given the different populations studied, and the different criteria for classification adopted, it is difficult to compare the rates reported. Nonetheless, it is clear that mathematical learning difficulties occur quite frequently and are often associated with reading difficulties. They also commonly co-occur with attention problems; Gross-Tsur, Manor, & Shalev, (1996) reported that 26% of children with mathematics disorder also had ADHD.

Cognitive Explanations of Arithmetic Difficulties

There is a relatively small literature investigating the cognitive impairments associated with mathematical difficulty in children who do not have comorbid reading impairments. Most of the evidence comes from arithmetic tasks (rather than mathematical problem-solving) and is therefore limited.

Deficits in Number Processing

Dehaene (1997) has argued that the basis of numerical cognition is a "number sense" – a preverbal system involving the ability to understand physical magnitudes and numerical quantities. It is possible that many of the problems observed in children with mathematics difficulties stem from a basic impairment in a number sense system that develops early and forms the foundation for later acquired verbally mediated mathematical skills (such as addition; Geary, 1993).

In line with this, Geary, Hoard, and Hamson (1999) found that children with arithmetic problems were less accurate than controls at comparing the magnitudes of Arabic digits. Landerl, Bevan, & Butterworth, (2004) found that children with arithmetic difficulties, either alone or comorbid with reading difficulties, were slower than controls at number naming, number reading, number comparisons and verbal counting. Thus, basic number processing has been shown to be impaired in children with specific arithmetic difficulties, and is to some degree independent of other abilities (Dehaene, 1997; Gelman & Butterworth, 2005). In children with intact number sense, other cognitive resources that are used in mathematics seem to be deficient.

Working Memory and Speed of Processing Impairments

During calculation, subcomponents of an arithmetic problem must be held in temporary storage while processing proceeds. With multidigit problems, it is necessary to monitor the calculation process, to inhibit numbers from the initial calculation and to hold in mind the products of different steps in the calculation. Thus, arithmetic skills carry both simple and complex working memory demands and also tap executive function. It is therefore not surprising that working memory deficits are associated with arithmetic difficulties.

Children with arithmetic difficulties perform poorly on complex working memory tasks, such as backward digit span (which has an executive component) and counting span (Geary, Hoard, & Hamson, 1999; Hitch & McAuley, 1991; Passolunghi & Siegal, 2001) but not typically on simple tests of verbal short-term or phonological memory unless the task has a numerical component (Geary, Brown, & Samaranayake, 1991; Hitch & McAuley, 1991).

According to Kail (1991), the amount of information that can be retained in memory depends on speed of processing, which in turn is related to the amount of attentional resources that can be directed to different tasks (Case, 1985). Bull and Johnston (1997) found that processing speed accounted for unique variance in arithmetic ability among 7-year-old children after controlling for differences in reading ability; children with lower arithmetic ability were slower than controls at number naming and sequencing, number matching, pegboard speed, one-syllable speech rate and reciting the alphabet. However, no IQ data were provided, and therefore processing speed may have been a proxy for general ability. Durand, Hulme, Larkin, and Snowling (2005) found that speed of information processing (as assessed by speed of visual search) was not a unique predictor of arithmetic skill after the effects of IQ and the speed of number comparison had been accounted for. This suggests that the speed of processing numerical information (rather than general information processing speed) may be critical for the development of arithmetic skills.

Executive Deficits

A body of evidence implicates executive deficits in arithmetic disability. McLean and Hitch (1999) found that 9-year-old children with specific arithmetic difficulties were impaired on the "Trail-Making" task where they were required to connect alternating sequences of numbers and letters (e.g., 1-A, 2-B) or numbers and colors (e.g., 1-yellow, 1-pink, 2-yellow, 2-pink). In a similar vein, Bull, Johnston, and Roy (1999) reported that children with high and low arithmetic ability differed on several aspects of the Wisconsin Card Sorting Test, notably perseveration (see also Bull & Scerif, 2001). The authors proposed that children with specific arithmetic difficulties have executive impairments that impair their ability to shift psychological set, plan action and judge the reasonableness of answers – all skills that are involved in mathematics. However, such difficulties may be attributable to comorbidities with other disorders (e.g., ADHD) that have not been controlled for in these studies.

Spatial Deficits

There is good evidence for associations between mathematical and spatial abilities (Dehaene, 1997; Hermelin & O'Connor,

1986). It is also common for children with non-verbal learning difficulties (typically associated with deficits on tests of spatial ability and performance IQ) to show mathematical difficulties (but not necessarily problems with number facts that are verbal). Such associations may reflect the anatomical proximity of brain systems subserving number sense and spatial processing. Alternatively, they may reflect a more fundamental association; the number sense system is itself a spatial system involving a spatially arranged "number line" (Dehaene, 1997). More basically, dealing with place values in arithmetic requires that we keep track of the spatial arrangements of numbers.

Verbal Impairments

Some aspects of arithmetic involve verbal skills. Learning to count is a verbal skill and problems with learning the count sequence are common in children with mathematics disorder. Similarly, arithmetic problems may place heavy demands on verbal working memory systems and these in turn place heavy demands on phonological (speech-based) coding. The frequent co-occurrence of reading and mathematics difficulties indicates that many children with mathematics difficulties will have phonological problems, and such problems might well be expected to compromise learning to count and the manipulation of numerical information in verbal working memory tasks.

To summarize, the nature of mathematics difficulties is much less well understood than reading difficulties, and this reflects the fact that much less is understood about the mechanisms of mathematic skills and their development than for reading skills and their development. Mathematical skills depend upon a complex interplay between non-verbal and verbal cognitive systems, and mathematical skills are arguably more diverse and more complex than reading skills. It seems likely from a cognitive perspective that mathematical difficulties may result from a number of underlying deficits, including deficits in a non-verbal "number sense" system located in parietal brain areas as well as verbal systems that interact with this system. Further progress in this area is likely to depend upon longitudinal studies that attempt to focus on more well-defined arithmetical skills.

Etiology

Genetic Effects

There is evidence indicating substantial genetic and environmental influences on the development of mathematical skills generally, and more specifically on the development of mathematics difficulties. There is good evidence that mathematical difficulties tend to run in families but this may reflect either shared environment or genetic effects. In a large-scale UK twin study, Kovas, Harlaar, Petrill, and Plomin (2005) found evidence for substantial heritability for normal variations in mathematical skills. There were substantial overlaps between the genes responsible for arithmetic and general intelligence, and arithmetic and reading, although the degree of overlap was far from perfect, suggesting that there are specific genetic effects on the development of arithmetic skills.

There are very few studies that have directly assessed possible genetic influences on mathematical difficulties (as opposed to normal variations in mathematical skills). In a study with a large sample size (Oliver, Harlaar, Hayiou-Thomas *et al.*, 2004), the heritability of mathematical difficulties was assessed by selecting children in the bottom 15% of the population on teacher ratings of children's mathematical abilities. This study yielded a high group heritability estimate for mathematical difficulties of 0.65 (compared to the estimate of 0.38 reported by Alarcón, DeFries, Light, & Pennington, 1997, based on a smaller sample). These results are compatible with the same genetic influences operating to produce the group deficits in mathematics as well as the range of individual differences in mathematical skills observed within the population as a whole (Plomin & Kovas, 2005).

In summary, current evidence suggests that there are substantial genetic influences on mathematical difficulties and that these same genetic influences may also operate to influence individual differences among people in the normal range of mathematical ability. It has also been reported that the co-morbidity between mathematical and reading difficulties is in part brought about by common genetic influences operating on both disorders (Knopik, Alarcón, & DeFries, 1997).

Brain Bases of Arithmetic Disorders

Neuroscientific studies suggest that the neural substrate of the number sense system depends critically upon bilateral areas of the horizontal intraparietal sulcus (HIPS) (Dehaene & Cohen, 1997). Dehaene, Piazza, Pinel, and Cohen (2003) have proposed that there are three parietal circuits for numerical processing. Problems in the development of such brain systems may be fundamental to the problems observed in children with mathematical difficulties, although as yet direct evidence for this is lacking (Wilson & Dehaene, 2006). Consistent with the idea of mathematical difficulties being associated with parietal dysfunction, Isaacs, Edmonds, Lucas, and Gadian (2001) reported a specific reduction in gray matter in the left HIPS in a group of adolescents with mathematical difficulties (without reading problems) who had been born prematurely, compared with a control group without mathematical difficulties who had been born equally prematurely. This difference in the left HIPS was only found for children with problems with calculation, and not for another group of children who had problems with mathematical reasoning. Also, several studies have shown parietal deficits in Turner's syndrome, a syndrome associated with arithmetic deficits (Reiss, Mazzocco, Greenlaw, Freund, & Ross, 1995).

Developmental Co-ordination Disorder

Nature, Classification and Incidence

Developmental co-ordination disorder (sometimes referred to as "dyspraxia") is a disorder of motor skills and is included here because problems with motor skills can adversely affect children's educational achievements and self-esteem. Formally, the diagnosis of developmental co-ordination disorder (DCD) is used to describe problems of motor co-ordination that occur in otherwise normal children and significantly affect the activities of daily living. In practice, such problems often signify risk factors for other disorders, and DCD is commonly found in association with developmental disorders such as language impairment (Hill, 2001) or autism, and the overlap with attention problems is high (Gillberg, 1999).

Population estimates of the incidence of DCD vary widely (5–18%) and these estimates depend both on the tests and the cut-offs used for diagnosis (Geuze, Jongmans, Schoemaker, & Sit-Englesman, 2001). Arguably, tests for the assessment of motor difficulties are less thoroughly developed and less well standardized than tests of reading, arithmetic and IQ but teacher and parent ratings are useful screening tools (Chambers & Sugden, 2006; Green, Bishop, Wilson *et al.*, 2005). It has been reported that there is a ratio of at least two boys to each girl with DCD (Wright & Sugden, 1996), although data on sex ratios may be hard to interpret because some of the tasks used to assess motor skills are gender-biased (e.g., throwing a ball) and there is little agreement among professionals about how to diagnose DCD (Sugden & Chambers, 2005). The symptoms of DCD can vary considerably and may include gross motor difficulties, such as problems running, hopping, jumping, catching a ball and balancing, and fine motor difficulties including a lack of manual dexterity, difficulty in doing up buttons and laces, in dressing and in using eating utensils. Speech-motor skills can be affected and problems of pencil control are widespread. When DCD occurs in pure form, such children have been reported to have normal reading skills and only minor spelling problems (Lord & Hulme, 1987a) even though their handwriting is usually very poor.

A mistaken view is that children with DCD grow out of their clumsiness; follow-up studies are rare but evidence suggests that such children remain less physically competent throughout adolescence (Gillberg, Gillberg, & Groth, 1989) and the difficulties they have at secondary school include problems with handwriting and the presentation of work, and difficulties in science, art, design and technology (Losse, Henderson, Elliman *et al.*, 1991). However, the coupling between motor impairments and academic achievement may not be causal and is likely mediated by comorbidities and/or psychosocial problems.

Explanations of Developmental Co-ordination Disorder

A dominant approach to explaining the motor deficits found in children with DCD has been in terms of perceptual impairments, particularly in terms of problems with kinesthetic or visual perception. (An earlier term used to refer to this group of children was developmental apraxia and agnosia which captures the central role of perceptual disorders in the clinical profile of these children.)

Problems of Kinesthetic Perception

Kinesthesis refers to an awareness of the position, location and velocity of movement of the limbs and the forces exerted by the muscles. Poor kinesthetic sensitivity has been reported among children with DCD (Laszlo, Bairstow, & Bartripp, 1988) but this finding has not been widely replicated (Lord & Hulme, 1987b) and a meta-analysis found only a weak association between kinesthetic sensitivity and poor motor skills (Wilson & McKenzie, 1998).

Visual Perceptual Deficits

Stronger evidence exists for an association between visual perceptual problems and motor disorders (in the absence of problems with visual acuity; Henderson, Barnett, & Henderson, 1994; Lord & Hulme, 1987a), with the greatest deficiency being observed in visuospatial tasks, regardless of whether they have a motor component. It has been proposed that guidance of our movements in space depends upon a sensorimotor map that serves to translate visually perceived locations to spatially appropriate action patterns (Held & Hein, 1963). It could be argued that a deficit in the visual perception of spatial information will inevitably lead to problems in the guidance of movements and problems in "calibrating" and "recalibrating" the sensorimotor map during development. Clinically, occupational therapists often use visual perceptual training programs with these children (Cermak & Larkin, 2002).

Balance and Postural Control

More proximal causes of DCD have been proposed in balance and postural control, movement planning and preparation, and execution and feedback processes (Geuze, 2005). In addition, limitations of memory and attention and reduced muscle strength may have a role to play. It should be noted that in principle some of these difficulties might arise as a consequence of the perceptual impairments discussed above.

Etiology

There is evidence that low birth weight or prematurity increases the risk of developing the disorder (Jongmans, Demetre, Dubowitz, & Henderson, 1996; Marlow, Roberts, & Cooke, 1989), suggesting links with neurodevelopmental immaturity. Furthermore, as noted in ICD-10 (WHO, 1996), a careful clinical examination may reveal neurological symptoms such as choreiform movements of unsupported limbs in such children. More generally, the comorbidity of DCD with impairments of reading and language, as well as with ADHD and autism spectrum disorder suggests shared genetic risk with these other developmental disorders (see chapter 3; Chambers & Sugden, 2006). A recent behavioral genetic study using questionnaire-based measures of DCD and ADHD with a large sample of twins (Martin, Piek, & Hay, 2006) indicates a substantial heritable influence on each disorder, as well as a substantial shared genetic influence.

Non-verbal Learning Disabilities

Definition

A diagnosis of non-verbal learning disabilities (NLD) is sometimes given to a child who displays difficulties with visual-perceptual-organizational abilities, motor skills, tactile perception, and non-verbal problem-solving in the absence of basic decoding or spelling impairments (Rourke, 1989, 1995). However, non-verbal learning difficulty syndrome is not a disorder with validated clinical criteria and therefore the diagnosis is controversial; rather it cuts across taxonomies such as reading and mathematical disorders that classify children according to patterns of impairment in the academic arena. Although described as a non-verbal difficulty, many children with NLD experience speech-language difficulties including pragmatic deficits (Semrud-Clikeman & Hynd, 1990). Worling, Humphries, and Tannock (1999) reported that children with NLD had difficulties making inferences despite apparently good verbal skills, and Klin, Volkmar, Sparrow, Cicchetti, and Rourke (1995) found a strikingly high degree of concordance between Asperger's syndrome and NLD but not between NLD and high-functioning autism.

Cognitive Deficits in Non-verbal Learning Disabilities

Most studies of NLD involve clinical samples and epidemiological data are not available. Moreover, few research studies have included adequate control groups and findings regarding the cognitive deficits in NLD are often tautological in that they reflect diagnostic or recruitment criteria. For example, although it is possible that deficits in spatial cognition are at the core of the syndrome, it must be remembered that the diagnosis may have been given to children who in particular gain lower performance than verbal IQs. Similar criticisms can be leveled at studies that test Rourke's (1995) hypothesis that the primary deficits are in visual and tactile perception, dealing with novel stimuli, and analogical reasoning (e.g., Chow & Skuy, 1999; Cornoldi, Dalla Vecchia, & Tressoldi, 1995).

It seems likely that, as theoretical understanding of the different components of NLD and their cognitive causes improves, the syndrome will be reconceptualized. At the present time, positing an overarching syndrome of NLD has little value and it is more productive clinically to assess and treat the diverse problems that are brought together under this heading.

Emotional and Behavioral Adjustment in Learning Difficulties

Reading Difficulties

There is evidence of a link between reading difficulties and both disruptive behavior (Hinshaw, 1992; Maughan, Pickles, Hagell, Rutter, & Yule, 1996) and emotional disorders (Maughan, Rowe, Loeber, & Stouthamer-Loeber, 2003; Willcutt & Pennington, 2000). However, the processes responsible for these outcomes are not understood. An influential hypothesis has been that behavior problems associated with reading difficulties may result from progressive school failure and lowered self-esteem (Chapman & Tunmer, 1997). An alternative causal model of the relationship is that disruptive behavior at school is the result of attention problems which are comorbid with poor reading and may interfere with the acquisition of reading skills. However, the causal relationships between reading, behavior and emotion are complex, and may differ between boys and girls and depend upon the stage of development that is considered (Williams & McGee, 1994).

In a study of 289 9- to 15-year-olds identified as having specific literacy difficulties from a representative sample of some 5000 UK children, Carroll, Maughan, Goodman, and Meltzer (2005) reported that children with reading difficulties are at increased risk of attention problems, conduct disorder, anxiety disorders and depressed mood. However, they argued that the mediating mechanisms differ. The association between literacy difficulties and behavior problems was mediated by inattention (rather than hyperactivity), whereas the link with heightened levels of anxiety was direct. A similar conclusion was reached from a twin study of literacy difficulties by Willcutt and Pennington (2000). These investigators reported an increased risk of attention and conduct difficulties in probands as well as cotwins; however, anxiety was reported only in those with reading difficulties, suggesting that such difficulties may arise as the result of stresses associated with educational difficulties. Regarding the link between poor reading and low mood, Willcutt and Pennington (2000) reported heightened levels of depression in girls mediated by ADHD, whereas Carroll, Snowling, Hulme *et al.* (2003) found that self-reported low mood was more common in boys than girls, and primarily in the 11- to 12-year-old age group.

Longitudinal data are required to test hypotheses regarding the psychosocial sequelae of reading difficulties. Snowling, Muter, & Carroll, (2007) assessed the outcomes of children at family risk of dyslexia at 12 years. There was an elevated risk of attentional and emotional problems in those who had reading problems (according to parental report); however, the children rated themselves as positively as did normal readers, except in the academic arena. Maughan, Pickles, Hagell *et al.* (1996) followed 127 poor readers from the age of 10 years into early adulthood. There was a tendency for reading difficulties to be associated with poor attention and overactivity, which in turn placed poor readers at risk of behavior problems (see also Fergusson & Lynskey, 1997). However, behavior problems at 14 years reflected earlier behavior problems rather than reading difficulties, and social adversity was found to increase the risk of antisocial behavior among girls but not among boys (for whom increased rates of offending were associated with poor school attendance).

As young adults, about 25% of this sample remained severely impaired in reading (Maughan & Hagell, 1996). Nonetheless, relatively positive self-reports suggested that many had gained employment in which there were restricted literacy demands and their reading problems were no longer of functional significance. In the majority of areas, those with a history of specific reading difficulties were functioning comparably to peers. However, young women with a history of specific reading retardation were at increased risk of psychiatric disorder, possibly related to a high rate of relationship breakdown. Male poor readers, in contrast, had more difficulty in gaining independence. However, these difficulties were the consequence of comorbid difficulties with peer relationships rather than reading problems.

Other Learning Difficulties

Relatively little attention has been paid to the outcomes of specific learning difficulties other than reading although there is evidence that anxiety specific to the subject at school increases with time among poor mathematicians and in turn affects maths attainments.

A little evidence suggests that the psychosocial outcomes of children with developmental co-ordination disorder can be reasonably good with low self-esteem restricted to the motor domain (Losse, Henderson, Elliman *et al.*, 1991), although poor social competence has also been reported. A frequent observation has been that rates of depression and suicidal behavior or ideation in adolescents and young adults with NLD are relatively high. However, studies suffer from the lack of representative samples and appropriate control groups (Little, 1993), and mediating mechanisms are unclear. In particular, the role of comorbid disorders in determining outcomes has not been addressed.

In summary, although it is generally believed that specific learning difficulties can cause psychosocial problems, the evidence for this view is sparse. The literature suggests that the majority of children with specific difficulties in literacy, numeracy or motor skills are relatively free of mental health problems. The heightened susceptibility to psychiatric disorder reported for children with NLD may reflect its comorbid nature.

Clinical Implications

Assessment

Children with specific learning difficulties will rarely be referred to child psychiatrists unless such difficulties have contributed to emotional or behavioral difficulties. However, it may be easy to miss a specific learning difficulty in a child with a mental health problem (particularly in a child referred for ADHD).

Children's Reading Difficulties

If a referred child reports a failure to learn to read, has dyspraxic tendencies or is seriously underachieving, the most appropriate strategy is to refer this child to an agency within the school system for assessment. A comprehensive assessment should include assessment of general cognitive ability (IQ), single word reading and spelling, reading comprehension, expressive writing and number skills (the Wechsler scales provide tools for comprehensive assessment of these skills; WISC-IV, Wechsler, 2004; WIAT-II, Wechsler, 2005). The assessment will have more value if it proceeds to assess phonological skills and the reading strategies the child is currently using with a view to prescribing appropriate intervention. In addition, tests of speed of processing and working memory, and in-depth investigation of oral language skills may be appropriate (Snowling & Stackhouse, 2006). In the past such assessments were the domain of educational psychologists; however, now it is often a teacher with specialist qualifications who would undertake such assessments, replacing IQ testing with assessment of language and/or non-verbal reasoning.

Other Learning Difficulties

Given the substantial overlap between reading difficulties and difficulties with mathematics, an assessment of mathematical performance using standardized tests should ideally be part of a comprehensive literacy assessment. However, time constraints often preclude this and a regrettable fact is that most referrals are from parents or teachers who are more concerned with planning literacy rather than numeracy support.

It can be difficult for clinicians to provide parents with the answer to the question foremost in their mind, "Is my child dyslexic?" Current diagnostic practice varies considerably, and although the term "dyslexia" is more widely accepted in educational circles than in the past, it may be used in a general sense to convey "reading difficulties with a phonological basis," irrespective of IQ. It is also important for clinicians to be aware that the label dyslexia may be used differently by different agencies. As with all developmental disorders, clinicians need to emphasize to families the dimensional nature of dyslexia; it can vary from mild to severe, there may be individuals who show some but not all of the symptoms (likely in families with dyslexia) and the problems that the child experiences may change through development with compensation possible in favorable circumstances (Snowling & Maughan, 2006).

A number of different practitioners, including physiotherapists, occupational therapists, specialist teachers and pediatricians, have a role in the assessment of DCD. It is generally agreed that such assessments should incorporate the evaluation of a range of movements as well as the impact of motor difficulties on everyday skills and psychosocial functioning. Individually administered tests of gross and fine motor skills, incorporating ball skills, manipulative skills and balance, are commonly used (Henderson & Sugden, 1992) and parent and teacher completed checklists and self-report questionnaires can be useful (Chambers & Sugden, 2006; Green, Bishop, Wilson *et al.*, 2005). It is also recommended that prior to an intervention program, physical fitness should be assessed.

Interventions

At the time of writing, there are few randomized controlled trials evaluating educational interventions; however, calls have been made that these should become the "gold-standard" methodology for informing educational policy and practice (Torgerson & Torgerson, 2001).

Children who have a family history of dyslexia or a history of speech-language difficulties are at high risk of reading difficulties, and motor delays appear to be part of an inherited form of dyslexia. If speech production deficits persist to school age, the likelihood of literacy problems is high. It is therefore important that such children receive appropriate support during the preschool period, including speech and language therapy, and, more generally, parental support with literacy can be helpful (Hewison, 1988). However, it is important to be mindful that many children with preschool speech and language impairments may make a good start in learning to read but fail later as the demands of reading increase. Careful monitoring of high-risk children is therefore advisable throughout the primary school years to ensure the effects of early interventions do not wash out.

Reading Intervention

Theoretical knowledge of the relationship between phonological skills and learning to read, and phonological deficits in dyslexia has led to the development of effective reading intervention programs that promote phonological skills in the context of reading (Brooks, 2002; National Reading Panel, 2000; Troia, 1999). For children with reading difficulties, such programs are best delivered by trained personnel who understand how to tune a program to a child's specific needs. The main elements of such approaches (e.g., Hatcher, Hulme, & Ellis, 1994) include:

- Training in letter knowledge;
- Teaching concepts of print;
- Training to manipulate the phonemes in words;
- Applying letter and sound knowledge to word reading and writing (phonics);
- Reading text;
- Writing activities.

Recently, the approach has been adapted for delivery by mainstream teachers to whole classes, and by teaching assistants to small groups (Hatcher, 2006). In a randomized controlled trial, the approach has been shown to be effective with reading gains of on average 0.23 standard score points per hour of intervention, an educationally significant improvement (Hatcher, Hulme, Miles *et al.*, 2006). These findings converge with those of other research groups and have direct policy implications for the treatment of children with dyslexia in the school system (Torgesen, 2005).

However, it is important to emphasize that children with dyslexia can respond very slowly even to the most effective of teaching approaches (Hindson, Byrne, Fielding-Barnsley *et al.*, 2005). An important issue therefore is the problem of "*treatment resistors*" – those children who, despite high-quality intervention, do not respond to teaching and continue to have persistent reading impairments (Torgesen, 2000). These "difficult to remediate" children tend to have the most severe phonological deficits (Vellutino, Scanlon, Sipay *et al.*, 1996), are often socially disadvantaged and many experience emotional and behavioral difficulties. Because of the intractable nature of the disorder in some cases, some families turn to alternative or complementary therapies. The evidence base for the efficacy of such therapies is almost totally lacking (Muter, 2003). For children who do not respond to conventional treatments, the best advice at the present time is to consider more intensive therapies, including placement in special units. In addition, information technologies have a lot to offer. Ideally, students with dyslexia should be taught to become fluent keyboard users, with special instruction in the use of a spell-checker. In addition, some children with dyslexia can use voice-recognition technology as an aid to written work. In formal assessments and examinations, people with dyslexia should normally be eligible for concessions. The most common arrangement is extra time in written examinations, and dispensation for spelling errors. If the student has particularly poor reading and writing skills, then they may be allowed someone to read the questions to them or an amanuensis.

In contrast to what is known about how to teach word-level reading skills, far less is known about how to promote reading comprehension effectively (for review see Westby, 2004). A meta-analysis of reading comprehension interventions designed for typically developing children reported that the eight most effective methods for improving text comprehension were comprehension monitoring, co-operative learning, graphic/semantic organizers for learning new vocabulary, story structure training, question answering, question generation, summarization and multiple strategy teaching (National Reading Panel, 2000). Also, the collaborative practice of speech and language therapists with teachers is likely to provide useful strategies for these children to learn.

Maths Intervention

Evidence regarding effective interventions for children's mathematical difficulties is sparse. In the USA, there has been some limited evaluation of preschool programs for the prevention of mathematical difficulties (Starkey & Klein, 2000) and in the UK, evaluations of individualized programs of instruction for children with poor mathematical skills are in progress (Dowker, 2004). So far, to our knowledge, there are no studies that have investigated the effectiveness of interventions for older children who have developed mathematical difficulties. This is clearly an important area for further research. To date, the received view is that interventions are best targeted at specific arithmetic processes that are weak or impaired; however, there is as yet no evidence regarding specifically what works for which children.

Interventions for Developmental Co-ordination Disorder

Evidence regarding effective interventions for DCD is sparse (Mandich, Polatajko, Macnab, & Miller, 2001). Broadly speaking, there are two approaches to intervention for such children: process-oriented and task-oriented approaches (Sugden & Chambers, 2005; Wilson, 2005). Process-oriented approaches begin with an analysis of the underlying components of the task to be achieved and aim to train these processes. Examples include sensory integration methods and kinesthetic approaches but neither has met with much success when compared with control interventions. Task-oriented approaches are more functional and aim to teach skills that are deficient, for example, eating, dressing, ball catching or writing. Most practitioners aim to harness the support of parents and teachers when implementing such programs. This is one way of circumventing a possible disadvantage of such approaches which is lack of transfer to related activities.

Conclusions and Future Directions

Understanding of the nature and causes of children's reading difficulties is well advanced as is knowledge about appropriate interventions for word-level decoding difficulties. In this domain, cognitive models of reading acquisition have had a positive effect on progress. Although less is known about children's arithmetic difficulties, the influence of cognitive models is beginning to bear fruit on methods of assessment and intervention. An advantage of the cognitive approach to learning difficulties is that it makes contact with what is know about normal development; furthermore, an understanding of the cognitive phenotype of disorders can foster understanding of links between genes, brain and behavior. Future research is needed to understand the causes and treatments of motor impairments and to better understand how comorbidity changes the nature, developmental course and outcomes of specific learning difficulties.

Acknowledgment

This chapter was prepared with the support of a British Academy Research Readership to the first author.

References

Alarcón, M., DeFries, J., Light, J., & Pennington, B. (1997). A twin study of mathematics disability. *Journal of Learning Disabilities*, *30*, 617–623.

American Psychiatric Association. (2000). *Diagnostic and Statistical Manual of Mental Disorders* (4th edn.). Text revision. Washington DC: American Psychiatric Association.

Ashcraft, M. H., & Kirk, E. P. (2001). The relationships among working memory, math anxiety, and performance. *Journal of Experimental Psychology: General*, *130*, 224–237.

Bailey, P. J., & Snowling, M. J. (2002). Auditory processing and the development of language and literacy. *British Medical Bulletin*, *63*, 135–146.

Baker, L., & Cantwell, D. P. (1985). Developmental arithmetic disorder. In H. I. Kaplan, & B. J. Sadock (Eds.), *Comprehensive textbook of psychiatry* (pp. 1697–1700). Baltimore: Williams & Wilkins.

Bird, J., Bishop, D. V. M., & Freeman, N. H. (1995). Phonological awareness and literacy development in children with expressive phonological impairments. *Journal of Speech and Hearing Research*, *38*, 446–462.

Bishop, D. V. M. (2001). Genetic influences on language impairment and literacy problems in children: Same or different? *Journal of Child Psychology and Psychiatry*, *42*, 189–198.

Bishop, D. V. M., & Adams, C. (1990). A prospective study of the relationship between specific language impairment, phonological disorders and reading retardation. *Journal of Child Psychology and Psychiatry*, 31, 1027–1050.

Bishop, D. V. M., & Snowling, M. J. (2004). Developmental dyslexia and specific language impairment: Same or different? *Psychological Bulletin*, *130*, 858–888.

Blomert, L. (2005). *Dyslexie in Nederland, theorie, praktijk en beleid*. Amsterdam: Nieuwezijds.

Bowey, J. A. (2005). Predicting individual differences in learning to read. In M. J. Snowling, & C. Hulme (Eds.), *The Science of Reading: A Handbook* (pp. 155–172). Oxford: Blackwell.

Brooks, G. (2002). *What works for children with literacy difficulties? The effectiveness of intervention schemes* (No. RR380). London: Department for Education & Skills. www.dfes.gov.uk/research

Bull, R., & Johnston, R. S. (1997). Children's arithmetical difficulties: contributions from processing speed, item identification and short-term memory. *Journal of Experimental Child Psychology*, *65*, 1–24.

Bull, R., Johnston, R., & Roy, J. (1999). Exploring the roles of the visual-spatial sketch pad and central executive in children's arithmetic skills: views from cognition and developmental neuropsychology. *Developmental Neuropsychology*, *15*, 421–442.

Bull, R., & Scerif, G. (2001). Executive functioning as a predictor of children's mathematical ability: Inhibition, switching, and working memory. *Developmental Neuropsychology*, *19*, 273–293.

Byrne, B. (1998). *The foundation of literacy: The child's acquisition of the alphabetic principle*. Hove: Psychology Press.

Cain, K., Oakhill, J. V., Barnes, M. A., & Bryant, P. E. (2001). Comprehension skill, inference-making ability, and their relation to knowledge. *Memory and Cognition*, *29*, 850–859.

Cain, K., Oakhill, J., & Bryant, P. E. (2004). Children's reading comprehension ability: Concurrent prediction by working memory, verbal ability, and component skills. *Journal of Educational Psychology*, *96*, 31–42.

Caravolas, M. (2005). The nature and causes of dyslexia in different languages. In M. J. Snowling, & C. Hulme (Eds.), *The science of reading: A handbook* (pp. 336–356). Oxford: Blackwell.

Caravolas, M., Volín, J., & Hulme, C. (2005). Phoneme awareness is a key component of alphabetic literacy skills in consistent and inconsistent orthographies: Evidence from Czech and English children. *Journal of Experimental Child Psychology*, *92*, 107–139.

Carroll, J., Maughan, B., Goodman, R., & Meltzer, H. (2005). Literacy difficulties and psychiatric disorders: Evidence for co-morbidity. *Journal of Child Psychology and Psychiatry*, *46*, 524–532.

Carroll, J., Snowling, M. J., Hulme, C., & Stevenson, J. (2003). The development of phonological awareness in pre-school children. *Developmental Psychology*, *39*, 913–923.

Case, R. (1985). *Intellectual development: Birth to adulthood*. New York: Academic Press.

Catts, H. W., Adlof, S. M., Hogan, T. P., & Weismer, S. E. (2005). Are specific language impairment and dyslexia distinct disorders? *Journal of Speech, Language and Hearing Research*, *48*, 1378–1396.

Catts, H. W., Fey, M. E., Zhang, X., & Tomblin, J. B. (1999). Language basis of reading and reading disabilities: Evidence from a longitudinal investigation. *Scientific Studies of Reading*, *3*, 331–361.

Cermak, S. A., & Larkin D. (2002). *Developmental coordination disorder*. Albany, New York: Delmar Thompson Learning.

Chambers, M., & Sugden, D. (2006). *Early years movement skills: description, diagnosis and intervention*. Chichester, Sussex: Wiley.

Chapman, J. W., & Tunmer, W. E. (1997). A longitudinal study of beginning reading achievement and reading self-concept. *British Journal of Educational Psychology*, *67*, 279–291.

Chow, D., & Skuy, M. (1999). Simultaneous and successive cognitive processing in children with nonverbal learning disabilities. *School Psychology International*, *20*, 219–231.

Cope, N., Harold, D., Hill, G., Moskvina, V., Stevenson, J., Holmans, P., *et al.* (2005). Strong evidence that *KIAA0319* on chromosome 6p is a susceptibility gene for developmental dyslexia. *American Journal of Human Genetics*, *76*, 581–591.

Cornoldi, C., Dalla Vecchia, R., & Tressoldi, P. (1995). Visuo-spatial working memory limitations in low visuo-spatial high verbal intelligence. *Journal of Child Psychology and Psychiatry*, *36*, 1051–1064.

Cunningham, A., & Stanovich, K. (1990). Assessing print exposure and orthographic processing skill in children: A quick measure of reading experience. *Journal of Educational Psychology*, *82*, 733–740.

Dehaene, S. (1997). *The number sense: How the mind creates mathematics*. New York: Oxford University Press.

Dehaene, S., & Cohen, L. (1997). Cerebral pathways for calculation: Double dissociation between rote verbal and quantitative knowledge of arithmetic. *Cortex*, *33*, 219–250.

Dehaene, S., Piazza, M., Pinel, P., & Cohen, L. (2003). Three parietal circuits for number processing. *Cognitive Neuropsychology*, *20*, 487–506.

Dowker, A. (2004). *What works for children with mathematical difficulties?* Nottingham: Department for Education and Skills.

Durand, M., Hulme, C., Larkin, R., & Snowling, M. J. (2005). The cognitive foundation of reading and arithmetic skills. *Journal of Experimental Child Psychology*, *91*, 113–136.

Eckert, M. A. (2004). Neuroanatomical markers for dyslexia: A review of dyslexia structural imaging studies. *Neuroscientist*, *10*, 362–371.

Facoetti, A., Turatto, M. L., & Mascetti, G. G. (2001). Orienting of visual attention in dyslexia: Evidence for asymmetric hemispheric control of attention. *Experimental Brain Research*, *138*, 46–53.

Fergusson, D. M., & Lynsky, M. T. (1997). Early reading difficulties and later conduct problems. *Journal of Child Psychology and Psychiatry*, *38*, 899–907.

Fisher, S. E., & DeFries, J. C. (2002). Developmental dyslexia: Genetic dissociation of a complex trait. *Nature Neuroscience*, *3*, 767–780.

Frith, U. (1980). *Cognitive processes in spelling*. London: Academic Press.

Galaburda, A. (1994). Developmental dyslexia and animal studies: At the interface between cognition and neurology. *Cognition*, *50*, 133–149.

Galaburda, A. M., & Kemper, T. L. (1978). Cytoarchitectonic abnormalities in developmental dyslexia: A case study. *Annals of Neurology*, *6*, 94–100.

Geary, D. C. (1990). A componential analysis of an early learning deficit in mathematics. *Journal of Experimental Child Psychology*, *49*, 363–383.

Geary, D. C. (1993). Mathematical disabilities: Cognitive, neuropsychological and genetic components. *Psychological Bulletin*, *114*, 345–362.

Geary, D. C., Bow-Thomas, C. C., & Yao, Y. (1992). Counting knowledge and skill in cognitive addition: A comparison of normal and mathematically disabled children. *Journal of Experimental Child Psychology*, *54*, 372–391.

Geary, D. C., Brown, S., & Samaranayake, V. (1991). Cognitive addition: A short longitudinal study of strategy choice and speed of processing differences in normal and mathematically disabled children. *Journal of Experimental Child Psychology*, *27*, 787–797.

Geary, D. C., Hoard, M. K., & Hamson, C. O. (1999). Numerical and arithmetical cognition: Patterns of functions and deficits in children at risk for a mathematical disability. *Journal of Experimental Child Psychology*, *74*, 213–239.

Geary, D. C., Hoard, M. K., Byrd-Craven, J., & DeSoto, M. C. (2004). Strategy choices in simple and complex addition: Contributions of working memory and counting knowledge for children with mathematical disability. *Journal of Experimental Child Psychology*, *88*, 121–151.

Gelman, R., & Butterworth, B. (2005). Number and language: How are they related? *Trends in Cognitive Sciences*, *9*, 6–10.

Geuze, R. H. (2005). Motor impairment in DCD and activities of daily living. In D. Sugden, & M. Chambers (Eds.), *Children with developmental coordination disorder* (pp. 19–46). London: Whurr.

Geuze, R. H., Jongmans, M., Schoemaker, M., & Sit-Englesman, B. (2001). Clinical and research diagnostic criteria for developmental coordination disorder: A review and discussion. *Human Movement Science*, *20*, 7–47.

Gillberg, C. (1999). *Clinical child neuropsychiatry*. Cambridge: Cambridge University Press.

Gillberg, I., Gillberg, C., & Groth, J. (1989). Children with preschool minor neurodevelopmental disorders IV: behaviour and school achievement at age 13. *Developmental Medical Child Neurology*, *31*, 14–24.

Goswami, U., Thomson, J., Richardson, U., Stainthorp, R., Hughes, D., Rosen, S., *et al.* (2002). Amplitude envelope onsets and developmental dyslexia: A new hypothesis. *Proceedings of the National Academy of Sciences of the United States of America*, *99*, 10911–10916.

Goulandris, N. (Ed.). (2003). *Dyslexia in different languages: A cross-linguistic comparison*. London: Whurr.

Goulandris, N., & Snowling, M. J. (1991). Visual memory deficits: A plausible cause of developmental dyslexia? Evidence from a single case study. *Cognitive Neuropsychology*, *8*, 127–154.

Green, D., Bishop, T., Wilson, B., Crawford, S., Hooper, R., Kaplan, B., *et al.* (2005). Is questionnaire based screening part of the solution to waiting lists for children with Developmental Coordination Disorder? *British Journal of Occupational Therapy*, *68*, 2–10.

Grigorenko, E. L. (2005). A conservative meta-analysis of linkage and linkage-association studies of developmental dyslexia. *Scientific Studies of Reading*, *9*, 285–316.

Gross Tsur, V., Manor, O., & Shalev, R. S. (1996). Developmental dyscalculia: Prevalence and demographic features. *Developmental Medicine and Child Neurology*, *38*, 25–33.

Guttorm, T. K., Leppänen, P. H. T., Poikkeus, A.-M., Eklund, K. M., Lyytinen, P., & Lyttinen, H. (2005). Brain event-related potentials (ERPs) measured at birth predict later language development in children with and without familial risk for dyslexia. *Cortex*, *41*, 291–303.

Hanley, J. R. (2005). Learning to read in Chinese. In M. Snowling, & C. Hulme (Eds.), *The science of reading: A handbook* (pp. 316–335). Oxford: Blackwell Publishing.

Hari, R., Renvall, H., & Tanskanen, T. (2001). Left mini-neglect in dyslexic adults. *Brain*, *124*, 1373–1380.

Harm, M. W., & Seidenberg, M. S. (1999). Phonology, reading acquisition and dyslexia: Insights from connectionist models. *Psychological Review*, *106*, 491–528.

Harris, M., & Hatano, G. (2000). *Learning to read and write: A cross-linguistic perspective*. Cambridge: Cambridge University Press.

Hatcher, P. (2006). Phonological awareness and reading intervention. In M. J. Snowling, & J. Stackhouse (Eds.), *Dyslexia, speech and language: A practitioner's handbook* (2nd edn., pp. 167–197). London: Whurr.

Hatcher, P. J., & Hulme, C. (1999). Phonemes, rhymes and intelligence as predictors of children's responsiveness to remedial reading instruction: Evidence from a longitudinal intervention study. *Journal of Experimental Child Psychology*, *72*, 130–153.

Hatcher, P., Hulme, C., & Ellis, A. W. (1994). Ameliorating early reading failure by integrating the teaching of reading and phonological skills: The phonological linkage hypothesis. *Child Development*, *65*, 41–57.

Hatcher, P. J., Hulme, C., Miles, J. N. V., Carroll, J. M., Hatcher, J., Gibbs, S., *et al.* (2006). Efficacy of small group reading intervention for beginning readers with reading-delay: A randomized controlled trial. *Journal of Child Psychology and Psychiatry*, *47*, 820–827.

Hecht, S. A., Burgess, S. R., Torgesen, J. K., Wagner, R. K., & Rashotte, C. A. (2000). Explaining social class differences in growth of reading skills from beginning kindergarten through fourth grade: The role of phonological awareness, rate of access, and print knowledge. *Reading and Writing*, *12*, 99–127.

Held, R. & Hein, A. (1963). Movement produced stimulation in the development of visually guided reaching. *Journal of Comparative and Physiological Psychology*, *56*, 872–876.

Henderson, S., & Sugden, D. (1992). *Movement Assessment Battery for Children*. London: Psychological Corporation.

Henderson, S., Barnett, A., & Henderson, L. (1994). Visual-spatial problems and clumsiness: On the interpretation of conjoined deficits. *Journal of Child Psychology and Psychiatry*, *35*, 961–967.

Hermelin, B., & O'Connor, N. (1986). Spatial representations in mathematically and in artistically gifted children. *British Journal of Educational Psychology*, *56*, 150–157.

Hewison, J. (1988). The long term effectiveness of parental involvement in reading: A follow-up to the Haringey reading project. *British Journal of Educational Psychology*, *58*, 184–190.

Hill, E. L. (2001). Non-specific nature of specific language impairment: A review of the literature with regard to concomitant motor impairments. *International Journal of Language and Communication Disorders*, *36*, 149–171.

Hindson, B., Byrne, B., Fielding-Barnsley, R., Newman, C., Hine, D. W., & Shankweiler, D. (2005). Assessment and early instruction of pre-school children at risk for reading disability. *Journal of Educational Psychology*, *97*, 687–704.

Hinshaw, S. P. (1992). Externalizing behaviour problems and academic underachievement in childhood and adolescence: Causal relationships and underlying mechanisms. *Psychological Bulletin*, *111*, 127–155.

Hitch, G. J., & McAuley, E. (1991). Working memory in children with specific arithmetical learning difficulties. *British Journal of Psychology*, *82*, 375–386.

Hulslander, J., Talcott, J., Witton, C., DeFries, J., Pennington, B., Wadsworth, S., *et al.* (2004). Sensory processing, reading, IQ and attention. *Journal of Experimental Child Psychology*, *88*, 274–295.

International Dyslexia Association. (2002). *Definition of dyslexia http://www.interdys.org/* Adopted by the IDA Board of Directors, Nov. 12, 2002, and used by the National Institute of Child Health and Human Development (NICHD).

Isaacs, E., Edmonds, C., Lucas, A., & Gadian, D. (2001). Calculation difficulties in children of very low birth weight: A neural correlate. *Brain*, *124*, 1701–1707.

Joanisse, M. F., Manis, F. R., Keating, P., & Seidenberg, M. S. (2000). Language deficits in dyslexic children: Speech perception, phonology and morphology. *Journal of Experimental Child Psychology*, *77*, 30–60.

Johnson, M. (2005). *Developmental cognitive neuroscience* (2nd edn.). Oxford: Blackwell.

Jongmans, M., Demetre, J., Dubowitz, L., & Henderson, S. E. (1996). How local is the impact of a specific learning difficulty on premature children's evaluation of their own competence? *Journal of Child Psychology and Psychiatry*, *37*, 565–568.

Kail, R. (1991). Developmental change in speed of processing during childhood and adolescence. *Psychological Bulletin*, *109*, 490–501.

Klin, A., Volkmar, F. R., Sparrow, S. S., Cicchetti, D. V., & Rourke, B. P. (1995). Validity and neuropsychological characterization of Asperger syndrome: Convergence with nonverbal learning disabilities syndrome. *Journal of Child Psychology and Psychiatry*, *36*, 1127–1140.

Knopik, V., Alarcón, M., & DeFries, J. (1997). Comorbidity of mathematics and reading deficits: Evidence for a genetic etiology. *Behavior Genetics*, *27*, 447–453.

Kovas, Y., Harlaar, N., Petrill, S. A., & Plomin, R. (2005). 'Generalist genes' and mathematics in 7-year-old twins. *Intelligence*, *33*, 473–489.

Landerl, K., Bevan, A., & Butterworth, B. (2004). Developmental dyscalculia and basic numerical capacities: A study of 8–9-year-old students. *Cognition*, *93*, 99–125.

Landerl, K., Wimmer, H., & Frith, U. (1997). The impact of orthographic consistency on dyslexia: A German-English comparison. *Cognition*, *63*, 315–334.

Lazlo, J. L., Bairstow, P. J., & Bartrip, J. (1988). A new approach to treatment of perceptuo-motor dysfunction, previously called 'clumsiness'. *Support for Learning*, *3*, 35–40.

Leonard, C. M., Eckert, M. A., Lombardino, L. J., Oakland, T., Kranzler, J., Mohr, C. M., *et al.* (2001). Anatomical risk factors for phonological dyslexia. *Cerebral Cortex*, *11*, 148–157.

Leonard, C. M., Eckert, M., Given, B., Berninger,V., & Eden, G. (2006). Individual differences in anatomy predict reading and oral language impairments in children. *Brain*, *129*, 3329–3342.

Leppänen, P. H. T., Eklund, K. M., & Lyytinen, H. (1997). Event-related brain potentials to change in rapidly presented acoustic stimuli in new borns. *Developmental Neuropsychology*, *13*, 175–204.

Lewis, C., Hitch, G. J., & Walker, P. (1994). The prevalence of specific arithmetic difficulties and specific reading difficulties in 9- to 10-year old boys and girls. *Journal of Child Psychology and Psychiatry*, *35*, 283–292.

Little, S. S. (1993). Nonverbal learning disabilities and socioemotional functioning: A review of recent literature. *Journal of Learning Disabilities*, *26*, 653–665.

Lord, R. & Hulme, C. (1987a). Perceptual judgements in normal and clumsy children. *Developmental Medicine and Child Neurology*, *29*, 250–257.

Lord, R. & Hulme, C. (1987b). Kinaesthetic sensitivity in normal and clumsy children. *Developmental Medicine and Child Neurology*, *29*, 720–725.

Losse, A., Henderson, S., Elliman, D., Hall, D., Knight, E., & Jongmans, M. (1991). Clumsiness in children: Do they grow out of it? A 10-year follow-up study. *Developmental Medicine and Child Neurology*, *33*, 55–68.

Lovegrove, W., Martin, F., & Slaghuis, W. (1986). The theoretical and experimental case for a visual deficit in specific reading disability. *Cognitive Neuropsychology*, *3*, 225–267.

Lovett, M. W., Ransby, M. J., & Barron, R. W. (1988). Treatment, sybtype and word-type effects in dyslexic children's response to remediation. *Brain and Language*, *34*, 328–349.

Lyytinen, H., Erskine, J. M., Tolvanen, A., Torppa, M., Poikkeus, A.-M., & Lyytinen, P. (2006). Trajectories of reading development: A follow-up from birth to school age of children with and without risk for dyslexia. *Merrill-Palmer Quarterly*, *52*, 514–546.

Mandich, A., Polatajko, H., Macnab, J., & Miller, L. (2001). Treatment of children with Developmental Coordination Disorder: What is the evidence? *Physical Occupational Therapy in Pediatrics*, *20*, 51–68.

Manis, F. R., McBride-Chang, C., Seidenberg, M. S., Keating, P., Doi, L. M., Munson, B., *et al.* (1997). Are speech perception deficits associated with developmental dyslexia? *Journal of Experimental Child Psychology*, *66*, 211–235.

Marlow, N., Roberts, B., & Cooke, R. (1989). Motor skills in extremely low birth weight children at the age of 6 years. *Archives of Disease in Childhood*, *64*, 839–847.

Martin, N. C., Piek, J. P., & Hay, D. (2006). DCD and ADHD: A genetic study of their shared aetiology. *Human Movement Science*, *25*, 110–124.

Maughan, B., Messer, J., Collishaw, S., Pickles, A., Yule, W., Snowling, M., *et al.* (submitted). Persistence of literacy problems: Spelling in adolescence and at mid-life.

Maughan, B., & Hagell, A. (1996). Poor readers in adulthood: Psychosocial functioning. *Development and Psychopathology*, *8*, 457–476.

Maughan, B., Pickles, A., Hagell, A., Rutter, M., & Yule, W. (1996). Reading problems and antisocial behaviour: Developmental trends in comorbidity. *Journal of Child Psychology and Psychiatry*, *37*, 405–418.

Maughan, B., Rowe, R., Loeber, R., & Stouthamer-Loeber, M. (2003). Reading problems and depressed mood. *Journal of Abnormal Child Psychology*, *31*, 219–229.

McCloskey, M., Caramazza, A., & Basili, A. (1985). Cognitive mechanisms in number processing and calculation: Evidence from dyscalculia. *Brain and Cognition*, *4*, 171–196.

McLean, J. F., & Hitch, G. J. (1999). Working memory impairments in children with specific arithmetic learning difficulties. *Journal of Experimental Child Psychology*, *74*, 240–260.

Mody, M. (2003). Rapid auditory processing deficits in dyslexia: A commentary on two differing views. *Journal of Phonetics*, *31*, 529–539.

Muter, V. (2003). *Early reading development and dyslexia*. London: Whurr.

Muter, V., Hulme, C., Snowling, M. J., & Stevenson, J. (2004). Phonemes, rimes, vocabulary, and grammatical skills as foundations of early reading development: Evidence from a longitudinal study. *Developmental Psychology*, *40*, 665–681.

Nathan, L., Stackhouse, J., Goulandris, N., & Snowling, M. J. (2004). Literacy skills and children with speech difficulties. *Journal of Speech, Hearing, and Language Research*, *47*, 377–391.

Nation, K. (2005). Children's reading comprehension difficulties. In M. J. Snowing, & C. Hulme (Eds.), *The science of reading: a handbook* (pp. 248–266). Oxford: Blackwell.

Nation, K., Clarke, P., Marshall, C., & Durand, M. (2004). Hidden language impairments in children: Parallels between poor reading comprehension and specific language impairment? *Journal of Speech, Language, and Hearing Research*, *47*, 199–211.

National Reading Panel. (2000). *Report of the National Reading Panel: Reports of the subgroups*. Washington, DC: National Institute of Child Health and Human Development Clearing House.

Nelson, H., & Warrington, E. K. (1974). Developmental spelling retardation and its relation to other cognitive abilities. *British Journal of Psychology*, *65*, 265–274.

Nicolson, R. I., & Fawcett, A. J. (1990). Automaticity: A new framework for dyslexia research. *Cognition*, *35*, 159–182.

Nicolson, R. I., Fawcett, A. J., & Dean, P. (2001). Developmental dyslexia: The cerebellar deficit hypothesis. *Trends in Neurological Sciences*, *24*, 508–511.

Oliver, B., Harlaar, N., Hayiou-Thomas, M. E., Kovas, Y., Walker, S. O., Petrill, S. A., *et al*. (2004). A twin study of teacher-reported mathematics performance and low performance in 7-year-olds. *Journal of Educational Psychology*, *96*, 504–517.

Olson, R. K., Datta, H. J. G., & DeFries, J. C. (1999). A behavior-genetic analysis of reading disabilities and component processes. In R. M. Klein, & P. McMullen (Eds.), *Converging methods for understanding reading and dyslexia* (pp. 133–152). Cambridge, MA: MIT Press.

Passolunghi, C. M., & Siegal, L. S. (2001). Short-term memory, working memory, and inhibitory control in children with difficulties in arithmetic problem solving. *Journal of Experimental Child Psychology*, *80*, 44–57.

Pennington, B. F. (2006). From single to multiple deficit models of developmental disorders. *Cognition*, *101*, 385–413.

Pennington, B. F., & Lefly, D. L. (2001). Early reading development in children at family risk for dyslexia. *Child Development*, *72*, 816–833.

Pennington, B. F., & Olson, R. K. (2005). Genetics of dyslexia. In M. J. Snowling, & C. Hulme (Eds.), *The science of reading: A handbook* (pp. 453–472). Oxford: Blackwell.

Petrill, S. A., Deater-Deckard, K., Schatschneider, C., & Davis, C. (2005). Measured environmental influences on early reading: evidence from an adoption study. *Scientific Studies of Reading*, *9*, 237–259.

Phillips, B. M., & Lonigan, C. J. (2005). Social correlates of emergent literacy. In M. J. Snowling, & C. Hulme (Eds.), *The science of reading: A handbook* (pp. 173–187). Oxford: Blackwell.

Plaut, D. C., McClelland, J. L., Seidenberg, M. S., & Patterson, K. (1996). Understanding normal and impaired word reading: Computational principles in quasi-regular domains. *Psychological Review*, *103*, 56–115.

Plomin, R., & Kovas, Y. (2005). Generalist genes and learning disabilities. *Psychological Bulletin*, *131*, 592–617.

Price, C. J., & McCrory, E. (2005). Functional brain imaging studies of skilled reading and developmental dyslexia. In M. J. Snowling, & C. Hulme (Eds.), *The science of reading: A handbook* (pp. 473–496). Oxford: Blackwell.

Raitano, N. A., Pennington, B. F., Tunick, R. A., & Boada, R. (2004). Pre-literacy skills of subgroups of children with phonological disorder. *Journal of Child Psychology and Psychiatry*, *45*, 821–835.

Ramus, F., Rosen, S., Dakin, S. C., Day, B. L., Castellote, J. M., White, S., *et al*. (2003). Theories of developmental dyslexia: Insights from a multiple case study of dyslexic adults. *Brain*, *126*, 1–25.

Reiss, A. L., Mazzocco, M. M., Greenlaw, R., Freund, L. S., & Ross, J. L. (1995). Neurodevelopmental effects of X monosomy: A volumetric imaging study. *Annals of Neurology*, *38*, 731–738.

Riddick, B. (2006). Dyslexia-friendly schools in the UK. *Topics in language disorders: Dyslexia in the current context*, *26*, 144–156.

Roach, N. W., & Hogben, J. H. (2004). Attentional modulation of visual processing in adult dyslexia: A spatial cuing deficit. *Psychological Science*, *15*, 650–654.

Romani, C., Olson, A., & Di Betta, A. M. (2005). Spelling disorders. In M. J. Snowling, & C. Hulme (Eds.), *The science of reading: A handbook* (pp. 431–448). Oxford: Blackwell.

Romani, C., Ward, J., & Olson, A. (1999). Developmental surface dysgraphia: What is the underlying cognitive impairment? *Quarterly Journal of Experimental Psychology*, *52*, 97–128.

Rourke, B. P. (1989). *Nonverbal learning disabilities. The syndrome and the model*. New York: Guilford.

Rourke, B. P. (Ed.). (1995). *Syndrome of nonverbal learning disabilities: Neuro-developmental manifestations*. New York: Guilford.

Rutter, M. (2006). *Genes and behavior: Nature-nurture interplay explained*. Oxford: Blackwell.

Rutter, M., Caspi, A., Fergusson, D., Horwood, L. J., Goodman, R., Maughan, B., *et al*. (2004). Sex differences in developmental reading disability: New findings from 4 epidemiological studies. *Journal of the American Medical Association*, *291*, 2007–2012.

Rutter, M., & Maughan, B. (2002). School effectiveness findings 1979–2002. *Journal of School Psychology*, *40*, 451–475.

Rutter, M., & Maughan, B. (2005). Dyslexia: 1965–2005. *Behavioural and Cognitive Psychotherapy*, *33*, 389–402.

Rutter, M., & Yule, W. (1975). The concept of specific reading retardation. *Journal of Child Psychology and Psychiatry*, *16*, 181–197.

Scarborough, H. S. (1990). Very early language deficits in dyslexic children. *Child Development*, *61*, 1728–1743.

Seidenberg, M. S., & McClelland, J. (1989). A distributed, developmental model of word recognition. *Psychological Review*, *96*, 523–568.

Semrud-Clikeman, M., & Hynd, G. (1990). Right hemispheric dysfunction in nonverbal learning disabilities: Social, academic and adaptive functioning in adults and children. *Psychological Bulletin*, *107*, 196–209.

Serniclaes, W., Van Heghe, S., Mousty, P., Carré, R., & Sprenger-Charolles, L. (2004). Allophonic mode of speech perception in dyslexia. *Journal of Experimental Child Psychology*, *87*, 336–361.

Seymour, P. H. K. (2005). Early reading development in European orthographies. In M. J. Snowling, & C. Hulme (Eds.), *The science of reading: A handbook* (pp. 296–315). Oxford: Blackwell.

Share, D. L. (1995). Phonological recoding and self-teaching: Sine qua non of reading acquisition. *Cognition*, *55*, 151–218.

Share, D. L., Moffitt, T. E., & Silva, P. A. (1988). Factors associated with arithmetic-and-reading disability and specific arithmetic disability. *Journal of Learning Disabilities*, *21*, 313–320.

Shaywitz, B. A., Fletcher, J. M., Holahan, J. M., & Shaywitz, S. E. (1992a). Discrepancy compared to low achievement definitions of reading disability: Results from the Connecticut longitudinal study. *Journal of Learning Disabilities*, *25*, 639–648.

Shaywitz, B. A., Shaywitz, S. E., Blachman, B. A., Pugh, K. R., Fulbright, R. K., Skudlarski, P., *et al*. (2004). Development of left occipito-temporal systems for skilled reading in children after a phonologically-based intervention. *Biological Psychiatry*, *55*, 926–933.

Shaywitz, S. E., Escobar, M. D., Shaywitz, B. A., Fletcher, J. M., & Makugh, R. (1992b). Evidence that dyslexia may represent the lower tail of a normal distribution of reading ability. *New England Journal of Medicine*, *326*, 145–150.

Shaywitz, S. E., Shaywitz, B. A., Fletcher, J. M., & Escobar, M. D. (1990). Prevalence of reading disability in boys and girls: Results of the Connecticut longitudinal study. *Journal of the American Medical Association*, *264*, 998–1002.

Simos, P. G., Fletcher, J. M., Bergman, E., Breir, J. I., Foorman, B. R., Castillo, E. M., *et al.* (2002). Dyslexia-specific brain activation profile becomes normal following successful remedial training. *Neurology*, *58*, 1203–1213.

Skoyles, J., & Skottun, B. (2004). On the prevalence of magnocellular deficits in the visual system of non-dyslexic individuals. *Brain and Language*, *88*, 79–82.

SLI Consortium. (2002). A genome-wide scan identifies two novel loci involved in specific language impairment (SLI). *American Journal of Human Genetics*, *70*, 384–398.

SLI Consortium. (2004). Highly significant linkage to SLI1 locus in an expanded sample of individuals affected by Specific Language Impairment (SLI). *American Journal of Human Genetics*, *74*, 1225–1238.

Snowling, M. J. (2000). *Dyslexia* (2nd edn.). Blackwell: Oxford.

Snowling, M. J., Bishop, D. V. M., & Stothard, S. E. (2000). Is preschool language impairment a risk factor for dyslexia in adolescence? *Journal of Child Psychology & Psychiatry*, *41*, 587–600.

Snowling, M. J., Gallagher, A., & Frith, U. (2003). Family risk of dyslexia is continuous: Individual differences in the precursors of reading skill. *Child Development*, *74*, 358–373.

Snowling, M. J., & Maughan, B. (2006). Reading and other learning disabilities. In C. Gillberg, R. Harrington, & H.-C. Steinhausen (Eds.), *Clinician's deskbook of child and adolescent psychiatry* (pp. 417–446). New York: Cambridge University Press.

Snowling, M., Muter, V., & Carroll, J. (2007). Children at family-risk of dyslexia: A follow-up in adolescence. *Journal of Child Psychology and Psychiatry*, *48*, 609–618.

Snowling, M. J., & Stackhouse, J. (Eds.). (2006). *Dyslexia, speech and language: A practitioner's handbook* (2nd edn.). London: Whurr.

Stanovich, K. E., & Siegel, L. S. (1994). The phenotypic performance profile of reading-disabled children: A regression-based test of the phonological-core variable-difference model. *Journal of Educational Psychology*, *86*, 24–53.

Starkey, P., & Klein, A. (2000). Fostering parental support for children's mathematical development. *Early Education and Development*, *11*, 659–680.

Stein, J., & Talcott, J. (1999). Impaired neuronal timing in developmental dyslexia: The magnocellular hypothesis. *Dyslexia*, *5*, 59–77.

Stevenson, J., & Fredman, G. (1990). The social environmental correlates of reading ability. *Journal of Child Psychology and Psychiatry and Allied Disciplines*, *31*, 681–698.

Stevenson, J., Graham, P., Fredman, G., & McLoughlin, V. (1987). A twin study of genetic influences on reading and spelling ability and disability. *Journal of Child Psychology and Psychiatry*, *28*, 229–247.

Sugden, D., & Chambers, M. (2005). *Children with developmental coordination disorder*. London: Whurr.

Taipale, M., Kaminen, N., Nopola-Hemmi, J., Haltia, T., Myllyluoma, B., & Lyytinen, H. (2003). A candidate gene for developmental dyslexia encodes a nuclear tetratricopeptide repeat domain protein dynamically regulated in brain. *Proceedings of the National Academy of Sciences of the United States of America*, *100*, 11553–11558.

Tallal, P. (1980). Auditory-temporal perception, phonics and reading disabilities in children. *Brain and Language*, *9*, 182–198.

Temple, C. M. (1994). The cognitive neuropsychology of the developmental dyscalculias. *Cahiers de Psychologie Cognitive*, *13*, 351–370.

Torgerson, C., & Torgerson, D. (2001). The need for randomised controlled trials in educational research. *British Journal of Educational Studies*, *25*, 129–143.

Torgesen, J. K. (2000). Individual differences in response to early interventions in reading: The lingering problem of treatment registers. *Learning Disabilities Research and Practice*, *15*, 55–64.

Torgesen, J. K. (2005). Recent discoveries on remedial interventions for children with dyslexia. In M. J. Snowling, & C. Hulme (Eds.), *The science of reading: A handbook* (pp. 521–537). Oxford: Blackwell.

Troia, G. A. (1999). Phonological awareness intervention research: A critical review of the experimental methodology. *Reading Research Quarterly*, *34*, 28–52.

Valdois, S., Bosse, M.-L., & Tainturier, M.-J. (2004). The cognitive deficits responsible for developmental dyslexia: Review of evidence for a selective visual attentional disorder. *Dyslexia*, *10*, 339–363.

Vellutino, F. R., Fletcher, J. M., Snowling, M. J., & Scanlon, D. M. (2004). Specific reading disability (dyslexia): what have we learned in the past four decades? *Journal of Child Psychology and Psychiatry*, *45*, 2–40.

Vellutino, F. R., Scanlon, D. M., Sipay, E., Small, S., Pratt, A., Chen, R., *et al.* (1996). Cognitive profiles of difficult-to-remediate and readily-remediated poor readers: Early intervention as a vehicle for distinguishing between cognitive and experiential deficits as basic causes of specific reading disability. *Journal of Educational Psychology*, *88*, 601–638.

Wechsler, D. (2004). *Wechsler Intelligence Scale for Children® – Fourth UK Edition (WISC-IV[UK])*. London: Harcourt Assessment.

Wechsler, D. (2005). *Wechsler Individual Achievement Test – Second UK Edition (WIAT-II[UK])*. London: Harcourt Assessment.

Westby, C. E. (2004). Assessing and remediating text comprehension problems. In H. W. Catts, & A. G. Kamhi (Eds.), *Lanugage and reading disabilities* (2nd edn., pp. 157–232). Boston, MA: Pearson Education.

White, S., Milne, E., Rosen, S., Hansen, P., Swettenham, J., Frith, U., *et al.* (2006). The role of sensorimotor impairments in dyslexia: A multiple case study of dyslexic children. *Developmental Science*, *9*, 237–269.

Whitehurst, G. J., & Lonigan, C. J. (1998). Child development and emergent literacy. *Child Development*, *69*, 848–872.

Willcutt, E., & Pennington, B. (2000). Psychiatry co-morbidity in children and adolescents with reading disability. *Journal of Child Psychology and Psychiatry*, *41*, 1039–1048.

Williams, S., & McGee, R. (1994). Reading attainment and juvenile delinquency. *Journal of Child Psychology and Psychiatry*, *35*, 441–461.

Wilson, A., & Dehaene, S. (2006). Number sense and developmental dyscalculia. In D. Coch, G. Dawson, & K. Fischer (Eds.), *Human behaviour, and the developing brain*. New York: Guilford.

Wilson, P. (2005). Practitioner review: approaches to assessment and treatment of children with DCD: an evaluative review. *Journal of Child Psychology and Psychiatry*, *46*, 806–823.

Wilson, P., & McKenzie, B. (1998). Information processing deficits associated with developmental coordination disorder: A meta-analysis of research findings. *Journal of Child Psychology and Psychiatry*, *39*, 829–840.

Wimmer, H., Mayringer, H., & Landerl, K. (2000). The double-deficit hypothesis and difficulties in learning to read a regular orthography. *Journal of Educational Psychology*, 92, 668–680.

Wolf, M., & Bowers, P. G. (1999). The double-deficit hypothesis for the developmental dyslexias. *Journal of Educational Psychology*, *91*, 415–438.

World Health Organization (WHO). (1996). *Multiaxial classification of child and adolescent psychiatric disorders: The ICD-10 classification of mental and behavioural disorders in children and adolescents*. Cambridge, UK: Cambridge University Press.

Worling, D. E., Humphries, T., & Tannock, R. (1999). Spatial and emotional aspects of language inferencing in nonverbal learning disabilities. *Brain and Language*, *70*, 220–239.

Wright, H., & Sugden, D. (1996). A two-step procedure for the identification of children with developmental coordination disorder in Singapore. *Developmental Medicine and Child Neurology*, *38*, 1099–1105.

Yuill, N., & Oakhill, J. (1991). *Children's problems in text comprehension*. Cambridge: Cambridge University Press.

Yule, W., Rutter, M., Berger, M., & Thompson, J. (1974). Over- and under-achievement in reading: Distribution in the general population. *British Journal of Educational Psychology*, *44*, 1–12.

49 Intellectual Disability

Stewart Einfeld and Eric Emerson

Terminology and Definitions

The terms used to refer to intellectual disability have undergone numerous changes over the last century. As terms used to describe socially devalued groups enter the common vocabulary, they quickly acquire disparaging connotations. Today's scientific terminology quickly becomes tomorrow's terms of abuse. "Idiots," "imbeciles," "morons," "subnormals" and "retards" are nowadays nothing more than terms of denigration.

In this chapter we use the term intellectual disability in preference to the synonymous terms "mental retardation" (used in the ICD-10 and DSM-IV-TR classificatory systems) and "learning disability" (often used in the UK). Our choice reflects intellectual disability having become the preferred terminology within the international scientific community. It also has the value of avoiding confusion arising from the use of terms that have very different meanings in different countries (e.g., learning disability).

The definition of intellectual disability involves two core components: a general deficit in cognitive functioning, which emerges during childhood (American Psychiatric Association, 2000; World Health Organization, 1996). A "general deficit in cognitive functioning" is usually operationalized as a score of less than 2 standard deviations (SD) below the mean on a standardized IQ test. (Given that most IQ tests are constructed to have a mean of 100 and standard deviation of 15, this is ordinarily equivalent to a score below 70.) However, intelligence is not a unitary construct. As such, individuals whose test performance places them within this range may have markedly different profiles across the wide range of cognitive skills and abilities that are assessed by IQ tests. The definition is important in discriminating between people with significant deficits in multiple areas of cognitive functioning and people with very specific cognitive deficits (or specific learning difficulties).

The second component of the definition (emergence during childhood, typically before the age of 18) is important in distinguishing people with intellectual disability from people with cognitive deficits acquired in later life; in particular, deficits associated with dementia.

Rutter's Child and Adolescent Psychiatry, 5th edition. Edited by M. Rutter, D. Bishop, D. Pine, S. Scott, J. Stevenson, E. Taylor and A. Thapar. ISBN: 978-1-4051-4549-7.

A third component, deficit in adaptive behavior, is sometimes added to the definition although this is more controversial. First, classificatory systems differ in the extent to which such deficits are seen as an inherent characteristic of the deficit in cognitive functioning or as an independent characteristic whose presence needs to be determined for the classification to apply. For example, ICD-10 guidance suggests that "adaptive behavior is *always impaired*, but in protected social environments where support is available this impairment may not be at all obvious in subjects with mild mental retardation" (World Health Organization, 1996, p. 1, italics added). In contrast, adaptive behavior is considered as an independent criterion in the commonly used definition advocated by the American Association on Intellectual and Developmental Disabilities (AAIDD, formerly the American Association on Mental Retardation; AAMR). Second, at present there is no consensus on how such "impairments" or "deficits" in social functioning and/or adaptive behavior should be operationalized.

Finally, a strong scientific case can be made for considering social functioning and adaptive behavior in terms of the conjunction between impairments in cognitive ability and prevailing social arrangements (rather than as a defining characteristic of intellectual disability). Such an approach is consistent with the World Health Organization's International Classification of Functioning, Disability and Health (ICF; World Health Organization, 2001). The ICF represents an attempt to integrate medical and social models of disability by describing the interplay between changes or impairments in body functions or structures (e.g., intellectual ability) and the person's potential capacity and actual performance in a range of activities in specific environmental, cultural and personal contexts. Domains of activity/participation considered under the ICF include: learning and applying knowledge; general tasks and demands; communication; movement; self-care; domestic life; interpersonal interactions; major life areas such as participation in education and employment; community, social and civic life.

Typology of Intellectual Disability

Intellectual disability (ID) can be considered to comprise two distinct groups. The first represents the lower end of the normal distribution of intelligence in the population. As a consequence, this group predominantly comprises individuals with mild ID with little evidence of identifiable brain disorder. ID is presumed to result from both genetic and environmental influences. There is a strong correlation between the intellectual function of the child and that of first-degree relatives (Bundey, Thake, & Todd, 1989). The heritability of ID in this group is about 0.5 (Spinath, Harlaar, Ronald, & Plomin, 2004). Genetic influences are presumed to be polygenic, although some specific gene loci have recently been identified as influential (Butcher, Meaburn, Knight *et al.*, 2005). Fertility in this group is normal or near-normal (Maughan, Collishaw, & Pickles, 1999), as is life expectancy (Patja, Iivanainen, Vesala, Oksanen, & Ruoppila, 2000). There is a strong association with lower socioeconomic status (see p. 822; Birch, Richardson, Baird, Horobin, & Illsley, 1970). That this association is at least partly mediated by environmental effects is apparent from the results of adoptee studies (Capron & Duyme, 1989). General health is usually unimpaired. Adaptive function and adult capacity to work and live independently are relatively mildly impaired.

The second group comprises ID as a consequence of identifiable or apparent brain disorders, of genetic or environmental origin (see p. 823). In this group, ID is typically more severe. There are more comorbid neurological problems such as epilepsy, and sensory or motor deficits, evidence of the greater degree of brain impairment. In this group, overt brain pathology is evident postmortem in most cases (Crome & Stern, 1972). Given that the majority of individuals in this group have a sporadic cause for ID, there is little or no correlation between the intellectual level of the affected child and their siblings or parents (Simonoff, Bolton, & Rutter, 1996). Stereotypic behaviors including self-injury and autistic symptoms are common (Einfeld, Piccinin, Mackinnon *et al.*, 2006). In the developed world, there is also little or no correlation with socioeconomic status (Roeleveld, Zielhuis, & Gabreels, 1997). Fertility is regarded as substantially reduced and life expectancy is significantly lower than that of the community (Lavin, Mcguire, & Hogan, 2006). Given the more severe intellectual impairment, eventual adaptive capacity to fill normal adult roles is substantially more impaired.

However, there are several important caveats to this typology. First, a minority of individuals with mild ID have identifiable causes. These may include acquired brain injuries, (e.g., from infection or trauma) or genetic disorders such as Prader–Willi or velocardiofacial syndromes (see p. 825). Second, a minor proportion of more severe ID will represent the group more than 3 SD below the mean on the normal distribution for intelligence. Third, it is important to recognize that there is substantial variation in level of function *within* each of these broad groupings.

Functional Levels of Intellectual Disability

Four levels of severity of ID, defined by ranges on standardized IQ tests, are described by both the ICD-10 and the DSM-IV. These are mild (approximate IQ 50–70), moderate (35–50), severe (20–35) and profound (below 20). However, it is important to note that individuals can vary considerably in their attainments across different developmental domains, often reflecting varied degrees of brain impairment to different cortical areas.

The following descriptions are derived from the ICD-10 Guide for Mental Retardation (World Health Organization, 1996) and Harris (2006) and describe functional abilities at the end of adolescence. More detailed descriptions of attainments at different functional levels are provided by standardized measures of adaptive behavior, such as the Vineland Adaptive Behavior Scales (Sparrow, Balla, & Cicchetti, 1984). Individuals with mild ID typically have impaired literacy but normal language. There may be some emotional and social immaturity. Some young people with mild ID will develop a capacity for open or partially supported employment, albeit with unsophisticated task roles. They may marry and have children. However, as adults, rates of employment and independent living away from the family are lower in those with mild ID than in the general community (Hall, Strydom, Richards *et al.*, 2005; Maughan, Collishaw, & Pickles, 1999).

Those with moderate ID typically have impaired language. For example, Carr (2000) found that a cohort of adults with Down syndrome, with a mean IQ in the moderate range, had on average language development at the 5-year level. Basic self-care skills are achieved. Social relationships such as friendships can be well developed. As adults, such individuals can eventually work productively in a special workplace setting with structured tasks and supervision. Fully independent living, marriage and parenting are very unusual.

In severe ID, language may be absent or limited to individual words or phrases, or a limited range of signs may be used in communication. Elementary self-care may be achieved but assistance is usually needed with most basic living activities. Mobility may be normal. Daytime recreational activity programs are usual rather than work placement (Tesio, Valsecchi, Sala, Guzzon, & Battaglia, 2002). Profound ID is often a consequence of catastrophic brain damage, with multisensory and major motor impairments accompanying limited cortical cerebral function. Some comprehension of basic commands is attainable. Assistance, often through nursing care, may be required for nearly all activities.

Incidence and Prevalence of Intellectual Disability

Most epidemiological studies of ID have sought to estimate prevalence rates – the total number of cases existing in a population at a given point in time (Roeleveld, Zielhuis, & Gabreels, 1997). These studies typically use IQ assessments (see chapter 21) to classify a person as having either mild (IQ 50 or 55–70) or severe (IQ <50 or 55) ID, rather than a combination of IQ and adaptive behavior.

In high-income countries in North America, Europe and Australia, studies have produced broadly consistent overall prevalence rates for severe ID of 3–4 per 1000 of the general population, although studies that have screened entire populations tend to yield slightly higher prevalence rates (approximately 6 people with severe ID per 1000; Roeleveld, Zielhuis, & Gabreels, 1997).

Studies that have sought to ascertain the prevalence of mild ID have reported much more diverse prevalence rates. This is likely to reflect at least two factors. First, most adults with mild ID do not use specialist services for people with ID. As a result, prevalence studies based on administratively defined adult populations will significantly underestimate prevalence rates of mild ID. Second, given that there is a strong association between socioeconomic deprivation and the prevalence of mild ID (see below), the level of socioeconomic deprivation in the communities sampled would be expected to have an impact on ascertained prevalence rates for mild ID. Studies that have screened entire populations have yielded prevalence rates of 25–80 people with mild ID per 1000 general population (Roeleveld, Zielhuis, & Gabreels, 1997; Simonoff, Pickles, Chadwick *et al.*, 2006).

Few studies have sought to ascertain the incidence of ID (the number of new cases arising in a population in a given period of time). A US study reported a cumulative incidence at age 8 years of 4.9 children with severe learning disabilities per 1000 births and 4.3 children with mild ID per 1000 births (Katusic, Colligan, Beard *et al.*, 1996). Similar rates have been reported in Northern European research (Rantakallio & von Wendt, 1986). The low incidence of mild ID reported in these studies is likely to reflect the reliance on biased, administratively defined (rather than "true" population-based) samples of people with ID.

There is no reliable information available on the global distribution of ID (Institute of Medicine, 2001). There is reason to believe that the incidence of severe ID in low-income countries is at least double that in high-income countries (Durkin, 2002). It has been estimated that the impact of undernutrition (as evidenced by severe to moderate stunting) alone may be responsible for a 31–43% elevation in the incidence of ID during childhood in low-income countries (Emerson, Fujiura, & Hatton, 2007). The prevalence and incidence of ID vary according to gender, age, ethnicity and socioeconomic circumstances.

Gender

Most studies report that males are more likely than females to have both severe ID (average male : female ratio 1.2:1) and mild ID (average male : female ratio 1.6:1), although gender ratios vary widely across studies (Roeleveld, Zielhuis, & Gabreels, 1997). It has been suggested that sex-linked genetic factors (Partington, Mowat, Einfeld, Tonge, & Turner, 2000), male vulnerability to insult and social processes in labeling and classification partly account for the majority of males with ID (Roeleveld, Zielhuis, & Gabreels, 1997). The latter are likely to be particularly relevant in studies that have relied on administratively defined populations of people with ID.

Age

Estimates of age-specific prevalence rates are highly influenced by methods of case identification (e.g., population screening versus the use of administrative samples). Most studies have reported an increase in the prevalence of both severe and mild ID throughout childhood, with prevalence peaking at 10–20 years of age (Roeleveld, Zielhuis, & Gabreels, 1997). While this may be because of the increasing "visibility" of ID in later school years, there is also evidence of IQ decline in some disorders. For example, Fisch, Simensen, and Schroer (2002) found evidence of declining IQ scores in children with fragile X syndrome, and this decline was greater than in children with autism.

Ethnicity

Estimating the impact of ethnicity on the prevalence and incidence of ID is difficult as other important factors also vary among ethnic groups. These include poverty, access to health care, lifestyles, communication barriers and uptake of specialist services (Modood, Berthoud, Lakey *et al.*, 1997). However, research in the USA, UK and Australia has found tentative evidence to suggest higher prevalence rates of mild ID amongst some minority ethnic groups, such as African-American groups in the USA (Fujiura & Yamaki, 1997) and Aboriginal groups in Australia (Leonard, Petterson, De Klerk *et al.*, 2005). In the UK, higher prevalence rates in South Asian communities have been reported for children and young adults with severe ID (Hatton & Emerson, 2004). However, it is unclear whether these higher rates are biologically or genetically linked with ethnicity (e.g., as a result of consanguinity), or are the result of other factors that have an impact upon minority ethnic groups, such as socioeconomic status or classification practices (e.g., through the use of culturally biased assessment methods).

Socioeconomic Circumstances

There is a strong association between lower socioeconomic position and higher prevalence rates of mild, but probably not severe, ID (Hatton & Emerson, 2004; Leonard, Petterson, De Klerk *et al.*, 2005; Roeleveld, Zielhuis, & Gabreels, 1997). For example, children in the most socioeconomically disadvantaged 10% of Western Australian families had more than five times the risk of mild and moder-ate ID when compared with those in the least disadvantaged 10% (Leonard, Petterson, De Klerk *et al.*, 2005). In Britain, children in the most socioeconomically disadvantaged 20% of families had more than four times the risk of ID when compared with those in the least disadvantaged 20% (Emerson, Graham, & Hatton, 2006). These associations have also been reported in middle- and low-income countries (Durkin, 2002).

Possible changes in Prevalence

The prevalence and incidence of ID are likely to change over time as a result of complex changes in society and the provision of education, health and social care. In high-income countries, factors that are likely to lead to an increase in the incidence of ID include: increases in maternal age (associated with higher risk factors for some conditions associated with

ID, such as Down syndrome); increased survival of "at risk" infants, such as very low birth weight infants or very preterm deliveries; increasing levels of HIV and AIDS in children; and increased rates of assisted conception. Factors that are likely to lead to a decrease in incidence include: increasing availability of prenatal screening for Down syndrome; improving health care and support resulting in fewer "at risk" infants developing ID. The net effect of these competing pressures on the overall incidence of ID is not known. However, there is a perception among practitioners that the rate of profound ID may have increased significantly over the past decade.

Social and Health Impact of Intellectual Disability

The social impact of ID can be considered at the level of the individual, their relatives and the wider society. As children, and later as adults, people with both mild and more severe ID are at significantly increased risk of facing discrimination, social exclusion and abuse (Department of Health, 2001; Grant, Goward, Richardson, & Ramcharan, 2005). In England, only 44% of the 95,000 children with a Statement of Special Educational Need for ID are educated in mainstream schools, a percentage that drops to just 20% for children with severe ID (Department for Education and Skills, 2005). As adults, people with both mild and severe ID are significantly less likely than their non-disabled peers to move out of their family home, have long-term intimate relationships, be employed, have friends and participate in the life of their communities (Emerson, Malam, Davies, & Spencer, 2005; Maughan, Collishaw, & Pickles, 1999). These trends toward extensive social exclusion appear to transcend national boundaries (Emerson, Fujiura, & Hatton, 2007) and be particularly exacerbated in people with more severe ID (Emerson, Malam, Davies *et al.*, 2005).

There is also extensive evidence that mothers (and to a much lesser extent fathers) of children with ID are more likely to shows signs of psychological distress and have lower well-being than parents of "typically developing" children (Baker, Blacher, Kopp, & Kraemer, 1997; Blacher & Baker, 2002; Blacher & Mink, 2004; Emerson, 2003). In addition to the health burden imposed on a vulnerable subgroup of parents, these findings are of concern as distress among mothers has been linked to a wide range of adverse outcomes for children, including less than optimal parenting, failure to engage with services, decisions to seek out-of-home care for their disabled child, impeded child development, and higher rates of child psychopathology and antisocial behavior (Llewellyn, McConnell, Thompson, & Whybrow, 2005; Zahn-Waxler, Duggal, & Gruber, 2002). Marriages in families with children with ID are only a little more likely to end in divorce (Risdal & Singer, 2004).

It is perhaps surprising that severity of ID per se is not the major determinant of family stress (Baker, McIntyre, Blacher *et al.*, 2003). The response of families to the presence of a chronically ill or disabled child is partly determined by parents' ways of thinking about the child. There is evidence that mothers with a high sense of locus of control and a belief in chance feel less burdened by caregiving than those with the opposite cognitive set (Green, 2004).

Other factors predicting high levels of stress for parents are increased rate of psychopathology among children with ID (Baker, McIntyre, Blacher *et al.*, 2003; Eisenhower, Baker, & Blacher, 2005; Emerson, 2003; Hastings & Beck, 2004; Tonge & Einfeld, 2003) and the poorer socioeconomic circumstances of families supporting children with ID (Emerson, 2003; Emerson, Hatton, Blacher, Llewellyn, & Graham, 2006). Problematic or "challenging" behaviors are one of the main predictors of whether parents will seek a residential placement for their son or daughter (Llewellyn, Dunn, Fante, Turnbull, & Grace, 1999; Llewellyn, McConnell, Thompson *et al.*, 2005). Daily care requirements on account of lack of mobility and incontinence of children with ID are also burdensome for parents, but do not cause as much stress in parents as behavior problems (Tonge & Einfeld, 2003). Siblings of children with ID in general do not show increased levels of distress or other psychopathology. There is some evidence that such siblings have more secure attachment styles and higher levels of emotional maturity (Levy-Wasser & Katz, 2004).

At the clinical level, there is wide variation in the way families respond to the experience of having a child or sibling with ID. One approach that is helpful in counseling such families is to support effective grieving for the loss of the wished-for healthy child. Families who are not unduly burdened by anger, guilt, shame or sadness are best able to have a realistic appreciation of their disabled child. In such families, the child with the disability is given the same value as other family members. Where this is not achieved, scapegoating of the affected child at one extreme, or overenmeshment with the disabled child at the other extreme is sometimes seen. In such families, "survivor guilt" may be apparent in siblings.

There is evidence that parental stress can be ameliorated by group interventions. Tonge, Brereton, Kiomall *et al.* (2006) used a randomized control design in demonstrating that parent education and behavior management training, or parental counseling alone were effective in reducing parental distress in parents of children with autism. Hastings and Beck (2004) reviewed a range of controlled parent intervention studies and found most support for the effectiveness of cognitive–behavioral techniques in reducing parental stress, although effects were of small to medium size.

The primary impact of ID on the wider society is financial. Current expenditure in England on health and social care services for people with ID is approximately £4 billion per annum (Association of Directors of Social Services, 2005). Increased rates of psychopathology among people with ID (see p. 827) also add major costs to care. Adolescents with ID who could gain vocational training through supported employment programs are unable to do so (Hupalo, 1997). Injuries to care workers are a major source of expense from compensation and occupational health and safety claims (Lowe, 1999) and the costs of supported accommodation services are significantly influenced by the extent of psychopathology exhibited by residents (Hallam & Emerson, 1999).

Causes of Intellectual Disability

Any pathogenic process that significantly impairs cognitive processing during childhood can cause ID. The most widely used classification of such causes is that of the AAIDD (Luckasson, Coulter, Polloway *et al.*, 1992, Luckasson, Borthwick-Duffy, Buntinx *et al.*, 2002). This groups causes into prenatal, perinatal and postnatal in origin. Prenatal causes include chromosome disorders, various dysmorphic syndrome disorders, inborn errors of metabolism and developmental disorders of brain formation, such as hydrocephalus or spina bifida, toxic and teratogenic influences such as fetal alcohol exposure and malnutrition. The second group, perinatal causes, includes placental insufficiency and neonatal disorders such as septicemia. Postnatal causes include head injuries, infections such as meningitis, and degenerative disorders such as the leukodystrophies, ID associated with seizures, toxic disorders such as lead poisoning, malnutrition and chronic social and sensory deprivation.

In surveys of individuals with more severe ID (Curry, Stevenson, Aughton *et al.*, 1997; Partington, Mowat, Einfeld *et al.*, 2000), chromosomal abnormalities are identifiable in 20%, about three-quarters of whom have Down syndrome. Monogenic disorders, either autosomal or X-linked, account for about 3–4% each. Recognizable or provisional genetic syndromes are found in about a further 5%. Environmental causes have been estimated as responsible for about 8% of cases. The causal link in some of these cases is clearly apparent (e.g., herpes encephalitis in childhood). However, it is important to appreciate that some conditions apparent perinatally or postnatally have uncertain prenatal origins (Nelson, 2003). These include structural abnormalities of the central nervous system (5%) and complications of prematurity (5%). No cause is currently identifiable in 45–50%.

There is reason to believe that the prevalence of severe ID in low-income countries is at least double that in high-income countries and that the distribution of causes is different (Durkin, 2002). Because of the lack of epidemiological studies it is not easy to distinguish cognitive impairments leading to specific learning disorders from those leading to ID. In low-income countries, undernutrition accounts for a larger proportion of at least mild ID (Olness, 2003). The most critical impact on brain development for undernutrition appears to be between the second trimester of pregnancy and age 2 years.

Endemic iodine deficiency occurs in up to 10% of the population in some areas of the world, particularly parts of China, the Congo, South America and mountainous areas of South-East Asia (Olness, 2003). Deficiency in thyroid hormone during pregnancy or in the newborn period impairs development of cortical neurons and retards myelinization (Pharoah, Buttfield, & Hetzel, 1971). Infectious diseases continue to be prominent causes of ID in low-income countries. Important infections include tuberculous meningitis, hemophilias, influenza and type B meningitis. Given the failure to achieve widespread immunization, insect-borne viruses such as Western Nile virus, cerebral malaria and congenital human immunodeficiency virus infection are increasingly prevalent in low-income countries and the brain impairment as a consequence has been documented (Drotar, Olness, Wiznitzer, *et al.*, 1997). The wider use of antiviral agents to treat AIDS may result in large numbers of survivors with ID. Many conditions leading to cognitive impairment occur concurrently, increasing the risk for ID (Olness, 2003). For example, low-birth-weight babies may also have malnutrition and malaria.

There is also some evidence to suggest that some genetic causes of developmental disabilities may also be unequally distributed (Institute of Medicine, 2001). For example, thalassemia, which is prevalent in 2–3% of all children in West Africa, has been linked to high rates of mild ID (Steen, Xiong, Mulhern, Langston, & Wang, 1999). In low-income countries, a higher proportion of births are to mothers aged over 35, possibly increasing the incidence of Down syndrome (Steen, Xiong, Mulhern *et al.*, 1999). Finally, high rates of cosanguineous marriage have been associated with increased rates of child disabilities (Institute of Medicine, 2001; Teebi & El-Shanti, 2006). The causes of ID vary with the severity of intellectual impairment (see chapter 30).

Down syndrome

The genetic basis of Down syndrome is discussed in chapter 24; here we focus on the clinical characteristics. Down syndrome is the most common genetic cause of ID, occurring in approximately 1 in 800 live births. The risk for Down syndrome increases with increasing maternal age. Down syndrome is characterized by upturned outward slanting eyes, a wide nasal bridge, a large posterior fontanelle, a single transverse palmar crease and hypotonia. Congenital heart disease and duodenal atresia are common (Harris, 2006). Hearing impairments, hypothyroidism and atlantoaxial instability and an increased vulnerability to leukemia are also characteristic. Guidelines for the management of the general health of children with Down syndrome have been formulated by the Committee on Genetics (American Academy of Pediatrics Committee on Genetics, 2001). Severity of ID covers a broad range, but is most commonly moderate or severe. It is also associated with earlier onset of menopause in Down syndrome women (Schupf, Pang, Patel *et al.*, 2003). Down syndrome is striking among genetic disorders causing ID in that it is associated with relatively low levels of psychopathology (Carr, 2002). There is some evidence to support the notion that children with Down syndrome have a stubborn temperament, but this is not problematic for most parents (Carr, 1994). Alzheimer-type dementia occurs at an increased rate and at an earlier age (mean of around 50 years) in Down syndrome. Early signs of dementia are a sustained increase in behavioral problems and a decline in independence and adaptive behavior skills (Carr,

2002). However, early dementia is occasionally apparent in young adulthood.

Fragile X syndrome

Fragile X syndrome (FXS) is caused by an expansion of the CGG trinucleotide sequence at Xq27.3 on the X chromosome (see chapter 24). Approximately one-third of boys with FXS have mild to moderate ID. One-third of carrier females have mild ID and the other two-thirds an IQ in the average range. The physical phenotype is characterized by a long face with protruding ears, a large jaw, hyperextensible joints and enlarged testes in postpubertal males (Hagerman, 1999).

ID is usually mild to moderate and the degree correlates inversely to the level of fragile X mental retardation protein (FMRP) (Loesch, Huggins, & Hagerman, 2004). Verbal intelligence often exceeds performance abilities in both affected males and non-learning disabled female carriers. The IQ may decline in childhood and adolescence, with an average adult IQ in males at the low end of the moderate range. Approximately 70% of females with the full mutation have an IQ of less than 85. Verbal dyspraxia is common (Spinelli, Rocha, Giacheti, & Richieri-Costa, 1995).

Children with FXS typically have initial social anxiety with aversion to eye contact, hand flapping and stereotypic behavior, but usually are socially responsive and affectionate with an interest in social interactions (Turk & Cornish, 1998). Self-injury, notably hand biting and scratching provoked by frustration, anxiety and excitement is common. Some children with FXS have autistic behaviors in childhood.

Prader–Willi syndrome

Prader–Willi syndrome has a prevalence of about 1 in 10,000–15,000 live births. It results from the failure of the paternally imprinted genes in the region 15q11–q13 (see chapter 24). Physical characteristics of Prader–Willi syndrome include hypotonia and poor feeding in infancy followed by hyperphagia and consequent obesity and its cardiopulmonary complications from early childhood, hypogonadism and small hands and feet and short stature. There is a characteristic, although subtle, facial appearance. Most individuals with Prader–Willi syndrome function in the mild ID range, although a few have more severe ID impairment and some have average intelligence.

Behavioral characteristics include marked hyperphagia, pica, gorging and stealing food. In addition, there are severe temper tantrums or episodes of rage. Insensitivity to pain, skin-picking or rectal gouging and impaired temperature regulation, hypersomnolence and reduced motor activity are also features (Einfeld, Smith, Durvasula, Florio, & Tonge, 1999b). Obsessional symptoms have also been noted (Dykens, 2004). There appears to be an increased vulnerability to psychosis in Prader–Willi syndrome. Although psychosis has been noted in both the deletion and uniparental disomy (UPD) forms, it is about six times more common in the UPD derived cases. There is evidence of hypothalamic disturbance from both post-mortem and functional magnetic resonance imaging (fMRI) studies (Shapira, Lessig, He *et al.*, 2005).

Neither surgery nor medications have been found effective in managing the hyperphagia. Instead, strict control of food intake is necessary. Sometimes this requires locking cupboards or refrigerators to prevent access to food (Holland, Whittington, & Butler, 2002). Medical management of the complications of obesity is required. Behavioral difficulties continue into young adulthood, but there is evidence that they decline in the 4th and 5th decades (Dykens, 2004).

Williams syndrome

Williams syndrome is caused by a chromosome deletion at 7q11.23 (see chapter 24). Around 95% of children with the condition have the same deletion, but a few individuals have partial deletions. Williams syndrome is characterized by short stature; hypercalcemia in infancy and subsequent abnormal dentition; vascular abnormalities, particularly supervalvular aortic stenosis; a stellate pattern in the iris; atypical face, sometimes described as "elfin-like"; and ID, generally in the low/mild or upper moderate range. Psychometric testing usually identifies language function significantly better than visuospatial function (Howlin, Davies, & Udwin, 1998).

Children with Williams syndrome show more noise sensitivity, sleep disturbance and anxiety than other children with ID (Einfeld, Tonge, & Rees, 2001). The anxiety pattern is quite distinct. Children with Williams syndrome have a high phobic anxiety but not social anxiety. Indeed, they have an absence of social anxiety. This has led to a substantial rate of sexual abuse of girls with Williams syndrome (Davies, Udwin, & Howlin, 1998; Dykens, 2003). Although the behavioral difficulties remain evident in young adulthood, they are less prominent (Tonge & Einfeld, 2003).

Angelman syndrome

Angelman syndrome involves a deficit in the same region on chromosome 15 as Prader–Willi syndrome. However, Angelman syndrome is caused by a deficit in the region inherited from the mother, whereas Prader–Willi syndrome is a consequence of a deficit in the same region inherited from the father (see chapter 24). Individuals with Angelman syndrome have a characteristic face with a wide mouth, a thin upper lip and a prominent tongue. The head is small. Most are fair with blue eyes. Feeding problems are common in the neonatal period. Children with Angelman syndrome have a characteristic ataxic gait with arms upheld and flexed. They have frequent laughing, which is mainly in response to social stimuli (Horsler & Oliver, 2006). Fascination for water, hand flapping, abnormal food-related behaviors and sleep disturbance occur more commonly than in IQ-matched controls (Barry, Leitner, Clarke, & Einfeld, 2005). Epilepsy is usual and often severe. ID is in the severe or profound range with little speech, although some affected children use a limited range of signs to communicate (Holland, Whittington, & Butler, 2002).

Velocardiofacial Syndrome

Velocardiofacial syndrome (VCFS) is a consequence of a deletion at 22q11.2 (see chapter 24). The physical phenotype includes congenital heart disease, cleft palate or other palatal anomalies, and a characteristic facial appearance including a long narrow face and a prominent nasal tip. Abnormalities of calcium metabolism and immune function are common. Individuals with VCFS often have mild ID but may have intelligence in the normal range. Particular difficulties with mathematics are common. As children, they are commonly shy and withdrawn with a bland affect. In adolescence or young adulthood, psychosis emerges in a high proportion of cases. In a large series, Murphy, Jones and Owen (1999) found a prevalence of psychosis of 30%, the majority of which was schizophrenia. At present, there is no known way of preventing the onset of psychosis. One series reported a poor response to antipsychotics (Gothelf & Lombroso, 2001), but another series suggested outcomes similar to schizophrenia in general (Murphy, 2005).

Prevention of Intellectual Disability

The prevention of ID raises a complex set of ethical issues (Louhiala, 2004). Least contentious among approaches to prevention are those that seek to avoid exposure to social and environmental risk factors for ID such as poverty, undernutrition, environmental toxins, infections, poor obstetric care, understimulating home environments, intrafamilial marriage, child abuse or low maternal education. It has been estimated, for example, that reducing the proportion of children living in poverty who are exposed to environmental deprivation could decrease the prevalence of ID in the USA by approximately 10% (McDermot & Altekrusse, 1994).

Recently, the International Child Development Steering Group have reviewed the evidence relating to risk factors for adverse developmental outcomes for children in low and middle income economies (Engle, Black, Behrman *et al.*, 2007; Walker, Wachs, Gardner *et al.*, 2007). While not specifically related to ID, there is a clear overlap between risk factors for not attaining general developmental potential and risk factors for ID. They identified four key risk factors where existing evidence suggested that the need for intervention was "urgent" (stunting as a result of inadequate nutrition, inadequate cognitive stimulation, iodine deficiency and iron deficiency anemia) and five areas where sufficient evidence existed to "warrant intervention" (malaria, intrauterine growth restriction, maternal depression, exposure to violence, and exposure to heavy metals; Walker, Wachs, Gardner *et al.*, 2007). They suggested that the most effective early child development programs "provide direct learning experiences to children and families, are targeted toward younger and disadvantaged children, are of longer duration, high quality, and high intensity, and are integrated with family support, health, nutrition, or educational systems and services" (Engle, Black, Behrman *et al.*, 2007).

Although there has been progress towards reduction of iodine deficiency in many countries, the WHO still estimates that in 2003, 36.5% of school-age children had insufficient iodine intake. Iodine deficiency actually increased in Europe between 1993 and 2003. Salt iodization continues to be an effective strategy (Andersson, Takkouche, Egli, Allen, & de Benoist, 2005). Folate supplementation reduces the rate of neural tube defects (Stoll, Alembik, & Dott, 2006). Lead poisoning can be prevented through screening children living near lead industries, the elimination of lead in petrol, old paint removal and replacement of lead water pipes. Some programs to reduce antenatal exposure to alcohol have been successful but others have been disappointing (Hankin, 2002). Reduction of head injuries through improved road safety and compulsory wearing of bicycle helmets and reductions in near-drowning morbidity are feasible. A number of studies have reported effective primary prevention programs to reduce injuries through child abuse, but secondary prevention to reduce repeat abuse has been less successful (Vandeven & Newton, 2006).

Concerning genetic causes of ID, genetic counseling provides information to guide reproductive choice (see chapter 73). Reducing the rate of consanguineous marriages can be a target of public health education (Alwan & Modell, 2003). The best candidates for prenatal gene therapy have been studied for glycogen, lipid and mucopolysaccharide storage diseases. However, successful prenatal gene therapy has not yet been demonstrated successfully in animals and there are a number of bioethical concerns about developing technology that can potentially manipulate the human genome (Ye, Mitchell, Newman, & Batshaw, 2001).

The contemporary rarity of once common causes such as congenital rubella and kernicterus demonstrate what can be achieved. Reduction of the prevalence of ID remains a viable goal.

Health Complications of Intellectual Disability

General Health

People with ID are more likely to experience poor general health and have a decreased life expectancy (Ouellette-Kuntz, 2005). While much remains to be learned about the causes of these disparities in health outcomes, existing research has drawn attention to the potential importance of a number of factors including the impact on health of the genetic and biological bases of ID, for example, thyroid impairment and atlantoaxial instability in Down syndrome (Cohen, 2006; Dykens, 1999, 2000; Hodapp & Dykens, 2004); increased risk of exposure to socioeconomic disadvantage (Emerson & Hatton, 2007a,b), behavioral or lifestyle factors (Emerson, 2005b; Robertson, Emerson, Gregory *et al.*, 2000); and the quality of existing health care support provided to people with ID (Webb & Rogers, 1999; Whitfield, Langan, & Russell, 1996).

The evidence pertaining to the potential importance of socioeconomic, behavioral or lifestyle factors and the quality of health care support suggests that the health status of people with ID could be improved and that the disparity in health outcomes between people with ID and their non-disabled peers may be reduced (Department of Health, 2001; Disability Rights Commission, 2004; Einfeld, Smith, Durvasula *et al.*, 1999b; Meijer, Carpenter, & Scholte, 2004; US Department of Health and Human Services, 2005). To the extent that the poorer health status of people with ID is *avoidable* and *unjust*, it can be considered to constitute an example of health inequity or inequality (Whitehead, 1992).

Guidelines have been developed to guide health care practitioners in addressing the particular health needs of individuals with ID (e.g., monitoring thyroid status in individuals with Down syndrome; Beange, Lennox, & Parmenter, 1999). These have been developed in response to research showing high rates of undiagnosed common health problems in persons with ID. It is important to consider intercurrent or chronic physical ill health as potential causes of behavioral disturbances in those with ID. For example, esophageal reflux is a common covert cause of agitation and distress in children and adolescents with severe and profound ID.

Epilepsy

Around 30% of children with ID have epilepsy. The prevalence varies substantially between causes of ID. For example, those with Down syndrome have low levels of seizures, whereas for those with tuberous sclerosis or cerebral palsy, epilepsy is common. In some disorders (e.g., autism and FXS), epilepsy often begins for the first time in adolescence. Epilepsy can be associated with psychopathology in young people with ID in a number of ways. Complex partial seizure disorder (previously known as temporal lobe epilepsy) may manifest only with behavioral manifestations, such as undirected aggression or olfactory or dissociative phenomena. Second, anticonvulsants can have an impact on the behavior of children with ID (see chapter 30). In general, children with ID and seizures do not have higher rates of psychopathology than children with ID but without seizures (Lewis, Tonge, Mowat *et al.*, 2000).

Sensorimotor impairments

Abnormalities of vision, hearing and motor function are common accompaniments of ID, but are often overlooked (Beckung, Steffenburg, & Uvebrant, 1997). Around 25% of children with idiopathic ID had visual impairments in one large study (Ghose & Chandra Sekhar, 1986). The prevalence of hearing impairment in children with ID is twice that found in typically developing children (Karjalainen, Kaariainen, & Vohlonen, 1983). Some conditions such as congenital rubella or severe anoxic brain injury can cause impairment of multiple senses.

Psychopathology

Psychopathology is a common and important feature of ID. Whereas methodological differences produce differing rates (for a review see Dykens, 2004), most studies find an increased rate two to four times that in the general population. The Isle of Wight studies of Rutter, Tizard, Yule, Graham, and Whitmore (1976) found that 7% of 10- to 12-year-old children in the community had psychiatric disorders, but for children with ID, the rate was 30%. Einfeld & Tonge (1996a,b) assessed psychopathology in an epidemiologically derived cohort of children and adolescents with more severe ID and identified 40% of the children aged between 4 and 18 years as meeting criteria as a psychiatric case. In comparison, 14% of Australian children without ID in a random community sample were found to have a psychiatric disorder (Sawyer, Arney, Baghurst *et al.*, 2001). In Britain, it has been estimated that 39% of 5- to 15-year-old children with ID had a diagnosable psychiatric disorder, compared to 8% among children without ID (Emerson, 2003).

Major psychopathology affects over 40% of young people with ID (Einfeld & Tonge, 1996b), therefore the number of persons affected by ID and severe psychopathology is approximately equal to the number with schizophrenia.

Factors Contributing to the High Prevalence of Psychopathology

These may be grouped as biological, psychological and social risk factors. Biological factors include particular genetic causes of ID that lend vulnerability to particular syndromes of psychopathology. Einfeld, Tonge, Turner, Parmenter, and Smith (1999a) found that children with Prader–Willi and Williams syndromes had considerably higher levels of psychopathology than did children with FXS or an epidemiological control group. Those with Down syndrome had significantly lower levels than controls. Various concomitant brain impairments that may accompany ID may increase the risk of behavior disturbance, such as complex partial seizures, or frontal lobe damage causing impulsivity. Sensory impairments are frequent in children with ID, and these are known to increase the risk of psychopathology (Sisson, Van Hasselt, & Hersen, 1993).

Psychological factors include the reduction in capacity for finding creative and adaptive solutions to life challenges. This is the corollary of the observation that children and adolescents of high intelligence have greater resilience to psychopathology (Goodman, 1995; Tiet, Bird, Davies *et al.*, 1998). Family dysfunction and parental mental health problems are associated with increased psychopathology in children with ID (Wallander, Koot, & Dekker, 2006), but the direction of causality is unclear.

Social disadvantage and poverty are an increased risk for children and adolescents with ID; social conditions that have been linked to risk of psychopathology (BMA Board of Science, 2006; Hatton & Emerson, 2004). They also experience higher rates of stressful life events, such as abuse, school failure and peer rejection, than children without ID (Ammerman, Hersen, van Hasselt, Lubetsky, & Sieck, 1994; Hatton & Emerson, 2004). It has been estimated that 20–33% of the increased risk of psychopathology among children with mild ID can be attributed to the impact of social disadvantage mediated by an increased risk of exposure to a range of adverse life events (Emerson & Hatton, 2007b).

Conceptual Issues and Classification of Psychopathology

Historically, the concepts of ID and mental illness have had a confused relationship. Mental health professionals have tended to view emotional and behavioral disturbances in the presence of ID as a "behavioral" manifestation of ID, rather than evidence of mental illness. At the same time, disability advocates have been keen to distance ID from the perceived stigma and overly medicalized concept of mental illness (Einfeld, 1992). More recently, there has been an increasing awareness that psychopathology is distinct from, but can co-occur with ID. An exception to this would occur, for example, where a 14-year-old boy with a mental age of 2 years may have tantrums which are appropriate for his mental age, which nevertheless, because of the boy's physical size, constitute a serious behavioral problem.

Taxonometric or "bottom-up" models of psychopathology were examined by Aman (1991). He identified seven syndromes common to the factor analyses of several symptom-based inventories of psychopathology used in individuals with ID: aggressive/antisocial, social withdrawal, stereotypic behavior, hyperactivity, repetitive verbalization, anxious/tense/fearful and self-injurious.

Standard DSM and ICD classifications are of limited value in individuals with the more severe levels of ID (Cooper, Melville, & Einfeld, 2003; Einfeld & Aman, 1995). Most specific diagnoses have not been subject to studies of interrater agreement. However, Einfeld, Tonge, Chapman *et al.* (2007) found the interrater agreement for the diagnoses of psychosis (any psychotic disorder) and depression (of any type) in a group of young people with ID to be high among clinicians who were trained in both psychiatry and ID. With the exception of autism, few diagnoses have had demonstrated concurrent, predictive or postdictive validity in individuals with more severe ID.

Case reports and epidemiological studies suggest that the range of psychiatric syndromes seen in the general population also occur in the presence of ID (Emerson, 2003; Menolascino, Levitas, & Greiner, 1986). Some writers have identified a "pathoplastic" effect of cognitive impairment on symptoms (e.g., depression presenting with agitation or increase in stereotypic behavior; Smiley & Cooper, 2003).

Children and adolescents with mild ID display psychopathology similar to that seen in others of the same mental age (Menolascino, 1971). The moderately and severely intellectually disabled are also subject to the psychiatric disorders seen in normal populations, albeit with modified symptoms, but also have a range of symptoms that are uncommon or rare in those without ID (Quine, 1986). Of those psychiatric problems that are closely associated with moderate and severe ID, and are unusual in the general population, the best studied syndrome is that of autism (see chapter 46). A further syndrome is that of stereotypic repetitive movements, such as rocking, head banging, or face slapping. These are most prevalent in those with severe ID, especially when accompanied by sensory deficits (Oliver, Murphy, & Corbett, 1987). These repetitive movements can cause tissue damage, when they are often termed "self-injurious behaviors."

Influences on and Course of Psychopathology

High rates of significant psychopathology are present in children with ID by the age of 4 (Baker, Blacher, & Olsson, 2005; Chadwick, Kusel, Cuddy, & Taylor, 2005; Einfeld & Tonge, 1996b; Quine & Pahl, 1989). Two longitudinal cohort studies of mainly untreated young people with ID, the Aberdeen Study (Richardson & Koller, 1996) and the Australian Child to Adult Development (ACAD) Study (Einfeld, Piccinin, Mackinnon *et al.*, 2006; Tonge & Einfeld, 2003) have shown that the severity of overall behavioral and emotional problems declines slowly through to young adulthood but still remains higher than for normally developing young people. The ACAD study found that all psychopathology syndromes declined over 14 years apart from social relating problems, which increased in severity. While the overall severity of psychopathology was similar across the mild to severe range of ID, the type of psychopathology that was most prominent varied. Those with mild ID were more likely to have antisocial and disruptive behaviors, while those with moderate or severe ID had more self-absorbed and social relating problems. Those with profound ID had lower overall levels of disturbed behavior. The genetic cause of ID had the most influence on severity of psychopathology, and this is largely consistent over time.

Assessment of Behavioral and Emotional Disturbance

Given that adolescent emotional development continues through the third decade for many young people with ID, child and adolescent mental health professionals are often consulted about young adults with ID. Therefore, the following discussion includes issues pertinent to that age group. The care of children and adolescents with ID often takes place within a matrix of environments, such as home, school, respite care facility, and vocational training placements. It is best to obtain information from as many of these sources as possible. This compensates for the often poor verbal skills of the patient, and enables one to determine if disordered behaviors are limited to one or pervasive through many contexts.

As a general guide, the interviewer may use language that would be understood by a child of equivalent mental age. Guided assessment techniques especially with visual cues are also useful, such as a mood thermometer or "COOP" pictograms (Nelson, Wasson, Kirk *et al.*, 1987), and drawing a picture of the family, or the people in his or her group home, if one suspects that these are areas of concern to the patient. This general guide requires several caveats, which derive from the discrepancy that can be present between expressive language, comprehension and emotional maturity. For example, individuals whose ID is a consequence of Williams syndrome may have relatively sophisticated verbal skills that belie a significantly lower level of comprehension and performance skill (Bennett, La Veck, & Sells, 1978). Adolescents with Prader–Willi syndrome often have a more immature level of empathy with others' needs than would be suggested by their level of verbal expression. On the other hand, many young adults or older adolescents with ID reach a level of emotional maturity, perhaps through life experience, which is greater than that suggested by a mental age derived from IQ tests. Such a person might regard an invitation to play with toys as devaluing or demeaning.

The interviewer should be aware of a general tendency on the part of some patients to answer "yes" to any question about symptoms. There is some evidence to suggest that this "yea-saying" phenomenon occurs with a higher prevalence in individuals with ID than in the general population (Finlay & Lyons, 2002; Sigelman, Budd, Spankel, & Schoenrock, 1981). Some, although fewer, have the opposite response bias, the "nay-saying" response (Sigelman, Schoenrock, Wiver *et al.*, 1979). Given the limitations in applying DSM or ICD diagnoses, formulation is often limited to an assessment of problems operating at the level of symptoms rather than at the level of disorders.

A number of questionnaires have been developed with the goal of supporting clinical assessment of children and adolescents with ID. Two in common use are the Aberrant Behavior Checklist (ABC; Aman, Singh, Stewart, & Field, 1985) and the Developmental Behavior Checklist (DBC; Einfeld & Tonge, 2002).

The ABC is an informant-based 58-item questionnaire suitable for people with moderate to profound levels of intellectual disability aged 5 and over. The checklist was designed to measure the effects of interventions and levels of maladaptive behavior. The checklist consists of five subscales.

The DBC-Parent/Primary Carer and DBC-Teacher versions are 96-item inventories used with young people aged 4–18 years, and measure the Total Behavior Problem Score as well as scores on five subscales: disruptive/antisocial, self-absorbed, communication disturbance, anxiety and social relating. Cases of disorder can be determined by a score of 46 or more on the Total Behavior Problem Score. The instrument is designed to supplement clinician assessment for use in treatment studies. It has been used in epidemiological studies because of the availability of norms from Australia, the UK and the Netherlands. A short form has recently been developed (Taffe, Gray, Einfeld *et al.*, 2007).

Issues in the Assessment of Some Particular Psychopathology Syndromes

Psychotic disorders are estimated to occur with increased frequency among adults with ID, with a prevalence of about 3–6% (Shedlack, Hennen, Magee, & Cheron, 2005), but the prevalence in children and adolescents is unknown. Despite this, there is evidence that psychosis is overdiagnosed (Aman, 1985). This may derive from the misdiagnosis of hallucinations. For example, care providers often describe a patient as conducting conversations while no-one else is present, or admitting to hearing voices of absent persons. However, if sufficient time is spent questioning and observing the young person, they may explain that they are remembering conversations or just thinking about them. These memories often center on troubling relationships or events and the patient has no difficulty in distinguishing between the remembered conversations and current reality. Such conversations with absent persons may be a behavioral habit, albeit a socially inappropriate one, but they do not constitute hallucinations. Similar caution needs to be exercised in the assessment of possible delusions. A common report is that a young person with ID is unjustifiably complaining that staff or peers are threatening him or her. It should be remembered that young people with ID actually do experience a good deal of devaluation, mockery, rejection and are victims of assaults, so it is not surprising that some individuals develop a sensitivity to communications from others that could be interpreted as critical. A patient interview will often reveal that the individual has not understood what was said and that the "persecutory" ideas resolve with explanation. Where delusions or hallucinations are truly present, the sophistication of their content is appropriate for the mental age. The consequence of uncritical diagnosis of psychotic illness is the overprescription of antipsychotics with serious consequences of impairment of adaptive function, akathisia and long-term risk of tardive dyskinesia.

Epilepsy syndromes are frequently associated with behavior disturbances in children and adolescents with ID, especially complex partial seizures and cyclical aggression and epilepsy (see chapter 30). Disinhibition and irritability with clonazepam are common. Given the presence of brain pathology, children and adolescents with ID are susceptible to delirium, and a search should be made for intercurrent physical illness as a cause for a recent onset of behavioral disturbance.

Various manifestations of inflexibility in cognitive processing are commonly associated with ID, manifesting as autistic rituals, preoccupations with particular topics, and anxiety with changes in routine or arrangement of objects in the environment. Preoccupations usually are not related to ideas of contamination or harm and lack the "magical" quality of true obsessions.

Ascertaining the cause of ID where possible is an important part of assessment, as psychological symptoms can be a consequence of localized or generalized brain pathology. For example, in tuberous sclerosis focal space-occupying lesions or "tubers" are present or develop, often in the limbic system, with consequent production of a wide range of psychiatric symptoms (Roach, 1988).

Developmental Issues

Key issues presenting to clinicians vary with the mental age of the young person. The birth of a disabled child presents a major crisis for parents. The psychiatrist may be consulted to assist with various aspects of the bereavement process (e.g., parental rejection of the handicapped child, or sudden marital separation). In infancy and childhood, the psychiatrist may be consulted to assist families with manifestations of unresolved grief, such as excessive denial of handicap, as the extent of disability becomes more apparent in the moderately to severely handicapped. As schooling progresses, the academic handicap of the child with mild ID becomes apparent. Parents of these children must face a grief, which is sometimes more difficult to accept as the cause of handicap is less often identified. Family relationship issues, such as sibling anger consequent to disturbances of family roles, often present in this phase. Autistic and hyperactive symptoms may also lead to psychiatric consultation at this stage. In adolescence, increased size adds to the stress of care of the physically dependent child. Handicapped teenagers with aggressive behaviors may become frightening to mothers or other carers. The emerging sexual drive of teenagers may lead to psychiatric referral for assistance with inappropriate sexual behaviors in both boys and girls. In general, those issues facing the normal adolescent continue through the twenties or thirties for many young people with ID. Psychotic disorders mainly present in early adulthood, but may be earlier in velocardiofacial syndrome and Prader–Willi syndrome. Adaptive decline may appear in this period in individuals with Down syndrome, but manifest dementia is unusual before age 30.

Pharmacological Treatment

There have been many reports documenting high levels of prescription of psychotropic medications to adults with ID (for a review see Spreat, Conroy, & Fullerton, 2004) but no contemporary surveys for children and adolescents. The surveys of adults with ID have commonly found poor prescribing practice. For example, Holden and Gitelson (2004) found that 37% of people with ID in one Norwegian county were using psychotropics, and that prescriptions frequently violated current guidelines, especially when given by general practitioners. For example, many prescriptions had not been indicated by a diagnosis, alternatives to medications had rarely been explored, and evaluations of effects and side effects were exceptions. Clinical experience suggests that these problems may also apply to children and adolescents with ID. Consequently, it is important for prescribers to consider the use of drugs in children with ID in a systematic way. Such approaches have been described by Einfeld (1990) and Szymanski and King (1999), and are summarized below. Prescribing for children with autism is considered in chapter 46.

Mental health professionals are frequently presented with crisis situations, with pressure to prescribe to immediately control disturbed behaviors. However, psychotropic medication will be most beneficial if it follows comprehensive assessment of the individual's emotional and behavioral disturbance, allowing the formulation of precipitating and ameliorating factors and an assessment of the efficacy of all the past modes of treatment. Where psychotropic medications are urgently required, they should be seen as a short-term intervention to allow full assessment to take place.

Proper consideration should be given to the issue of informed consent, particularly with respect to legal requirements (see chapter 8). For most children and adolescents with ID, legal requirements will be the same as for other children, but for older adolescents consent requirements may be different. Frequently, the practitioner is required to make an all-or-none decision with respect to the person's capacity to consent. In fact, capacity will be quite variable. For example, a person with mild ID may be able to understand that an anxiolytic may make them feel calmer, but not be able to weigh up the risk of longer-term side effects. Fischer (2003) and Clegg (1999) provide useful discussions of consent issues.

Pharmacological treatment needs to be an integrated part of other concurrent treatments, and this frequently requires good communication with colleagues providing the other treatments. The precise target symptoms for which the psychotropic medication is being prescribed should be stated. It is very difficult to gain valid information from global impressions, such as "child will be less disruptive" or "more compliant." It is better to use specific descriptions such as "frequency of child hitting others will be less." In order to assess this, a method for reliably and validly documenting changes in the target symptoms during the course of treatment is needed. One such method is the Developmental Behavior Checklist-Monitoring module (Einfeld & Tonge, 2002). The use of structured records of behavior is particularly important for children and adolescents with ID, because their care often takes place in a variety of settings (e.g., home, school and respite care). Conflicting information may be received from various carers who attend consultations, each of whom will have a different experience of the patient and different interpretations of behaviors manifested. It is also useful to have two independent carers in a setting (e.g., both parents, or teacher and teacher's aide) completing such charts independently to provide a basic measure of inter-rater reliability.

This record should note whether target symptoms have had a positive response to the medication before the psychotropic medication is continued. It is common for adult patients to be seen who have been receiving large doses of antipsychotics since adolescence without any evidence of benefit. When target symptoms have been reduced or absent for a reasonable period then an attempt should be made to reduce the dosage being prescribed, and structured measures of the effect of this dosage change should be used. Similarly, children and adolescents are frequently maintained on medication long after symptoms have resolved, out of fear that the behaviors will recur, despite developmental or environmental changes.

When a psychotropic medication is withdrawn, a proper withdrawal regime should be designed. Withdrawal symptoms appear commonly in individuals with ID if long-standing treatments are terminated suddenly. Because of the presence of organic brain dysfunction, the response to psychotropic drugs is often idiosyncratic. Therefore, the minimum dosage should be used initially with close attention paid to the emergence of side effects. Adverse effects may be more common in individuals with ID, partly because communication difficulties may impede reporting of symptoms (Aman, Paxton, Field, & Foote, 1986). Issues of compliance, pharmacokinetics and drug interactions need consideration also (see chapter 16).

Antipsychotics

The "typical" antipsychotics (see chapter 16) are the most researched medications in the ID field, but few studies have been rigorous enough to allow conclusions as to their value for the treatment of psychosis or disruptive behavior. The few exceptions have failed to identify any specific impact of antipsychotic medication on the treatment of challenging or problematic behaviors (Brylewski & Duggan, 2004). Aman, De Smedt, Derivan *et al.* (2002) and Snyder, Turgay, Aman *et al.* (2002) have reported double-blind placebo controlled trials of risperidone in children and adolescents with ID, using regimens of 0.02–0.06 $mg{\cdot}kg^{-1}{\cdot}day^{-1}$. These studies demonstrated an approximately 50% reduction in conduct disorder symptoms, significantly greater than placebo. Somnolence was transient and there was no impairment of cognition. However, weight gain was common, and prolactin levels were persistently elevated. While these agents cause lower levels of short-term extrapyramidal side effects, there is only limited evidence that the risk of tardive dyskinesia is lessened (Beasley, Dellva, Tamura *et al.*, 1999).

There is now substantial evidence that atypical antipsychotics are associated with an increased risk of metabolic syndrome and diabetes (De Hert, van Eyck, & De Nayer, 2006). There is no substantive evidence that the newer antipsychotics have greater efficacy than the traditional ones in individuals with ID. Buzan, Dubovsky, Firestone, and Dal Pozzo (1998) have reviewed 84 published cases of clozapine use in adults with ID. They concluded that clozapine was both efficacious and well tolerated. However, the occasional serious hematological side effects of clozapine warrant caution in using this medication. Antipsychotic medications frequently cause sedation and compromise cognitive functions and self-help skills. In addition, extrapyramidal side effects are common. Tremors and other movement disorders are common in individuals with ID who have taken antipsychotic medication (Sachdev, 1991). Campbell, Armenteros, Malone *et al.* (1997) found that 34% of autistic children who were receiving haloperidol over a prolonged period developed dyskinesias, mostly associated with withdrawal. Akathisia is an important side effect of antipsychotics to consider in persons with ID. Persons with limited verbal skills frequently are unable to describe the sense of restlessness and irritability, which can be very distressing. This can lead to increased agitation, which may mistakenly be seen as an indication for increased doses of antipsychotics, making the problem worse. Carers are sometimes very surprised to see a decline in agitation or aggression when antipsychotic dose is reduced.

Another rare but important complication of antipsychotic medication is neuroleptic malignant syndrome. Boyd (1993; as cited in Reiss & Aman, 1998) found the fatality rate (21%) to be double that occurring in persons without ID.

Antidepressants

Depression can be difficult to diagnose with confidence in people with limited verbal skills. However, given the relative safety of selective serotonin reuptake inhibitors (SSRIs), a low threshold for instigation of an antidepressant trial is reasonable. SSRIs (see chapter 16) have largely supplanted the tricyclic antidepressants in the treatment of depression in this population, given the lesser impact of side effects. Agitation and nausea are the most common. The evidence that one SSRI has any greater efficacy than another is inconclusive. It is important to start with small doses and for this reason SSRIs that are available in liquid form present advantages in that titration of small doses is possible.

SSRIs have also been widely used in the field to treat perseverative and repetitive behaviors including rituals of autism, preoccupations in Asperger's disorder and self-injurious behavior. Singh, Kleynhans, and Hersen (1998) found marked reductions in self-injurious behavior in 10 out of 12 individuals treated with fluoxetine or fluvoxamine. Janowsky, Shetty, Barnhill, Elamir, and Davis (2005) found statistically significant decreases in the ratings of aggression, self-injurious behavior, destruction/disruption and depression/dysphoria in institutionalized adults. Controlled studies in children and adolescents have not been reported.

Anxiolytics

There have been no specific studies of the treatment of anxiety in persons with ID. Clinicians have reported improvements in phobic or generalized anxiety disorders as well as obsessive-compulsive disorder with treatment with SSRIs similar to that seen in the general population. Moclobemide is an alternative, but, in the authors' experience, has less efficacy than the SSRIs. Buspirone has been described in case reports as of assistance. There is little or no indication for the use of benzodiazapines for the treatment of behavioral and emotional disturbance, although they are commonly used in the treatment of epilepsy. Benzodiazapines, particularly clonazepam, frequently cause disinhibition and irritability in persons with organic brain impairments (Kalachnik, Hanzel, Sevenich, & Harder, 2002). When a patient with ID taking benzodiazepines presents with these symptoms, it is always worth asking the patient's neurologist to consider an alternative anticonvulsant if possible.

Mood Stabilizers

Typical bipolar illness is occasionally seen, but more frequently people with ID present with instability of mood, that is to say rapid fluctuations between excitement, irritability and high levels of activity alternating with withdrawal and loss of interest. Langee's (1990) retrospective file study found 42% of individuals treated with lithium for a range of behavior disorders improved significantly. Lithium has also been widely used particularly for impulsive aggressive behavior although evidence for a particular efficacy for this presentation is equivocal.

It should be noted that hypothyroidism is common in Down syndrome, so particular care is needed to monitor for the side effects of lithium. Carbamazepine and valproate have been widely used as mood stabilizers in children and adolescents with ID and have lower toxicity risks than lithium. Despite their wide use there are surprisingly few studies of their use, predominantly case reports. Carbamazepine has the disadvantage of requiring more frequent monitoring of serum level.

Stimulants

The principal indication is for the same purpose as in children without ID, for the treatment of ADHD. There is some evidence to suggest that those with moderate and severe ID do not respond as well to stimulants as those with mild ID (Aman, Marks, Turbott, Wilsher, & Merry, 1991). ICD-10 includes overactive disorder associated with intellectual disability and stereotyped movements, a category of uncertain validity. Stimulants may worsen epilepsy, anxiety and tics, all of which are more common in children with ID. Curiously, there have been no systematic studies of which this author is aware studying stimulants in Prader–Willi syndrome, despite their appetite suppressant properties.

Atomoxetine, a noradrenergic reuptake inhibitor, has been shown in randomized controlled trials to be effective in the treatment of ADHD in children with autism (Arnold, Aman, Cook *et al.*, 2006). Clonidine has been shown in a randomized controlled trial to reduce symptoms in children with ADHD and ID (Agarwal, Sitholey, Kumar, & Prasad, 2001) but at the cost of sedation, tolerance development and requirements to monitor blood pressure.

Anticonvulsants

Anticonvulsants are frequently prescribed for persons with ID, given the high prevalence of epilepsy. They are also prescribed as mood stabilizers as above.

Antilibidinal agents

Inappropriate sexual behaviors of some adolescents with ID can cause considerable concern to others and restriction for the individual. Consequently, there has been a growth in the use of testosterone antagonists to reduce libido. Cyproterone is now widely favored as it is active orally, but causes weight gain. Luteinizing hormone-releasing hormone (LHRH) analogs (e.g., leuprorelin) are the most effective and safest method for reducing testosterone levels over prolonged periods but are expensive and of limited availability. The pharmacology of these medications and protocols for their use in paraphilias are described by Reilly, Delva, and Hudson (2000). The pharmacological reduction of libido is potentially of some ethical concern. Prescription to this end should only follow efforts to redirect inappropriate sexual behavior through behavioral and educative means. It may then be that the best interest of the adolescent with ID is served by suppression of a natural aspect of human function. These issues are discussed in greater detail by Clarke (1989).

Psychological Treatment

There is extensive evidence to support the efficacy of applied behavior analytic approaches in the treatment of problematic or challenging behaviors shown by both children and adults with ID (Ball, Bush, & Emerson, 2004; Emerson, 2001; Lucyshyn, Dunlap, & Albin, 2002; O'Reilly, Sigafoos, Lancioni *et al.*, 2007). While there is significantly less direct evidence, it is likely that some "talking therapies" (e.g., cognitive–behavior therapy) may be efficacious for some children with ID who have acquired more complex language skills (Dagnan, Joahoda, & Kroese, 2007). Detailed guidelines are available with regard to the implementation of behavioral approaches (Ball, Bush, & Emerson, 2004; Bush & Emerson, in press; Luiselli, 2006).

Contemporary behavioral approaches (often referred to as positive behavior support) tend to share three key underlying characteristics in that they strive to be functional, constructional and socially valid (Emerson, 2001). A *functional* approach assumes that it is necessary to identify the specific psychological processes that maintain a person's challenging behavior in order to maximize the efficacy of interventions. *Constructional* approaches seek to build competencies, rather than eliminate behaviors. Thus, the key question asked by any constructional intervention is "What should this person be doing in this context (instead of showing challenging behavior)?" rather than "How can we prevent the person engaging in challenging behavior in this context?" *Socially valid* approaches employ methods that are acceptable to the main constituencies involved to generate socially significant change in the person's behavior and life opportunities.

Behavioral approaches view challenging behavior as an example of *operant behavior*. That is, challenging behavior is seen as functional and (in a general sense) adaptive. It can be thought of as a way through which the person exercises some degree of control or power over key aspects of their world (see chapter 62).

One important aspect of the application of behavioral analytic methods in relation to children with ID is the attention given to the analysis and modification of antecedent and contextual factors. Contextual factors operate in two ways. First, and most importantly, they may *establish the motivational base* that underlies behavior. Second, they may *provide information or cues* to the individual concerning the probability of particular behaviors being reinforced.

Behavioral Assessment

Behavioral assessment has four distinct aims (Emerson, 2005a). These are to:

- Identify what it is that the person does that is challenging;
- Describe the impact of challenging behavior upon the person's quality of life;
- Attempt to understand the processes underlying the person's challenging behavior;
- Identify possible alternatives to replace challenging behavior.

Challenging behaviors are often described by carers and care staff in very general terms. The first step in any process of assessment therefore is to clarify the "How, what, where and when" of challenging behavior. Usually, the information needed to answer these questions will come from interviews with people who are in close contact with the person (e.g., family members, care staff). It may also be useful, both as a prompt during interviewing and as a basis for evaluating change, to use an existing checklist of challenging behavior. If the behavior is very frequent or highly predictable it is also important to spend some time observing the behavior.

Describing what the person does that is challenging has two aims. First, it provides a *detailed* description of the *different forms* of challenging behavior shown by the person (most people who show challenging behavior do so in several different ways). Second, we need to know about the *sequence of behaviors* that lead up to an episode of challenging behavior. Challenging behaviors rarely occur "out of the blue." More commonly, they follow a sequence during which the person's behavior escalates from more appropriate (e.g., turning away) to less appropriate (e.g., hitting out) ways of attempting to exercise control. Knowledge about sequences can be helpful in:

1 Developing guidelines for managing challenging behavior; and

2 Identifying possible alternatives that could replace challenging behavior.

Determining the impact that the person's challenging behavior has on their life opportunities is important for two reasons. First, it helps prioritize targets for intervention. Second, it provides a basis for evaluating the social validity of future interventions. Practical guidelines for this task are available (Ball, Bush, & Emerson, 2004; Fox & Emerson, 2002).

The component of the assessment process that seeks to identify the processes underlying a person's challenging behavior is commonly referred to as functional assessment. The primary focus of functional assessment is to describe the *immediate* social and environmental impact of the person's challenging behavior and in doing so to attempt to identify:

1 *Reinforcement contingencies* that are maintaining the behavior(s) (see chapter 62); and

2 *Setting events* or *establishing operations* that provide the motivational basis for challenging behavior.

This descriptive information is often gathered through a combination of structured interview, rating scales and observation (Emerson, 2005a).

The aim of constructional interventions is to replace challenging behavior with other (more appropriate) behaviors. The final aim of the assessment process therefore is to identify possible alternatives to challenging behavior. Possible strategies include:

1 Building upon behaviors that already occur earlier in the chain of events leading up to an episode of challenging behavior;

2 Soliciting the views of carers and care staff regarding appropriate alternatives in that particular setting;

3 Undertaking a general assessment of the person's existing skills and, in particular, their methods of communication.

Behavioral Interventions

A large array of specific behavioral techniques has been demonstrated to have some degree of efficacy in reducing the rate or severity of challenging behaviors (Ball, Bush, & Emerson, 2004; Emerson, 2001; Lucyshyn, Dunlap, & Albin, 2002; O'Reilly, Sigafoos, Lancioni *et al.*, 2007).

The results of a behavioral assessment should identify:

1 Contexts or settings in which challenging behavior is significantly more likely to occur;

2 Establishing operations that may either activate or abolish the contingencies maintaining the person's challenging behavior.

This knowledge opens up possibilities for either preventing or reducing the occurrence of challenging behaviors by the *manipulation of antecedent variables*. Examples of such approaches include:

- Modification of biobehavioral states (e.g., alertness, fatigue, sleep–wake patterns, hormonal changes, drug effects, seizure activity, psychiatric disorders, mood and illness or pain) that are correlated with the occurrence of challenging behavior.
- Changing the nature of activities that precede situations in which challenging behavior is more common (e.g., the use of *behavioral momentum* to increasing compliance and reduce challenging behaviors associated with non-compliance; increasing opportunities for choice making; increasing task variety and physical exercise).
- Changing the nature of activities that are concurrent with situations in which challenging behavior is more common through, for example, redesigning curricula to increase preferred activities, generally enriching the person's environment and providing non-contingent reinforcement and by embedding requests that may elicit challenging behaviors in a more positive prosocial context.

Behavioral theory suggests that decreases in challenging behavior may be brought about indirectly through processes of *behavioral competition or response covariation*. Two sets of procedures that share this common aim are the use of *functional displacement* and procedures involving the *differential reinforcement* of other alternative or incompatible behaviors.

Intervention through functional displacement (typically referred to as functional communication training) seeks to introduce a new behavior (or increase the rate of a pre-existing behavior) that serves exactly the same function as the person's challenging behavior. If this alternative is more efficient than the challenging behavior, it should displace the challenging behavior in the person's behavioral repertoire (Carr, Levin, McConnachie *et al.*, 1994). For example, if a child's aggression in the classroom serves the function of enabling them to escape from non-preferred activities, teaching the child an alternative method of escape (e.g., verbally requesting a change of activities) will displace aggression as long as it is a more efficient option (i.e., takes less effort and is just as or is more "successful" than aggression in delivering the desired consequences). A number of studies have demonstrated the viability of the procedure across a number of settings, participants and challenging behaviors and have indicated that treatment gains may generalize across settings and therapists and may be maintained over time (Emerson, 2001).

A more general set of approaches based on the notion of differential reinforcement also seek to intervene indirectly in challenging behavior by increasing the rate of other behaviors: the *differential reinforcement of other* behavior (DRO); and the *differential reinforcement of alternative* (DRA) or *incompatible* (DRI) behavior. The available evidence suggests that such procedures may not be particularly effective in reducing severely challenging behaviors (Didden, Duker, & Korzilius, 1997).

A third set of procedures seek to intervene by directly changing the contingencies of reinforcement that maintain the person's challenging behavior. These are primarily based upon variants of *extinction* (preventing the maintaining contingency from occurring). Whereas extinction may constitute a useful component of an intervention package (e.g., in combination with functional communication training), evidence and consensus suggests it should never form the primary mode of intervention (Ball, Bush, & Emerson, 2004; Emerson, 2001).

Finally, there exist a number of "default" or "last resort" approaches based on variations of *punishment* (including *time out*), which may be given consideration when more functional and constructional approaches have failed. While they can be effective in temporarily suppressing severe challenging behaviors, their use raises a number of significant ethical issues (Ball, Bush, & Emerson, 2004).

In addition to specific treatments, there is also evidence to suggest that programs of family-focused early intervention may have a significant and lasting impact on the cognitive and social development of children with ID (Anderson, Lakin, Hill, & Chen, 1992; Baker & Feinfield, 2007; Guralnick, 2005). This evidence has raised the possibility for the design and delivery of approaches to the prevention of or early intervention for psychopathology among children with ID (Powell, Dunlap, & Fox, 2005). As yet, the effectiveness of such approaches has still to be demonstrated.

Mental Health Services for Children and Adolescents with Intellectual Disability

Whereas child and adolescent mental health professionals may be well-equipped by training to provide help for children and adolescents with ID, the service settings in which they work have not always welcomed requests to assist such patients. At the same time, carers of those with ID have not always readily sought mental health assistance. In Australia, the USA and other countries, the uncritical application of the normalization principle interpreted mental health interventions as "restrictive" and expressive of the "medical model," which was seen as devaluing. On the mental health side, the fear grew that, as institutions for people with ID were closed, those with behavioral problems could be "dumped" on the mental health system (Bradley, Summers, Brereton *et al.*, 2007). While this was more apparent in services for adults, child and adolescent mental health services sometimes also reflected this reluctance. As a consequence, families were sometimes told by disability services that their child's problems were "psychiatric" and needed mental health services, while mental health services told families that the problems were "behavioral" and therefore not the province of mental health.

One key dilemma in service design is the extent to which mental health services for children and adolescents with ID should be "mainstreamed" within general child and adolescent mental health systems, or should exist as separate specialized teams. One approach is for generic child and adolescent mental health services to provide initial care, with support available from a specialized resource.

In the UK there exist explicit policy objectives to provide comprehensive child and adolescent mental health services in all localities (Department of Health, 2004b) and supposedly to ensure that such services are also responsive to the needs of children and adolescents with ID (BMA Board of Science, 2006; Department of Health, 2004a). Thus, for example, the recent *National Service Framework for Children, Young People and Maternity Services* states that "All children and young people with both a learning disability and a mental health disorder have access to appropriate child and adolescent mental health services" (Department of Health, 2004b).

These policy initiatives reflect a growing understanding of the importance of addressing the mental health needs of children and adolescents more generally (BMA Board of Science, 2006; Department of Health, 2004b), and an appreciation that mental health services for children and adolescents with ID were often of poor quality and highly variable in their availability (Foundation for People with Learning Difficulties, 2003; McCarthy & Boyd, 2002; YoungMinds, 2006). Since the publication of the National Serevice Framework, the percentage of specialist child and adolescent mental health services that also provide support to children and adolescents with ID has risen from 33% to 45% (Barnes, Wistow, Dean *et al.*, 2005). No data are available on the effectiveness or efficiency of these services for children and adolescents with ID. In some service contexts, mental health practitioners may find themselves responsible for ensuring that children and adolescents with ID receive appropriate service for the physical as well as mental health of their patients.

Service Issues Across Developmental Phases

In the antenatal period, parents may need mental health support in the face of prenatal detection in the fetus of conditions causing ID. The birth of a newborn with obvious congenital abnormalities, especially affecting the brain, precipitates a profound crisis for parents. Child and adolescent mental health professionals are needed either to assist parents with severe difficulty in coping with this crisis, or to support other health professionals who are working with families. The same crisis will be manifest at whatever age ID is first diagnosed. To resolve this crisis, families need to achieve a healthy bereavement in the face of the loss of the wished-for child. Typically, such bereavement recurs as each delayed major developmental milestone is experienced as a loss. During infancy and childhood, the parental focus is often on the acquisition of basic developmental tasks such as mobility, toileting and speech. Despite the evidence described above that behavioral and emotional problems are already apparent in early childhood, parents see these as containable as the child is still physically small. This can make it difficult to ensure parental interest in early intervention programs to prevent psychopathology.

The relationships between the child with ID and their siblings are important for mental health professionals to consider. If the child with ID is older, he or she may become aware over time that his or her younger siblings are granted more independence than he or she is. This reversal of the norm can lead to considerable sibling tension. The normal siblings will often have to contend with the stigma engendered by the presence of their disabled brother or sister. Groups aiming to support siblings of children with ID have been used to address this need (Evans, Jones, & Mansell, 2001).

Adolescence is often accompanied by new requests for mental health assistance, frequently on account of the increased size of the child. For example, a large 14-year-old with severe ID whose tantrums are precipitated by the same circumstances as earlier may be difficult to prevent from injuring themselves or others. In young adulthood, individuals with mild ID may still be struggling with adolescent independence and identity issues left behind by their normally developing peers. It is thus appropriate for child and adolescent mental health professionals to continue care for some years into the adult chronological age period.

Mental health practitioners will need to interact effectively with a range of other services and these will change with the patient's development. As the young person with ID grows, the focus of inter-agency collaboration may shift from maternal and infant services, through stages of the preschool and education system, to transitional vocational or day activity programs to degrees of independent living. The state of the young person's mental health will have a substantial impact on the success of this development.

Future Directions

Future research and practice hold out the possibility of advances on three fronts: furthering our understanding of the biological bases of ID; strengthening the evidence-base for specific interventions; and developing a more preventative approach to addressing psychopathology in children and adolescents with ID.

Prospects for substantial advances in understanding the biology of ID are likely to arise from advances in human genetics. In particular, microarray techniques promise to identify new small aneuploidies underlying ID. Lewis (2005) provides a useful review of these technologies in ID research. We also anticipate continuing advances in mapping gene–behavior pathways in the behavior phenotypes of genetic disorders causing ID (see chapter 24). These advances offer the prospect of prevention through prenatal molecular karyotyping (Larrabee, Johnson, Pestova *et al.*, 2004).

The evidence-base relating to interventions for reducing psychopathology primarily addresses issues of efficacy. There is a dearth of evidence relating to effectiveness or the factors associated in successfully scaling up existing interventions, and no evidence relating to efficiency (see chapter 18; Emerson, 2006). Such evidence is a prerequisite for evidence-based policy and practice.

The high prevalence and persistence of psychopathology among children and adolescents with ID, when combined with existing knowledge regarding risk factors and possible underlying mechanisms, open up the possibility of developing more preventative approaches. These are likely to encompass a range of possibilities including primary prevention through reducing exposure to risk factors associated with the development of psychopathology (e.g., poverty reduction, enhanced child protection, reduced exposure to unresponsive communicative environments) and developing resilience in the face of exposure to these risk factors, through to increased investment in targeted early intervention.

Further Reading

Emerson, E., & Einfeld, S. L. (in press). Challenging behaviours: Analysis and intervention in people with intellectual disabilities (3rd ed.). Cambridge: Cambridge University Press.

Harris, J. C. (2006). *Intellectual disability: Understanding its development, causes, classification, evaluation and treatment.* New York: Oxford University Press.

References

Agarwal, V., Sitholey, P., Kumar, S., & Prasad, M. (2001). Double-blind, placebo-controlled trial of clonidine in hyperactive children with mental retardation. *Mental Retardation*, *39*, 259–267.

Alwan, A., & Modell, B. (2003). Recommendations for introducing genetics services in developing countries. *Nature Reviews. Genetics*, *4*, 61–68.

Aman, M. (1991). *Assessing psychopathology and behavior problems in persons with mental retardation: A review of available instruments.* Rockville, MD: US Department of Health and Human Services.

Aman, M. G. (1985). Drugs in mental retardation: treatment or tragedy? *Australian and New Zealand Journal of Developmental Disabilities*, *10*, 215–226.

Aman, M. G., De Smedt, G., Derivan, A., Lyons, B., Findling, R. L., & The Risperidone Disruptive Behavior Study Group. (2002). Risperidone treatment of children with disruptive behavior symptoms and subaverage IQ: A double-blind, placebo-controlled study. *American Journal of Psychiatry*, *159*, 1337–1346.

Aman, M. G., Marks, R. E., Turbott, S. H., Wilsher, C. P., & Merry, S. N. (1991). Clinical effects of methylphenidate and thioridazine in intellectually subaverage children. *Journal of the American Academy of Child and Adolescent Psychiatry*, *30*, 246–256.

Aman, M. G., Paxton, J. W., Field, C. J., & Foote, S. E. (1986). Prevalence of toxic anticonvulsant drug concentrations in mentally retarded persons with epilepsy. *American Journal of Mental Deficiency*, *90*, 643–650.

Aman, M. G., Singh, N. N., Stewart, A. W., & Field, C. J. (1985). The Aberrant Behaviour Checklist: A behavior rating scale for the assessment of treatment effects. *American Journal of Mental Deficiency*, *5*, 485–491.

American Academy of Pediatrics Committee on Genetics. (2001). American Academy of Pediatrics: Health supervision for children with Down syndrome. *Pediatrics*, *107*, 442–450.

American Psychiatric Association. (2000). *Diagnostic and Statistical Manual of Mental Disorders* (4th edn.). Text revision. Washington, DC: American Psychiatric Association.

Ammerman, R. T., Hersen, M., van Hasselt, V. B., Lubetsky, M. J., & Sieck, W. R. (1994). Maltreatment in psychiatrically hospitalized children and adolescents with developmental disabilities: Prevalence and correlates. *Journal of the American Academy of Child and Adolescent Psychiatry*, *33*, 567–576.

Anderson, D. J., Lakin, K. C., Hill, B. K., & Chen, T. H. (1992). Social integration of older persons with mental retardation in residential facilities. *American Journal of Mental Retardation*, *96*, 488–501.

Andersson, M., Takkouche, B., Egli, I., Allen, H. E., & de Benoist, B. (2005). Current global iodine status and progress over the last decade towards the elimination of iodine deficiency. *Bulletin of the World Health Organization*, *83*, 518–525.

Arnold, L. E., Aman, M. G., Cook, A. M., Witwer, A. N., Hall, K. L., Thompson, S., *et al.* (2006). Atomoxetine for hyperactivity in autism spectrum disorders: Placebo-controlled crossover pilot trial. *Journal of the American Academy of Child and Adolescent Psychiatry*, *45*, 1196–1205.

Association of Directors of Social Services (ADSS). (2005). *Pressures on learning disability services: The case for review by Government of current funding*. London: ADSS.

Baker, B. L., Blacher, J., Kopp, C. B., & Kraemer, B. (1997). Parenting children with mental retardation. In N. W. Bray (Ed.), *International Review of Research in Mental Retardation*. Orlando, FL: Academic Press.

Baker, B. L., Blacher, J., & Olsson, M. B. (2005). Preschool children with and without developmental delay: Behaviour problems, parents' optimism and well-being. *Journal of Intellectual Disability Research*, *49*, 575–590.

Baker, B. L., & Feinfield, K. A. (2007). Early intervention and parent education. In A. Carr, G. O'Reilly, P. N. Walsh, & J. McEvoy (Eds.), *The handbook of intellectual disability and clinical psychology practice*. London: Routledge (pp. 336–370).

Baker, B. L., McIntyre, L. L., Blacher, J., Crnic, K., Edelbrock, C., & Low, C. (2003). Pre-school children with and without developmental delay: Behaviour problems and parenting stress over time. *Journal of Intellectual Disability Research*, *47*, 217–230.

Ball, T., Bush, A., & Emerson, E. (2004). *Psychological interventions for severely challenging behaviours shown by people with learning disabilities*. Leicester: British Psychological Society.

Barnes, D., Wistow, R., Dean, R., Appleby, C., Glover, G., & Bradley, S. (2005). *National Child and Adolescent Mental Health Service Mapping Exercise 2004*. Durham: School of Applied Social Sciences, Durham University.

Barry, R. J., Leitner, R. P., Clarke, A. R., & Einfeld, S. L. (2005). Behavioral aspects of Angelman syndrome: A case–control study. *American Journal of Medical Genetics. Part A*, *132*, 8–12.

Beange, H., Lennox, N., & Parmenter, T. (1999). Health targets for people with an intellectual disability. *Journal of Intellectual and Developmental Disability*, *24*, 283–297.

Beasley, C., Dellva, M., Tamura, R., Morgenstern, H., Glazer, W., Ferguson, K., *et al.* (1999). Randomised double-blind comparison of the incidence of tardive dyskinesia in patients with schizophrenia during long-term treatment with olanzapine or haloperidol. *British Journal of Psychiatry*, *174*, 23–30.

Beckung, E., Steffenburg, U., & Uvebrant, P. (1997). Motor and sensory dysfunctions in children with mental retardation and epilepsy. *Seizure*, *6*, 43–50.

Bennett, F. C., La Veck, B., & Sells, C. J. (1978). The Williams elfin facies syndrome: The psychological profile as an aid in syndrome identification. *Paediatrics*, *61*, 303–306.

Birch, H. G., Richardson, S. A., Baird, D., Horobin, G., & Illsley, R. (1970). *Mental subnormality in the community: A clinical and epidemiological study*. Baltimore: Williams & Wilkins.

Blacher, J., & Baker, B. L. (Eds.). (2002). *The best of AAMR: Families and mental retardation: A collection of notable AAMR journal articles across the 20th century*. Washington, DC: American Association on Mental Retardation.

Blacher, J., & Mink, I. T. (2004). Interviewing family members and careproviders: Concepts, methodologies, and cultures. In E. Emerson, C. Hatton, T. Thompson, & T. Parmenter (Eds.), *Handbook of applied research in intellectual disabilities*. Chichester: Wiley.

BMA Board of Science. (2006). *Child and adolescent mental health: A guide for healthcare professionals*. London: BMA.

Boyd, R. D. (1993). Antipsychotic malignant syndrome and mental retardation: Review and analysis of 29 cases. *American Journal of Mental Retardation*, *98*, 143–155.

Bradley, E., Summers, J., Brereton, A., Einfeld, S., Havercamp, S., Holt, G., *et al.* (2007). Intellectual disabilities and behavioral, emotional and psychiatric disturbances. In I. Ivan Brown, & M. Percy (Eds.), *A comprehensive guide to intellectual and developmental disabilities* (pp. 645–666). Baltimore: Brookes Publishing.

Brylewski, J., & Duggan, L. (2004). Antipsychotic medication for challenging behaviour in people with learning disability. *Cochrane Database of Systematic Reviews*, CD000377.

Bundey, S., Thake, A., & Todd, J. (1989). The recurrence risks for mild idiopathic mental retardation. *Journal of Medical Genetics*, *26*, 260–266.

Bush, A., & Emerson, E. (in press). Working with people with challenging behaviour. In E. Emerson, C. Hatton, J. Bromley, A. Caine, R. Gone, & K. Dickson (Eds.), *Clinical psychology and people with intellectual disabilities*. Chichester: Wiley.

Butcher, L. M., Meaburn, E., Knight, J., Sham, P. C., Schalkwyk, L. C., Craig, I. W., *et al.* (2005). SNPs, microarrays and pooled DNA: Identification of four loci associated with mild mental impairment in a sample of 6000 children. *Human Molecular Genetics*, *14*, 1315–1325.

Buzan, R. D., Dubovsky, S. L., Firestone, D., & Dal Pozzo, E. (1998). Use of clozapine in 10 mentally retarded adults. *Journal of Neuropsychiatry and Clinical Neurosciences*, *10*, 93–95.

Campbell, M., Armenteros, J. L., Malone, R. P., Adams, P. B., Eisenberg, Z. W., & Overall, J. E. (1997). Antipsychotic-related dyskinesias in autistic children: A prospective, longitudinal study. *Journal of the American Academy of Child and Adolescent Psychiatry*, *36*, 835–843.

Capron, C., & Duyme, M. (1989). Assessment of effects of socio-economic status on IQ in a full cross-fostering study. *Nature*, *340*, 552–554.

Carr, E. G., Levin, L., McConnachie, G., Carlson, J. I., Kemp, D. C., & Smith, C. (1994). *Communication-based intervention for problem behavior: A user's guide for producing positive change*. Baltimore: Brookes.

Carr, J. (1994). Long-term outcome for people with Down syndrome. *Journal of Child Psychology and Psychiatry and Allied Disciplines*, *35*, 425–439.

Carr, J. (2000). Intellectual and daily living skills of 30-year-olds with Down syndrome: Continuation of a longitudinal study. *Journal of Applied Research in Intellectual Disabilities*, *13*, 1–16.

Carr, J. (2002). Down syndrome. In P. Howlin, & O. Udwin (Eds.), *Outcomes in neurodevelopmental and genetic disorders* (pp. 169–197). Cambridge: Cambridge University Press.

Chadwick, O., Kusel, Y., Cuddy, M., & Taylor, E. (2005). Psychiatric diagnoses and behaviour problems from childhood to early adolescence in young people with severe intellectual disabilities. *Psychological Medicine*, *35*, 751–760.

Clarke, D. J. (1989). Antilibidinal drugs and mental retardation: A review. *Medicine, Science and the Law*, *29*, 136–146.

Clegg, J. (1999). Ethics and intellectual disability. *Current Opinion in Psychiatry*, *12*, 537–541.

Cohen, W. I. (2006). Current dilemmas in Down syndrome clinical care: Celiac disease, thyroid disorders, and atlanto-axial instability. *American Journal of Medical Genetics. Part C, Seminars in Medical Genetics*, *142*, 141–148.

Cooper, S. A., Melville, C. A., & Einfeld, S. L. (2003). Psychiatric diagnosis, intellectual disabilities and diagnostic criteria for psychiatric disorders for use with adults with learning disabilities/mental retardation (DC-LD). *Journal of Intellectual Disability Research*, *47*, 3–15.

Crome, L. S., & Stern, J. (1972). *Pathology of Mental Retardation*. London: Churchill Livingstone.

Curry, C. J., Stevenson, R. E., Aughton, D., Byrne, J., Carey, J. C., Cassidy, S., *et al.* (1997). Evaluation of mental retardation: Recommendations of a consensus conference. American College of Medical Genetics. *American Journal of Medical Genetics*, *72*, 468–477.

Dagnan, D., & Joahoda, A., Kroese, D. S. (2007). Cognitive behaviour therapy. In A. Corr, G. O'Reilly, P. N. Walsh, & J. McEvoy (Eds), The handbook of intellectual disability and clinical psychology practice (pp. 281–299). London: Routledge.

Davies, M., Udwin, O., & Howlin, P. (1998). Adults with Williams Syndrome. Preliminary study of social, emotional and behavioural difficulties. *The British Journal of Psychiatry*, *172*, 273–276.

De Hert, M., van Eyck, D., & De Nayer, A. (2006). Metabolic abnormalities associated with second generation antipsychotics: Fact or fiction? Development of guidelines for screening and monitoring. *International Clinical Psychopharmacology*, *21*, S11–S15.

Department for Education and Skills. (2005). *Special educational needs in England 2005*. London: Department for Education and Skills.

Department of Health. (2001). *Valuing people: A new strategy for learning disability for the 21st century*. London: Department of Health.

Department of Health. (2004a). *National service framework for children, young people and maternity services: Disabled children and young people and those with complex health needs*. London: Department of Health.

Department of Health. (2004b). *National service framework for children, young people and maternity services: The mental health and psychological well-being of children and young people*. London: Department of Health.

Didden, R., Duker, P. C., & Korzilius, H. (1997). Meta-analytic study on treatment effectiveness for problem behaviors with individuals who have mental retardation. *American Journal of Mental Retardation*, *101*, 387–399.

Disability Rights Commission. (2004). *Equal treatment: Closing the gap*. http://www.equalityhumanrights.com/en/publicationsandresource/Disability/Pages/Formalinvestigations.aspx. Accessed 12 November 2007.

Drotar, D., Olness, K., Wiznitzer, M., Guay, L., Marum, L., Svilar, G., *et al.* (1997). Neurodevelopmental outcomes of Ugandan infants with human immunodeficiency virus type 1 infection. *Pediatrics*, *100*, E5.

Durkin, M. (2002). The epidemiology of developmental disabilities in low-income countries. *Mental Retardation and Developmental Disabilities Research Reviews*, *8*, 206–211.

Dykens, E. M. (1999). Direct effects of genetic mental retardation syndromes: Maladaptive behavior and psychopathology. In L. M. Glidden (Ed.), *International review of research on mental retardation* (Vol. 22, pp. 1–26). New York: Academic Press.

Dykens, E. M. (2000). Psychopathology in children with intellectual disability. *Journal of Child Psychology and Psychiatry and Allied Disciplines*, *41*, 407–417.

Dykens, E. M. (2004). Maladaptive and compulsive behavior in Prader–Willi syndrome: New insights from older adults. *American Journal of Mental Retardation*, *109*, 142–153.

Einfeld, S., Tonge, B., Chapman, L., Mohr, C., Taffe, J., & Horstead, S. (2007). Inter-rater reliability of the diagnoses of psychosis and depression in individuals with intellectual disabilities. *Journal of Applied Research in Intellectual Disabilities*, *20*, 384–390.

Einfeld, S., Tonge, B., Turner, G., Parmenter, T., & Smith, A. (1999a). Longitudinal course of behavioural and emotional problems of young persons with Prader–Willi, Fragile X, Williams and Down syndromes. *Journal of Intellectual and Developmental Disability*, *24*, 349–354.

Einfeld, S. L. (1990). Guidelines for the use of psychotropic medication in patients with intellectual handicaps. *Australian and New Zealand Journal of Developmental Disabilities*, *16*, 71–73.

Einfeld, S. L. (1992). Clinical assessment of psychiatric symptoms in mentally retarded individuals. *Australian and New Zealand Journal of Psychiatry*, *26*, 48–63.

Einfeld, S. L., & Aman, M. (1995). Issues in the taxonomy of psychopathology in mental retardation. *Journal of Autism and Developmental Disorders*, *25*, 143–167.

Einfeld, S. L., Piccinin, A. M., Mackinnon, A., Hofer, S. M., Taffe, J., Gray, K. M., *et al.* (2006). Psychopathology in young people with intellectual disability. *Journal of the American Medical Association*, *296*, 1981–1989.

Einfeld, S. L., Smith, A., Durvasula, S., Florio, T., & Tonge, B. J. (1999b). Behavior and emotional disturbance in Prader–Willi syndrome. *American Journal of Medical Genetics*, *82*, 123–127.

Einfeld, S. L., & Tonge, B. J. (1996a). Population prevalence of psychopathology in children and adolescents with intellectual disability. I. Rationale and methods. *Journal of Intellectual Disability Research*, *40*, 91–98.

Einfeld, S. L., & Tonge, B. J. (1996b). Population prevalence of psychopathology in children and adolescents with intellectual disability. II. Epidemiological findings. *Journal of Intellectual Disability Research*, *40*, 99–109.

Einfeld, S. L., & Tonge, B. J. (2002). *Manual for the Developmental Behaviour Checklist. Primary Carer version (DBC-P) & Teacher version (DBC-T)* (2nd edn.). Sydney and Clayton: University of New South Wales and Monash University.

Einfeld, S. L., Tonge, B. J., & Rees, V. W. (2001). Longitudinal course of behavioral and emotional problems in Williams syndrome. *American Journal of Mental Retardation*, *106*, 73–81.

Eisenhower, A., Baker, B. L., & Blacher, J. (2005). Preschool children with intellectual disability: Syndrome specificity, behavior problems, and maternal well-being. *Journal of Intellectual Disability Research*, *49*, 657–671.

Emerson, E. (2001). *Challenging behaviour: Analysis and intervention in people with severe intellectual disabilities* (2nd edn.). Cambridge: Cambridge University Press.

Emerson, E. (2003). Mothers of children and adolescents with intellectual disability: Social and economic situation, mental health status, and the self-assessed social and psychological impact of the child's difficulties. *Journal of Intellectual Disability Research*, *47*, 385–399.

Emerson, E. (2005a). Issues in the assessment of challenging behaviour. In J. Hogg, & A. Langa (Eds.), *Assessing adults with intellectual disabilities: A service providers' guide*. Oxford: Blackwell.

Emerson, E. (2005b). Underweight, obesity and physical activity in adults with intellectual disability in supported accommodation in Northern England. *Journal of Intellectual Disability Research*, *49*, 134–143.

Emerson, E. (2006). The need for credible evidence: Comments on "On some recent claims for the efficacy of cognitive therapy for people with intellectual disabilities". *Journal of Applied Research in Intellectual Disabilities*, *19*, 21–23.

Emerson, E., Fujiura, G. T., & Hatton, C. (2007). International perspectives. In S. L. Odom, R. H. Horner, M. E. Snell, & J. Blacher (Eds.), *Handbook of developmental disabilities* (pp. 593–613). New York: Guilford Press.

Emerson, E., Graham, H., & Hatton, C. (2006). Household income and health status in children and adolescents: Cross-sectional study. *European Journal of Public Health*, *16*, 354–360.

Emerson, E., & Hatton, C. (2007a). Socioeconomic disadvantage, social participation and networks and the self-rated health of English men and women with mild and moderate intellectual disabilities: Cross-sectional survey. *European Journal of Public Health*, May 7, 2007 epub ahead of publication.

Emerson, E., & Hatton, C. (2007b). Contribution of socioeconomic position to health inequalities of British children and adolescents with intellectual disabilities. *American Journal of Mental Retardation*, *112*, 140–150.

Emerson, E., Hatton, C., Blacher, J., Llewellyn, G., & Graham, H. (2006). Socio-economic position, household composition, health status and indicators of the well-being of mothers of children with and without intellectual disability. *Journal of Intellectual Disability Research*, *50*, 862–873.

Emerson, E., Malam, S., Davies, I., & Spencer, K. (2005). *Adults with learning difficulties in England 2003/4*. Leeds: Health & Social Care Information Centre.

Engle, P. L., Black, M. M., Behrman, J. R., de Mello, M. C., Gertler, P. J., Kapiriri, L., *et al.* (2007). Strategies to avoid the loss of developmental potential in more than 200 million children in the developing world. *Lancet*, *369*, 229–242.

Evans, J., Jones, J., & Mansell, I. (2001). Supporting siblings: Evaluation of support groups for brothers and sisters of children with learning disabilities and challenging behaviour. *Journal of Learning Disabilities*, *5*, 69–78.

Finlay, W. M. L., & Lyons, E. (2002). Acquiesence in interviews with people who have mental retardation. *Mental Retardation*, *40*, 14–29.

Fisch, G. S., Simensen, R. J., & Schroer, R. J. (2002). Longitudinal changes in cognitive and adaptive behavior scores in children and adolescents with fragile X mutation or autism. *Journal of Autism and Developmental Disorders*, *32*, 107–114.

Fisher, C. B. (2003). Goodness-of-fit ethic for informed consent to research involving adults with mental retardation and developmental disabilities. *Mental Retardation and Developmental Disabilities Research Reviews*, *9*, 27–31.

Foundation for People with Learning Difficulties. (2003). *Count us in: Meeting the mental health needs of children with learning difficulties*. London: Foundation for People with Learning Difficulties.

Fox, P., & Emerson, E. (2002). *Positive outcomes*. Brighton: Pavillion Press.

Fujiura, G. T., & Yamaki, K. (1997). Analysis of ethnic variations in developmental disability prevalence and household economic status. *Mental Retardation*, *35*, 286–294.

Ghose, S., & Chandra Sekhar, G. (1986). The eye in idiopathic mental retardation. *Japanese Journal of Ophthalmology*, *30*, 431–435.

Goodman, R. (1995). The relationship between normal variation in IQ and common childhood psychopathology: A clinical study. *European Child and Adolescent Psychiatry*, *4*, 187–196.

Gothelf, D., & Lombroso, P. J. (2001). Genetics of childhood disorders. XXV. Velocardiofacial syndrome. *Journal of the American Academy of Child and Adolescent Psychiatry*, *40*, 489–491.

Grant, G., Goward, P., Richardson, M., & Ramcharan, P. (Eds.). (2005). *Learning disability: A life cycle approach to valuing people*. Maidenhead: Open University Press.

Green, S. E. (2004). Attitudes toward control in uncontrollable situations: The multidimensional impact of health locus of control on the well-being of mothers of children with disabilities. *Sociological Inquiry*, *74*, 20–49.

Guralnick, M. J. (2005). Early intervention for children with intellectual disabilities: Current knowledge and future prospects. *Journal of Applied Research in Intellectual Disabilities*, *18*, 313–323.

Hagerman, R. J. (1999). *Neurodevelopmental disorders, diagnosis and treatment*. New York: Oxford University Press.

Hall, I., Strydom, A., Richards, M., Hardy, R., Bernal, J., & Wadsworth, M. (2005). Social outcomes in adulthood of children with intellectual impairment: Evidence from a birth cohort. *Journal of Intellectual Disability Research*, *49*, 171–182.

Hallam, A., & Emerson, E. (1999). Costs of residential supports for people with learning disabilities. In A. Netten, J. Dennett, & J. Knight (Eds.), *Unit costs of health and social care* (pp. 53–58). Canterbury: PSSRU, University of Kent at Canterbury.

Hankin, J. R. (2002). Fetal alcohol syndrome prevention research. *Alcohol Research and Health*, *26*, 58.

Harris, J. C. (2006). *Intellectual disability: Understanding its development, causes, classification, evaluation, and treatment*. New York: Oxford University Press.

Hastings, R. P., & Beck, A. (2004). Practitioner review: Stress intervention for parents of children with intellectual disabilities. *Journal of Child Psychology and Psychiatry*, *45*, 1338–1349.

Hatton, C., & Emerson, E. (2004). The relationship between life events and psychopathology amongst children with intellectual disabilities. *Journal of Applied Research in Intellectual Disabilities*, *17*, 109–117.

Hodapp, R. M., & Dykens, E. M. (2004). Studying behavioural phenotypes: Issues, benefits, challenges. In E. Emerson, C. Hatton, T. Thompson, & T. Parmenter (Eds.), *International handbook of applied research in intellectual disabilities (pp. 203–220)*. Chichester: Wiley.

Holden, B., & Gitlesen, J. P. (2004). Psychotropic medication in adults with mental retardation: Prevalence, and prescription practices. *Research in Developmental Disabilities*, *25*, 509–521.

Holland, A., Whittington, J., & Butler, J. (2002). Prader–Willi and Angelman syndromes: From childhood to adult life. In P. Howlin, & O. Udwin (Eds.), *Outcomes in neurodevelopmental and genetic disorders* (pp. 220–240). Cambridge: Cambridge University Press.

Horsler, K., & Oliver, C. (2006). Environmental influences on the behavioral phenotype of Angelman syndrome. *American Journal of Mental Retardation*, *111*, 311–321.

Howlin, P., Davies, M., & Udwin, O. (1998). Cognitive functioning in adults with Williams syndrome. *Journal of Child Psychology and Psychiatry*, *39*, 183–190.

Hupalo, P. (1997). *Factors assisting the employment of people with disabilities*. Canberra: Department of Social Security.

Institute of Medicine. (2001). *Neurological, psychiatric and developmental disorders: Meeting the challenge in the developing world*. Washington, DC: National Academy Press.

Janowsky, D. S., Shetty, M., Barnhill, J., Elamir, B., & Davis, J. M. (2005). Serotonergic antidepressant effects on aggressive, self-injurious and destructive/disruptive behaviours in intellectually disabled adults: A retrospective, open-label, naturalistic trial. *International Journal of Neuropsychopharmacology*, *8*, 37–48.

Kalachnik, J. E., Hanzel, T. E., Sevenich, R., & Harder, S. R. (2002). Benzodiazepine behavioral side effects: Review and implications for individuals with mental retardation. *American Journal of Mental Retardation*, *107*, 376–410.

Karjalainen, S., Kääriäinen, R., & Vohlonen, I. (1983). Ear disease and hearing sensitivity in mentally retarded children. *International Journal of Pediatric Otorhinolaryngology*, *5*, 235–241.

Katusic, S. K., Colligan, R. C., Beard, C. M., O'Fallon, W. M., Bergstralh, E. J., Jacobsen, S. J., *et al.* (1996). Mental retardation in a birth cohort, 1976–1980, Rochester, Minnesota. *American Journal of Mental Retardation*, *100*, 335–344.

Langee, H. R. (1990). Retrospective study of lithium use for institutionalized mentally retarded individuals with behavior disorders. *American Journal of Mental Retardation*, *94*, 448–452.

Larrabee, P. B., Johnson, K. L., Pestova, E., Lucas, M., Wilber, K., LeShane, E. S., *et al.* (2004). Microarray analysis of cell-free fetal DNA in amniotic fluid: A prenatal molecular karyotype. *American Journal of Human Genetics*, *75*, 485–491.

Lavin, E. K., Mcguire, B. E., & Hogan, M. J. (2006). Age at death of people with an intellectual disability in Ireland. *Journal of Intellectual Disabilities*, *10*, 155–164.

Leonard, H., Petterson, B., De Klerk, N., Zubrick, S. R., Glasson, E., Sanders, R., *et al.* (2005). Association of sociodemographic characteristics of children with intellectual disability in Western Australia. *Social Science and Medicine*, *60*, 1499–1513.

Levy-Wasser, N., & Katz, S. (2004). The relationship between attachment style, birth order and adjustment in children who grow up with a sibling with mental retardation. *British Journal of Developmental Disability*, *50*, 89–98.

Lewis, J. N., Tonge, B. J., Mowat, D. R., Einfeld, S. L., Siddons, H. M., & Rees, V. W. (2000). Epilepsy and associated psychopathology in young people with intellectual disability. *Journal of Paediatrics and Child Health*, *36*, 172–175.

Lewis, S. M. E. (2005). Higher resolution solutions for mapping the mystery of idiopathic intellectual disability. *Clinical Genetics*, *67*, 155–157.

Llewellyn, G., Dunn, P., Fante, M., Turnbull, L., & Grace, R. (1999). Family factors influencing out-of-home placement decisions. *Journal of Intellectual Disability Research*, *43*, 219–241.

Llewellyn, G., McConnell, D., Thompson, K., & Whybrow, S. (2005). Out-of-home placement of school age children with disabilities. *Journal of Applied Research in Intellectual Disabilities*, *18*, 1–16.

Loesch, D. Z., Huggins, R. M., & Hagerman, R. J. (2004). Phenotypic variation and FMRP levels in fragile X. *Mental Retardation and Developmental Disabilities Research Reviews*, *10*, 31–41.

Louhiala, P. (2004). *Preventing intellectual disability: Ethical and clinical issues*. Cambridge: Cambridge University Press.

Lowe, K. (1999). *Report on compensation and workers' OH&S claims*. Canberra: Department of Community Services.

Luckasson, R., Borthwick-Duffy, S., Buntinx, W. H. E., Coulter, D. L., Craig, E. M., Reeve, A., *et al.* (2002). *Mental retardation: Definition, classification, and systems of support* (10th edn.). Washington, DC: American Association on Mental Retardation.

Luckasson, R., Coulter, D. L., Polloway, E. A., Reiss, S., Schalock, R. L., Snell, M. E., *et al.* (1992). *Mental retardation: Definition, classification, and systems of support* (9th edn.). Washington, DC: American Association on Mental Retardation.

Lucyshyn, J. M., Dunlap, G., & Albin, R. W. (Eds.). (2002). *Families and positive behavior support*. Baltimore: Brookes.

Luiselli, J. (Ed.). (2006). *Antecedent assessment and intervention: Supporting children and adults with developmental disabilities in community settings*. Baltimore: Brookes.

Maughan, B., Collishaw, S., & Pickles, A. (1999). Mild mental retardation: Psychosocial functioning in adulthood. *Psychological Medicine*, *29*, 351–366.

McCarthy, J., & Boyd, J. (2002). Mental health services and young people with intellectual disability: Is it time to do better? *Journal of Intellectual Disability Research*, *46*, 250–256.

McDermot, S. W., & Altekrusse, J. M. (1994). Dynamic model for preventing mental retardation in the population: The importance of poverty and deprivation. *Research in Developmental Disabilities*, *15*, 49–65.

Meijer, M., Carpenter, S., & Scholte, F. (2004). European manifesto on basic standards of health care for people with intellectual disabilities. *Journal of Policy and Practice in Intellectual Disabilities*, *1*, 10–15.

Menolascino, F. J. (1971). *Psychiatric aspects of diagnosis and treatment of mental retardation*. Seattle: Special Child Publications.

Menolascino, F. J., Levitas, A., & Greiner, C. (1986). The nature and types of mental illness in the mentally retarded. *Psychopharmacology Bulletin*, *22*, 1060–1071.

Modood, T., Berthoud, R., Lakey, J., Nazroo, J., Smith, P., Virdee, S., *et al.* (1997). *Ethnic minorities in Britain: Diversity and disadvantage*. London: Policy Studies Institute.

Murphy, K. C. (2005). Annotation: velo-cardio-facial syndrome. *Journal of Child Psychology and Psychiatry and Allied Disciplines*, *46*, 563–571.

Murphy, K. C., Jones, L. A., & Owen, M. L. (1999). High rates of schizophrenia in adults with Velo-Cardio Facial Syndrome. *Archives of General Psychiatry*, *56*, 940–945.

Nelson, K. B. (2003). Can we prevent cerebral palsy? *New England Journal of Medicine*, *349*, 1765–1769.

Nelson, E., Wasson, J., Kirk, J., Keller, A., Clark, D., Dietrich, A., *et al.* (1987). Assessment of function in routine clinical practice: Description of the COOP chart method and preliminary findings. *Journal of Chronic Diseases*, *40*, 55S–63S.

O'Reilly, M. F., Sigafoos, J., Lancioni, G. E., Green, V., Olive, M., Lacey, C., *et al.* (2007). Applied behaviour analysis. In A. Carr, G. O'Reilly, P. N. Walsh, & J. McEvoy (Eds.), *The handbook of intellectual disability and clinical psychology practice*. London: Routledge (pp. 253–280).

Oliver, C., Murphy, G. H., & Corbett, J. A. (1987). Self-injurious behaviour in people with mental handicap: a total population study. *Journal of Mental Deficiency Research*, *31*, 147–162.

Olness, K. (2003). Effects on brain development leading to cognitive impairment: A worldwide epidemic. *Journal of Developmental and Behavioral Pediatrics*, *24*, 120–130.

Ouellette-Kuntz, H. (2005). Understanding health disparities and inequities faced by individuals with intellectual disabilities. *Journal of Applied Research in Intellectual Disabilities*, *18*, 113–121.

Partington, M., Mowat, D., Einfeld, S., Tonge, B., & Turner, G. (2000). Genes on the X chromosome are important in undiagnosed mental retardation. *American Journal of Medical Genetics*, *92*, 57–61.

Patja, K., Iivanainen, M., Vesala, H., Oksanen, H., & Ruoppila, I. (2000). Life expectancy of people with intellectual disability: A 35-year follow-up study. *Journal of Intellectual Disability Research*, *44*, 591–599.

Pharoah, P. O., Buttfield, I. H., & Hetzel, B. S. (1971). Neurological damage to the fetus resulting from severe iodine deficiency during pregnancy. *Lancet*, *1*, 308–310.

Powell, D., Dunlap, G., & Fox, L. (2005). Prevention and intervention for challenging behaviors of toddlers and preschoolers. *Infants and Young Children*, *19*, 25–35.

Quine, L. (1986). Behaviour problems in severely mentally handicapped children. *Psychological Medicine*, *16*, 895–907.

Quine, L., & Pahl, J. (1989). *Stress and coping in families caring for a child with severe mental retardation: A longitudinal study*. Canterbury, England: University of Kent at Canterbury.

Rantakallio, P., & von Wendt, L. (1986). Mental retardation and subnormality in a birth cohort of 12,000 children in Northern Finland. *American Journal of Mental Deficiency*, *90*, 380–387.

Reilly, D. R., Delva, N. J., & Hudson, R. W. (2000). Protocols for the use of cyproterone, mexdroxyprogesterone, and leuprolide in the treatment of paraphilia. *Canadian Journal of Psychiatry, Revue Canadienne de Psychiatre*, *45*, 559–563.

Reiss, S., & Aman, M. (Eds.). (1998). *Psychotropic medication and developmental disabilities: The international consensus handbook*. Calumbus, Ohio: Ohio State University Nisonger Center.

Richardson, S. A., & Koller, H. (1996). *Twenty-two years: Causes and consequences of mental retardation*. Cambridge, MA: Harvard University Press.

Risdal, D., & Singer, G. H. S. (2004). Marital adjustment in parents of children with disabilities: A historical review and meta-analysis. *Research and Practice for Persons with Severe Disabilities. Special Family and Disability*, *29*, 95–103.

Roach, E. S. (1988). Diagnosis and management of neurocutaneous syndromes. *Seminars in Neurology*, *8*, 83–86.

Robertson, J., Emerson, E., Gregory, N., Hatton, C., Turner, S., Kessissoglou, S., *et al.* (2000). Lifestyle related risk factors for poor health in residential settings for people with intellectual disabilities. *Research in Developmental Disabilities*, *21*, 469–486.

Roeleveld, N., Zielhuis, G. A., & Gabreels, F. (1997). The prevalence of mental retardation: A critical review of recent literature. *Developmental Medicine and Child Neurology*, *39*, 125–132.

Rutter, M., Tizard, J., Yule, W., Graham, P., & Whitmore, K. (1976). Research report: Isle of Wight Studies, 1964–1974. *Psychological Medicine*, *6*, 313–332.

Sachdev, S. (1991). Psychoactive drug use in an institution for handicapped persons. *Medical Journal of Australia*, *155*, 75–79.

Sawyer, M. G., Arney, F. M., Baghurst, P. A., Clark, J. J., Graetz, B. W., Kosky, R. J., *et al.* (2001). The mental health of young people in Australia: Key findings from the child and adolescent component of the national survey of mental health and well-being. *Australian and New Zealand Journal of Psychiatry*, *35*, 806–814.

Schupf, N., Pang, D., Patel, B. N., Silverman, W., Schubert, R., Lai, F., *et al.* (2003). Onset of dementia is associated with age at menopause in women with Down syndrome. *Annals of Neurology*, *54*, 433–438.

Shapira, N. A., Lessig, M. C., He, A. G., James, G. A., Driscoll, D. J., & Liu, Y. (2005). Satiety dysfunction in Prader–Willi syndrome demonstrated by fMRI. *Journal of Neurology, Neurosurgery and Psychiatry*, *76*, 260–262.

Shedlack, K. J., Hennen, J., Magee, C., & Cheron, D. M. (2005). Assessing the utility of atypical antipsychotic medication in adults with mild mental retardation and comorbid psychiatric disorders. *Journal of Clinical Psychiatry*, *66*, 52–62.

Sigelman, C. K., Budd, E. C., Spankel, C. L., & Schoenrock, C. J. (1981). When in doubt say yes: Acquiescence in interviews with mentally retarded persons. *Mental Retardation*, *19*, 53–58.

Sigelman, C. K., Schoenrock, C. J., Wiver, J. L., Spankel, C. L., Hromas, S. E., Martin, P. W., *et al.* (1979). *Issues in interviewing mentally retarded persons: An empirical study*. Lubbock, TX: Research and Training Center in Mental Retardation, Texas Tech. University.

Simonoff, E., Bolton, P., & Rutter, M. (1996). Mental retardation: Genetic findings, clinical implications and research agenda. *Journal of Child Psychology and Psychiatry and Allied Disciplines*, *37*, 259–280.

Simonoff, E., Pickles, A., Chadwick, O., Gringras, P., Wood, N., Higgins, S., *et al.* (2006). The Croydon Assessment of Learning Study: Prevalence and educational identification of mild mental retardation. *Journal of Child Psychology and Psychiatry*, *47*, 828–839.

Singh, A., Kleynhans, D., & Barton, G. (1998). Selective serotonin re-uptake inhibitors in the treatment of self-injurious behaviour in adults with mental retardation. *Human Psychopharmacology*, *13*, 267–270.

Sisson, L. A., Van Hasselt, V. B., & Hersen, M. (1993). Behavioral interventions to reduce maladaptive responding in youth with dual sensory impairment: An analysis of direct and concurrent effects. *Behavior Modification*, *17*, 164–188.

Smiley, E., & Cooper, S.-A. (2003). Intellectual disabilities, depressive episode, diagnostic criteria and Diagnostic Criteria for Psychiatric Disorders for Use with Adults with Learning Disabilities/Mental Retardation (DC-LD). *Journal of Intellectual Disability Research*, *47*, 62–71.

Snyder, R., Turgay, A., Aman, M., Binder, C., Fisman, S., Carroll, A., *et al.* (2002). Effects of risperidone on conduct and disruptive behavior disorders in children with subaverage IQs. *Journal of the American Academy of Child and Adolescent Psychiatry*, *41*, 1026–1036.

Sparrow, S., Balla, D., & Cicchetti, D. V. (1984). *Vineland Adaptive Behavior Scales*. Minnesota: American Guidance Service.

Spinath, F., Harlaar, N., Ronald, A., & Plomin, R. (2004). Substantial genetic influence on mild mental impairment in early childhood. *American Journal of Mental Retardation*, *109*, 34–43.

Spinelli, M., Rocha, A. C., Giacheti, C. M., & Richieri-Costa, A. (1995). Word-finding difficulties, verbal paraphasias, and verbal dyspraxia in ten individuals with fragile X syndrome. *American Journal of Medical Genetics*, *60*, 39–43.

Spreat, S., Conroy, J. W., & Fullerton, A. (2004). Statewide longitudinal survey of psychotropic medication use for persons with mental retardation: 1994 to 2000. *American Journal of Mental Retardation*, *109*, 322–331.

Steen, R. G., Xiong, X., Mulhern, R. K., Langston, J. W., & Wang, W. C. (1999). Subtle brain abnormalities in children with sickle cell disease: Relationship to blood hematocrit. *Annals of Neurology*, *45*, 279–286.

Stoll, C., Alembik, Y., & Dott, B. (2006). Are the recommendations on the prevention of neural tube defects working? *European Journal of Medical Genetics*, *49*, 461–465.

Szymanski, L., & King, B. (1999). Summary of the practice parameters for the assessment and treatment of children, adolescents, and adults with mental retardation and comorbid mental disorders. *Journal of the American Academy of Child and Adolescent Psychiatry*, *38*, 1606–1610.

Taffe, J. R., Gray, K. M., Einfeld, S. L., Dekker, M. C., Koot, H. M., Emerson, E., *et al.* (2007). Short form of the Developmental Behaviour Checklist. *American Journal of Mental Retardation*, *112*, 31–39.

Teebi, A. S., & El-Shanti, H. (2006). Consanguinity: Implications for practice, research, and policy. *Lancet*, *367*, 970–971.

Tesio, L., Valsecchi, M. R., Sala, M., Guzzon, P., & Battaglia, M. A. (2002). Level of activity in profound/severe mental retardation (LAPMER): A Rasch-derived scale of disability. *Journal of Applied Measurement*, *3*, 50–84.

Tiet, Q. Q., Bird, H. R., Davies, M., Hoven, C., Cohen, P., Jensen, P. S., *et al.* (1998). Adverse life events and resilience. *Journal of American Academy of Child and Adolescent Psychiatry*, *37*, 1191–1200.

Tonge, B., Brereton, A., Kiomall, M., MacKinnon, A., King, N., & Rinehart, N. (2006). Effects on parental mental health of an education and skills training program for parents of young children with autism: A randomized controlled trial. *Journal of the American Academy of Child and Adolescent Psychiatry*, *45*, 561–569.

Tonge, B. J., & Einfeld, S. L. (2003). Psychopathology and intellectual disability. The Australian child to adult longitudinal study. In L. Masters Glidden (Ed.), *International review of research in mental retardation* (Vol. 26, pp. 61–91). California, USA: Academic Press.

Turk, J., & Cornish, K. (1998). Face recognition and emotion perception in boys with fragile-X syndrome. *Journal of Intellectual Disability Research*, *42*, 490–499.

US Department of Health and Human Services. (2005). *Closing the gap: A national blueprint to improve the health of persons with mental retardation*. Rockville, MD: US Department of Health and Human Services.

Vandeven, A. M., & Newton, A. W. (2006). Update on child physical abuse, sexual abuse and prevention. *Current Opinion in Pediatrics*, *18*, 201–205.

Walker, S. P., Wachs, T. D., Gardner, J. M., Lozoff, B., Wasserman, G. A., Pollitt, E., *et al.* (2007). Child development: Risk factors for adverse outcomes in developing countries. *Lancet*, *369*, 145–157.

Wallander, J. L., Dekker, M. C., & Koot, H. M. (2006). Risk factors for psychopathology in children with intellectual disability: A prospective longitudinal population-based study. *Journal of Intellectual Disability Research*, *50*, 259–268.

Webb, O. J., & Rogers, L. (1999). Health screening for people with intellectual disability: The New Zealand experience. *Journal of Intellectual Disability Research*, *43*, 497–503.

Whitehead, M. (1992). The concepts and principles of equity and health. *International Journal of Health Services*, *22*, 429–445.

Whitfield, M., Langan, J., & Russell, O. (1996). Assessing general practitioners' care of adult patients with learning disability: Case–control study. *Quality in Health Care*, *5*, 31–55.

World Health Organization. (1996). *Multiaxial classification of child and adolescent psychiatric disorders: The ICD-10 Classification of mental and behavioural disorders in children and adolescents*. Cambridge: Cambridge University Press.

World Health Organization. (2001). *International classification of functioning, disability and health*. Geneva: World Health Organization.

Ye, X., Mitchell, M., Newman, K., & Batshaw, M. L. (2001). Prospects for prenatal gene therapy in disorders causing mental retardation. *Mental Retardation and Developmental Disabilities Research Reviews*, *7*, 65–72.

YoungMinds. (2006). *Stressed out and struggling project. Report 1. Service-mapping*. London: YoungMinds.

Zahn-Waxler, C., Duggal, S., & Gruber, R. (2002). Parental psychopathology. In M. Bornstein (Ed.), *Handbook of parenting* (Vol. 4), *Social conditions and applied parenting* (pp. 295–327). Mahwah, NJ: Lawrence Erlbaum.

50 Disorders of Personality

Jonathan Hill

The concept of personality disorder in adult life is important and elusive. It is important because the problems it encompasses are a major cause of burden to patients, to the adults and children with whom they have relationships, and to society. It is elusive because there is relatively little agreement on basic issues such as whether there is one overarching disorder or many, and what the core defining features of a personality disorder are. Nevertheless, there is broad agreement that the concept must include stability of behaviors over substantial periods of time, and extensive or pervasive dysfunction encompassing a range of psychological, behavioral and interpersonal capacities. Prima facie it seems likely that such stable and severe problems will have started before adult life, and there is evidence that in many instances analogous disorders or their antecedents start in childhood, and that childhood experiences may affect risk for subsequent personality disorder. Accordingly, it seems crucial to consider what is known about personality disorders, with special reference to two key questions for child psychiatrists and child mental health practitioners more widely: the extent to which there is continuity in personality disturbance between childhood and adult life, and on whether it is useful to apply the diagnosis in childhood and adolescence.

Concepts of Personality Disorder

Attempts to classify personality types and dimensions go back to antiquity but concepts of personality disorder are of much more recent origin (Frances & Widiger, 1986; Rutter, 1987; Tyrer, Casey, & Ferguson, 1991). Although there are numerous variations on the specifics, the unifying notion is the idea that there are pervasive and persistent abnormalities of overall personality functioning that cause social impairment and/or subjective distress, which are not caused by episodic disorders of mental state. The basic assumption is that, in some way, personality disorders are different from other psychiatric conditions, such as schizophrenia, depression or anxiety states.

Most personality disorder research has made use of the American Psychiatric Association (2000) DSM classification which put forward four diagnostic criteria. There were first enduring patterns of inner experience and behaviours that deviated markedly from cultural expectations (specifying that they should be manifest in at least two of cognition affectivity, interpersonal functioning or impulse control). Second, this enduring pattern had to be inflexible and pervasive across a broad range of personal and social situations. Third, it had to lead to clinically significant distress or impairment. Fourth, the pattern must be stable over time with an onset by adolescence or early adult life.

Several attempts to provide a unified concept have been made, notably using the idea that personality disorder represents an extreme of normal personality. One approach, based on the proposal that there are five major domains of personality – the Five Factor Model – (Widiger & Costa, 1994), argues that "Personality disorders are not qualitatively distinct from normal personality functioning. They are maladaptive, extreme variants of common personality traits" (see chapter 14). In discussions of models such as these, two issues are commonly conflated: whether categorical or dimensional approaches to personality disorder are more useful, and what is "normal personality functioning?" The categorical versus dimensional dilemma is discussed later in the chapter. The identity of the key elements of personality remains a matter of debate. In the Five Factor Model, the higher-order traits extraversion/positive emotionality, neuroticism/negative emotionality, conscientiousness/constraint, agreeableness and openness-to-experience are proposed as providing a succinct yet comprehensive summary of personality dimensions. However, from the perspective of personality development several questions require attention. How coherent or homogenous are the hypothesized traits? Although the big five are characterized as "higher-order," each includes "lower-order" traits, some of which differ substantially. This issue is reviewed by Caspi, Roberts, and Shiner (2005) (see chapter 14). For example, the higher-order trait neuroticism is well validated and highly predictive in childhood and adult life, but includes both proneness to anxious distress and to anger. These different emotions motivate different behaviors, they are mediated via different neurological substrates, and they have different implications for development and psychopathology (Frick & Morris, 2004; Lemerise & Arsenio, 2000). Some of the personality traits also resemble temperamental characteristics. Thus, proneness to fearfulness and to anger are two aspects of temperament commonly assessed in infancy (Robinson & Acevedo, 2001). More generally, the overlap between temperament and

Rutter's Child and Adolescent Psychiatry, 5th edition. Edited by M. Rutter, D. Bishop, D. Pine, S. Scott, J. Stevenson, E. Taylor and A. Thapar. © 2008 Blackwell Publishing, ISBN: 978-1-4051-4549-7.

personality traits requires further attention (Caspi, Roberts, & Shiner, 2005). Big five personality traits are determined by the frequency of behaviors across context and time; however, traits can be conceptualized in other ways. In particular, coherence across context and time may occur at the level of the organization of behaviors (e.g., from the interplay between social information processing and context; Mischel, 2004). Personality development entails the development of the person as a social organism. Personality traits such as neuroticism undoubtedly influence social relationships (Robins, Caspi, & Moffitt, 2002), but there are also aspects of personality functioning such as social cognitive processes that are inherently social and entail dedicated neuronal networks (Johnson, Griffin, Csibra *et al.*, 2005). The capacity to regulate behaviors and emotions according to the demands of different kinds of social domain (e.g., contrasting teachers and parents) is key to effective personality development. Personality develops in interaction with the environment so that its features are likely to reflect more or less successful adaptations than any simple manifestation of stable traits.

An alternative view of personality disorders proposes that the key features entail limitations of social role performance. Studies of adult personality disorders consistently find that they are associated with social dysfunction (Hill, Fudge, Harrington, Pickles, & Rutter, 2000; Seivewright, Tyrer, & Johnson, 2004; Skodol, Pagano, Bender *et al.*, 2005a) and "the characteristic that seems to define them all is a pervasive persistent abnormality in maintaining social relationships" (Rutter, 1987). Causes of social dysfunction may include extremes of personality traits, such as those identified in the big five, and also deficits or biases in social processes including mentalization, attachment and the capacity for social domain management (Hill, Pilkonis, Morse *et al.*, 2008).

While these frameworks are promising, it should be borne in mind that the concept of personality disorder did not originate from a model of normal personality, and indeed descriptions of different personality disorder types have come about through several contrasting routes. First, there are those that derive from the clinical observation that there are individuals who show enduring patterns of inflexible and seriously maladaptive behavior that seem to fall outside the traditional criteria for mental illness or psychiatric syndrome. The need to have a term to describe these patterns of abnormal behavior led to the concepts of psychopathy put forward by writers such as Hare (1970), Henderson (1939) and Cleckley (1941) (see chapter 51). Second, there are the categories of personality disorder that identify individuals who are thought to be most prone to episodic mental disorders. Schneider's (1923, 1950) notion of psychopathic personality (defined quite differently from the psychopathy formulations of Hare, of Henderson and of Cleckley) provides the main historic notion of this approach. Many of the ICD-10 specific personality disorder categories (e.g., paranoid, anankastic and anxious) represent this tradition (World Health Organization, 1996). Third, some categories have their origins in empirical observations of the continuities between psychopathological disorders in childhood, and pervasive social malfunction in adult lifestyle. The DSM-IV (American Psychiatric Association, 2000) diagnosis of antisocial personality disorder is the obvious example of this type, with its starting point in the findings of the long-term longitudinal studies pioneered by Robins (1966, 1978). Fourth, some categories stem fairly directly from theoretical, especially psychoanalytic, notions. The concept of borderline personality organization (Kernberg, 1967, 1975) underlies specification of the DSM-IV diagnosis of borderline personality disorder (Gunderson, Kolb, & Austin, 1981). Finally, a few categories have come, at least in part, from genetic findings. Meehl (1962) coined the term schizotypy to describe the postulated characteristics of schizophrenia-prone individuals. The Danish adoption study showed that the biological families of adopted schizophrenic probands included a raised rate of personality disorders that seemed to exhibit some features reminiscent of schizophrenia (Kety, Rosenthal, & Wender, 1971). Spitzer, Endicott, and Gibbon (1979) developed more explicit criteria for this type of personality syndrome, which has come to be termed "schizotypal personality disorder."

The differences in the origins of personality disorder have contributed to substantial heterogeneity in the balance between behaviors and psychological states that are included in the subtypes of personality disorder. For instance, DSM-IV antisocial personality disorder is based primarily on antisocial behaviors and interpersonal difficulties, and includes only one state of mind item "lack of remorse" which is closely tied to behavior. By contrast, the borderline personality disorder category includes three items "identity disturbance," "chronic feelings of emptiness" and "transient paranoid ideation" referring solely to states of mind.

Validation

Stability and Separation from Episodic Disorders

It is assumed that the personality disorders should show substantial stability over time. However, there is surprisingly little evidence that this is the case. Several studies of referred adults have found low to moderate stability (Ferro, Klein, Schwartz, Casch, & Leader, 1998). There is increasing evidence that some personality disorders may remit over relatively short periods of time. In a follow-up every 2 years of 290 patients meeting DSM-IV criteria for borderline personality disorder, 74% had remitted after 6 years, and only 6% had remitted and then relapsed (Zanarini, Frankenburg, Hennen, Reich, & Silk, 2005).

The distinction between episodic disorders and personality disorder is enshrined in the DSM distinction between Axis I and Axis II. Axis II disorders should show persistence over a period in which there is either recovery from, or onset of, Axis I disorder. It is important to note that this distinction is not made for childhood disorders. Thus, DSM oppositional defiant disorder and conduct disorder are classified on Axis I even though they show strong continuities, and probably share causal mechanisms, with both Axis I and Axis II disorders in adult life. Remarkably few studies have been carried out to test the stability of personality disorder after accounting for episodic disorders in adults. Loranger, Lenzenweger, Gartner *et al.* (1991) examined changes in the diagnosis of personality disorder (on a standardized interview) in a series of 84 psychiatric patients over 1–6 weeks and found no effect of change in mental state on the diagnosis of personality disorder, supporting the personality disorder/episodic disorder distinction. Nevertheless, remission was associated with some fall in personality disorder symptoms and the diagnosis of personality disorder showed only moderate temporal stability (K = 0.55). Studies over greater time periods have used social dysfunction as the index of personality disorder at baseline and follow-up (Quinton, Gulliver, & Rutter, 1995; Rutter & Quinton, 1984) or a trait-based assessment of personality disorder at baseline and social dysfunction at follow-up (Seivewright, Tyrer, & Johnson, 2004). All reported substantial stability of personality dysfunction after accounting for duration or severity of symptoms of episodic disorders.

While these findings support the distinction between episodic and personality disorders, the two are strongly associated. There are very high rates of personality disorder in patients with episodic disorders – nearly half in in-patient samples and 20–40% in out-patient groups (Docherty, Fister, & Shea, 1986; Tyrer, Casey, & Ferguson, 1991). These figures are much higher than the rates of 6–13% that are typical of general population samples (Casey & Tyrer, 1986; Merikangas & Weissman, 1986). The meaning of these associations is not clear. It is likely that to a certain extent they are artifacts arising from difficulties in distinguishing Axis I and Axis II items. In clinical and research practice it is often difficult to disentangle symptoms associated with episodes and those that reflect personality disorder.

However, this is unlikely to be the whole explanation. There are three main ways in which the associations may arise. First, personality disorder may constitute a risk factor for episodic conditions. This could occur through direct mechanisms whereby a feature of the disorder, such as poor coping (Vollrath, Alnaes, & Torgersen, 1994), leads to helplessness and hence depression or indirect mechanisms in which the personality disorder increases the likelihood of psychosocial stressors that in turn are associated with a disorder such as depression (Daley, Hamman, Davila, & Burge, 1998). Second, episodic conditions may create the conditions in which personality disorders develop because a chain of maladaptive behaviors and adverse environmental responses is set in motion that fosters more persistent psychopathology (Kasen, Cohen, Skodol, Johnson, & Brook, 1999). Third, both the personality disorder and the episodic disorder could reflect one underlying liability. Malone, Taylor, Marmorstein, McGue, and Iacono (2004) assessed antisocial personality disorder and alcohol dependence in 289 twin pairs at ages 17, 20 and 24. There were moderate genetic influences on each disorder at each age, and a substantial proportion of these influences was common to the two disorders.

It might be expected that whatever the relationship between episodic disorders and personality disorder, the combination should in some sense reflect a more severe variant, with implications for treatment outcome. However, the evidence has been mixed. One recent review concluded there was no effect of personality disorder on treatment outcomes for depression (Mulder, 2002). Newton-Howes, Tyrer, and Johnson (2006) conducted a meta-analysis of all depression treatment studies in which personality disorder had been assessed and concluded that personality disorder was associated with a doubling of the risk of a poor outcome for depression (Newton-Howes, Tyrer, & Johnson, 2006). The authors point out that even the largest studies reviewed had inadequate statistical power to detect a difference of this size. Very little is known about the ways in which personality disorder may be associated with a poor outcome. Possibilities include that it may be associated with poor treatment compliance, with greater severity of overall psychopathology or with more psychosocial adversities and fewer interpersonal resources.

Differentiations Among Personality Disorders

The World Health Organization (1996) classification, ICD-10, makes a basic differentiation between organic personality disorders (meaning those resulting from severe head injury, encephalitis and other forms of overt brain damage); enduring personality changes deriving from some catastrophic experience (see chapter 42); personality abnormalities that reflect the residue of some mental illness (e.g., residual schizophrenia); and what they term personality disorders. The American Psychiatric Association (2000) scheme makes broadly comparable distinctions. This chapter is concerned with this last group of specific personality disorders, because the others have only an extremely limited application in childhood and adolescence.

The ICD classification specifies nine personality disorder types, and the DSM system eleven. To a certain extent the different categories reflect the different origins referred to earlier. The DSM classification has received a lot of attention and, in spite of the operational definitions of each of the categories, the evidence for the discriminant validity of the majority is not strong. Consistently, studies have shown that individuals who receive one DSM Axis II diagnosis often receive several (Morey, 1988; Oldham, Skodol, Kellman *et al.*, 1992; Pfohl, Coryell, Zimmerman, & Tsangl, 1986). Although there is evidence that the DSM categories cluster into three broad bands of the odd/eccentric, the dramatic/emotional/erratic and the anxious/fearful (Kass, Skodol, Charles, Spitzer, & Williams, 1985), combinations of personality disorders that cross these bands are common (Oldham, Skodol, Kellman *et al.*, 1992).

Support for the discriminant validity of particular personality disorders would be provided if it were possible to show differential association with other psychiatric conditions, family clustering, or associations with genetic or environmental influences. Studies of the association of borderline personality disorder with other episodic and personality disorders have provided some support for its discriminant validity. Zanarini, Frankenburg, Dubo *et al.* (1998) compared patients with borderline personality disorder with patients with other persoality disorders. Those with borderline disorder had higher rates of associated paranoid, avoidant and dependent personality disorders, and higher rates of mood, anxiety and eating disorders.

The most clear-cut finding from family studies is the association between schizophrenia and a loading of schizotypal personality disorders in the biological relatives (Kendler, Gruenberg, & Strauss, 1981, Kendler, Gruenberg, & Strauss, 1984). The evidence for a link between schizotypal personality disorder and schizophrenia is further supported by findings that there are similarities in magnetic resonance imaging appearances (Dickey, Shenton, Hirayasu *et al.*, 2000) and in deficits of attention and information processing (Cadenhead, Light, Geyer, & Braff, 2000). A significant but weaker association with schizophrenia has been found with paranoid personality disorders (Kendler & Gruenberg, 1982; Kendler, Masterson, & Davis, 1985).

There are very few family and genetic data on other personality disorders (Maier, Franke, & Hawallek, 1998; McGuffin & Thapar, 1992). There is some evidence that borderline personality disorders cluster in families and also are associated with affective disorders in other family members, but it remains quite uncertain whether the family loading has a genetic basis. Joyce, McHugh, McKenzie *et al.* (2006) reported a significant association between a 9-repeat allele of a dopamine transporter gene variant and borderline personality disorder in depressed patients entered into two treatment trials. This requires replication. There is consistent evidence for genetic influences on adult antisocial behaviors (Langbehn, Caderet, Yates, Troughton, & Stewart, 1998), but not adult violence (Carey & Goldman, 1997).

Most studies of the association between adverse childhood experiences and personality disorders have reported associations with a wide range of episodic and personality disorders (Johnson, Cohen, Brown, Smailes, & Bernstein, 1999). It should be borne in mind that such associations can reflect genetic as well as environmental influences; nevertheless, specificity with particular disorders would support their validity. Bezirganian, Cohen, and Brook (1993) found that the combination of maternal inconsistency and high maternal overinvolvement assessed in adolescence was associated with the persistence or emergence of borderline personality disorder, and no other episodic or personality disorders. Parker, Roy, Wilhelm *et al.* (1999) reported that dysfunctional parenting in childhood was associated with the dramatic and anxious DSM clusters, but not the odd/eccentric cluster.

Categorical versus Dimensional Characterizations of Personality Disorders

Diagnostic systems treat psychopathology as a categorical entity; however, it is evident that in most, and perhaps all, instances there are no natural cut-offs demarcating disorder from absence of disorder (see chapter 2; Pickles & Angold, 2003). The majority of early studies treated personality disorders as categories; however, the advantages of considering personality disorders dimensionally are becoming increasingly apparent. Simply from a measurement perspective, better interreliablity is achieved using symptom counts. Evidence for validity tends to be stronger for dimensional methods. Personality disorder symptoms scores show greater stability than diagnoses (Skodol, Gunderson, Shea *et al.*, 2005b) and there is a greater elevation of borderline symptoms than borderline personality disorder diagnoses in the first-degree relatives of borderline probands (Zanarini, Frankenburg, Yong *et al.*, 2004). Furthermore, there is no evidence that there is a natural diagnostic cut-off (Daley, Burge, & Hammen, 2000). Diagnoses may also lump together symptoms that reflect different processes. Zanarini, Frankenburg, Hennen *et al.* (2005) have suggested that borderline personality disorder comprises acute symptoms that wax and wane and may be affected by life events, and others are chronic or "temperamental." Such a proposal requires further investigation. However, it illustrates the advantages of a dimensional framework in relation to the personality disorders. In community studies, increasing personality disorder symptoms below a diagnostic threshold are associated with increasing social dysfunction (Daley, Burge, & Hammen, 2000; Hill, Hope, Lorenz *et al.*, unpublished data). This is of great clinical importance because it suggests that even among patients who do not meet criteria for a diagnosis, personality disorder symptoms may be associated with processes that influence course and treatment responsiveness in common presentations such as adolescent deliberate self-harm. It is also possible that in the same individual, symptoms below the diagnostic threshold from more than one disorder may each have prognostic significance.

Specific Personality Disorders

In view of the lack of good discriminant validity among the many specific personality disorders, only those particularly relevant in childhood and adolescence are covered in this chapter. Antisocial personality disorder (ASPD) is well validated and important because of its association with conduct disorders in childhood, particularly those with early onset, and because of its implications for the next generation via parenting difficulties and domestic violence (Moffitt, 2006). Psychopathic disorder is identified in a smaller group of antisocial adults, most of whom have ASPD, and is associated with distinctive patterns of offending and neurobiological correlates. In childhood, there appears to be a subset of antisocial children with "callous unemotional" traits with distinctive genetic and neurobiological contributions that may be the precursors of adult psychopathic disorder (Blair, Peschardt, Budhani *et al.*, 2006). Childhood conduct disorders and callous unemotional traits, and ASPD and psychopathic disorder are described in chapter 51. In this chapter we review borderline, schizotypal and schizoid disorders.

Borderline Personality Disorder

The overall concept of borderline personality disorder (BPD) is of a pervasive pattern of instability of interpersonal relationships, self-image, affects and control over impulses. The operationalization of this concept has varied somewhat over the years but the criteria have usually included a pattern of unstable and intense interpersonal relationships with alternating idealization and devaluation, frantic efforts to avoid real or imagined abandonment, an unstable or distorted self-image, impulsiveness, recurrent suicidal behavior, affective instability with intense episodic dysphoria, chronic feelings of emptiness and a lack of control over anger. In contrast to ASPD, BPD is more commonly diagnosed in females.

Very little is known about the childhood antecedents of BPD. Many individuals have both antisocial and borderline features, and some traits such as impulsivity are core to both disorders (Paris, 2005). It is possible that there is a common origin in early-onset disruptive behavior problems, with a gender-based divergence in adolescence or early adult life. Equally, borderline personality difficulties may emerge during early adolescence without a history of overt antisocial behavior problems. Retrospective studies suggest that, as children, adults with BPD may have had difficulties in separating from emotionally important people and show high mood reactivity (Reich & Zanarini, 2001) and that many started to self-harm before the age of 12 (Zanarini, Frankenburg, Ridolfi *et al.*, 2006).

Many theories of the origins of BPD have proposed a central role for adverse, and in particular traumatic, experiences in childhood. If this were the case there would be a particularly important preventative role for child care and mental health professionals. It is important to re-emphasize that both genetic and environmental mechanisms may be implicated in associations with childhood adversities, and genetic designs are usually required to tease them out. Moreover, in their meta-analysis covering 21 studies into possible associations between child sexual abuse and BPD, Fossati, Madeddu, and Maffei (1999) found there was only a moderate pooled effect size. It is difficult to disentangle the effects of child maltreatment from other family environmental and genetic risk factors, to identify which aspects of maltreatment may be relevant to BPD, and to determine the specific association with borderline as opposed to other conditions commonly comorbid with BPD. For example, it may be that particular kinds of child maltreatment are specific to BPD (see chapter 28). In a comparison of borderline patients and those with other personality disorders, those in the borderline group were more likely to have been abused by a male non-caretaker, to have experienced denial of their thoughts and feelings by a male caretaker and to have experienced inconsistent treatment by a female caretaker (Zanarini, Ruser, Frankenburg, Hennen, & Gunderson, 2000). We referred earlier to the particular patterns of mother-child interactions found in a general population study of adolescent predictors of borderline personality disorder (Bezirganian, Cohen, & Brook, 1993). There may also be specificities between type of maltreatment and features of BPD. For example, individuals with BPD also report more dissociative experiences (Jones, Heard, Startup *et al.*, 1999). Zanarini, Ruser, Frankeburg *et al.* (2000) found that dissociative experiences among BPD patients were associated with particular experiences that included inconsistent behavior by a caretaker and sexual abuse by a caretaker. Finally, some effects of childhood maltreatment on BPD may be evident only in subgroups with genetically influenced susceptibilities to experiences (see chapter 23).

Theories regarding mechanisms in BPD have focused on impulsivity (Paris, 2005), emotion dysregulation (Putnam & Silk, 2005), unresolved or insecure attachment (Levy, 2005) and failure of mentalization (Bateman & Fonagy, 2004). Some of the features of BPD, including suicide attempts, self-mutilation, substance misuse and sexual promiscuity, may reflect a more general trait of impulsivity. Impulsive spectrum disorders, such as ASPD and substance misuse, are elevated in the first-degree relatives of borderline patients (White, Gunderson, Zanarini, & Hudson, 2002), and levels of impulsivity predict clinical outcomes in BPD (Links, Heslegrave, & van Reekum, 1999). However, disorders other than BPD are also characterized by impulsivity, notably ASPD, and although there is substantial overlap between the disorders, there are important differences.

Emotion dysregulation is likely to be one of the keys to the difference between BPD and ASPD. "The inability to sustain positive affect coupled with the pervasive and unremitting distress as experienced by patients with BPD can become a veritable prison to those with the disorder and often as well to those who attempt to treat the individual with BPD" (Putnam & Silk, 2005, p. 900). Borderline individuals commonly have a low threshold for reacting to events, or to anticipated events (such as abandonment), with intense negative emotion. According to Linehan (1993), BPD arises from an interaction between temperamental emotional reactivity and an "invalidating" environment in which the child's communication about inner emotional experience is regarded as reflecting an inaccurate perception of themselves and others. One of the major consequences of this response is thought to be that children raised in these environments do not learn to identify emotional states accurately, nor do they learn to regulate affect, as it is more often than not denied. In addition, invalidating environments also intermittently reinforce escalations of emotional displays. This results in two opposing responses to affect being shaped. The first is the inhibition or denial of emotional states, and the second is an extreme response, which often appears to be inappropriate to the level of the stimulus that elicited it.

Instability of family and romantic relationships characterized by highly intense interactions, fear of abandonment and emotionally charged breakdown, are also common in individuals with BPD. Several studies have linked this to disturbances of attachment (Levy, 2005), although very few have tested whether attachment difficulties are associated specifically with BPD, as opposed to other personality disorders. Bateman and Fonagy (2004) argued that individuals with BPD have an impoverished model of their own and others' mental function (mentalization). "Their schematic, rigid and at times extreme ideas about their own and others' states of mind make them vulnerable to powerful emotional storms and apparently impulsive actions, and create profound problems of behavioral and affect regulation" (Fonagy & Bateman, 2004, p. 2). They also argue that these limitations in mentalization are seen particularly in relation to attachment relationships, thus leading to particular difficulties in close relationships.

The clinical picture of BPD may arise from interacting processes. For example, the combination of intrusive and inconsistent mother–child interactions associated specifically with BPD (Bezirganian, Cohen, & Brook, 1993) may contribute to affect dysregulation and a failure of mentalization. Intrusive parenting is likely to lead to intense negative affect from which the child takes evasive action, hence leading to extremes of high and low emotional intensity, and also to a reduced capacity to monitor mental states when highly aroused. Inconsistent mother–child interactions may inhibit the child's capacity to read the intentions or states of mind of the parent, and hence limit his or her ability to think of others' behaviors in mental state terms.

Repeated self-injury, cutting, burning or hitting, is frequently observed in individuals with severe personality disorders, and is one of the diagnostic items for BPD. It is a serious and puzzling phenomenon. There is a wide range of theories concerning the motivation for self-injury, and themes that are common to most of them are of regulation of emotions, communication and social reinforcement (Kemperman, Russ, & Shearin, 1997). Linehan (1993) has proposed that self-injury directly relieves painful emotions, and is reinforced by the attention and care given by others. Several studies have supported the role of self-injury in reducing painful affect, although most have used retrospective measures with samples that in different ways were unrepresentative. Proposals have been made that the mechanisms may entail effects on endogenous opioids or serotonin regulation, but results from a small number of investigations have been inconsistent (see chapter 40; Kemperman, Russ, & Shearin, 1997).

Dissociative Identity Disorder

The category multiple personality disorder (MPD), renamed dissociative identity disorder (DID) in DSM-IV, has provoked considerable controversy. The diagnosis is rarely made outside of the USA and Canada (Merskey, 1995), and in the USA only a minority of psychiatrists believe that DID is supported by strong evidence of scientific validity (Pope, Oliva, Hudson, Bodkin, & Gruber, 1999). Nevertheless, the phenomenon has been described in a range of scientific and clinical publications, and the case has been made that the symptoms can be corroborated, and that in offenders there is a strong association with documented severe abuse in childhood (Lewis, Yeager, Swica, Pincus, & Lewis, 1997). It is likely that this specific manifestation of personality disorder is culturally determined and to a certain extent iatrogenic, but it is possible that disorders of similar severity and with the same risk factors are seen more widely.

Schizotypal Personality Disorder

The general concept of schizotypal personality disorder is that of a pervasive pattern of social and interpersonal deficits marked by acute discomfort with, and reduced capacity for, close relationships, as well as by cognitive or perceptual distortions and eccentricities of behavior, beginning by early adulthood. It is likely that the concept of a spectrum of schizophrenic disorders, including schizotypal personality disorder, applies in the pre-adult years, as well as later. However, there have been only a small number of attempts to apply the criteria in childhood. One study suggested an overlap with pervasive developmental disorders, although not autism as such (Nagy & Szatmari, 1986); another suggested a course similar to that of schizophrenia arising in childhood (Asarnow & Ben-Meir, 1988); and a third suggested that there was a pattern of communication deficits similar to, but milder than, those found in schizophrenia (Caplin & Guthrie, 1992). Olin, Raine, Cannon *et al.* (1997) gathered prospective questionnaire data from teachers on 15-year-olds who subsequently developed schizotypal personality disorder. Compared with a range of other groups at varying levels of risk for psychiatric disorder other than schizophrenia, the schizotypal individuals as adolescents had been more passive and unengaged and more hypersensitive to criticism.

Schizoid Personality Disorder

The usual concept of schizoid personality disorder is of a pervasive pattern of detachment from social relationships and a restricted range of expression of emotions in interpersonal settings (American Psychiatric Association, DSM-IV, 2000). Thus, ICD-10 criteria (World Health Organization, 1996) include a lack of pleasure in activities, emotional coldness, apparent indifference to praise or criticism, a limited capacity to express either positive or negative emotions, a lack of close friends, a preference for solitary activities, a marked insensitivity to prevailing social norms and an excessive preoccupation with fantasy and introspection. The literature on the syndrome is almost confined to adults. However, since the 1970s, Wolff has pressed the case for the application of the diagnosis in childhood (Wolff & Barlow, 1979). Unfortunately for comparative purposes, her criteria differ in several key respects from those generally applied with adults. Thus, she has specified increased sensitivity and paranoid ideas, whereas ICD-10 and DSM-IV indicate marked insensitivity, and she has included an unusually odd style of communicating which would ordinarily be part of schizotypal, not schizoid, personality disorders (Wolff, 1991a,b; Wolff & Chick, 1980). The initial findings in childhood suggested some similarities with autism (Wolff & Barlow, 1979) and the follow-up showed substantial continuity with schizotypal personality disorder in adult life (Wolff, Townshend, McGuire *et al.*, 1991). However, a study of psychophysiological responses of adults who in childhood met Wolff's criteria for schizoid disorder failed to find abnormalities previously documented in the relatives of schizophrenic patients and adults with schizotypal personality disorder (Blackwood, Muir, Roxborough *et al.*, 1994).

Utility of Personality Disorder Diagnosis in Childhood and Adolescence

In the light of these considerations, is there an argument for applying the concept of personality disorder in adolescence or even in childhood? Clearly, given the probable heterogeneity of the personality disorders, it is unlikely that there will be one answer to this question.

There would be a strong case if it could be shown that the category unified diverse symptoms with a common cause, prognosis or response to treatment. It is for example clearly the case that the diagnosis of autism, which meets most of the requirements for personality disorder, provides an effective unifying diagnosis for diverse social and behavioral abnormalities. Might this be true also for childhood conditions such as oppositional defiant disorder or conduct disorder? Angold and Costello (2001) reviewed the DSM criteria for personality disorder outlined earlier and concluded that early-onset antisocial behaviors in children satisfy all the DSM requirements. Childhood oppositional and conduct problems associated with poor peer relationships are more likely to persist (Vitaro, Brendgen, & Tremblay, 2000), and adult antisocial outcomes are most common in children with multiple and diverse oppositional, social and educational difficulties (Stattin & Magnusson, 1996).

However, the use of the personality disorder designation could introduce the limitations of the adult categories into childhood. Crucially, it might reduce our scope for investigating the links between different types of dysfunction. Vitaro, Brendgen, & Tremblay, (2000) found that, in boys, although having a best friend who was deviant at age 10 predicted delinquency at age 14, this was much less the case among those with warm relationships with their parents. Such a specific mechanism could not be investigated within a personality disorder framework if poor peer relationships was simply one of a number of items within a childhood ASPD. Similarly, notwithstanding the strong association of conduct disorder and ADHD and evidence that ADHD in the presence of conduct disorder increases the likelihood of persistence (Loeber, Green, Keenan, & Lahey, 1995), important genetic and neuropsychological differences would not have been identified if they had been included in a hyperactivity–conduct personality disorder. Whatever the pros and cons of creating childhood personality disorders, or of other kinds of solution such as dissolving the Axis I–Axis II demarcation, the placement of disruptive disorders of childhood on DSM Axis I, and antisocial personality disorder on Axis II, is an anomaly and does not reflect a fundamental distinction between them.

Is there a case for applying adult personality disorder criteria in adolescence? Studies of hospital patients, mainly with BPD, have suggested that adolescent personality disorders may be less distinct and less stable than adult disorders, but the profile of symptoms is largely similar (Becker, Grilo, Edell, & McGlashan, 2004). There is a case for using a dimensional approach to personality disorders in adult life, and this is likely to be the case also in adolescence. The stability of personality disorder symptoms is no less during adolescence, and from adolescence to adult life, than it is in adult life (Cohen, Crawford, Johnson *et al.*, 2005). Correlation coefficients of 0.5–0.7 are commonly reported between adolescent and adult measures and over periods of up to 10 years. Equally, there can be informative developmental sequences involving personality disorder symptoms. Hamigami, McArdle, and Cohen (2000) showed that there were reciprocal effects of narcissistic and borderline symptoms on each other from early adolescence into the mid-twenties. Borderline symptoms predicted increasing narcissistic symptoms over time, but narcissistic symptoms predicted lower borderline symptoms! This may indicate that the appearance of borderline symptoms in early adolescence reflects substantial underlying pathology, whereas early narcissistic symptoms may be more developmentally benign. Later narcissistic symptoms, by contrast, may also reflect more problematic functioning, perhaps particularly when associated with borderline features.

Borderline Personality Disorder in Adolescence

Many of the studies of personality disorder in adolescence have focused on BPD. A substantial proportion of adolescent psychiatric in-patients in the USA and the UK can be diagnosed with the disorder using adult criteria. It resembles the adult diagnosis in that there is a strong association with episodic disorders, particularly depression, and its stability is low. In adolescents, the BPD diagnosis picks out a group who, compared with other adolescent psychiatric patients, have experienced high levels of maternal neglect and rejection, grossly inappropriate parental behavior and a number of parental surrogates, sexual abuse (Ludolph, Westen, Misle *et al.*, 1990) and higher levels of angry irritable interactions in the family (James, Berelowitz, & Verker, 1996). Associations of inconsistent and intrusive parenting with the emergence of BPD were found in the longitudinal study of a general population sample referred to earlier (Bezirganian, Cohen, & Brook, 1993).

Clinical Implications

In the light of the varied, and in many respects limited, body of research, should we make use of personality diagnoses in adolescence in clinical practice? The answer is, as is often the case, it depends on the purpose. It can serve the purpose of ensuring that attention is drawn to types of persistent dysfunction that are not reflected in the episodic diagnoses such as depression. For example, among adolescents assessed for suicidal behaviors, a substantial minority is depressed and a smaller group has borderline personality disorder. There are implications for treatment depending on the presence both of depression and of BPD. However, current evidence and clinical experience would suggest that the key issue is not whether the threshold for BPD is crossed but how many features of BPD are present. Similarly, the extent to which these are accompanied by symptoms of other disorders, notably ASPD, is equally important.

It should be emphasized that the evidence linking different personality disorders to treatment needs is limited in both adults and adolescents. In relation to ASPD, while there is some evidence for the efficacy of treatments such as multi-systemic therapy (MST) for juvenile offending, the studies have not assessed ASPD nor have they examined outcomes in relation to symptoms of other personality disorders such as BPD (see chapters 35 and 62).

Dialectical behaviour therapy (DBT) is increasingly being used as an approach with suicidal adolescents, many of whom are likely to have BPD symptoms (Katz, Cox, Gunasekara, & Miller, 2004). The "dialectic" refers to helping the adolescent to change what needs to be changed, while accepting what is a valid response to circumstances (Hill, Swales, & Byatt, 2006). Treatment is delivered by a team, and has several elements. *Capability enhancement* aims to increase the adolescent's basic capabilities of affect regulation, distress tolerance and interpersonal skills. This function is most often delivered by a skills training group. *Motivational enhancement* involves assisting adolescents to apply their new-found skills to their own life problems, in particular attending to cognitions, emotions or reinforcement contingencies that interfere with the implementation of skillful behavior. This function is most commonly delivered via individual psychotherapy. Explicit coaching in the application of problem-solutions to the adolescent's real world situations is designed to increase generalization of skills learned in the program. This may be delivered by between-session skills coaching, by telephone, by case management or by training family members in the same skills that the adolescents are learning. Considerable attention is also paid to supervision by and support of therapists and to the family and wider environment of the adolescent, including social services and education.

Studies of adult populations in relation to BPD and chronic self-harm may provide some pointers to provide support for the effectiveness of DBT and other psychosocial treatments in BPD in adolescents. Perry, Bannon, and Ianni (1999) reviewed the results of 15 studies, and Bateman and Fonagy (2000) reviewed 25 reports of a range of psychotherapeutic approaches in adult personality disorders. Both reviews concluded that there was evidence for short- to medium-term effectiveness in a number of indices of disorder including depression and interpersonal problems, as well as personality disorder diagnosis. However, there have been very few randomized controlled studies. By 2004 there had been seven randomized controlled trials of DBT, but only two had sample sizes of greater than 60 (Lieb, Zanarini, Yen *et al.*, 2004). These suggest a major effect on suicidal behaviors sustained for up to 1 year. Bateman and Fonagy (2001) conducted a randomized controlled trial of psychoanalytically oriented partial hospitalization with 38 borderline patients, based on their theory of impaired mentalization in BPD. The treated group had a lower frequency of self-harm, suicide attempts, hospital admissions, use of medication and depression, and better social adjustment over an 18-month treatment period. Generally, studies of effectiveness of treatment of personality disorders have used outcomes such as service utilization or depression levels as proxies for measures of changes in personality functioning. Tackling the difficulties associated with the current conceptualization and measurement of personality disorder should lead to improved treatment and more refined measurement of outcomes.

Bateman and Fonagy have summarized the principal features of treatments for which there is some evidence of effectiveness. The approach is active and structured with clear focus, in the context of a strong relationship between therapist and patient over a substantial period of time. The treatment is well integrated with other services available to the patient. Effective treatments for adolescents who have extensive dysfunction, paralleling that of the adult personality disorders, may well require an approach with these features, coupled with active involvement of the family and attention to educational or vocational needs.

Studies have been conducted of tricyclic antidepressants, selective serotonin reuptake inhibitors, neuroleptics and mood stabilizers in BPD (Lieb, Zanarini, Yen *et al.*, 2004). Most have shown some evidence of efficacy but with small sample sizes. Of the 16 studies reviewed by Lieb, Zanarini, Yen *et al.*, only two had a sample size of greater than 60, and in most cases they were substantially smaller. Soler, Pascual, Campins *et al.* (2005) randomized 60 patients with BPD to placebo or to olanzapine together with DBT. In assessments after 4 months, the combined DBT plus drug group had lower affective symptoms and impulsivity/aggression than the DBT only group.

Conclusions

Much remains to be discovered regarding the forms of dysfunction that best characterize the personality disorders. This will inform, and be informed by, increasing knowledge of childhood antecedents, developmental pathways, the interaction between individual and environmental processes, and basic psychopathological processes in the personality disorders. For all its shortcomings, the concept of personality has endured because it adds to our understanding of risk and psychopathology and, increasingly, research in this area highlights individuals with distinctive treatment needs. Patterns of symptomatology resembling adult personality disorders are seen during adolescence and also indicate distinctive and generally intensive treatment needs.

References

American Psychiatric Association. (2000). *Diagnostic and statistical manual of mental disorders* (4th edn.). Text Revision. Washington, DC: American Psychiatric Association.

Angold, A., & Costello, J. (2001). The epidemiology of disorders of conduct: Nosological issues and comorbidity. In J. Hill, & B. Maughan (Eds.), *Conduct disorders in childhood and adolescence* (pp. 126–168). Cambridge: Cambridge University Press.

Asarnow, J. R., & Ben-Meir, S. (1988). Children with schizophrenia spectrum and depressive disorders: A comparative study of premorbid adjustment, onset pattern and severity of impairment. *Journal of Child Psychology and Psychiatry*, *29*, 477–488.

Bateman, A. W., & Fonagy, P. (2000). Effectiveness of psychotherapeutic treatment of personality disorder. *British Journal of Psychiatry*, *177*, 138–143.

Bateman, A. W., & Fonagy, P. (2001). Treatment of borderline personality disorder with psychoanalytically oriented partial hospitalization: An 18-month follow-up. *American Journal of Psychiatry*, *158*, 36–42.

Bateman, A. W., & Fonagy, P. (2004). *Psychotherapy for borderline personality disorder: Mentalization based treatment.* Oxford: Oxford University Press.

Becker, D. F., Grilo, C. M., Edell, W. S., & McGlashan, T. H. (2002). Diagnostic efficiency of borderline personality disorder criteria in hospitalized adolescents: Comparison with hospitalized adults. *American Journal of Psychiatry*, *159*, 2042–2047.

Bezirganian, S., Cohen, P., & Brook, J. S. (1993). The impact of mother–child interaction on the development of Borderline Personality Disorder. *American Journal of Psychiatry*, *150*, 1836–1842.

Blackwood, D. H., Muir, W. J., Roxborough, H. M., Walker, M. R., Townsend, R., Glabus, M. F., *et al.* (1994). "Schizoid" personality in childhood: Auditory P300 and eye tracking responses at follow-up in adult life. *Journal of Autism and Developmental Disorders*, *24*, 487–500.

Blair, R. J., Peschardt, K. S., Budhani, S., Mitchell, D. G., & Pine, D. S. (2006). The development of psychopathy. *Journal of Child Psychology and Psychiatry*, 47, 262–276.

Cadenhead, K. S., Light, G. A., Geyer, M. O., & Braff, L. (2000). Sensory gaiting deficits assessed by the P50 events-related potential in subjects with schizotypal personality disorder. *American Journal of Psychiatry*, *157*, 55–59.

Caplin, R., & Guthrie, D. (1992). Communication deficits in childhood schizotypal personality disorder. *Journal of the American Academy of Child and Adolescent Psychiatry*, *31*, 961–967.

Carey, G., & Goldman, D. (1997). The genetics of antisocial behavior. In D. M. Stoff, J. Breilling, & J. Maser (Eds.), *Handbook of antisocial behavior* (pp. 243–254). New York: Wiley.

Casey, P. R., & Tyrer, P. J. (1986). Personality, functioning, and symptomatology. *Journal of Psychiatric Research*, *20*, 363–374.

Caspi, A., Roberts, B. W., & Shiner, R. L. (2005). Personality development: stability and change. *Annual Review of Psychology, 56*, 453–484.

Cleckley, H. (1941). *The mask of sanity*. London: Henry Kimpton.

Cohen, P., Crawford, T. N., Johnson, J. G., & Kasen, S. (2005). The children in the community study of developmental course of personality disorder. *Journal of Personality Disorders, 19*, 466–486.

Daley, S. E., Hammen, C., Davila, J., & Burge, D. (1998). Axis II symptomatology, depression, and life stress during the transition from adolescence to adulthood. *Journal of Consulting and Clinical Psychology*, *66*, 595–603.

Daley, S. E., Burge, D., & Hammen, C. (2000). Borderline personality disorder symptoms as predictors of four-year romantic relationship dysfunctioning young women: Addressing issues of specificity. *Journal of Abnormal Psychology*, *109*, 451–460.

Dickey, C. C., Shenton, M. E., Hirayasu, Y., Fischer, I., Voglmaier, M. M., Niznikiewicz, M. A., *et al.* (2000). Large CSF volume not attributable to ventricular volume in schizotypal personality disorder. *American Journal of Psychiatry*, *157*, 48–54.

Docherty, J. P., Fister, S. J., & Shea, T. (1986). Syndrome diagnosis and personality disorder. In A. J. Frances, & R. E. Hales (Eds.), *American Psychiatric Association Annual Review* (Vol. 5, pp. 315–355). Washington, DC: American Psychiatric Press.

Ferro, T., Klein, D. N., Schwartz, J. E., Casch, K. L., & Leader, J. D. (1998). Thirty-months' stability of personality disorder diagnoses in depressed out-patients. *American Journal of Psychiatry*, *155*, 653–659.

Fossati, A., Madeddu, F., & Maffei, C. (1999). Borderline personality disorder and childhood sexual abuse: A meta-analytic study. *Journal of Personality Disorders*, *13*, 268–280.

Frances, A. J., & Widiger, T. (1986). The classification of personality disorder: An overview of problems and solutions. In A. J. Frances, & R. E. Hales (Eds.), *American Psychiatric Association annual review* (Vol. 5, pp. 240–258). Washington, DC: American Psychiatric Press.

Frick, P. J., & Morris, A. S. (2004). Temperament and developmental pathways to conduct problems. *Journal of Clinical Child and Adolescent Psychology*, *33*, 54–68.

Gunderson, J. G., Kolb, J. E., & Austin, V. (1981). The diagnostic interview for borderline patients. *American Journal of Psychiatry*, *138*, 896–903.

Hamigami, F., McArdle, J. J., & Cohen P. (2000). A new approach to modelling bivariate dynamic relationships applied to evaluation of DSM-III personality disorder symptoms. In V. J. Molfese (Ed.), *Temperament and personality development across the life-span* (pp. 253–280). Mahwah, NJ: Lawrence Erlbaum.

Hare, R. D. (1970). *Psychopathy: Theory and research*. New York: John Wiley.

Henderson, D. K. (1939). *Psychopathic states*. New York: Norton.

Henry, B., Caspi, A., Moffitt, T. E., & Silva, P. A. (1996). Temperamental and familial predictors of violent and non-violent criminal convictions: Age three to eighteen. *Developmental Psychology*, *32*, 614–623.

Hill, J., Fudge, H., Harrington, R., Pickles, A., & Rutter, M. (2000). Complementary approaches to the assessment of personality disorder: The Personality Assessment Schedule and Adult Personality Functioning Assessment compared. *British Journal of Psychiatry*, *176*, 434–439.

Hill, J., Pilkonis, P., Morse, J., Feske, U., Reynolds, S., Hope, H., *et al.* (2008). Social domain dysfunction and disorganization in borderline personality disorder. *Psychological Medicine*, *38*, 1, 135–146.

Hill, J., Swales, M., & Byatt, M. (2006). Personality disorders. In C. Gillberg, R. Harrington, & H-C. Steinhausen (Eds.), *A clinician's handbook of child and adolescent psychiatry* (pp. 339–364). Cambridge: Cambridge University Press.

James, A., Berelowitz, M., & Verker, M. (1996). Borderline personality disorder: Study in adolescence. *European Child and Adolescent Psychiatry*, *5*, 11–17.

Johnson, J. G., Cohen, P., Brown, J., Smailes, E. M., & Bernstein, D. P. (1999). Childhood maltreatment increases risk for personality disorders during adulthood. *Archives of General Psychiatry*, *56*, 600–606.

Johnson, M. H., Griffin, R., Csibra, G., Halit, H., Farroni, T., de Haan, M., *et al.* (2005). The emergence of the social brain network: evidence from typical and atypical development. *Development and Psychopathology*, *17*, 599–619.

Jones, B., Heard, H., Startup, M., Swales, M., Williams, J. M., & Jones, R. F. (1999). Autobiographical memory and dissociation in borderline personality disorder. *Psychological Medicine*, *29*, 1397–1404.

Joyce, P. R., McHugh, P. C., McKenzie, J. M., Sullivan, P. F., Mulder, R. T., Luty, S. E., *et al.* (2006). A dopamine transporter polymorphism is a risk factor for borderline personality disorder in depressed patients. *Psychological Medicine*, *36*, 807–813.

Kasen, S., Cohen, P., Skodol, A. E., Johnson, J. G., & Brook, J. F. (1999). Influence of child and adolescent psychiatric disorders on young adult personality disorder. *American Journal of Pychiatry*, *56*, 1529–1535.

Kass, F., Skodol, A. E., Charles, E., Spitzer, R. L., & Williams, J. B. W. (1985). Scaled ratings of DSM-II personality disorders. *American Journal of Psychiatry*, *142*, 627–630.

Katz, L. Y., Cox, B. J., Gunasekara, S., & Miller, A. L. (2004). Feasibility of dialectical behavior therapy for suicidal adolescent inpatients. *Journal of the American Academy of Child and Adolescent Psychiatry*, *43*, 276–282.

Kemperman, I., Russ, M. J., & Shearin, E. (1997). Self-injurious behaviour and mood regulation in borderline patients. *Journal of Personality Disorder*, 11, 146–157.

Kendler, K. S., & Gruenberg, A. M. (1982). Genetic relationship between paranoid personality disorder and the "schizophrenic spectrum" disorder. *American Journal of Psychiatry*, *139*, 1185–1186.

Kendler, K. S., Gruenberg, A. M., & Strauss, J. S. (1981). An independent analysis of the Copenhagen sample of the Danish Adoption Study of Schizophrenia. II. The relationship between schizotypal personality disorders and schizophrenia. *Archives of General Psychiatry*, *38*, 928–984.

Kendler, K. S., Masterson, C. C., & Davis, K. L. (1985). Psychiatric illness in first-degree relatives of patients with paranoid psychosis, schizophrenia and medical illness. *British Journal of Psychiatry*, *147*, 524–532.

Kendler, K. S., Masterson, C. C., Ungaro, O. R., & Davis, K. L. (1984). A family history study of schizophrenia-related personality disorder. *American Journal of Psychiatry*, *141*, 424–427.

Kernberg, O. F. (1967). Borderline personality organization. *Journal of the American Psychoanalytic Association (New York)*, *15*, 641–685.

Kernberg, O. F. (1975). *Borderline conditions and pathological narcissism*. New York: Jason Ellinson.

Kety, S. S., Rosenthal, D., & Wender, P. H. (1971). Mental illness in the biological and adoptive families of adopted schizophrenics. *American Journal of Psychiatry*, *128*, 302–306.

Langbehn, D. R., Caderet, R. J., Yates, W. R., Troughton, E. P., & Stewart, M. A. (1998). *Archives of General Psychiatry*, *55*, 821–829.

Lemerise, E. A., & Arsenio, W. F. (2000). An integrated model of emotion processes and cognition in social information processing. *Child Development*, *71*, 107–118.

Levy, K. N. (2005). The implications of attachment theory and research for understanding borderline personality disorder. *Development and Psychopathology*, *17*, 959–986.

Lewis, D. O., Yeager, C. A., Swica, Y., Pincus, J. H., & Lewis, M. (1997). Objective documentation of child abuse and dissociation in twelve murderers with dissociative identity disorder. *American Journal of Psychiatry*, *154*, 1703–1710.

Lieb, K., Zanarini, M. C., Yen, S., Schmahl, C., Linehan, M. M., & Bohus, M. (2004). Borderline personality disorder. *Lancet*, *364*, 453–461.

Linehan, M. M. (1993). *Cognitive behavioral therapy of borderline personality disorder*. New York, NY: Guilford Press.

Links, P. S., Heslegrave, R., & van Reekum, R. (1999). Impulsivity: core aspect of borderline personality disorder. *Journal of Personality Disorders*, *13*, 1–9.

Loeber, R., Green, S. M., Keenan, K., & Lahey, B. B. (1995). Which boys will fare worse? Early predictors of the onset of conduct disorder in a six-year longitudinal study. *Journal of the American Academy of Child and Adolescent Psychiatry*, *34*, 499–509.

Loranger, A. W., Lenzenweger, M. F., Gartner, A. F., Susman, V. L., Herzig, J., Zammit, G. K., *et al.* (1991). Trait–state artifacts and the diagnosis of personality disorders. *Archives of General Psychiatry*, *48*, 720–728.

Ludolph, P. S., Westen, D., Misle, B., Jackson, A., Wixom, M. A., & Wiss, C. (1990). The borderline diagnosis in adolescence: Symptoms and developmental history. *Archives of General Psychiatry*, *147*, 470–476.

Maier, W., Franke, P., & Hawallek, B. (1998). Special feature: Family-genetic research strategies for personality disorders. *Journal of Personality Disorders*, *12*, 262–276.

Malone, S. M., Taylor, J., Marmorstein, N. R., McGue, M., & Iacono, W. G. (2004). Genetic and environmental influences on antisocial behavior and alcohol dependence from adolescence to early adulthood. *Development and Psychopathology*, *16*, 943–966.

McGuffin, P., & Thapar, A. (1992). The genetics of personality disorder. *British Journal of Psychiatry*, *160*, 12–23.

Meehl, P. E. (1962). Schizotaxia, schizotypy, schizophrenia. *American Psychologist*, *17*, 827–838.

Merikangas, K. R., & Weissman, M. M. (1986). Epidemiology of DSM-III Axis II personality disorders. In A. J. Frances, & R. E. Hales (Eds.), *American Psychiatric Association Annual Review* (Vol. 5, pp. 258–278). Washington, DC: American Psychiatric Press.

Merskey, H. (1995). Multiple personality disorder and false memory syndrome. *British Journal of Psychiatry*, *166*, 281–283.

Mischel, W. (2004). Toward an integrative science of the person. *Annual Review of Psychology*, *55*, 1–22.

Moffitt, T. E. (2006). Life-course persistent versus adolescence-limited antisocial behavior. In D. Cicchetti, & D. Cohen (Eds.), *Developmental psychopathology* (2nd edn.). New York: Wiley.

Morey, L. C. (1988). Personality disorders in DSM-III and DSM-III-R: Convergence, coverage and internal consistency. *American Journal of Psychiatry*, *145*, 573–577.

Mulder, R. (2002). Personality pathology and treatment outcome in major depression: A review. *American Journal of Psychiatry*, *159*, 359–371.

Nagy, J., & Szatmari, P. (1986). A chart review of schizotypal personality disorders in children. *Journal of Autism and Developmental Disorders*, *16*, 351–367.

Newton-Howes, G., Tyrer, P., & Johnson, T. (2006). Personality disorder and the outcome of depression: Meta-analysis of published studies. *British Journal of Psychiatry*, *188*, 13–20.

Oldham, J. M., Skodol, A. E., Kellman, H. D., Hyler, S. E., Rosnick, L., & Davies, M. (1992). Diagnosis of DSM-III-R personality disorders and two structured interviews: Patterns of comorbidity. *American Journal of Psychiatry*, *149*, 213–220.

Olin, S. S., Raine, A., Cannon, T. D., Parnas, J., Schulsinger, F., & Mednick, F. A. (1997). *Schizophrenia Bulletin*, *23*, 93–103.

Paris, J. (2005). The development of impulsivity and suicidality in borderline personality disorder. *Development and Psychopathology*, *17*, 1091–1104.

Parker, G., Roy, K., Wilhelm, K., Mitchell, P., Austin, M. P., & Hadzi-Pavlovic, D. (1999). An exploration of links between early parenting experiences and personality disorder type and disordered personality functioning. *Journal of Personality Disorders*, *13*, 361–374.

Perry, J. C., Bannon, E., & Ianni, F. (1999). Effectiveness or psychotherapy for personality disorders. *American Journal of Psychiatry*, *156*, 1312–1321.

Pfohl, B., Coryell, W., Zimmerman, M., & Tsangl, D. A. (1986). DSM-III personality disorders: Diagnostic overlap and internal consistency of individual DSM-III criteria. *Comprehensive Psychiatry*, *27*, 21–34.

Pickles, A., & Angold, A. (2003). Natural categories or fundamental dimensions: On carving nature at the joints and the rearticulation of psychopathology. *Development and Psychopathology*, *15*, 529–552.

Pope, H. G., Oliva, P. F., Hudson, J. I., Bodkin, J. A., & Gruber, A. J. (1999). Attitudes toward DSM-IV dissociative disorders diagnoses among board-certified American Psychiatrists. *American Journal of Psychiatry*, *156*, 321–323.

Putnam, K. M., & Silk, K. R. (2005). Emotion dysregulation and the development of borderline personality disorder. *Development and Psychopathology*, *17*, 899–926.

Quinton D., Gulliver L., & Rutter M. (1995). A 15–20 year follow-up of adult psychiatric patients: Psychiatric disorder and social functioning. *British Journal of Psychiatry*, *167*, 315–323.

Reich, D. B., & Zanarini, M. C. (2001). Developmental aspects of borderline personality disorder. *Harvard Review of Psychiatry*, *9*, 294–301.

Robins, L. N. (1996). *Deviant children grown up*. Baltimore, MD: Williams and Wilkins.

Robins, L. N. (1978). Sturdy childhood predictors of adult antisocial behaviour: Replications from longitudinal studies. *Psychological Medicine*, *8*, 611–622.

Robins, R. W., Caspi, A., & Moffitt, T. E. (2002). It's not just who you're with, it's who you are: personality and relationship experiences across multiple relationships. *Journal of Personality*, *70*, 925–964.

Robinson, J. L., & Acevedo, M. C. (2001). Infant reactivity and reliance on mother during emotion challenges: prediction of cognition and language skills in a low-income sample. *Child Development*, *72*, 402–415.

Rutter, M. (1987). Temperament, personality and personality disorder. *British Journal of Psychiatry*, *150*, 433–458.

Rutter, M., & Quinton, D. (1984). Parental psychiatric disorder: Effects on children. *Psychological Medicine*, *14*, 853–880.

Schneider, K. (1923). *Diepsychopathischen personlichkeiten.* Berlin: Springer.

Schneider, K. (1950). *Psychopathic personalities* (9th edn.). (English Translation, 1958). London: Cassell.

Seivewright, H., Tyrer, P., & Johnson, T. (2004). Persistent social dysfunction in anxious and depressed patients with personality disorder. *Acta Psychiatrica Scandanavica, 109*, 104–109.

Skodol, A. E., Pagano, M. E., Bender, D. S., Shea, M. T., Gunderson, J. G., Yen, S., *et al.* (2005a). Stability of functional impairment in patients with schizotypal, borderline, avoidant, or obsessive-compulsive personality disorder over two years. *Psychological Medicine, 35*, 443–451.

Skodol, A. E., Gunderson, J. G., Shea, M. T., McGlashan, T. H., Morey, L. C., Sanislow, C. A., *et al.* (2005b). The Collaborative Longitudinal Personality Disorders Study (CLPS): overview and implications. *Journal of Personality Disorders, 19*, 487–504.

Soler, J., Pascual, J. C., Campins, J., Barrachina, J., Puigdemont, D., Alvarez, E., *et al.* (2005). Double-blind, placebo-controlled study of dialectical behavior therapy plus olanzapine for borderline personality disorder. *American Journal of Psychiatry, 162*, 1221–1224.

Spitzer, R. L., Endicott, J., & Gibbon, A. M. (1979). Crossing the border into borderline personality and borderline schizophrenia: The development of criteria. *Archives of General Psychiatry, 36*, 17–24.

Stattin, H., & Magnusson, D. (1996). Antisocial development: A holistic approach. *Development and Psychopathology, 8*, 617–645.

Tyrer, P., Casey, P., & Ferguson, B. (1991). Personality disorder in perspective. *British Journal of Psychiatry, 159*, 463–472.

Vitaro, F., Brendgen, M., & Tremblay, R. E. (2000). Influence of deviant friends on delinquency: Searching for moderator variables. *Journal of Abnormal Psychology, 28*, 313–326.

Vollrath, M., Alnaes, R., & Torgersen, S. (1994). Coping and MCMI-II personality disorders. *Journal of Personality Disorders, 8*, 53–63.

Widiger, T. A., & Costa, P. T. (1994). Personality and personality disorders. *Journal of Abnormal Psychology, 103*, 78–91.

White, C. N., Gunderson, J. G., Zanarini, M. C., & Hudson, J. I. (2002). Family studies of borderline personality disorder: A review. *Harvard Review of Psychiatry, 12*, 118–119.

Wolff, S., Townshend, R., McGuire, R. J., & Weeks, D. J. (1991). 'Schizoid' personality in childhood and adult life. II: Adult adjustment and the continuity with schizotypal personality disorder. *British Journal of Psychiatry, 159*, 620–625.

Wolff, S. (1991a). "Schizoid" personality in childhood and adult life. I. The vagaries of diagnostic labelling. *British Journal of Psychiatry, 159*, 615–619.

Wolff, S. (1991b). "Schizoid" personality in childhood and adult life. III. The childhood picture. *British Journal of Psychiatry, 159*, 629–635.

Wolff, S., & Chick, J. (1980). Schizoid personality in childhood: A controlled follow-up study. *Psychological Medicine, 10*, 85–100.

Wolff, S., & Barlow, A. (1979). Schizoid personality in childhood: A comparative study of schizoid, autistic and normal children. *Journal of Child Psychology and Psychiatry, 20*, 29–46.

World Health Organization (WHO). (1996). *Multiaxial classification of child and adolescent psychiatric disorders: The ICD-10 classification of mental and behavioural disorders in children and adolescents.* Cambridge, UK: Cambridge University Press.

Zanarini, M. C., Ruser, T. F., Frankeburg, F. R., Hennen, J., & Gunderson, J. G. (2000). Risk factors associated with the dissociative experiences of borderline patients. *Journal of Nervous and Mental Disease, 188*, 26–30.

Zanarini, M. C., Frankenburg, F. R., Dubo, E. D., Sickel, A. E., Trikha, A., Levin, A., *et al.* (1998). Axis II comorbidity of borderline personality disorder. *Comprehensive Psychiatry, 39*, 296–302.

Zanarini, M. C., Frankenburg, F. R., Reich, D. B., Marino, M. S., Lewis, R. E., Williams, A. A., *et al.* (2000). Bi-parental failure in the childhood experiences of borderline patients. *Journal of Personality Disorders, 14*, 264–273.

Zanarini, M. C., Frankenburg, F. R., Yong, L., Raviola, G., Bradford Reich, D., Hennen, J., *et al.* (2004). Borderline psychopathology in the first-degree relatives of borderline and Axis II comparison probands. *Journal of Personality Disorders, 18*, 439–447.

Zanarini, M. C., Frankenburg, F. R., Hennen, J., Reich, D. B., & Silk, K. R. (2005). The McLean Study of Adult Development (MSAD). *Journal of Personality Disorders, 19*, 505–523.

Zanarini, M. C., Frankenburg, F. R., Ridolfi, M. E., Jager-Hyman, S., Hennen, J., & Gunderson, J. G. (2006). Reported childhood onset of self-mutilation among borderline patients. *Journal of Personality Disorders, 20*, 9–15.

51 Psychopathy

R. James Blair and Essi Viding

Psychopathy as a Clinical Entity

Classification of Psychopathy

The origins of the current description of the psychopathy syndrome can be traced back to the work of Cleckley (1941) and his book, *The Mask of Sanity*. Some of the key features of psychopathy recorded by Cleckley (1941) included: absence of nervousness, interpersonal charm, lack of shame, impoverished affect and poorly motivated antisocial behavior. From the criteria delineated by Cleckley, and his own clinical impressions, Hare (1980) developed the original Psychopathy Checklist (PCL), a formalized tool for the assessment of psychopathy in incarcerated adults. On the basis of considerable empirical work, this has been revised: first in 1991, the Psychopathy Checklist–Revised (PCL-R; Hare, 1991), and then again in 2003 (Hare, 2003). The first extension of the psychopathy concept to children was Bowlby's (1946) description of "affectionless psychopathy." It mirrored some of the key features introduced by Cleckley (such as lack of responsiveness to the suffering of others), but lay forgotten for a long time until the extension of the psychopathy construct to children was proposed again by Frick, O'Brien, Wootton, and McBurnett (1994). This chapter considers how far neuropsychological formulations about psychopathy in adult life may be useful for understanding related characteristics in childhood.

The current definitions of psychopathy comprise both ratings of emotional dysfunction and ratings of overt antisocial behavior. The emotional dysfunction definition involves reduced guilt and empathy as well as reduced attachment to significant others. The antisocial behavior definition involves a predisposition to antisocial behavior from an early age and comprises overt behavioral problems also manifest in those individuals with antisocial behavior who do not have psychopathy (e.g., adults with antisocial personality disorder [ASPD] and children with conduct disorder [CD]). This two-component structure was identified through factor analysis in samples of clinic children and incarcerated adults (Frick, O'Brien, Wootton *et al.*, 1994; Hart, Forth, & Hare, 1990).

Emotional dysfunction is often considered be the core distinctive feature of psychopathy (Blair, Mitchell, & Blair, 2005). However, most of the existing research has concentrated on criminal psychopathy and in order to qualify for the syndrome of psychopathy at the present, an individual must present with both emotional dysfunction and antisocial behavior (Hare, 2003). This has led to the notion of psychopathy as a subgroup within the antisocial behavior diagnoses in childhood and adulthood. Limited research suggests that "successful psychopaths" (i.e., those who manifest the emotional dysfunction, but do not engage in antisocial behavior) do exist and as such psychopathy may not invariably need to be accompanied by antisocial behavior. However, this chapter concentrates on reviewing research on psychopaths for whom the emotional dysfunction is combined with antisocial behavior.

Psychopathy is not part of the DSM-IV diagnostic system (see chapter 2). Given the current definition of psychopathy syndrome that comprises both the emotional dysfunction and antisocial behavior, most individuals with psychopathy would receive a childhood diagnosis of CD or adulthood diagnosis of ASPD (see chapters 35 and 50, respectively). The diagnosis of CD groups individuals together because they engage in antisocial behavior. Thus, children with CD can be found whose antisocial behavior is associated with the specific form of reduced emotional responsiveness characteristic of psychopathy as well as children whose antisocial behavior is associated with heightened emotional responsiveness or dysregulated emotional responding (Blair, Mitchell, & Blair, 2005). In short, the DSM-IV CD diagnosis identifies a heterogeneous population who do not appear to share a common etiology and have some distinct clinical features (with resulting troubling implications for successful treatment). In contrast, the available evidence points towards a core neurocognitive profile shared by a number of individuals with psychopathy.

Assessment of Psychopathy

Following the development of the adult PCL-R, tools for the assessment of psychopathy in childhood and adolescence have also been developed. Here we briefly highlight those measures that directly stem from the PCL-R. These include the Psychopathy Checklist: Youth Version (PCL-YV; Forth, Kosson, & Hare, 2003; Kosson, Cyterski, Steuerwald, Neumann, & Walker-Matthews, 2002) and the Antisocial Process Screening Device (APSD; Frick & Hare, 2001). There is evidence of substantial convergence among these measures (Salekin, Leistico, Trobst, Schrum, & Lochman, 2005).

The assessment techniques (PCL-R, PCL-YV and APSD) all involve 20 behavioral items. Both the PCL-R and PCL-YV are

Rutter's Child and Adolescent Psychiatry, 5th edition. Edited by M. Rutter, D. Bishop, D. Pine, S. Scott, J. Stevenson, E. Taylor and A. Thapar. © 2008 Blackwell Publishing, ISBN: 978-1-4051-4549-7.

scored on the basis of an extensive file review and a semi-structured interview. The APSD takes the format of a parent or teacher-rated questionnaire. For each behavioral item, an individual can score between 0 and 2 points. The individual's total score can therefore vary from 0 to 40 points. Adults scoring 30 or above on the PCL-R are generally considered as having psychopathy, at least in the USA, while those scoring less than 20 are considered as not having psychopathy. There are less-well-established criteria for considering whether a child has psychopathy. Typically, in empirical studies, cut-offs of 20+ scores have been used. Given that emotional dysfunction is what sets psychopaths apart, any APSD scoring criteria should ensure a high score on the emotional dysfunction index (i.e., the callous–unemotional scale of the APSD). The inter-rater reliability for the PCL-R (Hare, 1991) and APSD is comparable with other instruments assessing psychopathology (Frick & Hare, 2001; Frick, Kimonis, Dandreaux, & Farell, 2003).

At the present, callous–unemotional traits are not routinely assessed when making a clinical diagnosis of CD. The assessment of callous–unemotional traits in research settings has generally relied on parent and teacher ratings. Such assessments could be easily adapted for clinical use to supplement standard diagnostic interviews.

Utility and Validity of the Classification

Evidence for the validity of the psychopathy construct is extensive for clinic and criminal populations. Much research has been devoted to relating psychopathy construct to other instruments and scales, collecting data on recidivism and violence as well as laboratory measures involving behavioral, psychophysiological and functional magnetic resonance imaging (fMRI) indices (see Patrick, 2006). One of the major strengths of the construct has been its utility in risk assessment. Considerable work has shown the predictive power of scores on the PCL-R with respect to recidivism (for a review of this literature see Douglas, Vincent, & Edens, 2006). Moreover, this work has shown that the correlation between recidivism and psychopathy is significantly higher than that of the DSM diagnoses (Hare, 2006). The evidence of the success of the psychopathy construct in risk assessment has been almost exclusively conducted in adult samples (for data with adolescent samples see Frick & Marsee, 2006; Frick, Stickle, Dandreaux, Farell, & Kimonis, 2005). The available data indicate that children with psychopathy show more conduct problems, more severe aggression, poorer prognosis and more instrumental aggression than other children with conduct problems (see chapter 35; Frick & Marsee, 2006).

For children, considerable stability ($r > 0.70$ across all time points) of the core emotional dysfunction has been demonstrated over a 4-year period (Frick *et al.*, 2003). A long-term follow-up study measuring psychopathy at age 13 years demonstrated that the construct showed moderate stability to age 24 years ($r = 0.32$), despite different informants and assessment instruments used across the two age periods (Lynam, Caspi, Moffitt, Loeber, & Stouthamer-Loeber, 2007). This 11-year correlation is equivalent to that typically seen when different informants use the same instrument at the same time-point to rate an individual's behavior on a construct.

Importantly, recent data have shown that differentiating children who receive the DSM diagnoses of CD or oppositional defiant disorder (ODD) on the basis of the callous–unemotional (the emotional dysfunction component of psychopathy) traits has clear implications for treatment prognosis (Hawes & Dadds, 2005). Boys with high callous–unemotional traits were less responsive to treatment, and callous–unemotional traits uniquely predicted clinical outcomes when analyzed in relation to CD/ODD severity, other predictors of antisocial behavior, and parents' implementation of treatment (Hawes & Dadds, 2005). Moreover, children with psychopathy appear more difficult to socialize through standard socialization techniques (Oxford, Cavell, & Hughes, 2003; Wootton, Frick, Shelton, & Silverthorn, 1997).

As most of the research on psychopathy has concentrated on clinic or incarcerated populations, or has focused on the impact of psychopathy on antisocial outcomes, much less is known about the utility and validity of psychopathy construct in predicting other outcomes aside from antisocial behavior.

Co-occurrence With Other Syndromes

Attention Deficit/Hyperactivity Disorder

Considerable work has demonstrated that CD and attention deficit/hyperactivity disorder (ADHD) often co-occur (Hinshaw, 1987; Taylor, Schachar, Thorley, & Wieselberg, 1986). More recent work has suggested that psychopathy and ADHD also frequently co-occur (Barry, Frick, DeShazo *et al.*, 2000; Colledge & Blair, 2001; Lynam, 1996). However, it remains unclear whether the ADHD seen in the context of psychopathy can be considered equivalent to that seen in the absence of psychopathy symptoms or whether it should be considered as a behavioral phenocopy with a divergent neurocognitive signature (Blair, Mitchell, & Blair, 2005).

Autism and Asperger's Syndrome

Both autism and Asperger's syndrome are, like psychopathy, associated with problems in "empathy" (see chapter 46). However, the nature of the empathy impairment appears very different between the two populations (Blair, 2003a). Individuals with autism and Asperger's syndrome, as a group, tend to show impairment in Theory of Mind, the ability to represent the mental states of others (Baron-Cohen, Leslie, & Frith, 1985; Frith & Happé, 2005). Individuals with psychopathy do not (Blair, Sellars, Strickland *et al.*, 1996; Richell, Mitchell, Newman *et al.*, 2003). Individuals with psychopathy show impairment in processing the fearful and sad expressions of others and are poor at feeling for others, while capable of representing mental states (Blair, 2005; Blair, Colledge, Murray, & Mitchell, 2001). Individuals with autism or Asperger's syndrome, while potentially showing a global impairment in processing emotions, do not show indications of specific impairment for fear and sadness and appear to find others' distress aversive (Adolphs, Sears, & Piven, 2001;

Blair, 1999; Rogers, Viding, Blair, Frith, & Happé, 2006). To date there have been no reports of comorbid psychopathy and either autism or Asperger's syndrome although there have been isolated reports of individuals showing some of the emotion dysfunction associated with psychopathy (Fine, Lumsden, & Blair, 2001; Rogers, Viding, Blair *et al.*, 2006). As pointed out by Rutter (2005), unlike for psychopathy, the impaired socioemotional responsiveness found in autism spectrum disorders does not seem to be generally linked to increased risk for antisocial behavior. In support of this, Hippler & Klicpera (2003), in their study of 177 cases originally diagnosed by Asperger, found no raised incidence of criminal offences compared with general population rates. In contrast, Frick, Stickle, Dandreaux *et al.* (2005) have demonstrated that elevated levels of psychopathy predict increased antisocial behavior at a later time-point, even in children who do not start off as being antisocial. It thus appears that although both psychopaths and individuals with autism spectrum disorders can appear emotionally blunted, there are likely to be different roots to their emotional problems, which also explains the lack of increased risk for antisocial behavior in people with autism spectrum disorders. However, more research is needed that provides direct comparison of individuals with psychopathy and individuals with autism spectrum disorders.

Anxiety and Mood Disorders

Individuals presenting with anxiety and mood disorders (e.g., post-traumatic stress disorder and depression; see chapters 42 and 37, respectively) are at elevated risk for aggression at the time of this presentation (Silva, Derecho, Leong, Weinstock, & Ferrari, 2001; Zoccolillo, 1992). For example, in a recent community sample of almost 6000 individuals, over half (54.33%) of the 3.3% of adults with ASPD had a comorbid anxiety disorder (lifetime; Goodwin & Hamilton, 2003). Similarly, 42.31% of adults with a history of CD (9.4%) but who did not meet criteria for ASPD had a lifetime anxiety disorder.

In contrast to ASPD, psychopathy has been traditionally considered to be marked by reduced anxiety levels (Cleckley, 1941; Hare, 1970; Lykken, 1957). Moreover, studies have shown that anxiety level is *inversely* associated with the callous and unemotional/emotional dysfunction dimension of psychopathy (Frick, Lilienfeld, Ellis, Loney, & Silverthorn, 1999; Patrick, 1994; Verona, Patrick, & Joiner, 2001). In short, increases in anxiety are associated with increases in antisocial behavior but decreases in the emotional dysfunction component of psychopathy (for further discussion of this issue see Blair, Mitchell, & Blair, 2005).

Epidemiology of Psychopathy

The prevalence rates of CD are very high (6–16% for males and 2–9% for females, according to DSM-IV). The prevalence rate of psychopathy is far lower although full epidemiological studies have not been conducted. However, preliminary work conducted by Frick using the APSD, and using a cut-off for psychopathy commonly used in the literature, results in a prevalence rate of psychopathy of 1–3.5% (Frick & Hare, 2001). Using what we know about prevalence rates of ASPD from epidemiological studies and the proportion of psychopaths in the prison ASPD group, we can conservatively estimate the incidence of adult psychopathy at 0.75% (Blair, Mitchell, & Blair, 2005).

There is very little known with respect to prevalence and gender. Work on psychopathy has been conducted largely on males and relatively little is known about psychopathy in females (for a review see Verona & Vitale, 2006).

Development of the Behavioral Manifestation

There are few longitudinal data on the development of psychopathy, making it impossible to effectively describe how its behavioral manifestation varies with age. However, a recent study does suggest that cruelty to animals may be a potent indicator of early callous–unemotional predisposition (Dadds, Whiting, & Hawes, 2006). There is also some suggestion that fearlessness in early childhood may be one index of risk for callous–unemotional traits and conduct problems (Frick & Marsee, 2006; Kochanska, Gross, Lin, & Nichols, 2002). The importance of assessing age-appropriate behavioral features was recognized during the development of assessment instruments such as the APSD and PCL-YV. For example, attention is given to whether a child keeps the same friends rather than whether they have multiple marital partners (Frick & Hare, 2001). However, the extent to which individual components of the psychopathy are associated with the syndrome across time-points remains unknown. The few existent data indicate reasonable stability of callous–unemotional traits from middle childhood to early adolescence (see Frick & Marsee, 2006 p. 853). Also, it is worth noting the literature on fearlessness. While it is not an explicit measure of psychopathy, it has long been associated with the disorder (Cleckley, 1941; Patrick, 1994). This is interesting because fearlessness also shows moderate stability in early childhood, as well as a clear relationship with empathic and moral development (Kochanska, Gross, Lin *et al.*, 2002).

Does Psychopathy Extend into the Normal Distribution?

There has been some debate as to whether psychopathy is best characterized as a taxon or a constellation of normal personality traits (Edens, Marcus, Lilienfeld, & Poythress, 2006; Lynam, Caspi, Moffitt *et al.*, 2005; Vasey, Kotov, Frick, & Loney, 2005). This debate remains unresolved. What is clear is that psychopathy can be mapped as a mixture of normal personality dimensions (see chapters 14 and 50; Lynam, Caspi, Moffitt *et al.*, 2005). In addition, differences in brain function relevant to psychopathy can be identified within the healthy population and related to subclinical features of psychopathy (Gordon, Baird, & End, 2004). Although psychopathy can be mapped to a mixture of normal personality dimensions, and community samples high on psychopathic traits can display functional brain differences similar to those seen in incarcerated psychopaths, this does not suggest that psychopathy should necessarily be viewed as "normal." Cleckley (1941) strongly asserted that psychopathy represented something distinct from normal variations of personality. As pointed out by Rutter (2005), none of the existing measures of normal personality functioning set out to characterize the emotional dysfunction that defines psychopathy. In addition, we have no data addressing the question of whether the differences in brain function that are relevant to psychopathy need to reach a certain quantitative threshold before we see a true risk for the extreme psychopathic personality that might qualify as a taxon.

Origins of Psychopathy

Genetic Factors

A recent comprehensive meta-analysis of behavioral genetic studies on antisocial behavior concluded that antisocial behavior is moderately heritable (Rhee & Waldman, 2002). Work on psychopathy, a major risk factor for antisocial behavior marked by both reactive and instrumental acts, has revealed, using self-report measures in adult and adolescent populations, moderate heritability of callous–unemotional related traits, no shared environmental influence and moderate non-shared environmental influence (Blonigen, Hicks, Krueger, Patrick, & Iacono, 2005; Larsson, Andershed, & Lichtenstein, 2006; Taylor, Loney, Bobadilla, Iacono, & McGue, 2003). The heritability estimates were similar or slightly higher than typically found for self-report personality questionnaires (Loehlin, 1992). However, the sample sizes in these adult and adolescent samples were either relatively small or at best moderate. In recent work with around 3500 twin pairs, we have shown that callous–unemotional traits are strongly heritable (67% heritability) at both 7 and 9 years (Viding, Blair, Moffitt, & Plomin, 2005). Moreover, antisocial behavior in the presence of elevated levels of callous–unemotional traits is strongly heritable (81%). However, heritability of antisocial behavior without callous–unemotional traits was only moderate (30%; Viding, Blair, Moffitt *et al.*, 2005). Importantly, in addition, the high heritability of antisocial behavior in children with callous–unemotional traits has been shown to be independent of co-occurring ADHD pathology (Viding, Jones, Frick *et al.*, 2008).

Genes regulating serotonergic neurotransmission, in particular monoamine oxidase A (*MAOA*), have been highlighted in the search for a genetic predisposition to antisocial behavior (Lesch, 2003). The *MAOA* gene contains a well-characterized functional polymorphism consisting of a variable number of tandem repeats in the promoter region, with high- (*MAOA-H*) and low-activity (*MAOA-L*) allelic variants. The *MAOA-H* variant is associated with lower concentration of intracellular serotonin, whereas the *MAOA-L* variant is associated with higher concentration of intracellular serotonin. Recent research suggests that genetic vulnerability to antisocial behavior conferred by *MAOA-L* may only become evident in the presence of an environmental trigger, such as maltreatment (Caspi, McClay, Moffitt *et al.*, 2002; Kim-Cohen, Caspi, Taylor *et al.*, 2006). Despite the demonstration of genetic influences on individual differences in antisocial behavior, it is important to note that no genes *for* antisocial behavior exist. Instead, genes code for proteins that influence characteristics such as neurocognitive vulnerabilities which may in turn increase risk for antisocial behavior. Thus, although genetic risk alone may be of little consequence for behavior in favorable conditions, the genetic vulnerability may still manifest at the level of brain or cognition. Imaging genetics studies attest to genotype differences being associated with variation in brain structure and function in non-clinical samples (Meyer-Lindenberg & Weinberger, 2006). We can think of this as the neural fingerprint; ready to translate into disordered behavior in the presence of unfortunate environmental triggers.

Meyer-Lindenberg, Buckholtz, Kolachana *et al.* (2006) recently provided the first demonstration of the *MAOA-L* genotype being associated with a pattern of neural hypersensitivity to emotional stimuli. Specifically, they reported increased amygdala activity coupled with lesser activity in the frontal regulatory regions in *MAOA-L* compared to *MAOA-H* carriers. Meyer-Lindenberg, Buckholtz, Kolachana *et al.* (2006) speculated that their brain imaging findings of poor emotion regulation in *MAOA-L* carriers relate to threat reactive and impulsive, rather than psychopathic antisocial behavior. They based this speculation on the findings of individuals with psychopathy displaying under-reactivity of the brain's emotional circuit, particularly the amygdala (Birbaumer, Veit, Lotze *et al.*, 2005; Kiehl, Smith, Hare *et al.*, 2001).

Currently, while the behavioral genetics data suggest heritability of the emotional component of psychopathy, a molecular level account of the disorder remains in its infancy. Suggestions have been made that psychopathy might be related to anomalies in noradrenergic neurotransmission (Blair, Mitchell, & Blair, 2005). It is also interesting to note that a small number of studies have reported increased vulnerability to antisocial behavior in the presence of the *MAOA-H* allele (Manuck, Flory, Ferrell, Mann, & Muldoon, 2000). These may reflect false positive findings, but it is also possible to speculate that the amygdala hyporeactivity as opposed to hyper-reactivity seen in individuals with psychopathy could be influenced by *MAOA-H*, rather than *MAOA-L* genotype. This suggestion remains highly speculative, and as for any behavior, the genetic influences will not be limited to a single candidate gene. Other genes influencing amygdala reactivity, such as genes encoding 5-HTT, could also have a role in psychopathy.

Environmental Factors

Many environmental causes have been suggested for an increased risk for aggression and, at least in the lay population, psychopathy. We will consider four sets of potential causes: exposure to extreme threats (e.g., in the context of childhood abuse and/or chronic exposure to violence), incompetent parenting, environmental insults and environmental motivators (e.g., a lack of money; see chapter 25).

Exposure to Extreme Threats and Incompetent Parenting

There are considerable data that exposure to extreme threats increases the risk for aggression or being diagnosed with CD.

This is seen as a result of physical and sexual abuse (Dodge, Pettit, Bates, & Valente, 1995; Farrington & Loeber, 2000) as well as a result of exposure to violence in the home or neighborhood (Miller, Wasserman, Neugebauer, Gorman-Smith, & Kamboukos, 1999; Schwab-Stone, Chen, Greenberger *et al.*, 1999). There are also considerable data that exposure to poor parenting increases the risk for aggression or being diagnosed with CD (Snyder, Cramer, Afrank *et al.*, 2005). Moreover, Bowlby attributed "affectionless psychopathy" to family adversity that especially involved family disruption (Bowlby, 1946) and "impaired empathy" is considered an aspect of the "disinhibited attachment" that is characteristic of some children experiencing profound early institutional deprivation (O'Connor & Rutter, 2000; Rutter, 2005). Parental abuse is also frequently reported in forensic samples, including individuals diagnosed with psychopathy (Hare, 2003). A recent study specifically addressed the effect of childhood maltreatment on the different facets of psychopathy and found that maltreatment increases the risk for impulsive and irresponsible lifestyle, but does not have an effect on the core emotional dysfunction in psychopathy (Poythress, Skeem, & Lilienfeld, 2006).

The preliminary work by Poythress Skeem, & Lilienfeld (2006) suggests that the core emotional dysfunction of psychopathy may not be affected by maltreatment. In addition, work by Pollak and colleagues suggests that maltreated children show hyper-reactivity to anger, which is in contrast to hyporeactivity to fear and sadness seen in psychopaths (Pollak & Sinha, 2002). Animal studies can also provide some clues about the effects of maltreatment on emotional reactivity, although such work has to be interpreted with caution with regard to humans. Animal studies clearly show that prolonged threat or stress leads to a long-term potentiation of the neural and neurochemical systems that respond to threat (i.e., the individual becomes more responsive to aversive stimuli; Bremner & Vermetten, 2001; King, 1999). Moreover, animal studies also show that poor parenting is also associated with increased responsiveness to aversive stimuli (Rilling, Winslow, O'Brien *et al.*, 2001; Sanchez, Noble, Lyon *et al.*, 2005). Importantly, this concurs with much of the human literature (Pollak & Sinha, 2002). Thus, traumatic exposure, including exposure to violence in the home or neighborhood, appears to increase the risk for mood and anxiety disorders in general, although not all exposed to trauma will go on to develop these disorders (Charney, 2003; Gorman-Smith & Tolan, 1998; Schwab-Stone, Chen, Greenberger *et al.*, 1999). In other words, animal and much human work indicates that trauma and poor parenting increase emotional responsiveness to aversive stimuli (for an account of why this increased emotional responsiveness to aversive stimuli should be a risk factor for increased levels of reactive aggression and some forms of CD see Blair, Mitchell, & Blair, 2005), whereas a defining feature of psychopathy is the reduction, not elevation, in the individual's responsiveness to threat (Cleckley, 1941; Hare, 1970). More research is needed to investigate whether maltreated and neglected children displaying poor empathy and attachment problems show a similar neurocognitive profile to that seen in psychopathy. Current literature suggests that for the majority of cases, maltreatment produces a neural and behavioral signature that is different from that commonly observed in individuals with psychopathy. However, it is plausible that both biologically and environmentally "weighted" routes to the same pathophysiology can take place, even if one route is considerably more common than the other (for a discussion of this issue with respect to autism spectrum disorders see chapter 12).

Environmental Insults

Birth complications such as anoxia (lack of oxygen) and pre-eclampsia (hypertension leading to anoxia) are environmental factors that can give rise to brain damage. Minor physical anomalies (MPAs) are relatively minor physical abnormalities consisting of such features as low-seated ears and a furrowed tongue that are associated with disorders of pregnancy and are thought to be a marker for fetal neural maldevelopment towards the end of the first 3 months of pregnancy. They can be caused by environmental factors acting on the fetus such as anoxia and infection (Guy, Majorski, Wallace, & Guy, 1983) or can also indicate genetic liability. Several studies have shown that babies who have birth complications or present with MPAs are more likely to develop CD and delinquency and commit violence in adulthood, particularly when other psychosocial risk factors are present (Hodgins, Kratzer, & McNeil, 2001; Pine, Shaffer, Schonfeld, & Davies, 1997; Raine, 2002; although see, for example, Laucht, Esser, Baving *et al.*, 2000).

Unfortunately, the literature has not considered whether birth complications or MPAs are a risk factor for the emergence of psychopathy or syndromes linked to heightened levels of reactive aggression. However, there is no reason to believe that such environmental insults could not detrimentally affect neural systems associated with the disorder (i.e., they could be causal for the disorder). Future research is needed to clarify this issue.

Environmental Motivation

Lower socioeconomic status (SES) and lower IQ are both associated with an increased risk for antisocial behavior, including the antisocial behavior component of psychopathy (Frick, O'Brien, Wootton *et al.*, 1994; Hare, 2003). The SES data suggest a social contribution to at least the behavioral manifestation of psychopathy. Importantly, some antisocial behavior shown by individuals with psychopathy is instrumental in nature: it has the goal of gaining another's money, sexual favors or "respect" (Cornell, Warren, Hawk *et al.*, 1996; Williamson, Hare, & Wong, 1987). Individuals can attempt to achieve these goals through a variety of means. Having a higher SES (or for that matter intelligence) enables a wider choice of available routes for achieving these goals than having a lower SES or IQ. Lower SES or IQ limits the behavioral options. A healthy individual of limited SES or IQ may also have a narrow range of behavioral options but will exclude antisocial behavior because of aversion to this behavior formed during socialization. In contrast, individuals with psychopathy may entertain the antisocial option because they do not find the required antisocial behavior aversive. SES is also likely to impact on the probability of displaying instrumental aggressions by determining relative reward levels for particular actions. If the individual already has $100,000, the subjective value of the $50 that could be gained if the individual mugged another person on the street is low. In contrast, if the individual has only 50 cents, the subjective value of the $50 will be very high indeed (for a discussion of subjective value see Tversky & Kahneman, 1981).

Pathophysiology of Psychopathy

Two levels of accounts are considered: neural (which systems are dysfunctional in individuals with psychopathy) and cognitive (what functional impairments are seen in psychopathy and why should they give rise to symptoms).

Accounts at the Neural System Level

Frontal Lobes

There have long been suggestions that frontal lobe executive function dysfunction is causally related to psychopathy in particular or antisocial behavior more generally (Gorenstein, 1982; Moffitt, 1993; Raine, 2002). Three main strands of data support this contention:

1 Neuropsychological data indicate that individuals with antisocial behavior show impaired performance on classic measures of executive functioning (for reviews of this literature see Kandel & Freed, 1989; Morgan & Lilienfeld, 2000);

2 Neuroimaging data indicate that aggressive individuals are marked by reduced frontal functioning (Goyer, Andreason, Semple *et al.*, 1994; Raine, Meloy, Bihrle *et al.*, 1998; Volkow, Tancredi, Grant *et al.*, 1995);

3 Neurological patients with lesions of orbital frontal cortex, whether these occur early in life or adulthood, present with a heightened risk for aggression (Anderson, Bechara, Damasio, Tranel, & Damasio, 1999; Grafman, Schwab, Warden, Pridgen, & Brown, 1996).

However:

1 Individuals with psychopathy, unlike more general antisocial populations, show no impairment on measures of executive functioning linked to either dorsolateral prefrontal cortex or regions of medial frontal cortex including dorsal regions of anterior cingulate (Blair, Newman, Mitchell *et al.*, 2006; Kandel & Freed, 1989; LaPierre, Braun, & Hodgins, 1995). Impairment, when seen, is seen strictly for measures of executive functioning linked to orbital and inferior frontal cortex (e.g., response reversal; Blair Newman, Mitchell *et al.*, 2006; LaPierre, Braun, & Hodgins, 1995).

2 The neuroimaging data reveal a complex pattern with respect to frontal cortex and psychopathy. The results of early work indexing activity during rest in generally antisocial populations (Goyer, Andreason, Semple *et al.*, 1994; Raine, Meloy, Bihrle *et al.*, 1998; Volkow, Tancredi, Grant *et al.*, 1995) have not been borne out with more recent event-related fMRI studies. More recent studies have indicated the possibility of dysfunction in orbital frontal cortex and anterior cingulate (Birbaumer, Veit, Lotze *et al.*, 2005; Kiehl, Smith, Hare *et al.*, 2001).

3 Many of the functional impairments shown by neurological patients with acquired lesions of orbital frontal cortex are markedly different from those shown by individuals with psychopathy (Blair & Cipolotti, 2000). Moreover, clinically, while neurological patients with acquired lesions of orbital frontal cortex present with an increased risk for reactive aggression but not instrumental aggression (Anderson, Bechara, Damasio *et al.*, 1999; Grafman, Schwab, Warden *et al.*, 1996), individuals with psychopathy are at increased risk for both forms of aggression (Cornell, Warren, Hawk *et al.*, 1996; Williamson, Hare, & Wong, 1987).

We have argued elsewhere that "frontal lobe" explanations of psychopathy need greater specification (Blair, 2004). The current data indicate no impairment in executive functions reliant on dorsolateral prefrontal cortex and medial frontal cortex. However, there are reasons to believe that there may be impairment in executive functions reliant on orbital and inferior frontal cortex. This may indicate orbital and/or inferior frontal cortex dysfunction (Blair, Newman, Mitchell *et al.*, 2006; LaPierre, Braun, & Hodgins, 1995). However, it is worth noting that it may also indicate dysfunction in systems that feed information to orbital and/or inferior frontal cortex. Currently, the fMRI studies that have indicated reduced activity in these regions in adults with psychopathy have all used tasks where there is also reduced amygdala activity and where the amygdala is necessarily involved in the transmission of information to these frontal regions (Birbaumer, Veit, Lotze *et al.*, 2005; Kiehl, Smith, Hare *et al.*, 2001). Therefore, studies that employ tasks that do not recruit amygdala are needed to ascertain whether the differences in orbital and/or inferior frontal cortex are independent from amygdala input.

It is important to note that the executive function consistently identified as impaired in individuals with psychopathy is response reversal (Budhani & Blair, 2005). Response reversal is the ability to make a new response to gain a reward when the old behavior that previously gave rise to the reward no longer does so (Rolls, 1997). It is unlikely that impairment in this executive function is causally related to psychopathy per se. This is because impairment in response reversal is seen in other clinical populations, in particular children with bipolar disorder (Gorrindo, Blair, Budhani *et al.*, 2005). Importantly though, a common feature of both childhood bipolar disorder and psychopathy is an increased risk for reactive aggression (Frick, Cornell, Barry, Bodin, & Dane, 2003; Leibenluft, Blair, Charney, & Pine, 2003). Reactive aggression can be associated with frustration, as well as perceived threat. An individual who cannot change their behavior to accommodate to changing real-life contingencies, an individual who cannot perform response reversal, is someone at increased risk for reactive aggression. It therefore appears plausible that while response reversal impairment is not causally related to the development of the full syndrome of psychopathy, it is causally related to the increased risk for reactive aggression and that this is also seen in other childhood psychiatric conditions (Blair, Mitchell, & Blair, 2005).

Amygdala

Patrick (1994) originally suggested that amygdala dysfunction might be causally related to the development of psychopathy, and Blair, Mitchell, & Blair (2005) have developed and extended this position. Two main strands of data support the suggestion of amygdala dysfunction in psychopathy:

1 Neuropsychological data indicate that individuals with psychopathy show impairment on tasks indexing the functional integrity of the amygdala. Thus, individuals with psychopathy show impairment in aversive conditioning (Flor, Birbaumer, Hermann, Ziegler, & Patrick, 2002), the augmentation of the startle reflex by visual threat primes (Levenston, Patrick, Bradley, & Lang, 2000), passive avoidance learning (Newman & Kosson, 1986) and fearful expression recognition (Blair Colledge, Murray *et al.*, 2001); and

2 Neuroimaging data indicate that adults with the disorder are marked by reduced amygdala responsiveness during emotional memory (Kiehl, Smith, Hare *et al.*, 2001) and aversive conditioning tasks (Birbaumer, Veit, Lotze *et al.*, 2005; although see Muller, Sommer, Wagner *et al.*, 2003).

Importantly, the impairments seen in individuals with psychopathy closely mirror those seen in patients with amygdala damage. Thus, lesions of the amygdala disrupt aversive conditioning (Bechara, Tranel, Damasio *et al.*, 1995), the augmentation of the startle reflex by visual threat primes (Angrilli, Mauri, Palomba *et al.*, 1996), passive avoidance learning (Ambrogi Lorenzini, Baldi, Bucherelli, Sacchetti, & Tassoni, 1999) and fearful expression recognition (Adolphs, 2002). However, there is a caveat. Patients with acquired damage to the amygdala do not typically show increased levels of aggression. This dissociation between the clinical implications of acquired amygdala damage and psychopathy likely relates to the developmental trajectory of the disorder (Blair, Mitchell, & Blair, 2005).

The Paralimbic Hypothesis

On the basis of neuroimaging data, Kiehl (2006) has argued that, in individuals with psychopathy, there is dysfunction within paralimbic cortex (i.e., amygdala, anterior superior temporal gyrus, rostral and caudal anterior cingulate, posterior cingulate, ventromedial frontal cortex and parahippocampal regions). However, neuroimaging data are notoriously unable to localize deficits; impairment in any region will lead to anomalous activity in any region reliant on the dysfunctional region for input. We can only be sure that an area is dysfunctional in a population if both neuroimaging and neuropsychological data indicate impairment. Indeed, anterior cingulate, at least, does not appear globally impaired in individuals with psychopathy. Damage to anterior cingulate is known to increase the Stroop effect (i.e., the interference by distracter information; Stuss, Floden, Alexander, Levine, & Katz, 2001). However, individuals with psychopathy show no evidence of increases in the Stroop effect; if anything the opposite (Blair, Newman, Mitchell *et al.*, 2006; Hiatt, Schmitt, & Newman, 2004).

Specificity

It is important to note that for any of the brain areas of proposed involvement in psychopathy (e.g., orbitofrontal cortex and amygdala), associations with other psychopathologies also exist. For example, autism has been claimed to reflect, at least in part, aberrant functioning of the orbitofrontal–amygdala circuit to much the same direction as is seen in psychopathy (Bachevalier & Loveland, 2006). As another example, major depressive disorder is also associated with orbitofrontal cortex underactivity (Steele, Currie, Lawrie, & Reid, 2007). Clearly, these two disorders are not synonymous with psychopathy, although they share some features at the neural level and may even share overlapping behaviors. As we highlighted above, it is clearly important to combine information from both neuroimaging and neuropsychology to gain a more thorough understanding of a specific deficit profile. In addition, any other brain abnormalities associated with a given disorder, and which can potentially influence behavioral outcome, must be accounted for. Thus, with regard to autism, several other key regions, in addition to the orbitofrontal–amygdala circuitry, have emerged as important in providing explanations for the behavioral manifestations of the disorder. Finally, cognitive accounts of the disorder may work hand in hand with the neural system level of explanations to provide differentiation between disorders.

Accounts at the Level of Cognitive Function

Executive Accounts

Executive dysfunction in psychopathy has been linked to impulsivity (Miller, Flory, Lynam, & Leukefeld, 2003; Whiteside & Lynam, 2001). This in turn has been conceptualized as the lack of premeditation (i.e., the "inability to inhibit previously rewarded behavior when presented with changing contingencies") and the lack of perseverance (the "inability to ignore distracting stimuli or to remain focused on a particular task"; Whiteside & Lynam, 2001). In addition, it can be linked to response set modulation. This is characterized as the "rapid and relatively automatic (i.e., non-effortful or involuntary) shift of attention from the effortful organization and implementation of goal-directed behavior to its evaluation" (Newman, 1998).

Both Lynam's impulse control and Newman's response set modulation models can be considered executive accounts because they suggest the existence of general systems operating on multiple domains. These accounts suggest that the emotional deficits seen in individuals with psychopathy are secondary to executive deficits. Both positions should predict that individuals with psychopathy would be impaired on a broad range of tasks; many tasks can be considered to involve inhibition or response set modulation. However, more recent data suggest that there are finer empirical cuts to be made than those predicted by such general models. Thus, for example, dorsolateral prefrontal cortex is involved in processes that allow the alternation of responding to different conceptual categories (shapes versus lines) or spatial locations as a function of contingency change while inferior frontal cortex is involved in processes that allow the alternation of responding to different objects within the same conceptual category as a function of contingency change (Roberts, Robbins, & Weiskrantz, 1998). The functions of both these regions of frontal cortex have been characterized in terms similar to those proposed by the impulse control and response set modulation positions. However, whereas individuals with psychopathy show impairment on measures of inferior frontal cortex functioning, they show no impairment for tasks that index the functional integrity of dorsolateral prefrontal cortex (Blair, Newman, Mitchell *et al.*, 2006; LaPierre, Braun, & Hodgins, 1995). In short, even if a characterization of the impairment in individuals with psychopathy in terms of inhibition or response modulation was correct, we argue that it would be necessary to constrain such accounts such that they were not domain general but rather specific to particular neurocognitive systems.

Stimulus–Reinforcement Associations, Fear, Empathy, Moral Socialization and Instrumental Antisocial Behavior

A considerable animal literature shows that the amygdala is necessary for the formation of stimulus–reinforcement associations (Baxter & Murray, 2002; Everitt, Cardinal, Parkinson, & Robbins, 2003). With respect to psychopathy, it has been argued that individuals with psychopathy are impaired in the formation of stimulus–reinforcement associations (Blair, 2004). Impairment in the formation of aversive stimulus–reinforcement associations would give rise to the observed deficits in individuals with psychopathy in aversive conditioning, the augmentation of the startle reflex following the presentation of visual threat primes and passive avoidance learning (Flor, Birbaumer, Hermann, Ziegler, & Patrick, 2002; Levenston, Patrick, Bradley, & Lang, 2000; Newman & Kosson, 1986). In short, this impairment would give rise to the deficits consistent with previous suggestions that there is fear system dysfunction in psychopathy (Lykken, 1957; Patrick, 1994); for a re-evaluation of this literature see Blair (2004) and Blair, Mitchell, & Blair (2005).

One important class of aversive stimuli for socialization is the distress of other individuals, the expressions of fear and sadness (Blair, 2003b). The amygdala is crucially involved in the response to these stimuli (Adolphs, 2002; Blair, 2003b). In line with suggestions of a specific form of empathy deficit, individuals with psychopathy show reduced autonomic responses to the distress cues of other individuals and impaired fearful facial and vocal expression recognition (for a review see Blair, 2003b).

The argument has been made that the expressions of fear and sadness serve as social reinforcers allowing conspecifics to teach the societal valence of objects and actions to the developing individual (Blair, 2003b); actions/objects associated with the sadness/fear of others acquire, in healthy developing children, negative valence. Because of their impairment in the response to the sadness and fear of other individuals and in the formation of aversive stimulus–reinforcement associations, individuals with psychopathy are less able to take advantage of this "moral" social referencing. They should be, and are (Oxford, Cavell, & Hughes, 2003; Wootton, Frick, Shelton *et al.*, 1997), more difficult to socialize through standard parenting techniques. They will not learn to avoid using instrumental antisocial behavior to achieve their goals. This is because of relative in-difference to the "punishment" of the victim's distress and impairment in learning the association between this "punishment" and the representation of the action that caused the victim's distress. If confirmed, this observation should have fundamental implications for treatment. In the future, the nature of interventions directed to children with severe conduct problems could come to vary based on the degree to which the specific child exhibits the emotional features of psychopathy.

Treatment of Psychopathy

Critics express concern about labeling children as having psychopathy. This concern emerges mainly because adult psychopaths are presumed to be untreatable (see chapter 50; Hare, 2003). Clinicians rightly wish to avoid applying a label to children that implies they cannot be treated. However, identifying the emotional dysfunction early on can offer an important opportunity for prevention (for a discussion of this issue see Lynam, Caspi, Moffitt *et al.*, 2007). The concern about labeling should not curb clinical research that may lead to treatment options for this vulnerable group of youngsters.

The behavioral manifestation of psychopathy is not always resistant to change. Most clinicians familiar with individuals with psychopathy will have had experience with individuals substantially modifying their behavior to achieve particular goals in institutional settings. This change in behavioral manifestation does not necessarily imply modification of the disorder's core features, the emotional dysfunction (for a review see Harris & Rice, 2006). However, socially desirable responding could be achieved in individuals with psychopathy even if the core emotional dysfunction is resistant to complete amelioration. Individuals with psychopathy value status, power and dominance and are strong on self-interest and short-term rewards. They are poor at acting on long-term interest and low on empathy and altruism. Despite the demonstrated amygdala dysfunction in this population, several other brain areas, including most of frontal cortex, appear to function normally in psychopaths. It is thus possible to devise cognitive–behavioral intervention programs that capitalize on what is spared in terms of brain function and behavioral goal setting.

Intervention programs for at-risk, generally impoverished children, even those not developed specifically to address childhood aggression and antisocial behaviors, have had long-term effects on reducing the occurrence of conduct problems (New *et al.*, 2002; Zigler, Taussig, & Black, 1992). These programs have provided a mix of child care, family support, parental educational and job training, parent–child education and parent management training, and preschool education to high-risk families with children 0–5 years old (Connor, Carlson, Chang *et al.*, 2006). Only one study to date has investigated how the emotion dysfunction component of psychopathy mediates the success of parent training (Hawes & Dadds, 2005). This study found that the emotional dysfunction is associated with poorer treatment success. Frick (2001) has suggested that many of the current intervention programs do not incorporate elements that would be particularly important for treating psychopathic antisocial behavior. As such, it is possible to speculate that at least some of the current treatment success statistics may be marred by not accounting for the presence of children who have psychopathy and who may dilute the estimated effect of overall treatment success. Categorizing children with CD into those with and without psychopathy is highly desirable in developing appropriate intervention approaches.

Studies suggest that it is predominantly reactive, impulsive, affective aggression that responds to medication (for a review see Connor, Carlson, Chang *et al.*, 2006). However, most studies do not separate reactive from instrumental forms of aggression and no studies as yet have examined pharmacological interventions on the emotional dysfunction (and the potential consequence of instrumental aggression) seen in psychopathy. In addition to the development of new cognitive–behavioral treatment approaches, this is an area in urgent need of research.

Conclusions

In conclusion, current definitions of psychopathy categorize individuals with psychopathy as a subset of individuals with CD/ASPD. It is thought that their pathological development is related to a specific form of emotional dysfunction: callous and unemotional traits. Behaviorally, individuals with psychopathy are marked by an increased risk for both reactive *and* instrumental aggression. Importantly, the psychopathy construct has been extremely successful in predicting long-term prognosis, particularly in adult samples. Perhaps the greatest current importance of this construct for child psychiatrists is that it identifies a sample of children who are unlikely to benefit from standard treatment strategies for children with CD/ODD (Hawes & Dadds, 2005).

Behavioral genetic work indicates that callous and unemotional traits are strongly heritable and that antisocial behavior of callous–unemotional children is under considerable genetic influence. However, the corresponding molecular work remains in its infancy. What can be suggested is that the genetic contribution influences at the very minimum the functional integrity of the amygdala and the related circuitry. Because of the amygdala's important roles in responding to distress cues, fear expressions and the formation of stimulus–reinforcement associations, the capacity of the developing child to acquire morality is severely compromised. The child is able to learn the rewards associated with antisocial behavior but is less sensitive to the punishments (the distress of the victims), increasing the risk that antisocial behavior will be used instrumentally by the child to achieve goals.

Currently, there are no adequate treatment options for this disorder. This should be an area of urgent concern and translational research should focus on capitalizing on the emerging research findings from the cognitive neuroscience of psychopathy.

Acknowledgments

The authors' research into psychopathy is supported by the Intramural Research Program of the National Institutes of Health: National Institute of Mental Health (R.J.R.B.), UK Department of Health and Medical Research Council (E.V.).

Further Reading and Sources of Additional Information

Blair, R. J. R., Mitchell, D. G. V., & Blair, K. S. (2005). *The psychopath: Emotion and the brain.* Oxford: Blackwell.

Patrick, C. J. (2006). *Handbook of psychopathy.* New York: Guilford Press.

Robert Hare's home page: http://www.hare.org/

Rutter, M. (2005). Commentary: What is the meaning and utility of the psychopathy concept? *Journal of Abnormal Child Psychology*, *33*, 499–503.

References

Adolphs, R. (2002). Neural systems for recognizing emotion. *Current Opinion in Neurobiology*, *12*, 169–177.

Adolphs, R., Sears, L., & Piven, J. (2001). Abnormal processing of social information from faces in autism. *Journal of Cognitive Neuroscience*, *13*, 232–240.

Ambrogi Lorenzini, C. G., Baldi, E., Bucherelli, C., Sacchetti, B., & Tassoni, G. (1999). Neural topography and chronology of memory consolidation: A review of functional inactivation findings. *Neurobiology of Learning and Memory*, *71*, 1–18.

Anderson, S. W., Bechara, A., Damasio, H., Tranel, D., & Damasio, A. R. (1999). Impairment of social and moral behaviour related to early damage in human prefrontal cortex. *Nature Neuroscience*, *2*, 1032–1037.

Angrilli, A., Mauri, A., Palomba, D., Flor, H., Birhaumer, N., Sartori, G., *et al.* (1996). Startle reflex and emotion modulation impairment after a right amygdala lesion. *Brain*, *119*, 1991–2000.

Bachevalier, J., & Loveland, K. A. (2006). The orbitofrontal–amygdala circuit and self-regulation of social-emotional behavior in autism. *Neuroscience and Biobehavioural Reviews*, *30*, 97–117.

Baron-Cohen, S., Leslie, A. M., & Frith, U. (1985). Does the autistic child have a "theory of mind"? *Cognition*, *21*, 37–46.

Barry, C. T., Frick, P. J., DeShazo, T. M., McCoy, M. G., Ellis, M., & Loney, B. R. (2000). The importance of callous–unemotional traits for extending the concept of psychopathy to children. *Journal of Abnormal Psychology*, *109*, 335–340.

Baxter, M. G., & Murray, E. A. (2002). The amygdala and reward. *Nature Reviews Neuroscience*, *3*, 563–573.

Bechara, A., Tranel, D., Damasio, H., Adolphs, R., Rockland, C., & Damasio, A. R. (1995). Double dissociation of conditioning and declarative knowledge relative to the amygdala and hippocampus in humans. *Science*, *269*, 1115–1118.

Birbaumer, N., Veit, R., Lotze, M., Erb, M., Hermann, C., Grodd, W., *et al.* (2005). Deficient fear conditioning in psychopathy: A functional magnetic resonance imaging study. *Archives of General Psychiatry*, *62*, 799–805.

Blair, K. S., Newman, C., Mitchell, D. G., Richell, R. A., Leonard, A., Morton, J., *et al.* (2006). Differentiating among prefrontal substrates in psychopathy: neuropsychological test findings. *Neuropsychology*, *20*, 153–165.

Blair, R. J. (1999). Psychophysiological responsiveness to the distress of others in children with autism. *Personality and Individual Differences*, *26*, 477–485.

Blair, R. J. R. (2003a). Did Cain fail to represent the thoughts of Abel before he killed him? The relationship between theory of mind and aggression. In B. Repacholi, & V. Slaughter (Eds.), *Individual differences in theory of mind* (pp. 143–169). Hove, UK: Psychology Press.

Blair, R. J. R. (2003b). Facial expressions, their communicatory functions and neuro-cognitive substrates. *Philosophical Transactions of the Royal Society of London. Series B, Biological Sciences*, *358*, 561–572.

Blair, R. J. R. (2004). The roles of orbital frontal cortex in the modulation of antisocial behavior. *Brain and Cognition*, *55*, 198–208.

Blair, R. J. R. (2005). Applying a cognitive neuroscience perspective to the disorder of psychopathy. *Development and Psychopathology*, *17*, 865–891.

Blair, R. J. R., & Cipolotti, L. (2000). Impaired social response reversal: A case of "acquired sociopathy". *Brain*, *123*, 1122–1141.

Blair, R. J. R., Colledge, E., Murray, L., & Mitchell, D. G. (2001). A selective impairment in the processing of sad and fearful expressions in children with psychopathic tendencies. *Journal of Abnormal Child Psychology*, *29*, 491–498.

Blair, R. J. R., Mitchell, D. G. V., & Blair, K. S. (2005). *The psychopath: Emotion and the brain*. Oxford: Blackwell.

Blair, R. J. R., Sellars, C., Strickland, I., Clark, F., Williams, A., Smith, M., *et al.* (1996). Theory of Mind in the psychopath. *Journal of Forensic Psychiatry*, *7*, 15–25.

Blonigen, D. M., Hicks, B. M., Krueger, R. F., Patrick, C. J., & Iacono, W. G. (2005). Psychopathic personality traits: Heritability and genetic overlap with internalizing and externalizing psychopathology. *Psychological Medicine*, *35*, 637–648.

Bowlby, J. (1946). *Forty-four juvenile thieves: Their home life*. London: Bailliere, Tindall & Cox.

Bremner, J. D., & Vermetten, E. (2001). Stress and development: Behavioral and biological consequences. *Development and Psychopathology*, *13*, 473–489.

Budhani, S., & Blair, R. J. (2005). Response reversal and children with psychopathic tendencies: Success is a function of salience of contingency change. *Journal of Child Psychology and Psychiatry*, *46*, 972–981.

Caspi, A., McClay, J., Moffitt, T. E., Mill, J., Martin, J., Craig, I. W., *et al.* (2002). Role of genotype in the cycle of violence in maltreated children. *Science*, *297*, 851–854.

Charney, D. S. (2003). Neuroanatomical circuits modulating fear and anxiety behaviors. *Acta Psychiatrica Scandinavica Supplement*, *417*, 38–50.

Cleckley, H. (1941). *The mask of sanity*. St Louis, MO: Mosby.

Colledge, E., & Blair, R. J. R. (2001). Relationship between attention-deficit-hyperactivity disorder and psychopathic tendencies in children. *Personality and Individual Differences*, *30*, 1175–1187.

Connor, D. F., Carlson, G. A., Chang, K. D., Daniolos, P. T., Ferziger, R., Findling, R. L., *et al.* (2006). Juvenile maladaptive aggression: a review of prevention, treatment, and service configuration and a proposed research agenda. *Journal of Clinical Psychiatry*, *67*, 808–820.

Cornell, D. G., Warren, J., Hawk, G., Stafford, E., Oram, G., & Pine, D. (1996). Psychopathy in instrumental and reactive violent offenders. *Journal of Consulting and Clinical Psychology*, *64*, 783–790.

Dadds, M. R., Whiting, C., & Hawes, D. (2006). Associations among cruelty to animals, family conflict, and psychopathic traits in childhood. *Journal of Interpersonal Violence*, *21*, 411–429.

Dodge, K. A., Pettit, G. S., Bates, J. E., & Valente, E. (1995). Social information-processing patterns partially mediate the effect of early physical abuse on later conduct problems. *Journal of Abnormal Psychology*, *104*, 632–643.

Douglas, K. S., Vincent, G. M., & Edens, J. F. (2006). Risk for criminal recidivism: The role of psychopathy. In C. J. Patrick (Ed.), *Handbook of psychopathy* (pp. 533–554). New York: Guilford Press.

Edens, J. F., Marcus, D. K., Lilienfeld, S. O., & Poythress, N. G. Jr. (2006). Psychopathic, not psychopath: taxometric evidence for the dimensional structure of psychopathy. *Journal of Abnormal Psychology*, *115*, 131–144.

Everitt, B. J., Cardinal, R. N., Parkinson, J. A., & Robbins, T. W. (2003). Appetitive behavior: impact of amygdala-dependent mechanisms of emotional learning. *Annals of the New York Academy of Sciences*, *985*, 233–250.

Farrington, D. P., & Loeber, R. (2000). Epidemiology of juvenile violence. *Child and Adolescent Psychiatric Clinics of North America*, *9*, 733–748.

Fine, C., Lumsden, J., & Blair, R. J. (2001). Dissociation between "theory of mind" and executive functions in a patient with early left amygdala damage. *Brain*, *124*, 287–298.

Flor, H., Birbaumer, N., Hermann, C., Ziegler, S., & Patrick, C. J. (2002). Aversive Pavlovian conditioning in psychopaths: Peripheral and central correlates. *Psychophysiology*, *39*, 505–518.

Forth, A. E., Kosson, D. S., & Hare, R. D. (2003). *The Psychopathy Checklist: Youth Version*. Toronto, Ontario, Canada: Multi-Health Systems.

Frick, P. J. (2001). Effective interventions for children and adolescents with conduct disorder. *Canadian Journal of Psychiatry*, *46*, 597–608.

Frick, P. J., Cornell, A. H., Barry, C. T., Bodin, S. D., & Dane, H. E. (2003). Callous–unemotional traits and conduct problems in the prediction of conduct problem severity, aggression, and self-report delinquency. *Journal of Abnormal Child Psychology*, *31*, 457–470.

Frick, P. J., & Hare, R. D. (2001). *The antisocial process screening device*. Toronto: Multi-Health Systems.

Frick, P. J., Kimonis, E. R., Dandreaux, D. M., & Farell, J. M. (2003). The 4 year stability of psychopathic traits in non-referred youth. *Behavioral Sciences and the Law*, *21*, 713–736.

Frick, P. J., Lilienfeld, S. O., Ellis, M., Loney, B., & Silverthorn, P. (1999). The association between anxiety and psychopathy dimensions in children. *Journal of Abnormal Child Psychology*, *27*, 383–392.

Frick, P. J., & Marsee, M. A. (2006). Psychopathy and developmental pathways to antisocial behavior in youth. In C. J. Patrick (Ed.), *Handbook of psychopathy* (pp. 353–374). New York: Guilford.

Frick, P. J., O'Brien, B. S., Wootton, J. M., & McBurnett, K. (1994). Psychopathy and conduct problems in children. *Journal of Abnormal Psychology*, *103*, 700–707.

Frick, P. J., Stickle, T. R., Dandreaux, D. M., Farell, J. M., & Kimonis, E. R. (2005). Callous–unemotional traits in predicting the severity and stability of conduct problems and delinquency. *Journal of Abnormal Child Psychology*, *33*, 471–487.

Frith, U., & Happé, F. (2005). Autism spectrum disorder. *Current Biology*, *15*, R786–790.

Goodwin, R. D., & Hamilton, S. P. (2003). Lifetime comorbidity of antisocial personality disorder and anxiety disorders among adults in the community. *Psychiatry Research*, *117*, 159–166.

Gordon, H. L., Baird, A. A., & End, A. (2004). Functional differences among those high and low on a trait measure of psychopathy. *Biological Psychiatry*, *56*, 516–521.

Gorenstein, E. E. (1982). Frontal lobe functions in psychopaths. *Journal of Abnormal Psychology*, *91*, 368–379.

Gorman-Smith, D., & Tolan, P. (1998). The role of exposure to community violence and developmental problems among inner-city youth. *Development and Psychopathology*, *10*, 101–116.

Gorrindo, T., Blair, R. J., Budhani, S., Dickstein, D. P., Pine, D. S., & Leibenluft, E. (2005). Deficits on a probabilistic response-reversal task in patients with pediatric bipolar disorder. *American Journal of Psychiatry*, *162*, 1975–1977.

Goyer, P. F., Andreason, P. J., Semple, W. E., Clayton, A. H., King, A. C., Compton-Toth, B. A., *et al.* (1994). Positron-emission tomography and personality disorders. *Neuropsychopharmacology*, *10*, 21–28.

Grafman, J., Schwab, K., Warden, D., Pridgen, B. S., & Brown, H. R. (1996). Frontal lobe injuries, violence, and aggression: A report of the Vietnam head injury study. *Neurology*, *46*, 1231–1238.

Guy, J. D., Majorski, L. V., Wallace, C. J., & Guy, M. P. (1983). The incidence of minor physical anomalies in adult male schizophrenics. *Schizophrenia Bulletin*, *9*, 571–582.

Hare, R. D. (1970). *Psychopathy: Theory and research*. New York: Wiley.

Hare, R. D. (1980). A research scale for the assessment of psychopathy in criminal populations. *Personality and Individual Differences*, *1*, 111–119.

Hare, R. D. (1991). *The Hare Psychopathy Checklist–Revised*. Toronto, Ontario: Multi-Health Systems.

Hare, R. D. (2003). *Hare Psychopathy Checklist–Revised (PCL-R; 2nd Edn)*. Toronto: Multi-Health Systems.

Hare, R. D. (2006). Psychopathy: A clinical and forensic overview. *Psychiatric Clinics of North America*, *29*, 709–724.

Harris, G. T., & Rice, M. E. (2006). Treatment of psychopathy: A review of empirical findings. In C. J. Patrick (Ed.), *Handbook of Psychopathy* (pp. 555–572). New York: Guilford Press.

Hart, S. D., Forth, A. E., & Hare, R. D. (1990). Performance of criminal psychopaths on selected neuropsychological tests. *Journal of Abnormal Psychology*, *99*, 374–379.

Hawes, D. J., & Dadds, M. R. (2005). The treatment of conduct problems in children with callous–unemotional traits. *Journal of Consulting and Clinical Psychology*, *73*, 737–741.

Hiatt, K. D., Schmitt, W. A., & Newman, J. P. (2004). Stroop tasks reveal abnormal selective attention among psychopathic offenders. *Neuropsychology*, *18*, 50–59.

Hinshaw, S. P. (1987). On the distinction between attentional deficits/hyperactivity and conduct problems/aggression in child psychopathology. *Psychological Bulletin*, *101*, 443–463.

Hippler, K. & Klicpera, C. (2003). A retrospective analysis of the clinical case records of 'autistic psychopaths' diagnosed by Hans Asperger and his team at the University Children's Hospital, Vienna. *Philosophical Transactions of the Royal Society of London. Series B, Biological Sciences*, *358*, 291–301.

Hodgins, S., Kratzer, L., & McNeil, T. F. (2001). Obstetric complications, parenting, and risk of criminal behavior. *Archives of General Psychiatry*, *58*, 746–752.

Kandel, E., & Freed, D. (1989). Frontal lobe dysfunction and antisocial behavior: A review. *Journal of Clinical Psychology*, *45*, 404–413.

Kiehl, K. A. (2006). A cognitive neuroscience perspective on psychopathy: Evidence for paralimbic system dysfunction. *Psychiatry Research*, 142, 107–128.

Kiehl, K. A., Smith, A. M., Hare, R. D., Mendrek, A., Forster, B. B., Brink, J., *et al.* (2001). Limbic abnormalities in affective processing by criminal psychopaths as revealed by functional magnetic resonance imaging. *Biological Psychiatry*, *50*, 677–684.

Kim-Cohen, J., Caspi, A., Taylor, A., Williams, B., Newcombe, R., Craig, I. W., *et al.* (2006). MAOA, maltreatment, and gene-environment interaction predicting children's mental health: new evidence and a meta-analysis. *Molecular Psychiatry*, *11*, 903–913.

King, S. M. (1999). Escape-related behaviours in an unstable, elevated and exposed environment. II. Long-term sensitization after repetitive electrical stimulation of the rodent midbrain defence system. *Behavioural Brain Research*, *98*, 127–142.

Kochanska, G., Gross, J. N., Lin, M. H., & Nichols, K. E. (2002). Guilt in young children: Development, determinants, and relations with a broader system of standards. *Child Development*, *73*, 461–482.

Kosson, D. S., Cyterski, T. D., Steuerwald, B. L., Neumann, C. S., & Walker-Matthews, S. (2002). The reliability and validity of the psychopathy checklist: Youth version (PCL:YV) in nonincarcerated adolescent males. *Psychological Assessment*, *14*, 97–109.

LaPierre, D., Braun, C. M. J., & Hodgins, S. (1995). Ventral frontal deficits in psychopathy: Neuropsychological test findings. *Neuropsychologia*, *33*, 139–151.

Larsson, H., Andershed, H., & Lichtenstein, P. (2006). A genetic factor explains most of the variation in the psychopathic personality. *Journal of Abnormal Psychology*, *115*, 221–260.

Laucht, M., Esser, G., Baving, L., Gerhold, M., Hoesch, I., Ihle, W., *et al.* (2000). Behavioral sequelae of perinatal insults and early family adversity at 8 years of age. *Journal of the American Academy of Child and Adolescent Psychiatry*, *39*, 1229–1237.

Leibenluft, E., Blair, R. J., Charney, D. S., & Pine, D. S. (2003). Irritability in pediatric mania and other childhood psychopathology. *Annals of the New York Academy of Sciences*, *1008*, 201–218.

Lesch, K. P. (2003). The serotonergic dimension of aggression and violence. In Mattson M. P. (Ed.), *Neurobiology of Aggression*. Totowa, NJ, Humana Press.

Levenston, G. K., Patrick, C. J., Bradley, M. M., & Lang, P. J. (2000). The psychopath as observer: Emotion and attention in picture processing. *Journal of Abnormal Psychology*, *109*, 373–386.

Loehlin, J. C. (1992). *Genes and environment in personality development*. Newbury Park, CA: Sage Publications.

Lykken, D. T. (1957). A study of anxiety in the sociopathic personality. *Journal of Abnormal and Social Psychology*, *55*, 6–10.

Lynam, D. R. (1996). Early identification of chronic offenders: Who is the fledgling psychopath? *Psychological Bulletin*, *120*, 209–234.

Lynam, D. R., Caspi, A., Moffitt, T. E., Loeber, R., & Stouthamer-Loeber, M. (2007). Longitudinal evidence that psychopathy scores in early adolescence predict adult psychopathy. *Journal of Abnormal Psychology*, 116, 155–165.

Lynam, D. R., Caspi, A., Moffitt, T. E., Raine, A., Loeber, R., & Stouthamer-Loeber, M. (2005). Adolescent psychopathy and the Big Five: Results from two samples. *Journal of Abnormal Child Psychology*, *33*, 431–443.

Manuck, S. B., Flory, J. D., Ferrell, R. E., Dent, K. M., Mann, J. J., & Muldoon, M. F. (1999). Aggression and anger-related traits associated with a polymorphism of the tryptophan hydroxylase gene. *Biological Psychiatry*, *45*, 603–614.

Meyer-Lindenberg, A., Buckholtz, J. W., Kolachana, B., Hariri, A. R., Pezawas, L., Blasi, G., *et al.* (2006). Neural mechanisms of genetic risk for impulsivity and violence in humans. *Proceedings of the National Academy of Sciences of the USA*, *103*, 6269–6274.

Meyer-Lindenberg, A., & Weinberger, D. (2006). Intermediate phenotypes and genetic mechanisms of psychiatric disorders. *Nature Review Neuroscience*, *7*, 818–827.

Miller, J. D., Flory, K., Lynam, D. R., & Leukefeld, C. (2003). A test of the four-factor model of impulsivity-related traits. *Personality and Individual Differences*, *34*, 1403–1418.

Miller, L. S., Wasserman, G. A., Neugebauer, R., Gorman-Smith, D., & Kamboukos, D. (1999). Witnessed community violence and antisocial behavior in high-risk, urban boys. *Journal of Clinical Child Psychology*, *28*, 2–11.

Moffitt, T. E. (1993). The neuropsychology of conduct disorder. *Development and Psychopathology*, *5*, 135–152.

Morgan, A. B., & Lilienfeld, S. O. (2000). A meta-analytic review of the relation between antisocial behavior and neuropsychological measures of executive function. *Clinical Psychology Review*, *20*, 113–136.

Muller, J. L., Sommer, M., Wagner, V., Lange, K., Taschler, H., Roder, C. H., *et al.* (2003). Abnormalities in emotion processing within cortical and subcortical regions in criminal psychopaths: Evidence from a functional magnetic resonance imaging study using pictures with emotional content. *Biological Psychiatry*, *15*, 152–162.

New, A. S., Hazlett, E. A., Buchsbaum, M. S., Goodman, M., Reynolds, D., Mitropoulou, V., *et al.* (2002). Blunted prefrontal cortical 18fluorodeoxyglucose positron emission tomography response to meta-chlorophenylpiperazine in impulsive aggression. *Archives of General Psychiatry*, *59*, 621–629.

Newman, J. P. (1998). Psychopathic behaviour: An information processing perspective. In D. J. Cooke, A. E. Forth, & R. D. Hare (Eds.), *Psychopathy: Theory, research and implications for society* (pp. 81–105). Dordrecht, The Netherlands: Kluwer Academic Publishers.

Newman, J. P., & Kosson, D. S. (1986). Passive avoidance learning in psychopathic and nonpsychopathic offenders. *Journal of Abnormal Psychology, 95*, 252–256.

O'Connor, T. G., & Rutter, M. (2000). Attachment disorder behavior following early severe deprivation: Extension and longitudinal follow-up. English and Romanian Adoptees Study Team. *Journal of the American Academy of Child and Adolescent Psychiatry, 39*, 703–712.

Oxford, M., Cavell, T. A., & Hughes, J. N. (2003). Callous–unemotional traits moderate the relation between ineffective parenting and child externalizing problems: A partial replication and extension. *Journal of Clinical Child and Adolescent Psychology, 32*, 577–585.

Patrick, C. J. (1994). Emotion and psychopathy: Startling new insights. *Psychophysiology, 31*, 319–330.

Patrick, C. J. (2006). *Handbook of psychopathy*. New York: Guilford Press.

Pine, D. S., Shaffer, D., Schonfeld, I. S., & Davies, M. (1997). Minor physical anomalies: modifiers of environmental risks for psychiatric impairment? *Journal of the American Academy of Child and Adolescent Psychiatry, 36*, 395–403.

Pollak, S. D., & Sinha, P. (2002). Effects of early experience on children's recognition of facial displays of emotion. *Developmental Psychology, 38*, 784–791.

Poythress, N. G., Skeem, J. L., & Lilienfeld, S. O. (2006). Associations among early abuse, dissociation, and psychopathy in an offender sample. *Journal of Abnormal Psychology, 115*, 288–297.

Raine, A. (2002). Annotation: The role of prefrontal deficits, low autonomic arousal, and early health factors in the development of antisocial and aggressive behavior in children. *Journal of Child Psychology and Psychiatry, 43*, 417–434.

Raine, A., Meloy, J. R., Bihrle, S., Stoddard, J., LaCasse, L., & Buchsbaum, M. S. (1998). Reduced prefrontal and increased subcortical brain functioning assessed using positron emission tomography in predatory and affective murderers. *Behavioral Sciences and the Law, 16*, 319–332.

Rhee, S. H., & I. D. Waldman (2002). Genetic and environmental influences on antisocial behavior: a meta-analysis of twin and adoption studies. *Psychological Bulletin, 12*, 490–529.

Richell, R. A., Mitchell, D. G., Newman, C., Leonard, A., Baron-Cohen, S., & Blair, R. J. (2003). Theory of mind and psychopathy: Can psychopathic individuals read the 'language of the eyes'? *Neuropsychologia, 41*, 523–526.

Rilling, J. K., Winslow, J. T., O'Brien, D., Gutman, D. A., Hoffman, J. M., & Kilts, C. D. (2001). Neural correlates of maternal separation in rhesus monkeys. *Biological Psychiatry, 49*, 146–157.

Roberts, A. C., Robbins, T. W., & Weiskrantz, L. (1998). *The prefrontal cortex: Executive and cognitive functions*. Oxford, UK: Oxford University Press.

Rogers, J., Viding, E., Blair, R. J., Frith, U., & Happé, F. (2006). Autism spectrum disorder and psychopathy: Shared cognitive underpinnings or double hit? *Psychological Medicine*, 36, 1789–1798.

Rolls, E. T. (1997). The orbitofrontal cortex. *Philosophical Transactions of the Royal Society of London. Series B, Biological Sciences, 351*, 1433–1443.

Rutter, M. (2005). Commentary: What is the meaning and utility of the psychopathy concept? *Journal of Abnormal Child Psychology, 33*, 499–503.

Salekin, R. T., Leistico, A. M., Trobst, K. K., Schrum, C. L., & Lochman, J. E. (2005). Adolescent psychopathy and personality theory – the interpersonal circumplex: Expanding evidence of a nomological net. *Journal of Abnormal Child Psychology, 33*, 445–460.

Sanchez, M. M., Noble, P. M., Lyon, C. K., Plotsky, P. M., Davis, M., Nemeroff, C. B., *et al.* (2005). Alterations in diurnal cortisol rhythm and acoustic startle response in nonhuman primates with adverse rearing. *Biological Psychiatry, 57*, 373–381.

Schwab-Stone, M., Chen, C., Greenberger, E., Silver, D., Lichtman, J., & Voyce, C. (1999). No safe haven. II. The effects of violence exposure on urban youth. *Journal of the American Academy of Child and Adolescent Psychiatry, 38*, 359–367.

Silva, J. A., Derecho, D. V., Leong, G. B., Weinstock, R., & Ferrari, M. M. (2001). A classification of psychological factors leading to violent behavior in posttraumatic stress disorder. *Journal of Forensic Sciences, 46*, 309–316.

Snyder, J., Cramer, A., Afrank, J., & Patterson, G. R. (2005). The contributions of ineffective discipline and parental hostile attributions of child misbehaviour to the development of conduct problems at home and school. *Developmental Psychology, 41*, 30–41.

Steele, J. D., Currie, J., Lawrie, S. M., & Reid, I. (2007). Prefrontal cortical functional abnormality in major depressive disorder: A stereotactic meta-analysis. *Journal of Affective Disorders, 101*, 1–11.

Stuss, D. T., Floden, D., Alexander, M. P., Levine, B., & Katz, D. (2001). Stroop performance in focal lesion patients: dissociation of processes and frontal lobe lesion location. *Neuropsychologia, 39*, 771–786.

Taylor, E. A., Schachar, R., Thorley, G., & Wieselberg, M. (1986). Conduct disorder and hyperactivity. I. Separation of hyperactivity and antisocial conduct in British child psychiatric patients. *British Journal of Psychiatry, 149*, 760–767.

Taylor, J., Loney, B. R., Bobadilla, L., Iacono, W. G., & McGue, M. (2003). Genetic and environmental influences on psychopathy trait dimensions in a community sample of male twins. *Journal of Abnormal Child Psychology, 31*, 633–645.

Tversky, A., & Kahneman, D. (1981). The framing of decisions and the psychology of choice. *Science, 211*, 453–458.

Vasey, M. W., Kotov, R., Frick, P. J., & Loney, B. R. (2005). The latent structure of psychopathy in youth: a taxometric investigation. *Journal Abnormal Child Psychology, 33*, 411–429.

Verona, E., Patrick, C. J., & Joiner, T. E. (2001). Psychopathy, antisocial personality, and suicide risk. *Journal of Abnormal Psychology, 110*, 462–470.

Verona, E., & Vitale, J. (2006). Psychopathy in women: Assessment, manifestations, and etiology. In C. J. Patrick (Ed.), *Handbook of psychopathy* (pp. 415–436). New York: Guilford Press.

Viding, E., Blair, R. J. R., Moffitt, T. E., & Plomin, R. (2005). Evidence for substantial genetic risk for psychopathy in 7-year-olds. *Journal of Child Psychology and Psychiatry, 46*, 592–597.

Viding, E., Jones, A. P., Frick, P. J., Moffitt, T. E., & Plomin, R. (2008). Heritability of antisocial behaviour at 9: do callous-unemotional traits matter? *Developmental Science, 11*, 17–22.

Volkow, N. D., Tancredi, L. R., Grant, C., Gillespie, H., Valentine, A., Mullani, N., *et al.* (1995). Brain glucose metabolism in violent psychiatric patients: A preliminary study. *Psychiatry Research, 61*, 243–253.

Whiteside, S. P., & Lynam, D. R. (2001). The five factor model and impulsivity: Using a structural model of personality to understand impulsivity. *Personality and Individual Differences, 30*, 669–689.

Williamson, S., Hare, R. D., & Wong, S. (1987). Violence: Criminal psychopaths and their victims. *Canadian Journal of Behavioral Science, 19*, 454–462.

Wootton, J. M., Frick, P. J., Shelton, K. K., & Silverthorn, P. (1997). Ineffective parenting and childhood conduct problems: The moderating role of callous–unemotional traits. *Journal of Consulting and Clinical Psychology, 65*, 292–300.

Zigler, E., Taussig, C., & Black, K. (1992). Early childhood intervention: A promising preventative for juvenile delinquency. *American Psychologist, 47*, 997–1006.

Zoccolillo, M. (1992). Co-occurrence of conduct disorder and its adult outcomes with depressive and anxiety disorders: A review. *Journal of the American Academy of Child and Adolescent Psychiatry, 31*, 547–556.

52 Gender Identity and Sexual Disorders

Kenneth J. Zucker and Michael C. Seto

This chapter consists of two parts. First, we provide an overview on gender identity disorder (GID) in children and adolescents; second, we provide an overview on the paraphilias, with an emphasis on pedophilia because this diagnostic category is common among adolescents with sexual misconduct.

Gender Identity Disorder

Phenomenology

Boys and girls diagnosed with GID display an array of sex-typed behavior signaling a strong psychological identification with the opposite sex (Cohen-Kettenis & Pfäfflin, 2003; Green, 1974; Zucker & Bradley, 1995). Most of the behaviors that characterize GID begin during the preschool years (2–4 years), i.e., during the same period that more typical sex-dimorphic behaviors can be observed in young children (Ruble, Martin, & Berenbaum, 2006).

Epidemiology

Prevalence

Contemporary epidemiological studies on the prevalence of psychiatric disorders in children and youth have not examined GID. Accordingly, estimates of prevalence have had to rely on less sophisticated approaches. It has been suggested that prevalence might be inferred from the number of persons attending clinics for adults that serve as gateways for hormonal and surgical sex reassignment. Because not all gender-dysphoric adults may attend such clinics, this method may well underestimate the prevalence of GID; in any case, the number of adult transsexuals is small – one estimate from the Netherlands suggested a prevalence of 1 in 11,000 men and 1 in 30,400 women (Bakker, van Kesteren, Gooren, & Bezemer, 1993).

More liberal estimates of prevalence can be judged from studies of children in whom specific cross-gender behaviors have been assessed. For example, the standardization study of the Child Behavior Checklist (CBCL; Achenbach & Edelbrock, 1983), a parent-report questionnaire of behavior problems, includes two items that pertain to cross-gender identification: "behaves like opposite sex" and "wishes to be of opposite sex." In the standardization study, endorsement of both items was more common for girls than for boys, regardless of age and clinical status (referred versus non-referred).

Among non-referred boys (ages 4–11 years), 3.8% received a rating of 1 (somewhat true) and 1.0% received a rating of 2 (very true) for the item "behaves like opposite sex," but only 1.0% received a rating of 1 and 0.0% received a rating of 2 for the item "wishes to be of opposite sex" (Zucker, Bradley, & Sanikhani, 1997a). The comparable percentages among non-referred girls were 8.3%, 2.3%, 2.5% and 1.0%, respectively. Thus, there appears to be a sex difference in the occurrence of mild displays of cross-gender behavior, but not with regard to more extreme cross-gender behavior. These findings were largely replicated in a large-scale study of Dutch twins at ages 7 and 10 (van Beijsterveldt, Hudziak, & Boomsma, 2006).

Sex Differences in Referral Rates

Among children between the ages of 3 and 12 years, boys are referred clinically more often than girls for concerns regarding gender identity. From one specialty clinic in Toronto, Canada, Cohen-Kettenis, Owen, Kaijser, Bradley, and Zucker (2003) reported a sex ratio of 5.75:1 ($n = 358$) of boys to girls based on consecutive referrals 1975–2000. Comparative data from the sole gender identity clinic for children in Utrecht, the Netherlands, also favored referral of boys over girls (sex ratio of 2.93:1, $n = 130$).

The skewed sex ratio favoring boys may reflect bona fide sex differences in prevalence, but social factors may also have a role. Parents, teachers and peers are less tolerant of cross-gender behavior in boys than in girls, which might result in a sex-differential in clinical referral (Zucker & Bradley, 1995).

In support of this viewpoint, two studies found that girls may need to display more cross-gender behavior than boys before a referral is initiated (Cohen-Kettenis, Owen, Kaijser *et al.*, 2003; Zucker, Bradley, & Sanikhani, 1997a). In both the Toronto and Utrecht clinics, girls were referred at a slightly older age than boys (means 8.1 versus 7.3 years, respectively), despite the fact that the girls showed, on average, higher levels of cross-gender behavior than the boys (Cohen-Kettenis, Owen, Kaijser *et al.*, 2003). However, the sexes did not differ in the percentage who met the complete DSM criteria for GID; thus, there was no evidence for a sex difference in false positive referrals.

Another factor that could affect sex differences in referral rates pertains to the relative salience of cross-gender behavior

Rutter's Child and Adolescent Psychiatry, 5th edition. Edited by M. Rutter, D. Bishop, D. Pine, S. Scott, J. Stevenson, E. Taylor and A. Thapar. ISBN: 978-1-4051-4549-7.

in boys versus girls. For behaviors showing significant between-sex variation, it is almost always the case that girls are more likely to engage in masculine behaviors than boys are likely to engage in feminine behaviors (Zucker, 2005a). Thus, the base rates for cross-gender behavior, at least within the range of normative variation, may well differ between the sexes.

Diagnosis and Assessment

DSM-IV Diagnosis of Gender Identity Disorder

In DSM-IV-TR (American Psychiatric Association, 2000) there were some changes in the conceptualization of GID and in the diagnostic criteria. The DSM-IV Subcommittee on Gender Identity Disorders (Bradley, Blanchard, Coates *et al.*, 1991) took the position that the DSM-III-R diagnoses of gender identity disorder of childhood, transsexualism and gender identity disorder of adolescence or adulthood, non-transsexual type were not qualitatively distinct disorders, but reflected differences in both developmental and severity parameters. As a result, the DSM-IV Subcommittee recommended one overarching diagnosis, gender identity disorder, that could be used, with appropriate variations in criteria, across the life cycle.

In the DSM-IV, there are three criteria required for the diagnosis and there is also one exclusion criterion. The Point A criteria reflect the child's cross-gender identification, indexed by five behavioral characteristics, of which at least four must be present. The Point B criteria reflect the child's rejection of his or her anatomic status and/or rejection of same-sex stereotypical activities and behaviors. Point D specifies that the "disturbance . . . causes clinically significant distress or impairment in social, occupational, or other important areas of functioning." Point C is an exclusion criterion and pertains to the presence of a physical intersex condition (when the clinical signs of GID are present in individuals with a physical intersex condition, the DSM-IV specifies that the residual diagnosis, Gender Identity Disorder Not Otherwise Specified, can be used).

Reliability and Validity

The clinical research literature has paid little attention to reliability of diagnosis for GID. One study showed that, for children, clinicians can reliably make the diagnosis (Zucker, Finegan, Doering, & Bradley, 1984) but, to our knowledge, no study has evaluated the reliability of the diagnosis for adolescents (for further discussion see Zucker, 2006a).

There is a much more extensive literature on the discriminant validity of the GID diagnosis. Over the past 30-plus years, a variety of measurement approaches have been developed to assess the sex-typed behavior in children referred clinically for GID: observation of sex-typed behavior in free play tasks, on semi-projective or projective tasks and on a structured Gender Identity Interview schedule. In addition, several parent-report questionnaires pertaining to sex-typed behavior have been developed. In this line of research, several comparison groups have typically been utilized: siblings of GID probands, clinical controls and non-referred (or "normal") controls (for a summary and review of measures see Zucker, 1992, 2005a). These studies have demonstrated strong evidence for the discriminant validity of the various measures, with good evidence for sensitivity and specificity. Many of these measures can be used to complement the ordinary clinical assessment involving children and their parents.

Gender Identity Disorder as a Disorder?

In psychiatric nosology, it is common for there to be debate regarding the number of symptoms required for a diagnosis, the exact wording of indicators, validational evidence and so on. Although this has occurred for GID (Langer & Martin, 2004; Wilson, Griffin, & Wren, 2002; cf. Zucker, 2006b), the more common debate is over the general legitimacy of GID as a disorder (Isay, 1997). Critics of the GID diagnosis have made several claims:

1 GID is nothing more than normal variation, albeit extreme, in gender-related behavior (Hill, Rozanski, Carfagnini, & Willoughby, 2007);

2 Children with GID show little evidence of distress and/or impairment and, if they do, it is not inherent to the condition, but merely a reaction to social disapproval (Bartlett, Vasey, & Bukowski, 2000); and

3 Because GID in children is strongly predictive of a homosexual sexual orientation in adulthood, its inclusion in DSM-III was nothing more than a veiled backdoor maneuver to prevent later homosexuality.

As this last claim has been addressed elsewhere (Zucker & Spitzer, 2005), we will appraise here only the first two criticisms and suggest ways in which the diagnostic criteria for GID might be reformed in DSM-V.

GID as Normal Variation in Gender-Related Behavior

Because of the putative conflation of gender identity dysphoria and gender role behavior, particularly in the Point A criterion, one could argue that reform of the criteria is called for. One relatively simple reform would be to raise the threshold for the Point A criterion and require the presence of all five indicators. Thus, it would be necessary for the child to systematically verbalize the wish to be of the opposite sex in order for the Point A criterion to be met.

A more radical reform would be to relegate the indicators of extreme cross-gender role behavior (A2–A5) to the text description of GID, with an explanation that they may not be sufficient, on their own, to indicate the presence of gender dysphoria. The diagnostic criteria could then be modified by the inclusion of multiple indicators of gender dysphoria. To explore this, new psychometric studies would be required: factor analysis can be used to establish the coherence of these putative indicators of gender dysphoria; this would be followed by tests of discriminant validity; and then an empirical determination of the appropriate cutpoint for high sensitivity and specificity.

If such an enterprise proved successful, perhaps this would allay concerns that children with extreme gender non-conformity, but who are not truly gender dysphoric, are being inappropriately diagnosed.

Distress and Impairment

The DSM-III-R did not provide guidelines regarding the assessment of distress in the Point A criterion ("persistent and intense distress" about being a boy or a girl) or the ways in which it might be distinct from other operationalized components in the criteria (i.e., the "desire" to be of the other sex; Zucker, 1992). In the DSM-IV, this problem persists, except that it is now located in Point D, and there is the additional problem of defining impairment.

Some critics have argued that the distress and/or impairment that clinicians observe in people with GID are merely a response to the reaction of others (Bartlett, Vasey, & Bukowski, 2000). Consistent with this critique, Stoller (1968) argued that GID in boys was ego-syntonic and that they became distressed only when their cross-gender fantasies and behaviors were interfered with. However, Stoller's conceptualization was a *psychodynamic* formulation: he believed that GID was ego-syntonic because the familial conditions that produced it were systemically syntonic. Thus, it is likely that Stoller would have argued that the DSM's conceptualization of distress was, and is, too narrow.

Other theorists have argued otherwise. For example, Coates and Person (1985) claimed that GID was a "solution" to specific forms of psychopathology in the child, particularly separation anxiety and "annihilation" anxiety, which were induced by familial psychopathology. It is conceivable that both the "primary" and "secondary" views are correct or that one or the other better fits individual cases.

If one considers the developmental adolescent or adult "end-state" of GID (i.e., the strong desire to align the body via contrasex hormones and sex-reassignment surgery: in females, mastectomy, phalloplasty; in males, penectomy/castration, vaginoplasty), it is difficult to argue that cross-gender feelings and behaviors simply constitute normative variation or do not constitute an example of impairment. The required physical interventions are simply too radical to be thought about otherwise.

One indication of impairment is that children with GID have trouble with basic cognitive concepts concerning gender. They are more likely than other children to misclassify their own gender (Zucker, Bradley, Lowry Sullivan *et al.*, 1993), and they appear to have a "developmental lag" in the acquisition of gender constancy (Zucker, Bradley, Kuksis *et al.*, 1999). Given the ubiquity of gender as a social category, this may well lead to affective confusion in self-representation and in social interactions. As noted in the next section, there is evidence that children with GID have poor peer relations and more general behavioral problems, which are possible indices of impairment.

Associated Psychopathology

The most systematic information on general behavior problems in children with GID comes from parent-report data using the CBCL. Clinic-referred boys and girls with GID show, on average, significantly more general behavior problems than do their siblings and non-referred children (Cohen-Kettenis, Owen, Kaijser *et al.*, 2003; Zucker & Bradley, 1995). On the CBCL, boys with GID have a predominance of emotional difficulties whereas girls with GID do not (Cohen-Kettenis, Owen, Kaijser *et al.*, 2003; Zucker & Bradley, 1995).

Psychopathological problems increase with age in boys with GID (Cohen-Kettenis, Owen, Kaijser *et al.*, 2003; Zucker & Bradley, 1995). This could be influenced by peer ostracism. Children with GID experience significant difficulties within the peer group (Cohen-Kettenis, Owen, Kaijser *et al.*, 2003; Zucker, Bradley, & Sanikhani *et al.*, 1997a). Cohen-Kettenis, Owen, Kaijser *et al.* (2003) found that poor peer relations were the strongest predictor of CBCL behavior problems in both boys and girls with GID, accounting for 32% and 24% of the variance, respectively. Thus, social ostracism may be a potential mediator between cross-gender behavior and behavior problems. It seems likely that marked cross-gender behavior is particularly salient in eliciting negative reactions from peers.

Although we have shown that poor peer relations is an important correlate of general behavior problems in children with GID, this is not meant to imply that it is the only source of these difficulties. Other research has shown that CBCL-measured problems in boys with GID are associated with a composite index of maternal psychopathology, which may reflect generic non-specific familial risk factors in producing psychopathology in general (Zucker & Bradley, 1995) and the predominance of emotional psychopathology may reflect familial risk for affective disorders and temperamental features of the boys (Marantz & Coates, 1991). Thus, it is likely that there are both specific and general risk factors involved in the general psychological problems of children with GID.

Etiological Influences

Biological Mechanisms

The role of prenatal sex hormones in causing the postnatal display of various sex-dimorphic behaviors has been the focus of detailed experimental animal research for almost 50 years (Baum, 2006). In humans, the influence of normative sex differences in prenatal sex hormone exposure is hard to disentangle from normative sex-of-rearing effects; accordingly, researchers have relied on children born with various disorders of sex development (DSDs), previously referred to as physical intersex conditions, to separate the relative influence of biological and psychosocial processes on psychosexual differentiation.

This research provides considerable evidence for an influence of prenatal sex hormones on postnatal sex-dimorphic behavior. For example, chromosomal females with congenital adrenal hyperplasia (CAH), who are exposed to sex-atypical levels of prenatal androgen, show more masculinized gender role behavior in childhood and adolescence and a higher rate of a bisexual and/or homosexual sexual orientation in adulthood (for review see Cohen-Bendahan, van de Beek, & Berenbaum, 2005; Hines, 2004; Zucker, 1999). Nevertheless, most females with CAH show a sex-typical gender identity (e.g., Dessens, Slijper, & Drop, 2005; Meyer-Bahlburg, Dolezal, Baker *et al.*, 2004). It appears therefore that prenatal sex hormones may have a relatively stronger impact on some components of psychosexual differentiation (e.g., gender role behavior and sexual orientation) than on others (e.g., gender identity).

One of the most dramatic cases in this field was of a biologically normal male (one of a pair of identical twins), whose penis was accidentally ablated during a circumcision at the age of 7 months. Known in the literature as the John-Joan case (and then as David Reimer, the patient's name), this infant was gender-reassigned to female at the age of 17 months and gonadectomy was performed at age 22 months. Early reports indicated that the patient had differentiated a female gender identity (suggesting a crucial role for socialization influences on gender identity), although she was described as tomboyish in comportment (Money, 1975). However, a longer-term follow-up reported that the patient experienced profound conflict as a girl and, in early adolescence, "returned" to living as a boy and, in adulthood, married a woman and adopted her three children (Colapinto, 2000; Diamond & Sigmundson, 1997). Sadly, Mr. Reimer committed suicide in 2004 at the age of 38 (Agrell, 2004). His death followed the suicide of his cotwin 2 years earlier (Jang & Smith, 2004).

The David Reimer case has been used to highlight the importance of biological factors on psychosexual differentiation. Indeed, some have argued that a "normal" male sexual biology cannot be countered by socialization efforts to raise a male as a girl (even with gonadectomy, the use of female sex hormones to induce a feminizing puberty, feminizing surgery on the genitalia, etc.) and that the Reimer case was "proof" for the role of prenatal androgen "imprinting" of a male gender identity.

However, a counter to this position comes from another case of penile ablation reported on by Bradley, Oliver, Chernick, and Zucker (1998). In this case, the circumcision accident occurred at the age of 2 months and the patient was gender-reassigned, along with gonadectomy, at the age of 7 months. In adolescence, the patient began feminizing hormonal and surgical treatment. A follow-up at the age of 26 years showed that the patient had a female-typical gender identity; however, her gender role interests were conventionally masculine and she reported a bisexual sexual orientation in both fantasy and behavior.

Although the Reimer case has had a profound impact on the field, some authors have cautioned against extrapolating too much from it (Meyer-Bahlburg, 2005) and noted that the case has raised as many questions as answers.

When it comes to children with GID, one must appreciate that they invariably do not show signs of a DSD, which would appear to rule out an etiology that involves a marked prenatal hormonal anomaly (Meyer-Bahlburg, 2005). Thus, the search for biological influences on the development of GID must focus on factors that do not affect the configuration of the external genitalia. Prenatal hormonal influences may have a role, but there would have to be some kind of brain–genital dissociation in their impact (e.g., perhaps resulting from timing effects; Gooren, 2006; Goy, Bercovitch, & McBrair, 1988). Given that there are no postmortem studies on brain neuroanatomy in GID children or youth, research has focused either on indirect markers of putative prenatal hormonal influences or on other biological factors. A selective review of relevant studies is provided here.

Molecular and Behavior Genetics

There have been no molecular genetic studies of GID, but several behavioral genetic studies have shown that the liability for cross-gender behavior in the general population has a strong heritable component (van Beijsterveldt, Hudziak, & Boomsma *et al.*, 2006). Another twin study also identified strong shared environmental influences (Knafo, Iervolino, & Plomin, 2005). Such environmental influences could, of course, pertain to non-genetic biological factors but could also involve postnatal psychosocial factors, some of which may be specific to twins. In any case, it should be recognized that these studies have not identified the specific genetic and environmental factors, or the gene × environmental interactions, underlying the liability to cross-gender behavior. That genetic factors do not account for all of the variance in the liability to cross-gender behavior is demonstrated quite clearly from detailed clinical case reports of identical twins discordant for GID (Segal, 2006).

Activity Level

Activity level (AL) is a dimension of temperament with some evidence for a genetic basis and possibly prenatal hormonal influences (Campbell & Eaton, 1999). In general, boys have a higher AL than girls.

Parents report lower levels of AL in boys with GID compared to controls (Bates, Bentler, & Thompson, 1979; Zucker & Bradley, 1995). Zucker and Bradley also found that girls with GID had a higher AL than control girls.

It is possible that a sex-atypical AL is a temperamental factor that predisposes to the development of GID. For example, a low-active boy with GID may find the typical play behavior of other boys to be incompatible with his own behavioral style, which might make it difficult for him to integrate successfully into a male peer group.

Sibling Sex Ratio and Birth Order

Boys with GID have an excess of brothers to sisters (sibling sex ratio) and a later birth order. Some additional evidence shows that boys with GID are born later primarily in relation to the number of older brothers, but not sisters (Blanchard, Zucker, Bradley, & Hume, 1995; Zucker, Green, Coates *et al.*, 1997b). In the Blanchard *et al.* study, clinical control boys showed no evidence for an altered sibling sex ratio or a late birth order. These findings mesh nicely with studies of adult males with GID with a homosexual sexual orientation, who also have an excess of brothers to sisters and a later birth order (Blanchard, 2001).

One biological explanation that has been offered to account for these results pertains to maternal immune reactions during pregnancy. The male fetus is experienced by the mother as more "foreign" (antigenic) than the female fetus. Accordingly, it has been suggested that one consequence of this is that the mother produces antibodies that have the consequence of demasculinizing or feminizing the male fetus, but no corresponding masculinizing or defeminizing of the female fetus (Blanchard, 2001). This model would predict that males born later in a sibship might be more affected, because the mother's antigenicity increases with each successive male pregnancy, which is consistent with the empirical evidence on sibling sex ratio and birth order among GID probands. At present, this proposed mechanism has not been formally tested in humans.

Psychosocial Mechanisms

Psychosocial factors, to truly merit causal status, must be shown to influence the emergence of marked cross-gender behavior in the first few years of life. Otherwise, such factors would be better conceptualized as perpetuating rather than predisposing.

Sex Assignment at Birth

In some DSDs, sex assignment is delayed and, on occasion, changed from the initial sex assignment. It has been argued that prolonged delay or uncertainty about the child's "true" sex can contribute to gender identity conflict in affected individuals (Meyer-Bahlburg, Gruen, New *et al.*, 1996). Because most children with GID do not have a co-occurring DSD, this does not appear to be a relevant psychosocial factor.

Prenatal Gender Preference

It is common for parents to express a prenatal preference for the gender of the expected baby. However, there is no evidence that parents of children with GID are more likely than control parents to report having had a desire for a child of the opposite sex (Zucker, Green, Garofano *et al.*, 1994).

Social Reinforcement of Cross-Gender Behavior

The parental response to early cross-gender behavior in children with GID is typically neutral (tolerance) or even encouraging (Mitchell, 1991; Roberts, Green, Williams, & Goodman, 1987; Zucker & Bradley, 1995). Green (1974) concluded that "What comes closest so far to being a *necessary* variable is that, as any feminine behavior begins to emerge, there is *no* discouragement of that behavior by the child's principal caretaker" (p. 238, italics in original).

The reasons why parents might tolerate, if not encourage, early cross-gender behaviors appear to be quite diverse. Some report being influenced by ideas regarding non-sexist child rearing. In others, the antecedents seem to be rooted in pervasive conflict that revolves around gender issues, including what Zucker and Bradley (1995) characterized as *pathologic gender mourning*.

General Psychopathology

The role of maternal psychopathology in the genesis and perpetuation of GID has received a great deal of clinical and theoretical attention but, unfortunately, only limited empirical evaluation. All the available empirical studies have been confined to the mothers of boys with GID – comparable studies are not available regarding the mothers of girls with GID.

Marantz and Coates (1991) found that the mothers of boys with GID showed more signs of psychopathology than did the mothers of demographically matched normal boys, including more pathologic ratings on the Diagnostic Interview for Borderline Patients (Gunderson, Kolb, & Austin, 1981) and more symptoms of depression on the Beck Depression Inventory. In a similarly designed study, Zucker (2005b) reported that almost half of mothers of boys with GID ($n = 245$) met criteria for two or more diagnoses on the Diagnostic Interview Schedule, of whom over 30% had three or more diagnoses. The most common diagnoses were major depressive episode and recurrent major depression.

Although rates of emotional distress and psychiatric impairment are elevated in the mothers of boys with GID, these maternal characteristics are not unique to the mothers of boys with GID, but common to the mothers of clinic-referred boys in general. Accordingly, maternal emotional distress and/or impairment functions, at most, only as a non-specific risk factor in the development of GID.

The role of paternal influences in the genesis and perpetuation of GID has also received a great deal of clinical and theoretical attention but, again, only limited empirical evaluation and only for boys with GID. One account implicates the father's role by virtue of his absence from the family matrix. Across 10 samples of boys with GID, the rate of father absence was 34.5% (Zucker & Bradley, 1995). It is unlikely that this rate would differ significantly from the rate found in clinical populations in general, if not the general population. Green (1987) found that paternal separations occurred earlier in the families of boys with GID than normal control boys; therefore it is possible that timing is an additional variable to consider. Green also found that the fathers of boys with GID (both father-present and father-absent) recalled spending less time with their sons than did the fathers of control boys during preschool years and at the time of assessment. The inclusion of a clinical control group would be helpful in gauging the specificity of this finding.

Long-Term Follow-Up

The "natural history" of GID in children has been confined to clinic-referred samples. Because there are no natural history studies of such children taken from epidemiological samples, one has to be cautious in drawing any broad generalizations from this literature.

Follow-up Studies of Boys

Green's (1987) study constitutes the most comprehensive long-term follow-up of behaviorally feminine boys, the majority of whom would likely have met DSM criteria for GID. His study contained 66 feminine and 56 control boys, assessed initially at a mean age of 7.1 years (range, 4–12). Forty-four feminine boys and 30 control boys were available for follow-up at a mean age of 18.9 years (range, 14–24). The majority of the boys were not in therapy between assessment and follow-up. Sexual orientation in fantasy and behavior was assessed by means of a semi-structured interview. Of the previously feminine boys, 75–80% were either bisexual or homosexual at follow-up versus 0–4% of the control boys. Only one youth, at the age of 18 years, was gender-dysphoric to the extent of considering sex-reassignment surgery.

Data from six other follow-up reports on 55 boys with GID were summarized by Zucker and Bradley (1995). At follow-up (range, 13–26 years), if one excludes 13 uncertain cases, then 27 (64.3%) of the remaining 42 cases had "atypical" (i.e., homosexual, transsexual or transvestitic) outcomes. In these studies, the percentage of boys who showed persistent GID was higher than that reported by Green (11.9% vs. 2.2%, respectively), but the percentage who were homosexual (62.1%) was somewhat lower.

Zucker and Bradley (1995) reported preliminary follow-up data, at mean age 16 years, on their own sample of boys first seen in childhood (mean age at assessment, 8.2 years; range, 3–12). Of the 40 boys, 8 (20%) were classified as gender-dysphoric at follow-up. The remaining 80% had a "normal" gender identity. Regarding sexual orientation in fantasy, 20 (50%) were classified as heterosexual, 17 (42.5%) were classified as bisexual/homosexual and 3 (7.5%) were classified as "asexual" (i.e., they did not report any sexual fantasies). Regarding sexual orientation in behavior, 9 (22.5%) were classified as heterosexual, 11 (27.5%) were classified as bisexual/homosexual and 20 (50.0%) were classified as "asexual" (i.e., they did not report any interpersonal sexual experiences).

Cohen-Kettenis (2001) reported preliminary data on a sample of 56 boys first seen in childhood (mean age at assessment, 9 years; range, 6–12) and who had now reached adolescence. Of these, 9 (16.1%) requested sex-reassignment, and all 9 had a homosexual sexual orientation (P. T. Cohen-Kettenis, personal communication, February 1, 2003). Thus, the rate of GID persistence, at least into adolescence, was higher than that reported by Green (1987) and comparable with the rate obtained by Zucker and Bradley (1995).

In taking stock of these outcome data, Green's study shows that boys with GID were disproportionately, and substantially, more likely than the control boys to differentiate a bisexual/homosexual sexual orientation. The other follow-up studies yielded somewhat lower estimates of a bisexual/homosexual sexual orientation. In this regard, at least one caveat is in order. In the Zucker and Bradley follow-up, the boys were somewhat younger than were the boys followed-up by Green, so their lower rate of a bisexual/homosexual sexual orientation outcome should be interpreted cautiously, especially as one would expect that social desirability considerations would lead to underreporting of atypical sexual orientation. However, even these lower rates of a bisexual/homosexual sexual orientation are substantially higher than the currently accepted base rate of about 2–3% of a homosexual sexual orientation in men (Laumann, Gagnon, Michael, & Michaels, 1994).

A more substantive difference between Green's study and the other follow-up reports pertains to the persistence of gender dysphoria. Both Zucker and Bradley, and Cohen-Kettenis, for example, found higher rates of persistence than Green. At present, the explanations for this are unclear. One possibility pertains to sampling differences. Green's study was carried out in the context of an advertised research study whereas the Zucker and Bradley and Cohen-Kettenis samples were clinic-referred. Thus, it is conceivable that their samples may have included more extreme cases of childhood GID than the sample ascertained by Green. Because the Toronto and Dutch groups now have substantially larger samples on which to complete outcome studies, it should be possible to carry out within-group analyses to identify predictor variables (e.g., with regard to persistent GID versus desistent GID).

Follow-up Studies of Girls

Unfortunately, the long-term follow-up of girls with GID remains very patchy. In part, this reflects the comparatively lower rate of referred girls than referred boys with GID in child samples (Cohen-Kettenis, Owen, Kaijser *et al.*, 2003). Since the last edition of this volume, the first systematic follow-up of girls with GID has become available. Drummond, Bradley, Badali-Peterson, and Zucker (in press) evaluated 25 girls, originally assessed in our clinic at a mean age of 8.8 years (range, 3–12), at a follow-up mean age of 23.2 years (range, 15–36). Of these 25 girls, three (12%) had persistent GID (at follow-up ages of 17, 21 and 23 years, respectively), two of whom had a homosexual sexual orientation and the third was asexual. The remaining 22 (88%) girls had a "normal" gender identity.

Regarding sexual orientation in fantasy (Kinsey ratings) for the 12 months preceding the follow-up assessment, 15 (60%) girls were classified as exclusively heterosexual, 8 (32%) were classified as bisexual/homosexual and 2 (8%) were classified as "asexual" (i.e., they did not report any sexual fantasies). Regarding sexual orientation in behavior, 11 (44%) girls were classified as exclusively heterosexual, 6 (24%) were classified as bisexual/homosexual and 8 (32%) were classified as "asexual" (i.e., they did not report any interpersonal sexual experiences).

Although these data are preliminary, it appears that there is a range of outcomes, but it is clear that the rates of GID and a bisexual/homosexual sexual orientation without co-occurring gender dysphoria are likely to be higher than the base rates of these two aspects of psychosexual differentiation in an unselected population of women. Using Bakker, van Kesteren, Gooren *et al.*s' (1993) estimation of GID prevalence in females, the odds of persistent gender dysphoria in Drummond, Bradley, Badali-Peterson *et al.* was 4084 times the odds of gender dysphoria in the general population. Using prevalence estimates of bisexuality/homosexuality in fantasy among biological females (anywhere between 2% and 5%), the odds of reporting bisexuality/homosexuality in fantasy were 8.9–23.1 times higher than in the general population. The odds of reporting bisexuality/homosexuality in behavior were 6.7–15.5 times higher than in the general population.

In another study, Cohen-Kettenis (2001) reported preliminary data on a sample of 18 girls first seen in childhood (mean age at assessment, 9 years; range, 6–12) and who had now reached adolescence. Of these, 8 (44.4%) requested sex-reassignment and all had a homosexual sexual orientation (P. T. Cohen-Kettenis, personal communication, February 1, 2003). Thus, the rate of GID persistence, at least into adolescence, was high (and much higher than the rate of persistence for her boys with GID).

Persistence and Desistance in a Comparative-Developmental Perspective

A key challenge for developmental theories of psychosexual differentiation is to account for the disjunction between retrospective and prospective data with regard to GID persistence: it is clear that only a minority of children followed prospectively show a persistence of GID into adolescence and young adulthood.

Regarding children with GID then, we need to understand why, for the majority, the disorder apparently remits by adolescence, if not earlier. One possible explanation concerns referral bias. Green (1974) argued that children with GID who are referred for clinical assessment (and then, in some cases, therapy) may come from families in which there is more concern than is the case for adolescents and adults, the majority of whom did not receive a clinical evaluation and treatment during childhood. Thus, a clinical evaluation and subsequent therapeutic intervention during childhood may alter the natural history of GID. Of course, this is only one account of the disjunction and there may well be additional factors that might distinguish those children who are more strongly at risk for the disorder's continuation from those who are not.

One such explanation pertains to the concepts of developmental malleability and plasticity. It is possible that gender identity shows relative malleability during childhood, with a gradual narrowing of plasticity as the gendered sense of self consolidates as one approaches adolescence. Some support for this idea comes from follow-up studies of adolescents with GID, who appear to show a much higher rate of GID persistence as they are followed into young adulthood.

The best data on long-term outcome on adolescents come from the Dutch group. Cohen-Kettenis and van Goozen (1997) reported that 22 (66.7%) of 33 adolescents went on to receive sexual reassignment surgery (SRS). At initial assessment, the mean age of the 22 adolescents who received SRS was 17.5 years (range, 15–20). Of the 11 who did not receive SRS, 8 were not recommended for it because they were not diagnosed with transsexualism (presumably the DSM-IV diagnosis of GID); the three remaining patients were given a diagnosis of transsexualism but the "real-life test" (i.e., living for a time as the opposite sex prior to the institution of contrasex hormonal treatment and surgery) was postponed because of severe concurrent psychopathology and/or adverse social circumstances. Similar findings were reported by Smith, van Goozen, and Cohen-Kettenis (2002). These data suggest a very high rate of GID persistence, which is eventually treated by SRS.

Therapeutics

Ethical Considerations

Consider the following clinical scenarios:

1 A mother of a 4-year-old boy contacts a well-known clinic that specializes in sexuality throughout the lifespan. She describes behaviors consistent with the DSM diagnosis of GID. A clinician tells the mother: "Well, we don't consider 'it' to be a problem." The mother then contacts a specialty clinic for children and adolescents and asks "What should I do?"

2 A mother of a 4-year-old boy contacts a well-known clinic that specializes in gender identity problems. She describes behaviors consistent with the DSM diagnosis of GID. She says that she would like her child treated so he does not grow up to be gay. She also worries that her child will be ostracized within the peer group because of his pervasive cross-gender behavior. What should the clinician say to this mother?

3 The parents of a 6-year-old boy (somatically male) conclude that their son is really a girl, so they seek the help of an attorney to institute a legal name change (from Zachary to Aurora) and inform the school principal that their son will attend school as a girl. The local child protection agency is notified and the child removed from his parents' care (Cloud, 2000). If a clinician was asked to evaluate the situation, what would be in the best interests of the child and family?

4 A 15-year-old adolescent girl with GID asks to be seen for treatment. She would like cross-sex hormones and a mastectomy immediately. If refused, the patient threatens to kill herself. What should the clinician do?

5 A 16-year-old adolescent boy with GID asks for SRS. He states that he is sexually attracted to biological males and wants a sex-change because that will make his sexual feelings for males "normal." He states that homosexuality is against his religious beliefs and is taboo in his culture of origin. What should the clinician do?

Any contemporary developmental clinician responsible for the therapeutic care of children and adolescents with GID will quickly be introduced to these kinds of complex social and ethical scenarios and will have to think them through carefully in formulating a therapeutic plan.

Treatment of Children

In summarizing the treatment literature on GID, one will find not a single randomized controlled treatment trial. However, there have been some treatment effectiveness studies, although much is lacking in these investigations. In general, the practitioner must rely largely on the "clinical wisdom" that has accumulated in the case report literature and the conceptual underpinnings that inform the various approaches to intervention. In an era that emphasizes evidence-based therapeutics, the relatively meager empirical database is a source of frustration for many clinicians.

Behavioral Therapy

There are 13 published single-case reports that employed a behavioral therapy approach to the treatment of GID in children (for review see Zucker, 1985). One type of intervention employed has been termed *differential social attention* or *social reinforcement*. This type of intervention has been applied in clinic settings, particularly to sex-typed play behaviors. The therapist first establishes with baseline measures that the child (either when alone or in the presence of a non-interacting adult) prefers playing with cross-sex toys or dress-up apparel rather than same-sex toys or dress-up apparel. A parent or stranger is then introduced into the playroom and instructed to attend to the child's same-sex play (e.g., by looking, smiling and verbal praise) and to ignore the child's cross-sex play (e.g., by looking away and pretending to read). Such adult responses seem to elicit rather sharp changes in play behavior.

There have been two main limitations to the use of social attention or reinforcement in treating cross-gender behavior. First, at least some of the children studied reverted to cross-sex play patterns in the adult's absence or in other environments, such as the home; second, there was little generalization to untreated cross-sex behaviors (Rekers, 1975).

Such problems have led behavior therapists to seek more effective strategies of promoting generalization. One such strategy, *self-regulation* or *self-monitoring*, has the child reinforce himself or herself when engaging in a sex-typical behavior. Although self-monitoring also resulted in substantial decreases in cross-sex play, the evidence is weak that generalization is better promoted by self-regulation than by social attention (Zucker, 1985).

The behavior-therapy literature has produced no new case reports for over 20 years although its principles are often used in broader treatment approaches that involve the parents. This void is rather curious, because contemporary behavioral approaches, such as cognitive–behavioral therapy, are now used so widely with other disorders.

Behavior therapy with an emphasis on the child's cognitive structures regarding gender could be an interesting and novel approach to treatment. There is now a fairly large literature on the development of cognitive gender-schemas in typically developing children (Martin, Ruble, & Szkrybalo, 2002). It is possible that children with GID have more elaborately developed cross-gender schemas than same-gender schemas and that more positive affective appraisals are differentiated for the former than for the latter (e.g., in boys, "girls get to wear prettier clothes" versus "boys are too rough"). A cognitive approach to treatment might help children with GID to develop more flexible and realistic notions about gender-related traits (e.g., "boys can wear pretty cool clothes too" or "there are lots of boys who don't like to be rough"), which may result in more positive gender feelings about being a boy or being a girl.

Psychotherapy

There is a large case report literature on the treatment of children with GID using psychoanalysis, psychoanalytic psychotherapy or psychotherapy (for references see Zucker, 2001, 2007). The psychoanalytic treatment literature is more diverse than the behavior therapy literature, including varied theoretical approaches to understanding the putative etiology of GID (e.g., classic object relations and self-psychology). Unfortunately, this literature has not developed very far in providing systematic documentation of therapeutic effectiveness.

Apart from the general developmental perspective inherent in a psychoanalytic understanding of psychopathology, one might add to this a gender-specific perspective on development (Martin, Ruble, & Szkrybalo, 2002). Many developmentalists note that the first signs of normative gender development appear during the toddler years, including the ability to correctly self-label oneself as a boy or a girl. Money, Hampson, and Hampson (1957) postulated a sensitive period for gender identity formation, which suggests a period of time in which there is a greater malleability or plasticity in the direction that gender identity can move. Thus, early gender identity formation intersects quite neatly with analytic views on the early development of the sense of self in more global terms. It is likely therefore that the putative pathogenic mechanisms identified in the development of GID are likely to have a greater impact only if they occur during the alleged sensitive period for gender identity formation.

Treatment of the Parents

Two rationales have been offered for parental involvement in treatment. The first emphasizes the hypothesized role of parental dynamics and psychopathology in the genesis or maintenance of the disorder. From this perspective, individual therapy with the child will probably proceed more smoothly and quickly if the parents are able to gain some insight into their own contribution to their child's difficulties. Many clinicians who have worked extensively with gender-disturbed children subscribe to this rationale (Newman, 1976; Zucker, 2001, 2007). In this context, a treatment plan requires as much of an assessment of the parents as it does of the child, as is the case with many child psychiatric disorders. Assessment of psychopathology and the marital relationship in the parents of children with GID reveals great variability in adaptive functioning, which may well prove to be a prognostic factor.

The second rationale is that parents will benefit from regular formalized contact with the therapist to discuss day-to-day management issues that arise in carrying out the overall therapeutic plan. Work with parents can focus on the setting of limits with regard to cross-gender behavior, such as cross-dressing, cross-gender role and fantasy play, and cross-gender toy play and, at the same time, attempting to provide alternative activities (e.g., encouragement of same-sex peer relations and involvement in more gender-typical and neutral activities). In addition, parents can work on conveying to their child that they are trying to help him or her feel better about being a boy or a girl and that they want their child to be happier in this regard.

Although many contemporary clinicians have stressed the important role of working with the parents of children with GID, there is scanty empirical evidence on efficacy. The most relevant study found some evidence that parental involvement in therapy was significantly correlated with a greater degree of behavioral change in the child at a 1-year follow-up, but this study did not make random assignment to different treatment protocols, so one has to interpret the findings with caution (Zucker, Bradley, Doering, & Lozinski, 1985).

Supportive Treatments

In the past few years, clinicians critical of conceptualizing marked cross-gender behavior in children as a disorder have provided a dissenting perspective to the treatment approaches described so far (Menvielle & Tuerk, 2002; Menvielle, Tuerk, & Perrin, 2005). These clinicians conceptualize GID or pervasive gender-variant behavior from an essentialist perspective (i.e., that it is fully constitutional or congenital in origin) and are skeptical about the role of psychosocial or psychodynamic factors. For example, Menvielle and Tuerk (2002) noted that, while it might be helpful to set limits on pervasive cross-gender behaviors that may contribute to social ostracism, their primary treatment goal was "not at changing the children's behavior, but helping parents to be supportive and to maximize opportunities for the children's adjustment" (p. 2002). This perspective therefore appears to encourage some parents to take an approach that is rather different from the more "traditional" therapeutic models: there are now several examples reported on in the media in which parents of very young children enforce a social gender change (e.g., registering a biological male child in school as a girl; Brown, 2006; Santiago, 2006).

Because comparative treatment approaches are not available, it is not possible to say whether or not this supportive or "cross-gender affirming" approach will result in both short-term and long-term outcomes any different from the more traditional approaches to treatment.

Treatment of Adolescents

In adolescents with GID, there are three broad clinical issues that require evaluation:

1 Phenomenology pertaining to the GID itself;

2 Sexual orientation; and

3 Psychiatric comorbidity.

Apart from the GID itself, gender-dysphoric adolescents with a childhood onset of cross-gender behavior typically have a homosexual orientation (i.e., they are attracted to members of their own "birth sex"). Some such adolescents may not report any sexual feelings, but follow-up will typically find the emergence of same-sex attractions. Thus, the clinician must evaluate simultaneously two dimensions of the patient's psychosexual development: current gender identity and current sexual orientation.

The psychotherapy treatment literature on adolescents with GID has been very poorly developed and is confined to a few case reports (Zucker, 2006a; Zucker & Bradley, 1995). In general, the prognosis for adolescents resolving the GID is more guarded than it is for children. From a clinical management point of view, two key issues need to be considered:

1 Some adolescents with GID are not particularly good candidates for therapy because of comorbid disorders and general life circumstances;

2 Some adolescents with GID have little interest in psychologically oriented treatment and are quite adamant about proceeding with hormonal and surgical sex reassignment.

Prior to recommending hormonal and surgical interventions, many clinicians encourage adolescents with GID to consider alternatives to this invasive and expensive treatment. One area of inquiry can therefore explore the meaning behind the adolescent's desire for sex reassignment and if there are viable alternative lifestyle adaptations. The most common area of exploration in this regard pertains to the patient's sexual orientation. Some adolescents with GID recall that they always felt uncomfortable growing up as boys or as girls, but that the idea of "sex change" did not occur until they became aware of homoerotic attractions. For some of these youngsters, the idea that they might be gay or homosexual is abhorrent.

For adolescents in whom the gender dysphoria appears chronic, there is considerable evidence that it interferes with general social adaptation, including general psychiatric impairment, conflicted family relations and dropping out of school. For these youngsters, the treating clinician can consider two main options:

1 Management until the adolescent turns 18 and can be referred to an adult gender identity clinic; or

2 "Early" institution of contrasex hormonal treatment.

Gooren and Delemarre-van de Waal (1996) and Cohen-Kettenis and van Goozen (1998) recommended that one option with gender-dysphoric adolescents is to prescribe puberty-blocking luteinizing hormone-release agonists (e.g., depot leuprolide or triptorelin) that make it easier to pass as the opposite sex. Thus, in male adolescents such medication can suppress the development of secondary sex characteristics, such as facial hair growth and voice deepening, which make it more difficult to pass in the female social role. Cohen-Kettenis and van Goozen (1997) and Smith, van Goozen, & Cohen-Kettenis *et al.* (2002) reported that early cross-sex hormone treatment for adolescents under the age of 18 years, who were free of gross psychiatric comorbidity, facilitated the complex psychosexual and psychosocial transition to living as a member of the opposite sex and resulted in a lessening of the gender dysphoria. Although such early hormonal treatment is controversial (Beh & Diamond, 2005), it may well be the treatment of choice once the clinician is confident that other options have been exhausted (Cohen-Kettenis, 2005).

Paraphilic Sexual Disorders

Diagnosis

Paraphilias can broadly be classified into those that involve atypical sexual targets or those that involve atypical sexual activities. Atypical sexual targets include sexually immature persons (pedophilia), non-human animals (zoophilia) and inanimate objects (fetishism); atypical activities include the infliction of pain or humiliation on another (sadism), experiencing pain or humiliation (masochism) or exposing one's genitals to unsuspecting strangers (exhibitionism). A wide variety of paraphilias have been described in the clinical and research literatures, but most are rare. The most commonly seen paraphilias in clinical or correctional settings are those that involve illegal behavior if they are acted upon, such as pedophilia and the commission of sexual offences against children, or sadism and the commission of violent sexual offenses.

The DSM-IV-TR lists a number of the more commonly known paraphilias, including pedophilia, sadism and fetishism;

the paraphilias listed in the 10th revision of the ICD-10 are quite similar in content (World Health Organization, 1997). For example, the ICD-10 defines pedophilia as "a sexual preference for children, usually of prepubertal or early pubertal age" while the DSM-IV-TR elaborates by defining sexual preference in terms of timeline and manifestation, and adding criteria regarding the age difference between the person and the child or children (the person is at least age 16 years and at least 5 years older than the child or children).

Epidemiology

Neither the incidence nor prevalence of paraphilias is known. Epidemiological surveys of the general population, with the specific questions that are needed to identify paraphilias – particularly questions about the persistence and intensity of sexual thoughts, fantasies, urges, arousal or behavior involving the paraphilic target or activity – have not yet been conducted. Almost all of the research on paraphilias has been conducted with clinical or correctional samples, and most of that work has involved adult sex offenders rather than adolescent sex offenders, or other minors. Surveys of convenience samples of young adults suggest that paraphilias are rare (Templeman & Stinnett, 1991). Researchers have not asked similar questions of adolescents.

Assessment

Interviews and Questionnaires

In order to diagnose a paraphilic sexual disorder, a thorough sexual history is needed. Such histories are typically obtained through clinical interview. Respondents are asked questions about their sexual thoughts, interests and behaviors, especially with regard to atypical sexual targets or activities. Comprehensive interviews also include questions intended to help clinicians rule out other explanations for atypical sexual thoughts, urges, fantasies or behavior. For example, some individuals with obsessive-compulsive disorder may report being disturbed by thoughts about molesting a child (see, e.g., Gordon, 2002). The differential diagnosis is made by determining if the thoughts are associated with sexual arousal or pleasure and by inquiring about other symptoms of obsessive-compulsive disorder.

Interviews can be very informative, but there are potential problems with recall and other biases in gathering data on sexual behavior in this way (Wiederman, 2002). Questions about sexual history are sensitive and many interviewees may minimize or deny certain sexual interests or behaviors, especially those that could result in social ostracism. For example, a study found that male adolescents were more willing to disclose criminal acts they have committed than the fact that they have masturbated, even though many of them had engaged in both behaviors (Halpern, Udry, Suchindran, & Campbell, 2000). The validity of self-report may be increased if a rapport is established, as can occur after involvement in treatment (Worling & Curwen, 2000).

One way to reduce the reluctance of individuals to disclose sexual interests or behavior in interviews is to administer questionnaires. For example, Koss and Gidycz (1985) found that male respondents were more likely to admit engaging in sexually coercive acts on a questionnaire than in an interview. Using questionnaires also addresses the potential problem of interviewers who skip or forget important questions. An example of a measure that has been developed for adolescents is the Sexual Fantasy Questionnaire, which contains items about atypical sexual fantasies (Daleidin, Kaufman, Hilliker, & O'Neil, 1998).

Other Sources of Information

Sexual history information can also be obtained from other sources, including interviews with an adolescent's present sexual partner, if available, and a parent or guardian of children or younger adolescents. However, such information is usually limited because the minor will often be reluctant to disclose sexual urges, fantasies or thoughts to others, even with intimate others and even when such urges involve conventional targets or activities. A review of clinical or criminal justice records can also be very helpful. Clinicians can use information about sexual victim characteristics to make the diagnosis of pedophilia, because pedophilia is more likely to be present among sex offenders who have very young victims, boy victims and victims outside the offender's immediate family (Seto, Murphy, Page, & Ennis, 2003).

Data on the sexual behavior problems of children can be collected from maternal observations through the Child Sexual Behavior Inventory, which lists a variety of both typical and atypical sexual behaviors and asks mothers or other female caregivers to rate their frequency (Friedrich, 1997; Friedrich, Fisher, Dittner *et al.*, 2001). Childhood sexual behavior problems are positively correlated with non-sexual behavior problems as measured by the CBCL. Some sexual behaviors are common among young children (e.g., touching sex parts at home, undressing in front of others), but aggressive sexual behaviors and more intrusive behaviors are rare.

Phallometry and Viewing Time

Phallometry involves the measurement of penile responses to sexual stimuli that systematically vary on the dimensions of interest, such as the age and sex of the figures in a set of slides depicting female children, adolescents and adults, and male children, adolescents and adults. Phallometry was developed as an assessment method by Freund (1963). Phallometric responses are recorded as increases in either penile circumference or penile volume; bigger increases in circumference or volume are interpreted as evidence of greater sexual arousal to the presented stimulus. Erectile response (except for erections that occur during sleep) is a specifically sexual measure, unlike other psychophysiological responses, such as pupillary dilation, heart rate, viewing time and skin conductance (Zuckerman, 1971). Phallometric indices of responding discriminate sex offenders from men who have not committed sexual offences and predict sexual recidivism. Other investigators have shown that phallometry can similarly distinguish men who admit to sadistic fantasies, cross-dress or expose their genitals in public from men who do not (Freund, Seto, & Kuban, 1996; Marshall, Payne, Barbaree, & Eccles, 1991; Seto & Kuban, 1996).

Seto, Lalumière, and Blanchard (2000) evaluated the use of phallometric testing for adolescent sex offenders with child victims. Because an age-matched comparison group was not available, these adolescents were compared with young adults between the ages of 18 and 21 who had not committed sexual offences involving children. As a group, adolescents with male victims had relatively higher responses to pictures of children than the young adult comparison participants. Adolescents with both male and female children as victims responded more to pictures of children than to pictures of adults. Further evidence for the validity of phallometry in adolescent sex offenders comes from Blanchard and Barbaree (2005), Gretton, McBride, O'Shaughnessy, and Kumka (2001) and Robinson, Rouleau, and Madrigano (1997).

Another objective measure that is increasingly used with adolescent sex offenders is viewing time. The procedure involves showing a series of pictures depicting girls, boys, women or men; these pictures can depict clothed, semi-clothed or nude figures. Respondents are either asked to examine the pictures to answer later questions or they are asked to rate each picture (e.g., how attractive the depicted person is). Respondents are instructed to proceed to the next picture at their own pace and are expected to be unaware that the key dependent measure is the amount of time they spend looking at each picture. Viewing time is correlated with self-reported sexual interest and phallometric responding among non-offending volunteers recruited from the community (Quinsey, Ketsetsis, Earls, & Karamanoukian, 1996).

Several studies have shown that adult sex offenders with child victims can be distinguished from other men by the amount of time they spend looking at pictures of children relative to pictures of adults (Harris, Rice, Quinsey, & Chaplin, 1996) or by a combination of viewing time and additional questionnaire responses (Abel, Jordan, Hand, Holland, & Phipps, 2001). However, Smith and Fischer (1999) were not able to demonstrate discriminative validity in a study of adolescent sex offenders and non-offenders using viewing time without additional questionnaire responses. No published studies have yet demonstrated that scores on viewing time measures, whether alone or in combination with self-report, predict recidivism among adolescent (or adult) sex offenders. Another potential problem for viewing time measures is that they may become vulnerable to faking once the client finds out that viewing time is the key variable of interest.

Associated Psychopathology

Kafka (1997, 2003) noted that paraphilias and related sexual disorders are often comorbid with mood disorders. In conjunction with evidence on the impact of antidepressant medications on sexual behavior, Kafka (1997) suggested that there is evidence that paraphilias and mood disorders share a common serotonergic diathesis. Consistent with this idea, we recently completed a meta-analysis of studies that compared adolescent sex offenders with adolescents who committed other kinds of offences (Seto & Lalumière, 2004). We found that adolescent sex offenders reported significantly more anxiety or depression than other offenders, suggesting variables in this domain might have a unique role in explaining sexual offending. However, the timing of symptoms was not clearly distinguished in the studies that we reviewed. The symptoms could have preceded the sexual offences, but they could also be a consequence of being identified as a sex offender (e.g., becoming more anxious and depressed after being arrested and charged for a sexual offence), given the extremely negative social views about sexual offending, even when compared to other forms of crime. Research on the association between paraphilias and mood disorders in samples outside of clinical or correctional settings is needed to determine if this link is an artifact of where the research has been conducted.

There is also evidence that sexual behavior problems are frequently comorbid with non-sexual behavior problems (Friedrich, Grambsch, Broughton *et al.*, 1991; Friedrich, Fisher, Dittner *et al.*, 2001). Thus, children with sexual behavior problems and adolescent sex offenders may meet diagnostic criteria for attention deficit/hyperactivity disorder, oppositional defiant disorder or conduct disorder (Seto & Lalumière, 2004). France and Hudson (1993) reviewed studies on this topic and concluded that up to half of adolescent sex offenders would meet diagnostic criteria for conduct disorder.

Paraphilias are often comorbid, such that engaging in one form of paraphilic behavior greatly increases the likelihood of engaging in another (Abel, Becker, Cunningham-Rathner, Mittelman, & Rouleau, 1988; Bradford, Boulet, & Pawlak, 1992). We have recently demonstrated that exhibitionistic and voyeuristic behavior also co-occurred more often than expected by chance in a nationally representative sample of young men between the ages of 18 and 21 from Sweden (Långström & Seto, 2006). The co-occurrence of paraphilic behaviors suggests there may be a common cause to the paraphilias (which does not rule out specific factors). There are no data of this kind for adolescents.

Etiology

Different theories have been proposed to explain the etiology of paraphilias. We focus here on theories that posit conditioning has a role, and theories that suggest paraphilias are the result of neurological perturbations. We then discuss the implications of recent findings on the association between childhood sexual abuse and pedophilia.

Conditioning

It has been proposed that masturbatory conditioning has a role in the development of paraphilias (McGuire, Carlisle, & Young, 1965). Some individuals, for unspecified reasons, pair cues of unusual initial sexual experiences with the sexual pleasure elicited by these early experiences, and learn to associate these cues with the powerful reinforcement of orgasm. However, there is equivocal evidence about the ability to condition increases in sexual arousal in humans. Rachman and Hodgson (1968) reported significantly increased sexual arousal to pictures of boots among normal volunteers in a set of frequently cited experimental studies examining the development of boot fetishism, but these studies did not have control conditions. Lalumière and Quinsey (1998) and Hoffmann, Janssen, and Turner (2004) found a significant effect of conditioning on sexual arousal among male volunteers, while Plaud and Martini (1999) reported mixed results in a conditioning study of nine male volunteers.

The efficacy of conditioning approaches for changing sexual arousal patterns has been reviewed elsewhere (Barbaree & Seto, 1997). Overall, this research suggests that conditioning can have an effect on the suppression of sexual arousal of adolescent or adult sex offenders, but it is unclear how long these changes are maintained, what mechanisms are actually responsible for the changes in sexual arousal patterns and whether the changes reflect an actual shift in sexual interests or greater voluntary control over sexual arousal when assessed in the laboratory (Lalumière & Earls, 1992).

Conditioning might have a role in maintaining rather than initiating paraphilic sexual arousal. Dandescu and Wolfe (2003) found that atypical sexual fantasies preceded and accompanied the first sexual offence reported by a sample of 57 sex offenders with child victims; the sexual fantasies then increased in frequency after the first sexual offence. Approximately two-thirds of the offenders reported having any "deviant sexual fantasies" prior to their first contact with a child, while 81% reported having such fantasies afterwards. This finding suggests that the sexual arousal and gratification experienced during the first sexual offence increased the frequency of sexual fantasies among men who already had such fantasies.

These research findings suggest that conditioning is unlikely to have a significant role in the onset of paraphilias. Experimental efforts to increase sexual arousal have produced small effects, and it is unclear how long conditioned changes in sexual responding (e.g., suppression of sexual arousal to child stimuli through aversive conditioning) can be maintained. If conditioning does have a role in the development of paraphilia, as suggested by Dandescu and Wolfe's (2003) study, then there is probably an interaction between conditioning experiences and other predisposing factors.

Neurological Perturbations

Brain abnormalities have long been suspected as a cause of paraphilias. Information on brain functioning can be obtained both directly and indirectly. Indirectly, investigators have compared the performance of sex offenders with child victims with other groups of men on measures of intelligence and other aspects of cognitive functioning. Cantor, Blanchard, Robichaud, and Christensen (2005) conducted a meta-analysis of 165 adult samples and 71 adolescent samples. For the adults, there was a significant difference between sex offenders and others, with sex offenders scoring lower on measures of intelligence than other offenders, who, in turn, scored lower than non-offending controls. For the adolescents, there was a significant difference between sex offenders and other offenders. Among the sex offenders, Cantor *et al.* found that intelligence scores appeared to be related to the proportion of the sample who were pedophilic, because sex offenders with child victims scored lower than sex offenders without any child victims, and there was a positive relationship between the age cut-off used to define child victims and mean intelligence score; in other words, samples composed of men who offended against younger children tended to produce lower mean IQ scores than samples composed of men who offended against older children.

In earlier studies, this same research group also found that pedophilic sex offenders were more likely to report experiencing head injuries before age 13, but did not differ in reports of head injuries after age 13 (Blanchard, Christensen, Strong *et al.*, 2002; Blanchard, Kuban, Klassen *et al.*, 2003). The fact that there was no difference in reports of head injuries after age 13 counters the alternative explanation that pedophiles have a retrospective reporting bias in recalling head injuries, because there would be no reason to think that head injuries before the age of 13 are more socially acceptable than head injuries later in life. The fact that there was no difference after age 13 also suggests there is a critical age window in terms of the impact of head injury on the development of pedophilia (and perhaps other paraphilias). This is an intriguing possibility because of other work that suggests the time before and during puberty is critical in the development of sexual preferences. Of course, this assumes that the relationship between head injury and pedophilia is causal. It is possible that a third variable explains both the higher incidence of head injury and pedophilia; for example, prenatal neurological perturbations may both increase accident-proneness, resulting in a higher risk for head injury, as well as increase the likelihood that an individual will be pedophilic.

Researchers have also attempted to assess brain structure directly, especially in the frontal (associated with executive control) and temporal regions (associated with emotional processing and regulation of sexual behavior). Recently, Cantor, Kabani, Christensen *et al.* (2007) discovered a significant difference in white matter, such that pedophiles have less white matter than non-pedophilic men, particularly in two tracts: the right superior occipitofrontal fasciculus and the right arcuate fasciculus. These white matter tracts connect areas that are involved in determining if a stimulus is sexually relevant, suggesting that pedophiles are somehow deficient in how they process and integrate sexual cues.

Cycle of Sexual Abuse

The most frequently discussed factor in explanations of adolescent sexual offending is sexual abuse history (Knight & Sims-Knight, 2003). Seto and Lalumière (2004) conducted a meta-analysis of studies that compared adolescent sex offenders with other adolescent offenders, and found that adolescent sex offenders were almost five times as likely to have a history of sexual abuse. This was found whether the analysis involved studies that relied on self-report or on other sources of information (e.g., clinical files, official records). Moreover, adolescent sex offenders who have been sexually abused show relatively greater sexual arousal to children or coercive sex than those who have not been abused (Becker, Hunter, Stein, & Kaplan, 1989). Among children, Friedrich, Grambsch, Damon *et al.* (1992) showed that scores on the Child Sexual Behavior Inventory could discriminate children who had been sexually abused from those who had not. Hall, Matthews, and Pearce (1998) found, in a sample of 99 sexually abused boys and girls between the ages of 3 and 7, that those who became sexually aroused during the sexual abuse were more likely to engage in sexual behavior problems involving others ($n = 62$) than those who did not ($n = 37$).

The sexually abused–sexual abuser hypothesis suggests that male children who are sexually abused are more likely to engage in sexual offending later in life. Burton (2003) described plausible mechanisms linking sexual abuse and later sexual offending: modeling of the perpetrator's behavior, conditioning as a result of pairing any sexual stimulation caused by the sexual abuse with cues such as the type of acts that occurred, and changing cognitions about the acceptability of adult–child sex.

The mechanisms underlying the association between childhood sexual abuse and sexual behavior problems among children and adolescent sexual offending are not known (Widom & Ames, 1994). A number of investigators have suggested that aspects of the sexual abuse such as the victim–perpetrator relationship, nature of sexual abuse, duration and timing of the sexual abuse are important (Burton, 2003). There must be individual characteristics that increase both vulnerability to childhood sexual abuse and the likelihood of adolescent sexual offending, because many sexually abused children do not go on to commit sexual offenses later in life, and many adolescent sex offenders have no known history of sexual abuse.

Developmental Course

A developmental perspective is important because there are myriad differences between children, adolescents and adults, and because there is both persistence and desistance in sexual offending across the lifespan. Retrospective studies suggest approximately half of adult sex offenders report that their first sexual offense was committed as a juvenile (Abel, Osborn, & Twigg, 1993), and up to half of adolescent sex offenders have engaged in sexual misconduct under the age of 12 (Burton, 2000; Ryan, Miyoshi, Metzner, Krugman, & Fryer, 1996; Zolondek, Abel, Northey, & Jordan, 2001). In prospective studies, however, only a minority (perhaps 10–15%) of adolescent sex offenders commit another sexual offense over 5 years of opportunity (for review see Caldwell, 2002). The proportion of children with sexual behavior problems who persist and commit a sexual offense as an adolescent is also relatively small (Carpentier, Silovsky, & Chaffin, 2006). Taken together, these data indicate that many children with sexual behavior problems and many adolescent sex offenders desist. For many children, their sexual behavior problems may represent a reaction to sexual abuse they have experienced, sexual precocity and normative sexual play. For many adolescents, their sexual offenses may represent opportunistic and relatively transient antisocial behavior. A small group of children and adolescents, however, will persist in committing sexual offenses into adulthood. The adolescents who will develop paraphilias are more likely to persist.

Of particular relevance is a study reported by Zolondek, Abel, Northey *et al.* (2001) of 485 adolescent males between the ages of 11 and 17, referred for assessment or treatment of possibly paraphilic interests or behavior. The youths completed a questionnaire with questions regarding sexual interests and experiences as part of their assessment. Twenty-six percent acknowledged engaging in fetishistic behavior, 17% acknowledged voyeuristic acts and 12% acknowledged exhibitionistic behavior. The average age of onset across paraphilic behaviors was between 10 and 12 years, which is younger than the average age of onset found in retrospective studies of adults (Abel, Becker, Mittelman *et al.*, 1987). These data are consistent with the idea that the onset of paraphilias is likely around the time of puberty, just as many people are becoming aware of their sexual preference for males or females.

Treatment

Pharmacological Treatment

The common aim of drug therapies in the treatment of pedophilia is to suppress sexual response involving children. Much of the initial interest was in antiandrogens to reduce sexual response, but clinicians and researchers have more recently focused on serotonergic agents. Because of the impact of reducing androgens on physical development, antiandrogens are very rarely prescribed for minors, except in cases where the sexual behavior is very problematic (e.g., very violent sexual assaults on young children) and cannot be controlled by other means.

It is a logical hypothesis that antiandrogens would have an impact on paraphilic sexual responses, because testosterone has a critical role in male mammalian sexuality (Davidson, Smith, & Damassa, 1977). The earliest clinical study was reported by Laschet and Laschet (1971), who treated more than 100 paraphilic men; most were pedophiles or exhibitionists. Today, the most commonly prescribed agents are cyproterone acetate (CPA) or medroxyprogesterone acetate (MPA), both of which interfere with the action of testosterone. CPA blocks intracellular testosterone uptake and thus reduces plasma testosterone, while MPA reduces gonadotropin secretion. The use of either drug in the treatment of paraphilias is off-label, meaning it is not specifically approved by regulatory bodies for this purpose. Side effects of antiandrogens include headaches, dizziness, nausea, gynecomastia, depression and osteoporosis. As a result of these potentially serious side effects, and the fact that some patients do not want to experience a massive reduction in their sex drive, treatment attrition and compliance are significant issues in antiandrogen treatment. For example, in Hucker, Langevin, and Bain (1988), only 11 of 18 men completed the 12-week trial.

There is some support for the efficacy of antiandrogens in reducing the frequency or intensity of sexual urges and arousal, but there has been a dearth of larger, better controlled outcome studies. Gijs and Gooren (1996) reviewed the literature evaluating the effects of CPA and MPA, focusing on methodologically stronger studies that included features such as random assignment, a placebo condition and double-blinding. They identified four controlled studies of CPA and six such studies of MPA. All four studies of CPA reported that treated men had a significant reduction in sexual response, while only one of the six MPA studies showed a significant difference between men in the treatment and comparison conditions.

Serotonin is involved in the regulation of human sexual behavior, and antidepressant medications that have a serotonergic effect have long been known to reduce sexual desire and delay ejaculation in males (for a review see Meston & Gorzalka, 1992). Some clinical investigators have gone further and suggested, with little evidence, that selective serotonin reuptake inhibitors (SSRIs), such as fluoxetine and buspirone, can specifically affect sexual arousal to children without affecting sexual arousal to adults (Kafka, 1991).

The interest in serotonergic agents for the treatment of paraphilias appears to be almost entirely based on uncontrolled case studies or open trials (Gijs & Gooren, 1996); there has been only one experimental study that compared desipramine and chloripramine in a double-blind crossover trial that was preceded by a single-blind placebo condition (Kruesi, Fine, Valladares, Phillips, & Rapoport, 1992). Kruesi, Fine, Valladares *et al.* reported a significant reduction of self-reported paraphilic behavior (predominantly exhibitionism, transvestic fetishism, telephone scatalogia and fetishism) with either drug, but their result was difficult to interpret because only 8 of 15 paraphilic men completed the trial; four patients were dropped because they responded to the placebo and three did not complete the drug trial. Including the patients who responded to placebo would have attenuated, and perhaps eliminated, the apparent effect of the drugs on self-reported paraphilic behavior.

Despite the intuitive appeal of pharmacological interventions to reduce sexual drive and thus the likelihood of (illegal) paraphilic behavior, reviews of outcome studies suggest that there is no strong empirical support for the idea that such interventions can reduce sexual recidivism.

Psychosocial

Aversive conditioning techniques were used as early as the 1950s and 1960s for paraphilic interests such as fetishism and transvestic fetishism (Raymond, 1956). In the behavioral treatment of paraphilias, aversion techniques are used to suppress sexual arousal to the atypical target or activity, while masturbatory reconditioning techniques are used to increase sexual arousal to acceptable targets (peers or adults) and activities (consenting sexual activities). In aversion procedures, unpleasant stimuli such as mild electric shock or ammonia odors are paired with repeated presentations of sexual stimuli depicting the paraphilic target or activity. In a variation called covert sensitization, the aversive stimulus is imagined (e.g., being discovered by family, friends or coworkers while engaging in paraphilic behavior). Overall, the existing research suggests that behavioral techniques can have an effect on sexual arousal patterns, but it is unclear how long these changes are maintained and whether they result in actual changes in interests, as opposed to greater voluntary control over pedophilic sexual arousal (Lalumière & Earls, 1992).

Cognitive–behavioral treatments (CBT) aim to teach individuals how to manage their sexual urges. Published evaluations have reported promising results. Carpentier, Silovsky, & Chaffin (2006) reported on a long-term evaluation of 135 children with sexual behavior problems, compared with 156 children from the same out-patient clinic. The children with sexual behavior problems were randomly assigned to a play therapy group or a CBT group. Both treatments were manualized and ran for 12 hour-long sessions. The CBT group was highly structured and focused on education and behavior management. The play therapy group was less structured and more reflective, although it focused on many of the same themes: sexual behavior problems, boundaries, parenting skills and sex education. Children assigned to the CBT group were significantly less likely than children assigned to the play therapy group to sexually offend (defined as an arrest for a sexual offence or a child welfare report of sexual abuse perpetration) during the 10-year follow-up period. In fact, the rate of sexual offending among children in the CBT group was not significantly different from the comparison group without any sexual behavior problems.

Borduin, Henggeler, Blaske, and Stein (1990) reported a significant effect of treatment in a small sample of adolescent sex offenders, using a multisystemic treatment that targeted factors associated with criminal behavior, including antisocial attitudes and beliefs, associations with antisocial peers and substance abuse (for a review see Andrews & Bonta, 2002). Multisystemic treatment is also distinguished by being skills-focused, involving both the adolescent and his or her family, and paying careful attention to program fidelity and individualization. Multiple studies have shown that multisystemic treatment can significantly reduce recidivism and other negative outcomes among serious adolescent offenders (Henggeler, Schoenwald, Borduin, Rowland, & Cunningham, 1998). Borduin and Schaeffer (2001) replicated the Borduin, Henggeler, Blaske *et al.* (1990) study by showing that this multisystemic treatment had a large impact on sexual recidivism in a larger sample of 48 juvenile sex offenders, even though it was not designed specifically for this group.

Conclusions

There are many unanswered questions about the onset, development and prognosis of paraphilias. There has been relatively little research conducted on adolescents, perhaps reflecting a discomfort with the idea that some adolescents and older children engage in problematic sexual behavior as a result of atypical sexual interests that are very likely to be stable. As a result, this chapter has drawn upon relevant studies of adult sex offenders. This is not to suggest that children with sexual behavior problems or adolescent sex offenders are likely to have paraphilias. In fact, it is likely that most do not, given the high rate of desistance from childhood to adolescence, and from adolescence to adulthood. A small minority do persist, however, and are likely to continue engaging in problematic sexual behavior without intervention.

There is emerging evidence to support the idea that there may be neurodevelopmental or neurological risk factors for pedophilia. Given the high comorbidity of paraphilias, it is likely that other paraphilias are similarly influenced.

As for many other disorders, we know more about the assessment than the treatment of paraphilias. Further research on paraphilias will be expedited by the development of age-appropriate measures of sexual interests. Viewing time is a particularly promising technology.

Unlike the adult literature, however, there are some promising results in the treatment of sexual behavior problems in children and sexual offending among adolescents. These treatments share a common focus on skills, behavior and problem-solving, and involve parents or other caregivers. Further advances in treatment will benefit from a greater undestanding of the etiology and developmental course of paraphilias.

Further Reading

Barbaree, H. E., & Marshall, W. L. (Eds.). (2006). *The juvenile sex offender* (2nd edn.). New York: Guilford Press.

Cohen-Kettenis, P. T., & Pfäfflin, F. (2003). *Transgenderism and intersexuality in childhood and adolescence: Making choices*. Thousand Oaks, CA: Sage Publications.

Laws, D. R., & O'Donohue, W. T. (Eds.). (1997). *Sexual deviance: Theory, assessment and treatment*. New York: Guilford Press.

Zucker, K. J., & Bradley, S. J. (2005). *Gender identity disorder and psychosexual problems in children and adolescents*. New York: Guilford Press.

References

Abel, G. G., Becker, J. V., Cunningham-Rathner, J., Mittelman, M., & Rouleau, J. L. (1988). Multiple paraphilic diagnoses among sex offenders. *Bulletin of the American Academy of Psychiatry and the Law*, *16*, 153–168.

Abel, G. G., Becker, J. V., Mittelman, M., Cunningham-Rathner, J., Rouleau, J. L., & Murphy, W. D. (1987). Self-reported sex crimes of nonincarcerated paraphiliacs. *Journal of Interpersonal Violence*, *2*, 3–25.

Abel, G. G., Jordan, A. D., Hand, C. G., Holland, L. A., & Phipps, A. (2001). Classification models of child molesters utilizing the Abel Assessment for Sexual Interest. *Child Abuse and Neglect*, *25*, 703–718.

Abel, G., Osborn, C., & Twigg, D. (1993). Sexual assault through the life span: Adult offenders with juvenile histories. In H. E. Barbaree, W. L. Marshall, & S. M. Hudson (Eds.), *The juvenile sex offender* (pp. 104–117). New York: Guilford Press.

Achenbach, T. M., & Edelbrock, C. (1983). *Manual for the Child Behavior Checklist and Revised Child Behavior Profile*. Burlington, VT: University of Vermont, Department of Psychiatry.

Agrell, S. (2004, May 11). Born a boy, raised as a girl, he dies a man. *National Post*, A1, A10.

American Psychiatric Association. (2000). *Diagnostic and statistical manual of mental disorders* (4th edn.). Text revision. Washington, DC: American Psychiatric Association.

Andrews, D. A., & Bonta, J. (2002). *The psychology of criminal conduct* (3rd edn.). Cincinnati, OH: Anderson.

Bakker, A., van Kesteren, P. J. M., Gooren, L. J. G., & Bezemer, P. D. (1993). The prevalence of transsexualism in the Netherlands. *Acta Psychiatrica Scandinavica*, *87*, 237–238.

Barbaree, H. E., & Seto, M. C. (1997). Pedophilia: Assessment and treatment. In D. R. Laws, & W. T. O'Donohue (Eds.), *Sexual deviance: Theory, assessment and treatment* (pp. 175–193). New York: Guilford Press.

Bartlett, N. H., Vasey, P. L., & Bukowski, W. M. (2000). Is gender identity disorder in children a mental disorder? *Sex Roles*, *43*, 753–785.

Bates, J. E., Bentler, P. M., & Thompson, S. K. (1979). Gender-deviant boys compared with normal and clinical control boys. *Journal of Abnormal Child Psychology*, *7*, 243–259.

Baum, M. J. (2006). Mammalian animal models of psychosexual differentiation: When is "translation" to the human situation possible? *Hormones and Behavior*, *50*, 579–588.

Becker, J. V., Hunter, J., Stein, R., & Kaplan, M. S. (1989). Factors associated with erectile response in adolescent sex offenders. *Journal of Psychopathology and Behavioral Assessment*, *11*, 353–362.

Beh, H., & Diamond, M. (2005). Ethical concerns related to treating gender nonconformity in childhood and adolescence: Lessons from the Family Court of Australia. *Health Matrix: Journal of Law–Medicine*, *15*, 239–283.

Blanchard, R. (2001). Fraternal birth order and the maternal immune hypothesis of male homosexuality. *Hormones and Behavior*, *40*, 105–114.

Blanchard, R., & Barbaree, H. E. (2005). The strength of sexual arousal as a function of the age of the sex offender: Comparisons among pedophiles, hebephiles, and teleiophiles. *Sexual Abuse: A Journal of Research and Treatment*, *17*, 441–456.

Blanchard, R., Christensen, B. K., Strong, S. M., Cantor, J. M., Kuban, M. E., Klassen, P., *et al.* (2002). Retrospective self-reports of childhood accidents causing unconsciousness in phallometrically diagnosed pedophiles. *Archives of Sexual Behavior*, *31*, 511–526.

Blanchard, R., Kuban, M. E., Klassen, P., Dickey, R., Christensen, B. K., Cantor, J. M., *et al.* (2003). Self-reported head injuries before and after age 13 in pedophilic and nonpedophilic men referred for clinical assessment. *Archives of Sexual Behavior*, *32*, 573–581.

Blanchard, R., Zucker, K. J., Bradley, S. J., & Hume, C. S. (1995). Birth order and sibling sex ratio in homosexual male adolescents and probably prehomosexual feminine boys. *Developmental Psychology*, *31*, 22–30.

Borduin, C. M., Henggeler, S. W., Blaske, D. M., & Stein, R. J. (1990). Multisystemic treatment of adolescent sexual offenders. *International Journal of Offender Therapy and Comparative Criminology*, *34*, 105–113.

Borduin, C. M., & Schaeffer, C. M. (2001). Multisystemic treatment of juvenile sexual offenders: A progress report. *Journal of Psychology and Human Sexuality*, *13*, 25–42.

Bradford, J. M., Boulet, J., & Pawlak, A. (1992). The paraphilias: A multiplicity of deviant behaviours. *Canadian Journal of Psychiatry*, *37*, 104–108.

Bradley, S. J., Blanchard, R., Coates, S., Green, R., Levine, S. B., Meyer-Bahlburg, H. F. L., *et al.* (1991). Interim report of the DSM-IV subcommittee for gender identity disorders. *Archives of Sexual Behavior*, *20*, 333–343.

Bradley, S. J., Oliver, G. D., Chernick, A. B., & Zucker, K. J. (1998). Experiment of nurture: Ablatio penis at 2 months, sex reassignment at 7 months, and a psychosexual follow-up in young adulthood. *Pediatrics*, *102*, E91–E95. (Available at http://www.pediatrics.org/cgi/content/full/102/1/e9)

Brown, P. L. (2006, December 2). Supporting boys or girls when the line isn't clear. *New York Times*, pp. A1, A11.

Burton, D. L. (2000). Were adolescent sexual offenders children with sexual behavior problems? *Sexual Abuse: Journal of Research and Treatment*, *12*, 37–48.

Burton, D. L. (2003). Male adolescents: Sexual victimization and subsequent sexual abuse. *Child and Adolescent Social Work Journal*, *20*, 277–296.

Caldwell, M. F. (2002). What we do not know about juvenile sexual reoffense risk. *Child Maltreatment*, *7*, 291–302.

Campbell D. W., & Eaton W. O. (1999). Sex differences in the activity level of infants. *Infant and Child Development*, *8*, 1–17.

Cantor, J. M., Blanchard, R., Robichaud, L. K., & Christensen, B. K. (2005). Quantitative reanalysis of aggregate data on IQ in sexual offenders. *Psychological Bulletin*, *131*, 555–568.

Cantor, J. M., Kabani, N., Christensen, B. K., Zipursky, R. B., Barbaree, H. E., Dickey, R., *et al.* (2007). Cerebral white matter deficiencies in pedophilic men. *Journal of Psychiatric Research*, doi:10.1016/j.psychires.2007.10.013.

Carpentier, M. Y., Silovsky, J., & Chaffin, M. (2006). Randomized trial of treatment for children with sexual behavior problems: Ten-year follow-up. *Journal of Consulting and Clinical Psychology*, *74*, 482–488.

Cloud, J. (2000, September 25). His name is Aurora. *Time*, pp. 90–91.

Coates, S., & Person, E. S. (1985). Extreme boyhood femininity: Isolated behavior or pervasive disorder? *Journal of the American Academy of Child Psychiatry*, *24*, 702–709.

Cohen-Bendahan, C. C. C., van de Beek, C., & Berenbaum, S. A. (2005). Prenatal sex hormone effects on child and adult sex-typed behavior: Methods and findings. *Neuroscience and Biobehavioral Reviews*, *29*, 353–384.

Cohen-Kettenis, P. T. (2001). Gender identity disorder in *DSM*? [Letter]. *Journal of the American Academy of Child and Adolescent Psychiatry*, *40*, 391.

Cohen-Kettenis, P. T. (2005). Gender identity disorders. In C. Gillberg, R. Harrington, & H.-C. Steinhausen (Eds.), *A clinician's handbook of child and adolescent psychiatry* (pp. 695–725). Cambridge: Cambridge University Press.

Cohen-Kettenis, P. T., Owen, A., Kaijser, V. G., Bradley, S. J., & Zucker, K. J. (2003). Demographic characteristics, social competence, and behavior problems in children with gender identity disorder: A cross-national, cross-clinic comparative analysis. *Journal of Abnormal Child Psychology*, *31*, 41–53.

Cohen-Kettenis, P. T., & Pfäfflin, F. (2003). *Transgenderism and intersexuality in childhood and adolescence: Making choices*. Thousand Oaks, CA: Sage Publications.

Cohen-Kettenis, P. T., & van Goozen, S. H. M. (1997). Sex reassignment of adolescent transsexuals: A follow-up study. *Journal of the American Academy of Child and Adolescent Psychiatry*, *36*, 263–271.

Cohen-Kettenis, P. T., & van Goozen, S. H. M. (1998). Pubertal delay as an aid in diagnosis and treatment of a transsexual adolescent. *European Child and Adolescent Psychiatry*, *7*, 246–248.

Colapinto, J. (2000). *As nature made him: The boy who was raised as a girl*. Toronto: Harper Collins.

Daleiden, E. L., Kaufman, K. L., Hilliker, D. R., & O'Neil, J. N. (1998). The sexual histories and fantasies of youthful males: A comparison of sexual offending, nonsexual offending, and nonoffending groups. *Sexual Abuse: A Journal of Research and Treatment*, *10*, 195–209.

Dandescu, A., & Wolfe, R. (2003). Considerations on fantasy use by child molesters and exhibitionists. *Sexual Abuse: Journal of Research and Treatment*, *15*, 297–305.

Davidson, J. M., Smith, E. R., & Damassa, D. A. (1977). Comparative analysis of the roles of androgen in the feedback mechanisms and sexual behavior. In L. Martini & M. Motta (Eds.), *Androgens and antiandrogens* (pp. 137–149). New York: Raven.

Dessens, A. B., Slijper, F. M. E., & Drop, S. L. S. (2005). Gender dysphoria and gender change in chromosomal females with congenital adrenal hyperplasia. *Archives of Sexual Behavior*, *34*, 389–397.

Diamond, M., & Sigmundson, H. K. (1997). Sex reassignment at birth: Long-term review and clinical implications. *Archives of Pediatrics and Adolescent Medicine*, *151*, 298–304.

Drummond, K. D., Bradley, S. J., Badali-Peterson, M., & Zucker, K. J. (in press). A follow-up study of girls with gender identity disorder. *Developmental Psychology*.

France, K. G., & Hudson, S. M. (1993). The conduct disorders and the juvenile sex offender. In H. E. Barbaree, W. L. Marshall, & S. M. Hudson (Eds.), *The juvenile sex offender* (pp. 225–234). New York: Guilford Press.

Freund, K. (1963). A laboratory method of diagnosing predominance of homo- and hetero-erotic interest in the male. *Behaviour Research and Therapy*, *1*, 85–93.

Freund, K., Seto, M. C., & Kuban, M. (1996). Two types of fetishism. *Behaviour Research and Therapy*, *34*, 687–694.

Friedrich, W. N. (1997). *Child sexual behavior inventory: Professional manual*. Odessa, FL: Psychological Assessment Resources.

Friedrich, W. N., Fisher, J. L., Dittner, C. A., Acton, R., Berliner, L., Butler, J., *et al.* (2001). Child Sexual Behavior Inventory: Normative, psychiatric, and sexual abuse comparisons. *Child Maltreatment*, *6*, 37–49.

Friedrich, W. N., Grambsch, P., Broughton, D., Kuiper, J., & Beilke, R. L. (1991). Normative sexual behavior in children. *Pediatrics*, *88*, 456–464.

Friedrich, W. N., Grambsch, P., Damon, L., Hewitt, S. K., Koverola, C., Lang, R. A., *et al.* (1992). Child Sexual Behavior Inventory: Normative and clinical comparisons. *Psychological Assessment*, *4*, 303–311.

Gijs, L., & Gooren, L. (1996). Hormonal and psychopharmacological interventions in the treatment of paraphilias: An update. *Journal of Sex Research*, *33*, 273–290.

Gooren, L. (2006). The biology of human psychosexual differentiation. *Hormones and Behavior*, *50*, 589–601.

Gooren, L., & Delemarre-van de Waal, H. (1996). The feasibility of endocrine interventions in juvenile transsexuals. *Journal of Psychology and Human Sexuality*, *8*, 69–84.

Gordon, W. M. (2002). Sexual obsessions and OCD. *Sexual and Relationship Therapy*, *17*, 343–354.

Goy, R. W., Bercovitch, F. B., & McBrair, M. C. (1988). Behavioral masculinization is independent of genital masculinization in prenatally androgenized female rhesus macaques. *Hormones and Behavior*, *22*, 552–571.

Green, R. (1974). *Sexual identity conflict in children and adults*. New York: Basic Books.

Green, R. (1987). *The "sissy boy syndrome" and the development of homosexuality*. New Haven, CT: Yale University Press.

Gretton, H. M., McBride, M., Hare, R. D., O'Shaughnessy, R., & Kumka, G. (2001). Psychopathy and recidivism in adolescent sex offenders. *Criminal Justice and Behavior*, *28*, 427–449.

Gunderson, J. G., Kolb, J. E., & Austin, V. (1981). The Diagnostic Interview for Borderline Patients. *American Journal of Psychiatry*, *138*, 896–903.

Hall, D. K., Mathews, F., & Pearce, J. (1998). Factors associated with sexual behavior problems in young sexually abused children. *Child Abuse and Neglect*, *22*, 1045–1063.

Halpern, C. J. T., Udry, J. R., Suchindran, C., & Campbell, B. (2000). Adolescent males' willingness to report masturbation. *Journal of Sex Research*, *37*, 327–332.

Harris, G. T., Rice, M. E., Quinsey, V. L., & Chaplin, T. C. (1996). Viewing time as a measure of sexual interest among child molesters and normal heterosexual men. *Behaviour Research and Therapy*, *34*, 389–394.

Henggeler, S. W., Schoenwald, S. K., Borduin, C. M., Rowland, M. D., & Cunningham, P. B. (1998). *Multisystemic treatment of antisocial behavior in children and adolescents*. New York: Guilford Press.

Hill, D. B., Rozanski, C., Carfagnini, J., & Willoughby, B. (2007). Gender identity disorders in childhood and adolescence: A critical inquiry. *International Journal of Sexual Health*, *19*, 57–75.

Hines, M. (2004). *Brain gender*. Oxford: Oxford University Press.

Hoffmann, H. Janssen, E., & Turner, S. L. (2004). Classical conditioning of sexual arousal in women and men: Effects of varying awareness and biological relevance of the conditioned stimulus. *Archives of Sexual Behavior*, *33*, 43–53.

Hucker, S. J., Langevin, B., & Bain, J. (1988). A double blind trial of sex drive reducing medication in pedophiles. *Annals of Sex Research*, *1*, 227–242.

Isay, R. A. (1997). Remove gender identity disorder in DSM. *Psychiatric News*, *32*, 13.

Jang, B., & Smith, G. (2004, May 12). Troubled man "felt like a failure." *The Globe and Mail*, p. AX.

Kafka, M. P. (1991). Successful antidepressant treatment of non-paraphilic sexual addictions and paraphilias in men. *Journal of Clinical Psychiatry*, *52*, 60–65.

Kafka, M. P. (1997). A monoamine hypothesis for the pathophysiology of paraphilic disorders. *Archives of Sexual Behavior*, *26*, 343–358.

Kafka, M. P. (2003). The monoamine hypothesis for the pathophysiology of paraphilic disorders: An update. *Annals of the New York Academy of Sciences*, *989*, 86–94.

Knafo, A., Iervolino, A. C., & Plomin, R. (2005). Masculine girls and feminine boys: Genetic and environmental contributions to atypical gender development in early childhood. *Journal of Personality and Social Psychology*, *88*, 400–412.

Knight, R. A., & Sims-Knight, J. E. (2003). The developmental antecedents of sexual coercion against women: Testing alternative hypotheses with structural equation modeling. *Annals of the New York Academy of Sciences*, *989*, 72–85.

Koss, M. P., & Gidycz, C. A. (1985). Sexual experiences survey: Reliability and validity. *Journal of Consulting and Clinical Psychology*, *53*, 422–423.

Kruesi, M. P. J., Fine, S., Valladares, L., Phillips, R. A., & Rapoport, J. (1992). Paraphilias: A double blind cross-over comparison of clomipramine versus desipramine. *Archives of Sexual Behavior*, *21*, 587–593.

Lalumière, M. L., & Earls, C. M. (1992). Voluntary control of penile responses as a function of stimulus duration and instructions. *Behavioral Assessment*, *14*, 121–132.

Lalumière, M. L., & Quinsey, V. L. (1998). Pavlovian conditioning of sexual interests in human males. *Archives of Sexual Behavior*, *27*, 241–252.

Langer, S. J., & Martin, J. I. (2004). How dresses can make you mentally ill: Examining gender identity disorder in children. *Child and Adolescent Social Work Journal*, *21*, 5–23.

Långström, N., & Seto, M. C. (2006). Exhibitionistic and voyeuristic behavior in a Swedish national population survey. *Archives of Sexual Behavior*, *35*, 427–435.

Laschet, U., & Laschet, L. (1971). Psychopharmacotherapy of sex offenders with cyproterone acetate. *Pharmakopsychiatrie Neuro-psychopharmakologic*, *4*, 99–104.

Laumann, E. O., Gagnon, J. H., Michael, R. T., & Michaels, S. (1994). *The social organization of sexuality: Sexual practices in the United States*. Chicago, IL: University of Chicago Press.

Marantz, S., & Coates, S. (1991). Mothers of boys with gender identity disorder: A comparison of matched controls. *Journal of the American Academy of Child and Adolescent Psychiatry*, *30*, 310–315.

Marshall, W. L., Payne, K., Barbaree, H. E., & Eccles, A. (1991). Exhibitionists: Sexual preferences for exposing. *Behaviour Research and Therapy*, *29*, 37–40.

Martin, C. L., Ruble, D. N., & Szkrybalo, J. (2002). Cognitive theories of early gender development. *Psychological Bulletin*, *128*, 903–933.

McGuire, R. J., Carlisle, J. M., & Young, B. G. (1965). Sexual deviations as conditioned behavior: A hypothesis. *Behaviour Research and Therapy*, *2*, 185–190.

Menvielle, E. J., & Tuerk, C. (2002). A support group for parents of gender non-conforming boys. *Journal of the American Academy of Child and Adolescent Psychiatry*, *41*, 1010–1013.

Menvielle, E. J., Tuerk, C., & Perrin, E. C. (2005). To the beat of a different drummer: The gender-variant child. *Contemporary Pediatrics*, *22*, 38–39, 41, 43, 45–46.

Meston, C. M., & Gorzalka, B. B. (1992). Psychoactive drugs and human sexual behavior: The role of serotonergic activity. *Journal of Psychoactive Drugs*, *24*, 1–40.

Meyer-Bahlburg, H. F. L. (2005). Gender identity outcome in female-raised 46, XY persons with penile agenesis, cloacal exstrophy of the bladder, or penile ablation. *Archives of Sexual Behavior*, *34*, 423–438.

Meyer-Bahlburg, H. F. L., Gruen, R. S., New, M. I., Bell, J. J., Morishima, A., Shimshi, M., *et al.* (1996). Gender change from female to male in classical congenital adrenal hyperplasia. *Hormones and Behavior*, *30*, 319–332.

Meyer-Bahlburg, H. F. L., Dolezal, C., Baker, S. W., Carlson, A. D., Obeid, J. S., & New, M. I. (2004). Prenatal androgenization affects gender-related behavior but not gender identity in 5–12-year-old girls with congenital adrenal hyperplasia. *Archives of Sexual Behavior*, *33*, 97–104.

Mitchell, J. N. (1991). Maternal influences on gender identity disorder in boys: Searching for specificity. Unpublished doctoral dissertation, York University, Downsview, Ontario.

Money, J. (1975). Ablatio penis: Normal male infant sex-reassigned as a girl. *Archives of Sexual Behavior*, *4*, 65–71.

Money, J., Hampson, J. G., & Hampson, J. L. (1957). Imprinting and the establishment of gender role. *Archives of Neurology and Psychiatry*, *77*, 333–336.

Newman, L. E. (1976). Treatment for the parents of feminine boys. *American Journal of Psychiatry*, *133*, 683–687.

Plaud, J. J., & Martini, J. R. (1999). The respondent conditioning of male sexual arousal. *Behavior Modification*, *23*, 254–268.

Quinsey, V. L., Ketsetzis, M., Earls, C., & Karamanoukian, A. (1996). Viewing time as a measure of sexual interest. *Ethology and Sociobiology*, *17*, 341–354.

Rachman, S., & Hodgson, R. J. (1968). Experimentally-induced "sexual fetishism": Replication and development. *Psychological Record*, *18*, 25–27.

Raymond, M. (1956). Case of fetishism treated by aversion therapy. *British Medical Journal*, *2*, 854–856.

Rekers, G. A. (1975). Stimulus control over sex-typed play in cross-gender identified boys. *Journal of Experimental Child Psychology*, *20*, 136–148.

Roberts, C., Green, R., Williams, K., & Goodman, M. (1987). Boyhood gender identity development: A statistical contrast of two family groups. *Developmental Psychology*, *23*, 544–557.

Robinson, M.-C., Rouleau, J.-L., & Madrigano, G. (1997). Validation of penile plethysmography as a psychophysiological measure of the sexual interests of adolescent sex offenders [Validation de la pléthysmographie pénienne comme mesure psychophysiologique des intérêts sexuels des agresseurs adolescents]. *Revue Québécoise de Psychologie*, *18*, 111–124.

Ruble, D. N., Martin, C. L., & Berenbaum, S. A. (2006). Gender development. In W. Damon & R. M. Lerner (Series Eds.), & N. Eisenberg (Vol. Ed.), *Handbook of child psychology* (6th ed., Vol. 3) *Social, emotional, and personality development* (pp. 858–932). New York: Wiley.

Ryan, G., Miyoshi, T. J., Metzner, J. L., Krugman, R. D., & Fryer, G. E. (1996). Trends in a national sample of sexually abusive youths. *Journal of the American Academy of Child and Adolescent Psychiatry*, *35*, 17–25.

Santiago R. (2006). 5-year-old "girl" starting school is really a boy. *The Miami Herald*. Accessed July 11, 2006 from http://www.miami.com/mld/miamiherald/living/education/15003026.htm

Segal, N. L. (2006). Two monozygotic twin pairs discordant for female-to-male transsexualism. *Archives of Sexual Behavior*, *35*, 347–358.

Seto, M. C., & Kuban, M. (1996). Criterion-related validity of a phallometric test for paraphilic rape and sadism. *Behaviour Research and Therapy*, *34*, 175–183.

Seto, M. C., & Lalumière, M. L. (2004, October). The social and clinical functioning of juvenile sex offenders. In M. C. Seto (Chair), *The uniqueness of juvenile sex offenders: A meta-analysis*. Symposium conducted at the 23rd Annual Conference of the Association for the Treatment of Sexual Abusers, Albuquerque, New Mexico.

Seto, M. C., Lalumière, M. L., & Blanchard, R. (2000). The discriminative validity of a phallometric test for pedophilic interests among adolescent sex offenders against children. *Psychological Assessment*, *12*, 319–327.

Seto, M. C., Murphy, W. D., Page, J., & Ennis, L. (2003). Detecting anomalous sexual interests among juvenile sex offenders. *Annals of the New York Academy of Sciences*, *989*, 118–130.

Smith, G., & Fischer, L. (1999). Assessment of juvenile sexual offenders: Reliability and validity of the Abel Assessment for Interest in Paraphilias. *Sexual Abuse: A Journal of Research and Treatment*, *11*, 207–216.

Smith, Y. L. S., van Goozen, S. H. M., & Cohen-Kettenis, P. T. (2002). Adolescents with gender identity disorder who were accepted or rejected for sex reassignment surgery: A prospective follow-up study. *Journal of the American Academy of Child and Adolescent Psychiatry*, *40*, 472–481.

Stoller, R. J. (1968). *Sex and gender* (Vol. 1). *The development of masculinity and femininity*. New York: Jason Aronson.

Templeman, T. L., & Stinnett, R. D. (1991). Patterns of sexual arousal and history in a "normal" sample of young men. *Archives of Sexual Behavior*, *20*, 137–150.

van Beijsterveldt, C. E. M., Hudziak, J. J., & Boomsma, D. I. (2006). Genetic and environmental influences on cross-gender behavior and relations to psychopathology: A study of Dutch twins at ages 7 and 10 years. *Archives of Sexual Behavior*, *35*, 647–658.

Widom, C. S., & Ames, M. A. (1994). Criminal consequences of childhood sexual victimization. *Child Abuse & Neglect*, *18*, 303–318.

Wiederman, M. W. (2002). Reliability and validity of measurement. In M. W. Wiederman & B. E. Whitley (Eds.), *Handbook for conducting research on human sexuality* (pp. 25–50). Mahwah, NJ: Lawrence Erlbaum.

Wilson, I., Griffin, C., & Wren, B. (2002). The validity of the diagnosis of gender identity disorder (child and adolescent criteria). *Clinical Child Psychology and Psychiatry*, *7*, 335–351.

World Health Organization (WHO). (2000). *Multiaxial classification of child and adolescent psychiatric disorders: The ICD-10 classification of mental and behavioural disorders in children and adolescents*. Cambridge, UK: Cambridge University Press.

Worling, J. R., & Curwen T. (2000). Adolescent sexual offender recidivism: Success of specialized treatment and implications for risk prediction. *Child Abuse and Neglect*, *24*, 965–982.

Zolondek, S. C., Abel, G. G., Northey, W. F., & Jordan, A. D. (2001). The self-reported behaviors of juvenile sexual offenders. *Journal of Interpersonal Violence*, *16*, 73–85.

Zucker, K. J. (1985). Cross-gender identified children. In B. W. Steiner (Ed.), *Gender dysphoria: Development, research, management* (pp. 75–174). New York: Plenum.

Zucker, K. J. (1992). Gender identity disorder. In S. R. Hooper, G. W. Hynd, & R. E. Mattison (Eds.), *Child psychopathology: Diagnostic criteria and clinical assessment* (pp. 305–342). Hillsdale, NJ: Erlbaum.

Zucker, K. J. (1999). Intersexuality and gender identity differentiation. *Annual Review of Sex Research*, *10*, 1–69.

Zucker, K. J. (2001). Gender identity disorder in children and adolescents. In G. O. Gabbard (Ed.), *Treatments of psychiatric disorders* (3rd edn., Vol. 2, pp. 2069–2094). Washington, DC: American Psychiatric Press.

Zucker, K. J. (2005a). Measurement of psychosexual differentiation. *Archives of Sexual Behavior*, *34*, 375–388.

Zucker, K. J. (2005b, October). *Patterns of psychopathology in boys with gender identity disorder*. Paper presented at the joint meeting of the American Academy of Child Psychiatry and the Canadian Academy of Child Psychiatry, Toronto.

Zucker, K. J. (2006a). Gender identity disorder. In D. A. Wolfe & E. J. Mash (Eds.), *Behavioral and emotional disorders in adolescents: Nature, assessment, and treatment* (pp. 535–562). New York: Guilford Press.

Zucker, K. J. (2006b). Commentary on Langer and Martin's (2004) How dresses can make you mentally ill: Examining gender identity disorder in children. *Child and Adolescent Social Work Journal*, *23*, 533–555.

Zucker, K. J. (2007). Gender identity disorder in children, adolescents, and adults. In G. O. Gabbard (Ed.), *Gabbard's treatments of psychiatric disorders* (4th edn., pp. 683–701). Washington, DC: American Psychiatric Press.

Zucker, K. J., & Bradley, S. J. (1995). *Gender identity disorder and psychosexual problems in children and adolescents*. New York: Guilford Press.

Zucker, K. J., Bradley, S. J., Doering, R. W., & Lozinski, J. A. (1985). Sex-typed behavior in cross-gender-identified children: Stability and change at a one-year follow-up. *Journal of the American Academy of Child Psychiatry*, *24*, 710–719.

Zucker, K. J., Bradley, S. J., Kuksis, M., Pecore, K., Birkenfeld-Adams, A., Doering, R. W., *et al.* (1999). Gender constancy judgments in children with gender identity disorder: Evidence for a developmental lag. *Archives of Sexual Behavior*, *28*, 475–502.

Zucker, K. J., Bradley, S. J., Lowry Sullivan, C. B., Kuksis, M., Birkenfeld-Adams, A., & Mitchell, J. N. (1993). A gender identity interview for children. *Journal of Personality Assessment*, *61*, 443–456.

Zucker, K. J., Bradley, S. J., & Sanikhani, M. (1997a). Sex differences in referral rates of children with gender identity disorder: Some hypotheses. *Journal of Abnormal Child Psychology*, *25*, 217–227.

Zucker, K. J., Finegan, J. K., Doering, R. W., & Bradley, S. J. (1984). Two subgroups of gender-problem children. *Archives of Sexual Behavior*, *13*, 27–39.

Zucker, K. J., Green, R., Coates, S., Zuger, B., Cohen-Kettenis, P. T., Zecca, G. M., *et al.* (1997b). Sibling sex ratio of boys with gender identity disorder. *Journal of Child Psychology and Psychiatry*, *38*, 543–551.

Zucker, K. J., Green, R., Garofano, C., Bradley, S. J., Williams, K., Rebach, H. M., *et al.* (1994). Prenatal gender preference of mothers of feminine and masculine boys: Relation to sibling sex composition and birth order. *Journal of Abnormal Child Psychology*, *22*, 1–13.

Zucker, K. J., & Spitzer, R. L. (2005). Was the Gender Identity Disorder of Childhood diagnosis introduced into DSM-III as a backdoor maneuver to replace homosexuality? An historical note. *Journal of Sex and Marital Therapy*, *31*, 31–42.

Zuckerman, M. (1971). Physiological measures of sexual arousal in the human. *Psychological Bulletin*, *75*, 297–329.

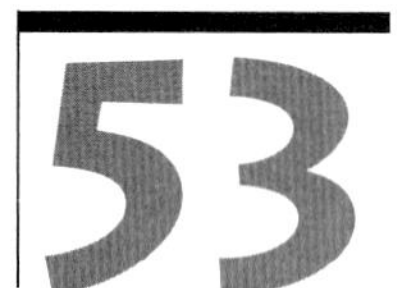

Behavioral Problems of Infancy and Preschool Children (0–5)

Frances Gardner and Daniel S. Shaw

This chapter covers disruptive behavior problems, including oppositional and attentional difficulties; emotional problems such as fears, phobias and depression; and feeding problems in the age period 0–5 years. It will begin by considering common developmental aspects and causal explanations of early behavioral problems, followed by describing, for each type of disorder, classification, prevalence and stability. Finally, we discuss treatment. Other problems common in the early years are discussed in chapters on sleep (see chapter 54), attachment disorder (see chapter 55) and developmental disorders (see chapters 3, 34, 46 and 47). Cross-reference is also made to chapters on similar disorders in older children.

The term "disorder" is used cautiously in this age group, with some skepticism about its validity (Campbell, 2002). Evidence for stability and prognostic significance of preschool problems is not particularly strong, especially in the underthrees. Comorbidity is very high, and there are also concerns about distinguishing normal from abnormal behavior in this period of rapid developmental change, and about labeling very young children with disorders. However, there may also be disadvantages of not defining disorders in young children, including failure to recognize distress and provide appropriate help (Carter, Briggs-Gowan, & Davis, 2004; Egger & Angold, 2006). The latter is particularly important, given that there is a good deal of evidence about effective interventions for this age group, particularly for disruptive behavior problems.

In view of these uncertainties about defining disorders, most studies in the 0–5 age group use dimensional approaches to defining and measuring problem behavior. Accordingly, we use the term "disruptive problems" to refer to a constellation of oppositional or attentional symptoms, and the term "emotional problems" to refer to depressive and anxious-type symptoms. Studies based on dimensional approaches include children with severe or milder problems, often defined by clinical cutoff on symptom questionnaires. Where studies use diagnostic criteria, we use DSM and/or ICD disorder terminology. The period of infancy refers to 0–1 years, toddlerhood 1–3 years and preschool 3–5 years.

Rutter's Child and Adolescent Psychiatry, 5th edition. Edited by M. Rutter, D. Bishop, D. Pine, S. Scott, J. Stevenson, E. Taylor and A. Thapar. © 2008 Blackwell Publishing, ISBN: 978-1-4051-4549-7.

Developmental Perspectives on Problem Behavior in Early Childhood

It is important to recognize the rapid pace of growth and maturation that takes place from birth to age 5, which has multiple implications for assessment and treatment. For the primary types of problem behavior discussed in this chapter (i.e., disruptive and emotional problems), identification and diagnosis based purely on child behavior have been shown to have limited stability and prognostic implications until at least 24 months of age (Campbell, Shaw, & Gilliom, 2000; Keenan, Shaw, Walsh, Delliquadri, & Giovannelli, 1997). For assessing risk of clinically significant child problem behavior in the 0–2 age group, greater emphasis has been placed on parenting and factors that might compromise parental functioning (e.g., depression, social support, teen parenthood; Shaw, Dishion Supplee *et al.*, 2006), as well as factors that might compromise the developing brain (e.g., prematurity; prenatal drug use). Child problem behavior shows increasing stability beginning in the toddler period. Whereas a substantial percentage of children will "outgrow" these problems, longitudinal studies suggest that 50–60% of children showing high rates of disruptive behavior at age 3–4 will continue to show these problems at school age (Campbell, Szumowski, Ewing *et al.*, 1982; Campbell, Pierce, Moore *et al.*, 1996; Campbell, Shaw, & Gilliom, 2000; Richman, Stevenson, & Graham, 1982). In a recent study of low-income boys, among those identified above the 90th percentile on disruptive symptoms at age 2, 60% remained above the 90th percentile and 100% (all 18) remained above the median at age 6 (Shaw, Gilliom, & Giovannelli, 2000; Shaw, Gilliom, Ingoldsby *et al.*, 2003).

The low stability of behavior problems between toddlerhood and later childhood has implications for using the term "disorder" in referring to these problems in very early childhood (Campbell, 2002; Egger & Angold, 2006). It may be somewhat less problematic in the preschool range. There is currently much debate about the appropriateness of using traditional diagnostic categories, particularly for infants and toddlers. Rapid developmental change within the period 0–5 makes it particularly hard to distinguish normal from abnormal behavior, and to set age-appropriate criteria for classification systems. Thus, having six temper tantrums a day might be bothersome but normal at 22 months, but could contribute to a diagnosis of oppositional defiant disorder (ODD) in a 4-year-old. Similarly, a 2-year-old showing difficulty separating from a parent in the first week of daycare would be less worrisome than a 5-year-old showing similar reactions over many weeks.

Clearly, diagnostic systems need to be able to take these developmental variations into account. Systems for assessing preschoolers go some way to solving this problem, using criteria that are more age-appropriate, and basing assessments on observations and reports of child behavior in multiple settings (i.e., home and preschool, from parents and teachers). Recent advances in the field include the Research Diagnostic Criteria–Preschool Age (RDC-PA) which has attempted to modify DSM criteria to be suitable for preschoolers (Task Force on Research Diagnostic Criteria, 2003), and the Preschool Age Psychiatric Assessment (PAPA; Egger & Angold, 2004), which is a structured parent-interview schedule for ages 2–5. However, these systems cannot easily solve the problem that meaning and significance of problem behavior shift rapidly even within this period, and within a given cultural or family setting. Systems for very young children, such as the diagnostic classification: 0–3 (DC: 0–3) (Zero to Three, 1994), tend to place more emphasis on aspects of the parent–child relationship, rather that focusing solely on child behavior, with an increasing focus on behavior as children approach school age. However, evidence for validity of 0–3 diagnostic categories, including stability and, in some cases, links to later disorders of the same name (e.g., infantile "anorexia"; Chatoor & Ganiban, 2004) is not strong.

Based on the relative instability of problem behavior during early childhood, it should not be surprising to learn that many children demonstrate multiple types of problem behavior, including co-occurring disruptive and emotional problems (e.g., oppositionality coupled with depression or attention deficit/hyperactivity disorder [ADHD]). Egger and Angold (2006) reported that 50% of preschoolers showing a disorder in their community sample also showed one or more co-occurring disorders. Similar rates of comorbidity were found by Lavigne, Gibbons, Christoffel *et al.* (1996) and Keenan, Shaw, Walsh *et al.* (1997). Arguably, very high rates of comorbidity could be seen as a reason for caution in using diagnostic systems in this age group. However, this problem is not specific to the 0–5 range, as high rates of comorbidity are typical of childhood disorders in general (see chapter 2; Angold, Costello, & Erkanli, 1999).

Because of these rapid changes in development, and instability across time and context, problems may manifest themselves in different ways in under-fives compared to older children. For example, toddler fears and worries may manifest as irritable or oppositional behavior (e.g., tantrums). These may be harder to detect than in older children because of young children's limited ability to communicate emotions to adults. Equally, superficially similar behaviors in toddlers may reflect quite different underlying problems. Thus, if a toddler is isolated from peers in the nursery, it is important to assess whether this is a temporary reaction to a new environment, or related to aggression, social anxiety or to a more profound problem in communication (e.g., severe learning disability, autism spectrum disorder; see chapters 46 and 49). In a school-aged child, pervasive learning problems would be more apparent and, in most cases, already identified.

Theoretical perspectives

Preschool behavior problems are influenced by both biological and environmental factors, as manifest in individual differences in child characteristics (e.g., temperamental dimensions of activity, sociability, attention) and the quality of the caregiving environment. Genetic and prenatal environmental factors are influential in this age period (see chapters 23 and 30). We distinguish between *risk factors*, in the presence of which the probability of showing a disorder is raised; *precursors*, where there is continuity between an early problem (e.g., preschool disruptive problems) and a later one (e.g., conduct disorder); and the presence of formal *disorder*. Extreme difficult temperament is often viewed as a risk factor for later behavior problems (Hill, 2002), although at moderate levels of difficulty and without other indicators of child or family risk, such individual differences are likely to reflect developmentally normative patterns rather than necessarily implying risk for disorder.

In recent years, there has been increasing recognition of the multiple interacting factors that contribute to divergence in outcomes of infants who demonstrate early problems in feeding, emotionality or disruptive behavior (Campbell, Shaw, & Gilliom, 2000). This change in focus can be traced to the pioneering efforts of Thomas, Chess, and Birch (1968), who emphasized the goodness-of-fit between parent and child temperament, to Bell's (1968) work on children's effects on parents, and Sameroff and Chandler's (1975) transactional model of parent–child interaction. Thus, assessment and intervention efforts across problem behavior types have focused on changing child behavior, parent behavior and resources, and the quality of parent–child interaction. As children under 5 years are so dependent on their caregiving environment, there is an emphasis on identifying risk factors in the family and the wider caregiving context (e.g., quality of daycare or non-parental caregiving) which moderate the course of early problem behavior.

In early childhood intervention, similar parent management strategies are often used to manage apparently dissimilar problems (e.g., infant feeding or sleeping problems, preschool disruptive behavior). That similar intervention strategies are used to treat these various problem behaviors should not be surprising, as self-regulation skills develop rapidly during this age period. Self-regulation involves the ability to control impulses and expressions of emotion; thus, children with difficulties in self-regulation might show a range of problems, including higher rates of tantrums, irritable mood and oppositionality, and disturbances in sleep, eating, activity or attention. Despite the range of symptoms, there may be common maintaining mechanisms. All of these problems might elicit similar levels of frustration in parents, their responses leading to a worsening of child symptoms, in a cycle of coercive interaction (Patterson, 1982; Shaw & Bell, 1993).

In recent decades, there has been much speculation about the need to ensure that children's early years are not marked by environmental adversity, because of the fear of irreversible harm, as evidenced in animal studies. Unfortunately, relevant human data are limited. There is some evidence to suggest that exposure to psychosocial adversity during the toddler period shows stronger predictions to later outcomes than exposure in later periods (Appleyard, Egeland, van Dulmen, & Sroufe, 2005; Shaw, Gilliom, & Giovannelli, 2000). Thus, in the study by Appleyard *et al.* (2005) of children from low-income families, a cumulative index of contextual adversity in early childhood continued to be associated with adolescent antisocial behavior after accounting for the effects of contextual risk in middle childhood. However, in most cases, study designs have not permitted examination of whether there are critical periods for the operation of risk factors, where, based on timing of exposure, there might be differential effects on child adjustment.

Clinical Problems

Disruptive Behavior

Disruptive behavior, sometimes referred to as externalizing or "acting-out" problems, includes attentional and oppositional problems and their corresponding disorders, ADHD and ODD (Lahey, Loeber, Quay, Frick, & Grimm, 1992). As conduct disorder (CD) includes more serious forms of aggression, property destruction and theft, it is rarely applied to preschoolers. Disruptive problems represent the most frequent type of problem behavior in early childhood, particularly after the second year when parental expectations for children to comply with rules and contain aggressive behavior increase. Tremblay (1998) reported that by age 17 months, 70% of children take toys away from other children, 46% push others to obtain what they want and 21–27% engage in one or more of the following with peers: biting, kicking, fighting or physically attacking. Tremblay also reported that aggression occurs more frequently for infants with siblings, especially for girls, providing daily opportunities for conflicts over possessions. Relative to emotional problems, much more research has been conducted on the stability, course and predictors of disruptive problems in early childhood and about 50% of oppositional 3-year-olds continue to have these problems in the school years (Campbell, Shaw, & Gilliom, 2000).

Using DSM-IV criteria, generated from a structured interview with parents, the prevalence of preschool ODD in a US sample was estimated at 7%, and ADHD at 3% (Egger & Angold, 2006). Other studies broadly concur, although some questionnaire studies arrive at higher estimates, depending, not surprisingly, on the choice of definition, cut-off and informant (Koot, 1993; Richman, Stevenson, & Graham, 1982). In the toddler and preschool years, sex differences are not as marked as in older children. Boys' higher rates of disruptive behavior seem to emerge during the later preschool period, with studies documenting absence of sex differences from ages 1 to 3 (Achenbach, 1992; Keenan & Shaw, 1994; Richman, Stevenson, & Graham, 1982), followed by increasing sex differences from age 4 to 5 (Lavigne, Gibbons, Christoffel *et al.*, 1996; Rose, Rose, & Feldman, 1989), although this was not found for ODD by Egger and Angold (2006).

Attention Deficit/Hyperactivity Disorder

Core features include inattention, impulsivity and hyperactivity (Barkley, 1998). In terms of etiology, models tend to focus on different biological factors, including activity, impulse and attention control (see chapter 34; Barkley, 1997; Rothbart, Ellis, Rueda, & Posner, 2003). As with older children, most preschoolers with ADHD show other difficulties, most typically conduct problems (Barkley, 1997; Shaw, LaCourse, & Nagin, 2005). This co-occurrence carries risk for more severe and chronic adjustment problems in adolescence and adulthood (Moffitt, 1990; Weiss & Hechtman, 1993).

Oppositional Problems

These include defiant, angry, annoying, non-compliant and sometimes aggressive behaviors. For a diagnosis of ODD, behaviors need to occur more commonly than is typical for that age, persist for more than 6 months, and impair the child's functioning (American Psychiatric Association, 2000; Campbell, 2002). During toddlerhood, despite the high frequency of aggressive-like and oppositional behavior, many of these behaviors tend to be tolerated by parents because of children's limited ability to understand the consequences of their actions. However, with emerging cognitive maturation during this period, parental tolerance for disruptive behavior decreases, particularly when children cannot refrain from showing this behavior with peers and adults outside of the home (e.g., in daycare).

Causes and Correlates of Disruptive Behavior Problems

Causal models emphasize the dynamic interplay of child, parenting and contextual factors (Sameroff & Chandler, 1975), with individual differences in disruptive behavior often being magnified by ineffective parent management strategies (Campbell, Pierce, Moore *et al.*, 1996; Shaw, Gilliom, Ingoldsby *et al.*, 2003). Most of this research has focused on early predictors of conduct problems rather than ADHD, but one recent study found similar types of predictors for both conduct problems and ADHD (Shaw, Lacourse, & Nagin, 2005). Predictive validity for early child markers of more serious disruptive behavior begins to emerge around age 2 (Keenan, Shaw, Walsh *et al.*, 1997; Shaw, Gilliom, Ingoldsby *et al.*, 2003), with clearer predictions from age 3 to later, more serious forms of antisocial behavior (Caspi, Henry, McGee, Moffitt, & Silva, 1995; Henry, Caspi, Moffitt, & Silva, 1996).

Parenting models have been developed from attachment and social learning perspectives, with attachment models emphasizing unresponsive caregiving during infancy (Greenberg, Speltz, & DeKlyen, 1993; Sroufe, 1997), and social learning models focusing on the development of coercive cycles in which parents unwittingly reinforce and maintain child disruptive behavior by using inconsistent and harsh management strategies

(Patterson, 1982; Shaw & Bell, 1993). Research has consistently validated associations among low-quality parent–child relationships in the early years, the use of unresponsive or harsh parenting practices, and disruptive behavior in preschool and later years (Loeber & Dishion, 1983; Lyons-Ruth, 1996; Shaw, Keenan, & Vondra, 1994; Shaw, Winslow, Owens *et al.*, 1998). Positive parenting skills (e.g., anticipating the child's troublesome moments, providing joint play activities) may be particularly important in the toddler years, as they can help to divert children from problem behavior at an age when children have limited skills for self-management of boredom and tempting impulses (Gardner, 1994; Gardner, Sonuga-Barke, & Sayal, 1999; Gardner, Ward, Burton *et al.*, 2003; Gardner, Shaw, Dishion *et al.*, 2007; Martin, 1981). Rather different parenting skills become important in middle childhood, where increasing independence requires greater monitoring of children across multiple settings, and planning for preventing problems that may occur in the parent's absence.

The wider family and caregiving environment can also influence the development of early emotional and behavioral problems. The nature of sibling relationships, for example, appears to be influenced by factors such as the temperament of each child, and the quality of other relationships in the family, such as parent–child and marital relationships (Dunn, 1993). Sibling relationships often encompass a complex mix of supportive and conflictual dimensions, and appear to be important for development. For example, Garcia, Shaw, Winslow, and Yaggi (2000) found that sibling conflict at age 5 was predictive of later disruptive problems at home and school, after accounting for earlier parenting and child behavior.

As young children spend more time outside the home, researchers have addressed whether and how daycare might affect early problem behavior. Early studies of daycare were mixed in quality of the methods used, quality of the daycare studied and the results found. A recent US study of daycare effects (over 1000 children) found that more hours spent in any kind of non-maternal care from infancy to age 54 months was associated with higher ratings of oppositional problems, more so for ratings made by alternative caregivers and teachers than parents (NICHD Early Child Care Research Network, 2003). These effects, albeit statistically significant, tended to be modest in magnitude and did not predict trajectories of clinically meaningful problem behavior. The quality of early child care has also bee found to discriminate conduct problems in a large sample of children from low-income families (Votruba–Drzal, Coley, & Chase-Landsdale, 2004). Results indicated that many hours of low-quality care was associated with higher oppositional problems at school entry, whereas high-quality care served a protective function. Fewer behavior problems have also been found in children in high-quality day care, compared to home care, in Sweden, even at 10-year follow-up (Andersson, 1992). Overall, quality and, to some extent, amount of care, have been found to influence the course of early disruptive problems.

In general, risk factors for early disruptive behavior are similar to those for later CD (see chapter 35), including parental attributes (e.g., mental illness; see chapter 27) and contextual factors (e.g., socioeconomic status; Shaw, Keenan, & Vondra, 1994; Shaw, Winslow, Owens *et al.*, 1998; Tremblay, Nagin, Seguin *et al.*, 2004). Cumulatively, these data suggest that several targets have been established for prevention and intervention studies (see chapter 61; Olds, 2002), some of which might be appropriate before a child is born.

Emotional Problems

Emotional problems such as anxiety, depression and post-traumatic stress in preschoolers have been much less studied than disruptive problems. There are a number of reasons for this, including the inability of young children easily to communicate about their emotions, or for adults to notice them as problematic. Furthermore, there are difficulties in distinguishing developmentally normal emotions (e.g., fears, crying) from more severe and prolonged anxiety or misery that might constitute a disorder. This is especially difficult in the early years, when children undergo rapid changes in the development of emotions, and in their ability to communicate these to others. There is probably insufficient evidence at present to decide whether diagnosing emotional disorders is valid and useful in the 0–5 year range.

Classification Systems

Many DSM categories, including social phobia, generalized anxiety and depression apply across the range of child to adulthood, and are therefore not designed to take preschool developmental factors into account. One exception is Separation Anxiety Disorder, which applies only to children. It is defined as "developmentally inappropriate and excessive anxiety concerning separation from home or from those the child is attached to" (APA, 2000). However, there are still problems in applying this diagnosis to very young children because normative expectations of responses to separation from caregivers change so much across the first 3 years. Thus, in the 0–3 system, this constellation is not considered abnormal and therefore is not included as a disorder. In all cases it is important to take into account the child's developmental stage in assessing whether a problem is of concern. The majority of children show fears at some stage in development, and typical fears change with age. Thus, fear of strangers is very common in late infancy, and fear of animals in toddlerhood. Whether they constitute a clinical problem (Campbell, 2002) depends also on factors such as persistence, and how much they impair the child's and family's well-being, for example if the child is persistently unable to engage in normal activities (e.g., going to daycare or the park).

Stability

Many emotional problems in this age range are thought to represent transient reactions to stressful life events, rather than disorders per se. Relative to studies of disruptive problems, there is a paucity of research on the stability of early emotional problems for young children. In one study, stability of preschool depression over 6 months was high among 3- to

5-year-olds (Luby, Heffelfinger, Mrakotsky *et al.*, 2002), but there are no data on the long-term prognosis for these children. Both predictive validity and functional impairment are important in validating a diagnostic category, and in the case of depressed preschoolers, there is preliminary evidence that these children show moderate to high levels of impairment in their daily functioning (Egger & Angold, 2006).

Prevalence

Studies of preschool children using DSM-III and DSM-IV criteria have estimated prevalence of emotional disorder diagnoses; these tend to be low for each category: separation anxiety (0.3–5%), social phobia (2–4%), specific phobia (0–2%) and depression (0–2%; Egger & Angold, 2006; Lavigne, Gibbons, Christoffel *et al.*, 1996). However, in Egger and Angold's study, which included multiple types of problem behavior, rates of any emotional disorder were as high as for disruptive disorders, both around 10%. As found in middle childhood, prevalence of depression and anxiety did not differ by gender (Keenan, Shaw, Walsh *et al.*, 1997). Sex differences tend to emerge around puberty. Comorbidity between depression and ODD was very high in one study of 2- to 5-year-olds (Egger & Angold, 2006), raising questions about whether these are separate disorders.

Causes and Correlates of Emotional Problems

As with disruptive behaviors, causes are likely to be multifaceted, and to reflect the interplay between child and parent genetic factors, parenting and the wider social environment around the child. As with other aspects of emotional problems, there have been few studies of multiple etiological factors, especially in preschool children. Studies have suggested quite high heritability for some preschool emotional problems (Eley, Bolton, O'Connor *et al.*, 2003). Where risk factors have been studied in preschoolers, broadly these appear similar to those found in studies of older children (Luby, Heffelfinger, Mrakotsky *et al.*, 2003). Maternal transmission of anxiety also seems to be an important factor, not only via genetic factors, but also through processes such as modeling and an anxious style of parenting (see chapter 27). Individual differences in children's temperament (see chapter 14) also have been linked to early emotional problems, most notably for children who are behaviorally inhibited (Hirshfeld-Becker, Biederman, & Rosenbaum, 2004). Behavioral inhibition is defined as the tendency to react to novelty with unusual fear, cautiousness and withdrawal, and appears to be moderately stable across early childhood (Kagan, 1999; Kagan, Reznick, & Snidman, 1988). Biederman, Hirshfeld-Becker, Rosenbaum *et al.* (2001) found that behavioral inhibition assessed during early childhood was associated with increased risk for anxiety disorders 5 years later. Another recent study examined predictors of trajectories of boys' anxiety from ages 2 to 10 years, and subsequent emotional disorders in early adolescence (Feng, Shaw, Lane, Alarcon, & Skuban, 2006). Consistent with Kagan's work, shy temperament at age 2 tended to differentiate between initial high- and low-anxiety trajectory groups, whereas early maternal negative control and maternal depression were associated with increasing trajectories and elevated anxiety symptoms in middle childhood. Follow-up to adolescence indicated that child factors such as temperament contributed strongly to diagnoses of anxiety disorders, whereas both child and parent factors (e.g., negative control) contributed to boys' depression.

Eating and Feeding Problems

Normal patterns of feeding change greatly between individuals and across time in the developmental period 0–5. The same can be said for disorders of eating and feeding, which present in a wide variety of ways (Stein & Barnes, 2002). Thus, in the early months, babies may fail to thrive for a number of reasons, or show signs of infantile colic. In the preschool years, food refusal or excess fussiness may be linked to other toddler oppositional behaviors, and intervention may need to consider parental management of child behavior more broadly. Feeding problems are common, but are more prevalent in children with developmental disabilities, pointing to the combination of physical health, family factors and developmental delay that are often involved in feeding problems. Their multifactorial origins can make it hard to define which problems belong within the realm of child psychiatry, rather than pediatrics, as many feeding problems that are primarily physical (e.g., failure to thrive [FTT] as a result of oral–motor dysfunction in cerebral palsy) may or may not have a substantial component exacerbated by family stress or poor parenting skills. The picture is further complicated by the fact that etiology is often unknown (e.g., in FTT, colic). While bearing in mind this caution, we will focus on problems thought to have a primarily psychosocial cause.

Classification and Prevalence

There is no standard system for classifying all types of feeding problems in the 0–5 period. DSM-IV includes the categories pica, rumination and "feeding disorder of infancy and early childhood," defined as persistent failure to eat adequately, with weight loss or failure to gain weight that is not caused by physical illness, and onset before age 6. Various systems of classification have been proposed, but some make unwarranted assumptions about etiology, for example Chatoor & Ganiban (2004), who classify disorders by psychogenic or other cause (e.g., "feeding disorder of caregiver–infant reciprocity," or "post-traumatic feeding disorder"). This chapter covers the most common problems in this age group, including colic, FTT and food refusal. Feeding problems have been estimated to affect up to 30% of infants (Jenkins, Bax, & Hart, 1980). However, given the lack of standard criteria for definition, figures vary quite widely across studies. Similarly, investigation of prognosis and causes of feeding problems is hampered by lack of a clear classification system.

Infant Colic

The causes of colic are unclear and, as a result, it has been classified variously as a feeding, regulatory or crying problem. Wessel, Cobb, Jackson, Harris, and Detweiler's (1954) classic "rule of three" definition involves "paroxysms of irritability, fussing, crying lasting more than 3 hours a day, on more than 3 days in 1 week" and continuing for more than 3 weeks, between the ages of 1 and 4 months. Colic is common, reported as occurring in 10–20% of babies in large community surveys (Crowcroft & Stachan, 1997). There may be little justification for using the term "colic" for a phenomenon that might be more parsimoniously viewed as persistent unexplained infant crying (St. James-Roberts, 2004). There are a number of theories of etiology, focusing on gastrointestinal dysfunction, central nervous system immaturity, and parental stress and anxiety. However, there is very little conclusive evidence to support these theories (Stifter & Wiggins, 2004), or to validate treatments that follow from them (Garrison & Christakis, 2000). Irrespective of cause, colic is a significant cause of parental stress and low confidence. A recent working party (Barr, St. James-Roberts, & Keefe, 2001) concluded that colic could most usefully be seen as a problem resulting from early individual differences in reactivity and the development of regulation. Although colic is seen by parents and professionals as a physical problem, rarely is there any known underlying condition, such as gastrointestinal disorder.

Failure to Thrive

Historically, there has been little agreement on a precise definition of the term "failure to thrive" (FTT). It has been defined in several ways, including by weight centile, by weight-for-height and by growth faltering over time (Benoit, 2000). Traditionally, FTT was divided into two subgroups: organic and non-organic, the latter term carrying connotations of psychosocial causation, such as parental neglect, abuse or poor management of feeding. However, more recently the assumption of a clear-cut distinction between organic and non-organic FTT has been called into question (Boddy & Skuse, 1994; Chatoor & Ganiban, 2004). Absence of a physical explanation does not mean that poor parenting is necessarily the cause. However, attributing growth delay to parental neglect may be unhelpful (Skuse, 1985), and in some cases may have harmful consequences. Furthermore, many children with non-organic FTT turn out later to have undiagnosed illnesses or impairments in oral–motor skills. One population survey (Reilly, Skuse, Wolke, & Stevenson, 1999) found oral–motor dysfunction in 35% of children with non-organic FTT, suggesting that assumptions about parental causes may often be unwarranted. Finally, as discussed in relation to other early behavior problems, FTT is now thought likely to have multifactorial causes, where factors such as temperament, developmental delay and poor feeding skills interact with parental stress and poor management of feeding. In a UK population survey of growth delay (Skuse, Reilly, & Wolke, 1994), a prevalence rate of 3–4% was found. However, it was also noted that there was considerable variation between ethnic groups, with higher rates among South Asian and lower rates in African groups. We should be cautious about assuming that these are related to cultural differences in early feeding patterns; it is also possible that norms are inadequate for defining growth faltering in minority groups.

Food Refusal

Food refusal is a general term for a range of feeding problems, broader than DSM "Feeding disorder of infancy and early childhood," as it focuses on child behavior rather than requiring growth failure. It includes children of normal weight who consistently or selectively refuse to eat. Selective refusal may be unpredictable, or may be specific to certain foods or situations (Chatoor & Ganniban, 2004; Douglas, 2002). In toddlers, it may be linked to other behavioral problems, or may be limited to feeding contexts. It may be related to long-standing early feeding problems or arise anew in the "terrible twos." Again, causes are likely to be multifactorial, including combinations of temperament, family stress and poor parenting skills, as for other oppositional problems. In many cases, there may be more specific contributing factors related to food, including feeding experiences, parental anxiety about food and body shape or prior health problems that might initiate the feeding problem (e.g., pain or anxiety about vomiting or reflux), which may then be unwittingly reinforced by parental reactions (Douglas, 2002; Stein & Barnes, 2002).

Treatment

General Principles for Selecting Treatments

From earlier discussions of multiple interacting factors that contribute to behavioral problems in the 0–5 period, it will be clear that intervention requires assessment of the presenting problems in the context of family and caregiver influences, as well as the child's development and physical health. Thus, factors such as fussy temperament, parental inconsistency, stress of poverty, early illness and oral–motor delay may all combine to produce toddler eating problems. Knowing the causes of a problem can be helpful for understanding and selecting treatment; however, at the same time it is vital that clinicians use, wherever possible, interventions that have a strong evidence-base, and that they keep up to date with this knowledge as new trials and systematic reviews appear. Thus, knowing that oral–motor dysfunction is contributing to a long-standing eating problem in a toddler born very prematurely is helpful in making sense of a problem, and for reducing parental blame and guilt; however, arguably it is not useful information for treatment if there is no evidence of effectiveness of available speech therapy for oral–motor delay. However, there is better evidence about the effectiveness of parenting interventions for food refusal and other mealtime behavior problems (Kerwin, 1999; Turner, Sanders, & Wall, 1994). Parent management difficulties are only one of several causal factors contributing to early eating, sleep, oppositional or attentional problems, but parenting intervention might nevertheless be the treatment of choice. In this age group, it is developmentally appropriate and has the strongest evidence-base from randomized trials. This is the case even for preschool ADHD, where there is a clear genetic contribution to etiology.

Given these considerations, this section focuses on common principles behind evidence-based approaches, particularly parent management of toddler behavior problems, as well as including specific guidance for clinicians. We concentrate on interventions with an evidence-base from high-quality systematic reviews, such as those published by the Cochrane Collaboration, and randomized controlled trials (RCTs). Some of these cover a wide age range but, where possible, we have sought effectiveness data applicable to the 0–5 age group. Readers are referred to other chapters for fuller details on particular problems and interventions.

Overview of Evidence

We begin with a brief overview of evidence on intervention effectiveness. A systematic review of interventions for early conduct problems age 3–8 (Barlow & Stewart-Brown, 2000) concluded that behaviorally based parent-training is effective. Several recent trials that comprise entirely, or high proportions of, preschoolers reach similar conclusions (Gardner, Burton, & Klimes, 2006; Hutchings, Bywater, Daley *et al.*, 2007; Sanders, Markie-Dadds, Tully, & Bor, 2000; Scott, Spender, Doolan, Jacobs, & Aspland, 2001; Webster-Stratton, 1998a), suggesting that interventions are translatable across countries and varied service settings. Some programs appear to be equally effective across ethnic groups; a secondary analysis of 630 preschoolers in trials of the Webster-Stratton preventive parenting program found no differences by ethnicity on any parent or child outcome measures, or on parent engagement and satisfaction (Reid, Webster-Stratton, & Beauchaine, 2001). For sleeping problems, systematic reviews suggest that behavioral parent management of settling and night-waking problems is effective (Mindell, 1999; Ramchandani, Wiggs, Webb, & Stores, 2000). For toddler and preschool eating problems, evidence from two very small RCTs and several case series leads to the tentative conclusion that parent management approaches may be effective (Turner, Sanders, & Wall, 1994). Kerwin's (1999) review reached a similar conclusion for severe infant feeding problems. The picture is much less clear for early emotional disorders, as very few treatment trials include children under 5.

Medication is controversial in this age group, and practice varies between USA and Europe. For ADHD, stimulant medication is not licensed for preschoolers because of worries about safety, and parenting interventions have been found to be as effective in this age group as stimulant drugs are in older children (Sonuga-Barke, Daley, Thompson, Laver-Bradbury, & Weeks, 2001). Nevertheless, one trial claimed methylphenidate may be effective in preschoolers (Greenhill, Kollins, Abikoff *et al.*, 2006), although it should be noted that the trial only included children for whom parent-training approaches were not effective, and there was quite a high rate of side effects. Tricyclic antidepressants are not recommended in prepubertal children (Hazell, O'Connell, Heathcote, & Henry, 2002), and there are considerable doubts about the effectiveness of selective serotonin reuptake inhibitors (SSRIs) in children of all ages (Whittington, Kendall, Fonagy *et al.*, 2004).

Interventions for Disruptive Behavior Problems

We begin with principles of parenting interventions for early oppositional and attentional problems, while noting that these broad principles are also applicable to toddler eating and sleeping problems, particularly given the frequent comorbidity and common causes for these problems. Specific interventions for feeding problems follow. (For fuller details on parenting interventions see chapter 64. For useful detailed guides to carrying out parenting interventions in young children see Sutton, 1999; Webster-Stratton, 1992; Webster-Stratton & Herbert, 1994.)

Intervention begins with broad assessment of the child's health, development and temperament, the overall family and caregiving setting, and a detailed evaluation of the frequency, duration and situational determinants of the presenting problems. In particular, assessment should focus on parenting strategies and other situational factors that may be triggering or maintaining the problem on a day-to-day basis. Equally important is examination of parenting strengths and competencies that can be built on in treatment. What are the positive features of the relationship between child and parents? Under what conditions does the problem fail to occur, or how have parents succeeded in preventing or alleviating it? Parenting strategies are best assessed through a combination of parent diary records, direct observation of parent–child interaction and careful interviewing. Observational methods are particularly useful for preschoolers (see chapter 19), who tend to be less reactive to being observed. There is increasing evidence that learning and putting into practice new parenting skills, carefully tailored to the child's needs, is a critical intervening mechanism (Rutter, 2005) underlying successful interventions for early conduct problems (Forgatch & DeGarmo, 1999; Gardner, Burton, & Klimes, 2006; Gardner, Shaw, Dishion *et al.*, 2007; Hutchings, Lane, & Gardner, 2004). Hence, this parenting assessment information is central to planning the main active ingredients of the intervention. Providing systematic sensitive feedback to parents about the findings of assessment may be helpful for several reasons (Dishion & Kavanagh, 2003; Shaw, Dishion, Gardner *et al.*, 2006), including to motivate parents' engagement with challenging interventions; to reach a shared formulation and plan for treatment (rather than one that is imposed by the clinician); and to aid later skills coaching.

Although enhancing parenting skills is a key part of intervention for behavior problems, it is important to help the parents understand that they are not necessarily the main cause of the problem, rather that they are the best solution. Helping parents understand how the child's temperament and development (e.g., language or cognitive impairment; see chapters 47 and 49) contribute to parenting and conflict can be very helpful in formulating a problem, and preparing the ground for skills-based work. A preschool ADHD intervention provides an excellent example of this approach (Sonuga-Barke, Daley, Thompson *et al.*, 2001; Thompson, Weeks, & Laver-Bradbury, 1999). The first part of the intervention involves helping parents to understand and empathize with the individual temperamental characteristics of the child with ADHD, and considering how some of the parents' expectations and skills may need to be adapted to fit better with the child. Following this, parents work on setting new expectations and limits, and practice strategies to manage the child and change symptomatic behavior. As the majority of children with ADHD show comorbid conduct problems, such approaches are also applicable to changing oppositional behavior (Sonuga-Barke, Daley, Thompson *et al.*, 2001).

Following assessment, intervention focuses on applying cognitive–behavioral parenting principles in an individualized manner to the child and family. An example of a well-specified effective parenting intervention is Webster-Stratton's (1998a,b; Webster-Stratton & Herbert, 1994) "Incredible Years" program (see chapter 64), which employs a collaborative approach, building on parents' strengths and expertise. Principles covered include parent–child play, praise, incentives, limit-setting, problem-solving and discipline. Video clips are used to encourage problem-solving around strategies to manage their child, and to illustrate their varying effects on child behavior. Role plays and homework are used to find solutions and practice parenting skills. In each session, homework successes and problems are discussed, and used as further problem-solving examples. Although this program is designed to be delivered to groups of parents, these principles are equally important in individual work with families of young children. Similar effective programs, aimed particularly at 2- to 5-year-olds, and designed to be carried out in a home or clinic setting with individual families, include Sanders, Markie-Dadds, Tully *et al.*s' (2000) Triple-P program, and Forgatch and DeGarmo's (1999) Parent Management Training.

When advising parents about disruptive behavior, it is helpful to encourage them to observe and record their child's behavior, the situations that trigger it, and their reactions and attempts at managing the behavior. It is important to help parents build a warm cooperative relationship with the child, especially if this appears to be lacking, by advising a regular daily joint play session, say 5–10 min, using an age-appropriate calm activity. Co-operative play should be encouraged and rewarded. Meanwhile, it is important for parents to explain simple ground rules to the child (behavior that is expected or prohibited, in key situations), and then to reward the child using praise, and token rewards (e.g., sticker or star charts) for behaving well, especially in situations that commonly lead to troublesome behavior. Planning ahead for how to deal with the most difficult situations is an important element. It is possible to plan to ignore milder problem behaviors, and use mild consequences for more severe problems (e.g., aggression, repeated defiance about important issues), such as time out (for 2–3 min at age 2–5) or brief immediate withdrawal of enjoyable activities. For milder problems, a Cochrane review suggests that self-help materials can improve disruptive problem behavior (Montgomery, Bjornstad, & Dennis, 2006). For example, books explaining evidence-based principles for managing early behavior problems (e.g., Sanders, 2004; Webster-Stratton, 1992) can be useful for parents, or for clinicians to work through with parents.

Non-attendance is a common problem in treatment services, and it behoves clinicians to find ways to overcome barriers to engagement, especially for distressed and disadvantaged families. Webster-Stratton (1998a,b) achieves this by offering flexible timing of intervention, transport and child care, which are particularly important for families with preschoolers. Other strategies include home-visiting, or using community locations, such as primary healthcare clinics (Stewart-Brown, Patterson, Mockford *et al.*, 2004; Turner & Sanders, 2006). Others have developed specific strategies to enhance parent motivation (Dishion & Kavanagh, 2003; Dishion, Shaw, Connell *et al.* (in press)). It is undoubtedly challenging to be flexible to parents' needs when working in a clinic setting; without attention to these issues, attendance rates may remain low and the most troubled children may be unable to access services.

Interventions for Emotional Problems

There is a good deal of evidence from systematic reviews and randomized trials (Ollendick & King, 1998) to support the use of cognitive–behavioral interventions for anxiety and depression in school-age children, but few treatment trials include children under 5 years. However, there is some evidence from single-case studies and small trials (Ollendick & King, 1998) that the same techniques may be applied to 3- to 5-year-olds, provided the intervention is carefully matched to the children's developmental level. There is also important evidence emerging about cognitive–behavioral interventions from studies aimed primarily at helping preschool conduct problems, namely Webster-Stratton and Hammond's (1997) child-focused "Dinosaur" program. They find that cognitive–behavioral techniques, delivered using developmentally appropriate games and puppets, to groups of preschoolers, can reduce comorbid emotional symptoms as well as disruptive problems. Parental involvement in cognitive–behavioral interventions is useful in older children, especially where parents are very anxious, and may well prove to be helpful with younger children, pending further empirical validation (Barrett, Dadds, & Rapee, 1996). Chapter 63 describes detailed principles of cognitive–behavioral interventions for anxiety. These intervention principles can be adapted for the developmental level of preschoolers (Hirshfeld-Becker & Biederman, 2002); for example, using pictures to help with discussions about emotions, and by a greater focus on behavioral strategies, such as graded exposure and modeling to deal with phobias.

Interventions for Feeding Problems

Colic

A systematic review by Garrison and Christakis (2000) found 22 randomized trials of interventions for colic. Most trials were of poor quality, and the reviewers concluded that there was little clear evidence for efficacy of the various interventions tested. Medication did not appear to be effective; nor did infant carrying (although this has been found to be effective for other, less persistent forms of crying). There was slightly more promising support for helping parents to manage crying by reducing stimulation or improving communication skills, and some support for dietary interventions, including four small trials of hypoallergenic diets. Lactase was not effective. Because of methodological weaknesses, these results need to be treated with a great deal of caution, as putting infants on restricted diets, although potentially beneficial, could cause harm to the infant and unnecessary stress to the family. A recent trial of 600 neonates tested whether persistent crying could be prevented with behavioral interventions (St. James-Roberts & Gillham, 2001). Only modest effects on sleeping and crying were found, representing an increase of 10% in the number of babies sleeping through the night. Given the evidence from many trials suggesting that most interventions are ineffective for colic, including parental management strategies (e.g., carrying) and dietary change, advice needs to be based on reassurance and information, coupled with acknowledgment and management of parents' understandably high levels of stress. Parents can be advised that there are no significant long-term consequences of early colic, that it normally peaks around 6 weeks and stops at 3–4 months (Stifter & Wiggins, 2004; St. James-Roberts, 2004), and that the child is not ill, nor necessarily in pain.

Failure to Thrive

Intervention should aim to assess the contribution of parent management and child feeding skills to mealtime and food intake problems, in order to reduce tense cycles of coercive interaction that often prevail (Skuse, 1985). Direct observations of mealtime interaction (see chapter 19), ideally at home, may be particularly useful for analyzing factors that contribute to maintaining conflict over food. There is some evidence for effectiveness of parent-focused interventions from a small number of trials. Wright, Callum, Birks, and Jarvis' (1998) RCT of a primary care-based, health visitor-led multidisciplinary intervention for under-twos, involving dietary advice and some parent-management work, found positive effects on growth 1 year later compared to usual health visitor care. Black, Dubowitz, Hutcheson *et al.* (1995) found more mixed effects for a combined intervention involving clinic-based dietary advice and home-based parenting skills. For under-twos with non-organic FTT from low-income families, there were no effects on growth; rather, both intervention and control group children improved over the trial period. However, beneficial intervention effects were found in the quality of the home environment and on child language development, suggesting that such interventions may alleviate some of the concomitant psychosocial problems found with FTT.

Food Refusal

Careful assessment is needed to establish whether food refusal is linked to weight loss, and to reveal the situations in which it occurs, and in toddlers whether it is linked to other oppositional behaviors. In the latter case, feeding problems need to be assessed and managed in the context of other toddler non-compliant behaviors. If assessment reveals that parents are very anxious about food intake, then this may be a factor contributing to mealtime conflict (Stein & Barnes, 2002). Where appropriate, reassuring parents about physical health and growth of the child is important, coupled with advice on strategies for setting reasonable limits on the child and for reducing mealtime conflict (Douglas, 2002; Turner, Sanders, & Wall, 1994).

There is modest evidence of effectiveness of interventions for food refusal. No Cochrane or other rigorous systematic review was found. We can draw tentative conclusions from a narrative review by Kerwin (1999), which found two very small RCTs (Turner, Sanders, & Wall, 1994) and 27 single-case designs with quantitative outcome measurement, suggesting that behavioral parent management interventions may be effective. Searching did not reveal further RCTs since 1999. When dealing with food refusal and other problem behavior at mealtime in 2- to 5-year-olds, clinicians need to adapt the broad principles outlined for disruptive behavior. Additionally, it is important with mealtime problems to plan how to help eating to become a positive experience and how to reduce stress and conflict over food, particularly by taking a graduated approach to changing the specific problem. Douglas (2002) provided very helpful advice to clinicians. For example, to help food refusal and fussy eating, parents should cease force-feeding and angry responses, and instead take small steps to introduce new habits. It is important to switch to providing praise and attention for eating, and to reduce parents' natural response, which is to attend to a child when they refuse to eat. Where child anxiety appears to be factor, modeling pleasure in eating and even playing with food can be helpful in establishing enjoyment and reducing anxiety around meals. This may be particularly difficult for parents who feel very anxious around food and its mess, and they may need a good deal of support and encouragement to change (see chapter 27).

Conclusions

It will be apparent that the state of knowledge about preschool behavior problems is quite uneven. A good deal is known about preschool disruptive behavior, and about effective preventive and treatment interventions for this age group. This is particularly true for oppositional problems, and somewhat less so for ADHD. There is a growing literature on how interventions for early disruptive behavior that have been tested in specialized settings (i.e., "efficacy" trials) can be translated to other settings and cultures, and how they might be disseminated on a wider scale. In contrast, little is known about preschool emotional problems, with poor agreement on classification and little evidence about causes and treatment. To some extent, the same applies to childhood emotional disorders in general. This area should be a priority for future basic and treatment research, especially if it can be confirmed that these problems are stable and significant from an early age. Feeding problems have a longer history of treatment research, much of it from pediatric multidisciplinary teams, but work in this area is still hampered by lack of an agreed classification. Furthermore, understanding diagnosis and causes is complicated by great clinical variability in children who may have accompanying disabilities and developmental delays, combined with psychogenic feeding problems. At the younger end of the 0–5 range, in the specialty known as infant psychiatry, diagnosis is much more controversial and there is a need to establish validity or otherwise of categories and, eventually, effectiveness of treatments that follow from diagnosis. To further understand causal mechanisms, and to delineate the active ingredients of interventions in this age group, work is needed on intervention mechanisms, including gene–environment interactions (Caspi, McClay, Moffitt *et al.*, 2002), to address questions about whether interventions operate in different or similar ways in early childhood compared to older ages.

References

Achenbach, T. M. (1992). *Manual for the Child Behavior Checklist 2/3 and 1992 profile*. Burlington, VT: University of Vermont Department of Psychiatry.

American Psychiatric Association (APA). (2000). *Diagnostic and statistical manual for mental disorders* (4th edn.). Text Revision. Washington, DC: American Psychiatric Association.

Andersson, B-E. (1992). Effects of day-care on cognitive and socio-emotional competence of thirteen-year-old Swedish schoolchildren. *Child Development*, *63*, 20–36.

Appleyard, K., Egeland, B., van Dulmen, M., & Sroufe, A. (2005). When more is not better: The role of cumulative risk in child behavior outcomes. *Journal of Child Psychology and Psychiatry*, *46*, 235–245.

Angold, A., Costello, E. J., & Erkanli, A. (1999). Comorbidity. *Journal of Child Psychology and Psychiatry*, *40*, 57–87.

Barkley, R. (1997). Behavioral inhibition, sustained attention, and executive function: Constructing a unifying theory of ADHD. *Psychological Bulletin*, *121*, 65–94.

Barkley, R. (1998). *Attention-deficit hyperactivity disorder: A handbook for diagnosis and treatment*. New York: Guilford Press.

Barlow, J., & Stewart-Brown, S. (2000). Review article: Behavior problems and parent training programs. *Journal of Developmental and Behavioral Pediatrics*, *21*, 356–370.

Barr, R. G., St. James-Roberts, I., & Keefe, M. (2001). *New evidence on unexplained early infant crying*. Calverton, NY: Johnson & Johnson Pediatric Institute.

Barrett, P. M., Dadds, M.. & Rapee, R. (1996). Family treatment of childhood anxiety: A controlled trial. *Journal of Consulting and Clinical Psychology*, *64*, 333–342.

Bell, R. Q. (1968). A reinterpretation of the direction of effects in studies of socialization. *Psychological Review*, *75*, 81–95.

Benoit, D. (2000). Feeding disorders, failure to thrive, and obesity. In C. H. Zeanah Jr. (Ed.), *Handbook of infant mental health* (Vol. 2, pp. 339–352). NY: Guilford Press.

Biederman, J., Hirshfeld-Becker, D. R., Rosenbaum, J. F., Friedman, D., Snidman, N., Kagan, J., *et al.* (2001). Further evidence of association between behavioral inhibition and social anxiety in children. *American Journal of Psychiatry*, *158*, 1673–1679.

Black, M., Dubowitz, H., Hutcheson, J., Berenson-Howard, J., & Starr, R. (1995). Randomized clinical trial of home intervention for children with Failure to Thrive. *Pediatrics*, *95*, 807–814.

Boddy, J. M., & Skuse, D. (1994). Annotation: The process of parenting in failure to thrive. *Journal of Child Psychology and Psychiatry*, *35*, 401–424.

Campbell, S. B. (2002). *Behavior problems in preschool children: Clinical development issues*. New York/London: Guilford Press.

Campbell, S. B., Pierce, E. W., Moore, G., Marakovitz, S., & Newby, K. (1996). Boys' externalizing problems at elementary school: Pathways from early behavior problems, maternal control, and family stress. *Development and Psychopathology*, *8*, 701–720.

Campbell, S. B., Shaw, D. S., & Gilliom, M. (2000). Early externalizing behavior problems: Toddlers and preschoolers at risk for later maladjustment. *Development and Psychopathology*, *12*, 467–488.

Campbell, S. B., Szumowski, E. K., Ewing, L. J., Gluck, D. S., & Breaux, A. M. (1982). A multidimensional assessment of parent-identified behavior problem toddlers. *Journal of Abnormal Child Psychology*, *10*, 569–592.

Carter, A. S., Briggs-Gowan, M. J., & Davis, N. O. (2004). Assessment of young children's social-emotional development and psychopathology: Recent advances and recommendations for practice. *Journal of Child Psychology and Psychiatry*, *45*, 109–134.

Caspi, A., Henry, B., McGee, R. O., Moffitt, T., & Silva, P. A. (1995). Temperamental origins of child and adolescent behavior problems: From age three to age fifteen. *Child Development*, *66*, 55–68.

Caspi, A., McClay, J., Moffitt, T. E., Mill, J., Martin, J., Craig, I. W., *et al.* (2002). Role of genotype in the cycle of violence in maltreated children. *Science*, *297*, 851–854.

Chatoor, I., & Ganiban, J. (2004). The diagnostic assessment and classification of feeding disorders. In R. DelCarmen-Wiggins, & A. Carter (Eds.), *Handbook of infant, toddler, and preschool mental health assessment* (pp. 289–305). NY: Oxford University Press.

Crowcroft, N. S., & Strachan, D. P. (1997). The social origins of infantile colic: Questionnaire study covering 76,747 infants. *Bitish Medical Journal*, *314*, 1325–1328.

Dishion, T., & Kavanagh, K. (2003). *Intervening in adolescent problem behavior: A family-centered approach*. New York: Guilford Press.

Dishion, T. J., Shaw, D. S., Connell, A., Gardner, F., Wilson, M., & Weaver, C. (in press). The family check-up with high-risk indigent families: Preventing problem behaviour by increasing parents' positive behaviour support in early childhood. *Child Development*.

Douglas, J. (2002). Psychological treatment of food refusal in young children. *Child and Adolescent Mental Health*, *7*, 173–180.

Dunn, J. (1993). *Young children's relationships: Beyond attachment*. Newbury Park, CA: Sage.

Egger, H., & Angold, A. (2004). The Preschool age Psychiatric Assessment (PAPA): A structured parent interview for diagnosing disorders in preschool children. In R. DelCarmen-Wiggins, & A. Carter (Eds.), *Handbook of infant, toddler, and preschool mental health assessment* (pp. 223–243). NY: Oxford University Press.

Egger, H., & Angold, A. (2006). Common emotional and behavioral disorders in preschool children: Presentation, nosology and epidemiology. *Journal of Child Psychology and Psychiatry*, *47*, 313–337.

Eley, T. C., Bolton, D., O'Connor, T. G., Perrin, S., Smith, P., & Plomin, R. (2003). A twin study of anxiety-related behaviours in pre-school children. *Journal of Child Psychology and Psychiatry*, *44*, 945–960.

Feng, X., Shaw, D. S., Lane, T., Alarcon, J., & Skuban, E. (2006, July). *Positive and negative affectivity of mother-child dyads: Stability, mutual influence, and effects of maternal depression and child inhibition*. Presented at the biennial meeting of the International Society for the Study of Behavioral Development, Melbourne, Australia.

Forgatch, M., & DeGarmo, D. (1999). Parenting through change: An effective parenting training program for single mothers. *Journal of Consulting and Clinical Psychology*, *67*, 711–724.

Garcia, M., Shaw, D. S., Winslow, E. B., & Yaggi, K. (2000). Destructive sibling conflict and the development of conduct problems in young boys. *Developmental Psychology*, *36*, 44–53.

Gardner, F. (1994). The quality of joint activity between mothers and their children with conduct problems. *Journal of Child Psychology and Psychiatry*, *35*, 935–949.

Gardner, F., Sonuga-Barke, E., & Sayal, K. (1999). Parents anticipating misbehaviour: An observational study of strategies parents use to prevent conflict with behaviour problem children. *Journal of Child Psychology and Psychiatry*, *40*, 1185–1196.

Gardner, F., Ward, S., Burton, J., & Wilson, C. (2003). The role of mother–child joint play in the early development of children's conduct problems: A longitudinal observational study. *Social Development*, *12*, 361–379.

Gardner, F., Burton, J., & Klimes, I. (2006). Randomised controlled trial of a parenting intervention in the voluntary sector for reducing child conduct problems: Outcomes and mechanisms of change. *Journal of Child Psychology and Psychiatry*, *47*, 1123–1132.

Gardner, F., Shaw, D., Dishion, T., Burton, J., & Supplee, L. (2007). Randomized prevention trial for early conduct problems: Effects on proactive parenting and links to toddler disruptive behavior. *Journal of Family Psychology*, *21*, 398–406.

Garrison, M. M., & Christakis, D. A. (2000). A systematic review of treatments for infant colic. *Pediatrics*, *106*, 184–190.

Greenberg, M. T., Speltz, M. L., & DeKlyen, M. (1993). The role of attachment in the early development of disruptive behavior problems. *Development and Psychopathology*, *5*, 191–213.

Greenhill, L., Kollins, S., Abikoff, H., McCracken, J., Riddle, M., Swanson, J., *et al.* (2006). Efficacy and safety of immediate-release methylphenidate treatment for preschoolers with ADHD. *Journal of the American Academy of Child and Adolescent Psychiatry*, *45*, 1284–1293.

Hazell, P., O'Connell, D., Heathcote, D., & Henry D. (2002). Tricyclic drugs for depression in children and adolescents. *Cochrane Database of Systematic Reviews*. 2002, CD002317.

Henry, B., Caspi, A., Moffitt, T., & Silva, P. (1996). Temperamental and familial predictors of violent and nonviolent criminal convictions: Age 3 to age 18. *Developmental Psychology*, *32*, 614–623.

Hill, J. (2002). Biological, psychological and social processes in the conduct disorders. *Journal of Child Psychology and Psychiatry*, *43*, 133–165.

Hirshfeld-Becker, D. R., & Biederman, J. (2002). Rationale and principles for early intervention with young children at risk for anxiety disorders. *Clinical Child and Family Psychology Review*, *5*, 161–172.

Hirshfeld-Becker, D. R., Biederman, J., & Rosenbaum, J. F. (2004). Behavioral inhibition. In T. L. Morris, & J. S. March (Eds.), *Anxiety disorders in children and adolescents* (2nd edn., pp. 27–58). New York: Guilford Press.

Hutchings, J., Bywater, T., Daley, D., Gardner, F., Jones K., Eames, K., *et al.* (2007). Parenting intervention in Sure Start Services for children at risk of developing conduct disorder: A pragmatic randomised controlled trial. *British Medical Journal*, *31*, 678.

Hutchings, J., Lane, E., & Gardner, F. (2004). Making evidence-based interventions work. In Farrington, D., Sutton, C., & Utting, D. (Eds.), *Support from the start: Working with young children and families to reduce risks of crime and antisocial behaviour*. London: DFES.

Jenkins, S., Bax, M., & Hart, H. (1980). Behaviour problems in preschool children. *Journal of Child Psychology and Psychiatry*, *21*, 5–17.

Kagan, J. (1999). The concept of behavioral inhibition. In L. A. Schmidt, & J. Schulkin (Eds.), *Extreme fear, shyness, and social phobia: Origins, biological mechanisms, and clinical outcomes* (pp. 14–29). New York: Oxford University Press.

Kagan, J., Reznick, J. S., & Snidman, N. (1988). The physiology and psychology of behavioral inhibition in children. *Science*, *240*, 167–171.

Keenan, K., & Shaw, D. S. (1994). The development of aggression in toddlers: A study of low-income families. *Journal of Abnormal Child Psychology*, *22*, 53–77.

Keenan, K., Shaw, D. S., Walsh, B., Delliquadri, E., & Giovannelli, J. (1997). DSM-III-R disorders in preschoolers from low-income families. *Journal of the American Academy of Child and Adolescent Psychiatry*, *36*, 620–627.

Kerwin, M. (1999). Empiricially supported treatments in pediatric psychology: Severe feeding problems. *Journal of Pediatric Psychology*, *24*, 193–214.

Koot, H. M. (1993). *Problem behaviour in Dutch preschoolers*. Rotterdam: Erasmus University.

Lahey, B. B., Loeber, R., Quay, H. C., Frick, P. J., & Grimm, S. (1992). Oppositional defiant and conduct disorders: Issues to be resolved for DSM-IV. *Journal of the American Academy of Child and Adolescent Psychiatry*, *31*, 539–546.

Lavigne, J. V., Gibbons, R. D., Christoffel, K. K., Arend., R., Rosenbaum, D., Binns, H., *et al.* (1996). Prevalence rates and correlates of psychiatric disorders among preschool children. *Journal of the American Academy of Child and Adolescent Psychiatry*, *35*, 204–214.

Loeber, R., & Dishion, T. J. (1983). Early predictors of male delinquency: A review. *Psychological Bulletin*, *94*, 68–99.

Luby, J. L., Heffelfinger, A. K., Mrakotsky, C., Hessler, M. J., Brown, K. & Hildebrand, T. (2002). Preschool major depressive disorder (MDD): Preliminary validation for developmentally modified DSM-IV criteria. *Journal of the American Academy of Child and Adolescent Psychiatry*, *41*, 928–937.

Luby, J. L., Heffelfinger, A. K., Mrakotsky, C., Brown, K., Hessler, M., Wallis, J., *et al.* (2003). The clinical picture of depression in preschool children. *Journal of the American Academy of Child and Adolescent Psychiatry*, *42*, 340–348.

Lyons-Ruth, K. (1996). Attachment relationships among children with aggressive behavior problems: The role of disorganized early attachment patterns. *Journal of Consulting and Clinical Psychology*, *64*, 572–585.

Martin, J. (1981). A longitudinal study of the consequences of early mother–infant interaction: A microanalytic approach. *Monographs of the Society for Research in Child Development*, *46*.

Mindell, J. A. (1999). Empirically supported treatments in pediatric psychology: Bedtime refusal and night wakings in young children. *Journal of Pediatric Psychology*, *24*, 465–481.

Moffitt, T. E. (1990). Juvenile delinquency and Attention Deficit Disorder: Boys' developmental trajectories from age 3 to age 15. *Child Development*, *61*, 893–910.

Montgomery, P., Bjornstad, G., & Dennis, J. (2006). Media-based behavioural treatments for behavioural problems in children. *Cochrane Database of Systematic Reviews*, CD002206.

NICHD Early Child Care Research Network. (2003). Does the amount of time spent in child care predict socioemotional adjustment during the transition to kindergarten? *Child Development*, *74*, 976–1005.

Olds, D. (2002). Prenatal and infancy home visiting by nurses: From randomized trials to community replication. *Prevention Science*, *3*, 153–172.

Ollendick, T. H., & King, N. J. (1998). Empirically supported treatments for children with phobic and anxiety disorders: current status. *Journal of Clinical Child Psychology and Psychiatry*, *27*, 156–167.

Patterson, G. R. (1982). *A social learning approach: 3. Coercive family process*. Eugene, OR: Castalia.

Ramchandani, P., Wiggs, L., Webb, V., & Stores, G. (2000). A systematic review of treatments for settling problems and night waking in young children. *British Medical Journal*, *320*, 209–213.

Reid, M. J., Webster-Stratton, C., & Beauchaine, T. (2001). Parent training in Head Start: A comparison of program response among African American, Asian American, Caucasian, and Hispanic mothers. *Prevention Science*, *2*, 209–227.

Reilly, S. M., Skuse, D. H., Wolke, D., & Stevenson, J. (1999). Oral–motor dysfunction of children who fail to thrive: Organic or non-organic? *Developmental Medicine and Child Neurology*, *41*, 115–122.

Richman, M., Stevenson, J., & Graham, P. J. (1982). *Preschool to school: A behavioral study*. London: Academic Press.

Rose, S. L., Rose, S. A., & Feldman, J. F. (1989). Stability of behavior problems in very young children. *Development and Psychopathology*, *1*, 5–19.

Rothbart, M. K., Ellis, L. K., Rueda, M. R., & Posner, M. I. (2003). Developing mechanisms of temperamental effortful control. *Journal of Personality*, *71*, 1113–1143.

Rutter, M. (2005). Environmentally mediated risks for psychopathology: Research strategies and findings. *Journal of the American Academy of Child and Adolescent Psychiatry*, 44, 3–18.

Sameroff, A. J., & Chandler, M. J. (1975). Reproductive risk and the continuum of caretaking casualty. In F. D. Horowitz (Ed.), *Review of child development research* (Vol. 4., pp. 187–241). Chicago: University of Chicago Press.

Sanders, M. R. (2004). *Every parent: A positive approach to children's behaviour* (2nd edn.). Melbourne: Penguin.

Sanders, M. R., Markie-Dadds, C., Tully, L., & Bor, W. (2000). The Triple P Positive Parenting Program: A comparison of enhanced, standard, and self-directed behavioral family intervention. *Journal of Consulting and Clinical Psychology*, *68*, 624–640.

Scott, S., Spender, Q., Doolan, M., Jacobs, B., & Aspland, H. C. (2001). Multicentre controlled trial of parenting groups for childhood antisocial behaviour in clinical practice. *British Medical Journal*, *323*, 194–203.

Shaw, D. S., & Bell, R. Q. (1993). Developmental theories of parental contributors to antisocial behavior. *Journal of Abnormal Child Psychology*, *21*, 493–518.

Shaw, D. S., Gilliom, M., & Giovannelli, J. (2000). Aggressive behavior disorders. In C. H. Zeanah (Ed.), *Handbook of infant mental health* (2nd edn., pp. 397–411). New York: Guilford.

Shaw, D. S., Gilliom, M., Ingoldsby, E. M., & Nagin, D. (2003). Trajectories leading to school-age conduct problems. *Developmental Psychology*, *39*, 189–200.

Shaw, D.S., Keenan, K., & Vondra, J. I. (1994). Developmental precursors of externalizing behavior: Ages 1 to 3. *Developmental Psychology*, *30*, 355–364.

Shaw, D. S., Lacourse, E., & Nagin, D. (2005). Developmental trajectories of conduct problems and hyperactivity from ages 2 to 10. *Journal of Child Psychology and Psychiatry*, *46*, 931–942.

Shaw, D. S., Winslow, E. B., Owens, E. B., & Hood, N. (1998). Young children's adjustment to chronic family adversity: A longitudinal study of low-income families. *Journal of the American Academy of Child and Adolescent Psychiatry*, *37*, 545–553.

Shaw, D. S., Dishion, T. J., Supplee, L., Gardner, F., & Arnds, K. (2006). Randomized trial of a family-centered approach to the prevention of early conduct problems: 2-year effects of the family check-up in early childhood. *Journal of Consulting and Clinical Psychology*, *74*, 1–9.

Skuse, D. (1985). Non-organic failure to thrive: A reappraisal. *Archives of Disease in Childhood*, *60*, 173–178.

Skuse, D., Reilly, S., & Wolke, D. (1994). Psychosocial adversity and growth during infancy. *European Journal of Clinical Nutrition*, *48*, 113–130.

Sonuga-Barke, E. J., Daley, D., Thompson, M., Laver-Bradbury, C., & Weeks, A. (2001). Parent-based therapies for preschool attention-deficit/hyperactivity disorder: A randomized controlled trial with a community sample. *Journal of the American Academy of Child and Adolescent Psychiatry*, *40*, 402–408.

Sroufe, L. A. (1997). Psychopathology as an outcome of development. *Development and Psychopathology*, *9*, 251–268.

Stein, A., & Barnes, J. (2002). Feeding and sleeping disorders. In M. Rutter, & E. Taylor (Eds.), *Child and adolescent psychiatry: Modern approaches* (4th edn.). Oxford, UK: Blackwell.

Stewart-Brown, S., Patterson, J., Mockford, C., Barlow, J., Klimes, I., & Pyper, C. (2004). Impact of a general practice-based group parenting programme: Quantitative and qualitative results from a controlled trial at 12 months. *Archives of Disease in Childhood*, *89*, 519–525.

Stifter, C. A., & Wiggins, C. N. (2004). Assessment of disturbances in emotion regulation and temperament. In R. DelCarmen-Wiggins, & A. Carter (Eds.), *Handbook of infant, toddler, and preschool mental health assessment* (pp. 70–103). NY: Oxford University Press.

St. James-Roberts, I. (2004). Effective services for managing infant crying disorders and their impact on the social and emotional development of young children. In R. Tremblay, R. Barr, & R. Peters (Eds.), *Encyclopedia on early childhood development* [online]. Montreal, Quebec: Centre of Excellence for Early Childhood Development 1–6. Accessed December 2, 2006 from http://www.excellence-earlychildhood.ca/documents/StJames-RobertANGxp.pdf

St. James-Roberts, I., & Gillham, P. (2001). Use of a behavioural programme in the first 3 months to prevent infant crying and sleeping problems. *Journal of Paediatrics and Child Health*, *37*, 289–297.

Sutton, C. (1999). *Helping families with troubled children: A preventive approach.* Chichester: Wiley.

Task Force on Research Diagnostic Criteria. (2003). Research diagnostic criteria for infants and preschool children: The process and empirical support. *Journal of the American Academy of Child and Adolescent Psychiatry*, *42*, 1504–1512.

Thomas, A., Chess, S., & Birch, H. H. (1968). *Temperament and behavior disorders in children.* New York: New York University Press.

Thompson, M., Weeks, C., & Laver-Bradbury, C. (1999). *Information manual for professionals working with families with hyperactive children aged 2–9 years.* Hampshire, UK: Ashurst Child and Family Guidance Centre.

Tremblay, R. (2000). The development of aggressive behavior during childhood: What have we learned in the past century? *International Journal of Behavioral Development*, *24*, 129–141.

Tremblay, R. E., Nagin, D. S., Seguin, J. R., Zoccolillo, M., Zelazo, P., Boivin, M., *et al.* (2004). Physical aggression during early childhood: Trajectories and predictors. *Pediatrics*, *114*, 43–50.

Turner, K., & Sanders, M. (2006). Help when it's needed first: a controlled evaluation of brief, preventive behavioural family intervention in a primary care setting. *Behavior Therapy*, *37*, 131–142.

Turner, K. M. T., Sanders, M. R., & Wall, C. R. (1994). Behavioural parent training versus dietary education in the treatment of children with persistent feeding difficulties. *Behaviour Change*, *11*, 242–258.

Votruba-Drzal, E., Coley, R. L., & Chase-Landsdale, P. L. (2004). Child care and low-income children's development: Direct and moderated effects. *Child Development*, *75*, 296–312.

Webster-Stratton, C. (1998a). Preventing conduct problems in Head Start children: Strengthening parenting competencies. *Journal of Consulting and Clinical Psychology*, *66*, 715–730.

Webster-Stratton, C. (1998b). Parent training with low-income clients: Promoting parental engagement through a collaborative approach. In J. Lutzker (Ed.), *Handbook of child abuse research and treatment* (pp. 183–210). NY: Plenum.

Webster-Stratton, C. (1992). *The incredible years: A trouble-shooting guide for parents of children ages 3–8 years.* Toronto: Umbrella Press.

Webster-Stratton, C., & Hammond, M. (1997). Treating children with early-onset conduct problems: A comparison of child and parent training interventions. *Journal of Consulting and Clinical Psychology*, *65*, 93–109.

Webster-Stratton, C., & Herbert, M. (1994). *Troubled families – problem children. Working with parents: A collaborative process.* Chichester: Wiley.

Weiss, G., & Hechtman, L. T. (1993). *Hyperactive children grown up: ADHD in children, adolescents and adults* (2nd edn.). New York: Guilford Press.

Wessel, M. A., Cobb, J. C., Jackson, E. B., Harris, G. S., & Detwiler, A. C. (1954). Paroxysmal fussing in infancy, sometimes called "colic". *Pediatrics*, *14*, 421–434.

Whittington, C., Kendall, T., Fonagy, P., Cottrell, D., Cotgrove, A., & Boddington, E. (2004). Selective serotonin reuptake inhibitors in childhood depression: Systematic review of published versus unpublished data. *Lancet*, *363*, 1341–1345.

Widom, C. S., & Ames, M. A. (1994). Criminal consequences of childhood sexual victimization. *Child Abuse & Neglect*, *18*, 303–318.

Wright, C. M, Callum, J., Birks, E., & Jarvis, S. (1998). Effect of community based management in failure to thrive: Randomised controlled trial. *British Medical Journal*, *317*, 571–574.

Zero to Three. (1994). *Diagnostic classification: 0–3. Diagnostic classification of mental health and developmental disorders of infancy and early childhood.* Arlington, VA: National Center for Clinical Infant Program.

54 Sleep Disorders

Ronald E. Dahl and Allison G. Harvey

Sleep problems occur frequently in children and adolescents – particularly among youth with behavioral and/or emotional disorders. Moreover, difficulties related to sleep often overlap with psychiatric problems, making sleep an important domain of symptoms relevant to the diagnosis and treatment of psychopathology. For example, sleep difficulties are a common symptom of depression and improving sleep can contribute positively to the management of mood disorders (Dahl, 1996a,b). A second example is illustrated by the way sleep deprivation can create irritability and difficulties with focused attention that mimic or exacerbate symptoms of attention deficit/hyperactivity disorder (ADHD) and improvements in sleep can have a positive impact on attentional functioning (Chervin, Archbold, Dillon *et al.*, 2002; Dahl, Pelham, & Wierson, 1991). Thus, not only is a knowledge about the assessment, diagnosis and treatment of sleep problems in youth an important clinical domain, but acquiring a solid knowledge of sleep – including its development and disorders – provides a critical foundation of expertise relevant to understanding (and effectively intervening in) a broad range of clinical problems in child and adolescent psychiatry.

At a pragmatic level, pediatric sleep problems in children range from highly specific disorders such as narcolepsy where the pathophysiology involves alterations in specific neural systems underpinning sleep–wake regulation to simple behavioral difficulties such as bedtime resistance and late erratic schedules (for estimates of prevalence rates see Table 54.1). However, it is important to recognize that even simple and seemingly minor behavioral sleep problems can become a source of major distress and conflict in children and their families, and these can have serious health consequences. There is increasing evidence that sleep has an important role in basic aspects of learning and memory consolidation as well as impacting on the regulation of behavior and emotions. Therefore, inadequate or disturbed sleep in childhood and adolescence may have long-term consequences on learning and the development of self-regulation that have major clinical implications for child and adolescent psychiatry – crucial questions at the forefront of current research.

For the clinician wanting to provide effective prevention, diagnosis and treatment of sleep problems or appropriate referral for the evaluation of more serious disorders, knowledge and clinical skills are needed in four areas:

1 Understanding normal sleep physiology and the normal development of sleep patterns in children and adolescents.

2 Knowledge of common sleep disorders, including aspects of the etiology, pathophysiology and differential diagnoses for common symptoms.

3 Clinical skills and knowledge relevant to assessing sleep habits and symptoms and diagnosing sleep disorders.

4 Knowledge of the relevant treatment principles – particularly behavioral interventions.

Accordingly, in this chapter we provide an overview of sleep physiology, organization and function, including emerging findings on the role of sleep in learning and regulatory control in the developing brain, and discuss five key examples of sleep disorders in youth, including assessment, diagnosis and approach to treatment.

Physiology, Organization and the Function of Sleep during Human Development

Beginning in infancy, the brain cycles through stages of neural activity/behavioral states which correspond to periods of wakefulness and different stages of sleep. Sleep is divided into two major categories: rapid eye movement (REM) sleep and non-REM (NREM) sleep. REM sleep is characterized by high levels of desynchronized cortical electroencephalogram (EEG) activity (mixed frequencies, relatively low voltage), absence of muscle tone, irregular heart rate and respiratory patterns, and episodic bursts of phasic eye movements. NREM sleep is characterized by low-frequency, high-voltage EEG activity, low muscle tone and absence of eye movements. NREM sleep is subdivided into four stages: stage 1 occurs at transitions of sleep and wakefulness; stage 2 is characterized by frequent bursts of rhythmic EEG activity, called sleep spindles, and high-voltage slow spikes, called K-complexes; stages 3 and 4 (also called slow wave sleep [SWS] or delta sleep), represent the deepest stages of sleep and are comprised largely of high-voltage EEG activity in the slowest (delta) frequency range.

Two independent regulatory processes appear to interact in regulating the timing, intensity and duration of sleep: a *homeostatic sleep process* and a *circadian sleep process* (Borbély, 1982; Borbély & Achermann, 2005). The first, often called

Rutter's Child and Adolescent Psychiatry, 5th edition. Edited by M. Rutter, D. Bishop, D. Pine, S. Scott, J. Stevenson, E. Taylor and A. Thapar. © 2008 Blackwell Publishing, ISBN: 978-1-4051-4549-7.

Table 54.1 Prevalence estimates for sleep disturbance in children and adolescents.

Sleep disorder or behavior	Prevalence estimate (%)	Reference
Behavioral insomnia of children (including bedtime refusals and night wakings)	10–30	AASM (2005)
Sleep talking	55	Owens *et al.* (2003)
Bruxism	28	Owens *et al.* (2003)
Night terrors	17	Owens *et al.* (2003)
Rhythmic movements	17	Owens *et al.* (2003)
Confusional arousals	17	Littner *et al.* (2005)
Sleepwalking	14	Owens *et al.* (2003)
Nightmares	10–50	Sheldon *et al.* (2005)
Insomnia		
Children	1–6	AASM (2005)
Adolescents	11	Hoban & Chervin (2005)
Delayed sleep phase	7–17	Lu, Manthena & Zee (2006)
Restless leg syndrome/PLMD	1–17	Chervin *et al.* (2002)
Narcolepsy	0.05	Dauvilliers *et al.* (2003)

AASM, American Academy of Sleep Medicine; PLMD, period limb movement disorder.

"Process S," represents a sleep–wake dependent homeostatic component of sleep that increases as a function of previous wakefulness and gradually decreases over the course of a sleep period. Process S has been associated with basic restorative processes of the brain. Intriguing from a developmental neuroscience perspective is the recent evidence that sleep homeostasis is involved in learning and neural plasticity – the progressive strengthening of neural circuits that occurs through use during wakefulness (Tononi & Cirelli, 2003, 2006). It appears that the progressive increase in synaptic strength from daytime activity must be "downscaled" during sleep to maintain synaptic homeostasis. This homeostatic aspect of sleep also appears to correlate with the deep stages 3 and 4 (slow-wave) sleep, which is particularly strong early in development.

The second process, often called "Process C," is the circadian or "biological clock" component. The neurobehavioral underpinnings of this circadian system have been well delineated, including the identification of specific neuroanatomical and molecular components (Carskadon, Acebo, & Jenni, 2004).

From a developmental perspective, both the homeostatic and the circadian processes undergo significant maturational changes (Jenni & LeBourgeois, 2006). Some of these developmental changes have important clinical implications. For example, the circadian phase marker, melatonin, correlates with pubertal stage such that more mature adolescents show a delay in the melatonin excretion pattern, even after controlling for psychosocial influences on sleep–wake patterns in adolescence (Carskadon, 2002). This contributes to the tendency to stay up later and sleep in later among adolescents (see p. 898). Furthermore, evidence is accumulating that the dynamics of sleep homeostatic processes slow down over the course of childhood (i.e., sleep pressure accumulates more slowly with increasing age), enabling children to be awake for consolidated periods during the day (Jenni & Carskadon, 2005; Jenni & LeBourgeois, 2006).

Recent progress in understanding the neural mechanisms involved in key aspects of the basic regulation of sleep and wakefulness (Saper, Cano, & Scammell, 2005; Saper, Scammell, & Lu, 2005) has focused on complex interactions across a number of different cell groups involved in cortical arousal, with a key part being played by sleep-inducing structures in the ventrolateral preoptic nucleus in the hypothalamus. These regulatory systems are becoming understood in greater detail in ways that are likely to inform clinically relevant aspects of sleep problems. Two specific examples discussed briefly include the role of *sleep in learning* and *sleep and emotion regulation.*

Sleep, Learning and the Developing Brain

One of the most intriguing lines of sleep research with clinical relevance to child and adolescent psychiatry is the growing understanding of the role of sleep in the consolidation of learning (Hobson & Pace-Schott, 2002; Peigneux, Laureys, Delbeuck, & Maquet, 2001; Stickgold, 2005; Stickgold & Walker, 2005; Walker & Stickgold, 2004). A central hypothesis is that sleep facilitates brain plasticity – the ability to constantly modify cerebral structures and functions depending on specific experience and environmental inputs. This view is supported by studies showing impaired memory consolidation following episodes with sleep loss (Pilcher & Huffcut, 1996), and recently there have been findings suggesting such a link at the cellular and molecular levels (Benington & Frank, 2003; Steriade, 1999). Studies have shown the influence of sleep on post-training consolidation, as well as initial memory encoding (Walker & Stickgold, 2006). One recent study demonstrated that sleep can enhance specific components of language learning in infants (Gomez, Bootzin, & Nadel, 2006).

These data indicate that adequate sleep may be essential to making enduring neural changes through learning. This role of sleep in learning may be particularly important during periods of rapid brain maturation in childhood and adolescence.

These findings have implications regarding the importance of sleep to educational goals as well as clinical relevance, because learning (and its consolidation) underpins many clinical interventions such as cognitive–behavioral therapy.

Sleep and Emotion Regulation

Over the past decade there has been increasing interest in understanding the bidirectional relationships between sleep disturbances and problems with emotion regulation in children and adolescents. There is growing evidence that problems with sleep can create and/or exacerbate emotional problems and that emotional difficulties can interfere with sleep. These bidirectional interactions (and the potential for a vicious cycle of negative effects) may have particular clinical relevance in several clinical domains including anxiety, depression and bipolar disorders in youth (Dahl, 1996a; Harvey, Mullin & Hinshaw, 2006) and with aggression, anger and impulse control (Haynes, Bootzin, Smith *et al.*, 2006).

With respect to sleep and mood, evidence from the sleep deprivation literature suggests that one of the strongest adverse effects of sleep deprivation is increased negative mood (Dinges, Pack, Williams *et al.*, 1997; Pilcher & Huffcutt, 1996; Van Dongen, Maislin, Mullington, & Dinges, 2003). This makes sense given evidence suggesting that REM sleep has an emotional processing and mood regulation function (Stickgold, Hobson, Fosse, & Fosse, 2001). In adults with bipolar disorder, the case for sleep contributing to mood disturbance is fairly compelling: sleep loss is highly correlated with daily manic symptoms (Barbini, Bertelli, Colombo, & Smeraldi, 1996); among patients with bipolar disorder, sleep disturbance is the most common prodrome of mania and the sixth most common prodrome of depression (Jackson, Cavanagh, & Scott, 2003); and induced sleep deprivation triggers hypomania or mania in a proportion of patients (Colombo, Benedetti, Barbini, Campori, & Smeraldi, 1999; Kasper & Wehr, 1992; Leibenluft, Albert, Rosenthal, & Wehr, 1996; Wehr, Sack, & Rosenthal, 1987; Wu & Bunney, 1990; Zwi, Shawe-Taylor, & Murray, 2005). In youth with bipolar disorder, rates of significant sleep disturbance range from 35 to 45% (for review see Harvey, Mullin, & Hinshaw, 2006). However, in these younger samples, research and clinical questions relating to a possible link between sleep disturbance and mood are yet to be addressed.

With respect to sleep and aggression, there are both human and animal data showing increased aggression and impulsivity following experimental sleep loss. For example, rats show increases in aggression and defensive fighting after sleep deprivation. One recent study found that animals who were easy to handle at baseline became irritable and aggressive following modest amounts of sleep deprivation, with evidence of related changes in synaptic plasticity associated with these behavioral changes (Marks & Wayner, 2005). Clinical studies of children and adolescents also have revealed associations between sleep deprivation and irritability/aggression and difficulties with self-regulation in youth (Chervin, Dillon, Archbold, & Ruzicka, 2003; Dahl, 1996b; Ireland & Culpin, 2005). Most relevant is a recent study by Haynes, Bootzin, Smith *et al.* (2006) which examined behavioral and emotional changes in adolescents with substance-related difficulties undergoing a behavioral sleep treatment. This study reported that improvements in sleep time were associated with significant decreases in the reporting of aggressive thoughts and actions. Taken together, these data suggest that inadequate sleep in adolescence may contribute to aggressive thoughts and actions and that increased or improved sleep may reduce problematic aggression, at least in some cases.

While the clinical *research* questions about the interrelationships between sleep and emotional regulation in children are compelling, it is also important to acknowledge that from a clinical *practice* perspective, traditional polysomnographic studies have not yielded clear evidence of specific sleep abnormalities associated with particular psychopathologies in youth (e.g., ADHD, major depressive disorder [MDD]). Thus, polysomnographic studies are best utilized clinically when a specific sleep disorder is suspected.

Genetic Contributions

To date, scant attention has been paid to investigations of possible genetic contributions to sleep disturbance in children and adolescents. The exception is a study by Gruber, Grizenko, Schwartz *et al.* (2006), who investigated the hypothesis that the catecholamine-O-methyltransferase (COMT) polymorphism modulates disturbance in children with ADHD. Sleep was measured over 2 weeks with actigraphy. The rationale for investigating COMT is its association with sleep in narcolepsy and Parkinson's disease and disorders related to dopamine dysfunction. Gruber, Grizenko, Schwartz *et al.* found that children who had the COMT high-activity allele, val (i.e., val/val or val/met) exhibited greater sleep disturbance compared with children who were met homozygous genotypes (i.e., met/met). The authors interpreted these findings as adding to the accruing evidence base suggesting that sleep disturbance is core to the pathology underpinning ADHD and that there may be a genetic basis for the association between ADHD and sleep disturbance.

Specific Clinical Problems

Problems Going to Sleep and Staying Asleep

Bedtime struggles and middle of the night wakings are not only a source of sleep disruption for children and their parents, but also can be a source of conflict and negative emotion among family members, contributing to negative parent–child interactions, marital discord and, in some rare cases, child abuse. One aspect of the difficulty is that young children often show a "paradoxical" reaction when obtaining insufficient or inadequate sleep. That is, sleep-deprived young children (whether from insufficient or disrupted sleep) often look irritable and impulsive, with some symptoms of distractibility and emotional lability, and may seem overly active. The three most important principles for treating bedtime resistance in young children are: (i) creating an emotional state of calmness and safety; (ii) consistent limit setting; and (iii) establishing good habits. Bedtime habits include a wind-down period and a sequence of activities that begin 30–60 min before bedtime. If a child continues to test limits and not to respond to strategies to reward desirable behaviors, it may become necessary to set consequences for the undesirable behaviors. However, this can still be done within a positive framework to avoid the escalating emotional arousals of yelling, screaming and flaring tempers.

Insomnia is a common complaint among older children and adolescents, particularly sleep-onset insomnia. Two theoretical perspectives are helpful for conceptualizing insomnia in children and adolescents. First, a vigilance–avoidance model has particular relevance to understanding sleep problems in childhood and adolescence (Dahl, 1996b). At the most fundamental level, sleep and vigilance represent *opponent* processes. Physiologically, going to sleep *requires* turning-off awareness and responsiveness to threats in the external environment. Because of this loss of vigilance and responsiveness, sleep is naturally restricted to "safe" times and places (e.g., animals and birds tend to sleep in safe burrows, nests or temporal niches that minimize dangers). In humans, one important domain for assessing the safe conditions that permit and promote sleep focuses on *social and emotional appraisals of threat* (Dahl, 1996b; Worthman & Melby, 2002). Individuals experiencing high levels of anxiety, vigilance and perceived threats often have difficulties going to sleep. While these tendencies have adaptive advantages (inhibiting sleep in truly dangerous environments), they also have costs: high levels of anxiety and vigilance based on *perceived* threats can lead to chronic sleep difficulties. A major source of difficulty for children and adolescents is rooted in presleep onset worries and ruminative thinking at bedtime – which naturally increase vigilance and interfere with going to sleep. Yet, it can be equally problematic if anxious youth *avoid* these distressing bedtime worries by staying up (or getting back out of bed) to engage in very late hours of school work, watching TV or socializing (via the Internet or cell phones). These patterns of behavior often lead to difficulty getting to sleep until very late on school nights and thus insufficient sleep because of the need to get up early for school. Without effective intervention, this pattern of vigilance and avoidance can lead to extremely problematic sleep habits and patterns in adolescents with anxiety disorders.

Second, a conditioning model of insomnia (Bootzin, 1979; Perlis, Giles, Mendelson, Bootzin, & Wyatt, 1997) emphasizes the contribution to insomnia of multiple pairings of the bed and not sleeping. This set of associations likely results in conditioning between the bedroom environment and heightened arousal, which serves to maintain the sleep disturbance.

The initial assessment of youth with insomnia should start with a thorough clinical interview with the patient and their family members to obtain information about the duration, frequency and severity of night-time sleep disturbance, including estimates of the key sleep parameters: sleep onset latency (SOL), number of awakenings after sleep onset (NWAKE), total amount of time awake after sleep onset (WASO), total sleep time (TST) and an estimate of sleep quality (SQ). This information should encompass both weekday and weekend schedules and should assess the regularity of the schedule as well as the average schedule. The onset and duration of the insomnia and type of symptoms (i.e., sleep onset, sleep maintenance, early morning or late morning awaking problem or combinations of these) should be assessed. A description of the daytime correlates and consequences of insomnia is a key domain of importance as is gauging parental responses to the insomnia. In addition, it is crucial to obtain information about medications (prescription and over-the-counter) and conduct a screen for the presence of psychiatric disorders and medical problems (including other sleep disorders). Asking the patient to complete a sleep diary each morning, as soon as possible after waking, for 1–2 weeks provides a wealth of information including an insight into the night-to-night variability in sleeping difficulty and sleep–wake patterns and the presence of circadian rhythm disorders, such as delayed sleep phase disorder. An assessment of insomnia in youth should include an exploration of the child's fears, because fear, distress or any cognitive or emotional cue that prevents an overall sense of safety can be antithetical to sleep (because sleep onset requires turning off awareness, responsiveness and vigilance). Children and adolescents can often get into the habit of mentally reviewing or replaying worrisome thoughts or memories of stressful events. Some youth with stressful memories or specific fears manage to avoid these during the day through distracting activities, but at night – especially when trying to fall asleep – the lack of distracters can result in rumination on these thoughts.

The treatment principles are threefold. First, helping the child *feel* emotionally and physically safe is often a critical component. (The emphasis on the word feel is because the affective appraisal of being safe appears to be extremely important for some youth – they may logically understand the absence of specific threats but unless they have an emotional sense of safety they may experience heightened vigilance that interferes with sleep.) Depending on the age and inclinations of the child, this can involve creative imagery, self-hypnosis techniques or systematic relaxation exercises. In addition, parents are encouraged to contribute to an emotional sense of safety, positive emotions and good associations at bedtime.

The second treatment principle is to establish a regular bedtime routine and consistent sequences of steps and habits. In children, this can involve a bedtime story, special quiet time with the parent and pleasant wind-down time. In adolescence, multiple sleep-interfering factors (e.g., cell phones, the Internet) interact with the pubertal phase delay in the circadian system causing a tendency to shift toward later bedtimes and increased autonomy to decide on bedtimes. Hence, the intervention is to identify sleep-interfering behaviors and work collaboratively with the young person to assist them to find internal motivations for enhancing their sleep by reducing the use of sleep-interfering technologies around bedtime. In addition, derived from the conditioning theory just discussed, there is preliminary evidence that the stimulus control intervention that has been so successful for adult insomnia (Morin, Bootzin, Buysse *et al.*, 2006) can also be helpful for youth (Bootzin & Stevens, 2005). The therapist provides a detailed rationale for and assists the patient to achieve the following:

1 Use the bed and bedroom only for sleep (i.e., no TV watching or text messaging).

2 Get out of bed and go to another room whenever you are unable to fall asleep or return to sleep within approximately 15–20 min and return to bed only when sleepy again.

3 Arise in the morning at the same time (no later than plus 2 hours on weekends) and gradually move closer to a regular schedule 7 days a week.

Third, based on the vigilance–avoidance model, there is a clear need to address bedtime worry, rumination and vigilance (Dahl, 2002). Interventions for worry and rumination include: diary writing or scheduling a "worry period" to encourage the processing of worries several hours prior to bedtime, creating a "to do" list prior to getting into bed to reduce worrying about future plans or events, training to disengage from presleep worry and redirect attention to pleasant (distracting) imagery, demonstrating the adverse consequences of thought suppression while in bed and scheduling a presleep "wind-down" period prior to bedtime.

The Adolescent with Daytime Sleepiness/ Difficulty Waking up for School

After the onset of puberty and throughout the adolescent period, the most prevalent sleep complaints tend to center on difficulty waking up for school in the morning and the associated difficulties with daytime sleepiness, tiredness and irritability. It is important to emphasize that there is a broad continuum of severity. This ranges from normative or mild difficulties that appear to affect up to half of all high-school students in the USA and result in at least some symptoms (National Sleep Foundation, 2006), to a much smaller subset of adolescents with severe difficulties with sleep and schedules that result in significant impairments (such as failures in school) and often meet full criteria for a delayed sleep phase syndrome (DSPS). At the current time, there is an absence of empirical data to help delineate precisely when to diagnose adolescents as having DSPS from the much larger set of youth with mild to moderate problems with erratic and late sleep schedules.

One pragmatic approach advocated in this chapter is that clinicians understand both the physiological and social influences that contribute to these problems, and apply sound behavioral principles aimed at improving and increasing sleep in any adolescent who shows evidence of suboptimal sleep as a result of late nights and erratic schedules. In other words, many of the simple behavioral interventions to regularize sleep–wake schedules and increase total sleep can be tried even in the case of mild to moderate problems (because these interventions have little to no risks or side effects and can result in improved alertness as well as improved mood regulation).

It is important to understand the interaction between biological and social processes underpinning these common problems. Biological changes in the circadian system at puberty shift sleep timing preferences in the direction of *delayed sleep phase* (Carskadon, 2005; Lee, Hummer, & Jechura, 2004). Unfortunately, these biological changes interact with early school start times, increase in paid work responsibilities and increased amounts of time devoted to socializing in a way that can spiral quickly into a pattern of extreme sleep deprivation. Then most "catch-up" sleep occurs on weekends and holidays on an extremely phase-delayed schedule. The human circadian system adapts more easily to phase delays as endogenous rhythms of body temperature and neuroendocrine function are able to reset quickly to later bed and wake times. However, the circadian system has more difficulty accommodating to phase advances (*earlier* sleep schedules). This creates an effect that is a bit like "jet-lag" on Monday morning; students try to adjust to a sudden phase advance in which they need to get up for school at a time that is often 3–4 hours (or more) earlier than their biological clock "expects" to wake up.

A thorough and detailed history is essential to evaluate and to characterize the nature of the sleepiness. This should include an assessment of whether the young person is fatigued or unable to stay awake, the frequency and duration of symptoms and whether the symptoms occur at particular times of day or only in certain situations. A family history of increased sleep needs and sleepiness can be important in the consideration of narcolepsy.

In adolescents with true sleepiness (not simply complaints of fatigue), two main categories of problems should be considered:

1 Inadequate amounts of sleep; and

2 Circadian and scheduling disorders.

Inadequate Amounts of Sleep

The most common cause of mild to moderate sleepiness in adolescents is an inadequate number of hours in bed. A combination of social schedules leading to late nights with early morning school requirements can significantly compress the number of hours of sleep. Part-time jobs, sports activities, hobbies and active social lives can exacerbate this problem. The catch-up sleep of naps, weekends and holidays can also contribute to the problem by leading to erratic schedules and even later nights. In taking a sleep history, it is important to ask specific questions about bedtime schedules. Many families will say the adolescent "usually" goes to bed at a certain time, but when asked for an exact time covering the previous few nights, a much later hour is reported. When assessing the amount of sleep an adolescent is getting, it is important to obtain details of bedtime (such as when the child gets into bed as well as lights-out time), estimates of sleep latency, nighttime arousals, time of getting up in the morning, difficulty getting up, and the frequency, timing and duration of daytime naps. It is also essential to get details of sleep–wake schedules on weekends, as well as during the school week. When this type of specific information is obtained either by interview or by having the family maintain a sleep diary, evidence of inadequate sleep is often apparent. A prospective detailed sleep diary provides the most reliable information.

When inadequate sleep is identified, simply recommending that the adolescent go to bed earlier is not likely to be effective. Often, the primary role of the clinician is to help the entire family understand and acknowledge the consequences resulting from the inadequate sleep. Sleep deprivation frequently contributes to many factors that the family identifies as problems, including falling asleep in school, oversleeping in the morning, fatigue and irritability. In cases in which the adolescent's school or social functioning is significantly impaired by sleep problems, a strict behavioral contract that is agreed upon by the family can be essential. The contract should specify hours in bed (with only *small* deviations on the weekends) and should target the specific behaviors contributing to bad sleep habits, such as specific late-night activities, erratic napping or oversleeping for school. The choice of rewards for successes and negative consequences for failures, as well as an accurate method of assessing compliance, are essential components of the contract.

Circadian and Scheduling Disorders

The most common specific problem that is relevant to adolescents is delayed sleep phase syndrome (DSPS). DSPS often begins with a tendency to stay up late at night, sleeping in late and/or taking a late afternoon nap. This process often begins on weekends, holidays or summer vacations. Problems become apparent when school schedules result in morning wake-up battles and difficulties in getting to school. Often, these adolescents cope by taking afternoon naps and getting catch-up sleep on the weekends. Although some of these behaviors occur in many normal adolescents, in extreme cases the circadian system can become set to such a late time that even highly motivated adolescents can have difficulty shifting their sleep back to an earlier time. In some instances, the attempts by the adolescent (and their families) to correct the problem go against circadian principles. For example, an adolescent who has been going to bed at 3 AM and getting up at noon during a vacation tries to go bed at 10 PM the Sunday night before the first day back at school, and finds that her physiology is quite resistant to sleep. For a few days, she manages to get up for school by overriding the system (despite inadequate sleep) but then takes a long nap after school. Despite numerous nights of trying to go to bed at 10 PM she is unable to shift her temperature cycle and circadian system back to an earlier phase.

There is a subgroup of adolescents who appear to have trouble following an early schedule but are not particularly troubled by their late schedule. These adolescents are not motivated to correct the problem, are not particularly troubled by their recurrent experiences of being late for or missing school, and do not show great motivation to change their late-night habits. These adolescents are essentially choosing a late-night schedule. Unless the clinician is able to alter the larger realm of priorities and motivators, these adolescents are very unlikely to respond to any treatment of a sleep schedule problem.

The treatment of DSPS consists of two parts. The first is *gradually* to align the sleep system to the desired schedule. The second is to maintain that alignment. The process of alignment consists of gradual consistent advances in bedtime and wake-up time (15 min per day). It is often best to begin from the time the adolescent usually goes to sleep without difficulty. It is important during this process to avoid any naps and to be consistent across weekends and holidays. In severe cases, some adolescents on very late schedules respond more favorably to going around the clock with successive delays in bedtime. This process has been described as phase delay "chronotherapy." As already highlighted, because the biological clock tends to run on a 25-hour cycle, it accommodates phase delays more easily than phase advances. Hence, the schedule changes can proceed with larger (2–3 hour) delays per day. An example is described for an adolescent who has been falling asleep at 3 AM and getting up at noon. On day 1, he stays up until 6 AM then sleeps until 3 PM. On day 2, he goes to bed at 9 AM and sleeps until 6 PM. On day 3, he sleeps from noon until 9 PM; day 4, from 3 PM until midnight; day 5, from 6 PM until 3 AM; day 6 from 9 PM until 6 AM; and day 7, from 10 PM until 7 AM. It is important that the adolescent take no naps during the chronotherapy. Upon waking up, he or she should be active and, if possible, during the day have bright light exposure, such as walking outdoors.

Although many adolescents do very well with this type of phase-delay chronotherapy, the first weekend or vacation of returning to old habits can undo a lot of hard work. Particularly in the first 2–3 weeks following chronotherapy, rigid requirements should be set about wake-up time. Maintenance of the new circadian phase is based on the same principles but usually can be somewhat less rigorous. For example, if the adolescent wants to stay up late on an occasional weekend night, he or she may be able to do so but should not be permitted to sleep more than 1–2 hours later than the usual wake-up time for school. Strict behavioral contracts worked out with the parents, having specific rewards for success and serious consequences for failures, are essential in this type of intervention.

Before moving to the consideration of bright light or melatonin therapy for DSPS in adolescents, it is important to place these comments in a larger context. In our experience, if an adolescent complies with the behavioral program the additional use of a light box or evening melatonin is often not necessary. Moreover, if the adolescent does not comply with the behavioral contract, light and melatonin alone are extremely unlikely to be successful. If the adolescent remains asleep in bed with eyes closed, the bright light beside the bed is not going to exert the needed physiological effect, and if adolescents are continuing to engage in arousing social activities or use of electronic media late at night, taking melatonin is not going to make them go to sleep any earlier. Thus, we conceptualize the use of light or melatonin as a way to augment the (primary) behavioral intervention. For example, an adolescent living in a far northern latitude may experience a complete absence of morning bright light exposure during the winter, awakening and travelling to school in darkness or dim light.

The use of melatonin has also been suggested as a potential treatment for this problem. Currently, there are some preliminary data supporting the use of low-dose melatonin in the evening to assist with sleep-onset insomnia, presumably resetting of the timing of sleep to an earlier phase (Smits, Nagtegaal, van der Heijden, Coenen, & Kerkhof, 2001; Smits, van Stel, van der Heijden *et al.*, 2003). In some ways, melatonin appears to act as "chemical darkness" to offset the effects of late-night artificial lights in influencing the biological clock. It is important to note the lack of any safety data regarding melatonin use in adolescents. Others have argued that direct control over exposure to light (darkness in the evening and bright light exposure on awakening) can be more effective than melatonin.

Use of Medications for Treating Insomnia and DSPS in Youth

One of the most contentious issues in the domain of treating sleep problems in children and adolescents with difficulty going to sleep is the use of medications to promote sleep onset (Owens, Rosen, & Mindell, 2003). Indeed, there are large numbers of medications prescribed by pediatricians, child psychiatrists and family practitioners for children of all ages in attempts to hasten sleep onset. The medications include an unusual array, ranging from relatively ineffective choices like antihistamines to powerfully sedating medications with an absence of any empirical data on risks or benefits in children and adolescents. Some of the most common agents, such as chloral hydrate and clonidine, not only lack empirical data, but would be regarded by adult sleep clinicians as poor choices regarding the relative degree of somnogenic properties compared to potential side effects (e.g., the dose of clonidine needed to induce sleepiness is relatively close to the dose that lowers blood pressure). Adult sleep pharmacology has seen numerous advances, including new generation agents with a much better specificity for sleep, duration of action, and relatively low risk and side effects *in adults*. Therefore, one might logically argue that some of these medications might represent better treatment options for insomnia in children and adolescents. However, until we have empirical data and controlled trials using these medications in youth (including dosing, side effects and efficacy), we are reluctant to advocate any specific medication at this time.

Weiss, Wasdell, Bomben, Rea, and Freeman (2006) have reported data on a small sample of stimulant-treated children with ADHD ($n = 27$) and sleep onset difficulty. A sleep hygiene intervention was administered first (effect size = 0.67). This intervention involved regularizing the sleep–wake schedule (negotiating a consistent bed and wake time), addressing parental unrealistic expectations about the child's sleep, and reducing caffeine and naps. Those who did not respond were then randomized to a double-blind cross-over design of 10 days of 5 mg melatonin or placebo. There was a reduction in sleep onset latency of 16 min during melatonin use, relative to placebo (effect size = 0.6). The effect size for the combination of sleep hygiene and melatonin was 1.7. An important next step in evaluating the use of sleep hygiene and melatonin for sleep disturbance in ADHD will be to assess the longevity of the reported improvements in sleep.

Ramchandani, Wiggs, Webb, and Stores (2000) published a systematic review of treatments for settling problems in children aged 5 years or younger. Nine studies met the inclusion criteria: four testing a drug, four testing a behavioral treatment and one testing non-directive education. Although the drugs appeared to reduce sleep disturbance in the short term, long-term effects were considered by the authors to be questionable. In contrast, behavioral interventions showed both short-term and longer-term efficacy. The behavioral interventions included positive routines and graduated extinction of parental involvement in resettling across the night.

The Child with Parasomnias

Parasomnias occur commonly in children as sudden partial awakenings from deep NREM sleep into a mixed state which has some aspects of being awake and some aspects of being in a deep sleep. There appear to be at least two routes to this mixed state:

1. Difficulty leaving deep sleep (stage 4) at the end of the first sleep cycle; or
2. A sudden disturbance or disruption during the middle of deep sleep.

The events include sleepwalking, night terrors and confused partial arousals (some enuretic events can also occur as partial arousals). Although the specific types of arousal (sleepwalking versus night terror) are sometimes considered as separate entities, these behaviors represent a spectrum of related phenomena with respect to sleep physiology. The *intense* events (with screaming, agitated flailing and running) represent the extreme *end* of a spectrum of partial arousal behaviors that occur in mild forms (such as calm mumbling or a few awkward movements) in many children. The events can last from a few seconds to 20 min, with an average duration of about 3 min. The termination is usually as sudden as the initiation, with a rapid return to deep sleep. During the events, the children may seem confused, often not recognizing their parents, being inconsolable and often appearing incoherent.

Overtiredness from any source (whether sleep deprivation, sleep disruption or erratic schedule) can increase or precipitate partial arousals. Any time a child is adjusting to getting less sleep, or has disturbed night-time sleep, the physiological compensation is to get deeper sleep (especially in the first 1–2 hours after sleep onset). This deep "recovery" sleep appears to be fertile ground for partial arousal events. A second theme of associated features is in the realm of psychological and emotional factors. Particularly with respect to night terrors, much has been written about the association with particular psychological states, such as anxiety, trauma, stressful events and repressed aggression (Ferber, 1989; Klackenberg, 1982). These psychological factors may contribute to sleep loss. For example, emotional and behavioral problems are also associated with difficulty falling asleep, as occurs with depression and anxiety in children (Dahl & Puig-Antich, 1990; Ryan, Puig-Antich, Ambrosini *et al.*, 1987). Likewise, disruptive disorders, such as ADHD and conduct disorder, can be accompanied by oppositional behaviors around bedtime, which may delay sleep onset, as well as occasional difficulties falling asleep (Dahl & Puig-Antich, 1990).

When a parasomnia is suspected, the clinical interview should include obtaining a careful history of all sleep-related habits, as well as the characteristics, pattern and frequency of the events. The pattern of events should also be assessed. Occurrence in the first third of the night and an increased frequency corresponding to periods of being overly tired are strongly suggestive of typical partial arousal events.

Given the wide range of intensity and clinical significance of these nocturnal partial arousals, the key to therapy is matching the appropriate intervention to the degree of problem. Mild sleepwalking or an occasional night terror in a young child requires only some parental reassurance with general suggestions regarding improved sleep habits and the likelihood that the events will decrease over time. In contrast, frequent, repetitive, intense and agitated arousals in an older child may require very aggressive treatments, because of the risk of self-injury during the events and the possibility of associated pathology. There are three broad principles that guide intervention.

First, educate the family about the events (and what to do during the actual partial arousal event). For mild to moderate events, the parents should try to direct the child to go back to bed and back to sleep. Physically taking the child by the hand and leading him or her back to bed during a mild event can also be effective. Usually, the event needs to take its course and will end spontaneously. During more agitated arousals, interventions trying to direct the child back to bed can result in increased arousal and can inadvertently prolong the event. In general, if mild directing of the child does not work, the parents should let the episode run its course. One very important caveat to this advice is with respect to the *need to prevent self-injury*. Eliminating factors such as sleeping on the top bunk bed, having a bedroom near the top of the stairs or having windows or dangerous objects in the room are major considerations. In severe cases, in which partial arousals are frequent and not responding to treatment, it may be necessary to install window guards or Plexiglas.

Second, encourage a regular sleep–wake schedule with good sleep habits. Parents should consider an earlier bedtime if there is any evidence that the child is getting inadequate sleep. Specific causes of delayed bedtime or difficulty falling asleep should also be directly addressed. It is important to try to improve the overall quantity and/or quality of sleep of the child when applicable.

Third, help the child feel safe, secure and relaxed at bedtime and to identify and express sources of anxiety and fear in a supportive environment. If there is evidence that anxiety and unexpressed anger may contribute to the frequency of these partial arousal events, the family should be encouraged to facilitate their child expressing sources of anxieties, fears, anger and conflicts in healthy ways while awake. Age-appropriate suggestions of positive family interactions within this realm can be very helpful. Also, helping children focus on positive images and positive relaxation exercises can help to foster feelings of safety and security at bedtime.

Tricyclic antidepressants and benzodiazepines have been shown to have positive effects on partial arousal events. Both medications decrease arousals from sleep, and lighten the deepest stage 4 sleep. Difficulties with pharmacological interventions include tolerance effects, withdrawal effects and questions concerning possible long-term detrimental effects on sleep.

Sleep-Disordered Breathing

It is important for child and adolescent psychiatrists to understand how sleep apnea and a related set of problems called sleep-disordered breathing can contribute to fragmented sleep (and possibly intermittent hypoxia; Gozal & Kheirandish, 2006; Kheirandish & Gozal, 2006), which can contribute to daytime difficulties with cognitive and affective functioning. In particular, difficulties with irritability, attentional difficulties and emotional lability can be created or exacerbated by sleep-disordered breathing in children.

During sleep, and particularly in REM sleep, there is a considerable drop in muscle tone. This decreased tone affects the musculature maintaining the airway and the muscles assisting in respiration. In susceptible individuals, these physiological changes can lead to obstructive sleep apnea syndrome (OSAS). In adults, the clinical picture of OSAS is typically an obese hypersomnolent lethargic individual. In children, the clinical appearance is quite different. The most common cause of OSAS in children is hypertrophy of adenoids and tonsils. Many of these children have little difficulty breathing when awake; however, with decreased muscle tone during sleep, the airway becomes smaller, airway resistance increases and the work of breathing increases. Brief arousals from sleep increase the muscle tone to the neck and pharyngeal muscles, open the airway and allow the child to resume breathing. Although the actual number of minutes of arousal during the night may be small, the repeated chronic but brief disruptions in sleep can lead to significant daytime symptoms in children. It is important to note that the child is usually unaware of waking up, and the parent often describes very restless sleep but usually does not describe the child's waking up completely. The most frequent symptoms reported by families include loud chronic snoring (or noisy breathing), restless sleep with unusual sleeping positions (attempts by the child to move and open the airway), a history of problems with tonsils, adenoids and/or ear infections, and signs of inadequate nighttime sleep.

There is still a great deal of uncertainty and controversy about the exact clinical threshold for performing formal sleep studies. Treatment decisions and options are also complex clinical decisions. In medical centers with pediatric sleep facilities, consultation with a child sleep specialist can be extremely helpful in making decisions in these cases. Some recent studies provide excellent reviews of these complex issues (Ferber, 1996; Marcus, 1997).

A similar (and even more controversial) situation exists regarding restless legs syndrome (RLS) and periodic limb movement disorder (PLMD) in children. Periodic limb movement in sleep (PLMS) is characterized by periodic episodes of repetitive and highly stereotypic limb movements during sleep (American Academy of Sleep Medicine, 2005). PLMD is defined by the presence of periodic limb movement during sleep associated with symptoms of insomnia or excessive daytime sleepiness (Chesson, Wise, Davila *et al.*, 1999). RLS is a clinical diagnosis characterized by disagreeable leg sensations that usually occur prior to sleep onset. PLMD and RLS are distinct entities but can coexist. Most patients with PLMD do not manifest RLS symptoms; however, approximately 80% of patients with RLS have PLMS (Montplaisir, Boucher, Poirier *et al.*, 1997).

PLMD has been described in children with somewhat different clinical presentations. Children with PLMD may present with non-specific symptoms such as growing pains, restless sleep and hyperactivity (Picchietti & Walters, 1999). These symptoms are most often unnoticed by their parents, although a family history of RLS and PLMD is common. In a series of studies, Picchietti, England, Walters, Willis, and Verrico (1998) suggested an increased prevalence of PLMD among children with ADHD.

Other studies have suggested that the sleep fragmentation secondary to these disorders is an important contribution to ADHD and that, particularly in the context of symptoms and/or a positive family history of RLS/PLMS, sleep studies should be performed if there is any question that sleep fragmentation is contributing to daytime impairments with attentional control (Cortese, Konofal, Lecendreus *et al.*, 2005; Hoban & Chervin, 2005).

Treatment

The guideline from the Standard of Practice Committee of the American Academy of Sleep Medicine states that no specific recommendation can be made regarding treatment of children with RLS or PLMD (Littner, Kushida, Wise *et al.*, 2005). There is limited information on the dopaminergic medications in children and other medications have not been adequately studied in children. There is some evidence that children with PLMD may have low iron storage as evidenced by low serum ferritin and iron. Children with low serum ferritin (<50 μg/L) have been reported to respond favorably to iron therapy (Simakajornboon, Gozal, Vlasic *et al.*, 2003). However, currently, there are no long-term data on the use of iron treatment. These children also appear to benefit from avoiding caffeine and behavioral interventions to improve sleep habits.

Narcolepsy

Narcolepsy is a chronic neurological disorder characterized by excessive daytime sleepiness. The classic tetrad of symptoms in narcolepsy comprises:

1 Sleep attacks;

2 Cataplexy (sudden loss of muscle tone without change of consciousness);

3 Sleep paralysis (inability to move after waking up); and

4 Hypnogogic hallucinations (dream-like imagery before falling asleep).

These symptoms do not all occur together or consistently in many cases of narcolepsy. Particularly in younger patients, signs of sleepiness may be the only initial symptom. Cataplexy is typically provoked by laughter, anger or sudden emotional changes. It may be as subtle as a slight weakness in the legs, or as dramatic as a patient falling to the floor limp and unable to move. If cataplectic attacks last long enough, full sleep can occur.

It is not a rare disorder, affecting approximately 1 in 10,000 people in the USA. Narcolepsy is a neurological disorder that appears to be caused by an abnormality in the hypocretin–orexin system – often by a loss of hypocretin neurons in the lateral hypothalamus and usually low cerebrospinal fluid (CSF) levels of hypocretin. About 10% of narcoleptics are members of familial clusters; however, genetic factors alone are apparently insufficient to cause the disease. A mutation on chromosome 6 affecting a human leukocyte antigen ([HLA] DR2/DQ6 [DQB1*0602]) is seen in 90–100% of patients; however, this also occurs in as many as 50% of people without narcolepsy. Hence, obtaining a family history of narcolepsy or excessive sleepiness can be helpful, although it is negative in many cases. Traditionally, the onset of narcolepsy is thought to occur in late adolescence and adulthood, but there are well-documented cases that begin in early childhood.

The diagnosis of narcolepsy requires evaluation in a sleep laboratory. Patients with narcolepsy show early REM periods near sleep onset, fragmented night-time sleep, excessive daytime sleepiness in objective nap studies during the day and sleep-onset REM periods in naps. In prepubertal children, this diagnosis can be very difficult to establish (Kotagal, Hartse, & Walsh, 1990). Repeat studies may be necessary before reaching a final diagnosis. At this time, neither HLA typing nor CSF hypocretin levels are routinely indicated in the clinical evaluation of narcolepsy; however, in unusual cases CSF hypocretins can be helpful.

Treatment of narcolepsy is generally focused on:

1 Education and counseling of the patient and family;

2 Adherence to a regular schedule to obtain optimal sleep with good sleep habits (often including scheduled naps);

3 Use of short-acting stimulant medication for treatment of daytime sleepiness (with drug holidays to avoid build-up of tolerance); and

4 Use of REM-suppressant medications (such as protriptyline) when symptoms of cataplexy are problematic.

The differential diagnosis of narcolepsy includes consideration of the following two sleep disorders.

Idiopathic Hypersomnolence

Some patients have significantly increased sleep needs without evidence of the REM abnormalities seen in narcolepsy. This condition has been called *idiopathic hypersomnolence*. There is often a familial history of excessive sleep needs, and these individuals show clear objective sleepiness in nap studies despite having obtained what appears to be adequate amounts of night-time sleep. These disorders are also frequently treated with stimulant medication when the diagnosis is definitively established and daytime functioning is impaired.

Kleine–Levin Syndrome

Symptoms of excessive somnolence, hypersexuality and compulsive overeating were first described in adolescent boys by Kleine (1925) and Levin (1929). Mental disturbances (irritability, confusion and occasional auditory or visual hallucinations) have also been reported in these cases. This syndrome (with more than 100 published cases) occurs more frequently in males (3:1). Typically, symptoms start during adolescence, either gradually or abruptly, and in about half of cases the onset follows a flu-like illness or injury with loss of consciousness. Frequently, there is an episodic nature to the symptoms, with cycles lasting from 1 to 30 days. The syndrome usually disappears spontaneously during late adolescence or early adulthood. Laboratory tests, imaging studies, EEGs and endocrine measures do not appear to be helpful in making the specific diagnosis of Kleine–Levin syndrome. It is important to rule out other organic causes of similar symptoms such as a hypothalamic tumor, localized CNS infection or vascular accident. The presence of neurological signs, evidence of increased CNS pressure, abnormalities in temperature regulation, abnormalities in water regulation or other endocrine abnormalities point to an organically based abnormality. A family history of bipolar illness or other signs suggesting an early onset bipolar illness should also be ruled out. Although stimulant medication or use of lithium carbonate has been reported to be helpful in individual cases, there is no clear consensus on treatment.

Conclusions

In this chapter we reviewed several important principles relevant to the assessment, diagnosis and treatment of sleep problems in children and adolescents. We have underscored the evidence for interactions between sleep and the regulation of behavior, emotion and learning and the importance of sleep disturbance to many aspects of child psychiatry (and behavioral pediatrics). We have consistently emphasized behavioral principles and behavioral approaches to these problems because we believe that there is great pragmatic value in understanding and implementing these in many domains of clinical practice. There are few risks – and potentially many benefits – from increasing and enhancing sleep in youth through cognitive–behavioral interventions. There is also a clear need for more studies to provide stronger empirical support and further insight into the benefit of these interventions.

Finally, it is important to emphasize the exciting advances in research in neuroscience, genetics and development in understanding the role of sleep in the developing brain. It is extremely likely that these rapid advances will continue to provide expanding areas of understanding with even greater clinical relevance to child and adolescent psychiatry in the near future.

References

American Academy of Sleep Medicine (AASM). (2005). *International classification of sleep disorders (ICSD): Diagnostic and coding manual* (2nd edn.). Westchester, IL: American Academy of Sleep Medicine.

Barbini, B., Bertelli, S., Colombo, C., & Smeraldi, E. (1996). Sleep loss, a possible factor in augmenting manic episode. *Psychiatry Research*, *65*, 121–125.

Benington, J. H., & Frank, M. G. (2003). Cellular and molecular connections between sleep and synaptic plasticity. *Progress in Neurobiology*, *69*, 71–101.

Bootzin, R. R. (1979). Effects of self-control procedures for insomnia. *American Journal of Clinical Biofeedback*, *2*, 70–77.

Bootzin, R. R., & Stevens, S. J. (2005). Adolescents, substance abuse, and the treatment of insomnia and daytime sleepiness. *Clinical Psychology Review*, *25*, 629–644.

Borbély, A. A. (1982). A two-process model of sleep regulation. *Human Neurobiology*, *1*, 195–204.

Borbély, A. A., & Achermann, P. (2005). Sleep homeostasis and models of sleep regulation. In M. H. Kryger, T. Roth, & W. C. Dement (Eds.), *Principles and practice of sleep medicine* (3rd edn., pp. 405–417). Philadelphia: Elsevier Saunders.

Carskadon, M. A. (Ed.). (2002). *Adolescent sleep patterns: Biological, social, and psychological influences*. Cambridge: Cambridge University Press.

Carskadon, M. A. (2005). Sleep and circadian rhythms in children and adolescents: Relevance for athletic performance of young people. *Clinics in Sports Medicine*, *24*, 319–328.

Carskadon, M. A., Acebo, C., & Jenni, O. G. (2004). Regulation of adolescent sleep: Implications for behavior. *Annals of the New York Academy of Sciences*, *1021*, 276–291.

Chervin, R. D., Archbold, K. H., Dillon, J. E., Panahi, P., Pituch, K. J., Dahl, R. E., *et al.* (2002). Inattention, hyperactivity, and symptoms of sleep-disordered breathing. *Pediatrics*, *109*, 449–456.

Chervin, R. D., Dillon, J. E., Archbold, K. H., & Ruzicka, D. L. (2003). Conduct problems and symptoms of sleep disorders in children. *Journal of the American Academy of Child and Adolescent Psychiatry*, *42*, 201–208.

Chesson, A. L. Jr., Wise, M., Davila, D., Johnson, S., Littner, M., Anderson, W. M., *et al.* (1999). Practice parameters for the treatment of restless legs syndrome and periodic limb movement disorder. An American Academy of Sleep Medicine Report. Standards of Practice Committee of the American Academy of Sleep Medicine. *Sleep*, *22*, 961–968.

Colombo, C., Benedetti, F., Barbini, B., Campori, E., & Smeraldi, E. (1999). Rate of switch from depression into mania after therapeutic sleep deprivation in bipolar depression. *Psychiatry Research*, *86*, 267–270.

Cortese, S., Konofal, E., Lecendreux, M., Arnulf, I., Mouren, M. C., Darra, F., & Dalla Bernadina, B. (2005). Restless legs syndrome and attention-deficit/hyperactivity disorder: A review of the literature. *Sleep*, *28*, 1007–1013.

Dahl, R. E. (1996a). The impact of inadequate sleep on children's daytime cognitive function. *Seminars in Pediatric Neurology*, *3*, 44–50.

Dahl, R. E. (1996b). The regulation of sleep and arousal: Development and psychopathology. *Development and Psychopathology*, *8*, 3–27.

Dahl, R. E. (2002). The regulation of sleep-arousal, affect, and attention in adolescence: Some questions and speculations. In M. A. Carskadon (Ed.), *Adolescent sleep patterns: Biological, social and psychological influences* (pp. 269–284). Cambridge: Cambridge University Press.

Dahl, R. E., Pelham, W. E., & Wierson, M. (1991). The role of sleep disturbances in attention deficit disorder symptoms: A case study. *Journal of Pediatric Psychology*, *16*, 229–239.

Dahl, R. E., & Puig-Antich, J. (1990). Sleep disturbances in child and adolescent psychiatric disorders. *Pediatrician*, *17*, 32–37.

Dauvilliers, Y., Baumann, C. R., Carlander, B., Bischof, M., Blatter, T., Lecendreux, M., *et al.* (2003). CSF hypocretin-1 levels in narcolepsy, Kleine–Levin syndrome, and other hypersomnias and neurological conditions. *Journal of Neurology, Neurosurgery and Psychiatry*, *74*, 1667–1673.

Dinges, D. F., Pack, F., Williams, K., Gillen, K. A., Powell, J. W., Ott, G. E., *et al.* (1997). Cumulative sleepiness, mood disturbance, and psychomotor vigilance performance decrements during a week of sleep restricted to 4–5 hours per night. *Sleep*, *20*, 267–277.

Ferber, R. (1989). Sleeplessness in the child. In M. H. Kryger, T. Roth, & W. C. Dement (Eds.), *Principles and practice of sleep medicine* (pp. 633–639). Philadelphia: W. B. Saunders.

Ferber, R. (1996). Clinical assessment of child and adolescent sleep disorders. In R. E. Dahl (Ed.), *Child and adolescent psychiatric clinics of North America* (pp. 569–580). Philadelphia: W. B. Saunders.

Gomez, R. L., Bootzin, R. R., & Nadel, L. (2006). Naps promote abstraction in language-learning infants. *Psychological Science*, *17*, 670–674.

Gozal, D., & Kheirandish, L. (2006). Oxidant stress and inflammation in the snoring child: Confluent pathways to upper airway pathogenesis and end-organ morbidity. *Sleep medicine Reviews*, *10*, 83–96.

Gruber, R., Grizenko, N., Schwartz, G., Ben Amor, L., Gauthier, J., de Guzman, R., *et al.* (2006). Sleep and COMT polymorphism in ADHD children: Preliminary actigraphic data. *Journal of the American Academy of Child and Adolescent Psychiatry*, *45*, 982–989.

Harvey, A. G., Mullin, B. C., & Hinshaw, S. P. (2006). Sleep and circadian rhythms in children and adolescents with bipolar disorder. *Development and Psychopathology*, *18*, 1147–1168.

Haynes, P. L., Bootzin, R. R., Smith, L., Cousins, J., Cameron, M., & Stevens, S. (2006). Sleep and aggression in substance-abusing adolescents: results from an integrative behavioral sleep-treatment pilot program. *Sleep*, *29*, 512–520.

Hoban, T. F., & Chervin, R. D. (2005). Pediatric sleep-related breathing disorders and restless legs syndrome: How children are different. *Neurologist*, *11*, 325–337.

Hobson, J. A., & Pace-Schott, E. F. (2002). The cognitive neuroscience of sleep: Neuronal systems, consciousness, and learning. *Nature Reviews. Neuroscience*, *3*, 679–693.

Ireland, J. L., & Culpin, V. (2006). The relationship between sleeping problems and aggression, anger, and impulsivity in a population of juvenile and young offenders. *Journal of Adolescent Health*, *38*, 649–655.

Jackson, A., Cavanagh, J., & Scott, J. (2003). A systematic review of manic and depressive prodromes. *Journal of Affective Disorders*, *74*, 209–217.

Jenni, O. G., & Carskadon, M. A. (2005). Normal human sleep at different ages: Infants to adolescents. In *SRS Basics of Sleep Guide*. Westchester, IL: Sleep Research Society.

Jenni, O. G., & LeBourgeois, M. K. (2006). Understanding sleep–wake regulation and sleep disorders during childhood: The value of a model. *Current Opinion in Psychiatry*, *19*, 282–287.

Kasper, S., & Wehr, T. A. (1992). The role of sleep and wakefulness in the genesis of depression and mania. *Encephale*, *18*, 45–50.

Kheirandish, L., & Gozal, D. (2006). Neurocognitive dysfunction in children with sleep disorders. *Developmental Science*, *9*, 388–399.

Klackenberg, G. (1982). Somnambulism in childhood: Prevalence, course and behavioral correlations. A prospective longitudinal study (6–16 years). *Acta Paediatrica Scandinavica*, *71*, 495–499.

Kleine, W. (1925). Periodische schlafsucht. *Monatsschrift für Psychiatrie und Neurologie*, *57*, 285.

Kotagal, S., Hartse, K. M., & Walsh, J. K. (1990). Characteristics of narcolepsy in preteenaged children. *Pediatrics*, *85*, 205–209.

Lee, T. M., Hummer, D. L., & Jechura, T. J. (2004). Pubertal development of sex differences in circadian function: An animal model. *Annals of the New York Academy of Sciences*, *1021*, 262–275.

Leibenluft, E., Albert, P. S., Rosenthal, N. E., & Wehr, T. A. (1996). Relationship between sleep and mood in patients with rapid-cycling bipolar disorder. *Psychiatry Research*, *63*, 161–168.

Levin, M. (1929). Narcolepsy and other varieties of morbid somnolence. *Archives of Neurology and Psychiatry*, *22*, 1172.

Littner, M. R., Kushida, C., Wise, M., Davila, D. G., Morgenthaler, T., Lee-Chiong, T., *et al.* (2005). Practice parameters for clinical use of the multiple sleep latency test and the maintenance of wakefulness test. *Sleep*, *28*, 113–121.

Lu, B. S., Manthena, P., Zee, P. C. (2006). Circadian Rhythm Sleep Disorders. In A. Y. Avidan & P. C. Zee (Eds.), *Handbook of Sleep Medicine* (pp. 137–164). Lippincott Williams & Wilkins.

Marcus, C. L. (1997). Management of obstructive sleep apnea in childhood. *Current Opinion in Pulmonary Medicine*, *3*, 464–469.

Marks, C. A., & Wayner, M. J. (2005). Effects of sleep disruption on rat dentate granule cell LTP *in vivo*. *Brain Research Bulletin*, *66*, 114–119.

Montplaisir, J., Boucher, S., Poirier, G., Lavigne, G., Lapierre, O., & Lesperance, P. (1997). Clinical, polysomnographic, and genetic characteristics of restless legs syndrome: A study of 133 patients diagnosed with new standard criteria. *Movement Disorders*, *12*, 61–65.

Morin, C. M., Bootzin, R. R., Buysse, D. J., Edinger, J., D., Espie, C. A., & Lichstein, K. L. (2006). Psychological and behavioral treatment of insomnia: An update of recent evidence (1998–2004). *Sleep*, *29*, 1398–1414.

National Sleep Foundation. (2006). *Adolescent sleep needs and patterns: Research report and resource guide*. Washington, DC: National Sleep Foundation.

Owens, J. A., Rosen, C. L., & Mindell, J. A. (2003). Medication use in the treatment of pediatric insomnia: Results of a survey of community-based pediatricians. *Pediatrics*, *111*, 628–635.

Peigneux, P., Laureys, S., Delbeuck, X., & Maquet, P. (2001). Sleeping brain, learning brain: The role of sleep for memory systems. *Neuroreport*, *12*, A111–124.

Perlis, M. L., Giles, D. E., Mendelson, W. B., Bootzin, R. R., & Wyatt, J. K. (1997). Psychophysiological insomnia: The behavioural model and a neurocognitive perspective. *Journal of Sleep Research*, *6*, 179–188.

Picchietti, D. L., England, S. J., Walters, A. S., Willis, K., & Verrico, T. (1998). Periodic limb movement disorder and restless legs syndrome in children with attention-deficit hyperactivity disorder. *Journal of Child Neurology*, *13*, 588–594.

Picchietti, D. L., & Walters, A. S. (1999). Moderate to severe periodic limb movement disorder in childhood and adolescence. *Sleep*, *22*, 297–300.

Pilcher, J. J., & Huffcut, A. I. (1996). Effects of sleep deprivation on performance: A meta-analysis. *Sleep*, *19*, 318–326.

Ramchandani, P., Wiggs, L., Webb, V., & Stores, G. (2000). A systematic review of treatments for settling problems and night waking in young children. *British Medical Journal*, *320*, 209–213.

Ryan, N. D., Puig-Antich, J., Ambrosini, P., Rabinovich, H., Robinson, D., Nelson, B., *et al.* (1987). The clinical picture of major depression in children and adolescents. *Archives of General Psychiatry*, *44*, 854–861.

Saper, C. B., Cano, G., & Scammell, T. E. (2005). Homeostatic, circadian, and emotional regulation of sleep. *Journal of Comparative Neurology*, *493*, 92–98.

Saper, C. B., Scammell, T. E., & Lu, J. (2005). Hypothalamic regulation of sleep and circadian rhythms. *Nature*, *437*, 1257–1263.

Sheldon, S., Ferber, R., & Kryger, M., (Eds.). (2005). *Principles and practice of sleep medicine*. Philadelphia, PA: Elsevier Saunders.

Simakajornboon, N., Gozal, D., Vlasic, V., Mack, C., Sharon, D., & McGinley, B. M. (2003). Periodic limb movements in sleep and iron status in children. *Sleep*, *26*, 735–738.

Smits, M. G., Nagtegaal, E. E., van der Heijden, J., Coenen, A. M., & Kerkhof, G. A. (2001). Melatonin for chronic sleep onset insomnia in children: A randomized placebo-controlled trial. *Journal of Child Neurology*, *16*, 86–92.

Smits, M. G., van Stel, H., van der Heijden, K. B., Meijer, A. M., Coenen, A. M., & Kerkhof, G. A. (2003). Melatonin improves health status and sleep in children with idiopathic chronic sleep-onset insomnia: a randomized placebo-controlled trial. *Journal of the American Academy of Child and Adolescent Psychiatry*, *42*, 1286–1293.

Steriade, M. (1999). Coherent oscillations and short-term plasticity in corticothalamic networks. *Trends in Neurosciences*, *22*, 337–345.

Stickgold, R. (2005). Sleep-dependent memory consolidation. *Nature*, *437*, 1272–1278.

Stickgold, R., Hobson, J. A., Fosse, R., & Fosse, M. (2001). Sleep, learning, and dreams: Off-line memory reprocessing. *Science*, *294*, 1052–1057.

Stickgold, R., & Walker, M. P. (2005). Memory consolidation and reconsolidation: What is the role of sleep? *Trends in Neurosciences*, *28*, 408–415.

Tononi, G., & Cirelli, C. (2003). Sleep and synaptic homeostasis: A hypothesis. *Brain Research Bulletin*, *62*, 143–150.

Tononi, G., & Cirelli, C. (2006). Sleep function and synaptic homeostasis. *Sleep Medicine Reviews*, *10*, 49–62.

Van Dongen, H. P. A., Maislin, G., Mullington, J. M., & Dinges, D. F. (2003). The cumulative cost of additional wakefulness: Dose–response effects on neurobehavioral functions and sleep physiology from chronic sleep restriction and total sleep deprivation. *Sleep*, *26*, 117–126.

Walker, M. P., & Stickgold, R. (2004). Sleep-dependent learning and memory consolidation. *Neuron*, *44*, 121–133.

Walker, M. P., & Stickgold, R. (2006). Sleep, memory, and plasticity. *Annual Review of Psychology*, *57*, 139–166.

Wehr, T. A., Sack, D. A., & Rosenthal, N. E. (1987). Sleep reduction as a final common pathway in the genesis of mania. *American Journal of Psychiatry*, *144*, 201–204.

Weiss, M. D., Wasdell, M. B., Bomben, M. M., Rea, K. J., & Freeman, M. D. (2006). Sleep hygiene and melatonin treatment for children and adolescents with ADHD and initial insomnia. *Journal of the American Academy of Child and Adolescent Psychiatry*, *45*, 512–518.

Worthman, C., & Melby, M. K. (2002). Toward a comparative developmental ecology of human sleep. In M. A. Carskadon (Ed.), *Adolescent sleep patterns: Biological, social, and psychological influences* (pp. 69–117). Cambridge: Cambridge University Press.

Wu, J. C., & Bunney, W. E. (1990). The biological basis of an antidepressant response to sleep deprivation and relapse: Review and hypothesis. *American Journal of Psychiatry*, *147*, 14–21.

Zwi, R., Shawe-Taylor, M., & Murray, J. (2005). Cognitive processes in the maintenance of insomnia and co-morbid anxiety. *Behavioural and Cognitive Psychotherapy*, *33*, 333–342.

Attachment Disorders in Relation to Deprivation

Charles H. Zeanah and Anna T. Smyke

Although attachment disorders have received increased attention in contemporary literature, there have been more reviews of these kinds of disorders published than systematic studies. In fact, although these disorders have been described for more than 50 years in the literature and have been defined by specified criteria in psychiatric nosologies for nearly 25 years, they have been studied directly only in the past decade. There is now a small but growing database, allowing for a beginning consensus on some points and clearer questions about areas of controversy.

The purpose of this chapter is to review attachment disorders, especially in the context of severe deprivation, and in light of what has been learned in recent investigations. Although different or more expanded versions of attachment disorders have been proposed by some (Minnis, Marwick, Arthur, & McLaughlin, 2006; van IJzendoorn & Bakermans-Kranenburg, 2002; Zeanah & Boris, 2000), these alternative approaches have not been well studied, and we have limited our review to the traditional conceptualization of the disorder, as defined in contemporary nosologies.

Definitional Challenges

The term "attachment" itself has been used variably to refer to somewhat different constructs, and this has led to confusion in the literature. Bowlby, who developed attachment theory, asserted that attachment referred to the young child's strong disposition "to seek proximity to and contact with a specific figure and to do so in certain situations, notably when . . . frightened, tired, or ill. The disposition to behave in this way is an attribute of the child, an attribute which changes only slowly over time and which is unaffected by the situation of the moment" (Bowlby, 1982, p. 371).

In addition to this description of behaviors, it is often useful to consider attachment as a relational construct. We have suggested, using Emde's (1989) model, that functions of the parent–child attachment relationship include:

1 Providing and seeking comfort for distress;

2 Providing and experiencing warmth, empathy and nurturance;

3 Providing emotional availability and regulating emotion; and

4 Providing and seeking physical and psychological protection (Zeanah, Mammen, & Lieberman, 1993).

Because the relationship is asymmetrical, the young child is the seeker and the adult caregiver or parent is the provider.

A significant challenge to the definition of attachment disorders is the very ubiquity of attachment in young children. Under species-typical rearing conditions, virtually all children form selected attachments to their caregivers. In children with clinical disturbances of a variety of types, attachment formation or expression may be compromised. Thus, an important question is when the disturbed attachment is the primary problem, in which case it comprises an attachment disorder, and when attachment is merely one of a number of developmental domains that is compromised, in which case it may be an associated feature of some other disorder. An appreciation of the development of attachment under usual circumstances provides a useful foundation from which to begin to answer this question.

Development of Attachment

Parents' affiliative feelings for their infants often begin prenatally. Studies have indicated that parents are willing to describe a sense of who the baby is and assert that they have a relationship with the baby even before the baby is born (Benoit, Parker, & Zeanah, 1997).

However, infants are not born attached to their caregivers. In fact, two conditions appear to be necessary for infants to become attached. First, they must have a significant amount of interaction on a regular basis with the caregiver and, second, they must reach a cognitive age of about 7–9 months. Phases in the development of attachment, modified slightly from Bowlby's (1982) original formulation, are described in Table 55.1.

By the end of the first year of life, it is possible to assess the quality of the young child's attachment to a particular caregiver. Usually, this is accomplished by means of a laboratory paradigm known as the Strange Situation Procedure (Ainsworth, Blehar, Waters, & Wall, 1978). Alternating episodes of separations and reunions between a young child and a familiar caregiver and an unfamiliar adult or stranger, the procedure yields classification of a young child's pattern of attachment to the caregiver with whom he or she is assessed as secure, insecure/avoidant, insecure/resistant or disorganized. Although secure attachment appears to confer some protection

Rutter's Child and Adolescent Psychiatry, 5th edition. Edited by M. Rutter, D. Bishop, D. Pine, S. Scott, J. Stevenson, E. Taylor and A. Thapar. © 2008 Blackwell Publishing, ISBN: 978-1-4051-4549-7.

Table 55.1 Development of attachment in early childhood.

Age	Phase	Characteristics
Newborn to 2 months	Limited discrimination	Ability to discriminate among different caregivers is limited and preferences are not readily observable
2–8 months	Discrimination with limited preference	Clearly discriminates different caregivers as evident by different patterns of interacting but usually engages readily with strangers as well as familiar caregivers
8–12 months	Focused attachment	Begins when separation protest and stranger wariness appear. Infant becomes notably more wary of interacting with strangers and protests readily if he or she anticipates or experiences separation from a preferred caregiver (i.e., attachment figure). In typical rearing circumstances, infants attach to more than one caregiver and demonstrate a hierarchy of preferences evident when stressed, fatigued or frightened
12–20 months	Secure base	Independent ambulation ushers in increasing exploratory forays away from the attachment figure, alternating with returns in which proximity is sought. Different patterns of attachment reflect differences in balance between exploration and secure base behavior
20 months and beyond	Goal corrected partnership	Attachment relationship shifts from nearly complete dependency on the caregiver to one in which the preschooler becomes aware that others, including the caregiver, have intentions and wishes different from their own

for young children in high-risk environments, the major risks for psychopathology appear to be associated with disorganized attachments (Green & Goldwyn, 2002).

Attachment Classifications and Psychopathology

Infant behaviors in the presence of the parent or caregiver suggesting fearfulness, freezing or other contradictory attachment behaviors (e.g., initial approach followed by avoidance while in close contact with the caregiver) during the Strange Situation Procedure are indices of a disorganized attachment classification. Although disorganized attachment has a prevalence of 14% in low-risk samples (van IJzendoorn, Schuengel, & Bakermans-Kranenberg, 1999), it is as high as 75–80% in maltreated and institutionalized samples (Carlson, Cicchetti, & Barnett, 1989; Vorria, Papaligoura, Dunn *et al.*, 2003; Zeanah, Smyke, Koga, & Carlson, 2005). Furthermore, disorganized attachment is associated with various disturbances in caregiving behavior, including frightening/frightened behavior, as well as antagonism, role confusion, withdrawal and contradictory cues (Lyons-Ruth, Bronfin, & Parsons, 1999; Schuengel, Bakermans-Kranenburg, & van IJzendoorn, 1999).

Of the attachment classifications, disorganized attachment has the strongest links to subsequent psychopathology, including social difficulties, role-inappropriate parent–child interactive behavior, peer rejection and poor social adjustment, aggression and disruptive behavior in middle childhood, in addition to emotional problems, low self-esteem and dissociative disorders in adolescence (Green & Goldwyn, 2002).

At least one group has suggested that because disorganized attachment represents failure of a stage-salient developmental task, is strongly linked to concurrent and subsequent psychopathology, is reliably identified in a laboratory procedure and is associated with "pathogenic" patterns of caregiving (e.g., frightening/frightened patterns), it should be considered a disorder of attachment (van IJzendoorn & Bakermans-Kranenburg, 2002). There are a number of problems with this suggestion, including the high prevalence of disorganized attachment in low-risk samples, identification based only on a child's behaviors (perhaps lasting only a few seconds) in a laboratory paradigm with no established connection to conventional signs or symptoms, an uncertain relation to impairment and the relationship specificity of the disorganized classification. That is, the child's attachment to one caregiver may be classified disorganized and the child's attachment to another caregiver as another attachment classification, meaning that the classification is a characteristic of the relationship rather than the child. Therefore, the prevailing consensus is that disorganized attachment is a risk factor rather than a clinical diagnostic category (for a discussion of the relationship between attachment and psychopathology see chapter 13).

Most descriptions of attachment as a clinical disorder have derived from studies of the effects on social and emotional development in young children who have experienced severe deprivation, such as that associated with institutional rearing. Because of that, we turn next to a brief review of the association between institutional care and attachment disorders and consider how studies of institutionalized children informed psychiatric nosologies.

Historical Considerations

Institutional Care and Deprivation

Maternal deprivation and the material deprivation that often accompanies it have long been recognized as important risk factors to development in humans (Bowlby, 1965; Chapin, 1915; Rutter, 1981; Spitz, 1945), primates (Suomi, Collins, Harlow, & Rupenthal, 1976) and rodents (Hofer, 2006; Zhang, Levine,

Dent *et al.*, 2002). For the past 50 years, children raised in institutions have been studied to assess the risks associated with this atypical rearing environment because it has been associated with deprivation. A series of small-scale descriptive studies began to raise questions about the consequences of institutionalization in the 1940s. Early studies focused on behavioral and cognitive manifestations of the effects of poor rearing environments (Goldfarb, 1945; Levy, 1947). In addition to disturbances of growth, cognitive development and language, these studies also documented that children who had been institutionalized during the first 3 years of life demonstrated consistently greater levels of problem behaviors, including feeding and sleeping difficulties, aggressive behavior and hyperactivity, and excessive attention-seeking and sociability with strangers when compared with children in foster care.

A recent resurgence in studies of children adopted out of Romania has demonstrated some significant problems across a range of outcomes, including disturbed attachment (Zeanah, 2000). In spite of these problems, Romanian children who have been adopted following institutional care have demonstrated varied developmental effects from their institutional experience (Kreppner, Rutter, Beckett *et al.*, 2007; Rutter, Beckett, Castle *et al.*, 2007), and many children seem to have recovered fully.

Tizard's Study

Tizard's (1977) landmark study deconstructed the institutional experience by removing the material deprivation often associated with institutional care and focusing on the variable of caregiver–child relationship. She described the cognitive and socioemotional development of a group of children who experienced varying lengths of institutional care in residential nurseries in Great Britain. Caregiver to child ratios were substantially better than those found in older studies (Goldfarb, 1945; Provence & Lipton, 1962). Children were maintained in small, mixed age groups, in a stimulating environment which included books, toys and instruction during the preschool years (Tizard, 1977).

Three groups of children with histories of early institutional rearing were studied at age 4 years: 24 children who were adopted between 2 and 4 years of age, 15 children who were restored to their biological families (often despite marked ambivalence on the part of the mother) and 26 children who remained institutionalized (Tizard, 1977). By age 4, this latter group had experienced an average of 50 different caregivers who had cared for the child for at least a week. Of the 26 children who remained in the residential nurseries, eight had developed a preferred attachment, eight were withdrawn and unresponsive and 10 were indiscriminate, attention-seeking and socially superficial (Tizard & Rees, 1975). The latter two groups, which had been noted in previous studies and were replicated in subsequent studies, formed the basis of reactive attachment disorder in contemporary nosologies.

Attachment Disorders in Nosologies

Reactive Attachment Disorder of Infancy first appeared in the DSM-III (American Psychiatric Association, 1980). Disordered social and emotional development was a hallmark of the disorder which was signaled also by the presence of failure to thrive. Inexplicably, there also was a requirement that the disorder be manifest prior to 8 months of age; that is, prior to the age at which preferred attachment ordinarily emerges (Zeanah, 1996).

Subsequent versions of the DSM removed this curious requirement and made the age of onset below 5 years of age. However, in DSM-IV-TR (American Psychiatric Association, 2000), a specified etiology – the child's signs of disturbed attachment are in response to "pathogenic care" – is included. ICD-10 (World Health Organization, 1996) criteria are generally consistent with DSM criteria. ICD-10 criteria do not specify pathogenic care, but they do caution against making the diagnosis in the absence of a history of maltreatment.

All revisions in criteria through 2000 occurred in the absence of systematic research of the disorders; in fact, such research is only beginning to appear. In addition to DSM-IV-TR and ICD-10, two other sets of criteria for disorders of attachment have been published recently. The Research Diagnostic Criteria–Preschool Age (RDC-PA; Task Force on Research Diagnostic Criteria: Infancy and Preschool, 2003) and the Diagnostic Classification: 0–3, Revised criteria (Zero to Three, 2005) are quite similar, although they differ from DSM-IV-TR and ICD-10 in focusing more explicitly on disturbed attachment behaviors rather than disturbed social behaviors more generally.

Clinical Disorders of Attachment: The Phenotype

Attachment disorders describe a constellation of aberrant attachment behaviors and other social behavioral anomalies apparent in early childhood which are believed to result from limited opportunities to form selected attachments. Historically, attachment disorders have been linked to deprivation or social neglect. The diagnosis is excluded in the presence of pervasive developmental disorders to distinguish social abnormalities associated with those disorders. Consistent with the notion of a disorder, both DSM-IV and ICD-10 require that the signs of disorder be evident across situations and relationships.

Two clinical patterns of attachment disorders have been described: (i) an emotionally withdrawn/inhibited pattern, in which the child exhibits limited or absent initiation or response to social interactions with caregivers, and a variety of aberrant social behaviors, such as inhibited, hypervigilant, or highly ambivalent reactions; and (ii) an indiscriminately social/disinhibited pattern, in which the child exhibits lack of expectable selectivity in seeking comfort, support and nurturance, with lack of social reticence with unfamiliar adults, including a willingness to "go off" with strangers.

Emotionally Withdrawn/Inhibited

Core features of this subtype of attachment disorder include lack of social and emotional responses, an absence or near-absence of attachment behaviors even in times of stress, and serious problems of emotion regulation. Most strikingly, the emotionally withdrawn subtype of attachment disorder involves a paucity of positive affect responses. It also often includes bouts of fear or irritability that are seemingly unprovoked, or at least out of proportion to the putative stimulus. Social and emotional reciprocal interactions are absent or at least severely dampened. Although few data have addressed the issue directly, cognitive delays are an expected associated feature, given that the conditions of neglect believed to lead to this pattern of attachment disorder also are associated with developmental delays.

These signs have been described in young children with a history of severe maltreatment (Zeanah, Scheeringa, Boris *et al.*, 2004) and those being raised in institutions (Smyke, Dumitrescu, & Zeanah, 2002; Zeanah, Smyke, Koga *et al.*, 2005). Interestingly, they have been much less noted in children adopted out of institutions (Chisholm, 1998; Chisholm, Carter, Ames, & Morison, 1995; O'Connor, Bredenkamp, & Rutter, 1999; O'Connor & Rutter, 2000).

Indiscriminately Social/Disinhibited

Core behavioral features of disinhibited/indiscriminately social attachment disorder in young children include inappropriate approach to unfamiliar adults, a lack of wariness of strangers, failure to check back with a caregiver in unfamiliar settings, and a willingness to accompany a stranger and wander away from a familiar caregiver. Indiscriminate behavior also may be associated with lack of appropriate physical boundaries, so that children may interact with strangers intrusively and aggressively and may even seek out physical contact (O'Connor & Zeanah, 2003).

In comparing three different investigative teams' approaches to indiscriminate behavior, Zeanah, Smyke, and Dumitrescu (2002) were able to show that despite differences in definition, there was overall a substantial convergence about how this type of disorder is identified. Nevertheless, the signs of this type of attachment disorder are not particularly clearly described in DSM-IV-TR or in ICD-10, and concerns remain about the heterogeneity of what we mean by indiscriminate behavior.

For example, some investigators have referred to "indiscriminately friendly" behavior (Chisholm, 1998; Chisholm, Carter, Ames *et al.*, 1995), but others have suggested that these terms imply more than is actually known about the nature of the child's behavior (O'Connor, 2002; O'Connor & Zeanah, 2003; Zeanah, 2000). Some children exhibit passive lack of reticence and willingness to accompany a stranger, but this may be quite distinct from children who eagerly accompany a stranger without even checking back with their putative attachment figure. Other behaviors subsumed under this description include lack of initial reticence around unfamiliar adults (e.g., sitting in the lap of an unfamiliar adult after just meeting him or her), actively choosing to approach an unfamiliar adult over an attachment figure in times of need, failing to monitor the whereabouts of the attachment figure in unfamiliar settings, displaying inappropriate social boundaries (e.g., making eye contact for too long or asking overly personal questions on initial meeting), or verbally or physically aggressive engagement of unfamiliar adults. These behaviors are not experienced as sociable or friendly by those on the receiving end, and they are not always indiscriminate either (O'Connor & Zeanah, 2003). There is much room for more precise delineation of behaviors subsumed by this term.

Measurement Issues and Differential Diagnosis

Attachment disorders have been assessed both continuously and categorically. Boris, Zeanah, Larrieu, Scheeringa, and Heller (1998) were the first to examine the reliability of categorical diagnostic criteria. This and subsequent categorical studies have demonstrated that attachment disorders can be reliably diagnosed in young children (Boris, Hinshaw-Fuselier, Smyke *et al.*, 2004; Zeanah, Scheeringa, Boris *et al.*, 2004). Studies using continuous measures of disordered attachment also have demonstrated adequate inter-rater reliability in identifying signs of both the emotionally withdrawn/inhibited and the indiscriminately social/disinhibited types of disorder (O'Connor, Bredenkamp, & Rutter, 1999; O'Connor, Marvin, Rutter *et al.*, 2003; Smyke, Dumitrescu, & Zeanah, 2002; Zeanah, Smyke, & Dumitrescu, 2002; Zeanah, Scheeringa, Boris *et al.*, 2004; Zeanah, Smyke, Koga *et al.*, 2005). The two patterns have been reliably identified in extreme populations, such as severely neglected children and those being raised in institutional settings, and they appear to be extremely rare in other populations of children (Boris, Hinshaw-Fuselier, Smyke *et al.*, 2004; Roy, Rutter, & Pickles, 2004).

Regarding convergent validity, Boris, Zeanah, Larrieu *et al.* (1998) demonstrated more severe parent–child relationship impairments in children with attachment disorders compared to children with other clinical problems. More specifically, Zeanah, Smyke, Koga *et al.* (2005) showed a moderate convergence between ratings of young children's attachment behaviors in the Strange Situation with their caregivers and caregivers' reports of signs of emotionally withdrawn/inhibited attachment disorder in the children. Also, the same group reported convergence of caregiver reports of signs of indiscriminately social/disinhibited attachment behavior and a procedure demonstrating the child's willingness to "go off" with a stranger (Zeanah, 2006). These preliminary findings are encouraging that there is reasonable convergence among different methods used to identify attachment disorders. Nevertheless, it must be acknowledged that there remains no gold standard method of identification at this point.

Given the earlier noted ubiquity of attachment as a developmental issue, it seems useful to explore whether putative attachment disorders can be distinguished from other types of disturbance. In fact, both types of attachment disorder have been shown to be only modestly or moderately correlated with aggressive behavior problems, language delays and stereotypies

(O'Connor & Rutter, 2000; Smyke, Dumitrescu, & Zeanah, 2002).

The emotionally withdrawn/inhibited type of attachment disorder shares some features with autistic spectrum disorders, including disturbances in emotion regulation, impaired or absent social and emotional reciprocity and, often, cognitive delays. However, children with reactive attachment disorder should not have a selective impairment in pretend play, repetitive preoccupations or language abnormalities other than delays. In addition, they should have a history of seriously adverse caregiving.

Because both the inhibited/emotionally withdrawn subtype and cognitive delays have been associated with severe deprivation (Zeanah, Smyke, & Settles, 2006), it is reasonable to assume that the emotionally withdrawn/inhibited type also may be confused with intellectual disability. Young children with emotionally withdrawn/inhibited attachment disorder should be distinguishable from children with intellectual disability because the latter group have social and emotional behaviors that are consistent with their developmental age, whereas children with emotionally withdrawn/inhibited attachment disorder have clear evidence of deviance in their social responsiveness and regulation of emotion. Clearly, both conditions may co-occur.

Disinhibited attachment may share features of attention deficit/hyperactivity disorder, particularly social impulsivity. Roy, Rutter, & Pickles (2004) found that school-age children with a history of institutional rearing had high levels of both disinhibited attachment behavior and inattention/hyperactivity, as well as a strong association between the two. In addition to lack of selectivity in relationships with caregivers, the children also showed lack of selectivity with peers, echoing the findings of Hodges and Tizard (1989) with adolescents who had formerly been indiscriminate with caregivers. Because both inattention/hyperactivity and disinhibited behavior have been reported as sequelae of institutional rearing, these findings raise questions about whether they may be part of a unitary "post-institutional" syndrome, at least in a subset of cases, or whether they are distinct disorders that occur comorbidly. Of note, in Roy, Rutter, & Pickles (2004), the combination of lack of selectivity in relationships and inattention/hyperactivity occurred only in boys, whereas there has been no gender specificity reported in other studies of disinhibited attachment.

Prevalence

Signs of attachment disorders and prevalence of attachment disorders are greater in more extreme populations; that is, in young children who have experienced severe deprivation (Boris, Hinshaw-Fuselier, Smyke *et al.*, 2004; Chisholm, 1998; O'Connor, Marvin, Rutter *et al.*, 2003; Smyke, Dumitrescu, & Zeanah, 2002; Zeanah, Scheeringa, Boris *et al.*, 2004). Still, there is a consensus that attachment disorders are rare, even though there have been no careful epidemiological studies.

In a sample of 300 children aged 2–5 years recruited from pediatric clinics in Durham, North Carolina, Egger, Erkanli, Keeler *et al.* (2006) found no cases of attachment disorders using DSM-IV or the RDC-PA criteria (Boris & Zeanah, 2005). Several recent studies of clinic-referred and high-risk children have assessed signs of disordered attachment using structured interviews and observational assessments. These studies have found that, even among maltreated children, few met criteria for attachment disorders, with the exception of maltreated children in foster care (Boris, Zeanah, Larrieu *et al.*, 1998; Boris, Hinshaw-Fuselier, Smyke *et al.*, 2004; Zeanah, Scheeringa, Boris *et al.*, 2004). In a sample of 12- to 30-month-old children living in institutions in Bucharest, Romania, 10% met criteria for emotionally withdrawn/inhibited attachment disorders and 24% for indiscriminate/disinhibited attachment disorder (Zeanah, 2006). Thus, although signs of the disorder may be common in extreme populations, a minority of children seem to reach the threshold of disorder.

Etiology

Together with post-traumatic stress disorder (PTSD), attachment disorders are one of the few psychiatric disorders in which the etiology is specified as one of the diagnostic criteria. A requirement of DSM-IV is that the signs and symptoms of attachment disorder be brought about by "pathogenic care." Although pathogenic care is not defined, maltreatment and multiple moves are cited as examples. Although ICD-10 is less insistent on requiring pathogenic care, the clinician is cautioned against making the diagnosis in the absence of a history of maltreatment.

Many questions about the nature of the caregiving compromise necessary to produce attachment disorders remain unanswered. For example, it seems reasonable to presume that neglect is the key feature, but the question of whether physical or sexual abuse alone could lead to a similar clinical picture has not been examined carefully, in part because of the difficulty of determining the nature of maltreatment in preverbal or barely verbal children. There does seem to be some component of institutional rearing that is specifically implicated in underlying indiscriminate behavior. In Roy, Rutter, & Pickles (2004), indiscriminate behavior occurred only in children with a history of institutional rearing and not in those placed in foster care, and in O'Connor, Marvin, Rutter *et al.* (2003) only in those with a history of institutional rearing and not those adopted within the UK. Because these studies involved institutional experiences that ranged in quality, it appears that even in better quality institutions, children remain at risk. It is also notable that the lone study to consider age at entry into institutions found that only children placed in institutions *early* showed a pattern of indiscriminate behavior (Wolkind, 1974).

However, anecdotal evidence suggests that even in the absence of pathogenic care, some young children display signs of disinhibited/indiscriminate attachment behavior. For example, individuals with Williams syndrome have been reported to show high levels of indiscriminate behavior (Jones, Bellugi, Lai *et al.*, 2002). Williams syndrome, a microdeletion on chromosome 7q11.23, is characterized by a tendency for affected individuals to approach persons they do not know and interact with them verbally. Parents of young children with Williams syndrome expend much effort to monitor their children's whereabouts and teach them to refrain from approaching strangers (Plesa-Skwerer, personal communication). Compared with non-affected individuals, they are unable to distinguish threatening faces, considering them just as trustworthy as non-threatening faces (Jones, Bellugi, Lai *et al.*, 2002).

Fetal alcohol syndrome (FAS) may be associated with indiscriminate behavior in the absence of pathogenic care. Alcohol acts as a central nervous system poison, and FAS results from prenatal exposure to high levels of alcohol. Signs of the syndrome in young children include a specific pattern of facial features as well as cognitive and socioemotional abnormalities, including children being talkative, affectionate, outgoing and overly friendly to strangers (see chapter 30; Jacobson & Jacobson, 2003). FAS has been associated both with increased risk of disorganized attachment (O'Connor, Sigman, & Brill, 1987) and with increased risk of reactive attachment disorder.

Course Over Time

The major impediment to understanding the course of attachment disorders is the paucity of longitudinal data available for review. Based upon preliminary results from several studies, however, it is possible to suggest that the two types of attachment disorder generally have different courses.

Studies of children adopted out of institutions have not reported evidence of the emotionally withdrawn/inhibited type following adoption (Chisholm, 1998; Tizard & Hodges, 1978; O'Connor, Marvin, Rutter *et al.*, 2003). Furthermore, the Bucharest Early Intervention Project (BEIP), the first randomized controlled trial to evaluate an intervention for attachment disorders, included baseline assessments and follow-up at 30, 42 and 54 months of age (Zeanah, Nelson, Fox *et al.*, 2003). At baseline, quality of caregiving, defined by parental sensitivity, stimulation of development, positive regard towards child, absence of detachment, absence of flat affect and absence of intrusiveness, was inversely related to signs of emotionally withdrawn/inhibited attachment disorder, although it was unrelated to signs of indiscriminate/disinhibited attachment disorder (Zeanah, Smyke, Koga *et al.*, 2005). Preliminary results from this study indicate that foster care leads to significant reductions in signs of attachment disorder in young children who had signs of the disorder when they were living in institutions. In the group of young children randomized to foster care following early institutional rearing, such placement effectively eliminated emotionally withdrawn/inhibited attachment disorder and reduced indiscriminately social/disinhibited attachment disorder, whereas both persisted in children who remained in institutions (Zeanah, 2006).

Over a 2-year period in the BEIP, there was no significant reduction in signs of inhibited/emotionally withdrawn reactive attachment disorder for young children who remained in institutions. This latter finding is important, as it represents preliminary evidence of persistence of the disorder in children who remain in an adverse caregiving environment.

In contrast, there is reasonably clear evidence demonstrating that indiscriminate behavior persists over time – sometimes even after improvements in the caregiving environment. This was demonstrated originally in the work of Tizard and colleagues, who showed that young children who had been indiscriminate with caregivers at age 4 years were more likely to have serious peer disturbances at 16 years, including superficial and even indiscriminate behavior with peers (Hodges & Tizard, 1989). Subsequent studies of children adopted into Canada and the UK from Romanian institutions have also demonstrated a tendency for indiscriminate behavior to persist even after the child forms attachments to the adopted family (Chisholm, 1998; O'Connor, Marvin, Rutter *et al.*, 2003). In fact, of those children adopted into the UK from Romanian institutions who had high levels of indiscriminate behavior at age 6 years, more than half continued to show high levels at age 11 years (Rutter, Colvert, Kreppner *et al.*, 2006). Furthermore, in the same randomized controlled trial of foster care described above, indiscriminate behavior was only weakly responsive to removal from institutions and placement in foster care, and persistence was noted in all children who had been reared in institutions (Zeanah, 2006).

Clinical Assessment

In keeping with recent trends in the assessment of early childhood psychopathology (delCarmen-Wiggins & Carter, 2004), attachment disorders are best identified through a combination of caregiver interview and observed interactions. In our view, there are no gold standard interviews nor observational paradigms of interactions between parents and children that must be included, but several useful approaches have been described.

Interviews

Structured interviews specifically focused on the child's attachment behaviors and signs of disordered attachment (Boris, Hinshaw-Fuselier, Smyke *et al.*, 2004; O'Connor, Bredenkamp, & Rutter, 1999; Smyke, Dumitrescu, & Zeanah, 2002; Zeanah, Scheeringa, Boris *et al.*, 2004) are more likely to be useful than interviews that are less specifically focused. At least two structured psychiatric interviews, the Psychiatric Assessment Preschool Age (Egger & Angold, 2004) and the Diagnostic Infant/Preschool Structured Interview (Scheeringa, 2005) include modules on attachment disorders. These approaches have been able to characterize attachment disorders both categorically and continuously.

Observations

Observations of parent and child together include procedures designed specifically to examine attachment behaviors (Boris, Hinshaw-Fuselier, Smyke *et al.*, 2004; Marvin, Cooper, Hoffman, & Powell, 2002; O'Connor, Marvin, Rutter *et al.*, 2003), or those in which other aspects of parent–child interaction are also assessed (Zeanah, Larrieu, Valliere, & Heller, 2000). It is generally useful to include in the observation some degree of distress that is likely to activate the child's need for the attachment figure. Conventionally, this has involved brief separations followed by reunions, but other approaches such as a novel (i.e., scary) toy also have been used (Boris, Hinshaw-Fuselier, Smyke *et al.*, 2004). Although it is neither necessary nor necessarily advisable to use the Strange Situation Procedure in clinical assessments, in some circumstances, it may be helpful. The Circle of Security Intervention, for example, includes review of videotaped recordings of a child's Strange Situation behavior with the parent as a part of the intervention (Marvin, Cooper, Hoffman *et al.*, 2002). What is important clinically is not to confuse attachment classifications derived from the Strange Situation with attachment disorder diagnoses. Although systematic observations of the child's behavior in paradigms designed to elicit attachment behaviors are often clinically valuable, naturalistic observations of a child's attachment behaviors also may yield important data.

Interventions

Given that the database on disordered attachment is so small and so recent, it is not surprising that studies of intervention efforts for reactive attachment disorder are limited. Intervention efforts to date have been guided by the principle that enhancing the caregiving environment will ameliorate signs of attachment disorder. There are case reports documenting substantial improvements in young children removed from severely neglecting environments and placed in foster care (Hinshaw-Fuselier, Boris, & Zeanah, 1999; Zeanah & Boris, 2000; Zeanah, Mammen, & Lieberman, 1993). Stovall and Dozier (2000) also reported a descriptive study indicating that attachment behaviors in a small sample of young children became organized towards their new caregivers within days to weeks of placement in foster care.

Studies of children raised in institutions have also begun to appear. Smyke, Dumitrescu, & Zeanah (2002) studied signs of attachment disorder in young children being raised in a large institution for young children in Bucharest. This institution had implemented a pilot unit designed to reduce the number of caregivers responsible for each child. In fact, compared to the more standard units, which included large numbers of rotating caregivers, on the pilot unit no more than four caregivers were responsible for each child on the day and evening shifts. Caregivers on the pilot unit reported that children had significantly fewer signs of both emotionally withdrawn/inhibited attachment disorder and indiscriminately social/disinhibited attachment disorder. Importantly, this reduction was evident even though the ratio of caregivers to children remained at 1:12 on the pilot unit (the same as on the standard units).

Studies of young children adopted out of institutions are also useful to examine because they represent such a dramatic change in caregiving environments. Two longitudinal studies of young children adopted out of Romanian institutions are particularly instructive.

A longitudinal study of young children adopted into Canada from Romanian institutions used parent reports of attachment and indiscriminate behavior. They found significant increases in attachment to adoptive parents during the first several years following adoption, although indiscriminate behavior persisted in a minority of children (Chisholm, 1998; Chisholm, Carter, Ames *et al.*, 1995).

Another longitudinal study of children adopted from Romanian institutions into families in the UK assessed signs of disordered attachment from parent reports at ages 4, 6 and 11 years (O'Connor & Rutter, 2000; O'Connor, Marvin, Rutter *et al.*, 2003; Rutter, Colvert, Kreppner *et al.*, 2006). They reported little change in the numbers of children with high levels of indiscriminate behaviors between 4 and 6 years, but some decline by age 11 years (O'Connor & Rutter, 2000; Rutter, Colvert, Kreppner *et al.*, 2006). To date, however, there has been no demonstration that quality of care in adoptive homes is inversely related to signs of indiscriminately social/disinhibited attachment in children.

In summary, findings from studies of children living in institutions and those adopted out of institutions suggest that signs of the indiscriminate/disinhibited type are remediated by enhanced caregiving only in *some* children. It is unclear whether this represents individual differences among children or partial remediation with persistence in those most severely affected initially. To date, adoption studies have not included assessments of children in the institutions prior to adoption, making it difficult to explain individual differences in response.

The only contemporary intervention study that included assessments of children's attachment prior to removal from institutions and placement in an enhanced caregiving environment is the BEIP, described earlier. Preliminary results from this study indicate that foster care leads to significant reductions in signs of attachment disorder in young children who had had signs of the disorder when they were living in institutions (Zeanah, 2006).

At this stage, clinicians must be guided by data indicating that secure attachment is fostered by caregivers who are emotionally available and sensitively responsive, who know and value the child as an individual, and who place the needs of the child ahead of their own needs. Preliminary data indicate that psychoeducational approaches involving training parents to respond sensitively to their child (van den Boom, 1995) and to understand their own and their child's attachment pattern (Hoffman, Marvin, Cooper, & Powell, 2006) have been shown to promote attachment security in the child. These interventions are reasonable starting points for developing an evidence base about intervening in disordered attachments.

Conclusions

Our understanding of attachment disorders has deepened considerably in the past decade as a result of the publication of a number of systematic studies of children with histories of severe neglect or institutional rearing. These studies have affirmed the reliable identification of both the emotionally withdrawn/inhibited and the indiscriminately social/disinhibited types of attachment disorder described in contemporary nosologies. They also have supported the link between pathogenic care and attachment disorders, and have suggested that the specific "pathogen" is any environment in which young children have limited opportunities to form selective attachments, as happens in cases of severe social neglect or in settings in which the child lacks regular and consistent contact with an emotionally involved caregiver (e.g., institutional settings).

These studies have suggested that although the two types of attachment disorder arise from similar conditions of risk, they have different correlates and different courses. In particular, placement in enhanced caregiving environments seems to lead to rapid and complete elimination of signs of emotionally withdrawn/inhibited attachment disorder, but the indiscriminately social/disinhibited attachment disorder remains persistent in some children, apparently for years.

However, a number of questions remain to be addressed. First, nothing is known about individual vulnerabilities to the disorder – in particular why such phenomenologically distinct syndromes arise from similar conditions of risk. Genetic polymorphisms, temperamental dispositions and differential caregiving experiences should all be examined. In addition, the relationship between the two types of disorder – if any – needs to be clarified. Second, why some children with indiscriminately social/disinhibited attachment disorder seem to respond to enhanced caregiving and others do not is unclear. Third, the specific components of enhanced caregiving that are crucial for amelioration of signs of the disorder are unclear. This is especially important given the heterogeneity of outcomes in post-adoption studies. Fourth, the putative social cognitive abnormalities that characterize indiscriminate behavior need to be delineated. It seems reasonable that such abnormalities are the most concerning aspect of the disorder from the standpoint of functional impairment. Finally, the underlying neurobiology of these disorders is largely unexplored. The links between indiscriminate behavior and Williams syndrome and FAS, each of which has begun to be explored neurobiologically, may suggest hypotheses about functional impairments to be examined in children with deprivation-induced indiscriminate behavior. Answers to these questions will assist clinicians concerned with helping children recover from the long-term effects of early adversity.

References

Ainsworth, M. D. S., Blehar, M. C., Waters, E., & Wall, S. (1978). *Patterns of attachment*. Hillsdale, NJ: Erlbaum.

American Psychiatric Association. (1980). *Diagnostic and statistical manual of mental disorders* (3rd edn.). Washington, DC: American Psychiatric Association.

American Psychiatric Association. (2000). *Diagnostic and statistical manual of mental disorders* (4th edn.). Text revision. Washington, DC: American Psychiatric Association.

Benoit, D., Parker, K. C. H., & Zeanah, C. H. (1997). Mothers' representations of their infants assessed prenatally: Stability and association with infants' attachment classifications. *Journal of Child Psychology, Psychiatry and Allied Disciplines*, *38*, 307–313.

Boris, N. W., Hinshaw-Fuselier, S. S., Smyke, A. T., Scheeringa, M., Heller, S. S. & Zeanah, C. H. (2004). Comparing criteria for attachment disorders: Establishing reliability and validity in high-risk samples. *Journal of the American Academy of Child and Adolescent Psychiatry*, *43*, 568–577.

Boris, N. W., & Zeanah, C. H.; Work Group on Quality Issues. (2005). Practice parameter for the assessment and treatment of children and adolescents with reactive attachment disorder of infancy and early childhood. *Journal of the American Academy of Child and Adolescent Psychiatry*, *44*, 1206–1219.

Boris, N. W., Zeanah, C. H., Larrieu, J. A., Scheeringa, M. S., & Heller, S. S. (1998). Attachment disorders in infancy and early childhood: A preliminary investigation of diagnostic criteria. *American Journal of Psychiatry*, *155*, 295–297.

Bowlby, J. (1965). *Child care and the growth of love*. London: Penguin.

Bowlby, J. (1982). *Attachment and loss*. Vol. 1. *Attachment* (2nd edn.). New York: Basic Books.

Carlson, V., Cicchetti, D., & Barnett, D. (1989). Finding order in disorganization: Lessons from research on maltreated infants' attachments to their caregivers. In D. Cicchetti & V. Carlson (Eds.), *Child maltreatment: Theory and research on the causes and consequences of child abuse and neglect* (pp. 494–528). New York: Cambridge University Press.

Chapin, H. D. (1915). Are institutions for infants necessary? *Journal of the American Medical Association*, *64*, 1–3.

Chisholm, K. (1998). A three year follow-up of attachment and indiscriminate friendliness in children adopted from Romanian orphanages. *Child Development*, *69*, 1092–1106.

Chisholm, K., Carter, M. C., Ames, E. W., & Morison, S. J. (1995). Attachment security and indiscriminately friendly behavior in children adopted from Romanian orphanages. *Development and Psychopathology*, *7*, 283–294.

delCarmen-Wiggins, R., & Carter, A. (2004). *Handbook of infant, toddler, and preschool mental health assessment*. New York: Oxford University Press.

Egger, H. L., & Angold, A. (2004). The Preschool Age Psychiatric Assessment (PAPA): A structured parent interview for diagnosing psychiatric disorders in preschool children. In R. DelCarmen-Wiggins & A. Carter (Eds.), *Handbook of infant, toddler, and preschool mental health assessment* (pp. 223–243). New York: Oxford University Press.

Egger, H. L., Erkanli, A., Keeler, G., Potts, E., Walter, B. K., & Angold, A. (2006). Test–retest reliability of the Preschool Age Psychiatric Assessment (PAPA). *Journal of the American Academy of Child and Adolescent Psychiatry*, *45*, 538–549.

Emde, R. N. (1989). The infant's relationship experience: Developmental and affective aspects. In A. J. Sameroff, & R. N. Emde (Eds.), *Relationship disturbances in early childhood: A developmental approach* (pp. 33–51). New York: Basic Books.

Goldfarb, W. (1945). Effects of psychological deprivation in infancy and subsequent stimulation. *American Journal of Psychiatry*, *102*, 18–33.

Green, J., & Goldwyn, R. (2002). Annotation: Attachment disorganisation and psychopathology: New findings in attachment research and their potential implications for developmental psychopathology in childhood. *Journal of Child Psychology and Psychiatry*, *43*, 835–846.

Hinshaw-Fuselier, S., Boris, N. W., & Zeanah, C. H. (1999). Reactive attachment disorder in maltreated twins. *Infant Mental Health Journal*, *20*, 42–59.

Hodges, J., & Tizard, B. (1989). Social and family relationships of ex-institutional adolescents. *Journal of Child Psychology, Psychiatry, and Allied Disciplines*, *30*, 77–97.

Hofer, M. A. (2006). Psychobiological roots of early attachment. *Current Directions in Psychological Science*, *15*, 84–88.

Hoffman, K., Marvin, R., Cooper, G., & Powell, B. (2006). Changing toddlers' and preschoolers' attachment classifications: The Circle of Security intervention. *Journal of Consulting and Clinical Psychology*, *74*, 1017–1026.

Jacobson, S., & Jacobson, J. (2003). FAS/FAE and its impact on psychosocial child development. In R. E. Tremblay, R. G. Barr, & R. D. V. Peters (Eds.), *Encyclopedia on early childhood development* [online]. Montreal, Quebec: Centre of Excellence for Early Childhood Development (pp. 1–7). Accessed June 15, 2006 from http://www.excellence-earlychildhood.ca/documents/JacobsonANGxp.pdf.

Jones, W., Bellugi, U., Lai, Z., Chiles, M., Reilly, J., Lincoln, A., *et al.* (2000). Hypersociability in Williams syndrome. *Journal of Cognitive Neuroscience*, *12*, 30–46.

Kreppner, J., Rutter, M., Beckett, C., Castle, J., Colvert, E., Groothues, C., *et al.* (2007). Normality and impairment following profound early institutional deprivation: A longitudinal follow-up into early adolescence. *Developmental Psychology*, *43*, 931–946.

Levy, R. J. (1947). Effects of institutional vs. boarding home care on a group of infants. *Journal of Personality*, *15*, 233–241.

Lyons-Ruth, K., Bronfin, E., & Parsons, E. (1999). Atypical attachment in early childhood among children at developmental risk. IV. Maternal disrupted affective communications, maternal frightening or frightened behavior, and infant disorganized attachment strategies. *Monographs of the Society for Research in Child Development*, *64*, 172–192.

Marvin, R. S., Cooper, G., Hoffman, K., & Powell, B. (2002). The Circle of Security project: Attachment-based intervention with caregiver–pre-school child dyads. *Attachment and Human Development*, *4*, 107–124.

Minnis, H., Marwick, H., Arthur, J., & McLaughlin, A. (2006). Reactive attachment disorder: A theoretical model beyond attachment. *European Journal of Child and Adolescent Psychiatry*, *15*, 336–342.

O'Connor, M. J., Sigman, M., & Brill, N. (1987). Disorganization of attachment in relation to maternal alcohol consumption. *Journal of Consulting and Clinical Psychology*, *81*, 231–236.

O'Connor, T. G. (2002). Attachment disorders in infancy and childhood. In M. Rutter, & E. Taylor (Eds.), *Child and adolescent psychiatry: Modern approaches* (4th edn., pp. 776–792). Oxford, UK: Blackwell Scientific.

O'Connor, T. G., Bredenkamp, D., & Rutter, M. (1999). Attachment disturbances and disorders in children exposed to early severe deprivation. *Infant Mental Health Journal*, *20*, 10–29.

O'Connor, T. G., Marvin, R. S., Rutter, M., Olrick, J. T., & Britner, P. A. (2003). Child–parent attachment following early institutional deprivation. *Development and Psychopathology*, *15*, 19–38.

O'Connor, T. G., & Rutter, M. (2000). Attachment disorder behavior following early severe deprivation: Extension and longitudinal follow-up. *Journal of the American Academy of Child and Adolescent Psychiatry*, *39*, 703–712.

O'Connor, T. G., & Zeanah, C. H. (2003). Assessment strategies and treatment approaches. *Attachment and Human Development*, *5*, 223–244.

Provence, S., & Lipton, R. C. (1962). *Infants in institutions*. New York: International Universities Press.

Roy, P., Rutter, M., & Pickles, A. (2004). Institutional care: Associations between overactivity and lack of selectivity in social relationships. *Journal of Child Psychology and Psychiatry*, *45*, 866–873.

Rutter, M. (1981). *Maternal deprivation reassessed* (2nd edn.). Harmondsworth: Penguin Books.

Rutter, M., Beckett, C., Castle, J., Colvert, E., Kreppner, J., Mehta, M., *et al.* (2007). Effects of profound early institutional deprivation: An overview of findings from a UK longitudinal study of Romanian adoptees. *European Journal of Developmental Psychology*, *4*, 332–350.

Rutter, M., Colvert, E., Kreppner, J., Beckett, C., Castle, J., Groothues, C., *et al.* (2006). Early adolescent outcomes for institutionally-deprived and non-deprived adoptees. I. Disinhibited attachment. *Journal of Child Psychology, Psychiatry and Allied Disciplines*, *48*, 17–30.

Scheeringa, M. (2005). *Diagnostic Infant/Preschool Structured Interview*. Unpublished manuscript, Tulane University.

Schuengel, C., Bakermans-Kranenburg, M. J., & van IJzendoorn, M. H. (1999). Frightening maternal behavior linking unresolved loss and disorganized infant attachment. *Journal of Consulting and Clinical Psychology*, *67*, 54–63.

Smyke, A. T., Dumitrescu, A., & Zeanah, C. H. (2002). Disturbances of attachment in young children. I. The continuum of caretaking casualty. *Journal of the American Academy of Child and Adolescent Psychiatry*, *41*, 972–982.

Spitz, R. A. (1945). Hospitalism: An inquiry into the genesis of psychiatric conditions in early childhood. *Psychoanalytic Study of the Child*, *1*, 53–74.

Stovall, K. C., & Dozier, M. (2000). The development of attachment in new relationships: Single subject analyses for ten foster infants. *Development and Psychopathology*, *12*, 133–156.

Suomi, S. J., Collins, M. L., Harlow, H. F., & Ruppenthal, G. C. (1976). Effects of maternal and peer separation on young monkeys. *Journal of Child Psychology and Psychiatry*, *17*, 101–112.

Task Force on Research Diagnostic Criteria: Infancy and Preschool. (2003). Research diagnostic criteria for infants and preschool children: The process and empirical support. *Journal of the American Academy of Child and Adolescent Psychiatry*, *42*, 1504–1512.

Tizard, B. (1977). *Adoption: A second chance*. London: Open Books.

Tizard, B., & Hodges, J. (1978). The effect of early institutional rearing on the development of eight year old children. *Journal of Child Psychology and Psychiatry*, *19*, 99–118.

Tizard, B., & Rees, J. (1975). The effect of early institutional rearing on the behaviour problems and affectional relationships of four-year-old children. *Journal of Child Psychology and Psychiatry*, *16*, 61–73.

van den Boom, D. (1995). Do first-year intervention effects endure? Follow-up during toddlerhood of a sample of Dutch irritable infants. *Child Development*, *66*, 1798–1816.

van IJzendoorn, M. H., & Bakermans-Kranenburg, M. J. (2002). Disorganized attachment and the dysregulation of negative emotions. In B. Zuckerman, A. Lieberman, & N. Fox (Eds.), *Emotion regulation and developmental health: Infancy and early childhood* (pp. 159–179). Somerville, NJ: Johnson and Johnson Pediatric Institute.

van IJzendoorn, M. H., Schuengel, C., & Bakermans-Kranenburg, M. J. (1999). Disorganized attachment in early childhood: Meta-analysis of precursors, concomitants, and sequelae. *Development and Psychopathology*, *11*, 225–249.

Vorria, P., Papaligoura, Z., Dunn, J., van IJzendoorn, M. H., Steele, H., Kontopoulou, A., *et al.* (2003). Early experiences and attachment relationships of Greek infants raised in residential group care. *Journal of Child Psychology and Psychiatry*, *44*, 1208–1220.

Wolkind, S. N. (1974). The components of "affectionless psychopathy" in institutionalized children. *Journal of Child Psychology and Psychiatry*, *15*, 215–220.

World Health Organization. (1996). *Multiaxial classification of child and adolescent psychiatric disorders: The ICD-10 classification of mental and behavioural disorders in children and adolescents*. Cambridge, UK: Cambridge University Press.

Zeanah, C. H. (1996). Beyond insecurity: A reconceptualization of attachment disorders of infancy. *Journal of Consulting and Clinical Psychology*, *64*, 42–52.

Zeanah, C. H. (2000). Disturbances of attachment in young children adopted from institutions. *Journal of Developmental and Behavioral Pediatrics*, *21*, 230–236.

Zeanah, C. H. (2006, February). *Bucharest Early Intervention Project: Psychiatric outcomes*. Presented at the American Association for Advancement of Science Annual Meeting, St. Louis, MO.

Zeanah, C. H., & Boris, N. W. (2000). Disturbances and disorders of attachment in early childhood. In C. H. Zeanah (Ed.), *Handbook of infant mental health* (2nd edn., pp. 353–368). New York: Guilford Press.

Zeanah, C. H., Larrieu, J. A., Valliere, J., & Heller, S. S. (2000). Infant–parent relationship assessment. In C. H. Zeanah (Ed.), *Handbook of infant mental health* (2nd ed., pp. 222–235). New York: Guilford Press.

Zeanah, C. H., Mammen, O., & Lieberman, A. (1993). Disorders of attachment. In C. H. Zeanah (Ed.), *Handbook of infant mental health* (pp. 332–349). New York: Guilford Press.

Zeanah, C. H., Nelson, C. A., Fox, N. A., Smyke, A. T., Marshall, P., Parker, S. *et al.* (2003). Effects of institutionalization on brain and behavioral development: The Bucharest Early Intervention Project. *Development and Psychopathology*, *15*, 885–907.

Zeanah, C. H., Scheeringa, M. S., Boris, N. W., Heller, S. S., Smyke, A. T., & Trapani, J. (2004). Reactive attachment disorder in maltreated toddlers. *Child Abuse and Neglect*, *28*, 877–888.

Zeanah, C. H., Smyke, A. T., & Settles, L. (2006). Children in orphanages. In K. McCartney, & D. Phillips (Eds.), *Blackwell handbook of early childhood development* (pp. 224–254). Malden, MA: Blackwell Publishing.

Zeanah, C. H., Smyke, A. T., & Dumitrescu, A. (2002). Disturbances of attachment in young children. II. Indiscriminate behavior and institutional care. *Journal of the American Academy of Child and Adolescent Psychiatry*, *41*, 983–989.

Zeanah, C. H., Smyke, A. T., Koga, S. F. M., Carlson, E., & the BEIP Core Group. (2005). Attachment in institutionalized and non-institutionalized Romanian children. *Child Development*, *76*, 1015–1028.

Zero to Three. (2005). *Diagnostic classification: 0–3R: the Diagnostic classification of mental health and developmental disorders of infancy and early childhood*, Revised edition. Washington, DC: Zero to Three Press.

Zhang, L. X., Levine, S., Dent, G., Zhan, Y., Xing, G., Okimoto, D., *et al.* (2002). Maternal deprivation increases cell death in the infant rat brain. *Developmental Brain Research*, *133*, 1–11.

56 Wetting and Soiling

Richard J. Butler

Wetting and soiling are widespread, and can be distressing. A recent epidemiological study of over 13,000 English children (Avon Longitudinal Study of Parents and Children [ALSPAC]) found from parental reports that at 7 years of age 15.5% children wet the bed sometimes, 7.7% sometimes wet during the day, 6.8% had daytime soiling and only 0.8% had night-time soiling (Butler, Golding, Northstone *et al.*, 2005a). There is an overall reduction in prevalence with age: by late adolescence 1–2% continue bedwetting (Verhulst, van der Lee, Akkerhuis *et al.*, 1985), 1% day wet (Hellström, Hanson, Hansson, Hjälmås, & Jodal, 1990) and very few soil (Bellman, 1966). However, the picture is not one of universal improvement. Children with the severest form of wetting or soiling (at least twice a week, in line with the DSM-IV diagnostic criteria) are much less prevalent (2.6% for bedwetting at age 7, 1% for daytime wetting and 0.8% soiling; Butler, Golding, Northstone *et al.*, 2005a), but an epidemiological survey by Yeung, Sreedhar, Sihoe, Sit, and Lau (2006) suggested that for these more severely affected individuals the prevalence profile remains flat, with enuresis tending to continue into late adolescence.

There is accordingly a complex issue about the point at which these forms of incontinence should be defined as problematic. One way of answering is developmental: to define an age at which there is a discontinuity and a sudden increase in the proportion becoming dry or clean. On this basis, Verhulst, van der Lee, Akkerhuis *et al.* (1985) identified a rapid decrease in the prevalence of nocturnal enuresis at about age 5 for girls and 8 for boys. A definition on this basis, however, would overlook the psychological distress for families with children (especially boys) who are enuretic but younger than the age of rapid decrease. A different approach, in line with recent evidence, suggests intervention to meet the child's needs. Both Yeung, Sreedhar, Sihoe *et al.* (2006) and Butler, Golding, Northstone *et al.* (2005a) suggest that those wetting less frequently than the DSM-IV definition of twice a week, now termed "infrequent wetters," will fairly quickly achieve dryness, and so are inappropriate for evidence-based treatment interventions, and are best supported in terms of management (e.g., regular drinking, regular toileting). However, children meeting the DSM-IV definition (wet at least twice a week) appear likely to continue wetting throughout childhood and need to be identified early and treated appropriately.

This chapter follows the DSM-IV approach of definitions based on both chronological age and frequency of occurrence, as set out in the following sections; but with the option of recognizing that treatment may be appropriate for some children who are distressed or impaired by the symptom even if they do not meet all the other criteria.

Children with wetting and soiling are usually seen in primary care or in community-based clinics, with more complex problems referred into pediatric or child mental health services. Wetting and soiling become of particular interest to clinical psychology and psychiatry in the context of comorbidity, family dynamics and lack of response to treatment intervention. Coexistence of the problems is common; in the ALSPAC study, the small proportion (2.6%) with severe bedwetting (more than twice per week) also had a substantially increased rate of severe day wetting and a few also showed daytime soiling (Butler, Golding, Northstone *et al.*, 2005a). Behavioral problems, including attention deficit/hyperactivity disorder (ADHD), are often identified as coexisting with nocturnal enuresis (von Gontard, Pluck, Berner, & Lehmkuhl, 1999). Urinary tract infection (UTI) can provoke overactivity of the detrusor muscles leading to painful voiding, urgency and day wetting (Hellström, Hanson, Hansson *et al.*, 1990). An accumulation of fecal mass in constipation can compress the bladder, leading to uninhibited bladder contractions and day wetting (Kodman-Jones, Hawkins, & Schulman, 2001).

Girls present a variable epidemiological profile (Verhulst, van der Lee, Akkerhuis *et al.*, 1985) with a higher likelihood of secondary wetting (a return of wetting after being dry for at least 6 months). Secondary enuresis has repeatedly been found to be associated with a high incidence of distressing events, including parental separation and disharmony (Jarvelin, Moilanen, Vikevainen-Tervonen, & Huttunen, 1990; von Gontard, Hollmann, Eiberg *et al.*, 1997). A minority of parents may hold the belief that wetting or soiling is under the child's control, leading to intolerance, and such reactions seem antagonistic to some of the treatments available.

An awareness of the heterogeneity of each problem can prove beneficial, both in terms of understanding the psychological ramifications and deciding on the apposite intervention. Nocturnal enuresis is divisible into monosymptomatic or polysymptomatic forms (based on the absence or presence of

Rutter's Child and Adolescent Psychiatry, 5th edition. Edited by M. Rutter, D. Bishop, D. Pine, S. Scott, J. Stevenson, E. Taylor and A. Thapar. © 2008 Blackwell Publishing, ISBN: 978-1-4051-4549-7.

bladder overactivity); day wetting can be considered as either urge incontinence, voiding postponement or detrusor–sphincter dyscoordination; and soiling can reflect a lack of bowel control, intentional inappropriate deposition or constipation with overflow. Clinicians enhance their effectiveness by assessing a child's particular needs, applying evidence-based treatment interventions and drawing, where possible, on a knowledge of pretreatment predictors of outcome (Butler & Stenberg, 2001).

Nocturnal Enuresis

Although parental concern and child distress should undoubtedly be considered in determining clinical significance, nocturnal enuresis is defined as an involuntary voiding of urine during sleep in children over 5 years with a severity of at least twice a week for at least 3 consecutive months when not provoked by congenital or acquired defects of the central nervous system (American Psychiatric Association, 2000).

The psychological associations of bedwetting have been reviewed by Butler (2001) and although the diversity of methodology hinders firm conclusions, the ALSPAC study suggests a tendency towards social avoidance, vulnerability to victimization and increased activity and impulsivity at 7 years compared with controls (Joinson, Heron, Emond, & Butler, 2007a). However, as a group, there are few differences between those with primary nocturnal enuresis (in the absence of daytime wetting) and controls in terms of emotional adjustment, self-construing (Butler, Redfern, & Holland, 1994; Joinson, Heron, Emond *et al.*, 2007a) or behavioral presentation (Friman, Handwerk, Swearer, McGinnis, & Warzak, 1998; Hirasing, Van Leerdam, Bolk-Bennink, & Bosch, 1997).

However, children with more complex presentations appear more psychologically vulnerable than controls. Emotional vulnerability and behavior problems have both been linked to secondary nocturnal enuresis (von Gontard, Hollmann, Eiberg *et al.*, 1997) and associated daytime wetting. There are probably several developmental pathways accounting for the associations between wetting and mental disturbances. The epidemiological basis of the findings makes it clear that referral bias is not the explanation. The timing of associations is an important clue: Rutter, Yule, and Graham (1973) drew on epidemiological data and reported that children who developed secondary enuresis were more likely to have shown psychological deviance before the enuresis started. This indicated that the psychological symptoms did not wholly result from the impact of wetting; rather, they either led to the wetting or resulted from a common cause, such as stressful life events and social adversity (see Chapters 25 and 26).

There may well be a further pathway from enuresis to psychological symptoms. Fergusson and Horwood (1994) reported longitudinal epidemiological data showing a predictive effect of childhood wetting on later adolescent disturbance. The effect survived allowance for potentially confounding factors, but its size was small. Clinically, it is common to find that children are upset by both the experience of wetting and the reaction of other people; specific treatment of enuresis, such as the alarm, has reduced psychological symptoms in randomized trials (Longstaffe, Moffatt, & Whalen, 2000). The higher rates of disturbance when daytime wetting is present suggest that the public nature of the problem may provoke a troublesome dilemma (Feehan, McGee, Stanton, & Silva, 1990). While most parents remain tolerant towards the wetting, a notable proportion become intolerant and punitive (Tissier, 1983), which can lead to early withdrawal from alarm-based treatment. Where parental intolerance is apparent, a package of interventions is advocated – designed to maintain contact with the family, immediately reduce hostile feelings and challenge parental attributions of controllability (Butler & McKenna, 2002).

Assessment

Physical examination should exclude organic causes such as neurological incontinence. Urine analysis is necessary to check for infection (UTI; Mikkelsen, 2001). A primary clinical objective is the identification of bedwetting as either monosymptomatic (MSNE) or polysymptomatic (PSNE) based on the absence or presence of bladder overactivity, respectively (Table 56.1). The three systems approach (Butler, 2004; Butler & Holland, 2000), a conceptual formulation drawing on empirical evidence, offers an explanatory model for children while aiding practitioners in selecting apposite treatment interventions.

Urine volume is normally reduced and concentrated through arginine vasopressin (AVP) secretion, enabling continuous sleep throughout the night. However, children with MSNE appear to lack circadian rhythmicity of AVP leading to urine volumes that exceed bladder capacity (Nørgaard, Pedersen, & Djurhuus, 1985; Rittig, Knudsen, Nørgaard, Pedersen, & Djurhuus, 1989). Clinical identifiers of low AVP include wetting soon after going to sleep and large wet patches (Butler & Holland, 2000; Nørgaard, Rittig, & Djurhuus, 1989). Studies of overnight cystometry recordings of children with nocturnal enuresis suggest 30–32% have uninhibited bladder contractions during sleep with small functional bladder capacities at the point of wetting (Kruse, Hellström, & Hjälmås, 1999; Watanabe, Imada, Kawauchi, Koyama, & Shirakawa, 1997). Such children are regarded as having PSNE and are identified by daytime urgency, frequent daytime voiding (more than 7 times per day), low voided volumes, variability in size of the wet patch and waking during or immediately after wetting (Butler, Robinson, Holland, & Doherty-Williams, 2004a; Yeung, Chiu, & Sit, 1999). Voided volumes are assessed by inviting the child to void into a measuring jug when the bladder "feels full," avoiding the first void of the morning (Watanabe & Kawauchi, 1995). The highest measurement provides an estimate of maximum voided volume, which is compared with expected voided volume, by employing the formula (up to 14 years), age $\times$ 30 + 30 (mL).

Approximately 80% of non-enuretic children sleep through the night without waking to toilet, yet they are more likely to wake spontaneously to void compared to enuretic children (Bower, Moore, Shepherd, & Adams, 1996), leading both

Table 56.1 Types of nocturnal enuresis.

	Monosymptomatic (MSNE)	Polysymptomatic (PSNE)	Key references
Definition	Normal, complete, coordinated void occurring when bladder filling has reached its capacity. Diuresis dependent	Bedwetting precipitated by increased frequency and amplitude of unstable detrusor contractions. Detrusor dependent	Butler & Holland (2000) Neveus (2001) Nijman *et al.* (2002)
Proportion of the enuretic population	Approx 2/3	Approx 1/3	Butler *et al.* (2006)
Assessment: signs	Large wet patches Wets soon after sleep Dilute urine on wetting Normal voided volumes	Daytime urgency Frequent day time toileting (>7/day) Low voided volumes Variable wet patch Wake after wetting	Nørgaard *et al.* (1989) Yeung *et al.* (1999) Butler *et al.* (2004a)
Comorbidity	Few related problems	Day time wetting Fecal soiling	Joinson *et al.* (2007a)
Treatment	Enuresis alarm Desmopressin	Bladder training Anticholinergic medication	Butler & Holland (2000)

children and parents to believe bedwetting is a deep sleep phenomenon. However, electroencephalography (EEG) investigations of sleep physiology suggest similar sleep architecture to that of non-enuretic children (Mikkelsen, Rapoport, Nee *et al.*, 1980; Neveus, Stenberg, Lackgren, Tuvemo, & Hetta, 1999). Wetting episodes occur during all sleep stages in proportion to the amount of time spent in that stage (Wolfish, 1999) and occur when the bladder is filled to the equivalent of maximal voided volume (Nørgaard & Djurhuus, 1993). Further, there are no apparent differences in sleep pattern on dry compared with wet nights (Gillin, Rapoport, Mikkelsen *et al.*, 1982). What appears problematic for bedwetting children is being unable to arouse from sleep to bladder signals (Watanabe, Imada, Kawauchi *et al.*, 1997).

Etiology

The heterogeneity of nocturnal enuresis suggests the possibility of differing etiologies. Arguably, the influential effect of any etiological determinant is through increasing vulnerability towards suboptimal nocturnal AVP secretion, bladder overactivity and/or reduced arousal response to bladder signals during sleep. Genetic influences play a part. Community surveys have shown high rates of enuresis in the families of people who are slow to acquire continence of urine at night (Fergusson, Horwood, & Shannon, 1986; Jarvelin, Moilanen, Kangas *et al.*, 1991). Familiality by itself does not imply heritability, but the rate of nocturnal enuresis in the identical twins of bedwetters is much higher than in non-identical, suggesting a genetic contribution (Bakwin, 1971); and a genetic contribution to the acquisition of night-time dryness is clear from twin studies even in 3-year-olds (Butler, Galsworthy, Rijsdijk, & Plomin, 2001a) and 4-year-olds (Hublin, Kaprio, Partinen, & Koskenvuo, 1998).

Psychosocial theories of etiology are supported by findings indicating the coexistence of bedwetting with low socioeconomic status (Chiozza, Bernardinelli, Caione *et al.*, 1998), families in overcrowded housing (Foxman, Valdez, & Brook, 1986), unemployment of father (Devlin, 1991), large family size (Hanafin, 1998) and, interestingly, the absence of breastfeeding (Kalo & Bella, 1996; Liu, Sun, Uchiyama, Li, & Okawa, 2000). A well-conducted study with matched controls drawn from an unselected population (Jarvelin, Moilanen, Vikevainen-Tervonen *et al.*, 1990) found that disruptive experiences (particularly splitting of the family through separation or divorce) during a sensitive stage in the development of bladder control (around 2–3 years) were related to the later development of nocturnal enuresis. Such disruptions may contribute to other potentially adverse experiences, including poorer living conditions, emotional turmoil and adaptation to new family dynamics and structures. The consequent anxiety could interrupt either the acquisition of co-ordinated muscular responses, leading to bladder overactivity, or the inhibition of AVP secretion (Houts, 1991).

Management

Facilitating an understanding of the three systems, often through pictures, enables an awareness of cause and the direction of treatment and emphasizes the importance of not attaching blame. Many parents adopt strategies for helping their child, with lifting and fluid restriction (Haque, Ellerstein, Gundy *et al.*, 1981; Butler, 1987) being the most frequently reported. However, both may inadvertently prolong bedwetting. Lifting (toileting at night, usually without waking the child) in effect encourages children to empty the bladder while asleep, while fluid restriction may precipitate bladder overactivity. Good clinical practice encourages regular daytime drinking and invites the child to test what fluid intake (both volume and type) is appropriate before bedtime. The only parental strategy that appears effective is the adoption of regular daytime toileting (Butler, Golding, Heron *et al.*, 2005b), which encourages development of control over the bladder.

Effective Treatment

Treatments for nocturnal enuresis are broadly categorized as either psychological, which typically aim for complete cessation, or pharmacological, which usually aim for wetting reduction. The three systems approach (Butler & Holland, 2000) encourages consideration of the child's needs, with desmopressin or the enuresis alarm being appropriate for MSNE, and bladder training, usually combined with anticholinergic medication, being applicable for PSNE (Table 56.1).

Desmopressin

Desmopressin, a synthetic analog of vasopressin, is considerably more resistant to metabolic degradation than natural AVP. The mode of action is antidiuretic, with decreased urine production and increased urine concentration (Rushton, Belman, Skoog, Zaontz, & Sihelnik, 1995). An excellent review of randomized controlled trials found 70% response rate with 24.5% complete cessation of bedwetting while taking desmopressin (Moffatt, Harlos, Kirshen, & Burd, 1993). When employed specifically with MSNE, higher response rates are reported (Caione, Arena, Biraghi *et al.*, 1997; Devitt, Holland, Butler *et al.*, 1999). With the correct dose, dry nights are realized immediately. Thus, where a rapid response is desired (e.g., sleepover, parental intolerance), desmopressin is preferable to the enuresis alarm. Because desmopressin has no detectable effect on endogenous AVP release (van Kerrebroeck, 2002), relapse is often evident with removal of medication. Thus, long-term treatment is often advocated. Pretreatment predictors of success include older children, less severe nocturnal enuresis and no bladder overactivity (Butler & Stenberg, 2001).

There are nasal spray, tablet and melt formulations with doses of 20–40 μg, 200–400 μg and 120–240 μg, respectively, taken just before bedtime with a break after 3 months to check if further treatment is indicated (Rittig, Knudsen, Nørgaard *et al.*, 1989). Very few side effects, even with long-term treatment, are reported (Hjälmås, Hanson, Hellström, Kruse, & Sillen, 1998; Miller, Goldberg, & Atkin, 1989) provided the child does not drink excessively before bedtime or throughout the night. However, there are rare reported cases of hyponatremia although of 11 cases reported, 6 were caused by excess fluid intake (Robson, Leung, & Bloom, 1996).

Enuresis Alarm

The enuresis alarm is considered the optimal intervention for MSNE (Mellon & McGrath, 2000). The essential principle is to alert and sensitize the child to respond quickly and appropriately to full bladder signals, converting the signal from one of urination to that of inhibition of urination and waking (Butler, 1994). A key to success is not stimulus intensity of alarm triggering, but the child's preparedness to wake and respond to the signal (Wolfish, 1999, 2001). Reviews of controlled studies with undifferentiated samples indicate 65–75% success with duration of 5–12 weeks and relapse of 30–45% in the 6 months following treatment (Butler & Gasson, 2005; Forsythe & Butler, 1989). Compared with desmopressin, rate of response with alarm treatment is slower but relapse less likely (Houts, Berman, & Abramson, 1994; Monda & Husmann, 1995).

The expanding literature pertaining to pretreatment predictors of outcome should enhance clinical efficacy. Failure is associated with multiple wetting at night, associated daytime wetting, lack of motivation, family distress and concomitant behavioral or psychiatric problems (Devlin & O'Cathain, 1990; Moffatt & Cheang, 1995). Early withdrawal has repeatedly been found where there is parental intolerance (Butler, Brewin, & Forsythe, 1988) and relapse tends to occur with multiple wetting, associated daytime wetting and secondary enuresis. With regards to within-treatment variables, failure is associated with lack of waking to alarm triggering (Butler & Robinson, 2002).

The mode of action remains open to conjecture, particularly as the majority of children who become dry sleep through the night, although theoretically it is assumed they learn to arouse to full bladder sensations (Butler & Robinson, 2002). Possible explanations include avoidance conditioning whereby alarm triggering is avoided by inhibition of micturition, increased functional bladder capacity or increased production of AVP in response to waking to the alarm (Butler & Stenberg, 2001).

Bladder Training

Bladder training aims to promote voluntary control over voiding, generating a change from unstable to stable bladder functioning at night. Fundamentally, children are encouraged to drink regularly (6–7 times per day), void at predetermined times, deal with urgency by voiding immediately if the sensations persist and keep regular checks of voided volumes. An uncontrolled clinical trial of children with PSNE found 68% response (>50% reduction in bedwetting) after 1 month of bladder training (Kruse, Hellström, & Hjälmås, 1999).

Anticholinergic Medication

Oxybutynin is a smooth muscle relaxant specifically targeting the detrusor muscles, both reducing overactivity and increasing functional bladder capacity (Kosar, Arikan, & Dincel, 1998). With unselected samples, oxybutynin has proved ineffective (Lovering, Tallett, & McKendry, 1988), yet in selected groups of children with PSNE, in uncontrolled case studies, success rates of 67–90% are reported (Kosar, Arikan, & Dincel, 1998; Watanabe, Kawauchi, Kiramori, & Azuma, 1994). Potential side effects include dry mouth, constipation and flushing.

Relapse Prevention

Although there are no published reports on relapse prevention with anticholinergic medication, clinical practice suggests removal is effective once the voided volume is age appropriate. Traditionally, overlearning, which involves increased drinking in the hour before bed, has been advocated with the enuresis alarm although there are both theoretical (regarding the mechanism of action) and clinical concerns (children being dispirited by emergence of wetting). With desmopressin, gradual reduction of dosage is advocated, but reduction is prolonged (up to 3 years) and emphasizes medication as the effective agent, and at best only 50% of children remain dry (Miller, Goldberg, & Atkin, 1989).

In becoming dry, children tend to attribute success to treatment (alarm or medication) so, in effect, externalize success. Relapse may arise through removal of what the child believes to be the effective agent. Recently, Butler, Holland, and Robinson (2001b) have reported a program specifically designed to prevent relapse after removal of medication, with 75% success. The program focuses on engaging the child in a process of internalizing success and highlighting the effective process by which this is accomplished, whether it is increased arousability or improved AVP release.

Daytime Wetting

According to DSM-IV, daytime wetting is considered an involuntary voiding of urine into clothing, with a severity of at least twice a week, in children over 5 years when not provoked by congenital or acquired defects of the central nervous system. The age criterion is not based on secure evidence, and Robson, Leung, & Bloom (1996) contended that daytime wetting is problematic at 4 years.

Assessment

All children deserve a careful history, pediatric physical examination, urinalysis to detect UTI and abdominal examination to rule out fecal impaction. Children with a difficulty initiating voiding, interruptions of the stream or constant dribbling require urological investigation. Von Gontard (1998) suggested non-invasive techniques should include a 24 h diary of fluid intake and urinary output; ultrasound to detect structural

Table 56.2 Types of daytime wetting.

	Urge incontinence	Voiding postponement	Detrusor–sphincter dyscoordination	Key reference
Other terms	Bladder–detrusor instability		Hinman's syndrome	
Definition	Wetting accompanied by sudden, unexpected urge symptoms	Wetting following postponement of micturition with urinary retention	Dysfunctional voiding with contraction instead of relaxation of the external urethral sphincter during micturition	van Gool & de Jonge (1989)
Proportion	Most common 82% girls; 74% boys		Rare	Hellström *et al.* (1990)
Gender	More common in girls	More common in boys	More common in girls	
Impact	Emotional disturbance	Disruptive behavior		von Gontard *et al.* (1998)
Presentation	Wetting of small volumes Worse in the afternoon	Wetting with large volumes Normal urodynamics	Voiding only possible with straining Prolonged micturition time Flow rate partially or completely interrupted	van Gool & de Jonge (1989)
Phase	Filling phase	Full bladder	Voiding phase	
Assessment: signs	Sudden urge to void Frequent micturition (>7/day) Holding maneuvers Small voided volumes	Infrequent urination (<5/day) Holding maneuvers Fidgeting	Normal micturition frequency Straining on voiding Staccato voiding Residual urine	von Gontard (1998)
Comorbidity	UTI PSNE	Stool retention Soiling Behavioral problems ADHD	Constipation Soiling	von Gontard *et al.* (1998)
Treatment	Cognitive–behavioral with anticholinergic medication	Cognitive–behavioral Non-directive prompts Bladder awareness	Biofeedback	

ADHD, attention deficit/hyperactivity disorder, PSNE, polysymptomatic nocturnal enuresis; UTI, urinary tract infection.

anomalies and residual urine; and uroflowmetry to identify detrusor–sphincter dyscoordination, although some clinicians rely on listening to the stream. Table 56.2 outlines the three main forms of daytime wetting.

Urge Incontinence

Urge incontinence results from sudden unexpected detrusor contractions. When access to a toilet is restricted children are unable to hold and countering the urge to void with pelvic floor contraction may lead to small voided volumes, inappropriate postponement of defecation and constipation. Wetting tends to occur when playing outdoors, shopping or walking home from school (van Gool & de Jonge, 1989).

Voiding Postponement

Voiding postponement is common in preschool children (Robson, Leung, & Bloom, 1996) although there are no reliable epidemiological estimates. During absorbing activities (play, television, computers), children ignore (or fail to register) a need to void, with bladder pressure building until the detrusor contracts and wetting occurs.

Dysfunctional Voiding

Several patterns are apparent, with overactivity of the pelvic floor muscles during micturition being a common denominator. Detrusor–sphincter dyscoordination is the most common. Although rare, because of potentially severe medical consequences, diagnosis and specific treatment are vital. Epidemiological data are lacking, although von Gontard (1998) suggested relatively high rates in psychiatric settings.

Less common forms of day wetting include the following:

Giggle Micturition

This is sudden involuntary complete bladder emptying, usually provoked by laughter, tickling or excitement. Of the few cases reported, 70% are girls. It may resolve in adolescence but can persist into adulthood. There are no evidence-based treatments but Schmitt (1982) advocated stream interruption exercises.

Stress Incontinence

Involuntary loss of urine when, in the absence of detrusor contractions, intravesical pressure exceeds the maximum urethral pressure (Nørgaard, van Gool, Hjälmås, Djurhuus, & Hellström, 1998). Voiding may be provoked through coughing and exertion such as running, jumping and gymnastics.

Resistive Wetting

Schmitt (1982) suggests that some children become resistive about using the toilet and deliberately wet themselves. Usually occurring with boys, with a history of pressurized or punitive toilet training, there is often non-retentive soiling. There is a need to reduce tension within the parent–child relationship, foster praise for appropriate toileting and encourage the child to take positive responsibility for bladder functioning.

Etiology

From inconclusive evidence, von Gontard, Schaumburg, Hollman, Eiberg, and Rittig (2001) suggested an autosomal mode of inheritance in urge incontinence; environmental and psychological determinants with voiding postponement, whereas dysfunctional voiding was considered to have a genetic predisposition in the form of a delayed development of sphincter–detrusor coordination.

Management

Although lacking empirical evidence, many strategies continue to be adopted by clinicians. These include explanation of bladder function; regular daytime fluid intake; keeping records of voiding; sitting on the whole seat when voiding with feet supported; voiding with a relaxed pelvic floor, bending slightly forwards; completely emptying the bladder; voiding in one go, listening to the sound; developing bladder awareness through linking behaviors (e.g., fidgeting) with a desire to void; measuring voided volumes; undertaking action replay (waiting a short while after voiding and trying again, to prevent residual urine); reinforcing all actions that improve the chances of staying dry; remaining calm as a parent as over-eager toileting may foster anxiety and fear over the toilet; and treating any wetting as a matter of fact and a chance for both renewed efforts and an opportunity to learn about what provoked wetting.

Effective Treatment

Cognitive–Behavioral Therapy

For children with urge incontinence, bladder training as described for nocturnal enuresis is the preferred intervention, with the aim of establishing a sense of voluntary control over bladder functioning. Briefly, it consists of regular drinks (6–7 times per day), regular toileting (approximately 6 times per day), coupled with toileting rather than holding when urgency is experienced. Non-directive prompts to assist a child in making decisions to use the toilet regularly are preferable to direct prompts where parents are often construed as "nagging." For children with voiding postponement, the goal is to increase frequency of daytime voiding with a watch triggering every 2 h to aid remembering.

Body Worn Alarm

Halliday, Meadow, and Berg (1987) reported 66% success although a non-contingent alarm schedule was equally as effective as triggering contingent on wetting, suggesting that regular toileting, rather than conditioning bladder signals, is the important factor (in contrast with nocturnal enuresis, where alarm triggering contingent with wetting is important).

Biofeedback

Van Gool, Vijverberg, and de Jong (1992) employed a program embracing bladder training (voiding at first sensation of urge, decreasing number of voids) with biofeedback involving visual (uroflow) and acoustic (electromyography [EMG]) readings of flow curves displayed for the child, who is encouraged to urinate with a steady flow. They reported 60% success in disappearance of urge syndrome and voiding dysfunction.

Medication

There is little evidence of medication being helpful for children with daytime wetting, although good controlled trials are lacking. Anticholinergic medication (oxybutynin), with a specific action on reducing detrusor overactivity, is regularly employed for children with urge incontinence. Oxybutynin is usually prescribed at 5 mg twice a day, with slow-release preparations administered only once a day (Hjälmås, Passerini-Glazel, & Chiozza, 1992). Side effects include dry mouth, constipation, skin flushing, blurred vision and headache (Robson, Leung, & Bloom, 1996).

Combination Therapy

Hellerstein and Zguta (2003) used bladder training coupled with anticholinergic medication with urge incontinence and found 47% complete recovery and 42% improvement. Vijverberg, Elzinga-Plomp, Messer, van Gool, and de Jong (1997) described a 10-day in-patient program for both urge incontinence and dysfunctional voiding involving biofeedback with uroflowmetry to display good (smooth curve) or poor (interrupted curve) micturition patterns; bladder training (regular fluid intake, voiding to a regular pattern and reacting appropriately to urge signals); and goal setting (six voids per day). They reported 68% success, especially with older children. The challenge is to develop similar programs for out-patients and discover the effective components of the program.

Fecal Soiling

According to DSM-IV (American Psychiatric Association, 2000), this is the repeated passage of feces into inappropriate places, after the chronological or mental age of 4 years, at least once a month for 3 months without any structural abnormality or physical cause. I would prefer to reduce the age criterion to 3 years to avoid excluding such youngsters in need of treatment.

In terms of the usual development, Clayden (2001) suggested the sensation to defecate occurs when rectal contents impinge on the upper part of the temporarily relaxed anal canal. With increasing rectal filling and distension, defecation is postponed by contraction of the external sphincter and pelvic floor muscles. The rectum contracts every 1–2 min and the sensation to defecate increases in intensity until the rectum is emptied. The sensation may be diminished where there is either sensory nerve loss (neuropathic rectum) or where the rectum is persistently full, especially where the fecal mass is firm (constipation) and prevents all but loose or liquidized feces passing through (overflow incontinence). The strength of the anal sphincter is likely to be affected by trauma such as abuse.

Appropriate defecation is dependent on this physiological response and is assisted where there is sufficient diet (fiber and fluid) to promote movement of feces through the bowel. The child needs to attend and respond to bodily cues related to peristalsis, rather than ignore them, to discriminate between appropriate and inappropriate places for defecation, have an inclination to use the toilet and to relax and tighten the stomach muscles to eliminate feces. Thus, the physiology is aided by behavioral responses. Stein and Susser (1967) showed bowel control was achieved by 50% of children at 24 months and by almost all children (both day and night) by 2.5 years.

Findings relating to impact of fecal soiling are equivocal. There is a need to clarify type of soiling in future empirical work. The clinical impression is that children with fecal soiling often live in fear of discovery, have poor peer relationships, tend to withdraw socially and avoid social events (Landman, Rappaport, Fenton, & Levine, 1986). The ALSPAC study showed that those soiling more frequently have greater levels of emotional problems (e.g., separation anxiety, social fears, general anxiety and sadness) and were more likely both to report being victimized and to bully others compared with controls (Joinson, Heron, Butler *et al.*, 2007b). Parental ratings of behavior can be influenced by the fact of soiling (halo effects), but an association between soiling and psychological disturbance is still present when the latter is rated by teachers (Rutter, Tizard, & Whitmore, 1970).

With respect to behavior, studies with strict inclusion criteria have found increased rates of behavior problems in those with fecal soiling compared with controls (Benninga, Bueller, & Heymans, 1994; Loening-Baucke, Cruikshank, & Savage, 1987). Foreman and Thambirajah (1996) reported more behavioral problems in those with secondary encopresis compared to primary encopresis. Other behavioral issues found to be associated with fecal soiling are obsessive compulsiveness and attention and activity problems (Joinson, Heron, Butler *et al.*, 2007b). Both Landman, Rappaport, Fenton *et al.* (1986) and Joinson, Heron, Butler *et al.* (2007b) reported reduced self-esteem in children with soiling problems.

Psychologically, vicious cycles are likely to develop as a result of soiling (Levine, 1982). Parents may attribute avoidance of toileting as willful or controlling, and diarrhoea-like soiling as laziness. With the resultant blame and admonishment, children experience hostile parental reactions despite being unable to feel a need to toilet. Consequently, they may hide soiled underclothes to avoid detection and humiliation. Children may fail to notice the resultant smell as the olfactory apparatus accommodates to incessant odors and thus children may have limited awareness of soiling and the consequences. It is also possible that soiling can result from pre-existent disturbance or from stresses (like those affecting wetting, see above) on the child that may be linked to psychological problems.

Assessment

Possible physical and organic factors need screening. The list of rare organic conditions involving soiling is long and well elucidated by Loening-Baucke (2002). Urinalysis and urine culture are necessary in the evaluation with girls because of a susceptibility to UTI. Clayden (2001) suggests the more normal the consistency of the stool in the clothing, the less likely there is to be a structural abnormality of the anus or rectum. Levine (1982) favored X-ray of the lower abdomen for the detection of abundant retained feces, or a clinical examination may reveal a constipated colon.

Careful history-taking is imperative to elucidate the type of soiling. Areas to cover include:

1 Precipitating factors: life events such as parental separation, birth of siblings, traumatic accidents, abuse, starting school, hospitalization;
2 History of soiling including age of onset;
3 History of toilet training;
4 Current toilet use, which defines pattern of toileting, and parental and child motivation;
5 Antecedents of soiling accidents;
6 The child's attitude and access to toilet/s (at home and school) and reasons for avoidance;
7 Severity of soiling, eliciting the intervals, amount and consistency of bowel movements (with the aid of the Bristol Stool Chart) deposited into the toilet and clothing;
8 Dietary habits;
9 Co-occurring problems;
10 Family attitudes to the child;
11 Family dynamics and coping strategies;
12 How accidents are dealt with: parental reactions, responsibility, denial, hiding underwear;
13 The child's understanding of the problem; and
14 Exceptions: are there times when motions and toileting are appropriate and what defines such episodes?

Empirically validated subtypes of fecal soiling have yet to be established (Mellon, Houts, & Lazar, 1996) leaving classification dependent on clinical acumen. There is potential confusion arising from interchangeable terminology yet a functional classification proves valuable in differentiating treatment. Clayden (2001) provided a useful three-way clinical classification (Table 56.3) based on descriptions of soiling behavior and proposed underlying psychological mechanisms.

This chapter used "*encopresis*" to define one pattern of secondary non-retentive soiling in which children control the physiological process of defecation but deposit normal motions in unusual places (e.g., behind sofa, in the deep freeze, parents'

Table 56.3 Types of fecal soiling.

	Lack of bowel control	Encopresis	Constipation with overflow	Key references
Other terms	Primary non-retentive encopresis	Secondary non-retentive encopresis	Soiling Retentive encopresis	
Definition	Passage of normal stools into clothing Child is either unaware of soiling, or unable to control the bowel	Passage of normal stools in socially unacceptable places	Continuous overflow of incomplete stools into clothing	Benninga & Taminiau (2001) Loening-Baucke (2002)
History	Never achieved bowel control	Bowel control established and lost	Toilet avoidance leading to constipation	
Gender		Usually boys		
Presentation	Normal stools Deposited randomly in clothing	Normal stools	Liquid or loose stools (odorous, thin and ribbon-like)	
Assessment: signs	No constipation	No constipation	Poor appetite Functional constipation (<3 stools/week) Painful passage Infrequent bowel movement Abdominal pain	Clayden (2001)
Comorbidity	May be neurological (e.g., cerebral palsy) or cognitive (intellectual disability) which impairs ability to learn bowel control	Smearing feces	Nocturnal enuresis Day wetting	
Treatment	Bowel training Contingent reinforcement Attention to the wider social climate	Understanding the particular stresses on the child	Stimulant laxative Stool softener Bowel training	

bed). It is hypothesized that this form of soiling is provoked by psychological events including sexual abuse (Boon & Singh, 1991), family stress and punitive reactions. Encopresis is of particular importance to mental health professionals, who may need to consider family dynamics in order to fully understand the presentation.

Constipation with overflow accounts for approximately 85% of fecal soiling (Loening-Baucke, 2002). A typical pattern may involve either physical or psychological factors:

1 Avoidance or fear of the toilet, either because of painful defecation (e.g., hard feces; anal fissure) or tension around toileting (e.g., overdemanding or punitive parental reactions);

2 Stools are held back, the rectal wall is stretched affecting contractibility and sensory feedback from the bowel is reduced with a loss of feeling and diminution in the normal call to stool;

3 With increased water absorption from the fecal matter, feces become larger and harder, leading to constipation and impaction;

4 The functioning of the external and internal sphincters become compromised, allowing seepage of soft diarrhoea-like feces around the impaction; and

5 Further toilet avoidance increases constipation, leading to more concerted efforts and/or punitive reactions on the part of parents.

Etiology

Primary soiling has been found to be related to developmental delay, whereas secondary soiling is associated with more psychosocial adversity and behavioral problems (Foreman & Thambirajah, 1996). Clinically, fecal soiling is best understood as an interaction of physiological and psychological factors, with differing influences depending on type of soiling. Clayden (2001) outlines the main pediatric causes:

- Developmental delay as a result of learning difficulty or social deprivation;
- Neuropathic rectum and sensory deficiency as a result of spinal cord defects;
- Abnormal internal sphincter as a result of anorectal anomaly or trauma such as abuse;
- Inhibited internal sphincter as a result of rectal fecal retention – fear of pain on passing motions is a major factor in constipation (Bernard-Bonnin, Haley, Belanger, & Nadeau, 1993);
- Increased motility and diminished awareness of sensation as a result of psychological distress.

The "encopresis" subtype particularly can reflect psychological causes, and family interactions need special consideration.

Management

There are a raft of clinically useful suggestions that appear to help both children and parents understand and approach the problem in a more enlightened manner. Many clinicians now suggest avoidance of early introduction to potty training unless the child makes clear signals they are ready to try. Levine (1982) appropriately discusses the prevalence of soiling, to counter any sense of isolation. Promoting an understanding, through drawings and diagrams, of normal bowel functioning and how constipation leads to soiling is important. Children are often relieved to discover their lack of control is understood, by hearing how a distended colon becomes less sensitive, leading to a lack of a warning of the need to defecate and ultimately to seepage.

Discussions with child and parent may highlight that no-one is perceived as being at fault or accused of causing the problem. Parents need to refrain from attributing blame or expressing anger and frustration towards the child. Soiling episodes are best handled in a matter-of-fact way, with an older child expected to clean up and place soiled clothing in the laundry. Maintaining a positive focus is imperative with parents encouraged to praise appropriate effort and toileting (e.g., trying; passing motions in toilet).

Promoting realistic expectations is important, given that treatment may be prolonged and that success is dependent on the bowel regaining muscle tone. The theme of treatment might be described as similar to a training program an athlete might use to develop better muscles and skills. It is important to enhance the appeal of the toilet at home (with décor, reading matter) and ensure access to toilets at school. Keeping a record of toilet sitting (prompted or child initiated), passage of motions, soiling accident (small stain; small formed bowel movement; full formed bowel movement) is considered useful (Houts, Mellon, & Whelan, 1988; Stark, Opipari, Donaldson *et al.*, 1997).

Effective Treatment

Few prospective controlled studies have been undertaken, limiting an understanding of effective treatment interventions. McGrath, Mellon, and Murphy (2000) found only 42 well-designed studies, of which 13 were single-case designs. Often, studies failed to specify characteristics of the population, creating problems in knowing whether children had constipation with overflow or encopresis. Treatment aims and interventions evidently differ according to the type of soiling, something future research needs to address before a good clinically relevant evidence base is established. McGrath, Mellon, & Murphy (2000) provided an excellent review of treatment interventions. Although most approaches involve a package of techniques and approaches, interventions will be discussed here in relation to the specified aim.

Medical Interventions

Regimes for initial clear-out of impacted fecal matter and removal of pain vary across studies but usually include suppositories, enemas, laxatives, mineral oil and stool softeners. Arguably, oral methods of bowel clean-out are preferable, given that enemas may be considered psychologically unsuitable. There is a need to seek an understanding from children as to the impact of various forms of bowel clean-out.

For prevention of reaccumulation of stools, long-term laxatives are likely to be required, with the dosage gradually decreased once regular bowel movements (once or twice per day) are established. On their own, enemas, laxatives and mineral oils may increase soiling initially in an effort to correct constipation. The mechanism of action is assumed to relate to the debulking effect of chronically retained stools, although it is possible that the stimulation of colonic smooth muscle not only increases colonic motility itself, but also increases awareness of motility and rectal filling (Nolan, Debelle, Oberklaid, & Coffey, 1991). Medical interventions are rarely employed on their own, with Cox, Sutphen, Ling, Quillan, and Borowitz (1996) finding that only 9% were significantly helped with just a laxative.

Diet

Diet theoretically offers an alternative means of correcting constipation that, although slower, has a more lasting solution than laxatives. The combination of fiber and water promotes bowel movement. Increased dietary fiber includes fruit, cereals containing bran, brown rice, baked beans, vegetables, baked potato and avoidance of milk products. Houts, Mellon, & Whelan (1988) and Mellon, Houts, & Lazar (1996) outlined an appropriate fiber intake, using points linked to amount of fiber. However, there is little evidence that dietary factors alleviate functional constipation once stool withholding becomes a problem (Loening-Baucke, 2002). Mellon, Houts, & Lazar (1996) found a dietary program to improve fiber intake was no more effective and took longer to take effect than mineral oil.

Behavioral Interventions

These aim to increase appropriate toilet use and encourage regular bowel movement but do not address the problem of constipation.

Bowel training, a customary intervention, consists of regular toilet sitting some 15 min after meals to coincide with the gastrocolic reflex which stimulates movement of feces through the bowel. As toilet sitting twice a day may be construed as tedious, the length of sitting should be a maximum of 5 min and contingent praise and rewards offered for the passage of stools. Children need to perceive the process as training not punitive. Cox, Sutphen, Ling, Quillian, and Borowitz (1998) found bowel training, coupled with medical intervention and positive reinforcement, to be 85% successful. Nolan, Debelle, Oberklaid *et al.* (1991) found the addition of laxative to bowel training improved success rates, although they found 12.5% failed to comply with bowel training.

Other behavioral approaches, often enmeshed within bowel training, include reinforcement (tangible or star charts) contingent on behaviors the child can control (e.g., increased fiber intake, self-initiated toileting, motions in toilet); differential attention (Stark, Opipari, Donaldson *et al.*, 1997), where soiling is treated in a neutral matter-of-fact way; overcorrection or cleanliness training, where the children are involved in washing the soiled clothing and cleaning themselves up; and awareness techniques, where children are encouraged to identify bowel sensations and behaviors as cues for toileting.

Biofeedback

Children with chronic constipation and encopresis are thought to have abnormal defecation dynamics with an inability to relax the external anal sphincter during attempted defecation. As this sphincter is striated muscle, theoretically amenable to modulation, biofeedback aims to enhance relaxation of the sphincter during defecation. Loening-Baucke (1990) employed a balloon, inserted in the anus at the level of internal and external sphincter, which transmitted pressure changes to an oscilloscope. Children were trained to alter their sphincter responses voluntarily using anal and buttock muscles. With reported success of 86% in relaxing the external anal sphincter and recovery from constipation in 55–60%, it was suggested that biofeedback was a promising intervention, complementary to good conventional treatment. However, being labor intensive, biofeedback may be reserved for those who have failed to respond to conventional treatment. There remains a question of clinical applicability for children and Cox, Sutphen, Ling *et al.* (1996) described a more convenient and accessible procedure involving electromyographic (EMG) biofeedback of the external anal sphincter. However, Loening-Baucke (1996) and Cox, Sutphen, Ling *et al.* (1996) reported no advantage of biofeedback over bowel training in randomized controlled studies. Further, van der Plas, Benninga, Buller *et al.* (1996) found that the addition of five sessions of biofeedback to the normal medical intervention plus bowel training did not improve success rates. They concluded that abnormal defecation dynamics do not have a crucial role in the pathogenesis of childhood constipation.

Psychotherapeutic Interventions

For children with non-retentive forms of fecal soiling, a raft of psychotherapeutic interventions have been advocated including play therapy, child psychotherapy and family therapy to reduce guilt, shame and anxiety. However, empirical investigations of such approaches are still required.

Pretreatment and Treatment Predictors

Treatment failure has been found to occur with children with severe constipation with overflow; when soiling happens in school or during sleep; and with associated behavioral problems, intellectual disability or psychiatric problems (Boon & Singh, 1991; Levine & Bakow, 1976; Stark, Spirito, Lewis, & Hart, 1990). There are few treatment predictors, but both lack of compliance in treatment (Levine & Bakow, 1976; Nolan, Debelle, Oberklaid *et al.*, 1991) and lack of initial progress in the first 2 weeks (Cox, Sutphen, Ling *et al.*, 1996) have been associated with failure.

Composite Programs

Treatment of fecal soiling should involve the employment of a package of interventions; accordingly, comparative studies are limited and could conceal the impact of any one component. Taking those studies with the largest samples, Nolan, Debelle, Oberklaid *et al.* (1991) with $n = 83$ found that a combination of medical intervention, diet, bowel training and contingent reinforcement produced 51% success at 12 months. Van der Plas, Benninga, Buller *et al.* (1996) applied a similar composite program to 94 children, with 33% success after 6 weeks, 52%

at 6 months and 59% at 1-year follow-up. Stark, Opipari, Donaldson *et al.* (1997), employing a similar package for 52 children with retentive encopresis, found soiling decreased by 85%, with 67% considered a success (one or fewer soils per week).

On a cautionary note, McGrath, Mellon, & Murphy (2000) suggest that adding components to a treatment package does not necessarily improve outcome, and may indeed decrease efficacy. Dietary recommendations and biofeedback have both been found to reduce efficacy when attached to medical interventions and bowel training (van der Plas, Benninga, Buller *et al.*, 1996).

Relapse Prevention

When relapse rates are reported, they tend to be high. Nolan, Debelle, Oberklaid *et al.* (1991) found 51% relapse with laxative treatment, while 37% of those treated with bowel training relapsed. Once soiling is relieved there may remain dynamics of family involvement that recreate the problem. Children with fecal soiling may therefore need continued support for a protracted time.

Conclusions

Nocturnal enuresis, daytime wetting and soiling often coexist, but are clinically best considered as discrete, each having heterogeneity. A differentiation between subtypes is imperative in both clinical and research contexts. The clinician is faced with an array of potential management and treatment interventions, many of which require an evidence base. However, there are proven treatments for all three problems, both medical and psychological, and with a thorough understanding of the child's problem the clinician is now well placed to determine an apposite treatment. Pretreatment predictors are potentially useful in fine tuning treatment options although many need replication. Parsimony of treatment is important and combination programs should therefore integrate interventions to meet a child's particular needs. Composite treatment packages are often applied in clinical practice, but require clarification; component analysis would prove beneficial in determining effective and redundant aspects.

There is a need to clarify outcome measures, as has been done with nocturnal enuresis (Butler, Robinson, Holland, & Doherty-Williams, 2004b), and develop consistency across studies. Methodology tends to employ "convenience" samples and, apart from a few notable exceptions, randomization into different treatment groups is lacking. Relapse following treatment is readily apparent and yet methods to help prevent relapse are lacking – particularly in relation to daytime wetting and fecal soiling.

Once children overcome wetting and soiling problems there are demonstrated improvements in psychological functioning. For example, successfully treated children with nocturnal enuresis exhibit an increase in self-esteem (Moffatt, Kato, & Pless, 1987) and develop into young adults no different psychologically from adults who were never enuretic (Stromgren & Thomson, 1990). For psychologists and psychiatrists, wetting and soiling provide interesting areas of study, because with clearly defined dependent variables, there is an ideal opportunity to test out particular theories and models. As Houts, Berman, & Abramson (1994) suggest, for most problems mental health workers confront, the therapeutic goal is management and improvement. However, wetting and soiling are exceptions – complete recovery is a realistic goal.

Acknowledgments

I am extremely grateful to Leeds Primary Care Trust, Dr. Philip Holland, Professor Eric Taylor and Leeds Mental Health Library for the support and assistance they kindly provided in the writing of this chapter.

References

American Psychiatric Association. (2000). *Diagnostic and statistical manual of mental disorders. DSM-IV* (4th edn.). Text Revision. Washington, DC: American Psychiatry Press.

Bakwin, H. (1971). Enuresis in twins. *American Journal of Diseases in Childhood*, *121*, 222–225.

Bellman, M. (1966). Studies on encopresis. *Acta Paediatrica Scandinavica*, *55*, 1–151.

Benninga, M. A., & Taminiau, J. A. (2001). Diagnosis and treatment efficacy of functional non-retentive fecal soiling in childhood. *Journal of Pediatric Gastroenterology and Nutrition*, *32 Suppl.*, S42–S43.

Benninga, M. A., Bueller, H. A., & Heymans, H. S. (1994). Is encopresis always the result of constipation? *Archives of Disease in Childhood*, *71*, 186–193.

Bernard-Bonnin, A., Haley, N., Belanger, S., & Nadeau, D. (1993). Parental and patient perceptions about encopresis and its treatment. *Developmental and Behavioral Pediatrics*, *14*, 397–400.

Boon, F. F. L., & Singh, N. N. (1991). A model for the treatment of encopresis. *Behavior Modification*, *15*, 355–371.

Bower, W. F., Moore, K. H., Shepherd, R. B., & Adams, R. D. (1996). The epidemiology of childhood enuresis in Australia. *British Journal of Urology*, *78*, 602–606.

Butler, R. J. (1987). *Nocturnal enuresis: Psychological perspectives.* Bristol: Wright.

Butler, R. J. (1994). *Nocturnal enuresis: The child's experience.* Oxford: Butterworth Heinemann.

Butler, R. J. (2001). Impact of nocturnal enuresis on children and young people. *Scandinavian Journal of Urology and Nephrology*, *35*, 169–176.

Butler, R. J. (2004). Childhood nocturnal enuresis: Developing a conceptual framework. *Clinical Psychology Review*, *24*, 909–931.

Butler, R. J., & Gasson, S. L. (2005). Enuresis alarm treatment. *Scandinavian Journal of Urology and Nephrology*, *39*, 349–357.

Butler, R. J., & Holland, P. (2000). The three systems: A conceptual way of understanding nocturnal enuresis. *Scandinavian Journal of Urology and Nephrology*, 34, 270–277.

Butler, R., & McKenna, S. (2002). Overcoming parental intolerance in childhood nocturnal enuresis: A survey of professional opinion. *British Journal of Urology International*, *89*, 295–297.

Butler, R., & Stenberg, A. (2001). Treatment of childhood nocturnal enuresis: An examination of clinically relevant principles. *British Journal of Urology International*, *88*, 563–571.

Butler, R. J., Brewin, C. R., & Forsythe, W. I. (1988). A comparison of two approaches to the treatment of nocturnal enuresis and the prediction of effectiveness using pre-treatment variables. *Journal of Child Psychology and Psychiatry*, *29*, 501–509.

Butler, R. J., Galsworthy, M. J., Rijsdijk, F., & Plomin, R. (2001a). Genetic and gender influences on nocturnal bladder control: A study of 2900 3-year-old twin pairs. *Scandinavian Journal of Urology and Nephrology*, *35*, 177–183.

Butler, R. J., Golding, J., Northstone, K., & the ALSPAC team (2005a). Nocturnal enuresis at 7.5 years old: Prevalence and analysis of clinical signs. *British Journal of Urology International*, *96*, 404–410.

Butler, R. J., Golding, J., Heron, J., & the ALSPAC Study Team. (2005b). Nocturnal enuresis: A survey of parental coping strategies at 7½ years. *Child: Care, Health and Development*, *31*, 659–667.

Butler, R. J., Heron, J., & the ALSPAC team. (2006). Exploring the differences between mono- and polysymptomatic nocturnal enuresis. *Scandinavian Journal of Urology and Nephrology*, *40*, 313–319.

Butler, R. J., Holland, P., & Robinson, J. (2001b). Examination of the structured withdrawal program to prevent relapse of nocturnal enuresis. *Journal of Urology*, *166*, 1–4.

Butler, R. J., Redfern, E. J., & Holland, P. (1994). Children's notions about enuresis and the implications for treatment. *Scandinavian Journal of Urology and Nephrology, Supplement*, *163*, 39–47.

Butler, R. J., & Robinson, J. C. (2002). Alarm treatment for childhood nocturnal enuresis: An investigation of within-treatment variables. *Scandinavian Journal of Urology and Nephrology*, *36*, 268–272.

Butler, R. J., Robinson, J. C., Holland, P., & Doherty-Williams, D. (2004a). Investigating the three systems approach to complex childhood nocturnal enuresis. *Scandinavian Journal of Urology and Nephrology*, *38*, 117–121.

Butler, R. J., Robinson, J. C., Holland, P., & Doherty-Williams, D. (2004b). An exploration of outcome criteria in nocturnal enuresis treatment. *Scandinavian Journal of Urology and Nephrology*, *38*, 196–206.

Caione, P., Arena, F., Biraghi, M., Cigna, R. M., Chendi, D., & Chiozza, M. L., *et al.* (1997). Nocturnal enuresis and daytime wetting: A multicentric trial with oxybutynin and desmopressin. *European Urology*, *31*, 459–463.

Chiozza, M. L., Bernardinelli, L., Caione, P., Del Gado, R., Ferrara, P., Giorgi, P. L., *et al.* (1998). An Italian epidemiological multicentre study of nocturnal enuresis. *British Journal of Urology*, *81*, 86–89.

Clayden, G. (2001). The child who soils. *Current Paediatrics*, *11*, 130–134.

Cox, D. J., Sutphen, J., Borowitz, S., Kovatchev, B., & Ling, W. (1998). Contribution of behavior therapy and bio-feedback to laxative therapy in the treatment of pediatric encopresis. *Annals of Behavioral Medicine*, *20*, 70–76.

Cox, D. J., Sutphen, J., Ling, W., Quillian, W., & Borowitz, S. (1996). Additive benefits of laxative, toilet training and biofeedback therapies in the treatment of pediatric encopresis. *Journal of Pediatric Psychology*, *21*, 659–670.

Devitt, H., Holland, P., Butler, R., Redfern, E., Hiley, E., & Roberts, G. (1999). Plasma vasopressin and response to treatment in primary nocturnal enuresis. *Archives of Disease in Childhood*, *80*, 448–451.

Devlin, J. B. (1991). Prevalence and risk factors for childhood nocturnal enuresis. *Irish Medical Journal*, *84*, 118–120.

Devlin, J. B., & O'Caithan, C. (1990). Predicting treatment outcome in nocturnal enuresis. *Archives of Disease in Childhood*, *65*, 1158–1161.

Feehan, M., McGee, R., Stanton, W., & Silva, P. A. (1990). A 6 year follow-up of childhood enuresis: Prevalence in adolescence and consequences for mental health. *Journal of Paediatrics and Child Health*, *26*, 75–79.

Fergusson, D. M., & Horwood, L. J. (1994). Nocturnal enuresis and behavioral problems in adolescence: A 15-year longitudinal study. *Pediatrics*, *94*, 662–668.

Fergusson, D. M., Horwood, L. J., & Shannon, F. T. (1986). Factors related to the age of attainment of nocturnal bladder control: an 8-year longitudinal study. *Pediatrics*, *78*, 884–890.

Foreman, D. M., & Thambirajah, M. S. (1996). Conduct disorder, enuresis, and specific developmental delays in two types of encopresis: A case note of 63 boys. *European Journal of Child and Adolescent Psychiatry*, *5*, 33–37.

Forsythe, W. I., & Butler, R. J. (1989). Fifty years of enuretic alarms. *Archives of Disease in Childhood*, *64*, 879–885.

Foxman, B., Valdez, R. B., & Brook, R. H. (1986). Childhood enuresis: Prevalence, perceived impact and prescribed treatments. *Pediatrics*, *77*, 482–487.

Friman, P. C., Handwerk, M. L., Swearer, S. M., McGinnis, J. C., & Warzak, W. J. (1998). Do children with primary nocturnal enuresis have clinically significant behavior problems? *Archives of Pediatric and Adolescent Medicine*, *152*, 537–539.

Gillin, J. C., Rapoport, J. L., Mikkelsen, E. J., Langer, D., Vanskiver, C., & Mendelson, W. (1982). EEG sleep patterns in enuresis: A further analysis and comparison with normal controls. *Biological Psychiatry*, *17*, 947–953.

Halliday, S., Meadow, S. R., & Berg, I. (1987). Successful management of daytime enuresis using alarm procedures: A randomly controlled trial. *Archives of Disease in Childhood*, *62*, 132–137.

Hanafin, S. (1998). Socio-demographic factors associated with nocturnal enuresis. *British Journal of Nursing*, *7*, 403–408.

Haque, M., Ellerstein, N. S., Gundy, J. H., Shelov, S. P., Weiss, J. C., McIntire, M. S., *et al.* (1981). Parental perceptions of enuresis. *American Journal of Diseases in Childhood*, *135*, 809–811.

Hellerstein, S., & Zguta, A. A. (2003). Outcome of overactive bladder in children. *Clinical Pediatrics*, *42*, 553–556.

Hellström, A. L., Hanson, E., Hansson, S., Hjälmås, K., & Jodal, U. (1990). Micturition habits and incontinence in 7-year-old Swedish school entrants. *European Journal of Paediatrics*, *149*, 434–437.

Hirasing, R. A., Van Leerdam, F. J., Bolk-Bennink, L. B., & Bosch, J. D. (1997). Bedwetting and behavioural and/or emotional problems. *Acta Paediatrica*, *86*, 1131–1134.

Hjälmås, K., Hanson, E., Hellström, A. L., Kruse, S., & Sillen, U. (1998). Long-term treatment with desmopressin in children with primary mono-symptomatic nocturnal enuresis: An open multicentre study. *British Journal of Urology*, *82*, 704–709.

Hjälmås, K., Passerini-Glazel, G., & Chiozza, M. L. (1992). Functional daytime incontinence: Pharmacological treatment. *Scandinavian Journal of Urology and Nephrology*, *141*, 108–116.

Houts, A. C. (1991). Nocturnal enuresis as a bio-behavioural problem. *Behaviour Therapy*, *22*, 133–151.

Houts, A. C., Mellon, M. W., & Whelan, J. P. (1988). Use of dietary fiber and stimulus control to treat retentive encopresis: A multiple baseline investigation. *Journal of Pediatric Psychology*, *13*, 435–445.

Houts, A. C., Berman, J. S., & Abramson, H. (1994). Effectiveness of psychological and pharmacological treatments for nocturnal enuresis. *Journal of Consulting and Clinical Psychology*, *62*, 737–745.

Hublin, C., Kaprio, J., Partinen, M., & Koskenvuo, M. (1998). Nocturnal enuresis in a nationwide twin cohort. *Sleep*, *21*, 579–585.

Jarvelin, M. J., Moilanen, I., Vikevainen-Tervonen, L., & Huttunen, N. P. (1990). Life changes and protective capacities in enuretic and non-enuretic children. *Journal of Child Psychology and Psychiatry*, *31*, 763–774.

Jarvelin, M. R., Moilanen, I., Kangas, P., Moring, K., Vikevainen-Tervonen, L., Huttunen, N. P., *et al.* (1991). Aetiological and precipitating factors for childhood enuresis. *Acta Paediatrica Scandinavica*, *80*, 361–369.

Joinson, C. J., Heron, J., Butler, U., von Gontard, A., & the Avon Longitudinal Study of Parents and Children Study Team (2007b). Psychological differences between children with and without soiling problems. *Pediatrics*, *117*, 1575–1584.

Joinson, C. J., Heron, J., Emond, A., & Butler, R. J. (2007a). Psychological problems in children with bedwetting and combined (day and night) wetting: A UK population-based study. *Journal of Pediatric Psychology*, *32*, 605–616.

Kalo, B. B., & Bella, H. (1996). Enuresis: Prevalence and associated factors among primary school children in Saudi Arabia. *Acta Paediatrica*, *85*, 1217–1222.

Kodman-Jones, C., Hawkins, L., & Schulman, S. L. (2001). Behavioral characteristics of children with daytime wetting. *Journal of Urology*, *166*, 2392–2395.

Kosar, A., Arikan, N., & Dincel, C. (1998). Effectiveness of oxybutynin hydrochloride in the treatment of enuresis nocturna. *Scandinavian Journal of Urology and Nephrology*, *33*, 115–118.

Kruse, S., Hellström, A. L., & Hjälmås, K. (1999). Daytime bladder dysfunction in therapy-resistant nocturnal enuresis. A pilot study in urotherapy. *Scandinavian Journal of Urology and Nephrology*, *33*, 49–52.

Landman, G. B., Rappaport, L., Fenton, T., & Levine, M. D. (1986). Locus of control and self-esteem in children with encopresis. *Journal of Developmental and Behavioral Pediatrics*, *7*, 111–113.

Levine, M. D. (1982). Encopresis: Its potentiation, evaluation and alleviation. *Pediatric Clinics of North America*, *29*, 315–330.

Levine, M. D., & Bakow, H. (1976). Children with encopresis: A study of treatment outcome. *Pediatrics*, *58*, 845–852.

Liu, X., Sun, Z., Uchiyama, M., Li, Y., & Okawa, M. (2000). Attaining nocturnal urinary control: Nocturnal enuresis and behavioral problems in Chinese children aged 6 through 16 years. *Journal of the American Academy of Child and Adolescent Psychiatry*, *39*, 1557–1564.

Loening-Baucke, V. (1990). Modulation of abnormal defecation dynamics by biofeedback treatment in chronically constipated children with encopresis. *Journal of Pediatrics*, *116*, 214–222.

Loening-Baucke, V. (1996). Biofeedback training in children with functional constipation. A critical review. *Digestive Diseases and Sciences*, *41*, 65–71.

Loening-Baucke, V. (2002). Encopresis. *Current Opinion in Pediatrics*, *14*, 570–575.

Loening-Baucke, V., Cruickshank, B., & Savage, C. (1987). Defecation dynamics and behavior profiles in encopretic children. *Pediatrics*, *80*, 672–679.

Longstaffe, S., Moffatt, M. E., & Whalen, J. C. (2000). Behavioral and self-concept changes after six months of enuresis treatment: A randomized, controlled trial. *Pediatrics*, *105*, 935–940.

Lovering, J. S., Tallett, S. E., & McKendry, J. B. (1988). Oxybutynin efficacy in the treatment of primary enuresis. *Pediatrics*, *82*, 104–106.

Mellon, M. W., Houts, A. C., & Lazar, L. F. (1996). Treatment of retentive encopresis with diet modification and scheduled toileting vs. mineral oil and rewards for toileting: a clinical decision. *Ambulatory Child Health*, *1*, 214–222.

McGrath, M. L., Mellon, M. W., & Murphy, L. (2000). Empirically supported treatments in pediatric psychology: Constipation and encopresis. *Journal of Pediatric Psychology*, *25*, 225–254.

Mellon, M. W., & McGrath, M. L. (2000). Empirically supported treatments in pediatric psychology: Nocturnal enuresis. *Journal of Pediatric Psychology*, *25*, 193–214.

Mikkelsen, E. J. (2001). Enuresis and encopresis: Ten years of progress. *Journal of the American Academy of Child and Adolescent Psychiatry*, *40*, 1146–1158.

Mikkelsen, E. J., Rapoport, J. L., Nee, L., Gruenau, C., Mendelson, W., & Gillin, C. (1980). Child enuresis: Sleep patterns and psychopathology. *Archives of General Psychiatry*, *37*, 1139–1144.

Miller, K., Goldberg, S., & Atkin, B. (1989). Nocturnal enuresis: Experience with long-term use of intranasally administered desmopressin. *Journal of Pediatrics*, *114*, 723–726.

Moffatt, M. E. K., Harlos, S., Kirshen, A. J., & Burd, L. (1993). Desmopressin acetate and nocturnal enuresis: How much do we know? *Pediatrics*, *92*, 420–425.

Moffatt, M. E. K., Kato, C., & Pless, I. V. (1987). Improvements in self-concept after treatment of nocturnal enuresis: Randomized controlled trial. *Journal of Pediatrics*, *110*, 647–652.

Moffat, M. E. K., & Cheang, M. (1995). Predicting treatment outcome with conditioning alarms. *Scandinavian Journal of Urology and Nephrology, Supplement*, *173*, 119–122.

Monda, J. M., & Husmann, D. A. (1995). Primary nocturnal enuresis: A comparison among observation, imipramine, desmopressin acetate and bedwetting alarm systems. *Journal of Urology*, *154*, 745–748.

Neveus, T. (2001). Oxybutynin, desmopressin and enuresis. *Journal of Urology*, *166*, 2459–2462.

Neveus, T., Stenberg, A., Lackgren, G., Tuvemo, T., & Hetta, J. (1999). Sleep of children with enuresis: A polysomnographic study. *Pediatrics*, *103*, 1193–1197.

Nijman, R. J., Butler, R. J., van Gool, J., Yeung, C. K., Bower, W., & Hjälmås, K. (2002). Conservative management of urinary incontinence in childhood. In P. Abrams, L. Cardozo, S. Khoury, & A. Wein (Eds.), *Incontinence* (2nd edn., pp. 515–551). Plymouth: World Health Publications.

Nolan, T., Debelle, G., Oberklaid, F., & Coffey, C. (1991). Randomised trial of laxatives in the treatment of childhood encopresis. *Lancet*, *338*, 523–527.

Nørgaard, J. P., & Djurhuus, J. C. (1993). The pathophysiology of enuresis in children and young adults. *Clinical Pediatrics*, *91*, 5–9.

Nørgaard, J. P., Pedersen, E. B., & Djurhuus, J. C. (1985). Diurnal anti-diuretic hormone levels in enuretics. *Journal of Urology*, *134*, 1029–1031.

Nørgaard, J. P., Rittig, S., & Djurhuus, J. C. (1989). Nocturnal enuresis: An approach to treatment based on pathogenesis. *Journal of Pediatrics*, *114*, 705–710.

Nørgaard, J. P., van Gool, J. D., Hjälmås, K., Djurhuus, J. C., & Hellström, A-L. (1998). Standardization and definitions in lower urinary tract dysfunction in children. International Children's Continence Society. *British Journal of Urology*, *81*, 1–16.

Rittig, S., Knudsen, U. B., Norgaard, J. P., Pedersen, E. B., & Djurhuus, J. C. (1989). Abnormal diurnal rhythm of plasma vasopressin and urinary output in patients with enuresis. *American Physiological Society*, *256*, 664–667.

Robson, W. L., Leung, A. K., & Bloom, D. A. (1996). Daytime wetting in childhood. *Clinical Pediatrics*, *31*, 91–98.

Rushton, H. G., Belman, A. B., Skoog, S., Zaontz, M. R., & Sihelnik, S. (1995). Predictors of response to desmopressin in children and adolescents with mono-symptomatic nocturnal enuresis. *Scandinavian Journal of Urology and Nephrology, Supplement*, *173*, 109–111.

Rutter, M., Tizard, J., & Whitmore, K. (Eds.). (1970). *Education, health and behaviour*. London: Longman.

Rutter, M. L., Yule, W., Graham, P. J. (1973). Enuresis and behavioural deviance: some epidemiological considerations. In I. Kolvin, R. C. MacKeith, & S. R. Meadows (Eds.), *Bladder control and enuresis: Clinics in developmental medicine* (pp. 137–147). London: William Heinemann/Spastics International Medical Publications.

Schmitt, B. D. (1982). Daytime wetting (diurnal enuresis). *Pediatric Clinics of North America*, *29*, 9–20.

Stark, L. J., Spirito, A., Lewis, A. V., & Hart, K. J. (1990). Encopresis: Behavioral parameters associated with children who fail medical management. *Child Psychiatry and Human Behavior*, *20*, 169–179.

Stark, L. J., Opipari, L. C., Donaldson, D. L., Danovsky, M. B., Rasile, D. A., & DelSanto, A. F. (1997). Evaluation of a standard protocol for retentive encopresis: A replication. *Journal of Pediatric Psychology*, *22*, 619–633.

Stein, Z., & Susser, M. (1967). Social factors in the development of sphincter control. *Developmental Medicine and Child Neurology*, *9*, 692–706.

Stromgren, A., & Thomson, P. H. (1990). Personality traits in young adults with a history of conditioning-treated childhood enuresis. *Acta Psychiatrica Scandinavica*, *81*, 538–541.

Tissier, G. (1983). Bedwetting at five years of age. *Health Visitor*, *56*, 333–335.

van der Plas, R. N., Benninga, M. A., Buller, H. A., Bossuyt, P. M., Akkermans, L. M., Redekop, W. K., *et al.* (1996). Biofeedback training in the treatment of childhood constipation: A randomised controlled study. *Lancet*, *348*, 776–778.

van Gool, J. D., & de Jonge, G. A. (1989). Urge syndrome and urge incontinence. *Archives of Disease in Childhood*, *64*, 1629–1634.

van Gool, J. D., Vijverberg, M. A., & de Jong, T. P. (1992). Functional daytime incontinence: Clinical and uro-dynamic assessment. *Scandinavian Journal of Urology and Nephrology*, *141*, 58–69.

van Kerrebroeck, P. E. (2002). Experience with the long-term use of desmopressin for nocturnal enuresis in children and adolescents. *British Journal of Urology International*, *89*, 420–425.

Verhulst, F. C., van der Lee, J. H., Akkerhuis, G. W., Sanders-Woudstra, J. A., Timmer, F. C., & Donkhorst, I. D. (1985). The prevalence of nocturnal enuresis: Do DSM III criteria need to be changed? A brief research report. *Journal of Child Psychology and Psychiatry*, *26*, 989–993.

Vijverberg, M. A., Elzinga-Plomp, A., Messer, A. P., van Gool, J. D., & de Jong, T. P. (1997). Bladder rehabilitation, the effect of a cognitive training programme on urge incontinence. *European Urology*, *31*, 68–72.

von Gontard, A. (1998). Annotation: Day and night wetting in children: A paediatric and child psychiatric perspective. *Journal of Child Psychology and Psychiatry*, *39*, 439–451.

von Gontard, A., Hollmann, E., Eiberg, H., Benden, B., Rittig, S., & Lehmkuhl, G. (1997). Clinical enuresis phenotypes in familial nocturnal enuresis. *Scandinavian Journal of Urology and Nephrology*, *31* (Supplement 183), 11–16.

von Gontard, A., Lettgen, B., Olbing, H., Heiken-Lowenua, C., Gaebel, E., & Schmitz, I. (1998). Behavioural problems in children with urge incontinence and voiding postponement: A comparison of a paediatric and child psychiatric sample. *British Journal of Urology*, *81*, 100–106.

von Gontard, A., Mauer-Mucke, K., Plück, J., Berner, W., & Lehmkuhl, G. (1999). Clinical behavioral problems in day- and night-wetting children. *Pediatric Nephrology*, *13*, 662–667.

von Gontard, A., Schaumburg, H., Hollmann, E., Eiberg, H., & Rittig, S. (2001). The genetics of enuresis: A review. *Journal of Urology*, *166*, 2438–2443.

Wagner, W. G., & Matthews, R. (1985). The treatment of nocturnal enuresis: A controlled comparison of two models of urine alarm. *Journal of Developmental and Behavioral Pediatrics*, *6*, 22–26.

Watanabe, H., & Kawauchi, A. (1995). Is small bladder capacity a cause of enuresis? *Scandinavian Journal of Urology and Nephrology, Supplement*, *173*, 37–41.

Watanabe, H., Kawauchi, A., Kiramori, T., & Azuma, Y. (1994). Treatment system for nocturnal enuresis according to an original classification system. *European Urology*, *23*, 43–50.

Watanabe, H., Imada, N., Kawauchi, A., Koyama, Y., & Shirakawa, S. (1997). Physiological background of enuresis Type I: A preliminary report. *Scandinavian Journal of Urology and Nephrology*, *31*, 7–10.

Wolfish, N. (1999). Sleep arousal function in enuretic males. *Scandinavian Journal of Urology and Nephrology*, *33*, 24–26.

Wolfish, N. (2001). Sleep/arousal and enuresis subtypes. *Journal of Urology*, *166*, 2444–2447.

Yeung, C. K., Chiu, H. N., & Sit, F. K. (1999). Bladder dysfunction in children with refractory mono-symptomatic primary nocturnal enuresis. *Journal of Urology*, *162*, 1049–1054.

Yeung, C. K., Sreedhar, B., Sihoe, J. D., Sit, F. K., & Lau, J. (2006). Differences in characteristics of nocturnal enuresis between children and adolescents: A critical appraisal from a large epidemiological study. *British Journal of Urology International*, *97*, 1069–1073.

Psychiatric Aspects of Somatic Disease

Seija Sandberg and Jim Stevenson

Chronic somatic disease affects an estimated 10–20% of all children during childhood or adolescence (Abraham, Silber, & Lyon, 1999; Northam, 1997). Pediatric chronic diseases are illnesses that affect a person for an extended period of time, often for life, and that require medical care and attention above and beyond the normal requirements for a child or adolescent. Improved medical outcomes for many childhood diseases mean that a vast majority survive into adulthood, thus emphasizing psychosocial and quality of life issues. This chapter studies both the contribution of psychological factors to physical ill health and the consequences for mental health of physical illness. The approach to the latter topic is that of Wallander and Varni (1998). This differentiates between non-categorical (i.e., general) and categorical (i.e., illness-specific effects).

Psychological and Psychosocial Factors in Development of Somatic Disease

Evidence of Effects

Children with psychosocial stress are significantly more likely to experience illness and hospitalizations as well as use health services more frequently than other children (Haavet & Grünfeld, 1997). Stress as a precipitating factor has been implicated for asthma, appendicitis, rheumatoid arthritis and leukemia. Prospective and experimental studies have also shown that adverse life events and other stressful experiences significantly increase a person's susceptibility to acute and recurrent respiratory infections (Cobb & Steptoe, 1998), and often precede acute exacerbations of asthma (Sandberg, Paton, Ahola *et al.*, 2000; Sandberg, Järvenpää, Penttinen *et al.*, 2004).

Mechanisms Producing Risk

The mechanisms by which psychosocial stress increases the risk of somatic disease involve cognitive, psychological, physiological and immune functions. It has been postulated that the mediators of stress response (glucocorticoids and catecholamines) have an immediate protective function (allostasis). However, when repeatedly activated they generate what has been called allostatic load, which itself creates risk of later diseases (McEwen, 2000; Turner-Cobb, 2005). For example, in the cardiovascular system, catecholamines promote adaptation by modifying heart rate and blood pressure to sleeping, waking and physical exertion. However, a concerted repetition of such blood pressure changes in response to stress can accelerate atherosclerosis and, acting jointly with metabolic hormones, can produce type 2 diabetes (McEwen, 1998).

Stress may compromise the body's immune responses to viral infection, with the individual differences in susceptibility possibly explained by differences in psychobiological reactivity (for review see Segerstrom & Miller, 2004). The immune system and the central nervous system form a bidirectional communication network (Heim, Ehlert, & Hellhammer, 2000) in which proinflammatory cytokines have a pivotal role.

Role of Somatic Disease in Increasing the Risk of Psychiatric Illness

Evidence of Effects

Chronic or life-threatening illness increases the risk of psychiatric disorder in children and adolescents. The risk is highest in conditions affecting the central nervous system or impairing motor functioning (Eiser, 1990). A meta-analysis by Lavigne and Faier-Routman (1992) confirmed the above, with those having a chronic somatic disease showing twice the rate of psychopathology as children in the comparison groups. However, in spite of the higher prevalence, only a minority of children with chronic disorders appeared maladjusted.

Few studies have addressed the specific types of mental health problems in children associated with somatic illness. Consequently, the evidence remains non-specific, although it points to anxiety and other emotional disorders being more common than behavior disorders (Thompson & Gustafson, 1996; Wallander & Varni, 1998). Even more notable is the paucity of longitudinal research to allow examination of individual differences in vulnerability and resistance.

Mechanisms Producing Risk

As searches for distinctive behavioral features or personality characteristics within individual illness groups have been unsuccessful, studies of psychosocial aspects of specific diseases have increasingly been replaced by the examination of various psychological and psychosocial effects associated with

Rutter's Child and Adolescent Psychiatry, 5th edition. Edited by M. Rutter, D. Bishop, D. Pine, S. Scott, J. Stevenson, E. Taylor and A. Thapar. © 2008 Blackwell Publishing, ISBN: 978-1-4051-4549-7.

somatic disease in general (Geist, Grdisa, & Otley, 2003; LeBlanc, Goldsmith, & Patel, 2003; Lewis & Vitulano, 2003; Stewart, 2003).

According to Wallander and Varni (1998), chronic physical disorders are most usefully conceptualized as sources of ongoing chronic strain for both the children and their families. Chronic strains are defined as persistent objective conditions requiring continual readjustment and repeatedly interfering with the performance of ordinary role-related activities. Their impact is determined by the nature of the onset and course of the illness, its potential fatality and the degree of incapacitation caused.

Complex vulnerability and protective mechanisms are also involved. These need to be considered in relation to a child's individual characteristics as well as to their contextual properties. In the context of a child's chronic physical illness, family stress is negatively associated with child adjustment. However, the effect will vary depending on the presence of other mediating factors. The strength or the direction of the relationship may depend on the type of coping used and a significant association may only emerge when a parent or child copes in a maladaptive manner.

Non-categorical Illness, Child- and Family-Related Factors Increasing Risk of Psychiatric Disorder

Age of Child at Time of Illness

It is important to view the onset of the illness in a developmental context. Early studies of hospitalization suggested that those necessitating separation from primary attachment figures are particularly difficult for children in their second to fourth year of life. Hospitalizations at an even earlier age, especially if reoccurring, have been shown to be associated with increased later behavior problems (Quinton & Rutter, 1976). However, for a school-age child, illnesses that disrupt participation in normal family and school life can become sources of stress (Vitulano, 2003). During this period gender differences also begin to emerge. For boys, illnesses that impair sports abilities are more difficult to cope with, while girls appear more sensitive to health problems that prevent accessing peer group support. In adolescence, illnesses interfering with the strive for greater independence are especially problematic, as belonging to a peer group and developing intimate relationships become critical developmental challenges (Greydanus, Rimsza, & Newhouse, 2002; Meijer, Sinnema, Bijstra *et al.*, 2002).

Accuracy and Timeliness of the Establishment of the Diagnosis

The process by which the diagnosis is established can affect the child's and parents' ability to adapt. Here, important factors include the duration of time required to reach the diagnosis and the certainty with which it can be made, as well as the sensitivity with which the diagnosis and its implications are conveyed. A rapid and accurate diagnosis can facilitate forming a "partnership of care" and improve the prognosis. Conversely, a misdiagnosis can lead to an acutely adversarial situation.

However, some illnesses are more easily recognized than others. Prodromal symptoms of some forms of leukemia, for example, can remain vague and their significance minimized for some time. In cases where malignancies are discovered at relatively advanced stages, answering the question why appropriate early investigations were not ordered is always difficult, but avoiding the issue may jeopardize subsequent treatment.

Communicating a confirmed grave or terminal diagnosis to a child is a challenging responsibility (Young, Dixon-Woods, Findlay, & Heney, 2002; Young, Dixon-Woods, Windridge, & Heney, 2003). The task can become even more intricate if the physician, or parent, is ambivalent about the need to share the prognosis with the child. When faced with a grave diagnosis to share, many physicians try to cope by focusing on treatment while avoiding addressing the crucial emotional issues. An opportunity to consult a psychologist or child psychiatrist is often helpful in such situations.

Interference with Function

There is a strong association between the level of disability and the severity of the illness, but there also exists great variability in types and levels of disability (Morad, Kandel, Hyam, & Merrick, 2004). However, this variability in functional capacity is frequently ignored as an independent risk factor despite clear links with long-term adaptation (Vitulano, 2003). Likewise, differences in the impact of the same disability with regard to the child's developmental level may get overlooked. Illness-related interference with cognitive processing has a negative effect at all stages of development, but cognitive deficits have even wider implications for a child facing academic examinations, for example.

Impact on Physical Appearance

Some somatic diseases can involve extensive physical disfigurements (e.g., atopic dermatitis), while others, although serious or incapacitating, usually have no effect on the physical appearance (e.g., diabetes or asthma). Some diseases, such as cystic fibrosis, involve complex dietary and medication regimes that older children, and especially adolescents, may perceive as socially stigmatizing. Given the importance of a positive physical appearance to the sense of self-worth, it is not surprising that stigmatizing illnesses are associated with emotional vulnerability (Breslau & Marshall, 1985).

Anxiety about being physically different from their peers is a common concern of chronically ill children. This becomes progressively more important during school years and reaches its peak in adolescence. With the peer group assuming greater importance, emotional rejection based on negative response from others can precipitate depression or lead to other emotional problems. Despite the obvious importance of these issues, little systematic research has been carried out on this topic.

Persistence of Symptoms

Childhood diseases vary in their pattern of symptom expression and consequent impact on the child's life. Asthma and epilepsy can involve long symptom-free periods and thus allow the child extended opportunities to lead a near-normal life. Diabetes and cystic fibrosis, however, demand strict daily adherence to special diets and medication routines, and in spite of these remain unremitting or result in gradual worsening and disability.

Illnesses with persistent or unremitting symptoms would be expected to have greater negative impact on psychological adaptation. Surprisingly, little evidence that this is so exists. However, it is also true that some children with chronic illness cope with their situation by getting compensatory rewards from academic achievement, or by excelling in music, art or some other skill.

Hope for Recovery

A brief encounter with a serious illness that results in complete recovery is unlikely to have significant impact on emotional health but children with a more precarious prognosis live with persistent uncertainty about their long-term survival. The primary concern for the mental health of children with a terminal prognosis is helping them not to lose hope prematurely or succumb to depression, with a likely detrimental effect on their illness. Some children manage to maintain strong optimism about their eventual recovery even in the face of the gravest of odds. Another core aspect of work with children who have a terminal prognosis is to help them and their family to reach some level of acceptance of the inevitability of their impending death.

Child's Personality Attributes Modifying or Mediating Risk

Many studies comparing children with even a severe physical illness with healthy peers have failed to find differences (Hocking & Lochman, 2005; Meijer, Sinnema, Bijstra *et al.*, 2002; Phipps & Steele, 2002). The same studies have also established that the lack of apparent anxiety even in a gravely ill child with cancer, for example, is explainable by the child's style of coping. Avoidant coping has been shown to predict poor adjustment characterized by low self-esteem and high social anxiety, whereas confrontation and readiness to seek social support predict positive adjustment (Meijer, Sinnema, Bijstra *et al.*, 2002), and defensive coping is associated with low generalized anxiety (Phipps & Steele, 2002). Tendency to repress feelings, especially anger, is another commonly found characteristic of children with serious physical illness. However, there is no evidence that any particular coping style is uniformly the best protection against psychological problems. Rather, it depends on the child's personality or temperament and social situation, including the availability of emotional support.

Psychiatric Aspects of the Child's Reactions to Somatic Disease

Functional impairment may result from psychological distress or psychiatric illness presenting itself in covert forms. Geist, Grdisa, & Otley (2003) list four common presentations, found singly or in combination, often indicating underlying psychosocial issues: medical symptoms unexplainable by organic factors alone; poor adherence to treatment recommendations; school refusal; and engagement in risky behaviors involving sex/sexuality or use of substances.

A change in a child's overall functioning can alert parents and professionals to possible difficulties in the disease management, treatment adherence or adjustment to illness. However, few assessment tools specific to pediatric populations exist, and measures developed for healthy children, or modifications of adult assessments, are often used instead. The questionnaire "Living with Chronic Illness" (LCI; Adams, Streisand, Zawacki, & Joseph, 2002), represents one exception. It provides an assessment from both a parent's and the patient's perspective across a variety of chronic conditions and has the advantage of distinguishing between social difficulties related to the illness and those resulting from other factors. Of the therapeutic approaches, cognitive–behavioral methods and psychoeducational interventions have proved most helpful (Barlow & Ellard, 2004; Christie & Wilson, 2005).

Parental Responsibility for the Treatment of the Illness

Parental response to the illness can affect the child's adaptation in many ways (Madden, Hastings, & Vant-Hoff, 2002; Wray & Sensky, 2004). Sensitive and effective parenting promotes optimal outcome, but inconsistent parenting (e.g., because of stress or depression) promotes poor adaptation. Age and developmental stage also determine the level of parental responsibility and degree of supervision of the child's treatment. Protective parenting may be appropriate in the case of a young child, but highly attentive and controlling parental behavior can be problematic for a teenager. Their growing need for independence includes increased responsibility for their treatments – a responsibility that is also open to exploitation. Chronic illness is a stressor that can negatively impact on the parents' mental health and marital relationship, and impair their ability to parent not only the sick child, but also the non-affected siblings. The increased risk for psychological problems in the siblings of chronically ill children has been well highlighted (Houtzager, Oort, Hoekstra-Weebers *et al.*, 2004; Sharpe & Rossiter, 2002; Van-Riper, 2003). Interventions combining educational and psychological approaches have proved helpful in reducing family stress and promoting better mental health in parents and siblings (Barrera, Fleming, & Khan, 2004; Williams, Williams, Graff *et al.*, 2003).

Role of Non-illness-related Psychosocial Stress

Children with somatic illness, like any other children, are vulnerable to the effects of psychosocial stressors, both acute life events and long-term adversities. These stresses may stem from the child's family life (e.g., parental ill health/deviance or marital conflicts/separations), school environment (e.g., academic pressures), peer group (e.g., being a victim of bullying), or result from acute life events (e.g., accidents or loss of someone close). For discussion of the mechanisms through which psychosocial stressors exert their influence see chapters 25 and 26.

Protective Factors and Mechanisms

Compared with the volume of research on the effects of negative experiences on children's health, far fewer studies focusing on protective factors exist. A confiding relationship with a close adult relative has been shown to protect children from a psychiatric disorder when faced with stressful life events and chronic psychosocial adversity (Sandberg, Rutter, Giles *et al.*, 1993). It is reasonable to believe that this would also be the case in children with somatic disease, although no empirical evidence so far exists. In children with asthma, family rituals and routines, as a proxy measure of good parenting, have been shown to protect against anxiety in the context of high parental stress (Markson & Fiese, 2000). Positive life events, such as the child's personal achievements, and minor rebelliousness also protected against the increased risk of new asthma attacks associated with stressful life events (Sandberg, McCann, Ahola *et al.*, 2002; Sandberg, Taskinen, Oja *et al.*, 2003).

Specific Conditions

Asthma

Of the chronic diseases of childhood, asthma is probably the most common, with up to one child in four being affected. Reports from different countries are consistent in indicating an increase in the prevalence of asthma and allergies, especially in industrialized societies (Asher, Montefort, Björkstén *et al.*, 2006).

Most childhood asthma begins in infancy. Adverse events in early life, allergen exposure, suboptimal feeding practices, viral infections and environmental pollutants seem important precipitating factors (Wright, Cohen, & Cohen, 2005), with gene–environment interactions determining illness manifestation (Hoffjan, Nicolae, Ostrovnaya *et al.*, 2005). Lately, research has focused on the potential link between exposures to microbial sources and the development of allergic diseases (for review see Schaub, Lauener, & von Mutius, 2006). The term "hygiene hypothesis" refers to a theory attempting to encompass the complex associations between viral and bacterial infections, exposure to substances produced by microbes in the environment, immune responses and the person's genetic background.

A growing body of evidence suggests that psychosocial stress contributes to the development of wheezing illnesses and asthma, especially during early childhood, and predicts greater morbidity in children who already have asthma (Bloomberg & Chen, 2005). Prospective studies of genetically predisposed infants have highlighted the role of early caregiver stress. It has been shown to predict repeated wheeze in the first year and was associated with an atopic immune profile (Wright, Cohen, Carey *et al.*, 2002; Wright, Finn, Contreras *et al.*, 2004) and, together with early parenting difficulties, the onset of asthma by age 3 (Mrazek, Klinnert, Mrazek *et al.*, 1999), and occurrence of asthma up to age 8 (Klinnert, Nelson, Price *et al.*, 2001).

Many clinicians also hold the view that asthma frequently gets worse following a stressful experience. That this is so was shown in a prospective study (Sandberg, Paton, Ahola *et al.*, 2000; Sandberg, Järvenpää, Penttinen *et al.*, 2004) involving children with chronic asthma. Severely negative life events significantly increased the risk of a new asthma attack both immediately and in the coming few weeks. The magnitude and timing of the maximum risk were influenced by the presence or absence of chronic psychosocial stress. Subsequently, a molecular genetic study by Miller and Chen (2006) showed that, in children with asthma, concurrent experience of acute and chronic stress alters the properties of genes responsible for fighting infection and keeping airways open.

Emotional arousal itself can act as a potential precursor of asthmatic symptoms (for review see Lehrer, Feldman, Giardino, Song, & Schmaling, 2002). The main focus has been on negative emotions such as anger, sadness and depression (Rietveld, Everaerd, & Creer, 2000; Ritz, George, & Dahme, 2000a). A non-reciprocal pattern of autonomic functioning has been proposed as the underlying physiological mechanism (Ritz, Steptoe, DeWilde, & Costa, 2000b), with the immediate and delayed effects of stress likely to involve different processes (Klinnert, 2003). In the presence of chronic or repeated stress, the physiological response to acute stress appears to result in more sustained effects on the immune system (Chen, Hanson, Paterson *et al.*, 2006). A less active hypothalamic–pituitary–adrenal (HPA) system in combination with high stress has been proposed as another explanation for the delayed effects (Ball, Anderson, Minto, & Halonen, 2006; Heim, Ehlert, & Hellhammer, 2000).

An association has been demonstrated between asthma severity and the child's ability to regulate negative emotions (Klinnert, McQuaid, McCormic, Adinoff, & Bryant, 2000), possibly reflecting wider physiological dysregulation indicating a common genetic vulnerability (Mrazek, 2003). These conclusions are supported by the Early Treatment of the Atopic Child study (ETAC; Stevenson, 2003) and a UK birth cohort study (Calam, Gregg, Simpson *et al.*, 2005). Behavior problems, as possible markers for stress, preceded the development of asthma.

Regarding psychiatric morbidity, emotional disorders, especially anxiety (separation anxiety being the most common) and depression, has been the most consistent finding (Feldman, Ortega, McQuaid, & Canino, 2006; Klinnert, Nelson, Price *et al.*, 2001; McQuaid, Kopel, & Nassau, 2001). Prior emotional problems also predicted a further increase in the risk of new asthma attacks associated with stressful life events (Sandberg, Taskinen, Oja *et al.*, 2003).

Of late, experimental intervention programs have been implemented in school settings with encouraging results. In a controlled study, McCann, McWhirter, Coleman, Calvert, and Warner (2006) showed that an intervention delivered as part science curriculum combined with staff training resulted in significant improvements of subjective well-being and less need for prescribed medication (for a review of psychological interventions see Lehrer, Feldman, Giardino *et al.*, 2002).

Atopic Dermatitis

Atopic dermatitis, commonly known as eczema, is an allergic skin condition that nearly always begins in infancy, and usually resolves during childhood, often even in the second year of life. It is a familial illness with evidence for a genetic etiology involving heritable hypersensitive immunoglobulin E (IgE) response (Ball, Anderson, Minto *et al.*, 2006; Wright, Cohen, & Cohen, 2005).

Studies in the fields of psychoimmunology have highlighted a probable connection between atopy and emotional dysregulation, possibly reflecting a common genetic vulnerability (Wright, Cohen, & Cohen, 2005). An increased rate of behavior problems in young children with atopic dermatitis (Stevenson, 2003), and a genetic association between atopy and emotional disorders in school-age children (Wamboldt, Schmidt, & Mrazek, 1998), indicate early difficulties in emotional regulation. Caring for a young child with atopic dermatitis can be a distressing task for parents as the child is often in discomfort, and therefore miserable, for long periods of time. This situation has the potential for major disruption of the early caregiving relationship. Because of a lack of systematic studies, however, little is known about the long-term psychological consequences of severe eczema in the early years of life.

Cystic Fibrosis

Cystic fibrosis (CF) is a complex multisystem disease with the patients often facing a number of physical and psychological problems (Bourke, 2003). It is caused by a defective gene, leading to thick sticky mucus that obstructs the airways, the digestive system and other organs, resulting in chronic infections and inflammation of the lungs and difficulty in digesting food and nutrients. CF is usually diagnosed in infancy or early childhood and prenatal screening now enables intrauterine detection.

Medical treatment has led to a substantial increase in life expectancy, and more children with CF are surviving into adulthood. Despite this promising outlook, children and adolescents with CF continue to live with a life-limiting disease, with CF influencing their relationships, education and plans for future employment, marriage, etc. Progress in the medical aspects of care has not been matched by comparable advances in psychological interventions.

The treatment regimens, involving strict adherence to special diets, multiple administrations of medicines and nutrition replacements, as well as "aggressive" daily physiotherapy, restrict the daily lives of the children and parents and may become a source of stress. "Successful" adherence to these regimens can also promote developmentally inappropriate dependence in the child and make negotiating the inevitable adolescent challenges problematic. Along with adolescence comes a transition to adult medical care with expectations for the patient to take responsibility for their disease management. To many adolescents with CF, moving to an adult clinic means taking a step closer to their death. Clinical problems associated with impending mortality are often challenging to manage. As the disease progresses, the young people and their families need extra support to cope with their feelings of anticipated loss and frustrations associated with the limitations of therapeutic interventions.

A full range of psychiatric problems has been reported in children and adolescents with CF, with depression and eating disorders specifically noted (for review see Christian, 2003), and family interactions – especially during mealtimes – are often strained (Janicke, Mitchell, & Stark, 2005). Avoidance and denial are common psychological coping mechanisms. Such coping strategies may be viewed as "negative" or maladaptive by professionals if they include non-compliance with treatments, but from a young person's perspective they may be adaptive, as a means of escaping from the world of CF for a while.

Juvenile Onset Diabetes Mellitus

Diabetes mellitus affects approximately 2% of the population in the UK and refers to a group of metabolic diseases characterized by hyperglycemia occurring as a result of defects in insulin secretion, insulin action or both. Long-term hyperglycemia is a serious problem and can lead to dysfunction of a number of organs including eyes, kidneys and the circulatory system. A distinction is made between types 1 and 2 diabetes, with the first requiring the administration of insulin to maintain health. Type 2 diabetes has usually been seen as a condition with onset in middle age. However, there is a substantial increase in type 2 diabetes amongst children and young people. This occurrence of type 2 diabetes in young people is of relatively recent origin and its clinical management is less well understood (Gungor, Hannon, Libman, Bacha, & Arslanian, 2005). The most obvious reason for the rapidly rising rate of type 2 diabetes in children and adolescents is a combination of low physical activity and the absence of a well-balanced low-fat and high-fiber diet. Action to prevent obesity in this age group is the only satisfactory way in which this alarming rise in type 2 diabetes can be controlled (Vivian, 2006). The psychological consequences of type 2 diabetes in children and young people are not well understood. There is some evidence that boys experiencing this condition are at increased risk of depressed mood compared with boys with type 1 diabetes. In turn, depressed mood is related to relatively poor metabolic control as indicated by mean glycosylated hemoglobin (HbA1c; Lawrence, Standiford, Loots *et al.*, 2006).

The care of children with type 1 diabetes is well established (Silverstein, Klingensmith, Copeland *et al.*, 2005). It is important to recognize, however, that the care of these children needs to take into account differences in the way in which the disease needs to be managed at different ages.

It has long been recognized that psychological factors can play a significant part in the course of diabetic illness (Wysochi, Buckloh, Lochrie, & Antel, 2005). Type 1 diabetes is a condition that arises from the interaction of genetic and environmental risks (Haller, Atkinson, & Schatz, 2005). The significance of emotional stresses in the onset of the disease is equivocal. However, it is clear that the management and course of the disease are strongly influenced by psychosocial factors.

For both children and adults, diabetes has been a major area of the application of behavioral science to medicine. The range of analyses and applications of psychobehavioral approaches to the condition has been reviewed by Gonder-Frederick, Cox, and Ritterband (2002). The significance of the specific association between type 1 diabetes and depression is given particular weight by the finding that suicidal ideation was a feature shortly after the onset of type 1 diabetes symptoms. Although relatively few attempted suicide, the misuse of insulin in the suicide attempts should be noted (Goldston, Kovacs, Ho, Pharrone, & Stiffler, 1994).

In addition to the association between the illness and psychiatric disorder, which the above findings suggest have a reciprocal effect on each other, the presence of type 1 diabetes has an adverse effect on family functioning more broadly. In a study of children between the ages of 1 and 14 years, Northam, Anderson, Adler, Werther, and Warne (1996) found that during the immediate period after diagnosis both children and parents exhibited a mild degree of psychological distress. Within 1 year this had largely resolved and the residual impact on the family was largely seen in terms of families becoming less flexible in their functioning. These complex interactions between the course of the disease and family and individual functioning led to an emphasis on psychological interventions to support children and their families with type 1 diabetes.

There is an extensive number of studies of efforts to intervene to enhance the psychological health of the children and their families (Northam, Todd, & Cameron, 2005). Many of these studies have suffered from methodological inadequacies including low participation rates, small unrepresentative samples and the use of unstandardized measures (Northam, Todd, & Cameron, 2005). They have tended to use interventions focused on increasing compliance rather than targeting a broader range of psychological distress. There have also been few attempts to evaluate interventions with younger children. Nevertheless, across the adult and child age range, the evidence suggests that interventions can be effective both in terms of enhancing the psychological well-being of individuals with type 1 diabetes and also, but to a lesser extent, promoting good metabolic control (Hampson, Skinner, Hart *et al.*, 2000).

Cancer

There are a number of childhood cancers, the most common of which is acute lymphoblastic leukemia (ALL). This comprises about 25% of childhood cancers and 75% of leukemias. It is a malignant disease of the lymphoid cells and the bone marrow, which are carried in the blood to most organs including the central nervous system. Brain tumors are the second most frequently diagnosed cancer of childhood (Strother, Pollack, Fisher *et al.*, 2002). Advances in medical treatment have substantially improved the survival rates for children with ALL to about 75%, with higher rates in Hodgkin's disease and lower rates in other cancers (Eiser, 1998). In considering the physical and psychological consequences of childhood cancer, the following conclusion has been drawn by Patenaude and Kupst (2005, p. 11): "From these studies emerging over the past 2 decades, we have learnt with increasing specificity that no child with cancer remains unchanged by the experience."

The level of adjustment difficulties in pediatric cancer patients is near to the levels of normal healthy children (Patenaude & Kupst, 2005). However, there appear to be about 25–30% of children and families who experience considerable psychological or social difficulties. These include low academic achievement, impaired social relationships and poor self-concept and low self-esteem. It needs to be recognized that for some children and families the experience of childhood cancer has a positive effect on psychological health with increased resilience and enhanced social relationships (Eiser, Hill, & Vance, 2000). Patenaude and Kupst (2005) were able to identify a number of factors that were associated with a worse psychological outcome. Among the disease and treatment factors were diagnoses of cancer involving the central nervous system (CNS), bone tumors, CNS irradiation and intense chemotherapy, shorter time since diagnosis and a shorter period of treatment. The personal characteristics associated with a worse psychosocial outcome were younger age at diagnosis, poor psychological health before diagnosis, higher levels of perceived stress and lower cognitive ability. Those family and environment factors that have a role were low adaptability and cohesiveness, a lack of open communication, low social support and fewer socioeconomic resources.

There are a number of instruments that have been developed to measure psychosocial outcome in pediatric cancer patients. An appraisal of the merits of alternative measures of health-related quality of life, including measures specifically targeted at pediatric cancer, can be found in Eiser and Morse (2001).

There are still unresolved issues concerning the neurocognitive consequences of some aspects of the treatment of childhood cancers. Waber, Carpentieri, Klar *et al.* (2000) found that children treated for ALL with dexamethasone performed less well on cognitive tests than those on prednisone. Chemotherapy for children with ALL has also been implicated in generating attentional deficits (Buizer, de Sonneville, Van Den Heuvel-Eibrink, & Verman, 2005). However, others have suggested that treatment for leukemia that does not involve the use of cranial irradiation does not produce cognitive losses or attentional deficits (Rodgers, Marckus, Kearns, & Windebank, 2003). Indeed, Eiser, Davies, Jenney, Stride, and Glaser (2006) suggest that dexamethasone does not have an adverse effect on the health-related quality of life of children. There is some evidence that methylphenidate may help reduce any attentional and social difficulties experienced by children being treated for childhood cancer (Mulhern, Khan, Kaplan *et al.*, 2004).

Chronic Fatigue Syndrome

The definition of chronic fatigue syndrome (CFS) in children is usually taken to be the same as for adults, and it is generally accepted that the key features are also similar (Garralda & Chalder, 2005; Garralda & Rangel, 2002). These consist of incapacitating chronic fatigue after comparatively little effort, unimproved by rest and unexplained by physical or psychiatric illness. Besides fatigue, CFS involves a characteristic constellation of physical symptoms such as headaches, a variety of other bodily pains and altered sleep and eating patterns. CFS commonly starts with an acute illness episode, such as "flu" or glandular fever, but it can also have insidious gradual onset. The condition can be intensely debilitating and follows a chronic, sometimes fluctuating, course. Children with CFS often receive repeated specialist medical consultations, and a variety of diagnoses, as the parents seek explanations for their ailments. Controversy has surrounded CFS stemming from strong beliefs held by patients and their advocates that the condition has a medical cause. For this reason, some prefer the term ME (myalgic encephalitis). It is also possible that the terms such as fibromyalgia, neurasthenia and post-viral fatigue syndrome are used to refer to the same condition.

Emotional distress and mood changes are common associated psychological problems, and psychiatric comorbidity, especially anxiety and depressive disorders, as well as personality problems, are identified in 50–75% of children and adolescents severely affected with CFS (Rangel, Garralda, Levin *et al.*, 2000b; Richards, Turk, & White, 2005), with some of this probably secondary to CFS (Garralda & Rangel, 2005). Independent genetic etiologies for depression and unexplained disabling fatigue were also indicated in a study by Fowler, Rice, Thapar, and Farmer (2006).

A variety of interventions have been used in the treatment and management of CFS, with considerable differences of opinion about the most appropriate and effective management. According to a systematic review (Whiting, Bagnall, Sowden *et al.*, 2001) of 44 controlled trials (36 of these randomized), involving 2801 mainly adult participants, the interventions with the most promising results included cognitive–behavioral therapy (CBT) and graded exercise therapy. A controlled clinical study of children and adolescents with CFS similarly demonstrated a clear superiority of active rehabilitation programs over traditional supportive care (Viner, Gregorowski, Wine *et al.*, 2004).

Outcome studies have at best involved a few dozen children and adolescents with CFS. Nevertheless, they have produced surprisingly uniform findings, showing that a distinct majority of severely affected young people eventually make a complete recovery, and many more improve sufficiently to lead near-normal lives (Rangel, Garralda, Levin *et al.*, 2000a).

Failure to thrive/deprivation dwarfism

Failure to thrive (FTT) can be defined as weight for age below the third percentile for a protracted period of time during the first year of life. Children falling into this group may do so for a variety of reasons, and historically a distinction was made between those with a known organic basis for growth faltering and those deemed to be non-organic. This differentiation is far from straightforward (Reilly, Skuse, Wolke, & Stevenson, 1999). The key question is whether such a group, even if heterogeneous in the origins of their FTT, are at risk for continuing developmental difficulties. That this may not be the case is highlighted by the marked developmental catch-up children can demonstrate even having experienced severe early deprivation (Rutter, 1998).

The prevalence rate of FTT has been estimated to be 3.5% and it is a relatively common cause of referral to pediatricians (Skuse, 1993). Such children are likely to present with a wide array of associated medical conditions. These will reflect both factors leading to their growth deficiency and the consequences of acute or chronic malnutrition.

The treatment of FTT will often require the joint expertise of a team of social workers and nutritionists as well as psychiatrists (Iwaniec, 2004). The value of a wide-ranging psychosocial intervention for children with FTT was shown in a study by Black, Dubowitz, Hutcheson, Berenson-Howard, & Starr (1995). They randomized 130 children (mean age, 12.7 months) recruited from low-income families into two groups: clinic plus home intervention or clinic only. All children received services in a multidisciplinary growth and nutrition clinic. Families in the home intervention group received weekly home visits for 1 year by lay home visitors, supervised by a community health nurse. Children's weight for age, weight for height and height for age improved significantly during the 12-month study period, regardless of intervention status. However, the enhanced cognitive and behavioral changes in the home intervention group led Black, Dubowitz, Hutcheson *et al.* (1995) to conclude that early home intervention can promote a nurturant home environment effectively and can reduce the developmental delays often experienced by low-income urban infants with FTT.

A meta-analysis of the extent to which FTT was associated with later poor cognitive development was produced by Corbett and Drewett (2004). They suggest that the adverse effect of FTT to later cognitive ability was −0.28 standard deviation (95% confidence interval [CI], −0.16 to −0.41), equivalent to 4.2 IQ points. This overall pattern of results is also illustrated by the findings from Boddy, Skuse, and Andrews (2000). Their longitudinal study of children who had FTT (defined as being at 3 months at least below the 3rd percentile of weight) indicated a diminishing effect of early malnutrition on cognitive ability as the children became older.

This pattern of emerging results, suggesting a relative benign outcome for children with FTT during early infancy, has led Rudolf and Logan (2005) to suggest that an "aggressive approach to the identification and management of failure to thrive needs reassessing." The key issue is that of identifying which of the children within this group might benefit from intervention. This is particularly significant given what they suggest are the equivocal results that have emerged from randomized controlled trials of intervention directed at this group as a whole. As yet there is no clear evidence of which children with FTT might benefit most from such intervention.

Sickle Cell Disease

Sickle cell disease (SCD) is a common blood disorder of genetic origin. It results in red blood cells that when partially or totally deoxygenated form into sickle-shaped cells that may obstruct blood vessels. This may cause a lack of oxygen in tissues in a wide variety of locations. The medical complications include delayed growth and sexual maturation, pulmonary dysfunction, stroke retinopathy and chronic pain (Edwards, Scales, Loghlin *et al.*, 2005). The condition therefore comprises pain, anemia, organ failure and a variety of other comorbid conditions.

Pain is a core feature of SCD. The psychological difficulties this creates have been reviewed by Anie (2005). The ability of the child with SCD to cope with pain is crucial to their quality of life. A specific measure has been developed to assess these coping mechanisms (Coping Strategies Questionnaire – SCD; Gil, Abrams, Phillips, & Keefe, 1989). Using this measure, Anie, Steptoe, Ball, Dick, and Smalling (2002) were able to show that there were three coping patterns:

1 Active coping (e.g., distraction or increased activity);
2 Affective coping (e.g., positive thoughts and feelings); and
3 Passive adherence coping (e.g., taking rests and fluids).

Pain severity was related to the use of passive adherence coping independently of other clinical markers of severity of SCD.

The risks of developing behavioral problems and poor psychological health were higher for children (Hurtig & White, 1986) than for adolescents (Hurtig & Park, 1989). The evidence for an elevated rate of clinical cases of anxiety disorders or depression in SCD is equivocal when compared with non-affected sibling controls (Anie, 2005). There is stronger evidence of neuropsychological deficits arising as a consequence of the cerebral infarcts associated with SCD (Kral, Brown, & Hynd, 2001). Some children develop overt strokes and the associated deficit is determined by the site of the consequent lesion. For those experiencing silent infarcts identified only by brain imaging, the area primarily affected is the frontal lobes and the cognitive problems are usually associated with attention and executive function (Anie, 2005).

Burns

SCD is a condition where the child is faced with the problem of chronic pain. For children who experience burns there may be sudden onset acute pain followed by an extended period of subsequent pain. There are a range of psychological methods that can augment pharmacological pain relief (Stoddard, Sheridan, Saxe *et al.*, 2002). The subsequent emergence of acute stress symptoms 1 month after experiencing a burn (primarily a scalding) was examined by Stoddard, Saxe, Ronfeldt *et al.* (2006) in a sample of 64 children aged 1–4 years. They found that there were two routes to acute stress symptoms. One was a direct reflection of burn severity (total body surface area [TBSA]). The other was via the parents' stress reactions in response to the child's demonstrated pain symptoms. There are clear clinical implications of these findings whereby attention to pain management and relieving stress in parents of children with burns of large body areas are likely to be effective.

To identify the factors that predict how well a child will be functioning 6 months after a burn, Tyack and Ziviani (2003) studied 68 children experiencing 1–35% burns of TBSA. They found that injury factors (e.g., TBSA), premorbid child factors (e.g., psychiatric problems or learning disability), parenting factors (e.g., anxiety and depression) and demographic factors (e.g., age and gender) each made a significant independent contribution to functional outcome 6 months after the burn. A more detailed study of the emergence of post-traumatic stress disorder (PTSD) in children experiencing burns was undertaken by Saxe, Stoddard, Hall *et al.* (2005). They suggested that PTSD could arise via two routes. The first was via the impact of size of burn and the amount of pain experienced on acute separation anxiety in the children. The second was via dissociation, again being more marked the larger the size of the burn. These two psychological mechanisms could explain over half of the variance in PTSD symptomatology 3 months after the burn.

Organ Transplantation

There have been a number of studies on psychiatric aspects of organ transplantation (e.g., liver and kidney) in children (for a review see Qvist, Jalanko, & Holmberg, 2003). The main set of studies are those concerning children receiving heart or heart–lung transplants. Survival rates for heart transplantation are improving and attention has therefore turned to psychosocial aspect of their functioning and to later quality of life (Mintzer, Stuber, Seacord *et al.*, 2005). Investigations into the cognitive development and psychological well-being of children after heart transplantation were reviewed by Todaro, Femmell, Sears, Rodrigue, and Roche (2000), who concluded that in general there was no adverse impact of surgery on the neuropsychological function of children receiving transplantation. A later study suggested that for younger children rather than adolescents, transplantation may indeed have some adverse effects on cognitive development (Wray & Radley-Smith, 2005). Moreover, a subset of studies suggest that those experiencing a more complex course of treatment, recurrent surgery or organ rejection may show more adverse effects of cognitive functioning. In addition, academic performance is adversely affected by recurrent hospitalization in these children.

The pattern of findings also suggests that most children receiving transplants have good psychological adjustment 1 year after transplantation; however, there is a subgroup of about 25% of children who show emotional and behavioral difficulties. Todaro, Femmell, Sears *et al.* (2000) suggest that it is the stresses associated with transplantation, such as intense medical treatment and the reduced opportunities to socialize with peers, that result in negative affect, decreased social competence and behavioral problems in this minority of transplant recipients. These emotional and behavioral difficulties may adversely affect adherence and thereby influence the long-term health of children (for recommendations on how to increase medical compliance in these circumstances see Griffin & Elkin, 2001).

Physical Symptoms Without Evidence of Somatic Etiology

Complaints of physical symptoms unexplainable by known somatic etiology are common presentations in children and adolescents. These mostly involve stomach aches, headaches and joint pains, manifest in a range of severity, and are associated with functional impairments interfering with normal social interactions (Eminson, 2001a; Garralda, 1999; Taylor, Szatmari, Boyle, & Offord, 1996). They can cause the child to avoid school, attend repeated medical appointments and undergo painful investigations. The parents, or even the whole family, may become adapted to the notion that the child has an organic illness, and thus reinforce the child's tendency to communicate by physical symptoms.

The children are often shy and compliant outside the home and somatic complaints are used to express emotional distress, usually in a long-standing pattern, accompanied by family traits of anxiety, overprotectiveness and somatization. The underlying psychosocial issues, however, may be difficult to identify and treat. Depression and anxiety disorders are the most common associated psychiatric disorders (Egger, Costello, Erkanli, & Angold, 1999; Eminson, 2001a,b; Garralda, 1999).

The etiology of somatizing disorders is complicated by the difficulty of distinguishing between factors relevant to the experience of physical symptoms and those contributing to illness behavior (Brown, Schrag, & Trimble, 2005). There is also a shortage of good-quality etiological studies. A variety of predisposing, precipitating and maintaining factors has been noted, although none is either necessary or sufficient on its own (Eminson, 2001a). A combination of vulnerability and trigger factors relates to issues unique to each child and family. The families are often characterized by a tendency to experience many somatic symptoms, limited verbal communication about emotional issues, including conflict, and parental history of somatoform illness or anxiety/depression. Conscientiousness, emotional lability or low self-esteem serve as predisposing factors in the children themselves. There may also be a history of abuse. Stressful life events, an episode of physical illness, peer group problems or academic pressures often precipitate the onset, and chronically stressful family situations or school-related problems may contribute to symptom maintenance.

Lately, the concept of somatization has been subjected to a major review in the light of psychoneuroimmunological research (Dantzer, 2005; Rief & Barsky, 2005; Thayer & Brosschot, 2005). It has been proposed that the brain cytokine system can become sensitized to repeated activation or exposure to environmental stressors in response to stimulation in the early stages of development. When sensitized, the system is less likely to turn off when the danger is over, and more likely to be triggered by extrinsic non-immune stimuli. This results in a sickness response along with its subjective, behavioral and metabolic components. Future research will no doubt either confirm or refute these propositions.

Factitious Illness by Proxy

The condition labeled Munchausen syndrome by proxy was formulated by Meadow (1977). Since that time there has been considerable controversy over the veracity of this concept, how frequently it occurs and its status within legislation and professional practice concerning child abuse. The current view is that this should be seen as a specific form of abnormal illness behavior (Pilowsky, 1997). This is shown by abnormalities in care-eliciting behaviors and relationships with health care professionals. By extension, this abnormal illness behavior can be generated by proxy via the manipulation of the health symptoms of a child. The term factitious illness by proxy has now been adopted.

The current criteria (American Psychiatric Association, 2000) for identifying factitious disorder by proxy are as follows:

1 Intentional production or feigning of physical signs or symptoms in another person who is under the individual's care.

2 The motivation for the perpetrator's behavior is to assume the sick role by proxy.

3 External incentives for the behavior, such as economic gain, are absent.

4 The behavior is not better accounted for by another mental disorder.

One of the most salient features of factitious illness by proxy is a history of abnormal illness behavior in the parent. For example, in a series of 37 families studied by Gray and Bentovim (1996), 18% of the mothers who had induced an illness in their child also had a history of factitious illness. In this sample, a total of 49% of the mothers presented with a psychiatric history. Very similar figures were obtained by Adshead and Bluglass (2005), with 21% showing a history of behaviors indicating personality disorder and 10% having a diagnosis of somatizing disorder. There was a history of psychiatric treatment in 52% of the mothers.

These findings by Adshead and Bluglass (2005) came from a study making a detailed examination of the attachment representations of mothers with factitious illness by proxy using the Adult Attachment Interview. The sample had been referred for medicolegal assessment to a psychiatrist with a specialist practice in this area. They found a very high rate of insecure attachment representation (85%). They conclude that "mothers with factitious illness by proxy are more like a clinical group than not and therefore are likely to have unmet treatment needs, which may be relevant to future risk."

The reoccurrence of instances of unexplained deaths of young children led to the claim by Meadow that the parents may have murdered their children (Meadow, 1999). The evidence to support this conclusion and the flawed logic adopted have been extensively criticized. The principles governing expert witness testimony highlighted by this case have been outlined by Butler-Sloss and Hall (2002).

An extensive collation of material on cases of factitious illness by proxy was produced by Sheridan (2003). The characteristics of 451 cases were described based on reports in journal papers. A substantial majority of the perpetrators were mothers (just over 75%). Gender was not related to the risk victim status. The average age at diagnosis was 48 months but with a wide range extending up to 204 months. Just fewer than 10% had long-term or permanent disability with a further 6% with fatalities. Of the known siblings, a substantial proportion were either dead or had symptoms similar to the victims'. The most common conditions and symptoms that are created or faked by parents are apnea (27%), feeding difficulties (25%), diarrhea (20%), seizures (17%), cyanosis (12%), asthma (9%) and allergy (9%). The age of the child involved in factitious illness by proxy is an important consideration. The issues in older children have been reviewed by Awadallah, Vaughan, Franco *et al.* (2005) and include the collusion of the older child with the perpetrator and the fear of the consequences of disclosure.

The difficulties in establishing parental involvement in factitious illness by proxy have led some pediatricians to advocate the use of covert video-recordings (Southall, Plunkett, Banks, Falkov, & Samuels, 1997). The dilemmas for clinicians have been clearly set out in a paper by Morley (1998) and its associated commentary. He concluded that, "Covert video surveillance is an infringement of the liberty of the parent and child and should be undertaken only as a last resort – when a group of people has assessed the case and no other way exists to diagnose the child's problem."

Presentation of Psychiatric Disorders in the Form of Somatic Symptoms

Dissociative Disorders

Dissociative disorders, also known as conversion disorders, are characterized by a loss of function in any modality, suggesting a neurological or other physical condition, which is in fact not present (Goodyer, 1981; Leary, 2003). They appear from middle childhood onwards. An apparent loss of motor function is the most common presentation. Loss of sight, hearing, sensation and consciousness (as in a pseudoseizure), or partial loss (as in fugue state), have also been reported.

These are not uncommon disorders although little is known about their true prevalence. This is mainly because the most transient disorders are not necessarily brought to medical attention or, if taken to an accident and emergency department or clinic, will often remit quickly with reassurance. Prolonged reactions usually lead to a referral to child and adolescent mental health services. However, a psychiatric referral does not necessarily exclude organic pathology, as demonstrated by a survey of over 10,000 patient records by Caplan (1970). One-third of the 28 children given the diagnosis of "conversion hysteria" were subsequently found to have an organic illness.

Precipitating factors include life stresses of all types, involving either the child directly, or the whole family. The family characteristics follow two broad patterns: chaotic social circumstances with multiple symptomatic family members, and those with high expectations for achievement and high anxiety about illness and loss (Grattan-Smith, Fairly, & Procopis, 1988). The children themselves are often described as unusually good and compliant, with anxiety or depression as a predisposing factor (Kozlowska, 2001). Taylor (1986) articulated four key elements of childhood conversion disorder: an intolerable predicament for which all solutions are blocked; a presence of an ally to promote sickness; an available model for sickness; and possession of the necessary social skills.

The diagnosis involves reviewing existing medical investigations and conveying to the child and parents that there is no physical illness. Gaining their confidence to explore alternative explanations, such as feelings and life stresses, is a key task in establishing therapeutic alliance. Intervention begins with an acknowledgment that the young person has a real illness seriously disrupting their life. The presenting disability may be explained in terms of the body's physical functions with a person's feelings/emotions and social/interpersonal situation interacting with one another. Of the therapeutic approaches, both behavior therapy and graded physiotherapy programs have proved effective (Leary, 2003). Prognosis varies from good to poor. Favorable prognostic features include a recent onset and monosymptomatic manifestation, whereas conditions associated with a history of sexual abuse or pre-existing anxiety disorder or depression may become chronic.

Epidemic Hysteria

Apart from "hysterical conversion" disorders that occur in individual children, there is the rather different variety of "epidemic hysteria" (McEvedy, Griffith, & Hall, 1966; Moss & McEvedy, 1966). The topic was succinctly reviewed by Hersov (1997), who noted that, unlike the individual form, which is equally common in both sexes, epidemic hysteria much more frequently affects girls. It typically occurs among adolescents or pre-adolescents in a relatively closed community such as a boarding school or hospital. The phenomenon commonly involves a pattern of events with one person first developing "hysterical" attacks of falling or convulsions, overbreathing or some similar phenomenon; then another does, and soon the hysteria spreads to involve a large number of youngsters in the community. The individuals first to develop the hysterical attacks are usually found to have severe psychological disturbances, but this is less often the case with the later affected ones, who may be more dependent and show more neurotic traits than average, but are otherwise fairly ordinary youngsters. The reasons for the spread of disorder relate to the social milieu as much as to the personality features of the affected individuals. Usually, those who start the epidemic have a dominant and influential position within their peer group, and the epidemic starts at a time when group anxieties (e.g., sexual activities, worries about pregnancy, work stresses or the death of a classmate) create an emotional vulnerability. Stresses relating to the youngsters' families of origin, such as parental divorce or death of a close relative, may also be behind the symptoms of the first affected individuals (Small & Nicholi, 1982). Outlining the main principles of managing mass hysteria, Hersov (1997) emphasized the need to first isolate the key initiating individuals. Following that, attention then needs to be paid to both the group tensions and emotions, and to the personal problems of the main instigators.

Pseudoepilepsy

Pseudoseizures or psychogenic seizures present as epileptic seizures but are not accompanied by abnormal patterns of electroencephalogram (EEG) activity. The prevalence rate is not known accurately but there are far fewer reports of psychogenic seizures in children than in adults. In a review of 883 patients assessed over a 6-year period in one pediatric epilepsy monitoring unit, 15% were classified as having paroxysmal non-epileptic events. Of these, the proportion with psychogenic seizures increased from 3% in the preschool years, to 43% and to 87% in the age ranges 5–12 and 12–18 years, respectively (Kotagal, Cota, Wyllie, & Wolgamuth, 2002). There is a concomitant decline with age in the proportion of these paroxysmal non-epileptic disorders that are physiological or organic in origin. Often, psychiatric disorders are found concomitant with pseudoepilepsy. For example, Papavasiliou, Vassilkai, Paraskevoulakos *et al.* (2004) reported depression, anxiety, obsessive-compulsive disorder and PTSD in a series of child and adolescent patients. In general, across all ages, depression is the psychiatric condition most commonly associated with pseudoepilepsy (Thompson, Osorio, & Hunter, 2005). There is an increased rate of epilepsy and of developmental delay in these children. However, those with pseudoepilepsy as well as epilepsy form only a small proportion of those with true epilepsy – Kotagal, Cota, Wyllie *et al.* (2002) estimate that they constitute just 1.5% of those with epilepsy.

Families where Psychological Factors are Seen as Important for Child's Somatic Symptoms

When assessing a child with somatic symptoms, a greater than usual level of attention may be required to engage the young person and their parents with psychiatric services. A careful narrative approach to the history of the illness, its impact and management is often helpful (Eminson, 2001b). Understanding the family's beliefs about the illness, the level of conviction that there is a physical cause, satisfaction with investigations already carried out and views about psychiatric referral is critical for successfully engaging the child and family (Garralda, 1999).

It may also be helpful to canvass the family's medical history more widely to establish whether other family members have had similar physical symptoms, whether a serious illness was the cause for them and whether the symptoms remained unexplained, as well as the outcome of the illness. A past failure of medical colleagues to find the cause of a family member's complaints (sometimes with serious consequences) may undermine parental confidence in medical opinions.

The individual assessment of the child or adolescent should proceed as normally, taking note of somatic symptoms, physical state and functional mobility, mental state and ability to relate and engage, as well as sleep, appetite, relationships, school attendance and ability to perform academic work. It is important also to enquire about the young person's views about the cause of the illness, although these usually quite closely mirror parental views.

Conclusions

The child psychiatrist has a significant part to play in the care of children with a range of physical illness. There is also an increasing involvement of specialists from other disciplines. Pediatric psychology is maturing as a research field in its own right and as a specialism in clinical and health psychology. The application of both child psychiatry and psychology expertise is developing more effective and evidence-based methods of intervention in pediatric settings (Drotar & Lemanek, 2001).

References

Abraham, A., Silber, T. J., & Lyon, M. (1999). Psychosocial aspects of chronic illness in adolescence. *Indian Journal of Pediatrics*, *66*, 447–453.

Adams, C. D., Streisand, R. M., Zawacki, T., & Joseph, K. E. (2002). Living with a chronic illness: A measure of social functioning for children and adolescents. *Journal of Pediatric Psychology*, *27*, 593–605.

Adshead, G., & Bluglass, K. (2005). Attachment representations in mothers with abnormal illness behaviour by proxy. *British Journal of Psychiatry*, *187*, 328–333.

American Psychiatric Association. (2000). *Diagnostic and statistical manual of mental disorders* (4th edn.). Text revision. Washington, DC: American Psychiatric Association.

Anie, K. A. (2005). Psychological complications in sickle cell disease. *British Journal of Haematology*, *129*, 723–729.

Anie, K. A., Steptoe, A., Ball, S., Dick, M., & Smalling, B. M. (2002). Coping and health service utilisation in a UK study of paediatric sickle cell pain. *Archives of Disease in Childhood*, *86*, 325–329.

Asher, M. I., Montefort, S., Björkstén, B., Lai, C. K. W., Strachan, D. P., Weiland, S. K., *et al.*, & the ISAAC Phase Three Study Group. (2006). Worldwide time trends in the prevalence of symptoms of asthma, allergic rhinoconjunctivitis, and eczema in childhood: ISAAC Phases One and Three repeat multicountry cross-sectional surveys. *Lancet*, *368*, 733–743.

Awadallah, N., Vaughan, A., Franco, K., Munir, F., Sharaby, N., & Goldfarb, J. (2005). Munchausen by proxy: A case, child series and literature review of older victims. *Child Abuse and Neglect*, *29*, 931–941.

Ball, T. M., Anderson, D., Minto, J., & Halonen, M. (2006). Cortisol circadian rhythms and stress responses in infants at risk of allergic disease. *Journal of Allergy and Clinical Immunology*, *117*, 306–311.

Barlow, J. H., & Ellard, D. R. (2004). Psycho-educational interventions for children with chronic disease, parents and siblings: an overview of the research evidence base. *Child: Care, Health & Development*, *30*, 637–645.

Barrera, M., Fleming, C. F., & Khan, F. S. (2004). The role of emotional social support in the psychological adjustment of siblings of children with cancer. *Child: Care, Health and Development*, *30*, 103–111.

Black, M. M., Dubowitz, H., Hutcheson, J., Berenson-Howard, J., & Starr, R. H. (1995). A randomized clinical trial of home intervention for children with failure to thrive. *Pediatrics*, *95*, 807–814.

Bloomberg, G. R., & Chen, E. (2005). The relationship of psychologic stress with childhood asthma. *Immunology and Allergy Clinics of North America*, *25*, 83–105.

Boddy, J., Skuse, D., & Andrews, B. (2000). The developmental sequelae of non-organic failure to thrive. *Journal of Child Psychology and Psychiatry*, *41*, 1003–1014.

Bourke, S. J. (2003). *Cystic fibrosis in respiratory medicine* (6th edn.). Oxford: Blackwell Publishing.

Breslau, N., & Marshall, I. A. (1985). Psychological disturbance in children with physical disabilities: Continuity and change in a 5-year follow-up. *Journal of Abnormal Child Psychology*, *13*, 199–216.

Brown, R. J., Schrag, A., & Trimble, M. R. (2005). Dissociation, childhood interpersonal trauma, and family functioning in patients with somatization disorder. *American Journal of Psychiatry*, *162*, 899–905.

Buizer, A.I., de Sonneville, L. M. J., Van Den Heuvel-Eibrink, M. M., & Verman, A. J. P. (2005). Chemotherapy and attentional dysfunction in survivors of childhood acute lymphoblastic leukaemia: An effect of treatment intensity. *Pediatric Blood and Cancer*, *45*, 281–290.

Butler-Sloss, E., & Hall, A. (2002). Expert witnesses, courts and the law. *Journal of the Royal Society of Medicine*, *95*, 431–434.

Calam, R., Gregg, L., Simpson, A., Simpson, B., Woodcock, A., & Custovic, A. (2005). Behavior problems antecede the development of wheeze in childhood: A birth cohort study. *American Journal of Respiratory and Critical Care Medicine*, *171*, 323–327.

Caplan, H. L. (1970). *Hysterical 'conversion' symptoms in childhood.* M. Phil. Thesis, University of London.

Chen, E., Hanson, M. D., Paterson, L. Q., Griffin, M. J., Walker, H. A., & Miller, G. E. (2006). Socioeconomic status, stress, and inflammatory processes in childhood asthma: The role of psychological stress. *Journal of Allergy and Clinical Immunology*, *117*, 1014–1020.

Christian, B. (2003). Growing up with chronic illness: Psychosocial adjustment of children and adolescents with cystic fibrosis. *Annual Review of Nursing Research*, *21*, 151–172.

Christie, D., & Wilson, C. (2005). CBT in paediatric and adolescent health settings: a review of practice-based evidence. *Pediatric Rehabilitation*, *8*, 241–247.

Cobb, J. M. T., & Steptoe, A. (1998). Psychosocial influences on upper respiratory infections in children. *Journal of Psychosomatic Research*, *45*, 319–330.

Corbett, S. S., & Drewett, R. F. (2004). To what extent is failure to thrive in infancy associated with poorer cognitive development? A review and meta-analysis. *Journal of Child Psychology and Psychiatry*, *45*, 641–654.

Dantzer, R. (2005). Somatization: A psychoneuroimmune perspective. *Psychoneuroendocrinology*, *30*, 947–952.

Drotar, D., & Lemanek, K. (2001). Steps toward a clinically relevant science of intervention in pediatric settings: Introduction to the special issue. *Journal of Pediatric Psychology*, *26*, 385–394.

Edwards, C. L., Scales, M. T., Loghlin, C., Bennett, G. G., Harris-Peterson, S., De Castro, L. M., *et al.* (2005). A brief review of the pathophysiology, associated pain and psychosocial issues in sickle cell disease. *International Journal of Behavioural Medicine*, *12*, 171–179.

Egger, H. L., Costello, E. J., Erkanli, A., & Angold, A. (1999). Somatic complaints and psychopathology in children and adolescents: Stomach aches, muscular-skeletal pains and headaches. *Journal of the American Academy of Child and Adolescent Psychiatry*, *38*, 852–860.

Eiser, C. (1990). Psychological effects of chronic disease. *Journal of Child Psychology and Psychiatry*, *31*, 85–98.

Eiser, C. (1998). Practitioner review: Long-term consequences of childhood cancer. *Journal of Child Psychology and Psychiatry*, *39*, 621–633.

Eiser, C., Davies, H., Jenney, M., Stride, C., & Glaser, A. (2006). HRQOL implications of treatment with dexamethasone for children with acute lymphoblastic leukaemia (ALL). *Pediatric Blood and Cancer*, *46*, 35–39.

Eiser, C., Hill, J. J., & Vance, Y. H. (2000). Examining the psychological consequences of surviving childhood cancer: Systematic review as a research method in pediatric psychology. *Journal of Pediatric Psychology*, *25*, 449–460.

Eiser, C., & Morse, R. (2001). A review of measures of quality of life for children with chronic illness. *Archives of Disease in Childhood*, *84*, 205–211.

Eminson, D. M. (2001a). Somatising in children and adolescents. 1. Clinical presentations and aetiological factors. *Advances in Psychiatric Treatment*, *7*, 266–274.

Eminson, D. M. (2001b). Somatising in children and adolescents. 2. Management and outcomes. *Advances in Psychiatric Treatment*, *7*, 388–398.

Feldman, J. M., Ortega, A. N., McQuaid, E. L., & Canino, G. (2006). Comorbidity between asthma attacks and internalizing disorders among Puerto Rican children at one-year follow-up. *Psychosomatics*, *47*, 333–339.

Fowler, T. A., Rice, F., Thapar, A., & Farmer, A. (2006). Relationship between disabling fatigue and depression in children. *British Journal of Psychiatry*, *189*, 247–253.

Garralda, M. E. (1999). Practitioner review. Assessment and management of somatisation in childhood and adolescence: A practical perspective. *Journal of Child Psychology and Psychiatry*, *40*, 1159–1167.

Garralda, M. E., & Chalder, T. (2005). Practitioner review: Chronic fatigue syndrome in childhood. *Journal of Child Psychology and Psychiatry*, *46*, 1143–1151.

Garralda, M. E., & Rangel, L. (2002). Annotation: Chronic fatigue syndrome in children and adolescents. *Journal of Child Psychology and Psychiatry*, *43*, 169–176.

Garralda, M. E., & Rangel, L. (2005). Chronic fatigue syndrome of childhood: Comparative study with emotional disorders. *European Child and Adolescent Psychiatry*, *14*, 424–430.

Geist, R., Grdisa, V., & Otley, A. (2003). Psychosocial issues in the child with chronic conditions: Best practice and research. *Clinical Gastroenterology*, *17*, 141–152.

Gil, K. M., Abrams, M. R., Phillips, G., & Keefe, F. J. (1989). Sickle cell disease pain: Relation of coping strategies to adjustment. *Journal of Consulting and Clinical Psychology*, *57*, 725–731.

Goldston, D. B., Kovacs, M., Ho, V. Y., Pharrone, P. L., & Stiffler, L. (1994). Suicidal ideation and suicide attempts among youth with insulin-dependent diabetes mellitus. *Journal of the American Academy of Child and Adolescent Psychiatry*, *33*, 240–246.

Gonder-Frederick, L. A., Cox, D. J., & Ritterband, L. M. (2002). Diabetes and behavioral medicine: The second decade. *Journal of Consulting and Clinical Psychology*, *70*, 611–625.

Goodyer, I. (1981). Hysterical conversion reactions in childhood. *Journal of Child Psychology and Psychiatry*, *22*, 179–188.

Grattan-Smith, P., Fairly, M., & Procopis, P. (1988). Clinical features of conversion disorder. *Archives of Disease in Childhood*, *63*, 408–414.

Gray, J., & Bentovim, A. (1996). Illness induction syndrome. *Child Abuse and Neglect*, *20*, 655–673.

Greydanus, D. E., Rimsza, M. E., & Newhouse, P. A. (2002). Adolescent sexuality and disability. *Adolescent Medicine (Philadelphia)*, *13*, 223–247.

Griffin, K. J., & Elkin, T. D. (2001). Non-adherence in pediatric transplantation: A review of the existing literature. *Pediatric Transplantation*, *5*, 246–249.

Gungor, N., Hannon, T., Libman, I., Bacha, F., & Arslanian, S. (2005). Type 2 diabetes mellitus in youth: Complete picture to date. *Pediatric Clinics of North America*, *52*, 1579–1609.

Haavet, O. R., & Grünfeld, B. (1997). Are life experiences of children significant for the development of somatic disease? A literature review. *Tidsskrift for den Norske Laegeforening*, *117*, 3644–3647.

Haller, M. J., Atkinson, M. A., & Schatz, D. (2005). Type 1 diabetes mellitus: Etiology, presentation and management. *Pediatric Clinics of North America*, *52*, 1553–1578.

Hampson, S. E., Skinner, T. C., Hart, J., Storey, L., Gage, H., Foxcroft, D., *et al.* (2000). Behavioral interventions for adolescents with type 1 diabetes: how effective are they? *Diabetes Care*, *23*, 1416–1422.

Heim, C., Ehlert, U., & Hellhammer, D. H. (2000). The potential role of hypocorticolism in the pathophysiology of stress-related bodily disorders. *Psychoneuroendocrinology*, *25*, 1–35.

Hersov, L. (1997). Emotional disorders. In M. Rutter, & L. Hersov (Eds.), *Child and Adolescent Psychiatry: Modern approaches* (2nd edn., pp. 368–381). Oxford: Blackwell.

Hocking, M. C., & Lochman, J. E. (2005). Applying the transactional stress and coping model to sickle cell disorder and insulin-dependent diabetes mellitus: Identifying psychosocial variables related to adjustment and intervention. *Clinical Child and Family Psychology Review*, *8*, 221–246.

Hoffjan, S., Nicolae, D., Ostrovnaya, I., Roberg, K., Evans, M., Mirel, D., *et al.* (2005). Gene–environment interaction effects on the development of immune responses in the 1st year of life. *American Journal of Human Genetics*, *76*, 696–704.

Houtzager, B. A., Oort, F. J., Hoekstra-Weebers, J. E. H. M., Caron, H. N., Grootenhuis, M. A., & Last, B. F. (2004). Coping and family functioning predict longitudinal psychological adaptation of siblings of childhood cancer patients. *Journal of Pediatric Psychology*, *29*, 591–605.

Hurtig, A. L., & Park, K. B. (1989). Adjustment and coping in adolescents with sickle cell disease. *Annals of the New York Academy of Sciences*, *565*, 172–182.

Hurtig, A. L., & White, L. S. (1986). Psychosocial adjustment in children and adolescents with sickle cell disease. *Journal of Pediatric Psychology*, *11*, 411–427.

Iwaniec, D. (2004). *Children who fail to thrive: A practice guide*. Chichester: Wiley.

Janicke, D. M., Mitchell, M. J., & Stark, L. J. (2005). Family functioning in school-age children with cystic fibrosis: An observational assessment of family interactions in the mealtime environment. *Journal of Pediatric Psychology*, *30*, 179–186.

Klinnert, M. D. (2003). Evaluating the effects of stress on asthma: A paradoxical challenge. *European Respiratory Journal*, *22*, 574–575.

Klinnert, M. D., McQuaid, E. L., McCormic, D., Adinoff, A. D., & Bryant, N. E. (2000). A multimethod assessment of behavioral and emotional adjustment in children with asthma. *Journal of Pediatric Psychology*, *25*, 35–46.

Klinnert, M. D., Nelson, H. S., Price, M. R., Adinoff, A. D., Leung, D. Y. M., & Mrazek, D. (2001). Onset and persistence of childhood asthma: Predictors from infancy. *Pediatrics*, *108*, 69–76.

Kotagal, P., Cota, M., Wyllie, E., & Wolgamuth, B. (2002). Paroxysmal nonepileptic events in children and adolescents. *Pediatrics*, *110*, e46.

Kozlowska, K. (2001). Good children presenting with conversion disorder. *Clinical Child Psychology and Psychiatry*, *6*, 575–591.

Kral, M. C., Brown, R. T., & Hynd, G. W. (2001). Neuropsychological aspects of pediatric sickle cell disease. *Neuropsychology Review*, *11*, 179–196.

Lavigne, J. V., & Faier-Routman, J. (1992). Psychological adjustment to pediatric physical disorders: A meta-analytic review. *Journal of Pediatric Psychology*, *17*, 133–157.

Lawrence, J. N., Standiford, D. A., Loots, B., Klingensmith, G. J., Williams, D. E., Ruggiero, A., *et al.* (2006). Prevalence and correlates of depressed mood among youth with diabetes: The SEARCH for Diabetes in Youth Study. *Pediatrics*, *117*, 1348–1358.

LeBlanc, L. A., Goldsmith, T., & Patel, D. R. (2003). Behavioral aspects of chronic illness in children and adolescents. *Pediatric Clinics of North America*, *50*, 859–878.

Leary, P. M. (2003). Conversion disorder in childhood: Diagnosed too late, investigated too much? *Journal of the Royal Society of Medicine*, *96*, 436–438.

Lehrer, P., Feldman, J., Giardino, N., Song, H-S., & Schmaling, K. (2002). Psychological aspects of asthma. *Journal of Consulting and Clinical Psychology*, *70*, 691–711.

Lewis, M., & Vitulano, L. A. (2003). Biopsychosocial issues and risk factors in the family when the child has a chronic illness. *Child and Adolescent Psychiatric Clinics of North America*, *12*, 389–399.

Madden, S. J., Hastings, R. P., & Vant-Hoff, W. (2002). Psychological adjustment in children with end stage renal disease: The impact of maternal stress and coping. *Child: Care, Health and Development*, *28*, 323–330.

Markson, S., & Fiese, B. H. (2000). Family rituals as a protective factor for children with asthma. *Journal of Pediatric Psychology*, *25*, 471–479.

McCann, D. C., McWhirter, J., Coleman, H., Calvert, M., & Warner, J. O. (2006). A controlled trial of a school-based intervention to improve asthma management. *European Respiratory Journal*, *27*, 921–928.

McEvedy, C. P., Griffith, A., & Hall, T. (1966). Two school epidemics. *British Medical Journal*, *2*, 1300–1302.

McEwen, B. S. (1998). Protective and damaging effects of stress mediators. *New England Journal of Medicine*, *338*, 171–179.

McEwen, B. S. (2000). Allostasis and allostatic load: Implications for neuropsychopharmacology. *Neuropsychopharmacology*, *22*, 108–124.

McQuaid, E. L., Kopel, S. J., & Nassau, J. H. (2001). Behavioral adjustment in children with asthma: A meta-analysis. *Developmental and Behavioral Pediatrics*, *22*, 430–439.

Meadow, R. (1977). Munchausen syndrome by proxy: Hinterland of child abuse. *Lancet*, *2*, 343–345.

Meadow, R. (1999). Unnatural sudden infant death. *Archives of Disease in Childhood*, *80*, 7–14.

Meijer, S. A., Sinnema, G., Bijstra, J. O., Mellenbergh, G. J., & Wolters, W. H. (2002). Coping styles and locus of control as predictors for psychological adjustment of adolescents with chronic illness. *Social Science and Medicine*, *54*, 1453–1461.

Miller, G. E., & Chen, E. (2006). Life stress and diminished expression of genes encoding glucocorticoid receptor and β2-adrenergic receptor in children with asthma. *Proceedings of the National Academy of Sciences of the USA*, *103*, 5496–5501.

Mintzer, L. L., Stuber, M. L., Seacord, D., Castaneda, M., Masrkhani, V., & Glover, D. (2005). Traumatic stress symptoms in adolescent organ transplant recipients. *Pediatrics*, *115*, 1640–1644.

Morad, M., Kandel, I., Hyam, E., & Merrick, J. (2004). Adolescence, chronic illness and disability. *International Journal of Adolescent Medicine and Health*, *16*, 21–27.

Morley, C. (1998). Concerns about using and interpreting covert video surveillance. *British Medical Journal*, *316*, 1603–1605.

Moss, P. D., & McEvedy, C. (1966). An epidemic of overbreathing among schoolgirls. *British Medical Journal*, *2*, 1295–1300.

Mrazek, D. A. (2003). Psychiatric symptoms in patients with asthma: Causality, comorbidity or shared genetic etiology. *Child and Adolescent Psychiatric Clinics of North America*, *12*, 459–471.

Mrazek, D. A., Klinnert, M., Mrazek, P. J., Brower, A., McGormick, D., Rubin, B., *et al.* (1999). Prediction of early-onset asthma in genetically at-risk children. *Pediatric Pulmonology*, *27*, 85–94.

Mulhern, R. K., Khan, R. B., Kaplan, S., Helton, S., Christensen, R., Bonner, M., *et al.* (2004). Short-term efficacy of methylphenidate: A randomized, double-blind, placebo-controlled trial among survivors of childhood cancer. *Journal of Clinical Oncology*, *22*, 4795–4803.

Northam, E. A. (1997). Psychosocial impact of chronic illness in children. *Journal of Paediatrics and Child Health*, *33*, 369–372.

Northam, E., Anderson, P., Adler, R., Werther, G., & Warne, G. (1996). Psychosocial and family functioning in children with insulin-dependent diabetes at diagnosis and one year later. *Journal of Pediatric Psychology*, *21*, 699–717.

Northam, E. A., Todd, S., & Cameron, F. J. (2005). Interventions to promote optimal health outcomes in children with type 1 diabetes – are they effective? *Diabetic Medicine*, *23*, 113–121.

Papavasiliou, A., Vassilkai, N., Paraskevoulakos, E., Kotsalis, C., Bazigou, H., & Bardani, I. (2004). Psychogenic status epilepticus in children. *Epilepsy and Behavior*, *5*, 539–546.

Patenaude, A. F., & Kupst, M. J. (2005). Psychosocial functioning in pediatric cancer. *Journal of Pediatric Psychology*, *30*, 9–27.

Phipps, S., & Steele, R. (2002). Repressive adaptive style in children with chronic illness. *Psychosomatic Medicine*, *64*, 34–42.

Pilowsky, I. (1997). *Abnormal illness behaviour*. Chichester: Wiley.

Quinton, D., & Rutter, M. (1976). Early hospital admissions and later disturbances of behaviour: An attempted replication of Douglas' findings. *Developmental Medicine and Child Neurology*, *18*, 447–459.

Qvist, E., Jalanko, H., & Holmberg, C. (2003). Psychosocial adaptation after solid organ transplantation in children. *Pediatric Clinics of North America*, *50*, 1505–1519.

Rangel, L. A., Garralda, M. E., Levin, M., & Roberts, H. (2000a). The course of chronic fatigue syndrome. *Journal of the Royal Society of Medicine*, *93*, 129–134.

Rangel, L. A., Garralda, M. E., Levin, M., & Roberts, H. (2000b). Personality in adolescents with chronic fatigue syndrome. *European Child and Adolescent Psychiatry*, *9*, 39–45.

Reilly, S. M., Skuse, D. H., Wolke, D., & Stevenson, J. (1999). Oral-motor dysfunction in children who fail to thrive: Organic or non-organic? *Developmental Medicine and Child Neurology*, *41*, 115–122.

Rief, W., & Barsky, A. J. (2005). Psychobiological perspectives on somatoform disorders. *Psychoneuroendocrinology*, *30*, 996–1002.

Richards, J., Turk, J., & White, S. (2005). Children and adolescents with Chronic Fatigue Syndrome in non-specialist settings: beliefs, functional impairment and psychiatric disturbance. *European Child and Adolescent Psychiatry*, *14*, 310–318.

Rietveld, S., Everaerd, W., & Creer, T. L. (2000). Stress-induced asthma: A review of research and potential mechanisms. *Clinical and Experimental Allergy*, *30*, 1058–1066.

Ritz, T., George, C., & Dahme, B. (2000a). Respiratory resistance during emotional stimulation: Evidence for a non-specific effect of experienced arousal? *Biological Psychology*, *52*, 143–160.

Ritz, T., Steptoe, A., DeWilde, S., & Costa, M. (2000b). Emotions and stress increase respiratory resistance in asthma. *Psychosomatic Medicine*, *62*, 401–412.

Rodgers, J., Marckus, R., Kearns, P., & Windebank, K. (2003). Attentional ability among surviviors of leukaemia treated without cranial irradiation. *Archives of Disease in Childhood*, *88*, 147–150.

Rudof, M. C. J., & Logan, S. (2005). What is the long term outcome for children who fail to thrive? A systematic review. *Archives of Disease in Childhood*, *90*, 925–931.

Rutter, M. (1998). Developmental catch-up, and deficit, following adoption after severe global early deprivation. *Journal of Child Psychology and Psychiatry*, *39*, 465–476.

Sandberg, S., Järvenpää, S., Penttinen, A., Paton, J. Y., & McCann, D. C. (2004). Asthma exacerbations in children immediately following stressful life events: A Cox's Hierarchical Regression. *Thorax*, *59*, 1046–1051.

Sandberg, S., McCann, D. C., Ahola, S., Oja, H., Paton, J. Y., & McGuinness, D. (2002). Positive experiences and the relationship between stress and asthma in children. *Acta Paediatrica*, *91*, 152–158.

Sandberg, S., Paton, J. Y., Ahola, S., MacCann, D. C., McGuinness, D., Hillary, C. R., *et al.* (2000). The role of acute and chronic stress in asthma attacks in children. *Lancet*, *356*, 982–987.

Sandberg, S., Rutter, M., Giles, S., Owen, A., Champion, L., Nicholls, J., *et al.* (1993). Assessment of psychosocial experiences in childhood: Methodological issues and some illustrative findings. *Journal of Child Psychology and Psychiatry*, *34*, 879–897.

Sandberg, S., Taskinen, S., Oja, H., & Paton, J. Y. (2003). Personality and behaviour moderating the stress–asthma relationship in children. *European Child and Adolescent Psychiatry*, *12*, 230.

Saxe, G. M., Stoddard, F., Hall, E., Chawla, N., Lopez, C., Sheridan, R., *et al.* (2005). Pathways to PTSD. 1. Children with burns. *American Journal of Psychiatry*, *162*, 1299–1304.

Schaub, B., Lauener, R., & von Mutius, E. (2006). The many faces of the hygiene hypothesis. *Journal of Allergy and Clinical Immunology*, *117*, 969–977.

Segerstrom, S. C., & Miller, G. E. (2004). Psychological stress and the human immune system: A meta-analytic study of 30 years of inquiry. *Psychological Bulletin*, *130*, 601–630.

Sharpe, D., & Rossiter, L. (2002). Siblings of children with a chronic illness: A meta-analysis. *Journal of Pediatric Psychology*, *27*, 699–710.

Sheridan, M. S. (2003). The deceit continues: An updated literature review of Munchausen syndrome by proxy. *Child Abuse and Neglect*, *27*, 431–451.

Silverstein, J., Klingensmith, G., Copeland, K., Plotnick, L., Kaufman, F., Laffel, L., *et al.* (2005). Care of children and adolescents with type 1 diabetes: A Statement of the American Diabetics Association. *Diabetes Care*, *28*, 186–212.

Skuse, D. (1993). Epidemiologic and definitional issues in failure to thrive. *Child and Adolescent Psychiatric Clinics of North America*, *2*, 37–59.

Small, G. W., & Nicholi, A. M. (1982). Mass hysteria among schoolchildren. *Archives of General Psychiatry*, *39*, 721–724.

Southall, D., Plunkett, M. C. B., Banks, M. W., Falkov, A. F., & Samuels, M. P. (1997). Covert video recordings of life-threatening child abuse: Lessons for child protection. *Pediatrics*, *100*, 735–760.

Stevenson, J. (2003). Relationship between behavior and asthma in children with atopic dermatitis. *Psychosomatic Medicine*, *65*, 971–975.

Stewart, J. L. (2003). Children living with chronic illness: An examination of their stressors, coping responses, and health outcomes. *Annual Review of Nursing Research*, *21*, 203–243.

Stoddard, F. J., Saxe, G., Ronfeldt, H., Drake, J. E., Burns, J., Edgren, C., *et al.* (2006). Acute stress symptoms in young children with burns. *Journal of the American Academy of Child and Adolescent Psychiatry*, *45*, 87–93.

Stoddard, F. J., Sheridan, R. L., Saxe, G. N., King, B. S., King, B. H., Chedekel, D. S., *et al.* (2002). Treatment of pain in acutely burned children. *Journal of Burn Care and Rehabilitation*, *23*, 135–156.

Strother, D. R., Pollack, I. F., Fisher, P. G., Hunter, J. V., Woo, S. Y., Pomeroy, S. L., *et al.* (2002). Tumors of the central nervous system. In P. A. Pizzo, & D. G. Poplack (Eds.), *Principles and practise of pediatric oncology* (pp. 751–824). Philadelphia: Lippincott Williams and Wilkins.

Taylor, D. C. (1986). Hysteria, play-acting and courage. *British Journal of Psychiatry*, *149*, 37–41.

Taylor, D. C., Szatmari, P., Boyle, M., & Offord, D. R. (1996). Somatization and the vocabulary of everyday bodily experiences and health concerns: A community study of adolescents. *Journal of the American Academy of Child and Adolescent Psychiatry*, *35*, 491–499.

Thayer, J. F., & Brosschot, J. F. (2005). Psychosomatics and psychopathology: Looking up and down from the brain. *Psychoneuroendocrinology*, *30*, 1050–1058.

Thompson, N. C., Osorio, I., & Hunter, E. E. (2005). Nonepileptic seizures: Reframing the diagnosis. *Perspectives in Psychiatric Care*, *41*, 71–78.

Thompson, R. J., & Gustafson, K. E. (1996). *Adaptation to chronic childhood illness*. Washington, DC: American Psychological Association.

Todaro, J. F., Femmell, E. B., Sears, S. F., Rodrigue, J. R., & Roche, A. K. (2000). Review: Cognitive and psychological outcomes in pediatric heart transplantation. *Journal of Pediatric Psychology*, *25*, 567–576.

Turner-Cobb, J. M. (2005). Psychological and stress hormone correlates in early life: A key to HPA-axis dysregulation and normalisation. *Stress*, *8*, 47–57.

Tyack, Z. F., & Ziviani, J. (2003). What influences the functional outcome of children at 6 months post burn? *Burns*, *29*, 433–444.

Van-Riper, M. (2003). The sibling experience of living with childhood chronic illness and disability. *Annual Review of Nursing Research*, *21*, 279–302.

Viner, R., Gregorowski, A., Wine, C., Bladen, M., Fisher, D., Miller, M., *et al.* (2004). Outpatient rehabilitative treatment of chronic fatigue syndrome (CFS/ME). *Archives of Disease in Childhood*, *89*, 615–619.

Vitulano, L. A. (2003). Psychosocial issues for children and adolescents with chronic illness: Self-esteem, school functioning and sports participation. *Child and Adolescent Psychiatric Clinics of North America*, *12*, 585–592.

Vivian, E. N. (2006). Type 2 diabetes in children and adolescents: The next epidemic? *Current Medical Research and Opinion*, *22*, 297–306.

Waber, D. P., Carpentieri, S. C., Klar, N., Silverman, L. B., Schwenn, M., Hurwitz, C. A., *et al.* (2000). Cognitive sequelae in children treated for acute lymphoblastic leukaemia with dexamethasone or prednisone. *Journal of Pediatric Hematology and Oncology*, *22*, 206–213.

Wallander, J. L., & Varni, J. W. (1998). Effects of pediatric chronic physical disorders on child and family adjustment. *Journal of Child Psychology and Psychiatry*, *39*, 29–46.

Wamboldt, M. Z., Schmitz, S., & Mrazek, D. (1998). Genetic association between atopy and behavioral symptoms in middle childhood. *Journal of Child Psychology and Psychiatry*, *39*, 1007–1016.

Whiting, P., Bagnall, A. M., Sowden, A. J., Cornell, J. E., Mulrow, C. D., & Ramirez, G. (2001). Interventions for the treatment and management of chronic fatigue syndrome: A systematic review. *Journal of the American Medical Association*, *286*, 1360–1368.

Williams, P. D., Williams, A. R., Graff, J. C., Hanson, S., Stanton, A., Hafeman, C., *et al.* (2003). A community-based intervention for siblings and parents of children with chronic illness or disability: ISEE study. *Journal of Pediatrics*, *143*, 386–393.

Wray, J., & Radley-Smith, R. (2005). Beyond the first year after pediatric heart or heart–lung transplantation: Changes in cognitive function and behaviour. *Pediatric Transplantation*, *9*, 170–177.

Wray, J., & Sensky, T. (2004). Psychological functioning in parents of children undergoing elective cardiac surgery. *Cardiology in the Young*, *14*, 131–139.

Wright, R. J., Cohen, S., Carey, V., Weiss, S. T., & Gold, D. R. (2002). Parental stress as a predictor of wheezing in infancy. A prospective birth-cohort study. *American Journal of Respiratory and Critical Care Medicine*, *165*, 358–365.

Wright, R. J., Cohen, R. T., & Cohen, S. (2005). The impact of stress on the development and expression of atopy. *Current Opinion in Allergy and Clinical Immunology*, *5*, 23–29.

Wright, R. J., Finn, P., Contreras, J. P., Cohen, S., Wright, R. O., Staudenmayer, J., *et al.* (2004). Chronic caregiver stress and IgE expression, allergen-induced proliferation, and cytokine profiles in a birth cohort predisposed to atopy. *Journal of Allergy and Clinical Immunology*, *113*, 1051–1057.

Wysocki, T., Buckloh, L. M., Lochrie, A. S., & Antel, H. (2005). The psychologic context of pediatric diabetes. *Pediatric Clinics of North America*, *52*, 1755–1778.

Young, B., Dixon-Woods, M., Findlay, M., & Heney, D. (2002). Parenting in a crisis: Conceptualising mothers of children with cancer. *Social Science and Medicine*, *55*, 1835–1847.

Young, B., Dixon-Woods, M., Windridge, K. C., & Heney, D. (2003). Managing communication with young people who have a potentially life threatening chronic illness: Qualitative study of patients and parents. *British Medical Journal, Research Edition*, *326*, 305.

58 Psychiatric Aspects of HIV/AIDS

Jennifer F. Havens and Claude Ann Mellins

Because of the steadily increasing rates of HIV infection in women of childbearing age, HIV/AIDS has become a major worldwide threat to the health and psychosocial well-being of children and adolescents, particularly in low-resource countries with limited access to antiretroviral treatment (ART). Even in high-resource countries where the use of ART has dramatically reduced rates of morbidity and mortality, many children and adolescents continue to live either with their own or a parent's HIV illness as a highly stigmatized, chronic or fatal transmittable illness with dramatic implications for their health, mental health and general well-being.

This chapter provides a review of the mental health and neurodevelopmental issues associated with perinatal or maternal HIV infection in children and adolescents. The majority of research on mental health issues has come from the USA and European countries. Until recently, most research on children from low-resource regions such as Africa has focused on the economic, material and health care needs considered most critical to survival (Foster, 2002). Psychosocial factors have been neglected or seen as secondary to other life-threatening issues. However, there is an increasing awareness that ignoring these psychosocial factors may ultimately hinder children's ability to obtain economic, material and basic health care resources and thus, their overall well-being (Foster, 2002).

Epidemiological Overview of the HIV Epidemic as it Affects Children and Adolescents

By the end of 2005, across the world, 40.3 million people were living with HIV/AIDS; 17.5 million were women and 2.3 million were children under the age of 15 years (UNAIDS, 2005a). Despite improved medical treatment options and ongoing prevention efforts, the death rate from AIDS continues to grow and new infections continue to emerge, particularly in women and children in low-resource countries. In 2005, 1.1 million women and 570,000 children died from AIDS (56% of the total deaths from AIDS) and 2.3 million women and 700,000 children under the age of 15 years were newly infected with HIV. In addition to the direct effects of HIV infection, millions of children worldwide are affected by HIV illness in their family members. Recent estimates of HIV-related orphaning in the USA were that 51,473 women have died from AIDS leaving 97,376 children motherless (Lee & Fleming, 2003). By the end of 2004, 15 million children across the globe, most significantly in sub-Saharan Africa, had lost one or both parents to AIDS (UNAIDS, 2005a).

Over 90% of children with HIV/AIDS worldwide acquire the virus through mother–infant (vertical) transmission either during birth or through their mother's breast milk (UNAIDS, 2005b). In high-resource countries such as the USA, widespread HIV counseling and testing, prophylaxis against opportunistic infections and the use of ART, including during pregnancy (Abrams, Weedon, Bertolli *et al.*, 2001) have significantly reduced both the incidence of and mortality associated with HIV/AIDS. Overall, the estimated numbers of deaths among persons with AIDS in the USA decreased by 8% from 2000 through 2004. In the USA, and in other developed countries, perinatal transmission of HIV infection has been substantially reduced by the use of ART by women during pregnancy and birth. For example, in the USA there were 1750 HIV-infected infants born each year during the early to mid-1990s; in 2004, there were just 47 cases (CDC, 2006).

Unfortunately, standard medical treatments utilized in the developed world for the treatment of HIV infection and the prevention of vertical transmission have only recently begun to reach much of the developing world, where the vast majority of new HIV infections occur. In developing countries, economic conditions and health infrastructure inadequacies have limited access to ART, including women's access to ART during pregnancy. This is a particular problem in sub-Saharan Africa, where over 75% of the world's HIV/AIDS cases exist, and HIV rates in pregnant women in antenatal clinics have been estimated to be as high as 40% (UNAIDS, 2005b). In the absence of ART treatment, vertical transmission rates are estimated at 25% (NIAID, 2004).

Whereas pharmacological advances in the treatment of HIV may reduce overall mortality, there is still a risk for poor health and mental health outcomes. Women and children infected and affected by HIV/AIDS in the USA are disproportionately ethnic minorities living in impoverished urban communities (CDC, 2004) who have been found to receive fewer health care services, including treatment with ART, and to have a greater risk of death (CDC, 2004; Cunningham, Hays, Duan

Rutter's Child and Adolescent Psychiatry, 5th edition. Edited by M. Rutter, D. Bishop, D. Pine, S. Scott, J. Stevenson, E. Taylor and A. Thapar. © 2008 Blackwell Publishing, ISBN: 978-1-4051-4549-7.

et al., 2005; Shapiro, Morton, McCaffrey *et al.*, 1999). Furthermore, although heterosexual contact is now the primary risk factor for HIV infection in women with AIDS in the USA (43%), 37% of women acquire AIDS through intravenous drug use (IDU; CDC, 2004). In the USA, 51% of children under 13 years with AIDS were born to women whose risk factor for HIV infection was IDU by themselves or their partner (CDC, 2004). As mortality decreases in HIV-infected adults, many continue or reinitiate substance use (Rotheram-Borus, Lee, Leonard *et al.*, 2003) and thus their children are not only coping with parental HIV, but also the detrimental effects of parental substance abuse (see chapter 36).

In low-resource areas, such as sub-Saharan Africa, the huge numbers of children infected and affected by HIV/AIDS represent a major threat to the stability of the region. South Africa, which has one of the highest rates of HIV-infection in the world (UNAIDS, 2005a), also has one of the highest poverty rates; 60% of its children live in extreme poverty (Giese & Hussey, 2002). Many Black children in South African cities live in informal settlements, exposed to violence, environmental degradation, racism and poor school districts; many also grow up in single-parent homes (Barbarin, Richter, & deWet, 2001; Richter, 2003), and as a consequence of poverty are subject to material scarcity and disruptions in caregiving (Werner & Smith, 2001; Williamson, 2006).

Because of the marked discrepancies in access to health care, the medical trajectories of the HIV/AIDS epidemics now differ significantly between the developed and the developing world. However, there remain striking commonalities in the psychosocial vulnerabilities of HIV-infected women and children across the globe, with poverty, minority status, family reconfiguration and exposure to violence and substance abuse complicating children's and families' adjustment to HIV/AIDS-related illness.

Perinatal HIV Infection in Children and Adolescents

Medical Treatment Issues

Prior to the advent of ART, the rate of disease progression among children with HIV varied considerably, but was typically more rapid in children than in adults, regardless of the mode of infection (Abrams & Kuhn, 2003). In the first decade of the HIV epidemic, perinatally HIV-infected children had a considerably shortened life expectancy. In 1995 in the USA, 75–90% of infected children were expected to have symptoms by 1 year of age; 25–30% would have clinical AIDS. Two relatively distinct courses were described: a rapidly progressive course occurring in 20% of children and a more common, slowly progressive course. The death rate was greatest during the first year of life (more than 15%) but slowed after 2 years, with many children remaining stable throughout their first 10 years of life (Abrams & Kuhn, 2003).

In the USA, the introduction of protease inhibitors in 1996, and the development of combination ART regimens with superior efficacy in viral suppression, provided substantial clinical benefits to HIV-infected children (Kline, 2005). These advances in ART led to substantial improvements in neurodevelopment, growth and immunological and virological status. Combination therapy is now recommended for all infants, children and adolescents who are being treated with antiretroviral agents (HIV/ATIS, 1999). By 1999, the median lifespan for perinatally HIV-infected children in the USA was 8.6–13 years (American Academy of Pediatrics, 1999). By 2005, 46% of pediatric HIV/AIDS cases in New York City, one of the epicenters of the US epidemic, were 13–19 years of age and 9% were 20 years and older (NYCDOH, 2005). Thus, in high-resource countries such as the USA in which new cases of pediatric HIV are increasingly rare, pediatric HIV infection is evolving into an adolescent disease.

In spite of enormous successes in decreasing morbidity and mortality in the USA, ART is not uniformly beneficial. Recent US studies indicate that standard combination ART regimens are effective in only 50% of children, most likely because of multidrug resistance associated with prior exposure to less than optimal HIV treatment, and poor adherence (Yogev, 2005). However, recent advances in new ART treatments have the potential to ameliorate the effects of drug resistance. Unfortunately, the toxicity of long-term ART use resulting in significant side effects (e.g., insulin resistance, cardiomyopathy, lipodystrophy) may still influence adherence. It is possible that in low-resource countries, where children and adolescents have had limited exposure to prior HIV treatments associated with drug resistance, recent trends in increasing availability of superior ART regimens (Domek, 2006) have the potential to improve outcomes significantly for children.

Neurodevelopmental Sequelae of HIV Infection

From the beginning of the epidemic, there have been consistent findings of significant neurological, developmental, cognitive and language deficits in HIV-infected children (Belman, Muenz, Marcus *et al.*, 1996; Brouwers, Belman, & Epstein, 1991; Coplan, Contello, Cunningham *et al.*, 1998; Drotar, Olness, Wiznitzer *et al.*, 1999; Epstein, Sharer, & Goudsmit, 1988; Mellins, Levenson, Zawadzki, Kairam, & Weston, 1994). In general, the severity of neurological and neuropsychological compromise increases with the severity of HIV-related illness; specifically higher viral loads and the most severe non-neurological health-related symptoms (Jeremy, Kim, Nozyce *et al.*, 2005; Pulsifer & Aylward, 2000).

HIV-Associated Encephalopathy

Prior to the advent of ART, two relatively distinct neurodevelopmental patterns were described in largely untreated HIV-infected infants and children: progressive encephalopathy and static encephalopathy (Brouwers, Belman, & Epstein, 1991; Epstein, Sharer, & Goudsmit, 1988). Static encephalopathy, characterized by non-progressive deficits in cognitive, motor and/or language function, is not considered to be directly attributable to HIV and is most likely associated with non-HIV risk factors such as prenatal drug exposure, prematurity, low birth weight and genetic risk factors (Epstein, Sharer, & Goudsmit, 1988; Mellins, Levenson, Zawadzki *et al.*, 1994). Progressive encephalopathy, corresponding with the AIDS dementia complex in adults, is characterized by the loss of developmental mile-stones in young children, declining IQ scores and increasing difficulties with language, attention, concentration and memory in older children. Encephalopathic children also manifest apathy, decreased social behavior and symptoms of depression and irritability compared to non-encephalopathic children (Moss, Brouwers, Wolters *et al.*, 1994; Moss, Wolters, Brouwers *et al.*, 1996). This neurodevelopmental pattern is considered to be a direct effect of HIV on the central nervous system (CNS) and has been associated with a poor overall health prognosis. Before the development of ART, HIV-related encephalopathy was a common sequela, reported in 35–50% of children with pediatric AIDS (Cooper, Hanson, Diaz *et al.*, 1998; Lobato, Caldwell, Ng, & Oxtoby, 1995; Rigardetto, Vigliano, Boffi *et al.*, 1999).

ART and Neurodevelopment

Early reports indicated that ART had the potential to ameliorate the development and progression of HIV-related CNS compromise. Zidovudine treatment alone was shown to be associated with improvements in cognitive and neuropsychological functioning (Brady, McGrath, Brouwers *et al.*, 1996; Brouwers, Moss, Wolters *et al.*, 1990; McKinney, Maha, Connor *et al.*, 1991; Pizzo, Eddy, Fallon *et al.*, 1988). Current treatments, which combine several antiviral agents to achieve near total viral suppression, have the potential to reduce the prevalence and severity of CNS disease in that they prevent HIV progression. Since the advent of ART, the rate of HIV encephalopathy has declined markedly. In a study of neurobehavioral outcomes in 126 children perinatally infected with HIV, the rate of progressive HIV encephalopathy was 1.6% (Chiriboga, Fleishman, Champion, Gaye-Robinson, & Abrams, 2005). Progressive HIV encephalopathy, which historically was considered a poor prognostic sign, was found to respond to ART. Yet, in spite of better prognosis, those children who experienced progressive encephalopathy showed higher rates of residual neurological, cognitive and academic difficulties (Chiriboga, Fleishman, Champion *et al.*, 2005). In a recent study of more subtle neuropsychological outcomes (e.g., vocabulary), treatment with ART, consisting of a protease inhibitor regimen for 48 weeks, did not significantly affect performance, even when the treatment reduced HIV RNA viral load significantly (Jeremy, Kim, Nozyce *et al.*, 2005).

Differential Diagnosis of Neuropsychological Deficits in HIV-Infected Children and Adolescents

More recent studies in the USA have evaluated the neuropsychological functioning of larger samples of older HIV-infected children, most of whom have had some experience with ART (Nozyce, Lee, Wiznia *et al.*, 2006; Smith, Malee, Leighty *et al.*, 2006). These studies generally report cognitive delays and deficits when comparing HIV-infected children to population norms. However, in US studies utilizing appropriate comparison groups (such as perinatally HIV-exposed but uninfected children), investigators have failed to find differences between the HIV-infected and comparison groups (Fishkin, Armstrong, Routh *et al.*, 2000). In a sample of HIV-infected, long-term surviving and ART-naïve Ugandan children, HIV-infected children did not differ significantly in neurological and cognitive assessments when compared with gender-matched HIV-exposed but uninfected and HIV-negative children (Bagenda, Nassali, Kalyesubula *et al.*, 2006). However, when studies consider severity of illness as a variable affecting neuropsychological outcomes, progression to AIDS has been consistently associated with poorer outcomes (Nozyce, Lee, Wiznia *et al.*, 2006; Smith, Malee, Leighty *et al.*, 2006). In conclusion, because of the high-risk backgrounds of HIV-exposed children, both in the USA and internationally, the effects of HIV infection on cognitive functioning, in the absence of disease progression, are often difficult to disentangle from other background characteristics that are also know to affect neuropsychological outcomes.

Emotional and Behavioral Disorder in HIV-Infected Children and Adolescents

Rates of Mental Health Problems and HIV Causality

In general, high rates of emotional and behavioral disorders have been reported in HIV-infected children and adolescents (Havens, Whitaker, Feldman, & Ehrhardt, 1994; Mellins, Brackis-Cott, Abrams, & Dolezal, 2006a; Moss, Bose, Wolters, & Brouwers, 1998; Nozyce, Lee, Wiznia *et al.*, 2006; Papola, Alvarez, & Cohen, 1994), although determining whether HIV infection has a causal effect on children's emotional and behavioral functioning is difficult.

There have been very few studies utilizing appropriate comparison groups and no large-scale epidemiological studies are available. Havens, Whitaker, Feldman *et al.* (1994) found that 21% of a small sample of HIV-infected children met criteria for attention deficit/hyperactivity disorder (ADHD). However, these rates were no different from those in a matched control group of children from similar backgrounds (children living in foster care who had been born to women who had used drugs during pregnancy). Similarly, Mellins, Kang, Leu, Havens, and Chesney (2003) in one of the largest controlled prospective longitudinal studies following perinatally HIV-exposed children (96 HIV-infected children and 211 seroreverters) also found high rates of emotional and behavioral problems, but failed to find an association between either HIV status or prenatal drug exposure and poor emotional and behavioral outcomes. The strongest correlates of increased behavioral symptoms were demographic characteristics (gender, ethnicity, maternal education).

Given the results of the above studies, caution is warranted in attributing HIV causality to the high rates of behavioral problems found in studies that do not include appropriate control groups (Nozyce, Lee, Wiznia *et al.*, 2006) given the association of HIV with other risk factors. Features associated with prenatal drug exposure and parental substance abuse, such as prematurity, low birth weight, exposure to trauma, abuse and neglect, and parental psychopathology may actually be more potent mediators of mental health problems in HIV-infected children than HIV itself (Campbell, 1997; Havens, Whitaker, Feldman *et al.*, 1994; Mellins, Levenson, Zawadzki *et al.*, 1994; Merikangas, Dierker, & Szatmari, 1998; Singer, Farkas, & Kliegman, 1992; Walsh, Macmillan, & Jamieson, 2003; Whitaker, Orzol, & Kahn, 2006; Wilens, Hahesy, Biederman *et al.*, 2005).

Psychotherapeutic Issues in Helping Perinatally Infected Children Cope with HIV

Regardless of causality, HIV-infected children are at risk for neurodevelopmental and mental health problems which need to be considered by mental health providers. These factors tend to differentiate HIV disease from other chronic illness of childhood and adolescence and frequently complicate young people's adjustment to HIV infection.

Communication About Health

HIV disclosure to the perinatally infected child remains one of the most clinically challenging issues for families and providers, in part because of the tremendous stigma that still exists. In general, age and developmental level dictate the child's capacity to understand the meaning of their illness. Across illnesses, preschoolers and young school-age children generally cannot grasp the concept of chronic illness and understand episodes of HIV-related illness as discrete and unconnected events (Bibace & Walsh, 1980; Wiener, Mellins, Marhefka, & Battles, 2007). Because of the stigma and young children's inability to contain information discretely, they are usually not informed about their HIV infection. Most providers agree that as children age, communication about their health problems becomes more important, both to secure their participation in health regimes and to facilitate adjustment to living with HIV. Often older school-age children who are not directly informed of their diagnosis will deduce it from clues in the medical care environment or elsewhere. A lack of open communication in these cases may isolate the child from adult help with issues related to HIV. These issues include coping with secrecy, stigma and potential peer rejection, coping with chronic illness, and anxiety about the future (Wiener, Mellins, Marhefka *et al.*, 2007).

Studies with HIV-infected children indicate that parents or other family caregivers often resist communication with the HIV-positive child about his or her health in an effort to protect the child from emotional distress (Mellins, Brackis-Cott, Dolezal *et al.*, 2002). Other reasons include the adult's fear of experiencing more pain about the child's diagnosis; biological parents' fears about disclosing their own HIV infection through disclosure of the child's infection and parental guilt about having transmitted the virus to the child and their own HIV risk behaviors (e.g., sexual behavior, drug use) and concerns that the child will disclose family secrets about HIV in undesirable ways (Wiener, Mellins, Marhefka *et al.*, 2007).

In 1999, the American Academy of Pediatrics published guidelines stating that all adolescents should know their HIV status and that disclosure should be considered for school-age children (American Academy of Pediatrics, 1999). Clinical reports have indicated positive outcomes associated with disclosure including the promotion of trust, improved adherence to treatment, enhanced access to support, open family communication and better long-term health outcomes (Wiener, Mellins, Marhefka *et al.*, 2007). However, disclosure of HIV to children still remains a difficult and controversial issue for families and providers, and relatively few research studies have been conducted to evaluate the following:

1 Most appropriate timing and determinants of disclosure;
2 Psychosocial effects of HIV disclosure;
3 Impact of disclosure on adherence and sexual behavior; and
4 Most effective strategies for full disclosure.

Lessons learned from pediatric oncology are applied to HIV disclosure, even though the population of children affected by HIV differs dramatically, in terms of socioeconomic and cultural variation, and the incomparable social stigma that surrounds HIV/AIDS. The few studies that have actually been conducted were recently reviewed (Wiener, Mellins, Marhefka *et al.*, 2007) with mixed findings: some showed psychological benefits of disclosure, others risks and still others showed no mental health differences between youth who knew and those who did not know their diagnosis.

Whereas for adults the specific diagnosis of HIV is often a highly charged, overwhelming element in their efforts to communicate to the child about health issues, it is in fact only a single component, which may in part explain differences in study findings. The child may be more concerned about medications, medical appointments and procedures associated with a chronic health condition, or with impingement on functioning. Establishment of effective communication with the child on the broad range of health-related issues is of great importance. What is most critical to remember is that disclosure is a process and that process must reflect a child's developmental understanding of illness and death. It is not a discrete event that can be forgotten once it occurs (Lipson, 1994). Children's needs for information and emotional response to the information change over time, as has been shown in the pediatric oncology literature (Spinetta, 1980).

Adherence to Medical Regimens

HIV-infected children need to adhere to complicated medication regimens, attend numerous medical appointments and undergo frequent diagnostic procedures. Optimism about the success of treatment has been tempered by the significant challenges to maintaining long-term adherence to these multi-drug ART regimens (Chesney, 2003; Mellins, Brackis-Cott, Dolezal, & Abrams, 2004). A number of studies of pediatric adherence to ART indicate that adherence ranges from 57%

to 81% (Mellins, Brackis-Cott, Dolezal *et al.*, 2004), comparable to results from adult HIV studies (Chesney, 2003). Although 80% adherence may be sufficient for some health conditions, it is well below what is necessary for successful HIV treatment. Even brief episodes of missed medication can permanently undermine efforts to suppress HIV RNA viral load (Macilwain, 1997).

In studies of other chronic childhood diseases (e.g., asthma, cancer, diabetes), a combination of child, caregiver and provider psychosocial characteristics has been associated with adherence (see chapters 57 and 70). For HIV-infected children, the possibility of stigma and discrimination may complicate adherence to medications that must be taken throughout the day, often when the child is in school (Armistad, Forehand, Steele, & Kotchick, 1998). Given that HIV-infected children are not always told their diagnosis, they may not cooperate with treatment, particularly given that HIV medications often have unpleasant tastes and significant medical side effects. Variables associated with increased non-adherence include older child age, female gender, worse parent–child communication, worse child and caregiver cognitive or educational function, stressful life events, youth mental health problems, parent–child relationship factors including less supervision and monitoring and less parent–child involvement, caregiver HIV status, and youth engagement in other risk behaviors (e.g., sexual intercourse; Mellins, Brackis-Cott, Dolezal *et al.*, 2004; Mellins, Brackis-Cott, Dolezal *et al.*, 2006b; Williams, Storm, & Montepiedra, 2006).

These data suggest that efforts to improve children's adherence to ART would benefit from behavioral and mental health interventions addressing psychosocial and familial issues, although intervention studies are only now under way. Based on clinical experience, many families will need support administering the complex regimen of medication for the child, and in managing the child's potential opposition to taking medication. Behavioral treatment may be helpful to families (see chapter 62). Finally, caregivers may give children too much responsibility for taking their medications before they are ready to manage the regimens effectively. Working with families to develop realistic expectations of older children's ability to manage their medication independently is important.

Promotion of Optimal Development and Education

The mental health issues for infected children change over the course of the disease. There are an increasing number of HIV-infected children who remain relatively symptom free for long periods of time. They may not know their diagnosis and their lives may be relatively unaffected by illness. However, they may be very stressed by the illness of a parent, substance abuse in the family, disrupted placements and ruptured attachments, or other problems faced by families at highest risk for HIV. Interventions for these problems and attention to promotion of the child's optimal development may be of more relevance in his or her mental health care than a narrow focus on HIV (Rosen, Mellins, Ryan, & Havens, 1997; Ryan, Havens, & Mellins, 1997).

A part of optimal development is the capacity for adequate school functioning. Often, the various systems that should serve the HIV-infected child – the family, child welfare agencies, foster agencies, public school and health care institutions – fail to ensure that the child's education needs are met. HIV-infected children are at high risk for school-related problems given neuropsychological deficits, frequent absence because of health problems and multiple medical appointments. Thus, HIV-infected children require regular psychoeducational evaluations to monitor possible deterioration. Teachers may not know about a child's HIV infection, given rules of confidentiality. They may misinterpret frequent absence and potential lack of motivation as reflecting a lack of interest or commitment to school. HIV-infected children may require special education resources. As their health deteriorates, home-based education may become necessary. It is important to the general well-being of these children that as normal an education experience as possible be maintained.

Issues in Adolescence

In the USA and other countries with widespread access to ART, perinatal HIV infection has become an adolescent epidemic. Adolescence is a developmental stage that poses many challenges for youth without chronic health conditions. Perinatally infected adolescents must confront the social ramifications of having a chronic and stigmatizing disease, including disclosure of illness and ostracism and possible transmission of the virus to others.

Many perinatally infected youth have delays in physical development, including the onset of puberty. These delays, as well as threats to body self-image posed by having a chronic health condition, present another risk factor for poor outcomes, given that adolescence is a time of increasing interest in body image, and several studies link body image with mental health and sexual risk outcomes in both boys and girls (Benjet & Hernandez-Guzman, 2002; Wingood, Diclemente, Harrington, & Davies, 2002).

Because ART did not become routinely available to children in the USA until 1998, many perinatally infected adolescents were exposed to years of less than optimal treatment and thus, active HIV disease (De Martino, Tovo, Balducci *et al.*, 2000; Gortmaker, Hughes, Cervia *et al.*, 2001), which in turn may have led to CNS insult and neurodevelopmental and cognitive deficits. Furthermore, adolescence is a time when certain psychiatric disorders may emerge. One study reported that over 50% of 9- to 16-year-old perinatally infected youth from a New York City medical clinic sample met criteria for a psychiatric disorder (Mellins, Brackis-Cott, Abrams *et al.*, 2006a).

As congenitally infected children move through adolescence and young adulthood and become sexually active, they require significant support in managing the complex issues of integrating healthy sexual development with their HIV infection. Because many of these youth were not expected to live until adolescence, their caregivers and providers have not necessarily engaged them in conversations about sexual health and sexual risk behavior. Open and honest communication around patterns of sexual behavior, disclosure to sexual partners and strategies for the prevention of the spread of HIV are essential. Secondary prevention among HIV-infected youth must be addressed, so that these youth do not re-expose themselves or infect others.

Other notable issues for HIV-infected adolescents include high rates of non-adherence (Mellins, Brackis-Cott, Dolezal *et al.*, 2006b). Non-adherence has not only individual health consequences (e.g., development of drug-resistant strains of HIV; poor immune function), but also public health consequences given the possibility of transmission of drug-resistant strains of the virus to potential partners. Again, this suggests that there is a need for interventions to promote healthy development and reduce risk in this population.

Reliance on parents or other adult family members for health care may lead to regression and difficulty seeing oneself as a young adult. One major goal is to help an effective transition into independent adulthood. Helping youth develop strategies to deal with their illness, the stressful life events that they experience and will encounter in the future, develop a support system, and navigate adolescence are critical tasks for therapeutic interventions.

Unfortunately, to date there have been very few interventions aimed at promoting optimum development and reducing risk behavior in the transition from childhood to adulthood. In one of the few examples, CHAMP+ (McKay, Block, Mellins *et al.*, 2006), multiple family groups are brought together to promote family communication, increase parental supervision and support of children, reduce youth sexual risk behavior and promote adherence and general well-being. It is clear from the experience of the investigators that interventions are needed to help parents and children communicate about adolescent issues, negotiate changing roles and youth autonomy in appropriate ways, and consider reduction of risk behaviors.

Psychopharmacological Management of HIV-Infected Children and Adolescents

Psychopharmacological management of psychiatric disorder, delirium and dementia in HIV-infected children is often a necessary component of adequate treatment. However, it is complicated by drug–drug interactions with ART medications used to treat HIV disease (an issue in all HIV-infected children undergoing such treatment) and potential CNS impairment secondary to HIV infection (a particular issue in those children with advanced HIV disease). Psychotropic medications in pediatric HIV should be initiated at doses lower than standard treatment and titration upward should be slow and carefully monitored.

When evaluating children with behavioral syndromes who are treated with antimicrobial, antifungal and/or antiviral agents, potential neuropsychiatric side effects must be included in the differential diagnosis. When planning pharmacological treatment of HIV-infected children on antiretroviral medication, potential drug interactions must be taken into consideration (Sahai, 1996). Of particular importance in drug interactions is the family of cytochrome P450 isoenzymes, which are responsible for the metabolism of many psychotropic medications and antiretrovirals, especially the protease inhibitors. Other HIV-related medications, including antimicrobial and antifungal medications used in treatment and prophylaxis, also interact with cytochrome P450 isoenzymes. It is important when initiating treatment with psychoactive medications to review the metabolism of the medication(s) with the entire treatment regimen to identify interactions and contraindications. As little is known on treating HIV-infected children with psychotropic medication, treatment should proceed cautiously and with frequent monitoring (Fauci, Bartlett, & Goosby, 1999; Heylen & Miller, 1996a,b; Oleske & Scott, 1999).

In a case series, Havens and McCaskill (1999) described the psychostimulant treatment of 12 HIV-infected children and adolescents, eight with ADHD and four with HIV-related dementia. Two-thirds of the children tolerated psychostimulants with good efficacy as measured by the Efficacy Index of the Clinical Global Impressions. The maintenance dosage of methylphenidate was in the range 0.2–1.2 $mg \cdot kg^{-1}$, and the one child on dextroamphetamine required 0.6 $mg \cdot kg^{-1}$. Four of the 12 children treated (three out of the ADHD sample) experienced adverse side effects precluding their continuation of methylphenidate. While the neuropsychiatric adverse effects argue for caution in the psychostimulant treatment of this population, such treatment should not be withheld when clinically indicated. Two out of the three children who could not tolerate methylphenidate were managed with clonidine.

Therapeutic Support for the Child and Family with End-stage Disease

There has been limited research on this topic in HIV-infected children. However, much of the work conducted on other terminal illnesses such as cancer is most likely applicable (Hurwitz, Duncan, & Wolfe, 2004). With disease progression, children must confront the physical and mental decline associated with AIDS. As they approach late-stage illness, they and their families must confront the terminal nature of the disease. Often, families are overwhelmed at this stage and have difficulty communicating with the child about issues related to prognosis and death. Sensitive mental health intervention by clinicians with an ongoing relationship with the child and their family can provide a place for the child to express the inevitable anxieties and fears about separation from family members and dying, and to help the child, if old enough, to communicate their wishes about medical treatment. Special attention must be paid to issues of pain management at this stage, particularly for young children with limited ability to communicate information to health care providers effectively (Havens, Ryan, & Mellins, 1999).

As children approach the end of life, they may experience confusion and great anxiety. Parents or other caregivers and perhaps even health care providers may find communicating with the child about the approach of death so difficult and overwhelming that they avoid it. Dying children need a venue in which death can be discussed with the opportunity to express their thoughts and fears, and receive reassurance. For many children, separation from family is the most worrisome aspect of death. A therapist may be able to draw on elements in the family's spiritual or religious belief system to sustain hope of continuity of attachment between the deceased and surviving family members (Havens, Ryan, & Mellins, 1999; Ryan, Havens, & Mellins, 1997).

Mental Health Issues in Children Living with Parental HIV Illness

There is a growing US literature suggesting that uninfected children and adolescents of HIV-infected parents show higher rates of depression, anxiety, learning problems, criminal activity, poor school functioning, diminished family and social support, risky sexual behavior and substance use than youth with unaffected parents (Esposito, Musetti, Musetti *et al.*, 1999; Forehand, Jones, Kotchick *et al.*, 2002; Rotheram-Borus, Leonard, Lightfoot *et al.*, 2002; Rotheram-Borus, Lee, Leonard *et al.*, 2003).

The mental health issues associated with HIV illness in families evolve over the dynamic course of HIV illness and vary depending on the stage of their parents' illness (Havens, Mellins, & Pilowski, 1996). The stages begin with diagnosis of HIV infection and include asymptomatic illness, illness progression, late-stage illness, death and reconfiguration of the family with the children in new care arrangements. With the development of effective ART, at least in the developed world, the inevitability of the linear progression through these stages has been reduced.

Children exhibit a variety of responses to parental HIV diagnosis, illness or loss at any stage in this process. These responses may be characterized as one or more of the following:

1 Normative responses requiring supportive counseling and/or increased access to existing social supports;

2 Responses complicated by developmental histories of poor or disrupted attachment and/or trauma (particularly common in children also affected by parental drug addiction), indicating a need for individual or family psychotherapy; and

3 Exacerbations of pre-existing psychiatric disorder or precipitations of new-onset disorder, in which syndrome-specific treatment must be among the interventions (Havens, Ryan, & Mellins, 1999; Ryan, Havens, & Mellins, 1997).

Issues in differential diagnosis within the stage model of HIV illness are reviewed below.

Diagnosis and Disclosure of HIV

Infected parents frequently withhold information about their HIV diagnosis from their children. The majority do not tell children prior to early or even middle adolescence (Lee & Rotheram-Borus, 2002; Mellins, Brackis-Cott, Dolezal *et al.*, 2002). Parents are often concerned about the child's negative emotional response, anger and inability to maintain the secret (Pilowski, Sohler, & Susser, 2000; Vallerand, Hough, Pittiglio, & Marvicsin, 2005). Even in the absence of direct communication, many children and teenagers develop their own suspicions about the parent's health problems from clues such as medications, symptoms or multiple medical appointments. Children experience a great deal of distress suspecting that a parent is struggling with HIV-related illness, yet because they are not "supposed to know" they remain unable to reach out for adult support and reassurance.

Research on disclosure of parental HIV has resulted in mixed findings, with some studies suggesting that children do worse after learning about parental HIV and other studies showing no difference (Mellins, Brackis-Cott, Dolezal, & Meyer-Bahlburg, 2005; Murphy, Marelich, & Hoffman, 2002; Vallerand, Hough, Pittiglio *et al.*, 2005). In part this may be because of variations in the ages of the children, the outcomes being studied, the length of time since disclosure occurred and the availability of support for the child and family. Also, as noted above, disclosure is often misunderstood as a discrete event that can be accomplished as a single communication. It is more appropriately handled as an ongoing process, with new information provided with any change in parental health status.

Parents and other adult caregivers of the HIV-affected child should be counseled about the importance of developmentally appropriate communication about the parent's health. The family's established style of communication about emotionally charged information may not be sufficiently flexible to allow for complete disclosure, but may be able to tolerate communication of part of the truth without specifying the precise diagnosis ("Mommy has an infection in her blood. She's taking medicine to keep her healthy."). Adults should be counseled to provide children with realistic reassurance about the parent's health, and about their own future care and security. HIV-negative children may worry that they themselves are infected because their parent is, and should be assured that they and their siblings are uninfected. In cases where there is uncertainty about a child's serostatus or where additional reassurance is indicated, HIV testing can be very helpful.

Progression of HIV Illness

When parental HIV disease progresses, children are confronted with deterioration in the parent's ability to function as well as separations resulting from hospitalizations. Use of ART means that parental death is no longer inevitable and parents often experience episodes of severe HIV-related illness with subsequent recovery with changes in their medication regimen. The importance of communication with children about parental illness increases as HIV disease progresses. Responding to a parent's physical, cognitive or functional decline without accurate information about illness and prognosis is very difficult for a child. The normal sadness, anger and anxiety experienced by children living with an ill parent can be exacerbated by the need to manage these feeling without support from adults who are unable to allow open communication about their illness.

Given the high-risk backgrounds of many HIV-affected families, children's responses to the parent's illness may also be complicated by underlying psychiatric disorder, developmental difficulties in the child's attachment to the parent, and difficulties in the family environment. When working with families affected by both drug use and HIV, it is important to carefully assess children presenting with symptoms in response to parental illness; the attribution of symptomatology to HIV-related stressors alone is often clinically inappropriate (Havens, Mellins, & Pilowski, 1996).

Permanency Planning

With ongoing progression of HIV disease in the parent, caregivers may require counseling about planning for the placement of children following parental death. Communication about HIV illness and permanency planning tend to be closely intertwined, with difficulties in one area being reflected in the other. Family-based permanency planning that actively involves the children, particularly teenagers, is more likely to have a successful outcome than that which excludes the affected young people. Effective permanency planning can be undermined by active substance abuse and untreated psychiatric disorder in family members, as well as by family dynamics related to substance abuse.

Bereavement and Family Reconfiguration

Loss of a parent can lead to adverse consequences (see chapters 26 and 27). A positive relationship between the parents prior to the death and a strong surviving parent to keep the family intact have been identified as protective against elevated risk of mental health problems (Harris, Brown, & Bifulco, 1986; Kranzler, Shaffer, Wasserman, & Davies, 1990). Among the predictors of complicated bereavement are prior child emotional difficulties, emotional lability and poor impulse control (Kranzler, Shaffer, Wasserman *et al.*, 1990). Many of the factors associated with complicated bereavement in childhood are present in HIV-affected children and adolescents. Furthermore, the effect of parental death in this population is exacerbated by the stigma associated with losing a parent to AIDS, which can lead to secrecy and social isolation, limiting the extent to which children and their families are able to access support (Draimin, Hudis, Segura, & Shire, 1999).

Grieving HIV-affected children and adolescents most commonly move into reconfigured families with extended family members also mourning the loss of the loved one. In countries with well-developed health services, the social and concrete service supports available to the families by virtue of the parent's AIDS diagnosis generally diminish or disappear following the parent's death. Generally, children and adolescents orphaned by AIDS are moving from one situation of poverty to another, with the responsibility for the care of these children falling on financially limited and often overwhelmed extended family members. In those cases where children and adolescents move into non-relative foster care, they must make the difficult adaptation to new family members and often very different family lifestyles.

Education for the grieving child and counseling for his or her adult caregivers are very useful in many families. It is helpful to distinguish the usual course of mourning of adults (a sustained period of dysphoria, followed by a gradual return to normal mood) from that more typical of children, especially pre-adolescents (immediate periods of dysphoria punctuated by apparently normal play or socializing, with periods of grieving throughout the developmental trajectory). When a child's deceased parent has been absent or otherwise deficient in their role with the child, adult caregivers may be puzzled by the child's mourning over the loss: they need an explanation that the loss of inadequate parenting may in fact complicate rather than minimize the child's grieving process.

Issues of Bereavement in Low-Resource Countries

Internationally, one of the most significant effects of the HIV epidemic is the staggering number of children with very few resources who are or will become orphaned because of HIV. Multiple losses, stigma and chronic social vulnerability hinder a therapeutic bereavement process among AIDS orphans. Also, because of high death rates in AIDS-affected African communities, orphans experience multiple losses (Foster, 2002). Studies from African countries have found that compared with non-orphans, AIDS orphans (defined as children who have lost at least one parent to AIDS) had more unmet basic living needs, less access to school and more psychological problems, including negative mood and pessimism (Atwine, Cantor-Grae, & Bajunirwe, 2005; Makame, Ani, & Grantham-McGregor, 2002; Sendengo & Nambi, 1997; UNAIDS, 2004). Given the devastating effects of family and community destruction resulting from years of poverty, racism, family relocation and migration, violence and famine, many African children orphaned by AIDS are at great risk for poor mental health and health outcomes given limited resources, stigma, exploitation by new caregivers and a dearth of appropriate caregivers.

Conclusions

Over 25 years into the HIV epidemic, HIV/AIDS continues to affect millions of children and adolescents worldwide. In the developed world, medical advances in both ART and prevention of vertical transmission have decreased morbidity and mortality in infected children and in their infected family members. In the developing world, the cost of ART and health infrastucture inadequacies have made widespread implementation of treatment advances difficult, leaving millions of children and adolescents without parents and at risk for their own HIV infection and illness. Although clinical trials are underway, there is no currently available vaccine against HIV (D'Souza, Cairnes, & Plaeger, 2000).

Continued targeted prevention efforts and more equitable distribution of health care resources are essential elements in the global fight against HIV/AIDS. In the meantime, effective therapeutic interventions to address the mental health consequences of individual and familial HIV disease have an essential part to play in maximizing the outcome for children and adolescents affected by HIV/AIDS.

References

Abrams, E. J., & Kuhn, L. (2003). Should treatment be started among all HIV-infected children and then stopped? *Lancet*, *362*, 1605–1611.

Abrams, E. J., Weedon, J., Bertolli, J., Bornschlegel, K., Cervia, J., Mendez, H., *et al.*, New York City Pediatric Surveillance of Disease Consortium. Centers for Disease Control and Prevention. (2001). Aging cohort of perinatally human immunodeficiency virus-infected children in New York City. New York City Pediatric Surveillance of Disease Consortium. *Pediatric Infectious Disease Journal*, *20*, 511–517.

American Academy of Pediatrics. (1999). Disclosure of illness status to children and adolescents with HIV infection. *Pediatrics*, *103*, 164–166.

Armistead, L., Forehand, R., Steele, R., & Kotchick, B. (1998). Pediatric AIDS. In T. H. Ollendick, & M. Hersen (Eds.), *Handbook of child psychopathology* (3rd edn., pp. 463–482). New York: Plenum Press.

Atwine, B., Cantor-Grae, E., & Bajunirwe, F. (2005). Psychological distress among AIDS orphans in rural Uganda. *Social Science and Medicine*, *61*, 555–564.

Bagenda, D., Nassali, A., Kalyesubula, I., Sherman, B., Drotar, D., Boivin, M. J., *et al.* (2006). Health, neurologic, and cognitive status of HIV-infected, long-surviving, and antiretroviral-naïve Ugandan children. *Pediatrics*, *117*, 729–740.

Barbarin, O., Richter, L., & deWet, T. (2001). Exposure to violence, coping resources, and psychological adjustment of South African children. *American Journal of Orthopsychiatry*, *71*, 16–25.

Belman, A. L., Muenz, L. R., Marcus, J. C., Goedert, J. J., Landesman, S., Rubenstein, A., *et al.* (1996). Neurologic status of human immunodeficiency virus 1-infected infants and their controls: A prospective study from birth to 2 years. *Pediatrics*, *98*, 1109–1118.

Benjet, C., & Hernandez-Guzman, L. (2002). A short-term longitudinal study of pubertal change, gender, and psychological well-being of Mexican early adolescents. *Journal of Youth and Adolescence*, *31*, 429–442.

Bibace, R., & Walsh, M. E. (1980). Development of children's concepts of illness. *Pediatrics*, *66*, 912–917.

Brady, M. T., McGrath, N., Brouwers, P., Gelber, R., Fowler, M. G., Yogev, R., *et al.* (1996). Randomized study of the tolerance and efficacy of high- versus low-dose zidovudine in human immunodeficiency virus-infected children with mild to moderate symptoms (AIDS Clinical Trial Group 128). *Journal of Infectious Disease*, *173*, 1097–1106.

Brouwers, P., Belman, A. L., & Epstein, L. G. (1991). Central nervous system involvement: Manifestations and evaluation. In P. Pizzo, & C. Wilfert (Eds.), *Pediatric AIDS: The challenge of HIV infection in infants, children and adolescents* (pp. 318–335). Baltimore, MD: Williams & Wilkins.

Brouwers, P., Moss, H., Wolters, P., Eddy, J., Balis, F., Poplack, D., *et al.* (1990). Effect of continuous-infusion zidovudine therapy on neuropsychologic functioning in children with symptomatic human immunodeficiency virus infection. *Journal of Pediatrics*, *117*, 980–985.

Campbell, T. (1997). A review of the psychological effects of vertically acquired HIV infection in infants and children. *British Journal of Health Psychology*, *2*, 1–13.

Centers for Disease Control and Prevention (CDC). (2004). *HIV/AIDS Surveillance Report: HIV Infection and AIDS in the United States*. Accessed from http://www.cdc.gov/hiv/topics/surveillance/resources/reports/2004report/pdf/2004SurveillanceReport.pdf May 31, 2006.

Centers for Disease Control and Prevention (CDC). (2006). CDC HIV/AIDS Fact Sheet. *Mother-to-child (perinatal) HIV transmission and prevention*. Centers for Disease Control and Prevention.

Chesney, M. (2003). Adherence to HAART regimens. *AIDS Patient Care and STDs*, *17*, 169–177.

Chiriboga, C. A., Fleishman, S., Champion, S., Gaye-Robinson, L., & Abrams, E. J. (2005). Incidence and prevalence of HIV encephalopathy in children with HIV infection receiving highly active antiretroviral therapy (HAART). *Journal of Pediatrics*, *146*, 402–407.

Cooper, E. R., Hanson, C., Diaz, C., Mendez H., Abboud, R., Nugent, R., *et al.* (1998). Encephalopathy and progression of human immunodeficiency virus disease in a cohort of children with perinatally acquired human immunodeficiency virus infection. *Journal of Pediatrics*, *132*, 808–812.

Coplan, J., Contello, K. A., Cunningham, C. K., Weiner, L. B., Dye, T. D., Roberge, L., *et al.* (1998). Early language development in children exposed to or infected with human immunodeficiency virus. *Pediatrics*, *102*, e8.

Cunningham, W., Hays, R., Duan, N., Andersen, R., Nakazono, T., Bozzett, S. A., *et al.* (2005). The effect of socioeconomic status on the survival of people receiving care for HIV infection in the United States. *Journal of Health Care for the Poor and Underserved*, *16*, 655–676.

De Martino, M., Tovo, P. A., Balducci, M., Galli, L., Gabiano, C., Rezza, G., *et al.* (2000). Reduction in mortality with availability of antiretroviral therapy for children with perinatal HIV-1 infection. *Journal of the American Medical Association*, *284*, 190–197.

Domek, G. (2006). Social consequences of antiretroviral therapy: Preparing for the unexpected futures of HIV-positive children. *Lancet*, *367*, 1367–1369.

Draimin, B. H., Hudis, J., Segura, A., & Shire, A. (1999). A troubled present, an uncertain future: Well adolescents in families with AIDS. In S. Taylor-Brown & A. Garcia (Eds.), *HIV affected and vulnerable youth* (pp. 37–50). New York: Haworth Press.

Drotar, D., Olness, K., Wiznitzer, M., Schatschneider, C., Marum, L., Guay, L., *et al.* (1999). Neurodevelopmental outcomes of Ugandan infants with HIV infection: An application of growth curve analysis. *Health Psychology*, *18*, 114–121.

D'Souza, M. P., Cairnes, J. S., & Plaeger, S. F. (2000). Current evidence and future directions for targeting HIV entry: Therapeutic and prophylactic strategies. *Journal of the American Medical Association*, *284*, 215–222.

Epstein, L. G., Sharer, L. R., & Goudsmit, J. (1988). Neurological and neuropathological features of human immunodeficiency virus infection in children. *Annals of Neurology*, *23*, S19–S23.

Esposito, S., Musetti, L., Musetti, M. C., Tornaghi, R., Corbella, S., Massirone, E., *et al.* (1999). Behavioral and psychological disorders in uninfected children 6 to 11 years born to human immunodeficiency virus-seropositive mothers. *Journal of Developmental and Behavioral Pediatrics*, *20*, 411–417.

Fauci, A. D., Bartlett, J. G., Goosby, E. P., *et al.* (1999). Guidelines for the use of antiretroviral agents in HIV-infected adults and adolescents. *Panel of clinical practices for treatment of HIV infection: The living document*. Accessed May 5, 1999 from www.hivatis.org/trtgdlns.html.

Fishkin P. E., Armstrong D., Routh D. K., Harris L., Thompson W., Miloslavich K., *et al.* (2000). Brief report: Relationship between HIV infection and WPPSI-R performance in preschool-age children. *Journal of Pediatric Psychology*, *25*, 347–351.

Forehand, R., Jones, D. J., Kotchick, B. A., Armistead, L., Morse, E., Morse, P. S., *et al.* (2002). Noninfected children of HIV-infected mothers: A 4-year longitudinal study of child psychosocial adjustment and parenting. *Behavior Therapy*, *33*, 579–600.

Foster, G. (2002). Beyond education and food: Psychosocial well-being of orphans in Africa. *Acta Paediatrica*, *91*, 502–504.

Giese, H., & Hussey, G. (2002). *Rapid appraisal of primary level health care services for HIV-positive children at public sector clinics in South Africa*. Cape Town: University of Cape Town, Child Health United Children's Institute.

Gortmaker, S. L., Hughes, M., Cervia, J., Brady, M., Johnson, G. M., Seage, G. R., *et al.* (2001). Effect of combination therapy including protease inhibitors on mortality among children and adolescents infected with HIV. *New England Journal of Medicine*, *345*, 1522–1528.

Harris, T., Brown, G. W., & Bifulco, A. (1986). Loss of parents in childhood and adult psychiatric disorder: The role of lack of adequate parental care. *Psychological Medicine*, *16*, 641–659.

Havens, J. F., & McCaskill, E. O. (1999). Psychostimulants in HIV-infected children and adolescents: A case series. In L. L. Greenhill, & B. B. Osman (Eds.), *Ritalin theory and practice* (2nd edn., pp. 165–173). Larchmont, NY: Mary Ann Liebert.

Havens, J., Mellins, C. A., & Pilowski, D. (1996). Mental health issues in HIV-affected women and children. *International Review of Psychiatry*, *8*, 217–225.

Havens, J., Ryan, S., & Mellins, C. A. (1999). Child psychiatry: Areas of special interest/psychiatric sequelae of HIV and AIDS. In H. Kaplan, & B. Saddock (Eds.), *Comprehensive textbook of psychiatry* (7th edn., pp. 2897–2902). Philadelphia, PA: Lipincott Williams & Wilkins.

Havens, J., Whitaker, A., Feldman, J., & Ehrhardt, A. (1994). Psychiatric morbidity in school-age children with congenital HIV-infection: A pilot study. *Journal of Developmental and Behavioral Pediatrics*, *15*, S18–S25.

Heylen, R., & Miller, R. (1996). Adverse effects and drug interactions of medications commonly used in the treatment of adult HIV positive patients. *Genitourinary Medicine*, *72*, 237–246.

Heylen, R., & Miller, R. (1997). Adverse effects and drug interactions of medications commonly used in the treatment of adult HIV positive patients. Part 2. *Genitourinary Medicine*, *73*, 6–11.

HIV/AIDS Treatment Information Services (HIVATIS). (1999). Accessed from http://hivatis.org May 31, 2006.

Hurwitz, C. A., Duncan, J., & Wolfe, J. (2004). Caring for the child with cancer at the close of life: "There are people who make it, and I'm hoping I'm one of them." *Journal of the American Medical Association*, *292*, 2141–2149.

Jeremy, R. J., Kim, S., Nozyce, M., Nachman, S., McIntosh, K., Pelton, S. I., *et al.* (2005). Neuropsychological functioning and viral load in stable antiretroviral therapy-experienced HIV-infected children. *Pediatrics*, *115*, 380–387.

Kline, M. W. (2005). Pediatric and adult HIV/AIDS treatment: still worlds apart. *Research Initiative, Treatment Action: Rita*, *11*, 22–23.

Kranzler, E. M., Shaffer, D., Wasserman, G., & Davies, M. (1990). Early childhood bereavement. *Journal of the American Academy of Child and Adolescent Psychiatry*, *29*, 513–520.

Lee, L., & Fleming, P. (2003). Estimated number of children left motherless by AIDS in the United States, 1978–1998. *Journal of AIDS*, *24*, 231–236.

Lee, M. B., & Rotheram-Borus, M. J. (2002). Parents' disclosure of HIV to their children. *AIDS*, *16*, 2201–2207.

Lipson, M. (1994). Disclosure of diagnosis to children with human immunodeficiency virus or acquired immunodeficiency syndrome. *Journal of Developmental and Behavioral Pediatrics*, *15*, S61–65.

Lobato, M. N., Caldwell, M. B., Ng, P., & Oxtoby, M. J. (1995). Encephalopathy in children with perinatally acquired human immunodeficiency virus infection. Pediatric Spectrum of Disease Clinical Consortium. *Journal of Pediatrics*, *126*, 710–715.

Macilwain, C. (1997). Better adherence vital in AIDS therapies. *Nature*, *390*, 326.

Makame, V., Ani, C., & Grantham-McGregor, S. (2002). Psychological well-being of orphans in Dar El Salaam, Tanzania. *Acta Paediatrica*, *91*, 459–465.

McKay, M., Block, M., Mellins, C., Traube, D., Brackis-Cott, E., Minott, D., *et al.* (2006). Adapting a family-based HIV prevention program for HIV-infected preadolescents and their families: Youth, families and health care providers coming together to address complex needs. In M. McKay, & R. L. Paikoff (Eds.), *Community collaborative partnerships*. Foundation for HIV Prevention Research Efforts.

McKinney, R. E., Maha, M. A., Connor, E. M., Feinberg, J., Scott, G. B., Wulfsohn, M., *et al.* (1991). A multicenter trial of oral zidovudine in children with advanced human immunodeficiency virus disease. The Protocol 043 Study Group. *New England Journal of Medicine*, *324*, 1018–1025.

Mellins, C., Brackis-Cott, E., Dolezal, C., Abrams, E., Wiznia, A., Bamji, M., *et al.* (2006b). Predictors of non-adherence in perinatally HIV-infected youths. NIMH/IAPAC International Conference on HIV Treatment and Adherence. Jersey City, NJ. Accessed from http://www.iapac.org/home.asp?pid=7639. May 21, 2006.

Mellins, C. A., Brackis-Cott, E., Abrams, E. J., & Dolezal, C. (2006a). Rates of psychiatric disorder in perinatally HIV-infected youth. *Pediatric Infectious Disease Journal*, *25*, 432–437.

Mellins C. A., Brackis-Cott, E., Dolezal, C., & Abrams, E. J. (2004). Adherence to antiretroviral treatment in HIV-infected children: The critical role of psychosocial factors. *Pediatric Infectious Disease Journal*, *23*, 1035–1041.

Mellins, C. A., Brackis-Cott, E., Dolezal, C., & Meyer-Bahlburg, H. F. L. (2005). Behavioral risk in early adolescents with HIV+ mothers. *Journal of Adolescent Health*, *36*, 342–351.

Mellins, C. A., Brackis-Cott, E., Dolezal, C., Richards, A., Nicholas, A., & Abrams, E. (2002). Patterns of HIV status disclosure to perinatally infected HIV-positive children and subsequent mental health outcomes. *Clinical Child Psychology and Psychiatry*, *7*, 101–114.

Mellins, C. A., Kang, E., Leu, C., Havens, J. F., & Chesney, M. A. (2003). Longitudinal study of mental health and psychosocial predictors of medical treatment adherence in mothers living with HIV disease. *AIDS Patient Care and STDs*, *17*, 407–416.

Mellins, C. A., Levenson, R. L., Zawadzki, R., Kairam, R., & Weston, M. (1994). Effects of pediatric HIV infection and prenatal drug exposure on mental and psychomotor development. *Journal of Pediatric Psychology*, *19*, 617–628.

Moss, H. A., Bose, S., Wolters, P., & Brouwers, P. (1998). A preliminary study of factors associated with psychological adjustment and disease course in school-age children infected with human immunodeficiency virus. *Journal of Developmental and Behavioral Pediatrics*, *19*, 18–25.

Moss, H. A., Brouwers, P., Wolters, P. L., Wiener, L., Hersh, S., & Pizzo, P. A. (1994). The development of a Q-sort behavioral rating procedure for pediatric HIV patients. *Journal of Pediatric Psychology*, *19*, 27–46.

Moss, H. A., Wolters, P. L., Brouwers, P., Hendricks, M. L., & Pizzo, P. A. (1996). Impairment of expressive behavior in pediatric HIV-infected patients with evidence of CNS disease. *Journal of Pediatric Psychology*, *21*, 379–400.

Murphy, D. A., Marelich, W. D., & Hoffman, D. (2002). A longitudinal study of the impact on young children of maternal HIV serostatus disclosure. *Clinical Child Psychology and Psychiatry*, *7*, 55–70.

National Institute of Allergy and Infectious Disease (NIAID). (2004). NIAID Fact Sheet: HIV Infection in Infants and Children. Accessed July 2004 from http://www.niaid.nih.gov/factsheets/hivchildren.htm.

New York City Department of Health (NYCDOH). (2005). *Pediatric and Adolescent HIV/AIDS Surveillance Update* (p. 5). Semi-annual Report, December, 2005.

Nozyce, M. L., Lee, S. S., Wiznia, A., Nachman, S., Mofenson, L. M., Smith, M. E., *et al.* (2006). A behavioral and cognitive profile of clinically stable HIV-infected children. *Pediatrics*, *117*, 763–770.

Oleske, J., Scott, G. B., *et al.* (1999). 1999 Guidelines for the use of antiretroviral agents in pediatric HIV infection. Working group on antiretroviral therapy and medical management of HIV-infected children. *The Living Document*. Accessed April 15, 1999 from www.hivatis.org/trtgdlns.html.

Papola, P., Alvarez, M., & Cohen, H. J. (1994). Developmental and service needs of school-age children with human immunodeficiency virus infection: A descriptive study. *Pediatrics*, *94*, 914–918.

Pilowski, D. J., Sohler, N., & Susser, E. (2000). Reasons given for disclosure of maternal HIV status to children. *Journal of Urban Health: Bulletin of the New York Academy of Medicine*, *77*, 723–734.

Pizzo, P., Eddy, J., Fallon, J., Balis, F., Murphy, R., Moss, H., *et al.* (1988). Effect of continuous intravenous infusion of zidovudine (AZT) in children with symptomatic HIV infection. *New England Journal of Medicine*, *319*, 889–896.

Pulsifer, M. B., & Aylward, E. H. (2000). Human immunodeficiency virus. In K. O. Yeates., M. D. Ris, & H. G. Taylor (Eds.), *Pediatric neuropsychology: Research, theory, and practice* (pp. 381–402). New York: Guilford Press.

Richter, L. M. (2003). Poverty, underdevelopment and infant mental health. *Journal of Pediatrics and Child Health*, *39*, 243–248.

Rigardetto, R., Vigliano, P., Boffi, P., Marotta, C., Raino, E., Arfelli, P., *et al.* (1999). Evolution of HIV-1 encephalopathy in children. *Panminerva Medica*, *41*, 221–226.

Rosen, L., Mellins, C., Ryan, S., & Havens, J. (1997). Family therapy with HIV/AIDS affected family. In L. Wicks (Ed.), *Psychotherapy and AIDS*. Washington, DC: Taylor & Francis (pp. 115–141).

Rotheram-Borus, M. J., Lee, M., Leonard, N., Lin, Y. Y., Franzke, L., Turner, E., *et al.* (2003). Four-year behavioral outcomes of an intervention for parents living with HIV and their adolescent children. *AIDS*, *17*, 1217–1225.

Rotheram-Borus, M., Leonard, N. R., Lightfoot, M., Franzke, L. H., Tottenham, N., & Lee, S. (2002). Picking up the pieces: Caregivers of adolescents bereaved by parental AIDS. *Clinical Child Psychology and Psychiatry*, *7*, 115–124.

Ryan, S., Havens, J., & Mellins, C. (1997). Psychotherapy with HIV-affected adolescents. In L. Wicks (Ed.), *Psychotherapy and AIDS* (pp. 143–164). Washington, DC: Taylor & Francis.

Sahai, J. (1996). Risks and synergies from drug interactions. *AIDS*, *10* (Supplement 1), S21–S25.

Sendengo, J., & Nambi, J. (1997). The psychological effect of orphanhood: A study of orphans in Rakai district. *Health Transition Review*, *7*, 105–124.

Shapiro, M. F., Morton, S. C., McCaffrey, D. F., Senterfitt, J. W., Fleishman, J. A., Perlman, J. F., *et al.* (1999). Variations in the care of HIV-infected adults in the United States: Results from the HIV cost and services utilization study. *Journal of the American Medical Association*, *281*, 2305–2315.

Singer, L., Farkas, K., & Kliegman, R. (1992). Childhood medical and behavioral consequences of maternal cocaine use. *Journal of Pediatric Psychology*, *17*, 389–406.

Smith, R., Malee, K., Leighty, R., Brouwers, P., Mellins, C., Hittelman, J., *et al.* for the Women and Infants Transmission Study Group. (2006). The effect of perinatal HIV infection and associated risk factors on cognitive development in children. *Pediatrics*, *117*, 851–862.

Spinetta, J. J. (1980). Disease-related communication: how to tell. In J. Kellerman (Ed.), *Psychological aspects of childhood cancer* (pp. 257–269). Springfield, IL: Charles C. Thomas.

UNAIDS/UNICEF/USAID. (2004). *Children on the Brink 2004: A Joint Report of New Orphan Estimates and a Framework for Action*. Accessed from UNICEF. http://www.unicef.org/publications/files/cob_layout6-013.pdf October 3, 2006

UNAIDS. (2005a). *AIDS Epidemic Update, December 2005*. World Health Organization, Joint United Nations Programme on HIV/AIDS, UNAIDS. Accesssed from http://www.unaids.org/epi/2005/doc/EPIupdate2005_pdf_en/epi-update2005_en.pdf October 3, 2006

UNAIDS. (2005b). *A call to action: Children, the missing faces of AIDS*. New York: United Nations Children's Fund October 3, 2006.

Vallerand, A. H., Hough, E., Pittiglio, L., & Marvicsin, D. (2005). The process of disclosing HIV serostatus between HIV-positive mothers and their HIV-negative children. *AIDS Patient Care and STDs*, *19*, 100–109.

Walsh, C., Macmillan, H. L., & Jamieson, E. (2003). The relationship between parental substance abuse and child maltreatment: Findings from the Ontario Health Supplement. *Child Abuse and Neglect*, *27*, 1409–1425.

Werner, E. E., Smith, R. S. (2001). *Journeys from Childhood to Midlife: Risk, Resilience and Recovery*. Ithaca, NY: Cornell University Press.

Whitaker, R. C., Orzol, S. M., & Kahn, R. S. (2006). Maternal mental health, substance use and domestic violence in the year after delivery and subsequent behavior problems in children at age 3 years. *Archives of General Psychiatry*, *63*, 551–560.

Wiener, L., Mellins, C. A., Marhefka, S., & Battles, H. B. (2007). Disclosure of an HIV diagnosis to children: History, current research and future directions. *Journal of Developmental and Behavioral Pediatrics*, *28*, 155–166.

Wilens, T. E., Hahesy, A. L., Biederman, J., Bredin, E., Tanguay, S., Kwon, A., *et al.* (2005). Influence of parental SUD and ADHD on ADHD in their offspring: preliminary results from a pilot-controlled family study. *American Journal on Addictions*, *14*, 179–187.

Williams, P. L., Storm, D., Montepiedra, G., *et al.* (2006). *Predictors of adherence to antiretroviral medications in children and adolescents with HIV infection*. International AIDS Conference. Toronto, Canada, August 13–19, 2006.

Williamson, J. (2005). Finding a way forward: reducing the impacts of HIV/AIDS on vulnerable children and families. In G. Foster, C. Levine, & J. Williamson (Eds.), *A generation at risk: the global impact of HIV/AIDS on orphans and vulnerable children*. Cambridge: Cambridge University Press (pp. 254–277).

Wingood, G. M., Diclemente, R. J., Harrington, K., & Davies, S. L. (2002). Body image and African American females' sexual health. *Journal of Women's Health and Gender-Based Medicine*, *11*, 433–439.

Yogev, R. (2005). Balancing the upside and downside of antiretroviral therapy in children. *Journal of the American Medical Association*, *293*, 2272–2274.

59 Mental Health in Children with Specific Sensory Impairments

Helen McConachie and Gwen Carr

Children with impairments of vision or hearing are reported to have higher rates of problems in psychosocial adjustment and of psychiatric disorder than typically developing children. However, potentially the only thing a deaf child cannot do is hear, and a blind child cannot see. In order to understand the sources of children's vulnerability, it is necessary to consider how impairment may link to mental health outcomes. Therefore, this chapter is structured in terms of impairments, functional limitations, mediating variables and outcomes including social participation (WHO, 2004).

Our intention is to provide an overview of the issues that most affect children's development and well-being, based on the research literature, and to offer a source of guidance for professionals on how to interpret the needs and behaviors of children appropriately. However, one of the main challenges lies in evaluating the validity of the picture presented in past literature. Currently, much received wisdom is being challenged. Therefore it is necessary to keep in mind throughout this chapter the question: To what extent have reported problems in psychosocial adjustment arisen from late identification of impairment, lack of appropriate guidance to parents and limitations in education and opportunity for children?

Sensory Impairments

Definitions and Prevalence

Prevalence figures for sensory impairments in childhood depend on the various definitions used. In the developed world, about 10–20 in 10,000 children have a severe visual impairment that has educational implications (Rahi & Dezateux, 1998; Walker, Tobin, & McKennell, 1992). Around one-quarter of these have only light perception or less, and are thus "blind" (profound visual impairment). Around 12 in 10,000 children per year are born with a hearing loss of 40 dB or more, with around half of these having a severe (over 70 dB) or profound loss (over 95 dB), these groupings hereafter referred to as "deaf" (Davis, Wood, Healy, Webb, & Rowe, 1995). In less developed countries, both types of sensory impairment are more common, with a larger range of causes.

Rutter's Child and Adolescent Psychiatry, 5th edition. Edited by M. Rutter, D. Bishop, D. Pine, S. Scott, J. Stevenson, E. Taylor and A. Thapar. © 2008 Blackwell Publishing, ISBN: 978-1-4051-4549-7.

In classifying types and causes of sensory impairment, it is helpful to use the site of origin. Congenital visual disorders are cerebral or peripheral. Much of the developmental research referred to in this chapter concentrates on blind children with simple disorders of the peripheral nervous system (such as anophthalmia, Norrie's disease and Leber's amaurosis); i.e., children likely to have no other impairments (Dale & Sonksen, 2002). Nevertheless, where neuroimaging is available, it is clear that at least half of these children are likely to have brain lesions that may affect broader development in subtle ways (Waugh, Chong, & Sonksen, 1998).

The main types of hearing loss are conductive and sensorineural; the latter has a genetic cause in at least half of cases. In most cases the gene is recessive, and one or both parents of about 10% of deaf children are themselves deaf. The other main causes of sensorineural deafness are maternal rubella, prematurity and infections of the nervous system, all of which are more likely to result in additional impairments (Freeman & Groenveld, 2000). The main cause of conductive deafness is otitis media with effusion (OME), with a prevalence of 12–14% in preschool children (Kvaerner, Nafstad, & Jaakkola, 2000). Conductive hearing loss tends to be mild to moderate, with a median of 25 dB (Klein, 2001).

For some children there are early interventions that aim to ameliorate the nature of the functional impairment. Timing may be critical, as there are sensitive periods for recovery from lack of vision (Lewis & Maurer, 2005), or for deaf children to be able to combine visual and auditory information (Schorr, Fox, van Wassenhove, & Knudsen, 2005) and thus to have more effective speech understanding and language development (Harrison, Gordon, & Mount, 2005). Thus, early cataract surgery coupled with visual training can radically improve a child's potential for functional vision. The introduction of hearing aids and cochlear implants makes an important difference to the sounds a child can hear, although again these must be appropriately supported. A major opportunity for transformation in professional practice has occurred recently with the introduction of the universal Newborn Hearing Screening Programme (NHSP). Infants can now be fitted with hearing aids as early as 2 months after birth, rather than on average at 2.5 years of age (UK data: Davis, Bamford, Wilson *et al.*, 1997). For those deaf infants who do not derive useful benefit from hearing aids, the age at which cochlear implantation is considered is increasingly early. With the introduction of early intervention programs, including very early support for communication development (orally or through sign), the prospects for deaf children are now radically improved (Davis & Hind, 2003; Yoshinaga-Itano, 2003).

The estimate for the prevalence of multisensory impairment in school-age children in developed countries is 1 in 10,000, a large proportion of whom will also have intellectual impairments (Bond, 2000; Nikolopoulos, Lioumi, Stamataki, & O'Donoghue, 2006). Given their heterogeneity, the chapter does not attempt to include children with multisensory impairment, nor those with later-acquired sensory impairments.

Function

Before we consider how impairment in vision or hearing may affect children's development and functional abilities, some limitations of the descriptive and experimental literature must be acknowledged. First, as there are few psychometrically adequate assessment measures developed specifically for children with sensory impairments, some comparisons that suggest poorer levels of ability in children who are blind or deaf may instead reflect inappropriate questions or greater cognitive challenges for the child. Second, the circumstances of the assessment need to be considered, as young children with impairments are disproportionately disadvantaged by being asked to carry out unfamiliar tasks by an unfamiliar person (McConachie, 1995; Pérez-Pereira & Conti-Ramsden, 1999). Furthermore, most studies with deaf children who sign are presented by a hearing examiner accompanied by an interpreter, which is likely to lead to less than optimal presentation and be inhibiting for the child (Austen & Crocker, 2004; Hindley, 1997). The third limitation is the inevitable one of small numbers, given the low prevalence of severe levels of hearing and visual loss and the concentration on children without apparent evidence of additional neurological impairment.

Early Language Development

Deafness is expected to lead to delay in language development. However, considerable evidence suggests that deaf children brought up by fluent signing parents have the potential for early language development that parallels the spoken language development of hearing children (Bonvillian, Richards, & Dooley, 1997). Furthermore, for many children who have an early cochlear implant, there is evidence of speedy learning of first words (Nott, Cowan, Brown, & Wigglesworth, 2003; Spencer, 2004; Tomblin, Barker, Spencer, Zhang, & Gantz, 2005) whatever the cause of deafness (Nikolopoulos, Archbold, & O'Donoghue, 2006). There is continuing debate concerning the best approach to facilitating the early language development of deaf children, and difficulty in drawing conclusions from studies that are usually cross-sectional and underpowered. Nicholas and Geers (2003) conducted one of the better observational studies of parent–child interaction and conclude "There is clearly more than one path to successful language development in severe to profoundly deaf children" (p. 435).

Following the widespread introduction of NHSP, along with early support and intervention, evidence suggests that, on average, language outcomes for children without other impairments are within the low normal range, and correlated with the children's non-verbal cognitive level. Yoshinaga-Itano, Sedey, Coulter, and Mehl (1998) compared 72 deaf and moderately hearing impaired children who had been identified between birth and 6 months, with 78 children identified after the age of 6 months. The early identified children had better receptive and expressive language skills by 36 months of age than later identified children (with a large effect size). As the research has expanded, the results suggest that children (without cognitive impairment) overall have an 80% probability of having language development in the normal range by 5 years (Yoshinaga-Itano, Coulter, & Thomson, 2001). What seems to matter in such studies is age of identification and early intervention, rather than socioeconomic status, the particular method of communication or degree of hearing loss (Moeller, 2000; Yoshinaga-Itano, 2003).

What about fluctuating hearing loss? A detailed prospective study from New Zealand (Chalmers, Stewart, Silva, & Mulvena, 1989) was widely accepted as confirmation of parents' and professionals' concerns about the consequences of chronic fluctuating conductive hearing loss, as it found reduced verbal comprehension and expression scores, and raised levels of behavior problems, in comparison with controls. However, recent systematic review of randomized clinical trials suggests none to very small negative associations of otitis media with children's later speech and language development (Roberts, Rosenfeld, & Zeisel, 2004). Undoubtedly, there are some children with recurrent infections and hearing loss for whom language outcomes are not good, such as children in low-quality daycare (Vernon-Feagans, Hurley, & Yont, 2002) but it seems that socioeconomic indicators are predictive both of language outcome and of duration of middle ear infections (Feldman, Dollaghan, Campbell *et al.*, 2003). Therefore, the evidence suggests that fluctuating levels of hearing loss are not in themselves predictive of poor language and other functions in the longer term.

Recent reviews (Lewis, 2003; Pérez-Pereira & Conti-Ramsden, 1999) concluded that blind children are not delayed in acquiring first words in comparison with sighted children. However, much of the evidence is from case studies (Mulford, 1988) and more representative group studies suggest some delay (McConachie & Moore, 1994). Differences in the content of the early vocabularies of blind and sighted children can be readily understood; for example, blind children's first words include actions and tactile experience (e.g., bath, swing, poo; McConachie & Moore, 1994). Many blind children appear to learn language as "chunks" (Andersen, Dunlea, & Kekelis, 1984), which may lead to better apparent expressive language skills than their assessed level of comprehension in the first 3 years (McConachie, 1990). Although they may take atypical routes in language learning, for blind children "Language seems to have an important compensatory function, allowing the children access to the external world and social information that they could not obtain by other means" (Pérez-Pereira & Conti-Ramsden, 1999, p. 8).

Emotional Development

It is clear that sensory impairment is no barrier to the formation of attachment by infants to their parents. At the time expected in sighted babies, blind babies are likely to smile when they hear their parent's voice (Fraiberg, 1977). Once they start to reach with their hands, they explore faces and discriminate between parent and a stranger. Protest when the parent leaves takes somewhat longer in blind babies than in sighted babies, and this may be related to delay in understanding object permanence, as blind babies cannot keep track of people easily (Tröster & Brambring, 1992).

Despite the primacy of the visual channel in the establishment of attachment (Stern, 1985), there are aspects of deaf babies' experience that might have been expected to affect attachment. Before the introduction of NHSP, most hearing mothers would not have been aware of their infant's hearing problem until later in the first year of life, and so would not have made adjustments in terms of touch, body postures and facial expression during interaction. However, experimental studies using the Strange Situation paradigm (Ainsworth, 1973) have not found a difference in security of attachment (Lederberg & Mobley, 1990).

How do children acquire an understanding of the perceptions of others, a key skill in emotional and social development? For deaf and for blind children, research suggests that this understanding is delayed. However, some evidence is questionable. To assess understanding of false belief in blind children, McAlpine and Moore (1995) used a hamburger box containing a sock, and Minter, Hobson, and Bishop (1998) used a warm teapot filled with sand. As Pérez-Pereira and Conti-Ramsen (2005) pointed out, these materials are inappropriately confusing; children will have been discouraged from touching a teapot (if the family even has one) and the box will not smell of hamburger. When verbal tasks involving false belief are used (Peterson, Peterson, & Webb, 2000), children are able to succeed, even though at a later age than is usual for sighted children. Given blind children's greater cognitive challenge in following key changes in the environment, and their need for conversational language skills in order to understand how events are experienced by others, some delay seems inevitable.

The finding of delay in development of theory of mind in deaf children has been widely replicated (Peterson & Siegal, 2000). Children of parents who are fluent signers, and deaf children with moderate to severe loss who are successfully using spoken language, show less delay (Courtin & Melot, 2005; Jackson, 2001), indicating the importance of early effective communication. One factor that facilitates development of theory of mind is the extent to which mothers include talk about mental states in play with their deaf child (Moeller & Schick, 2006). Theory of mind understanding can be expected by adolescence, as shown by Rhys-Jones and Ellis (2000) in a study of the spontaneous use of mental state expressions in telling stories from pictures. These deaf adolescents also showed no difference from a hearing comparison group on a social judgment test. Nevertheless, subtle differences may persist, such as difficulties in taking account of another person's perspective in negotiations (Terwogt & Rieffe, 2004).

Play

The development of symbolic play skills is closely related to the development of language. Spencer and Meadow-Orleans (1996) have shown appropriate play with toys such as a toolbox, dolls and a tea-set by deaf and hearing children at 18 months of age, although some deaf children with smaller vocabularies were not yet substituting one object for another. For blind children, understanding of objects and development of symbolic play is complicated. In the absence of vision, a doll is an irregularly shaped piece of hard plastic with strange-textured string at one end – not a "baby." Therefore, the repeated report (Tröster & Brambring, 1994) and observation (Hughes, Dote-Kwan, & Dolendo, 1998) that blind children have limitations in symbolic play requires careful unpicking. In some circumstances, such as having a helpful play partner, blind children do play symbolically, as was found for twin girls (one sighted, one blind) studied by Pérez-Pereira and Castro (1992). Lewis, Norgate, Collis, and Reynolds (2000) found no difference between blind and sighted children 2–7 years old on the Test of Pretend Play, except for fewer object substitutions made by the blind children. Other blind children prefer talking play, acting out pretend dialogues between themselves and others (Lewis & Collis, 2005).

Observations of blind children in nurseries suggest that they often play alone or rely on adults (Preisler, 1997; Skellenger, Rosenblum, & Jager, 1997). They have particular difficulty with outdoor play settings, where it is even more difficult to establish where other children are, and the boundaries of the space. McGaha and Farran (2001) found that blind children played more in parallel outdoors, and their initiations to other children in an inclusive preschool were less successful than indoors, in terms of number of conversational turns. Therefore, blind children clearly need skilfully planned support in order to develop successful interactions with other children in group settings at an early age (Webster & Roe, 1998).

For deaf children, successful play with others is dependent on level of communication skills. Observing social play in preschool settings, Lederberg, Ryan, and Robbins (1986) found that deaf children tended to swap play materials with hearing children but were more likely to use a variety of communication functions with other deaf children. The children with better communication skills were able to play successfully in groups, to interact with teachers and to make and receive more communicative initiations. In order to succeed in inclusive settings, deaf children may need to have superior social skills (Marschark, 1993); for example, to overcome hearing children's lack of awareness that they have to attract the deaf child's attention before speaking. Martin and Bat-Chava (2003) have described the parent-reported coping strategies of 35 children aged 5–11 years in inclusive education settings.

The children had either a cochlear implant or hearing aids and mostly used speech in communicating. Encouragingly, about half of the children were described as confident in socializing with hearing children, and only five children were rated as having poor relationships with others (not related to type of aid).

"Autistic Features" in Blind Children

Association between sensory impairment and diagnosis of mental health disorders, including autism, is discussed below (see p. 963). However, it is appropriate to consider at this point "autistic-like features" in the behavior of blind children, such as frequent verbal imitations and formulaic speech, reversed use of personal pronouns, difficulties with symbolic play, and repetitive behaviours such as eye-poking and rocking (Lewis, 2003; Pérez-Pereira & Conti-Ramsden, 2005; Tröster, Brambring, & Beelman, 1991a; Wing & Wing, 1971).

Many of these behaviors have an understandable function. For example, repeated head turning and rocking can give proprioceptive feedback to the blind child. Some behaviors seem to occur more when the child is bored (Tröster, Brambring, & Beelmann, 1991a) and they decrease between the ages of 3 and 6 years (Tröster, Brambring, & Beelman, 1991b). Formulaic speech seems to be useful to blind children, repeating whole phrases in order to explore how they apply, given that they have fewer other cues (Pérez-Pereira & Conti-Ramsden, 2005). Children may use repeated questions to keep in contact with others, and adults themselves use language more repetitively when talking with blind children (Kitzinger, 1984; Pérez-Pereira & Conti-Ramsden, 1999). The reported errors in the use of personal pronouns (Dunlea, 1989) may also arise in part from blind children's tendency to learn language in chunks. Finally, we have already examined the problems in research assumptions about blind children's symbolic play and theory of mind. Therefore, there is a persuasive argument to be made that "autistic-like" features in the early development of blind children without other impairments show no more than a surface similarity to autism.

Ability and Achievement

There is considerable concern that deaf children have poor academic achievements: is this related to ability or to other factors? The longitudinal study of Gregory, Bishop, and Sheldon (1995) found that 46% of young deaf adults had left school with no examination qualifications. Powers (1998) documented that only 18% of deaf children obtained the higher grades in GCSE (UK school leaving exams at 16 years) compared to 45% of hearing children. A good start with communication seems to be key to later achievement (Preisler, 1999). Long-term follow-up of 30 children with cochlear implants suggests a significantly better picture for young people's studying and employment than previously (Beadle, McKinley, Nikolopoulos *et al.*, 2005). The results of recent studies conducted on early identified deaf children using hearing aids and speech would point to the same possible conclusion (Yoshinaga-Itano, 2003) but longitudinal follow-up will give better indications of what deaf children in general can achieve with good educational support, and appropriate access to public examinations.

Standardized assessment of the ability of children with sensory impairments poses many difficulties in administration and interpretation of results. The limitations of assessing deaf children's ability with only one scale of an intelligence test, such as the Wechsler Intelligence Scale for Children (WISC), are considerable given the verbal component required to understand the instructions. Tests developed specifically for deaf children include the Snijders–Oomen Non-verbal Intelligence Scale (SON-R) for ages 2–17 years (Snijders, Tellegen, & Laros, 1989; Tellegen, Winkel, Wijnberg-Williams, & Laros, 1996). The SON-R is not simply a non-verbal test as it includes abstract and concrete reasoning. The Leiter International Performance Scale–Revised (Roid & Miller, 1997) does not have deaf norms, but is presented without language and used frequently in research.

There are few instruments developed specifically to assess ability in blind children, and their norms tend to be older than would be considered valid in the assessment of sighted children. The Reynell–Zinkin Developmental Scales for Young Visually Handicapped Children (Reynell, 1979) cover social adaptation, sensorimotor understanding, exploration of the environment, verbal comprehension, expressive language structure and vocabulary, with norms for blind, severely visually impaired and sighted children aged up to 5 years. For older children, the Intelligence Test for Visually Impaired Children (Dekker, 1993) has four main factors: orientation, reasoning, spatial ability and verbal ability. Otherwise, assessors usually rely on a verbal scale of measures such as the WISC, although this may be of more use in understanding a profile of skills and difficulties rather than deducing absolute levels of ability. Some studies have suggested that blind children may be less good at tasks that involve making comparisons or relating different pieces of information, while having better than expected short-term memory (Lewis, 2003).

Mediating Variables in the Child's Environment

Children's developmental course is affected by their relationships, environment and experiences. In this section, we consider some of the mediating variables that affect outcome, with particular emphasis on parenting. Obviously, children's educational environment, including the quality and frequency of support teaching, is important, but beyond the scope of this chapter.

Early Parenting

How do parents adapt to their child's sensory impairment? Many studies have charted the impact of a child's impairment on parents' emotions and on levels of stress in the family (Jackson & Turnbull, 2004; Singer, 2006; Tröster, 2001), and how parents cope has been shown to be important for child outcomes (Kurtzer-White & Luterman, 2003). Parents of blind children have usually learned of their baby's impairment early, but with the advent of NHSP, concerns have been raised about the impact on parents of being told early that their child is deaf. Evidence so far suggests that, with appropriate intervention, mothers' stress levels on average are low (Pipp-Siegel, Sedey, & Yoshinaga-Itano, 2002; Yoshinaga-Itano, 2001).

Sighted parents are very likely to have no prior knowledge of blindness, and have to become particularly adept at "reading" the cues; the infant becomes still when listening and leans toward an object (rather than reaching). Parents need to adapt their communication habits; for example, giving emotional feedback through vocalizing when smiling, and by mirroring the infant's movements (Fraiberg, 1977; Preisler, 1991). After the first 6 months, interest in objects means that sighted infants spend much less time in face-to-face interaction with their parents. The challenge for parents of blind infants is to judge their child's focus of attention (Fraiberg, 1977; Preisler, 2001). Some research with sighted parents of blind children suggests that they may use language in less than optimal ways, giving children directions, asking what they want (when the children have few words) and labeling rather than talking about objects and experiences (Andersen, Dunlea, & Kekelis, 1993; Moore & McConachie, 1994; Preisler, 1997). A style of commenting on what the child does, involving objects in rhymes and routines, providing descriptions and joining with the emotional content of the child's behavior seems to facilitate development (Dote-Kwan, Hughes & Taylor, 1997; Norgate, Collis, & Lewis, 1998; Pérez-Pereira & Conti-Ramsden, 1999; Preisler, 1997).

Early successful interaction is vital for deaf infants and their parents. When establishing joint attention to an object, deaf parents seem well attuned and tend to wait until the infant has looked at an object of interest, and then to them, before signing its name or a comment about the object. Hearing parents who are learning signing may make more signing attempts than deaf parents do, but either these are not seen by the child or the child's focus of attention may be interrupted by the parent (Lewis, 2003; Spencer, 2000). Luterman, Kurtzer-White, and Seewald (1999) refer to the impact of deafness on these early natural processes of interaction as causing "the system to crash" (p. 107) and cite the child's inability to hear and respond to parents' signals as a demotivating factor. Nevertheless, many hearing parents do adapt sensitively to their child's needs, and this process will be aided by early identification of the infant's impairment. The degree of emotional connectedness of mothers has been shown to be a significant predictor of deaf children's early language gains (Moeller, 2000), even more so than for hearing children (Pressman, Pipp-Siegel, Yoshinaga-Itano, & Deas, 1999). At an early stage in language development, it may be appropriate for parents to be quite controlling in order to encourage communication from their child; but it is then important for parents not to continue with a "teaching" style but instead to have the sensitivity to hang back from asking questions and requesting clarification, so that children can take the initiative in conversation (Lewis, 2003; Luterman, Kurtzer-White, & Seewald, 1999; Power, Wood, Wood & MacDougall, 1990). In a detailed longitudinal study of 22 preschool children with cochlear implants, Preisler, Tvingstedt, and Ahlström (2002) found no clear relationship between their communicative, social and emotional development and cause of deafness, but did show the importance of a child-centered communication style by parents and teachers.

There is considerable emphasis on problematic parenting in the older literature on young deaf children. For example, in an experimental study of problem-solving with 5-year-old children (Jamieson & Pedersen, 1993), it was notable that deaf children of deaf parents (and hearing children of hearing parents) succeeded in doing the puzzle alone after a joint attempt. Hearing parents tended to intervene even when their deaf child was succeeding, and the children requested help more often, as if they had learned to rely on others. Given the challenges to be faced by children with sensory impairments in becoming independent, parents' style in building up their self-reliance is of great importance. Some studies (Gregory, 1976; Lederberg, 1993) have also suggested that parents respond quickly to children's demands for attention because it may be difficult to explain the need to wait; children may then not learn how to take turns in social situations. For similar reasons of difficulties in communication, parents may be more ready to resort to physical punishment (Knutson, Johnson, & Sullivan, 2004; Schlesinger & Meadow, 1972). Thus, hearing parents of deaf children may need wide-ranging support in facilitating their child's early development.

Support and Training for Parents

As soon as hearing loss is identified, parents need information and support to help them make informed choices about communication options, and this requires appropriately skilled and knowledgeable staff within effective early intervention programs. The Nebraska Diagnostic Early Intervention Program and the Colorado Home Intervention Program have had the most extensive evaluations (Moeller, 2000; Yoshinaga-Itano, 2003). Research has shown the importance of family-focused services in harnessing parents' full involvement in early intervention programs, with level of involvement a strong predictor of outcomes for children at age 5 years (Moeller, 2000). Similarly for blind children, early programs help parents to stimulate the child's capacity for vision, as well as to develop a mutually rewarding relationship. There is generally a lack of objective evaluation, although one program (Sonksen & Stiff, 1991) has demonstrated effectiveness through a partially randomized controlled trial (Sonksen, Petrie, & Drew, 1991).

The UK government has published booklets for parents on visual impairment, on deafness and on multisensory impairment (Early Support, 2004). These are accompanied by *Developmental Journals* (2006), which allow parents and professionals to track developmental progress from birth to about 3 years of age, accompanied by Ideas and Activity suggestions, including sections on how to help the child who has "got stuck" in his or her development. There are many other website resources for both parents and professionals containing a wide range of materials (e.g., www.ed.arizona.

edu/dvi; www.tsbvi.edu/bib/early.htm; www.babyhearing.org; www.deafnessatbirth.org.uk).

Socioemotional Interventions for Children

For both blind and deaf children, social interaction in school poses challenges. "Co-operative learning" is one approach to supporting social development that has been evaluated with both groups. Teachers are trained to set up learning activities in such a way that completion is impossible unless everyone participates. Co-operative learning strategies have been shown to promote self-esteem, socialization skills and positive interactions amongst children, including visually impaired 4-year-olds (D'Allura, 2002) and deaf 8-year-olds (Johnson & Johnson, 1986) with their peers.

The PATHS (Promoting Alternative Thinking Strategies) Curriculum for deaf children (Greenberg, 2000; Greenberg & Kusché, 1998) is built on a model of social competence that emphasizes, from a foundation of good communication, the need for skills such as anticipation, reflection and imagination, as well as tolerance for ambiguity and for frustration. Thus, the program teaches children how to develop and maintain self-control, increase awareness of their feelings and ability to communicate about feelings, and improve problem-solving skills. Controlled evaluation of the program as implemented by teachers with 6- to 12-year-olds has indicated significant and sustained improvements in socioemotional adjustment, frustration tolerance and distractibility, with additional improvement in reading comprehension (Greenberg & Kusché, 1998).

For blind children, the literature has a wealth of single case studies and small-scale descriptive interventions, which lack information about generalizability and maintenance of gains, but contain useful clinical suggestions. For example, Jindal-Snape (2005) described a behavioral program designed to improve social interaction of a blind child through self-evaluation of his facial orientation to others, and through feedback by peers. Peavey and Leff (2002) described an evaluation of "friendship groups" in school, designed to increase trust and open communication. Visually impaired students were able to talk about their difficulties and sighted students learned how to include the visually impaired student.

Deaf Culture

Within a predominantly hearing world, deafness is seen most commonly as an impairment or disability; in other words, within a "medical model." A more general "social model" of disability, however, construes disability "as a consequence of society's failure to make proper provisions for disabled people" (Gregory, 2002, p. 2). Members of the deaf community, who use a sign language as their preferred language, regard themselves as a linguistic minority group with a rich worldwide culture (Ladd, 2002), disabled only by a hearing-oriented society. The format "Deaf" rather than "deaf" is used in recognition of this status. Mental health professionals need to be aware of these differing models and sensitive to both the culture and the belief frameworks that exist around them and the issues raised as a consequence. For some young people there is a tension around their identity as Deaf or deaf (Skelton & Valentine, 2003).

Adjustment and Vulnerability

Having considered the effects of impairment of hearing or vision upon children's development, and some mediating factors for development, we turn now to outcomes. For adolescents and young adults with sensory impairments do we expect to see a resolution of the different routes they may have taken through development, or is their healthy progress still at risk?

The striking impression gained from studies of adolescents is of a generally good outcome. The one available population longitudinal study painted a picture of young adults with visual impairment having few friends, with less than half employed (Freeman, Goetz, Richards, & Groenveld, 1991). However, more recent cross-sectional surveys give some indication of how well blind children are able to achieve with early intervention to families, good support in inclusive school settings and legislation to combat disability discrimination. Large-scale surveys in the USA, Finland and the Netherlands have shown no significant differences from controls in self-esteem, locus of control, happiness, physical and psychological symptoms, relationships with parents and siblings, and self-reported empathy for others (Griffin-Shirley & Nes, 2005; Huurre & Aro, 1998; Kef, 2002). Visually impaired adolescents are less likely than controls to describe themselves as having many friends (Huurre & Aro, 1998; RNIB, 2001), but the smaller social networks of visually impaired adolescents seem to provide quality support (Kef, Hox, & Habekothé, 2000; Rosenblum, 2000) and act as a helpful buffer against feeling an outsider in school. Young people who are blind still report problems with access to some leisure activities, independent travel and attitudes of others (RNIB, 2001).

For deaf adolescents, the issue of school placement may have more of a role in their social experience, maturity and self-esteem. For deaf students who sign and are at a specialist college, self-esteem is generally high (Crowe, 2003) and even higher for those who have at least one deaf parent who acts as a role model (Woolfe & Smith, 2001). However, the picture from older studies and those with mixed samples of children attending a variety of schools is more complex. Kluwin, Stinson, and Colarossi (2002) reviewed 33 studies published since 1980 and concluded that deaf students were generally less socially mature than hearing students, interacted with other deaf classmates more than with hearing ones and were only somewhat accepted by their hearing classmates. The effect of mainstream educational placement depended on the characteristics of the individual and on the support offered (Van Gurp, 2001). If children do not have adequate support to participate in the classroom then both academic achievement and social integration will suffer (Stinson & Antia, 1999). Several studies suggest that adolescents in mainstream settings have problems with loneliness, rejection and social isolation (Nunes, Pretzlik, & Olsson, 2001; Obrzut, Maddock, & Lee, 1999).

However, a recent Australian study of adolescents educated in fully inclusive settings found no difference between hearing and hearing-impaired students in self-reported loneliness and social participation (Punch & Hyde, 2005). Qualitative analysis revealed some difficulties such as self-consciousness and feelings of awkwardness, not related to level of impairment. New technology such as text-messaging has been shown to have benefits in terms of supporting social independence of deaf adolescents (Akamatsu, Mayer, & Farrelly, 2006).

There are accumulating indications that very early intervention may have positive effects in terms of deaf children's social outcomes. Five-year-olds identified by newborn screening have significantly higher levels of personal social skill development than later-identified children (Yoshinaga-Itano, 2003). Furthermore, children (mean age 10) using hearing aids or cochlear implants for several years have been found to have, on average, age-appropriate levels of communication and socialization skills on the Vineland Adaptive Behavior Scales (Bat-Chava, Martin & Kosciw, 2005). Such findings underline the importance of communication competence for positive adaptation.

There are perhaps unexpected findings in relation to the severity of impairment. It has long been suggested, counter-intuitively, that moderate hearing impairment is more problematic than deafness for psychosocial functioning (Myklebust, 1960). Recently, it has been shown that late identification has greater adverse implications for the personal social skills of children with mild hearing loss than for those with moderate to profound loss (Yoshinaga-Itano, 2003) and this may relate to the greater degrees of stress brought about by parent–child dysfunctional interactions found for parents of children with less severe degrees of loss (Pipp-Siegel, Sedey, & Yoshinaga-Itano, 2002). Kurtzer-White and Luterman (2003) suggested one reason is that children with less severe loss respond inconsistently to sound, and have an ambiguous prognosis, thus increasing parents' stress. A similar discussion can be found in literature on blind children. There is some evidence that for mothers of young children with severe visual impairment (i.e., with some form perception) stress is greater (Tröster, 2001), perhaps because they underestimate their children's specific problems. Kef (2002) noted that adolescents with severe visual impairment had less positive adjustment than those who were blind. One specific educational issue was not being able to read print, yet not using Braille. Thus, problems may be greater for those who have more expectations put upon them to "fit in" or who try to "pass" as non-disabled (Freeman, Goetz, Richards *et al.*, 1991).

Mental Health Disorders

For some children with sensory impairments, behavioral and emotional problems go beyond loneliness and frustration. However, a major difficulty in understanding the nature, degree and prevalence of mental health disorders is to disentangle what may arise from associated neurological damage rather than be attributable to sensory impairment (Carvill, 2001). Furthermore, there is evidence that young people with sensory impairments are at risk of emotional, physical and sexual abuse (Freeman, Goetz, Richards *et al.*, 1991; Kvam, 2004; Sullivan, Brookhouser, & Scanlan, 2000). However, as the evidence largely comes from adults looking back, and special educational settings were noted to increase risk, protection may now be much greater.

Prevalence of Emotional and Behavioral Problems

Since 1994, there have been five studies giving estimates of the rate of mental health problems in deaf children (Hindley, Hill, McGuigan, & Kitson, 1994; Sinkkonen, 1994, cited in Hindley, 1997; Van Eldik, Treffers, Veerman, & Verhulst, 2004; Van Gent, 2003; Vostanis, Hayes, Du Feu, & Warren, 1997). Two included interviews with young people themselves, and elicited information about emotional disorders that had hitherto been underestimated. Hindley, Hill, McGuigan *et al.* (1994) used scales developed specifically for screening mental health problems in deaf children, the Parents' Checklist (PCL) and Teachers' Checklist, followed by interviews with a proportion of parents and children aged 11–16 years. The reported estimated prevalence of disorder was 43%. However, the study was not population-based, and Vostanis, Hayes, Du Feu *et al.* (1997) found that the PCL overestimated problems.

Studies using the Achenbach Child Behaviour Checklist (CBCL) have suggested that 27–41% of deaf children have problems in the borderline or clinical range. The highest estimate was by Van Eldik, Treffers, Veerman *et al.* (2004), who compared the rates of total problems in children aged 4–18 years with Dutch CBCL norms (17%); however, as three-quarters of the children attended one regional educational institute, and total problems were related to parents' report of poor communication with the family, the results may be subject to some confounding. Only one questionnaire study had a contemporary control (Sinkkonen, 1994); in contrast to the findings of the other four studies, teacher report of behavior problems showed no significant difference between deaf children and young people aged 6–21 years (19%) and controls (16%), although low communication ability was associated with raised scores on hyperactivity. The pattern of problems in deaf children that might present to a mental health service is similar to that in hearing children (Hindley, 2000), but some of the medical causes associated with deafness (such as extreme prematurity) may also be associated with raised rates of autism spectrum disorder and attention deficit/hyperactivity disorder (ADHD; Hindley, 2005). A practitioner review by Roberts and Hindley (1999) gives useful case examples of specific mental health disorders, and the management strategies adopted.

Although most studies have demonstrated a higher rate of emotional and behavioral problems in deaf children and adolescents than in the hearing population, there remains some uncertainty about how much higher once factors such as additional impairments and validity of measures are taken into account. The evidence suggests that, where adequate language development has been achieved, a high rate of problems may not be inevitable. In Wallis, Musselman, and MacKay's (2004) longitudinal study of deaf adolescents' mental health (using an adaptation of the Achenbach Youth Self-Report), the three groupings consisted of those who always used oral communication, those who had used sign from early childhood and a "sign mismatch" group who had learned to sign later or whose parent had not signed to them in early childhood. The oral group had the most positive self-report (only 20% in the borderline or clinical range), with the sign mismatch group the most problematic (63%). The total population study in Finland by Sinkkonen (1994) reported that all the mothers and almost all fathers had sign language skills. Thus, effective early communication, and community support, may underpin that study's finding of a lack of difference in rate of behavioral problems. In this time of rapid change, only close follow-up of children given good support after NHSP will show what degree of emotional and behavioral problems are really a consequence of deafness itself.

There appear to be no recent population-based studies in blind children or adolescents. Clinic-based studies suggest that some children are particularly vulnerable. Around one-third of 102 blind children from a clinic population, who had had apparently typical development in the first 16 months of life, showed developmental setback (plateauing or regression) in their second or third year (Cass, Sonksen, & McConachie, 1994). Only one child with severe visual impairment showed a similar developmental pattern. In addition to probable neurological involvement, 60% of the children with setback had adverse social or medical histories. In some of the children, the developmental pattern was of increasingly disordered social communication and they were likely to meet criteria for a diagnosis of autism.

The only study to suggest an overall rate of disorders in blind and severely visually impaired preschool children without other disabilities is by Ophir-Cohen, Ashkenazy, Cohen, and Tirosh (2005). They considered 74 children who attended a specialist unit between 1975 and 1993, and recorded a disorder in 21%, defined when problems were still evident after 6 months in the early intervention program. How generalizable this finding might be is unclear as the authors comment that the children's difficulties in insecurity, withdrawal, attachment problems, inattentiveness, impulsive or hyperactive oppositional-defiant behavior, and temper tantrums could not easily be classified within DSM-IV (and a validated alternative such as Zero-to-Three, 1994, was not used). Sleep problems are common in blind children, at 40–50% (Stores & Ramchandani, 1999). Nevertheless, given the picture from surveys of adaptation in adolescents, it seems possible that the developmental and social difficulties encountered early on by blind children without neurological impairment may not progress to serious emotional and behavioral disorders at school age.

Autism

Population-based estimates for autism in blind and in deaf children are lacking. In a large series of hearing impaired children attending audiology clinics, Juré, Rapin, and Tuchman (1991) estimated a prevalence of autism of 5.3% and noted that, with co-occurrence, both late diagnosis and inappropriate educational management can ensue. For blind children there are no comparable large-scale studies, but the co-occurrence of autism is suggested to be much higher (Pring, 2005). Hobson, Lee, and Brown (1999) carefully matched sighted children with autism to nine blind children with autism, and found some differences in the patterning of clinical features. The blind children showed more abnormality in the use of objects and in motor stereotypies, but less abnormality in the degree of engagement with others and in pretend play. Hobson (2005) speculated that long-term follow-up of blind children with autism may indicate that they have a less severe primary social incapacity than sighted children with autism, and therefore may have a better overall outcome.

Issues in Mental Health Assessment

When assessing a child who has severe hearing or visual impairment, a number of factors will require consideration. The child will need to take time to get used to new people and the room; a blind child will be likely to ask questions about what is happening and why, and want to touch any assessment toys. For deaf children, effective communication is vital. Clinicians cannot expect to rely on writing, as deaf children are likely to have significant reading comprehension difficulties even if their word identification is good (Wauters, van Bon, & Tellings, 2006). Where the child's preference is for sign, clinicians with no or limited signing skills will need to work with an interpreter, which introduces several new dimensions to the assessment. First, families like to have advance notice of who is interpreting as they may know the person already. Teachers and parents are not appropriate as interpreters, both because they may inhibit what the child wants to communicate, but also because they are not trained as interpreters and may miss out important information. It is important to explain that the interpreter will abide by rules of confidentiality. Second, there must be a rule in the session that only one person speaks at once, and it is important to look at the child rather than at the interpreter. Sufficient time must be allowed, including time for the interpreter to take breaks. Third, it is unlikely that the interpreter will have had any training in child mental health or in language development. Their training has been in adult use of sign, and they may not understand child development of sign and how children express themselves. It is vital to brief the interpreter about the purpose and techniques of the session; interpreters are trained to enhance meaning, but the clinician will want at times to know if communications are unusual or disordered. It is important to distinguish grammar differences for those who use sign language from language disorder, and from thought disorder (Hindley, 2005; Roberts & Hindley, 1999).

In addition to previously mentioned socio-emotional measures validated for use with deaf children (e.g., PCL; Hindley), clinicians may use the Meadow–Kendall Social and Emotional Adjustment Inventory (Meadow, 1983) with 59 items completed by school staff. Sullivan, Brookhouser, & Scanlan (2000) provide a protocol for interviewing deaf children about abuse (pp. 435–443) and include a recommendation that deaf children respond best to direct questions rather than free recall.

For blind children, fewer adaptations are required for mental health assessment. It will be important for the clinician to translate into words information that might usually be conveyed non-verbally. It will also be important not to over-interpret elements of the child's behavior such as posture, facial orientation or expression, as well as "autistic-like" behaviors. There appear to be no recent adaptations of mental health assessment tools for blind children; as for deaf children, many research studies utilize the Achenbach CBCL and the Vineland Adaptive Behavior Scales. For sleep disorders, it is certainly the case that difficulties in light perception may lead to alteration of sleep–wake cycles. However, problems in parental inconsistency, overprotectiveness, not setting limits and not establishing routines are more of a determinant, and require assessment through interview and parent diaries (Stores & Ramchandani, 1999).

Interventions and Services for Children with Mental Health Disorders

This chapter has indicated that deaf children have been at particular risk of developing mental health problems, yet they experience significant delays in access to services (NDCS, 2005). The UK National Deaf Children's Society recommended, in addition to early programs of structured intervention for families of deaf children: local intervention programs in schools to promote positive mental health, and build self-confidence and problem-solving skills among deaf children; school anti-bullying policies and practice; a specialist child protection service; and primary mental health care workers specifically for deaf children and young people. A national specialist service in London uses outreach with other child and adolescent mental health services, and also video-link to consult with some young people who use sign. The above recommendations and developments build on the Department of Health best practice guidance for Mental Health and Deafness published in 2005, and the Deaf Mental Health Charter produced by the Mental Health Foundation and the National Society for Mental Health and Deafness (DoH, 2005; Sign, 2005). Similar strategies and standards are being pursued by generic and specialist mental health services for deaf children and young people in other developed countries (e.g., from the Boys Town National Research Hospital, and the Laurent Clerc National Deaf Education Center, Gallaudet University, USA; from the European Society for Mental Health and Deafness).

Conclusions

The development of children with sensory impairments does not allow easy generalizations. This chapter focuses on children apparently without other neurological disorder, but even their course of development needs to be viewed in the context of the range of severity of impairment, the quality and timing (or lack) of early intervention and support to parents, and changes in technological aids, educational practice and legislation. What seems clear is the central importance of language in enabling all other areas of cognitive, emotional and social development in both deaf and blind children. Given a good start with communication and social interaction, we have many reasons to be optimistic that mental health outcomes will be better in future, and that the general picture painted by past research studies, particularly for deaf children, has been overstated. The challenge for mental health professionals is to unpick for an individual referred child who has a sensory impairment how the various risk and protective factors have interacted, and to adapt their practice to the culture and communication needs of that child and their family. Because this is what we do for any referred child, the challenge is not insurmountable. It is important to ensure that all children, including those who have sensory impairments, have access to mental health services according to need.

References

Ainsworth, M. D. S. (1973). The development of infant–mother attachment. In B. M. Caldwell, & H. N. Ricciuti (Eds.), *Review of child development research*, Vol. 3. *Child development and social policy* (pp. 21–94). Chicago: University Press.

Akamatsu, C. T., Mayer, C., & Farrelly, S. (2006). An investigation of two-way text messaging use with deaf students at the secondary level. *Journal of Deaf Studies and Deaf Education*, *11*, 120–131.

Andersen, E. S., Dunlea, A., & Kekelis, L. S. (1984). Blind children's language: Resolving some differences. *Journal of Child Language*, *11*, 645–664.

Andersen, E. S., Dunlea, A., & Kekelis, L. (1993). The impact of input: Language acquisition in the visually impaired. *First Language*, *13*, 23–49.

Austen, S., & Crocker, S. (2004). *Deafness in mind. Working psychologically with deaf people across the lifespan.* London: Whurr Publishers.

Bat-Chava, Y., Martin, D., & Kosciw, J. G. (2005). Longitudinal improvements in communication and socialization of deaf children with cochlear implants and hearing aids: Evidence from parental reports. *Journal of Child Psychology and Psychiatry*, *46*, 1287–1296.

Beadle, E. A., McKinley, D. J., Nikolopoulos, T. P., Brough, J., O'Donoghue, G. M., & Archbold, S. M. (2005). Long-term functional outcomes and academic-occupational status in implanted children after 10 to 14 years of cochlear implant use. *Otology and Neurotology*, *26*, 1152–1160.

Bond, D. E. (2000). Mental health in children who are deaf and have multiple disabilities. In P. Hindley, & N. Kitson (Eds.), *Mental health and deafness* (pp. 127–148). London: Whurr Publishers.

Bonvillian, J. D., Richards, H. C., & Dooley, T. T. (1997). Early sign language acquisition and the development of hand preference in young children. *Brain and Language*, *58*, 1–22.

Carvill, S. (2001). Sensory impairments, intellectual disability and psychiatry. *Journal of Intellectual Disability Research*, *45*, 467–483.

Cass, H. D., Sonksen, P. M., & McConachie, H. (1994). Developmental setback in severe visual impairment. *Archives of Disease in Childhood*, *70*, 192–196.

Chalmers, D., Stewart, I., Silva, P., & Mulvena, A. (1989). Otitis media with effusion in children: The Dunedin study. *Clinics in Developmental Medicine*, 108. London: MacKeith Press.

Courtin, C., & Melot, A. M. (2005). Metacognitive development of deaf children: Lessons from the appearance-reality and false belief tasks. *Developmental Science*, *8*, 16–25.

Crowe, T. V. (2003). Self-esteem scores among deaf college students: An examination of gender and parents' hearing status and signing ability. *Journal of Deaf Studies and Deaf Education*, *8*, 199–206.

Dale, N., & Sonksen, P. (2002). Developmental outcome, including setback, in young children with severe visual impairment. *Developmental Medicine and Child Neurology*, *44*, 613–622.

D'Allura, T. (2002). Enhancing the social interaction skills of preschoolers with visual impairments. *Journal of Visual Impairment and Blindness*, *96*, 576–584.

Davis, A., Bamford, J., Wilson, I., Ramkalawan, T., Forshaw, M., & Wright, S. (1997). A critical review of the role of neonatal hearing screening in the detection of congenital hearing impairment. *Health Technology Assessment*, Vol. 1, No. 10.

Davis, A., & Hind, S. (2003). The newborn hearing screening programme in England. *International Journal of Pediatric Otorhinolaryngology, 67 (Suppl. 1)*, S193–S196.

Davis, A., Wood, S., Healy, R., Webb, H., & Rowe, S. (1995). Risk factors for hearing disorders: Epidemiological evidence of change over time in the UK. *Journal of the American Academy of Audiology*, 6, 365–370.

Dekker, R. (1993). Visually impaired children and haptic intelligence test scores: Intelligence test for visually impaired children (ITVIC). *Developmental Medicine and Child Neurology*, *35*, 478–489.

Department of Health (DoH). (2005). *Mental health and deafness: Towards equity and access*. London: Central Office for Information.

Dote-Kwan, J., Hughes, M., & Taylor, S. L. (1997). Impact of early experiences on the development of young children with visual impairments: Revisited. *Journal of Visual Impairment and Blindness*, *91*, 131–144.

Dunlea, A. (1989). *Vision and the emergence of meaning*. Cambridge: Cambridge University Press.

Early Support. (2004). *Information for parents: Visual impairment. Information for parents: Deafness. Information for Parents: Multi-sensory impairment.* Accessed July 30, 2006 from www.earlysupport.org.uk.

Feldman, H. M., Dollaghan, C. A., Campbell, T. F., Colborn, D. K., Janosky, J., Kurs-Lasky, M., *et al.* (2003). Parent-reported language skills in relation to otitis media during the first 3 years of life. *Journal of Speech, Language, and Hearing Research*, *46*, 273–287.

Fraiberg, S. (1977). *Insights from the blind*. London: Souvenir Press.

Freeman, R. D., Goetz, E., Richards, D. P., & Groenveld, M. (1991). Defiers of negative prediction: A 14-year follow-up study of legally blind children. *Journal of Visual Impairment and Blindness*, *85*, 365–370.

Freeman, R. D., & Groenveld, M. (2000). The behaviour of children and youth with visual and hearing disability. In C. Gillberg, & G. O'Brien (Eds.), *Developmental disability and behaviour* (pp. 27–42). *Clinics in developmental medicine*, No. 149. London: Mac Keith Press.

Greenberg, M. T. (2000). Educational interventions: Prevention and promotion of competence. In P. Hindley, & N. Kitson (Eds.), *Mental health and deafness* (pp. 311–336). London: Whurr Publishers.

Greenberg, M. T., & Kusché, C. A. (1998). Preventive intervention for school-age deaf children: The PATHS curriculum. *Journal of Deaf Studies and Deaf Education*, *3*, 49–63.

Gregory, S. (1976). *The deaf child and his family*. London: George Allen & Unwin.

Gregory, S. (2002). *Models of deafness and the implications for families of deaf children*. Accessed June 30, 2006 from www.deafnessatbirth.org.uk.

Gregory, S., Bishop, J., & Sheldon, L. (1995). *Deaf young people and their families: Developing understanding*. Cambridge: Cambridge University Press.

Griffin-Shirley, N., & Nes, S. L. (2005). Self-esteem and empathy in sighted and visually impaired preadolescents. *Journal of Visual Impairment and Blindness*, *99*, 276–285.

Harrison, R. V., Gordon, K. A., & Mount, R. J. (2005). Is there a critical period for cochlear implantation in congenitally deaf children? Analyses of hearing and speech perception performance after implantation. *Developmental Psychobiology*, *46*, 252–261.

Hindley, P. (1997). Psychiatric aspects of hearing impairments. *Journal of Child Psychology and Psychiatry*, *38*, 101–117.

Hindley, P. (2000). Child and adolescent psychiatry. In P. Hindley, & N. Kitson (Eds.), *Mental health and deafness* (pp. 42–74). London: Whurr Publishers.

Hindley, P. A. (2005). Mental health problems in deaf children. *Current Paediatrics*, *15*, 114–119.

Hindley, P. A., Hill, P. D., McGuigan, S., & Kitson, N. (1994). Psychiatric disorder in deaf and hearing impaired children and young people: A prevalence study. *Journal of Child Psychology and Psychiatry*, *35*, 917–934.

Hobson, R. P. (2005). Why connect? On the relation between autism and blindness. In L. Pring (Ed.), *Autism and blindness: Research and reflections* (pp. 10–25). London: Whurr Publishers.

Hobson, R. P., Lee, A., & Brown, R. (1999). Autism and congenital blindness. *Journal of Autism and Developmental Disorders*, *29*, 45–56.

Hughes, M., Dote-Kwan, J., & Dolendo, J. (1998). A close look at the cognitive play of preschoolers with visual impairments in the home. *Exceptional Children*, *64*, 451–462.

Huurre, T. M., & Aro, H. M. (1998). Psychosocial development among adolescents with visual impairment. *European Child and Adolescent Psychiatry*, *7*, 73–78.

Jackson, A. L. (2001). Language facility and theory of mind development in deaf children. *Journal of Deaf Studies and Deaf Education*, *6*, 161–176.

Jackson, C. W., & Turnbull, A. (2004). Impact of deafness on family life: A review of the literature. *Topics in Early Childhood Special Education*, *24*, 15–29.

Jamieson, J. R., & Pedersen, E. D. (1993). Deafness and mother–child interaction: Scaffolded instruction and the learning of problem-solving skills. *Early Development and Parenting*, *2*, 229–242.

Jindal-Snape, D. (2005). Use of feedback from sighted peers in promoting social interaction skills. *Journal of Visual Impairment and Blindness*, *99*, 403–412.

Johnson, D., & Johnson, R. (1986). Mainstreaming hearing-impaired students: The effect of effort in communicating on cooperation and interpersonal attraction. *Journal of Psychology*, *119*, 31–44.

Juré, R., Rapin, I., & Tuchman, R. F. (1991). Hearing-impaired autistic children. *Developmental Medicine and Child Neurology*, *33*, 1062–1072.

Kef, S. (2002). Psychosocial adjustment and the meaning of social support for visually impaired adolescents. *Journal of Visual Impairment and Blindness*, *96*, 22–37.

Kef, S., Hox, J. J., & Habekothé, H. T. (2000). Social networks of visually impaired and blind adolescents. Structure and effect on well-being. *Social Networks*, *22*, 73–91.

Kitzinger, M. (1984). The role of repeated and echoed utterances in communication with a blind child. *British Journal of Disorders of Communication*, *19*, 135–146.

Klein, J. O. (2001). The burden of otitis media. *Vaccine*, *19*, S2–S8.

Kluwin, T. N., Stinson, M. S., & Colarossi, G. M. (2002). Social processes and outcomes of in-school contact between deaf and hearing peers. *Journal of Deaf Studies and Deaf Education*, *7*, 200–213.

Knutson, J. F., Johnson, C. R., & Sullivan, P. M. (2004). Disciplinary choices of mothers of deaf children and mothers of normally hearing children. *Child Abuse and Neglect*, *28*, 925–937.

Kurtzer-White, E., & Luterman, D. (2003). Families and children with hearing loss: Grief and coping. *Mental Retardation and Developmental Disabilities Research Reviews*, *9*, 232–235.

Kvaerner, K. J., Nafstad, P., & Jaakkola, J. J. (2000). Upper respiratory morbidity in preschool children: A cross-sectional study. *Archives of Otolaryngology – Head and Neck Surgery*, *126*, 1201–1206.

Kvam, M. H. (2004). Sexual abuse of deaf children. A retrospective analysis of the prevalence and characteristics of childhood sexual abuse among deaf adults in Norway. *Child Abuse and Neglect*, *28*, 241–251.

Ladd, P. (2002). *Understanding deaf culture*. Clevedon, Somerset: Multilingual Matters.

Ledeberg, A. R. (1993). The impact of child deafness on social relationships. In M. Marschark, & D. Clark (Eds.), *Psychological perspectives on deafness* (pp. 93–199). Hillsdale, NJ: Lawrence Erlbaum.

Lederberg, A. R., & Mobley, C. E. (1990). The effect of hearing impairment on the quality of attachment and mother–toddler interaction. *Child Development*, *61*, 1596–1604.

Lederberg, A. R., Ryan, H. B., & Robbins, B. L. (1986). Peer interaction in young deaf children: The effect of partner hearing status and familiarity. *Developmental Psychology*, *22*, 691–700.

Lewis, T. L., & Maurer, D. (2005). Multiple sensitive periods in human visual development: Evidence from visually deprived children. *Developmental Psychobiology*, *46*, 163–183.

Lewis, V. (2003). *Development and disability* (2nd edn.). Oxford: Blackwell Publishing.

Lewis, V., & Collis, G. (2005). Research methods fit for purpose. In L. Pring (Ed.), *Autism and blindness: Research and reflections* (pp. 128–141). London: Whurr Publishers.

Lewis, V., Norgate, S., Collis, G., & Reynolds, R. (2000). The consequences of visual impairment for children's symbolic and functional play. *British Journal of Developmental Psychology*, *18*, 449–464.

Luterman, D. M., Kurtzer-White, E., & Seewald, R. C. (1999). *The young deaf child*. Baltimore, MD: York Press.

Marschark, M. (1993). *Psychological development of deaf children*. Oxford: Oxford University Press.

Martin, D., & Bat-Chava, Y. (2003). Negotiating deaf-hearing friendships: coping strategies of deaf boys and girls in mainstream schools. *Child: Care, Health and Development*, *29*, 511–521.

McAlpine, L. M., & Moore, C. L. (1995). The development of social understanding in children with visual impairments. *Journal of Visual Impairment and Blindness*, *89*, 349–358.

McConachie, H. (1990). Early language development and severe visual impairment. *Child: Care, Health and Development*, *16*, 55–61.

McConachie, H. (1995). Critique of current practices in assessment of children. In P. Zinkin, & H. McConachie (Eds.), *Disabled children and developing countries*. Clinics in Developmental Medicine No. 136 (pp. 110–130). London: MacKeith Press.

McConachie, H., & Moore, V. (1994). Early expressive language of severely visually impaired children. *Developmental Medicine and Child Neurology*, *36*, 230–240.

McGaha, C. G., & Farran, D. C. (2001). Interactions in an inclusive classroom: The effects of visual status and setting. *Journal of Visual Impairment and Blindness*, *95*, 80–94.

Meadow, K. P. (1983). *Meadow–Kendall Social–Emotional Assessment Inventory for Deaf and Hearing-Impaired Students Manual*. Washington, DC: Gallaudet College.

Minter, M., Hobson, R. P., & Bishop, M. (1998). Congenital visual impairment and theory of mind. *British Journal of Developmental Psychology*, *16*, 183–196.

Moeller, M. P. (2000). Early intervention and language development in children who are deaf and hard of hearing. *Pediatrics*, *106*, E43.

Moeller, M. P., & Schick, B. (2006). Relations between maternal input and theory of mind understanding in deaf children. *Child Development*, *7*, 751–766.

Moore, V., & McConachie, H. (1994). Communication between blind and severely visually impaired children and their parents. *British Journal of Developmental Psychology*, *12*, 491–502.

Mulford, R. (1988). First words of the blind child. In M. D. Smith, & J. L. Locke (Eds.), *The emergent lexicon: The child's development of a linguistic vocabulary* (pp. 293–338). London: Academic Press.

Mylkebust, H. R. (1960). *Psychology of deafness: Sensory deprivation, learning and adjustment*. New York: Grune & Stratton.

National Deaf Children's Society (NDCS). (2005). *Developing mental health services for deaf children and young people in Northern Ireland*. London: NDCS.

Nicholas, J. G., & Geers, A. E. (2003). Hearing status, language modality, and young children's communicative and linguistic behaviour. *Journal of Deaf Studies and Deaf Education*, *8*, 422–437.

Nikolopoulos, T. P., Archbold, S. M., & O'Donoghue, G. M. (2006). Does cause of deafness influence outcome after cochlear implantation in children? *Pediatrics*, *118*, 1350–1356.

Nikolopoulos, T. P., Lioumi, D., Stamataki, S., & O'Donoghue, G. M. (2006). Evidence-based overview of ophthalmic disorders in deaf children: a literature update. *Otology and Neurotology*, *27*, S1–24.

Norgate, S., Collis, G. M., & Lewis, V. (1998). The developmental role of rhymes and routines for congenitally blind children. *Current Psychology of Cognition*, *17*, 451–477.

Nott, P., Cowan, R., Brown, P. M., & Wigglesworth, G. (2003). Assessment of language skills in young children with profound hearing loss under two years of age. *Journal of Deaf Studies and Deaf Education*, *8*, 401–421.

Nunes, T., Pretzlik, U., & Olsson, J. (2001). Deaf children's social relationships in mainstream schools. *Deafness and Education International*, *3*, 123–136.

Obrzut, J. E., Maddock, G. J., & Lee, C. P. (1999). Determinants of self-concept in deaf and hard of hearing children. *Journal of Developmental and Physical Disabilities*, *11*, 237–251.

Ophir-Cohen, M., Ashkenazy, E., Cohen, A., & Tirosh, E. (2005). Emotional status and development in children who are visually impaired. *Journal of Visual Impairment and Blindness*, *99*, 478–485.

Peavey, K. O., & Leff, D. (2002). Social acceptance of adolescent mainstreamed students with visual impairments. *Journal of Visual Impairment and Blindness*, *96*, 808–811.

Pérez-Pereira, M., & Castro, J. (1992). Pragmatic functions of blind and sighted children's language: A twin case study. *First Language*, *12*, 17–37.

Pérez-Pereira, M., & Conti-Ramsden, G. (1999). *Language development and social interaction in blind children*. Hove, East Sussex: Psychology Press.

Pérez-Pereira, M., & Conti-Ramsden, G. (2005). Do blind children show autistic features? In L. Pring (Ed.), *Autism and blindness: Research and reflections* (pp. 99–127). London: Whurr Publishers.

Peterson, C. C., Peterson, J. L., & Webb, J. (2000). Factors influencing the development of a theory of mind in blind children. *British Journal of Developmental Psychology*, *18*, 431–447.

Peterson, C. C., & Siegal, M. (2000). Insights into a theory of mind from deafness and autism. *Mind and Language*, *15*, 123–145.

Pipp-Siegel, S., Sedey, A. L., & Yoshinaga-Itano, C. (2002). Predictors of parental stress in mothers of young children with hearing loss. *Journal of Deaf Studies and Deaf Education*, *7*, 1–17.

Power, D. J., Wood, D. J., Wood, H. A., & MacDougall, J. (1990). Maternal control over conversations with hearing and deaf infants and young children. *First Language*, *10*, 19–35.

Powers, S. (1998). An analysis of deaf pupils' examination results in ordinary schools in 1996. *Deafness and Education*, *22*, 30–36.

Preisler, G. M. (1991). Early patterns of interaction between blind infants and their sighted mothers. *Child: Care, Health and Development*, *17*, 65–90.

Preisler, G. M. (1997). Social and emotional development of blind children: A longitudinal study. In V. Lewis, & G. Collis (Eds.), *Blindness and psychological development in young children* (pp. 69–85). Leicester: BPS Books.

Preisler, G. M. (1999). The development of communication and language in deaf and severely hard of hearing children: Implications for the future. *International Journal of Pediatric Otorhinolaryngology*, *49*, S39–S44.

Preisler, G. (2001). Sensory deficits. In G. Bremner & A. Fogel (Eds.), *Blackwell handbook of infant development* (pp. 617–638). Oxford: Blackwell Publishers.

Preisler, G., Tvingstedt, A. L., & Ahlström, M. (2002). A psychosocial follow-up study of deaf preschool children using cochlear implants. *Child: Care, Health and Development*, *28*, 403–418.

Pressman, L., Pipp-Siegel, S., Yoshinaga-Itano, C., & Deas, A. (1999). Maternal sensitivity predicts language gain in preschool children who are deaf and hard of hearing. *Journal of Deaf Studies and Deaf Education*, *4*, 294–304.

Pring, L. (2005). *Autism and blindness: Research and reflections.* London: Whurr Publishers.

Punch, R., & Hyde, M. (2005). The social participation and career decision-making of hard-of-hearing adolescents in regular classes. *Deafness and Education International*, *7*, 122–138.

Rahi, J. S., & Dezateux, C. (1998). Epidemiology of visual impairment in Britain. *Archives of Disease in Childhood*, *78*, 381–386.

Reynell, J. (1979). *Manual for the Reynell–Zinkin Developmental Scales for Young Visually Handicapped Children.* Part 1. Windsor: NFER-Nelson.

Rhys-Jones, S. L., & Ellis, H. D. (2000). Theory of mind: Deaf and hearing children's comprehension of picture stories and judgments of social situations. *Journal of Deaf Studies and Deaf Education*, *5*, 248–261.

Roberts, C., & Hindley, P. (1999). Practitioner review: The assessment and treatment of deaf children with psychiatric disorders. *Journal of Child Psychology and Psychiatry*, *40*, 151–167.

Roberts, J. E., Rosenfeld, R. M., & Zeisel, S. A. (2004). Otitis media and speech and language: A meta-analysis of prospective studies. *Pediatrics*, *113*, 238–248.

Roid, G., & Miller, L. (1997). *Leiter International Performance Scale–Revised Examiner's Manual.* Wood Dale, IL: Stoelting.

Rosenblum, L. P. (2000). Perception of the impact of visual impairment on the lives of adolescents. *Journal of Visual Impairment and Blindness*, *94*, 434–445.

Royal National Institute for the Blind (RNIB). (2001). *The social life and leisure activities of blind and partially sighted children and young people aged 5 to 25.* London: RNIB.

Schlesinger, H. S., & Meadow, K. P. (1972). *Sound and sign: Childhood deafness and mental health.* Berkeley, CA: University of California Press.

Schorr, E. A., Fox, N. A., van Wassenhove, V., & Knudsen, E. I. (2005). Auditory-visual fusion in speech perception in children with cochlear implants. *Proceedings of the National Academy of Sciences of the USA*, *102*, 18748–18750.

Sign. (2005). *Deaf mental health charter.* Beaconsfield: National Society for Mental Health and Deafness. Accessed July 31, 2006 from www.signcharity.org.uk.

Singer, G. H. S. (2006). Meta-analysis of comparative studies of depression in mother of children with and without developmental disabilities. *American Journal of Mental Retardation*, *111*, 155–169.

Sinkkonen, J. (1994). *Hearing impairment, communication and personality development.* Helsinki: Department of Child Psychiatry, University of Helsinki (cited by Hindley, 1997).

Skellenger, A. C., Rosenblum, L. P., & Jager, B. K. (1997). Behaviors of preschoolers with visual impairments in indoor play settings. *Journal of Visual Impairment & Blindness*, *91*, 519–530.

Skelton, T., & Valentine, G. (2003). "It feels like being Deaf is normal": An exploration into the complexities of defining D/deafness and young D/deaf people's identities. *Canadian Geographer*, *47*, 451–466.

Snijders, J. T., Tellegen, P. J., & Laros, J. A. (1989). *Snijders–Oomen non-verbal intelligence test: SON-R 5.5–17. Manual and research report.* Groningen: Wolters-Noordhoff.

Sonksen, P. M., Petrie, A., & Drew, K. J. (1991). Promotion of visual development of severely visually impaired babies: Evaluation of a developmentally based programme. *Developmental Medicine and Child Neurology*, *33*, 320–335.

Sonksen, P. M., & Stiff, B. (1991). *Show me what my friends can see: A developmental guide for parents of babies with severely impaired sight and their professional advisors.* London: Wolfson Centre.

Spencer, P. E. (2000). Looking without listening: Is audition a prerequisite for normal development of visual attention during infancy? *Journal of Deaf Studies and Deaf Education*, *5*, 291–302.

Spencer, P. E. (2004). Individual differences in language performance after cochlear implantation at one to three years of age: child, family, and linguistic factors. *Journal of Deaf Studies and Deaf Education*, *9*, 395–412.

Spencer, P. E., & Meadow-Orlans, K. P. (1996). Play, language and maternal responsiveness: A longitudinal study of deaf and hearing infants. *Child Development*, *67*, 3176–3191.

Stern, D. (1985). *The interpersonal world of the infant.* New York: Basic Books.

Stinson, M. S., & Antia, S. D. (1999). Considerations in educating deaf and hard-of-hearing students in inclusive settings. *Journal of Deaf Studies and Deaf Education*, *4*, 163–175.

Stores, G., & Ramchandani, P. (1999). Sleep disorders in visually impaired children. *Developmental Medicine & Child Neurology*, *41*, 348–352.

Sullivan, P., Brookhouser, P., & Scanlan, M. (2000). Maltreatment of deaf and hard of hearing children. In P. Hindley, & N. Kitson (Eds.), *Mental health and deafness* (pp. 149–184). London: Whurr Publishers.

Tellegen, P. J., Winkel, M., Wijnberg-Williams, B. J., & Laros, J. A. (1996). *Snijders–Oomen non-verbal intelligence scale SON-R 2.5-7.* Lisse: Swets Test Publishers.

Terwogt, M. M., & Rieffe, C. (2004). Deaf children's use of beliefs and desires in negotiation. *Journal of Deaf Studies and Deaf Education*, *9*, 27–38.

Tomblin, J. B., Barker, B. A., Spencer, L. J., Zhang, X., & Gantz, B. J. (2005). The effect of age at cochlear implant initial stimulation on expressive language growth in infants and toddlers. *Journal of Speech, Language, and Hearing Research*, *48*, 853–867.

Tröster, H. (2001). Sources of stress in mothers of young children with visual impairments. *Journal of Visual Impairment and Blindness*, *94*, 623–637.

Tröster, H., & Brambring, M. (1992). Early social-emotional development in blind infants. *Child: Care, Health and Development*, *18*, 207–227.

Tröster, H., & Brambring, M. (1994). The play behaviour and play materials of blind and sighted infants and preschoolers. *Journal of Visual Impairment and Blindness*, *88*, 421–432.

Tröster, H., Brambring, M., & Beelmann, A. (1991a). Prevalence and situational causes of stereotyped behaviours in blind infants and preschoolers. *Journal of Abnormal Child Psychology*, *19*, 569–590.

Tröster, H., Brambring, M., & Beelmann, A. (1991b). The age dependence of stereotyped behaviours in blind infants and preschoolers. *Child: Care, Health and Development*, *17*, 137–157.

Van Eldik, T., Treffers, P. D. A., Veerman, J. W., & Verhulst, F. C. (2004). Mental health problems of deaf Dutch children as indicated by parents' responses to the Child Behavior Checklist. *American Annals of the Deaf*, *148*, 390–394.

Van Gent, T. (2003). *Assessment and diagnosis of behavioural disorders in deaf children and adolescents: Challenges and issues.* Plenary presentation, European Federation of Associations of Teachers of the Deaf (FEAPDA) Congress, Cardiff, October.

Van Gurp, S. (2001). Self-concept of deaf secondary school students in different educational settings. *Journal of Deaf Studies and Deaf Education*, *6*, 54–69.

Vernon-Feagans, L., Hurley, M., & Yont, K. (2002). The effect of otitis media and daycare quality on mother/child book reading and language use at 48 months of age. *Journal of Applied Developmental Psychology*, *23*, 113–133.

Vostanis, P., Hayes, M., Du Feu, M., & Warren, J. (1997). Detection of behavioural and emotional problems in deaf children and adolescents: Comparison of two rating scales. *Child: Care, Health and Development*, *23*, 233–246.

Walker, E. C., Tobin, M. J., & McKennell, A. C. (1992). *Blind and partially-sighted children in Britain: The RNIB survey*, *2*. London: HMSO.

Wallis, D., Musselman, C., & KacKay, S. (2004). Hearing mothers and their deaf children: The relationship between early, ongoing mode match and subsequent mental health functioning in adolescence. *Journal of Deaf Studies and Deaf Education*, *9*, 2–14.

Waugh, M. C., Chong, W. K., & Sonksen, P. M. (1998). Neuroimaging in children with congenital disorders of the peripheral visual system. *Developmental Medicine and Child Neurology*, *40*, 812–819.

Wauters, L. N., van Bon, W. H. J., & Tellings, A. E. J. M. (2006). Reading comprehension of Dutch deaf children. *Reading and Writing*, *19*, 49–76.

Webster, A., & Roe, J. (1998). *Children with visual impairments: Social interaction, language and learning*. London: Routledge.

Wing, L., & Wing, J. K. (1971). Multiple impairments in early childhood autism. *Journal of Autism and Childhood Schizophrenia*, *1*, 256–266.

Woolfe, T., & Smith, P. K. (2001). The self-esteem and cohesion to family members of deaf children in relation to the hearing status of their parents and siblings. *Deafness and Education International*, *3*, 80–96.

World Health Organization (WHO). (2004). *International classification of functioning, disability and health: Version for children and youth*. Geneva: WHO.

Yoshinaga-Itano, C. (2001). The social-emotional ramifications of universal newborn hearing screening, early identification and intervention of children who are deaf or hard of hearing. In R. C. Seewold, & J. S. Gravel (Eds.), *A sound foundation through early amplification*. Proceedings of the Second International Phonak Conference, Chicago (pp. 221–231). Accessed October 27, 2006 from www.phonak.com/professional/informationpool/proceedings.

Yoshinaga-Itano, C. (2003). From screening to early identification and intervention: discovering predictors to successful outcomes for children with significant hearing loss. *Journal of Deaf Studies and Deaf Education*, *8*, 11–30.

Yoshinaga-Itano, C., Coulter, D., & Thomson, V. (2001). Developmental outcomes of children with hearing loss born in Colorado hospitals with and without universal newborn hearing screening programs. *Seminars in Neonatology*, *6*, 521–529.

Yoshinaga-Itano, C., Sedey, A. L., Coulter, D. K., & Mehl, A. L. (1998). Language of early- and later-identified children with hearing loss. *Pediatrics*, *102*, 1161–1171.

Zero-to-Three. (1994). *Diagnostic classification, 0–3: Diagnostic classification of mental health and developmental disorders of infancy and early childhood*. Arlington, VA: National Center for Clinical Infant Programs.

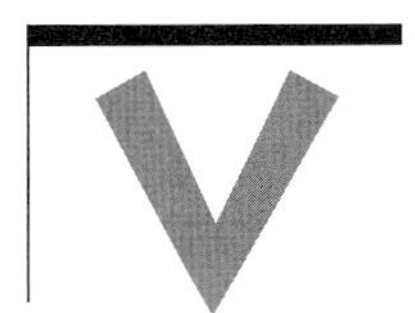

Approaches to Treatment

Community-Based Interventions and Services

Christina J. Groark and Robert B. McCall

The purpose of this chapter is to summarize the process by which one can conceive, design, implement, monitor, evaluate and sustain empirically based community-operated interventions and services. The focus is on the *process*, not the content, of such interventions and services. As such, the discussion accepts (and does not cover) the existing literature on the problem or target behaviors as well as on approaches to preventing or treating those behaviors as the starting point of the process.

There is relatively little scholarly analysis and even less empirical validation of this process *per se* (see Fixsen, Naoom, Blase *et al.*, 2005). Consequently, this chapter relies to a greater extent than is typical on the experience of the authors together with those of others and what scholarly work does exist.

Scope and Definition

The scope of this chapter can be further specified by considering the working definitions of certain key concepts.

Community-based

Community-based interventions and services are those that are implemented and operated by service professionals in the community. Often, but not always, such services are part of a demonstration and evaluation project investigating whether the intervention or service can be created, organized, implemented and produce benefits in participants. If successful, the same type of professionals will provide the service in the community on a routine basis. In contrast, innovative or experimental services conducted in a specialized environment (e.g., laboratory, school) by specialized practitioners (e.g., academic educators or social workers) do not fall in the chapter's purview. Thus, community-based services represent the most ecologically valid version of the service and the last step in the basic–applied research continuum.

Interventions and Services

The services to be considered consist of organized supports and activities designed to promote the health, education and welfare of children, youth and families. They focus on target behaviors that tend to be public rather than strictly intrapsychic. As such, they consist of problem behaviors that come to public attention and that require public resources to prevent or treat (e.g., abuse and neglect; drug and alcohol problems; antisocial behavior and delinquency; poverty, unemployment and public assistance; poor parenting; and mental health prevention, detection, diagnosis and referral). While participants may receive services individually or in groups, the services of concern do not include traditional private or group psychotherapy (APA Presidential Task Force on Evidence-Based Practice, 2006; Weisz, Jensen-Doss, & Hawley, 2006). Instead, they are closer to services within the domains of community psychology and psychiatry, social work, public health and education.

Prevention and Treatment/Remediation

The services include both prevention and treatment/remediation, although the distinction between these categories often blurs. For example, individuals come to public attention and are referred to services because they have already displayed certain problematic behaviors or are substantially at risk of doing so; the services focus on treating/remediating the manifest behaviors, preventing additional or more extreme undesirable behaviors, and promoting more positive behavioral alternatives.

Evidence-based

Services that are evidence-based have some research supporting their potential or actual effectiveness. While some people reserve the phrase "evidence-based program" for a well-articulated service program that has been empirically shown to be effective and could be replicated, we also use the term to refer to new programs based on principles or consisting of components that have theory and evidence that support their likely effectiveness. Unfortunately, no clear standard prescribes how much or what kind of evidence is required to substantiate the claim of "evidence-based" (see p. 975) so that use of the phrase has become commonplace and less meaningful in an era in which policy-makers and practitioners value and require evidence-based practices (Groark & McCall, 2005; McCall, submitted).

Universal, Quasi-universal and Targeted Services

Strictly speaking, *universal* services are available to everyone. For example, public education and some form of social security

Rutter's Child and Adolescent Psychiatry, 5th edition. Edited by M. Rutter, D. Bishop, D. Pine, S. Scott, J. Stevenson, E. Taylor and A. Thapar. © 2008 Blackwell Publishing, ISBN: 978-1-4051-4549-7.

or public retirement benefits are universal in many countries. Universal programs tend to be most appropriate when everyone in society can benefit (e.g., public education, retirement benefits) or when the target group is broadly dispersed in the population (e.g., smokers, automobile drivers, obese children) or not readily identifiable and/or without clear predictive risk factors (e.g., abusive parents). They often have the advantages of reaching large numbers of people, some of whom otherwise would not be identifiable, and satisfying broad crucial social needs (e.g., education). However, only a few social needs merit the cost of very intense services (e.g., education); some are inefficient because many people are reached or served who do not need the service; and some programs benefit the educationally, financially and behaviorally advantaged members of society more than those of relative disadvantage, because such individuals are more likely to take advantage of the program and already have a head start on achieving its goals (Ceci & Papierno, 2005). Truly universal programs are not within the focus of this chapter.

Instead, we will emphasize "*quasi-universal*" programs, which are ones that are available to all individuals within a geographical area (e.g., neighborhood, town) or institution (e.g., an entire school, orphanage), and such programs may or may not have additional eligibility criteria, such as income level (e.g., Head Start early childhood care and education programs in the USA). These programs tend to have broad goals (e.g., improvement of family functioning, parental psychological and economic self-sufficiency; improvement of child development, school readiness, and life success), but some have more specific aims (e.g., school readiness).

Conversely, *targeted* programs (see chapter 61) are often restricted to participants having certain specific characteristics that may exist in relatively small percentages of the population (e.g., drug addiction, blindness, physical disabilities) and may require intense (e.g., detoxification) or extensive services (e.g., for children with severe disabilities).

Quasi-universal programs tend to be most appropriate for conditions and services in between those for truly universal and highly targeted programs; for example, when the target group is concentrated in low-income neighborhoods and when the needed service is moderately intense or extensive and clearly needs to be targeted to some extent to be cost-efficient and to benefit those most in need (e.g., Sure Start in the UK, Head Start and offered to all in low-income neighborhoods in the USA). They have the advantage of having a large percentage of participants who need the service, but they may not serve all in society who need it (e.g., low-income families who live in unserved neighborhoods).

Examples of Different Quasi-Universal Programs

We describe several examples of quasi-universal programs that illustrate some of their commonalities and differences, many of which will be discussed more fully later.

Nurse–Family Partnership (formerly Nurse Home Visitation Program)

The Nurse–Family Partnership (NFP) program (Olds, Henderson, Kitzman *et al.*, 1999) is aimed at first time, low-income, higher risk mothers to improve pregnancy outcomes by reducing health-related adverse behaviors (e.g., smoking, alcohol consumption, drug use); improve child health and development by teaching parents to provide more responsible and competent health and behavioral care; and promote the economic self-sufficiency of families by encouraging planned pregnancies (i.e., fewer and more widely spaced) and supporting education, secure employment and linkages with other health and human services within the community. The program is being implemented in nearly half of the states of the USA and some other countries. It is quasi-universal for high-risk first-birth women located in the geographical region in which it is offered.

The program relies on nurses to visit the homes of participants, preferably during pregnancy and throughout the child's first 2 years. The program is heavily centrally prescribed, with specific and concrete goals and activities, although some tailoring to the needs of individual families must occur. The focus on small concrete specific goals from visit to visit and throughout the program likely contributes to the ease of implementing the program and positive outcomes.

The program was evaluated in three sequential studies in three USA cities (Olds, Henderson, Kitzman *et al.*, 1999). Pregnant women who had not previously given birth and who had at least one additional risk factor (e.g., low-income, unmarried, low education, unemployment) were randomly assigned to a treatment group (nurse home visitors, transportation to periodic health visits and home visits until the child's second birthday) versus a variety of control conditions that included fewer or shorter services. Samples ranged from 400 to 1139 with a predominance of either White, African-American or Hispanic women in different cities. Results showed benefits to mothers and children, but these were not pervasive and tended to occur under specific experimental and non-randomized circumstances: if nurses rather than paraprofessionals did the home visiting, if home visiting lasted until the child's second birthday and especially if the mother was at higher risk (e.g., unmarried, smoker, very low income/education). For these groups, NFP mothers were more likely to be employed and have better life skills, fewer problem behaviors, better reproductive histories, improved parenting and less abuse; their children improved in health, socioemotional, language and cognitive development as children and with reduced criminal and behavioral problems, sexual activity and substance use as teenagers. A similar but more intensive and extensive home visiting program in New Zealand produced similar (but not identical) results (Fergusson, Grant, Horwood, & Ridder, 2005, 2006).

Early Head Start

Early Head Start (EHS) is an attempt by the US government to provide health care, child care, family support and parent education to primarily low-income families. EHS is quasi-universal in that its services are available to all low-income families with at least one child approximately from birth to 3 years of age in the geographical area in which the program is located. A small percentage of families who are not low income and others who have children with disabilities are also enrolled.

The program is a combination of a centralized set of program requirements and standards for implementation with some local flexibility to create a program that matches the needs of local participants. For example, child development services are required, but they can be provided in centers, in the homes of participants through home visiting, or in a mixture of the two.

Seventeen programs were selected from applicants to provide EHS services and to participate in a research and evaluation consortium. The total evaluation followed 3001 families who were randomly assigned to EHS or whatever other program parents chose. EHS was unusual in having local evaluation specialists at each site supervise data collection, consisting of core assessments common across the 17 sites plus additional assessments to answer specific research and evaluation questions pertinent to that site. The consortium met periodically to advise the cross-site evaluation team and participate in subsets of sites that had similar programs and similar research interests (e.g., the role of fathers).

When EHS children were 3 years old, they performed better on measures of cognition, language and socioemotional functioning than control peers, and EHS parents were more supportive of children's emotional, cognitive and language development and more likely to be in education or job training. However, the benefits of EHS varied with non-randomized characteristics of participants and implementation. For example, benefits were greater for African-American families, families who enrolled during pregnancy versus after delivery, and families with a moderate rather than a substantial number of demographic risk factors. Further, programs with a mixed center and home visiting approach and those that more fully implemented the comprehensive performance standards had a wider range of larger benefits. Also, children who transitioned from EHS to formal early care and education programs between ages 3 and 5 had better early reading-related skills at age 5 (Administration for Children and Families, 2002; Love, Kisker, Ross *et al.*, 2005; http://www.acf.hhs.gov/programs/OPRE/EHS/EHS_resrch/index/htlm).

Comprehensive Child Development Program

The Comprehensive Child Development Program (CCDP) was a multisited demonstration project in 34 sites around the USA to provide comprehensive health, education, mental health and welfare services to low-income families with children from birth to 1 year of age at the beginning until the child reached approximately 5 years. Its purpose was to increase the financial and psychological self-sufficiency of those families and improve the children's development. It was quasi-universal, allowing all community members to participate, but sites were targeted to low-income areas.

The program was a combination of central prescription and local innovation. Services were required to be comprehensive, because high-risk families tend to have a variety of different needs, including obtaining basic necessities (shelter, food, medical care), preparation for employment (education, training), mental health services (e.g., drug and alcohol), child care and parenting education (for further information about parent-based programs in general see chapter 64). While specific services were to be tailored to the needs of each family and thus could vary between families and sites, certain procedures, such as the frequency of contact and devising individual family plans, were specified by the federal government.

A central evaluator conducted an evaluation on 21 sites, which had randomly assigned either individuals or site locations within their area. An intent-to-treat strategy was employed. However, the government awarded separate contracts for the central evaluator and the management information system developer, and these two databases were never merged across sites so that the nature and extent of services as well as specific family goals could not be related to outcomes. Results indicated that twice as many mothers in CCDP treatment sites became employed and improved their financial status as comparison mothers, but there were few other benefits for parents or children (St. Pierre, Layzer, Goodson, & Bernstein, 1997a,b). However, sites varied substantially in the nature and extent of the services they provided, families in the comparison group obtained on their own behalf almost as many services as those in the CCDP groups, families differed in their individual goals and the services they used but the intent-to-treat strategy assessed each outcome on all participants, regardless of their individual goals, nature and extent of services, or length of participation in the program (Gilliam, Ripple, Zigler, & Leiter, 2000; McCall, Ryan, & Plemons, 2003).

School Development Program

Comer's School Development Program (SDP) seeks to improve schools, primarily in low-income neighborhoods, and student academic performance and skills by mobilizing adults to support student learning and development (Comer, 1988; Comer, Haynes, Joyner, & Ben-Avie, 1996; Joyner, Comer, & Ben-Avie, 2004). It is quasi-universal because an entire school – administrators, teachers, students, parents and local organizations – and increasingly an entire school system may be involved. SDP is operating in hundreds of schools in dozens of USA states and other countries.

The program is planned and implemented within each school or school system, rather than by some central body. The program consists of a structure and process, rather than a set of specified actions, services or directions. Three structures comprise the basic system on which the Comer process is built. The *School Planning and Management Team* is composed of administrators, teachers, support staff and parents. It is responsible for developing a comprehensive school plan; setting academic, social, and community relations goals; co-ordinating all school activities, including staff development programs; and monitoring the progress to identify needed changes. The *Student and Staff Support Team* consists of the principal and professionals in child development and mental health, such as school counselors, social workers, psychologists and nurses. It promotes the social conditions and relationships necessary to connect all of the school's student services; it facilitates the sharing of information and advice; and it addresses individual student needs, obtains resources outside the school and develops prevention programs. The *Parent Team* is composed of parents. It selects representatives to serve on the School Planning and Management Team and develops activities for the parents to support the school's social and academic programs. Central to the process are three school operations including development of a comprehensive school plan, provision of staff development opportunities, and assessment and modification.

Evaluations conducted by SDP and independent professionals have shown that the program can improve school climate, student behavior and student achievement (e.g., Cook, Hunt, & Murphy, 1998; Haynes, 1995), but results have not been uniformly positive (Cook, Habib, Phillips *et al.*, 2000; Neufield & LaBue, 1994). Success seems to depend on how extensively and vigorously the process is pursued and implemented. This result is concordant with research conducted years earlier (Maughan, Pickles, Rutter, & Ouston, 1990; Ouston, Maughan, & Rutter, 1991) revealing that non-experimental changes that produced better attendance and school performance in students rested heavily on the extent to which there was a clear vision of and process to guide change and a focus by all of its administrators, staff, students and parents on improving the entire school – precisely what SDP intends to guide.

Sure Start Local Programmes

Sure Start Local Programmes (SSLPs) is an attempt to reduce child poverty and social exclusion in the UK (the gap between rich and poor) with a quasi-universal program within certain geographical areas that are relatively disadvantaged (Rutter, 2006). It is aimed at infants or young children. Support for the program is widely available, and numerous sites have been continued, modified or created across the UK.

Programs and services were largely locally created and unspecified. The central government required five core service themes:

1 Outreach and home visiting;
2 Support for families and parents;
3 High-quality play, learning and child care;
4 Primary and community health care, including advice about child and family health; and
5 Support for children and parents with special needs.

Services within these domains were to be "evidence-based" but their nature and extent were up to local agencies. It was expected that existing services would be improved and co-ordinated, and that facilities for early childhood care and education would be expanded, remodeled and otherwise improved. The government's rationale was that a minimally targeted program open to all in the area would minimize any stigma associated with using the program, and localities should have the opportunity to tailor services within the five areas to fit the needs of their local participants and existing services.

An extensive national evaluation (National Evaluation of Sure Start Team, 2005a,b) was conducted, but with at least two constraints imposed by government: first, neither families nor sites could be randomly assigned to Sure Start or a comparison condition because Sure Start was expected to be successful, and random assignment would unnecessarily deny services to certain families, and, second, that the services would not be "manualized," which meant that no site was required to specify, and no monitoring information would be gathered on, the nature and extent of services provided. These constraints meant that there was no uniform Sure Start program, sites were extremely heterogeneous in the nature and extent of services provided, it was nearly impossible to relate any characteristics of the nature and extent of services to outcomes, and the opportunities for a comparison group were limited.

Nevertheless, the national evaluation was able to study 150 SSLP sites in which the program had been initiated for at least 3 years and 50 comparison sites that had not yet begun to implement SSLP. Extensive data were collected on participants, administrative and broad characteristics of the SSLP services, and parental report, observations and developmental assessments on a variety of family and child (9–36 months old) outcomes. The evaluation used an intent-to-treat strategy (see p. 984) in which all families eligible within an SSLP area with 9- to 36-month-old children were included in the sample regardless of the nature and extent of services received.

Given the large number of possible outcomes for parents and children, SSLP was associated with consistent benefits for very few. For example, SSLP sites operated by health agencies and other local authority agencies did better than those led by voluntary agencies. In contrast to the NFP, there were some adverse effects the more disadvantaged the family (e.g., mothers who were teenagers, single parents, unemployed parents), including slightly lower scores of children on verbal ability, social competence and more behavioral problems. Similar to EHS, there were slight benefits for families who were not so disadvantaged, including fewer behavioral problems, more social competence and less negative parenting (Belsky, Melhuish, Barnes, Leyland, & Romaniuk, 2006; National Evaluation of Sure Start Team, 2005b).

Summary

While not intended to be representative of quasi-universal programs, these projects varied in how specifically and concretely the program was prescribed centrally versus the amount of local flexibility allowed and in how the programs were implemented and evaluated. The remainder of this chapter focuses on these aspects of program development, implementation and evaluation.

The next section of the chapter considers various issues in bringing evidence to the creation of evidence-based programs in the community. Then, principles of collaboration are offered, because most community-based programs are or should be developed, implemented and evaluated by a collaborative team whose members are often unaccustomed to working with each other and whose values and roles may conflict.

We next consider program design, which may occur at the national, state/province or local level and be very specific and detailed or consist of broad principles or service domains. We consider how such programs may be implemented, followed by a discussion of certain issues in their monitoring and evaluation. Finally, we discuss sustainability, which includes maintaining program effectiveness year after year as well sustaining funding.

Evidence and Evidence-Based Interventions and Services

Policy-makers and funders in many countries demand that the services they initiate or support be "evidence-based," that is, be rooted in empirically supported principles and preferably have already been demonstrated to produce benefits for participants (for an overview of treatment evaluation see chapter 18). The simplest and presumably most expeditious and effective strategy for creating and implementing service programs is to replicate "proven programs." Indeed, for some policy-makers, this is the only definition of an "evidence-based program."

Requirements for Services Replication

While the rationale for service replication is straightforward, it makes certain assumptions that must be met for this strategy to be effective, and such premises are often not fulfilled (Groark & McCall, 2005; McCall, submitted; McCall, Groark, & Nelkin, 2004).

• *One or more programs must have been demonstrated to have been effective.* Obviously, there must be a service program that has been implemented, evaluated and found to be effective to be a candidate for replication. Such demonstrated programs exist for teenage problem behaviors including school failure, risky sexual activity, substance abuse, delinquency and violence (Weissberg & Kumpfer, 2003) and for lowering rates of abuse and improving parenting skills for high-risk mothers (Olds & Kitzman, 1993), but this is not the case for many areas needing services. For example, nearly 50 years of research on early childhood education indicates such programs are beneficial, but much less research exists on specific curricula that might be replicated.

• *The service must be packaged in detail.* Relatively few service programs, even demonstration programs intended to be replicated if found successful, have a "manual" describing all of the elements of the program and its implementation that practice professionals elsewhere can use to replicate the program.

• *Local service providers must be willing to replicate the original service.* A major tenet of good therapeutic practice is to match the treatment to the specific characteristics of the client, so it is not surprising that agencies often want to adapt a model program to fit their own specific type of clientele, local social and policy circumstances, and each individual client. Indeed, a major principle of family support programs is that each individual family specifies their strengths and needs and a program of referrals, services and supports is tailored to their individual profile. But, even for services that are comprehensively and specifically prescribed, the service program may differ substantially from one incarnation to another (Gilliam, Ripple, Zigler *et al.*, 2000; McCall & Green, 2004), and often no research exists suggesting whether such modifications improve, harm or have no influence on program effectiveness.

• *Will a replicated program also replicate the benefits of the original demonstration?* Even if the program is as faithfully replicated as possible, it is not clear that it will have the same benefits for participants in its replicated incarnation as it did in its original demonstration (Green, 2001). Demonstration projects are typically implemented by professionals who are highly energized, passionate and committed to the new program and who may have substantial expertise in creating relationships with clients and motivating them to participate and persist in the service regimen. However, the practitioners who volunteer or are assigned to replicate the program may not possess the same level of motivation, commitment and interpersonal expertise. Also, the intended participants may differ from those in the original demonstration, and some services are not equally effective with all types of participants. For example, physical punishment is often discouraged in parenting improvement programs but is very common among African-American families, and research suggests that it is not as deleterious to African-American as it is to middle- and upper-class Caucasian children (Baumrind, Larzelere, & Cowan, 2002).

For these reasons, replicating proven programs may not produce replicated benefits; often the original demonstration is more effective than its replicates, which is why policy-makers and funders should evaluate replications and not assume that the program has already been shown to be effective and its replication does not need evaluation.

Nature of the Evidence

From a practical standpoint, a service program is never "proven"; rather, the evidence for its effectiveness will always be more or less "persuasive." Further, not all research studies and demonstrations are equally persuasive; some designs and results are more compelling than others. From the perspective of a policy-maker or practitioner faced with a mounting behavioral or social problem, one picks the "best available service approach" almost regardless of the persuasiveness of evidence.

Assessing the Evidence

It would be ideal to have a simple scheme to assess the research literature on a service program, and such a scheme has been proposed (Chambless & Hollon, 1998; Mrazek & Haggerty, 1994) which literally provides a "grade" from 1 to 7 (1 is highest) for the persuasiveness of the evidence. But this particular approach seems too narrow, considers only a few types of research designs (e.g., randomized trials and replications), emphasizes internal over external validity and ignores a great deal of information (e.g., effect size, cost : benefit ratio) that would be valuable in making policy and service program decisions (Groark & McCall, 2005; McCall & Green, 2004; McCall, Groark, & Nelkin, 2004).

Table 60.1 presents an alternative scheme (McCall, submitted) based on a broader representation of the standards of program evaluation research methodology. It has the advantages of being substantially more comprehensive, but it has the apparent disadvantages of being much more complex and not providing a simple grade for the research literature as a whole (although such a numerical rating scheme could be developed). In practice, the disadvantages may not be important, because research literatures are typically uneven and contain gaps, and they are best evaluated by academic research specialists who are capable of weighing different kinds of evidence and making judgments regarding the persuasiveness of the corpus of research.

Some groups, such as the Campbell Collaboration (C2; Co-oper, 1998) and the US Centers for Disease Control (2006),

Table 60.1 Elements of a scheme for assessing the research evidence in support of a service program.

1 Program effectiveness (internal validity) To what extent does the research demonstrate that the program *per se* produces its intended benefits in participants? (Generally a > b > c in persuasiveness).

(a) *Randomized experimental and quasi-randomized evidence* Studies using random assignment of individuals or larger units to program versus comparison conditions plus experimenter-selected units that are arbitrarily assigned to treatment versus comparison conditions

(b) *Non-randomized quasi-experimental designs* (Cook & Campbell, 1979; Rossi, Lipsey, & Freeman, 2004). Studies lacking random or experimenter-controlled assignment (i.e., participants self-select to conditions) with some comparison provision (e.g., comparison groups, propensity score comparison individuals, instrumental variable estimation) that supports the inference of causality. Also, interrupted time series with three or more time points before and after the program

(c) *Non-random single-group designs with a pre- and post-program assessment* These studies are more persuasive if they provide some additional evidence consistent with causality (e.g., dose–response effect; relations between program elements hypothesized to be causal mediators, such as fidelity of implementation or success of program implementation in individuals, and outcome benefits)

2 Elements of persuasive research design To what extent is the literature within each of the three design categories characterized by the following (the more characteristics the better):

(a) A theory or cause-and-effect conceptualization that is well-supported by a variety of other research?

(b) Large numbers and limited dropout?

(c) Preprogram as well as post-program assessments to demonstrate change within individuals?

(d) Assessment of program implementation that demonstrates the program was faithfully and completely implemented in the program group and less so or not at all in the comparison group?

(e) Monitoring and assessment of participant exposure to program elements (e.g., number of service hours experienced, number of participants completing the entire program) and immediate effects of program on participants (e.g., training produced learning gains; program experience improved participants' self-esteem) which are hypothesized to produce immediate or long-term outcomes?

(f) Various participant characteristics otherwise thought to influence outcome are assessed, covaried or examined as moderators in all groups?

3 Replication To what extent has the program been shown to be effective in each of the three design categories in two or more different studies (separate groups of participants), especially (in order of increasing persuasiveness) if they were:

(a) Conducted by the same investigators and providers but on different participants?

(b) Conducted by the same investigators but using different providers and participants?

(c) Conducted by different investigators using different providers and participants?

4 Effect size To what extent in each of the three design categories are the effect sizes associated with the program, measured in terms of odds ratios (Scott, Mason, & Chapman, 1999) and cost : benefit ratios, sufficient to justify replication?

5 Generality To what extent has the program been shown to be effective within each of the three design categories using as many of the following:

(a) *Participants* varying in gender, age, education, income, race and ethnicity, severity of risk or problem condition, and other characteristics thought to be related to outcome and program effectiveness?

(b) *Providers* who vary in education, training and experience in general and specifically related to this program?

(c) *Program characteristics* that vary, such as budgets, facilities and tangible and personnel resources and other aspects that may influence outcome (e.g., size of program, number of participants per provider, hours of service per participant)?

6 External validity specific to the replication circumstances To what extent has the program been shown to be effective within each of the three design categories using program characteristics as described in 5 above that are similar to those likely to characterize the replicated projects?

7 Feasibility of replication Are the program and its implementation process described comprehensively and packaged in a way that providers new to the program can faithfully replicate the program?

Characteristics of successful programs Does the literature support one or more characteristics that may be important to producing beneficial outcomes, because they are common components of programs that were successful, especially if they are not common components of programs that were not successful (such characteristics may be participant, provider and program characteristics [see 5 above] or the characteristics listed in Table 60.2)? Is there a strong theory of change and evidence on how or why the program is effective?

provide reviews of evidence on services for a variety of physical and behavioral health programs, and governments and foundations often operate consensus groups that bring together academic authorities to review literature and make specific recommendations regarding treatment approaches and services. The scheme in Table 60.1 makes more explicit the types of evidence and to some extent the standards that might be used by such groups to evaluate the literature.

When the Evidence is Not Sufficient

Except for the most thoroughly researched service programs (e.g., NFP), the research literature is not likely to cover all of the elements necessary to decide what kind of service will be most effective and how it should be implemented and operated. There may be gaps, uncertainties and technical limitations; no specific program may have a persuasive research track record; and doubts may emerge about how a program will need to be modified to fit the local clientele, service staff and circumstances.

An alternative to prescribing a specific service program is to provide *guidelines* for service creation and operation that are supported by research and that permit creativity and flexibility in matching the service to local circumstances. Sure Start was extreme in this regard, requiring only domains of services and the admonition that they be evidence-based. Fortunately, the general characteristics of successful service programs are remarkably similar across services aimed at preventing or treating a variety of different problems of children, youth and families. Table 60.2 (Groark & McCall, 2005) presents an integration across several lists of characteristics of successful programs in early childhood care and education (McCall, Larsen, & Ingram, 2003), family support (Layzer, Goodson, Bernstein, & Price, 2001; Schorr, 2003) and the prevention of adolescent problem behavior (Kumpfer & Alvarado, 2003; Nation, Crusto, Wandersman *et al.*, 2003). This list represents the beginning of a set of general guidelines which could be supplemented with additional characteristics unique to a specific type of service and problem area.

While such characteristics are useful as guidelines to local service professionals and funders, the characteristics themselves are rarely researched directly to assess their role in contributing to service effectiveness (but see Olds, Henderson, Kitzman *et al.*, 1999). Instead, they tend to be common characteristics of programs that have been demonstrated to produce benefits in participants. Nevertheless, coupled with other characteristics supported by research and best practices of service professionals,

Table 60.2 Characteristics of successful collaborations among diverse professionals. [Based upon Butterfoss, Goodman, & Wandersman, 1996; Grobe *et al.*, 1993; Kegerise, 1999; Mattessich & Monsey, 1992; Wandersman & Goodman, 1993. Table originally published in Groark & McCall (2005), reproduced with permission of the publisher.]

A common purpose A collaboration is beneficial and likely to succeed if it is created to accomplish a purpose that each of the participants needs or wants but that none of the participants alone or in smaller groups can attain. The common goal is necessary so that each participant focuses on a single set of criteria, and the mutual dependency keeps the coalition together and lays the ground work for mutual respect

Clear, concrete, achievable, specific goals A collaboration must identify common, clear, achievable and specific goals, both short-term process goals and long-term outcomes, plus a plan with concrete and realistic steps and a time schedule for achieving them

Selection of participants The collaboration should bring together at the outset all individuals and/or organizations that are necessary to accomplish the goals, even though the contribution of some may not be necessary until the final stage. Collaborations may be small, consisting of a scholar and a service agency (e.g., school, hospital, early childhood center) or much larger, involving several organizations of the same or different kinds (e.g., family support centers, early childhood centers, schools, public and private funders, elected officials, media representatives). Early and continuous involvement of key players (e.g., policy-makers) creates feelings of ownership and loyalty which may be needed later

Team players Participants must be selected for the resources and influence they may bring as well as for several personal characteristics, including the ability to get along with diverse people and groups, attend every meeting, represent their organization and commit its resources to the project, listen and understand divergent points of view as well as communicate clearly and honestly their own perspective, and accept a group decision even if it conflicts with their own self-interest

Diversity The diversity of participants that is needed can present challenges. Some participants may hold stereotypic attitudes towards others, but such beliefs do not always apply to the particular individuals and organizations represented in a collaboration. Ultimately, the members of each group need to learn the skills that each participant can contribute regardless of stereotypic roles

Strong, balanced, sensitive leadership Although all of the participants of a collaboration are necessary and should share in the rights, responsibilities and credit for the collaboration's activities and products, strong leadership is essential for any collaboration to function smoothly, efficiently and productively. The leader must be neither dictatorial nor a benign chairperson; instead, he or she must be strong enough to structure the process and activities of the collaboration, move the group in the appropriate direction, encourage participants to be appropriate to the group's process and goals, be sensitive to the needs and characteristics of each member without unnecessary accommodation, recognize and respect the contributions of each participant, and deal in a balanced and fair manner with disagreements and even conflicts within the group. It is a tall order; few people, especially scholars, excel in these characteristics; and occasionally collaborations must change leadership if necessary to preserve the collaboration and to achieve their goals such guidelines can communicate what research and professional practice have learned and permit modifications to fit local needs.

Consensus Groups

To produce such guidelines, consensus groups need to be composed not only of relevant scholars to assess the available research literature, but also service professionals, policy-makers and representatives of the intended clientele, and they need to be able to fill in the gaps in the research literature and come out with an action plan based upon the best available evidence and practice.

The Pathways Mapping Initiative (PMI) developed by Schorr (2003) represents a structured process by which such a group can create a "map" or set of recommended guidelines for the processes and characteristics that are effective in reaching the outcome under consideration. PMI recognizes that the traditional knowledge regarding a service program or a type of service is typically too limited, comes from a small number of interventions that have been adequately evaluated, and usually fails to identify all of the elements that actually make the service effective. The PMI process broadens the knowledge base by permitting reasonable judgments and plausible interpretations of a preponderance of evidence based on professional experience as well as program evaluations coupled with strong theory. The process also attempts to curb idiosyncratic opinion by insisting upon broad consensus among its diverse members. The product consists of a combination of actions needed to produce the desired outcome, the key ingredients that are likely to make those actions effective and the community contexts that will influence program effectiveness (for examples see www.PathwaysToOutcomes.org).

Proven Program or Principles?

In practice, the best solution may be somewhere between replicating a well-specified proven program (e.g., NFP) and a set of broad service domains (e.g., Sure Start), a structure and process (e.g., School Development Program) or principles of successful programs (Table 60.2). True replication of a highly specified program is likely a myth (Friesen & Koroloff, 1990; Green, Rodgers, & Johnson, 1999; McCall & Green, 2004) – it does not really take place – but vague or unspecified characteristics, such as in Sure Start, permit too much local variation and unsubstantiated program characteristics. A compromise of as much specification as research substantiates coupled with reasonable local flexibility is most desirable (and is likely to occur anyway).

Limits on the Transfer of Research and Best Practices to Communities

Whereas a set of guidelines reflecting the research literature and professional best practices may represent a necessary first step in creating and implementing effective service programs at a local level, it is not likely to be sufficient. First, simply communicating this information has not resulted in localities adopting the most effective program strategies (Ringwalt, Ennett, Vincus *et al.*, 2002; Wandersman & Florin, 2003). For example, until recently, the DARE program to prevent drug abuse had been adopted in 80% of school districts in the USA despite a research literature that showed it to be relatively ineffective (Ennett, Tobler, Ringwalt, & Fewling, 1994; General Accounting Office, 2003).

Research-to-Practice Gap

This gap may occur for several reasons.

1 The research knowledge is generated and communicated unidirectionally from researchers to practitioners and thus may be less relevant to the policy and practice context than is necessary.

2 The research and practice knowledge may be inadequately and ineffectively communicated to local practitioners and policy-makers.

3 Factors other than research and best practice contribute to service selection and effectiveness, such as the availability of a packaged program, ease of implementation, unique characteristics of local clientele, and local personnel and financial resources.

Chinman, Hannah, Wandersman *et al.* (2005) identified four broad factors that influence whether communities adopt, create and implement evidence-based services.

1 Implementing high-quality service programs is a complex process that requires considerably more knowledge and skill than is needed to simply follow a program manual.

2 Systems factors pertaining to co-ordination among different agencies and community readiness to adopt and maintain new strategies need to be considered.

3 Communities must have sufficient financial, technical and personnel resources.

4 Local clienteles and other circumstances may pose unique difficulties.

Technology Transfer

One approach to building such community capacity is technology transfer (Backer, David, & Soucy, 1995), which emphasizes training and technical assistance. However, these strategies alone have been only partly successful. Chinman, Hannah, Wandersman *et al.* (2005) reviewed a variety of training programs in substance abuse prevention, for example, and concluded that while such programs were helpful, their content was not always appropriate to the specific local context and there were often local barriers to incorporating the information into practice. Alternatively, having an intermediate set of professionals provide direct hands-on technical assistance similarly had limited effectiveness (Chinman, Hannah, Wandersman *et al.*, 2005). Such technical assistance, even when provided without cost, was not always welcomed at the local level; some minimal level of community capacity was required to make full use of such assistance, and community organizations seemed better able to utilize some forms of assistance (e.g., planning, implementation, organizational maintenance) than others (e.g., evaluation procedures, data analysis). While these results are based on experience with training and technical assistance in one area – substance abuse prevention – and their generality to other areas is unknown, many funders and service professionals believe that training and technical assistance as typically provided may be necessary but are not often sufficient to improve or create service programs.

Toward Effective Community Processes

The ability of local communities to adopt, create and implement effective services often requires a collaborative community process (Green, 2001), not simply technology transfer or a ready-made program to be replicated. Chinman, Hannah, Wandersman *et al.* (2005) suggest that this process must have genuine community involvement and commitment: the community must possess skills in a variety of domains; resources must be identified, acquired, and managed; and there must be a collective sense of community efficacy or power to manage the skills and resources and direct them toward successful outcomes. More specifically, such a community process requires:

1 Collaboration among a variety of stakeholders;
2 A strategy for designing services that fit local needs and circumstances;
3 Effective implementation and operational strategies;
4 Appropriate monitoring and evaluation; and
5 A plan to sustain the effectiveness and financing of services.

We consider each of these elements below.

Collaboration

While a specific service may be adopted or created by a single agency, many contemporary services are multi-sited or comprehensive, requiring collaboration across agencies and involving policy-makers, funders, academics, evaluators, the media and members of the intended clientele in their planning, implementation and operation. Such diverse collaborations have the potential benefit of converging the complementary expertise of such individuals to produce a better and more comprehensive service and to create involvement (i.e., "buy in") of major participants and groups that are necessary for the successful funding, roll-out, operation and sustainability of the service. Conversely, collaborations may take more time, require skilled leadership and sometimes involve individuals who obstruct progress for a variety of personal and professional reasons.

Membership

The members of a collaboration are typically *stakeholders* in the service to be created, that is, individuals who have an interest in the project, something to gain or lose as a function of its success or failure, and can contribute in some manner to its creation, implementation, operation and sustainability. Ideally, every member of the collaboration should be necessary to its success, and no smaller subset of the collaborators would be sufficient to carry out the project. Even collaborators whose contribution occurs late in the process should nevertheless be present from the beginning so they are knowledgeable about and involved in the project. Members of a community planning and implementation collaboration could include:

- Relevant service professionals representing key agencies to be involved in the future service;
- Policy-makers and funders, who have administrative responsibility for the type of proposed service, who will or could help to fund it, and who will be necessary to overcome local political barriers the service may face;
- Academics with the research and professional knowledge behind the guidelines, who can be used to steer the creation of the service;
- Evaluators, who will work with service providers to monitor and evaluate the implementation, service delivery process and outcomes for participants;
- Potential participants in the service, who can provide the perspective of the client in designing a user-friendly service; and
- Others who may be necessary for success (e.g., the media if public awareness is needed, celebrities if a public spokesperson would be helpful, business leaders if the service is to be integrated with or benefit private enterprise, and community leaders if the service will influence the wider community or will need community support to operate).

Members should be selected for their ability to fulfill their specific roles in the project and for their personal ability to function in a collaborative group. Collaborations often leave individual members with less control over the process and product than they are accustomed to exercising and require them to make compromises with cherished values and principles (e.g., evaluators not having random assignment). They should be committed to attend every meeting, represent their organization, bring its resources to the project, listen and understand divergent points of view, communicate their perspective honestly and accept a group decision even if it conflicts with their own self-interest.

Models of University–Community Relations

In the past, academics and program evaluators, generally from a local college or university, have often not been part of this process, but in the era of evidence-based practices and increased emphasis on evaluation, they have become more crucial to the planning and implementation processes. While each member of the collaboration is likely to have his or her own professional values and attitudes, those of academics and program evaluators may be less similar to, even at odds with, the values and attitudes of other collaborators (Groark & McCall, 1993, 1996, 2005; Mattessich & Monsey, 1992; McCall, Green, Strauss, & Groark, 1997; Shonkoff, 2000).

Historically, academics have worked with community professionals in different ways (Denner, Cooper, Lopez, & Dunbar, 1999). Often, academics simply serve as *expert consultants*. In this case, academics provide their knowledge in a rather unidirectional fashion. Sometimes, the *community sets the agenda*. In this case, the community tends to pick the problem, the methods and the services, selectively taking what information the academic provides that is useful to its purposes. The result is highly relevant to the community and thereby ecologically valid, but it tends to marginalize the role of evidence, monitoring and evaluation, making it less scientifically valid and difficult to replicate.

A better approach is the *true collaboration among stakeholders*, in which university and community members develop the project together, blending evidence and program evaluation with practitioner expertise and the resources and limits of the community. The interventions are developed in the community context with the community using its own resources, but research and evaluation priorities are selected collaboratively. In addition, consideration is given to broader policies and processes so that findings are relevant for general theory development. This model also requires the inclusion of various disciplines and diverse groups, thereby being more relevant to the ordinary lives of a wide variety of clientele.

One example of this collaborative approach is practiced by the University of Pittsburgh Office of Child Development (OCD; Groark & McCall, 1993, 1996, 2005; McCall, Green, Strauss *et al.*, 1997; McCall, Green, Groark *et al.*, 1999; McCall, Groark, & Nelkin, 2004). OCD employs:

1 Academic specialists in various aspects of child development who can bring research knowledge to the process;

2 Service professionals who are experienced in creating, implementing and managing innovative service demonstrations in collaboration with community agencies;

3 Program evaluation specialists who train service providers in monitoring and evaluation and who conduct evaluations on community-based programs in a collaborative and participatory manner with the service agency; and

4 Specialists experienced in policy and governmental service administration who work with policy-makers to create better policies and administrative services for children and families.

Some or all of these types of OCD staff may work on a specific project in collaboration with other academics, community service agencies and professionals, and administrators and policy-makers; each component of this team influences the others. The essential ingredient, however, is an attitude that emphasizes partnership – sharing of responsibility, power, control and credit among all stakeholders, who collaborate to achieve a common goal.

Characteristics of Successful Collaborations

Successful collaborations tend to have certain characteristics in common (Butterfoss, Goodman, & Wandersman, 1996; Grobe, Curnan, Melchior *et al.*, 1993; Kegerise, 1999; Mattessich & Monsey, 1992; Wandersman & Goodman, 1993). First, they have a *common purpose*. Each participant must value the main common purpose of the collaboration, which focuses each participant on a single set of criteria, and the mutual dependency helps to keep the coalition together and produce mutual respect. The common purpose must be articulated early and clearly so that it becomes the touchstone that helps members focus on the reason for the collaboration during debates. Therefore, it is helpful to write down the common purpose in the manner of a vision or mission statement which can be reviewed periodically to keep members operating in the same direction and also to constitute criteria for deciding whether each major decision contributes to accomplishing the stated purpose.

Further, the collaboration should establish *common, clear, achievable and specific goals*; *a plan with concrete and realistic steps*; and a *timetable for achieving them*. This plan becomes the roadmap for all future activities, and a monitoring method that helps institute controls on priorities for each partner by specifying who is responsible for which tasks and how they will be measured.

Strong, balanced, sensitive leadership is required. Although all participants should share in the rights, responsibilities and credit for the collaboration's activities and products, strong leadership is required to make the process work. The leader may be a local participant or an independent facilitator, but he or she needs to have or earn the respect and trust of all group members. The ideal leader needs to be sensitive and fair, hearing all sides of a debate, but at the same time be neither dictatorial nor benign. The leader must structure the process and move it along at an appropriate pace without restricting participation by each member and by encouraging participation by all. Further, the leader needs to deal in a balanced and fair manner with disagreements and conflicts within the group while respecting the diverse contribution of each participant. Few people have all these characteristics, yet such leadership is crucial to an effective collaboration (Groark & McCall, 2005; McCall, Green, Strauss *et al.*, 1997).

Program Development and Design

Effective program development requires establishing and operating a successful collaboration, preparing and planning, and then conducting a logic model program development process. Many of the principles described in this section appear obvious or common sense, but in our experience they are not always followed.

Operating Successful Collaborations

Successful collaborations tend to operate in a specific way (Butterfoss, Goodman, & Wandersman, 1996; Groark & McCall, 2005; Grobe, Curnan, Melchior *et al.*, 1993; Kegerise, 1999; Mattessich & Monsey, 1992; Wandersman & Goodman, 1993). They have regular meetings with required attendance, and they begin by identifying the values and perspectives of each participant and what they bring to the collaboration. The skills, resources, roles and responsibilities of each participant should be identified, as well as major resources and time commitments that will be needed.

If the collaboration is large and complex, written policies or even bylaws and procedures should be considered. The group should decide how decisions will be made, whether votes will be taken and how ties will be resolved. Ultimately, the collaboration should develop a "business plan" that specifies potential resources and expenses as well as goals, procedures, responsibilities, and legislative, legal and administrative needs. Finally, the collaboration itself may need to be monitored and periodically reviewed. Occasionally, procedures need to be modified, and sometimes even the leadership needs to change.

Planning and Preparation

An initial step in preparing to develop a new service program is to *understand the current situation*; namely, the nature of the intended participant group and its cultural and social values, political opportunities and constraints, and the history of the problem and previous attempts to remediate it (for service planning in general see chapter 71). For example, in the case of an intervention project to improve caregiving in the orphanages of St. Petersburg, Russian Federation Groark, Muhamedrahimov, Palmov, Nikiforova, & McCall, 2005; Muhamedrahimov, Palmov, Nikiforova, Groark, & McCall, 2004), this meant understanding the following:

1 How caregiving was currently provided, the rules and regulations governing the orphanage;
2 Why various practices exist (e.g., caregivers do not get socio-emotionally close to children to avoid the pain of separation later);
3 That caregivers work 24-h shifts to minimize transportation expenses and to have 3 days off to be with their own children or work in other jobs; and
4 There is a long tradition of adult-directed teaching.

Next, *learn what has been tried before, both locally and nationally*. This step includes a review of the service literature, which may focus on the guidelines offered by a consensus group or brief reviews provided by local scholars plus knowledge of what has been tried specifically in the target locale. In the case of the orphanage project, there were few precedents, but there was a literature on early socioemotional development (e.g., attachment) and on the components of early childhood care and education programs that correlate with children's development.

A *needs assessment*, conducted community-wide or specific to a particular location, agency, or program is very useful. Community needs assessments can be conducted by an independent organization with the assistance of a diverse committee of practice professionals, funders, policy-makers, scholars and service participants, or it could be the collaborative community group conducting this program development process. The needs assessment consists of reviewing the scholarly literature on the issue (e.g., after-school programming, adolescent crime prevention, comprehensive family services); determining the frequency and severity of the problems to be prevented or remediated in the target area; and specifying the short- and long-term consequences to individuals and costs to society if nothing is done or current services were continued, the nature and extent of existing services, the geographic distribution of problems versus services, available personnel and their training and preparation, and resources available or needed.

Creating the Planning Document

The program planning process should produce a written planning document. This is sometimes a grant proposal in which a government or private funder has issued a request for proposals that specifies the target population, goals and services it wants to fund. Alternatively, the diverse community-collaborative group may plan the services with or without a set of guidelines or request for proposals.

Several structured formats are available to facilitate program development. For example, the Strengths, Weaknesses, Opportunities, and Threats (SWOT) analysis (Kearns, 1992) provides an organized approach for general strategic planning, perhaps for an entire service agency. More specific to program development is the logic model. While research on the effectiveness of the logic model approach is limited, those who use it recommend it and it is widely advocated. For example, the Kellogg Foundation (1998, 2000) provided a detailed guide for conducting a generic logic model that could be applied to any service need. Benson (1997) presented an asset-based needs assessment pertaining to adolescents, and Catalano and Hawkins (1996) described risk and protective factors and suggestions for program development for preventing adolescent antisocial behavior. More recently, the logic model concept has been packaged into the Getting to Outcomes (GTO) process (Wandersman, Imm, Chinman, & Kaftarian, 1999, 2000), which is available in several formats pertinent to particular problems (Chinman, Imm, & Wandersman, 2004; Fisher, Imm, Chinman, & Wandersman, 2006; http://www.RAND.org/publications/TR/TR101). The GTO approach will soon be available in an interactive web-based technology system, *i*GTO.

Logic Model Approach

The logic model approach consists of a series of questions that provide a structure and logic to the program planning process. The logic model process is common sense, but not commonly conducted. It forces the collaborative to think clearly, specifically and realistically about needs, goals, participants, services, rationale, measures of process and outcome, and resources, and to make sure these components are aligned. Proponents of the logic model approach argue that it produces a clear integrated logical program that is more likely to be effective plus an evaluation that is more likely to be relevant and to contribute to program improvement and understanding how the program works (Armstrong & Barsion, 2006; Axford, Berry, & Little, 2006; W. K. Kellogg Foundation, 1998, 2000). Whereas the specific questions vary from one approach to another, generally logic models address the following questions (Groark & McCall, 2005).

What is the Ultimate Goal of the Services?

Specifically, what is the problem or need and what should be the situation if the new intervention or services were completely successful? This is the "blue sky question" – in the ideal case, what should the intervention or services accomplish? In the case of the orphanage project, the ultimate goal was that children should develop at typical levels in all domains.

What Measures Would Indicate that this Long-term Goal has been Achieved?

Often, the goal stated is phrased in very general terms (e.g., children develop typically) so in this step that goal must be specified in measurable terms. For example, the measurable long-term goal for the orphanage children was for them to reach heights, weights, and developmental scores (across personal, social, communication and cognition dimensions) comparable to non-orphanage parent-reared children.

Care must be taken to ensure that the indices of success indeed reflect the long-term goal and are reasonable and potentially attainable. Some policy-makers and funders prefer aggressive goals, such as "cutting the teenage pregnancy rate by 50%." The goal is worthwhile, but likely not attainable; should a program that cuts the rate by 25% be deemed a failure relative to such a lofty goal? Instead, determine both the minimum level of improvement that would be considered "success" as well as the maximum level likely to be attained. Thus, a goal of reducing the rate by 20–40% might be appropriate (no one will be upset if the program achieves a 45% reduction). The goal should also be well-specified – a reduction of 20–40% relative to what (e.g., current levels, a comparison group), in what length of time (e.g., 2 years, 5 years), for what ages of adolescents? Measuring instruments should also be specified when different assessment tools, reflecting different emphases, are available.

Who are the Targeted Participants?

Who do you want to help, how will they be identified, what are their characteristics and how many are there? In the orphanage project the participants were all caregivers and children in three orphanages, but in the case of Sure Start the services would be located in low-income neighborhoods and serve anyone living there. Should outreach efforts be made to recruit families, who should be employed to do this and how should it be done? For instance, should workers be hired from the neighborhood to recruit families because target families can relate to them, or would that cross the line of privacy?

What Services Can be Provided that will Produce the Long-term Goal?

First, determine a promising theory of change (Chen & Rossi, 1983, 1987), then identify services that follow from the theory that have been tried by others and found to be successful. This is the step in which theory, research evidence and best practice guidelines enter the process. What are the elements and characteristics of successful services, and what modifications need to be made to fit the local clientele and social and political circumstances? This step should have at least two major characteristics: first, there needs to be a clear rationale for why the proposed services should produce the intended outcome (i.e., theory of change), and, second, there should be some level of evidence (e.g., Table 60.1) to justify the potential effectiveness of the services, service components and characteristics. What frequency and intensity of services are sufficient to produce the intended benefits? Do the services match the risk level of participants? In the orphanage project, attachment theory provided a theoretical rationale for reducing the number of caregivers, making them more consistent in the lives of children and having them behave in a warm, caring, sensitive and responsive manner. Also, there was an empirical rationale for smaller group size, better caregiver : child ratios, age and disability integration, and child-directed caregiver–child interactions. Together, these changes should promote all aspects of children's development.

How Will You Know that the Intended Services are Actually Delivered and Match the Plan in Character and Intensity?

This step requires a plan to monitor the delivery of services, not just how many participants receive which services but whether the nature and extent of the services are consistent with the plan (i.e., "program fidelity"). Perhaps a management information system (MIS) needs to be developed. In the case of the CCDP, did the case manager work with the family to identify their strengths, did the family identify their needs and put them into a priority sequence, did the case manager develop a relationship of trust and support with the family and did the family participate in services relevant to the family's goals?

What are the Short-term Goals and Measures?

What should be the first beneficial outcomes of such services, and is there evidence that achieving the short-term outcomes predicts achieving the long-term outcomes? In the orphanage project, did HOME Inventory scores of caregivers' behavior on the wards increase, because there is evidence that higher scores are related to better developmental outcomes for children? Short-term goals should be laddered from goals that are obvious and easily attained to goals that are more difficult to achieve, so that the project will have some success.

What is an Appropriate Timeline Both to Deliver Services and to Expect Outcomes?

It is important to be realistic in planning the timeline for both implementation and when short- and long-term outcomes are likely to be achieved. Sometimes, a neighborhood is not ready for a needed service, and this should be anticipated. For example, a funder may suggest establishing a family support center in a particular low-income community. To do so, there must be community "will" for such a center, a recognized and respected leader, an agency willing to administer the program and other resources. If not, program developers may need a year or more to hold town meetings to assess the community's true interest and capacity and provide recreational services to gain trust.

What is a Reasonable Budget to Deliver These Services and Measure Their Implementation and Effectiveness?

This step begins with assigning costs to all of the elements in the previous steps, determining if the total budget is feasible and, if not, revisiting each of the above steps and making modifications to meet a specified budget. Ultimately, the group needs to decide whether a program that is likely to be effective can be operated for the amount of money available. This is also one of several reasons why it is helpful to have policy-makers and funders at the table during this planning process.

Implementation

Implementation is as crucial a process to successful services as program development, but it is often forgotten and rarely studied. Further, implementing new services in new communities may require months or even years to build trust among potential participants, and several cohorts of participants and much trial and error may transpire before even experienced teams of providers refine procedures sufficiently to produce benefits in participants (Fixsen, Naoom, Blase *et al.*, 2005).

Community Collaborative

The same community collaborative that designs the program may also be used to oversee its implementation. Such a committee should have the characteristics of, and operate according to the principles for, collaborations described above, and implementation should strive to have the characteristics of successful programs given in Table 60.2.

Characteristics of Good Implementation

Crucial to good implementation is to have a strong leader who relates to the diverse organizing committee plus a well-educated, trained and experienced staff who are supervised in a supportive and encouraging manner on a regular basis. Studies show that training alone is relatively ineffective unless it is accompanied by such supervision (Morrow, Townsend, & Pickering, 1991). Management needs to involve the staff in understanding the purpose of the services, their roles and the intended outcomes, perhaps by involving some of them in the logic model process described above or reviewing that process so that they can contribute modifications in the design of the services. If staff collect data, they need to understand why it is necessary and how they can use the data to guide and improve their services.

Staff also need structural supports, including reasonable work loads and the availability of resources such as technology, consultants and training necessary to do their jobs. Studies also show that teacher education and training tend not to be related to positive outcomes for children in early care and education settings, for example, unless group size and teacher : child ratios are small enough so that teachers can exercise the best practices of their training (Love, Schochet, & Meckstroth, 1996).

A management information system may be needed for large and multi-sited projects that systematizes in a uniform manner participant information, services delivered, and short- and long-term outcome measures. Directors and supervisors need to monitor such information to determine that the services are being delivered according to plan, including whether the participants are those who were originally targeted; whether services are delivered in a timely and consistent way and at an intensity or frequency sufficient to produce benefits; and whether short-term goals are being achieved.

Mid-course corrections may be necessary. For example, one program aimed at providing services and support to drug and alcohol abusing adolescent mothers found after 2 years of operation that the average age of the mothers was 26 years, not the adolescents the program was designed to target. Staff reported that drug and alcohol abusing adolescents did not perceive that they had a problem, because drug and alcohol use and abuse were rampant in their peer group; it seemed to take nearly 10 years for such mothers to recognize that they had a problem and to seek help. The project could change its target group to older mothers who were motivated to use the services and/or it could make greater efforts to recruit adolescents. It was decided to do both, using the older mothers to convince the adolescents that they needed help and enroll them in the service.

Evaluation

Most large comprehensive multi-sited services have a required monitoring and evaluation program. The funder may contract with a central and independent evaluation team, which may prescribe and conduct monitoring and evaluation for all sites, such as in Sure Start and CCDP. Smaller programs should also have a monitoring and evaluation plan, and select appropriate indices of participants, services and outcomes during the logic model process.

Program evaluation is a specialized skill, and relatively few service professionals have the appropriate training. Furthermore, simply providing local service professionals with technical assistance in evaluation does not work very well (Chinman, Hannah, Wandersman *et al.*, 2005). Consequently, large-scale and multi-sited service projects often have a central team of independent evaluators who should be part of the diverse community planning and implementation group and contribute to the program guidelines as well as collaboratively design the monitoring and evaluation plan, specify measurements, conduct the assessments, analyze the data, and report on the process and outcome effectiveness of the project. Alternatively, some communities have local evaluation teams that work with local agencies to design and conduct local evaluations, even the evaluation of the local site of a multi-sited national intervention, such as in Early Head Start (McCall, Green, Strauss *et al.*, 1997; McCall, Green, Groark *et al.*, 1999).

Modern service programs, especially services that are tailored to client needs and characteristics at both the site and individual participant levels, pose several issues for traditional methods of evaluation. We consider a few such issues below.

Independent Versus Participant/Collaborative Evaluation

Historically, innovative services were often created by a university scholar who both implemented the intervention and evaluated its effectiveness. Conversely, funders feel it is a conflict of interest for the people who create and implement a service to evaluate it, so they prefer an independent evaluation team.

In the past, independent evaluators have sometimes been distant from the program and the services staff, have "done the evaluation to the project," and sometimes issued reports that policy-makers and practitioners regarded as having missed the point of the service program. A modern and compromise strategy is participatory or empowerment evaluation (Fetterman, 1993; Fetterman, Kaftarian, & Wandersman, 1996; McCall, Green, Strauss *et al.*, 1997; McCall, Green, Groark *et al.*, 1999), in which evaluators and service professionals work together from the beginning of program development to monitor and evaluate the process and outcome of the service program. Participatory evaluation is more likely to produce useful results, because the measures and design are determined collaboratively with service professionals.

Central Versus Decentralized Evaluations

Large multi-sited service programs have often had a single evaluation team that designs and collects the data for all sites (e.g., Sure Start, CCDP). Such an approach has the benefit of a uniform evaluation of all sites, and it works best when the service program is prescribed in great detail and expected to be implemented in a uniform manner at each site. However, many modern service programs permit flexibility and modification to fit local circumstances, and even programs intended to be uniform across sites nevertheless are often implemented in different ways at different sites (Gilliam, Ripple, Zigler *et al.*, 2000; McCall, Larsen, & Ingram, 2003). A compromise strategy was used by the Early Head Start Research Consortium, which had a common core of service themes and a central evaluator, but each site had local evaluators who conducted the core assessments plus measures more pertinent to their local program emphases (Administration for Children and Families, 2002; Love Kisker, Ross *et al.*, 2005).

The Rush to Evaluate Outcomes

Understandably, funders and policy-makers are anxious to determine the effectiveness of programs they fund, and often there is an emphasis on assessing outcomes (i.e., benefits to participants) in the first cohort of participants. But the first "outcome" of any program should be that the services were implemented as planned for the targeted participants with the frequency and intensity that are likely to produce benefits. Until the services are delivered with such "fidelity," it is unreasonable to expect outcome benefits to participants; and it may well take two or three cohorts of participants before the program operates smoothly and according to plan. This fact prompted Campbell (1987), a patriarch of program evaluation, to admonish: "Evaluate no program before it's proud."

Overemphasis on Gold Standard Methodology

Scholars, policy-makers, funders and practice professionals have come to value the randomized clinical trial as the gold standard of applied research and program evaluation, so much so that often entire literatures using other methodological approaches are completely dismissed (e.g., as in review articles that only include randomized trials). While in some fields (e.g., education) there has been an avoidance of randomized trials, and some scholars (Cook, 2002) have called for greater use of this gold standard, in other fields randomized trials are overemphasized (McCall & Green, 2004).

While acknowledging the potential benefits of random assignment, McCall and Green (2004) argue that randomized trials work best in a double-blind design in which participants do not know which treatment they are being given and have relatively little influence over the success of the treatment (e.g., drug versus placebo studies). However, in behavioral interventions, participants are almost never blind to which treatment group they have been assigned, and participants' values and perceptions of the treatment can have substantial influence on how effective the treatment is for them. As a result, some participants display "reactive disappointment" to being in the control group and acquire the treatment services for themselves, shrinking the difference between the "treatment" and the "control/comparison" groups. For example, in one evaluation of the SDP (Millsap, Chase, Obeidallah *et al.*, 2000, reported by Datta, 2003) in which schools were assigned to treatment versus control conditions, several of the control schools implemented some or all of the Comer principles on their own. The result was that there was minimum difference between treatment and control schools in the amount of SDP "treatment" and in outcomes. However, the extent to which schools implemented the SDP principles within the control group was related to outcome. A gold standard purist would discount this finding because the beneficial outcomes were confounded with school motivation. Technically true, but a policy-maker or superintendent might be sufficiently persuaded to adopt the SDP strategy if it could be effectively implemented.

Further, after a demonstration project is completed successfully and services are offered routinely, they are never randomly assigned. So "participant bias" will always be in effect; from a practical standpoint, the "biased" demonstration sample is the group from which generalizations to future clients should be made (of course, one wants to know if such people would improve without a service program).

Also, such "bias" might be critical for program success. For example, if divorcing couples are randomly assigned to divorce mediation versus court-ordered settlements, it is possible that some couples cannot co-operate sufficiently for mediation to work whereas other couples would be dissatisfied with a divorce arrangement that was prescribed for them by a judge. The result of a strictly randomized trial might be no difference in parental satisfaction and adjustment of children between these two approaches. However, if couples were allowed to choose which approach they wanted, both strategies might be shown to be effective for those who choose them, more effective than for those who are randomly assigned to each approach. Notice that this is a case in which the randomized design produced a low effect size, contrary to those who sometimes claim that randomized designs provide a maximum effect size.

Consequently, McCall and Green (2004) advocated a greater balance of and respect for different methodological approaches which provide different kinds of information about an intervention or service. Results from a comprehensive set of approaches are more likely to provide a more complete and better understanding of the effectiveness of that service. Different research designs and statistical strategies are described elsewhere (McCall & Green, 2004; Rossi, Lipsey, & Freeman, 2004).

Intent-to-Treat Analyses

Another gold standard approach to program evaluation is to conduct intent-to-treat analyses in which the outcomes are assessed on all participants who were *assigned* to the treatment conditions regardless of whether they actually *experienced* them, such as in Sure Start. This approach preserves the random assignment feature; it "avoids" the problem of selective dropouts, which is common among the high-risk populations that many services target, by including the dropouts as if they were treated participants. This strategy works well when the treatment program is uniformly delivered to all participants and the number of actual dropouts is small.

However, including dropouts inflates the error within the treatment but not the control condition; and as the number of dropouts and partially treated participants increases, detecting significant differences between treatment and comparison groups becomes less likely. Further, it is logically absurd to pretend that dropouts received the treatment when they did not. In this case, it seems reasonable to conduct both the intent-to-treat analysis as well as an analysis that is restricted to fully treated subjects (perhaps limiting the control subjects to those who were similar to the fully treated participants through propensity score analysis; Rosenbaum & Rubin, 1983).

The intent-to-treat strategy also seems limited if not inappropriate when the treatment itself is different from participant to participant. In the CCDP, families chose their goals, and only approximately 15% of the treatment families chose more education and 10% of the control families decided on their own to undertake more education. Yet the evaluation asked the percentage of *all* participants in both treatment and control groups who attained more education. Not surprisingly, few did (i.e., certainly less than 15–10%), and there was a very small and insignificant difference in the rates between the two groups (McCall, Ryan, & Plemons, 2003; St. Pierre, Layzer, Goodson, & Bernstein, 1994, 1997a,b). Clearly, evaluation analyses must consider different goals and services delivered within the treatment and control groups with designs and analyses that consider that modern services are often individualized (McCall & Green, 2004).

Sustainability and Replication

Sustainability refers to at least two outcomes:

1 Maintaining the quality of services and benefit to participants over time; and

2 Keeping the service funded after the initial demonstration grant expires.

Replication refers to attempts to reproduce the program in new sites with similar populations with the intent of replicating the original benefits and outcomes.

Sustaining Program Benefits

It is not uncommon for there to be unusual passion, commitment and dedication among program directors and staff during the implementation of a new service program, and such commitment often wanes over subsequent years. Also, staff turnover and changes in the participant group may also lessen the effectiveness of the services over time.

An MIS and a good plan for monitoring participants and services can provide feedback to directors regarding changes in the characteristics of participants and the manner and intensity with which services are being delivered. The director and supervisory staff need to provide continuous supervision and monitoring, even of highly experienced staff, to maintain standards and program effectiveness. Supervision must be formative and reflective (Johnson & Tittnich, 2004) so that continuing improvements are made in services with staff input and enthusiasm for the program is maintained.

It also helps to design the original demonstration in such a way that the intervention can be maintained. Building intellectual and skill capacity in the community is essential in sustaining the quality of services. For example, the St. Petersburg (Russia) orphanage project (Groark, Muhamedrahimov, Palmov *et al.*, 2005; Muhamedrahimov, Palmov, Nikiforova *et al.*, 2004) used a train-the-trainer approach in which a written curriculum was produced and a specialist trained the professionals in each orphanage. Those professionals were available to train new caregivers who replaced those who left and thus keep the level of performance high in the orphanage over time.

Sustaining Funding

Many interventions and services are initiated with a demonstration project, which is often funded at relatively generous levels. However, once the demonstration is completed, it can be much more difficult to obtain funding to continue the program, even when the evaluation has clearly demonstrated program benefits to participants. Also, when governments assume funding after demonstration programs, it is often at substantially lower levels but with the same expectations for success – it is the government's penchant to expect champagne benefits on a beer budget.

Programs that must be trimmed to fit smaller budgets need to analyze and break down the program into its components, including personnel, participants, the types and extent of services provided, as well as the costs involved. The research literature on this type of service and characteristics of successful programs should be used as the criteria for determining which aspects of the service are likely to be crucial and which aspects appear less important and are likely candidates for trimming. Sometimes, the number of participants may need to be reduced to maintain program quality within the available budget. This is always a very difficult choice for service professionals, but it seems obvious that it is better to be effective with fewer participants than to be ineffective with many.

One strategy in sustaining programs after their initial demonstration is to invite potential long-term funders (e.g., the director of children and youth services for the geographical area in which the service program resides) to be on the community collaborative committee that designs, implements and oversees the management of the demonstration program. By involving such funders at the beginning, they are more likely to be committed and to feel a sense of ownership of the program after the initial demonstration and therefore more likely to provide funds to sustain it.

The results of a successful evaluation should be disseminated widely and specifically to potential funders. Further, results need to be packaged differently for different audiences, from detailed technical reports for scholarly journals to one-page summaries for policy-makers.

It is also helpful to have cultivated one or more "champions," who may be policy-makers, funders, influential citizens, celebrities or media professionals. They also should be part of the community collaborative that designs and oversees the project from the beginning, so they are fully informed and feel partial ownership of the service. Eventually, their job is to "sell" the program to policy-makers, funders and the general public.

Sometimes, successful participants can be the most powerful advocates for sustaining a service. Consider a drug and alcohol abusing mother of two young children who is assisted by a family support program to become substance free, develop marketable skills, become employed, and whose children wind up in honors classes. If she is willing to tell her story publicly, she can do more to sell a program than all the carefully collected evaluation results. It is difficult for legislators to see such a success story and then vote against funds to offer the same opportunities to others.

Replication

Replicating a program in a new locale with new staff and clientele requires the same planning process and ingredients for successful implementation as for the original (i.e., leadership, committed staff, perceived need for change, program development with the logic model process). Does the new director have sufficient commitment, energy and confidence to "pull this off"? Is the staff capable and receptive to change? Are the local social, cultural and economic conditions conducive to change? If not, these elements need to be resolved before or during the program planning process.

Conclusions

There is no "silver bullet" or step-by-step manual that will guarantee that community-based interventions services will be successful. However, there are principles and strategies suggested by research that help to create highly effective programs. They start with a thorough process of planning that customizes the service and its delivery to the clientele and context. It includes developing a solid collaboration of diverse but relevant stakeholders who become knowledgeable loyal partners. Together these stakeholders develop a common purpose, goals, and clearly agreed-upon rules, and are led by a fair, balanced and respected leader. They employ a structured planning process that designs a program founded on theoretical and practice evidence and based on characteristics that work, while always being sensitive to future sustainability and replication issues. The program is continuously monitored for service improvement and evaluated for interim and long-term outcomes. Moreover, all steps are documented and frequently reviewed by senior management and the diverse oversight group for "lessons learned." Finally, outcomes and lessons learned are disseminated to policy-makers and practitioners for sustainability in the current sites and replications to improve services and lives elsewhere.

References

Administration for Children and Families. (2002). *Making a difference in the lives of infants and toddlers and their families: The impacts of Early Head Start*. Washington, DC: US Department of Health and Human Services.

APA Presidential Task Force on Evidence-Based Practice. (2006). Evidence-based practice in psychology. *American Psychologist*, *61*, 271–285.

Armstrong, E. G., & Barsion, S. J. (2006). Using an outcomes-logic-model approach to evaluate a faculty development program for medical educators. *Journal of the Association of American Medical Colleges*, *51*, 483–488.

Axford, N., Berry, V., & Little, M. (2006). Enhancing service evaluability: Lessons learned from a programme for disaffected young people. *Children and Society*, *14*, 287–298.

Backer, T., David, S., & Soucy, G. (Eds.). (1995). *Reviewing the behavioral science knowledge base on technology transfer*. Washington, DC: National Institute of Drug Abuse.

Baumrind, D., Larzelere, R. E., & Cowen, P. A. (2002). Ordinary physical punishment: Is it harmful? Comment on Gershoff, 2002. *Psychological Bulletin*, *128*, 588–589.

Belksy, J., Melhuish, E. Barnes, J., Leyland, A. H., & Romaniuk, H. (2006). Effects of Sure Start local programmes on children and families: Early findings from a quasi-experimental, cross-sectional study. *British Medical Journal*, *332*, 1476.

Benson, P. (1997). *All kids are our kids: What communities must do to raise caring and responsible children and adolescents*. San Francisco, CA: Jossey-Bass.

Butterfoss, F. D., Goodman, R. M., & Wandersman, A. (1996). Community coalitions for prevention and health promotion: Factors predicting satisfaction, participation and planning. *Health Education Quarterly*, *23*, 65–79.

Campbell, D. T. (1987). Problems for the experimenting society in the interface between evaluations and service providers. In S. L. Kagan, D. R. Powell, B. Weissbourd, & E. F. Zigler (Eds.), *America's family support programs* (pp. 345–351). New Haven, CT: Yale University Press.

Catalano, R., & Hawkins, J. D. (1996). The social development model: A theory of antisocial behavior. In J. D. Hawkins (Ed.), *Delinquency and crime: Current theories* (pp. 149–197). New York, NY: Cambridge University Press.

Ceci, S. J., & Papierno, P. B. (2005). The rhetoric and reality of gap closing: When the "have nots " gain but the "haves" gain even more. *American Psychologist*, *60*, 149–160.

Centers for Disease Control. (2006). Guide to community preventive services. Accessed from www.thecommunityguide.org. (January 4, 2008).

Chambless, D. L., & Hollon, S. D. (1998). Defining empirically supported therapies. *Journal of Consulting and Clinical Psychology*, *66*, 7–18.

Chen, H., & Rossi, P. (1983). Evaluating with sense: The theory-driven approach. *Evaluation Review*, *7*, 283–302.

Chen, H., & Rossi, P. (1987). The theory-driven approach to validity. *Evaluation and Program Planning*, *10*, 95–103.

Chinman, M., Hannah, G., Wandersman, A., Ebener, P., Hunter, S. B., & Imm, P. (2005). Developing a community science research agenda for building community capacity for effective preventive interventions. *American Journal of Community Psychology*, *35*, 143–157.

Chinman, M., Imm, P., & Wandersman, A. (2004). *Getting to Outcomes 2004: Promoting accountability through methods and tools for planning, implementation, and evaluation*. Santa Monica, CA: RAND Corporation Technical Report. Accessed from http://www.rand.org/publs/technical-reports/TR101/. (January 4, 2008).

Comer, J. P. (1988). Educating poor minority children. *Scientific American*, *259*, 42–48.

Comer, J. P., Haynes, N. M., Joyner, E. T., & Ben Avie, M. (1996). *Rallying the whole village: The Comer process for reforming education*. New York: Teachers College Press.

Cook, T. D. (2002). Randomized experiments in educational policy research: A critical examination of the reasons the educational evaluation community has offered for not doing them. *Educational Evaluation and Policy Analysis*, *24*, 175–199.

Cook, T. D., & Campbell, D. T. (1979). *Quasi-experimentation: Design and analysis issues for field settings*. Chicago, IL: Rand McNally.

Cook, T. D., Hunt, H.D., & Murphy, R. F. (1998). *Comer's School Development Program in Chicago: A theory-based evaluation*. Evanston, IL: Northwestern University Institute for Policy Research.

Cook, T. D., Habib, F. N., Phillips, M., Settersten, R. A., Shagle, S. C., & Degirmencioglu, S. M. (2000). Comer's School Development Program in Prince George's County, Maryland: A theory-based evaluation. *American Educational Research Journal*, *36*, 543–597.

Cooper, H. (1998). *Synthesizing research: A guide for literature reviews*. Thousand Oaks, CA: Sage.

Datta, L. E. (2003). Avoiding unwarranted death by evaluation. *Evaluation Exchange*, *9*, 5.

Denner, J., Cooper, C. R., Lopez, E. M., & Dunbar, N. (1999). Beyond "giving science away": How university-community partnerships inform youth programs, research, and policy. *Society for Research in Child Development Social Policy Report*, *13*.

Early Head Start. www.acf.hhs.gov/programs/OPRE/EHS/EHS/. (January 4, 2008).

Ennett, S. T., Tobler, N. S., Ringwalt, C. L., & Fewling, R. L. (1994). How effective is drug abuse resistance education? A meta-analysis of Project DARE outcome evaluations. *American Journal of Public Health*, *84*, 1394–1401.

Fergusson, D. M., Grant, H., Horwood, L. J., & Ridder, E. M. (2005). Randomized trial of the Early Start Program of Home Visitation. *Pediatrics*, *116*, 803–809.

Fergusson, D. M., Grant, H., Horwood, L. J., & Ridder, E. M. (2006). Randomized trial of the Early Start Program of Home Visitation: Parent and family outcomes. *Pediatrics*, *117*, 781–786.

Fetterman, D. M. (1993). Empowerment evaluation. *Evaluation Practice*, *15*, 1–15.

Fetterman, D. M., Kaftarian, S. J., & Wandersman, A. (1996). *Empowerment evaluation: Knowledge and tools for self-assessment and accountability*. Thousand Oaks, CA: Sage.

Fisher, D., Imm, P., Chinman, M., & Wandersman, A. (2006). *Getting to outcomes with developmental assets: Ten steps to measuring success in youth programs and communities*. Minneapolis, MN: Search Institute. Accessed from www.search-institute.org. (January 4, 2008).

Fixsen, D. L., Naoom, S. F., Blase, K. A., Friedman, R. M., & Wallace, F. (2005). Implementation research: A synthesis of the literature. Tampa, FL: University of South Florida, Louis de la Parte Florida Mental Health Institute, the National Implementation Research Network (FMHI Publication #231).

Friesen, B. J., & Koroloff, N. M. (1990). Family-centered services: Implications for mental health administration and research. *Journal of Mental Health Administration*, *17*, 13–25.

General Accounting Office. (2003, January 15). *Youth illicit drug use prevention: DARE long-term evaluations and federal efforts to identify effective programs* (GAO-03-172R).

Gilliam, W. S., Ripple, C. H., Zigler, E. F., & Leiter, V. (2000). The Comprehensive Child Development Program: What went wrong? *Early Childhood Research Quarterly*, *15*, 41–59.

Green, L. W. (2001). From research to "best practices" in other settings and populations. *American Journal of Health Behavior*, *25*, 165–178.

Green, B., Rodgers, A., & Johnson, S. (1999). Understanding patterns of service delivery and participation in community-based family support programs. *Children's Services: Social Policy, Research, and Practice*, *2*, 1–22.

Groark, C. J., & McCall, R. B. (1993). Building mutually beneficial collaborations between researchers and community service professionals. *Newsletter of the Society for Research in Child Development, Spring*, 6–14.

Groark, C. J., & McCall, R. B. (1996). Building successful university–community human service agency collaborations. In C. D. Fisher, J. P. Murray, & I. E. Sigel (Eds.), *Applied developmental science: Graduate training for diverse disciplines and educational settings* (pp. 237–251). Norwood, NJ: Ablex.

Groark, C. J., & McCall, R. B. (2005). Integrating developmental scholarship into practice and policy. In M. H. Bornstein, & M. E. Lamb (Eds.), *Developmental psychology: An advanced textbook* (5th edn., pp. 570–601). Mahwah, NJ: Lawrence Erlbaum Associates.

Groark, C. J., Muhamedrahimov, R. J., Palmov, O. I., Nikiforova, N. V., & McCall, R. B. (2005). Improvements in early care in Russian orphanages and their relationship to observed behaviors. *Infant Mental Health Journal*, *26*, 96–109.

Grobe, T., Curnan, S., Melchior, A., & The Center for Human Resources. (1993, October). *Synthesis of existing knowledge and practice in the field of education partnerships*. Washington, DC: US Department of Education Office of Educational Research and Improvement.

Haynes, N. M. (Ed.). (1995). *School Development Program research monograph*. ERIC document ED 371 091.

Johnson, B., & Tittnich, E. (2004). Are you ready for an infant mental health consultant? *Zero to Three*, *24*, 39–46.

Joyner, E. T., Comer, J. P., & Ben-Avie, M. (Eds.). (2004). *Transforming school leadership and management to support student learning and development*. Thousand Oaks, CA: Corwin Press.

Kearns, K. P. (1992). From comparative advantage to damage control: Clarifying strategic issues using SWOT analysis. *Nonprofit Management and Leadership*, *3*, 3–22.

Kegerise, K. E. (1999, March). Keys to successful collaboration. *Developments, Special Report*. Pittsburgh, PA: University of Pittsburgh Office of Child Development.

W. K. Kellogg Foundation (1998). *W. K. Kellogg Foundation evaluation handbook*. Battle Creek, MI: W. K. Kellogg Foundation.

W. K. Kellogg Foundation (2000). *W. K. Kellogg Foundation logic model development guide*. Battle Creek, MI: W. K. Kellogg Foundation.

Kumpfer, K. L., & Alvarado, R. (2003). Family-strengthening approaches for the prevention of youth problem behaviors. *American Psychologist*, *58*, 457–465.

Layzer, J. I., Goodson, R. D., Bernstein, L., & Price, C. (2001). *National evaluation of family support programs*. Vol. A. *The meta analysis*. Cambridge, MA: Abt Associates.

Love, J. M., Kisker, E. E., Ross, C., Raikes, H., Constantine, J., Boller, K., *et al.* (2005). The effectiveness of Early Head Start for 3-year-old children and their parents: Lessons for policy and programs. *Developmental Psychology*, *41*, 885–901.

Love, J. M., Schochet, P. Z., & Meckstroth, A. L. (1996). Are they in real danger? What research does and doesn't tell us about child care quality and children's well-being. *Child Care Research and Policy Papers*. Princeton, NJ: Mathematica Policy Research.

Mattessich, P. W., & Monsey, B. R. (1992). *Collaboration: What makes it work? A review of research literature on factors influencing successful collaborations*. St. Paul, MN: Amherst H. Wilder Foundation.

Maughan, B., Pickles, A., Rutter, M., & Ouston, J. (1990). Can schools change? I. Outcomes at six London secondary schools. *School Effectiveness and School Improvement*, *1*, 188–210.

McCall, R. B. (submitted). Toward more realistic evidence-based programming and policies.

McCall, R. B., & Green, B. L. (2004). Beyond the methodological gold standards of behavioral research: Considerations for practice and policy. *Society for Research in Child Development Social Policy Reports*, *18*, 1–19.

McCall, R. B., Green, B. L., Groark, C. J., Strauss, M. S., & Farber, A. E. (1999). An interdisciplinary, university-community, applied developmental science partnership. *Journal of Applied Developmental Psychology*, *20*, 207–226.

McCall, R. B., Green, B. L., Strauss, M. S., & Groark, C. J. (1997). Issues in community-based research and program evaluation. In I. E. Sigel, & K. A. Renninger (Eds.), *Handbook of child psychology*, Vol. 4, 5th edn. (pp. 955–997). New York: Wiley.

McCall, R. B., Groark, C. J., & Nelkin, R. (2004). Integrating developmental scholarship and society: From dissemination and accountability to evidence-based programming and policies. *Merrill–Palmer Quarterly*, *50*, 326–340.

McCall, R. B., Larsen, L., & Ingram, A. (2003). The science and policy of early childhood education and family services. In A. J. Reynolds, M. C. Wang, & H. J. Walberg (Eds.), *Early childhood programs for a new century: Issues in children's and families' lives* (pp. 255–298). The University of Illinois at Chicago Series on Children and Youth. Washington, DC: CWLA Press.

McCall, R. B., Ryan, C. S., & Plemons, B. W. (2003). Some lessons learned on evaluating community-based, two-generation service programs: The case of the Comprehensive Child Development Program (CCDP). *Journal of Applied Developmental Psychology*, *24*, 125–141.

Millsap, M. A., Chase, A., Obeidallah, D., Perez-Smith, A., Brigham, N., & Johnston, K. (2000). *Evaluation of Detroit's Comer schools and families initiative*. Cambridge, MA: Abt Associates.

Morrow, A. L., Townsend, I. T., & Pickering, L. K. (1991). Risk of enteric infection associated with early child day care. *Pediatric Annals*, *20*, 427–433.

Mrazek, P. J., & Haggerty, R. J. (Eds.). (1994). *Reducing risks for mental disorders: Frontiers for prevention intervention research*. Washington, DC: National Academy Press.

Muhamedrahimov, R. J., Palmov, O. I., Nikiforova, N. V., Groark, C. J., & McCall, R. B. (2004). Institution-based early intervention program. *Infant Mental Health Journal*, *25*, 488–501.

Nation, M., Crusto, C., Wandersman, A., Kumpfer, K. L., Seybolt, D., Morrissey-Kane, E., *et al.* (2003). What works in prevention: Principles of effective prevention programs. *American Psychologist*, *58*, 449–456.

National Evaluation of Sure Start Team. (2005a). *Report for team: Variation in Sure Start local programme effectiveness: Early preliminary findings*. London, UK: HMSO.

National Evaluation of Sure Start Team. (2005b). *Report 13: Early impacts of Sure Start local programmes on children and families*. London, UK: HMSO.

Neufield, B., & LaBue, M. (1994). *The implementation of the School Development Program in Hartford: Final evaluation report*. Cambridge, MA: Education Matters.

Olds, D. L., & Kitzman, H. (1993). Review of research on home visiting for pregnant women and parents of young children. In R. E. Behrman (Ed.), *Home visiting: The future of children* (Vol. 3, pp. 53–92). Los Angeles, CA: David and Lucile Packard Foundation.

Olds, D. L., Henderson, C. R. Jr., Kitzman, H. J., Eckenrode, J. J., Cote, R. E., & Tatelbaum, R. C. (1999). In R. E. Behrman (Ed.), *Home visiting: Recent program evaluations. The Future of Children* (Vol. 9, pp. 44–65). Los Angeles, CA: David and Lucile Packard Foundation.

Ouston, J., Maughan, B., & Rutter, M. (1991). Can schools change? II. Practice in six London secondary schools. *School Effectiveness and School Improvement*, *2*, 3–13.

Ringwalt, C. L., Ennett, S., Vincus, A., Thorne, J., Rohrbach, L. A., & Simons-Rudolph, A. (2002). The prevalence of effective substance use prevention curricula in US middle schools. *Prevention Science*, *3*, 257–265.

Rosenbam, P. R., & Rubin, D. (1983). The central role of the propensity score in observational studies for causal effects. *Biometrika*, *70*, 41–55.

Rossi, P. H., Lipsey, M. W., & Freeman, H. E. (2004). *Evaluation: A systematic approach* (7th edn.). Thousand Oaks, CA: Sage.

Rutter, M. (2006). Is Sure Start an effective preventive intervention? *Child and Adolescent Mental Health*, *11*, 135–141.

Schorr, L. B. (2003). Determining "what works" in social programs and social policies: Toward a more inclusive knowledge base. Accessed February 2003 from www.brookings.edu/views/papers/sawhill/20030226.htm.

Scott, K. G., Mason, C. A., & Chapman, D. A. (1999). The use of epidemiological methodology as a means of influencing public policy. *Child Development*, *70*, 1263–1272.

Shonkoff, J. P. (2000). Science, policy, and practice: Three cultures in search of a shared mission. *Child Development*, *71*, 181–187.

St. Pierre, R. G., Layzer, J. I., Goodson, B. D., & Bernstein. L. S. (1994). *National evaluation of the Comprehensive Child Development Program: Interim report*. Cambridge, MA: Abt Associates.

St. Pierre, R. G., Layzer, J. I., Goodson, B. D. & Bernstein, L. S. (1997a, September). *The effectiveness of comprehensive case management interventions: Findings from the national evaluation of the Comprehensive Child Development Program*. Cambridge, MA: Abt Associates.

St. Pierre, R. G., Layzer, J. I., Goodson, B. D. & Bernstein, L. S. (1997b, June). *National impact evaluation of the Comprehensive Child Development Program: Final Report*. Cambridge, MA: Abt Associates.

Wandersman, A., & Florin, P. (2003). Community interventions and effective prevention. *American Psychologist*, *58*, 441–448.

Wandersman, A., & Goodman, R. (1993). *Understanding coalitions and how they operate: An "open systems" organizational perspective*. W. K. Kellogg Foundation Community-Based Public Health Initiative.

Wandersman, A., Imm, P., Chinman, M., & Kaftarian, S. (1999). *Getting to outcomes: Methods and tools for planning, evaluation and accountability*. Rockville, MD: Center for Substance Abuse Prevention.

Wandersman, A., Imm, P., Chinman, M., & Kaftarian, S. (2000). Getting to Outcomes: A results-based approach to accountability. *Evaluation and Program Planning*, *23*, 389–395.

Weissberg, R. P., & Kumpfer, K. L. (Eds.). (2003). Prevention that works for children and youth. Special Issue. *American Psychologist*, *58*, 425–490.

Weisz, J. R., Jensen-Doss, A., & Hawley, K. M. (2006). Evidence-based youth psychotherapies versus usual clinical care: A meta-analysis of direct comparisons. *American Psychologist*, *61*, 671–689.

www.surestart.gov.uk (January 4, 2008).

61 Clarifying and Maximizing the Usefulness of Targeted Preventive Interventions

Frank Vitaro and Richard E. Tremblay

Objectives and Overview

This chapter covers targeted preventive interventions as applied to the psychosocial domain and is divided into three parts. In the first part, we examine *who* should be the focus of preventive interventions. In doing so, we critically review past and current classification systems of prevention programs in light of the Science of Prevention concepts (Coie, Miller-Johnson, & Bagwell, 2000; Coie, Watt, West *et al.*, 1993) as well as new knowledge accumulated over the last decade in the area of developmental psychopathology (Cicchetti & Cohen, 2006; Masten, Burt, & Coatsworth, 2006). The second part focuses on *what* should be targeted for change, *how* such targeting should be accomplished and *when such targeting should occur*. Finally, we review practical and clinical issues related to recruitment and retention of participants, timing and components of preventive interventions, assessment of results, cost-effectiveness and dissemination. Throughout the chapter, we refer to past or ongoing preventive interventions to illustrate our points. We assume that most readers are aware of the theoretical and practical advantages of preventive interventions over treatment. These are well described by Coie, Miller-Johnson, & Bagwell (2000) and Offord and Bennett (2002) (see also chapter 60).

Who Should be Targeted?

Based on the Science of Prevention concept, preventive interventions are a series of organized, theoretically driven efforts to break the developmental pathways linking early risk factors to later adjustment problems. As illustrated in Fig. 61.1, the disruption of this psychopathological process can be achieved by:

1 Eliminating the initial risk factors or their subsequent mediators;

2 Adding beneficial factors to the developmental chain to compensate for risk factors; or

3 Putting in place protective factors (i.e., moderators) that mitigate the links between risk factors and their associated outcomes (for the distinction between risk factors, mediators and moderators see Kraemer, 2003).

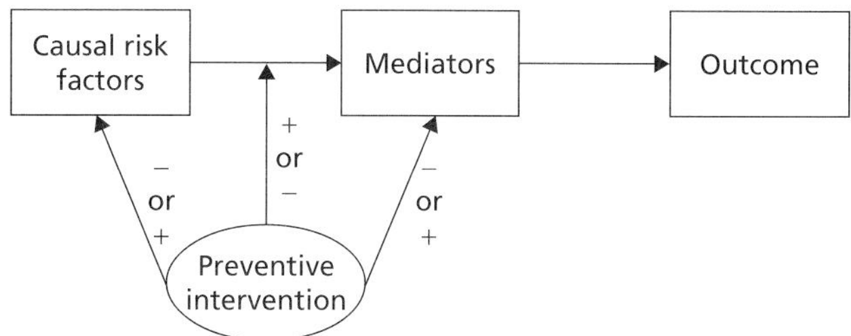

Fig. 61.1 Simplified developmental chain illustrating the targets and the functions of a preventive intervention. The signs – or + on the oblique lines indicate that a preventive intervention can either eliminate a risk factor or put in place a resource factor (which is often the opposite of a risk factor) with respect to main effects (i.e., causal risk factors and mediators). Alternatively, the signs + or – on the vertical line indicate that a preventive intervention can, instead or in addition, be designed to put in place protective factors or reduce vulnerability factors with respect to moderators.

In this context, developmental psychopathology provides a comprehensive framework for constructing "theories of the emerging problem," whereas the Science of Prevention can be seen as a comprehensive framework to construct "theories of the appropriate solutions" to prevent problems from emerging.

Brief Historical Overview

The first conceptualization of prevention into *primary*, *secondary* and *tertiary* interventions was proposed by Caplan (1964). Caplan's conceptualization emphasized the timing of intervention relative to the problem to be prevented: before onset (i.e., primary prevention), during early or preclinical manifestations (i.e., secondary prevention) or after the full-blown clinical establishment to prevent relapse or further complications (i.e., tertiary prevention). Caplan's model has been criticized on the basis that it is problematic to assume that the development of a problem follows three easily identifiable and conceptually distinct phases (Kraemer, Stice, Kazdin, Offord, & Kupfer, 2001). Indeed, for most psychopathological problems, frequency and severity of symptoms occur on a continuum, even though specific clusters can be identified (Maughan, 2005; Offord & Bennett, 2002).

Rutter's Child and Adolescent Psychiatry, 5th edition. Edited by M. Rutter, D. Bishop, D. Pine, S. Scott, J. Stevenson, E. Taylor and A. Thapar. © 2008 Blackwell Publishing, ISBN: 978-1-4051-4549-7.

A new classification system was proposed in the 1990s which remains in vogue (Mrazek & Haggerty, 1994; Offord & Bennett, 2002). In the current two-level classification system, prevention initiatives are classified according to *who* is offered the intervention (Gordon, 1983; Institute of Medicine, 1994; Offord, Kraemer, Kazdin, Jensen, & Harrington, 1998). At the first level are *universal preventive interventions* (UPI) in which all members of a geographical unit (e.g., a residential area, a school) or a social unit (e.g., kindergarteners, adolescents) are offered new activities or new services aimed at helping them overcome current or future challenges, but without targeting anyone in particular (see chapter 60). According to some authors, UPI encompasses the notion of *health promotion* (Cowen, 1991), although others do not agree with this view (Institute of Medicine, 1994). In UPI, intervention can occur in the absence of any sign of the problem to be prevented or any visible (i.e., quantifiable) risk, although risk for some individuals is suspected. UPI can also occur in the presence of identified risk factors as long as these factors might affect the entire population (e.g., the availability and acceptability of drugs that seem to be linked to an elevated rate of substance use in the entire adolescent population; Bachman, Johnson, & O'Malley, 1998).

The second level includes *targeted preventive interventions* (TPI). In the case of TPI, only individuals at risk for a problem are targeted. If the individuals are at risk for environmental reasons, as in the case of children born from teenage mothers, then the TPI is called *selective*. If instead, the children are at risk on the basis of personal dispositions such as early signs of persisting physical aggression, then the TPI is termed *indicated*. TPI is deployed in the context of risk factors or early precursors of the problem to be prevented. These risk factors or early precursors need to occur at the level of the individual or his or her immediate environment (i.e., family), not at the level of the entire community as in the case of UPI. This distinction may explain in part why TPI-oriented researchers and practitioners usually deploy their efforts at the level of the individual and his or her immediate social environment (i.e., family, teacher, peers). In contrast, UPI-oriented colleagues attempt to establish services and resources at the level of the community. More details about the distinctions between universal, selective and indicated preventive interventions can be found in Mrazek and Brown (2002).

Who is At Risk and to What Extent are They At Risk?

Traditionally, TPI involves a dichotomous view of those at risk (who should get the full TPI) and those not at risk (who do not need any preventive intervention). In most cases, risk is not a binary category but a continuum of probabilities, although this continuum may not be normally distributed (Meehl, 1992). Hence, it is inaccurate to think of individuals as being either at risk (and thus deserving TPI) or not at risk or not yet at risk. Given the multifactorial and developmental determination of most psychosocial problems, individual variation with respect to risk is most often a variation in degree, not in kind. In consequence, we advocate a continuous approach towards risk. This continuous approach also needs to be multivariate.

Three strategies can be used to help determine the degree of risk according to a continuous multivariate perspective. The first strategy was proposed by Burgess (1928). It is a *cumulative* strategy in which the total number of risk factors is calculated after establishing their individual presence (or absence) using a dichotomous approach. This approach is based on the traditional 2 × 2 epidemiology tables that are used to establish risk status based on its relationship with ulterior psychopathology status (Kraemer, Kazdin, Offord *et al.*, 1999; Offord, 1996; Rice & Harris, 1995). A second strategy is to use the results of a multivariate regression, either linear or logistic, to determine the weights of each risk factor before summing them. This method is known as the *weighted additive* approach. Some authors have claimed that the weighted additive and the cumulative methods are equally effective in determining the degree of risk (Farrington, 1985). However, others report divergent results. For example, Deater-Deckard, Dodge, Bates, and Pettit (1998) showed that a cumulative risk index based on four childhood risk factors (i.e., child characteristics, sociocultural level, parenting and caregiving, and peer victimization/rejection) correlated only modestly with later externalizing problems (i.e., 0.32–0.39 depending on whether parent, teacher or peer reports were used). In contrast, the predictive coefficients between the four risk factors and the outcome varied between 0.60 and 0.67 when using a weighted additive approach.

One important advantage of the regression approach on which the weighted additive method rests is that it can be expanded into the *interactive* approach, which is our favored strategy. Most developmental models include not only risk factors with main effects (either direct or indirect, via mediators), but also moderators that qualify these main effects, sometimes in dramatic ways (Coie, Watt, West *et al.*, 1993; Rutter, Giller, & Hagell, 1998). For example, child maltreatment leads to violent behavior, more so in children with the short allele of a variant in the gene coding for the neurotransmitter metabolizing enzyme monoamine oxidase A (MAOA; Caspi, McClay, Moffitt *et al.*, 2002). These findings correspond to a person × environment interaction model which is now becoming generally accepted in developmental psychopathology research (see chapter 23; Plomin & Crabbe, 2000; Sameroff & Mackenzie, 2003). This interactive model allows for the integration of moderating factors to determine the degree of risk. These moderators can reflect either protection or vulnerability. Contrary to resource (or compensatory) factors that have main effects opposite to risk factors, protection factors mitigate the relationship between risk factors and later outcomes. Conversely, vulnerability factors exacerbate the link between risk factors and later outcome; they can also reduce the link between resource factors and later outcomes (Fergusson, Vitaro, Wanner, & Brendgen, 2007; Luthar, Cicchetti, & Becker, 2000; Rutter, Giller, & Hagell, 1998).

It follows that the identification of at-risk individuals should result from a combination of environmental and personal factors that can operate additively or interactively, and not only on background factors or on personal vulnerabilities. An important consequence of such a multivariate interactive strategy is to minimize the distinction between *selective* and *indicated* TPI because this distinction requires that participants be selected on the basis of either background or personal factors. Already, some prevention programs target at-risk individuals on the basis of both personal and background characteristics. For example, the promoters of Fast Track, one of the major TPIs in the USA (Conduct Problems Prevention Research Group, 1999a,b), selected the participating children on the basis of neighborhood crime and poverty level *and* parent and teacher-rated disruptiveness scores.

To summarize, a risk score can be derived for each individual or each community by combining risk/resource factors and vulnerability/protective factors derived from multivariate analyses. Of course, one should not rely on only one study to establish which risk and protective factors are relevant. Meta-analyses and averaged effect sizes of the *r* type (i.e., beta weights or odds ratios) can also be used in this context (Lipsey, 1995; McCartney & Rosenthal, 2000). However, the value of the risk score may need to be adjusted depending on cultural or geographical variations (seen here as additional putative moderators). For example, children's anxiety may not be linked to depressive feelings in China as much as in Canada because anxious Chinese children are not ostracized by their peers as much as their anxious Canadian counterparts, a consequence of the differences in the ways anxiety is perceived in the two cultures (Chen, Rubin, & Sun, 1992). One must also be aware of possible non-linear relationships between risk factors and developmental outcomes. In addition, the risk score should be based on risk factors that are easy to measure, reducing the cost of the screening process and increasing its chance for widespread use. If necessary, the continuous risk score can be split into segments to reflect the degree of risk and possibly the nature of the risk faced by the individuals and the communities from each segment. The cut-off scores used to identify the different segments as well as their respective sets of risk and protective factors can take advantage of traditional or recent clustering techniques (Nagin, 2005; Pickles & Angold, 2003).

Note that this segmentation approach is different from the traditional epidemiological approach because: (i) it is based on the full information derived from additive and interactive statistical models; and (ii) in most cases, it generates more than the traditional two segments (i.e., one at risk and one not at risk). Ideally, each segment would receive a program with content and dosage tailored to its specific constellation and level of risk/resource and vulnerability/protective factors. This suggestion is in line with the *adaptive preventive intervention approach* proposed by Collins, Murphy, and Bierman (2004). According to this approach, different dosages of certain program components, including zero dosages, are assigned across individuals and/or within individuals across time in accordance with the individuals' needs or response to the program. Clear and well-informed decision rules help link specific levels and types of program components to the characteristics of the individuals in each segment. The latter are called *tailored variables*. Tailored variables refer essentially to pretest variables that might exert a moderating effect on the impact of a preventive intervention and/or participants' progress toward a prespecified threshold representing a successful outcome. To illustrate, in the Fast Track multicomponent program (see pp. 993–4), the number of home visits during the first years of the program (i.e., monthly, biweekly, weekly) was determined based upon ratings of parental functioning, which included empirically validated risk factors. A similar approach was used for the reading tutoring component; only the children whose academic performance was below the 33rd percentile received that component. Parental functioning and academic performance were selected because they were hypothesized to moderate the impact of the core elements of the Fast Track program, although they can also be seen as proximal outcomes and putative mediators. Given that the appropriate dosage depends on the tailored variables, these variables should be selected and measured with care. It is also important that they are stringently operationalized according to well-documented decision rules, which also help in the evaluation of these adaptive preventive interventions.

What? When? and How?

Now that we have clarified *who* should be targeted in preventive interventions, we turn to *what* should be targeted and *when*, and *how* preventive interventions should take place.

What Should be Targeted and When Should They be Targeted?

Not all risk/resource factors and not all vulnerability/protective factors are equally important or relevant for TPI. The risk/resource factors and the vulnerability/protective factors that should be targeted by TPI are those that are:

1 Theoretically relevant and empirically active;
2 High in predictive power and in causal plausibility;
3 Potent and generative;
4 Chronologically, culturally and geographically relevant; and
5 Modifiable in a cost-effective way.

Indeed, only variables and processes that have an active role as main effects or moderators in the developmental pathways leading to the emergence of maladaptation should be targeted by TPI (Felner, Yates Felner, & Silverman, 2000; Rutter, 2003). Hence, risk indicators such as factor B_1 in Fig. 61.2 (also called markers, proxies or incidental correlates) need to be distinguished from risk factors with unique main effects such as factors A_1 and A_2, mediators such as factors B_2 and B_3, and moderators such as factors B_4 and C_5. As acknowledged by Rutter (2003), this is not an easy task given that most knowledge about risk factors is derived from correlational studies. However, it is an important task if we want TPI to impact on factors that make an active and possibly causal contribution

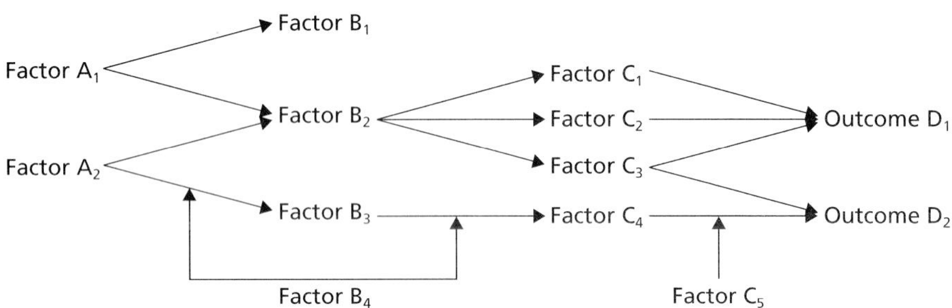

Fig. 61.2 Different roles of risk factors in developmental pathways.

to the complex chain of events leading to maladaptation. Causal plausibility is increased further when the probable mechanisms of these active factors are well documented.

Some risk/resource and vulnerability/protective factors may have an active role in a developmental pathway and their operating mode may be well documented, but their effect size may be small in terms of partial correlations and odds ratios resulting from multivariate analyses. These are not potent risk factors and may not be worth targeting through preventive efforts. Instead, priority should be given to risk/resource factors that are more potent in terms of their effect size relative to the outcome to be prevented. Similarly, priority should be given to protective and vulnerability factors that have a high multiplicative power with respect to the link between risk or resource factors and the outcome (Kraemer, Stice, Kazdin *et al.*, 2001). Protective factors with buffering effects should be the primary target of prevention efforts, especially if risk factors are difficult to modify.

Generativity of risk/resource factors and of vulnerability/protective factors is also important in determining which factors deserve to be targeted by TPI. The notion of generativity refers to the number of mediators with potentially additional unique effects of their own that are triggered by a single risk/resource factor according to a cascade model (i.e., such as factor B_2 in Fig. 61.2; Masten, Burt, & Coatworth, 2006). It also refers to the number of risk factors that can be moderated by a single protective factor (such as factor B_4 in Fig. 61.2) or the number of adjustment problems resulting from a single risk factor according to the principle of multifinality described by developmental psychopathologists (Cicchetti & Hinshaw, 2002; i.e., such as factor C_3 in Fig. 61.2). Hence, cost-effective TPI would target generic risk factors in order to "kill several birds with a few stones." Many, if not most, of these generic risk factors may be found early in life. As a result, early TPI during the prenatal and preschool periods may be the most (cost) effective, as results from preventive interventions during the prenatal and preschool years indicate (Aos, Lieb, Mayfield, Miller, & Pennucci, 2004; Carneiro, & Heckman, 2003; Olds, Henderson, Kitzman, & Eckenrode, 1998; Schweinhart, 2006). Interventions targeting these periods may also receive public and government support more easily because it makes common sense to try to prevent the complex chain of events that leads to later maladjustment in children by targeting the initial elements of the chain (that have a high generic power). Of course, these early risk factors must be ethically modifiable. They should also be easily modifiable. For example, low socioeconomic status (SES) and tobacco exposure during pregnancy are independent risk factors for later disruptive behavior (Maughan, Taylor, Taylor, Butler, & Bynner, 2001; Wakschlag & Hans, 2002). Low SES may be modifiable (Leventhal & Brooks-Gunn, 2004), but not by health professionals, at least not directly. In contrast, prenatal exposure to nicotine is easily modifiable, at least in principle. However, modifying prenatal nicotine exposure requires the right timing; after the first months of pregnancy, it may be too late to effect change. Other risk factors, although modifiable, may not be relevant because of the participants' characteristics such as age, sex, ethnicity or cultural background.

To conclude, trying to change factors that cannot be changed or, when changed, do not affect the incidence of the outcome because the factors are markers and not causal antecedents is a waste of time and valuable resources. Trying to change factors that, although causal, are not potent, not generic, not well-timed or not culturally relevant will also prove to be a waste of resources. In designing preventive interventions, the emphasis should be placed on active, independent, causal, generic, early, modifiable and culturally approved or important risk/resource and vulnerability/protective factors.

How do we Achieve the Maximum Impact of TPI?

One first step toward answering this question is to identity effective prevention strategies with respect to a specific problem. Narrative (e.g., Greenberg, Domitrovich, & Bumbarger, 2001) and quantitative (LeMarquand, Tremblay, & Vitaro, 2001) reviews of existing prevention programs are a good starting point. Meta-analyses are particularly useful because of the comparative statistics they generate in the form of effect sizes. As illustrated in Table 61.1, several meta-analyses of effective and ineffective prevention programs in different areas of adjustment have become available over the past decade. Above and beyond summary statistics such as the effect size, the usefulness of meta-analyses is to categorize original studies according to their theoretical background, methodological rigor, intervention components or participants' characteristics.

Also useful in the identification of the most effective programs are the hit lists of best preventive programs prepared by different groups of researchers. One such list was prepared by the Center for the Study and Prevention of Violence (http://www.colorado.edu/cspv/blueprints). The first part of this list

Table 61.1 Examples of meta-analyses about targeted preventive programs in regard to the prevention of different outcomes. Only meta-analyses that included primary studies with strong evaluation designs (i.e., either experimental or quasi-experimental) are considered here. Some meta-analyses include both universal and targeted prevention programs. One reason for including them was to compare the effect sizes of the two categories of prevention programs.

Author	Outcome	Number of primary studies	Participants	Effect size (range and average)
Ang & Hugues (2002)	Behavior problems	38	Disruptive children and adolescents (aged 6–18 years)	−0.83 to 2.51 (0.62)
Franklin, Grant, Corcoran, Miller, & Bultman (1997)	Early pregnancies	32	Adolescents (aged 11–20 years)	−0.25 to 0.47 (0.15)
DuPaul & Eckert (1997)	ADHD	63	Hyperactive children (aged 5–15 years)	None available (0.45)
Farrington & Welsh (2003)	Delinquency, violence, criminality	40	Mixed (from birth through adolescence)	−0.10 to 1.88 (0.22)
Grossman & Hugues (1992)	Internalized problems (anxiety and depression)	22	Anxious children and adolescents	0.25 to 1.54 (0.74)
Horowitz & Garber (2006)	Depression	30 (18 targeted)	Mixed (children and adolescents)	−0.62 to 1.151 (0.27 at post-intervention; 0.32 at follow-up)
LeMarquand, Tremblay, & Vitaro (2001)	Conduct disorder/delinquency	20	At-risk children	−0.31 to 0.87 (0.14)
Lipsey & Wilson (1998)	Delinquency relapse	200	Juvenile delinquents (aged 14–18 years)	None available (0.12)
Lösel & Beelmann (2003)	Antisocial behavior	84	Mixed (children and adolescents)	−2.39 to 2.79 (0.38 at post-intervention; 0.28 at follow-up)
Serketich & Dumas (1996)	Antisociality	26	Disruptive children and adolescents	None available (0.86)

includes 12 prevention programs considered "blueprints" according to a series of well-defined criteria. These programs mainly target substance abuse, aggression and delinquency. The second part of the list contains 16 programs that are considered promising.

In addition to narrative and meta-analytic reviews of prevention programs *in one problem outcome area*, some authors compared the results of several prevention programs *across different problem outcome areas* in order to identify key characteristics associated with successful programs that might transcend specific content areas. Nation, Crusto, Wandersman *et al.* (2003) identified nine principles after reviewing 35, mostly narrative, reviews of universal and selective prevention programs that targeted five problem areas: substance use, risky sexual behavior, delinquency, violence and school failure. Nation, Crusto, Wandersman *et al.* concluded that effective programs are:

1 Theory driven;
2 Appropriately timed;
3 Comprehensive;
4 Oriented towards opportunities for positive relationships;
5 Open to varied teaching methods;
6 Sufficiently potent with respect to dosage and duration;
7 Well integrated in delivery services;
8 Socioculturally relevant; and
9 Effective in triggering strategic mediators.

These principles are illustrated and discussed further through the examination of a number of targeted prevention programs.

Theory Driven

Prevention programs need to rest on clear theoretical grounds and strong empirical evidence. To illustrate, promoters of Fast Track, a multicomponent multitarget TPI for low SES disruptive children and their caregivers, elaborated a clear theoretical rationale for every component of their program and attached each component to specific objectives with regard to risk and protective factors (Conduct Problems Prevention Research Group, 1992, 2004). Hence, each component was first justified by the important part played by that component in the etiology of conduct disorder (the distal outcome in this study). Each component was also justified by its evidence-based effectiveness. The six components were as follows:

1 Group parent training aimed at improving parenting skills and parent–child interactions;

2 Home visits designed to ensure that parenting skills were implemented and to inspire feelings of confidence in parents;
3 Group-based social skills training with the children aimed at improving their social-cognitive skills;
4 Peer-pairing, in which a target child and a no-risk peer participated in guided play sessions designed to capitalize on positive modeling from the no-risk peer and to change the no-risk peer's likely negative perception of the target child;
5 Academic tutoring designed to prevent academic problems; and
6 Teacher support for effective management designed to help reduce the general level of disruptive behaviors in the classroom.

Despite the theoretical and empirical "cutting edge" nature of Fast Track, the evaluation results are at best moderate, with effects sizes varying between 0.2 and 0.5 for the children most at risk (i.e., above the 90th percentile on the disruptiveness screening scores) after the first 3 years. After 5 years (by age 11 or grade 5), 37% of the randomly assigned Fast Track children had no conduct problem dysfunction compared with 27% of control children (Conduct Problems Prevention Research Group, 2002). Interestingly, and importantly, mediation analyses indicated that these results were partially explained by gains in the domains targeted by the program (i.e., parenting, peer relations and social-cognitive skills). The most recent data available show that the children above the 90th percentile were significantly better off with respect to important outcomes such as a DSM diagnosis for conduct disorder, index criminal offenses and interpersonal violence, although the effect sizes remain moderate (Conduct Problems Prevention Research Group, 2005). To illustrate, 72% of the control children had committed an index crime by grade 10 compared to 28% of the intervention children (the percentages for conduct disorder and interpersonal violence were 14 and 43% in the control group versus 6 and 20% in the intervention group, respectively). However, for the lower-risk children (i.e., those between the 70th and the 90th percentiles), the differences between the two groups were non-significant.

Appropriately Timed and Developmentally Sensitive

Preventive interventions should be initiated early enough to have an impact on the development of the problem behavior to be prevented. There is empirical evidence to suggest that the timing of a preventive intervention may be as important as its content. To illustrate, the Metropolitan Area Child Study Research Group (2002) randomly assigned schools to one of four conditions: a universal 2-year general classroom enhancement program, a universal general enhancement plus small-group peer skills training program, a universal general enhancement plus small-group peer skills plus family intervention, and a care-as-usual control condition. The authors also examined whether the results pertaining to aggressive behaviors and school achievement differed according to the timing of implementation (i.e., grades 2 and 3 only, grades 5 and 6 only, or grades 2, 3, 5 and 6). Globally, the results of this complex factorial study with the high-risk children (defined according to their baseline aggression scores) revealed that the most comprehensive condition produced the best results when aggression scores were examined. Specifically, the improvement in the behavior doubled when the initial 2-year intervention in grades 2 and 3 was followed by a second 2-year intervention in grades 5 and 6. Perhaps even more important, however, were the findings that none of the interventions were effective in preventing aggression when implemented only in grades 5 and 6. In fact, an iatrogenic effect was found whereby children in the control condition decreased in aggression whereas the intervention participants, particularly those in the small-group peer-skills training condition, did not.

Comprehensive

Because risk is multifactorial, prevention programs must include several components that address as many risk and protective factors in as many systems as possible in order to maximally influence development and the behaviors to be prevented. This rationale guided several of the most recent prevention programs described here (e.g., Fast Track and the Metropolitan Area Child Study) as well as older TPIs (e.g., the Cambridge Somerville Youth Study; McCord, 1978). The evidence in support of this intuitively logical principle, however, is inconsistent. Reid, Webster-Stratton, and Hammond (2003) and Webster-Stratton and Hammond (1997) compared different combinations of their Incredible Years Parent Training Program, their Incredible Years Teacher Program and their Child Training Program within a sample of 159, 4- to 7-year-old children with oppositional-defiant disorder (in order to prevent later conduct disorder, substance abuse and school dropout, which represent more serious outcomes than ODD) (for further material on parenting programs see chapter 64). More specifically, the authors randomly assigned the children to one of the following conditions: the parent program only, the child program only, the parent and teacher programs, the child and teacher programs, and the child, parent and teacher programs. These five conditions were compared to a waitlist control condition.

In the parent program only condition, the parents watched a series of 17 videotapes depicting ways parents can effectively manage problematic behaviors or situations with their children. The rationale, efficacy and content of these weekly 2-h group training sessions at the clinic are described in detail by Webster-Stratton, Mihalic, Fagan *et al.* (2001a).

The child program consisted of 18–19 weekly 2-h sessions with two therapists and 6–7 target children. Through the use of puppets, the therapists illustrated a series of interpersonal skills that are usually absent or in excess in ODD children's repertoires. These included conflict resolution skills, negative attributions, perspective taking and empathy, complying with teacher or parent requests, and communicating and co-operatively playing with other children. In addition, parents and teachers were asked to reinforce the targeted skills (e.g., sharing, teamwork, friendly talk, listening, compliance with requests, feeling talk and problem-solving) whenever they noticed the child using them in the home or the school. Children were also given weekly homework assignments to complete with their parents. A more complete description of the videotape training curriculum and leader manuals is provided by Webster-Stratton (1990).

The teacher program comprised 4 full days group training sequenced throughout the school year. Through illustrations and discussion, the teacher program promoted the use of praise and encouragement for positive behaviors, proactive teaching, using of incentives to motivate children, techniques to decrease disruptive behavior and collaborative strategies with parents. The teacher workshops also included topics such as prevention of peer rejection, acknowledgment of individual differences and strategies to prevent playground aggression. Two individual appointments with each teacher were scheduled to develop an individual behavior plan for the targeted child.

At the end of the 6-month intervention period, children manifested improvements in comparison to controls that were consistent with the treatment condition. Hence, children in the three conditions with the child program showed more prosocial skills with peers than the children in the control condition. No difference between treatment and control was observed for children in the two conditions without the child program. Similarly, parents in the three parent program conditions manifested less negative and more positive parenting and reported fewer child behavior problems than parents in the control condition and parents in the two conditions without parent training. Children's behavior problems at school were reduced for those whose teacher participated in the teacher program relative to the control children. Overall, the conditions that included all three programs produced the best results after 6 months.

However, at 2-year follow-up the results were less clear-cut. Teachers reported an equal proportion of children with behavior problems across all five treatment conditions (i.e., around 50%). Parents in the parent + teacher programs reported fewer cases of behaviorally disordered children relative to only one other condition – the parent program only condition. Unfortunately, the waitlist control group was not available for comparison at the 2-year follow-up.

Results from the Early Risers program (August, Egan, Realmuto, & Hektner, 2003; August, Realmuto, Hektner, & Bloomquist, 2001) further illustrate the lack of evidence in support of the notion that more is necessarily better in the context of a TPI. In their first study, August, Realmuto, Hektner *et al.* (2001), August, Hektner, Egan *et al.* (2002) implemented a 2-year program aimed at altering the developmental trajectories of young children with early-onset aggressive behavior. The Early Risers multicomponent program included five CORE components: a child social skills group training that used Webster-Stratton, Mihalic, Fagan *et al.*s' (2001a) protocol, a parent education and skills training program that also used the parent training protocol of Webster-Stratton *et al.*, a teacher behavior management program, a student mentoring program focused on academic learning and an annual 6-week summer school program that included non-targeted children. In addition, it also included a FLEX family support component tailored to address the unique needs of families. Intent-to-treat analyses revealed that, compared to controls, program participants showed greater gains in academic functioning. The most severely aggressive children, but not the others, also progressed on measures of self-regulation.

In a second study, August, Egan, Realmuto *et al.* (2003) tested whether the FLEX component increased the impact of their program as expected. The authors randomly assigned a new group of aggressive children and their families to three groups. One group received both the CORE (applied in the same manner to all participants and their families) and the FLEX (tailored to families' specific needs) components of their Early Risers program. The second group received the CORE component only. The third group received care as usual. Implementation results showed that CORE + FLEX participants attended more program sessions than their CORE-only counterparts. However, the two experimental conditions did not differ from each other in reducing children's disruptive behaviors and parents' levels of stress, although both were superior to the care-as-usual condition; these results suggest that the FLEX component, although intuitively appealing, did not seem to improve upon the basic CORE program.

Consistent with the idea of creating a synergy between different prevention components, one strategy that might optimize the effects of a TPI is to combine targeted and universal components within the same program. Fast Track illustrates how such a combination of targeted and universal components can be achieved (Conduct Problems Prevention Research Group, 1999b). In addition to the six targeted components already described, a series of socioemotional skills training sessions (i.e., the Promoting Alternative Thinking Strategies or PATHS curriculum; Greenberg, Kusche, Cook, & Quamma, 1995) were implemented in the classrooms of participating children. The PATHS lessons were intended to teach all the classroom children such social and personal skills as self-regulation, emotional awareness and social problem-solving.

Combining universal and targeted prevention components in a single program may be more likely to mobilize and prepare the child's whole social environment, changing the local norms for appropriate behavior. These positive changes in social norms may support the positive changes that the targeted components can achieve with the at-risk children, promoting their maintenance and generalization to other contexts. Combining universal and targeted prevention also ensures that the "false negative" cases (i.e., children not considered at-risk who will nevertheless develop a problem) receive minimal preventive help through the universal component. Similarly, combined programs minimize the "Matthew effect" (Ceci & Papierno, 2005). The term "Matthew effect" refers to the possible outcome of a universal intervention in which children who are not at risk benefit more from the intervention than do those at risk, thus increasing the gap between the two groups. However, these are only speculations because to our knowledge no author has compared the results of a combined program with a TPI only or UPI only program.

Sufficient Dosage and Intensity

A related issue is the necessary and sufficient dosage and intensity of a TPI. Dosage and intensity refer to aspects of a TPI such as length and number of sessions, spacing of sessions and the duration of the total program. Most prevention programs offer all-or-none packages in which some children receive every component of an intervention and other children receive no treatment or treatment-as-usual. However, we believe that dosage of a program should be gauged to the level of risk faced by the targeted individuals or groups and program content should match the nature of the risk factors faced by those individuals or groups. Hence, different groups of at-risk individuals may require different combinations of program components. Ideally, preventionists should develop programs with different modules that address specific risk/protective factors. For example, a child at high risk for a certain problem outcome may receive modules, A, B, C and D whereas another child at a lower risk level may receive only modules A and B. Alternatively, as in the Early Risers program, a basic package can be complemented with supplementary activities tailored to the participants' needs. Another strategy is to train to criterion (i.e., until a desired threshold is reached).

Also of concern are the questions of when to start a TPI and for how long the TPI should last. These are important questions at the clinical, practical and financial levels that have not been addressed adequately until now. As a result, a wide variety of prevention programs of varying lengths have been devised to target the same risky outcomes. Among the prevention programs that start at birth and target children from disadvantaged families, some last for a period of 2 years (e.g., home visiting program; Olds, Eckenrode, Henderson *et al.*, 1997) and some for periods of 4 years (e.g., Sure Start, a large-scale preventive program currently deployed in the UK for young children in disadvantaged areas and their families; National Evaluation of the Sure Start Team, 2004). Similarly, among prevention programs that advocate high-quality childcare during the preschool period for at-risk children, some cover a period of 2 years (e.g., from age 3 to age 5 in the Perry Preschool Project; Schweinhart, Barnes, & Weikart, 1993), whereas others cover periods twice as long (e.g., from age 1 to age 5 in the Abecederian Project; Campbell & Ramey, 1995). Finally, programs targeting schoolchildren or early adolescents with behavior problems vary from 12 weeks (Dishion & Andrews, 1995) to 6 months (Webster-Stratton, Reid, & Hammond, 2001b), 1–2 years (e.g., Early Risers; August, Realmuto, Hektner *et al.*, 2001) or a decade (e.g., Fast Track; Conduct Problems Prevention Research Group, 2002). Some programs include booster sessions at transition periods (e.g., Early Alliance; Dumas, Prinz, Smith, & Laughlin, 1999), others do not.

More importantly, the reasoning behind the prevention researchers' choice of program duration and timing is often missing or unsubstantiated. Indeed, the only way to identify the most effective length and timing of a prevention program is through studies that compare different durations and different starting points with similarly at-risk children. Very few studies of this type are currently under way. Meta-analytical reviews that examine intervention dosage or timing as potential moderators of the impact of a prevention program offer a temporary alternative to clarify this question. The results of such reviews are not always in accordance with what one might expect. For example, a meta-analysis of the impact of 70 attachment-based interventions designed to improve maternal sensitivity (a known risk factor for later adjustment problems) concluded that the most effective interventions last between 5 and 16 sessions and are applied during the second half of the first year of life, when problems become visible but problematic child–parent relationships are not yet firmly established (Bakermans-Kranenburg, van IJzendoorn, & Juffer, 2003). Thus, effective interventions need not last many years – but they do need to be intensive and well timed.

Until experimental manipulations of timing and duration through factorial designs become available (i.e., experimental conditions × dosage or duration), some interventionists rely on dosage–effect analyses or instrumental variables to extract as much information as possible from their studies (Angrist, Imbens, & Rubin, 1996). It is important to keep in mind that these strategies use quasi-experimental designs and their results should be interpreted with caution. This comment also applies to results from meta-analyses.

Modes of Intervention and Teaching Methods

The necessary dosage and intensity of a TPI to achieve a goal can depend on the quality, effectiveness and appropriateness of the modalities used to implement the desired changes. Tobler, Roona, Ochshorn *et al.* (2000) concluded their meta-analysis on school-based drug use prevention programs by stressing that interactive programs were more effective than non-interactive lecture-oriented programs. Actually, non-interactive programs were ineffective, with average effect sizes of about 0.10. This finding suggests that effective prevention programs involve interactive teaching methods, such as role-playing, corrective feedback, instructions and modeling, and active learning of the desired skills. Such a strategy seems more likely to ensure that actual behaviors are learned – in addition to changes in knowledge and perceptions – by facilitating generalization from the training sessions to the real world.

Other researchers have found that teaching methods and modalities for change significantly impact a program's ability to achieve the desired objectives. For example, in their meta-analytical review of programs designed to prevent delinquency, Farrington and Welsh (2003) noted that the programs that use behavioral parent training (similar to Webster-Stratton's parent program) are the most effective, with a mean effect size of 0.40. The least effective types – with a mean effect size of 0.07 – are based solely in schools. These authors also found that home visiting, day care/preschool, home/community and multisystemic therapy programs tended to be modestly effective, with mean effect sizes in the mid 0.20s.

Ensure Potent Causal Mediators are Set in Motion

It is indeed important that by the end of a program, mediating processes have been triggered that will ensure the maintenance, and possibly the progress, of behavior change. The Urban Institute's Children at Risk program (Harrell, Cavanagh,

Harmon, Koper, & Sridharan, 1997; Harrell, Cavanagh, & Sridharan, 1999) serves to illustrate this point. Children at Risk targeted high-risk early adolescents from poor neighborhoods in five cities across the USA in an effort to prevent delinquency. The program included case management and family counseling, family skills training, academic tutoring, adult mentoring, after-school activities and community policing. In addition, the components of the program could be adjusted depending on the specific risk factors in each neighborhood in accordance with the adaptive prevention approach described earlier (Collins, Murphy, & Bierman, 2004). To explain the weak and inconsistent results reported at both post-intervention and at a 1-year follow-up with respect to delinquent behaviors, the authors noted that few individual, family and community factors were changed, although some peer-related factors were (i.e., program youth affiliated with less delinquent peers and had more positive peer support). If affiliation with deviant peers were the only causal risk factor or mediator of risk factors for delinquency (i.e., both necessary and sufficient), then the Urban Institute's Children at Risk program should have been successful at preventing delinquency even if it failed to influence other important risk factors. As suggested by most prominent theoretical models of delinquency, deviant peer affiliation is not likely to be the only causal risk factor for this outcome (for the possible role of deviant peers in delinquency see Vitaro, Tremblay, & Bukowski, 2001b). Therefore, it may prove important to trigger the necessary (i.e., potent and causal) and sufficient mediators identified in prominent developmental models in order to impact on an outcome at the endpoint of a long developmental chain formed by a series of mediators. Vitaro, Brendgen, and Tremblay (2001a) showed that delinquent behaviors could be prevented in their high-risk sample of low SES, disruptive boys provided that several mediators – each of which corresponded to the proximal objectives of their targeted preventive program – were changed. These mediators included the child's disruptiveness, parental supervision, academic performance and deviant peer affiliation.

The difficulty of triggering the important mediators (which often correspond to the proximal objectives of a TPI) may explain some of the so-called "sleeper effects" that seem to characterize some TPIs. One TPI in which sleeper effects were observed was the Queensland Early Intervention and Prevention of Anxiety Project. This program targeted anxious schoolchildren who did not yet reach the threshold for a clinical disorder (Dadds, Spence, Holland, Barrett, & Laurens, 1997). The program included 10 weekly group training sessions at school. Through modeling and behavioral rehearsal, the children were taught cognitive–behavioral coping strategies to overcome anxiety-arousing situations. They were also taught relaxation techniques to counteract their physiological discomfort. The parents of the anxious children were also taught how to support their child in the use of the coping strategies and how to use similar coping strategies to face their own anxiety. This short-term TPI, which also involved homework for both children and parents, may have required prolonged practice of the new coping skills by both parents and children before producing its optimal effects. Indeed, the experimental children differed from their control counterparts on a series of child- and parent-rated measures not at the immediate posttest but only at later follow-ups. At the 6-month follow-up, only 16% of the experimental group manifested anxiety problems, compared to 54% of the control group. Significant differences were again observed at the 1- and 2-year follow-ups (Dadds, Holland, Laurens *et al.*, 1999).

Well-Coordinated and Integrated Prevention Services

To ensure effective change on as many potent causal risk or protective factors as possible, comprehensive multimodal prevention programs rely on different categories of prevention agents (e.g., school personnel, childcare workers, physical and mental health professionals, nurses, community leaders, policymakers). As a result, the programs should rest on a well-coordinated and integrated prevention delivery infrastructure. The Nurse Home Visitation program, first developed for the Elmira project (Olds, Henderson, Tatelbaum *et al.*, 1986; Olds, Henderson, Kitzman *et al.*, 1998), is a good example of a program with such an infrastructure. In this program, a nurse visits primiparous pregnant women who have a high-risk profile. Specifically, the pregnant women are young, unmarried and poor. Nurses visit the women approximately 32 times between 24 weeks' gestation and the child's second birthday. Nurses give support to the mothers in three areas of their life:

1 Personal development, including education, workforce integration and family planning;

2 Health-related behavior, including smoking prevention and adequate nutrition for the mother and child; and

3 Competent care of the child.

The nurses also link mother and child with community services. This program has been shown to reduce child abuse and neglect (Olds, Henderson, Tatelbaum *et al.*, 1986) as well as maternal and child delinquency. This program has also revealed the importance of a well-trained clinician to the effectiveness of a prevention effort. In a randomized controlled trial, nurses were found to have significantly greater impact on most of the outcomes studied than trained paraprofessionals. The outcomes ranged from reduced smoking in pregnancy and increased workforce integration among the mothers, to improved emotional and cognitive development among the children (Olds, Henderson, Kitzman *et al.*, 1999).

Socioculturally Relevant and Engaging

Prevention programs need to be tailored to the cultural norms of the participants and the community (for a violence prevention program that specifically addresses cultural diversity see Alkon, Tschann, Ruane, Wolff, & Hittner, 2001). Community representatives should be consulted when planning the objectives and the implementation of a prevention program. The content of the program and the strategies used to ensure implementation may also need to be adjusted to the local norms. Interestingly, models and methods for cultural adaptation of empirically based prevention programs are available (Martinez, 2006).

Social Acceptability and Cost-Effectiveness

Finally, to ensure that prevention programs become part of standard practice and are disseminated, they need to be acceptable to – or even desired by – potential recipients and practitioners. They should also be cost-effective. These last two issues are discussed next.

Practical and Sociopolitical Issues

Strategies to Mobilize Program Recipients, Program Deliverers and Decision-makers

The most effective prevention program is useless if it is not attractive to program recipients or if it is not adopted into everyday practice by program deliverers (for a discussion of these topics in relation to treatment see chapter 18). Indeed, one challenge of preventive interventions, compared to curative interventions, is to engage eligible participants not just during an evaluation trial but also during widespread implementation. Several groups of researchers have noted that, in general, recruitment and retention rates for targeted preventive intervention trials are low, often below 50% (Coie, Underwood, & Lochman, 1991; Fontana, Fleischman, McCarton, Meltzer, & Ruff, 1988; Garvey, Wrenetha, Fogg, Kratovil, & Gross, 2006). Low participation has important consequences for efficacy and effectiveness demonstration trials. First, low participation is a threat to external validity because little or no information is usually available on non-participants. Second, low participation can result in a Matthew effect in which the less at-risk cases benefit more from the program than those at higher risk because the former tend to participate more than the latter (Ceci & Papierno, 2005). Third, low engagement may result in a highly selective sample of participants. This decreased diversity in the sample makes it more difficult to identify participant characteristics that amplify or attenuate the impact of a preventive intervention (i.e., moderators). Fourth, low participation can seriously limit the statistical significance of program effect size in the context of an intention-to-treat analysis. Such an analysis includes all of the assigned participants, regardless of level of participation. Finally, low participation rates (often compounded by low retention rates) may threaten the utility of the program as a tool for social change because sustained funding may not be achieved without a critical mass of participants. Therefore, as stated by Mrazek and Haggerty (1994), "A plan to successfully engage and retain targeted participants is needed."

Because of their key role in most prevention programs targeting child behavior, either as active participants or legal guardians of their children, parents should be at the center of this plan to engage participants. The key role of parents has been acknowledged by many of the successful or promising TPIs reviewed here. Indeed, almost all TPIs that target the prevention of externalized (i.e., violence, delinquency, conduct disorder, school dropout) or internalized (i.e., anxiety) problems include a parent-targeted program component, which is considered the most effective strategy to date (Kazdin, 1985). In contrast, few TPIs that target children and adolescents at risk for major depression (either because of their preclinical levels of depressive symptoms or their experience with divorce or death of a family member) include a parent-targeted component. Most TPIs for major depression adopt a cognitive–behavioral approach to teach youths coping strategies in 10–15 group sessions (e.g., Coping with Depression Course for Adolescents: Clarke, Hawkins, Murphy, & Sheeber, 1995; Penn Prevention/Resiliency program: Cardemil, Reivich, Beevers, Seligman, & James, 2007; Jaycox, Reivich, Gillham, & Seligman, 1994; Cognitive Psychoeducational Intervention program: Beardslee, Salt, Porterfield *et al.*, 1993). The few depression prevention programs that target parents tend to devote only a few sessions to this program component (e.g., three information meetings with the parents in the Clarke, Hornbrook, Lynch *et al.*, 2001, study). Not surprisingly, the effect sizes observed in most depression prevention programs are considered modest by current standards (with values in the low 0.30s at the immediate post-test and in the low 0.20s at follow-up). Similarly, the few TPIs intended to prevent suicide in at-risk individuals also rarely incorporate a parental or family component (Eggert, Thompson, Herting, & Nicholas, 1995; LaFromboise & Howard-Pitney, 1995). The results of these studies are even more mixed and inconclusive than in the case of TPIs to prevent depression.

Still, programs that include a parent component are not always successful in actually engaging parents. Hence, given that a parent component seems desirable, knowledge of how to successfully engage parents is needed. This knowledge can be derived from three sources:

1 Studies that examine the factors predicting engagement and perseverance in a prevention program;

2 Narrative or meta-analytical reviews that compare studies that address similar problems but result in different recruitment or retention rates; and

3 Studies that experimentally manipulate factors in order to directly examine the causal impact of those factors on recruitment and retention rates.

A combination of efforts in these three areas has revealed a number of factors that predict engagement and retention. These factors can be grouped into five categories. The first category is comprised of sociodemographic factors. The empirical evidence regarding this category is mixed. Some studies report that ethnicity, socioeconomic adversity and child age influence recruitment and retention whereas other studies do not (Holden, Lavigne, & Cameron, 1990; Prinz & Miller, 1994). Still, and although sociodemographic factors cannot be manipulated directly, these factors can have a key role through careful and strategic matching of participants' and trainers' characteristics. For example, using nurses to recruit young parents with a history of conduct disorder into a prevention program may be less threatening to the parents than using social care workers.

The second category of predictors includes parents' beliefs about child behavior problems and about the benefits the child will derive from participating in a prevention program. More specifically, the parents' perception of the benefits the child will receive from a prevention program is influenced by the parents' perception of the prevalence of the targeted problem and the likelihood that their child might experience that problem. These perceived benefits, in turn, predict the parents' enrollment in the program (Spoth & Redmond, 1995). Therefore, focusing a prevention program too narrowly on one specific problem may not attract many parents. First, the parents may think that their child is not at risk (even if they acknowledge that prevalence rates are high). Second, parents may think that they can deal with the problem themselves. Without alarming them unnecessarily, parents may need to be informed of their child's level of risk (if that child is facing many or more severe risk factors) and that the prevention program may help the parents with their own preventive efforts. In order to maximize parents' motivation to participate in a prevention program, some authors offer a self-screening questionnaire with respect to risk and protective factors. Dishion, Nelson, and Kavanagh (2003) use a "Family Check-up" assessment to enhance parents' motivation by providing them with feedback about the strengths and the weaknesses of their parent–child relational strategies and their child's functioning as well as a menu of intervention strategies from which to choose.

Once a child and his or her parents are involved in a prevention program, retention is predicted by the extent to which the participants benefit from the program. Improvement in the child's behavioral repertoire during the first months of a multimodal prevention program for disruptive boys predicted which families would remain involved in a 3-year prevention program and which families would drop out before the end of the first year (Charlebois, Vitaro, Normandeau, & Rondeau, 2001).

Another aspect to consider with respect to parents' beliefs is whether the parents deem the prevention strategies and targeted behaviors to be appropriate. Spoth, Ball, Klose, and Redmond (1996) used "conjoint analysis" (i.e., a marketing data collection strategy designed to tap into consumer choices and needs) to examine parents' preferences for different intervention strategies (e.g., child-only, family-only or combined child–family skills training) and different practical arrangements (i.e., home visits vs. group meetings, weekdays evening sessions vs. weekend sessions). Interestingly, Spoth, Ball, Klose *et al.* found that different clusters of parents preferred different arrangements and different strategies. Notably, some parents were open to address personal and sociofamilial issues whereas others were focused mainly on the child's problems.

Using an experimental approach, Miller and Prinz (2003) also found that assignment to a treatment condition that did not match parents' motivations and expectations was predictive of premature termination. More specifically, premature termination was higher in a parent-only treatment condition than in child-only and combined parent–child conditions. Prinz and Miller (1994) have also shown that adding supportive discussions not directly related to child behavior to a series of parent training sessions targeting children's disruptiveness resulted in less attrition than focusing exclusively on parenting and parent–child interactions during the sessions.

The third category of factors affecting engagement and retention of participants represents practical barriers to participation, including the scheduling of program activities. In general, flexibility in program delivery has been found to be related to retention rates (Prinz & Miller, 1996; Weisz, Weiss, Alicke, & Klotz, 1987). Of special interest is whether home delivery of services produces better engagement and recruitment than flexible out-of-home services. Unfortunately, no study has directly compared the two strategies. However, the relative effectiveness of these two strategies in enhancing participation and retention may vary depending on the child's age (e.g., newborns vs. early adolescents) and parent characteristics. Facilitating participation by offering transportation, daycare services for the target child and any siblings, or supplementing training sessions for the target child with fun activities may help overcome resistance if the out-of-home delivery service is chosen.

Another critical element with respect to participation and retention is the temporal spacing of the prevention activities. If program activities are spaced too far apart, participants may lose interest in the program. Activities spaced too close together may lead participants to feel overloaded. For example, during the Fast Track trial, parents "rebelled" during the third year when session spacing was changed to once every 3 months from once a week during the first year and twice a month during the second year. Based on parents' reactions, the Fast Track researchers reinstituted more frequent sessions of once a month. In addition, potential recipients who feel that they do not need some program components may refuse participation or become bored and withdraw from the study. In this situation, a differential approach to the spacing and number of sessions – similar to the adaptive approach described above (Collins, Murphy, & Bierman, 2004) – may increase compliance and retention of participants.

Parents' characteristics are another important category of factors that may affect participation in prevention programs. There is empirical evidence showing that fathers are less inclined to participate in prevention programs than mothers (Spoth, Ball, Klose *et al.*, 1996). In consequence, some authors tried to compensate for parents' low motivation by offering incentives in the form of tangible rewards, such as money and meals (Conduct Problems Prevention Research Group, 2002; St. Pierre, Mark, Kaltreider, & Aikin, 1997; Webster-Stratton, Mihalic, Fagan *et al.*, 2001a), or social rewards, including giving parents a role as co-therapists or co-trainers (Conduct Problems Prevention Research Group, 2002; Cunningham, Bremner, & Boyle, 1995; St. Pierre, Mark, Kaltreider *et al.*, 1997).

The final category of factors that might affect participation refers to the manner in which and the moment at which parental participation is requested. Personalized recruitment seems more effective than a generic and impersonal approach (Schlernitzauer, Bierhals, Geary *et al.*, 1998). Even the manner in which the initial invitation to participate is formulated may affect participation. Spoth and Redmond (1994) compared two different letter solicitation strategies for recruiting families of early adolescents to participate in a family-based drug prevention program. In one strategy, families were invited first to participate in an assessment session and next to the full program. In the other strategy, the families were offered full participation right away. Not surprisingly, the first strategy produced higher recruitment, but lower retention rates. Linking the program to an official and respected institution may also increase its credibility and, consequently, enhance participation rates of parents as well as of prevention service deliverers (i.e., teachers and mental health professionals). Promotion of the program by esteemed persons or the media may also help increase the participation of key stakeholders. Finally, the description of the program's objectives is also important. Because most prevention programs, including the targeted ones, focus at least as much on promoting skills and opportunities as on reducing risk factors, the objectives should emphasize health and competence promotion.

The timing of the offer to become involved in a prevention program may also affect participation. Transition periods may be particularly good points of entry because of the anxiety and the uncertainty experienced by many parents and children at these times of change. Some transition periods at which interventions are commonly directed include the birth of the child, beginning of preschool, transition to high school and transition to adulthood. Other, less normative experiences may also be considered important transitions (e.g., divorce of parents).

Finally, it is essential that the recruiters and trainers possess appropriate skills and knowledge of the targeted families' cultural and linguistic backgrounds. The recruiters and trainers should also establish a positive bond with the families. Low staff turnover may help ensure such a positive bond (Prinz, Smith, Dumas *et al.*, 2001).

In sum, many of the factors reviewed here are controlled or influenced by the individuals responsible for the prevention program. However, although participation rates may be dramatically affected by such factors, the experimental studies that have assessed the impact of these factors on participation remain scarce. Indeed, rates of engagement and retention should be included among the outcomes assessed in any prevention program.

How to Optimize Cost-Effectiveness

One important argument often used in support of prevention is its cost-effectiveness in comparison to treatment (for a description of cost-effectiveness analysis see chapter 10; Chatterji, Caffray, Jones, Lillie-Blanton, & Werthamer, 2001). However, effective prevention programs addressing psychoemotional problems are not cheap. Indeed, most prevention programs for high-risk individuals or communities need to target several domains of functioning (i.e., different systems) and deploy different intervention strategies over several years to hope for more than modest effect sizes (for an overall consideration of issues of service planning see chapter 71; Greenberg, Domitrovich, & Bumbarger, 2001; Yoshikawa, 1994).

One way to reduce the cost of a prevention program is to deliver as many components as possible, such as parent and child training sessions, in a group format. Such a strategy has resulted in at least one cost-effective program – a prevention program for adolescents at risk for major depression (Clarke, Hornbrook, Lynch *et al.*, 2001; Lynch, Hornbrook, Clarke *et al.*, 2005). Notably, the cost-effectiveness of this TPI was comparable to most treatments for adult depression.

Still, there is a risk that the economy of scale that results from group sessions may impact adversely on the program's effectiveness. Ang and Hugues (2002) concluded their meta-analysis by showing that individual social skills-training sessions are more effective in teaching social skills to children than group sessions, probably because of the additional attention a child receives and the additional opportunities to practice the learned skills. Moreover, prevention programs that aggregate at-risk children, such as those with externalizing problems, appear less effective than programs that mix at-risk children with prosocial peers. Group interventions that aggregate only at-risk children may even result in iatrogenic effects through a process known as deviancy training (Boxer, Guerra, Huesmann, & Morales, 2005; Dishion, McCord, & Poulin, 1999; Dodge, Dishion, & Lansford, 2006). However, iatrogenic effects do not invariably result from aggregating at-risk individuals because deviancy training depends on a host of circumstances, including the children's age and trainer's competence (Gifford-Smith, Dodge, Dishion, & McCord, 2005).

Another strategy to reduce costs during the training and the implementation phases of a prevention program is to manualize the program components as much as possible (van de Wiel, Matthys, Cohen-Kettenis, & van Engeland, 2003). However, it is important that the staff do not lose track of the theoretical principles behind the intervention, as was the case in an unsuccessful dissemination effort of the Prenatal/Infancy Project (Olds, Henderson, Tatelbaum *et al.*, 1986), which had been found to reduce abuse and promote health in children on many previous occasions.

If costs cannot be reduced without negative consequences, then either efficiency or effectiveness – or possibly both – need to be improved. Efficiency refers to the ability to produce optimal effects with the available resources and time. The adaptive approach is one promising strategy to increase efficiency. The resources saved when less at-risk participants receive fewer program components can be transferred to those who have greater need. This increases the potential for optimal impact with the available resources – and may even reduce costs relative to a fixed approach in which all participants receive all components (Collins, Murphy, & Bierman, 2004). There are no studies manipulating dosage or comparing an adaptive approach to a fixed approach.

Effectiveness may be increased in at least two ways. First, effectiveness may be enhanced by adding new innovative intervention strategies (such as Fast Track's peer pairing and academic tutoring components) to more traditional prevention strategies (such as parent training and social-cognitive skills training). Second, combining a universal with a targeted approach may also improve the targeted program's effectiveness. Adding new prevention components, such as the innovative components or a universal component, makes sense only if they target risk or protective factors not already targeted by the more traditional components. In other words, it is important to avoid redundancy and increase coverage of new targets such that enough – and the most potent – risk and protective factors are modified. This, in turn, increases the probability of enhanced effect sizes and notable and durable benefits.

Another aspect to consider in cost-effectiveness analysis is whether a prevention program is capable of helping the most at-risk and most costly cases. In the area of disruptive behavior, longitudinal studies have found that 5–10% of the children displaying conduct problems account for at least half of all adolescent and adult crimes (Moffitt, 1990; Nagin & Tremblay, 1999; Stattin & Magnusson, 1991). Each individual persistently involved in crime represents a $2 million lifetime cost (in today's dollars) to society (Cohen, 1998). This cost does not even include the expenses related to the collateral problems – such as a failure to complete high school and pathological dependence on substances – for which this small group of children is also at higher risk. To develop a full and accurate picture of the cost-effectiveness of a prevention program, investigators should include the cost of all possible problems that the program could prevent. Costly but moderately effective (i.e., effects size of 0.20–0.50 in the short term) prevention programs that impact on the most extreme cases, such as Fast Track, then seem particularly cost-effective (Foster & Jones, 2006). Cost-effectiveness analysis of a number of other targeted prevention programs, such as the Coping Power Program for aggressive children (van de Wiel, Matthys, Cohen-Kettenis *et al.*, 2003) or the Perry Preschool program for disadvantaged children and their families (Barnett, 1985; Schweinhart, Barnes, & Weikart, 1993) shows that these also appear to be cost-effective.

Importance of Dissemination, its Challenges, and Some Possible Solutions

Large-scale dissemination of evidence-based and cost-effective targeted prevention programs is important. The essential prerequisite before dissemination is a strong test of the program's validity and efficacy. Lists of model programs that are ready for large-scale implementation are available. However, given the diversity of prevention programs, even among programs targeting the same outcome, direct comparisons between competing prevention programs are needed in order to determine which is most cost-effective. Second, it is essential to replicate the original (effective) prevention programs in different socioeconomic contexts and different cultures in order to identify the program's limits. Such replications may also explain why the results of evidence-based interventions are often not as strong when disseminated to real-world settings (i.e., the so-called "effect erosion" problem; Lochman, 2001). To address the problem of "effect erosion" when going to scale, preventionists should conduct both efficacy and effectiveness trials for any given program. Contrary to efficacy trials, in which the "maximum" impact of a prevention program is assessed under optimal conditions, an effectiveness trial evaluates the "true" or actual impact of a prevention program under real-world conditions. Both are important preliminary steps that should be taken before large-scale implementation occurs. Only when both efficacy and effectiveness are assessed is it possible to understand the conditions that produce the maximum impact of the program.

Performing both efficacy and effectiveness trials may reduce – but not necessarily eliminate – the risk of inadequate dissemination. In order to further reduce or eliminate this risk, researchers need to turn their attention to what Dodge (2001) referred to as the science of dissemination towards practitioners and policy-makers. Elliott and Mihalic (2004) listed a six-step process for achieving successful dissemination of a prevention program: select the sites that are ready, train the practitioners, provide them with technical assistance, monitor and reflect on program fidelity, and assure sustainability through continuous funding and permanent changes in the service delivery system. Other researchers examined the ways to make scientific knowledge more usable and used more frequently by policy-makers and practitioners (Dodge, 2006; Huston, 2005). Among the proposed strategies is the use of the media through press releases or public briefings presenting research findings that are likely to be of interest to the public. Another interesting strategy is to create two-way communication forums in which policy-makers, practitioners and researchers share and debate their research questions, methodologies, cost–benefit analyses and conclusions. Research questions should be framed in such a way that evaluation results will clearly inform about:

1 The chain of factors that lead to change in at-risk individuals or communities;

2 The most cost-effective intervention strategies; and

3 Moderators of program effectiveness.

Conversely, preventive intervention evaluation results may also aid researchers in refining the theoretical models that served as the foundation for that intervention.

How Preventive Interventions can Inform Theory

TPIs can help to clarify the role of the risk and protective factors and processes that were initially selected as proximal outcomes or putative mediators of the intervention effects. They can also help to identify new factors that, although not targeted initially, may have an important role with respect to the program's impact. Finally, TPIs can help to validate the principles for change that were used to guide the development of the intervention strategies. Hence, a TPI evaluation can illuminate the theory behind the development of the problem to be prevented and the theory behind the process leading to more positive outcomes (Cicchetti & Hinshaw, 2002).

To illustrate, Vitaro, Brendgen, & Tremblay (2001a) showed that the Montreal longitudinal prevention program targeting young low SES disruptive boys achieved its impact on later delinquency in two ways. First, the program improved children's behavioral repertoire and parental supervision (i.e., proximal effects). Second, the program reduced affiliation with deviant peers and school problems (i.e., intermediate effects).

More specifically, improved social competence and parental supervision and reduced affiliation with deviant friends and school problems mediated, in a two-step sequential process, the impact of the prevention program on later delinquency. These findings enhance the plausibility that these mediators have a causal role in the chain of events leading disruptive boys to become involved in delinquency. They also point to the importance of targeting these mediators through booster sessions if necessary. However, most TPIs cannot clearly establish the causal role of risk factors because more than the putative mediators may have been triggered by the prevention program (Howe, Reiss, & Yuh, 2002). One solution to this problem would be to specify and measure all relevant mediators and control for their effects, a task rarely achieved or even achievable.

TPIs can also contribute to developmental models of psychopathology in other ways. Prevention programs can help uncover or verify mechanisms of influence, even when the programs result in iatrogenic effects. Dishion, Spracklen, Andrews, and Patterson (1996) used an experimental design to determine that a group-based social skills prevention program resulted in iatrogenic effects. Dishion, Spracklen, & Andrews *et al.* were able to confirm the causal role of deviancy training (discovered earlier through the coding of the interactions between the participating at-risk adolescents and their friends in the context of a correlational study). Deviancy training results from positive reinforcement through laughter or positive nonverbal feedback of rule-breaking talk and deviant acts as well as from ignoring or punishing normative behaviors through principles of operant conditioning.

Conclusions and Future Directions

To conclude, we offer suggestions for the next generation of TPIs.

Through narrative or quantitative reviews (i.e., meta-analysis) of prospective longitudinal studies, we need to establish more clearly which risk and protective factors should be used to identify individual levels of risk and categories of at-risk individuals. We favor an interactional approach over a cumulative approach. We also believe that more than two groups exist (i.e., more than simply the at-risk and the low-risk groups), although the number of relevant groups may depend on the type of outcome considered and a host of other factors.

Through narrative and quantitative reviews, we need to identify the best prevention practices and program models that match the evolving criteria for efficacy, effectiveness and dissemination. The Society for Prevention Research (2004) proposed a series of clear criteria with respect to each of these three elements that can serve as guidelines, although these criteria are likely to evolve over the coming years. The Institute of Medicine Committee on Prevention of Mental Disorders (Mrazek & Haggerty, 1994) has also issued a seven-level scale to judge the quality of a prevention program from the characteristics of that program's evaluation protocol.

Studies that compare different versions of the same program are needed (i.e., programs that differ with respect to the number of components or duration of the intervention). After experimenting with single or bimodal prevention programs during the 1980s (often social skills and/or family-based programs), prevention scientists started experimenting with multimodal comprehensive programs during the 1990s (e.g., Fast Track). These programs were often compared only with a control condition, a strategy that was well-justified at the time (Coie, Miller-Johnson, & Bagwell, 2000). However, we believe the time has come for factorial designs in which different sets of components, different durations or different programs are compared, taking into account their possible interactions with participants' characteristics and contextual factors (i.e., moderators). This factorial approach would help refine and possibly increase the power of current and future prevention programs in an optimal cost-effective manner by identifying necessary and sufficient components or important new elements of those programs. Indeed, it would be interesting to see whether targeted prevention programs that are embedded in universal prevention programs bring the multiplicative effects expected in comparison to targeted-only or universal-only programs. It would also be interesting to compare an adaptive approach (Collins, Murphy, & Bierman, 2004) to a fixed approach. Such a comparison could be achieved by comparing two randomly assigned groups of participants: one receiving a fixed dosage of a preventive package and one receiving different combinations and different dosages of the same package. However, costs and resources should be kept equivalent across the two conditions or be taken into account when comparing effect sizes. A randomly assigned no-intervention/care-as-usual control group could also be included. Small-scale experimental studies that compare the efficacy of different modes of intervention or teaching methods to achieve specific desired goals, both with respect to process variables and with respect to outcomes, are also needed. These experimental studies will advance our knowledge about effective strategies for change and their underlying theoretical principles.

Programmatic comparative studies are also needed to explore the most effective strategies to engage and retain potential participants, practitioners and decision-makers. The science of prevention took form during the past decade. Currently, a science of dissemination and social policy-making is taking form (Huston, 2005). In order to ensure that the best programs are disseminated and form the basis for social policy, valid and convincing cost-effectiveness studies need to be conducted. Luckily, more and more such studies are available (Foster & Jones, 2006; Lynch, Hornbrook, Clarke *et al.*, 2005; van de Wiel, Matthys, Cohen-Kettenis *et al.*, 2003; see also Cuijpers, 2003; Romeo, Byford, & Knapp, 2005). Business models can also contribute to the promotion and dissemination of the best prevention programs (Rotheram-Borus & Duan, 2003).

We need more process-oriented prevention research that documents mediators of change both during and after the prevention trial. This type of prevention research can have both theoretical and practical implications. Understanding mediating factors and processes can help to clarify and validate theoretical models. A greater understanding of the role of mediators can also enhance the intervention process by guiding program content and program duration until the potent, pertinent and plausibly causal mediators are sufficiently modified to ensure that the distal outcomes are affected. In the case of an unsuccessful prevention program, being able to pinpoint unchanged important mediators will inform the next wave of prevention programs so that they can target these mediators more effectively.

We also need to verify which preventive intervention program works best under which conditions and for which population. Interesting suggestions and examples of context-specific preventive interventions have been described by a number of researchers (Allen & Philliber, 2001; Beauchaine, Webster-Stratton, & Reid, 2005; Gillham, Shatté, & Reivich, 2001). It is particularly important to document the conditions under which a program previously observed to be effective may fail when applied to new populations (MacMillan, Thomas, Jamieson *et al.*, 2005).

The impact of TPIs should be assessed with respect to the distal outcomes they are designed to prevent. Short- and mid-term effects on important mediators, although promising, do not always guarantee the final result. In addition to including randomly assigned control participants to guard against spurious results or iatrogenic effects, a group of normative children should also be included to probe the clinical significance of the effects of the TPI (Kendall, Marrs-Garcia, Nath, & Sheldrick, 1999). Despite the statistically significant improvements demonstrated by program children on a number of measures, it is rarely the case that these children function "normally" (i.e., within 0.5 SD of the normative mean or without any clinical symptom) even after the intervention. Only a few TPIs reviewed in this chapter included a normative group (e.g., Early Risers, Fast Track, the Montreal longitudinal prevention program). Short-term results produced by these three high-intensity multicomponent preventive interventions show that none of them was able to move the targeted high-risk children into a normative range on important measures, despite significant overall differences between them and their counterparts in the control condition. In addition, long-term follow-ups show that many targeted children manifest serious adjustment problems, although proportionately less than their control counterparts (Boisjoli, Vitaro, Lacourse, & Tremblay, 2007; Conduct Problems Prevention Research Group, 2002, 2005). This finding alone calls for a renewed strategy with respect to our current prevention efforts.

We believe that the diverse and often competing prevention programs targeting different outcomes at different periods in development should become the building blocks of an integrated prevention system. These different programs should be linked to each other at three levels in addition to being delivered in accordance with an adaptive approach at each level. First, at the *chronological* level, the perinatal programs would be the first to be deployed. If the proximal results are satisfactory, these perinatal programs would be sufficient, as will undoubtedly be the case for some participants and problems. Participants still at risk for problems left unchanged by a perinatal program would be exposed to a second wave of prevention strategies during the preschool years. These may take place in the childcare setting, for example. This *cumulative modular strategy* would be repeated until the risk factors are dissipated or the protective factors are solid enough to ensure a highly probable positive trajectory. The early prevention programs should target as many *potent generic causal* factors as possible to achieve an optimal impact. However, because new risk factors may appear with development, booster programs might be needed at later transition periods to address these new and often *specific* risk factors. These booster programs would also capitalize on the malleability of participants' behavior during periods of transition. Periods of transition often correspond to the changing phase between two developmental stages which are particularly sensitive to new learning because of the disequilibrium created both at the cognitive and the emotional levels and the new opportunities that become available (Dahlberg & Potter, 2001; Pickles & Angold, 2003).

Second, at the *service delivery* level, different services which often involve different personnel in different contexts need to be integrated into a coherent prevention system. Finally, at the *outcome* level, it is important to acknowledge that many prevention programs target the same risk factors and use similar strategies to achieve change even though their stated intention is to prevent different adjustment problems (e.g., school dropout vs. delinquency). As a result, programs with different stated goals may also have an important impact on other aspects of development – a probable consequence of their many common risk factors. Hence, most TPIs should assess several types of outcome, independent of their initial goals. This is particularly true for TPIs that adopt a generic perspective. This strategy might help increase the cost-effectiveness of TPIs. In addition, assessing change in different types of problem makes sense given the surprising similarities in the components and strategies used in TPIs targeting children at risk for different types of outcome (e.g., conduct disorder, substance use and depression).

Despite our enthusiasm for prevention, we nevertheless wish to conclude by raising concern about several iatrogenic effects that have been reported sporadically in the literature and may represent only the tip of the iceberg (Dishion, McCord, & Poulin, 1999; Dodge, Dishion, & Lansford, 2006; Werch & Owen, 2001). One well-known TPI that produced spectacular iatrogenic effects is the Cambridge Somerville Youth Study (Dishion, McCord, & Poulin, 1999; McCord, 1978). After 30 years, boys who participated in a multimodal program throughout early adolescence which included academic tutoring, family counseling, medical attention, summer camps and contact with community organizations had worse outcomes in several domains of functioning (i.e., criminal behavior, alcoholism, mental and physical problems, death) than matched controls who did not participate in the program. We believe that the planners and the disseminators of prevention programs should be extremely sensitive and responsive to this issue. We need to learn about the conditions and the processes that are responsible for such iatrogenic effects as much as we need to learn about the conditions and processes responsible for positive and hopefully long-term effects of current and future targeted prevention programs.

Complementary References and Websites

Because the focus of this chapter is on the underlying principles, the number of prevention programs that were used for illustration purposes is necessarily limited. The reader can find a more complete and detailed list of targeted preventive programs in narrative reviews mentioned below. The reviews by Greenberg, Domitrovich, & Bumbarger (2001) and by Mrazek and Brown (2002) cover most programs targeting children aged 5–18 or 0–6 years, respectively. The reader can also consult the meta-analytical reviews reported in Table 61.1 and several of the other chapters in this volume for a more complete overview of preventive interventions targeting different areas of functioning.

Finally, some universal preventive interventions document their results for the most at-risk children in addition to the whole population of children. These findings may be relevant for targeted preventionists even if they are derived from universal programs. One such program is the Good Behavior Game (Kellam, Rebok, Ialongo, & Mayer, 1994), a team-based classroom program that uses group reinforcement and competition to promote appropriate behavior in first grade. At 6-year follow-up, experimental boys who were the most aggressive in first grade manifested less aggression according to teachers than their control counterparts, whereas the other children did not.

Further Information and Reading

Crill Russell, C. (2002). *The state of knowledge about prevention/early intervention*. Toronto, ON: Invest in Kids Foundation.

Greenberg, M. T., Domitrovich, C., & Bumbarger, B. (2001). The prevention of mental disorders in school-aged children: Current state of the field. *Prevention and Treatment*, *4*.

Mrazek, P. J., & Brown, C. H. (2002). An evidence-based literature review regarding outcomes in psychosocial prevention and early intervention in young children. In C. C. Russell (Ed.), *The state of knowledge about prevention/early intervention* (pp. 42–165). Toronto, ON: Invest in Kids Foundation.

National Institutes of Health State of the Science Conference Statement. (2006). Preventing violence and related health-risking, social behaviors in adolescents, October 13–15, 2004. *Journal of Abnormal Child Psychology*, *34*, 457–470.

Society for Prevention Research (SPR). Accessed from http://www.preventionresearch.org

University of Colorado Center for the Study and Prevention of Violence. Accessed from http://www.colorado.edu/cspv/blueprints

References

Alkon, A., Tschann, J. M., Ruane, S. H., Wolff, M., & Hittner, A. (2001). A violence-prevention and evaluation project with ethnically diverse populations. *American Journal of Preventive Medicine*, *20*, 48–55.

Allen, J. P., & Philliber, S. (2001). Who benefits most from a broadly targeted prevention program? Differential efficacy across populations in the Teen Outreach program. *Journal of Community Psychology*, *29*, 637–655.

Ang, R. P., & Hugues, J. N. (2002). Differential benefits of skills training with antisocial youth based on group composition: A meta-analytic investigation. *School Psychology Review*, *31*, 164–185.

Angrist, J. D., Imbens, G. W., & Rubin, D. B. (1996). Identification of causal effects using instrumental variables. *Journal of the American Statistical Association*, *91*, 444–455.

Aos, S., Lieb, R., Mayfield, J., Miller, M., & Pennucci, A. (2004). *Benefits and costs of prevention and early intervention programs for youth*. Seattle, WA: Washington State Public Policy Institute.

August, G. J., Egan, E. A., Realmuto, G. M., & Hektner, J. M. (2003). Four years of the early risers early-age-targeted preventive intervention: Effects on aggressive children's peer relations. *Behavior Therapy*, *34*, 453–470.

August, G. J., Hektner, J. M., Egan, E. E., Realmuto, G. M., & Bloomquist, M. L. (2002). The Early Risers longitudinal prevention trial: Examination of three year outcomes in aggressive children with intent-to-treat and as-intended analyses. *Psychology of Addictive Behaviors*, *16*, 27–39.

August, G. J., Realmuto, G. M., Hektner, J. M., & Bloomquist, M. L. (2001). An integrated components preventive intervention for aggressive elementary school children: The Early Risers Program. *Journal of Consulting and Clinical Psychology*, *69*, 614–626.

Bachman, J. G., Johnston, L. D., & O'Malley, P. M. (1998). Explaining recent increases in students' marijuana use: Impacts of perceived risks and disapproval, 1976 through 1996. *American Journal of Public Health*, *88*, 887–892.

Bakermans-Kranenburg, M. J., van IJzendoorn, M. H., & Juffer, F. (2003). Less is more: Meta-analyses of sensitivity and attachment interventions in early childhood. *Psychological Bulletin*, *129*, 195–215.

Barnett, W. S. (1985). *The Perry Preschool Program and its long-term effects: A benefit–cost analysis*. Ypsilanti, MI: High/Scope Educational Research Foundation.

Beardslee, W. R., Salt, P., Porterfield, K., Rothberg, P. C., van de Velde, P., Swatling, S., *et al.* (1993). Comparison of preventive interventions for families with parental affective disorder. *Journal of the American Academy of Child and Adolescent Psychiatry*, *32*, 254–263.

Beauchaine, T. P., Webster-Stratton, C., & Reid, M. J. (2005). Mediators, moderators, and predictors of 1-year outcomes among children treated for early-onset conduct problems: A latent growth curve analysis. *Journal of Consulting and Clinical Psychology*, *73*, 371–388.

Boisjoli, R., Vitaro, F., Lacourse, E., Barker, E. D., & Tremblay, R. E. (2007). Impact and clinical significance of a preventive intervention for disruptive boys: 15-year follow-up. *British Journal of Psychiatry*, *191*, 415–419.

Boxer, P., Guerra, N. G., Huesmann, L. R., & Morales, J. (2005). Proximal peer-level effects of a small-group selected prevention on aggression in elementary school children: An investigation of the peer contagion hypothesis. *Journal of Abnormal Child Psychology*, *33*, 325–338.

Burgess, E. W. (1928). Factors determining success or failure on parole. In A. A. Bruce, A. J. Harno, E. W. Burgess, & J. Landesco (Eds.), *The workings of the indeterminate-sentence law and the parole systems in Illinois* (pp. 221–234). Springfield, IL: Illinois State Board of Parole.

Campbell, F. A., & Ramey, C. T. (1995). Cognitive and school outcomes for high-risk African-American students at middle adolescence: Positive effects of early intervention. *American Educational Research Journal*, *32*, 743–772.

Caplan, G. (1964). *Principles of preventive psychology*. New York, NY: Basic Books.

Cardemil, E. V., Reivich, K. J., Beevers, C. G., Seligman, M. E. P., & James, J. (2007). The prevention of depressive symptoms in low-income, minority children: Two-year follow-up. *Behaviour Research and Therapy*, *45*, 313–327.

Carneiro, P., & Heckman, J. (2003). Human capital policy. In J. Heckman, & A. B. Krueger (Eds.), *Inequality in America: What role for Human Capital Policies?* (pp. 77–240). Boston, MA: MIT Press.

Caspi, A., McClay, J., Moffitt, T. E., Mill, J., Martin, J., Craig, I. W., *et al.* (2002). Role of genotype in the cycle of violence in maltreated children. *Science*, *297*, 851–854.

Ceci, S. J., & Papierno, P. B. (2005). The rhetoric and reality of gap closing: When the "Have-nots" gain but the "Haves" gain even more. *American Psychologist*, *60*, 149–160.

Charlebois, P., Vitaro, F., Normandeau, S., & Rondeau, N. (2001). Predictors of persistence in a longitudinal preventive intervention program for young disruptive boys. *Prevention Science*, *2*, 133–143.

Chatterji, P., Caffray, C. M., Jones, A. S., Lillie-Blanton, M., & Werthamer, L. (2001). Applying cost analysis methods to school-based prevention programs. *Prevention Science*, *2*, 45–55.

Chen, X. Y., Rubin, K. H., & Sun, Y. R. (1992). Social reputation and peer relationships in Chinese and Canadian children: A cross-cultural study. *Child Development*, *63*, 1336–1343.

Cicchetti, D., & Cohen, D. J. (2006). *Developmental psychopathology*, Vol. 1. *Theory and methods* (2nd edn.). New York, NY: Wiley.

Cicchetti, D., & Hinshaw, S. P. (2002). Editorial: Prevention and intervention science: Contributions to developmental theory. *Development and Psychopathology*, *14*, 667–671.

Clarke, G. N., Hawkins, W., Murphy, M., & Sheeber, L. B. (1995). Targeted prevention of unipolar depressive disorder in an at-risk sample of high school adolescents: A randomized trial of group cognitive intervention. *Journal of the American Academy of Child and Adolescent Psychiatry*, *34*, 312–321.

Clarke, G. N., Hornbrook, M., Lynch, F., Polen, M., Gale, J., Beardslee, W., *et al.* (2001). A randomized trial of a group cognitive intervention for preventing depression in adolescent offspring of depressed parents. *Archives of General Psychiatry*, *58*, 1127–1134.

Cohen, M. A. (1998). The monetary value of saving a high-risk youth. *Journal of Quantitative Criminology*, *4*, 5–33.

Coie, J. D., Miller-Johnson, S., & Bagwell, C. (2000). Prevention science. In A. J. Sameroff, M. Lewis, & S. M. Miller (Eds.), *Handbook of developmental psychopathology* (2nd edn., pp. 93–112). New York, NY: Kluwer Academic/Plenum.

Coie, J. D., Underwood, M., & Lochman, J. E. (1991). Programmatic intervention with aggressive children in the school setting. In D. J. Pepler, & K. H. Rubin (Eds.), *The development and treatment of childhood aggression* (pp. 389–410). Hillsdale, NJ: Lawrence Erlbaum Associates.

Coie, J. D., Watt, N. F., West, S. G., Hawkins, J. D., Asarnow, J. R., Markman, H. J., *et al.* (1993). The science of prevention: A conceptual framework and some directions for a national research program. *American Psychologist*, *48*, 1013–1022.

Collins, L. M., Murphy, S. A., & Bierman, K. L. (2004). A conceptual framework for adaptive preventive interventions. *Prevention Science*, *5*, 185–196.

Conduct Problems Prevention Research Group. (1992). A developmental and clinical model for the prevention of conduct disorder: The Fast Track Program. *Development and Psychopathology*, *4*, 509–527.

Conduct Problems Prevention Research Group. (1999a). Initial impact of the Fast Track prevention trial for conduct problems. I. The high-risk sample. *Journal of Consulting and Clinical Psychology*, *67*, 631–647.

Conduct Problems Prevention Research Group. (1999b). Initial impact of the Fast Track prevention trial for conduct problems. II. Classroom effects. *Journal of Consulting and Clinical Psychology*, *67*, 648–657.

Conduct Problems Prevention Research Group. (2002). Evaluation of the first 3 years of the Fast Track prevention trial with children at high risk for adolescent conduct problems. *Journal of Abnormal Child Psychology*, *30*, 19–35.

Conduct Problems Prevention Research Group. (2004). The effects of the Fast Track program on serious problem outcomes at the end of elementary school. *Journal of Clinical Child and Adolescent Psychology*, *33*, 650–661.

Conduct Problems Prevention Research Group. (2005). *The long-term prevention of serious conduct disorder, interpersonal violence, and violent crime* (No. 05–78. Technical Report). University Park, PA: Pennsylvania State University, Methodology Center.

Cowen, E. L. (1991). In pursuit of wellness. *American Psychologist*, *46*, 404–408.

Cuijpers, P. (2003). Examining the effects of prevention programs on the incidence of new cases of mental disorders: The lack of statistical power. *American Journal of Psychiatry*, *160*, 1385–1391.

Cunningham, C. E., Bremner, R., & Boyle, M. (1995). Large group community-based parenting programs for families of preschoolers at risk for disruptive behaviour disorders: Utilization, cost effectiveness, and outcome. *Journal of Child Psychology and Psychiatry, and Allied Disciplines*, *36*, 1141–1159.

Dadds, M. R., Holland, D. E., Laurens, K. R., Mullins, M., Barrett, P. M., & Spence, S. H. (1999). Early intervention and prevention of anxiety disorders in children: Results at 2-year follow-up. *Journal of Consulting and Clinical Psychology*, *67*, 145–150.

Dadds, M. R., Spence, S. H., Holland, D. E., Barrett, P. M., & Laurens, K. R. (1997). Prevention and early intervention for anxiety disorders: A controlled trial. *Journal of Consulting and Clinical Psychology*, *65*, 627–635.

Dahlberg, L. L., & Potter, L. B. (2001). Youth violence: Developmental pathways and prevention challenges. *American Journal of Preventive Medicine*, *20*, 3–14.

Deater-Deckard, K., Dodge, K. A., Bates, J. E., & Pettit, G. S. (1998). Multiple risk factors in the development of externalizing behavior problems: Group and individual differences. *Development and Psychopathology*, *10*, 469–493.

Dishion, T. J., & Andrews, D. W. (1995). Preventing escalation in problem behaviors with high-risk young adolescents: Immediate and 1-year outcomes. *Journal of Consulting and Clinical Psychology*, *63*, 538–548.

Dishion, T. J., McCord, J., & Poulin, F. (1999). When interventions harm: Peer groups and problem behavior. *American Psychologist*, *54*, 755–764.

Dishion, T. J., Nelson, S. E., & Kavanagh, K. (2003). The family check-up with high-risk young adolescents: Preventing early-onset substance use by parent monitoring. *Behavior Therapy*, *34*, 553–571.

Dishion, T. J., Spracklen, K. M., Andrews, D. W., & Patterson, G. R. (1996). Deviancy training in male adolescent friendships. *Behavior Therapy*, *27*, 373–390.

Dodge, K. A. (2001). The science of youth violence prevention: Progressing from developmental epidemiology to efficacy to effectiveness to public policy. *American Journal of Preventive Medicine*, *20*, 63–70.

Dodge, K. A. (2006). Professionalizing the practice of public policy in the prevention of violence. *Journal of Abnormal Child Psychology*, *34*, 475–479.

Dodge, K. A., Dishion, T. J., & Lansford, J. E. (2006). *Deviant peer influences in intervention and public policy for youth*. New York, NY: Guilford Press.

Dumas, J. E., Prinz, R. J., Smith, E. P., & Laughlin, J. (1999). The EARLY ALLIANCE prevention trial: An integrated set of interventions to promote competence and reduce risk for conduct disorder, substance abuse, and school failure. *Clinical Child and Family Psychology Review*, *2*, 37–53.

DuPaul, G., & Eckert, T. L. (1997). The effects of school-based interventions for attention deficit hyperactivity disorder: A meta-analysis. *School Psychology Review*, *26*, 5–27.

Eggert, L. L., Thompson, E. A., Herting, J. R., & Nicholas, L. J. (1995). Reducing suicide potential among high-risk youth: Tests of a school-based prevention program. *Suicide and Life-Threatening Behavior*, *25*, 276–296.

Elliott, D. S., & Mihalic, S. (2004). Issues in disseminating and replicating effective prevention programs. *Prevention Science*, *5*, 47–53.

Farrington, D. P. (1985). Delinquency prevention in the 1980s. *Journal of Adolescence*, *8*, 3–16.

Farrington, D. P., & Welsh, B. C. (2003). Family-based prevention of offending: A meta-analysis. *The Australian and New Zealand Journal of Criminology*, *36*, 127–151.

Felner, R. D., Yates Felner, T., & Silverman, M. M. (2000). Prevention in mental health and social intervention: Conceptual and methodological issues in the evolution of the science and practice of prevention. In J. Rappaport, & E. Seidman (Eds.), *Handbook of community psychology* (pp. 9–42). New York, NY: Kluwer Academic/Plenum.

Fergusson, D. M., Vitaro, F., Wanner, B., & Brendgen, M. (2007). Protective and compensatory factors mitigating the influence of deviant friends on delinquent behaviors during early adolescence. *Journal of Adolescence*, *30*, 33–50.

Fontana, C. A., Fleischman, A. R., McCarton, C., Meltzer, A., & Ruff, H. (1988). A neonatal preventative intervention study: Issues of recruitment and retention. *Journal of Primary Prevention*, *9*, 164–176.

Foster, E. M., Jones, D., and the Conduct Problem Prevention Research Group (2006). Can a costly intervention be cost-effective? An analysis of violence prevention. *Archives of General Psychiatry* *63*, 1284–1291.

Franklin, C., Grant, D., Corcoran, J., Miller, P., & Bultman, L. (1997). Effectiveness of prevention programs for adolescent pregnancy: A meta-analysis. *Journal of Marriage and the Family*, *59*, 551–567.

Garvey, C., Wrenetha, J., Fogg, L., Kratovil, A., & Gross, D. (2006). Measuring participation in a prevention trial with parents of young children. *Research in Nursing and Health*, *29*, 212–222.

Gifford-Smith, M., Dodge, K. A., Dishion, T. J., & McCord, J. (2005). Peer influence in children and adolescents: Crossing the bridge from developmental to intervention science. *Journal of Abnormal Child Psychology*, *33*, 255–265.

Gillham, J. E., Shatté, A. J., & Reivich, K. (2001). Needed for prevention research: Long-term follow up and the evaluation of mediators, moderators, and lay providers. Commentary on Greenberg, Domitrovich, & Bumbarger (2001). The prevention of mental disorders in school-age children: Current state of the field. *Prevention and Treatment*, *4*, Article 9.

Gordon, R. S. (1983). An operational classification of disease prevention. *Public Health Reports*, *98*, 107–109.

Greenberg, M. T., Domitrovich, C., & Bumbarger, B. (2001). The prevention of mental disorders in school-aged children: Current state of the field. *Prevention and Treatment*, *4*, Article 9.

Greenberg, M. T., Kusche, C. A., Cook, E. T., & Quamma, J. P. (1995). Promoting emotional competence in school-aged children: The effects of the PATHS curriculum. *Development and Psychopathology*, *7*, 117–136.

Grossman, P. B., & Hugues, J. N. (1992). Self-control interventions with internalizing disorders: A review and analysis. *School Psychology Review*, *21*, 229–245.

Harrell, A. V., Cavanagh, S. E., Harmon, M. A., Koper, C. S., & Sridharan, S. (1997). *Impact of the children at risk program: Comprehensive final report*. Vol. 1. Washington, DC: The Urban Institute.

Harrell, A. V., Cavanagh, S. E., & Sridharan, S. (1999). *Evaluation of the children at risk program: Results 1 year after the end of the program. Research in brief (November)*. Washington, DC: National Institute of Justice, US Department of Justice.

Holden, G. W., Lavigne, V. V., & Cameron, A. M. (1990). Probing the continuum of effectiveness in parent training: Characteristics of parents and preschoolers. *Journal of Clinical Child Psychology*, *19*, 2–8.

Horowitz, J. L., & Garber, J. (2006). The prevention of depressive symptoms in children and adolescents: A meta-analytic review. *Journal of Consulting and Clinical Psychology*, *74*, 401–415.

Howe, G. W., Reiss, D., & Yuh, J. (2002). Can prevention trials test theories of etiology? *Development and Psychopathology*, *14*, 673–694.

Huston, A. C. (2005). Connecting the science of child development to public policy. *SRCD Social Policy Report, XIX* (IV).

Institute of Medicine. (1994). *Reducing risks for mental disorders: Frontiers for preventive intervention research*. Washington, DC: National Academy Press.

Jaycox, L. H., Reivich, K. J., Gillham, J., & Seligman, M. E. (1994). Prevention of depressive symptoms in school children. *Behaviour Research and Therapy*, *32*, 801–816.

Kazdin, A. (1985). *Treatment of antisocial behavior in children and adolescents*. Homewood, IL: Dorsey.

Kellam, S. G., Rebok, G. W., Ialongo, N., & Mayer, L. S. (1994). The course and malleability of aggressive behavior from early 1st grade into middle school: Results of a developmental epidemiologically-based preventive trial. *Journal of Child Psychology and Psychiatry*, *35*, 259–281. [Published erratum appears in *Journal of Child Psychology and Psychiatry* 1994, *35*, 983.]

Kendall, P. C., Marrs-Garcia, A., Nath, S. R., & Sheldrick, R. C. (1999). Normative comparisons for the evaluation of clinical significance. *Journal of Consulting & Clinical Psychology*, *67*, 285–299.

Kraemer, H. C. (2003). Current concepts of risk in psychiatric disorders. *Current Opinion in Psychiatry*, *16*, 421–430.

Kraemer, H. C., Kazdin, A. E., Offord, D. R., Kessler, R. C., Jensen, P. S., & Kupfer, D. J. (1999). Measuring the potency of risk factors for clinical or policy significance. *Psychological Methods*, *4*, 257–271.

Kraemer, H. C., Stice, E., Kazdin, A., Offord, D., & Kupfer, D. (2001). How do risk factors work together? Mediators, moderators, and independent, overlapping, and proxy risk factors. *American Journal of Psychiatry*, *158*, 848–856.

LaFromboise, T., & Howard-Pitney, B. (1995). The Zuni life skills development curriculum: Description and evaluation of a suicide prevention program. *Journal of Counseling Psychology*, *42*, 479–486.

LeMarquand, D., Tremblay, R. E., & Vitaro, F. (2001). The prevention of conduct disorder: A review of successful and unsuccessful experiments. In J. Hill, & B. Maughan (Eds.), *Conduct disorder in childhood* (pp. 449–477). Cambridge: Cambridge University Press.

Leventhal, T., & Brooks-Gunn, J. (2004). A randomized study of neighborhood effects on low-income children's educational outcomes. *Developmental Psychology*, *40*, 488–507.

Lipsey, M. W. (1995). What do we learn from 400 research studies on the effectiveness of treatment with juvenile delinquents? In J. McGuire (Ed.), *What works: Reducing reoffending. Guidelines from research and practice* (pp. 63–78). New York, NY: John Wiley and Sons.

Lipsey, M. W., & Wilson, D. B. (1998). Effective intervention for serious juvenile offenders: A synthesis of research. In R. Loeber, & D. P. Farrington (Eds.), *Serious and violent juvenile offenders: Risk factors and successful interventions* (pp. 313–345). Thousand Oaks, CA: Sage.

Lochman, J. E. (2001). Issues in prevention with school-aged children: Ongoing intervention refinement, developmental theory, prediction and moderation, and implementation and dissemination. *Prevention and Treatment*, *4*, Article 4.

Lösel, F., & Beelmann, A. (2003). Effects of child skill training in preventing antisocial behavior: A systematic review of randomized evaluations. *Annals of the American Academy of Political and Social Science*, *587*, 84–109.

Luthar, S. S., Cicchetti, D., & Becker, B. (2000). The construct of resilience: A critical evaluation and guidelines for future work. *Child Development*, *71*, 543–562.

Lynch, F. L., Hornbrook, M., Clarke, G. N., Perrin, N., Polen, M. R., O'Connor, E., *et al.* (2005). Cost-effectiveness of an intervention to prevent depression in at-risk teens. *Archives of General Psychiatry*, *62*, 1241–1248.

MacMillan, H. L., Thomas, B. H., Jamieson, E., Walsh, C. A., Boyle, M. H., Shannon, H. S., *et al.* (2005). Effectiveness of home visitation by public-health nurses in prevention of the recurrence of child physical abuse and neglect: A randomised controlled trial. *Lancet*, *365*, 1786–1793.

Martinez, C. R. (2006, May). *Models and methods for cultural adaptation of prevention programs*, Pre-conference at the Annual meeting of the Society for Prevention Research, San Antonio, TX.

Masten, A. S., Burt, K. B., & Coatworth, J. D. (2006). Competence and psychopathology in development. In D. Cicchetti, & D. Cohen (Eds.), *Developmental psychopathology*. Vol 3. *Risk, disorder and adaptation* (2nd edn., pp. 696–738). New York, NY: Wiley.

Maughan, B. (2005). Developmental trajectory modeling: A view from developmental psychopathology. *Annals of the American Academy of Political and Social Science*, *602*, 118–130.

Maughan, B., Taylor, C., Taylor, A., Butler, N., & Bynner, J. (2001). Pregnancy smoking and childhood conduct problems: A causal association? *Journal of Child Psychology and Psychiatry and Allied Disciplines*, *42*, 1021–1028.

McCartney, K., & Rosenthal, R. (2000). Effect size, practical importance, and social policy for children. *Child Development*, *71*, 173–180.

McCord, J. (1978). A thirty-year follow-up of treatment effects. *American Psychologist*, *33*, 284–289.

Meehl, P. E. (1992). Factors and taxa, traits and types, differences of degree and differences in kind. *Journal of Personality*, *60*, 117–174.

Metropolitan Area Child Study Research Group. (2002). A cognitive–ecological approach to preventing aggression in urban settings: Initial outcomes for high-risk children. *Journal of Consulting and Clinical Psychology*, *70*, 179–194.

Miller, G. E., & Prinz, R. J. (2003). Engagement of families in treatment for childhood conduct problems. *Behavior Therapy*, *34*, 517–534.

Moffitt, T. E. (1990). The neuropsychology of juvenile delinquency: A critical review. In M. Tonry, & N. Morris (Eds.), *Crime and justice: A review of research* (Vol. 112, pp. 99–169). Chicago: University of Chicago Press.

Mrazek, P. J., & Brown, C. H. (2002). An evidence-based literature review regarding outcomes in psychosocial prevention and early intervention in young children. In C. C. Russell (Ed.), *The state of knowledge about prevention/early intervention* (pp. 42–165). Toronto, ON: Invest in Kids Foundation.

Mrazek, P. J., & Haggerty, R. J. (1994). *Reducing risk for mental disorders: Frontiers for preventive intervention research*. Washington, DC: National Academy Press.

Nagin, D. S. (2005). *Group-based modeling of development*. Cambridge, MA: Harvard University Press.

Nagin, D. S., & Tremblay, R. E. (1999). Trajectories of boys' physical aggression, opposition, and hyperactivity on the path to physically violent and non violent juvenile delinquency. *Child Development*, *70*, 1181–1196.

Nation, M., Crusto, C., Wandersman, A., Kumpfer, K. L., Seybolt, D., Morrissey-Kane, E., *et al.* (2003). What works in prevention: Principles of effective prevention programs. *American Psychologist*, *58*, 449–456.

National Evaluation of Sure Start Team. (2004). *The impact of Sure Start local programs on child development and family functioning: A report on preliminary findings*. Report by the Institute for the Study of Children Families and Social Issues, Birbeck University of London.

Offord, D. R. (1996). The state of prevention and early intervention. In R. D. Peters, & R. J. McMahon (Eds.), *Preventing childhood disorders, substance abuse, and delinquency* (pp. 329–344). Thousand Oaks, CA: Sage.

Offord, D. R., & Bennett, K. J. (2002). Prevention. In M. Rutter, & E. Taylor (Eds.), *Child and adolescent psychiatry* (4th edn., pp. 881–899). Oxford, UK: Blackwell Science.

Offord, D. R., Kraemer, H. C., Kazdin, A. E., Jensen, P. S., & Harrington, R. (1998). Lowering the burden of suffering from child psychiatric disorder: Trade-offs among clinical, targeted, and universal interventions. *Journal of the American Academy of Child and Adolescent Psychiatry*, *37*, 686–694.

Olds, D. L., Eckenrode, J., Henderson, C. R. J., Kitzman, H., Powers, J., Cole, R., *et al.* (1997). Long-term effects of home visitation on maternal life course and child abuse and neglect: Fifteen-year follow-up of a randomized trial. *Journal of the American Medical Association*, *278*, 637–643.

Olds, D. L., Henderson, C. R., Kitzman, H., & Eckenrode, J. (1998). Prenatal and home visitation by nurses: A program of research. In I. C. Rovee-Collier, P. Lipsitt, & H. Hayne (Eds.), *Advances in infancy research* (pp. 79–130). Stamford: Ablex.

Olds, D. L., Henderson, C. R., Kitzman, H., Eckenrode, J., Cole, R., & Tatelbaum, R. C. (1999). Prenatal and infancy home visitation by nurses: Recent findings. *Future of Children*, *9*, 44–65.

Olds, D. L., Henderson, C. R., Tatelbaum, R., & Chamberlin, R. (1986). Improving the delivery of prenatal care and outcomes of pregnancy: A randomized trial of nurse home visitation. *Pediatrics*, *77*, 16–28.

Pickles, A., & Angold, A. (2003). Natural categories or fundamental dimensions: On carving nature at the joints and the rearticulation of psychopathology. *Development and Psychopathology*, *15*, 529–551.

Plomin, R., & Crabbe, J. (2000). DNA. *Psychological Bulletin*, *126*, 806–828.

Prinz, R. J., & Miller, G. E. (1994). Family-based treatment for childhood antisocial behavior: Experimental influences on dropout and engagement. *Journal of Consulting and Clinical Psychology*, *62*, 645–650.

Prinz, R. J., & Miller, G. E. (1996). Parental engagement in interventions for children at risk for conduct disorder. In R. D. Peters, & R. J. McMahon (Eds.), *Preventing childhood disorders, substance abuse, and delinquency* (pp. 161–183). Thousand Oaks, CA: Sage.

Prinz, R. J., Smith, E. P., Dumas, J. E., Laughlin, J. E., White, D. W., & Barron, R. (2001). Recruitment and retention of participants in prevention trials involving family-based interventions. *American Journal of Preventive Medicine*, *20*, 31–37.

Reid, M. J., Webster-Stratton, C., & Hammond, M. (2003). Follow-up of children who received the Incredible Years intervention for oppositional-defiant disorder: Maintenance and prediction of 2-year outcome. *Behavior Therapy*, *34*, 471–491.

Rice, M. E., & Harris, G. T. (1995). Psychopathy, schizophrenia, alcohol abuse, and violent recidivism. *International Journal of Law and Psychiatry*, *18*, 333–342.

Romeo, R., Byford, S., & Knapp, M. (2005). Annotation: Economic evaluations of child and adolescent mental health interventions: A systematic review. *Journal of Child Psychology and Psychiatry*, *46*, 919–930.

Rotheram-Borus, M. J., & Duan, N. (2003). Next generation of preventive interventions. *Journal of the American Academy of Child and Adolescent Psychiatry*, *42*, 518–526.

Rutter, M. (2003). Crucial paths from risk indicator to causal mechanism. In B. B. Lahey, T. E. Moffitt, & A. Caspi (Eds.), *Causes of conduct disorder and juvenile delinquency* (pp. 3–24). New York, NY: Guilford Press.

Rutter, M., Giller, H., & Hagell, A. (1998). *Antisocial behavior by young people*. New York: Cambridge University Press.

Sameroff, A. J., & Mackenzie, M. J. (2003). Research strategies for capturing transactional models of development: The limits of the possible. *Development and Psychopathology*, *15*, 613–640.

Schlernitzauer, M., Bierhals, A. J., Geary, M. D., Prigerson, H. G., Stack, J. A., Miller, M. D., *et al.* (1998). Recruitment methods for intervention research in bereavement-related depression: Five years' experience. *American Journal of Geriatric Psychiatry*, 6, 67–74.

Schweinhart, L. J. (2006). The High/Scope approach: Evidence that participatory learning in early childhood contributes to human development. In N. F. Watt, C. Ayoub, R. H. Bradley, J. E. Puma, & W. LeBoeuf (Eds.), *The crisis in youth mental health: Critical issues and effective programs*, Vol. 4. *Early intervention programs and policies* (pp. 207–227). Westport, CT: Praeger Publishers/Greenwood Publishing Group.

Schweinhart, L. L., Barnes, H. V., & Weikart, D. P. (1993). *Significant benefits: The High/Scope Perry School Study through age 27*. Ypsilanti, MI: High/Scope Press.

Serketich, W. J., & Dumas, J. E. (1996). The effectiveness of behavioral parent training to modify antisocial behavior in children: A meta-analysis. *Behavior Therapy*, *27*, 171–186.

Society for Prevention Research. (2004). *Standards of evidence: Criteria for efficacy, effectiveness, and dissemination*. Falls Church, VA: Society for Prevention Research.

Society for Prevention Research. http://www.preventionresearch.org.

Spoth, R., Ball, A. D., Klose, A., & Redmond, C. (1996). Illustration of a market segmentation technique using family-focused prevention program preference data. *Health Education Research*, *11*, 259–267.

Spoth, R., & Redmond, C. (1994). Effective recruitment of parents into family-focused prevention research: A comparison of strategies. *Psychology and Health*, *9*, 353–370.

Spoth, R., & Redmond, C. (1995). Parent motivation to enroll in parenting skills programs: A model of family context and health belief predictors. *Journal of Family Psychology*, *9*, 294–310.

St. Pierre, T. L., Mark, M. M., Kaltreider, D. L., & Aikin, K. J. (1997). Involving parents of high-risk youth in drug prevention: A three-year longitudinal study in boys and girls clubs. *Journal of Early Adolescence*, *17*, 21–50.

Stattin, H., & Magnusson, D. (1991). Stability and change in criminal behaviour up to age 30. *British Journal of Criminology*, *31*, 327–346.

Tobler, N. S., Roona, M. R., Ochshorn, P., Marshall, D. G., Streke, A. V., & Stackpole, K. M. (2000). School-based adolescent drug prevention programs: 1998 Meta-analysis. *Journal of Primary Prevention*, *20*, 275–336.

University of Colorado Center for the Study and Prevention of Violence. http://www.colorado.edu/cspv/blueprints.

van de Wiel, N. M. H., Matthys, W., Cohen-Kettenis, P., & van Engeland, H. (2003). Application of the Utrecht Coping Power Program and care as usual to children with disruptive behavior disorders in outpatient clinics: A comparative study of cost and course of treatment. *Behavior Therapy*, *34*, 421–436.

Vitaro, F., Brendgen, M., & Tremblay, R. E. (2001a). Preventive intervention: Assessing its effects on the trajectories of delinquency and testing for mediational processes. *Applied Developmental Science*, *5*, 201–213.

Vitaro, F., Tremblay, R. E., & Bukowski, W. M. (2001b). Friends, friendships, and conduct disorders. In J. Hill, & B. Maughan (Eds.), *Conduct disorder in childhood* (pp. 346–378). Cambridge: Cambridge University Press.

Wakschlag, L. S., & Hans, S. L. (2002). Maternal smoking during pregnancy and conduct problems in high-risk youth: A developmental framework. *Development and Psychopathology*, *14*, 351–369.

Webster-Stratton, C. (1990). Long-term follow-up of families with young conduct-problem children: From preschool to grade school. *Journal of Consulting and Clinical Psychology*, *19*, 1344–1349.

Webster-Stratton, C., & Hammond, M. (1997). Treating children with early-onset conduct problems: A comparison of child and parent training interventions. *Journal of Consulting and Clinical Psychology*, *65*, 93–109.

Webster-Stratton, C., Mihalic, S., Fagan, A., Arnold, D., Taylor, T., & Tingley, C. (2001a). *Blueprints for violence prevention, book eleven: the incredible years: Parent, teacher, and child training series*. Boulder, CO: Center for the Study and Prevention of Violence.

Webster-Stratton, C., Reid, M. J., & Hammond, M. (2001b). Preventing conduct problems, promoting social competence: A parent and teacher training partnership in Head Start. *Journal of Clinical Child Psychology*, *30*, 283–302.

Weisz, J. R., Weiss, B., Alicke, M. D., & Klotz, M. L. (1987). Effectiveness of psychotherapy with children and adolescents: A meta-analysis for clinicians. *Journal of Consulting and Clinical Psychology*, *55*, 542–549.

Werch, C. E., & Owen, D. M. (2001). Iatrogenic effects of alcohol and drug prevention programs. *Journal of Studies on Alcohol*, *63*, 581–590.

Yoshikawa, H. (1994). Prevention as cumulative protection: Effects of early family support and education on chronic delinquency and its risks. *Psychological Bulletin*, *115*, 28–54.

62 Behavioral Therapies

Stephen Scott and William Yule

Background

Origins

Behaviorism began to take hold as a major influence in psychology in the early 20th century. John B. Watson finished his doctoral thesis on the behavior of the white rat in 1903, in which he acknowledged the powerful effects of innate capabilities, but showed that early experience, in a way that could be carefully measured, had a clear strong effect on current behavior. In 1913, in his article "Psychology as the behaviorist sees it," he drew attention to the limitations of psychological theories current at the time and proposed behaviorism as an objective natural science with a progressive pragmatic agenda that could be applied to humans as well as animals. The article has a lengthy footnote on the nature of thinking, and Watson believed that complex emotional reactions in humans were derived from the newborn's unlearned reactions of fear, rage and love. Thus, contrary to some current concerns, from the outset, major mainstream behaviorists recognized the importance of innate inherited traits, accepted the existence of complex emotional states and had theories about the role of cognitions. However, while recognizing these influences, behaviorists showed that for a given individual, many particular behaviors could be substantially altered by changing the immediately preceding events, and those that immediately followed.

Watson's ideas were developed by Skinner, who gave more emphasis to the influence of events subsequent to a given behavior than to antecedent stimuli. Skinner was especially skeptical of psychological explanations for behavior based on introspections, which he called "mental fictions." Skinner expanded his approach beyond the individual level to suggest a model society based on behavioral principles for returning US war veterans in *Walden Two* (Skinner, 1948), and applied behaviorist principles to language, in his classic *Verbal Behavior* (Skinner, 1957). However, the limitations of a behaviorist approach to language were set out by the young Chomsky (1959), who was scathing of Skinner's approach, pointing out that language learning occurs independently of external rewards.

Rutter's Child and Adolescent Psychiatry, 5th edition. Edited by M. Rutter, D. Bishop, D. Pine, S. Scott, J. Stevenson, E. Taylor and A. Thapar. © 2008 Blackwell Publishing, ISBN: 978-1-4051-4549-7.

Soon there were clinical applications, and in 1952 Eysenck coined the term "behavior therapy" to capture the application of behavioral principles to treatment of patients, and Wolpe began developing treatments based on classic conditioning theory. The 1960s saw the heyday of pure behaviorism, with the founding of several journals such as the *Journal for the Experimental Analysis of Behavior*, *Journal of Applied Behavioral Analysis*, *Behavior Therapy* and *Behavior Research and Therapy*, in which a plethora of articles explored the application of behavioral principles to a wide range of situations, from animal behavior to business management. Many clinical applications were developed for adults. In the 1970s, many treatments were developed for children and adolescents. These covered all the main disorder groupings, with, for example, exposure treatments with relaxation for fears and anxiety, contingency management through parent training for disruptive disorders and functional analysis for challenging behaviors in children with intellectual disability. In this era, evaluations showed that the new treatments were generally notably effective; typically, they used relatively small numbers (4–10 cases) in single-case designs, plus some group trials, typically with 15–40 participants.

In the last 25 years behavioral therapies have continued to be refined, and large-scale randomized controlled trials comparing behavioral therapy with controls or in combination with medications with 100–800 participants have generally attested to their effectiveness (Conduct Problems Research Group, 1999; MTA Cooperative Group, 1999). In addition to modifications along purely behavioral lines, other therapies have grafted different approaches onto a behavioral base. Cognitive–behavioral therapies (CBT; see chapter 63) address thoughts as well as actions, but not in a loose introspective way, instead applying to cognitions the same concepts espoused by behaviorists of precise measurement, pragmatic individual formulation of phenomena in the present time and experimental trying out of what works with each patient and modifying it according to its effectiveness. A number of family systems approaches have taken up behavioral ideas and methods; for example, Functional Family Therapy (Alexander, Pugh, Parsons, & Sexton, 2000) and Multisystemic Therapy (Henggeler, Schoenwald, Liao, Letourneau, & Edwards, 2002). Problem-solving and social skills therapies use behavioral methods within the context of impaired relationships (see chapter 63). Therapies for those with post-traumatic stress disorder (PTSD) in the context of wider personal violations such as war or sexual abuse have broadened behavioral therapies to include addressing the profound impact on the patient's sense of self and identity (e.g., using narrative approaches; Schauer, Neuner, Elbert *et al.*, 2004). In the last 10 years, a "third generation" of behaviorally-based cognitive therapies has emerged following traditional behavior therapy and CBT. Examples include Acceptance and Commitment Therapy (ACT; Hayes, Luomaa, Bond, Masudaa, & Lillisa, 2006), Dialectical Behavior Therapy (DBT; Linehan, 1993) and Mindfulness-Based Cognitive Therapy (MBCT; Segal, Williams, & Teasdale, 2001). Although based on behavioral principles, these therapies take cognitive issues further, by acknowledging that sometimes unpleasant thoughts and feelings cannot be changed, but can be accepted as less concerning; to date child and adolescent versions are only just emerging.

Basic Tenets

Classic Conditioning

Pavlov described classic conditioning, whereby unconditioned stimuli (e.g., food) that led to unconditioned responses (salivation) could be presented at the same time with other (conditioned) stimuli (e.g., a bell), which then led to similar, but not identical, conditioned responses. Watson showed that classic conditioning had wide applicability. Understanding this mechanism has led to several applications; for example, dogs given food as they smell explosives learn to associate the smell of explosives with a reward, and can be trained to sniff airline luggage. A clinical application was developed by Wolpe (1958) when he suggested that in phobias the unconditioned response of overwhelming fear to a stimulus could be replaced by a competing conditioned response of relaxation through sufficient exposure, so that habituation occurred, a process he named systematic desensitization. This mechanism continues to underpin many current treatments for anxiety, phobias and PTSD.

Operant Conditioning

Skinner was concerned that most everyday behaviors were not related to simple unconditioned responses such as fear or hunger, but rather were often emitted spontaneously, and if they were followed by rewards or punishment then their form and frequency were adapted. Thus, children starting school soon learn that speaking to their friends in class may be punished by disapproval and a consequence such as detention, but that putting their hands up to answer a teacher's question is likely to be rewarded by approval. Skinner termed behaviors that led to rewards or punishments *operants* because they operated to change the environment for the individual. Others have argued that this description of events is the wrong way round, because it is the events subsequent to the original behavior that control its future emission.

Both classic and operant approaches do not concern themselves with the inner motives of the individual, but instead address the antecedent stimuli and consequent responses. This is in contrast to psychotherapies that primarily aim to change the inner world. Some of the differences between behavioral therapies and traditional psychotherapies are outlined in Table 62.1. Private thoughts and feelings are not ignored by behavior therapists, but they take a very different approach to them from traditional therapists, because they believe the same principles can be applied to them as to behavior (e.g., precise operational definition, quantifiable measurement, modification through learning principles). In short, thoughts and feelings are not seen as belonging to a different world (Phillips, 1981).

Methods

Behavioral Assessment

A core tool is behavioral assessment. This can vary in intensity, from a behaviorally-based interview, supplemented with a chart or diary if necessary, using a reliable and valid rating scale, to adding direct observation, additionally carrying out a full functional analysis which includes experimental manipulation of key variables, where possible.

Interview

In the interview, a thorough and detailed description of the behavior in question is elicited, including its frequency, duration and severity. Usually, the account is from the parents or the teacher, who may need help in moving from a generalized concern such as "He's a rude boy" to specifics such as "He shouts at me in a loud voice for 3–4 minutes every day." The general setting should be explored, such as "He's only started doing it since his Dad left me 3 months ago," moving on to clarify the antecedents, "It's when I'm on the telephone," and the consequences, "I have to stop chatting to my friend and tell him off."

Diary

Where the picture is unclear, parents can be asked to keep a diary and note each day what happens over, say, a 2-week period. This may reveal exceptions, when the problem behavior is not shown; then the clinician will work closely with the parents to elucidate what else differed on those days.

Rating Scales

A standardized rating scale is helpful in ensuring that a systematic approach is taken to measuring the extent and severity of the problem domain. It can provide a useful talking point when an item has been checked, and can act as a baseline measurement of severity, to be given at different points of treatment to monitor progress. It is preferable to have at least two informants (e.g., parent and teacher for attention deficit/hyperactivity disorder [ADHD] symptoms, or parent and child for obsessive-compulsive disorder [OCD]). Some useful examples include the Conner's rating scales for ADHD symptoms, the Eyberg Inventory for conduct problems, the Mood and Feelings Questionnaire for depression, the Child Impact of Traumatic Events Scale Revised for PTSD, and the Yale–Brown Obsessive-Compulsive Scale for OCD (more details of rating scales are given in chapter 20).

Table 62.1 Behavior therapy contrasted with traditional psychotherapy.

	Behavior therapy	**Traditional psychotherapy**
Problem definition	Precisely measurable externally observable events	May be general concern about feelings (e.g., inner disquiet)
Assessment	Careful recording (e.g., by diary) of problem frequency and severity, with explicit noting of setting context, immediately preceding external events, and real-world consequences of the behavior	General review of patient's view of world and meanings attributed
Measurement type	Formal, often with diaries, charts and numbered rating scales	Not undertaken formally
Measurement frequency	Often repeated at each treatment session, so failure to progress picked up early and addressed by reappraisal and change of strategy	Formal reassessment may not be carried out; treatment may need to last months until improvement expected
Theory of problem causation	How problem arises not especially central; more important are the external contingencies that maintain it	Inner turmoil arises because of conflict between incompatible beliefs and desires
Treatment principle	Modification of current external contingencies leads to the learning of new, more adaptive behavior	Making covert desires and beliefs explicit leads to resolution of conflicts; it may or may not lead to changed behavior
Postulated mechanism of change	External context has to change and/or new behavior be learned; action is required, new responses have to be practiced; homework between sessions may be set to enable this to happen	Working through of conflicts occurs unconsciously between sessions
Empirical research base	Wide range of studies testing and experimentally altering variables including contingencies, form and duration of treatment, mechanisms	Wide range of theories and case studies; relatively few systematic studies of mechanisms or outcomes
Role of motivation	Not necessary to know patient's motives in order to treat (e.g., challenging behavior)	Necessary for patient to want to change and be ready for this; therapy helps uncover true drives and passions
Role of meanings	Therapy can successfully be given with no knowledge of child's personal meanings and understanding of events (e.g., by changing external contingencies) or with children with intellectual disability	Personal meanings and the patient's understanding of events core to therapy
Role of parent and teacher in therapy	Central figures for changing the environment around the child, crucial allies in delivering the therapy	May do little beyond referring or bringing the child
Treatment content	Often programmatic, stepwise application of principles to the problem; manual often available	Follows what patient reveals; no manual
Treatment duration	Weeks to months	Months to years
Relationship with therapist	Therapist is vehicle for delivery, which may also be self-administered by book or computer	Core to therapy. Therapist may use self as measuring instrument for feelings evoked by patient, and reflect these back
Transactions with therapist	After assessment, therapist sets agenda; may suggest courses of action, may praise patient	Therapist waits to see what patient brings up; interpretations offered; patient not directed, judged or praised: neutrality preserved

Direct Observation

Direct observation, preferably "live" in the context where the behavior occurs, is often revealing. For example, the same complaint "hits other children in school" might in one child be observed only to occur when other children speak to him while he is engrossed in schoolwork, and in another when she is taunted about her weight and told by her peers to go away. The first case might be triggered by too close proximity of others, in a child who is fairly solitary and wants to be left alone; the second by anger at being belittled and excluded by "friends."

Functional Analysis

Functional analysis goes a step further so that after generating hypotheses, they are tested experimentally. Thus, in the first example above, children might be asked to approach the boy and see whether indeed he then lashes out; it might emerge that he does so when boys approach and not girls. The hypothesis might be refined to state that the behavior has the function of keeping boys at a distance. In this way of thinking, causation in the pure sense is eschewed for practical functions, so that the hypothesized "cause":

1 Covaries with the behavior;
2 Is in principle changeable; and
3 When changed, leads to an alteration in behavior.

In many cases, interview and diary keeping are sufficient to formulate an effective plan. However, in secondary referrals for complex cases, observation is invaluable. Functional analysis is especially useful when children have intellectual disabilities with challenging behavior that is hard to make sense of, such as head banging.

Case Formulation

This should go considerably further than behavioral assessment to incorporate all relevant psychiatric factors. As well as determining triggering and maintaining factors, defining positive behaviors to train up is usually more important than simply eliminating negative behaviors in one context (Herbert, 1987).

Intervention Techniques to Increase Behavior

What follows is a broad account of techniques. Readers seeking a detailed manual are referred to Herbert (1987) and to Hersen (2005).

Positive Reinforcement

This should be used when a new behavior is to be incorporated into the child's repertoire, or when an existing behavior is desired more frequently or across more situations. It can also be used to increase the strength of an existing behavior so that an undesirable incompatible response diminishes. The method is to identify what is desired, and arrange matters so an immediate reward follows the performance of the behavior; in the words of one adage "Catch them being good" (and then reward them).

Social Rewards

Reinforcers may be social or tangible. In the social domain, attention is most powerful with younger children, but it is often also very effective for adolescents. It is often enough to say a few words showing that the behavior has been appreciated (e.g., describing what they did). To add power, it may be combined with words of praise or physical expressions of affection such as a hug. Positive attention is a two-way process in that children's positive behavior reinforces adults; a happy relationship results from many mutually reinforcing interactions. As the child grows up, attention from peers, when present, may be far more influential than attention from parents. Attention that is associated with criticism or punishment will usually not be reinforcing; however, there is an exception. For children raised with very little attention, negative attention (such as being told off in a disapproving tone of voice) may be more reinforcing than being ignored completely. In this way, a parent who mainly ignores their child and then only scolds them may unwittingly be reinforcing bad behavior.

Tangible Rewards

These include items such as food (from single sweets to a trip to a restaurant), leisure activities (time on the computer or the telephone, going swimming) and privileges (staying up late, having a friend over). For more frequently occurring behaviors, tokens such as stars on a chart, or points can be given and later exchanged for a tangible reward; money can be given too.

Application of Rewards

Reinforcers can be provided by adults such as parents and teachers, other children such as siblings or peers, or the child themselves. The person doing the reinforcing will need coaching in each case – one cannot automatically assume that a parent or teacher has a large repertoire of praising comments that they use freely and warmly; and a child may need to rehearse congratulating themselves for, say, doing their homework or not losing their temper. Praise in front of others (e.g., peers and siblings) can have a particularly strong effect. Reinforcers should be given for trying and for steps in the right direction – not withheld until a perfect performance is given. Praise is given for the behavior, and so needs to be labeled – it is not for the child in general. Rewards should be given often, and not mixed with criticism. "Well done for getting two A grades – if you hadn't been lazy, you'd have got three" is going to completely undo the effect of the praise element.

In practice, rules for rewards must be clear and simple; the therapist must check with the child that they understand them, and check that the parent implements them fairly and consistently. Rewards need to be changed every week or so to avoid satiation. Non-contingent general praise will not improve specific behaviors and can lead the child to be "spoiled" (i.e., believe they are approved of whatever they do). Reinforcers need to be carefully selected for the individual – they need to be something that the child wants.

Differential attention is where appropriate behavior is attended to, whereas inappropriate behavior is ignored (e.g., minor irritations, whining; hitting and destruction cannot be ignored). In practice, the difficulty here is to get the parent to switch back to attending to the desirable behavior after ignoring the undesirable behavior, because by now the parent is often irritated. Application of differential attention takes practice, and often some reattributions may need to be rehearsed with the parent (e.g., "He's only doing it for attention, I shan't give in!"). If assessment fails to show any relationship between attention and the behavior in question, it may not be appropriate to use this technique.

Schedules of Reinforcement

These may be continuous (i.e., after each behavior) or variable, either by time (interval) or after a certain number of behaviors (ratio). Rewards set up expectancies within the individual, and help them predict their world. Their effects will depend on what the child is previously used to; if they already receive a great deal of praise then adding more may not be a powerful reinforcer and a tangible reward may be more effective. Conversely, where there has previously been little or no praising, some children may take a while to accept it – parents may need to persist for a few weeks to be believed. Variable schedules establish behaviors that are hard to extinguish (the individual's experience is that reward may still come, even after a long time without).

Negative Reinforcement

This refers to the removal of something unpleasant, with the consequence that the procedure is reinforcing (the term is sometimes mistakenly used to refer to receiving reinforcement for negative behavior; e.g., through attention). Negative reinforcement can be used to increase wanted behavior through removing a mildly aversive situation after the child behaves as desired (e.g., a parent may threaten to turn off the TV unless the child takes his feet off the table, and remove the threat after he does). Inappropriate negative reinforcement may unwittingly lead parents to encourage antisocial behavior (e.g., by giving in). Thus, if a parent tells a child to go to bed (when the child wants to continue playing a video game), the child responds by whining and being defiant and the parent then backs off for 5 min, the child is learning that if they are defiant the aversive stimulus is removed.

Positive and negative reinforcement can be further divided into:

1 *Reward training:* "If you make the response, you will get a reward";

2 *Privation training:* "If you don't make the response, I will withdraw a reward";

3 *Escape training:* "If you make the response I will withdraw a punishment";

4 *Avoidance training:* "If you don't make the response you will be punished."

All serve to increase the frequency of a desired behavior.

In practice, parents need to be very clear about which behavior is to be rewarded and to ensure the child is also clear. This can be achieved by the parent devising a chart with the child, and placing it in a prominent position such as above the child's bed or on the refrigerator door.

Token Systems

These allow instant rewards to be given, and so maintain performance over a time when reward cannot be given without delay. Later, they can be exchanged for substantive rewards such as a special meal, going to the park or having a friend round. Useful applications apply in classrooms and in foster homes. Token systems can be helpful where adult social rewards such as attention or praise are for some reason less effective. An example would be in classrooms where peer pressures compete with adult attention. The Good Behavior Game is an evidence-based token system that makes use of peer influences, rather than fighting against them. Groups of children in a classroom earn points for good behavior, and the winning group gets rewarded; children monitor and control their peer group's behavior to ensure their group wins. This has proven effective in trials (Kellam, Rebok, Ialongo, & Mayer, 1994). A second example would be promoting peer friendship behaviors, for example by giving tokens for good gamesmanship such as praising a team-mate's efforts, which has also been proven effective in randomized controlled trials (RCTs; Frankel & Myatt, 2003). Some children are not responsive to social rewards because they have been abused and so do not trust adults. The Multidimensional Treatment Foster Care program uses token systems to improve behavior in the home and at school; it too is supported by RCT evidence (Chamberlain & Reid, 1998). Like other behavioral techniques, token systems are not a magical solution to be applied in a mechanical way, but require thought and skill.

Shaping

Here one reinforces small steps in the right direction of a behavior the individual has not done before. It is a popular technique with animal trainers, who can train two naïve pigeons to play ping-pong in half an hour! Shaping is especially helpful for children if they cannot imagine what is required, the behavior cannot be modeled for them or they will not understand it. Shaping is especially useful with children with intellectual disability.

The Premack Principle

Premack (1965) was concerned to identify effective reinforcers where obvious ones did not appear to work. He suggested that observing what an individual liked to do with high frequency when left to their own devices would be a good reinforcer for a targeted low-frequency behavior – thus, actually it is a *response* that is rewarding. This can be especially helpful for children with severe learning disability (e.g., one might let them suck a favorite toy for 2 min after they have learned a step towards a new behavior).

Modeling

This technique is useful for learning new complex behaviors or for learning more appropriate responses (e.g., a fearless response to a dog). It assumes the child can observe the model and internalize it, and that externally (or through internal motivation) one can reward it. If the model has characteristics the child respects or desires, this will aid effectiveness. One can use filmed modeling for children (e.g., of other children being brave when confronted by feared situations) or to show parents other ways of responding to their children (Webster-Stratton, Hibbs, & Jenson, 2005).

Prompting

A prompt is a stimulus that may help a behavior pattern be initiated, and is especially useful at the beginning of a program. When giving a command it may help to hold up the reward (say, a token) to the child to prompt him or her. For prompting to work, it is crucial to have rewarding consequences in place – parents and teachers often use multiple prompts ineffectively (nagging) without setting up the consequences likely to ensure that the desired behavior occurs. Written prompts are prevalent in everyday life ("Drive slowly!" "Now wash your hands").

Intervention Techniques to Decrease Behavior

Extinction

This refers to the withholding of reinforcements for behavior so that it is eliminated from the child's repertoire. It requires careful analysis of all possible reinforcers (e.g., attention from parents, siblings and peers) and then ensuring no source of reinforcement is available – in this example, asking all parties not to respond to the behavior in question. As ever, to succeed one has to be very clear and specific about the behavior to target, and rehearse with parents and teachers how to avoid responding. This may be hard; if the behavior in question is rude remarks from the child, the adult has to learn to withhold responding. Initially, the child may "strive" even harder to elicit the reinforcer and so behave more badly than ever, the so-called "extinction burst"; one needs to persevere to overcome this. For extinction to work, the behavior in question has actually to occur and the link with reward be weakened, so the procedure is not suitable for behaviors that are dangerous or seriously disruptive of others. In these cases, other strategies such as punishment may be necessary. The cutting out of reinforcers needs to be almost total, because if intermittent reinforcement is available, the behavior may be maintained indefinitely.

Extinction can work well in the classroom, although teachers may find it hard to ignore or only attend briefly to poor behavior. Thus, Walker and Buckley (1974) found that 18% of teachers' attention to non-problem children was for inappropriate behavior, whereas 89% of that paid to children with behavioral difficulties was for undesirable classroom behavior. Overall, 77% of all teachers' individual attention was directed at children with problem behavior. This state of affairs is likely to maintain difficult behavior. To extinguish it, teachers can be taught to give very brief, quiet warnings that are rapidly followed by a consequence if the behavior is repeated (Webster-Stratton, 2005). Extinction works especially well when combined with differential reinforcement of other behavior (DRO), so the teacher ignores the child looking out of the window but praises her when she is doing her bookwork.

Stimulus Control

Here the aim is to remove a stimulus that leads to a difficult behavior, rather than changing the consequences. Turning off the TV may help a child get to bed by removing the competing stimulus of the program; removing a boy from a place in class beside his chatty neighbor may stop him talking in class; halting access visits of a maltreated child to her abusive father may prevent the episodes of self-harm that used to follow. Older children can learn to self-regulate stimuli (e.g., avoiding going to parts of town where they are likely to be tempted by the offer of drugs).

Punishment

This can be the withdrawal of something reinforcing (i.e., extinction), or the contingent application of something aversive; at times one may shade into the other. Hitting and hurting are types of punishment that have been associated with more traditional cultures and families. Apart from the inhumanity and potential for abuse of such methods of discipline, they tend to suppress or inhibit behavior through fear, pain or humiliation, without necessarily extinguishing it or teaching a mutually incompatible constructive alternative. Punishment alone reduces the chance of the child learning prosocial alternatives. Excessive painful punishment may have undesirable side effects such as inducing general fearfulness of the parent or teacher, the promotion of aggressive responding to frustrating situations through modeling by the adult and the induction of resentment in the child, thus leading to cycles of retaliation, withdrawal and non-cooperation.

Punishment can be popular with parents and teachers because of its reinforcing characteristics for them – prompt cessation of the unwanted behavior by the child, even though it may recur relatively soon – and, for some, the feeling of having given the child their just desserts and "taught them a lesson." Even if it is not effective in the long term, these short-term reinforcers for the adult may help make it a frequently-used strategy unless other alternatives are taught. Studies suggest that punishing children is especially harmful when given in a painful, humiliating way that is ill-timed, irregular, inconsistent and retaliatory, with no accompanying choices for the child, or encouragement of more positive behaviors (Kazdin & Benjet, 2003). To be effective, punishment does not need to be intense or physical, but it does need to be applied quickly and consistently when the inappropriate behavior is displayed (Kazdin & Benjet, 2003). Time out is a good example of an appropriate way to administer punishment.

Time Out

The full term is time out from positive reinforcement. To be effective, before the punishment is given, the child has to be in a context that is positively reinforcing. Typically, the child is sent to a boring place such as the end of the corridor, a toilet or the bottom of the stairs. In time out there is general removal from a wide range of stimuli, as well as the reinforcing ones and removal from the context where undesirable behavior took place, so preventing further harm or damage to the surroundings or other people. In both these characteristics it differs from extinction, which is removal from specific, previously identified reinforcers. If the context around the child is not reinforcing – say, a boring lesson or a harsh parent – then being sent to time out will not be a punishment but may be a relief, and so will not be effective in reducing inappropriate behavior. As for other techniques, time out is less likely to work on its own than if combined with reinforcement of desired behaviors and extinction procedures.

The technique provides a useful alternative to smacking or spanking. It also has an advantage in terms of emotional control, because it provides a time for both the young person and the parent to cool down. It is especially useful for teachers as it removes the child from being an aggravating stimulus to other pupils, and to teachers and parents too. Adults need to be taught how to implement time out effectively; the time should not be longer than a maximum of around 5 min, with the proviso that the child has to be quiet for the last minute of the time (so a complaining child may need to be in time out for 40 min on the first occasion if it takes him that long to quieten down). The space used must be cleared of breakable objects as far as possible (e.g., perfume bottles in toilets) as the child may continue an angry tantrum and try escalating behavior before calming down. It is suitable for children aged around 3–10 years; older children may be too strong to be made to go, in which case a back-up strategy should be used, such as response cost strategies (e.g., "Because you have refused to go to time out, you will not be going to the football game tomorrow").

Response Cost

This refers to the withdrawal of specified amounts of reinforcement (e.g., points, tokens, money, privileges) immediately following a previously defined unwanted behavior. Thus, for responding in a way that violates rules, the child promptly loses out. Response cost tends to be used with tangible, rather than social rewards, and consequently is especially helpful when social rewards are not likely to work: for example, in the context of a relationship that the child does not particularly care about, say a disliked teacher whose disapproval would not matter; for children for whom social rewards are generally less effective (e.g., abused children); looked after children who have had several sets of carers and become mistrustful; or children with psychopathic traits.

There are a number of practice points to bear in mind when setting up a response cost regime:

1 By definition, there has to be some level of positive rewards (e.g., points or money) or else there is nothing to withdraw.

2 The value of points or tokens has to be agreed in advance and be individually tailored to the child.

3 As for any consequence, the cost has to be applied immediately and consistently; giving feedback to child so they learn to make the connection helps.

4 It is important to avoid making the costs too high (the child may give up out of frustration).

5 Wherever possible, after removal of points, it helps to arrange for the child to be able to earn them back soon through a reparative positive behavior.

In contrast to time out, immediately after losing points, the child can gain positive reinforcement. He also remains in the presence of the stimulus that triggered the unwanted behavior, which can help learning towards self-control, or provoke the inappropriate behavior again, depending on the circumstances. Response cost is easier to implement than time out, as there is no need to take the child physically to another place; in school, the child continues to be exposed to class learning material. Because there are set rules, response cost is helpful in situations where it is important to avoid lengthy emotional interchanges and nagging, for example with oppositional teenagers in a foster home (Chamberlain & Reid, 1998).

Overcorrection

Here the child is subjected not only to a response cost, but also to an additional penalty to "overcorrect" for their misbehavior; the idea being to make the child especially aware of the punishment that will follow the unwanted behavior. Thus, a child who throws down litter may be made not only to tidy up his or her own rubbish, but to clear up a whole field.

Differential Reinforcement of Other Behavior or Incompatible Behavior

DRO refers to reinforcement of any other behavior; incompatible behavior takes the principle further by selecting a behavior that is specifically impossible to perform at the same time as the undesirable behavior. Both strategies are enormously helpful in reducing undesirable behavior. A noisy child can be given tokens for keeping quiet, an obsessive child rewarded for not enacting rituals, and so on.

Graded Exposure/Systematic Desensitization

This procedure is typically used where there is avoidance (e.g., because of phobias or anxiety states, or events experienced as traumatic). It can be combined with other techniques such as participant modeling (see p. 1013; e.g., the child watches the therapist stroke a frightening dog). The method is to make a hierarchy of the feared stimuli, starting with imagined ones, moving up systematically to reproductions such as pictures, to being at a distance from the real stimulus and finally to being close to the frightening object. The child defines the hierarchy, with help from the therapist. The child is trained in incompatible responses – typically relatively pleasant ones, for example imagining a favorite place, or training the child in relaxation techniques, or simply reassuring the child, or another pleasant activity such as eating or playing. When the child is comfortable, he is exposed to the stimuli, for long enough to overcome an anxious or fearful response so that this is replaced with a relaxed one. Over a number of sessions, the stimulus strength is increased by ascending the hierarchy, and supports are withdrawn. Encouraging active participation by the child enhances the procedure. During exposure, the child can rank their fear response on, say, a 1–100 scale; as the level of fear goes up, they practice the techniques. In this way the procedure effectively includes a coping element, with the child achieving mastery. It is crucial not to stop too soon during the procedure, because adequate exposure for long enough is key to getting anxiety levels eventually to subside. A variation of exposure is response prevention, whereby steps are taken to stop the child responding to the feared stimulus by acting inappropriately, as occurs in obsessive-compulsive disorder.

Flooding

This is an extreme form of exposure, whereby the child is

brought into contact with the most feared item on the inventory, and kept in contact with it until the fear is extinguished. Because it is initially very frightening, this procedure is seldom used with children; it could be seen as abusive, especially in maltreated children, and adds little to graded exposure.

Modeling

Here a model is exposed to the feared stimuli while the child watches – thus it is a form of exposure whereby the child can identify and learn from the model that the stimuli are in fact safe and can be coped with. For example, a child can be shown a film of medical procedures, or a teddy bear can be given a blood test. Such procedures have been shown to reduce fear and anxiety (Melamed & Siegal, 1975). Live modeling is generally more effective than symbolic modeling. If anxiety is severe, it can be combined with relaxation, and repeated several times in a graded way. Modeling can be used to develop a whole range of prosocial skills, and is especially effective if combined with other techniques such as role play. It is more effective if the model gets rewarded for the new (e.g., prosocial) behavior. Complex behaviors may need to be broken down into component steps, as in problem-solving (see chapter 63).

Role Playing

By enacting behaviors rather than just talking about them, the child gets to practice the new responses in a favorable environment with fewer distracting stimuli than in real life. This is particularly helpful when emotional reactions may supervene (e.g., when a child with anger management problems is trying to stay calm while being provoked). For parents who cannot imagine the impact of their harsh practices on a child, it can be helpful to set up a role play with the parent playing the child, and another person behaving the way the parent usually does.

Fading and Generalization

After setting up a relatively intense reinforcement program, assuming it works, then the issues of generalization and withdrawal arise. Too abrupt a withdrawal of the reinforcement schedule is equivalent to introducing an extinction program for the new desired behavior. Fading procedures gradually change the environmental stimuli so they approximate, as far as possible, the natural conditions that will prevail following treatment. Methods include reducing reinforcement to an intermittent schedule, arranging for the artificial rewards such as tokens to be replaced by social ones such as praise from close adults – in real life these rewards are likely to be given only intermittently. If during fading the desired behavior diminishes or the undesired one recurs, then one should go back to the preceding reinforcement schedule for longer. Another approach is to widen the rewards and the people giving them, thus increasing generalization. Overlearning is a useful approach for more chaotic, conduct problem families where parents find it difficult to maintain consistency. Promoting the child to self-direct is a powerful way to promote generalization, whereby the child evaluates and directs their own behavior.

Application and Effectiveness in Specific Conditions

Emotional disorders

Anxiety Disorders

Anxiety disorders respond well to behavioral approaches, which are a mainstay of treatment, although medication can be effective too, at least in the short term (see chapter 39). The underlying principle is to expose the child to the feared stimulus and teach an alternative conditioned response characterized by calm and relaxation. Graded exposure and systematic desensitization are used as described above. Nowadays, the children's cognitions will be worked on as well, with an element teaching them to monitor their thoughts and challenge their erroneous beliefs ("Maybe I'm dying," "Everyone can see I'm going to faint"). These interventions would therefore be classified as cognitive–behavioral, but there is a strong behavioral element and cognitions are addressed using behavioral principles. The treatments work well, but then the question arises as to what is the active ingredient. Three studies have addressed this, using control groups that received various forms of non-specific supportive counseling or psychoeducation (Beidel, Turner, & Morris, 2000; Last, Hansen, & Franco, 1998; Silverman, Kurtines, Ginsburg *et al.*, 1999). Only the last of these showed CBT was more effective than active control. Further studies are needed to determine what mediated a good treatment response – for example, it may be that in the control conditions educating children about fears and supporting them about their anxieties gave sufficient mental exposure to allow them to learn more adaptive behavioral, cognitive and emotional responses. Additionally, trials are needed with long-term follow-up that directly compare medication with behavioral treatments.

Earlier trials of behavioral therapy for anxiety took an adult model of treatment, with the therapist seeing the child only. However, there are several reasons for involving parents in treatment. First, from the earliest months, infants look to their mothers to "read" whether situation are dangerous and anxiety provoking, as shown in Gibson's experiment where infants looked to their mothers to see if it was safe to walk across a glass plate with a drop beneath it (the "visual cliff"; Gibson & Walk, 1960). Therefore, helping parents to show a calm response rather than colluding with anxious responses should help to reduce child anxiety. Second, parents can support the therapeutic endeavor by ensuring that the child gets exposed to feared situations, and by helping with coping responses. The effectiveness of adding family involvement was tested by Barrett, Dadds, and Rapee (1996), who found it gave a significant advantage in reducing child anxiety, which was maintained at 1-year follow-up.

Obsessive-Compulsive Disorder

In childhood OCD, anxiety is a major feature, and the behavioral treatment is based on similar graded exposure to the feared object or context (say, dirt). During exposure (E) to the phobic stimulus, it is important to prevent the child from carrying out the obsessive response, which acts as a negative reinforcer for the child by reducing anxiety. Response prevention (RP) involves stopping the child carrying out rituals; for example, they must touch "germy things" but refrain from washing until their anxiety is reduced. A third element in addition to E and RP is stopping parental reassurance, to ensure full exposure effects (March, Franklin, & Foa, 2005). The efficacy of E and RP has been demonstrated in multiple open studies and two RCTs (Barrett, Healey-Farrell, & March, 2004; POTS, 2004). Cognitive components may be added if there are substantial obsessive thoughts, but these are absent in up to half of cases (Swedo, Rapoport, Leonard, Lenane, & Cheslow, 1989), and to date there have been no studies comparing the effectiveness of adding cognitive components with none.

As for other anxiety therapies, studies are now beginning to examine different parameters of delivery of E and RP. Involving families is now standard practice, but an RCT demonstrated that it is equally efficacious when conducted in a group setting as with individual families, an important consideration for cost-effective service delivery (Barrett, Healy-Farrell, & March, 2004). Futhermore, in adults, computer-based E and RP delivery with minimal therapist contact time is effective (Kenwright, Marks, Graham, Franses, & Mataix-Cols, 2005); a similar study with children is now needed. The necessary "dose" of behavior therapy for children has been studied by Franklin, Kozak, Cashman *et al.* (1998), who compared once weekly with daily therapy; no significant difference in outcome was found, although the study was not randomized, so conclusions now need confirmation in an RCT. The meta-analysis by the UK National Institute of Clinical Excellence (NICE, 2005) suggested that while more therapist-intensive approaches were more efficacious, even those involving relatively little therapist contact time (less than 10 h) were also effective (NICE, 2005).

Behavioral and pharmacological treatments were directly compared in the Pediatric OCD Treatment (POTS) multicenter study that randomized children to sertraline, CBT, both treatments combined, or pill placebo for 12 weeks (POTS, 2004). All active treatments were superior to pill placebo, and CBT alone was as efficacious as sertraline, but combined treatment was more effective than either alone. This finding of the superiority of combined psychological treatment and medication was also found in a small study (Neziroglu, Yaryhura-Tobias, Walz, & McKay, 2000); a direct comparison of behavior therapy with clomipramine found a non-significant advantage for psychotherapy (de Haan, Hoogduin, Buitelaar, & Keijsers, 1998), suggesting the POTS study findings broadly agreed with others.

Post-Traumatic Stress Disorder

As for other anxiety-related conditions, the core of behavioral treatment for PTSD is exposure, in this case to vivid recollection of the traumatic event. In a non-randomized design, Goenjian, Karayan, Pynoos *et al.* (1997) reported that a seven-session school-based CBT intervention for young people with PTSD over a year after an earthquake resulted in symptom reduction, whereas an untreated control group showed no such improvement. March, Biederman, Wolkow *et al.* (1998) used a single-case design and several measures to evaluate an 18-session group CBT intervention for 17 young people who had developed PTSD following a variety of trauma (road traffic accidents, accidental injury, gunshot injury and fires). After treatment, there were significant reductions in PTSD symptoms and associated psychopathology (anxiety, depression and anger).

Three RCTs of psychological interventions with children who developed PTSD symptoms as a result of single-event traumas have been reported. Chemtob, Nakashima, and Hamada (2002) randomly assigned 248 children at high risk of PTSD after a hurricane hit Hawaii to four sessions of CBT delivered individually, or in groups; or to a control group. Both individual and group treatment had equally good results compared to controls by an effect size of 0.76; more children dropped out of individual than group treatment. Stein, Jaycox, Kataoka *et al.* (2003) randomized 126 children who had been exposed to violence to 10 sessions of group CBT or a waitlist control. Three months post-treatment, the treated group had significantly lower scores on PTSD, depression and psychosocial dysfunction measures, although teacher-rated behavioral difficulties did not reflect improvement.

Using Ehlers and Clark's (2000) more cognitive model of PTSD, Smith, Yule, Perrin *et al.* (2007) randomized 24 clinically referred children with a diagnosis of PTSD (rather than a population-based sample screened for symptoms) following assault or a road traffic accident to trauma-focused CBT or waitlist control. After treatment, 92% of the CBT group no longer met criteria for PTSD, compared to 42% on the waitlist; treated children also showed significant reductions in symptoms of depression and anxiety. The effect size was 2.2 on the self-report measure and 1.6 on the clinician-rated instrument. The differences remained at 6-month follow-up. This study was innovative because it measured a potential mediator, maladaptive cognitions, which did indeed turn out to mediate treatment effectiveness.

Finally, the question arises whether a cognitive element adds anything to imaginal exposure. Tarrier and Sommerfield (2004) found no difference at 1-year follow-up in a trial comparing the two approaches in adults, but at 5-year follow-up 29% of the imaginal exposure group still had PTSD whereas none of the cognitive group did. Similar trials for children are now called for.

PTSD and Child Sexual Abuse

In recent years, some of the reactions some children develop after sexual abuse have been recognized as fulfilling some or all criteria for PTSD. This has resulted in a number of therapeutic trials of CBT to treat these reactions, including full PTSD. There are many other sequelae of abuse, and only PTSD-type outcomes in trials of CBT are reviewed here. Generally speaking, studies favor CBT. Thus, Deblinger, Stauffer, and Steer (2001) randomized 67 children aged 2–8 years to group

CBT or a support group; the CBT group had better outcomes. Cohen, Deblinger, Mannarino, and Steer's (2004) multi-site RCT also favored CBT, but Celano, Hazzard, Webb, and McCall (1996) compared 15 girls in an abuse-specific program with 17 given a parallel set of eight non-directive supportive sessions and found no differences in outcomes. To investigate different approaches to delivery, King, Tonge, Mullen *et al.* (2000) allocated 36 sexually abused children aged 5–17 years who met criteria for PTSD to CBT with child and family, CBT with child alone, or waitlist control. Both ways of delivering CBT (which lasted 20 sessions) were equally effective in reducing PTSD and anxiety more than in controls.

Disruptive Disorders

Conduct Disorders

Behavioral methods and the social learning approach revolutionized the treatment of conduct problems. In the late 1960s and through the 1970s, clinical researchers such as Patterson at the Oregon Social Learning Center, Wahler in Tennessee, Forehand in Georgia and Eyberg in Washington State tested and refined methods for parents to apply to disruptive children. By reducing attention for inappropriate behavior, giving it for desired responses and combining this with calm consistent discipline, antisocial behavior was considerably reduced. Over 100 trials attest to their effectiveness (Kazdin, 2005), and meta-analyses show mean effect sizes of around 0.4–1.0 standard deviations (SD; Barlow, 1999). More recent developments include similar programs for teachers to apply at school, because generalization of parenting programs to that setting is unreliable (Scott, 2002). Anger management programs working directly with children and adolescents are also based on behavioral theory, to which a self-control cognitive element has been added (see chapters 35 and 63). They are a useful adjunct to parent and teacher programs, helping temper control not only at home and in school, but also out in the community with peers (see chapters 35 and 63). The question arises whether parent, teacher and child interventions should ideally all be given.

Kazdin, Siegel, and Bass (1992) compared parent training alone with child social skills training alone, and both combined. All groups improved substantially, with improvements seen not only by parents at home, but also by teachers at school and self-reported offending by the young people. However, the combined treatment had greater effectiveness on nearly all measures, notably 0.5–1.1 SD greater effect than parent training alone on antisocial behavior. Webster-Stratton and Hammond (1997) used a group format with videotapes to compare parent training only with child training only, both parent training plus child training, and a waitlist control group. A total of 97 children aged 4–8 years specifically referred to a parenting clinic were studied with a thorough set of measures including direct observation at home and observation of interaction with a friend. The intervention was relatively long (22 weekly sessions of 2 h) and attendance was excellent, with all cases attending at least half of the sessions and most attending nearly all. There were no dropouts. There were several important findings. On parent questionnaire, children in all three intervention conditions did considerably better than waitlist controls, who did not improve significantly. The fact that *child training alone* led to improvements in child behavior is important practically because there will always be some parents who are unable or unwilling to attend for intervention. All interventions had an effect in reducing observed directive parenting behavior. From a theoretical standpoint, it is interesting that child training led to less coercive parenting behavior, confirming the hypothesis that for children with clinically significant antisocial behavior (as for non-clinical children) child as well as parent factors are involved in driving parenting style; it shows that the coercive cycle of negative parenting and child defiance can be interrupted from either end.

Parent training led to greater changes in parent-reported child behavior problems than child training, whereas child training led to better improvements in the ratio of positive to negative strategies used by children when interacting with a friend on direct observation, and on laboratory tests of social problem-solving. The combined parent–child intervention led to similar effect sizes as one would predict from either intervention alone in the domain in which they were most effective, but did not act synergistically. Thus, parent-rated child behavior was no more improved in the combined condition than for child training alone, and observed child–peer behavior was no more improved in the combined condition than with parent training alone. The exception was observed antisocial behavior in the home at 1-year follow-up, where the combined condition had a greater effect than either alone. Unfortunately, although in all intervention conditions there was a good effect compared to controls for observed reduction in child behavior at home (ES 0.7–0.8), total deviant behavior reduced to half original levels whereas controls did not change, the variance was large (standard deviations greater than means in all cases), so none was statistically significant.

All gains were maintained at 1-year follow-up, suggesting that the reduction in antisocial behavior is lasting. Unfortunately, further follow-up to test longer-term persistence of benefits will not be possible from this study as the control group were treated after the waiting period for ethical reasons. No intervention made any difference to teacher-rated child behavior in either the short or longer term. This was partly because some of the children had no significant problems at school, but nonetheless it suggests that child behavior may be fairly context specific, and supports adding a teacher element.

Attention Deficit/Hyperactivity Disorder

Behavior therapy for ADHD has tended to be similar to that for conduct disorders, with parents and teachers giving rewards for prosocial behavior and punishments for rule infringements and antisocial behavior. This is not unreasonable, given that it is often the comorbid conduct problems that are more troublesome than inattention and hyperactivity *per se*. Laboratory studies indicate that children with ADHD respond better to immediate rewards – delays beyond a few seconds lead to diminished responses; but, like other children, they will work to maximize the total reward on offer (Scheres, Dijkstra, Ainslie *et al.*, 2006). Modifications to standard behavioral programs should include giving rewards more rapidly and frequently, changing them more often to avoid boredom, and giving directions more clearly. Generally speaking, core symptoms of ADHD change less in behavioral programs than do conduct symptoms. Generalization outside the immediate situation where the reward system is being operated may be limited (e.g., in the playground when there is a teacher-administered reward system only in class); nonetheless, even after regimes are faded, there are some enduring effects (Arnold, Chuang, Davies *et al.*, 2004). The presence of ADHD does not prevent specific methods being effective. For example, Fabiano, Pelham, Manos *et al.* (2004) compared the effectiveness of short (5 min) and long (15 min) time out sessions versus none in a cross-over design with 71 6- to 12-year-olds with ADHD. Both time out regimes were more effective than none in reducing aggression, destructiveness and repeated non-compliance, with an effect size of 0.32 SD; longer time out was no more effective, confirming other findings that 5 min is sufficient.

In the MTA Cooperative Group trial (1999), behavioral therapy was compared to medication and both in combination; there was also a treatment-as-usual arm (which was mainly lower doses of medication). In the behavioral-treatment-only arm, ADHD symptoms improved only modestly but conduct symptoms more so; the mechanism here appears to be child insensitivity to the changed contingencies, because direct observation of the parents showed that they did indeed change their responses to the children (Wells, Chi, Hinshaw *et al.*, 2006). Behavioral treatment worked equally well irrespective of potential moderators, whereas in the medication arm, parental depression and more severe child ADHD symptoms moderated a poorer response (Owens, Hinshaw, Kraemer *et al.*, 2003). The question arises whether medication potentiates the effects of behavior therapy – it might be expected that because there is a central nervous system deficit in ADHD, correcting this through medication would then enable the behavior therapy to work much better. However, this was not found to be a large tendency in the MTA trial, where once medication had been given, adding behavior therapy did not improve outcomes much further – the main improvements in core ADHD symptoms came from the drug. However, adding behavior therapy increased the proportion of children brought into the normal range, and improved aggression at home (MTA Cooperaive Group, 1999). Also, in the arm with both behavior therapy and medication, substantially lower doses of medication were used while getting similar overall results – thus, behavior therapy allowed less medication to be used.

A final point to remember is that reasonably well-conducted intervention studies from 20–30 years ago that used relaxation training procedures alone or in combination with other treatments generated larger effect sizes than did CBT interventions (Benson, Beary, & Carol, 1974; Budzynski & Stovay, 1969; Kratter, 1983). More studies are needed that directly compare different treatments while measuring potential mediators.

Developmental Disorders

Nocturnal Enuresis

This is a good example of the great success behavioral methods can bring. Mowrer (1980) recounts how, despite being a professor at Yale, during the great depression in the 1930s to supplement his salary he and his wife took a job in a residential home for misfit boys, most of whom wet the bed every night. Based on classic conditioning, they devised an aversive conditioned response triggered by the stimulus of wetness in pads worn in underpants. Initially, the aversive response was provided by a spring-loaded metal bed that catapulted the child across the room, but soon a loud bell was used instead (Mowrer & Mowrer, 1938). This has repeatedly been shown to be effective in simple nocturnal enuresis (von Gontard, 2005). The Cochrane review of alarm interventions for nocturnal enuresis (Glazener, Evans, & Peto, 2005) found 55 trials involving 3152 children. Immediately after treatment, two-thirds were dry at night, with half remaining so in the long term (compared to no untreated controls ever becoming dry). Adding overlearning (e.g., by increasing fluid intake at night – for details see Houts' 2003 account) reduced the long-term relapse rate further to around 20%, but adding penalties for wet beds was positively counterproductive. Alarms were better than tricyclics during treatment, and while desmopressin achieved dryness in most cases while it was taken, a meta-analysis of studies has shown that almost all cases relapsed after it was stopped (Glazener & Evans, 2007).

The mechanism of action of alarms has been debated. Mowrer was clear that classic conditioning was involved as outlined above. Subsequent physiological studies (Norgaard, 1989) suggest that bladder detrusor muscle contractions that lead to urination are inhibited by pelvic floor muscle contractions. The alarm promotes these, and then the child does not wake up. However, nocturnal enuretics have learned to habituate to the aversive stimulus of a wet bed, and have relaxed pelvic floors during nocturnal micturition. The classic aversion account was challenged by Azrin, Sneed, and Foxx (1973), who claimed that the mechanism of effective treatment was that the child was operantly rewarded by dryness. He developed so-called "dry-bed" procedures with the parents waking up the child at regular intervals in the night and taking them to the toilet so they remained dry; no alarm was used. This procedure is demanding on parents, but results showed it was indeed as effective as simple alarm training (61% vs. 59% success at 2 years in the trial by Bollard, 1982). It seems therefore that both accounts of the mechanism of action of each treatment may hold true; at times it is a fine line between "classic" learning of conditioned responses to clearly identifiable stimuli, and "operant" learning whereby the individual responds because certain apparently spontaneous actions are rewarding.

Pervasive Developmental Disorders

Behavioral methods can help some specific problems in autistic spectrum disorders (ASD), but should only be part of an overall package. This should aim to stimulate, as far as possible, normal development of language and socialization, and to reduce the particular maladaptive behaviors such as rigidity, stereotypies and inflexibility as well as general ones such as hyperactivity and tantrums. Behavior therapy needs to be adapted to this client group in a number of ways. First, changes need to be introduced gradually, within a framework that is predictable and structured in terms of daily routines – otherwise anxiety, social isolation and rigidities may emerge rapidly. Second, instructions need to be concrete, specific and calmly delivered, because metaphorical expressions and using tone of voice to convey meanings may lead to misunderstandings. Third, the intensity of social stimulation will need to be titrated to the level that can be handled, which may be quite low in some cases. Fourth, training and interventions should be performed as much as possible in daily-life situations, to overcome the problems in the transfer of skills mastered in one setting to another.

There is a modest amount of research suggesting intensive early interventions for children with ASD are more likely to be successful than low-intensity treatment later on. A well-known approach is that taken by Lovaas and Smith (2003) in the Young Autism Project at the University of California in Los Angeles. This is a comprehensive teaching and rearing program, rather than just treatment for particular problems. There is an introductory phase of establishing a teaching relationship where basic directions such as "sit" or "come here" are established and interfering behaviors such as tantrums reduced. This is followed by several months of developing communication and social skills, culminating in peer relationship training; depending on the rate of progress, the program may take 1–3 years or longer, terminating when the child goes to elementary school. Lovaas (1987) and McEachin, Smith, and Lovaas (1993) published a comparison of 59 children non-randomly allocated to intensive treatment, minimal treatment or special education. By age 7 the mean IQ of the intensive-treatment group was 83 while those of the two comparison groups were 52 and 59; by age 12 the percent with an IQ over 85 who were in a normal school was 42% in the intensive-treatment group and 0% in the minimal-treatment group. An independent replication (Smith, Groen, & Wynn, 2000) that was less intensive (25 h per week rather than 40) but fully randomized found at follow-up that the intensive-intervention group had an IQ 16 points higher than controls. Other replications have yielded comparable results (Smith, 1999); thus, Eikeseth, Smith, Jahr, and Eldevik (2002) tried the method with older children (4 years and above) but still obtained good results, including an IQ gain of 13 points. Since then, reviews of more recent evaluations indicate that although this approach is certainly effective, the overall results are neither as marked nor as universal as initially claimed (Shea, 2004).

Is such intensive intervention by fully qualified professionals necessary, or can parents be taught to deliver it as effectively? Bibby, Eikeseth, Martin, Mudford, and Reeves (2001) studied 66 children treated through their parents using consultants, but the results were disappointing – although there were gains of 9 points on an adaptive behavior scale, there were no intelligence or language gains. Kabot, Masi, and Segal (2003) have suggested that for maximal gains, both intensive professional daycare and high-quality parent training are needed. Such a model is incorporated in the school-based Treatment and Education of Autistic and Communication Handicapped Children program (TEACCH; Mesibov, Shea, & Schopeler, 2005). This uses parents as co-therapists to ensure that the same principles are enacted at home; to date there has not been an RCT evaluation, although a small-scale study (Pancrai, Ferrante, & Zingale, 2002) reported significant gains in educational and adaptive behaviors compared to progress in an integrated classroom.

More specific interventions are available (e.g., social skills training programs, delivered on an individual or on a group basis), and are increasingly being offered to children and adolescents with ASD (Bauminger, 2002). However, the merits on a long-term basis are often disappointing because of a lack of generalization of skills.

Intellectual Disability (Mental Retardation)

Behavioral methods are a major part of treatment regimes in children with intellectual disability. While children with IQs above 60 or so may be able to participate to some extent in using cognitive techniques (Turk, 2005), this is seldom the case for those with lower IQs, for whom behavioral approaches are key. Challenging behaviors such as tantrums and self-injury are especially common in this group, and a thorough functional analysis should be carried out. Depending on what this shows, a range of techniques may be applied (Ball, Bush, & Emerson, 2004). Stimulus control and manipulation of antecedent variables are often especially helpful. These can include changing routines so the child is in a better biological state (e.g., less hungry, tired, or constipated); changing activities that precede the challenging behavior (e.g., by providing more varied activities and curricula to avert boredom and frustration); and changing triggers that in the functional analysis appear to lead immediately to the behavior (e.g., transition points in the daily routine, too close facial contact).

Teaching alternative responses can also be very effective. Functional communication training is a form of functional displacement, whereby a child is taught a more appropriate alternative. For example, if a child's aggression in class serves the function of enabling them to escape disliked activities, they can be taught to request an alternative activity instead. This will work so long as the child finds it is effective in getting the result, and is easy for the child to implement (Carr, Levin, McConnachie *et al.*, 1994). More generally, DRO, which is often a very effective technique in typically developing children, is often less effective in children with intellectual disability, who may find it hard to learn relatively complex alternatives (Didden, Duker, & Korzilius, 1997). Punishments such as time out can be effective, but should not be used frequently in this group as they could become abusive.

General Issues

Indications and Limitations

As the above review has shown, behavioral therapies have offered mainstream interventions for many conditions. However, they may not be especially helpful where the primary problem is an inner mood or belief state without pressing behavioral manifestations. Thus, there is no purely behavioral method for the treatment of the core symptoms of depression, although the approach can be used to tackle some of the manifestations (e.g., lack of physical activity), and some of the postulated maintaining factors (e.g., low self-esteem because of a lack of friends arising from poor social skills). In contrast, behavioral approaches offer unique strengths for conditions where the child's problems cannot easily be changed effectively by a cognitive approach, for example in babies and young infants (e.g., feeding and sleeping problems), in children with severe learning disabilities (e.g., challenging behavior) and more generally where the behavior is not very amenable to conscious control (e.g., hyperactivity and aggression). More widely, behavioral techniques are helpful for any condition where changes in the external environment can make a difference, and behavioral analysis can reveal where this is the case. Even where little can be done to change externally the main features of the environment such as a hostile family or a dangerous neighborhood, often children can be instructed in techniques that will enable them to mitigate its worst aspects or select better contexts (e.g., by learning what leads parents to become hostile, or learning to avoid bullies).

The absence of any theory about what is happening in the child's inner world and the failure to address it directly inevitably bring with them some limitations. While learning is expected to occur in an unconscious way, in certain conditions this does not always hold. Thus, there is the issue of generalization, which requires the individual to be able to extract the rules regarding both the context when they behave a certain way and the rewards. Many children learn new habits from the rewards, and these will persist after the rewards are withdrawn. If no lasting connection is made, then extinction will occur as the rewards are withdrawn. This can occur if material rewards such as sweets are given and then withdrawn, and particularly for children who may be poor at generalizing and so need ongoing rewards, such as those with autism. Rewards that can always be easily given such as social rewards (smiles, praise) may lead to better control in these cases. Likewise, newly learned behaviors may not persist in antisocial children once the context is changed – thus, delinquents may behave very well while in controlled settings such as "boot camps" but the rate of relapse is over 80% after they are released back into the community (Stinchcomb, 2005). The issue here is to change the contingencies in the child's natural environment (e.g., praise at home and close supervision in the community).

A further criticism of behavioral approaches arises from the apparent failure to take the individual's past or personal vulnerabilities and liabilities to a condition into account. While it is true that certain individuals may be more at risk than others, there is abundant evidence that for many problems and disorders, the dynamic interplay between the context and the individual is crucial in determining the expression of the difficulty in any particular case (e.g., life events in depression, or coercive parenting in antisocial behavior). A good therapist will take a very detailed history of the predicament of the child and check carefully what the triggers are for them – so that the resulting program will be entirely individualized and will not fit another child. Arguably, this is a much more personalized approach than, say, prescribing medication.

Has Adding Cognitive Elements to Behavior Therapy Improved Outcomes?

More trials are needed to explore this issue, in addition to the few reviewed above. Certainly, clinically there are often scenarios where the beliefs seem to prevent behavior change; for example, the parent who thinks it is militaristic to set limits, or who cannot bear to ignore a child crying at night. Adding cognitive components would be worth evaluating in these contexts. In the adult literature, CBT techniques have produced impressive outcomes in many areas but it is not clear how much of this is brought about by what was added to traditional behavior therapy. Component analysis studies have often failed to find support for the importance of direct cognitive change strategies, which was the common sense lynchpin of CBT (Jacobson, Dobson, Truax *et al.*, 1996). The response to traditional cognitive therapy often occurs before cognitive change techniques have been implemented (Ilardi & Craighead, 1994), and support for the hypothesized mediators of change in CBT is often weak (Burns & Spangler, 2001; Morgenstern & Longabaugh, 2000). Well-known cognitive therapists have been forced to conclude that in some important areas there is "no additive benefit to providing cognitive interventions in cognitive therapy" (Dobson & Khatri, 2000, p. 913).

This overall picture presents an anomaly. On the one hand, most empirical clinicians agree that traditional behavior therapy was simply not adequate and that better methods of dealing with thoughts and feelings were needed. CBT is widely understood to have been a step forward in freeing up the behavior therapy tradition to work directly with cognition, and the outcomes for CBT protocols are generally quite good compared to work outside of behavior therapy writ large. On the other hand, the core concept of traditional cognitive and CBT – that direct cognitive change is necessary for clinical improvement – is still only partially supported.

Therapist variables

Does it matter how well behavioral therapies are delivered? Therapist variables can be divided into:

1 The *alliance* which, put simply, refers to how well therapist and client get on together, including sharing of goals of treatment;

2 *Fidelity* or *adherence*, which refers to whether the therapist carried out specific procedures; and

3 The *skill* or *competence* with which the therapy was carried out.

The Alliance

A meta-analysis of studies of the alliance over a range of treatment modalities with children found an effect size of 0.21 for the effect of the alliance, and found it was important across treatment types (including giving medication), and across child, parent or family treatment approaches (Shirk & Karver, 2003). Kazdin, Whitley, and Marciano (2006) found about 7% of the variance in outcome of treatment for antisocial children was related to the alliance, although findings varied by informant.

Fidelity or Adherence

Fidelity or adherence concerns the extent to which the therapist follows the actions prescribed in the manual. Studies of child therapies have found equivocal effects. In a study of multisystemic therapy for delinquency, Henggeler, Melton, Brondino, Scherer, and Hanley (1997) compared a total of 15 parent, therapist and youth-rated fidelity scales with 7 youth outcomes, and found significant effects for only 7 out of 42 parent-rated associations, 4 out of 35 therapist-rated and 1 out of 28 adolescent-rated; moreover, some effects went the "wrong" way, with better fidelity leading to worse outcomes. The same group (Huey, Henggeler, Brondino, & Pickrel, 2000) found that when they used a latent variable approach, therapist-rated fidelity improved family functioning and parent monitoring, both of which in turn reduced youth delinquency, but that parent- and youth-rated fidelity had no effect. These somewhat modest findings for the role of adherence or fidelity raise the question of whether applying the treatment according to the manual is necessary or sufficient to bring about change.

Skill or Competence

It is possible that a more important and relevant influence on effectiveness is the skill or competence with which tasks are carried out; put simply, skill concerns how well the therapist performs the actions. Thus, two behavior therapists might each carry out a functional assessment, set up a behavioral program, choose targets and rewards, and issue homework. However, the more skilled one might do this in a more sensitive way with greater complexity, and so characterize the child's problems more accurately and be more proficient in overcoming barriers to doing homework, thus leading to more change.

Researchers from the Treatment of Depression Collaborative Research Program (TDCRP) reported that therapist variables had substantial effects on a clinician-rated outcome of depression (Shaw, Elkin, Yamaguchi *et al.*, 1999). The quality of the alliance accounted for 5% of outcome variability, but therapist adherence had no effect. Competence added a further 15%, although when this was decomposed into how well the sessions were structured and how skillfully the sessions were run, skill had no effect if structure was entered first in a multiple regression. Amongst childhood studies, Forgatch, Patterson, and DeGarmo (2005) developed an observer-based instrument to assess therapist variables that included skill in a parenting program for recently divorced parents. They measured knowledge, structure, teaching skill, clinical skill and overall effectiveness. The outcome they assessed was the proximal one of observed parenting practices, rather than child behavior; greater therapist skill led to more change in parenting. Finally, Scott, Carby, and Rendu (unpublished data) examined the effect of therapist skill in a multi-site trial of parent training for children with severe conduct problems. Skill correlated 0.7 with improvement in child antisocial behavior. The practitioners in the top third level of skill achieved twice the change of the bottom third, and the lowest level of skill actually made the children slightly worse. If further research supports these findings, then it will provide evidence for the need for more high-quality training.

Service Issues

In some countries and in some professions, behavioral approaches are poorly understood and poorly taught. They may be seen as mechanical and not addressing feelings and relationships, which some practitioners feel is core to their work. Further, there are still many practitioners in education, social work and mental health professions who pay scant attention to the evidence of what treatments work. In fact, the effectiveness of behavioral therapies means they often have a powerful effect on children's happiness, and the children have more fulfilling relationships with their families, friends and teachers. Behavioral methods can be combined well with other therapeutic modalities (e.g., with family therapy in disruptive disorders, with medication as reviewed above, or with life story and other work in war-affected refugees who have PTSD). Delivery may need to be commissioned at different levels of skill, with self-administered behavioral therapy being tried first for less severe cases with families judged to be able to handle this, ranging up to deployment of highly skilled therapists for complex cases.

Conclusions

In the last 40 years or so, behavioral therapies have revolutionized the treatment of emotional and behavioral disorders in children, and have offered effective interventions to improve social and intellectual functioning. Purely behavioral treatments have continued to be refined and expanded, in content, mode of application and large-scale evaluations. Behavioral approaches based on the same method of empirical scientific enquiry and experimental testing have strongly influenced the development of cognitive elements in CBT, in a manner that is entirely consistent with the thinking of the founders of behaviorism. Future research needs to clarify mechanisms of action and modes of delivery, and to compare behavioral therapies with plausible alternatives. Wider training is required in what behavioral techniques have to offer, and how to deliver them.

References

Alexander, J., Pugh, C., Parsons, B., & Sexton, T. (2000). *Blueprints for violence prevention: Functional family therapy*. University of Colorado: Institute of Behavioral Science.

Arnold, L. E., Chuang, S., Davies, M., Abikoff, H. B., Conners, C. K., Elliott, G. R., *et al.* (2004). Nine months of multicomponent behavioral treatment for ADHD and effectiveness of MTA fading procedures. *Journal of Abnormal Child Psychology*, *32*, 39–51.

Azrin, N. H., Sneed, T. J., & Foxx, R. M. (1973). Dry bed: A rapid method of eliminating bedwetting (enuresis) of the retarded. *Behavioral Research and Therapy*, *11*, 427–434.

Ball, T., Bush, A., & Emerson, F. (2004). *Psychological interventions for severely challenging behaviours shown by people with learning disabilities*. Leicester: British Psychological Society.

Barlow, J. (1999). *Systematic review of the effectiveness of parent-training programmes in improving behaviour problems in children aged 3–10 years* (2nd edn.). *A review of the literature on parent-training programmes and child behaviour outcome measures*. University of Oxford: Health Services Research Unit.

Barrett, P., Healy-Farrell, L., & March, J. S. (2004). Cognitive–behavioral family treatment of childhood obsessive-compulsive disorder: A controlled trial. *Journal of the American Academy of Child and Adolescent Psychiatry*, *43*, 46–62.

Barrett, P. M., Dadds, M. R., & Rapee, R. M. (1996). Family treatment of childhood anxiety: A controlled trial. *Journal of Consulting and Clinical Psychology*, *64*, 333–342.

Bauminger, N. (2002). The facilitation of social-emotional understanding and social interaction in high-functioning children with autism: Intervention outcomes. *Journal of Autism and Developmental Disorders*, *32*, 283–298.

Beidel, D. C., Turner, S. M., & Morris, T. L. (2000). Behavioral treatment of childhood social phobia. *Journal of Consulting and Clinical Psychology*, *68*, 1072–1080.

Benson, H., Beary, J. F., & Carol, M. P. (1974). The relaxation response. *Psychiatry: Journal for the Study of Interpersonal Processes*, *37*, 37–46.

Bibby, P., Eikeseth, S., Martin, N. T., Mudford, O. C., & Reeves, D. (2001). Progress and out comes for children with autism receiving parent-managed intensive interventions. *Research in Developmental Disabilities*, *22*, 425–447.

Bollard, J. (1982). A two year follow up of bedwetters treated with dry bed training and standard conditioning. *Behavioral Research and Therapy*, *20*, 571–580.

Budzynski, T. H., & Stoyva, J. M. (1969). An instrument for producing deep muscle relaxation by means of analog information feedback. *Journal of Applied Behavior Analysis*, *2*, 231–237.

Burns, D. D., & Spangler, D. L. (2001). Do changes in dysfunctional attitudes mediate changes in depression and anxiety in cognitive behavioral therapy? *Behavior Therapy*, *32*, 337–369.

Carr, E. G., Levin, L., McConnachie, G., Carlson, J. I., Kemp, D. C., & Smith, C. E. (1994). *Communication-based interventions for problem behavior: A user's guide for producing positive change*. Baltimore: Brookes.

Celano, M., Hazzard, A., Webb, C., & McCall, C. (1996). Treatment of traumagenic beliefs among sexually abused girls and their mothers: An evaluation study. *Journal of Abnormal Child Psychology*, *24*, 1–17.

Chamberlain, P., & Reid, J. B. (1998). Comparison of two community alternatives to incarceration for chronic juvenile offenders. *Journal of Consulting and Clinical Psychology*, *66*, 624–633.

Chemtob, C. M., Nakashima, J. P., & Hamada, R. S. (2002). Psychosocial intervention for postdisaster trauma symptoms in elementary school children: A controlled community field study. *Archives of Pediatrics and Adolescent Medicine*, *156*, 211–216.

Chomsky, N. (1959). Review of Skinner, 1957. *Language*, *35*, 26–58.

Cohen, J. A., Deblinger, E., Mannarino, A. P., & Steer, R. A. (2004). A multisite, randomized controlled trial for children with sexual abuse-related PTSD symptoms. *Journal of the American Academy of Child and Adolescent Psychiatry*, *43*, 393–402.

Conduct Problems Prevention Research Group. (1999). Initial impact of the Fast Track prevention trial for conduct problems. 1. The high-risk sample. *Journal of Consulting and Clinical Psychology*, *67*, 631–647.

de Haan, E., Hoogduin, K. A., Buitelaar, J. K., & Keijsers, G. P. (1998). Behavior therapy versus clomipramine for the treatment of obsessive-compulsive disorder in children and adolescents. *Journal of the American Academy of Child and Adolescent Psychiatry*, *37*, 1022–1029.

Deblinger, E., Stauffer, L. B., & Steer, R. A. (2001). Comparative efficacies of supportive and cognitive–behavioral group therapies for young children who have been sexually abused and their non-offending mothers. *Child Maltreatment: Journal of the American Professional Society on the Abuse of Children*, *6*, 332–343.

Didden, R., Duker, P. C., & Korzilius, H. (1997). Meta-analytic study on treatment effectiveness for problem behaviors with individuals who have mental retardation. *American Journal of Mental Retardation*, *101*, 387–399.

Dobson, K. S., & Khatri, N. (2000). Cognitive therapy: Looking backward, looking forward. *Journal of Clinical Psychology*, *56*, 907–923.

Ehlers, A., & Clark, D. M. (2000). A cognitive model of posttraumatic stress disorder. *Behaviour Research and Therapy*, *38*, 319–345.

Eikeseth, S., Smith, T., Jahr, E., & Eldevik, S. (2002). Intensive behavioral treatment at school for 4- to 7-year-old children with autism: A 1-year comparison controlled study. *Behavior Modification*, *26*, 49–68.

Fabiano, G. A., Pelham, W. E., Manos, M. J., Gnagy, E. M., Chronis, A. M., Onyango, A. N., *et al.* (2004). An evaluation of three time-out procedures for children with attention deficit/hyperactivity disorder. *Behavior Therapy*, *35*, 449–469.

Forgatch, M. S., Patterson, G. R., & DeGarmo, D. S. (2005). Evaluating fidelity: Predictive validity for a measure of competent adherence to the Oregon model of parent management training. *Behavior Therapy*, *36*, 3–13.

Frankel, F., & Myatt, R. (2003). *Children's friendship training*. Brunner-Routledge. New York.

Franklin, M. E., Kozak, M. J., Cashman, L. A., Coles, M. E., Rheingold, A. A., & Foa, E. B. (1998). Cognitive–behavioral treatment of pediatric obsessive-compulsive disorder: An open clinical trial. *Journal of the American Academy of Child and Adolescent Psychiatry*, *37*, 412–419.

Gibson, E. J., & Walk, R. D. (1960). The visual cliff. *Scientific American*, *202*, 64–71.

Glazener, C. M. A., Evans, J. H. C., & Peto, R. E. (2005). Alarm interventions for nocturnal enuresis in children. *Cochrane Database of Systematic Reviews*, CD01567, 1.

Glazener, C. M. A., & Evans, J. H. C. (2007). Desmopressin for nocturnal enuresis in children. *Cochrane Database of Systematic Reviews*, CD002911, 2.

Goenjian, A. K., Karayan, I., Pynoos, R. S., Minassian, D., Najarian, L. M., Steinberg, A. M., *et al.* (1997). Outcome of psychotherapy among early adolescents after trauma. *American Journal of Psychiatry*, *154*, 536–542.

Hayes, S. C., Luomaa, J. B., Bond, F. W., Masudaa, A., & Lillisa, J. (2006). Acceptance and commitment therapy: Model, processes and outcomes. *Behaviour Research and Therapy*, *44*, 1–25.

Henggeler, S. W., Melton, G. B., Brondino, M. J., Scherer, D. G., & Hanley, J. H. (1997). Multisystemic therapy with violent and chronic juvenile offenders and their families: The role of treatment fidelity in successful dissemination. *Journal of Consulting and Clinical Psychology*, *65*, 821–833.

Henggeler, S. W., Schoenwald, S. K., Liao, J. G., Letourneau, E. J., & Edwards, D. L. (2002). Transporting efficacious treatments to field settings: The link between supervisory practices and therapist fidelity in MST programs. *Journal of Clinical Child and Adolescent Psychology*, *31*, 155–167.

Herbert, M. (1987). *Behavioural treatment of children with problems: A practical manual* (2nd edn.). London: Academic Press.

Hersen, M. (2005). *Encyclopedia of behavior modification and cognitive behavior therapy*. Vol. 2. *Clinical child applications*. Thousand Oaks, CA: Sage.

Houts, A. C. (2003). Behavioral treatments for enuresis. In A. Kazdin, & J. Weisz (Eds.), *Evidence-based psychotherapies for children and adolescents* (pp. 389–406). New York: Guilford Press.

Huey, S. J., Henggeler, S. W., Brondino, M. J., & Pickrel, S. G. (2000). Mechanisms of change in multisystemic therapy: Reducing delinquent behavior through therapist adherence and improved family and peer functioning. *Journal of Consulting and Clinical Psychology*, *68*, 451–467.

Ilardi, S. S., & Craighead, W. E. (1994). The role of nonspecific factors in cognitive-behavior therapy for depression. *Clinical Psychology: Science and Practice*, *1*, 138–156.

Jacobson, N. S., Dobson, K. S., Truax, P. A., Addis, M. E., Koerner, K., Gollan, J. K., *et al.* (1996). A component analysis of cognitive behavioral treatment for depression. *Journal of Consulting and Clinical Psychology*, *64*, 295–304.

Kabot, S., Masi, W., & Segal, M. (2003). Advances in the diagnosis and treatment of autism spectrum disorders. *Professional Psychology: Research and Practice*, *34*, 26–33.

Kazdin, A. E. (2005). *Parent management training*. Oxford: Oxford University Press.

Kazdin, A. E., & Benjet, C. (2003). Spanking children: Evidence and issues. *Current Directions in Psychological Science*, *12*, 99–103.

Kazdin, A. E., Siegel, T. C., & Bass, D. (1992). Cognitive problem-solving skills training and parent management training in the treatment of antisocial behavior in children. *Journal of Consulting and Clinical Psychology*, *60*, 733–747.

Kazdin, A. E., Whitley, M., & Marciano, P. L. (2006). Child–therapist and parent–therapist alliance and therapeutic change in the treatment of children referred for oppositional, aggressive, and antisocial behavior. *Journal of Child Psychology and Psychiatry*, *47*, 436–445.

Kellam, S. G., Rebok, G. W., Ialongo, N., & Mayer, L. S. (1994). The course and malleability of aggressive behavior from early first grade into middle school: Results of a developmental epidemiology-based preventive trial. *Journal of Child Psychology and Psychiatry*, *35*, 259–281.

Kenwright, M., Marks, I., Graham, C., Franses, A., & Mataix-Cols, D. (2005). Brief scheduled phone support from a clinician to enhance computer-aided self-help for obsessive-compulsive disorder: Randomized controlled trial. *Journal of Clinical Psychology*, *61*, 1499–1508.

King, N. J., Tonge, B. J., Mullen, P., Myerson, N., Heyne, D., Rollings, S., *et al.* (2000). Treating sexually abused children with posttraumatic stress symptoms: A randomized clinical trial. *Journal of the American Academy of Child and Adolescent Psychiatry*, *39*, 1347–1355.

Kratter, J. (1983). The use of meditation in the treatment of attention deficit disorder with hyperactivity. *Dissertation Abstracts International*, *44*, 1965.

Last, C. G., Hansen, C., & Franco, N. (1998). Cognitive–behavioral treatment of school phobia. *Journal of the American Academy of Child and Adolescent Psychiatry*, *37*, 404–411.

Linehan, M. M. (1993). *Cognitive–behavioral treatment of borderline personality disorder*. New York: Guilford Press.

Lovaas, O. I. (1987). Behavioural treatment and normal educational and intellectual functioning in young autistic children. *Journal of Consulting and Clinical Psychology*, *55*, 3–9.

Lovaas, O. I., & Smith, T. (2003). Early and intensive behavioral intervention in autism. In: A. E. Kazdin and J. Weisz (Eds.), *Evidence-based psychotherapies for children and adolescents*. New York: Guilford Press, pp. 325–340.

March, J. S., Biederman, J., Wolkow, R., Safferman, A., Mardekian, J., Cook, E. H., *et al.* (1998). Sertraline in children and adolescents with obsessive-compulsive disorder: A multicenter randomized controlled trial [see comment]. *Journal of the American Medical Association*, *280*, 1752–1756. [Erratum appears in *Journal of the American Medical Association* (2000) *283*, 1293.]

March, J. S., Franklin, M., & Foa, E. (2005). Cognitive behavioural psychotherapy for obsessive-compulsive disorders. In P. Graham (Ed.), *Cognitive–behaviour therapy for children and families* (pp. 281–300). Cambridge, UK: Cambridge University Press.

McEachin, J. J., Smith, T., & Lovaas, O. I. (1993). Long-term outcome for children with autism who received early intensive behavioral treatment. *American Journal of Mental Retardation*, *97*, 359–372.

Melamed, B. G., & Siegel, L. J. (1975). Reduction of anxiety in children facing surgery by modeling. *Journal of Consulting and Clinical Psychology*, *43*, 511–521.

Mesibov, G. B., Shea, V., & Schopler, E. (2005). *The TEACCH approach to autism spectrum disorders*. New York: Springer Science & Business Media.

Morgenstern, J., & Longabaugh, R. (2000). Cognitive–behavioral treatment for alcohol dependence: A review of evidence for its hypothesized mechanisms of action. *Addiction*, *95*, 1475–1490.

Mowrer, O. H. (1980). Enuresis: The beginning work: What really happened. *Journal of the History of the Behavioral Sciences*, *16*, 25–30.

Mowrer, O. H., & Mowrer, W. M. (1938). Enuresis: A method for its study and treatment. *American Journal of Orthopsychiatry*, *8*, 436–459.

MTA Cooperative Group. (1999). A 14-month randomized clinical trial of treatment strategies for attention-deficit/hyperactivity disorder. Multimodal Treatment Study of Children with ADHD. *Archives of General Psychiatry*, *56*, 1073–1086.

National Institute of Clinical Excellence (NICE). (2005). *Obsessive-compulsive disorder: Clinical guidelines 31*. London: National Institute for Health and Clinical Excellence.

Neziroglu, F., Yaryura-Tobias, J. A., Walz, J., & McKay, D. (2000). The effect of fluvoxamine and behavior therapy on children and adolescents with obsessive-compulsive disorder. *Journal of Child and Adolescent Psychopharmacology*, *10*, 295–306.

Norgaard, J. P. (1989). Urodynamics in enuretics. I. Reservoir function. *Neurology and Urodynamics*, *8*, 199–211.

Owens, E. B., Hinshaw, S. P., Kraemer, H. C., Arnold, L. E., Abikoff, H. B., Cantwell, D. P., *et al.* (2003). Which treatment for whom for ADHD? Moderators of treatment response in the MTA. *Journal of Consulting and Clinical Psychology*, *71*, 540–552.

Panerai, S., Ferrante, L., & Zingale, M. (2002). Benefits of the Treatment and Education of Autistic and Communication Handicapped Children (TEACCH) programme as compared with a non-specific approach. *Journal of Intellectual Disability Research*, *46*, 318–327.

Pediatric OCD Treatment Study (POTS). (2004). Cognitive–behavior therapy, sertraline, and their combination for children and adolescents with obsessive-compulsive disorder: The Pediatric OCD Treatment Study (POTS) randomized controlled trial. *Journal of the American Medical Association*, *292*, 1969–1976.

Phillips, L.W. (1981). Roots and branches of behavioral and cognitive practice. *Journal of Behavior Therapy and Experimental Psychiatry*, *12*, 5–17.

Premack, D. (1965). Reinforcement theory. In D. Levine (Ed.), *Nebraska symposium on motivation* (pp. 123–180). Lincoln, NE: University of Nebraska Press.

Schauer, E., Neuner, F., Elbert, T., Ertl, V., Onyut, L. P., Odenwald, M., *et al.* (2004). Narrative exposure therapy in children: A case study. *Intervention: International Journal of Mental Health, Psychosocial Work and Counselling in Areas of Armed Conflict*, *2*, 18–32.

Scheres, A., Dijkstra, M., Ainslie, E., Balkan, J., Reynolds, B., Sonuga-Barke, E., *et al.* (2006). Temporal and probabilistic discounting of rewards in children and adolescents: Effects of age and ADHD symptoms. *Neuropsychologia*, *44*, 2092–2103.

Scott, S. (2002). Parent training programmes. In M. Rutter, & E. Taylor (Eds.), *Child and adolescent psychiatry* (4th edn., pp. 949–967). Oxford: Blackwell.

Segal, Z. V., Williams, J. M. G., & Teasdale, J. T. (2001). *Mindfulness-based cognitive therapy for depression: A new approach to preventing relapse*. New York: Guilford Press.

Shaw, B. F., Elkin, I., Yamaguchi, J., Olmsted, M., Vallis, T. M., Dobson, K. S., *et al.* (1999). Therapist competence ratings in relation to clinical outcome in cognitive therapy of depression. *Journal of Consulting and Clinical Psychology*, *67*, 837–846.

Shea, V. (2004). A perspective on the research literature related to early intensive behavioral intervention (Lovaas) for young children with autism. *Autism*, *8*, 349–367.

Shirk, S. R., & Karver, M. (2003). Prediction of treatment outcome from relationship variables in child and adolescent therapy: A meta-analytic review. *Journal of Consulting and Clinical Psychology*, *71*, 452–464.

Silverman, W. K., Kurtines, W. M., Ginsburg, G. S., Weems, C. F., Rabian, B., & Serafini, L.T. (1999). Contingency management, self-control, and education support in the treatment of childhood phobic disorders: A randomized clinical trial. *Journal of Consulting and Clinical Psychology*, *67*, 675–687.

Skinner, B. F. (1948). *Walden Two*. New York: Macmillan.

Skinner, B. F. (1957). *Verbal behavior*. New York: Appleton-Century-Croft.

Smith, T. (1999). Outcome of early intervention for children with autism. *Clinical Psychology: Science and Practice*, 6, 33–49.

Smith, P., Yule, W., Perrin, S., Tranah, T., Dalgleish, T., & Clark, D. M. (2007). Cognitive–behavior therapy for PTSD in children and adolescents: A preliminary randomized controlled trial. *Journal of the American Academy of Child and Adolescent Psychiatry*, *46*, 1051–1061.

Smith, T., Groen A., & Wynn, J. W. (2000). Randomized trial of intensive early intervention for children with pervasive developmental disorder. *American Journal of Mental Retardation*, *105*, 269–285.

Stein, B. D., Jaycox, L. H., Kataoka, S. H., Wong, M., Tu, W., Elliott, M. N., *et al.* (2003). A mental health intervention for schoolchildren exposed to violence: A randomized controlled trial. *Journal of the American Medical Association*, *290*, 603–611.

Stinchcomb, J. B. (2005). From optimistic policies to pessimistic outcomes: Why won't boot camps either succeed pragmatically or succumb politically? In B. B. Benda, & N. J. Pallone (Eds.), *Rehabilitation issues, problems, and prospects in boot camp* (pp. 27–52). New York, NY: Haworth Press.

Swedo, S., Rapoport, J., Leonard, H., Lenane, M., & Cheslow, D. (1989). Obsessive compulsive disorder in children and adolescents. Clinical phenomenology of 70 consecutive cases. *Archives of General Psychiatry*, *46*, 335–341.

Tarrier, N., & Sommerfield, C. (2004). Treatment of chronic PTSD by cognitive therapy and exposure: 5-year follow-up. *Behavior Therapy*, *35*, 231–246.

Turk, J. (2005). Children with developmental disabilities and their parents. In P. Graham (Ed.), *Cognitive behaviour therapy for children and families* (pp. 244–262). Cambridge, UK: Cambridge University Press.

von Gontard, A. (2005). Elimination disorders: enuresis and encopresis. In C. Gillberg, R. Harrington, & H. C. Steinhausen (Eds.), *A clinician's handbook of child and adolescent psychiatry* (pp. 625–654). Cambridge, UK: Cambridge University Press.

Walker, H. M., & Buckley, N. K. (1974). *Token reinforcement techniques*. Eugene, OR: Engelmann-Becker.

Webster-Stratton, C., & Hammond, M. (1997). Treating children with early-onset conduct problems: A comparison of child and parent training interventions. *Journal of Consulting and Clinical Psychology*, *65*, 93–109.

Webster-Stratton, C. (2005). The Incredible Years: A training program for the prevention and treatment of conduct problems in young children. In E. D. Hibbs and P. S. Jensen (Eds.), Psychological Treatments for Child and Adolescent Disorders: Empirically-based Strategies for Clinical Practice (2nd edn). pp. 507–555. Washington DC: *American Psychological Association*.

Wells, K. C., Chi, T. C., Hinshaw, S. P., Epstein, J. N., Pfiffner, L., Nebel-Schwalm, M., *et al.* (2006). Treatment-related changes in objectively measured parenting behaviors in the multimodal treatment study of children with attention deficit/hyperactivity disorder. *Journal of Consulting and Clinical Psychology*, *74*, 649–657.

Wolpe, J. (1958). *Psychotherapy by reciprocal inhibition*. Stanford, CA: Stanford University Press.

Cognitive–Behavioral Therapies

John E. Lochman and Dustin A. Pardini

Cognitive–behavioral therapies represent a large portion of empirically supported treatments for child and adolescent psychiatric disorders (Kazdin & Weisz, 1998). Cognitive–behavioral therapy (CBT) is based on the premise that cognitions or thoughts can influence emotions and behaviors across a variety of situations, and thus altering maladaptive, distorted or deficient cognitions can be effective in treating various forms of psychopathology. While the widespread application of CBT to emotional and behavioral problems in youth began in the mid 1980s (Graham, 2005), often using problem-solving interventions, the theoretical and empirical underpinnings of these treatments began as early as the 1950s. In this chapter we provide an overview of the development of cognitive–behavioral interventions, as well as their current application in treating various disorders in childhood and adolescence.

Historical Cognitive Processing Models

Social Learning Theory

The application of CBT to the treatment of child and adolescent disorders is based upon social and cognitive learning theories proposed over 40 years ago. Rotter (1954) developed one of the first social learning models of early child development and psychological disorders, drawing on studies of animal learning (Hull, 1943) and conceptualizations of personality development as a dynamic process (Jones & Burks, 1936). Rotter noted that behavioral theories that focused on innate drives and reinforcement contingencies were insufficient for understanding individual differences in human behavior. He stressed that behavior was also influenced by cognitive processes, such as the subjective value individuals placed on reinforcers and their expectations that specific behaviors would result in rewards. Whereas these expectancy contingencies were influenced by previous experiences, they were not necessarily equivalent to objective probabilities (Rotter, Seeman, & Liverant, 1962), and were believed to impact on behavior across a wide variety of social situations (Jessor, 1954). As a result, this model expanded upon existing behavioral theories by introducing cognitive representations of social information and reinforcement contingencies as mediating processes.

Rutter's Child and Adolescent Psychiatry, 5th edition. Edited by M. Rutter, D. Bishop, D. Pine, S. Scott, J. Stevenson, E. Taylor and A. Thapar. © 2008 Blackwell Publishing, ISBN: 978-1-4051-4549-7.

Observational Learning

Early observation learning theories also stressed the importance of cognitions by recognizing that a child's observations of real-life and symbolic models could influence subjective reward contingencies and decision-making processes. The processes initially proposed for acquiring a behavioral pattern through observational learning included attending to a model, cognitively retaining relevant aspects of the model's behavior, enacting the observed behavior and then being reinforced for the reproduced behavior (Miller & Dollard, 1941). Early studies in this area found that children tended to imitate aggressive behavior when they observed a model being reinforced for aggression, and were less likely to imitate aggressive behavior when they observed a model being punished for aggression (Bandura, Ross, & Ross, 1963). Subsequent studies demonstrated that observational learning could be used to promote morality development (Bandura & McDonald, 1963) and delayed gratification (Bandura & Mischel, 1965). In addition, several factors were found to impact on the extent to which observational learning occurred in children, including characteristics of the model, the observer and the social context (Bandura, 1973). These early studies provided evidence that modeling could be used to influence children's cognitions and promote positive behavioral change.

Cognitive Social Learning

Mischel (1973) proposed a cognitive social learning model of human behavior that combined developments in social learning theory (Bandura, 1969) with research on cognitive processing and symbolic mental representations (Neisser, 1967) in an attempt to explain the complex and dynamic interactions between children and their environment. He posited that the relation between environmental stimuli and behavior was mediated by individual difference characteristics such as construction competencies, encoding strategies, outcome expectancies and values, behavioral regulation systems and planning abilities. Environmental characteristics were believed to influence future behavior in so far as they changed an individual's cognitive perceptions at these various stages or levels. In addition, Mischel (1973) theorized that children's overt behavior could modify the amount and type of situations they experienced. As a result, children were viewed as active participants in their social environment, with the ability to influence social exchanges and reinforcement contingencies, as well as be influenced by them.

Cognitive Problem-Solving Models

In conjunction with the development of cognitive social learning models, researchers also began stressing the importance of deficient cognitive problem-solving in the development of emotional and behavioral problems in children. These early models suggested that ineffective interpersonal problem-solving in daily life could produce a wide variety of social and emotional adjustment difficulties (Jahoda, 1953, 1958). Along these lines, Shure, Spivack, and Jaeger (1971, p. 1792) noted that a well-adjusted person "is one who thinks through ways of solving real-life problems and has an appreciation of the potential consequences which could ensue from an act." Early theoretical models of effective problem-solving often described five basic steps:

1 Recognizing there is a problem that requires a novel solution;
2 Defining the nature of the problem;
3 Generating possible solutions to the problem;
4 Evaluating the proposed solutions to determine which has the greatest chance of a favorable outcome; and
5 Evaluating the outcome that results from the chosen solution (D'Zurilla & Goldfried, 1971).

The last stage allows the individual to make self-corrections in future problem-solving scenarios in the event that the chosen solution was less than optimal. While outlined as distinct and sequential stages, researchers acknowledged that in real-life problem-solving situations these stages likely overlap and influence one another in a bidirectional manner (D'Zurilla & Goldfried, 1971). However, these stages have proven to be a useful heuristic for understanding the components of effective problem-solving and facilitating the teaching of these components to others.

Early research supported the notion that deficits in problem-solving may be driving conduct problems in youths. For example, elementary school children with disruptive behavior problems developed fewer logical strategies to solve problems and were less likely to foresee obstacles associated with implementing solutions in comparison with their non-externalizing peers (Shure & Spivack, 1972). In preschool children, poorer school adjustment was also associated with the generation of fewer solutions to problems and a narrower range of possible solutions (Shure & Spivack, 1970). Importantly, early research suggested that the link between poor problem-solving and disruptive behavior problems could not be accounted for by differences in intellectual functioning (Shure & Spivack, 1972; Shure, Spivack, & Jaeger, 1971). However, later studies have found mixed support for the notion that children with disruptive behavior generate fewer possible solutions to social problems (Quiggle, Garber, Panak, & Dodge, 1992; Youngstrom, Wolpaw, Kogos *et al.*, 2000). Instead, finer-grained analysis suggests that disruptive behavior is more consistently associated with the generation of specific types of solutions (Lochman & Dodge, 1994; Lochman & Lampron, 1986). For example, children exhibiting disruptive behavior tend to generate a greater proportion of forceful solutions (Youngstrom, Wolpaw, Kogos *et al.*, 2000), are more likely to choose an aggressive solution to solve the problem and indicate that an aggressive solution would be easy to implement (Quiggle, Garber, Panak *et al.*, 1992) than children without these problems.

Research on problem-solving skills in children and adolescents exhibiting emotional problems also revealed relatively circumscribed deficits. Several studies indicate that children with emotional problems do not seem to have significant difficulties generating alternative solutions to hypothetical problems involving social interactions (Mullins, Siegal, & Hodgens, 1985; Quiggle, Garber, Panak *et al.*, 1992; Youngstrom, Wolpaw, Kogos *et al.*, 2000). However, depressed adolescents tend to be less confident in their ability to solve problems (Sacco & Graves, 1984), and are more likely to report making snap judgments in problem situations than non-depressed adolescents (Marcotte, Alain, & Gosselin, 1999). Depressed children were also more likely to evaluate withdrawal positively as a solution to conflict situations (Spence, Sheffield, & Donovan, 2003), and were more likely to expect that with-drawal would lead to positive outcomes than non-depressed youth (Quiggle, Garber, Panak *et al.*, 1992). Taken together, this suggests that children with emotional problems tend to "cope by withdrawing from other children and from problems they cannot solve" (Shure, 1993, p. 50).

One of the earliest and best researched programs designed to teach children and adolescents problem-solving skills was Interpersonal Cognitive Problem Solving (ICPS) developed by Spivack and Shure (for a review of early studies see Urbain & Kendall, 1980). An early study on the preschool version of the training program was conducted with 219 African-American children (113 intervention, 106 no intervention) attending a federally funded daycare program (Spivack & Shure, 1974; Shure & Spivack, 1980). This version of the ICPS intervention consisted of 46 daily lessons implemented by the teacher, with each daily session lasting 20 minutes. The initial sessions focused on teaching children the basic word concepts necessary for consequential and causal thinking. The remaining sessions focused on developing three problem-solving abilities: alternative thinking, consequential thinking and causal thinking. Using both hypothetical and real-life interpersonal conflict situations, alternative thinking sessions focused on teaching children how to generate multiple possible solutions to a problem. Sessions on consequential thinking had children consider both the immediate and long-range consequences of the multitude of possible solutions to a problem. The final sessions of the intervention involved teaching children causal thinking, such as linking specific solutions with their consequences to identify the solution that would best help them reach a desired outcome or goal. All sessions were taught using techniques such as role plays, games and puppet demonstrations.

Findings from this early study suggested that children who received the intervention showed improvements in alternative, consequential and causal thinking, as well as behavioral improvements, in comparison to a no-treatment control group at post-treatment (Shure & Spivack, 1980). Consistent with the theoretical underpinnings of the program, children who showed improvements in problem-solving skills were more likely to exhibit sustained behavioral improvements 1 year later. Over the years, Shure (1992a,b) has further developed the program (now called "I Can Problem Solve") for use as either a primary prevention or preventative–intervention program during the preschool and elementary school years.

While problem-solving therapies can be included under the broad umbrella of cognitive–behavioral interventions, a defining feature of these therapies is that they focus on teaching the process of successful problem-solving, rather than targeting specific behavioral responses or distorted cognitive processes (D'Zurilla & Goldfried, 1971). The primary goal of problem-solving skills interventions is to teach children *how* to think, rather than telling them *what* to think (Youngstrom, Wolpaw, Kogos *et al.*, 2000). For example, solutions to problems are not evaluated as being good or bad, even if the solution involves engaging in aggressive behavior (Shure, 1993). However, many problem-solving therapies do include sessions devoted to teaching children social skills such as emotion recognition (Shure, 1992a,b) and some include sessions devoted to challenging negative or irrational beliefs (Spence, Sheffield, & Donovan, 2003). Similarly, nearly all cognitive–behavioral interventions targeting disruptive and emotional problems in children and adolescents include a problem-solving component.

Early Cognitive–Behavioral Treatments

Whereas Beck (1963) began publishing on the use of cognitive therapy to treat adult depression in the 1960s, the earliest cognitive–behavioral treatments for children focused on problems of self-control. The downward extension of adult cognitive therapies to children was largely influenced by early models of cognitive development in healthy children. Specifically, Piaget described children as developing an increasingly sophisticated set of mental representations and logical structures in order to master their own behavior and the environment (for review see Thomas, 1996). According to Piaget, children initially perceived the world through simple cause and effect relationships driven by their own overt actions. However, children quickly learned to represent objects and events using symbols (e.g., words, mental imagery) and then began performing logical operations on these symbols to represent cause and effect relationships in the real world, helping to facilitate behavioral planning and effortful self-control. In concert with Piaget, developmental theorists Vygotsky and Luria also proposed that children learned to master their behavior in a predictable pattern contingent upon early cognitive development (for review see Akhutina, 1997). Their model of self-mastery asserted that the behavior of preverbal children was initially directed and controlled by the verbalizations of adults, but as children developed the ability to speak, they began using overt self-verbalizations, and later internalized self-talk, to master their own behavior. Based on these early theories, impulsive children were believed to have difficulties using mental operations (e.g., internalized verbalizations) to guide and regulate their behavior (Meichenbaum & Goodman, 1969).

Inspired by the use of cognitive therapies to treat adult depression and guided by studies of child cognitive development, Meichenbaum developed the first cognitive self-guidance treatment program for impulsive children (Meichenbaum & Goodman, 1971). The program taught children to control their own behavior by modeling self-control verbalizations and instructing children on how to engage in private self-speech while performing sustained attention tasks. Findings suggested that impulsive children who underwent this treatment improved their ability to use private self-speech to orient attention and think carefully when making important decisions. Kendall and Braswell (1982) developed a more comprehensive cognitive therapy that taught impulsive children the general steps to problem-solving and how to use internalized coping statements to deal with frustration and failures when engaged in goal-directed behaviors. Children who received this intervention were shown to have better school compliance at a 10-week follow-up than children who received behavioral training alone. While relatively simplistic, these studies demonstrated that children could be taught cognitive strategies to help improve their behavioral functioning.

Uniqueness of Cognitive–Behavioral Therapy

A core feature underlying all cognitive–behavioral therapies is the idea that altering dysfunctional or deficient thoughts that accompany or precede problematic emotions or behaviors can be effective in treating various disorders (Graham, 2005). Whereas this concept may seem mundane given the widespread adoption of cognitive–behavioral approaches, it is important to recognize that cognitive therapies received substantial criticism from pure behaviorists as late as the 1970s. During this period, some behavioral journals were refusing to publish the word "cognition" in articles, and presentations on cognitive factors were banned from the American Association of Behavior Therapy (Meichenbaum, 2003). However, in contrast to purely cognitive therapies, interventions that are cognitive–behavioral in nature are more likely to incorporate techniques based on basic behavioral principles when appropriate (see chapter 62). For example, cognitive–behavioral interventions for very young children with conduct problems often teach parents how to use the behavioral principals of reinforcement, extinction and shaping to change their child's behavior (Brestan & Eyberg, 1998). It is also important to note that contemporary cognitive–behavioral interventions often include elements of problem-solving therapy and parent-training interventions (Graham, 2005), which are described in greater detail within other chapters in this text. However, all cognitive–behavioral interventions seek to integrate these strategies into an overarching treatment model that emphasizes the influence of both cognitive factors and behavioral contingencies in the development of problematic emotions and behaviors.

Contemporary Cognitive Processing Models

Because various forms of social maladjustment are often the focus of cognitive–behavioral interventions with children and adolescents, social information processing models have been developed as a framework for understanding and treating both externalizing and internalizing problems in youth. Contemporary models have attempted to delineate the primary cognitive processing steps associated with encoding and interpreting social information, as well as generating and enacting solutions during social conflicts, as a mean of understanding the drivers of social maladjustment. In addition, research on the relative influence that cognitive schemas and emotional arousal have on social information processing guides contemporary cognitive–behavioral therapies for youth. The importance of distinguishing automatic from deliberate cognitive processing and distorted cognitions from cognitive deficits is also implicit in many cognitive–behavioral therapies.

Social Information Processing Model

Arguably the most influential and comprehensive social information processing model relevant for cognitive–behavioral interventions with children and adolescents was developed by Dodge (1993; Crick & Dodge, 1994). The model explicitly describes the "online" cognitive process steps that occur when children are engaged in social interactions and social problem-solving. In the most recent version of this model, a series of six sequential steps are outlined:

1 Encoding of external and internal cues;
2 Interpretation of these cues;
3 Determining goals or desired outcomes for the situation;
4 Generating possible responses;
5 Evaluating and selecting a response; and
6 Enacting and evaluating the chosen response.

Social adjustment problems in youth are believed to arise because of difficulties at one or more of these information processing steps. Whereas certain problem behaviors (e.g., aggression, depression) have been associated with specific social information processing problems, this framework is also useful for understanding heterogeneity among children exhibiting the same problem behavior. For example, the aggressive behavior of one child may be driven by a propensity to misinterpret others' benign behaviors as hostile (stage 2), whereas a second aggressive child may be able to accurately interpret others' intentions, but have particular difficulties generating non-aggressive solutions to social conflicts (stage 4). Understanding this heterogeneity in the context of CBT is important because the most efficient and effective treatment plans for these two children would focus on ameliorating fundamentally different social information processing problems.

Although it is important to recognize that there are individual differences within groups of children exhibiting the same problem behavior, there is considerable research indicating that children with disruptive behavior problems (e.g., aggression, conduct problems) tend to exhibit a general pattern of social information processing difficulties. At encoding, disruptive children recall fewer relevant cues about events (Lochman & Dodge, 1994) and overattend to hostile cues (Gouze, 1987; Milich & Dodge, 1984) than non-disruptive controls. In the interpretation stage, they are also more likely to infer that others are acting in an aggressive or hostile manner (Burgess, Wojsalawowicz, Rubin, Rose-Krasnor, & Booth-LaForce, 2006; Dodge, Petit, McClaskey, & Brown, 1986). When clarifying goals in conflict situations, disruptive and seriously antisocial youth tend to focus on dominance and self-centered rewards, and are less concerned with avoiding punishment and the suffering of others (Lochman, Wayland, & White, 1993; Pardini, Lochman, & Frick, 2003). In conflict situations, aggressive and disruptive children also tend to generate fewer verbal assertions (Asarnow & Callan, 1985; Lochman & Lampron, 1986) and compromise solutions (Lochman & Dodge, 1994), and generate more physically aggressive solutions (Pepler, Craig, & Roberts, 1998; Waas & French, 1989). When evaluating possible responses to social conflicts, children with disruptive behavior problems rate aggressive solutions more positively than children without these difficulties (Crick & Werner, 1998). Even when they choose prosocial responses, children with disruptive behavior problems tend to be less adept at enacting them (Dodge, Petit, McClaskey *et al.*, 1986).

There is also emerging evidence suggesting that children with emotional problems (e.g., depression, anxiety) tend to exhibit a unique pattern of social information processing problems. At the encoding stage, depressed children tend to recall more negative cues in the environment (Hammen & Zupan, 1984), whereas anxious children seem to have an attentional bias associated with processing environmental cues of potential threat (Ehrenreich & Gross, 2002). During the interpretation phase, both depressed and anxious children are more likely to attribute negative events to internal, stable and global characteristics (Jacobs & Joseph, 1997; Quiggle, Garber, Panak *et al.*, 1992). There is also evidence suggesting that children with emotional problems may be less likely to generate assertive solutions to social conflicts (Quiggle, Garber, Panak *et al.*, 1992) and tend to understate their own social competence (Rudolph & Clark, 2001). When choosing solutions to social problems, both depressed and shy or withdrawn children tend to adopt avoidant strategies and depressed children tend to view assertive social solutions as resulting in fewer positive and more negative outcomes (Burgess, Wojslawowicz, Rubin *et al.*, 2006; Quiggle, Garber, Panak *et al.*, 1992).

Role of Schemas

Recent revisions of social cognitive models have more explicitly introduced the role that children's cognitive schemas have on information processing (Crick & Dodge, 1994; Lochman, Wayland, & White, 1993). Schemas are commonly regarded as patterns of thinking or beliefs that remain relatively consistent across social situations (Lochman & Lenhart, 1995). These latent cognitive structures are believed to promote the filtering of incoming information and can distort self and other perceptions (Fiske & Taylor, 1984). While schemas allow people to operate efficiently in their social worlds by providing prototypes for how to interpret social cues and manage social conflicts, dysfunctional schemas can perpetuate emotional and behavioral problems by negatively influencing several social information processing steps (Lochman & Dodge, 1998).

When encoding social cues, schemas can narrow children's attention to specific facets of the social environment at the expense of other social cues (Lochman, Nelson, & Sims, 1981). For example, a child with a general expectancy that others will try to dominate him, may be hypervigilant to verbal and non-verbal signals about a peer's control efforts, while missing signs of the peer's friend-liness or attempts to negotiate. Children's schemas can also influence the interpretation of encoded social cues, such as the tendency for a depressed or anxious child to attribute negative social events to internal, stable and global characteristics (Jacobs & Joseph, 1997; Quiggle, Garber, Panak *et al.*, 1992). Schemas can also play a significant part at the end stages of information processing, as the child anticipates consequences for different problem solutions, and decides which strategy will be enacted. In this regard, social goals and outcome expectations that are consistently endorsed in social situations of a particular theme (e.g., social conflicts with peers) are often conceptualized as schemas (Mischel, 1990; Rotter, Chance, & Phares, 1972).

Emotional Arousal and Social Information Processing

It is important to recognize that social information processing might both influence, and be adversely impacted by, heightened levels of negative affect and emotional arousal. Emotions have been hypothesized to mediate the relationship between attributions and behavior (Weiner, 1990) and serve as an adaptive system that motivates individuals to solve their perceived problems (Smith & Lazarus, 1990). For example, when a child attributes blame for a social conflict to another person's hostility, the child will tend to experience frustration or anger, but when the child attributes a social conflict to personal flaws or imperfections, the child will tend to experience sadness or depression (Weiner, 1990). These attribution–emotion linkages can then result in different decisions about social goals (e.g., revenge vs. conflict avoidance) and appropriate behavioral responses in interpersonal situations (e.g., aggression vs. withdrawal). In addition, emotional reactions in the early stages of interactions often persist across time, which can negatively influence social attributions and response styles throughout an extended social exchange (Dodge & Somberg, 1987; Lochman, 1987). Along these lines, a recent laboratory investigation found that young boys who experience increased heart rate as the result of provocation also experience increases in hostile attributional biases (Williams, Lochman, Phillips, & Barry, 2003). Whereas the temporal ordering of these relations (increased heart rate influences attributions or vice versa) could not be determined based on the design of the study, this study provides convincing evidence that changes in negative emotional arousal and dysfunctional cognitions are closely linked.

Distinguishing Automatic and Controlled Information Processing

When evaluating the social information processing of children and adolescents, it is often useful to differentiate between more automatic and more controlled processing problems (Lazarus, 1991). Automatic processing is commonly described as occurring outside of conscious awareness and is fast, effortless and unintentional. Effortful processing, on the other hand, occurs within conscious awareness and is depicted as slow, effortful and deliberate. At each stage of social information processing, the difficulties exhibited by children and adolescents with various emotional and behavioral problems can be conceptualized as being on a continuum from relatively automatic to more controlled (Daleiden & Vasey, 1997). Although a vast majority of research with children and adolescents has focused on effortful social information processing, studies have begun to examine the association between emotional problems and more automatic processing of social stimuli. For example, trait anxiety in adults has been associated with increased skin conductance responses to threatening pictures in comparison with neutral pictures, even when these stimuli are presented outside of conscious awareness (Najström & Jansson, 2006). Whereas this suggests that relatively automatic attentional biases to fear and threat cues may be associated with anxiety problems in adults, studies examining how automatic processes are related to children's and adolescents' anxiety, as well as other forms of psychopathology, are needed.

Differentiating Cognitive Distortions from Cognitive Skills Deficits

Cognitive–behavioral therapies with youth often make distinctions between cognitive distortions and cognitive skills deficits when treating social information processing problems. Cognitive distortions are self-defeating interpretations of people or events that do not accurately represent reality (Daleiden & Vasey, 1997). These thinking errors are believed to help maintain negative emotions and often result in dysfunctional social interactions and poor social problem-solving. A common cognitive distortion is an overgeneralization, in which an individual assumes that a specific negative event is part of a continual or pervasive pattern. For example, a depressed child may think "All people I care about will leave me" when a friend moves out of town, or an aggressive child my think "Everyone is out to get me" after being ridiculed by a single peer. Other common forms of cognitive distortion include jumping to conclusions about the intentions of others, catastrophizing relative minor setbacks, personalizing negative events and discounting positive events (Dodge, 1993). Within the context of cognitive–behavioral therapies, children and adolescents are often taught to recognize and refute these distortions, which is a process commonly referred to as cognitive restructuring. Replacing these distorted cognitions with more realistic and adaptive thinking patterns is designed to reduce negative emotional reactions to adverse social events and promote more competent social problem-solving.

Although negative appraisals of the self and social environment may be caused by cognitive distortions, it is also possible that these perceptions are actually accurate representations of reality that may arise from cognitive skills deficits. For example, a depressed child may accurately endorse having no friends at school because of an inability to start appropriate conversations with others. In this instance, the child is describing a deficiency in the cognitive skills necessary to develop peer friendships, rather than engaging in cognitive distortions by exaggerating a complete absence of friends or lack of social skills. CBT with a child or adolescent exhibiting cognitive deficits focuses primarily on skill building, such as practicing how to start and maintain conversations. Often, it may be difficult to determine from the youth's self-report alone whether social difficulties are the result of cognitive distortions, cognitive skills deficits or some other factor. As a result, it is often necessary to gather information from collateral informants (e.g., parents, teachers, peers) to garner an accurate depiction of the problem (Pardini, Barry, Barth, Lochman, & Wells, 2006). It is also important to keep in mind that cognitive distortions and deficits are not mutually exclusive categories. For example, Ruldolph and Clark (2001) found that depressed children not only have greater difficulties engaging in skillful social interactions with peers than non-depressed children (cognitive deficit), but also tend to exaggerate the extent of their social problems (cognitive distortion). In addition, there are cases in which children's emotional difficulties are brought about by life circumstances beyond their control (e.g., death in the family, victimization, physical deformity) rather than a cognitive deficit or distortion, in which case it may be more appropriate to focus on teaching children skills for coping with stressful life events.

Areas of Application

Conduct Problems

The largest application of CBT to child and adolescent psychopathology has focused on the treatment of conduct problems (e.g., aggression, defiance, oppositional behaviors, rule-breaking). Whereas cognitive–behavioral therapies for conduct problems differ based on the developmental level of the target population (e.g., preschool children vs. adolescents) and the severity of the behavior problems being targeted (e.g., treatment for conduct disorder vs. preventative–intervention for minor aggressive behavior), common elements pervade most empirically supported cognitive–behavioral approaches (for descriptions see Lochman, Phillips, McElroy, & Pardini, 2005; Pardini & Lochman, 2003). Nearly all of these treatments involve a child–parent intervention component, and there are several topic areas that are commonly addressed in these interventions. As a result, a prototypical cognitive–behavioral intervention for treating conduct problems in youth is described, followed by empirical evidence supporting the efficacy of these interventions with various populations.

Prototypical Youth Intervention for Conduct Problems

Most youth interventions for conduct problems are performed with small groups of 4–6 individuals over the course of several weeks to a year. There is typically an emphasis on anger management, social problem-solving and social skills development, and prosocial goal-setting. Anger management sessions involve assisting children in recognizing the level of arousal and anger they experience in difficult interpersonal situations and identifying the triggers that lead to these high arousal reactions. Perspective-taking sessions are commonly used to help participants understand how others can have a range of intentions in a given situation that are often unclear. This is done in an attempt to prevent children from assuming that other people are always trying to be cruel or mean in conflict situations, which often triggers increased anger. Coping techniques to manage anger arousal and to avoid impulsive rage-filled responses are often the focus of several sessions, including the use of distraction, relaxation and self-talk techniques. Children often practise using coping self-instructions and distraction techniques within the group, sometimes while being teased directly by other group members or by using puppets. Children are reinforced for creating a repertoire of coping self-statements that are relevant and useful for them, and are encouraged to use these strategies in real-life social situations. Parents and teachers are often taught to cue and assist the youth in using anger management strategies at home and school, and are instructed to reinforce the successful implementation of these skills.

Cognitive–behavioral interventions for conduct problems also focus on teaching youth appropriate social problem-solving strategies and social skills. Consistent with Dodge's (1993; Crick & Dodge, 1994) social information processing model, participants are commonly taught to engage in a series of cognitive processing steps when solving social problems. In most interventions, youth learn to:

1 Identify the problem and their emotional reaction to it;
2 Analyze the possible intentions of the other party;
3 Come up with potential solutions to the conflict;
4 Analyze the short- and long-term consequences of each solution;
5 Choose and enact a final plan; and
6 Evaluate the effectiveness of the plan after it is implemented.

In addition, children are often taught basic social skills that are important for making friends: empathizing and co-operating with others, and successfully resolving interpersonal conflicts. These skills are often taught through a combination of verbal instructions, modeling and in-session role plays. The in-session role plays frequently focus on dealing with interpersonal conflicts experienced by youth (e.g., being teased by a peer), as well as other social situations that are difficult for youth with conduct problems, such as making new friends. As therapy progresses, children are often given homework assignments in which they are asked to apply their newly learned problem-solving and social skills to real-life interpersonal situations of increasing complexity. Parents and teachers are often taught to cue and assist the youth in using these problem-solving strategies and social skills, as well as to reinforce their successful implementation.

Another facet of cognitive–behavioral treatments for conduct problems involves having the youth identify and work on goals designed to improve their behavior. In order to help facilitate this process, teachers or parents are often asked to identify four or five behavioral goals designed to reduce problematic behaviors. Because initial successes are important in motivating children to work on challenging issues, children are often encouraged to select goals initially that are of low to moderate difficulty. Progress in meeting these goals is monitored regularly, and children receive rewards or privileges for reaching agreed-upon levels of goal completion.

Prototypical Parent Intervention for Conduct Problems

Most efficacious cognitive–behavioral programs for child and adolescent conduct problems involve a parent-training component. Cognitive–behavioral parenting interventions have received the most consistent empirical support for the successful treatment of conduct problems in youth, both in isolation and when combined with child interventions (Brestan & Eyberg, 1998). As a result, it is strongly recommended that cognitive–behavioral interventions for child and adolescent conduct problems involve a parenting component whenever possible. Typically, these sessions are conducted during several group sessions lasting approximately 2 h, with periodic individual contacts through home visits and telephone contacts to promote generalization of skills learned in group sessions. In order to lay a foundation for positive parent–child interactions, parents are initially encouraged to initiate non-threatening play sessions with their child in a manner that shows a genuine interest in and appreciation of their ideas. This typically includes using skills such as reflecting the child's statements, describing and praising the child's behavior, ignoring undesirable behaviors and avoiding the tendency to direct the play or criticize the child. Parents are coached on ways in which they can verbally and non-verbally express acceptance, warmth and caring toward their child. The purpose of this component is to strengthen a positive parent–child relationship and extinguish maladaptive behaviors that are reinforced by parental attention. Most interventions have parents practice these skills in session as the therapist provides feedback and suggestions for improvement.

Another common component of parenting interventions involves learning to analyze child behavior problems from a cognitive–behavioral mindset, and implement discipline strategies that target the drivers of conduct problems from a cognitive–behavioral perspective. Along these lines, parents are taught to use positive reinforcement to increase the frequency of their child's prosocial behaviors, while using non-abusive, yet consistent, methods of discipline to deal with disruptive behaviors. The appropriate use of time out, verbal reprimands, negotiation and behavioral contracting is often discussed, as well as using a naturally occurring consequence for inappropriate behavior, such as giving children an earlier bedtime when they refuse to get up on time for school in the morning. Sessions also focus on teaching parents to use problem-solving strategies similar to those taught to their children to manage crises within the family.

After a home behavioral program is started, parents are encouraged to begin a school-based reinforcement program to help improve their child's academic and behavioral compliance. The school program consists of negotiating certain school goals and monitoring the child's progress in meeting these goals through the use of a home–school behavioral report card. Children are typically given reinforcement for achieving specific goals (e.g., special activities, privileges) and are frequently given feedback regarding their behavioral progress.

Outcome Research

Reviews of Efficacy of Cognitive–Behavioral Therapy for Conduct Problems

Several reviews have examined the efficacy of psychosocial treatments for conduct problems in children and adolescents in comparison to no treatment or waitlist control conditions. These reviews indicate that a vast majority of the empirically supported treatments for conduct problems in youth are based upon a CBT framework (Brestan & Eyberg, 1998; Farmer, Compton, Burns, & Robertson, 2002; Kazdin & Weisz, 1998; Nock, 2003). Meta-analytic studies suggest that the effect sizes for cognitive–behavioral interventions targeting conduct problems range from medium to large, i.e., 0.47–0.90 (for review see Nock, 2003). In addition, research suggests that cognitive–behavioral interventions that include a child component focusing on social problem-solving and social skills development together with a parent-training component produce broader positive effects and better maintenance of behavioral improvements over time than interventions with either component in isolation (Kazdin, Siegel & Bass, 1992; Nock, 2003; Webster-Stratton & Hammond, 1997). However, the parenting component of these interventions has been shown to produce particularly robust reductions in conduct problems and delinquent behaviors (Beauchaine, Webster-Stratton, & Reid, 2005; Lochman & Wells, 2004).

Two exemplars: The Incredible Years and Coping Power Programs

Two examples of intervention programs that have received empirical support for the treatment of conduct problems are the Incredible Years program and the Coping Power program. The Incredible Years program primarily consists of a parent and child intervention designed for children aged 4–7 who have conduct problems significant enough to warrant a diagnosis of either oppositional defiant disorder or conduct disorder (Webster-Stratton, Reid, & Hammond, 2004). Research findings regarding the effectiveness of the child and parent training interventions alone and in combination are impressive. The parent-training component has repeatedly been show to produce significant reductions in child conduct problems at home and school, decreases in negative parenting and increases in positive parenting in comparison with waitlist control conditions (Webster-Stratton, 1984; Webster-Stratton & Hammond, 1997; Webster-Stratton, Kolpacoff, & Hollinsworth, 1988; Webster-Stratton, Reid, & Hammond, 2004). In addition, evidence suggests that overall improvements in children's behavior problems as the result of the parenting intervention can still be seen at 3-year follow-up (Webster-Stratton, 1990).

The Incredible Years child intervention has also been shown to produce significant reductions in the amount of conduct problems children exhibit at home and school, as well as produce increases in social problem-solving skills in comparison with wait-list controls (Webster-Stratton & Hammond, 1997; Webster-Stratton, Reid, & Hammond, 2004). There is also evidence indicating that at 1-year follow-up approximately two-thirds of children who participated in the intervention have parent ratings of behavioral problems in the normal rather than clinically significant range (Webster-Stratton & Hammond, 1997).

In contrast to the Incredible Years program, the Coping Power program was developed as a preventative intervention to assist aggressive elementary schoolchildren in making a successful transition to middle school. The efficacy of the Coping Power program in comparison with no treatment has also been demonstrated in several studies. For example, aggressive boys randomly assigned to an early version of the program (i.e., anger coping) displayed less parent-reported aggressive behavior, fewer behavior problems in the classroom and higher levels of self-esteem at post-treatment than aggressive boys who did not receive treatment (Lochman, Burch, Curry, & Lampoon, 1984). At a 3-year follow-up, the intervention boys exhibited lower substance use involvement and increased self-esteem and social problem-solving skills than controls (Lochman, 1992). Aggressive children who have participated in the expanded Coping Power program have been shown to exhibit post-treatment reductions in self-reported substance use, proactive aggression, as well as improved social competence and teacher-rated behavioral improvements in comparison with non-treated controls (Lochman & Wells, 2004). The intervention has also been found to reduce several maladaptive cognitions related to aggressive behavior by post-treatment, such as hostile attributions, expectations that aggression will result in positive outcomes and an external locus of control regarding positive outcomes (Lochman & Wells, 2002a). At 1-year follow-up, findings indicate that aggressive boys who have participated in the Coping Power program exhibit lower levels of self-reported delinquency and parent-reported substance use, as well as higher levels of teacher-rated behavioral improvements than non-treated controls (Lochman & Wells, 2002a). The Coping Power effects on children's self-reported delinquency and substance use, and teacher-reported aggressive behavior at the time of a 1-year follow-up, compared with a randomly assigned control condition, were replicated in a second sample (Lochman & Wells, 2003).

Moderators and Mediators of Treatment Efficacy

Whereas cognitive–behavioral treatments are generally effective for treating conduct problems in youth, it is also clear that some children's behavior problems do not improve as the result of treatment. Along these lines, research has been increasingly focused on answering the question: "What child, parent, family, and contextual features influence (moderate) outcome?" (Kazdin, 2003). Although there has been some historical speculation that preschool children and youth with learning problems may not benefit from CBT for disruptive behavior, recent evidence suggests that this may not be the case. For example, children as young as 4 years old (Beauchaine, Webster-Stratton, & Reid, 2005; Webster-Stratton, Reid, & Hammond, 2004), and youth with mild cognitive impairments (e.g., learning problems, mild intellectual disability) have shown significant behavioral improvements as the result of developmentally appropriate cognitive–behavioral interventions (Kam, Greenberg, & Kusché, 2004; Kazdin & Crowley, 1997). More recently, researchers have suggested that conduct problem youth with a callous and unemotional (CU) interpersonal style may exhibit a particularly severe and recalcitrant form of antisocial behavior that is resistant to traditional treatments (see chapter 51; Frick, Cornell, Barry, Bodin, & Dane, 2003; Pardini, 2006). Along these lines, one study found that increased CU traits were associated with lower levels of behavioral improvements following a cognitive–behavioral parenting intervention for youth with conduct problems (Hawes & Dadds, 2005). However, this effect was relatively small in magnitude, suggesting that youth with CU traits may benefit from empirically supported CBT.

Many studies examining moderators of CBT for youth with disruptive behavior have produced contradictory or counterintuitive findings. Whereas early studies suggested that children with more global psychiatric impairment were less likely to benefit from CBT for disruptive behavior (Kazdin & Wassell, 1999), more recent evidence suggests that comorbidity and case complexity may not significantly influence therapeutic change (Kazdin & Whitely, 2006a). Similarly, lower socioeconomic status and increased parental psychopathology and stress have been found to predict poorer treatment outcomes in some studies (Dumas & Wahler, 1983; Kazdin & Wassell, 1999; Reyno & McGrath, 2006; Webster-Stratton & Hammond, 1990), but not in others (Beauchaine, Webster-Stratton, & Reid, 2005; Hartman, Stage, & Webster-Stratton, 2003). Recently, a large and comprehensive examination of treatment moderators was conducted with 514 children who participated in six randomized trials of the empirically supported Incredible Years program (Beauchaine, Webster-Stratton, & Reid, 2005). Findings indicated that children whose parents had a history of substance abuse and those with co-occurring emotional disturbance showed greater improvements in disruptive behaviors by 1-year follow-up. Children of parents who exhibited lower levels of critical, harsh and ineffective discipline at baseline also exhibited greater behavioral improvements. In addition, the parent-training component of the program (in comparison with the other components) produced greater improvements in children's disruptive behavior at 1-year follow-up for single mothers, mothers who reported low levels of marital satisfaction and children low on emotional disturbance. In contrast to theoretical conjecture (Lynam, 1996), the intervention was equally effective in reducing conduct problems among children with elevated levels of attention deficit/hyperactivity disorder (ADHD) symptoms as in those without these problems (Beauchaine, Webster-Stratton, & Reid, 2005; Hartman, Stage, & Webster-Stratton, 2003). However, evidence does suggest that CBT may not be effective for reducing core ADHD symptoms in youth (MTA Cooperative Group, 1999). Although these studies have begun providing insights into possible moderators of treatment efficacy, there remains a lack of understanding about why these factors lead to differential responses to treatment (Nock, 2003). This issue seems particularly important given that research in this area has produced counterintuitive (e.g., parental substance use history positively influences treatment outcome) and contradictory findings.

An under-studied area involves examining the mechanisms through which CBT influences reductions in child and adolescent conduct problems (i.e., mediators). Evidence suggests that reductions in critical, harsh and ineffective parenting practices tend to co-occur with improvements in disruptive behavior problems at post-treatment and 1-year follow-up (Beauchaine, Webster-Stratton, & Reid, 2005). In addition, Lochman and Wells (2002b) found evidence indicating that intervention-related reductions in delinquency at 1-year follow-up were at least partially mediated by reductions in inconsistent parenting from pre- to post-treatment. However, evidence supporting the assertion that modifying maladaptive or deficient cognitions in children leads to subsequent changes in their problem behavior was limited.

Depression

Depressed youth have certain common social–cognitive characteristics. Depressed youth display both cognitive distortions and cognitive deficits, evident in their core symptoms of feelings of worthlessness, associated negative beliefs about themselves and their future, attributions of failures, and having an external locus of control (Gladstone & Kaslow, 1995). The onset of youth depression is often preceded by family conflict, physical illness, the break-up of romantic relationships or the loss of a friendship (Weersing & Brent, 2003). Depressed pre-adolescent children have similar causal attributions for the positive and negative events that they experience, which is quite different from non-depressed children, who perceive the causes of negative events to be external to themselves (Kaslow, Rehm, Pollack, & Siegel, 1988). These attribution distortions become even more apparent with adolescent in-patient samples, where the depressed adolescents attribute the cause of positive events to external, unstable and specific causes, consistent with findings that adolescents experience more anhedonia than younger depressed children (Curry & Craighead, 1990).

Depressed children's distorted schemas and internal working models have been found to be linked to insecure attachment to parent figures (Cowan, Cohn, Cowan, & Peterson, 1996; Stark, Sander, Hauser *et al.*, 2006b). In addition to these problems in their habits of thought, they often show problems in their low rates of social acceptance and high rates of isolation from their peers, caused by poor social skills and poor problem-solving skills. Garber, Braafladt, and Zeman (1991) found that depressed children had certain specific social information processing difficulties, evident in their patterns of generating avoidant and aggressive strategies to handle social difficulties, rather than using more adaptive strategies involving active problem-solving and distraction.

Contents of a Typical Cognitive–Behavioral Therapy Approach

Common treatment components across different CBT programs include:

1 Self-control skills, self-consequation (reinforcing themselves more, punishing themselves less), self-monitoring (paying attention to positive things they do), self-evaluation (setting less perfectionistic standards for their performance) and assertiveness training;

2 Social skills, including methods of initiating interactions, maintaining interactions, handling conflict, and using relaxation and imagery; and

3 Cognitive restructuring, involving confronting children about the lack of evidence for their distorted perceptions (Stark, Hargrave, Sander *et al.*, 2006a).

An example of how the cognitive skills are separated from the behavioral skills is evident in the CBT program for adolescents developed by Weersing and Brent (2003). This program consisted of 15 sessions, 10 of which were manualized and structured, and 5 of which were highly individualized for the particular client's strengths and abilities. In addition to the work in the session with the adolescent, there was take home work from a practice book, and there was some parent involvement. The skills were separated into two sets for the ACT behavioral skills (activities that solve problems, activities that the youth enjoys, being calm and confident, using one's talents) and the THINK cognitive skills (think positive, get help from a friend, identify the silver lining, don't replay bad thoughts, keep thinking and don't give up). The youth develops a coping plan with sequential steps, and the skills are actively practiced in role plays and *in vivo* activities. CBT with depressed children can also be given in a group format, where the CBT sessions are typically carefully structured, going through a regular sequence of activities, each session including: rapport building, set agenda, goal attainment check-in, review of previous meeting and homework, coping skills activity, skill building, review, positive behavior review and assignment of therapeutic homework (Stark, Hargrave, Sander *et al.*, 2006a).

Outcome Research

Reviews of Evidence-based Cognitive–Behavioral Therapy Approaches

Meta-analytic reviews indicate that children and adolescents benefit from CBT interventions regardless of severity of depressive symptoms, and that adolescents have larger effect-size improvements from CBT intervention than do younger children (Michael & Crowley, 2002; Stark, Hargrave, Sander *et al.*, 2006a). Overall, CBT interventions have had similar effects for mildly to severely depressed adolescents in these reviews, but recent research has suggested that the beneficial effects of CBT may be most apparent with mild to moderate depression in youth (Melvin, Tonge, King *et al.*, 2006). Treated youths' reductions in depressive symptoms are maintained over time, and effect sizes at the end of treatment are in the moderate to large range across studies (Reinecke, Ryan, & DuBois, 1998).

Two Exemplars: CBT for Adolescents and the TADS Study

Typical of the positive results that have been reported from CBT programs for depressed youth, Weersing and Brent (2003)

described the results from the series of CBT studies conducted at the Western Psychiatric Institute Mood and Anxiety Disorders Clinic. In the 1997 clinical trial (Brent, Holder, Kolko *et al.*, 1997), 107 youth were screened for major depressive disorder, were required to have at least borderline Beck Depression Inventory scores, and did not have psychosis, bipolar disorder, obsessive-compulsive disorder, eating disorders or substance abuse. The youth were randomly assigned to CBT, systemic behavioral family therapy (SBFT) or non-specific therapy (NST). SBFT was based on models of the effects of negative life events and family conflict on youth depression, and included a problem definition stage, in which adolescents' problems were redefined as being problems for the entire family system and in which dysfunctional interactions and alliances were identified, and a problem-solving stage. NST controlled for the non-specific aspects of therapy by having adolescents express feelings with warm and non-directive therapists. At post-treatment, CBT had significantly higher rates of youth being diagnosis-free (CBT 83%, SBFT 38%, NST 39%), but these treatment group differences had become non-significant by the time of a 2-year follow-up (Birmaher, Brent, Kolko *et al.*, 2000).

However, the utility of the CBT as a stand-alone treatment for depression has become less clear with the results of the large multi-site TADS study (March, Silva, Petrycki *et al.*, 2004). A total of 351 adolescents who had received primary diagnoses of moderate to severe major depressive disorder were randomly assigned to fluoxetine, CBT, the combination of fluoxetine and CBT, or placebo. The CBT intervention included six structured skill-building sessions and six modular or optional sessions, to permit more careful tailoring of interventions to specific adolescents' needs with regard to social engagement, communication, negotiation, compromise or assertion. The CBT intervention used in TADS did not have as many intensive cognitive elements as was evident in the Brent, Holder, Kolko *et al.* (1979) study (Stark, Sander, Hanser *et al.*, 2006b). The greatest decreases in symptoms in the TADS study were evident in the condition that included both CBT and fluoxetine, followed by the fluoxetine-only condition. Both of these conditions were more effective than CBT only or placebo. Thus, CBT used in the TADS study was found to be useful in accompaniment to medication, and was found to produce greater reduction in the likelihood of suicidal ideation and behavior than the fluoxetine-only condition. However, CBT alone was less effective than fluoxetine in reducing depression symptoms among those adolescents with major depressive disorder. The findings of the lack of intervention effects for CBT alone may have been because of the inclusion of fewer cognitive treatment elements in the TADS CBT intervention, or to the use of less-experienced therapists.

Mediation and Moderation

Kolko, Brent, Baugher, Bridge, and Birmaher (2000) examined whether the CBT and SBFT conditions in the Brent, Holder, Kolko *et al.* (1997) study produced differential improvements in cognitive distortions. As anticipated, CBT was uniquely able to change adolescents' cognitive distortions, unlike the SBFT condition, and was able to produce changes in general family functioning to a similar degree as the SBFT condition, suggesting that a mechanism of action in CBT is the ability to alter cognitive distortions.

In terms of predictors of outcomes, youth with more severe and chronic depression, evident in the presence of double depression and more severe cognitive distortions, have poorer outcomes after any form of treatment in the Brent, Holder, Kolko *et al.* (1997) study of CBT. Youth with serious suicidality were more responsive to CBT than to non-CBT treatment, with equal levels of CBT effectiveness for suicidal and non-suicidal youth (Barbe, Bridge, Birmaher, Kolke, & Brent, 2004). Youth with greater numbers of depressive episodes and younger age at first onset had the best outcomes in the Adolescents Coping With Depression program (Clarke, DeBar, & Lewinsohn, 2003). Thus, there is mixed evidence at this time about whether CBT would have its best effects with less severe or chronic depressive children.

Anxiety

CBT for anxiety disorders integrates cognitive and behavioral perspectives on the origin and maintenance of anxiety symptoms (Stark, Sander, Hauser *et al.*, 2006b). There is a focus on the children's internal and external environments, addressing behavioral, cognitive, affective and social factors. Children with anxiety disorders have been found to have certain information processing and emotional experiencing styles.

The children's interpersonal contexts within their family and peer groups have also been linked to their experience of anxiety, and have implications for treatment. There is considerable correspondence between serious levels of child and maternal anxiety (Frick, Silverthorn, & Evans, 1994). Family factors that are linked to child anxiety include parental over-control, parental reinforcement of avoidant strategies, the presence of parental anxiety and the presence of anxiety in siblings. Interestingly, some parental anxiety has been found to decrease when mothers have been included as coaches to assist their children's use of comforting self-talk, cue controlled relaxation and pleasant imagery in the management of their anxiety symptoms (Peterson & Shigetomi, 1981). Parents have benefitted by using the same skills themselves, and their anxiety may decline as children have reduced levels of symptoms.

Contents of a Typical Cognitive–Behavioral Therapy Approach

The Coping Model underlying Kendall's Coping Cat program (Kendall & Suveg, 2006) emphasizes that the goal is not to alleviate anxiety entirely, but to assist the child to learn skills to better manage or cope with anxiety in the future. Three of the primary treatment targets are:

1 To identify physiological cues related to anxiety and to use relaxation skills to manage this arousal, because anxiety is associated with manifest physiological arousal;

2 To identify automatic thoughts and to learn countervailing coping thoughts, because children have cognitive distortions that lead them to overestimate the chance of negative events occurring and the impact of those events; and

3 To be exposed to the feared situations as the child learns and actively practices problem-solving skills.

The Coping Cat program consists of 16–18 sessions, with the first eight sessions focusing on teaching the components of the FEAR plan. In the FEAR plan, "F" refers to assisting children to becoming better aware of their feelings of being frightened, emphasizing greater awareness of physical symptoms as a cue to respond, and using deep breaths and muscle relaxation to teach the child that he or she has control over physical reactions. "E" refers to children's identification of their incorrect expectations and self-statements that bad things will happen. Through modeling and role play, the child identifies his or her thoughts in anxiety-provoking situations, and learns to test out the negative expectations. "A" is a problem-solving step in which the child develops his or her confidence and ability to clearly define the problem situation and goals, and to generate alternative solutions to the anxiety-provoking situation. The idea of needing to deal with problems is normalized as part of everyday life, and the importance of not relying on initial reactions in problem situations is stressed. Finally, "R" reminds children to reward themselves and to take credit for the results they achieve. The critical aspect of self-evaluation for these children is to help them perceive that perfection is not the goal, because many of these children have unrealistically high achievement standards.

Exposure to the feared situation is an important part of the treatment process, and children move through exposure experiences in structured stepwise ways, starting with imaginal in-office exercises with low levels of anxiety, then moving to *in vivo* situations that have low levels of anxiety, and then moving to increasingly anxiety-provoking situations in imaginal and *in vivo* practice. In addition to the direct work with children, periodic meetings are held with parents to maintain their support and to collaborate on treatment plans.

The Coping Cat program has led to several other similar evidence-based programs such as Coping Koala and the FRIENDS program (Barrett & Shortt, 2003). Some of these more recent programs, such as FRIENDS, have a more substantial focus on working with parents. In group meetings, parents learn to deal with their own anxiety and to use behavioral reward skills with their children.

Outcome Research

Reviews of Evidence-based Cognitive–Behavioral Approaches

Reviews of empirically supported treatments for children with anxiety disorders conclude that behavioral and cognitive–behavioral procedures have more empirical support than do other approaches (Chorpita & Southam-Gerow, 2006; Kazdin & Weisz, 1998). Behavioral techniques (including imaginal and *in vivo* desensitization) are especially efficacious for phobias, and cognitive–behavioral procedures have been determined to be well-established and probably efficacious for other anxiety disorders (Kendall & Suveg, 2006).

Two Exemplars: Coping Cat and FRIENDS Programs

The Coping Cat program has been evaluated in a series of studies, beginning with Kendall's (1994) study of 47 9- to 13-year-old youth diagnosed as having separation anxiety disorder, overanxious disorder or avoidant disorder. At post-treatment, 64% of those who had received Coping Cat no longer met diagnostic criteria for one of these disorders, in comparison to a 5% diagnosis-free rate for waitlist controls, and these gains were maintained at a 1-year follow-up. A longer-term follow-up of this sample, at a point over 3 years after the end of intervention, indicated that these intervention gains were long-lasting (Kendall & Southam-Gerow, 1996).

In a second sample, Kendall, Flannery-Schroeder, Panichelli-Mindel *et al.* (1997) followed 94 9- to 13-year-old children who were randomly assigned to Coping Cat or to waitlist control, and found that 50% of Coping Cat children were diagnosis-free at post-treatment, and for those who still had diagnoses there was a significant decrease in the severity of their conditions. These significant intervention effects were maintained at 1-year and 7.4-year follow-ups, and the intervention children had reduced risk for other related sequelae of the anxiety disorder, such as substance abuse.

In an effort to compare the different forms for delivering the intervention, Flannery-Schroeder and Kendall (2000) randomly assigned 37 8- to 14-year-old children to group CBT, individually delivered CBT or a waitlist control. At post-intervention, both intervention conditions demonstrated significant improvement, but the rate of improvement was stronger in children who had been seen individually (73% diagnosis-free in individual CBT, 50% in group CBT and 8% in the control condition).

The Coping Cat program was adapted in Australia as the Coping Koala program, and a first evaluation study randomly assigned 79 7- to 14-year-olds to child CBT, child + family CBT or to a waitlist control (Barrett, Dadds, & Rapes, 1996). Children had been diagnosed with separation anxiety disorder, overanxious disorder or social phobia. The combined intervention was somewhat more effective at post-intervention than the child-only intervention (88% diagnosis-free for child + family intervention, 61% diagnosis-free for child-only intervention), but both were more effective than the waitlist control condition (less than 30% diagnosis-free), and both had a similar rate of continued effectiveness at a follow-up that occurred 5–7 years after intervention ended (87% diagnosis-free for child CBT only and 86% for the combined intervention).

In a study of the FRIENDS program, Barrett (1998) randomly assigned 60 7- to 14-year-old children to either group CBT, group CBT plus family intervention or to waitlist control. The results favored the combined intervention at post-intervention (56% diagnosis-free for child group CBT, 71% for group CBT + family, 25% for control) and at a 1-year follow-up (65% diagnosis-free for group CBT, 85% for group CBT + family), indicating the added value of also working with parents in these CBT approaches for anxious children.

Mediation and Moderation

Variables that have been found to be predictive of poorer responses to the Coping Cat intervention are:

1 Higher levels of children's internalizing problems, using teacher or maternal reports;

2 Higher rates of maternal self-reported depressive symptoms; and

3 Older ages (Southam-Gerow, Kendall, & Weersing, 2001).

In contrast, variables that have not been found to moderate CBT intervention outcomes for children with anxiety problems are ethnicity, gender, family income, family composition, maternal-rated externalizing problems or child-reported internalizing problems. The family component of the Barrett, Dadds, & Rapee (1996) program is most effective with younger children, consistent with prior findings of moderators of child-oriented CBT programs, and with girls and with families that have parents with anxiety problems. Thus, child-focused CBT appears to be more appropriate for older and more seriously anxious children, and for children with depressed mothers. In contrast, parent-focused CBT is more effective with younger children.

Examining mediation effects, Treadwell and Kendall (1996) examined longitudinal changes in 8- to 13-year-olds who had received CBT intervention. Children's reductions in negative cognitions and state-of-mind ratio were found to mediate the effects of intervention on children's subsequent improvement in anxiety after treatment.

Factors that Influence Outcomes

Treatment Fidelity and Adaptation

Psychotherapy with children and adolescents has traditionally been a field in which many empirically unsupported approaches have been used (Roberts, Lazicki-Puddy, Puddy, & Johnson, 2003), and typical community-based care had consistently poor outcomes (Bickman, 2002). There was a scarcity of evidence-based research on child interventions until recent years (Rubenstein, 2003). However, in the past decade there has been a tremendous increase in efforts to identify and disseminate evidence-based treatments, many of them based on cognitive–behavioral models (Bickman, 2002; Hawley & Weisz, 2002). Efforts to study systematically the dissemination process of evidence-based interventions for children has only recently begun (Schoenwald & Hoagwood, 2001; Silverman & Kurtines, 2004).

Although intervention developers may often insist on complete adherence to protocols, innovations inevitably change as development proceeds (Berwick, 2003), including adjustments made to program materials to address participants' educational developmental and motivational levels. Arguments can be made for both sides of debates about whether adaptations to evidence-based prevention protocols promote effective use of the programs or not. On the one hand, careful use of the intervention protocol, with high intervention integrity, would be expected to produce outcomes similar to those obtained in rigorous efficacy trials with that intervention. On the other hand, innovative interventions often need to be adapted to the realities of intervening with children in applied settings (Stirman, Crits-Christoph, & DeRubeis, 2004). When exporting interventions from research laboratories to clinical practice settings, refinements can be made to fit clinic conditions (Weisz, Donenberg, Han, & Kauneckis, 1995a), and to make strategies appropriate for the target audiences. As long as rigid adherence to manuals is avoided (Henry, 1998) then clinicians may not regard a manual as a "required cookie cutter approach" (Kendall, 2002). The creative flexible use of CBT manual-based interventions can permit individualization of intervention and increases the likely transportability of the intervention to new settings (Kendall, Chu, Gifford, Hayes, & Nauta, 1998). Thus, manuals derived from intervention research may not be expected to be followed word-for-word in applied practice, but could instead provide a *guide* for core skills and concepts to be covered (Connor-Smith & Weisz, 2003).

Despite the likelihood of adaptation of programs over time, and the possibility that rigid inflexible use of manuals may lead to less effective outcomes when interventions are disseminated to applied settings, little research has examined the effects of program adaptations. Research on the overall usefulness of manuals in treatments with adults have had mixed results (Herschell, McNeil, & McNeil, 2004). Although some studies with adults have found the use of a manual to be related to better outcomes (DeRubeis & Feeley, 1990), other studies of the use of intervention manuals with adult clients have had negative outcomes (Castonguay, Goldfried, Wiser, Raue, & Hayes, 1996).

Only two studies have directly addressed this issue with child interventions (Harnett & Dadds, 2004; Kendall & Chu, 2000). Harnett and Dadds (2004) asked facilitators in a school-based dissemination of a universal prevention program for depression to complete checklists on intervention integrity and on their degree of deviation from the manual's instructions for specific activities. Prior analyses had found that facilitators' ratings on this checklist were generally, although not completely, correlated with the ratings of independent observers ($r = 0.65$ for changes on activities; $r = 0.73$ for the percentage of core concepts presented). The program was not found to have an influence on outcomes in this dissemination study, and facilitators' degree of deviation from session activities was not found to be significantly associated with program outcomes.

Kendall and Chu (2000) asked therapists who had used a structured evidence-based cognitive–behavioral intervention manual with 148 children (aged 9–13) who had primary anxiety disorders, what kinds of intervention adaptations they made. Therapists made retrospective ratings using the Flexibility Questionnaire. This measure had 7-point rating scales, and assessed the therapists' degree of flexibility in using seven techniques and activities, and their flexibility in the scope of material discussed. The Flexibility Questionnaire had strong internal consistency (alpha = 0.83). Prior research with these samples had found very high treatment integrity, with 100% adherence to session goals. The study found that the therapists' ratings of flexible adaptation of intervention activities were not related to intervention outcome. In addition, flexible adaptation was not found to be related to client characteristics such as their age, sex, race, family income, specific anxiety diagnosis or comorbid diagnoses. Thus, it appears that the combination of requiring strict adherence to session goals while permitting careful flexibility in adapting specific activities meant to address the session goals can lead to successful implementation of programs in "real-world" settings.

Therapeutic Alliance

Later studies have suggested that a rigid adherence to a manual could have a negative effect on the therapeutic alliance, because as therapists' technical competence increased their attention to the relationship decreased (Herschell, McNeil, & McNeil, 2004). The therapeutic alliance has been found in a meta-analysis to be significantly, albeit modestly, associated with outcomes in child and adolescent therapy (Shirk & Karver, 2003).

Historically, the therapeutic relationship has been viewed as a key change mechanism in child psychotherapy (Shirk & Karver, 2003). Currently, the majority of child psychologists and psychiatrists report in surveys that the therapeutic alliance and other non-specific processes are critical for change in child treatment (Chu, Choudhury, Shortt *et al.*, 2004; Kazdin, Siegel, & Bass, 1990). Therapeutic alliance can be conceptualized as (Chu, Choudhury, Shortt *et al.*, 2004):

1 A means to an end, such as the working alliance in psychoanalytic therapy;
2 A necessary and sufficient mechanism for therapeutic change, as in play therapy and client-centered therapy; or
3 In CBT, the therapist serves as an active "coach," with an emphasis on a collaborative process.

Thus, therapeutic alliance is assumed to be necessary but not sufficient in CBT. Therapeutic alliance may be especially important in child intervention, because children do not initiate treatment. The *affiliative bond between client and therapist* and the *agreement and involvement in intervention tasks* may be key in child interventions. These dimensions are expected to be inter-related (Shirk & Saiz, 1992), and are assessed in one of the few therapeutic alliance measures available for children (Shirk & Russell, 1996).

There is minimal research to date, but a meta-analysis (Shirk & Karver, 2003) and literature review (Green, 2006) indicated:

1 A small but significant effect for therapeutic alliance (0.21), with somewhat greater effect for disruptive behavior (0.30) than emotional (0.10) problems;
2 Measures of therapeutic alliance taken late in treatment are more strongly associated with outcome than measures taken early in treatment; and
3 There was little support for the *predictive* effect of therapeutic alliance.

However, recent research has found that a positive alliance between parents and therapists in parent management training for antisocial children has predicted improvements in parenting practices (Kazdin & Whitley, 2006b) and positive child–therapist alliance has predicted improvements in children's behavior (Kazdin, Whitley, & Marciano, 2006). To address a lack of examination of therapeutic alliance in group forms of CBT, Lochman, Barth, and Czopp (2005, June) examined therapeutic alliance in a sample of 80 children screened as being in the top 30% of children according to 4th grade teachers. The children received the Coping Power group CBT program. Findings indicated that children's baseline behavior problems predicted poor therapeutic alliances, and weak therapeutic alliances are related to higher levels of children's problem behaviors at the end of intervention. However, the therapeutic alliance was not a very good predictor of *change* in children's disruptive behavior during intervention, suggesting that therapeutic alliance was not the primary mechanism accounting for CBT effects in group interventions with children.

Potential Iatrogenic Effects: The Example of Deviancy Training

Before widespread dissemination of evidence-based CBT interventions occurs, it is critical to understand who the interventions successfully influence, and whether there are intervention characteristics that can produce iatrogenic effects or subgroups of youth who are vulnerable to iatrogenic effects of a given intervention program. Within the field of youth violence prevention, a critical such concern that has arisen is the potential iatrogenic effect resulting from working with antisocial children in group formats where they may escalate, rather than reduce, their behavior problems. Research results were sufficiently alarming to lead some researchers to recommend that practitioners must be cautious in how they provide group-based interventions (Dishion, McCord, & Poulin, 1999).

In one of the seminal articles on this form of iatrogenic effect, Dishion and Andrews (1995) randomly assigned high-risk young adolescents to one of four conditions varying in whether the youths received 12 youth-only sessions, their parents received 12 parent-only sessions, the youths and the parents both received combined intervention, or the youths and parents received no intervention. All three of the Adolescent Transition program (ATP) intervention cells had some positive effects at post-intervention, and the conditions providing youth intervention produced reductions in negative family interactions and good acquisition of the concepts presented in the intervention. However, by the time of a 1-year follow-up, the youths who had received youth sessions had higher rates of tobacco use and of teacher-rated delinquent behaviors than did the control children, and these iatrogenic effects were evident even if the parents had also received intervention in the combined condition. At a 3-year follow-up, the teen intervention conditions continued to have more tobacco use and delinquency (Poulin, Dishion, & Burraston, 2001). Analyses of the iatrogenic group conditions revealed that subtle dynamics of deviancy training during unstructured transitions in the groups predicted growth in self-reported smoking and growth in teacher ratings of delinquency.

A recent meta-analysis by Weiss, Caron, Ball *et al.* (2005) concluded that the risk for iatrogenic effects may currently be overstated. Weiss, Caron, Ball *et al.* (2005) updated their prior treatment metaanalysis datasets with new studies, and found that there was no difference in effect size for group versus individual treatment (group effect size 0.79, individual effect size 0.68). Surprisingly, group intervention studies had a significantly lower likelihood of creating negative effect sizes than did individual intervention studies, although the log odds for having a negative effect size peaked at age 11 for children in groups versus age 8.6 for individual interventions. This suggests that groups tend to have worse effects as children approach adolescence, consistent with prior concerns that group iatrogenic effects may be most noticeable as children move into early adolescence. This meta-analysis suggests that iatrogenic effects of group interventions are not universal effects, and suggests that it is critically important to research further the potential iatrogenic effects of group interventions at key developmental points. In addition to developmental issues, the therapists' behaviors may have a key role in whether deviancy training emerges in CBT groups. Carefully managed and supervised groups may avoid iatrogenic effects (Dishion & Dodge, 2006). The adult group leaders' abilities to manage and structure peer interactions can assist in redirecting or stopping peers' reinforcement of deviant behaviors. The deviancy effects may be substantially reduced or eliminated if group leaders exercise adequate control over deviancy training behaviors in the group sessions.

Implications for Training and Implementation in Clinic and School Settings

An issue that increases the difficulty of detecting the effects of interventions, especially cognitive–behavioral preventive interventions, is that they are typically implemented at a number of sites (Raudenbush & Willms, 1991). The degree to which the intervention is implemented fully, and the context in which the intervention is embedded, can vary markedly from site to site. With school interventions, contextual factors such as the characteristics of the schools and the school climate can be markedly different across schools. Raudenbush and Willms (1991) argue that this variation, rather than being a nuisance which must be controlled in analyses, can provide critical information and is more important than the overall average effectiveness of the intervention. Variations in the adoption, success and maintenance of interventions across sites can have major implications for the effective dissemination of preventive interventions. In studies of organizational structure and climate, the level of analysis of organization effects should be both at the group level (i.e., school level) and at the individual level (i.e., individual school staff implementing the intervention; Rowan, Raudenbush, & Kang, 1991).

Organizational Influences at the School Level

New interventions and programs need organizational support to be adequately implemented (Berwick, 2003; Henggeler, Lee, & Burns, 2002). One of the central influences within Rogers' (1995) model of the diffusion of innovations involves characteristics of the social system in which the innovation will be embedded, including how decisions are made to adopt innovations and the organizational norms of the setting. The social environment of the organization, and the relationships between individuals in the work setting, are critical characteristics of the organization and are evident in the patterns of leadership, control, autonomy and communication among workers and supervisors (Mowdy & Sutton, 1993; O'Reilly, 1991; Pfeffer, 1983; Porras & Robertson, 1992; Turnipseed, 1994; Weich & Quinn, 1999; Wilport, 1995). The work environment can be conceptualized as having certain systematic characteristics (Moos, 1974, 2002; Trickett & Moos, 1973), consisting of a relationship dimension (involvement, peer cohesion, staff support), a personal growth and development dimension (autonomy, task orientation, work pressure) and a system maintenance and change dimension (clarity, control, innovation, physical comfort). School personnel who perceive that their school climate is negative have been found to think that innovations introduced into their schools are burdens, and they have more burn out (McClure, 1980). In contrast, positively perceived school climate has been found to lead to successful implementation of new reforms in schools (Bulach & Malone, 1994), and collegiality, shared authority among colleagues and positive leadership by principals have been linked to the ability to facilitate change in schools and to continue school improvements (Peterson, 1997). In addition, school-level factors that have been found to influence those perceived environment factors that operate at the school level, and which can affect the implementation of interventions and students' behavior, are school size, school-wide achievement levels, the ethnic composition of schools, the socioeconomic level of the student body and school-wide aggression levels among students (Barth, Dunlap, Dane, Lochman, & Wells, 2004; Kellam, Ling, Merisca, Brown, & Ialongo, 1998; Rowan, Raudenbush, & Kang, 1991).

Effects of Training

The characteristics of the training process and the integrity of the intervention implementation can influence the outcomes of intervention and can contribute to weaker effects of an intervention when it is transported to new settings (Henggeler, Melton, Brondino, Scherer, & Hanley, 1997; Henggeler, Schoenwald, Borduin, Rowland, & Cunningham, 1998). Meta-analyses of the child treatment literature have found that a higher degree of provision of structure (through intervention manuals) and monitoring (through review of intervention session tapes) in treatments offered in a variety of university and community settings were directly linked to superior intervention effectiveness (Weisz, Donenberg, Han *et al.*, 1995a; Weisz, Donenberg, Han *et al.*, 1995b).

Although rarely examined in the intervention literature, the degree of intensity of training can be anticipated to affect intervention outcomes. Henggeler, Schoenwald, Borduin *et al.* (1998) have advocated that Multisystemic Therapy (MST) can only have maximal impact when training is both intense (5-day initial training), ongoing (weekly supervision by MST trained supervisors) and carefully specified. With sufficient intensity, training can achieve its primary purpose of enabling high levels of adherence to the intervention protocol, and producing high levels of intervention integrity (Henggeler, Schoenwald, Borduin *et al.*, 1998). For example, adherence to MST intervention principles has been found to be an important predictor of key outcomes of criminal activity, incarceration and psychiatric symptoms for adolescents receiving MST (Henggeler, Schoenwald, Borduin *et al.*, 1998).

Future Development and Refinement of Cognitive–Behavioral Interventions

Comorbidity

Structured manualized CBT may ignore the complexities of individual cases and neglect the individual idiographic nature of each client (Henry, 1998; Herschell, McNeil, & McNeil, 2004). Thus, the manual may be targeted at the average client with the particular disorder being addressed, but it may not permit a focus on comorbid problems or on individuals with extremely serious versions of the disorder (Weisz, Donenberg, Han *et al.*, 1995b).

Range of Acceptable Adaptation

The clinician may perceive that a CBT manual's predetermined intervention components have to be presented in a linear, invariant order, limiting the efficiency of the program (Weisz, Donenberg, Han *et al.*, 1995b). If so, a manual may limit the clinician's flexibility in addressing issues that go beyond the scope of the portion of the manual currently being used in a given session, but that are still relevant to the treatment plan and the specific issues being raised in the session (Kendall & Chu, 2000; Weissman, Rounsaville, & Chevron, 1982).

Booster Interventions

The current intervention literature indicates that one of the greatest difficulties with interventions for children with disruptive behavior problems is that the children's improved changes in behavior tend to erode over time (McMahon & Wells, 1998), because following intervention the children remain in the same peer, family and neighborhood settings that may have contributed to the child's baseline level of problems. Thus, gains are not positively reinforced, and others, such as teachers, still expect that the formerly aggressive child will continue to behave in antisocial ways. One solution to this problem has been to consider the use of booster interventions, which have been found to assist in maintaining intervention effects (Bry, Catalano, Kumpfer, Lochman, & Szapocznik, 1998). In research on the Anger Coping program, Lochman (1992) found that earlier intervention-produced reductions in children's disruptive off-task behavior in school settings was maintained at a 3-year follow-up only for aggressive children who had received a booster intervention.

Technology and Internet Use

Empirical evidence indicates that individuals pay more attention to and learn more deeply from multimedia presentations than from verbal-only messages, resulting in greater problem-solving transfer (Eveland, Seo, & Marton, 2002; Lieberman, 2001; Mayer, 2003; van der Molen & van der Voort, 2000). Given this and the popularity of computers and video games among children and adolescents (Vorderer & Ritterfeld, 2003), it is not surprising that electronic media have become a popular modality for youth preventive interventions. Indeed, children and adolescents indicate that their preferred method of learning involves interactive multimedia (Lieberman, 2001). Multimedia programs have been developed to prevent youth violence. One such program, SMART Talk (Students Managing Anger and Resolution Together) aims to teach middle school students anger management and conflict resolution skills through a similar set of computer-based activities. While no significant changes in the frequency of aggressive behavior were found in a randomized controlled study of SMART Talk, significant effects were observed on several mediating factors associated with violence. In particular, students in the intervention condition were less likely to value violence as a solution to conflict, were more likely to report intentions to use non-violent strategies and reported more self-awareness about their response to anger in conflict situations than students in the control group (Bosworth, Espelage, & DuBay, 2000). Thus, multimedia programs display promising effects on risk and protective factors for negative youth outcomes, and may have effects on their actual behavior, especially for children already motivated to change. Research will need to explore whether multimedia programs can produce effective behavior change in children without a therapist, and without a therapeutic alliance, or whether multimedia programs can best be considered to be adjuncts to therapist-provided CBT.

References

Akhutina, T. V. (1997). The remediation of executive functions in children with cognitive disorders: The Vygotsky–Luria neuropsychological approach. *Journal of Intellectual Disability Research*, *41*, 144–151.

Asarnow, J. R., & Callan, J. W. (1985). Boys with peer adjustment problems: Social cognitive processes. *Journal of Consulting and Clinical Psychology*, *53*, 80–87.

Bandura, A. (1969). *Principles of behavior modification*. New York: Holt, Rinehart & Winston.

Bandura, A. (1973). *Aggression: A social learning analysis*. Englewood Cliffs, NJ: Prentice Hall.

Bandura, A., & McDonald, F. J. (1963). The influence of social reinforcement and the behavior of models in shaping children's moral judgments. *Journal of Abnormal and Social Psychology*, *67*, 274–281.

Bandura, A., & Mischel, W. (1965). Modification of self-imposed delay of gratification through exposure to live and symbolic models. *Journal of Personality and Social Psychology*, *2*, 698–705.

Bandura, A., Ross, D., & Ross, S. A. (1963). Vicarious reinforcement and imitative social learning. *Journal of Abnormal and Social Psychology*, *67*, 601–607.

Barbe, R. P., Bridge, J., Birmaher, B., Kolko, D. J., & Brent, D. A. (2004). Suicidality and its relationship to treatment outcome in depressed adolescents. *Suicide and Life Threatening Behavior*, *34*, 44–55.

Barrett, P. M. (1998). Evaluation of cognitive–behavioral group treatments for childhood anxiety disorders. *Journal of Clinical Child Psychology*, *27*, 459–468.

Barrett, P. M., Dadds, M. R., & Rapee, R. M. (1996). Family treatment of childhood anxiety: A controlled trial. *Journal of Consulting and Clinical Psychology*, *64*, 333–342.

Barrett, P. M., & Shortt, A. L. (2003). Parental involvement in the treatment of anxious children. In A. E. Kazdin, & J. R. Weisz (Eds.), *Evidence-based psychotherapies for children and adolescents* (pp. 101–119). New York: Guilford.

Barth, J. M., Dunlap, S. T., Dane, H., Lochman, J. E., & Wells, K. (2004). Classroom environment influences on aggression, peer relations, and academic focus. *Journal of School Psychology*, *42*, 115–133.

Beauchaine, T. P., Webster-Stratton, C., & Reid, M. J. (2005). Mediators, moderators, and predictors of 1-year outcomes among children treated for early-onset conduct problems: A latent growth curve analysis. *Journal of Consulting and Clinical Psychology*, *73*, 371–388.

Beck, A. (1963). Thinking and depression. *Archives of General Psychiatry*, *49*, 681–689.

Berwick, D. M. (2003). Disseminating innovations in health care. *Journal of the American Medical Association*, *289*, 1969–1975.

Bickman, L. (2002). The death of treatment as usual: An excellent first step on a long road. *Clinical Psychology: Science and Practice*, *9*, 195–199.

Birmaher, B., Brent, D. A., Kolko, D., Baugher, M., Bridge, J., Iyengar, S., *et al.* (2000). Clinical outcome after short-term psychotherapy for adolescents with major depressive disorder. *Archives of general Psychiatry*, *57*, 29–36.

Bosworth, K., Espelage, D., & DuBay, T. (2000). Preliminary evaluation of a multimedia violence prevention program for adolescents. *American Journal of Health Behavior*, *24*, 268–280.

Brent, D. A., Holder, D., Kolko, D., Birmaher, B., Baugher, M., Roth, C., *et al.* (1997). A clinical psychotherapy trial for adolescent depression comparing cognitive, family, and supportive treatments. *Archives of General Psychiatry*, *54*, 877–885.

Brestan, E. V., & Eyberg, S. M. (1998). Effective psychosocial treatments of conduct-disordered children and adolescents: 29 years, 82 studies, and 5,272 kids. *Journal of Clinical Child Psychology*, *27*, 180–189.

Bry, B. H., Catalano, R. F., Kumpfer, K., Lochman, J. E., & Szapocznik, J. (1998). Scientific findings from family prevention intervention research. In R. Ashery (Ed.), *Family-based prevention interventions* (pp. 103–129). Rockville, MD: National Institute of Drug Abuse.

Bulach, C., & Malone, B. (1994). The relationship of school climate to the implementation of school reform. *ERS Spectrum*, *12*, 3–8.

Burgess, K. B., Wojslawowicz, J. C., Rubin, K. H., Rose-Krasnor, L., & Booth-LaForce, C. (2006). Social information processing and coping strategies of shy/withdrawn and aggressive children: Does friendship matter? *Child Development*, *77*, 371–383.

Castonguay, L. G., Goldfried, M. R., Wiser, S., Raue, P. J., & Hayes, A. M. (1996). Predicting the effects of cognitive therapy for depression: A study of unique and common factors. *Journal of Consulting and Clinical Psychology*, *64*, 497–504.

Chorpita, B. F., & Southam-Gerow, M. A. (2006). Fears and anxieties. In E. J. Mash, & R. A. Barkley (Eds.), *Treatment of childhood disorders* (3rd edn., pp. 271–335). New York: Guilford.

Chu, B. C., Choudhury, M. S., Shortt, A. L., Pncus, D. B., Creed, T. A., & Kendall, P. C. (2004). Alliance, technology, and outcome in the treatment of anxious youth. *Cognitive and Behavioral Practice*, *11*, 44–55.

Clarke, G. N., DeBar, L. L., & Lewinsohn, P. M. (2003). Cognitive-behavioral group treatment for adolescent depression. In A. E. Kazdin, & J. R. Weisz (Eds.), *Evidence-based psychotherapies for children and adolescents* (pp. 120–134). New York: Guilford.

Connor-Smith, J. K., & Weisz, J. R. (2003). Applying treatment outcome research in clinical practice: Techniques for adapting interventions to the real world. *Child and Adolescent Mental Health*, *8*, 3–10.

Cowan, P. A., Cohn, D. A., Cowan, C. P., & Pearson, J. L. (1996). Parents' attachment histories and children's externalizing and internalizing behaviors: Exploring family systems models of linkage. *Journal of Consulting and Clinical Psychology*, *64*, 53–63.

Crick, N. R., & Dodge, K. A. (1994). A review and reformulation of social information-processing mechanisms in children's social adjustment. *Psychological Bulletin*, *115*, 74–101.

Crick, N. R., & Werner, N. E. (1998). Response decision processes in relational and overt aggression. *Child Development*, *69*, 1630–1639.

Curry, J. F., & Craighead, W. E. (1990). Attributional style in clinic depressed and conduct disordered adolescents. *Journal of Consulting and Clinical Psychology*, *58*, 109–116.

Daleiden, E. L., & Vasey, M. W. (1997). An information-processing perspective on childhood anxiety. *Clinical Psychology Review*, *4*, 407–429.

DeRubeis, R. J., & Feeley, M. J. V. (1990). Determinants of change in cognitive therapy for depression. *Cognitive Therapy and Research*, *14*, 469–482.

Dishion, T. J., & Andrews, D. W. (1995). Preventing escalation in problem behaviors with high-risk young adolescents: Immediate and 1-year outcomes. *Journal of Consulting and Clinical Psychology*, *63*, 538–548.

Dishion, T. J., & Dodge, K. A. (2006). Deviant peer contagion in interventions and programs: An ecological framework for understanding influence mechanisms. In K. A. Dodge, T. J. Dishion, & J. E. Lansford (Eds.), *Deviant peer influences in programs for youth* (pp. 14–43). New York: Guilford Publications.

Dishion, T. J., McCord, J., & Poulin, F. (1999). When interventions harm: Peer groups and problem behavior. *American Psychologist*, *54*, 755–764.

Dodge, K. A. (1993). Social cognitive mechanisms in the development of conduct disorder and depression. *Annual Review of Psychology*, *44*, 558–584.

Dodge, K. A., Petit, G. S., McClaskey, C. L., & Brown, M. M. (1986). Social competence in children. *Monographs of the Society for Research in Child Development 51* (2, Serial No. 213).

Dumas, J. E., & Wahler, R. G. (1983). Predictors of treatment outcome in parent training: Mother insularity and socioeconomic disadvantage. *Behavioral Assessment*, *5*, 301–313.

D'Zurilla, T. J., & Goldfried, M. R. (1971). Problem solving and behavior modification. *Journal of Abnormal Psychology*, *78*, 107–126.

Ehrenreich, J. T., & Gross, A. M. (2002). Biased attentional behavior in childhood anxiety: A review of theory and current empirical investigation. *Clinical Psychology Review*, *22*, 991–1008.

Eveland, W. P., Seo, M., & Marton, K. (2002). Learning from the news in campaign 2002: An experimental comparison of TV news, newspapers, and online news. *Media Psychology*, *4*, 355–380.

Farmer, E. M. Z., Compton, S. N., Burns, B., & Robertson, E. (2002). Review of evidence base for treatment of childhood psychopathology: Externalizing disorders. *Journal of Consulting and Clinical Psychology*, *70*, 1267–1302.

Fiske, S. T., & Taylor, S. E. (1984). *Social cognition*. Reading, MA: Addison-Wesley.

Flannery-Schroeder, E., & Kendall, P. C. (2000). Group and individual cognitive–behavioral treatments for youth with anxiety disorders: A randomized clinical trial. *Cognitive Therapy and Research*, *24*, 251–278.

Frick, P. J., Cornell, A. H., Barry, C. T., Bodin, S. D., & Dane, H. E. (2003). Callous-unemotional traits and conduct problems in the prediction of conduct problem severity, aggression, and self-report of delinquency. *Journal of Abnormal Child Psychology*, *31*, 457–470.

Frick, P. J., Silverthorn, P., & Evans, C. (1994). Assessment of childhood anxiety using structured interviews: Patterns of agreement among informants and association with maternal anxiety. *Psychological Assessment*, *6*, 372–379.

Garber, J., Braafladt, N., & Zeman, J. (1991). The regulation of sad affect: An information-processing perspective. In J. Garber, & K. Dodge (Eds.), *The development of emotional regulation and dysregulation* (pp. 208–240). New York: CUP.

Gladstone, T. R. G., & Kaslow, N. J. (1995). Depression and attributions in children and adolescents: A meta-analytic review. *Journal of Abnormal Child Psychology*, *23*, 597–606.

Gouze, K. R. (1987). Attention and social problem solving as correlates of aggression in preschool males. *Journal of Abnormal Child Psychology*, *15*, 181–197.

Graham, P. (2005). Jack Tizard lecture. Cognitive–behavior therapies for children: Passing fashion or here to stay? *Child and Adolescent Mental Health*, *10*, 57–62.

Green, J. (2006). Annotation. The therapeutic alliance: A significant but neglected variable in child mental health treatment studies. *Journal of Child Psychology and Psychiatry*, *47*, 425–435.

Hammen, C., & Zupan, B. A. (1984). Self-schemas, depression, social problem solving and social competence in preadolescence: Is inconsistency the hobgoblin of little minds? *Cognitive Therapy and Research*, *9*, 685–702.

Harnett, P. H., & Dadds, M. R. (2004). Training school personnel to implement a universal school-based prevention of depression program under real-world conditions. *Journal of School Psychology*, *42*, 343–357.

Hartman, R. R., Stage, S. A., & Webster-Stratton, C. (2003). A growth curve analysis of parent training outcomes: Examining the influence of child risk factors (inattention, impulsivity, and hyperactivity problems), parental and family risk factors. *Journal of Child Psychology and Psychiatry*, *44*, 388–398.

Hawes, D. J., & Dadds, M. R. (2005). The treatment of conduct problems in children with callous-unemotional traits. *Journal of Consulting and Clinical Psychology*, *73*, 737–741.

Hawley, K. M., & Weisz, J. R. (2002). Increasing the relevance of evidence-based treatment review to practitioners and consumers. *Clinical Psychology: Science and Practice*, *9*, 225–230.

Henggeler, S. W., Lee, T., & Burns, J. A. (2002). What happens after the innovation is identified? *Clinical Psychology: Science and Practice*, *9*, 191–194.

Henggeler, S. W., Melton, G. B., Brondino, M. J., Scherer, D. G., & Hanley, J. H. (1997). Multisystemic therapy with violent and chronic juvenile offenders and their families: The role of treatment fidelity in successful dissemination. *Journal of Consulting and Clinical Psychology*, *65*, 821–833.

Henggeler, S. W., Schoenwald, S. K., Borduin, C. M., Rowland, M. D., & Cunningham, P. B. (1998). *Multisystemic treatment of antisocial behavior in children and adolescents*. New York: Guilford.

Henry, W. P. (1998). Science, politics, and the politics of science: The use and misuse of empirically validated treatment research. *Psychotherapy Research*, *8*, 126–140.

Herschell, A. D., McNeil, C. B., & McNeil, D. W. (2004). Clinical child psychology's progress in disseminating empirically supported treatments. *Clinical Psychology: Science and Practice*, *11*, 267–288.

Hull, C. L. (1943). *Principles of behavior: An introduction to behavior theory*. New York: Appleton-Century Crofts.

Jacobs, L., & Joseph, S. (1997). Cognitive Triad Inventory and its association with symptoms of depression and anxiety in adolescents. *Personality and Individual Differences*, *22*, 769–770.

Jahoda, M. (1953). The meaning of psychological health. *Social Casework*, *34*, 349–354.

Jahoda, M. (1958). *Current concepts of positive mental health*. New York, NY: Basic Books.

Jessor, R. (1954). The generalization of expectancies. *Journal of Abnormal Social Psychology*, *49*, 196–200.

Jones, N. C., & Burks, B. S. (1936). Personality development in childhood. *Social Research in Child Development Monogram*, *1*, 1–205.

Kam, C., Greenberg, M. T., & Kusché, C. A. (2004). Sustained effects of the PATHS curriculum on the social and psychological adjustment of children in special education. *Journal of Emotional and Behavioral Disorders*, *12*, 66–78.

Kaslow, N. J., Rehm, L. P., Pollack, S. L., & Siegel, A. W. (1988). Attributional style and self-control behavior in depressed and non-depressed children and their parents. *Journal of Abnormal Child Psychology*, *16*, 163–175.

Kazdin, A. E. (2003). Psychotherapy for children and adolescents. *Annual Review of Psychology*, *54*, 253–276.

Kazdin, A. E., & Crowley, M. (1997). Moderators of treatment outcome in cognitively based treatment of antisocial children. *Cognitive Therapy and Research*, *21*, 185–207.

Kazdin, A. E., Siegel, T. C., & Bass, D. (1990). Drawing on clinical practice to inform research on child and adolescent psychotherapy: Survey of practitioners. *Journal of Consulting and Clinical Psychology*, *21*, 189–198.

Kazdin, A. E., Siegel, T. C., & Bass, D. (1992). Cognitive problem solving skills training and parent management training in the treatment of antisocial behavior in children. *Journal of Consulting and Clinical Psychology*, *60*, 733–747.

Kazdin, A. E., & Wassell, G. (1999). Barriers to treatment participation and therapeutic change among children referred for conduct disorder. *Journal of Clinical Child Psychology*, *28*, 160–172.

Kazdin, A. E., & Weisz, J. R. (1998). Identifying and developing empirically supported child and adolescent treatments. *Journal of Consulting and Clinical Psychology*, *66*, 19–36.

Kazdin, A. E., & Whitley, M. K. (2006a). Comorbidity, case complexity, and effects of evidence-based treatment for children referred for disruptive behavior. *Journal of Consulting and Clinical Psychology*, *74*, 455–467.

Kazdin, A. E., & Whitley, M. K. (2006b). Pretreatment social relations, therapeutic alliance, and improvements in parenting practices in parent management training. *Journal of Consulting and Clinical Psychology*, *74*, 346–355.

Kazdin, A. E., Whitley, M., & Marciano, P. L. (2006). Child–therapist and parent–therapist alliance and therapeutic change in the treatment of children referred for oppositional, aggressive, and antisocial behavior. *Journal of Child Psychology and Psychiatry*, *47*, 436–445.

Kellam, S. G., Ling, X., Mersica, R., Brown, C. H., & Ialongo, N. (1998). The effect of the level of aggression in the first grade classroom on the course of malleability of aggressive behavior into middle school. *Development and Psychopathology*, *10*, 165–185.

Kendall, P.C. (1994). Treating anxiety disorders in children: Results of a randomized clinical trial. *Journal of Consulting and Clinical Psychology*, *62*, 100–110.

Kendall, P. (2002). Toward a research-practice–community partnership: Goin' fishing and showing slides. *Clinical Psychology: Science and Practice*, *9*, 214–216.

Kendall, P. C., & Braswell, L. (1982). Cognitive–behavioral self-control therapy for children: A components analysis. *Journal of Consulting and Clinical Psychology*, *5*, 672–689.

Kendall, P. C., & Chu, B. C. (2000). Retrospective self-reports of therapist flexibility in a manual-based treatment for youths with anxiety disorders. *Journal of Clinical Child Psychology*, *29*, 209–220.

Kendall, P. C., Chu, B., Gifford, A., Hayes, C., & Nauta, M. (1998). Breathing life into a manual: Flexibility and creativity with manual-based treatments. *Cognitive and Behavioral Practice*, *5*, 177–198.

Kendall, P. C., Flannery-Schroeder, E., Panichelli-Mindel, S., Southam-Gerow, M., Henin, A., & Warman, M. (1997). Therapy for youths with anxiety disorders: A second randomized clinical trial. *Journal of Consulting and Clinical Psychology*, *65*, 366–380.

Kendall, P. C., & Southam-Gerow, M. (1996). Long-term follow-up of treatment for anxiety disordered youth. *Journal of Consulting and Clinical Psychology*, *65*, 883–888.

Kendall, P. C., & Suveg, C. (2006). Treating anxiety disorders in youth. In P. Kendall (Ed.), *Child and adolescent therapy: Cognitive–behavioral procedures* (3rd edn., pp. 243–294). New York: Guilford.

Kolko, D. J., Brent, D. A., Baugher, M., Bridge, J., & Birmaher, B. (2000). Cognitive and family therapies for adolescent depression: Treatment specificity, mediation, and moderation. *Journal of Consulting and Clinical Psychology*, *68*, 603–614.

Lazarus, R. (1991). Cognition and motivation in emotion. *American Psychologist*, *46*, 352–367.

Lieberman, D. A. (2001). Using interactive media in communication campaigns for children and adolescents. In R. E. Rice, & C. K. Atkin (Eds.), *Public communication campaigns* (3rd edn., pp. 373–388). Thousand Oaks, CA: Sage.

Lochman, J. E. (1987). Self and peer perceptions and attributional biases of aggressive and non-aggressive boys in dyadic interactions. *Journal of Consulting and Clinical Psychology*, *55*, 404–410.

Lochman, J. E. (1992). Cognitive–behavioral intervention with aggressive boys: Three-year follow-up and preventive effects. *Journal of Consulting and Clinical Psychology*, *60*, 426–432.

Lochman, J. E., Barth, J. M., & Czopp, W. (2005, June). Effects of therapeutic alliance in preventive intervention with aggressive children. Paper presented in a symposium (I. Granic, Chair) at the Twelfth Scientific Meeting of the International Society for Research in Child and Adolescent Psychopathology, New York, NY.

Lochman, J. E., Burch, P. P., Curry, J. F., & Lampron, L. B. (1984). Treatment and generalization effects of cognitive–behavioral and goal setting interventions with aggressive boys. *Journal of Consulting and Clinical Psychology*, *52*, 915–916.

Lochman, J. E., & Dodge, K. A. (1994). Social cognitive processes of severely violent, moderately aggressive, and nonaggressive boys. *Journal of Consulting and Clinical Psychology*, *62*, 366–374.

Lochman, J. E., & Dodge, K. A. (1998). Distorted perceptions in dyadic interactions of aggressive and nonaggressive boys: Effects of prior expectations, context, and boys' age. *Development and Psychopathology*, *10*, 495–512.

Lochman J. E., & Lampron, L. B. (1986). Situational social problem-solving skills and self-esteem of aggressive and nonaggressive boys. *Journal of Abnormal Child Psychology*, *14*, 605–617.

Lochman, J. E., & Lenhart, L. A. (1995). Cognitive behavioral therapy of aggressive children: Effects of schemas. In H. P. J. G. van Bilsen, P. C. Kendall, & J. H. Slavenbury (Eds.), *Behavioral approaches for children and adolescents: Challenges for the next century* (pp. 145–166). New York, NY: Plenum Press.

Lochman, J. E., Nelson, W. M., & Sims, J. P. (1981). A cognitive behavioral program for use with aggressive children. *Journal of Clinical Child Psychology*, *13*, 146–148.

Lochman, J. E., Phillips, N. C., McElroy, H. K., & Pardini, D. A. (2005). Conduct disorder in adolescence. In P. Graham (Ed.), *Cognitive behaviour therapy for children and families* (2nd edn., pp. 443–458). Cambridge, England: Cambridge University Press.

Lochman, J. E., Wayland, K. K., & White, K. J. (1993). Social goals: Relationship to adolescent adjustment and to social problem solving. *Journal of Abnormal Child Psychology*, *21*, 135–151.

Lochman, J. E., & Wells, K. C. (2002a). The Coping Power Program at the middle school transition: Universal and indicated prevention effects. *Psychology of Addictive Behaviors*, *16*, S40–S54.

Lochman, J. E., & Wells, K. C. (2002b). Contextual social-cognitive mediators and child outcome: A test of the theoretical model in the Coping Power program. *Development and Psychopathology*, *14*, 945–967.

Lochman, J. E., & Wells, K. C. (2003). Effectiveness study of Coping Power and classroom intention with aggressive children: Outcomes at a 1-year follow-up. *Behavior Therapy*, *34*, 493–515.

Lochman, J. E., & Wells, K. C. (2004). The Coping Power Program for preadolescent aggressive boys and their parents: Outcome effects at the 1-year follow-up. *Journal of Consulting and Clinical Psychology*, *72*, 571–578.

Lynam, D. R. (1996). Early identification of chronic offenders: Who is the fledgling psychopath? *Psychological Bulletin*, *120*, 209–234.

March, J. S., Silva, S., Petrycki, S., Curry, J., Wells, K., Fairbank, J., *et al.* (2004). The Treatment for Adolescents with Depression Study (TADS): Short-term effectiveness and safety outcomes. *Journal of the American Medical Association*, *292*, 807–820.

Marcotte, D., Alain, M., & Gosselin, M. J. (1999). Gender differences in adolescent depression: Gender-typed characteristics or problem-solving skills deficits? *Sex Roles*, *41*, 31–48.

Mash, E. J. (1998). Treatment of child and family disturbance: A behavioral-systems perspective. In E. J. Mash, & R. A. Barkley (Eds.), *Treatment of childhood disorders* (2nd edn., pp. 3–51). New York, NY: Guilford Press.

Mayer, R. E. (2003). The promise of multimedia learning: Using the same instructional design methods across different media. *Learning and Instruction*, *13*, 125–139.

McClure, L. (1980). Community psychology concepts and research base: Promise and product. *American Psychologist*, *35*, 1000–1011.

McMahon, R. J., & Wells, K. C. (1998). Conduct problems. In E. J. Mash, & R. A. Barkley (Eds.), *Treatment of childhood disorders* (2nd edn., pp. 111–207). New York: Guilford.

Meichenbaum, D. (2003). Cognitive–behavior therapy: Folktales and the unexpurgated history. *Cognitive Therapy and Research*, *27*, 125–129.

Meichenbaum, D. H., & Goodman, J. (1969). The developmental control of operant motor responding by verbal operants. *Journal of Experimental Child Psychology*, *7*, 553–565.

Meichenbaum, D. H., & Goodman, J. (1971). Training impulsive children to talk to themselves: A means for developing self-control. *Journal of Abnormal Psychology*, *77*, 115–125.

Melvin, G. A., Tonge, B. J., King, N. J., Heyne, D., Gordon, M. S., & Klimkeit, E. (2006). A comparison of cognitive–behavioral therapy, sertraline, and their combination for adolescent depression. *Journal of the American Academy of Child and Adolescent Psychiatry*, *45*, 1151–1161.

Michael, K. D., & Crowley, S. L. (2002). How effective are treatments for child and adolescent depression? A meta-analytic review. *Clinical Psychology Review*, *22*, 247–269.

Milich, R., & Dodge, K. A. (1984). Social information processing in child psychiatric populations. *Journal of Abnormal Child Psychology*, *12*, 471–490.

Miller, N. E., & Dollard, J. (1941). *Social learning and imitation.* New Haven: Yale University Press.

Mischel, W. (1973). Toward a cognitive social learning conceptualization of personality. *Psychological Review*, *80*, 252–283.

Mischel, W. (1990). Personality disposition revisited and revised: A view after three decades. In L. Pervin (Ed.), *Handbook of personality: Theory and research* (pp. 111–134). New York: Guilford.

Moos, R. H. (1974). *The social climate scales: An overview.* Palo Alto, CA: Consulting Psychologists Press.

Moos, R. H. (2002). The mystery of human context and coping: An unraveling of clues. *American Journal of Community Psychology*, *30*, 67–88.

Mowday, R. T., & Sutton, R. I. (1993). Organizational behavior: Linking individuals and groups to organizational contexts. In L. W. Porter, & M. R. Rosenzweig (Eds.), *Annual review of psychology* (Vol. 44, pp. 195–229). Palo Alto, CA: Annual Reviews.

MTA Cooperative Group. (1999). A 14-month randomized clinical trial of treatment strategies for attention-deficit/hyperactivity disorder. Multimodal Treatment Study of Children with ADHD. *Archives of General Psychiatry*, *56*, 1073–1086.

Mullins, L. L., Siegel, L. J., & Hodges, K. (1985). Cognitive problem-solving and life event correlates of depressive symptoms in children. *Journal of Abnormal Child Psychology*, *12*, 471–490.

Najström, M., & Jansson, B. (2006). Unconscious responses to threatening pictures: Interactive effect of trait anxiety and social desirability on skin conductance responses. *Cognitive Behaviour Therapy*, *35*, 11–18.

Neisser, U. (1967). *Cognitive psychology*. New York, NY: Appleton-Century Crofts.

Nock, M. K. (2003). Progress review of the psychosocial treatment of child conduct problems. *Clinical Psychology: Science and Practice*, *10*, 1–28.

O'Reilly, C. A. (1991). Organizational behavior: Where we've been, where we're going. In M. R. Rozenzweig, & L. W. Porter (Eds.), *Annual review of psychology* (Vol. 42, pp. 427–458). Palo Alto, CA: Annual Reviews.

Pardini, D. A. (2006). The callousness pathway to severe violent delinquency. *Aggressive Behavior*, *32*, 590–598.

Pardini, D. A., Barry, T. D., Barth, J. M., Lochman, J. E., & Wells, K. C. (2006). Self-perceived social acceptance and peer social standing in children with aggressive-disruptive behaviors. *Social Development*, *15*, 46–64.

Pardini, D. A., & Lochman, J. E. (2003). Treatment for Oppositional Defiant Disorder. In M. A. Reinecke, F. M. Dattilio, & A. Freeman (Eds.), *Cognitive therapy with children and adolescents* (2nd edn., pp. 43–69). New York: Guilford.

Pardini, D. A., Lochman, J. E., & Frick, P. J. (2003). Callous/unemotional traits and social-cognitive processes in adjudicated youths. *Journal of the American Academy of Child and Adolescent Psychiatry*, *42*, 364–371.

Pepler, D. J., Craig, W. M., & Roverts, W. I. (1998). Observations of aggressive and nonaggressive children on the school playground. *Merrill Palmer Quarterly*, *44*, 55–76.

Peterson, A. M. (1997). Aspects of school climate: A review of the literature. *ERS Spectrum*, *15*, 36–42.

Peterson, L., & Shigetomi, C. (1981). The use of coping techniques to minimize anxiety in hospitalized children. *Behavior Therapy*, *12*, 1–14.

Pfeffer, J. (1983). Organizational demography. *Research on Organizational Behavior*, *5*, 299–357.

Porras, J. I., & Robertson, P. J. (1992). Organizational development: Theory, practice, and research. In M. D. Dunnette, & L. M. Hough (Eds.), *Handbook of organizational psychology* (2nd edn., pp. 719–822). Palo Alto, CA: Consulting Psychology Press.

Poulin, F., Dishion, T. J., & Burraston, B. (2001). 3-year iatrogenic effects associated with aggregating high-risk adolescents in cognitive-behavioral interventions. *Applied Developmental Science*, *5*, 214–224.

Quiggle, N. L., Garber, W. F., Panak, W. F., & Dodge, K. A. (1992). Social information processing in aggressive and depressed children. *Child Development*, *63*, 1305–1320.

Raudenbush, S. W., & Willms, J. D. (1991). The organization of schooling and its methodological implications. In S. W. Raudenbush, & J. D. Willms (Eds.), *Schools, classrooms, and pupils: International studies of schooling from a multilevel perspective* (pp. 1–12). San Diego, CA: Academic Press.

Reinecke, M. A., Ryan, N. E., & DuBois, D. L. (1998). Cognitive–behavioral therapy of depression and depressive symptoms during adolescence: A review and meta-analysis. *Journal of the American Academy of Child and Adolescent Psychiatry*, *37*, 26–34.

Reyno, S. M., & McGrath, P. J. (2006). Predictors of parent training efficacy for child externalizing behavior problems: A meta-analytic review. *Journal of Child Psychology and Psychiatry*, *47*, 99–111.

Roberts, M. C., Lazicki-Puddy, T. A., Puddy, R. W., & Johnson, R. J. (2003). The outcomes of psychotherapy with adolescents: A practitioner-friendly research review. *Journal of Clinical Psychology*, *59*, 1177–1191.

Rogers, E. (1995). *Diffusion of innovations* (4th edn.). New York: The Free Press.

Rotter, J. B. (1954). *Social learning and clinical psychology*. New York: Prentice-Hall.

Rotter, J. B., Chance, J. E., & Phares, E. J. (1972). *Applications of a social learning theory of personality*. New York: Holt, Rinehart, and Winston.

Rotter, J., Seeman, M., & Liverant, S. (1962). Internal versus external control of reinforcement: A major variable in behavior theory. In N. F. Washburne (Ed.), *Decisions, values and groups* (Vol. 2). London: Pergamon Press (pp. 473–516).

Rowan, B., Raudenbush, S. W., & Kang, S. J. (1991). School climate in secondary schools. In S. W. Raudenbush, & J. D. Willms (Eds.), *Schools, classrooms, and pupils: International studies of schooling from a multilevel perspective* (pp. 203–223). San Diego, CA: Academic Press.

Rubenstein, A. K. (2003). Adolescent psychotherapy: An introduction. *Journal of Clinical Psychology*, *59*, 1169–1175.

Rudolph, K. D., & Clark, A. G. (2001). Conceptions of relationships in children with depressive and aggressive symptoms: Social-cognitive distortion or reality? *Journal of Abnormal Child Psychology*, *29*, 41–56.

Sacco, W. P., & Graves, D. J. (1984). Childhood depression, interpersonal problem-solving, and self-ratings of performance. *Journal of Clinical Child Psychology*, *13*, 10–15.

Schoenwald, S. K., & Hoagwood, K. (2001). Effectiveness, transportability, and dissemination of interventions: What matters when? *Psychiatric Services*, *52*, 1190–1196.

Shirk, S. R., & Karver, M. (2003). Prediction of treatment outcome from relationship variables in child and adolescent therapy: A meta-analytic review. *Journal of Consulting and Clinical Psychology*, *71*, 452–464.

Shirk, S., & Russell, R. L. (1996). *Change processes in child psychotherapy: Revitalizing treatment and research*. New York: Guilford Press.

Shirk, S., & Saiz, C. (1992). Clinical, empirical, and developmental perspectives on the relationship in child psychotherapy. *Development and Psychopathology*, *4*, 713–728.

Shure, M. B. (1992a). *I Can Problem Solve (ICPS): An interpersonal problem-solving program (preschool)*. Champaign, IL: Research Press.

Shure, M. B. (1992b). *I Can Problem Solve (ICPS): An interpersonal problem-solving program. Kindergarten and primary grades*. Champaign, IL: Research Press.

Shure, M. B. (1993). I Can Problem Solve (ICPS): Interpersonal cognitive problem solving for young children. *Early Child Development and Care*, *96*, 49–64.

Shure, M. B. & Spivack, G. (1970).*Cognitive problem-solving skills, adjustment and social class* (Research and Evaluation Report no. 26). Philadelphia: Department of Mental Health Sciences, Hahnemann Community Mental Health/Mental Retardation Center.

Shure, M. B., & Spivack, G. (1972). Means-ends thinking, adjustment, and social class among elementary-school-aged children. *Journal of Consulting and Clinical Psychology*, *38*, 348–353.

Shure, M. B., & Spivack, G. (1980). Interpersonal problem solving as a mediator of behavioral adjustment in preschool and kindergarten children. *Journal of Applied Developmental Psychology*, *1*, 29–44.

Shure, M. B., Spivack, G., & Jaeger, M. (1971). Problem-solving thinking and adjustment among disadvantaged preschool children. *Child Development*, *42*, 1791–1803.

Silverman, W. K., & Kurtines, W. M. (2004). Research progress on effectiveness, transportability, and dissemination of empirically supported treatments: Integrating theory and research. *Clinical Psychology: Science and Practice*, *11*, 295–299.

Smith, C. A., & Lazarus, R. W. (1990). Emotion and adaptation. In L. Previn (Ed.), *Handbook of personality: Theory and research* (pp. 609–637). New York: Guilford.

Southam-Gerow, M., Kendall, P. C., & Weersing, V. R. (2002). Examining outcome variability: Correlates of treatment response in a child and adolescent anxiety clinic. *Journal of Clinical Child Psychology*, *30*, 422–436.

Spence, S. H., Sheffield, J. K., & Donovan, C. L. (2003). Preventing adolescent depression: An evaluation of the problem solving for life program. *Journal of Consulting and Clinical Psychology*, *71*, 3–13.

Spivack, G., & Shure, M. B. (1974). *Social adjustment of young children*. San Francisco: Jossey-Bass.

Stark, K. D., Hargrave, J., Sander, J., Custer, G., Schnoebelen, S., Simpson, J., *et al.* (2006a). Treatment of childhood depression: The ACTION treatment program. In P. Kendall (Ed.), *Child and adolescent therapy: Cognitive–behavioral procedures* (3rd edn., pp. 169–216). New York: Guilford.

Stark, K. D., Sander, J., Hauser, M., Simpson, J., Schnoebelen, S., Glenn, R., *et al.* (2006b). Depressive disorders during adolescence. In E. J. Mash, & R. A. Barkley (Eds.), *Treatment of childhood disorders* (3rd edn., pp. 336–407). New York: Guilford.

Stirman, S. W., Crits-Christoph, P., & DeRubeis, R. J. (2004). Achieving successful dissemination of empirically supported psychotherapies: A synthesis of dissemination theory. *Clinical Psychology: Science and Practice*, *11*, 343–359.

Thomas, R. M. (1996). *Comparing theories of child development* (4th edn.). Pacific Grove, CA: Brooks/Coles Publishing Company.

Treadwell, K. H., & Kendall, P. C. (1996). Self-talk in anxiety-disordered youth: States-of-mind, content specificity, and treatment outcome. *Journal of Consulting and Clinical Psychology*, *64*, 941–950.

Trickett, E. J., & Moos, R. H. (1973). Social environment of junior high and high school classrooms. *Journal of Educational Psychology*, *65*, 93–102.

Turnipseed, D. (1994). The relationship between the social environment of organizations and the climate for innovation and creativity. *Journal of Applied Social Psychology*, *24*, 782–800.

Urbain, E. S, & Kendall, P. C. (1980). Review of social-cognitive problem-solving interventions with children. *Psychological Bulletin*, *88*, 109–143.

van de Molen, J. H. W., & van der Voort, T. H. A. (2000). Children's and adults' recall of television and print news in children's and adult news formats. *Communication Research*, *27*, 132–160.

Vorderer, P., & Ritterfeld, U. (2003). Children's future programming and media use between entertainment and education. In E. L. Palmer, & B. M. Young (Eds.), *Faces of televisual media: Teaching, violence, selling to children* (2nd edn., pp. 241–262). Mahwah, NJ: Lawrence Erlbaum Associates.

Waas, G. A., & French, D. C. (1989). Children's social problem solving: Comparison of the open middle interview and children's assertive behavior scale. *Behavioral Assessment*, *11*, 219–230.

Webster-Stratton, C. (1984). Randomized trial of two parent-training programs for families with conduct-disordered children. *Journal of Consulting and Clinical Psychology*, *52*, 666–678.

Webster-Stratton, C. (1990). Long-term follow-up of families with young conduct-problem children: From preschool to grade school. *Journal of Consulting and Clinical Psychology*, *19*, 1344–1349.

Webster-Stratton, C., & Hammond, M. (1990). Predictors of treatment outcome in parent training for families with conduct-problem children. *Behavior Therapy*, *21*, 319–337.

Webster-Stratton, C., & Hammond, M. (1997). Treating children with early-onset conduct problems: A comparison of child and parent training interventions. *Journal of Consulting and Clinical Psychology*, *65*, 93–109.

Webster-Stratton, C., Kolpacoff, M., & Hollinsworth, T. (1988). Self-administered videotape therapy for families with conduct-problem children: Comparison with two cost-effective treatments and a control group. *Journal of Consulting and Clinical Psychology*, *56*, 558–566.

Webster-Stratton, C., Reid, M. J., & Hammond, M. (2004). Treating children with early-onset conduct problems: Intervention outcomes for parent, child and teacher training. *Journal of Clinical Child and Adolescent Psychology*, *33*, 105–124.

Weersing, V. R., & Brent, D. A. (2003). Cognitive–behavioral therapy for adolescent depression: Comparative efficacy, mediation, moderation, and effectiveness. In A. E. Kazdin, & J. R. Weisz (Eds.), *Evidence-based psychotherapies for children and adolescents* (pp. 135–147). New York: Guilford.

Weich, K. E., & Quinn, R. E. (1999). Organizational change and development. In J. T. Spence, J. M. Darley, & D. J. Foss (Eds.), *Annual review of psychology* (Vol. 50, pp. 361–386). Palo Alto, CA: Annual Reviews.

Weiner, B. (1990). Attribution in personality psychology. In L. Pervin (Ed.), *Handbook of personality: Theory and research* (pp. 609–637). New York: Guilford.

Weiss, B., Caron, A., Ball, S., Tapp, J., Johnson, M., & Weisz, J. R. (2005). Iatrogenic effects of group treatment for antisocial youths. *Journal of Consulting and Clinical Psychology*, *73*, 1036–1044.

Weissman, M. M., Rounsaville, B. J., & Chevron, E. (1982). Training psychotherapists to participate in psychotherapy outcome studies. *American Journal of Psychiatry*, *139*, 1442–1446.

Weisz, J. R., Donenberg, G. R., Han, S. S., & Kauneckis, D. (1995a). Child and adolescent psychotherapy outcomes in experiments versus clinics: Why the disparity? *Journal of Abnormal Child Psychology*, *23*, 83–106.

Weisz, J. R., Donenberg, G. R., Han, S. S., & Weiss, B. (1995b). Bridging the gap between laboratory and clinic in child and adolescent psychotherapy. *Journal of Consulting and Clinical Psychology*, *63*, 688–701.

Williams, S. C., Lochman, J. E., Phillips, N. C., & Barry, T. D. (2003). Aggressive and nonaggressive boys' physiological and cognitive processes in response to peer provocations. *Journal of Clinical Child & Adolescent Psychology*, *32*, 568–576.

Wilpert, B. (1995). Organizational behavior. In J. T. Spence, J. M. Darley, & D. J. Foss (Eds.), *Annual review of psychology* (Vol. 46, pp. 59–90). Palo Alto, CA: Annual Reviews.

Youngstrom, E., Wolpaw, J. M., Kogos, J. L., Schoff, K., Ackerman, B., & Izard, C. (2000). Interpersonal problem solving in preschool and first grade: Developmental change and ecological validity. *Journal of Clinical Child Psychology*, *29*, 589–602.

64 Parenting Programs

Stephen Scott

Advice on how to rear children has been around for a long time. Socrates (435 BC) reports on how a girl should be brought up "so she might see, hear, and speak as little as possible"; both sexes should be brought up to be schooled in modesty and self-control, a girl's physique is designed for indoor work (childcare, breadmaking and woolworking), whereas a boy's was designed for outdoor activity (ploughing, planting and herding) so their rearing should be focused towards these skills. Thus, from early on we have a notion of raising children to function well in their future worlds, taking into account their characteristics. This is usually believed to be reasonably successful – in the Bible it is written "Train up a child in the way he should go: and when he is old, he will not depart from it" (Proverbs 22:6). However, the question is how best to do this: should one use plenty of physical chastisement "Spare the rod and spoil the child" (Samuel Butler, 1660); or should one believe in the virtue of rewards, "And he who gives a child a treat/makes joy-bells ring in Heaven's street" (John Masefield, 1908). Beliefs about how children should be raised vary enormously, within the same culture over time, and across differing cultures at any one time, including the present. Designing materials for parenting programs for disruptive children is not new; Jonathan Swift (1708) stated: "I conceived some scattered notions about a superior power to be of singular use for the common people, as furnishing excellent materials to keep children quiet when they grow peevish."

Because of the wide range of theoretical ideas about how children should be brought up, this chapter first reviews evidence concerning parenting styles in relation to child outcomes. Then programs based on attachment theory and social learning theory are described in detail, and their effectiveness reviewed. Finally, factors that affect their effectiveness are discussed, including what predicts outcome, what are the mechanisms of change and the role of therapist factors in making programs work.

Theoretical Basis

Theories Linking Parenting to Child Outcomes

Whereas many theories link parenting to child outcomes, two perspectives – attachment theory and social learning theory – have been especially influential in recent times and have led to rather different types of parenting programs. Attachment theory has led to interventions mainly for babies and infants, and social learning theory has led to interventions mainly for children from around 3 years upwards.

Attachment Theory

Attachment theorists (Ainsworth, Blehar, Waters, & Wall, 1978; Bowlby, 1969/1982; Cassidy & Shaver, 1999) developed a model of parent–child relationships from a broad theoretical base, including ethology, cognitive psychology and control systems (see chapter 55). Bowlby was particularly interested in identifying the nature, significance and function of a child's (or animal offspring's) tie to his or her parent. Although the theory had its roots in clinical observations of children who experienced severely compromised, disrupted or deprived caregiving arrangements, it has been applied as a model for normal and abnormal development. "Parent–child attachment" is not synonymous with "parent–child relationship" insofar as the former was conceptualized as being far more limited in scope. Attachment theory is concerned with fundamental issues of safety and protection; in psychological terms, attachment theory focuses on the extent to which the relationship provides the child with protection against harm and with a sense of emotional security or, to use the term made famous by Bowlby, a "secure base" for exploration. Many components of the parent–child relationship are not central to an attachment assessment, such as cognitive stimulation or discipline.

The theory proposes that the quality of care provided to the child, particularly sensitivity and responsiveness, leads to a secure or insecure attachment. Attachment theorists use the term "pathway" to make explicit that early attachment experiences do not shape subsequent development in a fixed deterministic manner (Bowlby, 1988). Insecure attachment is not synonymous with disturbance, and neither is a secure attachment a guarantee against disturbance. Indeed, long-term follow-up studies suggest that it is family relationships that are more important for child functioning than attachment insecurity *per se* (Grossman, Grossman, & Waters, 2005). However, we now know that a particular form of non-secure attachment in infants and young children termed "disorganized" is strongly related to risk for psychopathology and is a marker of particular risk in the caregiving environment (Greenberg, 1999; Lyons-Ruth, 1996), although it is important to note that it occurs in 15% or more of normal populations. Attachment

Rutter's Child and Adolescent Psychiatry, 5th edition. Edited by M. Rutter, D. Bishop, D. Pine, S. Scott, J. Stevenson, E. Taylor and A. Thapar. © 2008 Blackwell Publishing, ISBN: 978-1-4051-4549-7.

relationships are, it is suggested, internalized and carried forward to influence expectations for other important relationships, a process mediated by what Bowlby referred to as an "internal working model." A history of consistent and sensitive care with the parent is therefore expected to lead to the child developing a model of self and others as lovable and loving and helpful. Effective attachment-based interventions have been developed and validated for a range of clinical problems (Bakermans-Kranenburg, van Ijzendoorn, & Juffer, 2003; Cicchetti, Rogosch, & Toth, 2000).

Social Learning Theory

Social learning theory evolved from different roots in general learning theory and behaviorism (Bandura, 1977). Broadly put, the notion behind social learning theory is that children's real-life experiences and exposures directly or indirectly shape behavior; processes by which this learning occurs can be diverse. For many, there is a focus on traditional behavioral principles of reinforcement and conditioning, and so there is a near-exclusive focus on observed behavior (Patterson, 1969, 1996). The fundamental tenet is that moment-to-moment exchanges are crucial; if a child receives an immediate reward for their behavior, such as getting parental attention or approval, then they are likely to do the behavior again, whereas if they are ignored (or punished) then they are less likely to do it again. Other advocates of social learning models have expanded this focus to consider the cognitive or "mindful" processes such as attributions and expectations that underlie the parent's behavior (Bugental, Blue, & Cruzcosa, 1989; Dix, 1992) and its effects on children (Dodge, Pettit, Bates, & Valente, 1995). Thus, social learning theory can be applied to behavior, cognitions, or both. Whether the assessment and conceptual focus is on behavior or cognitions, the model suggests that children learn strategies about managing emotions, resolving disputes and engaging with others, not only from their experiences, but also from the way their own reactions were responded to. For younger children especially, the primary source of these experiences is in the context of the parent–child relationship and the family environment. Furthermore, children take these strategies and apply them to other settings, for example to relationships with peers and teachers. This means that there will be a carrying forward of the effects of parent–child relationships across setting and time.

Given its historical emphasis on altering negative, aggressive behavior in the child, social learning theory-based models of parenting traditionally emphasized the harmful effects of parent–child conflict, coercion and inconsistent discipline. The focus was on the extent to which children's aggressive behaviors were learned from and reinforced by parallel negative behaviors by the parents. More recently, social learning theory has explicitly incorporated positive dimensions of parenting as a way of promoting child positive behavior and affect, improving the pleasurable nature of parents' and children's interactions with one another, and providing a more positive and effective relationship context for parental disciplinary interventions (Gardner, 1987).

Research on social learning theory-based approaches to parenting interventions, especially as applied to antisocial children, is most closely associated with the work of Patterson (1969), founder of the Oregon Social Learning Center. Also influential was Hanf (1969), who developed play therapy based on rewarding child behavior through attention. Many leading current interventions directly incorporate social learning principles, notably the programs of McMahon and Forehand (2003), Brinkmeyer and Eyberg (2003), Forgatch and DeGarmo (1999) and Webster-Stratton (1981). Several interventionists expanded the social learning model to incorporate consideration of the parents' social setting that may contribute to poor parenting, including Wahler, Winkel, Peterson, and Morrison (1965), whose program recognized the particular needs of isolated "insular" mothers. They were instrumental in showing, with hard evidence, that "insular" mothers were harsher to their children on those days when the few other adults with whom they had contact – such as local government officials or their own mothers – had been rejecting of them.

Parenting Styles

There are many other theories of parenting, some with a considerable evidence base. One is mentioned here, as it has been influential, even though to date it has not led to specific interventions. This is what can broadly be described as the parenting styles approach, and is associated with the work of Baumrind (e.g., 1991) and elaborated by others (Hetherington, Henderson, & Reiss, 1999; Maccoby & Martin, 1983; Steinberg, Lamborn, Darling, Mounts, & Dournbusch, 1994).

Baumrind observed interactions between parents and young children. Several important dimensions of parenting were measured and repeatedly found in subsequent studies carried out by successive generations of researchers. Core dimensions were warmth (versus conflict or neglect) and control strategies. Parenting typologies were thus constructed from a cross of warmth/conflict and control: authoritative (high warmth, positive/assertive control, and in adolescence high expectations), authoritarian (low warmth, high conflict, and coercive, punitive control attempts), permissive (high warmth coupled with low control attempts) and neglectful/disengaged (low warmth and low control). These four typologies have proved to be surprisingly robust and have been repeatedly associated with child outcomes. Children and adolescents of authoritative parents are consistently found to be more prosocial, academically and socially competent, and less symptomatic. Children whose parents are described as authoritarian, permissive or disengaged show significantly worse outcomes, with children of authoritarian parents showing typically the most disturbed adjustment of the four parenting types. As discussed below, these associations may be in part brought about by child characteristics shaping parental responses, but nonetheless there are likely to be substantial parent to child effects. Although some parenting programs may make parents more authoritative, they have not been conceptualized in these terms – it would be interesting to see the effectiveness of a new program developed on these principles.

Evidence Linking Parenting to Child Psychopathology

Aggression, Conduct Disorder and Delinquency

The finding that parent–child relationship quality is associated with aggressive behavior, conduct disorder and delinquency is one of the most widely reported findings in the literature, repeatedly found in:

1 Large-scale epidemiological investigations, such as the Cambridge and Isle of Wight studies in the UK, and the Dunedin and Christchurch studies in New Zealand;

2 Intensive clinical investigations, such as the work of Patterson and colleagues; and

3 Numerous naturalistic studies of diverse samples using a mixture of methods (Denham, Workman, Cole *et al.*, 2000; Dodge, Pettit, Bates *et al.*, 1995; Dunn, Deater-Deckard, Pickering *et al.*, 1998; Gardner, Sonuga-Barke, & Sayal, 1999; Hetherington, Henderson, & Reiss, 1999; Kilgore, Snyder, & Lentz, 2000; Lyons-Ruth, 1996; Steinberg, Lamborn, Darling *et al.*, 1994). The sort of parenting behaviors associated with these outcomes are high criticism and hostility, harsh punishment, inconsistent discipline, low warmth, low involvement, low encouragement and poor supervision.

More recent research has begun to disentangle different aspects of parenting that may be associated with antisocial behavior; for example, after controlling for the effects of conflict in the relationship, the amount of warmth or type of control predict additional variance in externalizing problems (Fletcher, Steinberg, & Williams-Wheeler, 2004; Kerr & Stattin, 2000). The main take-home message is that several aspects of the parent–child relationship are important. An implication for parenting programs is that they should not be simplistic and focus only on one dimension of parenting. The connection between parent–child relationships and disruptive behavior holds for variation within the normal range as well as for clinical disturbance. That is so both for parenting (e.g., harsh parenting versus documented maltreatment) and child outcome (e.g., moderate aggression to conviction for minor and serious offenses; Lansford, Dodge, Pettit *et al.*, 2002; Patterson & Bank, 1989). An implication for parenting programs is that the same principles (albeit differently applied) are important for preventive work and less severe populations, and for "hard-end" cases.

Depression, Anxiety and Other Emotional Problems

Evidence supporting a link between quality of parent–child relationships and depression, anxiety and other emotional problems (e.g., somatic complaints, social withdrawal) is clear although weaker than that found for disruptive outcomes. Here again, the association is obtained from large-scale epidemiological investigations as well as clinical and normative developmental studies, and is evident in a range of samples and according to diverse methods (Dadds, Barrett, Rapee, & Ryan, 1996; Garber, Little, Hilsman, & Weaver, 1998; Wood, McLeod, Sigman, Hwang, & Chu, 2003). Just as it is the case for disruptive behavior, there is mounting evidence that individual variation in emotional symptoms is not specifically associated with a single dimension of the parent–child relationship. Low warmth and conflict are both reliably linked with depression and anxiety; however, the influence of control strategies is generally much weaker. Additionally, emotional symptoms in children are linked with overprotectiveness (Dadds, Barrett, Rapee *et al.*, 1996). Therefore, parenting programs for emotional symptoms, of which there are few, should probably address overinvolvement and autonomy granting.

Social Competence and Peer Relationships

Family–Peer Links

Evidence supporting a link between quality of relationships in the family and social competence – most commonly studied within peer relationships – is substantial and supported by both attachment and social learning approaches. Several studies from an attachment perspective demonstrate that the quality of child–parent attachment in infancy and early childhood predicts relationship quality with peers concurrently, although longitudinal associations are weak (Cassidy, Kirs, Scolton, & Parke, 1996; Moss, Rousseau, Parent, St-Laurant, & Saintonge, 1998; Sroufe, Egeland, & Carlson, 1999). In general, these studies show that, compared with children who were judged to have an insecure attachment relationship with parents, children with a secure attachment relationship are more likely to be rated as popular and accepted by their peers, and to be rated as having more prosocial skills which promote positive peer interactions (Greenberg, Siegel, & Leitch, 1983; Lieberman, Doyle, & Markiewicz, 1999).

In the social learning model, the connection between parenting and peer relationships is believed to be mediated by social cognitions and behavioral strategies (e.g., concerning the effectiveness of aggressive behavior) learned from interacting with parents. Social learning researchers and those adopting the parenting typology approach have also emphasized the importance of parental monitoring and control in preventing the child from developing affiliations with deviant peers and poor role models (Brown, Mounts, Lamborn, & Steinberg, 1993). Empirical research using the social learning approach has established linkages between parenting and peer relationships (Dishion, 1990; Petit, Dodge, & Brown, 1988; Vuchinich, Bank, & Patterson, 1992). A related approach proposes that social-cognitive capacities important for positive peer relationships, such as emotional understanding, perspective-taking and emotional regulation, are developed in the context of the early parent–child relationship and are carried forward or generalized to later social relationships, including those with peers (Carson & Parke, 1996; Dunn, 1992; Parke, MacDonald, Burks *et al.*, 1989).

There is some uncertainty as to which theoretical position is strongest or which dimensions of the parent–child relationship are most relevant. As with the areas noted above, existing models of parent–child relationships converge in expecting that optimal parent–child relationships would be strongly linked with social competence and positive peer relationships, and that multiple components of the relationship, including warmth, conflict, and control and monitoring, have an important role.

Again, parenting programs may be more likely to be successful if they attend to all these dimensions.

Impact of Abusive Parenting on Physiological Functioning

Rutter (1981) in his book *Maternal deprivation reassessed* concluded that it was not separation *per se* that necessarily was very harmful; rather, more important for child well-being was the quality of parenting that had preceded the separation, and in particular the quality of parenting and other experiences that then followed it. Research on animal models has illuminated some of the physiological concomitants of the stress that can arise from particular types of separation and poor parenting. For example, the work of Meaney and colleagues (Kaffman & Meaney, 2007) showed that after infant rats were separated from their mothers for short periods (less than 15 min) in the first 2 weeks of their lives, they showed much more marked rises in stress hormones (on the hypothalamic–pituitary–adrenal axis [HPA]), leading to sharp rises in cortisol in response to aversive stimuli, but that this overreactivity went back to normal after a few days. However, longer separations (3 h per day) during this period led to large and lasting over-reactivity to stress, physiologically with six-fold increases in adrenocorticotropic hormone (ACTH) and cortisol production a year later in response to a mildly aversive stress (a puff of air in the eye), and behaviorally with far greater fearfulness, emotional arousal and poorer sociability with other rats. The core component is likely not to be the separation, but the treatment of the infant rat on reunion by the mother, who largely ignores it, seldom licking or grooming it, and sometimes trampling over it.

Moreover, differences in physiological and behavioral responses to stress are not confined to cases of relatively extreme abuse. Amongst mother rats who have undisturbed access to their infants, there are marked differences in the prevalence of licking and grooming (L/G). Infants exposed to higher L/G grow up to have lower physiological reactivity, less fearful behavior and more prosocial behavior (Francis, Caldji, Champagne, Plotsky, & Meaney, 1999). This also affects brain growth, with offspring of high L/G mothers showing increased neural growth factors, specific receptors and cholinergic innervation of the hippocampus, which correlates with improved spatial learning and memory (Liu, Diorio, Day, Francis, & Meaney, 2000; Zhang, Chretien, Meaney, & Gratton, 2005); in contrast, pups of low L/G mothers show increased hippocampal cell death (apostosis). The mechanism is environmental because cross-fostering studies show that infants of low L/G mothers develop normally when reared by high L/G mothers (Caldji, Diorio, & Meaney, 2000). Various interventions can mitigate the effects of poor early rearing, including gentle handling by humans, provision of a more stimulating environment and even antidepressants. Each of these interventions was reasonably successful in both physiological and behavioral terms (Bredy, Humpartzoomian, Cain, & Meaney, 2003). Broadly similar findings apply to primates, who have more similar developmental trajectories to humans; they provide good models for examining how much is a result of genetic susceptibility and how much is due to rearing, and for examining gene–environment interactions in the development of psychopathology (Barr, Newman, Becker *et al.*, 2003).

These findings are likely to obtain for humans too. Thus, Nemeroff and colleagues found that, compared with controls, women who had a history of child maltreatment showed a six-fold increase in HPA axis reactivity to laboratory-induced stress (Heim, Newport, Bonsall, Miller, & Nemeroff, 2001). The child and adolescent literature is emerging (see chapter 28), but as yet there have been few studies.

These studies have implications for parenting programs. First, children who have experienced repeated deprivation and abuse are likely to be biologically affected. The emotional over-reactivity seen in some is not likely to be caused solely by learned habits in a background of typical physiology. Rather, some abused children may have been "set" to have far stronger reactions to stressors. This has implications for how they are seen, whether they are blamed for their reactions and may account for possible slowness to change behavior and "treatment resistance" compared with more appropriately raised children. Treatment implications are, compared with most children who had adequate parenting:

1 They need to be managed with understanding – reacting explosively in response to difficulties or frustrating situations may be far harder for them to control;

2 They should be managed in as calm and non-stressful a way as possible, to avoid setting off over-arousal with its concomitant outbursts of destructive aggression; and

3 They may take more learning trials to achieve goals, and may achieve less.

Second, the biological data suggest that prevention and early intervention may be even more important than previously appreciated, in that children are not, as it were "only" psychologically affected by poor early experiences that can then be "corrected" by psychological therapy, but rather their experience may have lasting physiological and brain effects (Heim, Newport, Bonsall *et al.*, 2001). Further research is now needed to determine the type, severity and duration of harmful experiences, how these interact with individual susceptibility and, crucially, how far early and later benign experiences and therapeutic interventions can modify not only behavioral responses, but also physiological responses. Helpful interventions worth investigating include biological and pharmaceutical ones in addition to psychosocial interventions.

Limitations of Parenting Effects on Child Outcomes and Psychopathology

Although there is increasing interest in the public and in government in promoting parent-based initiatives to improve the well-being of children, this is based on the assumption that improving parenting will lead to improvements in children's well-being. However, the link is not a straightforward unidirectional one of simple cause and effect. If this is not understood, then parenting programs will be expected to deliver more than is possible, and disappointment will follow. Concerns about these limitations have been expressed in no uncertain terms in some quarters. Thus, Scarr (1992) asserted that for most children, parenting had little influence on their outcomes. By this she meant that apart from abusive parenting, the new behavioral genetic research alluded to below was showing that most of the variability in children's outcomes was brought about by genetic factors, implying that so long as parenting was reasonable and "good enough," differences in children's developmental trajectories would be brought about by inherent factors. That parenting is not irrelevant is shown by the evidence of solid links provided in preceding sections, but it is nonetheless important to consider the limits of parenting effects.

Genetic Influences on Parenting

Genetically informed designs such as adoption studies can help tease out direction of effect. Parenting itself is not a purely socially determined activity. Results from several samples and methods show genetic mediation (Kendler & Baker, 2007; Neiderhiser, Reiss, Pedersen *et al.*, 2004). Parents who are monozygotic (MZ) twins report engaging in more similar patterns of child-rearing with their children than do parents who are dizygotic (DZ) twins; this is also true for directly observed, dynamic, moment to moment, close interchanges in the parent–child relationship (Plomin, Reiss, Hetherington, & Howe, 1994). This has implications for those interventionists who believe parenting behavior is entirely socially determined.

One consistent exception to the pattern of moderate to large genetic mediation of parent–child relationship quality is attachment. Studies of attachment in twins find similar rates of attachment security in MZ and DZ twins, suggesting only a small part is played by genetic factors in child attachment security (Bokhorst, Bakermans-Kranenburg, Fearon *et al.*, 2003; O'Connor & Croft, 2001). Why genetic factors in attachment security exert considerably less effect than for other aspects of parent–child relationship quality is not readily apparent, but it is a replicated finding.

Genetic designs can also help show environmental effects. In a unique "cross-fostering" study, in which adoptive parents of high and low socioeconomic status (SES) adopted children who were born into high and low SES families, Duyme, Dumaret, and Tomkiewicz (1999) found that low SES children adopted into high SES families exhibited a higher IQ than children who were adopted into low SES families, a difference of approximately 8 IQ points. By using a behavioral genetic "tool," these researchers have provided some of the strongest evidence that an improved home environment can indeed have a causal link with children's intellectual ability.

Broader Social Influences

There is a substantial covariation of risk factors in the child's environment, such as marital discord, lack of money and poor schools; the same may be so for protective factors. Studies that fail to account for these environmental risks may overestimate the importance of the link between parenting and child outcomes. Further, the same parenting practice may have different effects in different contexts. For example, Pettit, Bates, Dodge, and Meece (1999) reported that parental monitoring of a child (e.g., knowing who he or she is with and what he or she is doing) played a particularly important part in preventing delinquency in adolescents living in violent and high-risk neighborhoods. The effect of similar levels of monitoring in low-risk environments was less. Thus, the larger social context moderates the patterns of associations and likely causal processes that operate more proximally to the parent–child relationship.

A second example of research on contextualizing parenting focused on the child's temperament. Kochanska (1997) reported that, for temperamentally fearful children, gentle parental control was associated with optimal behavioral/emotional regulation whereas temperamentally more aggressive ("fearless") children required more firm control to achieve the same positive results. Other studies have similarly shown that children with difficult/irritable temperament may be less likely to develop behavioral problems under conditions of firm compared with lax or less restrictive control (Bates, Pettit, Dodge, & Ridge, 1998). Belsky (1997) has taken this view further in suggesting that children differ from one another in how susceptible they are to rearing influence. In his model, those children who are more irritable may be more susceptible to rearing influence. The implication for parenting programs is that they should not follow a "one size fits all children" rigid manualized approach, but rather should vary their recommendations according to child characteristics and the wider social context.

Influence of Child Characteristics on Parenting

The notion that there are "child effects" on parenting behavior is hardly new. Indeed, Bell and Harper's (1977) book summarized numerous studies of several types showing the myriad ways in which child characteristics shape the parenting they receive. Key child characteristics included gender, age, temperament and presence of physical or intellectual or behavioral disability. In one classic study, Anderson, Lytton, and Romney (1986) crossed parent–child dyads in which the child was antisocial with parent–child dyads in which the child was not antisocial. Observations of parent–child interactions across the mixed pairings demonstrated that parents of non-antisocial children exhibited increased negativity toward the antisocial child, but parents of the antisocial children did not exhibit elevated conflict toward the non-antisocial child. In other words, it appeared to be the child's behavior that was driving the interaction and not the parent's.

Another study used a longitudinal follow-up of a sample of adopted children (Croft, O'Connor, Keaveney *et al.*, 2001). When the parent–child interactions were observed at age 4, the researchers found that child developmental status, indexed by lower cognitive ability, was associated with lower levels of parental positive interactions and higher levels of parental negative behavior. Two years later, many of the children had shown a significant improvement in cognitive ability. However, this developmental catch-up was not predicted by earlier parenting;

instead, gains in the children's cognitive ability predicted positive changes in the parents' behavior between assessments.

Intervention strategies with children with disorders can illuminate child effects on parenting. Compared with other mothers, mothers of children with attention deficit/hyperactivity disorder (ADHD) exhibit more negative control and less warmth. However, giving children medication for ADHD leads to positive changes in their parents' behavior (Barkley, 1988). Thus, improvements in parenting behavior can be made without targeting the parent but merely improving children's behavior. As well as making the theoretical point that child characteristics affect parenting behavior, this process has practical implications. In families where a child is overwhelming their parents' parenting capacity, in addition to targeting parenting skills, changing child characteristics directly may also enable parenting to be better.

In summary, recent research suggests that parenting styles are to some extent genetically influenced; parenting effects will vary in their impact on the child according to the context in which they live; and children with different temperaments will elicit different parenting styles and will have different parenting needs. All these considerations have implications for parenting programs, including the need for a careful assessment prior to commencing treatment, which should then be tailored accordingly.

Programs for Infants Based on Attachment Theory

In the last decade or so, many new parenting programs have sprung up that directly use attachment theory. Some use it in a very focused way, whereas others use it more loosely and incorporate other concepts. The core notion is that parents should increase sensitive responding to provide a secure base. For a review of the effects of disrupted early attachments, see Dozier and Rutter (in press).

Content of Typical Programs

Focused interventions typically last 5–20 sessions and videotape mother–infant interactions and then replay them. During replay the idea of recognizing the infant's signals is brought out – in early stages, even if a mother is usually ignoring her infant, the therapist will try to find one bit of videotape where nonetheless she does respond. Perhaps the infant will smile and she will smile back, leading the infant to gurgle with pleasure. The therapist might say "Look, when he smiled you smiled back so warmly that he showed he loved it by gurgling!" In later sessions, when the mother's confidence has been gained (over 95% of participants are mothers, but the principle is the same for fathers or other carers), a less satisfactory piece of interaction may be examined. When a mother is not responding, the therapist can point this out, and ask "What was going through your mind at that moment?" This may elicit many interesting responses, from preoccupation with the mother's own needs or hassles ("I was wondering how to pay off my debt") to misperception of cues ("I thought he was trying to wind me up" said of a messy eater), to strong negative emotions arising from her past experience ("When he does that I think he's just like his father, who ruined my life"). The great strength of this approach is that:

1 It gives parents an accurate picture of what is actually happening (rather than just talking about their perception of their relationship with their infant, as in traditional parent–infant psychotherapies);

2 It enables them to see for themselves that when they change their behavior, this impacts on their infant;

3 It allows simultaneous exploration of the mother's mental state, so that mental blocks to more sensitive responding can be explored and often overcome.

Examples of focused programs include that by the Leiden group (Velderman, Bakermans-Kranenburg, Juffer *et al.*, 2006).

Broader attachment-based therapies have been developed for infants and children who have been abused and who may have been transferred to foster families. This provides an interesting context in which to apply attachment theory because by definition these children have experienced disruption of attachment figures, and almost always suffered abuse or neglect at their hands. These include the program devised by Dozier, Lindheim, and Acierman (2005), which is used with both birth and foster-parents. It lasts 10 sessions and is based on the following (empirically based) notions.

1 Like parents in intact families, foster-carers may have their own insecure (unresolved or dismissing) attachment representations which will predispose them to be insensitive to their foster-children, who will have elevated need in terms of disorganized attachment patterns. Dozier concludes that because of their states of mind, some carers may find that providing nurturance does not come naturally. Thus, the first goal of the intervention is to help foster-carers provide care even if it does not come naturally to them.

2 Infants in foster care often fail to elicit nurturance. Dozier's group showed that fostered children fail to elicit nurturance from carers who would normally provide it. For example, after falling from a chair, such an infant may turn away; even an autonomous mother might say "Oh, I'm glad you're OK" and tidy up the toys without picking the infant up and comforting him, as she would have had he shown distress. The intervention therefore aims to train foster-mothers to act in nurturing ways even in the absence of cues from the infant.

3 Abused infants are often poorly regulated at physiological, emotional and behavioral levels. This means they sleep poorly, often eat sporadically, show disruptive behavior and abnormal arousal patterns. The response by Dozier's group is to teach parents to follow the child's lead. Others might counsel that parents should stay especially calm so as not to over-arouse the child, be more patient and turn away from conflicts, but be quick to soothe the child and look assiduously for ways to do this.

4 Abused infants often have experienced threatening situations. This may lead them to cut off or dissociate or have other maladaptive interactions. Foster-parents are therefore trained to avoid being threatening, either emotionally through being angry, or by threatening the security of the relationship (e.g., saying they will return the child to social services). Other attachment-based programs include the Circle of Security program developed by Cooper, Hoffman, Powell, and Marvin (2005) for at-risk children in birth families.

All three programs mentioned so far use video-feedback. Other interventions that do not use video-feedback include that developed by Zeanah and Smyke (2005) for children who were severely deprived in institutions such as Romanian orphanages, and more lengthy and intensive psychodynamic ones such as that of Slade, Sadler, and Mayes (2005). Olds (2006), in contrast, developed a home visiting program delivered by nurses (Nurse–Family Partnership) that is not based on attachment theory but on systematic evaluation of and evidence-based interventions for risk factors from pregnancy onwards. Thus, parents are encouraged to reduce cigarette and alcohol consumption in pregnancy through understanding the effects on their babies; once the baby is born, parent–child interaction is coached, including how to stimulate the baby appropriately, and wider issues such as partner violence and further general education for the mother are addressed.

Effectiveness

There have been several trials for attachment-based approaches. The meta-analysis by Bakermans-Kranenburg, van Ijzendoorn, & Juffer (2003) found 81 studies with a total of over 7000 parent–infant pairs assessed. Overall, they improved parental sensitivity by 0.33 standard deviations (SD) and attachment security by 0.20 SD. However, there were large variations between approaches used. Perhaps surprisingly, the most effective interventions were relatively short (under 26 sessions) and started later (after the infant was 6 months). Both of these finding go against cherished notions that early intervention must be better, and that more effort should lead to more change (in fact, the mean effect size for long interventions was –0.03). However, were the findings true for disorganized attachment patterns, which carry a worse prognosis? A separate meta-analysis of this group again found the more focused interventions still worked better (Bakermans-Kranenburg, van Ijzendoorn, & Juffer, 2005). Was it the case that short interventions were not effective for multi-problem families? Again, this was not the case, the short interventions still worked better than long ones (effect size 0.48).

Possible reasons for these findings are that the short interventions focus more specifically on sensitive responding and mostly use video-feedback in a pragmatic behavioral way, rather than taking a more counseling or traditionally psychotherapeutic approach. Is it then the case that the longer interventions have a broader impact on a wider range of outcomes? There is rather limited information on this issue, but again the data do not appear to support this (van IJzendoorn, Bakermans-Kranenburg, & Juffer, 2005).

What about parenting programs that do not rely heavily on attachment theory? Some use a general notion that if the parents are supported, then they in turn will relate better to their infants. For example, in a trial of the home visiting program Homestart, which involved a mean of 97 h of face-to-face contact with mothers, none of the many mother or child variables measured changed (McAuley, Knapp, Beecham, McCurry, & Sleed, 2004); a similar lack of effectiveness was found for the Oxfordshire Home Visiting project (Barlow, Parsons, & Stewart-Brown, 2005). In contrast, interventions that focus precisely on specified risk factors, even when these are many, seem to fare much better. Thus, the Nurse–Family Partnership (NFP) approach has been evaluated in three randomized controlled trials involving over 1000 mother–infant pairs. This has shown benefits for the children in terms of improved cognitive and emotional development and fewer accidents and injuries, and for the mothers in terms of fewer harmful health behaviors (e.g., smoking) and higher take-up of further education, less use of public handouts and a longer interval until subsequent pregnancy (Olds, 2006). Interestingly, in the third NFP trial (in Denver), mothers were randomized to receive the program from volunteer paraprofessionals or nurses. Both were given the same amount of training in the program, but overall the paraprofessionals failed to change the child or parent outcomes, whereas the nurses did. The problems of making early parenting interventions work under field conditions rather than in university trials was underlined by Spieker, Nelson, Deklyen, and Staerkel (2005), who embedded a trial of video-feedback with high-risk mothers in a Head Start preventive program in the USA, but there were no changes in parenting or child attachment status.

Current Status of Attachment-based Interventions

A number of conclusions seem warranted. First, interventions that only offer "support" for parents do not appear to improve quality of parenting or child attachment status, even though they are appreciated by parents. Second, the more specifically focused interventions that target particular parental behaviors such as sensitive responding lead to greater effect sizes on parenting and child attachment status. Third, the same is true of interventions that target broader risk factors such as maternal alcohol intake and further education; those with specific goals that make use of previously tested methods are more effective than less focused interventions. Fourth, it seems likely that using more skilled staff leads to larger effects.

There are a number of unanswered questions that future studies could address. How important is increasing child attachment security, in itself? If the interventions only improve attachment security but not other outcomes, that will be of limited interest. Generally, long-term follow-up studies suggest that infants brought up in favorable circumstances who have insecure attachment patterns nonetheless do well in terms of later relationship quality and attainment, whereas those brought up with harsh parenting and disadvantaged circumstances do relatively poorly irrespective of attachment status (see summaries of the major longitudinal studies in Grossman, Grossman, & Waters, 2005). This is not to say that attachment patterns are not important, but rather to say that the research needs to broaden out to embrace other aspects of parent and child functioning.

Programs for Children Based on Social Learning Theory

Programs based on social learning theory have evolved over 40 years and there is a large evidence base. The vast majority are aimed at antisocial behavior as their proximal target outcome. The content and delivery of a typical program are shown in Table 64.1.

Most basic programs take 8–12 sessions lasting 1.5–2 h each. Full accounts of programs are given by the developers (e.g., *Triple P*, Markie-Dadds & Sanders, 2006; *Helping the Noncompliant Child*, McMahon & Forehand, 2003; *Parent–Child Interaction Therapy*, Brinkmeyer & Eyberg, 2003; *Defiant Children*, Mash & Barkley, 2006; and *The Incredible Years*, Webster-Stratton & Reid, 2003).

Format of a Typical Social Learning Program

A typical individual program might run as follows.

Part 1. Techniques for Promoting a Child-Centered Approach

The first session covers play. This is seen as a fundamental aspect of improving the relationship with the child. Parents are asked to follow the child's lead rather than impose their own ideas. Instead of giving directions, teaching and asking questions during play, parents are instructed simply to describe what the child is doing, to give a running commentary on their child's actions. The target is to give at least four of these "descriptive comments" per minute. If the parent has difficulty in getting going, the practitioner suggests precisely what they should do, for example by saying "I'd like you to say to Johnny 'You've put the car in the garage'." As soon as the parent complies, the practitioner gives feedback, "That was a good descriptive comment."

After 10–15 min, this directly supervised play ends and the parent is "debriefed" for half an hour or more alone with the clinician. How the parent felt during the session is explored, and reservations and difficulties that arose are addressed. Usually, the effect of their behavior on the child during the training session is soon observed by the parent. Experiencing this close non-judgmental attention is surprisingly powerful for children, who at best feel they are "the apple of their parent's eye." For cases where virtually all communication with the child has become nagging and complaining, play is an important first step in mending the relationship. It often helps the parent to have fun with the child and begin to have some positive feelings towards them. Parents are asked to practice these techniques for 10 min every day.

The second session involves elaboration of play skills. For the first 20 min, the previous week's "homework" of playing at home is gone over with the parent in considerable detail. Often there are practical reasons for not doing it ("I have to look after the other children" or "I've got no help") and parents are then encouraged to solve the problem and find ways around the difficulty. Solutions arrived at might include doing the play after the younger sibling has gone to bed or getting the oldest child to look after the baby while the parent plays with the toddler. For some parents there may be emotional blocks ("It feels wrong – no one ever played with me as a child") which need to be overcome before they feel able to practice the homework.

After this discussion, live practice with the child is carried out. This time the parent is encouraged to go beyond describing

Table 64.1 Features of effective social learning theory-based parenting programs.

Content
Structured sequence of topics, introduced in set order over 10–12 weeks
Curriculum includes play, praise, rewards, setting limits and discipline
Parenting seen as a set of skills to be deployed in the relationship
Emphasis on promoting sociable self-reliant child behavior and calm parenting
Constant reference to parent's own experience and predicament
Theoretical basis informed by extensive empirical research and made explicit
Plentiful practice, either live or role-played during sessions
Homework set to promote generalization
Accurate but encouraging feedback given to parent at each stage
Self-reliance prompted (e.g., through giving parents tip sheets or book)
Emphasis on parent's own thoughts and feelings varies from little to considerable
Detailed manual available to enable replicability
Delivery
Strong efforts made to engage parents (e.g., home visits if necessary)
Collaborative approach, typically acknowledging parents' feelings and beliefs
Difficulties normalized, humor and fun encouraged
Parents supported to practice new approaches during session and through homework
Parent and child can be seen together, or parents only seen in some group programs
Crèche, good-quality refreshments and transport provided if necessary
Therapists supervise regularly to ensure adherence and to develop skills

the child's behavior and to make comments describing the child's likely mood state (e.g., "You're really trying hard making that tower" or "That puzzle is making you really fed up"). This process has benefits for both the parent and the child. The parent gets better at observing the fine details of the child's behavior, which makes them more sensitive to the child's mood. The child gradually gets better at understanding and labeling their own emotional states, a crucial step in gaining self-control in frustrating situations.

Subsequent sessions follow the same pattern:

1 Reviewing the previous week's homework;
2 Direct training of interaction with the child; and
3 Discussion afterwards of how it went.

The speed at which the content is covered depends on progress. Later sessions cover the following ground.

Part 2. Increasing Acceptable Child Behavior

Praise and rewards are covered here. The parent is required to praise their child for lots of simple everyday behaviors such as playing quietly on their own, eating nicely, getting dressed the first time they are asked, and so on. In this way the frequency of desired behavior increases. However, many parents find this difficult. They may say "But he *should* be doing these things anyway, without being praised for it – there's really no need." When their child has misbehaved earlier in the day they are still cross, and this prevents them praising good behavior when it occurs. Some parents find that even when they want to praise their child, the whole process feels alien to them. Often, they never experienced praise themselves as a child. Usually, with directly coached practice, it becomes easier. Later sessions go through the use of reward charts.

Part 3. Setting Clear Expectations

Clear commands are covered next. A hallmark of ineffective parenting is a continuing stream of ineffectual nagging demands for the child to do something. In the program, parents are taught to reduce the number but make them much more authoritative. This is achieved through altering both the manner in which they are given, and what is said. The manner should be forceful (not sitting down, timidly requesting from the other end of the room; instead, standing over the child, fixing him in the eye and in a clear firm voice giving the instruction). The emotional tone should be calm, without shouting and criticism. The content should be phrased directly ("I want you to . . .") and not indirectly or as a question ("Wouldn't you like to . . ."). It should be specific, labeling the desired behavior which the child can understand, so it is clear to him when he has complied ("Keep the sand in the box") rather than vague ("Do be tidy"). It should be simple (one action at a time, not a chain of orders), and performable immediately. Commands should be phrased as what the parent *does* want the child to do, not as what he should *stop* doing ("Please speak quietly" rather than "Stop shouting"). If a child is in the middle of an activity, rather than abruptly ordering a stop, a warning should be given ("In two minutes you'll have to go to bed"). Rather than threatening the child with vague, dire consequences ("You're going to be sorry you did that"), *when–then* commands should be given ("When you've laid the table, then you can watch TV").

Part 4. Reducing Unacceptable Child Behavior

Consequences for disobedience are covered next. They should be applied as soon as possible. They must always be followed through – children quickly learn to calculate the probability they will be applied, and if a sanction is only given on every third occasion, a child is being taught he can misbehave the rest of the time. Simple logical consequences should be devised and enforced for everyday situations. If water is splashed out of the bath, the bath will end; if a child refuses to eat dinner, there will be no pudding. The consequences should "fit the crime," should not be punitive and should not be long-term (e.g., no bike riding for a month), as this will lead to a sense of hopelessness in the child, who may see no point in behaving well if it seems there is nothing to gain. Consistency of enforcement is central.

Ignoring is an important additional technique. This sounds easy but is a hard skill to teach parents. Whining, arguing, swearing and tantrums are not dangerous to children and other people and can usually safely be ignored. The technique is very effective. Children soon realize they are getting no pay-off for the behaviors and soon stop. Vice versa, if acting this way gets attention and shows them they can annoy and wind-up their parents, they will continue to hone their skills in so doing. Ignoring means avoiding discussion, avoiding eye-contact, turning away, but staying in the room to monitor. As soon as the child begins to behave appropriately, it is essential to attend and give praise. This is central to shaping up desirable behavior. Many parents find this difficult as they are often still angry with the child.

Time out from positive reinforcement remains the final "big one" as a sanction for unacceptable behavior. The point here is to put the child in some boring place away from a reasonably pleasant context. This will not be the case if the home is generally negative, when being sent to a room alone will be a relief and not a punishment. Equally, if the room has lots of interesting toys it will also not be a punishment. Time out should be for a previously agreed reason (hitting, breaking things – not minor infringements) for a short time (say 1 min for each year of age). However, the child must be quiet for the last minute – if he is still screaming, he stays in for as long as it takes until he's been quiet for a minute. Parents must resist responding to taunts and cries from the child during time out, as this will reinforce the child by giving attention. Time out provides a break for the adult to calm down too.

Part 5. Strategies for Avoiding Trouble

These include planning ahead to avoid troublesome times of day and situations, negotiating with the child how to accommodate their wishes while fitting in with the family goals, and developing a problem-solving approach with the child to promote independence, along the lines of problem-solving approaches taught directly by professionals to children (Kazdin, 2005).

Effectiveness of Social Learning Programs

Outcomes

Research has predominantly looked at children with antisocial behavior. This is a reasonable target because it indexes a wide range of poor outcomes, and because parenting is implicated as a major contributory factor (see review above, and chapter 35). A decade or so ago there was still a question as to whether parenting programs improved child antisocial behavior. Since then systematic reviews and meta-analyses of scores of studies usually with no-treatment controls have confirmed that they do indeed generally work well for children aged 3–10 (Lundahl, Nimer, & Parsons, 2006; Maughan, Denita, Christiansen *et al.*, 2005; McCart, Priester, Davies, & Azen, 2006; for a narrative review including comparison of individual versus group based studies see Scott, 2002). Mean effect sizes across studies vary from around 0.4 to 1.0 according to outcome, showing reasonably good effectiveness. The field has moved on to consider further questions, including comparison with active controls such as non-behavioral programs, investigation of predictors of treatment response and mechanisms of change.

Comparison with Non-behavioral Programs

There have been a number of head-to-head comparisons of non-behavioral humanistic approaches with behavioral programs, although most trials have been on relatively well-functioning volunteer samples. Humanistic approaches are usually based on the notion that supporting the parent in a non-judgmental accepting way will make them feel better and parent more effectively. Pinsker and Geoffrey (1981) compared a behavioral group with a humanistic approach, Parent Effectiveness Training (PET). On parent report, the behavioral group showed a significant reduction in child problem behavior whereas PET and controls did not; on direct observation, both treatment groups did better than controls. Bernal, Kinnert, and Schultz (1980) compared a client-centered group with behavioral management and waitlist controls, and found on parent report the behavioral group did better than the other two, but on direct observation no group changed. With a clinical sample, Nichol, Smith, Kay *et al.* (1988) studied families referred by local social services for active physical abuse and allocated them to individual play therapy for the child plus support from social worker for the mother, or home-based work that offered parent training plus parent support through casework. Parent training led to a greater reduction in parental coerciveness and aversive behavior towards their children, measured using direct observation. In summary, behaviorally based programs appear to improve child outcomes more reliably.

What Makes Parenting Programs Work?

Predictors and Moderators of Outcome

In a controlled trial, if a characteristic of the participants such as child age or severity of symptoms predicts outcome in both the intervention and control groups, then it is a predictor. However, if after allowing for this there is additionally an interaction with treatment, so that one subgroup (say, younger children) do better than another (older children) in the intervention group only, then the characteristic is operating as a moderator. Until recently, analyses have mainly been at the level of predictors only, with one or two exceptions. A number of predictors have been identified.

Child Age and Gender

Clinicians often gain the impression that boys and older children, especially adolescents, do worse. Indeed, adolescents are generally found to do less well in parenting programs for antisocial behavior. Bank, Marlowe, Reid, Patterson, and Weinrott (1991) found a far smaller effect size when using parent training with adolescents than with younger children at the same institution. More generally, the meta-analyses of interventions for antisocial behavior and juvenile delinquency (see chapter 68) find that their effectiveness was considerably smaller than parent-training studies on younger children. However, studies on adolescents generally have the most severe, persistent cases. When cases of similar severity are compared directly, there is no age effect; Ruma, Burke, and Thompson (1996) compared response to treatment using the parent Child Behavior Checklist (CBCL) score for groups in early childhood (2–5 years), middle childhood (6–11 years) and adolescence (12–16 years). The adolescent group did slightly less well, but the difference disappeared on multiple regression analysis, which showed that greater initial severity was the only significant predictor of poorer response. Within the prepubertal age group, Dishion and Patterson (1992) had expected to find parent training more effective for younger (2.5–6.5 years) than older children (6.5–12.5 years) assessed by direct observation. However, they found it was of similar effectiveness for both age groups, a finding replicated by Beauchaine, Webster-Stratton, and Reid (2005). The meta-analysis by Serekitch and Dumas (1996) found that across 36 studies (not within them), effectiveness was greater in older children, within the range 3–10 years.

In summary, it appears that age is not a clear determinant of outcome. Naturally, in adolescence different approaches are needed, with more emphasis on negotiation, and close supervision when the young person is out of the house, but the belief that adolescents are inevitably very difficult to change is not supported by the evidence. Likewise, boys are as likely to improve as girls (Beauchaine, Webster-Stratton, & Reid, 2005; Scott, 2005). There is therefore room for some optimism when treating adolescents, so long as evidence-based approaches are skillfully applied.

Child Psychopathology

The meta-analysis by Reyno and McGrath (2006) found that more severe initial antisocial behavior predicted less change, but this was a bivariate association with no controlling for related factors such as family adversity. In contrast, taking such factors into account, Scott, 2005) found the opposite: those with higher initial levels improved more. Further studies that address this issue using multivariate statistics are needed. Child ADHD generally predicts a less good response (MTA

Cooperative Group, 1999; Scott, 2005), although some investigators find it is no bar to improvement (Beauchaine, Webster-Stratton, & Reid, 2005). The MTA study is informative about possible mechanisms, because direct observations of the parents in the psychological treatment-only arm showed that they had changed their behavior, whereas using the same measure, child ADHD symptoms did not (Wells, Chi, Hinshaw *et al.*, 2006). This would suggest that it is the characteristics of the child with ADHD that make them less sensitive to change, rather than alternative mechanisms such as, say, the parents themselves having ADHD so not implementing more effective parenting practices. In contrast, when studied, comorbid anxiety appears to predict better treatment response (Beauchaine, Webster-Stratton, & Reid, 2005).

Family Factors

Demographic indicators such as single parenthood, lower maternal education, lower family income and larger family size have all been found to have a small but negative effect on outcomes (Reyno & McGrath, 2006). Most studies find that parental psychopathology, especially maternal depression, predicts worse outcomes, as do life events and harsher initial parenting practices (Reyno & McGrath, 2006). Doolan (2006) found that for mothers with the most negative beliefs about their children (especially when they felt persecuted by them), their children's behavior did not change at all. The implications of how programs may be modified to take into account these findings are discussed below. For a review of how parenting programs have been developed to address difficulties that prevent change in parenting, such as discordant partner relationships, depression and substance abuse, see Scott (2002).

Mediators of Change

In recent years, researchers have begun to investigate what mediates outcome, as recommended by Rutter (2005). To mediate treatment outcome:

1 The treatment has to change outcome;
2 Treatment has to change the mediator;
3 The mediator has to correlate with outcome; and
4 The effect of treatment on outcome has to reduce or disappear after controlling for the mediator (Baron & Kenny, 1986; Kraemer, Wilson, Fairburn, & Agras, 2002).

In other words, the treatment does not work unless it changes the mediator. It would seem likely that for parenting programs to change child behavior, some aspect of parenting would first have to change. This is worth testing as it might not be the case – for example, the parenting program could make a couple realize that they should, say, stop arguing in front of their child, but still spend the same amount of time in play and joint activities and use the same disciplinary strategies; or the parenting might stay the same but as a result of the program, the parents may have changed the child's school. These wider aspects of a child's world are typically not measured in parenting intervention studies.

Beauchaine, Webster-Stratton, & Reid (2005) found that changes in critical, harsh and ineffective parenting both predicted and mediated child change in antisocial behavior. Similarly, Tein, Irwin, MacKinnon, and Wolchik (2004) found that parental discipline and mother–child relationship quality mediated reduction in antisocial behavior in post-divorce children, whereas Gardner, Burton, and Klimes (2006) found that positive parenting also mediated change. In adolescents, there have been two high-quality studies. Eddy and Chamberlain (2000) investigated mediators of change in seriously antisocial adolescents (average 13 police contacts at age 15) looked after by specially trained foster-parents. They found that all three measured parenting constructs mediated change, namely effectiveness of discipline (fairness, punitiveness, use of positive reinforcement); quality of supervision (youth reports of supervision and of doing things the foster-parent did not know about, difference between fosterer's and youth's accounts of problem behavior, percentage of time spent by youth in the presence of an adult); and an overall positive adult–youth relationship (how much they liked each other). Additionally, the amount of time spent with deviant peers including the degree of their influence also mediated outcome. Taken together, these four factors accounted for 32% of variance in subsequent antisocial behavior – a substantial amount. Similarly, Huey, Henggeler, Brondino, and Pickrel (2000) in a trial of multisystemic therapy for delinquency showed that a positive relationship and firm discipline mediated outcome, and good supervision mediated deviant peer association, which in turn mediated subsequent antisocial behavior. Recent studies are beginning to investigate the extent to which parental beliefs, rather than just behavior, need to change – Doolan (2006) found that improvement in the positive view of the child mediated reduction in antisocial behavior.

These studies have moved the field on, because they indicate not just which dimensions are associated with antisocial behavior in longitudinal studies, nor baldly whether treatment works, but rather show which variables need to change for a good outcome, thus helping to understand how treatment works (Rutter, 2005). This is turn has led to changes in programs. Thus, there is now a much stronger emphasis on preventing deviant peer association – for example, the Oregon Social Learning Center (OSLC) foster program penalizes youth for every minute they cannot verifiably account for their where-abouts. Future program modifications may include specifically cognitive elements to address negative cognitions that appear to stop change occurring (Sanders, Pidgeon, Gravestock *et al.*, 2004).

Future studies will need to take measures of mediators at several time points, to determine the sequence of changes – to answer, for example, whether parenting must change before child behavior can change; whether all aspects of the parenting relationship need to change to get most child improvement, or just those that are poorly practiced; how much parenting change is necessary for child change to occur; and what systematic interactions are there between parenting styles and child psychopathology that could inform how best to improve outcomes.

Dissemination: The Role of Therapist Skill

Many of the cited trials have taken place in university clinics run by highly motivated originators of programs, who supervise carefully chosen therapists intensively in demonstration projects. In the meta-analysis of child psychotherapy trials by Weisz, Donenberg, and Han (1995) those conducted in university clinics had a large mean effect size of 0.7 SD. In stark contrast, all the clinic-based studies reviewed since 1950 did not have any significant effects. This has enormous implications for service delivery, as it is of little use if interventions do not work under "real-life" conditions. Reasons postulated include:

1 Children with comorbid conditions are typically excluded from trials;

2 Therapists in trials deliver evidence-based programs for the condition under study only, whereas in real life therapists see many diverse conditions and do not deliver evidence-based programs – they have to be "jacks of all trades" (and so perhaps "masters of none");

3 Even where therapists in everyday clinics do deliver evidence-based approaches, they do not receive good quality ongoing supervision.

Therefore, for a therapeutic approach to be considered useful, findings need to be replicated in ordinary clinical settings by therapists who are part of the routine service and independent of the program originator. Weisz noted that fewer than 1% of published child psychotherapy trials met all three of the following criteria:

1 Carried out by teams independent of the program developer;

2 Delivered by clinicians employed in regular clinical practice; and

3 Used clinically referred children as participants.

To address these concerns Scott, Spender, Doolan, Jacobs, and Aspland (2001) carried out a trial of Webster-Stratton's Incredible Years program on regular clinical referrals for severe conduct problems (98th percentile), most of whom had comorbid ADHD (mean hyperactivity percentile 90th). Therapists were local clinicians given additional training. Despite these constraints, the effect size was large (over 1 SD) and maintained 1 year after the end of treatment (Scott, 2005). The authors suggested that the effectiveness was related to having skilled staff who, despite having regular clinical jobs, made time to come to supervision each week, when videotapes of practice were examined and alternative therapeutic approaches rehearsed. This approach to supervision is in contrast to traditional supervision, where therapists recount what they think went on, and are given advice.

Therapist Variables

Therapist performance can be divided into the following:

1 The *alliance*, which could be defined as how well, both personally and collaboratively, client and therapist get on together;

2 *Fidelity* or adherence to specific components of a model, which concerns the extent to which the therapist follows the actions prescribed in the manual;

3 The *skill* or competence with which the therapist carries out the tasks (i.e., how well the therapist performs the actions).

A meta-analysis of youth studies of the alliance found it contributed on average an effect size of 0.21 SD to outcome; this held across treatment types, and across youth, parent and family approaches (Shirk & Carver, 2003). Kazdin, Whitley, and Marciano (2006) found about 7% of the variance in outcome of treatment for antisocial children was related to the alliance, although findings varied by informant.

Given the importance of these qualities that are therapy type independent, does it matter what the warm and genuine therapist who makes a strong alliance does during the sessions? One might expect fidelity would be central, because if the "wrong" therapy is given, it should be less effective. However, studies are somewhat equivocal, thus Henggeler, Melton, Brondino, Scherer, and Hanley (1997) compared a total of 15 parent, therapist and youth-rated fidelity scales with seven youth outcomes in a trial of multisystemic therapy, and found statistically significant effects for only 11 out of 105 associations. The same group (Huey, Henggeler, Brondino *et al.*, 2000) found that when they used a latent variable approach, therapist-rated fidelity improved family functioning and parent monitoring, both of which in turn reduced youth delinquency, but that parent- and youth-rated fidelity had no effect. This last finding could be because it requires a therapist to appreciate the complexity of fidelity, and also because therapists working across cases will be more consistent in their ratings than parents and youths, who may differ widely in their rating of the same phenomena.

These somewhat modest findings for the role of adherence or fidelity raise the question whether applying the treatment according to the manual is necessary or sufficient to bring about change. Often adherence and fidelity ratings concern the extent to which certain actions specific to the therapy were carried out, such as following sequences as laid down in the manual during sessions, using certain questioning techniques, issuing homework, and so on.

It is possible that a more important and relevant influence on effectiveness is the skill or competence with which these tasks are carried out. Thus, for example, two therapists running a parenting group might to the same extent discuss punishment, explore parents' beliefs, teach time out as an alternative to spanking, rehearse it and issue homework. However, the more skilled one might do this in a more sensitive way with greater complexity, and so characterize the client's mental state more accurately and be more proficient in overcoming barriers to rehearsal and homework, thus leading to more change. Supporting this notion, Forgatch, Patterson, and DeGarmo (2005) developed an observer-based instrument to assess therapist variables which included skill in a parenting program for recently divorced parents. They measured knowledge, structure, teaching skill, clinical skill and overall effectiveness. The outcome assessed was the proximal one of observed parenting practices, rather than child behavior; greater therapist skill led to more change in parenting. Likewise, in their trial under regular clinical conditions described above, Scott, Carby, & Rendu (2006a) found that therapist skill had a large effect on child outcomes; the worst therapist made outcomes slightly worse. If replicated, these findings have major implications for service delivery, because they suggest that at least for multiproblem clinical cases, a high level of therapist skill is required; staff training will need to reflect this.

Conclusions

Parenting programs have developed considerably in recent years. The best now incorporate modern empirical findings from developmental studies and use these to alter dimensions of parenting shown to improve specified child outcomes. Future developments may include better assessments of parenting so that programs can be tailored to specific needs rather than "one size fits all." Studies are needed of the mechanisms that mediate changes in parenting behavior; for example, whether is it necessary for parental beliefs about the child to change, or whether it is sufficient for parents to learn better habits. Then how changes in parenting mediate child change and interact with different types of child temperament and behavior problems needs clarifying. Finally, how therapy works and the degree of therapist skill needed to bring about change are beginning to be worked out. Future studies will be able to help service delivery by elucidating which families can improve sufficiently using computer-based self-instruction, allowing scarce resources to be targeted on those who most need them.

References

Ainsworth, M. D. S., Blehar, M. C., Waters, E., & Wall, S. (1978). *Patterns of attachment: A psychological study of the Strange Situation*. Hillsdale, NJ: Erlbaum.

Anderson, K. E., Lytton, H., & Romney, D. M. (1986). Mothers' interactions with normal and conduct-disordered boys: Who affects whom? *Developmental Psychology*, *22*, 604–609.

Bakermans-Kranenburg, M. J., van Ijzendoorn, M. H., & Juffer, F. (2003). Less is more: Meta-analyses of sensitivity and attachment interventions in early childhood. *Psychological Bulletin*, *129*, 195–215.

Bakermans-Kranenburg, M. J., van Ijzendoorn, M. H., & Juffer, F. (2005). The importance of parenting in the development of disorganized attachment: Evidence from a preventive intervention study in adoptive families. *Journal of Child Psychology and Psychiatry*, *46*, 263–274.

Bandura, A. (1977). *Social learning theory*. New York: General Learning Press.

Bank, L., Marlowe, J. H., Reid, J. B., Patterson, G. R., & Weinrott, M. R. (1991). A comparative evaluation of parent-training interventions for families of chronic delinquents. *Journal of Abnormal Child Psychology*, *19*, 15–33.

Barkley, R. A. (1988). Child behavior rating scales and checklists. In R. Rutter, A. H. Tuma, & I. S. Lann (Eds.), *Assessment and diagnosis in child psychopathology* (pp. 113–155). New York: Guilford Press.

Barlow, J., Parsons, J., & Stewart-Brown, S. (2005). Preventing emotional and behavioral problems: The effectiveness of parenting programmes with children less than 3 years of age. *Child: Care, Health and Development*, *31*, 33–42.

Baron, R., & Kenny, D. (1986). The moderator–mediator variable distinction in social psychological research: Conceptual, strategic, and statistical considerations. *Journal of Personality and Social Psychology*, *51*, 1173–1182.

Barr, C. S., Newman, T. K., Becker, M. L., Parker, C., Champoux, M., Lesch, K. P., *et al.* (2003). The utility of the non-human primate model for studying gene by environment interactions in behavioral research. *Genes, Brain and Behavior*, *2*, 336–340.

Bates, J. E., Pettit, G. S., Dodge, K. A., & Ridge, B. (1998). Interaction of temperament resistance to control and restrictive parenting in the development of externalizing behavior. *Developmental Psychology*, *34*, 982–995.

Baumrind, D. (1991). Effective parenting during the early adolescent transition. In P. Cowan, & E. M. Hetherington (Eds.), *Family transitions* (pp. 111–163). Hillsdale, NJ: Erlbaum.

Beauchaine, T. P., Webster-Stratton, C., & Reid, M. J. (2005). Mediators, moderators and predictors of 1-year outcomes among children treated for early-onset problems: A latent growth curve analysis. *Journal of Consulting and Clinical Psychology*, *75*, 371–388.

Bell, R. Q., & Harper, L. V. (1977). *Child effects on adults*. Lincoln, NE: University of Nebraska Press.

Belsky, J. (1997). Theory testing, effect-size evaluation, and differential susceptibility to rearing influence: the case of mothering and attachment. *Child Development*, *68*, 598–600.

Bernal, M. E., Klinnert, M. D., & Schultz, L. A. (1980). Outcome evaluations of behavioral parent training and client-centered parent counseling for children with conduct problems. *Journal of Applied Behavior Analysis*, *13*, 677–691.

Bokhorst, C. L., Bakermans-Kranenburg, M. J., Fearon, R. M., van Ijzendoorn, M. H., Fonagy, P., & Schuengel, C. (2003). The importance of shared environment in mother-infant attachment security: a behavioral genetic study. *Child Development*, *74*, 1769–1782.

Bowlby, J. (1969). *Attachment and loss*. Vol. 1. *Attachment*. New York: Basic Books.

Bowlby, J. (1988). Developmental psychiatry comes of age. *American Journal of Psychiatry*, *145*, 1–10.

Bredy, T. W., Humpartzoomian, R. A., Cain, D. P., & Meaney, M. J. (2003). Partial reversal of the effect of maternal care on cognitive function through environmental enrichment. *Neuroscience*, *118*, 571–576.

Brinkmeyer, M. Y., & Eyberg, S. M. (2003). Parent–child interaction therapy for oppositional children. In A. E. Kazdin, & J. R. Weisz (Eds.), *Evidence-based psychotherapies for children and adolescents* (pp. 204–223). New York: Guilford.

Brown, B. B., Mounts, N., Lamborn, S. D., & Steinberg, L. (1993). Parenting practices and peer group affiliation in adolescence. *Child Development*, *64*, 467–482.

Bugental, D. B., Blue, J. B., & Cruzcosa, M. (1989). Perceived control over caregiving outcomes: Implications for child abuse. *Developmental Psychology*, *25*, 532–539.

Butler, Samuel. (1660). *Hudibras*. Cited in *The Oxford dictionary of quotations* (3rd edn., line 844). 1986. Oxford: Oxford University Press.

Caldji, C., Diorio, J., & Meaney, M. J. (2000). Variations in maternal care in infancy regulate the development of stress reactivity. *Biological Psychiatry*, *48*, 1164–1174.

Carson, J. L., & Parke, R. D. (1996). Reciprocal negative affect in parent–child interactions and children's peer competency. *Child Development*, *67*, 2217–2226.

Cassidy, J., Kirsh, S. J., Scolton, K. L., & Parke, R. D. (1996). Attachment and representations of peers relationships. *Developmental Psychology*, *32*, 892–904.

Cassidy, J., & Shaver, P. (Eds.). (1999). *Handbook of attachment*. New York: Guilford.

Cicchetti, D., Rogosch, F. A., & Toth, S. L. (2000). The efficacy of toddler–parent psychotherapy for fostering cognitive development in offspring of depressed mothers. *Journal of Abnormal Child Psychology*, *28*, 135–148.

Cooper, G., Hoffman, K., Powell, B., & Marvin, R. (2005). In The Circle of Security Intervention L. J. Berlin, Y. Ziv, L. M. Amaya-Jackson, & M. T. Greenberg (Eds.), *Enhancing early attachment: Theory, research, intervention and policy*. New York, London: Guilford Press (pp. 127–151).

Croft, C. M., O'Connor, T. G., Keaveney, L., Groothues, C., & Rutter. M., and the English and Romanian Adoptee study team. (2001). Longitudinal change in parenting associated with developmental delay and catch-up. *Journal of Child Psychology and Psychiatry*, *42*, 649–659.

Dadds, M. R., Barrett, P. M., Rapee, R. M., & Ryan, S. (1996). Family process and child anxiety and aggression: An observational analysis. *Journal of Abnormal Child Psychology*, *24*, 715–734.

Denham, S. A., Workman, E., Cole, P. M., Weissbrod, C., Kendziora, K. T., & Zahn-Waxler, C. (2000). Prediction of externalizing behavior problems from early to middle childhood: The role of parental socialization and emotion expression. *Development and Psychopathology*, *12*, 23–45.

Dishion, T. (1990). The family ecology of boys' peer relations in middle childhood. *Child Development*, *61*, 874–892.

Dishion, T. J., & Patterson, G. R. (1992). Age effects in parent training outcome. *Journal of Behavior Therapy*, *23*, 719–729.

Dix, T. (1992). Parenting on behalf of the child: Empathic goals in the regulation of responsive parenting. In E. Sigel, A. V. McGillicuddy-Delisi, & J. J. Goodnow (Eds.), *Parental belief systems: The psychological consequences for children* (2nd edn., pp. 319–346). Hillsdale, NJ: Erlbaum.

Dodge, K. A., Pettit, G. S., Bates, J. E., & Valente, E. (1995). Social information-processing patterns partially mediate the effect of early physical abuse on later conduct problems. *Journal of Abnormal Psychology*, *104*, 632–643.

Doolan, M. (2006). Mothers' care giving appraisals and emotional valence representations of their young children with antisocial behaviour and their role in treatment outcome. PhD Thesis, King's College London.

Dozier, M., Lindheim, O., & Acierman, J. P. (2005). In Attachment and Biobehavioral catch-up: an intervention targeting empirically identified needs of foster children L. J. Berlin, Y. Ziv, L. M. Amaya-Jackson, & M. T. Greenberg (Eds.), *Enhancing early attachment: Theory, research, intervention and policy* (pp. 178–194). New York, London: Guilford Press.

Dozier, M., & Rutter, M. (in press). Challenges to the development of attachment relationships faced by young children in foster and adoptive care. In J. Cassidy, & P. Shaver (Eds.), *Handbook of attachment* (2nd edn.). New York: Guilford Press.

Dunn, J. (1992). *Young children's close relationships: Beyond attachment*. Newbury Park, CA: Sage.

Dunn, J., Deater-Deckard, K., Pickering, K., O'Connor, T. G., & Golding, J., and the ALSPAC Study Team. (1998). Children's adjustment and prosocial behavior in step-, single, and nonstep-family settings: Findings from a community study. *Journal of Child Psychology and Psychiatry*, *39*, 1083–1095.

Duyme, M., Dumaret, A. C., & Tomkiewicz, T. C. (1999). How can we boost IQs of "dull children"?: A late adoption study. *Proceedings of the National Academy of Sciences of the USA*, 96, 8790–8794.

Eddy, M. J., & Chamberlain, P. (2000). Family management and deviant peer association as mediators of the impact of treatment condition on youth antisocial behavior. *Journal of Consulting and Clinical Psychology*, *68*, 857–863.

Fletcher, A. C., Steinberg, L., & Williams-Wheeler, M. (2004). Parental influences on adolescent problem behavior: Revisiting Stattin and Kerr. *Child Development*, *75*, 781–796.

Forgatch, M., & DeGarmo, D. S. (1999). Parenting through change: An effective prevention program for single mothers. *Journal of Consulting and Clinical Psychology*, *67*, 711–724.

Forgatch, M. S., Patterson, G. R., & DeGarmo, D. S. (2005). Evaluating fidelity: Predictive validity for a measure of competent adherence to the Oregon model of parent management training. *Behavior Therapy*, *36*, 3–13.

Francis, D. D., Caldji, C., Champagne, F., Plotsky, P. M., & Meaney, M. J. (1999). The role of corticotrophin-releasing factor–norepinephrine systems in mediating the effects of early experience on the development of behavioral and endocrine responses to stress. *Biological Psychiatry*, *46*, 1153–1166.

Garber, J., Little, S., Hilsman, R., & Weaver, K. R. (1998). Family predictors of suicidal symptoms in young adolescents. *Journal of Adolescence*, *21*, 445–457.

Gardner, F. M. E. (1987). Positive interaction between mothers and conduct-problem children: Is there training for harmony as well as fighting? *Journal of Abnormal Child Psychology*, *15*, 283–293.

Gardner, F., Burton, J., & Klimes, I. (2006). Randomised controlled trial of a parenting intervention in the voluntary sector for reducing child conduct problems: outcomes and mechanisms of change. *Journal of Child Psychology and Psychiatry*, *47*, 1123–1132.

Gardner, F. E., Sonuga-Barke, E. J., & Sayal, K. (1999). Parents anticipating misbehaviour: An observational study of strategies parents use to prevent conflict with behaviour problem children. *Journal of Child Psychology and Psychiatry*, *40*, 1185–1196.

Greenberg, M. T. (1999). Attachment and psychopathology in childhood. In J. Cassidy, & P. Shaver (Eds.), *Handbook of attachment* (pp. 469–496). New York: Guilford.

Greenberg, M. T., Siegel, J. M., & Leitch, C. J. (1983). The nature and importance of attachment relationships to parents and peers during adolescence. *Journal of Youth and Adolescence*, *12*, 373–386.

Grossman, K. E., Grossman, K., & Waters, E. (2005). *Attachment from infancy to adulthood: The major longitudinal studies*. New York, London: Guilford Press.

Hanf, C. (1969). *A two stage program for modifying maternal controlling during mother-child (M-C) interaction*. Vancouver, British Columbia: Western Psychological Association.

Heim, C. D., Newport, D. J., Bonsall, R., Miller, A. H., & Nemeroff, C. B. (2001). Altered pituitary–adrenal axis responses to provocative challenge tests in adult survivors of childhood abuse. *American Journal of Psychiatry*, *158*, 575–581.

Henggeler, S. W., Melton, G. B., Brondino, M. J., Scherer, D. G., & Hanley, J. H. (1997). Multisystemic therapy with violent and chronic juvenile offenders and their families: The role of treatment fidelity in successful dissemination. *Journal of Consulting and Clinical Psychology*, *65*, 821–833.

Hetherington, E. M., Henderson, S., & Reiss, D. (1999). Family functioning and adolescent adjustment of siblings in nondivorced families and diverse types of stepfamilies. *Monographs of the Society for Research in Child Development*, *64*, 4, Serial no. 259.

Huey, S. J., Henggeler, S. W., Brondino, M. J., & Pickrel, S. G. (2000). Mechanisms of change in multisystemic therapy: Reducing delinquent behavior through therapist adherence and improved family and peer functioning. *Journal of Consulting and Clinical Psychology*, *68*, 451–467.

Kaffman, A., & Meaney, M. (2007). Neurodevelopmental sequelae of postnatal maternal care in rodents: Clinical and research implications of molecular insights. *Journal of Child Psychology and Psychiatry*, *48*, 224–244.

Kazdin, A. E. (2005). *Parent management training*. New York: Oxford University Press.

Kazdin, A. E., Whitley, M., & Marciano, P. L. (2006). Child–therapist and parent–therapist alliance and therapeutic change in the treatment of children referred for oppositional, aggressive, and antisocial behavior. *Journal of Child Psychology and Psychiatry*, *47*, 436–445.

Kendler, K. S. & Baker, J. H. (2007). Genetic influence on measures of the environment: A systematic review. *Psychological Medicine*, *37*, 615–626.

Kerr, M., & Stattin, H. (2000). What parents know, how they know it, and several forms of adolescent adjustment: further support for a reinterpretation of monitoring. *Developmental Psychology*, *36*, 366–380.

Kilgore, K., Snyder, J., & Lentz, C. (2000). The contribution of parental discipline, parental monitoring, and school risk to early-onset conduct problems in African American boys and girls. *Developmental Psychology*, *36*, 835–845.

Kochanska, G. (1997). Multiple pathways to conscience for children with different temperaments: From toddlerhood to age 5. *Developmental Psychology*, *33*, 228–240.

Kraemer, H., Wilson, G., Fairburn, C., & Agras, W. (2002). Mediators and moderators of treatment effects. *Archives of General Psychiatry*, *59*, 877–883.

Lansford, J. E., Dodge, K. A., Pettit, G. S., Bates, J. E., Crozier, J., & Kaplow, J. (2002). A 12-year prospective study of the long-term effects of early child physical maltreatment on psychological, behavioral, and academic problems in adolescence. *Archives of Pediatric and Adolescent Medicine*, *156*, 824–830.

Lieberman, M., Doyle, A. B., & Markiewicz, D. (1999). Developmental patterns in security of attachment to mother and father in late childhood and early adolescence: Associations with peer relations. *Child Development*, *70*, 202–213.

Liu, D., Diorio, D., Day, J. C., Francis, D. D., & Meaney, M. J. (2000). Maternal care, hippocampal synaptogenesis and cognitive development in rats. *Nature Neuroscience*, *3*, 799–806.

Lundahl, B. W., Nimer, J., & Parsons, B. (2006). Preventing child abuse: A meta-analysis of parent training programs. *Research on Social Work Practice*, *16*, 251–262.

Lyons-Ruth, K. (1996). Attachment relationships among children with aggressive behavior problems: The role of disorganized early attachment patterns. *Journal of Clinical and Consulting Psychology*, *64*, 64–73.

Maccoby, E. E., & Martin, J. A. (1983). Socialization in the context of the family: Parent–child interaction. In E.M. Hetherington (Ed.), *Mussen manual of child psychology* (Vol. 4, pp. 1–102). New York: Wiley.

Markie-Dadds, C., & Sanders, M. R. (2006). Self-directed Triple P (Positive Parenting Program) for mothers with children at-risk of developing conduct problems. *Behavioural and Cognitive Pyschotherapy*, *34*, 259–275.

Masefield J. (1908). Pompey the Great. Quoted in the Oxford Dictionary of Quotations (3rd edition), p. 333. Oxford: Oxford University Press.

Mash, E. J., & Barkley, R. (2006). *Treatment of childhood disorders*. New York: Guilford Press.

Maughan, B., Denita, R., Christiansen, E., Jenson, W. R., Olympia, D., & Clark, E. (2005). Behavioral parent training as a treatment for externalizing behaviors and disruptive behavior disorders: A meta-analysis. *School Psychology Review*, *34*, 267–286.

McCart, M. R., Priester, P. E., Davies, W. H., & Azen, R. (2006). Differential effectiveness of behavioral parent-training and cognitive–behavioral therapy for antisocial youth: A meta-analysis. *Journal of Abnormal Child Psychology*, 34, 527–543.

McCauley, C., Knapp, M., Beecham, J., McCurry, N., & Sleed, M. (2004). *Young families under stress: Outcomes and costs of the Home-Start support*. York: Joseph Rowntree Foundation.

McMahon, R. J., & Forehand, R. L. (2003). *Helping the noncompliant child: Family-based treatment for oppositional behavior* (2nd edn.). New York: Guilford Press.

Moss, E., Rousseau, D., Parent, S., St-Laurant, D., & Saintonge, J. (1998). Correlates of attachment at school age: Maternal reported stress, mother–child interaction, and behavior problems. *Child Development*, *69*, 1390–1405.

MTA Cooperative Group. (1999). A 14-month randomized clinical trial of treatment strategies for attention-deficit/hyperactivity disorder. Multimodal Treatment Study of Children with ADHD. *Archives of General Psychiatry*, *56*, 1073–1086.

Neiderhiser, J. M., Reiss, D., Pedersen, N. L., Lichtenstein, P., Spotts, E. L., Hansson, K., *et al.* (2004). Genetic and environmental influences on mothering of adolescents: a comparison of two samples. *Developmental Psychology*, *40*, 335–351.

Nichol, A. R., Smith, J., Kay, B., Hall, D., Barlow, J., & Williams, B. (1988). A focused casework approach to the treatment of child abuse: a controlled comparison. *Journal of Child Psychology and Psychiatry*, *29*, 703–711.

O'Connor, T. G., & Croft, C. M. (2001). A twin study of attachment in pre-school children. *Child Development*, *72*, 1501–1511.

Olds, D. (2006). The Nurse–Family Partnership: An evidence-based preventive intervention. *Infant Mental Health Journal*, *27*, 5–25.

Parke, R. D., MacDonald, K. B., Burks, V. M., Carson, J., Bhvnagri, N., Barth, J. M., *et al.* (1989). Family and peer systems: In search of the linkages. In K. Kreppner, & R. M. Lerner (Eds.), *Family systems and life-span development*. Hillsdale, NJ: Erlbaum (pp. 65–92).

Patterson, G. P. (1996). Some characteristics of a developmental theory for early onset delinquency. In M. F. Lenzenweger, & J. J. Haugaard (Eds.), *Frontiers of developmental psychopathology* (pp. 81–124). New York: Oxford University Press.

Patterson, G. P., & Bank, L. (1989). Some amplifying mechanisms for pathological processes in families. In M. Gunnar, & E. Thelan (Eds.), *Systems and development: The Minnesota symposium on child psychology* (Vol. 22, pp. 167–209). Hillsdale, NJ: Erlbaum.

Patterson, G. R. (1969). Behavioral techniques based upon social learning: An additional base for developing behavior modification technologies. In C. Franks (Ed.), *Behavior therapy: Appraisal and status*. New York: McGraw Hill (pp. 57–74).

Pettit, G. S., Bates, J. E., Dodge, K. A., & Meece, D. W. (1999). The impact of after-school peer contact on early adolescent externalizing problems is moderated by parental monitoring, perceived neighborhood safety, and prior adjustment. *Child Development*, *70*, 768–778.

Pettit, G. S., Dodge, K. A., & Brown, M. M. (1988). Early family experience, social problem solving patterns, and children's social competence. *Child Development*, *59*, 107–120.

Pinsker, M., & Geoffrey, K. (1981). A comparison of parent-effectiveness training and behavior modification training. *Family Relations*, *30*, 61–68.

Plomin, R., Reiss, D., Hetherington, E. M., & Howe, G. (1994). Nature and nurture: Genetic contributions to measures of the family environment. *Developmental Psychology*, *30*, 32–43.

Reyno, S. M., & McGrath, P. J. (2006). Predictors of parent training efficacy for child externalizing behavior problems: A meta-analytic review. *Journal of Child Psychology and Psychiatry*, *47*, 99–111.

Ruma, P. R., Burke, R., & Thompson, R. W. (1996). Group parent training: is it effective for children of all ages? *Behaviour Therapy*, *27*, 159–169.

Rutter, M. (1981). *Maternal deprivation re-assessed* (2nd edn.). Harmondsworth: Penguin Books.

Rutter, M. (2005). Environmentally mediated risks for psychopathology: Research strategies and findings. *Journal of the American Academy of Child and Adolescent Psychiatry*, *44*, 3–18.

Sanders, M. R., Pidgeon, A. M., Gravestock, F., Connors, M. D., Brown, S., & Young, R. W. (2004). Does parental attributional retraining and anger management enhance the effects of the Triple P-Positive Parenting Program with parents at risk of child maltreatment? *Behavior Therapy*, *35*, 513–535.

Scarr, S. (1992). Developmental theories for the 1990s: development and individual differences. *Child Development*, *63*, 1–19.

Scott, S. (2002). Parent training programmes. In M. Rutter, & E. Taylor (Eds.), *Child and Adolescent Psychiatry* (4th edn.). Oxford: Blackwell Publishing (pp. 949–967).

Scott, S. (2005). Do parenting programmes for severe child antisocial behaviour work over the longer term, and for whom? One year follow-up of a multicentre controlled trial. *Behavioural and Cognitive Psychotherapy*, *33*, 403–421.

Scott, S., Carby, A., & Rendu, A. (2006a). Does it matter what therapists do? The impact of treatment fidelity in parent training. Unpublished work.

Scott, S., O'Connor, T., & Futh, A. (2006b). *What makes parenting programmes work in disadvantaged areas? The PALS Trial.* The Joseph Rowntree Foundation.

Scott, S., Spender, Q., Doolan, M., Jacobs, B., & Aspland, H. (2001). Multicentre controlled trial of parenting groups for childhood antisocial behaviour in clinical practice. *British Medical Journal*, *323*, 1–7.

Scott, S., Sylva, K., Doolan, M., Jacobs, B., Price, J., Crook, C., & Landau, S. (in press) Randomized controlled trial of parenting groups for child antisocial behavior targeting multiple risk factors: The SPOKES project. *Journal of the American Academy of Child and Adolescent Psychiatry*,

Serketich, W. J., & Dumas, J. E. (1996). The effectiveness of behavioral parent training to modify antisocial behavior in children: A meta-analysis. *Journal of Behavior Therapy*, *27*, 171–186.

Shirk, S. R., & Karver, M. (2003). Prediction of treatment outcome from relationship variables in child and adolescent therapy: A meta-analytic review. *Journal of Consulting and Clinical Psychology*, *71*, 452–464.

Slade, A., Sadler, L. S., & Mayes, L. C. (2005). Minding the baby: enhancing parental reflective functioning in a nursing/home-visiting program. In L. J. Berlin, Y. Ziv, L. M. Amaya-Jackson, & M. T. Greenberg (Eds.), *Enhancing Early Attachment: Theory, research, intervention and policy*. New York, London: Guilford Press (pp. 152–177).

Socrates (435 BC). Cited in Cartledge (1998). *Cambridge history of Ancient Greece* (p. 132). Cambridge: Cambridge University Press.

Spieker, S., Nelson, D., Deklyen, M., & Staerkel, F. (2005). Enhancing early attachments in the context of early head start. In L. J. Berlin, Y. Ziv, L. M. Amaya-Jackson, & M. T. Greenberg (Eds.), *Enhancing Early Attachment: Theory, research, intervention and policy* (pp. 250–275). New York, London: Guilford Press.

Sroufe, L. A., Egeland, B., & Carlson, E. A. (1999). One social world. In W. A. Collins, & B. Laursen (Eds.), *Minnesota symposium on child psychology* (Vol. 30, pp. 241–262). Hillsdale, NJ: Erlbaum.

Steinberg, L., Lamborn, S. D., Darling, N., Mounts, N. S., & Dournbusch, S. M. (1994). Over-time changes in adjustment and competence among adolescents from authoritative, authoritarian, indulgent, and neglectful families. *Child Development*, *65*, 754–770.

Swift, Jonathan. (1708). *An argument against abolishing Christianity.* Cited in *The Oxford dictionary of quotations* (3rd edn.), 1986. Oxford: Oxford University Press.

Tein, J. Y., Irwin, N. S., MacKinnon, D. P., & Wolchik, S. A. (2004). How did it work? Who did it work for? Mediation in the context of a moderated prevention effect for children of divorce. *Journal of Consulting and Clinical Psychology*, *72*, 617–624.

Van IJzendoorn, M., Bakermans-Kranenburg, M. J., & Juffer, F. (2005). Why less is more: From the dodo bird verdict to evidence-based interventions on sensitivity and early attachments. In L. J. Berlin, Y. Ziv, L. M. Amaya-Jackson, & M. T. Greenberg (Eds.), *Enhancing Early Attachment: Theory, research, intervention and policy* (pp. 297–312). New York, London: Guilford Press.

Velderman, M. K., Bakermans-Kranenburg, M. J., Juffer, F., van Ijzendoorn, M. H., Mangelsdorf, S. C., & Zevalkink, J. (2006). Preventing preschool externalizing behavior problems through video-feedback intervention in infancy. *Infant Mental Health Journal*, *27*, 466–493.

Vuchinich, S., Bank, L., & Patterson, G. R. (1992). Parenting, peers, and the stability of antisocial behavior in preadolescent boys. *Developmental Psychology*, *28*, 510–521.

Wahler, R. G., Winkel, G. H., Peterson, R. F., & Morrison, D. C. (1965). Mothers as behavior therapists for their own children. *Behavior Research and Therapy*, *3*, 113–124.

Webster-Stratton, C. (1981). Modification of mothers' behaviours and attitudes through videotape modelling group discussion. *Behavior Therapy*, *12*, 634–642.

Webster-Stratton, C., & Reid, J. M. (2003). The Incredible years Parent, Teacher, and Children Training Series. In A. E. Kadin, & J. R. Weisz (Eds.), *Evidence-based psychotherapies for children and adolescents* (pp. 224–240). New York: Guilford Press.

Weisz, J. R., Donenberg, G. R., & Han, S. S. (1995). Bridging the gap between laboratory and clinic in child and adolescent pyschotherapy. *Journal of Consulting and Clinical Psychology*, *63*, 688–701.

Wells, K. C., Chi, T. C., Hinshaw, S. P., Epstein, J. N., Pfiffner, L., Nebel-Schwalm, M., *et al.* (2006). Treatment related changes in objectively measured parent behaviors in the multimodal treatment study of children with Attention-Deficit/Hyperactivity Disorder. *Journal of Consulting and Clinical Psychology*, *74*, 649–657.

Wood, J. J., McLeod, B. D., Sigman, M., Hwang, W. C., & Chu, B. C. (2003). Parenting and childhood anxiety: theory, empirical findings, and future directions. *Journal of Child Psychology and Psychiatry*, *44*, 134–151.

Zeanah, C. H., & Smyke, A. T. (2005). Building attachment relationships following maltreatment and severe deprivation. In L. J. Berlin, Y. Ziv, L. M. Amaya-Jackson, & M. T. Greenberg (Eds.), *Enhancing Early Attachment: Theory, research, intervention and policy* (pp. 195–216). New York, London: Guilford Press.

Zhang, T. Y., Chretien, P., Meaney, M. J., & Gratton, A. (2005). Influence of naturally occurring variations in maternal care on prepulse inhibition of acoustic startle and the medial prefrontal cortical dopamine response to stress in adult rats. *Journal of Neuroscience*, *25*, 1493–1502.

Family Interviewing and Family Therapy

Ivan Eisler and Judith Lask

Family therapy, like other psychotherapies, has evolved over several decades and today includes a broad range of ideas that are often described as representing discrete theoretical models or schools (e.g., structural, strategic, Milan systemic, narrative; Carr, 2006). Different approaches to family therapy tend to focus on one particular aspect of change (e.g., the structural model on the need for change in relationships, or the Milan approach on the need to change beliefs) and are usually associated with particular groups or centers. In practice, the conceptual ideas as well as the techniques associated with each of them tend to be adopted quite widely and most family therapists integrate ideas from different approaches in their work, as single theoretical models often do not provide sufficient conceptual breadth or choice of treatment techniques to address the wide range of difficulties presented to clinicians.

The boundary lines between family therapy and other therapeutic approaches are also indistinct and there are many overlaps. The distinctions are often more about historical developments and professional and philosophical allegiances than clearly defined conceptual differences. This is reinforced by research on common factors in psychotherapy, which suggests that they may account for as much as 90% of outcome variance (Asay & Lambert, 2000; Wampold, 2001), although the actual role of common factors is subject to much debate (Sexton & Ridley, 2004; Sexton, Ridley, & Kleiner, 2004; Simon, 2006; Sprenkle & Blow, 2004, 2007). Alongside this, the growing body of research on evidence-based practice identifies a number of clearly defined family treatments as effective (Lundahl, Risser, & Lovejoy, 2006; Shaddish & Baldwin, 2003; Stanton & Shaddish, 1997; Woolfenden, Williams, & Peat, 2007). Taken together they suggest that while there may be common factors across all psychotherapeutic approaches, particular problems may respond well to very specific treatment *components* which may be incorporated in a number of different treatment models, albeit sometimes conceptualized in different ways. At the same time, the research also indicates that successful treatments are united at another level by factors such as empathy or warmth of the therapist or the level of motivation of the client (Beutler, Malik, Alimohamed *et al.*, 2004; Clarkin & Levy, 2004; but see chapter 18 for a somewhat different conclusion). Part of the effectiveness of family therapy will be the skill of the therapist to use the most appropriate approach and interventions and to maintain the engagement and motivation of family members.

Rutter's Child and Adolescent Psychiatry, 5th edition. Edited by M. Rutter, D. Bishop, D. Pine, S. Scott, J. Stevenson, E. Taylor and A. Thapar. © 2008 Blackwell Publishing, ISBN: 978-1-4051-4549-7.

Theoretical and Empirical Developments

The Family as a System

Family Systems Theory, the conceptual framework for much of the thinking about working with families, has evolved considerably over the years. The original notion of the family as a system (Ackerman, 1938; Burgess, 1926), strongly influenced by cybernetic concepts (von Bertalanffy, 1968), described a number of features such as the recursive nature of relationships, the multilevel nature of communication (Bateson, 1972; Bateson & Ruesch, 1951), the development of recognizable patterns of interaction, the role of relationships and beliefs, and the allocation of family roles (Bateson, Jackson, Haley, & Weakland, 1956; Palazzoli, Boscolo, Cecchin, & Prata, 1978). More recent theoretical developments in family therapy theory have come from social constructionism (Berger & Luckman, 1966) and in particular narrative therapy (White & Epston, 1989). This emphasizes that what we consider as objective everyday reality is derived from and maintained by social experiences and that through social interactions we develop narratives to make sense of our own lived experience. Later in the chapter we discuss the impact that the incorporation of social constructionist ideas has had on the field.

The second main strand in family therapy theory is the Family Life Cycle model (Carter & McGoldrick, 1999), which provides a "developmental lens" for understanding the way the family as a system evolves over time. Families need to provide stability and predictability but they also have to be able to change in order to adapt to new circumstances and the developmental demands of individual family members (Byng-Hall, 1991; Eisler, 1993). For instance, the child's need for dependence and attachment requires a degree of stability and constancy in the family but, as the child develops, the family must find ways of meeting his or her needs for independence and separation too. As the family evolves through the predictable stages of the family life cycle, it needs to be able to adapt and change its habitual style of functioning. These expected stages of the family life cycle can be complicated by unexpected events such as illness, death, family separation or migration and the combined stress can contribute to the development of problems. There is evidence that at these transitional times there is an increased vulnerability and increased psychological morbidity (Gorell Barnes, Thompson, Daniel, & Burchardt, 1998; Hetherington, 1989; Kendler & Prescott, 1999; Ritsner & Ponizovsky, 1999; Sartorius, 1996; Varnik, Kolves, & Wasserman, 2005). The way the family responds to an emerging problem is a crucial factor in determining the extent of individual vulnerability to such pressures (Walsh, 1997).

Role of the Family in the Development and Maintenance of Psychological Difficulties

Early theorizing assumed that particular types of family organization or patterns of family interaction would be connected with specific presenting problems. Explanatory models such as the "double-bind" theory of schizophrenia (Bateson, Jackson, Haley *et al.*, 1956) or the "psychosomatic family" model of anorexia nervosa (Minuchin, Rosman, & Baker, 1978) were highly influential and led to important clinical innovations. Paradoxically, while many of the treatments developed in this way seem to be efficacious, the theoretical models themselves have generally proved to be flawed (Eisler, 1995; Kog, Vandereycken, & Vertommen, 1985; Olson, 1972). This has resulted in a somewhat unfortunate legacy. On the one hand, there are those who still see family therapy in its original guise (i.e., a treatment that aims to correct family dysfunction which was thought to lie at the heart of individual problems). Although few family therapists would today subscribe to this notion, outside of the field the view is still held quite widely. On the other hand, many within the field of family therapy, partly as a reaction to concerns about families being blamed by the early theoretical models, argue that the impact of family factors on child development is part of such a complex matrix of influences that any explanation that focuses on them is bound to be misleading. While we have some sympathy with the latter view, it clearly does not take into account the large body of research that now exists on the role of family factors in the development of the child. These include a range of adversities from prenatal factors such as being an unwanted child (David, Dytrych, & Matejcek, 2003; Kubicka, Roth, Dytrych, & Matejcek, 2002) or maternal stress (Huizink, Robles De Medina, Mulder, Visser, & Buitelaar, 2002), the consequences of growing up in an environment characterized by negative emotion, harsh parenting, high levels of discord or hostility (Fergusson & Lynskey, 1996; Fergusson, Horwood, & Lynskey, 1992; Moffitt, Caspi, Harrington, & Milne, 2002; Riggins-Casper, Cadoret, Knutson, & Langbehn, 2003) or the impact of neglect (Rutter & O'Connor, 2004). Equally, there are factors in the family that may have a protective role or promote resilience (Rutter, 1999, 2006).

There are three reasons why one has to be cautious about how these findings are interpreted in relation to clinical practice. First is the often-made point that there is a complex interaction over time between the effect of the family environment, personality and temperamental characteristics of the child, the impact of the developing disorder on the family, and resilience factors as well as mediating genetic factors (Fergusson & Lynskey, 1996; Rutter, 1999). This is highlighted by behavior genetic research showing the differential impact of the family environment on children within the same family (Dunn & Plomin, 1990; Reiss, Hetherington, & Plomin, 1995; Rutter, Silberg, O'Connor, & Simonoff, 1999). The second is the reciprocity of influences between parents and children, which is well documented empirically (Crockenberg & Leerkes, 2003; Crockenberg, Leerkes, & Lekka, 2007; Deater-Deckard, Atzaba-Poria, & Pike, 2004; Scaramella & Leve, 2004). The third and probably most important is the variability of the findings showing that the impact of even the most powerful factors is anything but uniform (O'Connor, Rutter, Beckett *et al.*, 2000). There are many examples but perhaps the best way of illustrating our point is to use a specific example of how research findings of this kind do not easily translate into practice.

There are a number of clinical and research accounts of the possible adverse effects of maternal eating disorder on the infant or young child (Lacey & Smith, 1987; Park, Senior, & Stein, 2003a; Russell, Treasure, & Eisler, 1998) showing obstetric complications, low birth weight, poorer physical development and in some cases the development of an eating disorder in the offspring when they reach adolescence. A series of observational studies by Stein and colleagues (Park, Lee, Woolley, Murray, & Stein, 2003b; Stein, Woolley, Cooper *et al.*, 1994; Stein, Woolley, Cooper *et al.*, 2006) has shown that mothers with a history of an eating disorder tended to be more intrusive and express more negative emotion with their infants during mealtimes and the children themselves had a more negative emotional tone and their mealtimes were more conflictual compared with controls. The children tended to be lighter than controls and their weight was related to the amount of conflict during mealtimes and the extent of the mother's concern about her own body shape. The problematic interaction around mealtimes persisted at 5 years and when followed-up at 10 years the index children showed increased levels of shape and weight concerns and greater dietary restraint compared with controls (although at a considerably lower level than would be found in children with early-onset anorexia nervosa). A further study in the form of a randomized controlled trial (Stein, Woolley, Cooper *et al.*, 2006) showed that a video-feedback intervention was effective in improving mother–infant interaction at mealtimes. Thus, we have research that identifies not only risk factors, but also some likely mechanisms through which these might operate and a possible effective preventive intervention derived from this.

In spite of this, the clinical implications are much less straightforward than may seem at first sight. First, although the group effects in comparison with controls are strong, the findings apply only to a minority of the children in the index group. For instance, 27% of the index group was below the 25th centile for weight. This is much higher than the 4% in the control group but is still only a quarter of the sample. At age 10 there were no differences in the children's weights. Similarly, there is considerable variability in the findings of mother–child interaction within the index group, both in the initial study and at follow-up, and at 10 years there was no difference in levels of criticism or intrusive behaviors on the part of the mothers compared with controls. Second, while there is an association between the degree of a mother's psychopathology and the disturbed interactional pattern, it is not clear what mechanism underpins this. Thus, it is unclear to what extent it is a direct consequence of the mother's eating disorder (e.g., fearing that her infant might put on too much weight) or if the problems arise out of her lack of confidence in her parenting, resulting in being unnecessarily controlling with the child. The point we want to emphasize, however, is the complexity of the process through which adversity operates over time in individual cases. While it is clear that although as a group the children were at increased risk of developing disturbed eating attitudes, most in fact did not.

Consider now the opposite scenario when as a clinician we see an adolescent with an eating disorder whose mother also had an eating disorder. Stein's work would indicate that the two might be linked but actually tells us very little about how this potential link may have operated for these individuals and even less about what the target of our intervention would need to be. Knowing what factors may have a negative impact on a child's development is of course useful, but without knowing if these are still operating and if so how they operate, our clinical interventions remain blunt instruments. The current emphasis by most family therapy approaches on family strengths and resilience (Walsh, 1997), and on trying to optimize the family's own resources, may be no better in terms of the science that informs it but it has the merit of engaging families in positive ways instead of adding to their sense of failure and self-blame.

Impact of Individual Problems on Family Life

When one member of a family begins to develop a problem it affects other members and also the relationships within that system (Rolland, 1999). Some of the effects may be readily apparent such as bullying or aggression from a young person with attention deficit/hyperactivity disorder (ADHD), at other times the impact may be less obvious and not immediately apparent (e.g., "well" siblings receiving less attention from parents). The stress of dealing with difficulties may put a strain on the parents' relationship or the relationships with wider family. For the clinician, the crucial issue is to understand the gradual process of reorganization of the family in response to the problem to the point where it becomes the "central organizing principle" in the family's life (Eisler, 2005; Steinglass, 1998). The process will often start through the activation of protective and supportive processes in the family but can in time become part of what reinforces or maintains the problem. For example, what may start as supportive reassurance of an anxious and perhaps somewhat perfectionist child may with hindsight turn out to be the start of a process of parents being drawn into the emerging rituals of a developing obsessive-compulsive disorder (OCD; Amir, Freshman, & Foa, 2000; Calvocoressi, Mazure, & Kasl, 1999). Useful models for understanding the process through which the family accommodates to the child's problem can be found in the studies of the impact on the family of serious and enduring physical illness and disability (Rolland, 1987, 1994; Steinglass, 1998) and anorexia nervosa (Eisler, 2005; Neilsen & Bara-Carril, 2003). Understanding how families respond to emerging problems is an area demanding further research.

The way families respond to this invasion into their lives will vary, but there is a tendency for the problem to magnify certain aspects of the family's dynamics and narrow the range of their adaptive behaviors (Whitney & Eisler, 2005). As the symptomatic behavior increasingly takes a central role in family life what may be normal variations in family functioning may become more pronounced and take on new meanings. Concern may begin to feel like overprotection and intrusiveness, while attempts to promote independence may feel like lack of care. For the clinician, the important thing to be aware of is that much of what is observed in families is, at least in part, an outcome of the process of family accommodation to the problem and should not be too readily labeled as dysfunctional.

Family Interviewing and Family Therapy

Interviewing Families as Part of the Assessment Process

The family interview is an important component in a comprehensive assessment. It provides the clinician with an opportunity to observe the family in direct interaction, to assess patterns of relationships, the emotional climate of the family and a chance to see how the family is organized around the symptoms presented by the child. Interviewing the family for purposes of assessment is a good starting point for making an effective treatment alliance with the family. Hearing the concerns of family members and their hopes for the future is as important as gathering information and making an assessment of the problem and can determine the most effective ways of helping the family to promote change.

Observing Patterns of Interaction

From the first contact with the family the clinician has opportunities to observe patterns of interaction, both immediately and over time (Byng Hall, 1995; Minuchin, 1974), which provide information about family structure and the nature of relationships in the family. Who presents the problem, how others respond, who finds it easy or difficult to have their say and how disagreements are handled will all provide initial impressions about the family's preferred style. Careful observation of the interaction process will provide information that may confirm or contradict the content of what is being said. For instance, a mother may describe her relationship with her teenage daughter as difficult or conflictual. This may be supported by observing regular clashes or irritable responses between the two but at the same time one may notice that there are also many warm and supportive interactions taking place.

When making observations it is important not to draw conclusions too readily as to what the observed patterns might "mean" or how they might be related to the presenting problem. While certain interactions may be clearly unhelpful (e.g., a parent, perhaps unwittingly, reinforcing the challenging behavior of a 6-year-old or frequent changes of topic preventing the discussion of difficult emotional issues), there may be a range of different (often overlapping) explanations for the observed behaviors. It is important to explore the family members' own perceptions of such patterns and how they are connected to the beliefs and expectations of the family and how much flexibility or rigidity there is around them. Some patterns may reflect family beliefs, often strongly influenced by cultural or specific family traditions about the nature of family life, gender roles and parenting tasks, and may include patterns of which the family members themselves may not be aware.

Family Beliefs and Meanings Attached to Behaviors

These can be useful in making sense of behavior and relationships but also aid the process of engagement so that a family feels more understood. Beliefs relating to the presenting problem are particularly important. Future therapy may focus on exploring those beliefs and questioning them so that new meanings can develop. It may be possible to identify strong individual and family narratives that cloud the possibility of other options for change (Parry & Doan, 1994). One of the central aims of interviewing families is to explore alternative perceptions and meanings. This will include giving space to family members whose voices are not readily heard but also looking for different ways of framing the family narrative in a way that may provide a more constructive way forward. For instance, when a family is invited to a clinical meeting only one parent (e.g., mother) might attend the session. A variety of explanations may be given (dad is too busy; mum normally deals with doctors' appointments; he doesn't really understand). Implicit in such explanations is often a suggestion that the father is somewhat detached or does not really care. Often the most effective way of getting the father to attend the next session is to explore possible alternative reasons for his non-attendance ("Is he not here because he doesn't care or is it because he does not believe he can help?" "If he believed that coming here would make a difference to you, would he come?" "If he thought that coming here would help him understand better, would he want to be here?"). The value of such questioning is that it creates a new frame of reference for familiar behaviors and may allow new conversations to develop.

Social and Cultural Contexts

One of the criticisms of some of the earlier models of family therapy is that they were based on a normative western model of the family and did not take sufficient account of the diversity of family life across cultures and the considerable change that families have undergone in most societies. The notion of what family life means in terms of the nature of relationships within the family, the expectations of the way in which families change over the life cycle or the roles of different family members varies hugely. Children may grow up in foster and adoptive families or a succession of different families or may be part of more than one family constellation following marriage break-up. Single-parent families, same-sex parent partnerships and friendship networks provide different forms of family life. While much of this may seem self-evident, it is crucial to be open to the different experiences and expectations that families bring with them. We also have to be aware that as professionals our own personal and cultural contexts will inevitably color our observations and assessments.

Exploring the family's social and cultural contexts will help to give meaning to specific behaviors, beliefs and relationships, but it may also provide information on stresses (e.g., specific social expectations in the community) and resources such as sources of networking and support (Falicov, 1995). An evaluation of the role of professionals in the referral process and the history and relationship of the family with other helping systems is important, particularly where there has been multi-agency involvement, which may itself have become disabling for the family (Asen, 2002).

Exploration of the Presenting Problem in the Context of Individual and Family Development

An understanding of current life cycle and developmental demands and how the family is meeting these can be very helpful (Carter & McGoldrick, 1999). Sometimes, outside pressures such as illness or bereavement or internal changes such as separation and divorce add extra demands for change in addition to and sometimes contradictory to developmental demands. For instance, when an adolescent develops psychosis the normal developmental need for greater autonomy may be countered by the need for greater care and supervision. Accommodating to the needs of the illness is an understandable (and generally positive) response, although over time it may itself become unhelpful and limit the possibilities for change. Enquiring about the impact of the problem on family life is a good way of understanding the way the family is functioning and can often also reveal areas of strength and resilience that are not at first evident.

Assessing the Family's Style of Dealing with Problems and Identifying Strengths and Weaknesses

This should help to address the important question about how best to work with a family, identify transferable skills and also aid the engagement process. The therapist will draw from the evidence relating to positive parenting and resilience factors to identify areas of strength which can be developed. For example, the capacity for reflection and empathy can be developed through sensitive and skillful questioning. The ability to make sense of past experiences can also be developed through the therapeutic process. Completing a family genogram (Bloch, Hafner, Harari, & Szmukler, 1994; McGoldrick & Gerson, 1985) is a useful way of learning about the way in which the family has dealt with other problems, family traditions and beliefs about family coping with adversity.

Family Interview Techniques

It is beyond the scope of this chapter to cover in depth the variety of techniques that have been developed for interviewing families (Dallos & Draper, 2005; Palazzoli, Boscolo, Cecchin, & Prata, 1980; Tomm, 1988). Much of this literature is concerned with the way in which different types of question can shape the therapeutic relationship and the importance of questioning (as opposed to information giving) in general, in maintaining a position of curiosity which aims to keep the therapist and the family open to new information and new meanings. The following is a brief outline of some of the different styles of questioning that have proved useful in family interviews. Tomm (1988) suggests the following classification.

Lineal Questions

All interviews will include some questions of this type (e.g., "What is the problem that you have come with?" "How long has it been going on for?"). The disadvantage of lineal questions is that they tend to elicit a rather well-rehearsed way of presenting the problem which may be quite fixed, and not only expresses the family's belief about the nature of the problem but also often connects with feelings of helplessness, guilt, blame and resentment.

Circular Questions

These differ from lineal questions not only in form but also in their underlying assumption. They draw on the assumption that individual problems are connected or embedded in patterns of relationships, and the aim of these questions is to illuminate or make visible what these patterns are. So, instead of simply asking "What is the problem?" one might ask "How would different people in the family describe your problem?" "Who worries about it?" "When people get worried about how unhappy you are, does it make you more or less depressed?" Other questions might require family members to describe what they make of behaviors that they observe, or speculate about thoughts and feelings of other family members. For instance, instead of asking just about the duration of the problem, the therapist might ask "When did your family first notice that you had a problem?" or "What effect did it have on you when your parents started talking about the problem?" Additional questions might be asked about the way different people in the family responded to the problem and what interactions this might lead to "When your mother shows her worry, what does your father do?"

Asking circular questions starts to provide a basis for describing the problem in a more contextual way and also allows for alternative descriptions to be heard. For instance, the family might explain that "Mum worries a lot whereas father does not show his feelings much," implying that mother is too anxious and father too detached. Useful questions to develop alternative aspects of this might be "How do you know when your husband is getting worried?" and "When your dad tries to reassure your mum, what effect does it have on her worry?" This may lead to a discussion of the differences between experiencing and showing feelings, and the interplay within the family between behaviors and emotion of different family members. It may also be an opportunity to talk about individual and gender differences and perhaps the different expectations that each parent brings with them from their own family of origin.

One way of organizing the use of circular questions is to connect them to a systemic hypothesis. The therapist links information about the family to form a hypothesis about the family and their relationship to the presenting problem. This hypothesis is then tested through circular questions and continually revised in the light of feedback until an idea is arrived at that fits well enough with the family to provide some useful new information for them. For example, a systemic hypothesis might suggest that when a child feels sad his mother becomes anxious that she is not a good mother and hands over the care to her husband, who worries about his wife and criticizes his son, who finds that self-harming is a way of bringing his parents back into a caring contact with him. This hypothesis could be tested with reflexive questions such as "What would happen if your father was not at home?" or to the mother "If you felt more confident in yourself as a mother what might you do differently?"

Strategic Questions

These are questions that are used with the primary aim of influencing the family in a particular way rather than obtaining information and are analogous to giving instructions but because they are formulated as questions this may not always be immediately apparent. "Why do you let your mother speak for you?" is as much a statement that implies that it would be better for the adolescent to speak for him or herself as a question asking for an explanation. Challenging interventions of this kind can be useful at times but should be used sparingly, as they can induce feelings of guilt and they may also undermine the therapeutic relationship with the family (Tomm, 1988).

Reflexive Questions

These are questions that are also intended to influence the family but are less directive, instead requiring family members to reflect on how things might be different under changed circumstances, or if they took a different course of action: "What would happen if you were able to hide your worry when your daughter got depressed?" "If your mother didn't try to help next time you have a row with your father, which one of you would be more likely to find a way of ending the argument; who would be the one to suggest a compromise solution?" Reflexive questions will typically introduce an alternative way of framing a particular behavior, opening up new possibilities and challenging the assumptions that may underlie a particular pattern of behavior. They may address an emotion or an aspect of behavior that is not being expressed overtly and may only be guessed at. They may include an implicit assumption: "What will you argue about with your mother when you are no longer bulimic?" – implying both that there will be change and that arguments between adolescents and parents are normal. Reflexive questions, like circular questions, assume that behaviors and the meanings that we attach to them are part of the relational context of the family and that there may be more than one meaning that might be attached to a particular behavior. The aim is for the family to reflect on this context and to explore the way in which thoughts, feelings and behaviors of different family members connect and how they might change.

Relative Influence Questions

These are specifically linked with the technique of externalizing the problem and explore the influence the problem has had on the person(s) and, more importantly, the influence the person has had on the problem. Through the process (e.g., of exploring how the family has helped a young child with fears or anxiety) it may be possible to establish exceptions or unique outcomes when there has been some control over the problem and how these can be developed further.

It is important for the clinician to be able to use a range of interview styles with families and to have a repertoire of different types of question. Circular questions can be extremely useful in illuminating patterns of relationships in the family and this in itself may be an important and powerful part of the therapeutic process. However, such questions are most usefully applied when the interviewer has developed a clear hypothesis about the nature of the family relationships and the part played by the symptomatic behavior in the family organization (Burnham, 1986). When the interviewer has a clear focus, one question will naturally lead to the next one, helping to confirm or disconfirm the particular hypothesis. However, if such questions are used without a clear focus they are more likely to create confusion and a sense of alienation (Reimers, 1999; Strickland-Clark, Campbell, & Dallos, 2000).

Intervening in the Family Interaction Process

Careful and sensitive observation of the processes within the family allows the therapist to assess the nature of the relationships, provides opportunities for joining the family but is also the basis for introducing change in more active ways. There are numerous techniques (Minuchin & Fishman, 1981) for this, including blocking repetitive patterns (e.g., when one person in the family regularly acts as a peacemaker), reinforcing behaviors such as positive parenting, setting rules to prevent repetitive escalation of arguments or encouraging a family member whose voice tends to get lost to make sure they are heard. Interventions may range from fairly unobtrusive non-verbal ones (fixing the gaze of the person who is speaking, making it more difficult for others to interrupt) to much more overt, even dramatic gestures ("Why don't you go and sit next to your dad and try to work out a compromise with him without getting mum to help you?") and may include specific suggestions or homework tasks. Alternatively, the therapist may ask a question or make a comment in a way that draws attention to what is happening. When commenting on family process it is always important to recognize that the same phenomenon can be described in a number of ways ranging from neutral, through ascribing agency to one or other participant in the interaction, to overtly critical. Even quite neutral comments from the therapist may appear critical to family members. The clinician therefore has to be careful in choosing an appropriate style of comment or question. Andersen (1987) recommends that reflections of this kind are best carried out in a tentative way rather than being pronouncements or authoritative interpretations which are likely to come across as being judgmental.

Involving Children and Adolescents in Family Interviews

Even very young children can be effectively included in family interviews, provided they are engaged in an age-appropriate way. All too often, however, such interviews end up simply as an adult conversation in the presence of the child. It is helpful to provide appropriate toys and drawing materials, and use creative and play techniques in a similar way that they would be used in individual interviews with a child. Engaging a child effectively is often reassuring for parents, who may be concerned whether bringing the child to a psychiatric setting is the right thing to do. The choice of language in talking to parents about their child's problems is also important with young children present as it may be difficult for the child to understand what is being said. Often it is better to ask the parents to explain things to the child, rather than the clinician doing this directly as this may be less threatening for the child, and reinforces the sense that the parents are the experts for their own child.

With very lively active children the first task is to create a working environment in which what family members have to say can be attended to. This is best achieved by actively collaborating with the parents. Asking the parents for advice on how best to occupy young children will reinforce the parents' sense that they are being respected and also may make it easier for the child to listen and join in spontaneously at some point during the interview. Children may not be too keen to take part in discussions at first. Making it clear at the start of the session that everyone in the room will have an opportunity to have their say, while stressing that it is also OK to sit and listen, is important for some children, to avoid making them feel that they are being put on the spot. When the pressure on them to join in is removed, children will often join in spontaneously. Joining with a child in creative play or talking about a drawing he or she has made can also provide an opportunity for the child to have a voice in the session (see also Dare & Lindsey, 1979; Larner, 1996; Wilson, 1998).

A similar situation can sometimes arise with adolescents who may be reluctant to talk, while the parents may have an expectation that the "experts" will succeed where they have failed. Sometimes, such an adolescent may be more willing to talk when seen individually, but this is by no means always the case. The advantage of a family interview is that even a reluctant or unwilling participant can be included in an interview through indirect means. Making it clear that the therapist respects the adolescent's right not to speak can help avoid an unhelpful battle. This can be done in a way that respects the adolescent's autonomy while at the same time making sure that he or she is not simply being ignored. One might encourage the adolescent to listen but also to correct other family members if he or she thinks they have misunderstood or got things wrong. The therapist can check this out from time to time.

Who to See and When

Although it is always useful to see the whole family interacting together, conjoint interviews also have their limitations in both the assessment and treatment phases. During assessment there may be indications that some individuals do not have an effective voice in the family group or the presence of the whole family may seriously inhibit some aspect of discussion. For example, an adolescent may not want his or her parents to know about drug use or there may be concern that a child has been abused and may not want to talk about this in front of their parents. Similarly, there may be issues that parents may not wish to discuss with the child present (e.g., to do with marital issues or perhaps when parents of a child with disability may not be able to share negative feelings in front of the child). For these reasons it is generally useful to make at least some separate sessions a routine part of practice even when family therapy is indicated as the main mode of treatment.

There are several other considerations that should be taken into account when deciding on individual or conjoint sessions. For instance, we might decide that it is age-appropriate to see an adolescent on their own, particularly if they express a wish for this. We should consider (and enquire about) to what extent this is determined by a wish to avoid talking about a painful or upsetting issue, which may not necessarily be a helpful thing to do. Some topics may seem difficult to address in a conjoint meeting although the discomfort may be largely to do with the clinician's own uncertainty about how or whether to raise the issue. Asking questions about what is acceptable or usual in the particular family will tell the clinician what can or cannot be easily talked about and may open up the topic for discussion. Questions such as "If your parents thought you were smoking dope, what would they do?" or "Some teenagers are very up-front about what they get up to, others keep things closer to their chest – what is your son like?" may quickly lead to frank and open conversations. More importantly, this kind of discussion will clarify what the actual boundaries in the family are rather than being assumed by the therapist.

In families where there is much hostility, criticism or open conflict, conjoint meetings may not always be helpful particularly if the hostility or conflict simply escalates in sessions. There is evidence that families with high parental scores on criticism are more likely to drop out of treatment (Szmukler, Eisler, Russell, & Dare, 1985). In a study comparing conjoint therapy with separated therapy (i.e., separate meetings with parents and the adolescent) for adolescent anorexia nervosa, critical families did better in separated therapy (Eisler, Dare, Hodes *et al.*, 2000). It is sometimes assumed that family dysfunction should be the main indication for family therapy. In fact, the opposite is the case. Several studies have shown (Barrett, Healey-Farrell, & March, 2004; Eisler, Dare, Hodes *et al.*, 2000; Hampson & Beavers, 1996a) that the quality of family functioning moderates the effect of family therapy, with poorly functioning families gaining less benefit. This should not be interpreted as simply showing that more dysfunction leads to poor outcome, as there is evidence that these effects might be specific to particular types of family intervention. For instance, collaborative approaches to treatment (which are often favored by therapists) are less effective with disorganized families (Hampson & Beavers, 1996b), who tend to respond better to a more directive and less open style whereas the opposite is true of more balanced type families. Our own study of separated and conjoint therapy was interesting in this context in showing a three-way interaction between level of criticism at the beginning of treatment, type of treatment and long-term outcome, but somewhat surprisingly this effect disappeared when end of treatment level of criticism was considered (Eisler, Simic, Russell, & Dare, 2007). This suggests that it may be an effect that is operating at the level of treatment engagement rather then a persistent effect of criticism itself.

In general, it is often useful to try to separate the question of how and when to involve the family in treatment to help deal with the child's problem from the question of how to address possible problems in the family. This is partly to avoid reinforcing disabling feelings of guilt and blame and partly that, as we discussed earlier, much of what may appear dysfunctional is part of the way the family has accommodated to the problem. Most importantly, it is seldom going to be the case that resolving a family difficulty is itself going to resolve the child's problem.

The Family Therapist in the Multidisciplinary Team

Most clinicians working with children and adolescents will to a greater or lesser degree include families in their work. This is sometimes referred to as "family work" to distinguish it from "family therapy" although the divide between the two is somewhat artificial. Family therapists by virtue of their training will have developed specialist skills in working with families and may therefore take on more complex work but where there is an indication for family interventions the same principles should apply whether the work is carried out by the specialist family therapist or the non-specialist. The role of the family therapist within the multidisciplinary team is of course much wider than just seeing families. They will have to be able to identify when a family approach is likely to be helpful and the different styles of work that might be best suited for the specific problem or a particular family. The family therapist can provide support and supervision for other team members working with families which may involve using a one-way screen or video link. This can have a number of purposes. It allows for "live supervision" for less experienced therapists and provides a training environment in which other team members can learn new skills. It can provide a rich team experience in which professionals pool their ideas and thinking in order to understand the family and move forward with the therapy. As in all clinical work, there is a need to attend carefully to ethical issues. These can be more complicated when a number of people are being worked with at the same time and members of the team are observing through one-way screens.

Frameworks for Intervention

This section sets out a framework for grouping treatment approaches for working therapeutically with families under several conceptual headings and describes some basic interventions that arise from them. We believe that this is more useful than to focus on models of family therapy which provide a somewhat artificial categorization and do not reflect day-to-day practice particularly well. This also provides a way of grouping the empirical evidence for effectiveness of family interventions for different types of disorder.

Maintenance Frameworks

Much of the early theoretical work informing family therapy was concerned with the idea of the family as a self-regulating social system (Jackson, 1957) and the way in which family interactions and family structures maintain problems. Two influential strands of family therapy (*structural* and *behavioral*) have drawn heavily on these notions. As a number of authors have argued (Kraemer, Stice, Kazdin, Offord, & Kupfer, 2001; Schmidt & Treasure, 2006; Stice, 2002), a focus on maintenance mechanisms provides one of the strongest way of gaining an understanding of what makes treatments work and, perhaps not surprisingly, the strongest body of empirical evidence for the effectiveness of family therapy is found in this area.

Structural Family Therapy

Structural family therapy, developed by Minuchin and colleagues (Minuchin, 1974), originally derived from work with deprived families of delinquent boys (Minuchin, Montalvo, Guerney, Rosman, & Schumer, 1967) and was later applied to work with psychosomatic problems, particularly anorexia nervosa (Minuchin, Rosman, & Baker, 1978). The model assumes that well-functioning families have a number of specific features such as clear and flexible boundaries between individuals and subsystems and well-defined roles within the family, and that they provide an appropriate balance between closeness and independence. Individual problems were seen to be embedded in self-perpetuating dysfunctional family structures. The model, because of its emphasis on family relationship and interaction, relies to a great extent on interventions into transactional patterns in the "here and now" – that is, within the therapeutic session. Interventions include *strengthening the "parental subsystem"*, where the therapist encourages the parents to work together to find a way of jointly managing the difficulty. This includes actively intervening in the process of discussion with encouraging language, highlighting success and framing the role of the parents as responsible and "in charge" of the children. During *enactments*, families are encouraged to demonstrate their usual family processes and interactions within the therapeutic session to provide an opportunity for the therapist to help the family to "do it differently" and to assess the impact of following a different pattern. In *boundary making* the therapist enquires about rules (or boundaries) defining the roles of different family members and the degree of flexibility with which they are maintained. The family are helped to redefine boundaries, increase flexibility by encouragement to "talk more" or "make clearer rules" within the safe environment of the session. Sometimes, the intervention is to "de-triangulate" a particular family member (e.g., when an adolescent becomes involved in helping parents to stop arguing).

Behavioral Family Therapy

Behavioral family therapy approaches draw on similar ideas as structural family therapy. They focus on the behavioral sequences that occur in family life (Patterson, 1971, 1982) and interventions are aimed at interrupting unhelpful patterns and strengthening positive ones. As in structural therapy, the therapist tends to work with observed processes within the therapy session, often focusing on specific areas such as communication skills, problem-solving or interrupting escalating patterns of symmetrical communication. Behavioral approaches include interventions aimed primarily at parents in the form of *Parent Management Training (PMT)*, by far the best researched of all family interventions (for a full account see chapter 64).

Evidence for Effectiveness

Structural and behavioral approaches have been the most widely researched of all family interventions. The largest body of evidence is for behavioral family therapy and in particular parenting interventions for child and adolescent behavior problems (Brosnan & Carr, 2000; Kazdin, 2004) with PMT alone being evaluated in over 60 high-quality randomized controlled trials (Lundahl, Risser, & Lovejoy *et al.*, 2006). There is also persuasive evidence for structural and behavioral approaches in the treatment of anorexia nervosa (but see chapter 41 for some reservations). A series of randomized controlled trials at the Maudsley Hospital, London, compared family therapy with individual supportive therapy following hospitalization for anorexia nervosa (Russell, Szmukler, Dare, & Eisler, 1987) and also compared two forms of out-patient family therapy (Eisler, Dare, Hodes *et al.*, 2000; Le Grange, Eisler, Dare, & Hodes, 1992), demonstrating the efficacy of family therapy with continued improvement post-treatment for up to 5 years (Eisler, Dare, Russell *et al.*, 1997; Eisler, Simic, Russell *et al.*, 2007).

The research has led to a gradual refinement of the treatment approach (Dare, Eisler, Colahan *et al.*, 1995; Eisler, 2005; Rhodes, Gosbee, Madden, & Brown, 2005) from the original structural model described by Minuchin, Rosman, & Baker, (1978) but has retained as a central feature the empowerment of parents in helping their child tackle his or her eating problems. Similar results were obtained in the USA by Robin, Siegal, Koepke, Moye, and Trice (1994) using behavioral systems therapy and Lock, Agras, Bryson *et al.* (2005), Lock, Couturier, & Agras (2006), who adapted the Maudsley approach (Lock, Le Grange, Agras, & Dare, 2001). Several studies (Barrett, 1998; Barrett, Dadds, & Rapee, 1996; Barrett, Healey-Farrell, & March, 2004; King, Tonge, Heyne *et al.*, 1998; Mendlowitz, Manassis, Bradley *et al.*, 1999; Silverman, Kurtines, Ginsburg *et al.*, 1998) have shown that behaviorally based family therapy was effective in treating children with OCD and anxiety disorders. An interesting addition to these findings comes from Cobham, Dadds, and Spence's (1998) study comparing cognitive–behavioral therapy (CBT) and CBT combined with PMT for children with anxiety problems. For children of non-anxious parents, both CBT and CBT + PMT resulted in good outcome in about 80% of cases. However, for children with anxious parents, individual CBT resulted in good outcome in approximately 40% of cases compared with 80% good outcome for CBT + PMT.

Influencing Frameworks

All psychotherapies are concerned with bringing about change but what characterizes the family therapy approaches that we discuss under this heading is that they have focused primarily on *how change* is brought about while being agnostic to the question of how the problems might have arisen. The two groups of therapies that are most clearly defined by an influencing framework are *Strategic therapies* (Haley, 1963, 1976) and *Brief therapies* (Watzlawick, Weakland, & Fisch *et al.*, 1974) developed by the group at the Mental Research Institute (MRI) in Palo Alto, the latter eventually developing into what is now known as *Solution-focused therapy* (de Shazer, 1985). Similarly to the originators of the approaches described in the previous section, the Palo Alto group were interested in the way in which symptoms became part of the family regulatory system but also introduced the idea that repeated ineffective attempts at solutions could themselves maintain the problem. Their focus was on the interactive process that interfered with change, rather than the processes that maintained problems. They assumed that the process that blocked change would be specific to each individual or each family and, unlike structural therapy for example, did not assume that the family organization or family structure needed to be changed in a specific predetermined way.

While there is obvious overlap with the structural and behavioral approaches described earlier, the main interest in the strategic approaches has been in how change happens rather than the kind of change that should be achieved. *Brief solution-focused* therapy (de Shazer, 1985) has some overlaps with *Motivational interviewing* approaches (Miller & Rollnick, 2002) in developing differential strategies depending on the level of motivation of family members, who are classified as "clients" (ready for change), "visitors" (do not see themselves as having a problem) or "complainants" (have a problem but not sure they want to do anything to change).

The following example may serve as an illustration of a strategic intervention. In an early family session with an adolescent with anorexia nervosa the therapist asks the following question: "Have you reached the stage when you feel that people trying to encourage you to eat are on your side and helping you fight anorexia or do you still always feel that they are against you?" The girl thought for a bit before responding: "Sometimes, but not very often at the moment." The therapist nodded and added: "It is important that you go on noticing these instances. As they become more frequent it will make it easier for you to deal with the times when you feel that everyone is against you."

One can see several ideas underlying this intervention. The therapist had noted that the young woman and her parents were regularly locked in repetitive battles at mealtimes which resulted in the daughter partly giving in and the parents backing off. The daughter acknowledged that she had a problem and wanted to get better but after every meal felt resentful and angry with her parents. Asking the above question had a number of goals:

1 To establish an exception to the disabling family belief that *every* mealtime is inevitably a battle of wills;

2 To imply that when an exception happens, it is an indication of the start of a process of recovery; and

3 To imply that the exceptions will increase in frequency.

The therapist was also using his position as an expert who had been through a similar process with many other families. While the discussion was with the daughter, it was important that it was witnessed by the parents, who were perhaps as much paralyzed by seeing their daughter's despair as they were by their own sense of helplessness.

Strategic ideas were also the basis of the early work of the Milan group. The Milan associates developed a stylized form of interviewing the family in which a co-therapist pair was supported by a team behind a one-way screen. The central assumption that guided the therapy was that the symptomatic behavior was part of a paradoxical bind that prevented the family system from changing and the aim of the therapeutic team was to devise an intervention that would counter the paradox of the symptom (Palazzoli, Boscolo, Cecchin *et al.*, 1978). The therapeutic team developed hypotheses that were explored with the family through the use a "circular interview" (Bertrando, 2006). The observation of the family's response to these questions was used during a mid-session discussion of the team to gain other perspectives and the therapist (especially in the earlier versions of the approach) would deliver a message aimed at "perturbing" what were thought to be stuck patterns of interaction and fixed beliefs (Palazzoli, Boscolo, Cecchin *et al.*, 1980).

Evidence for Effectiveness

The therapies that we have grouped under this heading are relatively poorly researched. The strongest evidence has come from the work of Szapocznik and Kurtines (1989), who have systematically and over many years evaluated Brief strategic therapy for substance misusing adolescents. In addition to demonstrating the effectiveness of their treatment approach in a number of randomized controlled trials (Szapocznik & Williams, 2000), they have also shown the specific value of strategic techniques in engaging difficult-to-reach families (Coatsworth, Santisteban, McBridge, & Szapocznik, 2001; Santisteban, Suarez-Morales, Robbins, & Szapocznik, 2004). Many of the treatment components developed by Szapocznik and colleagues have been incorporated into the well-researched multidimensional treatments described later.

Meaning Creating Frameworks

An important idea that underpins all family therapy approaches is that all problems are embedded and shaped by their social context and to a lesser extent help to shape the context. If we try to understand the interpersonal nature of problems it is almost inevitable that we become concerned with language, beliefs, cognitions and narratives because these are central to understanding the process of social interaction. In the early developments of the family therapy field, these ideas were focused primarily on the exploration of interpersonal communication and in particular the way in which the overt content of communication was given different meanings by communication at another (meta) level (e.g., tone of voice, non-verbal cues).

The ideas about the importance of beliefs in shaping behavior have been developed by a number of authors in the field. Following their split from the original Milan team in the early 1980s, Boscolo and Cecchin started developing a style of work that abandoned much of the early strategic components and focused on the process of the interview and the way it could bring forward new perceptions, unexplored stories and hidden meanings (Bertrando, 2006; Boscolo, Cecchin, Hoffman, & Penn, 1987). This was accompanied by a change in the understanding of the therapist's role in bringing about change and a shift in emphasis away from behaviors to beliefs and narratives.

The Therapist as Participant Observer

Up until the early 1980s the therapist was invariably seen as an outside observer of the family process who could use his or her "metaposition" to gain an understanding of the family dynamic and intervene in a purposeful way to bring about change. This was challenged first by von Foerster (1979), who argued that the act of observation (and the describing of the observation) make the observer part of the system. The implication for the clinician was the need to recognize not only that any observations being made are influenced by the subjectivity of the observer's perceptions, but also that they become part of a recursive pattern of mutual influences between clinician and family. This shift has had a major impact on the practice of family therapy. The first was a change in the conceptualization of family therapy from a treatment *of* families (with the implication that the family was problematic or dysfunctional) to a treatment *with* families, where the meetings with families provide the context for change rather than the target of change. Secondly, thinking about the therapist as being part of the system also led to the re-examination of issues of power and control (Hoffman, 1985) and to a more collaborative and less "expert" role for the therapist. Where a team was used, its role also changed and became a more open and transparent vehicle for bringing alternative perspectives on the work, for instance by making sure that families meet the team rather than always keeping the team invisible behind a one-way screen. Other developments leading to greater respectfulness and collaboration with families was the practice of inviting families to observe the team reflecting on the session in front of them (Andersen, 1987) or therapists developing their hypotheses jointly with families (Bertrando & Arcelloni, 2006).

Language and Narratives

The interest in meaning systems and their influences on shaping family interactions have always had their place in the family therapy field (Ferreira, 1963; Palazzoli, Boscolo, Cecchin *et al.*, 1978; Watzlawick, Beavin, & Jackson, 1967). However, the more recent developments have placed language and narratives center stage for several influential therapy approaches, in particular *narrative therapies* (Parry & Doane, 1994; White & Epston, 1989) and the *collaborative language approaches* (Anderson & Goolishan, 1988; Goolishan & Anderson, 1987). These approaches have been the most overtly embedded in a social constructionist understanding which emphasizes the relativity of observed reality and which sees language and narratives as the vehicle through which people acquire their definitions of self. Individual problems are understood to be, at least in part, the result of the filtering of experiences through narratives that people have about themselves. These individual narratives are seen as being embedded in wider systems narratives such as cultural, political or educational narratives (Paré, 1995; White, 2005).

Although the narrative and language approaches are theoretically distinct, there is a clear overlap with cognitive therapies both at a conceptual level (i.e., in seeing beliefs and meanings attached to problems as central targets of treatment) and borrowing each others' intervention techniques (e.g., the use of behavioral scaling techniques by narrative therapists or the use of externalization of the problem in some CBT approaches).

Evidence for Effectiveness

The evidence for the value of approaches that have been described in this section is limited. There are a small number of studies that have directly evaluated treatments such as narrative therapy. Seymour and Epston (1989) followed up 45 cases of childhood stealing where the family intervention used a narrative approach and found that over 80% of cases were treated successfully. Carr (1991) reviewed 10 studies using a Milan systemic approach and concluded that they provided evidence for the effectiveness of the treatments. However, only four of the studies were randomized controlled trials and the samples were mostly small with a mixture of problems. More recently, there have been several studies evaluating family therapy for depression (Campbell, Bianco, Dowling *et al.*, 2003; Diamond, Reis, Diamond, Siqueland, & Isaacs, 2002; Trowell, Joffe, Campbell *et al.*, 2007), in which the family approach had as a main focus addressing cognitions, beliefs and narratives that showed evidence for the efficacy of these approaches. The most recent of these studies (Trowell, Joffe, Campbell *et al.*, 2007), which compared family therapy with brief psychodynamic psychotherapy, was notable in two respects. Both treatments achieved around 75% remission by the end of treatment (with an average of 11 sessions of family therapy or 25 sessions of individual psychotherapy) and both treatments showed a continuing improvement at 6-month follow-up.

Multidimensional and Integrative Frameworks

In recent years there has been a growing move towards integrating different approaches, both from within the family therapy field and outside it (Norcross & Goldfield, 2005). In clinical practice it is not uncommon to find clinicians drawing on a number of conceptual models and using intervention techniques developed within a different approach than the one they see as their primary treatment approach. As Fraenkel and Pinsof (2001) point out, this happens in one of two ways. Clinicians include techniques or ideas from other approaches and incorporate them into their own conceptual framework, which Fraenkel and Pinsof describe as "technical eclecticism" (or "assimilative integration" following Messer, 1992). This can be contrasted with integration at a theoretical level or "theoretical eclecticism" (Fraenkel & Pinsof, 2001), in which different conceptualizations of the therapy process are drawn on and applied depending on the nature of the problem, stage of treatment or difficulties encountered in treatment.

In this section we briefly describe four treatment models (Functional Family Therapy, Multisystemic Therapy, Multidimensional Family Therapy and Multidimensional Treatment Foster Care) that have integrated several family therapy approaches and have been well researched, and a model that has integrated systemic, cognitive–behavioral and psychodynamic approaches (Integrative Problem-Centered Therapy). Finally, we describe recent developments in using multi-family approaches with child and adolescent problems which also draw on a number of different conceptual frameworks.

Functional Family Therapy

This is an approach developed by Alexander and Parsons (1982) and Alexander and Sexton (2002) combining aspects of behavioral and structural approaches with strategic family therapy. Functional family therapy starts from the assumption that problem behaviors and symptoms (whatever their origin) take on a functional role in the way that relationships and family hierarchies are maintained and aim to replace problem behaviors with more appropriate behaviors that can serve the same function but in a positive way in the family organization. For example, in a family with a child with OCD the child may have a very close and intense relationship with mother centered on assurance seeking/receiving behaviors, and a more distant relationship with father, who tends to respond dismissively to requests for reassurance. The family might be encouraged to find alternative activities that would meet the need for closeness and assurance but not of symptom-related behaviors and would also seek to involve the father in spending time with the child in such activities.

Multisystemic Therapy and Multidimensional Family Therapy

Multisystemic Therapy (MST; Henggeler, 1999; Henggeler & Borduin, 1990) and Multidimensional Family Therapy (MDFT; Liddle, 1992; Liddle & Hogue, 2001) are two well-researched treatments that have been designed to include interventions at several different levels, drawing on conceptualizations from strategic, structural and behavioral family therapy. Both have been designed with a fairly specific target population in mind (delinquent and substance misusing adolescents). The integration of conceptual ideas from other approaches is based on an analysis of the target problem which both MST and MDFT see as needing to be addressed at individual and family as well as social levels. Interventions are targeted at several levels which aim to address individual and contextual issues around the problem behavior but also motivational and engagement issues, recognizing that the adolescent with the problem may be the least motivated person in the system. For both MST and MDFT, the analysis of the nature of the problems (delinquency and substance misuse) is central and provides the framework within which the integration of conceptual ideas from different treatment approaches takes place (which differentiates them, for instance, from Functional Family Therapy). A further treatment program could be added to this group, *Multidimensional Treatment Foster Care* (MTFC; Chamberlain, 2003). Although distinct in some ways (not least in the fact that the youth offenders enrolled in the program are placed in foster families) there are many overlaps with MST and MDFT in the structure and intensity of the treatment interventions as well as in many of the conceptual ideas that inform it.

Multiple Family Approaches

Multiple family approaches have also developed with a focus on particular problems and draw on multiple theoretical frameworks. They have a history in adult psychiatry, particularly in the treatment of schizophrenia (Lacquer, La Burt, & Morong, 1964; McFarlane, 2005; Strelnick, 1977), but in more recent years have increasingly been utilized with child and adolescent mental health problems (Asen, 2002; Asen & Schuff, 2006; Eisler, 2005; Saayman, Saayman, & Weins, 2006). The initial impetus for working with several families at the same time was partly pragmatic (i.e., to maximize the use of limited resources and to address the social isolation that patients and their families were experiencing). Theoretically, they drew on a mixture of systemic, group and psychodynamic ideas, and most multi-family groups also include a significant psychoeducational component. The practical experience of bringing together several families very quickly brought forward new ideas about the nature of the therapeutic relationship, the importance of maximizing family resources in dealing with individual problems and ways in which clinicians can facilitate change through providing a structured setting in which families can interact and learn from each other. Seeing several families together is not simply a matter of pragmatic or economic convenience. The multi-family group format affords many opportunities for helping families to learn from each others' strengths, to reduce the sense of isolation and stigma and to use the group as a resource for problem-solving (Asen, 2002; Eisler, 2005).

The most common form of multi-family work has 5–7 families meeting weekly or fortnightly for 1.5–2 h. Groups of this kind have now been developed for a growing range of problems including mood disorders (Fristad, Goldberg-Arnold, & Gavazzi, 2002; Goldberg-Arnold, Fristad, & Gavazzi, 1999), eating disorders (Geist, Heinmaa, Stephens, Davis, & Gavazzi, 2000), behavior problems (McKay, Harrison, Gonzales, Kim, & Quintana, 2002), schizophrenia (Asen & Shuff, 2006; Schepp, O'Connor, Kennedy, & Tsai, 2003), learning difficulties (Russell, John, Lakshmanan, Russell, & Lakshmidevi, 2004) and school problems (Kratochwill, McDonald, Levin, Bear-Tibbetts, & Demaray, 2004). In the UK a more intensive format of multi-family treatment has been developed by Asen, Dawson, and McHugh (2001) in which families take part in a brief multi-family day program. Originally developed for work with multi-problem "multi-agency" families (Cooklin, Miller, & McHugh, 1983), it has been modified for treatment of anorexia nervosa (Eisler, 2005; Scholz, Rix, Scholz, Gantchev, & Thomke, 2005) and for school problems (Dawson & McHugh, 1994, 2006).

Integrative Family Therapy Approaches

A different approach to integration of treatment approaches is found in the work of authors who start from an analysis of the conceptual overlaps between different psychotherapeutic models (Breunlin, Schwartz, & MacKune-Karrer, 1997; Fraenkel & Pinsof, 2001; Lebow, 1987; Pinsof, 1994, 2005). Pinsof's (2005) Integrative Problem-Centered Therapy (IPCT) provides a good example. IPCT integrates six different therapeutic orientations (behavioral, biobehavioral, experiential, family of origin, psychodynamic, self-psychology) and three treatment contexts or modalities (family/community, couple, individual). The underlying assumption of IPCT is that individual problems are maintained by a set of constraints (social/organizational, biological, meaning, transgenerational, object relations, self) which roughly correspond to the therapeutic orientations. IPCT starts from a premise that individuals and families can usually resolve problems with minimal interventions aimed at reinforcing and building upon existing individual and family strengths. A brief problem-focused behavioral family intervention is recommended as an appropriate starting point for most child and adolescent problems and only when these have failed would the therapist need to start exploring potential deficits and constraints at other levels.

The strength of IPCT (like that of other integrative approaches) is that it attempts to find common conceptual ground between different therapies and to maximize their potential by targeting different levels of difficulties by appropriate interventions. The disadvantage is that it assumes that the framework can be fitted to any kind of problem and that the way that treatments are tailored to individual needs comes purely from an analysis of the different levels of constraints that particular individuals and their families are faced with. This is theoretically attractive but difficult to evaluate empirically. It is notable that approaches such as MST, MDFT and MTFC have generated considerable outcome research whereas integrative approaches such as IPCT have not.

Evidence for Effectiveness

The strongest evidence for treatment approaches described in this section come from studies of multidimensional approaches used for treatment of youth offenders (Curtis, Ronan, & Borduin, 2004; Littell, Popo, & Forsythe, 2007; Woolfenden, Williams, & Peat, 2007) and substance misuse (Stanton & Shaddish, 1997). The meta-analyses in the above studies included mainly treatments using a multidimensional approach and these were also the studies producing the clearest results (although none of the meta-analyses compared multidimensional with other family therapy approaches). The evidence for the efficacy of multifamily therapy with child and adolescent problems is sparse so far. There have been few randomized studies and while they provide positive support (Barrett, Healey-Farrell, & March, 2004; Kratochwill, McDonald, Levin *et al.*, 2004), the current overall conclusion has to be "promising but unproven" (McDonell & Dyck, 2004).

Overview and Conclusions

Family therapy, in our account, covers a broad range of approaches. Many of the things that apparently differentiate treatments are a matter of what is emphasized and inevitably there will be large overlaps with other approaches. We have suggested a way of conceptualizing different frameworks of treatments as a way of understanding some of the differences and similarities both within the family therapy field and outside of it. The empirical evidence in support of family therapy in the broadest sense is considerable. There have been more than 20 meta-analyses of family interventions, approximately half of which either included or were solely concerned with child and adolescent problems (for a review see Shadish & Baldwin, 2003). The findings are consistent in showing family therapy to be effective when compared to no treatment or waitlist controls (with an average effect size of 0.65) and to do at least as well as, or better than, alternative treatments, although the differences here are generally small. However, the quality of the evidence is variable depending on the type of problem being considered. In some areas (such as the treatment of substance misuse, anorexia nervosa, delinquency and behavior problems) the evidence for the effectiveness of family therapy of one kind or another makes it currently the treatment of choice. In other areas (depression, anxiety disorders, OCD) there is more limited evidence but nevertheless it points to family-based treatments being effective. When one takes a look across the field as a whole, perhaps the most striking thing is that taking a broad definition of family therapy (as any family-based or family-oriented treatment) then for most if not all child and adolescent problems it is shown to be effective. However, what is also clear is that for different kinds of problem often quite different types of family intervention have been shown to be useful. To what extent this is really a result of the specificity of treatment needs generated by particular problems or simply a reflection of the particular interests of researchers who have investigated these problems is unclear, as very little research exists at present comparing different family therapy approaches and what comparisons do exist are quite general and do not focus on specific components that might be needed when dealing with specific types of problem.

In the treatment of conduct disorder, juvenile delinquency and substance misuse there is considerable conceptual as well as technical overlap between the best-researched treatments

(MST, MDFT, MTFC and, to a lesser degree, Functional Family Therapy) although the proponents of these approaches do not always acknowledge the similarities. One of the negative consequences of the current emphasis on developing evidence-based practice is that it encourages treatments to be viewed as complete and competing packages, which tends to obscure the common ground between treatment models. The family therapy field has been particularly prone to this malaise and is awash with differently labeled (similar) treatments with little attempt to compare them at either a theoretical or an empirical level.

The other downside of the focus on evaluating treatment models has been the dearth of research on factors that might act as mediators and moderators of treatment. At present, the evidence is thin on the ground but nevertheless indicates that these are clinically crucial areas to investigate. We discussed earlier the moderating effect of disorganization in the family (Hampson & Beavers, 1996b) and high levels of criticism (Eisler, Simic, Russell *et al.*, 2007) which has implications for the style of family therapy best suited for these types of family. Such findings are rare at present yet they have important implications for clinical practice. Even less is known about family factors that might act as mediators of treatment (i.e., those that might be amenable to treatment and might need to change in order for treatment to be effective). This may well include variables that have been well researched from a developmental or etiological perspective such as attachment but that need to be looked at from a different angle. For instance, our clinical experience suggests that parent(s) with insecure attachment patterns can sometimes be difficult to engage in treatment and may feel they are being covertly blamed when asked to take quite an active role in their child's treatment. Of course, this may be because of the particular way in which we work with families and it is possible that for such families an attachment-oriented family therapy (Byng-Hall, 1991; Diamond, Reis, Diamond *et al.*, 2002) may be able to engage them more effectively in treatment regardless of whether attachment is shown to have a role in the development of the particular problem their child has.

In order for these issues to be addressed by empirical study two major shifts are needed in the conceptual ideas informing family therapy research and indeed psychotherapy research in general. The first is the recognition that much more work is needed to find the common ground between treatments in order to highlight the specific aspects that differentiate them. This will allow outcome research to target much more focused questions about core ingredients of treatments and how these might interact with other factors. The second requires a re-examination of the theoretical models of change underpinning different family therapy approaches and testing these empirically. While our knowledge of *what* works has increased considerably in recent years, our understanding of *how* treatments work is still extremely limited. We should not assume that the process of change will necessarily follow the same path for everyone or that the role that the family will play in this process will be the same.

References

Ackerman, N. W. (1938). The unity of the family. *Archives of Pediatrics, 55*, 51–62.

Alexander, J., & Parsons, B. (1982). *Functional family therapy.* Monterey, CA: Brooks Cole.

Alexander, J., & Sexton, T. L. (2002). Functional family therapy: A model for treating high risk, acting out youth. In F. Kaslow (Ed.), *Comprehensive handbook of psychotherapy: Integrative/eclectic.* (Vol. 4, pp. 111–132). New Jersey: John Wiley & Sons.

Amir, N., Freshman, M., & Foa, E. B. (2000). Family distress and involvement in relatives of obsessive-compulsive disorder patients. *Journal of Anxiety Disorders, 14*, 209–217.

Andersen, T. (1987). The reflecting team: Dialogues and meta-dialogues in clinical work. *Family Process, 26*, 415–428.

Anderson, H., & Goolishian, H. (1988). Human systems as linguistic systems: Evolving ideas for the implications in theory and practice. *Family Process, 27*, 371–393.

Asay, T. P., & Lambert, M. J. (2000). The empirical case for common factors in therapy: Quantitative findings. In M. A. Hubble, B. L. Duncan, & S. D. Miller (Eds.), *The heart and soul of change* (pp. 33–55). Washington, DC: American Psychological Association.

Asen, E. (2002). Multiple family therapy: An overview. *Journal of Family Therapy, 24*, 3–16.

Asen, E., & Schuff, H. (2006). Psychosis and multiple family group therapy. *Journal of Family Therapy, 28*, 56–72.

Asen, K. E., Dawson, N., & McHugh, B. (2001). *Multiple family therapy: The Marlborough model and its wider applications.* London and New York: Karnac.

Barrett, P., Healey-Farrell, L., & March, J. S. (2004). Cognitive–behavioral family treatment of childhood obsessive compulsive disorder: A controlled trial. *Journal of the American Academy of Child and Adolescent Psychiatry, 34*, 46–62.

Barrett, P. M. (1998). Evaluation of cognitive–behavioral group treatments for childhood anxiety disorders. *Journal of Clinical Child Psychology, 27*, 459–468.

Barrett, P. M., Dadds, M. R., & Rapee, R. M. (1996). Family treatment of childhood anxiety: A controlled trial. *Journal of Consulting and Clinical Psychology, 64*, 333–342.

Bateson, G. (1972). *Steps to an ecology of mind.* New York: Ballentine.

Bateson, G., Jackson, D. D., Haley, J., & Weakland, J. H. (1956). Towards a theory of schizophrenia. *Behavioral Science, 1*, 251–265.

Bateson, G., & Ruesch, J. (1951). *Communication: The social matrix of psychiatry.* New York: Norton.

Berger, P., & Luckman, T. (1966). *The social construction of reality: A treatise in the sociology of knowledge.* Garden City, NY: Doubleday.

Bertrando, P. (2006). The evolution of family interventions for schizophrenia: A tribute to Gianfranco Cecchin. *Journal of Family Therapy, 28*, 4–22.

Bertrando, P., & Arcelloni, T. (2006). Hypotheses are dialogues: Sharing hypotheses with clients. *Journal of Family Therapy, 28*, 370–387.

Beutler, L. E., Malik, M., Alimohamed, S., Harwood, T. M., Talebi, H., Noble, S., *et al.* (2004). Therapist variables. In M. J. Lambert (Ed.), *Bergin and Garfield's handbook of psychotherapy and behavior change* (pp. 227–306). New York: John Wiley & Sons.

Bloch, S., Hafner, J., Harari, E., & Szmukler, G. I. (1994). *The family in clinical psychiatry.* Oxford: Oxford University Press.

Boscolo, L., Cecchin, G., Hoffman, L., & Penn, P. (1987). *Milan system family therapy: Conversations in theory and practice.* New York: Basic Books.

Breunlin, D. C., Schwartz, R. C., & MacKune-Karrer, B. (1997). *Metaframeworks: Transcending the models of family therapy.* San Francisco, CA: Jossey-Bass.

Brosnan, R., & Carr, A. (2000). Adolescent conduct problems. In A. Carr (Ed.), *What works with children and adolescents? A critical review of psychological interventions with children, adolescents and their families* (pp. 131–154). London: Routledge.

Burgess, E. W. (1926). The family as a unity of interacting personalities. *The Family*, *7*, 3–9.

Burnham, J. (1986). *Family therapy*. London: Routledge.

Byng-Hall, J. (1991). The application of attachment theory to understanding and treatment in family therapy. In C. M. Parkes, J. Stevenson-Hinde, & P. Marris (Eds.), *Attachment across the family life-cycle* (pp. 199–215). London: Routledge.

Byng-Hall, J. (1995). Creating a secure base: Some implications of attachment theory for family therapy. *Family Relations*, *34*, 45–58.

Calvocoressi, L., Mazure, C. M., & Kasl, S. V. (1999). Family accommodation of obsessive-compulsive symptoms: Instrument development and assessment of family behavior. *Journal of Nervous and Mental Disease*, *187*, 636–642.

Campbell, D., Bianco, V., Dowling, E., Goldberg, H., McNab, S., & Pentecost, D. (2003). Family therapy for childhood depression: researching significant moments. *Journal of Family Therapy*, *25*, 417–435.

Carr, A. (1991). Milan systemic family therapy: A review of 10 empirical investigations. *Journal of Family Therapy*, *13*, 237–264.

Carr, A. (2006). *Family therapy: Concepts, process and practice* (2nd edn.). Chichester: John Wiley and Sons.

Carter, B. & McGoldrick, M. (1999). *The expanded family lifecycle: Individual, family and social perspectives*. Boston: Allyn & Bacon.

Chamberlain, P. (2003). *Treating chronic juvenile offenders: Advances made through the Oregon multidimensional treatment/foster care model*. Washington, DC: American Psychological Association.

Clarkin, J. F., & Levy, K. N. (2004). The influence of client variables on psychotherapy. In M. J. Lambert (Ed.), *Bergin and Garfield's handbook of psychotherapy and behavior change* (Part ii, ch 6). New York: John Wiley & Sons.

Coatsworth, J. D., Santisteban, D. A., McBridge, C. K., & Szapocznik, J. (2001). Brief strategic family therapy versus community control: Engagement, retention, and an exploration of the moderating role of adolescent symptom severity. *Family Process*, *40*, 313–332.

Cobham, J. E., Dadds, M. R., & Spence, S. H. (1998). The role of parental anxiety in the treatment of childhood anxiety. *Journal of Consulting and Clinical Psychology*, *66*, 893–905.

Cooklin, A., Miller, A., & McHugh, B. (1983). An institution for change: Developing a family day unit. *Family Process*, *22*, 453–468.

Crockenberg, S. C., & Leerkes, E. M. (2003). Parental acceptance, postpartum depression and maternal sensitivity: Mediating and moderating processes. *Journal of Family Psychology*, *17*, 80–93.

Crockenberg, S. C., Leerkes, E. M., & Lekka, S. K. (2007). Pathways from marital aggression to infant emotion regulation: The development of withdrawal in infancy. *Infant Behavior and Development*, *30*, 97–113.

Curtis, N. M., Ronan, K. R., & Borduin, C. M. (2004). Multisystemic treatment: A meta-analysis of outcome studies. *Journal of Family Psychology*, *18*, 411–419.

Dallos, R., & Draper, R. (2005). *An introduction to family therapy and systemic practice*. Maidenhead: Open University Press.

Dare, C., & Lindsey, C. (1979). Children in family therapy. *Journal of Family Therapy*, 1, 253–269.

Dare, C., Eisler, I., Colahan, M., Crowther, C., Senior, R., & Asen E. (1995). The listening heart and the chi square: Clinical and empirical perceptions in the family therapy of anorexia nervosa. *Journal of Family Therapy*, *17*, 31–57.

David, H. P., Dytrych, Z., & Matejcek, Z. (2003). Born unwanted: Observations from Prague study. *American Psychologist*, *58*, 224–229.

Dawson, N., & McHugh, B. (1994). Parents and children: Participants in change. In E. Dowling, & E. Osborne (Eds.), *The family and school: A joint systems approach to problems with children*. London: Routledge.

Dawson, N., & McHugh, B. (2006). A systemic response to school based violence from a UK perspective. *Journal of Family Therapy*, *28*, 267–271.

Deater-Deckard, K., Atzaba-Poria, N., & Pike, A. (2004). Mother- and father–child mutuality in Anglo and Indian British families: A link with lower externalizing problems. *Journal of Abnormal Child Psychology*, *32*, 609–620.

de Shazer, S. (1985). *Keys to solutions in brief therapy*. New York: Norton.

Diamond, G. S., Reis, B. F., Diamond, G. M., Siqueland, L., & Isaacs, L. (2002). Attachment-based family therapy for depressed adolescents: A treatment development study. *Journal of the American Academy of Child and Adolescent Psychiatry*, *41*, 1190–1196.

Dunn, J., & Plomin, R. (1990). *Separate lives: Why siblings are so different*. New York: Basic Books.

Eisler, I. (1993). Families, family therapy and psychosomatic illness. In S. Moorey, & M. Hodes (Eds.), *Psychological treatments in human disease and illness* (pp. 42–62). London: Gaskill.

Eisler, I. (1995). Family models of eating disorders. In G. I. Szmukler, C. Dare, & J. Treasure (Eds.), *Handbook of eating disorders: Theory, treatment and research* (pp. 155–176). London: Wiley.

Eisler, I. (2005). The empirical and theoretical base of family therapy and multiple family day therapy for adolescent anorexia nervosa. *Journal of Family Therapy*, *27*, 104–131.

Eisler, I., Dare, C., Hodes, M., Russell, G. F. M., Dodge, E., & Le Grange, D. (2000). Family therapy for adolescent anorexia nervosa: The results of a controlled comparison of two family interventions. *Journal of Child Psychology and Psychiatry*, *41*, 727–736.

Eisler, I., Dare, C., Russell, G. F. M., Szmukler, G. I., Dodge, E., & le Grange, D. (1997). Family and individual therapy for anorexia nervosa: A 5-year follow-up. *Archives of General Psychiatry*, *54*, 1025–1030.

Eisler, I., Simic, M., Russell, G. F. M., & Dare, C. (2007). A randomized controlled treatment trial of two forms of family therapy in adolescent anorexia nervosa: A five-year follow-up. *Journal of Child Psychology and Psychiatry*, *48*, 552–560.

Falicov, C. (1995). Training to think culturally: A multidimensional comparative framework. *Family Process*, *34*, 373–388.

Fergusson, D. M., Horwood, L. J., & Lynskey, M. T. (1992). Family change, parental discord and early offending. *Journal of Child Psychology and Psychiatry*, *33*, 1059–1075.

Fergusson, D. M., & Lynskey, M. T. (1996). Adolescent resiliency to family adversity. *Journal of Child Psychology and Psychiatry*, *37*, 281–292.

Ferreira, A. J. (1963). Family myth and homoeostasis. *Archives of General Psychiatry*, *9*, 457–463.

Fraenkel, P., & Pinsof, W. (2001). Teaching family therapy-centred integration: Assimilation and beyond. *Journal of Psychotherapy Integration*, *11*, 59–86.

Fristad, M. A., Goldberg-Arnold, J. S., & Gavazzi, S. M. (2002). Multifamily psychoeducation groups (MFPG) for families with bipolar disorder. *Bipolar Disorders*, *4*, 254–262.

Geist, R., Heinmaa, M., Stephens, D., Davis, R., & Katzman, D. K. (2000). Comparison of family therapy and family group psychoeducation in adolescents with anorexia nervosa. *Canadian Journal of Psychiatry*, *45*, 173–178.

Goldberg-Arnold, J. S., Fristad, M. A., & Gavazzi, S. M. (1999). Family psychoeducation: Giving caregivers what they want and need. *Family Relations*, *48*, 411–417.

Goolishian, H., & Anderson, H. (1987). Language systems and therapy: An evolving idea. *Psychotherapy*, *24*, 529–538.

Gorrell Barnes, G., Thompson, P., Daniel, G., & Burchardt, N. (1998). *Growing up in step-families*. Oxford: Clarendon Press.

Haley, J. (1963). *Strategies of psychotherapy*. New York: Grune & Stratton.

Haley, J. (1976). *Problem solving therapy*. San Francisco, CA: Jossey Bass.

Hampson, R. B., & Beavers, R. (1996a). Family therapy and outcome: Relationships between therapists and family styles. *Contemporary Family Therapy*, *18*, 345–370.

Hampson, R. B., & Beavers, R. (1996b). Measuring family therapy outcome in a clinical setting. *Family Process*, *35*, 347–360.

Henggeler, S. W. (1999). Multisystemic therapy: An overview of clinical procedures, outcomes and policy implications. *Child Psychology and Psychiatry Review*, *4*, 2–10.

Henggeler, S. W., & Borduin, C. M. (1990). *Family therapy and beyond: A multidimensional approach to treating the behaviour problems of children and adolescents*. Pacirc Grove, CA: Brooks Cole.

Hetherington, M. E. (1989). Coping with family transitions: Winners, losers and survivors. *Child Development*, *60*, 1–14.

Hoffman, L. (1985). Beyond power and control: Towards a "second order" family systems therapy. *Family Systems Medicine*, *3*, 381–396.

Huizink, A. C., Robles De Medina, P. G., Mulder, E. J. H., Visser, G. H. A., & Buitelaar, J. K. (2002). Psychological measures of prenatal stress as predictors of infant temperament. *Journal of the American Academy of Child and Adolescent Psychiatry*, *41*, 1078–1085.

Jackson, D. (1957). The question of family homeostasis. *Psychiatric Quarterly*, *31 (Suppl 1)*, 79–90.

Kazdin, A. (2004). Evidence based treatments: Challenges and priorities for practice and research. *Child and Adolescent Psychiatric Clinics of North America*, *13*, 923–940.

Kendler, K. S., & Prescott, C. A. (1999). A population-based twin study of lifetime major depression in men and women. *Archives of General Psychiatry*, *56*, 39–44.

King, N., Tonge, B. J., Heyne, D., Pritchard, M., Rollings, S., Young, D., *et al.* (1998). Cognitive–behavioral treatment of school refusing children: A controlled evaluation. *Journal of American Child and Adolescent Psychiatry*, *37*, 395–403.

Kog, E., Vandereycken, W., & Vertommen, H. (1985). The psychosomatic family model: A critical analysis of family interaction concepts. *Journal of Family Therapy*, *7*, 31–44.

Kraemer, H. C., Stice, E., Kazdin, A., Offord, O., & Kupfer, D. (2001). How do risk factors work together? Mediators, moderators and independent overlapping and proxy risk factors. *American Journal of Psychiatry*, *158*, 848–856.

Kratochwill, T., McDonald, L., Levin, J., Bear-Tibbetts, H., & Demaray, M. (2004). Families and schools together: An experimental analysis of a parent mediated multi-family group program for American Indian children. *Journal of School Psychology*, *42*, 359–383.

Kubicka, L., Roth, Z., Dytrych, Z., & Matějcek, Z. (2002). The mental health of adults born of unwanted pregnancies, their siblings, and matched controls: A 35-year follow-up study from Prague, Czech Republic. *Journal of Nervous and Mental Disease*, *190*, 653–662.

Lacey, J. H., & Smith, G. (1987). Bulimia nervosa: The impact of pregnancy on mother and baby. *British Journal of Psychiatry*, 150, 777–781.

Laqueur, H. P., Laburt, H. A., Morong, E. (1964). Multiple family therapy. *Current Psychiatric Therapies*, *4*, 150–154.

Larner, G. (1996). Narrative child family therapy. *Family Process*, *35*, 423–440.

Lebow, J. L. (1987). Developing a personal integration in family therapy: Principles for model construction and practice. *Journal of Marital and Family Therapy*, *13*, 1–14.

Le Grange, D., Eisler, I., Dare, C., & Hodes, M. (1992). Family criticism and self-starvation: A study of expressed emotion. *Journal of Family Therapy*, *14*, 177–192.

Liddle, H. A. (1992). A multidimensional model for the adolescent who is abusing drugs and alcohol. In F. Snyder, & T. Ooms (Eds.), *Empowering families, helping adolescents: Family centered treatments of adolescents with alcohol, drug and other mental health problems*. Washington, DC: US Government Printing Office.

Liddle, H. A., & Hogue, A. (2001). Multidimensional family therapy: pursuing empirical support through planful treatment development. In E. Wagner, & H. Waldron (Eds.), *Adolescent substance abuse*. Needham Heights, MA: Allyn and Bacon.

Littell, J. H., Popa, M., & Forsythe, B. (2007). *Multisystemic therapy for social, emotional, and behavioural problems in youth aged 10–17*. London: John Wiley & Sons.

Lock, J., Le Grange, D., Agras, W., & Dare, C. (2001). *Treatment manual for anorexia nervosa: A family based approach*. New York: Guilford.

Lock, J., Agras, W. S., Bryson, S., & Kraemer, H. C. (2005). A comparison of short- and long-term family therapy for adolescent anorexia nervosa. *Journal of the American Academy of Child and Adolescent Psychiatry*, *44*, 632–639.

Lock, J., Couturier, J., & Agras, W. S. (2006). Comparison of long-term outcomes in adolescents with anorexia nervosa treated with family therapy. *Journal of the American Academy of Child and Adolescent Psychiatry*, *45*, 666–672.

Lundahl, B., Risser, H. J., & Lovejoy, C. (2006). A meta-analysis of parent training: Moderators and follow-up effects. *Clinical Psychology Review*, *26*, 86–104.

McDonell, M. G., & Dyck, D. G. (2004). Multifamily group treatment as an effective intervention for children with psychological disorders. *Clinical Psychology Review*, *24*, 685–706.

McFarlane, W. (2005). Psychoeducational multifamily groups for families with persons with severe mental illness. In J. Lebow (Ed.), *Handbook of clinical family therapy*. New Jersey: John Wiley & Sons.

McGoldrick, M., & Gerson, R. (1985). *Genograms in family assessment*. New York: Norton.

McKay, M. M., Harrison, M. E., Gonzales, J., Kim, L., & Quintana, E. (2002). Multiple family groups for urban children with conduct difficulties and their families. *Psychiatric Services*, *53*, 1467–1468.

Mendlowitz, S., Manassis, K., Bradley, S., Scapillto, D., Mieztis, S., & Shaw, B. F. (1999). Cognitive–behavioral group treatments in childhood anxiety disorders: The role of parental involvement. *Journal of the American Academy of Child and Adolescent Psychiatry*, *38*, 1223–1229.

Messer, S. (1992). A critical examination of belief structures in integrative and eclectic psychotherapy. In J. C. Norcross, & M. R. Goldfried (Eds.), *Handbook of psychotherapy integration* (pp. 130–168). New York: Basic Books.

Miller, W. R., & Rollnick, S. (2002). *Motivational interviewing: Preparing people for change*. New York: Guilford Press.

Minuchin, S. (1974). *Families and family therapy*. Cambridge, MA: Harvard University Press.

Minuchin, S., & Fishman, H. C. (1981). *Family therapy techniques*. Cambridge, MA: Harvard University Press.

Minuchin, S., Montalvo, B., Guerney, B., Rosman, B., & Schumer, F. (1967). *Families of the slums*. New York: Basic Books.

Minuchin, S., Rosman, B. L., & Baker, L. (1978). *Psychosomatic families: Anorexia nervosa in context*. Cambridge, MA: Harvard University Press.

Moffitt, T. E., Caspi, A., Harrington, H., & Milne, B. J. (2002). Males on the life-course-persistent and adolescence-limited antisocial pathways: Follow-up at age 26 years. *Development and Psychopathology*, *14*, 179–207.

Neilsen, S., & Bara-Carril, N. (2003). Family, burden of care and social consequences. In J. Treasure, U. Schmidt, & E. van Furth (Eds.), *Handbook of eating disorders* (2nd edn., pp. 75–90). London: John Wiley & Sons.

Norcross, J., & Goldfried, M. (2005). *Handbook of psychotherapy integration* (2nd edn.). New York: Oxford University Press.

O'Connor, T. G., Rutter, M., Beckett, C., Keaveney, L., Kreppner, J., & the English and Romanian Adoptees Study Team. (2000). The effects of global severe privation on cognitive competence: Extension and longitudinal follow-up. *Child Development*, *71*, 376–390.

Olson, D. H. (1972). Empirically unbinding the double bind: Review of research and conceptual reformulations. *Family Process*, *18*, 3–28.

Palazzoli, M. S., Boscolo, L., Cecchin, G., & Prata, G. (1978). *Paradox and counterparadox*. New York: Aronson.

Palazzoli, M. S., Boscolo, L., Cecchin, G., & Prata, G. (1980). Hypothesizing–circularity–neutrality: Three guidelines for the conductor of the session. *Family Process*, *19*, 3–12.

Pare, D. A. (1995). Of families and other cultures: The shifting paradigm of family therapy. *Family Process*, *34*, 1–19.

Park, R. J., Senior, R., & Stein, A. (2003a). The offspring of mothers with eating disorders. *European Child and Adolescent Psychiatry*, *12*, 110–119.

Park, R. J., Lee, A., Woolley, H., Murray, L., & Stein, A. (2003b). Children's representation of family mealtime in the context of maternal eating disorders. *Child: Care, Health and Development*, *29*, 111–119.

Parry, A., & Doane, R. (1994). *Story re-visions: Narrative therapy in the postmodern world*. New York: Guilford.

Patterson, G. (1971). *Families: Applications of social learning to family life*. Champaign, IL: Research Press.

Patterson, G. (1982). *Coercive family process*. Eugene, OR: Castalia.

Pinsof, W. (1994). An overview of integrative problem centred therapy: A synthesis of family and individual psychotherapies. *Journal of Family Therapy*, *16*, 103–120.

Pinsof, W. (2005). Integrative problem centred therapy. In J. Norcross, & M. Goldfried (Eds.), *Handbook of psychotherapy integration* (2nd edn., pp. 282–402). New York: Oxford University Press.

Reimers, S. (1999). "Good morning Sir!", axe handle: Talking at cross-purposes in family therapy. *Journal of Family Therapy*, *21*, 360–376.

Reiss, D., Hetherington, E. M., & Plomin, R. (1995). Genetic questions for environmental studies: Differential parenting and psychopathology in adolescence. *Archives of General Psychiatry*, *52*, 925–936.

Rhodes, P., Gosbee, M., Madden, S., & Brown, J. (2005). "Communities of concern" in the family based treatment of anorexia nervosa: Toward a consensus in the Maudsley model. *European Eating Disorders Review*, *13*, 392–398.

Riggins-Caspers, K., Cadoret, R. J., Knutson, J. F., & Langbehn, D. (2003). Biology–environment interaction and evocative biology–environment correlation: Contributions of harsh discipline and parental psychopathology to problem adolescent behaviors. *Behavior Genetics*, *33*, 205–220.

Ritsner, M., & Ponizovsky, A. (1999). Psychological distress through immigration: The two-phase temporal pattern? *International Journal of Social Psychiatry*, *45*, 125–139.

Robin, A. L., Siegal, P. T., Koepke, T., Moye, A. W., & Tice, S. (1994). Family therapy versus individual therapy for adolescent females with anorexia nervosa. *Developmental and Behavioural Paediatrics*, *15*, 111–116.

Rolland, J. (1987). Chronic illness and life cycle: A conceptual framework. *Family Processes*, *26*, 203–221.

Rolland, J. S. (1994). *Families, illness and disability: An integrative treatment model*. New York: Basic Books.

Rolland, J. S. (1999). Parental illness and disability: A family systems framework. *Journal of Family Therapy*, *21*, 242–266.

Russell, G. F. M., Szmukler, G. I., Dare, C., & Eisler, I. (1987). An evaluation of family therapy in anorexia nervosa and bulimia nervosa. *Archives of General Psychiatry*, *44*, 1047–1056.

Russell, G. F. M., Treasure, J., & Eisler, I. (1998). Mothers with anorexia nervosa who underfeed their children: Their recognition and management. *Psychological Medicine*, *28*, 93–108.

Russell, P. S. S., John, J. K., Lakshmanan J., Russell, S., & Lakshmidevi, K. M. (2004). Family intervention and acquisition of adaptive behavior among intellectually disabled children. *Journal of Intellectual Disabilities*, *8*, 383–395.

Rutter, M. (1999). Resilience concepts and findings: Implications for family therapy. *Journal of Family Therapy*, *21*, 119–144.

Rutter, M. (2006). The promotion of resilience in the face of adversity. In A. Clarke-Stewart, & J. Dunn (Eds.), *Families count: Effects on child and adolescent development* (pp. 26–52). Cambridge: Cambridge University Press.

Rutter, M., O'Connor, T., and the English and Romanian Adoptees Research Team. (2004). Are there biological programming effects for psychological development? Findings from a study of Romanian adoptees. *Developmental Psychology*, *40*, 81–94.

Rutter, M., Silberg, J., O'Connor, T., & Simonoff, E. (1999). Genetics and child psychiatry. I. Advances in quantitative and molecular genetics. *Journal of Child Psychology and Psychiatry*, *40*, 3–18.

Saayman, R. V., Saayman, G. S., & Weins, S. M. (2006). Training staff in multiple family therapy in a children's psychiatric hospital: From theory to practice. *Journal of Family Therapy*, *28*, 404–419.

Santisteban, D. A., Suarez-Morales, L., Robbins, M. S., & Szapocznik, J. (2006). Brief strategic family therapy: Lessons learned in efficacy research and challenges to blending research and practice. *Family Process*, *45*, 259–271.

Sartorius, N. (1996). Recent changes in suicide rates in selected Eastern European and other European Countries. *International Psychogeriatrics*, *7*, 301–308.

Scaramella, L. V., & Leve, L. D. (2004). Clarifying parent–child reciprocities during early childhood: The early childhood coercion model. *Clinical Child and Family Psychology Review*, *7*, 89–107.

Schepp, K. G., O'Connor, F., Kennedy, M. G., & Tsai, J. H. (2003). *Book of abstracts: Family centered program for adolescents with mental illness*. Seattle, WA: Department of Psychosocial and Community Health, University of Washington.

Schmidt, U., & Treasure, J. (2006). Anorexia nervosa: Valued and visible. A cognitive interpersonal maintenance model and its implications for research and practice. *British Journal of Clinical Psychology*, *45*, 343–366.

Scholz, M., Rix, M., Scholz, K., Gantchev, K., & Thomke, T. (2005). Multiple family therapy for anorexia nervosa: Concepts, experiences and results. *Journal of Family Therapy*, *27*, 132–141.

Sexton, T. L., & Ridley, C. R. (2004). Implications of a moderated common factors approach: Does it move the field forward? *Journal of Marital and Family Therapy*, *30*, 159–163.

Sexton, T. L., Ridley, C. R., & Kleiner, A. J. (2004). Beyond common factors: Multilevel process models of therapeutic change in marriage and family therapy. *Journal of Marital and Family Therapy*, *30*, 131–149.

Seymour, F. W., & Epston, D. (1989). An approach to childhood stealing with evaluation of 45 cases. *Australian and New Zealand Journal of Family Therapy*, *10*, 137–143.

Shadish, W. R., & Baldwin, S. A. (2003). Meta-analysis of MFT interventions. *Journal of Marital and Family Therapy*, *29*, 547–570.

Silverman, K., Kurtines, W., Ginsburg, G., Weems, C., Lumpkin, P., & Carmichael, D. (1998). Treating anxiety disorders in children with group cognitive behavioural therapy: A randomized clinical trial. *Journal of Consulting and Clinical Psychology*, *67*, 995–1003.

Simon, G. M. (2006). The heart of the matter: A proposal for placing the self of the therapist at the center of family therapy research and training. *Family Process*, *45*, 331–344.

Sprenkle, D. H., & Blow, A. J. (2004). Common factors and our sacred model. *Journal of Marital and Family Therapy*, *30*, 113–129.

Sprenkle, D. H., &. Blow A. J. (2007). The role of the therapist as the bridge between common factors and therapeutic change: More complex than congruency with a worldview. *Journal of Family Therapy*, *29*, 109–113.

Stanton, M., & Shadish, W. (1997). Outcome, attrition, and family-couples treatment for drug abuse: A meta-analysis and review of the controlled, comparative studies. *Psychological Bulletin*, *122*, 170–191.

Stein, A., Woolley, H., Cooper, S., & Fairburn, C. G. (1994). An observational study of mothers with eating disorders and their infants. *Journal of Child Psychology and Psychiatry*, *35*, 733–748.

Stein, A., Woolley, H., Cooper, S., Winterbottom, J., Fairburn, C. G., & Cortina-Borja, M. (2006). Eating habits and attitudes among 10-year-old children of mothers with eating disorders: Longitudinal study. *British Journal of Psychiatry*, *189*, 324–329.

Steinglass, P. (1998). Multiple family discussion groups for patients with chronic medical illness. *Families, Systems and Health*, *16*, 55–70.

Stice, E. (2002). Risk and maintenance factors for eating pathology: A meta-analytic review. *Psychological Bulletin*, *128*, 825–848.

Strelnick, A. H. J. (1977). Multiple family group therapy: A review of the literature. *Family Process*, *16*, 307–325.

Strickland-Clark, L., Campbell, D., & Dallos, R. (2000). Children's and adolescents' views on family therapy. *Journal of Family Therapy*, *22*, 324–341.

Szapocznik, J., & Kurtines, W. (1989). *Breakthroughs in family therapy with drug abusing and problem youth*. New York: Springer.

Szapocznik, J., & Williams, R. (2000). Brief strategic family therapy: Twenty-five years of interplay among theory, research and practice in adolescent behavior problems and drug abuse. *Clinical Child and Family Psychology Review*, *3*, 117–134.

Szmukler, G. I., Eisler, I., Russell, G. F. M., & Dare, C. (1985). Anorexia nervosa, parental "expressed emotion" and dropping out of treatment. *British Journal of Psychiatry*, *147*, 265–271.

Tomm, K. (1988). Interventive interviewing. III. Intending to ask linear, circular, strategic and reflexive questions. *Family Process*, *27*, 1–15.

Trowell, J., Joffe, I., Campbell, J., Clemente, C., Almqvist, F., Soininen, M., *et al.* (2007). Childhood depression: A place for psychotherapy. An outcome study comparing individual psychodynamic psychotherapy and family therapy. *European Child and Adolescent Psychiatry*, 16, 157–167.

Varnik, A., Kolves, K., & Wasserman, D. (2005). Suicide among Russians in Estonia: Database study before and after independence. *British Medical Journal*, *330*, 176–177.

von Bertalanffy, L. (1968). *General system theory*. New York: Braziller.

von Foerster, H. (1979). "Cybernetics of cybernetics". In K. K. Krippendorff (Ed.), *Communication and control in society* (pp. 5–8). New York: Gordon and Breach.

Walsh, F. (1997). The concept of family resilience: Crisis and challenge. *Family Process*, *35*, 261–281.

Wampold, B. E. (2001). *The great psychotherapy debate: Models, methods, and findings*. Mahwah, NJ: Lawrence Erlbaum.

Watzlawick, P., Beavin, J., & Jackson, D. (1967). *The pragmatics of human communication*. New York: W. W. Norton.

Watzlawick, P., Weakland, J., & Fisch, R. (1974). *Change: Principles of problem formation and problem resolution*. New York: W. W. Norton.

White, M. (2005). *Narrative practice and exotic lives: Resurrecting diversity in everyday life*. Adelaide: Dulwich Centre Publications.

White, M. & Epston, D. (1989). *Literate means to therapeutic ends*. Adelaide: Dulwich Centre Publications.

Whitney, J., & Eisler, I. (2005). Theoretical and empirical models around caring for someone with an eating disorder: The reorganization of family life and interpersonal maintenance factors. *Journal of Mental Health*, *14*, 575–585.

Wilson, J. (1998). *Child-focused practice: A collaborative systemic approach*. London: Karnac Books.

Woolfenden, S. R., Williams, K., & Peat, J. (2007). *Family and parenting interventions in children and adolescents with conduct disorder and delinquency aged 10–17*. The Cochrane Library. London: John Wiley and Sons.

66 Psychodynamic Treatments

Peter Fonagy and Mary Target

What is Psychodynamic Psychotherapy?

The term "dynamic" first began to be used in the late 19th century by Leibniz, Herbart, Fechner and Hughlings-Jackson to highlight the distinction between a psychological and a fixed organic neurological impairment model of mental disorder. Dynamic approaches offer an alternative perspective to descriptive phenomenological psychiatry with the latter's focus on accurate categorization of mental disorders; in contrast, dynamic approaches emphasize the way mental processes interact to generate problems of subjective experience and behavior. Such interactions can occur consciously as well as unconsciously, but the psychodynamic model has historically been understood as a model of the mind that emphasizes wishes and ideas that have been defensively excluded from conscious experience. In our view this is a narrow and somewhat misleading definition of psychodynamic concepts. The psychodynamic approach is better understood as a comprehensive account of human subjectivity that aims to understand *all* aspects of an individual's relationship with their environment, external and internal.

Freud's great discovery was the power of the conscious mind to alter its position radically with respect to aspects of its own functions. In our view, psychodynamic should refer to this potential for dynamic self-alteration. All psychodynamic therapies aim to strengthen patients' capacity to understand the motivations and meanings of their own and others' subjective experiences, behavior and relationships. In this sense there is overlap with cognitive therapy, which of course also has psychodynamic origins, but at least classically focuses more narrowly on particular aspects of subjectivity (e.g., particular types of cognitive distortion) and is more targeted at specific behaviors or problems. By contrast, psychodynamic therapists strive to understand the organization of the child's mind in its full complexity, the social influences on the child's emotional experience and the ways in which the child's subjectivity has adapted to internal and external pressures. The therapist aims to expand the child's and parents' conscious awareness of these mechanisms and influences, so that they are better able to use their increased emotional awareness to manage continuing pressures. It assumes that once the mechanisms are made conscious, the individual will be able to change their inner world or their behavior to improve matters.

Psychodynamic psychotherapy can take a variety of forms; correspondingly, this chapter covers a number of therapeutic modalities. These include child psychoanalysis, individual and group psychotherapy, together with (using the above definition) certain family-based approaches, interpersonal approaches and psychodrama. Techniques differ in the extent to which they make use of play, supportive versus expressive techniques, or structured directive (group) work. Many current cognitive–behavioral therapies share with traditional psychodynamic approaches concerns such as the developmental and relational origin of particular ways of thinking, and use the relationship with the therapist as an example of broader patterns of relating (Beck, Davis, & Freeman, 2004). The following eight assumptions may be considered core to modern psychodynamic therapy. While some are shared by other approaches, as a set other orientations would be unlikely to embrace them wholeheartedly:

Common Assumptions

Notion of Psychological Causation

The child's problems are understood in terms of their thoughts and feelings. The emphasis is more on the child's interpretation of events and the world than on its external reality. It is assumed that mental disorders can be adequately comprehended as specific organizations of a child's conscious or unconscious beliefs, thoughts and feelings, whatever the root cause of such maladaptive organizations might be. The individual's motivations (wishes and anxieties, including expectations of others) are assumed to underlie experience, mental functioning and behavior. Alternative explanations such as genetic predispositions or chance are not prominent.

Limitations of Consciousness and the Influence of Non-conscious Mental States

Psychodynamic clinicians generally assume that to understand conscious experiences we need to refer to other mental states of which the individual is unaware. Psychodynamic models assume that non-conscious narrative-like experiences, analogous to conscious fantasies, profoundly influence children's behavior, capacity to manage their emotions and their social interactions. For example, attachment theory assumes that a mental representation of distress soothed by the parent is internalized as an unconscious expectation of future caregiving,

Rutter's Child and Adolescent Psychiatry, 5th edition. Edited by M. Rutter, D. Bishop, D. Pine, S. Scott, J. Stevenson, E. Taylor and A. Thapar. © 2008 Blackwell Publishing, ISBN: 978-1-4051-4549-7.

and becomes the foundation for a sense of the self as having understandable feelings that are deserving of care. This unconscious expectation guides the infant to seek soothing. Through the repetition of such experiences the capacity to self-soothe emerges without undue recourse to denial or amplification of distress.

There is substantial empirical support for Freud's suggestion that human consciousness cannot account for its maladaptive actions (Westen & Gabbard, 2002), but this should not be taken to imply a diminution of the emphasis placed on consciousness. Helping the child and caregivers to become aware of the unconscious expectations underlying the child's behavior can help them to gain control of previously unmanageable emotions and behavior. For example, when working with young people who apparently deliberately mismanage their diabetes, helping them elaborate their subjective experiences of peers and parents turns out to help them bring their diabetes under control (Moran, Fonagy, Kurtz *et al.*, 1991). It was helpful, for example, when the therapist could help a girl to understand that throwing away her insulin could be seen as an attempt to escape the intrusiveness of her overconcerned father, who used to listen outside her bedroom door in case she had a hypoglycemic attack. Once this was understood, more space could be created within the relationship without the need for her self-destructive protest.

Assumption of Internal Representations of Interpersonal Relationships

Psychodynamic clinicians consider interpersonal relationships, particularly attachment relationships, to be central to the organization of personality, and that representations of these intense relationship experiences are aggregated across time to form schematic mental structures, perhaps metaphorically represented as neural networks. These structures are seen as shaping interpersonal expectations and self-representations. Within many models self–other relationship representations are also viewed as organizers of emotion: certain feelings come to characterize particular patterns of interpersonal relating (e.g., sadness and disappointment at the anticipated loss of a person).

Ubiquity of Psychological Conflict

Psychodynamic approaches assume that wishes, affects and ideas will sometimes be in conflict. These conflicts are seen as key causes of distress, undermining a sense of safety and leading to maladaptive attempts to overcome this. Experientially insurmountable conflicts are commonly associated with adverse environmental conditions. For example, neglect or abuse is likely to aggravate an arguably natural ambivalence of the child towards the (in this case maltreating or neglectful) caregiver, who is nevertheless perceived as vital to the child's continuing existence. Psychodynamic techniques often aim to identify and elaborate perceived inconsistencies, conscious or unconscious, in feelings, beliefs and wishes in order to reduce the individual's distress when conflicts have become entrenched. Not only are conflicts thought to cause distress, they are also considered potentially to undermine the normal development of key psychological capacities that in turn reduce the child's ability to resolve incompatible ideas. At times psychodynamic models attempt to contrast conflict and development-focused approaches, but the reality of developmental trajectories means that the two are most often seen together in the same individual.

Assumption of Psychic Defenses

Historically, the psychodynamic approach has been particularly concerned with defenses: mental operations that distort conscious mental states to reduce their potential to generate anxiety. The term may risk reification and anthropomorphism (who is defending whom against what?) yet it is generally accepted that self-serving distortions of mental states relative to an external or internal reality take place. Classifications of defenses have been frequently attempted, often in order to categorize individuals or mental disorders (Kaye & Shea, 2000), but few of these approaches have achieved general acceptance. Nevertheless, most might agree that mental operations such as projection (attribution of a self-state to the other), denial (refusal to acknowledge self-states) or splitting (simultaneously holding self-states with opposite valence but experiencing them only sequentially) are characteristic of an early phase of development and are more commonly found in individuals with more severe mental disorder diagnoses. By contrast, intellectualization (elaborating a self-serving but inaccurate rationale for one's actions) or sublimation (diverting mental energy from drive-oriented to more constructive activity) are relatively mature and, when not used to excess, non-pathological forms. Aside from such broad categorizations, the cognitive and socio-cognitive strategies associated with reducing anxiety or displeasure and enhancing safety are perhaps better thought of not as independent classes of mental activity or psychological entities, but as a pervasive dynamic aspect of complex cognition interfacing with emotional experience.

Assumption of Complex Meanings

Psychodynamic approaches assume that behavior can be understood in terms of mental states that are not explicit in action or within the awareness of the person concerned. Symptoms of mental disorder are classically considered as condensations of wishes in conflict with one another, alongside the defense against recognition of that wish. It is striking that different psychodynamic orientations find different types of meanings "concealed" behind the same symptomatic behaviors. Some clinicians focus on unexpressed aggression or sexual impulses, others on a fear of not being validated, yet others on anxieties about abandonment and isolation. Within a contemporary context it is the effort of seeking further personal meaning that would be considered most significant therapeutically. Elaborating and clarifying implicit meaning structures rather than giving the patient insight in the terms of any particular meaning structure may turn out to be the essence of psychodynamic psychotherapy (Allen & Fonagy, 2006).

Emphasis on the Therapeutic Relationship

There is consensus that it is helpful to establish an attachment relationship with a clinician. Different therapeutic schools explain this differently, but converging theorization and research data suggest that engagement with an understanding adult will trigger a basic set of human capacities for relatedness that appears therapeutic, apparently almost regardless of content (PDM Task Force, 2006). Controlled trials have repeatedly demonstrated that therapeutic alliance without theoretical content is insufficient (Dew & Bickman, 2005); however, the importance of the therapeutic alliance has been found across a wide range of therapeutic approaches, including counseling and cognitive therapies (Beutler, Malik, Alimohamed *et al.*, 2004). Therapeutic technique varies in the degree of emphasis placed on: (i) the "transference" relationship, in which non-conscious relationship expectations, repudiated wishes, etc. are assumed to be played out and can be better understood through the shared experience of their enactment in a new context; and (ii) the "real" relationship, which captures the generic factor referred to above, of the therapeutic impact of having a relationship with an understanding adult, which may be a new experience for some young people. Therapists then vary in focusing mainly on interpretation of the "transference," or on gaining a broader understanding of the child's relationships and difficulties.

A Developmental Perspective

In common with many child therapists, psychodynamic psychotherapists are invariably oriented to the developmental aspects of their patients' problems (when and how they started, how they relate to an idealized "normal" developmental sequence), and work at least in part to optimize developmental processes. Varying assumptions are made concerning normal and abnormal child and adolescent development. Importantly, the outcome of interventions is often evaluated in developmental terms, less in terms of reduction of problem behaviors associated with a disorder and more in terms of what emotional, social and behavioral characteristics may be expected of a particular child at a particular age. There are developmentally sensitive measures of social adjustment that have operationalized Anna Freud's ideas concerning lines of emotional and social development (Fonagy & Target, 1994); how these map on to mainstream measures of social and emotional functioning needs to be researched.

Outdated Assumptions

Some features of the original psychodynamic model are no longer shared by all contemporary psychodynamic approaches. A good example concerns insight. Classically, psychotherapists regarded the patient's insight into their repressed unconscious as central to the process of change. It is now clear that improvements commonly occur in the absence of insight into non-conscious processes (Gabbard & Westen, 2003). Insight does not guarantee improvement even if the two sometimes occur together. Modern psychodynamic psychotherapy focuses on (mixed) feelings, confusing interpersonal expectations, the complexity of relationship experiences and much less on identifying derivatives of unconscious drives. Whereas some therapists remain committed to the insight-oriented interpretive approach, most feel that uncovering repressed unconscious content is less important than engaging with children and helping them to think about their experience in a psychological way.

Similarly, not all psychodynamic psychotherapists see a focus on *transference* as a key component of therapeutic work. However, it is commonly accepted that the relationship that the child creates in the therapeutic setting, either with the therapist or with other children in a group, can serve as a window on the child's inner world. Modern, especially relational, psychodynamic psychotherapists often rely on their subjective reactions to help them understand the parts the child implicitly asks them to play. By this indirect route they hope to gain an understanding of the child's internal struggles and the child's representations of themselves and others. This is very different from the use of such understanding as part of an interpretive process.

It may also be misleading to think of psychodynamic therapies as being invariably about *"the unconscious."* Uncovering neurotic motivations that have been dynamically defended against is no longer the defining feature of the psychodynamic approach. Psychodynamic therapies are often about increasing mental coherence, and randomized controlled trials of the treatment of borderline personality-disordered adults show that improvement in psychodynamic psychotherapy is specifically associated with increased coherence of attachment narratives (Levy, Meehan, Kelly *et al.*, 2006). It is postulated that having one's attention drawn to an aspect of one's experience that one is unaware of may increase this coherence. For example, if a child is continually failing at school to his parents' distress, drawing his attention to his ambivalent feelings may help him recognize a secret wish to upset his parents. This may enable him to find ways to stand up to his parents without damaging his own prospects. However, under certain circumstances, such insight may undermine coherence, increasing the child's confusion with iatrogenic consequences. For example, interpreting the masochistic wishes of a child who has been abused within the family may only add self-loathing and self-blame to his distress, making it harder for him to recover.

Risks of Psychodynamic Psychotherapy

Whereas pharmacological studies routinely test for the possibility of adverse reaction, psychological therapists mostly assume that their treatment is at worst inert. There are few systematic studies of adverse reactions. There may be particular disorders where psychotherapy represents significant risk to a patient. Irrespective of the assumed mechanism of change, most psychotherapists assume that the client is capable of considering their experience of their own mental states alongside the psychotherapist's representation of these. We have recently drawn attention to the fact that this may be an unrealistic expectation in cases where the client's capacity to represent their own mental states with any degree of coherence is very limited (Fonagy & Bateman, 2006). Such individuals may react to a therapist's attempts to teach them about the "true" contents of their mind by either breaking off the therapy or playing along without real understanding. It is possible that the difficulties psychodynamic therapists have in the past reported in relation to conduct problems may be associated with limitations in the ability of young people with severe behavioral problems to represent their own mental states (mentalize). Adolescents' resistance to psychodynamic therapy could also be explained by age-specific limitations in social cognition (Blakemore & Choudhury, 2006). In general, it seems to us that modifications to classic psychodynamic technique along the lines described above may be necessary for these techniques to be appropriately used with young people whose mental disorder is associated with limitations in their mentalizing capacity. Also, psychodynamic therapists who continue to give their therapy alone when it is ineffective while failing to recognize and refer on conditions for which there is a solid evidence base (e.g., attention deficit/hyperactivity disorder [ADHD] or obsessive-compulsive disorder [OCD]) are allowing unnecessary harm to befall their patients.

Theoretical Frameworks in Psychodynamic Therapy

Developmental Considerations in Psychodynamic Thinking

The theoretical bases for psychodynamic psychotherapy are rooted in Freud's establishment of his developmental approach to the understanding of psychopathology. In Freud's view, personality types and neurotic symptoms could be best understood in terms of fixations at and regressions to specific points of development; this has not been supported by any empirical evidence. Psychoanalysts following Freud have continued the developmental motif while taking radically different perspectives on both child development and psychopathology. Recent psychoanalytic models, such as relational theories (Mitchell, 2000) or psychoanalytic schema theories (Stern, 1993) focus their explanations on psychosocial development and the parent–child relationship.

Despite this unequivocally developmental perspective, most psychoanalytic theorists have done little directly to explore the nature of early development through research or to incorporate empirically tested modern findings into their approaches, preferring instead to speculate about infancy on the basis of largely adult clinical experience.

Historical and Current Traditions

The field of psychodynamic child psychotherapy was historically established by Melanie Klein (1932) and Anna Freud (1946). Klein assumed that play in the consulting room was motivated by unconscious fantasy, activated by the child's relationship to the analyst (the transference). This generated deep anxiety which required verbalization if it was to be addressed. The child's relationship with external figures (e.g., parents, teachers) was considered far less relevant. By understanding the child's perception of him or herself as a person, the clinician could gain an understanding of children's experience of themselves. A highly influential psychoanalyst working in this tradition, Bion (1959) described how such projections could be evocative: they could impact upon the "container." The capacity of the container of the projection to understand and accept these is seen by Kleinian analysts as critical to successful therapy as well as normal development.

A highly influential psychodynamic therapist emerging from the Kleinian tradition was the pediatrician Donald Winnicott. Winnicott (1971) introduced drawing techniques into child psychotherapy, highlighting his interest in what was beyond verbal experience. The idea of an intermediate space between the subjective and the interpersonal has become a central notion in the work of relational therapists. Winnicott elaborated a developmental model within which the caregiver is committed to the infant but imperfectly, so that the child has gradually to sacrifice infantile omnipotence. This gave rise to a therapeutic attitude where the therapist's constancy and tolerance create a sense of being understood and accepted that provides the patient with an important figure for internalization and identification.

At the other end of the spectrum, Anna Freud introduced only minor modifications to Freud's classic theories but dramatically reorganized the clinical situation of child psychotherapy, focusing on the child's developmental struggle with the social as well as the internal environment (Edgcumbe, 2000). She viewed pathology as a disturbance of normal developmental processes and therapy with children as aimed at returning to normal developmental lines. Not in content but in structure, Anna Freud's approach shares some ideas with modern developmental psychopathology. The aims of the developmental psychodynamic approach have some similarities with cognitive therapy; however, the means by which these improvements are considered to be most readily achieved are often quite different. For example, a psychodynamic psychotherapist working to enhance affect regulation may feel that working with the child's feelings about his or her therapist is the best way to assist the child in acquiring the capacity to regulate emotion in the context of intense attachment relationships. Similarly, clarifying the child's thoughts and feelings in relation to the therapist has the effect of strengthening mentalizing or reflective function.

Modern Psychodynamic Therapy: Relational and Attachment Theory Approaches

More recently, the Kleinian, Winnicottian and Anna Freudian traditions have all to some degree been superseded, especially in the USA, by an interpersonal relational perspective (Altman, Briggs, Frankel, Gensler, & Pantone, 2002). In a relational approach, conflict is no longer seen as within the individual but as produced by conflictual and contradictory signals and values in the environment. The relational therapist, like the therapist offering developmental help, does not work to impart understanding. The relational therapist's style is more active and participatory and aims to explore and correct maladaptive patterns of relating.

Importantly, the intersubjective relational approach does not privilege early developmental periods at the risk of overlooking current relationship needs (Greenberg, 1991). Interpersonal therapists therefore tend to be active, to work with current relationships of the client, rather than focusing on a deeper layer of reality beyond the surface. Relational ideas form the basis of the psychodynamic model underpinning interpersonal therapy (IPT), which has a strong evidence base in the adult literature on depression and a somewhat more meager one for its adolescent adaptation (Mufson, Dorta, Wickramaratne *et al.*, 2004; Young, Mufson, & Davies, 2006). In some people's eyes, IPT might have moved too far from its origins to be genuinely considered a psychodynamic approach, yet the clearly psychoanalytic adaptations of the interpersonal psychodynamic tradition retain the focus on the relationship-seeking aspect of human character and a pragmatic focus to the child's life and the therapeutic relationship in the context of this.

Attachment theory (Bowlby, 1980) overlaps with both the relational tradition and Winnicottian object relations theories. Attachment theory implements selected aspects of psychoanalytic theory, using a general systems model and an ethological approach, with the additional virtue of openness to empirical scrutiny. Bowlby's work on separation and loss focused developmentalists' attention on the importance of the security (safety and predictability) of the earliest relationships. It is postulated that safety and predictability give the child the capacity for relatively problem-free later interpersonal relationships. Bowlby assumed that representational systems (internal working models) evolve based on a template created by the earliest relationship of the infant to the caregiver. If the expectation that need and distress will be met by comforting is encoded into these models, the child will be able to approach relationships in a relatively non-defensive way. If this is not the case, if the child's caregivers lacked sensitivity, the child's representational system will be defensively distorted to either minimize or heighten experiences of arousal, and dismiss or become entangled in the response of others. Longitudinal work confirmed Bowlby's emphasis on the formative nature of early relationships and the pathological significance of the disorganization of the attachment system (Lyons-Ruth, 2003; Sroufe, Egeland, Carlson, & Collins, 2005), although the child's subsequent experience is also important in determining outcome (Rutter, 1987). Further, recent work has also demonstrated the relative independence of the attachment system from genetic influence (Fearon, van IJzendoorn, Fonagy *et al.*, 2006; O'Connor & Croft, 2001). However, clinical approaches rooted in attachment theory are only beginning to emerge.

Recently, a group of workers have focused on an application of attachment theory that goes beyond Bowlby's original rationale framed in the context of the quality of the infant–caregiver relationship. It is suggested that the attachment relationship has a key role in the development of social intelligence and meaning-making. The key evolutionary role of attachment in human development is in the opportunity that it confers for the development of social cognition (Fonagy, 2003). The relationship to the attachment figure has a long-term developmental impact through facilitating the emergence of complex psychological processes. In interaction with the infant, the caregiver tends to "reflect" the infant's emotional states back to him, instinctively "mirroring" his feelings in a way that helps the child to feel that they are contained and not out of control. Such interactions enable the child to learn how to represent his own thoughts and feelings. The capacity for mentalization builds upon affect regulation as well as attentional control. For example, the capacity for pretend play has been found to be associated longitudinally with the mother's ability to mirror the infant's affects (Koos & Gergely, 2001). Weak affect regulation, attentional control and mentalization leave infants vulnerable to the impact of trauma (maltreatment), which undermines mentalizing capacities (Cicchetti, Rogosch, Maughan, Toth, & Bruce, 2003). The therapeutic approach to emanate from this developmental model may be particularly appropriate for more severe conditions, such as emerging personality disorder and multiple comorbidities that include an emotional disorder diagnosis. The therapeutic focus is no longer on enhancing insight but rather on strengthening social-cognitive capacities, particularly mentalization.

Brief Psychotherapy, Group, Dyadic and Family Psychodynamic Therapy

In the child literature, brief therapy has not been systematically studied even though this may be the form of individual dynamic therapy that is most commonly delivered in community settings (Kennedy, 2004). The one exception to this is interpersonal psychotherapy for adolescent depression (Young & Mufson, 2004), which is based on identifying maladaptive interpersonal patterns, making these patterns explicit and helping the patient to disrupt these patterns during the course of the treatment. These generally fall into one of five categories: grief, interpersonal disputes, role transitions, interpersonal deficits or single-parent families (Young & Mufson, 2004). There are some open trials and randomized controlled trials (Mufson, Dorta, Wickramaratne *et al.*, 2004; Young, Mufson, & Davies, 2006) showing the effectiveness of the technique.

Group therapy is frequently employed for children and adolescents, particularly in school and residential settings. Group therapy offers several advantages beyond economy. For children and adolescents the group format reflects the developmental priority of finding and integrating into a peer group. Process research in group therapy (Schechtman, 2001) suggests that children benefit from cathartic experiences and sharing. In adolescence, the group process may help with separation–individuation and identity formation. A range of processes that take place in group therapy facilitate developmental goals: identification through recognizing commonalities, a refinement and calibration of social perceptions, a benefit from social support, a counteracting of social isolation and improved feedback to enhance self-esteem. There is some evidence that group therapy with medically ill children is beneficial (see systematic review by Plante, Lobato, & Engel, 2001). Many other factors may assist change: the instillment of hope; altruism through assisting others; corrective recapitulation of the primary family group;

the development of social skills; group cohesiveness; and interpersonal learning through developing positive relationships with another. The improvements seen can also be accounted for within other theoretical frameworks such as cognitive–behavioral or social learning models. Although psychodynamic psychotherapy groups are quite heterogeneous in character, in most group work it is assumed that conflicts and concerns within the group in some ways mirror those in the children's lives outside of the group. Further, group members are frequently exposed to discussions that may foster new ways of dealing with personal or interpersonal issues and they are afforded an opportunity to exercise empathy capacity and perspective taking. Psychodrama offers a frame for group treatments and a method for creating a structured awareness-producing milieu. It has been used with a range of problems including middle school girls coping with trauma (Carbonelli & Partelno-Bareehmi, 1999), adolescents with developmental problems (Oezbay, Goeka, Oeztuerk, & Guengoer, 1993) and as an adjunct to family therapy (Blatner, 1994). The efficacy of these forms of group therapy needs to be evaluated through properly conducted randomized controlled trials.

Increasing recognition of the formative character of aspects of early childhood has led to increasing concern with child mental health issues. Epidemiological and prevention studies have highlighted the prevalence of early maltreatment and other trauma that may impact on subsequent mental health (Pynoos, Steinberg, & Piacentini, 1999). The now generally accepted transactional model of early childhood development (Sameroff & Fiese, 2000), highlighting the complexity of the early caregiving environment, has offered a focus for therapeutic interventions in the child–caregiver relationship. Therapeutic interventions are directed not at the child who is presented as bringing a problem but at the child–caregiver relationship and its entire cultural, social, family, marital and parent context.

Child–parent psychotherapy (CPP; Lieberman, 2004) is based on the premise that the attachment system is the main organizer of children's responses to danger and safety in the first years of life and a therapeutic relationship can be mutative. Weekly joint child–parent sessions over 1 year are interspersed with individual sessions for the mother, with the aim of changing maladaptive parenting behaviors and supporting developmentally appropriate interactions while guiding the child–parent couple to create a joint narrative of traumatic events working towards their resolution. Two randomized controlled trials have demonstrated the effectiveness of this method (Lieberman, Weston, & Pawl, 1991; Lieberman, Van Horn, & Ippen, 2005). When compared with case management, including community referral for individual treatment, child–parent psychotherapy was associated with significantly more improvement in parent-rated measures of child symptomatology (Effect Size = 0.840). This runs counter to the finding of van IJzendoorn, Juffer, and Duyvesteyn (1995) in their review of attachment-oriented interventions with relatively low-risk samples without major psychiatric symptomatology. This review suggested that brief treatment was more effective than long-term treatment in increasing attachment security, but psychiatric symptomatology was not assessed. A dyadic narrative-oriented therapeutic approach similar to Lieberman *et al.*s' has been demonstrated to be effective for toddlers of depressed mothers (Cicchetti, Rogosch, & Toth, 2000) and neglected and maltreated preschoolers (Toth, Maughan, Manly, Spagnola, & Cicchetti, 2002).

Psychodynamic psychotherapy now normally includes some "family work" or help for the parents. This is of course not the same as formal family therapy, which has a theoretical frame that is often antagonistic to or at least divergent from psychodynamic approaches. However, there are psychodynamically oriented implementations of family therapy that combine systemic approaches with psychodynamic ideas (Johnson & Lee, 2000). There is a move from both sides towards an integration between family and psychodynamic therapy. Thus, many more recent variants of structural family therapy recognize the relevance of aspects of the psychodynamic approach (e.g., attachment theory) as a core component of systemic family interventions. There is a spectrum, from more clearly psychodynamic approaches such as attachment-based family therapy (Diamond, Diamond, & Siqueland, unpublished data), to those that have taken only particular aspects of a psychodynamic perspective, such as multidimensional family therapy (Liddle, Dakof, Parker *et al.*, 2001) and the biobehavioral family model (Wood, Klebba, & Miller, 2000).

From the other direction, there are examples of traditional psychodynamic therapy taking on a family dimension. In the psychodynamic implementation of family therapy, intrapersonal problems are considered alongside characteristic family dynamics. The family is viewed as a system whose process determines adolescent development. Psychodynamic family therapy focuses on communication and negotiation, challenges problematic coalitions and supports the appropriate roles of parents and children in a family hierarchy. It also concerns itself with family narratives, helping families to understand the way they deal with the child's problems at both conscious and unconscious levels (Lock, 2004). Treatment focuses on increasing parental self-efficacy but also on diminishing parental guilt. This is postulated to help parents to become more authoritative and able to manage problems while still being both warm and understanding. The therapist acts as a consultant, there to empower family members to solve their own problems. In narrative family therapy, the therapist relies on the creativity and playfulness of children with words and other activities. The therapist can facilitate the creation of coherent and lasting alternative stories by, for example, eliciting and developing a counterplot to a problem-saturated story. In emotion-focused family therapy (Johnson & Lee, 2000) techniques such as the family puppet interview, mutual storytelling and different forms of art therapy are used to set up a safe environment in which attachment needs can be identified and expressed. There is evidence for the effectiveness of emotion-focused family therapy, principally from couples research (Dunn & Schwebel, 1995). There is also empirical support for the efficacy of explicitly psychodynamic family therapy from studies with anorexia nervosa (see p. 1086).

Empirical Basis of Psychodynamic Child Psychotherapy

Randomized Controlled Trials

Comprehensive reviews of outcome studies of psychodynamic approaches to child and adolescent mental health difficulties are few. Surveys focus on the treatment of children with mental health problems in general (Fonagy, Target, Cottrell, Phillips, & Kurtz, 2002; Kazdin, 2004; Target & Fonagy, 2005) or psychosocial interventions limited to "evidence-based treatments" (Hibbs, 2004; Weisz, 2004). The most comprehensive survey of outcome studies specifically concerned with psychoanalytic approaches was that undertaken by Kennedy 2004. The conclusions are more optimistic than the current state of empirical evidence justifies, which is reviewed below.

There are no really good randomized controlled trials of psychodynamic psychotherapy with children. The few controlled trials are underpowered and suffer from other methodological limitations (Robin, Siegel, Moye *et al.*, 1999; Sinha & Kapur, 1999; Smyrnios & Kirkby, 1993; Szapocznik, Rio, Murray *et al.*, 1989; Trowell, Kolvin, Weeramanthri *et al.*, 2002; Trowell, Joffe, Campbell 2007). All but one of these trials contrasted individual child psychotherapy with another treatment. In no case did child psychotherapy emerge as superior to the contrast treatment. These trials are all considered further below. Several studies employed quasi-randomized methods of assignment such as postcode (Moran, Fonagy, Kurtz *et al.*, 1991) or therapist vacancy (Muratori, Picchi, Casella *et al.*, 2001, Muratori, Picchi, Bruni *et al.*, 2003). Six studies reported on findings with matched comparison groups (Fonagy & Target, 1994; Heinicke & Ramsey-Klee, 1986; Reid, Alvarez, & Lee, 2001; Target & Fonagy, 1994a,b). Three studies used experimental single-case methodology (Fonagy & Moran, 1990; Lush, Boston, Morgam, & Kolvin, 1998; Moran & Fonagy, 1987). On the basis of these studies, the evidence base for child psychotherapy is quite poor.

Indications of Differential Effectiveness of Psychodynamic Approaches for Specific Clinical Problems

Anxiety disorders

There is only very preliminary evidence that psychodynamic psychotherapy may be effective in the treatment of anxiety disorders (Target & Fonagy, 1994). In this chart review study, children with anxiety disorders (with or without comorbidity) showed greater improvements than those with other conditions, and greater improvements than would have been expected on the basis of studies of untreated outcome. Muratori, Picchi, Casella *et al.* (2001) examined the efficacy among 58 children with depression and anxiety, of 11 sessions of psychodynamic therapy based on the Parent–Child Model involving work with the parents for 6 of the 11 sessions. This was contrasted with treatment as usual in the community (poorly described in the report). Allocation was based on therapist vacancy at referral. At 2-year follow-up only 34% of the treated group were in the clinical range on the Child Behavior Checklist (CBCL), compared with 65% of the controls. Unusually for trials of psychotherapy, treatment effects increased during the 2-year follow-up period (the so-called "*sleeper effect*"): the average child with emotional problems moved from the clinical to the non-clinical range in the psychodynamically treated group only (Muratori, Picchi, Bruni *et al.*, 2003). In the control group, the average child remained at the same level of severity through the follow-up period. The conclusions from this trial are limited because of the small sample size and the lack of random allocation. However, it is encouraging that psychodynamic psychotherapy patients sought mental health services at a significantly lower rate than those in the treatment as usual comparison condition over the 2-year follow-up period.

A very small randomized controlled trial ($n = 30$) of adolescents showed a surprisingly strong statistically significant benefit from 10 sessions of psychodynamic psychotherapy in a school setting in India. The vast majority of young people improved in psychodynamic psychotherapy (over 90%, reported effect size 1.8; Sinha & Kapur, 1999). Notably, young people with disruptive behavior were specifically excluded from this sample. Therapy outcome was independently, but not blindly, assessed by teachers.

Childhood Depression

A multicenter European trial compared family therapy with brief individual psychodynamic psychotherapy (Trowell, Joffe, Campbell *et al.*, 2007). At 7-month follow-up none of the moderately to severely depressed young people who received psychotherapy met diagnostic criteria, whereas 29% in the family therapy group did. This trial did not have an untreated control group, so it is uncertain how far these results are superior to no treatment, although the results with individual treatment are comparable to children treated with a combination of fluoxetine and cognitive–behavior therapy (Goodyer, Dubicka, Wilkinson *et al.*, 2007).

Smyrnios and Kirkby (1993) investigated the therapeutic effects of a therapy combining psychodynamic and systemic principles with 30 school-age children. The children were randomly divided into three groups of 10:

1 One group received "time-unlimited" psychoanalytic therapy using a Kleinian model (on average 28 sessions, with a range of 3–62 sessions);

2 Another group received short-term therapy (on average 10.5 sessions, with a range of 5–12 sessions); and

3 A third group was offered a three-session consultation.

All three groups showed significant improvements from pre-test to post-test on a number of individual and family ratings, but the effect size was greatest for the time-unlimited treatment. Effect sizes for target complaints at post-treatment, relative to consultation: 0.76 (95% confidence interval [CI], 0.28–1.3) for time-limited; 1.23 (95% CI, 0.84–1.6) for time-unlimited. At 4-year follow-up, the effect sizes for target complaints were no longer significantly different from the control group, who are likely to have had other treatments. In line with this, the consultation group caught up with the treated groups and reported significant improvement relative to post-treatment on follow-up, severity of target problems and measure of family functioning. However, a high proportion (up to 50%) of the very small numbers in the original groups was lost to follow-up.

Disruptive Disorders

In the Anna Freud Centre retrospective study (Fonagy & Target, 1994), whereas children and young people treated for major depression were likely to improve even if they remained in the dysfunctional range after treatment, diagnoses related to conduct problems appeared particularly resistant to psychodynamic therapy (CD and ODD).

Family Involvement

In a comparison of family therapy and individual psychodynamic psychotherapy with a mixed behaviorally and emotionally disordered sample of Hispanic children, both treatments were found to be effective in reducing behavioral and emotional problems, relative to a no-treatment control group (Szapocznik, Rio, Murray *et al.*, 1989). The symptomatic improvements were maintained at 1-year follow-up, but the control group caught up with these improvements over the follow-up period. It should be noted that there was considerable attrition in the control group and the analysis was not on the basis of intent-to-treat. A total of 16% of families dropped out of family therapy compared with 4% who abandoned individual psychodynamic therapy, but family functioning improved following family therapy and deteriorated following individual psychodynamic psychotherapy (i.e., between end of treatment and follow-up).

Individual child psychotherapy is now rarely carried out without family work. In the Anna Freud Centre retrospective study, concurrent work with parents was a predictor of good outcome (Target & Fonagy, 1994). With younger children, particularly preschool age, a mother–child dyadic therapy where the parent and child are jointly seen appears to be an effective psychodynamic intervention. For example, in Lieberman, Van Horn, & Ippen (2005) study, 75 children who had been exposed to marital violence were treated in child–parent psychotherapy weekly for 1 year and this was contrasted with individual treatment and case management. The dyadic work yielded superior outcomes in terms of behavioral problems, traumatic stress symptoms and diagnostic status and post-traumatic stress disorder (PTSD) symptoms and general distress for the mother.

Pervasive Developmental Problems

Non-directive play is often used to try to promote communication skills in children with autism (Cogher, 1999). Although such interventions have common components they are not specifically psychodynamic. The Tavistock Clinic has developed a specialized psychodynamic approach to the treatment of individuals with autism (Reid, Alvarez, & Lee, 2001), but this has not been evaluated in a controlled trial.

Eating Disorders

A further specific diagnostic group for which some trial data are available is anorexia nervosa. Randomized controlled trials of behavioral family systems therapy aimed to contrast this therapy with an "inert" treatment and they chose ego-oriented individual therapy, a specially designed treatment with a clear psychodynamic basis (Robin, Siegel, & Moye, 1995; Robin, Siegel, Moye *et al.*, 1999). Each patient received 10–16 months of therapy and was assessed at post-therapy, and followed up at 1, 2.5 and 4 years. Improvements were equivalent in both treatments; two-thirds of the girls reached their target weights by the end of treatment, and at 1-year follow-up 80% of those receiving family therapy and 69% of those treated individually had reached their target weights (a difference that was not statistically significant). As is often found, the non-psychodynamic approach produced changes faster but in this instance carried the cost of a somewhat higher rate of hospitalization. Both therapies produced equally large improvements in attitudes to eating, depressed affect and family functioning (Robin, Siegel, & Moye, 1995). Robin *et al.* concluded that parental involvement was essential to the success of their interventions for younger adolescents with anorexia nervosa.

The comparability of the effectiveness of family and individual approaches in the above studies is somewhat in contrast to the long-term superiority of family therapy for a group of young adult anorexics using a similar psychodynamic approach (Dare, Eisler, Russell, Treasure, & Dodge, 2001; Eisler, Dare, Russell *et al.*, 1997; Eisler, Dare, Hodes *et al.*, 2000; Russell, Szmukler, Dare, & Eisler, 1987). In these studies at the Maudsley Hospital, individuals who were relatively older generally benefitted more from individual treatment while younger individuals benefitted more from family-based approaches (for further details of these studies see chapter 41).

Chronic Physical Illness

There is a tradition of psychodynamic work with individuals with chronic physical conditions such as asthma and diabetes (Shaw & Palmer, 2004) but trial data are hard to come by. In a series of experimental single-case studies, individual psychodynamic therapy was found to improve several growth parameters probably associated with improvement of diabetic control (Fonagy & Moran, 1990).

Trauma

Goenjian, Karayan, Pynoos *et al.* (1997) reported a naturalistic study on the outcome of psychotherapeutically treated and untreated earthquake victims at 1.5 years (pre-treatment) and 3 years (post-treatment) after the earthquake. While the severity of PTSD symptoms significantly decreased among recipients of trauma/grief-focused brief psychotherapy, symptoms significantly worsened among untreated subjects. Layne, Pynoos, and Cardenas (2001) have developed a program for adolescents who experienced or witnessed violence. The UCLA School-Based Trauma/Grief Intervention Program for children and adolescents includes a systematic method for screening students, a manualized 16–20 week group psychotherapy protocol which addresses current stresses and conflicts not limited to the trauma exposure, and adjunctive individual and family therapy. As a package, the protocol is a skills-based cognitive–behavioral therapy program and is very far from a prototypical unfocused insight-oriented group psychotherapy, but the attention to developmental considerations and the model of traumatic stress within which the treatment is rooted (Pynoos, Steinberg, & Wraith, 1995) make the intervention deserving of consideration under a general psychodynamic heading. Controlled trials are now needed.

More directly relevant is a multicenter randomized trial of the treatment of sexually abused girls treated in individual psychotherapy and psychoeducational group therapy (Trowell, Kolvin, Weeramanthri *et al.*, 2002). A total of 71 sexually abused girls were randomized to either 30 sessions of individual psychoanalytic psychotherapy or 18 sessions of group psychotherapy with psychoeducational components. These young people presented with a range of psychiatric problems, most commonly PTSD and depression. Psychodynamic treatment was no different from psychoeducation in terms of overall levels of psychopathology measures and psychosocial functioning measures. In relation to PTSD, however, there were greater gains in the individual psychotherapy group; the between-treatments effect size ranged from 0.6–0.79 for specific symptoms. Trials are now needed comparing dynamic psychotherapy with other proven treatments such as cognitive–behavioral therapy and exposure.

Summary

The empirical status of all psychodynamic approaches remains controversial. The body of rigorous research supporting psychodynamic therapies for both adults and children for most disorders remains limited, particularly relative to research supporting pharmaceutical treatments and even other psychosocial approaches such as cognitive–behavioral therapy (Roth & Fonagy, 2005). There are both practical and theoretical difficulties in mounting trials of dynamic therapies, which go some way to explaining the lack of evidence. These include, for example, the bias against research by many practitioners of psychodynamic therapies, their epistemological problems with accepting the canons of modern scientific studies, the reluctance of funding bodies to invest in research on clinical problems considered "solved" by a combination of drug and cognitive–behavioral treatments, the expense of mounting trials sufficiently powered to yield information on what treatments are appropriate for which disorder and the failure to manualize psychodynamic treatments. Currently, there is some modest evidence to support the use of psychodynamic psychotherapy for children whose problems are either emotional or mixed. There is also evidence that the support and inclusion of parents are important aspects of this treatment, that effects tend to increase following the end of treatment and that behavioral problems are more resistant – at least to a classic insight-oriented psychodynamic approach.

Those who argue (correctly in our view) for continued investment in this approach point to the limitations of the evidence base in childhood supporting cognitive–behavioral therapy (Westen, Novotny, & Thompson-Brenner, 2004) or pharmacological approaches (Whittington, Kendall, Fonagy *et al.*, 2004). Notwith-standing the general weakness of the evidence base of mental health treatments for children, this weakness is particularly strong for psychodynamic treatments and the shortage of research studies needs to be addressed urgently. In the light of the limitations of cognitive–behavioral therapy with severe disorders in comparison with medication (Goodyer, Dubicka, Wilkinson *et al.*, 2007; March, Silva, Petrycki *et al.*, 2004; Swanson, Arnold, Vitiello *et al.*, 2002), it behoves us to investigate the effectiveness of alternative treatment approaches.

Integration of Psychodynamic Psychotherapy into Child and Adolescent Mental Health Services

This section addresses the place of psychodynamic child psychotherapy within child and adolescent mental health services (CAMHS). This will be described from the UK perspective, in which child psychotherapy is delivered mainly within the National Health Service (NHS), but many of the principles probably also apply elsewhere.

In the UK, psychoanalytic psychotherapy for children and young people is usually delivered within a multidisciplinary CAMHS. A considerable part of child psychotherapists' work is consultation with and supervision of other CAMHS professionals and paraprofessional staff, as well as contributing to thinking within the team and the network about the situations and emotional development of children referred. Working long-term and/or intensively with individual children has been shown to occupy only about one-third of the employed time of these specialized staff. Their perspective should complement rather than compete with systemic, biological, cognitive–behavioral or other frameworks. The range of contexts for child psychotherapy work has also very much extended, particularly the proportion of work focused on children who are being looked after by local authorities (child protective services); other areas to which child psychotherapists contribute include education, forensic services, pediatric liaison, perinatal services and parent–infant community settings.

The perspective of psychoanalytic psychotherapy appears to be used in several distinct ways; the following approximate proportions of time are based on consistent data from three large-scale surveys (Rance, 2003):

1 To treat individual children (usually once weekly; 36%);

2 To provide training, supervision (8%), assessment (14%) and consultation (14%) using a psychoanalytic framework (e.g., to support treatment carried out by other professionals in a team or their trainees);

3 Working using a variety of techniques other than individual psychotherapy (e.g., family therapy, work on parenting, group therapy with young people, parent–infant therapy); this is often joint work with colleagues in other disciplines (18%); and

4 To inform discussion and understanding of a child's behavior and the impact a child or family is having on relationships between the agencies involved (approximately 10%).

Individual psychotherapy is often carried out by other staff with teaching and supervision from a child psychotherapist. Medium- or long-term one-to-one work is a scarce, intensive and expensive resource that tends to be reserved for situations where other perspectives have been tried or are ongoing, but there are still serious problems. This is commonly where there are chronic and complex difficulties, often in the context of trauma and disrupted or abusive caregiving. Qualified child therapists can often help another colleague to do this work in the relatively less disturbed and disturbing cases. An interesting study by Kam and Midgley (2006) of one large inner city service found that almost all children referred for individual child psychotherapy were referred by other members of the CAMHS team after an average of 3 years of contact with the service and input from an average of 3–4 other CAMHS professionals. They tended to have the most complex developmental and social problems (e.g., parental mental illness, maltreatment histories). Individual therapy is often a last resort for children who are particularly hard to help.

Surveys and audits show that parent, foster carer and whole family work is usually carried out while therapy is provided for an individual child; this is not routine in the treatment of older adolescents. The parent or family work may be carried out by a colleague from another discipline, another child psychotherapist or the therapist who is treating the child. There are very often concerns about child protection in cases considered for referral to a child psychotherapist and this can raise difficult issues; psychotherapy for a child currently being emotionally, physically or sexually abused is clearly not a solution to the abuse. The first priority then is the child's safety. Some therapists may look for that to have been achieved before beginning therapy, while others may try to establish a relationship with the child while steps are being taken to make sure that the child is safe. However, this risks disruption of the new therapeutic relationship if the child is removed from the current home or care environment to live outside the area. Child psychotherapists often carry out assessment work with the courts, and mostly carry out their ongoing therapeutic work with children who – even if still in unsatisfactory or disrupted care arrangements – are at least in a safe environment. The therapist may sometimes be the only consistent figure in the child's life over a considerable period, and may effectively become an advocate for the child's feelings and perspective.

We suggest that, in general, child psychotherapists – who are relatively few in number and expensive to train – should be kept for the more intractable cases where a briefer symptom-focused approach has been tried and failed or seems inappropriate. This is particularly important when the child's attachment history places them beyond the reach of therapists without extensive relational training. However, to sustain this position will require controlled trials assessing effectiveness and cost-effectiveness.

A developmental psychodynamic approach includes a model of attachment processes and the ways in which the development of (for example) the social cognitive capacities of regulation of emotion and attention, and social understanding are shaped by early experiences particularly within the family. This framework also gives a rationale for relatively long-term work with a child to help build more positive capacities and to help the child to develop more coherent and effective social and mental functioning, and to increase resilience to cope with often ongoing trauma and dislocation (e.g., from disrupted care placements). Research needs to be designed that can include the type of children often seen by child psychotherapists, and that can follow up their outcomes in the longer term.

Finally, we come to issues of training, treatment integrity and monitoring. In the UK, psychoanalytic child psychotherapists have a 4-year full-time training, usually based in a multidisciplinary CAMHS team, which includes supervised clinical practice, theoretical work and intensive personal psychotherapy. Trainees are required to have considerable work experience with children prior to starting. A masters-level pre-clinical course is followed by 4 years of clinical training. Most available training courses are accredited as professional doctorate programs. Personal therapy is required because child psychotherapists' work with profoundly disturbed and disturbing children and parents will often be distressing or unnerving to the therapist. The therapist is thought to gain two advantages from personal therapy: the first is resolution of disturbances in the therapist's own personality, which might complicate the relationship with patients, and the second is to give an intensive and direct experience of the process that the patient will later experience. Without such personal experience, intensive work with highly vulnerable and disturbed children could be damaging rather than therapeutic. Close awareness of the phenomena involved not only helps the qualified therapist to tolerate, conceptualize and work with profound disturbances of development and functioning, but also helps him or her to teach and supervise other workers who have not had psychoanalytic training or therapy but who wish to gain experience with the techniques.

Every child psychotherapy post in the NHS has a set of skills and competencies (covering clinical, management and research knowledge) established within the knowledge and skills framework. This skill-set is individually reviewed annually and modified as needed. Maintenance of competence is through the registration requirements for continuing supervision and continuing professional development.

Conclusions

Psychodynamic psychotherapy is one of the oldest theory-driven forms of psychological treatment of mental disorders. The personal meaning of the discourse concerning the subjective world behind behavior has inspired many generations of clinicians. Psychodynamic ideas are applied in contexts well beyond the treatment of psychiatric disorders, including psychology, other social sciences, literature and the arts. Sadly, empirical investigations of both its underlying constructs and its therapeutic outcomes are still in their infancy.

The shortcomings of the psychodynamic approach are considerable and include:

1 Shortage of operationalization;

2 Uncritical application of a relatively uniform approach to a wide range of disorders;

3 Limited amount of good evidence supporting its efficacy;

4 Over-reliance on individual case reports for helping theory and technique develop;

5 Common vagueness of treatment goals;

6 Possibility of unnecessarily prolonged treatment and even iatrogenic effects;

7 Significant heterogeneity of theoretical and linked clinical approaches calling themselves psychodynamic almost defying integration and rationalization; and

8 Antagonism on the part of many psychodynamic practitioners to the idea of systematic evaluation and scrutiny.

Notwithstanding these limitations, we remain convinced of the unique value of the psychodynamic approach, not only as a methodology for the study of the psychological difficulties of childhood, but also as a method of clinical intervention with children who are hard to reach using other methods. Considerable work remains to be done but a new culture of research is now emerging within the psychoanalytic community. It is, we believe, a realistic hope that over the next decade a substantial evidence base will emerge for child treatment. This would delineate the specific value of the approach for the long-term development of children with psychological disorders. Work is already under way at a number of centers internationally and will in time show whether psychodynamic treatment works for children and, if so, for whom.

References

Allen, J. G., & Fonagy, P. (Eds.). (2006). *Handbook of Mentalization-based treatment*. New York: Wiley.

Altman, N., Briggs, R., Frankel, J., Gensler, D., & Pantone, P. (2002). *Relational child psychotherapy*. New York: Springer.

Beck, A. T., Davis, D. D., & Freeman, A. M. (2004). *Cognitive therapy of personality disorders* (Vol. 2). New York: Guilford Press.

Beutler, L. E., Malik, M., Alimohamed, S., Harwood, T. M., Talebi, H., Noble, S., *et al.* (2004). Therapist variables. In M. J. Lambert (Ed.), *Bergin and Garfield's handbook of psychotherapy and behavior* (pp. 227–306). New York: John Wiley and Sons.

Bion, W. R. (1959). Attacks on linking. *International Journal of Psychoanalysis*, *40*, 308–315.

Blakemore, S. J., & Choudhury, S. (2006). Development of the adolescent brain: Implications for executive function and social cognition. *Journal of Child Psychology and Psychiatry*, *47*, 296–312.

Blatner, H. A. (1994). Psychodramatic methods in family therapy. In C. E. Schaefer, & L. J. Carey (Eds.), *Family play therapy*. Northvale, NJ: Aronson.

Bowlby, J. (1980). *Attachment and loss*, Vol. 3. *Loss: Sadness and depression*. London: Hogarth Press and Institute of Psycho-Analysis.

Carbonelli, D. M., & Partelno-Bareehmi, C. (1999). Psychodrama groups for girls coping with trauma. *International Journal of Group Psychotherapy*, *49*, 285–306.

Cicchetti, D., Rogosch, F. A., Maughan, A., Toth, S. L., & Bruce, J. (2003). False belief understanding in maltreated children. *Development and Psychopathology*, *15*, 1067–1091.

Cicchetti, D., Rogosch, F. A., & Toth, S. L. (2000). The efficacy of toddler–parent psychotherapy for fostering cognitive development in offspring of depressed mothers. *Journal of Abnormal Child Psychology*, *28*, 135–148.

Cogher, L. (1999). The use of non-directive play in speech and language therapy. *Child Language Teaching and Therapy*, *15*, 7–15.

Dare, C., Eisler, I., Russell, G., Treasure, J., & Dodge, L. (2001). Psychological therapies for adults with anorexia nervosa: Randomised controlled trial of out-patient treatments. *British Journal of Psychiatry*, *178*, 216–221.

Dew, S. E., & Bickman, L. (2005). Client expectancies about therapy. *Mental Health Services Research*, *7*, 21–33.

Dunn, R. L., & Schwebel, A. I. (1995). Meta-analysis of marital therapy outcome research. *Journal of Family Psychology*, *9*, 58–68.

Edgcumbe, R. (2000). *Anna Freud: A view of development, disturbance and therapeutic techniques*. London: Routledge.

Eisler, I., Dare, C., Hodes, M., Russell, G., Dodge, E., & Le Grange, D. (2000). Family therapy for adolescent anorexia nervosa: The results of a controlled comparison of two family interventions. *Journal of Child Psychology and Psychiatry*, *41*, 727–736.

Eisler, I., Dare, C., Russell, G. F. M., Szmukler, G., le Grange, D., & Dodge, E. (1997). Family and individual therapy in anorexia nervosa: A 5-year follow-up. *Archives of General Psychiatry*, *54*, 1025–1030.

Fearon, P., van IJzendoorn, M. H., Fonagy, P., Bakermans-Kranenburg, M. J., Schuengel, C. & Bokhorst, C. L. (2006). In search of shared and non-shared environmental factors in security of attachment: A behavior–genetic study of the association between sensitivity and attachment security. *Developmental Psychology*, *42*, 1026–1040.

Fonagy, P. (2003). The development of psychopathology from infancy to adulthood: The mysterious unfolding of disturbance in time. *Infant Mental Health Journal*, *24*, 212–239.

Fonagy, P., & Bateman, A. (2006). Progress in the treatment of borderline personality disorder. *British Journal of Psychiatry*, *188*, 1–3.

Fonagy, P., & Moran, G. S. (1990). Studies on the efficacy of child psychoanalysis. *Journal of Consulting and Clinical Psychology*, *58*, 684–695.

Fonagy, P., & Target, M. (1994). The efficacy of psychoanalysis for children with disruptive disorders. *Journal of the American Academy of Child and Adolescent Psychiatry*, *33*, 45–55.

Fonagy, P., & Target, M. (1996). Predictors of outcome in child psychoanalysis: A retrospective study of 763 cases at the Anna Freud Centre. *Journal of the American Psychoanalytic Association*, *44*, 27–77.

Fonagy, P., Target, M., Cottrell, D., Phillips, J., & Kurtz, Z. (2002). *What works for whom? A critical review of treatments for children and adolescents*. New York: Guilford.

Freud, A. (1946). *The psychoanalytic treatment of children*. London: Imago Publishing.

Gabbard, G. O., & Westen, D. (2003). Rethinking therapeutic action. *International Journal of Psychoanalysis*, *84*, 823–841.

Goenjian, A. K., Karayan, I., Pynoos, R. S., Minassian, D., Najarian, L. M., Steinberg, A. M., *et al.* (1997). Outcome of psychotherapy among early adolescents after trauma. *American Journal of Psychiatry*, *154*, 536–542.

Goodyer, I., Dubicka, B., Wilkinson, P., Kelvin, K., Roberts, C., Byford, S., *et al.* (2007). Selective serotonin reuptake inhibitors (SSRIs) and routine specialist care with and without cognitive behaviour therapy in adolescents with major depression: Randomised controlled trial. *British Medical Journal*, *335*, 142–150.

Greenberg, J. (1991). *Oedipus and beyond: A clinical theory*. Cambridge, MA: Harvard University Press.

Heinicke, C. M., & Ramsey-Klee, D. M. (1986). Outcome of child psychotherapy as a function of frequency of session. *Journal of the American Academy of Child Psychiatry*, 25, 247–253.

Hibbs, E. D. (Ed.). (2004). *Psychosocial treatments for child and adolescent disorders: Empirically based strategies for clinical practice* (2nd edn.). Washington, DC: American Psychological Association.

Johnson, S. M., & Lee, A. C. (2000). Emotionally focused family therapy: Restructuring attachment. In C. E. Bailey (Ed.), *Children in therapy: Using the family as a resource* (pp. 112–133). New York: Norton.

Kam, S.-E., & Midgley, N. (2006). Exploring "clinical judgement": How do child and adolescent mental health professionals decide whether a young person needs individual psychotherapy? *Clinical Child Psychology and Psychiatry*, *11*, 27–44.

Kaye, A. L., & Shea, M. T. (2000). Personality disorders, personality traits, and defense mechanisms. In Task Force for the Handbook of Psychiatric Measures (Eds.), *Handbook of psychiatric measures* (pp. 713–749). Washington, DC: American Psychiatric Association.

Kazdin, A. E. (2004). Psychotherapy for children and adolescents. In M. Lambert (Ed.), *Bergin and Garfield's handbook of psychotherapy and behavior change* (5th edn., pp. 543–589). New York: Wiley.

Kennedy, E. (2004). Child and Adolescent Psychotherapy: a Systematic Review of Psychoanalytic Approaches. London: North Central London Strategic Health Authority.

Klein, M. (1932). *The psycho-analysis of children*. London: Hogarth Press.

Koos, O., & Gergely, G. (2001). A contingency-based approach to the etiology of "disorganized" attachment: The "flickering switch" hypothesis. *Bulletin of the Menninger Clinic*, *65*, 397–410.

Layne, C. M., Pynoos, R. S., & Cardenas, J. (2001). Wounded adolescence: School-based group psychotherapy for adolescents who sustained or witnessed violent injury. In M. Shafii, & S. L. Shafii (Eds.), *School violence: Assessment, management, prevention* (pp. 163–186). Washington, DC: American Psychiatric Association.

Levy, K. N., Meehan, K. B., Kelly, K. M., Reynoso, J. S., Weber, M., Clarkin, J. F., *et al.* (2006). Change in attachment patterns and reflective function in a randomized control trial of transference-focused psychotherapy for borderline personality disorder. *Journal of Consulting and Clinical Psychology*, *74*, 1027–1040.

Liddle, H. A., Dakof, G. A., Parker, K., Diamond, G. S., Barrett, K., & Tejeda, M. (2001). Multidimensional family therapy for adolescent drug abuse: Results of a randomized clinical trial. *American Journal of Drug and Alcohol Abuse*, *27*, 651–688.

Lieberman, A. F. (2004). Traumatic stress and quality of attachment: reality and internalization in disorders of infant mental health. *Infant Mental Health Journal*, *25*, 336–351.

Lieberman, A. F., Van Horn, P., & Ippen, C. G. (2005). Toward evidence-based treatment: Child–parent psychotherapy with preschoolers exposed to marital violence. *Journal of the American Academy of Child and Adolescent Psychiatry*, *44*, 1241–1248.

Lieberman, A. F., Weston, D. R., & Pawl, J. H. (1991). Preventive intervention and outcome with anxiously attached dyads. *Child Development*, *62*, 199–209.

Lock, J. (2004). Empowering the family as a resource for recovery: An example of family-based treatment for anorexia nervosa. In H. Steiner (Ed.), *Handbook of mental health interventions in children and adolescents: An integrated developmental approach*. San Francisco, CA: Jossey Bass.

Lush, D., Boston, M., Morgan, J., & Kolvin, I. (1998). Psychoanalytic psychotherapy with disturbed adopted and foster children: A single case follow-up study. *Clinical Child Psychology and Psychiatry*, *3*, 51–69.

Lyons-Ruth, K. (2003). Dissociation and the parent-infant dialogue: A longitudinal perspective from attachment research. *Journal of the American Psychoanalytic Association*, *51*, 883–911.

March, J., Silva, S., Petrycki, S., Curry, J., Wells, K., Fairbank, J., *et al.* (2004). Fluoxetine, cognitive–behavioral therapy, and their combination for adolescents with depression: Treatment for Adolescents with Depression Study (TADS) randomized controlled trial. *Journal of the American Medical Association*, *292*, 807–820.

Mitchell, S. A. (2000). *Relationality: From attachment to intersubjectivity*. Hillsdale, NJ: Analytic Press.

Moran, G., & Fonagy, P. (1987). Psycho-analysis and diabetic control: A single-case study. *British Journal of Medical Psychology*, *60*, 357–372.

Moran, G., Fonagy, P., Kurtz, A., Bolton, A., & Brook, C. (1991). A controlled study of the psychoanalytic treatment of brittle diabetes. *Journal of the American Academy of Child and Adolescent Psychiatry*, *30*, 926–935.

Mufson, L., Dorta, K. P., Wickramaratne, P., Nomura, Y., Olfson, M., & Weissman, M. M. (2004). A randomized effectiveness trial of interpersonal psychotherapy for depressed adolescents. *Archives of General Psychiatry*, *61*, 577–584.

Muratori, F., Picchi, L., Bruni, G., Patarnello, M., & Romagnoli, G. (2003). A two-year follow-up of psychodynamic psychotherapy for internalizing disorders in children. *Journal of the American Academy of Child and Adolescent Psychiatry*, *42*, 331–339.

Muratori, F., Picchi, L., Casella, C., Tancredi, R., Milone, A., & Patarnello, M. G. (2001). Efficacy of brief dynamic psychotherapy for children with emotional disorders. *Psychotherapy and Psychosomatics*, *71*, 28–38.

O'Connor, T. G., & Croft, C. M. (2001). A twin study of attachment in preschool children. *Child Development*, *72*, 1501–1511.

Oezbay, H., Goeka, E., Oeztuerk, E., & Guengoer, S. (1993). Therapeutic factors in an adolescent psychodrama group. *Journal of Group Psychotherapy, Psychodrama and Sociometry*, *46*, 3–11.

PDM Task Force. (2006). *Psychodynamic diagnostic manual*. Silver Spring, MD: Alliance of Psychoanalytic Organizations.

Plante, W., Lobato, D., & Engel, R. (2001). Review of group interventions for pediatric chronic conditions. *Journal of Pediatric Psychology*, *26*, 435–453.

Pynoos, R., Steinberg, A., & Wraith, R. (1995). A developmental model of childhood traumatic stress. In D. Cicchetti, & D. J. Cohen (Eds.), *Developmental psychopathology* (Vol. 2, pp. 72–95). New York: Wiley.

Pynoos, R. S., Steinberg, A. M., & Piacentini, J. C. (1999). A developmental psychopathology model of childhood traumatic stress and intersection with anxiety disorders. *Biological Psychiatry*, *46*, 1542–1554.

Rance, S. (2003). Report on the survey of ACP members about the outcome study. II. Summary of therapist activity and child data. *Bulletin of the Association of Child Psychotherapists*, *133*, 25–32.

Reid, S., Alvarez, A., & Lee, A. (2001). The Tavistock autism workshop approach. In J. Richer, & S. Coates (Eds.), *Autism: The search for coherence* (pp. 182–192). London: Jessica Kingsley.

Robin, A. L., Siegel, P. T., & Moye, A. (1995). Family versus individual therapy for anorexia: Impact on family conflict. *International Journal of Eating Disorders*, *17*, 313–322.

Robin, A. L., Siegel, P. T., Moye, A. W., Gilroy, M., Baker-Dennis, A., & Sikard, A. (1999). A controlled comparison of family versus individual therapy for adolescents with anorexia nervosa. *Journal of the American Academy of Child and Adolescent Psychiatry*, *38*, 1482–1489.

Roth, A., & Fonagy, P. (2005). *What works for whom? A critical review of psychotherapy research* (2nd edn.). New York: Guilford Press.

Russell, G. F. M., Szmukler, G., Dare, C., & Eisler, I. (1987). An evaluation of family therapy in anorexia nervosa and bulimia nervosa. *Archives of General Psychiatry*, *44*, 1047–1056.

Rutter, M. L. (1987). The role of cognition in child development and disorder. *British Journal of Medical Psychology*, *60*, 1–16.

Sameroff, A. J., & Fiese, B. H. (2000). Models of development and developmental risk. In C. H. Zeanah (Ed.), *Handbook of infant mental health* (pp. 3–19). New York: Guilford.

Schechtman, Z. (2001, Feb/March). Process research in child group counseling/therapy. *The Group Circle*.

Shaw, R. J., & Palmer, L. (2004). Consultation in the medical setting: A model to enhance treatment adherence. In H. Steiner (Ed.), *Handbook of mental health interventions in children and adolescents* (pp. 917–941). San Francisco, CA: Jossey-Bass.

Sinha, U. K., & Kapur, M. (1999). Psychotherapy with emotionally disturbed adolescent boys: Outcome and process study. *NIMHANS Journal*, *17*, 113–130.

Smyrnios, K. X., & Kirkby, R. J. (1993). Long-term comparison of brief versus unlimited psychodynamic treatments with children and their parents. *Journal of Consulting and Clinical Psychology*, *61*, 1020–1027.

Sroufe, L. A., Egeland, B., Carlson, E., & Collins, W. A. (2005). *The development of the person: The Minnesota study of risk and adaptation from birth to adulthood*. New York: Guilford.

Stern, D. (1993). Acting versus remembering and transference-love and infantile love. In E. Person, A. Hagelin, & P. Fonagy (Eds.), *On Freud's "Observations and transference-love"*. New Haven, CT: Yale University Press.

Swanson, J. M., Arnold, L. E., Vitiello, B., Abikoff, H. B., Wells, K. C., Pelham, W. E., *et al.* (2002). Response to commentary on the multimodal treatment study of ADHD (MTA): Mining the meaning of the MTA. *Journal of Abnormal Child Psychology*, *30*, 327–332.

Szapocznik, J., Rio, A., Murray, E., Cohen, R., Scopetta, M., Rivas-Valquez, A., *et al.* (1989). Structural family versus psychodynamic child therapy for problematic Hispanic boys. *Journal of Consulting and Clinical Psychology*, *57*, 571–578.

Target, M., & Fonagy, P. (1994a). The efficacy of psychoanalysis for children with emotional disorders. *Journal of the American Academy of Child and Adolescent Psychiatry*, *33*, 361–371.

Target, M., & Fonagy, P. (1994b) The efficacy of psychoanalysis for children: Developmental considerations. *Journal of the American Academy of Child and Adolescent Psychiatry*, *33*, 1134–1144.

Target, M., & Fonagy, P. (2005). The psychological treatment of child and adolescent psychological disorders. In A. Roth, & P. Fonagy (Eds.), *What works for whom? A critical review of psychotherapy research* (2nd edn., pp. 385–424). New York: Guilford Press.

Toth, S. L., Maughan, A., Manly, J. T., Spagnola, M., & Cicchetti, D. (2002). The relative efficacy of two interventions in altering maltreated preschool children's representational models: Implications for attachment theory. *Developmental Psychopathology*, *14*, 877–908.

Trowell, J., Joffe, I., Campbell, J., Clemente, C., Almqvist, F., Soininen, M., *et al.* (2007). Childhood depression: A place for psychotherapy. An outcome study comparing individual psychodynamic psychotherapy and family therapy. *European Child and Adolescent Psychiatry*, 16, 157–167.

Trowell, J., Kolvin, I., Weeramanthri, T., Sadowski, H., Berelowitz, M., Glaser, D., *et al.* (2002). Psychotherapy for sexually abused girls: psychopathological outcome findings and patterns of change. *British Journal of Psychiatry*, *180*, 234–247.

van IJzendoorn, M. H., Juffer, F., & Duyvesteyn, M. G. C. (1995). Breaking the intergenerational cycle of insecure attachment: A review of the effects of attachment-based interventions on maternal sensitivity and infant security. *Journal of Child Psychology and Psychiatry*, *36*, 225–248.

Weisz, J. R. (2004). *Psychotherapy for children and adolescents: Evidence-based treatments and case examples*. Cambridge: Cambridge University Press.

Westen, D., & Gabbard, G. O. (2002). Developments in cognitive neuroscience. I. Conflict, compromise, and connectionism. *Journal of the American Psychoanalytic Association*, *50*, 53–98.

Westen, D., Novotny, C. M., & Thompson-Brenner, H. (2004). The empirical status of empirically supported psychotherapies: assumptions, findings, and reporting in controlled clinical trials. *Psychological Bulletin*, *130*, 631–663.

Whittington, C. J., Kendall, T., Fonagy, P., Cottrell, D., Cotgrove, A., & Boddington, E. (2004). Selective serotonin reuptake inhibitors in childhood depression: Systematic review of published versus unpublished data. *Lancet*, *363*, 1341–1345.

Winnicott, D. W. (1971). Transitional objects and transitional phenomena. In D. W. Winnicott (Ed.), *Playing and reality* (pp. 1–25). London: Tavistock.

Wood, B. L., Klebba, K. B., & Miller, B. D. (2000). Evolving the biobehavioral family model: The fit of attachment. *Family Process*, *39*, 319–344.

Young, J. F., & Mufson, L. (2004). Interpersonal psychotherapy for the treatment of adolescent depression: A guide to techniques and implementation. In H. Steiner (Ed.), *Handbook of mental health interventions in children and adolescents* (pp. 685–703). San Francisco, CA: Jossey Bass.

Young, J. F., Mufson, L., & Davies, M. (2006). Impact of comorbid anxiety in an effectiveness study of interpersonal psychotherapy for depressed adolescents. *Journal of the American Academy of Child and Adolescent Psychiatry*, *45*, 904–912.

67 Physical Treatments

Stanley Kutcher and Sonia Chehil

In the final analysis, all psychiatric treatments are biological. That is, whatever their mode of delivery, theoretical basis or assumed mode of effect, they modulate, change or otherwise alter the brain functions of behavior, cognition or affect. They do so in many ways, directly through their impact on neural networks (see chapter 16), and indirectly through altering attitudes and ideas.

There is no ascribed nobility, precedence or honor to either psychological or physical interventions. There is only the moral imperative to improve the lives of those who suffer, to do more good than harm and to adhere to three fundamentals of knowledge acquisition and application: developmental neurobiology, evidence-based care and the systematic application of sound therapeutic principles. Thus, although this chapter deals with physical (predominantly chemical) treatments, they hold no *a priori* primacy of place over non-physical interventions.

This chapter addresses the third of these fundamentals – the systematic application of sound therapeutic principles – using physical interventions as the model. Developmental neurobiology (see chapter 12) can be expected to inform our understanding of both patho-etiology and therapeutic response. Evidence-based care is woven into each of the chapters of this book in which interventions for specific disorders are discussed, and the details of somatic treatments for specific disorders are dealt with there. This chapter provides the clinician with a useful framework that can be applied to any therapeutic intervention. This framework has five components: selecting a treatment target; selecting a treatment; assessment and measurement; evaluating and maximizing treatment outcome; and the human interface.

Selecting a Treatment Target

Medical treatments are usually applied to three target conditions: illnesses/disorders, symptoms or risk factors. The target condition may be simply the illness/disorder (e.g., hypertension), it may be a symptom, such as pain (e.g., a "tension" headache), or it may be both (e.g., pain associated with arthritis). In some cases, treatment may be targeted towards a risk factor or constellation of factors, the effective treatment of which may prevent the onset of a known mental illness. Psychiatric treatments share the same contingencies. The target condition may be an illness/disorder (e.g., panic disorder), it may be simply a symptom (e.g., self-injurious behavior) or it may be both (e.g., panic attacks occurring only in the context of a major depressive disorder). In other cases, treating a risk factor (or constellation of risk factors) may prevent the onset of a mental illness (e.g., the prodrome in schizophrenia).

It is imperative that the clinician (and by extension the patient, family or responsible caregiver) understands what the treatment target is. Otherwise, treatments may be wrongly prescribed, wrongly understood or wrongly expected to produce a particular outcome. Furthermore, efforts should be made to ensure that all treatment participants (patient, clinician and others) agree on what the treatment target(s) is/are. Often there may be more than one treatment target, but at least one of these targets needs to be of significant importance to the patient. Put simply – if the patient does not buy into a treatment target it is not a treatment target.

The first step in the identification of a treatment target is determining if the patient has a psychiatric diagnosis. This is performed using standard DSM or ICD criteria, applied by a trained clinician in a systematic and reliable manner. The use of idiosyncratic diagnostic criteria makes it impossible to use the generalized experience of the profession. While interviewing creativity and the use of clinically suitable yet personally unique methods of data collection are to be encouraged, in the final analysis the information collected by the clinician must allow for a reliable application to determine diagnostic classification so that other clinicians obtaining information from the patient will arrive at similar diagnostic conclusions most of the time.

As psychiatric diagnoses are syndromal and are not yet based on independent objective methods of validation (e.g., laboratory tests), the clinician must be aware of the problems inherent in their use. These problems fall into two categories: composition and threshold problems. Composition difficulties arise when diagnostic categories can be realized by different combinations of their components. For example, in major depression, the DSM demands that five of nine components be present in order for the category to be confirmed. The difficulty that arises is that the composition of the category can be quite different, depending on the combination of the components being used. It is not yet clear that in all cases, similar

Rutter's Child and Adolescent Psychiatry, 5th edition. Edited by M. Rutter, D. Bishop, D. Pine, S. Scott, J. Stevenson, E. Taylor and A. Thapar. © 2008 Blackwell Publishing, ISBN: 978-1-4051-4549-7.

therapeutic interventions are useful for all combinations. In child and adolescent psychiatry, this potential confounding effect may be even greater as developmentally determined expression of individual components (symptoms) may differ depending on age, pubertal status or cognitive capacity.

Threshold problems occur at the level of the components (symptoms) of the category (diagnosis). For example, sleep difficulties, such as problems falling asleep, are a symptom used to make a diagnosis of depression. The issue facing the clinician is how much sleep difficulty must be present for that problem to be considered a symptom. This is obviously a crucial issue as difficulty falling asleep can be part of usual life, a response to a stressor or a symptom of a disorder. Thus, threshold considerations must be kept in mind whenever a diagnostic interview is being conducted. If the threshold is set too low, too many components will be classified as symptoms and individuals will be diagnosed as having a disorder when the reality is rather that they may be distressed or dysphoric. In these cases, unnecessary somatic interventions may be applied. If the threshold is set too high, individuals may be incorrectly classified as not requiring medical intervention.

These problems can be alleviated somewhat by the use of standardized diagnostic interviews; for example, the Kiddie Schedule for Affective Disorders and Schizophrenia (K-SADS), the Diagnostic Interview for Children and Adolescents (DICA) and others (see chapter 19). However, these standardized interviews are too cumbersome for everyday application and are unlikely to be used in most clinical settings. An alternative approach is to utilize a simple diagnostic checklist, to ensure that each of the components of the diagnostic category has been addressed and occasionally to apply one of the diagnostic interviews (e.g., K-SADS) to ensure continued reliable use of threshold criteria.

However, the determination of a diagnosis is not an act of clinical finality. A diagnosis is merely a hypothesis that predicts a particular outcome and leads to a specific intervention. As new information becomes available the hypothesis may need refinement or revision, or may even need to be completely discarded. As much treatment research is based on diagnostic categories, diagnostic classification can assist the clinician in choosing a particular treatment by referencing their patient's condition to the research data. Similarly, diagnostic classification can assist the clinician in the risk–benefit evaluation pertaining to treatment. Simply put, does the risk–benefit ratio of the treatment available for the condition outweigh the risk posed by not treating the condition? The diagnosis then helps the clinician to select a particular intervention, one that has been demonstrated to be effective in ameliorating the problems for which the intervention is being sought.

However, choosing a diagnosis as a treatment target, while useful and necessary, is not without problems. Given that diagnoses are syndromal, it is possible that any particular intervention may improve some components of the syndrome while not affecting others, or perhaps even worsening some. For example, a particular medication taken to treat major depressive disorder may improve mood but may worsen sleep and enhance anxiety. Furthermore, some components of the syndrome may exhibit different phase effects in response to the same intervention. For example, in a young psychotic patient, an antipsychotic medication may show a positive effect on agitation within 3 days but not demonstrate a positive effect on delusions until 3 weeks of continued treatment.

Additionally, some patients may have significant problems that in and of themselves may be legitimate treatment targets, regardless of diagnosis. For example, aggressive outbursts or self-harming behaviors may be treatment targets in an individual with autism, although neither of these symptoms is necessary for the diagnostic category. In other cases such as borderline personality disorder one component of the diagnostic category (e.g., self-harming behavior) may be a target for medication treatment while another component (e.g., chronic feelings of emptiness) may not. In other words, both diagnoses and symptoms can be legitimate treatment targets. It is essential that both the clinician and the patient know and agree on what the treatment targets are.

Whatever the choice for the intervention target, the physician must be aware of the social and regulatory issues surrounding the use of medications for treatment of disorders or symptoms that are "off-label." This means that the physician elects to use medications to treat disorders or symptoms, although the particular medication has not been approved by the regulatory agency in that particular country. In some cases, this will be because of procedural or work load delays at the level of the regulatory agency or because of decisions by manufacturers to differentially submit products for registration. These factors lead to a medication being registered for a particular indication in one jurisdiction (e.g., the EU) but not in another (e.g., the USA). In other situations, medications may not have been studied in youth and are therefore not registered for use in that age group although they are registered for use in adults. In other situations, medications will not have been studied in enough detail to be considered for registration – and if the medication is used for the control of specific symptoms, and if registration is disease-specific then by definition it will not have been registered for the purpose of specific symptom control. In child and adolescent psychiatric care, most medication interventions are "off-label" (as are all psychological interventions as there is no regulatory process for those). This does not mean that medications should not be used for "off-label" purposes. It does mean that the clinician should have reasonable evidence to support the use of "off-label" prescribing and that the rationale for this use should be clearly communicated to the patient and family and noted in the medical record.

The choice of treatment target depends on three factors: patient need, clinician knowledge and weight of therapeutic evidence.

Patient Need

Patient need may be expressed in syndromal or symptomatic terms. A young person with a major depressive disorder requires an intervention that will address the entire syndrome.

A young person with Tourette's syndrome complicated by severe obsessive-compulsive symptoms may require an intervention directed not only at the Tourette's syndrome but also at the obsessive-compulsive symptoms. A young person with autism complicated by aggressive outbursts may benefit significantly from a treatment directed towards the aggressive outbursts alone. In some cases, treatment targets can be simultaneously syndromal and symptomatic (e.g., significant depressive symptoms in a schizoaffective disorder) and both somatic and non-somatic interventions may be used – alone, concurrently or sequentially.

Clinician Knowledge

Clinicians must be informed about the unique strengths and weaknesses of each physical intervention, and of possible interactions (both therapeutic and adverse) amongst them. These include both pharmacodynamic (what the drug does to the body) and pharmacokinetic (what the body does to the drug) interactions (see chapter 16). For example, does adding an antipsychotic medication to a selective serotonin reuptake inhibitor (SSRI) enhance the treatment response in a young person with OCD? What are the potential drug–drug interactions associated with such a combination? How does the addition of the antipsychotic drug alter the serum levels and the half-life of the antidepressant?

Weight of Therapeutic Evidence

The field of physical treatments for child and adolescent psychiatric disorders is rapidly developing and reports of potentially effective somatic interventions for numerous syndromes or symptoms are frequently found in the literature. However, not all evidence is of similar value. Case studies and naturalistic studies (particularly those with small sample sizes) do not provide sufficient scientifically sound evidence to guide treatments. Meta-analyses that are based on inadequately conducted studies may lead to erroneous conclusions.

Additionally, as the field is early in its development, few properly conducted studies have been carried out so absence of evidence cannot be equated with evidence of absence. Efficacy studies in homogeneous patient groups do not always positively translate into large heterogeneous populations – where effectiveness studies are needed. Acute results cannot be extrapolated into long-term conclusions, and studies of relapse prevention and length of remission are required to answer important duration-of-treatment questions. Some adverse and therapeutic effects (particularly those that are rare or require long-term use for expression) can only be identified using population surveillance techniques for which large numbers of patients treated for long durations are needed.

Given this developing database it is sometimes difficult to address the issue of therapeutic evidence with complete confidence, and guidelines and algorithms for assisting the clinician have been devised (Emslie, Hughes, Crismon *et al.*, 2004). Generally, these guidelines use levels of evidence, ranging from high to low, based on the quality of scientifically conducted research. Data from double-blind placebo-controlled studies are usually considered to be more robust evidence than data from naturalistic studies, which in turn are considered to be more robust than the opinions of "experts." However, the thresholds used to define these levels of evidence can vary across guidelines and different authorities may support different guidelines.

Guidelines along these lines (evidence-based medicine) have been developed for some conditions by national agencies (e.g., the UK National Institute of Health and Clinical Excellence [NICE]) and professional bodies (e.g., American Academy of Child and Adolescent Psychiatry). These can be helpful to the practitioner but, as recent history has shown, they are not always free from ideological bias that colors their interpretation of the available scientific evidence. For example, the NICE recommendations for the treatment of depression in young people differ significantly from the guideline standards used in their own literature review. Levels of evidence that are meant to inform the recommendations are not consistently applied. For example, interventions for which there is no evidence (such as watchful waiting) are recommended over an intervention for which there is the highest level of evidence (fluoxetine) (NICE, 2005). Multiple factors come into play when choosing if and how to treat (see p. 1092), but the evidence for efficacy, the probability and type of treatment emergent adverse effects, and the severity of the condition always need to be considered by the clinician, and his or her own experience used in the risk–benefit interpretation of any guidelines.

Additionally, in a rapidly evolving field such as child and adolescent psychopharmacology, guidelines may lose their relevance not long after their publication. New compounds for a specific disorder may come on the market in rapid succession or new indications for older medications may be defined. Clinicians must therefore be able to apply basic principles of psychopharmacology to their practice of therapeutics and not rely simply on algorithms or guidelines to direct their practice (see chapter 16).

Social factors (such as stigma against mental illness, strongly embedded belief systems regarding the effectiveness or danger of somatic interventions, belief-driven organizations or groups who are advancing unique political agendas, the over-enthusiastic uptake of somatic interventions by professionals unskilled in their use prior to their systematic evaluation, pharmaceutical company marketing methods) combine with the deficiencies of the syndromal classification system of psychiatric medicine and with long-standing ideological differences amongst child and adolescent mental health practitioners may create situations that at times are confusing not only to patients and family members but also to practitioners. This situation can only be effectively addressed by frank, honest and open discussion between clinicians and their patients and their families about what is and what is not known about various somatic interventions for syndromes and for symptoms. The weight of scientific evidence, with all forms of possible interventions being equally evaluated (e.g., it is not valid to expect that somatic treatments be evaluated at the highest standard of evidence while non-somatic treatments are evaluated using a lower standard of evidence), must be reviewed by clinicians and discussed with patients and their families. The decision to choose any treatment, somatic or not, must be the result of a joint decision-making process which recognizes the strengths and weaknesses of the available scientific evidence and which is not driven by preconceived ideological frameworks or professional biases.

Addressing Treatment Needs – Physical or Non-physical Treatments

Physical treatments are not provided in a vacuum but are always provided within a specific social context – the relationship between the clinician and the patient. In many cases, this social contract between provider and recipient of the treatment is complicated by the legitimate interests of third parties (e.g., parents and institutions). The impact of all of these different interests on the application, operationalization and outcome of any physical treatment must be taken into consideration at every intervention stage. Additionally, there may well be non-specific "healing" impacts in the clinician–patient interaction, and this also needs to be recognized.

In some cases, physical treatments will clearly be much more useful in addressing symptoms than non-physical treatments. In other cases, non-physical treatments may be as effective or even more effective. If the latter are available, then the preference may be to use them, because, in general, adverse effects are less common. In many circles it has become almost fashionable to "prescribe" non-physical treatments for disorders in which the evidence for the effectiveness of physical treatments is high – particularly if the disorder is judged to be "mild." However, in many cases, such as the NICE guidelines for the treatment of depression in youth, there is little or no evidence that the suggested non-physical interventions are any better than placebo or the standard non-specific healing properties inherent in the clinician–client relationship. While such arguments are not without merit, it is important not to oversimplify the complexities of treatment effects. For example, depression is regarded by some as a degenerative disorder involving the hippocampus perhaps through an altered expression of brain-derived neurotropic factor, with antidepressants but not other interventions slowing down or reversing that process (Hashimoto, Shimizu, & Iyo, 2004; Swaab, Bao, & Lucassen, 2005). If that were to be the case (and it is not yet established), then not providing the physical treatment even to "mild" cases would have negative long-term effects on the progression of the disease. Generally, just as we are usually better at ascribing causality to proximal rather than distal causes, so we may be equally poorly prepared to consider long-term outcomes rather than immediate effects of treatments.

This dilemma has no simple solution. It becomes a particularly vexing problem if our commitment to "first do no harm" has to challenge us with different types of possible harm, expressed in different ways at different points in time. How does the clinician address the difference between "harm" from tolerable but unpleasant side-effects (short-term effects) and "harm" from not intervening in the disease process (long-term effects)? To date, the research evidence to help address these concerns is still quite limited, but it would be professionally improper not to consider these complexities carefully, albeit in the face of imperfect data.

In many cases, providing a particular physical treatment together with a specific non-physical treatment (such as fluoxetine plus cognitive–behavioral therapy [CBT] in adolescent depression) may lead to a better outcome than either one alone. In other cases, providing interventions designed to enhance learning, social or other skills when physical treatments have brought symptoms under control is necessary to improve outcomes over the use of the physical treatment alone (e.g., mathematics tutoring or social skills training for children with ADHD effectively treated with methylphenidate). At other times, physical treatments may be used to enable non-physical interventions to be more effectively applied (e.g., short-term benzodiazepines in the behavioral treatment of phobia when excessive anxiety prevents the application of a desensitization procedure from being initiated). Judicious application of physical treatments includes knowing when to use them and when not to use them; both are equally important.

In the future, the ability of the clinician to select treatments – whether physical or non-physical – or to choose amongst various types of physical or non-physical treatments on the basis of genetic or other biological variables may supersede our currently imperfect and opinion-laden approaches to these topics. There is some promise in that direction, but for now there are no objective physiological guideposts to assist us; and best available evidence, clinical judgment and trial and monitoring still provide the decision-making triad from which we usually operate. Given this climate of uncertainty, it is necessary to address patient need using the best evidence we have, with humility and the willingness to modify or change our approach as science catches up with clinical care.

Selecting a Physical Treatment

Once the scientific evidence base has been reviewed, a target or targets selected and a treatment or treatments that meet(s) acceptable criteria for use has been identified, a further process of selection occurs. This process is driven by the following considerations: practitioner familiarity with the specific treatment; patient acceptability; comparative risk–benefit profile; ease of administration; cost and availability.

Practitioner Familiarity

Given all the possible somatic treatments available, it is not likely that the average clinician can become proficient in the use of every one of them. At the same time, it is essential that clinicians become very familiar with the treatment that they are using. It is therefore reasonable for the clinician to choose one or two compounds that will become his or her "personal" medication choices, which will be used in most cases in which that class of medication is indicated. This is also known as the "Personal" or "P drug" selection. This approach to therapeutic medication selection is essential for primary or even secondary care, but even tertiary care physicians may find this approach useful (WHO, 2000; 2001).

The "P drug" should have the following characteristics:

1 It should have good experimental evidence (placebo-controlled trials) supporting its therapeutic effect;
2 Its side-effect profile should be well known;
3 It should be relatively well tolerated by most patients;
4 It should be reasonably priced;
5 It should not have any significant disadvantages compared with other medications in its class;
6 It should be readily available; and
7 It should be relatively familiar to most clinicians.

Applying these criteria to medications in every class or subclass should allow the clinician to select a "P drug" for any target syndrome or target symptom. For example, and as illustration only, fluoxetine would be a reasonable "P drug" for adolescent depression; methylphenidate would be a reasonable "P drug" for childhood ADHD; and risperidone would be a reasonable "P drug" for youth-onset schizophrenia.

Once the "P drug" is selected, the clinician should become fully versed in its pharmacodynamics and pharmacokinetics. Repeated usage of the "P drug" will increase familiarity with its unique characteristics. Physicians in both primary and secondary care settings may find it useful to select two or three "P drugs" for each commonly treated condition using similar criteria to those noted above. This will allow greater flexibility in dealing with patients who may not have experienced therapeutic success with a previously used medication or who wish to have options in their choice of medications. Knowledge of the "P drug" also entails knowing its limitations, when others may be preferable and when a tertiary center should be consulted. Tertiary care physicians need to have a much wider familiarity with various therapeutic modalities.

Patient Acceptability

Patients and their families (as appropriate) should be active partners in their care and their acceptability of any treatment is important, not only for adherence but possibly also for therapeutic outcome. Patient (and family) participation in the choice of treatment (see p. 1104) is an important process of treatment selection. Patient preference for a specific intervention should be carefully considered whenever reasonable and may be driven by one or more of the following: previous experience with a medication (positive or negative); experience of a friend or relative with a medication; cost; and media coverage. Many young patients may find it difficult to swallow medications. For them, the type of preparation (tablet or capsule) or size of tablet is often an important consideration.

Comparative Risk–Benefit Profile

No medical treatment is risk-free. Every choice of medical treatment uses a risk–benefit approach. Risk–benefit can be analyzed by comparing the number needed to treat (NNT) with the number needed to harm (NNH). This creates a method for assessing the risk–benefit ratio of any treatment – regardless of its type. Such information may not be easily available for all somatic interventions (and is not available for most non-somatic interventions) but when it is, it should be used to guide treatment choice. As a rule of thumb, the number 10 is often taken as a "cut-off point" in treatment decisions using the NNT. How many individuals does the clinician need to treat with a given intervention before he or she can be sure that at least one individual is getting better because of the intervention and not because of other reasons? In the Treatment of Adolescent Depression Study (TADS), the NNT was calculated for each of the four treatment arms. The combined fluoxetine and CBT treatment arm was found to have an NNT of 4, compared with fluoxetine alone which was 5 and CBT alone which was 12 (TADS, 2004). (Of course, single studies cannot by themselves provide sufficient assurance that NNT or NNH calculations based on their results alone are representative.) Clinicians should assess risk–benefit on the basis of likely therapeutic effect; likely adverse effects; rare adverse effects; likely outcome without treatment; and other available treatments. While there is no simple statistical or other method by which the individual practitioner can calculate the risk–benefit ratio for any single treatment for any single patient, the process of addressing the various domains will in itself raise issues that will need to be considered by both clinician and patient.

For some individuals, certain treatments may be contraindicated (they should not be used because their risk far outweighs their potential benefit) or contra-advised (they should generally not be used but for some specific patient reason they may be considered). For example, a medication that is known to demonstrate significant negative interactions with another medicine that is being used would be a contraindication for treatment. Treating an agitated psychotic manic male with a history of ADHD with methylphenidate alone would be contraindicated. Contra-advised selection would be a treatment that may raise the risk for an untoward outcome because of patient or treatment characteristics (or both). For example, the use of benzodiazepines to treat anxiety in a young person who has a strong family history of alcohol addiction would be contra-advised (Evans, Levin, & Fischman, 2000).

Ease of Administration

Ease of administration is a vital criterion for treatment selection. The easier a treatment is to administer, the more likely adherence is to be high. Considerations include the number of times the treatment is given (e.g., number of doses per day) and method of delivery (oral, parenteral, rectal). Additionally, the presence or absence of other associated features such as the necessity for periodic venipunctures (to monitor serum levels) and ancillary investigations because of possible negative drug effects (e.g., electrocardiograms [ECG]; lipid and glucose monitoring) need to be considered in treatment selection. As a general "rule of thumb," when effectiveness and adverse events are similar, medications that are more convenient for the patient to use are preferred to those that carry greater inconveniences.

Cost and Availability

The cost of somatic treatments is an important factor in treatment selection. In this assessment, the availability of personal insurance or public health system coverage) should be considered. As many pharmacological treatments will be long term (a year or longer), clinicians and patients should consider the cumulative and not just the single-dose costs of a treatment. In situations where individuals do not have coverage of costs, careful consideration needs to be given to the assessment of comparative benefits between medications that are less costly but "traditional" and those that are more costly and novel. Higher cost does not always mean better medication.

Additionally, the indirect costs of any specific medication must also be considered. For example, a medication may increase the likelihood of other medical problems for which later treatment will be needed (e.g., tardive dyskinesia or metabolic syndromes), or which entail frequent laboratory monitoring, either for serum levels of the medication (e.g., carbamazepine) or for medication-induced changes in physiology (e.g., prolactin, glucose or lipid levels which may be induced by some "atypical" antipsychotics). These "indirect" medication costs can have a substantial cumulative impact in both private and public payment systems.

In some settings, medication availability is an important issue. In many low-income countries, the supply chain of psychotropic medications is vulnerable to a variety of negative impacts often not considered by practitioners working in wealthy countries. A patient who cannot rely on a consistent supply of needed medications may be at risk for a variety of negative outcomes associated with supply discontinuation – including but not limited to relapse and withdrawal. If that is the case, then the clinician may choose to treat using a medication that in circumstances of reliable supply may not be preferred. For example, a long-acting injectable antipsychotic may be chosen instead of lithium carbonate for the maintenance therapy of a patient with bipolar disorder.

Assessment and Measurement

Once treatment targets have been identified, treatment goals (amount of expected change and expected timeline for change) need to be defined. These will vary depending on the treatment target and the intervention chosen. For example, panic disorder may be selected as a syndromal treatment target. Within that framework, panic attacks may be selected as a specific symptom target, with anticipatory anxiety and phobic avoidance also being chosen as symptom targets. In this case, assessment and measurement will need to be directed at both the syndromal and the symptom targets. This will lead the clinician to select a number of different measurement tools. For example, the syndrome can be assessed using ICD or DSM criteria; the panic attacks can be assessed using a diary that captures the number and severity of attacks weekly; the anticipatory anxiety and phobic avoidance can be assessed using a visual analog scale.

The expected timeline of effect will vary with the drug; not all treatment targets can be expected to show similar time courses of improvement. For example, in panic disorder, expected decreases in anticipatory anxiety may require 2–3 times longer to achieve than expected decreases in panic attack frequency. Phobic avoidance may similarly require a longer duration for a similar proportional improvement. In some cases, application of complementary concurrent interventions (e.g., behavioral therapy) may be required to achieve the treatment goals.

Treatment goals may be response or remission. Response can be defined as symptomatic improvement that is clearly experienced by the patient accompanied by functional improvement across a variety of domains (e.g., interpersonal, vocational, academic). Remission can be defined as a return to premorbid conditions (both symptomatic and functional). These outcomes may vary amongst treatment targets, as not all syndromes or symptoms show equal potential for response or remission with currently available somatic interventions. In some cases, addition of non-somatic interventions (e.g., CBT added to SSRIs for youth with OCD) may enhance the probability of improved outcomes.

Relapse prevention is also a treatment goal. Exacerbation of initial symptoms after treatment discontinuation is known as *rebound*, and the emergence of previously not experienced symptoms is known as *withdrawal*. Neither rebound nor withdrawal is synonymous with addiction, but either can occur in addictive states.

One of the many areas of therapeutics that require extensive additional research is that of the continued effectiveness of interventions that have shown positive short-term effects with acute treatment (e.g., methylphenidate in ADHD). There is a dearth of long-term studies of continued effectiveness of treatments (both physical and psychological) that can be used to guide clinical practice. So, in many cases (e.g., in the treatment of depression) we have to use data extrapolated from studies in adults. While this is not optimal information (and depression in adolescents does not follow the same expectations for treatment as in adults), it often is the only treatment available and so is still used to inform clinical practice for young people. It is hoped that future editions of this textbook will be able to draw on child- and adolescent-specific research that can address this issue.

Treatment emergent adverse events (commonly known as side-effects) are also treatment targets. However, here the target is to avoid or mitigate treatment emergent adverse events, not to achieve them. Treatment emergent adverse events are defined as any phenomena that have their onset during a treatment and are directly attributable to that treatment. For example, a specific medication can cause physical side-effects (e.g., nausea or diarrhea) by its effect on either the digestive system or the central nervous system. Similarly, behavioral side-effects (e.g., agitation, impulsivity), cognitive/perceptual side-effects (e.g., suicidal ideation or hallucinations) and affective side-effects (e.g., depressed mood) may occur as treatment emergent adverse events.

At times it may be difficult for the clinician to determine if patient complaints of adverse events are truly side-effects (i.e., they occur during treatment as a direct result of that treatment), or if they are reflections of another phenomenon. One such potentially confusing scenario is the onset of concurrent but unrelated events (e.g., the patient develops a flu-like illness during the flu season). Another potentially confusing scenario is attributional in nature. For example, the patient has had a long history of headaches, for which no cause has been established, but now is convinced that it is the treatment that is "causing" the headaches. In addition, negative outcomes occurring during treatment may also be the result of the natural history of the disorder and may be serendipitously linked to treatment application. For example, an increase in depressed mood that occurs a week after beginning an antidepressant may be a result of the natural progression of the illness prior to the onset of the therapeutic action of the treatment rather than a result of the application of the treatment. In such cases, the propensity for patients and clinicians alike to ascribe causality to proximal rather than distal factors may lead to the termination of a potentially effective intervention.

Thus, prior to any somatic intervention, a thorough assessment of treatment targets (syndrome, symptom, side-effect) must be conducted by the clinician. The initial application of this comprehensive evaluation is commonly known as the "baseline assessment."

Baseline Assessment and Measurements

The baseline assessment takes place during a specified period of time prior to the initiation of a specific somatic treatment. It is carried on concurrently with patient (and where appropriate, family or responsible other) education about the disorder and its treatment (see p. 1103). In psychiatric treatments, emergency or life-saving interventions are usually not the norm and in most cases an appropriate window of time exists for the baseline assessment to be properly conducted. The baseline assessment addresses all of the treatment targets, provides specific measurements of those targets and sets outcome and evaluation process expectations.

Treatment targets can be syndromal, symptomatic, adverse effect or overall functioning. Syndromal targets are predefined by syndromal criteria (either ICD or DSM). Symptomatic targets can be directly defined by the disorder (e.g., hyperactivity, panic attacks, hopelessness). Functioning targets can be defined by assessing the effect of the disorder or symptom(s) on the individual's functioning (e.g., interpersonal conflict, academic success). Adverse effects can be somatic, behavioral, cognitive/perceptual or affective.

Measurements of targets have three complementary components: frequency, severity and duration. For each target on which a measurement is conducted, each of these components should be noted. For example, for an aggressive boy: how many fist-fights (frequency) occurred during the last week (duration); and how intense were they (pushing, hitting, using a weapon at three different levels of severity)? Each of these components should be consistently noted at each measurement point.

Syndromal targets tend to be binary – that is, the syndrome is either present or it is not. They are therefore measured categorically. Syndromes may be measured in a variety of manners including the use of diagnostic rating scales such as the K-SADS and the DICA. These measurement tools are generally thought to be too cumbersome and time-consuming for routine clinical use but extensive training in their use may be associated with more comprehensive clinical assessments even when they are not being directly applied. Therefore, clinician training in one or more of these diagnostic instruments may be useful in a general sense for assessment and measurement purposes. Some authors suggest that syndromal checklists are a reasonable tool that can assist the clinician both in validating a clinical interview (does the patient clearly meet a syndromal diagnosis?) and in improving rater reliability over time (repeated application of the diagnostic checklist at designated intervals may enhance certainty in diagnostic outcome monitoring by ensuring that all the components of the diagnosis are appropriately considered each time the tool is applied). Application of a symptom checklist, which can be created directly from the diagnostic manuals for any psychiatric disorder, should be conducted at baseline.

Symptom treatment targets can often be ordinarily defined and thus lend themselves to measurement by scales. Sometimes these can be measured as symptom clusters which relate strongly to diagnostic categories (e.g., depression rating scales which include many of the symptoms found in major depressive disorder or obsessive-compulsive symptom rating scales). At other times, one or two symptoms will be the target of treatment (e.g., tics, aggressive outbursts; Storch, Murphy, Geffken *et al.*, 2005). In many of these cases, a well-validated scale such as the Yale Global Tic Severity Scale (Storch, Murphy, Geffken *et al.*, 2005) may not be available, or the clinician may prefer to use simple clinically useful measurement tools such as a Visual Analog Scale or an ordinal 0–3 scale where 0 equals none, 1 equals mild, 2 equals moderate and 3 equals severe. If this type of "shorthand" clinical measurement is used, the clinician must ensure that both he or she and the patient (or responsible other) understand the meaning of the different measurement points on the scale.

Symptom measurement tools can be either self- or other-administered, with the "other" being a clinician, parent or a specified responsible observer (e.g., a classroom teacher). There are pros and cons associated with the use of each type of tool and different informants may rate differently. When parents and patients rate differently on similar instruments (e.g., for ADHD symptoms), the astute clinician may use the occasion to explore the different perceptions of the problem, its treatment and the hoped for results. Thus, quantitative tools may also facilitate qualitative assessment.

For many mental disorders in children and adolescents, a variety of validated symptom rating scales are available. These often come complete with instructions for use and some may be commercially available. The choice of measurement tool will depend on the realities of the clinician's practice, the costs associated with their use and the acceptance of patients and responsible others. The routine application of 2–4 h of rating scales prior to therapeutic prescription is unlikely to find favor amongst patients and their families (nor is it necessary) outside of tertiary care or clinical research settings. However, routine application of some clinically useful standardized measurement tools at baseline and at appropriate times thereafter will improve clinical care.

As functional improvement should be a target of every somatic intervention, there must be some baseline assessment and measurement of functioning in various domains. The Global Assessment of Functioning Scale found in the DSM is helpful in this regard but different clinicians may prefer to use different tools. Some functional assessment tools have been developed for specific syndromes (e.g., the Kutcher scale for Social Anxiety Disorder; Brooks & Kutcher, 2004). In many cases, application of the Visual Analog Scale methodology to one or more functional targets will suffice. For example, level of family discord in the past week, success in getting homework completed prior to class. For some targets, simple counting is appropriate (e.g., number of fist-fights in the past week). The "best" choice of measurement tool will depend on the target.

Side-effects should be measured using standardized techniques that cover a wide variety of somatic dimensions (for examples see Kutcher, 1997) and must be applied at baseline before a somatic intervention is initiated. This will allow for appropriate identification of treatment emergent adverse effects, which can be either phenomena that arise for the first time during treatment or exacerbations of phenomena already existing at the onset of treatment.

Appropriate medical assessments may also be indicated at baseline. These include laboratory and other investigations, which may be diagnostic of a medical condition (such as a thyroid-stimulating hormone [TSH] test for hypothyroidism or a magnetic resonance imaging [MRI] scan for pituitary adenoma) suggested by information obtained during the history and functional enquiry (see chapter 22). Routine laboratory screening is not indicated given its low positive predictive value. Additionally, those laboratory or other physiological parameters (such as heart rate/rhythm) that can be affected by the somatic treatment used (e.g., thyroid function for lithium, prolactin for risperidone, metabolic indices for olanzepine, ECG for tricyclics) should be assessed at baseline. Pubertal females should have a pregnancy test and high-risk teenagers may be strongly considered for sexually transmitted disease (STD) investigations.

Evaluating and Maximizing Treatment Outcome

Following the baseline and at the time of expected outcomes, evaluation of each target should be conducted, using the same measurements that were obtained at baseline. The timing of these will vary depending on the target being evaluated, the treatment being applied and the expected time course for change to occur. For example, if syndromal outcome is being measured in a teenager with major depressive disorder, a checklist for major depressive disorder should be repeated following 8–10 consecutive weeks of treatment if an SSRI is being used. Syndromal assessment for ADHD in a 9-year-old boy could be conducted following 2–4 weeks if a psychostimulant is being used. For panic disorder (PD) it is reasonable to conduct a syndromal evaluation following 4–6 weeks if a benzodiazepine is being used. Conversely, depressive symptoms in major depressive disorder measured using either a self-rating or clinician-rating scale should be conducted at week 4 and weekly thereafter, while both ADHD and PD symptoms should be monitored weekly following treatment initiation. Side-effects should usually be evaluated within 2 days of initiation of treatment and weekly thereafter.

In acute agitated psychotic states, both therapeutic and side-effects may need to be evaluated hourly if clinically indicated. School functioning in OCD may be next assessed at 3 months and every 2 months thereafter. Serum carbamazepine levels can be assessed weekly for 4 weeks and then every 6–8 weeks following hepatic calibration to steady state levels.

In chronic treatments, similar criteria apply. For institutionalized children or teenagers, frequent evaluation of all target conditions will help ensure that appropriate clinical care is being provided, and institutional policies and procedures should be developed to ensure that such careful and standardized ongoing evaluation is in place.

Once maximal treatment outcome has been obtained (remission or recovery), treatment evaluation becomes treatment monitoring. In this scenario, regularly scheduled visits should be structured to ensure that syndromal, symptomatic, functioning and side-effect targets can be parsimoniously evaluated. Additionally, qualitative evaluation becomes increasingly important in the face of insufficient scientific data on the potential risks and benefits of long-term treatments. Evaluation tools should therefore be supplemented by more open-ended dialog. Patients and their families should be instructed to report any untoward adverse events immediately. Always check with the treating physician if other medications are being prescribed (in case of drug–drug interactions). Patients and families should be instructed in the earliest signs of relapse so that potentially useful interventions are not delayed.

Maximizing Treatment Outcome

The ideal goal of treatment outcome is recovery, which is remission followed by a prolonged sense of well-being. Unfortunately, our therapeutics are not perfect and in many cases, because of either individual or therapeutics reasons, neither recovery nor remission occurs. The aim is then an optimal outcome – achieving the best improvements possible in all treatment targets. For this purpose, somatic treatments are often necessary but insufficient, and should be linked with various other interventions, including psychological, social and vocational components, guided by the same principles of evidence and application as are used to direct somatic treatments. They should be chosen on the basis of patient need rather than clinician preference or ideological commitment.

In many cases, somatic treatments may differentially affect chosen targets in a manner that limits their ability to address patient needs effectively. For example, the same dose of a "P" medication that maximizes symptomatic improvement may lead to intolerable side-effects, thus limiting its dose. This may require the use of a different medication or "layering" of medications (the use of a lower dose of the "P" medicine with the addition of another medication, usually from a different class of drug). These different strategies are known as *substitution* and *augmentation*. While there is often anecdotal evidence for these strategies, and in some cases there is reasonable scientifically supported evidence from adult populations, neither of these two sources of information provides the necessary weight of scientific evidence required to clearly guide clinical practice in young people. In such situations, clinicians will need to rely on their best judgment and must discuss the limits of evidence and the basis for their further treatment advice with their patient and his or her family or responsible caretaker. The rationale for choosing either substitution or augmentation strategies should be noted in the clinical file.

Achieving therapeutic outcome with the initial "P" drug is based on two factors – dose and duration of treatment. The dose must be one that provides the greatest positive benefit with the fewest side-effects and it must be maintained for the necessary length of time – in both acute and long-term conditions. In dose determination, three factors are important: dose initiation, dose target and dose duration. The dose must be properly initiated; doses that are too high to begin with or which are raised too rapidly will not usually hasten symptomatic improvement but will often lead to significant side-effects. Sometimes there is a significant possibility of an individual showing adverse effects at an ordinary dose. For example, some individuals are slow metabolizers of atomoxetine (see chapter 16). A low dose may then be given as a check on sensitivity, with patient and family aware of the rationale. Choosing an initial dose target that is too low is unlikely to lead to optimal benefit, while choosing an initial dose target that is too high is unlikely to improve outcome over side-effects. Up-titration, the process of dose increases to achieve the initial target dose, should be carried out slowly – giving time for the patient to acclimatize to each stepped increase.

Medications that achieve their initial dosing targets but are not maintained for a sufficient length of time are unlikely to provide optimal treatment response. It is essential that the clinician allow sufficient time for the treatment to demonstrate its effect. This time to response will differ depending on the condition and the medication used. For example, a young person treated with an SSRI for major depressive disorder should be maintained at the initial target dose for a period of 8 weeks. For a youth with OCD being treated with an SSRI the time to response is about 12 weeks. Discontinuation of treatment prior to the expected time to response may not only negate the therapeutic effects of an effective treatment, but may also lead to negative perspectives about the value of a particular intervention on the part of patient, family and clinician alike.

Both dose initiation and dose duration must be based on the pharmacokinetics and pharmacodynamics of the medication chosen and the known response of a syndrome or symptom to the medication. For example, an SSRI used to treat OCD may require a higher therapeutic target dose level for a longer duration than the same SSRI used in the treatment of major depressive disorder. However, both will require similar rates of dose titration to reach the initial target dose. In general, for most medications, a "start low and go slow" dose titration model is to be preferred. Of particular importance in acute psychosis is that the expected course of clinical outcomes should be used to inform dose titration. For example, initial dosing strategies should target agitation and restore a "normal" sleep–wake cycle. Improvement in socialization and psychotic thinking can be expected later in the treatment course. Over-medicating by using higher doses of antipsychotics to treat agitation and sleep difficulties is to be avoided. The layering of medications (such as adding short-acting benzodiazepines to address agitation) is preferred to using larger (and potentially more problematic) doses of non-sedating antipsychotics.

Possible drug–drug interactions must be considered whenever multiple medications are being used in the same individual. While it is unlikely that any clinician can remember all such interactions, it is possible to keep in mind the most common that could be expected for children and adolescents. Up-to-date resources containing P450 level drug–drug interaction tables are readily available and any physician treating young people with medications should routinely consult these references. Some are free of charge (Flokhart, 2007) and others require a subscription (GeneMedRx, 2007). Every patient and responsible caregiver should be informed about the possibility of drug–drug interactions and asked to notify the treating physician before beginning any new medication. Over-the-counter and herbal compounds may also interact with prescribed medicines (Hu, Yang, Chan *et al.*, 2005). Therefore, as a general rule, patients and responsible others should be informed (and repeatedly reminded) that *any* medication (including cold remedies, pain modulators and oral contraceptives) should be discussed prior to their use. Encouraging patients to have their prescriptions filled at reputable pharmacy outlets that maintain personal medication profiles is recommended.

At a predetermined time (set by the known expected time course for therapeutic improvement) the therapeutic intervention should be systematically evaluated. Ideally, this should include a comprehensive review of the initial presentation, all treatment targets, the outcome in every target, newly emerging problems (including side-effects), functioning and a diagnostic re-evaluation. At that time one of three outcomes can be determined:

1 Remission has occurred;

2 Response has occurred but some difficulties remain; or

3 Insufficient therapeutic response has occurred or the situation has worsened.

If the outcome is recovery, the usual strategy is to continue the somatic treatment for an appropriate length of time following remission prior to deciding if treatment discontinuation is warranted. Although insufficient scientific literature exists to direct clinical decision-making on this point, practice should in general be guided by the answers to the following questions: what are the known or suspected negative outcomes of continuing medication treatment; what are the known or suspected positive outcomes of continuing medication treatment; what is the evidence for relapse if medication treatment is discontinued? Open discussion of these issues with a patient and responsible others can be used to guide continued treatment.

In the situation where response has occurred but some significant problems remain, the clinician should reconsider the treatment targets and the known therapeutic gains that can be expected with available somatic interventions. For example, in cases of severe OCD treated with an SSRI, a 75% response in OCD symptoms may be the best that can be expected (see for example March, Biederman, Wolkow *et al.*, 1998). Additionally, a search for other factors that could contribute to insufficient improvements such as treatment adherence difficulties; the presence of significant comorbid conditions; the effect of ongoing psychosocial stressors or the possibility of heretofore unrecognized substance misuse should be explored. Following from that, the initial treatment should be optimized.

Pharmacologically, treatment optimization may require increasing the dose beyond the initial target dose. If adverse effects are tolerable, this may be initiated using dose increments similar to those used during the period of up-titration to the initial target dose. Once a new target dose is reached, this should be maintained for a reasonable period of time to determine if therapeutic response improves. This pattern of gradual step increases, interspersed with appropriate periods of waiting, can continue until either the patient no longer continues to demonstrate expected treatment gains or side-effects that are not tolerable to the patient occur.

In some cases, the patient may be genetically predisposed to rapid metabolism of the medication. These "ultra-rapid metabolizers" are more common in African and Middle Eastern populations and demonstrate highly efficient CYP2D6 hepatic enzyme activity. Such individuals may rapidly metabolize various antidepressant and antipsychotic medications. However, a small percentage of the population demonstrates slower than usual metabolism of medications. These "poor metabolizers" as they are called, may have genetic differences of either the CYP2D6 or CYP2C19 hepatic enzyme systems (Desta, Zhao, Shin, & Flockhart, 2002). Now that a relatively simple test for genotyping of 2D6 and 2C19 has received Food and Drug Agency (FDA) approval, patients whose clinical presentation suggests a problem with drug metabolism could be tested in locations where that test is available (de Leon, Armstrong, & Cozza, 2006).

Optimization of response may also be achieved with the addition of psychological treatments with well-demonstrated efficacy, such as CBT added to fluoxetine in depressed adolescents (TADS, 2004) or CBT added to sertraline in OCD patients (POTS, 2004). In other cases, augmentation with another class of medication (e.g., adding lithium to an antidepressant in the treatment of depression) may be indicated (Hughes, Emslie, Crismon *et al.*, 1999). Another alternative is to switch medications, either to a compound in a similar class or to a compound from a different class (Hughes, Emslie, Crismon *et al.*, 1999). In some circumstances, the clinician may choose to substitute a non-somatic intervention for a physical treatment that has not led to good therapeutic results. This should only be considered where the research evidence for the effectiveness of the non-somatic is substantial and if the patient and/or family concurs (e.g., in OCD; O'Kearney, Anstey, & von Sanden, 2006). If this course of action is contemplated, then a graduated medication withdrawal strategy should be put into place to minimize the potential for a withdrawal syndrome.

Given the lack of substantive scientific evidence for any of the above strategies in the child and adolescent literature, treatment options will need to be discussed with the patient and responsible others and a jointly acceptable decision will need to be made as to the direction taken. Once that decision has been made, similarly rigorous assessments and treatment target selection and monitoring are necessary.

In cases where improvement has been unsatisfactory or the situation has worsened, the diagnosis should be critically reviewed and the social ecology of the therapeutic situation critically addressed (including treatment adherence, family and peer factors, and possible substance abuse). Then a new conceptualization of the problems and treatment targets needs to be undertaken and the systematic assessment, measurement and application once again initiated. A consultation with an experienced colleague is often useful in such situations.

The "N of One" Assessment Methodology

For some conditions and with some medications, an "N of One" treatment trial can be effectively and relatively simply initiated (Kutcher, 1986). This approach has stood the test of time and is appreciated by patients and families alike (Kent, Camfield, & Camfield, 1999) and can be implemented over the telephone (Nikles, Mitchell, Del Mar, Clavarino, & McNairn, 2006). Ideally, the medication should be paired with an identical placebo which can be made up by a pharmacist (or a non-identical comparison with blind raters). Then an on–off cycle (3–5 days on the medication followed by a similar length of time on the placebo) is initiated. Ideally, this cycle should be repeated so that an ABAB model is applied (A = medication phase; B = placebo phase). Ideally, multiple raters of the patient's symptoms, blind to the treatment condition and all using the same rating scale in the same manner across the entire ABAB sequence provide the assessments on which therapeutic decisions will be made. A positive trial demonstrates a repeated therapeutic effect of the medicine that is not found with the placebo.

This assessment method is well suited for a medication that demonstrates a rapid therapeutic onset and rapid therapeutic offset. Of all the child and adolescent disorders, ADHD is most amenable to this type of evaluation, using immediate-action medications and standard measures such as the SNAP (Pelham, Gnagy, Burrows-Maclean *et al.*, 2001; Swanson, 1992) with a methylphenidate specific side-effects scale (Kutcher, 1997). If therapeutic response is limited or side-effects are substantial, the "N of One" can suggest that a non-stimulant alternative be considered, thus saving the time and expense of an initial unsuccessful clinical trial.

Variations on this design can be used to answer other important clinical questions – for instance, of the need for different doses as a child with ADHD grows. Other, less rigorous "N of One" approaches to test hypotheses about medication treatments are less well supported by evidence and less well grounded in scientific validity. For example, some clinicians may choose to stop a medication to "see if it is still working." While the intent may be honest this suggests that the initial approach to the treatment was weak on assessment and evaluation. It is not necessary to stop a treatment to see if it is working. That question can be answered by comparing current assessments of symptoms and functioning against the baseline. Furthermore, discontinuation of treatment is not without its risks – for example, in bipolar patients, continuation of lithium treatment is highly correlated with lower rates of suicide (Baldessarini, Tondo, Davis *et al.*, 2006).

Polypharmacy

The increasing rate of psychotropic medication use in young people has been well documented (Thomas, Conrad, Casler, & Goodman, 2006). In some jurisdictions those increases (e.g., the use of SSRIs to treat depression) may be reasonably justified (Hunkeler, Fireman, Lee *et al.*, 2005) while in other jurisdictions the choice of medications used (e.g., the use of tricyclic anti-depressants and herbal preparations to treat depression) is not supported by the available data on safety and efficacy (Fegert, Kolch, Glaeske, & Janhsen, 2006). Many reasons to explain this increase have been suggested, including but not limited to: changes in clinical practice (from inpatient to out-patient care); increased treatment of heretofore untreated populations; better diagnosis and case identification of mental disorders in young people; availability of less toxic and less dangerous medications; pharmaceutical industry promotion of medication use; and better data on the effectiveness of medication treatment. Given the complexities of this issue, it is reasonable to conclude that multiple factors have come together to create this phenomenon.

As part of this increase, there is a general perspective that polypharmacy – the use of many medications concurrently – has become relatively commonplace, up to half of the populations studied in some reports (Russell, George, & Mammen, 2006), even though the evidence to support this use is not always robust (Lopez-Larson & Frazier, 2006). There may be a number of reasons for this increase. For example, some medications are routinely prescribed to counter possible adverse events caused by others (e.g., anticholinergic medicines used concurrently with "typical" antipsychotic compounds to limit extrapyramidal side-effects). Such clinical use is reasonable and consistent with both the pharmacodynamics and pharmacokinetics of the concurrently prescribed compounds. Another example of rational polypharmacy is the combined short-term use of a sedating benzodiazepine with an antipsychotic in the initial stages of an acute agitated psychosis.

However, there are a number of concerns about the use of polypharmacy. These include but are not limited to: an increased risk of side-effects caused by drug–drug interactions; decreased treatment adherence; increased treatment cost; and using two medications when one will do in the treatment of comorbid conditions (e.g., depression and panic attacks). Therefore, it is necessary to consider carefully the rationale for combining psychotropic medications and to monitor their use closely.

The following are issues that the clinician should consider prior to combining medications:

1 Why is the combination being considered? If it is for subtherapeutic response to a monotherapy, has the necessary review of the case and monotherapeutic optimization been conducted?
2 Is there a clinical and pathophysiological rationale for the combination?
3 Is there a scientific literature that addresses the combination being considered?
4 Are there known or likely drug–drug interactions?
5 If the combination is being used to treat a number of different symptoms or conditions, is there one medication that can be used instead?
6 How long will the combination be used and what are the evaluations that will be put into place to monitor therapeutic outcomes and adverse events?

When combining medications (and when changing medications) it is advisable to add (or subtract) only one compound at a time, ensuring that enough time passes to allow for appropriate evaluation of the effects of the medication addition (or subtraction). Careful monitoring will also be necessary as insufficient research data are available on possible adverse reactions to medication combinations.

The Human Interface

No medical treatment takes place in a social vacuum. Every interaction includes a host of individual, group and society factors, which influence, color and impact on the interaction between clinician and patient. Indeed, this interaction in and of itself may have therapeutic effect and thus, by implication, may have a negative effect. In some disorders, specific psychological or social therapies may extend some of the activities found in the clinician–patient interface but do not substantively alter or necessarily even improve on them. For example, the best estimation of the effect size of CBT for major depressive disorder in adolescents is 0.3–0.4 (Weersing & Brent, 2006; Weisz, McCarty, & Valeri, 2006), which is strikingly similar to the placebo rate found in strictly conducted studies of somatic therapies (Cheung, Emlie, & Mayes, 2006). In other disorders (such as OCD), however, a similar type of psychotherapeutic intervention shows a greater effect size, suggesting a unique positive effect of that specific treatment.

The foundation of the clinician–patient interaction is based on two important principles: clinician responsibility to the patient and respect for the autonomy and rights of the patient. Each of these principles can be used to inform and direct the clinician–patient interaction in the delivery of somatic treatments.

Clinician Responsibility to the Patient

This value is arguably the basis for all physician–patient interaction, has its roots in centuries of medical history and is the framework on which the Hippocratic oath is built. In the provision of somatic treatments this value has certain specific applications.

First, the clinician is obligated to provide the therapeutic intervention for which the best and strongest scientific evidence for safety and effectiveness is available. This means that in some cases the clinician may advise against the use of somatic interventions if equally effective, inexpensive, safer and readily available non-somatic modalities are available. Conversely, it means that any responsible clinician should advise the use of somatic treatments when these are clearly indicated. Personal adherence to a particular "school" of therapeutics is not the criterion upon which patient care is based. Ideology should not trump science. The tradition of offering the "least restrictive" treatment as the preferred intervention in child psychiatry is still very strong and has important human rights foundations which should not be ignored. In days when therapeutic interventions were both all very much of a kind and all with a minimal evidence base, that framework as the primary guide to treatment selection was at least partly defensible. Currently, it is not a sufficient criterion for treatment selection. Not only must treatment be as minimally restrictive as possible, but it must also be as safe and effective as possible.

Additionally, clinicians must be honest with the patient and family about the strength of the scientific evidence used to guide their interventions. In a rapidly changing and imperfect world clinicians work with the best evidence that is available, not necessarily with the best evidence that should be available. Often therapeutic decisions need to be made on the basis of weak or even contradictory evidence. Sometimes, the available evidence is inconsistent. For example, we have a reasonable understanding of the acute therapeutic and side-effects of antidepressants but limited knowledge about their long-term therapeutic and side-effects. Long-term safety information can only be obtained from long-term use with ongoing surveillance. Apart from methylphenidate in the treatment of ADHD, this level of uncertainty is actually the norm and not the exception. A fair and reasonable discussion about the limits of the scientific knowledge is to be preferred to dogmatic statements about the prescriptions being offered. This of course applies to all therapeutic interventions, not just somatic treatments. Best clinical judgment means applying best available evidence to address the needs of the patient. Physicians are expected to ply their craft at the limits of certainty.

Second, clinicians are obligated to be as up-to-date as possible regarding all aspects of the diagnosis and treatments for the population that they are serving. There is no excuse for "not knowing." If the clinician is unsure, or uninformed, then referral should be made to a colleague who has the up-to-date knowledge needed to provide proper patient care. In child and adolescent psychiatry, it is still too common to find practitioners who practice what they learned as residents or house officers. Every clinician treating mentally ill children and adolescents either needs to have a solid working knowledge of diagnosis and somatic treatments, or else must discharge the obligation to the patient by referral to one who does. Furthermore, this requirement of life-long learning must be driven by appropriate educational activities. It is not appropriate to base one's understanding of somatic treatments on information solely supplied by the pharmaceutical industry. Similarly, it is not appropriate to base this understanding on the basis of the opinions of colleagues alone. Ongoing critical reading of the evidence and constructive, unbiased peer discussion of the scientific literature form the foundation of continuing self-education.

Third, the clinician is obligated to inform others, often within the wider society, of the values, risks and benefits of somatic treatments for child and adolescent mental disorders. Societies are complex organizations, comprised of many subgroupings, some of which are more certain of the truth than others. In some situations, social criticism of medical practice is well warranted and provides an independent and necessary counterpoint to medical tradition and self-certainty. In other situations, social criticism of medical practice is the result of certain ideologies or socioeconomic agendas, which may make great theater and sell newspapers or lead to wealth accumulation in some of the members of the legal profession. Responsible physicians need to become involved in proactively countering such negatively driven social discourse, as the outcome of some of these social processes, if not appropriately addressed, may lead to negative outcomes for patients and their families. At times, clinicians must discharge their obligation to their patients by active participation in the public debates of civil society. Here again this participation is to be driven by the scientific and not the ideological prerogative.

Fourth, clinicians must discharge their obligation by doing no harm. This does not mean "Do not treat." Nor does it mean "Do not treat using an intervention that may be harmful if used incorrectly or if inappropriately applied." As chemists, alchemists and sorcerers have known for centuries, toxicity is mostly an issue of dose! The obligation is to ensure that the therapeutic intervention does not do more harm than good and that it does not do more harm than the unchecked progression of the disease and that it does not do more harm than an available, equally effective intervention. The clinician is obligated to use treatments that have a positive benefit–risk ratio, and to use them in a way that maximizes benefits and minimizes risks. In order to do this properly, the three obligations described above must be effectively discharged.

Clinician Respect for the Autonomy and Rights of the Patient

In many religious and philosophical traditions, the "golden rule" is "Do unto others as you would have them do unto you." This is a useful dictum for clinicians to follow, regardless of their personal beliefs. Treating your patient as you would like to be treated means that you respect the autonomy and rights of your patient. In practical consideration this includes such activities as ensuring that the patient provides informed consent to treatment. Younger patients (perhaps as young as 7–8 years of age) may be able to provide informed assent while all patients under the age of majority should (apart from exceptional circumstances that could be professionally or legally defended) receive parental or responsible other's consent prior to treatment (De Lourdes, Larcher, & Kurz, 2003).

The treatment contract between care provider and patient includes the framework of active patient participation in decision-making pertaining to care. This means that treatment decisions need to be shared with patients and responsible others and that treatment choices should be made mutually. There may be exceptional circumstances in which such collaborative decision-making may not be possible – such as a psychotic disorder with no insight from the patient – and in those cases, the legal framework governing physician–patient interaction must be followed. Psychoeducation, the provision and comprehensive review of information pertaining to the illness, its treatments and its treatment options should be provided to patients and their families in language that they can understand. Many such resources (including web-based materials) are easily available from reputable sources – such as the American Academy of Child and Adolescent Psychiatry and the National Institutes of Mental Health (or, e.g., World Health Organization, 1998). The patient and family should be given hard copies of "best information" and referred to other sources that they can review on their own. Following this, time should be spent answering questions and addressing specific concerns. This educational process should be ongoing and may require additional time at both baseline and follow-up visits.

It is not clear whether good psychoeducational interventions can improve adherence to treatments, which may be especially problematic during the adolescent years (Staples & Bravender, 2002). Compared with adults, treatment adherence issues may be more complex in children and adolescents (Gau, Shen, Chou *et al.*, 2006) for many reasons, including but not limited to: the input of parents; input of teachers or other institutional representatives; family conflicts; and peer pressures. The importance of treatment adherence is not to be overlooked, as it may not only impact on therapeutic outcome, but may also be linked to adverse effects – such as suicidality in depressed youth treated with antidepressants, in which it has been postulated that poor treatment adherence may explain "suicidality" (Weiss & Gorman, 2005).

Additionally, the clinician and any others participating in the care of the mentally ill young person must be aware of the sociocultural aspects of their interaction. In this multicultural and global environment, not to understand and consciously consider the cultural, religious and social frameworks that the patient and family bring to the care interaction is to be disrespectful to the patient and his or her sense of self. Thus, the clinician cannot prescribe somatic treatments by "giving a prescription." Somatic treatments are a science, dispensed in the form of an art.

References

Baldessarini, R. J., Tondo, L., Davis, P., Pompili, M., Goodwin, F. K., & Hennen, J. (2006). Decreased risk of suicides and attempts during long-term lithium treatment: A meta-analytic review. *Bipolar Disorders*, *8*, 625–639.

Brooks, S. J., & Kutcher, S. (2004). The Kutcher Generalized Social Anxiety Disorder Scale for Adolescents: Assessment of its evaluative properties over the course of a 16-week pediatric psychopharmacotherapy trial. *Journal of Child and Adolescent Psychopharmacology*, *14*, 273–286.

Cheung, A. H., Emslie, G. J., & Mayes, T. L. (2006). The use of antidepressants to treat depression in children and adolescents. *Canadian Medical Association Journal*, *174*, 193–200.

de Leon, J., Armstrong, S. C., & Cozza, K. L. (2006). Clinical guidelines for psychiatrists for the use of pharmacogenetic testing for CYP450 2D and CYP450 2C19. *Psychosomatics*, *47*, 75–85.

De Lourdes, L. M., Larcher, V., & Kurz, R. (2003). Informed consent/assent in children. Statement of the Ethics Working Group of the Confederation of European Specialists in Paediatrics (CESP). *European Journal of Pediatrics*, *162*, 629–633.

Desta, Z., Zhao, X., Shin, J. G., & Flockhart, D. A. (2002). Clinical significance of the cytochrome P450 2C19 genetic polymorphism. *Clinical Pharmacokinetics*, *41*, 913–958.

Emslie, G. J., Hughes, C. W., Crismon, M. L., Lopez, M., Pliszka, S., Toprac, M. G., *et al.* (2004). A feasibility study of the childhood depression medication algorithm: the Texas Children's Medication Algorithm Project (CMAP). *Journal of the American Academy of Child and Adolescent Psychiatry*, *43*, 519–527.

Evans, S. M., Levin, F. R., & Fischman, M. W. (2000). Increased sensitivity to alprazolam in females with a paternal history of alcoholism. *Psychopharmacology*, *150*, 150–162.

Fegert, J. M., Kolch, M., Glaeske, G., & Janhsen, K. (2006). Antidepressant use in children and adolescents in Germany. *Child and Adolescent Psychopharmacology*, *16*, 197–206.

Flokhart, D. (2007). Drug interactions. Accessed March 14, 2007 from http://medicine.iupui.edu/flockhart/.

Gau, S. S., Shen, H. Y., Chou, M. C., Tang, C. S., Chiu, Y. N., & Gau, C. S. (2006). Determinants of adherence to methylphenidate and the impact of poor adherence on maternal and family measures. *Journal of Child and Adolescent Psychopharmacology*, *16*, 286–297.

GeneMedRx. (2007). Accessed March 14, 2007 from http://www.genemedrx.com/Drhome.html.

Hashimoto, K., Shimizu, E., & Iyo, M. (2004). Critical role of brain-derived neurotrophic factor in mood disorders. *Brain Research Reviews*, *45*, 104–114.

Hu, Z., Yang, X., Chan, S. Y., Heng, P. W., Chan, E., Duan, W., *et al.* (2005). Herb–drug interactions: A literature review. *Drugs*, *65*, 1239–1282.

Hughes, C. W., Emslie, G. J., Crismon, M. L., Wagner, K. D., Birmaher, B., Geller, B., *et al.* (1999). The Texas children's medication algorithm project: Report of the Texas consensus conference panel on medication treatment of childhood major depressive disorder. *Journal of the American Academy of Child and Adolescent Psychiatry*, *38*, 1442–1454.

Hunkeler, E. M., Fireman, B., Lee, J., Diamond, R., Hamilton, J., He, C. X., *et al.* (2005). Trends in use of antidepressants, lithium and anticonvulsants in Kaiser Permanente-insured youths, 1994–2003. *Child and Adolescent Psychopharmacology*, *15*, 26–37.

Kent, M. A., Camfield, C. S., & Camfield, P. R. (1999). Double-blind methylphenidate trials: Practical, useful, and highly endorsed by families. *Archives of Pediatric and Adolescent Medicine*, *153*, 1292–1296.

Kutcher, S. P. (1986). Assessing and treating attention deficit disorder in adolescents. The clinical application of a single-case research design. *British Journal of Psychiatry*, *149*, 710–715.

Kutcher, S. (1997). *Child and adolescent psychopharmacology*. Toronto, Ontario, Canada: W. B. Saunders Company.

Lopez-Larson, M., & Frazier, J. A. (2006). Empirical evidence for the use of lithium and anticonvulsants in children with psychiatric disorders. *Harvard Review of Psychiatry*, *14*, 285–304.

March, J. S., Biederman, J., Wolkow, R., Safferman, A., Mardekian, J., Cook, E. H., *et al.* (1998). Sertraline in children and adolescents with obsessive compulsive disorder: A multicenter randomized controlled trial. *Journal of the American Medical Association*, *280*, 1752–1756.

National Institute for Health and Clinical Excellence (NICE). (2005). *Depression in children and young people: Identification and management in primary, community and secondary care*. Accessed March 15, 2007 from http:www.nice.org.uk/pdf/CG028NICEguideline.pdf.

Nikles, C. J., Mitchell, G. K., Del Mar, C. B., Clavarino, A., & McNairn, N. (2006). An n-of-1 trial service in clinical practice: Testing the effectiveness of stimulants for attention-deficit/hyperactivity disorder. *Pediatrics*, *117*, 2040–2046.

O'Kearney, R. T., Anstey, K. J., & von Sanden, C. (2006). Behavioural and cognitive–behavioural therapy for obsessive-compulsive disorder in children and adolescents. *Cochrane Database System Review*, Oct 18 (4): CD004856.

Pelham, W. E., Gnagy, E. M., Burrows-Maclean, L., Williams, A., Fabiano, G. A., Morrisey, S. M., *et al.* (2001). Once-a-day Concerta methylphenidate versus three-times-daily methylphenidate in laboratory and natural settings. *Pediatrics*, *107*, E105.

Pediatric OCD Treatment Study (POTS) Team. (2004). Cognitive–behavior therapy, sertraline and their combination for children and adolescents with obsessive-compulsive disorder: The Pediatric OCD Treatment Study (POTS) randomized controlled trial. *Journal of the American Medical Association*, *292*, 1969–1976.

Russell, P. S., George, C., & Mammen, P. (2006). Predictive factors for polypharmacy among child and adolescent psychiatry inpatients. *Clinical Practice and Epidemiology in Mental Health*, *2*, 22–25.

Staples, B., & Bravender, T. (2002). Drug compliance in adolescents: Assessing and managing modifiable risk factors. *Paediatric Drugs*, *4*, 503–513.

Storch, E. A., Murphy, T. K., Geffken, G. R., Sajid, M., Allen, P., Roberti, J. S., *et al.* (2005). Reliability and validity of the Yale Global Tic Severity Scale. *Psychological Assessment*, *17*, 486–491.

Swaab, D., Bao, A., & Lucassen, P. J. (2005). The stress system in the human brain in depression and neurodegeneration. *Ageing Research Reviews*, *4*, 141–194.

Swanson, J. M. (1992). *School-based assessments for ADD students*. Irvine, CA: K. C. Publications.

Thomas, C. P., Conrad, P., Casler, R., & Goodman, E. (2006). Trends in the use of psychotropic medications among adolescents, 1994 to 2001. *Psychiatric Services*, *57*, 63–69.

Treatment for Adolescents with Depression Study (TADS). (2004). Fluoxetine, cognitive–behavioral therapy, and their combination for adolescents with depression: Treatment for Adolescents with Depression Study (TADS) randomized controlled trial. *Journal of the American Medical Association*, *292*, 807–820.

Weersing, V. R., & Brent, D. A. (2006). Cognitive–behavioral therapy for depression in youth. *Child and Adolescent Psychiatric Clinics of North America*, *15*, 939–957.

Weiss, J. J., & Gorman, J. M. (2005). Antidepressant adherence and suicide risk in depressed youth. *American Journal of Psychiatry*, *162*, 1756–1757.

Weisz, J. R., McCarty, C. A., & Valeri, S. M. (2006). Effects of psychotherapy for depression in children and adolescents: A meta-analysis. *Psychological Bulletin*, *132*, 132–149.

World Health Organization (WHO). (1994). *Guide to good prescribing: A practical manual*. WHO Action Program on Essential Drugs. Geneva: WHO. WHO/DAP/94.11.

World Health Organization (WHO). (2000). *Progress in Essential Drugs and Medicines Policy 1998–1999*. WHO Health Technology and Pharmaceuticals Cluster. Geneva: WHO. WHO/EDM/2000.2.

World Health Organization (WHO). (2001). *Teacher's Guide to Good Prescribing*. WHO Essential Drugs and Medicines Policy. Geneva: WHO. WHO/EDM/PAR/2001.2.

68 Juvenile Delinquency

Sue Bailey and Stephen Scott

The term *delinquency* is a legal one and refers to antisocial acts that could result in conviction, although most do not. The term *juvenile* refers to the age of the perpetrator. This extends from the age when they are first deemed able to be criminally responsible, through an age range when they are processed in a legal system for youths, until an upper age when they are dealt with in courts for adult crimes (see chapter 8). These ages vary between countries and states, and also may vary according to the offense (Cavadino & Allen, 2000; Justice, 1996). In England and Wales the juvenile age range is currently 10–18 years, although some have proposed the minimum age should be older (e.g., 14 years). Juvenile delinquency is a major public concern because of the damage inflicted on property and people, and the wasted unproductive lives of the young people themselves (Surgeon General, 2001).

The legal term delinquency should be distinguished from scientific concepts in developmental psychopathology such as antisocial behavior and aggression, and from clinical psychiatric diagnoses such as conduct disorder (see chapter 35; Frick, 2006). There is a considerable degree of overlap because all involve antisocial behaviors that fail to conform to societal norms. However, they are not the same; for example, a child under 10 with conduct disorder in England cannot be a delinquent, and a single delinquent act by an otherwise well-adjusted 15-year-old would not qualify for a diagnosis of conduct disorder. A major role of the forensic psychiatrist in the youth justice system is to bring the benefits of modern developmental psychopathology to illuminate the assessment and management of offenders.

This task is helped by important advances in understanding the epidemiology, longitudinal course and treatment of antisocial behavior in recent years. Understanding is growing of how risk factors combine to both precipitate and maintain antisocial behavior (see chapter 35). Progress has been made in the development of validated screening, needs assessment and risk assessment tools for this specific population (Bailey, Doreleijers, & Tarbuck, 2006; Grisso, Vincent, & Seagrave, 2005) and in the development of promising interventions (Harrington & Bailey, 2003).

This chapter has three sections. First, the contribution of psychiatric disorders to delinquency is reviewed. Second, three aspects of assessment are covered: determining the personal needs of delinquents; assessing the risks they pose to others; and judging their mental capacity with regard to their fitness to stand trial. Third, treatment of special groups is covered, and interventions for youths displaying delinquent behaviors are reviewed. Because of the trend to treat antisocial youth outside of expensive formal court proceedings where possible (AACAP, 2005; Bailey & Williams, 2005), this last section includes general treatment of offending youths whether or not they have come to the attention of justice systems.

Rutter's Child and Adolescent Psychiatry, 5th edition. Edited by M. Rutter, D. Bishop, D. Pine, S. Scott, J. Stevenson, E. Taylor and A. Thapar. © 2008 Blackwell Publishing, ISBN: 978-1-4051-4549-7.

Historical Context

The need to control a small group of very persistent recalcitrant youth, perhaps 1–2% of the population, is perennial. In the 18th and 19th centuries, offending children were seldom distinguished from adults and were placed in prison. In the England of 1823, boys as young as 9 years were held in solitary confinement in ships retired from the Battle of Trafalgar. Over the last 50 years, both community and secure residential interventions in youth justice have been characterized by a pattern of reforming zeal, followed by gradual disappointment as the results of evaluations have become available (Hagell, Hazel, & Shaw, 2000).

Throughout the 20th century, concern about levels of juvenile offending has absorbed the attention of the public, politicians, practitioners and researchers (Burt, 1925; Glover, 1960; Rutter, Giller, & Hagell, 1998). Throughout the western world (Junger-Tas, 1994) there has been a widespread and growing perception that juvenile crime is inevitable, a fact of life in an increasingly violent society (Shepherd & Farrington, 1993). However, this has been accompanied by increasing urgency to curb the spread of serious juvenile crime. A century ago, the plan underlying the juvenile justice system in the USA had as its purpose, through the juvenile court, the creation of a whole new system of law for responding to youthful offending based on the developmental premise that young people were still malleable and could be saved from a life of crime. This philosophy held its ground for nearly 100 years, until the USA experienced an increasing tide of youth violence from the late 1980s (Zimring, 1998). Grisso (1996) commented that in its wake the "rehabilitative approach to juvenile justice has all but disappeared in the USA in an avalanche of massive legislative efforts to transform it." These changes are echoed in the overhaul of the youth justice system in England and Wales (Bailey, 1999).

This more sobering view of whether delinquents naturally improve is supported by recent advances in developmental psychopathology. Increased understanding of the continuities between child and adult life (see chapter 13; Maughan & Kim-Cohen, 2005) has served as a timely reminder that many childhood disorders once thought to resolve with age are known to cast long shadows over later development (Moffitt, 2005). This is especially true with regard to the trajectory from antisocial behavior in childhood, through adolescence and on into antisocial personality disorder (ASPD) in adult life where the prevalence is approximately 2% (Coid, 2003; Torgersen, Kringlen, & Cramer, 2001). ASPD is associated with a high degree of social handicap and increased risk of death through accidents, suicide, substance abuse and murder (Robins & Rutter, 1990; Tremblay & Pare, 2003). Once established, it is very hard to treat. Nonetheless, recent studies suggest that there are several promising interventions for juvenile offending, as reviewed below.

Psychiatric Disorders and Offending

Rates of psychiatric disorder in detained juveniles vary, according to study, from 50% to 100% (Lader, Singleton, & Meltzer, 2003; Lederman, Dakof, Larrea, & Li, 2004; Sailas, Feodoroff, Virkkunen, & Wahlbeck, 2005; Vermeiren, De Clippele, & Deboutte, 2000; Vreugdenhill, Vermeiren, Wouters, Doreleijers, & van den Brink, 2004). A survey in England and Wales by the Office of National Statistics (ONS) of 590 young offenders (aged 16–20 years) found that 80% had two or more disorders (Lader, Singleton, & Meltzer, 2003); broadly comparable figures were found in two large Finnish cohorts (Sailas, Feodoroff, Virkkunen *et al.*, 2005). The most common disorders, unsurprisingly, are conduct disorders (CD), but other disorders such as substance abuse disorders, attention deficit/hyperactivity disorder (ADHD), mood and anxiety disorders and post-traumatic stress disorder (PTSD) are common; psychoses are significant, and autistic spectrum disorders are being increasingly recognized.

Conduct Disorders and Attention Deficit/Hyperactivity Disorder

High rates of physically aggressive behavior are found in children and adolescents with CD, and particularly those with comorbid CD and ADHD. They are at substantially greater risk of delinquent acts in adolescence and continued violence and offending into adulthood; many develop ASPD (Loeber, Pardini, Homish *et al.*, 2005; Seagrove & Grisso, 2002; Soderstrom, Sjodin, Carlstedt & Forsman, 2004; Sourander, Elonheimo, Niemela *et al.*, 2006). Factors that may be protective for other outcomes may not necessarily reduce offending; thus, having a partner in itself does not appear to reduce criminality (indeed, juvenile delinquents with a partner commit more offenses); however, if the partner is supportive, this is associated with less offending (Meeus, Branje, & Overbeek, 2004). CD are discussed in more detail in chapter 35.

Psychopathic Traits and Antisocial Personality Disorder

Psychopathic traits are being increasingly recognized in children and adolescents (see chapter 51). Youths with these traits are commonly seen in justice systems as a result of the combination of deceptiveness and antisocial behavior. Factor analyses typically find three sets of characteristics (Cooke & Michie, 2001):

1 An arrogant, deceitful interpersonal style, involving dishonesty, manipulation, grandiosity and glibness;

2 Defective emotional experience, involving lack of remorse, poor empathy, shallow emotions and a lack of responsibility for one's own actions; and

3 Behavioral manifestations of impulsiveness, irresponsibility and sensation-seeking.

Delinquent offenders with these psychopathic traits have an earlier onset of offending, commit more crimes, re-offend more often (Forth & Burke, 1998) and more violently (Spain, Douglas, Poythress, & Epstein, 2004) than non-psychopathic criminal youth. In addition, they exhibit insensitivity to punishment cues irrespective of whether or not they have conduct problems, making them especially hard to treat (O'Brien & Frick, 1996). ASPD (using DSM-IV criteria) was found in 81% of sentenced 16- to 20-year-old males in the ONS survey (Lader, Singleton, & Meltzer, 2003). However, overconfident predictions about poor outcomes for youth with these traits should be avoided, as knowledge about the nature, stability and consequences of juvenile psychopathy is still very limited. There is only one published longitudinal study of its stability and it remains unclear to what degree the antisocial behaviors in callous-unemotional youths change over time.

Autistic Spectrum Disorders

Autistic spectrum disorders are being increasingly recognized in general populations (Baird, Simonoff, Pickles *et al.*, 2006), and at a clinical level in adolescent forensic populations, although there have not yet been thorough surveys. Jones, Forster, and Skuse (2007) found high rates of impaired social cognition in young offenders, but they did not fully assess autistic spectrum disorders. Suspicion should be raised if an offense or assault is bizarre in nature, the degree or nature of aggression is unaccountable or there is a stereotypic pattern of offending. Howlin (1997) proposed four reasons for offending and aggression in autistic persons:

1 Their social naivety may allow them to be led into criminal acts by others;

2 Aggression may arise from a disruption of routines;

3 Antisocial behavior may stem from a lack of understanding or misinterpretation of social cues; and

4 Crimes may reflect obsessions, especially when these involve morbid fascination with violence – there are similarities with the intense and obsessional nature of fantasies described by some adult sadists (Bailey, 2002).

Autistic spectrum traits share some characteristics with the callous-unemotional and interpersonal aspects of psychopathy: in both a lack of appreciation of, or concern for the feelings of others is prominent. Future studies need not only to disentangle these emotional dimensions of autistic spectrum disorders and psychopathy, but also to determine how the behavioral dimensions of impulsiveness and recklessness of psychopathy overlap with the same traits in ADHD. We need phenomenological, etiological and longitudinal studies to characterize these symptom clusters, and intervention trials to see what works in ameliorating them, and how they moderate response to treatment.

Substance Misuse

Drug and alcohol misuse are strongly associated with offending. The ONS survey (Lader, Singleton, & Meltzer, 2003) found that 70% of male and 51% of female young offenders had misused alcohol in the year before coming to prison (Alcohol Use Disorders Identification Test scores over 8), and that in the same period 30% of men and 26% of women had used heroin. Rutter, Giller, & Hagell (1998) describe three mechanisms that operate. First, both sets of behaviors share common antecedent risk factors, including individual characteristics such as impulsiveness with lower IQ, environmental characteristics such as harsh parenting with poor supervision, and associating with a deviant peer group. Second, while under the influence of substances, youths are more disinhibited and commit more offenses, including violent assault and driving offenses. Third, once addicted, some youths commit crimes to pay for their habits; for the same reason, a substantial proportion of female addicts turn to prostitution. Additionally, use of cannabis is associated with psychosis, which also increases the likelihood of offending (Arseneault, Moffitt, & Caspi, 2002; Henquet, Krabbendam, Spauwen *et al.*, 2005).

Early Onset Psychosis

Of the juvenile population in the youth justice system, 5–10% have psychoses (Chitsabesan, Kroll, Bailey *et al.*, 2006; Lader, Singleton, & Meltzer, 2003) compared with around 1% of the general juvenile population. As in adult life (Taylor & Gunn, 1999), most young people with schizophrenia are non-delinquent and non-violent. However, about 10% of adults with psychoses commit offenses (Soyka, Morhart-Klute, & Schoech, 2004) and the juvenile proportion is likely to be similar. Non-psychotic prodromal behavioral disturbances precede full-blown psychotic symptoms in about half of cases of early-onset schizophrenia, and can last between 1 and 7 years. They include disruptive behaviors, ADHD and CD. Therefore, the forensic psychiatrist needs to carry out mental health assessments repeatedly over time, to be able to detect changes in social functioning (often from an already disorganized baseline level) and mental state changes including perceptual distortion, ideas of reference and delusional mood.

There is an increased risk of violence to others when youths with psychoses have active symptoms, especially when exacerbated by misuse of drugs or alcohol. The risk of violent acts is related to subjective feelings of tension, ideas of violence, delusional symptoms that incorporate named persons known to the individual, persecutory delusions, command hallucinations, fear of imminent attack, feelings of sustained anger, and fear and passivity experiences that reduce the youth's sense of self-control. Protective factors include responding to and ongoing compliance with physical and psychosocial treatments, good social networks, a valued home environment, no interest in or knowledge of weapons as a means of violence, good insight into the psychiatric illness and any previous violent aggressive behavior, and a fear of their own potential for violence. These features require particular attention during assessment, but full general psychiatric assessment remains essential, as the best predictors of future violent offending in young people with mental disorder are the same as those in the general adolescent population (Clare, Bailey, & Clark, 2000).

Depression, Anxiety and Post-Traumatic Stress Disorder

These disorders are also very common in young offenders. The ONS survey, using the Clinical Interview Schedule, found 41% of men and 67% of women scored above the cut-off score of 12 for symptoms of "neurotic" (emotional) disorders, compared with 11% of the general population. The combination of depression, anxiety and severe PTSD is being increasingly recognized in the child literature as one pathway into adult ASPD (Harrington & Bailey, 2003; Pliszka, Stienman, Barrow, & Frick, 2000). In depression, as well as feelings of low mood, there may also be irritability, hostility and anger, which increase the risk of defensive aggression (Harrington, 2001), a pattern seen in juvenile justice populations (Harrington, Kroll, Rothwell *et al.*, 2005).

Anxiety and PTSD (see chapter 42) are relatively common in children who have experienced violence in war-torn countries and those who live in a context of "urban war zones" (Fletcher, 2003). Exposure to brutalizing violence can then lead the victims to be violent themselves. Garbarino (2001) has set out an ecological framework to explain the process and conditions that transform the "developmental challenge" of coping with violence into the "developmental harm" of meting it out to others. He proposed an accumulation of risk factors for understanding how and when children who suffer the most adverse consequences of exposure to community violence then have the limits of their resilience overwhelmed. Emotional symptoms such as these can easily be missed, so it is essential to enquire about them during the mental state examination.

Suicide and Deliberate Self-Harm

Deliberate self-harm and completed suicide are particular problems for both out-patient and incarcerated young offenders. In the community, youths with more severe conduct symptoms are more likely to have comorbid depressive symptoms, and rates of deliberate self-harm have long been recognized to be elevated to levels higher than in either condition alone. Thus, Kovacs, Goldston, and Gatsonis (1993) found 22% of adolescents with depression, 9% with CD, but 45% of those with both had attempted suicide; Fombonne, Wostear, Cooper, Harrington, and Rutter (2001) found a similar pattern. Mechanisms to explain this include a higher genetic loading and also increased psychosocial risk factors.

Rates are especially high amongst incarcerated youths. Because they are a more severely antisocial subsample, they tend to have more of the genetic and environmental risk factors mentioned above. Additionally, immediate proximal risk factors are elevated: self-harm is often a serious attempt to escape from unbearable feelings or situations (see chapter 40), and youths in prison often feel, and are, powerless and trapped. In England and Wales, the number of self-inflicted deaths in prison in 2006 was 99 per 100,000 prisoners per year, compared with 18 in the general community (Safer Custody Group, 2007). A total of 20% were by under twenties, 95% were by males (reflecting the prison population make-up), and over 90% were by hanging, with half occurring within the first month of imprisonment (Safer Custody Group, 2007). Violent and sexual offenders are at highest risk. Triggering factors include being bullied and being locked in a cell for long periods. These worryingly high rates led in 2004 to the Safer Custody Group being formed for England and Wales, and attempts are being made to ameliorate the risk factors within prisons. However, there is still a long way to go. It is incumbent on psychiatrists working with these youths to assess suicidal tendencies thoroughly and plan interventions accordingly; this can be overlooked when the focus is on the offending record.

Assessment

General Principles

Assessment of need and risk are two separate but intertwined processes. The former has improving the health of the young person as its goal, the latter concerns the danger the young person poses to others, and is often more prominent in public debates about policy and legislation. Both types of assessment contribute to risk-management procedures (Bailey & Dolan, 2004).

Needs Assessment

While carrying out a traditional clinical psychiatric assessment with multiaxial diagnosis should form the backbone of a needs assessment, additionally using a formal needs assessment instrument can help because there are specific issues for the forensic population, and often a formal report is required for court in which it is essential to demonstrate that all key issues have been addressed (Bailey, Doreleijers, & Tarbuck, 2006). As there is rather little literature about needs assessment instruments for adolescent offenders (Knight, Goodman, Pulerwitz, & DuRant, 2001), the first author (S.B.), with colleagues, developed a new interview-based instrument called the Salford Needs Assessment Schedule for Adolescents (SNASA; Kroll, Woodham, Rothwell *et al.*, 1999). This follows the design of the Cardinal Needs Schedule (Marshall, Hogg, Gath, & Lockwood, 1995), which is widely used with adult populations and has well-established reliability and validity. It covers 21 different domains, including individual behaviors (such as aggression), social relations and living situation (Kroll, Rothwell, Bradley *et al.*, 2002). A clinical version is available, as is a shortened form (including a screening questionnaire) developed for use by youth offending teams (Youth Justice Board, 2007).

A recent study in the UK used the SNASA. It adopted a cross-sectional design and investigated 301 young offenders: 151 in custody and 150 in the community. Participants were found to have high levels of need in a number of different areas, including mental health (31%), education/work (48%) and social relationships (36%), but these needs were often unmet because they were not recognized. One in five young offenders were identified as having intellectual disability (IQ <70; Chitsabesan, Kroll, Bailey *et al.*, 2006).

Risk Assessment

Risk assessment has a theory and methodology separate from needs assessment. Most instruments combine factors from various areas of risk (e.g., individual, family, neighborhood) in order to predict the probability of future offending. A number of instruments have been designed for application in the juvenile justice system (Barnoski & Markussen, 2005; Borum & Grisso, 2007; Corrado, 2002; Desai, Goulet, Robbins *et al.*, 2006; Odgers, Burnette, Chauhan, Moretti, & Reppucci, 2005). For better reliability and validity, items should refer to multiple contexts of behavior and use multiple sources of independent information (Farrington & Loeber, 1999). They should tap into not only static risks, but also dynamic factors that can be changed by interventions. To maximize predictive power, information on risks should be complemented by data on protective factors and strengths; however, this is rarely done.

Fitness to Stand Trial

In the UK, a young person's age, level of maturity and intellectual and emotional capacities must be taken into account when they are charged with a criminal offense, and appropriate steps taken in order to promote their ability to understand and participate in the court proceedings (T&V v United Kingdom, 1993). A responsibility therefore falls on the defense lawyer to be aware of the possibility that a young person may not be able to participate effectively in the trial process, particularly if they are under 14 years old, or have learning problems or a history of absence from school (Ashford, Chard, & Redhouse, 2006). Ashford and Bailey (2004) stated that all young defendants, regardless of the offenses they are charged with, should be tried in youth courts with permission for adult sanctions for older youths if certain conditions are met. The idea was to enable a mode of trial for young defendants that would be subject to safeguards that can enhance their understanding and participation.

Assessment of cognitive and emotional capacities should occur before any decisions on venue and mode of trial take place. It needs to be borne in mind that a distinction is made in criminal law between conditions that negate criminal liability and those that mitigate the punishment deserved (see chapter 8). Very young and mentally immature children, and the profoundly mentally ill, may lack the minimum capacity necessary to be criminally liable. Those exhibiting less profound impairments may meet the minimum conditions for some punishment but qualify for a lesser level. It should also be borne in mind that capacity is not a generic skill that a person either has or lacks; rather, it is specific to the issues in question and is multifaceted, with four key elements:

1 The capacity to understand information relevant to the specific decision at issue (understanding);
2 The capacity to appreciate one's situation as the defendant when confronted with a specific legal decision (appreciation);
3 The capacity to think rationally about alternative courses of action (reasoning); and
4 The capacity to express a choice among alternatives (choice).

In addition to these facets, capacity is also situation-specific, and open to influence.

Evaluation of capacity should include assessment of all possibly relevant psychopathology, emotional understanding as well as cognitive level, the child's experiences and appreciation of situations comparable to the one relevant to the crime and to the trial, and any particular features that may be pertinent to this individual in this particular set of circumstances (Barnum, 2000; Grisso, 1997). Particular attention needs to be paid to developmental background, emotional and cognitive maturity, trauma exposure and substance misuse. Appropriate sources for obtaining information relevant to assessment of a juvenile's competence to stand trial will include a variety of historical records, a range of interviews, a variety of other observations and, in some cases, specialized tests. Records of the child's school functioning, past clinical assessment, treatment history and previous legal involvements need to be obtained. In coming to an overall formulation, there should be a particular focus on how both developmental and psychopathological features may be relevant to the forensic issues that have to be addressed. Potentially relevant problems include: inattention, depression, disorganization of thought processes that interfered with the ability to consider alternatives, hopelessness, such that the decision is felt not to matter, delusion or other fixed beliefs that distort understanding of options (or their likely outcomes), maturity of judgment and the developmental challenges of adolescence (Ashford, Chard, & Redhouse, 2006).

Interventions for Particular Crimes and Groups

Juvenile Homicide

Youths who have been prosecuted for murder or manslaughter are similar in background to other juvenile delinquents on points such as age, gender and ethnic background, but usually have more risk factors (Crespi & Rigazio-DiGili, 1996; Myers & Scott, 1998). However, there are differences – murder and manslaughter are more often committed alone rather than in a gang, and on average the perpetrators start their criminal activities at a later age and are much less likely to have previous convictions than other minors taken into judicial youth institutions. Nevertheless, there is great variety in terms of motives, victims and modus operandi – each case stands on its own.

The majority of young persons who have killed initially dissociate themselves from the reality of their act, but gradually experience a progression of reactions and feelings akin to a grief reaction. In these early stages, while the young person is still facing an adversarial and public trial process, they may move through processes of disbelief, denial, loss, grief and anger/blame.

Therapeutic work with juveniles who have killed needs to include an understanding of the role of violence and sadism in a young person's life. The therapist has to understand the depth of the young person's sensitivity and reaction to perceived threat, and how their past maladaptive behaviors may have allowed them to feel in control of their lives. There may be expression of considerable anger and distress in sessions as the young person comes to terms with their rage, and also when they are exploring feeling empathy for their victim and saying sorry for their actions and reattributing blame. PTSD arising from the participation in sadistic acts (either directly or observing the actions of co-defendants) has to be treated, as does any trauma arising from past personal emotional, physical or sexual abuse. Later, considerable work is likely to be needed to prepare the young person for the transition from long-term incarceration to re-entry into the community; preferably, this should be followed by extended aftercare (Heide, 1999).

Sexually Abusive Behavior

Sexually inappropriate behavior in children and adolescents constitutes a substantial health and social problem (Quinsey, Harris, Rice, & Cormier, 2006). Young abusers who have been charged come within the criminal justice system but should also be considered in their own right within the child protection framework (see chapter 32). Most, but not all, abusers are male, often come from disadvantaged backgrounds with a history of victimization, sexual and physical abuse (Bentovim & Williams, 1998; Skuse, Bentovim, Hodges *et al.*, 1998) and show high rates of psychopathology (Hummel, Thomke, Oldenburger, & Specht, 2000; van Outsem, Beckett, Bullens *et al.*, 2006). Of particular concern are a significant subgroup with mild learning disability, for whom treatment programs have to be tailored to their level of development and cognitive ability. Most adult sexual abusers of children started their abuse when adolescents, yet neither ICD–10 nor DSM-IV has a diagnostic category for pedophilia in those under 16 years (see chapter 52). Langstrom, Grann, and Lindblad (2000) advocated the development of empirically based typologies for this offender group.

A structured, carefully planned multiagency approach is required when working with sexually aggressive younger children and sexually abusive adolescents (Becker, 1998; Vizard, Wynick, Hawkes, Woods, & Jenkins, 1996). The treatment process includes managing the crisis of the disclosure, assessing the family, therapeutic work in a protective context for the victim, separate therapeutic work for the offender, and work around the reconstruction and reunification of the victim's family.

To date, there have been few methodologically sound trials of sexually abusing children and adolescents, so it is of interest to note the results of adult studies. Lösel and Schmucker (2005) carried out a meta-analysis of 69 trials of treatments for adult sexual offenders involving 22,181cases. Despite a wide range of positive and negative effect sizes, the majority of trials confirmed the benefits of treatment with on average 37% less sexual recidivism than controls. Somatic treatments (surgical castration and hormonal medication) showed larger effects than psychosocial interventions, amongst which cognitive–behavioral approaches revealed the most robust effect. Non-behavioral treatments did not demonstrate a significant impact.

New approaches to cognitive–behavioral therapy (CBT) with sexually abusing youth have recently been described within the context of relapse prevention (Steen, 2007). CBT group work with sexually abusing children and young people is widely practiced in the UK (Hackett, Masson, & Phillips, 2006), but there are few rigorous evaluations. In contrast to CBT, dynamic psychotherapy aims to work at an unconscious level with the sexually abusive young person to explore and understand the reasons for his or her persistent behavior. However, evidence-based treatment outcome studies have not yet been undertaken for dynamic therapy with juvenile sexual abusers.

It is plausible that interventions carried out as early as possible with young oversexualized children, before their patterns of sexually aggressive behaviors become entrenched, may be more effective. However, there is a dearth of randomized trials and follow-up studies looking at treatment outcomes with this group of younger children. Recidivism as a sole outcome measure for treatment is often used in forensic studies of sexually offending adults, but is unlikely to be reliable with children and adolescents because persistent sexual behavior problems in children under the age of criminal responsibility will not appear in crime statistics, and conviction statistics for sex offenders of all ages are notoriously unreliable for a variety of reasons, including failure to report victimization experiences, failure to proceed with charges and a high rate of trial failures. More studies in this area are therefore needed.

Firesetting/Arson

Arson can have a devastating impact on the victim and more widely. Juvenile arsonists are not a homogeneous group, with a wide range of familial (Fineman, 1980), social (Patterson, 1982), developmental, interpersonal (Vreeland & Lowin, 1980), clinical and "legal" needs. Kolko and Kazdin (1992) highlighted the importance of attraction to fire, heightened arousal, impulsivity and limited social competence. Compared with one-off firesetters, recidivists show more covert antisocial behavior, have greater interest in fire and fire-related activities, are more likely to be male and have poorer social skills and more family dysfunction (Kennedy, Vale, Khan, & McAnaney, 2006; MacKay, Henderson, Del Bove *et al.*, 2006). In addition to the general assessment of antisocial behavior, the specific domains to be considered include: history of fireplay; history of hoax telephone calls; social context of firesetting (whether alone or with peers); where the fires were set; previous threats/targets; type of fire, single/multiple seats of fire setting; motivation (e.g., anger resolution, boredom, rejection, cry for help, thrill-seeking, fire-fighting, crime concealment, no motivation, curiosity and peer pressure).

As with other forms of serious antisocial behavior, no single standard treatment approach is appropriate for all individuals (Repo & Virkunnen, 1997). For recidivistic firesetters, therapy may include psychotherapy to increase the understanding of the behavior, including antecedents defining the problem behavior and the environmental or intrapersonal triggers, and establishing the behavioral reinforcers. Skills training may help to promote adaptive coping mechanisms, and carers will need to be trained in how to supervise the adolescent closely. However, to date there have been no randomized controlled trials of treatments.

Female Delinquents

Any framework offering treatment for young offenders must consider appropriate provision for the special needs of young females who constitute an important minority of offenders (Bailey, 2000a; Miller, Trapani, Fejes-Mendoza, Eggleston, & Dwiggins, 1995; Zoccolillo, 1993). Whereas the overall level of offending is far lower in girls, in general similar risk factors operate (Gorman-Smith & Loeber, 2005; Moffitt, Caspi, Rutter, & Silva, 2001) although early physical aggression seems not to predict later delinquency in girls (Broidy, Nagin, Tremblay *et al.*, 2003). As well as external risk factors, the thinking patterns of violent girls are similar to those of violent boys (Jasper, Smith, & Bailey, 1998; Lenssen, Doreleijers, Van Dijk, & Hartman, 2000). Longitudinal data demonstrate that girlhood aggression often contributes to a cascading set of negative outcomes as young women move into adolescence and adulthood. Young girls who engage in disruptive behavior and fight are at risk for several negative outcomes, including being rejected by peers and feeling alienated and unsupported in their relationships with peers and adults; struggling academically; affiliating with other peers prone to deviant behavior and with them becoming involved in more serious antisocial behaviors; choosing antisocial romantic partners, and hence initiating and receiving partner violence; becoming adolescent mothers who are less sensitive and responsive as parents, and who have children with increased physical and mental health problems. A downward spiral can ensue in those who are sufficiently antisocial and violent; for example, if they are incarcerated, opportunities for stable employment and relationships may be much diminished. If they are also mothers they may lose custody of their children.

In treatment, while similar general principles should be applied as for boys, specific consideration should be given to sexual and reproductive health – including education, contraceptive advice, information about help for sexually transmitted diseases, appropriate support for problems around menstruation, and support and access to relevant resources in the event of a pregnancy. For those who have been abused, when the adolescent female is ready to engage in it, post-abuse counseling from an appropriate adult should take into account the gender of the therapist. Where there is parasuicidal behavior, medical and psychiatric assessment should be followed by appropriate treatment, remembering that the distraction and attention provided by the emergency may be an important component in reinforcing the use of this behavior as a coping strategy. Recognizing that eating problems are far more common in girls is important. Girls seem to respond as well as boys to evidence-based treatments. The trial of Multidimensional Treatment Foster Care (MTFC) by Leve, Chamberlain, and Reid (2005) randomized 81 girls to MTFC or usual care and found 1 year later that those in the experimental group had fewer days locked up and 42% fewer criminal referrals, a similar success rate to that in boys.

Early identification of girls at risk is an important step for prevention and intervention programs but can get overlooked given the low base rates of girls engaging in physical aggression and violence. As well as the usual risk factors, high-risk groups of girls to consider for early intervention include those girls who are temperamentally overactive as well as antisocial as toddlers and preschoolers (fewer than boys) and those who have early pubertal development.

Interventions for Offending Behavior

A large number of different treatments have been used to try to reduce antisocial and offending behavior. These include psychotherapy, pharmacotherapy, school interventions, residential programs and social treatments. A decade and a half ago, Kazdin (1993) documented over 230 psychotherapies that were available, the great majority of which had not been systematically studied. In this review, focus is on treatments with a testable scientific basis and which have been evaluated in randomized trials (Sukhodolsky & Ruchkin, 2006) and applied to populations of young offenders. This section is concerned with the treatment of youth who offend, whether or not they have been formally apprehended by the criminal justice system. There is increasing interest in using community-based interventions for young offenders, because incarceration on its own is barely effective in the longer term, and for intervention to be effective, the young person has to learn not to offend once released back into the home environment. Prevention is covered in chapter 61, and treatment of younger children with CD is covered in chapter 35.

Rational Targets for Intervention Derived From Longitudinal and Causal Research

There is an abundance of research describing risk and protective factors influencing delinquency (Loeber, Pardini, Homish *et al.*, 2005; Rutter, Giller, & Hagell, 1998), so a rational starting point when considering intervention is to consider the main causal factors and processes, and then design interventions around them. However, in practice many other considerations have shaped interventions, from the desire to punish offending youths, to making use of what is currently available at relatively low cost. These different motives may conflict with what is effective for the young person and what works in reducing the damage they cause to society. One of the best examples of this is shock incarceration in military style boot camps, which, although recommended in the 1990s by the US Office of Juvenile Justice and Delinquency Prevention, and satisfying the desire for retribution and somewhat lower running costs, have repeatedly proven at best ineffective, and often positively harmful (see p. 1119; Benda, 2005). We now turn to consider factors that may be modifiable.

Factors Within the Young Person

On their own, temperamental and personality factors with high heritability and little malleability would seem poor candidates for intervention (e.g., being male or having a low IQ). However, even when this is the case, treatability is not ruled out. Thus, part of the effect of being male on delinquency is associating with more violent peers, which is potentially treatable; low IQ has many effects such as poorer understanding of social situations, lower empathy (Jolliffe & Farrington, 2004) and lower academic attainments, which in turn affect, for example, propensity to violence and employability. Social skills training and remedial education may moderate some of the impact of low IQ. There are other individual risk factors for which there is good evidence of modifiability; for example, hyperactivity and inattention are eminently treatable (see chapter 34), and hostile attributional styles can be changed (see chapter 63). Even psychopathic traits can be improved through treatment (Hawes & Dadds, 2007).

Factors in the Environment

Family factors have repeatedly been associated with delinquency (see chapter 25). Parenting styles are characterized by low warmth and involvement, high hostility, inept discipline and poor supervision (Stouthamer-Loeber, Loeber, Wei, Farrington, & Wikstrom, 2002), and these are not just reactive to irritating child behavior, but also have a causal role (Patterson, 2002; Snyder & Stoolmiller, 2002) and are modifiable (see chapter 64). More distal parental characteristics such as having a criminal record and being alcoholic may be impossible or hard to treat, but the mechanism through which they convey risk is likely to be partly through inherited temperament, and partly through parenting style and values (Rutter & Quinton, 1987), which may be modifiable.

Beyond the family, peers have an important role through two mechanisms: peer rejection and deviant peer association (Gifford-Smith, Dodge, Dishion, & McCord, 2005). Again, both of these are potentially modifiable. A particularly harmful aspect of the latter is membership of a gang, although the evidence suggests that part of the poor prognosis accrues from gang members being worse than other antisocial youths before they join, but nevertheless being in a gang promotes further antisocial acts (Gatti, Tremblay, Vitaro, & McDuff, 2005). The neighborhood a youth lives in can exacerbate delinquent tendencies, with low ties to the neighborhood, poor social control of irregular behavior and exposure to risky activities such as drug-taking (Sampson, Morenoff, & Gannon-Rowley, 2002). Whereas community-wide interventions to improve neighborhoods are beyond the scope of this chapter, they are mentioned because they are a potentially modifiable risk factor.

Implications for Treatment of Mechanisms Through Which Risk Factors are Postulated to Work

Social learning theory proponents (Patterson, 1982) suggest that the immediate proximal environment is crucial in engendering antisocial behavior, with the contingencies provided by parents, and then later peers, shaping delinquency. By ignoring prosocial overtures, and inadvertently rewarding aggression (e.g., by giving in to threats or tantrums), parents and peers reinforce deviant behavior. This has formed the basis of parenting programs for antisocial behavior (see chapter 64) that try to change these contingencies; some peer-relationship programs also take this approach (Frankel & Myatt, 2003). Other processes implicated by social learning theorists are imitation and identification (Bandura, 2004), although interventions addressing these mechanisms are not well developed. Parenting also involves the transmission of values, and some treatment approaches specifically address these (e.g., attempting to dissuade parents from believing in the effectiveness of excessive corporal punishment).

Within the individual at a psychological level, different theories lead to different intervention approaches. Thus, cognitive theory has led to cognitive therapies that concentrate on the way the youth perceives threats and cues; whereas if the causal theory postulates that the fundamental problem is one of emotional over-reactivity, then teaching youth to become more aware of their own emotions and develop strategies to control these may be tried, as in anger-management programs. Likewise, where a deficit in empathy has been postulated, "restorative justice" programs have attempted to reduce recidivism by confronting perpetrators with their victims, so they have sympathy for what they have done. Each of these treatment approaches is discussed below.

Within the individual at a biological level, rather few findings on mechanisms have led to treatment approaches so far. Low autonomic reactivity (as seen in resting and reactive pulse rates) has not led to any well-validated drug treatment, and no neurotransmitter abnormalities have been identified, so the use of neuroleptics is not based on solid etiological theory.

At a simple level, risk factors appear to operate in a cumulative fashion that is not simply additive, so that increasing numbers of risk factors appear to confer disproportionately higher risk. The Minnesota group (Appleyard, Egeland, van Dulmen, & Sroufe, 2005) recently reconfirmed Rutter's (1979) findings that multiple risks had a disproportionately harmful association with poor outcomes and, taking a cluster analytic approach, Stattin and Magnusson (1996) found that antisocial behavior alone did not carry substantial risks unless accompanied by several other risk factors. A clinical implication of this would be that to get a reasonable effect, several risk factors need to be tackled or, alternatively, tackling only one is unlikely to lead to much change. At a rather more sophisticated level, risk factors also do not co-occur randomly. Moving a child experiencing harsh parenting to a different family with parents who are calm, could reduce his or her experience of hostility. However, impulsive children evoke harsher, more critical parenting than controls (Schachar, Taylor, Wieselberg, Thorley, & Rutter, 1987), so this mechanism needs to be borne in mind when planning interventions. Even if there is placement within a foster family, the new parents may need training in techniques of delivering calm discipline. Finally, there may be active selection of environments, so that an impulsive youth might, for example, positively seek out peers and neighborhoods where drugs are sold. Understanding these mechanisms has practical implications, because simply removing a youth from a high-risk neighborhood in the hope that he or she will not get into trouble will not help if the child actively seeks the troublespots.

Beyond this, interactions between environmental and constitutional factors may play a part, rather than risk factors operating in a linear fashion. Thus, the *MAOA* gene confers an increased risk of antisocial behavior only in the presence of adverse parenting (Kim-Cohen, Caspi, Taylor *et al.*, 2006), and adoption studies indicate that whereas having biological parents who are criminal or alcoholic raises the risk of delinquency two- or three-fold, the odds increase to four to five times if the adoptive parents are also criminal or alcoholic (Bohman, 1996). The implication then is that children who are constitutionally at risk may be more susceptible to adverse environments. A therapeutic sequel of this is the potentially optimistic point that if the environment can be substantially changed, youths with greater constitutional risk factors may show the greatest improvements.

Intervention is not solely the removal of risk, but also the enhancement of protective factors. Simply conceived, a protective factor may only be the positive end of a risk factor. However, in clinical intervention terms, conceptualizing a factor as protective can lead to a different approach from directly reducing risk factors for antisocial behavior. This could take the form of encouraging parents to build a positive relationship for the young person outside the home, or helping the youth find an activity or hobby in which they can take pride and develop self-esteem. Longitudinal studies suggest that protective factors may be especially important in high-risk individuals. Stattin, Romelsjo, and Stenbacka (1997) found that having physical, emotional, social and cognitive personal resources at age 18 was associated with far lower later conviction rates in high-risk individuals, but made little difference in low-risk cases. Other experiences along the life path found to be protective in the follow-up of delinquents to age 70 by Laub and Sampson (2003) included marriage and military service; in both cases it seemed the changes in practical external circumstances and contingencies were the crucial change agent, rather than any shift in internal motivation or intention. Although not immediately relevant for the treatment of delinquents, perhaps a learning point is that it can be effective to change the context and contingencies around these youths.

Given these theoretical considerations, treatment is more likely to be effective if it alters several risk variables for the youth. It follows that, ideally, these risk mechanisms should be measured during treatment to see if they alter. In the past, therapy has often been carried out with only one approach, for several months, and then progress in achieving the end goal (e.g., offending) has been reviewed. It would be preferable to measure progress regularly (say, weekly or monthly) and include risk mechanisms such as quality of parental monitoring and school attendance so that the proximal mechanisms as well as end targets of treatment can be monitored. Then, if there is no change in the youth offending, it would be possible to see whether this was because the mechanisms had been changed and the youth failed to respond, or whether no change in mechanism had occurred. For example, hostile cognitions or negative parenting or teacher rewards could be monitored. If they do not change, they can be addressed and more therapeutic effort directed at them; if they do change, but the youth is not changing, then other barriers to improvement can be explored and a different formulation made. A number of the interventions described below do this more or less formally.

Interventions in Practice

Political and Social Context

The major challenge of altering the trajectories of persistent young offenders has to be met in the context of satisfying public demands for retribution, together with welfare and civil liberties considerations. Treatment of delinquents in institutional settings has to meet the sometimes contradictory needs to control young people, to remove their liberty and to maintain good order in the institution, at the same time as offering education and training to foster future prosocial participation in society and meeting their welfare needs. In England and Wales, over 3000 juveniles aged 13–18 are locked up at any one time, out of a total population of around 3.5 million, a rate approaching 1 in 1000 overall but around 1 in 300 late teenage boys. In 1998, the Crime and Disorder Act led to an overhaul of youth justice systems, mandating practitioners to improve community treatments and so fill the gap before and after institutional detainment by involving families in the use of new Youth Offending Teams (YOTs). The use of empirically validated interventions by YOTs is gradually increasing but still has a long way to go. As well as leading to better provision of community treatment, the 1998 Act introduced instruments to enable magistrates to make control orders for lower level disruptive behavior in the community, called Antisocial Behaviour Orders (ASBOs).

Prevention

Prevention is discussed more fully in chapter 60. This chapter does not discuss crime prevention, which is a wide subject. However, it is worth noting that as well as prevention being aimed at individual propensities, environmental factors can also be altered. For example, target hardening refers to the strengthening of the security of premises with a view to minimizing the risk of attack. Such deterrence aims to reduce the opportunity for the juvenile to steal from or vandalize the premises. Examples include fitting grilles over windows, installing cables on computers or fitting stronger locks on doors. Evaluations show that these simple measures can be relatively cost-effective (Bowers, Johnson, & Hirshfield, 2004).

Need for Assessment

Because multiple factors affect antisocial behavior, and each case is different, giving the same treatment to all cases would seem likely to be less effective, although there do not seem to be studies comparing "one size fits all" interventions with those in which a thorough assessment has been conducted. Nonetheless, it seems logical to know which youths have a low IQ or a high one, particular skills to build on, comorbid depression or hyperactivity, parents needing treatment for alcoholism before they can set limits, and so on. In contrast, if the family is taking all steps to manage their adolescent well, then an approach based on family management might not be very effective.

Overviews of Intervention Effectiveness

Belief in the effectiveness of treatments for offending behavior has oscillated between modest hope and downright pessimism. In the 1950s and 1960s, practitioners and scholars were optimistic about interventions. However, in 1974, Martinson reviewed the literature of the time and concluded "nothing works." The early controlled studies later in the 1970s were more optimistic (Gendreau & Ross, 1979). The first meta-analysis of outcomes in residential or community settings was of studies between 1960 and 1983 in the USA. It found that psychoanalytically oriented residential treatment had an effect size of 0.01 on recidivism, behavioral approaches 0.18 and educational approaches 0.28 (Garrett, 1985); by 1990 it was possible to conclude "Some things work in some settings with some people" (Izzo & Ross, 1990). Lipsey and Wilson (1998) in their classic meta-analysis included nearly 400 programs with around 40,000 juveniles. The effect size for institutionalized offenders was 0.10, and 0.14 for non-residential or non-institutional (community) settings. Behavioral programs and those training interpersonal skills produced the highest effects, whereas group counseling, milieu therapy and programs focusing only on employment produced little or no effect.

An updated meta-analysis by Wilson, Lipsey, and Soydan (2003) concluded that the programs were equally effective for those from ethnic minorities as for White people. Lösel and Köferl (1989) carried out the first meta-analysis of studies outside the USA, focusing on 16 studies of sociotherapeutic prisons in Germany with around 3500 juvenile offenders. The aim of these is social training and encouragement of contacts in the outside world with preparation for release. Compared with normal prisons, the mean effect size was 0.21. Dowden and Andrews (2000) included US and Canadian studies published after 1990 in their meta-analysis. Although the overall effect size was 0.09, effects were greater for high-risk (0.12) than for low-risk offenders (0.03); programs targeted at personal needs (e.g., academic achievement, enhancing self-esteem, supervision, affection from family members) were more effective (0.22) than those that were not (–0.01); those with behavioral methods (e.g., role play, modeling) had larger effects (0.24) than those that did not (0.04). An overview of meta-analyses is provided by Grietens and Hellinckx (2004), and in 2001 the Campbell Collaboration Crime and Justice Group was set up to make available reviews of criminological interventions (Farrington, 2001). Further work is needed using stricter inclusion criteria, because there is evidence that if one only includes the highest methodological quality, effect sizes reduce, sometimes to zero (Dowden & Andrews, 2003; Latimer, 2001).

What principles should guide interventions? Over a decade ago, McGuire and Priestley (1995) identified six principles for effective programs which still hold:

1 The intensity should match the extent of the risk posed by the offender;
2 There should be a focus on active collaboration, which is not too didactic or unstructured;
3 There should be close integration with the community from which the offender came;
4 There should be an emphasis on behavioral or cognitive approaches;
5 The program should be delivered with high quality and the staff should be trained adequately and monitored; and
6 There should be a focus on the proximal causes of offending behavior rather than distal causes.

In other words, the program should focus on peer groups, promoting current family communication, and enhancing self-management and problem-solving skills. There should not be a focus on early childhood or other distal causes of delinquency.

All of the reviews suggest that there are a number of promising targets for treatment programs, which include antisocial thoughts, antisocial peer associations, promotion of family communication and affection, promotion of family supervision, identification of positive role models, improving problem-solving skills, reducing chemical dependencies, provision of adequate living conditions and helping the young offender to identify high-risk situations for antisocial behaviors. Conversely, the systematic reviews have also suggested a number of approaches that are unlikely to be promising. For instance, improving self-esteem without reducing antisocial cognitions is unlikely to be of value. Similarly, it is unlikely that a focus on emotional symptoms that is not clearly linked to criminal conduct will be of great benefit.

Psychological Interventions with Individual Youths

On theoretical grounds, working with youths to control anger and promote more sociable interactions would seem a plausible approach. There are a number of programs, broadly based on cognitive–behavioral principles. Elements include:

1 Attributional retraining;
2 Anger management;
3 Social problem-solving;
4 Social skills training; and
5 Helping the youth set targets for desirable behavior and negotiate rewards for achieving them.

While each of these elements can be separated out, most modern programs incorporate a number of these themes blended together.

Attributional retraining helps correct the cognitive distortions identified by Dodge (1993) whereby the youths tend to perceive threat and hostile intent even in neutral scenarios; work is done to help understand others' points of view. The anger management aspect usually lasts several sessions and provides techniques to slow down instant angry arousal. Techniques include coping self-talk, distraction and relaxation; plenty of *in vivo* practice is needed because otherwise what is learned as a good idea in the clinic often does not generalize to the more emotionally arousing scenarios on the street (Kazdin, Siegel, & Bass, 1992). Social problem-solving programs follow classic lines:

1 Defining the problem;
2 Analyzing the intentions of the other party;
3 Generating a range of solutions;
4 Evaluating them;
5 Selecting the best and putting it into action; then
6 Reviewing how well it worked (see chapter 63 for further details).

The social skills element involves lots of practice in role plays and in real life, whereby the youth practices conversations, asking teachers for guidance, expressing disappointment, declining drugs without getting angry, and so on. The target setting is usually agreed in negotiation with teachers or parents, and involves starting with small achievable goals with strong immediate rewards to promote success.

Two of the best validated programs of the type described above are Problem Solving Skills Training (PSST), which lasts 22 weeks (Kazdin, Siegel, & Bass, 1992) and the Coping Power (CP) program, which lasts 18 weeks (Lochman & Wells, 2004). PSST was found to be effective in a randomized controlled trial with in-patients with severe conduct problems (Kazdin, Siegel, & Bass, 1992), but now needs independent replication. CP has been shown to have effects that lasted both at home and in school at 1-year follow-up (Lochman & Wells, 2004); independent replications in Holland and Germany are under way. More generally, a meta-analysis of randomized controlled trials of social skills training confirmed its usefulness, although studies with larger samples led to smaller effect sizes (Lösel & Beelman, 2003). Likewise, a meta-analysis of CBT with offenders found that it worked, and better effects were obtained for higher-risk offenders, higher-quality treatment implementation and a CBT program that included anger control and interpersonal problem-solving but not victim impact or behavior modification components (Landenburger & Lipsey, 2005).

More directly within the justice system, individual offenders have had to take part in victim–offender mediation sessions, so-called "restorative justice" (Latimer, Dowden, & Muise, 2005). A meta-analysis of 15 studies concluded the approach was effective, with a rate of re-offending 70% of that of controls (Nugent, Williams, & Umbreit, 2004). Similarly, a meta-analysis of "reasoning and rehabilitation" programs by Tong and Farrington (2006) concluded that these reduced offending by 14%.

Special Education

Approaches to special education are covered in chapter 74. Here we simply note that because of the high rates of poor literacy and educational attainments in offenders, this is a crucial component of interventions. If formerly offending youths are expected to conform to societal norms and become employed and work within the system, then they need sufficient educational attainments and work skills to succeed in getting and holding down jobs. Without these, it is far harder even for well-motivated youths to avoid the apparently quick rewards crime appears to offer them (Hawkins, Herrenkohl, Farrington *et al.*, 1998).

Family-Based Interventions

These typically attempt to alter the structure and functioning of the family unit, being based on systemic family therapy theories (see chapter 65). The best known in the context of delinquency is Functional Family Therapy (FFT), brought into being in 1969 by James Alexander and colleagues. It is designed to be practicable and relatively inexpensive: 8–12 1-h sessions are given in the family home to overcome attendance problems common in this client group; for more intractable cases, 26–30 h are offered, usually over 3 months. The target age range is 11–18 years. One of the attractive aspects of FFT is that it has evolved and changed over four decades. Thus, there is now a standardized assessment, including separate family and therapist perspectives on the issues, which the therapist monitors and updates regularly. Following assessment, there are four phases to treatment. The first two are the *engagement* and *motivation* phases. Here the therapist works hard to enhance the perception that change is possible, and to minimize perceptions that might signify insensitivity or inappropriateness (e.g., poor program image, difficult to access, insensitive referral). The aim is to keep the family in treatment, and then to move on to find what precisely the family wants. Techniques include reframing, whereby positive attributes are enhanced (e.g., a youth who offends a lot but does not get caught is labeled as bright), and the emotional motivation is brought out (e.g., a mother who continually nags may be labeled as caring, upset and hurt).

Families are encouraged to see themselves as doing the best they can under the circumstances. Problem-solving and behavior change are not commenced until motivation is enhanced, negativity decreased and a positive alliance established. Explicit attempts are made to reduce negative spirals in family interactions, by interrupting and diverting the flow of negative blaming speeches. Reframes do not belittle the impact of the negative behavior, but each family member should feel at the end of these two initial stages that:

1 They are not inherently bad, it is the way they have done things that has not worked;

2 Even though they have made mistakes, the therapist "sided" with them as much as with everybody else;

3 Even though they experience the problems differently, each family member must contribute to the solution;

4 Even though they may have a lot to change, the therapist will work hard to protect them and everyone else in the family; and

5 They want to come back to the next session because it finally seems that things might get better.

The third phase of FFT targets *behavior change*. There are two main elements to this: communication training and parent training. The success of this stage is dependent on the first two having been achieved, and is not commenced unless they have been (this differs from some programs where a predetermined number of sessions is allocated to each topic irrespective of the rate of family progress). This stage is applied flexibly according to family needs. Thus, if there are two parents who continually argue and this is impinging on the adolescent, the "marital subsystem" will be addressed, using standard techniques. These include using the first person voice rather than the second (instead of "you are a lazy slob," "I find it upsets me when you leave your socks on the floor"), being direct (instead of complaining to partner "he never . . . ," say it directly to the youth), brevity instead of long speeches, behavioral specificity about what is desired, offering alternatives to the young person and active listening. Parent training techniques are similar to those found in standard approaches, and include praise, rewards (called contracting in FFT; e.g., "If you come home by 6pm each night, I will take you to the cinema on Saturday"), limit setting, consequences and response-cost (e.g., losing TV time for swearing; for more details of these techniques see chapter 64).

The fourth and final phase of FFT is *generalization*. Here, the goal is to get the improvements made in a few specific situations to generalize to other similar family situations; to help the youth and family negotiate positively with community agencies such as school, and help them get the resources they need. Sometimes, this latter goal may require the therapist to be a case manager for the family. To do this therefore requires that the therapist knows the community agencies and how the system works, and be prepared to spend time engaging it – these characteristics are specified in the model. This is a very different approach from traditional therapies in which the therapist stays neutral with regard to outside agencies.

Beyond specifying the intervention, FFT has a formal schedule for training professionals, which over and above the initial 3 days, requires three 2-day follow-up visits in the ensuing year and supervision for 4 h per month with FFT supervisors for the first 2 years. There are four levels of worker: functional family therapist, FFT clinical team leader (who coordinates a site), FFT clinical supervisor (who takes clinical responsibility for therapists' cases and provides individual and group surpervision) and FFT trainer, who is officially certified to run training. These personal training approaches to maintaining treatment fidelity are backed up by a tracking system of questionnaires filled in by the clients as well as the therapist. However, there is no insistence that supervision is by showing video or audio tapes of actual sessions, although the three on-site visits per year offer an opportunity for the developers to do this. The effectiveness of FFT is well established; there have been over 10 replication studies (Alexander, Pugh, Parsons, & Sexton, 2000), of which over half have been independent of the developers, and four are under way in Sweden. The trials published to date have all been positive, with typical recidivism rates being 20–30% lower than in controls.

Family programs can be delivered within school settings (e.g., as part of after-school programs). Thus, "Project Back-on-Track" included family therapy and diversionary projects for only 4 weeks (although for 4 days a week, giving 32 h contact time) and led to significant reductions in offenses 1 year later (Myers, Burton, Sanders *et al.*, 2000).

Multiple Component Interventions

The example of Multisystemic Therapy (MST) is taken as it is one of the best developed treatments of this kind. MST was developed by Henggeler, Rowland, Randall *et al.* (1999) in the USA. There are nine treatment principles:

1 An assessment should be made to determine the fit between the problems and the wider environment: difficulties are understood as a reaction to a specific context, not seen as necessarily intrinsic deficits.

2 Therapeutic contacts emphasize the positive and use systemic strengths as levers for change. Already, the assessment will have identified strengths (e.g., being good at sports, getting on well with grandmother, the presence of prosocial peers in grandmother's neighborhood), and the implementation of this principle means that each contact should acknowledge and work on these. The strengths may be in the young person (competencies and abilities), the parent (skills, friendliness, motivation), the family (practical resources such as nice house, affection between members, some good parenting practices, supportive friends locally, and so on), peers (any with prosocial activities or hobbies, with parents who monitor well), at the school (good classroom management, understanding of youth's special needs, drama, music or sports facilities) and in the community (organized activities by voluntary or church organizations, parks, well-functioning social services departments, children's centers). Each contact should reinforce these strengths and use a problem-solving approach to mobilize them.

3 Interventions are designed to promote responsible behavior and decrease irresponsible behavior. This principle is similar to other parenting programs, and is core: by increasing prosocial behavior and the amount of time during which it is carried out, then inevitably antisocial behavior is not being carried out. Eventually, the objective is more than the elimination of antisocial behavior, it is to help the youth become independent and to have prosocial life skills to make relationships, contribute effectively in work and so stay out of trouble and have a productive life. However, this goal is not just for the youth; parents too have their role in changing their practices and beliefs, which includes taking more responsibility for their youth's behavior and making life changes to enable this to happen – which could include giving up a second job or helping with school work.

4 Interventions are focused in the present and are action oriented, and have specific well-defined goals. The approach is what can be done in the here and now, in contrast to some therapies which emphasize the need to understand the family's and the youth's past. By having clear targets, all family members are aware of the direction of treatment and the criteria that will be used to measure success. This also means that effectiveness can be monitored effectively and accurately, and there are clear treatment termination points when targets are met. In this respect MST is similar to behavioral and some other therapies, but differs from counseling and psychoanalytic approaches.

5 Interventions target sequences of behavior in multiple systems that maintain problems. This is an approach similar to systemic family therapy (see chapter 65), in that change is postulated to be mediated by interpersonal transactions rather than insight. What is different is that multiple arenas are explicitly assessed and, where appropriate, targeted (e.g., the youth's peer group, extended family, school).

6 Interventions are developmentally appropriate. They should fit the life stage and personal level of the family members.

7 Interventions require daily or weekly effort by family members. This enables frequent practice of new skills and frequent positive feedback for efforts made; non-adherence to treatment agreements rapidly becomes apparent.

8 Intervention effectiveness is evaluated continuously from multiple perspectives, with the intervention team assuming responsibility for overcoming barriers to successful outcomes.

9 Interventions are designed to promote treatment generalization by empowering parents to address youth needs across multiple contexts.

Interestingly, the precise nature of the moment-to-moment content of intervention is not tightly prescribed, although in practice the greater part is not dissimilar to the approach used in behavioral family therapy. However, MST is not limited to work on psychosocial interactions; for example, when the program developers found that despite influencing the more distal risk factors for drug-taking, such as parental supervision and school attendance, drug use was not diminishing as much as they had hoped, they instituted daily urine tests and paid the young people if they were clear of drugs. What is noticeably different from many therapies is the explicit recognition of the multiple contexts in which difficulties may occur, and the need to influence these. In a sense, MST is a set of operating principles that draw on the evidence for whatever works (e.g., CBT, close monitoring of association with deviant peers, constructive teaching) rather than one specific therapy.

The way the therapy is delivered is closely controlled. Because of the weekly monitoring of progress, if there are barriers to improvement these should be rapidly addressed, and the hypotheses of what is going on in the family and systems around the youth should be revised in the light of progress. Clinicians only take on 4–6 cases because the work is intensive; there is close attention to quality control by weekly supervision along prescribed lines, and parents and youths fill in weekly questionnaires on whether they have been receiving therapy as planned. Therapy is given for 3 months and then stopped.

Given that MST makes good use of up-to-date evidence on the causes of antisocial behavior, and good use of effective treatment principles such as close measurement of effectiveness during treatment and close attention to implementation quality, one might hope that results would be encouraging. Indeed, the first raft of outcome studies by the program developers were positive. Thus, the meta-analysis of papers up to and including 2002 by authors that include one of the program developers, Charles Borduin, found that in seven outcome studies comparing MST with treatment as usual or an alternative with 708 youths by 35 therapists, the mean overall effective size across several domains was 0.55 (Curtis, Ronan, & Bourduin, 2004). Outcome domains ranged from offending (arrests, days in prison, self-reported criminality, self-reported drug use), where the mean effect size was 0.50, peer relations (ES 0.11), family relations (self-reported 0.57, observed 0.76), and individual youth and parent psychopathology symptoms (0.28). When these studies were subdivided into chronic offenders versus the remainder (youths who were abusing drugs, sex offenders and psychiatrically disturbed youths), no differences were found. However, the three studies using the developers' own graduate students as therapists obtained noticeably larger effect sizes (mean 0.81) than when the developers were supervising local community therapists, where the mean effect size was 0.26. Long-term follow-up 14 years later (when the individuals' mean age was 29 years) by the developers of one of the first trials, with 176 cases allocated to MST or usual individual therapy, gave recidivism rates of 50% versus 81%, respectively.

There have been at least 27 published reviews of MST (Littell, 2005), and the sorts of findings cited above have led MST to be cited as an effective evidence-based treatment by the US National Institute on Drug Abuse, the National Institute of Mental Health, the Office of Juvenile Justice and Delinquency Prevention, and others. However, in the process of evaluation, the next test of any therapy is its effectiveness when carried out by teams who have no financial or employment ties with the developers (although they may pay the developers for materials and supervision), with an independent evaluation team. The only independent evaluation was also the only one to use proper intent-to-treat analyses (rather than exclude treatment refusers, etc.), and it found, with a large sample ($n = 409$) in Ontario, Canada, that MST gave no improvement on treatment as usual on any outcome, either immediately or by 3-year follow-up (Leschied & Cunningham, 2002). A smaller independent study in Norway ($n = 75$; Ogden & Hagen, 2006) was more positive, and found effect sizes of 0.26 for self-reported delinquency, 0.50 for parent-rated and 0.68 for teacher-rated, although here there was 40% missing data. Likewise, a totally independent trial by Timmons-Mitchell, Bender, Kishna, and Mitchell (2006) in the USA randomized 93 delinquents and also obtained substantial beneficial effects. The Canadian study (not published in a peer-reviewed journal but of high quality) was included in the Cochrane Library's review of MST (2005), but the other two independent Norwegian and US studies were not. The Cochrane conclusion that "Evidence suggests that MST is not consistently more effective than other alternatives" is thus in our view unduly harsh; its general tone was very conservative, thus it also concluded that MST had no harmful effects and that nothing else was proven better than MST.

This conclusion is more cautious than the previously established view. A number of reasons are possible. First, the developers' own studies did not do full intent-to-treat analyses, and may have been more favorable because some cases with worse outcomes (the dropouts) were excluded. Second, the degree of skill with which the intervention was delivered may have been higher in the developers' sites. Evidence on treatment fidelity for MST is mixed – in the independent Ontario study, fidelity as rated on-site was unrelated to outcomes. Henggeler, Rowland, Randall *et al.* state that fidelity is crucial for effectiveness, and in their first paper on the subject they made 105 correlations between fidelity and outcomes, but only 11 were significant, with some being in the opposite direction to that predicted (i.e., better adherence leading to worse results). However, the same group (Huey, Henggeler, Brondino, & Pickrel, 2000) found that when they used a latent variable approach, therapist-rated fidelity improved family functioning and parent monitoring, both of which reduced youth delinquency, but that parent- and youth-rated fidelity had no effect. This rater effect could be because it requires a therapist to appreciate the complexity of fidelity, and also because therapists working across cases will be more consistent in their ratings than parents and youths, who may differ widely in their rating of the same phenomena. Third, the financial conflict of interest may have consciously or unconsciously led the developers to bias their results favorably. Henggeler and his associates direct and hold stock in MST Services Inc., which has the exclusive licensing agreement for MST. It serves around 10,000 families a year and total fees amount to around $500 per youth served (Littell, 2006). Fourth, the comparison treatment may have been different in Canada, where the justice system is perhaps better organized; however, the Cochrane reviewers (2005) point out that their conclusions would have been largely the same even without this study.

Given that MST is predicated on sound modern principles, why is it often hard to obtain consistently reliable effects? A further possibility is that 3 months of treatment is too short a duration. To disentangle possible explanations, we need good measures of mediators during treatment and, crucially, after the end of treatment. This would enable, for example, one to see whether parenting practices continue to be strong after the intervention ceases, and whether this mediates relapse; or is it deviant peer association that leads to more offending? Some conclusions are in order. We need more randomized controlled trials independent of the program developers. They should use intent-to-treat analyses, develop therapist adherence and skill to as high a level as possible and measure it, and be of sufficient power to measure moderators and mediators, so that variations in outcomes can, where possible, be accounted for.

Interventions with Multiple Components that Put Youths into Foster Families

The best example of this approach is Multidimensional Treatment Foster Care (MTFC). It evolved at the Oregon Social Learning Center (OSLC), beginning in 1983 (Chamberlain, 2003), where parent training with families of delinquents proved extremely difficult, although reasonably effective (Bank, Marlowe, Reid, Patterson, & Weinrott, 1991), because of the inability of the family to cope with the extreme demands of having a delinquent youth. This led to the idea of placing them in a specially trained foster family. It has a number of similarities with MST: it is based on an interactive model, whereby the moment-to-moment interactions are seen as the key to change. However, it differs in that the regime in the foster home is based on the youth earning points from the moment they get up. They have to earn 100 points a day for privileges such as going to bed later, having time on the computer or extra time to phone friends. Points are awarded for day-to-day living and social skills, such as making the bed, being polite, getting to school on time. While at school points are awarded for good behavior in class.

Unlike some programs, in MTFC points are also taken away (e.g., for swearing or being unhelpful). Foster carers are carefully trained to take away points with the minimum of negative affect, and to quickly offer the young person the opportunity to make up points by doing a small chore. For the youth, the immediacy of experiencing a contingent response to their behavior is often a stark contrast to being left alone or having long coercive interchanges with their parents. In addition to close liaison with the school, close supervision is key – the young person loses a point a minute for all the time when they cannot verify their whereabouts, a sizeable fine. There is a relatively large team to carry out MTFC. The program supervisor oversees the case, and has a maximum caseload of 10. An individual therapist sees the youth once or twice a week, for problem-solving and to develop skills-based coaching of how to negotiate everyday situations – not for traditional psychotherapy. When the youth is in the community, there is a skills trainer, usually a young graduate, to help them negotiate prosocial activities and avoid dangerous situations.

MTFC lasts for around 6 months and then the young person returns to their birth family. However, crucial to the model is the birth family therapist who, while the youth is in the foster family, works with the birth family to inculcate the same regime. While the youth is in foster care, there is a weekly clinical meeting for all team members, and a weekly foster carer meeting attended by the program supervisor and other team members at which progress is discussed, support given to foster carers and the day-to-day management regime carefully adjusted. However, each youth's progress is even more closely monitored, because every morning a team member calls the foster carer and goes through the Parent Daily Report, a simple 36-item checklist of antisocial behaviors requiring a yes/no answer. The clinical team plot progress graphically, so that any deterioration is quickly detected and remedial action put in place.

There have been two main trials completed with MTFC for delinquency: one in boys and one in girls, both by the program developers. With boys ($n = 79$), MTFC compared with group care led to a reduction in the number of arrests at 2-year follow-up (for two or more arrests, 5% versus 24%) and reduced self-reports of aggression and fighting (Eddy, Whaley, & Chamberlain, 2004). With girls at 1-year follow-up ($n = 81$), criminal referrals showed a trend (mean 0.76 referrals in MTFC, 1.3 for group care; $P = 0.10$), 22 versus 56 days locked up ($P < 0.05$) and a reduction on Child Behavior Checklist (CBCL) delinquency but none on Elliott delinquency. No report of CBCL aggression scales or other measures such as the Parent Daily Report (PDR) are given (Leve, Chamberlain, & Reid, 2005). Clearly, independent replications of MTFC are now needed, and are in progress. The model is being extended to younger children, and to less intensive forms.

Rather few intervention studies measure mediators of effectiveness, but the Oregon Social Learning Center (OSLC) staff did this for the male delinquency study (Eddy & Chamberlain, 2000). Three family process mediators and one relating to the youth's peer group were found to be relevant. The three family mediators were harsh and inappropriate discipline, quality of the parent–youth relationship and supervision of the youth's whereabouts; the peer dimension was association with deviant peers. When these variables were changed by treatment, then delinquency reduced. Here then is a model of how to measure mediators during treatment. Not only can these findings guide treatment targets, but they confirm important information about the causes and maintenance of antisocial behavior.

Interventions That Do Not Work

Harsh, military style, shock incarceration, so-called "boot camps" are still popular for young offenders in the USA, and were promoted by the Office of Juvenile Justice and Delinquency Prevention in 1992 when three pilot programs were set up. However, several reviews have concluded that they are ineffective (Benda, 2005; Cullen, Blevins, Trager, & Gendreau, 2005; Stinchcomb, 2005; Tyler, Darville, & Stalnaker, 2001), and a randomized controlled trial by the California Youth Authority that included long-term arrest data found no difference between boot camp and standard custody and parole (Bottcher & Ezell, 2005). In contrast, a meta-analysis of 28 studies of wilderness programs found an overall effect size of 0.18, with recidivism rates of 29% versus 37% for controls (Wilson & Lipsey, 2000). Programs with intense physical activity and a distinct therapeutic component were the most effective. Another approach is to attempt to frighten delinquents with visits to prisons in an attempt to deter them, as for example in the "Scared Straight" program. However, a meta-analysis of nine controlled trials found that on average the intervention is more harmful than doing nothing, as it led to worse outcomes in participants (Petrosino, Turpin-Petrosino, & Buehler, 2003).

Peer group work can also be harmful. In an evaluation of the Adolescent Transitions Program, Dishion and Andrews (1995) studied 120 families with an antisocial youth who were randomized to one of four conditions: parent only, youth only, parent and youth, and control. The parents attended standard parent-training sessions, but the youths attended in groups of 4–6. At 1- and 3-year follow-up, adolescents allocated to the youth group intervention fared significantly worse on a number of outcomes, including teacher-rated delinquency and self-reported antisocial behavior and substance use. Those allocated to the parent-only condition in contrast showed reduced teacher-(but not parent-) rated delinquency, and less negative family interaction patterns as assessed by direct observation. Videotapes of the group process revealed that despite the group leaders supporting a reduction in deviant talk and promoting positive peer support for prosocial behavior, in fact youth engaged in surreptitious deviant talk both during sessions and in intervals. Subsequent analyses proved that those youths who took part in increasing amounts of deviant talk predicted poor outcomes 3 years later, such as expulsion from school, arrests and drug use (Granic & Dishion, 2003). Over 40 years ago Patterson had shown that within residential institutions for antisocial youths, for every one positive behavior reinforced by an adult, nine deviant behaviors were reinforced by peers (Buehler, Patterson, & Furniss, 1966).

The famous Cambridge–Somerville delinquency project studied 400 youths, half of whom were offered a range of interventions for 4 years which were state of the art at the time in the early 1940s, but 30-year follow-up showed increased criminal activity, drug, cigarette and alcohol use by the intervention group compared with controls (McCord, 1978). Dishion encouraged her to reanalyze the data, and she concluded that those who had done poorly were those who had been sent on summer camp twice, where she hypothesized "deviancy training" occurred amongst delinquent peers; subsequent deviant acts were 10 times more likely (Dishion, McCord, & Poulin, 1999; McCord, 1997). These lines of evidence have led the group (Gifford-Smith, Dodge, Dishion *et al.*, 2005) to warn against "peer contagion" in a whole range of settings. However, Weiss, Caron, Ball *et al.* (2005) have questioned these findings and, in a fresh meta-analysis to address the question, found that in 17 of 18 studies group treatments for antisocial behavior did not support iatrogenic or deviancy training effects. In conclusion, it seems likely that unsupervised and prolonged contact with deviant peers is harmful, but well-supervised and well-supported contact during which youths are actively taught new skills can be effective.

Pharmacological Therapies

As for non-offenders, medication may be helpful in juvenile delinquents with diagnosed mental disorders for which it has been shown to be effective, such as schizophrenia, bipolar disorder and ADHD (for details of appropriate treatment see the chapter covering the relevant disorder). The question arises whether medication has any role in the management of long-standing antisocial or aggressive behavior in offenders. Most authorities agree that, on present evidence, psychopharmacological treatments alone are unlikely to be an effective and acceptable treatment for behavioral problems in adolescents. However, in younger children with more unpredictable explosive aggression there has been a recent trend by some clinicians to prescribing a range of drugs, from mood stabilizers such as carbamazepine and lithium to newer antispsychotics such as risperidone; certainly reviews by employees of the drug manufacturers argue for their effectiveness and acceptability (Pandina, Aman, & Findling, 2006). However, the evidence for the effectiveness of these medications in straightforward antisocial behavior without comorbid diagnoses or intellectual disability over the medium to long term is minimal (for review see chapter 35); most trials to date have lasted under 2 months and have not been undertaken with teenage offenders (Pappadopulos, Woolston, Chait *et al.*, 2006).

Conclusions

There is now a considerable body of knowledge about the causes of delinquency, how to assess the young people and what interventions are likely to be effective. Recent advances in genetics at a molecular and behavioral level have shown that certain genotypes predispose to antisocial behavior, but that it is likely that in many cases these interact with adverse environmental conditions to lead individuals towards antisocial and offending behavior. In future, genetic and longitudinal studies should further elucidate not only the mechanisms through which individuals embark on a pathway of crime, but also what is the crucial combination of influences leading to desistance in particular groups of cases. Person-centered analyses such as cluster analysis and its longitudinal variants should illuminate what is likely to be a heterogeneous picture, and take forward the majority of current findings, which have often lumped whole samples together when using multivariate statistics. Thus, the causal factors influencing a child born with callous-unemotional traits who is brought up in favorable circumstances may be very different from a child with hyperactive traits who is subjected to prolonged abuse and rejection. Studies will need to combine such an approach with consideration of wider societal influences such as the effects of valuing violence and criminal behavior that predominate in some youth subcultures.

It is to be hoped that treatments will be developed in tandem with increasing specificity according to the youth's needs. For example, while at present psychopathic traits have the reputation of being associated with untreatable offending behavior, this needs to be tested out using treatments tailored to the psychopathology – thus, if these individuals are, as experimental studies suggest, punishment insensitive but reasonably responsive to rewards, then intensive reward programs need to be devised and then subjected to trials. For the established treatments for general delinquency, again greater differentiation according to youth need is required, rather than a "one size fits all" approach. This should include trials where the intervention is given for reasonably long periods if necessary (say, 9–12 months) rather than for the more typical 3 months.

While the studies envisaged above may lead to potential further improvements in outcomes for young offenders, there will be little improvement in their prospects unless high-quality services are implemented. To clarify what difference this could make, it would help to have trials of model forensic services. These would include preventive community services, thorough assessments of all apprehended youths and high-quality interventions based on the assessments. The issue of implementation quality is important, because with highly motivated and skilled teams, good effect sizes are repeatedly achieved with the better interventions. Such trials of model services would need thorough economic evaluations so that potential economic gains of good services could be clarified. Armed with the results of such trials, it might be easier to persuade policy-makers to invest in adequate services. In the meantime, there is a need for a change in culture at local and national governmental levels so that evidence-based interventions are demanded and their effectiveness regularly monitored. At present there are considerable opportunities in most countries to switch from currently used interventions to more effective ones without incurring extra expenditure. Finally, by way of prevention, we need further studies of how to better identify, screen and effectively intervene with young children at risk of antisocial behavior. If such studies are completed, and if (and only if) service improvements are made, there are grounds for definite optimism for the outlook for delinquent youths.

References

Alexander, J., Pugh, C., Parsons, B., & Sexton, T. (2000). *Blueprints for violence prevention: Functional family therapy*. University of Colorado: Institute of Behavioral Science.

American Academy of Child and Adolescent Psychiatry (AACAP). (2005). Practice parameter for the assessment and treatment of youth in juvenile detention and correctional facilities. *Journal of the American Academy of Child and Adolescent Psychiatry*, *14*, 1085–1086.

Appleyard, K., Egeland, B., van Dulmen, M. H. M., & Sroufe, L. A. (2005). When more is not better: The role of cumulative risk in child behavior outcomes. *Journal of Child Psychology and Psychiatry*, *46*, 235–245.

Arsenault, L., Moffitt, T., & Caspi, A. (2002). The targets of violence committed by young offenders with alcohol dependence, marijuana dependence and schizophrenia-spectrum disorders: Findings from a birth cohort. *Criminal Behaviour and Mental Health*, *12*, 155–168.

Ashford, M., & Bailey, S. (2004). The Youth Justice System in England & Wales. In S. Bailey, & M. Dolan (Eds.), *Adolescent forensic psychiatry* (pp. 409–416). London: Arnold.

Ashford, M., Chard, A., & Redhouse, N. (2006). *Defending young people in the criminal justice system* (3rd edn.). Glasgow: Legal Action Groups.

Bailey, S. (1999). The interface between mental health, criminal justice and forensic mental health services for children and adolescents. *Current Opinion in Psychiatry*, *12*, 425–432.

Bailey, S. (2000a). European perspectives on young offenders and mental health. *Journal of Adolescence*, *23*, 237–241.

Bailey, S. (2000b). *Juvenile homicide, criminal behavior and mental health* (Vol. 10, pp. 149–154). London: Whurr Publishers.

Bailey, S. (2002). Violent children: A framework for assessment. *Advances in Psychiatric Treatment*, *8*, 97–106.

Bailey, S., & Dolan, M. (2004). Violence. In S. Bailey, & M. Dolan (Eds.), *Adolescent forensic psychiatry* (pp. 213–227). London: Arnold Publishing.

Bailey, S., Doreleijers, T., & Tarbuck, P. (2006). Recent developments in mental health screening and assessment in juvenile justice systems. *Psychiatric Clinics of North America*, *15*, 391–406.

Bailey, S., & Williams, R. (2005). Forensic mental health services for children and adolescents. In R. Williams, & M. Kerfoot (Eds.), *Child and adolescent mental health service: Strategy, planning, delivery and evaluation* (pp. 271–295). Oxford: Oxford University Press.

Baird, G., Simonoff, E., Pickles, A., Chandler, S., Loucas, T., Meldrum, D., *et al.* (2006). Prevalence of disorders of the autism spectrum in a population cohort of children in South Thames: the Special Needs and Autism Project (SNAP). *Lancet*, *368*, 210–215.

Bandura, A. (2004). Model of causality in social learning theory. In A. Freeman, M. J. Mahoney, P. DeVito, & D. Martin (Eds.), *Cognition and psychotherapy* (2nd edn., pp. 25–44). New York: Springer.

Bank, L., Marlowe, J. H., Reid, J. B., Patterson, G. R., & Weinrott, M. R. (1991). A comparative evaluation of parent-training interventions for families of chronic delinquents. *Journal of Abnormal Child Psychology*, *19*, 15–33.

Barnoski, R., & Markussen, S. (2005). Washington State Juvenile Court Assessment. In T. Grisso, G. Vincent, & D. Seagrave (Eds.), *Mental health screening and assessment in juvenile justice* (pp. 271–282). New York, NY: Guilford Press.

Barnum, R. (2000). Clinical and forensic evaluation of competence to stand trial in juvenile defendants. In T. Grisso, & R. G. Schwartz (Eds.), *Youth on trial: A developmental perspective in juvenile justice* (pp. 193–224). Chicago: University of Chicago Press.

Becker, J. V. (1998). The assessment of adolescent perpetrators of childhood sexual abuse. *Irish Journal of Psychology*, *19*, 68–81.

Benda, B. B. (2005). Introduction. Boot camps revisited: Issues, problems, prospects. In B. B. Benda, & N. J. Pallone (Eds.), *Rehabilitation issues, problems, and prospects in boot camp* (pp. 1–25). New York, NY: Haworth Press.

Bentovim, A., & Williams, B. (1998). Children and adolescents: Victims who become perpetrators. *Advances in Psychiatric Treatment*, *4*, 101–107.

Bohman, M. (1996). Predisposition to criminality: Swedish adoption studies in retrospect. In G. R. Bock & J. A. Goode (Eds.), *Genetics of criminal and antisocial behavior: Ciba Foundation Symposium 194* (pp. 99–114). Chichester: John Wiley & Sons.

Borum, R., & Grisso, T. (2007). Developmental considerations for forensic assessment in delinquency cases. In A. Goldstein (Ed.), *Forensic psychology: Emerging topics and expanding roles* (pp. 553–570). Hoboken, NJ: John Wiley & Sons.

Bottcher, J., & Ezell, M. E. (2005). Examining the effectiveness of boot camps: A randomized experiment with a long-term follow up. *Journal of Research in Crime and Delinquency*, *42*, 309–332.

Bowers, K., Johnson, S., & Hirshfield, A. (2004). The measurement of crime prevention intensity and its impact on levels of crime. *British Journal of Criminology*, *44*, 419–440.

Broidy, L. M., Nagin, D. S., Tremblay, R. E., Bates, J. E., Brame, B., Dodge, K. A., *et al.* (2003). Developmental trajectories of childhood disruptive behaviors and adolescent delinquency: A six-site, cross-national study. *Developmental Psychology*, *39*, 222–245.

Buehler, R. E., Patterson, G. R., & Furniss, J. M. (1966). The reinforcement of behavior in institutional settings. *Behavior Research and Therapy*, *4*, 157–167.

Burt, C. (1925). *The young delinquent*. London: University of London Press.

Cavadino, P., & Allen, R. (2000). Children who kill: Trends, reasons and procedures. In G. Boswell (Ed.), *Violent children and adolescents: Asking the question why* (pp. 16–17). London: Whurr Publishers.

Chamberlain, P. (2003). *Treating chronic juvenile offenders: Advances made through the Oregon Multidimensional Treatment Foster Care*. Washington, DC: American Psychological Association.

Chitsabesan, P., Kroll, L., Bailey, S., Kenning, C., Sneider, S., Macdonald, W., *et al.* (2006). Mental health needs of young offenders in custody and in the community. *British Journal of Psychiatry*, *188*, 534–540.

Clare, P., Bailey, S., & Clark, A. (2000). Relationship between psychotic disorders in adolescence and criminally violent behavior. *British Journal of Psychiatry*, *177*, 275–279.

Coid, J. W. (2003). The co-morbidity of personality disorder and lifetime clinical syndromes in dangerous offenders. *Journal of Forensic Psychiatry and Psychology*, *14*, 341–366.

Cooke, D. J., & Michie, C. (2001). Refining the construct of psychopathy: Towards a hierarchical model. *Psychological Assessment*, *13*, 171–188.

Corrado, R. (2002). An introduction to the risk–needs case management instrument for children and youth at risk for violence: The Cracow Instrument. In R. Corrado, R. Roesch, S. Hart, & J. Gierowski (Eds.), *Multi-problem violent youth: A foundation for comparative research on needs, interventions and outcomes* (pp. 295–301). Amsterdam, Netherlands: IOS Press.

Crespi, T. D., & Rigazio-DiGili, S. A. (1996). Adolescent homicide and family pathology: Implications for research and treatment with adolescents. *Adolescence*, *31*, 353–366.

Cullen, F. T., Blevins, K. R., Trager, J. S., & Gendreau, P. (2005). The rise and fall of boot camps: A case study in common-sense corrections. *Journal of Offender Rehabilitation*, *40*, 53–70.

Curtis, N. M., Ronan, K. R., & Borduin, C. M. (2004). Multisystemic treatment: A meta-analysis of outcome studies. *Journal of Family Psychology*, *18*, 411–419.

Desai, R. A., Goulet, J. L., Robbins, J., Chapman, J. F., Migdole, S. J., & Hoge, M. A. (2006). Mental health care in juvenile detention facilities: A review. *Journal of the American Academy of Psychiatry and the Law*, *34*, 204–214.

Dishion, T. J., & Andrews, D. W. (1995). Preventing escalation in problem behaviors with high-risk young adolescents: Immediate and 1-year outcomes. *Journal of Consulting and Clinical Psychology*, *63*, 538–548.

Dishion, T. J., McCord, J., & Poulin, F. (1999). When interventions harm: Peer groups and problem behavior. *American Psychologist*, *54*, 755–764.

Dodge, K. A. (1993). Social-cognitive mechanisms in the development of conduct disorder and depression. *Annual Review of Psychology*, *44*, 559–584.

Dowden, C., & Andrews, D. A. (2000). Effective correctional treatment and violent reoffending: A meta-analysis. *Canadian Journal of Criminology*, *42*, 449–467.

Dowden, C., & Andrews, D. A. (2003). Does family intervention work for delinquents? Results of a meta-analysis. *Canadian Journal of Criminology and Criminal Justice*, *45*, 327–342.

Eddy, J. M., & Chamberlain, P. (2000). Family management and deviant peer association as mediators of the impact of treatment condition on youth antisocial behavior. *Journal of Consulting and Clinical Psychology*, *68*, 857–863.

Eddy, J. M., Whaley, R B., & Chamberlain, P. (2004). The prevention of violent behavior by chronic and serious male juvenile offenders: A 2-year follow-up of a randomized clinical trial. *Journal of Emotional and Behavioral Disorders*, *12*, 2–8.

Farrington, D. P. (2001). Systematic reviews of criminological interventions. *Criminal Behavior and Mental Health*, *11*, 127–130.

Farrington, D. P., & Loeber, R. (1999). Transatlantic replicability of risk factors in the development of delinquency. In P. Cohen, C. Slomkowski, & L. N. Robins (Eds.), *Historical and geographical influences on psychopathology* (pp. 299–329). Mahwah, NJ: Lawrence Erlbaum Associates.

Fletcher, K. E. (2003). Childhood posttraumatic stress disorder. In E. Mash, & R. Barkley (Eds.), *Child psychopathology* (2nd edn., pp. 330–371). New York, NY: Guilford Press.

Fineman, K. R. (1980). Firesetting in childhood and adolescence. *Psychiatric Clinics of North America*, *3*, 483–500.

Fombonne, E., Wostear, G., Cooper, V., Harrington, R., & Rutter, M. (2001). The Maudsley long-term follow-up of child and adolescent depression. II. Suicidality, criminality and social dysfunction in adulthood. *British Journal of Psychiatry*, *179*, 218–223.

Forth, A. E., & Burke, H. C. (1998). Psychopathy in adolescence: Assessment, violence and developmental precursors. In D. Cooke, A. Forth, & R. Hare (Eds.), *Psychopathy: Theory, research and implications for society* (pp. 205–230). Dordrecht: Kluwer.

Frankel, F., & Myatt, R. (2003). *Children's friendship training*. Hove, UK: Brunner-Routledge.

Frick, P. J. (2006). Developmental pathways to conduct disorder. *Child and Adolescent Psychiatric Clinics of North America*, *15*, 311–331.

Garbarino, J. (2001). An ecological perspective on the effects of violence on children. *Journal of Community Psychology*, *29*, 361–378.

Garrett, C. J. (1985). Effects of residential treatment on adjudicated delinquents: A meta-analysis. *Journal of Research in Crime and Delinquency*, *22*, 287–308.

Gatti, U., Tremblay, R. E., Vitaro, F., & McDuff, P. (2005). Youth gangs, delinquency and drug use: A test of the selection, facilitation, and enhancement hypotheses. *Journal of Child Psychology and Psychiatry*, *46*, 1178–1190.

Gendreau, P., & Ross, R. R. (1979). Effective correctional treatment: Bibliotherapy for cynics. *Crime and Delinquency*, *22*, 463–489.

Gifford-Smith, M., Dodge, K. A., Dishion, T. J., & McCord, J. (2005). Peer influence in children and adolescents: Crossing the bridge from developmental to intervention science. *Journal of Abnormal Child Psychology*, *33*, 255–265.

Glover, E. (1960). The Roots of Crime. New York: International University Press.

Gorman-Smith, D., & Loeber, R. (2005). Are developmental pathways in disruptive behaviors the same for girls and boys? *Journal of Child and Family Studies*, *14*, 15–27.

Granic, I., & Dishion, T. J. (2003). Deviant talk in adolescent friendships: A step toward measuring a pathogenic attractor process. *Social Development*, *12*, 314–334.

Grietens, H., & Hellinckx, W. (2004). Evaluating effects of residential treatment for juvenile offenders by statistical meta-analysis: A review. *Aggression and Violent Behavior*, *9*, 401–415.

Grisso, T. (1996). Society's retributive response to juvenile violence. A developmental perspective. *Law and Human Behavior*, *20*, 229–247.

Grisso, T. (1997). The competence of adolescents as trial defendants. *Psychology, Public Policy and Law*, *3*, 3–32.

Grisso, T., Vincent, G., & Seagrave, D. (Eds.). (2005). *Mental health screening and assessment in juvenile justice*. London: Guilford Press.

Hackett, S., Masson, H., & Phillips, S. (2006). Exploring consensus in practice with youth who are sexually abusive: Findings from a Delphi study of practitioner views in the United Kingdom and the Republic of Ireland. *Child Maltreatment*, *11*, 146–156.

Hagell, A., Hazel, N., & Shaw, C. (2000). *Evaluation of Medway Secure Training Centre* (pp. 1–13). London: Home Office.

Harrington, C. (2001). Childhood depression and conduct disorder: Different routes to the same outcome? *Archives of General Psychiatry*, *58*, 237–238.

Harrington, R., & Bailey, S. (2003). *Expert Paper: The scope for preventing antisocial personality disorder by intervening in adolescence.*

NHS National Programme on Forensic Mental Health Research and Development.

Harrington, R. C., Kroll, L., Rothwell, J., McCarthy, K., Bradley, D., & Bailey, S. (2005). Psychosocial needs of boys in secure care for serious or persistent offending. *Journal of Child Psychology and Psychiatry*, *46*, 859–866.

Hawes, D. J., & Dadd, M. R. (2007). Stability and malleability of callous-unemotional traits during treatment for childhood conduct problems. *Journal of Consulting and Clinical Psychology*, *36*, 347–355.

Hawkins, J. D., Herrenkohl, T., Farrington, D. P., Brewer, D., Catalano, R. F., & Harachi, T. W. (1998). A review of predictors of youth violence. In R. Loeber, & D. P. Farrington (Eds.), *Serious and violent juvenile offenders: Risk factors and successful interventions* (pp. 106–146). Thousand Oaks, CA: Sage Publications.

Heide, K. M. (1999). *Young killers: The challenge of juvenile homicide* (pp. 219–238). Thousand Oaks, CA: Sage Publications.

Henggeler, S. W., Rowland, M. D., Randall, J., Ward, D. M., Pickrel, S. G., Cunningham, P. B., *et al.* (1999). Home-based multisystemic therapy as an alternative to the hospitalization of youths in psychiatric crisis: Clinical outcomes. *Journal of the American Academy of Child and Adolescent Psychiatry*, *38*, 1331–1339.

Henquet, C., Krabbendam, L., Spauwen, J., Kaplan, C., Lieb, R., Witchen, H. U., & Vanos, J. (2005). Prospective cohort study of cannabis use, predisposition for psychosis and psychotic symptoms in young people. *British Medical Journal*, *330*, 11–14.

Howlin, P. (1997). *Autism: Preparing for adulthood*. London: Routledge.

Huey, S. J., Henggeler, S. W., Brondino, M. J., & Pickrel, S. G. (2000). Mechanisms of change in multisystemic therapy: Reducing delinquent behavior through therapist adherence and improved family and peer functioning. *Journal of Consulting and Clinical Psychology*, *68*, 451–467.

Hummel, P., Thomke, V., Oldenburger, H. A., & Specht, F. (2000). Male adolescent sex offenders against children: Similarities and differences between those offenders with and those without a history of sexual abuse. *Journal of Adolescence*, *23*, 305–317.

Izzo, R. L., & Ross, R. R. (1990). Meta-analysis of rehabilitation programs for juvenile delinquents: A brief report. *Criminal Justice and Behavior*, *17*, 134–142.

Jasper, A., Smith, C., & Bailey, S. (1998). One hundred girls in care referred to an adolescent forensic mental health service. *Journal of Adolescence*, *21*, 555–568.

Jolliffe, D., & Farrington, D. P. (2004). Empathy and offending: A systematic review and meta-analysis. *Aggression and Violent Behavior*, *9*, 441–476.

Jones, A., Forster, A., & Skuse, D. (2007). What do you think you're looking at? Investigating social cognition in young offenders. *Criminal Behaviour and Mental Health*, *17*, 101–106.

Junger-Tas, J. (1994). *Delinquent behavior among young people in the western world*. Amsterdam: Kugler.

Justice. (1996). *Children and homicide: Appropriate procedures for juveniles in murder and manslaughter cases*. London: Justice.

Kazdin, A. E. (1993). Treatment of conduct disorder: Progress and directions in psychotherapy research. *Developmental Psychopathology*, *5*, 277–310.

Kazdin, A. E., Siegel, T. C., & Bass, D. (1992). Cognitive problem-solving skills training and parent management training in the treatment of antisocial behavior in children. *Journal of Consulting and Clinical Psychology*, *60*, 733–747.

Kennedy, P. J., Vale, E. L. E., Khan, S., J., & McAnaney, A. (2006). Factors predicting recidivism in child and adolescent fire-setters: A systematic review of the literature. *Journal of Forensic Psychiatry and Psychology*, *17*, 151–164.

Kim-Cohen, J., Caspi, A., Taylor, A., Williams, B., Newcombe, R., Craig, I. W., *et al.* (2006). MAOA, maltreatment, and gene–environment interaction predicting children's mental health: New evidence and a meta-analysis. *Molecular Psychiatry*, *11*, 903–913.

Knight, J. R., Goodman, E., Pulerwitz, T., & DuRant, R. H. (2001). Reliability of the Problem Orientated Screening Instrument for Teenagers (POSIT) in adolescent medical practice. *Journal of Adolescent Health*, *29*, 125–130.

Kolko, D. J., & Kazdin, A. E. (1992). The emergence and re-occurrence of child firesetting. A one-year prospective study. *Journal of Abnormal Child Psychology*, *20*, 17–37.

Kovacs, M., Goldston, D., & Gatsonis, C. (1993). Suicidal behaviors and childhood-onset depressive disorders: A longitudinal investigation. *Journal of the American Academy of Child and Adolescent Psychiatry*, *32*, 8–20.

Kroll, L., Rothwell, J., Bradley, D., Bailey, S., Shah, P., & Harrington, R. C. (2002). Mental health needs of boys in secure care for serious or persistent offending: A prospective, longitudinal study. *Lancet*, *359*, 1975–1979.

Kroll, L., Woodham, A., Rothwell, J., Bailey, S., Tobias, C., Harrington, R., *et al.* (1999). Reliability of the Salford needs assessment schedule for adolescents. *Psychological Medicine*, *29*, 891–902.

Lader, D., Singleton, N., & Meltzer, H. (2003). Psychiatric morbidity among young offenders in England and Wales. *International Review of Psychiatry*, *15*, 144–147.

Landenberger, N. A., & Lipsey, M. W. (2005). The positive effects of cognitive–behavioral programs for offenders: A meta-analysis of factors associated with effective treatment. *Journal of Experimental Criminology*, *1*, 451–476.

Langstrom, N., Grann, M., & Lindblad, F. (2000). A preliminary typology of young sex offenders. *Journal of Adolescence*, *23*, 319–329.

Latimer, J. (2001). A meta-analytic examination of youth delinquency, family treatment, and recidivism. *Canadian Journal of Criminology*, *43*, 237–253.

Latimer, J., Dowden, C., & Muise, D. (2005). The effectiveness of restorative justice practices: A meta-analysis. *Prison Journal*, *85*, 127–144.

Laub, J. H., & Sampson, R. J. (2003). *Shared beginnings, divergent lives: Delinquent boys to age 70*. Cambridge, MA: Harvard University Press.

Lederman, C., Dakof, G., Larrea, M., & Li, H. (2004). Characteristics of adolescent females in juvenile detention. *International Journal of Law and Psychiatry*, *27*, 321–337.

Lenssen, S. A. M., Doreleijers, T. A. H., Van Dijk, M. E., & Hartman, C. A. (2000). Girls in detention: what are their characteristics? A project to explore and document the character of this target group and the significant ways in which it differs from one consisting of boys. *Journal of Adolescence*, *23*, 287–303.

Leschied, A. W., & Cunningham, A. (2002). *Seeking effective interventions for serious young offenders: Interim results of a four-year randomized study of Multisystemic Therapy in Ontario, Canada*. London, Ontario: Centre for Children and Families in the Justice System.

Leve, L. D., Chamberlain, P., & Reid, J. B. (2005). Intervention outcomes for girls referred from juvenile justice: Effects on delinquency. *Journal of Consulting and Clinical Psychology*, *73*, 1181–1185.

Lipsey, M. W., & Wilson D. B. (1998). Effective intervention for serious juvenile offenders: A synthesis of research. In R. Loeber, & D. P. Farrington (Eds.), *Serious and violent juvenile offenders: Risk factors and successful interventions*. Thousand Oaks, CA: Sage Publications.

Littell, J. H. (2005). Lessons from a systematic review of effects of multisystemic therapy. *Children and Youth Services Review*, *27*, 445–463.

Littell, J. H. (2006). The case for multisystemic therapy: Evidence or orthodoxy? *Children and Youth Services Review*, *28*, 458–472.

Lochman, J. E., & Wells, K. C. (2004). The coping power program for preadolescent aggressive boys and their parents: Outcome effects at the 1-year follow-up. *Journal of Consulting and Clinical Psychology*, *72*, 571–578.

Loeber, R., Pardini, D., Homish, D. L., Wei, E. H., Crawford, A. M., Farrington, D. P., *et al.* (2005). The prediction of violence and homicide in young males. *Journal of Consulting and Clinical Psychology*, *73*, 1074–1088.

Lösel, F., & Beelmann, A. (2003). Effects of child skills training in preventing antisocial behavior: A systematic review of randomized evaluations. *Annals of the American Academy of Political and Social Science*, *587*, 84–109.

Lösel, F., & Köferl, P. (1989). Evaluation research on correctional treatment in West Germany: A meta-analysis. In H. Wegener, F. Lösel, & J. Haisch (Eds.), *Criminal behavior and the justice system: Psychological perspectives* (pp. 334–355). New York: Springer-Verlag.

Lösel, F., & Schmucker, M. (2005). The effectiveness of treatment for sexual offenders: A comprehensive meta-analysis. *Journal of Experimental Criminology*, *1*, 114–146.

McCord, J. (1997). On discipline. *Psychological Inquiry*, *8*, 215–217.

McCord, J. (1978). A thirty-year follow-up of treatment effects. *American Psychologist*, *33*, 284–289.

McGuire, J., & Priestley, P. (1995). Reviewing "what works": Past, present and future. In J. McGuire (Ed.), *What works: Reducing reoffending: Guidelines from research and practice* (pp. 3–34). Chichester: Wiley.

MacKay, S., Henderson, J., Del Bove, G., Marton, P., Warling, D., & Root, C. (2006). Fire interest and antisociality as risk factors in the severity and persistence of juvenile firesetting. *Journal of the American Academy of Child and Adolescent Psychiatry*, *45*, 1077–1084.

Marshall, M., Hogg, L. I., Gath, D. H., & Lockwood, A. (1995). The cardinal needs schedule: A modified version of the MRC needs for care assessment schedule. *Psychological Medicine*, *25*, 605–617.

Maughan, B., & Kim-Cohen, J. (2005). Continuities between childhood and adult life. *British Journal of Psychiatry*, *187*, 301–303.

Meeus, W., Branje, S., & Overbeek, G. J. (2004). Parents and partners in crime: A six-year longitudinal study on changes in supportive relationships and delinquency in adolescence and young adulthood. *Journal of Child Psychology and Psychiatry*, *45*, 1288–1298.

Miller, D., Trapani, C., Fejes-Mendoza, K., Eggleston, C., & Dwiggins, D. (1995). Adolescent female offenders: Unique consideration. *Adolescence*, *30*, 429–435.

Moffitt, T. E. (2005). The new look of behavioral genetics in developmental psychopathology: gene–environment interplay in antisocial behaviors. *Psychological Bulletin*, *131*, 533–554.

Moffitt, T. E., Caspi, A., Rutter, M., & Silva, P. (2001). *Sex differences in antisocial behaviour*. Cambridge, UK: Cambridge University Press.

Myers, W. C., Burton, P. R. S., Sanders, P. D., Donat, K. M., Cheney, J., Fitzpatrick, T. M., *et al.* (2000). Project Back-on-Track at 1 year: A delinquency treatment program for early-career juvenile offenders. *Journal of the American Academy of Child and Adolescent Psychiatry*, *39*, 1127–1134.

Myers, W. C., & Scott, K. (1998). Psychotic and conduct disorder symptoms in juvenile murderers. *Journal of Homicide Studies*, *2*, 160–175.

Nugent, W. R., Williams, M., & Umbreit, M. S. (2004). Participation in victim-offender mediation and the prevalence of subsequent delinquent behavior: A meta-analysis. *Research on Social Work Practice*, *14*, 408–416.

O'Brien, B. S., & Frick, P. J. (1996). Reward dominance associations with anxiety conduct problems and psychopathy in children. *Journal of Abnormal Child Psychology*, *24*, 223–240.

Odgers, C. L., Burnette, M. L., Chauhan, P., Moretti, M. M., & Reppucci, N. D. (2005). Misdiagnosing the problem: Mental health profiles of incarcerated juveniles. *Canadian Child and Adolescent Psychiatry Review*, *14*, 26–29.

Ogden, T., & Hagen K. A. (2006). Multisytemic treatment of serious behaviour problems in youth: Sustainability of effectiveness two years after intake. *Child and Adolescent Mental Health*, *11*, 142–149.

Pandina, G. J., Aman, M. G., & Findling, R. L. (2006). Risperidone in the management of disruptive behavior disorders. *Journal of Child and Adolescent Psychopharmacology*, *16*, 379–392.

Pappadopulos, E., Woolston, S., Chait, A., Perkins, M., Connor, D., & Jensen, P. (2006). Pharmacotherapy of aggression in children and adolescents: Efficacy and effect size. *Journal of the Canadian Academy of Child and Adolescent Psychiatry*, *15*, 27–39.

Patterson, G. R. (1982). *Coercive family process*. Eugene, OR, USA: Castalia Publishing.

Patterson, G. R. (2002). Future extensions of the model. In J. B. Reid, G. R. Patterson, & J. Snyder (Eds.), *Antisocial behavior in children and adolescents: A developmental analysis and model for intervention*. (pp. 273–283). Washington, DC: American Psychological Association.

Petrosino, A., Turpin-Petrosino, C., & Buehler, J. (2003). Scared Straight and other juvenile awareness programs for preventing juvenile delinquency: A systematic review of the randomized experimental evidence. *Annals of the American Academy of Political and Social Science*, *589*, 41–62.

Pliszka, S., Stienman, J., Barrow, V., & Frick, S. (2000). Affective disorders in juvenile offenders. A preliminary study. *American Journal of Psychiatry*, *157*, 130–132.

Quinsey, V. L., Harris, G. T., Rice, E., & Cormier, C. A. (2006). Sex offenders. In V. L. Quinsey, G. T. Harris, M. E. Rice, & C. A. Cormier (Eds.), *Violent offenders: Appraising and managing risk* (2nd edn., pp. 131–151). Washington, DC: American Psychological Association.

Repo, E., & Virkunnen, M. (1997). Young arsonists, history of conduct disorder, psychiatric diagnosis, and criminal recidivism. *Journal of Forensic Psychiatry*, *8*, 311–320.

Robins, L. N., & Rutter, M. (Eds.). (1990). *Straight and devious pathways from childhood to adulthood*. New York, NY: Cambridge University Press.

Rutter, M. (1979). Protective factors in children's responses to stress and disadvantage. In M. W. Kent, & J. E. Rolf (Eds.), *Primary prevention of psychopathology* (pp. 49–74). Hanover, NH: University of New England Press.

Rutter, M., Giller, H., & Hagell, A. (1998). *Antisocial behavior by young people*. Cambridge: Cambridge University Press.

Rutter, M., & Quinton, D. (1987). Parental mental illness as a risk factor for psychiatric disorders in childhood. In D. Magnusson, & A. Ohman (Eds.), *Psychopathology: An interactional perspective* (pp. 199–219). San Diego, CA: Academic Press.

Safer Custody Group. (2007). *Self-inflicted deaths annual report: 2006*. London: National Offender Management Group. Accessed from http://www.phrn.nhs.uk/workstreams/mentalhealth/SCGAnnualReport.doc. Accessed March 15 2007.

Sailas, E. S., Feodoroff, B., Virkkunen, M., & Wahlbeck, K. (2005). Mental disorders in prison populations aged 15–21: National register study of two cohorts in Finland. *British Medical Journal*, *330*, 1364–1365.

Sampson, R. J., Morenoff, J. D., & Gannon-Rowley, T. (2002). Assessing "neighborhood effects": Social processes and new directions in research. *Annual Review of Sociology*, *28*, 443–478.

Schachar, R., Taylor, E., Wieselberg, M., Thorley, G., & Rutter, M. (1987). Changes in family function and relationships in children who respond to methylphenidate. *Journal of the American Academy of Child and Adolescent Psychiatry*, *26*, 728–732.

Seagrave, D., & Grisso, T. (2002). Adolescent development and the measurement of juvenile psychopathy. *Law and Human Behavior*, *26*, 219–239.

Shepherd, J. P., & Farrington, D. P. (1993). Assault as a public health problem: Discussion paper. *Journal of the Royal Society of Medicine*, *86*, 89–92.

Skuse, D., Bentovim, A., Hodges, J., Stevenson, C., Andreou, M., Lanyado, M., *et al.* (1998). Risk factors for development of sexually abusive behavior in sexually victimized adolescent boys: Cross-sectional study. *British Medical Journal*, *317*, 175–179.

Snyder, J., & Stoolmiller, M. (2002). Reinforcement and coercion mechanisms in the development of antisocial behavior: The family. In J. B. Reid, G. R. Patterson, & J. Snyder (Eds.), *Antisocial behavior in children and adolescents: A developmental analysis and model for intervention* (pp. 65–100). Washington, DC: American Psychological Association.

Soderstrom, H., Sjodin, A.-K., Carlstedt, A. F., & Forsman, A. (2004). Adult psychopathic personality with childhood-onset hyperactivity and conduct disorder: A central problem constellation in forensic psychiatry. *Psychiatry Research*, *121*, 271–280.

Sourander, A., Elonheimo, H., Niemela, S., Nuutila, A. M., Helenius, H., Sillanmaki, L., *et al.* (2006). Childhood predictors of male criminality: A prospective population-based follow-up study from age 8 to late adolescence. *Journal of the American Academy of Child and Adolescent Psychiatry*, *45*, 578–586.

Soyka, M., Morhart-Klute, V., & Schoech, H. (2004). Delinquency and criminal offenses in former schizophrenic inpatients 7–12 years following discharge. *European Archives of Psychiatry and Clinical Neuroscience*, *254*, 289–294.

Spain, S. E., Douglas, K. S., Poythress, N. G., & Epstein, M. (2004). The relationship between psychopathic features, violence and treatment outcomes: the comparison of three youth measures of psychopathic features. *Behavioral Sciences and the Law*, *22*, 85–102.

Stattin, H., & Magnusson, D. (1996). Antisocial development: A holistic approach. *Development and Psychopathology*, *8*, 617–645.

Stattin, H., Romelsjo, A., & Stenbacka, M. (1997). Personal resources as modifiers of the risk for future criminality: An analysis of protective factors in relation to 18-year-old boys. *British Journal of Criminology*, *37*, 198–223.

Steen, S. (2007). Conferring sameness: Institutional management of juvenile sex offenders. *Journal of Contemporary Ethnography*, *36*, 31–49.

Stinchcomb, J. B. (2005). From optimistic policies to pessimistic outcomes: Why won't boot camps either succeed pragmatically or succumb politically? In B. B. Benda, & N. J. Pallone (Eds.), *Rehabilitation issues, problems, and prospects in boot camp* (pp. 27–52). New York, NY: Haworth Press.

Stouthamer-Loeber, M., Loeber, R., Wei, E., Farrington, D. P., & Wikstrom, P. O. H. (2002). Risk and promotive effects in the explanation of persistent serious delinquency in boys. *Journal of Consulting and Clinical Psychology*, *70*, 111–123.

Sukhodolsky, D. G., & Ruchkin, V. (2006). Evidence-based psychosocial treatments in the juvenile justice system. *Child and Adolescent Psychiatric Clinics of North America*, *15*, 501–516.

Surgeon General. (2001). *Youth violence: a report of the Surgeon General.* Washington, DC: Department of Health and Human Services. Accessed from http://www.surgeongeneral.gov/library/youthviolence/summary.htm Accessed March 15 2007.

Taylor, P. J., Gunn, J., (1999). Homicides by people with mental illness, myth and reality. *British Journal of Psychiatry*, *174*, 9–14.

Timmons-Mitchell, J., Bender, M. B., Kishna, M. A., & Mitchell, C. C. (2006). An independent effectiveness trial of multisystemic therapy with juvenile justice youth. *Journal of Clinical Child and Adolescent Psychology*, *35*, 227–236.

Tong, L. S. J., & Farrington, D. P. (2006). How effective is the "Reasoning and Rehabilitation" program in reducing reoffending? A meta-analysis of evaluations in four countries. *Psychology, Crime and Law*, *12*, 3–24.

Torgersen, S., Kringlen, E., & Cramer, V. (2001). The prevalence of personality disorders in a community sample. *Archives of General Psychiatry*, *58*, 590–596.

Tremblay, P., & Pare, P. (2003). Crime and destiny: Patterns in serious offenders' mortality rates. *Canadian Journal of Criminology and Criminal Justice*, *45*, 299–326.

Tyler, J., Darville, R., & Stalnaker, K. (2001). Juvenile boot camps: A descriptive analysis of program diversity and effectiveness. *Social Science Journal*, *38*, 445–460.

Van Outsem, R., Beckett, R., Bullens, R., Vermeiren, R., van Horn, J., & Doreleijers, T. (2006). The Adolescent Sexual Abuser Project (ASAP) Assessment Measures-Dutch Revised Version: A comparison of personality characteristics between juvenile sex offenders, juvenile perpetrators of non-sexual violent offences and non-delinquent youth in the Netherlands. *Journal of Sexual Aggression*, *12*, 127–141.

Vermeiren, R., De Clippele, A., & Deboutte, D. (2000). A descriptive survey of Flemish delinquent adolescents. *Journal of Adolescence*, *23*, 277–285.

Vizard, E., Wynick, S., Hawkes, C., Woods, J., & Jenkins, J. (1996). Juvenile sexual offenders. *British Journal of Psychiatry*, *168*, 259–262.

Vreeland, R. G., & Lowin, B. M. (1980). Psychological aspects of firesetting. In D. Canter (Ed.), *Fires and human behavior*. New York, NY: Wiley.

Vreugdenhil, C., Vermeiren, R., Wouters, L., Doreleijers, T., & van den Brink, W. (2004). Psychotic symptoms among male adolescent detainees in the Netherlands. *Schizophrenia Bulletin*, *30*, 73–86.

Weiss, B., Caron, A., Ball, S., Tapp, J., Johnson, M., & Weisz, J. R. (2005). Iatrogenic effects of group treatment for antisocial youths. *Journal of Consulting and Clinical Psychology*, *73*, 1036–1044.

Wilson, S. J., & Lipsey, M. W. (2000). Wilderness challenge programs for delinquent youth: A meta-analysis of outcome evaluations. *Evaluation and Program Planning*, *23*, 1–12.

Wilson, S. J., Lipsey, M. W., & Soydan, H. (2003). Are mainstream programs for juvenile delinquency less effective with minority youth than majority youth? A meta-analysis of outcomes research. *Research on Social Work Practice*, *13*, 3–26.

Youth Justice Board. (2007). *ASSET: A structured assessment tool for Youth Offending Teams to use on all young offenders who come into contact with the criminal justice system.* London: Youth Justice Board. Accessed from www.yjb.gov.uk. Accessed March 15 2007.

Zimring, F. (1998). *The challenge of youth violence*. Cambridge: Cambridge University Press.

Zoccolillo, M. (1993). Gender and the development of conduct disorder. *Development and Psychopathology*, 5, 65–78.

Provision of Intensive Treatment: In-patient Units, Day Units and Intensive Outreach

Jonathan Green and Anne Worrall-Davies

The last decade has seen a rapid evolution in the structure and delivery of mental health services in many countries. The use of in-patient beds has generally declined in developed countries and there is an increasing interest in alternative models of intensive service delivery such as day provision or intensive outreach. In parallel, the context within which children's mental health disorders are seen has progressively widened to encompass the context of family, school and wider community. The stage emphasis in personality and social development, which provided a rationale for intensive episodic interventions, has largely been replaced by a new appreciation of chronicity and long-term pathways in the evolution of many disorders (see chapter 13). Acute episodes of intensive treatment have therefore to be considered now in the wider contexts of family and local environment as well as in the longitudinal context of what is known about the natural history of particular disorders. This chapter reviews new developments in intensive mental health treatments for young people, the evidence base for intensive treatments in the light of these considerations and prospects for the future.

In-patient Treatment

Historical Roots

Two broad forms of residential mental health care for young people emerged in the early 20th century. The first was based on the idea that a self-contained environment could act as a "therapeutic milieu," effecting personality and behavior change (Kennard, 1983). Examples in the UK were Homer Lane's "Little Commonwealth" (Bazeley, 1928) and residential therapeutic schools such as the Mulberry Bush; in the USA, there was the work of Bettelheim (1955). The second historical root was the adaptations made for children within the asylums of the 19th century (Parry Jones, 1998) and the accelerated development of specialized medically based psychiatric units for children following the encephalitis epidemic in the USA in the 1920s (Beskind, 1962). Such hospital units developed to provide a comprehensive approach to assessment and treatment based on a biopsychosocial model (Cameron, 1949). Here, the hospital environment was the *location* for assessment and treatment rather than its *primary agent*. The decades after World War II saw a rapid expansion of in-patient units, usually combining elements of both models. Recent decades have seen a plateauing or reduction in numbers of units and increasing specialization, alongside an awareness of the potential negative effects of residential treatment (Wolkind, 1974). However, the two historical themes remain a useful way of conceptualizing the in-patient treatment process.

Rutter's Child and Adolescent Psychiatry, 5th edition. Edited by M. Rutter, D. Bishop, D. Pine, S. Scott, J. Stevenson, E. Taylor and A. Thapar. © 2008 Blackwell Publishing, ISBN: 978-1-4051-4549-7.

The Ward as a Therapeutic Milieu

The "therapeutic milieu" is a term subject to numerous reinterpretations but little research (Green & Burke, 1998). Early psychodynamic formulations (Bettelheim, 1955) contained an assumption that the milieu substituted for a lack in the child's previous experience – particularly, sensitive parental care. There was an emphasis on a closed environment and long treatments. Later, systemic models (Woolston, 1989) emphasized the ward as an "open system" mediating the "goodness of fit" between young person and their environment through collaboration with other agencies and the family; parents often taking an active part in the ward caregiving. Other models have emphasized the ward environment as a shorter-term "corrective emotional experience" with high levels of warm staff communication, peer contact and active behavioral control (Cotton, 1993). A few specialized developments have involved admitting whole families (Lynch, Steinberg, & Ounsted, 1975); these then can have some convergent roles with mother and baby units. Five-day residential patterns have become common (Green & Jacobs, 1998). Recent developments – notably driven by managed care in the USA (Nurcombe, 1989) – have in contrast reduced the ward environment to its most minimal form. The emphasis here is on symptom stabilization and "minimum necessary change" before rapid discharge. Stays are often under 2 weeks; a radically different form of milieu from the 3-year or more stays described by earlier writers. In this recent model, the "therapeutic milieu" as historically understood has essentially disappeared and in-patient care has returned to its root in acute hospital practice.

What are the components of a successful milieu? Systematic research into the comparative effectiveness of different types of milieu has been identified as a priority in a number of reviews (Pfeiffer & Strzelecki, 1990; Pottick, Hansell, Gaboda, & Gutterman, 1993). Work in adult psychiatry addressed the character and effect of different forms of residential milieu (Moos, Shelton & Petty, 1973) and Steiner, Marx, and Walton (1991) applied similar methods to a study of an adolescent unit. The clinical literature, as one might expect, identifies the importance of a combination of appropriate physical environment, space design, adequate staff numbers, skill mix, therapeutic culture and leadership (Green & Burke, 1998). The creation of a coherent therapeutic culture – "like a well-conducted orchestra" – is found in meta-analysis to be strongly related to therapeutic outcome (Pfeiffer & Strzelecki, 1990) but there has been little research into its component parts until recently (Green, Jacobs, Beecham *et al.*, 2007). A necessary condition clearly is shared values and complementary theoretical approaches within the multiprofessional team. Other important and related indicators are staff morale, consistency, good communication and self-confidence. A milieu has above all to remain functionally intact in the face of staff and patient turnover, disruption and conflict, and challenges from the patients, individually and as a group. Self-confidence will communicate itself to the children and increase their ability to trust. The instilling of hope is one of the first outcomes of successful treatment and the milieu is no exception. Recently, a national comparative study of UK in-patient units measured the variation of ward atmosphere between units (Green, Jacobs, Beecham *et al.*, 2007) and showed the negative effect of patient aggression on atmosphere and reduced length of stay.

Social Functioning and Education

By the time of admission, a young person's social adaptation in their community has often broken down, sometimes in all areas of school, family and community life. Widespread social difficulties were found in 58 consecutive general admissions in New Zealand, including a moderate to severe language handicap in 40% of cases (Paterson, Bauer, McDonald, & McDermott, 1997). In the USA, Luthar, Woolston, Sparrow, and Zimmerman (1995) similarly found severe impairments on Vineland social competency scores in 126 patients admitted with disruptive and mixed emotional–disruptive disorders. Social competency was associated with specific reading scores rather than broad intelligence quotient. These findings have practical implications. The traditional therapeutic milieu contains elements of group living, peer relationships and intensive staff–patient contact. Removal from social difficulties in the external environment and exposure to such a milieu can produce rapid gains in functioning and self-esteem. Nevertheless, young people with significant social impairments may not be able to make effective use of such a socially orientated therapeutic environment. Assessing and targeting social difficulties more precisely and defining the effective milieu characteristics for different problems are important tasks for future developments in milieu treatment.

Similarly, many in-patients have a history of school failure or acute school breakdown. The individualized assessment and intensive educational input possible within the in-patient unit can make a radical impact (French & Tate, 1998). Recent studies (Green, Kroll, Imre *et al.*, 2001; Green, Jacobs, Beecham *et al.*, 2007) have shown rapid reduction in teacher ratings of behavioral disturbance in the classroom from pre-admission to early admission. Green, Kroll, Imre *et al.* (2001) showed that these persisted when reassessed in a 6-month follow-up.

Rapid gains in socialization and academic achievement represent two of the potential therapeutic strengths of residential treatment. They can be used as a platform from which to reintegrate patients into their own communities with enhanced resilience, as long as there is good linkage into aftercare. However, such targeted interventions take time and are not compatible with ultrashort in-patient stays.

Admission Practice

Admission rates into in-patient care differ greatly between countries. A national survey of young people receiving mental health treatment in the USA during 1986 (Pottick, Hansell, Gaboda *et al.*, 1993) found 5% of the children (6–12 years) and 30% of the adolescents (13–18 years) were being treated in in-patient facilities (combined proportion 20%). More recent UK admission rates are much lower, estimated at around 1% of the clinical pool of children in one area (Maskey, 1998). Costello, Dulcan, and Kalas (1991) studied 389 children between 2 and 12 years referred for in-patient evaluation in the USA. Factors leading to admission included deterioration despite out-patient treatment; increasing aggressiveness; difficulties with assessment or diagnosis; family difficulties in the context of psychiatric disorder making treatment impossible; and the need for 24 h observational nursing care. A prospective study of 276 admissions to UK adolescent units (Wrate, Rothery, McCabe, & Aspin, 1994) characterized diagnostic formulation as the key factor accounting for most admissions. However, Pottick, Hansell, Gutterman, and White (1995) found that the strongest influence on admission in the USA was the presence of insurance cover: a cut in insurance benefit between 1978 and 1983 coincided with a significant drop in US in-patient usage (Patrick, Padgett, Burns, Schlesinger, & Cohen, 1993). Proximity to a specialist center increases referral rates in developed countries (Gutterman, Markovitz, LoConte, & Beier, 1993) and Blanz and Schmidt (2000) describe how devolution of in-patient care to smaller local units in Germany reduced admission times and changed admission practice. On the other hand, it may be that sparsely distributed or generally poorly provided populations might tend to use concentrated in-patient provision more.

Pragmatically, admission is often a negotiation between referrer, family and admitting unit around which the specific needs of each party can be met by admission (Bruggen & O'Brien, 1987). In the future it is to be hoped that an increasing part of such decision-making will be the empirical evidence regarding the effectiveness of in-patient treatments in particular situations and for particular disorders (see pp. 1132–1133). Whereas the in-patient resource is rightly held in reserve for the most complex and severe cases, referral should not be overdelayed: a well-timed intensive treatment may often prevent further deterioration in an acute disorder.

Admissions generally fall into a number of broad categories:

1 The need for detailed assessment in complex cases where the formulation is unclear. The combination of the medical setting with the range of health professionals makes the ward particularly well able to address the interaction of biological, psychological and social aspects of disorders.

2 Assessment or treatment away from the family. This can be crucial when the role of family in a presentation may be unclear – for instance, in possible factitious presentations (see chapter 57), or when complex symptoms seem confined to home.

3 When psychiatric symptomatology is escalating despite the most intensive out-patient treatment available. This includes acute risk management of self-harm or family disruption associated with psychiatric disorder.

4 For controlled trials of specific interventions.

Pre-admission evaluation is a crucial area. The admission must be seen within the context of a continuum of service use and the developmental trajectory of the child, because it will be a brief episode in both these areas. Many of the key predictors of in-patient outcome lie in details of previous family adaptation, child social functioning and child symptomatology (see p. 1132); assessment should thus focus on these aspects as well as the needs and motivation of patient and family. Pre-admission evaluation may lead to a decision not to admit. For instance, many children with social and behavioral difficulties may be more appropriately cared for within the social care system with psychiatric input.

Emergency Admission

Studies of referrer attitudes emphasize the high priority given to the specialist unit's responsiveness and capacity to admit emergencies (Gowers & Kushlick, 1992; Worrall & O'Herlihy, 2001). This is particularly the case in situations of acute risk management. Responsive consultation around the emergency may meet referrer needs without admission (Cotgrove, 1997). However, provision of emergency beds is likely to be an increasing priority and will shape service provision. Street (2000) found that even with a clear agreement between referrer, admitting in-patient unit and family, the time taken to actually acquire a UK child and adolescent mental health services (CAMHS) bed from time of acute referral averaged 3 days. Where facilities are not immediately available, young people may have to be temporarily cared for in inappropriate environments such as pediatric wards, adult psychiatric wards or out-of-district facilities (Street, 2000).

Discharge and Aftercare

Discharge planning should receive equal attention to admission planning. Many studies point to the crucial role of aftercare in the maintenance of treatment gains made during admission (Pfeiffer & Strzelecki, 1990). In a minority of cases, admission may prove to be a stepping stone towards longer-term alternative care or residential schooling. Because of the multifaceted nature of in-patient problems, the team liaises with a wide variety of local services in education, social services and mental health. A "care program approach" may be used along lines developed in adult mental health as an aid to transition into adult services. Hoagwood, Jensen, Wigal *et al.* (2000) showed that a limited period of intensive specialist treatment resulted in a more effective use of other services thereafter; this may explain some "sleeper" effects in outcome. There is evidence (Green, Jacobs, Beecham *et al.*, 2007) that in-patient treatment can have a similar effect, but provision of post-discharge services is vital, and the same study showed that in the majority of cases the discharge plan recommendations were not carried out.

Potential Unwanted Effects

Theoretically, unwanted effects could derive from:

1 Loss of support from the child's local environment;

2 Presence of adverse effects within the in-patient environment; and

3 The effects of admission on family life (Green & Jones, 1998).

However, there is no convincing research into their prevalence.

Losses Consequent on Admission

Reporting bias towards acute problems during pre-admission assessment could obscure hidden sources of support and resilience in the local environment – within the extended family, peers or school. Pre-admission assessment should therefore actively focus on strengths as well as difficulties and identify key areas of individual resilience. Admission may also result in the loss of important local professional input, which should be ameliorated by good communication between unit, referring teams and local services. These factors need particular attention from in-patient clinicians because they may be less obvious than active effects from within the in-patient environment itself.

Impact of the In-patient Environment

Some young people may enter the ward with a profound sense of relief but others may find it at least initially frightening or bewildering. Patient ratings after in-patient psychiatric care (usually collected by the units themselves) generally show positive evaluation of the treatment. However, parents are often concerned that their child may be negatively affected ("contaminated") by other patients' problems. There is additionally the stigma that is often attached to the prospect of in-patient psychiatric treatment. Units must be constantly vigilant to the possibility of the negative impact of peers on each other, the pooling of problems or abuse. To counter such potential problems, Newbold and Jones (1998) suggested a proactive emphasis on child welfare and rights, embodied in the appointment of a "welfare co-ordinator," with a role to investigate any complaints. This is done in the context of procedural agreements with local child protection agencies and a continuing program of awareness training and education of staff.

There have been no specific studies into institutionalization in child or adolescent psychiatry units. Well-publicized episodes of abuse in residential social care environments (Levy & Kahan, 1991) may be unreasonably generalized into attitudes towards residential psychiatry treatments by families, although the intensity of monitoring and supervision in the latter hopefully makes such disasters less likely.

Effect on Families

Some professional concern has focused on the effect of admission on family dynamics, for instance the reinforcement of "scapegoating." This may indeed be a contraindication to admission, although equally a scapegoated child has a right to the best possible assessment and care – and this may involve admission. As the child engages with the ward there can also be a danger that the parents feel deskilled (Green, 1994). Good family contracting pre-admission and sustained family work can counteract these negative effects. A family's commitment to intensive treatments can be disruptive and expensive. In a study of eight UK units, Green, Jacobs, Beecham *et al.* (2007) found that family-borne costs averaged £2400 per admission, a good proportion of the average annual wage. It is essential to anticipate this by building support for family travel into the contracting around the case and actively to support the family in relation to employers.

However, there is a need for systematic study of unwanted effects rather than reliance on theoretical concerns or anecdote. Along with general standards of good practice, systematic procedures of anticipation, prevention, recognition and repair should minimize unwanted effects (Green & Jones, 1998).

Day Units

The concept of psychiatric day care developed in the USA in the 1940s with the therapeutic nursery school for very young children (Zimet & Farley, 1985). Relieved of the need to provide residential aspects of care, day unit environments have been able to evolve in a host of different directions. These have ranged from specific day programs for young children with developmental problems, as an adjunct to specialist school provision, to intensive 5 day a week treatment interventions with whole families. The range is now too great to summarize neatly and this is a difficulty in appraising the effectiveness of day units from published literature. Day hospital units are often associated with in-patient units in the UK (Green & Jacobs, 1998), Germany and Switzerland. In Finland, there is a high number of in-patient beds but only 8% of these units offered a day program (Ellila, Sourander, Valimaki, & Piha, 2005). Integrated in-patient and day units can share programming, staff and infrastructure; the advantages of independent day units relate to flexibility. The reduced need for a shift system to cover nights allows ward staff to work predictable hours and be available regularly for liaison sessions and outreach work. Partial attendance also means that staff can have days free for supervision and continuing education. Flexibility of in-patient, day and outreach is emerging as a priority; Street (2004) highlighted the need for more CAMHS to be able to offer outreach and/or day care before and after admission.

Amid the variety of day unit functioning, a number of broad themes may be distinguished:

1 Day units for the treatment of disruptive behavior. A number of programs have been developed, usually using multimodal treatment packages with a combination of individual family and liaison intervention alongside psychopharmacology. Grizenko (1997) and Rey, Denshire, Wever, and Apollonov (1998) reported the outcome of such programs.

2 Units have specialized in the management of younger children with developmental disorders such as autism, speech and language disorders or attention deficit/hyperactivity disorder (ADHD). These provide centers for comprehensive assessment and initiation of treatment management involving family and school liaison.

3 Units whose prime aim is to influence family functioning in situations of family breakdown or child maltreatment. A number of influential programs of this kind have been described (Asen, Stein, Stevens *et al.*, 1982).

The partial milieu of the day unit shares care with family or local school to a greater extent than residential units. Thus, liaison takes up correspondingly more time and contact with parents may be more frequent. The day unit has the opportunity to generate treatment programs that link closely with parental care. The emphasis on education means that the academic focus of the milieu in day care can be fully exploited. Educationally, therefore, in-patient and day unit treatment can be identical. There are also opportunities to transfer learned skills into the community and family setting (McCarthy, Baker, Betts *et al.*, 2006) or to provide outreach into the community (http://www.swindonmarlborough.nhs.uk/departments/child/beacon_under_8's.htm).

Disadvantages of the day unit milieu mirror these advantages. Many stand alone day units do not have the critical mass of staff to mount a full educational program and make do with sessional teacher inputs. This may not in itself be enough to achieve the key academic goals necessary for a child failing in school. The day unit has to achieve a balance between adequate intense academic input on the one hand and the socialization and therapeutic experience on the other; they may find that they have insufficient time to do both properly with children with complex problems. The child may have to make multiple adaptations to different environments during the week and in many areas the daily transport to and from the unit can be complex and tiring. The opportunities for completeness and intensity of treatment and observation are less. There are some multiagency collaborative units (http://www.tavi-port.org/patient/tavistock-clinic/patient-services-and-departments/mulberrysvc.html?no_cache=1&sword_list%5B%5D=bush) using facilities from education, health or social care services to meet complex needs.

Common Aspects of Day Unit and In-patient Treatment

Therapeutic Alliance

Therapeutic alliance is poorly researched in child psychiatry when compared with adult mental health treatments (Green, 2006), yet proxy measures of therapeutic alliance such as "parental co-operation" commonly provide the most significant predictor of in-patient and day patient outcome (Grizenko, 1997; Sourander, Helenius, Leijala *et al.*, 1996). Kroll and Green (1997) reviewed the complexity of the therapeutic alliance in in-patient and day patient care. Alliances are necessary between child and parents separately and a complex in-patient team. The team acts in a number of different roles, ranging from a quasi-parenting role in relation to a child's basic needs to a therapeutic role while undertaking specific programs; from a "collaborative" role with parents to a "patient" status for adults within family therapy. Adult studies find that therapeutic alliance relates to pretreatment social adaptation (Hougaard, 1994) and social competency is found to be a key variable predicting adaptation into an adolescent in-patient treatment environment (Luthar, Woolston, Sparrow *et al.*, 1995). Such findings emphasize the importance of pre-admission work for building a therapeutic alliance. Techniques for maximizing alliance independently with both child and parent need consideration. Two studies (Green, Kroll, Imre *et al.*, 2001; Green, Jacobs, Beecham *et al.*, 2007) found that child and parental alliances were independent of each other and that the child alliance was a main predictor of health gain during admission.

Assessment Strategies

The ward environment creates opportunities for detailed assessment of biological and psychological aspects of disorder. Covert causes of behavioral difficulties can be elucidated – for instance, a study of unselected adolescent admissions (Szabo & Magnus, 1999) revealed 4% of patients with undiagnosed complex partial seizures. Wards need ready access to the full range of biological investigations, including scanning, electroencephalography (EEG) and clinical chemistry; a range of developmental assessments such as detailed speech pathology, occupational therapy and psychometric evaluation; and the opportunity for pediatric and neurological liaison. There are unique opportunities for observational studies in settings ranging from highly structured individual assessments to naturalistic observations during ward and school activities. Making best use of these opportunities requires good planning because important observations are often made by the least experienced staff and multiple assessments have to be integrated into a whole. One solution is to have structured assessment protocols for particular problems in which different staff have defined tasks towards a common end (Green, 1996). Assessments carried out in this way are always challenging – initial assumptions based on limited information can be examined critically in the light of different staff perspectives: this is one of the strengths of multidisciplinary working in the ward environment. Staff use specific skills from their core profession as well as skills developed within the team to serve these tasks – the team thus needs a program of generic skill development to meet the priorities of the unit.

Planning Treatment Goals

The concept of treatment goal planning was elegantly outlined by Shaw (1998) and has many attractive features. It acts to organize thinking and focus treatment in complex cases and counters therapeutic drift. However, it is deceptively simple and needs significant assessment and engagement with the family. Shaw suggested that treatment goals should be understandable, ideally framed in the child's own words, achievable and measurable; they are distinguished from the *staff hypothesis* (a professional formulation of the case) and the *treatment plan* established by the staff group on the basis of this hypothesis. Rothery, Wrate, McCabe, and Aspin (1995) made an audit of treatment goals in admissions to four adolescent units. They found that the majority of treatment goals reflected relationship and maturational aims rather than symptom change alone. Improvement across such goals was noted during treatment. Goals should be flexible enough to be able to evolve in potentially unexpected directions when necessary during treatment.

Adapting Treatments to the In-patient and Day Patient Settings

In addition to individualized treatments, there remain generic aspects of ward management. Behavioral management on any unit is a key area, requiring ward policies on the management of aggression, use of seclusion or restraint, bullying and runaway behavior (AACAP, 2000). Minimization of problems begins with a thorough initial risk assessment and treatment planning, but equal emphasis needs to be placed on the overall culture of the unit, staff behavior and the ongoing use of social skills and anger-management programs (Cotton, 1993; Higgins & Burke, 1998). The AACAP review commented that the trend to brief treatment stays can undermine such a culture. Luiselli, Bastien, and Putnam (1998) applied a behavioral analysis to incidents of mechanical restraint in a US unit and concluded that such extreme measures were often the result of a failure of preplanning, unit policy or staff awareness. Antecedents to restraint were commonly an escalation of conflict initiated by staff behavior rather than child behavior and based on unrealistic staff expectations of child compliance. The authors advocated a comprehensive functional assessment, proactive treatment planning and the use of short time-out procedures in which the child has control as to duration. When prevention fails, crisis intervention techniques can range from de-escalation strategies and seclusion to brief carefully trained physical holding. More controversial techniques include use of medication and mechanical restraint (papoose boards or holding blankets) but these are contraindicated for younger children or when there is previous trauma related to confinement (AACAP, 2000). There are no comparative studies of the relative value of these techniques and the whole area is relatively under-researched and subject to clinical fashion (Angold & Pickles, 1993). However, careful reviews of available evidence and explicit clinical guidelines such as those from the AACAP form the best current safeguard for patients and professionals alike.

Individual treatments such as cognitive–behavioral therapy (CBT) and individual psychotherapy are incorporated into individualized treatment planning. The trend towards shorter treatment stays favors brief and focal treatments such as CBT. The detailed assessments provided by individual psychotherapy have continuing value but there are particular challenges in adapting psychotherapeutic treatment techniques to the modern treatment milieu when stays are relatively short (Leibenluft, Tasman, & Green, 1993; Magnagna, 1998). The challenge of mounting family therapy in the context of a busy in-patient unit has been reviewed by Lask and Maynerd (1998). Pre-admission family functioning has been found to be a predictor of health gain during treatment in a number of studies (Pfeiffer & Strzelecki, 1990) but Green, Kroll, Imre *et al.* (2001) found in one study that family functioning did not improve during admission. An option may be for the formal family therapy to take place at the local site of referral in partnership with the in-patient team. The ward staff provide a form of psychological care which inevitably has elements of substitute parenting, especially for younger children, and have the opportunity to pioneer the development of specialized forms of care for extreme difficulties. In wards taking multiple diagnostic groups, flexibility and thoughtfulness are needed; the management of a behaviorally disturbed child with attachment disorder will be very different to superficially similar behaviors in a child with pervasive developmental disorder or obsessive-compulsive disorder (OCD).

Consent and Motivation

The United Nations Convention on the Rights of the Child (UNICEF, 1995) and national legislation with regard to children (e.g., the UK Children Act; White, Carr, & Lowe, 1990) have significant implications for practice. The trend is for consent to be increasingly explicit, treatment-specific and involving of the child. Developmental issues around competency have been reviewed (Shaw, 1998). Within residential units, the social and linguistic impairments of patients, described elsewhere in this chapter, need to be carefully considered. In a useful study of competency in a consecutive series of 25 psychiatric child in-patients, Billick, Edwards, Burget, Serlen, and Bruni (1998) found that "legal competency" (the ability to understand legal rights and the principle of consent) was associated with the achievement of a 5th or 6th grade (year 12 equivalent) reading level.

Another principle of consent should be collaboration with parents. A generic consent to treatment can be obtained early in admission in conjunction with treatment goal planning, based on what is likely to happen within a particular program of care. Such an approach combines the best principles of both consent and treatment goal planning. In the case of enforced treatment, there is debate as to whether it is best to use various aspects of children's legislation or adult-orientated mental health legislation in particular circumstances (see chapter 8).

The Staff Team

As treatment approaches become more sophisticated, the staff team in both in-patient and day patient care have increasingly complex tasks to perform. In many countries, nurses with mental health and/or pediatric qualifications form the main ward staff group but play specialists, trainee psychologists and volunteers can also usefully add to the skill mix. Guidance from both the USA (AACAP, 1990) and the UK (Royal College of Psychiatrists, 1999) emphasized the wide variety of other professionals that should be represented in well-run in-patient or day patient units: consultant child and adolescent psychiatrists; social workers; psychologists; speech and language therapists; occupational therapists; family therapists; and psychotherapists. Attempts to operate with too few staff are a recipe for stress, burnout and institutional decay. Staff numbers are best discussed in "shift ratios" (number of staff per shift) or in sessional terms, because this allows application to diverse unit functioning. For nursing staff, factors influencing the shift ratio include skill mix, the task demands of a particular shift (from low-intensity observation at night to high-intensity active therapy) and patient dependency (Table 69.1). Units caring for those with diverse disorders need more intensive staff ratios. Furlong and Ward (1997) piloted a dependency measure that shows predictable weekly fluctuations and interactions with staffing levels and quality of care. American and UK guidelines (AACAP, 1990; Royal College of Psychiatrists, 1999) recommend nursing shift ratios of 1:3 for low-intensity activities rising to 1:2 for active treatment and 1:1 for intensive care. Recommendations for other staff include 1 whole time equivalent (WTE) consultant per 10–12 bedded unit, up to 1 WTE in clinical psychology and up to 0.5 WTE sessional inputs from social work, psychotherapy, family therapy and occupational therapy. The UK recommendation for specialized teaching is 1 teacher to 4 students per lesson.

Table 69.1 Factors indicating the need for higher shift ratios. [After Cotton, 1993 with permission.]

1 Patient heterogeneity
   - Greater number of patients
   - Broader range of ages
   - Variation in levels of developmental functioning and diagnosis (e.g., combining cognitively impaired or psychotic children with brighter, behaviorally disordered children)
2 Case severity
   - Greater severity and pervasiveness of impairments
   - Severity of symptoms, such as suicidality, aggressiveness, sexualization
3 Lack of family or support systems outside the hospital
4 Poor therapeutic alliance (e.g., families with statutory orders or referred from courts)
5 Frequent staff turnover
6 Shorter lengths of stay (more acute admissions and an inability to develop routines and relationships)

Models of team management and functioning vary with the style of the unit. A popular current style is a model of "matrix management," which combines different disciplines with multiple tasks in a flat hierarchy with task-focused "mini teams" (Maskey, 1998). Whatever the organization, responsive and adequate staff supervision is vital.

Effectiveness of In-patient and Day Patient Treatment

Generic Outcomes

In-patient and day units are considered as a single entity for the purposes of administrative planning and therapeutic organization, and most studies have investigated generic outcomes across a range of disorders. Pfeiffer and Strzelecki (1990) reported a meta-analysis of 34 such in-patient outcome studies; there have been subsequent reviews (Curry, 1991; Pottick, Hansell, Gaboda *et al.*, 1993) and individual reports. These studies pointed to the overall efficacy of in-patient care and have been able to identify predictors of outcome. However, the reviews have also highlighted significant methodological limitations. Few early studies included control groups or standardized outcome measures and sample sizes have often been insufficient to overcome problems of patient heterogeneity. Pottick, Hansell, Gaboda *et al.* (1993) argued for more experimental designs to investigate the value of the residential component of care against other components, and prospective randomized trials of in-patient versus other forms of treatment for particular disorders are now beginning to appear (see p. 1136). Outcome measurement is also becoming more sophisticated with "triangulation" methods to measure multiple perspectives on outcome (Jensen, Hoagwood, & Petti, 1996). Use of change-sensitive common methodologies in the future will greatly help the field. It will also be necessary to be creative in the variables measured; markers such as social competency may be more relevant for treatment and outcome than diagnostic groupings *per se*. Grizenko, Papineau, and Sayegh (1993), in a study of multimodal day treatment for children with disruptive behavior problems, found that compared with a waitlist control group, day treatment produced significantly greater improvement in behavior, and that this was maintained at 6-month follow-up.

Predictors of Outcome

Pfeiffer and Strzelecki (1990) identified a number of predictors of in-patient outcome in their meta-analysis, which have received support and extension in subsequent studies. However, the design limitation of these studies must again be emphasized. By contemporary standards of evidence, these older studies do not robustly establish the causal link between admission and outcome or test predictor variables against other possible explanations. More recent study designs have begun to address these limitations. High levels of aggressive antisocial behavior and "organicity" of *symptoms*, as in schizophrenia, predict poor outcome; emotional disorders do better. *Well-organized treatment*, *multimodal treatment*, *positive alliance* and good *aftercare* are common predictors (Grizenko, Papineau, & Sayegh, 1993). *Intelligence* measured as IQ shows a moderate positive effect, but the study of Luthar, Woolston, Sparrow *et al.* (1995) suggested that functional achievement may be a more critical variable than IQ per se. Pretreatment *family functioning* is a strong predictor of outcome but the effects may be complex and disorder-specific. In a study of anorexia nervosa, North, Gowers, and Byram (1997) found that the child's perception of family functioning was prognostic but parents' perception was not. *Gender*, *age* and *emergency or elective admission* were found to have little predictive value.

Length of Stay (LOS) had only a modest association with outcome in Pfeiffer and Strzelecki's (1990) review. However, interest in treatment lengths has been increased by the rapid progress in the USA and elsewhere towards managed care and very short hospital stays. Influences on LOS are complex. A retrospective case note study of pre-admission variables in 100 children in one private US unit (Gold, Shera, & Clarkson, 1993) found that longer LOS was predicted by greater global impairment, post-traumatic symptoms and psychosocial stressors; diagnosis of adjustment disorder predicted shorter stays. In contrast, Christ, Tsernberis, and Andrew (1989) found that LOS was predicted by funding constraints or unit philosophy rather than diagnosis. In a multi-unit study, Green, Jacobs, Beecham *et al.* (2007) showed that longer treatment stays were associated with improved outcome independent of diagnosis and when other factors were controlled using robust standard errors. Because of the size of the sample ($n = 155$) and the variation in LOS between the units, this may be a salient finding. The clinical lore that symptoms often decline rapidly early in an admission and then worsen – the "honeymoon" effect – was supported by LaBarbera and Dozier (1985), who showed symptom increase from early to late in admission. No measure of preadmission symptomatology was made here but the authors argued that shortening admissions beyond a certain limit might well produce spurious health gains based on symptom inhibition early in admission. Alternatively, the fact of admission may relieve contextual causes of symptoms in the young person's environment and the early symptom reduction may be a valid effect – but the work needed to maintain these positive changes into discharge will take longer.

Outcome for Specific Disorders

Eating Disorders

There is unresolved debate on the value of in-patient treatment for eating disorders. The anxiety that these disorders induce, the issues around control and the significant mortality often combine to produce a desire for admission as a safe option. Adolescents themselves often resist admission and some of the extreme behavioral methods previously used on units to promote eating continue to cause anger when patients recount their experiences (Shelley, 1997). On the other hand, the residential experience can be therapeutically powerful. Studies of the outcome of in-patient treatment show widely differing results. Steinhausen and Seidel (1993) followed 50 patients over 5 years and found a 68% recovery rate, with 14% still diagnosable with eating disorder. Saccomani, Savoini, Cirrincione, Vercellino, and Ravera (1998) followed 81 children over 9 years and found a 53% good outcome. A comparison of out-patient and in-patient treatment (Crisp, Norton, Gowers *et al.*, 1991; Gowers, Weetman, Shore, Hossain, & Elvins, 2000) showed little additional benefit from in-patient care, and in a recent large randomized study no significant difference was found between in-patient and assertive out-patient arms in weight outcomes (Gowers, Weetman, Shore *et al.*, personal communication).

Depression and Suicidality

Admission practice following suicide attempts shows great regional variation. A recent large study found that, for similar presentations, 39% of cases in the USA were admitted compared with 12% in Europe (Safer, 1996). There are no studies directly comparing hospitalization with other forms of post-overdose care although an evidence-based review (Hawton, Arensman, & Townsend, 1998) recommended that psychiatric admission should *not* be the intervention of first choice for self-harm (see chapter 40).

A number of recent uncontrolled studies have investigated suicide risk following in-patient treatment of depression or suicidality. Of 111 emergency admissions, 20% remained depressed and suicidal at 2–4-year follow-up (Ivarsson, Larsson, & Gillberg, 1998), 18% of 100 patients admitted with depression reported suicidal behavior at 6-month follow-up (King, Segal, Kaminski, & Naylor, 1995) and 25% of 180 similar admissions attempted suicide within 5 years of discharge (Goldston, Sergent-Daniel, Reboussin *et al.*, 1999). Predictors of ongoing symptoms were suicide attempts prior to hospitalization, high levels of depressive symptomatology and family dysfunction at in-patient assessment.

Psychosis

Adolescents with first-onset psychotic illness will commonly be admitted but there are no studies comparing admission with alternative forms of treatment at this stage. One study of 58 adolescents admitted with psychotic disorder showed that 78% were continuously ill at follow-up after 2 years (Cawthron, James, Dell, & Seagroatt, 1994).

Conduct Disorder

The presence of unsocialized aggressive or disruptive behaviors at presentation is a consistent predictor of poor outcome for in-patient treatment (Green, Jacobs, Beecham *et al.*, 2007; Pfeiffer & Strzelecki, 1990). However, this reflects the general prognosis for these disorders. Conduct disorder is a specific exclusion criterion in some units but accounted for 25% of child admissions overall in a study of UK child psychiatry units (Green & Jacobs, 1998) and 15% of children and adolescents referred to Finnish in-patient units in 1990 and 1993 (Sourander & Turunen, 1999). In a recent UK study of eight units, conduct and aggression were associated with worsened ward milieu and shorter stays. Current evidence suggests that the management of conduct disorder is best seen in terms of long-term maintenance rather than episodes of care and the contextual basis of much of the symptomatology supports community intervention as a first-choice treatment. In spite of these arguments, and the often disruptive effect of such children on the milieu, there is good indication for admitting selected patients: for assessment when there are concerns about covert underlying comorbidity relevant to treatment (e.g., ADHD, emotional disorder, pervasive developmental disorder, specific learning disability or subclinical seizures; Jacobs, 1998); or when a trial of treatment is needed within a controlled setting.

Children with disruptive disorders receiving a multimodal day program showed improvements in adjustment at 5-year follow-up (Grizenko, 1997). Another multimodal day program (Rey, Denshire, Wever *et al.*, 1998) also showed improvement over matched controls who had received other treatments; however, both groups showed poor outcome. In a study of in-patient treatment of adolescents with emotional and conduct disorder, patients who completed the treatment showed more progress 1 month post-discharge than patients who were early dropouts, but these differences had become insignificant at 1- and 2-year follow-up (Wells & Faragher, 1993).

Substance Misuse

A number of in-patient and day patient addiction programs have been evaluated. Of 280 adolescents treated in a substance abuse in-patient program (Dobkin, Chabot, Maliantovitch, & Craig, 1998), 67 subjects completed 1-month follow-up questionnaires; 19 had improved and 48 had not. The improvers tended to be older with better motivation for social adjustment and less emotional symptomatology; those who did worse were distinguished by more mental state abnormalities at admission. Cornwall and Blood (1998) compared in-patient with day patient programs in this area and found they showed similar outcomes. A random allocation trial comparing in-patient with intensive community treatment of adolescents with substance misuse and juvenile offending (Schoenwald, Ward, Henggeler, & Pickrel, 1996) showed additional benefits for the community treatment. Freeman, Garrick, Kreisher *et al.* (1993) report a matched study comparing long-term out-patient treatment with short-term in-patient treatment and found benefits in the longer-term out-patient treatment.

Obsessive-Compulsive Disorder

In a prospective naturalistic study, Wever and Rey (1997) examined the effectiveness of combined CBT and psychopharmacology in a group of 57 children and adolescents first diagnosed with OCD, 20% of whom received in-patient treatment. Factors leading to admission included the severity and type of OCD symptoms, the failure of past therapy, comorbidity, family factors and geographical isolation. The in-patient group had double the rate of comorbid diagnoses compared with the out-patient group and showed a poorer outcome.

Alternatives to In-patient Care

Historical Development

Over the last 40 years changing philosophical beliefs among educators and health professionals (Bracken & Thomas, 2002) have led to a movement away from residential psychiatric care in the UK, Europe and North America (Smyth & Hoult, 2000). Reforms in US mental health policy (including the introduction of Medicare, Medicaid and the Supplemental Security Income program) encouraged policy-makers to discharge patients to the community and transfer state mental health costs to the federal government. Systemization of the Child and Adolescent Service System Program (England & Cole, 1992) opened up discussion among in-patient service providers about how best to meet the complex needs of children and young people (Burns & Friedman, 1990). A range of alternative community-based services were then developed, many now systematically evaluated (Henggeler, Rodick, Borduin *et al.*, 1986). In general, evidence-based changes to mental health care have underpinned reform of psychiatric service provision for adults and young people, and intensive home-based treatments are central to these changes (McGorry, 2005).

In the UK, the development and evaluation of psychiatric intensive home treatment has somewhat lagged behind the US developments (Smyth & Hoult, 2000). However, a commitment to tackling the links between mental illness and social deprivation has been made explicit in the National Service Frameworks for Mental Health (Department of Health, 1999) and for Children (Department of Health, 2003), which challenge health professionals to widen their approaches to care. A review of home-treatment studies (Joy, Adams, & Rice, 2004) found that patient and relative satisfaction was higher in home care compared with admission in adults and that carers found home care less disruptive and burdensome. Recent surveys showed that young people and families want CAMHS to be delivered flexibly (Baruch & James, 2003) and in a variety of settings, including the home (National Service Framework for Children, 2004).

Current Developments

In adult mental health services a range of treatment models are now used, sometimes specifically to reduce the need for hospitalization, sometimes to allow more patient choice and active involvement in care (Department of Health, 1999; Priebe, Fakhoury, White *et al.*, 2004). These include assertive community treatment (Wright, Burns, James *et al.*, 2003), case management (Burns, Fioritti, Holloway, Malm, & Rossler, 2001a) and home treatment (Burns, Knapp, Catty *et al.*, 2001b), all of which have the aim of providing increased support and care for the mentally ill within their own homes so that hospitalization can be avoided where possible. However, the disorders for which young people – especially children – are admitted vary greatly from those in adults, as does the developmental context. Thus, direct comparisons with adult psychiatry can be misleading. Assertive outreach, case management and wraparound models have been adapted for use in child services but there has also been the development of developmentally specific models, such as treatment foster care and multisystemic therapy. The heterogeneity of these initiatives makes comparison difficult, although they tend to share common features (e.g., the importance of the family and social context, the complex needs of young people and families, multimodal interventions and the understanding of outcomes as being multifaceted). The services with which home treatment is compared are often poorly defined as "standard care," which can vary enormously from study to study (Burns, Knapp, Catty *et al.*, 2001b). Furthermore, the majority of the studies focus on young people not at the highest risk (often the acutely suicidal or psychotic are excluded) and therefore results may not be generalizable outside of a specific and narrow patient group. While most studies report that effective systems of care can be developed in the community (Henggeler, Rodick, Borduin *et al.*, 1986), other work suggests that outcomes may not always be substantially improved (Burns, Farmer, Angold, Costello, & Behar, 1996).

Models of Out-of-Hospital Care

Family Preservation

Family Preservation is a home-based intensive service for families who need additional support beyond typical out-patient services. It can be used as a transitional service for families with children returning home from psychiatric admission, or to prevent admission. The aims are to improve parenting skills, promote healthy child development, prevent out-of-home placement of children and provide or co-ordinate services needed to maintain family stability. The therapists make contact with the family several times a week, providing assessment and treatment, and access to educational and practical resources. Family Preservation services are usually limited to weeks in duration. However, family contact with therapists is intensive during this time, almost double that in residential units (Wilmshurst, 2002). A randomized controlled trial of young people allocated to either Family Preservation or a 5-day residential program found that at 1-year follow-up more of the Family Preservation group had sustained the improvements in behavior and the symptom reduction than had those in the residential program (Wilmshurst, 2002).

Home Treatment

Home treatment can be summarized as a service for young people with mental illness who are in crisis and are eligible for hospital admission. Features of an effective home treatment team are 24 h a day, 7 days a week availability; rapid response time; and the ability to work flexibly with families and their networks (Smyth & Hoult, 2000). In a series of studies from Germany, home treatment was compared with "standard" in-patient treatment. The first study (Remschmidt, Schmidt, Mattejat, Eisert, & Eisert, 1988) randomly allocated young people to home treatment or admission; it found that the baseline severity of symptoms was similar for both treatment groups, and that immediate treatment effects were similar. However, only about 15% of young people could safely be diverted from in-patient to home treatment, exclusion criteria for the home treatment arm being severe psychosis, life-threatening eating disorders, families living more than 30 km from the therapeutic unit and risk-taking behavior. Mattejat, Hirt, Wilken, Schmidt, and Remschmidt (2001) conducted a re-analysis and 3-year follow-up of these data. They contacted 68 of the original 92 families (in-patient $n = 33$, home treatment $n = 35$). Baseline symptom scores and psychosocial functioning were similar for both groups. Home treatment was found to be as effective as in-patient treatment across diagnoses in reducing symptom scores and improving psychosocial functioning, both immediately after treatment and at 3-year follow-up. The longer-term treatment effect declined somewhat, to an equal extent in both groups. Compliance of the child with the therapeutic regime and the skill of the therapist were the most important predictors of treatment outcome. The study suggested that, even if community treatment is an effective alternative to admission, it could only be used for a small proportion of all possible admissions, a finding also reported by others (Woolston, Berkowitz, Schaefer, & Adnopoz, 1998).

Case Management

Case management encompasses a number of approaches including assertive outreach, assertive community treatment, wraparound and intensive community treatments. It can be defined as "a commonly used strategy for increasing access to and coordination of services within the care system" (Farmer, Dorsey, & Mustillo, 2004). Case management in a child and adolescent mental health setting assigns the coordination and responsibility of care for an individual young person with a serious mental illness to a single person (or team). Case managers may be responsible for a variety of tasks, ranging from linking young people and families to services to providing intensive clinical or rehabilitative services. Other core functions include outreach to engage clients in services, assessing individual needs, arranging support services (such as education, careers advice, family benefits), monitoring medication and advocating for young people's rights. Case management is not a time-limited service, but is intended to be ongoing, providing clients with whatever they need whenever they need it, for as long as necessary. This is a controversial point, as some authors feel that the "never discharge" philosophy encourages pathologizing of normal behaviors and re-invention of some of the worst practices of the old asylums, a *de facto* "institutionalization" in the community (Smith, 1999). Case management has been adopted in the UK, Germany and Sweden, but not in all European countries (Burns, Fioritti, Holloway *et al.*, 2001a).

The two models of case management described most often are assertive community treatment (ACT) and intensive case management. A third model, clinical case management, refers to a program where the case manager assigned to a client also functions as their primary therapist, generally considered to be less effective (Burns, Farmer, Angold *et al.*, 1996).

The *assertive outreach/community treatment model* for adults originated in an in-patient research unit at Mendota State Hospital, Madison, Wisconsin in the late 1960s (Stein & Test, 1980) in an attempt to create a "hospital without walls." In the UK, it is now part of the national mental health policy for adults (Department of Health, 2003) with over 200 teams, but in Europe it has not developed to the same extent (Bonsack, Adam, Haefliger, Besson, & Conus, 2005). The key features of ACT are multidisciplinary teams, 24 h a day, 365 days a year care; low client : staff ratios; an emphasis on assertive outreach; provision of *in vivo* services (in the client's own setting); an emphasis on assisting the client in managing their illness; assistance with activities of daily living (ADL) skills; emphasis on relationship building; and crisis intervention. The interventions are strengths-based and focused on promoting symptom stability, increasing the individual's ability to cope and relate to others. Adult patients are rarely discharged (Smith, 1999) and this may lead to everyday difficulties being reframed as symptoms or dissuade commissioners and providers from developing ACT services (Bonsack, Adam, Haefliger *et al.*, 2005).

In the UK, assertive outreach is a requirement for adults of working age only (Office of the Deputy Prime Minister, 2004) although as Early Intervention in Psychosis teams become more common and report on their outcomes this situation will change. Much of the evidence for the effectiveness of assertive outreach is from studies with overlapping age groups of young people and working age adults. Broadly, assertive outreach in young and working age adults is effective (Marshall & Lockwood, 2004; Minghella, Ford, Freeman *et al.*, 1999) despite concerns that fidelity to the model is not always adhered to. Good quality assertive outreach studies have shown that assertive outreach is effective with young adults with early psychosis, the treatment effect size is similar to that of in-patient care, in-patient admission can often be avoided without increasing risk of critical incidents, and it can be highly cost-effective (Craig, Garety, Power *et al.*, 2004). Whether it is more effective than "standard" community care is debatable, with mixed findings perhaps related to many community mental health teams being able to provide the "assertive" component for young adults when required. Two randomized studies of only young people report that compared with those who received standard community care, young people who received assertive outreach were more likely to access and continue using services, had better family relationships and fewer psychiatric symptoms (Evans, Boothroyd, Armstrong *et al.*, 2003; Godley, Godley, Dennis, Funk, & Passetti, 2002). Service user views of young people and their families suggest that assertive community treatment is useful and valued (White, Godley, & Passetti, 2004), although this should be taken with caution as it was based on young people with substance abuse problems and may not be generalizable.

Intensive case management typically targets young people with the greatest service needs. It shares many key features with ACT, but relies more on an individual than team approach. In addition, intensive case managers are more likely to "broker" treatment and rehabilitation services rather than provide them directly. Finally, intensive case management focuses more on family strengths and empowering families. Case managers act as advocates and brokers between services, and coordinate, plan and implement services.

Clinical case management is one of the intensive case management models but has the weakest effect of the models. An aggregation of studies comparing ACT with clinical case management found that while the generic approach resulted in increased hospital admissions, it significantly decreased the length of stay. This suggests that the overall impact of clinical case management is positive but might result in "revolving door" admissions. However, randomized trials have shown full-time case manager models to be perceived as more satisfactory and allow young people to access community rather than residential-based services, compared with treatment models where the primary worker or therapist also acts as case manager (Burns, Farmer, Angold *et al.*, 1996).

Wraparound helps families develop a plan to address the child's individual needs at home and school (Burns, Schoenwald, Burchard, Faw, & Santos, 2000). Research on the effectiveness of this model is still at an early stage. Wraparound addresses a child's individual needs and builds on the child's and family's strengths, so the exact services vary. The services are provided through teams that link children, families and foster parents and their support networks with child welfare, health, mental health, education and the criminal justice services to develop and implement comprehensive support plans. Findings suggest that this broker/advocacy model results in behavioral improvements and fewer days in hospital. A randomized controlled trial of treatment foster care versus case management (with wraparound components) found that outcomes were better for young people in case management interventions than for treatment foster care and at one-third of the cost (Evans, Armstrong, Kuppinger, Huz, & Johnson, 1998). More radically, families or volunteers sometimes act as case managers in wraparound care, although this is probably more as a result of lack of support and funding than a philosophical step forward.

Multisystemic Therapy

Multisystemic therapy (MST) was developed as an intensive approach to juvenile offenders presenting with serious antisocial behaviors and who were at risk of being placed out-of-home (see chapter 68). It is an intensive family and community-based treatment program (Henggeler, Rodick, Borduin *et al.*, 1986) designed to make positive changes in the various social systems (home, school, community, peers) that contribute to the serious antisocial behaviors of children and adolescents. It is based on the work of systems theorists such as Haley and Minuchin. Time-limited (4–6 months), it adheres strictly to a treatment manual with nine treatment principles, and relies for success on adherence to the treatment model and ongoing training of staff to this end (Henggeler, Schoenwald, Borduin, Rowland, & Cunningham, 1998). The main purpose of assessment is to understand the fit between the identified problems and their broader systemic context (Henggeler, Schoenwald, Borduin *et al.*, 1998). Interventions are designed to promote treatment generalization and long-term maintenance of therapeutic change by empowering caregivers to address family members' needs across multiple systemic contexts. Outcome studies show that staff adherence to the treatment model correlates to strong case outcomes (Henggeler, Rowland, Halliday-Boykins *et al.*, 2003).

MST has a relatively strong evidence base (Farmer, Dorsey & Mustillo, 2004). Consistently positive outcomes are reported for young offenders compared with standard out-patient treatment (reduced offending, fewer out-of-home placements, less substance-related offending). Randomized controlled trials and pooling of previously conducted studies demonstrated significant symptom improvement in psychiatrically ill young people receiving MST compared with standard care (Curtis, Ronan & Bourdin, 2004; Henggeler, Rowland, Halliday-Boykins *et al.*, 2003; Schoenwald, Ward, Henggeler, & Rowland, 2000). However, at 12-month follow-up, the two treatment approaches yielded similar results. Schoenwald, Ward, Henggeler *et al.* (1996) randomized MST against service as usual for adolescent substance abusers. The MST treatment resulted in a 46% decrease in the need for residential care at 1-year follow-up and succeeded in reducing dramatically the rate of imprisonment for substance abuse and abuse-related in-patient stays. The cost savings made through this almost compensated for the increased cost of the MST treatment.

A recent randomized trial (Henggeler, Rowland, Randall *et al.*, 1999) compared MST with brief hospitalization for a diverse group of adolescent psychiatric emergencies in a relatively disadvantaged population. MST was given for 4 months whereas hospitalization was for 2 weeks only, followed by standard community aftercare. The MST condition involved a mean of 97.1 h of therapy contact time during the study and 24 h, 7 days a week availability of staff. Staff had a caseload of three cases each and there was high-frequency psychiatric supervision. By comparison, the hospitalization condition had a mean contact time of 8.5 h subsequent to the admission period. Nearly half of the young people in the MST condition in fact needed psychiatric admission in the initial period and MST only had the effect of reducing out-of-home placement by 50% through the whole study. Given these methodological qualifications, the MST had a significantly greater effect than hospitalization on disruptive behavior and targeted social outcomes such as enhanced family cohesion, structure and school attendance. Family and youth satisfaction was also higher. The hospital condition showed a significantly greater impact on youth self-esteem – a result that may reflect the individually orientated treatment model in the hospital group. No follow-up data beyond 4 months are reported. The study concluded that even this highly intense form of ecologically focused care does not substitute for the need for in-patient provision – but it can reduce the need, and results in enhanced outcomes over treatment as usual. It was unfortunate for the design of the study that there was such an imbalance between the treatment intensity in the two conditions. The study – important as it is – does not yet address the question of the relative value of the residential component *per se*.

Treatment Foster Care

Treatment foster care (TFC) is one of the least restrictive treatment-based residential options for young people with emotional or disruptive disorders (Farmer, Dorsey, & Mustillo, 2004). It comprises structured therapy within a foster family setting, delivered with a multiagency approach. Theoretically, TFC is largely based on social learning theory. TFC programs recruit, train and support foster families, who usually only look after one fostered child. The families are closely supervised and supported, and receive a monthly salary. TFC specialists work with the child and foster parent on identified goals 1–2 h per week. This work is supervised by a mental health practitioner, who also meets with the foster-care family frequently (every 1 to 2 weeks) to coordinate services and ensure the treatment plan is being followed. TFC programs also prepare the child for successful transition to return home. TFC differs from standard foster care in three ways:

1 Substantial training and supervision of foster parents by experienced case managers;
2 Detailed functional assessment and close monitoring of behaviors, their antecedents and consequences; and
3 Emphasis on "therapy."

The evidence base comes mainly from two well-reported randomized controlled trials undertaken by those who deliver the Oregon model (Chamberlain, 2002). Outcomes (improved behavior, reduced offending behavior) for both psychiatrically ill and offending young people were significantly better for those who received TFC than group home or hospital care. Outcomes were dependent on four main factors: the amount and type of supervision received by the young person; consistency of parental discipline; presence of a close, confiding relationship with a trusted adult; and not being closely linked with delinquent or deviant peers (Chamberlain, 2002).

Although most of the evidence base for TFC comes from its original proponents in Oregon, it has translated across the Atlantic successfully, albeit in an altered format (Brady, Harwin, Pugh, Scott, & Sinclair, 2005). Outcomes reported for young people in this project include: a greater stability in placements; an increase from 14% (on admission) to 71% in young people attending school. 21% showed significant improvements in their behavior and a further 25% some behavioral improvement. There was also a significant decrease in young people being cautioned or convicted of offenses with less than 1% receiving a custodial sentence. 21% young people returned home to their birth family and 10% moved to independent living. However, the level of professional and financial risk involved in a TFC project could only be sustained if it is based on a partnership agreement with one or more local authorities and CAMHS teams. A modified form of TFC is currently being implemented in the UK for looked-after children at risk of multiple placement breakdowns and is being systematically evaluated. Projects are also under way in Sweden, Finland and Holland.

Staffing

These intensive outreach models need much skilled professional time. In Woolston's (1998) model between three and five professional teams, consisting of two senior clinicians or counselors, provide the home-based assessment and therapeutic input. They are backed up by a multidisciplinary infrastructure described in the model as a program director and medical director, a child psychiatrist, a clinical program co-ordinator, two senior clinicians and an administrator. This staff level is quoted as sufficient for a caseload of 25 patients. The intensity of the involvement can vary according to need and expense but a 24 h, 7 day on-call crisis intervention service is provided throughout the duration of the input. In one study of MST (Schoenwald, Ward, Henggeler *et al.*, 1996), the average duration of treatment was 130 days (standard deviation [SD] 32 days), during which there was an average of 40 direct contact hours between professionals and family (range 12–187 h, SD 28 h). Woolston emphasized that the intensive home-based services are considered as supplementary to an array of more traditional services including in-patient and day patient hospitalization and out-patient programs.

Conclusions

There is now research evidence supporting the use of alternatives to in-patient care for certain groups of young people with mental health problems. The evidence suggests that, within these groups, treatment effects of several outreach models of care can be of similar size to those obtained through residential treatment, and may be sustained as long after follow-up. MST, TFC and assertive outreach have the strongest evidence bases, wraparound care the weakest. However, it should be remembered that the evidence for TFC is largely based on the model as delivered in Oregon solely, clearly limiting generalizability of the findings. Assertive outreach work is largely based on older adolescents and young adults, and comparisons with "standard" treatment do not reflect a fair comparison with CAMHS "standard" treatments, which arguably are already more "assertive" and "outreach" than standard adult mental health services. The evidence surrounding MST is now extending beyond use with antisocial behavior but still needs further work to demonstrate effectiveness in other disorders.

Therefore, there is not always the evidence to decide which model is best for which group of young people, and funding and service provision issues may not allow development of the chosen model, requiring pragmatic choices to be made by commissioners and providers. Little, Kohm, and Thompson (2005) rightly called for less ideology and more science. Comparative studies are needed to allow an informed decision about which type of care best fits the needs of which group of young people.

Future Directions

A number of contemporary themes and future directions may be summarized. The trend for shorter in-patient stays and the development of intensive care alternatives to residential treatment is likely to continue but there may well also emerge a reactive emphasis on the value of intensive residential treatment experience for selected conditions. The demand for adolescent units to respond to acute emergencies is likely to continue to grow as the severity of presenting psychopathology moves down the age range. In well-provided health services there may be increasing growth of specialist environments such as specialized eating disorder or forensic units. Referral to intensive care facilities is often thought to follow a bimodal pattern: high when there are relatively few out-patient services, lower as out-patient services are more developed, and higher again when out-patient provision becomes still better and more complex need is identified. This should not imply that the potential demand for intensive services is endless: epidemiological surveys of children with complex needs suggest that the pool of these problems in communities is finite and measurable (Kurtz, 1994).

At the complex end of the spectrum, young people are likely to be involved with multiple agencies (Kurtz, 1994). This implies another necessary development; a more sophisticated integration between mental health care, education and social services to form complementary and mutually supporting provision. Some children who now are admitted to in-patient psychiatric units may be better placed in residential social care institutions with psychiatric input or in specialist residential schools; some children in these other institutions may be better placed in primarily mental health facilities. Case management approaches have much to offer in coordinating these complex care pathways and need to be systematically tested.

The development of robust alternatives to in-patient care will make possible the ethical use of randomized controlled trials to compare residential, intensive day and outreach alternatives for particular groups or severity of problems. Along with this we can hope for an increasing delineation of methodologies to measure treatment process. The result of these two developments may be further clarification of the specific value of the different components of intensive treatment – for instance, the specific indications for admission. The current evidence suggests that the residential milieu has a particular ability to provide stabilization and rapid reduction of symptomatology and risk. In medium-term treatments it provides an environment in which treatment and rehabilitation can occur outside the demands of the home environment – this is the historical function of respite. Notwithstanding the efforts that have been made in recent years to engage effectively with families, the residential unit is inevitably largely focused on the individual and individual pathology. This can prove highly advantageous in situations where assessment or treatment of complex individual psychopathology is at a premium but needs to be complemented by an emphasis on the environmental context during pre-admission and follow-up. Reduction of in-patient stays beyond a certain minimum negates any value of the in-patient milieu as a treatment in its own right, but the very fact of removal from a noxious mental environment in the community of origin may still result in temporary benefit.

Intensive outreach programs have already generated impressive levels of rigorous treatment programming and evaluation. The face validity of this theory of intervention is strong and in keeping with recent research in the developmental psychopathology of a number of disorders. The emphasis on changing presumed maintaining factors in the young person's environment may result in longer stabilization of treatment gains – although this has not yet been tested. On the other hand, it should be quite apparent that these outreach solutions are no easy option, either financially or in terms of professional expertise. The first randomized trial including costing shows that the extra cost of the service only approaches being met if non-health cost savings are taken into account and there is evidence that the efficacy of the intervention drops if the intensity of the intervention is not adhered to (Henggeler, Schoenwald, Pickrel *et al.*, 1994). Nevertheless, early studies of intensive outreach models are impressive and are undergoing replication outside the developing centers. Most of the comparative studies suggest that intensive outreach does not replace the need for the in-patient option but can certainly reduce its usage. The emphasis in this treatment on the social context of psychopathology is a strength and complementary to in-patient care but runs the risk of overlooking intrinsic problems in the patient. There is no evidence to support the development of intensive services for young people with a specific disorder over the development of generic intensive services, although many of the studies of intensive work have focused on broad unitary disorder services, such as those working with young people with psychosis or substance misuse. The flexibility of intensive services to cross over traditional age ranges should be encouraged, running alongside the move in traditional out-patient CAMHS to extend the client age covered.

Day unit care may seem to be a compromise between these two extremes and may often usefully be so. For the most severe problems, however, it may fall between the two and offer insufficient containment for safety or intensive outreach for effectiveness. The great strength of the day unit resource is its flexibility to adapt to different disorders and circumstances. It is unrealistic to believe that the day unit provision can substitute for other intensive treatment modalities.

Thus, in an ideal future there would be a set of flexible and complementary platforms for the delivery of intensive care for acute and complex disorders. Service providers would identify themselves as "serious disorder" or "intensive care" services offering a variety of different modes of delivery. In practice, organization and financial constraints will inevitably lead health services to have to make preferred choices. There is now a greater likelihood that in the future an increased evidence base may inform such decisions.

References

American Academy of Child and Adolescent Psychiatry (AACAP). (1990). *Model for minimum staffing patterns for hospitals providing acute inpatient treatment for children and adolescents with psychiatric illnesses.* Washington, DC: American Academy of Child and Adolescent Psychiatry.

American Academy of Child and Adolescent Psychiatry (AACAP). (2000). *Practice parameter for the prevention and management of aggressive behavior in child and adolescent psychiatric institutions with special reference to seclusion and restraint. Draft 9.* Washington, DC: American Academy of Child and Adolescent Psychiatry.

Angold, A., & Pickles, A. (1993). Seclusion on an adolescent unit. *Journal of Child Psychology and Psychiatry, 34*, 975–990.

Asen, K., Stein, R., Stevens, A., McHugh, B., Greenwood, J., & Cooklin, A. (1982). A day unit for families. *Journal of Family Therapy, 4*, 345–358.

Baruch, G., & James, C. (2003). *The national framework for children, young people and maternity services: The mental health and psychological well-being of children and young people.* Report from Consultation with Users of Children and Adolescent Mental Health Services. London: Department of Health.

Bazeley, E. T. (1928). *Homer Lane and the Little Commonwealth.* London: George, Allen & Unwin.

Beskind, H. (1962). Psychiatric inpatient treatment of adolescents: A review of clinical experience. *Comprehensive Psychiatry, 3*, 354–369.

Bettelheim, B. (1955). *Truants from life.* New York: Free Press.

Billick, S. B., Edwards, J. L., Burget, W., Serlen, J. R., & Bruni, M. S. (1998). A clinical study of competency in child psychiatric in patients. *Journal of the American Academy of Psychiatry and the Law, 26*, 587–594.

Blanz, B., & Schmidt, M. H. (2000). Practitioner review: Preconditions and outcome of inpatient treatment in child and adolescent psychiatry. *Journal of Child Psychology and Psychiatry, 41*, 703–712.

Bonsack, C., Adam, L., Haefliger, T., Besson, J., & Conus, P. (2005). Difficult-to-engage patients: A specific target for time-limited assertive outreach in a Swiss setting. *Canadian Journal of Psychiatry, Revue Canadienne de Psychiatrie, 50*, 845–850.

Bracken, P., & Thomas, P. (2002). Editorial. Time to move beyond the mind–body split. *British Medical Journal, 325*, 1433–1434.

Brady, L., Harwin, J., Pugh, G., Scott, J., & Sinclair, R. (2005). *Specialist fostering for young people with challenging behaviour: Coram family's fostering new links project.* London: Coram Family with Brunel University and National Children's Bureau.

Bruggen, P., & O'Brien, C. (1987). *Helping families: Systems, residential and agency responsibility.* London: Faber & Faber.

Burns, B., Farmer, E., Angold, A., Costello, E., & Behar, L. (1996). A randomized trial of case management for youths with serious emotional disturbance. *Journal of Child Psychology and Psychiatry, 25*, 476–486.

Burns, B., & Friedman, R. (1990). Examining the research base for child mental health services and policy. *Journal of Mental Health Administration, 17*, 87–98.

Burns, B., Schoenwald, S., Burchard, J., Faw, L., & Santos, A. (2000). Comprehensive community-based interventions for youth with severe emotional disorders: Multisystemic therapy and the wrap-around process. *Journal of Child and Family Studies, 9*, 283–314.

Burns, T., Fioritti, A., Holloway, F., Malm, U., & Rossler, W. (2001a). Case management and assertive community treatment in Europe. *Psychiatric Services, 52*, 631–636.

Burns, T., Knapp, M., Catty, J., Healey, A., Henderson, J., Watt, H., *et al.* (2001b). Home treatment for mental health problems: A systematic review. *Health Technology Assessment, 5*, 1–139.

Cameron, K. A. (1949). A psychiatric inpatient department for children. *Journal of Mental Science, 95*, 560–566.

Cawthron, P., James, A., Dell, D., & Seagroatt, V. (1994). Adolescent onset psychosis: A clinical and outcome study. *Journal of Child Psychology and Psychiatry and Allied Disciplines, 35*, 1321–1332.

Chamberlain, P. (2002). Treatment foster care. In B. Burns, & K. Hoagwood (Eds.), *Community treatment for youth: Evidence-based interventions for severe emotional and behavioral disorders* (pp. 117–138). New York: Oxford University Press.

Christ, A., Tsernberis, S., & Andrew, H. (1989). Fiscal implications of a childhood disorder DRG. *Journal of the American Academy of Child and Adolescent Psychiatry, 28*, 729–733.

Cornwall, A., & Blood, L. (1998). Inpatient versus day treatment for substance abusing adolescents. *Journal of Nervous and Mental Disease, 186*, 580–582.

Costello, A. J., Dulcan, M. K., & Kalas, R. (1991). A checklist of hospitalisation criteria for use with children. *Hospital and Community Psychiatry, 42*, 823–828.

Cotgrove, A. (1997). Emergency admissions to a regional adolescent unit: Piloting a new service. *Psychiatric Bulletin, 21*, 604–608.

Cotton, N. S. (1993). *Lessons from the lion's den: Therapeutic management of children in psychiatric hospitals and treatment centers.* San Francisco, CA: Jossey-Bass.

Crisp, A. H., Norton, K., Gowers, S., Halek, C., Bowyer, C., Yeldham, D., *et al.* (1991). A controlled study of the effects of therapies aimed at adolescent and family psychopathology in anorexia nervosa. *British Journal of Psychiatry, 159*, 325–333.

Craig, T. J. K., Garety, P., Power, P., Rahaman, N., Colbert, S., Fornells-Ambrojo, M., *et al.* (2004). The Lambeth Early Onset (LEO) team: Randomised controlled trial of the effectiveness of specialised care for early psychosis. *British Medical Journal, 329*, 1067.

Curry, J. E. (1991). Outcome research on residential treatment: Implications and suggested directions. *American Journal of Psychiatry, 621*, 348–357.

Curtis, N. M., Ronan, K. R., & Bourdin, C. M. (2004). Multisystemic treatment: A meta-analysis of outcome studies. *Journal of Family Psychology, 18*, 411–419.

Department of Health. (1999). *The National Service Framework for Mental Health.* London: Department of Health.

Department of Health. (2003). *Getting the Right Start: National Service Framework for Children. Emerging Findings.* London: Department of Health.

Department of Health/Department for Education and Skills. (2004). *National Service Framework for Children, Young People and Maternity Services.* London: DH/DfES.

Dobkin, P. L., Chabot, L., Maliantovitch, K., & Craig, W. (1998). Predictors of outcome in drug treatment of adolescent inpatients. *Psychological Reports, 83*, 175–186.

Ellila, H., Sourander, A., Valimaki, M., & Piha, J. (2005). Characteristics and staff resources of child and adolescent psychiatric hospital wards in Finland. *Journal of Psychiatric and Mental Health Nursing, 12*, 209–214.

England, M., & Cole, R. (1992). Building systems of care for youth with serious mental illness. *Hospital and Community Psychiatry, 43*, 630–633.

Evans, M. E., Armstrong, M., Kuppinger, A., Huz, S., & Johnson, S. (1998). *A randomized trial of family-centered intensive case management and family-based treatment: Final report.* Tampa, FL: University of South Florida.

Evans, M., Boothroyd, R., Armstrong, M., Greenbaum, P., Borwn, E., & Kuppinger, A. (2003). An experimental study of the effectiveness of intensive in-home crisis services for children and their families: Program outcomes. *Journal of Emotional and Behavioural Disorders, 11*, 93–104.

Farmer, E. M. Z., Dorsey, S., & Mustillo, S. A. (2004). Intensive home and community interventions. *Child and Adolescent Psychiatric Clinics of North America*, *13*, 857–884.

Friedman, A. S., Granick, S., Kreisher, C., & Terras, A. (1993). Addiction and treatment. *American Journal of Addictions*, 2, 232–237.

French, W., & Tate, A. (1998). Educational management. In J. M. Green, & B. W. Jacobs (Eds.), *Inpatient child psychiatry: Modern practice research and the future* (pp. 143–155). London: Routledge.

Furlong, S., & Ward, M. (1997). Assessing patient dependency and staff skill mix. *Nursing Standard*, *11*, 33–38.

Godley, M., Godley, S., Dennis, M., Funk, R., & Passetti, L. (2002). Preliminary outcomes from the assertive continuing care experiment for adolescents discharged from residential treatment. *Journal of Substance Abuse Treatment*, *23*, 21–32.

Gold, J., Shera, D., & Clarkson, B. (1993). Private psychiatric hospitalization of children: Predictors of length of stay. *Journal of the American Academy of Child and Adolescent Psychiatry*, *32*, 135–144.

Goldston, D. B., Sergent-Daniel, S., Reboussin, D. M., Reboussin, B. A., Frazier, P. H., & Kelley, A. E. (1999). Suicide attempts among formerly hospitalized adolescents: A prospective naturalistic study of risk during the first 5 years. *Journal of the American Academy of Child and Adolescent Psychiatry*, *38*, 660–671.

Gowers, S. G., & Kushlick, A. (1992). Customer satisfaction in adolescent psychiatry. *Journal of Mental Health*, *1*, 353–362.

Gowers, S. G., Weetman, J., Shore, A., Hossain, F., & Elvins, R. (2000). Impact of hospitalisation on the outcome of adolescent anorexia nervosa. *British Journal of Psychiatry*, *176*, 138–141.

Green, J. M. (1994). Child in-patient treatment and family relationships. *Psychiatric Bulletin*, *18*, 744–747.

Green, J. M. (1996). A structured assessment of parenting based on attachment theory: Theoretical background, description and initial clinical experience. *European Journal of Child and Adolescent Psychiatry*, *5*, 133–138.

Green, J. M. (2006). The therapeutic alliance: A significant but neglected variable in child mental health treatment studies. *Journal of Child Psychology and Psychiatry*, *47*, 425–435.

Green, J. M., & Burke, M. (1998). The ward as a therapeutic agent. In J. M. Green, & B. W. Jacobs (Eds.), *Inpatient child psychiatry: Modern practice, research and the future* (pp. 93–110). London: Routledge.

Green, J. M., & Jacobs, B. W. (1998). Current practice: A questionnaire survey of inpatient child psychiatry in the UK. In J. M. Green, & B. W. Jacobs (Eds.), *Inpatient child psychiatry: Modern practice, research and the future* (pp. 9–22). London: Routledge.

Green, J. M., & Jones, D. (1998). Unwanted effects of inpatient treatment: Anticipation, prevention, repair. In J. M. Green, & B. W. Jacobs (Eds.), *Inpatient child psychiatry: Modern practice, research and the future* (pp. 212–220). London: Routledge.

Green, J. M., Jacobs, B. W., Beecham, J., Dunn, G., Kroll, L., Tobias, C., *et al.* (2007). Inpatient treatment in child and adolescent psychiatry: A prospective study of health gain and costs. *Journal of Child Psychology and Psychiatry, and Allied Disciplines*, *48*, 1259–1267.

Green, J. M., Kroll, I., Imre, D., Frances, F. M., Begum, K., Gannon, L., *et al.* (2001). Health gain and predictors of outcome in inpatient and day patient child psychiatry treatment. *Journal of the American Academy of Child and Adolescent Psychiatry*, *40*, 325–332.

Grizenko, N. (1997). Outcome of multimodal day treatment for children with severe behavior problems: A five-year follow-up. *Journal of the American Academy of Child and Adolescent Psychiatry*, *36*, 989–997.

Grizenko, N., Papineau, D., & Sayegh, L. (1993). Effectiveness of a multimodal day treatment program for children with disruptive behavior problems. *Journal of the American Academy of Child and Adolescent Psychiatry*, *32*, 127–134.

Gutterman, E. N., Markovitz, J. S., LoConte, J. S., & Beier, J. (1993). Determinants for hospitalization from an emergency mental heath service. *Journal of the American Academy of Child and Adolescent Psychiatry*, *32*, 114–122.

Hawton, K., Arensman, E., Townsend, E., Bremner, S., Feldman, E., Goldney, R., *et al.* (1998). Deliberate self-harm: A systematic review of efficacy of psychosocial and pharmacological treatments in preventing repetition. *British Medical Journal*, *317*, 441–447.

Henggeler, S., Rodick, J., Borduin, C., Hanson, C., Watson, S., & Urey, J. (1986). Multisytemic treatment of juvenile offenders: Effects on adolescent behavior and family interaction. *Developmental Psychology*, *22*, 132–141.

Henggeler, S., Rowland, M., Halliday-Boykins, C., Sheidow, A. J., Ward, D. M., Randall, J., *et al.* (2003). One-year follow-up of multisystemic therapy as an alternative to the hospitalization of youths in psychiatric crisis. *Journal of the American Academy of Child and Adolescent Psychiatry*, *42*, 543–551.

Henggeler, S. W., Rowland, M. D., Randall, J., Ward, D. M., Pickrel, S. G., Cunningham, P. B., *et al.* (1999). Home-based multisystemic therapy as an alternative to the hospitalization of youths in psychiatric crisis: Clinical outcomes. *Journal of the American Academy of Child and Adolescent Psychiatry*, *38*, 1331–1339.

Henggeler, S. W., Schoenwald, S. K., Pickrel, S. G., Brondino, M. J., Borduin, C. M., & Hall, A. A. (1994). *Treatment manual for Family Preservation using multisystemic therapy*. Columbia, SC: State of Columbia Health and Human Services Finance Commission.

Henggeler, S. W., Schoenwald, S. K., Borduin, C. M., Rowland, M. D., & Cunningham, P. B. (1998). *Multisystemic treatment of antisocial behavior in children and adolescents*. New York: Guilford Press.

Higgins, I., & Burke, M. (1998). Managing oppositional and aggressive behaviour. In J. M. Green, & B. W. Jacobs (Eds.), *Inpatient child psychiatry: Modern practice, research and the future* (pp. 189–201). London: Routledge.

Hoagwood, K., Jensen, P., Wigal, T., March, J., Roper, M., & Odbert, C. (2000). Impact of ADHD treatments on subsequent use of services. *Presentation at the Annual meeting of the American Academy of Child and Adolescent Psychiatry*, October 2000, New York.

Hougaard, E. (1994). The therapeutic alliance: A conceptual analysis. *Scandinavian Journal of Psychology*, *35*, 67–85.

Ivarsson, T., Larsson, B., & Gillberg, C. (1998). A 2–4 year follow up of depressive symptoms, suicidal ideation, and suicide attempts among adolescent psychiatric inpatients. *European Child and Adolescent Psychiatry*, *7*, 96–104.

Jacobs, B. W. (1998). Externalising disorders: Conduct disorder and hyperkinetic disorder. In J. M. Green and B. W. Jacobs (Eds.), *Inpatient child psychiatry: Modern practice, research and the future* (pp. 220–232). London: Routledge.

Jensen, P. S., Hoagwood, K., & Petti, T. (1996). Outcomes of mental health care for children and adolescents. 2. Literature review and application of a comprehensive model. *Journal of the American Academy of Child and Adolescent Psychiatry*, *35*, 1064–1077.

Joy, C. B., Adams, C. E., & Rice, K. (2004). Crisis intervention for people with severe mental illnesses (Cochrane Review). In: *The Cochrane Library*, Issue 4. Chichester, UK: John Wiley & Sons, Ltd.

Kennard, D. (1983). *An introduction to therapeutic communities*. London: Routledge & Kegan Paul.

King, C. A., Segal, H., Kaminski, K., & Naylor, M. W. (1995). A prospective study of adolescent suicidal behaviour following hospitalisation. *Suicide and Life Threatening Behaviour*, *25*, 327–338.

Kroll, L., & Green, J. M. (1997). Therapeutic alliance in inpatient child psychiatry. Development and initial validation of the Family Engagement Questionnaire. *Clinical Child Psychology and Psychiatry*, *2*, 431–447.

Kurtz, Z. (1994). *Treating children well*. London: Mental Health Foundation.

LaBarbera, J. D., & Dozier, J. E. (1985). A honeymoon effect in child psychiatric hospitalization: A research note. *Journal of Child Psychology and Psychiatry*, *26*, 479–483.

Lask, J., & Maynerd, C. (1998). Engaging and working with the family. In J. M. Green & B. W. Jacobs (Eds.), *Inpatient child psychiatry: Modern practice, research and the future* (pp. 75–93). London: Routledge.

Leibenluft, E., Tasman, A., & Green, S. A. (Eds.). (1993). *Less time to do more: Psychotherapy on the short-term inpatient unit.* Washington, DC: American Psychiatric Press.

Levy, A., & Kahan, B. (1991). *The Pindown experience and the protection of children. Report of the Staffordshire child care inquiry.* Staffordshire County Council.

Little, M., Kohm, A., & Thompson, R. (2005). The impact of residential placement on child development: Research and policy implications. *International Journal of Social Welfare*, *14*, 200–209.

Luisielli, J. K., Bastien, J. S., & Putnam, R. F. (1998). Behavioral assessment and analysis of mechanical restraint utilization on a psychiatric, child and adolescent inpatient setting. *Behavioral Interventions*, *13*, 147–155.

Luthar, S. S., Woolston, J. L., Sparrow, S. S., & Zimmerman, L. D. (1995). Adaptive behaviors among psychiatrically hospitalized children: The role of intelligence and related attributes. *Journal of Clinical Child Psychology*, *24*, 98–108.

Lynch, M., Steinberg, D., & Ounsted, C. (1975). A family unit in a children's psychiatric hospital. *British Medical Journal*, *2*, 127–129.

Magnagna, J. (1998). Psychodynamic psychotherapy. In J. M. Green, & B. W. Jacobs (Eds.), *Inpatient child psychiatry: Modern practice, research and the future* (pp. 124–143). London: Routledge.

Marshall, M., & Lockwood, A. (2004). Assertive community treatment for people with severe mental disorders. *Cochrane Database of Systematic Reviews*, *4*.

Maskey, S. (1998). The process of admission. In J. M. Green, & B. W. Jacobs (Eds.), *Inpatient child psychiatry: Modern practice, research and the future* (pp. 39–50). London: Routledge.

Mattejat, F., Hirt, B. R., Wilken, J., Schmidt, M. H., & Remschmidt, H. (2001). Efficacy of inpatient and home treatment in psychiatrically disturbed children and adolescents. Follow-up assessment of the results of a controlled treatment study. *European Child and Adolescent Psychiatry*, *10*, 171–179.

McCarthy, G., Baker, S., Betts, K., Bernard, D., Dove, J., Elliot, M., *et al.* (2006). The development of a new day treatment program for older children (8–11 years) with behavioural problems: The Go-Zone. *Clinical Child Psychology and Psychiatry*, *11*, 156–166.

McGorry, P. D. (2005). Evidence based reform of mental health care. *British Medical Journal*, *331*, 586–587.

Minghella, E., Ford, R., Freeman, T., Hoult, J., McGlynn, P., & O'Halloran, P. (1998). *Open all hours: 24-hour response for people with mental health emergencies.* London: Sainsbury Centre for Mental Health.

Moos, R., Shelton, R., & Petty, C. (1973). Perceived ward climate and treatment outcome. *Journal of Abnormal Psychology*, *82*, 291–298.

Newbold, C., & Jones, D. (1998). Child maltreatment and inpatient unit. In J. M. Green, & B. W. Jacobs (Eds.), *Inpatient child psychiatry: Modern practice, research and the future* (pp. 201–211). London: Routledge.

North, C., Gowers, S., & Byram, V. (1997). Family functioning and life events in the outcome of adolescent anorexia nervosa. *British Journal of Psychiatry*, *171*, 545–549.

Nurcombe, B. (1989). Goal-directed treatment planning and the principles of brief hospitalization. *Journal of the American Academy of Child and Adolescent Psychiatry*, *28*, 26–30.

Office of the Deputy Prime Minister, Social Exclusion Unit. (2004). *Mental health and social exclusion report.* Norwich: HMSO.

Parry-Jones, W. (1998). Historical Themes. In J. M. Green, & B. W. Jacobs (Eds.), *Inpatient child psychiatry: Modern practice, research and the future* (pp. 22–36). London: Routledge.

Paterson, R., Bauer, P., McDonald, C. A., & McDermott, B. (1997). A profile of children and adolescents in a psychiatric unit: Multi-domain impairment and research implications. *Australian and New Zealand Journal of Psychiatry*, *31*, 682–690.

Patrick, C., Padgett, D. K., Burns, B. J., Schlesinger, H. J., & Cohen, J. (1993). Use of inpatient services by a national population: Do benefits make a difference? *Journal of the American Academy of Child and Adolescent Psychiatry*, *32*, 144–152.

Pfeiffer, S. I., & Strzelecki, S. C. (1990). Inpatient psychiatric treatment of children and adolescents: A review of outcome studies. *Journal of the American Academy of Child and Adolescent Psychiatry*, *29*, 847–853.

Pottick, K., Hansell, S., Gaboda, D., & Gutterman, E. (1993). Child and adolescent outcomes of inpatient psychiatric services: A research agenda. *Children and Youth Services Review*, *15*, 371–384.

Pottick, K., Hansell, S., Gutterman, E., & White, R. H. (1995). Factors associated with inpatient and outpatient treatment for children and adolescents with serious mental illness. *Journal of the American Academy of Child and Adolescent Psychiatry*, *34*, 425–433.

Priebe, S., Fakhoury, W., White, I., Watts, J., Bebbington, P., Billings, J., *et al.* (2004). Pan-London Assertive Outreach Study Group. Characteristics of teams, staff and patients: associations with outcomes of patients in assertive outreach. *British Journal of Psychiatry*, *185*, 306–311.

Remschmidt, H., Schmidt, M. H., Mattejat, F., Eisert, H. G., & Eisert, M. (1988). Therapie-evaluation in der Kinder- und Jungendpsychiatrie: Stationäre Behandlung, tagesklinische Behandlung und Home treatment im Vergleich. *Zeitscrift für Kinder- und Jungendpsychiatrie*, *16*, 124–134.

Rey, J. M., Denshire, E., Wever, C., & Apollonov, I. (1998). Three-year outcome of disruptive adolescents treated in a day program. *European Child and Adolescent Psychiatry*, *7*, 42–48.

Rothery, D., Wrate, R., McCabe, R., & Aspin, J. (1995). Treatment goal planning: Outcome findings of a British prospective multi-centre study of adolescent inpatient units. *European Child and Adolescent Psychiatry*, *4*, 209–220.

Royal College of Psychiatrists. (1999). *Guidance for the staffing of child and adolescent inpatient units. Council Report 62.* London: Royal College of Psychiatrists.

Saccomani, L., Savoini, M., Cirrincione, M., Vercellino, F., & Ravera, G. (1998). Long-term outcome of children and adolescents with anorexia nervosa: Study of comorbidity. *Journal of Psychosomatic Research*, *44*, 565–571.

Safer, D. J. (1996). A comparison of studies from the United States and Western Europe on psychiatric hospitalization referrals for youths exhibiting suicidal behavior. *Annals of Clinical Psychiatry*, *8*, 161–168.

Schoenwald, S. K., Ward, D. M., Henggeler, S. W., Pickrel, S. G., & Patel, H. (1996). Multisystemic therapy treatment of substance abusing or dependent adolescent offenders: Costs of reducing incarceration, inpatient, and residential placement. *Journal of Child and Family Studies*, *5*, 431–444.

Schoenwald, S. K., Ward, D. M., Henggeler, S. W., & Rowland, M. D. (2000). Multisystemic therapy versus hospitalization for crisis stabilization of youth: Placement outcomes 4 months post referral. *Mental Health Services Research*, *2*, 3–12.

Shaw, M. (1998). Childhood mental health and the law. In J. M. Green, & B. W. Jacobs (Eds.), *Inpatient child psychiatry: Modern practice, research and the future* (pp. 349–362). London: Routledge.

Shelley, R. (1997). *Anorexics on anorexia.* London: Jessica Kingsley.

Smith, M. (1999). Assertive outreach: a step backwards. *Nursing Times*, *95*, 46–47.

Smyth, M. G., & Hoult, J. (2000). The home treatment enigma. *British Medical Journal*, *320*, 305–309.

Sourander, A., Helenius, H., Leijala, H., Heikkila, T., Bergroth, L., & Piha, J. (1996). Predictors of outcome of short-term child psychiatric inpatient treatment. *European Child and Adolescent Psychiatry*, *5*, 75–82.

Sourander, A., & Turunen, M. M. (1999). Psychiatric hospital care among children and adolescents in Finland: A nationwide register study. *Social Psychiatry and Psychiatric Epidemiology*, *34*, 105–110.

Stein, L. I., & Test, M. A. (1980). An alternative to mental hospital treatment: Conceptual model, treatment program and clinical evaluation. *Archives of General Psychiatry*, *37*, 392–397.

Steiner, H., Marx, L., & Walton, C. (1991). The ward atmosphere of a child psychosomatic unit: a ten-year follow-up. *General Hospital Psychiatry*, *13*, 246–252.

Steinhausen, H. C., & Seidel, R. (1993). Outcome in adolescent eating disorders. *International Journal of Eating Disorders*, *14*, 487–496.

Street, C. (2000). Whose crisis?: Responding to children and young people in an emergency. *Young Minds Magazine*, *49*, 14–16.

Street, C. (2004). In-patient mental health services for young people: Changing to meet new needs? *The Journal of the Royal Society for the Promotion of Health*, *124*, 115–118.

Szabo, C. P., & Magnus, C. (1999). Complex partial seizures in an adolescent psychiatric inpatient setting. *Journal of the American Academy of Child and Adolescent Psychiatry*, *38*, 477–479.

United Nations Children's Fund (UNICEF). (1995). *The Convention on the Rights of the Child*. London.

Wells, P., & Faragher, B. (1993). Inpatient treatment of 165 adolescents with emotional and conduct disorders: A study of outcome. *British Journal of Psychiatry*, *162*, 345–352.

Wever, C., & Rey, J. (1997). Juvenile obsessive-compulsive disorder. *Australian and New Zealand Journal of Psychiatry*, *31*, 105–113.

White, M. K., Godley, S. H., & Passetti, L. L. (2004). Adolescent and parent perceptions of outpatient substance abuse treatment: A qualitative study. *Journal of Psychoactive Drugs*, *36*, 65–74.

White, R., Carr, P., & Lowe, N. (1990). *A Guide to the Children Act 1989*. London: Routledge.

Wilmshurst, L. (2002). Treatment programs for youth with emotional and behavioral disorders: An outcome study of two alternate approaches. *Mental Health Services Research*, *4*, 85–96.

Wolkind, S. N. (1974). The components of affectionless psychopathy in institutionalized children. *Journal of Child Psychology and Psychiatry*, *15*, 215–220.

Woolston, J. L. (1989). Transactional risk model for short and intermediate term psychiatric inpatient treatment of children. *Journal of the American Academy of Child and Adolescent Psychiatry*, *28*, 38–41.

Woolston, J. L., Berkowitz, S. J., Schaefer, M. C., & Adnopoz, J. A. (1998). Intensive, integrated in-home psychiatric services: The catalyst to enhancing outpatient intervention. *Child and Adolescent Psychiatric Clinics of North America*, *7*, 615–633.

Worrall, A., & O'Herlihy, A. (2001). Psychiatrists' views of in-patient child and adolescent mental health services: A survey of members of the child and adolescent faculty of the Royal College of Psychiatrists. *Psychiatric Bulletin of the Royal College of Psychiatrists*, *25*, 219–222.

Wrate, R. M., Rothery, D. J., McCabe, R. J. R., & Aspin, J. (1994). A prospective multi-centre study of admissions to adolescent inpatient units. *Journal of Adolescence*, *17*, 221–237.

Wright, C., Burns, T., James, P., Billings, J., Johnson, S., Muijen, M., *et al.* (2003). Assertive outreach teams in London: Models of operation. Pan-London Assertive Outreach Study, Part 1. *British Journal of Psychiatry*, *183*, 132–138.

Zimet, S. G., & Farley, G. K. (1985). Day treatment for children in the United States. *Journal of the American Academy of Child Psychiatry*, *24*, 732–738.

70 Pediatric Consultation

Annah N. Abrams and Paula K. Rauch

The child mental health consultant[1] assesses the psychiatric status of an ill child in a hospital environment. The child's phase of development, temperament, type and stage of illness, family dynamics and level of pain and anxiety are among the multitude of contributing factors determining the complexity of clinical care and research in the pediatric consultation population. Every consultation encompasses aspects of biology, mediating influences of family and community, and the primacy of personal meaning in defining an experience as bearable or traumatizing (Eisenberg, 1995).

Mental health consultants assess the following:

1 Children with primary psychiatric illnesses leading to medical conditions;
2 Psychiatric manifestations of medical illnesses or treatments;
3 Adjustment to a chronic or life-threatening illness; and
4 Differential diagnosis of psychosomatic illness.

The consultant's scope includes working with anxious or difficult parents and liaison with the ward staff. The child mental health consultant's role may include offering didactic lectures for medical staff or parents. The consultant should also be an advocate for children, working with hospital leadership to develop more psychologically attuned standard practices. It is hoped that research in best practices for the medically ill child will increasingly guide future practice, but the limits of current evidence-based practice leave us relying on clinical experience, practice parameters and smaller research studies which are commonly disease-specific (AACAP, in press; for a fuller clinical approach see Rauch & Jellinek, 2002).

History

Adult consultation psychiatry arose in general hospitals during the 1930s, with the recognition that a mind–body dichotomy was an inadequate approach to providing quality medical care. Best practice demanded attention be paid to the psychological issues that were acknowledged to impact on medical illness and treatment (Ortiz, 1997). As the integral role of psychological factors was established in adult medical care, similar attention was focused on the needs of children.

Although a role for psychiatry with the medically ill child dates back to the 1930s (Lask, 1994; Work, 1989), consultation psychiatry by no means exists in every pediatric medical and surgical setting today. Recent articles continue to tout the benefit of collaboration between child psychiatrists and pediatricians, pediatric surgeons and pediatric nursing staff (Fritz, 2003; Watson, 2006), and encourage the establishment of consultation services and recommend their increased utilization.

Consultation services require financial support. In the USA, the National Institute of Mental Health (NIMH) provided grant money in the 1970s to support interdisciplinary pediatric and psychiatric clinical collaborations, thus increasing the number of consultation services nationwide. This seed money supported unreimbursed activities such as comprehensive evaluation and interdisciplinary team meetings. As this support ended in the 1980s, most consultation services were forced to downsize and decrease the range of activities and services offered (Shaw, Wamboldt, Bursch, & Stuber, 2006; Wright, Eaton, Butterfield *et al.*, 1987). In the USA, managed care has carved out psychiatric services from medical services provided to patients. As a result, consultation liaison services face barriers to reimbursement for psychological care. A recent report found that 60% of programs received lower rates than previously for service provided and collection rates for services covered averaged only 30% (Shaw, Wamboldt, Bursch *et al.*, 2006). Throughout Europe, consultation resources are limited, and they are virtually unavailable in many developing countries.

Clinically, the approach to consultations has seen attention shift away from looking at the mother–child dyad as the source of psychopathology and toward appreciating the impact of pediatric illness on the entire family (Labay & Walco, 2004; Svavarsdottir & Sigurdardottis, 2005). As the medical care of children, like that of adults, is moving toward shorter hospital stays and greater utilization of out-patient settings for treatment of chronic and life-threatening illness, mental health consultants will be called upon to shift their availability to encompass these out-patient settings. This chapter focuses on the medical in-patient setting, but it is important to recognize that child psychiatry consultation liaison covers a much broader terrain.

[1] In this chapter, the term mental health consultant refers to a child psychiatrist or child psychologist who is a mental health professional providing psychological and/or psychiatric care to medically ill children in an in-patient hospital setting.

Rutter's Child and Adolescent Psychiatry, 5th edition. Edited by M. Rutter, D. Bishop, D. Pine, S. Scott, J. Stevenson, E. Taylor and A. Thapar. © 2008 Blackwell Publishing, ISBN: 978-1-4051-4549-7.

Psychological Distress in the Pediatric Population

Children with medical illnesses serious enough to warrant hospitalization are recognized as at increased risk for emotional disorders (AACAP, in press). Those conditions that result in long-term physical disabilities or impact on the central nervous system pose additional risk (Meyer, Blakeney, Russell *et al.*, 2004; Poggi, Liscio, Adduci *et al.*, 2005a; Poggi, Liscio, Galbiati *et al.*, 2005b), as may certain symptoms and challenges associated with specific diseases (AACAP, in press).

Disease-specific rates of psychological symptomatology are found elsewhere in this textbook. Estimates of psychological distress in hospitalized children and adolescents vary and range from 20% to more than 35% (Loutherenoo, Sittipreechacharn, Thanarattanakorn, & Sanguansermsri, 2002; Stoppelbein, Greening, Jordon *et al.*, 2005). These rates reflect the particular medically ill and socioeconomic populations found in any given pediatric hospital and so vary substantially.

Collaboration Between Pediatricians and Mental Health Consultants

Pediatricians, nurses and parents caring for a child with behavioral, adjustment or coping difficulties often see the benefit in their improved ability to manage a child's illness when a child psychiatrist or psychologist is part of the medical team (Carter, Kronenberger, Baker *et al.*, 2003). Dissatisfaction with mental health consultations has been linked to a perception that the child psychiatrist was not available quickly enough or did not communicate findings adequately, or that findings were not tailored to the needs and realities of the referring pediatrician (Burket & Hodgin, 1993). Older studies also suggested that lifelong consultation practices may begin with access during training (Bergman & Fritz, 1985). In a study from the same era, mental health consultants for their part expressed frustration that consultations were requested too late in the course of the hospital stay instead of seeking a psychiatric assessment as an integral part of the initial work-up (Fritz, Pumariega, & Fischhoff, 1987).

Barriers to Requesting Consultation

Barriers to child mental health consultation include discomfort with talking to the patient and family about psychiatric consultation, lack of availability of child mental health consultants or the lack of their availability in a timely manner. Funding for child mental health services as well as misperceptions about the role of child psychiatrists in the care of medically ill children are additional obstacles. Hospital financial priorities and national health care policy as well as educational initiatives between clinicians and within hospital units are necessary to address some of these issues.

Consultation Models

Consultation service models are determined by the size of the patient group served, the illness severity of treatment populations and the availability of child mental health consultants. When consultants are available only for a limited number of hours, they need to utilize some of their time to supervise nurse clinicians, social workers or others, who are available to do more direct clinical service, reserving the remaining consultation time for seeing the most challenging cases. In many pediatric settings, child psychologists are the primary child mental health consultants, with child psychiatrists limited to acting as pediatric psychopharmacologists (Shaw, Wamboldt, Bursch *et al.*, 2006). Mental health consultants, regardless of their training discipline, need understanding of the disease process, medical management of relevant illnesses and a skill set that includes behavioral interventions such as desensitization, hypnotherapy and behavior modification.

Consultations can be initiated on a case-by-case basis, by protocol or a combination. In the case-by-case model, the pediatrician requests a consultation after assessing an individual patient, whereas consultation by protocol systematizes psychiatric consultation for children with certain diagnoses or risk factors. Examples of protocol-driven consultation include routine consultation for patients who are candidates for transplant or have been admitted after suicide attempts. Protocols can be based on factors other than the diagnosis, such as hospitalization lasting more than 2 weeks or injury requiring intensive care unit (ICU) admission. In the setting of short hospital stays, protocols maximize early identification of need and minimize time before consultation is initiated. When possible, for continuity the same consultant should follow a child over multiple hospitalizations or from in-patient to an outpatient specialty clinic.

In an older study of several hundred consultations, one-third of the consultation requests were ascribed to staff-related conflict (Hengeveld & Rooysman, 1983). Arguably, no consultation for a hospitalized child can be carried out effectively without the integral "liaison" component of understanding the child's condition in the context of the concerns arising from members of the treatment team (Hengeveld & Rooysman, 1983; Tarnow & Gutstein, 1982). Liaison requires understanding and respect for the roles of each member of the multidisciplinary treatment team as well as sensitivity to particular challenges inherent in each discipline's treatment demands. Unfortunately, the important liaison role of mental health consultants has decreased in many institutions because of lack of funding (Shaw, Wamboldt, Bursch *et al.*, 2006).

Psychiatric consultation requests routinely differ according to the particular hospital setting. Consultations for children on the wards often deal with behavioral and adjustment issues, in many cases present prior to hospitalization (Carter,

Kronenberger, Baker *et al.*, 2003). Psychiatric consultation for the pediatric ICU tends to be more acute and requires the consultant to make assessments and recommendations more rapidly (DeMaso & Meyer, 1996).

Work with medically ill children is rewarding, but it can also arouse powerful feelings of sadness, frustration and helplessness. Pediatric units may seek to address the emotional challenges experienced by the medical team. The goal is to provide staff support that will assist them in their ability to provide the best care for patients and may prevent long-term burnout (Levi, Thomas, Green *et al.*, 2004; Maytum, Heiman, & Garwick, 2004). For example, an emergency department or ICU may institute a time to meet together as a team after a traumatic case or upsetting outcome. A pediatric ward may institute bereavement rounds following the death of a patient to address the emotional toll of caring for terminally ill children and to share remembrances of the child.

When a member of the multidisciplinary medical team faces a personal or professional challenge that interferes with the ability to provide quality care, the consultant may be asked, in a liaison role, to facilitate referral to psychiatric treatment for the team member. The consultant should not personally provide treatment for a team member, as this would be crossing an essential boundary in a long-term working relationship. If a team member is believed by others to be impaired but seems unaware of his or her problem, concerned colleagues may approach the mental health consultant for direction on how to help this individual. The consultant can encourage the concerned colleague to share observations with the appropriate supervisor and may meet separately with the supervisor or director to share relevant personal observations. Behaviors that put patients at risk are mandated to be reported to the appropriate overseeing body such as the chief of service, a regional board of medical or nursing registration or hospital-based board.

Approach to Consultation Requests

The first task for the consultant is to understand what concerns have led to the consultation request by speaking with the consulting pediatrician or staff member, listening to the expressed concerns and asking for elaboration about concerns that seem present but not disclosed. It is helpful to work together to establish realistic goals for the initial consultation, with a plan to set additional goals after the initial meetings with the child and parents. The consultant should seek supporting information available from other members of the treatment team and from the hospital chart. It is useful to gather observations from several individuals as the child may behave differently in different settings, or may have established warmer relationships with some team members than with others. After the initial assessment, and with permission from the parents or guardian, the consultant may seek input provided by sources outside of the medical arena such as an out-patient psychotherapist, school professionals or members of other involved social agencies such as the department of social services, or the court system.

While the consultant will gather data from many sources, a basic tenet of consultation work is being clear about with whom the consultant is consulting. Ultimately, the goal of consultation is to facilitate the child's receipt of optimum care, but the consultant may be serving the primary pediatrician, a subspecialist or a subspecialty team. Usually, what serves the child best is helpful to many team members and to the family, but there may be conflicts. For example, the consultant to the pediatrician may recommend that an aggressive interventional gastroenterologist chosen by the parents may not be the best choice for a somatizing child with recurrent abdominal pain.

It is best if the pediatrician or subspecialist, with whom the family already has a relationship, informs the parents of the decision to obtain a psychiatric consultation and its purpose. Psychiatric consultation may be presented as part of the diagnostic protocol, a way to help the team understand how the child is feeling and to help the child cope with the difficult circumstance that led to hospitalization or as a response to the challenges that hospitalization has presented. The mental health consultant may be asked to help the referring pediatrician articulate the reason for the consultation in a positive manner. Some parents and children are uncomfortable with the idea of a psychiatric consultation, and yet appreciate the intervention upon finding the child mental health consultant respectful, knowledgeable and attuned to the needs of the child and family. Other parents will be resistant, reluctantly agree under some pressure from the referring pediatrician, and perhaps remain ambivalent about the benefit of the assessment or come to appreciate its value. For those families who refuse consultation, the consultant may meet with the team in a liaison capacity and assist the team without directly interviewing the child. If the psychiatric consultation is deemed urgent, the pediatrician should seek input from the hospital legal counsel about the appropriate way to proceed within the legal system in which he or she practices. The British Medical Association and the American Academy of Pediatrics address the issues of consent and the right to refuse treatment in persons under the age of 18 and provide very helpful guides for the clinician in practice (AAP, 1995; BMA, 2001).

Depending on the age and circumstances of the child's condition, the consultant will decide whether to meet with the parents first, the child first or both together. Meeting with older children without a parent present at some point in the initial work-up allows them to voice private concerns that may be censored when a parent is present. Even young children may not want to say things in front of parents that they believe the parent will find upsetting. Children under 6 years may be more comfortable meeting the consultant with a parent. Because the goal is to facilitate the child being most forthcoming in talk and play, it is key to respond to the child's preferences for the initial interview.

The parents of young children are likely to want time alone with the consultant to share observations and concerns that are not appropriate to share in the child's presence. Similarly, many parents of older children find it easier to be candid about their worries in the absence of the child. Older children may be uncomfortable knowing that their parents are talking to the consultant without knowing what is being said. Nonetheless, it remains key to the initial assessment to provide an interview setting that facilitates the child and parent being independently able to express feelings freely, and this goal can be articulated to the child and parent.

Assessing the Child

Premorbid Functioning of the Child and Family

When assessing a hospitalized child, the consultant is seeing only "a snapshot" out of the child's life. Some families are confronting a new diagnosis or change in the prognosis, while others may have had time to develop an ongoing coping strategy in the face of a chronic illness or a lengthy treatment protocol. Assessment should recognize the potential for wide variation in coping at different points in the unfolding medical experience.

It may be helpful to utilize a biopsychosocial model to understand the child's coping and family's functioning prior to the hospitalization. Under the "bio" heading, the consultant will want to understand the particular challenges presented by the child's medical condition and interplay of medications. Under the "psych" heading, the consultant will want to learn about depression and anxiety preceding the medical condition as well as psychological strengths and resiliency. In the "social" arena, the consultant wants to know about the child's relationship with peers and his or her functioning at school.

Developmental Perspective

Development is an important lens through which a childhood medical illness can be seen. A full review of the interplay of development and medical illness is beyond the scope of this chapter, but a few key developmental points are highlighted to illustrate common issues.

Infants and toddlers cannot understand the gravity of a given diagnosis. They live in the moment, experiencing the medical condition and treatment according to the physical limitations and discomforts imposed. Infants rely on key caretakers to hold and soothe them and to make the hospital environment feel safe. It is important for the hospital staff to support infant–parent attachment, and not allow treatments and technologies to interfere with this key emotional milestone. The pediatric unit can provide a milieu that supports breastfeeding mothers, and allows rooming-in by parents.

Very young children (3–6 years) are egocentric (i.e., they understand all events as occurring in relation to them). They have associative logic, which means that for them any two unrelated things can be understood as if one is causing or explaining the other. The combination of egocentricity and associative logic leads to magical thinking. Magical thinking is the weaving together of fantasy and logic to explain how the young child caused something to happen. In the medical setting, it is frequently the child's misconception that having a "bad illness" means he or she did something wrong and is being punished. It is helpful to get young children (and older children as well) to elaborate their understanding of the etiology of their medical conditions to uncover self-blaming misconceptions and correct them. When young children have a life-threatening illness, parents often wonder if the child is worrying about dying. At this age, children do not yet have the cognitive capacity to comprehend forever, and envision death as a reversible event. The young child is likely to demonstrate the most affect around separations, such as having anxiety about going to sleep at night in his or her own bed, or wanting a parent to promise to be there when they wake up from surgery.

At this age, children cannot localize a medical condition to a specific body part, so they feel particularly physically vulnerable when ill. Faced with needlesticks, intravenous medication and surgical procedures, they are often fearful. They rely on parents and medical staff to prepare them for procedures.

Older children (7–12 years) can understand simple functional explanations of medical conditions. Many will pride themselves on mastering the names of medicines, illness-related terminology and how to use hospital equipment. Children of this age look for simple cause and effect etiologies for illnesses. They can understand viral illnesses being caused by "germs," but are perplexed when there is no clear causal explanation (e.g., why they have cancer without having smoked cigarettes). It is important to explain illness and treatment simply and clearly. In the context of understanding why a treatment plan is being initiated, the medical staff should seek the child's assent to procedures and treatments. In this age group, "rules rule" and it is troubling to the child that so often medical illness does not follow the rules (e.g., the child avoids asthma triggers and has an asthmatic attack anyway). One of the challenges of working with the preteens is to capitalize on the children's pride in trying hard and their wish for competency, while keeping them from getting too disappointed by setbacks that occur in spite of their own best efforts.

Adolescents have the capacity for abstract thinking, and thus are able to understand the chance bad luck of having an uncommon, life-threatening or chronic illness with the same cognitive complexity as adults. Education is a prerequisite for behavioral change, but on its own is not sufficient. Commonly, teenagers do not have the maturity to incorporate the consistently health-promoting behaviors they know they should engage in into appropriate changes in lifestyle. Turning cognitive understanding into behavioral change is the common battleground of adolescent and authority figure – parent or physician. Assent for medical treatments is sought from the younger child, while consent is sought from adolescents who have the cognitive ability to comprehend the purpose of treatment and the ramifications of refusing treatment (BMA, 2001). Although some physicians may view seeking consent from an adolescent for treatments and procedures as time-consuming and burdensome, knowing that parents must give legal consent to proceed, these discussions foster trust and build a valuable alliance between patient and clinician.

Adolescence is a self-conscious time, with the emergence of sexual interests and heightened reliance on peer group norms for style and status. Medical illnesses or treatments that affect appearance are particularly difficult (e.g., becoming Cushingoid on steroids or bald with chemotherapy). The medical staff is challenged to find ways to respect the teenager's age-appropriate wish to be more independent in the face of illness that so often increases dependency.

As children with chronic illnesses live into adulthood, the transition to young adulthood and understanding of associated issues become relevant. Young adults negotiate intimate relationships, career decisions, independence from parents, and sometimes relocation or parenthood. One challenge that the treatment team and patient may face is whether to transition care from a pediatric into an adult setting, which often necessitates a new treatment team. Some patients may prefer to be on an adult ward or waiting room, but may find it very difficult to leave lifelong caretakers and the pediatric model of care.

Specific Challenges Associated with a Given Medical Condition

Each medical condition carries its own specific challenges. When the consultant is familiar with common frustrations or limitations imposed by a particular illness, this can provide a kind of credibility in the process of acquiring a child's and parent's trust as they relate what is hardest for them. Routine consultation to the same pediatric unit leads to the consultant becoming familiar with technology, treatment protocols and terminology, all of which makes it easier for the child and family to tell their medical story and feel understood.

Mental Status Examination

Hospitalized children have many reasons for an altered mental status including delirium, CNS changes secondary to medical conditions, effects of medications and trauma. A formal mental status examination should be part of the medical record including observations of appearance, gross and fine motor function, speech, mood, affect, thought, suicidal ideation, memory and cognition. By performing a mental status assessment, the consultant may uncover significant mental impairment that has gone undetected in spite of multiple specialists seeing the child.

Medically ill children may be developmentally delayed or emotionally immature. It is helpful for the consultant to integrate the information from the mental status examination and premorbid school and developmental information to assist the medical team in understanding the child's ability to comprehend medical information.

The Family

No child can be understood independently of his or her family. In the initial evaluation it is therefore essential to assess the family's level of functioning and their ability to support the child in the hospital and through the anticipated treatment and outcome. During hospitalization, parents often have to cope with new and anxiety-provoking information. Information presented by multiple caregivers is common on a medical unit and may lead to inconsistencies: one person emphasizing a particular laboratory value but another devaluing its importance, one suggesting discharge is imminent but another indicating it may be many days away. Parents and older children may find these inconsistencies confusing and upsetting. Many parents identify the continuous feelings of uncertainty as the hardest aspect of adapting to the child's illness. The focus of the uncertainty changes during the course of the hospitalization as the challenges of the treatment evolve from the time of diagnosis to the child's changing appearance and ultimately to when will the illness recur or what follow-up is necessary (Diaz-Caneja, Gledhill, Weaver, Nadel, & Garralda, 2005). Some parents derive support from other parents on the pediatric unit whereas others report feeling further traumatized by witnessing other families in crisis. Parental anxiety and distress are associated with a child's psychological adjustment and capacity to cope (Bonner, Hardy, Guill *et al.*, 2006; Sawyer, Streiner, Antoniou, Toogood, & Rice, 1998; Wagner, Chaney, Hommel *et al.*, 2003). The consultant can help the medical team be mindful of the importance of addressing the anxiety around uncertainty and facilitating consistent communication.

Asking parents to share the history of the current illness, from the first symptoms through to the present hospital stay, allows the consultant to learn about the parents' experience of the medical care (i.e., to what extent have they felt responded to or ignored in the process of diagnosis and treatment). It is helpful to understand the parents' views of past and present medical caregivers as well as their experience of their own role in the child's medical condition. The stress of a child's illness and treatment may uncover parental discord and perhaps coincide with divorce although it should not be assumed to be causal. In a recent study, the rates of divorce after a child has died from cancer were not found to be increased relative to the general population (Kreicbergs, Valdimarsdottir, Onelov *et al.*, 2005).

An assessment of the family should include psychiatric history (including use of substances). It is helpful to ask questions about depression symptoms for each parent and the siblings. Some parents may increase their own risk-taking behavior including use of alcohol or driving with less care. Many parents benefit from being reminded of the importance of eating and sleeping so that they do not compromise their own health during what may be a long period in which the sick child will need their additional care.

The family's experience is affected by past experiences with illness and loss. The consultant will want to know if any other family members have had the same or similar illnesses, what the experience was of their care and the outcome. Helping the parent differentiate the current medical situation from past experiences helps the parent be more attuned to the child's actual needs.

Siblings are often the forgotten sufferers (Murray, 2002; Wilkins & Woodgate, 2005). The sick child is commonly the object of everyone's attention and recipient of many gifts; while the siblings often live with disrupted schedules, few gifts and often absent, less emotionally available parents. The consultant and social worker can model important empathy for the plight of the siblings, and help parents with ways of addressing the needs of their well children.

Pediatric hospital staff members may have a harder time working with some parents than with their child. The consultant can help the team understand the family better and feel more empathy for difficult behaviors. Difficult parents often cannot bear the feelings of helplessness, and vent their anger and frustration on hospital staff by being critical and devaluing (Groves & Beresin, 1999).

Presenting the Assessment to the Treatment Team

After meeting with the child and family for the initial assessment, the consultant will share observations and recommendations with the referring pediatrician and available team members, and write a note in the hospital chart. The preliminary formulation and recommendations should avoid the use of psychiatric jargon. Clear practical recommendations to improve coping, address behavioral problems, treat primary psychiatric disorders and maintain safety are most helpful. Hospital records are permanent documents and should not be used for private or informal communications between clinicians. One should assume that patients and parents will read the record, as can hospital staff and insurers. No one should write pejorative comments about other clinicians, patients or families in the hospital record. The consultant should be thoughtful about including personal information about the patient or family members, avoiding what is not germane to the care of the patient, such as a past history of parental substance abuse or marital infidelity.

When presenting recommendations, safety must be addressed first and an understanding of the urgency and time frame in which the referring doctor needs assistance must be attended to by the consultant. Sharing an understanding of motivations that may underlie maladaptive behaviors can increase empathy for the child and family, but the consultant must work with the team to arrive at concrete suggestions that can be implemented by the team in order for the consultation to be experienced as valuable.

Emergency Consultations

The most common emergency consultations relate to the suicidal or self-abusive child. The consultant's first recommendations focus on the child's immediate safety, recognizing that hospital units are not designed with the safety of a self-injurious child in mind. There is potentially dangerous medical equipment throughout the unit. It is therefore necessary to assess carefully the child's risk for self-harm in this setting. After having made an impulsive suicide attempt or gesture, some children are frightened, regret their actions, feel supported by their families and may be assessed as being at low risk for self-injury while hospitalized. Others regret that the suicide attempt was unsuccessful or are uncommunicative, leaving the consultant unsure of their mental state. When unsure, one must err on the side of safety, providing continuous observation of these children on the pediatric unit. Once safety has been assured, the consultant can assess the precipitants for the acts of self-harm and recommend appropriate treatment in the hospital and disposition (see chapter 40).

Behavior that disrupts essential medical treatment also requires immediate intervention. Such behavior may be driven by extreme anxiety, delirium, disinhibition following head injury or as a side-effect of medication use. Angry threatening behavior in a child with a clear sensorium, but who views the essential medical treatment as an unnecessary assault can also create an emergency situation. Assessment of the etiology of the difficult behavior will determine the appropriate intervention.

Parental behavior may be the reason for an urgent consultation with the mental health consultant or the team social worker. Parents may be refusing essential medical treatment for the child or acting bizarrely. The reason for the parental actions may be unclear or may be revealed to be beliefs at odds with standard medical practice, mistrust of the hospital staff, psychiatric illness in the parent or extreme anxiety. Hostile parents can interfere with critical care by frightening the medical staff. Interventions will be determined by an understanding of the etiology of the parents' behavior and may include the appropriate use of hospital security personnel.

The consultant may be asked to interact directly with the parent to help the referring physician work with the family or to recommend further assessment, including social services or court interventions. Often, parents who are obstructing necessary care for their child are doing so because they are themselves overwhelmed with helplessness and are trying to control what they see as uncontrollable. By helping the parent to feel that he or she is an essential member of the decision-making process and thus has some control in productive ways, many parents will step out of a combative stance and into a more collaborative one. There are specific legal interventions that are implemented when parents prevent a life-sustaining treatment, such as a blood transfusion for a child with life-threatening blood loss. These interventions are determined by the legal parameters of the place of practice.

Primary Psychiatric Illnesses

Depression

Depression is common in the hospitalized child. It may be a secondary response to the stress of acute or chronic illness, or it may be the primary presenting symptom of psychosomatic illness or behavioral problems including self-harm. Practice patterns vary from country to country (see chapter 37). One barrier to the appropriate treatment of depression in hospitalized children is the misconception that depressed mood and symptoms are an appropriate response to serious illness. Another barrier to treatment is the difficulty of making the diagnosis of depression in a medically ill child given the overlap of somatic symptoms and depressive symptoms (Shemesh, Yehuda, Rockmore *et al.*, 2005a). Individual and family therapy, play therapy, behavioral therapy and medication are useful modalities in the hospital setting. Our clinical experience supports the use of antidepressants for depression in the medically ill older child or adolescent. Selective serotonergic reuptake inhibitors have become the antidepressant of choice as they are generally well tolerated, have limited interactions with other medications and present a lower risk of intentional or accidental overdose (see chapter 37).

Anxiety

Anxiety can be secondary to the stresses of the medical condition and treatment or be pre-existing. Children with pre-existing generalized anxiety or specific fear of doctors, needles or shots are likely to have more difficulty adjusting to medical assessment and treatment. In addition to the obvious discomfort severe anxiety causes the child and parents, anxiety can interfere with procedures and complicate history-taking and symptom assessment.

Age-appropriate explanation of medical interventions for older children, and medical play with explanation for younger children, can decrease anxiety. Children from around 6 years of age can learn a variety of coping techniques to help them with anxiety-provoking procedures. Many children will respond to distraction, breathing exercises, visualization or hypnotherapy (Butler, Symons, Henderson, Shortliffe, & Spiegel, 2005; Gershon, Zimand, Pickering, Rothbaum, & Hodges, 2004; Mundy, DuHamel, & Montgomery, 2003).

Clinicians must pay attention to minimizing pain for every child (Greco & Berde, 2005). Effective interventions including preparation, relaxation, distraction, use of anesthetic creams before procedures, and treating chronic and acute pain with analgesics, significantly reduce the amount of stress experienced by the child (Schiff, Holts, Peterson, & Rakusan, 2001; Young, 2005). For young children, all painful procedures should occur in a treatment room and not in the child's bed nor in the playroom. Protecting the child's bed and the playroom as safe havens helps the young child relax in these settings.

Even with quality pain management, relaxation techniques and preparation for procedures, some children will continue to be too anxious to comply with treatment and may experience sleepless nights, be nauseated or frantic during the hospital stay or in anticipation of visits to the hospital. Benzodiazepines may be helpful adjuncts for lessening debilitating anxiety. In young children, one must be aware of the potential for benzodiazepines to disinhibit children and thus worsen coping difficulties.

Anorexia Nervosa

Anorexia nervosa is characterized by significant weight loss or the absence of appropriate weight gain for age and height in the setting of distorted body image and fear of gaining weight (see chapter 41). Pediatric hospitalization usually occurs when there has been rapid or profound weight loss, cardiovascular abnormalities, electrolyte imbalance and hypothermia. The goal of pediatric hospitalization is medical stabilization with nutritional assessment and treatment, psychological assessment of the child and family, and recommendation for level of psychiatric intervention after medical stabilization (Andersen, Bowers, & Evans, 1997). If the anorexic patient has been in out-patient psychotherapy, it is important to seek input from the out-patient therapist. Medical hospitalization often represents failure of the out-patient treatment for the child or adolescent.

It is often helpful to institute a detailed anorexia protocol with very restricted activity, including bed rest, observation during and directly after meal times, bathroom privileges only after weight gain has begun, and limited phone contact and visitation with family. As the child demonstrates that he or she is able to meet nutritional goals, privileges are added. Once the child is medically stable recommendations about disposition can be initiated as outlined in chapter 41.

Pediatric and nursing staff may feel frustrated and angry at anorexic patients, whom they may see as making themselves ill. This is in stark contrast to other children on the pediatric unit who are viewed as struggling to overcome "real" illnesses. Regular team meetings provide an opportunity for staff members to voice the feelings engendered by the patient, ensure that the protocol is being instituted consistently, unify the team in providing quality and compassionate care and provide an opportunity to give consistent information to the patient and their family.

Psychosomatic Illness (see chapter 57)

Some children are admitted to pediatric units with intense persistent somatic complaints such as headaches, abdominal pains, bowel complaints, neurological symptoms or fatigue. The pediatrician may suspect that the intensity of the symptoms or the combination of complaints exceeds what can be explained by a medical condition and reflects underlying emotional factors and may thus seek a psychiatric consultation. The pediatrician's assessment that psychological factors are influencing the somatic presentation is usually at odds with the child's and parents' understanding of the etiology of the condition. Often the child and parents are seen as overly invested in an exhaustive medical work-up to prove a purely medical etiology. In psychosomatic illness, the somatic complaints are an unconscious expression of emotional issues, thus the child and parents believe that the child is seriously ill and needs this work-up despite its risks.

Commonly, psychiatric consultation is resisted, because it is viewed as evidence that the medical team either does not believe the symptoms or medical condition to be "real" or is unwilling to investigate fully all the medical possibilities. It is common for the family to seek multiple medical opinions, and often to choose the most aggressive specialists (e.g., those who perform the most diagnostic testing or prescribe the most medications). Diagnostic tests may be repeated to satisfy parental demands for action or in an attempt to decrease persistent patient and parental anxiety about undetected serious illness. Parents may overvalue insignificant positive findings from the diagnostic work-ups to vindicate their belief that a yet undiscovered medical etiology exists.

Hospitalization can be viewed as evidence of more serious psychosomatic illness and may be an important opportunity for a coordinated care plan addressing psychological and medical issues together. The psychiatric consultant must be willing to listen to the somatic symptoms and associated medical hypotheses in order to establish an alliance with the patient and family. Presenting the consultant's role as one of helping the child cope with chronic symptoms that are interfering with school, peer activities or family life is less threatening than suggesting that the consultant has been sought because the symptom intensity reflects psychological issues. The child and family must be reassured that the presence of the child mental health consultant will not be associated with reduced access to the medical team, but is truly an adjunct to ongoing medical care. The pediatrician has the important role of re-examining the child regularly, reassuring the patient and family that no worrying new findings exist and not acquiescing to unnecessary testing.

Non-compliance

Non-compliance with medical treatments is common, ranging from estimates of 50% to as high as 88%. Surprisingly, confidence in the efficacy and importance of the treatment does not always translate into improved compliance rates (Van Sciver, D'Angelo, Rappaport, & Woolf, 1995). However, physicians should recognize that education and an alliance with parents and children can improve patient compliance rates (Cork, Britton, Butler *et al.*, 2003; Feinstein, Keich, Becker-Cohen *et al.*, 2005). Furthermore, beliefs about why a medication is *not* adequately treating an illness also need to be addressed to improve compliance (Rubin, 2004). The impact of non-compliance ranges from essentially harmless to life-threatening. Medical non-compliance in a particular child is multi-determined, associated with medical education, active versus passive coping style, pride versus embarrassment with respect to self-care, impulsivity, family support, peer support and relationship with medical providers (Dinwiddie & Muller, 2002). It may also be a function of underlying psychiatric illness including depression, anxiety, oppositional defiant disorder and attention deficit disorder. When consultation is sought for non-compliance, usually it is because of risk to the child's health, escalating conflict in the family or frustration with inappropriate use of medical resources.

The consultant's task is to understand why the child is non-compliant and to work with the team to modify aspects of treatments that trouble the child where possible, while working to help the child and family adopt strategies that support clinically important treatments. Treatable psychiatric disorders need to be identified and addressed. Treatment-promoting supports – including disease-specific support groups, more frequent meetings with clinicians, and psychoeducation groups – can be helpful.

Child Abuse (see chapters 28 and 29)

In the consultation setting, it is appropriate to restate the importance of suspecting abuse. Without educated suspicion, abuse will often go undetected. Injuries to body surfaces that do not commonly bear the brunt of an accidental fall, multiple broken bones or bruises in various stages of healing, bruises that resemble finger marks, belts or cords are highly suspicious. Implausible or inconsistent stories from caretakers, and inappropriate delay in bringing a child for medical care should raise suspicion, as should caretakers who ascribe the injury to siblings or self-inflicted injuries.

Suspicion of abuse must be reported to the appropriate social agency. When abuse is suspected, the child should be fully examined for other physical signs. It is important to notify authorities of other children known to be in a potentially unsafe home. The pediatric unit may serve as a safe haven for a child while allegations are being investigated.

Coping with Chronic Illness

Chronically ill children should not be defined by their illnesses (i.e., there is no typical child with diabetes or classic child with asthma). On the contrary, chronically ill children have the same range of personalities and coping styles seen in healthy children, and are engaged in mastering the developmental milestones and challenges they share with their peers.

Estimates of psychological morbidity associated with chronic illnesses in childhood range 10–30% (Bauman, Drotar, Leventhal, Perrin, & Pless, 1997), which is only slightly higher than the general pediatric population (Barlow & Ellard, 2006). Greater morbidity is associated with multiple admissions to hospital (Geist, 1977). Other documented risk factors for adaptation to chronic illness include physical disability and brain dysfunction, pain frequency, younger age, poverty, single-parent family and increased psychological symptoms in the parents (Knapp & Harris, 1998).

Specific illnesses present unique challenges, such as the dietary restrictions in diabetes (Patton, Dolan, & Powers, 2006) or the decreased exercise endurance in advancing cystic fibrosis. However, many factors influence how problematic a disease-specific challenge is for an individual child. It is the consultant's job to understand the unique meaning of the illness to the child and family, and to assist in the process of adaptation. Disease-specific research in common chronic illnesses can inform clinical approaches with these illnesses and can offer useful guidance for approaches to children with other medical conditions.

The consultant needs to elucidate the child's subjective experience of the illness, such as what is the hardest aspect of the illness or treatment from the child's perspective, how does it affect the child's image of themself, and are there specific worries about the future? Enquiries about the impact on peer interactions, and favorite activities, areas of conflict between the child and parent or the child and physician in relation to the illness, and the child's perception of the parents' worries may be useful. Variations of these questions can be asked of the parents and siblings.

Chronic illness requires adjustment on the part of the child, the family, and sometimes the school, friends and organizers of activities. Efforts should be made to assist a child's ability to continue with age-appropriate activities and special interests. Children with personal strengths – whether in academics, sports, music or interpersonal skills – may have an easier time accommodating to the limits imposed by the illness and treatment. Temperament can affect a child's ability to adapt, with more flexible and outgoing children likely to bear the uncertainty and limitations imposed by illness more easily. Parental support, warmth and attitude toward the illness and the child's adaptive style are key. Parental anxiety, anger, sadness, guilt or blame can impede adjustment (Vance & Eiser, 2004; Wagner, Chaney, Hommel *et al.*, 2003).

Asthma

Asthma is the most common chronic illness of childhood, with a pediatric population prevalence of 5–10% and an increasing mortality rate from 1980 to 1998 that appears to have reached a plateau (Akinbami & Schoendorf, 2002). Racial and ethnic disparities account for much of the increase in morbidity (McDaniel, Paxson, & Waldfogel, 2006). Recent studies have sought to understand the factors that affect adherence and compliance, delineate common psychosocial stresses that may act as triggers for asthma attacks, and devise psychoeducational programs, combined medical and psychological treatment strategies, and teach stress management skills to improve compliance and decrease morbidity (Bender, 2006; Hockemeyer & Smyth, 2002; Self, Chrisman, Mason, & Rumbak, 2005; Teach, Crain, Quint, Hylan, & Joseph, 2006).

Hospitalization is an opportunity to emphasize education. Clear guidelines on when to call the pediatrician for appropriate timely guidance can be established along with seeking input from the family about barriers to these contacts. Triggers in the home can be addressed realistically and empathically in light of the exacerbation that led to admission. Common triggers, such as smoking and pets, require a major commitment from family members in order to change. School-related issues need to be explored from the perspective of the child (e.g., embarrassment associated with going to the school nurse) and the school (e.g., access to inhalers in the classroom). Strategies to improve parent and child anxiety and to address parent–child conflicts around compliance are valuable.

Diabetes

Adaptation to insulin-dependent (type 1) diabetes presents special challenges associated with the need for tight control of blood sugar, the primary role of food as a source of nurturance and soothing, the meaning to a parent of providing or limiting access to desirable foods, and the complexity of monitoring blood sugars and delivering insulin involving needlesticks and thus pain. The acute consequences of blood sugar abnormalities include symptomatic hypoglycemia, hyperglycemia and ketoacidosis and may lead to hospitalization. The long-term sequelae include effects on vision, renal function and neuropathy. Symptoms associated with hypoglycemia are often difficult for parents to differentiate from common irritability in young children or for older children to recognize as different from anxiety. This leads to either more frequent blood testing or a tendency to keep the blood sugars at a higher level than the physician would recommend. Some children have considerable anxiety about hypoglycemia, either in response to an actual episode or arising independently. It is key to treat anxiety disorders in order to improve compliance as well as recognize emerging eating disorders in the female teenage population as a factor in non-compliance (Hamilton & Daneman, 2002; Jacobson, 1996; Strauss, 1996).

Parents of children with diabetes may benefit from the support of the child mental health consultant as well as parent support groups to help achieve a healthy family attitude towards eating. Concrete ways to minimize the child's experience of being deprived of popular food treats are useful, such as having sugar-free desserts at school and at home, altering insulin to accommodate special events, and supporting the child's understanding of how insulin helps him or her grow bigger and stronger.

When patterns of conflict between parent and child around non-compliance arise (e.g., lying about foods eaten, hiding sweets and refusing blood monitoring), psychotherapeutic input should be initiated early. Family conflict is strongly related to adherence (Lewin, Heidgerken, Geffken *et al.*, 2006). Children who enter adolescence with pre-existing parent–child conflict around health maintenance can be expected to have greater difficulty during their teenage years. Non-compliance in type 1 diabetes can be life-threatening, so the full range of psychotherapeutic, educational and family supports should be utilized. Blood testing (hemoglobin A1C) enables the pediatrician to assess the child's compliance over an extended period and may be considered an appropriate factor for protocol-driven mental health consultation.

Cancer

Childhood cancer presents numerous challenges to adaptation and development, fortunately however most studies suggest that childhood cancer survivors adapt well following treatment (Kazak, 2005; Zebrack, Zevon, Turk *et al.*, 2007). There are predictable high stress points in the course of an illness which often coincide with hospitalization including diagnosis, onset of treatment and treatment completion, as well as for some recurrence, renewed treatment and end-of-life care. Psychological support for the child and parents is particularly beneficial at these critical points. Siblings also benefit from support at the various transitions during the course of the illness (Wilkins & Woodgate, 2005).

Diagnosis of a life-threatening illness is understandably frightening to parents and older children, creating a family crisis. Some children and parents respond to diagnosis and aspects of treatment by exhibiting symptoms seen in post-traumatic stress syndrome (Stuber, Kazak, Meeske, & Baraket, 1998).

Frequently, children and families will face the child's cancer diagnosis with past experiences of cancer in a family member, or close friend, coloring their understanding of what lies ahead for their child (Hoekstra-Weebers, Jaspers, Kamps, & Klip, 1999). It is helpful to invite the child to share his or her understanding of the diagnosis as an opportunity to differentiate the child's situation from that of others, while potentially uncovering misconceptions about the illness.

Challenges to psychological adaptation include persistent pain, whether as a result of the cancer or of the procedures (Ljungman, Gordh, Sorensen, & Kreuger, 1999), persistent debilitating side-effects of treatment such as nausea, alteration in body image, school disruptions, compromised peer relationships, interference with ability to engage in favorite activities and conflicts in the family. Adolescents may worry about future health status, sexual function and reproductive capacities, and future career choices (Kazak, 2005; Patenaude & Kupst, 2005). Awareness of these challenges may guide the consultant in addressing concerns and adapting treatments whenever possible.

During the course of cancer treatment, many children develop strong positive relationships with members of the medical team, experience a special closeness with supportive parents and maintain key pre-existing peer friendships while acquiring new friends in the hospital. Many children will report feeling a special sense of purpose for living as a result of the cancer diagnosis and most will be treated with special status as a result of the illness. Resiliency and positive life change are also part of the cancer experience (Woodgate, 1999).

Organ Transplantation

Liver, kidney and lung transplantation are well-established practices in the pediatric population and intestinal transplantation is beginning to be undertaken. Transplantation centers in the USA are required to include psychological assessment in order to receive accreditation. Data on criteria for approval of candidacy for transplant are vague. The serious disease process leading up to transplantation, risks of surgery, long-term medical management of organ rejection post-transplantation, threat to survival, and the vast array of medical personnel involved should place these children in the highest of high-risk populations. It is noteworthy therefore that the data on adjustment to liver and renal transplantation suggest that overall these children view themselves as healthy and competent (Karrfelt, Lindblad, Crafoord, & Berg, 2003; Mastroyannopoulou, Sclere, Baker, & Mowat, 1998; Tonquist, Van Broeck, Finkenauer *et al.*, 1999). Not surprisingly, some children and parents are vulnerable to anxiety and experience distress post-transplant (Mintzer, Stuber, Seacord *et al.*, 2005; Shemesh, Annunziato, Shneider *et al.*, 2005b). It is therefore important that transplant centers involve mental health consultants and provide emotional support (Ullrich, Meyke, Haase *et al.*, 1997; Walker, Harris, Baker, Kelly, & Houghton, 1999).

Dying in Hospital

The death of a child is an enormous tragedy affecting every member of the child's family. There is no way to protect a child or family from the unique pain of the loss of a child, but sensitive care at this difficult time may serve to lessen regrets and support bereavement. Careful attention to the child's quality of life in the last days or hours is essential. Attending to pain, anxiety and privacy/dignity needs is key. Adapting the medical setting to allow parents to nurture the dying child within the limitations of the setting or facilitating a child's return home to die can play a significant part in the family's experience of the death and the subsequent bereavement (American Academy of Pediatrics, 2000).

The emotional impact on the medical team deserves careful attention in order to best preserve team members' ability to continue to deliver quality care into the future. The grieving process of the staff warrants recognition. Some units have staff meetings including the child mental health consultant or other facilitator after every death or after those deaths that are most troubling to staff members, such as a patient with chronic disease, a trauma-related death or an unanticipated death.

Many of the hospital-based pediatric deaths occur in neonatal ICUs or during infancy. Key to supporting the family of a dying infant is respecting the infant's full status as a loved child. This may include facilitating religious ceremonies such as a naming or christening, creating mementos such as photographs, footprints or a lock of hair, and creating the most loving situation possible for the moment of dying such as providing a private room and allowing a parent to hold the infant at the time life support is disconnected.

From age 3 years onwards, the child's personal experience of impending death should be considered. The child should be offered developmentally appropriate opportunities to express thoughts and fears associated with dying either with words, drawings or through play. It is not uncommon for even 3- or 4-year-olds to verbalize explicit thoughts of joining dead grandparents and seeing angels, but it is also common for dying children to focus only on wanting parents with them at all times, and exhibiting a shift in behavior with more resistance to medical treatment, loss of interest in activities and food, but without any explicit verbalization of an awareness of dying.

Children of all ages, but especially younger children, are likely to take their cues about whether explicit discussion of death is permissible from parents and caregivers. When parents invite this dialog it is more like to occur. When parents signal that such discussion would be unbearable, the child is likely either not to speak about dying or to talk with a medical staff member when the parent is not present.

Child mental health consultants may help ready parents for discussions with their dying child. Asking the parents for observations about shifts in the child's behavior may help the parents recognize that they would not be introducing a new frightening idea to the child in talking about death, but would rather be accompanying the child in the thoughts that he or she is already engaged in. Asking open-ended questions about worries, enquiring whether the child has questions that he or she is afraid to say aloud, or asking if he or she thinks about peers from the hospital who have died, may serve as invitations to begin the dialog. Reminding children that articulating worries does not make them happen may free some children who are worrying silently to speak. Many parents will feel more comfortable embarking on end-of-life conversations with a child if they are told that they can welcome the child's questions warmly without having specific answers. "I am interested in your ideas." "What got you wondering about that?" "Your good questions deserve good answers. I want to think about that or talk to our minister or the doctor." These are examples of reasonable responses to a child's existential or medical questions. In the role of child mental health consultant, one of the most useful comments in response to questions about death is to tell a child, "I don't know what it is like to be dead, because I have never been dead. But I am always interested to hear children's ideas about it."

Children from age 7 onward may talk about the life experiences that they will not get to enjoy. These discussions challenge a parent's or professional's ability to bear the sadness of facing an untimely death as well as whether to talk directly with a child about their death (Kreicbergs, Valdimarsdottir, Onelov, Henter, & Steinek, 2004). The child may talk about not getting to attend the 5th grade, never being able to drive a car or not growing up to be a doctor or a teacher. It is often the specificity of the opportunities lost in the words of a child that is so evocative. There is a sense of privilege that one experiences in listening to children as they face the end of their lives that is as special as it is sad.

Often, children will talk about being tired of the fight against the disease and will look to parents for permission to give up. When the surviving family members can support each other in the painful process of letting go of the beloved child, believing that everything that could be done was done, and that further treatment would be unfair to the child, the final phase of dying seems more peaceful. In the setting of a long battle against an illness, it is easier to get to this difficult emotional state. In the setting of an acute event with little time for adjustment, or when parental discord interferes with the parents' ability to grieve together, such peace is harder to achieve.

The consultant should encourage hospital staff to follow up with parents 6 months to a year after the death of a child. Parents are appreciative when staff attend memorial services and funerals, write sympathy cards and make telephone calls (Bedell, Cadenhead, & Graboys, 2001; Macdonald, Liven, Carnevale *et al.*, 2005). Telephone calls provide an opportunity to assess the parents' grieving and need for referral as well as help the staff member connect with the family.

Conclusions

Child mental health consultants must stay attuned to the changes in the field of pediatrics. Advances in pharmacology, genomics and technology offer new hope and new challenges to psychosocial adaptation. Patterns of access to consultation will need to reflect shorter hospital stays and utilization of outpatient venues. New technology, such as telemedicine, can offer novel access to consultative expertise. Research in compliancy outcomes, efficacy and quality of life become increasingly important as the financial pressures of modern medicine force the consultant to justify the value of their work.

However, many of the key features of quality consultation remain unchanged. The consultant will continue to bring to the multidisciplinary medical team the combined expertise of psychodynamic understanding, psychopharmacology, a developmental perspective on the meaning of illness, adaptation to trauma, knowledge of psychiatric conditions, behavioral interventions, and CNS influences in medical illness and as a result of medical treatment. The goal remains to answer the consultation request in a thoughtful timely fashion which respects the needs of the child, the family and the treatment team while facilitating quality of care and quality of life.

References

Akinbami, L. J., & Schoendorf, K. C. (2002). Trends in childhood asthma: Prevalence, health care utilization, and mortality. *Pediatrics*, *110*, 315–322.

American Academy of Child and Adolescent Psychiatry (AACAP). (in press). Practice parameter for the psychiatric assessment and management of physically ill children and adolescents. *Journal of Clinical Child and Adolescent Psychology*,

American Academy of Pediatrics (AAP), Committee on Bioethics. (1995). Informed consent, parental permission, and assent in pediatric practice. *Pediatrics*, *95*, 314–317.

American Academy of Pediatrics (AAP), Committee on Bioethics and Committee on Hospital Care. (2000). Palliative care for children. *Pediatrics*, *106*, 351–357.

Andersen, A., Bowers, W., & Evans, K. (1997). Inpatient treatment of anorexia nervosa. In D. M. Garner, & P. E. Garfinkel (Eds.), *Handbook of treatment for eating disorders* (2nd edn., pp. 327–353). New York: Guilford Press.

Barlow, J. H., & Ellard, D. R. (2006). The psychosocial well-being of children with chronic disease, their parents and siblings: An overview of the research evidence base. *Child: Care, Health and Development*, *32*, 19–31.

Bauman, L., Drotar, D., Leventhal, J., Perrin, E., & Pless, I. (1997). A review of psychosocial interventions for children with chronic health conditions. *Pediatrics*, *100*, 244–251.

Bedell, S. E., Cadenhead, K., & Graboys, T. B. (2001). The doctor's letter of condolence. *New England Journal of Medicine*, *344*, 1162–1164.

Bender, B. G. (2006). Risk taking, depression, adherence, and symptom control in adolescents and young adults with asthma. *American Journal of Respiratory and Critical Care Medicine*, *173*, 953–957.

Bergman, A., & Fritz, G. (1985). Pediatricians and mental health professionals: Patterns of collaboration and utilization. *American Journal of Diseases in Children*, *139*, 155–159.

Bonner, M. J., Hardy, K. K., Guill, A. B., McLaughlin, C., Schweitzer, H., & Carter, K. (2006). Development and validation of the parent experience of child illness. *Journal of Pediatric Psychology*, *31*, 310–321.

British Medical Association. (2001). *Consent, rights and choices in health care for children and young people*. London: BMJ Books.

Burket, R. C., & Hodgin, J. D. (1993). Pediatricians' perceptions of child psychiatry consultations. *Psychosomatics*, *34*, 402–408.

Butler, L. D., Symons, B. K., Henderson, S. L., Shortliffe, L. D., & Spiegel, D. (2005). Hypnosis reduces distress and duration of an invasive medical procedure for children. *Pediatrics*, *115*, 77–85.

Carter, B. D., Kronenberger, W. G., Baker, J., Grimes, L. M., Crabtree, V. M., Smith, C., *et al.* (2003). Inpatient pediatric consultation-liaison: A case-controlled study. *Journal of Pediatric Psychology*, *28*, 423–432.

Cork, M. J., Britton, J., Butler, L., Young, S., Murphy, R., & Keohane, S. G. (2003). Comparison of parent knowledge, therapy utilization and severity of atopic eczema before and after explanation and demonstration of topical therapies by a specialist dermatology nurse. *British Journal of Dermatology*, *149*, 582–589.

DeMaso, D. R., & Meyer, E. C. (1996). A psychiatric consultant's survival guide to the pediatric intensive care unit. *Journal of the American Academy of Child and Adolescent Psychiatry*, *35*, 1411–1413.

Diaz-Caneja, A., Gledhill, J., Weaver, T., Nadel, S., & Garralda, E. (2005). A child's admission to hospital: A qualitative study examining the experiences of parents. *Intensive Care Medicine*, *31*, 1248–1254.

Dinwiddie, R., & Muller, W. G. (2002). Adolescent treatment compliance in asthma. *Journal of the Royal Society of Medicine*, *95*, 68–71.

Eisenberg, L. (1995). The social construction of the human brain. *American Journal of Psychiatry*, *152*, 1563–1575.

Feinstein, S., Keich, R., Becker-Cohen, R., Rinat, C., Schwartz, S. B., & Frishberg, Y. (2005). Is noncompliance among adolescent renal transplant recipients inevitable? *Pediatrics*, *115*, 969–973.

Fritz, G., Pumariega, A., & Fischhoff, J. (1987). Child psychiatrists' perceptions of timing and frequency of consultation requests. *Journal of the American Academy of Child and Adolescent Psychiatry*, *26*, 425–427.

Fritz, G. K. (2003). Promoting effective collaboration between pediatricians and child and adolescent psychiatrists. *Pediatric Annals*, *32*, 387–389.

Geist, R. (1977). Consultation on a pediatric surgical ward: Creating an empathic climate. *American Journal of Orthopsychiatry*, *47*, 432–444.

Gershon, J., Zimand, E., Pickering, M., Rothbaum, B. O., & Hodges, L. (2004). A pilot and feasibility study of virtual reality as a distraction for children with cancer. *Journal of the American Academy of Child and Adolescent Psychiatry*, *43*, 1243–1249.

Greco, C., & Berde, C. (2005). Pain management for the hospitalized pediatric patient. *Pediatric Clinics of North America*, *52*, 995–1027, vii–viii.

Groves, J., & Beresin, E. (1999). Difficult patients, difficult families. *New Horizons*, *6*, 331–343.

Hamilton, J., & Daneman, D. (2002). Deteriorating diabetes control during adolescence: Physiological or psychosocial? *Journal of Pediatric Endocrinology*, *15*, 115–126.

Hengeveld, M., & Rooysman, H. (1983). The relevance of a staff-oriented approach in consultation psychiatry: A preliminary study. *General Hospital Psychiatry*, *5*, 259–264.

Hockemeyer, J., & Smyth, J. (2002). Evaluating the feasibility and efficacy of a self-administered manual-based stress management intervention for individuals with asthma: Results from a controlled study. *Behavioral Medicine*, *27*, 161–172.

Hoekstra-Weebers, J., Jaspers, J., Kamps, W., & Klip, E. (1999). Risk factors for psychological maladjustment of parents of children with cancer. *Journal of the American Academy of Child and Adolescent Psychiatry*, *38*, 1526–1535.

Jacobson, A. (1996). The psychological care of patients with insulin-dependent diabetes mellitus. *New England Journal of Medicine*, *334*, 1249–1253.

Karrfelt, H. M. E., Lindblad, F. I. E., Crafoord, J., & Berg, U. B. (2003). Renal transplantation: Long-term adaptation and the children's own reflections. *Pediatric Transplantation*, *7*, 69–75.

Kazak, A. E. (2005). Evidence-based interventions for survivors of childhood cancer and their families. *Journal of Pediatric Psychology*, *30*, 29–39.

Knapp, P., & Harris, E. (1998). Consultation-liaison in child psychiatry: A review of the past 10 years. *Journal of the American Academy of Child and Adolescent Psychiatry*, *37*, 139–146.

Kreicbergs, U., Valdimarsdottir, U., Onelov, E., Bjork, O., Steineck, G., & Henter, J. I. (2005). Care-related distress: A nationwide study of parents who lost their child to cancer. *Journal of Clinical Oncology*, *23*, 9162–9171.

Kreicbergs, U., Valdimarsdottir, U., Onelov, E., Henter, J. I., & Steinek, G. (2004). Talking about death with children who have severe malignant disease. *New England Journal of Medicine*, *351*, 1251–1253.

Labay, L. E., & Walco, G. A. (2004). Brief report: Empathy and psychological adjustment in siblings of children with cancer. *Journal of Pediatric Psychology*, *29*, 309–314.

Lask, B. (1994). Paediatric liaison work. In M. Rutter, E. Taylor, & L. Hersov (Eds.), *Child and adolescent psychiatry: Modern approaches* (3rd edn., pp. 996–1005). Oxford: Blackwell Science.

Levi, B. H., Thomas, N. J., Green, M. J., Rentmeester, C. A., & Ceneviva, G. D. (2004). Jading in the pediatric intensive care unit: Implications for healthcare providers of medically complex children. *Pediatric Critical Care Medicine*, *5*, 275–277.

Lewin, A. B., Heidgerken, A. D., Geffken, G. R., Williams, L. B., Storch, E. A., Gelfand, K. M., *et al.* (2006). The relation between family factors and metabolic control: The role of diabetes adherence. *Journal of Pediatric Psychology*, *31*, 174–183.

Ljungman, G., Gordh, T., Sorensen, S., & Kreuger, A. (1999). Pain in paediatric oncology: Interviews with children, adolescents and their parents. *Acta Paediatrica Scandinavica*, *88*, 623–630.

Louthrenoo, O., Sittipreechacharn, S., Thanarattanakorn, P., & Sanguansermsri, T. (2002). Psychosocial problems in children with thalassemia and their siblings. *Journal of the Medical Association of Thailand*, *85*, 881–885.

Macdonald, M. E., Liven, S., Carnevale, F. A., Rennick, J. E., Wolf, S. L., Meloche, D., *et al.* (2005). Parental perspectives on hospital staff members' acts of kindness and commemoration after a child's death. *Pediatrics*, *116*, 884–890.

Mastroyannopoulou, K., Sclare, I., Baker, A., & Mowat, A. (1998). Psychological effects of liver disease and transplantation. *European Journal of Pediatrics*, *157*, 856–860.

Maytum, J. C., Heiman, M. B., & Garwick, A. W. (2004). Compassion fatigue and burnout in nurses who work with children with chronic conditions and their families. *Journal of Pediatric Health Care*, *18*, 171–179.

McDaniel, M., Paxson, C., & Waldfogel, J. (2006). Racial disparities in childhood asthma in the United States: Evidence from the national health interview survey, 1997 to 2003. *Pediatrics*, *117*, 868–877.

Meyer, W. J. 3rd, Blakeney, P., Russell, W., Thomas, C., Robert, R., Berniger, F., *et al.* (2004). Psychological problems reported by young adults who were burned as children. *Journal of Burn Care and Rehabilitation*, *25*, 98–106.

Mintzer, L. L., Stuber, M. L., Seacord, D., Castaneda, M., Mesrkhani, V., & Glover, D. (2005). Traumatic stress symptoms in adolescent organ transplant recipients. *Pediatrics*, *115*, 1640–1644.

Mundy, E. A., DuHamel, K. N., & Montgomery, G. H. (2003). The efficacy of behavioral interventions for cancer treatment-related side effects. *Seminars in Clinical Neuropsychiatry*, *8*, 253–275.

Murray, J. S. (2002). A qualitative exploration of psychosocial support for siblings of children with cancer. *Journal of Pediatric Nursing*, *17*, 327–337.

Ortiz, P. (1997). General principles in child liaison consultation services: A literature review. *European Child and Adolescent Psychiatry*, *6*, 1–6.

Patenaude, A. F., & Kupst, M. J. (2005). Psychosocial functioning in pediatric cancer. *Journal of Pediatric Psychology*, *30*, 9–27.

Patton, S. R., Dolan, L. M., & Powers, S. W. (2006). Parent report of mealtime behaviors in young children with type 1 diabetes mellitus: Implications for better assessment of dietary adherence problems in the clinic. *Journal of Developmental and Behavioral Pediatrics*, *27*, 202–208.

Poggi, G., Liscio, M., Adduci, A., Galbiati, S., Massimino, M., Sommovigo, M., *et al.* (2005a). Psychological and adjustment problems due to acquired brain lesions in childhood: A comparison between post-traumatic patients and brain tumour survivors. *Brain Injury*, *19*, 777–785.

Poggi, G., Liscio, M., Galbiati, S., Adduci, A., Massimino, M., Gandola, L., *et al.* (2005b). Brain tumors in children and adolescents: Cognitive and psychological disorders at different ages. *Psycho-Oncology*, *14*, 386–395.

Rauch, P., & Jellinek, M. (2002). Pediatric consultation. In M. Rutter, & E. Taylor (Eds.), *Child and adolescent psychiatry* (4th edn., pp. 1051–1066). Oxford: Blackwell Publishing.

Rubin, B. K. (2004). What does it mean when a patient says, "My asthma medication is not working?". *Chest*, *126*, 972–981.

Sawyer, M. G., Streiner, D. L., Antoniou, G., Toogood, I., & Rice, M. (1998). Influence of parental and family adjustment on the later psychological adjustment of children treated for cancer. *Journal of the American Academy of Child and Adolescent Psychiatry*, *37*, 815–822.

Schiff, W. B., Holtz, K. D., Peterson, N., & Rakusan, T. (2001). Effect of an intervention to reduce procedural pain and distress for children with HIV infection. *Journal of Pediatric Psychology*, *26*, 417–427.

Self, T. H., Chrisman, C. R., Mason, D. L., & Rumbak, M. J. (2005). Reducing emergency department visits and hospitalizations in African American and Hispanic patients with asthma: A 15-year review. *Journal of Asthma*, *42*, 807–812.

Shaw, R. J., Wamboldt, M., Bursch, B., & Stuber, M. (2006). Practice patterns in pediatric consultation-liaison psychiatry. *Psychosomatics*, *47*, 43–49.

Shemesh, E., Yehuda, R., Rockmore, L., Shneider, B. L., Emre, S., Bartell, A. S., *et al.* (2005a). Assessment of depression in medically ill children presenting to pediatric specialty clinics. *Journal of the American Academy of Child and Adolescent Psychiatry*, *44*, 1249–1257.

Shemesh, E., Annunziato, R. A., Shneider, B. L., Newcorn, J. H., Warshaw, J. K., Dugan, C. A., *et al.* (2005b). Parents and clinicans underestimate distress and depression in children who had a transplant. *Pediatric Transplantation*, *9*, 673–679.

Stoppelbein, L., Greening, L., Jordon, S. S., Elkin, T. D., Moll, G., & Pullen, J. (2005). Factor analysis of the pediatric symptom checklist with a chronically ill pediatric population. *Journal of Developmental and Behavioral Pediatrics*, *26*, 349–355.

Strauss, G. (1996). Psychological factors in intensive management of insulin-dependent diabetes mellitus. *Nursing Clinics of North America*, *31*, 737–745.

Stuber, M., Kazak, A., Meeske, K., & Baraket, L. (1998). Is post traumatic stress a viable model for understanding response to childhood cancer? *Child and Adolescent Psychiatric Clinics of North America*, *7*, 169–182.

Svavarsdottis, E. K., & Sigurdardottis, A. (2005). The feasibility of offering a family level intervention to parents of children with cancer. *Scandinavian Journal of Caring Sciences*, *19*, 368–372.

Tarnow, J., & Gutstein, S. (1982). Systemic consultation in a general hospital. *International Journal of Psychiatry and Medicine*, *12*, 161–186.

Teach, S. J., Crain, E. F., Quint, D. M., Hylan, M. L., & Joseph, J. G. (2006). Improved asthma outcomes in a high-morbidity pediatric population: Results of an emergency department-based randomized clinical trial. *Archives of Pediatrics and Adolescent Medicine*, *160*, 535–541.

Tonquist, J., Van Broeck, N., Finkenauer, C., Rosati, R., Schwering, K. L., Hayez, J. Y., *et al.* (1999). Long-term psychosocial adjustment following pediatric liver transplatation. *Pediatric Transplantation*, *3*, 115–125.

Ullrich, G., Meyke, A., Haase, H., Erzfeld, C., Beckmann, S., Schmidt-Schaller, S., *et al.* (1997). Psychological support of children undergoing liver transplantation and their parents: a single-centre experience. *Pediatric Rehabilitation*, *1*, 19–24.

Vance, Y., & Eiser, C. (2004). Caring for a child with cancer: A systematic review. *Pediatric Blood and Cancer*, *42*, 249–253.

Van Sciver, M., D'Angelo, E., Rappaport, L., & Woolf, A. (1995). Pediatric compliance and the roles of distinct treatment characteristics, treatment attitudes, and family stress: A preliminary report. *Journal of Developmental and Behavioral Pediatrics*, *16*, 350–358.

Wagner, J. L., Chaney, J. M., Hommel, K. A., Page, M. C., Mullins, L. L., White, M. M., *et al.* (2003). The influence of parental distress on child depressive symptoms in juvenile rheumatic diseases: The moderating effect of illness intrusiveness. *Journal of Pediatric Psychology*, *28*, 453–462.

Walker, A., Harris, G., Baker, A., Kelly, D., & Houghton, J. (1999). Post-traumatic stress response following liver transplantation in older children. *Journal of Child Psychology and Psychiatry*, *40*, 363–374.

Watson, E. (2006). CAMHS liaison: Supporting care in general paediatric settings. *Paediatric Nursing*, *18*, 30–33.

Wilkins, K. L., & Woodgate, R. L. (2005). A review of qualitative research on the childhood cancer experience from the perspective of siblings: A need to give them a voice [review]. *Journal of Pediatric Oncology Nursing*, *22*, 305–319.

Woodgate, R. (1999). Conceptual understanding of resilience in the adolescent with cancer: Part I. *Journal of Pediatric Oncology Nursing*, *16*, 35–43.

Woodgate, R. (1999). A review of the literature on resilience in the adolescent with cancer: Part II. *Journal of Pediatric Oncology Nursing*, *16*, 78–89.

Work, H. (1989). The "menace of psychiatry" revisited: The evolving relationship between pediatrics and child psychiatry. *Psychosomatics*, *30*, 86–93.

Wright, H., Eaton, J., Butterfield, P., Snellgrove, N., Hanna, K., & Cole, E. (1987). Financing of child psychiatry pediatric consultation-liaison programs. *Journal of Developmental and Behavioral Pediatrics*, *8*, 221–228.

Young, K. D. (2005). Pediatric procedural pain. *Annals of Emergency Medicine*, *45*, 160–171.

Zebrack, B. J., Zevon, M. A., Turk, N., Nagarajan, R., Whitton, J., Robison, L. L., *et al.* (2007). Psychological distress in long-term survivors of solid tumors diagnosed in childhood: A report from the childhood cancer survivor study. *Pediatric Blood and Cancer*, *49*, 47–51.

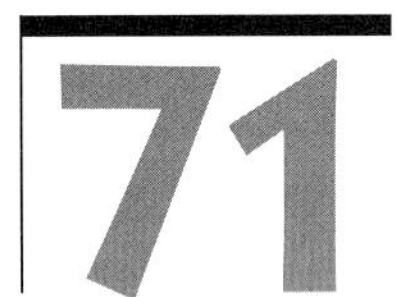

Organization of Services for Children and Adolescents with Mental Health Problems

Miranda Wolpert

Only a handful of countries have an articulated national policy in relation to services for children and young people with mental health problems. Of 191 countries sampled in 2003, 14 (7%) had produced policy in this area (World Health Organization [WHO], 2005). The vision for the future is that it will become possible to agree a clear and coherent approach to service provision, based on a growing evidence base, underpinned by a comprehensive assessment of need and in line with the core values and priorities of a given society.

This chapter offers an approach to thinking about the organization of services across a range of contexts. It will not attempt to put forward one ideal model to fit all, nor attempt a comprehensive review of existing models of provision,[2] but will try to develop a systematic way of considering the different aspects of service organization, trying to take into consideration some of the different factors that may present particular challenges in different countries.

The topic is examined in terms of the following five key domains, which are taken to represent crucial building blocks for thinking about service organization:

1 Responding to need;
2 Understanding the evidence base;
3 Developing a workforce;
4 Ensuring accessibility; and
5 Assuring quality.

Responding to Need

The issues of what counts as a "mental health problem" and whose needs should be the legitimate focus of service provision are far from settled. Clearly, there should be provision for children with diagnosable mental health problems that are causing a significant degree of impairment where there are effective treatments, but beyond that there is much room for debate (for an important but controversial discussion of these issues in relation to services in England see Goodman, 1997).

An ever-expanding conceptualization of what constitutes children's "mental health needs" has rendered the concept of children's "mental health problems" increasingly open to interpretation. At least four groups of children with "mental health needs" are routinely referred to in the discussions about developing national policy:

1 Children and young people in difficult (and often terrible) circumstances;
2 Children at risk of developing diagnosable mental health problems;
3 Children with diagnosable mental health problems; and
4 Children with levels of impairment resulting from mental health issues that make it difficult for them to function within their community or culture.

These groups of children are sometimes discussed (Remschmidt, Belfer, & Goodyer, 2004) as if they exist in the relation to each other shown in Fig. 71.1. In fact, it may be more appropriate

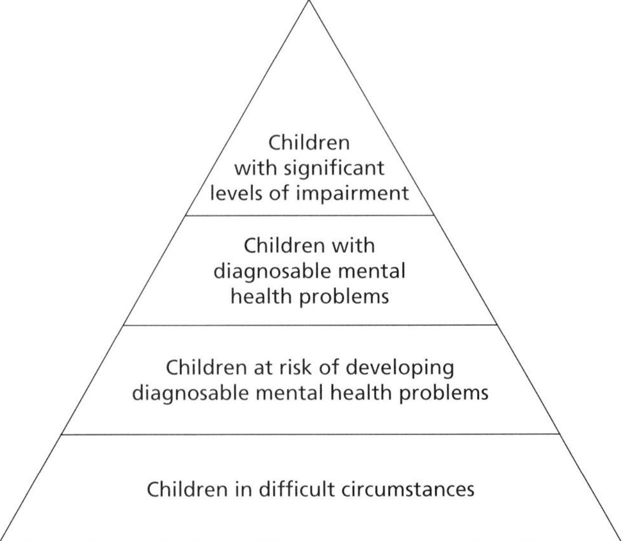

Fig. 71.1 Relationship of groups of children with mental health needs.

[1] For brevity from now on the terms "children" and "child" will be used to refer to "children and young people."
[2] For an excellent source book on provision across the world see Remschmidt, Belfer and Goodyer (Eds.). (2004). *Facilitating Pathways: Care treatment and prevention in child and adolescent mental health*. Berlin: Springer.

Rutter's Child and Adolescent Psychiatry, 5th edition. Edited by M. Rutter, D. Bishop, D. Pine, S. Scott, J. Stevenson, E. Taylor and A. Thapar. © 2008 Blackwell Publishing, ISBN: 978-1-4051-4549-7.

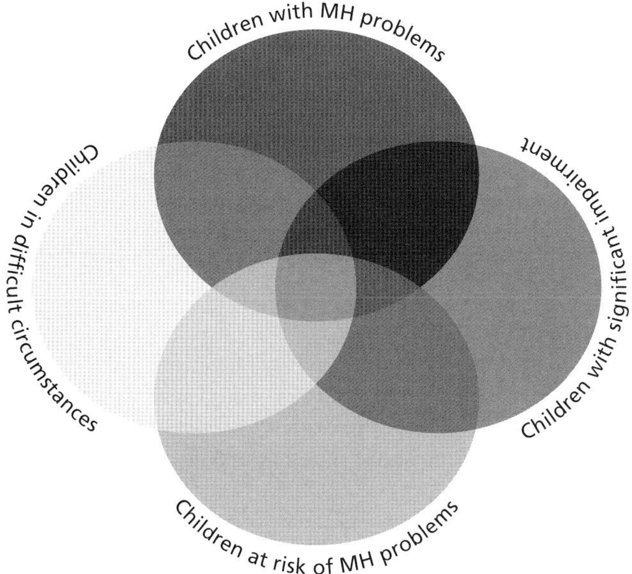

Fig. 71.2 Alternative view of groups of children with mental health needs as highly overlapping but distinct groups. MH, mental health.

to think of these four groups as highly overlapping but potentially distinct populations of children (Fig. 71.2). Lack of clarity when discussing the needs of the different groups can obscure the fact that different groups may be a priority for different communities and lead to misunderstandings between service developers when discussing their common commitment to services based on "needs assessment."

Children in Difficult Circumstances

Definitions of "difficult circumstances" vary with national context. The estimated 14 million AIDS orphans (concentrated largely in Africa) would fall into this category, as would the 12 million children in the USA living below the poverty line, along with all those children who are in contexts of war, famine or abuse (WHO, 2005). Although child mental health services are unlikely to be the main provider for the majority, this group is likely to include those children with high and complex mental health needs who are the hardest to reach and who are an increasing policy priority in many countries (Belfer, 2004). However, it may also include children who do not have specific mental health needs (Robertson, Mandlhate, Seif El Din, & Seck, 2004). Determining the most pressing needs of these children and determining the most effective contribution of mental health provision within this group are likely to be key tasks in terms of service organization.

Children "At Risk"

Risk factors for developing diagnosable mental health problems include some aspect of difficult circumstances (e.g., violent environments, lack of warm family environments) but risk is also heightened by other individual and interpersonal factors such as brain injury, low birth weight, poor parental mental health, low IQ, irritable temperament, family dysfunction and the lack of a key supportive relationship with an adult (Goodman & Scott, 2005). For children identified as "at risk," the focus for mental health provision is likely to be on how to enhance resilience. There may be key opportunities for intervention, such as when the child is born or at key transition points (e.g., starting school, changing school, leaving school). There is an argument for targeting particular groups such as children of parents with mental health problems (Falkov, Phillips, Brady, Stathis, & Finney, 2003). However, promotion of resilience may best be achieved by agencies other than child mental health specialists, such as welfare sectors creating greater neighborhood cohesion, perinatal services reducing risk of low birth weight and educational services implementing appropriate programs to promote emotional well-being and support children in times of stress.

Children with Diagnosable Mental Health Problems

Epidemiological data from Europe and the USA suggest that around 10–20% of children have diagnosable mental health problems (using ICD-10 or DSM-IV criteria; Goodman & Scott, 2005). There are indications of differences between countries, with slightly lower rates found in India and Norway, for example (Heiervang, Stormark, Lundervold *et al.*, 2007; Malhotra, Kohli, & Arun, 2002), and slightly higher in Brazil, Bangladesh and Russia (Fleitlich-Bilyk & Goodman, 2004; Mullick & Goodman, 2005). There is a need both for more international epidemiological data and for greater international consensus on some broad definitions of difficulties which would allow a common language to develop that could underpin appropriate policy development (Belfer, 2004).

Some diagnosable mental health problems in children may get better without intervention (such as depression in mild forms), suggesting it may be counterproductive to rush to provide services for all diagnosable difficulties in all circumstances. For these reasons, amongst others (in particular the fact that not all current treatments are proven to do more good than harm; see p. 1160), it may be unwise to go down the route recently suggested by the American Psychiatric Association of screening all children in schools and treating all diagnosable difficulties (American Psychiatric Association [APA], 2002).

Children with Impairment Caused by Mental Health Difficulties

This category covers children with a wide range of difficulties ranging from enuresis to psychosis, including those with chronic and multiple difficulties and those with discrete and defined difficulties. It includes those with difficulties where there are known to be effective interventions and those presenting with problems where the best course of action is much less clear. It may also include some children who do not meet the diagnostic criteria but still have significant impairment. Angold, Messer, Strangl *et al.* (1998) found that 50% of children attending one US clinic did not meet diagnostic criteria, but half of these were significantly functionally impaired.

The impact of significant and impairing mental health difficulties, if not effectively treated, can be substantial. Worldwide, suicide is the third leading cause of death amongst adolescents; major depressive disorder, often starting in adolescence, is associated with substantial psychosocial impairment; conduct disorders amongst children tend to persist into adult life and are reflected in later drug abuse, antisocial behavior and poor physical health (Broidy, Nagin, Tremblay *et al.*, 2003). Attempts to calculate the cost to society of unresolved difficulties are still in their infancy (Romeo, Byford, & Knapp, 2006), but some figures are being estimated. The additional public expenditure on a child with conduct disorder over a 7-year period in the USA was estimated to exceed $70,000, largely in costs related to criminal behavior (Foster & Jones, 2005).

Access to Provision

Since Rutter's seminal work in this area in the UK in the 1970s, suggesting only 1 in 10 children identified with problems warranting specialist intervention actually accessed services, further studies have suggested that it has remained the case that the majority of children and young people with significant mental health needs do not reach services (Ford, Hamilton, Goodman, & Meltzer, 2005; Green, McGinnity, Meltzer, Ford, & Goodman, 2005; Rutter, Tizard, & Whitmore, 1970). In the developing world, access to specialist services is likely to be far more limited and for those children also in difficult circumstances access is likely to be even harder. Access is limited not just by levels of resources available, but also in many countries by alternative beliefs about the best way to understand and treat problems and the stigma associated with seeking specialist "mental health" help (Eapen & Ghubash, 2004; Nikapota, 2002).

Prioritizing Needs

Each community will have to determine its own way to resolve the tension between the needs of these different groups. In some countries this may make independent child mental health provision an unaffordable luxury when pitted against other basic needs (Robertson, Mandlhate, Seif El Din *et al.*, 2004). Where some resources are available, then the country will need to balance the desire to put resources into mental health promotion and prevention of mental ill health (to meet the needs of the first two groups above) with the need to ensure that adequate resources are available to provide services for the most impaired and troubled children (the latter two groups above). While there is as yet no easy metric to determine what the ratio should be, the World Health Organization suggested that where resources are particularly limited, priority for funds for child mental health provision should be given to those children with existing difficulties that occur frequently (and/or have highest cost implications); cause a high degree of impairment and the greatest long-term care/cost consequences; have an evidence base for treatment; and (particularly in those countries with the most limited resources) where the difficulties can be dealt with in primary care or universal services such as schools or GPs (WHO, 2003). In such circumstances, the best that can be suggested for promotion is to encourage positive activity in terms of universal service provision that does not require additional resource allocation.

In countries with greater resources, there is more opportunity to support a range of provision. In such countries, child mental health professionals' input can be conceptualized as being provided at universal, targeted and specialist levels. This involves supporting and working alongside universal provision to promote emotional well-being whether in schools or via primary care health workers. Targeted provision aims to promote emotional well-being in those deemed either at most risk (group 2 above) or in most need (group 1 above), with the groups being determined by policy imperatives. Here, specialist mental health professionals will work alongside workers from other sectors who take a lead in relation to the needs of these groups as a whole, such as social welfare workers and primary care staff. Specialist provision aims to support group 4 above, and can be provided at a local community level, although more rare and specialized resources may be provided at a regional or even a national level.

In planning response to "need," however, it is important to consider the potential negative and even harmful impact of increased specialist mental health services. Mental health professionals are frequently in danger of assuming that more specialist mental health provision is unquestionably an unalloyed good. The need for more provision must be set in the context of other (sometimes competing) "needs," such as the primary need of children to be nourished, sheltered and protected; their need not to be stigmatized or miss education; and their need not to receive inappropriate, ineffective or harmful treatment. At times, an inappropriate mental health focus can be an unhelpful drain on resources (Shooter, 2005). One documented example is when well-meaning voluntary groups enter a country following a disaster to provide "interventions for post-traumatic stress disorder (PTSD)" that were not linked to other relief efforts and actually interfered with and undermined key initiatives (WHO, 2005). While the costs of not providing effective specialist mental health inputs can be high, it is important to remember there are also costs to providing unhelpful services.

Understanding the Evidence Base

The arguments for trying to promote evidence-based service development are compelling. Natural biases in reasoning mean that people tend to make decisions based more on things that fit their assumptive world view than those that challenge it and are more influenced by the charisma of those promoting a particular approach than by evidence for its effectiveness (Garb, 1997; Kahnemann, Slovix, & Tvmersky, 1982). When the evidence base is not used as the basis for service development, it makes it more likely that seemingly plausible but ineffective and/or harmful interventions may be introduced or continued and that new interventions that have been shown to do more good than harm may never be introduced (Muir Gray, 2001).

As yet, few services have been developed on the basis of considered evidence. This may in part be because of a lack of effective dissemination of evidence and a lack of effective means of supporting implementation (Woolgar & Scott, 2005). However, a major limiting factor remains the sheer lack of relevant evidence, and the difficulties of agreeing the meaning of what is there, despite huge strides in recent years.

The short-comings of the evidence base in relation to child mental health interventions generally will not be analyzed in detail here – an overview can be found elsewhere (Fonagy, Target, Cottrell, Jeanette, & Kurtz, 2002) – but five key areas of limitation of particular relevance when looking to the evidence base to underpin service development should be highlighted.

The first, most obvious, problem is the sheer paucity of high-quality research. Even in the most extensively researched area in relation to child mental health service provision (exploring which interventions work in controlled conditions) studies are limited. There is even more limited research activity in relation to key questions about service design itself. This partly reflects the difficulty of designing studies that are rigorous, feasible and meaningful in this area.

The second key limitation is that the vast majority of service-related research so far conducted has been produced in the West, and the majority of this in the USA. The question is how far these findings can be generalized to other contexts, particularly those with very different cultural backgrounds and traditions (Hackett & Hackett, 1999).

The third key limitation is the lack of agreement as to appropriate outcomes to use to evaluate services. There is an emerging appreciation of the need to look at outcomes from a range of perspectives and across a range of domains (Kazdin & Kendall, 1998; Wolpert, Bartholomew, Domb *et al.*, 2005a). However, there is as yet no consensus as to how to weigh the different outcomes that might arise from these different perspectives or across different domains. Thus, there is no agreement as to which type of outcome should be regarded as most important (e.g., change in symptoms, social adaptation, experience of care, or some other dimension) nor whose view should be prioritized where views differ (e.g., child, parent, practitioner or others). The issue of how to make valid comparisons across studies where different outcomes have been used is yet to be resolved (Weisz, Chu, & Polo, 2004).

Fourthly, there is inevitably a complex interaction between the emerging evidence base and the political priorities and pre-occupations within a given country, both in terms of which topics are funded to be explored and in terms of the credence given to any findings that emerge. The pressure to implement a favored policy before it has been formally evaluated can mean that attempts to establish meaningful evaluation may be compromised (Rutter, 2006).

Finally, the way research is funded and the resources available for this from different groups may also crucially shape the nature of the "evidence" available. The financial resources available to pharmaceutical companies, for example, mean that disproportionately large amounts of research are carried out on "drug trials" as opposed to comparing different forms of psychological intervention.

Bearing these limitations in mind, the evidence will be considered in terms of how far it can contribute to answering two key questions:

1 "What interventions should be prioritized?"

2 "What organizational structures should be prioritized?"

What Interventions Should be Prioritized?

Attempts are starting to be made to summarize the existing evidence base to make it more accessible to practitioners and service developers. Table 71.1 offers an attempt to summarize some of the key findings in relation to interventions for children with diagnosable difficulties drawn from Goodman & Scott (2005) and Wolpert, Fuggle, Cottrell *et al.* (2006).[3]

The implications for service design might at first sight appear to be straightforward: that the interventions in the left-hand column of Table 71.1 should definitely be offered, those in the middle column should be at least considered and those in the right-hand column should be discontinued. However, caution must be exercised. No matter how rigorous the process used, any attempt at summary of the evidence will inevitably involve delicate judgments in determining what conclusions it may be appropriate to draw from existing studies. As alluded to above, much current research is flawed and limited. Any summary will need revision in the light of new evidence as it emerges. Moreover, even for the most well-designed studies, the evidence for the applicability of research findings to other contexts remains mixed. Research that looks at the impact of services using routine clinical practice, even where that could be anticipated to be relatively independent of context (such as when medication is prescribed), generally find lower effectiveness than is indicated in the studies informing Table 71.1 (MTA Co-operative Group, 1999; Weisz, Donenberg, Han, & Weiss, 1995). This difference may be because of differences in the populations of children seen, types of interventions made and/or outcomes assessed (Kendall & Southam-Gerow, 1995). Outcome-focused intervention studies are generally conducted with controlled groups of children in academic settings, so the relevance of any findings for children from different cultural backgrounds with complex overlapping difficulties needs to be established (Murray, Fayyad, Jensen *et al.*, 2006); moreover, the role of non-specific factors such as therapeutic engagement, expectations of change and therapist warmth may need to be taken into account (Jensen, Weersing, Hoagwood, & Goldman, 2005).

It is hoped that as the evidence base develops so too should the sophistication with which it might be interrogated. For every intervention listed as having "good evidence" to support it, the following questions should be asked (modified from Kazdin, 2004, p. 113):

1 What are the costs, risks and benefits of this intervention relative to no intervention?

2 What are the costs, risks and benefits of this intervention relative to other interventions?

Table 71.1 Selected evidence-based examples. (After Wolpert *et al.*, 2006 and Goodman & Scott, 2005.)

Mental health problem	Interventions with good evidence	Interventions with some evidence	Interventions with evidence of no effect or harmful
Disturbances of Attention and Activity	Stimulant drugs Atomoxetine	Behaviour therapy used alongside parent training	Cognitive Therapy
Disturbances of Conduct	Parent training for under 10s where the difficulties are not too severe Parent training combined with problem solving/social skills training for 8–12 year olds Multi-systemic therapy or therapeutic foster care for those with severe long term difficulties	Family therapy including focused behavioral advice	Large group therapy Unfocused therapy
Deliberate Self Harm		Focused group therapy for those who have harmed several times Family therapy focused on solving key problem areas	General education based prevention programmes in schools
Substance abuse	Family therapy focused on changing behaviours	Multi-systemic therapy where there are multiple problems Motivational interviewing	Family psycho-education Unstructured family support groups

3 What are the key components that appear to contribute to positive outcomes?
4 What parameters can be varied to improve outcomes (e.g., including addition of other interventions, non-specific clinical skills)?
5 To what extent are effects of interventions generalizable across: (i) problem areas; (ii) settings; (iii) populations of children; and (iv) other relevant domains?
We are a long way from being able to answer these questions in relation to the majority of interventions in child mental health.

It is likely that more sophisticated models are going to need to be developed to allow such analysis. Current metrics available to compare financial costs and benefits for example include quality adjusted life years (QALYs) and disability adjusted life years (DALYs). These are based on adult populations and are thought to dramatically under-represent burden related to conditions such as attention deficit/hyperactivity disorder (ADHD), conduct disorders and learning disorders (Remschmidt, Belfer, & Goodyer, 2004).

Weighing mental health promotion initiatives against interventions for those with existing impairments may require particularly careful analysis. The evidence base for prevention and promotion programs is discussed in depth elsewhere in this volume, but it would appear that while there is evidence that such programs may promote emotional well-being (Barnes, 1998), research to date has not proved that this will reduce levels of significant disturbance and thus impact on specialist services, nor that such programs are necessarily the most effective approach (Harrington & Clark, 1998; McLellan, MacMillan, & Jamieson, 2004).

Similarly, the evidence base for in-patient provision is unclear (Offord, 2005). Examples of well-researched alternatives to in-patient care are now emerging that suggest viable opportunities for effective treatment for even the most disturbed and disturbing groups without the need for hospitalization (Hewson, 2002). However, it should be noted that these are not necessarily any cheaper than in-patient provision (Baruch & Cannon, 2006).

One clear inference that can be drawn from current evidence is that it makes sense to start by decommissioning ineffective interventions. Unstructured work for conduct disordered young people is still prevalent despite evidence of its ineffectiveness and even potentially harmful effects. More effort should perhaps go into stopping unhelpful interventions than currently.

What Organizational Structures Should be Prioritized?

The Fort Bragg study (and the subsequent Stark County study) conducted by Bickman *et al.* in the USA (in 1995 and 1999, respectively) perhaps warrants particular attention as it generated such high levels of interest and controversy. This study evaluated a large-scale system change project designed to improve outcomes by providing an unrestricted set of coordinated inputs from a range of services. Results were compared with other sites using traditional services. Information was collected on service use, cost, satisfaction, clinical and functional data over the course of the 3-year study and at follow-up since.

The study found greater access and increased rates of satisfaction and less use of in-patient services, but no differences in behavioral–emotional functioning overall and the cost was much greater at Fort Bragg. The subsequent Stark County study also found that a multiagency system for care led to no significant difference in clinical outcomes when compared with routine services (Bickman, Summerfelt, Firth, & Douglas, 1997). Bickman, Lambert, Andrade *et al.* (2000) concluded: "The current national policy of large investments in systems of care infrastructure is unlikely to affect children in the manner intended . . . we need to focus on the services or treatments themselves to improve outcomes" (Bickman, Lambert, Andrade, & Penaloza, 2000).

This conclusion has been hotly contested. Flaws in the study design, implementation and interpretation have been pointed out (Friedman & Burns, 1996; Mordock, 1997; Saxe & Cross, 1997). It was argued that services were overwhelmed in the early months and provided less effective interventions, that the researchers failed to take account of some of the positive outcomes on some of the measures used and so on. It has been suggested that there is evidence that "wraparound services" (whereby a range of services are provided in a coordinated fashion to children and families based on their needs and not those of the services) do produce better outcomes and that the poor results above may have been a result of lack of fidelity to this model (Bruns, Burchard, Suter, & Force, 2005).

There is some evidence that shared understandings at the highest level and pooled budgets seem to be crucial to positive multiagency collaboration (Robinson, Anning, Cottrell, Frost, & Green, 2004). "MHSPY" in the USA is an initiative that involves five public and two private agencies that have come together with blended funding to provide a coordinated approach to focus on a group of "at risk" and ill children and where outcomes look positive, although lacking a control group or clear cost-effectiveness data as yet (Grimes, 2004).

It can be hypothesized on the basis of the current evidence that integral to creating joined up services may be the ability for state departments, or their equivalent, to agree joined up policy (rather than diverting resources into costly service reorganization). Thus, clear and shared agreements about protocols around information sharing, prioritized outcomes and agreed child protection arrangements are crucial, although often sadly lacking. The indications are that a key aspect is continuity of intent, reflected in a "shared mission through both administrative and clinical aspects of the system" (Grimes, 2004, p. 38).

There is little evidence available currently to guide service developers as to the best way to structure services in relation to a number of other key issues, such as what age group of children should be seen by different services; is it best to structure services around particular problems or around different age groups? In the light of lack of evidence and the fact that whichever way services are organized boundary issues arise, whether across age groups or specialisms, it may make sense to see the onus as being on service providers and developers to ensure that they work meaningfully across divisions rather than trying to create an ideal service structure. It may be hypothesized that, here too, non-specific factors are likely to be relevant. Thus, strength of the commitment of service providers to a particular shape of service and the ability of key individuals to collaborate across whatever boundaries are inevitably created, may impact as much, if not more, than the specifics of different forms of service structure.

Building a Workforce

The international literature has traditionally discussed child mental health workforce issues largely in relation to numbers of child psychiatrists. This may reflect the fact that in many countries, such as those in Europe, systems of care often developed in close conjunction with adolescent and child psychiatry as a speciality and as part of the health sector. However, increasingly research and policy highlight the importance of the input of a range of possible groups in relation to child mental health provision (Hansen, Litzelman, Marsh, & Milspaw, 2004; Homonoff & Maltz, 1991).

Schools are recognized as perhaps the most influential place in relation to help seeking and efforts are being put into training education staff to recognize and work with mental health difficulties (Remschmidt, Belfer, & Goodyer, 2004). Some promotion programs in schools are showing positive results in terms of emotional well-being and academic performance, such as the international FRIENDs program and the Roots of Empathy in Canada (Weare & Markham, 2005; Wyn, Cahill, Holdsworth, Rowling, & Carson, 2000). However, care must be taken not to overload schools and there is likely to remain a need for more specialist and health-focused provision for some children.

Pediatricians often work with some of the most difficult and complex children with a range of behavioral and psychological needs, particularly in the younger age range. In some European countries, such as Austria, Finland and Germany, links between pediatrics and child mental health services are particularly strong (Rydelius, 2004). Other health workers, such as health visitors in the UK who work as part of the primary care system working with mothers and babies in the early months and years, and primary care workers in India, have been found to have a positive impact as part of mental health initiatives (Davis & Spurr, 1998; Nikapota, 2002). In the developing world, the ability to engage a workforce that also links with relevant belief systems of the community, such as traditional healers, ayurvedic treatment and yoga, may be crucial and the use of extended networks of informal and formal sources of support can be of great benefit (Robertson, Mandlhate, Seif El Din *et al.*, 2004; Thara, Padmavati, & Srinivasan, 2004).

There have been a number of attempts to agree a common framework for assessing and understanding difficulties across different sectors. Some specialist assessment tools have been developed, such as the Child and Adolescent Psychiatry Assessment (CAPA; Angold & Costello, 2000) and the Development and Wellbeing Assessment (DAWBA), which can be filled in over the Internet (Goodman, Ford, Simmons, Gatward, & Meltzer, 2003). However, national consensus as to the key items of information to collect has been hampered by professional disagreement about the appropriate conceptual model and approach to adopt. It is hoped that a consensus view of typology emerges that will allow enough agreement in the future for a common assessment approach to be used across child mental health.

In terms of the key staff to provide specialist mental health provision, while there is much assertion and rhetoric there is in fact very little hard evidence as to what form an ideal workforce should take, although some attempts are now being developed to model extent of need for specialist staff based on calculations of the amount and types of input required for particular difficulties (Goodman, 1997; Kelvin, 2005).

Traditionally, training of specialists in relation to mental health, on top of any core professional training, has been undertaken according to theoretical models. Thus, people are trained in "family therapy," "play therapy," "psychodynamic psychotherapy," "cognitive–behavioral therapy" and "group therapy" to name a few. This has meant that when people come to practice they often come with an allegiance to a particular theoretical model and belief system.

It is perhaps not too fanciful to speculate that what is called for is a different sort of specialist training, built not around allegiance to models of therapy but founded instead on a commitment to act on the best available research and evidence base, drawing on a range of models and approaches, as appropriate, and an ability to review options in the light of emerging evidence. This is perhaps starting to emerge in some countries as training for new members of the workforce – variously termed generic child and adolescent mental health workers – is starting to be developed. This initiative might usefully be advanced by specific training for support staff to become expert in particular evidence-based interventions such as specialized providers of parent training.

Even allowing for any shifts in training approach, the accepted wisdom is that multiprofessional teams and multiagency working will remain the way forward (Department of Health, 2004; Stroul & Friedman, 1986). The idea is that complex problems need the combined expertise of specialists which can best be provided as part of a team and that by bringing different agencies together the necessity for individual children and families to negotiate their way through a variety of systems is reduced. However, these assumptions remain largely unproven. The amount of time necessary to promote effective team building and the degree of anxiety that can be created between team members in clarifying their different roles and responsibilities may use up precious resources and reduce capacity to carry out direct clinical work. More empirical research in this area is needed.

In most countries, specialist mental health professionals are perceived as a scarce resource. Figures are generally quoted for psychiatrists. Worldwide, the availability of psychiatrists varies from 1:5300 in Switzerland to 1:1 million in China and even greater ratios in parts of the developing world. Sometimes, lack of psychiatric provision is more a result of inadequate distribution of resources, with psychiatrists working mainly in academic institutions in large urban centers. This appears to be the case in parts of South America (Rohde, Celia, & Berganza, 2004). Figures for other professional groups are harder to come by but it is likely that similar issues pertain. Staff shortages, particularly in the developing world, are exacerbated by the brain drain – there are more Indian psychiatrists working in the USA than in India (WHO, 2005).

In those countries where key professionals are an expensive and limited resource, policy seeks to ensure more equitable distribution of specialists and/or adopt a cascade approach whereby most senior mental health professionals spend most time in consulting and training others, such as in Bosnia (Shooter, 2005). This can be achieved via a range of means such as telephone or video links (Pesämaa, Ebeling, Kuusimäki *et al.*, 2004).

Where resources are in particularly short supply, opportunities can be explored for mental health provision to piggyback on other sectors with more provision, such as HIV programs in Africa (Robertson, Mandlhate, Seif El Din *et al.*, 2004). Models of very rapid professional training for primary care staff and training of traditional healers or educational support personnel have been promoted as attempts to improve mental health provision where specialist input is lacking (Robertson, Mandlhate, Seif El Din *et al.*, 2004). However, research highlighting the importance of fidelity to model in terms of efficacy of interventions indicates that there may be a necessary threshold of amount of training combined with ongoing organizational support for subsequent interventions to be effective (Scott, 2004).

Even in the industrialized West it may be relevant to look to develop new workforces to extend capacity, such as by the use of support staff, technicians and volunteers. Models of encouraging family members to train as key workers are now being piloted in a range of contexts worldwide (US Department of Health and Human Services, 1999).

Ensuring Accessibility

Promoting Accessibility via Service Location

Wherever child mental health provision is located (either geographically or in terms of overarching management systems) boundary issues arise. Thus, age cut-offs, balance between regional and local provision and whether child mental health provision is located mainly within children's services generally or as primarily linked to adult mental health, vary across countries. In parts of Europe – such as Switzerland and Hungary – and in Egypt, child mental health services are primarily organized under the auspices of education. This has many advantages for younger children in terms of reducing stigma and increasing accessibility, but can increase difficulties of coordination for older adolescents and those with more severe mental illness. Countries have dealt with boundary issues in a variety of ways. In Australia and New Zealand, there is a deliberate 2-year overlap between youth and adult mental health service provision to try to help encourage flexibility for young people in this transitional age group (18–20 years; Hazell, 2005). In Finland, in-patient units for under-11-year-olds are located wherever possible nearer pediatric resources and those for adolescents nearer adult mental health provision (Piha & Almqvist, 1999). There is increased attention internationally to the need for services to be meaningfully linked across a range of sectors including the criminal justice system, substance abuse services and religious networks (Belfer, 2004).

Promoting Accessibility for the "Hard to Reach"

There is an increasing preoccupation with how to ensure that the most marginalized groups or communities in a given society can access services. As discussed above, attempts to make provision more accessible as well as less stigmatizing to these groups can include use of education and primary care workers, community and religious leaders, and family networks.

The work of voluntary organizations can be a source of innovation and energy, and communities need to find ways for statutory services to learn from them. For example, the walk-in community center Empilwent, South Africa, pioneered a more accessible drop-in approach (WHO, 2005).

There is currently a call for services to become more culturally competent, and widespread consensus on this aim, but it is unclear as yet what a culturally competent service would be like. Although there is a welter of innovative attempts to make services more culturally sensitive and appropriate, the evidence of the long-term impact of these initiatives is as yet limited (Nikapota, 2002).

Promoting Geographical Accessibility

It could be argued that child mental health services have been slow on the whole to "get out of the clinic" and in particular to embrace the impact of new technologies that might increase access. However, some interesting innovations are developing. These range from mobile services, such as the peripatetic child mental health team which travels across Germany providing, amongst other things, follow-up on previously hospitalized young people (Remschmidt, Belfer, & Goodyer, 2004) to increased use of telephone, Internet and text contact generally.

Telephone helplines such as KidsHelp in Australia, Childline and YoungMinds Parent Information Service in the UK are run by charities independent of statutory provision but it may be that greater links can be made between such resources and more traditional services in the future. Telefono Azzuro, Italy, shows the way these can be combined with other provision (Caffo, Forresi, Belaise *et al.*, 2004).

A range of websites have been developed by and for young people, some of which allow for discussions between young people, and others offer access to specialist advice and support (e.g., ru-ok.com). The use of emails and text messaging to communicate between professionals and young people is now increasing, as is the use of IT aids to assessment and treatment. The pace of innovation in this area is likely to accelerate sharply in the future.

Assuring Quality

Whatever organizational structures a society adopts and whatever workforce is in place to provide services, systems need to be put in place to ensure quality of provision, promote best practice and allow for change in practice in the light of increased knowledge and future policy imperatives.

A key dilemma for policy-makers is how to get the right balance between centralized and devolved decision-making in relation to service development. Too great an attempt to control all aspects of service organization from a national center is likely to lead to unwieldy bureaucratic decision-making, while too much devolution to local decision-making can lead to huge variations in type and quality of services. There is no clear solution to this tension. One approach is to try to ensure that, where decisions are devolved to agreed geographical units (accountable to local populations), those charged with decision-making have the necessary skills and resources to enable them to plan and develop services in line with best evidence, in line with national guidance, and are able to implement effective performance management arrangements.

One mechanism of quality assurance is to set standards to ensure that key activities are undertaken. Services may then be evaluated by inspectors to ensure compliance and a variety of incentives and penalties can be applied. However, real problems are presented by the danger of perverse incentives, as activity can easily become skewed. In an effort to meet waitlist targets, for example, other crucial activities may be neglected.

National (and international) guidelines can be used to shape practice. Different countries have developed systems to sift the evidence and pull together consensus statements to guide and inform practice (e.g., National Institute of Clinical Excellence in England, American Psychiatric Association Practice parameters in the USA). The danger remains of overprescription on a very narrow evidence base and the possibility that the implementation of poorly understood guidance may be every bit as distorting as inappropriate targets. Some countries have sought to overcome this by stressing that guidance is advisory only. For example, in New South Wales, Australia, model care packages for adolescents with severe problems are outlined. These include one 90-min family-orientated mental health assessment and six 45-min family-orientated community contacts. The aim is to inform service planning, not prescribe or proscribe clinical work (Hazell, 2005).

Some of the most successful initiatives involve collaborations between service providers to promote best practice and disseminate and share information. Organizations such as the International Association for Child and Adolescent Psychiatry and Allied Professionals (IACAPAP) have done much to promote sharing of the latest research, and more formal peer review groups have also been established whereby members agree standards and undertake peer monitoring and evaluation, such as the Quality Network for Inpatient Care in the UK (Royal College of Psychiatrists: College Research and Training Unit).

It is increasingly recognized that for tacit complex knowledge, as is likely to underpin best practice in child mental health, having face-to-face meetings and encouraging learning collaborations are likely to be more effective than circulating written information alone (Office for Public Management, 2000). A number of countries distribute awards for best practice in child mental health – although the impact of these on quality is as yet unknown.

In order to ensure that child mental health services develop into self-reflective and learning organizations, allowing for future development and innovation, providers must have feedback about their current outcomes. This requires functioning IT systems and a core dataset (Tingay & Stein, 2004; Wolpert, Thompson, & Tingay, 2005b), but even in the most developed countries, the promise of coherent IT systems remains more a hope than a reality. It is key that IT systems are developed that are capable of supporting decision-making by providing easy access to information for practitioners so that they can obtain feedback on their work and learn accordingly.

While in no country in the world are there data systematically gathered for the assessment of child and adolescent mental health service outcomes at a national level, some encouraging national and international collaborations are emerging. The CAMHS Outcome Research Consortium (CORC; chaired by the author) is a collaboration between over half of all services across the UK who are implementing an agreed model of routine outcome and have agreed ways to present the data in order to inform service providers and users and to help inform service developments (Wolpert, Bartholomew, Domb *et al.*, 2005a). The approach has parallels with that being employed in the USA (Ohio; Brower, 2003). In all cases, a small suite of measures is completed by service users and providers at initial contact and at some time later.

There is an increasing policy emphasis on the need for service users to inform service development priorities and to be part of any evaluation of services. Some innovative models have been tried, such as in Ohio, which has created outcome systems from a service user perspective, and in parts of the UK where young people are trained as service evaluators ("Investing in Children", Durham County Council, UK), although, once again, the impact of these on quality of services is yet to be researched. There are also increasing attempts to inform service users about different options so that they can make informed choices. For example, the current author and colleagues have recently produced a small booklet which sets out to summarize the evidence base for different interventions for children and young people – this is freely available from ebpu@annafreudcentre.org/ebpu (Wolpert, Goodman, Raby *et al.*, 2007).

Conclusions

There is no one ideal model for organizing services, but some key themes can be highlighted. It is helpful to start with an analysis of the range of anticipated needs, and to seek clarity at a policy level as to the current priorities for a given community. Where resources are limited, specialist mental health provision should be targeted foremost on those with greatest levels of impairment for whom there are available effective interventions. Implementation of effective models of prevention and promotion should be supported in so far as resources allow, but in the light of the current limited evidence base and likely resource constraints, providing treatment for people with existing difficulties should be seen as the highest priority. It is anticipated that the evidence base will grow and that while it is likely to continue to generate as many questions as answers, the emerging findings may increasingly guide practice, particularly in relation to decommissioning ineffective or harmful strategies. Signs of a shift in the professional culture for child mental health specialists have been noted, as they start to adopt a more evidence-based and an outcomes-focused world view and move away from firm allegiance to theoretical belief-based models. The range of innovative models of services, making increasingly good use of the new technologies and supported by increasingly mature collaborations and networks, may aid further the development of reflective, high-quality and accessible provision. Tension is likely to remain, however, between allowing for child mental heath specialists' creativity and innovation on the one hand and the increasing emphasis on the importance of fidelity to model and shared arrangements around initial assessments and outcomes on the other. How this tension is played out over the coming years may well determine the future shape of services for some time to come.

Acknowledgments

With thanks to Anula Nikapota, Robert Goodman, Rachel Jenkins and Eric Taylor for the benefits of their wisdom and advice and to Paula Lavis and Emma Svanberg for sourcing of information.

References

American Psychiatric Association (APA). (2002). *Quality indicators: Defining and measuring quality in psychiatric care for adults and children*. American Psychiatric Association.

Angold, A., & Costello, J. (2000). The Child and Adolescent Psychiatric Assessment (CAPA). *Journal of the American Academy of Child and Adolescent Psychiatry*, *39*, 39–48.

Angold, A., Messer, S. C., Strangl, D., Farmer, E. M. Z., Costello, E. J., & Burns, B. J. (1998). Perceived parental burden and service use for child and adolescent psychiatric disorders. *American Journal of Public Health*, *88*, 75–80.

Barnes, J. (1998). Mental health promotion: A developmental perspective. *Psychology, Health and Medicine*, *3*, 55–69.

Baruch, G., & Cannon, J. (2006). A study of multi-systemic therapy: A new type of help in the UK for young people in trouble with the law. In D. Robins, G. Baruch, & P. Fonagy (Eds.), *Reaching the hard to reach: Evidence-based funding priorities for intervention and research* (pp. 71–90). Chichester: Wiley.

Belfer, M. L. (2004). Systems of care: A global perspective. In H. Remschmidt, M. L. Belfer, & I. Goodyer (Eds.), *Facilitating pathways: Care, treatment and preventions in child and adolescent mental health*. Berlin: Springer-Verlag (pp. 16–26).

Bickman, L., Lambert, E. W., Andrade, A. R., & Penaloza, R. V. (2000). The Fort Bragg continuum of care for children and adolescents: Mental health outcomes over 5 years. *Journal of Consulting and Clinical Psychology*, *68*, 710–716.

Bickman, L., Summerfelt, W. T., Firth, J. M., & Douglas, S. M. (1997). The Stark County evaluation project: Baseline results of a randomized experiment. In C. Nixon, & D. A. Northrup (Eds.), *Evaluating mental health services: How do programs for children "work" in the real world?* (pp. 231–258). Thousand Oaks, CA: Sage.

Broidy, L. M., Nagin, D. S., Tremblay, R. E., Bates, J. E., Brame, B., Dodge, K. A., *et al.* (2003). Developmental trajectories of childhood disruptive behaviors and adolescent delinquency: A six-site, cross-national study. *Developmental Psychology*, *39*, 222–245.

Brower, L. A. (2003). The Ohio mental health consumer outcomes system: Reflections on a major policy initiative in the US. *Clinical Psychology and Psychotherapy*, *10*, 400–406.

Bruns, E. J., Burchard, J. D., Suter, J. C., & Force, M. D. (2005). Measuring fidelity within community treatments for children and families. In M. Epstein, A. Duchnowski, & K. Kutash (Eds.), *Outcomes for children and youth with emotional and behavioral disorders and their families*, Vol. 2. Austin, TX: Pro-ED.

Caffo, E., Forresi, B., Belaise, C., Nicolais, G., Laor, N., Wolmer, L., *et al.* (2004). Innovation intervention in the community. In H. Remschmidt, M. L. Belfer, & I. Goodyer (Eds.), *Facilitating pathways: Care, treatment and prevention in child and adolescent mental health* (pp. 187–207). Berlin: Springer-Verlag.

CAMHS Outcome Research Consortium (CORC). Accessed from http: www.corc.uk.net 2 January 2008.

Childline. Accessed from http://www.childline.org.uk/ 2 January 2008.

Davis, H., & Spurr, P. (1998). Parent counselling: An evaluation of a community child mental health service. *Journal of Child Psychology and Psychiatry*, *39*, 365–376.

Department of Health. (2004). *The mental health and psychological well-being of children and young people. Standard nine of the National Service Framework for Children, Young People and Maternity Services.* London: Department of Health.

Eapen, V., & Ghubash, R. (2004). Help-seeking for mental health problems of children: Preferences and attitudes in the United Arab Emirates. *Psychological Reports*, *94*, 663–667.

Falkov, A., Phillips, R., Brady, P., Stathis, B., & Finney, D. (2003). The COPMI (Children of parents with mental illness) clinic: A model of service provision linking adult and child mental health services. *Australian and New Zealand Journal of Psychiatry*, *37* (Supplement 1), A42.

Fleitlich-Bilyk, B., & Goodman, R. (2004). Prevalence of child and adolescent psychiatric disorders in Southeast Brazil. *Journal American Academy Child and Adolescent Psychiatry*, *43*, 727–34.

Fonagy, P., Target, M., Cottrell, D., Jeanette, P., & Kurtz, Z. (2002). *What works for whom? A critical review of treatments for children and adolescents.* London: Guilford Press.

Ford, T., Hamilton, H., Goodman, R., & Meltzer, H. (2005). Service contacts among the children participating in the British child and adolescent mental health surveys. *Child and Adolescent Mental Health*, *10*, 2–9.

Foster, E. M., Jones, D. E., & the Conduct Problems Prevention Research Group. (2005). The high costs of aggression: Public expenditures resulting from conduct disorder. *American Journal of Public Health*, *95*, 1767–1772.

Friedman, R. M., & Burns, B. J. T. (1996). The evaluation of the Fort Bragg demonstration project: An alternative interpretation of the findings. *Journal of Mental Health Administration*, *23*, 128–136.

Garb, H. N. (1997). Race bias, social class bias and gender bias in clinical judgement. *Clinical Psychology: Science and Practice*, *4*, 99–102.

Goodman, R. (1997). *Child and adolescent mental health services: Reasoned advice to commissioners and providers. Maudsley discussion paper no 4* (Discussion paper). London: Institute of Psychiatry.

Goodman, R., Ford, T., Simmons, H., Gatward, R., & Meltzer, H. (2003). Using the Strengths and Difficulties Questionnaire (SDQ) to screen for child psychiatric disorders in a community sample. *International Review of Psychiatry*, *15*, 166–172.

Goodman, R., & Scott, S. (2005). *Child psychiatry* (2nd edn.). Oxford: Blackwell.

Green, H., McGinnity, A., Meltzer, H., Ford, T., & Goodman, R. (2005). *Mental health of children and young people in Great Britain, 2004.* London: Palgrave.

Grimes, K. (2004). Systems of care in North America. In H. Remschmidt, M. L. Belfer, I. Goodyer (Eds.), *Facilitating pathways: Care, treatment and prevention in child and adolescent mental health* (pp. 35–41). Berlin: Springer-Verlag.

Hackett, R., & Hackett, L. (1999). Child psychiatry across cultures. *International Review of Psychiatry*, *11*, 225–235.

Hansen, M., Litzelman, A., Marsh, D. T., & Milspaw, A. (2004). Approaches to serious emotional disturbance: Involving multiple systems. *Professional Psychology: Research and Practice*, *35*, 457–465.

Harrington, R., & Clark, A. (1998). Prevention and early intervention for depression in adolescence and early adult life. *European Archives of Psychiatry*, *8*, 1–10.

Hazell, P. (2005). Child & adolescent mental health services in Australia and New Zealand; policy and development. In R. Williams, & M. Kerfoot (Eds.), *Child and adolescent mental health services. Strategy, planning, delivery and evaluation* (pp. 355–363). Oxford: Oxford University Press.

Heiervang, E., Stormark, K. M., Lundervold, A. J., Heimann, M., Goodman, R., Posserud, M., *et al.* (2007). Psychiatric disorders in Norwegian 8- to 10-year-olds: An epidemiological survey of prevalence, risk factors, and service use. *Journal of the American Academy of Child and Adolescent Psychiatry*, *46*, 438–447.

Hewson, L. (2002). Care begins at home: Reducing the use of inpatient beds. *YoungMinds Magazine*, *58*, 3–5.

Homonoff, E. E., & Maltz, P. F. (1991). Developing and maintaining a coordinated system of community-based services to children. *Community Mental Health Journal*, *27*, 347–358.

Jensen, P. S., Weersing, R., Hoagwood, K. E., & Goldman, E. (2005). What is the evidence for evidence-based treatments? A hard look at our soft underbelly. *Mental Health Services Research*, *7*, 53–74.

Kahnemann, D., Slovix, P., & Tvwersky, A. (Eds.). (1982). *Judgment under uncertainly: Heuristics and biases.* New York: Cambridge University Press.

Kazdin, A. E. (2004). Evidence-based psychotherapies for children and adolescents: Strategies, strengths and limitations. In H. Remschmidt, M. Belfer, & I. Goodyer (Eds.), *Facilitating pathways: Care, treatment and prevention in child and adolescent mental health* (pp. 103–118). Berlin: Springer-Verlag.

Kazdin, A. E., & Kendall, P. C. (1998). Current progress and future plans for developing effective treatments, comments and perspectives. *Journal of Clinical Child Psychology*, *27*, 217–226.

Kelvin, R. G. (2005). Capacity of tier 2/3 CAMHS and service specification: A model to enable evidence based service development. *Child and Adolescent Mental Health*, *10*, 63–73.

Kendall, P. C., & Southam-Gerow, M. A. (1995). Issues in the transportability of treatment: The case of anxiety disorders in youths. *Journal of Consulting and Clinical Psychology*, *63*, 702–708.

Kids Help Line. Accessed from http://www.kidshelp.com.au/home_KHL.aspx?s=6 2 January 2008.

Malhotra, S., Kohli, A., & Arun, P. (2002). Prevalence of psychiatric disorders in school children in Chandigarh, India. *Indian Journal of Medical Research*, 116, 21–28.

McLellan, J. D., MacMillan, H. L., & Jamieson, E. (2004). Canada's programs to prevent mental health problems in children: The research–practice gap. *Canadian Medical Association Journal*, *171*, 1069–1072.

Mordock, J. B. (1997). The Fort Bragg continuum of care demonstration project: The population served was unique and the outcomes are questionable. *Child Psychiatry and Human Development*, *29*, 241–254.

MTA Co-operative Group. (1999). Moderators and mediators of treatment response for children with attention deficit/hyperactivity disorder: The multimodal treatment study of children with attention deficit/hyperactivity disorder. *Archives of General Psychiatry*, *56*, 1088–1096.

Muir Gray, J. A. (2001). *Evidence-based healthcare: How to make health policy and management decisions*. Edinburgh: Churchill Livingstone.

Mullick, M. S., & Goodman, R. (2005). The prevalence of psychiatric disorders among 5–10 year olds in rural, urban and slum areas in Bangladesh: an exploratory study. *Social Psychiatry and Psychiatric Epidemiology*, *40*, 663–671.

Murray, L. K., Fayyad, J., Jensen, P. S., Hoagwood, K., Azer, M., & Integrated Services Program Task Force. (2006). An examination of cross-cultural systems implementing evidence-based assessment and intervention approaches. *Revista Brasileira de Psiquiatria*, *28*, 76–79.

Nikapota, A. (2002). Cultural and ethnic issues in service provision. In M. Rutter, & E. Taylor (Eds.), *Child and adolescent psychiatry* (4th edn., pp. 1148–1157). Oxford: Blackwell Publishing.

Office for Public Management. (2000). *The effectiveness of different mechanisms for spreading best practice*. London: Cabinet Office.

Offord, D. R. (2005). Comparative analyses: Challenges facing CAMHS in North America. In R. Williams, & M. Kerfoot (Eds.), *Child and adolescent mental health services: Strategy, planning, delivery and evaluation* (pp. 365–372). Oxford: Oxford University Press.

Pesämaa, L., Ebeling, H., Kuusimäki, M.-L., Winblad, I., Isohanni, M., & Moilanen, I. (2004). Videoconferencing in child and adolescent telepsychiatry: A systematic review of the literature. *Journal of Telemedicine and Telecare*, *10*, 187–192.

Piha, J., & Almqvist, F. (1999). Child and adolescent psychiatry in Finland. In H. Remschmidt, & H. van Engeland (Eds.), *Child and adolescent psychiatry in Europe* (pp. 93–103). New York: Steinkopff, Darmstadt & Springer.

Remschmidt, H., Belfer, M., & Goodyer, I. (Eds.). (2004). *Facilitating pathways: Care, treatment and prevention in child and adolescent mental health*. Berlin: Springer-Verlag.

Robertson, B., Mandlhate, C., Seif El Din, A., & Seck, B. (2004). Systems of care in Africa. In H. Remschmidt, M. Belfer, & I. Goodyer (Eds.), *Facilitating pathways: Care, treatment and prevention in child and adolescent mental health*. Berlin: Springer-Verlag.

Robinson, R. M., Anning, A., Cottrell, D., Frost, N., & Green, J. M. (2004). *New forms of professional knowledge in multi-agency delivery of services for children (The MATCh Project)*. Leeds: University of Leeds.

Rohde, L. A., Celia, S., & Berganza, C. G. (2004). Systems of care in South America. In H. Remschmidt, M. Belfer, & I. Goodyer (Eds.), *Facilitating pathways: Care, treatment and prevention in child and adolescent mental health* (pp. 42–52). Berlin: Springer-Verlag.

Romeo, R., Byford, S., & Knapp, M. (2005). Economic evaluations of child and adolescent mental health interventions: A systematic review. *Journal of Child Psychology and Psychiatry*, *46*, 919–930.

Royal College of Psychiatrists: College Research and Training Unit. *QNIC: A quality network for inpatient CAMHS*. Accessed from http://www.rcpsych.ac.uk/crtu/centreforqualityimprovement/qnic.aspx Accessed 2 January 2008.

RU-OK.Com. Accessed from http://www.ru-ok.com/ 2 January 2008.

Rutter, M. (2006). Is Sure Start an effective preventive intervention? *Child and Adolescent Mental Health*, *11*, 135–141.

Rutter, M., Tizard, J., & Whitmore, K. (1970). *Education, health and behaviour*. London: Longman.

Rydelius, P. (2004). Systems of care in Europe. In H. Remschmidt, M. Belfer, & I. Goodyer (Eds.), *Facilitating pathways: Care, treatment and prevention in child and adolescent mental health* (pp. 27–34). Berlin: Springer-Verlag.

Saxe, L., & Cross, T. (1997). Interpreting the Fort Bragg Children's Mental Health Demonstration Project: The cup is half full. *American Psychologist*, *52*, 553–556.

Scott, S. (2004). Outcomes of treatment. In H. Remschmidt, M. Belfer, & I. Goodyer (Eds.), *Facilitating pathways: Care, treatment and prevention in child and adolescent mental health* (pp. 222–231). Berlin: Springer-Verlag.

Shooter, M. (2005). European psychiatry: Construction, destruction and reconstruction. In R. Williams, & M. Kerfoot (Eds.), *Child and adolescent mental health services: Strategy, planning, delivery and evaluation* (pp. 341–350). Oxford: Oxford University Press.

Stroul, B., & Friedman, R. (1986). *A system of care for severely emotionally disturbed children and youth*. Wasington, DC: National Technical Assistance Center.

Thara, R., Padmavati, R., & Srinivasan, T. N. (2004). Focus on psychiatry in India. *British Journal of Psychiatry*, *184*, 366–373.

Tingay, K., & Stein, S. (2004). *National CAMHS dataset*. Dunstable: Durocobrivis.

US Department of Health and Human Services. (1999). *Mental health: A report of the Surgeon General*. Rockville, MD: Department of Health and Human Services.

Weare, K., & Markham, W. (2005). What do we know about promoting mental health through schools? *Promotion and Education*, *12*, 118–122.

Weisz, J. R., Chu, B. C., & Polo, A. J. (2004). Treatment dissemination and evidence-based practice: Strengthening intervention through clinician–researcher collaboration. *Clinical Psychology: Science and Practice*, *11*, 300–307.

Weisz, J. R., Donenberg, G. R., Han, S. S., & Weiss, B. J. (1995). Bridging the gap between laboratory and clinic in child and adolescent psychotherapy. *Journal of Consulting and Clinical Psychology*, *63*, 688–701.

Wolpert, M., Bartholomew, R., Domb, Y., Fonagy, P., Ford, T., Foster, B., *et al.* (2005a). *Collaborating to improve child mental health services: CAMHS Outcome Research Consortium Handbook* (Version 1). London: CORC.

Wolpert, M., Fuggle, P., Cottrell, D., Fonagy, P., Phillips, J., Pilling, S., *et al.* (2006). *Drawing on the evidence: Advice for mental health professionals working with children and adolescents* (Revised version). London: Child and Adolescent Mental Health Services Evidence Based Practice Unit, University College London.

Wolpert, M., Thompson, M., & Tingay, T. (2005b). Data collection, clinical audit and measuring outcomes. In R. Williams, & M. Kerfoot (Eds.), *Strategic approaches to planning and delivering child and adolescent mental health services* (pp. 519–533). Oxford: Oxford University Press.

Wolpert, M., Goodman, R., Raby, C., Cottrell, D., Lavis, P., Bureau, J., *et al.* (2007). *Choosing what's best for you: What scientists have found helps children and young people who are sad, worried or troubled*. London: CAMHS Publications.

Woolgar, M., & Scott, S. (2005). Evidence-based management of conduct disorders. *Current Opinion in Psychiatry*, *18*, 392–396.

World Health Organization (WHO). (2003). *Caring for children and adolescents with mental disorders: Setting WHO directions*. Geneva: World Health Organization.

World Health Organization (WHO). (2005). *Atlas: Child and adolescent mental health resources. Global concerns: Implications for the future*. Geneva: World Health Organization.

Wyn, J., Cahill, H., Holdsworth, R., Rowling, L., & Carson, S. (2000). MindMatters: A whole-school approach promoting mental health and wellbeing. *Australian and New Zealand Journal of Psychiatry*, *34*, 594–601.

YoungMinds. (2006). *Emerging practice: Examples of services for the 16–25 year age group*. London: YoungMinds.

YoungMinds' Parents Information Service. Accessed from http://www.youngminds.org.uk/parents 2 January 2008.

72 Primary Health Care Psychiatry

Tami Kramer and Elena Garralda

Primary care is the first point of contact for families seeking professional attention for health problems. It aims to clarify demand, diagnose disorder, offer information, advice, treatment and rehabilitation and coordinate care with other disciplines and sectors over time (Boerma, 2006). The relevance of primary health care to mental health has been highlighted, with emphasis on the need to enhance its central role and to build capacity, to reduce the global burden of suffering and impairment from mental and behavioral disorder (WHO, 2001, 2005). It offers scope for prevention and early intervention. The role within child and adolescent mental health has been less well documented but evidence is slowly accumulating, much of it from developed countries.

The chapter begins by describing different models of pediatric primary care service delivery. The relevance for child and adolescent mental health is then discussed in relation to the core roles of primary care. The mental health research literature on different age ranges (preschoolers, school-aged children and adolescents) and important disorders (depression, somatization, attention deficit/hyperactivity disorder [ADHD], behavioral problems) is considered as it pertains to the core primary care roles. Finally, the need and means for expanding capacity with future directions are discussed.

Primary Health Care Services for Children and Adolescents

Primary health care services across different countries vary widely in terms of setting, staffing, funding source and levels relative to the size of the population. Those for children and adolescents are delivered by a range of physicians (general practitioners/family physicians, general and community pediatricians) and non-physicians (nurses, health visitors, public health workers). They are based in primary care clinics, health centers, child health clinics, school medical services, emergency departments and ambulatory hospital/out-patient departments. Funding may be private, on the basis of insurance, or part of centrally organized national or regional health services.

A European survey demonstrated that 35% (12 of 34) of countries who took part had a system of pediatric primary care provided by pediatricians, 18% (6 of 34) by general practitioner/family doctor systems but the majority (47% or 16 of 34) had mixed systems (Katz, Rubino, Collier, Rosen, & Ehrich, 2002). Level, type and quality of care varied widely, with only 40% of countries having community pediatricians (defined as those concerned with recognition, prevention and treatment of community health problems such as child protection, children in need, behavior problems, teenager approach, growth and development, school medicine). Postgraduate training in pediatric primary care was available for the majority but not for all pediatric or family medicine trainees and levels of training in child protection were much lower, particularly for family medicine trainees.

Within the USA, both pediatricians and family physicians provide pediatric primary care. However, increasingly over the last 20 years these services have been provided by pediatricians (Freed, Nahra, & Wheeler, 2004). Particularly in more affluent areas, services often integrate well care and acute care. In many other countries, preventative services are offered in different settings from those providing acute illness care (Cheng, 2004). In contrast, in Canada, pediatric primary care is provided largely by general practitioners and public health units. In many developing countries, public health workers provide the point of first contact with health services and pediatricians provide specialized Western-type medical care (Cheng, 2004). Thus, globally, the differences in level of provision, structure of services and competencies of personnel delivering the services are important and likely to impact on the potential to provide mental health services for children and adolescents within the primary care setting. In addition to the nature and distribution of primary care services, this potential will be determined by patterns of attendance (i.e., who uses the service, how frequently and the nature of their needs).

Primary Care as a First Point of Contact for Child and Adolescent Mental Health Problems

Frequency of Contact

Contact with primary health care is a common experience in childhood. Over the course of 1 year, most parents take their children to primary care services, and work with children has been estimated to occupy one-quarter of the doctor's

Rutter's Child and Adolescent Psychiatry, 5th edition. Edited by M. Rutter, D. Bishop, D. Pine, S. Scott, J. Stevenson, E. Taylor and A. Thapar. © 2008 Blackwell Publishing, ISBN: 978-1-4051-4549-7.

time. There are age trends, with young preschool children being seen more often than older children. Within the UK, over 90% of preschool age children and about two-thirds of 5- to 14-year-olds will consult primary care at least once a year (OPCS, 1995). A study of a large London inner city practice demonstrated that over 50% of 13- to 17-year-olds who were registered had attended in 1 year (Kramer, Illife, Murray, & Waterman, 1997). Within the USA, it has been reported that more than 70% of adolescents see a physician at least once each year (Frankenfield, Keyl, Gielen *et al.*, 2000). This suggests a significant potential for attention to mental health within this context.

Modes of Presentation

The majority of the consultations are for physical health problems. Surveys in various countries have documented that 2–5% of children and adolescents attending primary care or general pediatric clinics present primarily for psychological problems (e.g., anxiety, behavioral problems and overactivity; Garralda & Bailey, 1986; Jacobson, Goldberg, Burns *et al.*, 1980; Kramer & Garralda, 1998; Starfield, Gross, Wood *et al.*, 1980). Higher rates of 10% for emotional–behavioral presentations have been given in some reports. Educational and social problems also feature as reasons for consultation.

Frequency and Nature of Associated Psychiatric Disorder

There is evidence that psychiatric disorders are present in a considerably higher number of children attending primary care than may be expected from the overt presenting complaint. Research interviews with children and parents, following primary care contact, have found disorders in one-tenth to one-quarter of children across different countries (Costello, Costello, Edelbrock *et al.*, 1988; Garralda & Bailey, 1986; Giel, de Arango, Climent *et al.*, 1981; Gureje, Omigbodun, Gater *et al.*, 1994), with higher rates in adolescents (40%; Kramer & Garralda, 1998) and in schoolchildren attending hospital pediatric out-patient departments (28%; Garralda & Bailey, 1989). Although the range of disorders is seen, in contrast with population surveys, emotional disorders predominate over conduct disorders (Garralda & Bailey, 1986; Kramer & Garralda, 1998), suggesting a specific role for primary care in identifying and managing anxiety and depressive disorders. In the UK, levels of depressive symptoms in adolescents attending primary care have been shown to be high in both urban and suburban areas (with significantly different levels of psychosocial disadvantage), reinforcing the relevance of primary care for adolescent depression across socioeconomic groups (Yates, Kramer, & Garralda, 2004). This study found that the presence of depressive symptoms in adolescents was associated with an increased risk of substance abuse and with parental psychiatric symptoms, while a study in the USA found links with school problems and substance abuse (Burns, Cottrell, Perkins *et al.*, 2004). These associations suggest that identification of psychopathology within primary care will provide an opportunity to identify and address a wider range of psychosocial difficulties.

Implications of the High Levels of Hidden Psychiatric Disorder

Do psychiatric disorders contribute to physical consultations in children and young people? Psychiatric symptoms have been found to be linked to high use of primary care and of other medical services by children and young people (Lavigne, Arend, Rosenbaum *et al.*, 1998; Meltzer, Gatward, Goodman, & Ford, 2000; Monck, Graham, Richman, & Dobbs, 1994; Offord, Boyle, Szatmari *et al.*, 1987; Richman, Stevenson & Graham, 1982; Yates, Kramer, & Garralda, 2004). Adolescent primary care attenders with associated psychiatric disorder describe greater frequency and more intense physical symptoms causing impairment than those without associated disorder (Kramer & Garralda, 1998). Children with psychiatric disorders who are frequent primary care attenders do not present with a particular physical problem. Nevertheless, their mothers view them as more lethargic, in poorer general health and more handicapped by their symptoms than mothers of frequent attending children without psychiatric disorder (Garralda, Bowman, & Mandalia, 1999).

In younger children who are brought to the surgery, maternal anxiety about the child is likely to be a factor leading to presentation. In a study of frequent surgery attenders (Garralda, Bowman, & Mandalia, 1999), mothers of children who had psychiatric disorders reported generally more stress in work, finances and relationships. However, what differentiated them most strongly from other mothers was the stress they felt about their child; over half of the mothers of children with disorder (compared with 10% of those without) felt highly stressed about them. Because they also saw these children as in comparatively poor physical health, it would seem logical to seek relief from this by focusing on symptoms for which help is available at the surgery. Nevertheless, this relief may be expected to be only partial, as it does not address the reasons that were presumably stressing mothers most and leading to frequent consulting, namely the child's psychological distress and its management. Primary care practitioners could be more helpful to the child and mother if attention was directed directly to these associated emotional difficulties.

Functional Somatic Symptoms and Psychosomatic Presentations

Addressing mental health issues is of special relevance in the primary care setting, first for children presenting with recurrent and impairing functional or unexplained medical symptoms; and, second, when clinicians suspect that problems in psychiatric adjustment affect the child's ability to manage physical problems effectively.

Recurrent unexplained functional physical symptoms (e.g., abdominal pains, aches and pains, and fatigue) are commonly seen in primary care. They can be an expression of the somatization of distress and are often seen in conjunction with psychiatric disorders (see chapter 57). Campo, Jansen-McWilliams, Comer *et al.* (1999) reported frequent complaints of aches and pains with no organic diagnosis in 2% of 11- to 15-year-old pediatric primary care attenders, and occasional complaints in 11%, with a ratio of two girls to one boy. In about half of the children – significantly more than in children attending with other complaints – doctors and parents identified psychosocial problems and impairment caused by the symptom, and about one-third were described as frequent health service users. In 8- to 15-year-olds with recurrent abdominal pain attending primary care, Campo, Bridge, Ehmann *et al.* (2004) identified a comorbid anxiety disorder in as many as 79% and a depressive disorder in 43%, as well as an excess of temperamental harm avoidance and functional impairment. The close links between emotional and functional physical symptoms in children is further supported by indications that parental anxiety in the first year of the child's life, together with reports of irregular feeding and sleeping habits in the child, can predict recurrent abdominal pains later in childhood (see chapter 57; Ramchandani, Stein, Hotopf *et al.*, 2006).

Psychosocial problems and psychiatric disorders can adversely affect the physical health of a broader group of children. When doctors are asked to note any physical presentation with associated or contributing psychological factors (e.g., asthma exacerbated by stress), such presentations are recorded for about one-fifth of schoolchildren attending primary care and for as many as half in out-patient pediatric clinics, indicating a high degree of sensitivity and vigilance by many clinicians to these issues (Bailey, Graham, & Boniface, 1978; Garralda & Bailey, 1987, 1990). Presenting symptoms in these cases tend to be those regarded traditionally as having psychosomatic components (e.g., aches and pains, incontinence, asthma and blackouts) but virtually all physical complaints are featured. These children have an excess of emotional and behavioral symptoms, including mood changes and relationship problems. However, most do not have a psychiatric disorder. Mothers' stress over parenting, and concerns over schooling have particularly been noted in primary care settings, suggesting the relevance of high academic and behavioral expectations.

Addressing the psychosocial concerns of families with children with psychosomatic presentations may have substantial consequences for medical service use. These families have a high tendency to focus on health issues, as shown by the fact that they are high users of primary care. The children themselves are given more hospital appointments, more referrals to specialist clinics and more follow-up appointments at the surgery than children with purely physical presentations (Campo, Jansen-McWilliams, Comer *et al.*, 1999; Garralda & Bailey, 1987).

Thus, at the first point of contact with primary care, professionals could maximize the impact of the contact if they are alert to looking for hidden or associated emotional and behavioral difficulties and recognize links with physical presentation.

Clarifying Demand and Diagnosing Disorder

Attention to mental health is only possible once need has been recognized and demand for intervention clarified. Rates of recognition within primary care have been shown to be poor (Brugman, Reijneveld, Verhulst, & Verloove-Vanhorick, 2001; Chang, Warner, & Weissman, 1988; Costello & Eddelbrock, 1985; Garralda & Bailey, 1986; Glazebrook, Hollis, Heussler, Goodman, & Coates, 2003; Kramer & Garralda, 1998; Sayal & Taylor, 2004), with poor sensitivity and high specificity (Brugman, Reijneveld, Verhulst *et al.*, 2001). Most affected children fail to receive any mental health services (Burns, Costello, Angold *et al.*, 1995; Rushton, Bruckman, & Kelleher, 2002; Verhulst & Van der Ende, 1997). Recognition has been linked to severity of disorders, age (best in 7- to 14-year-olds), male gender, the presence of social difficulties (being on welfare, broken homes), presenting symptoms (chronic conditions, digestive problems and ill-defined problems), type of consultation (to well child clinics rather than acute care visits), clinician relationship with the child and parental perception of difficulty (Goldberg, Regier, McInerny *et al.*, 1979; Horwitz, Leaf, Leventhal, Forsyth, & Speechley, 1992; Kramer & Garralda, 1998). Sayal and Taylor (2004) demonstrated that parental expression of concern during consultation increased the sensitivity of doctor recognition of mental health problems. In very young children (11–39 months), Ellingson, Briggs-Gowan, Carter, and Horwitz (2004) demonstrated that parental discussion with the primary care provider was associated with parental worry and perceived low socioemotional competence in the child, and with disruption to family routines. Nevertheless, even though many parents believe it is appropriate to express concerns about child behavior to a primary care provider, few parents who have concerns do so (Dulcan, Costello, Costello *et al.*, 1990; Ellingson, Briggs-Gowan, Carter *et al.*, 2004; Horwitz, Leaf, & Leventhal, 1998; Sayal & Taylor, 2004). Thus, education, which enables parents to identify their children's needs, express these within the consultation and understand the potential for intervention, is an important first step in promoting identification within the primary care setting.

The use of screening questionnaires has been considered as a potentially quick and easy method to improve primary care identification (see chapter 20) across the age range (Borowsky, Mozayeny, & Ireland, 2003; Briggs-Gowan, Carter, Irwin, Wachtel, & Cicchetti, 2004; Luby, Heffelfinger, Koenig-McNaught, Brown, & Spitznagel, 2004). Information was improved if collected from both parents and children (Wildman, 2000; Wren, Bridge, & Birmaher, 2004) and at all types of visit to the service (i.e., whether injury or illness related visits as opposed to routine screening visits alone; Borowsky, Mozayeny, & Ireland, 2003). However, questionnaires alone are likely to over-identify the number of children requiring further assessment and intervention, and burden the limited resources. The primary care professional will still need to use clarifying questions about the nature, severity and associated impairment of any symptoms before deciding on appropriate action. Question-naires may be best used to provide a guide as to when psychological, behavioral and psychosocial routes of inquiry should be followed.

Training for primary care physicians in the use of psychiatric diagnostic classifications such as ICD-10 or DSM-IV has been seen as a potential means of improving diagnostic reliability, treatment planning and communication between clinicians. In order to promote and facilitate the use of these classifications in primary care, versions specifically relevant to this setting have been developed, ICD-10 Primary Health Care and DSM-IV Primary Care (American Psychiatric Association, 1995; WHO, 1996) including advice on the management of children and adolescents with disorder (Jenkins, 2004). However, in the USA, Gardner, Kelleher, Pajer, and Campo (2004) demonstrated that primary care clinicians used DSM criteria in only 23% of visits where psychosocial problems were recognized, mostly for ADHD symptoms; in this survey half reported no use of DSM criteria whatsoever. The majority of primary care clinicians in the UK regularly use Read Codes to record patient signs, symptoms and interventions (www.connectingforhealth.nhs.uk/terminology/readcodes/faqs/index_html#6) whereas within the rest of Europe and Australia, use of the International Classification of Primary Care (ICPC-2; WONCA, 1998) is widespread. Although categories within both these systems have been linked with ICD-10 categories, evidence of practitioner knowledge and use of the criteria for psychiatric disorder in children and adolescents is lacking. A cluster randomized study of 30 primary care practices, following dissemination of Diagnostic and Management Guidelines for Mental Disorders in Primary Care: ICD-10 (WHO, 1996) in adult patients, failed to demonstrate improved sensitivity or specificity of diagnosis in clinicians who received the guidelines (Croudace, Evans, Harrison *et al.*, 2003). The potential of these guidelines for use with children and adolescents, and in developing countries with very scarce specialist resources, has not been documented.

Systematic mental health screening of all child and adolescent attenders (at well child and other visits) would reach a large proportion of the population and reveal many of the currently untreated cases. However, as well as training primary care providers to do this, additional resources for intervention will be required. Primary care providers are unlikely to identify needs unless they are able to intervene.

Offering Advice and Treatment

Thus, large numbers of children and adolescents presenting to primary care with physical complaints have concurrent emotional difficulties. Primary care is viewed by many service users as more accessible and less stigmatizing than mental health services. Even where child mental health services are well developed, only a small proportion of psychiatrically disordered young people currently access these services (Rushton, Bruckman, & Kelleher, 2002) and specialist child and adolescent mental health services are already often working to full capacity or overburdened with long waitlists for treatment (US Public Health Service, 2000). Thus, policy-makers in the UK (Health Advisory Service, 1995) and the USA (US Public Health Service, 2000) have highlighted the need for improved provision within the broad range of services already in contact with children and adolescents (e.g., preschool, childcare, education, health, welfare, juvenile justice). If services are to become more available within primary health care, it makes sense to conceptualize a stepped provision with improved primary care recognition, followed by advice and treatment within primary care of the less complex and severe difficulties. Limited consultation duration presents a potential barrier to such interventions. One US study of 2- to 18-year-olds found that pediatricians spent an average of 10.3 min in each well visit consultation (Reisinger & Bires, 1980). A study of adolescent consultation times in the UK (Jacobson, Wilkinson, & Owen, 1994) demonstrated that consultation duration of 11- to 19-year-olds was shorter than for any other age group. Also, little is known about which child and adolescent mental health interventions are appropriate and effective when offered within primary care.

Bower, Garralda, Kramer, Harrington, and Sibbald (2001) carried out a systematic review and identified three types of child mental health intervention offered within primary care: management by specialist mental health professionals based in primary care (often referred to as shifted out-patient clinics); treatments offered by the primary care team; and consultation liaison models. They documented that there were a limited number of studies, many of which were of poor quality, and concluded that a significant program of research was required if the potential for child and adolescent mental health services in primary care was to be realized in an effective and efficient way.

Shifted Out-patient Clinics

Most early work on children and adolescents with actual psychiatric disorders involved treatment by *specialist staff within primary care* (so-called shifted out-patient clinics). Interventions described were brief (6–12 sessions) and included a variety of techniques: cognitive–behavioral therapy, family therapy, non-directive counseling, dynamic therapy, psychiatric evaluation and guidance, parent education and counseling, group work and child education (Bower, Garralda, Kramer *et al.*, 2001). Studies consisted largely of simple before–after designs without control groups and often lacked details on the process of treatment delivery. Two large-scale studies that used randomization failed to demonstrate a marked effect on child health outcomes (Cooper & Murray, 1997; Nicol, Stretch, & Fundudis, 1993). Conclusions about effectiveness are therefore tentative. Moreover, provision of comprehensive coverage of this nature by specialist staff would require marked expansion of specialist services, is unlikely to be cost-effective and may not be achievable.

Treatment by the Primary Care Team

There is little information on the management of child emotional and behavioral difficulties offered by the actual primary care team. Bower, Garralda, Kramer *et al.* (2001) reviewed six studies of treatment offered by the primary care team, offering a variety of interventions for different problems. Of the four controlled studies, only the study by Cullen (1976) and Cullen and Cullen (1996), of preventative interviews with preschool children, demonstrated significant objectively improved outcomes.

Wren, Scholle, Heo, and Comer (2005) documented the practice of 395 primary care clinicians during consultation with 20,861 consecutive attenders aged 4–15 years in the USA, Puerto Rico and Canada. Children identified as having a mood or anxiety syndrome were no more likely to be counseled during the visit than those with other psychosocial problems, and – unless accompanied by a comorbid behavioral syndrome – they were offered fewer scheduled follow-up appointments. Rates of prescription of antidepressants or antianxiety agents were comparatively higher for the mood/anxiety groups but this was still uncommon (6.7%) and they were also more likely to be referred to mental health services. Thus, even when identified, active management by primary care was uncommon in this group. This may be because primary care clinicians feel more responsible for recognizing than for treating child and adolescent depression. In Olson, Kelleher, Kemper *et al.* (2001) survey, respondents reported providing a wide range of brief interventions to almost 80% of young people with depression and prescribing medication to approximately 20%, but they also reported referring a similar proportion to mental health professionals. Factors limiting diagnosis and management most frequently cited included time and training/knowledge and, less commonly, financial or patient issues. However, the response rate in this survey (55–63%) was modest, and it is unclear whether these findings are broadly representative.

Consultation Liaison Models

Consultation liaison, in which the specialist acts to support management by primary care rather than take responsibility for individual patients (Gask, Sibbald, & Creed, 1997), has traditionally been viewed as a means of increasing the capacity of primary care clinicians to offer mental health services, partly through improving their skills and knowledge. In their review, Bower, Garralda, Kramer *et al.* (2001) identified only one study of consultation liaison offered to primary care personnel by specialist child and adolescent mental health workers (Neira-Munoz & Ward, 1998). The intervention (which included reviewing referrals, running liaison clinics and seeing patients on their own) was associated with a reduction in the rate of referrals to specialist mental health services and an increase in appropriateness. The service was rated highly by primary care staff but only one-third of primary care doctors thought that the liaison clinics increased their knowledge and skills. Connor, McLaughlin, Jeffers-Terry *et al.* (2006) have described a similar model of collaboration, in the USA. A child psychiatrist or specialist nurse offers telephone consultation during office hours (139 primary care practitioners in 22 practices). A proportion of cases will then be managed within primary care while the rest are referred to the child psychiatrist for assessment within 4 weeks. During the first 18 months, the child psychiatrist offered direct evaluation of 329 (54%) patients. Time was also spent educating primary care practitioners in case conferences and informal consultations. Neither of these reports included data on patient outcomes and both models included specialist mental health clinicians working primarily on this "specialist" area, consultation liaison with primary care. A survey of all specialist child and adolescent mental health services in England demonstrated that collaborative work with primary care was significantly associated first with a developed "specialist" provision for this, and second with larger sized mental health services (Bradley, Kramer, Garralda *et al.*, 2003). This suggests that it is difficult for individual mental health clinicians to facilitate collaboration on their own when they have a broad range of other commitments. Furthermore, if there is an increase in collaboration, future work will need to address more clearly medicolegal responsibilities in those cases where primary care practitioners provide treatments on the advice of specialist clinicians, especially prescription of psychotropic medications, where primary care practitioners may have limited training and experience.

Use of Psychotropic Medication for Child and Adolescent Depression

There is evidence that prescribing of pediatric psychotropic drugs has increased over recent years across many countries (UK, USA, Canada, France, Germany, Spain, Argentina, Brazil and Mexico; Wong, Murray, Camilleri-Novak, & Stephens, 2004). More specifically, in the UK there has been an increase in prescriptions of antidepressants by primary care clinicians, between 1992 and 2002, especially of selective serotonin reuptake inhibitors (SSRIs) and venlafaxine rather than tricyclic antidepressants (Murray, de Vries, & Wong, 2004, Murray, Wong, & Thompson, 2005). However, treatment is often not sustained, with more than half of subjects discontinuing treatment after 2 months. Similarly, in the USA only 47% of youth continued out-patient treatment with anti-depressants at 3 months and 26% at 6 months, suggesting both inadequate duration of treatment and follow-up (Richardson, DiGiuseppe, Christakis, McCauley, & Katon, 2004). In a survey in North Carolina, 91% of family physicians ($n = 242$) and 58% of pediatricians ($n = 349$) had prescribed SSRIs for pediatric patients, most commonly for depression (Rushton, Clark, & Freed, 2000). In this study, very few physicians (8%) reported adequate training in the treatment of adolescent depression.

In a large community survey, approximately 1% of children and adolescents received out-patient treatment for depression, a rate below epidemiological prevalence estimates (2–8%) (Olfson, Gameroff, Marcus, & Waslick, 2003). Anhedonia was more common in adolescents receiving medication prescribed by psychiatrists, pediatricians or other physicians, but treatment was otherwise unrelated to measures of clinical severity (Olfson, Gameroff, Marcus *et al.*, 2003), despite the recommendation of the American Academy of Child and Adolescent Psychiatry that antidepressant use should be limited to those with severe or psychotherapy-resistant disorders

(American Academy of Child and Adolescent Psychiatry, 1998).

Following widely publicized safety concerns and recommendations about the use of SSRIs, and the recommended ban of those other than fluoxetine as a treatment in child and adolescent depression (CSM, 2005), fewer children and adolescents have been prescribed antidepressants in primary care (Murray, Wong, & Thompson, 2005). It is unclear whether this reduction in drug treatment has resulted in more psychotherapeutic treatments being offered as an alternative in the UK, but in the USA provision of psychotherapy/mental health counseling declined between 1995–1996 and 2001–2002 (Ma, Lee, & Stafford, 2005).

Thus, comprehensive treatment of depressive disorders within primary care will require improved education of primary care providers in the treatment of depression and will need to address a balance of psychotherapeutic and medical interventions in addition to approaches to improve compliance and follow-up.

Complex Interventions for Adolescent Depression in Primary Care

Systematic reviews of screening and intervention programs for adult depression in primary care have outlined a range of issues that are relevant to intervention with young people. Simple educational strategies for staff or passive dissemination of formal guidelines to improve recognition and management have had minimal effect, whereas multifaceted programs that integrate improvements in detection, treatment and follow-up are most effective (Gilbody, Whitty, Grimsha, & Thomas, 2003; Katon, Von, Lin *et al.*, 1999; Pignone, Gaynes, Rushton *et al.*, 2002; WHO, 2004). These include combinations of clinician and patient education, nurse case management, enhanced support from specialist services and monitoring of medication. Further research is needed to clarify which elements of these complex interventions are active ingredients, who benefits most from different elements of the interventions, and to what extent the programs can be translated between different settings in different countries.

In light of the adult findings, Asarnow, Jaycox, Duan *et al.* (2005b) carried out a landmark study of adolescents in six primary care centers in the USA. They included two public sector, two managed care and two academic health programs and enrolled 418 patients aged 13–21 years into a randomized controlled trial of a "quality improvement intervention" versus usual care. The quality improvement intervention included:

1 Expert leader teams at each site to implement and adapt the intervention;

2 Care managers to support primary care clinicians with evaluation, education, medication and psychosocial treatment, and with linkage with specialist mental health services;

3 Training care managers in manualized cognitive–behavioral therapy (CBT) for depression; and

4 Access to participant and clinician choice of treatment.

Treatment options included CBT, medication, combined CBT with medication, care manager follow-up, or specialist referral. Usual care was enhanced by providing primary care clinicians with training and educational materials on depression evaluation and treatment. Six months after assessment, quality improvement patients reported significantly fewer depressive symptoms, higher mental health-related quality of life and greater satisfaction with mental health care. They had also received significantly higher rates of mental health care and psychotherapy or counseling. Enhancement of usual care meant that the benefits detected are probably conservative. However, almost one-third of quality improvement patients continued to show severe depressive symptoms. Increased use of combined psychotherapy and medication might have led to improved outcomes in this group (March, Silva, Petrycki *et al.*, 2004). Moreover, screening and recruitment resulted in the loss of many young people from the study, indicating that this approach may benefit only a selected group and longer-term benefits require further study. Nevertheless, this study demonstrated improved quality of care, increased access to evidence-based treatments and favorable outcomes through increased support to primary care clinicians in naturalistic settings.

In the UK, Gledhill, Kramer, Iliffe, and Garralda (2003) have developed "therapeutic identification" techniques that incorporate training for general practitioners in the identification of depression with opportunistic intervention based on cognitive and interpersonal principles. In one large practice this was shown to be feasible in a pilot study, to lead to improved doctor detection rates and adolescent clinical outcomes, but it needs to be further evaluated and shown to be cost and clinically effective before it can become recommended practice. Approaches such as this that enhance the mental health care provided within primary care in contrast with traditional "shifted" out-patient specialist clinics, may offer the potential for more comprehensive and effective provision, but practically implementation requires investment in primary care and realignment of professional roles.

Intervention for depressive disorders is the most obvious focus for intervention by primary care workers with adolescents, because of the large contribution to hidden morbidity and the long-term adverse outcome (Asarnow, Jaycox, Duan *et al.*, 2005a). However, other important areas for future investigation include intervention for anxiety and somatization-related or somatoform disorders in children, and disruptive disorders (Lavigne, Binns, Christoffel *et al.*, 1993).

The development in primary care of appropriate techniques for the identification and management of functional or somatization-related somatic symptoms is especially relevant. Identification of these children can be aided by establishing the unexplained nature and impairment caused by the physical symptoms and taking notice of risk factors such as family social or structural problems, parental somatization and school problems (Konijnenberg, de Graeff-Meeder, van der Hoeven *et al.*, 2006). Discussion of psychosocial issues needs to take special account of sensitivities by many parents and children in addressing these issues, as some parents – especially those of the more severely affected children – may feel undermined and threatened when these are explored, which leads to their stressing the physical aspects of the child's presentation (Smart & Cottrell, 2005).

Coordinating Care

The primary care clinician has a central role in coordinating care. Coordination includes referral to specialist or other services, as well as long-term management of those with chronic or complex conditions with support from specialist services.

Referral to Specialist Services

The most frequent interface between primary care and child psychiatry or mental health services is through referral to specialist psychiatric services. This may follow less than 10–17% of psychiatric presentations to primary care practitioners (Brugman, Reijneveld, Verhulst *et al.*, 2001; Garralda & Bailey, 1988; OPCS, 1995). The psychiatric referral of schoolchildren by primary care practitioners has been found to be linked to the severity of the child's disorder, male gender, the presence of antisocial symptoms and/or relationship problems and to psychosocial disadvantage (i.e., family stress, unemployment; Garralda & Bailey, 1988). Higher severity and male gender have also been confirmed as factors in other studies (Laclave & Campbell, 1986; Lavigne, Arend, Rosenbaum *et al.*, 1998). One Dutch study found no link between referral and sociodemographic factors (Brugman, Reijneveld, Verhulst *et al.*, 2001). In this setting with a highly developed preventative child health system (90% of children and adolescents receive 3–4 preventative assessments during childhood and adolescence), referral was related to information regarding the mental health of the child *per se*. This may indicate practice that is directly focused on specific mental health need rather than on associated psychosocial risks. In most settings, parental request remains a central determinant for referral, the role of general practitioners and pediatricians tending to remain more passive (Bailey & Garralda, 1989; Briggs-Gowen, Horwitz, Schwab-Stone, Leventhal, & Leaf, 2000; Sayal, Taylor, Beecham, & Byrne, 2002). Parents' views on the passive role taken by practitioners remain unclear, although one study found most parents of referred children to be satisfied (Bailey & Garralda, 1989).

For clearly diagnosable psychiatric problems in children who are not already under the care of mental health services, the primary care clinician needs to make decisions about whether and how to refer. Although existing research indicates that psychiatric referrals by primary care doctors are generally appropriate, increasing awareness of child and adolescent psychiatric problems by parents and primary care teams is likely to result in more referrals than specialist services can possibly accommodate. Protocols refining the criteria for severity, psychosocial complexity and likely response to treatments will need to be developed and audited jointly by child and adolescent and primary care services. Consultation liaison activities by child and adolescent mental health services may be particularly helpful in developing this work.

Managing Chronic Conditions

For problems such as hyperkinetic disorder, it has been shown that once recognized by the general practitioner or family doctor a referral to specialist services usually follows (Sayal, Taylor, Beecham *et al.*, 2002). Other primary providers (e.g., pediatricians) are likely to initiate some treatment but mental health specialists will need to become involved in resistant cases or those with comorbidity (e.g., severe conduct disorder, tic disorders). As a chronic disorder with high levels of comorbidity, a comprehensive model of care could include long-term monitoring within the primary care setting with intermittent involvement of specialist services as appropriate for medication review or adjuvant behavior therapy. However, general practitioners have been shown to be skeptical about hyperkinetic disorder as a diagnostic entity (Klasen & Goodman, 2000). Adequate training and ongoing support are therefore necessities if such a model of joint working is to be developed. Traditional consultation–liaison work by specialist child and adolescent mental health staff provides a mechanism for this joint working but has been limited by a lack of capacity. More recent models of improved collaboration have been facilitated through the use of non-physician care managers/professionals with specialized clinical and behavioral skills, who prioritize frequent communication with primary care clinicians and also maintain strong links with specialist mental health services.

Prevention and Early Intervention

Primary care services provide the most widespread point of access to health services among both the better and the less developed health care systems. As such, they are crucially placed for a role in prevention and early intervention for mental health problems of children and adolescents.

Many broad public health programs relevant to primary care, impact on the *primary prevention* of mental distress and disorder in young people by targeting risk and resilience factors. Examples are family planning programs, prenatal care, promotion of adequate nutrition, child safety information and home visiting programs. These programs are implemented by a range of professionals including general/family practitioners, primary care pediatricians (e.g., in the USA), community pediatricians and health visitors (e.g., in the UK) or community nurses, all of whom are in an ideal position to disseminate information on child health, development, behavior and positive parenting (Bower, Macdonald, Sibbald *et al.*, 2003).

An early study of preventative general practitioner consultations during a child's first 4 years demonstrated favorable outcomes at 6 and 20 years later (Cullen, 1976; Cullen & Cullen, 1996). This study demonstrated that mental health promotion interventions can be carried out systematically by general practitioners or family doctors who, through regular supervision, may be able to influence parental actions and have some long-lasting effects on their children's behavior. However, it is unlikely that many general practitioners or pediatricians would be able to invest the time required into such an intervention.

It may be more practical and cost-effective to implement prenatal and infancy home visiting by trained nurses with mothers at high risk of difficulties (see chapter 61). Olds (2002) and Olds, Eckenrode, Henderson *et al.* 1997, Olds, Henderson, Cole *et al.* 1998, Olds, Kitzman, Cole *et al.* 2004), in a program whereby mothers were visited during pregnancy and up until the child's second birthday, have demonstrated in three large randomized controlled trials benefits for young, low-income, unmarried mothers and children. Improved parental care of the child included fewer injuries and accidental substance ingestions, which may in some cases reflect child abuse and neglect, fewer emergency visits and less use of punishment in the first 4 years. Further beneficial changes with regard to maternal life-course include fewer subsequent pregnancies, greater workforce participation and reduced use of public assistance and food stamps. In the first trial, the program also produced longer-term effects on the number of arrests, convictions, emergent substance use and promiscuous sexual activity of 15-year-old children. However, not all home visiting programs have been shown to be effective. A number of attempts at training primary care community nurses or health visitors to promote parenting in order to reduce behavioral problems in young children have reported inconsistent or equivocal results, and this remains an area requiring further exploration (Bower, Garralda, Kramer *et al.*, 2001). It is important to establish which elements of such interventions are the minimum required to achieve mental health gains for children (see chapter 61).

Secondary prevention, aimed at early detection and diagnosis, is integral to child surveillance programs, and can be implemented by professionals in a range of primary care settings across different countries. For example, community-based group parenting programs, addressing child behavioral difficulties, have been shown to improve parenting practices, parent–child interactions and child behavior through multiple, independently replicated, randomized controlled trials (Scott, Spender, Doolan *et al.*, 2001; Webster Stratton, 1989, 2001). In developing countries, where most of the health care is delivered by the primary or the general health care team, detection of developmental delays and epilepsy is also relevant. However, research is required to ascertain whether systematic early detection by primary care personnel would lead to better outcomes in the medium to long term.

The role of primary care personnel in suicide prevention has been well described (Gould, Greenberg, Velting, & Shaffer, 2003; Mann, Apter, Bertolote *et al.*, 2005). Many suicidal young people (aged 15–34 years) have contact with primary care in the month prior to suicide or self-harm (Luoma, Martin, & Pearson, 2002; Pfaff, Acres, & Wilson, 1999). However, a study of pediatricians and family physicians in the USA revealed that fewer than half reported that they routinely screened their adolescent patients for suicide risk (Frankenfield, Keyl, Gielen *et al.*, 2000). Although the Gotland study (in Sweden) demonstrated a decline in adult suicide rate following general practitioner education to improve diagnosis and treatment of depression, this was not maintained at follow-up (Rutz, von Knorring, & Walinder, 1992). A 1-day training course for general practitioners in Australia enhanced detection rates of adolescent psychological distress and suicidal ideation, but failed to lead to changes in patient management (Pfaff, Acres, & McKelvey, 2001). As with treatment for depression, educational approaches alone may prove insufficient to change the management of suicidal young people in primary care, and systematic screening may need to be integrated into more complex multifaceted approaches.

Parental Substance Misuse and Psychiatric Disorder

Children of parents with substance misuse problems and other psychiatric disorders such as depression and anxiety are at increased risk of developmental, emotional and behavioral difficulties (see chapter 27; Nomura, Wickramaratne, Warner, Mufson, & Weissman, 2002; Weissman, Feder, Pilowsky *et al.*, 2004; Whitaker, Orzol, & Kahn, 2006). Primary care clinicians may be treating these adults or be aware that they are receiving help from specialist services. They should be alert to the increased risks for these children and especially vigilant in relation to their general and mental health needs. Advice, support and guidance for mothers on child rearing may lead to more favorable outcomes for children. Increased support to improve access to specialist services may also be required.

Building Capacity in Primary Care

Integration of mental health provision for children and adolescents into primary care requires improved professional knowledge, skills and attitudes as well as changes to service delivery systems to support this.

Educational interventions should address health workers' undergraduate and postgraduate education. A number of initiatives have addressed this (Bernard, Garralda, Hughes, & Tylee, 1999; Bower, Garralda, Kramer *et al.*, 2001; de Jong, 1996; Dogra, Frake, Bretherton, Dwivedi, & Sharma, 2005; Hughes, Garralda, & Tylee, 1995; Sanci, Coffey, Patton, & Bowes, 2005). Evaluation tends to show benefits by increasing skills and confidence of primary health care staff, but few studies have been methodologically rigorous. Leaf, Owens, Leventhal *et al.* (2004) demonstrated that pediatricians with advanced training in psychosocial problems were more likely to identify children's psychosocial problems and use multiple management strategies compared with pediatricians without specialized training. However, not all general practitioners, pediatricians and other primary care staff wish to obtain training and implement potentially effective management techniques. Primary care is being expected to fulfill an ever-increasing number of preventative and curative interventions and some degree of prioritization is required. While some practitioners welcome the conceptual clarity and management guidance offered by psychiatric terminology and thinking, others have concern about medicalizing distress, especially in children and adolescents (Iliffe, Gledhill, daCunha, Kramer,

& Garralda, 2004). Future work may helpfully clarify which primary care practitioners are especially well suited to the task of promoting and managing child and adolescent mental health. Furthermore, clarification is needed about which specific components of evidence-based knowledge and skills should be included.

Improved training may not be enough to bring about the required change. Alteration to service delivery systems (Pincus, Pechura, Elinson, & Pettit, 2001) and the development of innovative roles for new workers may be required. This has recently been attempted within the UK. Policy aimed at improving access to child and adolescent mental health services led to the development of primary mental health workers (PMHWs) to work with both primary and specialist child and adolescent mental health services performing the following functions:

1 Consolidating the skills of existing workers in primary services;

2 Helping workers in primary services develop new skills and confidence through training and education;

3 Supporting recognition of disorders and their referral to more specialist services if appropriate; and

4 Assessing and treating some individuals (Department of Health, 2004).

Initially, posts were filled by a variety of professionals including a majority of nurses but also by social workers, psychologists and others with significant experience of working in child mental health services (Bradley, Kramer, Garralda *et al.*, 2003). Their presence has been shown to bridge the wide gap between primary care and specialist mental health services (Macdonald, Bradley, Bower *et al.*, 2004) and improve integration of primary and secondary services. However, subsequent expansion of the role, with a limited pool of experienced professionals available for recruitment, would have led to the recruitment of professionals with less experience, raising questions about their effectiveness. Shortages of appropriately skilled personnel are likely to be a limiting factor in any program aiming to expand provision in primary care, underlining the need for training. There has also been a rapid expansion of specialist liaison nurse posts with roles similar to those of the PMHW within other medical services (e.g., in palliative care, asthma, epilepsy, infection control, HIV/AIDS; Hobbs & Murray, 1999). Surveys reveal high levels of patient satisfaction but there have been few randomized controlled trials to look at clinical and cost-effectiveness. Where these have been undertaken, evidence of effectiveness is conflicting (Hobbs & Murray, 1999). Research is needed to evaluate the impact of PMHWs on patterns of service use and health outcomes.

Another program with similar features has been developed in the USA in a large rural pediatric practice (Campo, Shafer, Strohm *et al.*, 2005). After identification of emotional or behavioral problems by primary care clinicians, young people are offered an assessment of their clinical need by an advanced practice nurse (APN). Based on the level of impairment, complexity of the mental health problem, treatment history and needs, young people are triaged to routine care by primary care clinicians with APN support, to on-site mental health service for intervention or psychiatric consultation by the APN, psychiatric social worker and/or part time pediatric psychiatrist, or referred to specialist mental health or emergency mental health services. In the course of 1 year, 789 (2.5%) primary care visits were referred for triage. Of these 789 visits to the APN, 279 (35%) represented first-time or new mental health contacts. Of these 187 (67%) received routine care, 52 (19%) received on-site mental health services, 36 (13%) were referred to specialist mental health services and 4 (1%) were referred for emergency evaluation and admission. Although at 2.5% the overall proportion of children requiring triage was low, the vast majority of new mental health contacts were assessed to be treatable within primary care, with most receiving intervention from the primary care clinician with APN support.

Pillay and Lockhat (1997) described a community program in South Africa. As in many developing countries, South Africa has a large proportion of young people in its population, and mental health services are lacking in many areas. Two clinical psychologists who had been providing a clinical service within an urban teaching hospital to young people from a large geographical area (up to 300 km away), changed their model to include providing a monthly service, traveling to five centers in outlying areas, in line with a combined shifted out-patient/liaison-consultation model. They offered a day that combined training in the identification of problems and intervention techniques for frontline workers (e.g., primary care, school and psychiatric nurses, social workers and teachers), with their own clinical assessment of more complex cases. As with the other models described above across different national contexts, this again confirms that it is feasible to improve integration of services, but research is required to assess whether integration is clinically and cost-effective, and whether these models of service delivery lead to improved access to services, clinical outcomes and user satisfaction.

Large-scale improvement in access to interventions for child and adolescent mental health problems through integration with primary services will require commitment of resources to build capacity. A global lack of mental health policy pertaining to children and adolescents contributes to the barriers to service development, in spite of the significant progress made in policy development over the last 10 years (Shatkin & Belfer, 2004). This should include attention to research, professional training and public education, in conjunction with service developments based on locally determined, culturally sensitive needs assessment (Rahman, Mubbashar, Harrington, & Gater, 2000). Intersectoral collaboration across health, education and social care is important across settings, whether in poorly or well-developed systems, with priorities for development according to patterns and profiles of disorder in relation to available resources and the growing evidence base for interventions.

Future Directions

It may be expected that in future years there will be a continuing impetus to enhancing attention to the mental health of children and adolescents in primary care by the following developments:

- A better appreciation by the public and by health service providers of child psychiatric disorders such as ADHD and depression, with parallel increasing expectations of assistance and knowledge about these from professionals in primary care;
- Clearer identification of primary care staff with a special interest in child and adolescent mental health;
- More active "therapeutic identification" of child and adolescent mental health problems by primary care professionals, with the development of setting-appropriate information and well-informed advice providing techniques for children and families and halting the increase in the primary prescription of psychotropic medication in primary care;
- More attention to the appropriate management of functional somatic symptoms in the primary care setting;
- Development of general practice therapist posts to implement setting-appropriate therapeutic techniques; and
- Further development of liaison posts with clearer areas of expertise and enhanced training to help bridge the gap between primary and specialist mental health services.

On the research field, it may be expected that there will be further:

- Systematic description of innovative mental health informed interventions in countries with developing health services;
- In countries with better developed services, a trend for more evaluation of new setting-appropriate techniques for specific disorders using simple before–after controlled designs, followed by larger evaluations of complex interventions with the progressive elucidation of the more active treatment ingredients;
- Evaluation of new liaison services through the development of adequate outcome measures; and
- Evaluation of training to increase primary care workers' awareness, knowledge and skills in relation to child and adolescent mental health problems.

References

American Academy of Child and Adolescent Psychiatry. (1998). Practice parameters for the assessment and treatment of children and adolescents with depressive disorders. *Journal of the American Academy of Child and Adolescent Psychiatry*, *37* (Supplement), 63S–83S.

American Psychiatric Association. (1995). *Diagnostic and statistical manual of mental disorders* (4th edn.). Primary care. Washington, DC: American Psychiatric Association.

Asarnow, J. R., Jaycox, L. H., Duan, N., LaBorde, A. P., Rea, M. M., Tang, L., *et al.* (2005a). Depression and role impairment among adolescents in primary care clinics. *Journal of Adolescent Health*, *37*, 477–483.

Asarnow, J. R., Jaycox, L. H., Duan, N., LaBorde, A. P., Rea, M. M., Murray, P., *et al.* (2005b). Effectiveness of a quality improvement intervention for adolescent depression in primary care clinics: A randomized controlled trial. *Journal of the American Medical Association*, *293*, 311–319.

Bailey, D., & Garralda, M. E. (1989). Referral to child psychiatry: parent and doctor motives and expectations. *Journal of Child Psychology and Psychiatry*, *30*, 449–458.

Bailey, V., Graham, P., & Boniface, D. (1978). How much child psychiatry does a general practitioner do? *Journal of the Royal College of General Practitioners*, *28*, 621–626.

Bernard, P., Garralda, E., Hughes, T., & Tylee, A. (2006). Evaluation of a teaching package in adolescent psychiatry for general practitioners. *Education for General Practice*, *10*, 21–28.

Boerma, W. G. W. (2006). *Primary care in the driver's seat? Organisational reform in European primary care*. Buckingham: Open University Press.

Borowsky, I. W., Mozayeny, S., & Ireland, M. (2003). Brief psychosocial screening at health supervision and acute care visits. *Pediatrics*, *112*, 129–133.

Bower, P., Garralda, E., Kramer, T., Harrington, R., & Sibbald, B. (2001). The treatment of child and adolescent mental health problems in primary care: A systematic review. *Family Practice*, *18*, 373–382.

Bower, P., Macdonald, W., Sibbald, B., Bradley, S., Garralda, E., Kramer, T., *et al.* (2003). Postal survey of services for child and adolescent mental health problems in general practice in England. *Primary Care Mental Health*, *1*, 17–26.

Bradley, S., Kramer, T., Garralda, E., Bower, P., Macdonald, W., Sibbald, B., *et al.* (2003). Child and adolescent mental health interface work with primary services: A survey of NHS provider trusts. *Child and Adolescent Mental Health*, *8*, 170–176.

Briggs-Gowan, M. J., Carter, A. S., Irwin, J. R., Wachtel, K., & Cicchetti, D. V. (2004). The Brief Infant–Toddler Social and Emotional Assessment: Screening for social-emotional problems and delays in competence. *Journal of Pediatric Psychology*, *29*, 143–155.

Briggs-Gowan, M. J., Horwitz, S. M., Schwab-Stone, M. E., Leventhal, J. M., & Leaf, P. J. (2000). Mental health in pediatric settings: Distribution of disorders and factors related to service use. *Journal of the American Academy of Child and Adolescent Psychiatry*, *39*, 841–849.

Brugman, E., Reijneveld, S. A., Verhulst, F. C., & Verloove-Vanhorick, S. P. (2001). Identification and management of psychosocial problems by preventive child health care. *Archives of Pediatrics and Adolescent Medicine*, *155*, 462–469.

Burns, B. J., Costello, E. J., Angold, A., Tweed, D., Stangl, D., Farmer, E. M., *et al.* (1995). Children's mental health service use across service sectors. *Health Affairs (Millwood)*, *14*, 147–159.

Burns, J. J., Cottrell, L., Perkins, K., Pack, R., Stanton, B., Hobbs, G., *et al.* (2004). Depressive symptoms and health risk among rural adolescents. *Pediatrics*, *113*, 1313–1320.

Campo, J. V., Bridge, J., Ehmann, M., Altman, S., Lucas, A., Birmaher, B., *et al.* (2004). Recurrent abdominal pain, anxiety, and depression in primary care. *Pediatrics*, *113*, 817–824.

Campo, J. V., Jansen-McWilliams, L., Comer, D. M., Kelleher, K. J. (1999). Somatization in pediatric primary care: association with psychopathology, functional impairment, and use of services. *Journal of the American Academy of Child & Adolescent Psychiatry*, *38*, 1093–1101.

Campo, J. V., Shafer, S., Strohm, J., Lucas, A., Cassesse, C. G., Shaeffer, D., *et al.* (2005). Pediatric behavioral health in primary care: A collaborative approach. *Journal of the American Psychiatric Nurses Association*, *11*, 276–282.

Chang, G., Warner, V., & Weissman, M. M. (1988). Physicians' recognition of psychiatric disorders in children and adolescents. *Am J Dis Child*, *142*, 736–739.

Cheng, T. L. (2004). Primary care pediatrics: 2004 and beyond. *Pediatrics*, *113*, 1802–1809.

Connor, D. F., McLaughlin, T. J., Jeffers-Terry, M., O'Brien, W. H., Stille, C. J., Young, L. M., *et al.* (2006). Targeted child psychiatric services: A new model of pediatric primary clinician–child psychiatry collaborative care. *Clinical Pediatrics*, *45*, 423–434.

Cooper, P., & Murray, L. (1997). The impact of psychological treatments of postpartum depression on maternal mood and infant development. In L. Murray, & P. Cooper (Eds.), *Postpartum depression and child development* (pp. 201–220). New York: Guilford Press.

Costello, E. J., & Edelbrock, C. S. (1985). Detection of psychiatric disorders in pediatric primary care: A preliminary report. *Journal of the American Academy of Child Psychiatry*, *24*, 771–774.

Costello, E. J., Costello, A. J., Edelbrock, C., Burns, B. J., Dulcan, M. K., Brent, D., *et al.* (1988). Psychiatric disorders in pediatric primary care. Prevalence and risk factors. *Archives of General Psychiatry*, *45*, 1107–1116.

Croudace, T. I. M., Evans, J. O. N. A., Harrison, G. L. Y. N., Sharp, D. J., Wilkinson, E. L. L. E., Mccann, G. E. M. M., *et al.* (2003). Impact of the ICD-10 Primary Health Care (PHC) diagnostic and management guidelines for mental disorders on detection and outcome in primary care: Cluster randomized controlled trial. *British Journal of Psychiatry*, *182*, 20–30.

CSM. (2005). *Selective serotonin reuptake inhibitors (SSRI) overview of regulatory status and CSM advice relating to major depressive disorder in children and adolescents including a survey of safety and efficacy data.* Accessed October 10, 2003 from http://www.mhra.gov.uk/home/idcplg?IdcService=SS_GET_PAGE&useSecondary=true&ssDocName=CON019494&ssTargetNodeld=221 (Last viewed 9 December 2007).

Cullen, K. J. (1976). A six-year controlled trial of prevention of children's behavior disorders. *Journal of Pediatrics*, *88*, 662–667.

Cullen, K. J., & Cullen, A. M. (1996). Long-term follow-up of the Busselton six-year controlled trial of prevention of children's behavior disorders. *Journal of Pediatrics*, *129*, 136–139.

de Jong, J. T. (1996). A comprehensive public mental health programme in Guinea-Bissau: A useful model for African, Asian and Latin-American countries. *Psychological Medicine*, *26*, 97–108.

Department of Health and Department for Education and Skills (2004). *National Service Framework for Children, Young People and Maternity Services.* London: Department of Health.

Dogra, N., Frake, C., Bretherton, K., Dwivedi, K., & Sharma, I. (2005). Training CAMHS professionals in developing countries: An Indian case study. *Child and Adolescent Mental Health*, *10*, 74–79.

Dulcan, M. K., Costello, E. J., Costello, A. J., Edelbrock, C., Brent, D., & Janiszewski, S. (1990). The pediatrician as gatekeeper to mental health care for children: Do parents' concerns open the gate? *Journal of the American Academy of Child and Adolescent Psychiatry*, *29*, 453–458.

Ellingson, K. D., Briggs-Gowan, M. J., Carter, A. S., & Horwitz, S. M. (2004). Parent identification of early emerging child behavior problems: Predictors of sharing parental concern with health providers. *Archives of Pediatrics and Adolescent Medicine*, *158*, 766–772.

Frankenfield, D. L., Keyl, P. M., Gielen, A., Wissow, L. S., Werthamer, L., & Baker, S. P. (2000). Adolescent patients: Healthy or hurting? Missed opportunities to screen for suicide risk in the primary care setting. *Archives of Pediatrics and Adolescent Medicine*, *154*, 162–168.

Freed, G. L., Nahra, T. A., & Wheeler, J. R. C. (2004). Which physicians are providing health care to America's children? Trends and changes during the past 20 years. *Archives of Pediatrics and Adolescent Medicine*, *158*, 22–26.

Gardner, W., Kelleher, K. J., Pajer, K. A., & Campo, J. V. (2004). Primary care clinicians' use of standardized psychiatric diagnoses. *Child: Care, Health and Development*, *30*, 401–412.

Garralda, M. E., & Bailey, D. (1986). Children with psychiatric disorders in primary care. *Journal of Child Psychology and Psychiatry*, *27*, 611–624.

Garralda, M. E., & Bailey, D. (1987). Psychosomatic aspects of children's consultations in primary care. *European Archives of Psychiatry & Neurological Science*, *236*, 319–322.

Garralda, M. E., & Bailey, D. (1988). Child and family factors associated with referral to child psychiatrists. *British Journal of Psychiatry*, *153*, 81–89.

Garralda, M. E., & Bailey, D. (1989). Psychiatric disorders in general paediatric referrals. *Archives of Disease in Childhood*, *64*, 1727–1733.

Garralda, M. E., & Bailey, D. (1990). Paediatrician identification of psychological factors associated with general paediatric consultations. *Journal of Psychosomatic Research*, *34*, 303–312.

Garralda, M. E., Bowman, F. M., & Mandalia, S. (1999). Children with psychiatric disorders who are frequent attenders to primary care. *European Child and Adolescent Psychiatry*, *8*, 34–44.

Gask, L., Sibbald, B., & Creed, F. (1997). Evaluating models of working at the interface between mental health services and primary care. *British Journal of Psychiatry*, *170*, 6–11.

Giel, R., de Arango, M. V., Climent, C. E., Harding, T. W., Ibrahim, H. H., Ladrido-Ignacio, L., *et al.* (1981). Childhood mental disorders in primary health care: results of observations in four developing countries. A report from the WHO collaborative Study on Strategies for Extending Mental Health Care. *Pediatrics*, *68*, 677–683.

Gilbody, S., Whitty, P., Grimshaw, J., & Thomas, R. (2003). Educational and organizational interventions to improve the management of depression in primary care: A systematic review. *Journal of the American Medical Association*, *289*, 3145–3151.

Glazebrook, C., Hollis, C., Heussler, H., Goodman, R., & Coates, L. (2003). Detecting emotional and behavioural problems in paediatric clinics. *Child: Care, Health and Development*, *29*, 141–149.

Gledhill, J., Kramer, T., Iliffe, S., & Garralda, M. E. (2003). Training general practitioners in the identification and management of adolescent depression within the consultation: A feasibility study. *Journal of Adolescence*, *26*, 245–250.

Goldberg, I. D., Regier, D. A., McInerny, T. K., Pless, I. B., Roghmann, K. J. (1979). The role of the pediatrician in the delivery of mental health services to children. *Pediatrics*, *63*, 898–909.

Gould, M. S., Greenberg, T., Velting, D. M., & Shaffer, D. (2003). Youth suicide risk and preventative interventions: A review of the past 10 years. *Journal of the American Academy of Child and Adolescent Psychiatry*, *42*, 386–405.

Gureje, O., Omigbodun, O. O., Gater, R., Acha, R. A., Ikuesan, B. A., & Morris, J. (1994). Psychiatric disorders in a paediatric primary care clinic. *British Journal of Psychiatry*, *165*, 527–530.

Health Advisory Service. (1995). *Child and adolescent mental health services: Together we stand.* London: HMSO.

Hobbs, R., & Murray, E. T. (1999). Specialist liaison nurses. *British Medical Journal*, *318*, 683–684.

Horwitz, S. M., Leaf, P. J., & Leventhal, J. M. (1998). Identification of psychosocial problems in pediatric primary care: Do family attitudes make a difference? *Archives of Pediatrics and Adolescent Medicine*, *152*, 367–371.

Horwitz, S. M., Leaf, P. J., Leventhal, J. M., Forsyth, B., & Speechley, K. N. (1992). Identification and management of psychosocial and developmental problems in community-based, primary care pediatric practices. *Pediatrics*, *89*, 480–485.

Hughes, T., Garralda, E., & Tylee, A. (1995). *Child mental health problems.* London: St Mary's Hospital Medical School.

Iliffe, S., Gledhill, J., daCunha, F., Kramer, T., & Garralda, E. (2004). The recognition of adolescent depression in general practice: Issues in the acquisition of new skills. *Primary Care Psychiatry*, *9*, 51–56.

Jacobson, A. M., Goldberg, I. D., Burns, B. J., Hoeper, E. W., Hankin, J. R., & Hewitt, K. (1980). Diagnosed mental disorder in children and use of health services in four organized health care settings. *American Journal of Psychiatry*, *137*, 559–565.

Jacobson, L. D., Wilkinson, C. L. A. R., & Owen, P. A. (1994). Is the potential of teenage consultations being missed? A study of consultation times in primary care. *Family Practice*, *11*, 296–299.

Jenkins, R. (Ed.). (2004). *WHO guide to mental and neurological health in primary care.* London: Royal Society of Medicine Press.

Katon, W., Von, K. M., Lin, E., Simon, G., Walker, E., Unutzer, J., *et al.* (1999). Stepped collaborative care for primary care patients with persistent symptoms of depression: A randomized trial. *Archives of General Psychiatry*, *56*, 1109–1115.

Katz, M., Rubino, A., Collier, J., Rosen, J., & Ehrich, J. H. H. (2002). Demography of pediatric primary care in Europe: Delivery of care and training. *Pediatrics*, *109*, 788–796.

Klasen, H., & Goodman, R. (2000). Parents and GPs at cross-purposes over hyperactivity: A qualitative study of possible barriers to treatment. *British Journal of General Practice*, *50*, 199–202.

Konijnenberg, A. Y., de Graeff-Meeder, E. R., van der Hoeven, J., Kimpen, J. L., Buitelaar, J. K., & Uiterwaal, C. S. (2006). Psychiatric morbidity in children with medically unexplained chronic pain: Diagnosis from the pediatrician's perspective. *Pediatrics*, *117*, 889–897.

Kramer, T., & Garralda, M. E. (1998). Psychiatric disorders in adolescents in primary care. *British Journal of Psychiatry*, *173*, 508–513.

Kramer, T., Illife, S., Murray, E., & Waterman, S. (1997). Which adolescents attend the GP? The association with psychiatric and psychosomatic complaints. *British Journal of General Practice*, *47*, 327.

Laclave, L. J., & Campbell, J. L. (1986). Psychiatric intervention in children: Sex differences in referral rates. *Journal of the American Academy of Child and Adolescent Psychiatry*, *25*, 430–432.

Lavigne, J. V., Arend, R., Rosenbaum, D., Binns, H. J., Christoffel, K. K., Burns, A., *et al.* (1998). Mental health service use among young children receiving pediatric primary care. *Journal of the American Academy of Child and Adolescent Psychiatry*, *37*, 1175–1183.

Lavigne, J. V., Binns, H. J., Christoffel, K. K., Rosenbaum, D., Arend, R., Smith, K., *et al.* (1993). Behavioral and emotional problems among preschool children in pediatric primary care: Prevalence and pediatricians' recognition. Pediatric Practice Research Group. *Pediatrics*, *91*, 649–655.

Leaf, P. J., Owens, P. L., Leventhal, J. M., Forsyth, B. W. C., Vaden-Kiernan, M., Epstein, L. D., *et al.* (2004). Pediatricians' training and identification and management of psychosocial problems. *Clinical Pediatrics*, *43*, 355–365.

Luby, J. L., Heffelfinger, A., Koenig-McNaught, A. L., Brown, K., & Spitznagel, E. (2004). The Preschool Feelings Checklist: A brief and sensitive screening measure for depression in young children. *Journal of the American Academy of Child and Adolescent Psychiatry*, *43*, 708–717.

Luoma, J. B., Martin, C. E., & Pearson, J. L. (2002). Contact with mental health and primary care providers before suicide: A review of the evidence. *American Journal of Psychiatry*, *159*, 909–916.

Ma, J., Lee, K. V., & Stafford, R. S. (2005). Depression treatment during outpatient visits by US children and adolescents. *Journal of Adolescent Health*, *37*, 434–442.

Macdonald, W., Bradley, S., Bower, P., Kramer, T., Sibbald, B., Garralda, E., *et al.* (2004). Primary mental health workers in child and adolescent mental health services. *Journal of Advanced Nursing*, *46*, 78–87.

Mann, J. J., Apter, A., Bertolote, J., Beautrais, A., Currier, D., Haas, A., *et al.* (2005). Suicide prevention strategies: A systematic review. *Journal of the American Medical Association*, *294*, 2064–2074.

March, J., Silva, S., Petrycki, S., Curry, J., Wells, K., Fairbank, J., *et al.* (2004). Fluoxetine, cognitive–behavioral therapy, and their combination for adolescents with depression: Treatment for Adolescents with Depression Study (TADS) randomized controlled trial. *Journal of the American Medical Association*, *292*, 807–820.

Melzer, H., Gatward, R., Goodman, R., & Ford, T. (2000). *The mental health of children and adolescents in Great Britain*. London: HMSO.

Monck, E., Graham, P., Richman, N., & Dobbs, R. (1994). Adolescent girls. I. Self-reported mood disturbance in a community population. *British Journal of Psychiatry*, *165*, 760–769.

Murray, M. L., de Vries, C. S., & Wong, I. C. (2004). A drug utilization study of antidepressants in children and adolescents using the General Practice Research Database. *Archives of Disease in Childhood*, *89*, 1098–1102.

Murray, M. L., Wong, I. C. K., & Thompson, M. (2005). Do selective serotonin reuptake inhibitors cause suicide? Antidepressant prescribing to children and adolescents by GPs has fallen since CSM advice. *British Medical Journal*, *330*, 1151.

Neira-Munoz, E., & Ward, D. (1998). Child mental health services. Side by side. *Health Service Journal*, *108*, 26–27.

Nicol, R., Stretch, D., & Fundudis, T. (1993). *Preschool children in troubled families*. Chichester: John Wiley and Sons.

Nomura, Y., Wickramaratne, P. J., Warner, V., Mufson, L., & Weissman, M. M. (2002). Family discord, parental depression, and psychopathology in offspring: 10-year follow-up. *Journal of the American Academy of Child and Adolescent Psychiatry*, *41*, 402–409.

Offord, D. R., Boyle, M. H., Szatmari, P., Rae-Grant, N. I., Links, P. S., Cadman, D. T., *et al.* (1987). Ontario Child Health Study. II. Six-month prevalence of disorder and rates of service utilization. *Archives of General Psychiatry*, *44*, 832–836.

Olds, D. L. (2002). Prenatal and infancy home visiting by nurses: From randomized trials to community replication. *Prevention Science*, *3*, 153–172.

Olds, D. L., Eckenrode, J., Henderson, C. R., Kitzman, H., Powers, J., Cole, R., *et al.* (1997). Long-term effects of home visitation on maternal life course and child abuse and neglect. Fifteen-year follow-up of a randomized trial. *Journal of the American Medical Association*, *278*, 637–643.

Olds, D. L., Henderson, C. R., Cole, R., Eckenrode, J., Kitzman, H., Luckey, D., *et al.* (1998). Long-term effects of nurse home visitation on children's criminal and antisocial behavior: 15-year follow-up of a randomized trial. *Journal of the American Medical Association*, *280*, 1238–1244.

Olds, D. L., Kitzman, H., Cole, R., Robinson, J., Sidora, K., Luckey, D. W., *et al.* (2004). Effects of nurse home-visiting on maternal life course and child development: Age 6 follow-up results of a randomized trial. *Pediatrics*, *114*, 1550–1559.

Olfson, M., Gameroff, M. J., Marcus, S. C., & Waslick, B. D. (2003). Outpatient treatment of child and adolescent depression in the United States. *Archives of General Psychiatry*, *60*, 1236–1242.

Olson, A. L., Kelleher, K. J., Kemper, K. J., Zuckerman, B. S., Hammond, C. S., & Dietrich, A. J. (2001). Primary care pediatricians' roles and perceived responsibilities in the identification and management of depression in children and adolescents. *Ambululatory Pediatrics*, *1*, 91–98.

OPCS. (1995). *Morbidity statistics from general practice*. London: HMSO.

Pfaff, J. J., Acres, J. G., & McKelvey, R. S. (2001). Training general practitioners to recognise and respond to psychological distress and suicidal ideation in young people. *Medical Journal of Australia*, *174*, 222–226.

Pfaff, J. J., Acres, J., & Wilson, M. (1999). The role of general practitioners in parasuicide: A Western Australia perspective. *Archives of Suicide Research*, *5*, 207–214.

Pignone, M. P., Gaynes, B. N., Rushton, J. L., Burchell, C. M., Orleans, C. T., Mulrow, C. D., *et al.* (2002). Screening for depression in adults: A summary of the evidence for the US Preventive Services Task Force. *Annals of Internal Medicine*, *136*, 765–776.

Pillay, A. L., & Lockhat, M. R. (1997). Developing community mental health services for children in South Africa. *Social Science and Medicine*, *45*, 1493–1501.

Pincus, H. A., Pechura, C. M., Elinson, L., & Pettit, A. R. (2001). Depression in primary care: Linking clinical and systems strategies. *General Hospital Psychiatry*, *23*, 311–318.

Rahman, A., Mubbashar, M., Harrington, R., & Gater, R. (2000). Developing child mental health services in developing countries. *Journal of Child Psychology and Psychiatry*, *41*, 539–546.

Ramchandani, P. G., Stein, A., Hotopf, M., Wiles, N. J., & the ALSPAC Study Team. (2006). Early parental and child predictors of recurrent abdominal pain at school age: Results of a large population-based study. *Journal of the American Academy of Child and Adolescent Psychiatry*, *45*, 729–736.

Reisinger, K. S., & Bires, J. A. (1980). Anticipatory guidance in pediatric practice. *Pediatrics*, *66*, 889–892.

Richardson, L. P., DiGiuseppe, D., Christakis, D. A., McCauley, E., & Katon, W. (2004). Quality of care for Medicaid-covered youth treated with antidepressant therapy. *Archives of General Psychiatry*, *61*, 475–480.

Richman, N., Stevenson, J., & Graham, P. J. (1982). *Preschool to school: A behavioral study*. London: Academic Press.

Rushton, J. L., Clark, S. J., & Freed, G. L. (2000). Pediatrician and family physician prescription of selective serotonin reuptake inhibitors. *Pediatrics*, *105*, e82.

Rushton, J., Bruckman, D., & Kelleher, K. (2002). Primary care referral of children with psychosocial problems. *Archives of Pediatrics and Adolescent Medicine*, *156*, 592–598.

Rutz, W., von Knorring, L., & Walinder, J. (1992). Long-term effects of an educational program for general practitioners given by the Swedish Committee for the Prevention and Treatment of Depression. *Acta Psychiatrica Scandinavica*, *85*, 83–88.

Sanci, L., Coffey, C., Patton, G., & Bowes, G. (2005). Sustainability of change with quality general practitioner education in adolescent health: A 5-year follow-up. *Medical Education*, *39*, 557–560.

Sayal, K., & Taylor, E. (2004). Detection of child mental health disorders by general practitioners. *British Journal of General Practice*, *54*, 348–352.

Sayal, K., Taylor, E., Beecham, J., & Byrne, P. (2002). Pathways to care in children at risk of attention-deficit hyperactivity disorder. *British Journal of Psychiatry*, *181*, 43–48.

Scott, S., Spender, Q., Doolan, M., Jacobs, B., Aspland, H., & Webster-Stratton, C. (2001). Multicentre controlled trial of parenting groups for childhood antisocial behaviour in clinical practice. *British Medical Journal*, *323*, 194–198.

Shatkin, J., & Belfer, M. (2004). The global absence of child and adolescent mental health policy. *Child and Adolescent Mental Health*, *9*, 104–108.

Smart, S., & Cottrell, D. (2005). Going to the doctors: The views of mothers of children with recurrent abdominal pain. *Child: Care, Health and Development*, *31*, 265–273.

Starfield, B., Gross, E., Wood, M., Pantell, R., Allen, C., Bruce, I., *et al.* (1980). Psychosocial and psychosomatic diagnoses in primary care of children. *Pediatrics*, *66*, 159–167.

US Public Health Service. (2000). *Report of the Surgeon General's Conference on Children's Mental Health: A national action agenda*. Washington, DC: Department of Health and Human Services.

Verhulst, F. C., & van der Ende, J. (1997). Factors associated with child mental health service use in the community. *Journal of the American Academy of Child and Adolescent Psychiatry*, *36*, 901–909.

Webster-Stratton, C., Hollinsworth, T., & Kolpacoff, M. (1989). The long-term effectiveness and clinical significance of three cost-effective training programs for families with conduct-problem children. *Journal of Consulting and Clinical Psychology*, *57*, 550–553.

Webster-Stratton, C., Reid, M. J., & Hammond, M. (2001). Preventing conduct problems, promoting social competence: A parent and teacher training partnership in Head Start. *Journal of Clinical Child Psychology*, *30*, 283–302.

Weissman, M. M., Feder, A., Pilowsky, D. J., Olfson, M., Fuentes, M., Blanco, C., *et al.* (2004). Depressed mothers coming to primary care: Maternal reports of problems with their children. *Journal of Affective Disorders*, *78*, 93–100.

Whitaker, R. C., Orzol, S. M., & Kahn, R. S. (2006). Maternal mental health, substance use, and domestic violence in the year after delivery and subsequent behavior problems in children at age 3 years. *Archives of General Psychiatry*, *63*, 551–560.

Wildman, B. G., Kinsman, A. M., & Smucker, W. D. (2000). Use of child reports of daily functioning to facilitate identification of psychosocial problems in children. *Archives of Family Medicine*, *9*, 612–616.

WONCA: International Classification Committee. (1998). *ICPC-2 International Classification of Primary Care* (2nd edn.). Oxford: Oxford University Press.

Wong, I. C., Murray, M. L., Camilleri-Novak, D., & Stephens, P. (2004). Increased prescribing trends of paediatric psychotropic medications. *Archives of Disease in Childhood*, *89*, 1131–1132.

World Health Organization (WHO). (1996). *Diagnostic and management guidelines for mental disorders in primary care: ICD-10*. Göttingen: Hogrefe & Huber.

World Health Organization (WHO). (2001). *The world health report: 2001. Mental health: New understanding, new hope*. Geneva: World Health Organization.

World Health Organization. Regional Office for Europe's Health Evidence Network. (2004). *What is the evidence of capacity building of primary health care professionals in the detection, management and outcome of depression?* Geneva: World Health Organization.

World Health Organization (WHO). (2005). *Mental health: Facing the challenges, building solutions*. Denmark: World Health Organization.

Wren, F. J., Bridge, J. A., & Birmaher, B. (2004). Screening for childhood anxiety symptoms in primary care: Integrating child and parent reports. *Journal of the American Academy of Child and Adolescent Psychiatry*, *43*, 1364–1371.

Wren, F. J., Scholle, S. H., Heo, J., & Comer, D. M. (2005). How do primary care clinicians manage childhood mood and anxiety syndromes? *International Journal of Psychiatry in Medicine*, *35*, 1–12.

Yates, P., Kramer, T., & Garralda, E. (2004). Depressive symptoms amongst adolescent primary care attenders: Levels and associations. *Social Psychiatry and Psychiatric Epidemiology*, *39*, 588–594.

73 Genetic Counseling

Emily Simonoff

Genetic Counseling and the Role of the Genetic Counselor

Genetic counseling is the process of requesting and receiving information on genetic disorders, risk and possible interventions for oneself and one's relatives. Genetic counseling focuses on providing clients with information that will allow them to make informed decisions with regard to family planning and health care (Kelly, 1986). People presenting for genetic counseling may not have a health problem at the time of presentation. Although the term "counseling" is used, it differs from mental health counseling in being brief (usually 1–3 visits) and focusing on the communication of fact, with limited exploration of individual factors that may alter decisions about management of the information given.

Nature of Genetic Counseling in Child Psychiatry

The majority of child psychiatric disorders are complex in their inheritance in that multiple genes and environmental factors both influence the occurrence of disorder (see chapter 23). Susceptibility genes are usually common variants rather than rare mutations and co-act with environmental risk factors, which may also be common variations in experience or exposure. Single gene mutations, chromosomal anomalies and submicroscopic abnormalities *do* occur, predominantly but not exclusively in global intellectual disability, and these are important to be aware of, as intellectual disability may first be identified in child mental health services (see chapter 24). Genetic counseling in complex disorders raises a number of issues that usually do not apply in these other contexts. The first is that of deciding whether or not the disorder is present. A hallmark of many common complex disorders is the absence of a clear threshold between normality and disorder, whether this distinction is made by number or type of symptoms, degree of impairment, response to treatment or any of the other methods used in diagnostic classification systems. Most studies of recurrence risk of disorder start with probands who unambiguously meet full diagnostic criteria. Where the affected family member demonstrates milder symptoms or an atypical presentation, the genetic counselor must decide whether this person is "affected" with the full condition. For many psychiatric disorders, genetic liability confers a spectrum of abnormalities. For example, in autism, co-twins of individuals with autism may have autistic-like social and cognitive impairments that do not reach the diagnostic threshold for childhood autism (Bailey, Le Couteur, Gottesman *et al.*, 1995). However, it does not follow that all individuals showing the broader autistic phenotype have the full genetic liability for autism. Thus, it is not currently known how to estimate the risk of autism in family members of more mildly affected individuals.

Disorder boundaries are also unclear in relation to psychiatric comorbidity. The available evidence suggests that this may often be because of genetic influences that increase liability non-specifically for several disorders (i.e., that are risk factors for both disorders; Kendler, Heath, Martin, & Eaves, 1987; Silberg, Rutter, Meyer *et al.*, 1996). Such findings raise more questions than they answer for genetic counseling. For example, the finding of shared genetic risk factors between symptoms of attention deficit/hyperactivity disorder (ADHD) and conduct disorder highlights that some families with children with ADHD are also at risk of having children with conduct disorder, but at present there are no methods for identifying the different risks.

In some cases, such as ADHD, some of the susceptibility genes appear to have been identified, while in others, such as autism, none are yet confirmed. However, even where one or more susceptibility genes are identified, it is not currently possible to predict with any degree of certainty who will develop the disorder. To date, most genetic testing has occurred where the presence of a risk genotype is strongly associated with development of the disorder. The costs and benefits of testing for susceptibility genes that lead to relatively small alterations in risk have not yet been fully explored but it is almost certain that the negative effects will have a greater influence than is the case when testing for Mendelian disorders.

A further challenge with respect to complex disorders is how to incorporate environmental risk factors into counseling. The extent to which environmental risk is important will vary across disorders and may be underestimated in classic behavioral genetic studies, which assume that genetic and environmental factors act independently rather than in concert. Empirical recurrence rates are agnostic to the origin of familiality and are also helpful because they are easily understood concepts. However, empirical recurrence risks in psychiatry are disorderbased and do not take account of etiological and clinical heterogeneity and comorbidity so that they may

Rutter's Child and Adolescent Psychiatry, 5th edition. Edited by M. Rutter, D. Bishop, D. Pine, S. Scott, J. Stevenson, E. Taylor and A. Thapar. © 2008 Blackwell Publishing, ISBN: 978-1-4051-4549-7.

be imprecise for any individual. Even where environmental risk factors have been identified, it is not always clear how to use them within genetic counseling, either because the risk factor is inherently undesirable (e.g., child maltreatment) or difficult to avoid (e.g., life events). In other cases, knowledge of specific risk may be helpful, as in the interplay between catechol-O-methyltransferase (COMT) genotype and cannabis use (Caspi, Moffitt, Cannon *et al.*, 2005).

With the exception of disorders caused by single gene and chromosomal anomalies, the nature of genetic counseling for psychiatric disorders is probabilistic rather than based on predicting binary outcomes (affected or disorder-free). Whereas genetic counseling has always included situations in which there is uncertainty about affected status, these are decreasing for Mendelian disorders and chromosomal anomalies but not for complex disorders. Genetic counseling for complex disorders is likely to remain probabilistic even as susceptibility genes and environmental risk factors are identified. An ongoing challenge will be to communicate probabilistic risk and uncertainties in accurate and helpful ways.

Social Aspects of Genetic Counseling

The explosion in requests for genetic counseling has fuelled interest in alternative modes of delivery. Controlled trials comparing the outcomes of different methods of delivering genetic counseling are just beginning and include group-based counseling prior to prenatal diagnostic screening (Hunter, Cappelli, Humphreys *et al.*, 2005), the use of structured presentations (Baker, Uus, Bamford, & Marteau, 2004), interactive computer-based systems and CD-ROMs to deliver basic information (Green, Peterson, Baker *et al.*, 2005) and telemedicine (Coelho, Arnold, Nayler, Tischkowitz, & MacKay, 2005). Early results suggest these strategies are largely equally effective. These evaluations highlight the diversity of outcome measures employed, and uncertainty about what outcome measures are most appropriate. Outcome measures have included client satisfaction, enhanced knowledge of genetics and individual risk, anxiety reduction, help with decision-making and, where applicable, undergoing medical investigations and interventions. Perhaps the most important outcome to measure is whether clients can make informed choices, "based upon relevant knowledge, consistent with the decision-maker's values and behaviorally implemented" (Broadstock, Michie, & Marteau, 2000). In some situations, the results of genetic testing may appropriately increase anxiety, such as where it has led to identification of the cardiac disorder of long QT syndrome, with its increased risk of sudden death (van Langen, Hofman, Tan, & Wilde, 2004); here the outcome of choice may be compliance with recommended treatment.

Because genetic counseling has been considered optional, the health inequalities related to differential uptake have not previously been considered. However, racial, ethnic and cultural diversity in genetic counseling affects uptake and use of genetic counseling. There are also racial, ethnic and sociodemographic differences in personal knowledge about genetic risk, perceived genetic risk and knowledge about family history more generally (Dormandy, Michie, Hooper, & Marteau, 2005; Hall & Olopade, 2005), with women from ethnic minority and sociodemographically disadvantaged backgrounds being less likely to take up prenatal screening for Down syndrome or counseling for themselves in relation to breast cancer (Armstrong, Micco, Carney, Stopfer, & Putt, 2005). This difference is similar to that in the uptake of preventive health care more generally.

The results of genetic counseling can produce a conflict between the individual patient wishing to maintain confidentiality about results and the potential harm caused by not alerting other family members to their risk. While guidelines vary in the emphasis given to maintaining patient confidentiality versus informing relatives, all emphasize the importance of exploring such issues prior to genetic testing and of working with patients to help them communicate with family members (American Society of Human Genetics, 1998; Council on Ethical and Judicial Affairs of the American Medical Association, 2004; Taub, Morin, Spillman *et al.*, 2004). There is ongoing concern about the use that health insurance may make of the results of genetic testing.

Tasks of the Genetic Counselor

Professionals from different backgrounds are involved in genetic counseling: clinical geneticists (medical doctors with specialist training), non-medical geneticists, genetic counselors (who come from a range of backgrounds but undertake postgraduate training in genetic counseling) and medical and other health professionals with an interest in particular genetically influenced disorders. With respect to child psychiatric disorders, counseling may be undertaken in the mental health setting or by referral to clinical genetics with the option of holding joint clinics. Genetic counselors vary widely in their experience of counseling for genetically complex conditions and psychiatric disorders in particular. Professionals giving genetic counseling must have adequate knowledge and skills and this should dictate the choice of setting. Because genetic counseling deals with a wide range of situations, the tasks for the counselor vary.

Diagnosis of Genetic Disorders

Geneticists are called upon to help make a diagnosis of a genetic disorder, either prenatally or later. Within child psychiatry, this most often occurs in the context of intellectual disability or developmental delay where investigation for genetic causes forms part of an overall investigation for etiological causes, in which general population studies suggest approximately 40–50% will have an identifiable cause (Srour, Mazer, & Shevell, 2006). The extent to which genetic investigation should be undertaken depends in part on severity of intellectual disability, family history, physical examination and the pattern of symptoms. A history of multiple affected family members or consanguinity always warrants further investigation, as do findings on physical examination suggestive of a specific disorder or multiple dysmorphic features. Severe intellectual disability (IQ < 50) is more likely to be associated with identifiable medical causes. There is no firm consensus on when and how to investigate genetic causes of intellectual disability but routine chromosomal analysis is generally supported with either structural abnormalities or aneuploidy occurring in approximately 13% with moderate to severe intellectual disability and approximately 4% with mild to moderate intellectual disability (van Karnebeek, Scheper, Abeling *et al.*, 2005).

There is much interest in investigations to detect microscopic deletions or duplications, using either fluorescence *in situ* hybridization (FISH) for telomeric rearrangements or comparative genomic hybridization (CGH) array, which may be abnormal in 5–10% of individuals with intellectual disability (Sharkey, Maher, & FitzPatrick, 2005). Clinicians should remain cautious about their use and interpretation because of inadequate population-based studies to determine the base rate for such findings and uncertainties about the distinction between normal variation and abnormality. Factors supporting an etiological role for cytogenetic and submicroscopic genetic variations include previous reports of a similar clinical picture associated with the abnormality and either a failure to find the abnormality in the parents (*de novo* mutation) or the abnormality segregating with the clinical characteristics within the family. Clinical characteristics associated with submicroscopic abnormalities include: positive family history of intellectual disability, prenatal growth retardation, postnatal growth abnormalities (including tall and short stature and micro- and macrocephaly) and dysmorphic features (de Vries, White, Knight *et al.*, 2001).

Other investigations of intellectual disability are more focused and usually taken on by clinical geneticists or pediatricians (Cleary & Green, 2005; McDonald, Rennie, Tolmie, Galloway, & McWilliam, 2006; Sharkey, Maher, & FitzPatrick, 2005). Many of the investigations that may be undertaken do not involve a genetic test *per se* but, if positive, will diagnose a genetic disorder. Many genetic laboratories require evidence that the nature and possible implications of genetic tests have been discussed with patients or parents, but such a requirement is unusual for non-genetic investigations and clinicians must decide whether the genetic implications should be discussed prior to testing.

With respect to other child psychiatric disorders, clinicians must be alert to the rare but important instances in which genetic disorders may have a role in exactly the same way that other rare medical causes of psychiatric disorders need to be evaluated. Velocardiofacial syndrome (VCFS) should be considered in early-onset psychosis and Williams syndrome in ADHD and subaverage intelligence (see chapter 24). In general, protocols for investigating genetic causes of child psychiatric disorders do not exist at present and clinicians need to make individual decisions based on the clinical picture, including the presence of other features associated with the genetic disorder. Clinicians should also balance the possible benefits of an etiological diagnosis that may affect reproductive decisions for other family members against the cost of routine testing and the possible anxiety engendered while test results are awaited. An etiological diagnosis may have specific treatment implications and more commonly is helpful in highlighting other features of the genetic disorder, as well as giving patients and families a causal explanation.

Pre-conception Counseling for Couples At Risk

Couples present for genetic counseling because they believe themselves to be at risk of having a child affected with an intellectual disability or psychiatric disorder. This common genetic counseling situation is covered on p. 1185). Ensuring correct diagnosis in the affected family member is essential and may be difficult if direct examination and availability of contemporaneous records are not possible. It is important to obtain a full family history for both members of the couple, even when the affected person is related only on one side. Genetic testing of the unaffected couple should be considered but undertaken only where there is a specific question.

Prenatal Diagnosis

The aim of prenatal diagnosis is to detect abnormalities (both genetic and otherwise) at an early stage of fetal development, usually to allow parental choice whether to continue with the pregnancy or, rarely, to allow prenatal intervention. Prenatal diagnosis is considered in disorders resulting in severe disability not open to other treatment options, where there is an accurate diagnostic test and in instances where there is a reasonable chance the pregnancy will be affected (Harper, 1998). The boundaries in relation to what is considered a severe disability are not clear-cut and there is diversity across individuals, cultures and societies. Divergence in opinion is exemplified by the sex chromosome anomalies in which affected individuals frequently have subaverage intelligence and varying degrees of behavioral disturbance (Abramsky, Hall, Levitan, & Marteau, 2001; Ratcliffe, 1999). There has been debate about whether prenatal diagnosis should only be undertaken if couples wish to terminate an affected pregnancy. In population prenatal screening for common genetic disorders, such as the triple test for Down syndrome, it is common for the testing to be undertaken without ascertaining the couple's view about continuing an affected pregnancy. Prenatal diagnosis for severe late-onset disorders such as Huntington disease evokes controversy as many clinicians believe parents have the right to terminate an affected pregnancy but highlight that otherwise current guidance discourages testing of children for late-onset disorders until they are able to give consent (Duncan, Foddy, & Delatycki, 2006). Prenatal diagnosis is possible for chromosomal abnormalities, many Mendelian disorders and for those caused by identified microscopic deletions and/or duplications, but these are relevant only rarely in child psychiatric disorders. In child psychiatric disorders in which there is an excess of affected males but no specific prenatal diagnostic tests, the question of female sex selection arises. This is an imprecise method of altering the risk of an affected child as the majority of male offspring will be unaffected and female offspring may develop the disorder.

Pre-implantation Genetic Diagnosis

Pre-implantation genetic diagnosis (PGD) involves genetic analysis of the embryo *in vitro* and selection for implantation only of those appearing disease-free. PGD has been used to detect mutations responsible for Mendelian disorders in the embryos of at-risk couples (Sermon, Van Steirteghem, & Liebaers, 2004), and to screen for chromosomal abnormalities in the embryos of couples at greater risk or with a history of multiple miscarriages, infertility for unknown reason or male factor infertility, or *in vitro* fertilization (IVF) failures. In non-disclosure PGD, couples at risk themselves for a late-onset disorder, such as Huntington disease, can opt for the selection of disease-free embryos without knowing themselves whether they carry the mutation. Parents have also selected embryos on the basis of their HLA type, to provide stem-cell donation for a sick sibling (Devolder, 2005). In the latter instances, there has been considerable ethical debate about the circumstances in which such methods should be applied and the practice is determined in some but not all countries by regulatory authorities (Takeshita & Kubo, 2004). Because embryo selection is perceived as less drastic than termination of pregnancy, it may be used in the future to select in relation to susceptibility genes, which increase the risk of, but do not determine the presence of, complex disorders.

Presymptomatic Testing

Molecular genetic tests allow detection of mutations that will lead to a disorder in currently healthy persons. Such presymptomatic testing should be differentiated according to whether there are therapeutic implications of a positive test result. In some conditions, including the hereditary cancers, a positive presymptomatic result has direct implications for screening and surveillance while a negative test result obviates this need. For other conditions, such as Huntington disease, there are at present no treatment consequences of a positive result and the reasons for requesting testing are more complex. The uptake of presymptomatic testing has, not surprisingly, varied according to treatment implications of a positive result. Uptake for Huntington disease testing has been approximately 10–20% (Crauford, Dodge, Kerzin-Storrar, & Harris, 1989; Quaid & Morris, 1993), compared with approximately 50% for hereditary breast cancer, where the role of early treatment is uncertain, and 80% for familial adenomatous polyposis, for which early surgical intervention has a significant health impact (Harper, 1998).

With regard to presymptomatic testing of children, current guidance indicates that children should not be tested for disorders for which there are no therapeutic consequences, until they are of an age to give consent themselves, unless there is demonstrable medical or psychosocial benefit (Clarke *et al.*, 1994). Non-geneticists are more likely to offer presymptomatic and carrier testing of children at parental request; one commonly stated reason for testing was to reduce parental anxiety (Clarke, 1994). Although the impact has not been examined in children, studies of adults tested for late-onset disorders failed to find long-term anxiety reduction (Braidstock *et al.*, 2000). In relation to diseases such as cancers in which a positive test result may alter the screening practice, current guidelines propose that testing should be permitted at the earliest age of onset (Kodish, 1999). In some cases, this delays testing until an age at which children can participate in the consent process. This position stems from the bioethics paradigm adopted by most genetic counselors which places pre-eminence on the autonomy of the individual (child) over that of the wider social network (family), but such a view ignores the broader psychological and cultural diversity in which family needs could take precedence over individual autonomy (McConkie-Rosell & Spiridigliozzi, 2004).

Child psychiatrists and their colleagues may be called upon to advise on the child's ability to give informed consent to genetic testing or upon family issues thrown up by the genetic disorder and testing. Evaluating the child's ability to consent follows the same principles as those for any medical treatment but account should be taken of longer-term consequences of genetic testing such as discrimination, the impact on wider family relationships and that, unlike some treatments, once testing has been undertaken, the information cannot be withdrawn.

Presymptomatic assessment is beginning to include testing of susceptibility genes for complex disorders. The preliminary results suggest that inclusion of genetic data in risk results, in comparison to similar risks based only on empirical recurrence, reduces anxiety and risk perception in those receiving a low-risk result (LaRusse, Roberts, Marteau *et al.*, 2005) and does not alter risk perception in those receiving a high-risk genotypic result (Marteau, Roberts, LaRusse, & Green, 2005). Such presymptomatic testing is theoretically feasible for susceptibility genes in some child psychiatric disorders but is not routinely offered at present.

Carrier Detection

A carrier is someone who carries a single copy of a genetic mutation and is healthy at the time of study. With the exception of carriers of late-onset dominant disorders, carrier status is therefore of importance primarily for reproductive planning. Carrier status is a concern for families with affected members where healthy individuals are uncertain whether they may pass on the disorder to their offspring. The issues in relation to testing of minors overlap with those raised by presymptomatic testing (McConkie-Rosell, Spiridigliozzi, Rounds *et al.*, 1999). The benefits could include a reduction in parental concerns regarding the child's status, a longer time for the child and family to accommodate to the knowledge, an understanding of the genetic risks prior to any unplanned pregnancy and to consider alternatives regarding reproductive planning (McConkie-Rosell, Finucane, Cronister *et al.*, 2005). However, the drawbacks include the loss of the child's autonomy, possible labeling and differential (real or perceived) treatment of siblings according to genetic status, potential effects on the child's self-concept and adverse effects on their ability to form future relationships, and possible discrimination (e.g., from insurance companies). The extent to which self-concept and future relationships are adversely affected by genetic testing of minors is largely unknown. Although parents with one affected child may press to have other children tested for carrier status, current recommendations state this should be resisted until the children are of an age to give informed consent themselves (Clarke, Fielding, Kerzin-Storrer *et al.*, 1994). An effect of waiting until children are able to give informed consent is that uptake of testing may be lower. In cystic fibrosis, where genetic carrier testing has been available for some years, uptake amongst siblings of affected people has been poor. Several reasons have been cited, including poor communication with parents regarding genetic issues and feeling that affected siblings would have difficulty accepting their decision to be tested (Fanos & Johnson, 1995a). The finding that beliefs about carrier status were not influenced by educational or income level suggests that emotional factors may play an important part in attitudes about screening (Fanos & Johnson, 1995b).

Population Screening

Population screening involves identifying those with or at risk of having offspring with genetic disorders amongst the general population. Population screening aims to detect diseases for which early treatment improves prognosis and to identify untreatable severe disorders in fetuses to allow couples to make informed reproductive decisions. Population screening may occur at any stage from the prenatal period to later life and now includes testing for common genetic variants that may influence disease, both in a Mendelian pattern, such as hypercholesterolemia associated with low-density lipoprotein receptor abnormalities and as a susceptibility allele for a complex disorder, such as apolipoprotein E4 in late-onset Alzheimer's disease. Cascade screening is an intermediate strategy involving systematic contact of more distant at-risk family members with the offer of testing.

Genetic population screening differs from other forms of population screening because it detects disease of genetic origin, for which there may be implications for other family members. Unlike individual genetic testing, in population screening clients may have little knowledge of the disorder, raising uncertainty about the degree of informed consent. At present, population screening with respect to child psychiatric disorders is limited to conditions causing significant intellectual disability such as phenylketonuria and Down syndrome. There is debate over the merits of population screening for fragile X syndrome. As one of the most commonly inherited forms of intellectual disability, detection of the carrier state in mothers has the potential to promote greater reproductive choice. Current recommendations are that prenatal carrier screening for fragile X should be undertaken only in those at known risk (Sherman, Pletcher, & Driscoll, 2005). However, popular opinion does not fully support this strategy; women attending a prenatal diagnostic clinic for other purposes were strongly in favor of global screening (Fanos, Spangner, & Musci, 2006) as were parents of children affected with the disorder (Skinner, Sparkman, & Bailey, 2003), raising the question of who should decide which tests are available.

Multiplex genetic tests assess a person's genotype for a range of different genes, much in the way current laboratory tests examine a range of blood chemistries. Such tests may provide the simplest and least expensive way to assess risk for one condition, but they may also detect variations in other genes for which testing was not intended and no consent was obtained.

Pharmacogenomics

Pharmacogenomics is the study of the variability in genes relevant to disease susceptibility and drug response (see chapters 16 and 23). Genetic variations influence drug response in three ways:

1 Affecting the processing of drugs by the body (pharmacokinetics);

2 Modifying the proteins that are targeted by drugs (pharmacodynamics); and

3 Altering the risk of acquiring certain diseases.

In psychiatry, pharmacogenomics holds promises especially for more effective, individually tailored treatments with reduced adverse effects. However, a range of ethical concerns are raised, amongst them the concern that more personalized treatments may also increase health inequalities and jeopardize patient confidentiality and informed consent (Breckenridge, Lindpaintner, Lipton *et al.*, 2004; Nuffield Council on Bioethics, 2003; van Delden, Bolt, Kalis, Derijks, & Leufkens, 2004).

Counseling Prior to Adoption

Requests for pre-adoption genetic counseling occur when the biological parents are believed to have a genetically influenced disorder, especially as mental illness in parents is a common reason for childhood adoption. In considering such requests, one needs first to determine whether the individual requesting the information has the legal status to do so. In considering the child's rights, one needs to balance the abrogation of his or her right to decide whether or not to be the subject of genetic counseling against the possibility that, without genetic information, prospective parents may decline the adoption, which may not be in the child's interests. Alternatively, the results of genetic information may reverse a positive decision from prospective parents. In addition, one needs to consider the rights of adoptive parents to accurate information about the child's background and what problems they are likely to encounter in rearing the child. Although genetic counseling for potential adoptees is currently mainly requested in relation to severe mental illness in parents, the considerations in relation to which disorders should be the focus of genetic counseling (see p. 1185) apply here as they do to couples making enquiries on their own behalf. Genetic counseling may be hampered by vague information regarding biological parents, as giving accurate advice requires specific information about both parents. Where parental medical records are available, it is essential to ensure that these have been obtained through legal and ethical channels. When it is impossible to obtain adequate background history, the information imparted needs to reflect this uncertainty and should include the range of plausible levels of risk. Should genetic testing of a child be considered, an independent advocate for the child should be involved in the decision-making. It has been suggested that adopted children might be informed about known genetic risks from their birth parents at age 18, when they are able to request knowledge of the identity of their birth parents; otherwise, adopted children are at a disadvantage with respect to knowledge of their potential genetic risks (Nuffield Council on Bioethics, 1998).

Role of the Child Mental Health Specialist in Genetic Counseling

The considerable variation in uptake of genetic screening and counseling according to racial/ethnic and sociodemographic groups (Hall & Olopade, 2005) suggests it may constitute an area of a health inequality. The diagnosis of a disorder associated with a strong genetic risk places a responsibility on the professional to apprise family members of this risk and to assist with the provision of appropriate genetic counseling and investigation if desired. This requires the professional to have a good general understanding of the nature and importance of genetic risk factors. Only those able to interpret the results of a genetic test should order the investigation (Taub, Morin, Spillman *et al.*, 2004), so that referral to a geneticist or a joint consultation may be most appropriate.

Practical Aspects of Genetic Counseling

Referral for Genetic Counseling

Almost all child psychiatric disorders show some degree of genetic risk (Rutter, Silberg, O'Connor, & Simonoff, 1999), but this does not mean genetic counseling is necessarily appropriate. First, the quality and precision of the evidence in relation to genetic factors require consideration. The heritability of the disorder, the proportion of individual variation that is accounted for by genetic factors and the recurrence risk in relatives of those affected should be considered. Although the latter is the figure most directly relevant to families, it fails to distinguish genetic and environmental causes of familial aggregation. For many child psychiatric disorders, the current literature contains widely varying findings that make it impossible to give precise information to families. Another practical problem is that the empirical recurrence risk may be known for offspring and siblings, but not for other relationships.

A second consideration is the extent of impairment or disability caused by the problem. Traits such as emotionality and sociability are strongly genetic but infrequently impairing in their own right. Whereas professionals should not impose their view as to which traits or disorders warrant genetic counseling, issues of severity, impairment and treatability should be considered by families and professionals alike (Nuffield Council on Bioethics, 2002).

Autism is the child psychiatric disorder (other than intellectual disability) for which there is the strongest case for formal genetic counseling and it is therefore the template for what follows. Although formal genetic counseling may not be appropriate for all other child psychiatric disorders, it may be helpful for parents to know when genetic influences have a role in their child's difficulties, particularly if they have inappropriately blamed themselves or other causes for the problem.

Twin studies of autism show a high heritability of the disorder (Bailey, Le Couteur, Gottesman *et al.*, 1995) and family studies concur that the sibling recurrence risk is 5–6% for autism and pervasive developmental disorder (Rutter, Bailey, Simonoff, & Pickles, 1997). Although population rates of autism have increased (Baird, Simonoff, Pickles *et al.*, 2006), there is at present no evidence to suggest a similar change in the sibling recurrence risk. Autism is life-long, essentially incurable, severely impairing and creates a heavy burden on families. In the majority of cases, inheritance will be complex and is likely to involve a number of susceptibility genes and as yet unspecified environmental or random factors (see chapter 46). Although families may need some time to adjust to the diagnosis, it is important that they have access to genetic counseling before planning further children. If genetic counseling is to be offered by the clinician looking after affected family members, such counseling is best undertaken in an appointment specifically designated for this purpose.

Assessment

Genetic counseling should commence by confirming the diagnosis in the proband. The challenge of this task varies enormously depending on the information available, but is a necessary first step to ensure that genetic counseling is given for the correct disorder. This may raise at an early stage family issues of communication regarding illness and may delay the more formal aspects of genetic counseling until the necessary information has been obtained. In rare cases it is impossible to obtain adequate diagnostic information. Approaches vary but the clinician should usually go ahead with genetic counseling having apprised the clients of the uncertainty regarding diagnosis.

Consideration is given to etiological factors that may alter recurrence risk. In autism, 5–10% of cases are caused by a recognized medical disorder and these should ideally be excluded in the proband as they will alter the recurrence risk. The most common medical disorders causing autism are tuberous sclerosis and fragile X (Rutter, Bailey, Simonoff *et al.*, 1997) and, in such instances, the relevant disorder for genetic counseling is the underlying medical condition. Where cytogenetic or microscopic chromosomal abnormalities are present, there may be less certainty regarding their etiological role and a clinical genetics opinion should be sought, as well as testing other family members.

Rare environmental causes in the proband should also be excluded. Congenital rubella is the most common infectious cause of autism. There has been much debate as to whether association of obstetric complications with autism (usually with milder levels of adversity) indicates a causative role (Goodman, 1990); the further association of obstetric complications with congenital anomalies suggests that abnormal development in the fetus may be responsible for the obstetric complications (Bailey, Le Couteur, Gottesman *et al.*, 1995; Bolton, Murphy,

Macdonald *et al.*, 1997). However, it is likely that severe perinatal adversity, as well as other causes of brain injury, can cause autism. Where an "environmental" cause of brain injury is the likely cause of autism, the recurrence risk may be much lower and possibly the same as for the general population.

In gathering information, a systematic family history is essential. Multiple miscarriages and consanguinity should be excluded. In determining whether there are other family members affected, enquiry should include a broad range of psychiatric and neurological disorders. If a pattern suggestive of Mendelian inheritance emerges, it may be appropriate to review the original diagnosis and consider whether further investigation is required. In multifactorial disorders where heavier family loading is thought to indicate greater disease liability within the family and therefore predict a higher recurrence risk (Carter, 1976; Falconer, 1981), such information can be used to alter the recurrence risk information given to families. In practice, there are few empirical data from which to vary recurrence risk for any of the child psychiatric disorders.

It is important to enquire about both sides of the family even when the proband is related to only one member of the couple. In genetically complex disorders, individual susceptibility genes are likely to be common and the risk for a couple seeking counseling depends upon the genetic contribution of each side. Family history should also take account of maternal and paternal age, as there may be a risk of chromosomal disorders that have not been considered and should note other disorders that may place the couple at increased risk of having a child with a genetic disorder.

Communication

When families attend for genetic counseling, it is essential to clarify at the outset the questions they wish to address. It is helpful to find out who has sought the referral and, if not the family, how they view it. A small minority of families do not agree with the diagnosis; without addressing this first, genetic counseling is unlikely to be helpful. Clients may have additional questions about the risk for other family members; the usual policy is to give specific counseling only to the couple attending the clinic. A further question for families may be whether there was a causal role of environmental factors. Families may wish to know whether there are any measures they can take to reduce the chances of having an affected child.

In discussing risk, it is important to clarify the clinical spectrum of the disorder. With autism, this includes the broader phenotype of speech and language delay, literacy problems and social eccentricities. Although these are substantially more common, they are also much less impairing and this is important to emphasize to families (Rutter, Bailey, Simonoff *et al.*, 1997). Couples may be preoccupied with the risk of the disorder for which they have sought counseling and it can be helpful to remind them of the general population risk of 1 in 50 infants having a significant mental or physical handicap (Harper, 1998). Couples also find it helpful to compare their personal risk with that of the general population. It is important to ascertain that clients understand the risk information given to them; observational studies have suggested genetic counselors frequently fail to confirm this (Michie, Lester, Pinto, & Marteau, 2005).

There is a general view that genetic counseling should be non-directive, making information available to families but not advising them on how to proceed. In actual fact, this may be difficult to achieve. Michie, Bron, Bobrow, and Marteau (1997) found that counselors made an average of 5.8 pieces of "advice" and the same number of "evaluative" comments per counseling session, throwing into question the perception of the counseling process as non-directive. This may not be undesirable; in another study, 80% of clients at risk for having an offspring with a severe disorder reported that they wished to receive an opinion from their genetic counselor on what course of action to take (Furu, Kääriäinen, Sankila, & Norio, 1993). In another study, patients receiving non-directive counseling perceived their risk to be higher than those obtaining more directive counseling, possibly feeling in the former case that the neutral counselor was withholding information (Shiloh & Saxe, 1989). Families receiving the same recurrence risk for a child psychiatric disorder have widely varying opinions of whether the risk is high and may make different reproductive decisions.

A great deal of information is exchanged during genetic counseling and it is good practice to write directly to clients following the consultation to summarize the information they have been given. It may be appropriate to offer follow-up sessions to the clients, particularly if there is a large difference in how each member of the couple views the information they have been given.

Problems and Limitations in Counseling for Child Psychiatric Disorders

With increasing awareness of the role of genetic factors in common disorders, clients make more sophisticated requests of genetic counseling, many of which extend beyond present knowledge. A common difficulty arises when the proband does not fulfill the full diagnostic criteria upon which the relevant genetic studies were based. It is often unclear whether the findings can be generalized to diagnostic variant, subthreshold cases or individuals with other comorbidities. When there are no empirical recurrence risk data for the client's relationship to the proband, it is necessary to rely on genetic principles showing that for multifactorial disorders, there is a rapid fall-off in recurrence as the genetic relationship becomes more distant, to estimate risk. Whereas it is recognized that genetic heterogeneity will occur even within a homogeneous clinical picture and that the same genetic susceptibility can lead to marked clinical variation (Le Couteur, Bailey, Goode *et al.*, 1996), it is unlikely that this knowledge can be used to modify risk until the molecular genetic basis is better understood. This means the genetic information for individual families is likely to be very imprecise. Families seeking genetic counseling often want a way of knowing in advance whether a child will be affected. In multifactorial disorders, it remains to be seen how precise risk information will become.

Genetic Testing in Research Contexts

In the last two decades, genetic research has increased exponentially and many non-genetic studies have chosen to include a genetic component. The research may be exploratory and without clear implications for participants. Consent is therefore often non-specific, open-ended and not discussed in detail with participants. Frequently, researchers do not expect to obtain findings with clinical implications for the research participant. Research samples are frequently anonymized to ensure confidentiality but there is little information on whether participants fully understand the implications of this. As genetic research becomes increasingly relevant to clinical concerns, it is essential that the framework for consent and conduct is regularly reviewed.

Conclusions

The rapid pace of advances in psychiatric genetics requires genetic counseling to be flexible in relation to its scope, approach to investigation and conceptualization of disorders. Those delivering genetic counseling will need to communicate effectively with mental health professionals diagnosing and treating disorders to ensure that patients and their families have access to genetic investigation and counseling when it is appropriate. Research on genetic causes of psychiatric disorder must be matched by research on the ethical and social consequences of providing the different aspects of genetic testing and counseling with respect to disorders that show a complex pattern of inheritance.

References

Abramsky, L., Hall, S., Levitan, J., & Marteau, T. M. (2001). What parents are told after prenatal diagnosis of a sex chromosome abnormality: Interview and questionnaire study. *British Medical Journal*, *322*, 463–466.

American Society of Human Genetics. (1998). Professional disclosure of familial genetic information. *American Journal of Human Genetics*, *62*, 474–483.

Armstrong, K., Micco, E., Carney, A., Stopfer, J., & Putt, M. (2005). Racial differences in the use of BRCA1/2 testing among women with a family history of breast or ovarian cancer. *Journal of the American Medical Association*, *293*, 1729–1736.

Bailey, A. J., Le Couteur, A., Gottesman, I., Bolton, P., Simonoff, E., Yazda, E., *et al.* (1995). Autism as a strongly genetic disorder: Evidence from a British twin study. *Psychological Medicine*, *25*, 63–78.

Baird, G., Simonoff, E., Pickles, A., Chandler, S., Loucas, T., Meldrum, D., *et al.* (2006). Prevalence of disorders of the autism spectrum in a population cohort of children in South Thames: The Special Needs and Autism Project (SNAP). *Lancet*, *368*, 210–215.

Baker, H., Uus, K., Bamford, J., & Marteau, T. M. (2004). Increasing knowledge about a screening test: Preliminary evaluation of a structured, chart-based, screener presentation. *Patient Education and Counseling*, *52*, 55–59.

Bolton, P. F., Murphy, M., Macdonald, H., Whitlock, B., Pickles, A., & Rutter, M. (1997). Obstetric complications in autism: Consequences or causes of the condition? *Journal of the American Academy of Child and Adolescent Psychiatry*, *36*, 272–281.

Breckenridge, A., Lindpaintner, K., Lipton, P., McLeod, H., Rothstein, M., & Wallace, H. (2004). Pharmacogenetics: Ethical problems and solutions. *Nature Reviews Genetics*, *5*, 676–680.

Broadstock, M., Michie, S., & Marteau, T. (2000). The psychological consequences of predictive genetic testing: A systematic review. *European Journal of Human Genetics*, *8*, 731–738.

Carter, C. O. (1976). Genetics of common single malformations. *British Medical Bulletin*, *32*, 21–26.

Caspi, A., Moffitt, T. E., Cannon, M., McClay, J., Murray, R., Harrington, H., *et al.* (2005). Moderation of the effect of adolescent-onset cannabis use on adult psychosis by a functional polymorphism in the catechol-O-methyltransferase gene: Longitudinal evidence of a gene X environment interaction. *Biological Psychiatry*, *57*, 1117–1127.

Clarke, A. (1994). *Results of survey for report: The genetic testing of children*. Report of a Working Party of the Clinical Genetics Society.

Clarke, A., Fleming, D., Kerzin-Storrar, L., Middleton-Price, H., Montgomery, J., Payne, H., *et al.* (1994). The genetic testing of children. Report of a Working Party of the Clinical Genetics Society. *Journal of Medical Genetics*, *31*, 785–797.

Cleary, M. A., & Green, A. (2005). Developmental delay: When to suspect and how to investigate for an inborn error of metabolism. *Archives of Disease in Childhood*, *90*, 1128–1132.

Coelho, J. J., Arnold, A., Nayler, J., Tischkowitz, M., & MacKay, J. (2005). An assessment of the efficacy of cancer genetic counselling using real-time videoconferencing technology (telemedicine) compared to face-to-face consultations. *European Journal of Cancer*, *41*, 2257–2261.

Council on Ethical and Judicial Affairs of the American Medical Association. (2004). *Opinion 5.05:Confidentiality*. Chicago.

Crauford, D., Dodge, A., Kerzin-Storrar, L., & Harris, R. (1989). Uptake of presymptomatic predictive testing for Huntington disease. *Lancet*, *334*, 603–605.

de Vries, B. B. A., White, S. M., Knight, S. J. L., Regan, R., Homfray, T., Young, I. D., *et al.* (2001). Clinical studies on submicroscopic subtelomeric rearrangements: A checklist. *Journal of Medical Genetics*, *38*, 145–150.

Devolder, K. (2005). Preimplantation HLA typing: Having children to save our loved ones. *Journal of Medical Ethics*, *31*, 582–586.

Dormandy, E., Michie, S., Hooper, R., & Marteau, T. M. (2005). Low uptake of prenatal screening for Down syndrome in minority ethnic groups and socially deprived groups: A reflection of women's attitudes or a failure to facilitate informed choices? *International Journal of Epidemiology*, *34*, 346–352.

Duncan, R. E., Foddy, B., & Delatycki, M. B. (2006). Refusing to provide a prenatal test: Can it ever be ethical? [see comment]. *British Medical Journal*, *333*, 1066–1068.

Falconer, D. S. (1981). *Introduction to quantitative genetics*. London: Longman.

Fanos, J. H., & Johnson, J. P. (1995a). Barriers to carrier testing for adult cystic fibrosis sibs: The importance of not knowing. *American Journal of Medical Genetics*, *59*, 85–91.

Fanos, J. H., & Johnson, J. P. (1995b). Perception of carrier status by cystic fibrosis siblings. *American Journal of Human Genetics*, *57*, 431–438.

Fanos, J. H., Spangner, K. A., & Musci, T. J. (2006). Attitudes toward prenatal screening and testing for fragile X. *Genetics in Medicine*, *8*, 129–133.

Furu, T., Kääriäinen, H., Sankila, E. M., & Norio, R. (1993). Attitudes towards prenatal diagnosis and selective abortion among patients with retinitis pigmentosa or choroideremia as well as among their relatives. *Clinical Genetics*, *43*, 160–165.

Goodman, R. (1990). Technical note: Are perinatal complications causes or consequences of autism? *Journal of Child Psychology and Psychiatry*, *31*, 809–812.

Green, M. J., Peterson, S. K., Baker, M. W., Friedman, L. C., Harper, G. R., Rubinstein, W. S., *et al.* (2005). Use of an educational computer program before genetic counseling for breast cancer susceptibility: Effects on duration and content of counseling sessions. *Genetics in Medicine*, *7*, 221–229.

Hall, M., & Olopade, O. I. (2005). Confronting genetic testing disparities: Knowledge is power. *Journal of the American Medical Association*, *293*, 1783–1785.

Harper, P. S. (1998). *Practical genetic counselling*. Oxford: Butterworth-Heinemann.

Hunter, A. G. W., Cappelli, M., Humphreys, L., Allanson, J. E., Chiu, T. T., Peeters, C., *et al.* (2005). A randomized trial comparing alternative approaches to prenatal diagnosis counseling in advanced maternal age patients. *Clinical Genetics*, *67*, 303–313.

Kelly, T. E. (1986). *Clinical genetics and genetic counseling*. Chicago: Year Book.

Kendler, K. S., Heath, A. C., Martin, N. G., & Eaves, L. J. (1987). Symptoms of anxiety and symptoms of depression: Same genes, different environments? *Archives of General Psychiatry*, *44*, 451–457.

Kodish, E. D. (1999). Testing children for cancer genes: The rule of earliest onset. *Journal of Pediatrics*, *135*, 390–395.

LaRusse, S., Roberts, J. S., Marteau, T. M., Katzen, H., Linnenbringer, E. L., Barber, M., *et al.* (2005). Genetic susceptibility testing versus family history-based risk assessment: Impact on perceived risk of Alzheimer disease. *Genetics in Medicine*, *7*, 48–53.

Le Couteur, A., Bailey, A., Goode, S., Pickles, A., Robertson, S., Gottesman, I., *et al.* (1996). A broader phenotype of autism: The clinical spectrum in twins. *Journal of Child Psychology and Psychiatry and Allied Disciplines*, *37*, 785–801.

Marteau, T. M., Roberts, S., LaRusse, S., & Green, R. C. (2005). Predictive genetic testing for Alzheimer's disease: Impact upon risk perception. *Risk Analysis*, *25*, 397–404.

McConkie-Rosell, A., Finucane, B., Cronister, A., Abrams, L., Bennett, R. L., & Pettersen, B. J. (2005). Genetic counseling for fragile X syndrome: Updated recommendations of the national society of genetic counselors. *Journal of Genetic Counseling*, *14*, 249–270.

McConkie-Rosell, A., & Spiridigliozzi, G. A. (2004). "Family matters": A conceptual framework for genetic testing in children. *Journal of Genetic Counseling*, *13*, 9–29.

McConkie-Rosell, A., Spiridigliozzi, G. A., Rounds, K., Dawson, D. V., Sullivan, J. A., Burgess, D., *et al.* (1999). Parental attitudes regarding carrier testing in children at risk for fragile X syndrome. *American Journal of Medical Genetics*, *82*, 206–211.

McDonald, L., Rennie, A., Tolmie, J., Galloway, P., & McWilliam, R. (2006). Investigation of global developmental delay. *Archives of Disease in Childhood*, *91*, 701–705.

Michie, S., Bron, F., Bobrow, M., & Marteau, T. M. (1997). Nondirectiveness in genetic counseling: An empirical study. *American Journal of Human Genetics*, *60*, 40–47.

Michie, S., Lester, K., Pinto, J., & Marteau, T. M. (2005). Communicating risk information in genetic counseling: An observational study. *Health Education and Behavior*, *32*, 589–598.

Nuffield Council on Bioethics. (1998). *Mental disorders and genetics: The ethical context*. Oxford: Nuffield Foundation.

Nuffield Council on Bioethics. (2002). *Genetics and human behaviour: The ethical context*. London: Nuffield Foundation.

Nuffield Council on Bioethics. (2003). *Pharmacogenetics: Ethical issues*. London: Nuffield Foundation.

Quaid, K. A., & Morris, M. (1993). Reluctance to undergo predictive testing: The case of Huntington disease. *American Journal of Medical Genetics*, *43*, 41–45.

Ratcliffe, S. (1999). Long-term outcome in children of sex chromosome abnormalities. *Archives of Disease in Childhood*, *80*, 192–195.

Rutter, M., Bailey, A., Simonoff, E., & Pickles, A. (1997). Genetic influences and autism. In D. J. Cohen, & F. R. Volkmar (Eds.), *Handbook of autism* (2nd edn., pp. 370–387). New York: Wiley.

Rutter, M., Silberg, J., O'Connor, T., & Simonoff, E. (1999). Genetics and child psychiatry. 2. Empirical research findings. *Journal of Child Psychology and Psychiatry*, *40*, 19–55.

Sermon, K., Van Steirteghem, A., & Liebaers, I. (2004). Preimplantation genetic diagnosis. *Lancet*, *363*, 1633–1641.

Sharkey, F. H., Maher, E., & FitzPatrick, D. R. (2005). Chromosome analysis: What and when to request. *Archives of Disease in Childhood*, *90*, 1264–1269.

Sherman, S., Pletcher, B. A., & Driscoll, D. A. (2005). Fragile X syndrome: Diagnostic and carrier testing. *Genetics in Medicine*, *7*, 584–587.

Shiloh, S., & Saxe, L. (1989). Perception of risk in genetic counseling. *Psychology and Health*, *3*, 45–61.

Silberg, J., Rutter, M., Meyer, J., Simonoff, E., Hewitt, J., Loeber, R., *et al.* (1996). Genetic and environmental influences on the covariation between hyperactivity and conduct disturbance in juvenile twins. *Journal of Child Psychology and Psychiatry*, *37*, 803–816.

Skinner, D., Sparkman, K. L., & Bailey, D. B. (2003). Screening for fragile X syndrome: Parent attitudes and perspectives. *Genetics in Medicine*, *5*, 378–384.

Srour, M., Mazer, B., & Shevell, M. I. (2006). Analysis of clinical features predicting etiologic yield in the assessment of global developmental delay. *Pediatrics*, *118*, 139–145.

Takeshita, N., & Kubo, H. (2004). Regulating preimplantation genetic diagnosis: How to control PGD. *Journal of Assisted Reproduction and Genetics*, *21*, 19–25.

Taub, S., Morin, K., Spillman, M. A., Sade, R. M., Riddick, F. A., & Council on Ethical and Judicial Affairs of the American Medical Association. (2004). Managing familial risk in genetic testing. *Genetic Testing*, *8*, 356–359.

van Delden, J., Bolt, I., Kalis, A., Derijks, J., & Leufkens, H. (2004). Tailor-made pharmacotherapy: Future developments and ethical challenges in the field of pharmacogenomics. *Bioethics*, *18*, 303–321.

van Karnebeek, C. D. M., Scheper, F. Y., Abeling, N. G., Alders, M., Barth, P. G., Hoovers, J. M. N., *et al.* (2005). Etiology of mental retardation in children referred to a tertiary care center: A prospective study. *American Journal of Mental Retardation*, *110*, 253–267.

van Langen, I. M., Hofman, N., Tan, H. L., & Wilde, A. A. M. (2004). Family and population strategies for screening and counselling of inherited cardiac arrhythmias. *Annals of Medicine*, *36*, 116–124.

74

Special Education

Patricia Howlin

This chapter examines educational provision for those children who, at some stage in their school lives, experience difficulties that interfere with learning. These are children who, because of developmental delays or behavioral difficulties, lack the cognitive, linguistic, attentional or social skills needed to cope with ordinary schooling and who thus require special help in order to access the wider teaching curriculum. They include children with long-term and pervasive conditions such as intellectual impairments (intellectual disability), developmental language disorders or autism; more specific learning disabilities, such as dyslexia; sensory and physical impairments or chronic illnesses; and children with severe emotional and/or behavioral difficulties.

What are Special Educational Needs?

Many different definitions exist, but the Special Education Needs (SEN) Code of Practice (Special Educational Needs and Disability Act, 2001) defines children with special educational needs as those who, compared with their peer group, have:

1 A significantly greater difficulty in learning; or

2 A disability that prevents or hinders them from making use of educational facilities of a kind generally provided.

Further, "A child is defined as disabled if he is blind, deaf or dumb or suffers from a mental disorder of any kind or is substantially and permanently handicapped by illness, injury or congenital deformity or such other disability as may be prescribed."

The same document defines special educational provision as that "which is additional to, or otherwise different from, the educational provision made generally for children of their age in (state) maintained schools."

However, decisions about what constitutes a "significantly greater disability" vary across schools and education authorities and are influenced by the political and financial factors operating at any one time. Moreover, although the same Code of Practice notes that children with special educational needs "should have their needs met . . . and be offered full access to a broad, balanced and relevant education," how to achieve this remains unspecified.

Rutter's Child and Adolescent Psychiatry, 5th edition. Edited by M. Rutter, D. Bishop, D. Pine, S. Scott, J. Stevenson, E. Taylor and A. Thapar. © 2008 Blackwell Publishing, ISBN: 978-1-4051-4549-7.

What are the Goals of Special Education?

Educational goals are affected by the nature and extent of an individual's disabilities. Many children with sensory or physical impairments or chronic illnesses are of normal intellectual ability and, with appropriate support, should be able to progress within mainstream settings. Children with more pervasive developmental, learning or behavioral difficulties require more radical modifications to the educational environment and curriculum. For the majority of children with special needs, education should provide them with the skills required for social inclusion as adults so that they leave school with the skills needed to fit in with and be accepted by society, develop strategies to minimize their difficulties and achieve emotional stability and positive self-esteem. Although scholastic attainments and academic qualifications are important, these should be of an appropriate kind and level, and there must also be a focus on broader aspects of social, emotional and behavioral development. Moreover, some children, particularly those with severe to profound intellectual impairments, are unlikely ever to lead totally independent lives. For them, education should promote the development of effective means of communication, the acquisition of basic daily living and social skills and the minimization of behavioral problems.

Does Special Education Mean Inclusive Education?

During the 19th century, individuals concerned to improve education for children with special needs (Gordon, 1885; Lettsom, 1894) fought to establish specialist, disability-specific schools. However, by the latter half of the 20th century, there were increasing fears about the long-term effects of isolating these children from their typically developing peers. Pressure for integration was strengthened by significant changes in legislation. In the USA, the Education of All Handicapped Children Act, 1975 (Public Law 94-142; now the Individuals with Disabilities Education Act [IDEA], Public Law 101-476) required public schools to provide all students with special needs with access to a "free and appropriate education" in the "least restrictive environment." The Americans with Disabilities Act, 1990 (ADA, Public Law 101-336) further outlawed discrimination against any child with special needs. UNESCO's

Salamanca Statement (1994) called for all governments to "adopt as a matter of law or policy the principle of inclusive education." In the UK, the highly influential Warnock Committee report (1978) led to the widespread view that all pupils with special needs had a "right" to mainstream education (Department for Education and Employment, 1998).

However, although inclusion has often been interpreted as requiring the elimination of all segregated schooling, Public Law 94-142 states that there may be grounds for "special classes, separate schooling, or removal . . . from the regular education environment . . . (if) education in regular classes. . . . cannot be achieved satisfactorily." The UK Special Educational Needs and Disability Act (2001) also notes that pupils may be educated in alternative provision if their presence in mainstream is incompatible with the provision of efficient education for other children. Moreover, Warnock herself (2005) criticized the manner in which her original report was misinterpreted as espousing mainstreaming for all children, regardless of disability level, the impact on other pupils or the availability of adequate resources.

Empirical Evidence for Inclusion

Empirical research on the relative effectiveness of special versus integrated education is extremely limited. Indeed, it has been suggested that such research is inappropriate because the issue is one of rights, not evidence (Gallagher, 2001). Well-conducted comparative studies are rare, randomized controlled trials virtually non-existent and research methods and analysis vary from study to study (Lindsay, 2007). A major problem is that inclusion is not a simple unambiguous concept: "special educational needs" encompass specific learning disabilities, severe and pervasive developmental disorders, and disruptive and challenging behaviors. Programs range from the highly specific to a general (often poorly defined) "whole school inclusion policy"; and monitoring treatment fidelity presents major practical difficulties (Lindsay, 2003). Heterogeneity of samples and inadequate information on children's cognitive, linguistic, social and behavioral characteristics make it almost impossible to generalize from one study to another. Finding appropriate comparison groups also presents difficulties because children in specialist settings often tend to have more academic and behavioral problems than pupils of similar IQ in mainstream (Rafferty, Piscitelli, & Boettcher, 2003). Even terminology is a problem. Thus, "learning disability" refers to *specific* difficulties (e.g., reading, spelling, motor) in the USA but is used synonymously with mental retardation (now termed intellectual disability; see chapter 49) in the UK. In a review of 1373 published studies on inclusion from 2001–2005, Lindsay (2007) identified only nine that compared outcomes for children with special needs in specialized versus mainstream settings. There were no randomized controlled trials; the results of most studies were equivocal and the few that did find positive effects for mainstreaming all suffered from significant methodological limitations.

Alternatives to Full Inclusion

The UK Office for Standards in Education (Ofsted, 2004) recently noted that, despite the widespread policy of inclusion, the numbers of pupils being sent to referral units or special schools was rising as mainstream schools were finding it increasingly difficult to manage students with social and behavioral difficulties. Even when pupils with special educational needs were mainstreamed, much teaching was carried out by unqualified staff and the quality of education was poor, resulting in disruptive behavior, poor attendance and high staff turnover, especially in secondary school.

Because of the conflicts faced by teachers trying to cope with the demands of perhaps 30 other pupils, various alternatives to full-time integration have been explored. Although critics claim these lead to increased discrimination by excluding difficult pupils from the classroom, there is some evidence of their effectiveness.

Resource rooms are usually separate classrooms where children can be offered individual teaching for part of the school day. Some cater for children with specific difficulties, others for pupils with broader impairments, and a combination of resource room and regular classroom teaching has been found to improve educational progress (Marston, 1996). Placement on the same site as the mainstream school seems more likely to result in integration than placement in units that are geographically isolated (Burack, Root, & Zigler, 1997) and students with special educational needs themselves indicate a preference for receiving support in a separate environment while being able to mix with their peers at other times (Norwich & Kelly, 2004).

Dual placements – in which pupils are enrolled in both mainstream and a special placement – are currently recommended by the Department for Education and Skills (2001a) in the UK as an alternative means of supporting inclusion. Dual placements can help prepare pupils for mainstream education by providing them with skilled individualized support for areas of particular need while mainstream teachers profit from the input and advice of specialist staff. Although evaluation of the benefits of dual placements is still needed, this flexibility could potentially meet the requirements of many pupils, and provides a bridge between fully inclusive and full-time special education.

Specialist Teaching Programs

There are vast numbers of publications offering advice on "the making of the inclusive school," and how to improve the curriculum, environment, support structures and general attitudes. Co-operative learning (groups of students working together to achieve mutual goals) has been recommended in a number of studies although this seems to have more impact on social engagement than academic skills (Murphy, Grey, & Honan, 2005). Self-evaluation and self-monitoring programs (Sainato, Goldstein, & Strain, 1992), the Adaptive Learning Environment Model (ALEM; Wang & Walberg, 1993), Mediated Learning (Mills, Dale, Cole, & Jenkins, 1995), Instrumental Enrichment (Feuerstein, Rand, Hoffman, & Miller, 1980) and Creative Action

Planning techniques (Forest, Pearpoint, & O'Brien, 1996) all have their advocates, but either experimental evaluations are small in scale or their findings are equivocal (Dale, Jenkins, Mills, & Cole, 2005; Hornby, Atkinson, & Howard, 1997).

The following sections address issues related to special education for children with different types of difficulties. The earlier sections relate to children with relatively mild intellectual impairments, "specific" learning difficulties, or sensory or physical problems, for whom the crucial issue is how their needs can be *better* met in mainstream settings. The latter sections deal with those pupils for whom the merits of inclusive education are much less well established – children with severe emotional and behavioral problems and those with pervasive disabilities, such as developmental language problems, autism or severe intellectual disability.

Education for Children with Mild to Moderate Intellectual Impairments

The American Association on Mental Retardation (2002) defines intellectual disability as "characterized by significant limitations both in intellectual functioning (generally accepted as IQ below 70) and in adaptive behavior (and) refers to a particular state of functioning that begins in childhood, has many dimensions, and is affected positively by individualized supports."

Academic Attainments

The majority of studies on inclusion have focused on children with mild intellectual disabilities (IQ 50–70, DSM-IV-TR; American Psychiatric Association, 2000). Once they leave school, most of these individuals will be expected to live independently and be able to socialize with and work alongside their "typically developing" peers. Thus, it is important that they are provided with the skills needed for optimum social inclusion from the earliest years. In principle at least, helping them to learn with and from their peers should enhance academic skills, social adjustment and self-esteem. There is also evidence that once children are placed in segregated provision their chances of reintegration or of achieving age-appropriate educational standards diminish with age (Farrell & Tsakalidou, 1999). European statistics over the last 2–3 decades show a significant decline in the number of special schools for children with mild to moderate intellectual impairments (Meijer, Soriano, & Watkins, 2003) and those that remain tend to cater for children with more severe social and behavioral problems.

What is known about the educational progress of these pupils in inclusive settings? Baker, Wang, and Walberg (1994) summarized the findings of three meta-analyses of inclusive education 1970–1992 involving over 70 studies. The results provide only limited support for inclusion, with effect sizes for academic outcomes being generally small (range 0.08–0.44; average 0.22), albeit positive. Findings are also influenced by pupil characteristics. Mills, Cole, Jenkins, and Dale (1998) reported no main effect of classroom type for children with mild to moderate intellectual impairment but there was an interaction effect, with higher-functioning children gaining more from special integrated classes and lower-functioning children performing better in segregated classes. The choice of outcome measures further affects conclusions. Rafferty, Piscitelli, & Boettcher, (2003) found that although pupils with mild intellectual disabilities appeared to do equally well in segregated or inclusive classes, the subgroup with the lowest IQ made greater language and social progress in inclusive classes but showed higher rates of behavior problems than children in segregated classes.

A further experimental confound relates to the quality of the educational settings studied. Much research into the benefits of inclusive placements has been conducted, especially in the USA, in highly resourced university-based research settings, in small classrooms (often fewer than 15 children), and with preschool or elementary school pupils. In contrast, the poor progress of many pupils in special schools may be a result, not of segregation *per se*, but of the poor quality of teaching provided (Giangreco, 1997; Manset & Semmel, 1997).

Finally, conclusions are often limited by a lack of crucial information about the participants. One frequently cited study in support of inclusive compared with "pull-out" programs (Rea, McLaughlin, & Walther-Thomas, 2002) included only children of average IQ and provided very limited information on the preplacement skills of the pupils involved.

Social Integration and Self-Esteem

Writers espousing the human rights and equality arguments in favor of inclusion (Lipsky & Gartner, 1999) insist that this is essential for positive social development. Early reviews (Carlberg & Kavale, 1980; Cole & Meyer, 1991; Lakhen & Norwich, 1990) also claimed that inclusion led to more positive social outcomes and higher self-esteem. However, effect sizes for social improvements among children with mild intellectual disabilities in inclusive classrooms are typically even smaller than the effect sizes for academic attainments (range 0.11–0.28; average 0.19; Baker, Wang, & Walberg, 1994). A review of 14 studies (Nakken & Pijl, 2002) found some reported better social interactions and friendships among mainstreamed pupils; in others inclusion seemed to make little difference, whereas some reported negative effects. Other reviews (Burack, Root, & Zigler, 1997; Hornby, Atkinson, & Howard, 1997) have failed to find evidence of enhanced social skills, self-esteem or peer acceptance within inclusive settings. Moreover, for some pupils with mild to moderate intellectual impairments, the school experience can be very negative, with integrated schooling actually leading to lower self-esteem and increased stigmatization, bullying and rejection by peers (Bear, Clever, & Proctor, 1991; Norwich & Kelly, 2004).

Education for Children with "Specific" Learning Disabilities

Reading and spelling difficulties

Around 5% of school-aged pupils have persistent and significant reading difficulties and the adverse effects on many aspects of children's development, including emotional and behavioral disturbance, are well documented (see chapter 48).

Almost any type of intervention initially seems to produce short-term gains, although these are rarely well maintained. Overall, a combination of the "Reading Recovery" approach (intensive, structured, individualized reading programs; Clay, 1985) together with training in phonological awareness and explicit work on letter–sound correspondence, has proved most consistently effective (Troia, 1999). Computerized programs, allowing self-assessment of reading ability and providing clear and immediate feedback using synthesized speech, are also reported as successful (Vollands, Topping, & Ryka, 1999; Wise, Ring, & Olson, 2000). However, the gains may be very specific to the skills taught and often fail to generalize to other literacy problems or to new situations. Thus, a computer-based Colorado remediation project (Wise, Ring, & Olson, 2000) indicated that outcome may still depend on the amount of direct monitoring by adults. This study also reported an interaction between treatment response and the nature and severity of children's reading problems although, overall, meta-analyses have failed to demonstrate a clear relationship between basic aptitude and type of intervention (Norwich, 2003).

Given the complexity of the problems of many pupils with reading difficulties, factors other than the specific literacy intervention are likely to have an impact: teacher effectiveness, classroom organization, amount of time spent on reading and adequacy of resources (human, environmental and technical). Classroom assistants *can* have an important role, but only if they are fully trained to implement the program. Peer tutors may also prove an effective source of intervention (Topping, 2001). Specific homework tasks can be helpful and parental participation is also important (Topping, 2001), but only if parents are given appropriate guidance in what to do; simply encouraging them to *listen* to their child has little effect. A major problem is the poor maintenance of reading skills once intervention ceases and research is still needed to identify the factors required to ensure continuing long-term progress. Extra tuition for children with reading and/or spelling problems often continues to be provided outside the classroom or in privately funded centers, both of which limit opportunities for participating fully in school life.

Specific Language Impairments

Specific language impairments are among the most frequent of childhood developmental disorders, with epidemiological studies suggesting prevalence rates in 5-year-olds of around 6–7% (see chapter 47). Co-occurring scholastic problems, related to reading, spelling and mathematics, are common and there is a significant risk of later emotional, social, behavioral and psychiatric problems. Meta-analyses of speech and language therapy interventions indicate that, although these may be helpful for children with phonological and vocabulary difficulties, the evidence for their impact on expressive syntax disorders is variable, and there is little evidence of effectiveness for children with receptive disorders (Law, Garrett, & Nye, 2003).

In recent years, much of the focus of intervention programs for specific language impairments has been on the development of improved reciprocal communication strategies for parents and very young children (Pepper & Weitzman, 2004). The University of Kansas Language Acquisition Pre-school Program (Rice & Wilcox, 1991) indicated that this inclusive preschool model, involving parents and normal peers, significantly increases children's chances of remaining with their peer group once they reach school age. School-based programs for older children (e.g., Speech Foundation of Ontario, Hayden & Pukonen, 1996; or the ECLIPSE project, Schwartz, Garfinkle, & McBride, 1998) stress the need for individual assessment and involve the creation of an environment that is designed to elicit and enhance communication, the structuring of interactions with and by peers, and the use of naturalistic teaching strategies, together with specific techniques such as modeling, turn taking, topic manipulation, conversational repair, scripts and time delay. The FastForword program (Tallal, Miller, Bedi *et al.*, 1996) involves an intensive computer-based program designed to develop a range of language skills, although recent research has shown disappointing results (see chapter 47). Moreover, there are few interventions that can be readily used by class teachers, either in mainstream or specialist settings. The FastForword program, for example, requires a rigorous 100 min per day, 5 days per week for 4–8 weeks. Instead, for most children access to language therapy, of any kind, tends to be limited. Mainstream teachers frequently have little understanding of the wider needs and problems of these children (Lindsay, Dockrell, Mackie, & Letchford, 2005) and few receive any direct input from specialist therapists (Davison & Howlin, 1997).

Lindsay and Dockrell (2000) suggested that self-esteem may be higher in children with speech and language disorders educated in special rather than mainstream schools, but generally evidence for the benefits of different placements on academic, social or even language outcomes is lacking. Lindsay *et al.* (2005) found widely varying practices and very different degrees of inclusion and levels of classroom support in their study of specialist language provision for children in England and Wales. The criteria for admission to language units, integrated resources or special schools also differed so it was not possible to make direct comparisons between specialist or integrated provision – each seemed to have some advantages and drawbacks. Of particular concern is the lack of any specialist provision for most children, including those with severe language impairments, when they reach junior school (at around 8 years). Once *speech* improves (even though many other difficulties persist) children are often transferred to mainstream school, without any additional help (Davison & Howlin, 1997). Howlin, Mawhood, and Rutter (2000), in a follow-up study of 20 individuals with receptive language impairments, found that although half had required specialist (often residential) schooling during the primary years, by secondary age 50% were in mainstream schools with little or no additional support. The remainder were in a variety of non-language-specific placements, including schools for behavioral, learning and emotional disorders. The children also experienced frequent changes of school, often resulting in educational failure, exclusion, bullying, social rejection and low self-esteem.

Education for Children with Behavioral and Emotional Problems

Definitions of "emotional and behavioral disorders" (EBD) vary widely and encompass a host of different problems: conduct disorders, antisocial behaviors, hyperactivity, attention deficits, learning disabilities, psychiatric or mood disorders, or any combination of these. The US National Association of School Psychologists (2005) defines EBD as conditions in which "behavioral or emotional responses of an individual in school are so different from his or her generally accepted, age appropriate, ethnic or cultural norms that they adversely affect performance in such areas as self care, social relationships, personal adjustment, academic progress, classroom behavior, or work adjustment."

Low academic attainments, high rates of challenging behavior and increased dropout from school are typical and the controversy over segregated versus inclusive education for these pupils has been particularly marked because of the disruption they can cause in the classroom. However, the heterogeneity and complexity of problems involved make it impossible to identify any one specific form of effective educational intervention.

Ideally, any treatment program should be based on detailed assessments of the child's behavioral difficulties, family circumstances, social competence, learning strategies and academic capabilities. Successful interventions involve cognitive–behavioral therapy, interpersonal problem-solving, social skills training, counseling and play – or other individual therapies together with remedial input to enhance general academic skills, memory, auditory and visual processing, and sequencing (Cooper & Ideus, 1996; Hechtman, Kouri, & Respitz, 1996). Other approaches include preschool preventative programs and educational enrichment strategies; there are also studies indicating the importance of combining child-focused interventions with parent training (Frankel, Myatt, Cantwell, & Feinberg, 1997). Randomized controlled trials, conducted in *experimental* settings, indicate moderate effect sizes on reducing disruptive and/or aggressive behaviors for programs involving social competence training and cognitive–behavioral strategies. Relatively few of these programs have been successfully incorporated into *routine* educational *practice* (Wilson, Lipsey, & Derzon, 2003). However, interventions such as the "Dinosaur program" (Webster-Stratton & Reid, 2004) and Promoting Alternative Thinking Strategies (PATHS; Karn, Greenberg, & Kusché, 2004) have been shown to be effective in special education and preschool settings and to have lasting benefits.

It is also important to be aware that judgments as to whether a child has behavioral or emotional problems may depend as much on the attitudes, policies and practices of the school, or the tolerance level of individual teachers, as on the child's own characteristics. A child who shows very disruptive behavior in one setting may not do so elsewhere (Werthamer-Larsson, Kellam, & Wheeler, 1991) and the role of schools in maintaining or minimizing disruptive behaviors has been widely investigated (Reynolds, 1991; Rutter, 1983). In some cases, transfer to a different class, or a move to a school where teachers are more sensitive to the child's needs may be sufficient to significantly reduce the level of problems.

Management Techniques Within the Classroom

Although school-based programs alone are likely to have only a partial impact on the child's problems, strategies based on behavioral principles have been shown to be effective in many single-case and studies of small groups for improving disruptive, aggressive and on-task behaviors within the classroom (Gresham, Watson, & Skinner, 2001; Herbert, 1995). As with much behavioral intervention research, group sizes tend to be small and long-term follow-up or generalization measures are often lacking (Evans, Harden, Thomas, & Benefield, 2003). However, there is an increasing number of randomized controlled trials demonstrating the effectiveness of a range of classroom management techniques (e.g., Fast Track Program, Good Behavior Game and Webster-Stratton's Teacher program; for review see Greenberg, Domitrovich, & Bumberger, 2000; see also chapter 62).

Behavioral approaches have considerable advantages in that they do not require removal of the child from the class and, in principle, the basic techniques can be adapted to the particular needs of any individual child or classroom. On the whole, a focus on positive on-task behaviors is more effective than concentrating on disruptive behaviors (Barkley, 1997; Scott, 1998; Warner Rogers, 1998). Extinction and time out techniques, although extremely effective in controlled settings (Barkley, 1997), can be difficult to apply consistently in the classroom. Other pupils or staff may respond to activities that the class teacher is trying to ignore, or the behavior may escalate to such a level that ignoring is no longer an option. Time out is all too often interpreted as "time out from the classroom" – not necessarily a deterrent for many children – and there is a danger of exclusion periods becoming increasingly lengthy.

Cognitive–behavioral strategies are also effective (see chapter 63; Sawyer, MacMullin, Graetz *et al.*, 1997) but because of the variability of such programs it is generally not possible to identify which specific components are most crucial. Moreover, the more complex the program the more difficult it becomes to incorporate within the regular classroom. The use of other behavioral approaches, such as token economies, differential reinforcement or response-cost, has also been reported in many studies (Rutherford & Nelson, 1995). The most successful programs are based on a detailed functional analysis of the causes and nature of the problems involved but many of these more sophisticated studies have been conducted in specially designed or experimental classes (Gresham, Watson, & Skinner, 2001). The consistent use of such strategies is much more difficult for mainstream teachers coping with 30 or more pupils.

"Co-operative learning" programs, in which students with emotional and behavioral problems work together in groups with typically developing peers, have proved popular, particularly in the USA. A review of co-operative learning programs (Sutherland, Wehby, & Gunter, 2000) indicated some limited evidence for a positive effect on on-task behavior and social skills, but not disruptive behaviors. Nelson, Johnson, and Marchand-Martella (1996) also found that direct instruction was more effective in improving on-task engagement and behavior problems than co-operative learning. Other researchers caution that children with emotional and behavior problems may lack the social and communication understanding required to benefit from these programs (Sutherland, Wehby, & Gunter, 2000).

Sometimes, simple environmental modifications can have surprising effects. For example, the provision of specially designed study areas or changing sitting arrangements from groups to rows can significantly improve on-task behaviors (Hastings & Schwieso, 1995) and reduce classroom disruption (Ware, 1994). Morning teaching sessions tend to be more productive than teaching later in the day; visual aids and brightly colored materials increase attention, and the presentation of materials in small chunks, interspersed with brief breaks, is likely to improve concentration and co-operation (Warner-Rogers, 1998). Generally, however, in order to have a significant impact on severely disturbed or disruptive pupils, attention must also focus on factors outside the classroom, such as the wider school curriculum, organization and climate. Strategies for *avoiding* potentially high-risk situations (i.e., those when the setting, peer group or even a particular teacher is likely to exacerbate difficulties) also have an important role. Negotiating potentially difficult situations with children themselves, so that they feel part of the consultation and planning process, can increase appropriate behaviors, while remedial intervention for academic difficulties may prevent the escalation of secondary behavior problems. Finally, the involvement of parents is also crucial for the generalization and maintenance of behavior change (Desforges & Abouchaar, 2003).

Children Who are Excluded from Mainstream School

The push towards inclusion has coincided, in the UK at least, with government requirements for a rise in school standards, generally measured by formal examination results. However, the presence of one or more disruptive pupils in the classroom can affect the academic progress of other children and official exclusions from school on behavioral grounds have risen over recent years (from 3833 in 1991 to 9880 in 2003–2004; Department for Education and Skills, 2005). The rates of *unofficial* exclusions are unknown. Children registered as having special educational needs are nine times more likely to be excluded than other pupils, and exclusions from special schools are also rising (about 300 per year in the UK). Boys are almost five times more likely to be excluded than girls, with rates being highest among Afro-Caribbean boys and children in foster care. Most exclusions (around 60%) are for physical assault or persistent disruptive behavior; around 15% are for verbal abuse or threatening behavior; the remainder involve racist abuse, drugs and alcohol, theft, damage to property and bullying (Department for Education and Skills, 2005). Nevertheless, individual schools and local authorities differ widely in their reasons for and rates of exclusion, and headteachers' attitudes, school status, policies and practices may have a greater impact than a pupil's behavior (Hornby, Atkinson, & Howard, 1997).

Overall, the outlook for children excluded from mainstream school is bleak. Around 25% receive home tuition, usually for only a few hours a week; many others attend pupil referral units (over 14,500 children in 2002–2003; UK Department for Education and Skills, 2006). These placements are generally part-time and, as they are not required to offer the full national curriculum, pupils often fall even further behind academically. Moreover, other mainstream schools are often reluctant to accept a child who has been previously excluded. Once they reach their mid-teens, little effort is made to reintroduce these pupils back into school and as many also come from unsupportive and/or disrupted homes they risk drifting into a life of continuing social exclusion.

Although the cost of exclusion to pupils, their families and to society has been widely publicized, the issue of how to deal with it remains largely unsolved. There is general agreement that effective intervention requires better training and resources for teachers, together with the expertise and input of a network of interagency support (Department for Education and Skills, 2006). In practice, provision of such services is limited and many schools only seek specialist support when the classroom situation has totally broken down, rather than at an earlier stage when there is some chance of remediation.

Although some specialist day and boarding schools for children with emotional and behavioral problems survive (some offering intensive therapeutic as well as educational provision), critics claim that these placements are very expensive, isolate children from their home and community and are particularly unsuitable for children from ethnic minorities (Abbott, Morris, & Ward, 2001). However, although data on long-term academic or social benefits are lacking, they may be a helpful resource for some children and their parents (Crawford & Simonoff, 2003) and residential provision can offer a vital "break" for children whose difficulties are largely a result of a severely disturbed or deprived family environment.

Education for Children With Physical and Sensory Handicaps

Physical Disabilities

The desirability of integrating children with physical handicaps into normal classrooms has been recognized for well over a century (see Cole, 1989) but developments in medical technology now mean that increasing numbers of children are surviving with long-term and often highly complex needs. For example, children with cerebral palsy may also have incontinence or epilepsy; they may be unable to communicate effectively; sensory, behavioral, emotional and psychiatric problems are common; and 30–60% have some degree of intellectual disability (Harris, 1998). Kohn (1990) and Harris (1998) discuss the many components required for a comprehensive package of educational care but in practice "inclusion" frequently involves simply the provision of physical aids, some – often inadequate – adaptations to the school environment, and the use of support staff or classmates to assist the class teacher. Few mainstream schools have adequate access to trained nursing or physiotherapy help for children with chronic or complex physical problems and most teachers receive little guidance on how to help manage their difficulties. For example, augmentative and alternative communication systems (AAC) for children who are unable to use speech (because of physical or developmental difficulties) have improved significantly over recent years. These range from single-touch devices (e.g., a large colored square or circle that emits a prerecorded message when pressed) to multisymbol display boards, with extensive vocabularies personally tailored to individuals' own environments, needs or interests. The development of highly sensitive switch mechanisms and greatly improved speech output software has resulted in computers becoming far more effective means of communication than in the past (Howlin, 2006). There is also evidence that the attitudes of listeners and/or observers towards people with disabilities are more favorable when complex augmentative systems, such as computers, are used (Gorenflo & Gorenflo, 1991). However, effective use of these systems is often restricted by teachers' lack of training in their use, or awareness of the range and complexity of current AAC aids. Thus, most individuals with cerebral palsy tend to use only low-technology devices, despite much more sophisticated aids being available, and to use these only during limited periods of the day (Murphy, Markova, Collins, & Moodie, 1996).

Teachers are also often poorly prepared to deal with the social and emotional difficulties associated with chronic physical conditions, particularly those related to teasing, isolation or low self-esteem. Although inclusion in elementary school may be relatively easy to achieve, at secondary school real inclusion becomes far more difficult because of increasing social, physical and academic demands (Lightfoot, Wright, & Sloper, 1999).

Hearing Impairments (see chapter 59)

In developed countries, approximately 1 child in 1000 has a profound hearing loss and 3–5 per 1000 have mild to moderate hearing loss that can affect language acquisition. Deafness can have a profound effect on parent–child relationships and around 25% of children with severe hearing loss show additional emotional, intellectual, physical or sensory problems (Roberts & Hindley, 1999).

The issue of appropriate education for deaf children is complicated by opposing arguments within the deaf community. The poor signing skills of many hearing parents and teachers, and the fact that deaf children of deaf parents often make better academic and social progress than those of hearing parents, have led to claims that education should be provided in specialist settings (residential if necessary). Cochlear implants are criticized as depriving children of their "right" to belong to the deaf community, and fluency in signing, with its own grammar and idiom, is considered a primary educational goal (Balkaney, Hodges, & Goodman, 1996). However, studies of children with successful implants suggest that they are more likely to move into mainstream settings, are better able to communicate with hearing peers and continue to make good progress into secondary school and beyond (Beadle, McKinley, Nikolopoulos *et al.*, 2005; Geers & Brenner, 2003). There are no well-controlled comparative studies of different models of communication teaching (signing, lip reading + speech, cued speech, in which hand signs are used to assist lip reading, or speech alone). Because a focus on signing alone can result in isolating children from their families and neighborhood (Groenveld, 1998), "total communication" (the combination of a formal signing system with written and spoken language) has become widely adopted, both in special schools and some mainstream placements (Hindley & van Gent, 2002). The success of such programs is at least partly dependent on the adequacy of parents' signing skills: 20% of deaf children have no family members who sign and 40% have only one signing family member (Gravel & O'Gara, 2003; Preisler, Tvingstedt & Ahlstrom, 2002).

Early intervention programs involving a combined oral–visual approach are suggested as being crucial for avoiding the "cultural divide" that may otherwise develop between hearing parents and their deaf children (Hindley & van Gent, 2002). Massaro and Light (2004) reported on the use of "Baldi," a computerized talking head, which can teach children to control tongue, mouth and face movements and airflow, thereby improving both speech production and perception. Sample sizes have been small, and the effects are limited once training ceases, but this approach could potentially assist many children.

Hearing impaired children have many additional problems, and poor cognitive and educational attainments, and increasing isolation from their hearing peers with age, are of major concern (Antia, Stinson, & Gaustad, 2002; Martin & Bat-Chava, 2003). Although, academically, deaf children in regular schools seem to do better than those in specialist placements (Powers, Thoutenhoofd, & Gregory, 1999), it is also evident that their difficulties may be significantly underestimated by mainstream teachers. Thus, the choice of an appropriate placement depends not only on the extent of hearing loss, but on factors such as IQ, the presence of other impairments and, most importantly, on the quality of instruction offered (Roberts & Hindley, 1999; Watson, Gregory, & Powers, 1999).

Visual Problems (see chapter 59)

Around 14,000 children in the UK are estimated as having significant visual impairment, although only one-third of these are registered as blind or partially sighted (Keil & Clunies-Ross, 2003). Children with visual difficulties are also likely to have a range of additional problems including cerebral palsy, epilepsy, linguistic and hearing impairments, autism, intellectual disability, and emotional and psychiatric disturbance (Groenveld, 1998; Webster & Roe, 1998). The proportion educated in specialist provision has declined steadily in the UK – from 22% in 1998 to 5% in 2003 (Keil & Clunies-Ross, 2003) – and those special schools that still exist tend to cater for pupils with more complex physical or cognitive needs. For the remainder, education within mainstream settings is necessary to meet their educational and social needs and enhance future job prospects (Arter, Mason, McCall, McLinden, & Stone, 1999; Davis & Hopwood, 2002; Wagner & Blackorby, 1996). However, successful inclusion requires considerable modification to teaching materials and curriculum. Input from specialist staff is needed, with teachers, teaching assistants and specialist advisers working closely together. The teaching environment must be carefully structured in order to facilitate interactions with peers, and the successful integration of a severely visually impaired child requires careful preparation of all staff, sighted pupils and their parents.

Education for Children With Severe and Pervasive Intellectual Disabilities

(see chapter 49)

Many different teaching strategies have been reported as effective in enhancing inclusion for this group of children. These include peer-tutoring, co-operative learning, parallel instruction, behavioral and token programs, discrete trial learning, modeling, shaping, prompting and reinforcement techniques, naturalistic teaching, embedded instruction and many more (McDonnell, 1998). Much research in this area involves single-case or small case-series but there are some successful reports of implementing behavioral approaches within a "whole school" framework. Harris, Cook, and Upton (1996) utilized a combination of behavioral strategies, together with communication and social skills programs, to enhance overall functioning and reduce challenging behavior in pupils with severe intellectual disabilities in a mainstream school. Nevertheless, teachers found the program difficult to cope with, and many felt they lacked adequate support. Generalization to other settings or staff members was also limited.

The most successful inclusion programs have generally been conducted with very young children in settings that are unrepresentative of most mainstream schools (university-based experimental units; highly skilled educators; very small classes). For preschool children with severe intellectual disability, inclusive education may produce greater gains in language and social skills (Hundert, Mahoney, Mundy, & Vernon, 1998). However, other studies have found no social or cognitive advantages of inclusive preschools, and behavior problems may actually be more frequent in these settings (Rafferty, Piscitelli, & Boettcher, 2003). For older pupils with severe intellectual impairments there is no good evidence that inclusion enhances cognitive or social development (Kavale & Mostert, 2003; Lindsay, 2003). Acceptance by peers and teachers tends to decrease with age and few studies have reported on successful integration within secondary school (Beveridge, 1996; Booth, 1996). Moreover, unless there is adequate support, children with severe disabilities may receive significantly *less* individualized instruction in mainstream than in segregated classes.

Advocates of inclusive education for children with severe intellectual disabilities claim that it has a positive impact on both their social development and that of their typically developing peers. However, there is little evidence that simple exposure to non-handicapped peers improves either language or social skills (Lewis, 1995). Moreover, although guided contact with their disabled peers can have a positive impact on other pupils' *attitudes* (Farrell, 1996), joint spontaneous interactions remain limited and close, reciprocal friendships are very *unlikely* to develop, particularly at secondary school (Burack, Root, & Zigler, 1997).

Many studies in this area are compromised because of the tendency to treat children with severe intellectual disabilities as a homogenous group. It is thus difficult to reach conclusions on what types of inclusive setting work best for which children, at which stage of their lives and in which developmental domains. For example, in comparison with children of similar cognitive levels, pupils with Down syndrome seem to do better *academically* in mainstream, but social interactions are enhanced in specialist settings (Buckley, 2006). Kavale and Mostert (2003) suggest that "Empirical evidence, not existential exaggeration, should be the cornerstone of deciding where students with special needs should be served." They note that so-called "fully inclusive" classrooms may actually increase segregation and isolation. High self-esteem in pupils depends principally on the ability to achieve academically and socially in comparison with peers (Heward, 2003). If this is not attainable, children with special needs may have lower self-esteem and feel more stigmatized in "inclusive" than in specialist provision. The primary goal must be to improve existing provision and the quality of teaching to ensure maximum opportunities for inclusion for those children who will benefit, while providing high-quality segregated or partially integrated provision for those who may not. Resource bases within mainstream settings may provide the most flexible option for many students, allowing full-time inclusion (with support as necessary) for some, while providing others with the daily opportunity to mix with mainstream peers.

"Syndrome Specific" Approaches to Education for Children With Severe Intellectual Impairments

(see chapter 24)

There are now over 750 known genetic causes of intellectual disability (Dykens, 2000) and research into cognitive and behavioral phenotypes has greatly increased understanding of syndrome-specific deficits. Fragile X, for example, is associated with deficits in visuospatial abilities, abstract reasoning, motor coordination, memory and sequential processing. Vocabulary skills, simultaneous processing and ability to learn verbally based factual material are relatively unimpaired. Perceptual organization, visuospatial memory and fine motor skills are strengths in children with Cornelia De Lange syndrome (Kline, Stanley, Belevich-Brodsky, Barr, & Jackson, 2005). Expressive language skills are particularly poor in children with cri-du-chat syndrome (Cornish & Munir, 1998). Short-term auditory memory deficits are typical of children with Down syndrome (Jarrold, Baddeley, & Phillips, 2002). Smith–Magenis syndrome is characterized by difficulties with arithmetic, sequential processing and short-term memory; long-term memory for facts and information is relatively good (Udwin, Webber, & Horn, 2001). Individuals with Prader–Willi syndrome typically show deficits in arithmetic, writing, short-term memory and auditory attention but have strengths in visual organization and perception, long-term memory, reading and vocabulary (Cassidy & Morris, 2002). Understanding the underlying phenotype can help teachers adapt teaching strategies to suit specific profiles of skills and difficulties (Hodapp & Fidler, 1999). However, this requires acceptance by educational providers that a child's diagnostic "label" is of value in highlighting potential strengths and weaknesses *and* recognition of the need for detailed individual assessment, including the use of formal psychometric measures. (For examples of teaching guides to specific syndromes see Lorenz, 1998 for Down syndrome; Lewis & Wilson, 1998 for Rett's syndrome; Saunders, 2001 for fragile X; Waters, 1999 for Prader–Willi.)

Children With Autism Spectrum Disorders (see chapter 46)

Recent research indicates that not only is the prevalence of autism spectrum disorders (ASD) far higher than originally estimated, possibly as high as 1% of the population (Baird, Simonoff, Pickles *et al.*, 2006), but also that around 40–50% of all those affected are of normal IQ (Edelson, 2006). These figures have enormous service implications and specialist educational approaches for children with ASD have been studied in particular detail. Programs may be center-based (e.g., Waldon; LEAP; Douglass); home-based (e.g., Applied Behavioral Analysis; Pivotal Response Training) or school-based (e.g., TEACCH; Denver Model; Harris, Handleman, & Jennet, 2005). Although evaluative data are limited, highly structured, visually based approaches to teaching appear to be particularly helpful. The internationally used TEACCH program, for example (Marcus, Schopler, & Lord, 2001), emphasizes the need for structure, appropriate environmental organization and the use of visual cues to circumvent communication difficulties in autism. The program stresses the importance of individually based teaching, and incorporates developmental, behavioral and cognitive approaches. A recent small-scale study of TEACCH (Panerai, Ferrante, & Zingale, 2002) reported significant gains in educational and adaptive behaviors compared with progress in an integrated classroom.

Many other educational programs for children with ASD have been reported. Most are US-based, and include peer-tutoring programs to enhance social interactions and play; co-operative learning groups; the Bright Start Program, which concentrates on the development of cognitive and metacognitive abilities; and the STAR curriculum (for reviews see Arick, Krug, Fullerton, Loos, & Falco, 2005; Lord & McGee, 2001). The effectiveness of various developmental and behaviorally based programs has also been demonstrated (Harris, Handleman, & Jennet, 2005). In UK settings, Jordan and Jones (1999) describe a variety of innovative techniques that can be used in the classroom and Cumine, Leach, and Stevenson (1998, 1999) provide practical suggestions for teaching children with autism and Asperger syndrome within mainstream settings.

One program widely used throughout the USA, Europe and Australasia is the Picture Exchange Communication System (PECS; Bondy & Frost, 1996). PECS aims to increase communication skills by means of pictures or objects and claims to improve both verbal and non-verbal skills (for review see Howlin, 2006). A large randomized controlled trial (Howlin, Gordon, Pasco, Wade, & Charman, 2007) found that children exposed to formal PECS training showed significant increases in their use of PECS symbols and in spontaneous initiations, but little change in other forms of communication. Outcome also varied according to the characteristics of the children involved.

The approach that has given rise to most controversy in recent years, mainly because of claims of "recovery from autism," is the Early Intensive Behavioral Intervention program (EIBI) of Lovaas and colleagues (Lovaas, 1993, 1996; McEachin, Smith, & Lovaas, 1993). EIBI involves 40 h per week or more of behaviorally based teaching, starting at the age of 2–3 years and lasting for at least 2 years. Initial evaluations reported IQ gains of up to 30 points with 40% of participants becoming "indistinguishable from their normal peers." However, reanalysis of the early data, and reviews of more recent EIBI programs, indicate that although this approach is certainly effective, the overall results are neither as marked nor as universal as initially claimed (Shea, 2004).

For children with ASD of average IQ, full access to the normal school curriculum is crucial for their future academic and employment prospects. In contrast, fully inclusive schooling is unlikely to succeed for children with the most severe cognitive, behavioral and communication difficulties. Although some studies have found that cognitive and linguistic development in this more severely impaired group can be enhanced by inclusion, the educational settings involved tended to be experimental in nature and/or involved very young children (Harris, Handleman, Gordon *et al.*, 1991). Other research indicates that while mainstreaming does not necessarily improve cognitive or language skills, it may help to improve social and play behavior, at least in preschoolers (Handleman, Harris, & Martins, 2005).

A number of specialized programs in the USA (e.g., Denver model, Douglass Developmental Disabilities Center, LEAP, May Center for Early Childhood Education, TEACCH and Waldon; for reviews see Arick, Krug, Fullerton *et al.*, 2005; Handleman, Harris, & Martins, 2005; Harris, Handleman, & Jennet, 2005) now involve staged integration into inclusive schooling, together with training and support for mainstream class teachers. Harris, Handleman, & Jennet (2005) concluded that, as there is no good evidence in favor of any one specific model, the choice of program needs to be based on the needs of the individual child and his or her family. An educational program suitable for a child with Asperger syndrome, for example, is unlikely to suit a non-verbal pupil with autism and severe cognitive delays. Furthermore, children's needs change over time, and placements should be reviewed at regular intervals. Many very young children with ASD require specialist, one-to-one teaching, but once basic communication and social skills have been acquired a gradual program of integration can begin. For some children this will mean continuing support in mainstream, for others specialized help in some settings/classes but not in others, and for others full inclusion. However, unless the very specific needs and difficulties of pupils with ASD in mainstream are recognized, these children can become extremely isolated, suffering bullying and rejection from both children and teachers (Sainsbury, 2000).

General Approaches to Improving the Classroom Environment

Without appropriate resources, simply placing children with special educational needs (SEN) in mainstream settings will almost certainly result in educational deprivation and social alienation (Hornby, Atkinson, & Howard, 1997). Successful inclusion requires mainstream teachers to be appropriately trained and supported (Burack, Root, & Zigler, 1997); the curriculum and teaching programs should be appropriately individualized and structured; and teaching goals must be clear to both teachers and pupils (Farrell, 1997). Time spent on learning activities, the use of directive teaching methods, together with reinforcement, feedback and monitoring techniques, are all associated with improved classroom behavior. Several reviews (Farrell, 1997; Hunt & Goetz, 1997; King-Sears, 1997; Manset & Semmel, 1997; Wehmeyer, Lance, & Bashinski, 2002) concur in suggesting a number of specific strategies related to "best academic practice":

- *Co-operative learning* – teaching activities structured to ensure that typically developing children and students with AEN work and learn together;
- *Differentiated instruction and one-to-one provision* as necessary, according to individual needs and abilities;
- *Explicit instruction* – including step-by step teaching, feedback and reinforcement;
- *Generalization training* – to ensure that skills taught in one-to-one or small group sessions are maintained across the wider school;
- *Strategy instruction* – teaching pupils with SEN to acquire self-directed learning strategies;
- *Curriculum-based assessments* – to ensure that students with SEN continue to make progress in areas covered by the teaching curriculum; and
- *Training for teachers* in SEN awareness and in the use of techniques to modify problem behaviors and enhance learning.

Other factors related to "best practice" include a high staff: student ratio; help for pupils with special educational needs to acquire self-determination and self-advocacy skills; the development of social networks to facilitate peer support and friendships; collaboration between school staff, and between teachers, parents, other therapeutic agencies and the wider community.

The issue of class size has provoked considerable debate (Zarghami & Schnellert, 2004) but evidence that this directly affects outcome, either for regular or special needs pupils, is limited. Blatchford, Edmonds, and Martin (2003) found no impact of class size on the educational attainments of regular primary school children, but class size did affect teaching style and modes of learning, with children in smaller groups taking a more interactive role. A review by Wilson (2002) concluded that although, overall, class size had little direct influence on progress or behavior, smaller classes benefitted younger pupils and those from disadvantaged or minority groups; they also reduced teacher stress. Moreover, in almost all successful studies in inclusive settings, class size has been far smaller than in most state schools (the average class size in the EU is 20; many experimental classes comprise only 8–10 children). It is suggested that, to maintain an effective teacher: pupil ratio within inclusive classrooms, each child with special needs should be counted as the equivalent of six typically developing pupils (Pirrie, Head, & Bryna, 2006). Structured small group teaching also appears to enhance academic and social skills (Ainscow, 1995) and may also profit typically developing peers.

Improving Training and Support for Teachers

While mainstream classrooms and curricula *can* be adapted to meet the requirements of children with SEN, this is not an easy task for most teachers who are already working under considerable pressure. Although specialist training is crucial, full-time courses have been increasingly replaced by cheaper part-time modular courses and even the best-trained teachers are unlikely to be effective without adequate support. Collaborative teamwork, a shared framework for teaching, clear role relationships among professionals, procedures for evaluating teaching effectiveness, adequate training, administrative support and effective use of support staff are among the factors identified as important in maintaining positive teaching practices in inclusive settings (Giangreco, 1997; Salend & Duhaney, 1999; Villa, Thousand, Meyers, & Nevin, 1996).

Teachers' attitudes are also crucial. In a review of 28 studies, Scruggs and Mastropieri (1996) found that although two-thirds of teachers supported the general concept of inclusion, only one-third considered they had sufficient time, experience, training or resources to implement this successfully and 30% felt inclusion could have a negative impact on typically developing peers. Negative attitudes to inclusion are greater among teachers of older pupils or pupils with severe intellectual, physical or behavioral problems. Negative attitudes are also associated with poor collaboration between staff, inadequate support, larger class sizes and lack of confidence in their own teaching competence (Salend & Duhaney, 1999; Soodak, Podell, & Lehman, 1998).

Conflicts may also arise because the teaching strategies that are most effective for children with severe intellectual disabilities (i.e., highly structured and individualized) may be very different to those utilized in typical mainstream classrooms (i.e., experiential, group learning). Similarly, whereas the communication skills of children with severe language and/or cognitive impairments are enhanced by teaching styles that encourage initiations and spontaneous language, in mainstream classes the interactional styles of both teachers and other pupils are mainly directive (Bayliss, 1995). Moreover, because the educational goals for this group of pupils often involve developing very basic self-help and independence skills, it is difficult to accommodate these within the more academic National Curriculum, especially in secondary schools.

Role of Para-professionals

Almost by definition, children with special needs require some one-to-one teaching, especially when learning new skills. The role of para-professional support staff is crucial here but they are frequently assigned to students with the most challenging behavioral and learning needs. They are expected to: work collaboratively with other staff and pupils; foster the child's academic and social progress; plan and carry out individually tailored educational programs; teach basic life skills; take care of feeding and toileting; and deal with very difficult behaviors. Rarely are they adequately trained or supported to meet these demands and all too often their role focuses on the minimization of behavioral difficulties. Moreover, assigning the least powerful staff within the school hierarchy to the least powerful students may simply perpetuate the "underclass" status of both groups (Giangreco, Edelman, Broer, & Doyle, 2001). Working individually with a pupil with special needs in the corner of the classroom (or in the library or medical room) may actually increase rather than decrease segregation and without close liaison between teaching and support staff children can become over-dependent on the teaching assistant, which in turn becomes a further barrier to inclusion (Marks, Schrader, & Levine, 1999). Although it is clear that para-professionals can be trained successfully to carry out and monitor a range of different behavioral, educational and social interventions and that they gain personal satisfaction from so doing, if training and support are inadequate, both they and their pupils will be disadvantaged (Giangreco, Doyle, Halvorson, & Broer, 2004).

Consultation Services

Consultation by outside agencies may be required for a number of different reasons: to improve teachers' general skills in dealing with children who have special needs; to train them in the use of specific intervention techniques; or to assess or treat children directly, thereby reducing the need for referrals to external psychiatric or psychology agencies. Consultation services may be requested at times of crisis although increasingly they are part of a planned contractual service to schools. The relationship between the consultant and consultee is a complex one and requires careful clarification of the expectations and roles of all concerned. Effective consultation can have a positive effect on teachers, individual children and the classroom as a whole, resulting in a reduction in behavioral problems and in referrals to outside agencies (Dyson, 1990; Fuchs, Fuchs, & Bahr, 1990; Jordan, 1994). However, inadequate preparation may simply undermine teacher status and independence (Dockrell & Lindsay, 2001; Law, Dockrell, Williams, & Seeff, 2002). The quality of research on school-based consultancy for children with mental health problems is generally poor, but there is some evidence for the value of consultancy services in providing cognitive–behavioral therapy, social skills training and general support for teachers (Hoagwood & Erwin, 1997). Nevertheless, pupils themselves often indicate that they would prefer to receive additional help from their own teacher rather than from a specialist, because this makes them feel less conspicuous (Jenkins & Heinen, 1989). There is also a need to extend specialist support into the home setting if any advantages are to generalize. A report for the UK National Foundation for Educational Research (Fletcher-Campbell & Cullen, 2000) noted the very variable effects of introducing external support agencies into schools and cautions that, when collaboration between mainstream and specialist staff was weak, "it was the pupil who was disadvantaged." The benefits derived from consultancy services may also be short-lived. For example, in a randomized controlled trial, using specialist consultants to introduce the use of specific communication strategies into classrooms for non-speaking, low IQ children with autism, the positive treatment effects were not maintained once consultations ceased (Howlin, Gordon, Pasco, 2007). The provision of specialist support teachers (not untrained classroom assistants) working alongside the class teacher may be more beneficial in the longer term, but again, support teaching often fails because of inadequate liaison and planning (Thomas, 1992).

Parental Roles and Views

Ensuring generalization of treatment effects is a crucial issue for any intervention. Many of the more successful special educational or inclusion programs have actively involved parents (Desforges & Abouchaar, 2003; Frankel, Myatt, Cantwell *et al.*, 1997; McEachin, Smith, & Lovaas, 1993) and family-centered models for curriculum development have become increasingly popular (Skrtic, Sailor, & Gee, 1996). Without parent involvement, and often parent training, the benefits of intervention are unlikely to generalize to non-school settings, and inconsistent or ineffective parental strategies may weaken the impact of successful school programs. However, the involvement of parents, and indeed the wider community, in SEN programs cannot be expected to occur without adequate planning, resources and full understanding of the background of pupils with special needs.

There is little evidence to suggest that parents are either overwhelmingly for or against inclusive education and around 65–80% of parents of SEN children in *either* mainstream or segregated settings express satisfaction with the placement. Many parents of children in inclusive placements believe that this facilitates both social and academic progress but others express concerns about the lack of individualized instruction, inadequate support (for both pupils and teachers) and the risk of teasing or rejection by other children. Parental views are also likely to be affected by the age of their child, the nature of his or her disability and their own educational background (Duhaney & Salend, 2000).

Impact on Other Pupils

Overall, the available evidence does not support concerns that the progress of typically developing pupils is negatively affected by the presence of children with special needs. A review of 26 (mostly US-based) studies (Dyson, Farrell, Polat, Hutcheson, & Gallannaugh, 2004) found that 23% reported a positive academic and/or social impact on "typical" pupils; 15% suggested a negative impact; 53% a neutral impact; and 10% a mixed impact. Studies involving the inclusion of children with physical, sensory or communication difficulties were generally positive but there were more negative effects when pupils had behavioral or emotional problems. However, the authors noted that few data were available on secondary schools and they stressed the need to study the relationship between inclusion and the achievements of classmates over time. Data from British schools indicated a small but negative relationship between the level of inclusivity in schools and pupil attainments, but the schools with higher levels of inclusion tended to be those serving more disadvantaged, lower-achieving populations (Dyson, Farrell, Polat *et al.*, 2004).

Improving Acceptance by Peers

Without specific intervention, integration is unlikely to improve acceptance by peers. Social interactions may occur more frequently in integrated settings but children with developmental delays still remain relatively isolated, spontaneous joint play is infrequent, close friendships are rare and bullying is a significant problem (Burack, Root, & Zigler, 1997; Norwich & Kelly, 2004; Siperstein & Leffert, 1997). Programs that have focused on training typically developing peers to initiate interactions or implement co-operative learning strategies have been successful in increasing the frequency and quality of social responses and in enhancing academic skills (Hornby, Atkinson, & Howard, 1997). Peer tutoring appears to be more effective than attempts to change attitudes by indirect methods, such as teaching tapes, stories or simulations, and also improves peers' academic attainments, social maturity and empathy (Hornby, Atkinson, & Howard, 1997; Topping, 2001). "Circles of friends" or carefully structured pairings of typical pupils and children with special needs are also claimed to promote social inclusion, but evaluations are few and generalization is often limited (Newton, Taylor, & Wilson, 1996).

Early Prevention Programs

For children at risk of learning or behavioral problems because of social disadvantage, the best known, and best funded, community-based interventions are the Head Start and Early Headstart Programs. The short-term effects on children's cognitive, social and physical development are well established and early interventions of this kind can produce improvements in mother–child interaction and a reduction in problem behaviors (Bailey, Aytch, Odom, Symons, & Wolery, 1999; Barnett, 2004; Reid, Webster-Stratton, & Hammond, 2004). There is less agreement about the longer-term benefits. In a detailed review, Barnett and Hustedt (2005) noted the lack of adequately controlled, long-term follow-up studies and despite positive effects on academic achievements and social adjustment, effect sizes are smaller than for some other model programs, such as the Abecedarian Project (Campbell, Ramey, Pungello, Sparling, & Miller-Johnson, 2002) or the Chicago Child Parent Centers (Reynolds, Temple, Robertson, & Mann, 2002). Other criticisms include the very variable timespan and quality of these programs, the relatively small number of children involved (under 1.7% of the total infant population), the racial imbalance (poor Blacks are significantly more likely to be enrolled than poor Whites) and the often poor standards of teaching (fewer than 30% of teachers have a Bachelor's degree and salaries are far lower than in public school kindergartens). Sure Start is the UK version of Head Start, but variations in the quality and funding of programs in different areas, and arguments concerning the most appropriate means of delivery, mean that the findings remain inconclusive. The program seems to benefit those parents who are less socially disadvantaged or have greater personal resources, but there may be adverse effects for the most disadvantaged families (Belsky, Melhuish, Barnes, Leyland, & Romaniuk, 2006; Rutter, 2006). Moreover, recent government-directed changes in the focus of (and funding for) Head Start, Early Head Start and Sure Start mean that many questions remain about the effectiveness of their various components, the real long-term benefits and the types and ages of children for whom they prove most effective.

Post School

The difficulties and social exclusion experienced by many children with special educational needs frequently extend into adult life. Dropout rates from school are often double those of other students, and fewer than half obtain any formal qualifications or go on to further education. Outcome is particularly poor for pupils with intellectual disability, learning disability or emotional disturbance. Unemployment is as high as 60–70%, even for individuals with mild intellectual disability or sensory problems, and earnings, job status and stability are low (Lipsky & Gartner, 1996; Wagner & Blackorby, 1996). Long-term dependence on parental support is also typical (Howlin, 2004; Lipsky & Gartner, 1996). Although there has been an increase in post-school vocational training programs over recent years, few such courses are of an appropriate academic or vocational level. Many students may find it difficult to gain access to courses that adequately meet their needs

(Harrison, 1996) and improved transition services to facilitate the transition from school to college to work are essential for all pupils with special educational needs.

Clinical Recommendations

Education has a major influence on the life of any child but for pupils with disabilities the quality of schooling they receive is likely to have an even greater and longer lasting impact. Clinicians can play an important part in providing schools with guidance on how to help these children because failure to meet their educational needs will undermine the effects of any other forms of treatment. Attention to the following guidelines may be helpful.

• Placement in *appropriate* education from the earliest years is crucial. Early failure in mainstream settings can result in the need for much more expensive intervention subsequently, while early success in a specialist setting can provide children with greater chances of later inclusion. A "let's try it and see" approach to mainstream is unlikely to be helpful.

• Children with special educational needs are a broad and heterogenous group and require a range of different educational provision. This should include highly specialist placements for those with the most severe and handicapping conditions. For some older children, particularly those who will require residential care as adults, residential schooling may also be needed.

• Families need to be offered detailed information on the full range of educational and other provision available locally. Lack of information and the feeling that they have no choice in educational decisions are significant factors in leading parents to seek out alternative, expensive and often unproven therapies.

• Appropriate placement will depend on a thorough assessment of children's and families' needs, and of children's profiles of skills and difficulties. Standardized assessments of cognitive, linguistic and other abilities are *not* a waste of time, and can prove highly valid and reliable indicators of children's potential, as well as highlighting areas of deficit and skill.

• Understanding the nature of the underlying condition and any associated behavioral, social, emotional or cognitive impairments is crucial for optimal educational provision. The view that "We don't label children here" is of no help to the child, parents or teachers, and recognition of the characteristics associated with particular disorders can be of great help in informing educational practice.

• The number of children requiring specialist educational help and advice greatly outweighs the number of professionals who are able to offer this – educational psychologists, speech and language therapists and occupational therapists are particularly thin on the ground. Thus, professionals in child and adult mental health services (CAMHS) teams need to work together to develop a group expertise that can assist different children with different problems in a variety of different ways.

• Most of the conditions described in this chapter are both pervasive and persistent. Parents care more for professional consistency than professional background, and need to have long-term access to staff who can continue to offer individualized help or advice over the years.

• Similarly, these conditions do not disappear when children reach puberty or school leaving age – indeed, new problems may emerge at these times. Ongoing support for young people and their families at these transitional stages is vital, as are careful planning and close inter-professional liaison.

• Finally, when clinicians are involved in advising schools as to how pupils with special needs should, or should not, be managed, it is important that they are aware of the realities of the local situation – unrealistic and impractical recommendations will not enhance working relationships or benefit the children or families involved.

Conclusions

Warnock (2005, p. 38) suggested that the correct view of special education is one that: "Maximizes the entitlement of all pupils to a broad, relevant and stimulating curriculum. All schools whether special or mainstream should reflect a culture in which the institution adapts to the needs of its pupils. The most appropriate setting is . . . one in which children can be most fully included in the life of their school community and which gives them a sense of both belonging and achieving."

Warnock stressed that the pursuit of equality should be directed at ensuring that children with special needs have equal opportunities as adults – this does *not* mean that they should all be educated under one roof. Instead, the concept of "special school" should be replaced by "specialist school" along the lines of those now being designed for children with particular gifts in music, art or technology.

The goal should be to ensure that all children with special needs are provided with an education that enables them to make optimum academic, social and emotional progress and offers them the best chance of inclusion as adults. This will require a flexible continuum of provision, including special schools, resource units and special classes which, as far as possible, allow ready access to mainstream school and the normal curriculum. The perspective of the family, the teachers and other pupils should also be acknowledged and positive involvement with non-disabled peers fostered as early as possible.

References

Abbott, D., Morris, J., & Ward, L. (2001). *The best place to be? Policy, practice and the experiences of residential school placements for disabled children.* York: Joseph Rowntree Foundation.

Ainscow, M. (1995). Special needs through school improvement: School improvement through special needs. In C. Clark, A. Dyson, & A. Milward (Eds.), *Towards inclusive schools?* (pp. 63–77). London: David Fulton.

American Association on Mental Retardation (AAMR). (2002). *The AAMR definition of mental retardation.* Accessed from www.aamr.org 5 July 2005.

American Psychiatric Association. (2000). *Diagnostic and statistical manual of mental disorders* (4th edn.). Text revision. Washington, DC: American Psychiatric Association.

Americans with Disabilities Act. (1990). ADA, Public Law 101–336.

Antia, S. D., Stinson M. S., & Gaustad, M. A. (2002). Developing membership in the education of deaf and hard-of-hearing students in inclusive settings. *Journal of Deaf Studies and Deaf Education*, *7*, 214–229.

Arick, J. R., Krug, D. A., Fullerton, A., Loos, L., & Falco, R. (2005). School-based programs. In F. R. Volkmar, R. Paul, A. Klin, & D. Cohen (Eds.), *Handbook of autism and pervasive developmental disorders*. (3rd edn., pp. 1003–1028). New Jersey: Wiley.

Arter, C., Mason, H., McCall, S., McLinden, M., & Stone, J. (1999). *Children with a visual impairment in mainstream settings: A guide for teachers*. London: David Fulton.

Bailey, D. B., Aytch, L., Odom, S., Symons, F., & Wolery, M. (1999). Early intervention as we know it. *Mental Retardation and Developmental Disabilities Research Reviews*, *5*, 11–20.

Baird, G., Simonoff, S., Pickles, A., Chandler, S., Loucas, S., Meldrun, D., *et al.* (2006). Prevalence of disorders of the autism spectrum in a population cohort of children in South Thames: The Special Needs and Autism Project (SNAP). *Lancet*, *368*, 210–215.

Baker, E. T., Wang, M. C., & Walberg, H. J. (1994). The effects of inclusion on learning. *Educational Leadership*, *52*, 33–35.

Balkany, T., Hodges, A. V., & Goodman, K. W. (1996). Ethics of cochlear implantation in young children. *Otolaryngology, Head and Neck Surgery*, *114*, 748–755.

Barkley, R. A. (1997). *Defiant children: A clinician's manual for assessment and parent training* (2nd edn.). New York: Guilford Press.

Barnett, W. S. (2004). Does Head Start have lasting cognitive effects? The myth of fade-out. In E. Zigler, & S. Styfco (Eds.), *The Head Start debates* (pp. 221–249). Baltimore: Paul H. Brookes.

Barnett, W. S., & Hustedt, J. T. (2005). Head Start's lasting benefits. *Infants and Young Children*, *18*, 16–24.

Bayliss, M. (1995). Integration and interpersonal relations: Interactions between disabled children and their non-disabled peers. *British Journal of Special Education*, *22*, 131–140.

Beadle, E. A., McKinley, D. J., Nikolopoulos, T. P., Brough, J., O'Donoghue, G. M., & Archbold, S. M. (2005). Long-term functional outcomes and academic-occupational status in implanted children after 10–14 years of cochlear implant use. *Otology and Neurology*, *26*, 1152–1160.

Bear, G. G., Clever, A., & Proctor, W. A. (1991). Self-perceptions of non-handicapped children and children with learning disabilities in integrated classes. *Journal of Special Education*, *24*, 409–426.

Belsky, J., Melhlish, E., Barnes, J., Leyland, A. H., & Romaniuk, H. (2006). Effects of Sure Start local programmes on children and families: Early findings from a quasi-experimental, cross-sectional study. *British Medical Journal*, *332*, 1476.

Beveridge, S. (1996). Experiences of an integration link scheme: The perspectives of pupils with severe learning difficulties and their mainstream peers. *European Journal of Learning Disabilities*, *26*, 87–101.

Blatchford, P., Edmonds, S., & Martin, C. (2003). Class size, pupil attentiveness and peer relations. *British Journal of Educational Psychology*, *73*, 15–36.

Bondy, A., & Frost, L. (1996). Educational approaches in pre-school: Behavior techniques in a public school setting. In E. Schopler, & G. B. Mesibov (Eds.), *Learning and cognition in autism* (pp. 311–334). New York: Plenum Press.

Booth, T. (1996). A perspective on inclusion from England. *Cambridge Journal of Education*, *26*, 87–101.

Buckley, S. (2006). *The education of individuals with Down syndrome: A review of educational provision and outcomes in the United Kingdom*. Portsmouth: Down Syndrome Educational Trust.

Burack, J. A., Root, R., & Zigler, E. (1997). Inclusive education for children with autism: Reviewing ideological, empirical and community considerations. In D. Cohen, & F. Volkmar (Eds.), *Handbook of autism and pervasive developmental disorders* (2nd edn., pp. 796–807). New York: Wiley.

Campbell, F. A., Ramey, C. T., Pungello, E., Sparling, J., & Miller-Johnson, S. (2002). Early childhood education: Young adult outcomes from the Abecedarian Project. *Applied Developmental Science*, *6*, 42–57.

Carlberg, C., & Kavale, K. (1980). The efficacy of special versus regular class placement for exceptional children: A meta-analysis. *Journal of Special Education*, *14*, 295–309.

Cassidy, S. B., & Morris, C. A. (2002). Behavioral phenotypes in genetic syndromes: Genetic clues to human behavior. *Advances in Pediatrics*, *49*, 59–86.

Clay, M. (1985). *The early detection of reading difficulties* (3rd edn.). Auckland: Heinemann.

Cole, T. (1989). *Apart or A Part? Integration and the growth of British special education*. Milton Keynes: Open University Press.

Cole, T., & Meyer, L. (1991). Social integration and severe disabilities: A longitudinal analysis of child outcomes. *Journal of Special Education*, *25*, 340–351.

Cooper, P., & Ideus, K. (1996). *Attention deficit/hyperactivity disorder: A practical guide for teachers*. London: David Fulton.

Crawford, T., & Simonoff, E. (2003). Parental views about services for children attending schools for the emotionally and behaviourally disturbed (EBD): A qualitative analysis. *Child: Care, Health and Development*, *29*, 481–491.

Cornish K., & Munir, F. (1998). Receptive and expressive language skills in children with cri-du-chat syndrome. *Journal of Communication Disorders*, *31*, 73–81.

Cumine, V., Leach, J., & Stevenson, G. (1998). *Asperger syndrome: A practical guide for teachers*. London: David Fulton.

Cumine, V., Leach, J., & Stevenson, G. (1999). *Autism in the early years: A practical guide*. London: David Fulton.

Dale, P., Jenkins, J. R., Mills, P., & Cole, K. N. (2005). Follow-up of children from academic and cognitive preschool curricula at 12 and 16. *Exceptional Children*, *71*, 301–307.

Davis, P., & Hopwood, V. (2002). Including children with a visual impairment in the mainstream primary school classroom. *Journal of Research in Special Educational Needs*, *2*, 1–11.

Davison, F. M., & Howlin, P. (1997). A follow-up study of children attending a primary-age language unit. *European Journal of Disorders of Communication*, *32*, 19–36.

Department for Education and Employment. (1998). *Meeting special educational needs. A programme of action*. London: DfEE.

Department for Education and Skills. (2001a). *Special educational needs (SEN) code of practice*. London: DfES.

Department for Education and Skills. (2001b). *Inclusive schooling: Children with special educational needs*. London: DfES.

Department for Education and Skills. (2005). *Guidance for education improvement partnerships on improving behaviour and persistent truancy*. London: DfES.

Department for Education and Skills. (2006). *Behaviour improvement programme*. London: DfES.

Desforges, C., & Abouchaar, A. (2003). *The impact of parental involvement, parental support and family education on pupil achievements and adjustment*. London: Department for Education and Skills; Research Report No. 433.

Dockrell, J. E., & Lindsay, G. (2001). Children with specific speech and language difficulties: The teachers' perspective. *Oxford Review of Education*, *27*, 369–394.

Duhaney, L. M. G., & Salend, S. J. (2000). Parental perceptions of inclusive educational placements. *Remedial and Special Education*, *21*, 121–128.

Dykens, E. M. (2000). Annotation: Psychopathology in children with intellectual disability. *Journal of Child Psychology and Psychiatry*, *41*, 407–417.

Dyson, A. (1990). Effective learning consultancy: A future role for special needs coordinators? *Support for Learning*, *5*, 116–127.

Dyson, A., Farrell, P., Polat, F., Hutcheson, G., & Gallannaugh, F. (2004). *Inclusion and pupil achievement*. London: Department for Education and Skills Research Report No. 578.

Edelson, M. G. (2006). Are the majority of children with autism mentally retarded? A systematic evaluation of the data. *Focus on Autism and Other Developmental Disabilities*, *21*, 66–83.

Education of All Handicapped Children Act. (1975). Public Law 94-142.

Evans, J., Harden, A., Thomas, J., & Benefield, P. (2003). *Supporting pupils with emotional and behavioural difficulties in mainstream primary schools: A systematic review of recent research on strategy effectiveness (1999–2002)*. Windsor: National Foundation for Educational Research.

Farrell, P. (1996). Integration: Where do we go from here? In J. Coupe, O. Kane, & J. Goldbart (Eds.), *Whose choice? Contentious issues for those working with people with learning difficulties* (pp. 177–195). London: David Fulton.

Farrell, P. (1997). The integration of children with severe learning difficulties: A review of the recent literature. *Journal of Applied Research in Intellectual Disabilities*, *10*, 1–14.

Farrell, P., & Tsakalidou, K. (1999). Recent trends in the re-integration of pupils with emotional and behavioural difficulties in the United Kingdom. *School Psychology International*, *20*, 323–337.

Feuerstein, R., Rand, Y., Hoffman, N., & Miller, M. (1980). *Instrumental enrichment: An intervention program for cognitive modifiability*. Baltimore: University Park Press.

Fletcher-Campbell, F., & Cullen, M. A. (2000). Schools' perceptions of support services for Special Educational Needs. *Support for Learning*, *15*, 90–94.

Foorman, B. R., Rancis, D. J., Novy, D. M., & Liberman, D. (1991). How letter-sound instruction mediates progress in first-grade reading and spelling. *Journal of Educational Psychology*, *83*, 456–469.

Forest, M., Pearpoint, J., & O'Brien, J. (1996). "MPAS": Educators, parents, young people and their friends planning together. *Educational Psychology in Practice*, *11*, 35–40.

Frankel, F., Myatt, R., Cantwell, D. P., & Feinberg, D. T. (1997). Parent-assisted transfer of children's social skills training: Effects on children with and without Attention Deficit Hyperactivity Disorder. *Journal of the American Academy of Child and Adolescent Psychiatry*, *36*, 1056–1064.

Fuchs, D., Fuchs, L. S., & Bahr, M. W. (1990). Mainstream assistance teams: A scientific basis for the art of consultation. *Exceptional Children*, *57*, 128–134.

Gallagher, D. J. (2001). Neutrality as a moral standpoint, conceptual confusion and the full inclusion debate. *Disability and Society*, *16*, 637–654.

Geers, A., & Brenner, C. (2003). Background and educational characteristics of prelingually deaf children implanted by 5 years of age. *Ear and Hearing*, *24* (Supplement), 2S–14S.

Giangreco, M. F. (1997). Key lessons learned about inclusive education: Summary of the 1996 Schonell Memorial Lecture. *International Journal of Disability*, *44*, 193–206.

Giangreco, M. F., Doyle, M. B., Halvorson, A. T., & Broer, S. M. (2004). Alternatives to overreliance on paraprofessionals in inclusive schools. *Journal of Special Educational Leadership*, *17*, 82–90.

Giangreco, M. F., Edelman, S. W., Broer, S. M., & Doyle, M. B. (2001). Paraprofessional support of students with disabilities: Literature from the past decade. *Exceptional Children*, *68*, 45–63.

Gordon, J. C. (1885). Deaf-mutes and the public schools from 1815 to the present day. *American Annals of the Deaf*, 30, 137.

Gorenflo, C. W., & Gorenflo, D. W. (1991). The effects of information and augmentative communication technique on attitudes toward nonspeaking individuals. *Journal of Speech and Hearing Research*, *34*, 19–26.

Gravel, J. S., & O'Gara, J. (2003). Communication options for children with hearing loss. *Mental Retardation and Developmental Disabilities Research Reviews*, *9*, 243–251.

Greenberg, M. T., Domitrovich, C., & Bumberger, B. (2000). *Preventing mental disorder in school-age children: A review of the effectiveness of prevention programs*. Prevention Research Center for the Promotion of Human Development; College of Health and Human Development, Pennsylvania State University.

Gresham, F. M., Watson, T. S., & Skinner, C. H. (2001). Functional behavioral assessment: Principles, procedures, and future directions. *School Psychology Review*, *30*, 156–172.

Groenveld, M. (1998). Sensory difficulties. In P. Howlin (Ed.), *Behavioural approaches to problems in childhood* (pp. 114–135). London: MacKeith Press.

Handleman, J. S., Harris, S. L., & Martins, M. P. (2005). Helping children with autism enter the mainstream. In F. R. Volkmar, R. Paul, A. Klin, & D. Cohen (Eds.), *Handbook of autism and pervasive developmental disorders* (3rd edn., pp. 1029–1042). New Jersey: Wiley.

Harris, H. J., Cook, M., & Upton, G. (1996). *Pupils with severe learning disabilities who present challenging behaviour: A whole school approach to assessment and intervention*. Clevedon: BILD Publications.

Harris, J. (1998). Cerebral palsy. In P. Howlin (Ed.), *Behavioural approaches to problems in childhood* (pp. 136–151). London: MacKeith Press.

Harris, S. L., Handleman J. S., Gordon, R., Kristoff, B., Bass, L., & Fuentes, F. (1991). Changes in cognitive and language functioning of preschool children with autism. *Journal of Autism and Developmental Disorders*, *21*, 281–290.

Harris, S. L., Handleman, J. S., & Jennet, H. K. (2005). Models of educational intervention for students with autism: Home, center, and school-based programming. In F. R. Volkmar, R. Paul, A. Klin, & D. Cohen (Eds.), *Handbook of autism and pervasive developmental disorders* (3rd edn., pp. 1043–1054). New Jersey: Wiley.

Harrison, J. (1996). Accessing further education: Views and experiences of FE students with learning difficulties and/or disabilities. *British Journal of Special Education*, *23*, 187–196.

Hastings, N., & Schwieso, J. (1995). Tasks and tables: The effects of seating arrangements on task engagement in primary classrooms. *Educational Research*, *37*, 279–291.

Hayden, D. A., & Pukonen, M. (1996). Language intervention programming for preschool children with social and pragmatic disorders. In J. H. Beitchman, N. J. Cohen, M. M. Konstantareas, & R. Tannock (Eds.), *Language, learning, and behavior disorders: developmental, biological, and clinical perspectives* (pp. 436–465). Cambridge: Cambridge University Press.

Hechtman, L., Kouri, J., & Respitz, E. (1996). Multimodal treatment of the hyperactive child with and without learning disabilities. In J. H. Beitchman, N. J. Cohen, M. M. Konstantareas, & R. Tannock (Eds.), *Language, learning, and behavior disorders: developmental, biological, and clinical perspectives* (pp. 395–417). Cambridge: Cambridge University Press.

Herbert, M. (1995). A collaborative model of training for parents of children with disruptive behaviour disorders. *British Journal of Clinical Psychology*, *34*, 325–342.

Heward, W. L. (2003). Ten faulty notions about teaching and learning that hinder the effectiveness of special education. *Journal of Special Education*, *36*, 186–205.

Hindley, P. A., & van Gent, T. (2002). Psychiatric aspects of sensory impairment. In M. Rutter, & E. Taylor (Eds.), *Child and adolescent psychiatry: Modern approaches* (4th edn., pp. 720–736). Oxford: Blackwell.

Hoagwood, K., & Erwin, H. D. (1997). Effectiveness of school-based mental health services for children: A 10-year research review. *Journal of Child and Family Studies*, *6*, 435–451.

Hodapp, R. M., & Fidler, D. J. (1999). Special education and genetics: Connections for the 21st century. *Journal of Special Education*, *33*, 130–137.

Hornby, G., Atkinson, M., & Howard, J. (1997). *Controversial issues in special education*. London: David Fulton.

Howlin, P. (2004). *Autism and Asperger syndrome: Preparing for adulthood*. London: Routledge.

Howlin, P. (2006). Augmentative and alternative communication systems for children with autism. In T. Charman, & W. Stone (Eds.), *Early social communication in autism spectrum disorders.* New York: Guilford.

Howlin, P., Gordon, K., Pasco, G., Wade, A., & Charman, T. (2007). The effectiveness of Picture Exchange Communication System (PECS) training for teachers of children with autism: A pragmatic, group randomized controlled trial. *Journal of Child Psychology and Psychiatry, 48,* 473–481.

Howlin, P., Mawhood, L. M., & Rutter, M. (2000). Autism and developmental receptive language disorder: A follow-up comparison in early adult life. II. Social, behavioural and psychiatric outcomes. *Journal of Child Psychology and Psychiatry, 41,* 561–576.

Hundert, J., Mahoney, B., Mundy, F., & Vernon, M. L. (1998). A descriptive analysis of developmental and social gains of children with severe disabilities in segregated and inclusive preschools in southern Ontario. *Early Childhood Research Quarterly, 13,* 49–65.

Hunt, P., & Goetz, L. (1997). Research on inclusive educational programs, practices, and outcomes for students with severe disabilities. *Journal of Special Education, 31,* 13–29.

Individuals with Disabilities Education Act. (2004). IDEA; Public Law 101-476.

Jarrold, C., Baddeley, A. D., & Phillips, C. E. (2002). Verbal short-term memory in Down syndrome: a problem of memory, audition, or speech? *Journal of Speech, Language, and Hearing Research, 45,* 531–544.

Jenkins, J. R., & Heinen, A. (1989). Students' preferences for service delivery: Pull-Out, in-class or integrated models. *Exceptional Children, 55,* 516–523.

Jordan, A. (1994). *Skills in collaborative classroom consultation.* London: Routledge.

Jordan, R., & Jones, G. (1999). *Meeting the needs of children with autistic spectrum disorders.* London: David Fulton.

Karn, C. M., Greenberg, M. T., & Kusché, C. A. (2004). Sustained effects of the PATHS curriculum on the social and psychological adjustment of children in special education. *Journal of Emotional and Behavioral Disorders, 12,* 66–79.

Kavale, K., & Mostert, M. P. (2003). River of ideology, islands of evidence. *Exceptionality, 11,* 191–208.

Keil, S., & Clunies-Ross, L. (2003). *Survey of educational provision for blind and partially sighted children in England, Scotland and Wales in 2002.* London: RNIB.

King-Sears, M. E. (1997). Best academic practices for inclusive classrooms. *Focus on Exceptional Children, 29,* 1–21.

Kline, A. D., Stanley, C., Belevich-Brodsky, K., Barr, J., & Jackson, L. G. (2005). Developmental data on individuals with the Brachmann–de Lange syndrome. *American Journal of Medical Genetics, 7,* 1053–1058.

Kohn, J. G. (1990). Issues in the management of children with spastic cerebral palsy. *Pediatrician, 17,* 230–236.

Lakhen, Y., & Norwich, B. (1990). The self-concept and self-esteem of adolescents with physical impairments in integrated and special school settings. *European Journal of Special Needs Education, 5,* 1–12.

Law, J., Dockrell, J., Williams, K., & Seeff, B. (2002). Comparing specialist early years provision for speech and language impaired children with mainstream nursery provision in the UK: An application of the Early Childhood Environment Rating Scale (ECERS). *Child: Care, Health and Development, 30,* 177–184.

Law, J., Garret, Z., & Nye, C. (2003). Speech and language therapy interventions for children with primary speech and language delay or disorder. *Cochrane Database Systematic Review, 3,* CD004110.

Lettsom, J. C. (1801, 1894). *The blind: Hints designed to promote beneficence, temperance and medical science.* [Reprinted 1894 by Sampson Low, London.]

Lewis, A. (1995) *Primary special needs and the National Curriculum* (2nd edn.). London: Routledge.

Lewis, J., & Wilson, D. (1998). *Pathways to learning in Rett syndrome.* London: David Fulton.

Lightfoot, J., Wright, S., & Sloper, P. (1999). Supporting pupils in mainstream school with an illness or disability: Young people's views. *Child: Care, Health and Development, 25,* 267–283.

Lindsay, G. (2003). Inclusive education: A critical perspective. *British Journal of Special Education, 30,* 3–12.

Lindsay, G. (2007). Annual review: Educational psychology and the effectiveness of inclusive education/mainstreaming. *British Journal of Educational Psychology, 77,* 1–24.

Lindsay, G., & Dockrell, J. (2000). The behaviour and self-esteem of children with specific speech and language difficulties. *British Journal of Educational Psychology, 70,* 583–601.

Lindsay, G., Dockrell, J., Mackie, C., & Letchford, B. (2005). The roles of specialist provision for children with specific speech and language difficulties in England and Wales: A model for inclusion? *Journal of Research in Special Educational Needs, 5,* 88–96.

Lipsky, D., & Gartner, A. (1996). Inclusion, school restructuring and the making of American Society. *Harvard Educational Review, 66,* 762–796.

Lipsky, D., & Gartner, A. (1999). Inclusive education: A requirement of a democratic society. In H. Daniels, & P. Garner (Eds.), *World Year Book of Education 1999: Inclusive education* (pp. 12–23). London: Kogan Page.

Lord, C., & McGee, J. (2001). *Educating children with autism.* National Research Council. Washington: National Academies Press.

Lorenz, S. (1998). *Children with Down syndrome. A guide for teachers and learning support assistants in mainstream primary and secondary schools.* London: David Fulton.

Lovaas, O. I. (1993). The development of a treatment: Research project for developmentally disabled and autistic children. *Journal of Applied Behavior Analysis, 26,* 617–630.

Lovaas, O. I. (1996). The UCLA young autism model of service delivery. In C. Maurice (Ed.), *Behavioral intervention for young children with autism* (pp. 241–250). Austin, TX: Pro-Ed.

Manset, G., & Semmel, M. (1997). Are inclusive programs for students with mild disabilities effective? A comparative review of model programs. *Journal of Special Education, 31,* 155–180.

Marcus, L., Schopler, E., & Lord, C. (2001). TEACCH services for preschool children. In J. S. Handelman, & S. L. Harris (Eds.), *Preschool education programs for children with autism* (2nd edn., pp. 215–232). Austin, TX: Pro-Ed.

Marks, S. U., Schrader, C., & Levine, M. (1999). Para-educator experiences in inclusive settings: Helping, hovering or holding their own? *Exceptional Children, 65,* 315–328.

Marston, D. (1996). A comparison of inclusion only, pull-out only, and combined service models for students with mild disabilities. *Journal of Special Education, 30,* 121–132.

Martin, D., & Bat-Chava, Y. (2003). Negotiating deaf–hearing friendships: Coping strategies of deaf boys and girls in mainstream schools. *Child: Care, Health and Development, 29,* 511–521.

Massaro, D. W., & Light, J. (2004). Using visible speech to train perception and production of speech for individuals with hearing loss. *Journal of Speech, Language, and Hearing Research, 47,* 304–320.

McDonnell, J. (1998). Instruction for students with severe disabilities in general education settings. *Education and Training in Mental Retardation and Developmental Disabilities, 33,* 199–215.

McEachin, J. J., Smith, T., & Lovaas, O. I. (1993). Long-term outcome for children with autism who received early intensive behavioral treatment. *American Journal of Mental Retardation, 97,* 359–372.

Meijer, C., Soriano, V., & Watkins, A. (Eds.). (2003). *Special needs education in Europe.* Middelfart: European Agency for Development in Special Needs Education.

Mills, P., Cole, K. N., Jenkins, J. R., & Dale, P. (1998). Effects of differing levels of inclusion on preschoolers with disabilities. *Exceptional Children, 65,* 79–90.

Mills, P., Dale, P., Cole, K. N., & Jenkins, J. R. (1995). Follow-up of children from academic and cognitive preschool curricula at age 9. *Exceptional Children*, *69*, 378–393.

Murphy, E., Grey, I. M., & Honan, R. (2005). Co-operative learning for students with difficulties in learning: A description of models and guidelines for implementation. *British Journal of Special Education*, *32*, 157–164.

Murphy, J., Markova, I., Collins, S., & Moodie, E. (1996). AAC systems: Obstacles to effective use. *European Journal of Disorders of Communication*, *31*, 31–44.

Nakken, H., & Pijl, S. J. (2002). Getting along with classmates in regular schools: A review of the effects of integration on the development of social relationships. *International Journal of Inclusive Education*, *6*, 47–61.

National Association of School Psychologists, Bethesda, MD (2005). Position statement on students with emotional and behavioral disorders. Washington, DC: National Association of School Psychologists.

Nelson, J. R., Johnson, A., & Marchand-Martella, N. (1996). Effects of direct instruction, cooperative learning, and independent learning practices on the classroom behavior of students with behavioral disorders: A comparative analysis. *Journal of Emotional and Behavioral Disorders*, *4*, 43–62.

Newton, C., Taylor, H., & Wilson, D. (1996). Circles of friends: An inclusive approach to meeting emotional and behavioural needs. *Educational Psychology in Practice*, *11*, 41–48.

Norwich, B. (2003). Is there a distinctive pedagogy for learning difficulties? *Association for Child Psychology and Psychiatry Occasional Papers*, *20*, 25–37.

Norwich, B., & Kelly, N. (2004). Pupils' views on inclusion: Moderate learning difficulties and bullying in mainstream and special schools. *British Educational Research Journal*, *30*, 43–65.

Office for Standards in Education (Ofsted). (2004). *Special educational needs and disability: Towards inclusive schools.* London: Audit Office.

Panerai, S., Ferrante, L., & Zingale, M. (2002). Benefits of the Treatment and Education of Autistic and Communication Handicapped Children (TEACCH) programme as compared with a non-specific approach. *Journal of Intellectual Disability Research*, *46*, 318–327.

Pepper, J., & Weitzman, E. (2004). *It takes two to talk: A practical guide for parents of children with language delays.* Toronto: Hanen Center.

Pirrie, A., Head, G., & Bryna, P. (2006). *Mainstreaming pupils with special educational needs.* Edinburgh: Scottish Executive Education Department.

Powers, S., Thoutenhoofd, E. D., & Gregory, S. (1999). *The educational achievements of deaf children: A literature review (Research report).* London: Prentice Hall.

Preisler, G., Tvingstedt, A-L., & Ahlstrom, M. (2002). A psychosocial follow-up study of deaf preschool children using cochlear implants. *Child: Care, Health and Development*, *28*, 403–418.

Rafferty, Y., Piscitelli V., & Boettcher, C. (2003). The impact of inclusion on language development and social competence among pre-schoolers with disabilities. *Exceptional Children*, *69*, 467–479.

Rea, P. J., McLaughlin, V. L., & Walther-Thomas, C. (2002). Outcomes for students with learning disabilities in inclusive and pullout programs. *Exceptional Children*, *68*, 203–223.

Reid, M. J., Webster-Stratton, C., & Hammond, M. (2004). Halting the development of conduct problems in Head Start children: The effects of parent training. *Journal of Clinical Child and Adolescent Psychology*, *33*, 279–291.

Reynolds, A., Temple, J., Robertson, D., & Mann, E. (2002). *Age 21 cost–benefit analysis of the Chicago child–parent centers.* Institute for Research on Poverty Discussion Paper No. 1254-02. Madison: University of Wisconsin.

Reynolds, D. (1991). School effectiveness and school improvement in the 1990s. *Newsletter of the Association for Child Psychology and Psychiatry*, *13*, 5–9.

Rice, M. L., & Wilcox, K. A. (1991). *Language acquisition pre-school curriculum: Development and implementation.* Lawrence, KS: University of Kansas.

Roberts, C., & Hindley, P. (1999). The assessment and treatment of deaf children with psychiatric disorders. *Journal of Child Psychology and Psychiatry*, *40*, 151–167.

Rutherford, R. B., & Nelson, C. M. (1995). Management of aggressive and violent behavior in schools. *Focus on Exceptional Children*, *27*, 1–15.

Rutter, M. (1983). School effects on pupil progress: Research findings and policy implications. *Child Development*, *54*, 1–29.

Rutter, M. (2006). Is Sure Start an effective preventative intervention? *Child and Adolescent Mental Health*, *11*, 135–141.

Salend, S. J., & Duhaney, L. G. (1999). The impact of inclusion on students with and without disabilities and their educators. *Remedial and Special Education*, *20*, 114–127.

Sainato, D., Goldstein, H., & Strain, P. (1992). Effects of self-evaluation on preschool children's use of social interaction strategies with their classmates with autism. *Journal of Applied Behavior Analysis*, *25*, 127–141.

Sainsbury, C. (2000). *Martian in the playground: Understanding the schoolchild with Asperger's syndrome.* Bristol: Lucky Duck.

Saunders, S. (2001). *Fragile X syndrome. A guide for teachers.* London: David Fulton.

Sawyer, M. G., MacMullin, C., Graetz B., Said, J. A., Clark, J. J., & Baghurst P. (1997). Social skills training for primary school children: A 1-year follow-up study. *Journal of Paediatric Child Health*, *33*, 378–383.

Schwartz, I. S., Garfinkle, A. N., & McBride, B. J. (1998). Communication and language disorders. In P. Howlin (Ed.), *Behavioural approaches to problems in childhood.* London: MacKeith Press (pp. 95–113).

Scott, S. (1998). Conduct disorders. In P. Howlin (Ed.), *Behavioural approaches to problems in childhood.* (pp. 1–27). London: MacKeith Press.

Scruggs, T. E., & Mastropieri, M. A. (1996). Teacher perceptions of mainstreaming/inclusion, 1958–1995: a research synthesis. *Exceptional Children*, *63*, 59–74.

Shea, V. (2004). A perspective on the research literature related to early intensive behavioral intervention (Lovaas) for young children with autism. *Autism*, *8*, 349–367.

Siperstein, G. N., & Leffert, J. S. (1997). Comparison of socially accepted and rejected children with mental retardation. *American Journal of Mental Retardation*, *101*, 339–351.

Skrtic, T. M., Sailor, D., & Gee, K. (1996). Voice, collaboration and inclusion: Democratic themes in educational and social reform initiatives. *Remedial and Special Education*, *17*, 142–157.

Soodak, L. C., Podell, D. M., & Lehman, R. (1998). Teacher, student, and school attributes as predictors of teachers' responses to inclusion. *Journal of Special Education*, *31*, 480–497.

Special Educational Needs and Disability Act. (2001). London: HMSO.

Sutherland, K. S.,Wehby, J. H., & Gunter, P. L. (2000). The effectiveness of cooperative learning with students with emotional and behavioral disorders: A literature review. *Behavioral Disorders*, *25*, 225–238.

Tallal, P., Miller, S. L., Bedi, G., Byma, G., Wang, X., Nagarajan, S., *et al.* (1996). Language comprehension in language-learning impaired children improved with acoustically modified speech. *Science*, *271*, 81–84.

Thomas, G. (1992). *Effective classroom teamwork: Support or intrusion?* London: Routledge.

Topping, K. (2001). *Thinking, reading, writing: A practical guide to paired learning with peers, parents and volunteers.* New York and London: Continuum International.

Troia, G. A. (1999). Phonological awareness intervention research: A critical review of the experimental methodology. *Reading Research Quarterly*, *34*, 28–52.

Udwin, O., Webber, C., & Horn, I. (2001). Abilities and attainment in Smith–Magenis syndrome. *Developmental Medicine and Child Neurology*, *43*, 823–828.

United Nations Educational, Scientific and Cultural Organization (UNESCO). (1994). *The Salamanca Statement and Framework for Action on Special Needs Education*. Paris: UNESCO.

Villa, R., Thousand, J., Meyers, H., & Nevin, A. (1996). Teacher and administrator perceptions of heterogeneous education. *Exceptional Children*, *63*, 29–45.

Vollands, S., Topping, K. J., & Ryka, M. E. (1999). Computerized self-assessment of reading comprehension with the accelerated reader: action research. *Reading and Writing Quarterly*, *15*, 197–211.

Wagner, M. M., & Blackorby, J. (1996). Transition from high school to work or college: How special education students fare. *Special Education for Students with Disabilities*, 6, 103–119.

Wang, M. C., & Walberg, H. J. (1993). Adaptive instruction and classroom time. *American Educational Research Journal*, *20*, 601–626.

Ware, J. (1994). *Educating children with profound and multiple learning difficulties*. London: David Fulton.

Warner-Rogers, J. (1998). Attention deficit-hyperactivity disorder. In P. Howlin (Ed.), *Behavioural approaches to problems in childhood* (pp. 28–53). London: MacKeith Press.

Warnock, M. (2005). *Special educational needs: A new look*. London: Philosophy of Education Society of Great Britain.

Warnock Committee. (1978). *Special Educational Needs: The Warnock Report*. London: Department of Education and Science.

Waters, J. (1999). *Prader–Willi syndrome: A practical guide*. London: David Fulton.

Watson, L., Gregory, S., & Powers, S. (1999). *Deaf and hearing impaired pupils in mainstream schools*. London: David Fulton.

Webster, A., & Roe, J. (1998). *Children with visual impairments*. New York: Routledge.

Webster-Stratton, C., & Reid, M. J. (2004). Strengthening social and emotional competence in young children: The foundation for early school readiness and success: Incredible years classroom social skills and problem-solving curriculum. *Infants and Young Children*, *17*, 96–113.

Wehmeyer, M. L., Lance, G. D., & Bashinski, S. (2002). Promoting access to the general curriculum for students with mental retardation: A multi-level model. *Education and Training in Mental Retardation and Developmental Disabilities*, *37*, 223–234.

Werthamer-Larsson, L., Kellam, S. G., & Wheeler, L. (1991). Effect of classroom environment on shy behavior, aggressive behavior, and concentration problems. *American Journal of Community Psychology*, *19*, 585–602.

Wilson, S. J., Lipsey, M. W., & Derzon, J. H. (2003). The effects of school-based intervention programs on aggressive behavior: A meta-analysis. *Journal of Consulting and Clinical Psychology*, *71*, 136–149.

Wilson, V. (2002). *Does small really make a difference?* University of Glasgow: Scottish Council for Research in Education.

Wise, B. W., Ring, J., & Olson, R. K. (2000). Individual differences in gains from computer-assisted remedial reading. *Journal of Experimental Child Psychology*, *77*, 197–235.

Zarghami, F., & Schnellert, G. (2004). Class size reduction: No silver bullet for special education students' achievements. *International Journal of Special Education*, *19*, 89–96.

Index